2025

ICD-10-CM FOR HOSPITALS

Jackie L. Koesterman, CPC
Coding and Reimbursement Specialist
JDK Medical Coding EDU
Grand Forks, North Dakota

BUCK'S

INCLUDES NETTER'S ANATOMY ART

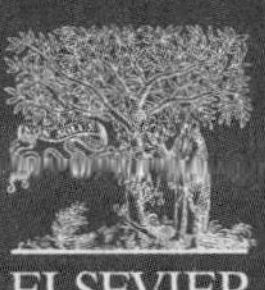

ELSEVIER

Elsevier
3251 Riverport Lane
St. Louis, Missouri 63043

BUCK'S 2025 ICD-10-CM FOR HOSPITALS ISBN: 978-0-443-24883-2

Notice

Practitioners and researchers must always rely on their own experience and knowledge in evaluating and using any information, methods, compounds or experiments described herein. Because of rapid advances in the medical sciences, in particular, independent verification of diagnoses and drug dosages should be made. To the fullest extent of the law, no responsibility is assumed by Elsevier, authors, editors or contributors for any injury and/or damage to persons or property as a matter of products liability, negligence or otherwise, or from any use or operation of any methods, products, instructions, or ideas contained in the material herein.

Previous editions copyrighted 2024, 2023, 2022, 2021, 2020, 2019, 2018, 2017, 2016, 2015, 2014, 2013, 2010

International Standard Book Number: 978-0-443-24883-2

Senior Content Strategist: Luke Held
Content Development Manager: Danielle Frazier
Senior Content Development Specialist: Joshua S. Rapplean
Publishing Services Manager: Deepthi Unni
Project Manager: Nayagi Anandan
Senior Book Designer: Maggie Reid

Printed in Canada

Last digit is the print number: 9 8 7 6 5 4 3 2 1

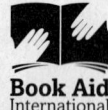

DEDICATION

To all who require of themselves the highest level of accuracy, integrity, and professionalism. You enhance our profession and are a tremendous asset to health care. May this manual be of assistance to you.

With Greatest Admiration.

Carol J. Buck, MS

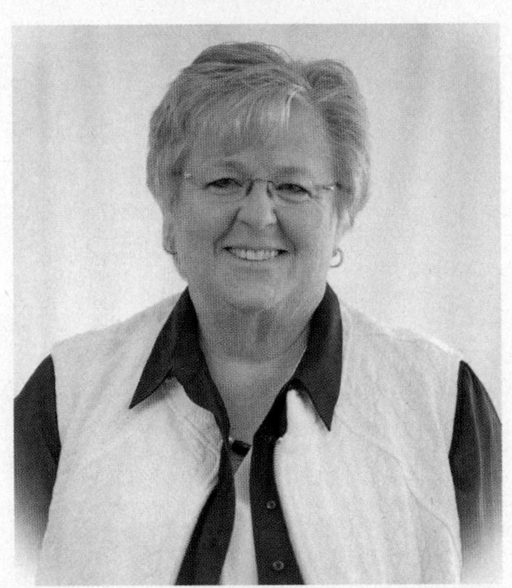

DEVELOPMENT OF THIS EDITION

Lead Technical Collaborator

Jackie L. Koesterman, CPC
Coding and Reimbursement Specialist
JDK Medical Coding EDU
Grand Forks, North Dakota

Query Team

Robin Linker, CHCA, CHCAS, CPC-I, COC, CCS-P, CPC-P, MCS-P, CHC
AAPC Approved Instructor
CEO, Robin Linker & Education Associates, Inc.; and
Association of Health Care Auditors and Educators
Aurora, Colorado

CONTENTS

ICD-10-CM

GUIDE TO USING THE 2025 ICD-10-CM FOR HOSPITALS

Medical coding has long been a part of the health care profession. Through the years medical coding systems have become more complex and extensive. Today, medical coding is an intricate and immense process that is present in every health care setting. The increased use of electronic submissions for health care services only increases the need for coders who understand the coding process.

2025 ICD-10-CM for Hospitals, Professional Edition was developed to help meet the needs of coding professionals at all levels by offering a comprehensive coding text at a reasonable price.

All material strictly adheres to the latest government versions available at the time of publication. Updates from the *Definitions of Medicare Code Edits* (MCE) will be posted to the companion website (www.codingupdates.com) when available.

Illustrations and Items

The ICD-10-CM Tabular List contains illustrations, pictures, and items to assist you in understanding difficult terminology, diseases/conditions, or coding in a specific category. Items are always shaded with ink so that the added material is not mistaken for official notations or instructions. shading is used for other annotations in the text. Your ideas on what other descriptions or illustrations should be in future editions of this text are always appreciated.

Instructional Notations

Includes Notes

Includes

The word "Includes" appears immediately under certain categories to further define, or give examples of, the content of the category.

Excludes Notes

The ICD-10-CM has two types of excludes notes. Each note has a different definition for use, but they are both similar in that they indicate that codes excluded from each other are independent of each other.

Excludes1

A type 1 Excludes note is a pure excludes. It means "NOT CODED HERE!" An Excludes1 note indicates that the code excluded should never be used at the same time as the code above the Excludes1 note. An Excludes1 is for use when two conditions cannot occur together, such as a congenital form versus an acquired form of the same condition.

Excludes2

A type 2 Excludes note represents "NOT INCLUDED HERE." An Excludes2 note indicates that the condition excluded is not part of the condition it is excluded from, but a patient may have both conditions at the same time. When an Excludes2 note appears under a code, it is acceptable to use both the code and the excluded code together.

Code First/Use Additional Code notes (etiology/manifestation paired codes)

Certain conditions have both an underlying etiology and multiple body system manifestations due to the underlying etiology. For such conditions the ICD-10-CM has a coding convention that requires the underlying condition be sequenced first, followed by the manifestation. Wherever such a combination exists, there is a "use additional code" note at the etiology code, and a "code first" note at the manifestation code. These instructional notes indicate the proper sequencing order of the codes, etiology followed by manifestation.

In most cases the manifestation codes will have in the code title, "in diseases classified elsewhere." Codes with this title are a component of the etiology/manifestation convention. The code title indicates that it is a manifestation code. "In diseases classified elsewhere" codes are never permitted to be used as first-listed or principal diagnosis codes. They must be used in conjunction with an underlying condition code, and they must be listed following the underlying condition.

Use additional

The words indicate an instructional note that another code may be needed.

Code first

The words indicate an instructional note that directs the coder to sequence the underlying condition before the manifestation.

Code also

A "code also" note instructs that two codes may be required to fully describe a condition, but the sequencing of the two codes is discretionary, depending on the severity of the conditions and the reason for the encounter.

7th characters and placeholder X

For codes less than 6 characters that require a 7th character, a placeholder X should be assigned for all characters less than 6. The 7th character must always be the 7th character of a code.

Annotated

Throughout the manual, revisions, additions, and deleted codes or words are indicated by the following symbols:

- **Revised:** Revisions within the line or code from the previous edition are indicated by the arrow.
- ▶ **New:** Additions to the previous edition are indicated by the triangle.
- ~~deleted~~ **Deleted:** Deletions from the previous edition are struck through.

ICD-10-CM Tabular List Symbols

● **Use Additional Character(s):** The red stop sign cautions that the code requires additional character(s) to ensure the greatest specificity.

X For codes less than 6 characters that require a 7th character, a placeholder X should be assigned for all characters less than 6. The 7th character must always be the 7th character of a code.

● **Unacceptable Principal Diagnosis:** These codes have a blue dot before them and give additional information or describe the circumstances affecting the health care encounter but are unacceptable as principal diagnosis in the *Definitions of Medicare Code Edits* (MCE) for inpatient admission.

OGCR The ***Official Guidelines for Coding and Reporting*** symbol includes the placement of a portion of a guideline as that guideline pertains to the code by which it is located. The complete OGCR are located in Part I.

Indicates **complications and comorbidities** and **major complications and comorbidities** according to the *Medicare Severity Diagnosis Related Groups (MS-DRGs), Definitions Manual.*

(Ex:) Indicates **exclusions** to complications and comorbidities (CC) and major complications and comorbidities (MCC) for both primary and secondary diagnoses, according to the *Medicare Severity Diagnosis Related Groups (MS-DRGs), Definitions Manual.* Each exclusion will indicate the corresponding PDX Collection unless the PDX Collection is noted earlier in the Category hierarchy. The collections that list all of the excluded codes will be posted to the companion website (www.codingupdates.com) when available.

PDX as its own CC/MCC Indicates a combination code that when assigned as the Principal Diagnosis, it includes a condition that also qualifies as a CC/MCC according to the *Medicare Severity Diagnosis Related Groups (MS-DRGs), Definitions Manual.*

HAC is a **Hospital-Acquired Condition** that, when present as a secondary diagnosis in an inpatient setting, is a higher cost, higher volume, or both and results in a higher MS-DRG assignment according to the *Medicare Severity Diagnosis Related Groups (MS-DRGs), Definitions Manual.*

The **Hierarchical condition category (HCC)** was initiated in 2004 for the reimbursement for patients with Medicare Advantage plans (Medicare Part C). HCC is based on a list of chronic or severity of illness diagnosis codes that CMS uses to determine reimbursements to Medicare Advantage plans. The HCC risk adjustment factor data is calculated for an entire year for encounters of the patient's care.

Manifestation Code: Describes the manifestation of an underlying disease, not the disease itself, and therefore should not be assigned as a principal diagnosis, according to the *Definitions of Medicare Code Edits* (MCE).

Age conflict: The *Definitions of Medicare Code Edits* (MCE) detects inconsistencies between a patient's age and diagnosis. For example, a 5-year-old patient with benign prostatic hypertrophy or a 78-year-old pregnant female.

The diagnosis is clinically and virtually impossible in a patient of the stated age. Therefore, either the diagnosis or the age is presumed to be incorrect. There are four age categories for diagnoses in the *Definitions of Medicare Code Edits* (MCE):

- **N** Newborn. Age of 0 years; a subset of diagnoses intended only for newborns and neonates (e.g., fetal distress, perinatal jaundice).
- **P** Pediatric. Age range is 0-17 years inclusive (e.g., Reye's syndrome, routine child health exam).
- **M** Maternity. Age range is 9-64 years inclusive (e.g., diabetes in pregnancy, antepartum pulmonary complication).
- **A** Adult. Age range is 15-124 years inclusive (e.g., senile delirium, mature cataract).

♀♂ **Sex conflict:** *Definitions of Medicare Code Edits* (MCE) detects inconsistencies between a patient's sex and any diagnosis or procedure on the patient's record. For example, a male patient with cervical cancer (diagnosis) or a female patient with a prostatectomy (procedure). In both instances, the indicated diagnosis or the procedure conflicts with the stated sex of the patient. Therefore, either the patient's diagnosis, procedure, or sex is presumed to be incorrect.

Key words
Highlight identifies key words within similar code descriptions in a particular category.

Coding Clinic Identifies the year, quarter, and page number that presents information about an ICD-10-CM code in the American Hospital Association's *Coding Clinic®* for ICD-10-CM.

Visit codingupdates.com for the full list of 2025 Present on Admission codes.

SYMBOLS AND CONVENTIONS

ICD-10-CM Tabular

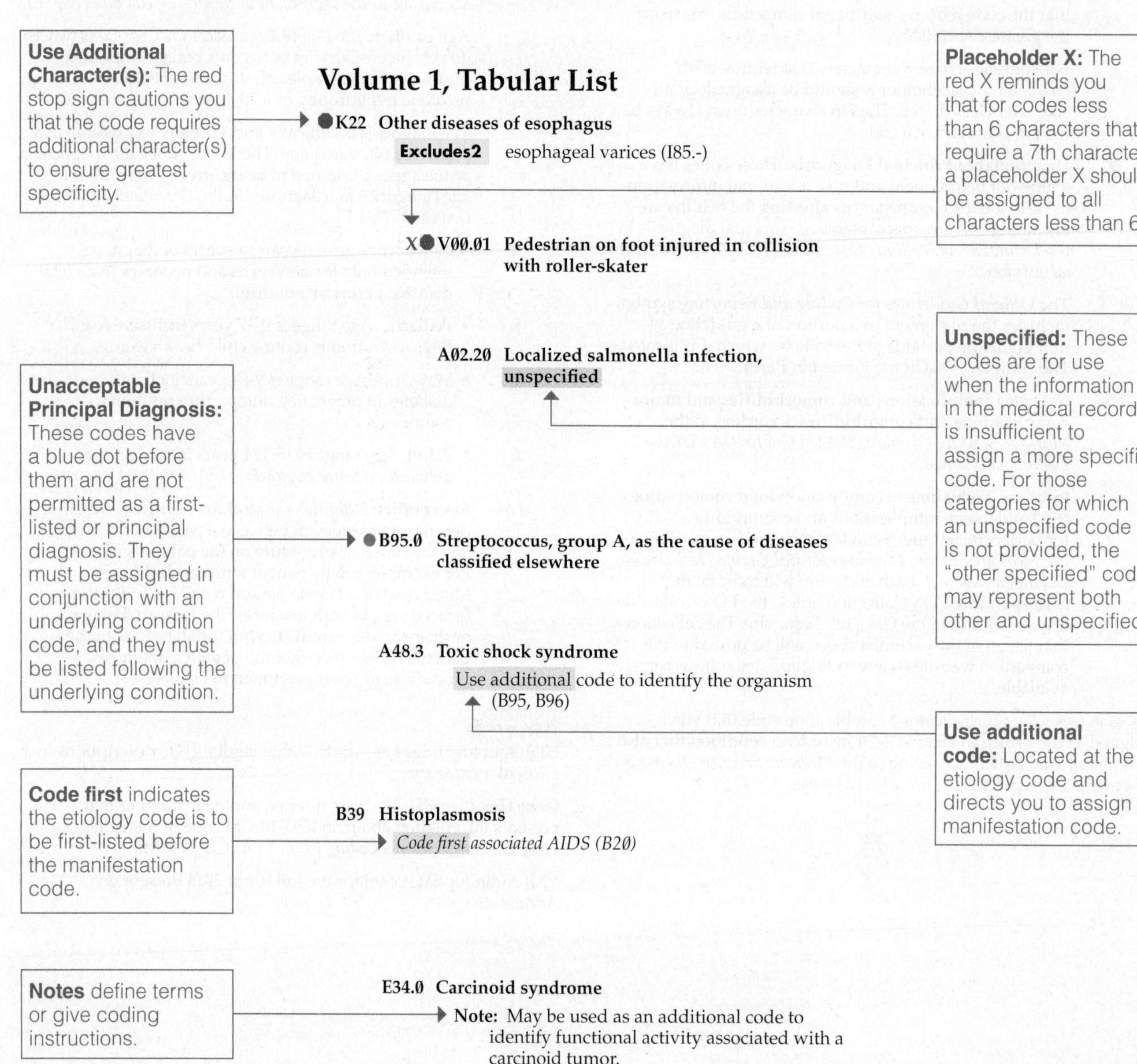
Use Additional Character(s): The red stop sign cautions you that the code requires additional character(s) to ensure greatest specificity.
Volume 1, Tabular List
K22 Other diseases of esophagus
Excludes2 esophageal varices (I85.-)
X V00.01 Pedestrian on foot injured in collision with roller-skater
Placeholder X: The red X reminds you that for codes less than 6 characters that require a 7th character, a placeholder X should be assigned to all characters less than 6.
A02.20 Localized salmonella infection, unspecified
Unspecified: These codes are for use when the information in the medical record is insufficient to assign a more specific code. For those categories for which an unspecified code is not provided, the "other specified" code may represent both other and unspecified.
Unacceptable Principal Diagnosis: These codes have a blue dot before them and are not permitted as a first-listed or principal diagnosis. They must be assigned in conjunction with an underlying condition code, and they must be listed following the underlying condition.
B95.0 Streptococcus, group A, as the cause of diseases classified elsewhere
A48.3 Toxic shock syndrome
Use additional code to identify the organism (B95, B96)
Use additional code: Located at the etiology code and directs you to assign a manifestation code.
Code first indicates the etiology code is to be first-listed before the manifestation code.
B39 Histoplasmosis
Code first associated AIDS (B20)
Notes define terms or give coding instructions.
E34.0 Carcinoid syndrome
Note: May be used as an additional code to identify functional activity associated with a carcinoid tumor.

Codes or index entries are for purposes of illustration only and may not be current.

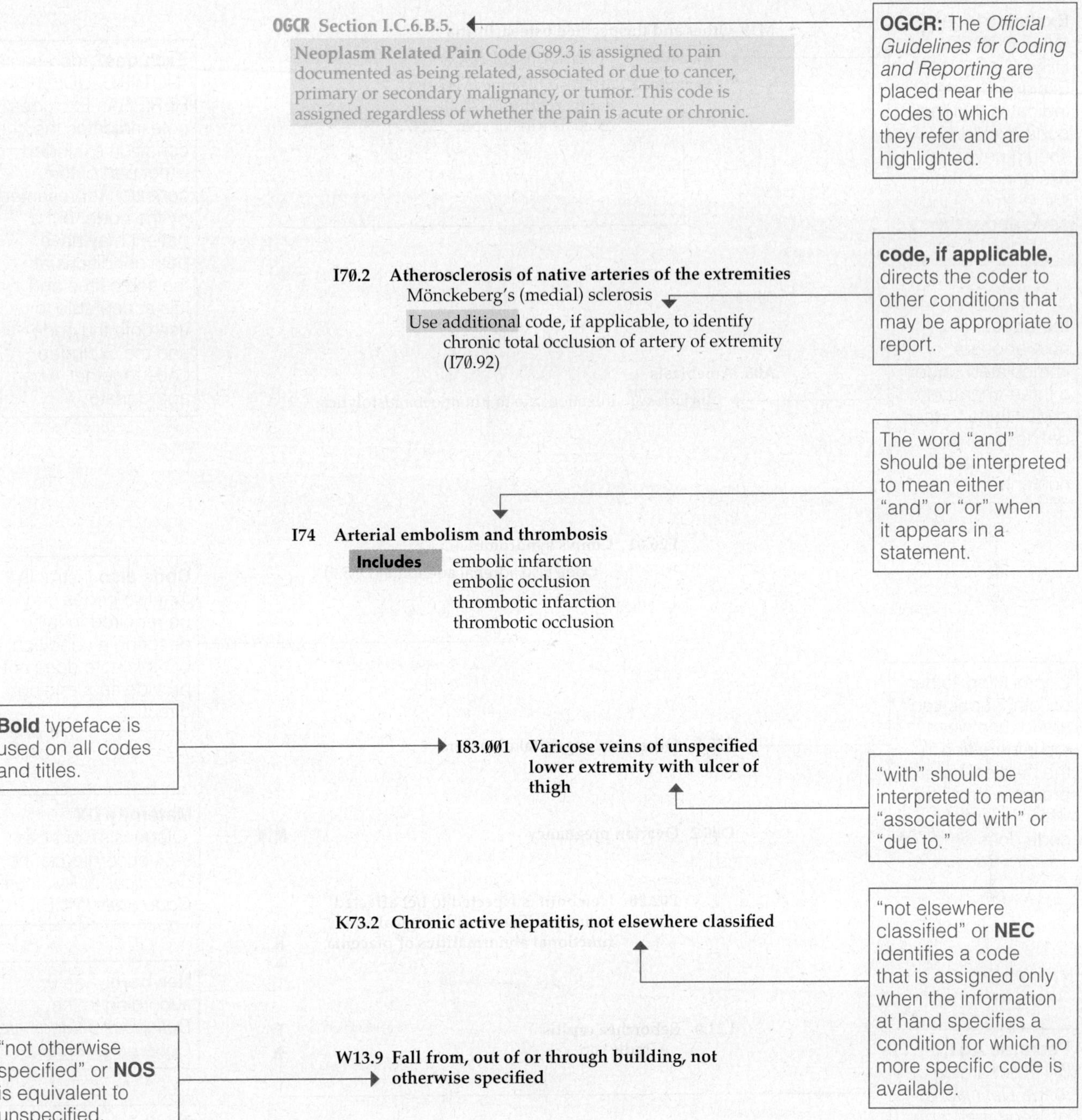
OGCR Section I.C.6.B.5.
Neoplasm Related Pain Code G89.3 is assigned to pain documented as being related, associated or due to cancer, primary or secondary malignancy, or tumor. This code is assigned regardless of whether the pain is acute or chronic.
OGCR: The Official Guidelines for Coding and Reporting are placed near the codes to which they refer and are highlighted.
I70.2 Atherosclerosis of native arteries of the extremities
Mönckeberg's (medial) sclerosis
Use additional code, if applicable, to identify chronic total occlusion of artery of extremity (I70.92)
code, if applicable, directs the coder to other conditions that may be appropriate to report.
The word "and" should be interpreted to mean either "and" or "or" when it appears in a statement.
I74 Arterial embolism and thrombosis
Includes
embolic infarction
embolic occlusion
thrombotic infarction
thrombotic occlusion
Bold typeface is used on all codes and titles.
I83.001 Varicose veins of unspecified lower extremity with ulcer of thigh
"with" should be interpreted to mean "associated with" or "due to."
K73.2 Chronic active hepatitis, not elsewhere classified
"not elsewhere classified" or NEC identifies a code that is assigned only when the information at hand specifies a condition for which no more specific code is available.
"not otherwise specified" or NOS is equivalent to unspecified.
W13.9 Fall from, out of or through building, not otherwise specified

Codes or index entries are for purposes of illustration only and may not be current.

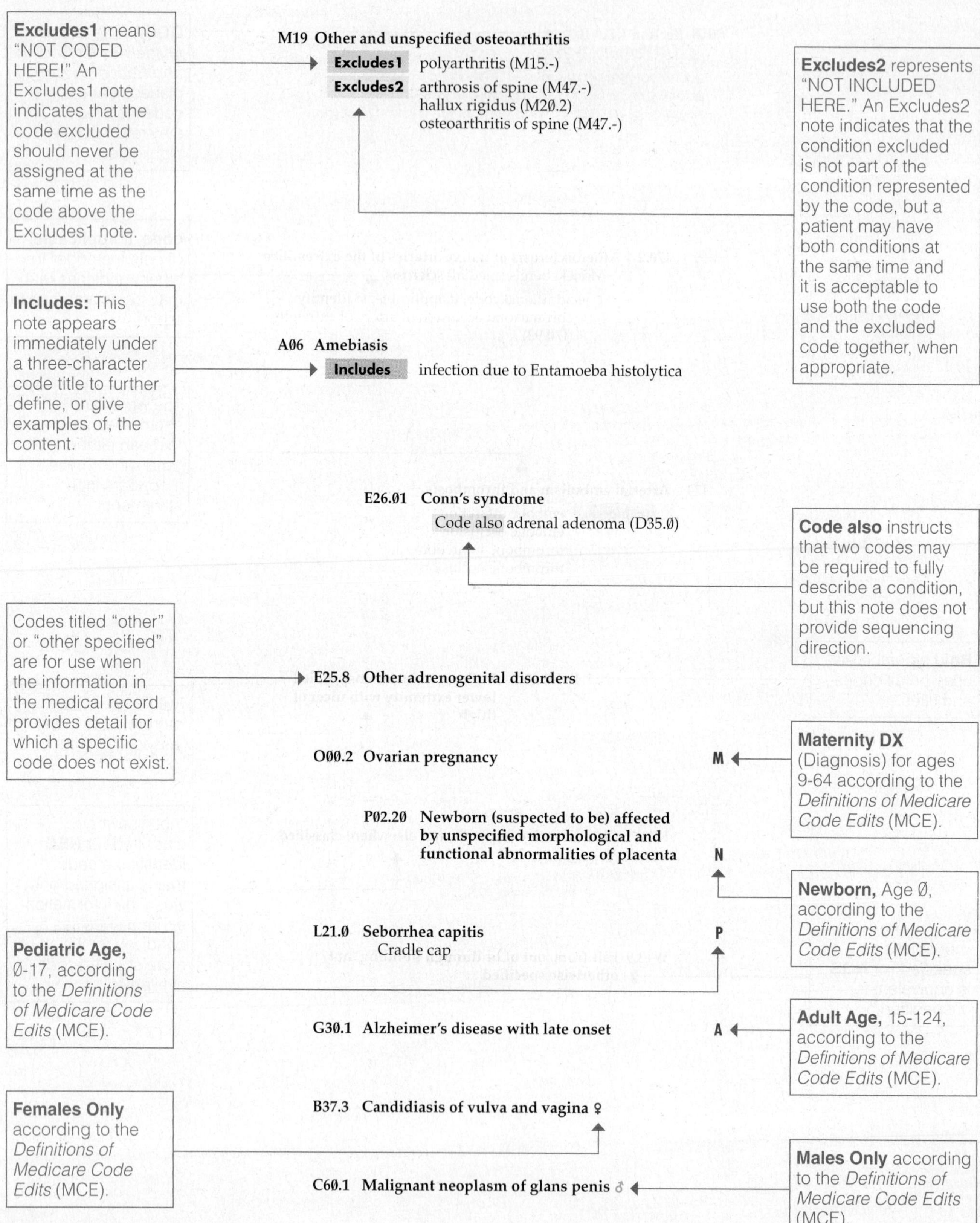

Excludes1 means "NOT CODED HERE!" An Excludes1 note indicates that the code excluded should never be assigned at the same time as the code above the Excludes1 note.
M19 Other and unspecified osteoarthritis
Excludes1 polyarthritis (M15.-)
Excludes2 arthrosis of spine (M47.-)
hallux rigidus (M20.2)
osteoarthritis of spine (M47.-)
Excludes2 represents "NOT INCLUDED HERE." An Excludes2 note indicates that the condition excluded is not part of the condition represented by the code, but a patient may have both conditions at the same time and it is acceptable to use both the code and the excluded code together, when appropriate.
Includes: This note appears immediately under a three-character code title to further define, or give examples of, the content.
A06 Amebiasis
Includes infection due to Entamoeba histolytica
E26.01 Conn's syndrome
Code also adrenal adenoma (D35.0)
Code also instructs that two codes may be required to fully describe a condition, but this note does not provide sequencing direction.
Codes titled "other" or "other specified" are for use when the information in the medical record provides detail for which a specific code does not exist.
E25.8 Other adrenogenital disorders
O00.2 Ovarian pregnancy
M
Maternity DX (Diagnosis) for ages 9-64 according to the Definitions of Medicare Code Edits (MCE).
P02.20 Newborn (suspected to be) affected by unspecified morphological and functional abnormalities of placenta
N
Newborn, Age 0, according to the Definitions of Medicare Code Edits (MCE).
L21.0 Seborrhea capitis
Cradle cap
P
Pediatric Age, 0-17, according to the Definitions of Medicare Code Edits (MCE).
G30.1 Alzheimer's disease with late onset
A
Adult Age, 15-124, according to the Definitions of Medicare Code Edits (MCE).
B37.3 Candidiasis of vulva and vagina ♀
Females Only according to the Definitions of Medicare Code Edits (MCE).
C60.1 Malignant neoplasm of glans penis ♂
Males Only according to the Definitions of Medicare Code Edits (MCE).

Codes or index entries are for purposes of illustration only and may not be current.

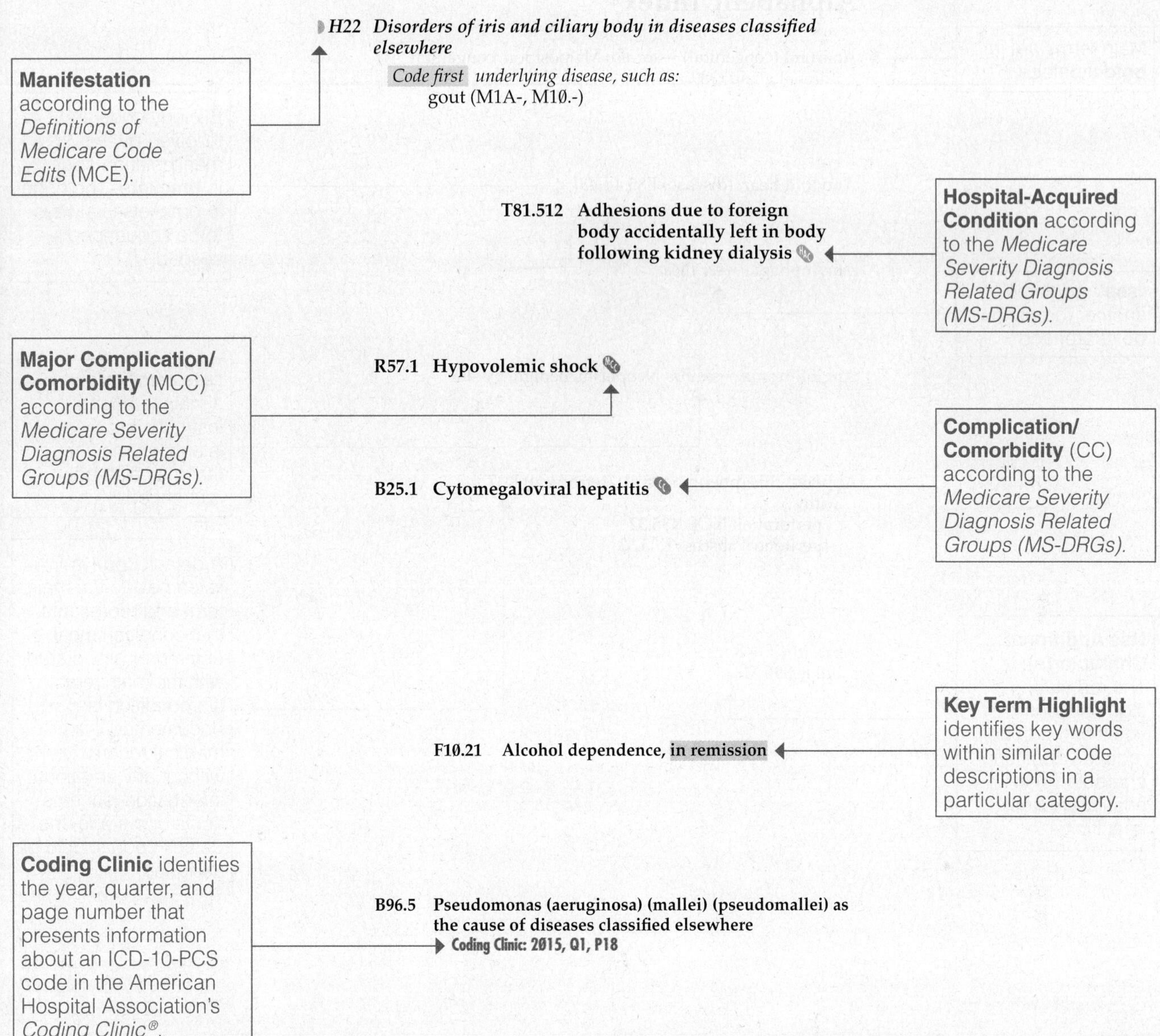
H22 Disorders of iris and ciliary body in diseases classified elsewhere
Code first underlying disease, such as:
gout (M1A-, M1Ø.-)
Manifestation according to the Definitions of Medicare Code Edits (MCE).
T81.512 Adhesions due to foreign body accidentally left in body following kidney dialysis
Hospital-Acquired Condition according to the Medicare Severity Diagnosis Related Groups (MS-DRGs).
Major Complication/ Comorbidity (MCC) according to the Medicare Severity Diagnosis Related Groups (MS-DRGs).
R57.1 Hypovolemic shock
B25.1 Cytomegaloviral hepatitis
Complication/ Comorbidity (CC) according to the Medicare Severity Diagnosis Related Groups (MS-DRGs).
Key Term Highlight identifies key words within similar code descriptions in a particular category.
F1Ø.21 Alcohol dependence, in remission
Coding Clinic identifies the year, quarter, and page number that presents information about an ICD-10-PCS code in the American Hospital Association's Coding Clinic®.
B96.5 Pseudomonas (aeruginosa) (mallei) (pseudomallei) as the cause of diseases classified elsewhere
Coding Clinic: 2015, Q1, P18

Codes or index entries are for purposes of illustration only and may not be current.

Alphabetic Index

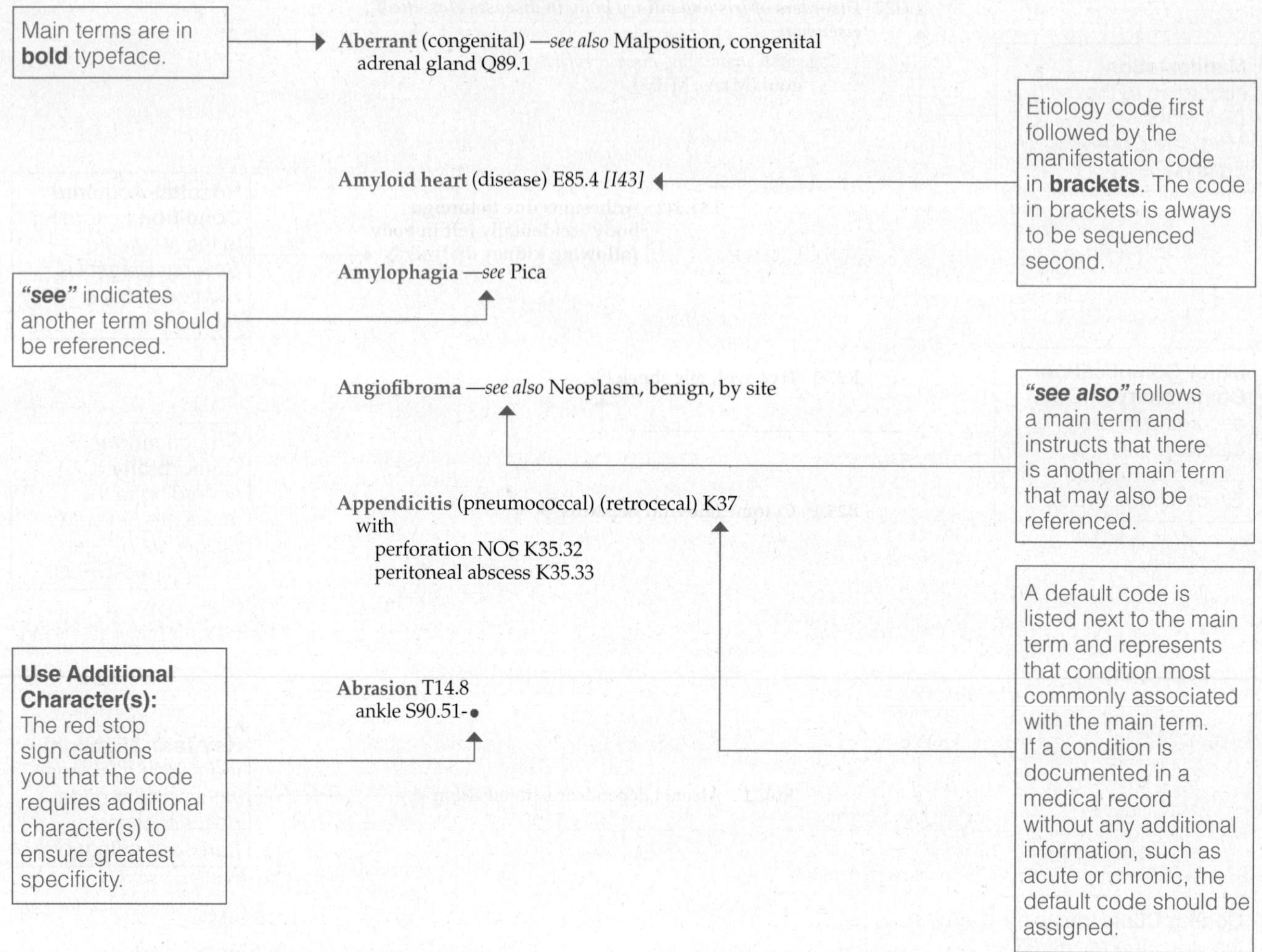
Main terms are in **bold** typeface.
Aberrant (congenital) —*see also* Malposition, congenital
adrenal gland Q89.1
Amyloid heart (disease) E85.4 *[I43]*
Etiology code first followed by the manifestation code in **brackets**. The code in brackets is always to be sequenced second.
Amylophagia —*see* Pica
"see" indicates another term should be referenced.
Angiofibroma —*see also* Neoplasm, benign, by site
"see also" follows a main term and instructs that there is another main term that may also be referenced.
Appendicitis (pneumococcal) (retrocecal) K37
with
perforation NOS K35.32
peritoneal abscess K35.33
A default code is listed next to the main term and represents that condition most commonly associated with the main term. If a condition is documented in a medical record without any additional information, such as acute or chronic, the default code should be assigned.
Abrasion T14.8
ankle S90.51-●
Use Additional Character(s): The red stop sign cautions you that the code requires additional character(s) to ensure greatest specificity.

Codes or index entries are for purposes of illustration only and may not be current.

GUIDE TO THE 2025 ICD-10-CM UPDATES

No Change **CHAPTER 1**

No Change **CERTAIN INFECTIOUS AND PARASITIC DISEASES (AØØ-B99)**

No Change **INTESTINAL INFECTIOUS DISEASES (AØØ-AØ9)**

No Change **AØ4 Other bacterial intestinal infections**
No Change **AØ4.7 Enterocolitis due to Clostridium difficile**
Add Clostridioides difficile colitis

No Change **TUBERCULOSIS (A15-A19)**

No Change **A18 Tuberculosis of other organs**
No Change **A18.4 Tuberculosis of skin and subcutaneous tissue**
Revise from Lupus excedens
Lupus exedens

No Change **INFECTIONS WITH A PREDOMINANTLY SEXUAL MODE OF TRANSMISSION (A5Ø-A64)**

No Change **A5Ø Congenital syphilis**
No Change **A5Ø.4 Late congenital neurosyphilis [juvenile neurosyphilis]**
No Change **A5Ø.45 Juvenile general paresis**
Revise from Juvenile tabetoparetic neurosyphilis
Juvenile taboparetic neurosyphilis

No Change **RICKETTSIOSES (A75-A79)**

No Change **A77 Spotted fever [tick-borne rickettsioses]**
No Change **A77.4 Ehrlichiosis**
Revise from **A77.41 Ehrlichiosis chafeensis [E. chafeensis]**
A77.41 Ehrlichiosis chaffeensis [E. chaffeensis]

No Change **CHAPTER 2**

No Change **NEOPLASMS (CØØ-D49)**

No Change **MALIGNANT NEOPLASMS OF BREAST (C5Ø)**

No Change **C5Ø Malignant neoplasm of breast**
No Change Use Additional
Revise from code to identify estrogen receptor status (Z17.Ø, Z17.1)
code to identify estrogen, and other hormones and factors receptor status (Z17.-)

No Change **MALIGNANT NEUROENDOCRINE TUMORS (C7A)**

No Change **C7A Malignant neuroendocrine tumors**
No Change Use Additional
Revise from carcinoid syndrome (E34.Ø)
carcinoid syndrome (E34.ØØ)

No Change **MALIGNANT NEOPLASMS OF LYMPHOID, HEMATOPOIETIC AND RELATED TISSUE (C81-C96)**

No Change **C81 Hodgkin lymphoma**
No Change **C81.Ø Nodular lymphocyte predominant Hodgkin lymphoma**
Add **C81.ØA Nodular lymphocyte predominant Hodgkin lymphoma, in remission**
No Change **C81.1 Nodular sclerosis Hodgkin lymphoma**
Add **C81.1A Nodular sclerosis Hodgkin lymphoma, in remission**
No Change **C81.2 Mixed cellularity Hodgkin lymphoma**
Add **C81.2A Mixed cellularity Hodgkin lymphoma, in remission**
No Change **C81.3 Lymphocyte depleted Hodgkin lymphoma**
Add **C81.3A Lymphocyte depleted Hodgkin lymphoma, in remission**
No Change **C81.4 Lymphocyte-rich Hodgkin lymphoma**
Add **C81.4A Lymphocyte-rich Hodgkin lymphoma, in remission**
No Change **C81.7 Other Hodgkin lymphoma**
Add **C81.7A Other Hodgkin lymphoma, in remission**
No Change **C81.9 Hodgkin lymphoma, unspecified**
Add **C81.9A Hodgkin lymphoma, unspecified, in remission**

No Change **C82 Follicular lymphoma**
No Change **C82.Ø Follicular lymphoma grade I**
Add **C82.ØA Follicular lymphoma grade I, in remission**
No Change **C82.1 Follicular lymphoma grade II**
Add **C82.1A Follicular lymphoma grade II, in remission**
No Change **C82.2 Follicular lymphoma grade III, unspecified**
Add **C82.2A Follicular lymphoma grade III, unspecified, in remission**
No Change **C82.3 Follicular lymphoma grade IIIa**
Add **C82.3A Follicular lymphoma grade IIIa, in remission**
No Change **C82.4 Follicular lymphoma grade IIIb**
Add **C82.4A Follicular lymphoma grade IIIb, in remission**
No Change **C82.5 Diffuse follicle center lymphoma**
Add **C82.5A Diffuse follicle center lymphoma, in remission**
No Change **C82.6 Cutaneous follicle center lymphoma**
Add **C82.6A Cutaneous follicle center lymphoma, in remission**
No Change **C82.8 Other types of follicular lymphoma**
Add **C82.8A Other types of follicular lymphoma, in remission**
No Change **C82.9 Follicular lymphoma, unspecified**
Add **C82.9A Follicular lymphoma, unspecified, in remission**

No Change C83 Non-follicular lymphoma
No Change C83.0 Small cell B-cell lymphoma
No Change **Excludes1**
Waldenström macroglobulinemia (C88.0)
Waldenström macroglobulinemia (C88.00)
Add C83.0A Small cell B-cell lymphoma, in remission
No Change C83.1 Mantle cell lymphoma
Add C83.1A Mantle cell lymphoma, in remission
Add Centrocytic lymphoma, in remission
No Change C83.3 Diffuse large B-cell lymphoma
Add Diffuse large B-cell lymphoma, subtype not specified
No Change C83.39 Diffuse large B-cell lymphoma, extranodal and solid organ sites
Add C83.390 Primary central nervous system lymphoma
Add PCNSL of brain
Add PCNSL of meninges
Add PCNSL of spinal cord
Add PCNSL NOS
Add **Excludes1** Primary central nervous system lymphoma, Burkitt (C83.79)
Add Primary central nervous system lymphoma, lymphoblastic (C83.59)
Add Primary central nervous system lymphoma, other (C83.89)
Add Primary central nervous system lymphoma, peripheral T-cell (C84.49)
Add C83.398 Diffuse large B-cell lymphoma of other extranodal and solid organ sites
Add C83.3A Diffuse large B-cell lymphoma, in remission
No Change C83.5 Lymphoblastic (diffuse) lymphoma
C83.5A Lymphoblastic (diffuse) lymphoma, in remission
No Change C83.7 Burkitt lymphoma
C83.7A Burkitt lymphoma, in remission
No Change C83.8 Other non-follicular lymphoma
C83.8A Other non-follicular lymphoma, in remission
No Change C83.9 Non-follicular (diffuse) lymphoma, unspecified
C83.9A Non-follicular (diffuse) lymphoma, unspecified, in remission

No Change C84 Mature T/NK-cell lymphomas
No Change C84.0 Mycosis fungoides
C84.0A Mycosis fungoides, in remission
No Change C84.1 Sézary disease
C84.1A Sézary disease, in remission
No Change C84.4 Peripheral T-cell lymphoma, not elsewhere classified
Add C84.4A Peripheral T-cell lymphoma, not elsewhere classified, in remission
No Change C84.6 Anaplastic large cell lymphoma, ALK-positive
Add C84.6A Anaplastic large cell lymphoma, ALK-positive, in remission
No Change C84.7 Anaplastic large cell lymphoma, ALK-negative
Add C84.7B Anaplastic large cell lymphoma, ALK-negative, in remission
No Change C84.A Cutaneous T-cell lymphoma, unspecified
Add C84.AA Cutaneous T-cell lymphoma, unspecified, in remission
No Change C84.Z Other mature T/NK-cell lymphomas
Excludes1
Revise from angioimmunoblastic T-cell lymphoma (C86.5)
Revise to angioimmunoblastic T-cell lymphoma (C86.50)
Revise from blastic NK-cell lymphoma (C86.4)
Revise to blastic NK-cell lymphoma (C86.40)
Revise from enteropathy-type T-cell lymphoma (C86.2)
Revise to enteropathy-type T-cell lymphoma (C86.20)
Revise from extranodal NK-cell lymphoma, nasal type (C86.0)
Revise to extranodal NK-cell lymphoma, nasal type (C86.00)
Revise from hepatosplenic T-cell lymphoma (C86.1)
Revise to hepatosplenic T-cell lymphoma (C86.10)
Revise from primary cutaneous CD30-positive T-cell proliferations (C86.6)
Revise to primary cutaneous CD30-positive T-cell proliferations (C86.60)
Revise from subcutaneous panniculitis-like T-cell lymphoma (C86.3)
Revise to subcutaneous panniculitis-like T-cell lymphoma (C86.30)
Add C84.ZA Other mature T/NK-cell lymphomas, in remission
No Change C84.9 Mature T/NK-cell lymphomas, unspecified
Add C84.9A Mature T/NK-cell lymphomas, unspecified, in remission

No Change C85 Other specified and unspecified types of non-Hodgkin lymphoma
No Change C85.1 Unspecified B-cell lymphoma
Add C85.1A Unspecified B-cell lymphoma, in remission
No Change C85.2 Mediastinal (thymic) large B-cell lymphoma
Add C85.2A Mediastinal (thymic) large B-cell lymphoma, in remission
No Change C85.8 Other specified types of non-Hodgkin lymphoma
Add C85.8A Other specified types of non-Hodgkin lymphoma, in remission
No Change C85.9 Non-Hodgkin lymphoma, unspecified
Add C85.9A Non-Hodgkin lymphoma, unspecified, in remission

No Change C86 **Other specified types of T/NK-cell lymphoma**
No Change C86.0 **Extranodal NK/T-cell lymphoma, nasal type**
Add C86.00 **Extranodal NK/T-cell lymphoma, nasal type not having achieved remission**
Add Extranodal NK/T-cell lymphoma, nasal type NOS
Add Extranodal NK/T-cell lymphoma, nasal type with failed remission
Add C86.01 **Extranodal NK/T-cell lymphoma, nasal type, in remission**
No Change C86.1 **Hepatosplenic T-cell lymphoma**
Add C86.10 **Hepatosplenic T-cell lymphoma not having achieved remission**
Add Hepatosplenic T-cell lymphoma NOS
Add Hepatosplenic T-cell lymphoma with failed remission
Add C86.11 **Hepatosplenic T-cell lymphoma, in remission**
No Change C86.2 **Enteropathy-type (intestinal) T-cell lymphoma**
Add C86.20 **Enteropathy-type (intestinal) T-cell lymphoma not having achieved remission**
Add Enteropathy associated T-cell lymphoma NOS
Add Enteropathy associated T-cell lymphoma not having achieved remission
Add Enteropathy associated T-cell lymphoma with failed remission
Add Enteropathy-type (intestinal) T-cell lymphoma NOS
Add Enteropathy-type (intestinal) T-cell lymphoma with failed remission
Add C86.21 **Enteropathy-type (intestinal) T-cell lymphoma, in remission**
Add Enteropathy associated T-cell lymphoma, in remission
No Change C86.3 **Subcutaneous panniculitis-like T-cell lymphoma**
Add C86.30 **Subcutaneous panniculitis-like T-cell lymphoma not having achieved remission**
Add Subcutaneous panniculitis-like T-cell lymphoma NOS
Add Subcutaneous panniculitis-like T-cell lymphoma with failed remission
C86.31 **Subcutaneous panniculitis-like T-cell lymphoma, in remission**
No Change C86.4 **Blastic NK-cell lymphoma**
Add C86.40 **Blastic NK-cell lymphoma not having achieved remission**
Add Blastic NK-cell lymphoma NOS
Add Blastic NK-cell lymphoma with failed remission
Add Blastic plasmacytoid dendritic cell neoplasm (BPDCN) NOS
Add Blastic plasmacytoid dendritic cell neoplasm (BPDCN) not having achieved remission
Add Blastic plasmacytoid dendritic cell neoplasm (BPDCN) with failed remission
Add C86.41 **Blastic NK-cell lymphoma, in remission**
Add Blastic plasmacytoid dendritic cell neoplasm (BPDCN), in remission

No Change C86.5 **Angioimmunoblastic T-cell lymphoma**
Add C86.50 **Angioimmunoblastic T-cell lymphoma not having achieved remission**
Add Angioimmunoblastic lymphadenopathy with dysproteinemia (AILD) NOS
Add Angioimmunoblastic lymphadenopathy with dysproteinemia (AILD) not having achieved remission
Add Angioimmunoblastic lymphadenopathy with dysproteinemia (AILD) with failed remission
Add Angioimmunoblastic T-cell lymphoma NOS
Add Angioimmunoblastic T-cell lymphoma with failed remission
Add C86.51 **Angioimmunoblastic T-cell lymphoma, in remission**
Add Angioimmunoblastic lymphadenopathy with dysproteinemia (AILD), in remission
No Change C86.6 **Primary cutaneous CD30-positive T-cell proliferations**
Add C86.60 **Primary cutaneous CD30-positive T-cell proliferations not having achieved remission**
Add Lymphomatoid papulosis NOS
Add Lymphomatoid papulosis not having achieved remission
Add Lymphomatoid papulosis with failed remission
Add Primary cutaneous anaplastic large cell lymphoma NOS
Add Primary cutaneous anaplastic large cell lymphoma not having achieved remission
Add Primary cutaneous anaplastic large cell lymphoma with failed remission
Add Primary cutaneous CD30-positive large T-cell lymphoma NOS
Add Primary cutaneous CD30-positive large T-cell lymphoma not having achieved remission
Add Primary cutaneous CD30-positive large T-cell lymphoma with failed remission
Add Primary cutaneous CD30-positive T-cell proliferations NOS
Add Primary cutaneous CD30-positive T-cell proliferations with failed remission
Add C86.61 **Primary cutaneous CD30-positive T-cell proliferations, in remission**
No Change C88 **Malignant immunoproliferative diseases and certain other B-cell lymphomas**
No Change C88.0 **Waldenström macroglobulinemia**
Add C88.00 **Waldenström macroglobulinemia not having achieved remission**
Add Lymphoplasmacytic lymphoma with IgM-production, NOS
Add Lymphoplasmacytic lymphoma with IgM-production not having achieved remission
Add Lymphoplasmacytic lymphoma with IgM-production with failed remission
Add Macroglobulinemia (idiopathic) (primary) NOS
Add Macroglobulinemia (idiopathic) (primary) not having achieved remission
Add Macroglobulinemia (idiopathic) (primary) with failed remission
Add Waldenström macroglobulinemia NOS
Add Waldenström macroglobulinemia with failed remission
Add C88.01 **Waldenström macroglobulinemia, in remission**

No Change C88.2 **Heavy chain disease**
Add C88.20 **Heavy chain disease not having achieved remission**
Add Franklin disease NOS
Add Franklin disease not having achieved remission
Add Franklin disease with failed remission
Add Gamma heavy chain disease NOS
Add Gamma heavy chain disease not having achieved remission
Add Gamma heavy chain disease with failed remission
Add Heavy chain disease NOS
Heavy chain disease with failed remissionMu heavy chain disease not having achieved remission
Add Mu heavy chain disease NOS
Add Mu heavy chain disease not having achieved remission
Add Mu heavy chain disease with failed remission
Add C88.21 **Heavy chain disease, in remission**
No Change C88.3 **Immunoproliferative small intestinal disease**
Add C88.30 **Immunoproliferative small intestinal disease not having achieved remission**
Add Alpha heavy chain disease NOS
Add Alpha heavy chain disease not having achieved remission
Add Alpha heavy chain disease with failed remission
Add Immunoproliferative small intestinal disease NOS
Add Immunoproliferative small intestinal disease with failed remission
Add Mediterranean lymphoma NOS
Add Mediterranean lymphoma not having achieved remission
Add Mediterranean lymphoma with failed remission
Add C88.31 **Immunoproliferative small intestinal disease, in remission**
No Change C88.4 **Extranodal marginal zone B-cell lymphoma of mucosa-associated lymphoid tissue [MALT-lymphoma]**
Add C88.40 **Extranodal marginal zone B-cell lymphoma of mucosa-associated lymphoid tissue [MALT-lymphoma] not having achieved remission**
Add Extranodal marginal zone B-cell lymphoma of mucosa-associated lymphoid tissue [MALT-lymphoma] NOS
Add Extranodal marginal zone B-cell lymphoma of mucosa-associated lymphoid tissue [MALT-lymphoma] with failed remission
Add Lymphoma of bronchial-associated lymphoid tissue [BALT-lymphoma] NOS
Add Lymphoma of bronchial-associated lymphoid tissue [BALT-lymphoma] not having achieved remission
Add Lymphoma of bronchial-associated lymphoid tissue [BALT-lymphoma] with failed remission
Add Lymphoma of skin-associated lymphoid tissue [SALT-lymphoma] NOS
Add Lymphoma of skin-associated lymphoid tissue [SALT-lymphoma] not having achieved remission
Add Lymphoma of skin-associated lymphoid tissue [SALT-lymphoma] with failed remission

Add C88.41 **Extranodal marginal zone B-cell lymphoma of mucosa-associated lymphoid tissue [MALT-lymphoma], in remission**
No Change C88.8 **Other malignant immunoproliferative diseases**
Add C88.80 **Other malignant immunoproliferative diseases not having achieved remission**
Add Other malignant immunoproliferative diseases NOS
Add Other malignant immunoproliferative diseases with failed remission
Add C88.81 **Other malignant immunoproliferative diseases, in remission**
No Change C88.9 **Malignant immunoproliferative disease, unspecified**
Add C88.90 **Malignant immunoproliferative disease, unspecified not having achieved remission**
Add Immunoproliferative disease NOS
Add Immunoproliferative disease NOS not having achieved remission
Add Immunoproliferative disease NOS with failed remission
Add Malignant immunoproliferative disease, unspecified NOS
Add Malignant immunoproliferative disease, unspecified with failed remission
Add C88.91 **Malignant immunoproliferative disease, unspecified, in remission**

No Change **IN SITU NEOPLASMS (D00-D09)**

No Change D05 **Carcinoma in situ of breast**
Add **Excludes2** malignant neoplasm of breast (C50.-)

No Change **BENIGN NEUROENDOCRINE TUMORS (D3A)**

No Change D3A **Benign neuroendocrine tumors**
No Change Use Additional
Revise from carcinoid syndrome (E34.0)
Revise to carcinoid syndrome (E34.00)

No Change **CHAPTER 3**

No Change **DISEASES OF THE BLOOD AND BLOOD-FORMING ORGANS AND CERTAIN DISORDERS INVOLVING THE IMMUNE MECHANISM (D50-D89)**

No Change **APLASTIC AND OTHER ANEMIAS AND OTHER BONE MARROW FAILURE SYNDROMES (D60-D64)**

No Change D61 **Other aplastic anemias and other bone marrow failure syndromes**
No Change D61.0 **Constitutional aplastic anemia**
Add D61.03 **Fanconi anemia**
Add Fanconi pancytopenia
Add Fanconi's anemia
Add **Excludes1** Fanconi syndrome (E72.0-)
No Change D61.09 **Other constitutional aplastic anemia**
Delete Fanconi's anemia

No Change **CERTAIN DISORDERS INVOLVING THE IMMUNE MECHANISM (D80-D89)**

No Change D89 **Other disorders involving the immune mechanism, not elsewhere classified**
No Change D89.8 **Other specified disorders involving the immune mechanism, not elsewhere classified**
No Change D89.83 **Cytokine release syndrome**
Add Use Additional code for adverse effect, if applicable, to identify immune checkpoint inhibitors and immunostimulant drugs (T45.AX5)

No Change **CHAPTER 4**

No Change **ENDOCRINE, NUTRITIONAL AND METABOLIC DISEASES (E00-E89)**

No Change **DISORDERS OF THYROID GLAND (E00-E07)**

No Change **E07 Other disorders of thyroid**

No Change **E07.1 Dyshormogenetic goiter**
Add Dyshormonogenetic goiter
Add Familial dyshormonogenetic goiter

No Change **DIABETES MELLITUS (E08-E13)**

No Change **E08 Diabetes mellitus due to underlying condition**
Add Use Additional injectable non-insulin antidiabetic drugs (Z79.85)

No Change **E08.6 Diabetes mellitus due to underlying condition with other specified complications**

No Change **E08.64 Diabetes mellitus due to underlying condition with hypoglycemia**
Add Use Additional code for hypoglycemia level, if applicable (E16.A-)

No Change **E09 Drug or chemical induced diabetes mellitus**
Add Use Additional injectable non-insulin antidiabetic drugs (Z79.85)

No Change **E09.6 Drug or chemical induced diabetes mellitus with other specified complications**

No Change **E09.64 Drug or chemical induced diabetes mellitus with hypoglycemia**
Add Use Additional code for hypoglycemia level, if applicable (E16.A-)

No Change **E10 Type 1 diabetes mellitus**

No Change **E10.6 Type 1 diabetes mellitus with other specified complications**

No Change **E10.64 Type 1 diabetes mellitus with hypoglycemia**
Add Use Additional code for hypoglycemia level, if applicable (E16.A-)

Add **E10.A Type 1 diabetes mellitus, presymptomatic**
Early-stage type 1 diabetes mellitus

Add **E10.A0 Type 1 diabetes mellitus, presymptomatic, unspecified**

Add **E10.A1 Type 1 diabetes mellitus, presymptomatic, Stage 1**
Add Multiple confirmed islet autoantibodies with normoglycemia

Add **E10.A2 Type 1 diabetes mellitus, presymptomatic, Stage 2**
Add Confirmed islet autoimmunity with dysglycemia

No Change **E11 Type 2 diabetes mellitus**
Add Use Additional injectable non-insulin antidiabetic drugs (Z79.85)

No Change **E11.6 Type 2 diabetes mellitus with other specified complications**

No Change **E11.64 Type 2 diabetes mellitus with hypoglycemia**
Add Use Additional code for hypoglycemia level, if applicable (E16.A-)

No Change **E13 Other specified diabetes mellitus**
Add Use Additional injectable non-insulin antidiabetic drugs (Z79.85)

No Change **E13.6 Other specified diabetes mellitus with other specified complications**

No Change **E13.64 Other specified diabetes mellitus with hypoglycemia**
Add Use Additional code for hypoglycemia level, if applicable (E16.A-)

No Change **OTHER DISORDERS OF GLUCOSE REGULATION AND PANCREATIC INTERNAL SECRETION (E15-E16)**

No Change **E16 Other disorders of pancreatic internal secretion**

No Change **E16.0 Drug-induced hypoglycemia without coma**
No Change Use Additional
Delete code for adverse effect, if applicable, to identify drug (T36-T50 with fifth or sixth character 5)
Add code for hypoglycemia level, if applicable (E16.A-)

No Change **E16.1 Other hypoglycemia**
Add Use Additional code for hypoglycemia level, if applicable (E16.A-)

No Change **E16.2 Hypoglycemia, unspecified**
Add Use Additional code for hypoglycemia level, if applicable (E16.A-)

No Change **E16.A Hypoglycemia level**
Add **E16.A1 Hypoglycemia level 1**
Add Decreased blood glucose level 1
Add **E16.A2 Hypoglycemia level 2**
Add Decreased blood glucose level 2
Add **E16.A3 Hypoglycemia level 3**
Add Decreased blood glucose level 3

No Change **DISORDERS OF OTHER ENDOCRINE GLANDS (E20-E35)**

No Change **E34 Other endocrine disorders**

No Change **E34.0 Carcinoid syndrome**
Delete **Note:** May be used as an Additional code to identify functional activity associated with a carcinoid tumor.
Add Code also the underlying disorder, such as:
Add primary neuroendocrine tumors (C7A.-)
Add secondary neuroendocrine tumors (C7B.-)
Add **E34.00 Carcinoid syndrome, unspecified**
Add Carcinoid disease, unspecified
Add **E34.01 Carcinoid heart syndrome**
Add Carcinoid heart disease
Add Hedinger syndrome
Add **E34.09 Other carcinoid syndrome**
Add Carcinoid disease NEC
Add Carcinoid syndrome NEC
Add Other carcinoid disease

No Change **OVERWEIGHT, OBESITY AND OTHER HYPERALIMENTATION (E65-E68)**

No Change **E66 Overweight and obesity**
No Change Use Additional
Revise from code to identify body mass index (BMI), if known (Z68.-)
Revise to code to identify body mass index (BMI), if known, for adults (Z68.1-Z68.45) or pediatrics (Z68.5-)
Delete **Excludes1** adiposogenital dystrophy (E23.6)
Delete lipomatosis NOS (E88.2)
Delete lipomatosis dolorosa [Dercum] (E88.2)
Delete Prader-Willi syndrome (Q87.11)
Add **Excludes2** adiposogenital dystrophy (E23.6)
Add lipomatosis dolorosa [Dercum] (E88.2)
Add lipomatosis NOS (E88.2)
Add Prader-Willi syndrome (Q87.11)

No Change **E66.8 Other obesity**
Add **E66.81 Obesity class**
Add **E66.811 Obesity, class 1**
Add **E66.812 Obesity, class 2**
Add **E66.813 Obesity, class 3**
Add **E66.89 Other obesity not elsewhere classified**

No Change **METABOLIC DISORDERS (E70-E88)**

No Change E74 **Other disorders of carbohydrate metabolism**

No Change E74.8 **Other specified disorders of carbohydrate metabolism**

Add E74.82 **Disorders of citrate metabolism**

Add E74.820 **SLC13A5 Citrate Transporter Disorder**

Add E74.829 **Other disorders of citrate metabolism**

No Change E87 **Other disorders of fluid, electrolyte and acid-base balance**

No Change E87.Ø **Hyperosmolality and hypernatremia**

Delete **Excludes1** diabetes with hyperosmolarity (EØ8, EØ9, E11, E13 with final characters .ØØ or .Ø1)

Add **Excludes2** diabetes with hyperosmolarity (EØ8, EØ9, E11, E13 with final characters .ØØ or .Ø1)

No Change E88 **Other and unspecified metabolic disorders**

No Change E88.Ø **Disorders of plasma-protein metabolism, not elsewhere classified**

No Change **Excludes1**

Revise from Waldenström macroglobulinemia (C88.Ø)

Revise to Waldenström macroglobulinemia (C88.ØØ)

No Change E88.8 **Other specified metabolic disorders**

Add E88.82 **Obesity due to disruption of MC4R pathway**

Add Use Additional code, if applicable, to identify associated manifestations, such as polyphagia (R63.2)

Add Use Additional code to identify body mass index (BMI), if known (Z68.-)

No Change CHAPTER 5

No Change MENTAL, BEHAVIORAL AND NEURODEVELOPMENTAL DISORDERS (FØ1-F99)

No Change **MENTAL DISORDERS DUE TO KNOWN PHYSIOLOGICAL CONDITIONS (FØ1-FØ9)**

No Change FØ1 **Vascular dementia**

No Change *Code first*

Delete the underlying physiological condition or sequelae of cerebrovascular disease.

Add , if applicable, any causal condition

No Change FØ2 **Dementia in other diseases classified elsewhere**

No Change *Code first*

Delete dementia with Lewy bodies (G31.83)

Delete dementia with Parkinsonism (G31.83)

Add neurocognitive disorder with Lewy bodies (G31.83)

Add other frontotemporal neurocognitive disorder (G31.9Ø)

No Change FØ3 **Unspecified dementia**

Delete **Excludes1** senility NOS (R41.81)

No Change **Excludes2**

Add dementia with delirium or acute confusional state (FØ5)

Delete senile dementia with delirium or acute confusional state (FØ5)

No Change FØ6 **Other mental disorders due to known physiological condition**

No Change **Excludes1**

Revise from unspecified dementia (FØ3)

Revise to unspecified dementia (FØ3.-)

No Change FØ6.7 **Mild neurocognitive disorder due to known physiological condition**

No Change *Code first*

Delete frontotemporal neurocognitive disorder (G31.Ø9)

Add other frontotemporal neurocognitive disorder (G31.Ø9)

No Change **Excludes1**

Revise from dementia (FØ1.-, FØ2.-, FØ3)

Revise to dementia (FØ1.-, FØ2.-, FØ3.-)

No Change **SCHIZOPHRENIA, SCHIZOTYPAL, DELUSIONAL, AND OTHER NON-MOOD PSYCHOTIC DISORDERS (F2Ø-F29)**

No Change F2Ø **Schizophrenia**

Add Use Additional code, if applicable, to identify:

Add other specified cognitive deficit (R41.84-)

No Change **ANXIETY, DISSOCIATIVE, STRESS-RELATED, SOMATOFORM AND OTHER NONPSYCHOTIC MENTAL DISORDERS (F4Ø-F48)**

No Change F45 **Somatoform disorders**

No Change F45.2 **Hypochondriacal disorders**

No Change F45.22 **Body dysmorphic disorder**

Add Bigorexia

Add Muscle dysmorphia

No Change **BEHAVIORAL SYNDROMES ASSOCIATED WITH PHYSIOLOGICAL DISTURBANCES AND PHYSICAL FACTORS (F5Ø-F59)**

No Change F5Ø **Eating disorders**

No Change F5Ø.Ø **Anorexia nervosa**

No Change F5Ø.Ø1 **Anorexia nervosa, restricting type**

Add F5Ø.Ø1Ø **Anorexia nervosa, restricting type, mild**

Add Anorexia nervosa, restricting type, with a body mass index greater than or equal to 17 kg/m2

Add F5Ø.Ø11 **Anorexia nervosa, restricting type, moderate**

Add Anorexia nervosa, restricting type, with a body mass index of 16.Ø-16.99 kg/m2

Add F5Ø.Ø12 **Anorexia nervosa, restricting type, severe**

Add Anorexia nervosa, restricting type, with a body mass index of 15.Ø-15.99 kg/m2

Add F5Ø.Ø13 **Anorexia nervosa, restricting type, extreme**

Add Anorexia nervosa, restricting type, with a body mass index of less than 15.Ø kg/m2

Add F5Ø.Ø14 **Anorexia nervosa, restricting type, in remission**

Add Anorexia nervosa, restricting type, in full remission

Add Anorexia nervosa, restricting type, in partial remission

Add F5Ø.Ø19 **Anorexia nervosa, restricting type, unspecified**

No Change **F50.02 Anorexia nervosa, binge eating/purging type**
No Change **Excludes1**
Revise from bulimia nervosa (F50.2)
Revise to bulimia nervosa (F50.2-)
Add **F50.020 Anorexia nervosa, binge eating/purging type, mild**
Add Anorexia nervosa, binge eating/purging type, with a body mass index greater than or equal to 17 kg/m2
Add **F50.021 Anorexia nervosa, binge eating/purging type, moderate**
Add Anorexia nervosa, binge eating/purging type, with a body mass index of 16.0-16.99 kg/m2
Add **F50.022 Anorexia nervosa, binge eating/purging type, severe**
Add Anorexia nervosa, binge eating/purging type, with a body mass index of 15.0-15.99 kg/m2
Add **F50.023 Anorexia nervosa, binge eating/purging type, extreme**
Add Anorexia nervosa, binge eating/purging type, with a body mass index of less than 15.0 kg/m2
Add **F50.024 Anorexia nervosa, binge eating/purging type, in remission**
Add Anorexia nervosa, binge eating/purging type, in full remission
Add Anorexia nervosa, binge eating/purging type, in partial remission
Add **F50.029 Anorexia nervosa, binge eating/purging type, unspecified**
No Change **F50.2 Bulimia nervosa**
No Change **Excludes1**
Revise from anorexia nervosa, binge eating/purging type (F50.02)
Revise to anorexia nervosa, binge eating/purging type (F50.02-)
Add **F50.20 Bulimia nervosa, unspecified**
Add **F50.21 Bulimia nervosa, mild**
Add Bulimia nervosa with 1-3 episodes of inappropriate compensatory behavior per week
Add **F50.22 Bulimia nervosa, moderate**
Add Bulimia nervosa with 4-7 episodes of inappropriate compensatory behavior per week
Add **F50.23 Bulimia nervosa, severe**
Add Bulimia nervosa with 8-13 episodes of inappropriate compensatory behavior per week
Add **F50.24 Bulimia nervosa, extreme**
Add Bulimia nervosa with 14 or more episodes of inappropriate compensatory behavior per week
Add **F50.25 Bulimia nervosa, in remission**
Add Bulimia nervosa, in full remission
Add Bulimia nervosa, in partial remission

No Change **F50.8 Other eating disorders**
Delete **Excludes2** pica of infancy and childhood (F98.3)
No Change **F50.81 Binge eating disorder**
Add **F50.810 Binge eating disorder, mild**
Add Binge eating disorder with 1-3 binge eating episodes per week
Add **F50.811 Binge eating disorder, moderate**
Add Binge eating disorder with 4-7 binge eating episodes per week
Add **F50.812 Binge eating disorder, severe**
Add Binge eating disorder with 8-13 binge eating episodes per week
Add **F50.813 Binge eating disorder, extreme**
Add Binge eating disorder with 14 or more eating episodes per week
Add **F50.814 Binge eating disorder, in remission**
Add Binge eating disorder, in full remission
Add Binge eating disorder, in partial remission
Add **F50.819 Binge eating disorder, unspecified**
No Change **F50.82 Avoidant/restrictive food intake disorder**
Add Avoidant/restrictive food intake disorder, in remission
Add **F50.83 Pica in adults**
Add Pica in adults, in remission
Add **Excludes1** pica in infancy and childhood (F98.3)
Add **F50.84 Rumination disorder in adults**
Add Rumination disorder in adults, in remission
Add **Excludes1** rumination disorder in infancy and childhood (F98.21)
No Change **F50.89 Other specified eating disorder**
Delete Pica in adults

No Change **BEHAVIORAL AND EMOTIONAL DISORDERS WITH ONSET USUALLY OCCURRING IN CHILDHOOD AND ADOLESCENCE (F90-F98)**

No Change **F98 Other behavioral and emotional disorders with onset usually occurring in childhood and adolescence**
No Change **F98.2 Other feeding disorders of infancy and childhood**
Revise from **F98.21 Rumination disorder of infancy**
Revise to **F98.21 Rumination disorder of infancy and childhood**
Add Rumination disorder in infancy or childhood, in remission
Add **Excludes1** rumination disorder in adults (F50.84)
No Change **F98.3 Pica of infancy and childhood**
Add Pica in infancy or childhood, in remission
Add **Excludes1** pica in adults (F50.83)

No Change CHAPTER 6

No Change **DISEASES OF THE NERVOUS SYSTEM (GØØ-G99)**

No Change **EXTRAPYRAMIDAL AND MOVEMENT DISORDERS (G2Ø-G26)**

No Change G21 **Secondary parkinsonism**
No Change **Excludes1**
Delete dementia with Parkinsonism (G31.83)
Add neurocognitive disorder with Lewy bodies (G31.83)

No Change **OTHER DEGENERATIVE DISEASES OF THE NERVOUS SYSTEM (G3Ø-G32)**

No Change G3Ø **Alzheimer's disease**
No Change **Excludes1**
Revise from senile dementia NOS (FØ3)
Revise to senile dementia NOS (FØ3.-)

No Change G31 **Other degenerative diseases of nervous system, not elsewhere classified**
No Change G31.8 **Other specified degenerative diseases of nervous system**
No Change G31.84 **Mild cognitive impairment of uncertain or unknown etiology**
No Change **Excludes1**
Revise from dementia (FØ1.-, FØ2.-, FØ3)
Revise to dementia (FØ1.-, FØ2.-, FØ3.-)

No Change **EPISODIC AND PAROXYSMAL DISORDERS (G4Ø-G47)**

No Change G4Ø **Epilepsy and recurrent seizures**
No Change G4Ø.8 **Other epilepsy and recurrent seizures**
Add G4Ø.84 **KCNQ2-related epilepsy**
Add G4Ø.841 **KCNQ2-related epilepsy, not intractable, with status epilepticus**
Add G4Ø.842 **KCNQ2-related epilepsy, not intractable, without status epilepticus**
Add KCNQ2-related epilepsy NOS
Add G4Ø.843 **KCNQ2-related epilepsy, intractable, with status epilepticus**
Add G4Ø.844 **KCNQ2-related epilepsy, intractable, without status epilepticus**

No Change **OTHER DISORDERS OF THE NERVOUS SYSTEM (G89-G99)**

No Change G9Ø **Disorders of autonomic nervous system**
No Change G9Ø.8 **Other disorders of autonomic nervous system**
Add G9Ø.81 **Serotonin syndrome**
Add Serotonin toxicity
Add *Code first poisoning due to drug or toxin, such as:*
Add linezolid (T36.8X- with sixth character 1-4)
Add monoamine oxidase inhibitors (T43.1X with sixth character 1-4)
Add selective serotonin and norepinephrine reuptake inhibitors [SSNRI] (T43.21 with sixth character 1-4)
Add selective serotonin reuptake inhibitors [SSRI] (T43.22 with sixth character 1-4)
Add Use Additional code for adverse effect, if applicable, to identify drug, such as:
Add linezolid (T36.8X5)
Add monoamine oxidase inhibitors (T43.1X5)
Add selective serotonin and norepinephrine reuptake inhibitors [SSNRI] (T43.215)
Add selective serotonin reuptake inhibitors [SSRI] (T43.225)
Add Use Additional code, if applicable, to identify:
Add disseminated intravascular coagulation (D65)
Add hypertensive crisis (I16.-)
Add metabolic acidosis (E87.2-)
Add shock, not elsewhere classified (R57.-)
Add toxic encephalopathy (G92.-)
Add ventricular tachycardia (I47.2-)
Add G9Ø.89 **Other disorders of autonomic nervous system**

No Change G93 **Other disorders of brain**
No Change G93.4 **Other and unspecified encephalopathy**
Revise from G93.42 **Megaloencephalic leukoencephalopathy with subcortical cysts**
Revise to G93.42 **Megalencephalic leukoencephalopathy with subcortical cysts**
Add G93.45 **Developmental and epileptic encephalopathy**
Add Early infantile epileptic encephalopathy
Add Code also, if applicable, associated disorders such as:
Add developmental disorders of scholastic skills (F81.-)
Add developmental disorder of speech and language (F8Ø.-)
Add epilepsy, by specific type (G4Ø.-)
Add intellectual disabilities (F7Ø-F79)
Add other neurodevelopmental disorder (F88)
Add pervasive developmental disorders (F84.-)

No Change **CHAPTER 7**

No Change **DISEASES OF THE EYE AND ADNEXA (H00-H59)**

No Change **GLAUCOMA (H40-H42)**

No Change **H42 Glaucoma in diseases classified elsewhere**
No Change *Code first*
Revise from Reiger's anomaly (Q13.81)
Revise to Rieger anomaly (Q13.81)

No Change **DISORDERS OF VITREOUS BODY AND GLOBE (H43-H44)**

No Change **H44 Disorders of globe**
No Change **H44.2 Degenerative myopia**
No Change **H44.2A Degenerative myopia with choroidal neovascularization**
Revise from **H44.2A3 Degenerative myopia with choroidal neovascularization, bilateral eye**
Revise to **H44.2A3 Degenerative myopia with choroidal neovascularization, bilateral**
No Change **H44.2B Degenerative myopia with macular hole**
Revise from **H44.2B3 Degenerative myopia with macular hole, bilateral eye**
Revise to **H44.2B3 Degenerative myopia with macular hole, bilateral**
No Change **H44.2C Degenerative myopia with retinal detachment**
Revise from **H44.2C3 Degenerative myopia with retinal detachment, bilateral eye**
Revise to **H44.2C3 Degenerative myopia with retinal detachment, bilateral**
No Change **H44.2D Degenerative myopia with foveoschisis**
Revise from **H44.2D3 Degenerative myopia with foveoschisis, bilateral eye**
Revise to **H44.2D3 Degenerative myopia with foveoschisis, bilateral**
No Change **H44.2E Degenerative myopia with other maculopathy**
Revise from **H44.2E3 Degenerative myopia with other maculopathy, bilateral eye**
Revise to **H44.2E3 Degenerative myopia with other maculopathy, bilateral**

No Change **CHAPTER 9**

No Change **DISEASES OF THE CIRCULATORY SYSTEM (I00-I99)**

No Change **CHRONIC RHEUMATIC HEART DISEASES (I05-I09)**

No Change **I08 Multiple valve diseases**
Delete **Excludes1** multiple valve disease specified a nonrheumatic (I34.-, I35.-, I36.-, I37.-, I38.-, Q22.-, Q23.-, Q24.8-)
Add **Excludes2** multiple valve disease specified as nonrheumatic (I34.-, I35.-, I36.-, I37.-, I38.-, Q22.-, Q23.-, Q24.8-)

No Change **HYPERTENSIVE DISEASES (I10-I1A)**

No Change **I16 Hypertensive crisis**
No Change **I16.1 Hypertensive emergency**
Add Use Additional code, if applicable, to identify specific organ dysfunction, such as:
Add acute kidney injury (N17.-)
Add acute myocardial infarction (I21.-)
Add acute pulmonary edema (left and/or right ventricular failure) (J81.0, I50.-)
Add aortic dissection (I71.0-)
Add cerebral hemorrhage (I60.-. I61.-, I62.-)
Add cerebral infarction (I63.-)
Add eclampsia (O15.-)
Add hypertensive encephalopathy (I67.4)
Add seizure (R56.9)

No Change **ISCHEMIC HEART DISEASES (I20-I25)**

No Change **I21 Acute myocardial infarction**
No Change **I21.A Other type of myocardial infarction**
No Change **I21.A1 Myocardial infarction type 2**
No Change *Code first*
Revise from the underlying cause, such as:
Revise to , if applicable, the underlying cause, such as:

No Change **PULMONARY HEART DISEASE AND DISEASES OF PULMONARY CIRCULATION (I26-I28)**

No Change **I26 Pulmonary embolism**
No Change **I26.0 Pulmonary embolism with acute cor pulmonale**
Add **I26.03 Cement embolism of pulmonary artery with acute cor pulmonale**
Add *Code first complication of other artery following a procedure (T81.718)*
Add **I26.04 Fat embolism of pulmonary artery with acute cor pulmonale**
Add *Code first, if applicable:*
Add complication of other artery following a procedure (T81.718)
Add traumatic fat embolism (T79.1)
No Change **I26.09 Other pulmonary embolism with acute cor pulmonale**
Add Other thrombotic pulmonary embolism with acute cor pulmonale
No Change **I26.9 Pulmonary embolism without acute cor pulmonale**
Revise from **I26.93 Single subsegmental pulmonary embolism without acute cor pulmonale**
Revise to **I26.93 Single subsegmental thrombotic pulmonary embolism without acute cor pulmonale**
Revise from **I26.94 Multiple subsegmental pulmonary emboli without acute cor pulmonale**
Revise to **I26.94 Multiple subsegmental thrombotic pulmonary emboli without acute cor pulmonale**
Add **I26.95 Cement embolism of pulmonary artery without acute cor pulmonale**
Add *Code first complication of other artery following a procedure (T81.718)*
Add **I26.96 Fat embolism of pulmonary artery without acute cor pulmonale**
Add *Code first, if applicable:*
complication of other artery following a procedure (T81.718)
Add traumatic fat embolism (T79.1)
No Change **I26.99 Other pulmonary embolism without acute cor pulmonale**
Add Other thrombotic pulmonary embolism without acute cor pulmonale

No Change **OTHER FORMS OF HEART DISEASE (I30-I5A)**

No Change **I30 Acute pericarditis**
No Change **Excludes1**
Revise from viral pericarditis due to Coxsakie virus (B33.23)
Revise to viral pericarditis due to Coxsackie virus (B33.23)

No Change **I35 Nonrheumatic aortic valve disorders**
Delete **Excludes1** aortic valve disorder of unspecified cause but with diseases of mitral and/or tricuspid valve(s) (I08.-)
Delete aortic valve disorder specified as congenital (Q23.0, Q23.1)
Delete aortic valve disorder specified as rheumatic (I06.-)
Delete hypertrophic subaortic stenosis (I42.1)
Add Code also, if applicable, bicuspid aortic valve (Q23.81)
Add **Excludes2** aortic valve disorder of unspecified cause but with diseases of mitral and/or tricuspid valve(s) (I08.-)
Add aortic valve disorder specified as congenital (Q23.0, Q23.1)
Add aortic valve disorder specified as rheumatic (I06.-)
Add hypertrophic subaortic stenosis (I42.1)

No Change **CHAPTER 10**

No Change **DISEASES OF THE RESPIRATORY SYSTEM (J00-J99)**

No Change **INFLUENZA AND PNEUMONIA (J09-J18)**

No Change **J13 Pneumonia due to Streptococcus pneumoniae**
No Change *Code first*
Revise from associated influenza, if applicable (J09.X1, J10.0-, J11.0-)
Revise from , if applicable, associated influenza (J09.X1, J10.0-, J11.0-)
No Change Code also
Delete associated abscess, if applicable (J85.1)
Add , if applicable, any associated condition such as:
Add abscess (J85.1)
Add aspiration pneumonia (J69.-)

No Change **J14 Pneumonia due to Hemophilus influenzae**
No Change *Code first*
Revise from associated influenza, if applicable (J09.X1, J10.0-, J11.0-)
Revise to , if applicable, associated influenza (J09.X1, J10.0-, J11.0-)
No Change Code also
Delete associated abscess, if applicable (J85.1)
Add , if applicable, any associated condition such as:
Add abscess (J85.1)
Add aspiration pneumonia (J69.-)

No Change **J15 Bacterial pneumonia, not elsewhere classified**
No Change *Code first*
Revise from associated influenza, if applicable (J09.X1, J10.0-, J11.0-)
Revise to , if applicable, associated influenza (J09.X1, J10.0-, J11.0-)
No Change Code also
Delete associated abscess, if applicable (J85.1)
Add , if applicable, any associated condition such as:
Add abscess (J85.1)
Add aspiration pneumonia (J69.-)

No Change **J16 Pneumonia due to other infectious organisms, not elsewhere classified**
No Change *Code first*
Revise from associated influenza, if applicable (J09.X1, J10.0-, J11.0-)
Revise to , if applicable, associated influenza (J09.X1, J10.0-, J11.0-)
No Change Code also
Delete associated abscess, if applicable (J85.1)
Add , if applicable, any associated condition such as:
Add abscess (J85.1)
Add aspiration pneumonia (J69.-)

No Change **J17 Pneumonia in diseases classified elsewhere**
Add Code also, if applicable, any associated condition such as:
Add abscess (J85.1)
Add aspiration pneumonia (J69.-)

No Change **J18 Pneumonia, unspecified organism**
No Change *Code first*
Revise from associated influenza, if applicable (J09.X1, J10.0-, J11.0-)
Revise to , if applicable, associated influenza (J09.X1, J10.0-, J11.0-)
Add Code also, if applicable, any associated condition such as:
Add aspiration pneumonia (J69.-)
Delete **Excludes1** abscess of lung with pneumonia (J85.1)
Delete aspiration pneumonia due to anesthesia during labor and delivery (O74.0)
Delete aspiration pneumonia due to anesthesia during pregnancy (O29)
Delete aspiration pneumonia due to anesthesia during puerperium (O89.0)
Delete aspiration pneumonia due to solids and liquids (J69.-)
Delete aspiration pneumonia NOS (J69.0)
Delete lipid pneumonia (J69.1)
Delete pneumonitis due to external agents (J67-J70)
Add **Excludes2** abscess of lung with pneumonia (J85.1)
Add aspiration pneumonia due to anesthesia during labor and delivery (O74.0)
Add aspiration pneumonia due to anesthesia during pregnancy (O29)
Add aspiration pneumonia due to anesthesia during puerperium (O89.0)
Add aspiration pneumonia due to solids and liquids (J69.-)
Add aspiration pneumonia NOS (J69.0)
Add lipid pneumonia (J69.1)
Add pneumonitis due to external agents (J67-J70)

No Change **OTHER ACUTE LOWER RESPIRATORY INFECTIONS (J20-J22)**

No Change **J21 Acute bronchiolitis**
No Change **J21.9 Acute bronchiolitis, unspecified**
No Change **Excludes1**
Revise from chronic bronchiolitis (J44.-)
Revise to chronic bronchiolitis (J44.89)

No Change **OTHER DISEASES OF UPPER RESPIRATORY TRACT (J3Ø-J39)**

No Change J34 **Other and unspecified disorders of nose and nasal sinuses**

No Change J34.8 **Other specified disorders of nose and nasal sinuses**

Add J34.82 **Nasal valve collapse**

Add Nasal valve compromise

Add Nasal valve stenosis

Add *Code first underlying cause, such as:* deviated nasal septum (J34.2)

Add J34.82Ø **Internal nasal valve collapse**

Add J34.82ØØ **Internal nasal valve collapse, unspecified**

Add J34.82Ø1 **Internal nasal valve collapse, static**

Add Narrowing of the septum, head of the inferior turbinate and the upper lateral cartilage

Add J34.82Ø2 **Internal nasal valve collapse, dynamic**

Add Collapse or falling of the upper, middle sidewall of the nose on inspiration

Add J34.821 **External nasal valve collapse**

Add J34.821Ø **External nasal valve collapse, unspecified**

Add J34.8211 **External nasal valve collapse, static**

Add Fixed narrowing of the caudal septum, lower lateral cartilage, alar rim and nasal sill

Add J34.8212 **External nasal valve collapse, dynamic**

Add Collapse or falling of the lower sidewall or nostril of the nose on inspiration

Add J34.829 **Nasal valve collapse, unspecified**

Add Nasal valve collapse, NOS

No Change **LUNG DISEASES DUE TO EXTERNAL AGENTS (J6Ø-J7Ø)**

No Change J69 **Pneumonitis due to solids and liquids**

Add Code also, if applicable, other types of pneumonias

No Change **OTHER RESPIRATORY DISEASES PRINCIPALLY AFFECTING THE INTERSTITIUM (J8Ø-J84)**

No Change J84 **Other interstitial pulmonary diseases**

Add Code also, if applicable, associated condition

No Change **SUPPURATIVE AND NECROTIC CONDITIONS OF THE LOWER RESPIRATORY TRACT (J85-J86)**

No Change J86 **Pyothorax**

No Change J86.Ø **Pyothorax with fistula**

Add Code also, if applicable, disruption of internal operation (surgical) wound (T81.32-)

No Change **CHAPTER 11**

No Change **DISEASES OF THE DIGESTIVE SYSTEM (KØØ-K95)**

No Change **DISEASES OF ORAL CAVITY AND SALIVARY GLANDS (KØØ-K14)**

No Change K14 **Diseases of tongue**

No Change **Excludes2**

Revise from leukedema of tongue (K13.29)

Revise to leukoedema of tongue (K13.29)

No Change **DISEASES OF ESOPHAGUS, STOMACH AND DUODENUM (K2Ø-K31)**

No Change K31 **Other diseases of stomach and duodenum**

No Change K31.6 **Fistula of stomach and duodenum**

Add Code also, if applicable, disruption of internal operation (surgical) wound (T81.32-)

No Change **NONINFECTIVE ENTERITIS AND COLITIS (K5Ø-K52)**

No Change K5Ø **Crohn's disease [regional enteritis]**

Add Use Additional code to identify any associated fistulas, if applicable:

Add anal fistula (K6Ø.3-)

Add anorectal fistula (K6Ø.5-)

Add rectal fistula (K6Ø.4-)

No Change K51 **Ulcerative colitis**

Add Use Additional code to identify any associated fistulas, if applicable:

Add anal fistula (K6Ø.3-)

Add anorectal fistula (K6Ø.5-)

Add rectal fistula (K6Ø.4-)

No Change **OTHER DISEASES OF INTESTINES (K55-K64)**

No Change K58 **Irritable bowel syndrome**

Revise from K58.9 **Irritable bowel syndrome without diarrhea**

Revise to K58.9 **Irritable bowel syndrome, unspecified**

No Change K6Ø **Fissure and fistula of anal and rectal regions**

Add **Excludes2** abscess or cellulitis of anal and rectal regions (K61.-)

No Change K6Ø.3 **Anal fistula**

Add *Code first, if applicable:*

Add Crohn's disease (K5Ø.-)

Add ulcerative colitis (K51.-)

Add **Excludes1** congenital fistula (Q43.6)

Add K6Ø.3Ø **Anal fistula, unspecified**

Add Anal fistula NOS

Add K6Ø.31 **Anal fistula, simple**

Add Low intersphincteric anal fistula

Add Superficial anal fistula

Add K6Ø.311 **Anal fistula, simple, initial**

Add Anal fistula, simple, new

Add K6Ø.312 **Anal fistula, simple, persistent**

Add Anal fistula, simple, chronic

Add K6Ø.313 **Anal fistula, simple, recurrent**

Add Anal fistula simple, occurring following complete healing

Add K6Ø.319 **Anal fistula, simple, unspecified**

Add K6Ø.32 **Anal fistula, complex**
Add Extrasphincteric anal fistula
Add High intersphincteric anal fistula
Add Suprasphincteric anal fistula
Add Transsphincteric anal fistula
Add Code also, if applicable:
perianal abscess (K61.Ø)
rectovaginal fistula (N82.3)
stenosis of anus and rectum (K62.4)
Add K6Ø.321 **Anal fistula, complex, initial**
Add Anal fistula, complex, new
Add K6Ø.322 **Anal fistula, complex, persistent**
Add Anal fistula, complex, chronic
Add K6Ø.323 **Anal fistula, complex, recurrent**
Add Anal fistula complex, occurring following complete healing
Add K6Ø.329 **Anal fistula, complex, unspecified**
No Change K6Ø.4 **Rectal fistula**
Add *Code first, if applicable:*
Add Crohn's disease (K5Ø.-)
Add ulcerative colitis (K51.-)
Add **Excludes1** congenital fistula (Q43.6)
Add K6Ø.4Ø **Rectal fistula, unspecified**
Add Rectal fistula NOS
Add K6Ø.41 **Rectal fistula, simple**
Add Low intersphincteric rectal fistula
Add Superficial rectal fistula
Add K6Ø.411 **Rectal fistula, simple, initial**
Add Rectal, fistula, simple, new
Add K6Ø.412 **Rectal fistula, simple, persistent**
Add Rectal fistula, simple, chronic
Add K6Ø.413 **Rectal fistula, simple, recurrent**
Add Rectal fistula simple, occurring following complete healing
Add K6Ø.419 **Rectal fistula, simple, unspecified**
Add K6Ø.42 **Rectal fistula, complex**
Add Extrasphincteric rectal fistula
Add High intersphincteric rectal fistula
Add Suprasphincteric rectal fistula
Add Transsphincteric rectal fistula
Add Code also, if applicable:
perianal abscess (K61.Ø)
rectovaginal fistula (N82.3)
stenosis of anus and rectum (K62.4)
Add K6Ø.421 **Rectal fistula, complex, initial**
Add Rectal fistula, complex, new
Add K6Ø.422 **Rectal fistula, complex, persistent**
Add Rectal fistula, complex, chronic
Add K6Ø.423 **Rectal fistula, complex, recurrent**
Add Rectal fistula complex occurring following complete healing
Add K6Ø.429 **Rectal fistula, complex, unspecified**
No Change K6Ø.5 **Anorectal fistula**
Add *Code first, if applicable:*
Add Crohn's disease (K5Ø.-)
Add ulcerative colitis (K51.-)
Add **Excludes1** congenital fistula (Q43.6)
Add K6Ø.5Ø **Anorectal fistula, unspecified**
Add Anorectal fistula NOS
Add K6Ø.51 **Anorectal fistula, simple**
Add Low intersphincteric anorectal fistula
Add Superficial anorectal fistula
Add K6Ø.511 **Anorectal fistula, simple, initial**
Add Anorectal fistula, simple, new
Add K6Ø.512 **Anorectal fistula, simple, persistent**
Add Anorectal fistula, simple, chronic
Add K6Ø.513 **Anorectal fistula, simple, recurrent**
Add Anorectal fistula simple, occurring following complete healing
Add K6Ø.519 **Anorectal fistula, simple, unspecified**
Add K6Ø.52 **Anorectal fistula, complex**
Add Extrasphincteric anorectal fistula
Add High intersphincteric anorectal fistula
Add Suprasphincteric anorectal fistula
Add Transsphincteric anorectal fistula
Add Code also, if applicable:
perianal abscess (K61.Ø)
rectovaginal fistula (N82.3)
stenosis of anus and rectum (K62.4)
Add K6Ø.521 **Anorectal fistula, complex, initial**
Add Anorectal fistula, complex, new
Add K6Ø.522 **Anorectal fistula, complex, persistent**
Add Anorectal fistula, complex, chronic
Add K6Ø.523 **Anorectal fistula, complex, recurrent**
Add Anorectal fistula complex, occurring following complete healing
Add K6Ø.529 **Anorectal fistula, complex, unspecified**

No Change K63 **Other diseases of intestine**
No Change K63.2 **Fistula of intestine**
Add Code also, if applicable, disruption of internal operation (surgical) wound (T81.32-)

No Change **DISORDERS OF GALLBLADDER, BILIARY TRACT AND PANCREAS (K8Ø-K87)**

No Change K82 **Other diseases of gallbladder**
No Change K82.3 **Fistula of gallbladder**
Add Code also, if applicable, disruption of internal operation (surgical) wound (T81.32-)

No Change **CHAPTER 12**

No Change **DISEASES OF THE SKIN AND SUBCUTANEOUS TISSUE (LØØ-L99)**

No Change **DERMATITIS AND ECZEMA (L2Ø-L3Ø)**

No Change L29 **Pruritus**
No Change L29.8 **Other pruritus**
Add L29.81 **Cholestatic pruritus**
Add Code also, if applicable, type of liver disease
Add Use Additional code for adverse effect, if applicable, to identify drug (T36-T5Ø with fifth or sixth character 5)
Add L29.89 **Other pruritus**

No Change **PAPULOSQUAMOUS DISORDERS (L40-L45)**

No Change L43 **Lichen planus**
No Change **Excludes1**
Revise from lichen planopilaris (L66.1)
Revise to lichen planopilaris (L66.1-)

No Change **DISORDERS OF SKIN APPENDAGES (L60-L75)**

No Change L66 **Cicatricial alopecia [scarring hair loss]**
No Change L66.1 **Lichen planopilaris**
Delete Follicular lichen planus
Add L66.10 **Lichen planopilaris, unspecified**
Add L66.11 **Classic lichen planopilaris**
Add Follicular lichen planus
Add L66.12 **Frontal fibrosing alopecia**
Add FFA
Add L66.19 **Other lichen planopilaris**
Add Lassueur Graham-Little Piccardi syndrome
No Change L66.8 **Other cicatricial alopecia**
Add L66.81 **Central centrifugal cicatricial alopecia**
Add CCCA
Add L66.89 **Other cicatricial alopecia**

No Change **CHAPTER 13**

No Change **DISEASES OF THE MUSCULOSKELETAL SYSTEM AND CONNECTIVE TISSUE (M00-M99)**

No Change **OTHER DORSOPATHIES (M50-M54)**

No Change M51 **Thoracic, thoracolumbar, and lumbosacral intervertebral disc disorders**
No Change M51.3 **Other thoracic, thoracolumbar and lumbosacral intervertebral disc degeneration**
No Change M51.36 **Other intervertebral disc degeneration, lumbar region**
Add M51.360 **Other intervertebral disc degeneration, lumbar region with discogenic back pain only**
Add Other intervertebral disc degeneration, lumbar region with axial back pain only
Add M51.361 **Other intervertebral disc degeneration, lumbar region with lower extremity pain only**
Add Other intervertebral disc degeneration, lumbar region with leg pain only
Add Other intervertebral disc degeneration, lumbar region with referred sclerotomal pain only
Add M51.362 **Other intervertebral disc degeneration, lumbar region with discogenic back pain and lower extremity pain**
Add Other intervertebral disc degeneration, lumbar region with discogenic back pain and leg pain
Add Other intervertebral disc degeneration, lumbar region with axial back pain and referred sclerotomal pain
Add M51.369 **Other intervertebral disc degeneration, lumbar region without mention of lumbar back pain or lower extremity pain**
Add Other intervertebral disc degeneration, lumbar region without mention of lumbar back pain or leg pain
Add Other intervertebral disc degeneration, lumbar region, NOS
No Change M51.37 **Other intervertebral disc degeneration, lumbosacral region**
Add M51.370 **Other intervertebral disc degeneration, lumbosacral region with discogenic back pain only**
Add Other intervertebral disc degeneration, lumbosacral region with axial back pain only
Add M51.371 **Other intervertebral disc degeneration, lumbosacral region with lower extremity pain only**
Add Other intervertebral disc degeneration, lumbosacral region with leg pain only
Add Other intervertebral disc degeneration, lumbosacral region with referred sclerotomal pain only
Add M51.372 **Other intervertebral disc degeneration, lumbosacral region with discogenic back pain and lower extremity pain**
Add Other intervertebral disc degeneration, lumbosacral region with discogenic back pain and leg pain
Add Other intervertebral disc degeneration, lumbosacral region with axial back pain and referred sclerotomal pain
Add M51.379 **Other intervertebral disc degeneration, lumbosacral region without mention of lumbar back pain or lower extremity pain**
Add Other intervertebral disc degeneration, lumbosacral region without mention of lumbar back pain or leg pain
Add Other intervertebral disc degeneration, lumbosacral region, NOS

No Change M54 Dorsalgia
No Change M54.3 Sciatica
Add **Excludes1** intervertebral disc degeneration, lumbar region with lower extremity pain only (M51.361)
Add intervertebral disc degeneration, lumbosacral region with lower extremity pain only (M51.371)
No Change M54.4 Lumbago with sciatica
Add **Excludes1** intervertebral disc degeneration, lumbar region with discogenic back pain and lower extremity pain (M51.362)
Add intervertebral disc degeneration, lumbosacral region with discogenic back pain and lower extremity pain (M51.372)
No Change M54.5 Low back pain
Add **Excludes1** intervertebral disc degeneration, lumbar region with discogenic back pain only (M51.36Ø)
Add intervertebral disc degeneration, lumbosacral region with discogenic back pain only (M51.37Ø)

No Change **DISORDERS OF MUSCLES (M6Ø-M63)**

No Change M62 Other disorders of muscle
No Change M62.8 Other specified disorders of muscle
Add M62.85 Dysfunction of the multifidus muscles, lumbar region

No Change **DISORDERS OF SYNOVIUM AND TENDON (M65-M67)**

No Change M65 Synovitis and tenosynovitis
No Change M65.9 Synovitis and tenosynovitis, unspecified
Add M65.9Ø Unspecified synovitis and tenosynovitis, unspecified site
Add M65.91 Unspecified synovitis and tenosynovitis, shoulder
Add M65.911 Unspecified synovitis and tenosynovitis, right shoulder
Add M65.912 Unspecified synovitis and tenosynovitis, left shoulder
Add M65.919 Unspecified synovitis and tenosynovitis, unspecified shoulder
Add M65.92 Unspecified synovitis and tenosynovitis, upper arm
Add M65.921 Unspecified synovitis and tenosynovitis, right upper arm
Add M65.922 Unspecified synovitis and tenosynovitis, left upper arm
Add M65.929 Unspecified synovitis and tenosynovitis, unspecified upper arm
Add M65.93 Unspecified synovitis and tenosynovitis, forearm
Add M65.931 Unspecified synovitis and tenosynovitis, right forearm
Add M65.932 Unspecified synovitis and tenosynovitis, left forearm
Add M65.939 Unspecified synovitis and tenosynovitis, unspecified forearm
Add M65.94 Unspecified synovitis and tenosynovitis, hand
Add M65.941 Unspecified synovitis and tenosynovitis, right hand
Add M65.942 Unspecified synovitis and tenosynovitis, left hand
Add M65.949 Unspecified synovitis and tenosynovitis, unspecified hand
Add M65.95 Unspecified synovitis and tenosynovitis, thigh
Add M65.951 Unspecified synovitis and tenosynovitis, right thigh
Add M65.952 Unspecified synovitis and tenosynovitis, left thigh
Add M65.959 Unspecified synovitis and tenosynovitis, unspecified thigh
Add M65.96 Unspecified synovitis and tenosynovitis, lower leg
Add M65.961 Unspecified synovitis and tenosynovitis, right lower leg
Add M65.962 Unspecified synovitis and tenosynovitis, left lower leg
Add M65.969 Unspecified synovitis and tenosynovitis, unspecified lower leg
Add M65.97 Unspecified synovitis and tenosynovitis, ankle and foot
Add M65.971 Unspecified synovitis and tenosynovitis, right ankle and foot
Add M65.972 Unspecified synovitis and tenosynovitis, left ankle and foot
Add M65.979 Unspecified synovitis and tenosynovitis, unspecified ankle and foot
Add M65.98 Unspecified synovitis and tenosynovitis, other site
Add M65.99 Unspecified synovitis and tenosynovitis, multiple sites

No Change **CHONDROPATHIES (M91-M94)**

No Change M92 Other juvenile osteochondrosis
No Change M92.8 Other specified juvenile osteochondrosis
Delete Calcaneal apophysitis

No Change **CHAPTER 14**

No Change **DISEASES OF THE GENITOURINARY SYSTEM (NØØ-N99)**

No Change **OTHER DISEASES OF THE URINARY SYSTEM (N3Ø-N39)**

No Change N39 Other disorders of urinary system
No Change N39.Ø Urinary tract infection, site not specified
Add **Excludes1** pyonephrosis (N13.6)

No Change CHAPTER 15

No Change **PREGNANCY, CHILDBIRTH AND THE PUERPERIUM (O00-O9A)**

No Change **OTHER MATERNAL DISORDERS PREDOMINANTLY RELATED TO PREGNANCY (O20-O29)**

No Change O24 **Diabetes mellitus in pregnancy, childbirth, and the puerperium**

No Change O24.1 **Pre-existing type 2 diabetes mellitus, in pregnancy, childbirth and the puerperium**

Add Use Additional injectable non-insulin antidiabetic drugs (Z79.85)

No Change O24.3 **Unspecified pre-existing diabetes mellitus in pregnancy, childbirth and the puerperium**

Add Use Additional injectable non-insulin antidiabetic drugs (Z79.85)

No Change O24.8 **Other pre-existing diabetes mellitus in pregnancy, childbirth, and the puerperium**

Add Use Additional injectable non-insulin antidiabetic drugs (Z79.85)

No Change O24.9 **Unspecified diabetes mellitus in pregnancy, childbirth and the puerperium**

Add Use Additional

Revise from code for long-term (current) use of insulin (Z79.4)

Revise to code (for):

Add from categories E08, E09 and E13 to further identify any manifestation

Add injectable non-insulin antidiabetic drugs (Z79.85)

Add long-term (current) use of insulin (Z79.4)

No Change CHAPTER 16

No Change **CERTAIN CONDITIONS ORIGINATING IN THE PERINATAL PERIOD (P00-P96)**

No Change **TRANSITORY ENDOCRINE AND METABOLIC DISORDERS SPECIFIC TO NEWBORN (P70-P74)**

No Change P72 **Other transitory neonatal endocrine disorders**

Add **Excludes1** dyshormonogenetic goiter (E07.1)

No Change CHAPTER 17

No Change **CONGENITAL MALFORMATIONS, DEFORMATIONS AND CHROMOSOMAL ABNORMALITIES (Q00-Q99)**

No Change **CONGENITAL MALFORMATIONS OF EYE, EAR, FACE AND NECK (Q10-Q18)**

No Change Q13 **Congenital malformations of anterior segment of eye**

No Change Q13.8 **Other congenital malformations of anterior segment of eye**

Revise from Q13.81 **Rieger's anomaly**

Revise to Q13.81 **Rieger anomaly**

Add Axenfeld-Rieger syndrome

Add Code also any other associated congenital malformations such as cardiac defects

No Change **CONGENITAL MALFORMATIONS OF THE CIRCULATORY SYSTEM (Q20-Q28)**

No Change Q23 **Congenital malformations of aortic and mitral valves**

No Change Q23.1 **Congenital insufficiency of aortic valve**

Delete Bicuspid aortic valve

No Change Q23.8 **Other congenital malformations of aortic and mitral valves**

Add Q23.81 **Bicuspid aortic valve**

Add Congenital bicuspid aortic valve

Add Unicuspid (congenital) aortic valve (at birth)

Add Code also, if applicable, acquired aortic valve disorders, such as:

Add aortic (valve) insufficiency (nonrheumatic) (I35.1)

Add aortic (valve) stenosis (nonrheumatic) (I35.0)

Add aortic (valve) stenosis with insufficiency (nonrheumatic) (I35.2)

Add Q23.82 **Congenital mitral valve cleft leaflet**

Add Cleft mitral valve leaflet at birth

Add Q23.88 **Other congenital malformations of aortic and mitral valves**

No Change **OTHER CONGENITAL MALFORMATIONS (Q80-Q89)**

No Change Q87 **Other specified congenital malformation syndromes affecting multiple systems**

No Change Q87.8 **Other specified congenital malformation syndromes, not elsewhere classified**

Add Q87.86 **Kleefstra syndrome**

No Change CHAPTER 18

No Change **SYMPTOMS, SIGNS AND ABNORMAL CLINICAL AND LABORATORY FINDINGS, NOT ELSEWHERE CLASSIFIED (R00-R99)**

No Change **SYMPTOMS AND SIGNS INVOLVING THE DIGESTIVE SYSTEM AND ABDOMEN (R10-R19)**

No Change R11 **Nausea and vomiting**

No Change **Excludes1**

Revise from vomiting associated with bulimia nervosa (F50.2)

Revise to vomiting associated with bulimia nervosa (F50.2-)

No Change R11.1 **Vomiting**

No Change R11.15 **Cyclical vomiting syndrome unrelated to migraine**

No Change **Excludes2**

Revise from bulimia nervosa (F50.2)

Revise to bulimia nervosa (F50.20)

No Change **SYMPTOMS AND SIGNS INVOLVING COGNITION, PERCEPTION, EMOTIONAL STATE AND BEHAVIOR (R4Ø-R46)**

No Change R41 **Other symptoms and signs involving cognitive functions and awareness**

No Change R41.Ø **Disorientation, unspecified**

Excludes1 delirium due to known

Add physiological condition (FØ5)

No Change R41.8 **Other symptoms and signs involving cognitive functions and awareness**

No Change R41.84 **Other specified cognitive deficit**

Code first the underlying condition, if

Add *known, such as:*

Add schizophrenia (F2Ø.-)

Add R41.85 **Anosognosia**

No Change R41.89 **Other symptoms and signs involving cognitive functions and awareness**

Delete Anosognosia

No Change **GENERAL SYMPTOMS AND SIGNS (R5Ø-R69)**

No Change R54 **Age-related physical debility**

No Change **Excludes1**

Revise from senile psychosis (FØ3)

Revise to senile psychosis (FØ3.-)

No Change R63 **Symptoms and signs concerning food and fluid intake**

No Change **Excludes1**

Revise from bulimia NOS (F5Ø.2)

Revise to bulimia NOS (F5Ø.2-)

No Change **ABNORMAL FINDINGS ON EXAMINATION OF BLOOD, WITHOUT DIAGNOSIS (R7Ø-R79)**

No Change R73 **Elevated blood glucose level**

No Change R73.Ø **Abnormal glucose**

Add **Excludes1** type 1 diabetes mellitus, presymptomatic (E1Ø.A-)

No Change **CHAPTER 19**

No Change **INJURY, POISONING AND CERTAIN OTHER CONSEQUENCES OF EXTERNAL CAUSES (SØØ-T88)**

No Change **INJURIES TO THE HEAD (SØØ-SØ9)**

No Change SØ6 **Intracranial injury**

No Change SØ6.3 **Focal traumatic brain injury**

No Change SØ6.34 **Traumatic hemorrhage of right cerebrum**

No Change SØ6.341 **Traumatic hemorrhage of right cerebrum with loss of consciousness of 3Ø minutes or less**

Revise from Traumatic hemorrhage of right cerebrum with loss of consciousness

Revise to Traumatic hemorrhage of right cerebrum with brief loss of consciousness

No Change **INJURIES TO THE THORAX (S2Ø-S29)**

No Change S22 **Fracture of rib(s), sternum and thoracic spine**

No Change Code also

Revise from , if applicable, any associated:

Revise from , if applicable, any associated condition such as:

Add traumatic hemopneumothorax (S27.2)

Add traumatic hemothorax (S27.1-)

Add traumatic pneumothorax (S27.Ø)

No Change **POISONING BY, ADVERSE EFFECTS OF AND UNDERDOSING OF DRUGS, MEDICAMENTS AND BIOLOGICAL SUBSTANCES (T36-T5Ø)**

No Change T45 **Poisoning by, adverse effect of and underdosing of primarily systemic and hematological agents, not elsewhere classified**

No Change T45.1 **Poisoning by, adverse effect of and underdosing of antineoplastic and immunosuppressive drugs**

Add **Excludes1** poisoning by, adverse effect of and underdosing of immune checkpoint inhibitors and immunostimulant drugs (T45.A)

Add T45.A **Poisoning by, adverse effect of and underdosing of immune checkpoint inhibitors and immunostimulant drugs**

Add **Excludes1** poisoning by, adverse effect of and underdosing of antineoplastic and immunosuppressive drug (T45.1)

Add T45.AX **Poisoning by, adverse effect of and underdosing of immune checkpoint inhibitors and immunostimulant drugs**

Add T45.AX1 **Poisoning by immune checkpoint inhibitors and immunostimulant drugs, accidental (unintentional)**

Add Poisoning by immune checkpoint inhibitors and immunosuppressive drugs NOS

Add T45.AX2 **Poisoning by immune checkpoint inhibitors and immunostimulant drugs, intentional self-harm**

Add T45.AX3 **Poisoning by immune checkpoint inhibitors and immunostimulant drugs, assault**

Add T45.AX4 **Poisoning by immune checkpoint inhibitors and immunostimulant drugs, undetermined**

Add T45.AX5 **Adverse effect of immune checkpoint inhibitors and immunostimulant drugs**

Add T45.AX6 **Underdosing of immune checkpoint inhibitors and immunostimulant drugs**

No Change **TOXIC EFFECTS OF SUBSTANCES CHIEFLY NONMEDICINAL AS TO SOURCE (T51-T65)**

No Change T63 **Toxic effect of contact with venomous animals and plants**

T63.4 **Toxic effect of venom of other arthropods**

Add Use Additional code, if applicable, for anaphylactic shock (T78.2)

No Change T65 **Toxic effect of other and unspecified substances**

No Change T65.3 **Toxic effect of nitroderivatives and aminoderivatives of benzene and its homologues**

Revise from Toxic effect of anilin [benzenamine]

Revise to Toxic effect of aniline [benzenamine]

No Change **COMPLICATIONS OF SURGICAL AND MEDICAL CARE, NOT ELSEWHERE CLASSIFIED (T80-T88)**

No Change **T80 Complications following infusion, transfusion and therapeutic injection**

No Change **T80.8 Other complications following infusion, transfusion and therapeutic injection**

No Change **T80.82 Complication of immune effector cellular therapy**

Add **Excludes2** adverse effect of immune checkpoint inhibitors and immunostimulant drugs (T45.AX5)

Add **T81 Complications of procedures, not elsewhere classified**

No Change **T81.3 Disruption of wound, not elsewhere classified**

No Change **T81.32 Disruption of internal operation (surgical) wound, not elsewhere classified**

Delete Deep disruption or dehiscence of operation wound NOS

Delete Disruption or dehiscence of closure of internal organ or other internal tissue

Delete Disruption or dehiscence of closure of muscle or muscle flap

Delete Disruption or dehiscence of closure of ribs or rib cage

Delete Disruption or dehiscence of closure of skull or craniotomy

Delete Disruption or dehiscence of closure of sternum or sternotomy

Delete Disruption or dehiscence of closure of tendon or ligament

Delete Disruption or dehiscence of closure of superficial or muscular fascia

Add **T81.320 Disruption or dehiscence of gastrointestinal tract anastomosis, repair, or closure**

Add **T81.321 Disruption or dehiscence of closure of internal operation (surgical) wound of abdominal wall muscle or fascia**

Add **T81.328 Disruption or dehiscence of closure of other specified internal operation (surgical) wound**

Add Disruption or dehiscence of closure of muscle or muscle flap (other than abdominal wall muscle)

Add Disruption or dehiscence of closure of ribs or rib cage

Add Disruption or dehiscence of closure of skull or craniotomy

Add Disruption or dehiscence of closure of sternum or sternotomy

Add Disruption or dehiscence of closure of tendon or ligament

Add Disruption or dehiscence of closure of superficial or muscular fascia (other than abdominal wall fascia)

Add **T81.329 Deep disruption or dehiscence of operation wound, unspecified**

Add Deep disruption or dehiscence of operation wound NOS

No Change **T81.4 Infection following a procedure**

Add Code also, if applicable, disruption of internal operation (surgical) wound (T81.32-)

No Change **T81.8 Other complications of procedures, not elsewhere classified**

No Change **T81.83 Persistent postprocedural fistula**

Add Code also, if applicable, disruption of internal operation (surgical) wound (T81.32-)

No Change Use Additional

Revise from anal fistula (K60.3)

Revise to anal fistula (K60.3-)

Revise from anorectal fistula (K60.5)

Revise to anorectal fistula (K60.5-)

No Change **CHAPTER 21**

No Change

FACTORS INFLUENCING HEALTH STATUS AND CONTACT WITH HEALTH SERVICES (Z00-Z99)

No Change This chapter contains the following blocks:

Revise from	Z17	Estrogen receptor status
Revise to	Z17	Estrogen, and other hormones and factors receptor status

No Change **GENETIC CARRIER AND GENETIC SUSCEPTIBILITY TO DISEASE (Z14-Z15)**

No Change **Z15 Genetic susceptibility to disease**

Add **Z15.1 Genetic susceptibility to epilepsy and neurodevelopmental disorders**

Add Code also, if applicable, related disorders such as:

Add developmental and epileptic encephalopathy (G93.45)

Add developmental disorder of speech and language (F80.-)

Add developmental disorders of scholastic skills (F81.-)

Add epilepsy, by specific type (G40.-)

Add intellectual disabilities (F70-F79)

Add other neurodevelopmental disorder (F88)

Add pervasive developmental disorders (F84.-)

Add **Z15.2 Genetic susceptibility to obesity**

Add Code also, if applicable, any associated manifestations, such as:

Add other obesity (E66.8-)

Add polyphagia (R63.2)

Add Use Additional code to identify body mass index (BMI), if known (Z68.-)

Revise from **ESTROGEN RECEPTOR STATUS (Z17)**

Revise to **ESTROGEN, AND OTHER HORMONES AND FACTORS RECEPTOR STATUS (Z17)**

Revise from **Z17 Estrogen receptor status**

Revise to **Z17 Estrogen, and other hormones and factors receptor status**

Add **Note:** Use one code, as available, for each receptor: Z17.0, Z17.1, Z17.2-, Z17.3-

Add *Code first* *malignant neoplasm, such as:* malignant neoplasm of ovary (C56.-)

Add **Z17.2 Progesterone receptor status**

Add **Z17.21 Progesterone receptor positive status** PR+

Add **Z17.22 Progesterone receptor negative status** PR-

Add **Z17.3 Human epidermal growth factor 2 receptor**

Add **Z17.31 Human epidermal growth factor receptor 2 positive status** HER2+

Add Z17.32 **Human epidermal growth factor receptor 2 negative status**
Add HER2-
Add Z17.4 **Combined receptor status**
Add **Note:** Assign a code from subcategory Z17.4- when only a combined receptor status is documented
Add Z17.41 **Hormone receptor positive**
Add HR+
Add Z17.410 **Hormone receptor positive with human epidermal growth factor receptor 2 positive status**
Add HR+ with HER2+
Add Z17.411 **Hormone receptor positive with human epidermal growth factor receptor 2 negative status**
Add HR+ with HER2-
Add Z17.42 **Hormone receptor negative**
Add HR-
Add Z17.420 **Hormone receptor negative with human epidermal growth factor receptor 2 positive status**
Add HR- with HER2+
Add Z17.421 **Hormone receptor negative with human epidermal growth factor receptor 2 negative status**
Add HR- with HER2-
Add TNBC
Add Triple negative breast cancer

No Change **ENCOUNTERS FOR OTHER SPECIFIC HEALTH CARE (Z40-Z53)**

No Change Z45 **Encounter for adjustment and management of implanted device**
No Change Z45.3 **Encounter for adjustment and management of implanted devices of the special senses**
No Change Z45.32 **Encounter for adjustment and management of implanted hearing device**
No Change **Excludes1**
Revise from Encounter for fitting and adjustment of hearing aide (Z46.1)
Revise to Encounter for fitting and adjustment of hearing aid (Z46.1)

No Change Z51 **Encounter for other aftercare and medical care**
Add Z51.A **Encounter for sepsis aftercare**

No Change **PERSONS WITH POTENTIAL HEALTH HAZARDS RELATED TO SOCIOECONOMIC AND PSYCHOSOCIAL CIRCUMSTANCES (Z55-Z65)**

No Change Z59 **Problems related to housing and economic circumstances**
No Change Z59.7 **Insufficient social insurance and welfare support**
Add Insufficient social and welfare insurance
Add Z59.71 **Insufficient health insurance coverage**
Add Inadequate social insurance
Add Insufficient social insurance
Add No health insurance coverage
Add Z59.72 **Insufficient welfare support**
Add Inadequate welfare support

No Change **BLOOD TYPE (Z67)**

No Change Z67 **Blood type**
Add Z67.A **Duffy phenotype**
Add Z67.A1 **Duffy null**
Add Duffy phenotype Fy(a-b-)
Add Z67.A2 **Duffy a positive**
Add Duffy phenotype Fy(a+b-)
Add Z67.A3 **Duffy b positive**
Add Duffy phenotype Fy(a-b+)
Add Z67.A4 **Duffy a and b positive**
Add Duffy phenotype Fy(a+b+)

No Change **BODY MASS INDEX [BMI] (Z68)**

No Change Z68 **Body mass index [BMI]**
No Change Z68.5 **Body mass index [BMI] pediatric**
Revise from Z68.54 **Body mass index [BMI] pediatric, greater than or equal to 95th percentile for age**
Revise to Z68.54 **Body mass index [BMI] pediatric, 95th percentile for age to less than 120% of the 95th percentile for age**
Add Z68.55 **Body mass index [BMI] pediatric, 120% of the 95th percentile for age to less than 140% of the 95th percentile for age**
Add Z68.56 **Body mass index [BMI] pediatric, greater than or equal to 140% of the 95th percentile for age**

No Change **PERSONS WITH POTENTIAL HEALTH HAZARDS RELATED TO FAMILY AND PERSONAL HISTORY AND CERTAIN CONDITIONS INFLUENCING HEALTH STATUS (Z77-Z99)**

No Change Z79 **Long term (current) drug therapy**
No Change Z79.6 **Long term (current) use of immunomodulators and immunosuppressants**
No Change Z79.62 **Long term (current) use of immunosuppressant**
No Change Z79.624 **Long term (current) use of inhibitors of nucleotide synthesis**
Revise from Long term (current) use omycophenolate
Revise to Long term (current) use of mycophenolate

No Change Z83 **Family history of other specific disorders**
No Change Z83.7 **Family history of diseases of the digestive system**
Add Z83.72 **Family history of familial adenomatous polyposis**

No Change Z86 **Personal history of certain other diseases**
No Change Z86.0 **Personal history of in-situ and benign neoplasms and neoplasms of uncertain behavior**
No Change Z86.01 **Personal history of benign neoplasm**
Revise from Z86.010 **Personal history of colonic polyps**
Revise to Z86.010 **Personal history of colon polyps**
Add Personal history of colorectal polyps
Add Personal history of rectal polyps
Add Z86.0100 **Personal history of colon polyps, unspecified**
Add Personal history of colon polyps NOS

Add **Z86.0101 Personal history of adenomatous and serrated colon polyps**
Personal history of tubular adenoma polyps
Add Personal history of sessile adenomatous colon polyp
Add Personal history of sessile serrated colon polyp
Add Personal history of tubulovillous adenoma polyps
Add Personal history of villous adenoma polyps
Add Personal history of traditional serrated adenoma polyps
Add **Z86.0102 Personal history of hyperplastic colon polyps**
Add **Z86.0109 Personal history of other colon polyps**

No Change **Z91 Personal risk factors, not elsewhere classified**
No Change **Z91.1 Patient's noncompliance with medical treatment and regimen**
No Change **Z91.12 Patient's intentional underdosing of medication regimen**
Excludes1 adverse effect of
Delete prescribed drug taken as directed-code to adverse effect
Delete poisoning (overdose) -code to poisoning

No Change **Z91.13 Patient's unintentional underdosing of medication regimen**
Delete **Excludes1** adverse effect of prescribed drug taken as directed-code to adverse effect
Delete poisoning (overdose) -code to poisoning
No Change **Z91.14 Patient's other noncompliance with medication regimen**
Add *Code first, if applicable, adverse effect of underdosing (T36-T50)*

No Change **Z92 Personal history of medical treatment**
No Change **Z92.2 Personal history of drug therapy**
No Change **Z92.22 Personal history of monoclonal drug therapy**
Excludes2 personal history of
Add immune checkpoint inhibitor therapy (Z92.26)
Add **Z92.26 Personal history of immune checkpoint inhibitor therapy**
Add Personal history of ICI drug therapy
No Change **Z92.8 Personal history of other medical treatment**
No Change **Z92.85 Personal history of cellular therapy**
Add **Excludes2** personal history of immune checkpoint inhibitor therapy (Z92.26)

No Change **Z93 Artificial opening status**
No Change **Z93.2 Ileostomy status**
Add Ileal pouch status
Add Kock pouch status

PART I

Introduction

ICD-10-CM Official Guidelines for Coding and Reporting FY2025 (October 1, 2024 - September 30, 2025)

Narrative changes appear in bold text

Items underlined have been moved within the guidelines since the 2024 version

***Italics* are used to indicate revisions to heading changes**

The Centers for Medicare and Medicaid Services (CMS) and the National Center for Health Statistics (NCHS), two departments within the U.S. Federal Government's Department of Health and Human Services (DHHS), provide the following guidelines for coding and reporting using the International Classification of Diseases, 10th Revision, Clinical Modification (ICD-10-CM). These guidelines should be used as a companion document to the official version of the ICD-10-CM as published on the NCHS website. The ICD-10-CM is a morbidity classification published by the United States for classifying diagnoses and reason for visits in all health care settings. The ICD-10-CM is based on the ICD-10, the statistical classification of disease published by the World Health Organization (WHO).

These guidelines have been approved by the four organizations that make up the Cooperating Parties for the ICD-10-CM: the American Hospital Association (AHA), the American Health Information Management Association (AHIMA), CMS, and NCHS.

These guidelines are a set of rules that have been developed to accompany and complement the official conventions and instructions provided within the ICD-10-CM itself. The instructions and conventions of the classification take precedence over guidelines. These guidelines are based on the coding and sequencing instructions in the Tabular List and Alphabetic Index of ICD-10-CM, but provide additional instruction. Adherence to these guidelines when assigning ICD-10-CM diagnosis codes is required under the Health Insurance Portability and Accountability Act (HIPAA). The diagnosis codes (Tabular List and Alphabetic Index) have been adopted under HIPAA for all health care settings. A joint effort between the health care provider and the coder is essential to achieve complete and accurate documentation, code assignment, and reporting of diagnoses and procedures. These guidelines have been developed to assist both the health care provider and the coder in identifying those diagnoses that are to be reported. The importance of consistent, complete documentation in the medical record cannot be overemphasized. Without such documentation accurate coding cannot be achieved. The entire record should be reviewed to determine the specific reason for the encounter and the conditions treated.

The term "encounter" is used for all settings, including hospital admissions. In the context of these guidelines, the term "provider" is used throughout the guidelines to mean physician or any qualified health care practitioner who is legally accountable for establishing the patient's diagnosis. Only this set of guidelines, approved by the Cooperating Parties, is official.

The guidelines are organized into sections. Section I includes the structure and conventions of the classification and general guidelines that apply to the entire classification, and chapter-specific guidelines that correspond to the chapters as they are arranged in the classification. Section II includes guidelines for selection of principal diagnosis for non-outpatient settings. Section III includes guidelines for reporting additional diagnoses in non-outpatient settings. Section IV is for outpatient coding and reporting. It is necessary to review all sections of the guidelines to fully understand all of the rules and instructions needed to code properly.

ICD-10-CM Official Guidelines for Coding and Reporting

Section I. Conventions, General Coding Guidelines and Chapter Specific Guidelines

GUIDELINES (ICD-10-CM)

7. Chapter 7: Diseases of the Eye and Adnexa (H00-H59)
   a. Glaucoma
   b. Blindness
8. Chapter 8: Diseases of the Ear and Mastoid Process (H60-H95)
9. Chapter 9: Diseases of the Circulatory System (I00-I99)
   a. Hypertension
   b. Atherosclerotic Coronary Artery Disease and Angina
   c. Intraoperative and Postprocedural Cerebrovascular Accident
   d. Sequelae of Cerebrovascular Disease
   e. Acute myocardial infarction (AMI)
10. Chapter 10: Diseases of the Respiratory System (J00-J99)
   a. Chronic Obstructive Pulmonary Disease [COPD] and Asthma
   b. Acute Respiratory Failure
   c. Influenza due to certain identified influenza viruses
   d. Ventilator associated Pneumonia
   e. Vaping-related disorders
11. Chapter 11: Diseases of the Digestive System (K00-K95)
12. Chapter 12: Diseases of the Skin and Subcutaneous Tissue (L00-L99)
   a. Pressure ulcer stage codes
   b. Non-Pressure Chronic Ulcers
13. Chapter 13: Diseases of the Musculoskeletal System and Connective Tissue (M00-M99)
   a. Site and laterality
   b. Acute traumatic versus chronic or recurrent musculoskeletal conditions
   c. Coding of Pathologic Fractures
   d. Osteoporosis
   e. Multisystem Inflammatory Syndrome
14. Chapter 14: Diseases of Genitourinary System (N00-N99)
   a. Chronic kidney disease
15. Chapter 15: Pregnancy, Childbirth, and the Puerperium (O00-O9A)
   a. General Rules for Obstetric Cases
   b. Selection of OB Principal or First-listed Diagnosis
   c. Pre-existing conditions versus conditions due to the pregnancy
   d. Pre-existing hypertension in pregnancy
   e. Fetal Conditions Affecting the Management of the Mother
   f. HIV Infection in Pregnancy, Childbirth and the Puerperium
   g. Diabetes mellitus in pregnancy
   h. Long term use of insulin and oral hypoglycemics
   i. Gestational (pregnancy induced) diabetes
   j. Sepsis and septic shock complicating abortion, pregnancy, childbirth and the puerperium
   k. Puerperal sepsis
   l. Alcohol, tobacco and drug use during pregnancy, childbirth and the puerperium
   m. Poisoning, toxic effects, adverse effects and underdosing in a pregnant patient
   n. Normal Delivery, Code O80
   o. The Peripartum and Postpartum Periods
   p. Code O94, Sequelae of complication of pregnancy, childbirth, and the puerperium
   q. Termination of Pregnancy and Spontaneous abortions
   r. Abuse in a pregnant patient
   s. COVID-19 infection in pregnancy, childbirth, and the puerperium
16. Chapter 16: Certain Conditions Originating in the Perinatal Period (P00-P96)
   a. General Perinatal Rules
   b. Observation and Evaluation of Newborns for Suspected Conditions not Found
   c. Coding Additional Perinatal Diagnoses
   d. Prematurity and Fetal Growth Retardation
   e. Low birth weight and immaturity status
   f. Bacterial Sepsis of Newborn
   g. Stillbirth
   h. COVID-19 Infection in Newborn
17. Chapter 17: Congenital Malformations, Deformations, and Chromosomal Abnormalities (Q00-Q99)
18. Chapter 18: Symptoms, Signs, and Abnormal Clinical and Laboratory Findings, Not Elsewhere Classified (R00-R99)
   a. Use of symptom codes
   b. Use of a symptom code with a definitive diagnosis code
   c. Combination codes that include symptoms
   d. Repeated falls
   e. Coma scale
   f. Functional quadriplegia
   g. SIRS due to Non-Infectious Process
   h. Death NOS
   i. NIHSS Stroke Scale
19. Chapter 19: Injury, Poisoning, and Certain Other Consequences of External Causes (S00-T88)
   a. Application of 7th Characters in Chapter 19
   b. Coding of Injuries
   c. Coding of Traumatic Fractures
   d. Coding of Burns and Corrosions
   e. Adverse Effects, Poisoning, Underdosing and Toxic Effects
   f. Adult and child abuse, neglect and other maltreatment
   g. Complications of care
20. Chapter 20: External Causes of Morbidity (V00-Y99)
   a. General External Cause Coding Guidelines
   b. Place of Occurrence Guideline
   c. Activity Code
   d. Place of Occurrence, Activity, and Status Codes Used with other External Cause Code
   e. If the Reporting Format Limits the Number of External Cause Codes
   f. Multiple External Cause Coding Guidelines
   g. Child and Adult Abuse Guideline
   h. Unknown or Undetermined Intent Guideline
   i. Sequelae (Late Effects) of External Cause Guidelines
   j. Terrorism Guidelines
   k. External Cause Status

21. Chapter 21: Factors Influencing Health Status and Contact with Health Services (Z00-Z99)
    a. Use of Z Codes in Any Healthcare Setting
    b. Z Codes Indicate a Reason for an Encounter or Provide Additional Information about a Patient Encounter
    c. Categories of Z Codes
22. Chapter 22: Codes for Special Purposes (U00-U85)

Section II. Selection of Principal Diagnosis

A. Codes for symptoms, signs, and ill-defined conditions
B. Two or more interrelated conditions, each potentially meeting the definition for principal diagnosis
C. Two or more diagnoses that equally meet the definition for principal diagnosis
D. Two or more comparative or contrasting conditions
E. A symptom(s) followed by contrasting/comparative diagnoses
F. Original treatment plan not carried out
G. Complications of surgery and other medical care
H. Uncertain Diagnosis
I. Admission from Observation Unit
   1. Admission Following Medical Observation
   2. Admission Following Post-Operative Observation
J. Admission from Outpatient Surgery
K. Admissions/Encounters for Rehabilitation

Section III. Reporting Additional Diagnoses

A. Previous conditions
B. Abnormal findings
C. Uncertain Diagnosis

Section IV. Diagnostic Coding and Reporting Guidelines for Outpatient Services

A. Selection of first-listed condition
   1. Outpatient Surgery
   2. Observation Stay
B. Codes from A00.0 through T88.9, Z00-Z99, U00-U85
C. Accurate reporting of ICD-10-CM diagnosis codes
D. Codes that describe symptoms and signs
E. Encounters for circumstances other than a disease or injury
F. Level of Detail in Coding
   1. ICD-10-CM codes with 3, 4, 5, 6, or 7 characters
   2. Use of full number of characters required for a code
   3. Highest level of specificity
G. ICD-10-CM code for the diagnosis, condition, problem, or other reason for encounter/visit
H. Uncertain diagnosis
I. Chronic diseases
J. Code all documented conditions that coexist
K. Patients receiving diagnostic services only
L. Patients receiving therapeutic services only
M. Patients receiving preoperative evaluations only
N. Ambulatory surgery
O. Routine outpatient prenatal visits
P. Encounters for general medical examinations with abnormal findings
Q. Encounters for routine health screenings

Appendix I: Present on Admission Reporting Guidelines

Section I. Conventions, General Coding Guidelines, and Chapter Specific Guidelines

The conventions, general guidelines, and chapter-specific guidelines are applicable to all health care settings unless otherwise indicated. The conventions and instructions of the classification take precedence over guidelines.

A. Conventions for the ICD-10-CM

The conventions for the ICD-10-CM are the general rules for use of the classification independent of the guidelines. These conventions are incorporated within the Alphabetic Index and Tabular List of the ICD-10-CM as instructional notes.

1. The Alphabetic Index and Tabular List

The ICD-10-CM is divided into the Alphabetic Index, an alphabetical list of terms and their corresponding code, and the Tabular List, a structured list of codes divided into chapters based on body system or condition. The Alphabetic Index consists of the following parts: the Index of Diseases and Injury, the Index of External Causes of Injury, the Table of Neoplasms, and the Table of Drugs and Chemicals.

See Section I.C.2. ***Neoplasms***

See Section I.C.19. Adverse effects, poisoning, underdosing and toxic effects

2. Format and Structure:

The ICD-10-CM Tabular List contains categories, subcategories and codes. Characters for categories, subcategories and codes may be either a letter or a number. All categories are 3 characters. A 3-character category that has no further subdivision is equivalent to a code. Subcategories are either 4 or 5 characters. Codes may be 3, 4, 5, 6 or 7 characters. That is, each level of subdivision after a category is a subcategory. The final level of subdivision is a code. Codes that have applicable 7th characters are still referred to as codes, not subcategories. A code that has an applicable 7th character is considered invalid without the 7th character.

The ICD-10-CM uses an indented format for ease in reference

3. Use of codes for reporting purposes

For reporting purposes only codes are permissible, not categories or subcategories, and any applicable 7th character is required.

4. Placeholder character

The ICD-10-CM utilizes a placeholder character "X". The "X" is used as a placeholder at certain codes to allow for future expansion. An example of this is at the poisoning, adverse effect and underdosing codes, categories T36-T50. Where a placeholder exists, the X must be used in order for the code to be considered a valid code.

5. 7th Characters

Certain ICD-10-CM categories have applicable 7th characters. The applicable 7th character is required for all codes within the category, or as the notes in the Tabular List instruct. The 7th character must always be the 7th character in the data field. If a code that requires a 7th character is not 6 characters, a placeholder X must be used to fill in the empty characters.

6. Abbreviations

a. Alphabetic Index abbreviations

NEC "Not elsewhere classifiable"

This abbreviation in the Alphabetic Index represents "other specified". When a specific code is not available for a condition the Alphabetic Index directs the coder to the "other specified" code in the Tabular List.

NOS "Not otherwise specified"

This abbreviation is the equivalent of unspecified.

b. Tabular List abbreviations

NEC "Not elsewhere classifiable"

This abbreviation in the Tabular List represents "other specified". When a specific code is not available for a condition, the Tabular List includes an NEC entry under a code to identify the code as the "other specified" code.

NOS "Not otherwise specified"

This abbreviation is the equivalent of unspecified.

7. Punctuation

[ ] Brackets are used in the Tabular List to enclose synonyms, alternative wording or explanatory phrases. Brackets are used in the Alphabetic Index to identify manifestation codes.

( ) Parentheses are used in both the Alphabetic Index and Tabular List to enclose supplementary words that may be present or absent in the statement of a disease or procedure without affecting the code number to which it is assigned. The terms within the parentheses are referred to as nonessential modifiers. The nonessential modifiers in the Alphabetic Index to Diseases apply to subterms following a main term except when a nonessential modifier and a subentry are mutually exclusive, the subentry takes precedence. For example, in the ICD-10-CM Alphabetic Index under the main term Enteritis, "acute" is a nonessential modifier and "chronic" is a subentry. In this case, the nonessential modifier "acute" does not apply to the subentry "chronic".

: Colons are used in the Tabular List after an incomplete term which needs one or more of the modifiers following the colon to make it assignable to a given category.

8. Use of "and".

See Section I.A.14. Use of the term "And"

9. Other and Unspecified codes

a. "Other" codes

Codes titled "other" or "other specified" are for use when the information in the medical record provides detail for which a specific code does not exist. Alphabetic Index entries with NEC in the line designate "other" codes in the Tabular List. These Alphabetic Index entries represent specific disease entities for which no specific code exists so the term is included within an "other" code.

b. "Unspecified" codes

Codes titled "unspecified" are for use when the information in the medical record is insufficient to assign a more specific code. For those categories for which an unspecified code is not provided, the "other specified" code may represent both other and unspecified.

See Section I.B.18 Use of signs/symptoms/unspecified codes

10. Includes Notes

This note appears immediately under a 3-character code title to further define, or give examples of, the content of the category.

11. Inclusion terms

List of terms is included under some codes. These terms are the conditions for which that code is to be used. The terms may be synonyms of the code title, or, in the case of "other specified" codes, the terms are a list of the various conditions assigned to that code. The inclusion terms are not necessarily exhaustive. Additional terms found only in the Alphabetic Index may also be assigned to a code.

12. Excludes Notes

The ICD-10-CM has two types of excludes notes. Each type of note has a different definition for use, but they are all similar in that they indicate that codes excluded from each other are independent of each other.

a. Excludes1

A type 1 Excludes note is a pure excludes note. It means "NOT CODED HERE!" An Excludes1 note indicates that the code excluded should never be used at the same time as the code above the Excludes1 note. An Excludes1 is used when two conditions cannot occur together, such as a congenital form versus an acquired form of the same condition.

An exception to the Excludes1 definition is the circumstance when the two conditions are unrelated to each other. If it is not clear whether the two conditions involving an Excludes1 note are related or not, query the provider. For example, code F45.8, Other somatoform disorders, has an Excludes1 note for "sleep related teeth grinding (G47.63)" because "teeth grinding" is an inclusion term under F45.8. Only one of these two codes should be assigned for teeth grinding. However, psychogenic dysmenorrhea is also an inclusion term under F45.8, and a patient could have both this condition and sleep-related teeth grinding. In this case, the two conditions are clearly unrelated to each other, and so it would be appropriate to report F45.8 and G47.63 together.

b. Excludes2

A Type 2 Excludes note represents "Not included here." An excludes2 note indicates that the condition excluded is not part of the condition represented by the code, but a patient may have both conditions at the same time. When an Excludes2 note appears under a code, it is acceptable to use both the code and the excluded code together, when appropriate.

13. **Etiology/manifestation convention ("code first", "use additional code" and "in diseases classified elsewhere" notes)**
Certain conditions have both an underlying etiology and multiple body system manifestations due to the underlying etiology. For such conditions, the ICD-10-CM has a coding convention that requires the underlying condition be sequenced first, if applicable, followed by the manifestation. Wherever such a combination exists, there is a "use additional code" note at the etiology code, and a "code first" note at the manifestation code. These instructional notes indicate the proper sequencing order of the codes, etiology followed by manifestation.
In most cases the manifestation codes will have in the code title, "in diseases classified elsewhere." Codes with this title are a component of the etiology/manifestation convention. The code title indicates that it is a manifestation code. "In diseases classified elsewhere" codes are never permitted to be used as first-listed or principal diagnosis codes. They must be used in conjunction with an underlying condition code and they must be listed following the underlying condition. See category F02, Dementia in other diseases classified elsewhere, for an example of this convention.
There are manifestation codes that do not have "in diseases classified elsewhere" in the title. For such codes, there is a "use additional code" note at the etiology code and a "code first" note at the manifestation code and the rules for sequencing apply.
In addition to the notes in the Tabular List, these conditions also have a specific Alphabetic Index entry structure. In the Alphabetic Index both conditions are listed together with the etiology code first followed by the manifestation codes in brackets. The code in brackets is always to be sequenced second.
An example of the etiology/manifestation convention is dementia with Parkinson's disease. In the Alphabetic Index, **a** code **from category** G20 is listed first, followed by code F02.80 or F02.81 in brackets. A code from category G20- represents the underlying etiology, Parkinson's disease, and must be sequenced first, whereas *codes* F02.80 and F02.81 represent the manifestation of dementia in diseases classified elsewhere, with or without behavioral disturbance.
"Code first" and "Use additional code" notes are also used as sequencing rules in the classification for certain codes that are not part of an etiology/manifestation combination.
See Section I.B.7. Multiple coding for a single condition.

14. **"And"**
The word "and" should be interpreted to mean either "and" or "or" when it appears in a title.
For example, cases of "tuberculosis of bones", "tuberculosis of joints" and "tuberculosis of bones and joints" are classified to subcategory A18.0, Tuberculosis of bones and joints.

15. **"With"**
The word "with" or "in" should be interpreted to mean "associated with" or "due to" when it appears in a code title, the Alphabetic Index, (either under a main term or subterm) or an instructional note in the Tabular List. The classification presumes a causal relationship between the two conditions linked by these terms in the Alphabetic Index or Tabular List. These conditions should be coded as related even in the absence of provider documentation explicitly linking them, unless the documentation clearly states the conditions are unrelated or when another guideline exists that specifically requires a documented linkage between two conditions (e.g., sepsis guideline for "acute organ dysfunction that is not clearly associated with the sepsis").
For conditions not specifically linked by these relational terms in the classification or when a guideline requires that a linkage between two conditions be explicitly documented provider documentation must link the conditions in order to code them as related.
The word "with" in the Alphabetic Index is sequenced immediately following the main term or subterm, not in alphabetical order.

16. **"See" and "See Also"**
The "see" instruction following a main term in the Alphabetic Index indicates that another term should be referenced. It is necessary to go to the main term referenced with the "see" note to locate the correct code.
A "see also" instruction following a main term in the Alphabetic Index instructs that there is another main term that may also be referenced that may provide additional Alphabetic Index entries that may be useful. It is not necessary to follow the "see also" note when the original main term provides the necessary code.

17. **"Code also" note**
A "code also" note instructs that two codes may be required to fully describe a condition, but this note does not provide sequencing direction. The sequencing depends on the circumstances of the encounter.

18. **Default codes**
A code listed next to a main term in the ICD-10-CM Alphabetic Index is referred to as a default code. The default code represents that condition that is most commonly associated with the main term, or is the unspecified code for the condition. If a condition is documented in a medical record (for example, appendicitis) without any additional information, such as acute or chronic, the default code should be assigned.

19. **Code assignment and Clinical Criteria**
The assignment of a diagnosis code is based on the provider's diagnostic statement that the condition exists. The provider's statement that the patient has a particular condition is sufficient. Code assignment is not based on clinical criteria used by the provider to establish the diagnosis. **If there is**

GUIDELINES (ICD-10-CM)

conflicting medical record documentation, query the provider.

B. General Coding Guidelines

1. Locating a code in the ICD-10-CM

To select a code in the classification that corresponds to a diagnosis or reason for visit documented in a medical record, first locate the term in the Alphabetic Index, and then verify the code in the Tabular List. Read and be guided by instructional notations that appear in both the Alphabetic Index and the Tabular List.

It is essential to use both the Alphabetic Index and Tabular List when locating and assigning a code. The Alphabetic Index does not always provide the full code. Selection of the full code, including laterality and any applicable 7th character can only be done in the Tabular List. A dash (-) at the end of an Alphabetic Index entry indicates that additional characters are required. Even if a dash is not included at the Alphabetic Index entry, it is necessary to refer to the Tabular List to verify that no 7th character is required.

2. Level of Detail in Coding

Diagnosis codes are to be used and reported at their highest number of characters available and to the highest level of specificity documented in the medical record.

ICD-10-CM diagnosis codes are composed of codes with 3, 4, 5, 6, or 7 characters. Codes with three characters are included in ICD-10-CM as the heading of a category of codes that may be further subdivided by the use of 4th and/or 5th characters and/or 6th characters, which provide greater detail.

A 3-character code is to be used only if it is not further subdivided. A code is invalid if it has not been coded to the full number of characters required for that code, including the 7th character, if applicable.

3. Code or codes from A00.0 through T88.9, Z00-Z99.8, U00-U85

The appropriate code or codes from A00.0 through T88.9, Z00-Z99.8 and U00-U85 must be used to identify diagnoses, symptoms, conditions, problems, complaints or other reason(s) for the encounter/visit.

4. Signs and symptoms

Codes that describe symptoms and signs, as opposed to diagnoses, are acceptable for reporting purposes when a related definitive diagnosis has not been established (confirmed) by the provider. Chapter 18 of ICD-10-CM, Symptoms, Signs, and Abnormal Clinical and Laboratory Findings, Not Elsewhere Classified (codes R00.0 - R99) contains many, but not all codes for symptoms.

See Section I.B.18 Use of signs/symptoms/unspecified codes

5. Conditions that are an integral part of a disease process

Signs and symptoms that are associated routinely with a disease process should not be assigned as additional codes, unless otherwise instructed by the classification.

6. Conditions that are not an integral part of a disease process

Additional signs and symptoms that may not be associated routinely with a disease process should be coded when present.

7. Multiple coding for a single condition

In addition to the etiology/manifestation convention that requires two codes to fully describe a single condition that affects multiple body systems, there are other single conditions that also require more than one code. "Use additional code" notes are found in the Tabular List at codes that are not part of an etiology/manifestation pair where a secondary code is useful to fully describe a condition. The sequencing rule is the same as the etiology/manifestation pair, "use additional code" indicates that a secondary code should be added, if known.

For example, for bacterial infections that are not included in Chapter 1, a secondary code from category B95, Streptococcus, Staphylococcus, and Enterococcus, as the cause of diseases classified elsewhere, or B96, Other bacterial agents as the cause of diseases classified elsewhere, may be required to identify the bacterial organism causing the infection. A "use additional code" note will normally be found at the infectious disease code, indicating a need for the organism code to be added as a secondary code.

"Code first" notes are also under certain codes that are not specifically manifestation codes but may be due to an underlying cause. When there is a "code first" note and an underlying condition is present, the underlying condition should be sequenced first, if known.

"Code, if applicable, any causal condition first," notes indicate that this code may be assigned as a principal diagnosis when the causal condition is unknown or not applicable. If a causal condition is known, then the code for that condition should be sequenced as the principal or first-listed diagnosis.

Multiple codes may be needed for sequela, complication codes and obstetric codes to more fully describe a condition. See the specific guidelines for these conditions for further instruction.

8. Acute and Chronic Conditions

If the same condition is described as both acute (subacute) and chronic, and separate subentries exist in the Alphabetic Index at the same indentation level, code both and sequence the acute (subacute) code first.

9. Combination Code

A combination code is a single code used to classify:

Two diagnoses, or

A diagnosis with an associated secondary process (manifestation)

A diagnosis with an associated complication

Combination codes are identified by referring to subterm entries in the Alphabetic Index and by reading the inclusion and exclusion notes in the Tabular List.

GUIDELINES (ICD-10-CM)

Assign only the combination code when that code fully identifies the diagnostic conditions involved or when the Alphabetic Index so directs. Multiple coding should not be used when the classification provides a combination code that clearly identifies all of the elements documented in the diagnosis. When the combination code lacks necessary specificity in describing the manifestation or complication, an additional code should be used as a secondary code.

10. Sequela (Late Effects)

A sequela is the residual effect (condition produced) after the acute phase of an illness or injury has terminated. There is no time limit on when a sequela code can be used. The residual may be apparent early, such as in cerebral infarction, or it may occur months or years later, such as that due to a previous injury. Examples of sequela include: scar formation resulting from a burn, deviated septum due to a nasal fracture, and infertility due to tubal occlusion from old tuberculosis. Coding of sequela generally requires two codes sequenced in the following order: the condition or nature of the sequela is sequenced first. The sequela code is sequenced second.

An exception to the above guidelines are those instances where the code for the sequela is followed by a manifestation code identified in the Tabular List and title, or the sequela code has been expanded (at the 4th, 5th, or 6th character levels) to include the manifestation(s). The code for the acute phase of an illness or injury that led to the sequela is never used with a code for the late effect.

See Section I.C.9. Sequelae of cerebrovascular disease

See Section I.C.15. Sequelae of complication of pregnancy, childbirth and the puerperium

See Section I.C.19. Application of 7th characters for Chapter 19

11. Impending or Threatened Condition

Code any condition described at the time of discharge as "impending" or "threatened" as follows:

If it did occur, code as confirmed diagnosis.

If it did not occur, reference the Alphabetic Index to determine if the condition has a subentry term for "impending" or "threatened" and also reference main term entries for "Impending" and for "Threatened."

If the subterms are listed, assign the given code.

If the subterms are not listed, code the existing underlying condition(s) and not the condition described as impending or threatened.

12. Reporting Same Diagnosis Code More Than Once

Each unique ICD-10-CM diagnosis code may be reported only once for an encounter. This applies to bilateral conditions when there are no distinct codes identifying laterality or two different conditions classified to the same ICD-10-CM diagnosis code.

13. Laterality

Some ICD-10-CM codes indicate laterality, specifying whether the condition occurs on the left, right or is bilateral. If no bilateral code is provided and the condition is bilateral, assign separate codes for both the left and right side. If the side is not identified in the medical record, assign the code for the unspecified side.

When a patient has a bilateral condition and each side is treated during separate encounters, assign the "bilateral" code (as the condition still exists on both sides), including for the encounter to treat the first side. For the second encounter for treatment after one side has previously been treated and the condition no longer exists on that side, assign the appropriate unilateral code for the side where the condition still exists (e.g., cataract surgery performed on each eye in separate encounters). The bilateral code would not be assigned for the subsequent encounter, as the patient no longer has the condition in the previously-treated site. If the treatment on the first side did not completely resolve the condition, then the bilateral code would still be appropriate.

When laterality is not documented by the patient's provider, code assignment for the affected side may be based on medical record documentation from other clinicians. If there is conflicting medical record documentation regarding the affected side, the patient's provider should be queried for clarification. Codes for "unspecified" side should rarely be used, such as when the documentation in the record is insufficient to determine the affected side and it is not possible to obtain clarification.

14. Documentation by Clinicians Other than the Patient's Provider

Code assignment is based on the documentation by the patient's provider (i.e., physician or other qualified healthcare practitioner legally accountable for establishing the patient's diagnosis). There are a few exceptions when code assignment may be based on medical record documentation from clinicians who are not the patient's provider (i.e., physician or other qualified healthcare practitioner legally accountable for establishing the patient's diagnosis).

In this context, "clinicians" other than the patient's provider refer to healthcare professionals permitted, based on regulatory or accreditation requirements or internal hospital policies, to document in a patient's official medical record.

These exceptions include codes for:

- Body Mass Index (BMI)
- Depth of non-pressure chronic ulcers
- Pressure ulcer stage
- Coma scale
- NIH stroke scale (NIHSS)
- Social determinants of health (SDOH) **classified to Chapter 21**
- Laterality
- Blood alcohol level

This information is typically, **or may be,** documented by other clinicians involved in the care of the patient (e.g., a dietitian often documents the BMI, a nurse often documents the pressure ulcer stages, and an emergency medical technician

GUIDELINES (ICD-10-CM)

often documents the coma scale). However, the associated diagnosis (such as overweight, obesity, acute stroke, pressure ulcer, or a condition classifiable to category F10, Alcohol related disorders) must be documented by the patient's provider. If there is conflicting medical record documentation, either from the same clinician or different clinicians, the patient's provider should be queried for clarification.

The BMI, coma scale, and NIHSS blood alcohol level codes, codes for social determinants of health **and underimmunization status** should only be reported as secondary diagnoses.

See Section I.C.21.c.17 for additional information regarding coding social determinants of health.

15. Syndromes

Follow the Alphabetic Index guidance when coding syndromes. In the absence of Alphabetic Index guidance, assign codes for the documented manifestations of the syndrome. Additional codes for manifestations that are not an integral part of the disease process may also be assigned when the condition does not have a unique code.

16. Documentation of Complications of Care

Code assignment is based on the provider's documentation of the relationship between the condition and the care or procedure, unless otherwise instructed by the classification. The guideline extends to any complications of care, regardless of the chapter the code is located in. It is important to note that not all conditions that occur during or following medical care or surgery are classified as complications. There must be a cause-and-effect relationship between the care provided and the condition, and **the documentation must support that the condition is clinically significant. It is not necessary for the provider to explicitly document the term "complication." For example, if the condition alters the course of the surgery as documented in the operative report, then it is would be appropriate to report a complication code.** Query the provider for clarification **if the documentation is not clear as to the relationship between the condition and the care or procedure.**

17. Borderline Diagnosis

If the provider documents a "borderline" diagnosis at the time of discharge, the diagnosis is coded as confirmed, unless the classification provides a specific entry (e.g., borderline diabetes). If a borderline condition has a specific index entry in ICD-10-CM, it should be coded as such. Since borderline conditions are not uncertain diagnoses, no distinction is made between the care setting (inpatient versus outpatient). Whenever the documentation is unclear regarding a borderline condition, coders are encouraged to query for clarification.

18. Use of Sign/Symptom/Unspecified Codes

Sign/symptom and "unspecified" codes have acceptable, even necessary, uses. While specific diagnosis codes should be reported when they are supported by the available medical record documentation and clinical knowledge of the patient's health condition, there are instances when signs/symptoms or unspecified codes are the best choices for accurately reflecting the healthcare encounter. Each healthcare encounter should be coded to the level of certainty known for that encounter.

As stated in the introductory section of these official coding guidelines, a joint effort between the healthcare provider and the coder is essential to achieve complete and accurate documentation, code assignment, and reporting of diagnoses and procedures. The importance of consistent, complete documentation in the medical record cannot be overemphasized. Without such documentation accurate coding cannot be achieved. The entire record should be reviewed to determine the specific reason for the encounter and the conditions treated.

If a definitive diagnosis has not been established by the end of the encounter, it is appropriate to report codes for sign(s) and/or symptom(s) in lieu of a definitive diagnosis. When sufficient clinical information isn't known or available about a particular health condition to assign a more specific code, it is acceptable to report the appropriate "unspecified" code (e.g., a diagnosis of pneumonia has been determined, but not the specific type). Unspecified codes should be reported when they are the codes that most accurately reflect what is known about the patient's condition at the time of that particular encounter. It would be inappropriate to select a specific code that is not supported by the medical record documentation or conduct medically unnecessary diagnostic testing in order to determine a more specific code.

19. Coding for Healthcare Encounters in Hurricane Aftermath

a. Use of External Cause of Morbidity Codes

An external cause of morbidity code should be assigned to identify the cause of the injury(ies) incurred as a result of the hurricane. The use of external cause of morbidity codes is supplemental to the application of ICD-10-CM codes. External cause of morbidity codes are never to be recorded as a principal diagnosis (first-listed in non-inpatient settings). The appropriate injury code should be sequenced before any external cause codes. The external cause of morbidity codes capture how the injury or health condition happened (cause), the intent (unintentional or accidental; or intentional, such as suicide or assault), the place where the event occurred, the activity of the patient at the time of the event, and the person's status (e.g., civilian, military). They should not be assigned for encounters to treat hurricane victims' medical conditions when no injury, adverse effect or poisoning is involved. External cause of morbidity codes should be assigned for each encounter for care and treatment of the injury. External cause of morbidity codes may be assigned in all health care settings. For the purpose of capturing complete and accurate ICD-10-CM data in the aftermath of the hurricane, a healthcare setting should be considered as any location where medical care is provided by licensed healthcare professionals.

b. Sequencing of External Causes of Morbidity Codes

Codes for cataclysmic events, such as a hurricane, take priority over all other external cause codes except child and adult abuse and terrorism and should be sequenced before other external cause of injury codes. Assign as many external cause of morbidity codes as necessary to fully explain each cause. For example, if an injury occurs as a result of a building collapse during the hurricane, external cause codes for both the hurricane and the building collapse should be assigned, with the external causes code for hurricane being sequenced as the first external cause code. For injuries incurred as a direct result of the hurricane, assign the appropriate code(s) for the injuries, followed by the code X37.0-, Hurricane (with the appropriate 7th character), and any other applicable external cause of injury codes. Code X37.0- also should be assigned when an injury is incurred as a result of flooding caused by a levee breaking related to the hurricane. Code X38.-, Flood (with the appropriate 7th character), should be assigned when an injury is from flooding resulting directly from the storm. Code X36.0.-, Collapse of dam or man-made structure, should not be assigned when the cause of the collapse is due to the hurricane. Use of code X36.0- is limited to collapses of man-made structures due to earth surface movements, not due to storm surges directly from a hurricane.

c. Other External Causes of Morbidity Code Issues

For injuries that are not a direct result of the hurricane, such as an evacuee that has incurred an injury as a result of a motor vehicle accident, assign the appropriate external cause of morbidity code(s) to describe the cause of the injury, but do not assign code X37.0-, Hurricane. If it is not clear whether the injury was a direct result of the hurricane, assume the injury is due to the hurricane and assign code X37.0-, Hurricane, as well as any other applicable external cause of morbidity codes. In addition to code X37.0-, Hurricane, other possible applicable external cause of morbidity codes include:

X30-	Exposure to excessive natural heat
X31-	Exposure to excessive natural cold
X38-	Flood

d. Use of Z codes

Z codes (other reasons for healthcare encounters) may be assigned as appropriate to further explain the reasons for presenting for healthcare services, including transfers between healthcare facilities or provide additional information relevant to a patient encounter. The ICD-10-CM Official Guidelines for Coding and Reporting identify which codes maybe assigned as principal or first-listed diagnosis only, secondary diagnosis only, or principal/first-listed or secondary (depending on the circumstances). Possible applicable Z codes include:

Z59.0-	Homelessness
Z59.1	Inadequate housing
Z59.5	Extreme poverty
Z75.1	Person awaiting admission to adequate facility elsewhere
Z75.3	Unavailability and inaccessibility of health-care facilities
Z75.4	Unavailability and inaccessibility of other helping agencies
Z76.2	Encounter for health supervision and care of other healthy infant and child
Z99.12	Encounter for respirator [ventilator] dependence during power failure

The external cause of morbidity codes and the Z codes listed above are not an all-inclusive list. Other codes may be applicable to the encounter based upon the documentation. Assign as many codes as necessary to fully explain each healthcare encounter. Since patient history information may be very limited, use any available documentation to assign the appropriate external cause of morbidity and Z codes.

C. Chapter-Specific Coding Guidelines

In addition to general coding guidelines, there are guidelines for specific diagnoses and/or conditions in the classification. Unless otherwise indicated, these guidelines apply to all health care settings. Please refer to Section II for guidelines on the selection of principal diagnosis.

1. Chapter 1: Certain Infectious and Parasitic Diseases (A00-B99, U07.1, U09.9)

a. Human Immunodeficiency Virus (HIV) Infections

1) Code only confirmed cases

Code only confirmed cases of HIV infection/illness. This is an exception to the hospital inpatient guideline Section II, H.

In this context, "confirmation" does not require documentation of positive serology or culture for HIV; the provider's diagnostic statement that the patient is HIV positive, or has an HIV-related illness is sufficient.

2) Selection and sequencing of HIV codes

(a) Patient admitted for HIV-related condition

If a patient is admitted for an HIV-related condition, the principal diagnosis should be B20, Human immunodeficiency virus [HIV] disease followed by additional diagnosis codes for all reported HIV-related conditions.

An exception to this guideline is if the reason for admission is hemolytic-uremic syndrome associated with HIV disease. Assign code D59.31, Infection-associated hemolytic-uremic syndrome, followed by code B20, Human immunodeficiency virus [HIV] disease.

GUIDELINES (ICD-10-CM)

(b) Patient with HIV disease admitted for unrelated condition

If a patient with HIV disease is admitted for an unrelated condition (such as a traumatic injury), the code for the unrelated condition (e.g., the nature of injury code) should be the principal diagnosis. Other diagnoses would be B20 followed by additional diagnosis codes for all reported HIV-related conditions.

(c) Whether the patient is newly diagnosed

Whether the patient is newly diagnosed or has had previous admissions/encounters for HIV conditions is irrelevant to the sequencing decision.

(d) Asymptomatic human immunodeficiency virus

Z21, Asymptomatic human immunodeficiency virus [HIV] infection status, is to be applied when the patient without any documentation of symptoms is listed as being "HIV positive," "known HIV," "HIV test positive," or similar terminology. Do not use this code if the term "AIDS" **or** "HIV disease" is used or if the patient is treated for any HIV-related illness or is described as having any condition(s) resulting from his/her HIV positive status; use B20 in these cases.

(e) Patients with inconclusive HIV serology

Patients with inconclusive HIV serology, but no definitive diagnosis or manifestations of the illness, may be assigned code R75, Inconclusive laboratory evidence of human immunodeficiency virus [HIV].

(f) Previously diagnosed HIV-related illness

Patients with any known prior diagnosis of an HIV-related illness should be coded to B20. Once a patient has developed an HIV-related illness, the patient should always be assigned code B20 on every subsequent admission/encounter. Patients previously diagnosed with any HIV illness (B20) should never be assigned to R75 or Z21, Asymptomatic human immunodeficiency virus [HIV] infection status.

(g) HIV Infection in Pregnancy, Childbirth and the Puerperium

During pregnancy, childbirth or the puerperium, a patient admitted (or presenting for a health care encounter) because of an HIV-related illness should receive a principal diagnosis code of O98.7-, Human immunodeficiency [HIV] disease complicating pregnancy, childbirth and the puerperium, followed by B20 and the code(s) for the HIV-related illness(es). Codes from Chapter 15 always take sequencing priority.

Patients with asymptomatic HIV infection status admitted (or presenting for a health care encounter) during pregnancy, childbirth, or the puerperium should receive codes of O98.7- and Z21.

(h) Encounters for testing for HIV

If a patient is being seen to determine his/her HIV status, use code Z11.4, Encounter for screening for human immunodeficiency virus [HIV]. Use additional codes for any associated high-risk behavior, if applicable.

If a patient with signs or symptoms is being seen for HIV testing, code the signs and symptoms. An additional counseling code Z71.7, Human immunodeficiency virus [HIV] counseling, may be used if counseling is provided during the encounter for the test.

When a patient returns to be informed of his/her HIV test results and the test result is negative, use code Z71.7, Human immunodeficiency virus [HIV] counseling.

If the results are positive, see previous guidelines and assign codes as appropriate.

(i) HIV managed by **antiretroviral** medication

If a patient with documented HIV disease, **HIV-related illness or AIDS** is currently managed on antiretroviral medications, assign code B20, Human immunodeficiency virus [HIV] disease. Code Z79.899, Other long term (current) drug therapy, may be assigned as an additional code to identify the long-term (current) use of antiretroviral medications.

(j) Encounter for HIV Prophylaxis Measures

When a patient is seen for administration of pre-exposure prophylaxis medication for HIV, assign code Z29.81, Encounter for HIV pre-exposure prophylaxis. Pre-exposure prophylaxis (PrEP) is intended to prevent infection in people who are at risk for getting HIV through sex or injection drug use. Any risk factors for HIV should also be coded.

b. Infectious agents as the cause of diseases classified to other chapters

Certain infections are classified in chapters other than Chapter 1 and no organism is identified as part of the infection code. In these instances, it is necessary to use an additional code from Chapter 1 to identify the organism. A code from category B95, Streptococcus, Staphylococcus, and Enterococcus as the cause of diseases classified to other chapters, B96, Other bacterial agents as the cause of diseases classified to other chapters, or B97, Viral agents as the cause of diseases classified to other chapters, is to be used as an additional code to identify the organism. An instructional note will be found at the infection code advising that an additional organism code is required.

c. Infections resistant to antibiotics

Many bacterial infections are resistant to current antibiotics. It is necessary to identify all infections documented as antibiotic resistant. Assign a code from category Z16, Resistance to antimicrobial drugs, following the infection code only if the infection code does not identify drug resistance.

d. Sepsis, Severe Sepsis, and Septic Shock

1) Coding of Sepsis and Severe Sepsis

(a) Sepsis

For a diagnosis of sepsis, assign the appropriate code for the underlying systemic infection. If the type of infection or causal organism is not further specified, assign code A41.9, Sepsis, unspecified organism.

A code from subcategory R65.2, Severe sepsis, should not be assigned unless severe sepsis or an associated acute organ dysfunction is documented.

(i) Negative or inconclusive blood cultures and sepsis

Negative or inconclusive blood cultures do not preclude a diagnosis of sepsis in patients with clinical evidence of the condition, however, the provider should be queried.

(ii) Urosepsis

The term urosepsis is a nonspecific term. It is not to be considered synonymous with sepsis. It has no default code in the Alphabetic Index. Should a provider use this term, he/she must be queried for clarification.

(iii) Sepsis with organ dysfunction

If a patient has sepsis and associated acute organ dysfunction or multiple organ dysfunction (MOD), follow the instructions for coding severe sepsis.

(iv) Acute organ dysfunction that is not clearly associated with the sepsis

If a patient has sepsis and an acute organ dysfunction, but the medical record documentation indicates that the acute organ dysfunction is related to a medical condition other than the sepsis, do not assign a code from subcategory R65.2, Severe sepsis. An acute organ dysfunction must be associated with the sepsis in order to assign the severe sepsis code. If the documentation is not clear as to whether an acute organ dysfunction is related to the sepsis or another medical condition, query the provider.

(b) Severe sepsis

The coding of severe sepsis requires a minimum of 2 codes: first a code for the underlying systemic infection, followed by a code from subcategory R65.2, Severe sepsis. If the causal organism is not documented, assign code A41.9, Sepsis, unspecified organism, for the infection. Additional code(s) for the associated acute organ dysfunction are also required.

Due to the complex nature of severe sepsis, some cases may require querying the provider prior to assignment of the codes.

2) Septic shock

(a) Septic shock generally refers to circulatory failure associated with severe sepsis, and therefore, it represents a type of acute organ dysfunction.

For all cases of septic shock, the code for the systemic infection should be sequenced first, followed by code R65.21, Severe sepsis with septic shock or code T81.12, Postprocedural septic shock. Any additional codes for the other acute organ dysfunctions should also be assigned. As noted in the sequencing instructions in the Tabular List, the code for septic shock cannot be assigned as a principal diagnosis.

3) Sequencing of severe sepsis

If severe sepsis is present on admission, and meets the definition of principal diagnosis, the underlying systemic infection should be assigned as principal diagnosis followed by the appropriate code from subcategory R65.2 as required by the sequencing rules in the Tabular List. A code from subcategory R65.2 can never be assigned as a principal diagnosis.

When severe sepsis develops during an encounter (it was not present on admission) the underlying systemic infection and the appropriate code from subcategory R65.2 should be assigned as secondary diagnoses.

Severe sepsis may be present on admission but the diagnosis may not be confirmed until sometime after admission. If the documentation is not clear whether severe sepsis was present on admission, the provider should be queried.

For infection-associated hemolytic-uremic syndrome with severe sepsis, see guideline I.C.1.d.9.

4) Sepsis or severe sepsis with a localized infection

If the reason for admission is sepsis or severe sepsis and a localized infection, such as pneumonia or cellulitis, a code(s) for the underlying systemic infection should be assigned first and the code for the localized infection should be assigned as a secondary diagnosis. If the patient has severe sepsis, a code from subcategory R65.2 should also be assigned as a secondary diagnosis. If the patient is admitted with a localized infection, such as pneumonia, and sepsis/severe sepsis doesn't develop until after admission, the localized infection should be assigned first, followed by the appropriate sepsis/severe sepsis codes.

For hemolytic-uremic syndrome associated with sepsis, see guideline I.C.1.d.9.

5) Sepsis due to a postprocedural infection

(a) Documentation of causal relationship

As with all postprocedural complications, code assignment is based on the provider's documentation of the relationship between the infection and the procedure.

(b) Sepsis due to a postprocedural infection

For **sepsis** following a **postprocedural wound (surgical site) infection**, a code from **T81.41** to T81.43, Infection following a procedure, or a code from O86.00 to O86.03, Infection of obstetric surgical wound, that identifies the site of the infection should be **sequenced** first, if known. Assign an additional code for sepsis following a procedure (T81.44) or sepsis following an obstetrical procedure (O86.04). Use an additional code to identify the infectious agent. If the patient has severe sepsis the appropriate code from subcategory R65.2 should also be assigned with the additional code(s) for any acute organ dysfunction.

For infections following infusion, transfusion, therapeutic injection, or immunization, a code from subcategory T80.2, Infections following infusion, transfusion, and therapeutic injection, or code T88.0-, Infection following immunization, should be coded first, followed by the code for the specific infection. If the patient has severe sepsis, the appropriate code from subcategory R65.2 should also be assigned, with the additional codes(s) for any acute organ dysfunction.

(c) Postprocedural infection and postprocedural septic shock

If a postprocedural infection has resulted in postprocedural septic shock, assign the codes indicated above for sepsis due to a postprocedural infection, followed by code T81.12-, Postprocedural septic shock. Do not assign code R65.21, Severe sepsis with septic shock. Additional code(s) should be assigned for any acute organ dysfunction.

6) Sepsis and severe sepsis associated with a noninfectious process (condition)

In some cases a noninfectious process (condition), such as trauma, may lead to an infection which can result in sepsis or severe sepsis. If sepsis or severe sepsis is documented as associated with a noninfectious condition, such as a burn or serious injury, and this condition meets the definition for principal diagnosis, the code for the noninfectious condition should be sequenced first, followed by the code for the resulting infection. If severe sepsis is present, a code from subcategory R65.2 should also be assigned with any associated organ dysfunction(s) codes. It is not necessary to assign a code from subcategory R65.1, Systemic inflammatory response syndrome (SIRS) of non-infectious origin, for these cases.

If the infection meets the definition of principal diagnosis it should be sequenced before the non-infectious condition. When both the associated non-infectious condition and the infection meet the definition of principal diagnosis either may be assigned as principal diagnosis.

Only one code from category R65, Symptoms and signs specifically associated with systemic inflammation and infection, should be assigned. Therefore, when a non-infectious condition leads to an infection resulting in severe sepsis, assign the appropriate code from subcategory R65.2, Severe sepsis. Do not additionally assign a code from subcategory R65.1, Systemic inflammatory response syndrome (SIRS) of non-infectious origin.

See Section I.C.18. SIRS due to non-infectious process

7) Sepsis and septic shock complicating abortion, pregnancy, childbirth, and the puerperium

See Section I.C.15. Sepsis and septic shock complicating abortion, pregnancy, childbirth and the puerperium

8) Newborn sepsis

See Section I.C.16. f. Bacterial sepsis of Newborn

9) Hemolytic-uremic syndrome associated with sepsis

If the reason for admission is hemolytic-uremic syndrome that is associated with sepsis, assign code D59.31, Infection-associated hemolytic-uremic syndrome, as the principal diagnosis. Codes for the underlying systemic infection and any other conditions (such as severe sepsis) should be assigned as secondary diagnoses.

e. Methicillin Resistant Staphylococcus aureus (MRSA) Conditions

1) Selection and sequencing of MRSA codes

(a) Combination codes for MRSA infection

When a patient is diagnosed with an infection that is due to methicillin resistant Staphylococcus aureus (MRSA), and that infection has a combination code that includes the causal organism (e.g., sepsis, pneumonia) assign the appropriate combination code for the condition (e.g., code A41.02, Sepsis due to Methicillin resistant Staphylococcus aureus or code J15.212, Pneumonia due to Methicillin resistant Staphylococcus aureus). Do not assign code B95.62, Methicillin resistant Staphylococcus aureus infection as the cause of diseases classified elsewhere, as an additional code because the combination code includes the type of infection and the MRSA organism. Do not assign a code from subcategory Z16.11, Resistance to penicillins, as an additional diagnosis.

See Section C.1. for instructions on coding and sequencing of sepsis and severe sepsis.

(b) Other codes for MRSA infection

When there is documentation of a current infection (e.g., wound infection, stitch abscess, urinary tract infection) due to MRSA, and that infection does not have a combination code that includes the causal organism, assign the appropriate code to identify the condition along with code B95.62, Methicillin resistant Staphylococcus aureus infection as the cause of diseases classified elsewhere for the MRSA infection. Do not assign a code from subcategory Z16.11, Resistance to penicillins.

(c) Methicillin susceptible Staphylococcus aureus (MSSA) and MRSA colonization

The condition or state of being colonized or carrying MSSA or MRSA is called colonization or carriage, while an individual person is described as being colonized or being a carrier. Colonization means that MSSA or MSRA is present on or in the body without necessarily causing illness. A positive MRSA colonization test might be documented by the provider as "MRSA screen positive" or "MRSA nasal swab positive".

Assign code Z22.322, Carrier or suspected carrier of Methicillin resistant Staphylococcus aureus, for patients documented as having MRSA colonization. Assign code Z22.321, Carrier or suspected carrier of Methicillin susceptible Staphylococcus aureus, for patients documented as having MSSA colonization. Colonization is not necessarily indicative of a disease process or as the cause of a specific condition the patient may have unless documented as such by the provider.

(d) MRSA colonization and infection

If a patient is documented as having both MRSA colonization and infection during a hospital admission, code Z22.322, Carrier or suspected carrier of Methicillin resistant Staphylococcus aureus, and a code for the MRSA infection may both be assigned.

f. Zika virus infections

1) Code only confirmed cases

Code only a confirmed diagnosis of Zika virus (A92.5, Zika virus disease) as documented by the provider. This is an exception to the hospital inpatient guideline Section II, H.

In this context, "confirmation" does not require documentation of the type of test performed; the provider's diagnostic statement that the condition is confirmed is sufficient. This code should be assigned regardless of the stated mode of transmission.

If the provider documents "suspected", "possible" or "probable" Zika, do not assign code A92.5. Assign a code(s) explaining the reason for encounter (such as fever, rash, or joint pain) or Z20.821, Contact with and (suspected) exposure to Zika virus.

g. Coronavirus infections

1) COVID-19 infection (infection due to SARS-CoV-2)

(a) Code only confirmed cases

Code only a confirmed diagnosis of the 2019 novel coronavirus disease (COVID-19) as documented by the provider, or documentation of a positive COVID-19 test result. For a confirmed diagnosis, assign code U07.1, COVID-19. This is an exception to the hospital inpatient guideline Section II, H. In this context, "confirmation" does not require documentation of a positive test result for COVID-19; the provider's documentation that the individual has COVID-19 is sufficient.

If the provider documents "suspected," "possible," "probable," or "inconclusive" COVID-19, do not assign code U07.1. Instead, code the signs and symptoms reported. *See guideline I.C.1.g.1.g.*

(b) Sequencing of codes

When COVID-19 meets the definition of principal diagnosis, code U07.1, COVID-19, should be sequenced first, followed by the appropriate codes for associated manifestations, except when another guideline requires that certain codes be sequenced first, such as obstetrics, sepsis, or transplant complications.

For a COVID-19 infection that progresses to sepsis, see Section I.C.1.d. Sepsis, Severe Sepsis, and Septic Shock

See Section I.C.15.s. for COVID-19 infection in pregnancy, childbirth, and the puerperium

See Section I.C.16.h. for COVID-19 infection in newborn

For a COVID-19 infection in a lung transplant patient, see Section I.C.19.g.3.a. Transplant complications other than kidney.

(c) Acute respiratory manifestations of COVID-19

When the reason for the encounter/admission is a respiratory manifestation of COVID-19, assign code U07.1, COVID-19, as the principal/first-listed diagnosis and assign code(s) for the respiratory manifestation(s) as additional diagnoses.

The following conditions are examples of common respiratory manifestations of COVID-19.

(i) Pneumonia

For a patient with pneumonia confirmed as due to COVID-19, assign codes U07.1, COVID-19, and J12.89, Other viral pneumonia.

(ii) Acute bronchitis

For a patient with acute bronchitis confirmed as due to COVID-19, assign codes U07.1, and J20.8, Acute bronchitis due to other specified organisms.

Bronchitis not otherwise specified (NOS) due to COVID-19 should be coded using code U07.1 and J40, Bronchitis, not specified as acute or chronic.

(iii) Lower respiratory infection

If the COVID-19 is documented as being associated with a lower respiratory infection, not otherwise specified (NOS), or an acute respiratory infection, NOS, codes U07.1 and J22, Unspecified acute lower respiratory infection, should be assigned.

If the COVID-19 is documented as being associated with a respiratory infection, NOS, codes U07.1 and J98.8, Other specified respiratory disorders, should be assigned.

(iv) Acute respiratory distress syndrome

For acute respiratory distress syndrome (ARDS) due to COVID-19, assign codes U07.1, and J80, Acute respiratory distress syndrome.

(v) Acute respiratory failure

For acute respiratory failure due to COVID-19, assign code U07.1, and code J96.0-, Acute respiratory failure.

(d) Non-respiratory manifestations of COVID-19

When the reason for the encounter/admission is a **nonrespiratory** manifestation (e.g., viral enteritis) of COVID-19, assign code U07.1, COVID-19, as the principal/first-listed diagnosis and assign code(s) for the manifestation(s) as additional diagnoses.

(e) Exposure to COVID-19

For asymptomatic individuals with actual or suspected exposure to COVID-19, assign code Z20.828, Contact with and (suspected) exposure to other viral communicable diseases.

For symptomatic individuals with actual or suspected exposure to COVID-19 and the infection has been ruled out, or test results are inconclusive or unknown, assign code Z20.828, Contact with and (suspected) exposure to other viral communicable diseases. See guideline I.C.21.c.1, Contact/Exposure, for additional guidance regarding the use of category Z20 codes.

If COVID-19 is confirmed, see guideline I.C.1.g.1.a.

(f) Screening for COVID-19

For screening for COVID-19, including preoperative testing, assign code Z11.52, Encounter for screening for COVID-19.

(g) Signs and symptoms without definitive diagnosis of **COVID19**

For patients presenting with any signs/symptoms associated with COVID-19 (such as fever, etc.) but a definitive diagnosis has not been established, assign the appropriate code(s) for each of the presenting signs and symptoms such as:

- R05.1, Acute cough, or R05.9, Cough, unspecified
- R06.02 Shortness of breath
- R50.9 Fever, unspecified

If a patient with signs/symptoms associated with COVID-19 also has an actual or suspected contact with or exposure to COVID-19, assign Z20.828, Contact with and (suspected) exposure to other viral communicable diseases, as an additional code.

(h) Asymptomatic individuals who test positive for COVID-19

For asymptomatic individuals who test positive for COVID-19, see guideline I.C.1.g.1.a. Although the individual is asymptomatic, the individual has tested positive and is considered to have the COVID-19 infection.

(i) Personal history of COVID-19

For patients with a history of COVID-19, assign code Z86.19, Personal history of other infectious and parasitic diseases.

(j) Follow-up visits after COVID-19 infection has resolved

For individuals who previously had COVID-19 without residual symptom(s) or condition(s), and are being seen for follow-up evaluation, and COVID-19 test results are negative, assign codes Z09, Encounter for follow-up examination after completed treatment for conditions other than malignant neoplasm, and Z86.19, Personal history of other infectious and parasitic diseases.

For follow-up visits for individuals with symptom(s) or condition(s) related to a previous COVID-19 infection, see guideline I.C.1.g.1.m.

See Section I.C.21.c.8, Factors influencing health states and contact with health services, Follow-up

(k) Encounter for antibody testing

For an encounter for antibody testing that is not being performed to confirm a current COVID-19 infection, nor is a follow-up test after resolution of COVID-19, assign Z01.84, Encounter for antibody response examination.

Follow the applicable guidelines above if the individual is being tested to confirm a current COVID-19 infection.

For follow-up testing after a COVID-19 infection, see guideline I.C.1.g.1.j.

(l) Multisystem Inflammatory Syndrome

For individuals with multisystem inflammatory syndrome (MIS) and COVID-19, assign code U07.1, COVID-19, as the principal/first-listed diagnosis and assign code M35.81, Multisystem inflammatory syndrome, as an additional diagnosis.

If an individual with a history of COVID-19 develops MIS, assign codes M35.81, Multisystem inflammatory syndrome, and U09.9, Post COVID-19 condition, unspecified.

If an individual with a known or suspected exposure to COVID-19, and no current COVID-19 infection or history of COVID-19, develops MIS, assign codes M35.81, Multisystem inflammatory syndrome, and Z20.822, Contact with and (suspected) exposure to COVID-19.

Additional codes should be assigned for any associated complications of MIS.

(m) Post COVID-19 Condition

For sequela of COVID-19, or associated symptoms or conditions that develop following a previous COVID-19 infection, assign a code(s) for the specific symptom(s) or condition(s) related to the previous COVID-19 infection, if known, and code U09.9, Post COVID-19 condition, unspecified.

Code U09.9 should not be assigned for manifestations of an active (current) COVID-19 infection.

If a patient has a condition(s) associated with a previous COVID-19 infection and develops a new active (current) COVID-19 infection, code U09.9 may be assigned in conjunction with code U07.1, COVID-19, to identify that the patient also has a condition(s) associated with a previous COVID-19 infection. Code(s) for the specific condition(s) associated with the previous COVID-19 infection and code(s) for manifestation(s) of the new active (current) COVID-19 infection should also be assigned.

(n) Underimmunization for COVID-19 Status

Code Z28.310, Unvaccinated for COVID-19, may be assigned when the patient has not received a COVID-19 vaccine of any type. Code

Z28.311, Partially vaccinated for COVID-19, may be assigned when the patient has been partially vaccinated for COVID-19 as per the recommendations of the Centers for Disease Control and Prevention (CDC) in place at the time of the encounter. For information, visit the CDC's website

https://www.cdc.gov/coronavirus/2019-ncov/vaccines/.

See Section I.B.14. for underimmunization documentation by clinicians other than patient's provider.

2. **Chapter 2: Neoplasms (C00-D49)**

General guidelines

Chapter 2 of the ICD-10-CM contains the codes for most benign and all malignant neoplasms. Certain benign neoplasms, such as prostatic adenomas, may be found in the specific body system chapters. To properly code a neoplasm it is necessary to determine from the record if the neoplasm is benign, in-situ, malignant, or of uncertain histologic behavior. If malignant, any secondary (metastatic) sites should also be determined.

Primary malignant neoplasms overlapping site boundaries

A primary malignant neoplasm that overlaps two or more contiguous (next to each other) sites should be classified to the subcategory/ code .8 ("overlapping lesion"), unless the combination is specifically indexed elsewhere. For multiple neoplasms of the same site that are not contiguous such as tumors in different quadrants of the same breast, codes for each site should be assigned.

Malignant neoplasm of ectopic tissue

Malignant neoplasms of ectopic tissue are to be coded to the site of origin mentioned (e.g., ectopic pancreatic malignant neoplasms involving the stomach are coded to malignant neoplasm of pancreas, unspecified) (C25.9).

The neoplasm table in the Alphabetic Index should be referenced first. However, if the histological term is documented, that term should be referenced first, rather than going immediately to the Neoplasm Table, in order to determine which column in the Neoplasm Table is appropriate. For example, if the documentation indicates "adenoma," refer to the term in the Alphabetic Index to review the entries under this term and the instructional note to "see also neoplasm, by site, benign." The table provides the proper code based on the type of neoplasm and the site. It is important to select the proper column in the table that corresponds to the type of neoplasm. The Tabular List should then be referenced to verify that the correct code has been selected from the table and that a more specific site code does not exist.

See Section I.C.21. Factors influencing health status and contact with health services, Status, for information regarding Z15.0, codes for genetic susceptibility to cancer.

a. *Admission/Encounter for treatment of primary site*

If the **malignancy is chiefly responsible for occasioning the patient admission/encounter and treatment is directed at the primary site,** designate the **primary** malignancy as the principal **/first-listed** diagnosis.

The only exception to this guideline is if the administration of chemotherapy, immunotherapy or external beam radiation therapy **is chiefly responsible for occasioning the admission/ encounter. In that case,** assign the appropriate Z51.— code as the first-listed or principal diagnosis, and the **underlying** diagnosis or problem for which the service is being performed as a secondary diagnosis.

b. *Admission/Encounter for* **treatment of secondary site**

When a patient is admitted because of a primary neoplasm with metastasis and treatment is directed toward the secondary site only, the secondary neoplasm is designated as the principal diagnosis even though the primary malignancy is still present.

c. **Coding and sequencing of complications**

Coding and sequencing of complications associated with the malignancies or with the therapy thereof are subject to the following guidelines:

1) **Anemia associated with malignancy**

When admission/encounter is for management of an anemia associated with the malignancy, and the treatment is only for anemia, the appropriate code for the malignancy is sequenced as the principal or first-listed diagnosis followed by the appropriate code for the anemia (such as code D63.0, Anemia in neoplastic disease).

2) **Anemia associated with chemotherapy, immunotherapy and radiation therapy**

When the admission/encounter is for management of an anemia associated with an adverse effect of the administration of chemotherapy or immunotherapy and the only treatment is for the anemia, the anemia code is sequenced first followed by the appropriate codes for the neoplasm and the adverse effect (T45.1X5, Adverse effect of antineoplastic and immunosuppressive drugs).

When the admission/encounter is for management of an anemia associated with an adverse effect of radiotherapy, the anemia code should be sequenced first, followed by the appropriate neoplasm code and code Y84.2, Radiological procedure and radiotherapy as the cause of abnormal reaction of the patient, or of later complication, without mention of misadventure at the time of the procedure.

3) **Management of dehydration due to the malignancy**

When the admission/encounter is for management of dehydration due to the malignancy and only the dehydration is being treated (intravenous rehydration), the dehydration is sequenced first, followed by the code(s) for the malignancy.

4) Treatment of a complication resulting from a surgical procedure

When the admission/encounter is for treatment of a complication resulting from a surgical procedure, designate the complication as the principal or first-listed diagnosis if treatment is directed at resolving the complication.

d. Primary malignancy previously excised

When a primary malignancy has been previously excised or eradicated from its site and there is no further treatment directed to that site and there is no evidence of any existing primary malignancy, at that site a code from category Z85, Personal history of malignant neoplasm, should be used to indicate the former site of the malignancy. Any mention of extension, invasion, or metastasis to another site is coded as a secondary malignant neoplasm to that site. The secondary site may be the principal or first-listed diagnosis with the Z85 code used as a secondary code.

See section I.C.2.t. Secondary malignant neoplasm of lymphoid tissue.

e. Admissions/Encounters involving chemotherapy, immunotherapy and radiation therapy

1) Episode of care involves surgical removal of neoplasm

When an episode of care involves the surgical removal of a neoplasm, primary or secondary site, followed by adjunct chemotherapy or radiation treatment during the same episode of care, the code for the neoplasm should be assigned as principal or first-listed diagnosis.

2) Patient admission/encounter chiefly for administration of chemotherapy, immunotherapy and radiation therapy

If a patient admission/encounter is **chiefly** for the administration of chemotherapy, immunotherapy or external beam radiation therapy assign code Z51.0, Encounter for antineoplastic radiation therapy, or Z51.11, Encounter for antineoplastic chemotherapy, or Z51.12, Encounter for antineoplastic immunotherapy as the first-listed or principal diagnosis. If a patient receives more than one of these therapies during the same admission, more than one of these codes may be assigned, in any sequence.

The malignancy for which the therapy is being administered should be assigned as a secondary diagnosis.

If a patient admission/encounter is for the insertion or implantation of radioactive elements (e.g., brachytherapy) the appropriate code for the malignancy is sequenced as the principal or first-listed diagnosis. Code Z51.0 should not be assigned.

3) Patient admitted for radiation therapy, chemotherapy or immunotherapy and develops complications

When a patient is admitted for the purpose of external beam radiotherapy, immunotherapy or chemotherapy and develops complications such as uncontrolled nausea and vomiting or dehydration, the principal or first-listed diagnosis is Z51.0, Encounter for antineoplastic radiation therapy, or Z51.11, Encounter for antineoplastic chemotherapy, or Z51.12, Encounter for antineoplastic immunotherapy followed by any codes for the complications.

When a patient is admitted for the purpose of insertion or implantation of radioactive elements (e.g., brachytherapy) and develops complications such as uncontrolled nausea and vomiting or dehydration, the principal or first-listed diagnosis is the appropriate code for the malignancy followed by any codes for the complications.

f. Admission/encounter to determine extent of malignancy

When the reason for admission/encounter is to determine the extent of the malignancy, or for a procedure such as paracentesis or thoracentesis, the primary malignancy or appropriate metastatic site is designated as the principal or first-listed diagnosis, even though chemotherapy or radiotherapy is administered.

g. Symptoms, signs, and abnormal findings listed in Chapter 18 associated with neoplasms

Symptoms, signs, and ill-defined conditions listed in Chapter 18 characteristic of, or associated with, an existing primary or secondary site malignancy cannot be used to replace the malignancy as principal or first-listed diagnosis, regardless of the number of admissions or encounters for treatment and care of the neoplasm.

See Section I.C.21. Factors influencing health status and contact with health services, Encounter for prophylactic organ removal.

h. Admission/encounter for pain control/management

See Section I.C.6. for information on coding admission/encounter for pain control/management.

i. Malignancy in two or more noncontiguous sites

A patient may have more than one malignant tumor in the same organ. These tumors may represent different primaries or metastatic disease, depending on the site. Should the documentation be unclear, the provider should be queried as to the status of each tumor so that the correct codes can be assigned.

j. Disseminated malignant neoplasm, unspecified

Code C80.0, Disseminated malignant neoplasm, unspecified, is for use only in those cases where the patient has advanced metastatic disease and no known primary or secondary sites are specified. It should not be used in place of assigning codes for the primary site and all known secondary sites.

k. Malignant neoplasm without specification of site

Code C80.1, Malignant (primary) neoplasm, unspecified, equates to Cancer, unspecified. This code should only be used when no determination can be made as to the primary site of a malignancy. This code should rarely be used in the inpatient setting.

l. Sequencing of neoplasm codes

1) Encounter for treatment of primary malignancy

If the reason for the encounter is for treatment of a primary malignancy, assign the malignancy as the principal/first-listed diagnosis. The primary site is to be sequenced first, followed by any metastatic sites.

2) Encounter for treatment of secondary malignancy

When an encounter is for a primary malignancy with metastasis and treatment is directed toward the metastatic (secondary) site(s) only, the metastatic site(s) is designated as the principal/first-listed diagnosis. The primary malignancy is coded as an additional code.

3) Malignant neoplasm in a pregnant patient

When a pregnant patient has a malignant neoplasm, a code from subcategory O9A.1-, Malignant neoplasm complicating pregnancy, childbirth, and the puerperium, should be sequenced first, followed by the appropriate code from Chapter 2 to indicate the type of neoplasm.

4) Encounter for complication associated with a neoplasm

When an encounter is for management of a complication associated with a neoplasm, such as dehydration, and the treatment is only for the complication, the complication is coded first, followed by the appropriate code(s) for the neoplasm.

The exception to this guideline is anemia. When the admission/encounter is for management of an anemia associated with the malignancy, and the treatment is only for anemia, the appropriate code for the malignancy is sequenced as the principal or first-listed diagnosis followed by code D63.0, Anemia in neoplastic disease.

5) Complication from surgical procedure for treatment of a neoplasm

When an encounter is for treatment of a complication resulting from a surgical procedure performed for the treatment of the neoplasm, designate the complication as the principal/first-listed diagnosis. See the guideline regarding the coding of a current malignancy versus personal history to determine if the code for the neoplasm should also be assigned.

6) Pathologic fracture due to a neoplasm

When an encounter is for a pathological fracture due to a neoplasm, and the focus of treatment is the fracture, a code from subcategory M84.5, Pathological fracture in neoplastic disease, should be sequenced first, followed by the code for the neoplasm.

If the focus of treatment is the neoplasm with an associated pathological fracture, the neoplasm code should be sequenced first, followed by a code from M84.5 for the pathological fracture.

m. Current malignancy versus personal history of malignancy

When a primary malignancy has been excised but further treatment, such as an additional surgery for the malignancy, radiation therapy or chemotherapy is directed to that site, the primary malignancy code should be used until treatment is completed.

When a primary malignancy has been previously excised or eradicated from its site, there is no further treatment (of the malignancy) directed to that site, and there is no evidence of any existing primary malignancy at that site, a code from category Z85, Personal history of malignant neoplasm, should be used to indicate the former site of the malignancy.

Codes from subcategories Z85.0 – Z85.85 should only be assigned for the former site of a primary malignancy, not the site of a secondary malignancy. Code Z85.89, may be assigned for the former site(s) of either a primary or secondary malignancy.

See Section I.C.21. Factors influencing health status and contact with health services, History (of)

n. Leukemia, Multiple Myeloma, and Malignant Plasma Cell Neoplasms in remission versus personal history

The categories for leukemia, and category C90, Multiple myeloma and malignant plasma cell neoplasms, have codes indicating whether or not the leukemia has achieved remission. There are also codes Z85.6, Personal history of leukemia, and Z85.79, Personal history of other malignant neoplasms of lymphoid, hematopoietic and related tissues. If the documentation is unclear, as to whether the leukemia has achieved remission, the provider should be queried.

See Section I.C.21. Factors influencing health status and contact with health services, History (of)

o. Aftercare following surgery for neoplasm

See Section I.C.21. Factors influencing health status and contact with health services, Aftercare

p. Follow-up care for completed treatment of a malignancy

See Section I.C.21. Factors influencing health status and contact with health services, Follow-up

q. Prophylactic organ removal for prevention of malignancy

See Section I.C. 21, Factors influencing health status and contact with health services, Prophylactic organ removal

r. Malignant neoplasm associated with transplanted organ

A malignant neoplasm of a transplanted organ should be coded as a transplant complication. Assign first the appropriate code from category T86.-, Complications of transplanted organs and tissue, followed by code C80.2, Malignant neoplasm associated with transplanted organ. Use an additional code for the specific malignancy.

s. Breast Implant Associated Anaplastic Large Cell Lymphoma

Breast implant associated anaplastic large cell lymphoma (BIA-ALCL) is a type of lymphoma that can develop around breast implants. Assign code C84.7A, Anaplastic large cell lymphoma, ALK-negative, breast, for BIA-ALCL or C84.7B, Anaplastic large cell lymphoma, ALK-negative, in remission, for BIA-ALCL in remission. Do not assign a complication code from chapter 19.

t. Secondary malignant neoplasm of lymphoid tissue

When a malignant neoplasm of lymphoid tissue metastasizes beyond the lymph nodes, a code from categories C81-C85 with a final character identifying "extranodal and solid organ sites" should be assigned rather than a code for the secondary neoplasm of the affected solid organ. For example, for metastasis of diffuse large B-cell lymphoma to the lung, brain and left adrenal gland, assign code C83.398, Diffuse large B-cell lymphoma of other extranodal and solid organ sites.

3. **Chapter 3: Disease of the blood and blood-forming organs and certain disorders involving the immune mechanism (D5Ø-D89)**
Reserved for future guideline expansion

4. **Chapter 4: Endocrine, Nutritional, and Metabolic Diseases (EØØ-E89)**

a. Diabetes mellitus

The diabetes mellitus codes are combination codes that include the type of diabetes mellitus, the body system affected, and the complications affecting that body system. As many codes within a particular category as are necessary to describe all of the complications of the disease may be used. They should be sequenced based on the reason for a particular encounter. Assign as many codes from categories EØ8 – E13 as needed to identify all of the associated conditions that the patient has.

1) Type of diabetes

The age of a patient is not the sole determining factor, though most type 1 diabetics develop the condition before reaching puberty. For this reason type 1 diabetes mellitus is also referred to as juvenile diabetes.

(a) Presymptomatic Type 1 Diabetes Mellitus Codes E1Ø.A-, Type 1 diabetes mellitus, presymptomatic, are assigned for early-stage type 1 diabetes that predates the onset of symptoms.

2) Type of diabetes mellitus not documented

If the type of diabetes mellitus is not documented in the medical record the default is E11.-, Type 2 diabetes mellitus.

3) Diabetes mellitus and the use of insulin, oral hypoglycemics, and injectable non-insulin drugs

If the documentation in a medical record does not indicate the type of diabetes but does indicate that the patient uses insulin, code E11, Type 2 diabetes mellitus, should be assigned. Additional code(s) should be assigned from category Z79 to identify the long-term (current) use of insulin or oral hypoglycemic drugs, or injectable non-insulin antidiabetic, as follows: If the patient is treated with both oral **hypoglycemic drugs** and insulin, both code Z79.4, Long term (current) use of insulin, and code Z79.84, Long term (current) use of oral hypoglycemic drugs, should be assigned. If the patient is treated with both insulin and an injectable non-insulin antidiabetic drug, assign codes Z79.4, Long-term (current) use of insulin, and **Z79.85, Long-term (current) use of injectable non-insulin antidiabetic drugs.** If the patient is treated with both oral hypoglycemic drugs and an injectable non-insulin antidiabetic drug, assign codes Z79.84, Long-term (current) use of oral hypoglycemic drugs, and **Z79.85, Long-term (current) use of injectable non-insulin antidiabetic drugs.** Code Z79.4 should not be assigned if insulin is given temporarily to bring a type 2 patient's blood sugar under control during an encounter.

4) Diabetes mellitus in pregnancy and gestational diabetes

See Section I.C.15. Diabetes mellitus in pregnancy.

See Section I.C.15. Gestational (pregnancy induced) diabetes

5) Complications due to insulin pump malfunction

(a) Underdose of insulin due to insulin pump failure

An underdose of insulin due to an insulin pump failure should be assigned to a code from subcategory T85.6, Mechanical complication of other specified internal and external prosthetic devices, implants and grafts, that specifies the type of pump malfunction, as the principal or first-listed code, followed by code T38.3X6-, Underdosing of insulin and oral hypoglycemic [antidiabetic] drugs. Additional codes for the type of diabetes mellitus and any associated complications due to the underdosing should also be assigned.

(b) Overdose of insulin due to insulin pump failure

The principal or first-listed code for an encounter due to an insulin pump malfunction resulting in an overdose of insulin, should also be T85.6-, Mechanical complication of other specified internal and external prosthetic devices, implants and grafts, followed by code T38.3X1-, Poisoning by insulin and oral hypoglycemic [antidiabetic] drugs, accidental (unintentional).

6) Secondary diabetes mellitus

Codes under categories EØ8, Diabetes mellitus due to underlying condition, EØ9, Drug or chemical induced diabetes mellitus and E13, Other specified diabetes mellitus, identify complications/manifestations associated with secondary diabetes mellitus. Secondary diabetes is always caused by another condition or event (e.g., cystic fibrosis, malignant neoplasm of pancreas, pancreatectomy, adverse effect of drug, or poisoning).

(a) Secondary diabetes mellitus and the use of insulin or hypoglycemic drugs

For patients with secondary diabetes mellitus who routinely use insulin or oral hypoglycemic drugs, or injectable non-insulin drugs, an additional code(s) from category Z79 should be assigned to identity the long-term (current) use of insulin or oral hypoglycemic drugs, or non-injectable non-insulin drugs as follows: If the patient is treated

GUIDELINES (ICD-10-CM)

with both oral **hypoglycemic drugs** and insulin, both code Z79.4, Long term (current) use of insulin, and code Z79.84, Long term (current) use of oral hypoglycemic drugs, should be assigned. If the patient is treated with both insulin and an injectable non-insulin antidiabetic drug, assign codes Z79.4, Long- term (current) use of insulin, and **Z79.85, Long-term (current) use of injectable non-insulin antidiabetic drugs.** If the patient is treated with both oral hypoglycemic drugs and an injectable non-insulin antidiabetic drug, assign codes Z79.84, Long-term (current) use of oral hypoglycemic drugs, and **Z79.85, Long-term (current) use of injectable non-insulin antidiabetic drugs.** Code Z79.4 should not be assigned if insulin is given temporarily to bring a type 2 patient's blood sugar under control during an encounter.

(b) Assigning and sequencing secondary diabetes codes and its causes

The sequencing of the secondary diabetes codes in relationship to codes for the cause of the diabetes is based on the Tabular List instructions for categories E08, E09 and E13.

(i) Secondary diabetes mellitus due to pancreatectomy For postpancreatectomy diabetes mellitus (lack of insulin due to the surgical removal of all or part of the pancreas), assign code E89.1, Postprocedural hypoinsulinemia. Assign a code from category E13 as the principal or firstlisted diagnosis and a code from subcategory Z90.41-, Acquired absence of pancreas, as additional codes.

(ii) Secondary diabetes due to drugs Secondary diabetes may be caused by an adverse effect of correctly administered medications, poisoning or sequela of poisoning.

See Section I.C.19.e for coding of adverse effects and poisoning, and Section I.C.20 for external cause code reporting.

5. Chapter 5: Mental, Behavioral and Neurodevelopmental disorders (F01 – F99)

a. Pain disorders related to psychological factors

Assign code F45.41, for pain that is exclusively related to psychological disorders. As indicated by the Excludes1 note under category G89, a code from category G89 should not be assigned with code F45.41

Code F45.42, Pain disorders with related psychological factors, should be used with a code from category G89, Pain, not elsewhere classified, if there is documentation of a psychological component for a patient with acute or chronic pain.

See Section I.C.6. Pain

b. Mental and behavioral disorders due to psychoactive substance use

1) In Remission

Selection of codes **describing** "in remission" for categories F10-F19, Mental and behavioral disorders due to psychoactive substance use (categories F10-F19 with -11, -.21, **-91**) requires the provider's clinical judgment **and** are assigned only on the basis of provider documentation (as defined in the Official Guidelines for Coding and Reporting), unless otherwise instructed by the classification.

Mild substance use disorders in early or sustained remission are classified to the appropriate codes for substance abuse in remission, and moderate or severe substance use disorders in early or sustained remission are classified to the appropriate codes for substance dependence in remission.

2) Psychoactive Substance Use, Abuse and Dependence

When the provider documentation refers to use, abuse and dependence of the same substance (e.g., alcohol, opioid, cannabis, etc.), only one code should be assigned to identify the pattern of use based on the following hierarchy:

- If both use and abuse are documented, assign only the code for abuse
- If both abuse and dependence are documented, assign only the code for dependence
- If use, abuse and dependence are all documented, assign only the code for dependence
- If both use and dependence are documented, assign only the code for dependence.

3) Psychoactive Substance Use, Unspecified

As with all other unspecified diagnoses, the codes for unspecified psychoactive substance use disorders (F10.9-, F11.9-, F12.9-, F13.9-, F14.9-, F15.9-, F16.9-, F18.9-, F19.9-) should only be assigned based on provider documentation and when they meet the definition of a reportable diagnosis (see Section III, Reporting Additional Diagnoses). These codes are to be used only when the psychoactive substance use is associated 1with a substance related disorder (chapter 5 such as sexual dysfunction and sleep disorder, or a mental or behavioral disorder) or medical condition, and such a relationship is documented by the provider.

4) Medical Conditions Due to Psychoactive Substance Use, Abuse and Dependence

Medical conditions due to substance use, abuse, and dependence are not classified as substance-induced disorders. Assign the diagnosis code for the medical condition as directed by the Alphabetical Index along with the appropriate psychoactive substance use, abuse or dependence code. For example, for alcoholic pancreatitis due to alcohol dependence, assign the appropriate code from subcategory K85.2, Alcohol induced acute pancreatitis, and the appropriate code from subcategory F10.2, such as code F10.20, Alcohol dependence, uncomplicated. It would not be appropriate to assign code F10.288, Alcohol dependence with other alcohol-induced disorder.

5) Blood Alcohol Level

A code from category Y90, Evidence of alcohol involvement determined by blood alcohol level, may be assigned when this information is documented and the patient's provider has documented a condition classifiable to category F10, Alcohol related disorders. The blood alcohol level does not need to be documented by the patient's provider in order for it to be coded.

See Section I.B.14. for blood alcohol level documentation by clinicians other than patient's provider.

c. Factitious Disorder

Factitious disorder imposed on self or Munchausen's syndrome is a disorder in which a person falsely reports or causes his or her own physical or psychological signs or symptoms. For patients with documented factitious disorder on self or Munchausen's syndrome, assign the appropriate code from subcategory F68.1-, Factitious disorder imposed on self.

Munchausen's syndrome by proxy (MSBP) is a disorder in which a caregiver (perpetrator) falsely reports or causes an illness or injury in another person (victim) under his or her care, such as a child, an elderly adult, or a person who has a disability. The condition is also referred to as "factitious disorder imposed on another" or "factitious disorder by proxy." The perpetrator, not the victim, receives this diagnosis. Assign code F68.A, Factitious disorder imposed on another, to the perpetrator's record. For the victim of a patient suffering from MSBP, assign the appropriate code from categories T74, Adult and child abuse, neglect and other maltreatment, confirmed, or T76, Adult and child abuse, neglect and other maltreatment, suspected.

See Section I.C.19.f. Adult and child abuse, neglect and other maltreatment

d. Dementia

The ICD-10-CM classifies dementia (categories F01, F02, and F03) on the basis of the etiology and severity (unspecified, mild, moderate or severe). Selection of the appropriate severity level requires the provider's clinical judgment and codes should be assigned only on the basis of provider documentation (as defined in the *Official Guidelines for Coding and Reporting*), unless otherwise instructed by the classification. If the documentation does not provide information about the severity of the dementia, assign the appropriate code for unspecified severity.

If a patient is admitted to an inpatient acute care hospital or other inpatient facility setting with dementia at one severity level and it progresses to a higher severity level, assign one code for the highest severity level reported during the stay.

6. Chapter 6: Diseases of the Nervous System (G00-G99)

a. Dominant/nondominant side

Codes from category G81, Hemiplegia and hemiparesis, and subcategories, G83.1, Monoplegia of lower limb, G83.2, Monoplegia of upper limb, and G83.3, Monoplegia, unspecified, identify whether the dominant or nondominant side is affected. Should the affected side be documented, but not specified as dominant or nondominant, and the classification system does not indicate a default, code selection is as follows:

- For ambidextrous patients, the default should be dominant.
- If the left side is affected, the default is non-dominant.
- If the right side is affected, the default is dominant.

b. Pain - Category G89

1) General coding information

Codes in category G89, Pain, not elsewhere classified, may be used in conjunction with codes from other categories and chapters to provide more detail about acute or chronic pain and neoplasm-related pain, unless otherwise indicated below.

If the pain is not specified as acute or chronic, post-thoracotomy, postprocedural, or neoplasm-related, do not assign codes from category G89.

A code from category G89 should not be assigned if the underlying (definitive) diagnosis is known, unless the reason for the encounter is pain control/management and not management of the underlying condition.

When an admission or encounter is for a procedure aimed at treating the underlying condition (e.g., spinal fusion, kyphoplasty), a code for the underlying condition (e.g., vertebral fracture, spinal stenosis) should be assigned as the principal diagnosis. No code from category G89 should be assigned.

(a) Category G89 Codes as Principal or First-Listed Diagnosis

Category G89 codes are acceptable as principal diagnosis or the first-listed code:

- When pain control or pain management is the reason for the admission/encounter (e.g., a patient with displaced intervertebral disc, nerve impingement and severe back pain presents for injection of steroid into the spinal canal). The underlying cause of the pain should be reported as an additional diagnosis, if known.
- When a patient is admitted for the insertion of a neurostimulator for pain control, assign the appropriate pain code as the principal or first-listed diagnosis. When an admission or encounter is for a procedure aimed at treating the underlying condition and a neurostimulator is inserted for pain control during the same admission/encounter, a code for the underlying condition should be assigned as the principal diagnosis and the appropriate pain code should be assigned as a secondary diagnosis.

(b) Use of Category G89 Codes in Conjunction with Site-Specific Pain Codes

(i) Assigning Category G89 and Site-Specific Pain Codes

Codes from category G89 may be used in conjunction with codes that identify the site of pain (including codes from Chapter 18) if the category G89 code provides additional information. For example, if the code describes the site of the pain, but does not fully describe whether the pain is acute or chronic, then both codes should be assigned.

(ii) Sequencing of Category G89 Codes with Site-Specific Pain Codes

The sequencing of category G89 codes with site-specific pain codes (including Chapter 18 codes), is dependent on the circumstances of the encounter/admission as follows:

- If the encounter is for pain control or pain management, assign the code from category G89 followed by the code identifying the specific site of pain (e.g., encounter for pain management for acute neck pain from trauma is assigned code G89.11, Acute pain due to trauma, followed by code M54.2, Cervicalgia, to identify the site of pain).
- If the encounter is for any other reason except pain control or pain management, and a related definitive diagnosis has not been established (confirmed) by the provider, assign the code for the specific site of pain first, followed by the appropriate code from category G89.

2) Pain due to devices, implants and grafts

See Section I.C.19. Pain due to medical devices

3) Postoperative Pain

The provider's documentation should be used to guide the coding of postoperative pain, as well as Section III. Reporting Additional Diagnoses and Section IV. Diagnostic Coding and Reporting in the Outpatient Setting.

The default for post-thoracotomy and other postoperative pain not specified as acute or chronic is the code for the acute form.

Routine or expected postoperative pain immediately after surgery should not be coded.

(a) Postoperative pain not associated with specific postoperative complication

Postoperative pain not associated with a specific postoperative complication is assigned to the appropriate postoperative pain code in category G89.

(b) Postoperative pain associated with specific postoperative complication

Postoperative pain associated with a specific postoperative complication (such as painful wire sutures) is assigned to the appropriate code(s) found in Chapter 19, Injury, poisoning, and certain other consequences of external causes. If appropriate, use additional code(s) from category G89 to identify acute or chronic pain (G89.18 or G89.28).

4) Chronic pain

Chronic pain is classified to subcategory G89.2. There is no time frame defining when pain becomes chronic pain. The provider's documentation should be used to guide use of these codes.

5) Neoplasm Related Pain

Code G89.3 is assigned to pain documented as being related, associated or due to cancer, primary or secondary malignancy, or tumor. This code is assigned regardless of whether the pain is acute or chronic.

This code may be assigned as the principal or first-listed code when the stated reason for the admission/encounter is documented as pain control/pain management. The underlying neoplasm should be reported as an additional diagnosis.

When the reason for the admission/encounter is management of the neoplasm and the pain associated with the neoplasm is also documented, code G89.3 may be assigned as an additional diagnosis. It is not necessary to assign an additional code for the site of the pain.

See Section I.C.2 for instructions on the sequencing of neoplasms for all other stated reasons for the admission/encounter (except for pain control/pain management).

6) Chronic pain syndrome

Central pain syndrome (G89.0) and chronic pain syndrome (G89.4) are different than the term "chronic pain," and therefore codes should only be used when the provider has specifically documented this condition.

See Section I.C.5. Pain disorders related to psychological factors

7. Chapter 7: Diseases of the Eye and Adnexa (H00-H59)

a. Glaucoma

1) Assigning Glaucoma Codes

Assign as many codes from category H40, Glaucoma, as needed to identify the type of glaucoma, the affected eye, and the glaucoma stage.

2) Bilateral glaucoma with same type and stage

When a patient has bilateral glaucoma and both eyes are documented as being the same type and stage, and there is a code for bilateral glaucoma, report only the code for the type of glaucoma, bilateral, with the seventh character for the stage.

When a patient has bilateral glaucoma and both eyes are documented as being the same type and stage, and the classification does not provide a code for bilateral glaucoma (i.e., subcategories H40.10, H40.11 and H40.20) report only one code for the type of glaucoma with the appropriate seventh character for the stage.

3) Bilateral glaucoma stage with different types or stages

When a patient has bilateral glaucoma and each eye is documented as having a different type or stage, and the classification distinguishes laterality, assign the appropriate code for each eye rather than the code for bilateral glaucoma.

When a patient has bilateral glaucoma and each eye is documented as having a different type, and the classification does not distinguish laterality (i.e., subcategories H40.10, H40.11 and H40.20), assign one code for each type of glaucoma with the appropriate 7th character for the stage.

When a patient has bilateral glaucoma and each eye is documented as having the same type, but different stage, and the classification does not distinguish laterality (i.e., subcategories H40.10, H40.11 and H40.20), assign a code for the type of glaucoma for each eye with the 7th character for the specific glaucoma stage documented for each eye.

4) Patient admitted with glaucoma and stage evolves during the admission

If a patient is admitted with glaucoma and the stage progresses during the admission, assign the code for highest stage documented.

5) Indeterminate stage glaucoma

Assignment of the 7th character "4" for "indeterminate stage" should be based on the clinical documentation. The 7th character "4" is used for glaucomas whose stage cannot be clinically determined. This 7th character should not be confused with the 7th character "0", unspecified, which should be assigned when there is no documentation regarding the stage of the glaucoma.

b. Blindness

If "blindness" or "low vision" of both eyes is documented but the visual impairment category is not documented, assign code H54.3, Unqualified visual loss, both eyes. If "blindness" or "low vision" in one eye is documented but the visual impairment category is not documented, assign a code from H54.6-, Unqualified visual loss, one eye. If "blindness" or "visual loss" is documented without any information about whether one or both eyes are affected, assign code H54.7, Unspecified visual loss.

8. Chapter 8: Diseases of the Ear and Mastoid Process (H60-H95)

Reserved for future guideline expansion

9. Chapter 9: Diseases of the Circulatory System (I00-I99)

a. Hypertension

The classification presumes a causal relationship between hypertension and heart involvement and between hypertension and kidney involvement, as the two conditions are linked by the term "with" in the Alphabetic Index. These conditions should be coded as related even in the absence of provider documentation explicitly linking them, unless the documentation clearly states the conditions are unrelated.

For hypertension and conditions not specifically linked by relational terms such as "with," "associated with" or "due to" in the classification, provider documentation must link the conditions in order to code them as related.

1) Hypertension with Heart Disease

Hypertension with heart conditions classified to I50.- or I51.4-I51.7, I51.89, I51.9, are assigned to, a code from category I11, Hypertensive heart disease. Use additional code(s) from category I50, Heart failure, to identify the type(s) of heart failure in those patients with heart failure.

The same heart conditions (I50.-, I51.4-I51.7, I51.89, I51.9) with hypertension are coded separately if the provider has documented they are unrelated to the hypertension. Sequence according to the circumstances of the admission/encounter.

2) Hypertensive Chronic Kidney Disease

Assign codes from category I12, Hypertensive chronic kidney disease, when both hypertension and a condition classifiable to category N18, Chronic kidney disease (CKD), are present. CKD should not be coded as hypertensive if the provider indicates the CKD is not related to the hypertension.

The appropriate code from category N18 should be used as a secondary code with a code from category I12 to identify the stage of chronic kidney disease.

See Section I.C.14. Chronic kidney disease.

If a patient has hypertensive chronic kidney disease and acute renal failure, the acute renal failure should also be coded. Sequence according to the circumstances of the admission/encounter.

3) Hypertensive Heart and Chronic Kidney Disease

Assign codes from combination category I13, Hypertensive heart and chronic kidney disease, when there is hypertension with both heart and kidney involvement. If heart failure is present, assign an additional code from category I50 to identify the type of heart failure.

The appropriate code from category N18, Chronic kidney disease, should be used as a secondary code with a code from category I13 to identify the stage of chronic kidney disease.

See Section I.C.14. Chronic kidney disease.

The codes in category I13, Hypertensive heart and chronic kidney disease, are combination codes that include hypertension, heart disease and chronic kidney disease. The Includes note at I13 specifies that the conditions included at I11 and I12 are included together in I13. If a patient has hypertension, heart disease and chronic kidney disease then a code from I13 should be used, not individual codes for hypertension, heart disease and chronic kidney disease, or codes from I11 or I12.

For patients with both acute renal failure and chronic kidney disease the acute renal failure should also be coded. Sequence according to the circumstances of the admission/encounter.

4) Hypertensive Cerebrovascular Disease

For hypertensive cerebrovascular disease, first assign the appropriate code from categories I60-I69, followed by the appropriate hypertension code.

5) Hypertensive Retinopathy

Subcategory H35.0, Background retinopathy and retinal vascular changes, should be used with a code from category I10 – I15, Hypertensive disease to include the systemic hypertension. The sequencing is based on the reason for the encounter.

GUIDELINES (ICD-10-CM)

6) Hypertension, Secondary

Secondary hypertension is due to an underlying condition. Two codes are required: one to identify the underlying etiology and one from category I15 to identify the hypertension. Sequencing of codes is determined by the reason for admission/encounter.

7) Hypertension, Transient

Assign code R03.0, Elevated blood pressure reading without diagnosis of hypertension, unless patient has an established diagnosis of hypertension. Assign code O13.-, Gestational [pregnancy-induced] hypertension without significant proteinuria, or O14.-, Pre-eclampsia, for transient hypertension of pregnancy.

8) Hypertension, Controlled

This diagnostic statement usually refers to an existing state of hypertension under control by therapy. Assign the appropriate code from categories I10-I15, Hypertensive diseases.

9) Hypertension, Uncontrolled

Uncontrolled hypertension may refer to untreated hypertension or hypertension not responding to current therapeutic regimen. In either case, assign the appropriate code from categories I10-I15, Hypertensive diseases.

10) Hypertensive Crisis

Assign a code from category I16, Hypertensive crisis, for documented hypertensive urgency, hypertensive emergency or unspecified hypertensive crisis. Code also any identified hypertensive disease (I10-I15). The sequencing is based on the reason for the encounter.

11) Pulmonary Hypertension

Pulmonary hypertension is classified to category I27, Other pulmonary heart diseases. For secondary pulmonary hypertension (I27.1, I27.2-), code also any associated conditions or adverse effects of drugs or toxins. The sequencing is based on the reason for the encounter, except for adverse effects of drugs.

See Section I.C.19.e

12) Hypertension, Resistant

Resistant hypertension refers to blood pressure of a patient with hypertension that remains above goal in spite of the use of antihypertensive medications. Assign code I1A.0, Resistant hypertension, as an additional code when apparent treatment resistant hypertension, treatment resistant hypertension, or true resistant hypertension is documented by the provider. A code for the specific type of existing hypertension is sequenced first, if known.

b. Atherosclerotic Coronary Artery Disease and Angina

ICD-10-CM has combination codes for atherosclerotic heart disease with angina pectoris. The subcategories for these codes are I25.11, Atherosclerotic heart disease of native coronary artery with angina pectoris and I25.7, Atherosclerosis of coronary artery bypass graft(s) and coronary artery of transplanted heart with angina pectoris.

When using one of these combination codes it is not necessary to use an additional code for angina pectoris. A causal relationship can be assumed in a patient with both atherosclerosis and angina pectoris, unless the documentation indicates the angina is due to something other than the atherosclerosis.

If a patient with coronary artery disease is admitted due to an acute myocardial infarction (AMI), the AMI should be sequenced before the coronary artery disease.

See Section I.C.9. Acute myocardial infarction (AMI)

c. Intraoperative and Postprocedural Cerebrovascular Accident

Medical record documentation should clearly specify the cause-and-effect relationship between the medical intervention and the cerebrovascular accident in order to assign a code for intraoperative or postprocedural cerebrovascular accident.

Proper code assignment depends on whether it was an infarction or hemorrhage and whether it occurred intraoperatively or postoperatively. If it was a cerebral hemorrhage, code assignment depends on the type of procedure performed.

d. Sequelae of Cerebrovascular Disease

1) Category I69, Sequelae of Cerebrovascular disease

Category I69 is used to indicate conditions classifiable to categories I60-I67 as the causes of sequela (neurologic deficits), themselves classified elsewhere. These "late effects" include neurologic deficits that persist after initial onset of conditions classifiable to categories I60-I67. The neurologic deficits caused by cerebrovascular disease may be present from the onset or may arise at any time after the onset of the condition classifiable to categories I60-I67.

Codes from category I69, Sequelae of cerebrovascular disease, that specify hemiplegia, hemiparesis and monoplegia identify whether the dominant or nondominant side is affected. Should the affected side be documented, but not specified as dominant or nondominant, and the classification system does not indicate a default, code selection is as follows:

- For ambidextrous patients, the default should be dominant.
- If the left side is affected, the default is non-dominant.
- If the right side is affected, the default is dominant.

2) Codes from category I69 with codes from I60-I67

Codes from category I69 may be assigned on a health care record with codes from I60-I67, if the patient has a current cerebrovascular disease and deficits from an old cerebrovascular disease.

3) Codes from category I69 and Personal history of transient ischemic attack (TIA) and cerebral infarction (Z86.73)

Codes from category I69 should not be assigned if the patient does not have neurologic deficits.

See Section I.C.21. 4. History (of) for use of personal history codes

GUIDELINES (ICD-10-CM)

e. Acute myocardial infarction (AMI)

1) Type 1 ST elevation myocardial infarction (STEMI) and non ST elevation myocardial infarction (NSTEMI)

The ICD-10-CM codes for type 1 acute myocardial infarction (AMI) identify the site, such as anterolateral wall or true posterior wall. Subcategories I21.0-I21.2 and code I21.3 are used for type 1 ST elevation myocardial infarction (STEMI). Code I21.4, Non-ST elevation (NSTEMI) myocardial infarction, is used for type 1 non ST elevation myocardial infarction (NSTEMI) and nontransmural MIs.

If a type 1 NSTEMI evolves to STEMI, assign the STEMI code. If a type 1 STEMI converts to NSTEMI due to thrombolytic therapy, it is still coded as STEMI.

For encounters occurring while the myocardial infarction is equal to, or less than, 4 weeks old, including transfers to another acute setting or a postacute setting, and the myocardial infarction meets the definition for "other diagnoses" (see Section III, Reporting Additional Diagnoses), codes from category I21 may continue to be reported. For encounters after the 4 week time frame and the patient is still receiving care related to the myocardial infarction, the appropriate aftercare code should be assigned, rather than a code from category I21. For old or healed myocardial infarctions not requiring further care, code I25.2, Old myocardial infarction, may be assigned.

2) Acute myocardial infarction, unspecified

Code I21.9, Acute myocardial infarction, unspecified, is the default for unspecified acute myocardial infarction or unspecified type. If only type 1 STEMI or transmural MI without the site is documented, assign code I21.3, ST elevation (STEMI) myocardial infarction of unspecified site.

3) AMI documented as nontransmural or subendocardial but site provided

If an AMI is documented as nontransmural or subendocardial, but the site is provided, it is still coded as a subendocardial AMI.

See Section I.C.21.3 for information on coding status post administration of tPA in a different facility within the last 24 hours.

4) Subsequent acute myocardial infarction

A code from category I22, Subsequent ST elevation (STEMI) and non ST elevation (NSTEMI) myocardial infarction, is to be used when a patient who has suffered a type 1 or unspecified AMI has a new AMI within the 4 week time frame of the initial AMI. A code from category I22 must be used in conjunction with a code from category I21. The sequencing of the I22 and I21 codes depends on the circumstances of the encounter.

Do not assign code I22 for subsequent myocardial infarctions other than type 1 or unspecified. For subsequent type 2 AMI assign only code I21.A1. For subsequent type 4 or type 5 AMI, assign only code I21.A9.

If a subsequent myocardial infarction of one type occurs within 4 weeks of a myocardial infarction of a different type, assign the appropriate codes from category I21 to identify each type. Do not assign a code from I22. Codes from category I22 should only be assigned if both the initial and subsequent myocardial infarctions are type 1 or unspecified.

5) Other Types of Myocardial Infarction

The ICD-10-CM provides codes for different types of myocardial infarction. Type 1 myocardial infarctions are assigned to codes I21.0-I21.4.

Type 2 myocardial infarction (myocardial infarction due to demand ischemia or secondary to ischemic imbalance) is assigned to code I21.A1, Myocardial infarction type 2 with the underlying cause coded first, if applicable. Do not assign code I24.8, Other forms of acute ischemic heart disease, for the demand ischemia. If a type 2 AMI is described as NSTEMI or STEMI, only assign code I21.A1. Codes I21.01-I21.4 should only be assigned for type 1 AMIs.

Acute myocardial infarctions type 3, 4a, 4b, 4c, and 5 are assigned to code I21.A9, Other myocardial infarction type.

The "Code also" and "Code first" notes should be followed related to complications, and for coding of postprocedural myocardial infarctions during or following cardiac surgery.

6) Myocardial Infarction with Coronary Microvascular Dysfunction

Coronary microvascular dysfunction (CMD) is a condition that impacts the microvasculature by restricting microvascular flow and increasing microvascular resistance. Code I21.B, Myocardial infarction with coronary microvascular dysfunction, is assigned for myocardial infarction with coronary microvascular disease, myocardial infarction with coronary microvascular dysfunction, and myocardial infarction with non-obstructive coronary arteries (MINOCA) with microvascular disease.

10. Chapter 10: Diseases of the Respiratory System (J00-J99, U07.1)

a. Chronic Obstructive Pulmonary Disease [COPD] and Asthma

1) Acute exacerbation of chronic obstructive bronchitis and asthma

The codes in categories J44 and J45 distinguish between uncomplicated cases and those in acute exacerbation. An acute exacerbation is a worsening or a decompensation of a chronic condition. An acute exacerbation is not equivalent to an infection superimposed on a chronic condition, though an exacerbation may be triggered by an infection.

b. Acute Respiratory Failure

1) Acute respiratory failure as principal diagnosis

A code from subcategory J96.0, Acute respiratory failure, or subcategory J96.2, Acute and chronic respiratory failure, may be assigned as a principal diagnosis when it is the condition established after study to be chiefly responsible for occasioning the admission to the hospital, and the selection is supported by the Alphabetic Index and Tabular List. However, chapter-specific coding guidelines (such as obstetrics, poisoning, HIV, newborn) that provide sequencing direction take precedence.

2) Acute respiratory failure as secondary diagnosis

Respiratory failure may be listed as a secondary diagnosis if it occurs after admission, or if it is present on admission, but does not meet the definition of principal diagnosis.

3) Sequencing of acute respiratory failure and another acute condition

When a patient is admitted with respiratory failure and another acute condition (e.g., myocardial infarction, cerebrovascular accident, aspiration pneumonia), the principal diagnosis will not be the same in every situation. This applies whether the other acute condition is a respiratory or nonrespiratory condition. Selection of the principal diagnosis will be dependent on the circumstances of admission. If both the respiratory failure and the other acute condition are equally responsible for occasioning the admission to the hospital, and there are no chapter-specific sequencing rules, the guideline regarding two or more diagnoses that equally meet the definition for principal diagnosis (Section II, C.) may be applied in these situations.

If the documentation is not clear as to whether acute respiratory failure and another condition are equally responsible for occasioning the admission, query the provider for clarification.

c. Influenza due to certain identified influenza viruses

Code only confirmed cases of influenza due to certain identified influenza viruses (category J09), and due to other identified influenza virus (category J10). This is an exception to the hospital inpatient guideline Section II, H. (Uncertain Diagnosis).

In this context, "confirmation" does not require documentation of positive laboratory testing specific for avian or other novel influenza A or other identified influenza virus. However, coding should be based on the provider's diagnostic statement that the patient has avian influenza, or other novel influenza A, for category J09, or has another particular identified strain of influenza, such as H1N1 or H3N2, but not identified as novel or variant, for category J10.

If the provider records "suspected" or "possible" or "probable" avian influenza, or novel influenza, or other identified influenza, then the appropriate influenza code from category J11, Influenza due to unidentified influenza virus, should be assigned. A code from category J09, Influenza due to certain identified influenza viruses, should not be assigned nor should a code from category J10, Influenza due to other identified influenza virus.

d. Ventilator associated Pneumonia

1) Documentation of Ventilator associated Pneumonia

As with all procedural or postprocedural complications, code assignment is based on the provider's documentation of the relationship between the condition and the procedure.

Code J95.851, Ventilator associated pneumonia, should be assigned only when the provider has documented ventilator associated pneumonia (VAP). An additional code to identify the organism (e.g., Pseudomonas aeruginosa, code B96.5) should also be assigned. Do not assign an additional code from categories J12-J18 to identify the type of pneumonia.

Code J95.851 should not be assigned for cases where the patient has pneumonia and is on a mechanical ventilator and the provider has not specifically stated that the pneumonia is ventilator-associated pneumonia. If the documentation is unclear as to whether the patient has a pneumonia that is a complication attributable to the mechanical ventilator, query the provider.

2) Ventilator associated Pneumonia Develops after Admission

A patient may be admitted with one type of pneumonia (e.g., code J13, Pneumonia due to Streptococcus pneumonia) and subsequently develop VAP. In this instance, the principal diagnosis would be the appropriate code from categories J12-J18 for the pneumonia diagnosed at the time of admission. Code J95.851, Ventilator associated pneumonia, would be assigned as an additional diagnosis when the provider has also documented the presence of ventilator associated pneumonia.

e. Vaping-related disorders

For patients presenting with condition(s) related to vaping, assign code U07.0, Vaping-related disorder, as the principal diagnosis. For lung injury due to vaping, assign only code U07.0. Assign additional codes for other manifestations, such as acute respiratory failure (subcategory J96.0-) or pneumonitis (code J68.0).

Associated respiratory signs and symptoms due to vaping, such as cough, shortness of breath, etc., are not coded separately, when a definitive diagnosis has been established. However, it would be appropriate to code separately any gastrointestinal symptoms, such as diarrhea and abdominal pain.

11. Chapter 11: Diseases of the Digestive System (K00-K95)

Reserved for future guideline expansion

12. Chapter 12: Diseases of the Skin and Subcutaneous Tissue (L00-L99)

a. Pressure ulcer stage codes

1) Pressure ulcer stages

Codes in category L89, Pressure ulcer, identify the site and stage of the pressure ulcer.

The ICD-10-CM classifies pressure ulcer stages based on severity, which is designated by stages 1-4, deep tissue pressure injury, unspecified stage, and unstageable.

Assign as many codes from category L89 as needed to identify all the pressure ulcers the patient has, if applicable.

See Section I.B.14 for pressure ulcer stage documentation by clinicians other than patient's provider

GUIDELINES (ICD-10-CM)

2) Unstageable pressure ulcers
Assignment of the code for unstageable pressure ulcer (L89.--0) should be based on the clinical documentation. These codes are used for pressure ulcers whose stage cannot be clinically determined (e.g., the ulcer is covered by eschar or has been treated with a skin or muscle graft). This code should not be confused with the codes for unspecified stage (L89.--9). When there is no documentation regarding the stage of the pressure ulcer, assign the appropriate code for unspecified stage (L89.9).

If during an encounter, the stage of an unstageable pressure ulcer is revealed after debridement, assign only the code for the stage revealed following debridement.

3) Documented pressure ulcer stage
Assignment of the pressure ulcer stage code should be guided by clinical documentation of the stage or documentation of the terms found in the Alphabetic Index. For clinical terms describing the stage that are not found in the Alphabetic Index, and there is no documentation of the stage, the provider should be queried.

4) Patients admitted with pressure ulcers documented as healed
No code is assigned if the documentation states that the pressure ulcer is completely healed at the time of admission.

5) Pressure ulcers documented as healing
Pressure ulcers described as healing should be assigned the appropriate pressure ulcer stage code based on the documentation in the medical record. If the documentation does not provide information about the stage of the healing pressure ulcer, assign the appropriate code for unspecified stage.

If the documentation is unclear as to whether the patient has a current (new) pressure ulcer or if the patient is being treated for a healing pressure ulcer, query the provider.

For ulcers that were present on admission but healed at the time of discharge, assign the code for the site and stage of the pressure ulcer at the time of admission.

6) Patient admitted with pressure ulcer evolving into another stage during the admission
If a patient is admitted to an inpatient hospital with a pressure ulcer at one stage and it progresses to a higher stage, two separate codes should be assigned: one code for the site and stage of the ulcer on admission and a second code for the same ulcer site and the highest stage reported during the stay.

7) Pressure-induced deep tissue damage
For pressure-induced deep tissue damage or deep tissue pressure injury, assign only the appropriate code for pressure-induced deep tissue damage (L89.--6).

b. Non-Pressure Chronic Ulcers

1) Patients admitted with non-pressure ulcers documented as healed
No code is assigned if the documentation states that the non-pressure ulcer is completely healed at the time of admission.

2) Non-pressure ulcers documented as healing
Non-pressure ulcers described as healing should be assigned the appropriate non-pressure ulcer code based on the documentation in the medical record. If the documentation does not provide information about the severity of the healing non-pressure ulcer, assign the appropriate code for unspecified severity.

If the documentation is unclear as to whether the patient has a current (new) non-pressure ulcer or if the patient is being treated for a healing non-pressure ulcer, query the provider.

For ulcers that were present on admission but healed at the time of discharge, assign the code for the site and severity of the non-pressure ulcer at the time of admission.

3) Patient admitted with non-pressure ulcer that progresses to another severity level during the admission
If a patient is admitted to an inpatient hospital with a non-pressure ulcer at one severity level and it progresses to a higher severity level, two separate codes should be assigned: one code for the site and severity level of the ulcer on admission and a second code for the same ulcer site and the highest severity level reported during the stay.

See Section I.B.14 for pressure ulcer stage documentation by clinicians other than patient's provider

13. Chapter 13: Diseases of the Musculoskeletal System and Connective Tissue (M00-M99)

a. Site and laterality
Most of the codes within Chapter 13 have site and laterality designations. The site represents the bone, joint or the muscle involved. For some conditions where more than one bone, joint or muscle is usually involved, such as osteoarthritis, there is a "multiple sites" code available. For categories where no multiple site code is provided and more than one bone, joint or muscle is involved, multiple codes should be used to indicate the different sites involved.

1) Bone versus joint
For certain conditions, the bone may be affected at the upper or lower end (e.g., avascular necrosis of bone, M87, Osteoporosis, M80, M81). Though the portion of the bone affected may be at the joint, the site designation will be the bone, not the joint.

b. Acute traumatic versus chronic or recurrent musculoskeletal conditions
Many musculoskeletal conditions are a result of previous injury or trauma to a site, or are recurrent conditions. Bone, joint or muscle conditions that are the result of a healed injury are usually found in Chapter 13. Recurrent bone, joint or muscle conditions are also usually found in Chapter 13. Any current, acute injury should be coded to the appropriate injury code from Chapter 19. Chronic or recurrent conditions should generally be coded with a code from Chapter 13. If it is difficult to determine from the documentation in the record which code is best to describe a condition, query the provider.

c. Coding of Pathologic Fractures
Seventh character A is for use as long as the patient is receiving active treatment for the

fracture. While the patient may be seen by a new or different provider over the course of treatment for a pathological fracture, assignment of the 7th character is based on whether the patient is undergoing active treatment and not whether the provider is seeing the patient for the first time.

Seventh character, D is to be used for encounters after the patient has completed active treatment for the fracture and is receiving routine care for the fracture during the healing or recovery phase. The other 7th characters, listed under each subcategory in the Tabular List, are to be used for subsequent encounters for treatment of problems associated with the healing, such as malunions, nonunions, and sequelae.

Care for complications of surgical treatment for fracture repairs during the healing or recovery phase should be coded with the appropriate complication codes.

See Section I.C.19. Coding of traumatic fractures

d. Osteoporosis

Osteoporosis is a systemic condition, meaning that all bones of the musculoskeletal system are affected. Therefore, site is not a component of the codes under category M81, Osteoporosis without current pathological fracture. The site codes under category M80, Osteoporosis with current pathological fracture, identify the site of the fracture, not the osteoporosis.

1) Osteoporosis without pathological fracture

Category M81, Osteoporosis without current pathological fracture, is for use for patients with osteoporosis who do not currently have a pathologic fracture due to the osteoporosis, even if they have had a fracture in the past. For patients with a history of osteoporosis fractures, status code Z87.310, Personal history of (healed) osteoporosis fracture, should follow the code from M81.

2) Osteoporosis with current pathological fracture

Category M80, Osteoporosis with current pathological fracture, is for patients who have a current pathologic fracture at the time of an encounter. The codes under M80 identify the site of the fracture. A code from category M80, not a traumatic fracture code, should be used for any patient with known osteoporosis who suffers a fracture, even if the patient had a minor fall or trauma, if that fall or trauma would not usually break a normal, healthy bone.

e. Multisystem Inflammatory Syndrome

See Section I.C.1.g.1.l for Multisystem Inflammatory Syndrome

14. Chapter 14: Diseases of Genitourinary System (N00-N99)

a. Chronic kidney disease

1) Stages of chronic kidney disease (CKD)

The ICD-10-CM classifies CKD based on severity. The severity of CKD is designated by stages 1-5. Stage 2, code N18.2, equates to mild CKD; stage 3, codes N18.30-N18.32, equate to moderate CKD; and stage 4, code N18.4, equates to severe CKD. Code N18.6, End stage renal disease (ESRD), is assigned when the provider has documented end-stage-renal disease (ESRD).

If both a stage of CKD and ESRD are documented, assign code N18.6 only.

2) Chronic kidney disease and kidney transplant status

Patients who have undergone kidney transplant may still have some form of chronic kidney disease (CKD) because the kidney transplant may not fully restore kidney function. Therefore, the presence of CKD alone does not constitute a transplant complication. Assign the appropriate N18 code for the patient's stage of CKD and code Z94.0, Kidney transplant status. If a transplant complication such as failure or rejection or other transplant complication is documented, see Section I.C.19.g for information on coding complications of a kidney transplant. If the documentation is unclear as to whether the patient has a complication of the transplant, query the provider.

3) Chronic kidney disease with other conditions

Patients with CKD may also suffer from other serious conditions, most commonly diabetes mellitus and hypertension. The sequencing of the CKD code in relationship to codes for other contributing conditions is based on the conventions in the Tabular List.

See I.C.9. Hypertensive chronic kidney disease.

See I.C.19. Chronic kidney disease and kidney transplant complications.

15. Chapter 15: Pregnancy, Childbirth, and the Puerperium (O00-O9A)

a. General Rules for Obstetric Cases

1) Codes from chapter 15 and sequencing priority

Obstetric cases require codes from chapter 15, codes in the range O00O9A, Pregnancy, Childbirth, and the Puerperium. Chapter 15 codes have sequencing priority over codes from other chapters. Additional codes from other chapters may be used in conjunction with chapter 15 codes to further specify conditions. Should the provider document that the pregnancy is incidental to the encounter, then code Z33.1, Pregnant state, incidental, should be used in place of any chapter 15 codes. It is the provider's responsibility to state that the condition being treated is not affecting the pregnancy.

2) Chapter 15 codes used only on the maternal record

Chapter 15 codes are to be used only on the maternal record, never on the record of the newborn.

3) Final character for trimester

The majority of codes in Chapter 15 have a final character indicating the trimester of pregnancy. The timeframes for the trimesters are indicated at the beginning of the chapter. If trimester is not a component of a code it is because the condition always occurs in a specific trimester, or the concept

GUIDELINES (ICD-10-CM)

of trimester of pregnancy is not applicable. Certain codes have characters for only certain trimesters because the condition does not occur in all trimesters, but it may occur in more than just one.

Assignment of the final character for trimester should be based on the provider's documentation of the trimester (or number of weeks) for the current admission/encounter. This applies to the assignment of trimester for pre-existing conditions as well as those that develop during or are due to the pregnancy. The provider's documentation of the number of weeks may be used to assign the appropriate code identifying the trimester.

Whenever delivery occurs during the current admission, and there is an "in childbirth" option for the obstetric complication being coded, the "in childbirth" code should be assigned.

When the classification does not provide an obstetric code with an "in childbirth" option, it is appropriate to assign a code describing the current trimester.

4) Selection of trimester for inpatient admissions that encompass more than one trimester

In instances when a patient is admitted to a hospital for complications of pregnancy during one trimester and remains in the hospital into a subsequent trimester, the trimester character for the antepartum complication code should be assigned on the basis of the trimester when the complication developed, not the trimester of the discharge. If the condition developed prior to the current admission/encounter or represents a pre-existing condition, the trimester character for the trimester at the time of the admission/encounter should be assigned.

5) Unspecified trimester

Each category that includes codes for trimester has a code for "unspecified trimester." The "unspecified trimester" code should rarely be used, such as when the documentation in the record is insufficient to determine the trimester and it is not possible to obtain clarification.

6) 7th character for fetus identification

Where applicable, a 7th character is to be assigned for certain categories (O31, O32, O33.3 - O33.6, O35, O36, O40, O41, O60.1, O60.2, O64, and O69) to identify the fetus for which the complication code applies.

Assign 7th character "0":

- For single gestations
- When the documentation in the record is insufficient to determine the fetus affected and it is not possible to obtain clarification.
- When it is not possible to clinically determine which fetus is affected.

7) Completed weeks of gestation

In ICD-10-CM, "completed" weeks of gestation refers to full weeks. For example, if the provider documents gestation at 39 weeks and 6 days, the code for 39 weeks of gestation should be assigned, as the patient has not yet reached 40 completed weeks.

b. Selection of OB Principal or First-listed Diagnosis

1) Routine outpatient prenatal visits

For routine outpatient prenatal visits when no complications are present, a code from category Z34, Encounter for supervision of normal pregnancy, should be used as the first-listed diagnosis. These codes should not be used in conjunction with chapter 15 codes.

2) Supervision of High-Risk Pregnancy

Codes from category O09, Supervision of high-risk pregnancy, are intended for use only during the prenatal period. For complications during the labor or delivery episode as a result of a high-risk pregnancy, assign the applicable complication codes from chapter 15. If there are no complications during the labor or delivery episode, assign code O80, Encounter for full-term uncomplicated delivery.

For routine prenatal outpatient visits for patients with high-risk pregnancies, a code from category O09, Supervision of high-risk pregnancy, should be used as the first-listed diagnosis. Secondary Chapter 15 codes may be used in conjunction with these codes if appropriate.

3) Episodes when no delivery occurs

In episodes when no delivery occurs, the principal diagnosis should correspond to the principal complication of the pregnancy which necessitated the encounter. Should more than one complication exist, all of which are treated or monitored, any of the complication codes may be sequenced first.

4) When a delivery occurs

When an obstetric patient is admitted and delivers during that admission, the condition that prompted the admission should be sequenced as the principal diagnosis. If multiple conditions prompted the admission, sequence the one most related to the delivery as the principal diagnosis. A code for any complication of the delivery should be assigned as an additional diagnosis. In cases of cesarean delivery, if the patient was admitted with a condition that resulted in the performance of a cesarean procedure, that condition should be selected as the principal diagnosis. If the reason for the admission was unrelated to the condition resulting in the cesarean delivery, the condition related to the reason for the admission should be selected as the principal diagnosis.

5) Outcome of delivery

A code from category Z37, Outcome of delivery, should be included on every maternal record when a delivery has occurred. These codes are not to be used on subsequent records or on the newborn record.

c. Pre-existing conditions versus conditions due to the pregnancy

Certain categories in Chapter 15 distinguish between conditions of the mother that existed prior to pregnancy (pre-existing) and those that are a direct result of pregnancy. When assigning codes from Chapter 15, it is important to assess if a condition was pre-existing prior to pregnancy or developed during or due to the pregnancy in order to assign the correct code.

Categories that do not distinguish between pre-existing and pregnancy-related conditions may be used for either. It is acceptable to use codes specifically for the puerperium with codes complicating pregnancy and childbirth if a condition arises postpartum during the delivery encounter.

d. Pre-existing hypertension in pregnancy

Category O10, Pre-existing hypertension complicating pregnancy, childbirth and the puerperium, includes codes for hypertensive heart and hypertensive chronic kidney disease. When assigning one of the O10 codes that includes hypertensive heart disease or hypertensive chronic kidney disease, it is necessary to add a secondary code from the appropriate hypertension category to specify the type of heart failure or chronic kidney disease.

See Section I.C.9. Hypertension.

e. Fetal Conditions Affecting the Management of the Mother

1) Codes from categories O35 and O36

Codes from categories O35, Maternal care for known or suspected fetal abnormality and damage, and O36, Maternal care for other fetal problems, are assigned only when the fetal condition is actually responsible for modifying the management of the mother, i.e., by requiring diagnostic studies, additional observation, special care, or termination of pregnancy. The fact that the fetal condition exists does not justify assigning a code from this series to the mother's record.

2) In utero surgery

In cases when surgery is performed on the fetus, a diagnosis code from category O35, Maternal care for known or suspected fetal abnormality and damage, should be assigned identifying the fetal condition. Assign the appropriate procedure code for the procedure performed.

No code from Chapter 16, the perinatal codes, should be used on the mother's record to identify fetal conditions. Surgery performed in utero on a fetus is still to be coded as an obstetric encounter.

f. HIV Infection in Pregnancy, Childbirth and the Puerperium

During pregnancy, childbirth or the puerperium, a patient admitted because of an HIV-related illness should receive a principal diagnosis from subcategory O98.7-, Human immunodeficiency [HIV] disease complicating pregnancy, childbirth and the puerperium, followed by the code(s) for the HIV-related illness(es).

Patients with asymptomatic HIV infection status admitted during pregnancy, childbirth, or the puerperium should receive codes of O98.7- and Z21, Asymptomatic human immunodeficiency virus [HIV] infection status.

g. Diabetes mellitus in pregnancy

Diabetes mellitus is a significant complicating factor in pregnancy. Pregnant patients who are diabetic should be assigned a code from category O24, Diabetes mellitus in pregnancy, childbirth, and the puerperium, first, followed by the appropriate diabetes code(s) (E08-E13) from Chapter 4.

h. Longterm use of insulin and oral hypoglycemics

See section I.C.4.a.3 for information on the longterm use of insulin and oral hypoglycemics.

i. Gestational (pregnancy induced) diabetes

Gestational (pregnancy induced) diabetes can occur during the second and third trimester of pregnancy in patients who were not diabetic prior to pregnancy. Gestational diabetes can cause complications in the pregnancy similar to those of pre-existing diabetes mellitus. It also puts the patient at greater risk of developing diabetes after the pregnancy. Codes for gestational diabetes are in subcategory O24.4, Gestational diabetes mellitus. No other code from category O24, Diabetes mellitus in pregnancy, childbirth, and the puerperium, should be used with a code from O24.4.

The codes under subcategory O24.4 include diet controlled, insulin controlled, and controlled by oral hypoglycemic drugs. If a patient with gestational diabetes is treated with both diet and insulin, only the code for insulin-controlled is required. If a patient with gestational diabetes is treated with both diet and oral hypoglycemic medications, only the code for "controlled by oral hypoglycemic drugs" is required. Codes Z79.4, Long-term (current) use of insulin, Z79.84, Long-term (current) use of oral hypoglycemic drugs, **and Z79.85, Long-term (current) use of injectable non-insulin antidiabetic drugs,** should not be assigned with codes from subcategory O24.4.

An abnormal glucose tolerance in pregnancy is assigned a code from subcategory O99.81, Abnormal glucose complicating pregnancy, childbirth, and the puerperium.

j. Sepsis and septic shock complicating abortion, pregnancy, childbirth and the puerperium

When assigning a chapter 15 code for sepsis complicating abortion, pregnancy, childbirth, and the puerperium, a code for the specific type of infection should be assigned as an additional diagnosis. If severe sepsis is present, a code from subcategory R65.2, Severe sepsis, and code(s) for associated organ dysfunction(s) should also be assigned as additional diagnoses.

k. Puerperal sepsis

Code O85, Puerperal sepsis, should be assigned with a secondary code to identify the causal organism (e.g., for a bacterial infection, assign a code from category B95-B96, Bacterial infections in conditions classified elsewhere). A code from category A40, Streptococcal sepsis, or A41, Other sepsis, should not be used for puerperal sepsis. If applicable, use additional codes to identify severe sepsis (R65.2-) and any associated acute organ dysfunction.

Code O85 should not be assigned for sepsis following an obstetrical procedure (See Section I.C.1.d.5.b., Sepsis due to a postprocedural infection).

l. Alcohol, tobacco and drug use during pregnancy, childbirth and the puerperium

1) Alcohol use during pregnancy, childbirth and the puerperium

Codes under subcategory O99.31, Alcohol use complicating pregnancy, childbirth, and the puerperium, should be assigned for any pregnancy case when a patient uses alcohol during the pregnancy or postpartum. A secondary code from category F10, Alcohol related disorders, should also be assigned to identify manifestations of the alcohol use.

2) Tobacco use during pregnancy, childbirth and the puerperium

Codes under subcategory O99.33, Smoking (tobacco) complicating pregnancy, childbirth, and the puerperium, should be assigned for any pregnancy case when a patient uses any type of tobacco product during the pregnancy or postpartum. A secondary code from category F17, Nicotine dependence, should also be assigned to identify the type of nicotine dependence.

3) Drug use during pregnancy, childbirth and the puerperium

Codes under subcategory O99.32, Drug use complicating pregnancy, childbirth, and the puerperium, should be assigned for any pregnancy case when a patient uses drugs during the pregnancy or postpartum. This can involve illegal drugs, or inappropriate use or abuse of prescription drugs. Secondary code(s) from categories F11-F16 and F18-F19 should also be assigned to identify manifestations of the drug use.

m. Poisoning, toxic effects, adverse effects and underdosing in a pregnant patient

A code from subcategory O9A.2, Injury, poisoning and certain other consequences of external causes complicating pregnancy, childbirth, and the puerperium, should be sequenced first, followed by the appropriate injury, poisoning, toxic effect, adverse effect or underdosing code, and then the additional code(s) that specifies the condition caused by the poisoning, toxic effect, adverse effect or underdosing.

See Section I.C.19. Adverse effects, poisoning, underdosing and toxic effects.

n. Normal Delivery, Code O80

1) Encounter for full term uncomplicated delivery

Code O80 should be assigned when a patient is admitted for a full-term normal delivery and delivers a single, healthy infant without any complications antepartum, during the delivery, or postpartum during the delivery episode. Code O80 is always a principal diagnosis. It is not to be used if any other code from chapter 15 is needed to describe a current complication of the antenatal, delivery, or postnatal period. Additional codes from other chapters may be used with code O80 if they are not related to or are in any way complicating the pregnancy.

2) Uncomplicated delivery with resolved antepartum complication

Code O80 may be used if the patient had a complication at some point during the pregnancy, but the complication is not present at the time of the admission for delivery.

3) Outcome of delivery for O80

Z37.0, Single live birth, is the only outcome of delivery code appropriate for use with O80.

o. The Peripartum and Postpartum Periods

1) Peripartum and Postpartum periods

The postpartum period begins immediately after delivery and continues for six weeks following delivery. The peripartum period is defined as the last month of pregnancy to five months postpartum.

2) Peripartum and postpartum complication

A postpartum complication is any complication occurring within the six week period.

3) Pregnancy-related complications after 6-week period

Chapter 15 codes may also be used to describe pregnancy-related complications after the peripartum or postpartum period if the provider documents that a condition is pregnancy related.

4) Admission for routine postpartum care following delivery outside hospital

When the mother delivers outside the hospital prior to admission and is admitted for routine postpartum care and no complications are noted, code Z39.0, Encounter for care and examination of mother immediately after delivery, should be assigned as the principal diagnosis.

5) Pregnancy associated cardiomyopathy

Pregnancy associated cardiomyopathy, code O90.3, is unique in that it may be diagnosed in the third trimester of pregnancy but may continue to progress months after delivery. For this reason, it is referred to as peripartum cardiomyopathy. Code O90.3 is only for use when the cardiomyopathy develops as a result of pregnancy in a patient who did not have pre-existing heart disease.

p. Code O94, Sequelae of complication of pregnancy, childbirth, and the puerperium

1) Code O94

Code O94, Sequelae of complication of pregnancy, childbirth, and the puerperium, is for use in those cases when an initial complication of a pregnancy develops a sequela or sequelae requiring care or treatment at a future date.

2) After the initial postpartum period

This code may be used at any time after the initial postpartum period.

3) Sequencing of Code O94

This code, like all sequela codes, is to be sequenced following the code describing the sequelae of the complication.

GUIDELINES (ICD-10-CM)

q. Termination of Pregnancy and Spontaneous abortions

1) Abortion with Liveborn Fetus

When an attempted termination of pregnancy results in a liveborn fetus assign code Z33.2, Encounter for elective termination of pregnancy and a code from category Z37, Outcome of Delivery.

2) Retained Products of Conception following an abortion

Subsequent encounters for retained products of conception following a spontaneous abortion or elective termination of pregnancy, without complications are assigned O03.4, Incomplete spontaneous abortion without complication or code O07.4, Failed attempted termination of pregnancy without complication. This advice is appropriate even when the patient was discharged previously with a discharge diagnosis of complete abortion. If the patient has a specific complication associated with the spontaneous abortion or elective termination of pregnancy in addition to retained products of conception, assign the appropriate complication code (e.g., O03.-, O04.-, O07.-) instead of code O03.4 or O07.4

3) Complications leading to abortion

Codes from chapter 15 may be used as additional codes to identify any documented complications of the pregnancy in conjunction with codes in categories in O04, O07 and O08.

4) Hemorrhage following elective abortion

For hemorrhage post elective abortion, assign code O04.6, Delayed or excessive hemorrhage following (induced) termination of pregnancy. Do not assign code O72.1, Other immediate postpartum hemorrhage, as this code should not be assigned for post abortion conditions.

r. Abuse in a pregnant patient

For suspected or confirmed cases of abuse of a pregnant patient, a code(s) from subcategories O9A.3, Physical abuse complicating pregnancy, childbirth, and the puerperium, O9A.4, Sexual abuse complicating pregnancy, childbirth, and the puerperium, and O9A.5, Psychological abuse complicating pregnancy, childbirth, and the puerperium, should be sequenced first, followed by the appropriate codes (if applicable) to identify any associated current injury due to physical abuse, sexual abuse, and the perpetrator of abuse.

See Section I.C.19. Adult and child abuse, neglect and other maltreatment.

s. COVID-19 infection in pregnancy, childbirth, and the puerperium

During pregnancy, childbirth or the puerperium, when COVID-19 is the reason for admission/encounter, code O98.5-, Other viral diseases complicating pregnancy, childbirth and the puerperium, should be sequenced as the principal/first-listed diagnosis, and code U07.1, COVID-19, and the appropriate codes for associated manifestation(s) should be assigned as additional diagnoses. Codes from Chapter 15 always take sequencing priority.

If the reason for admission/encounter is unrelated to COVID-19 but the patient tests positive for COVID-19 during the admission/encounter, the appropriate code for the reason for admission/encounter should be sequenced as the principal/first-listed diagnosis, and codes O98.5- and U07.1, as well as the appropriate codes for associated COVID-19 manifestations, should be assigned as additional diagnoses.

16. Chapter 16: Certain Conditions Originating in the Perinatal Period (P00-P96)

For coding and reporting purposes the perinatal period is defined as before birth through the 28th day following birth. The following guidelines are provided for reporting purposes

a. General Perinatal Rules

1) Use of Chapter 16 Codes

Codes in this chapter are never for use on the maternal record. Codes from Chapter 15, the obstetric chapter, are never permitted on the newborn record. Chapter 16 codes may be used throughout the life of the patient if the condition is still present.

2) Principal Diagnosis for Birth Record

When coding the birth episode in a newborn record, assign a code from category Z38, Liveborn infants according to place of birth and type of delivery, as the principal diagnosis. A code from category Z38 is assigned only once, to a newborn at the time of birth. If a newborn is transferred to another institution, a code from category Z38 should not be used at the receiving hospital.

A code from category Z38 is used only on the newborn record, not on the mother's record.

3) Use of Codes from other Chapters with Codes from Chapter 16

Codes from other chapters may be used with codes from chapter 16 if the codes from the other chapters provide more specific detail. Codes for signs and symptoms may be assigned when a definitive diagnosis has not been established. If the reason for the encounter is a perinatal condition, the code from chapter 16 should be sequenced first.

4) Use of Chapter 16 Codes after the Perinatal Period

Should a condition originate in the perinatal period, and continue throughout the life of the patient, the perinatal code should continue to be used regardless of the patient's age.

5) Birth process or community acquired conditions

If a newborn has a condition that may be either due to the birth process or community acquired and the documentation does not indicate which it is, the default is due to the birth process and the code from Chapter 16 should be used. If the condition is community-acquired, a code from Chapter 16 should not be assigned.

For COVID-19 infection in a newborn, see guideline I.C.16.h.

6) Code all clinically significant conditions
All clinically significant conditions noted on routine newborn examination should be coded. A condition is clinically significant if it requires:

- clinical evaluation; or
- therapeutic treatment; or
- diagnostic procedures; or
- extended length of hospital stay; or
- increased nursing care and/or monitoring; or
- has implications for future health care needs

Note: The perinatal guidelines listed above are the same as the general coding guidelines for "additional diagnoses," except for the final point regarding implications for future health care needs. Codes should be assigned for conditions that have been specified by the provider as having implications for future health care needs.

b. Observation and Evaluation of Newborns for Suspected Conditions not Found

1) Use of Z05 codes
Assign a code from category Z05, Observation and evaluation of newborn for suspected **diseases and** conditions ruled out, to identify those instances when a healthy newborn is evaluated for a suspected condition/**disease** that is determined after study not to be present. Do not use a code from category Z05 when the patient **is documented to have** signs or symptoms of a suspected problem; in such cases code the sign or symptom.

2) Z05 on other than the birth record
A code from category Z05 may also be assigned as a principal or firstlisted code for readmissions or encounters when the code from category Z38 code no longer applies. Codes from category Z05 are for use only for healthy newborns and infants for which no condition after study is found to be present.

3) Z05 on a birth record
A code from category Z05 is to be used as a secondary code after the code from category Z38, Liveborn infants according to place of birth and type of delivery.

c. Coding Additional Perinatal Diagnoses

1) Assigning codes for conditions that require treatment
Assign codes for conditions that require treatment or further investigation, prolong the length of stay, or require resource utilization.

2) Codes for conditions specified as having implications for future health care needs
Assign codes for conditions that have been specified by the provider as having implications for future health care needs.

Note: This guideline should not be used for adult patients.

d. Prematurity and Fetal Growth Retardation
Providers utilize different criteria in determining prematurity. A code for prematurity should not be assigned unless it is documented. Assignment of codes in categories P05, Disorders of newborn related to slow fetal growth and fetal malnutrition, and P07, Disorders of newborn related to short gestation and low birth weight, not elsewhere classified, should be based on the recorded birth weight and estimated gestational age.

When both birth weight and gestational age are available, two codes from category P07 should be assigned, with the code for birth weight sequenced before the code for gestational age.

e. Low birth weight and immaturity status
Codes from category P07, Disorders of newborn related to short gestation and low birth weight, not elsewhere classified, are for use for a child or adult who was premature or had a low birth weight as a newborn and this is affecting the patient's current health status.

See Section I.C.21. Factors influencing health status and contact with health services, Status.

f. Bacterial Sepsis of Newborn
Category P36, Bacterial sepsis of newborn, includes congenital sepsis. If a perinate is documented as having sepsis without documentation of congenital or community acquired, the default is congenital and a code from category P36 should be assigned. If the P36 code includes the causal organism, an additional code from category B95, Streptococcus, Staphylococcus, and Enterococcus as the cause of diseases classified elsewhere, or B96, Other bacterial agents as the cause of diseases classified elsewhere, should not be assigned. If the P36 code does not include the causal organism, assign an additional code from category B96. If applicable, use additional codes to identify severe sepsis (R65.2-) and any associated acute organ dysfunction.

g. Stillbirth
Code P95, Stillbirth, is only for use in institutions that maintain separate records for stillbirths. No other code should be used with P95. Code P95 should not be used on the mother's record.

h. COVID-19 Infection in Newborn
For a newborn that tests positive for COVID-19, assign code U07.1, COVID-19, and the appropriate codes for associated manifestation(s) in neonates/newborns in the absence of documentation indicating a specific type of transmission. For a newborn that tests positive for COVID-19 and the provider documents the condition was contracted in utero or during the birth process, assign codes P35.8, Other congenital viral diseases, and U07.1, COVID-19. When coding the birth episode in a newborn record, the appropriate code from category Z38, Liveborn infants according to place of birth and type of delivery, should be assigned as the principal diagnosis.

17. Chapter 17: Congenital malformations, deformations, and chromosomal abnormalities (Q00-Q99)
Assign an appropriate code(s) from categories Q00-Q99, Congenital malformations, deformations, and chromosomal abnormalities when a malformation/deformation or chromosomal abnormality is documented. A malformation/deformation/or chromosomal abnormality may be the principal/first-listed diagnosis on a record or a secondary diagnosis.

When a malformation/deformation/or chromosomal abnormality does not have a unique code assignment, assign additional code(s) for any manifestations that may be present.

When the code assignment specifically identifies the malformation/deformation/or chromosomal abnormality, manifestations that are an inherent component of the anomaly should not be coded separately. Additional codes should be assigned for manifestations that are not an inherent component.

Codes from Chapter 17 may be used throughout the life of the patient. If a congenital malformation or deformity has been corrected, a personal history code should be used to identify the history of the malformation or deformity. Although present at birth, a malformation/deformation/or chromosomal abnormality may not be identified until later in life. Whenever the condition is diagnosed by the provider, it is appropriate to assign a code from codes Q00-Q99.

For the birth admission, the appropriate code from category Z38, Liveborn infants, according to place of birth and type of delivery, should be sequenced as the principal diagnosis, followed by any congenital anomaly codes, Q00-Q99.

18. **Chapter 18: Symptoms, signs, and abnormal clinical and laboratory findings, not elsewhere classified (R00-R99)**

Chapter 18 includes symptoms, signs, abnormal results of clinical or other investigative procedures, and ill-defined conditions regarding which no diagnosis classifiable elsewhere is recorded. Signs and symptoms that point to a specific diagnosis have been assigned to a category in other chapters of the classification.

a. **Use of symptom codes**

Codes that describe symptoms and signs are acceptable for reporting purposes when a related definitive diagnosis has not been established (confirmed) by the provider.

b. **Use of a symptom code with a definitive diagnosis code**

Codes for signs and symptoms may be reported in addition to a related definitive diagnosis when the sign or symptom is not routinely associated with that diagnosis, such as the various signs and symptoms associated with complex syndromes. The definitive diagnosis code should be sequenced before the symptom code.

Signs or symptoms that are associated routinely with a disease process should not be assigned as additional codes, unless otherwise instructed by the classification.

c. **Combination codes that include symptoms**

ICD-10-CM contains a number of combination codes that identify both the definitive diagnosis and common symptoms of that diagnosis. When using one of these combination codes, an additional code should not be assigned for the symptom.

d. **Repeated falls**

Code R29.6, Repeated falls, is for use for encounters when a patient has recently fallen and the reason for the fall is being investigated.

Code Z91.81, History of falling, is for use when a patient has fallen in the past and is at risk for future falls. When appropriate, both codes R29.6 and Z91.81 may be assigned together.

e. **Coma**

Code R40.20, Unspecified coma, **should** be assigned **when the underlying cause of the coma is not known, or the cause is a traumatic brain injury and the coma scale is not documented in the medical record.**

Do not report codes for unspecified coma, individual or total Glasgow coma scale scores for a patient with a medically induced coma or a sedated patient.

1) Coma Scale

The coma scale codes (R40.21- to R40.24-) can be used in conjunction with traumatic brain injury codes. These codes **cannot be used with code R40.2A, Nontraumatic coma due to underlying condition. They** are primarily for use by trauma registries, but they may be used in any setting where this information is collected. The coma scale codes should be sequenced after the diagnosis code(s).

These codes, one from each subcategory, are needed to complete the scale. The 7th character indicates when the scale was recorded. The 7th character should match for all three codes.

At a minimum, report the initial score documented on presentation at your facility. This may be a score from the emergency medicine technician (EMT) or in the emergency department. If desired, a facility may choose to capture multiple coma scale scores.

Assign code R40.24-, Glasgow coma scale, total score, when only the total score is documented in the medical record and not the individual score(s).

If multiple coma scores are captured within the first 24 hours after hospital admission, assign only the code for the score at the time of admission. ICD-10-CM does not classify coma scores that are reported after admission but less than 24 hours later.

See Section I.B.14. for coma scale documentation by clinicians other than patient's provider

f. **Functional quadriplegia**

GUIDELINE HAS BEEN DELETED EFFECTIVE OCTOBER 1, 2017

g. **SIRS due to Non-Infectious Process**

The systemic inflammatory response syndrome (SIRS) can develop as a result of certain non-infectious disease processes, such as trauma, malignant neoplasm, or pancreatitis. When SIRS is documented with a noninfectious condition, and no subsequent infection is documented, the code for the underlying condition, such as an injury, should be assigned, followed by code R65.10, Systemic inflammatory response syndrome (SIRS) of non-infectious origin without acute organ dysfunction, or code R65.11, Systemic inflammatory response syndrome (SIRS) of non-infectious origin with acute organ dysfunction. If an associated acute organ dysfunction is documented, the appropriate code(s) for the specific type of organ dysfunction(s) should be assigned in addition to code R65.11. If acute organ dysfunction is documented, but it cannot be determined if the acute organ dysfunction is associated with SIRS or due to another condition (e.g., directly due to the trauma), the provider should be queried.

h. Death NOS

Code R99, Ill-defined and unknown cause of mortality, is only for use in the very limited circumstance when a patient who has already died is brought into an emergency department or other healthcare facility and is pronounced dead upon arrival. It does not represent the discharge disposition of death.

i. NIHSS Stroke Scale

The NIH stroke scale (NIHSS) codes (R29.7- -) can be used in conjunction with acute stroke codes **(I6Ø-I63)** to identify the patient's neurological status and the severity of the stroke. The stroke scale codes should be sequenced after the acute stroke diagnosis code(s).

At a minimum, report the initial score documented. If desired, a facility may choose to capture multiple stroke scale scores.

See Section I.B.14 for NIHSS stroke scale documentation by clinicians other than patient's provider

19. Chapter 19: Injury, poisoning, and certain other consequences of external causes (SØØ-T88)

a. Application of 7th Characters in Chapter 19

Most categories in chapter 19 have a 7th character requirement for each applicable code. Most categories in this chapter have three 7th character values (with the exception of fractures): A, initial encounter, D, subsequent encounter and S, sequela. Categories for traumatic fractures have additional 7th character values. While the patient may be seen by a new or different provider over the course of treatment for an injury, assignment of the 7th character is based on whether the patient is undergoing active treatment and not whether the provider is seeing the patient for the first time.

For complication codes, active treatment refers to treatment for the condition described by the code, even though it may be related to an earlier precipitating problem. For example, code T84.50XA, Infection and inflammatory reaction due to unspecified internal joint prosthesis, initial encounter, is used when active treatment is provided for the infection, even though the condition relates to the prosthetic device, implant or graft that was placed at a previous encounter.

7th character "A", initial encounter is used for each encounter where the patient is receiving active treatment for the condition.

7th character "D" subsequent encounter is used for encounters after the patient has completed active treatment of the condition and is receiving routine care for the condition during the healing or recovery phase.

The aftercare Z codes should not be used for aftercare for conditions such as injuries or poisonings, where 7th characters are provided to identify subsequent care. For example, for aftercare of an injury, assign the acute injury code with the 7th character "D" (subsequent encounter).

7th character "S", sequela, is for use for complications or conditions that arise as a direct result of a condition, such as scar formation after a burn. The scars are sequelae of the burn. When using 7th character "S", it is necessary to use both the injury code that precipitated the sequela and the code for the sequela itself. The "S" is added only to the injury code, not the sequela code. The 7th character "S" identifies the injury responsible for the sequela. The specific type of sequela (e.g., scar) is sequenced first, followed by the injury code.

See Section I.B.1Ø. Sequelae, (Late Effects)

b. Coding of Injuries

When coding injuries, assign separate codes for each injury unless a combination code is provided, in which case the combination code is assigned. Codes from category TØ7, Unspecified multiple injuries should not be assigned in the inpatient setting unless information for a more specific code is not available. Traumatic injury codes (SØØ-T14.9) are not to be used for normal, healing surgical wounds or to identify complications of surgical wounds.

The code for the most serious injury, as determined by the provider and the focus of treatment, is sequenced first.

1) Superficial injuries

Superficial injuries such as abrasions or contusions are not coded when associated with more severe injuries of the same site.

2) Primary injury with damage to nerves/ blood vessels

When a primary injury results in minor damage to peripheral nerves or blood vessels, the primary injury is sequenced first with additional code(s) for injuries to nerves and spinal cord (such as category SØ4), and/or injury to blood vessels (such as category S15). When the primary injury is to the blood vessels or nerves, that injury should be sequenced first.

3) Iatrogenic injuries

Injury codes from Chapter 19 should not be assigned for injuries that occur during, or as a result of, a medical intervention. Assign the appropriate complication code(s).

c. Coding of Traumatic Fractures

The principles of multiple coding of injuries should be followed in coding fractures. Fractures of specified sites are coded individually by site in accordance with both the provisions within categories SØ2, S12, S22, S32, S42, S49, S52, S59, S62, S72, S79, S82, S89, S92 and the level of detail furnished by medical record content.

A fracture not indicated as open or closed should be coded to closed. A fracture not indicated whether displaced or not displaced should be coded to displaced.

More specific guidelines are as follows:

1) Initial vs. subsequent encounter for fractures

Traumatic fractures are coded using the appropriate 7th character for initial encounter (A, B, C) for each encounter where the patient is receiving active treatment for the fracture. The appropriate 7th character for initial encounter should also be assigned for a patient who delayed seeking treatment for the fracture or nonunion.

Fractures are coded using the appropriate 7th character for subsequent care for encounters after the patient has completed active treatment of the fracture and is receiving routine care for the fracture during the healing or recovery phase.

Care for complications of surgical treatment for fracture repairs during the healing or recovery phase should be coded with the appropriate complication codes.

Care of complications of fractures, such as malunion and nonunion, should be reported with the appropriate 7th character for subsequent care with nonunion (K, M, N,) or subsequent care with malunion (P, Q, R).

Malunion/nonunion: The appropriate 7th character for initial encounter should also be assigned for a patient who delayed seeking treatment for the fracture or nonunion.

The open fracture designations in the assignment of the 7th character for fractures of the forearm, femur and lower leg, including ankle are based on the Gustilo open fracture classification. When the Gustilo classification type is not specified for an open fracture, the 7th character for open fracture type I or II should be assigned (B, E, H, M, Q).

A code from category M80, not a traumatic fracture code, should be used for any patient with known osteoporosis who suffers a fracture, even if the patient had a minor fall or trauma, if that fall or trauma would not usually break a normal, healthy bone.

See Section I.C.13. Osteoporosis.

The aftercare Z codes should not be used for aftercare for traumatic fractures. For aftercare of a traumatic fracture, assign the acute fracture code with the appropriate 7th character.

2) Multiple fractures sequencing

Multiple fractures are sequenced in accordance with the severity of the fracture.

3) Physeal fractures

For physeal fractures, assign only the code identifying the type of physeal fracture. Do not assign a separate code to identify the specific bone that is fractured.

d. Coding of Burns and Corrosions

The ICD-10-CM makes a distinction between burns and corrosions. The burn codes are for thermal burns, except sunburns, that come from a heat source, such as a fire or hot appliance. The burn codes are also for burns resulting from electricity and radiation. Corrosions are burns due to chemicals. The guidelines are the same for burns and corrosions.

Current burns (T20-T25) are classified by depth, extent and by agent (X code). Burns are classified by depth as first degree (erythema), second degree (blistering), and third degree (full-thickness involvement). Burns of the eye and internal organs (T26-T28) are classified by site, but not by degree.

1) Sequencing of burn and related condition codes

Sequence first the code that reflects the highest degree of burn when more than one burn is present.

a. When the reason for the admission or encounter is for treatment of external multiple burns, sequence first the code that reflects the burn of the highest degree.

b. When a patient has both internal and external burns, the circumstances of admission govern the selection of the principal diagnosis or first-listed diagnosis.

c. When a patient is admitted for burn injuries and other related conditions such as smoke inhalation and/or respiratory failure, the circumstances of admission govern the selection of the principal or first-listed diagnosis.

2) Burns of the same anatomic site

Classify burns of the same anatomic site and on the same side but of different degrees to the subcategory identifying the highest degree recorded in the diagnosis (e.g., for second and third degree burns of right thigh, assign only code T24.311-).

3) Non-healing burns

Non-healing burns are coded as acute burns.

Necrosis of burned skin should be coded as a non-healed burn.

4) Infected burn

For any documented infected burn site, use an additional code for the infection.

5) Assign separate codes for each burn site

When coding burns, assign separate codes for each burn site. Category T30, Burn and corrosion, body region unspecified is extremely vague and should rarely be used.

Codes for burns of "multiple sites" should only be assigned when the medical record documentation does not specify the individual sites.

6) Burns and corrosions classified according to extent of body surface involved

Assign codes from category T31, Burns classified according to extent of body surface involved, or T32, Corrosions classified according to extent of body surface involved, for acute burns or corrosions when the site of the burn or corrosion is not specified or when there is a need for additional data. It is advisable to use category T31 as additional coding when needed to provide data for evaluating burn mortality, such as that needed by burn units. It is also advisable to use category T31 as an additional code for reporting purposes when there is mention of a thirddegree burn involving 20 percent or more of the body surface. Codes from categories T31 and T32 should not be used for sequelae of burns or corrosions.

Categories T31 and T32 are based on the classic "rule of nines" in estimating body surface involved: head and neck are assigned nine percent, each arm nine percent, each leg 18 percent, the anterior trunk 18 percent, posterior trunk 18 percent, and genitalia one percent. Providers may change these percentage assignments where necessary to accommodate infants and children who have proportionately larger heads than adults, and patients who have large buttocks, thighs, or abdomen that involve burns.

7) Encounters for treatment of sequela of burns

Encounters for the treatment of the late effects of burns or corrosions (i.e., scars or joint contractures) should be coded with a burn or corrosion code with the 7th character "S" for sequela.

8) Sequelae with a late effect code and current burn

When appropriate, both a code for a current burn or corrosion with 7th character "A" or "D" and a burn or corrosion code with 7th character "S" may be assigned on the same record (when both a current burn and sequelae of an old burn exist). Burns and corrosions do not heal at the same rate and a current healing wound may still exist with sequela of a healed burn or corrosion.

See Section I.B.10. Sequela, (Late Effects)

9) Use of an external cause code with burns and corrosions

An external cause code should be used with burns and corrosions to identify the source and intent of the burn, as well as the place where it occurred.

e. Adverse Effects, Poisoning, Underdosing and Toxic Effects

Codes in categories T36-T65 are combination codes that include the substance that was taken as well as the intent. No additional external cause code is required for poisonings, toxic effects, adverse effects and underdosing codes.

1) Do not code directly from the Table of Drugs

Do not code directly from the Table of Drugs and Chemicals. Always refer back to the Tabular List.

2) Use as many codes as necessary to describe

Use as many codes as necessary to describe completely all drugs, medicinal or biological substances.

3) If the same code would describe the causative agent

If the same code would describe the causative agent for more than one adverse reaction, poisoning, toxic effect or underdosing, assign the code only once.

4) If two or more drugs, medicinal or biological substances

If two or more drugs, medicinal or biological substances are taken, code each individually unless a combination code is listed in the Table of Drugs and Chemicals.

If multiple unspecified drugs, medicinal or biological substances were taken, assign the appropriate code from subcategory T50.91, Poisoning by, adverse effect of and underdosing of multiple unspecified drugs, medicaments and biological substances.

5) The occurrence of drug toxicity is classified in ICD-10-CM as follows:

(a) Adverse Effect

When coding an adverse effect of a drug that has been correctly prescribed and properly administered, assign the appropriate code for the nature of the adverse effect followed by the appropriate code for the adverse effect of the drug (T36-T50). The code for the drug should have a 5th or 6th character "5" (for example T36.0X5-) Examples of the nature of an adverse effect are tachycardia, delirium, gastrointestinal hemorrhaging, vomiting, hypokalemia, hepatitis, renal failure, or respiratory failure.

(b) Poisoning

When coding a poisoning or reaction to the improper use of a medication (e.g., overdose, wrong substance given or taken in error, wrong route of administration), first assign the appropriate code from categories T36-T50. The poisoning codes have an associated intent as their 5th or 6th character (accidental, intentional self-harm, assault and undetermined). If the intent of the poisoning is unknown or unspecified, code the intent as accidental intent. The undetermined intent is only for use if the documentation in the record specifies that the intent cannot be determined. Use additional code(s) for all manifestations of poisonings.

If there is also a diagnosis of abuse or dependence of the substance, the abuse or dependence is assigned as an additional code.

Examples of poisoning include:

(i) Error was made in drug prescription Errors made in drug prescription or in the administration of the drug by provider, nurse, patient, or other person.

(ii) Overdose of a drug intentionally taken If an overdose of a drug was intentionally taken or administered and resulted in drug toxicity, it would be coded as a poisoning.

(iii) Nonprescribed drug taken with correctly prescribed and properly administered drug.
If a nonprescribed drug or medicinal agent was taken in combination with a correctly prescribed and properly administered drug, any drug toxicity or other reaction resulting from the interaction of the two drugs would be classified as a poisoning.

(iv) Interaction of drug(s) and alcohol.
When a reaction results from the interaction of a drug(s) and alcohol, this would be classified as poisoning.

See Section I.C.4. if poisoning is the result of insulin pump malfunctions.

For Sequela (Late Effects) see Section I.B.10.

(c) **Underdosing**

Underdosing refers to taking less of a medication than is prescribed by a provider or a manufacturer's instruction. Discontinuing the use of a prescribed medication on the patient's own initiative (not directed by the patient's provider) is also classified as an underdosing. For underdosing, assign the code from categories T36-T50 (fifth or sixth character "6").

Documentation of a change in the patient's condition is not required in order to assign an underdosing code.

Documentation that the patient is taking less of a medication than is prescribed or discontinued the prescribed medication is sufficient for code assignment.

Codes for underdosing should never be assigned as principal or first-listed codes. If a patient has a relapse or exacerbation of the medical condition for which the drug is prescribed because of the reduction in dose, then the medical condition itself should be coded.

Noncompliance (Z91.12-, Z91.13-, **Z91.14-** and **Z91.A4-**) or complication of care (Y63.6-Y63.9) codes are to be used with an underdosing code to indicate intent, if known.

(d) **Toxic Effects**

When a harmful substance is ingested or comes in contact with a person, this is classified as a toxic effect. The toxic effect codes are in categories T51-T65. **When coding a toxic effect, assign the toxic effect code first, followed by codes for all associated manifestations of the toxic effect.**

Toxic effect codes have an associated intent: accidental, intentional self-harm, assault and undetermined.

For Sequela (Late Effects) see Section I.B.10. Sequela

f. **Adult and child abuse, neglect and other maltreatment**

Sequence first the appropriate code from categories T74, Adult and child abuse, neglect and other maltreatment, confirmed, or T76, Adult and child abuse, neglect and other maltreatment, suspected, for abuse, neglect and other maltreatment, followed by any accompanying mental health or injury code(s).

If the documentation in the medical record states abuse or neglect it is coded as confirmed (T74.-). It is coded as suspected if it is documented as suspected (T76.-).

For cases of confirmed abuse or neglect an external cause code from the assault section (X92-Y09) should be added to identify the cause of any physical injuries. A perpetrator code (Y07) should be added when the perpetrator of the abuse is known. For suspected cases of abuse or neglect, do not report external cause or perpetrator code.

If a suspected case of abuse, neglect or mistreatment is ruled out during an encounter code Z04.71, Encounter for examination and observation following alleged physical adult abuse, ruled out, or code Z04.72, Encounter for examination and observation following alleged child physical abuse, ruled out, should be used, not a code from T76.

If a suspected case of alleged rape or sexual abuse is ruled out during an encounter code Z04.41, Encounter for examination and observation following alleged adult rape or code Z04.42, Encounter for examination and observation following alleged child rape, should be used, not a code from T76.

If a suspected case of forced sexual exploitation or forced labor exploitation is ruled out during an encounter, code Z04.81, Encounter for examination and observation of victim following forced sexual exploitation, or code Z04.82, Encounter for examination and observation of victim following forced labor exploitation, should be used, not a code from T76.

See Section I.C.15. Abuse in a pregnant patient.

g. **Complications of care**

1) **General guidelines for complications of care**

(a) **Documentation of complications of care**

See Section I.B.16. for information on documentation of complications of care.

2) **Pain due to medical devices**

Pain associated with devices, implants or grafts left in a surgical site (for example painful hip prosthesis) is assigned to the appropriate code(s) found in Chapter 19, Injury, poisoning, and certain other consequences of external causes. Specific codes for pain due to medical devices are found in the T code section of the ICD-10-CM. Use additional code(s) from category G89 to identify acute or chronic pain due to presence of the device, implant or graft (G89.18 or G89.28).

3) **Transplant complications**

(a) **Transplant complications other than kidney**

Codes under category T86, Complications of transplanted organs and tissues, are for use for both complications and rejection of transplanted organs. A transplant complication code is only assigned if the complication affects the function of the transplanted organ. Two codes are required to fully describe a transplant complication: the appropriate code from category T86 and a secondary code that identifies the complication.

Pre-existing conditions or conditions that develop after the transplant are not coded as complications unless they affect the function of the transplanted organs.

See Section I.C.21. for transplant organ removal status

See Section I.C.2. for malignant neoplasm associated with transplanted organ.

See I.C.1.d.4. for sequencing of sepsis due to infection in transplanted organ

(b) **Kidney transplant complications**

Patients who have undergone kidney transplant may still have some form of chronic kidney disease (CKD) because the kidney transplant may not fully restore kidney function. Code T86.1- should be assigned for documented complications of a kidney transplant, such as transplant failure or rejection or other transplant complication. Code T86.1- should not be assigned for post kidney transplant patients who have chronic kidney (CKD) unless a transplant complication such as transplant failure or rejection is documented. If the documentation is unclear as to whether the patient has a complication of the transplant, query the provider.

Conditions that affect the function of the transplanted kidney, other than CKD, should be assigned a code from subcategory T86.1, Complications of transplanted organ, Kidney, and a secondary code that identifies the complication.

For patients with CKD following a kidney transplant, but who do not have a complication such as failure or rejection, *see Section I.C.14. Chronic kidney disease and kidney transplant status.*

See I.C.1.d.4. for sequencing of sepsis due to infection in transplanted organ

4) Complication codes that include the external cause

As with certain other T codes, some of the complications of care codes have the external cause included in the code. The code includes the nature of the complication as well as the type of procedure that caused the complication. No external cause code indicating the type of procedure is necessary for these codes.

5) Complications of care codes within the body system chapters

Intraoperative and postprocedural complication codes are found within the body system chapters with codes specific to the organs and structures of that body system. These codes should be sequenced first, followed by a code(s) for the specific complication, if applicable.

Complication codes from the body system chapters should be assigned for intraoperative and postprocedural complications (e.g., the appropriate complication code from chapter 9 would be assigned for a vascular intraoperative or postprocedural complication) unless the complication is specifically indexed to a T code in chapter 19.

20. Chapter 20: External Causes of Morbidity (V00-Y99)

The external causes of morbidity codes should never be sequenced as the first-listed or principal diagnosis.

External cause codes are intended to provide data for injury research and evaluation of injury prevention strategies. These codes capture how the injury or health condition happened (cause), the intent (unintentional or accidental; or intentional, such as suicide or assault), the place where the event occurred the activity of the patient at the time of the event, and the person's status (e.g., civilian, military).

There is no national requirement for mandatory ICD-10-CM external cause code reporting. Unless a provider is subject to a state-based external cause code reporting mandate or these codes are required by a particular payer, reporting of ICD-10-CM codes in Chapter 20, External Causes of Morbidity, is not required. In the absence of a mandatory reporting requirement, providers are encouraged to voluntarily report external cause codes, as they provide valuable data for injury research and evaluation of injury prevention strategies.

a. General External Cause Coding Guidelines

1) Used with any code in the range of A00.0-T88.9, Z00-Z99

An external cause code may be used with any code in the range of A00.0-T88.9, Z00-Z99, classification that represents a health condition due to an external cause. Though they are most applicable to injuries, they are also valid for use with such things as infections or diseases due to an external source, and other health conditions, such as a heart attack that occurs during strenuous physical activity.

2) External cause code used for length of treatment

Assign the external cause code, with the appropriate 7th character (initial encounter, subsequent encounter or sequela) for each encounter for which the injury or condition is being treated.

Most categories in Chapter 20 have a 7th character requirement for each applicable code. Most categories in this chapter have three 7th character values: A, initial encounter, D, subsequent encounter and S, sequela. While the patient may be seen by a new or different provider over the course of treatment for an injury or condition, assignment of the 7th character for external cause should match the 7th character of the code assigned for the associated injury or condition for the encounter.

3) Use the full range of external cause codes

Use the full range of external cause codes to completely describe the cause, the intent, the place of occurrence, and if applicable, the activity of the patient at the time of the event, and the patient's status, for all injuries, and other health conditions due to an external cause.

4) Assign as many external cause codes as necessary

Assign as many external cause codes as necessary to fully explain each cause. If only one external code can be recorded, assign the code most related to the principal diagnosis.

5) The selection of the appropriate external cause code

The selection of the appropriate external cause code is guided by the Alphabetic Index of External Causes and by Inclusion and Exclusion notes in the Tabular List.

6) External cause code can never be a principal diagnosis

An external cause code can never be a principal (first-listed) diagnosis.

7) Combination external cause codes

Certain of the external cause codes are combination codes that identify sequential events that result in an injury, such as a fall which results in striking against an object. The injury may be due to either event or both. The combination external cause code used should correspond to the sequence of events regardless of which caused the most serious injury.

8) No external cause code needed in certain circumstances

No external cause code from Chapter 20 is needed if the external cause and intent are included in a code from another chapter (e.g., T36.0X1- Poisoning by penicillins, accidental (unintentional)).

b. Place of Occurrence Guideline

Codes from category Y92, Place of occurrence of the external cause, are secondary codes for use after other external cause codes to identify the location of the patient at the time of injury or other condition.

Generally, a place of occurrence code is assigned only once, at the initial encounter for treatment. However, in the rare instance that a new injury occurs during hospitalization, an additional place of occurrence code may be assigned. No 7th characters are used for Y92.

Do not use place of occurrence code Y92.9 if the place is not stated or is not applicable.

c. Activity Code

Assign a code from category Y93, Activity code, to describe the activity of the patient at the time the injury or other health condition occurred.

An activity code is used only once, at the initial encounter for treatment. Only one code from Y93 should be recorded on a medical record.

The activity codes are not applicable to poisonings, adverse effects, misadventures or sequela.

Do not assign Y93.9, Unspecified activity, if the activity is not stated.

A code from category Y93 is appropriate for use with external cause and intent codes if identifying the activity provides additional information about the event.

d. Place of Occurrence, Activity, and Status Codes Used with other External Cause Code

When applicable, place of occurrence, activity, and external cause status codes are sequenced after the main external cause code(s). Regardless of the number of external cause codes assigned, generally there should be only one place of occurrence code, one activity code, and one external cause status code assigned to an encounter. However, in the rare instance that a new injury occurs during hospitalization, an additional place of occurrence code may be assigned.

e. If the Reporting Format Limits the Number of External Cause Codes

If the reporting format limits the number of external cause codes that can be used in reporting clinical data, report the code for the cause/intent most related to the principal diagnosis. If the format permits capture of additional external cause codes, the cause/intent, including medical misadventures, of the additional events should be reported rather than the codes for place, activity, or external status.

f. Multiple External Cause Coding Guidelines

More than one external cause code is required to fully describe the external cause of an illness or injury. The assignment of external cause codes should be sequenced in the following priority:

If two or more events cause separate injuries, an external cause code should be assigned for each cause. The first-listed external cause code will be selected in the following order:

External codes for child and adult abuse take priority over all other external cause codes.

See Section I.C.19., Child and Adult abuse guidelines.

External cause codes for terrorism events take priority over all other external cause codes except child and adult abuse.

External cause codes for cataclysmic events take priority over all other external cause codes except child and adult abuse and terrorism.

External cause codes for transport accidents take priority over all other external cause codes except cataclysmic events, child and adult abuse and terrorism.

Activity and external cause status codes are assigned following all causal (intent) external cause codes.

The first-listed external cause code should correspond to the cause of the most serious diagnosis due to an assault, accident, or self-harm, following the order of hierarchy listed above.

g. Child and Adult Abuse Guideline

Adult and child abuse, neglect and maltreatment are classified as assault. Any of the assault codes may be used to indicate the external cause of any injury resulting from the confirmed abuse.

For confirmed cases of abuse, neglect and maltreatment, when the perpetrator is known, a code from Y07, Perpetrator of maltreatment and neglect, should accompany any other assault codes.

See Section I.C.19. Adult and child abuse, neglect and other maltreatment

h. Unknown or Undetermined Intent Guideline

If the intent (accident, self-harm, assault) of the cause of an injury or other condition is unknown or unspecified, code the intent as accidental intent. All transport accident categories assume accidental intent.

1) Use of undetermined intent

External cause codes for events of undetermined intent are only for use if the documentation in the record specifies that the intent cannot be determined.

i. Sequelae (Late Effects) of External Cause Guidelines

1) Sequelae external cause codes

Sequela are reported using the external cause code with the 7th character "S" for sequela. These codes should be used with any report of a late effect or sequela resulting from a previous injury.

See Section I.B.10. Sequela (Late Effects)

2) Sequela external cause code with a related current injury

A sequela external cause code should never be used with a related current nature of injury code.

3) Use of sequela external cause codes for subsequent visits

Use a late effect external cause code for subsequent visits when a late effect of the initial injury is being treated. Do not use a late effect external cause code for subsequent visits for follow-up care (e.g., to assess healing, to receive rehabilitative therapy) of the injury when no late effect of the injury has been documented.

j. Terrorism Guidelines

1) Cause of injury identified by the Federal Government (FBI) as terrorism

When the cause of an injury is identified by the Federal Government (FBI) as terrorism, the first-listed external cause code should be a code from category Y38, Terrorism. The definition of terrorism employed by the FBI is found at the inclusion note at the beginning of category Y38. Use additional code for place of occurrence (Y92.-). More than one Y38 code may be assigned if the injury is the result of more than one mechanism of terrorism.

2) Cause of an injury is suspected to be the result of terrorism

When the cause of an injury is suspected to be the result of terrorism a code from category Y38 should not be assigned. Suspected cases should be classified as assault.

3) Code Y38.9, Terrorism, secondary effects

Assign code Y38.9, Terrorism, secondary effects, for conditions occurring subsequent to the terrorist event. This code should not be assigned for conditions that are due to the initial terrorist act.

It is acceptable to assign code Y38.9 with another code from Y38 if there is an injury due to the initial terrorist event and an injury that is a subsequent result of the terrorist event.

k. External Cause Status

A code from category Y99, External cause status, should be assigned whenever any other external cause code is assigned for an encounter, including an Activity code, except for the events noted below. Assign a code from category Y99, External cause status, to indicate the work status of the person at the time the event occurred. The status code indicates whether the event occurred during military activity, whether a non-military person was at work, whether an individual including a student or volunteer was involved in a non-work activity at the time of the causal event.

A code from Y99, External cause status, should be assigned, when applicable, with other external cause codes, such as transport accidents and falls. The external cause status codes are not applicable to poisonings, adverse effects, misadventures or late effects.

Do not assign a code from category Y99 if no other external cause codes (cause, activity) are applicable for the encounter.

An external cause status code is used only once, at the initial encounter for treatment. Only one code from Y99 should be recorded on a medical record.

Do not assign code Y99.9, Unspecified external cause status, if the status is not stated.

21. Chapter 21: Factors influencing health status and contact with health services (Z00-Z99)

Note: The chapter-specific guidelines provide additional information about the use of Z codes for specified encounters.

a. Use of Z Codes in Any Healthcare Setting

Z codes are for use in any healthcare setting. Z codes may be used as either a first-listed (principal diagnosis code in the inpatient setting) or secondary code, depending on the circumstances of the encounter. Certain Z codes may only be used as first-listed or principal diagnosis.

b. Z Codes Indicate a Reason for an Encounter *or Provide Additional Information about a Patient Encounter*

Z codes are not procedure codes. A corresponding procedure code must accompany a Z code to describe any procedure performed.

c. Categories of Z Codes

1) Contact/Exposure

Category Z20 indicates contact with, and suspected exposure to, communicable diseases. These codes are for patients who are suspected to have been exposed to a disease by close personal contact with an infected individual or are in an area where a disease is epidemic.

Category Z77, Other contact with and (suspected) exposures hazardous to health, indicates contact with and suspected exposures hazardous to health.

Contact/exposure codes may be used as a first-listed code to explain an encounter for testing, or, more commonly, as a secondary code to identify a potential risk.

2) Inoculations and vaccinations

Code Z23 is for encounters for inoculations and vaccinations. It indicates that a patient is being seen to receive a prophylactic inoculation against a disease. Procedure codes are required to identify the actual administration of the injection and the type(s) of immunizations given. Code Z23 may be used as a secondary code if the inoculation is given as a routine part of preventive health care, such as a well-baby visit.

3) Status

Status codes indicate that a patient is either a carrier of a disease or has the sequelae or residual of a past disease or condition. This includes such things as the presence of prosthetic or mechanical devices resulting from past treatment. A status code is informative, because the status may affect the course of treatment and its outcome. A status code is distinct from a history code. The history code indicates that the patient no longer has the condition.

A status code should not be used with a diagnosis code from one of the body system chapters, if the diagnosis code includes the information provided by the status code. For example, code Z94.1, Heart transplant status, should not be used with a code from subcategory T86.2, Complications of heart transplant. The status code does not provide additional information. The complication code indicates that the patient is a heart transplant patient.

For encounters for weaning from a mechanical ventilator, assign a code from subcategory J96.1, Chronic respiratory failure, followed by code Z99.11, Dependence on respirator [ventilator] status.

The status Z codes/categories are:

Z14 Genetic carrier
Genetic carrier status indicates that a person carries a gene, associated with a particular disease, which may be passed to offspring who may develop that disease. The person does not have the disease and is not at risk of developing the disease.

Z15 Genetic susceptibility to disease Genetic susceptibility indicates that a person has a gene that increases the risk of that person developing the disease.

Codes from category Z15 should not be used as principal or first-listed codes. If the patient has the condition to which he/she is susceptible, and that condition is the reason for the encounter, the code for the current condition should be sequenced first. If the patient is being seen for follow-up after completed treatment for this condition, and the condition no longer exists, a follow-up code should be sequenced first, followed by the appropriate personal history and genetic susceptibility codes. If the purpose of the encounter is genetic counseling associated with procreative management, code Z31.5, Encounter for genetic counseling, should be assigned as the first-listed code, followed by a code from category Z15. Additional codes should be assigned for any applicable family or personal history.

Z16 Resistance to antimicrobial drugs
This code indicates that a patient has a condition that is resistant to antimicrobial drug treatment. Sequence the infection code first.

Z17 Estrogen, and other hormones and factors receptor status

Z18 Retained foreign body fragments

Z19 Hormone sensitivity malignancy status

Z21 Asymptomatic HIV infection status This code indicates that a patient has tested positive for HIV but has manifested no signs or symptoms of the disease.

Z22 Carrier of infectious disease Carrier status indicates that a person harbors the specific organisms of a disease without manifest symptoms and is capable of transmitting the infection.

Z28.3 Underimmunization status

See Section I.B.14. for underimmunization documentation by clinicians other than the patient's provider.

Z33.1 Pregnant state, incidental This code is a secondary code only for use when the pregnancy is in no way complicating the reason for visit. Otherwise, a code from the obstetric chapter is required.

Z66 Do not resuscitate

This code may be used when it is documented by the provider that a patient is on do not resuscitate status at any time during the stay.

Z67 Blood type

Z68 Body mass index (BMI)
BMI codes should only be assigned when there is an associated reportable diagnosis (such as obesity). Do not assign BMI codes during pregnancy.

See Section I.B.14 for BMI documentation by clinicians other than the patient's provider.

Z74.01 Bed confinement status

Z76.82 Awaiting organ transplant status

Z78 Other specified health status

Code Z78.1, Physical restraint status, may be used when it is documented by the provider that a patient has been put in restraints during the current encounter. Please note that this code should not be reported when it is documented by the provider that a patient is temporarily restrained during a procedure.

Z79 Long-term (current) drug therapy

Codes from this category indicate a patient's continuous use of a prescribed drug (including such things as aspirin therapy) for the long-term treatment of a condition or for prophylactic use. It is not for use for patients who have addictions to drugs. This subcategory is not for use of medications for detoxification or maintenance programs to prevent withdrawal symptoms (e.g., methadone maintenance for opiate dependence). Assign the appropriate code for the drug use, abuse, or dependence instead.

Assign a code from Z79 if the patient is receiving a medication for an extended period as a prophylactic measure (such as for the prevention of deep vein thrombosis) or as treatment of a chronic condition (such as arthritis) or a disease requiring a lengthy course of treatment (such as cancer). Do not assign a code from category Z79 for medication being administered for a brief period of time to treat an acute illness or injury (such as a course of antibiotics to treat acute bronchitis).

Z88 Allergy status to drugs, medicaments and biological substances Except: Z88.9, Allergy status to unspecified drugs, medicaments and biological substances status

Z89 Acquired absence of limb

Z90 Acquired absence of organs, not elsewhere classified

Z91.0- Allergy status, other than to drugs and biological substances

Z92.82 Status post administration of tPA (rtPA) in a different facility within the last 24 hours prior to admission to a current facility Assign code Z92.82, Status post administration of tPA (rtPA) in a different facility within the last 24 hours prior to admission to current facility, as a secondary diagnosis when a patient is received by transfer into a facility and documentation indicates they were administered tissue plasminogen activator (tPA) within the last 24 hours prior to admission to the current facility. This guideline applies even if the patient is still receiving the tPA at the time they are received into the current facility. The appropriate code for the condition for which the tPA was administered (such as cerebrovascular disease or myocardial infarction) should be assigned first. Code Z92.82 is only applicable to the receiving facility record and not to the transferring facility record.

Z93 Artificial opening status

Z94 Transplanted organ and tissue status

Z95 Presence of cardiac and vascular implants and grafts

Z96 Presence of other functional implants

Z97 Presence of other devices

Z98 Other postprocedural states

Assign code Z98.85, Transplanted organ removal status, to indicate that a transplanted organ has been previously removed. This code should not be assigned for the encounter in which the transplanted organ is removed. The complication necessitating removal of the transplant organ should be assigned for that encounter.

See Section I.C.19. for information on the coding of organ transplant complications.

Z99 Dependence on enabling machines and devices, not elsewhere classified

Note: Categories Z89-Z90 and Z93-Z99 are for use only if there are no complications or malfunctions of the organ or tissue replaced, the amputation site or the equipment on which the patient is dependent.

4) History (of)

There are two types of history Z codes, personal and family. Personal history codes explain a patient's past medical condition that no longer exists and is not receiving any treatment, but that has the potential for recurrence, and therefore may require continued monitoring.

Family history codes are for use when a patient has a family member(s) who has had a particular disease that causes the patient to be at higher risk of also contracting the disease.

Personal history codes may be used in conjunction with follow-up codes and family history codes may be used in conjunction with screening codes to explain the need for a test or procedure. History codes are also acceptable on any medical record regardless of the reason for visit. A history of an illness, even if no longer present, is important information that may alter the type of treatment ordered.

The reason for the encounter (for example, screening or counseling) should be sequenced first and the appropriate personal and/or family history code(s) should be assigned as additional diagnos(es).

The history Z code categories are:

Z80 Family history of primary malignant neoplasm

Z81 Family history of mental and behavioral disorders

Z82 Family history of certain disabilities and chronic diseases (leading to disablement)

Z83 Family history of other specific disorders

Z84 Family history of other conditions

Z85 Personal history of malignant neoplasm

Z86 Personal history of certain other diseases

Z87 Personal history of other diseases and conditions

Z91.4- Personal history of psychological trauma, not elsewhere classified

Z91.5 Personal history of self-harm

Z91.81 History of falling

Z91.82 Personal history of military deployment

Z91.85 Personal history of military service

Z92 Personal history of medical treatment Except: Z92.0, Personal history of contraception Except: Z92.82, Status post administration of tPA (rtPA) in a different facility within the last 24 hours prior to admission to a current facility

5) Screening

Screening is the testing for disease or disease precursors in seemingly well individuals so that early detection and treatment can be provided for those who test positive for the disease (e.g., screening mammogram).

The testing of a person to rule out or confirm a suspected diagnosis because the patient has some sign or symptom is a diagnostic examination, not a screening. In these cases, the sign or symptom is used to explain the reason for the test.

A screening code may be a first-listed code if the reason for the visit is specifically the screening exam. It may also be used as an additional code if the screening is done during an office visit for other health problems. A screening code is not necessary if the screening is inherent to a routine examination, such as a pap smear done during a routine pelvic examination.

Should a condition be discovered during the screening then the code for the condition may be assigned as an additional diagnosis.

The Z code indicates that a screening exam is planned. A procedure code is required to confirm that the screening was performed.

The screening Z codes/categories:

Z11	Encounter for screening for infectious and parasitic diseases
Z12	Encounter for screening for malignant neoplasms
Z13	Encounter for screening for other diseases and disorders Except: Z13.9, Encounter for screening, unspecified
Z36	Encounter for antenatal screening for mother

6) Observation

There are three observation Z code categories. They are for use in very limited circumstances when a person is being observed for a suspected condition that is ruled out. The observation codes are not for use if an injury or illness or any signs or symptoms related to the suspected condition are present. In such cases the diagnosis/symptom code is used with the corresponding external cause code.

The observation codes are primarily to be used as a principal/first-listed diagnosis. An observation code may be assigned as a secondary diagnosis code when the patient is being observed for a condition that is ruled out and is unrelated to the principal/first-listed diagnosis. Also, when the principal diagnosis is required to be a code from category Z38, Liveborn infants according to place of birth and type of delivery, then a code from category Z05, Encounter for observation and evaluation of newborn for suspected diseases and conditions ruled out, is sequenced after the Z38 code. Additional codes may be used in addition to the observation code, but only if they are unrelated to the suspected condition being observed.

Codes from subcategory Z03.7, Encounter for suspected maternal and fetal conditions ruled out, may either be used as a first-listed or as an additional code assignment depending on the case. They are for use in very limited circumstances on a maternal record when an encounter is for a suspected maternal or fetal condition that is ruled out during that encounter (for example, a maternal or fetal condition may be suspected due to an abnormal test result). These codes should not be used when the condition is confirmed. In those cases, the confirmed condition should be coded. In addition, these codes are not for use if an illness or any signs or symptoms related to the suspected condition or problem are present. In such cases the diagnosis/symptom code is used.

Additional codes may be used in addition to the code from subcategory Z03.7, but only if they are unrelated to the suspected condition being evaluated.

Codes from subcategory Z03.7, may not be used for encounters for antenatal screening of mother. *See Section I.C.21. Screening.*

For encounters for suspected fetal condition that are inconclusive following testing and evaluation, assign the appropriate code from category O35, O36, O40 or O41.

The observation Z code categories:

Z03	Encounter for medical observation for suspected diseases and conditions ruled out
Z04	Encounter for examination and observation for other reasons Except: Z04.9, Encounter for examination and observation for unspecified reason
Z05	Encounter for observation and evaluation of newborn for suspected diseases and conditions ruled out

7) Aftercare

Aftercare visit codes cover situations when the initial treatment of a disease has been performed and the patient requires continued care during the healing or recovery phase, or for the long-term consequences of the disease. The aftercare Z code should not be used if treatment is directed at a current, acute disease. The diagnosis code is to be used in these cases.

Exceptions to this rule are codes Z51.0, Encounter for antineoplastic radiation therapy, and codes from subcategory Z51.1, Encounter for antineoplastic chemotherapy and immunotherapy. These codes are to be first-listed, followed by the diagnosis code when a patient's encounter is solely to receive radiation therapy, chemotherapy, or immunotherapy for the treatment of a neoplasm. If the reason for the encounter is more than one type of antineoplastic therapy, code Z51.0 and a code from subcategory Z51.1 may be assigned together, in which case one of these codes would be reported as a secondary diagnosis.

The aftercare Z codes should also not be used for aftercare for injuries. For aftercare of an injury, assign the acute injury code with the appropriate 7th character (for subsequent encounter).

The aftercare codes are generally first-listed to explain the specific reason for the encounter. An aftercare code may be used as an additional code when some type of aftercare is provided in addition to the reason for admission and no diagnosis code is applicable. An example of this would be the closure of a colostomy during an encounter for treatment of another condition.

Aftercare codes should be used in conjunction with other aftercare codes or diagnosis codes to provide better detail on the specifics of an aftercare encounter visit, unless otherwise directed by the classification. The sequencing of multiple aftercare codes depends on the circumstances of the encounter.

Certain aftercare Z code categories need a secondary diagnosis code to describe the resolving condition or sequelae. For others, the condition is included in the code title.

Additional Z code aftercare category terms include fitting and adjustment, and attention to artificial openings.

Status Z codes may be used with aftercare Z codes to indicate the nature of the aftercare. For example code Z95.1, Presence of aortocoronary bypass graft, may be used with code Z48.812, Encounter for surgical aftercare following surgery on the circulatory system, to indicate the surgery for which the aftercare is being performed. A status code should not be used when the aftercare code indicates the type of status, such as using Z43.0, Encounter for attention to tracheostomy, with Z93.0, Tracheostomy status.

The aftercare Z category/codes:

Z42 Encounter for plastic and reconstructive surgery following medical procedure or healed injury
Z43 Encounter for attention to artificial openings
Z44 Encounter for fitting and adjustment of external prosthetic device
Z45 Encounter for adjustment and management of implanted device
Z46 Encounter for fitting and adjustment of other devices
Z47 Orthopedic aftercare
Z48 Encounter for other postprocedural aftercare
Z49 Encounter for care involving renal dialysis
Z51 Encounter for other aftercare and medical care

8) Follow-up

The follow-up codes are used to explain continuing surveillance following completed treatment of a disease, condition, or injury. They imply that the condition has been fully treated and no longer exists. They should not be confused with aftercare codes, or injury codes with a 7th character for subsequent encounter, that explain ongoing care of a healing condition or its sequelae. Follow-up codes may be used in conjunction with history codes to provide the full picture of the healed condition and its treatment. The follow-up code is sequenced first, followed by the history code.

A follow-up code may be used to explain multiple visits. Should a condition be found to have recurred on the follow-up visit, then the diagnosis code for the condition should be assigned in place of the follow-up code.

The follow-up Z **codes/**categories:

Z08 Encounter for follow-up examination after completed treatment for malignant neoplasm
Z09 Encounter for follow-up examination after completed treatment for conditions other than malignant neoplasm
Codes Z08, Encounter for follow-up examination after completed treatment for malignant neoplasm, and Z09, Encounter for follow up examination after completed treatment for conditions other than malignant neoplasm, may be assigned following any type of completed treatment modality (including both medical and surgical treatments).
Z39 Encounter for maternal postpartum care and examination

9) Donor

Codes in category Z52, Donors of organs and tissues, are used for living individuals who are donating blood or other body tissue. These codes are for individuals donating for others, as well as for self-donations. They are not used to identify cadaveric donations.

10) Counseling

Counseling Z codes are used when a patient or family member receives assistance in the aftermath of an illness or injury, or when support is required in coping with family or social problems.

The counseling Z codes/categories:

Z30.0- Encounter for general counseling and advice on contraception
Z31.5 Encounter for procreative genetic counseling
Z31.6- Encounter for general counseling and advice on procreation
Z32.2 Encounter for childbirth instruction
Z32.3 Encounter for childcare instruction
Z69 Encounter for mental health services for victim and perpetrator of abuse
Z70 Counseling related to sexual attitude, behavior and orientation
Z71 Persons encountering health services for other counseling and medical advice, not elsewhere classified
Note: Code Z71.84, Encounter for health counseling related to travel, is to be used for health risk and safety counseling for future travel purposes.
Code Z71.85, Encounter for immunization safety counseling, is to be used for counseling of the patient or caregiver regarding the safety of a vaccine. This code should not be used for the provision of general information regarding risks and potential side effects during routine encounters for the administration of vaccines.
Code Z71.87, Encounter for pediatric-to-adult transition counseling, should be assigned when pediatric-to-adult transition counseling is the sole reason for the encounter or when this counseling is provided in addition to other services, such as treatment of a chronic condition. If both transition counseling and treatment of a medical condition are provided during the same encounter, the code(s) for the medical condition(s) treated and code Z71.87 should be assigned, with sequencing depending on the circumstances of the encounter.
Z76.81 Expectant mother prebirth pediatrician visit

11) Encounters for Obstetrical and Reproductive Services

See Section I.C.15. Pregnancy, Childbirth, and the Puerperium, for further instruction on the use of these codes.

Z codes for pregnancy are for use in those circumstances when none of the problems or complications included in the codes from the Obstetrics chapter exist (a routine prenatal visit or postpartum care). Codes in category Z34, Encounter for supervision of normal pregnancy, are always first listed and are not to be used with any other code from the OB chapter.

Codes in category Z3A, Weeks of gestation, may be assigned to provide additional information about the pregnancy. Category Z3A codes should not be assigned for pregnancies with abortive outcomes (categories O00-O08), elective termination of pregnancy (code Z33.2), nor for postpartum conditions, as category Z3A is not applicable to these conditions. The date of the admission should be used to determine weeks of gestation for inpatient admissions that encompass more than one gestational week.

The outcome of delivery, category Z37, should be included on all maternal delivery records. It is always a secondary code. Codes in category Z37 should not be used on the newborn record.

Z codes for family planning (contraceptive) or procreative management and counseling should be included on an obstetric record either during the pregnancy or the postpartum stage, if applicable.

Z codes/categories for obstetrical and reproductive services:

Z30	Encounter for contraceptive management
Z31	Encounter for procreative management
Z32.2	Encounter for childbirth instruction
Z32.3	Encounter for childcare instruction
Z33	Pregnant state
Z34	Encounter for supervision of normal pregnancy
Z36	Encounter for antenatal screening of mother
Z3A	Weeks of gestation
Z37	Outcome of delivery
Z39	Encounter for maternal postpartum care and examination
Z76.81	Expectant mother prebirth pediatrician visit

12) Newborns and Infants

See Section I.C.16. Newborn (Perinatal) Guidelines, for further instruction on the use of these codes.

Newborn Z codes/categories:

Z76.1	Encounter for health supervision and care of foundling
Z00.1-	Encounter for routine child health examination
Z38	Liveborn infants according to place of birth and type of delivery

13) Routine and Administrative Examinations

The Z codes allow for the description of encounters for routine examinations, such as, a general check-up, or, examinations for administrative purposes, such as, a pre-employment physical. The codes are not to be used if the examination is for diagnosis of a suspected condition or for treatment purposes. In such cases the diagnosis code is used. During a routine exam, should a diagnosis or condition be discovered, it should be coded as an additional code. Pre-existing and chronic conditions and history codes may also be included as additional codes as long as the examination is for administrative purposes and not focused on any particular condition.

Some of the codes for routine health examinations distinguish between "with" and "without" abnormal findings. Code assignment depends on the information that is known at the time the encounter is being coded. For example, if no abnormal findings were found during the examination, but the encounter is being coded before test results are back, it is acceptable to assign the code for "without abnormal findings." When assigning a code for "with abnormal findings," additional code(s) should be assigned to identify the specific abnormal finding(s).

Pre-operative examination and pre-procedural laboratory examination Z codes are for use only in those situations when a patient is being cleared for a procedure or surgery and no treatment is given.

The Z codes/categories for routine and administrative examinations:

Z00	Encounter for general examination without complaint, suspected or reported diagnosis
Z01	Encounter for other special examination without complaint, suspected or reported diagnosis
Z02	Encounter for administrative examination Except: Z02.9, Encounter for administrative examinations, unspecified
Z32.0-	Encounter for pregnancy test

14) Miscellaneous Z Codes

The miscellaneous Z codes capture a number of other health care encounters that do not fall into one of the other categories. Some of these codes identify the reason for the encounter; others are for use as additional codes that provide useful information on circumstances that may affect a patient's care and treatment.

Prophylactic Organ Removal

For encounters specifically for prophylactic removal of an organ (such as prophylactic removal of breasts due to a genetic susceptibility to cancer or a family history of cancer), the principal or first-listed code should be a code from category Z40, Encounter for prophylactic surgery, followed by the appropriate codes to identify the associated risk factor (such as genetic susceptibility or family history).

If the patient has a malignancy of one site and is having prophylactic removal at another site to prevent either a new primary malignancy or metastatic disease, a code for the malignancy should also be assigned in addition to a code from subcategory Z40.0, Encounter for prophylactic surgery for risk factors related to malignant neoplasms. A Z40.0 code should not be assigned if the patient is having organ removal for treatment of a malignancy, such as the removal of the testes for the treatment of prostate cancer.

Miscellaneous Z codes/categories:

Z28 Immunization not carried out
Except: Z28.3, Underimmunization status

Z29 Encounter for other prophylactic measures

Z40 Encounter for prophylactic surgery

Z41 Encounter for procedures for purposes other than remedying health state
Except: Z41.9, Encounter for procedure for purposes other than remedying health state, unspecified

Z72 Problems related to lifestyle
Note: These codes should be assigned only when the documentation specifies that the patient has an associated problem

Z73 Problems related to life management difficulty
Note: These codes should be assigned only when the documentation specifies that the patient has an associated problem.

Z74 Problems related to care provider dependency Except: Z74.01, Bed confinement status

Z75 Problems related to medical facilities and other health care

Z76.0 Encounter for issue of repeat prescription

Z76.3 Healthy person accompanying sick person

Z76.4 Other boarder to healthcare facility

Z76.5 Malingerer [conscious simulation]

Z91.1- Patient's noncompliance with medical treatment and regimen

Z91.A- Caregiver's noncompliance with patient's medical treatment and regimen

Z91.83 Wandering in diseases classified elsewhere

Z91.84- Oral health risk factors

Z91.89 Other specified personal risk factors, not elsewhere classified

See Section I.B.14 for Z55-Z65 Persons with potential health hazards related to socioeconomic and psychosocial circumstances, documentation by clinicians other than the patient's provider

15) Nonspecific Z Codes

Certain Z codes are so non-specific, or potentially redundant with other codes in the classification, that there can be little justification for their use in the inpatient setting. Their use in the outpatient setting should be limited to those instances when there is no further documentation to permit more precise coding. Otherwise, any sign or symptom or any other reason for visit that is captured in another code should be used.

Nonspecific Z codes/categories:

Z02.9 Encounter for administrative examinations, unspecified

Z04.9 Encounter for examination and observation for unspecified reason

Z13.9 Encounter for screening, unspecified

Z41.9 Encounter for procedure for purposes other than remedying health state, unspecified

Z52.9 Donor of unspecified organ or tissue

Z86.59 Personal history of other mental and behavioral disorders

Z88.9 Allergy status to unspecified drugs, medicaments and biological substances status

Z92.0 Personal history of contraception

16) Z Codes That May Only be Principal/First-Listed Diagnosis

The following Z codes/categories may only be reported as the principal/first-listed diagnosis, except when there are multiple encounters on the same day and the medical records for the encounters are combined:

Z00 Encounter for general examination without complaint, suspected or reported diagnosis
Except: Z00.6

Z01 Encounter for other special examination without complaint, suspected or reported diagnosis

Z02 Encounter for administrative examination

Z04 Encounter for examination and observation for other reasons

Z33.2 Encounter for elective termination of pregnancy

Z31.81 Encounter for male factor infertility in female patient

Z31.83 Encounter for assisted reproductive fertility procedure cycle

Z31.84 Encounter for fertility preservation procedure

Z34 Encounter for supervision of normal pregnancy

Z39 Encounter for maternal postpartum care and examination

Z38 Liveborn infants according to place of birth and type of delivery

Z40 Encounter for prophylactic surgery

Z42 Encounter for plastic and reconstructive surgery following medical procedure or healed injury

Z51.0 Encounter for antineoplastic radiation therapy

Z51.1- Encounter for antineoplastic chemotherapy and immunotherapy

Z52 Donors of organs and tissues Except: Z52.9, Donor of unspecified organ or tissue

Z76.1 Encounter for health supervision and care of foundling

Z76.2 Encounter for health supervision and care of other healthy infant and child

Z99.12 Encounter for respirator [ventilator] dependence during power failure

17) Social Determinants of Health

Social determinants of health (SDOH) codes describing social problems, conditions, or risk factors that influence a patient's health should be assigned when this information is documented in the patient's medical record. Assign as many SDOH codes as are necessary to describe all of the social problems, conditions, or risk factors documented during the current episode of care. For example, a patient who lives alone may suffer an acute injury temporarily impacting their ability to perform routine activities of daily living. When documented as such, this would support assignment of code Z60.2, Problems related to living alone. However, merely living alone, without documentation of a risk or unmet need for assistance at home, would not support assignment of code Z60.2. Documentation by a clinician (or patient-reported information that is signed off by a clinician) that the patient expressed concerns with access and availability of food would support assignment of code Z59.41, Food insecurity. Similarly, medical record documentation indicating the patient is homeless would support assignment of a code from subcategory Z59.0-, Homelessness.

For social determinants of health **classified to chapter 21**, such as information found in categories Z55-Z65, Persons with potential health hazards related to socioeconomic and psychosocial circumstances, code assignment may be based on medical record documentation from clinicians involved in the care of the patient who are not the patient's provider since this information represents social information, rather than medical diagnoses.

For example, coding professionals may utilize documentation of social information from social workers, community health workers, case managers, or nurses, if their documentation is included in the official medical record.

Patient self-reported documentation may be used to assign codes for social determinants of health, as long as the patient self-reported information is signed-off by and incorporated into the medical record by either a clinician or provider.

Social determinants of health codes are located primarily in these Z code categories:

- Z55 Problems related to education and literacy
- Z56 Problems related to employment and unemployment
- Z57 Occupational exposure to risk factors
- Z58 Problems related to physical environment
- Z59 Problems related to housing and economic circumstances
- Z60 Problems related to social environment
- Z62 Problems related to upbringing
- Z63 Other problems related to primary support group, including family circumstances
- Z64 Problems related to certain psychosocial circumstances
- Z65 Problems related to other psychosocial circumstances

See Section I.B.14. Documentation by Clinicians Other than the Patient's Provider.

22. **Chapter 22: Codes for Special Purposes (U00-U85)**
    - U07.0 Vaping-related disorder (see Section I.C.10.e., Vaping-related disorders)
    - U07.1 COVID-19 (see Section I.C.1.g.1., COVID-19 infection)
    - U09.9 Post COVID-19 condition, unspecified (see Section I.C.1.g.1.m)

Section II. Selection of Principal Diagnosis

The circumstances of inpatient admission always govern the selection of principal diagnosis. The principal diagnosis is defined in the Uniform Hospital Discharge Data Set (UHDDS) as "that condition established after study to be chiefly responsible for occasioning the admission of the patient to the hospital for care."

The UHDDS definitions are used by hospitals to report inpatient data elements in a standardized manner. These data elements and their definitions can be found in the July 31, 1985, Federal Register (Vol. 50, No, 147), pp. 31038-40.

Since that time, the application of the UHDDS definitions has been expanded to include all nonoutpatient settings (acute care, short term, long-term care and psychiatric hospitals; home health agencies; rehab facilities; nursing homes, etc. . .). The UHDDS definitions also apply to hospice services (all levels of care).

In determining principal diagnosis, coding conventions in the ICD-10-CM, the Tabular List and Alphabetic Index take precedence over these official coding guidelines.

(See Section I.A., Conventions for the ICD-10-CM)

The importance of consistent, complete documentation in the medical record cannot be overemphasized. Without such documentation the application of all coding guidelines is a difficult, if not impossible, task.

A. **Codes for symptoms, signs, and ill-defined conditions**

   Codes for symptoms, signs, and ill-defined conditions from Chapter 18 are not to be used as principal diagnosis when a related definitive diagnosis has been established.

B. **Two or more interrelated conditions, each potentially meeting the definition for principal diagnosis**

   When there are two or more interrelated conditions (such as diseases in the same ICD-10-CM chapter or manifestations characteristically associated with a certain disease) potentially meeting the definition of principal diagnosis, either condition may be sequenced first, unless the circumstances of the admission, the therapy provided, the Tabular List, or the Alphabetic Index indicate otherwise.

C. **Two or more diagnoses that equally meet the definition for principal diagnosis**

   In the unusual instance when two or more diagnoses equally meet the criteria for principal

GUIDELINES (ICD-10-CM)

diagnosis as determined by the circumstances of admission, diagnostic workup and/or therapy provided, and the Alphabetic Index, Tabular List, or another coding guidelines does not provide sequencing direction, any one of the diagnoses may be sequenced first.

D. Two or more comparative or contrasting conditions.

In those rare instances when two or more contrasting or comparative diagnoses are documented as "either/or" (or similar terminology), they are coded as if the diagnoses were confirmed and the diagnoses are sequenced according to the circumstances of the admission. If no further determination can be made as to which diagnosis should be principal, either diagnosis may be sequenced first

E. A symptom(s) followed by contrasting/ comparative diagnoses

GUIDELINE HAS BEEN DELETED EFFECTIVE OCTOBER 1, 2014

F. Original treatment plan not carried out

Sequence as the principal diagnosis the condition, which after study occasioned the admission to the hospital, even though treatment may not have been carried out due to unforeseen circumstances.

G. Complications of surgery and other medical care

When the admission is for treatment of a complication resulting from surgery or other medical care, the complication code is sequenced as the principal diagnosis. If the complication is classified to the T80-T88 series and the code lacks the necessary specificity in describing the complication, an additional code for the specific complication should be assigned.

H. Uncertain Diagnosis

If the diagnosis documented at the time of discharge is qualified as "probable," "suspected," "likely," "questionable," "possible," or "still to be ruled out," "compatible with," "consistent with," or other similar terms indicating uncertainty, code the condition as if it existed or was established. The bases for these guidelines are the diagnostic workup, arrangements for further workup or observation, and initial therapeutic approach that correspond most closely with the established diagnosis.

Note: This guideline is applicable only to inpatient admissions to short-term, acute, long-term care and psychiatric hospitals.

I. Admission from Observation Unit

1. Admission Following Medical Observation

When a patient is admitted to an observation unit for a medical condition, which either worsens or does not improve, and is subsequently admitted as an inpatient of the same hospital for this same medical condition, the principal diagnosis would be the medical condition which led to the hospital admission.

2. Admission Following Post-Operative Observation

When a patient is admitted to an observation unit to monitor a condition (or complication) that develops following outpatient surgery, and then is subsequently admitted as an inpatient of the same hospital, hospitals should apply the Uniform Hospital Discharge Data Set (UHDDS) definition of principal diagnosis as "that condition established after study to be chiefly responsible for occasioning the admission of the patient to the hospital for care."

J. Admission from Outpatient Surgery

When a patient receives surgery in the hospital's outpatient surgery department and is subsequently admitted for continuing inpatient care at the same hospital, the following guidelines should be followed in selecting the principal diagnosis for the inpatient admission:

- If the reason for the inpatient admission is a complication, assign the complication as the principal diagnosis.
- If no complication, or other condition, is documented as the reason for the inpatient admission, assign the reason for the outpatient surgery as the principal diagnosis.
- If the reason for the inpatient admission is another condition unrelated to the surgery, assign the unrelated condition as the principal diagnosis.

K. Admissions/Encounters for Rehabilitation

When the purpose for the admission/encounter is rehabilitation, sequence first the code for the condition for which the service is being performed. For example, for an admission/encounter for rehabilitation for right-sided dominant hemiplegia following a cerebrovascular infarction, report code I69.351, Hemiplegia and hemiparesis following cerebral infarction affecting right dominant side, as the first-listed or principal diagnosis.

If the condition for which the rehabilitation service is being provided is no longer present, report the appropriate aftercare code as the first-listed or principal diagnosis, unless the rehabilitation service is being provided following an injury. For rehabilitation services following active treatment of an injury, assign the injury code with the appropriate seventh character for subsequent encounter as the first-listed or principal diagnosis. For example, if a patient with severe degenerative osteoarthritis of the hip, underwent hip replacement and the current encounter/admission is for rehabilitation, report code Z47.1, Aftercare following joint replacement surgery, as the first-listed or principal diagnosis. If the patient requires rehabilitation post hip replacement for right intertrochanteric femur fracture, report code S72.141D, Displaced intertrochanteric fracture of right femur, subsequent encounter for closed fracture with routine healing, as the first-listed or principal diagnosis.

See Section I.C.21.c.7., Factors influencing health states and contact with health services, Aftercare.

See Section I.C.19.a., for additional information about the use of 7th characters for injury codes.

Section III. Reporting Additional Diagnoses

GENERAL RULES FOR OTHER (ADDITIONAL) DIAGNOSES

For reporting purposes the definition for "other diagnoses" is interpreted as additional **clinically significant** conditions that affect patient care in terms of requiring:

clinical evaluation; or
therapeutic treatment; or
diagnostic procedures; or
extended length of hospital stay; or
increased nursing care and/or monitoring.

The UHDDS item #11-b defines Other Diagnoses as "all conditions that coexist at the time of admission, that develop subsequently, or that affect the treatment received and/or the length of stay. Diagnoses that relate to an earlier episode which have no bearing on the current hospital stay are to be excluded." UHDDS definitions apply to inpatients in acute care, short-term, long term care and psychiatric hospital setting. The UHDDS definitions are used by acute care short-term hospitals to report inpatient data elements in a standardized manner. These data elements and their definitions can be found in the July 31, 1985, Federal Register (Vol. 50, No, 147), pp. 31038-40.

Since that time, the application of the UHDDS definitions has been expanded to include all non-outpatient settings (acute care, short term, long term care and psychiatric hospitals; home health agencies; rehab facilities; nursing homes, etc. . .). The UHDDS definitions also apply to hospice services (all levels of care).

The following guidelines are to be applied in designating "other diagnoses" when neither the Alphabetic Index nor the Tabular List in ICD-10-CM provide direction. The listing of the diagnoses in the patient record is the responsibility of the provider.

A. **Previous conditions**

If the provider has included a diagnosis in the final diagnostic statement, such as the discharge summary or the face sheet, it should ordinarily be coded. Some providers include in the diagnostic statement resolved conditions or diagnoses and status-post procedures from previous admissions that have no bearing on the current stay. Such conditions are not to be reported and are coded only if required by hospital policy.

However, history codes (categories Z80-Z87) may be used as secondary codes if the historical condition or family history has an impact on current care or influences treatment.

B. **Abnormal findings**

Abnormal findings (laboratory, x-ray, pathologic, and other diagnostic results) are not coded and reported unless the provider indicates their clinical significance. If the findings are outside the normal range and the provider has ordered other tests to evaluate the condition or prescribed treatment, it is appropriate to ask the provider whether the abnormal finding should be added.

Please note: This differs from the coding practices in the outpatient setting for coding encounters for diagnostic tests that have been interpreted by a provider.

C. **Uncertain Diagnosis**

If the diagnosis documented at the time of discharge is qualified as "probable," "suspected," "likely," "questionable," "possible," or "still to be ruled out," "compatible with," "consistent with," or other similar terms indicating uncertainty, code the condition as if it existed or was established. The bases for these guidelines are the diagnostic workup, arrangements for further workup or observation, and initial therapeutic approach that correspond most closely with the established diagnosis.

Note: This guideline is applicable only to inpatient admissions to short-term, acute, long-term care and psychiatric hospitals.

Section IV. Diagnostic Coding and Reporting Guidelines for Outpatient Services

These coding guidelines for outpatient diagnoses have been approved for use by hospitals/ providers in coding and reporting hospital-based outpatient services and provider-based office visits. Guidelines in Section I, Conventions, general coding guidelines and chapter-specific guidelines, should also be applied for outpatient services and office visits.

Information about the use of certain abbreviations, punctuation, symbols, and other conventions used in the ICD-10-CM Tabular List (code numbers and titles), can be found in Section IA of these guidelines, under "Conventions Used in the Tabular List." Section I.B. contains general guidelines that apply to the entire classification. Section I.C. contains chapter-specific guidelines that correspond to the chapters as they are arranged in the classification. Information about the correct sequence to use in finding a code is also described in Section I.

The terms encounter and visit are often used interchangeably in describing outpatient service contacts and, therefore, appear together in these guidelines without distinguishing one from the other.

Though the conventions and general guidelines apply to all settings, coding guidelines for outpatient and provider reporting of diagnoses will vary in a number of instances from those for inpatient diagnoses, recognizing that:

The Uniform Hospital Discharge Data Set (UHDDS) definition of principal diagnosis does not apply to hospital-based outpatient services and provider-based office visits.

Coding guidelines for inconclusive diagnoses (probable, suspected, rule out, etc.) were developed for inpatient reporting and do not apply to outpatients.

A. **Selection of first-listed condition**

In the outpatient setting, the term first-listed diagnosis is used in lieu of principal diagnosis.

In determining the first-listed diagnosis the coding conventions of ICD-10-CM, as well as the general and disease specific guidelines take precedence over the outpatient guidelines.

Diagnoses often are not established at the time of the initial encounter/visit. It may take two or more visits before the diagnosis is confirmed.

The most critical rule involves beginning the search for the correct code assignment through the Alphabetic Index. Never begin searching initially in the Tabular List as this will lead to coding errors.

1. Outpatient Surgery
When a patient presents for outpatient surgery (same day surgery), code the reason for the surgery as the first-listed diagnosis (reason for the encounter), even if the surgery is not performed due to a contraindication.

2. Observation Stay
When a patient is admitted for observation for a medical condition, assign a code for the medical condition as the first-listed diagnosis.

When a patient presents for outpatient surgery and develops complications requiring admission to observation, code the reason for the surgery as the first reported diagnosis (reason for the encounter), followed by codes for the complications as secondary diagnoses.

B. Codes from A00.0 through T88.9, Z00-Z99, U00-U85
The appropriate code(s) from A00.0 through T88.9, Z00-Z99, and U00-U85 must be used to identify diagnoses, symptoms, conditions, problems, complaints, or other reason(s) for the encounter/visit.

C. Accurate reporting of ICD-10-CM diagnosis codes
For accurate reporting of ICD-10-CM diagnosis codes, the documentation should describe the patient's condition, using terminology which includes specific diagnoses as well as symptoms, problems, or reasons for the encounter. There are ICD-10-CM codes to describe all of these.

D. Codes that describe symptoms and signs
Codes that describe symptoms and signs, as opposed to diagnoses, are acceptable for reporting purposes when a diagnosis has not been established (confirmed) by the provider. Chapter 18 of ICD-10-CM, Symptoms, Signs, and Abnormal Clinical and Laboratory Findings Not Elsewhere Classified (codes R00-R99) contains many, but not all codes for symptoms.

E. Encounters for circumstances other than a disease or injury
ICD-10-CM provides codes to deal with encounters for circumstances other than a disease or injury. The Factors Influencing Health Status and Contact with Health Services codes (Z00-Z99) are provided to deal with occasions when circumstances other than a disease or injury are recorded as diagnosis or problems.

See Section I.C.21., Factors influencing health status and contact with health services.

F. Level of Detail in Coding

1. ICD-10-CM codes with 3, 4, 5, 6 or 7 characters
ICD-10-CM is composed of codes with 3, 4, 5, 6 or 7 characters. Codes with three characters are included in ICD-10-CM as the heading of a category of codes that may be further subdivided by the use of fourth, fifth, sixth or seventh characters to provide greater specificity.

2. Use of full number of characters required for a code
A 3-character code is to be used only if it is not further subdivided. A code is invalid if it has not been coded to the full number of characters required for that code, including the 7th character, if applicable.

3. Highest level of specificity
Code to the highest level of specificity when supported by the medical record documentation.

G. ICD-10-CM code for the diagnosis, condition, problem, or other reason for encounter/visit
List first the ICD-10-CM code for the diagnosis, condition, problem, or other reason for encounter/visit shown in the medical record to be chiefly responsible for the services provided. List additional codes that describe any coexisting conditions. In some cases the first-listed diagnosis may be a symptom when a diagnosis has not been established (confirmed) by the provider.

H. Uncertain diagnosis
Do not code diagnoses documented as "probable," "suspected," "questionable," "rule out," "compatible with," "consistent with," or "working diagnosis" or other similar terms indicating uncertainty. Rather, code the condition(s) to the highest degree of certainty for that encounter/visit, such as symptoms, signs, abnormal test results, or other reason for the visit.

Please note: This differs from the coding practices used by short-term, acute care, long-term care and psychiatric hospitals.

I. Chronic diseases
Chronic diseases treated on an ongoing basis may be coded and reported as many times as the patient receives treatment and care for the condition(s)

J. Code all documented conditions that coexist
Code all documented conditions that coexist at the time of the encounter/visit, and that require or affect patient care treatment or management. Do not code conditions that were previously treated and no longer exist. However, history codes (categories Z80-Z87) may be used as secondary codes if the historical condition or family history has an impact on current care or influences treatment.

K. Patients receiving diagnostic services only
For patients receiving diagnostic services only during an encounter/visit, sequence first the diagnosis, condition, problem, or other reason for encounter/visit shown in the medical record to be chiefly responsible for the outpatient services provided during the encounter/visit. Codes for other diagnoses (e.g., chronic conditions) may be sequenced as additional diagnoses.

For encounters for routine laboratory/radiology testing in the absence of any signs, symptoms, or associated diagnosis, assign Z01.89, Encounter for other specified special examinations. If routine testing is performed during the same encounter as a test to evaluate a sign, symptom, or diagnosis, it is appropriate to assign both the Z code and the code describing the reason for the non-routine test.

For outpatient encounters for diagnostic tests that have been interpreted by a physician, and the final report is available at the time of coding, code any confirmed or definitive diagnosis(es) documented in the interpretation. Do not code related signs and symptoms as additional diagnoses.

Please note: This differs from the coding practice in the hospital inpatient setting regarding abnormal findings on test results.

L. Patients receiving therapeutic services only

For patients receiving therapeutic services only during an encounter/visit, sequence first the diagnosis, condition, problem, or other reason for encounter/visit shown in the medical record to be chiefly responsible for the outpatient services provided during the encounter/visit. Codes for other diagnoses (e.g., chronic conditions) may be sequenced as additional diagnoses.

The only exception to this rule is that when the primary reason for the admission/encounter is chemotherapy or radiation therapy, the appropriate Z code for the service is listed first, and the diagnosis or problem for which the service is being performed listed second.

M. Patients receiving preoperative evaluations only

For patients receiving preoperative evaluations only, sequence first a code from subcategory Z01.81, Encounter for pre-procedural examinations, to describe the pre-op consultations. Assign a code for the condition to describe the reason for the surgery as an additional diagnosis. Code also any findings related to the pre-op evaluation.

N. Ambulatory surgery

For ambulatory surgery, code the diagnosis for which the surgery was performed. If the postoperative diagnosis is known to be different from the preoperative diagnosis at the time the diagnosis is confirmed, select the postoperative diagnosis for coding, since it is the most definitive.

O. Routine outpatient prenatal visits

See Section I.C.15., Routine outpatient prenatal visits.

P. Encounters for general medical examinations with abnormal findings

The subcategories for encounters for general medical examinations, Z00.0- and encounter for routine child health examination, Z00.12-, provide codes for with and without abnormal findings. Should a general medical examination result in an abnormal finding, the code for general medical examination with abnormal finding should be assigned as the first-listed diagnosis. An examination with abnormal findings refers to a condition/diagnosis that is newly identified or a change in severity of a chronic condition (such as uncontrolled hypertension, or an acute exacerbation of chronic obstructive pulmonary disease) during a routine physical examination. A secondary code for the abnormal finding should also be coded.

Q. Encounters for routine health screenings

See Section I.C.21., Factors influencing health status and contact with health services, Screening

GUIDELINES (ICD-10-CM)

Appendix I
Present on Admission Reporting Guidelines

Introduction

These guidelines are to be used as a supplement to the ICD-10-CM Official Guidelines for Coding and Reporting to facilitate the assignment of the Present on Admission (POA) indicator for each diagnosis and external cause of injury code reported on claim forms (UB-04 and 837 Institutional).

These guidelines are not intended to replace any guidelines in the main body of the ICD-10-CM Official Guidelines for Coding and Reporting. The POA guidelines are not intended to provide guidance on when a condition should be coded, but rather, how to apply the POA indicator to the final set of diagnosis codes that have been assigned in accordance with Sections I, II, and III of the official coding guidelines. Subsequent to the assignment of the ICD-10-CM codes, the POA indicator should then be assigned to those conditions that have been coded.

As stated in the Introduction to the ICD-10-CM Official Guidelines for Coding and Reporting, a joint effort between the healthcare provider and the coder is essential to achieve complete and accurate documentation, code assignment, and reporting of diagnoses and procedures. The importance of consistent, complete documentation in the medical record cannot be overemphasized. Medical record documentation from any provider involved in the care and treatment of the patient may be used to support the determination of whether a condition was present on admission or not. In the context of the official coding guidelines, the term "provider" means a physician or any qualified healthcare practitioner who is legally accountable for establishing the patient's diagnosis.

These guidelines are not a substitute for the provider's clinical judgment as to the determination of whether a condition was/was not present on admission. The provider should be queried regarding issues related to the linking of signs/symptoms, timing of test results, and the timing of findings.

Please see the CDC website for the detailed list of ICD-10-CM codes that do not require the use of a POA indicator (https://www.cdc.gov/nchs/icd/icd-10-cm/files.html). The codes and categories on this exempt list are for circumstances regarding the healthcare encounter or factors influencing health status that do not represent a current disease or injury or that describe conditions that are always present on admission.

General Reporting Requirements

All claims involving inpatient admissions to general acute care hospitals or other facilities that are subject to a law or regulation mandating collection of present on admission information.

Present on admission is defined as present at the time the order for inpatient admission occurs—conditions that develop during an outpatient encounter, including emergency department, observation, or outpatient surgery, are considered as present on admission.

POA indicator is assigned to principal and secondary diagnoses (as defined in Section II of the Official Guidelines for Coding and Reporting) and the external cause of injury codes.

Issues related to inconsistent, missing, conflicting or unclear documentation must still be resolved by the provider.

If a condition would not be coded and reported based on UHDDS definitions and current official coding guidelines, then the POA indicator would not be reported.

Reporting Options

Y - Yes

N - No

U - Unknown

W - Clinically undetermined

Unreported/Not used - (Exempt from POA reporting)

Reporting Definitions

Y = present at the time of inpatient admission

N = not present at the time of inpatient admission

U = documentation is insufficient to determine if condition is present on admission

W = provider is unable to clinically determine whether condition was present on admission or not

Timeframe for POA Identification and Documentation

There is no required timeframe as to when a provider (per the definition of "provider" used in these guidelines) must identify or document a condition to be present on admission. In some clinical situations, it may not be possible for a provider to make a definitive diagnosis (or a condition may not be recognized or reported by the patient) for a period of time after admission. In some cases it may be several days before the provider arrives at a definitive diagnosis. This does not mean that the condition was not present on admission. Determination of whether the condition was present on admission or not will be based on the applicable POA guideline as identified in this document, or on the provider's best clinical judgment.

If at the time of code assignment the documentation is unclear as to whether a condition was present on admission or not, it is appropriate to query the provider for clarification.

Assigning the POA Indicator

Condition is on the "Exempt from Reporting" list

Leave the "present on admission" field blank if the condition is on the list of ICD-10-CM codes for which this field is not applicable. This is the only circumstance in which the field may be left blank.

POA Explicitly Documented

Assign "Y" for any condition the provider explicitly documents as being present on admission.

Assign "N" for any condition the provider explicitly documents as not present at the time of admission.

Conditions diagnosed prior to inpatient admission

Assign "Y" for conditions that were diagnosed prior to admission (example: hypertension, diabetes mellitus, asthma)

Conditions diagnosed during the admission but clearly present before admission

Assign "Y" for conditions diagnosed during the admission that were clearly present but not diagnosed until after admission occurred.

Diagnoses subsequently confirmed after admission are considered present on admission if at the time of admission they are documented as suspected, possible, rule out, differential diagnosis, or constitute an underlying cause of a symptom that is present at the time of admission.

Condition develops during outpatient encounter prior to inpatient admission

Assign "Y" for any condition that develops during an outpatient encounter prior to a written order for inpatient admission.

Documentation does not indicate whether condition was present on admission

Assign "U" when the medical record documentation is unclear as to whether the condition was present on admission. "U" should not be routinely assigned and used only in very limited circumstances. Coders are encouraged to query the providers when the documentation is unclear.

Documentation states that it cannot be determined whether the condition was or was not present on admission

Assign "W" when the medical record documentation indicates that it cannot be clinically determined whether or not the condition was present on admission.

Chronic condition with acute exacerbation during the admission

If a single code identifies both the chronic condition and the acute exacerbation, see POA guidelines pertaining to codes that contain multiple clinical concepts.

If a single code only identifies the chronic condition and not the acute exacerbation (e.g., acute exacerbation of chronic leukemia), assign "Y."

Conditions documented as possible, probable, suspected, or rule out at the time of discharge

If the final diagnosis contains a possible, probable, suspected, or rule out diagnosis, and this diagnosis was based on signs, symptoms or clinical findings suspected at the time of inpatient admission, assign "Y."

If the final diagnosis contains a possible, probable, suspected, or rule out diagnosis, and this diagnosis was based on signs, symptoms or clinical findings that were not present on admission, assign "N".

Conditions documented as impending or threatened at the time of discharge

If the final diagnosis contains an impending or threatened diagnosis, and this diagnosis is based on symptoms or clinical findings that were present on admission, assign "Y".

If the final diagnosis contains an impending or threatened diagnosis, and this diagnosis is based on symptoms or clinical findings that were not present on admission, assign "N".

Acute and Chronic Conditions

Assign "Y" for acute conditions that are present at time of admission and "N" for acute conditions that are not present at time of admission.

Assign "Y" for chronic conditions, even though the condition may not be diagnosed until after admission.

If a single code identifies both an acute and chronic condition, see the POA guidelines for codes that contain multiple clinical concepts.

Codes That Contain Multiple Clinical Concepts

Assign "N" if at least one of the clinical concepts included in the code was not present on admission (e.g., COPD with acute exacerbation and the exacerbation was not present on admission; gastric ulcer that does not start bleeding until after admission; asthma patient develops status asthmaticus after admission).

Assign "Y" if all of the clinical concepts included in the code were present on admission (e.g., duodenal ulcer that perforates prior to admission).

For infection codes that include the causal organism, assign "Y" if the infection (or signs of the infection) were present on admission, even though the culture results may not be known until after admission (e.g., patient is admitted with pneumonia and the provider documents Pseudomonas as the causal organism a few days later).

Same Diagnosis Code for Two or More Conditions

When the same ICD-10-CM diagnosis code applies to two or more conditions during the same encounter (e.g., two separate conditions classified to the same ICD-10-CM diagnosis code):

Assign "Y" if all conditions represented by the single ICD-10-CM code were present on admission (e.g., bilateral unspecified age-related cataracts).

Assign "N" if any of the conditions represented by the single ICD-10-CM code was not present on admission (e.g., traumatic secondary and recurrent hemorrhage and seroma is assigned to a single code T79.2, but only one of the conditions was present on admission).

Obstetrical conditions

Whether or not the patient delivers during the current hospitalization does not affect assignment of the POA indicator. The determining factor for POA assignment is whether the pregnancy complication or obstetrical condition described by the code was present at the time of admission or not.

If the pregnancy complication or obstetrical condition was present on admission (e.g., patient admitted in preterm labor), assign "Y".

If the pregnancy complication or obstetrical condition was not present on admission (e.g., 2nd degree laceration during delivery, postpartum hemorrhage that occurred during current hospitalization, fetal distress develops after admission), assign "N".

If the obstetrical code includes more than one diagnosis and any of the diagnoses identified by the code were not present on admission assign "N".

(e.g., Category O11, Pre-existing hypertension with pre-eclampsia)

Perinatal conditions

Newborns are not considered to be admitted until after birth. Therefore, any condition present at birth or that developed in utero is considered present at admission and should be assigned "Y". This includes conditions that occur during delivery (e.g., injury during delivery, meconium aspiration, exposure to streptococcus B in the vaginal canal).

Congenital conditions and anomalies

Assign "Y" for congenital conditions and anomalies except for categories Q00-Q99, Congenital anomalies, which are on the exempt list. Congenital conditions are always considered present on admission.

External cause of injury codes

Assign "Y" for any external cause code representing an external cause of morbidity that occurred prior to inpatient admission (e.g., patient fell out of bed at home, patient fell out of bed in emergency room prior to admission).

Assign "N" for any external cause code representing an external cause of morbidity that occurred during inpatient hospitalization (e.g., patient fell out of hospital bed during hospital stay, patient experienced an adverse reaction to a medication administered after inpatient admission).

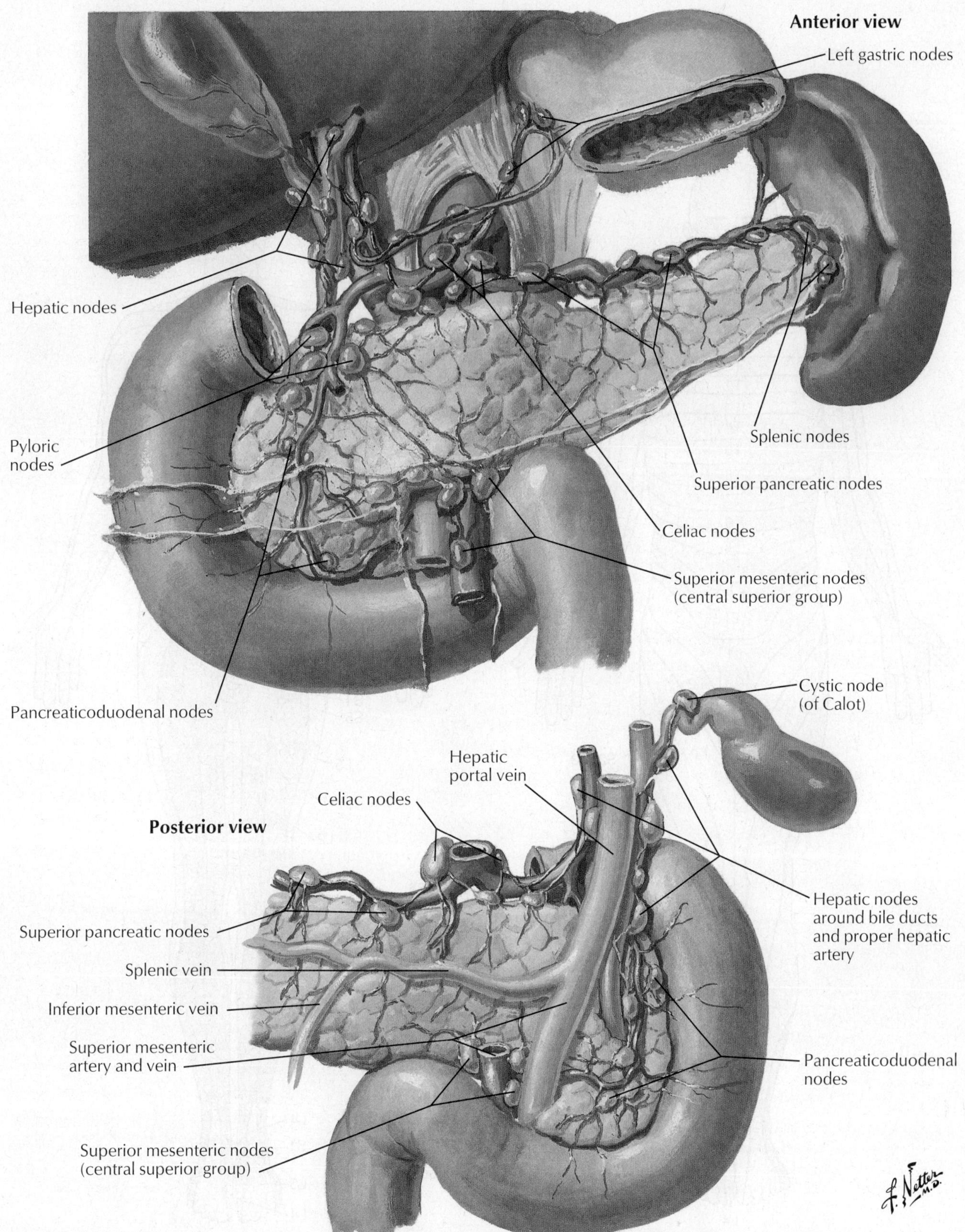

ANATOMY ILLUSTRATIONS

Plate 1 Lymph Vessels and Nodes of Pancreas.

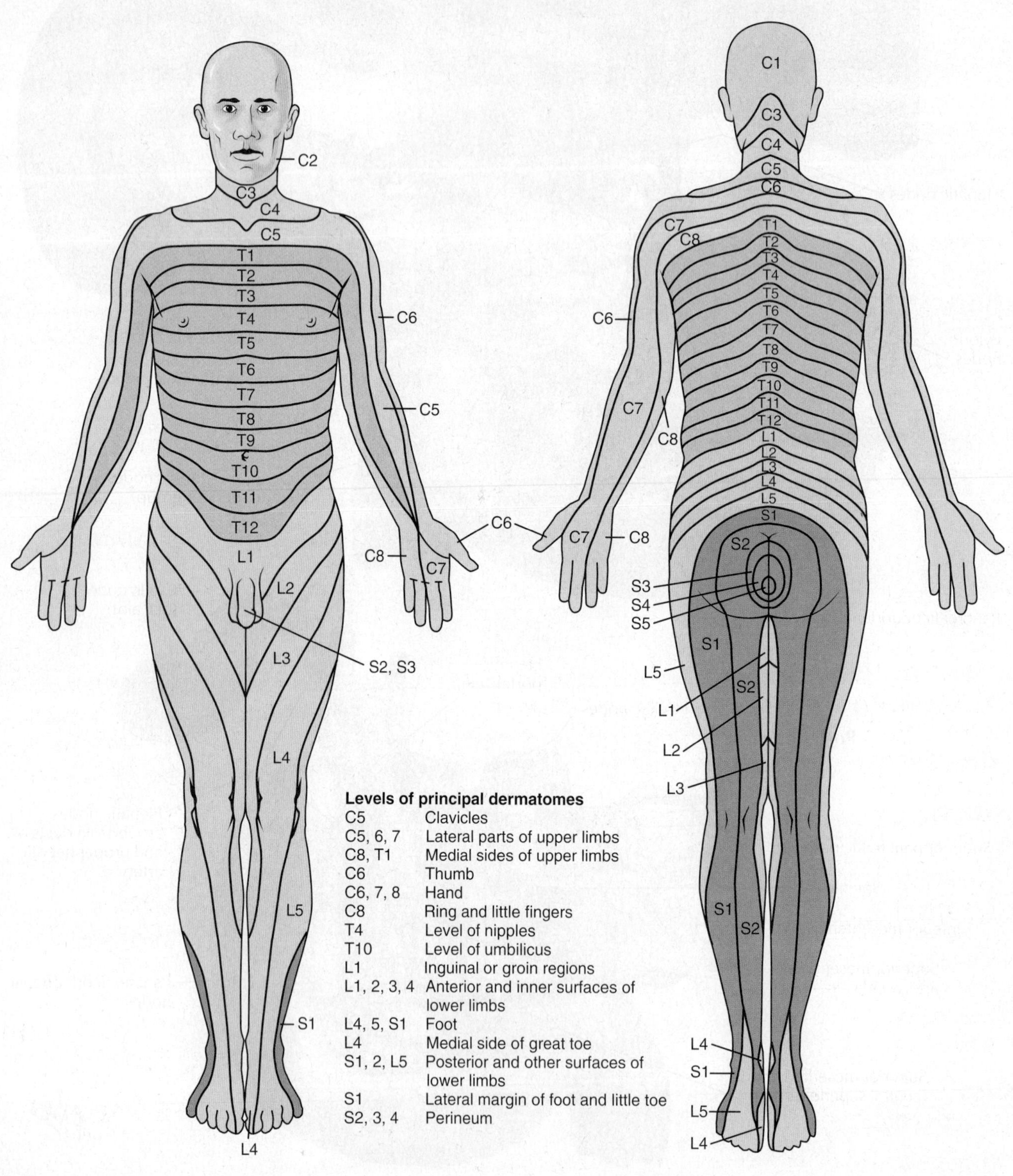

Plate 2 Schematic demarcation of Dermatomes. (Miller MD, Hart JA, MacKnight JM: Essential Orthopaedics, ed 2, Philadelphia, 2020, Elsevier.)

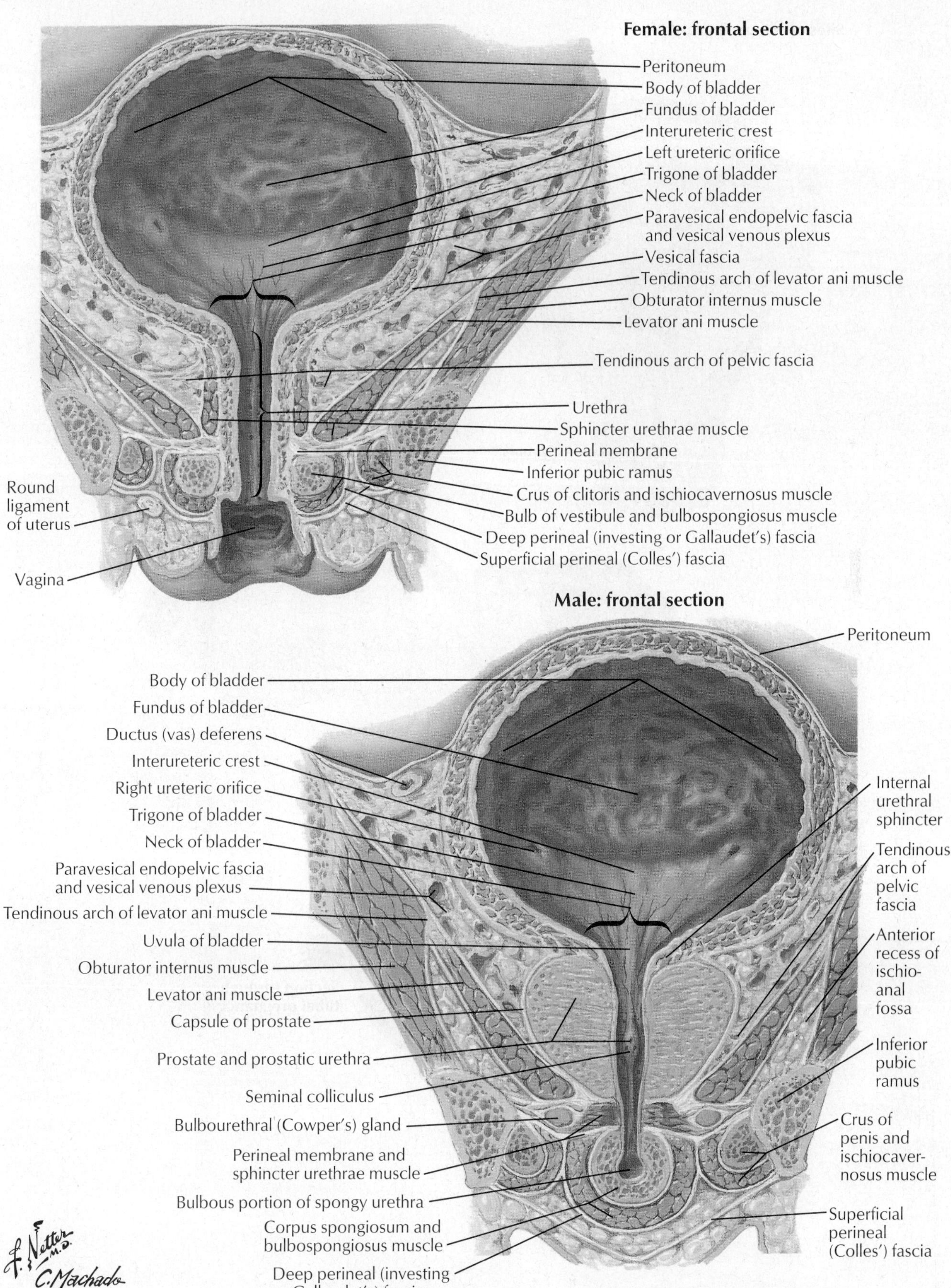
Female: frontal section
Peritoneum
Body of bladder
Fundus of bladder
Interureteric crest
Left ureteric orifice
Trigone of bladder
Neck of bladder
Paravesical endopelvic fascia and vesical venous plexus
Vesical fascia
Tendinous arch of levator ani muscle
Obturator internus muscle
Levator ani muscle
Tendinous arch of pelvic fascia
Urethra
Sphincter urethrae muscle
Perineal membrane
Inferior pubic ramus
Crus of clitoris and ischiocavernosus muscle
Bulb of vestibule and bulbospongiosus muscle
Deep perineal (investing or Gallaudet's) fascia
Superficial perineal (Colles') fascia
Round ligament of uterus
Vagina
Male: frontal section
Peritoneum
Body of bladder
Fundus of bladder
Ductus (vas) deferens
Interureteric crest
Right ureteric orifice
Trigone of bladder
Neck of bladder
Paravesical endopelvic fascia and vesical venous plexus
Tendinous arch of levator ani muscle
Uvula of bladder
Obturator internus muscle
Levator ani muscle
Capsule of prostate
Prostate and prostatic urethra
Seminal colliculus
Bulbourethral (Cowper's) gland
Perineal membrane and sphincter urethrae muscle
Bulbous portion of spongy urethra
Corpus spongiosum and bulbospongiosus muscle
Deep perineal (investing or Gallaudet's) fascia
Internal urethral sphincter
Tendinous arch of pelvic fascia
Anterior recess of ischio-anal fossa
Inferior pubic ramus
Crus of penis and ischiocavernosus muscle
Superficial perineal (Colles') fascia
F. Netter M.D.
C. Machado M.D.

Plate 3 Urinary Bladder: Female and Male.

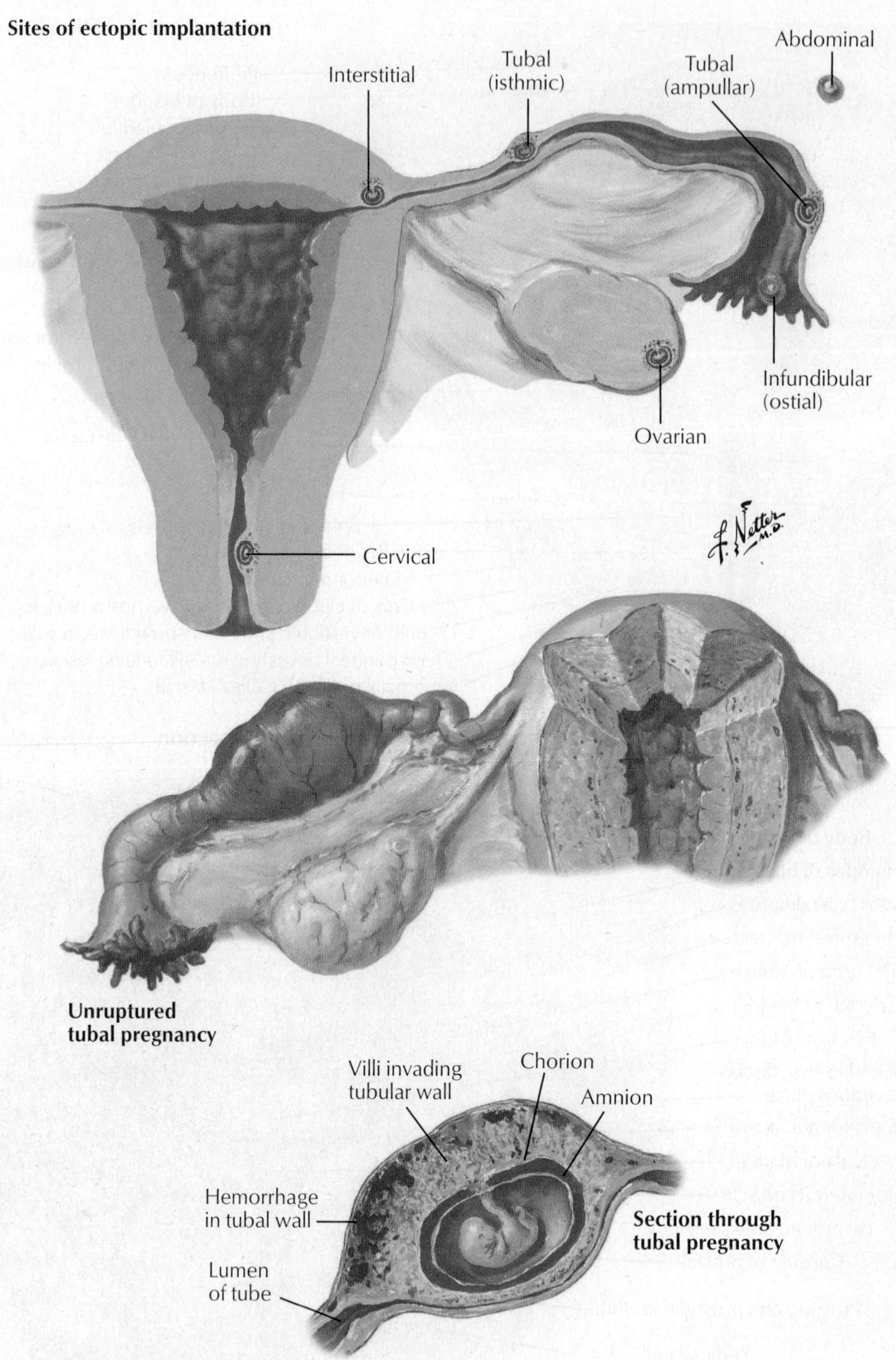

Plate 4 Ectopic Pregnancy. (www.netterimages.com. Image ID: 5148)

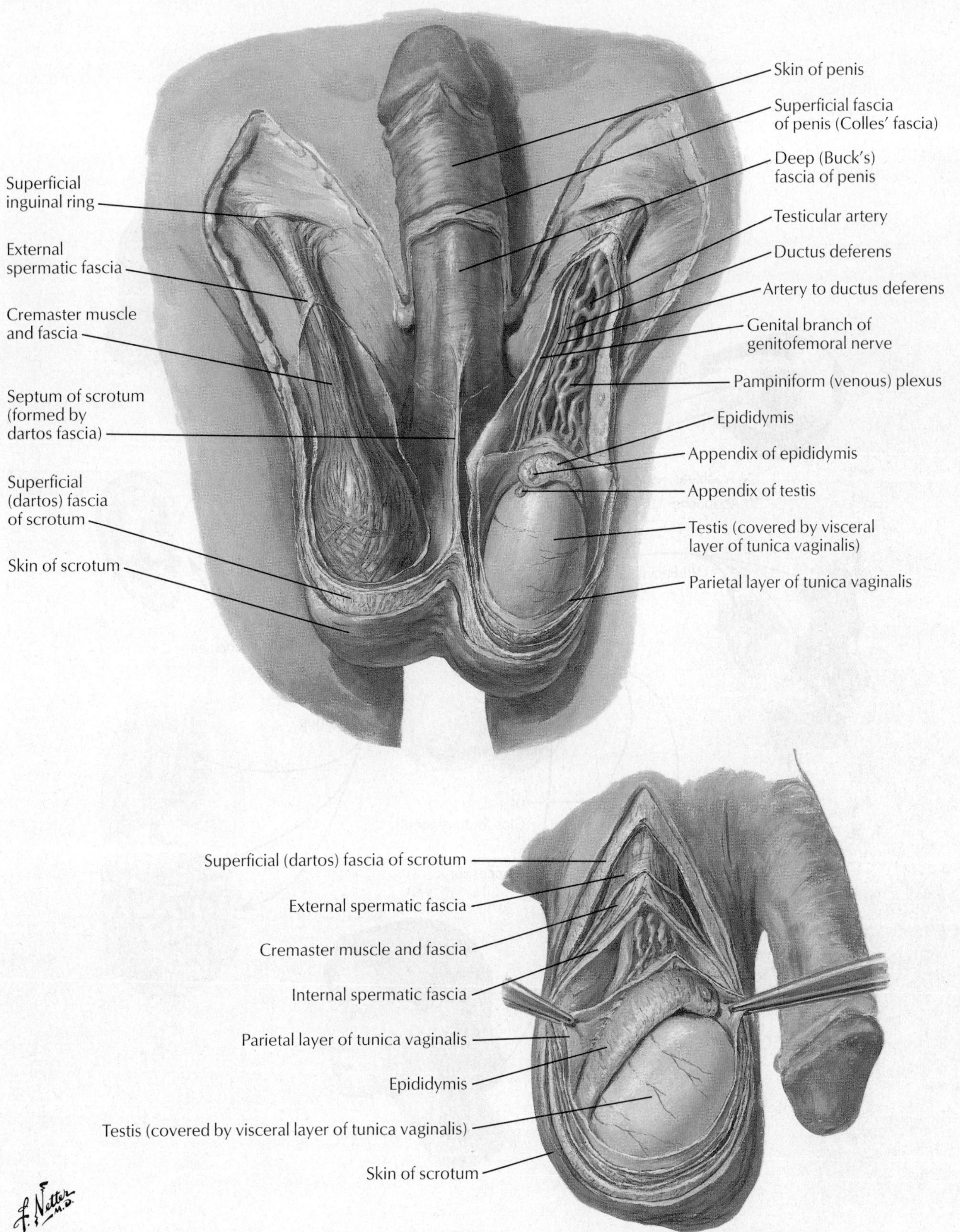
Skin of penis
Superficial fascia of penis (Colles' fascia)
Deep (Buck's) fascia of penis
Testicular artery
Ductus deferens
Artery to ductus deferens
Genital branch of genitofemoral nerve
Pampiniform (venous) plexus
Epididymis
Appendix of epididymis
Appendix of testis
Testis (covered by visceral layer of tunica vaginalis)
Parietal layer of tunica vaginalis
Superficial inguinal ring
External spermatic fascia
Cremaster muscle and fascia
Septum of scrotum (formed by dartos fascia)
Superficial (dartos) fascia of scrotum
Skin of scrotum
Superficial (dartos) fascia of scrotum
External spermatic fascia
Cremaster muscle and fascia
Internal spermatic fascia
Parietal layer of tunica vaginalis
Epididymis
Testis (covered by visceral layer of tunica vaginalis)
Skin of scrotum
F. Netter M.D.

Plate 5 Scrotum and Contents.

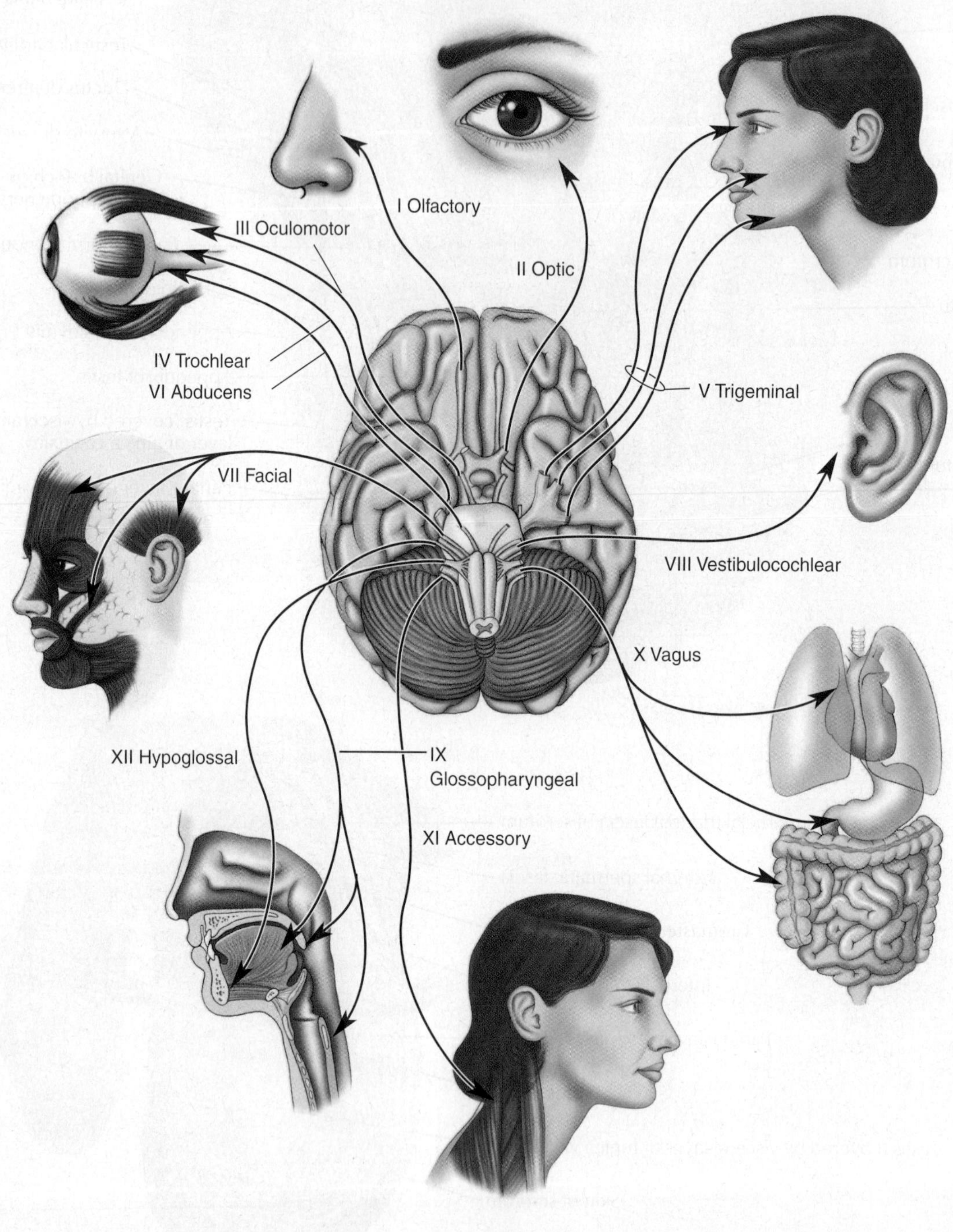

Plate 6 Cranial Nerves (12 pairs) are known by their numbers (Roman numerals) and names. (Herlihy BL: The Human Body in Health and Illness, ed 6, St. Louis, 2018, Elsevier.)

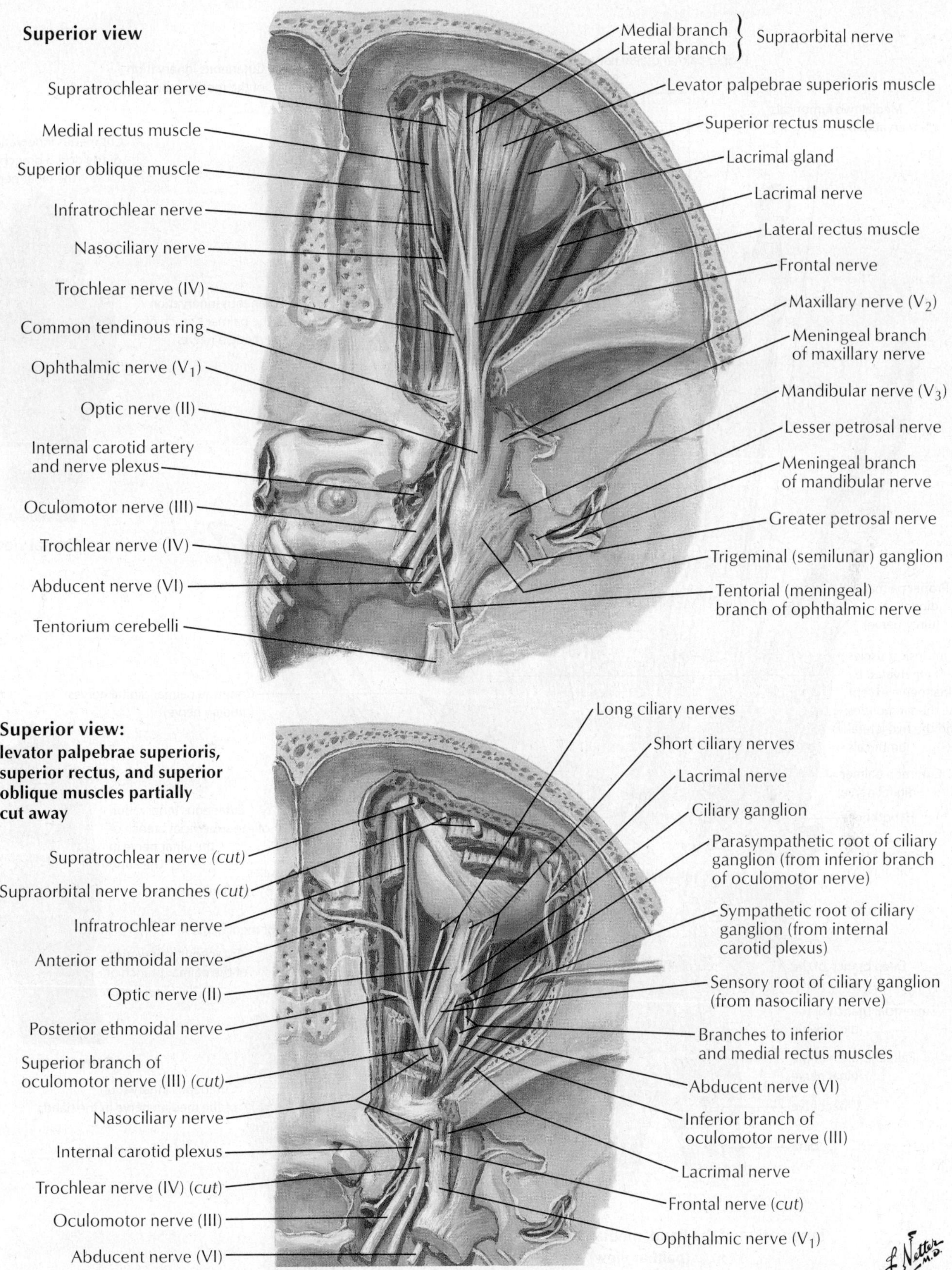
Superior view
Medial branch
Lateral branch
Supraorbital nerve
Supratrochlear nerve
Levator palpebrae superioris muscle
Medial rectus muscle
Superior rectus muscle
Superior oblique muscle
Lacrimal gland
Infratrochlear nerve
Lacrimal nerve
Nasociliary nerve
Lateral rectus muscle
Frontal nerve
Trochlear nerve (IV)
Maxillary nerve (V_2)
Common tendinous ring
Meningeal branch of maxillary nerve
Ophthalmic nerve (V_1)
Mandibular nerve (V_3)
Optic nerve (II)
Lesser petrosal nerve
Internal carotid artery and nerve plexus
Meningeal branch of mandibular nerve
Oculomotor nerve (III)
Greater petrosal nerve
Trochlear nerve (IV)
Trigeminal (semilunar) ganglion
Abducent nerve (VI)
Tentorial (meningeal) branch of ophthalmic nerve
Tentorium cerebelli
Superior view: levator palpebrae superioris, superior rectus, and superior oblique muscles partially cut away
Long ciliary nerves
Short ciliary nerves
Lacrimal nerve
Ciliary ganglion
Supratrochlear nerve (cut)
Parasympathetic root of ciliary ganglion (from inferior branch of oculomotor nerve)
Supraorbital nerve branches (cut)
Infratrochlear nerve
Sympathetic root of ciliary ganglion (from internal carotid plexus)
Anterior ethmoidal nerve
Optic nerve (II)
Sensory root of ciliary ganglion (from nasociliary nerve)
Posterior ethmoidal nerve
Branches to inferior and medial rectus muscles
Superior branch of oculomotor nerve (III) (cut)
Abducent nerve (VI)
Nasociliary nerve
Inferior branch of oculomotor nerve (III)
Internal carotid plexus
Lacrimal nerve
Trochlear nerve (IV) (cut)
Frontal nerve (cut)
Oculomotor nerve (III)
Ophthalmic nerve (V_1)
Abducent nerve (VI)
F. Netter M.D.

Plate 7 Nerves of Orbit.

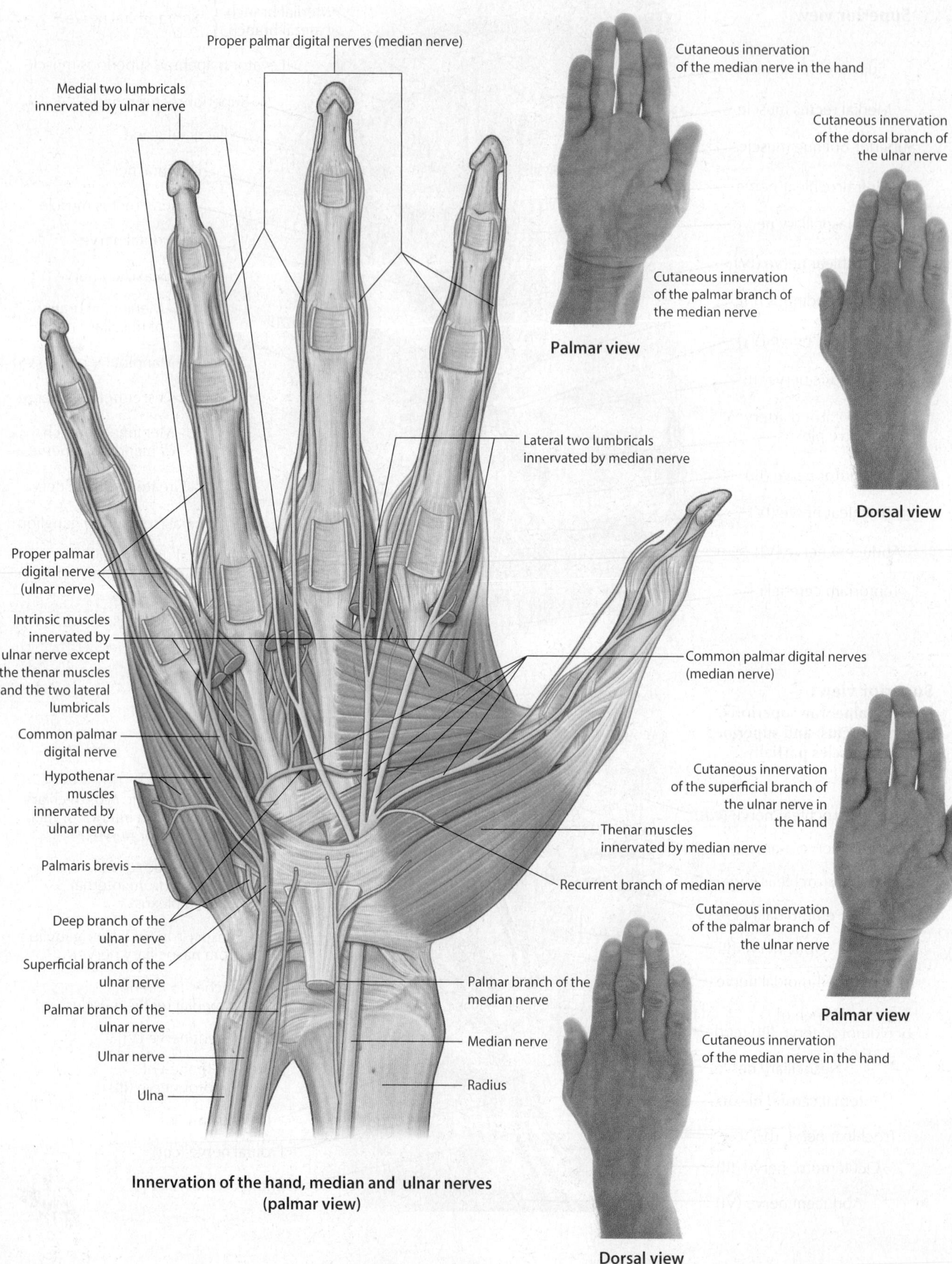

Plate 8 Innervation of the Hand: Median and Ulnar Nerves (From Drake RL, Vogl AW, Mitchell AWM, Tibbitts RM, Richardson PE: Gray's Atlas of Anatomy, ed 2, Philadelphia, 2015, Churchill Livingstone.)

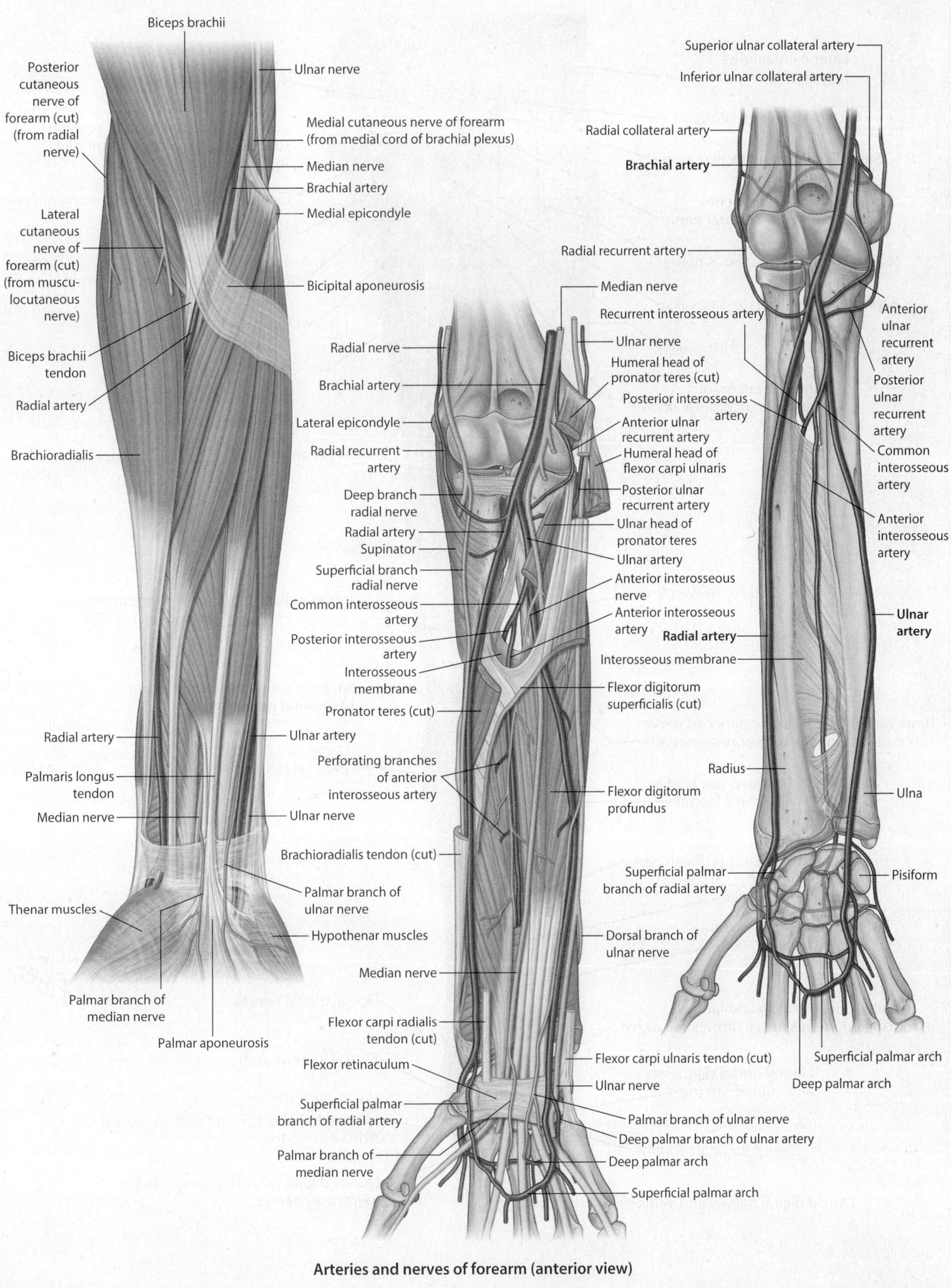

Biceps brachii

Posterior cutaneous nerve of forearm (cut) (from radial nerve)

Ulnar nerve

Medial cutaneous nerve of forearm (from medial cord of brachial plexus)

Median nerve

Brachial artery

Medial epicondyle

Lateral cutaneous nerve of forearm (cut) (from musculocutaneous nerve)

Bicipital aponeurosis

Biceps brachii tendon

Radial artery

Brachioradialis

Radial artery

Palmaris longus tendon

Median nerve

Thenar muscles

Palmar branch of median nerve

Palmar aponeurosis

Ulnar artery

Ulnar nerve

Brachioradialis tendon (cut)

Palmar branch of ulnar nerve

Hypothenar muscles

Median nerve

Flexor carpi radialis tendon (cut)

Flexor retinaculum

Superficial palmar branch of radial artery

Palmar branch of median nerve

Radial nerve

Brachial artery

Lateral epicondyle

Radial recurrent artery

Deep branch radial nerve

Radial artery

Supinator

Superficial branch radial nerve

Common interosseous artery

Posterior interosseous artery

Interosseous membrane

Pronator teres (cut)

Perforating branches of anterior interosseous artery

Median nerve

Recurrent interosseous artery

Ulnar nerve

Humeral head of pronator teres (cut)

Posterior interosseous artery

Anterior ulnar recurrent artery

Humeral head of flexor carpi ulnaris

Posterior ulnar recurrent artery

Ulnar head of pronator teres

Ulnar artery

Anterior interosseous nerve

Anterior interosseous artery

Interosseous membrane

Flexor digitorum superficialis (cut)

Flexor digitorum profundus

Superficial palmar branch of radial artery

Dorsal branch of ulnar nerve

Flexor carpi ulnaris tendon (cut)

Ulnar nerve

Palmar branch of ulnar nerve

Deep palmar branch of ulnar artery

Deep palmar arch

Superficial palmar arch

Superior ulnar collateral artery

Inferior ulnar collateral artery

Radial collateral artery

Brachial artery

Radial recurrent artery

Median nerve

Anterior ulnar recurrent artery

Posterior ulnar recurrent artery

Common interosseous artery

Anterior interosseous artery

Ulnar artery

Radial artery

Radius

Ulna

Superficial palmar branch of radial artery

Pisiform

Superficial palmar arch

Deep palmar arch

Arteries and nerves of forearm (anterior view)

Plate 9 Arteries and Nerves of the Forearm (Anterior View) (From Drake RL, Vogl AW, Mitchell AWM, Tibbitts RM, Richardson PE: Gray's Atlas of Anatomy, ed 2, Philadelphia, 2015, Churchill Livingstone.)

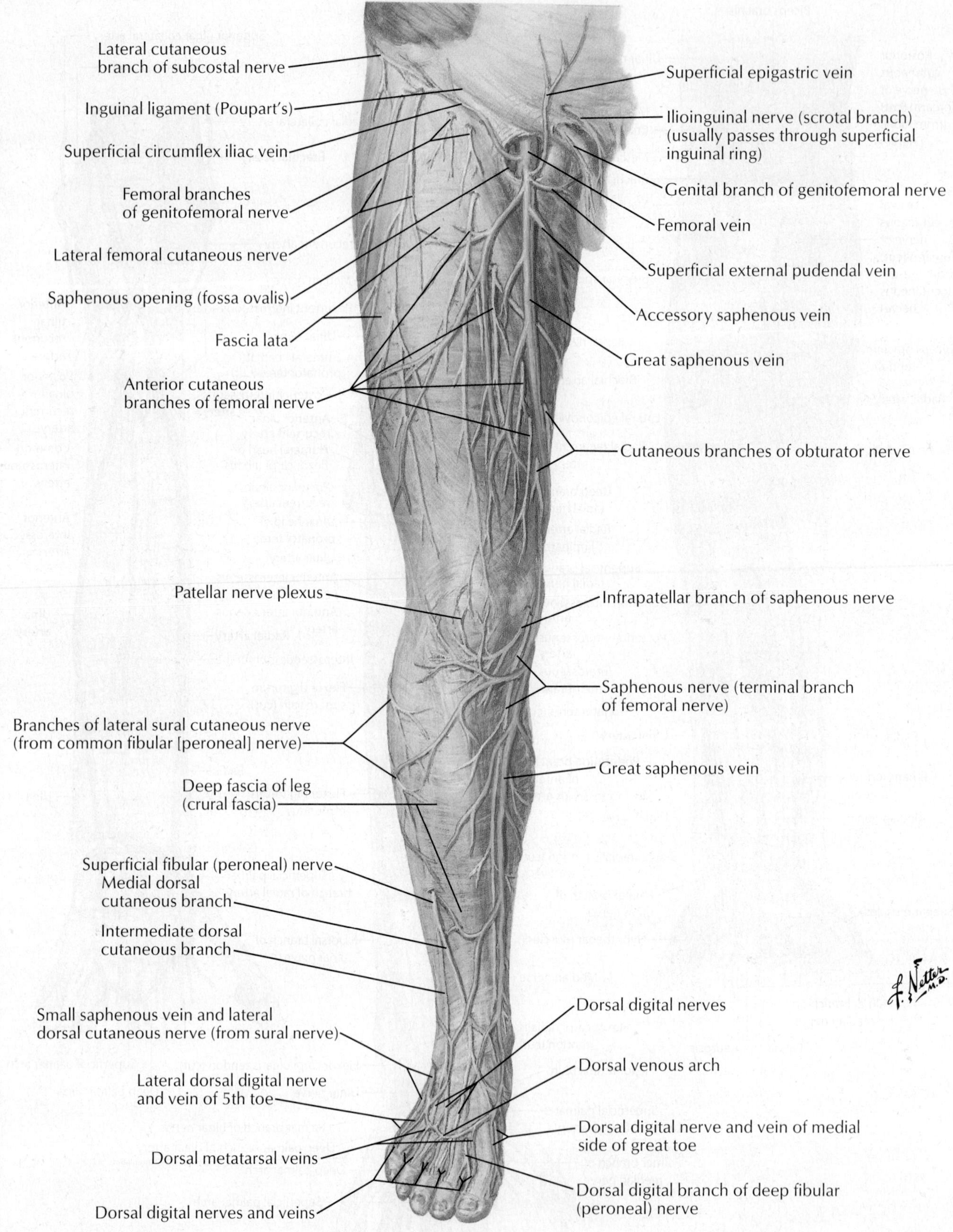
Lateral cutaneous branch of subcostal nerve
Inguinal ligament (Poupart's)
Superficial circumflex iliac vein
Femoral branches of genitofemoral nerve
Lateral femoral cutaneous nerve
Saphenous opening (fossa ovalis)
Fascia lata
Anterior cutaneous branches of femoral nerve
Superficial epigastric vein
Ilioinguinal nerve (scrotal branch) (usually passes through superficial inguinal ring)
Genital branch of genitofemoral nerve
Femoral vein
Superficial external pudendal vein
Accessory saphenous vein
Great saphenous vein
Cutaneous branches of obturator nerve
Patellar nerve plexus
Infrapatellar branch of saphenous nerve
Saphenous nerve (terminal branch of femoral nerve)
Branches of lateral sural cutaneous nerve (from common fibular [peroneal] nerve)
Great saphenous vein
Deep fascia of leg (crural fascia)
Superficial fibular (peroneal) nerve
Medial dorsal cutaneous branch
Intermediate dorsal cutaneous branch
Small saphenous vein and lateral dorsal cutaneous nerve (from sural nerve)
Lateral dorsal digital nerve and vein of 5th toe
Dorsal metatarsal veins
Dorsal digital nerves and veins
Dorsal digital nerves
Dorsal venous arch
Dorsal digital nerve and vein of medial side of great toe
Dorsal digital branch of deep fibular (peroneal) nerve
F. Netter M.D.

Plate 10 Superficial Nerves and Veins of Lower Limb: Anterior View.

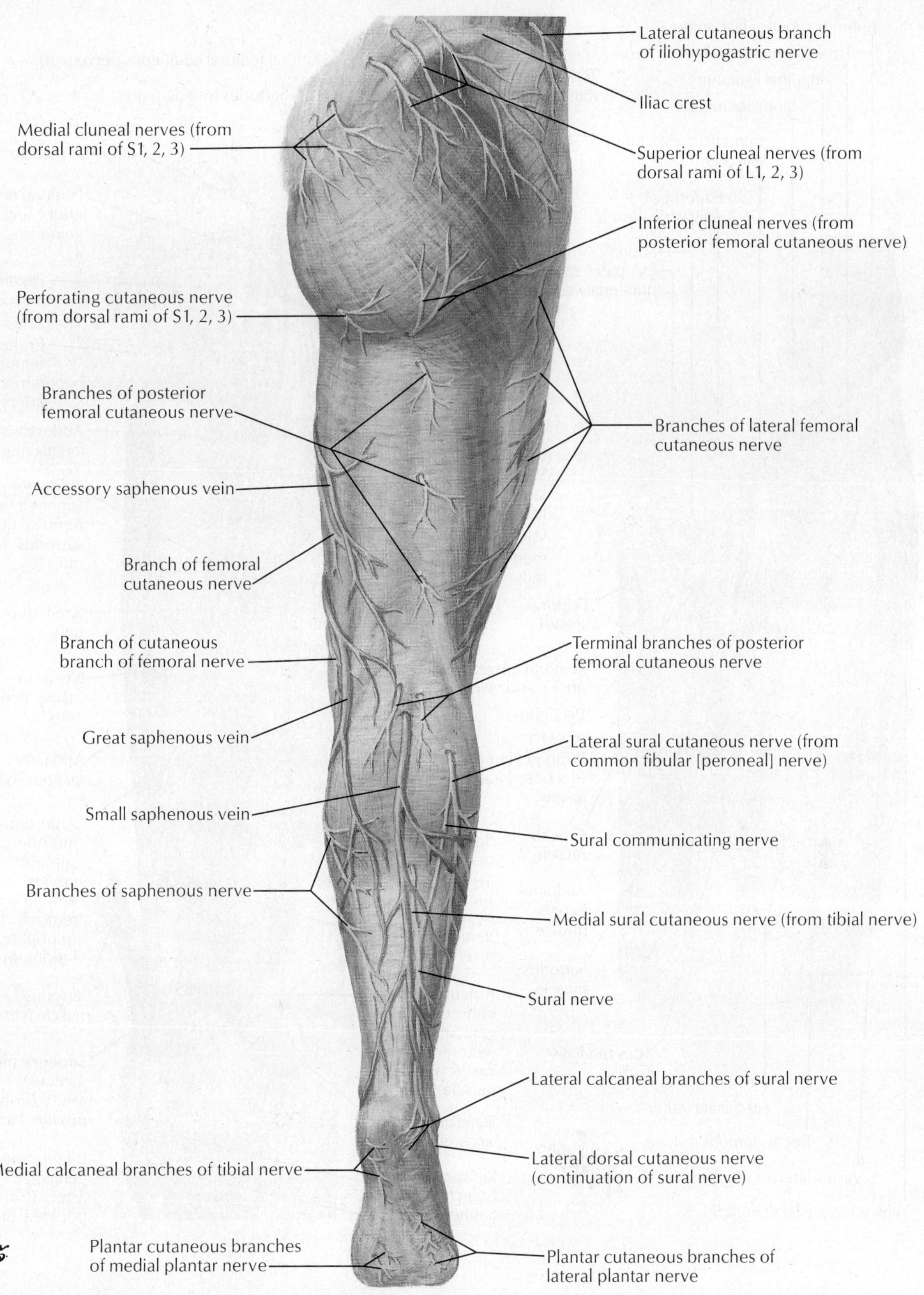

Plate 11 Superficial Nerves and Veins of Lower Limb: Posterior View. Image ID: 4669)

Lateral cutaneous branch of iliohypogastric nerve

Iliac crest

Superior cluneal nerves (from dorsal rami of L1, 2, 3)

Inferior cluneal nerves (from posterior femoral cutaneous nerve)

Medial cluneal nerves (from dorsal rami of S1, 2, 3)

Perforating cutaneous nerve (from dorsal rami of S1, 2, 3)

Branches of posterior femoral cutaneous nerve

Accessory saphenous vein

Branches of lateral femoral cutaneous nerve

Branch of femoral cutaneous nerve

Branch of cutaneous branch of femoral nerve

Terminal branches of posterior femoral cutaneous nerve

Great saphenous vein

Lateral sural cutaneous nerve (from common fibular [peroneal] nerve)

Small saphenous vein

Sural communicating nerve

Branches of saphenous nerve

Medial sural cutaneous nerve (from tibial nerve)

Sural nerve

Lateral calcaneal branches of sural nerve

Medial calcaneal branches of tibial nerve

Lateral dorsal cutaneous nerve (continuation of sural nerve)

Plantar cutaneous branches of medial plantar nerve

Plantar cutaneous branches of lateral plantar nerve

ANATOMY ILLUSTRATIONS

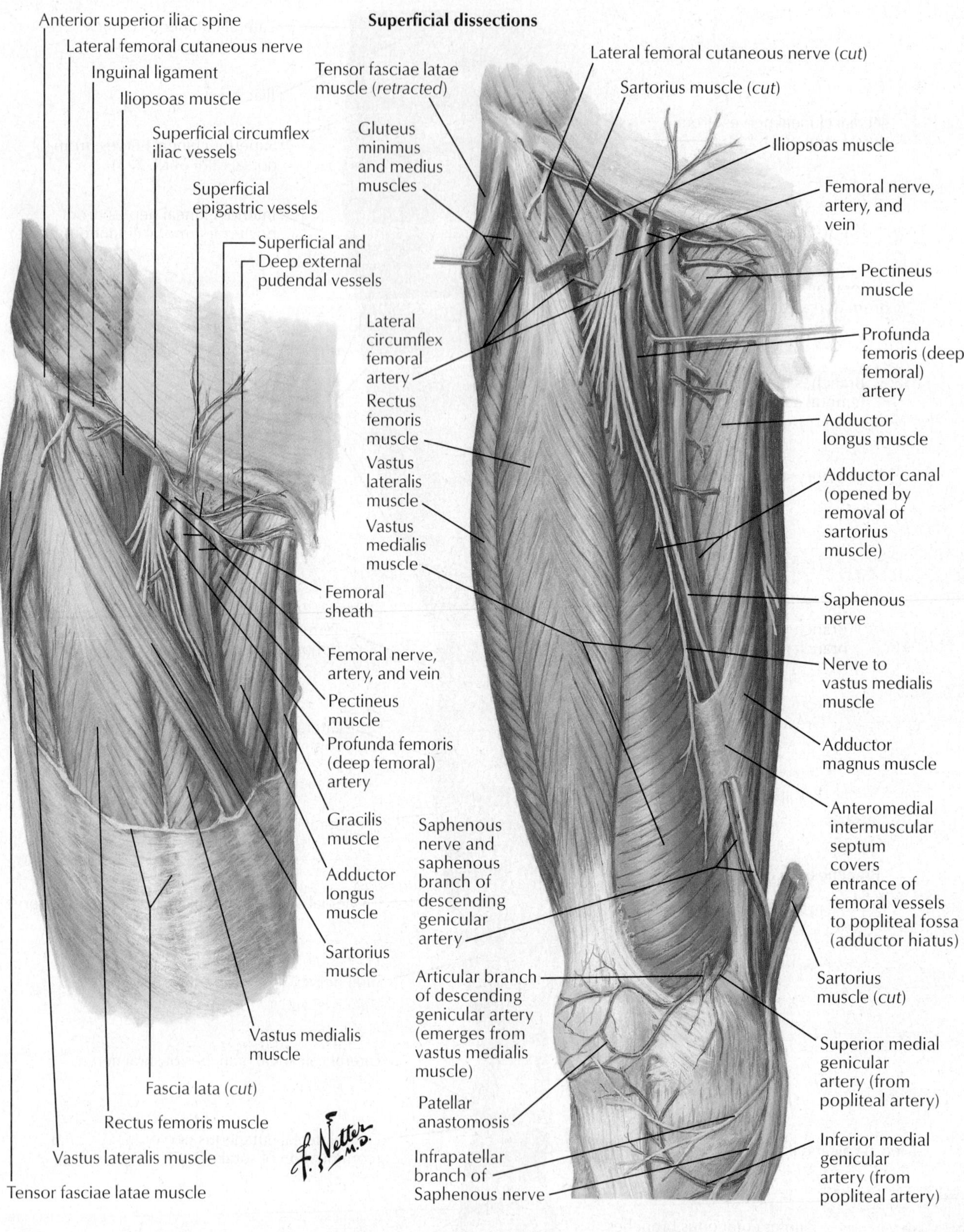
Superficial dissections
Anterior superior iliac spine
Lateral femoral cutaneous nerve
Inguinal ligament
Iliopsoas muscle
Superficial circumflex iliac vessels
Superficial epigastric vessels
Superficial and Deep external pudendal vessels
Femoral sheath
Femoral nerve, artery, and vein
Pectineus muscle
Profunda femoris (deep femoral) artery
Gracilis muscle
Adductor longus muscle
Sartorius muscle
Vastus medialis muscle
Fascia lata (cut)
Rectus femoris muscle
Vastus lateralis muscle
Tensor fasciae latae muscle
Tensor fasciae latae muscle (retracted)
Gluteus minimus and medius muscles
Lateral circumflex femoral artery
Rectus femoris muscle
Vastus lateralis muscle
Vastus medialis muscle
Saphenous nerve and saphenous branch of descending genicular artery
Articular branch of descending genicular artery (emerges from vastus medialis muscle)
Patellar anastomosis
Infrapatellar branch of Saphenous nerve
Lateral femoral cutaneous nerve (cut)
Sartorius muscle (cut)
Iliopsoas muscle
Femoral nerve, artery, and vein
Pectineus muscle
Profunda femoris (deep femoral) artery
Adductor longus muscle
Adductor canal (opened by removal of sartorius muscle)
Saphenous nerve
Nerve to vastus medialis muscle
Adductor magnus muscle
Anteromedial intermuscular septum covers entrance of femoral vessels to popliteal fossa (adductor hiatus)
Sartorius muscle (cut)
Superior medial genicular artery (from popliteal artery)
Inferior medial genicular artery (from popliteal artery)
F. Netter M.D.

Plate 12 Arteries and Nerves of Thigh: Anterior Views. Image ID: 4475)

Deep dissection

Deep circumflex iliac artery

Lateral femoral cutaneous nerve

Sartorius muscle (cut)

Iliopsoas muscle

Tensor fasciae latae muscle (retracted)

Gluteus medius and minimus muscles

Femoral nerve

Rectus femoris muscle (cut)

Ascending, transverse and descending branches of Lateral circumflex femoral artery

Medial circumflex femoral artery

Pectineus muscle (cut)

Profunda femoris (deep femoral) artery

Perforating branches

Adductor longus muscle (cut)

Vastus lateralis muscle

Vastus intermedius muscle

Rectus femoris muscle (cut)

Saphenous nerve

Anteromedial intermuscular septum (opened)

Vastus medialis muscle

Quadriceps femoris tendon

Patella and patellar anastomosis

Medial patellar retinaculum

Patellar ligament

External iliac artery and vein

Inguinal ligament (Poupart's)

Femoral artery and vein (cut)

Pectineus muscle (cut)

Obturator canal

Obturator externus muscle

Adductor longus muscle (cut)

Anterior branch and Posterior branch of obturator nerve

Quadratus femoris muscle

Adductor brevis muscle

Branches of posterior branch of obturator nerve

Adductor magnus muscle

Gracilis muscle

Cutaneous branch of obturator nerve

Femoral artery and vein (cut)

Descending genicular artery
Articular branch
Saphenous branch

Adductor hiatus

Sartorius muscle (cut)

Adductor magnus tendon

Adductor tubercle on medial epicondyle of femur

Superior medial genicular artery (from popliteal artery)

Infrapatellar branch of Saphenous nerve

Inferior medial genicular artery (from popliteal artery)

ANATOMY ILLUSTRATIONS

Plate 13 Arteries and Nerves of Thigh: Posterior View. (Copyright 2024 Elsevier Inc. All rights reserved. www.netterimages.com. Image ID: 49316)

ANATOMY ILLUSTRATIONS

Deep dissection

Superior cluneal nerves
Gluteus maximus muscle (*cut*)
Medial cluneal nerves
Inferior gluteal artery and nerve
Pudendal nerve
Nerve to obturator internus (and superior gemellus)
Posterior femoral cutaneous nerve
Sacrotuberous ligament
Ischial tuberosity
Inferior cluneal nerves (*cut*)
Adductor magnus muscle
Gracilis muscle
Sciatic nerve
Muscular branches of sciatic nerve
Semitendinosus muscle (*retracted*)
Semimembranosus muscle
Sciatic nerve
Articular branch
Adductor hiatus
Popliteal vein and artery
Superior medial genicular artery
Medial epicondyle of femur
Tibial nerve
Gastrocnemius muscle (medial head)
Medial sural cutaneous nerve
Small saphenous vein
Iliac crest
Gluteal aponeurosis and gluteus medius muscle (*cut*)
Superior gluteal artery and nerve
Gluteus minimus muscle
Tensor fasciae latae muscle
Piriformis muscle
Gluteus medius muscle (*cut*)
Superior gemellus muscle
Greater trochanter of femur
Obturator internus muscle
Inferior gemellus muscle
Gluteus maximus muscle (*cut*)
Quadratus femoris muscle
Medial circumflex femoral artery
Vastus lateralis muscle and iliotibial tract
Adductor minimus part of adductor magnus muscle
1st perforating artery (from profunda femoris artery)
Adductor magnus muscle
2nd and 3rd perforating arteries (from profunda femoris artery)
4th perforating artery (from profunda femoris artery)
Long head (*retracted*) } Biceps femoris muscle
Short head
Superior lateral genicular artery
Common fibular (peroneal) nerve
Plantaris muscle
Gastrocnemius muscle (lateral head)
Lateral sural cutaneous nerve
F. Netter M.D.

Plate 14 Arteries and Nerves of Thigh: Posterior View. Image ID: 49317)

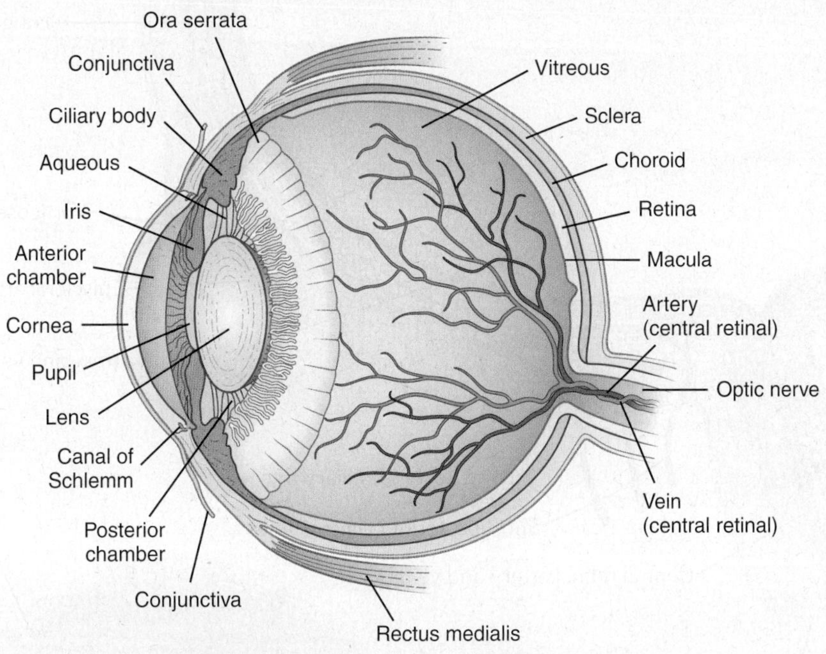

Plate 15 Anatomy of the eye. (Dehn RW, Asprey DP. Essential Clinical Procedures, ed 3, Philadelphia, 2013, Saunders.)

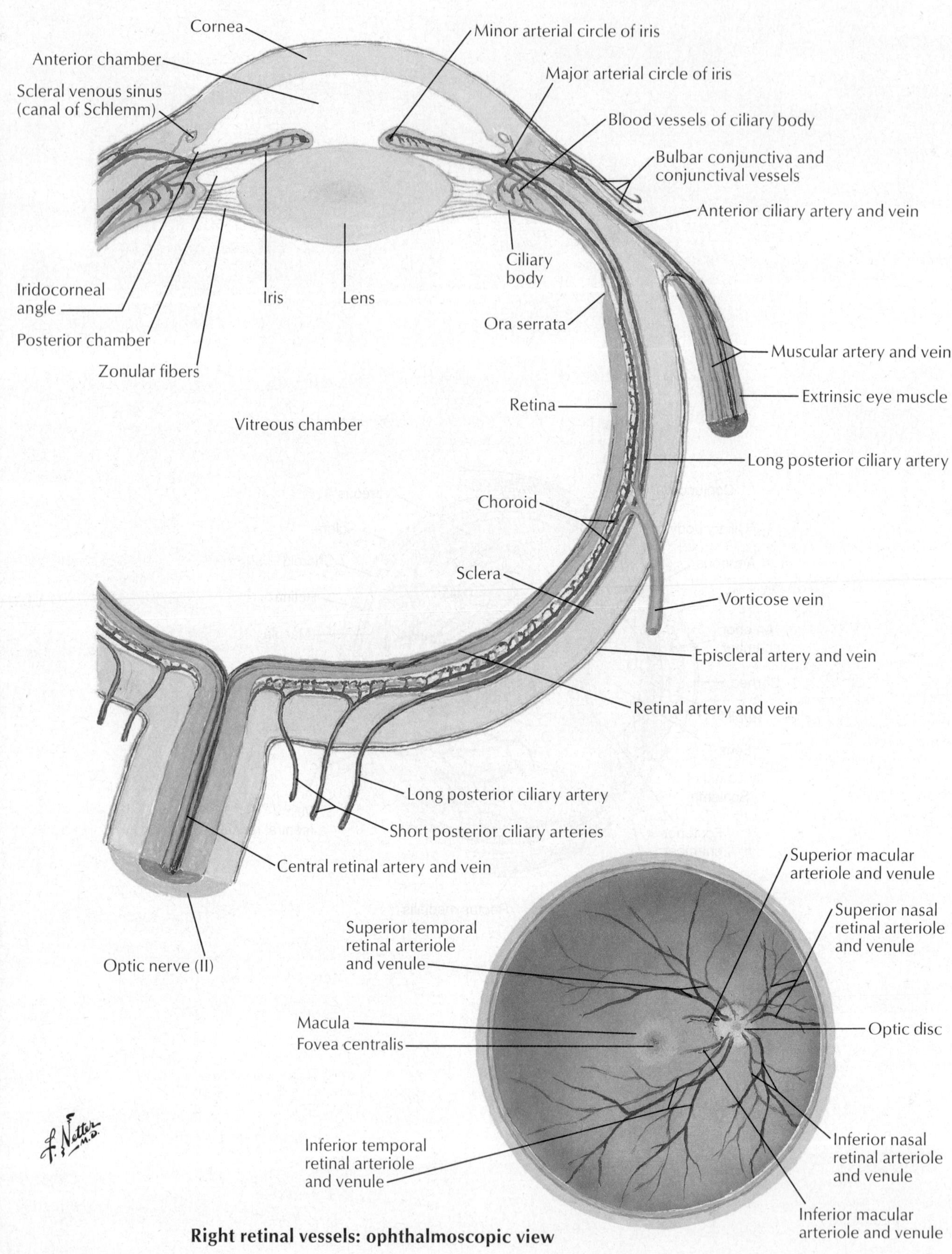

Cornea

Minor arterial circle of iris

Anterior chamber

Major arterial circle of iris

Scleral venous sinus
(canal of Schlemm)

Blood vessels of ciliary body

Bulbar conjunctiva and
conjunctival vessels

Anterior ciliary artery and vein

Iridocorneal
angle

Iris

Lens

Ciliary
body

Posterior chamber

Ora serrata

Muscular artery and vein

Zonular fibers

Extrinsic eye muscle

Vitreous chamber

Retina

Long posterior ciliary artery

Choroid

Sclera

Vorticose vein

Episcleral artery and vein

Retinal artery and vein

Long posterior ciliary artery

Short posterior ciliary arteries

Central retinal artery and vein

Optic nerve (II)

Superior temporal
retinal arteriole
and venule

Macula

Fovea centralis

Superior macular
arteriole and venule

Superior nasal
retinal arteriole
and venule

Optic disc

Inferior nasal
retinal arteriole
and venule

Inferior temporal
retinal arteriole
and venule

Inferior macular
arteriole and venule

Right retinal vessels: ophthalmoscopic view

Plate 16 Intrinsic Arteries and Veins of Eye.

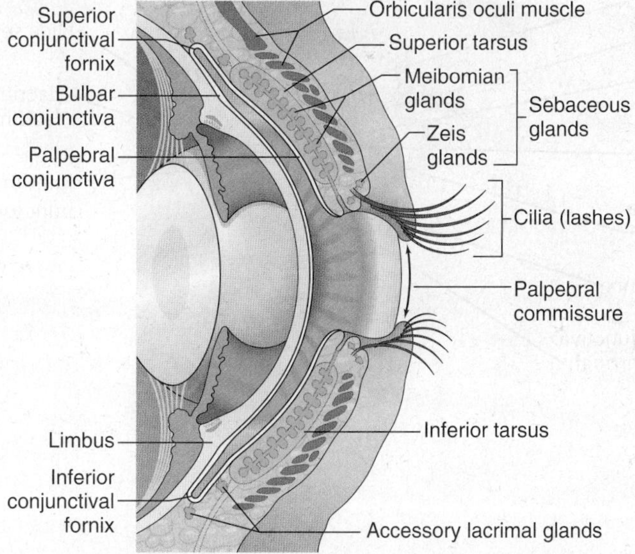

Plate 17 Anatomy of the conjunctiva and eyelids. (Kumar V, Abbas AK, Aster JC: Robbins and Cotran Pathologic Basis of Disease, ed 9, Philadelphia, 2013, Saunders.)

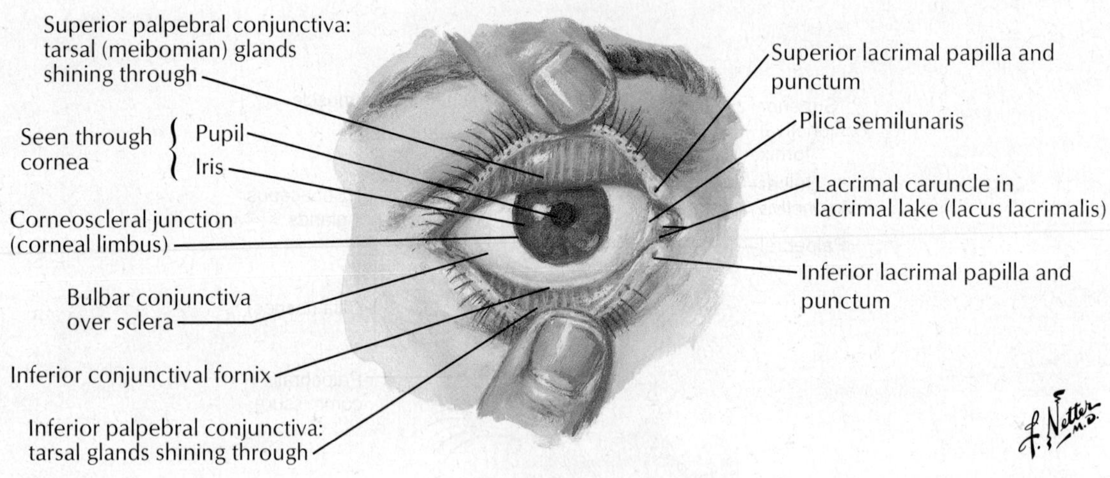
Superior palpebral conjunctiva: tarsal (meibomian) glands shining through
Seen through cornea
Pupil
Iris
Corneoscleral junction (corneal limbus)
Bulbar conjunctiva over sclera
Inferior conjunctival fornix
Inferior palpebral conjunctiva: tarsal glands shining through
Superior lacrimal papilla and punctum
Plica semilunaris
Lacrimal caruncle in lacrimal lake (lacus lacrimalis)
Inferior lacrimal papilla and punctum
F. Netter M.D.

Plate 18 Eyelid.

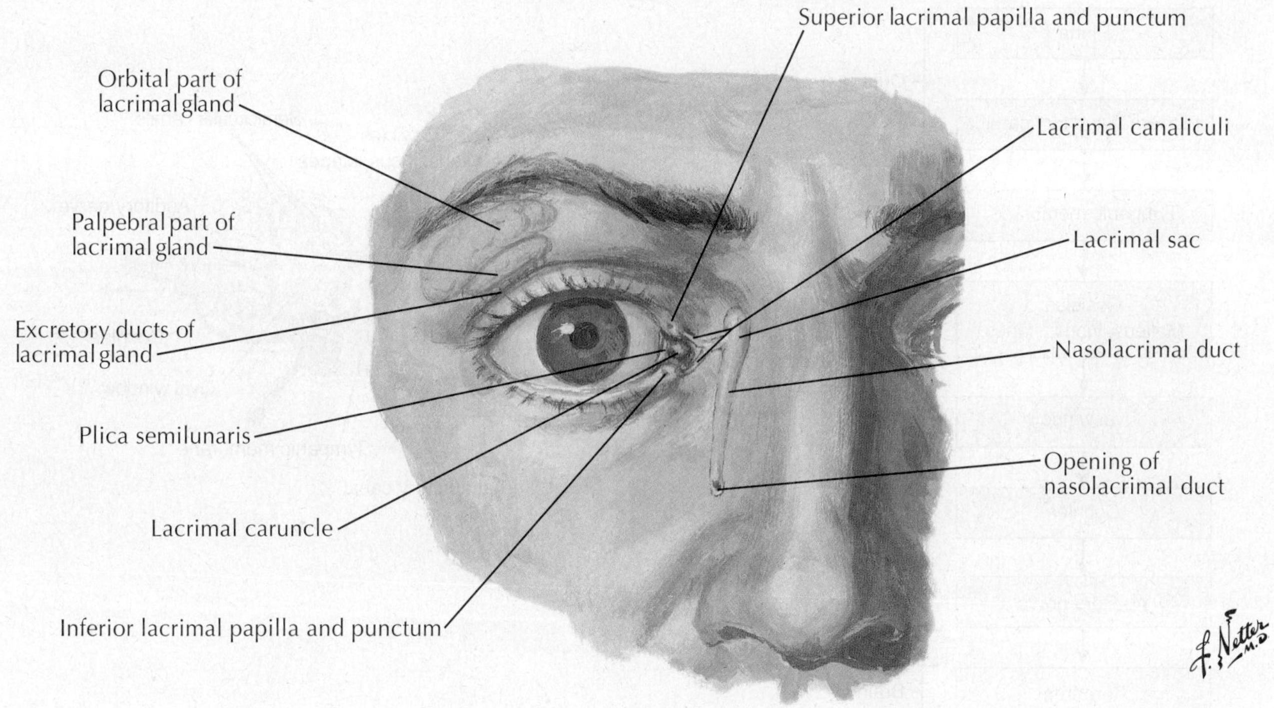

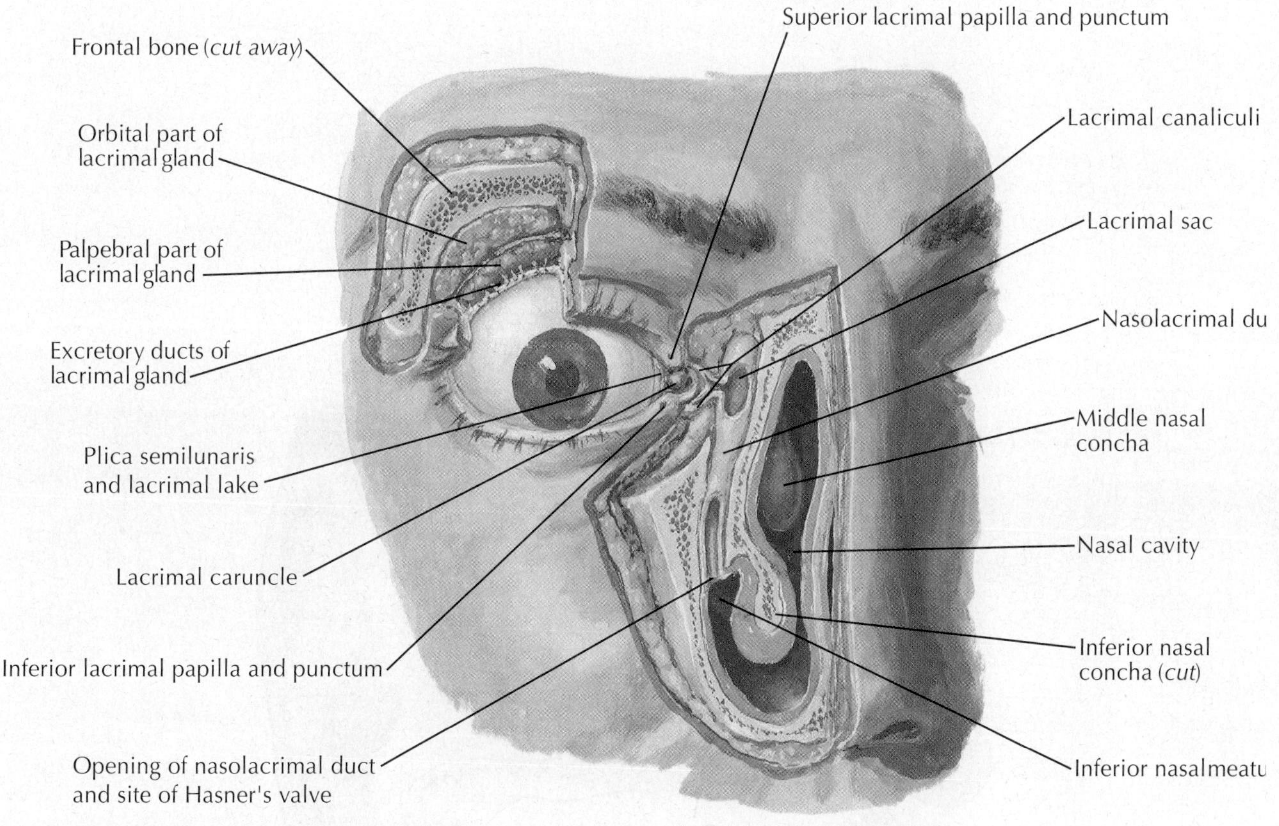

Plate 19 Lacrimal Apparatus.

Orbital part of lacrimal gland

Palpebral part of lacrimal gland

Excretory ducts of lacrimal gland

Plica semilunaris

Lacrimal caruncle

Inferior lacrimal papilla and punctum

Superior lacrimal papilla and punctum

Lacrimal canaliculi

Lacrimal sac

Nasolacrimal duct

Opening of nasolacrimal duct

Frontal bone (cut away)

Orbital part of lacrimal gland

Palpebral part of lacrimal gland

Excretory ducts of lacrimal gland

Plica semilunaris and lacrimal lake

Lacrimal caruncle

Inferior lacrimal papilla and punctum

Opening of nasolacrimal duct and site of Hasner's valve

Superior lacrimal papilla and punctum

Lacrimal canaliculi

Lacrimal sac

Nasolacrimal du

Middle nasal concha

Nasal cavity

Inferior nasal concha (cut)

Inferior nasalmeatu

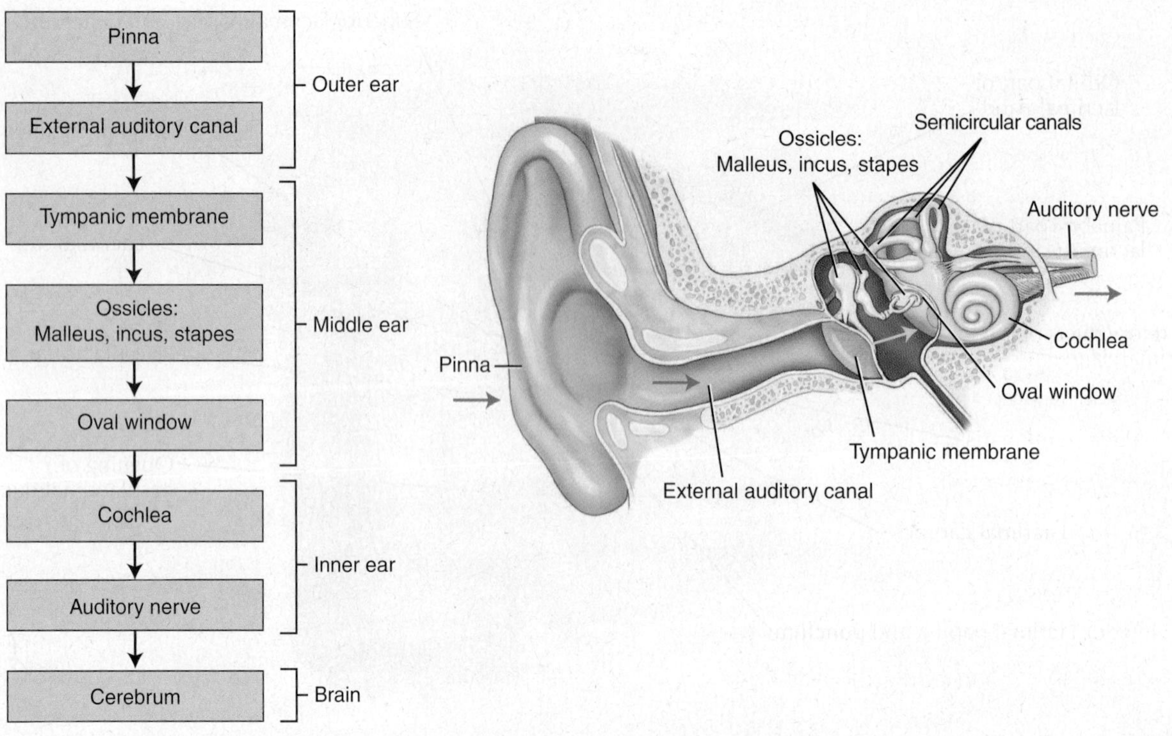

Plate 20 Pathway of Sound. (LaFleur Brooks D, LaFleur Brooks M: Basic Medical Language, ed 4, St. Louis, 2013, Mosby.)

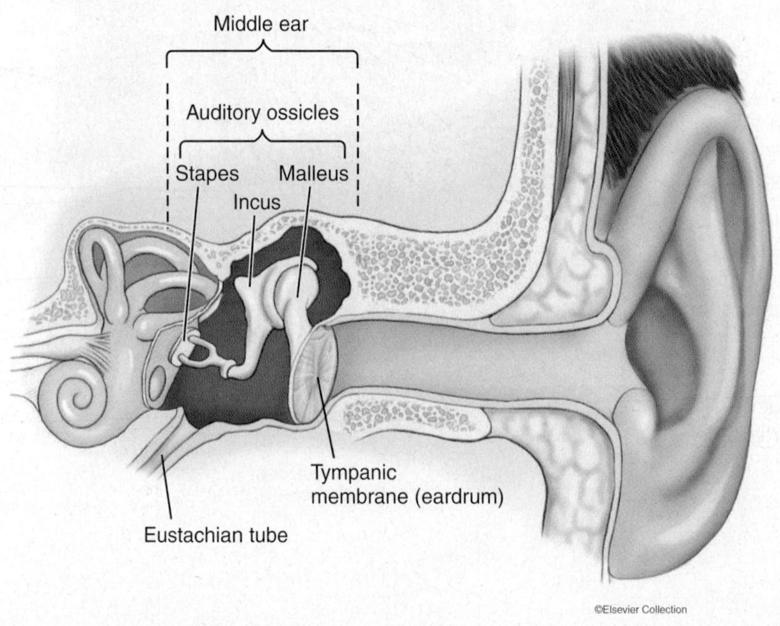

Plate 21 Middle ear structures. (©Elsevier Collection.)

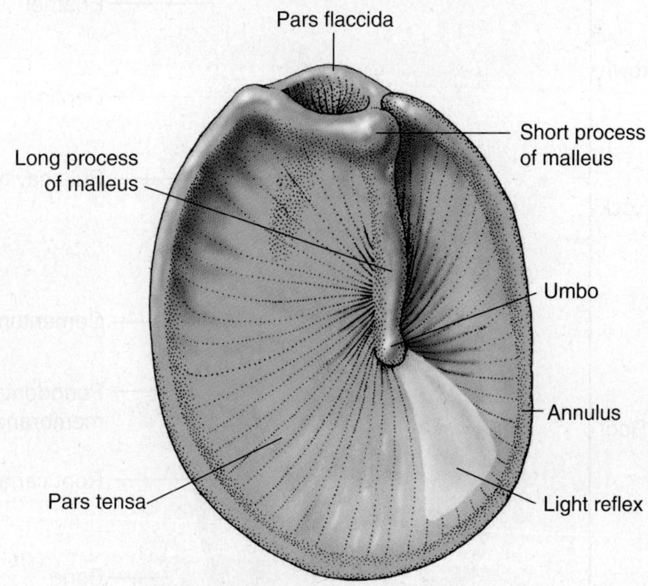

Plate 22 Structural landmarks of tympanic membrane. (Ignatavicius DD, Workman ML: Medical-Surgical Nursing: Patient-Centered Collaborative Care, ed 7, St. Louis, 2013, Saunders.)

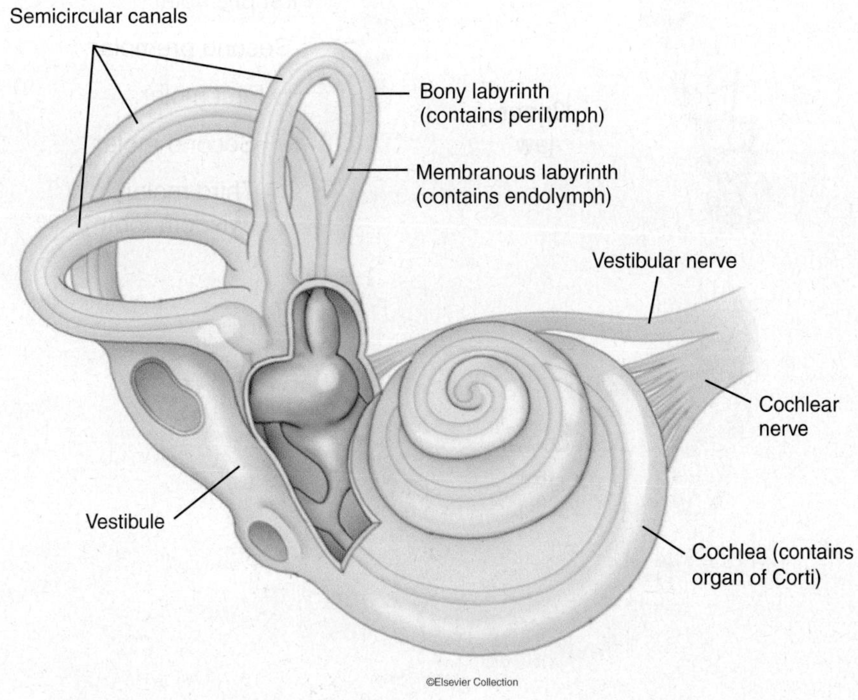

Plate 23 Inner ear structures. (©Elsevier Collection.)

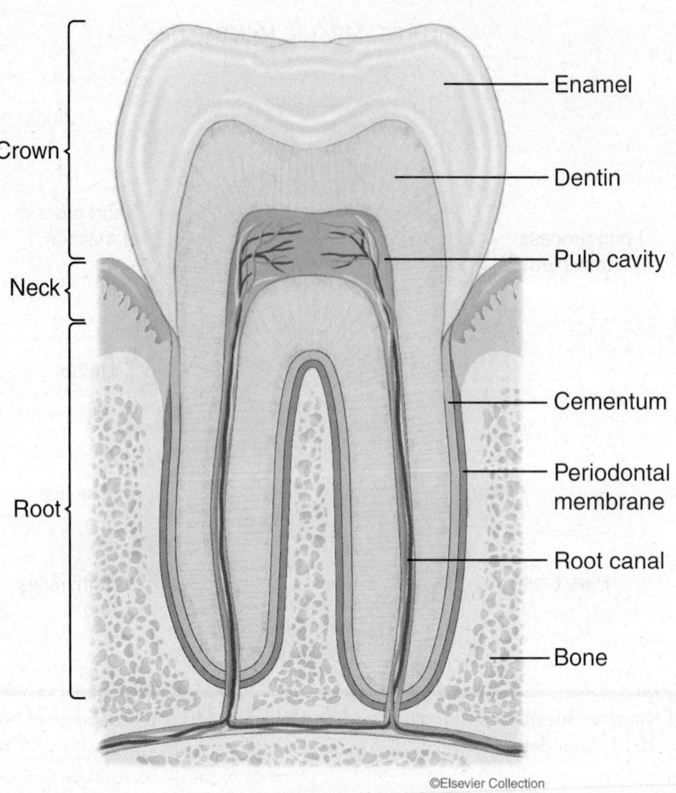

Plate 24 The Tooth. (©Elsevier Collection).

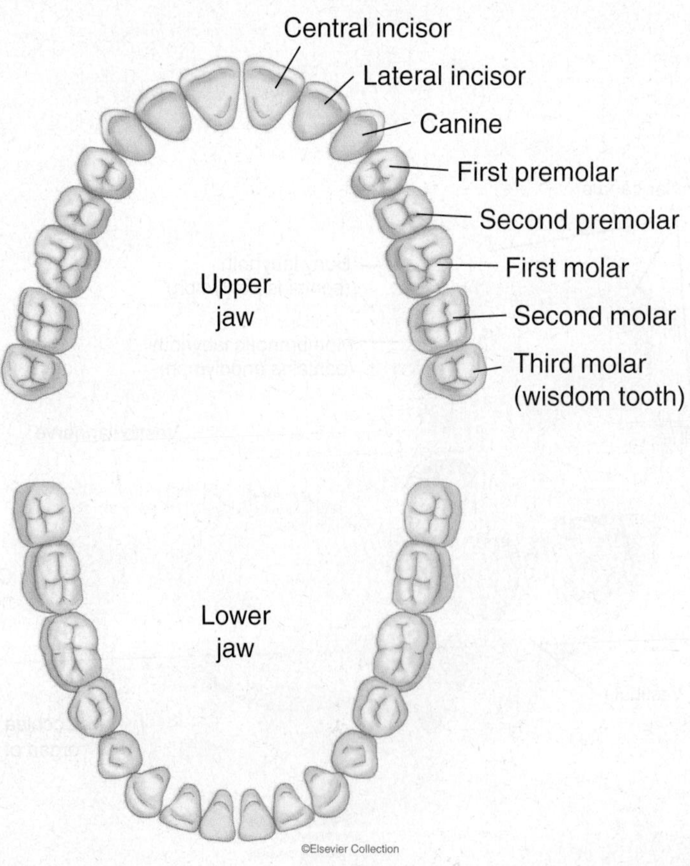

Plate 25 Adult Teeth. (©Elsevier Collection).

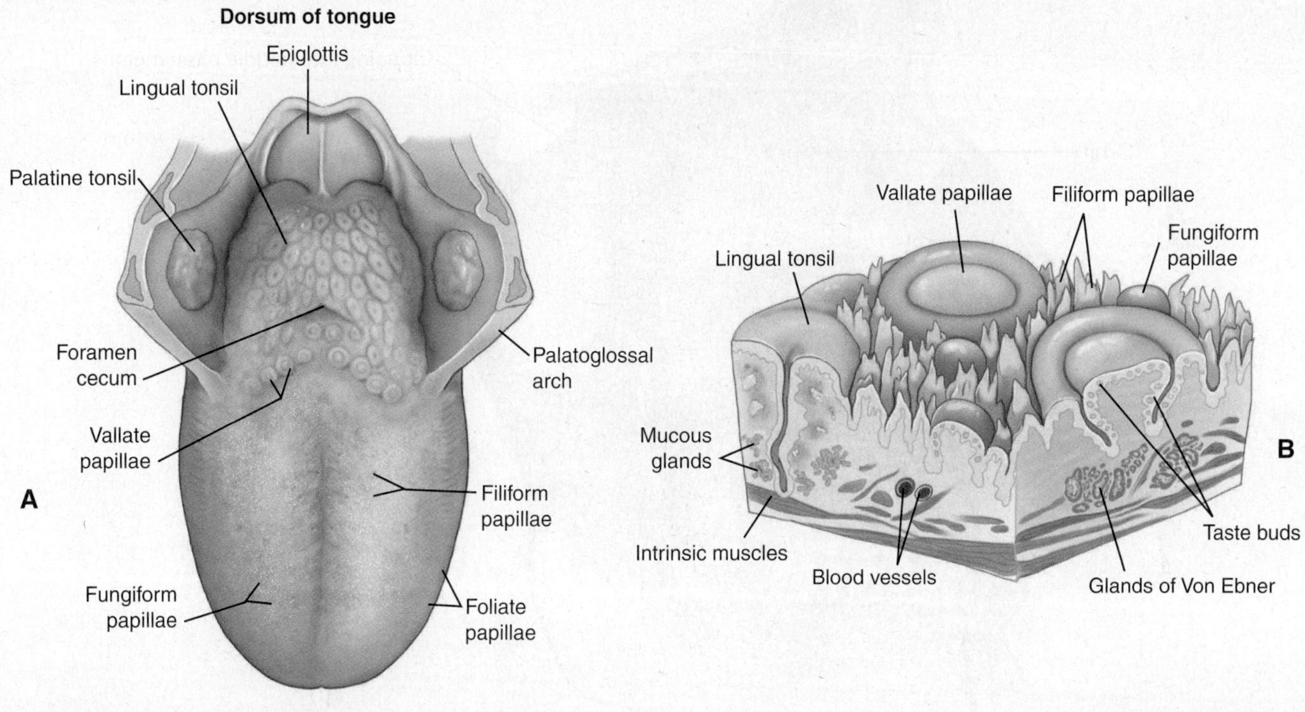

Plate 26 A, Dorsal view of tongue showing the roughened large lingual tonsils on the posterior of the tongue and the foliate papillae on the side. B, Section of dorsal of the tongue showing a cutaway through lingual papillae and showing von Ebner's glands at the base of the vallate papilla. (Brand RW, Isselhard DE: Anatomy of Orofacial Structures. A Comprehensive Approach, ed 8, St. Louis, 2019, Elsevier.)

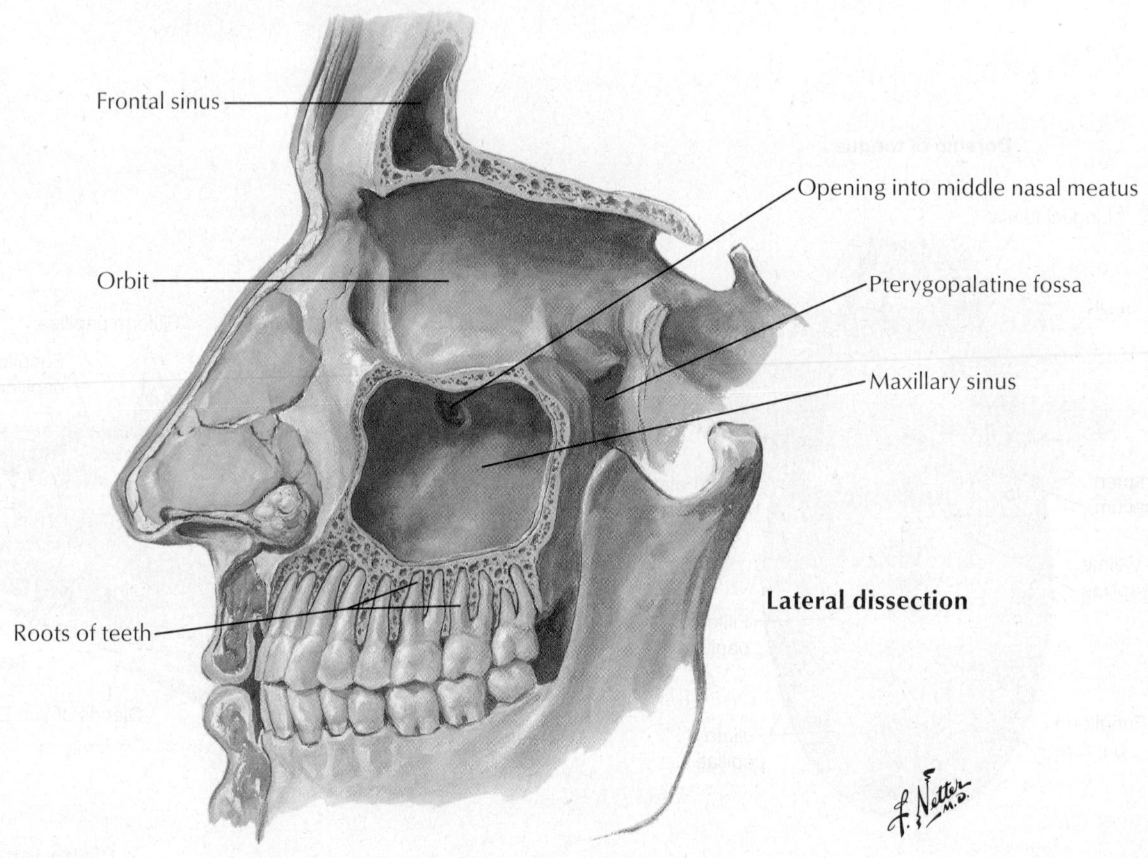

Plate 27 Paranasal Sinuses.

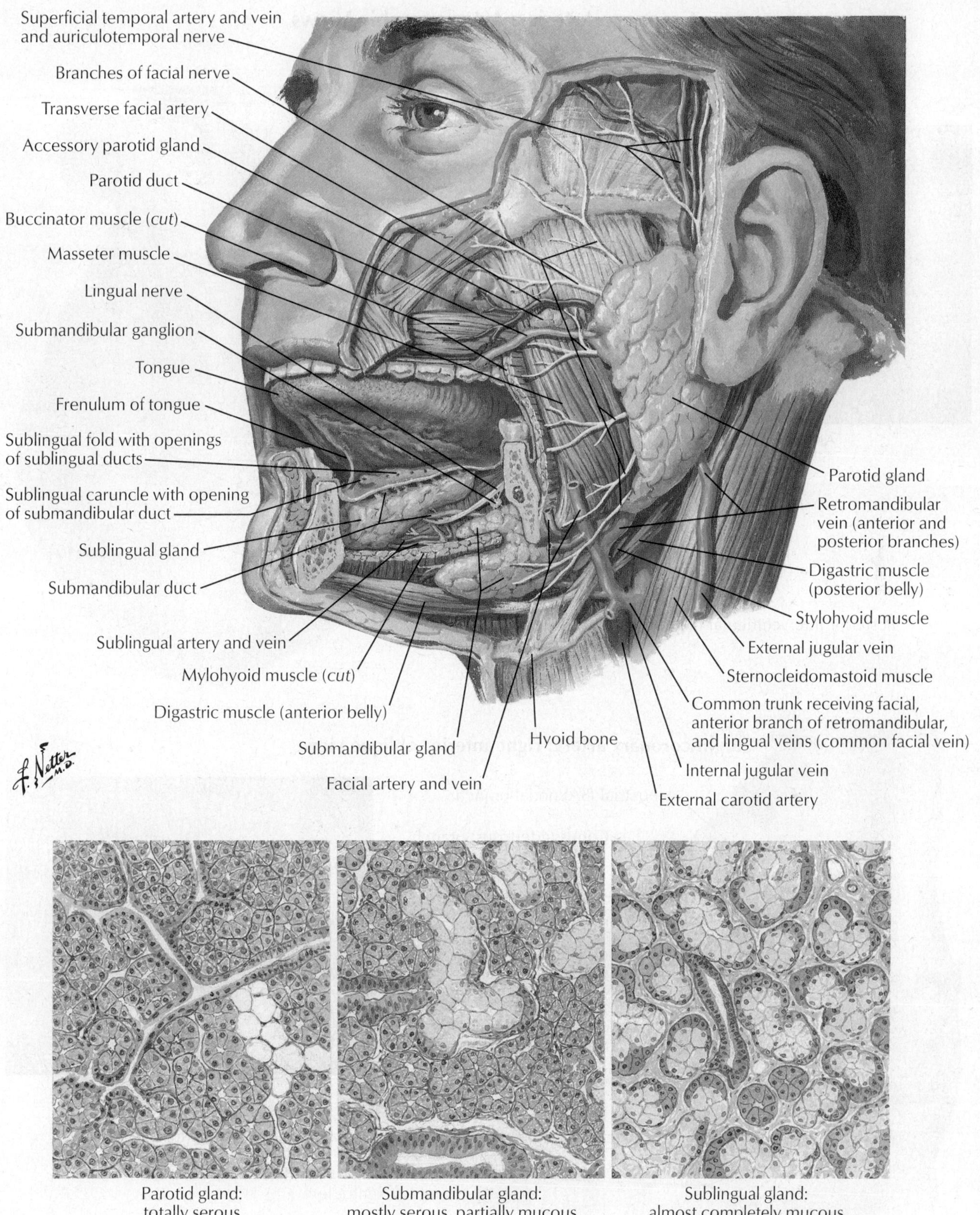

Parotid gland: totally serous

Submandibular gland: mostly serous, partially mucous

Sublingual gland: almost completely mucous

Plate 28 Salivary Glands.

Coronary Arteries: Arteriographic Views

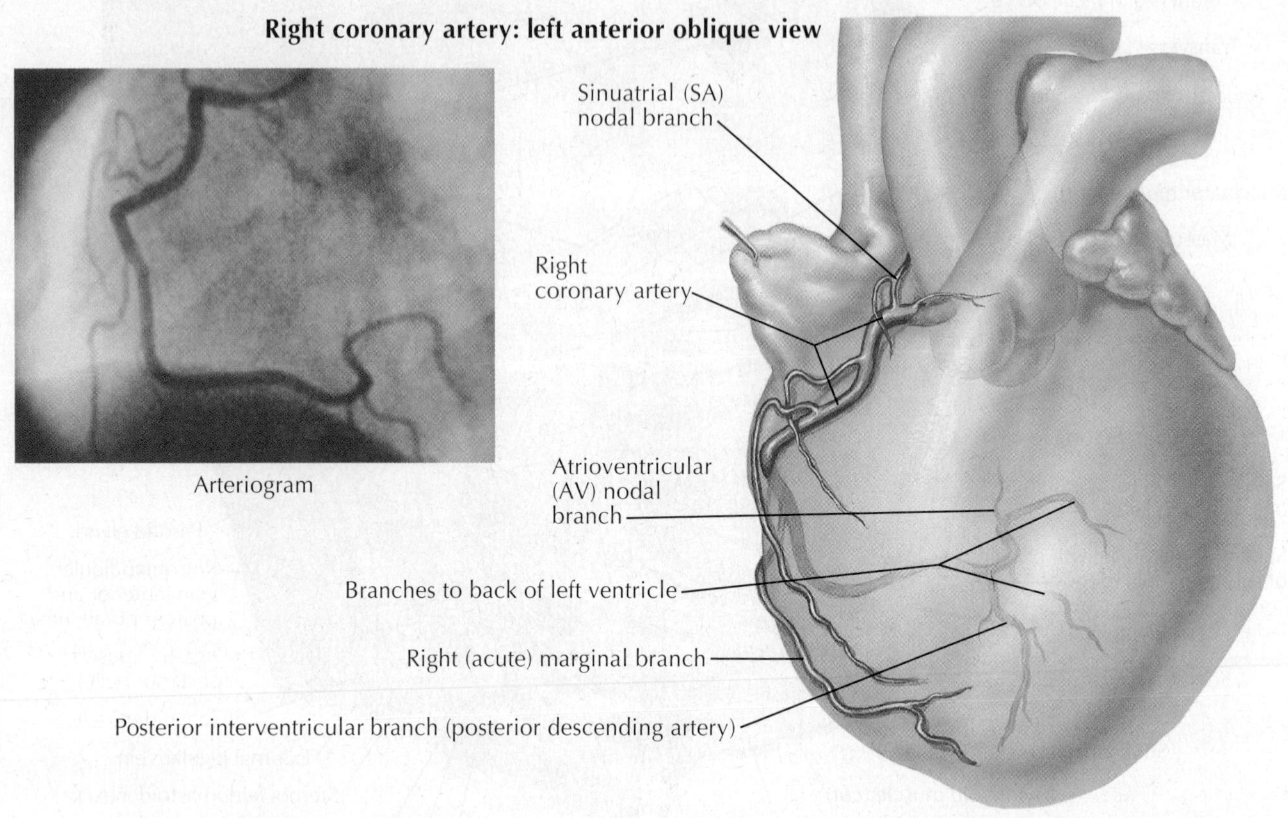

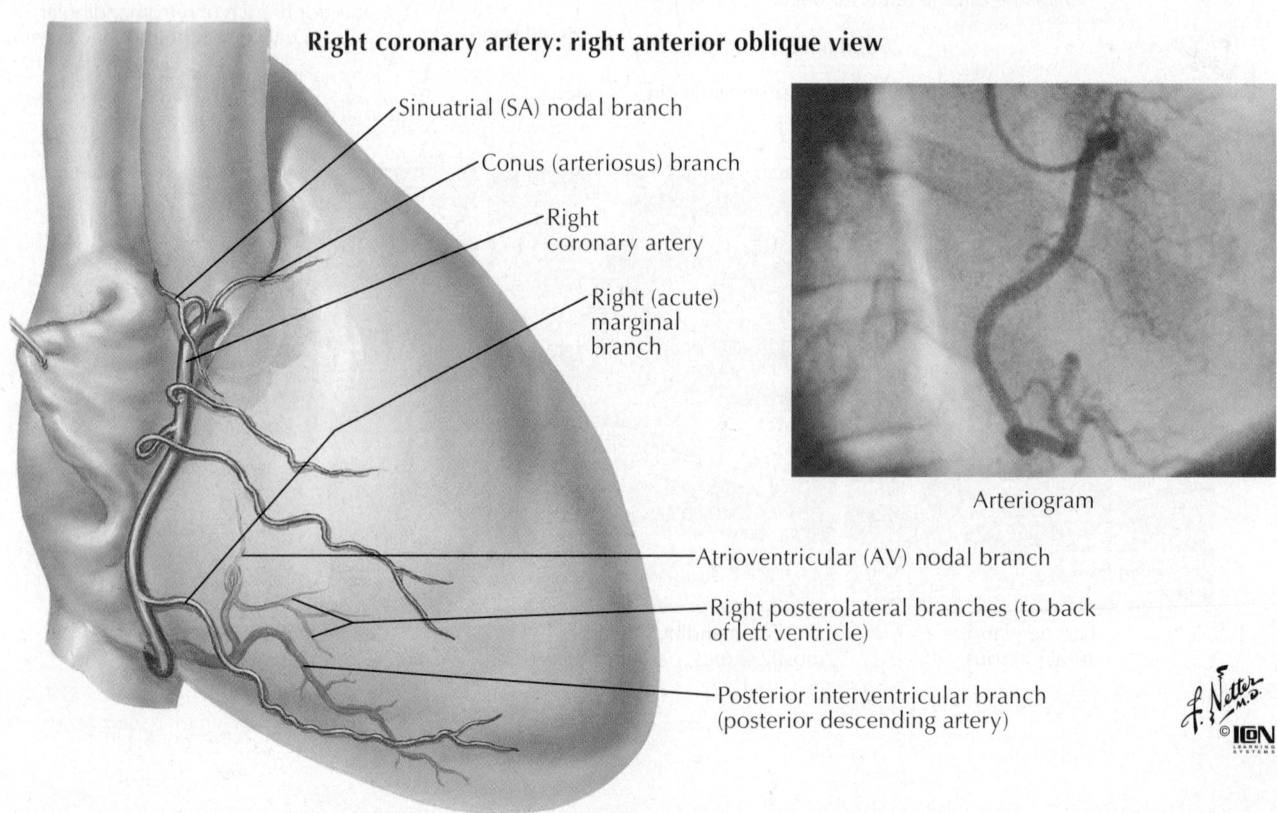

Plate 29 Coronary Arteries: Arteriographic Views.

Left coronary artery: left anterior oblique view

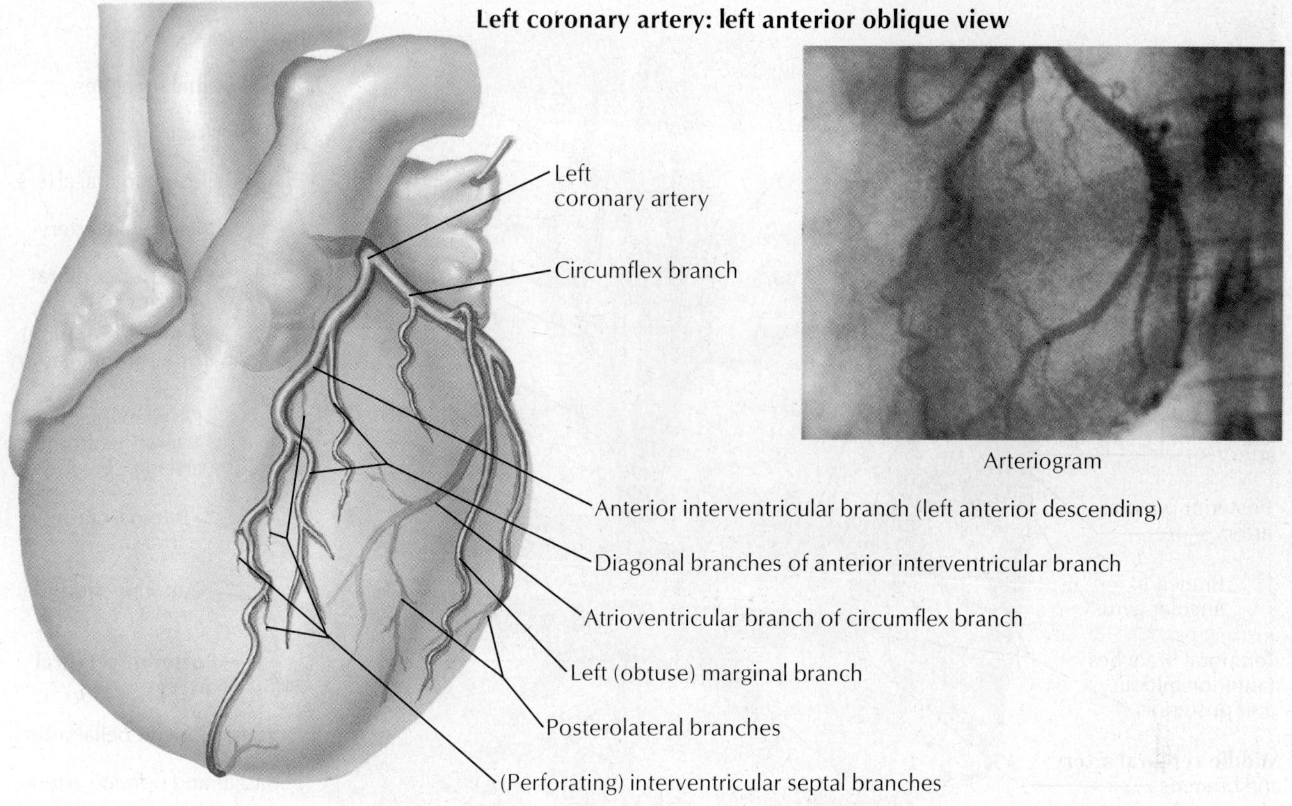

Left coronary artery: right anterior oblique view

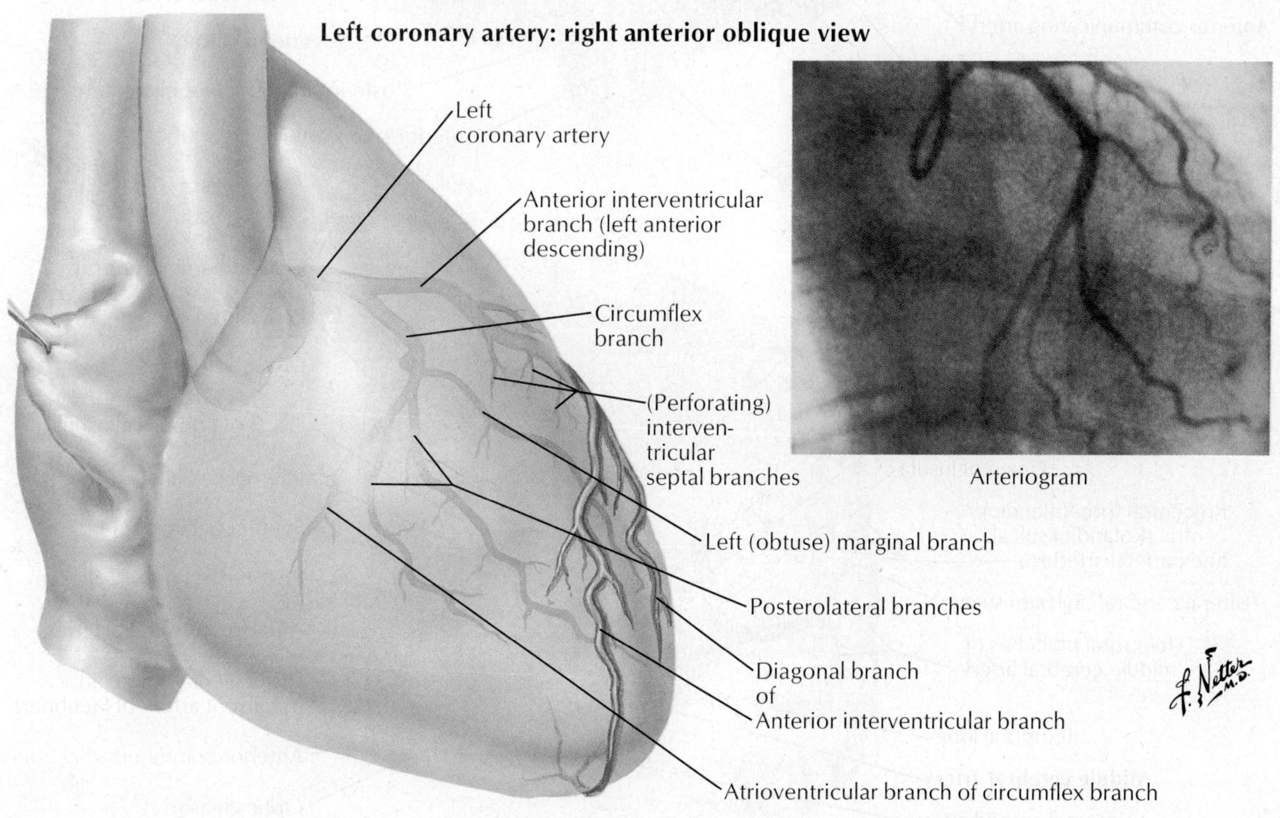

ANATOMY ILLUSTRATIONS

Plate 30 Coronary Arteries: Arteriographic Views.

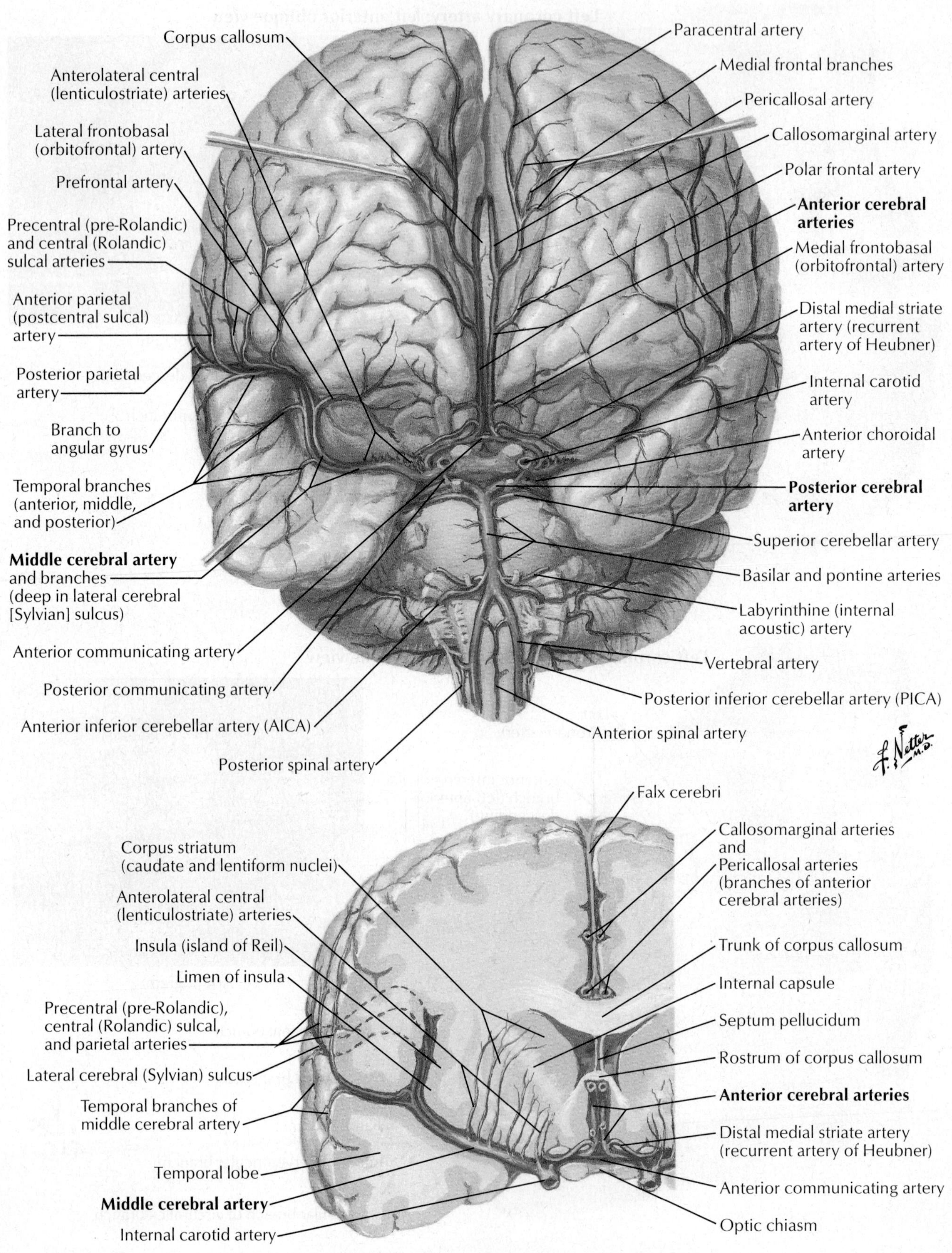
Corpus callosum
Anterolateral central (lenticulostriate) arteries
Lateral frontobasal (orbitofrontal) artery
Prefrontal artery
Precentral (pre-Rolandic) and central (Rolandic) sulcal arteries
Anterior parietal (postcentral sulcal) artery
Posterior parietal artery
Branch to angular gyrus
Temporal branches (anterior, middle, and posterior)
Middle cerebral artery and branches (deep in lateral cerebral [Sylvian] sulcus)
Anterior communicating artery
Posterior communicating artery
Anterior inferior cerebellar artery (AICA)
Posterior spinal artery
Paracentral artery
Medial frontal branches
Pericallosal artery
Callosomarginal artery
Polar frontal artery
Anterior cerebral arteries
Medial frontobasal (orbitofrontal) artery
Distal medial striate artery (recurrent artery of Heubner)
Internal carotid artery
Anterior choroidal artery
Posterior cerebral artery
Superior cerebellar artery
Basilar and pontine arteries
Labyrinthine (internal acoustic) artery
Vertebral artery
Posterior inferior cerebellar artery (PICA)
Anterior spinal artery
F. Netter M.D.
Falx cerebri
Corpus striatum (caudate and lentiform nuclei)
Anterolateral central (lenticulostriate) arteries
Insula (island of Reil)
Limen of insula
Precentral (pre-Rolandic), central (Rolandic) sulcal, and parietal arteries
Lateral cerebral (Sylvian) sulcus
Temporal branches of middle cerebral artery
Temporal lobe
Middle cerebral artery
Internal carotid artery
Callosomarginal arteries and Pericallosal arteries (branches of anterior cerebral arteries)
Trunk of corpus callosum
Internal capsule
Septum pellucidum
Rostrum of corpus callosum
Anterior cerebral arteries
Distal medial striate artery (recurrent artery of Heubner)
Anterior communicating artery
Optic chiasm

Plate 31 Arteries of Brain: Frontal View and Section. Image ID: 4588)

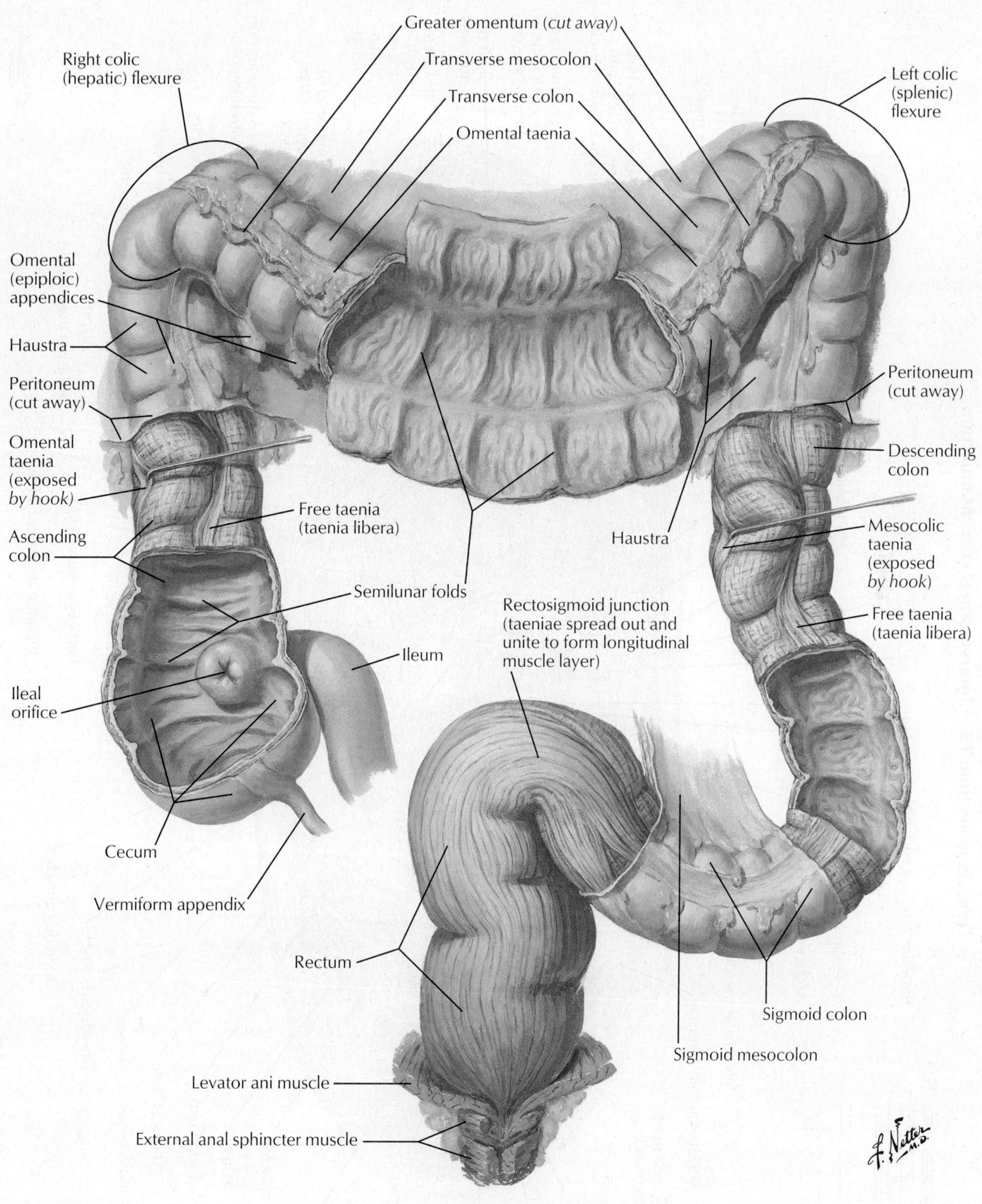

Greater omentum (cut away)
Transverse mesocolon
Transverse colon
Omental taenia
Right colic (hepatic) flexure
Left colic (splenic) flexure
Omental (epiploic) appendices
Haustra
Peritoneum (cut away)
Omental taenia (exposed by hook)
Free taenia (taenia libera)
Ascending colon
Semilunar folds
Haustra
Peritoneum (cut away)
Descending colon
Mesocolic taenia (exposed by hook)
Free taenia (taenia libera)
Rectosigmoid junction (taeniae spread out and unite to form longitudinal muscle layer)
Ileum
Ileal orifice
Cecum
Vermiform appendix
Rectum
Sigmoid colon
Sigmoid mesocolon
Levator ani muscle
External anal sphincter muscle
F. Netter M.D.

Plate 32 Mucosa and Musculature of Large Intestine. Image ID: 4778)

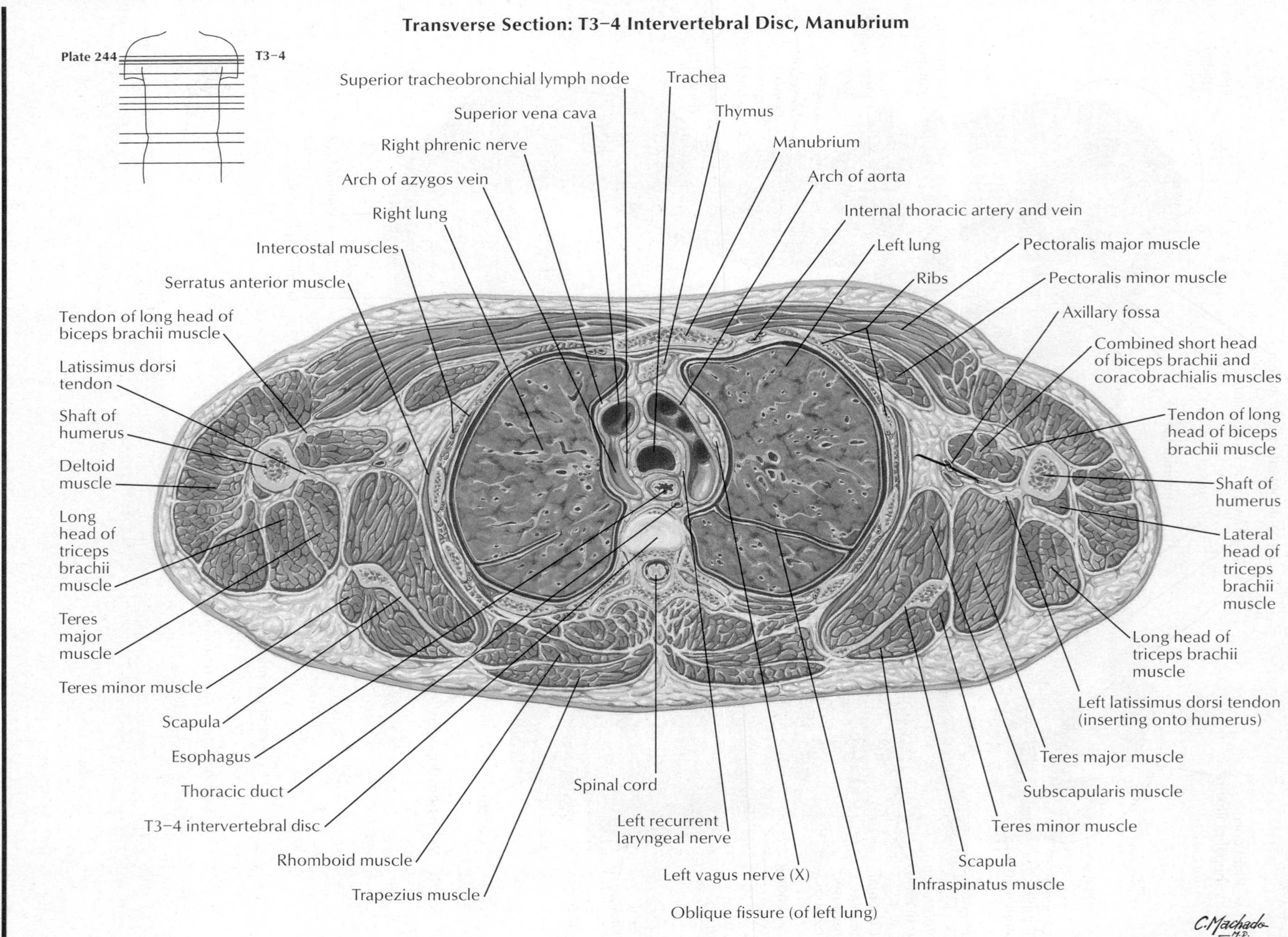
Transverse Section: T3–4 Intervertebral Disc, Manubrium
Plate 244
T3–4
Superior tracheobronchial lymph node
Trachea
Superior vena cava
Thymus
Right phrenic nerve
Manubrium
Arch of azygos vein
Arch of aorta
Right lung
Internal thoracic artery and vein
Intercostal muscles
Left lung
Pectoralis major muscle
Serratus anterior muscle
Ribs
Pectoralis minor muscle
Tendon of long head of biceps brachii muscle
Axillary fossa
Combined short head of biceps brachii and coracobrachialis muscles
Latissimus dorsi tendon
Shaft of humerus
Tendon of long head of biceps brachii muscle
Deltoid muscle
Shaft of humerus
Long head of triceps brachii muscle
Lateral head of triceps brachii muscle
Teres major muscle
Long head of triceps brachii muscle
Teres minor muscle
Scapula
Left latissimus dorsi tendon (inserting onto humerus)
Esophagus
Teres major muscle
Thoracic duct
Spinal cord
Subscapularis muscle
T3–4 intervertebral disc
Left recurrent laryngeal nerve
Teres minor muscle
Rhomboid muscle
Scapula
Left vagus nerve (X)
Infraspinatus muscle
Trapezius muscle
Oblique fissure (of left lung)
C. Machado M.D.

Plate 33 Cross Section of Thorax at T3-4 Disc Level. Image ID: 4880)

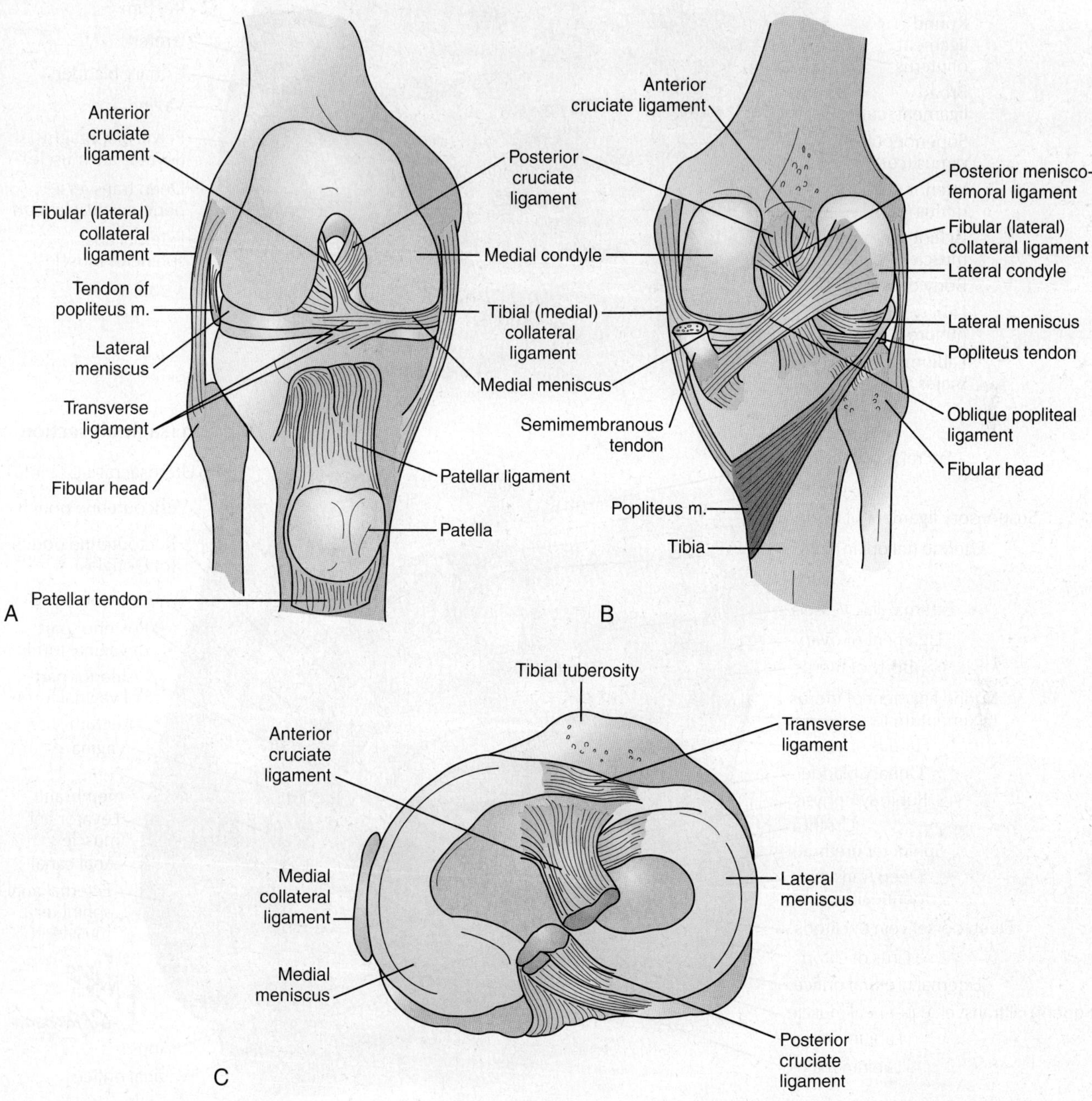

Plate 34 Knee joint opened; anterior, posterior, and proximal views. A, Anterior view of the knee joint, opened by folding the patella and patellar ligament inferiorly. On the lateral side is the fibular collateral ligament, separated by the popliteal tendon from the lateral meniscus. On the medial side, the tibial collateral ligament is attached to the medial meniscus. The anterior and posterior cruciate ligaments are seen between the femoral condyles. B, Posterior view of the opened knee joint with a more complete view of the posterior cruciate ligament. C, The femur is removed, showing the proximal (articular) end of the right tibia. On the medial side is the gently curved medial meniscus; on the lateral side is the more tightly curved lateral meniscus. The anterior end of the medial meniscus is anchored to the surface of the tibia by the transverse ligament. The cut ends of the anterior and posterior cruciate ligaments are shown, as well as the meniscofemoral ligament. (Fritz S: Mosby's Essential Sciences for Therapeutic Massage: Anatomy, Physiology, Biomechanics, and Pathology, ed 5, St. Louis, 2017, Elsevier.)

ANATOMY ILLUSTRATIONS

Paramedian (sagittal) dissection

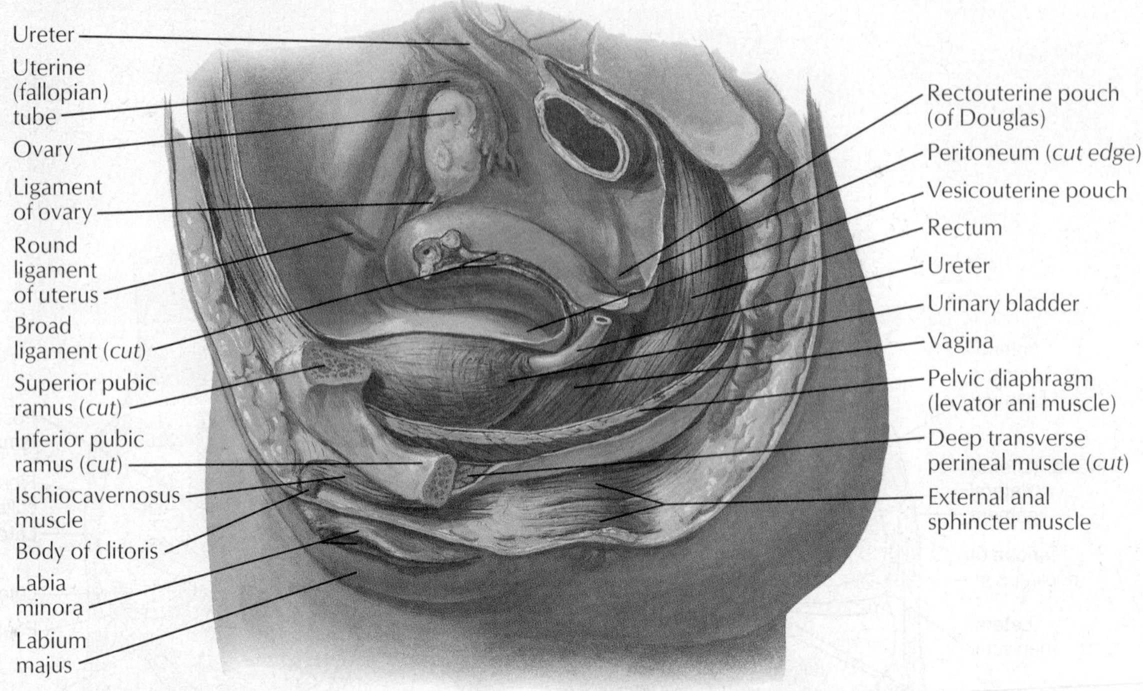
Ureter
Uterine (fallopian) tube
Ovary
Ligament of ovary
Round ligament of uterus
Broad ligament (*cut*)
Superior pubic ramus (*cut*)
Inferior pubic ramus (*cut*)
Ischiocavernosus muscle
Body of clitoris
Labia minora
Labium majus
Rectouterine pouch (of Douglas)
Peritoneum (*cut edge*)
Vesicouterine pouch
Rectum
Ureter
Urinary bladder
Vagina
Pelvic diaphragm (levator ani muscle)
Deep transverse perineal muscle (*cut*)
External anal sphincter muscle

Median (sagittal) section

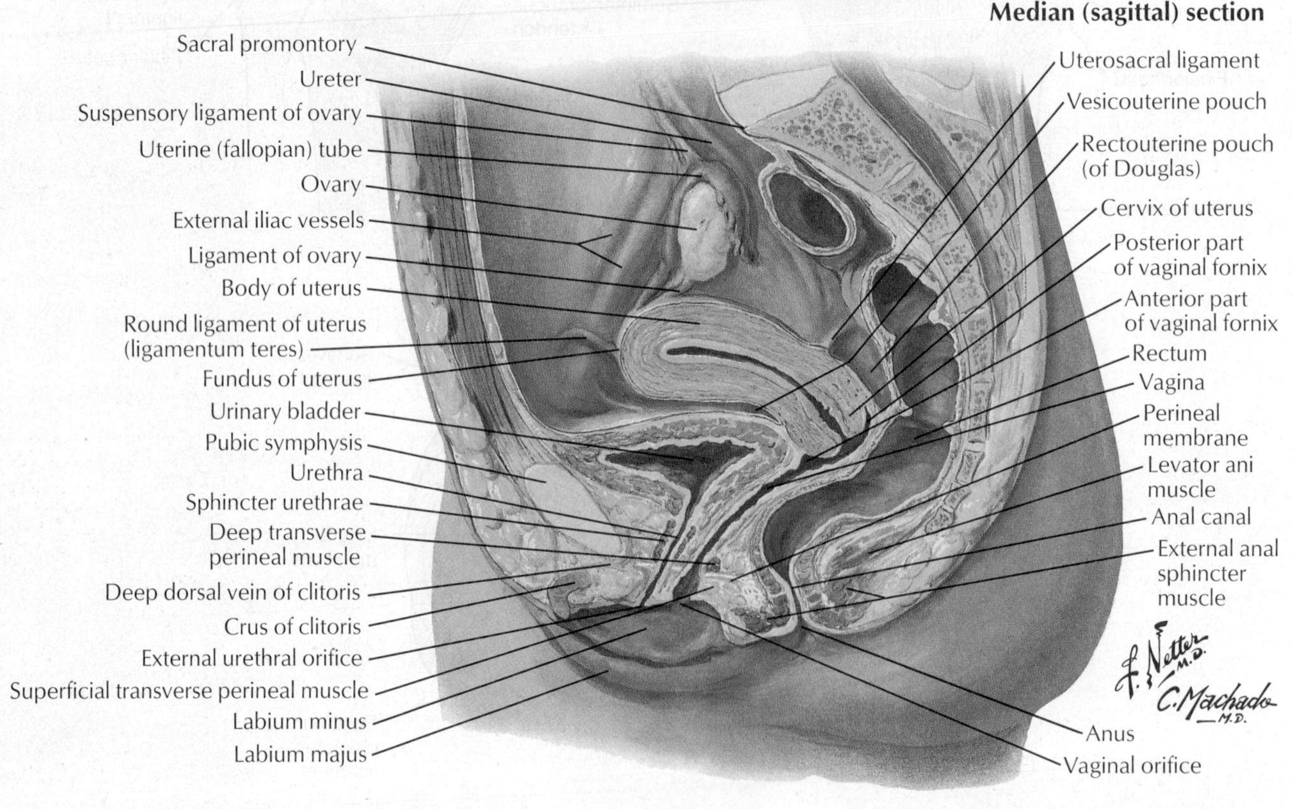
Sacral promontory
Ureter
Suspensory ligament of ovary
Uterine (fallopian) tube
Ovary
External iliac vessels
Ligament of ovary
Body of uterus
Round ligament of uterus (ligamentum teres)
Fundus of uterus
Urinary bladder
Pubic symphysis
Urethra
Sphincter urethrae
Deep transverse perineal muscle
Deep dorsal vein of clitoris
Crus of clitoris
External urethral orifice
Superficial transverse perineal muscle
Labium minus
Labium majus
Uterosacral ligament
Vesicouterine pouch
Rectouterine pouch (of Douglas)
Cervix of uterus
Posterior part of vaginal fornix
Anterior part of vaginal fornix
Rectum
Vagina
Perineal membrane
Levator ani muscle
Anal canal
External anal sphincter muscle
F. Netter M.D.
C. Machado M.D.
Anus
Vaginal orifice

Plate 35 Pelvic Viscera and Perineum: Female.

PART II

Alphabetic Index

ICD-10-CM INDEX TO DISEASES AND INJURIES

A

- **Aarskog's syndrome** Q87.19
- **Abandonment** —*see* Maltreatment
- **Abasia** (-astasia) (hysterical) F44.4
- **Abderhalden-Kaufmann-Lignac syndrome** (cystinosis) E72.Ø4
- **Abdomen, abdominal** —*see also* condition
  - acute R1Ø.Ø
  - angina K55.1
  - muscle deficiency syndrome Q79.4
- **Abdominalgia** —*see* Pain, abdominal
- **Abduction contracture, hip or other joint** —*see* Contraction, joint
- **Aberrant** (congenital) —*see also* Malposition, congenital
  - adrenal gland Q89.1
  - artery (peripheral) Q27.8
    - basilar NEC Q28.1
    - cerebral Q28.3
    - coronary Q24.5
    - digestive system Q27.8
    - eye Q15.8
    - lower limb Q27.8
    - precerebral Q28.1
    - pulmonary Q25.79
    - renal Q27.2
    - retina Q14.1
    - specified site NEC Q27.8
    - subclavian Q27.8
    - upper limb Q27.8
    - vertebral Q28.1
  - breast Q83.8
  - endocrine gland NEC Q89.2
  - hepatic duct Q44.5
  - pancreas Q45.3
  - parathyroid gland Q89.2
  - pituitary gland Q89.2
  - sebaceous glands, mucous membrane, mouth, congenital Q38.6
  - spleen Q89.Ø9
  - subclavian artery Q27.8
  - thymus (gland) Q89.2
  - thyroid gland Q89.2
  - vein (peripheral) NEC Q27.8
    - cerebral Q28.3
    - digestive system Q27.8
    - lower limb Q27.8
    - precerebral Q28.1
    - specified site NEC Q27.8
    - upper limb Q27.8
- **Aberration**
  - distantial —*see* Disturbance, visual
  - mental F99
- **Abetalipoproteinemia** E78.6
- **Abiotrophy** R68.89
- **Ablatio, ablation**
  - retinae —*see* Detachment, retina
- **Ablepharia, ablepharon** Q1Ø.3
- **Abnormal, abnormality, abnormalities** —*see also* Anomaly
  - acid-base balance (mixed) E87.4
  - albumin R77.Ø
  - alphafetoprotein R77.2
  - alveolar ridge KØ8.9
  - anatomical relationship Q89.9
  - apertures, congenital, diaphragm Q79.1
  - atrial septal, specified NEC Q21.19
  - auditory perception H93.29-●
    - diplacusis —*see* Diplacusis
    - hyperacusis —*see* Hyperacusis
    - recruitment —*see* Recruitment, auditory
    - threshold shift —*see* Shift, auditory threshold
  - autosomes Q99.9
    - fragile site Q95.5
  - basal metabolic rate R94.8
  - biosynthesis, testicular androgen E29.1
  - bleeding time R79.1
  - blood amino-acid level R79.83
  - blood level (of)
    - cobalt R79.Ø
    - copper R79.Ø
    - iron R79.Ø
    - lithium R78.89
    - magnesium R79.Ø
    - mineral NEC R79.Ø
    - zinc R79.Ø
  - blood pressure
    - elevated RØ3.Ø
    - low reading (nonspecific) RØ3.1

Abnormal, abnormality, abnormalities *(Continued)*

  - blood sugar R73.Ø9
  - blood-gas level R79.81
  - bowel sounds R19.15
    - absent R19.11
    - hyperactive R19.12
  - brain scan R94.Ø2
  - breathing RØ6.9
  - caloric test R94.138
  - cerebrospinal fluid R83.9
    - cytology R83.6
    - drug level R83.2
    - enzyme level R83.Ø
    - hormones R83.1
    - immunology R83.4
    - microbiology R83.5
    - nonmedicinal level R83.3
    - specified type NEC R83.8
  - chemistry, blood R79.9
    - C-reactive protein R79.82
    - drugs —*see* Findings, abnormal, in blood
    - gas level R79.81
    - minerals R79.Ø
    - pancytopenia D61.818
    - PTT R79.1
    - specified NEC R79.89
    - toxins —*see* Findings, abnormal, in blood
  - chest sounds (friction) (rales) RØ9.89
  - chromosome, chromosomal Q99.9
    - with more than three X chromosomes, female Q97.1
    - analysis result R89.8
      - bronchial washings R84.8
      - cerebrospinal fluid R83.8
      - cervix uteri NEC R87.89
      - nasal secretions R84.8
      - nipple discharge R89.8
      - peritoneal fluid R85.89
      - pleural fluid R84.8
      - prostatic secretions R86.8
      - saliva R85.89
      - seminal fluid R86.8
      - sputum R84.8
      - synovial fluid R89.8
      - throat scrapings R84.8
      - vagina R87.89
      - vulva R87.89
      - wound secretions R89.8
    - dicentric replacement Q93.2
    - ring replacement Q93.2
    - sex Q99.8
      - female phenotype Q97.9
        - specified NEC Q97.8
      - male phenotype Q98.9
        - specified NEC Q98.8
      - structural male Q98.6
    - specified NEC Q99.8
  - clinical findings NEC R68.89
  - coagulation D68.9
    - newborn, transient P61.6
    - profile R79.1
    - time R79.1
  - communication —*see* Fistula
  - conjunctiva, vascular H11.41-●
  - coronary artery Q24.5
  - cortisol-binding globulin E27.8
  - course, eustachian tube Q17.8
  - creatinine clearance R94.4
  - cytology
    - anus R85.619
      - atypical squamous cells cannot exclude high grade squamous intraepithelial lesion (ASC-H) R85.611
      - atypical squamous cells of undetermined significance (ASC-US) R85.61Ø
      - cytologic evidence of malignancy R85.614
      - high grade squamous intraepithelial lesion (HGSIL) R85.613
      - human papillomavirus (HPV) DNA test
        - high risk positive R85.81
        - low risk postive R85.82
      - inadequate smear R85.615
      - low grade squamous intraepithelial lesion (LGSIL) R85.612
      - satisfactory anal smear but lacking transformation zone R85.616
      - specified NEC R85.618
      - unsatisfactory smear R85.615
    - female genital organs —*see* Abnormal, Papanicolaou (smear)

Abnormal, abnormality, abnormalities *(Continued)*

  - dark adaptation curve H53.61
  - dentofacial NEC —*see* Anomaly, dentofacial
  - development, developmental Q89.9
    - central nervous system QØ7.9
  - diagnostic imaging
    - abdomen, abdominal region NEC R93.5
    - biliary tract R93.2
    - bladder R93.41
    - breast R92.8
    - central nervous system NEC R9Ø.89
    - cerebrovascular NEC R9Ø.89
    - coronary circulation R93.1
    - digestive tract NEC R93.3
    - gastrointestinal (tract) R93.3
    - genitourinary organs R93.89
    - head R93.Ø
    - heart R93.1
    - intrathoracic organ NEC R93.89
    - kidney R93.42-●
    - limbs R93.6
    - liver R93.2
    - lung (field) R91.8
    - musculoskeletal system NEC R93.7
    - renal pelvis R93.41
    - retroperitoneum R93.5
    - site specified NEC R93.89
    - skin and subcutaneous tissue R93.89
    - skull R93.Ø
    - testis R93.81-●
    - urinary organs specified NEC R93.49
    - ureter R93.41
  - direction, teeth, fully erupted M26.3Ø
  - ear ossicles, acquired NEC H74.39-●
    - ankylosis —*see* Ankylosis, ear ossicles
    - discontinuity —*see* Discontinuity, ossicles, ear
    - partial loss —*see* Loss, ossicles, ear (partial)
  - Ebstein Q22.5
  - echocardiogram R93.1
  - echoencephalogram R9Ø.81
  - echogram —*see* Abnormal, diagnostic imaging
  - electrocardiogram [ECG] [EKG] R94.31
  - electroencephalogram [EEG] R94.Ø1
  - electrolyte —*see* Imbalance, electrolyte
  - electromyogram [EMG] R94.131
  - electro-oculogram [EOG] R94.11Ø
  - electrophysiological intracardiac studies R94.39
  - electroretinogram [ERG] R94.111
  - erythrocytes
    - congenital, with perinatal jaundice D58.9
  - feces (color) (contents) (mucus) R19.5
  - finding —*see* Findings, abnormal, without diagnosis
  - fluid
    - amniotic —*see* Abnormal, specimen, specified
    - cerebrospinal —*see* Abnormal, cerebrospinal fluid
    - peritoneal —*see* Abnormal, specimen, digestive organs
    - pleural —*see* Abnormal, specimen, respiratory organs
    - synovial —*see* Abnormal, specimen, specified
    - thorax (bronchial washings) (pleural fluid) —*see* Abnormal, specimen, respiratory organs
    - vaginal —*see* Abnormal, specimen, female genital organs
  - form
    - teeth KØØ.2
    - uterus —*see* Anomaly, uterus
  - function studies
    - auditory R94.12Ø
    - bladder R94.8
    - brain R94.Ø9
    - cardiovascular R94.3Ø
    - ear R94.128
    - endocrine NEC R94.7
    - eye NEC R94.118
    - kidney R94.4
    - liver R94.5
    - nervous system
      - central NEC R94.Ø9
      - peripheral NEC R94.138
    - pancreas R94.8
    - placenta R94.8
    - pulmonary R94.2
    - special senses NEC R94.128
    - spleen R94.8
    - thyroid R94.6
    - vestibular R94.121

A

A

A

A

A

Absence *(Continued)*
- cricoid cartilage, congenital Q31.8
- diaphragm (with hernia), congenital Q79.1
- digestive organ(s) or tract, congenital Q45.8
  - acquired NEC Z90.49
  - upper Q40.8
- ductus arteriosus Q28.8
- duodenum (acquired) Z90.49
  - congenital Q41.0
- ear, congenital Q16.9
  - acquired H93.8-●
  - auricle Q16.0
  - external Q16.0
  - inner Q16.5
  - lobe, lobule Q17.8
  - middle, except ossicles Q16.4
    - ossicles Q16.3
  - ossicles Q16.3
- ejaculatory duct (congenital) Q55.4
- endocrine gland (congenital) NEC Q89.2
  - acquired E89.89
- epididymis (congenital) Q55.4
  - acquired Z90.79
- epiglottis, congenital Q31.8
- esophagus (congenital) Q39.8
  - acquired (partial) Z90.49
- eustachian tube (congenital) Q16.2
- extremity (acquired) Z89.9
  - congenital Q73.0
  - knee (following explantation of knee joint prosthesis) (joint) (with or without presence of antibiotic-impregnated cement spacer) Z89.52-●
  - lower (above knee) Z89.619
    - below knee Z89.51-●
  - upper *—see* Absence, arm
- eye (acquired) Z90.01
  - congenital Q11.1
  - muscle (congenital) Q10.3
- eyeball (acquired) Z90.01
- eyelid (fold) (congenital) Q10.3
  - acquired Z90.01
- face, specified part NEC Q18.8
- fallopian tube(s) (acquired) Z90.79
  - congenital Q50.6
- family member (causing problem in home) NEC *—see also* Disruption, family Z63.32
- femur, congenital *—see* Defect, reduction, lower limb, longitudinal, femur
- fibrinogen (congenital) D68.2
  - acquired D65
- finger(s) (acquired) Z89.02-●
  - congenital *—see* Agenesis, hand
- foot (acquired) Z89.43-●
  - congenital *—see* Agenesis, foot
- forearm (acquired) *—see* Absence, arm, below elbow
- gallbladder (acquired) Z90.49
  - congenital Q44.0
- gamma globulin in blood D80.1
  - hereditary D80.0
- genital organs
  - acquired (female) (male) Z90.79
  - female, congenital Q52.8
    - external Q52.71
    - internal NEC Q52.8
  - male, congenital Q55.8
- genitourinary organs, congenital NEC
  - female Q52.8
  - male Q55.8
- globe (acquired) Z90.01
  - congenital Q11.1
- glottis, congenital Q31.8
- hand and wrist (acquired) Z89.11-●
  - congenital *—see* Agenesis, hand
- head, part (acquired) NEC Z90.09
- heat sense R20.8
- hip (following explantation of hip joint prosthesis) (joint) (with or without presence of antibiotic-impregnated cement spacer) Z89.62-●
- hymen (congenital) Q52.4
- ileum (acquired) Z90.49
  - congenital Q41.2
- immunoglobulin, isolated NEC D80.3
  - IgA D80.2
  - IgG D80.3
  - IgM D80.4
- incus (acquired) *—see* Loss, ossicles, ear
  - congenital Q16.3
- inner ear, congenital Q16.5

Absence *(Continued)*
- intestine (acquired) (small) Z90.49
  - congenital Q41.9
    - specified NEC Q41.8
  - large Z90.49
    - congenital Q42.9
      - specified NEC Q42.8
- iris, congenital Q13.1
- jejunum (acquired) Z90.49
  - congenital Q41.1
- joint
  - acquired
    - hip (following explantation of hip joint prosthesis) (with or without presence of antibiotic-impregnated cement spacer) Z89.62-●
    - knee (following explantation of knee joint prosthesis) (with or without presence of antibiotic-impregnated cement spacer) Z89.52-●
    - shoulder (following explantation of shoulder joint prosthesis) (with or without presence of antibiotic-impregnated cement spacer) Z89.23-●
  - congenital NEC Q74.8
- kidney(s) (acquired) Z90.5
  - congenital Q60.2
    - bilateral Q60.1
    - unilateral Q60.0
- knee (following explantation of knee joint prosthesis) (joint) (with or without presence of antibiotic-impregnated cement spacer) Z89.52-●
- labyrinth, membranous Q16.5
- larynx (congenital) Q31.8
  - acquired Z90.02
- leg (acquired) (above knee) Z89.61-●
  - below knee (acquired) Z89.51-●
  - congenital *—see* Defect, reduction, lower limb
- lens (acquired) *—see also* Aphakia
  - congenital Q12.3
  - post cataract extraction Z98.4-●
- limb (acquired) *—see* Absence, extremity
- lip Q38.6
- liver (congenital) Q44.79
- lung (fissure) (lobe) (bilateral) (unilateral) (congenital) Q33.3
  - acquired (any part) Z90.2
- menstruation *—see* Amenorrhea
- muscle (congenital) (pectoral) Q79.8
  - ocular Q10.3
- neck, part Q18.8
- neutrophil *—see* Agranulocytosis
- nipple(s) (with breast(s)) (acquired) Z90.1-●
  - congenital Q83.2
- nose (congenital) Q30.1
  - acquired Z90.09
- organ
  - of Corti, congenital Q16.5
  - or site, congenital NEC Q89.8
    - acquired NEC Z90.89
- osseous meatus (ear) Q16.4
- ovary (acquired)
  - bilateral Z90.722
  - congenital
    - bilateral Q50.02
    - unilateral Q50.01
  - unilateral Z90.721
- oviduct (acquired)
  - bilateral Z90.722
  - congenital Q50.6
  - unilateral Z90.721
- pancreas (congenital) Q45.0
  - acquired Z90.410
    - complete Z90.410
    - partial Z90.411
    - total Z90.410
- parathyroid gland (acquired) E89.2
  - congenital Q89.2
- patella, congenital Q74.1
- penis (congenital) Q55.5
  - acquired Z90.79
- pericardium (congenital) Q24.8
- pituitary gland (congenital) Q89.2
  - acquired E89.3
- prostate (acquired) Z90.79
  - congenital Q55.4
- pulmonary valve Q22.0
- punctum lacrimale (congenital) Q10.4
- radius, congenital *—see* Defect, reduction, upper limb, longitudinal, radius

Absence *(Continued)*
- rectum (congenital) Q42.1
  - with fistula Q42.0
  - acquired Z90.49
- respiratory organ NOS Q34.9
- rib (acquired) Z90.89
  - congenital Q76.6
- sacrum, congenital Q76.49
- salivary gland(s), congenital Q38.4
- scrotum, congenital Q55.29
- seminal vesicles (congenital) Q55.4
  - acquired Z90.79
- septum
  - atrial (congenital) Q21.19
  - between aorta and pulmonary artery Q21.4
  - ventricular (congenital) Q20.4
- sex chromosome
  - female phenotype Q97.8
  - male phenotype Q98.8
- skull bone (congenital) Q75.8
  - with
    - anencephaly Q00.0
    - encephalocele *—see* Encephalocele
    - hydrocephalus Q03.9
      - with spina bifida *—see* Spina bifida, by site, with hydrocephalus
    - microcephaly Q02
- spermatic cord, congenital Q55.4
- spine, congenital Q76.49
- spleen (congenital) Q89.01
  - acquired Z90.81
- sternum, congenital Q76.7
- stomach (acquired) (partial) Z90.3
  - congenital Q40.2
- superior vena cava, congenital Q26.8
- teeth, tooth (congenital) K00.0
  - acquired (complete) K08.109
    - class I K08.101
    - class II K08.102
    - class III K08.103
    - class IV K08.104
    - due to
      - caries K08.139
        - class I K08.131
        - class II K08.132
        - class III K08.133
        - class IV K08.134
      - periodontal disease K08.129
        - class I K08.121
        - class II K08.122
        - class III K08.123
        - class IV K08.124
      - specified NEC K08.199
        - class I K08.191
        - class II K08.192
        - class III K08.193
        - class IV K08.194
      - trauma K08.119
        - class I K08.111
        - class II K08.112
        - class III K08.113
        - class IV K08.114
  - partial K08.409
    - class I K08.401
    - class II K08.402
    - class III K08.403
    - class IV K08.404
    - due to
      - caries K08.439
        - class I K08.431
        - class II K08.432
        - class III K08.433
        - class IV K08.434
      - periodontal disease K08.429
        - class I K08.421
        - class II K08.422
        - class III K08.423
        - class IV K08.424
      - specified NEC K08.499
        - class I K08.491
        - class II K08.492
        - class III K08.493
        - class IV K08.494
      - trauma K08.419
        - class I K08.411
        - class II K08.412
        - class III K08.413
        - class IV K08.414
- tendon (congenital) Q79.8
- testis (congenital) Q55.0
  - acquired Z90.79

A

▶ New ➡ Revised ~~deleted~~ Deleted • Use Additional Character(s)

- **Accretio cordis** (nonrheumatic) I31.Ø
- **Accretions, tooth, teeth** KØ3.6
- **Acculturation difficulty** Z6Ø.3
- **Accumulation secretion, prostate** N42.89
- **Acephalia, acephalism, acephalus, acephaly** QØØ.Ø
- **Acephalobrachia monster** Q89.8
- **Acephalochirus monster** Q89.8
- **Acephalogaster** Q89.8
- **Acephalostomus monster** Q89.8
- **Acephalothorax** Q89.8
- **Acerophobia** F4Ø.298
- **Acetonemia** R79.89
  - in Type 1 diabetes E1Ø.1Ø
    - with coma E1Ø.11
- **Acetonuria** R82.4
- **Achalasia** (cardia) (esophagus) K22.Ø
  - congenital Q39.5
  - pylorus Q4Ø.Ø
  - sphincteral NEC K59.89
- **Ache(s)** —*see* Pain
- **Acheilia** Q38.6
- **Achillobursitis** —*see* Tendinitis, Achilles
- **Achillodynia** —*see* Tendinitis, Achilles
- **Achlorhydria, achlorhydric** (neurogenic) K31.83
  - anemia D5Ø.8
  - diarrhea K31.83
  - psychogenic F45.8
  - secondary to vagotomy K91.1
- **Achluophobia** F4Ø.228
- **Acholia** K82.8
- **Acholuric jaundice** (familial) (splenomegalic) —*see also* Spherocytosis
  - acquired D59.8
- **Achondrogenesis** Q77.Ø
- **Achondroplasia** (osteosclerosis congenita) Q77.4
- **Achroma, cutis** L8Ø
- **Achromat** (ism), achromatopsia (acquired) (congenital) H53.51
- **Achromia, congenital** —*see* Albinism
- **Achromia parasitica** B36.Ø
- **Achylia gastrica** K31.89
  - psychogenic F45.8
- **Acid**
  - burn —*see* Corrosion
  - deficiency
    - amide nicotinic E52
    - ascorbic E54
    - folic E53.8
    - nicotinic E52
    - pantothenic E53.8
  - intoxication (*see also* Acidosis) E87.29
  - peptic disease K3Ø
  - phosphatase deficiency E83.39
  - stomach K3Ø
    - psychogenic F45.8
- **Acidemia** (*see also* Acidosis) E87.2Ø
  - argininosuccinic E72.22
  - isovaleric E71.11Ø
  - metabolic - *see also* Acidosis, metabolic
  - newborn P19.9
    - first noted before onset of labor P19.Ø
    - first noted during labor P19.1
    - noted at birth P19.2
  - methylmalonic E71.12Ø
  - pipecolic E72.3
  - propionic E71.121
- **Acidity, gastric** (high) K3Ø
  - psychogenic F45.8
- **Acidocytopenia** —*see* Agranulocytosis
- **Acidocytosis** D72.1Ø
- **Acidopenia** —*see* Agranulocytosis
- **Acidosis** (lactic) E87.2Ø
  - in Type 1 diabetes E1Ø.1Ø
    - with coma E1Ø.11
  - kidney, tubular N25.89
  - lactic E87.2Ø
    - acute E87.21
    - chronic E87.22
  - metabolic NEC E87.2Ø
    - acute E87.21
    - chronic E87.22
    - hyperchloremic, of newborn P74.421
      - with respiratory acidosis E87.4
    - late, of newborn P74.Ø
  - mixed metabolic and respiratory, newborn P84
  - newborn P84
  - renal (hyperchloremic) (tubular) N25.89
  - respiratory E87.29
    - acute J96.Ø2
    - chronic J96.12
    - complicated by

- **Acidosis** *(Continued)*
  - respiratory *(Continued)*
    - complicated by *(Continued)*
      - metabolic
        - acidosis E87.4
        - alkalosis E87.4
    - specified NEC E87.29
- **Aciduria**
  - 4-hydroxybutyric E72.81
  - argininosuccinic E72.22
  - gamma-hydroxybutyric E72.81
  - glutaric (type I) E72.3
    - type II E71.313
    - type III E71.5-●
  - orotic (congenital) (hereditary) (pyrimidine deficiency) E79.89
    - anemia D53.Ø
- **Acladiosis** (skin) B36.Ø
- **Aclasis, diaphyseal** Q78.6
- **Acleistocardia** Q21.19
- **Aclusion** —*see* Anomaly, dentofacial, malocclusion
- **Acne** L7Ø.9
  - artificialis L7Ø.8
  - atrophica L7Ø.2
  - cachecticorum (Hebra) L7Ø.8
  - conglobata L7Ø.1
  - cystic L7Ø.Ø
  - decalvans L66.2
  - excoriée (des jeunes filles) L7Ø.5
  - frontalis L7Ø.2
  - indurata L7Ø.Ø
  - infantile L7Ø.4
  - keloid L73.Ø
  - lupoid L7Ø.2
  - necrotic, necrotica (miliaris) L7Ø.2
  - neonatal L7Ø.4
  - nodular L7Ø.Ø
  - occupational L7Ø.8
  - picker's L7Ø.5
  - pustular L7Ø.Ø
  - rodens L7Ø.2
  - rosacea L71.9
  - specified NEC L7Ø.8
  - tropica L7Ø.3
  - varioliformis L7Ø.2
  - vulgaris L7Ø.Ø
- **Acnitis** (primary) A18.4
- **Acosta's disease** T7Ø.29
- **Acoustic** —*see* condition
- **Acousticophobia** F4Ø.298
- **ACPO** (acute colonic pseudo-obstruction) K59.81
- **Acquired** —*see also* condition
  - immunodeficiency syndrome (AIDS) B2Ø
- **Acrania** QØØ.Ø
- **Acroangiodermatitis** I78.9
- **Acroasphyxia, chronic** I73.89
- **Acrobystitis** N47.7
- **Acrocephalopolysyndactyly** Q87.Ø
- **Acrocephalosyndactyly** Q87.Ø
- **Acrocephaly** Q75.ØØ9
- **Acrochondrohyperplasia** —*see* Syndrome, Marfan
- **Acrocyanosis** I73.89
  - newborn P28.2
    - meaning transient blue hands and feet - omit code
- **Acrodermatitis** L3Ø.8
  - atrophicans (chronica) L9Ø.4
  - continua (Hallopeau) L4Ø.2
  - enteropathica (hereditary) E83.2
  - Hallopeau's L4Ø.2
  - infantile papular L44.4
  - perstans L4Ø.2
  - pustulosa continua L4Ø.2
  - recalcitrant pustular L4Ø.2
- **Acrodynia** —*see* Poisoning, mercury
- **Acromegaly, acromegalia** E22.Ø
- **Acromelalgia** I73.81
- **Acromicria, acromikria** Q79.8
- **Acronyx** L6Ø.Ø
- **Acropachy, thyroid** —*see* Thyrotoxicosis
- **Acroparesthesia** (simple) (vasomotor) I73.89
- **Acropathy, thyroid** —*see* Thyrotoxicosis
- **Acrophobia** F4Ø.241
- **Acroposthitis** N47.7
- **Acroscleriasis, acroscleroderma, acrosclerosis** —*see* Sclerosis, systemic
- **Acrosphacelus** I96
- **Acrospiroma, eccrine** —*see* Neoplasm, skin, benign
- **Acrostealgia** —*see* Osteochondropathy
- **Acrotrophodynia** —*see* Immersion
- **ACTH ectopic syndrome** E24.3
- **Actinic** —*see* condition

- **Actinobacillosis, actinobacillus** A28.8
  - mallei A24.Ø
  - muris A25.1
- **Actinomyces israelii** (infection) —*see* Actinomycosis
- **Actinomycetoma** (foot) B47.1
- **Actinomycosis, actinomycotic** A42.9
  - with pneumonia A42.Ø
  - abdominal A42.1
  - cervicofacial A42.2
  - cutaneous A42.89
  - gastrointestinal A42.1
  - pulmonary A42.Ø
  - sepsis A42.7
  - specified site NEC A42.89
- **Actinoneuritis** G62.82
- **Action, heart**
  - disorder I49.9
  - irregular I49.9
    - psychogenic F45.8
- **Activated protein C resistance** D68.51
- **Activation**
  - mast cell (disorder) (syndrome) D89.4Ø
    - idiopathic D89.42
    - monoclonal D89.41
    - secondary D89.43
    - specified type NEC D89.49
- **Active** —*see* condition
- **Acute** —*see also* condition
  - abdomen R1Ø.Ø
  - gallbladder —*see* Cholecystitis, acute
- **Acyanotic heart disease** (congenital) Q24.9
- **Acystia** Q64.5
- **Adair-Dighton syndrome** (brittle bones and blue sclera, deafness) Q78.Ø
- **Adamantinoblastoma** —*see* Ameloblastoma
- **Adamantinoma** —*see also* Cyst, calcifying odontogenic
  - long bones C4Ø.9Ø
    - lower limb C4Ø.2-●
    - upper limb C4Ø.Ø-●
  - malignant C41.1
    - jaw (bone) (lower) C41.1
      - upper C41.Ø
  - tibial C4Ø.2-●
- **Adamantoblastoma** —*see* Ameloblastoma
- **Adams-Stokes (-Morgagni) disease or syndrome** I45.9
- **Adaption reaction** —*see* Disorder, adjustment
- **Addiction** —*see also* Dependence F19.2Ø
  - alcohol, alcoholic (ethyl) (methyl) (wood) (without remission) F1Ø.2Ø
    - with remission F1Ø.21
  - drug —*see* Dependence, drug
  - ethyl alcohol (without remission) F1Ø.2Ø
    - with remission F1Ø.21
  - heroin —*see* Dependence, drug, opioid
  - methyl alcohol (without remission) F1Ø.2Ø
    - with remission F1Ø.21
  - methylated spirit (without remission) F1Ø.2Ø
    - with remission F1Ø.21
  - morphine(-like substances) —*see* Dependence, drug, opioid
  - nicotine —*see* Dependence, drug, nicotine
  - opium and opioids —*see* Dependence, drug, opioid
  - tobacco —*see* Dependence, drug, nicotine
- **Addisonian crisis** E27.2
- **Addison's**
  - anemia (pernicious) D51.Ø
  - disease (bronze) or syndrome E27.1
    - tuberculous A18.7
  - keloid L94.Ø
- **Addison-Biermer anemia** (pernicious) D51.Ø
- **Addison-Schilder complex** E71.528
- **Additional** —*see also* Accessory
  - chromosome(s) (*see also* Trisomy) Q99.8
    - 21 —*see* Trisomy, 21
    - marker —*see* Extra, marker chromosomes
    - sex —*see* Abnormal, chromosome, sex
- **Adduction contracture, hip or other joint** —*see* Contraction, joint
- **Adenitis** —*see also* Lymphadenitis
  - acute, unspecified site LØ4.9
  - axillary I88.9
    - acute LØ4.2
    - chronic or subacute I88.1
  - Bartholin's gland N75.8
  - bulbourethral gland —*see* Urethritis
  - cervical I88.9
    - acute LØ4.Ø
    - chronic or subacute I88.1

A

- **Adenitis** *(Continued)*
  - chancroid (Hemophilus ducreyi) A57
  - chronic, unspecified site I88.1
  - Cowper's gland —*see* Urethritis
  - due to Pasteurella multocida (P. septica) A28.Ø
  - epidemic, acute B27.Ø9
  - gangrenous LØ4.9
  - gonorrheal NEC A54.89
  - groin I88.9
    - acute LØ4.1
    - chronic or subacute I88.1
  - infectious (acute) (epidemic) B27.Ø9
  - inguinal I88.9
    - acute LØ4.1
    - chronic or subacute I88.1
  - lymph gland or node, except mesenteric I88.9
    - acute —*see* Lymphadenitis, acute
    - chronic or subacute I88.1
  - mesenteric (acute) (chronic) (nonspecific) (subacute) I88.Ø
  - parotid gland (suppurative) —*see* Sialoadenitis
  - salivary gland (any) (suppurative) —*see* Sialoadenitis
  - scrofulous (tuberculous) A18.2
  - Skene's duct or gland —*see* Urethritis
  - strumous, tuberculous A18.2
  - subacute, unspecified site I88.1
  - sublingual gland (suppurative) —*see* Sialoadenitis
  - submandibular gland (suppurative) —*see* Sialoadenitis
  - submaxillary gland (suppurative) —*see* Sialoadenitis
  - tuberculous —*see* Tuberculosis, lymph gland
  - urethral gland —*see* Urethritis
  - Wharton's duct (suppurative) —*see* Sialoadenitis
- **Adenoacanthoma** —*see* Neoplasm, malignant, by site
- **Adenoameloblastoma** —*see* Cyst, calcifying odontogenic
- **Adenocarcinoid** (tumor) —*see* Neoplasm, malignant, by site
- **Adenocarcinoma** —*see also* Neoplasm, malignant, by site
  - acidophil
    - specified site —*see* Neoplasm, malignant, by site
    - unspecified site C75.1
  - adrenal cortical C74.Ø-●
  - alveolar —*see* Neoplasm, lung, malignant
  - apocrine
    - breast —*see* Neoplasm, breast, malignant
    - in situ
      - breast DØ5.8-●
      - specified site NEC —*see* Neoplasm, skin, in situ
      - unspecified site DØ4.9
    - specified site NEC —*see* Neoplasm, skin, malignant
    - unspecified site C44.99
  - basal cell
    - specified site —*see* Neoplasm, skin, malignant
    - unspecified site CØ8.9
  - basophil
    - specified site —*see* Neoplasm, malignant, by site
    - unspecified site C75.1
  - bile duct type C22.1
    - liver C22.1
    - specified site NEC —*see* Neoplasm, malignant, by site
    - unspecified site C22.1
  - bronchiolar —*see* Neoplasm, lung, malignant
  - bronchioloalveolar —*see* Neoplasm, lung, malignant
  - ceruminous C44.29-●
  - cervix, in situ (*see also* Carcinoma, cervix uteri, in situ) DØ6.9
  - chromophobe
    - specified site —*see* Neoplasm, malignant, by site
    - unspecified site C75.1
  - diffuse type
    - specified site —*see* Neoplasm, malignant, by site
    - unspecified site C16.9
  - duct
    - infiltrating
      - with Paget's disease —*see* Neoplasm, breast, malignant
      - specified site —*see* Neoplasm, malignant, by site

- **Adenocarcinoma** *(Continued)*
  - duct *(Continued)*
    - infiltrating *(Continued)*
      - unspecified site (female) C5Ø.91-●
        - male C5Ø.92-●
    - specified site —*see* Neoplasm, malignant, by site
    - unspecified site
      - female C56.9
      - male C61
  - eosinophil
    - specified site —*see* Neoplasm, malignant, by site
    - unspecified site C75.1
  - follicular
    - with papillary C73
    - moderately differentiated C73
    - specified site —*see* Neoplasm, malignant, by site
    - trabecular C73
    - unspecified site C73
    - well differentiated C73
  - Hurthle cell C73
  - in
    - adenomatous
      - polyposis coli C18.9
  - infiltrating duct
    - with Paget's disease —*see* Neoplasm, breast, malignant
    - specified site —*see* Neoplasm, malignant, by site
    - unspecified site (female) C5Ø.91-●
      - male C5Ø.92-●
  - inflammatory
    - specified site —*see* Neoplasm, malignant, by site
    - unspecified site (female) C5Ø.91-●
      - male C5Ø.92-●
  - intestinal type
    - specified site —*see* Neoplasm, malignant, by site
    - unspecified site C16.9
  - intracystic papillary
  - intraductal
    - breast DØ5.1-●
    - noninfiltrating
      - breast DØ5.1-●
      - papillary
        - with invasion
          - specified site —*see* Neoplasm, malignant, by site
          - unspecified site (female) C5Ø.91-●
            - male C5Ø.92-●
        - breast DØ5.1-●
        - specified site NEC —*see* Neoplasm, in situ, by site
        - unspecified site DØ5.1-●
      - specified site NEC —*see* Neoplasm, in situ, by site
      - unspecified site DØ5.1-●
    - papillary
      - with invasion
        - specified site —*see* Neoplasm, malignant, by site
        - unspecified site (female) C5Ø.91-●
          - male C5Ø.92-●
      - breast DØ5.1-●
      - specified site —*see* Neoplasm, in situ, by site
      - unspecified site DØ5.1-●
    - specified site NEC —*see* Neoplasm, in situ, by site
    - unspecified site DØ5.1-●
  - islet cell
    - with exocrine, mixed
      - specified site —*see* Neoplasm, malignant, by site
      - unspecified site C25.9
    - pancreas C25.4
    - specified site NEC —*see* Neoplasm, malignant, by site
    - unspecified site C25.4
  - lobular
    - in situ
      - breast DØ5.Ø-●
      - specified site NEC —*see* Neoplasm, in situ, by site
      - unspecified site DØ5.Ø-●
    - specified site —*see* Neoplasm, malignant, by site
    - unspecified site (female) C5Ø.91-●
      - male C5Ø.92-●

- **Adenocarcinoma** *(Continued)*
  - mucoid —*see also* Neoplasm, malignant, by site
    - cell
      - specified site —*see* Neoplasm, malignant, by site
      - unspecified site C75.1
  - nonencapsulated sclerosing C73
  - papillary
    - with follicular C73
    - follicular variant C73
    - intraductal (noninfiltrating)
      - with invasion
        - specified site —*see* Neoplasm, malignant, by site
        - unspecified site (female) C5Ø.91-●
          - male C5Ø.92-●
      - breast DØ5.1-●
      - specified site NEC —*see* Neoplasm, in situ, by site
      - unspecified site DØ5.1-●
    - serous
      - specified site —*see* Neoplasm, malignant, by site
      - unspecified site C56.9
  - papillocystic
    - specified site —*see* Neoplasm, malignant, by site
    - unspecified site C56.9
  - pseudomucinous
    - specified site —*see* Neoplasm, malignant, by site
    - unspecified site C56.9
  - renal cell C64-●
  - sebaceous —*see* Neoplasm, skin, malignant, by site
  - serous —*see also* Neoplasm, malignant, by site
    - papillary
      - specified site —*see* Neoplasm, malignant, by site
      - unspecified site C56.9
  - sweat gland —*see* Neoplasm, skin, malignant
  - water-clear cell C75.Ø
- **Adenocarcinoma-in-situ** —*see also* Neoplasm, in situ, by site
  - breast DØ5.9-●
- **Adenofibroma**
  - clear cell —*see* Neoplasm, benign, by site
  - endometrioid D27.9
    - borderline malignancy D39.1Ø
    - malignant C56-●
  - mucinous
    - specified site —*see* Neoplasm, benign, by site
    - unspecified site D27.9
  - papillary
    - specified site —*see* Neoplasm, benign, by site
    - unspecified site D27.9
  - prostate —*see* Enlargement, enlarged, prostate
  - serous
    - specified site —*see* Neoplasm, benign, by site
    - unspecified site D27.9
  - specified site —*see* Neoplasm, benign, by site
  - unspecified site D27.9
- **Adenofibrosis**
  - breast —*see* Fibroadenosis, breast
  - endometrioid N8Ø.ØØ
- **Adenoiditis** (chronic) J35.Ø2
  - with tonsillitis J35.Ø3
  - acute JØ3.9Ø
    - recurrent JØ3.91
    - specified organism NEC JØ3.8Ø
      - recurrent JØ3.81
    - staphylococcal JØ3.8Ø
      - recurrent JØ3.81
    - streptococcal JØ3.ØØ
      - recurrent JØ3.Ø1
- **Adenoids** —*see* condition
- **Adenolipoma** —*see* Neoplasm, benign, by site
- **Adenolipomatosis, Launois-Bensaude** E88.89
- **Adenolymphoma**
  - specified site —*see* Neoplasm, benign, by site
  - unspecified site D11.9
- **Adenoma** —*see also* Neoplasm, benign, by site
  - acidophil
    - specified site —*see* Neoplasm, benign, by site
    - unspecified site D35.2
  - acidophil-basophil, mixed
    - specified site —*see* Neoplasm, benign, by site
    - unspecified site D35.2
  - adrenal (cortical) D35.ØØ
    - clear cell D35.ØØ
    - compact cell D35.ØØ

A

A

▶ New ➡ Revised ~~deleted~~ Deleted ● Use Additional Character(s)

A

A

- **Air** *(Continued)*
  - embolism *(Continued)*
    - due to implanted device NEC —*see* Complications, by site and type, specified NEC
    - following
      - abortion —*see* Abortion by type, complicated by, embolism
      - ectopic or molar pregnancy O08.2
      - infusion, therapeutic injection or transfusion T80.Ø
    - in pregnancy, childbirth or puerperium —*see* Embolism, obstetric
    - traumatic T79.Ø
  - hunger, psychogenic F45.8
  - rarefied, effects of —*see* Effect, adverse, high altitude
  - sickness T75.3
- **Airplane sickness** T75.3
- **Akathisia** (drug-induced) (treatment- induced) G25.71
  - neuroleptic induced (acute) G25.71
  - tardive G25.71
- **Akinesia** R29.898
- **Akinetic mutism** R41.89
- **Akureyri's disease** G93.39
- **Alactasia, congenital** E73.Ø
- **Alagille (-Watson) syndrome** Q44.71
- **Alastrim** BØ3
- **Albers-Schönberg syndrome** Q78.2
- **Albert's syndrome** —*see* Tendinitis, Achilles
- **Albinism, albino** E7Ø.3Ø
  - with hematologic abnormality E7Ø.339
    - Chédiak-Higashi syndrome E7Ø.33Ø
    - Hermansky-Pudlak syndrome E7Ø.331
    - other specified E7Ø.338
  - I E7Ø.32Ø
  - II E7Ø.321
  - ocular E7Ø.319
    - autosomal recessive E7Ø.311
    - other specified E7Ø.318
    - X-linked E7Ø.31Ø
  - oculocutaneous E7Ø.329
    - other specified E7Ø.328
    - tyrosinase (ty) negative E7Ø.32Ø
    - tyrosinase (ty) positive E7Ø.321
  - other specified E7Ø.39
- **Albinismus** E7Ø.3Ø
- **Albright** (-McCune)(-Sternberg) **syndrome** Q78.1
- **Albuminous** —*see* condition
- **Albuminuria, albuminuric** (acute) (chronic) (subacute) —*see also* Proteinuria R8Ø.9
  - complicating pregnancy —*see* Proteinuria, gestational
    - with
      - gestational hypertension —*see* Pre-eclampsia
      - pre-existing hypertension —*see* Hypertension, complicating pregnancy, pre-existing, with, pre-eclampsia
  - gestational —*see* Proteinuria, gestational
    - with
      - gestational hypertension —*see* Pre-eclampsia
      - pre-existing hypertension —*see* Hypertension, complicating pregnancy, pre-existing, with, pre-eclampsia
  - orthostatic R8Ø.2
  - postural R8Ø.2
  - pre-eclamptic —*see* Pre-eclampsia
  - scarlatinal A38.8
- **Albuminurophobia** F4Ø.298
- **Alcaptonuria** E7Ø.29
- **Alcohol, alcoholic, alcohol-induced**
  - addiction (without remission) F1Ø.2Ø
    - with remission F1Ø.21
  - amnestic disorder, persisting F1Ø.96
    - with dependence F1Ø.26
  - anxiety disorder F1Ø.98Ø
  - bipolar and related disorder F1Ø.94
  - brain syndrome, chronic F1Ø.97
    - with dependence F1Ø.27
  - cardiopathy I42.6
  - counseling and surveillance Z71.41
    - family member Z71.42
  - delirium (acute) (tremens) (withdrawal) F1Ø.921
    - abuse F1Ø.131
      - with intoxication F1Ø.121
    - with intoxication F1Ø.921

- **Alcohol, alcoholic, alcohol-induced** *(Continued)*
  - delirium *(Continued)*
    - with intoxication *(Continued)*
      - in
        - abuse F1Ø.121
        - dependence F1Ø.221
  - dementia F1Ø.97
    - with dependence F1Ø.27
  - dependence (acute) (tremens) (withdrawal) F1Ø.231
    - with intoxication F1Ø.221
      - use, unspecified F1Ø.931
      - with intoxication F1Ø.921
  - depressive disorder F1Ø.94
  - deterioration F1Ø.97
    - with dependence F1Ø.27
  - hallucinosis (acute) F1Ø.951
    - in
      - abuse F1Ø.151
      - dependence F1Ø.251
  - insanity F1Ø.959
  - intoxication (acute) (without dependence) F1Ø.129
    - with
      - delirium F1Ø.121
      - dependence F1Ø.229
        - with delirium F1Ø.221
        - uncomplicated F1Ø.22Ø
    - uncomplicated F1Ø.12Ø
  - jealousy F1Ø.988
  - Korsakoff's, Korsakov's, Korsakow's F1Ø.26
  - liver K7Ø.9
    - acute —*see* Disease, liver, alcoholic, hepatitis
  - major neurocognitive disorder, amnestic-confabulatory type F1Ø.96
  - major neurocognitive disorder, nonamnestic-confabulatory type F1Ø.97
  - mania (acute) (chronic) F1Ø.959
  - mild neurocognitive disorder F1Ø.988
  - paranoia, paranoid (type) psychosis F1Ø.95Ø
  - pellagra E52
  - poisoning, accidental (acute) NEC —*see* Table of Drugs and Chemicals, alcohol, poisoning
  - psychosis —*see* Psychosis, alcoholic
  - psychotic disorder F1Ø.959
  - sexual dysfunction F1Ø.981
  - sleep disorder F1Ø.982
  - withdrawal (without convulsions) F1Ø.239
    - with delirium F1Ø.231
- **Alcoholism** (chronic) (without remission) F1Ø.2Ø
  - with
    - psychosis —*see* Psychosis, alcoholic
    - remission F1Ø.21
  - Korsakov's F1Ø.96
    - with dependence F1Ø.26
- **Alder (-Reilly) anomaly or syndrome** (leukocyte granulation) D72.Ø
- **Aldosteronism** E26.9
  - familial (type I) E26.Ø2
  - glucocorticoid-remediable E26.Ø2
  - primary (due to (bilateral) adrenal hyperplasia) E26.Ø9
  - primary NEC E26.Ø9
  - secondary E26.1
  - specified NEC E26.89
- **Aldosteronoma** D44.1Ø
- **Aldrich(-Wiskott) syndrome** (eczema-thrombocytopenia) D82.Ø
- **Alektorophobia** F4Ø.218
- **Aleppo boil** B55.1
- **Aleukemic** —*see* condition Aleukia
  - congenital D7Ø.Ø
  - hemorrhagica D61.9
    - congenital D61.Ø9
  - splenica D73.1
- **Alexia** R48.Ø
  - developmental F81.Ø
  - secondary to organic lesion R48.Ø
- **Algoneurodystrophy** M89.ØØ
  - ankle M89.Ø7- ●
  - foot M89.Ø7- ●
  - forearm M89.Ø3- ●
  - hand M89.Ø4- ●
  - lower leg M89.Ø6- ●
  - multiple sites M89.Ø- ●
  - shoulder M89.Ø1- ●
  - specified site NEC M89.Ø8
  - thigh M89.Ø5- ●
  - upper arm M89.Ø2- ●
- **Algophobia** F4Ø.298
- **Alienation, mental** —*see* Psychosis

- **Alkalemia** E87.3
- **Alkalosis** E87.3
  - metabolic E87.3
    - with respiratory acidosis E87.4
  - of newborn P74.41
  - respiratory E87.3
- **Alkaptonuria** E7Ø.29
- **Allen-Masters syndrome** N83.8
- **Allergy, allergic** (reaction) (to) T78.4Ø
  - air-borne substance NEC (rhinitis) J3Ø.89
  - alveolitis (extrinsic) J67.9
    - due to
      - Aspergillus clavatus J67.4
      - Cryptostroma corticale J67.6
      - organisms (fungal, thermophilic actinomycete) growing in ventilation (air conditioning) systems J67.7
    - specified type NEC J67.8
  - anaphylactic reaction or shock T78.2
  - angioneurotic edema T78.3
  - animal (dander) (epidermal) (hair) (rhinitis) J3Ø.81
  - ➡ bee sting (anaphylactic shock) T63.44- ●
  - biological —*see* Allergy, drug
  - colitis —*see also* Colitis, allergic K52.29
  - dander (animal) (rhinitis) J3Ø.81
  - dandruff (rhinitis) J3Ø.81
  - dental restorative material (existing) KØ8.55
  - dermatitis —*see* Dermatitis, contact, allergic
  - diathesis —*see* History, allergy
  - drug, medicament & biological (any) (external) (internal) T78.4Ø
    - correct substance properly administered —*see* Table of Drugs and Chemicals, by drug, adverse effect
    - wrong substance given or taken NEC (by accident) —*see* Table of Drugs and Chemicals, by drug, poisoning
  - due to pollen J3Ø.1
  - dust (house) (stock) (rhinitis) J3Ø.89
    - with asthma —*see* Asthma, allergic extrinsic
  - eczema —*see* Dermatitis, contact, allergic
  - epidermal (animal) (rhinitis) J3Ø.81
  - feathers (rhinitis) J3Ø.89
  - food (any) (ingested) NEC T78.1
    - anaphylactic shock —*see* Shock, anaphylactic, due to food
    - dermatitis —*see* Dermatitis, due to, food
    - dietary counseling and surveillance Z71.3
    - in contact with skin L23.6
    - rhinitis J3Ø.5
    - status (without reaction) Z91.Ø18
      - beef Z91.Ø14
      - eggs Z91.Ø12
      - lamb Z91.Ø14
      - mammalian meats Z91.Ø14
      - milk products Z91.Ø11
      - peanuts Z91.Ø1Ø
      - pork Z91.Ø14
      - red meats Z91.Ø14
      - seafood Z91.Ø13
      - specified NEC Z91.Ø18
  - gastrointestinal —*see also* specific type of allergic reaction
    - meaning colitis —*see also* Colitis, allergic) K52.29
    - meaning gastroenteritis —*see also* Gastroenteritis, allergic) K52.29
    - meaning other adverse food reaction not elsewhere classified T78.1
  - grain J3Ø.1
  - grass (hay fever) (pollen) J3Ø.1
    - asthma —*see* Asthma, allergic extrinsic
  - hair (animal) (rhinitis) J3Ø.81
  - history (of) —*see* History, allergy
  - horse serum —*see* Allergy, serum
  - inhalant (rhinitis) J3Ø.89
    - pollen J3Ø.1
  - kapok (rhinitis) J3Ø.89
  - medicine —*see* Allergy, drug
  - milk protein —*see also* Allergy, food Z91.Ø11
    - anaphylactic reaction T78.Ø7
    - dermatitis L27.2
    - enterocolitis syndrome K52.21
    - enteropathy K52.22
    - gastroenteritis K52.29
    - gastroesophageal reflux —*see also* Reaction, adverse, food) K21.9
      - with esophagitis without bleeding K21.ØØ
        - with bleeding K21.Ø1
    - proctocolitis K52.29

Allergy, allergic *(Continued)*
nasal, seasonal due to pollen J30.1
pneumonia J82.89
pollen (any) (hay fever) J30.1
asthma —*see* Asthma, allergic extrinsic
primrose J30.1
primula J30.1
proctocolitis K52.29
purpura D69.0
ragweed (hay fever) (pollen) J30.1
asthma —*see* Asthma, allergic extrinsic
rose (pollen) J30.1
seasonal NEC J30.2
Senecio jacobae (pollen) J30.1
serum —*see also* Reaction, serum T80.69
anaphylactic shock T80.59
shock (anaphylactic) T78.2
due to
administration of blood and blood products T80.51
adverse effect of correct medicinal substance properly administered T88.6
immunization T80.52
serum NEC T80.59
vaccination T80.52
specific NEC T78.49
tree (any) (hay fever) (pollen) J30.1
asthma —*see* Asthma, allergic extrinsic
upper respiratory J30.9
urticaria L50.0
vaccine —*see* Allergy, serum
wheat —*see* Allergy, food
Allescheriasis B48.2
Alligator skin disease Q80.9
Allocheiria, allochiria R20.8
Almeida's disease —*see* Paracoccidioidomycosis
Alopecia (hereditaria) (seborrheica) L65.9
androgenic L64.9
drug-induced L64.0
specified NEC L64.8
areata L63.9
ophiasis L63.2
specified NEC L63.8
totalis L63.0
universalis L63.1
cicatricial L66.9
▶central centrifugal L66.81
➡specified NEC L66.89
circumscripta L63.9
congenital, congenitalis Q84.0
due to cytotoxic drugs NEC L65.8
▶frontal fibrosing L66.12
mucinosa L65.2
postinfective NEC L65.8
postpartum L65.0
premature L64.8
specific (syphilitic) A51.32
specified NEC L65.8
syphilitic (secondary) A51.32
totalis (capitis) L63.0
universalis (entire body) L63.1
X-ray L58.1
Alpers' disease G31.81
Alpine sickness T70.29
Alport syndrome Q87.81
ALTE (apparent life threatening event) in newborn and infant R68.13
Alteration (of), Altered
awareness
transient R40.4
unintended under general anesthesia, during procedure T88.53
mental status R41.82
pattern of family relationships affecting child Z62.898
sensation
following
cerebrovascular disease I69.998
cerebral infarction I69.398
intracerebral hemorrhage I69.198
nontraumatic intracranial hemorrhage NEC I69.298
specified disease NEC I69.898
subarachnoid hemorrhage I69.098
Alternating —*see* condition
Altitude, high (effects) —*see* Effect, adverse, high altitude
Aluminosis (of lung) J63.0
Alveolitis
allergic (extrinsic) —*see* Pneumonitis, hypersensitivity

Alveolitis *(Continued)*
due to
Aspergillus clavatus J67.4
Cryptostroma corticale J67.6
fibrosing (cryptogenic) (idiopathic) J84.112
jaw M27.3
sicca dolorosa M27.3
Alveolus, alveolar —*see* condition
Alymphocytosis D72.810
thymic (with immunodeficiency) D82.1
Alymphoplasia, thymic D82.1
Alzheimer's disease or sclerosis —*see* Disease, Alzheimer's
Amastia (with nipple present) Q83.8
with absent nipple Q83.0
Amathophobia F40.228
Amaurosis (acquired) (congenital) —*see also* Blindness
fugax G45.3
hysterical F44.6
Leber's congenital H35.50
uremic —*see* Uremia
Amaurotic idiocy (infantile) (juvenile) (late) E75.4
Amaxophobia F40.248
Ambiguous genitalia Q56.4
Amblyopia (congenital) (ex anopsia) (partial) (suppression) H53.00- •
anisometropic —*see* Amblyopia, refractive
deprivation H53.01- •
hysterical F44.6
nocturnal —*see also* Blindness, night
vitamin A deficiency E50.5
refractive H53.02- •
strabismic H53.03- •
suspect H53.04- •
tobacco H53.8
toxic NEC H53.8
uremic —*see* Uremia
Ameba, amebic (histolytica) —*see also* Amebiasis
abscess (liver) A06.4
Amebiasis A06.9
with abscess —*see* Abscess, amebic
acute A06.0
chronic (intestine) A06.1
with abscess —*see* Abscess, amebic
cutaneous A06.7
cutis A06.7
cystitis A06.81
genitourinary tract NEC A06.82
hepatic —*see* Abscess, liver, amebic
intestine A06.0
nondysenteric colitis A06.2
skin A06.7
specified site NEC A06.89
Ameboma (of intestine) A06.3
Amelia Q73.0
lower limb —*see* Agenesis, leg
upper limb —*see* Agenesis, arm
Ameloblastoma —*see also* Cyst, calcifying odontogenic
long bones C40.9- •
lower limb C40.2- •
upper limb C40.0- •
malignant C41.1
jaw (bone) (lower) C41.1
upper C41.0
tibial C40.2- •
Amelogenesis imperfecta K00.5
nonhereditaria (segmentalis) K00.4
Amenorrhea N91.2
hyperhormonal E28.8
primary N91.0
secondary N91.1
Amentia —*see* Disability, intellectual
Meynert's (nonalcoholic) F04
American
leishmaniasis B55.2
mountain tick fever A93.2
Ametropia —*see* Disorder, refraction
AMH (asymptomatic microscopic hematuria) R31.21
Amianthosis J61
Amimia R48.8
Amino-acid disorder E72.9
anemia D53.0
Aminoacidopathy E72.9
Aminoaciduria E72.9
Amnes (t)ic syndrome (post-traumatic) F04
induced by
alcohol F10.96
with dependence F10.26

Amnes (t)ic syndrome *(Continued)*
induced by *(Continued)*
psychoactive NEC F19.96
with
abuse F19.16
dependence F19.26
sedative F13.96
with dependence F13.26
Amnesia R41.3
anterograde R41.1
auditory R48.8
dissociative F44.0
with dissociative fugue F44.1
hysterical F44.0
postictal in epilepsy —*see* Epilepsy
psychogenic F44.0
retrograde R41.2
transient global G45.4
Amnion, amniotic —*see* condition
Amnionitis —*see* Pregnancy, complicated by
Amok F68.8
Amoral traits F60.89
Amphetamine (or other stimulant) —induced
anxiety disorder F15.980
bipolar and related disorder F15.94
delirium F15.921
depressive disorder F15.94
obsessive-compulsive and related disorder F15.988
psychotic disorder F15.959
sexual dysfunction F15.981
sleep disorder F15.982
stimulant withdrawal F15.23
Ampulla
lower esophagus K22.89
phrenic K22.89
Amputation —*see also* Absence, by site, acquired
neuroma (postoperative) (traumatic) —*see* Complications, amputation stump, neuroma
stump (surgical)
abnormal, painful, or with complication (late) —*see* Complications, amputation stump
healed or old NOS Z89.9
traumatic (complete) (partial)
arm (upper) (complete) S48.91- •
at
elbow S58.01- •
partial S58.02- •
shoulder joint (complete) S48.01- •
partial S48.02- •
between
elbow and wrist (complete) S58.11- •
partial S58.12- •
shoulder and elbow (complete) S48.11- •
partial S48.12- •
partial S48.92- •
breast (complete) S28.21- •
partial S28.22- •
clitoris (complete) S38.211
partial S38.212
ear (complete) S08.11- •
partial S08.12- •
finger (complete) (metacarpophalangeal) S68.11- •
index S68.11- •
little S68.11- •
middle S68.11- •
partial S68.12- •
index S68.12- •
little S68.12- •
middle S68.12- •
ring S68.12- •
ring S68.11- •
thumb —*see* Amputation, traumatic, thumb
transphalangeal (complete) S68.61- •
index S68.61- •
little S68.61- •
middle S68.61- •
partial S68.62- •
index S68.62- •
little S68.62- •
middle S68.62- •
ring S68.62- •
ring S68.61- •
foot (complete) S98.91- •
at ankle level S98.01- •
partial S98.02- •

A

Amputation *(Continued)*
- traumatic *(Continued)*
  - foot *(Continued)*
    - midfoot S98.31-●
      - partial S98.32-●
    - partial S98.92-●
  - forearm (complete) S58.91-●
    - at elbow level (complete) S58.01-●
      - partial S58.02-●
    - between elbow and wrist (complete) S58.11-●
      - partial S58.12-●
    - partial S58.92-●
  - genital organ(s) (external)
    - female (complete) S38.211
      - partial S38.212
    - male
      - penis (complete) S38.221
        - partial S38.222
      - scrotum (complete) S38.231
        - partial S38.232
      - testes (complete) S38.231
        - partial S38.232
  - hand (complete) (wrist level) S68.41-●
    - finger(s) alone —*see* Amputation, traumatic, finger
    - partial S68.42-●
    - thumb alone —*see* Amputation, traumatic, thumb
    - transmetacarpal (complete) S68.71-●
      - partial S68.72-●
  - head
    - ear —*see* Amputation, traumatic, ear
    - nose (partial) S08.812
      - complete S08.811
    - part S08.89
      - scalp S08.0
  - hip (and thigh) (complete) S78.91-●
    - at hip joint (complete) S78.01-●
      - partial S78.02-●
    - between hip and knee (complete) S78.11-●
      - partial S78.12-●
    - partial S78.92-●
  - labium (majus) (minus) (complete) S38.21-●
    - partial S38.21-●
  - leg (lower) S88.91-●
    - at knee level S88.01-●
      - partial S88.02-●
    - between knee and ankle S88.11-●
      - partial S88.12-●
    - partial S88.92-●
  - nose (partial) S08.812
    - complete S08.811
  - penis (complete) S38.221
    - partial S38.222
  - scrotum (complete) S38.231
    - partial S38.232
  - shoulder —*see* Amputation, traumatic, arm
    - at shoulder joint —*see* Amputation, traumatic, arm, at shoulder joint
  - testes (complete) S38.231
    - partial S38.232
  - thigh —*see* Amputation, traumatic, hip
  - thorax, part of S28.1
    - breast —*see* Amputation, traumatic, breast
  - thumb (complete) (metacarpophalangeal) S68.01-●
    - partial S68.02-●
    - transphalangeal (complete) S68.51-●
      - partial S68.52-●
  - toe (lesser) S98.13-●
    - great S98.11-●
      - partial S98.12-●
    - more than one S98.21-●
      - partial S98.22-●
    - partial S98.14-●
  - vulva (complete) S38.211
    - partial S38.212

Amputee (bilateral) (old) Z89.9

Amsterdam dwarfism Q87.19

Amusia R48.8
- developmental F80.89

Amyelencephalus, amyelencephaly Q00.0

Amyelia Q06.0

Amygdalitis —*see* Tonsillitis

Amygdalolith J35.8

Amyloid heart (disease) E85.4 *[I43]*

Amyloidosis (generalized) (primary) E85.9
- with lung involvement E85.4 *[J99]*
- familial E85.2

Amyloidosis *(Continued)*
- genetic E85.2
- heart E85.4 *[I43]*
- hemodialysis-associated E85.3
- light chain (AL) E85.81
- liver E85.4 *[K77]*
- localized E85.4
- neuropathic heredofamilial E85.1
- non-neuropathic heredofamilial E85.0
- organ limited E85.4
- Portuguese E85.1
- pulmonary E85.4 *[J99]*
- secondary systemic E85.3
- senile systemic (SSA) E85.82
- skin (lichen) (macular) E85.4 *[L99]*
- specified NEC E85.89
- subglottic E85.4 *[J99]*
- wild-type transthyretin-related (ATTR) E85.82

Amylopectinosis (brancher enzyme deficiency) E74.03

Amylophagia —*see* Pica

Amyoplasia congenita Q79.8

Amyotonia M62.89
- congenita G70.2

Amyotrophia, amyotrophy, amyotrophic G71.8
- congenita Q79.8
- diabetic —*see* Diabetes, amyotrophy
- lateral sclerosis G12.21
- neuralgic G54.5
- spinal progressive G12.25

Anacidity, gastric K31.83
- psychogenic F45.8

Anaerosis of newborn P28.89

Analbuminemia E88.09

Analgesia —*see* Anesthesia

Analphalipoproteinemia E78.6

Anaphylactic
- purpura D69.0
- shock or reaction —*see* Shock, anaphylactic

Anaphylactoid shock or reaction —*see* Shock, anaphylactic

Anaphylactoid syndrome of pregnancy O88.01-●

Anaphylaxis —*see* Shock, anaphylactic

Anaplasia cervix —*see also* Dysplasia, cervix N87.9

Anaplasmosis [A. phagocytophilum] (transfusion transmitted) A79.82
- human A77.49

Anarthria R47.1

Anasarca R60.1
- cardiac —*see* Failure, heart, congestive
- lung J18.2
- newborn P83.2
- nutritional E43
- pulmonary J18.2
- renal N04.9

Anastomosis
- aneurysmal —*see* Aneurysm
- arteriovenous ruptured brain I60.8
- intestinal K63.89
  - complicated NEC K91.89
    - involving urinary tract N99.89
- intracerebral I61.8
- intraparenchymal I61.8
- intraventricular I61.5
- retinal and choroidal vessels (congenital) Q14.8
- subarachnoid I60.8

Anatomical narrow angle H40.03-●

Ancylostoma, ancylostomiasis (braziliense) (caninum) (ceylanicum) (duodenale) B76.0
- Necator americanus B76.1

Andersen's disease (glycogen storage) E74.09

Anderson-Fabry disease E75.21

Andes disease T70.29

Andrews' disease (bacterid) L08.89

Androblastoma
- benign
  - specified site —*see* Neoplasm, benign, by site
  - unspecified site
    - female D27.9
    - male D29.20
- malignant
  - specified site —*see* Neoplasm, malignant, by site
  - unspecified site
    - female C56.9
    - male C62.90
- specified site —*see* Neoplasm, uncertain behavior, by site

Androblastoma *(Continued)*
- tubular
  - with lipid storage
    - specified site —*see* Neoplasm, benign, by site
    - unspecified site
      - female D27.9
      - male D29.20
  - specified site —*see* Neoplasm, benign, by site
  - unspecified site
    - female D27.9
    - male D29.20
- unspecified site
  - female D39.10
  - male D40.10

Androgen insensitivity syndrome —*see also* Syndrome, androgen insensitivity E34.50

Androgen resistance syndrome —*see also* Syndrome, androgen insensitivity E34.50

Android pelvis Q74.2
- with disproportion (fetopelvic) O33.3
  - causing obstructed labor O65.3

Androphobia F40.290

Anectasis, pulmonary (newborn) —*see* Atelectasis

Anemia (essential) (general) (hemoglobin deficiency) (infantile) (primary) (profound) D64.9
- with (due to) (in)
  - disorder of
    - anaerobic glycolysis D55.29
    - pentose phosphate pathway D55.1
  - koilonychia D50.9
- achlorhydric D50.8
- achrestic D53.1
- Addison (-Biermer) (pernicious) D51.0
- agranulocytic —*see* Agranulocytosis
- amino-acid-deficiency D53.0
- aplastic D61.9
  - congenital D61.09
  - drug-induced D61.1
  - due to
    - drugs D61.1
    - external agents NEC D61.2
    - infection D61.2
    - radiation D61.2
  - idiopathic D61.3
  - red cell (pure) D60.9
    - chronic D60.0
    - congenital D61.01
    - specified type NEC D60.8
    - transient D60.1
  - specified type NEC D61.89
  - toxic D61.2
- aregenerative
  - congenital D61.09
- asiderotic D50.9
- atypical (primary) D64.9
- Baghdad spring D55.0
- Balantidium coli A07.0
- Biermer's (pernicious) D51.0
- blood loss (chronic) D50.0
  - acute D62
- bothriocephalus B70.0 *[D63.8]*
- brickmaker's B76.9 *[D63.8]*
- cerebral I67.89
- childhood D58.9
- chlorotic D50.8
- chronic
  - blood loss D50.0
  - hemolytic D58.9
    - idiopathic D59.9
  - simple D53.9
- chronica congenita aregenerativa D61.09
- combined system disease NEC D51.0 *[G32.0]*
  - due to dietary vitamin B12 deficiency D51.3 *[G32.0]*
- complicating pregnancy, childbirth or puerperium —*see* Pregnancy, complicated by (management affected by), anemia
- congenital P61.4
  - aplastic D61.09
  - due to isoimmunization NOS P55.9
  - dyserythropoietic, dyshematopoietic D64.4
  - following fetal blood loss P61.3
  - Heinz body D58.2
  - hereditary hemolytic NOS D58.9
  - pernicious D51.0
  - spherocytic D58.0
- Cooley's (erythroblastic) D56.1
- cytogenic D51.0

A

Aneurysm *(Continued)*
congenital *(Continued)*
digestive system Q27.8
lower limb Q27.8
pulmonary Q25.79
retina Q14.1
specified site NEC Q27.8
upper limb Q27.8
conjunctiva —*see* Abnormality, conjunctiva, vascular
conus arteriosus —*see* Aneurysm, heart
coronary (arteriosclerotic) (artery) I25.41
arteriovenous, congenital Q24.5
congenital Q24.5
ruptured —*see* Infarct, myocardium
syphilitic A52.Ø6
vein I25.89
cylindroid (aorta) I71.9
ruptured I71.8
syphilitic A52.Ø1
ductus arteriosus Q25.Ø
endocardial, infective (any valve) I33.Ø
femoral (artery) (ruptured) I72.4
gastroduodenal I72.8
gastroepiploic I72.8
heart (wall) (chronic or with a stated duration of over 4 weeks) I25.3
valve —*see* Endocarditis
hepatic I72.8
iliac (common) (artery) (ruptured) I72.3
infective I72.9
endocardial (any valve) I33.Ø
innominate (nonsyphilitic) I72.8
syphilitic A52.Ø9
interauricular septum —*see* Aneurysm, heart
interventricular septum —*see* Aneurysm, heart
intrathoracic (nonsyphilitic) (*see also* Aneurysm, aorta, thorax) I71.2Ø
ruptured (*see also* Aneurysm, aorta, thorax, ruptured) I71.1Ø
syphilitic A52.Ø1
lower limb I72.4
lung (pulmonary artery) I28.1
mediastinal (nonsyphilitic) I72.8
syphilitic A52.Ø9
miliary (congenital) I67.1
ruptured —*see* Hemorrhage, intracerebral, subarachnoid, intracranial
mitral (heart) (valve) I34.89
mural —*see* Aneurysm, heart
mycotic I72.9
endocardial (any valve) I33.Ø
ruptured, brain —*see* Hemorrhage, intracerebral, subarachnoid
myocardium —*see* Aneurysm, heart
neck I72.Ø
pancreaticoduodenal I72.8
patent ductus arteriosus Q25.Ø
peripheral NEC I72.8
congenital Q27.8
digestive system Q27.8
lower limb Q27.8
specified site NEC Q27.8
upper limb Q27.8
popliteal (artery) (ruptured) I72.4
precerebral
congenital (nonruptured) Q28.1
specified site, NEC I72.5
pulmonary I28.1
arteriovenous Q25.72
acquired I28.Ø
syphilitic A52.Ø9
valve (heart) —*see* Endocarditis, pulmonary
racemose (peripheral) I72.9
congenital —*see* Aneurysm, congenital
radial I72.1
Rasmussen NEC A15.Ø
renal (artery) I72.2
retina —*see also* Disorder, retina, microaneurysms
congenital Q14.1
diabetic —*see* EØ8-E13 with .3-●
sinus of Valsalva Q25.43
specified NEC I72.8
spinal (cord) I72.8
syphilitic (hemorrhage) A52.Ø9
splenic I72.8
subclavian (artery) (ruptured) I72.8
syphilitic A52.Ø9
superior mesenteric I72.8

Aneurysm *(Continued)*
syphilitic (aorta) A52.Ø1
central nervous system A52.Ø5
congenital (late) A5Ø.54 *[I79.Ø]*
spine, spinal A52.Ø9
thoracoabdominal (aorta) I71.6Ø
ruptured I71.5Ø
syphilitic A52.Ø1
thorax, thoracic (aorta) (arch) (nonsyphilitic) —*see* Aneurysm, aorta, thorax
ruptured —*see* Aneurysm, aorta, thorax, ruptured
syphilitic A52.Ø1
traumatic (complication) (early), specified site —*see* Injury, blood vessel
tricuspid (heart) (valve) IØ7.8
ulnar I72.1
upper limb (ruptured) I72.1
valve, valvular —*see* Endocarditis
visceral NEC I72.8
venous —*see also* Varix I86.8
congenital Q27.8
digestive system Q27.8
lower limb Q27.8
specified site NEC Q27.8
upper limb Q27.8
ventricle —*see* Aneurysm, heart
vertebral artery I72.6
visceral NEC I72.8
Angelman syndrome Q93.51
Anger R45.4
Angiectasis, angiectopia I99.8
Angiitis I77.6
allergic granulomatous M3Ø.1
hypersensitivity M31.Ø
necrotizing M31.9
specified NEC M31.8
nervous system, granulomatous I67.7
Angina (attack) (cardiac) (chest) (heart) (pectoris) (syndrome) (vasomotor) I2Ø.9
with
atherosclerotic heart disease —*see* Arteriosclerosis, coronary (artery)
coronary microvascular disease I2Ø.81
coronary microvascular dysfunction I2Ø.81
documented spasm I2Ø.1
abdominal K55.1
accelerated —*see* Angina, unstable
agranulocytic —*see* Agranulocytosis
angiospastic —*see* Angina, with documented spasm
aphthous BØ8.5
crescendo —*see* Angina, unstable
croupous JØ5.Ø
cruris I73.9
de novo effort —*see* Angina, unstable
diphtheritic, membranous A36.Ø
equivalent I2Ø.89
exudative, chronic J37.Ø
following acute myocardial infarction I23.7
gangrenous diphtheritic A36.Ø
intestinal K55.1
Ludovici K12.2
Ludwig's K12.2
malignant diphtheritic A36.Ø
membranous JØ5.Ø
diphtheritic A36.Ø
Vincent's A69.1
mesenteric K55.1
monocytic —*see* Mononucleosis, infectious
of effort —*see* Angina, specified NEC
phlegmonous J36
diphtheritic A36.Ø
post-infarctional I23.7
pre-infarctional —*see* Angina, unstable
Prinzmetal —*see* Angina, with documented spasm
progressive —*see* Angina, unstable
pseudomembranous A69.1
pultaceous, diphtheritic A36.Ø
refractory I2Ø.2
spasm-induced —*see* Angina, with documented spasm
specified NEC I2Ø.89
stable I2Ø.89
stenocardia —*see* Angina, specified NEC
stridulous, diphtheritic A36.2
tonsil J36
trachealis JØ5.Ø
unstable I2Ø.Ø
variant —*see* Angina, with documented spasm

Angina *(Continued)*
Vincent's A69.1
worsening effort —*see* Angina, unstable
Angioblastoma —*see* Neoplasm, connective tissue, uncertain behavior
Angiocholecystitis —*see* Cholecystitis, acute
Angiocholitis —*see also* Cholecystitis, acute K83.Ø9
Angiodysgenesis spinalis G95.19
Angiodysplasia (cecum) (colon) K55.2Ø
with bleeding K55.21
duodenum (and stomach) K31.819
with bleeding K31.811
stomach (and duodenum) K31.819
with bleeding K31.811
Angioedema (allergic) (any site) (with urticaria) T78.3
episodic, with eosinophilia D72.118
hereditary D84.1
Angioendothelioma —*see* Neoplasm, uncertain behavior, by site
benign D18.ØØ
intra-abdominal D18.Ø3
intracranial D18.Ø2
skin D18.Ø1
specified site NEC D18.Ø9
bone —*see* Neoplasm, bone, malignant
Ewing's —*see* Neoplasm, bone, malignant
Angioendotheliomatosis C85.8-●
Angiofibroma —*see also* Neoplasm, benign, by site
juvenile
specified site —*see* Neoplasm, benign, by site
unspecified site D1Ø.6
Angiohemophilia (A) (B) —*see* Disease, von Willebrand
Angioid streaks (choroid) (macula) (retina) H35.33
Angiokeratoma —*see* Neoplasm, skin, benign
corporis diffusum E75.21
Angioleiomyoma —*see* Neoplasm, connective tissue, benign
Angiolipoma —*see also* Lipoma
infiltrating —*see* Lipoma
Angioma —*see also* Hemangioma, by site
capillary I78.1
hemorrhagicum hereditaria I78.Ø
intra-abdominal D18.Ø3
intracranial D18.Ø2
malignant —*see* Neoplasm, connective tissue, malignant
plexiform D18.ØØ
intra-abdominal D18.Ø3
intracranial D18.Ø2
skin D18.Ø1
specified site NEC D18.Ø9
senile I78.1
serpiginosum L81.7
skin D18.Ø1
specified site NEC D18.Ø9
spider I78.1
stellate I78.1
venous Q28.3
Angiomatosis Q82.8
bacillary A79.89
encephalotrigeminal Q85.89
hemorrhagic familial I78.Ø
hereditary familial I78.Ø
liver K76.4
Angiomyolipoma —*see* Lipoma
Angiomyoliposarcoma —*see* Neoplasm, connective tissue, malignant
Angiomyoma —*see* Neoplasm, connective tissue, benign
Angiomyosarcoma —*see* Neoplasm, connective tissue, malignant
Angiomyxoma —*see* Neoplasm, connective tissue, uncertain behavior
Angioneurosis F45.8
Angioneurotic edema (allergic) (any site) (with urticaria) T78.3
hereditary D84.1
Angiopathia, angiopathy I99.9
cerebral I67.9
amyloid E85.4 *[I68.Ø]*
diabetic (peripheral) —*see* Diabetes, angiopathy
peripheral I73.9
diabetic —*see* Diabetes, angiopathy
specified type NEC I73.89
retinae syphilitica A52.Ø5
retinalis (juvenilis)
diabetic —*see* Diabetes, retinopathy
proliferative —*see* Retinopathy, proliferative

A

A

Angiosarcoma —*see also* Neoplasm, connective
 tissue, malignant
 liver C22.3
Angiosclerosis —*see* Arteriosclerosis
Angiospasm (peripheral) (traumatic) (vessel) (see
 also Vasospasm) I73.9
 brachial plexus G54.0
 cerebral G45.9
 cervical plexus G54.2
 nerve
 arm —*see* Mononeuropathy, upper limb
 axillary G54.0
 median —*see* Lesion, nerve, median
 ulnar —*see* Lesion, nerve, ulnar
 axillary G54.0
 leg —*see* Mononeuropathy, lower limb
 median —*see* Lesion, nerve, median
 plantar —*see* Lesion, nerve, plantar
 ulnar —*see* Lesion, nerve, ulnar
Angiospastic disease or edema I73.9
Angiostrongyliasis
 due to
 Parastrongylus
 cantonensis B83.2
 costaricensis B81.3
 intestinal B81.3
Anguillulosis —*see* Strongyloidiasis
Angulation
 cecum —*see* Obstruction, intestine
 coccyx (acquired) —*see also* subcategory M43.8
 congenital NEC Q76.49
 femur (acquired) —*see also* Deformity, limb,
 specified type NEC, thigh
 congenital Q74.2
 intestine (large) (small) —*see* Obstruction,
 intestine
 sacrum (acquired) —*see also* subcategory M43.8
 congenital NEC Q76.49
 sigmoid (flexure) —*see* Obstruction, intestine
 spine —*see* Dorsopathy, deforming, specified NEC
 tibia (acquired) —*see also* Deformity, limb,
 specified type NEC, lower leg
 congenital Q74.2
 ureter N13.5
 with infection N13.6
 wrist (acquired) —*see also* Deformity, limb,
 specified type NEC, forearm
 congenital Q74.0
Angulus infectiosus (lips) K13.0
Anhedonia R45.84
 sexual F52.0
Anhidrosis L74.4
Anhydration E86.0
Anhydremia E86.0
Anidrosis L74.4
Aniridia (congenital) Q13.1
Anisakiasis (infection) (infestation) B81.0
Anisakis larvae infestation B81.0
Aniseikonia H52.32
Anisocoria (pupil) H57.02
 congenital Q13.2
Anisocytosis R71.8
Anisometropia (congenital) H52.31
Ankle —*see* condition
Ankyloblepharon (eyelid) (acquired) —*see also*
 Blepharophimosis
 filiforme (adnatum) (congenital) Q10.3
 total Q10.3
Ankyloglossia Q38.1
Ankylosis (fibrous) (osseous) (joint) M24.60
 ankle M24.67-●
 arthrodesis status Z98.1
 cricoarytenoid (cartilage) (joint) (larynx) J38.7
 dental K03.5
 ear ossicles H74.31-●
 elbow M24.62-●
 foot M24.67-●
 hand M24.64-●
 hip M24.65-●
 incostapedial joint (infectional) —*see* Ankylosis,
 ear ossicles
 jaw (temporomandibular) M26.61-●
 knee M24.66-●
 lumbosacral (joint) M43.27
 postoperative (status) Z98.1
 produced by surgical fusion, status Z98.1
 sacro-iliac (joint) M43.28
 shoulder M24.61-●
 specified site NEC M24.69
 spine (joint) —*see also* Fusion, spine
 spondylitic —*see* Spondylitis, ankylosing

Ankylosis *(Continued)*
 surgical Z98.1
 temporomandibular M26.61-●
 tooth, teeth (hard tissues) K03.5
 wrist M24.63-●
Ankylostoma —*see* Ancylostoma
Ankylostomiasis —*see* Ancylostomiasis
Ankylurethria —*see* Stricture, urethra
Annular —*see also* condition
 detachment, cervix N88.8
 organ or site, congenital NEC —*see* Distortion
 pancreas (congenital) Q45.1
Anoctaminopathy G71.035
Anodontia (complete) (partial) (vera) K00.0
 acquired K08.10
Anomaly, anomalous (congenital) (unspecified
 type) Q89.9
 abdominal wall NEC Q79.59
 acoustic nerve Q07.8
 adrenal (gland) Q89.1
 Alder (-Reilly) (leukocyte granulation)
 D72.0
 alimentary tract Q45.9
 upper Q40.9
 alveolar M26.70
 hyperplasia M26.79
 mandibular M26.72
 maxillary M26.71
 hypoplasia M26.79
 mandibular M26.74
 maxillary M26.73
 ridge (process) M26.79
 specified NEC M26.79
 ankle (joint) Q74.2
 anus Q43.9
 aorta (arch) NEC Q25.40
 coarctation (preductal) (postductal) Q25.1
 aortic cusp or valve Q23.9
 appendix Q43.8
 apple peel syndrome Q41.1
 aqueduct of Sylvius Q03.0
 with spina bifida —*see* Spina bifida, with
 hydrocephalus
 arm Q74.0
 arteriovenous NEC
 coronary Q24.5
 gastrointestinal Q27.33
 acquired —*see* Angiodysplasia
 artery (peripheral) Q27.9
 basilar NEC Q28.1
 cerebral Q28.3
 coronary Q24.5
 digestive system Q27.8
 eye Q15.8
 great Q25.9
 specified NEC Q25.8
 lower limb Q27.8
 peripheral Q27.9
 specified NEC Q27.8
 pulmonary NEC Q25.79
 renal Q27.2
 retina Q14.1
 specified site NEC Q27.8
 subclavian Q27.8
 origin Q25.48
 umbilical Q27.0
 upper limb Q27.8
 vertebral NEC Q28.1
 aryteno-epiglottic folds Q31.8
 atrial
 bands or folds Q20.8
 septa Q21.10
 atrioventricular
 excitation I45.6
 septum Q21.0
 auditory canal Q17.8
 auricle
 ear Q17.8
 causing impairment of hearing Q16.9
 heart Q20.8
 Axenfeld's Q15.0
 back Q89.9
 band
 atrial Q20.8
 heart Q24.8
 ventricular Q24.8
 Bartholin's duct Q38.4
 biliary duct or passage Q44.5
 bladder Q64.70
 absence Q64.5
 diverticulum Q64.6

Anomaly, anomalous *(Continued)*
 bladder *(Continued)*
 exstrophy Q64.10
 cloacal Q64.12
 extroversion Q64.19
 specified type NEC Q64.19
 supravesical fissure Q64.11
 neck obstruction Q64.31
 specified type NEC Q64.79
 bone Q79.9
 arm Q74.0
 face Q75.0
 leg Q74.2
 pelvic girdle Q74.2
 shoulder girdle Q74.0
 skull Q75.9
 with
 anencephaly Q00.0
 encephalocele —*see* Encephalocele
 hydrocephalus Q03.9
 with spina bifida —*see* Spina bifida, by
 site, with hydrocephalus
 microcephaly Q02
 brain (multiple) Q04.9
 vessel Q28.3
 breast Q83.9
 broad ligament Q50.6
 bronchus Q32.4
 bulbus cordis Q21.9
 bursa Q79.9
 canal of Nuck Q52.4
 canthus Q10.3
 capillary Q27.9
 cardiac Q24.9
 chambers Q20.9
 specified NEC Q20.8
 septal closure Q21.9
 specified NEC Q21.8
 valve NEC Q24.8
 pulmonary Q22.3
 cardiovascular system Q28.8
 carpus Q74.0
 caruncle, lacrimal Q10.6
 cascade stomach Q40.2
 cauda equina Q06.3
 cecum Q43.9
 cerebral Q04.9
 vessels Q28.3
 cervix Q51.9
 Chédiak-Higashi(-Steinbrinck) (congenital
 gigantism of peroxidase granules) E70.330
 cheek Q18.9
 chest wall Q67.8
 bones Q76.9
 chin Q18.9
 chordae tendineae Q24.8
 choroid Q14.3
 plexus Q07.8
 chromosomes, chromosomal Q99.9
 D (1) —*see* condition, chromosome 13
 E (3) —*see* condition, chromosome 18
 G —*see* condition, chromosome 21
 sex
 female phenotype Q97.8
 gonadal dysgenesis (pure) Q99.1
 Klinefelter's Q98.4
 male phenotype Q98.9
 Turner's Q96.9
 specified NEC Q99.8
 cilia Q10.3
 circulatory system Q28.9
 clavicle Q74.0
 clitoris Q52.6
 coccyx Q76.49
 colon Q43.9
 common duct Q44.5
 communication
 coronary artery Q24.5
 left ventricle with right atrium Q21.0
 concha (ear) Q17.3
 connection
 portal vein Q26.5
 pulmonary venous Q26.4
 partial Q26.3
 total Q26.2
 renal artery with kidney Q27.2
 cornea (shape) Q13.4
 coronary artery or vein Q24.5
 cranium —*see* Anomaly, skull
 cricoid cartilage Q31.8
 cystic duct Q44.5

A

▶ New ➡ Revised ~~deleted~~ Deleted ● Use Additional Character(s)

A

- **Apneumatosis, newborn** P28.Ø
- **Apocrine metaplasia** (breast) —*see* Dysplasia, mammary, specified type NEC
- **Apophysitis** (bone) —*see also* Osteochondropathy
  - calcaneus M92.6
  - juvenile M92.9
- **Apoplectiform convulsions** (cerebral ischemia) I67.82
- **Apoplexia, apoplexy, apoplectic**
  - adrenal A39.1
  - heart (auricle) (ventricle) —*see* Infarct, myocardium
  - heat T67.Ø1
  - hemorrhagic (stroke) —*see* Hemorrhage, intracranial
  - meninges, hemorrhagic —*see* Hemorrhage, intracranial, subarachnoid
  - uremic N18.9 *[I68.8]*
- **Appearance**
  - bizarre R46.1
  - specified NEC R46.89
  - very low level of personal hygiene R46.Ø
- **Appendage**
  - epididymal (organ of Morgagni) Q55.4
  - intestine (epiploic) Q43.8
  - preauricular Q17.Ø
  - testicular (organ of Morgagni) Q55.29
- **Appendicitis** (pneumococcal) (retrocecal) K37
  - with
    - gangrene K35.891
      - with localized peritonitis K35.31
    - perforation NOS K35.32
    - peritoneal abscess K35.33
    - peritonitis NEC K35.33
      - generalized K35.2Ø9
        - with
          - abscess K35.219
            - with perforation or rupture K35.211
            - following rupture or perforation of appendix NOS K35.211
            - without perforation or rupture K35.21Ø
            - perforation or rupture K35.2Ø1
        - following rupture or perforation of appendix NOS K35.2Ø1
        - without rupture or perforation of appendix K35.2ØØ
      - localized K35.3Ø
        - with
          - gangrene K35.32
          - perforation K35.32
            - and abscess K35.33
      - ruptured NOS (with localized peritonitis) K35.32
  - acute (catarrhal) (fulminating) (obstructive) (retrocecal) (suppurative) K35.8Ø
    - with
      - gangrene K35.891
      - peritoneal abscess K35.33
      - peritonitis NEC K35.33
        - generalized K35.2Ø9
          - with
            - abscess K35.219
              - with perforation or rupture K35.211
              - following rupture or perforation of appendix NOS K35.211
              - without perforation or rupture K35.21Ø
              - perforation or rupture K35.2Ø1
          - following rupture or perforation of appendix NOS K35.2Ø1
          - without rupture or perforation of appendix K35.2ØØ
        - localized K35.3Ø
          - with
            - gangrene K35.32
            - perforation K35.32
              - and abscess K35.33
    - specified NEC K35.89Ø
      - with gangrene K35.891
    - with localized peritonitis K35.31
  - amebic AØ6.89
  - chronic (recurrent) K36
  - exacerbation —*see* Appendicitis, with, gangrene
  - gangrenous —*see* Appendicitis, acute
  - healed (obliterative) K36
  - interval K36
  - neurogenic K36
  - obstructive K36
  - recurrent K36
- **Appendicitis** *(Continued)*
  - relapsing K36
    - ruptured NOS (with localized peritonitis) K35.32
  - subacute (adhesive) K36
  - subsiding K36
  - suppurative —*see* Appendicitis, acute
  - tuberculous A18.32
- **Appendicopathia oxyurica** B8Ø
- **Appendix, appendicular** —*see also* condition
  - epididymis Q55.4
  - Morgagni
    - female Q5Ø.5
    - male (epididymal) Q55.4
      - testicular Q55.29
  - testis Q55.29
- **Appetite**
  - depraved —*see* Pica
  - excessive R63.2
  - lack or loss —*see also* Anorexia R63.Ø
    - nonorganic origin F5Ø.89
    - psychogenic F5Ø.89
  - perverted (hysterical) —*see* Pica
- **Apple peel syndrome** Q41.1
- **Apprehension state** F41.1
- **Apprehensiveness, abnormal** F41.9
- **Approximal wear** KØ3.Ø
- **Apraxia** (classic) (ideational) (ideokinetic) (ideomotor) (motor) (verbal) R48.2
  - following
    - cerebrovascular disease I69.99Ø
      - cerebral infarction I69.39Ø
      - intracerebral hemorrhage I69.19Ø
      - nontraumatic intracranial hemorrhage NEC I69.29Ø
      - specified disease NEC I69.89Ø
      - subarachnoid hemorrhage I69.Ø9Ø
  - oculomotor, congenital H51.8
- **Aptyalism** K11.7
- **Apudoma** —*see* Neoplasm, uncertain behavior, by site
- **Aqueous misdirection** H4Ø.83-●
- **Arabicum elephantiasis** —*see* Infestation, filarial
- **Arachnitis** —*see* Meningitis
- **Arachnodactyly** —*see* Syndrome, Marfan
- **Arachnoiditis** (acute) (adhesive) (basal) (brain) (cerebrospinal) —*see* Meningitis
- **Arachnophobia** F4Ø.21Ø
- **Arboencephalitis, Australian** A83.4
- **Arborization block** (heart) I45.5
- **ARC** (AIDS-related complex) B2Ø
- **Arch**
  - aortic Q25.49
  - bovine Q25.49
- **Arches** —*see* condition
- **Arcuate uterus** Q51.81Ø
- **Arcuatus uterus** Q51.81Ø
- **Arcus** (cornea) **senilis** —*see* Degeneration, cornea, senile
- **Arc-welder's lung** J63.4
- **Areflexia** R29.2
- **Areola** —*see* condition
- **Argentaffinoma** —*see also* Neoplasm, uncertain behavior, by site
  - malignant —*see* Neoplasm, malignant, by site
  - syndrome E34.Ø9
- **Argininemia** E72.21
- **Argininosuccinic aciduria** E72.22
- **Argyll Robertson phenomenon, pupil or syndrome** (syphilitic) A52.19
  - atypical H57.Ø9
  - nonsyphilitic H57.Ø9
- **Argyria, argyriasis**
  - conjunctival H11.13-●
  - from drug or medicament —*see* Table of Drugs and Chemicals, by substance
- **Argyrosis, conjunctival** H11.13-●
- **Arhinencephaly** QØ4.1
- **Ariboflavinosis** E53.Ø
- **Arm** —*see* condition
- **Arnold-Chiari disease, obstruction or syndrome** (type II) QØ7.ØØ
  - with
    - hydrocephalus QØ7.Ø2
      - with spina bifida QØ7.Ø3
    - spina bifida QØ7.Ø1
      - with hydrocephalus QØ7.Ø3
  - type III —*see* Encephalocele
  - type IV QØ4.8
- **Aromatic amino-acid metabolism disorder** E7Ø.9
  - specified NEC E7Ø.89
- **Arousals, confusional** G47.51
- **Arrest, arrested**
  - cardiac I46.9
    - complicating
      - abortion —*see* Abortion, by type, complicated by, cardiac arrest
      - anesthesia (general) (local) or other sedation —*see* Table of Drugs and Chemicals, by drug
        - in labor and delivery O74.2
        - in pregnancy O29.11-●
        - postpartum, puerperal O89.1
      - delivery (cesarean) (instrumental) O75.4
    - due to
      - cardiac condition I46.2
      - specified condition NEC I46.8
    - intraoperative I97.71-●
    - newborn P29.81
    - personal history, successfully resuscitated Z86.74
    - postprocedural I97.12-●
      - obstetric procedure O75.4
  - cardiorespiratory —*see* Arrest, cardiac
  - circulatory —*see* Arrest, cardiac
  - deep transverse O64.Ø
  - development or growth
    - bone —*see* Disorder, bone, development or growth
    - child R62.5Ø
    - tracheal rings Q32.1
  - epiphyseal
    - complete
      - femur M89.15-●
      - humerus M89.12-●
      - tibia M89.16-●
      - ulna M89.13-●
    - forearm M89.13-●
      - specified NEC M89.13-●
      - ulna —*see* Arrest, epiphyseal, by type, ulna
    - lower leg M89.16-●
      - specified NEC M89.168
      - tibia —*see* Arrest, epiphyseal, by type, tibia
    - partial
      - femur M89.15-●
      - humerus M89.12-●
      - tibia M89.16-●
      - ulna M89.13-●
    - specified NEC M89.18
  - granulopoiesis —*see* Agranulocytosis
  - growth plate —*see* Arrest, epiphyseal
  - heart —*see* Arrest, cardiac
  - legal, anxiety concerning Z65.3
  - physeal —*see* Arrest, epiphyseal
  - respiratory RØ9.2
    - newborn P28.81
  - sinus I45.5
  - spermatogenesis (complete) —*see* Azoospermia
    - incomplete —*see* Oligospermia
  - transverse (deep) O64.Ø
- **Arrhenoblastoma**
  - benign
    - specified site —*see* Neoplasm, benign, by site
    - unspecified site
      - female D27.9
      - male D29.2Ø
  - malignant
    - specified site —*see* Neoplasm, malignant, by site
    - unspecified site
      - female C56.9
      - male C62.9Ø
  - specified site —*see* Neoplasm, uncertain behavior, by site
  - unspecified site
    - female D39.1Ø
    - male D4Ø.1Ø
- **Arrhythmia** (auricle)(cardiac) (juvenile)(nodal) (reflex)(supraventricular)(transitory) (ventricle) I49.9
  - block I45.9
  - extrasystolic I49.49
  - newborn
    - bradycardia P29.12
    - occurring before birth PØ3.819
      - before onset of labor PØ3.81Ø
      - during labor PØ3.811
    - tachycardia P29.11
  - psychogenic F45.8
  - sinus I49.8
  - specified NEC I49.8
  - vagal R55
  - ventricular re-entry I47.Ø

A

Arsenical pigmentation L81.8
 from drug or medicament —*see* Table of Drugs and Chemicals
Arsenism —*see* Poisoning, arsenic
Arterial —*see* condition
Arteriofibrosis —*see* Arteriosclerosis
Arteriolar sclerosis —*see* Arteriosclerosis
Arteriolith —*see* Arteriosclerosis
Arteriolitis I77.6
 necrotizing, kidney I77.5
 renal —*see* Hypertension, kidney
Arteriolosclerosis —*see* Arteriosclerosis
Arterionephrosclerosis —*see* Hypertension, kidney
leg I70.429
 with
 gangrene (and intermittent claudication, rest pain, and ulcer) I70.469
 rest pain (and intermittent claudication) I70.429
 bilateral I70.423
 with
 gangrene (and intermittent claudication, rest pain, and ulcer) I70.463
 rest pain (and intermittent claudication) I70.423
 left I70.422
 with
 gangrene (and intermittent claudication, rest pain, and ulcer) I70.462
 rest pain (and intermittent claudication) I70.422
 ulceration (and intermittent claudication and rest pain) I70.449
mid foot I70.444
 thigh I70.441
 right I70.421
 with
 gangrene (and intermittent claudication, rest pain, and ulcer) I70.461
 rest pain (and intermittent claudication) I70.421
 ulceration (and intermittent claudication and rest pain) I70.439
midfoot I70.434
 thigh I70.431
 leg I70.329
 with
 gangrene (and intermittent claudication, rest pain, and ulcer) I70.369
 rest pain (and intermittent claudication) I70.329
 bilateral I70.323
 with
 gangrene (and intermittent claudication, rest pain, and ulcer) I70.363
 rest pain (and intermittent claudication) I70.323

Arteriosclerosis, arteriosclerotic (*Continued*)
 with (*Continued*)
 critical limb ischemia (*Continued*)
 bypass graft (*Continued*)
 leg (*Continued*)
 left I70.322
 with
 rest pain (and intermittent claudication) I70.322
 ulceration (and intermittent claudication and rest pain) I70.349
 ankle I70.343
thigh I70.341
 right I70.321
 with
 gangrene (and intermittent claudication, rest pain, and ulcer) I70.361
 rest pain (and intermittent claudication) I70.321
 ulceration (and intermittent claudication and rest pain) I70.339
 ankle I70.333
 calf I70.332
 foot site NEC I70.335
 heel I70.334
 lower leg NEC I70.338
with
 gangrene (and intermittent claudication, rest pain, and ulcer) I70.569
 rest pain (and intermittent claudication) I70.529
 bilateral I70.523
 with
 gangrene (and intermittent claudication, rest pain, and ulcer) I70.563
 rest pain (and intermittent claudication) I70.523
 left I70.522
 with
 gangrene (and intermittent claudication, rest pain, and ulcer) I70.562
 rest pain (and intermittent claudication) I70.522
 ulceration (and intermittent claudication and rest pain) I70.549
gangrene (and intermittent claudication, rest pain, and ulcer) I70.669

Arteriosclerosis, arteriosclerotic (*Continued*)
 with (*Continued*)
 critical limb ischemia (*Continued*)
 bypass graft (*Continued*)
 nonbiological graf (*Continued*)
 leg (*Continued*)
 with (*Continued*)
 rest pain (and intermittent claudication) I70.629
 bilateral I70.623
 with
 gangrene (and intermittent claudication, rest pain, and ulcer) I70.663
 rest pain (and intermittent claudication) I70.623
 left I70.622
 with
 gangrene (and intermittent claudication, rest pain, and ulcer) I70.662
 rest pain (and intermittent claudication) I70.622
 ulceration (and intermittent claudication and rest pain) I70.649
midfoot I70.634
 thigh I70.631
 specified graft NEC I70.729
 leg I70.729
 with
 gangrene (and intermittent claudication, rest pain, and ulcer) I70.769
 rest pain (and intermittent claudication) I70.729
 bilateral I70.723
 with
 gangrene (and intermittent claudication, rest pain, and ulcer) I70.763
 rest pain (and intermittent claudication) I70.723
 left I70.722
 with
 gangrene (and intermittent claudication, rest pain, and ulcer) I70.762
 rest pain (and intermittent claudication) I70.722
 ulceration (and intermittent claudication and rest pain) I70.749
 ankle I70.743
 calf I70.742
 foot site NEC I70.745
 heel I70.744
 lower leg NEC I70.748
 midfoot I70.744
 thigh I70.741
 right I70.721
 with
 gangrene (and intermittent claudication, rest pain, and ulcer) I70.761

brain I67.2
 with infarction —*see* Occlusion, artery, brain or cerebral, with infarction
coronary —*see* Arteriosclerosis, coronary, bypass graft
 extremities —*see* Arteriosclerosis, extremities, bypass graft
 cardiac —*see* Disease, heart, ischemic, atherosclerotic

Arteriosclerosis, arteriosclerotic *(Continued)*
central nervous system I67.2
 with infarction —*see* Occlusion, artery, cerebral or precerebral, with infarction
 cerebral I67.2
 with infarction —*see* Occlusion, artery, brain or cerebral, with infarction
 cerebrovascular I67.2
 with infarction —*see* Occlusion, artery, brain or cerebral, with infarction
ischemic chest pain I25.759

Arteriosclerosis, arteriosclerotic *(Continued)*
autologous vein graft I70.409
 leg I70.409
 with
 gangrene (and intermittent claudication, rest pain and ulcer) I70.469
 intermittent claudication I70.419
 rest pain (and intermittent claudication) I70.429
 bilateral I70.403
 with
 gangrene (and intermittent claudication, rest pain and ulcer) I70.463
 intermittent claudication I70.413
 rest pain (and intermittent claudication) I70.423
 specified type NEC I70.493
 left I70.402
 with
 gangrene (and intermittent claudication, rest pain and ulcer) I70.462
 intermittent claudication I70.412
 rest pain (and intermittent claudication) I70.422
 ulceration (and intermittent claudication and rest pain) I70.449
 ankle I70.443
thigh I70.441
 specified type NEC I70.492
 right I70.401
 with
 gangrene (and intermittent claudication, rest pain and ulcer) I70.461
 intermittent claudication I70.411
 with
 rest pain (and intermittent claudication) I70.421
 ulceration (and intermittent claudication and rest pain) I70.439
 ankle I70.433
with
 gangrene (and intermittent claudication, rest pain and ulcer) I70.468
 intermittent claudication I70.418
 rest pain (and intermittent claudication) I70.428
 ulceration (and intermittent claudication and rest pain) I70.45
 specified type NEC I70.498

A

Arteriosclerosis, arteriosclerotic (Continued)
 coronary (artery) (Continued)
 bypass graft (Continued)
 leg I70.309
 with
 gangrene (and intermittent
 claudication, rest pain and ulcer)
 I70.369
 intermittent claudication I70.319
 rest pain (and intermittent
 claudication) I70.329
 bilateral I70.303
 with
 gangrene (and intermittent
 claudication, rest pain and
 ulcer) I70.363
 intermittent claudication I70.313
 rest pain (and intermittent
 claudication) I70.323
 specified type NEC I70.393
 left I70.302
 with
 gangrene (and intermittent
 claudication, rest pain and
 ulcer) I70.362
 intermittent claudication I70.312
 rest pain (and intermittent
 claudication) I70.322
 ulceration (and intermittent
 claudication and rest pain)
 I70.349
 ankle I70.343
 calf I70.342
 foot site NEC I70.345
right I70.301
 with
 gangrene (and intermittent
 claudication, rest pain and
 ulcer) I70.361
 intermittent claudication I70.311
 rest pain (and intermittent
 claudication) I70.321
 ulceration (and intermittent
 claudication and rest pain)
 I70.339
 ankle I70.333
 calf I70.332
 foot site NEC I70.335
 heel I70.334
 lower leg NEC I70.338
 midfoot I70.334
 thigh I70.331
 specified type NEC I70.391
 specified type NEC I70.399
claudication, rest pain and
 ulcer) I70.569
 intermittent claudication I70.519
 rest pain (and intermittent
 claudication) I70.529
 bilateral I70.503
 with
 gangrene (and intermittent
 claudication, rest pain and
 ulcer) I70.563
 intermittent claudication I70.513
 rest pain (and intermittent
 claudication) I70.523
 specified type NEC I70.593
 left I70.502
 with
 gangrene (and intermittent
 claudication, rest pain and
 ulcer) I70.562
 intermittent claudication I70.512
 rest pain (and intermittent
 claudication) I70.522
 ulceration (and intermittent
 claudication and rest pain)
 I70.549
 ankle I70.543
 calf I70.542
 foot site NEC I70.545

Arteriosclerosis, arteriosclerotic (Continued)
 coronary (artery) (Continued)
 bypass graft (Continued)
 nonautologous biological graft (Continued)
 leg (Continued)
 left (Continued)
 with (Continued)
 ulceration (Continued)
 heel I70.544
specified NEC I70.508
 with
 gangrene (and intermittent
 claudication, rest pain and
 ulcer) I70.568
 intermittent claudication I70.518
 rest pain (and intermittent
 claudication) I70.528
 ulceration (and intermittent
 claudication and rest pain)
gangrene (and intermittent
 claudication, rest pain and
 ulcer) I70.669
 intermittent claudication I70.619
 rest pain (and intermittent
 claudication) I70.629
 bilateral I70.603
 with
 gangrene (and intermittent
 claudication, rest pain and
 ulcer) I70.663
 intermittent claudication I70.613
 rest pain (and intermittent
 claudication) I70.623
 specified type NEC I70.693
 left I70.602
 with
 gangrene (and intermittent
 claudication, rest pain and
 ulcer) I70.662
 intermittent claudication
 I70.612
 rest pain (and intermittent
 claudication) I70.622
 ulceration (and intermittent
 claudication and rest pain)
 I70.649
 ankle I70.643
claudication, rest pain and
 ulcer) I70.661
 intermittent claudication I70.611
 rest pain (and intermittent
 claudication) I70.621

Arteriosclerosis, arteriosclerotic (Continued)
 coronary (artery) (Continued)
 bypass graft (Continued)
 nonbiological graft (Continued)
 leg (Continued)
 right (Continued)
 with (Continued)
 ulceration (and intermittent
leg I70.709
 with
 gangrene (and intermittent
 claudication, rest pain and
 ulcer) I70.769
 intermittent claudication I70.719
 rest pain (and intermittent
 claudication) I70.729
 bilateral I70.703
 with
 gangrene (and intermittent
 claudication, rest pain and
 ulcer) I70.763
 intermittent claudication
 I70.713
 rest pain (and intermittent
 claudication) I70.723
 specified type NEC I70.793
 left I70.702
 with
 gangrene (and intermittent
 claudication, rest pain and
 ulcer) I70.762
 intermittent claudication
 I70.712
 rest pain (and intermittent
 claudication) I70.722
 ulceration (and intermittent
 claudication and rest pain)
 I70.749
 ankle I70.743
 calf I70.742
 foot site NEC I70.745
right I70.701
 with
 gangrene (and intermittent
 claudication, rest pain and
 ulcer) I70.761
 intermittent claudication I70.711
 rest pain (and intermittent
 claudication) I70.721
 ulceration (and intermittent
 claudication and rest pain)
 I70.739
 ankle I70.733
 calf I70.732
 foot site NEC I70.735
 heel I70.734
 lower leg NEC I70.738

Arteriosclerosis, arteriosclerotic *(Continued)*
  coronary (artery) *(Continued)*
    bypass graft *(Continued)*
      specified graft NEC *(Continued)*
        specified NEC *(Continued)*
          with
            gangrene (and intermittent claudication, rest pain and ulcer) I70.768
            intermittent claudication I70.718
            rest pain (and intermittent claudication) I70.728
            ulceration (and intermittent claudication and rest pain) I70.75
          specified type NEC I70.798
      specified NEC I70.308
        with
          gangrene (and intermittent claudication, rest pain and ulcer) I70.368
          intermittent claudication I70.318
          rest pain (and intermittent claudication) I70.328
          ulceration (and intermittent claudication and rest pain) I70.35
        specified type NEC I70.398
    leg I70.209
      with
        gangrene (and intermittent claudication, rest pain and ulcer) I70.269
        intermittent claudication I70.219
        rest pain (and intermittent claudication) I70.229
      bilateral I70.203
        with
          gangrene (and intermittent claudication, rest pain and ulcer) I70.263
          intermittent claudication I70.213
          rest pain (and intermittent claudication) I70.223
        specified type NEC I70.293
      left I70.202
        with
          gangrene (and intermittent claudication, rest pain and ulcer) I70.262
          intermittent claudication I70.212
          rest pain (and intermittent claudication) I70.222
          ulceration (and intermittent claudication and rest pain) I70.249
            ankle I70.243
            calf I70.242
            foot site NEC I70.245
            heel I70.244
            lower leg NEC I70.248
            midfoot I70.244
            thigh I70.241
        specified type NEC I70.292
      right I70.201
        with
          gangrene (and intermittent claudication, rest pain and ulcer) I70.261
          intermittent claudication I70.211
          rest pain (and intermittent claudication) I70.221
          ulceration (and intermittent claudication and rest pain) I70.239
            ankle I70.233
            calf I70.232
            foot site NEC I70.235
            heel I70.234
            lower leg NEC I70.238
            midfoot I70.234
            thigh I70.231
        specified type NEC I70.291
      specified type NEC I70.299
    specified site NEC I70.208
      with
        gangrene (and intermittent claudication, rest pain and ulcer) I70.268
        intermittent claudication I70.218
        rest pain (and intermittent claudication) I70.228

rteriosclerosis, arteriosclerotic *(Continued)*
  coronary (artery) *(Continued)*
    specified site NEC *(Continued)*
      with *(Continued)*
        ulceration (and intermittent claudication and rest pain) I70.25
      specified type NEC I70.298
  generalized I70.91
  heart (disease) —*see* Arteriosclerosis, coronary (artery)
  kidney —*see* Hypertension, kidney
  medial —*see* Arteriosclerosis, extremities
  mesenteric (artery) K55.1
  Mönckeberg's —*see* Arteriosclerosis, extremities
  myocarditis I51.4
  peripheral (of extremities) —*see* Arteriosclerosis, extremities
  pulmonary (idiopathic) I27.0
  renal (arterioles) —*see also* Hypertension, kidney
    artery I70.1
  retina (vascular) I70.8 *[H35.0-●]*
  specified artery NEC I70.8
  spinal (cord) G95.19
  vertebral (artery) I67.2
    with infarction - *see* Occlusion, artery, vertebral, with infarction

Arteriospasm I73.9

Arteriovenous —*see* condition

Arteritis I77.6
  allergic M31.0
  aorta (nonsyphilitic) I77.6
    syphilitic A52.02
  aortic arch M31.4
  brachiocephalic M31.4
  brain I67.7
    syphilitic A52.04
  cerebral I67.7
    in
      diseases classified elsewhere I68.2
      systemic lupus erythematosus M32.19
    listerial A32.89
    syphilitic A52.04
    tuberculous A18.89
  coronary (artery) I25.89
    rheumatic I01.8
      chronic I09.89
    syphilitic A52.06
  cranial (left) (right), giant cell M31.6
  deformans —*see* Arteriosclerosis
  giant cell NEC M31.6
    with polymyalgia rheumatica M31.5
  necrosing or necrotizing M31.9
    specified NEC M31.8
  nodosa M30.0
  obliterans —*see* Arteriosclerosis
  pulmonary I28.8
  rheumatic —*see* Fever, rheumatic
  senile —*see* Arteriosclerosis
  suppurative I77.2
  syphilitic (general) A52.09
    brain A52.04
    coronary A52.06
    spinal A52.09
  temporal, giant cell M31.6
  young female aortic arch syndrome M31.4

Artery, arterial —*see also* condition
  abscess I77.89
  single umbilical Q27.0

Arthralgia (allergic) —*see also* Pain, joint
  in caisson disease T70.3
  temporomandibular M26.62

Arthritis, arthritic (acute) (chronic) (nonpyogenic) (subacute) M19.90
  allergic —*see* Arthritis, specified form NEC
  ankylosing (crippling) (spine) —*see also* Spondylitis, ankylosing
    sites other than spine —*see* Arthritis, specified form NEC
  atrophic —*see* Osteoarthritis
    spine —*see* Spondylitis, ankylosing
  back —*see* Spondylopathy, inflammatory
  blennorrhagic (gonococcal) A54.42
  Charcot's —*see* Arthropathy, neuropathic
    diabetic —*see* Diabetes, arthropathy, neuropathic
    syringomyelic G95.0
  chylous (filarial) —*see also* category M01 B74.9
  climacteric (any site) NEC —*see* Arthritis, specified form NEC
  crystal (-induced) —*see* Arthritis, in, crystals
  deformans —*see* Osteoarthritis

Arthritis, arthritic *(Continued)*
  degenerative —*see* Osteoarthritis
  due to or associated with
    acromegaly E22.0
    brucellosis —*see* Brucellosis
    caisson disease T70.3
    diabetes —*see* Diabetes, arthropathy
    dracontiasis —*see also* category M01 B72
    enteritis NEC
      regional —*see* Enteritis, regional
    erysipelas —*see also* category M01 A46
    erythema
      epidemic A25.1
      nodosum L52
    filariasis NOS B74.9
    glanders A24.0
    helminthiasis —*see also* category M01 B83.9
    hemophilia D66 *[M36.2]*
    Henoch-(Schönlein) purpura D69.0 *[M36.4]*
    human parvovirus —*see also* category M01 B97.6
    infectious disease NEC —*see* category M01
    leprosy (*see also* category M01) —*see also* Leprosy A30.9
    Lyme disease A69.23
    mycobacteria —*see also* category M01 A31.8
    parasitic disease NEC —*see also* category M01 B89
    paratyphoid fever (*see also* category M01)—*see also* Fever, paratyphoid A01.4
    rat bite fever —*see also* category M01 A25.1
    regional enteritis —*see* Enteritis, regional
    respiratory disorder NOS J98.9
    serum sickness —*see also* Reaction, serum T80.69
    syringomyelia G95.0
    typhoid fever A01.04
  epidemic erythema A25.1
  facet joint (*see also* Spondylosis) M47.819
  febrile —*see* Fever, rheumatic
  gonococcal A54.42
  gouty (acute) —*see* Gout
  in (due to)
    acromegaly —*see also* subcategory M14.8-● E22.0
    amyloidosis —*see also* subcategory M14.8-● E85.4
    bacterial disease —*see also* subcategory M01 A49.9
    Behçet's syndrome M35.2
    caisson disease —*see also* subcategory M14.8-● T70.3
    coliform bacilli (Escherichia coli) —*see* Arthritis, in, pyogenic organism NEC
    crystals M11.9
      dicalcium phosphate —*see* Arthritis, in, crystals, specified type NEC
      hydroxyapatite M11.0-●
      pyrophosphate —*see* Arthritis, in, crystals, specified type NEC
      specified type NEC M11.80
        ankle M11.87-●
        elbow M11.82-●
        foot joint M11.87-●
        hand joint M11.84-●
        hip M11.85-●
        knee M11.86-●
        multiple sites M11.8-●
        shoulder M11.81-●
        vertebrae M11.88
        wrist M11.83-●
    dermatoarthritis, lipoid E78.81
    dracontiasis (dracunculiasis) —*see also* category M01 B72
    endocrine disorder NEC —*see also* subcategory M14.8-● E34.9
    enteritis, infectious NEC —*see also* category M01 A09
      specified organism NEC —*see also* category M01 A08.8
    erythema
      multiforme —*see also* subcategory M14.8-● L51.9
      nodosum —*see also* subcategory M14.8-● L52
    gout —*see* Gout
    helminthiasis NEC —*see also* category M01 B83.9
    hemochromatosis —*see also* subcategory M14.8-● E83.118
    hemoglobinopathy NEC D58.2 *[M36.3]*

Arthritis, arthritic *(Continued)*
in *(Continued)*
hemophilia NEC D66 *[M36.2]*
Hemophilus influenzae M00.8-● *[B96.3]*
Henoch(-Schönlein) purpura D69.0 *[M36.4]*
hyperparathyroidism NEC —*see also* subcategory M14.8-● E21.3
hypersensitivity reaction NEC T78.49 *[M36.4]*
hypogammaglobulinemia —*see also* subcategory M14.8-● D80.1
hypothyroidism NEC —*see also* subcategory M14.8-● E03.9
infection —*see* Arthritis, pyogenic or pyemic
spine —*see* Spondylopathy, infective
infectious disease NEC —*see* category M01
leprosy —*see also* category M01 A30.9
leukemia NEC C95.9-● *[M36.1]*
lipoid dermatoarthritis E78.81
Lyme disease A69.23
Mediterranean fever, familial —*see also* subcategory M14.8-● M04.1
Meningococcus A39.83
metabolic disorder NEC —*see also* subcategory M14.8-● E88.9
multiple myelomatosis C90.0-● *[M36.1]*
mumps B26.85
mycosis NEC —*see also* category M01 B49
myelomatosis (multiple) C90.0-● *[M36.1]*
neurological disorder NEC G98.0
ochronosis —*see also* subcategory M14.8-● E70.29
O'nyong-nyong —*see also* category M01 A92.1
parasitic disease NEC —*see also* category M01 B89
paratyphoid fever —*see also* category M01 A01.4
Pseudomonas —*see* Arthritis, pyogenic, bacterial NEC
psoriasis L40.50
pyogenic organism NEC —*see* Arthritis, pyogenic, bacterial NEC
Reiter's disease —*see* Reiter's disease
respiratory disorder NEC —*see also* subcategory M14.8-● J98.9
reticulosis, malignant —*see also* subcategory M14.8-● C86.0-●
rubella B06.82
Salmonella (arizonae) (cholerae-suis) (enteritidis) (typhimurium) A02.23
sarcoidosis D86.86
specified bacteria NEC —*see* Arthritis, pyogenic, bacterial NEC
sporotrichosis B42.82
syringomyelia G95.0
thalassemia NEC D56.9 *[M36.3]*
tuberculosis —*see* Tuberculosis, arthritis
typhoid fever A01.04
urethritis, Reiter's —*see* Reiter's disease
viral disease NEC —*see also* category M01 B34.9
infectious or infective —*see also* Arthritis, pyogenic or pyemic
spine —*see* Spondylopathy, infective
juvenile M08.90
with systemic onset —*see* Still's disease
ankle M08.97-●
elbow M08.92-●
foot joint M08.97-●
hand joint M08.94-●
hip M08.95-●
knee M08.96-●
multiple site M08.99
pauciarticular M08.40
ankle M08.47-●
elbow M08.42-●
foot joint M08.47-●
hand joint M08.44-●
hip M08.45-●
knee M08.46-●
shoulder M08.41-●
specified site NEC M08.4A
vertebrae M08.48
wrist M08.43-●
psoriatic L40.54
rheumatoid —*see* Arthritis, rheumatoid, juvenile
shoulder M08.91-●
specified site NEC M08.9A
specified type NEC M08.80
ankle M08.87-●
elbow M08.82-●
foot joint M08.87-●

Arthritis, arthritic *(Continued)*
juvenile *(Continued)*
specified type NEC *(Continued)*
hand joint M08.84-●
hip M08.85-●
knee M08.86-●
multiple site M08.89
shoulder M08.81-●
specified joint NEC M08.88
vertebrae M08.88
wrist M08.83-●
vertebra M08.98
wrist M08.93-●
meaning osteoarthritis —*see* Osteoarthritis
meningococcal A39.83
menopausal (any site) NEC —*see* Arthritis, specified form NEC
mutilans (psoriatic) L40.52
mycotic NEC —*see also* category M01 B49
neuropathic (Charcot) —*see* Arthropathy, neuropathic
diabetic —*see* Diabetes, arthropathy, neuropathic
nonsyphilitic NEC G98.0
syringomyelic G95.0
ochronotic —*see also* subcategory M14.8-● E70.29
palindromic (any site) —*see* Rheumatism, palindromic
pneumococcal M00.10
ankle M00.17-●
elbow M00.12-●
foot joint —*see* Arthritis, pneumococcal, ankle
hand joint M00.14-●
hip M00.15-●
knee M00.16-●
multiple site M00.19
shoulder M00.11-●
vertebra M00.18
wrist M00.13-●
postdysenteric —*see* Arthropathy, postdysenteric
postmeningococcal A39.84
postrheumatic, chronic —*see* Arthropathy, postrheumatic, chronic
primary progressive —*see also* Arthritis, specified form NEC
spine —*see* Spondylitis, ankylosing
psoriatic L40.50
purulent (any site except spine) —*see* Arthritis, pyogenic or pyemic
spine —*see* Spondylopathy, infective
pyogenic or pyemic (any site except spine) M00.9
bacterial NEC M00.80
ankle M00.87-●
elbow M00.82-●
foot joint —*see* Arthritis, pyogenic, bacterial NEC, ankle
hand joint M00.84-●
hip M00.85-●
knee M00.86-●
multiple site M00.89
shoulder M00.81-●
vertebra M00.88
wrist M00.83-●
pneumococcal —*see* Arthritis, pneumococcal
spine —*see* Spondylopathy, infective
staphylococcal —*see* Arthritis, staphylococcal
streptococcal —*see* Arthritis, streptococcal NEC
pneumococcal —*see* Arthritis, pneumococcal
reactive —*see* Reiter's disease
rheumatic —*see also* Arthritis, rheumatoid
acute or subacute —*see* Fever, rheumatic
rheumatoid M06.9
with
carditis —*see* Rheumatoid, carditis
endocarditis —*see* Rheumatoid, carditis
heart involvement NEC —*see* Rheumatoid, carditis
lung involvement —*see* Rheumatoid, lung
myocarditis —*see* Rheumatoid, carditis
myopathy —*see* Rheumatoid, myopathy
pericarditis —*see* Rheumatoid, carditis
polyneuropathy —*see* Rheumatoid, polyneuropathy
rheumatoid factor —*see* Arthritis, rheumatoid, seropositive
splenoadenomegaly and leukopenia —*see* Felty's syndrome
vasculitis —*see* Rheumatoid, vasculitis
visceral involvement NEC —*see* Rheumatoid, arthritis, with involvement of organs NEC

Arthritis, arthritic *(Continued)*
rheumatoid *(Continued)*
juvenile (with or without rheumatoid factor) M08.00
with systemic onset —*see* Still's disease
ankle M08.07-●
elbow M08.02-●
foot joint M08.07-●
hand joint M08.04-●
hip M08.05-●
knee M08.06-●
multiple site M08.09
shoulder M08.01-●
specified site NEC M08.0A
vertebra M08.08
wrist M08.03-●
seronegative M06.00
ankle M06.07-●
elbow M06.02-●
foot joint M06.07-●
hand joint M06.04-●
hip M06.05-●
knee M06.06-●
multiple sites M06.09
shoulder M06.01-●
specified site NEC M06.0A
vertebra M06.08
wrist M06.03-●
seropositive M05.9
without organ involvement M05.70
ankle M05.77-●
elbow M05.72-●
foot joint M05.77-●
hand joint M05.74-●
hip M05.75-●
knee M05.76-●
multiple sites M05.79
shoulder M05.71-●
specified site NEC M05.7A
vertebra —*see* Spondylitis, ankylosing
wrist M05.73-●
specified NEC M05.80
ankle M05.87-●
elbow M05.82-●
foot joint M05.87-●
hand joint M05.84-●
hip M05.85-●
knee M05.86-●
multiple sites M05.89
specified site NEC M05.8A
shoulder M05.81-●
vertebra —*see* Spondylitis, ankylosing
wrist M05.83-●
specified type NEC M06.80
ankle M06.87-●
elbow M06.82-●
foot joint M06.87-●
hand joint M06.84-●
hip M06.85-●
knee M06.86-●
multiple site M06.89
shoulder M06.81-●
specified site NEC M06.8A
vertebra M06.88
wrist M06.83-●
spine —*see* Spondylitis, ankylosing
rubella B06.82
scorbutic —*see also* subcategory M14.8-● E54
senile or senescent —*see* Osteoarthritis
septic (any site except spine) —*see* Arthritis, pyogenic or pyemic
spine —*see* Spondylopathy, infective
serum (nontherapeutic) (therapeutic) —*see* Arthropathy, postimmunization
specified form NEC M13.80
ankle M13.87-●
elbow M13.82-●
foot joint M13.87-●
hand joint M13.84-●
hip M13.85-●
knee M13.86-●
multiple site M13.89
shoulder M13.81-●
specified joint NEC M13.88
wrist M13.83-●
spine —*see also* Spondylosis
infectious or infective NEC —*see* Spondylopathy, infective
Marie-Strümpell —*see* Spondylitis, ankylosing
pyogenic —*see* Spondylopathy, infective
rheumatoid —*see* Spondylitis, ankylosing

A

Arthritis, arthritic *(Continued)*
spine *(Continued)*
traumatic (old) —*see* Spondylopathy, traumatic
tuberculous A18.01
staphylococcal M00.00
ankle M00.07-•
elbow M00.02-•
foot joint —*see* Arthritis, staphylococcal, ankle
hand joint M00.04-•
hip M00.05-•
knee M00.06-•
multiple site M00.09
shoulder M00.01-•
vertebra M00.08
wrist M00.03-•
streptococcal NEC M00.20
ankle M00.27-•
elbow M00.22-•
foot joint —*see* Arthritis, streptococcal, ankle
hand joint M00.24-•
hip M00.25-•
knee M00.26-•
multiple site M00.29
shoulder M00.21-•
vertebra M00.28
wrist M00.23-•
suppurative —*see* Arthritis, pyogenic or pyemic
syphilitic (late) A52.16
congenital A50.55 *[M12.80]*
syphilitica deformans (Charcot) A52.16
temporomandibular joint M26.65-•
toxic of menopause (any site) —*see* Arthritis, specified form NEC
transient —*see* Arthropathy, specified form NEC
traumatic (chronic) —*see* Arthropathy, traumatic
tuberculous A18.02
spine A18.01
uratic —*see* Gout
urethritica (Reiter's) —*see* Reiter's disease
vertebral —*see* Spondylopathy, inflammatory
villous (any site) —*see* Arthropathy, specified form NEC
Arthrocele —*see* Effusion, joint
Arthrodesis status Z98.1
Arthrodynia —*see also* Pain, joint
Arthrodysplasia Q74.9
Arthrofibrosis, joint —*see* Ankylosis
Arthrogryposis (congenital) Q68.8
multiplex congenita Q74.3
Arthrokatadysis M24.7
Arthropathy (*see also* Arthritis) M12.9
Charcot's —*see* Arthropathy, neuropathic
diabetic —*see* Diabetes, arthropathy, neuropathic
syringomyelic G95.0
cricoarytenoid J38.7
crystal(-induced) —*see* Arthritis, in, crystals
diabetic NEC —*see* Diabetes, arthropathy
distal interphalangeal, psoriatic L40.51
enteropathic M07.60
ankle M07.67-•
elbow M07.62-•
foot joint M07.67-•
hand joint M07.64-•
hip M07.65-•
knee M07.66-•
multiple site M07.69
shoulder M07.61-•
vertebra M07.68
wrist M07.63-•
facet joint (*see also* Spondylosis) M47.819
following intestinal bypass M02.00
ankle M02.07-•
elbow M02.02-•
foot joint M02.07-•
hand joint M02.04-•
hip M02.05-•
knee M02.06-•
multiple site M02.09
shoulder M02.01-•
vertebra M02.08
wrist M02.03-•
gouty —*see also* Gout
in (due to)
Lesch-Nyhan syndrome E79.1 *[M14.8-•]*
sickle-cell disorders D57-• *[M14.8-•]*
hemophilic NEC D66 *[M36.2]*
in (due to)
hyperparathyroidism NEC E21.3 *[M14.8-•]*
metabolic disease NOS E88.9 *[M14.8-•]*

Arthropathy *(Continued)*
hemophilic NEC *(Continued)*
acromegaly E22.0 *[M14.8-•]*
amyloidosis E85.4 *[M14.8-•]*
blood disorder NOS D75.9 *[M36.3]*
diabetes —*see* Diabetes, arthropathy
endocrine disease NOS E34.9 *[M14.8-•]*
erythema
multiforme L51.9 *[M14.8-•]*
nodosum L52 *[M14.8-•]*
hemochromatosis E83.118 *[M14.8-•]*
hemoglobinopathy NEC D58.2 *[M36.3]*
hemophilia NEC D66 *[M36.2]*
Henoch-Schönlein purpura D69.0 *[M36.4]*
hyperthyroidism E05.90 *[M14.8-•]*
hypothyroidism E03.9 *[M14.8-•]*
infective endocarditis I33.0 *[M12.80]*
leukemia NEC C95.9-• *[M36.1]*
malignant histiocytosis C96.A *[M36.1]*
metabolic disease NOS E88.9 *[M14.8-•]*
multiple myeloma C90.0-• *[M36.1]*
neoplastic disease NOS (*see also* Neoplasm) D49.9 *[M36.1]*
nutritional deficiency —*see also* subcategory M14.8-• E63.9
psoriasis NOS L40.50
sarcoidosis D86.86
syphilis (late) A52.77
congenital A50.55 *[M12.80]*
thyrotoxicosis —*see also* subcategory M14.8-• E05.90
ulcerative colitis K51.90 *[M07.60]*
viral hepatitis (postinfectious) NEC B19.9 *[M12.80]*
Whipple's disease —*see also* subcategory M14.8-• K90.81
Jaccoud —*see* Arthropathy, postrheumatic, chronic
juvenile —*see* Arthritis, juvenile
psoriatic L40.54
mutilans (psoriatic) L40.52
neuropathic (Charcot) M14.60
ankle M14.67-•
diabetic —*see* Diabetes, arthropathy, neuropathic
elbow M14.62-•
foot joint M14.67-•
hand joint M14.64-•
hip M14.65-•
knee M14.66-•
multiple site M14.69
nonsyphilitic NEC G98.0
shoulder M14.61-•
syringomyelic G95.0
vertebra M14.68
wrist M14.63-•
osteopulmonary —*see* Osteoarthropathy, hypertrophic, specified NEC
postdysenteric M02.10
ankle M02.17-•
elbow M02.12-•
foot joint M02.17-•
hand joint M02.14-•
hip M02.15-•
knee M02.16-•
multiple site M02.19
shoulder M02.11-•
vertebra M02.18
wrist M02.13-•
postimmunization M02.20
ankle M02.27-•
elbow M02.22-•
foot joint M02.27-•
hand joint M02.24-•
hip M02.25-•
knee M02.26-•
multiple site M02.29
shoulder M02.21-•
vertebra M02.28
wrist M02.23-•
postinfectious NEC B99 *[M12.80]*
in (due to)
enteritis due to Yersinia enterocolitica A04.6 *[M12.80]*
syphilis A52.77
viral hepatitis NEC B19.9 *[M12.80]*
postrheumatic, chronic (Jaccoud) M12.00
ankle M12.07-•
elbow M12.02-•
foot joint M12.07-•
hand joint M12.04-•

Arthropathy *(Continued)*
postrheumatic, chronic *(Continued)*
hip M12.05-•
knee M12.06-•
multiple site M12.09
shoulder M12.01-•
specified joint NEC M12.08
vertebrae M12.08
wrist M12.03-•
psoriatic NEC L40.59
interphalangeal, distal L40.51
reactive M02.9
in (due to)
infective endocarditis I33.0 *[M02.9]*
specified type NEC M02.80
ankle M02.87-•
elbow M02.82-•
foot joint M02.87-•
hand joint M02.84-•
hip M02.85-•
knee M02.86-•
multiple site M02.89
shoulder M02.81-•
vertebra M02.88
wrist M02.83-•
specified form NEC M12.80
ankle M12.87-•
elbow M12.82-•
foot joint M12.87-•
hand joint M12.84-•
hip M12.85-•
knee M12.86-•
multiple site M12.89
shoulder M12.81-•
specified joint NEC M12.88
vertebrae M12.88
wrist M12.83-•
syringomyelic G95.0
tabes dorsalis A52.16
tabetic A52.16
temporomandibular joint M26.65-•
transient —*see* Arthropathy, specified form NEC
traumatic M12.50
ankle M12.57-•
elbow M12.52-•
foot joint M12.57-•
hand joint M12.54-•
hip M12.55-•
knee M12.56-•
multiple site M12.59
shoulder M12.51-•
specified joint NEC M12.58
vertebrae M12.58
wrist M12.53-•
Arthropyosis —*see* Arthritis, pyogenic or pyemic
Arthrosis (deformans) (degenerative) (localized) —*see also* Osteoarthritis M19.90
spine —*see* Spondylosis
Arthus' phenomenon or reaction T78.41
due to
drug —*see* Table of Drugs and Chemicals, by drug
Articular —*see* condition
Articulation, reverse (teeth) M26.24
Artificial
insemination complication —*see* Complications, artificial, fertilization
opening status (functioning) (without complication) Z93.9
anus (colostomy) Z93.3
colostomy Z93.3
cystostomy Z93.50
appendico-vesicostomy Z93.52
cutaneous Z93.51
specified NEC Z93.59
enterostomy Z93.4
gastrostomy Z93.1
➡ ileostomy (ileal pouch) (Kock pouch) Z93.2
intestinal tract NEC Z93.4
jejunostomy Z93.4
nephrostomy Z93.6
specified site NEC Z93.8
tracheostomy Z93.0
ureterostomy Z93.6
urethrostomy Z93.6
urinary tract NEC Z93.6
vagina Z93.8
vagina status Z93.8
Arytenoid —*see* condition
Asadollahi-Rauch syndrome Q87.85
Asbestosis (occupational) J61

A

A

ASC-H (atypical squamous cells cannot exclude high grade squamous intraepithelial lesion on cytologic smear)
 anus R85.611
 cervix R87.611
 vagina R87.621
ASC-US (atypical squamous cells of undetermined significance on cytologic smear)
 anus R85.610
 cervix R87.610
 vagina R87.620
Ascariasis B77.9
 with
 complications NEC B77.89
 intestinal complications B77.0
 pneumonia, pneumonitis B77.81
Ascaridosis, ascaridiasis —see Ascariasis
Ascaris (infection) (infestation) (lumbricoides) —see Ascariasis
Ascending —see condition
Aschoff's bodies —see Myocarditis, rheumatic
Ascites (abdominal) R18.8
 cardiac —see also Failure, heart, right I50.810
 chylous (nonfilarial) I89.8
 filarial —see Infestation, filarial
 due to
 cirrhosis, alcoholic K70.31
 hepatitis
 alcoholic K70.11
 chronic active K71.51
 S. japonicum B65.2
 heart —see also Failure, heart, right I50.810
 malignant R18.0
 pseudochylous R18.8
 syphilitic A52.74
 tuberculous A18.31
Aseptic —see condition
Asherman's syndrome N85.6
Asialia K11.7
Asiatic cholera —see Cholera
Asimultagnosia (simultanagnosia) R48.3
Askin's tumor —see Neoplasm, connective tissue, malignant
Asocial personality F60.2
Asomatognosia R41.4
Aspartylglucosaminuria E77.1
Asperger's disease or syndrome F84.5
Aspergilloma —see Aspergillosis
Aspergillosis (with pneumonia) B44.9
 bronchopulmonary, allergic B44.81
 disseminated B44.7
 generalized B44.7
 pulmonary NEC B44.1
 allergic B44.81
 invasive B44.0
 specified NEC B44.89
 tonsillar B44.2
Aspergillus (flavus) (fumigatus) (infection) (terreus) —see Aspergillosis
Aspermatogenesis —see Azoospermia
Aspermia (testis) —see Azoospermia
Asphyxia, asphyxiation (by) R09.01
 antenatal P84
 birth P84
 bunny bag —see Asphyxia, due to, mechanical threat to breathing, trapped in bed clothes
 crushing S28.0
 drowning T75.1
 gas, fumes, or vapor —see Table of Drugs and Chemicals
 inhalation —see Inhalation
 intrauterine P84
 local I73.00
 with gangrene I73.01
 mucus —see also Foreign body, respiratory tract, causing asphyxiation
 newborn P84
 pathological R09.01
 postnatal P84
 mechanical —see Asphyxia, due to, mechanical threat to breathing
 prenatal P84
 reticularis R23.1
 strangulation —see Asphyxia, due to, mechanical threat to breathing
 submersion T75.1
 traumatic T71.9
 due to
 crushed chest S28.0
 foreign body (in) —see Foreign body, respiratory tract, causing asphyxia

Asphyxia, asphyxiation (Continued)
 traumatic (Continued)
 due to (Continued)
 low oxygen content of ambient air T71.20
 due to
 being trapped in
 low oxygen environment T71.29
 in car trunk T71.221
 circumstances undetermined T71.224
 done with intent to harm by
 another person T71.223
 self T71.222
 in refrigerator T71.231
 circumstances undetermined T71.234
 done with intent to harm by
 another person T71.233
 self T71.232
 cave-in T71.21
 mechanical threat to breathing (accidental) T71.191
 circumstances undetermined T71.194
 done with intent to harm by
 another person T71.193
 self T71.192
 hanging T71.161
 circumstances undetermined T71.164
 done with intent to harm by
 another person T71.163
 self T71.162
 plastic bag T71.121
 circumstances undetermined T71.124
 done with intent to harm by
 another person T71.123
 self T71.122
 smothering
 in furniture T71.151
 circumstances undetermined T71.154
 done with intent to harm by
 another person T71.153
 self T71.152
 under
 another person's body T71.141
 circumstances undetermined T71.144
 done with intent to harm T71.143
 pillow T71.111
 circumstances undetermined T71.114
 done with intent to harm by
 another person T71.113
 self T71.112
 trapped in bed clothes T71.131
 circumstances undetermined T71.134
 done with intent to harm by
 another person T71.133
 self T71.132
 vomiting, vomitus —see Foreign body, respiratory tract, causing asphyxia
Aspiration
 amniotic (clear) fluid (newborn) P24.10
 with
 pneumonia (pneumonitis) P24.11
 respiratory symptoms P24.11
 blood
 newborn (without respiratory symptoms) P24.20
 with
 pneumonia (pneumonitis) P24.21
 respiratory symptoms P24.21
 specified age NEC —see Foreign body, respiratory tract
 bronchitis J69.0
 food or foreign body —see Foreign body, by site
 liquor (amnii) (newborn) P24.10
 with
 pneumonia (pneumonitis) P24.11
 respiratory symptoms P24.11
 meconium (newborn) (without respiratory symptoms) P24.00
 with
 pneumonitis (pneumonia) P24.01
 respiratory symptoms P24.01
 milk (newborn) (without respiratory symptoms) P24.30
 with
 pneumonia (pneumonitis) P24.31
 respiratory symptoms P24.31
 specified age NEC —see Foreign body, respiratory tract

Aspiration (Continued)
 mucus —see also Foreign body, by site, causing asphyxia
 newborn P24.10
 with
 pneumonia (pneumonitis) P24.11
 respiratory symptoms P24.11
 neonatal P24.9
 specific NEC (without respiratory symptoms) P24.80
 with
 pneumonia (pneumonitis) P24.81
 respiratory symptoms P24.81
 newborn P24.9
 specific NEC (without respiratory symptoms) P24.80
 with
 pneumonia (pneumonitis) P24.81
 respiratory symptoms P24.81
 pneumonia J69.0
 pneumonitis J69.0
 syndrome of newborn —see Aspiration, by substance, with pneumonia
 vernix caseosa (newborn) P24.80
 with
 pneumonia (pneumonitis) P24.81
 respiratory symptoms P24.81
 vomitus —see also Foreign body, respiratory tract
 newborn (without respiratory symptoms) P24.30
 with
 pneumonia (pneumonitis) P24.31
 respiratory symptoms P24.31
Asplenia (congenital) Q89.01
▶functional D73.0
 postsurgical Z90.81
Assam fever B55.0
Assault, sexual —see Maltreatment
Assmann's focus NEC A15.0
Astasia (-abasia) (hysterical) F44.4
Asteatosis cutis L85.3
Astereognosia, astereognosis R48.1
Asterixis R27.8
 in liver disease K71.3
Asteroid hyalitis —see Deposit, crystalline
Asthenia, asthenic R53.1
 cardiac —see also Failure, heart I50.9
 psychogenic F45.8
 cardiovascular —see also Failure, heart I50.9
 psychogenic F45.8
 heart —see also Failure, heart I50.9
 psychogenic F45.8
 hysterical F44.4
 myocardial —see also Failure, heart I50.9
 psychogenic F45.8
 nervous F48.8
 neurocirculatory F45.8
 neurotic F48.8
 psychogenic F48.8
 psychoneurotic F48.8
 psychophysiologic F48.8
 reaction (psychophysiologic) F48.8
 senile R54
Asthenopia —see also Discomfort, visual
 hysterical F44.6
 psychogenic F44.6
Asthenospermia —see Abnormal, specimen, male genital organs
Asthma, asthmatic (bronchial) (catarrh) (spasmodic) J45.909
 with
 chronic obstructive bronchitis J44.89
 with
 acute lower respiratory infection J44.0
 exacerbation (acute) J44.1
 chronic obstructive pulmonary disease J44.89
 with
 acute lower respiratory infection J44.0
 exacerbation (acute) J44.1
 exacerbation (acute) J45.901
 hay fever —see Asthma, allergic extrinsic
 rhinitis, allergic —see Asthma, allergic extrinsic
 status asthmaticus J45.902
 allergic extrinsic J45.909
 with
 exacerbation (acute) J45.901
 status asthmaticus J45.902
 atopic —see Asthma, allergic extrinsic
 cardiac —see Failure, ventricular, left
 cardiobronchial I50.1

A

A

B

▶ New ➠ Revised ~~deleted~~ Deleted ● Use Additional Character(s)

- **Bigeminal pulse** RØØ.8
- ▶ **Bigorexia** F45.22
- **Bilateral** —*see* condition
- **Bile**
  - duct —*see* condition
  - pigments in urine R82.2
- **Bilharziasis** —*see also* Schistosomiasis
  - chyluria B65.Ø
  - cutaneous B65.3
  - galacturia B65.Ø
  - hematochyluria B65.Ø
  - intestinal B65.1
  - lipemia B65.9
  - lipuria B65.Ø
  - oriental B65.2
  - piarhemia B65.9
  - pulmonary NOS B65.9 *[J99]*
    - pneumonia B65.9 *[J17]*
  - tropical hematuria B65.Ø
  - vesical B65.Ø
- **Biliary** —*see* condition
- **Bilirubin metabolism disorder** E8Ø.7
  - specified NEC E8Ø.6
- **Bilirubinemia, familial nonhemolytic** E8Ø.4
- **Bilirubinuria** R82.2
- **Biliuria** R82.2
- **Bilocular stomach** K31.2
- **Binswanger's disease** I67.3
- **Biparta, bipartite**
  - carpal scaphoid Q74.Ø
  - patella Q74.1
  - vagina Q52.1Ø
- **BI-RADS** —*see* Breast, Imaging Reporting and Data System
- **Bird**
  - face Q75.8
  - fancier's disease or lung J67.2
- **Birt-Hogg-Dube syndrome** Q87.89
- **Birth**
  - complications in mother —*see* Delivery, complicated
  - compression during NOS P15.9
  - defect —*see* Anomaly
  - immature (less than 37 completed weeks) —*see* Preterm, newborn
    - extremely (less than 28 completed weeks) —*see* Immaturity, extreme
  - inattention, at or after —*see* Maltreatment, child, neglect
  - injury NOS P15.9
    - basal ganglia P11.1
    - brachial plexus NEC P14.3
    - brain (compression) (pressure) P11.2
    - central nervous system NOS P11.9
    - cerebellum P11.1
    - cerebral hemorrhage P1Ø.1
    - external genitalia P15.5
    - eye P15.3
    - face P15.4
    - fracture
      - bone P13.9
        - specified NEC P13.8
      - clavicle P13.4
      - femur P13.2
      - humerus P13.3
      - long bone, except femur P13.3
      - radius and ulna P13.3
      - skull P13.Ø
      - spine P11.5
      - tibia and fibula P13.3
    - intracranial P11.2
      - laceration or hemorrhage P1Ø.9
        - specified NEC P1Ø.8
    - intraventricular hemorrhage P1Ø.2
    - laceration
      - brain P1Ø.1
      - by scalpel P15.8
      - peripheral nerve P14.9
    - liver P15.Ø
    - meninges
      - brain P11.1
      - spinal cord P11.5
    - nerve
      - brachial plexus P14.3
      - cranial NEC (except facial) P11.4
      - facial P11.3
      - peripheral P14.9
      - phrenic (paralysis) P14.2
    - paralysis
      - facial nerve P11.3
      - spinal P11.5

- **Birth** *(Continued)*
  - injury *(Continued)*
    - penis P15.5
    - rupture
      - spinal cord P11.5
    - scalp P12.9
    - scalpel wound P15.8
    - scrotum P15.5
    - skull NEC P13.1
      - fracture P13.Ø
    - specified type NEC P15.8
    - spinal cord P11.5
    - spine P11.5
    - spleen P15.1
    - sternomastoid (hematoma) P15.2
    - subarachnoid hemorrhage P1Ø.3
    - subcutaneous fat necrosis P15.6
    - subdural hemorrhage P1Ø.Ø
    - tentorial tear P1Ø.4
    - testes P15.5
    - vulva P15.5
  - lack of care, at or after —*see* Maltreatment, child, neglect
  - neglect, at or after —*see* Maltreatment, child, neglect
  - palsy or paralysis, newborn, NOS (birth injury) P14.9
  - premature (infant) —*see* Preterm, newborn
  - shock, newborn P96.89
  - trauma —*see* Birth, injury
  - weight
    - 4ØØØ grams to 4499 grams PØ8.1
    - 45ØØ grams or more PØ8.Ø
    - low (2499 grams or less) —*see* Low, birthweight
      - extremely (999 grams or less) —*see* Low, birthweight, extreme
- **Birthmark** Q82.5
- **Bisalbuminemia** E88.Ø9
- **Biskra's button** B55.1
- **Bite(s)** (animal) (human)
  - abdomen, abdominal
    - wall S31.159
      - with penetration into peritoneal cavity S31.659
      - epigastric region S31.152
        - with penetration into peritoneal cavity S31.652
      - left
        - lower quadrant S31.154
          - with penetration into peritoneal cavity S31.654
        - upper quadrant S31.151
          - with penetration into peritoneal cavity S31.651
      - periumbilic region S31.155
        - with penetration into peritoneal cavity S31.655
      - right
        - lower quadrant S31.153
          - with penetration into peritoneal cavity S31.653
        - upper quadrant S31.15Ø
          - with penetration into peritoneal cavity S31.65Ø
      - superficial NEC S3Ø.871
        - insect S3Ø.861
  - alveolar (process) —*see* Bite, oral cavity
  - amphibian (venomous) —*see* Venom, bite, amphibian
  - animal —*see also* Bite, by site
    - venomous —*see* Venom
  - ankle S91.Ø5-●
    - superficial NEC S9Ø.57-●
      - insect S9Ø.56-●
  - antecubital space —*see* Bite, elbow
  - anus S31.835
    - superficial NEC S3Ø.877
      - insect S3Ø.867
  - arm (upper) S41.15-●
    - lower —*see* Bite, forearm
    - superficial NEC S4Ø.87-●
      - insect S4Ø.86-●
  - arthropod NEC —*see* Venom, bite, arthropod
  - auditory canal (external) (meatus) —*see* Bite, ear
  - auricle, ear —*see* Bite, ear
  - axilla —*see* Bite, arm

- **Bite** *(Continued)*
  - back —*see also* Bite, thorax, back
    - lower S31.Ø5Ø
      - with penetration into retroperitoneal space S31.Ø51
      - superficial NEC S3Ø.87Ø
        - insect S3Ø.86Ø
  - bedbug —*see* Bite(s), by site, superficial, insect
  - breast S21.Ø5-●
    - superficial NEC S2Ø.17-●
      - insect S2Ø.16-●
  - brow —*see* Bite, head, specified site NEC
  - buttock S31.8Ø5
    - left S31.825
    - right S31.815
    - superficial NEC S3Ø.87Ø
      - insect S3Ø.86Ø
  - calf —*see* Bite, leg
  - canaliculus lacrimalis —*see* Bite, eyelid
  - canthus, eye —*see* Bite, eyelid
  - centipede —*see* Toxicity, venom, arthropod, centipede
  - cheek (external) SØ1.45-●
    - internal —*see* Bite, oral cavity
    - superficial NEC SØØ.87
      - insect SØØ.86
  - chest wall —*see* Bite, thorax
  - chigger B88.Ø
  - chin —*see* Bite, head, specified site NEC
  - clitoris —*see* Bite, vulva
  - costal region —*see* Bite, thorax
  - digit(s)
    - hand —*see* Bite, finger
    - toe —*see* Bite, toe
  - ear (canal) (external) SØ1.35-●
    - superficial NEC SØØ.47-●
      - insect SØØ.46-●
  - elbow S51.Ø5-●
    - superficial NEC S5Ø.37-●
      - insect S5Ø.36-●
  - epididymis —*see* Bite, testis
  - epigastric region —*see* Bite, abdomen
  - epiglottis —*see* Bite, neck, specified site NEC
  - esophagus, cervical S11.25
    - superficial NEC S1Ø.17
      - insect S1Ø.16
  - eyebrow —*see* Bite, eyelid
  - eyelid SØ1.15-●
    - superficial NEC SØØ.27-●
      - insect SØØ.26-●
  - face NEC —*see* Bite, head, specified site NEC
  - finger(s) S61.259
    - with
      - damage to nail S61.359
    - index S61.258
      - with
        - damage to nail S61.358
      - left S61.251
        - with
          - damage to nail S61.351
      - right S61.25Ø
        - with
          - damage to nail S61.35Ø
      - superficial NEC S6Ø.478
        - insect S6Ø.46-●
    - little S61.25-●
      - with
        - damage to nail S61.35-●
      - superficial NEC S6Ø.47-●
        - insect S6Ø.46-●
    - middle S61.25-●
      - with
        - damage to nail S61.35-●
      - superficial NEC S6Ø.47-●
        - insect S6Ø.46-●
    - ring S61.25-●
      - with
        - damage to nail S61.35-●
      - superficial NEC S6Ø.47-●
        - insect S6Ø.46-●
    - superficial NEC S6Ø.479
      - insect S6Ø.469
    - thumb —*see* Bite, thumb
  - flank —*see* Bite, abdomen, wall
  - flea —*see* Bite, by site, superficial, insect
  - foot (except toe(s) alone) S91.35-●
    - superficial NEC S9Ø.87-●
      - insect S9Ø.86-●
    - toe —*see* Bite, toe

Bite *(Continued)*
- forearm S51.85-●
  - elbow only —*see* Bite, elbow
  - superficial NEC S50.87-●
    - insect S50.86-●
- forehead —*see* Bite, head, specified site NEC
- genital organs, external
  - female S31.552
    - superficial NEC S30.876
      - insect S30.866
    - vagina and vulva —*see* Bite, vulva
  - male S31.551
    - penis —*see* Bite, penis
    - scrotum —*see* Bite, scrotum
    - superficial NEC S30.875
      - insect S30.865
    - testes —*see* Bite, testis
- groin —*see* Bite, abdomen, wall
- gum —*see* Bite, oral cavity
- hand S61.45-●
  - finger —*see* Bite, finger
  - superficial NEC S60.57-●
    - insect S60.56-●
  - thumb —*see* Bite, thumb
- head S01.95
  - cheek —*see* Bite, cheek
  - ear —*see* Bite, ear
  - eyelid —*see* Bite, eyelid
  - lip —*see* Bite, lip
  - nose —*see* Bite, nose
  - oral cavity —*see* Bite, oral cavity
  - scalp —*see* Bite, scalp
  - specified site NEC S01.85
    - superficial NEC S00.87
      - insect S00.86
  - superficial NEC S00.97
    - insect S00.96
  - temporomandibular area —*see* Bite, cheek
- heel —*see* Bite, foot
- hip S71.05-●
  - superficial NEC S70.27-●
    - insect S70.26-●
- hymen S31.45
- hypochondrium —*see* Bite, abdomen, wall
- hypogastric region —*see* Bite, abdomen, wall
- inguinal region —*see* Bite, abdomen, wall
- insect —*see* Bite, by site, superficial, insect
- instep —*see* Bite, foot
- interscapular region —*see* Bite, thorax, back
- jaw —*see* Bite, head, specified site NEC
- knee S81.05-●
  - superficial NEC S80.27-●
    - insect S80.26-●
- labium (majus) (minus) —*see* Bite, vulva
- lacrimal duct —*see* Bite, eyelid
- larynx S11.015
  - superficial NEC S10.17
    - insect S10.16
- leg (lower) S81.85-●
  - ankle —*see* Bite, ankle
  - foot —*see* Bite, foot
  - knee —*see* Bite, knee
  - superficial NEC S80.87-●
    - insect S80.86-●
  - toe —*see* Bite, toe
  - upper —*see* Bite, thigh
- lip S01.551
  - superficial NEC S00.571
    - insect S00.561
- lizard (venomous) —*see* Venom, bite, reptile
- loin —*see* Bite, abdomen, wall
- lower back —*see* Bite, back, lower
- lumbar region —*see* Bite, back, lower
- malar region —*see* Bite, head, specified site NEC
- mammary —*see* Bite, breast
- marine animals (venomous) —*see* Toxicity, venom, marine animal
- mastoid region —*see* Bite, head, specified site NEC
- mouth —*see* Bite, oral cavity
- nail
  - finger —*see* Bite, finger
  - toe —*see* Bite, toe
- nape —*see* Bite, neck, specified site NEC
- nasal (septum) (sinus) —*see* Bite, nose
- nasopharynx —*see* Bite, head, specified site NEC
- neck S11.95
  - involving
    - cervical esophagus —*see* Bite, esophagus, cervical
    - larynx —*see* Bite, larynx

Bite *(Continued)*
- neck *(Continued)*
  - involving *(Continued)*
    - pharynx —*see* Bite, pharynx
    - thyroid gland S11.15
    - trachea —*see* Bite, trachea
  - specified site NEC S11.85
    - superficial NEC S10.87
      - insect S10.86
  - superficial NEC S10.97
    - insect S10.96
  - throat S11.85
    - superficial NEC S10.17
      - insect S10.16
- nose (septum) (sinus) S01.25
  - superficial NEC S00.37
    - insect S00.36
- occipital region —*see* Bite, scalp
- oral cavity S01.552
  - superficial NEC S00.572
    - insect S00.562
- orbital region —*see* Bite, eyelid
- palate —*see* Bite, oral cavity
- palm —*see* Bite, hand
- parietal region —*see* Bite, scalp
- pelvis S31.050
  - with penetration into retroperitoneal space S31.051
  - superficial NEC S30.870
    - insect S30.860
- penis S31.25
  - superficial NEC S30.872
    - insect S30.862
- perineum
  - female —*see* Bite, vulva
  - male —*see* Bite, pelvis
- periocular area (with or without lacrimal passages) —*see* Bite, eyelid
- phalanges
  - finger —*see* Bite, finger
  - toe —*see* Bite, toe
- pharynx S11.25
  - superficial NEC S10.17
    - insect S10.16
- pinna —*see* Bite, ear
- poisonous —*see* Venom
- popliteal space —*see* Bite, knee
- prepuce —*see* Bite, penis
- pubic region —*see* Bite, abdomen, wall
- rectovaginal septum —*see* Bite, vulva
- red bug B88.0
- reptile NEC —*see also* Venom, bite, reptile
  - nonvenomous —*see* Bite, by site
  - snake —*see* Venom, bite, snake
- sacral region —*see* Bite, back, lower
- sacroiliac region —*see* Bite, back, lower
- salivary gland —*see* Bite, oral cavity
- scalp S01.05
  - superficial NEC S00.07
    - insect S00.06
- scapular region —*see* Bite, shoulder
- scrotum S31.35
  - superficial NEC S30.873
    - insect S30.863
- sea-snake (venomous) —*see* Toxicity, venom, snake, sea snake
- shin —*see* Bite, leg
- shoulder S41.05-●
  - superficial NEC S40.27-●
    - insect S40.26-●
- snake —*see also* Venom, bite, snake
  - nonvenomous —*see* Bite, by site
- spermatic cord —*see* Bite, testis
- spider (venomous) —*see* Toxicity, venom, spider
  - nonvenomous —*see* Bite, by site, superficial, insect
- sternal region —*see* Bite, thorax, front
- submaxillary region —*see* Bite, head, specified site NEC
- submental region —*see* Bite, head, specified site NEC
- subungual
  - finger(s) —*see* Bite, finger
  - toe —*see* Bite, toe
- superficial —*see* Bite, by site, superficial
- supraclavicular fossa S11.85
- supraorbital —*see* Bite, head, specified site NEC
- temple, temporal region —*see* Bite, head, specified site NEC

Bite *(Continued)*
- temporomandibular area —*see* Bite, cheek
- testis S31.35
  - superficial NEC S30.873
    - insect S30.863
- thigh S71.15-●
  - superficial NEC S70.37-●
    - insect S70.36-●
- thorax, thoracic (wall) S21.95
  - back S21.25-●
    - with penetration into thoracic cavity S21.45-●
  - breast —*see* Bite, breast
  - front S21.15-●
    - with penetration into thoracic cavity S21.35-●
  - superficial NEC S20.97
    - back S20.47-●
    - front S20.37-●
    - insect S20.96
      - back S20.46-●
      - front S20.36-●
- throat —*see* Bite, neck, throat
- thumb S61.05-●
  - with
    - damage to nail S61.15-●
  - superficial NEC S60.37-●
    - insect S60.36-●
- thyroid S11.15
  - superficial NEC S10.87
    - insect S10.86
- toe(s) S91.15-●
  - with
    - damage to nail S91.25-●
  - great S91.15-●
    - with
      - damage to nail S91.25-●
  - lesser S91.15-●
    - with
      - damage to nail S91.25-●
  - superficial NEC S90.47-●
    - great S90.47-●
    - insect S90.46-●
      - great S90.46-●
- tongue S01.552
- trachea S11.025
  - superficial NEC S10.17
    - insect S10.16
- tunica vaginalis —*see* Bite, testis
- tympanum, tympanic membrane —*see* Bite, ear
- umbilical region S31.155
- uvula —*see* Bite, oral cavity
- vagina —*see* Bite, vulva
- venomous —*see* Venom
- vocal cords S11.035
  - superficial NEC S10.17
    - insect S10.16
- vulva S31.45
  - superficial NEC S30.874
    - insect S30.864
- wrist S61.55-●
  - superficial NEC S60.87-●
    - insect S60.86-●

Biting, cheek or lip K13.1

Biventricular failure (heart) I50.82

Björck (-Thorson) syndrome (malignant carcinoid) E34.09

Black
- death A20.9
- eye S00.1-●
- hairy tongue K14.3
- heel (foot) S90.3-●
- lung (disease) J60
- palm (hand) S60.22-●

Blackfan-Diamond anemia or syndrome (congenital hypoplastic anemia) D61.01

Blackhead L70.0

Blackout R55

Bladder —*see* condition

Blast (air) (hydraulic) (immersion) (underwater)
- blindness S05.8X-●
- injury
  - abdomen or thorax —*see* Injury, by site
  - ear (acoustic nerve trauma) —*see* Injury, nerve, acoustic, specified type NEC
- syndrome NEC T70.8

Blastoma —*see* Neoplasm, malignant, by site
- pulmonary —*see* Neoplasm, lung, malignant

Blastomycosis, blastomycotic B40.9
- Brazilian —*see* Paracoccidioidomycosis
- cutaneous B40.3

INDEX TO DISEASES AND INJURIES / Blastomycosis, blastomycotic

Blastomycosis, blastomycotic *(Continued)*
disseminated B40.7
European —*see* Cryptococcosis
generalized B40.7
keloidal B48.0
North American B40.9
primary pulmonary B40.0
pulmonary B40.2
acute B40.0
chronic B40.1
skin B40.3
South American —*see* Paracoccidioidomycosis
specified NEC B40.89
Bleb(s) R23.8
emphysematous (lung) (solitary) J43.9
endophthalmitis H59.43
filtering (vitreous), after glaucoma surgery Z98.83
inflammed (infected), postprocedural H59.40
stage 1 H59.41
stage 2 H59.42
stage 3 H59.43
lung (ruptured) J43.9
congenital —*see* Atelectasis
newborn P25.8
subpleural (emphysematous) J43.9
Blebitis, postprocedural H59.40
stage 1 H59.41
stage 2 H59.42
stage 3 H59.43
Bleeder (familial) (hereditary) —*see* Hemophilia
Bleeding —*see also* Hemorrhage
anal K62.5
anovulatory N97.0
atonic, following delivery O72.1
capillary I78.8
puerperal O72.2
contact (postcoital) N93.0
due to uterine subinvolution N85.3
ear —*see* Otorrhagia
excessive, associated with menopausal onset N92.4
familial —*see* Defect, coagulation
following intercourse N93.0
gastrointestinal K92.2
hemorrhoids —*see* Hemorrhoids
intermenstrual (regular) N92.3
irregular N92.1
intraoperative —*see* Complication, intraoperative, hemorrhage
irregular N92.6
menopausal N92.4
newborn, intraventricular —*see* Newborn, affected by, hemorrhage, intraventricular
nipple N64.59
nose R04.0
ovulation N92.3
perimenopausal N92.4
postclimacteric N95.0
postcoital N93.0
postmenopausal N95.0
postoperative —*see* Complication, postprocedural, hemorrhage
preclimacteric N92.4
pre-pubertal vaginal N93.1
puberty (excessive, with onset of menstrual periods) N92.2
rectum, rectal K62.5
newborn P54.2
tendencies —*see* Defect, coagulation
throat R04.1
tooth socket (post-extraction) K91.840
umbilical stump P51.9
uterus, uterine NEC N93.9
climacteric N92.4
dysfunctional or functional N93.8
menopausal N92.4
preclimacteric or premenopausal N92.4
unrelated to menstrual cycle N93.9
vagina, vaginal (abnormal) N93.9
dysfunctional or functional N93.8
newborn P54.6
pre-pubertal N93.1
vicarious N94.89
Blennorrhagia, blennorrhagic —*see* Gonorrhea
Blennorrhea (acute) (chronic) —*see also* Gonorrhea
inclusion (neonatal) (newborn) P39.1
lower genitourinary tract (gonococcal) A54.00
neonatorum (gonococcal ophthalmia) A54.31
Blepharelosis —*see* Entropion
Blepharitis (angularis) (ciliaris) (eyelid) (marginal) (nonulcerative) H01.009
herpes zoster B02.39
left H01.006
lower H01.005
upper H01.004
upper and lower H01.00B
right H01.003
lower H01.002
upper H01.001
upper and lower H01.00A
squamous H01.029
left H01.026
lower H01.025
upper H01.024
upper and lower H01.02B
right H01.023
lower H01.022
upper H01.021
upper and lower H01.02A
ulcerative H01.019
left H01.016
lower H01.015
upper H01.014
upper and lower H01.01B
right H01.013
lower H01.012
upper H01.011
upper and lower H01.01B
Blepharochalasis H02.30
congenital Q10.0
left H02.36
lower H02.35
upper H02.34
right H02.33
lower H02.32
upper H02.31
Blepharoclonus H02.59
Blepharoconjunctivitis H10.50-●
angular H10.52-●
contact H10.53-●
ligneous H10.51-●
Blepharophimosis (eyelid) H02.529
congenital Q10.3
left H02.526
lower H02.525
upper H02.524
right H02.523
lower H02.522
upper H02.521
Blepharoptosis H02.40-●
congenital Q10.0
mechanical H02.41-●
myogenic H02.42-●
neurogenic H02.43-●
paralytic H02.43-●
Blepharopyorrhea, gonococcal A54.39
Blepharospasm G24.5
drug induced G24.01
Blighted ovum O02.0
Blind —*see also* Blindness
bronchus (congenital) Q32.4
loop syndrome K90.2
congenital Q43.8
sac, fallopian tube (congenital) Q50.6
spot, enlarged —*see* Defect, visual field, localized, scotoma, blind spot area
tract or tube, congenital NEC —*see* Atresia, by site
Blindness (acquired) (congenital) (both eyes) H54.0X-●
blast S05.8X-●
color —*see* Deficiency, color vision
concussion S05.8X-●
cortical H47.619
left brain H47.612
right brain H47.611
day H53.11
due to injury (current episode) S05.9-●
sequelae — code to injury with seventh character S
eclipse (total) —*see* Retinopathy, solar
emotional (hysterical) F44.6
face H53.16
hysterical F44.6
legal (both eyes) (USA definition) H54.8
mind R48.8
night H53.60
abnormal dark adaptation curve H53.61
acquired H53.62
congenital H53.63
Blindness *(Continued)*
night *(Continued)*
specified type NEC H53.69
vitamin A deficiency E50.5
one eye (other eye normal) H54.40
left (normal vision on right) H54.42-●
low vision on right H54.12-●
low vision, other eye H54.10
right (normal vision on left) H54.41-●
low vision on left H54.11-●
psychic R48.8
river B73.01
snow —*see* Photokeratitis
sun, solar —*see* Retinopathy, solar
transient —*see* Disturbance, vision, subjective, loss, transient
traumatic (current episode) S05.9-●
word (developmental) F81.0
acquired R48.0
secondary to organic lesion R48.0
Blister (nonthermal)
abdominal wall S30.821
alveolar process S00.522
ankle S90.52-●
antecubital space —*see* Blister, elbow
anus S30.827
arm (upper) S40.82-●
auditory canal —*see* Blister, ear
auricle —*see* Blister, ear
axilla —*see* Blister, arm
back, lower S30.820
beetle dermatitis L24.89
breast S20.12-●
brow S00.82
calf —*see* Blister, leg
canthus —*see* Blister, eyelid
cheek S00.82
internal S00.522
chest wall —*see* Blister, thorax
chin S00.82
costal region —*see* Blister, thorax
digit(s)
foot —*see* Blister, toe
hand —*see* Blister, finger
due to burn —*see* Burn, by site, second degree
ear S00.42-●
elbow S50.32-●
epiglottis S10.12
esophagus, cervical S10.12
eyebrow —*see* Blister, eyelid
eyelid S00.22-●
face S00.82
fever B00.1
finger(s) S60.429
index S60.42-●
little S60.42-●
middle S60.42-●
ring S60.42-●
foot (except toe(s) alone) S90.82-●
toe —*see* Blister, toe
forearm S50.82-●
elbow only —*see* Blister, elbow
forehead S00.82
fracture - omit code
genital organ
female S30.826
male S30.825
gum S00.522
hand S60.52-●
head S00.92
ear —*see* Blister, ear
eyelid —*see* Blister, eyelid
lip S00.521
nose S00.32
oral cavity S00.522
scalp S00.02
specified site NEC S00.82
heel —*see* Blister, foot
hip S70.22-●
interscapular region S20.429
jaw S00.82
knee S80.22-●
larynx S10.12
leg (lower) S80.82-●
knee —*see* Blister, knee
upper —*see* Blister, thigh
lip S00.521
malar region S00.82
mammary —*see* Blister, breast
mastoid region S00.82

130 ▶ New ➡ Revised ~~deleted~~ Deleted ● Use Additional Character(s)

Blister *(Continued)*
- mouth SØØ.522
- multiple, skin, nontraumatic R23.8
- nail
  - finger —*see* Blister, finger
  - toe —*see* Blister, toe
- nasal SØØ.32
- neck S1Ø.92
  - specified site NEC S1Ø.82
  - throat S1Ø.12
- nose SØØ.32
- occipital region SØØ.Ø2
- oral cavity SØØ.522
- orbital region —*see* Blister, eyelid
- palate SØØ.522
- palm —*see* Blister, hand
- parietal region SØØ.Ø2
- pelvis S3Ø.82Ø
- penis S3Ø.822
- periocular area —*see* Blister, eyelid
- phalanges
  - finger —*see* Blister, finger
  - toe —*see* Blister, toe
- pharynx S1Ø.12
- pinna —*see* Blister, ear
- popliteal space —*see* Blister, knee
- scalp SØØ.Ø2
- scapular region —*see* Blister, shoulder
- scrotum S3Ø.823
- shin —*see* Blister, leg
- shoulder S4Ø.22-●
- sternal region S2Ø.329
- submaxillary region SØØ.82
- submental region SØØ.82
- subungual
  - finger(s) —*see* Blister, finger
  - toe(s) —*see* Blister, toe
- supraclavicular fossa S1Ø.82
- supraorbital SØØ.82
- temple SØØ.82
- temporal region SØØ.82
- testis S3Ø.823
- thermal —*see* Burn, by site, second degree
- thigh S7Ø.32-●
- thorax, thoracic (wall) S2Ø.92
  - back S2Ø.42-●
  - front S2Ø.32-●
- throat S1Ø.12
- thumb S6Ø.32-●
- toe(s) S9Ø.42-●
  - great S9Ø.42-●
- tongue SØØ.522
- trachea S1Ø.12
- tympanum, tympanic membrane —*see* Blister, ear
- upper arm —*see* Blister, arm (upper)
- uvula SØØ.522
- vagina S3Ø.824
- vocal cords S1Ø.12
- vulva S3Ø.824
- wrist S6Ø.82-●

Bloating R14.Ø

Bloch-Sulzberger disease or syndrome Q82.3

Block, blocked
- alveolocapillary J84.1Ø
- arborization (heart) I45.5
- arrhythmic I45.9
- atrioventricular (incomplete) (partial) I44.3Ø
  - with atrioventricular dissociation I44.2
  - complete I44.2
    - congenital Q24.6
  - congenital Q24.6
  - first degree I44.Ø
  - second degree (types I and II) I44.1
  - specified NEC I44.39
  - third degree I44.2
  - types I and II I44.1
- auriculoventricular —*see* Block, atrioventricular
- bifascicular (cardiac) I45.2
- bundle-branch (complete) (false) (incomplete) I45.4
  - bilateral I45.2
  - left I44.7
    - with right bundle branch block I45.2
    - hemiblock I44.6Ø
      - anterior I44.4
      - posterior I44.5
    - incomplete I44.7
      - with right bundle branch block I45.2

Block, blocked *(Continued)*
- bundle-branc *(Continued)*
  - right I45.1Ø
    - with
      - left bundle branch block I45.2
      - left fascicular block I45.2
    - specified NEC I45.19
  - Wilson's type I45.19
- cardiac I45.9
- conduction I45.9
  - complete I44.2
- fascicular (left) I44.6Ø
  - anterior I44.4
  - posterior I44.5
  - right I45.Ø
  - specified NEC I44.69
- foramen Magendie (acquired) G91.1
  - congenital QØ3.1
    - with spina bifida —*see* Spina bifida, by site, with hydrocephalus
- heart I45.9
  - bundle branch I45.4
    - bilateral I45.2
  - complete (atrioventricular) I44.2
  - congenital Q24.6
  - first degree (atrioventricular) I44.Ø
  - second degree (atrioventricular) I44.1
  - specified type NEC I45.5
  - third degree (atrioventricular) I44.2
- hepatic vein I82.Ø
- intraventricular (nonspecific) I45.4
  - bundle branch
    - bilateral I45.2
- kidney N28.9
  - postcystoscopic or postprocedural N99.Ø
- Mobitz (types I and II) I44.1
- myocardial —*see* Block, heart
- nodal I45.5
- organ or site, congenital NEC —*see* Atresia, by site
- portal (vein) I81
- second degree (types I and II) I44.1
- sinoatrial I45.5
- sinoauricular I45.5
- third degree I44.2
- trifascicular I45.3
- tubal N97.1
- vein NOS I82.9Ø
- Wenckebach (types I and II) I44.1

Blockage —*see* Obstruction

Blocq's disease F44.4

Blood
- constituents, abnormal R78.9
- disease D75.9
- donor —*see* Donor, blood
- dyscrasia D75.9
  - with
    - abortion —*see* Abortion, by type, complicated by, hemorrhage
    - ectopic pregnancy OØ8.1
    - molar pregnancy OØ8.1
  - following ectopic or molar pregnancy OØ8.1
  - newborn P61.9
  - puerperal, postpartum O72.3
- flukes NEC —*see* Schistosomiasis
- in
  - feces K92.1
    - occult R19.5
  - urine —*see* Hematuria
- mole OØ2.Ø
- occult in feces R19.5
- pressure
  - decreased, due to shock following injury T79.4
  - examination only ZØ1.3Ø
  - fluctuating I99.8
  - high —*see* Hypertension
    - borderline RØ3.Ø
    - incidental reading, without diagnosis of hypertension RØ3.Ø
  - low —*see also* Hypotension
    - incidental reading, without diagnosis of hypotension RØ3.1
- spitting —*see* Hemoptysis
- staining cornea —*see* Pigmentation, cornea, stromal
- transfusion
  - reaction or complication —*see* Complications, transfusion
- type
  - A (Rh positive) Z67.1Ø
    - Rh negative Z67.11

Blood *(Continued)*
- type *(Continued)*
  - AB (Rh positive) Z67.3Ø
    - Rh negative Z67.31
  - B (Rh positive) Z67.2Ø
    - Rh negative Z67.21
  - O (Rh positive) Z67.4Ø
    - Rh negative Z67.41
  - Rh (positive) Z67.9Ø
    - negative Z67.91
- vessel rupture —*see* Hemorrhage
- vomiting —*see* Hematemesis

Blood-forming organs, disease D75.9

Bloodgood's disease —*see* Mastopathy, cystic

Bloom (-Machacek)(-Torre) syndrome Q82.8

Blount disease or osteochondrosis M92.51-●

Blue
- baby Q24.9
- diaper syndrome E72.Ø9
- dome cyst (breast) —*see* Cyst, breast
- dot cataract Q12.Ø
- nevus D22.9
- sclera Q13.5
  - with fragility of bone and deafness Q78.Ø
- toe syndrome I75.Ø2-●

Blueness —*see* Cyanosis

Blues, postpartal O9Ø.6
- baby O9Ø.6

Blurring, visual H53.8

Blushing (abnormal) (excessive) R23.2

BMI —*see* Body, mass index

Boarder, hospital NEC Z76.4
- accompanying sick person Z76.3
- healthy infant or child Z76.2
  - foundling Z76.1

Bockhart's impetigo LØ1.Ø2

Bodechtel-Guttman disease (subacute sclerosing panencephalitis) A81.1

Boder-Sedgwick syndrome (ataxia- telangiectasia) G11.3

Body, bodies
- Aschoff's —*see* Myocarditis, rheumatic
- asteroid, vitreous —*see* Deposit, crystalline
- cytoid (retina) —*see* Occlusion, artery, retina
- drusen (degenerative) (macula) (retinal) —*see also* Degeneration, macula, drusen
  - optic disc —*see* Drusen, optic disc
- foreign —*see* Foreign body
- loose
  - joint, except knee —*see* Loose, body, joint
    - knee M23.4-●
  - sheath, tendon —*see* Disorder, tendon, specified type NEC
- mass index (BMI)
  - adult
    - 19.9 or less Z68.1
    - 2Ø.Ø-2Ø.9 Z68.2Ø
    - 21.Ø-21.9 Z68.21
    - 22.Ø-22.9 Z68.22
    - 23.Ø-23.9 Z68.23
    - 24.Ø-24.9 Z68.24
    - 25.Ø-25.9 Z68.25
    - 26.Ø-26.9 Z68.26
    - 27.Ø-27.9 Z68.27
    - 28.Ø-28.9 Z68.28
    - 29.Ø-29.9 Z68.29
    - 3Ø.Ø-3Ø.9 Z68.3Ø
    - 31.Ø-31.9 Z68.31
    - 32.Ø-32.9 Z68.32
    - 33.Ø-33.9 Z68.33
    - 34.Ø-34.9 Z68.34
    - 35.Ø-35.9 Z68.35
    - 36.Ø-36.9 Z68.36
    - 37.Ø-37.9 Z68.37
    - 38.Ø-38.9 Z68.38
    - 39.Ø-39.9 Z68.39
    - 4Ø.Ø-44.9 Z68.41
    - 45.Ø-49.9 Z68.42
    - 5Ø.Ø-59.9 Z68.43
    - 6Ø.Ø-69.9 Z68.44
    - 7Ø and over Z68.45
  - pediatric
    - 5th percentile to less than 85th percentile for age Z68.52
    - 85th percentile to less than 95th percentile for age Z68.53
    - ~~greater than or equal to ninety-fifth percentile for age Z68.54~~
    - ▶95th percentile for age to less than 12Ø% of the 95th percentile for age Z68.54

B

Body, bodies *(Continued)*
mass index (BMI) *(Continued)*
pediatric *(Continued)*
▶120% of the 95th percentile for age to less than 140% of the 95th percentile for age Z68.55
▶greater than or equal to 140% of the 95th percentile for age Z68.56
less than fifth percentile for age Z68.51
Mooser's A75.2
rice —*see also* Loose, body, joint
knee M23.4-●
rocking F98.4
Boeck's
disease or sarcoid —*see* Sarcoidosis
lupoid (miliary) D86.3
Boerhaave's syndrome (spontaneous esophageal rupture) K22.3
Boggy
cervix N88.8
uterus N85.8
Boil —*see also* Furuncle, by site
Aleppo B55.1
Baghdad B55.1
Delhi B55.1
lacrimal
gland —*see* Dacryoadenitis
passages (duct) (sac) —*see* Inflammation, lacrimal, passages, acute
Natal B55.1
orbit, orbital —*see* Abscess, orbit
tropical B55.1
Bold hives —*see* Urticaria
Bombé, iris —*see* Membrane, pupillary
Bone —*see* condition
Bonnevie-Ullrich syndrome —*see also* Turner's syndrome Q87.19
Bonnier's syndrome —*see* subcategory H81.8
Bonvale dam fever T73.3
Bony block of joint —*see* Ankylosis
BOOP (bronchiolitis obliterans organized pneumonia) J84.89
Borderline
diabetes mellitus R73.03
hypertension R03.0
osteopenia M85.8-●
pelvis, with obstruction during labor O65.1
personality F60.3
Borna disease A83.9
Bornholm disease B33.0
Boston exanthem A88.0
Botalli, ductus (patent) (persistent) Q25.0
Bothriocephalus latus infestation B70.0
Botulism (foodborne intoxication) A05.1
infant A48.51
non-foodborne A48.52
wound A48.52
Bouba —*see* Yaws
Bouchard's nodes (with arthropathy) M15.2
Bouffée délirante F23
Bouillaud's disease or syndrome (rheumatic heart disease) I01.9
Bourneville's disease Q85.1
Boutonniere deformity (finger) —*see* Deformity, finger, boutonniere
Bouveret (-Hoffmann) syndrome (paroxysmal tachycardia) I47.9
Bovine heart —*see* Hypertrophy, cardiac
Bowel —*see* condition
Bowen's
dermatosis (precancerous) —*see* Neoplasm, skin, in situ
disease —*see* Neoplasm, skin, in situ
epithelioma —*see* Neoplasm, skin, in situ
type
epidermoid carcinoma-in-situ —*see* Neoplasm, skin, in situ
intraepidermal squamous cell carcinoma —*see* Neoplasm, skin, in situ
Bowing
femur —*see also* Deformity, limb, specified type NEC, thigh
congenital Q68.3
fibula —*see also* Deformity, limb, specified type NEC, lower leg
congenital Q68.4
forearm —*see* Deformity, limb, specified type NEC, forearm
leg(s), long bones, congenital Q68.5
radius —*see* Deformity, limb, specified type NEC, forearm

Bowing *(Continued)*
tibia —*see also* Deformity, limb, specified type NEC, lower leg
congenital Q68.4
Bowleg(s) (acquired) M21.16-●
congenital Q68.5
rachitic E64.3
Boyd's dysentery A03.2
Brachial —*see* condition
Brachycardia R00.1
Brachycephaly, non-deformational Q75.022
Bradley's disease A08.19
Bradyarrhythmia, cardiac I49.8
Bradycardia (sinoatrial) (sinus) (vagal) R00.1
neonatal P29.12
reflex G90.09
tachycardia syndrome I49.5
Bradykinesia R25.8
Bradypnea R06.89
Bradytachycardia I49.5
Brailsford's disease or osteochondrosis —*see* Osteochondrosis, juvenile, radius
Brain —*see also* condition
death G93.82
syndrome —*see* Syndrome, brain
Branched-chain amino-acid disorder E71.2
Branchial —*see* condition
cartilage, congenital Q18.2
Branchiogenic remnant (in neck) Q18.0
Brandt's syndrome (acrodermatitis enteropathica) E83.2
Brash (water) R12
Bravais-Jacksonian epilepsy —*see* Epilepsy, localization-related, symptomatic, with simple partial seizures
Braxton Hicks contractions —*see* False, labor
Brazilian leishmaniasis B55.2
BRBPR K62.5
Break, retina (without detachment) H33.30-●
with retinal detachment —*see* Detachment, retina
horseshoe tear H33.31-●
multiple H33.33-●
round hole H33.32-●
Breakdown
device, graft or implant —*see also* Complications, by site and type, mechanical T85.618
arterial graft NEC —*see* Complication, cardiovascular device, mechanical, vascular
breast (implant) T85.41
catheter NEC T85.618
cystostomy T83.010
dialysis (renal) T82.41
intraperitoneal T85.611
Hopkins T83.018
ileostomy T83.018
infusion NEC T82.514
cranial T85.610
epidural T85.610
intrathecal T85.610
spinal T85.610
subarachnoid T85.610
subdural T85.610
nephrostomy T83.012
urethral indwelling T83.011
urinary NEC T83.018
urostomy T83.018
electronic (electrode) (pulse generator) (stimulator)
bone T84.310
cardiac T82.119
electrode T82.110
pulse generator T82.111
specified type NEC T82.118
nervous system —*see* Complication, prosthetic device, mechanical, electronic nervous system stimulator
urinary —*see* Complication, genitourinary, device, urinary, mechanical
fixation, internal (orthopedic) NEC —*see* Complication, fixation device, mechanical
gastrointestinal —*see* Complications, prosthetic device, mechanical, gastrointestinal device
genital NEC T83.418
intrauterine contraceptive device T83.31
➡penile prosthesis (cylinder) (implanted) (pump) (reservoir) T83.410
testicular prosthesis T83.411

Breakdown *(Continued)*
device, graft or implant *(Continued)*
heart NEC —*see* Complication, cardiovascular device, mechanical
intrathecal infusion pump T85.615
joint prosthesis —*see* Complications..., joint prosthesis,internal, mechanical, by site
nervous system, specified device NEC T85.615
ocular NEC —*see* Complications, prosthetic device, mechanical, ocular device
orthopedic NEC —*see* Complication, orthopedic, device, mechanical
specified NEC T85.618
subcutaneous device pocket
nervous system prosthetic device, implant, or graft T85.890
other internal prosthetic device, implant, or graft T85.898
sutures, permanent T85.612
used in bone repair —*see* Complications, fixation device, internal (orthopedic), mechanical
urinary NEC T83.118
graft T83.21
sphincter, implanted T83.111
stent (ileal conduit) (nephroureteral) T83.113
ureteral indwelling T83.112
vascular NEC —*see* Complication, cardiovascular device, mechanical
ventricular intracranial shunt T85.01
nervous F48.8
perineum O90.1
respirator J95.850
specified NEC J95.859
ventilator J95.850
specified NEC J95.859
Breast —*see also* condition
buds E30.1
in newborn P96.89
dense R92.3-
Imaging Reporting and Data System (BI-RADS) : A R92.31-●
Imaging Reporting and Data System (BI-RADS) : B R92.32-●
Imaging Reporting and Data System (BI-RADS) : C R92.33-●
Imaging Reporting and Data System (BI-RADS) : D R92.34-●
Imaging Reporting and Data System (BI-RADS) : 1 R92.31-●
Imaging Reporting and Data System (BI-RADS) : 2 R92.32-●
Imaging Reporting and Data System (BI-RADS) : 3 R92.33-●
Imaging Reporting and Data System (BI-RADS) : 4 R92.34-●
nodule —*see also* Lump, breast N63.0
Breath
foul R19.6
holder, child R06.89
holding spell R06.89
shortness R06.02
Breathing
labored —*see* Hyperventilation
mouth R06.5
causing malocclusion M26.5
periodic R06.3
high altitude G47.32
Breathlessness R06.81
Breda's disease —*see* Yaws
Breech presentation (mother) O32.1
causing obstructed labor O64.1
footling O32.8
causing obstructed labor O64.8
incomplete O32.8
causing obstructed labor O64.8
Breisky's disease N90.4
Brennemann's syndrome I88.0
Brenner
tumor (benign) D27.9
borderline malignancy D39.1-●
malignant C56
proliferating D39.1
Bretonneau's disease or angina A36.0
Breus' mole O02.0
Brevicollis Q76.49
Brickmakers' anemia B76.9 *[D63.8]*
Bridge, myocardial Q24.5
Bright red blood per rectum (BRBPR) K62.5

Bright's disease —*see also* Nephritis
arteriosclerotic —*see* Hypertension, kidney
Brill (-Zinsser) disease (recrudescent typhus) A75.1
Brill-Symmers' disease C82.90
Brion-Kayser disease —*see* Fever, paratyphoid
Briquet's disorder or syndrome F45.0
Brissaud's
infantilism or dwarfism E23.0
motor-verbal tic F95.2
Brittle
bones disease Q78.0
nails L60.3
congenital Q84.6
Broad —*see also* condition
beta disease E78.2
ligament laceration syndrome N83.8
Broad- or floating-betalipoproteinemia E78.2
Brock's syndrome (atelectasis due to enlarged lymph nodes) J98.19
Brocq-Duhring disease (dermatitis herpetiformis) L13.0
Brodie's abscess or disease M86.8X-●
Broken
arches —*see also* Deformity, limb, flat foot
arm (meaning upper limb) —*see* Fracture, arm
back —*see* Fracture, vertebra
bone —*see* Fracture
implant or internal device —*see* Complications, by site and type, mechanical
leg (meaning lower limb) —*see* Fracture, leg
nose S02.2
tooth, teeth —*see* Fracture, tooth
Bromhidrosis, bromidrosis L75.0
Bromidism, bromism G92.8
chronic (dependence) F13.20
due to
correct substance properly administered —*see* Table of Drugs and Chemicals, by drug, adverse effect
overdose or wrong substance given or taken —*see* Table of Drugs and Chemicals, by drug, poisoning
Bromidrosiphobia F40.298
Bronchi, bronchial —*see* condition
Bronchiectasis (cylindrical) (diffuse) (fusiform) (localized) (saccular) J47.9
with
acute
bronchitis J47.0
lower respiratory infection J47.0
exacerbation (acute) J47.1
congenital Q33.4
tuberculous NEC —*see* Tuberculosis, pulmonary
Bronchiolectasis —*see* Bronchiectasis
Bronchiolitis (acute) (infective) (subacute) J21.9
with
bronchospasm or obstruction J21.9
influenza, flu or grippe —*see* Influenza, with, respiratory manifestations NEC
chemical (chronic) J68.4
acute J68.0
chronic (fibrosing) J44.89
obliterative J44.81
due to
external agent —*see* Bronchitis, acute, due to
human metapneumovirus J21.1
respiratory syncytial virus (RSV) J21.0
specified organism NEC J21.8
fibrosa obliterans J44.81
influenzal —*see* Influenza, with, respiratory manifestations NEC
obliterans (*see also* Bronchiolitis, obliterative) J44.81
with organizing pneumonia (BOOP) J84.89
syndrome J44.81
obliterative (chronic) (subacute) (*see also* Bronchiolitis, obliterans) J44.81
due to chemicals, gases, fumes or vapors (inhalation) (*see also* Disease, respiratory, chronic, due tochemicals, gases, fumes or vapors) J44.81
due to fumes or vapors (*see also* Disease, respiratory, chronic, due to chemicals, gases, fumes or vapors) J44.81
respiratory, interstitial lung disease J84.115
Bronchitis (diffuse) (fibrinous) (hypostatic) (infective) (membranous) J40
with
influenza, flu or grippe —*see* Influenza, with, respiratory manifestations NEC

Bronchitis *(Continued)*
with *(Continued)*
obstruction (airway) (lung) J44.89
tracheitis (15 years of age and above) J40
acute or subacute J20.9
chronic J42
under 15 years of age J20.9
acute or subacute (with bronchospasm or obstruction) J20.9
with
bronchiectasis J47.0
chronic obstructive pulmonary disease J44.0
chemical (due to gases, fumes or vapors) J68.0
due to
fumes or vapors J68.0
Haemophilus influenzae J20.1
Mycoplasma pneumoniae J20.0
radiation J70.0
specified organism NEC J20.8
Streptococcus J20.2
virus
coxsackie J20.3
echovirus J20.7
parainfluenzae J20.4
respiratory syncytial (RSV) J20.5
rhinovirus J20.6
viral NEC J20.8
allergic (acute) J45.909
with
exacerbation (acute) J45.901
status asthmaticus J45.902
arachidic T17.528
aspiration (due to food and vomit) J69.0
asthmatic J45.9
chronic J44.89
with
acute lower respiratory infection J44.0
exacerbation (acute) J44.1
capillary —*see* Pneumonia, broncho
caseous (tuberculous) A15.5
Castellani's A69.8
catarrhal (15 years of age and above) J40
acute —*see* Bronchitis, acute
chronic J41.0
under 15 years of age J20.9
chemical (acute) (subacute) J68.0
chronic (*see also* Disease, respiratory, chronic, due to chemicals, gases, fumes or vapors) J42
due to fumes or vapors (*see also* Disease, respiratory, chronic, due to chemicals, gases, fumes or vapors) J42
chronic J68.4
chronic J42
with
airways obstruction J44.89
tracheitis (chronic) J42
asthmatic (obstructive) J44.89
catarrhal J41.0
chemical (due to fumes or vapors) (*see also* Disease, respiratory, chronic, due to chemicals, gases, fumes or vapors) J42
due to
chemicals, gases, fumes or vapors (inhalation) (*see also* Disease, respiratory, chronic, due to chemicals, gases, fumes or vapors) J42
radiation J70.1
tobacco smoking J41.0
emphysematous J44.89
mucopurulent J41.1
non-obstructive J41.0
obliterans —*see* Bronchiolitis, obliterans
obstructive J44.89
purulent J41.1
simple J41.0
croupous —*see* Bronchitis, acute
due to gases, fumes or vapors (chemical) J68.0
emphysematous (obstructive) J44.89
exudative —*see* Bronchitis, acute
fetid J41.1
grippal —*see* Influenza, with, respiratory manifestations NEC
in those under 15 years age —*see* Bronchitis, acute
chronic —*see* Bronchitis, chronic
influenzal —*see* Influenza, with, respiratory manifestations NEC
mixed simple and mucopurulent J41.8
moulder's J62.8

Bronchitis *(Continued)*
mucopurulent (chronic) (recurrent) J41.1
acute or subacute J20.9
simple (mixed) J41.8
obliterans (chronic) —*see* Bronchiolitis, obliterans
obstructive (chronic) (diffuse) J44.89
pituitous J41.1
pneumococcal, acute or subacute J20.2
pseudomembranous, acute or subacute —*see* Bronchitis, acute
purulent (chronic) (recurrent) J41.1
acute or subacute —*see* Bronchitis, acute
putrid J41.1
senile (chronic) J42
simple and mucopurulent (mixed) J41.8
smokers' J41.0
spirochetal NEC A69.8
subacute —*see* Bronchitis, acute
suppurative (chronic) J41.1
acute or subacute —*see* Bronchitis, acute
tuberculous A15.5
under 15 years of age —*see* Bronchitis, acute
chronic —*see* Bronchitis, chronic
viral NEC, acute or subacute —*see also* Bronchitis, acute J20.8
Bronchoalveolitis J18.0
Bronchoaspergillosis B44.1
Bronchocele meaning goiter E04.0
Broncholithiasis J98.09
tuberculous NEC A15.5
Bronchomalacia J98.09
congenital Q32.2
Bronchomycosis NOS B49 *[J99]*
candidal B37.1
Bronchopleuropneumonia —*see* Pneumonia, broncho
Bronchopneumonia —*see* Pneumonia, broncho
Bronchopneumonitis —*see* Pneumonia, broncho
Bronchopulmonary —*see* condition
Bronchopulmonitis —*see* Pneumonia, broncho
Bronchorrhagia (*see* Hemoptysis)
Bronchorrhea J98.09
acute J20.9
chronic (infective) (purulent) J42
Bronchospasm (acute) J98.01
with
bronchiolitis, acute J21.9
bronchitis, acute (conditions in J20) —*see* Bronchitis, acute
due to external agent —*see* condition, respiratory, acute, due to
exercise induced J45.990
Bronchospirochetosis A69.8
Castellani A69.8
Bronchostenosis J98.09
Bronchus —*see* condition
Brontophobia F40.220
Bronze baby syndrome P83.88
Brooke's tumor —*see* Neoplasm, skin, benign
Brown enamel of teeth (hereditary) K00.5
Brown's sheath syndrome H50.61-●
Brown-Séquard disease, paralysis or syndrome G83.81
Bruce sepsis A23.0
Brucellosis (infection) A23.9
abortus A23.1
canis A23.3
dermatitis A23.9
melitensis A23.0
mixed A23.8
sepsis A23.9
melitensis A23.0
specified NEC A23.8
suis A23.2
Bruck-de Lange disease Q87.19
Bruck's disease —*see* Deformity, limb
BRUE (brief resolved unexplained event) R68.13
Brugsch's syndrome Q82.8
Bruise (skin surface intact) —*see also* Contusion
with
open wound —*see* Wound, open
internal organ —*see* Injury, by site
newborn P54.5
scalp, due to birth injury, newborn P12.3
umbilical cord O69.5
Bruit (arterial) R09.89
cardiac R01.1
Brush burn —*see* Abrasion, by site
Bruton's X-linked agammaglobulinemia D80.0

B

Bruxism
  psychogenic F45.8
  sleep related G47.63
Bubbly lung syndrome P27.Ø
Bubo I88.8
  blennorrhagic (gonococcal) A54.89
  chancroidal A57
  climatic A55
  due to Haemophilus ducreyi A57
  gonococcal A54.89
  indolent (nonspecific) I88.8
  inguinal (nonspecific) I88.8
    chancroidal A57
    climatic A55
    due to H. ducreyi A57
    infective I88.8
  scrofulous (tuberculous) A18.2
  soft chancre A57
  suppurating —*see* Lymphadenitis, acute
  syphilitic (primary) A51.Ø
    congenital A5Ø.Ø7
  tropical A55
  virulent (chancroidal) A57
Bubonic plague A2Ø.Ø
Bubonocele —*see* Hernia, inguinal
Buccal —*see* condition
Buchanan's disease or osteochondrosis M91.Ø
Buchem's syndrome (hyperostosis corticalis) M85.2
Bucket-handle fracture or tear (semilunar cartilage) —*see* Tear, meniscus
Budd-Chiari syndrome (hepatic vein thrombosis) I82.Ø
Budgerigar fancier's disease or lung J67.2
Buds
  breast E3Ø.1
    in newborn P96.89
Buerger's disease (thromboangiitis obliterans) I73.1
Bulbar —*see* condition
Bulbus cordis (left ventricle) (persistent) Q21.8
➡ **Bulimia** (nervosa) F5Ø.2-●
  atypical F5Ø.9
  normal weight F5Ø.9
Bulky
  stools R19.5
  uterus N85.2
Bulla (e) R23.8
  lung (emphysematous) (solitary) J43.9
    newborn P25.8
Bullet wound —*see also* Puncture
  fracture - code as Fracture, by site
  internal organ —*see* Injury, by site
Bundle
  branch block (complete) (false) (incomplete) —*see* Block, bundle-branch
  of His —*see* condition
Bunion M21.61-●
  tailor's M21.62-●
Bunionette M21.62-●
Buphthalmia, buphthalmos (congenital) Q15.Ø
Burdwan fever B55.Ø
Bürger-Grütz disease or syndrome E78.3
Buried
  penis (congenital) Q55.64
    acquired N48.83
  roots KØ8.3
Burke's syndrome K86.89
Burkholderia
  cepacia A49.8
  mallei A24.Ø
  pseudomallei —*see* Melioidosis
Burkitt
  cell leukemia C91.Ø-●
  lymphoma (malignant) C83.7-●
    small noncleaved, diffuse C83.7-●
    spleen C83.77
    undifferentiated C83.7-●
  tumor C83.7-●
  type
    acute lymphoblastic leukemia C91.Ø-●
    undifferentiated C83.7-●
Burn (electricity) (flame) (hot gas, liquid or hot object) (radiation) (steam) (thermal) T3Ø.Ø
  abdomen, abdominal (muscle) (wall) T21.Ø2
    first degree T21.12
    second degree T21.22
    third degree T21.32

Burn *(Continued)*
  above elbow T22.Ø39
    first degree T22.139
    left T22.Ø32
      first degree T22.132
      second degree T22.232
      third degree T22.332
    right T22.Ø31
      first degree T22.131
      second degree T22.231
      third degree T22.331
    second degree T22.239
    third degree T22.339
  acid (caustic) (external) (internal) —*see* Corrosion, by site
  alimentary tract NEC T28.2
    esophagus T28.1
    mouth T28.Ø
    pharynx T28.Ø
  alkaline (caustic) (external) (internal) —*see* Corrosion, by site
  ankle T25.Ø19
    first degree T25.119
    left T25.Ø12
      first degree T25.112
      second degree T25.212
      third degree T25.312
    multiple with foot —*see* Burn, lower, limb, multiple, ankle and foot
    right T25.Ø11
      first degree T25.111
      second degree T25.211
      third degree T25.311
    second degree T25.219
    third degree T25.319
  anus —*see* Burn, buttock
  arm (lower) (upper) —*see* Burn, upper, limb
  axilla T22.Ø49
    first degree T22.149
    left T22.Ø42
      first degree T22.142
      second degree T22.242
      third degree T22.342
    right T22.Ø41
      first degree T22.141
      second degree T22.241
      third degree T22.341
    second degree T22.249
    third degree T22.349
  back (lower) T21.Ø4
    first degree T21.14
    second degree T21.24
    third degree T21.34
    upper T21.Ø3
      first degree T21.13
      second degree T21.23
      third degree T21.33
  blisters - code as Burn, second degree, by site
  breast(s) —*see* Burn, chest wall
  buttock(s) T21.Ø5
    first degree T21.15
    second degree T21.25
    third degree T21.35
  calf T24.Ø39
    first degree T24.139
    left T24.Ø32
      first degree T24.132
      second degree T24.232
      third degree T24.332
    right T24.Ø31
      first degree T24.131
      second degree T24.231
      third degree T24.331
    second degree T24.239
    third degree T24.339
  canthus (eye) —*see* Burn, eyelid
  caustic acid or alkaline —*see* Corrosion, by site
  cervix T28.3
  cheek T2Ø.Ø6
    first degree T2Ø.16
    second degree T2Ø.26
    third degree T2Ø.36
  chemical (acids) (alkalines) (caustics) (external) (internal) —*see* Corrosion, by site
  chest wall T21.Ø1
    first degree T21.11
    second degree T21.21
    third degree T21.31

Burn *(Continued)*
  chin T2Ø.Ø3
    first degree T2Ø.13
    second degree T2Ø.23
    third degree T2Ø.33
  colon T28.2
  conjunctiva (and cornea) —*see* Burn, cornea
  cornea (and conjunctiva) T26.1-●
    chemical —*see* Corrosion, cornea
  corrosion (external) (internal) —*see* Corrosion, by site
  deep necrosis of underlying tissue - code as Burn, third degree, by site
  dorsum of hand T23.Ø69
    first degree T23.169
    left T23.Ø62
      first degree T23.162
      second degree T23.262
      third degree T23.362
    right T23.Ø61
      first degree T23.161
      second degree T23.261
      third degree T23.361
    second degree T23.269
    third degree T23.369
  due to ingested chemical agent —*see* Corrosion, by site
  ear (auricle) (external) (canal) T2Ø.Ø1
    first degree T2Ø.11
    second degree T2Ø.21
    third degree T2Ø.31
  elbow T22.Ø29
    first degree T22.129
    left T22.Ø22
      first degree T22.122
      second degree T22.222
      third degree T22.322
    right T22.Ø21
      first degree T22.121
      second degree T22.221
      third degree T22.321
    second degree T22.229
    third degree T22.329
  epidermal loss - code as Burn, second degree, by site
  erythema, erythematous - code as Burn, first degree, by site
  esophagus T28.1
  extent (percentage of body surface)
    less than 1Ø percent T31.Ø
    1Ø-19 percent T31.1Ø
      with Ø-9 percent third degree burns T31.1Ø
      with 1Ø-19 percent third degree burns T31.11
    2Ø-29 percent T31.2Ø
      with Ø-9 percent third degree burns T31.2Ø
      with 1Ø-19 percent third degree burns T31.21
      with 2Ø-29 percent third degree burns T31.22
    3Ø-39 percent T31.3Ø
      with Ø-9 percent third degree burns T31.3Ø
      with 1Ø-19 percent third degree burns T31.31
      with 2Ø-29 percent third degree burns T31.32
      with 3Ø-39 percent third degree burns T31.33
    4Ø-49 percent T31.4Ø
      with Ø-9 percent third degree burns T31.4Ø
      with 1Ø-19 percent third degree burns T31.41
      with 2Ø-29 percent third degree burns T31.42
      with 3Ø-39 percent third degree burns T31.43
      with 4Ø-49 percent third degree burns T31.44
    5Ø-59 percent T31.5Ø
      with Ø-9 percent third degree burns T31.5Ø
      with 1Ø-19 percent third degree burns T31.51
      with 2Ø-29 percent third degree burns T31.52
      with 3Ø-39 percent third degree burns T31.53
      with 4Ø-49 percent third degree burns T31.54
      with 5Ø-59 percent third degree burns T31.55
    6Ø-69 percent T31.6Ø
      with Ø-9 percent third degree burns T31.6Ø
      with 1Ø-19 percent third degree burns T31.61
      with 2Ø-29 percent third degree burns T31.62

B

- **Burn** *(Continued)*
  - extent *(Continued)*
    - 60-69 percent *(Continued)*
      - with 30-39 percent third degree burns T31.63
      - with 40-49 percent third degree burns T31.64
      - with 50-59 percent third degree burns T31.65
      - with 60-69 percent third degree burns T31.66
    - 70-79 percent T31.70
      - with 0-9 percent third degree burns T31.70
      - with 10-19 percent third degree burns T31.71
      - with 20-29 percent third degree burns T31.72
      - with 30-39 percent third degree burns T31.73
      - with 40-49 percent third degree burns T31.74
      - with 50-59 percent third degree burns T31.75
      - with 60-69 percent third degree burns T31.76
      - with 70-79 percent third degree burns T31.77
    - 80-89 percent T31.80
      - with 0-9 percent third degree burns T31.80
      - with 10-19 percent third degree burns T31.81
      - with 20-29 percent third degree burns T31.82
      - with 30-39 percent third degree burns T31.83
      - with 40-49 percent third degree burns T31.84
      - with 50-59 percent third degree burns T31.85
      - with 60-69 percent third degree burns T31.86
      - with 70-79 percent third degree burns T31.87
      - with 80-89 percent third degree burns T31.88
    - 90 percent or more T31.90
      - with 0-9 percent third degree burns T31.90
      - with 10-19 percent third degree burns T31.91
      - with 20-29 percent third degree burns T31.92
      - with 30-39 percent third degree burns T31.93
      - with 40-49 percent third degree burns T31.94
      - with 50-59 percent third degree burns T31.95
      - with 60-69 percent third degree burns T31.96
      - with 70-79 percent third degree burns T31.97
      - with 80-89 percent third degree burns T31.98
      - with 90 percent or more third degree burns T31.99
  - extremity —*see* Burn, limb
  - eye(s) and adnexa T26.4-●
    - with resulting rupture and destruction of eyeball T26.2-●
    - conjunctival sac —*see* Burn, cornea
    - cornea —*see* Burn, cornea
    - lid —*see* Burn, eyelid
    - periocular area —*see* Burn, eyelid
    - specified site NEC T26.3-●
  - eyeball —*see* Burn, eye
  - eyelid(s) T26.0-●
    - chemical —*see* Corrosion, eyelid
  - face —*see* Burn, head
  - finger T23.029
    - first degree T23.129
    - left T23.022
      - first degree T23.122
      - second degree T23.222
      - third degree T23.322
    - multiple sites (without thumb) T23.039
      - with thumb T23.049
        - first degree T23.149
        - left T23.042
          - first degree T23.142
          - second degree T23.242
          - third degree T23.342
        - right T23.041
          - first degree T23.141
          - second degree T23.241
          - third degree T23.341
        - second degree T23.249
        - third degree T23.349
      - first degree T23.139
      - left T23.032
        - first degree T23.132
        - second degree T23.232
        - third degree T23.332
      - right T23.031
        - first degree T23.131
        - second degree T23.231
        - third degree T23.331
      - second degree T23.239
      - third degree T23.339
    - right T23.021
      - first degree T23.121
      - second degree T23.221
      - third degree T23.321
    - second degree T23.229
    - third degree T23.329
- **Burn** *(Continued)*
  - flank —*see* Burn, abdominal wall
  - foot T25.029
    - first degree T25.129
    - left T25.022
      - first degree T25.122
      - second degree T25.222
      - third degree T25.322
    - multiple with ankle —*see* Burn, lower, limb, multiple, ankle and foot
    - right T25.021
      - first degree T25.121
      - second degree T25.221
      - third degree T25.321
    - second degree T25.229
    - third degree T25.329
  - forearm T22.019
    - first degree T22.119
    - left T22.012
      - first degree T22.112
      - second degree T22.212
      - third degree T22.312
    - right T22.011
      - first degree T22.111
      - second degree T22.211
      - third degree T22.311
    - second degree T22.219
    - third degree T22.319
  - forehead T20.06
    - first degree T20.16
    - second degree T20.26
    - third degree T20.36
  - fourth degree - code as Burn, third degree, by site
  - friction —*see* Burn, by site
  - from swallowing caustic or corrosive substance NEC —*see* Corrosion, by site
  - full thickness skin loss - code as Burn, third degree, by site
  - gastrointestinal tract NEC T28.2
    - from swallowing caustic or corrosive substance T28.7
  - genital organs
    - external
      - female T21.07
        - first degree T21.17
        - second degree T21.27
        - third degree T21.37
      - male T21.06
        - first degree T21.16
        - second degree T21.26
        - third degree T21.36
    - internal T28.3
      - from caustic or corrosive substance T28.8
  - groin —*see* Burn, abdominal wall
  - hand(s) T23.009
    - back —*see* Burn, dorsum of hand
    - finger —*see* Burn, finger
    - first degree T23.109
    - left T23.002
      - first degree T23.102
      - second degree T23.202
      - third degree T23.302
    - multiple sites with wrist T23.099
      - first degree T23.199
      - left T23.092
        - first degree T23.192
        - second degree T23.292
        - third degree T23.392
      - right T23.091
        - first degree T23.191
        - second degree T23.291
        - third degree T23.391
      - second degree T23.299
      - third degree T23.399
    - palm —*see* Burn, palm
    - right T23.001
      - first degree T23.101
      - second degree T23.201
      - third degree T23.301
    - second degree T23.209
    - third degree T23.309
    - thumb —*see* Burn, thumb
  - head (and face) (and neck) T20.00
    - cheek —*see* Burn, cheek
    - chin —*see* Burn, chin
    - ear —*see* Burn, ear
    - eye(s) only —*see* Burn, eye
    - first degree T20.10
- **Burn** *(Continued)*
  - head *(Continued)*
    - forehead —*see* Burn, forehead
    - lip —*see* Burn, lip
    - multiple sites T20.09
      - first degree T20.19
      - second degree T20.29
      - third degree T20.39
    - neck —*see* Burn, neck
    - nose —*see* Burn, nose
    - scalp —*see* Burn, scalp
    - second degree T20.20
    - third degree T20.30
  - hip(s) —*see* Burn, thigh
  - inhalation —*see* Burn, respiratory tract
    - caustic or corrosive substance (fumes) —*see* Corrosion, respiratory tract
  - internal organ(s) T28.40
    - alimentary tract T28.2
      - esophagus T28.1
    - eardrum T28.41
    - esophagus T28.1
    - from caustic or corrosive substance (swallowing) NEC —*see* Corrosion, by site
    - genitourinary T28.3
    - mouth T28.0
    - pharynx T28.0
    - respiratory tract —*see* Burn, respiratory tract
    - specified organ NEC T28.49
  - interscapular region —*see* Burn, back, upper
  - intestine (large) (small) T28.2
  - knee T24.029
    - first degree T24.129
    - left T24.022
      - first degree T24.122
      - second degree T24.222
      - third degree T24.322
    - right T24.021
      - first degree T24.121
      - second degree T24.221
      - third degree T24.321
    - second degree T24.229
    - third degree T24.329
  - labium (majus) (minus) —*see* Burn, genital organs, external, female
  - lacrimal apparatus, duct, gland or sac —*see* Burn, eye, specified site NEC
  - larynx T27.0
    - with lung T27.1
  - leg(s) (lower) (upper) —*see* Burn, lower, limb
  - lightning —*see* Burn, by site
  - limb(s)
    - lower (except ankle or foot alone) —*see* Burn, lower, limb
    - upper —*see* Burn, upper limb
  - lip(s) T20.02
    - first degree T20.12
    - second degree T20.22
    - third degree T20.32
  - lower
    - back —*see* Burn, back
    - limb T24.009
      - ankle —*see* Burn, ankle
      - calf —*see* Burn, calf
      - first degree T24.109
      - foot —*see* Burn, foot
      - hip —*see* Burn, thigh
      - knee —*see* Burn, knee
      - left T24.002
        - first degree T24.102
        - second degree T24.202
        - third degree T24.302
      - multiple sites, except ankle and foot T24.099
        - ankle and foot T25.099
          - first degree T25.199
          - left T25.092
            - first degree T25.192
            - second degree T25.292
            - third degree T25.392
          - right T25.091
            - first degree T25.191
            - second degree T25.291
            - third degree T25.391
          - second degree T25.299
          - third degree T25.399
      - first degree T24.199

B

- **Burn** *(Continued)*
  - lower *(Continued)*
    - limb *(Continued)*
      - multiple sites *(Continued)*
        - left T24.092
          - first degree T24.192
          - second degree T24.292
          - third degree T24.392
        - right T24.091
          - first degree T24.191
          - second degree T24.291
          - third degree T24.391
        - second degree T24.299
        - third degree T24.399
      - right T24.001
        - first degree T24.101
        - second degree T24.201
        - third degree T24.301
      - second degree T24.209
      - thigh —*see* Burn, thigh
      - third degree T24.309
      - toe —*see* Burn, toe
  - lung (with larynx and trachea) T27.1
  - mouth T28.0
  - neck T20.07
    - first degree T20.17
    - second degree T20.27
    - third degree T20.37
  - nose (septum) T20.04
    - first degree T20.14
    - second degree T20.24
    - third degree T20.34
  - ocular adnexa —*see* Burn, eye
  - orbit region —*see* Burn, eyelid
  - palm T23.059
    - first degree T23.159
    - left T23.052
      - first degree T23.152
      - second degree T23.252
      - third degree T23.352
    - right T23.051
      - first degree T23.151
      - second degree T23.251
      - third degree T23.351
    - second degree T23.259
    - third degree T23.359
  - partial thickness - code as Burn, by site, second degree
  - pelvis —*see* Burn, trunk
  - penis —*see* Burn, genital organs, external, male
  - perineum
    - female —*see* Burn, genital organs, external, female
    - male —*see* Burn, genital organs, external, male
  - periocular area —*see* Burn, eyelid
  - pharynx T28.0
  - rectum T28.2
  - respiratory tract T27.3
    - larynx —*see* Burn, larynx
    - specified part NEC T27.2
    - trachea —*see* Burn, trachea
  - sac, lacrimal —*see* Burn, eye, specified site NEC
  - scalp T20.05
    - first degree T20.15
    - second degree T20.25
    - third degree T20.35
  - scapular region T22.069
    - first degree T22.169
    - left T22.062
      - first degree T22.162
      - second degree T22.262
      - third degree T22.362
    - right T22.061
      - first degree T22.161
      - second degree T22.261
      - third degree T22.361
    - second degree T22.269
    - third degree T22.369
  - sclera —*see* Burn, eye, specified site NEC
  - scrotum —*see* Burn, genital organs, external, male
  - shoulder T22.059
    - first degree T22.159
    - left T22.052
      - first degree T22.152
      - second degree T22.252
      - third degree T22.352
    - right T22.051
      - first degree T22.151
      - second degree T22.251
      - third degree T22.351
    - second degree T22.259
    - third degree T22.359

- **Burn** *(Continued)*
  - stomach T28.2
  - temple —*see* Burn, head
  - testis —*see* Burn, genital organs, external, male
  - thigh T24.019
    - first degree T24.119
    - left T24.012
      - first degree T24.112
      - second degree T24.212
      - third degree T24.312
    - right T24.011
      - first degree T24.111
      - second degree T24.211
      - third degree T24.311
    - second degree T24.219
    - third degree T24.319
  - thorax (external) —*see* Burn, trunk
  - throat (meaning pharynx) T28.0
  - thumb(s) T23.019
    - first degree T23.119
    - left T23.012
      - first degree T23.112
      - second degree T23.212
      - third degree T23.312
    - multiple sites with fingers T23.049
      - first degree T23.149
      - left T23.042
        - first degree T23.142
        - second degree T23.242
        - third degree T23.342
      - right T23.041
        - first degree T23.141
        - second degree T23.241
        - third degree T23.341
      - second degree T23.249
      - third degree T23.349
    - right T23.011
      - first degree T23.111
      - second degree T23.211
      - third degree T23.311
    - second degree T23.219
    - third degree T23.319
  - toe T25.039
    - first degree T25.139
    - left T25.032
      - first degree T25.132
      - second degree T25.232
      - third degree T25.332
    - right T25.031
      - first degree T25.131
      - second degree T25.231
      - third degree T25.331
    - second degree T25.239
    - third degree T25.339
  - tongue T28.0
  - tonsil(s) T28.0
  - trachea T27.0
    - with lung T27.1
  - trunk T21.00
    - abdominal wall —*see* Burn, abdominal wall
    - anus —*see* Burn, buttock
    - axilla —*see* Burn, upper limb
    - back —*see* Burn, back
    - breast —*see* Burn, chest wall
    - buttock —*see* Burn, buttock
    - chest wall —*see* Burn, chest wall
    - first degree T21.10
    - flank —*see* Burn, abdominal wall
    - genital
      - female —*see* Burn, genital organs, external, female
      - male —*see* Burn, genital organs, external, male
    - groin —*see* Burn, abdominal wall
    - interscapular region —*see* Burn, back, upper
    - labia —*see* Burn, genital organs, external, female
    - lower back —*see* Burn, back
    - penis —*see* Burn, genital organs, external, male
    - perineum
      - female —*see* Burn, genital organs, external, female
      - male —*see* Burn, genital organs, external, male
    - scapula region —*see* Burn, scapular region
    - scrotum —*see* Burn, genital organs, external, male
    - second degree T21.20
    - specified site NEC T21.09
      - first degree T21.19
      - second degree T21.29
      - third degree T21.39

- **Burn** *(Continued)*
  - trunk *(Continued)*
    - testes —*see* Burn, genital organs, external, male
    - third degree T21.30
    - upper back —*see* Burn, back, upper
    - vulva —*see* Burn, genital organs, external, female
  - unspecified site with extent of body surface involved specified
    - less than 10 percent T31.0
    - 10-19 percent (0-9 percent third degree) T31.10
      - with 10-19 percent third degree T31.11
    - 20-29 percent (0-9 percent third degree) T31.20
      - with
        - 10-19 percent third degree T31.21
        - 20-29 percent third degree T31.22
    - 30-39 percent (0-9 percent third degree) T31.30
      - with
        - 10-19 percent third degree T31.31
        - 20-29 percent third degree T31.32
        - 30-39 percent third degree T31.33
  - unspecified site with extent of body surface 40-49 percent (0-9 percent third degree) T31.40
      - with
        - 10-19 percent third degree T31.41
        - 20-29 percent third degree T31.42
        - 30-39 percent third degree T31.43
        - 40-49 percent third degree T31.44
    - 50-59 percent (0-9 percent third degree) T31.50
      - with
        - 10-19 percent third degree T31.51
        - 20-29 percent third degree T31.52
        - 30-39 percent third degree T31.53
        - 40-49 percent third degree T31.54
        - 50-59 percent third degree T31.55
    - 60-69 percent (0-9 percent third degree) T31.60
      - with
        - 10-19 percent third degree T31.61
        - 20-29 percent third degree T31.62
        - 30-39 percent third degree T31.63
        - 40-49 percent third degree T31.64
        - 50-59 percent third degree T31.65
        - 60-69 percent third degree T31.66
    - 70-79 percent (0-9 percent third degree) T31.70
      - with
        - 10-19 percent third degree T31.71
        - 20-29 percent third degree T31.72
        - 30-39 percent third degree T31.73
        - 40-49 percent third degree T31.74
        - 50-59 percent third degree T31.75
        - 60-69 percent third degree T31.76
        - 70-79 percent third degree T31.77
    - 80-89 percent (0-9 percent third degree) T31.80
      - with
        - 10-19 percent third degree T31.81
        - 20-29 percent third degree T31.82
        - 30-39 percent third degree T31.83
        - 40-49 percent third degree T31.84
        - 50-59 percent third degree T31.85
        - 60-69 percent third degree T31.86
        - 70-79 percent third degree T31.87
        - 80-89 percent third degree T31.88
    - 90 percent or more (0-9 percent third degree) T31.90
      - with
        - 10-19 percent third degree T31.91
        - 20-29 percent third degree T31.92
        - 30-39 percent third degree T31.93
        - 40-49 percent third degree T31.94
        - 50-59 percent third degree T31.95
        - 60-69 percent third degree T31.96
        - 70-79 percent third degree T31.97
        - 80-89 percent third degree T31.98
        - 90-99 percent third degree T31.99
  - upper limb T22.00
    - above elbow —*see* Burn, above elbow
    - axilla —*see* Burn, axilla
    - elbow —*see* Burn, elbow
    - first degree T22.10
    - forearm —*see* Burn, forearm
    - hand —*see* Burn, hand
    - interscapular region —*see* Burn, back, upper
    - multiple sites T22.099
      - first degree T22.199
      - left T22.092
        - first degree T22.192
        - second degree T22.292
        - third degree T22.392

B

C

Canal *(Continued)*
- atrioventricular *(Continued)*
  - intermediate Q21.22
  - partial Q21.21
  - transitional Q21.22

Canaliculitis (lacrimal) (acute) (subacute) H04.33- •
- Actinomyces A42.89
- chronic H04.42- •

Canavan disease E75.28

Canceled procedure (surgical) Z53.9
- because of
  - contraindication Z53.09
    - smoking Z53.01
  - left against medical advice (AMA) Z53.29
  - patient's decision Z53.20
    - for reasons of belief or group pressure Z53.1
    - specified reason NEC Z53.29
  - specified reason NEC Z53.8

Cancer —*see also* Neoplasm, by site, malignant
- bile duct type, liver C22.1
- blood —*see* Leukemia
- breast —*see also* Neoplasm, breast, malignant C50.91- •
- hepatocellular C22.0
- lung —*see also* Neoplasm, lung, malignant C34.90- •
- ovarian —*see also* Neoplasm, ovary, malignant C56.9- •
- unspecified site (primary) C80.1

Cancer (o)phobia F45.29

Cancerous —*see* Neoplasm, malignant, by site

Cancrum oris A69.0

Candidiasis, candidal B37.9
- balanitis B37.42
- bronchitis B37.1
- cheilitis B37.83
- congenital P37.5
- cystitis B37.41
- disseminated B37.7
- endocarditis B37.6
- enteritis B37.82
- esophagitis B37.81
- intertrigo B37.2
- lung B37.1
- meningitis B37.5
- mouth B37.0
- nails B37.2
- neonatal P37.5
- onychia B37.2
- oral B37.0
- osteomyelitis B37.89
- otitis externa B37.84
- paronychia B37.2
- perionyxis B37.2
- pneumonia B37.1
- proctitis B37.82
- pulmonary B37.1
- pyelonephritis B37.49
- sepsis B37.7
- skin B37.2
- specified site NEC B37.89
- stomatitis B37.0
- systemic B37.7
- urethritis B37.41
- urogenital site NEC B37.49
- vagina (acute) B37.31
  - chronic (recurrent) B37.32
- vulva (acute) B37.31
  - chronic (recurrent) B37.32
- vulvovaginitis (acute) B37.31
  - chronic (recurrent) B37.32

Candidid L30.2

Candidosis —*see* Candidiasis

Candiru infection or infestation B88.8

Canities (premature) L67.1
- congenital Q84.2

Canker (mouth) (sore) K12.0
- rash A38.9

Cannabinosis J66.2

Cannabis induced
- anxiety disorder F12.980
- psychotic disorder F12.959
- sleep disorder F12.988

Canton fever A75.9

Cantrell's syndrome Q87.89

Capillariasis (intestinal) B81.1
- hepatic B83.8

Capillary —*see* condition

Caplan's syndrome —*see* Rheumatoid, lung

Capsule —*see* condition

Capsulitis (joint) —*see also* Enthesopathy
- adhesive (shoulder) M75.0- •
- hepatic K65.8
- labyrinthine —*see* Otosclerosis, specified NEC
- thyroid E06.9

Caput
- crepitus Q75.8
- medusae I86.8
- succedaneum P12.81

Car sickness T75.3

Carapata (disease) A68.0

Carate —*see* Pinta

Carbon lung J60

Carbuncle L02.93
- abdominal wall L02.231
- anus K61.0
- auditory canal, external —*see* Abscess, ear, external
- auricle ear —*see* Abscess, ear, external
- axilla L02.43- •
- back (any part) L02.232
- breast N61.1
- buttock L02.33
- cheek (external) L02.03
- chest wall L02.233
- chin L02.03
- corpus cavernosum N48.21
- ear (any part) (external) (middle) —*see* Abscess, ear, external
- external auditory canal —*see* Abscess, ear, external
- eyelid —*see* Abscess, eyelid
- face NEC L02.03
- femoral (region) —*see* Carbuncle, lower limb
- finger —*see* Carbuncle, hand
- flank L02.231
- foot L02.63- •
- forehead L02.03
- genital —*see* Abscess, genital
- gluteal (region) L02.33
- groin L02.234
- hand L02.53- •
- head NEC L02.831
- heel —*see* Carbuncle, foot
- hip —*see* Carbuncle, lower limb
- kidney —*see* Abscess, kidney
- knee —*see* Carbuncle, lower limb
- labium (majus) (minus) N76.4
- lacrimal
  - gland —*see* Dacryoadenitis
  - passages (duct) (sac) —*see* Inflammation, lacrimal, passages, acute
- leg —*see* Carbuncle, lower limb
- lower limb L02.43- •
- malignant A22.0
- navel L02.236
- neck L02.13
- nose (external) (septum) J34.0
- orbit, orbital —*see* Abscess, orbit
- palmar (space) —*see* Carbuncle, hand
- partes posteriores L02.33
- pectoral region L02.233
- penis N48.21
- perineum L02.235
- pinna —*see* Abscess, ear, external
- popliteal —*see* Carbuncle, lower limb
- scalp L02.831
- seminal vesicle N49.0
- shoulder —*see* Carbuncle, upper limb
- specified site NEC L02.838
- temple (region) L02.03
- thumb —*see* Carbuncle, hand
- toe —*see* Carbuncle, foot
- trunk L02.239
  - abdominal wall L02.231
  - back L02.232
  - chest wall L02.233
  - groin L02.234
  - perineum L02.235
  - umbilicus L02.236
- umbilicus L02.236
- upper limb L02.43- •
- urethra N34.0
- vulva N76.4

Carbunculus —*see* Carbuncle

Carcinoid (tumor) —*see* Tumor, carcinoid

Carcinoidosis E34.00
- heart E34.01

Carcinoma (malignant) —*see also* Neoplasm, by site, malignant
- acidophil
  - specified site —*see* Neoplasm, malignant, by site
  - unspecified site C75.1

Carcinoma *(Continued)*
- acidophil-basophil, mixed
  - specified site —*see* Neoplasm, malignant, by site
  - unspecified site C75.1
- adnexal (skin) —*see* Neoplasm, skin, malignant
- adrenal cortical C74.0- •
- alveolar —*see* Neoplasm, lung, malignant
  - cell —*see* Neoplasm, lung, malignant
- ameloblastic C41.1
  - upper jaw (bone) C41.0
- apocrine
  - breast —*see* Neoplasm, breast, malignant
  - specified site NEC —*see* Neoplasm, skin, malignant
  - unspecified site C44.99
- basal cell (pigmented) (*see also* Neoplasm, skin, malignant) C44.91
  - fibro-epithelial —*see* Neoplasm, skin, malignant
  - morphea —*see* Neoplasm, skin, malignant
  - multicentric —*see* Neoplasm, skin, malignant
- basaloid
- basal-squamous cell, mixed —*see* Neoplasm, skin, malignant
- basophil
  - specified site —*see* Neoplasm, malignant, by site
  - unspecified site C75.1
- basophil-acidophil, mixed
  - specified site —*see* Neoplasm, malignant, by site
  - unspecified site C75.1
- basosquamous —*see* Neoplasm, skin, malignant
- bile duct
  - with hepatocellular, mixed C22.0
  - liver C22.1
  - specified site NEC —*see* Neoplasm, malignant, by site
  - unspecified site C22.1
- branchial or branchiogenic C10.4
- bronchial or bronchogenic —*see* Neoplasm, lung, malignant
- bronchiolar —*see* Neoplasm, lung, malignant
- bronchioloalveolar —*see* Neoplasm, lung, malignant
- C cell
  - specified site —*see* Neoplasm, malignant, by site
  - unspecified site C73
- ceruminous C44.29- •
- cervix uteri
  - in situ D06.9
    - endocervix D06.0
    - exocervix D06.1
    - specified site NEC D06.7
- chorionic
  - specified site —*see* Neoplasm, malignant, by site
  - unspecified site
    - female C58
    - male C62.90
- chromophobe
  - specified site —*see* Neoplasm, malignant, by site
  - unspecified site C75.1
- cloacogenic
  - specified site —*see* Neoplasm, malignant, by site
  - unspecified site C21.2
- diffuse type
  - specified site —*see* Neoplasm, malignant, by site
  - unspecified site C16.9
- duct (cell)
  - with Paget's disease —*see* Neoplasm, breast, malignant
  - infiltrating
    - with lobular carcinoma (in situ)
      - specified site —*see* Neoplasm, malignant, by site
      - unspecified site (female) C50.91- •
        - male C50.92- •
    - specified site —*see* Neoplasm, malignant, by site
    - unspecified site (female) C50.91- •
      - male C50.92- •
- ductal
  - with lobular
    - specified site —*see* Neoplasm, malignant, by site
    - unspecified site (female) C50.91- •
      - male C50.92- •

- **Carcinoma** *(Continued)*
  - serous
    - papillary
      - specified site —*see* Neoplasm, malignant, by site
      - unspecified site C56.9
    - surface, papillary
      - specified site —*see* Neoplasm, malignant, by site
      - unspecified site C56.9
  - Sertoli cell
    - specified site —*see* Neoplasm, malignant, by site
    - unspecified site C62.9Ø
      - female C56.9
      - male C62.9Ø
  - skin appendage —*see* Neoplasm, skin, malignant
  - small cell
    - fusiform cell
      - specified site —*see* Neoplasm, malignant, by site
      - unspecified site C34.9Ø
    - intermediate cell
      - specified site —*see* Neoplasm, malignant, by site
      - unspecified site C34.9Ø
    - large cell
      - specified site —*see* Neoplasm, malignant, by site
      - unspecified site C34.9Ø
  - solid
    - with amyloid stroma
      - specified site —*see* Neoplasm, malignant, by site
      - unspecified site C73
    - microinvasive
      - specified site —*see* Neoplasm, malignant, by site
      - unspecified site C53.9
  - sweat gland —*see* Neoplasm, skin, malignant
  - theca cell C56.- ●
  - thymic C37
  - unspecified site (primary) C8Ø.1
  - water-clear cell C75.Ø
- **Carcinoma-in-situ** —*see also* Neoplasm, in situ, by site
  - breast NOS DØ5.9- ●
    - specified type NEC DØ5.8- ●
  - epidermoid —*see also* Neoplasm, in situ, by site
    - with questionable stromal invasion
      - cervix DØ6.9
      - specified site NEC —*see* Neoplasm, in situ, by site
      - unspecified site DØ6.9
    - Bowen's type —*see* Neoplasm, skin, in situ
  - intraductal
    - breast DØ5.1- ●
    - specified site NEC —*see* Neoplasm, in situ, by site
    - unspecified site DØ5.1- ●
  - lobular
    - with
      - infiltrating duct
        - breast (female) C5Ø.91- ●
          - male C5Ø.92- ●
        - specified site NEC —*see* Neoplasm, malignant
        - unspecified site (female) C5Ø.91- ●
          - male C5Ø.92- ●
      - intraductal
        - breast DØ5.8- ●
        - specified site NEC —*see* Neoplasm, in situ, by site
        - unspecified site (female) DØ5.8- ●
    - breast DØ5.Ø- ●
    - specified site NEC —*see* Neoplasm, in situ, by site
    - unspecified site DØ5.Ø- ●
  - squamous cell —*see also* Neoplasm, in situ, by site
    - with questionable stromal invasion
      - cervix DØ6.9
      - specified site NEC —*see* Neoplasm, in situ, by site
      - unspecified site DØ6.9
- **Carcinomaphobia** F45.29
- **Carcinomatosis** C8Ø.Ø
  - peritonei C78.6
  - unspecified site (primary) (secondary) C8Ø.Ø
- **Carcinosarcoma** —*see* Neoplasm, malignant, by site
  - embryonal —*see* Neoplasm, malignant, by site
- **Cardia, cardial** —*see* condition
- **Cardiac** —*see also* condition
  - death, sudden —*see* Arrest, cardiac
  - pacemaker
    - in situ Z95.Ø
    - management or adjustment Z45.Ø18
  - tamponade I31.4
- **Cardialgia** —*see* Pain, precordial
- **Cardiectasis** —*see* Hypertrophy, cardiac
- **Cardiochalasia** K21.9
- **Cardiomalacia** I51.5
- **Cardiomegalia glycogenica diffusa** E74.Ø2 *[I43]*
- **Cardiomegaly** —*see also* Hypertrophy, cardiac
  - congenital Q24.8
  - glycogen E74.Ø2 *[I43]*
  - idiopathic I51.7
- **Cardiomyoliposis** I51.5
- **Cardiomyopathy** (familial) (idiopathic) I42.9
  - alcoholic I42.6
  - amyloid E85.4 *[I43]*
    - transthyretin-related (ATTR) familial E85.4 *[I43]*
  - arteriosclerotic —*see* Disease, heart, ischemic, atherosclerotic
  - beriberi E51.12
  - cobalt-beer I42.6
  - congenital I42.4
  - congestive I42.Ø
  - constrictive NOS I42.5
  - dilated I42.Ø
  - due to
    - alcohol I42.6
    - beriberi E51.12
    - cardiac glycogenosis E74.Ø2 *[I43]*
    - drugs I42.7
    - external agents NEC I42.7
    - Friedreich's ataxia G11.11
    - myotonia atrophica G71.11 *[I43]*
    - progressive muscular dystrophy (*see also* Dystrophy, muscular, by type) G71.Ø9 *[I43]*
  - glycogen storage E74.Ø2 *[I43]*
  - hypertensive —*see* Hypertension, heart
  - hypertrophic (nonobstructive) I42.2
    - obstructive I42.1
      - congenital Q24.8
  - in
    - Chagas' disease (chronic) B57.2
      - acute B57.Ø
    - sarcoidosis D86.85
  - ischemic I25.5
  - metabolic E88.9 *[I43]*
    - thyrotoxic EØ5.9Ø *[I43]*
      - with thyroid storm EØ5.91 *[I43]*
  - newborn I42.8
    - congenital I42.4
  - non-ischemic (*see also* by cause) I42.8
  - nutritional E63.9 *[I43]*
    - beriberi E51.12
  - obscure of Africa I42.8
  - peripartum O9Ø.3
  - postpartum O9Ø.3
  - restrictive NEC I42.5
  - rheumatic IØ9.Ø
  - secondary I42.9
  - specified NEC I42.8
  - stress induced I51.81
  - takotsubo I51.81
  - thyrotoxic EØ5.9Ø *[I43]*
    - with thyroid storm EØ5.91 *[I43]*
  - toxic NEC I42.7
  - transthyretin-related (ATTR) familial amyloid E85.4
  - tuberculous A18.84
  - viral B33.24
- **Cardionephritis** —*see* Hypertension, cardiorenal
- **Cardionephropathy** —*see* Hypertension, cardiorenal
- **Cardionephrosis** —*see* Hypertension, cardiorenal
- **Cardiopathia nigra** I27.Ø
- **Cardiopathy** —*see also* Disease, heart I51.9
  - idiopathic I42.9
  - mucopolysaccharidosis E76.3 *[I52]*
- **Cardiopericarditis** —*see* Pericarditis
- **Cardiophobia** F45.29
- **Cardiorenal** —*see* condition
- **Cardiorrhexis** —*see* Infarct, myocardium
- **Cardiosclerosis** —*see* Disease, heart, ischemic, atherosclerotic
- **Cardiosis** —*see* Disease, heart
- **Cardiospasm** (esophagus) (reflex) (stomach) K22.Ø
  - congenital Q39.5
    - with megaesophagus Q39.5
- **Cardiostenosis** —*see* Disease, heart
- **Cardiosymphysis** I31.Ø
- **Cardiovascular** —*see* condition
- **Carditis** (acute) (bacterial) (chronic) (subacute) I51.89
  - meningococcal A39.5Ø
  - rheumatic —*see* Disease, heart, rheumatic
  - rheumatoid —*see* Rheumatoid, carditis
  - viral B33.2Ø
- **Care** (of) (for) (following)
  - child (routine) Z76.2
  - family member (handicapped) (sick)
    - creating problem for family Z63.6
    - provided away from home for holiday relief Z75.5
    - unavailable, due to
      - absence (person rendering care) (sufferer) Z74.2
      - inability (any reason) of person rendering care Z74.2
  - foundling Z76.1
  - holiday relief Z75.5
  - improper —*see* Maltreatment
  - lack of (at or after birth) (infant) —*see* Maltreatment, child, neglect
  - lactating mother Z39.1
  - palliative Z51.5
  - postpartum
    - immediately after delivery Z39.Ø
    - routine follow-up Z39.2
  - respite Z75.5
  - unavailable, due to
    - absence of person rendering care Z74.2
    - inability (any reason) of person rendering care Z74.2
  - well-baby Z76.2
- **Caries**
  - bone NEC A18.Ø3
  - dental (dentino enamel junction) (early childhood) (of dentine) (pre-eruptive) (recurrent) (to the pulp) KØ2.9
    - arrested (coronal) (root) KØ2.3
    - chewing surface
      - limited to enamel KØ2.51
      - penetrating into dentin KØ2.52
      - penetrating into pulp KØ2.53
    - coronal surface
      - chewing surface
        - limited to enamel KØ2.51
        - penetrating into dentin KØ2.52
        - penetrating into pulp KØ2.53
      - pit and fissure surface
        - limited to enamel KØ2.51
        - penetrating into dentin KØ2.52
        - penetrating into pulp KØ2.53
      - smooth surface
        - limited to enamel KØ2.61
        - penetrating into dentin KØ2.62
        - penetrating into pulp KØ2.63
    - pit and fissure surface
      - limited to enamel KØ2.51
      - penetrating into dentin KØ2.52
      - penetrating into pulp KØ2.53
    - primary, cervical origin KØ2.52
    - root KØ2.7
    - smooth surface
      - limited to enamel KØ2.61
      - penetrating into dentin KØ2.62
      - penetrating into pulp KØ2.63
  - external meatus —*see* Disorder, ear, external, specified type NEC
  - hip (tuberculous) A18.Ø2
  - initial (tooth)
    - chewing surface KØ2.51
    - pit and fissure surface KØ2.51
    - smooth surface KØ2.61
  - knee (tuberculous) A18.Ø2
  - labyrinth —*see* subcategory H83.8
  - limb NEC (tuberculous) A18.Ø3
  - mastoid process (chronic) —*see* Mastoiditis, chronic
    - tuberculous A18.Ø3
  - middle ear —*see* subcategory H74.8
  - nose (tuberculous) A18.Ø3
  - orbit (tuberculous) A18.Ø3
  - ossicles, ear —*see* Abnormal, ear ossicles

Chagas' disease *(Continued)*
- acute (with) B57.1
  - cardiovascular NEC B57.Ø
  - myocarditis B57.Ø

Chagres fever B5Ø.9
Chairridden Z74.Ø9
Chalasia (cardiac sphincter) K21.9
Chalazion HØØ.19
- left HØØ.16
  - lower HØØ.15
  - upper HØØ.14
- right HØØ.13
  - lower HØØ.12
  - upper HØØ.11

Chalcosis —*see also* Disorder, globe, degenerative, chalcosis
- cornea —*see* Deposit, cornea
- crystalline lens —*see* Cataract, complicated
- retina H35.89

Chalicosis (pulmonum) J62.8
Chancre (any genital site) (hard) (hunterian) (mixed) (primary) (seronegative) (seropositive) (syphilitic) A51.Ø
- congenital A5Ø.Ø7
- conjunctiva NEC A51.2
- ▶ducreyi A57
- Ducrey's A57
- extragenital A51.2
- eyelid A51.2
- lip A51.2
- nipple A51.2
- Nisbet's A57
- of
  - carate A67.Ø
  - pinta A67.Ø
  - yaws A66.Ø
- palate, soft A51.2
- phagedenic A57
- simple A57
- soft A57
  - bubo A57
  - palate A51.2
- urethra A51.Ø
- yaws A66.Ø

Chancroid (anus) (genital) (penis) (perineum) (rectum) (urethra) (vulva) A57
Chandler's disease (osteochondritis dissecans, hip) —*see* Osteochondritis, dissecans, hip
Change(s) (in) (of) —*see also* Removal
- arteriosclerotic —*see* Arteriosclerosis
- bone —*see also* Disorder, bone
  - diabetic —*see* Diabetes, bone change
- bowel habit R19.4
- cardiorenal (vascular) —*see* Hypertension, cardiorenal
- cardiovascular —*see* Disease, cardiovascular
- circulatory I99.9
- cognitive (mild) (organic) R41.89
- color, tooth, teeth
  - during formation KØØ.8
  - posteruptive KØ3.7
- contraceptive device Z3Ø.433
- corneal membrane H18.3Ø
  - Bowman's membrane fold or rupture H18.31-•
  - Descemet's membrane
    - fold H18.32-•
    - rupture H18.33-•
- coronary —*see* Disease, heart, ischemic
- degenerative, spine or vertebra —*see* Spondylosis
- dental pulp, regressive KØ4.2
- dressing (nonsurgical) Z48.ØØ
  - surgical Z48.Ø1
- heart —*see* Disease, heart
- hip joint —*see* Derangement, joint, hip
- hyperplastic larynx J38.7
- hypertrophic
  - nasal sinus J34.89
  - turbinate, nasal J34.3
  - upper respiratory tract J39.8
- indwelling catheter Z46.6
- inflammatory —*see also* Inflammation
  - sacroiliac M46.1
- job, anxiety concerning Z56.1
- joint —*see* Derangement, joint
- life —*see* Menopause
- mental status R41.82
- minimal (glomerular) —*see also* NØØ-NØ7 with fourth character .Ø NØ5.Ø
- myocardium, myocardial —*see* Degeneration, myocardial - of life —*see* Menopause

Change *(Continued)*
- pacemaker Z45.Ø18
  - pulse generator Z45.Ø1Ø
- personality (enduring) F68.8
  - due to (secondary to)
    - general medical condition FØ7.Ø
  - secondary (nonspecific) F6Ø.89
- regressive, dental pulp KØ4.2
- renal —*see* Disease, renal
- retina H35.9
  - myopic —*see also* Myopia, degenerative H44.2-•
- sacroiliac joint M53.3
- senile —*see also* condition R54
- sensory R2Ø.8
- skin R23.9
  - acute, due to ultraviolet radiation L56.9
    - specified NEC L56.8
  - chronic, due to nonionizing radiation L57.9
    - specified NEC L57.8
  - cyanosis R23.Ø
  - flushing R23.2
  - pallor R23.1
  - petechiae R23.3
  - specified change NEC R23.8
  - swelling —*see* Mass, localized
  - texture R23.4
- trophic
  - arm —*see* Mononeuropathy, upper limb
  - leg —*see* Mononeuropathy, lower limb
- vascular I99.9
- vasomotor I73.9
- voice R49.9
  - psychogenic F44.4
  - specified NEC R49.8

Changing sleep-work schedule, affecting sleep G47.26
Changuinola fever A93.1
Chapping skin T69.8
Charcot-Marie-Tooth disease, paralysis or syndrome G6Ø.Ø
Charcot's
- arthropathy —*see* Arthropathy, neuropathic
- cirrhosis K74.3
- disease (tabetic arthropathy) A52.16
- joint (disease) (tabetic) A52.16
  - diabetic —*see* Diabetes, with, arthropathy
  - syringomyelic G95.Ø
- syndrome (intermittent claudication) I73.9

CHARGE association Q89.8
Charley-horse (quadriceps) M62.831
- traumatic (quadriceps) S76.11-•

Charlouis' disease —*see* Yaws
Cheadle's disease E54
Checking (of)
- cardiac pacemaker (battery) (electrode(s)) Z45.Ø18
  - pulse generator Z45.Ø1Ø
- implantable subdermal contraceptive Z3Ø.46
- intrauterine contraceptive device Z3Ø.431
- wound Z48.Ø-•
  - due to injury - code to Injury, by site, using appropriate seventh character for subsequent encounter
  - postoperative - see Aftercare

Check-up —*see* Examination
Chédiak-Higashi (-Steinbrinck) **syndrome** (congenital gigantism of peroxidase granules) E7Ø.33Ø
Cheek —*see* condition
Cheese itch B88.Ø
Cheese-washer's lung J67.8
Cheese-worker's lung J67.8
Cheilitis (acute) (angular) (catarrhal) (chronic) (exfoliative) (gangrenous) (glandular) (infectional) (suppurative) (ulcerative) (vesicular) K13.Ø
- actinic (due to sun) L56.8
  - other than from sun L59.8
- candidal B37.83

Cheilodynia K13.Ø
Cheiloschisis —*see* Cleft, lip
Cheilosis (angular) K13.Ø
- with pellagra E52
- due to
  - vitamin B2 (riboflavin) deficiency E53.Ø

Cheiromegaly M79.89
Cheiropompholyx L3Ø.1
Cheloid —*see* Keloid
Chemical burn —*see* Corrosion, by site
Chemodectoma —*see* Paraganglioma, nonchromaffin
Chemosis, conjunctiva —*see* Edema, conjunctiva
Chemotherapy (session) (for)
- cancer Z51.11
- neoplasm Z51.11

Cherubism M27.8
Chest —*see* condition
Cheyne-Stokes breathing (respiration) RØ6.3
Chiari's
- disease or syndrome (hepatic vein thrombosis) I82.Ø
- malformation
  - type I G93.5
  - type II —*see* Spina bifida
- net Q24.8

Chicago disease B4Ø.9
Chickenpox —*see* Varicella
Chiclero ulcer or sore B55.1
Chigger (infestation) B88.Ø
Chignon (disease) B36.8
- newborn (from vacuum extraction) (birth injury) P12.1

Chilaiditi's syndrome (subphrenic displacement, colon) Q43.3
Chilblain(s) (lupus) T69.1
➡**Child** —*see also* Problem, child
- custody dispute Z65.3

Childbirth —*see* Delivery
Childhood
- cerebral X-linked adrenoleukodystrophy E71.52Ø
- period of rapid growth ZØØ.2

Chill(s) R68.83
- with fever R5Ø.9
- without fever R68.83
- congestive in malarial regions B54

Chilomastigiasis AØ7.8
Chimera 46,XX/46,XY Q99.Ø
Chin —*see* condition
Chinese dysentery AØ3.9
Chionophobia F4Ø.228
Chitral fever A93.1
Chlamydia, chlamydial A74.9
- cervicitis A56.Ø9
- conjunctivitis A74.Ø
- cystitis A56.Ø1
- endometritis A56.11
- epididymitis A56.19
- female
  - pelvic inflammatory disease A56.11
  - pelviperitonitis A56.11
- orchitis A56.19
- peritonitis A74.81
- pharyngitis A56.4
- proctitis A56.3
- psittaci (infection) A7Ø
- salpingitis A56.11
- sexually-transmitted infection NEC A56.8
- specified NEC A74.89
- urethritis A56.Ø1
- vulvovaginitis A56.Ø2

Chlamydiosis —*see* Chlamydia
Chloasma (skin) (idiopathic) (symptomatic) L81.1
- eyelid HØ2.719
  - hyperthyroid EØ5.9Ø *[HØ2.719]*
    - with thyroid storm EØ5.91 *[HØ2.719]*
  - left HØ2.716
    - lower HØ2.715
    - upper HØ2.714
  - right HØ2.713
    - lower HØ2.712
    - upper HØ2.711

Chloroma C92.3-•
Chlorosis D5Ø.9
- Egyptian B76.9 *[D63.8]*
- miner's B76.9 *[D63.8]*

Chlorotic anemia D5Ø.8
Chocolate cyst (ovary) N8Ø.1Ø-•
Choked
- disc or disk —*see* Papilledema
- on food, phlegm, or vomitus NOS —*see* Foreign body, by site
- while vomiting NOS —*see* Foreign body, by site

Chokes (resulting from bends) T7Ø.3
Choking sensation RØ9.89
Cholangiectasis K83.8
Cholangiocarcinoma
- with hepatocellular carcinoma, combined C22.Ø
- liver C22.1
- specified site NEC —*see* Neoplasm, malignant, by site
- unspecified site C22.1

C

Cholangiohepatitis K83.8
- due to fluke infestation B66.1

Cholangiohepatoma C22.0

Cholangiolitis (acute) (chronic) (extrahepatic) (gangrenous) (intrahepatic) K83.09
- paratyphoidal —*see* Fever, paratyphoid
- typhoidal A01.09

Cholangioma D13.4
- malignant —*see* Cholangiocarcinoma

Cholangitis (ascending) (primary) (recurrent) (sclerosing) (secondary) (stenosing) (suppurative) K83.09
- with calculus, bile duct —*see* Calculus, bile duct, with cholangitis
- chronic nonsuppurative destructive K74.3
- primary K83.09
  - sclerosing K83.01
- sclerosing K83.09

Cholecystectasia K82.8

Cholecystitis K81.9
- with
  - calculus, stones in
    - bile duct (common) (hepatic) —*see* Calculus, bile duct, with cholecystitis
    - cystic duct —*see* Calculus, gallbladder, with cholecystitis
    - gallbladder —*see* Calculus, gallbladder, with cholecystitis
  - choledocholithiasis —*see* Calculus, bile duct, with cholecystitis
  - cholelithiasis —*see* Calculus, gallbladder, with cholecystitis
  - gangrene of gallbladder K82.A1
  - perforation of gallbladder K82.A2
- acute (emphysematous) (gangrenous) (suppurative) K81.0
  - with
    - calculus, stones in
      - cystic duct —*see* Calculus, gallbladder, with cholecystitis, acute
      - gallbladder —*see* Calculus, gallbladder, with cholecystitis, acute
    - choledocholithiasis —*see* Calculus, bile duct, with cholecystitis, acute
    - cholelithiasis —*see* Calculus, gallbladder, with cholecystitis, acute
    - chronic cholecystitis K81.2
      - with gallbladder calculus K80.12
        - with obstruction K80.13
- chronic K81.1
  - with acute cholecystitis K81.2
    - with gallbladder calculus K80.12
      - with obstruction K80.13
- emphysematous (acute) —*see* Cholecystitis, acute
- gangrenous —*see* Cholecystitis, acute
- paratyphoidal, current A01.4
- suppurative —*see* Cholecystitis, acute
- typhoidal A01.09

Cholecystolithiasis —*see* Calculus, gallbladder

Choledochitis (suppurative) K83.09

Choledocholith —*see* Calculus, bile duct

Choledocholithiasis (common duct) (hepatic duct) —*see* Calculus, bile duct
- cystic —*see* Calculus, gallbladder
- typhoidal A01.09

Cholelithiasis (cystic duct) (gallbladder) (impacted) (multiple) —*see* Calculus, gallbladder
- bile duct (common) (hepatic) —*see* Calculus, bile duct
- hepatic duct —*see* Calculus, bile duct
- specified NEC K80.80
  - with obstruction K80.81

Cholemia —*see also* Jaundice
- familial (simple) (congenital) E80.4
- Gilbert's E80.4

Choleperitoneum, choleperitonitis K65.3

Cholera (Asiatic) (epidemic) (malignant) A00.9
- antimonial —*see* Poisoning, antimony
- classical A00.0
- due to Vibrio cholerae 01 A00.9
  - biovar cholerae A00.0
  - biovar eltor A00.1
  - el tor A00.1
- el tor A00.1

Cholerine —*see* Cholera

Cholestasis NEC K83.1
- with hepatocyte injury K71.0
- due to total parenteral nutrition (TPN) K76.89
- pure K71.0

Cholesteatoma (ear) (middle) (with reaction) H71.9-•
- attic H71.0-•
- external ear (canal) H60.4-•
- mastoid H71.2-•
- postmastoidectomy cavity (recurrent) —*see* Complications, postmastoidectomy, recurrent cholesteatoma
- recurrent (postmastoidectomy) —*see* Complications, postmastoidectomy, recurrent cholesteatoma
- tympanum H71.1-•

Cholesteatosis, diffuse H71.3-•

Cholesteremia E78.00

Cholesterin in vitreous —*see* Deposit, crystalline

Cholesterol
- deposit
  - retina H35.89
  - vitreous —*see* Deposit, crystalline
- elevated (high) E78.00
  - with elevated (high) triglycerides E78.2
  - screening for Z13.220
- imbibition of gallbladder K82.4

Cholesterolemia (essential) (pure) E78.00
- familial E78.01
- hereditary E78.01

Cholesterolosis, cholesterosis (gallbladder) K82.4
- cerebrotendinous E75.5

Cholocolic fistula K82.3

Choluria R82.2

Chondritis M94.8X9
- aurical H61.03-•
- costal (Tietze's) M94.0
- external ear H61.03-•
- patella, posttraumatic —*see* Chondromalacia, patella
- pinna H61.03-•
- purulent M94.8X-•
- tuberculous NEC A18.02
  - intervertebral A18.01

Chondroblastoma —*see also* Neoplasm, bone, benign
- malignant —*see* Neoplasm, bone, malignant

Chondrocalcinosis M11.20
- ankle M11.27-•
- elbow M11.22-•
- familial M11.10
  - ankle M11.17-•
  - elbow M11.12-•
  - foot joint M11.17-•
  - hand joint M11.14-•
  - hip M11.15-•
  - knee M11.16-•
  - multiple site M11.19
  - shoulder M11.11-•
  - vertebrae M11.18
  - wrist M11.13-•
- foot joint M11.27-•
- hand joint M11.24-•
- hip M11.25-•
- knee M11.26-•
- multiple site M11.29
- shoulder M11.21-•
- specified type NEC M11.20
  - ankle M11.27-•
  - elbow M11.22-•
  - foot joint M11.27-•
  - hand joint M11.24-•
  - hip M11.25-•
  - knee M11.26-•
  - multiple site M11.29
  - shoulder M11.21-•
  - vertebrae M11.28
  - wrist M11.23-•
- vertebrae M11.28
- wrist M11.23-•

Chondrodermatitis nodularis helicis or anthelicis —*see* Perichondritis, ear

Chondrodysplasia Q78.9
- with hemangioma Q78.4
- calcificans congenita Q77.3
- fetalis Q77.4
- metaphyseal (Jansen's) (McKusick's) (Schmid's) Q78.8
- punctata Q77.3

Chondrodystrophy, chondrodystrophia (familial) (fetalis) (hypoplastic) Q78.9
- calcificans congenita Q77.3
- myotonic (congenital) G71.13
- punctata Q77.3

Chondroectodermal dysplasia Q77.6

Chondrogenesis imperfecta Q77.4

Chondrolysis M94.35-•

Chondroma —*see also* Neoplasm, cartilage, benign
- juxtacortical —*see* Neoplasm, bone, benign
- periosteal —*see* Neoplasm, bone, benign

Chondromalacia (systemic) M94.20
- acromioclavicular joint M94.21-•
- ankle M94.27-•
- elbow M94.22-•
- foot joint M94.27-•
- glenohumeral joint M94.21-•
- hand joint M94.24-•
- hip M94.25-•
- knee M94.26-•
  - patella M22.4-•
- multiple sites M94.29
- patella M22.4-•
- rib M94.28
- sacroiliac joint M94.259
- shoulder M94.21-•
- sternoclavicular joint M94.21-•
- vertebral joint M94.28
- wrist M94.23-•

Chondromatosis —*see also* Neoplasm, cartilage, uncertain behavior
- internal Q78.4

Chondromyxosarcoma —*see* Neoplasm, cartilage, malignant

Chondro-osteodysplasia (Morquio-Brailsford type) E76.219

Chondro-osteodystrophy E76.29

Chondro-osteoma —*see* Neoplasm, bone, benign

Chondropathia tuberosa M94.0

Chondrosarcoma —*see* Neoplasm, cartilage, malignant
- juxtacortical —*see* Neoplasm, bone, malignant
- mesenchymal —*see* Neoplasm, connective tissue, malignant
- myxoid —*see* Neoplasm, cartilage, malignant

Chordee (nonvenereal) N48.89
- congenital Q54.4
- gonococcal A54.09

Chorditis (fibrinous) (nodosa) (tuberosa) J38.2

Chordoma —*see* Neoplasm, vertebral (column), malignant

Chorea (chronic) (gravis) (posthemiplegic) (senile) (spasmodic) G25.5
- with
  - heart involvement I02.0
    - active or acute (conditions in I01-•) I02.0
    - rheumatic I02.9
      - with valvular disorder I02.0
  - rheumatic heart disease (chronic) (inactive) (quiescent) — code to rheumatic heart condition involved
- drug-induced G25.4
- habit F95.8
- hereditary G10
- Huntington's G10
- hysterical F44.4
- minor I02.9
  - with heart involvement I02.0
- progressive G25.5
  - hereditary G10
- rheumatic (chronic) I02.9
  - with heart involvement I02.0
- Sydenham's I02.9
  - with heart involvement —*see* Chorea, with rheumatic heart disease
  - nonrheumatic G25.5

Choreoathetosis (paroxysmal) G25.5

Chorioadenoma (destruens) D39.2

Chorioamnionitis O41.12-•

Chorioangioma D26.7

Choriocarcinoma —*see* Neoplasm, malignant, by site
- combined with
  - embryonal carcinoma —*see* Neoplasm, malignant, by site
  - other germ cell elements —*see* Neoplasm, malignant, by site
  - teratoma —*see* Neoplasm, malignant, by site
- specified site —*see* Neoplasm, malignant, by site
- unspecified site
  - female C58
  - male C62.90

Chorioencephalitis (acute) (lymphocytic) (serous) A87.2

Chorioepithelioma —*see* Choriocarcinoma

Choriomeningitis (acute) (lymphocytic) (serous) A87.2

INDEX TO DISEASES AND INJURIES / Chorionepithelioma

Chorionepithelioma —*see* Choriocarcinoma
Chorioretinitis —*see also* Inflammation, chorioretinal
disseminated —*see also* Inflammation, chorioretinal, disseminated
in neurosyphilis A52.19
Egyptian B76.9 *[D63.8]*
focal —*see also* Inflammation, chorioretinal, focal
histoplasmic B39.9 *[H32]*
in (due to)
histoplasmosis B39.9 *[H32]*
syphilis (secondary) A51.43
late A52.71
toxoplasmosis (acquired) B58.01
congenital (active) P37.1 *[H32]*
tuberculosis A18.53
juxtapapillary, juxtapapillaris —*see* Inflammation, chorioretinal, focal, juxtapapillary
leprous A30.9 *[H32]*
miner's B76.9 *[D63.8]*
progressive myopia (degeneration) —*see also* Myopia, degenerative H44.2-●
syphilitic (secondary) A51.43
congenital (early) A50.01 *[H32]*
late A50.32
late A52.71
tuberculous A18.53
Chorioretinopathy, central serous H35.71-●
Choroid —*see* condition
Choroideremia H31.21
Choroiditis —*see* Chorioretinitis
Choroidopathy —*see* Disorder, choroid
Choroidoretinitis —*see* Chorioretinitis
Choroidoretinopathy, central serous —*see* Chorioretinopathy, central serous
Christian-Weber disease M35.6
Christmas disease D67
Chromaffinoma —*see also* Neoplasm, benign, by site
malignant —*see* Neoplasm, malignant, by site
Chromatopsia —*see* Deficiency, color vision
Chromhidrosis, chromidrosis L75.1
Chromoblastomycosis —*see* Chromomycosis
Chromoconversion R82.91
Chromomycosis B43.9
brain abscess B43.1
cerebral B43.1
cutaneous B43.0
skin B43.0
specified NEC B43.8
subcutaneous abscess or cyst B43.2
Chromophytosis B36.0
Chromosome —*see* condition by chromosome involved
D (1) —*see* condition, chromosome 13
E (3) —*see* condition, chromosome 18
G —*see* condition, chromosome 21
Chromotrichomycosis B36.8
Chronic —*see* condition
fracture —*see* Fracture, pathological
Churg-Strauss syndrome M30.1
Chyle cyst, mesentery I89.8
Chylocele (nonfilarial) I89.8
filarial —*see also* Infestation, filarial B74.9 *[N51]*
tunica vaginalis N50.89
filarial —*see also* Infestation, filarial B74.9 *[N51]*
Chylomicronemia (fasting) (with hyperprebetalipoproteinemia) E78.3
Chylopericardium I31.39
acute I30.9
Chylothorax (nonfilarial) J94.0
filarial —*see also* Infestation, filarial B74.9 *[J91.8]*
Chylous —*see* condition
Chyluria (nonfilarial) R82.0
due to
bilharziasis B65.0
Brugia (malayi) B74.1
timori B74.2
schistosomiasis (bilharziasis) B65.0
Wuchereria (bancrofti) B74.0
filarial —*see* Infestation, filarial
Cicatricial (deformity) —*see* Cicatrix
Cicatrix (adherent) (contracted) (painful) (vicious) —*see also* Scar L90.5
adenoid (and tonsil) J35.8
alveolar process M26.79
anus K62.89
auricle —*see* Disorder, pinna, specified type NEC

Cicatrix *(Continued)*
bile duct (common) (hepatic) K83.8
bladder N32.89
bone —*see* Disorder, bone, specified type NEC
brain G93.89
cervix (postoperative) (postpartal) N88.1
common duct K83.8
cornea H17.9
tuberculous A18.59
duodenum (bulb), obstructive K31.5
esophagus K22.2
eyelid —*see* Disorder, eyelid function
hypopharynx J39.2
lacrimal passages —*see* Obstruction, lacrimal
larynx J38.7
lung J98.4
middle ear —*see* subcategory H74.8
mouth K13.79
muscle M62.89
with contracture —*see* Contraction, muscle NEC
nasopharynx J39.2
palate (soft) K13.79
penis N48.89
pharynx J39.2
prostate N42.89
rectum K62.89
retina —*see* Scar, chorioretinal
semilunar cartilage —*see* Derangement, meniscus
seminal vesicle N50.89
skin L90.5
infected L08.89
postinfective L90.5
tuberculous B90.8
specified site NEC L90.5
throat J39.2
tongue K14.8
tonsil (and adenoid) J35.8
trachea J39.8
tuberculous NEC B90.9
urethra N36.8
uterus N85.8
vagina N89.8
postoperative N99.2
vocal cord J38.3
wrist, constricting (annular) L90.5
CIDP (chronic inflammatory demyelinating polyneuropathy) G61.81
CIN —*see* Neoplasia, intraepithelial, cervix
CINCA (chronic infantile neurological, cutaneous and articular syndrome) M04.2
Cinchonism —*see* Deafness, ototoxic
correct substance properly administered —*see* Table of Drugs and Chemicals, by drug, adverse effect
overdose or wrong substance given or taken —*see* Table of Drugs and Chemicals, by drug, poisoning
Circle of Willis —*see* condition
Circular —*see* condition
Circulating anticoagulants —*see also* - Disorder, hemorrhagic D68.318
due to drugs —*see also* - Disorder, hemorrhagic D68.32
following childbirth O72.3
Circulation
collateral, any site I99.8
defective (lower extremity) I99.9
congenital Q28.9
embryonic Q28.9
failure (peripheral) R57.9
newborn P29.89
fetal, persistent P29.38
heart, incomplete Q28.9
Circulatory system —*see* condition
Circulus senilis (cornea) —*see* Degeneration, cornea, senile
Circumcision (in absence of medical indication) (ritual) (routine) Z41.2
Circumscribed —*see* condition
Circumvallate placenta O43.11-●
Cirrhosis, cirrhotic (hepatic) (liver) K74.60
alcoholic K70.30
with ascites K70.31
atrophic —*see* Cirrhosis, liver
Baumgarten-Cruveilhier K74.69
biliary (cholangiolitic) (cholangitic) (hypertrophic) (obstructive) (pericholangiolitic) K74.5

Cirrhosis, cirrhotic *(Continued)*
biliary *(Continued)*
due to
Clonorchiasis B66.1
flukes B66.3
primary K74.3
secondary K74.4
cardiac (of liver) K76.1
Charcot's K74.3
cholangiolitic, cholangitic, cholostatic (primary) K74.3
congestive K76.1
Cruveilhier-Baumgarten K74.69
cryptogenic (liver) K74.69
due to
hepatolenticular degeneration E83.01
Wilson's disease E83.01
xanthomatosis E78.2
fatty K76.0
alcoholic K70.0
Hanot's (hypertrophic) K74.3
hepatic —*see* Cirrhosis, liver
hypertrophic K74.3
Indian childhood K74.69
kidney —*see* Sclerosis, renal
Laennec's K70.30
with ascites K70.31
alcoholic K70.30
with ascites K70.31
nonalcoholic K74.69
liver K74.60
alcoholic K70.30
with ascites K70.31
fatty K70.0
congenital P78.81
syphilitic A52.74
lung (chronic) J84.10
macronodular K74.69
alcoholic K70.30
with ascites K70.31
micronodular K74.69
alcoholic K70.30
with ascites K70.31
mixed type K74.69
monolobular K74.3
nephritis —*see* Sclerosis, renal
nutritional K74.69
alcoholic K70.30
with ascites K70.31
obstructive —*see* Cirrhosis, biliary
ovarian N83.8
pancreas (duct) K86.89
pigmentary E83.110
portal K74.69
alcoholic K70.30
with ascites K70.31
postnecrotic K74.69
alcoholic K70.30
with ascites K70.31
pulmonary J84.10
renal —*see* Sclerosis, renal
spleen D73.2
stasis K76.1
Todd's K74.3
unilobar K74.3
xanthomatous (biliary) K74.5
due to xanthomatosis (familial) (metabolic) (primary) E78.2
Cistern, subarachnoid R93.0
Citrullinemia E72.23
Citrullinuria E72.23
Civatte's disease or poikiloderma L57.3
CLAD —*see* Dysfunction, chronic, lung allograft
Clam digger's itch B65.3
Clammy skin R23.1
Clap —*see* Gonorrhea
Clarke-Hadfield syndrome (pancreatic infantilism) K86.89
Clark's paralysis G80.9
Clastothrix L67.8
Claude Bernard-Horner syndrome G90.2
traumatic —*see* Injury, nerve, cervical sympathetic
Claude's disease or syndrome G46.3
Claudicatio venosa intermittens I87.8
Claudication (intermittent) I73.9
cerebral (artery) G45.9
spinal cord (arteriosclerotic) G95.19
syphilitic A52.09
venous (axillary) I87.8
Claustrophobia F40.240

▶ New ➡ Revised ~~deleted~~ Deleted ● Use Additional Character(s)

Clavus (infected) L84
Clawfoot (congenital) Q66.89
acquired —*see* Deformity, limb, clawfoot
Clawhand (acquired) —*see also* Deformity, limb, clawhand
congenital Q68.1
Clawtoe (congenital) Q66.89
acquired —*see* Deformity, toe, specified NEC
Clay eating —*see* Pica
Cleansing of artificial opening —*see* Attention to, artificial, opening
Cleft (congenital) —*see also* Imperfect, closure
alveolar process M26.79
branchial (persistent) Q18.2
cyst Q18.Ø
fistula Q18.Ø
sinus Q18.Ø
cricoid cartilage, posterior Q31.8
foot Q72.7
hand Q71.6
lip (unilateral) Q36.9
with cleft palate Q37.9
hard Q37.1
with soft Q37.5
soft Q37.3
with hard Q37.5
bilateral Q36.Ø
with cleft palate Q37.8
hard Q37.Ø
with soft Q37.4
soft Q37.2
with hard Q37.4
median Q36.1
▶mitral valve leaflet (at birth) (congenital) Q23.82
nose Q3Ø.2
palate Q35.9
with cleft lip (unilateral) Q37.9
bilateral Q37.8
hard Q35.1
with
cleft lip (unilateral) Q37.1
bilateral Q37.Ø
soft Q35.5
with cleft lip (unilateral) Q37.5
bilateral Q37.4
medial Q35.5
soft Q35.3
with
cleft lip (unilateral) Q37.3
bilateral Q37.2
hard Q35.5
with cleft lip (unilateral) Q37.5
bilateral Q37.4
penis Q55.69
scrotum Q55.29
thyroid cartilage Q31.8
uvula Q35.7
Cleidocranial dysostosis Q74.Ø
Cleptomania F63.2
Clicking hip (newborn) R29.4
Climacteric (female) —*see also* Menopause
arthritis (any site) NEC —*see* Arthritis, specified form NEC
depression (single episode) F32.89
recurrent episode F33.8
male (symptoms) (syndrome) NEC N5Ø.89
melancholia (single episode) F32.89
recurrent episode F33.8
paranoid state F22
polyarthritis NEC —*see* Arthritis, specified form NEC
symptoms (female) N95.1
Clinical research investigation (clinical trial) (control subject) (normal comparison) (participant) ZØØ.6
Clitoris —*see* condition **Cloaca** (persistent) Q43.7
Clonorchiasis, clonorchis infection (liver) B66.1
Clonus R25.8
Closed bite M26.29
Clostridium (C.) perfringens, as cause of disease classified elsewhere B96.7
Closure
congenital, nose Q3Ø.Ø
cranial sutures, premature Q75.ØØ9
defective or imperfect NEC —*see* Imperfect, closure
fistula, delayed —*see* Fistula
foramen ovale, imperfect Q21.12
hymen N89.6
interauricular septum, defective Q21.19
interventricular septum, defective Q21.Ø
Closure *(Continued)*
lacrimal duct —*see also* Stenosis, lacrimal, duct
congenital Q1Ø.5
nose (congenital) Q3Ø.Ø
acquired M95.Ø
of artificial opening —*see* Attention to, artificial, opening
primary angle, without glaucoma damage H4Ø.Ø6-•
vagina N89.5
valve —*see* Endocarditis
vulva N9Ø.5
Clot (blood) —*see also* Embolism
artery (obstruction) (occlusion) —*see* Embolism
bladder N32.89
brain (intradural or extradural) —*see* Occlusion, artery, cerebral
circulation I74.9
heart —*see also* Infarct, myocardium
not resulting in infarction I51.3
vein —*see* Thrombosis
Clouded state R4Ø.1
epileptic —*see* Epilepsy, specified NEC
paroxysmal —*see* Epilepsy, specified NEC
Cloudy antrum, antra J32.Ø
Clouston's (hidrotic) **ectodermal dysplasia** Q82.4
Cloverleaf skull Q75.Ø51
Clubbed nail pachydermoperiostosis M89.4Ø *[L62]*
Clubbing of finger(s) (nails) R68.3
Clubfinger R68.3
congenital Q68.1
Clubfoot (congenital) Q66.89
acquired —*see* Deformity, limb, clubfoot
equinovarus Q66.Ø-•
paralytic —*see* Deformity, limb, clubfoot
Clubhand (congenital) (radial) Q71.4-•
acquired —*see* Deformity, limb, clubhand
Clubnail R68.3
congenital Q84.6
Clump, kidney Q63.1
Clumsiness, clumsy child syndrome F82
Cluttering F98.81
Clutton's joints A5Ø.51 *[M12.8Ø]*
Coagulation, intravascular (diffuse) (disseminated) —*see also* Defibrination syndrome
complicating abortion —*see* Abortion, by type, complicated by, intravascular coagulation
COVID-19 associated (see also COVID-19) D65
following ectopic or molar pregnancy OØ8.1
Coagulopathy —*see also* Defect, coagulation
consumption D65
intravascular D65
newborn P6Ø
Coalition
calcaneo-scaphoid Q66.89
tarsal Q66.89
Coalminer's
elbow —*see* Bursitis, elbow, olecranon
lung or pneumoconiosis J6Ø
Coalworker's lung or pneumoconiosis J6Ø
Coarctation
aorta (preductal) (postductal) Q25.1
pulmonary artery Q25.71
Coated tongue K14.3
Coats' disease (exudative retinopathy) —*see* Retinopathy, exudative
Cocaine-induced
anxiety disorder F14.98Ø
bipolar and related disorder F14.94
depressive disorder F14.94
obsessive-compulsive and related disorder F14.988
psychotic disorder F14.959
sleep disorder F14.982
sexual dysfunction F14.981
Cocainism —*see* Disorder, cocaine use
Coccidioidomycosis B38.9
cutaneous B38.3
disseminated B38.7
generalized B38.7
meninges B38.4
prostate B38.81
pulmonary B38.2
acute B38.Ø
chronic B38.1
skin B38.3
specified NEC B38.89
Coccidioidosis —*see* Coccidioidomycosis
Coccidiosis (intestinal) AØ7.3
Coccydynia, coccygodynia M53.3
Coccyx —*see* condition
Cochin-China diarrhea K9Ø.1
Cockayne's syndrome Q87.19
Cocked up toe —*see* Deformity, toe, specified NEC
Cock's peculiar tumor L72.3
Codman's tumor —*see* Neoplasm, bone, benign
Coenurosis B71.8
Coffee-worker's lung J67.8
Cogan's syndrome H16.32-•
oculomotor apraxia H51.8
Coitus, painful (female) N94.1Ø
male N53.12
psychogenic F52.6
Cold JØØ
with influenza, flu, or grippe —*see* Influenza, with, respiratory manifestations NEC
agglutinin disease or hemoglobinuria (chronic) D59.12
bronchial —*see* Bronchitis
chest —*see* Bronchitis
common (head) JØØ
effects of T69.9
specified effect NEC T69.8
excessive, effects of T69.9
specified effect NEC T69.8
exhaustion from T69.8
exposure to T69.9
specified effect NEC T69.8
head JØØ
injury syndrome (newborn) P8Ø.Ø
on lung —*see* Bronchitis
rose J3Ø.1
sensitivity, auto-immune D59.12
symptoms JØØ
virus JØØ
Coldsore BØØ.1
Colibacillosis A49.8
as the cause of other disease (*see also* Escherichia coli) B96.2Ø
generalized (*see also* Sepsis, Escherichia coli) A41.5Ø
Colic (bilious) (infantile) (intestinal) (recurrent) (spasmodic) R1Ø.83
abdomen R1Ø.83
psychogenic F45.8
appendix, appendicular K38.8
bile duct —*see* Calculus, bile duct
biliary —*see* Calculus, bile duct
common duct —*see* Calculus, bile duct
cystic duct —*see* Calculus, gallbladder
Devonshire NEC —*see* Poisoning, lead
gallbladder —*see* Calculus, gallbladder
gallstone —*see* Calculus, gallbladder
gallbladder or cystic duct —*see* Calculus, gallbladder
hepatic (duct) —*see* Calculus, bile duct
hysterical F45.8
kidney N23
lead NEC —*see* Poisoning, lead
mucous K58.9
with diarrhea K58.Ø
psychogenic F54
nephritic N23
painter's NEC —*see* Poisoning, lead
pancreas K86.89
psychogenic F45.8
renal N23
saturnine NEC —*see* Poisoning, lead
ureter N23
urethral N36.8
due to calculus N21.1
uterus NEC N94.89
menstrual —*see* Dysmenorrhea
worm NOS B83.9
Colicystitis —*see* Cystitis
Colitis (acute) (catarrhal) (chronic) (noninfective) (hemorrhagic) (*see also* Enteritis) K52.9
allergic K52.29
with
food protein-induced enterocolitis syndrome K52.21
proctocolitis K52.29
amebic (acute) —*see also* Amebiasis AØ6.Ø
nondysenteric AØ6.2
anthrax A22.2
bacillary —*see* Infection, Shigella
balantidial AØ7.Ø
▶Clostridioides difficile
▶not specified as recurrent AØ4.72
▶recurrent AØ4.71
Clostridium difficile
not specified as recurrent AØ4.72
recurrent AØ4.71

Colitis *(Continued)*
coccidial A07.3
collagenous K52.831
cystica superficialis K52.89
dietary counseling and surveillance (for) Z71.3
dietetic *—see also* Colitis, allergic K52.29
drug-induced K52.1
due to radiation K52.0
eosinophilic K52.82
food hypersensitivity *—see also* Colitis, allergic K52.29
giardial A07.1
granulomatous *—see* Enteritis, regional, large intestine
infectious *—see* Enteritis, infectious
indeterminate, so stated K52.3
ischemic K55.9
acute (subacute) *—see also* Ischemia, intestine, acute K55.039
chronic K55.1
due to mesenteric artery insufficiency K55.1
fulminant (acute) *—see also* Ischemia, intestine, acute K55.039
left sided K51.50
with
abscess K51.514
complication K51.519
specified NEC K51.518
fistula K51.513
obstruction K51.512
rectal bleeding K51.511
lymphocytic K52.832
membranous
psychogenic F54
microscopic K52.839
specified NEC K52.838
mucous *—see* Syndrome, irritable, bowel
psychogenic F54
noninfective K52.9
specified NEC K52.89
polyposa *—see* Polyp, colon, inflammatory
protozoal A07.9
pseudomembranous
not specified as recurrent A04.72
recurrent A04.71
pseudomucinous *—see* Syndrome, irritable, bowel
regional *—see* Enteritis, regional, large intestine
infectious A09
segmental *—see* Enteritis, regional, large intestine
septic *—see* Enteritis, infectious
spastic K58.9
with diarrhea K58.0
psychogenic F54
staphylococcal A04.8
foodborne A05.0
subacute ischemic *—see also* Ischemia, intestine, acute K55.039
thromboulcerative *—see also* Ischemia, intestine, acute K55.039
toxic NEC K52.1
~~due to Clostridium difficile~~
~~not specified as recurrent A04.72~~
~~recurrent A04.71~~
▶ due to
▶ Clostridioides difficile
▶ not specified as recurrent A04.72
▶ recurrent A04.71
▶ Clostridium difficile
▶ not specified as recurrent A04.72
▶ recurrent A04.71
transmural *—see* Enteritis, regional, large intestine
trichomonal A07.8
tuberculous (ulcerative) A18.32
ulcerative (chronic) K51.90
with
complication K51.919
abscess K51.914
fistula K51.913
obstruction K51.912
rectal bleeding K51.911
specified complication NEC K51.918
enterocolitis *—see* Enterocolitis, ulcerative
ileocolitis *—see* Ileocolitis, ulcerative
mucosal proctocolitis *—see* Proctocolitis, mucosal

Colitis *(Continued)*
ulcerative (chronic) *(Continued)*
proctitis *—see* Proctitis, ulcerative
pseudopolyposis *—see* Polyp, colon, inflammatory
psychogenic F54
rectosigmoiditis *—see* Rectosigmoiditis, ulcerative
specified type NEC K51.80
with
complication K51.819
abscess K51.814
fistula K51.813
obstruction K51.812
rectal bleeding K51.811
specified complication NEC K51.818
Collagenosis, collagen disease (nonvascular) (vascular) M35.9
cardiovascular I42.8
reactive perforating L87.1
specified NEC M35.89
Collapse R55
adrenal E27.2
cardiorespiratory R57.0
cardiovascular R57.0
newborn P29.89
circulatory (peripheral) R57.9
during or after labor and delivery O75.1
following ectopic or molar pregnancy O08.3
newborn P29.89
during or
after labor and delivery O75.1
resulting from a procedure, not elsewhere classified T81.10
external ear canal *—see* Stenosis, external ear canal
general R55
heart *—see* Disease, heart
heat T67.1
hysterical F44.89
labyrinth, membranous (congenital) Q16.5
lung (massive) *—see also* Atelectasis J98.19
pressure due to anesthesia (general) (local) or other sedation T88.2
during labor and delivery O74.1
in pregnancy O29.02-●
postpartum, puerperal O89.09
myocardial *—see* Disease, heart
▶ nasal valve J34.829
▶ external J34.8210
▶ dynamic J34.8212
▶ static J34.8211
▶ internal J34.8200
▶ dynamic J34.8202
▶ static J34.8201
nervous F48.8
neurocirculatory F45.8
nose M95.0
▶ lower sidewall or nostril, on inspiration J34.8212
▶ upper, middle sidewall, on inspiration J34.8202
postoperative T81.10
pulmonary *—see also* Atelectasis J98.19
newborn *—see* Atelectasis
trachea J39.8
tracheobronchial J98.09
valvular *—see* Endocarditis
vascular (peripheral) R57.9
during or after labor and delivery O75.1
following ectopic or molar pregnancy O08.3
newborn P29.89
vertebra M48.50-●
cervical region M48.52-●
cervicothoracic region M48.53-●
in (due to)
neoplasm (metastasis) M84.58-●
osteoporosis *—see also* Osteoporosis M80.88
cervical region M80.88
cervicothoracic region M80.88
lumbar region M80.88
lumbosacral region M80.88
multiple sites M80.88
occipito-atlanto-axial region M80.88
sacrococcygeal region M80.88
thoracic region M80.88
thoracolumbar region M80.88
specified disease NEC M48.50-●
cervical region M48.52-●
cervicothoracic region M48.53-●
lumbar region M48.56-●

Collapse *(Continued)*
vascular *(Continued)*
in (due to) *(Continued)*
specified disease *(Continued)*
lumbosacral region M48.57-●
occipito-atlanto-axial region M48.51-●
sacrococcygeal region M48.58-●
thoracic region M48.54-●
thoracolumbar region M48.55-●
lumbar region M48.56-●
lumbosacral region M48.57-●
occipito-atlanto-axial region M48.51-●
sacrococcygeal region M48.58-●
thoracic region M48.54-●
thoracolumbar region M48.55-●
Collateral *—see also* condition
circulation (venous) I87.8
dilation, veins I87.8
Colles' fracture S52.53-●
Collet (-Sicard) **syndrome** G52.7
Collier's asthma or lung J60
Collodion baby Q80.2
Colloid nodule (of thyroid) (cystic) E04.1
Coloboma (iris) Q13.0
eyelid Q10.3
fundus Q14.8
lens Q12.2
optic disc (congenital) Q14.2
acquired H47.31-●
Coloenteritis *—see* Enteritis
Colon *—see* condition
Colonization
MRSA (Methicillin resistant Staphylococcus aureus) Z22.322
MSSA (Methicillin susceptible Staphylococcus aureus) Z22.321
status *—see* Carrier (suspected) of
Coloptosis K63.4
Color blindness *—see* Deficiency, color vision
Colostomy
attention to Z43.3
fitting or adjustment Z46.89
malfunctioning K94.03
status Z93.3
Colpitis (acute) *—see* Vaginitis
Colpocele N81.5
Colpocystitis *—see* Vaginitis
Colpospasm N94.2
Column, spinal, vertebral *—see* condition
Coma R40.20
with
motor response (none) R40.231
abnormal R40.233
abnormal extensor posturing to pain or noxious stimuli (<2 years of age) R40.232
abnormal flexure posturing to pain or noxious stimuli (0-5 years of age) R40.233
extension R40.232
extensor posturing to pain or noxious stimuli (2-5 years of age) R40.232
flexion/decorticate posturing (<2 years of age) R40.233
flexion withdrawal R40.234
localizes pain (2-5 years of age) R40.235
normal or spontaneous movement (<2 years of age) R40.236
obeys commands (2-5 years of age) R40.236
score of
1 R40.231
2 R40.232
3 R40.233
4 R40.234
5 R40.235
6 R40.236
withdraws from pain or noxious stimuli (0-5 years of age) R40.234
withdraws to touch (<2 years of age) R40.235
opening of eyes (never) R40.211
in response to
pain R40.212
sound R40.213
score of
1 R40.211
2 R40.212
3 R40.213
4 R40.214
spontaneous R40.214

C

▶ New ▶ Revised ~~deleted~~ Deleted ● Use Additional Character(s)

Coma (Continued)
with (Continued)
verbal response (none) R40.221
confused conversation R40.224
cooing or babbling or crying appropriately (<2 years of age) R40.225
inappropriate crying or screaming (<2 years of age) R40.223
inappropriate words R40.223
inappropriate words (2-5 years of age) R40.224
incomprehensible sounds (2-5 years of age) R40.222
incomprehensible words R40.222
irritable cries (<2 years of age) R40.224
moans/grunts to pain; restless (<2 years old) R40.222
oriented R40.225
score of
1 R40.221
2 R40.222
3 R40.223
4 R40.224
5 R40.225
screaming (2-5 years of age) R40.223
uses appropriate words (2-5 years of age) R40.225
eclamptic —*see* Eclampsia
epileptic —*see* Epilepsy
Glasgow, scale score —*see* Glasgow coma scale
hepatic —*see* Failure, hepatic, by type, with coma
hyperglycemic (diabetic) —*see* Diabetes, by type, with hyperosmolarity, with coma
hyperosmolar (diabetic) —*see* Diabetes, by type, with hyperosmolarity, with coma
hypoglycemic (diabetic) —*see* Diabetes, by type, with hypoglycemia, with coma
nondiabetic E15
in diabetes —*see* Diabetes, coma
insulin-induced —*see* Coma, hypoglycemic
ketoacidotic (diabetic) —*see* Diabetes, by type, with ketoacidosis, with coma
myxedematous E03.5
newborn P91.5
nontraumatic, due to underlying condition R40.2A
persistent vegetative state R40.3
secondary R40.2A
specified NEC, without documented Glasgow coma scale score, or with partial Glasgow coma scale score reported R40.244
Comatose —*see* Coma
Combat fatigue F43.0
Combined —*see* condition
Comedo, comedones (giant) L70.0
Comedocarcinoma —*see also* Neoplasm, breast, malignant
noninfiltrating
breast D05.8-●
specified site —*see* Neoplasm, in situ, by site
unspecified site D05.8-●
Comedomastitis —*see* Ectasia, mammary duct
Comminuted fracture - code as Fracture, closed
Common
arterial trunk Q20.0
atrioventricular canal Q21.23
atrium Q21.19
cold (head) J00
truncus (arteriosus) Q20.0
variable immunodeficiency —*see* Immunodeficiency, common variable
ventricle Q20.4
Commotio, commotion (current)
brain —*see* Injury, intracranial, concussion
cerebri —*see* Injury, intracranial, concussion
retinae S05.8X-●
spinal cord —*see* Injury, spinal cord, by region
spinalis —*see* Injury, spinal cord, by region
Communication
between
base of aorta and pulmonary artery Q21.4
left ventricle and right atrium Q20.5
pericardial sac and pleural sac Q34.8
pulmonary artery and pulmonary vein, congenital Q25.72
congenital between uterus and digestive or urinary tract Q51.7
Compartment syndrome (deep) (posterior) (traumatic) T79.A0
abdomen T79.A3
lower extremity (hip, buttock, thigh, leg, foot, toes) T79.A2
Compartment syndrome (Continued)
nontraumatic
abdomen M79.A3
lower extremity (hip, buttock, thigh, leg, foot, toes) M79.A2-●
specified site NEC M79.A9
upper extremity (shoulder, arm, forearm, wrist, hand, fingers) M79.A1-●
specified site NEC T79.A9
upper extremity (shoulder, arm, forearm, wrist, hand, fingers) T79.A1
Compensation
failure —*see* Disease, heart
neurosis, psychoneurosis —*see* Disorder, factitious
Complaint —*see also* Disease
bowel, functional K59.9
psychogenic F45.8
intestine, functional K59.9
psychogenic F45.8
kidney —*see* Disease, renal
miners' J60
Complete —*see* condition
Complex
Addison-Schilder E71.528
cardiorenal —*see* Hypertension, cardiorenal
Costen's M26.69
disseminated mycobacterium avium-intracellulare (DMAC) A31.2
Eisenmenger's (ventricular septal defect) I27.83
hypersexual F52.8
jumped process, spine —*see* Dislocation, vertebra
primary, tuberculous A15.7
Schilder-Addison E71.528
subluxation (vertebral) M99.19
abdomen M99.19
acromioclavicular M99.17
cervical region M99.11
cervicothoracic M99.11
costochondral M99.18
costovertebral M99.18
head region M99.10
hip M99.15
lower extremity M99.16
lumbar region M99.13
lumbosacral M99.13
occipitocervical M99.10
pelvic region M99.15
pubic M99.15
rib cage M99.18
sacral region M99.14
sacrococcygeal M99.14
sacroiliac M99.14
specified NEC M99.19
sternochondral M99.18
sternoclavicular M99.17
thoracic region M99.12
thoracolumbar M99.12
upper extremity M99.17
Taussig-Bing (transposition, aorta and overriding pulmonary artery) Q20.1
Complication(s) (from) (of)
accidental puncture or laceration during a procedure (of) —*see* Complications, intraoperative (intraprocedural), puncture or laceration
amputation stump (surgical) (late) NEC T87.9
dehiscence T87.81
infection or inflammation T87.40
lower limb T87.4-●
upper limb T87.4-●
necrosis T87.50
lower limb T87.5-●
upper limb T87.5-●
neuroma T87.30
lower limb T87.3-●
upper limb T87.3-●
specified type NEC T87.89
anastomosis (and bypass) —*see also* Complications, prosthetic device or implant
intestinal (internal) NEC K91.89
involving urinary tract N99.89
urinary tract (involving intestinal tract) N99.89
vascular —*see* Complications, cardiovascular device or implant
anesthesia, anesthetic —*see also* Anesthesia, complication T88.59
brain, postpartum, puerperal O89.2
Complication (Continued)
anesthesia, anesthetic (Continued)
cardiac
in
labor and delivery O74.2
pregnancy O29.19-●
postpartum, puerperal O89.1
central nervous system
in
labor and delivery O74.3
pregnancy O29.29-●
postpartum, puerperal O89.2
difficult or failed intubation T88.4
in pregnancy O29.6-●
failed sedation (conscious) (moderate) during procedure T88.52
general, unintended awareness during procedure T88.53
hyperthermia, malignant T88.3
hypothermia T88.51
intubation failure T88.4
malignant hyperthermia T88.3
pulmonary
in
labor and delivery O74.1
pregnancy NEC O29.09-●
postpartum, puerperal O89.09
shock T88.2
spinal and epidural
in
labor and delivery NEC O74.6
headache O74.5
pregnancy NEC O29.5X-●
postpartum, puerperal NEC O89.5
headache O89.4
unintended awareness under general anesthesia during procedure T88.53
anti-reflux device —*see* Complications, esophageal anti-reflux device
aortic (bifurcation) graft —*see* Complications, graft, vascular
aortocoronary (bypass) graft —*see* Complications, coronary artery (bypass) graft
aortofemoral (bypass) graft —*see* Complications, extremity artery (bypass) graft
arteriovenous
fistula, surgically created T82.9
embolism T82.818
fibrosis T82.828
hemorrhage T82.838
infection or inflammation T82.7
mechanical
breakdown T82.510
displacement T82.520
leakage T82.530
malposition T82.520
obstruction T82.590
perforation T82.590
protrusion T82.590
pain T82.848
specified type NEC T82.898
stenosis T82.858
thrombosis T82.868
shunt, surgically created T82.9
embolism T82.818
fibrosis T82.828
hemorrhage T82.838
infection or inflammation T82.7
mechanical
breakdown T82.511
displacement T82.521
leakage T82.531
malposition T82.521
obstruction T82.591
perforation T82.591
protrusion T82.591
pain T82.848
specified type NEC T82.898
stenosis T82.858
thrombosis T82.868
arthroplasty —*see* Complications, joint prosthesis
artificial
fertilization or insemination N98.9
attempted introduction (of)
embryo in embryo transfer N98.3
ovum following in vitro fertilization N98.2
hyperstimulation of ovaries N98.1
infection N98.0
specified NEC N98.8

C

C

- **Complication** *(Continued)*
  - postprocedural *(Continued)*
    - hematoma *(Continued)*
      - musculoskeletal structure *(Continued)*
        - following non-orthopedic surgery M96.841
        - following orthopedic surgery M96.840
      - nervous system
        - following nervous system procedure G97.61
        - following other procedure G97.62
      - respiratory system
        - following other procedure J95.861
        - following procedure on respiratory system organ or structure J95.860
      - skin and subcutaneous tissue
        - following dermatologic procedure L76.31
        - following procedure on other organ L76.32
      - spleen
        - following procedure on other organ D78.32
        - following procedure on the spleen D78.31
    - hemorrhage (of)
      - circulatory system organ or structure
        - following cardiac bypass I97.611
        - following cardiac catheterization I97.610
        - following other circulatory system procedure I97.618
        - following other procedure I97.620
      - digestive system
        - following procedure on digestive system K91.840
        - following procedure on other organ K91.841
      - ear
        - following other procedure H95.42
        - following procedure on ear and mastoid process H95.41
      - endocrine system
        - following endocrine system procedure E89.810
        - following other procedure E89.811
      - eye and adnexa
        - following ophthalmic procedure H59.31-●
        - following other procedure H59.32-●
      - genitourinary organ or structure
        - following procedure on genitourinary organ or structure N99.820
        - following procedure on other organ N99.821
      - mastoid process
        - following other procedure H95.42
        - following procedure on ear and mastoid process H95.41
      - musculoskeletal structure
        - following musculoskeletal surgery M96.830
        - following non-orthopedic surgery M96.831
        - following orthopedic surgery M96.830
      - nervous system
        - following nervous system procedure G97.51
        - following other procedure G97.52
      - respiratory system
        - following other procedure J95.831
        - following procedure on respiratory system organ or structure J95.830
      - skin and subcutaneous tissue
        - following dermatologic procedure L76.21
        - following a procedure on other organ L76.22
      - spleen
        - following procedure on other organ D78.22
        - following procedure on the spleen D78.21
    - seroma (of)
      - circulatory system organ or structure
        - following cardiac bypass I97.641
        - following cardiac catheterization I97.640
        - following other circulatory system procedure I97.648
        - following other procedure I97.622
      - digestive system
        - following procedure on digestive system K91.872
        - following procedure on other organ K91.873

- **Complication** *(Continued)*
  - postprocedural *(Continued)*
    - seroma *(Continued)*
      - ear
        - following other procedure H95.54
        - following procedure on ear and mastoid process H95.53
      - endocrine system
        - following endocrine system procedure E89.822
        - following other procedure E89.823
      - eye and adnexa
        - following ophthalmic procedure H59.35-●
        - following other procedure H59.36-●
      - genitourinary organ or structure
        - following procedure on genitourinary organ or structure N99.842
        - following procedure on other organ N99.843
      - mastoid process
        - following other procedure H95.54
        - following procedure on ear and mastoid process H95.53
      - musculoskeletal structure
        - following musculoskeletal surgery M96.842
        - following non-orthopedic surgery M96.843
        - following orthopedic surgery M96.842
      - nervous system
        - following nervous system procedure G97.63
        - following other procedure G97.64
      - respiratory system
        - following other procedure J95.863
        - following procedure on respiratory system organ or structure J95.862
      - skin and subcutaneous tissue
        - following dermatologic procedure L76.33
        - following procedure on other organ L76.34
      - spleen
        - following procedure on other organ D78.34
        - following procedure on the spleen D78.33
    - specified NEC
      - circulatory system I97.89
      - digestive K91.89
      - ear H95.89
      - endocrine E89.89
      - eye and adnexa H59.89
      - genitourinary N99.89
      - mastoid process H95.89
      - metabolic E89.89
      - musculoskeletal structure M96.89
      - nervous system G97.82
      - respiratory system J95.89
      - skin and subcutaneous tissue L76.82
      - spleen D78.89
  - pregnancy NEC *—see* Pregnancy, complicated by
  - prosthetic device or implant T85.9
    - bile duct *—see* Complications, bile duct implant
    - breast *—see* Complications, breast implant
    - bulking agent
      - ureteral
        - erosion T83.714
        - exposure T83.724
      - urethral
        - erosion T83.713
        - exposure T83.723
    - cardiac and vascular NEC *—see* Complications, cardiovascular device or implant
    - corneal transplant *—see* Complications, graft, cornea
    - electronic nervous system stimulator *—see* Complications, electronic stimulator device
    - epidural infusion catheter *—see* Complications, catheter, epidural
    - esophageal anti-reflux device *—see* Complications, esophageal anti-reflux device
    - genital organ or tract *—see* Complications, genitourinary, device or implant, genital tract
      - specified NEC T83.79
    - heart valve *—see* Complications, heart, valve, prosthesis

- **Complication** *(Continued)*
  - prosthetic device or implant *(Continued)*
    - infection or inflammation T85.79
      - intestine transplant T86.852
      - liver transplant T86.43
      - lung transplant T86.812
      - pancreas transplant T86.892
      - skin graft T86.822
    - intraocular lens *—see* Complications, intraocular lens
    - intraperitoneal (dialysis) catheter *—see* Complication(s), catheter, intraperitoneal dialysis
    - joint *—see* Complications, joint prosthesis, internal
    - mechanical NEC T85.698
      - dialysis catheter (vascular) *—see also* Complication, catheter, dialysis, mechanical
        - peritoneal *—see* Complication(s), catheter, intraperitoneal dialysis
      - gastrointestinal device T85.598
      - ocular device T85.398
      - subdural (infusion) catheter T85.690
      - suture, permanent T85.692
        - that for bone repair *—see* Complications, fixation device, internal (orthopedic), mechanical
      - ventricular shunt
        - breakdown T85.01
        - displacement T85.02
        - leakage T85.03
        - malposition T85.02
        - obstruction T85.09
        - perforation T85.09
        - protrusion T85.09
        - specified NEC T85.09
    - mesh
      - erosion (to surrounding organ or tissue) T83.718
        - urethral (into pelvic floor muscles) T83.712
        - vaginal (into pelvic floor muscles) T83.711
      - exposure (into surrounding organ or tissue) T83.728
        - urethral (through urethral wall) T83.722
        - vaginal (into vagina) (through vaginal wall) T83.721
    - orbital *—see* Complications, orbital prosthesis
    - penile T83.9
      - embolism T83.81
      - fibrosis T83.82
      - hemorrhage T83.83
      - infection and inflammation T83.61
      - mechanical
        - breakdown T83.410
        - displacement T83.420
        - leakage T83.490
        - malposition T83.420
        - obstruction T83.490
        - perforation T83.490
        - protrusion T83.490
        - specified NEC T83.490
      - pain T83.84
      - specified type NEC T83.89
      - stenosis T83.85
      - thrombosis T83.86
    - prosthetic materials NEC
      - erosion (to surrounding organ or tissue) T83.718
      - exposure (into surrounding organ or tissue) T83.728
    - skin graft T86.829
      - artificial skin or decellularized allodermis
        - embolism T85.818
        - fibrosis T85.828
        - hemorrhage T85.838
        - infection and inflammation T85.79
        - mechanical
          - breakdown T85.613
          - displacement T85.623
          - malfunction T85.613
          - malposition T85.623
          - obstruction T85.693
          - perforation T85.693
          - protrusion T85.693
          - specified NEC T85.693
        - pain T85.848
        - specified type NEC T85.898
        - stenosis T85.858
        - thrombosis T85.868

- **Complication** *(Continued)*
  - prosthetic device or implant *(Continued)*
    - skin graft *(Continued)*
      - failure T86.821
      - infection T86.822
      - rejection T86.82Ø
      - specified NEC T86.828
    - sling
      - urethral (female) (male)
        - erosion T83.712
        - exposure T83.722
    - specified NEC T85.9
      - embolism T85.818
      - fibrosis T85.828
      - hemorrhage T85.838
      - infection and inflammation T85.79
      - mechanical
        - breakdown T85.618
        - displacement T85.628
        - leakage T85.638
        - malfunction T85.618
        - malposition T85.628
        - obstruction T85.698
        - perforation T85.698
        - protrusion T85.698
        - specified NEC T85.698
      - pain T85.848
      - specified type NEC T85.898
      - stenosis T85.858
      - thrombosis T85.868
    - subdural infusion catheter —*see* Complications, catheter, subdural
    - sutures —*see* Complications, sutures
    - urinary organ or tract NEC —*see* Complications, genitourinary, device or implant, urinary system
    - vascular —*see* Complications, cardiovascular device, graft or implant
    - ventricular shunt —*see* Complications, ventricular shunt (device)
  - puerperium —*see* Puerperal
  - puncture, spinal G97.1
    - cerebrospinal fluid leak G97.Ø
    - headache or reaction G97.1
  - pyelogram N99.89
  - radiation
    - kyphosis M96.2
    - scoliosis M96.5
  - reattached
    - extremity (infection) (rejection)
      - lower T87.1X-●
      - upper T87.ØX-●
    - specified body part NEC T87.2
  - reconstructed breast
    - asymmetry between native and reconstructed breast N65.1
    - deformity N65.Ø
    - disproportion between native and reconstructed breast N65.1
    - excess tissue N65.Ø
    - misshappen N65.Ø
  - reimplant NEC —*see also* Complications, prosthetic device or implant
    - limb (infection) (rejection) —*see* Complications, reattached, extremity
    - organ (partial) (total) —*see* Complications, transplant
    - prosthetic device NEC —*see* Complications, prosthetic device
  - renal N28.9
    - allograft —*see* Complications, transplant, kidney
    - dialysis —*see* Complications, dialysis
  - respirator
    - mechancial J95.85Ø
      - specified NEC J95.859
  - respiratory system J98.9
    - device, implant or graft —*see* Complication, prosthetic device or implant, specified NEC
    - lung transplant —*see* Complications, prosthetic device or implant, lung transplant
    - postoperative J95.89
      - air leak J95.812
      - Mendelson's syndrome (chemical pneumonitis) J95.4
      - pneumothorax J95.811
      - pulmonary insufficiency (acute) (after nonthoracic surgery) J95.2
        - chronic J95.3
        - following thoracic surgery J95.1

- **Complication** *(Continued)*
  - respiratory system *(Continued)*
    - postoperative *(Continued)*
      - respiratory failure (acute) J95.821
        - acute and chronic J95.822
      - specified NEC J95.89
      - subglottic stenosis J95.5
      - tracheostomy complication —*see* Complications, tracheostomy
    - therapy T81.89
  - sedation during labor and delivery O74.9
    - cardiac O74.2
    - central nervous system O74.3
    - pulmonary NEC O74.1
  - shunt —*see also* Complications, prosthetic device or implant
    - arteriovenous —*see* Complications, arteriovenous, shunt
    - ventricular (communicating) —*see* Complications, ventricular shunt
  - skin
    - graft T86.829
      - failure T86.821
      - infection T86.822
      - rejection T86.82Ø
      - specified type NEC T86.828
  - spinal
    - anesthesia —*see* Complications, anesthesia, spinal
    - catheter (epidural) (subdural) —*see* Complications, catheter
    - puncture or tap G97.1
      - cerebrospinal fluid leak G97.Ø
      - headache or reaction G97.1
  - stent
    - bile duct —*see* Complications, bile duct prosthesis
    - ureteral indwelling
      - breakdown T83.112
      - displacement T83.122
      - leakage T83.192
      - malposition T83.122
      - obstruction T83.192
      - perforation T83.192
      - protrusion T83.192
      - specified NEC T83.192
    - urinary (ileal conduit) (nephroureteral) T83.193
      - embolism T83.81
      - fibrosis T83.82
      - hemorrhage T83.83
      - infection and inflammation T83.593
      - mechanical
        - breakdown T83.113
        - displacement T83.123
        - leakage T83.193
        - malposition T83.123
        - obstruction T83.193
        - perforation T83.193
        - protrusion T83.193
        - specified NEC T83.193
      - pain T83.84
      - specified type NEC T83.89
      - stenosis T83.85
      - thrombosis T83.86
    - vascular
      - end stent stenosis —*see* Restenosis, stent
      - in stent stenosis —*see* Restenosis, stent
  - stoma
    - digestive tract
      - colostomy —*see* Complications, colostomy
      - enterostomy —*see* Complications, enterostomy
      - esophagostomy —*see* Complications, esophagostomy
      - gastrostomy —*see* Complications, gastrostomy
    - urinary tract N99.528
      - continent N99.538
        - hemorrhage N99.53Ø
        - herniation N99.533
        - infection N99.531
        - malfunction N99.532
        - specified type NEC N99.538
        - stenosis N99.534
      - cystostomy —*see* Complications, cystostomy
      - external NOS N99.528
      - hemorrhage N99.52Ø
      - herniation N99.523
      - incontinent N99.528
        - hemorrhage N99.52Ø
        - herniation N99.523

- **Complication** *(Continued)*
  - stoma *(Continued)*
    - urinary tracte *(Continued)*
      - incontinent *(Continued)*
        - infection N99.521
        - malfunction N99.522
        - specified type NEC N99.528
        - stenosis N99.524
      - infection N99.521
      - malfunction N99.522
      - specified type NEC N99.528
      - stenosis N99.524
  - stomach banding —*see* Complication(s), bariatric procedure
  - stomach stapling —*see* Complication(s), bariatric procedure
  - surgical material, nonabsorbable —*see* Complication, suture, permanent
  - surgical procedure (on) T81.9
    - amputation stump (late) —*see* Complications, amputation stump
    - cardiac —*see* Complications, circulatory system
    - cholesteatoma, recurrent —*see* Complications, postmastoidectomy, recurrent cholesteatoma
    - circulatory (early) —*see* Complications, circulatory system
    - digestive system —*see* Complications, gastrointestinal
    - dumping syndrome (postgastrectomy) K91.1
    - ear —*see* Complications, ear
    - elephantiasis or lymphedema I97.89
      - postmastectomy I97.2
    - emphysema (surgical) T81.82
    - endocrine —*see* Complications, endocrine
    - eye —*see* Complications, eye
    - fistula (persistent postoperative) T81.83
    - foreign body inadvertently left in wound (sponge) (suture) (swab) —*see* Foreign body, accidentally left during a procedure
    - gastrointestinal —*see* Complications, gastrointestinal
    - genitourinary NEC N99.89
    - hematoma
      - intraoperative —*see* Complication, intraoperative, hemorrhage
      - postprocedural —*see* Complication, postprocedural, hematoma
    - hemorrhage
      - intraoperative —*see* Complication, intraoperative, hemorrhage
      - postprocedural —*see* Complication, postprocedural, hemorrhage
    - hepatic failure K91.82
    - hyperglycemia (postpancreatectomy) E89.1
    - hypoinsulinemia (postpancreatectomy) E89.1
    - hypoparathyroidism (postparathyroidectomy) E89.2
    - hypopituitarism (posthypophysectomy) E89.3
    - hypothyroidism (post-thyroidectomy) E89.Ø
    - intestinal obstruction —*see also* Obstruction, intestine, postoperative K91.3Ø
    - intracranial hypotension following ventricular shunting (ventriculostomy) G97.2
    - lymphedema I97.89
      - postmastectomy I97.2
    - malabsorption (postsurgical) NEC K91.2
      - osteoporosis —*see* Osteoporosis, postsurgical malabsorption
    - mastoidectomy cavity NEC —*see* Complications, postmastoidectomy
    - metabolic E89.89
      - specified NEC E89.89
    - musculoskeletal —*see* Complications, musculoskeletal system
    - nervous system (central) (peripheral) —*see* Complications, nervous system
    - ovarian failure E89.4Ø
      - asymptomatic E89.4Ø
      - symptomatic E89.41
    - peripheral vascular —*see* Complications, surgical procedure, vascular
    - postcardiotomy syndrome I97.Ø
    - postcholecystectomy syndrome K91.5
    - postcommissurotomy syndrome I97.Ø

▶ New ➡ Revised ~~deleted~~ Deleted ● Use Additional Character(s)

C

▶ New ➡ Revised ~~deleted~~ Deleted ● Use Additional Character(s)

C

C

Contusion *(Continued)*
- intra-abdominal organ S36.92
  - colon —*see* Injury, intestine, large, contusion
  - liver S36.112
  - pancreas —*see* Contusion, pancreas
  - rectum S36.62
  - small intestine —*see* Injury, intestine, small, contusion
  - specified organ NEC S36.892
  - spleen —*see* Contusion, spleen
  - stomach S36.32
- iris (eye) —*see* Contusion, eyeball
- jaw S00.83
- jejunum S36.428
- kidney S37.01-•
  - major (greater than 2 cm) S37.02-•
  - minor (less than 2 cm) S37.01-•
- knee S80.0-•
- labium (majus) (minus) S30.23
- lacrimal apparatus, gland or sac S05.8X-•
- larynx S10.0
- leg (lower) S80.1-•
  - knee —*see* Contusion, knee
- lens —*see* Contusion, eyeball
- lip S00.531
- liver S36.112
- lower back S30.0
- lumbar region S30.0
- lung S27.329
  - bilateral S27.322
  - unilateral S27.321
- malar region S00.83
- mastoid region S00.83
- membrane, brain —*see* Injury, intracranial, diffuse
  - focal —*see* Injury, intracranial, focal
- mesentery S36.892
- mesosalpinx S37.892
- mouth S00.532
- muscle —*see* Contusion, by site
- nail
  - finger —*see* Contusion, finger, with damage to nail
  - toe —*see* Contusion, toe, with damage to nail
- nasal S00.33
- neck S10.93
  - specified site NEC S10.83
  - throat S10.0
- nerve —*see* Injury, nerve
- newborn P54.5
- nose S00.33
- occipital
  - lobe (brain) —*see* Injury, intracranial, diffuse
    - focal —*see* Injury, intracranial, focal
  - region (scalp) S00.03
- orbit (region) (tissues) S05.1-•
- ovary S37.429
  - bilateral S37.422
  - unilateral S37.421
- palate S00.532
- pancreas S36.229
  - body S36.221
  - head S36.220
  - tail S36.222
- parietal
  - lobe (brain) —*see* Injury, intracranial, diffuse
    - focal —*see* Injury, intracranial, focal
  - region (scalp) S00.03
- pelvic organ S37.92
  - adrenal gland S37.812
  - bladder S37.22
  - fallopian tube —*see* Contusion, fallopian tube
  - kidney —*see* Contusion, kidney
  - ovary —*see* Contusion, ovary
  - prostate S37.822
  - specified organ NEC S37.892
  - ureter S37.12
  - urethra S37.32
  - uterus S37.62
- pelvis S30.0
- penis S30.21
- perineum
  - female S30.23
  - male S30.0
- periocular area S00.1-•
- peritoneum S36.81
- periurethral tissue —*see* Contusion, urethra
- pharynx S10.0
- pinna —*see* Contusion, ear

Contusion *(Continued)*
- popliteal space —*see* Contusion, knee
- prepuce S30.21
- prostate S37.822
- pubic region S30.1
- pudendum
  - female S30.202
  - male S30.201
- quadriceps femoris —*see* Contusion, thigh
- rectum S36.62
- retroperitoneum S36.892
- round ligament S37.892
- sacral region S30.0
- scalp S00.03
  - due to birth injury P12.3
- scapular region —*see* Contusion, shoulder
- sclera —*see* Contusion, eyeball
- scrotum S30.22
- seminal vesicle S37.892
- shoulder S40.01-•
- skin NEC T14.8
- small intestine —*see* Injury, intestine, small, contusion
- spermatic cord S30.22
- spinal cord —*see* Injury, spinal cord, by region
  - cauda equina S34.3
  - conus medullaris S34.139
- spleen S36.029
  - major S36.021
  - minor S36.020
- sternal region S20.219
- stomach S36.32
- subconjunctival S05.1-•
- subcutaneous NEC T14.8
- submaxillary region S00.83
- submental region S00.83
- subperiosteal NEC T14.8
- subungual
  - finger —*see* Contusion, finger, with damage to nail
  - toe —*see* Contusion, toe, with damage to nail
- supraclavicular fossa S10.83
- supraorbital S00.83
- suprarenal gland S37.812
- temple (region) S00.83
- temporal
  - lobe (brain) —*see* Injury, intracranial, diffuse
    - focal —*see* Injury, intracranial, focal
  - region S00.83
- testis S30.22
- thigh S70.1-•
- thorax (wall) S20.20
  - back S20.22-•
  - front S20.21-•
- throat S10.0
- thumb S60.01-•
  - with damage to nail S60.11-•
- toe(s) (lesser) S90.12-•
  - with damage to nail S90.22-•
  - great S90.11-•
    - with damage to nail S90.21-•
- tongue S00.532
- trachea (cervical) S10.0
  - thoracic S27.52
- tunica vaginalis S30.22
- tympanum, tympanic membrane —*see* Contusion, ear
- ureter S37.12
- urethra S37.32
- urinary organ NEC S37.892
- uterus S37.62
- uvula S00.532
- vagina S30.23
- vas deferens S37.892
- vesical S37.22
- vocal cord(s) S10.0
- vulva S30.23
- wrist S60.21-•

Conus (congenital) (any type) Q14.8
- cornea —*see* Keratoconus
- medullaris syndrome G95.81

Conversion hysteria, neurosis or reaction F44.9

Converter, tuberculosis (test reaction) R76.11

Conviction (legal), anxiety concerning Z65.0
- with imprisonment Z65.1

Convulsions (idiopathic) —*see also* Seizure(s) R56.9
- apoplectiform (cerebral ischemia) I67.82
- dissociative F44.5

Convulsions *(Continued)*
- epileptic —*see* Epilepsy
- epileptiform, epileptoid —*see* Epilepsy
- ether (anesthetic) —*see* Table of Drugs and Chemicals, by drug
- febrile R56.00
  - with status epilepticus G40.901
  - complex R56.01
    - with status epilepticus G40.901
  - simple R56.00
- hysterical F44.5
- infantile P90
  - epilepsy —*see* Epilepsy
- jacksonian —*see* Epilepsy, localization-related, symptomatic, with simple partial seizures
- myoclonic G25.3
- newborn P90
- obstetrical (nephritic) (uremic) —*see* Eclampsia
- paretic A52.17
- post traumatic R56.1
- psychomotor —*see* Epilepsy, localization-related, symptomatic, with complex partial seizures
- recurrent R56.9
- reflex R25.8
- scarlatinal A38.8
- tetanus, tetanic —*see* Tetanus
- thymic E32.8

Convulsive —*see also* Convulsions

Cooley's anemia D56.1

Coolie itch B76.9

Cooper's
- disease —*see* Mastopathy, cystic
- hernia —*see* Hernia, abdomen, specified site NEC

Copra itch B88.0

Coprophagy F50.89

Coprophobia F40.298

Coproporphyria, hereditary E80.29

Cor
- biloculare Q20.8
- bovis, bovinum —*see* Hypertrophy, cardiac
- pulmonale I27.81
  - acute I26.09
    - without pulmonary embolism I27.81
  - chronic I27.81
    - with chronic pulmonary embolism I27.82
- triatriatum, triatrium Q24.2
- triloculare Q20.8
  - biatrium Q20.4
  - biventriculare Q21.19

Corbus' disease (gangrenous balanitis) N48.1

Cord —*see also* condition
- around neck
  - complicating delivery O69.81
    - with compression O69.1
- bladder G95.89
  - tabetic A52.19

Cordis ectopia Q24.8

Corditis (spermatic) N49.1

Corectopia Q13.2

Cori's disease (glycogen storage) E74.03

Corkhandler's disease or lung J67.3

Corkscrew esophagus K22.4

Corkworker's disease or lung J67.3

Corn (infected) L84

Cornea —*see also* condition
- donor Z52.5
- plana Q13.4

Cornelia de Lange syndrome Q87.19

Cornu cutaneum L85.8

Cornual gestation or pregnancy O00.80
- with intrauterine pregnancy O00.81

Coronary (artery) —*see* condition

Coronavirus (infection)
- as cause of disease classified elsewhere B97.29
- coronavirus-19 U07.1
- COVID-19 U07.1
- SARS-associated B97.21

Corpora —*see also* condition
- amylacea, prostate N42.89
- cavernosa —*see* condition

Corpulence —*see* Obesity

Corpus —*see* condition

Corrected transposition Q20.5

Corrosion (injury) (acid) (caustic) (chemical) (lime) (external) (internal) T30.4
- abdomen, abdominal (muscle) (wall) T21.42
  - first degree T21.52
  - second degree T21.62
  - third degree T21.72

C

C

Corrosion *(Continued)*
toe T25.439
first degree T25.539
left T25.432
first degree T25.532
second degree T25.632
third degree T25.732
right T25.431
first degree T25.531
second degree T25.631
third degree T25.731
second degree T25.639
third degree T25.739
tongue T28.5
tonsil(s) T28.5
total body —*see* Corrosion, multiple body regions
trachea T27.4
with lung T27.5
trunk T21.4Ø
abdominal wall —*see* Corrosion, abdominal wall
anus —*see* Corrosion, buttock
axilla —*see* Corrosion, upper limb
back —*see* Corrosion, back
breast —*see* Corrosion, chest wall
buttock —*see* Corrosion, buttock
chest wall —*see* Corrosion, chest wall
first degree T21.5Ø
flank —*see* Corrosion, abdominal wall
genital
female —*see* Corrosion, genital organs, external, female
male —*see* Corrosion, genital organs, external, male
groin —*see* Corrosion, abdominal wall
interscapular region —*see* Corrosion, back, upper
labia —*see* Corrosion, genital organs, external, female
lower back —*see* Corrosion, back
penis —*see* Corrosion, genital organs, external, male
perineum
female —*see* Corrosion, genital organs, external, female
male —*see* Corrosion, genital organs, external, male
scapular region —*see* Corrosion, upper limb
scrotum —*see* Corrosion, genital organs, external, male
second degree T21.6Ø
shoulder —*see* Corrosion, upper limb
specified site NEC T21.49
first degree T21.59
second degree T21.69
third degree T21.79
testes —*see* Corrosion, genital organs, external, male
third degree T21.7Ø
upper back —*see* Corrosion, back, upper
vagina T28.8
vulva —*see* Corrosion, genital organs, external, female
unspecified site with extent of body surface involved specified
less than 1Ø percent T32.Ø
1Ø-19 percent (Ø-9 percent third degree) T32.1Ø
with 1Ø-19 percent third degree T32.11
2Ø-29 percent (Ø-9 percent third degree) T32.2Ø
with
1Ø-19 percent third degree T32.21
2Ø-29 percent third degree T32.22
3Ø-39 percent (Ø-9 percent third degree) T32.3Ø
with
1Ø-19 percent third degree T32.31
2Ø-29 percent third degree T32.32
3Ø-39 percent third degree T32.33
4Ø-49 percent (Ø-9 percent third degree) T32.4Ø
with
1Ø-19 percent third degree T32.41
2Ø-29 percent third degree T32.42
3Ø-39 percent third degree T32.43
4Ø-49 percent third degree T32.44
5Ø-59 percent (Ø-9 percent third degree) T32.5Ø
with
1Ø-19 percent third degree T32.51
2Ø-29 percent third degree T32.52
3Ø-39 percent third degree T32.53
4Ø-49 percent third degree T32.54
5Ø-59 percent third degree T32.55

Corrosion *(Continued)*
unspecified site with extent of body surface involved specified *(Continued)*
6Ø-69 percent (Ø-9 percent third degree) T32.6Ø
with
1Ø-19 percent third degree T32.61
2Ø-29 percent third degree T32.62
3Ø-39 percent third degree T32.63
4Ø-49 percent third degree T32.64
5Ø-59 percent third degree T32.65
6Ø-69 percent third degree T32.66
7Ø-79 percent (Ø-9 percent third degree) T32.7Ø
with
1Ø-19 percent third degree T32.71
2Ø-29 percent third degree T32.72
3Ø-39 percent third degree T32.73
4Ø-49 percent third degree T32.74
5Ø-59 percent third degree T32.75
6Ø-69 percent third degree T32.76
7Ø-79 percent third degree T32.77
8Ø-89 percent (Ø-9 percent third degree) T32.8Ø
with
1Ø-19 percent third degree T32.81
2Ø-29 percent third degree T32.82
3Ø-39 percent third degree T32.83
4Ø-49 percent third degree T32.84
5Ø-59 percent third degree T32.85
6Ø-69 percent third degree T32.86
7Ø-79 percent third degree T32.87
8Ø-89 percent third degree T32.88
9Ø percent or more (Ø-9 percent third degree) T32.9Ø
with
1Ø-19 percent third degree T32.91
2Ø-29 percent third degree T32.92
3Ø-39 percent third degree T32.93
4Ø-49 percent third degree T32.94
5Ø-59 percent third degree T32.95
6Ø-69 percent third degree T32.96
7Ø-79 percent third degree T32.97
8Ø-89 percent third degree T32.98
9Ø-99 percent third degree T32.99
upper limb (axilla) (scapular region) T22.4Ø
above elbow —*see* Corrosion, above elbow
axilla —*see* Corrosion, axilla
elbow —*see* Corrosion, elbow
first degree T22.5Ø
forearm —*see* Corrosion, forearm
hand —*see* Corrosion, hand
interscapular region —*see* Corrosion, back, upper
multiple sites T22.499
first degree T22.599
left T22.492
first degree T22.592
second degree T22.692
third degree T22.792
right T22.491
first degree T22.591
second degree T22.691
third degree T22.791
second degree T22.699
third degree T22.799
scapular region —*see* Corrosion, scapular region
second degree T22.6Ø
shoulder —*see* Corrosion, shoulder
third degree T22.7Ø
wrist —*see* Corrosion, hand
uterus T28.8
vagina T28.8
vulva —*see* Corrosion, genital organs, external, female
wrist T23.479
first degree T23.579
left T23.472
first degree T23.572
second degree T23.672
third degree T23.772
multiple sites with hand T23.499
first degree T23.599
left T23.492
first degree T23.592
second degree T23.692
third degree T23.792
right T23.491
first degree T23.591
second degree T23.691
third degree T23.791
second degree T23.699
third degree T23.799

Corrosion *(Continued)*
wrist *(Continued)*
right T23.471
first degree T23.571
second degree T23.671
third degree T23.771
second degree T23.679
third degree T23.779
Corrosive burn —*see* Corrosion
Corsican fever —*see* Malaria
Cortical —*see* condition
Cortico-adrenal —*see* condition
Coryza (acute) JØØ
with grippe or influenza —*see* Influenza, with, respiratory manifestations NEC
syphilitic
congenital (chronic) A5Ø.Ø5
Co-sleeping, child-caregiver Z72.823
Costen's syndrome or complex M26.69
Costiveness —*see* Constipation
Costochondritis M94.Ø
Cot death R99
Cotard's syndrome F22
Cotia virus BØ8.8
Cotton wool spots (retinal) H35.81
~~Cotungo's disease —see Sciatica~~
▶ **Cotugno disease** —*see* Sciatica
Cough (affected) (epidemic) (nervous) RØ5.9
with hemorrhage —*see* Hemoptysis
acute RØ5.1
bronchial RØ5.8
with grippe or influenza —*see* Influenza, with, respiratory manifestations NEC
chronic RØ5.3
functional F45.8
hysterical F45.8
laryngeal, spasmodic RØ5.8
paroxysmal, due to Bordetella pertussis (without pneumonia) A37.ØØ
with pneumonia A37.Ø1
persistent RØ5.3
refractory RØ5.3
psychogenic F45.8
smokers' J41.Ø
specified NEC RØ5.8
subacute RØ5.2
syncope RØ5.4
tea taster's B49
unexplained RØ5.3
Counseling (for) Z71.9
abuse NEC
perpetrator Z69.82
victim Z69.81
alcohol abuser Z71.41
family Z71.42
child abuse
nonparental
perpetrator Z69.Ø21
victim Z69.Ø2Ø
parental
perpetrator Z69.Ø11
victim Z69.Ø1Ø
consanguinity Z71.89
contraceptive Z3Ø.Ø9
dietary Z71.3
drug abuser Z71.51
family member Z71.52
exercise Z71.82
family Z71.89
fertility preservation (prior to cancer therapy) (prior to removal of gonads) Z31.62
for non-attending third party Z71.Ø
related to sexual behavior or orientation Z7Ø.2
genetic
nonprocreative Z71.83
procreative NEC Z31.5
gestational carrier Z31.7
health (advice) (education) (instruction) —*see* Counseling, medical
risk for travel (international) Z71.84
human immunodeficiency virus (HIV) Z71.7
immunization safety Z71.85
impotence Z7Ø.1
insulin pump use Z46.81
medical (for) Z71.9
boarding school resident Z59.3
consanguinity Z71.89
feared complaint and no disease found Z71.1
human immunodeficiency virus (HIV) Z 71.7

Crush, crushed, crushing *(Continued)*
back, lower S38.1
buttock S38.1
cheek SØ7.Ø
chest S28.Ø
cranium SØ7.1
ear SØ7.Ø
elbow S57.Ø-●
extremity
lower
ankle —*see* Crush, ankle
below knee —*see* Crush, leg
foot —*see* Crush, foot
hip —*see* Crush, hip
knee —*see* Crush, knee
thigh —*see* Crush, thigh
toe —*see* Crush, toe
upper
below elbow S67.9-●
elbow —*see* Crush, elbow
finger —*see* Crush, finger
forearm —*see* Crush, forearm
hand —*see* Crush, hand
thumb —*see* Crush, thumb
upper arm —*see* Crush, arm
wrist —*see* Crush, wrist
face SØ7.Ø
finger(s) S67.1-●
with hand (and wrist) —*see* Crush, hand, specified site NEC
index S67.19-●
little S67.19-●
middle S67.19-●
ring S67.19-●
thumb —*see* Crush, thumb
foot S97.8-●
toe —*see* Crush, toe
forearm S57.8-●
genitalia, external
female S38.ØØ2
vagina S38.Ø3
vulva S38.Ø3
male S38.ØØ1
penis S38.Ø1
scrotum S38.Ø2
testis S38.Ø2
hand (except fingers alone) S67.2-●
with wrist S67.4-●
head SØ7.9
specified NEC SØ7.8
heel —*see* Crush, foot
hip S77.Ø-●
with thigh S77.2-●
internal organ (abdomen, chest, or pelvis) NEC T14.8
knee S87.Ø-●
labium (majus) (minus) S38.Ø3
larynx S17.Ø
leg (lower) S87.8-●
knee —*see* Crush, knee
lip SØ7.Ø
lower
back S38.1
leg —*see* Crush, leg
neck S17.9
nerve —*see* Injury, nerve
nose SØ7.Ø
pelvis S38.1
penis S38.Ø1
scalp SØ7.8
scapular region —*see* Crush, arm
scrotum S38.Ø2
severe, unspecified site T14.8
shoulder (and upper arm) —*see* Crush, arm
skull SØ7.1
syndrome (complication of trauma) T79.5
testis S38.Ø2
thigh S77.1-●
with hip S77.2-●
throat S17.8
thumb S67.Ø-●
with hand (and wrist) —*see* Crush, hand, specified site NEC
toe(s) S97.1Ø-●
great S97.11-●
lesser S97.12-●
trachea S17.Ø
vagina S38.Ø3
vulva S38.Ø3
wrist S67.3-●
with hand S67.4-●

Crusta lactea L21.Ø
Crusts R23.4
Crutch paralysis —*see* Injury, brachial plexus
Cruveilhier-Baumgarten cirrhosis, disease or syndrome K74.69
Cruveilhier's atrophy or disease G12.8
Crying (constant) (continuous) (excessive)
child, adolescent, or adult R45.83
infant (baby) (newborn) R68.11
Cryofibrinogenemia D89.2
Cryoglobulinemia (essential) (idiopathic) (mixed) (primary) (purpura) (secondary) (vasculitis) D89.1
with lung involvement D89.1 *[J99]*
Cryptitis (anal) (rectal) K62.89
Cryptococcosis, cryptococcus (infection) (neoformans) B45.9
bone B45.3
cerebral B45.1
cutaneous B45.2
disseminated B45.7
generalized B45.7
meningitis B45.1
meningocerebralis B45.1
osseous B45.3
pulmonary B45.Ø
skin B45.2
specified NEC B45.8
Cryptopapillitis (anus) K62.89
Cryptophthalmos Q11.2
syndrome Q87.Ø
Cryptorchid, cryptorchism, cryptorchidism Q53.9
bilateral Q53.2Ø
abdominal Q53.211
perineal Q53.22
unilateral Q53.1Ø
abdominal Q53.111
perineal Q53.12
Cryptosporidiosis AØ7.2
hepatobiliary B88.8
respiratory B88.8
Cryptostromosis J67.6
Crystalluria R82.998
Cubitus
congenital Q68.8
valgus (acquired) M21.Ø-●
congenital Q68.8
sequelae (late effect) of rickets E64.3
varus (acquired) M21.1-●
congenital Q68.8
sequelae (late effect) of rickets E64.3
Cultural deprivation or shock Z6Ø.3
Curling esophagus K22.4
Curling's ulcer —*see* Ulcer, peptic, acute
Curschmann (-Batten) (-Steinert) disease or syndrome G71.11
Curse, Ondine's —*see* Apnea, sleep
Curvature
organ or site, congenital NEC —*see* Distortion
penis (lateral) Q55.61
Pott's (spinal) A18.Ø1
radius, idiopathic, progressive (congenital) Q74.Ø
spine (acquired) (angular) (idiopathic) (incorrect) (postural) —*see* Dorsopathy, deforming
congenital Q67.5
due to or associated with
Charcot-Marie-Tooth disease —*see also* subcategory M49.8 G6Ø.Ø
osteitis
deformans M88.88
fibrosa cystica —*see also* subcategory M49.8 E21.Ø
tuberculosis (Pott's curvature) A18.Ø1
sequelae (late effect) of rickets E64.3
tuberculous A18.Ø1
Cushingoid due to steroid therapy E24.2
correct substance properly administered —*see* Table of Drugs and Chemicals, by drug, adverse effect
overdose or wrong substance given or taken —*see* Table of Drugs and Chemicals, by drug, poisoning
Cushing's
syndrome or disease E24.9
drug-induced E24.2
iatrogenic E24.2
pituitary-dependent E24.Ø
specified NEC E24.8
ulcer —*see* Ulcer, peptic, acute
Cusp, Carabelli - omit code

Cut (external) —*see also* Laceration
muscle —*see* Injury, muscle
Cutaneous —*see also* condition
hemorrhage R23.3
larva migrans B76.9
Cutis —*see also* condition
hyperelastica Q82.8
acquired L57.4
laxa (hyperelastica) —*see* Dermatolysis
marmorata R23.8
osteosis L94.2
pendula —*see* Dermatolysis
rhomboidalis nuchae L57.2
verticis gyrata Q82.8
acquired L91.8
Cyanosis R23.Ø
due to
patent foramen botalli Q21.12
persistent foramen ovale Q21.12
enterogenous D74.8
paroxysmal digital —*see* Raynaud's disease
with gangrene I73.Ø1
retina, retinal H35.89
Cyanotic heart disease I24.9
congenital Q24.9
Cycle
anovulatory N97.Ø
menstrual, irregular N92.6
Cyclencephaly QØ4.9
Cyclical vomiting, in migraine (*see also* Vomiting, cyclical) G43.AØ
psychogenic F5Ø.89
Cyclitis —*see also* Iridocyclitis H2Ø.9
chronic —*see* Iridocyclitis, chronic
Fuchs' heterochromic H2Ø.81-●
granulomatous —*see* Iridocyclitis, chronic
lens-induced —*see* Iridocyclitis, lens-induced
posterior H3Ø.2-●
Cycloid personality F34.Ø
Cyclophoria H5Ø.54
Cyclopia, cyclops Q87.Ø
Cyclopism Q87.Ø
Cyclosporiasis AØ7.4
Cyclothymia F34.Ø
Cyclothymic personality F34.Ø
Cyclotropia H5Ø.41-●
Cylindroma —*see also* Neoplasm, malignant, by site
eccrine dermal —*see* Neoplasm, skin, benign
skin —*see* Neoplasm, skin, benign
Cylindruria R82.998
Cynanche
diphtheritic A36.2
tonsillaris J36
Cynophobia F4Ø.218
Cynorexia R63.2
Cyphosis —*see* Kyphosis
Cyprus fever —*see* Brucellosis
Cyst (colloid) (mucous) (simple) (retention)
adenoid (infected) J35.8
adrenal gland E27.8
congenital Q89.1
air, lung J98.4
allantoic Q64.4
alveolar process (jaw bone) M27.4Ø
amnion, amniotic O41.8X-●
aneurysmal M27.49
anterior
chamber (eye) —*see* Cyst, iris
nasopalatine KØ9.1
antrum J34.1
anus K62.89
apical (tooth) (periodontal) KØ4.8
appendix K38.8
arachnoid, brain (acquired) G93.Ø
congenital QØ4.6
arytenoid J38.7
Baker's M71.2-●
ruptured M66.Ø
tuberculous A18.Ø2
Bartholin's gland N75.Ø
bile duct (common) (hepatic) K83.5
bladder (multiple) (trigone) N32.89
blue dome (breast) —*see* Cyst, breast
bone (local) NEC M85.6Ø
aneurysmal M85.5Ø
ankle M85.57-●
foot M85.57-●
forearm M85.53-●
hand M85.54-●
jaw M27.49

C

C

D

Cystitis (*Continued*)
 echinococcal
 granulosus B67.39
 multilocularis B67.69
 emphysematous —*see* Cystitis, specified type
 NEC
 encysted —*see* Cystitis, specified type NEC
 eosinophilic —*see* Cystitis, specified type NEC
 follicular —*see* Cystitis, of trigone
 gangrenous —*see* Cystitis, specified type NEC
 glandularis —*see* Cystitis, specified type NEC
 gonococcal A54.01
 incrusted —*see* Cystitis, specified type NEC
 interstitial (chronic) —*see* Cystitis, chronic,
 interstitial
 irradiation N30.40
 with hematuria N30.41
 irritation —*see* Cystitis, specified type NEC
 malignant —*see* Cystitis, specified type NEC
 of trigone N30.30
 with hematuria N30.31
 panmural —*see* Cystitis, chronic, interstitial
 polyposa —*see* Cystitis, specified type NEC
 prostatic N41.3
 puerperal (postpartum) O86.22
 radiation —*see* Cystitis, irradiation
 specified type NEC N30.80
 with hematuria N30.81
 subacute —*see* Cystitis, chronic
 submucous —*see* Cystitis, chronic, interstitial
 syphilitic (late) A52.76
 trichomonal A59.03
 tuberculous A18.12
 ulcerative —*see* Cystitis, chronic, interstitial
Cystocele (-urethrocele)
 female N81.10
 with prolapse of uterus —*see* Prolapse, uterus
 lateral N81.12
 midline N81.11
 paravaginal N81.12
 in pregnancy or childbirth O34.8-●
 causing obstructed labor O65.5
 male N32.89
Cystolithiasis N21.0
Cystoma —*see also* Neoplasm, benign, by site
 endometrial, ovary N80.10-●
 mucinous
 specified site —*see* Neoplasm, benign, by site
 unspecified site D27.9
 serous
 specified site —*see* Neoplasm, benign, by site
 unspecified site D27.9
 simple (ovary) N83.29-●
Cystoplegia N31.2
Cystoptosis N32.89
Cystopyelitis —*see* Pyelonephritis
Cystorrhagia N32.89
Cystosarcoma phyllodes D48.6-●
 benign D24-●
 malignant —*see* Neoplasm, breast, malignant
Cystostomy
 attention to Z43.5
 complication —*see* Complications, cystostomy
 status Z93.50
 appendico-vesicostomy Z93.52
 cutaneous Z93.51
 specified NEC Z93.59
Cystourethritis —*see* Urethritis
Cystourethrocele —*see also* Cystocele
 female N81.10
 with uterine prolapse —*see* Prolapse, uterus
 lateral N81.12
 midline N81.11
 paravaginal N81.12
 male N32.89
Cytomegalic inclusion disease
 congenital P35.1
Cytomegalovirus infection B25.9
Cytomycosis (reticuloendothelial) B39.4
Cytopenia D75.9
 refractory
 with multilineage dysplasia D46.A
 and ring sideroblasts (RCMD RS) D46.B
Czerny's disease (periodic hydrarthrosis of the
 knee) —*see* Effusion, joint, knee

Daae (-Finsen) disease (epidemic pleurodynia)
 B33.0
Dabney's grip B33.0
Da Costa's syndrome F45.8
Dacryoadenitis, dacryadenitis H04.00-●
 acute H04.01-●
 chronic H04.02-●
Dacryocystitis H04.30-●
 acute H04.32-●
 chronic H04.41-●
 neonatal P39.1
 phlegmonous H04.31-●
 syphilitic A52.71
 congenital (early) A50.01
 trachomatous, active A71.1
 sequelae (late effect) B94.0
~~Dacryocystoblennorrhea —see Inflammation, lacrimal, passages, chronic~~
▶Dacryocystoblennorrhea —*see* see Inflammation,
 lacrimal, passages, chronic
Dacryocystocele —*see* Disorder, lacrimal system,
 changes
Dacryolith, dacryolithiasis H04.51-●
Dacryoma —*see* Disorder, lacrimal system,
 changes
Dacryopericystitis —*see* Dacryocystitis
Dacryops H04.11-●
Dacryostenosis —*see also* Stenosis, lacrimal
 congenital Q10.5
Dactylitis
 bone —*see* Osteomyelitis
 sickle-cell D57.00
 Hb C D57.219
 Hb SS D57.00
 specified NEC D57.819
 skin L08.9
 syphilitic A52.77
 tuberculous A18.03
Dactylolysis spontanea (ainhum) L94.6
Dactylosymphysis Q70.9
 fingers —*see* Syndactylism, complex, fingers
 toes —*see* Syndactylism, complex, toes
Damage
 arteriosclerotic —*see* Arteriosclerosis
 brain (nontraumatic) G93.9
 anoxic, hypoxic G93.1
 resulting from a procedure G97.82
 child NEC G80.9
 due to birth injury P11.2
 cardiorenal (vascular) —*see* Hypertension,
 cardiorenal
 cerebral NEC —*see* Damage, brain
 coccyx, complicating delivery O71.6
 coronary —*see* Disease, heart, ischemic
 deep tissue, pressure-induced —*see also* L89 with
 final character .6
 eye, birth injury P15.3
 liver (nontraumatic) K76.9
 alcoholic K70.9
 due to drugs —*see* Disease, liver, toxic
 toxic —*see* Disease, liver, toxic
 lung
 dabbing (related) U07.0
 electronic cigarette (related) U07.0
 vaping (associated) (device) (product) (use)
 U07.0
 medication T88.7
 organ
 dabbing (related) U07.0
 electronic cigarette (related) U07.0
 vaping (associated) (device) (product) (use)
 U07.0
 pelvic
 joint or ligament, during delivery O71.6
 organ NEC
 during delivery O71.5
 following ectopic or molar pregnancy O08.6
 renal —*see* Disease, renal
 subendocardium, subendocardial —*see*
 Degeneration, myocardial
 vascular I99.9
Dana-Putnam syndrome (subacute combined
 sclerosis with pernicious anemia) —*see*
 Degeneration, combined
Danbolt (-Cross) syndrome (acrodermatitis
 enteropathica) E83.2
Dandruff L21.0
Dandy-Walker syndrome Q03.1
 with spina bifida —*see* Spina bifida

Danlos' syndrome (*see also* Syndrome, Ehler-
 Danlos) Q79.60
Darier (-White) disease (congenital) Q82.8
 meaning erythema annulare centrifugum L53.1
Darier-Roussy sarcoid D86.3
Darling's disease or histoplasmosis B39.4
Darwin's tubercle Q17.8
Dawson's (inclusion body) encephalitis A81.1
De Beurmann (-Gougerot) disease B42.1
De la Tourette's syndrome F95.2
De Lange's syndrome Q87.19
De Morgan's spots (senile angiomas) I78.1
De Quervain's
 disease (tendon sheath) M65.4
 syndrome E34.51
 thyroiditis (subacute granulomatous thyroiditis)
 E06.1
De Toni-Fanconi (-Debré) syndrome E72.09
 with cystinosis E72.04
Dead
 fetus, retained (mother) O36.4
 early pregnancy O02.1
 labyrinth —*see* subcategory H83.2
 ovum, retained O02.0
Deaf nonspeaking NEC H91.3
Deafmutism (acquired) (congenital) NEC H91.3
 hysterical F44.6
 syphilitic, congenital —*see also* subcategory
 H94.8 A50.09
Deafness (acquired) (complete) (hereditary)
 (partial) H91.9-●
 with blue sclera and fragility of bone Q78.0
 auditory fatigue —*see* Deafness, specified type NEC
 aviation T70.0
 nerve injury —*see* Injury, nerve, acoustic,
 specified type NEC
 boilermaker's —*see* subcategory H83.3
 central —*see* Deafness, sensorineural
 conductive H90.2
 and sensorineural
 mixed H90.8
 bilateral H90.6
 bilateral H90.0
 unilateral H90.1-●
 with restricted hearing on the contralateral
 side H90.A-●
 congenital H90.5
 with blue sclera and fragility of bone Q78.0
 due to toxic agents —*see* Deafness, ototoxic
 emotional (hysterical) F44.6
 functional (hysterical) F44.6
 high frequency H91.9-●
 hysterical F44.6
 low frequency H91.9-●
 mental R48.8
 mixed conductive and sensorineural H90.8
 bilateral H90.6
 unilateral H90.7-●
 nerve —*see* Deafness, sensorineural
 neural —*see* Deafness, sensorineural
 noise-induced —*see also* subcategory H83.3
 nerve injury —*see* Injury, nerve, acoustic,
 specified type NEC
 nonspeaking H91.3
 ototoxic —*see* subcategory H91.0
 perceptive —*see* Deafness, sensorineural
 psychogenic (hysterical) F44.6
 sensorineural H90.5
 and conductive
 mixed H90.8
 bilateral H90.6
 bilateral H90.3
 unilateral H90.4-●
 with restricted hearing on the contralateral
 side H90.A-●
 sensory —*see* Deafness, sensorineural
 specified type NEC —*see* subcategory H91.8
 sudden (idiopathic) H91.2-●
 syphilitic A52.15
 transient ischemic H93.01-●
 traumatic —*see* Injury, nerve, acoustic, specified
 type NEC
 word (developmental) H93.25
Death (cause unknown) (of) (unexplained)
 (unspecified cause) R99
 brain G93.82
 cardiac (sudden) (with successful
 resuscitation) —*see* Arrest, cardiac
 family history of Z82.41
 personal history of Z86.74
 family member (assumed) Z63.4

- **Defect, defective** *(Continued)*
  - osseous, major *(Continued)*
    - scapula M89.71-●
    - shoulder region M89.71-●
    - specified NEC M89.78
    - tarsus M89.77-●
    - thigh M89.75-●
    - tibia M89.76-●
    - toes M89.77-●
    - ulna M89.73-●
  - osteochondral NEC —*see also* Deformity M95.8-●
  - ostium
    - primum Q21.20
    - secundum Q21.11
  - peroxidase E80.3
  - placental blood supply —*see* Insufficiency, placental
  - platelets, qualitative D69.1
    - constitutional —*see* Disease, von Willebrand
  - postural NEC, spine —*see* Dorsopathy, deforming
  - qualitative, of von Willebrand factor
    - with
      - decreased platelet adhesion and selective deficiency of high-molecular-weight multimers (*see also* Disease, von Willebrand) D68.020
      - defective platelet adhesion with a normal size distribution of von Willebrand factor multimers (*see also* Disease, von Willebrand) D68.022
      - defective von Willebrand factor to factor VIII binding (*see also* Disease, von Willebrand) D68.023
      - high-molecular-weight von Willebrand factor loss (*see also* Disease, von Willebrand) D68.021
      - hyper-adhesive forms (*see also* Disease, von Willebrand) D68.021
      - increased affinity for platelet glycoprotein lb (*see also* Disease, von Willebrand) D68.021
      - markedly decreased affinity for factor VIII (*see also* Disease, von Willebrand) D68.023
    - in von Willebrand factor function, with no further subtyping (*see also* Disease, von Willebrand) D68.029
  - reduction
    - limb Q73.8
      - lower Q72.9-●
        - absence —*see* Agenesis, leg
          - foot —*see* Agenesis, foot
        - longitudinal
          - femur Q72.4-●
          - fibula Q72.6-●
          - tibia Q72.5-●
        - specified type NEC Q72.89-●
        - split foot Q72.7-●
      - specified type NEC Q73.8
      - upper Q71.9-●
        - absence —*see* Agenesis, arm
          - forearm —*see* Agenesis, forearm
          - hand —*see* Agenesis, hand
        - lobster-claw hand Q71.6-●
        - longitudinal
          - radius Q71.4-●
          - ulna Q71.5-●
        - specified type NEC Q71.89-●
  - renal pelvis Q63.8
    - obstructive Q62.39
  - respiratory system, congenital Q34.9
  - restoration, dental K08.50
    - specified NEC K08.59
  - retinal nerve bundle fibers H35.89
  - septal (heart) NOS Q21.9
    - acquired (atrial) (auricular) (ventricular) (old) I51.0
    - atrial (*see also* Defect, atrial septal) Q21.10
      - concurrent with acute myocardial infarction —*see* Infarct, myocardium
      - following acute myocardial infarction (current complication) I23.1
    - ventricular —*see also* Defect, ventricular septal Q21.0
  - sinus venosus (*see also* Defect, atrial septal, sinus venosus) Q21.16
  - speech —*see* Disorder, speech
    - developmental F80.9
    - specified NEC R47.89

- **Defect, defective** *(Continued)*
  - Taussig-Bing (aortic transposition and overriding pulmonary artery) Q20.1
  - teeth, wedge K03.1
  - vascular (local) I99.9
    - congenital Q27.9
  - ventricular septal Q21.0
    - concurrent with acute myocardial infarction —*see* Infarct, myocardium
    - following acute myocardial infarction (current complication) I23.2
    - in tetralogy of Fallot Q21.3
  - vision NEC H54.7
  - visual field H53.40
    - bilateral
      - heteronymous H53.47
      - homonymous H53.46-●
    - generalized contraction H53.48-●
    - localized
      - arcuate H53.43-●
      - scotoma (central area) H53.41-●
        - blind spot area H53.42-●
      - sector H53.43-●
      - specified type NEC H53.45-●
  - voice R49.9
    - specified NEC R49.8
  - wedge, tooth, teeth (abrasion) K03.1
- **Deferentitis** N49.1
  - gonorrheal (acute) (chronic) A54.23
- **Defibrination** (syndrome) D65
  - antepartum —*see* Hemorrhage, antepartum, with coagulation defect, disseminated intravascular coagulation
  - following ectopic or molar pregnancy O08.1
  - intrapartum O67.0
  - newborn P60
  - postpartum O72.3
- **Deficiency, deficient**
  - 3-beta hydroxysteroid dehydrogenase E25.0
  - 11-hydroxylase E25.0
  - 21-hydroxylase E25.0
  - 5-alpha reductase (with male pseudohermaphroditism) E29.1
  - AADC (aromatic L-amino acid decarboxylase) E70.81
  - abdominal muscle syndrome Q79.4
  - AC globulin (congenital) (hereditary) D68.2
    - acquired D68.4
  - accelerator globulin (Ac G) (blood) D68.2
  - acid phosphatase E83.39
  - acid sphingomyelinase (ASMD) E75.249
    - type
      - A E75.240
      - A/B E75.244
      - B E75.241
  - activating factor (blood) D68.2
  - ADA2 (adenosine deaminase 2) D81.32
  - adenosine deaminase (ADA) D81.30
    - with severe combined immunodeficiency (SCID) D81.31
    - partial (type 1) D81.39
    - specified NEC D81.39
    - type 1 (without SCID) (without severe combined immunodeficiency) D81.39
    - type 2 D81.32
  - aldolase (hereditary) E74.19
  - alpha-1-antitrypsin E88.01
  - amino-acids E72.9
  - anemia —*see* Anemia
  - aneurin E51.9
  - antibody with
    - hyperimmunoglobulinemia D80.6
    - near-normal immunoglobins D80.6
  - antidiuretic hormone E23.2
  - anti-hemophilic
    - factor (A) D66
      - B D67
      - C D68.1
    - globulin (AHG) NEC D66
  - antithrombin (antithrombin III) D68.59
  - aromatic L-amino acid decarboxylase (AADC) E70.81
  - ascorbic acid E54
  - attention (disorder) (syndrome) F98.8
    - with hyperactivity —*see* Disorder, attention-deficit hyperactivity
  - autoprothrombin
    - I D68.2
    - II D67
    - C D68.2
  - beta-glucuronidase E76.29

- **Deficiency, deficient** *(Continued)*
  - biotin E53.8
  - biotin-dependent carboxylase D81.819
  - biotinidase D81.810
  - brancher enzyme (amylopectinosis) E74.03
  - C1 esterase inhibitor (C1-INH) D84.1
  - calciferol E55.9
    - with
      - adult osteomalacia M83.8
      - rickets —*see* Rickets
  - calcium (dietary) E58
  - calorie, severe E43
    - with marasmus E41
      - and kwashiorkor E42
  - cardiac —*see* Insufficiency, myocardial
  - carnitine E71.40
    - due to
      - hemodialysis E71.43
      - inborn errors of metabolism E71.42
      - Valproic acid therapy E71.43
    - iatrogenic E71.43
    - muscle palmityltransferase E71.314
    - primary E71.41
    - secondary E71.448
  - carotene E50.9
  - central nervous system G96.89
  - ceruloplasmin (Wilson) E83.01
  - choline E53.8
  - Christmas factor D67
  - chromium E61.4
  - chronic neurovisceral acid sphingomyelinase E75.244
  - chronic visceral acid sphingomyelinase E75.241
  - clotting (blood) —*see also* Deficiency, coagulation factor D68.9
  - clotting factor NEC (hereditary) —*see also* Deficiency, factor D68.2
  - coagulation NOS D68.9
    - with
      - ectopic pregnancy O08.1
      - molar pregnancy O08.1
    - acquired (any) D68.4
    - antepartum hemorrhage —*see* Hemorrhage, antepartum, with coagulation defect
    - clotting factor NEC —*see also* Deficiency, factor D68.2
    - due to
      - hyperprothrombinemia D68.4
      - liver disease D68.4
      - vitamin K deficiency D68.4
    - newborn, transient P61.6
    - postpartum O72.3
    - specified NEC D68.8
  - cognitive F09
  - color vision H53.50
    - achromatopsia H53.51
    - acquired H53.52
    - deuteranomaly H53.53
    - protanomaly H53.54
    - specified type NEC H53.59
    - tritanomaly H53.55
  - combined glucocorticoid and mineralocorticoid E27.49
  - contact factor D68.2
  - copper (nutritional) E61.0
  - corticoadrenal E27.40
    - primary E27.1
  - craniofacial axis Q75.009
  - cyanocobalamin E53.8
  - debrancher enzyme (limit dextrinosis) E74.03
  - dehydrogenase
    - long chain/very long chain acyl CoA E71.310
    - medium chain acyl CoA E71.311
    - short chain acyl CoA E71.312
  - diet E63.9
  - dihydropyrimidine dehydrogenase (DPD) E88.89
  - disaccharidase E73.9
  - edema —*see* Malnutrition, severe
  - endocrine E34.9
  - energy-supply —*see* Malnutrition
  - enzymes, circulating NEC E88.09
  - ergosterol E55.9
    - with
      - adult osteomalacia M83.8
      - rickets —*see* Rickets
  - essential fatty acid (EFA) E63.0
  - eye movements
    - saccadic H55.81
    - smooth pursuit H55.82

Deficiency, deficient *(Continued)*
- factor —*see also* Deficiency, coagulation
  - Hageman D68.2
  - I (congenital) (hereditary) D68.2
  - II (congenital) (hereditary) D68.2
  - IX (congenital) (functional) (hereditary) (with functional defect) D67
  - multiple (congenital) D68.8
    - acquired D68.4
  - V (congenital) (hereditary) D68.2
  - Hageman D68.2
  - VII (congenital) (hereditary) D68.2
  - VIII (congenital) (functional) (hereditary) (with functional defect) D66
    - with vascular defect —*see* Disease, von Willebrand
  - X (congenital) (hereditary) D68.2
  - XI (congenital) (hereditary) D68.1
  - XII (congenital) (hereditary) D68.2
  - XIII (congenital) (hereditary) D68.2
- femoral, proximal focal (congenital) —*see* Defect, reduction, lower limb, longitudinal, femur
- fibrin-stabilizing factor (congenital) (hereditary) D68.2
  - acquired D68.4
- fibrinase D68.2
- fibrinogen (congenital) (hereditary) D68.2
  - acquired D65
- folate E53.8
- folic acid E53.8
- foreskin N47.3
- fructokinase E74.11
- fructose 1,6-diphosphatase E74.19
- fructose-1-phosphate aldolase E74.19
- GABA (gamma aminobutyric acid) transaminase E72.81
- GABA-T (gamma aminobutyric acid transaminase) E72.81
- galactokinase E74.29
- galactose-1-phosphate uridyl transferase E74.29
- gammaglobulin in blood D80.1
  - hereditary D80.0
- glass factor D68.2
- glucocorticoid E27.49
  - mineralocorticoid E27.49
- glucose-6-phosphatase E74.01
- glucose-6-phosphate dehydrogenase anemia
  - anemia D55.0
  - without anemia D75.A
- glucose transporter protein type 1 E74.810
- glucuronyl transferase E80.5
- Glut1 E74.810
- glycogen synthetase E74.09
- gonadotropin (isolated) E23.0
- growth hormone (idiopathic) (isolated) E23.0
- Hageman factor D68.2
- hemoglobin D64.9
- hepatophosphorylase E74.09
- homogentisate 1,2-dioxygenase E70.29
- hormone
  - anterior pituitary (partial) NEC E23.0
    - growth E23.0
  - growth (isolated) E23.0
  - pituitary E23.0
  - testicular E29.1
- hypoxanthine-(guanine)-phosphoribosyltransferase (HG-PRT) (total HG-PRT) E79.1
- immunity D84.9
  - cell-mediated D84.89
    - with thrombocytopenia and eczema D82.0
  - combined D81.9
  - humoral D80.9
  - IgA (secretory) D80.2
  - IgG D80.3
  - IgM D80.4
- immuno —*see* Immunodeficiency
- immunoglobulin, selective
  - A (IgA) D80.2
  - G (IgG) (subclasses) D80.3
  - M (IgM) D80.4
- infantile neurovisceral acid sphingomyelinase E75.240
- inositol (B complex) E53.8
- intrinsic
  - factor (congenital) D51.0
  - sphincter N36.42
    - with urethral hypermobility N36.43
- iodine E61.8
  - congenital syndrome —*see* Syndrome, iodine-deficiency, congenital

Deficiency, deficient *(Continued)*
- iron E61.1
  - anemia D50.9
- kalium E87.6
- kappa-light chain D80.8
- labile factor (congenital) (hereditary) D68.2
  - acquired D68.4
- lacrimal fluid (acquired) —*see also* Syndrome, dry eye
  - congenital Q10.6
- lactase
  - congenital E73.0
  - secondary E73.1
- Laki-Lorand factor D68.2
- LCAD (long chain acyl CoA dehydrogenase deficiency) E71.310
- lecithin cholesterol acyltransferase E78.6
- lipocaic K86.89
- lipoprotein (familial) (high density) E78.6
- liver phosphorylase E74.09
- lysosomal alpha-1, 4 glucosidase E74.02
- lysosome-associated membrane protein 2 [LAMP2] E74.05
- magnesium E61.2
- major histocompatibility complex
  - class I D81.6
  - class II D81.7
- manganese E61.3
- MCAD (medium chain acyl CoA dehydrogenase deficiency) E71.311
- menadione (vitamin K) E56.1
  - newborn P53
- mental (familial) (hereditary) —*see* Disability, intellectual
- methylenetetrahydrofolate reductase (MTHFR) E72.12
- mevalonate kinase M04.1
- mineral NEC E61.8
- mineralocorticoid E27.49
  - with glucocorticoid E27.49
- molybdenum (nutritional) E61.5
- moral F60.2
- multiple nutrient elements E61.7
- multiple sulfatase (MSD) E75.26
- muscle
  - carnitine (palmityltransferase) E71.314
  - phosphofructokinase E74.09
- myoadenylate deaminase E79.2
- myocardial —*see* Insufficiency, myocardial
- myophosphorylase E74.04
- NADH diaphorase or reductase (congenital) D74.0
- NADH-methemoglobin reductase (congenital) D74.0
- natrium E87.1
- niacin (amide) (-tryptophan) E52
- nicotinamide E52
- nicotinic acid E52
- number of teeth —*see* Anodontia
- nutrient element E61.9
  - multiple E61.7
  - specified NEC E61.8
- nutrition, nutritional (*see also* Nutrition deficient) E63.9
  - sequelae —*see* Sequelae, nutritional deficiency
  - specified NEC E63.8
- of interleukin 1 receptor antagonist [DIRA] M04.8
- ornithine transcarbamylase E72.4
- ovarian E28.39
- oxygen —*see* Anoxia
- pantothenic acid E53.8
- parathyroid (gland) E20.9
- perineum (female) N81.89
- phenylalanine hydroxylase E70.1
- phosphoenolpyruvate carboxykinase E74.4
- phosphofructokinase E74.19
- ~~phosphomannomutase E74.818~~
- ▶ phosphomannomutase E74.818
- phosphomannose isomerase E74.818
- phosphomannosyl mutase E74.818
- phosphorylase kinase, liver E74.09
- pituitary hormone (isolated) E23.0
- plasma thromboplastin
  - antecedent (PTA) D68.1
  - component (PTC) D67
- plasminogen (type 1) (type 2) E88.02
- platelet NEC D69.1
  - constitutional —*see* Disease, von Willebrand
- polyglandular E31.8
  - autoimmune E31.0

Deficiency, deficient *(Continued)*
- potassium (K) E87.6
- prepuce N47.3
- proaccelerin (congenital) (hereditary) D68.2
  - acquired D68.4
- proconvertin factor (congenital) (hereditary) D68.2
  - acquired D68.4
- protein —*see also* Malnutrition E46
  - anemia D53.0
  - C D68.59
  - S D68.59
- prothrombin (congenital) (hereditary) D68.2
  - acquired D68.4
- Prower factor D68.2
- pseudocholinesterase E88.09
- PTA (plasma thromboplastin antecedent) D68.1
- PTC (plasma thromboplastin component) D67
- purine nucleoside phosphorylase (PNP) D81.5
- pyracin (alpha) (beta) E53.1
- pyridoxal E53.1
- pyridoxamine E53.1
- pyridoxine (derivatives) E53.1
- pyruvate
  - carboxylase E74.4
  - dehydrogenase E74.4
- riboflavin (vitamin B2) E53.0
- salt E87.1
- SCAD (short chain acyl CoA dehydrogenase deficiency) E71.312
- secretion
  - ovary E28.39
  - salivary gland (any) K11.7
  - urine R34
- selenium (dietary) E59
- serum antitrypsin, familial E88.01
- short stature homeobox gene (SHOX)
  - with
    - dyschondrosteosis Q78.8
    - short stature (idiopathic) E34.328
    - Turner's syndrome Q96.9
- sodium (Na) E87.1
- SPCA (factor VII) D68.2
- sphincter, intrinsic N36.42
  - with urethral hypermobility N36.43
- stable factor (congenital) (hereditary) D68.2
  - acquired D68.4
- Stuart-Prower (factor X) D68.2
- succinic semialdehyde dehydrogenase E72.81
- sucrase E74.39
- sulfatase E75.26
- sulfite oxidase E72.19
- thiamin, thiaminic (chloride) E51.9
  - beriberi (dry) E51.11
    - wet E51.12
- thrombokinase D68.2
  - newborn P53
- thyroid (gland) —*see* Hypothyroidism
- tocopherol E56.0
- tooth bud K00.0
- transcobalamine II (anemia) D51.2
- vanadium E61.6
- vascular I99.9
- vasopressin E23.2
- vertical ridge K06.8
- viosterol —*see* Deficiency, calciferol
- vitamin (multiple) NOS E56.9
  - A E50.9
    - with
      - Bitot's spot (corneal) E50.1
      - follicular keratosis E50.8
      - keratomalacia E50.4
      - manifestations NEC E50.8
      - night blindness E50.5
      - scar of cornea, xerophthalmic E50.6
      - xeroderma E50.8
      - xerophthalmia E50.7
      - xerosis
        - conjunctival E50.0
          - and Bitot's spot E50.1
        - cornea E50.2
          - and ulceration E50.3
    - sequelae E64.1
  - B (complex) NOS E53.9
    - with
      - beriberi (dry) E51.11
        - wet E51.12
      - pellagra E52

D

Deformity *(Continued)*
nervous system (congenital) QØ7.9
nipple (congenital) Q83.9
acquired N64.89
nose (acquired) (cartilage) M95.Ø
bone (turbinate) M95.Ø
congenital Q3Ø.9
bent or squashed Q67.4
saddle M95.Ø
syphilitic A5Ø.57
septum (acquired) J34.2
congenital Q3Ø.8
sinus (wall) (congenital) Q3Ø.8
acquired M95.Ø
syphilitic (congenital) A5Ø.57
late A52.73
ocular muscle (congenital) Q1Ø.3
acquired *—see* Strabismus, mechanical
opticociliary vessels (congenital) Q13.2
orbit (eye) (acquired) HØ5.3Ø
atrophy *—see* Atrophy, orbit
congenital Q1Ø.7
due to
bone disease NEC HØ5.32-●
trauma or surgery HØ5.33-●
enlargement *—see* Enlargement, orbit
exostosis *—see* Exostosis, orbit
organ of Corti (congenital) Q16.5
ovary (congenital) Q5Ø.39
acquired N83.8
oviduct, acquired N83.8
palate (congenital) Q38.5
acquired M27.8
cleft (congenital) *—see* Cleft, palate
pancreas (congenital) Q45.3
acquired K86.89
parathyroid (gland) Q89.2
parotid (gland) (congenital) Q38.4
acquired K11.8
patella (acquired) *—see* Disorder, patella, specified NEC
pelvis, pelvic (acquired) (bony) M95.5
with disproportion (fetopelvic) O33.Ø
causing obstructed labor O65.Ø
congenital Q74.2
rachitic sequelae (late effect) E64.3
penis (glans) (congenital) Q55.69
acquired N48.89
pericardium (congenital) Q24.8
acquired *—see* Pericarditis
pharynx (congenital) Q38.8
acquired J39.2
pinna, acquired *—see also* Disorder, pinna, deformity
congenital Q17.9
pituitary (congenital) Q89.2
posture *—see* Dorsopathy, deforming
prepuce (congenital) Q55.69
acquired N47.8
prostate (congenital) Q55.4
acquired N42.89
pupil (congenital) Q13.2
acquired *—see* Abnormality, pupillary
pylorus (congenital) Q4Ø.3
acquired K31.89
rachitic (acquired), old or healed E64.3
radius (acquired) *—see also* Deformity, limb, forearm
congenital Q68.8
rectum (congenital) Q43.9
acquired K62.89
reduction (extremity) (limb), congenital (*see also* condition and site) Q73.8
brain QØ4.3
lower *—see* Defect, reduction, lower limb
upper *—see* Defect, reduction, upper limb
renal *—see* Deformity, kidney
respiratory system (congenital) Q34.9
rib (acquired) M95.4
congenital Q76.6
cervical Q76.5
rotation (joint) (acquired) *—see* Deformity, limb, specified site NEC
congenital Q74.9
hip *—see* Deformity, limb, specified type NEC, thigh
congenital Q65.89
sacroiliac joint (congenital) Q74.2
acquired *—see* subcategory M43.8
sacrum (acquired) *—see* subcategory M43.8

Deformity *(Continued)*
saddle
back *—see* Lordosis
nose M95.Ø
syphilitic A5Ø.57
salivary gland or duct (congenital) Q38.4
acquired K11.8
scapula (acquired) M95.8
congenital Q68.8
scrotum (congenital) *—see also* Malformation, testis and scrotum
acquired N5Ø.89
seminal vesicles (congenital) Q55.4
acquired N5Ø.89
septum, nasal (acquired) J34.2
shoulder (joint) (acquired) *—see* Deformity, limb, upper arm
congenital Q74.Ø
contraction *—see* Contraction, joint, shoulder
sigmoid (flexure) (congenital) Q43.9
acquired K63.89
skin (congenital) Q82.9
skull (acquired) M95.2
congenital Q75.8
with
anencephaly QØØ.Ø
encephalocele *—see* Encephalocele
hydrocephalus QØ3.9
with spina bifida *—see* Spina bifida, by site, with hydrocephalus
microcephaly QØ2
soft parts, organs or tissues (of pelvis)
in pregnancy or childbirth NEC O34.8-●
causing obstructed labor O65.5
spermatic cord (congenital) Q55.4
acquired N5Ø.89
torsion *—see* Torsion, spermatic cord
spinal *—see* Dorsopathy, deforming
column (acquired) *—see* Dorsopathy, deforming
congenital Q67.5
cord (congenital) QØ6.9
acquired G95.89
nerve root (congenital) QØ7.9
spine (acquired) *—see also* Dorsopathy, deforming
congenital Q67.5
rachitic E64.3
specified NEC *—see* Dorsopathy, deforming, specified NEC
spleen
acquired D73.89
congenital Q89.Ø9
Sprengel's (congenital) Q74.Ø
sternocleidomastoid (muscle), congenital Q68.Ø
sternum (acquired) M95.4
congenital NEC Q76.7
stomach (congenital) Q4Ø.3
acquired K31.89
submandibular gland (congenital) Q38.4
submaxillary gland (congenital) Q38.4
acquired K11.8
talipes *—see* Talipes
testis (congenital) *—see also* Malformation, testis and scrotum
acquired N44.8
torsion *—see* Torsion, testis
thigh (acquired) *—see also* Deformity, limb, thigh
congenital NEC Q68.8
thorax (acquired) (wall) M95.4
congenital Q67.8
sequelae of rickets E64.3
thumb (acquired) *—see also* Deformity, finger
congenital NEC Q68.1
thymus (tissue) (congenital) Q89.2
thyroid (gland) (congenital) Q89.2
cartilage Q31.8
acquired J38.7
tibia (acquired) *—see also* Deformity, limb, specified type NEC, lower leg
congenital NEC Q68.8
saber (syphilitic) A5Ø.56
toe (acquired) M2Ø.6-●
congenital Q66.9-●
hallux rigidus M2Ø.2-●
hallux valgus M2Ø.1-●
hallux varus M2Ø.3-●
hammer toe M2Ø.4-●
specified NEC M2Ø.5X-●
tongue (congenital) Q38.3
acquired K14.8

Deformity *(Continued)*
tooth, teeth KØØ.2
trachea (rings) (congenital) Q32.1
acquired J39.8
transverse aortic arch (congenital) Q25.49
tricuspid (leaflets) (valve) IØ7.8
atresia or stenosis Q22.4
Ebstein's Q22.5
trunk (acquired) M95.8
congenital Q89.9
ulna (acquired) *—see also* Deformity, limb, forearm
congenital NEC Q68.8
urachus, congenital Q64.4
ureter (opening) (congenital) Q62.8
acquired N28.89
urethra (congenital) Q64.79
acquired N36.8
urinary tract (congenital) Q64.9
urachus Q64.4
uterus (congenital) Q51.9
acquired N85.8
uvula (congenital) Q38.5
vagina (acquired) N89.8
congenital Q52.4
valgus NEC M21.ØØ
ankle M21.Ø7-●
elbow M21.Ø2-●
hip M21.Ø5-●
knee M21.Ø6-●
valve, valvular (congenital) (heart) Q24.8
acquired *—see* Endocarditis
varus NEC M21.1Ø
ankle M21.17-●
elbow M21.12-●
hip M21.15
knee M21.16-●
tibia *—see* Osteochondrosis, juvenile, tibia
vas deferens (congenital) Q55.4
acquired N5Ø.89
vein (congenital) Q27.9
great Q26.9
vertebra *—see* Dorsopathy, deforming
vertical talus (congenital) Q66.8Ø
left foot Q66.82
right foot Q66.81
vesicourethral orifice (acquired) N32.89
congenital NEC Q64.79
vessels of optic papilla (congenital) Q14.2
visual field (contraction) *—see* Defect, visual field
vitreous body, acquired H43.89
vulva (congenital) Q52.79
acquired N9Ø.89
wrist (joint) (acquired) *—see also* Deformity, limb, forearm
congenital Q68.8
contraction *—see* Contraction, joint, wrist

Degeneration, degenerative
adrenal (capsule) (fatty) (gland) (hyaline) (infectional) E27.8
amyloid *—see also* Amyloidosis E85.9
anterior cornua, spinal cord G12.29
anterior labral S43.49-●
aorta, aortic I7Ø.Ø
fatty I77.89
aortic valve (heart) *—see* Endocarditis, aortic
arteriovascular *—see* Arteriosclerosis
artery, arterial (atheromatous) (calcareous) *—see also* Arteriosclerosis
cerebral, amyloid E85.4 *[I68.Ø]*
medial *—see* Arteriosclerosis, extremities
articular cartilage NEC *—see* Derangement, joint, articular cartilage, by site
atheromatous *—see* Arteriosclerosis
basal nuclei or ganglia G23.9
specified NEC G23.8
bone NEC *—see* Disorder, bone, specified type NEC
brachial plexus G54.Ø
brain (cortical) (progressive) G31.9
alcoholic G31.2
arteriosclerotic I67.2
childhood G31.9
specified NEC G31.89
cystic G31.89
congenital QØ4.6
in
alcoholism G31.2
beriberi E51.2
cerebrovascular disease I67.9
congenital hydrocephalus QØ3.9
with spina bifida *—see also* Spina bifida

INDEX TO DISEASES AND INJURIES / Degeneration, degenerative

Degeneration, degenerative *(Continued)*
- brain *(Continued)*
  - in *(Continued)*
    - Fabry-Anderson disease E75.21
    - Gaucher's disease E75.22
    - Hunter's syndrome E76.1
    - lipidosis
      - cerebral E75.4
      - generalized E75.6
    - mucopolysaccharidosis *—see* Mucopolysaccharidosis
    - myxedema E03.9 *[G32.89]*
    - neoplastic disease *—see also* Neoplasm D49.6 *[G32.89]*
    - Niemann-Pick disease E75.249 *[G32.89]*
    - sphingolipidosis E75.3 *[G32.89]*
    - vitamin B12 deficiency E53.8 *[G32.89]*
  - senile NEC G31.1
- breast N64.89
- Bruch's membrane *—see* Degeneration, choroid
- capillaries (fatty) I78.8
  - amyloid E85.89 *[I79.8]*
- cardiac *—see also* Degeneration, myocardial
  - valve, valvular *—see* Endocarditis
- cardiorenal *—see* Hypertension, cardiorenal
- cardiovascular *—see also* Disease, cardiovascular
  - renal *—see* Hypertension, cardiorenal
- cerebellar NOS G31.9
  - alcoholic G31.2
  - primary (hereditary) (sporadic) G11.9
- cerebral *—see* Degeneration, brain
- cerebrovascular I67.9
  - due to hypertension I67.4
- cervical plexus G54.2
- cervix N88.8
  - due to radiation (intended effect) N88.8
    - adverse effect or misadventure N99.89
- chamber angle H21.21-●
- changes, spine or vertebra *—see* Spondylosis
- chorioretinal *—see also* Degeneration, choroid
  - hereditary H31.20
- choroid (colloid) (drusen) H31.10-●
  - atrophy *—see* Atrophy, choroidal
  - hereditary *—see* Dystrophy, choroidal, hereditary
- ciliary body H21.22-●
- cochlear *—see* subcategory H83.8
- combined (spinal cord) (subacute) E53.8 *[G32.0]*
  - with anemia (pernicious) D51.0 *[G32.0]*
    - due to dietary vitamin B12 deficiency D51.3 *[G32.0]*
  - in (due to)
    - vitamin B12 deficiency E53.8 *[G32.0]*
      - anemia D51.9 *[G32.0]*
- conjunctiva H11.10
  - concretions *—see* Concretion, conjunctiva
  - deposits *—see* Deposit, conjunctiva
  - pigmentations *—see* Pigmentation, conjunctiva
  - pinguecula *—see* Pinguecula
  - xerosis *—see* Xerosis, conjunctiva
- cornea H18.40
  - calcerous H18.43
    - band keratopathy H18.42-●
  - familial, hereditary *—see* Dystrophy, cornea
  - hyaline (of old scars) H18.49
  - keratomalacia *—see* Keratomalacia
  - nodular H18.45-●
  - peripheral H18.46-●
  - senile H18.41-●
  - specified type NEC H18.49
- cortical (cerebellar) (parenchymatous) G31.89
  - alcoholic G31.2
  - diffuse, due to arteriopathy I67.2
- corticobasal G31.85
- cutis L98.8
  - amyloid E85.4 *[L99]*
- dental pulp K04.2
- disc disease *—see* Degeneration, intervertebral disc, by site
- dorsolateral (spinal cord) *—see* Degeneration, combined
- extrapyramidal G25.9
- eye, macular *—see also* Degeneration, macula
  - congenital or hereditary *—see* Dystrophy, retina
- facet joints *—see* Spondylosis
- fatty
  - liver NEC K76.0
    - alcoholic K70.0
- grey matter (brain) (Alpers') G31.81

Degeneration, degenerative *(Continued)*
- heart *—see also* Degeneration, myocardial
  - amyloid E85.4 *[I43]*
  - atheromatous *—see* Disease, heart, ischemic, atherosclerotic
  - ischemic *—see* Disease, heart, ischemic
- hepatolenticular (Wilson's) E83.01
- hepatorenal K76.7
- hyaline (diffuse) (generalized)
  - localized *—see* Degeneration, by site
- infrapatellar fat pad M79.4
- intervertebral disc
  - with
    - myelopathy *—see* Disorder, disc, with, myelopathy
    - radiculitis or radiculopathy *—see* Disorder, disc, with, radiculopathy
  - cervical, cervicothoracic *—see* Disorder, disc, cervical, degeneration
    - with
      - myelopathy *—see* Disorder, disc, cervical, with myelopathy
      - neuritis, radiculitis or radiculopathy *—see* Disorder, disc, cervical, with neuritis
  - lumbar region M51.36-●
    - with
      - myelopathy M51.06
      - neuritis, radiculitis, radiculopathy or sciatica M51.16
  - lumbosacral region M51.37-●
    - with
      - neuritis, radiculitis, radiculopathy or sciatica M51.17
  - sacrococcygeal region M53.3
  - thoracic region M51.34
    - with
      - myelopathy M51.04
      - neuritis, radiculitis, radiculopathy M51.14
  - thoracolumbar region M51.35
    - with
      - myelopathy M51.05
      - neuritis, radiculitis, radiculopathy M51.15
- intestine, amyloid E85.4
- iris (pigmentary) H21.23-●
- ischemic *—see* Ischemia
- joint disease *—see* Osteoarthritis
- kidney N28.89
  - amyloid E85.4 *[N29]*
  - cystic, congenital Q61.9
  - fatty N28.89
  - polycystic Q61.3
    - adult type (autosomal dominant) Q61.2
    - infantile type (autosomal recessive) NEC Q61.19
      - collecting duct dilatation Q61.11
- Kuhnt-Junius *—see also* Degeneration, macula H35.32-●
- lens *—see* Cataract
- lenticular (familial) (progressive) (Wilson's) (with cirrhosis of liver) E83.01
- liver (diffuse) NEC K76.89
  - amyloid E85.4 *[K77]*
  - cystic K76.89
    - congenital Q44.6
  - fatty NEC K76.0
    - alcoholic K70.0
  - hypertrophic K76.89
  - parenchymatous, acute or subacute K72.00
    - with coma K72.01
  - pigmentary K76.89
  - toxic (acute) K71.9
- lung J98.4
- lymph gland I89.8
  - hyaline I89.8
- macula, macular (acquired) (age-related) (senile) H35.30
  - angioid streaks H35.33
  - atrophic age-related H35.31-●
  - congenital or hereditary *—see* Dystrophy, retina
  - cystoid H35.35-●
  - drusen H35.36-●
  - dry age-related H35.31-●
  - exudative H35.32-●
  - hole H35.34-●
  - nonexudative H35.31-●
  - puckering H35.37-●
  - toxic H35.38-●
  - wet age-related H35.32-●

Degeneration, degenerative *(Continued)*
- membranous labyrinth, congenital (causing impairment of hearing) Q16.5
- meniscus *—see* Derangement, meniscus
- mitral *—see* Insufficiency, mitral
- Mönckeberg's *—see* Arteriosclerosis, extremities
- motor centers, senile G31.1
- multi-system G90.3
- mural *—see* Degeneration, myocardial
- muscle (fatty) (fibrous) (hyaline) (progressive) M62.89
  - heart *—see* Degeneration, myocardial
- myelin, central nervous system G37.9
- myocardial, myocardium (fatty) (hyaline) (senile) I51.5
  - with rheumatic fever (conditions in I00) I09.0
    - active, acute or subacute I01.2
      - with chorea I02.0
    - inactive or quiescent (with chorea) I09.0
  - hypertensive *—see* Hypertension, heart
  - rheumatic *—see* Degeneration, myocardial, with rheumatic fever
  - syphilitic A52.06
- nasal sinus (mucosa) J32.9
  - frontal J32.1
  - maxillary J32.0
- nerve *—see* Disorder, nerve
- nervous system G31.9
  - alcoholic G31.2
  - amyloid E85.4 *[G99.8]*
  - autonomic G90.9
  - fatty G31.89
  - specified NEC G31.89
- nipple N64.89
- olivopontocerebellar (hereditary) (familial) G23.8
- osseous labyrinth *—see* subcategory H83.8
- ovary N83.8
  - cystic N83.20-●
  - microcystic N83.20-●
- pallidal pigmentary (progressive) G23.0
- pancreas K86.89
  - tuberculous A18.83
- penis N48.89
- pigmentary (diffuse) (general)
  - localized *—see* Degeneration, by site
  - pallidal (progressive) G23.0
- pineal gland E34.8
- pituitary (gland) E23.6
- popliteal fat pad M79.4
- posterolateral (spinal cord) *—see* Degeneration, combined
- pulmonary valve (heart) I37.8
- pulp (tooth) K04.2
- pupillary margin H21.24-●
- renal *—see* Degeneration, kidney
- retina H35.9
  - hereditary (cerebroretinal) (congenital) (juvenile) (macula) (peripheral) (pigmentary) *—see* Dystrophy, retina
  - Kuhnt-Junius *—see also* Degeneration, macula H35.32-●
  - macula (cystic) (exudative) (hole) (nonexudative) (pseudohole) (senile) (toxic) *—see* Degeneration, macula
  - peripheral H35.40
    - lattice H35.41-●
    - microcystoid H35.42-●
    - paving stone H35.43-●
    - secondary
      - pigmentary H35.45-●
      - vitreoretinal H35.46-●
    - senile reticular H35.44-●
  - pigmentary (primary) *—see also* Dystrophy, retina
    - secondary *—see* Degeneration, retina, peripheral, secondary
  - posterior pole *—see* Degeneration, macula
- saccule, congenital (causing impairment of hearing) Q16.5
- senile R54
  - brain G31.1
  - cardiac, heart or myocardium *—see* Degeneration, myocardial
  - motor centers G31.1
  - vascular *—see* Arteriosclerosis
- sinus (cystic) *—see also* Sinusitis
  - polypoid J33.1
- skin L98.8
  - amyloid E85.4 *[L99]*
  - colloid L98.8

- **Degeneration, degenerative** *(Continued)*
  - spinal (cord) G31.89
    - amyloid E85.4 *[G32.89]*
    - combined (subacute) —*see* Degeneration, combined
    - dorsolateral —*see* Degeneration, combined
    - familial NEC G31.89
    - fatty G31.89
    - funicular —*see* Degeneration, combined
    - posterolateral —*see* Degeneration, combined
    - subacute combined —*see* Degeneration, combined
    - tuberculous A17.81
  - spleen D73.0
    - amyloid E85.4 *[D77]*
  - stomach K31.89
  - striatonigral G23.2
  - suprarenal (capsule) (gland) E27.8
  - synovial membrane (pulpy) —*see* Disorder, synovium, specified type NEC
  - tapetoretinal —*see* Dystrophy, retina
  - thymus (gland) E32.8
    - fatty E32.8
  - thyroid (gland) E07.89
  - tricuspid (heart) (valve) I07.9
  - tuberculous NEC —*see* Tuberculosis
  - turbinate J34.89
  - uterus (cystic) N85.8
  - vascular (senile) —*see* Arteriosclerosis
    - hypertensive —*see* Hypertension
  - vitreoretinal, secondary —*see* Degeneration, retina, peripheral, secondary, vitreoretinal
  - vitreous (body) H43.81-●
  - Wallerian —*see* Disorder, nerve
  - Wilson's hepatolenticular E83.01
- **Deglutition**
  - paralysis R13.0
    - hysterical F44.4
  - pneumonia J69.0
- **Degos' disease** I77.89
- **Dehiscence (of)**
  - amputation stump T87.81
  - cesarean wound O90.0
  - closure of
    - ▶ abdominal wall muscle or fascia T81.321
    - cornea T81.31
    - ➡ craniotomy T81.328
    - ➡ fascia (muscular) (superficial) T81.328
    - ▶ gastrointestinal tract anastomosis, repair, or closure T81.320
    - ➡ internal organ or tissue T81.328
    - laceration (external) (internal) T81.33
    - ➡ ligament T81.328
    - mucosa T81.31
    - ➡ muscle or muscle flap T81.328
    - ➡ ribs or rib cage T81.328
    - skin and subcutaneous tissue (full-thickness) (superficial) T81.31
    - ➡ skull T81.328
    - ➡ sternum (sternotomy) T81.328
    - ➡ tendon T81.328
    - traumatic laceration (external) (internal) T81.33
  - episiotomy O90.1
  - operation wound NEC T81.31
    - ▶ deep T81.329
    - external operation wound (superficial) T81.31
    - ➡ internal operation wound (deep) T81.329
      - ▶ abdominal wall muscle or fascia T81.321
      - ▶ specified NEC T81.328
  - perineal wound (postpartum) O90.1
  - traumatic injury wound repair T81.33
  - wound T81.30
    - traumatic repair T81.33
- **Dehydration** E86.0
  - newborn P74.1
- **Déjérine-Roussy syndrome** G93.89
- **Déjérine-Sottas disease or neuropathy** (hypertrophic) G60.0
- **Déjérine-Thomas atrophy** G23.8
- **Delay, delayed**
  - any plane in pelvis
    - complicating delivery O66.9
  - birth or delivery NOS O63.9
  - closure, ductus arteriosus (Botalli) P29.38
  - coagulation —*see* Defect, coagulation
  - conduction (cardiac) (ventricular) I45.9
  - delivery, second twin, triplet, etc O63.2
- **Delay, delayed** *(Continued)*
  - development R62.50
    - global F88
    - intellectual (specific) F81.9
    - language F80.9
      - due to hearing loss F80.4
    - learning F81.9
    - milestone R62.0
    - pervasive F84.9
    - physiological R62.50
      - specified stage NEC R62.0
    - reading F81.0
    - sexual E30.0
    - speech F80.9
      - due to hearing loss F80.4
    - spelling F81.81
  - ejaculation F52.32
  - gastric emptying K30
  - menarche E30.0
  - menstruation (cause unknown) N91.0
  - milestone R62.0
  - passage of meconium (newborn) P76.0
  - primary respiration P28.9
  - puberty (constitutional) E30.0
  - separation of umbilical cord P96.82
  - sexual maturation, female E30.0
  - sleep phase syndrome G47.21
  - union, fracture —*see* Fracture, by site
  - vaccination Z28.9
- **Deletion(s)**
  - autosome Q93.9
    - identified by fluorescence in situ hybridization (FISH) Q93.89
    - identified by in situ hybridization (ISH) Q93.89
  - chromosome
    - with complex rearrangements NEC Q93.7
    - part of NEC Q93.59
    - seen only at prometaphase Q93.89
    - short arm
      - 4 Q93.3
      - 5p Q93.4
      - 22q11.2 Q93.81
    - specified NEC Q93.89
  - long arm chromosome 18 or 21 Q93.89
    - with complex rearrangements NEC Q93.7
  - microdeletions NEC Q93.88
- **Delhi boil or button** B55.1
- **Delinquency** (juvenile) (neurotic) F91.8
  - group Z72.810
- **Delinquent immunization status** Z28.3
- ➡ **Delirium, delirious** (acute or subacute) (not alcohol or drug-induced) R41.0
  - ▶ with
    - ▶ dementia (see also Dementia) F05
  - alcoholic (acute) (tremens) (withdrawal) F10.921
    - with intoxication F10.921
      - in
        - abuse F10.121
        - dependence F10.221
  - due to (secondary to)
    - alcohol
      - intoxication F10.921
        - in
          - abuse F10.121
          - dependence F10.221
      - withdrawal F10.231
    - amphetamine intoxication F15.921
      - in
        - abuse F15.121
        - dependence F15.221
    - anxiolytic
      - intoxication F13.921
        - in
          - abuse F13.121
          - dependence F13.221
      - withdrawal F13.231
    - cannabis intoxication (acute) F12.921
      - in
        - abuse F12.121
        - dependence F12.221
    - cocaine intoxication (acute) F14.921
      - in
        - abuse F14.121
        - dependence F14.221
    - general medical condition F05
    - hallucinogen intoxication F16.921
      - in
        - abuse F16.121
        - dependence F16.221
- **Delirium, delirious** *(Continued)*
  - due to *(Continued)*
    - hypnotic
      - intoxication F13.921
        - in
          - abuse F13.121
          - dependence F13.221
      - withdrawal F13.231
    - inhalant intoxication (acute) F18.921
      - in
        - abuse F18.121
        - dependence F18.221
    - multiple etiologies F05
    - opioid intoxication (acute) F11.921
      - in
        - abuse F11.121
        - dependence F11.221
    - other (or unknown) substance F19.921
    - phencyclidine intoxication (acute) F16.921
      - in
        - abuse F16.121
        - dependence F16.221
    - psychoactive substance NEC intoxication (acute) F19.921
      - in
        - abuse F19.121
        - dependence F19.221
    - sedative
      - intoxication F13.921
        - in
          - abuse F13.121
          - dependence F13.221
      - withdrawal F13.231
    - unknown etiology R41.0
  - exhaustion F43.0
  - hysterical F44.89
  - postprocedural (postoperative) F05
  - puerperal F05
  - thyroid —*see* Thyrotoxicosis with thyroid storm
  - traumatic —*see* Injury, intracranial
  - tremens (alcohol-induced) F10.231
    - sedative-induced F13.231
- **Delivery** (childbirth) (labor)
  - arrested active phase O62.1
  - cesarean (for)
    - without indication O82
    - abnormal
      - pelvis (bony) (deformity) (major) NEC with disproportion (fetopelvic) O33.0
        - with obstructed labor O65.0
      - presentation or position O32.9
    - abruptio placentae —*see also* Abruptio placentae 045.9-●
    - acromion presentation O32.2
    - atony, uterus O62.2
    - breech presentation O32.1
      - incomplete O32.8
    - brow presentation O32.3
    - cephalopelvic disproportion O33.9
    - cerclage O34.3-●
    - chin presentation O32.3
    - cicatrix of cervix O34.4-●
    - contracted pelvis (general)
      - inlet O33.2
      - outlet O33.3
    - cord presentation or prolapse O69.0
    - cystocele O34.8-●
    - deformity (acquired) (congenital)
      - pelvic organs or tissues NEC O34.8-●
      - pelvis (bony) NEC O33.0
    - disproportion NOS O33.9
    - eclampsia —*see* Eclampsia
    - face presentation O32.3
    - failed
      - forceps O66.5
      - induction of labor O61.9
        - instrumental O61.1
        - mechanical O61.1
        - medical O61.0
        - specified NEC O61.8
        - surgical O61.1
      - trial of labor NOS O66.40
        - following previous cesarean delivery O66.41
      - vacuum extraction O66.5
      - ventouse O66.5
    - fetal-maternal hemorrhage O43.01-●
    - hemorrhage (intrapartum) O67.9
      - with coagulation defect O67.0
      - specified cause NEC O67.8
    - high head at term O32.4

D

- Delivery *(Continued)*
  - cesarean *(Continued)*
    - hydrocephalic fetus O33.6
    - incarceration of uterus O34.51-●
    - incoordinate uterine action O62.4
    - increased size, fetus O33.5
    - inertia, uterus O62.2
      - primary O62.Ø
      - secondary O62.1
    - isthmocele O34.22
    - lateroversion, uterus O34.59-●
    - mal lie O32.9
    - malposition
      - fetus O32.9
      - pelvic organs or tissues NEC O34.8-●
      - uterus NEC O34.59-●
    - malpresentation NOS O32.9
    - oblique presentation O32.2
    - occurring after 37 completed weeks of gestation but before 39 completed weeks gestation due to (spontaneous) onset of labor O75.82
    - oversize fetus O33.5
    - pelvic tumor NEC O34.8-●
    - placenta previa O44.Ø-●
      - complete O44.Ø-●
        - with hemorrhage O44.1-●
    - placental insufficiency O36.51-●
    - planned, occurring after 37 completed weeks of gestation but before 39 completed weeks gestation due to (spontaneous) onset of labor O75.82
    - polyp, cervix O34.4-●
      - causing obstructed labor O65.5
    - poor dilatation, cervix O62.Ø
    - pre-eclampsia O14.94
      - mild O14.Ø4
      - moderate O14.Ø4
      - severe O14.14
        - with hemolysis, elevated liver enzymes and low platelet count (HELLP) O14.24
    - previous
      - cesarean delivery O34.219
        - classical (vertical) scar O34.212
        - isthmocele O34.22
        - low transverse scar O34.211
      - mid-transverse T incision O34.218
      - scar
        - defect (isthmocele) O34.22
        - specified type NEC O34.218
      - surgery (to)
        - cervix O34.4-●
        - gynecological NEC O34.8-●
        - rectum O34.7-●
        - uterus O34.29
        - vagina O34.6-●
    - prolapse
      - arm or hand O32.2
      - uterus O34.52-●
    - prolonged labor NOS O63.9
    - rectocele O34.8-●
    - retroversion
      - uterus O34.53-●
    - rigid
      - cervix O34.4-●
      - pelvic floor O34.8-●
      - perineum O34.7-●
      - vagina O34.6-●
      - vulva O34.7-●
    - sacculation, pregnant uterus O34.59-●
    - scar(s)
      - cervix O34.4-●
      - cesarean delivery O34.219
        - classical (vertical) O34.212
        - isthmocele O34.22
        - low transverse O34.211
        - mid-transverse T incision O34.218
        - scar
          - defect (isthmocele) O34.22
          - specified type NEC O34.218
      - defect (isthmocele) O34.22
      - transmural uterine O34.29
      - uterus O34.29
    - Shirodkar suture in situ O34.3-●
    - shoulder presentation O32.2
    - stenosis or stricture, cervix O34.4-●
    - streptococcus group B (GBS) carrier state O99.824
    - transmural uterine scar O34.29
    - transverse presentation or lie O32.2
    - tumor, pelvic organs or tissues NEC O34.8-●
      - cervix O34.4-●
    - umbilical cord presentation or prolapse O69.Ø
  - completely normal case O8Ø
  - complicated O75.9
    - by
      - abnormal, abnormality (of)
        - forces of labor O62.9
          - specified type NEC O62.8
        - glucose O99.814
        - uterine contractions NOS O62.9
      - abruptio placentae —*see also* Abruptio placentae O45.9-●
      - abuse
        - physical O9A.32
        - psychological O9A.52
        - sexual O9A.42
      - adherent placenta O72.Ø
        - without hemorrhage O73.Ø
      - alcohol use O99.314
      - anemia (pre-existing) O99.Ø2
      - anesthetic death O74.8
      - annular detachment of cervix O71.3
      - atony, uterus O62.2
      - attempted vacuum extraction and forceps O66.5
      - Bandl's ring O62.4
      - bariatric surgery status O99.844
      - biliary tract disorder O26.62
      - bleeding —*see* Delivery, complicated by, hemorrhage
      - blood disorder NEC O99.12
      - cervical dystocia (hypotonic) O62.2
        - primary O62.Ø
        - secondary O62.1
      - circulatory system disorder O99.42
      - compression of cord (umbilical) NEC O69.2
      - condition NEC O99.892
      - contraction, contracted ring O62.4
      - cord (umbilical)
        - around neck
          - with compression O69.1
          - without compression O69.81
        - bruising O69.5
        - complication O69.9
          - specified NEC O69.89
        - compression NEC O69.2
        - entanglement O69.2
          - without compression O69.82
        - hematoma O69.5
        - presentation O69.Ø
        - prolapse O69.Ø
        - short O69.3
        - thrombosis (vessels) O69.5
        - vascular lesion O69.5
      - Couvelaire uterus O45.8X-●
      - damage to (injury to) NEC
        - perineum O71.82
        - periurethral tissue O71.82
        - vulva O71.82
      - delay following rupture of membranes (spontaneous) —*see* Pregnancy, complicated by, premature rupture of membranes
      - depressed fetal heart tones O76
      - diabetes O24.92
        - gestational O24.429
          - diet controlled O24.42Ø
          - insulin controlled O24.424
          - oral drug controlled (antidiabetic) (hypoglycemic) O24.425
        - pre-existing O24.32
          - specified NEC O24.82
          - type 1 O24.Ø2
          - type 2 O24.12
      - diastasis recti (abdominis) O71.89
      - dilatation
        - bladder O66.8
        - cervix incomplete, poor or slow O62.Ø
      - disease NEC O99.892
      - disruptio uteri —*see* Delivery, complicated by, rupture, uterus
      - drug use O99.324
      - dysfunction, uterus NOS O62.9
        - hypertonic O62.4
        - hypotonic O62.2
          - primary O62.Ø
          - secondary O62.1
        - incoordinate O62.4
      - eclampsia O15.1
      - embolism (pulmonary) —*see* Embolism, obstetric
      - endocrine, nutritional or metabolic disease NEC O99.284
      - failed
        - attempted vaginal birth after previous cesarean delivery O66.41
        - induction of labor O61.9
          - instrumental O61.1
          - mechanical O61.1
          - medical O61.Ø
          - specified NEC O61.8
          - surgical O61.1
        - trial of labor O66.4Ø
      - female genital mutilation O65.5
      - fetal
        - abnormal acid-base balance O68
        - acidemia O68
        - acidosis O68
        - alkalosis O68
        - death, early OØ2.1
        - deformity O66.3
        - heart rate or rhythm (abnormal) (non-reassuring) O76
        - hypoxia O77.8
        - stress O77.9
          - due to drug administration O77.1
          - electrocardiographic evidence of O77.8
          - specified NEC O77.8
          - ultrasound evidence of O77.8
      - fever during labor O75.2
      - gastric banding status O99.844
      - gastric bypass status O99.844
      - gastrointestinal disease NEC O99.62
      - gestational
        - diabetes O24.429
          - diet controlled O24.42Ø
          - insulin (and diet) controlled O24.424
          - oral drug controlled (antidiabetic) (hypoglycemic) O24.425
        - edema O12.Ø4
          - with proteinuria O12.24
        - proteinuria O12.14
      - gonorrhea O98.22
      - hematoma O71.7
        - ischial spine O71.7
        - pelvic O71.7
        - vagina O71.7
        - vulva or perineum O71.7
      - hemorrhage (uterine) O67.9
        - associated with
          - afibrinogenemia O67.Ø
          - coagulation defect O67.Ø
          - hyperfibrinolysis O67.Ø
          - hypofibrinogenemia O67.Ø
        - due to
          - low implantation of placenta O44.5-●
          - low-lying placenta O44.5-●
          - placenta previa O44.1-●
            - marginal O44.3-●
            - partial O44.3-●
          - premature separation of placenta (normally implanted) (*see also* Abruptio placentae) O45.9-●
          - retained placenta O72.Ø
          - uterine leiomyoma O67.8
        - placenta NEC O67.8
        - postpartum NEC (atonic) (immediate) O72.1
          - with retained or trapped placenta O72.Ø
          - delayed O72.2
          - secondary O72.2
          - third stage O72.Ø
      - hourglass contraction, uterus O62.4
      - hypertension, hypertensive (pre-existing) —*see* Hypertension, complicated by, childbirth (labor)
      - hypotension O26.5-●
      - incomplete dilatation (cervix) O62.Ø
      - incoordinate uterus contractions O62.4
      - inertia, uterus O62.2
        - during latent phase of labor O62.Ø
        - primary O62.Ø
        - secondary O62.1

D

Delivery *(Continued)*
  complicated *(Continued)*
    by *(Continued)*
      infection (maternal) O98.92
        carrier state NEC O99.834
        gonorrhea O98.22
        human immunodeficiency virus (HIV) O98.72
        sexually transmitted NEC O98.32
        specified NEC O98.82
        syphilis O98.12
        tuberculosis O98.02
        viral hepatitis O98.42
        viral NEC O98.52
      injury (to mother) (*see also* Delivery, complicated, by, damage to) O71.9
        nonobstetric O9A.22
          caused by abuse —*see* Delivery, complicated by, abuse
      intrauterine fetal death, early O02.1
      inversion, uterus O71.2
      laceration (perineal) O70.9
        anus (sphincter) O70.4
          with third degree laceration —*see also* Delivery, complicated, by, laceration, perineum, third degree O70.20
            with mucosa O70.3
          without third degree laceration O70.4
        bladder (urinary) O71.5
        bowel O71.5
        cervix (uteri) O71.3
        fourchette O70.0
        hymen O70.0
        labia O70.0
        pelvic
          floor O70.1
          organ NEC O71.5
        perineum, perineal O70.9
          first degree O70.0
          fourth degree O70.3
          muscles O70.1
          second degree O70.1
          skin O70.0
          slight O70.0
          third degree O70.20
            with
              both external anal sphincter (EAS) and internal anal sphincter (IAS) torn (IIIc) O70.23
              less than 50% of external anal sphincter (EAS) thickness torn (IIIa) O70.21
              more than 50% external anal sphincter (EAS) thickness torn (IIIb) O70.22
            IIIa O70.21
            IIIb O70.22
            IIIc O70.23
        peritoneum (pelvic) O71.5
        rectovaginal (septum) (without perineal laceration) O71.4
          with perineum —*see also* Delivery, complicated, by, laceration, perineum, third degree O70.20
            with anal or rectal mucosa O70.3
        specified NEC O71.89
        sphincter ani —*see* Delivery, complicated, by, laceration, anus (sphincter)
        urethra O71.5
        uterus O71.81
          before labor O71.81
        vagina, vaginal (deep) (high) (without perineal laceration) O71.4
          with perineum O70.0
          muscles, with perineum O70.1
        vulva O70.0
      liver disorder O26.62
      malignancy O9A.12
      malnutrition O25.2
      malposition, malpresentation
        without obstruction O32.9 —*see also* Delivery, complicated by, obstruction
          breech O32.1
          compound O32.6
          face (brow) (chin) O32.3
          footling O32.8
          high head O32.4

Delivery *(Continued)*
  complicated *(Continued)*
    by *(Continued)*
      malposition, malpresentation *(Continued)*
        without obstruction *(Continued)*
          oblique O32.2
          specified NEC O32.8
          transverse O32.2
          unstable lie O32.0
        placenta O44.0-●
          with hemorrhage O44.1-●
        uterus or cervix O65.5
      meconium in amniotic fluid O77.0
      mental disorder NEC O99.344
      metrorrhexis —*see* Delivery, complicated by, rupture, uterus
      nervous system disorder O99.354
      obesity (pre-existing) O99.214
      obesity surgery status O99.844
      obstetric trauma O71.9
        specified NEC O71.89
      obstructed labor
        due to
          breech (complete) (frank) presentation O64.1
            incomplete O64.8
          brow presenation O64.3
          buttock presentation O64.1
          chin presentation O64.2
          compound presentation O64.5
          contracted pelvis O65.1
          deep transverse arrest O64.0
          deformed pelvis O65.0
          dystocia (fetal) O66.9
            due to
              conjoined twins O66.3
              fetal
                abnormality NEC O66.3
                ascites O66.3
                hydrops O66.3
                meningomyelocele O66.3
                sacral teratoma O66.3
                tumor O66.3
              hydrocephalic fetus O66.3
            shoulder O66.0
          face presentation O64.2
          fetopelvic disproportion O65.4
          footling presentation O64.8
          impacted shoulders O66.0
          incomplete rotation of fetal head O64.0
          large fetus O66.2
          locked twins O66.1
          malposition O64.9
            specified NEC O64.8
          malpresentation O64.9
            specified NEC O64.8
          multiple fetuses NEC O66.6
          pelvic
            abnormality (maternal) O65.9
              organ O65.5
              specified NEC O65.8
            contraction
              inlet O65.2
              mid-cavity O65.3
              outlet O65.3
          persistent (position)
            occipitoiliac O64.0
            occipitoposterior O64.0
            occipitosacral O64.0
            occipitotransverse O64.0
          prolapsed arm O64.4
          shoulder presentation O64.4
        specified NEC O66.8
      pathological retraction ring, uterus O62.4
      penetration, pregnant uterus by instrument O71.1
      perforation —*see* Delivery, complicated by, laceration
      placenta, placental
        ablatio —*see also* Abruptio placentae O45.9-●
        abnormality O43.9-●
          specified NEC O43.89-●
        abruptio —*see also* Abruptio placentae O45.9-●
        accreta O43.21-●
        adherent (with hemorrhage) O72.0
          without hemorrhage O73.0
        detachment (premature) —*see also* Abruptio placentae O45.9-●

Delivery *(Continued)*
  complicated *(Continued)*
    by *(Continued)*
      malposition, malpresentation *(Continued)*
        disorder O43.9-●
          specified NEC O43.89-●
        hemorrhage NEC O67.8
        increta O43.22-●
        low (implantation) (lying) O44.4-●
          with hemorrhage O44.5-●
        malformation O43.10-●
        malposition O44.0-●
          without hemorrhage O44.1-●
        percreta O43.23-●
        previa (central) (complete) (lateral) (total) O44.0-●
          with hemorrhage O44.1-●
            marginal O44.2-●
              with hemorrhage O44.3-●
            partial O44.2-●
              with hemorrhage O44.3-●
        retained (with hemorrhage) O72.0
          without hemorrhage O73.0
        separation (premature) O45.9-●
          specified NEC O45.8X-●
        vicious insertion O44.1-●
      precipitate labor O62.3
      premature rupture, membranes (*see also* Pregnancy, complicated by, premature rupture of membranes) O42.90
      prolapse
        arm or hand O32.2
        cord (umbilical) O69.0
        foot or leg O32.8
        uterus O34.52-●
      prolonged labor O63.9
        first stage O63.0
        second stage O63.1
      protozoal disease (maternal) O98.62
      respiratory disease NEC O99.52
      retained membranes or portions of placenta O72.2
        without hemorrhage O73.1
      retarded birth O63.9
      retention of secundines (with hemorrhage) O72.0
        without hemorrhage O73.0
        partial O72.2
          without hemorrhage O73.1
      rupture
        bladder (urinary) O71.5
        cervix O71.3
        pelvic organ NEC O71.5
        urethra O71.5
        uterus (during or after labor) O71.1
          before labor O71.0-●
      separation, pubic bone (symphysis pubis) O71.6
      shock O75.1
      shoulder presentation O64.4
      skin disorder NEC O99.72
      spasm, cervix O62.4
      stenosis or stricture, cervix O65.5
      streptococcus group B (GBS) carrier state O99.824
      subluxation of symphysis (pubis) O26.72
      syphilis (maternal) O98.12
      tear —*see* Delivery, complicated by, laceration
      tetanic uterus O62.4
      trauma (obstetrical) —*see also* Delivery, complicated, by, damage to O71.9
        non-obstetric O9A.22
        periurethral O71.82
        specified NEC O71.89
      tuberculosis (maternal) O98.02
      tumor, pelvic organs or tissues NEC O65.5
      umbilical cord around neck
        with compression O69.1
        without compression O69.81
      uterine inertia O62.2
        during latent phase of labor O62.0
        primary O62.0
        secondary O62.1
      vasa previa O69.4
      velamentous insertion of cord O43.12-●
    specified complication NEC O75.89
  delayed NOS O63.9
    following rupture of membranes
      artificial O75.5
    second twin, triplet, etc. O63.2

▶ New ➠ Revised ~~deleted~~ Deleted ● Use Additional Character(s) 183

Delivery *(Continued)*
- forceps, low following failed vacuum extraction O66.5
- missed (at or near term) O36.4
- normal O8Ø
- obstructed *—see* Delivery, complicated by, obstructed labor
- precipitate O62.3
- preterm *—see also* Pregnancy, complicated by, preterm labor O6Ø.1Ø
- spontaneous O8Ø
- term pregnancy NOS O8Ø
- uncomplicated O8Ø
- vaginal, following previous cesarean delivery O34.219
  - classical (vertical) scar O34.212
  - low transverse scar O34.211
  - mid-transverse T incision O34.218
  - scar
    - defect (isthmocele) O34.22
    - specified type NEC O34.218]

Delusions (paranoid) *—see* Disorder, delusional

➡ **Dementia** (degenerative (primary)) (persisting) (unspecified severity) (without behavioral disturbance, psychotic disturbance, mood disturbance, and anxiety) F03.9Ø
- with
  - aberrant motor behavior (exit-seeking) (pacing) (restlessness) (rocking) F03.911
  - ▶ acute confusional state F05
  - agitation F03.911
  - anxiety F03.94
  - behavioral disturbances (sexual disinhibition) (sleep disturbance) (social disinhibition) F03.918
    - specified NEC F03.918
  - Lewy bodies (*see also* Dementia, in, diseases specified elsewhere) G31.83 *[F02.80]*
    - with behavioral disturbance (*see also* Dementia, in, diseases specified elsewhere) G31.83 *[F02.81-●]*
  - mood disturbance (anhedonia) (apathy) (depression) F03.93
  - ▶ old age (senile) F03
    - ▶ Alzheimer's type *—see* Disease, Alzheimer's, late onset
  - Parkinson's disease (*see also* Dementia, in, diseases specified elsewhere) G2Ø.A1 *[F02.80]*
    - with behavioral disturbance G2Ø.A1 *[F02.81-●]*
  - Parkinsonism (*see also* Dementia, in, diseases specified elsewhere) G2Ø.C *[F02.80]*
    - with behavioral disturbance (*see also* Dementia, in, diseases specified elsewhere) G2Ø.C *[F02.81-●]*
  - psychotic disturbance (delusional state) (hallucinations) (paranoia) (suspiciousness) F03.92
  - verbal or physical behaviors (anger) (aggression) (combativeness) (profanity) (shouting) (threatening)(violence) F03.911
- alcoholic F1Ø.97
  - with dependence F1Ø.27
- Alzheimer's type *—see* Disease, Alzheimer's
- arteriosclerotic *—see* Dementia, vascular
- atypical, Alzheimer's type *—see* Disease, Alzheimer's, specified NEC
- congenital *—see* Disability, intellectual
- frontal (lobe) (*see also* Dementia, in, diseases specified elsewhere) G31.Ø9 *[F02.80]*
  - with behavioral disturbance (*see also* Dementia, in, diseases specified elsewhere) G31.Ø9 *[F02.81-●]*
- frontotemporal (*see also* Dementia, in, diseases specified elsewhere) G31.Ø9 *[F02.80]*
  - with behavioral disturbance (*see also* Dementia, in, diseases specified elsewhere) G31.Ø9 *[F02.81-●]*
  - specified NEC (*see also* Dementia, in, diseases specified elsewhere) G31.Ø9 *[F02.80]*
    - with behavioral disturbance (*see also* Dementia, in, diseases specified elsewhere) G31.Ø9 *[F02.81-●]*
- in (due to)
  - alcohol F1Ø.97
    - with dependence F1Ø.27
  - Alzheimer's disease *—see* Disease, Alzheimer's
  - arteriosclerotic brain disease *—see* Dementia, vascular

Dementia *(Continued)*
- in (due to) *(Continued)*
  - cerebral lipidoses (*see also* Dementia, in, diseases specified elsewhere) E75.-● *[F02.80]*
    - with behavioral disturbance (*see also* Dementia, in, diseases specified elsewhere) E75.-● *[F02.81-●]*
  - Creutzfeldt-Jakob disease *—see also* Creutzfeldt-Jakob disease or syndrome (with dementia) A81.ØØ
  - diseases specified elsewhere (unspecified severity) (without behavioral disturbance, psychotic disturbance, mood disturbance, and anxiety) F02.80
    - with
      - aberrant motor behavior (exit-seeking) (pacing) (restlessness) (rocking) F02.811
      - agitation F02.811
      - anxiety F02.84
      - behavioral disturbances (sexual disinhibition) (sleep disturbance) (social disinhibition) F02.818
        - specified NEC F02.818
      - mood disturbance (anhedonia) (apathy) (depression) F02.83
      - psychotic disturbance (delusional state) (hallucinations) (paranoia) (suspiciousness) F02.82
      - verbal or physical behaviors (anger) (aggression) (combativeness) (profanity) (shouting) (threatening) (violence) F02.811
    - mild F02.AØ
      - with
        - aberrant motor behavior (exit-seeking) (pacing) (restlessness) (rocking) F02.A11
        - agitation F02.A11
        - anxiety F02.A4
        - behavioral disturbances (sexual disinhibition) (sleep disturbance) (social disinhibition) F02.A18
          - specified NEC F02.A18
        - mood disturbance (anhedonia) (apathy) (depression) F02.A3
        - psychotic disturbance (delusional state) (hallucinations) (paranoia) (suspiciousness) F02.A2
        - verbal or physical behaviors (anger) (aggression) (combativeness) (profanity) (shouting) (threatening)(violence) F02.A11
    - moderate F02.BØ
      - with
        - aberrant motor behavior (exit-seeking) (pacing) (restlessness) (rocking) F02.B11
        - agitation F02.B11
        - anxiety F02.B4
        - behavioral disturbances (sexual disinhibition) (sleep disturbance) (social disinhibition) F02.B18
          - specified NEC F02.B18
        - mood disturbance (anhedonia) (apathy) (depression) F02.B3
        - psychotic disturbance (delusional state) (hallucinations) (paranoia) (suspiciousness) F02.B2
        - verbal or physical behaviors (anger) (aggression) (combativeness) (profanity) (shouting) (threatening)(violence) F02.B11
    - severe F02.CØ
      - with
        - aberrant motor behavior (exit-seeking) (pacing) (restlessness) (rocking) F02.C11
        - agitation F02.C11
        - anxiety F02.C4
        - behavioral disturbances (sexual disinhibition) (sleep disturbance) (social disinhibition) F02.C18
          - specified NEC F02.C18
        - mood disturbance (anhedonia) (apathy) (depression) F02.C3
        - psychotic disturbance (delusional state) (hallucinations) (paranoia) (suspiciousness) F02.C2

Dementia *(Continued)*
- in (due to) *(Continued)*
  - diseases specified elsewhere *(Continued)*
    - severe *(Continued)*
      - with *(Continued)*
        - verbal or physical behaviors (anger) (aggression) (combativeness) (profanity) (shouting) (threatening)(violence) F02.C11
  - epilepsy (*see also* Dementia, in, diseases specified elsewhere) G4Ø.-● *[F02.80]*
    - with behavioral disturbance (*see also* Dementia, in, diseases specified elsewhere) G4Ø.-● *[F02.81-●]*
  - hepatolenticular degeneration (*see also* Dementia, in, diseases specified elsewhere) E83.Ø1 *[F02.80]*
    - with behavioral disturbance (*see also* Dementia, in, diseases specified elsewhere) E83.Ø1 *[F02.81-●]*
  - human immunodeficiency virus (HIV) disease (*see also* Dementia, in, diseases specified elsewhere) B2Ø *[F02.80]*
    - with behavioral disturbance (*see also* Dementia, in, diseases specified elsewhere) B2Ø *[F02.81-●]*
  - Huntington's disease or chorea (*see also* Dementia, in, diseases specified elsewhere) G1Ø *[F02.80]*
    - with behavioral disturbance (*see also* Dementia, in, diseases specified elsewhere) G1Ø *[F02.81-●]*
  - hypercalcemia (*see also* Dementia, in, diseases specified elsewhere) E83.52 *[F02.80]*
    - with behavioral disturbance (*see also* Dementia, in, diseases specified elsewhere) E83.52 *[F02.81-●]*
  - hypothyroidism, acquired (*see also* Dementia, in, diseases specified elsewhere) E03.9 *[F02.80]*
    - with behavioral disturbance (*see also* Dementia, in, diseases specified elsewhere) E03.9 *[F02.81-●]*
    - due to iodine deficiency (*see also* Dementia, in, diseases specified elsewhere) EØ1.8 *[F02.80]*
      - with behavioral disturbance (*see also* Dementia, in, diseases specified elsewhere) EØ1.8 *[F02.81-●]*
  - inhalants F18.97
    - with dependence F18.27
  - multiple
    - etiologies F03
    - sclerosis (*see also* Dementia, in, diseases specified elsewhere) G35 *[F02.80]*
      - with behavioral disturbance (*see also* Dementia, in, diseases specified elsewhere) G35 *[F02.81-●]*
  - neurosyphilis (*see also* Dementia, in, diseases specified elsewhere) A52.17 *[F02.80]*
    - with behavioral disturbance (*see also* Dementia, in, diseases specified elsewhere) A52.17 *[F02.81-●]*
    - juvenile (*see also* Dementia, in, diseases specified elsewhere) A5Ø.49 *[F02.80]*
      - with behavioral disturbance (*see also* Dementia, in, diseases specified elsewhere) A5Ø.49 *[F02.81-●]*
  - niacin deficiency (*see also* Dementia, in, diseases specified elsewhere) E52 *[F02.80]*
    - with behavioral disturbance (*see also* Dementia, in, diseases specified elsewhere) E52 *[F02.81-●]*
  - paralysis agitans (*see also* Dementia, in, diseases specified elsewhere) G2Ø.C *[F02.80]*
    - with behavioral disturbance (*see also* Dementia, in, diseases specified elsewhere) G2Ø.C *[F02.81-●]*
  - Parkinson's disease (*see also* Dementia, in, diseases specified elsewhere) G2Ø.A1 *[F02.80]*
  - pellagra (*see also* Dementia, in, diseases specified elsewhere) E52 *[F02.80]*
    - with behavioral disturbance (*see also* Dementia, in, diseases specified elsewhere) E52 *[F02.81-●]*

D

Dementia *(Continued)*
in (due to) *(Continued)*
Pick's G31.Ø1 (*see also* Dementia, in, diseases specified elsewhere) *[FØ2.8Ø]*
with behavioral disturbance (*see also* Dementia, in, diseases specified elsewhere) G31.Ø1 *[FØ2.81-•]*
polyarteritis nodosa (*see also* Dementia, in, diseases specified elsewhere) M3Ø.Ø *[FØ2.8Ø]*
with behavioral disturbance (*see also* Dementia, in, diseases specified elsewhere) M3Ø.Ø *[FØ2.81-•]*
psychoactive drug F19.97
with dependence F19.27
inhalants F18.97
with dependence F18.27
sedatives, hypnotics or anxiolytics F13.97
with dependence F13.27
sedatives, hypnotics or anxiolytics F13.97
with dependence F13.27
systemic lupus erythematosus (*see also* Dementia, in, diseases specified elsewhere) M32.-• *[FØ2.8Ø]*
with behavioral disturbance (*see also* Dementia, in, diseases specified elsewhere) M32.-• *[FØ2.81-•]*
trypanosomiasis
African (*see also* Dementia, in, diseases specified elsewhere) B56.9 *[FØ2.8Ø]*
with behavioral disturbance (*see also* Dementia, in, diseases specified elsewhere) B56.9 *[FØ2.81-•]*
unknown etiology (*see also* Dementia, in, diseases specified elsewhere) FØ3.-•
vitamin B12 deficiency (*see also* Dementia, in, diseases specified elsewhere) E53.8 *[FØ2.8Ø]*
with behavioral disturbance (*see also* Dementia, in, diseases specified elsewhere) E53.8 *[FØ2.81-•]*
volatile solvents F18.97
with dependence F18.27
infantile, infantilis F84.3
Lewy body (*see also* Dementia, in, diseases specified elsewhere) G31.83 *[FØ2.8Ø]*
with behavioral disturbance (*see also* Dementia, in, diseases specified elsewhere) G31.83 *[FØ2.81-•]*
mild FØ2.AØ
with
aberrant motor behavior (exit-seeking) (pacing) (restlessness) (rocking) FØ2.A11
agitation FØ2.A11
anxiety FØ2.A4
behavioral disturbances (sexual disinhibition) (sleep disturbance) (social disinhibition) FØ2.A18
specified NEC FØ2.A18
mood disturbance (anhedonia) (apathy) (depression) FØ2.A3
psychotic disturbance (delusional state) (hallucinations) (paranoia) (suspiciousness) FØ2.A2
verbal or physical behaviors (anger) (aggression) (combativeness) (profanity) (shouting) (threatening) (violence) FØ2.A11
moderate FØ2.BØ
with
aberrant motor behavior (exit-seeking) (pacing) (restlessness) (rocking) FØ2.B11
agitation FØ2.B11
anxiety FØ2.B4
behavioral disturbances (sexual disinhibition) (sleep disturbance) (social disinhibition) FØ2.B18
specified NEC FØ2.B18
mood disturbance (anhedonia) (apathy) (depression) FØ2.B3
psychotic disturbance (delusional state) (hallucinations) (paranoia) (suspiciousness) FØ2.B2
verbal or physical behaviors (anger) (aggression) (combativeness) (profanity) (shouting) (threatening) (violence) FØ2.B11

Dementia *(Continued)*
multi-infarct —*see* Dementia, vascular
paralytica, paralytic (syphilitic) (*see also* Dementia, in, diseases specified elsewhere) A52.17 *[FØ2.8Ø]*
with behavioral disturbance (*see also* Dementia, in, diseases specified elsewhere) A52.17 *[FØ2.81-•]*
juvenilis A5Ø.45
paretic A52.17
praecox —*see* Schizophrenia
presenile FØ3
Alzheimer's type —*see* Disease, Alzheimer's, early onset
primary degenerative FØ3
progressive, syphilitic A52.17
senile FØ3
~~with acute confusional state FØ5~~
Alzheimer's type —*see* Disease, Alzheimer's, late onset
depressed or paranoid type FØ3
severe FØ2.CØ
with
aberrant motor behavior (exit-seeking) (pacing) (restlessness) (rocking) FØ2.C11
agitation FØ2.C11
anxiety FØ2.C4
behavioral disturbances (sexual disinhibition) (sleep disturbance) (social disinhibition) FØ2.C18
specified NEC FØ2.C18
mood disturbance (anhedonia) (apathy) (depression) FØ2.C3
psychotic disturbance (delusional state) (hallucinations) (paranoia) (suspiciousness) FØ2.C2
verbal or physical behaviors (anger) (aggression) (combativeness) (profanity) (shouting) (threatening) (violence) FØ2.C11
vascular (acute onset) (mixed) (multi-infarct) (subcortical) (unspecified severity) (without behavioral disturbance, psychotic disturbance, mood disturbance, and anxiety) FØ1.5Ø
with
aberrant motor behavior (exit-seeking) (pacing) (restlessness) (rocking) FØ1.511
agitation FØ1.511
anxiety FØ1.54
behavioral disturbances (sleep disturbance) (sexual disinhibition) (social disinhibition) FØ1.518
specified NEC FØ1.518
mood disturbance (anhedonia) (apathy) (depression) FØ1.53
psychotic disturbance (delusional state) (hallucinations) (paranoia) (suspiciousness) FØ1.52
verbal or physical behaviors (anger) (aggression) (combativeness) (profanity) (shouting) (threatening) (violence) FØ1.511
mild FØ1.AØ
with
aberrant motor behavior (exit-seeking) (pacing) (restlessness) (rocking) FØ1.A11
agitation FØ1.A11
anxiety FØ1.A4
behavioral disturbances (sleep disturbance) (sexual disinhibition) (social disinhibition) FØ1.A18
specified NEC FØ1.A18
mood disturbance (anhedonia) (apathy) (depression) FØ1.A3
psychotic disturbance (delusional state) (hallucinations) (paranoia) (suspiciousness) FØ1.A2
verbal or physical behaviors (anger) (aggression) (combativeness) (profanity) (shouting) (threatening) (violence) FØ1.A11
moderate FØ1.BØ
with
aberrant motor behavior (exit-seeking) (pacing) (restlessness) (rocking) FØ1.B11
agitation FØ1.B11

Dementia *(Continued)*
vascular *(Continued)*
moderate *(Continued)*
with *(Continued)*
anxiety FØ1.B4
behavioral disturbances (sleep disturbance) (sexual disinhibition) (social disinhibition) FØ1.B18
specified NEC FØ1.B18
mood disturbance (anhedonia) (apathy) (depression) FØ1.B3
psychotic disturbance (delusional state) (hallucinations) (paranoia) (suspiciousness) FØ1.B2
verbal or physical behaviors (anger) (aggression) (combativeness) (profanity) (shouting) (threatening) (violence) FØ1.B11
severe FØ1.CØ
with
aberrant motor behavior (exit-seeking) (pacing) (restlessness) (rocking) FØ1.C11
agitation FØ1.C11
anxiety FØ1.C4
behavioral disturbances (sleep disturbance) (sexual disinhibition) (social disinhibition) FØ1.C18
specified NEC FØ1.C18
mood disturbance (anhedonia) (apathy) (depression) FØ1.C3
psychotic disturbance (delusional state) (hallucinations) (paranoia) (suspiciousness) FØ1.C2
verbal or physical behaviors (anger) (aggression) (combativeness) (profanity) (shouting) (threatening) (violence) FØ1.C11
Demineralization, bone —*see* Osteoporosis
Demodex folliculorum (infestation) B88.Ø
Demophobia F4Ø.248
Demoralization R45.3
Demyelination, demyelinization
central nervous system G37.9
specified NEC G37.89
corpus callosum (central) G37.1
disseminated, acute G36.9
specified NEC G36.8
global G35
in optic neuritis G36.Ø
Dengue (classical) (fever) A9Ø
hemorrhagic A91
sandfly A93.1
Dennie-Marfan syphilitic syndrome A5Ø.45
Dens evaginatus, in dente or invaginatus KØØ.2
Dense breasts (*see also* Density, breast) R92.3Ø
Density
breast R92.3Ø•
mammographic•
extreme R92.34-•
fatty tissue R92.31-•
fibroglandular R92.32-•
heterogeneous R92.33-•
increased, bone (disseminated) (generalized) (spotted) —*see* Disorder, bone, density and structure, specified type NEC
low R92.3Ø•
lung (nodular) J98.4
Dental —*see also* condition
examination ZØ1.2Ø
with abnormal findings ZØ1.21
restoration
aesthetically inadequate or displeasing KØ8.56
defective KØ8.5Ø
specified NEC KØ8.59
failure of marginal integrity KØ8.51
failure of periodontal anatomical integrity KØ8.54
Dentia praecox KØØ.6
Denticles (pulp) KØ4.2
Dentigerous cyst KØ9.Ø
Dentin
irregular (in pulp) KØ4.3
opalescent KØØ.5
secondary (in pulp) KØ4.3
sensitive KØ3.89
Dentinogenesis imperfecta KØØ.5
Dentinoma —*see* Cyst, calcifying odontogenic
Dentition (syndrome) KØØ.7
delayed KØØ.6
difficult KØØ.7

D

Dentition (Continued)
 precocious K00.6
 premature K00.6
 retarded K00.6
Dependence (on) (syndrome) F19.20
 with remission F19.21
 alcohol (ethyl) (methyl) (without remission)
 F10.20
 with
 amnestic disorder, persisting F10.26
 anxiety disorder F10.280
 dementia, persisting F10.27
 intoxication F10.229
 with delirium F10.221
 uncomplicated F10.220
 mood disorder F10.24
 psychotic disorder F10.259
 with
 delusions F10.250
 hallucinations F10.251
 remission F10.21
 sexual dysfunction F10.281
 sleep disorder F10.282
 specified disorder NEC F10.288
 withdrawal F10.239
 with
 delirium F10.231
 perceptual disturbance F10.232
 uncomplicated F10.230
 counseling and surveillance Z71.41
 in remission F10.21
 amobarbital —see Dependence, drug, sedative
 amphetamine(s) (type) —see Dependence, drug,
 stimulant NEC
 amytal (sodium) —see Dependence, drug,
 sedative
 analgesic NEC F55.8
 anesthetic (agent) (gas) (general) (local) NEC —
 see Dependence, drug, psychoactive NEC
 anxiolytic NEC —see Dependence, drug, sedative
 barbital(s) —see Dependence, drug, sedative
 barbiturate(s) (compounds) (drugs classifiable to
 T42) —see Dependence, drug, sedative
 benzedrine —see Dependence, drug, stimulant
 NEC
 bhang —see Dependence, drug, cannabis
 bromide(s) NEC —see Dependence, drug,
 sedative
 caffeine —see Dependence, drug, stimulant NEC
 cannabis (sativa) (indica) (resin) (derivatives)
 (type) —see Dependence, drug, cannabis
 chloral (betaine) (hydrate) —see Dependence,
 drug, sedative
 chlordiazepoxide —see Dependence, drug,
 sedative
 coca (leaf) (derivatives) —see Dependence, drug,
 cocaine
 cocaine —see Dependence, drug, cocaine
 codeine —see Dependence, drug, opioid
 combinations of drugs F19.20
 dagga —see Dependence, drug, cannabis
 demerol —see Dependence, drug, opioid
 dexamphetamine —see Dependence, drug,
 stimulant NEC
 dexedrine —see Dependence, drug, stimulant
 NEC
 dextromethorphan —see Dependence, drug,
 opioid
 dextromoramide —see Dependence, drug, opioid
 dextro-nor-pseudo-ephedrine —see Dependence,
 drug, stimulant NEC
 dextrorphan —see Dependence, drug, opioid
 diazepam —see Dependence, drug,
 sedative
 dilaudid —see Dependence, drug, opioid
 D-lysergic acid diethylamide —see Dependence,
 drug, hallucinogen
 drug NEC F19.20
 with sleep disorder F19.282
 cannabis F12.20
 with
 anxiety disorder F12.280
 intoxication F12.229
 with
 delirium F12.221
 perceptual disturbance F12.222
 uncomplicated F12.220
 other specified disorder F12.288
 psychosis F12.259
 delusions F12.250
 hallucinations F12.251

Dependence (Continued)
 drug (Continued)
 cannabis (Continued)
 with (Continued)
 unspecified disorder F12.29
 withdrawal F12.23
 in remission F12.21
 cocaine F14.20
 with
 anxiety disorder F14.280
 intoxication F14.229
 with
 delirium F14.221
 perceptual disturbance F14.222
 uncomplicated F14.220
 mood disorder F14.24
 other specified disorder F14.288
 psychosis F14.259
 delusions F14.250
 hallucinations F14.251
 sexual dysfunction F14.281
 sleep disorder F14.282
 unspecified disorder F14.29
 withdrawal F14.23
 in remission F14.21
 withdrawal symptoms in newborn P96.1
 counseling and surveillance Z71.51
 hallucinogen F16.20
 with
 anxiety disorder F16.280
 flashbacks F16.283
 intoxication F16.229
 with delirium F16.221
 uncomplicated F16.220
 mood disorder F16.24
 other specified disorder F16.288
 perception disorder, persisting F16.283
 psychosis F16.259
 delusions F16.250
 hallucinations F16.251
 unspecified disorder F16.29
 in remission F16.21
 in remission F19.21
 inhalant F18.20
 with
 anxiety disorder F18.280
 dementia, persisting F18.27
 intoxication F18.229
 with delirium F18.221
 uncomplicated F18.220
 mood disorder F18.24
 other specified disorder F18.288
 psychosis F18.259
 delusions F18.250
 hallucinations F18.251
 unspecified disorder F18.29
 in remission F18.21
 nicotine F17.200
 with disorder F17.209
 in remission F17.201
 specified disorder NEC F17.208
 withdrawal F17.203
 chewing tobacco F17.220
 with disorder F17.229
 in remission F17.221
 specified disorder NEC F17.228
 withdrawal F17.223
 cigarettes F17.210
 with disorder F17.219
 in remission F17.211
 specified disorder NEC F17.218
 withdrawal F17.213
 specified product NEC F17.290
 with disorder F17.299
 remission F17.291
 specified disorder NEC F17.298
 withdrawal F17.293
 opioid F11.20
 with
 intoxication F11.229
 with
 delirium F11.221
 perceptual disturbance F11.222
 uncomplicated F11.220
 mood disorder F11.24
 opioid-associated amnestic syndrome
 F11.288
 other specified disorder F11.288
 psychosis F11.259
 delusions F11.250
 hallucinations F11.251

Dependence (Continued)
 drug (Continued)
 opioid (Continued)
 with (Continued)
 sexual dysfunction F11.281
 sleep disorder F11.282
 unspecified disorder F11.29
 withdrawal F11.23
 in remission F11.21
 psychoactive NEC F19.20
 with
 amnestic disorder F19.26
 anxiety disorder F19.280
 dementia F19.27
 intoxication F19.229
 with
 delirium F19.221
 perceptual disturbance F19.222
 uncomplicated F19.220
 mood disorder F19.24
 other specified disorder F19.288
 psychosis F19.259
 delusions F19.250
 hallucinations F19.251
 sexual dysfunction F19.281
 sleep disorder F19.282
 unspecified disorder F19.29
 withdrawal F19.239
 with
 delirium F19.231
 perceptual disturbance F19.232
 uncomplicated F19.230
 in remission F19.21
 sedative, hypnotic or anxiolytic F13.20
 with
 amnestic disorder F13.26
 anxiety disorder F13.280
 dementia, persisting F13.27
 intoxication F13.229
 with delirium F13.221
 uncomplicated F13.220
 mood disorder F13.24
 other specified disorder F13.288
 psychosis F13.259
 delusions F13.250
 hallucinations F13.251
 sexual dysfunction F13.281
 sleep disorder F13.282
 unspecified disorder F13.29
 withdrawal F13.239
 with
 delirium F13.231
 perceptual disturbance F13.232
 uncomplicated F13.230
 in remission F13.21
 stimulant NEC F15.20
 with
 anxiety disorder F15.280
 intoxication F15.229
 with
 delirium F15.221
 perceptual disturbance F15.222
 uncomplicated F15.220
 mood disorder F15.24
 other specified disorder F15.288
 psychosis F15.259
 delusions F15.250
 hallucinations F15.251
 sexual dysfunction F15.281
 sleep disorder F15.282
 unspecified disorder F15.29
 withdrawal F15.23
 in remission F15.21
 ethyl
 alcohol (without remission) F10.20
 with remission F10.21
 bromide —see Dependence, drug, sedative
 carbamate F19.20
 chloride F19.20
 morphine —see Dependence, drug, opioid
 ganja —see Dependence, drug, cannabis
 glue (airplane) (sniffing) —see Dependence,
 drug, inhalant
 glutethimide —see Dependence, drug, sedative
 hallucinogenics —see Dependence, drug,
 hallucinogen
 hashish —see Dependence, drug, cannabis
 hemp —see Dependence, drug, cannabis
 heroin (salt) (any) —see Dependence, drug,
 opioid
 hypnotic NEC —see Dependence, drug, sedative

 ▶ New ⇒ Revised ~~deleted~~ Deleted ● Use Additional Character(s)

- **Dependence** *(Continued)*
  - Indian hemp —*see* Dependence, drug, cannabis
  - inhalants —*see* Dependence, drug, inhalant
  - khat —*see* Dependence, drug, stimulant NEC
  - laudanum —*see* Dependence, drug, opioid
  - LSD (-25) (derivatives) —*see* Dependence, drug, hallucinogen
  - luminal —*see* Dependence, drug, sedative
  - lysergic acid —*see* Dependence, drug, hallucinogen
  - maconha —*see* Dependence, drug, cannabis
  - marihuana —*see* Dependence, drug, cannabis
  - meprobamate —*see* Dependence, drug, sedative
  - mescaline —*see* Dependence, drug, hallucinogen
  - methadone —*see* Dependence, drug, opioid
  - methamphetamine(s) —*see* Dependence, drug, stimulant NEC
  - methaqualone —*see* Dependence, drug, sedative
  - methyl
    - alcohol (without remission) F1Ø.2Ø
      - with remission F1Ø.21
    - bromide —*see* Dependence, drug, sedative
    - morphine —*see* Dependence, drug, opioid
    - phenidate —*see* Dependence, drug, stimulant NEC
    - sulfonal —*see* Dependence, drug, sedative
  - morphine (sulfate) (sulfite) (type) —*see* Dependence, drug, opioid
  - narcotic (drug) NEC —*see* Dependence, drug, opioid
  - nembutal —*see* Dependence, drug, sedative
  - neraval —*see* Dependence, drug, sedative
  - neravan —*see* Dependence, drug, sedative
  - neurobarb —*see* Dependence, drug, sedative
  - nicotine —*see* Dependence, drug, nicotine
  - nitrous oxide F19.2Ø
  - nonbarbiturate sedatives and tranquilizers with similar effect —*see* Dependence, drug, sedative
  - on
    - artificial heart (fully implantable) (mechanical) Z95.812
    - aspirator Z99.Ø
    - care provider (because of) Z74.9
      - impaired mobility Z74.Ø9
      - need for
        - assistance with personal care Z74.1
        - continuous supervision Z74.3
      - no other household member able to render care Z74.2
      - specified reason NEC Z74.8
    - machine Z99.89
      - enabling NEC Z99.89
      - specified type NEC Z99.89
    - renal dialysis (hemodialysis) (peritoneal) Z99.2
    - respirator Z99.11
    - ventilator Z99.11
    - wheelchair Z99.3
  - opiate —*see* Dependence, drug, opioid
  - opioids —*see* Dependence, drug, opioid
  - opium (alkaloids) (derivatives) (tincture) —*see* Dependence, drug, opioid
  - oxygen (long-term) (supplemental) Z99.81
  - paraldehyde —*see* Dependence, drug, sedative
  - paregoric —*see* Dependence, drug, opioid
  - PCP (phencyclidine) (or related substance) —*see* Dependence, drug, hallucinogen
  - pentobarbital —*see* Dependence, drug, sedative
  - pentobarbitone (sodium) —*see* Dependence, drug, sedative
  - pentothal —*see* Dependence, drug, sedative
  - peyote —*see* Dependence, drug, hallucinogen
  - phencyclidine (PCP) (or related substance) —*see* Dependence, drug, hallucinogen
  - phenmetrazine —*see* Dependence, drug, stimulant NEC
  - phenobarbital —*see* Dependence, drug, sedative
  - polysubstance F19.2Ø
  - psilocibin, psilocin, psilocyn, psilocyline —*see* Dependence, drug, hallucinogen
  - psychostimulant NEC —*see* Dependence, drug, stimulant NEC
  - secobarbital —*see* Dependence, drug, sedative
  - seconal —*see* Dependence, drug, sedative
  - sedative NEC —*see* Dependence, drug, sedative
  - specified drug NEC —*see* Dependence, drug
  - stimulant NEC —*see* Dependence, drug, stimulant NEC
  - substance NEC —*see* Dependence, drug
  - supplemental oxygen Z99.81
  - tobacco —*see* Dependence, drug, nicotine
    - counseling and surveillance Z71.6
  - tranquilizer NEC —*see* Dependence, drug, sedative
  - vitamin B6 E53.1
  - volatile solvents —*see* Dependence, drug, inhalant
- **Dependency**
  - care-provider Z74.9
  - passive F6Ø.7
  - reactions (persistent) F6Ø.7
- **Depersonalization** (in neurotic state) (neurotic) (syndrome) F48.1
- **Depletion**
  - extracellular fluid E86.9
  - plasma E86.1
  - potassium E87.6
    - nephropathy N25.89
  - salt or sodium E87.1
    - causing heat exhaustion or prostration T67.4
    - nephropathy N28.9
  - volume NOS E86.9
- **Deployment** (current) (military) status Z56.82
  - in theater or in support of military war, peacekeeping and humanitarian operations Z56.82
  - personal history of Z91.82
    - military war, peacekeeping and humanitarian deployment (current or past conflict) Z91.82
  - returned from Z91.82
- **Depolarization, premature** I49.4Ø
  - atrial I49.1
  - junctional I49.2
  - specified NEC I49.49
  - ventricular I49.3
- **Deposit**
  - bone in Boeck's sarcoid D86.89
  - calcareous, calcium —*see* Calcification
  - cholesterol
    - retina H35.89
    - vitreous (body) (humor) —*see* Deposit, crystalline
  - conjunctiva H11.11-•
  - cornea H18.ØØ-•
    - argentous H18.Ø2-•
    - due to metabolic disorder H18.Ø3-•
    - Kayser-Fleischer ring H18.Ø4-•
    - pigmentation —*see* Pigmentation, cornea
  - crystalline, vitreous (body) (humor) H43.2-•
  - hemosiderin in old scars of cornea —*see* Pigmentation, cornea, stromal
  - metallic in lens —*see* Cataract, specified NEC
  - skin R23.8
  - tooth, teeth (betel) (black) (green) (materia alba) (orange) (tobacco) KØ3.6
  - urate, kidney —*see* Calculus, kidney
- **Depraved appetite** —*see* Pica
- **Depressed**
  - HDL cholesterol E78.6
- **Depression** (acute) (mental) F32.A
  - agitated (single episode) F32.2
  - anaclitic —*see* Disorder, adjustment
  - anxiety F41.8
    - persistent F34.1
  - arches —*see also* Deformity, limb, flat foot
  - atypical (single episode) F32.89
    - recurrent episode F33.8
  - basal metabolic rate R94.8
  - bone marrow D75.89
  - central nervous system G98.8
  - cerebral R29.818
    - newborn P91.4
  - cerebrovascular I67.9
  - chest wall M95.4
  - climacteric (single episode) F32.89
    - recurrent episode F33.8
  - endogenous (without psychotic symptoms) F33.2
    - with psychotic symptoms F33.3
  - functional activity R68.89
  - hysterical F44.89
  - involutional (single episode) F32.89
    - recurrent episode F33.8
  - major F32.9
    - with psychotic symptoms F32.3
    - recurrent —*see* Disorder, depressive, recurrent
  - manic-depressive —*see* Disorder, depressive, recurrent
  - masked (single episode) F32.89
  - medullary G93.89
  - menopausal (single episode) F32.89
    - recurrent episode F33.8
  - metatarsus —*see* Depression, arches
  - monopolar F33.9
  - nervous F34.1
  - neurotic F34.1
  - nose M95.Ø
  - postnatal (NOS) F53.Ø
  - postpartum (NOS) F53.Ø
  - post-psychotic of schizophrenia F32.89
  - post-schizophrenic F32.89
  - psychogenic (reactive) (single episode) F32.9
  - psychoneurotic F34.1
  - psychotic (single episode) F32.3
    - recurrent F33.3
  - reactive (psychogenic) (single episode) F32.9
    - psychotic (single episode) F32.3
  - recurrent —*see* Disorder, depressive, recurrent
  - respiratory center G93.89
  - seasonal —*see* Disorder, depressive, recurrent
  - senile FØ3
  - severe, single episode F32.2
  - situational F43.21
  - skull Q67.4
  - specified NEC (single episode) F32.89
  - sternum M95.4
  - visual field —*see* Defect, visual field
  - vital (recurrent) (without psychotic symptoms) F33.2
    - with psychotic symptoms F33.3
    - single episode F32.2
- **Deprivation**
  - cultural Z6Ø.3
  - effects NOS T73.9
    - specified NEC T73.8
  - emotional NEC Z65.8
    - affecting infant or child —*see* Maltreatment, child, psychological
  - food T73.Ø
  - material due to limited financial resources, specified NEC Z59.87
  - protein —*see* Malnutrition
  - sleep Z72.82Ø
  - social Z6Ø.4
    - affecting infant or child —*see* Maltreatment, child, psychological
  - specified NEC T73.8
  - vitamins —*see* Deficiency, vitamin
  - water T73.1
- **Derangement**
  - ankle (internal) —*see* Derangement, joint, articular cartilage, ankle
  - cartilage (articular) NEC —*see* Derangement, joint, articular cartilage, by site
    - recurrent —*see* Dislocation, recurrent
  - cruciate ligament, anterior, current injury —*see* Sprain, knee, cruciate, anterior
  - elbow (internal) —*see* Derangement, joint, articular cartilage, elbow
  - hip (joint) (internal) (old) —*see* Derangement, joint, articular cartilage, hip
  - joint (internal) M24.9
    - ankylosis —*see* Ankylosis
    - articular cartilage M24.1Ø
      - ankle M24.17-•
      - elbow M24.12-•
      - foot M24.17-•
      - hand M24.14-•
      - hip M24.15-•
      - knee NEC M23.9-•
      - loose body —*see* Loose, body
      - shoulder M24.11-•
      - specified site NEC M24.19
      - wrist M24.13-•
    - contracture —*see* Contraction, joint
    - current injury —*see also* Dislocation
      - knee, meniscus or cartilage —*see* Tear, meniscus
    - dislocation
      - pathological —*see* Dislocation, pathological
      - recurrent —*see* Dislocation, recurrent
    - knee —*see* Derangement, knee
    - ligament —*see* Disorder, ligament
    - loose body —*see* Loose, body
    - recurrent —*see* Dislocation, recurrent
    - specified type NEC M24.8Ø
      - ankle M24.87-•
      - elbow M24.82-•
      - foot joint M24.87-•
      - hand joint M24.84-•

D

- **Dermatitis** *(Continued)*
  - due to *(Continued)*
    - radiation L59.8
      - nonionizing (chronic exposure) L57.8
      - sun NEC L57.8
        - acute L56.8
    - radioactive substance L58.9
      - acute L58.Ø
      - chronic L58.1
    - radium L58.9
      - acute L58.Ø
      - chronic L58.1
    - ragweed (allergic) (contact) L23.7
    - Rhus (allergic) (contact) (diversiloba) (radicans) (toxicodendron) (venenata) (verniciflua) L23.7
    - rubber (contact) L24.5
    - Senecio jacobaea (allergic) (contact) L23.7
    - solvents (contact) (irritant) (substances in categories T52) L24.2
    - specified agent NEC (contact) L25.8
      - allergic L23.89
      - irritant L24.89
    - sunshine NEC L57.8
      - acute L56.8
    - tetrachlorethylene (contact) (irritant) L24.2
    - toluene (contact) (irritant) L24.2
    - turpentine (contact) L24.2
    - ultraviolet rays (sun NEC) (chronic exposure) L57.8
      - acute L56.8
    - vaccine or vaccination L27.Ø
      - specified substance —*see* Table of Drugs and Chemicals
    - varicose veins —*see* Varix, leg, with, inflammation
    - X-rays L58.9
      - acute L58.Ø
      - chronic L58.1
  - dyshydrotic L3Ø.1
  - dysmenorrheica N94.6
  - escharotica —*see* Burn
  - exfoliative, exfoliativa (generalized) L26
    - neonatorum LØØ
  - eyelid —*(see also* Dermatosis, eyelid) HØ1.9
    - allergic HØ1.119
      - left HØ1.116
        - lower HØ1.115
        - upper HØ1.114
      - right HØ1.113
        - lower HØ1.112
        - upper HØ1.111
    - contact —*see* Dermatitis, eyelid, allergic
    - due to
      - Demodex species B88.Ø
      - herpes (zoster) BØ2.39
        - simplex BØØ.59
    - eczematous HØ1.139
      - left HØ1.136
        - lower HØ1.135
        - upper HØ1.134
      - right HØ1.133
        - lower HØ1.132
        - upper HØ1.131
    - specified NEC HØ1.8
  - facta, factitia, factitial L98.1
    - psychogenic F54
  - flexural NEC L2Ø.82
  - friction L3Ø.4
  - fungus B36.9
    - specified type NEC B36.8
  - gangrenosa, gangrenous infantum LØ8.Ø
  - harvest mite B88.Ø
  - heat L59.Ø
  - herpesviral, vesicular (ear) (lip) BØØ.1
  - herpetiformis (bullous) (erythematous) (pustular) (vesicular) L13.Ø
    - juvenile L12.2
    - senile L12.Ø
  - hiemalis L3Ø.8
  - hypostatic, hypostatica —*see* Varix, leg, with, inflammation
  - infectious eczematoid L3Ø.3
  - infective L3Ø.3
  - irritant —*see* Dermatitis, contact, irritant
  - Jacquet's (diaper dermatitis) L22
  - Leptus B88.Ø

- **Dermatitis** *(Continued)*
  - lichenified NEC L28.Ø
  - medicamentosa (generalized) (internal use) —*see* Dermatitis, due to drugs
  - mite B88.Ø
  - multiformis L13.Ø
    - juvenile L12.2
  - napkin L22
  - neurotica L13.Ø
  - nummular L3Ø.Ø
  - papillaris capillitii L73.Ø
  - pellagrous E52
  - perioral L71.Ø
  - photocontact L56.2
  - polymorpha dolorosa L13.Ø
  - pruriginosa L13.Ø
  - pruritic NEC L3Ø.8
  - psychogenic F54
  - purulent LØ8.Ø
  - pustular
    - contagious BØ8.Ø2
    - subcorneal L13.1
  - pyococcal LØ8.Ø
  - pyogenica LØ8.Ø
  - repens L4Ø.2
  - Ritter's (exfoliativa) LØØ
  - Schamberg's L81.7
  - schistosome B65.3
  - seasonal bullous L3Ø.8
  - seborrheic L21.9
    - infantile L21.1
    - specified NEC L21.8
  - sensitization NOS L23.9
  - septic LØ8.Ø
  - solare L57.8
  - specified NEC L3Ø.8
  - stasis I87.2
    - with
      - varicose ulcer —*see* Varix, leg, with ulcer, with inflammation
      - varicose veins —*see* Varix, leg, with, inflammation
    - due to postthrombotic syndrome —*see* Syndrome, postthrombotic
  - suppurative LØ8.Ø
  - traumatic NEC L3Ø.4
  - trophoneurotica L13.Ø
  - ultraviolet (sun) (chronic exposure) L57.8
    - acute L56.8
  - varicose —*see* Varix, leg, with, inflammation
  - vegetans L1Ø.1
  - verrucosa B43.Ø
  - vesicular, herpesviral BØØ.1
- **Dermatoarthritis, lipoid** E78.81
- **Dermatochalasis, eyelid** HØ2.839
  - left HØ2.836
    - lower HØ2.835
    - upper HØ2.834
  - right HØ2.833
    - lower HØ2.832
    - upper HØ2.831
- **Dermatofibroma** (lenticulare) —*see* Neoplasm, skin, benign
  - protuberans —*see* Neoplasm, skin, uncertain behavior
- **Dermatofibrosarcoma** (pigmented) (protuberans) —*see* Neoplasm, skin, malignant
- **Dermatographia** L5Ø.3
- **Dermatolysis** (exfoliativa) (congenital) Q82.8
  - acquired L57.4
  - eyelids —*see* Blepharochalasis
  - palpebrarum —*see* Blepharochalasis
  - senile L57.4
- **Dermatomegaly** NEC Q82.8
- **Dermatomucosomyositis** (*see also* Dermatomyositis) M33.1Ø
  - with
    - myopathy M33.12
    - respiratory involvement M33.11
    - specified organ involvement NEC M33.19
- **Dermatomycosis** B36.9
  - furfuracea B36.Ø
  - specified type NEC B36.8
- **Dermatomyositis** (acute) (chronic) —*see also* Dermatopolymyositis
  - adult —*see also* Dermatomyositis, specified NEC M33.1Ø
  - in (due to) neoplastic disease —*see also* Neoplasm D49.9 *[M36.Ø]*

- **Dermatomyositis** *(Continued)*
  - juvenile M33.ØØ
    - with
      - myopathy M33.Ø2
      - respiratory involvement M33.Ø1
      - specified organ involvement NEC M33.Ø9
        - amyopathic M33.Ø3
    - without myopathy M33.Ø3
  - specified NEC M33.1Ø
    - with
      - myopathy M33.12
      - respiratory involvement M33.11
      - specified organ involvement NEC M33.19
        - amyopathic M33.13
    - without myopathy M33.13
- **Dermatoneuritis of children** —*see* Poisoning, mercury
- **Dermatophilosis** A48.8
- **Dermatophytid** L3Ø.2
- **Dermatophytide** —*see* Dermatophytosis
- **Dermatophytosis** (epidermophyton) (infection) (Microsporum) (tinea) (Trichophyton) B35.9
  - beard B35.Ø
  - body B35.4
  - capitis B35.Ø
  - corporis B35.4
  - deep-seated B35.8
  - disseminated B35.8
  - foot B35.3
  - granulomatous B35.8
  - groin B35.6
  - hand B35.2
  - nail B35.1
  - perianal (area) B35.6
  - scalp B35.Ø
  - specified NEC B35.8
- **Dermatopolymyositis** M33.9Ø
  - with
    - myopathy M33.92
    - respiratory involvement M33.91
    - specified organ involvement NEC M33.99
      - amyopathic M33.93
  - in neoplastic disease —*see also* Neoplasm D49.9 *[M36.Ø]*
  - juvenile M33.ØØ
    - with
      - myopathy M33.Ø2
      - respiratory involvement M33.Ø1
      - specified organ involvement NEC M33.Ø9
        - amyopathic M33.Ø3
        - without myopathy M33.Ø3
  - specified NEC M33.1Ø
    - myopathy M33.12
    - respiratory involvement M33.11
    - specified organ involvement NEC M33.19
      - amyopathic M33.13
      - without myopathy M33.13
  - without myopathy M33.93
- **Dermatopolyneuritis** —*see* Poisoning, mercury
- **Dermatorrhexis** (*see also* Syndrome, Ehlers-Danlos) Q79.6Ø
  - acquired L57.4
- **Dermatosclerosis** —*see also* Scleroderma
  - localized L94.Ø
- **Dermatosis** L98.9
  - Andrews' LØ8.89
  - Bowen's —*see* Neoplasm, skin, in situ
  - bullous L13.9
    - specified NEC L13.8
  - exfoliativa L26
  - eyelid (noninfectious) (*see also* Dermatitis, eyelid) HØ1.9
    - discoid lupus erythematosus —*see* Lupus, erythematosus, eyelid
    - xeroderma —*see* Xeroderma, acquired, eyelid
  - factitial L98.1
  - febrile neutrophilic L98.2
  - gonococcal A54.89
  - herpetiformis L13.Ø
    - juvenile L12.2
  - linear IgA L13.8
  - menstrual NEC L98.8
  - neutrophilic, febrile L98.2
  - occupational —*see* Dermatitis, contact
  - papulosa nigra L82.1
  - pigmentary L81.9
    - progressive L81.7
    - Schamberg's L81.7

D

D

Diabetes, diabetic *(Continued)*
- specified type *(Continued)*
  - with *(Continued)*
    - skin complication NEC E13.628
    - skin ulcer NEC E13.622
- steroid-induced *—see* Diabetes, due to, drug or chemical
- type 1 E10.9
  - with
    - amyotrophy E10.44
    - arthropathy NEC E10.618
    - autonomic (poly)neuropathy E10.43
    - cataract E10.36
    - Charcot's joints E10.610
    - chronic kidney disease E10.22
    - circulatory complication NEC E10.59
    - coma due to
      - hypoglycemia E11.641
      - ketoacidosis E11.11
    - complication E10.8
      - specified NEC E10.69
    - dermatitis E10.620
    - foot ulcer E10.621
    - gangrene E10.52
    - gastroparalysis E10.43
    - gastroparesis E10.43
    - glomerulonephrosis, intracapillary E10.21
    - glomerulosclerosis, intercapillary E10.21
    - hyperglycemia E10.65
    - hypoglycemia E10.649
      - with coma E10.641
    - ketoacidosis E10.10
      - with coma E10.11
    - kidney complications NEC E10.29
    - Kimmelstiel-Wilson disease E10.21
    - mononeuropathy E10.41
    - myasthenia E10.44
    - necrobiosis lipoidica E10.620
    - nephropathy E10.21
    - neuralgia E10.42
    - neurologic complication NEC E10.49
    - neuropathic arthropathy E10.610
    - neuropathy E10.40
    - ophthalmic complication NEC E10.39
    - oral complication NEC E10.638
    - osteomyelitis E10.69
    - periodontal disease E10.630
    - peripheral angiopathy E10.51
      - with gangrene E10.52
    - polyneuropathy E10.42
    - renal complication NEC E10.29
    - renal tubular degeneration E10.29
    - retinopathy E10.319
      - with macular edema E10.311
        - resolved following treatment E10.37
      - nonproliferative E10.329
        - with macular edema E10.321
        - mild E10.329
          - with macular edema E10.321
        - moderate E10.339
          - with macular edema E10.331
        - severe E10.349
          - with macular edema E10.341
      - proliferative E10.359
        - with
          - combined traction retinal detachment and rhegmatogenous retinal detachment E13.354
          - macular edema E13.351
          - stable proliferative diabetic retinopathy E13.355
          - traction retinal detachment involving the macula E13.352
          - traction retinal detachment not involving the macula E13.353
    - skin complication NEC E10.628
    - skin ulcer NEC E10.622
  - ▶early-stage E10.A-●
  - ▶presymptomatic E10.A0
    - ▶Stage 1 E10.A1
    - ▶Stage 2 E10.A2
- type 2 E11.9
  - with
    - amyotrophy E11.44
    - arthropathy NEC E11.618
    - autonomic (poly)neuropathy E11.43
    - cataract E11.36
    - Charcot's joints E11.610
    - chronic kidney disease E11.22
    - circulatory complication NEC E11.59
    - coma due to
      - hyperosmolarity E11.01
      - hypoglycemia E11.641
      - ketoacidosis E11.1-●
    - complication E11.8
      - specified NEC E11.69
    - dermatitis E11.620
    - foot ulcer E11.621
    - gangrene E11.52
    - gastroparalysis E11.43
    - gastroparesis E11.43
    - glomerulonephrosis, intracapillary E11.21
    - glomerulosclerosis, intercapillary E11.21
    - hyperglycemia E11.65
    - hyperosmolarity E11.00
      - with coma E11.01
    - hypoglycemia E11.649
      - with coma E11.641
    - ketoacidosis E11.10
      - with coma E11.11
    - kidney complications NEC E11.29
    - Kimmelstiel-Wilson disease E11.21
    - mononeuropathy E11.41
    - myasthenia E11.44
    - necrobiosis lipoidica E11.620
    - nephropathy E11.21
    - neuralgia E11.42
    - neurologic complication NEC E11.49
    - neuropathic arthropathy E11.610
    - neuropathy E11.40
    - ophthalmic complication NEC E11.39
    - oral complication NEC E11.638
    - osteomyelitis E11.69
    - periodontal disease E11.630
    - peripheral angiopathy E11.51
      - with gangrene E11.52
    - polyneuropathy E11.42
    - renal complication NEC E11.29
    - renal tubular degeneration E11.29
    - retinopathy E11.319
      - with macular edema E11.311
        - resolved following treatment E11.37
      - nonproliferative E11.329
        - with macular edema E11.321
        - mild E11.329
          - with macular edema E11.321
        - moderate E11.339
          - with macular edema E11.331
        - severe E11.349
          - with macular edema E11.341
      - proliferative E11.359
        - with
          - combined traction retinal detachment and rhegmatogenous retinal detachment E11.354
          - macular edema E11.351
          - stable proliferative diabetic retinopathy E11.355
          - traction retinal detachment involving the macula E11.352
          - traction retinal detachment not involving the macula E11.353
    - skin complication NEC E11.628
    - skin ulcer NEC E11.622
- uncontrolled
  - meaning
    - hyperglycemia *—see* Diabetes, by type, with, hyperglycemia
    - hypoglycemia *—see* Diabetes, by type, with, hypoglycemia

Diacyclothrombopathia D69.1

Diagnosis deferred R69

Dialysis (intermittent) (treatment)
- noncompliance (with) Z91.158
  - due to financial hardship Z91.151
- renal (hemodialysis) (peritoneal), status Z99.2
- retina, retinal *—see* Detachment, retina, with retinal, dialysis

Diamond-Blackfan anemia (congenital hypoplastic) D61.01

Diamond-Gardener syndrome (autoerythrocyte sensitization) D69.2

Diaper rash L22

Diaphoresis (excessive) R61

Diaphragm *—see* condition

Diaphragmalgia R07.1

Diaphragmatitis, diaphragmitis J98.6

Diaphysial aclasis Q78.6

Diaphysitis *—see* Osteomyelitis, specified type NEC

Diarrhea, diarrheal (disease) (infantile) (inflammatory) R19.7
- achlorhydric K31.83
- allergic K52.29
  - due to
    - colitis *—see* Colitis, allergic
    - enteritis *—see* Enteritis, allergic
- amebic *—see also* Amebiasis A06.0
  - with abscess *—see* Abscess, amebic
  - acute A06.0
  - chronic A06.1
  - nondysenteric A06.2
- bacillary *—see* Dysentery, bacillary
- balantidial A07.0
- cachectic NEC K52.89
- Chilomastix A07.8
- choleriformis A00.1
- chronic (noninfectious) K52.9
- coccidial A07.3
- Cochin-China K90.1
  - strongyloidiasis B78.0
- Dientamoeba A07.8
- dietetic *—see also* Diarrhea, allergic K52.29
- drug-induced K52.1
- due to
  - bacteria A04.9
    - specified NEC A04.8
  - Campylobacter A04.5
  - Capillaria philippinensis B81.1
  - Clostridium difficile
    - not specified as recurrent A04.72
    - recurrent A04.71
  - Clostridium perfringens (C) (F) A04.8
  - Cryptosporidium A07.2
  - drugs K52.1
  - Escherichia coli A04.4
    - enteroaggregative A04.4
    - enterohemorrhagic A04.3
    - enteroinvasive A04.2
    - enteropathogenic A04.0
    - enterotoxigenic A04.1
    - specified NEC A04.4
  - food hypersensitivity *—see also* Diarrhea, allergic K52.29
  - Necator americanus B76.1
  - S. japonicum B65.2
  - specified organism NEC A08.8
    - bacterial A04.8
    - viral A08.39
  - Staphylococcus A04.8
  - Trichuris trichiuria B79
  - virus *—see* Enteritis, viral
  - Yersinia enterocolitica A04.6
- dysenteric A09
- endemic A09
- epidemic A09
- flagellate A07.9
- Flexner's (ulcerative) A03.1
- functional K59.1
  - following gastrointestinal surgery K91.89
  - psychogenic F45.8
- Giardia lamblia A07.1
- giardial A07.1
- hill K90.1
- infectious A09
- malarial *—see* Malaria
- mite B88.0
- mycotic NEC B49
- neonatal (noninfectious) P78.3
- nervous F45.8
- neurogenic K59.1
- noninfectious K52.9
- postgastrectomy K91.1
- postvagotomy K91.1
- protozoal A07.9
  - specified NEC A07.8
- psychogenic F45.8
- specified
  - bacterium NEC A04.8
  - virus NEC A08.39
- strongyloidiasis B78.0
- toxic K52.1
- trichomonal A07.8
- tropical K90.1
- tuberculous A18.32
- viral *—see* Enteritis, viral

Disease, diseased *(Continued)*
- bladder N32.9
  - in (due to)
    - schistosomiasis (bilharziasis) B65.0 *[N33]*
  - specified NEC N32.89
- bleeder's D66
- blood D75.9
  - forming organs D75.9
  - vessel I99.9
- Bloodgood's —*see* Mastopathy, cystic
- Blount M92.51- ●
- Bodechtel-Guttmann (subacute sclerosing panencephalitis) A81.1
- bone —*see also* Disorder, bone
  - aluminum M83.4
  - fibrocystic NEC
    - jaw M27.49
- bone-marrow D75.9
- Borna A83.9
- Bornholm (epidemic pleurodynia) B33.0
- Bouchard's (myopathic dilatation of the stomach) K31.0
- Bouillaud's (rheumatic heart disease) I01.9
- Bourneville (-Brissaud) (tuberous sclerosis) Q85.1
- Bouveret (-Hoffmann) (paroxysmal tachycardia) I47.9
- bowel K63.9
  - functional K59.9
    - psychogenic F45.8
- brain G93.9
  - arterial, artery I67.9
  - arteriosclerotic I67.2
  - congenital Q04.9
  - degenerative —*see* Degeneration, brain
  - inflammatory —*see* Encephalitis
  - organic G93.9
    - arteriosclerotic I67.2
  - parasitic NEC B71.9 *[G94]*
  - senile NEC G31.1
  - specified NEC G93.89
- breast (*see also* Disorder, breast) N64.9
  - cystic (chronic) —*see* Mastopathy, cystic
  - fibrocystic —*see* Mastopathy, cystic
  - Paget's
    - female, unspecified side C50.91- ●
    - male, unspecified side C50.92- ●
  - specified NEC N64.89
- Breda's —*see* Yaws
- Bretonneau's (diphtheritic malignant angina) A36.0
- Bright's —*see* Nephritis
  - arteriosclerotic —*see* Hypertension, kidney
- Brill's (recrudescent typhus) A75.1
- Brill-Zinsser (recrudescent typhus) A75.1
- Brion-Kayser —*see* Fever, paratyphoid
- broad
  - beta E78.2
  - ligament (noninflammatory) N83.9
    - inflammatory —*see* Disease, pelvis, inflammatory
    - specified NEC N83.8
- Brocq-Duhring (dermatitis herpetiformis) L13.0
- Brocq's
  - meaning
    - dermatitis herpetiformis L13.0
    - prurigo L28.2
- bronchopulmonary J98.4
- bronchus NEC J98.09
- bronze Addison's E27.1
  - tuberculous A18.7
- budgerigar fancier's J67.2
- Buerger's (thromboangiitis obliterans) I73.1
- bullous L13.9
  - chronic of childhood L12.2
  - specified NEC L13.8
- Bürger-Grütz (essential familial hyperlipemia) E78.3
- bursa —*see* Bursopathy
- caisson T70.3
- California —*see* Coccidioidomycosis
- Canavan E75.28
- capillaries I78.9
  - specified NEC I78.8
- Carapata A68.0
- ▶ carcinoid E34.00
  - ▶ heart E34.01
  - ▶ specified NEC E34.09
- cardiac —*see* Disease, heart
- cardiopulmonary, chronic I27.9

Disease, diseased *(Continued)*
- cardiorenal (hepatic) (hypertensive) (vascular) —*see* Hypertension, cardiorenal
- cardiovascular (atherosclerotic) I25.10
  - with angina pectoris —*see* Arteriosclerosis, coronary (artery),
  - congenital Q28.9
  - hypertensive —*see* Hypertension, heart
  - newborn P29.9
    - specified NEC P29.89
  - renal (hypertensive) —*see* Hypertension, cardiorenal
  - syphilitic (asymptomatic) A52.00
- cartilage —*see* Disorder, cartilage
- Castellani's A69.8
- Castleman (unicentric) (multicentric) D47.Z2
  - HHV-8-associated —*see also* Herpesvirus, human, 8 D47.Z2
- cat-scratch A28.1
- Cavare's (familial periodic paralysis) G72.3
- cecum K63.9
- celiac (adult) (infantile) (with steatorrhea) K90.0
- cellular tissue L98.9
- central core G71.29
- cerebellar, cerebellum —*see* Disease, brain
- cerebral —*see also* Disease, brain
  - degenerative —*see* Degeneration, brain
- cerebrospinal G96.9
- cerebrovascular I67.9
  - acute I67.89
    - embolic I63.4- ●
    - thrombotic I63.3- ●
  - arteriosclerotic I67.2
  - hereditary NEC I67.858
  - specified NEC I67.89
- cervix (uteri) (noninflammatory) N88.9
  - inflammatory —*see* Cervicitis
  - specified NEC N88.8
- Chabert's A22.9
- Chandler's (osteochondritis dissecans, hip) —*see* Osteochondritis, dissecans, hip
- Charlouis —*see* Yaws
- Chédiak-Steinbrinck (-Higashi) (congenital gigantism of peroxidase granules) E70.330
- chest J98.9
- Chiari's (hepatic vein thrombosis) I82.0
- Chicago B40.9
- Chignon B36.8
- chigo, chigoe B88.1
- childhood granulomatous D71
- Chinese liver fluke B66.1
- chlamydial A74.9
  - specified NEC A74.89
- cholecystic K82.9
- choroid H31.9
  - specified NEC H31.8
- Christmas D67
- chronic bullous of childhood L12.2
- chylomicron retention E78.3
- ciliary body H21.9
  - specified NEC H21.89
- circulatory (system) NEC I99.8
  - newborn P29.9
  - syphilitic A52.00
    - congenital A50.54
- coagulation factor deficiency (congenital) —*see* Defect, coagulation
- coccidioidal —*see* Coccidioidomycosis
- cold
  - agglutinin or hemoglobinuria D59.12
    - paroxysmal D59.6
  - hemagglutinin (chronic) D59.12
- collagen NOS (nonvascular) (vascular) M35.9
  - specified NEC M35.89
- colon K63.9
  - functional K59.9
    - congenital Q43.2
  - ischemic —*see also* Ischemia, intestine, acute K55.039
- colonic inflammatory bowel, unclassified (IBDU) K52.3
- combined system —*see* Degeneration, combined
- compressed air T70.3
- Concato's (pericardial polyserositis) A19.9
  - nontubercular I31.1
  - pleural —*see* Pleurisy, with effusion
- conjunctiva H11.9
  - chlamydial A74.0
  - specified NEC H11.89
  - viral B30.9
    - specified NEC B30.8

Disease, diseased *(Continued)*
- connective tissue, systemic (diffuse) M35.9
  - in (due to)
    - hypogammaglobulinemia D80.1 *[M36.8]*
    - ochronosis E70.29 *[M36.8]*
  - specified NEC M35.89
- Conor and Bruch's (boutonneuse fever) A77.1
- Cooper's —*see* Mastopathy, cystic
- Cori's (glycogenosis III) E74.03
- corkhandler's or corkworker's J67.3
- cornea H18.9
  - specified NEC H18.89- ●
- coronary (artery) —*see* Disease, heart, ischemic, atherosclerotic
  - congenital Q24.5
  - microvascular
    - with
      - angina pectoris I20.81
      - myocardial infarction I21.B
  - acute I24.81
  - chronic I25.85
  - ostial, syphilitic (aortic) (mitral) (pulmonary) A52.03
- corpus cavernosum N48.9
  - specified NEC N48.89
- ~~Cotugno's —see Sciatica~~
- ▶ Cotugno —*see* Sciatica
- COVID-19 U07.1
- coxsackie (virus) NEC B34.1
- cranial nerve NOS G52.9
- Creutzfeldt-Jakob —*see* Creutzfeldt-Jakob disease or syndrome
- Crocq's (acrocyanosis) I73.89
- Crohn's —*see* Enteritis, regional
- Curschmann G71.11
- cystic
  - breast (chronic) —*see* Mastopathy, cystic
  - kidney, congenital Q61.9
  - liver, congenital Q44.6
  - lung J98.4
    - congenital Q33.0
- cytomegalic inclusion (generalized) B25.9
  - with pneumonia B25.0
  - congenital P35.1
- cytomegaloviral B25.9
  - specified NEC B25.8
- Czerny's (periodic hydrarthrosis of the knee) —*see* Effusion, joint, knee
- Daae (-Finsen) (epidemic pleurodynia) B33.0
- Danon E74.05
- Darling's —*see* Histoplasmosis capsulati
- Débove's (splenomegaly) R16.1
- deer fly —*see* Tularemia
- Degos' I77.8
- demyelinating, demyelinizating (nervous system) G37.9
  - multiple sclerosis G35
  - specified NEC G37.89
- dense deposit —*see also* N00-N07 with fourth character .6 N05.6
- deposition, hydroxyapatite —*see* Disease, hydroxyapatite deposition
- de Quervain's (tendon sheath) M65.4
  - thyroid (subacute granulomatous thyroiditis) E06.1
- Devergie's (pityriasis rubra pilaris) L44.0
- Devic's G36.0
- diaphorase deficiency D74.0
- diaphragm J98.6
- diarrheal, infectious NEC A09
- digestive system K92.9
  - specified NEC K92.89
- disc, degenerative —*see* Degeneration, intervertebral disc
- discogenic —*see also* Displacement, intervertebral disc NEC
  - with myelopathy —*see* Disorder, disc, with, myelopathy
- diverticular —*see* Diverticula
- Dubois (thymus) A50.59 *[E35]*
- Duchenne-Griesinger G71.01
- Duchenne's
  - muscular dystrophy G71.01
  - pseudohypertrophy, muscles G71.01
- ductless glands E34.9
- Duhring's (dermatitis herpetiformis) L13.0
- duodenum K31.9
  - specified NEC K31.89
- Dupré's (meningism) R29.1
- Dupuytren's (muscle contracture) M72.0
- Durand-Nicholas-Favre (climatic bubo) A55

D

- **Disease, diseased** *(Continued)*
  - Morgagni-Adams-Stokes (syncope with heart block) I45.9
  - Morgagni's (syndrome) (hyperostosis frontalis interna) M85.2
  - Morton's (with metatarsalgia) —*see* Lesion, nerve, plantar
  - Morvan's G6Ø.8
  - motor neuron (bulbar) (mixed type) (spinal) G12.2Ø
    - amyotrophic lateral sclerosis G12.21
    - familial G12.24
    - progressive bulbar palsy G12.22
    - specified NEC G12.29
  - moyamoya I67.5
  - ➡ mu heavy chain disease C88.2- •
  - multicore G71.29
  - multiminicore G71.29
  - muscle —*see also* Disorder, muscle
    - inflammatory —*see* Myositis
    - ocular (external) —*see* Strabismus
  - musculoskeletal system, soft tissue —*see also* Disorder, soft tissue
    - specified NEC —*see* Disorder, soft tissue, specified type NEC
  - mushroom workers' J67.5
  - mycotic B49
  - myelin oligodendrocyte glycoprotein antibody G37.81
  - ➡ myelodysplastic (*see also* Syndrome, myelodysplastic) C94.6
  - myelodysplastic/myeloproliferative neoplasm, unclassifiable C94.6
  - myeloproliferative D47.1
    - chronic D47.1
    - not classified C94.6
    - specified NEC C94.6
    - unclassifiable C94.6
  - myocardium, myocardial —*see also* Degeneration, myocardial I51.5
    - primary (idiopathic) I42.9
  - myoneural G7Ø.9
  - Naegeli's D69.1
  - nails L6Ø.9
    - specified NEC L6Ø.8
  - Nairobi (sheep virus) A93.8
  - nasal J34.9
  - nemaline body G71.21
  - nerve —*see* Disorder, nerve
  - nervous system G98.8
    - autonomic G9Ø.9
    - central G96.9
      - specified NEC G96.89
    - congenital QØ7.9
    - parasympathetic G9Ø.9
    - specified NEC G98.8
    - sympathetic G9Ø.9
    - vegetative G9Ø.9
  - neuromuscular system G7Ø.9
  - Newcastle B3Ø.8
  - Nicolas (-Durand)-Favre (climatic bubo) A55
  - nipple N64.9
    - Paget's C5Ø.Ø1- •
      - female C5Ø.Ø1- •
      - male C5Ø.Ø2- •
  - Nishimoto (-Takeuchi) I67.5
  - nonarthropod-borne NOS (viral) B34.9
    - enterovirus NEC B34.1
  - nonautoimmune hemolytic D59.4
    - drug-induced D59.2
  - Nonne-Milroy-Meige (chronic hereditary edema) Q82.Ø
  - nose J34.9
  - nucleus pulposus —*see* Disorder, disc
  - nutritional E63.9
  - oast-house-urine E72.19
    - ocular
      - herpesviral BØØ.5Ø
      - zoster BØ2.3Ø
  - obliterative vascular I77.1
  - Ohara's —*see* Tularemia
  - Opitz's (congestive splenomegaly) D73.2
  - Oppenheim-Urbach (necrobiosis lipoidica diabeticorum) —*see* EØ8-E13 with .62Ø
  - optic nerve NEC —*see* Disorder, nerve, optic
    - orbit —*see* Disorder, orbit
  - organ
    - dabbing (related) UØ7.Ø
    - electronic cigarette (related) UØ7.Ø
    - vaping (associated) (device) (product) (use) UØ7.Ø
  - Oriental liver fluke B66.1
  - Oriental lung fluke B66.4
  - Ormond's N13.5
  - Oropouche virus A93.Ø
  - Osler-Rendu (familial hemorrhagic telangiectasia) I78.Ø
  - osteofibrocystic E21.Ø
  - Otto's M24.7
  - outer ear —*see* Disorder, ear, external
  - ovary (noninflammatory) N83.9
    - cystic N83.2Ø- •
    - inflammatory —*see* Salpingo-oophoritis
    - polycystic E28.2
    - specified NEC N83.8
  - Owren's (congenital) —*see* Defect, coagulation
  - p11Ød-activating mutation causing senescent T cells, lymphadenopathy, and immunodeficiency [PASLI] D81.82
  - pancreas K86.9
    - cystic K86.2
    - fibrocystic E84.9
    - specified NEC K86.89
  - panvalvular IØ8.9
    - specified NEC IØ8.8
  - parametrium (noninflammatory) N83.9
  - parasitic B89
    - cerebral NEC B71.9 *[G94]*
    - intestinal NOS B82.9
    - mouth B37.Ø
    - skin NOS B88.9
    - specified type —*see* Infestation
    - tongue B37.Ø
  - parathyroid (gland) E21.5
    - specified NEC E21.4
  - Parkinson's G2Ø.A1
    - with dyskinesia
      - with
        - fluctuations G2Ø.B2
        - OFF episodes G2Ø.B2
      - without mention of
        - fluctuations G2Ø.B1
        - OFF episodes G2Ø.B1
    - without dyskinesia
      - with
        - fluctuations G2Ø.A2
        - OFF episodes G2Ø.A2
      - without mention of
        - fluctuations G2Ø.A1
        - OFF episodes G2Ø.A1
  - parodontal KØ5.6
  - Parrot's (syphilitic osteochondritis) A5Ø.Ø2
  - Parry's (exophthalmic goiter) —*see* Hyperthyroidism, with, goiter (diffuse)
  - Parson's (exophthalmic goiter) —*see* Hyperthyroidism, with, goiter (diffuse)
  - Paxton's (white piedra) B36.2
  - pearl-worker's —*see* Osteomyelitis, specified type NEC
  - Pellegrini-Stieda (calcification, knee joint) —*see* Bursitis, tibial collateral
  - pelvis, pelvic
    - female NOS N94.9
      - specified NEC N94.89
    - gonococcal (acute) (chronic) A54.24
    - inflammatory (female) N73.9
      - acute N73.Ø
      - chlamydial A56.11
      - chronic N73.1
      - specified NEC N73.8
      - syphilitic (secondary) A51.42
        - late A52.76
      - tuberculous A18.17
    - organ, female N94.9
    - peritoneum, female NEC N94.89
  - penis N48.9
    - inflammatory N48.29
      - abscess N48.21
      - cellulitis N48.22
    - specified NEC N48.89
  - periapical tissues NOS KØ4.9Ø
  - periodontal KØ5.6
    - specified NEC KØ5.5
  - periosteum —*see* Disorder, bone, specified type NEC
  - peripheral
    - arterial I73.9
    - autonomic nervous system G9Ø.9
    - nerves —*see* Polyneuropathy
    - vascular NOS I73.9
      - in diabetes mellitus —*see* Diabetes, by type, with peripheral angiopathy
  - peritoneum K66.9
    - pelvic, female NEC N94.89
    - specified NEC K66.8
  - persistent mucosal (middle ear) H66.2Ø
    - left H66.22
      - with right H66.23
    - right H66.21
      - with left H66.23
  - Petit's —*see* Hernia, abdomen, specified site NEC
  - pharynx J39.2
    - specified NEC J39.2
  - Phocas' —*see* Mastopathy, cystic
  - photochromogenic (acid-fast bacilli) (pulmonary) A31.Ø
    - nonpulmonary A31.9
  - Pick's (*see also* Dementia, in, diseases specified elsewhere) G31.Ø1 *[FØ2.8Ø]*
    - with behavioral disturbance (*see also* Dementia, in, diseases specified elsewhere) G31.Ø1 *[FØ2.81-•]*
    - brain (*see also* Dementia, in, diseases specified elsewhere) G31.Ø1 *[FØ2.8Ø]*
      - with behavioral disturbance (*see also* Dementia, in, diseases specified elsewhere) G31.Ø1 *[FØ2.81-•]*
    - of pericardium (pericardial pseudocirrhosis of liver) I31.1
  - pigeon fancier's J67.2
  - pineal gland E34.8
  - pink —*see* Poisoning, mercury
  - Pinkus' (lichen nitidus) L44.1
  - pinworm B8Ø
  - Piry virus A93.8
  - pituitary (gland) E23.7
  - pituitary-snuff-taker's J67.8
  - pleura (cavity) J94.9
    - specified NEC J94.8
  - pneumatic drill (hammer) T75.21
  - Pollitzer's (hidradenitis suppurativa) L73.2
  - polycystic
    - kidney or renal Q61.3
      - adult type Q61.2
      - childhood type NEC Q61.19
        - collecting duct dilatation Q61.11
    - liver or hepatic Q44.6
    - lung or pulmonary J98.4
      - congenital Q33.Ø
    - ovary, ovaries E28.2
    - spleen Q89.Ø9
  - polyethylene T84.Ø5- •
  - Pompe's (glycogenosis II) E74.Ø2
  - Posadas-Wernicke B38.9
  - Potain's (pulmonary edema) —*see* Edema, lung
  - prepuce N47.8
    - inflammatory N47.7
      - balanoposthitis N47.6
  - Pringle's (tuberous sclerosis) Q85.1
  - prion, central nervous system A81.9
    - specified NEC A81.89
  - prostate N42.9
    - specified NEC N42.89
  - protozoal B64
    - acanthamebiasis —*see* Acanthamebiasis
    - African trypanosomiasis —*see* African trypanosomiasis
    - babesiosis —(*see also* Babesiosis) B6Ø.ØØ
    - Chagas disease —*see* Chagas disease
    - intestine, intestinal AØ7.9
    - leishmaniasis —*see* Leishmaniasis
    - malaria —*see* Malaria
    - naegleriasis B6Ø.2
    - pneumocystosis B59
    - specified organism NEC B6Ø.8
    - toxoplasmosis —*see* Toxoplasmosis
  - pseudo-Hurler's E77.Ø
  - psychiatric F99
  - psychotic —*see* Psychosis
  - Puente's (simple glandular cheilitis) K13.Ø
  - puerperal —*see also* Puerperal O9Ø.89
  - pulmonary —*see also* Disease, lung
    - artery I28.9
    - chronic obstructive J44.9
      - with
        - acute bronchitis J44.Ø
        - exacerbation (acute) J44.1
        - lower respiratory infection (acute) J44.Ø
      - decompensated J44.1
        - with
          - exacerbation (acute) J44.1

Disease, diseased *(Continued)*
- pulmonary *(Continued)*
  - heart I27.9
    - specified NEC I27.89
  - hypertensive (vascular) *—see also* Hypertension, pulmonary I27.2Ø
    - primary (idiopathic) I27.Ø
  - valve I37.9
    - rheumatic IØ9.89
- pulp (dental) NOS KØ4.9Ø
- pulseless M31.4
- Putnam's (subacute combined sclerosis with pernicious anemia) D51.Ø
- Pyle (-Cohn) (metaphyseal dysplasia) Q78.5
- ragpicker's or ragsorter's A22.1
- Raynaud's *—see* Raynaud's disease
- reactive airway *—see* Asthma
- Reclus' (cystic) *—see* Mastopathy, cystic
- rectum K62.9
  - specified NEC K62.89
- Refsum's (heredopathia atactica polyneuritiformis) G6Ø.1
- renal (functional) (pelvis) *—see also* Disease, kidney N28.9
  - with
    - edema *—see* Nephrosis
    - glomerular lesion *—see* Glomerulonephritis
      - with edema *—see* Nephrosis
    - interstitial nephritis N12
  - acute N28.9
  - chronic *—see also* Disease, kidney, chronic N18.9
  - cystic, congenital Q61.9
  - diabetic *—see* EØ8-E13 with .22
  - end-stage (failure) N18.6
    - due to hypertension I12.Ø
  - fibrocystic (congenital) Q61.8
  - hypertensive *—see* Hypertension, kidney
  - lupus M32.14
  - phosphate-losing (tubular) N25.Ø
  - polycystic (congenital) Q61.3
    - adult type Q61.2
    - childhood type NEC Q61.19
      - collecting duct dilatation Q61.11
  - rapidly progressive NØ1.9
  - subacute NØ1.9
- Rendu-Osler-Weber (familial hemorrhagic telangiectasia) I78.Ø
- renovascular (arteriosclerotic) *—see* Hypertension, kidney
- respiratory (tract) J98.9
  - acute or subacute NOS JØ6.9
    - due to
      - chemicals, gases, fumes or vapors (inhalation) J68.3
      - external agent J7Ø.9
        - specified NEC J7Ø.8
      - radiation J7Ø.Ø
      - smoke inhalation J7Ø.5
    - noninfectious J39.8
  - chronic NOS J98.9
    - due to
      - chemicals, gases, fumes or vapors J68.4
      - external agent J7Ø.9
        - specified NEC J7Ø.8
      - radiation J7Ø.1
    - newborn P27.9
      - specified NEC P27.8
  - due to
    - chemicals, gases, fumes or vapors J68.9
      - acute or subacute NEC J68.3
      - chronic J68.4
    - external agent J7Ø.9
      - specified NEC J7Ø.8
  - newborn P28.9
    - specified type NEC P28.89
  - upper J39.9
    - acute or subacute JØ6.9
    - noninfectious NEC J39.8
    - specified NEC J39.8
    - streptococcal JØ6.9
- retina, retinal H35.9
  - Batten's or Batten-Mayou E75.4 *[H36.89]*
  - specified NEC H35.89
- rheumatoid *—see* Arthritis, rheumatoid
- rickettsial NOS A79.9
  - specified type NEC A79.89
- Riga (-Fede) (cachectic aphthae) K14.Ø
- Riggs' (compound periodontitis) *—see* Periodontitis
- Ritter's LØØ

Disease, diseased *(Continued)*
- Rivalta's (cervicofacial actinomycosis) A42.2
- rod body G71.21
- Robles' (onchocerciasis) B73.Ø1
- Roger's (congenital interventricular septal defect) Q21.Ø
- Rosenthal's (factor XI deficiency) D68.1
- Ross River B33.1
- Rossbach's (hyperchlorhydria) K31.89
  - psychogenic F45.8
- Rotes Quérol *—see* Hyperostosis, ankylosing
- Roth (-Bernhardt) *—see* Mononeuropathy, lower limb, meralgia paresthetica
- Runeberg's (progressive pernicious anemia) D51.Ø
- sacroiliac NEC M53.3
- salivary gland or duct K11.9
  - inclusion B25.9
  - specified NEC K11.8
  - virus B25.9
- sandworm B76.9
- Schimmelbusch's *—see* Mastopathy, cystic
- Schmorl's *—see* Schmorl's disease or nodes
- Schönlein (-Henoch) (purpura rheumatica) D69.Ø
- Schottmüller's *—see* Fever, paratyphoid
- Schultz's (agranulocytosis) *—see* Agranulocytosis
- Schwalbe-Ziehen-Oppenheim G24.1
- Schwartz-Jampel G71.13
- sclera H15.9
  - specified NEC H15.89
- scrofulous (tuberculous) A18.2
- scrotum N5Ø.9
- sebaceous glands L73.9
- semilunar cartilage, cystic *—see also* Derangement, knee, meniscus, cystic
- seminal vesicle N5Ø.9
- serum NEC *—see also* Reaction, serum T8Ø.69
- sexually transmitted A64
  - anogenital
    - herpesviral infection *—see* Herpes, anogenital
    - warts A63.Ø
  - chancroid A57
  - chlamydial infection *—see* Chlamydia
  - gonorrhea *—see* Gonorrhea
  - granuloma inguinale A58
  - specified organism NEC A63.8
  - syphilis *—see* Syphilis
  - trichomoniasis *—see* Trichomoniasis
- Sézary C84.1-●
- shimamushi (scrub typhus) A75.3
- shipyard B3Ø.Ø
- sickle-cell D57.1
  - with
    - acute chest syndrome D57.Ø1
    - cerebral vascular involvement D57.Ø3
    - crisis (painful) D57.ØØ
      - with
        - complication specified NEC D57.Ø9
        - dactylitis D57.Ø4
    - dactylitis D57.Ø4
    - pain (vaso-occlusive) D57.ØØ
    - priapism D57.Ø9
    - splenic sequestration D57.Ø2
  - elliptocytosis D57.8-●
  - Hb-C D57.2Ø
    - with
      - acute chest syndrome D57.211
      - cerebral vascular involvement D57.213
      - crisis (painful) D57.219
        - with
          - dactylitis D57.214
          - specified complication NEC D57.218
      - dactylitis D57.214
      - pain (vaso-occlusive) D57.219
      - priapism D57.218
      - splenic sequestration D57.212
    - without crisis D57.2Ø
  - Hb-SD D57.8Ø
    - with
      - acute chest syndrome D57.811
      - cerebral vascular involvement D57.813
      - crisis (painful) D57.819
        - with
          - complication specified NEC D57.818
          - dactylitis D57.814
      - dactylitis D57.814
      - pain (vaso-occlusive) D57.819
      - splenic sequestration D57.812
    - without crisis D57.8Ø

Disease, diseased *(Continued)*
- sickle-cell *(Continued)*
  - Hb-SE D57.8Ø
    - with
      - acute chest syndrome D57.811
      - cerebral vascular involvement D57.813
      - crisis (painful) D57.819
        - with
          - complication specified NEC D57.818
          - dactylitis D57.814
      - dactylitis D57.814
      - pain (vaso-occlusive) D57.819
      - splenic sequestration D57.812
    - without crisis D57.8Ø
  - specified NEC D57.8Ø
    - with
      - acute chest syndrome D57.811
      - cerebral vascular involvement D57.813
      - crisis (painful) D57.819
        - with
          - complication specified NEC D57.818
          - dactylitis D57.814
      - dactylitis D57.814
      - pain (vaso-occlusive) D57.819
      - splenic sequestration D57.812
    - without crisis D57.8Ø
  - spherocytosis D57.8Ø
    - with
      - acute chest syndrome D57.811
      - cerebral vascular involvement D57.813
      - crisis (painful) D57.819
        - with complication specified NEC D57.818
      - pain (vaso-occlusive) D57.819
      - splenic sequestration D57.812
    - without crisis D57.8Ø
  - thalassemia D57.4Ø
    - with
      - acute chest syndrome D57.411
        - with dactylitis D57.414
        - with specified complication NEC D57.418
      - cerebral vascular involvement D57.413
      - crisis (painful) D57.419
        - with specified complication NEC D57.418
      - dactylitis D57.414
      - pain (vaso-occlusive) D57.419
      - splenic sequestration D57.412
    - beta plus D57.44
      - with
        - acute chest syndrome D57.451
          - with dactylitis D57.454
        - cerebral vascular involvement D57.453
        - crisis D57.459
          - with specified complication NEC D57.458
        - dactylitis D57.454
        - pain (vaso-occlusive) D57.459
        - splenic sequestration D57.452
      - without crisis D57.44
    - beta zero D57.42
      - with
        - acute chest syndrome D57.431
          - with dactylitis D57.434
        - cerebral vascular involvement D57.433
        - crisis D57.439
          - with specified complication NEC D57.438
        - dactylitis D57.434
        - pain (vaso-occlusive) D57.439
        - splenic sequestration D57.432
      - without crisis D57.42
- silo-filler's J68.8
  - bronchitis J68.Ø
  - pneumonitis J68.Ø
  - pulmonary edema J68.1
- simian B BØØ.4
- Simons' (progressive lipodystrophy) E88.1
- sin nombre virus B33.4
- sinus *—see* Sinusitis
- Sirkari's B55.Ø
- sixth BØ8.2Ø
  - due to human herpesvirus 6 BØ8.21
  - due to human herpesvirus 7 BØ8.22
- skin L98.9
  - due to metabolic disorder NEC E88.9 *[L99]*
  - specified NEC L98.8
- slim (HIV) B2Ø

D

Disease, diseased *(Continued)*
- small vessel I73.9
- Sneddon-Wilkinson (subcorneal pustular dermatosis) L13.1
- South African creeping B88.Ø
- spinal (cord) G95.9
  - congenital QØ6.9
  - specified NEC G95.89
- spine —*see also* Spondylopathy
  - joint —*see* Dorsopathy
  - tuberculous A18.Ø1
- spinocerebellar (hereditary) G11.9
  - specified NEC G11.8
- spleen D73.9
  - amyloid E85.4 *[D77]*
  - organic D73.9
  - polycystic Q89.Ø9
  - postinfectional D73.89
- sponge-diver's —*see* Toxicity, venom, marine animal, sea anemone
- Startle Q89.8
- Steinert's G71.11
- Sticker's (erythema infectiosum) BØ8.3
- Stieda's (calcification, knee joint) —*see* Bursitis, tibial collateral
- Stokes' (exophthalmic goiter) —*see* Hyperthyroidism, with, goiter (diffuse)
- Stokes-Adams (syncope with heart block) I45.9
- stomach K31.9
  - functional, psychogenic F45.8
  - specified NEC K31.89
- stonemason's J62.8
- storage
  - glycogen —*see* Disease, glycogen storage
  - mucopolysaccharide —*see* Mucopolysaccharidosis
- striatopallidal system NEC G25.89
- Stuart-Prower (congenital factor X deficiency) D68.2
- Stuart's (congenital factor X deficiency) D68.2
- subcutaneous tissue —*see* Disease, skin
- supporting structures of teeth KØ8.9
  - specified NEC KØ8.89
- suprarenal (capsule) (gland) E27.9
  - hyperfunction E27.Ø
  - specified NEC E27.8
- sweat glands L74.9
  - specified NEC L74.8
- Sweeley-Klionsky E75.21
- Swift (-Feer) —*see* Poisoning, mercury
- swimming-pool granuloma A31.1
- Sylvest's (epidemic pleurodynia) B33.Ø
- sympathetic nervous system G9Ø.9
- synovium —*see* Disorder, synovium
- syphilitic —*see* Syphilis
- systemic tissue mast cell D47.Ø2
- tanapox (virus) BØ8.71
- Tangier E78.6
- Tarral-Besnier (pityriasis rubra pilaris) L44.Ø
- Tauri's E74.Ø9
- tear duct —*see* Disorder, lacrimal system
- tendon, tendinous —*see also* Disorder, tendon
  - nodular —*see* Trigger finger
- terminal vessel I73.9
- testis N5Ø.9
- thalassemia Hb-S —*see* Disease, sickle-cell, thalassemia
- Thaysen-Gee (nontropical sprue) K9Ø.Ø
- Thomsen G71.12
- throat J39.2
  - septic JØ2.Ø
- thromboembolic —*see* Embolism
- thymus (gland) E32.9
  - specified NEC E32.8
- thyroid (gland) EØ7.9
  - heart —*see also* Hyperthyroidism EØ5.9Ø *[I43]*
    - with thyroid storm EØ5.91 *[I43]*
  - specified NEC EØ7.8
- Tietze's M94.Ø
- tongue K14.9
  - specified NEC K14.89
- tonsils, tonsillar (and adenoids) J35.9
- tooth, teeth KØ8.9
  - hard tissues KØ3.9
    - specified NEC KØ3.89
  - pulp NEC KØ4.99
  - specified NEC KØ8.89
- Tourette's F95.2
- trachea NEC J39.8
- tricuspid IØ7.9
  - nonrheumatic I36.9
- triglyceride-storage E75.5
- trophoblastic —*see* Mole, hydatidiform
- tsutsugamushi A75.3
- tube (fallopian) (noninflammatory) N83.9
  - inflammatory —*see* Salpingitis
  - specified NEC N83.8
- tuberculous NEC —*see* Tuberculosis
- tubo-ovarian (noninflammatory) N83.9
  - inflammatory —*see* Salpingo-oophoritis
  - specified NEC N83.8
- tubotympanic, chronic —*see* Otitis, media, suppurative, chronic, tubotympanic
- tubulo-interstitial N15.9
  - specified NEC N15.8
- tympanum —*see* Disorder, tympanic membrane
- Uhl's Q24.8
- Underwood's (sclerema neonatorum) P83.Ø
- Unverricht (-Lundborg) —*see* Epilepsy, generalized, idiopathic
- Urbach-Oppenheim (necrobiosis lipoidica diabeticorum) —*see* EØ8-E13 with .62Ø
- ureter N28.9
  - in (due to)
    - schistosomiasis (bilharziasis) B65.Ø *[N29]*
- urethra N36.9
  - specified NEC N36.8
- urinary (tract) N39.9
  - bladder N32.9
    - specified NEC N32.89
  - specified NEC N39.8
- uterus (noninflammatory) N85.9
  - infective —*see* Endometritis
  - inflammatory —*see* Endometritis
  - specified NEC N85.8
- uveal tract (anterior) H21.9
  - posterior H31.9
- vagabond's B85.1
- vagina, vaginal (noninflammatory) N89.9
  - inflammatory NEC N76.89
  - specified NEC N89.8
- valve, valvular I38
  - multiple IØ8.9
    - specified NEC IØ8.8
- van Creveld-von Gierke (glycogenosis I) E74.Ø1
- vas deferens N5Ø.9
- vascular I99.9
  - arteriosclerotic —*see* Arteriosclerosis
  - ciliary body NEC —*see* Disorder, iris, vascular
  - hypertensive —*see* Hypertension
  - iris NEC —*see* Disorder, iris, vascular
  - obliterative I77.1
    - peripheral I73.9
  - occlusive I99.8
  - peripheral (occlusive) I73.9
    - in diabetes mellitus —*see* EØ8-E13 with .51
- vasomotor I73.9
- vasospastic I73.9
- vein I87.9
- venereal —*see also* Disease, sexually transmitted A64
  - chlamydial NEC A56.8
    - anus A56.3
    - genitourinary NOS A56.2
    - pharynx A56.4
    - rectum A56.3
  - fifth A55
  - sixth A55
  - specified nature or type NEC A63.8
- vertebra, vertebral —*see also* Spondylopathy
  - disc —*see* Disorder, disc
- vibration —*see* Vibration, adverse effects
- viral, virus —*see also* Disease, by type of virus B34.9
  - arbovirus NOS A94
  - arthropod-borne NOS A94
  - congenital P35.9
    - specified NEC P35.8
  - Hanta (with renal manifestations) (Dobrava) (Puumala) (Seoul) A98.5
    - with pulmonary manifestations (Andes) (Bayou) (Bermejo) (Black Creek Canal) (Choclo) (Juquitiba) (Laguna negra) (Lechiguanas) (New York) (Oran) (Sin nombre) B33.4
  - Hantaan (Korean hemorrhagic fever) A98.5
  - human immunodeficiency (HIV) B2Ø
  - Kunjin A83.4
  - nonarthropod-borne NOS B34.9
  - Powassan A84.81
  - Rocio (encephalitis) A83.6

Disease, diseased *(Continued)*
- viral, virus *(Continued)*
  - Sin nombre (Hantavirus) (cardio)- pulmonary syndrome B33.4
  - Tahyna B33.8
  - vesicular stomatitis A93.8
- vitreous H43.9
  - specified NEC H43.89
- vocal cord J38.3
- Volkmann's, acquired T79.6
- von Eulenburg's (congenital paramyotonia) G71.19
- von Gierke's (glycogenosis I) E74.Ø1
- von Graefe's —*see* Strabismus, paralytic, ophthalmoplegia, progressive
- von Willebrand (-Jürgens) (angiohemophilia) D68.ØØ
  - acquired D68.Ø4
  - platelet-type D68.Ø9
  - pseudo D68.Ø9
  - specified NEC D68.Ø9
  - type 1 D68.Ø1
  - type 1C D68.01
  - type 2 D68.Ø29
    - type 2A D68.Ø2Ø
    - type 2B D68.Ø21
    - type 2M D68.Ø22
    - type 2N D68.Ø23
  - type 3 D68.Ø3
- Vrolik's (osteogenesis imperfecta) Q78.Ø
- vulva (noninflammatory) N9Ø.9
  - inflammatory NEC N76.89
  - specified NEC N9Ø.89
- Wallgren's (obstruction of splenic vein with collateral circulation) I87.8
- Wassilieff's (leptospiral jaundice) A27.Ø
- wasting NEC E88.A
  - due to
    - malnutrition E43
      - with marasmus E41
    - underlying condition E88.A
- Waterhouse-Friderichsen A39.1
- Wegner's (syphilitic osteochondritis) A5Ø.Ø2
- Weil's (leptospiral jaundice of lung) A27.Ø
- Weir Mitchell's (erythromelalgia) I73.81
- Werdnig-Hoffmann G12.Ø
- Wermer's E31.21
- Werner-His (trench fever) A79.Ø
- Werner-Schultz (neutropenic splenomegaly) D73.81
- Wernicke-Posadas B38.9
- whipworm B79
- white blood cells D72.9
  - specified NEC D72.89
- white matter R9Ø.82
- white-spot, meaning lichen sclerosus et atrophicus L9Ø.Ø
  - penis N48.Ø
  - vulva N9Ø.4
- Wilkie's K55.1
- Wilkinson-Sneddon (subcorneal pustular dermatosis) L13.1
- Willis' —*see* Diabetes
- Wilson's (hepatolenticular degeneration) E83.Ø1
- woolsorter's A22.1
- yaba monkey tumor BØ8.72
- yaba pox (virus) BØ8.72
- Zika virus A92.5
- zoonotic, bacterial A28.9
  - congenital P35.4
  - specified type NEC A28.8

Disfigurement (due to scar) L9Ø.5

Disgerminoma —*see* Dysgerminoma

DISH (diffuse idiopathic skeletal hyperostosis) —*see* Hyperostosis, ankylosing

Disinsertion, retina —*see* Detachment, retina

Dislocatable hip, congenital Q65.6

Dislocation (articular)
- with fracture —*see* Fracture
- acromioclavicular (joint) S43.1Ø- •
  - with displacement
    - 1ØØ%-2ØØ% S43.12- •
    - more than 2ØØ% S43.13- •
  - inferior S43.14- •
  - posterior S43.15- •
- ankle S93.Ø- •
- astragalus —*see* Dislocation, ankle
- atlantoaxial S13.121
- atlantooccipital S13.111
- atloidooccipital S13.111
- breast bone S23.29

D

D

▶ New ➡ Revised ~~deleted~~ Deleted ● Use Additional Character(s)

Disorder *(Continued)*
joint *(Continued)*
specified type *(Continued)*
foot joint M25.87-●
hand joint M25.84-●
hip M25.85-●
knee M25.86-●
shoulder M25.81-●
wrist M25.83-●
stiffness —*see* Stiffness, joint
ketone metabolism E71.32
kidney N28.9
functional (tubular) N25.9
in
schistosomiasis B65.9 *[N29]*
tubular function N25.9
specified NEC N25.89
lacrimal system H04.9
changes H04.69
fistula —*see* Fistula, lacrimal
gland H04.19
atrophy —*see* Atrophy, lacrimal gland
cyst —*see* Cyst, lacrimal, gland
dacryops —*see* Dacryops
dislocation —*see* Dislocation, lacrimal gland
dry eye syndrome —*see* Syndrome, dry eye
infection —*see* Dacryoadenitis
granuloma —*see* Granuloma, lacrimal
inflammation —*see* Inflammation, lacrimal
obstruction —*see* Obstruction, lacrimal
specified NEC H04.89
lactation NEC O92.79
language (developmental) F80.9
expressive F80.1
mixed receptive and expressive F80.2
receptive F80.2
late luteal phase dysphoric N94.89
learning (specific) F81.9
acalculia R48.8
alexia R48.0
mathematics F81.2
reading F81.0
specified
with impairment in
mathematics F81.2
reading F81.0
written expression F81.81
specified NEC F81.89
spelling F81.81
written expression F81.81
lens H27.9
aphakia —*see* Aphakia
cataract —*see* Cataract
dislocation —*see* Dislocation, lens
specified type NEC H27.8
ligament M24.20
ankle M24.27-●
attachment, spine —*see* Enthesopathy, spinal
elbow M24.22-●
foot joint M24.27-●
hand joint M24.24-●
hip M24.25-●
knee —*see* Derangement, knee, specified NEC
shoulder M24.21-●
specified site NEC M24.29
vertebra M24.28
wrist M24.23-●
ligamentous attachments —*see also* Enthesopathy
spine —*see* Enthesopathy, spinal
lipid
metabolism, congenital E78.9
storage E75.6
specified NEC E75.5
lipoprotein
deficiency (familial) E78.6
metabolism E78.9
specified NEC E78.89
liver K76.9
malarial B54 *[K77]*
low back —*see also* Dorsopathy, specified NEC
lumbosacral
plexus G54.1
root (nerve) NEC G54.4
lung, interstitial, drug-induced J70.4
acute J70.2
chronic J70.3
dabbing (related) U07.0
e-cigarette (related) U07.0
electronic cigarette (related) U07.0
vaping (associated) (device) (product) (related) (use) U07.0

Disorder *(Continued)*
lymphoproliferative, post-transplant (PTLD) D47.Z1
lysine and hydroxylysine metabolism E72.3
major neurocognitive (*see also* Dementia, in (due to)) F03-●
male
erectile (organic) —*see also* Dysfunction, sexual, male, erectile N52.9
nonorganic F52.21
hypoactive sexual desire F52.0
orgasmic F52.32
manic F30.9
organic F06.33
mast cell activation —*see* Activation, mast cell
mastoid —*see also* Disorder, ear, middle
postprocedural —*see* Complications, ear, procedure
meninges, specified type NEC G96.198
meniscus —*see* Derangement, knee, meniscus
menopausal N95.9
specified NEC N95.8
menstrual N92.6
psychogenic F45.8
specified NEC N92.5
mental (or behavioral) (nonpsychotic) F99
due to (secondary to)
amphetamine
due to drug abuse —*see* Abuse, drug, stimulant
due to drug dependence —*see* Dependence, drug, stimulant
brain disease, damage and dysfunction F09
caffeine use
due to drug abuse —*see* Abuse, drug, stimulant
due to drug dependence —*see* Dependence, drug, stimulant
cannabis use
due to drug abuse —*see* Abuse, drug, cannabis
due to drug dependence —*see* Dependence, drug, cannabis
general medical condition F09
sedative or hypnotic use
due to drug abuse —*see* Abuse, drug, sedative
due to drug dependence —*see* Dependence, drug, sedative
tobacco (nicotine) use —*see* Dependence, drug, nicotine
following organic brain damage F07.9
frontal lobe syndrome F07.0
personality change F07.0
postconcussional syndrome F07.81
specified NEC F07.89
infancy, childhood or adolescence F98.9
neurotic —*see* Neurosis
organic or symptomatic F09
presenile, psychotic F03
problem NEC
psychoneurotic —*see* Neurosis
psychotic —*see* Psychosis
puerperal F53.0
senile, psychotic NEC F03
metabolic, amino acid, transitory, newborn P74.8
metabolism NOS E88.9
amino-acid E72.9
aromatic E70.9
albinism —*see* Albinism
histidine E70.40
histidinemia E70.41
other specified E70.49
hyperphenylalaninemia E70.1
classical phenylketonuria E70.0
other specified E70.89
tryptophan E70.5
tyrosine E70.20
hypertyrosinemia E70.21
other specified E70.29
branched chain E71.2
3-methylglutaconic aciduria E71.111
hyperleucine-isoleucinemia E71.19
hypervalinemia E71.19
isovaleric acidemia E71.110
maple syrup urine disease E71.0
methylmalonic acidemia E71.120
organic aciduria NEC E71.118
other specified E71.19

Disorder *(Continued)*
metabolism *(Continued)*
amino-acid *(Continued)*
branched chain *(Continued)*
~~propionate NEC E71.128~~
~~proprionic acidemia E71.121~~
▶ propionate NEC E71.128
▶ propionic acidemia E71.121
glycine E72.50
d-glycericacidemia E72.59
hyperhydroxyprolinemia E72.59
hyperoxaluria R82.992
primary E72.53
hyperprolinemia E72.59
non-ketotic hyperglycinemia E72.51
other specified E72.59
sarcosinemia E72.59
trimethylaminuria E72.52
hydroxylysine E72.3
lysine E72.3
ornithine E72.4
other specified E72.89
beta-amino acid E72.89
gamma-glutamyl cycle E72.89
straight-chain E72.89
sulfur-bearing E72.10
homocystinuria E72.11
methylenetetrahydrofolate reductase deficiency E72.12
other specified E72.19
bile acid and cholesterol metabolism E78.70
bilirubin E80.7
specified NEC E80.6
calcium E83.50
hypercalcemia E83.52
hypocalcemia E83.51
other specified E83.59
carbohydrate E74.9
specified NEC E74.89
cholesterol and bile acid metabolism E78.70
▶ citrate NEC E74.829
congenital E88.9
copper E83.00
specified type NEC E83.09
Wilson's disease E83.01
cystinuria E72.01
fructose E74.10
galactose E74.20
glucosaminoglycan E76.9
mucopolysaccharidosis —*see* Mucopolysaccharidosis
specified NEC E76.8
glutamine E72.89
glycine E72.50
glycogen storage (hepatorenal) E74.09
glycoprotein E77.9
specified NEC E77.8
glycosaminoglycan E76.9
specified NEC E76.8
in labor and delivery O75.89
iron E83.10
isoleucine E71.19
leucine E71.19
lipoid E78.9
lipoprotein E78.9
specified NEC E78.89
magnesium E83.40
hypermagnesemia E83.41
hypomagnesemia E83.42
other specified E83.49
mineral E83.9
specified NEC E83.89
mitochondrial E88.40
MELAS syndrome E88.41
MERRF syndrome (myoclonic epilepsy associated with ragged-red fibers) E88.42
other specified E88.49
tRNA synthetases E88.43
ornithine E72.4
phosphatases E83.30
phosphorus E83.30
acid phosphatase deficiency E83.39
hypophosphatasia E83.39
hypophosphatemia E83.39
familial E83.31
other specified E83.39
pseudovitamin D deficiency E83.32
plasma protein NEC E88.09
porphyrin —*see* Porphyria

D

▶ New ➡ Revised ~~deleted~~ Deleted ● Use Additional Character(s)

Disorder *(Continued)*
- metabolism *(Continued)*
  - postprocedural E89.89
    - specified NEC E89.89
  - purine E79.9
    - specified NEC E79.89
  - pyrimidine E79.9
    - specified NEC E79.89
  - pyruvate E74.4
  - serine E72.89
  - sodium E87.8
  - specified NEC E88.89
  - threonine E72.89
  - valine E71.19
  - zinc E83.2
- methylmalonic acidemia E71.12Ø
- micturition NEC —*see also* Difficulty, micturition R39.198
  - feeling of incomplete emptying R39.14
  - hesitancy R39.11
  - poor stream R39.12
  - psychogenic F45.8
  - split stream R39.13
  - straining R39.16
  - urgency R39.15
- mild neurocognitive G31.84
  - due to known physiological condition (without behavioral disturbance) FØ6.7Ø
    - with behavioral disturbance FØ6.71
- mitochondrial metabolism E88.4Ø
- mitral (valve) —*see* Endocarditis, mitral
- mixed
  - anxiety and depressive F41.8
  - of scholastic skills (developmental) F81.89
  - receptive expressive language F8Ø.2
- mood F39
  - bipolar —*see* Disorder, bipolar
  - depressive —*see* Disorder, depressive
  - due to (secondary to)
    - alcohol F1Ø.94
    - amphetamine F15.94
      - in
        - abuse F15.14
        - dependence F15.24
    - anxiolytic F13.94
      - in
        - abuse F13.14
        - dependence F13.24
    - cocaine F14.94
      - in
        - abuse F14.14
        - dependence F14.24
    - general medical condition FØ6.3Ø
    - hallucinogen F16.94
      - in
        - abuse F16.14
        - dependence F16.24
    - hypnotic F13.94
      - in
        - abuse F13.14
        - dependence F13.24
    - inhalant F18.94
      - in
        - abuse F18.14
        - dependence F18.24
    - opioid F11.94
      - in
        - abuse F11.14
        - dependence F11.24
    - phencyclidine (PCP) F16.94
      - in
        - abuse F16.14
        - dependence F16.24
    - physiological condition FØ6.3Ø
      - with
        - depressive features FØ6.31
        - major depressive-like episode FØ6.32
        - manic features FØ6.33
        - mixed features FØ6.34
    - psychoactive substance NEC F19.94
      - in
        - abuse F19.14
        - dependence F19.24
    - sedative F13.94
      - in
        - abuse F13.14
        - dependence F13.24
    - volatile solvents F18.94
      - in
        - abuse F18.14
        - dependence F18.24

Disorder *(Continued)*
- mood *(Continued)*
  - manic episode F3Ø.9
    - with psychotic symptoms F3Ø.2
    - without psychotic symptoms F3Ø.1Ø
      - mild F3Ø.11
      - moderate F3Ø.12
      - severe F3Ø.13
    - in remission (full) F3Ø.4
      - partial F3Ø.3
    - specified type NEC F3Ø.8
  - organic FØ6.3Ø
    - right hemisphere FØ7.89
  - persistent F34.9
    - cyclothymia F34.Ø
    - dysthymia F34.1
    - specified type NEC F34.89
  - recurrent F39
  - right hemisphere organic FØ7.89
- movement G25.9
  - drug-induced G25.7Ø
    - akathisia G25.71
    - specified NEC G25.79
  - hysterical F44.4
  - in diseases classified elsewhere —*see* category G26
  - periodic limb G47.61
    - sleep related G47.61
  - sleep related NEC G47.69
  - specified NEC G25.89
  - stereotyped F98.4
  - treatment-induced G25.9
- multiple personality F44.81
- muscle M62.9
  - attachment, spine —*see* Enthesopathy, spinal
  - in trichinellosis —*see* Trichinellosis, with muscle disorder
  - psychogenic F45.8
  - specified type NEC M62.89
  - tone, newborn P94.9
    - specified NEC P94.8
- muscular
  - attachments —*see also* Enthesopathy
    - spine —*see* Enthesopathy, spinal
  - urethra N36.44
- musculoskeletal system, soft tissue —*see* Disorder, soft tissue
  - postprocedural M96.89
  - psychogenic F45.8
- myoneural G7Ø.9
  - due to lead G7Ø.1
  - specified NEC G7Ø.89
  - toxic G7Ø.1
- myotonic NEC G71.19
- nail, in diseases classified elsewhere L62
- neck region NEC —*see* Dorsopathy, specified NEC
- neonatal onset multisystemic inflammatory (NOMID) MØ4.2
- nerve G58.9
  - abducent NEC —*see* Strabismus, paralytic, sixth nerve
  - accessory G52.8
  - acoustic —*see* subcategory H93.3
  - auditory —*see* subcategory H93.3
  - auriculotemporal G5Ø.8
  - axillary G54.Ø
  - cerebral —*see* Disorder, nerve, cranial
  - cranial G52.9
    - eighth —*see* subcategory H93.3
    - eleventh G52.8
    - fifth G5Ø.9
    - first G52.Ø
    - fourth NEC —*see* Strabismus, paralytic, fourth nerve
    - multiple G52.7
    - ninth G52.1
    - second NEC —*see* Disorder, nerve, optic
    - seventh NEC G51.8
    - sixth NEC —*see* Strabismus, paralytic, sixth nerve
    - specified NEC G52.8
    - tenth G52.2
    - third NEC —*see* Strabismus, paralytic, third nerve
    - twelfth G52.3
  - entrapment —*see* Neuropathy, entrapment
  - facial G51.9
    - specified NEC G51.8
  - femoral —*see* Lesion, nerve, femoral
  - glossopharyngeal NEC G52.1

Disorder *(Continued)*
- nerve *(Continued)*
  - hypoglossal G52.3
  - intercostal G58.Ø
  - lateral
    - cutaneous of thigh —*see* Mononeuropathy, lower limb, meralgia paresthetica
    - popliteal —*see* Lesion, nerve, popliteal
  - lower limb —*see* Mononeuropathy, lower limb
  - medial popliteal —*see* Lesion, nerve, popliteal, medial
  - median NEC —*see* Lesion, nerve, median
  - multiple G58.7
  - oculomotor NEC —*see* Strabismus, paralytic, third nerve
  - olfactory G52.Ø
  - optic NEC H47.Ø9-●
    - hemorrhage into sheath —*see* Hemorrhage, optic nerve
    - ischemic H47.Ø1-●
  - peroneal —*see* Lesion, nerve, popliteal
  - phrenic G58.8
  - plantar —*see* Lesion, nerve, plantar
  - pneumogastric G52.2
  - posterior tibial —*see* Syndrome, tarsal tunnel
  - radial —*see* Lesion, nerve, radial
  - recurrent laryngeal G52.2
  - root G54.9
    - cervical G54.2
    - lumbosacral G54.1
    - specified NEC G54.8
    - thoracic G54.3
  - sciatic NEC —*see* Lesion, nerve, sciatic
  - specified NEC G58.8
    - lower limb —*see* Mononeuropathy, lower limb, specified NEC
    - upper limb —*see* Mononeuropathy, upper limb, specified NEC
  - sympathetic G9Ø.9
  - tibial —*see* Lesion, nerve, popliteal, medial
  - trigeminal G5Ø.9
    - specified NEC G5Ø.8
  - trochlear NEC —*see* Strabismus, paralytic, fourth nerve
  - ulnar —*see* Lesion, nerve, ulnar
  - upper limb —*see* Mononeuropathy, upper limb
  - vagus G52.2
- nervous system G98.8
  - autonomic (peripheral) G9Ø.9
    - ➡ specified NEC G9Ø.89
  - central G96.9
    - specified NEC G96.89
  - parasympathetic G9Ø.9
  - specified NEC G98.8
  - sympathetic G9Ø.9
  - vegetative G9Ø.9
- neurocognitive R41.9
  - with Lewy bodies (*see also* Dementia, in, diseases specified elsewhere) G31.83 [FØ2.-]
  - frontotemporal, specified NEC (*see also* Dementia, in, diseases specified elsewhere) G31.Ø9 [FØ2.-●]
  - major (*see also* Dementia) FØ3.-●
    - due to vascular disease —*see* Dementia, vascular
      - mild —*see* Dementia, vascular, mild
      - moderate —*see* Dementia, vascular, moderate
      - severe —*see* Dementia, vascular, severe
    - in (due to) (other diseases classified elsewhere) —*see also* Dementia, in (due to) FØ2.8Ø
    - with
      - aggressive behavior (*see also* Dementia, in (due to)) FØ2.81-●
      - combative behavior (*see also* Dementia, in (due to)) FØ2.81-●
      - violent behavior (*see also* Dementia, in (due to)) FØ2.81-●
  - mild (of uncertain or unknown etiology) (*see also* Disorder, mild neurocognitive) G31.84
- neurodevelopmental F89
  - specified NEC F88
- neurohypophysis NEC E23.3
- neurological NEC R29.818
- neuromuscular G7Ø.9
  - hereditary NEC G71.9
  - specified NEC G7Ø.89
  - toxic G7Ø.1

D

D

▶ New ➡ Revised ~~deleted~~ Deleted ● Use Additional Character(s)

- **Disorder** *(Continued)*
  - tubulo-interstitial *(Continued)*
    - lymphoma NEC C85.9-● *[N16]*
    - mixed cryoglobulinemia D89.1 *[N16]*
    - multiple myeloma C9Ø.Ø-● *[N16]*
    - Salmonella infection AØ2.25
    - sarcoidosis D86.84
    - sepsis A41.9 *[N16]*
      - streptococcal A4Ø.9 *[N16]*
    - systemic lupus erythematosus M32.15
    - toxoplasmosis B58.83
    - transplant rejection T86.91 *[N16]*
    - Wilson's disease E83.Ø1 *[N16]*
  - tubulo-renal function, impaired N25.9
    - specified NEC N25.89
  - tympanic membrane H73.9-●
    - atrophy *—see* Atrophy, tympanic membrane
    - infection *—see* Myringitis
    - perforation *—see* Perforation, tympanum
    - specified NEC H73.89-●
  - unsocialized aggressive F91.1
  - urea cycle metabolism E72.2Ø
    - argininemia E72.21
    - arginosuccinic aciduria E72.22
    - citrullinemia E72.23
    - ornithine transcarbamylase deficiency E72.4
    - other specified E72.29
  - ureter (in) N28.9
    - schistosomiasis B65.Ø *[N29]*
    - tuberculosis A18.11
  - urethra N36.9
    - specified NEC N36.8
  - urinary system N39.9
    - specified NEC N39.8
  - valve, heart
    - aortic *—see* Endocarditis, aortic
    - mitral *—see* Endocarditis, mitral
    - pulmonary *—see* Endocarditis, pulmonary
    - rheumatic
      - aortic *—see* Endocarditis, aortic, rheumatic
      - mitral *—see* Endocarditis, mitral
      - pulmonary *—see* Endocarditis, pulmonary, rheumatic
      - tricuspid *—see* Endocarditis, tricuspid
    - tricuspid *—see* Endocarditis, tricuspid
  - vestibular function H81.9-●
    - specified NEC *—see* subcategory H81.8
      - in diseases classified elsewhere H82.-●
    - vertigo *—see* Vertigo
  - vision, binocular H53.3Ø
    - abnormal retinal correspondence H53.31
    - diplopia H53.2
    - fusion with defective stereopsis H53.32
    - simultaneous perception H53.33
    - suppression H53.34
  - visual
    - cortex
      - blindness H47.619
        - left brain H47.612
        - right brain H47.611
      - due to
        - inflammatory disorder H47.629
          - left brain H47.622
          - right brain H47.621
        - neoplasm H47.639
          - left brain H47.632
          - right brain H47.631
        - vascular disorder H47.649
          - left brain H47.642
          - right brain H47.641
    - pathway H47.9
      - due to
        - inflammatory disorder H47.51-●
        - neoplasm H47.52-●
        - vascular disorder H47.53-●
      - optic chiasm *—see* Disorder, optic, chiasm
  - vitreous body H43.9
    - crystalline deposits *—see* Deposit, crystalline
    - degeneration *—see* Degeneration, vitreous
    - hemorrhage *—see* Hemorrhage, vitreous
    - opacities *—see* Opacity, vitreous
    - prolapse *—see* Prolapse, vitreous
    - specified type NEC H43.89
  - voice R49.9
    - specified type NEC R49.8
  - volatile solvent use
    - due to drug abuse *—see* Abuse, drug, inhalant
    - due to drug dependence *—see* Dependence, drug, inhalant
  - voyeuristic F65.3
- **Disorder** *(Continued)*
  - white blood cells D72.9
    - specified NEC D72.89
  - withdrawing, child or adolescent F4Ø.1Ø
- **Disorientation** R41.Ø
- **Displacement, displaced**
  - acquired traumatic of bone, cartilage, joint, tendon NEC *—see* Dislocation
  - adrenal gland (congenital) Q89.1
  - appendix, retrocecal (congenital) Q43.8
  - auricle (congenital) Q17.4
  - bladder (acquired) N32.89
    - congenital Q64.19
  - brachial plexus (congenital) QØ7.8
  - brain stem, caudal (congenital) QØ4.8
  - canaliculus (lacrimalis), congenital Q1Ø.6
  - cardia through esophageal hiatus (congenital) Q4Ø.1
  - cerebellum, caudal (congenital) QØ4.8
  - cervix *—see* Malposition, uterus
  - colon (congenital) Q43.3
  - device, implant or graft *—see also* Complications, by site and type, mechanical T85.628
    - arterial graft NEC *—see* Complication, cardiovascular device, mechanical, vascular
    - breast (implant) T85.42
    - catheter NEC T85.628
      - dialysis (renal) T82.42
        - intraperitoneal T85.621
      - infusion NEC T82.524
        - spinal (epidural) (subdural) T85.62Ø
      - urinary
        - cystostomy T83.Ø2Ø
        - Hopkins T83.Ø28
        - ileostomy T83.Ø28
        - indwelling T83.Ø21
        - nephrostomy T83.Ø22
        - specified NEC T83.Ø28
        - urostomy T83.Ø28
    - electronic (electrode) (pulse generator) (stimulator) *—see* Complication, electronic stimulator
    - fixation, internal (orthopedic) NEC *—see* Complication, fixation device, mechanical
    - gastrointestinal *—see* Complications, prosthetic device, mechanical, gastrointestinal device
    - genital NEC T83.428
      - intrauterine contraceptive device (string) T83.32
      - penile prosthesis (cylinder) (implanted) (pump) (reservoir) T83.42Ø
      - testicular prosthesis T83.421
    - heart NEC *—see* Complication, cardiovascular device, mechanical
    - joint prosthesis *—see* Complications, joint prosthesis, mechanical
    - ocular *—see* Complications, prosthetic device, mechanical, ocular device
    - orthopedic NEC *—see* Complication, orthopedic, device or graft, mechanical
    - specified NEC T85.628
    - urinary NEC T83.128
      - graft T83.22
      - sphincter, implanted T83.121
      - stent (ileal conduit) (nephroureteral) T83.123
      - ureteral indwelling T83.122
    - vascular NEC *—see* Complication, cardiovascular device, mechanical
    - ventricular intracranial shunt T85.Ø2
  - electronic stimulator
    - bone T84.32Ø
    - cardiac *—see* Complications, cardiac device, electronic
    - nervous system *—see* Complication, prosthetic device, mechanical, electronic nervous system stimulator
    - urinary *—see* Complications, electronic stimulator, urinary
  - esophageal mucosa into cardia of stomach, congenital Q39.8
  - esophagus (acquired) K22.89
    - congenital Q39.8
  - eyeball (acquired) (lateral) (old) *—see* Displacement, globe
    - congenital Q15.8
    - current *—see* Avulsion, eye
- **Displacement, displaced** *(Continued)*
  - fallopian tube (acquired) N83.4-●
    - congenital Q5Ø.6
    - opening (congenital) Q5Ø.6
  - gallbladder (congenital) Q44.1
  - gastric mucosa (congenital) Q4Ø.2
  - globe (acquired) (old) (lateral) HØ5.21-●
    - current *—see* Avulsion, eye
  - heart (congenital) Q24.8
    - acquired I51.89
  - hymen (upward) (congenital) Q52.4
  - intervertebral disc NEC
    - with myelopathy *—see* Disorder, disc, with, myelopathy
    - cervical, cervicothoracic (with) M5Ø.2Ø
      - myelopathy *—see* Disorder, disc, cervical, with myelopathy
      - neuritis, radiculitis or radiculopathy *—see* Disorder, disc, cervical, with neuritis
    - due to trauma *—see* Dislocation, vertebra
    - lumbar region M51.26
      - with
        - neuritis, radiculitis, radiculopathy or sciatica M51.16
    - lumbosacral region M51.27
      - with
        - myelopathy M51.Ø7
        - neuritis, radiculitis, radiculopathy or sciatica M51.17
    - sacrococcygeal region M53.3
    - thoracic region M51.24
      - with
        - myelopathy M51.Ø4
        - neuritis, radiculitis, radiculopathy M51.14
    - thoracolumbar region M51.25
      - with
        - myelopathy M51.Ø5
        - neuritis, radiculitis, radiculopathy M51.15
  - intrauterine device (string) T83.32
  - kidney (acquired) N28.83
    - congenital Q63.2
  - lachrymal, lacrimal apparatus or duct (congenital) Q1Ø.6
  - lens, congenital Q12.1
  - macula (congenital) Q14.1
  - Meckel's diverticulum Q43.Ø
    - malignant *—see* Table of Neoplasms, small intestine, malignant
  - nail (congenital) Q84.6
    - acquired L6Ø.8
  - opening of Wharton's duct in mouth Q38.4
  - organ or site, congenital NEC *—see* Malposition, congenital
  - ovary (acquired) N83.4-●
    - congenital Q5Ø.39
    - free in peritoneal cavity (congenital) Q5Ø.39
    - into hernial sac N83.4-●
  - oviduct (acquired) N83.4-●
    - congenital Q5Ø.6
  - parathyroid (gland) E21.4
  - parotid gland (congenital) Q38.4
  - punctum lacrimale (congenital) Q1Ø.6
  - sacro-iliac (joint) (congenital) Q74.2
    - current injury S33.2
    - old *—see* subcategory M53.2
  - salivary gland (any) (congenital) Q38.4
  - spleen (congenital) Q89.Ø9
  - stomach, congenital Q4Ø.2
  - sublingual duct Q38.4
  - tongue (downward) (congenital) Q38.3
  - tooth, teeth, fully erupted M26.3Ø
    - horizontal M26.33
    - vertical M26.34
  - trachea (congenital) Q32.1
  - ureter or ureteric opening or orifice (congenital) Q62.62
  - uterine opening of oviducts or fallopian tubes Q5Ø.6
  - uterus, uterine *—see* Malposition, uterus
  - ventricular septum Q21.Ø
    - with rudimentary ventricle Q2Ø.4
- **Disproportion**
  - between native and reconstructed breast N65.1
  - fiber-type G71.2Ø
    - congenital G71.29
- **Disruptio uteri** *—see* Rupture, uterus

D

D

D

Diverticulitis (Continued)
 intestine (Continued)
 congenital Q43.8
 large K57.32
 with
 abscess, perforation K57.20
 with bleeding K57.21
 bleeding K57.33
 small intestine K57.52
 with
 abscess, perforation K57.40
 with bleeding K57.41
 bleeding K57.53
 small K57.12
 with
 abscess, perforation K57.00
 with bleeding K57.01
 bleeding K57.13
 large intestine K57.52
 with
 abscess, perforation K57.40
 with bleeding K57.41
 bleeding K57.53
Diverticulosis K57.90
 with bleeding K57.91
 large intestine K57.30
 with
 bleeding K57.31
 small intestine K57.50
 with bleeding K57.51
 small intestine K57.10
 with
 bleeding K57.11
 large intestine K57.50
 with bleeding K57.51
Diverticulum, diverticula (multiple) K57.90
 appendix (noninflammatory) K38.2
 bladder (sphincter) N32.3
 congenital Q64.6
 bronchus (congenital) Q32.4
 acquired J98.09
 calyx, calyceal (kidney) N28.89
 cardia (stomach) K31.4
 cecum —see Diverticulosis, intestine, large
 congenital Q43.8
 colon —see Diverticulosis, intestine, large
 congenital Q43.8
 duodenum —see Diverticulosis, intestine, small
 congenital Q43.8
 epiphrenic (esophagus) K22.5
 esophagus (congenital) Q39.6
 acquired (epiphrenic) (pulsion) (traction)
 K22.5
 eustachian tube —see Disorder, eustachian tube,
 specified NEC
 fallopian tube N83.8
 gastric K31.4
 heart (congenital) Q24.8
 ileum —see Diverticulosis, intestine, small
 jejunum —see Diverticulosis, intestine, small
 kidney (pelvis) (calyces) N28.89
 with calculus —see Calculus, kidney
 Meckel's (displaced) (hypertrophic) Q43.0
 malignant —see Table of Neoplasms, small
 intestine, malignant
 midthoracic K22.5
 organ or site, congenital NEC —see Distortion
 pericardium (congenital) (cyst) Q24.8
 acquired I31.8
 pharyngoesophageal (congenital) Q39.6
 acquired K22.5
 pharynx (congenital) Q38.7
 rectosigmoid —see Diverticulosis, intestine, large
 congenital Q43.8
 rectum —see Diverticulosis, intestine, large
 Rokitansky's K22.5
 seminal vesicle N50.89
 sigmoid —see Diverticulosis, intestine, large
 congenital Q43.8
 stomach (acquired) K31.4
 congenital Q40.2
 trachea (acquired) J39.8
 ureter (acquired) N28.89
 congenital Q62.8
 ureterovesical orifice N28.89
 urethra (acquired) N36.1
 congenital Q64.79
 ventricle, left (congenital) Q24.8
 vesical N32.3
 congenital Q64.6
 Zenker's (esophagus) K22.5

Division
 cervix uteri (acquired) N88.8
 glans penis Q55.69
 labia minora (congenital) Q52.79
 ligament (partial or complete) (current) —see
 also Sprain
 with open wound —see Wound, open
 muscle (partial or complete) (current) —see also
 Injury, muscle
 with open wound —see Wound, open
 nerve (traumatic) —see Injury, nerve
 spinal cord —see Injury, spinal cord,
 by region
 vein I87.8
Divorce, causing family disruption Z63.5
Dix-Hallpike neurolabyrinthitis —see Neuronitis,
 vestibular
Dizziness R42
 hysterical F44.89
 psychogenic F45.8
DMAC (disseminated mycobacterium avium-
 intracellulare complex) A31.2
DNR (do not resuscitate) Z66
Doan-Wiseman syndrome (primary splenic
 neutropenia) —see Agranulocytosis
Doehle-Heller aortitis A52.02
Dog bite —see Bite
Dohle body panmyelopathic syndrome D72.0
Dolichocephaly Q67.2
 non-deformational Q75.01
Dolichocolon Q43.8
Dolichostenomelia —see Syndrome, Marfan
Donohue's syndrome E34.8
Donor (organ or tissue) Z52.9
 blood (whole) Z52.000
 autologous Z52.010
 specified component (lymphocytes) (platelets)
 NEC Z52.008
 autologous Z52.018
 specified donor NEC Z52.098
 specified donor NEC Z52.090
 stem cells Z52.001
 autologous Z52.011
 specified donor NEC Z52.091
 bone Z52.20
 autologous Z52.21
 marrow Z52.3
 specified type NEC Z52.29
 cornea Z52.5
 egg (Oocyte) Z52.819
 age 35 and over Z52.812
 anonymous recipient Z52.812
 designated recipient Z52.813
 under age 35 Z52.810
 anonymous recipient Z52.810
 designated recipient Z52.811
 kidney Z52.4
 liver Z52.6
 lung Z52.89
 lymphocyte —see Donor, blood, specified
 components NEC
 Oocyte —see Donor, egg
 platelets Z52.008
 potential, examination of Z00.5
 semen Z52.89
 skin Z52.10
 autologous Z52.11
 specified type NEC Z52.19
 specified organ or tissue NEC Z52.89
 sperm Z52.89
Donovanosis A58
Dorsalgia M54.9
 psychogenic F45.41
 specified NEC M54.89
Dorsopathy M53.9
 deforming M43.9
 specified NEC —see subcategory M43.8
 specified NEC M53.80
 cervical region M53.82
 cervicothoracic region M53.83
 lumbar region M53.86
 lumbosacral region M53.87
 occipito-atlanto-axial region M53.81
 sacrococcygeal region M53.88
 thoracic region M53.84
 thoracolumbar region M53.85
Double
 albumin E88.09
 aortic arch Q25.45
 auditory canal Q17.8
 auricle (heart) Q20.8

Double (Continued)
 bladder Q64.79
 cervix Q51.820
 with doubling of uterus (and vagina) Q51.10
 with obstruction Q51.11
 inlet ventricle Q20.4
 kidney with double pelvis (renal) Q63.0
 meatus urinarius Q64.75
 monster Q89.4
 outlet
 left ventricle Q20.2
 right ventricle Q20.1
 pelvis (renal) with double ureter Q62.5
 tongue Q38.3
 ureter (one or both sides) Q62.5
 with double pelvis (renal) Q62.5
 urethra Q64.74
 urinary meatus Q64.75
 uterus Q51.28
 with
 doubling of cervix (and vagina) Q51.10
 with obstruction Q51.11
 complete Q51.21
 in pregnancy or childbirth O34.0-●
 causing obstructed labor O65.5
 partial Q51.22
 specified NEC Q51.28
 vagina Q52.10
 with doubling of uterus (and cervix) Q51.10
 with obstruction Q51.11
 vision H53.2
 vulva Q52.79
Doubled up Z59.01
Douglas' pouch, cul-de-sac —see condition
Down syndrome Q90.9
 meiotic nondisjunction Q90.0
 mitotic nondisjunction Q90.1
 mosaicism Q90.1
 translocation Q90.2
DPD (dihydropyrimidine dehydrogenase
 deficiency) E88.89
Dracontiasis B72
Dracunculiasis, dracunculosis B72
Dream state, hysterical F44.89
Drepanocytic anemia —see Disease, sickle-cell
Dresbach's syndrome (elliptocytosis) D58.1
Dreschlera (hawaiiensis) (infection)
 B43.8
Dressler's syndrome I24.1
Drift, ulnar —see Deformity, limb, specified type
 NEC, forearm
Drinking (alcohol)
 excessive, to excess NEC (without dependence)
 F10.10
 habitual (continual) (without remission)
 F10.20
 with remission F10.21
Drip, postnasal (chronic) R09.82
 due to
 allergic rhinitis —see Rhinitis, allergic
 common cold J00
 gastroesophageal reflux —see Reflux,
 gastroesophageal
 nasopharyngitis —see Nasopharyngitis
 other known condition — code to condition
 sinusitis —see Sinusitis
Droop
 facial R29.810
 cerebrovascular disease I69.992
 cerebral infarction I69.392
 intracerebral hemorrhage I69.192
 nontraumatic intracranial hemorrhage NEC
 I69.292
 specified disease NEC I69.892
 subarachnoid hemorrhage I69.092
Drop (in)
 attack NEC R55
 finger —see Deformity, finger
 foot —see Deformity, limb, foot, drop
 hematocrit (precipitous) R71.0
 hemoglobin R71.0
 toe —see Deformity, toe, specified NEC
 wrist —see Deformity, limb, wrist drop
Dropped heart beats I45.9
Dropsy, dropsical —see also Hydrops
 abdomen R18.8
 brain —see Hydrocephalus
 cardiac, heart —see Failure, heart, congestive
 gangrenous —see Gangrene
 heart —see Failure, heart, congestive
 kidney —see Nephrosis

▶ New ➡ Revised ~~deleted~~ Deleted ● Use Additional Character(s)

D

D

E

▶ New ➠ Revised ~~deleted~~ Deleted ● Use Additional Character(s)

Elevated, elevation *(Continued)*
- GFR (glomerular filtration rate) —*see* Findings, abnormal, inconclusive, without diagnosis, by type of exam
- glucose tolerance (oral) R73.Ø2
- immunoglobulin level R76.8
- indoleacetic acid R82.5
- lactic acid dehydrogenase (LDH) level R74.Ø2
- leukocytes D72.829
- lipoprotein a (Lp(a)) level E78.41
- liver function
  - study R94.5
  - test R79.89
    - alkaline phosphatase R74.8
    - aminotransferase R74.Ø1
    - bilirubin R17
    - hepatic enzyme R74.8
    - lactate dehydrogenase R74.Ø2
- (Lp(a)) (lipoprotein(a)) E78.41
- lymphocytes D72.82Ø
- prostate specific antigen [PSA] R97.2Ø
- Rh titer —*see* Complication(s), transfusion, incompatibility reaction, Rh (factor)
- scapula, congenital Q74.Ø
- sedimentation rate R7Ø.Ø
- SGOT R74.Ø1
- SGPT R74.Ø1
- transaminase level R74.Ø1
- triglycerides E78.1
  - with high cholesterol E78.2
- troponin R79.89
- tumor associated antigens [TAA] NEC R97.8
- tumor specific antigens [TSA] NEC R97.8
- urine level of
  - 17-ketosteroids R82.5
  - catecholamine R82.5
  - indoleacetic acid R82.5
  - steroids R82.5
  - vanillylmandelic acid (VMA) R82.5
- venous pressure I87.8
- white blood cell count D72.829
  - specified NEC D72.828

Elliptocytosis (congenital) (hereditary) D58.1
- Hb C (disease) D58.1
- hemoglobin disease D58.1
- sickle-cell (disease) D57.8-●
  - trait D57.3

Ellison-Zollinger syndrome E16.4

Ellis-van Creveld syndrome (chondroectodermal dysplasia) Q77.6

Elongated, elongation (congenital) —*see also* Distortion
- bone Q79.9
- cervix (uteri) Q51.828
  - acquired N88.4
  - hypertrophic N88.4
- colon Q43.8
- common bile duct Q44.5
- cystic duct Q44.5
- frenulum, penis Q55.69
- labia minora (acquired) N9Ø.69
- ligamentum patellae Q74.1
- petiolus (epiglottidis) Q31.8
- tooth, teeth KØØ.2
- uvula Q38.6

Eltor cholera AØØ.1

Emaciation R64
- due to manutrition E43

Embadomoniasis AØ7.8

Embedded tooth, teeth KØ1.Ø
- root only KØ8.3

Embolic —*see* condition

Embolism (multiple) (paradoxical) I74.9
- air (any site) (traumatic) T79.Ø
  - following
    - abortion —*see* Abortion by type complicated by embolism
    - ectopic pregnancy OØ8.2
    - infusion, therapeutic injection or transfusion T8Ø.Ø
    - molar pregnancy OØ8.2
    - procedure NEC
      - artery T81.719
        - mesenteric T81.71Ø
        - renal T81.711
        - specified NEC T81.718
      - vein T81.72
  - in pregnancy, childbirth or puerperium —*see* Embolism, obstetric

Embolism *(Continued)*
- amniotic fluid (pulmonary) —*see also* Embolism, obstetric
  - following
    - abortion —*see* Abortion by type complicated by embolism
    - ectopic pregnancy OØ8.2
    - molar pregnancy OØ8.2
- aorta, aortic I74.1Ø
  - abdominal I74.Ø9
    - saddle I74.Ø1
  - bifurcation I74.Ø9
  - saddle I74.Ø1
  - thoracic I74.11
- artery I74.9
  - auditory, internal I65.8
  - basilar —*see* Occlusion, artery, basilar
  - carotid (common) (internal) —*see* Occlusion, artery, carotid
  - cerebellar (anterior inferior) (posterior inferior) (superior) I66.3
  - cerebral —*see* Occlusion, artery, cerebral
  - choroidal (anterior) I65.8
  - communicating posterior I65.8
  - coronary —*see also* Infarct, myocardium
    - not resulting in infarction I24.Ø
  - extremity I74.4
    - lower I74.3
    - upper I74.2
  - hypophyseal I65.8
  - iliac I74.5
  - limb I74.4
    - lower I74.3
    - upper I74.2
  - mesenteric (with gangrene) —*see also* Ischemia, intestine, acute K55.Ø9
  - ophthalmic —*see* Occlusion, artery, retina
  - peripheral I74.4
  - pontine I65.8
  - precerebral —*see* Occlusion, artery, precerebral
  - pulmonary —*see* Embolism, pulmonary
  - renal N28.Ø
  - retinal —*see* Occlusion, artery, retina
  - septic I76
  - specified NEC I74.8
  - vertebral —*see* Occlusion, artery, vertebral
- basilar (artery) I65.1
- blood clot
  - following
    - abortion —*see* Abortion by type complicated by embolism
    - ectopic or molar pregnancy OØ8.2
  - in pregnancy, childbirth or puerperium —*see* Embolism, obstetric
- brain —*see also* Occlusion, artery, cerebral
  - following
    - abortion —*see* Abortion by type complicated by embolism
    - ectopic or molar pregnancy OØ8.2
  - puerperal, postpartum, childbirth —*see* Embolism, obstetric
- capillary I78.8
- cardiac —*see also* Infarct, myocardium
  - not resulting in infarction I51.3
- carotid (artery) (common) (internal) —*see* Occlusion, artery, carotid
- ➡ cavernous sinus (venous) —*see* Embolism, intracranial, venous sinus
- ▶ cement
  - ▶ pulmonary artery I26.95
    - ▶ with acute cor pulmonale I26.Ø3
- cerebral —*see* Occlusion, artery, cerebral
- cholesterol —*see* Atheroembolism
- coronary (artery or vein) (systemic) —*see* Occlusion, coronary
- due to device, implant or graft —*see also* Complications, by site and type, specified NEC
  - arterial graft NEC T82.818
  - breast (implant) T85.818
  - catheter NEC T85.818
    - dialysis (renal) T82.818
      - intraperitoneal T85.818
    - infusion NEC T82.818
      - spinal (epidural) (subdural) T85.81Ø
    - urinary (indwelling) T83.81
  - electronic (electrode) (pulse generator) (stimulator)
    - bone T84.81
    - cardiac T82.817

Embolism *(Continued)*
- due to device, implant or graft *(Continued)*
  - electronic *(Continued)*
    - nervous system (brain) (peripheral nerve) (spinal) T85.81Ø
    - urinary T83.81
  - fixation, internal (orthopedic) NEC T84.81
  - gastrointestinal (bile duct) (esophagus) T85.818
  - genital NEC T83.81
  - heart (graft) (valve) T82.817
  - joint prosthesis T84.81
  - ocular (corneal graft) (orbital implant) T85.818
  - orthopedic (bone graft) NEC T86.838
  - specified NEC T85.818
  - urinary (graft) NEC T83.81
  - vascular NEC T82.818
  - ventricular intracranial shunt T85.81Ø
- extremities
  - lower —*see* Embolism, vein, lower extremity
    - arterial I74.3
  - upper I74.2
- eye H34.9
- fat (cerebral) (pulmonary) (systemic) T79.1
  - complicating delivery —*see* Embolism, obstetric
  - following
    - abortion —*see* Abortion by type complicated by embolism
    - ectopic or molar pregnancy OØ8.2
  - ▶ pulmonary artery I26.96
    - ▶ with acute cor pulmonale I26.Ø4
- following
  - abortion —*see* Abortion by type complicated by embolism
  - ectopic or molar pregnancy OØ8.2
  - infusion, therapeutic injection or transfusion
    - air T8Ø.Ø
- heart (fatty) —*see also* Infarct, myocardium
  - not resulting in infarction I51.3
- hepatic (vein) I82.Ø
- in pregnancy, childbirth or puerperium —*see* Embolism, obstetric
- intestine (artery) (vein) (with gangrene) —*see also* Ischemia, intestine, acute K55.Ø39
- intracranial —*see also* Occlusion, artery, cerebral
  - venous sinus (any) GØ8
    - nonpyogenic I67.6
- intraspinal venous sinuses or veins GØ8
  - nonpyogenic G95.19
- kidney (artery) N28.Ø
- lateral sinus (venous) —*see* Embolism, intracranial, venous sinus
- leg —*see* Embolism, vein, lower extremity
  - arterial I74.3
- longitudinal sinus (venous) —*see* Embolism, intracranial, venous sinus
- lung (massive) —*see* Embolism, pulmonary
- meninges I66.8
- mesenteric (artery) (vein) (with gangrene) —*see also* Ischemia, intestine, acute K55.Ø59
- obstetric (in) (pulmonary)
  - childbirth O88.22
    - air O88.Ø2
    - amniotic fluid O88.12
    - blood clot O88.22
    - fat O88.82
    - pyemic O88.32
    - septic O88.32
    - specified type NEC O88.82
  - pregnancy O88.21-●
    - air O88.Ø1-●
    - amniotic fluid O88.11-●
    - blood clot O88.21-●
    - fat O88.81-●
    - pyemic O88.31-●
    - septic O88.31-●
    - specified type NEC O88.81-●
  - puerperal O88.23
    - air O88.Ø3
    - amniotic fluid O88.13
    - blood clot O88.23
    - fat O88.83
    - pyemic O88.33
    - septic O88.33
    - specified type NEC O88.83
- ophthalmic —*see* Occlusion, artery, retina
- penis N48.81
- peripheral artery NOS I74.4
- pituitary E23.6
- popliteal (artery) I74.3

E

E

E

E

- **Endocarditis** *(Continued)*
  - acute or subacute I33.9
    - infective I33.Ø
    - rheumatic (aortic) (mitral) (pulmonary) (tricuspid) IØ1.1
      - with chorea (acute) (rheumatic) (Sydenham's) IØ2.Ø
  - aortic (heart) (nonrheumatic) (valve) I35.8
    - with
      - mitral disease IØ8.Ø
        - with tricuspid (valve) disease IØ8.3
        - active or acute IØ1.1
          - with chorea (acute) (rheumatic) (Sydenham's) IØ2.Ø
      - rheumatic fever (conditions in IØØ)
        - active —*see* Endocarditis, acute, rheumatic
        - inactive or quiescent (with chorea) IØ6.9
      - tricuspid (valve) disease IØ8.2
        - with mitral (valve) disease IØ8.3
    - acute or subacute I33.9
    - arteriosclerotic I35.8
    - rheumatic IØ6.9
      - with mitral disease IØ8.Ø
        - with tricuspid (valve) disease IØ8.3
        - active or acute IØ1.1
          - with chorea (acute) (rheumatic) (Sydenham's) IØ2.Ø
      - active or acute IØ1.1
        - with chorea (acute) (rheumatic) (Sydenham's) IØ2.Ø
      - specified NEC IØ6.8
    - specified cause NEC I35.8
    - syphilitic A52.Ø3
  - arteriosclerotic I38
  - atypical verrucous (Libman-Sacks) M32.11
  - bacterial (acute) (any valve) (subacute) I33.Ø
  - candidal B37.6
  - congenital Q24.8
  - constrictive I33.Ø
  - Coxiella burnetii A78 *[I39]*
  - Coxsackie B33.21
  - due to
    - prosthetic cardiac valve T82.6
    - Q fever A78 *[I39]*
    - Serratia marcescens I33.Ø
    - typhoid (fever) AØ1.Ø2
  - gonococcal A54.83
  - infectious or infective (acute) (any valve) (subacute) I33.Ø
  - lenta (acute) (any valve) (subacute) I33.Ø
  - Libman-Sacks M32.11
  - listerial A32.82
  - Löffler's I42.3
  - malignant (acute) (any valve) (subacute) I33.Ø
  - meningococcal A39.51
  - mitral (chronic) (double) (fibroid) (heart) (inactive) (valve) (with chorea) IØ5.9
    - with
      - aortic (valve) disease IØ8.Ø
        - with tricuspid (valve) disease IØ8.3
        - active or acute IØ1.1
          - with chorea (acute) (rheumatic) (Sydenham's) IØ2.Ø
      - rheumatic fever (conditions in IØØ)
        - active —*see* Endocarditis, acute, rheumatic
        - inactive or quiescent (with chorea) IØ5.9
      - tricuspid (valve) disease IØ8.1
        - with aortic (valve) disease IØ8.3
    - active or acute IØ1.1
      - with chorea (acute) (rheumatic) (Sydenham's) IØ2.Ø
      - bacterial I33.Ø
    - arteriosclerotic I34.89
    - nonrheumatic I34.89
      - acute or subacute I33.9
    - specified NEC IØ5.8
  - monilial B37.6
  - multiple valves IØ8.9
    - specified disorders IØ8.8
  - mycotic (acute) (any valve) (subacute) I33.Ø
  - pneumococcal (acute) (any valve) (subacute) I33.Ø
  - pulmonary (chronic) (heart) (valve) I37.8
    - with rheumatic fever (conditions in IØØ)
      - active —*see* Endocarditis, acute, rheumatic
      - inactive or quiescent (with chorea) IØ9.89
        - with aortic, mitral or tricuspid disease IØ8.8
    - acute or subacute I33.9
      - rheumatic IØ1.1
        - with chorea (acute) (rheumatic) (Sydenham's) IØ2.Ø

- **Endocarditis** *(Continued)*
  - pulmonary *(Continued)*
    - arteriosclerotic I37.8
    - congenital Q22.2
    - rheumatic (chronic) (inactive) (with chorea) IØ9.89
      - active or acute IØ1.1
        - with chorea (acute) (rheumatic) (Sydenham's) IØ2.Ø
    - syphilitic A52.Ø3
  - purulent (acute) (any valve) (subacute) I33.Ø
  - Q fever A78 *[I39]*
  - rheumatic (chronic) (inactive) (with chorea) IØ9.1
    - active or acute (aortic) (mitral) (pulmonary) (tricuspid) IØ1.1
      - with chorea (acute) (rheumatic) (Sydenham's) IØ2.Ø
  - rheumatoid —*see* Rheumatoid, carditis
  - septic (acute) (any valve) (subacute) I33.Ø
  - streptococcal (acute) (any valve) (subacute) I33.Ø
  - subacute —*see* Endocarditis, acute
  - suppurative (acute) (any valve) (subacute) I33.Ø
  - syphilitic A52.Ø3
  - toxic I33.9
  - tricuspid (chronic) (heart) (inactive) (rheumatic) (valve) (with chorea) IØ7.9
    - with
      - aortic (valve) disease IØ8.2
        - mitral (valve) disease IØ8.3
      - mitral (valve) disease IØ8.1
        - aortic (valve) disease IØ8.3
      - rheumatic fever (conditions in IØØ)
        - active —*see* Endocarditis, acute, rheumatic
        - inactive or quiescent (with chorea) IØ7.8
    - active or acute IØ1.1
      - with chorea (acute) (rheumatic) (Sydenham's) IØ2.Ø
    - arteriosclerotic I36.8
    - nonrheumatic I36.8
      - acute or subacute I33.9
    - specified cause, except rheumatic I36.8
  - tuberculous —*see* Tuberculosis, endocarditis
  - typhoid AØ1.Ø2
  - ulcerative (acute) (any valve) (subacute) I33.Ø
  - vegetative (acute) (any valve) (subacute) I33.Ø
  - verrucous (atypical) (nonbacterial) (nonrheumatic) M32.11
- **Endocardium, endocardial** —*see also* condition
  - cushion defect Q21.2Ø
- **Endocervicitis** —*see also* Cervicitis
  - due to intrauterine (contraceptive) device T83.69
  - hyperplastic N72
- **Endocrine** —*see* condition
- **Endocrinopathy, pluriglandular** E31.9
- **Endodontic**
  - overfill M27.52
  - underfill M27.53
- **Endodontitis** KØ4.Ø1
  - irreversible KØ4.Ø2
  - reversible KØ4.Ø1
- **Endomastoiditis** —*see* Mastoiditis
- **Endometrioma** N8Ø.12-•
- **Endometriosis** N8Ø.9
  - abdomen, abdominal N8Ø.CØ
    - specified site, NEC N8Ø.C9
    - wall N8Ø.C19
      - fascia and muscular layers N8Ø.C11
      - subcutaneous tissue N8Ø.C1Ø
      - unspecified depth N8Ø.C19
  - appendix N8Ø.549
    - deep N8Ø.542
    - superficial N8Ø.541
  - bladder (unspecified depth) N8Ø.AØ
    - deep N8Ø.A2
    - superficial N8Ø.A1
  - bowel N8Ø.5Ø
  - broad ligament N8Ø.3C
  - cardiothoracic space N8Ø.B6
  - cecum N8Ø.539
    - N8Ø.532
    - superficial N8Ø.531
  - cervix N8Ø.Ø-•
  - colon N8Ø.559
    - descending N8Ø.559
      - deep N8Ø.552
      - superficial N8Ø.551
    - sigmoid N8Ø.529
      - deep N8Ø.522
      - superficial N8Ø.521

- **Endometriosis** *(Continued)*
  - colon *(Continued)*
    - transverse N8Ø.559
      - deep N8Ø.552
      - superficial N8Ø.551
  - cul-de-sac (Douglas')
    - anterior (unspecified depth) N8Ø.319
      - deep N8Ø.312
      - superficial N8Ø.311
    - posterior (unspecified depth) N8Ø.329
      - deep N8Ø.322
      - superficial N8Ø.321
  - deep
    - involving muscular wall of fallopian tube N8Ø.22
    - retrocervical N8Ø.Ø2
  - diaphragm N8Ø.B39
    - deep N8Ø.B32
    - superficial N8Ø.B31
    - unspecified depth N8Ø.B39
  - exocervix N8Ø.Ø1
  - extra-pelvic abdominal peritoneum N8Ø.C4
  - fallopian tube (unspecified depth) N8Ø.2Ø-•
    - deep N8Ø.22-•
    - superficial N8Ø.21-•
  - female genital organ NEC N8Ø.8
  - gallbladder N8Ø.8
  - inguinal canal N8Ø.C3
  - in scar of skin N8Ø.6
  - internal N8Ø.Ø2
  - intestine N8Ø.5Ø
    - small N8Ø.569
      - deep (multifocal) N8Ø.562
      - superficial N8Ø.561
  - lung N8Ø.B2
  - mediastinal space N8Ø.B5
  - myometrium N8Ø.Ø3
  - nerve
    - femoral N8Ø.D6
    - obturator N8Ø.D3
    - pelvic N8Ø.DØ
      - splanchnic N8Ø.D1
    - pudendal N8Ø.D5
    - retroperitoneum, NEC N8Ø.D9
    - sacral splanchnic N8Ø.D1
    - sciatic N8Ø.D4
    - specified, NEC N8Ø.D9
  - ovary (unspecified depth) N8Ø.1Ø-•
    - deep N8Ø.12-•
    - superficial N8Ø.11-•
  - parametrium N8Ø.399
  - pelvic
    - brim N8Ø.38-•
      - deep N8Ø.37-•
      - superficial N8Ø.36-•
    - peritoneum N8Ø.3Ø
      - specified sites, NEC N8Ø.399
        - deep N8Ø.392
        - superficial N8Ø.391
    - sidewall N8Ø.35-•
      - deep N8Ø.34-•
      - superficial N8Ø.33-•
  - pericardial space N8Ø.B4
  - peritoneal (pelvic) N8Ø.3Ø
  - pleura N8Ø.B1
  - rectovaginal septum N8Ø.4Ø
    - with involvement of vagina N8Ø.42
    - without involvement of vagina N8Ø.41
  - rectum N8Ø.519
    - deep (multifocal) N8Ø.512
    - superficial N8Ø.511
  - retroperitoneum N8Ø.3Ø
  - round ligament N8Ø.3C9
  - sacral nerve roots N8Ø.D2
  - skin (scar) N8Ø.6
  - specified site NEC N8Ø.8
  - stromal D39.Ø
  - thorax N8Ø.B-•
  - umbilicus N8Ø.C2
  - ureter N8Ø.A69
    - deep N8Ø.A5-•
    - extrinsic N8Ø.A4-•
    - intrinsic N8Ø.A5-•
    - unspecified depth N8Ø.A6-•
  - uterosacral ligament(s) N8Ø.3C-•
    - deep N8Ø.3B-•
    - superficial N8Ø.3A-•
  - uterus N8Ø.ØØ
    - deep N8Ø.Ø2
    - internal N8Ø.Ø2
    - superficial N8Ø.Ø1

E

- **Enteritis** *(Continued)*
  - regional *(Continued)*
    - large intestine *(Continued)*
      - with *(Continued)*
        - complication *(Continued)*
          - intestinal obstruction K50.112
          - rectal bleeding K50.111
          - small intestine (duodenum) (ileum) (jejunum) involvement K50.80
            - with
              - complication K50.819
                - abscess K50.814
                - fistula K50.813
                - intestinal obstruction K50.812
                - rectal bleeding K50.811
                - specified complication NEC K50.818
          - specified complication NEC K50.118
    - rectum —*see* Enteritis, regional, large intestine
    - small intestine (duodenum) (ileum) (jejunum) K50.00
      - with
        - complication K50.019
          - abscess K50.014
          - fistula K50.013
          - intestinal obstruction K50.012
          - large intestine (colon) (rectum) involvement K50.80
            - with
              - complication K50.819
                - abscess K50.814
                - fistula K50.813
                - intestinal obstruction K50.812
                - rectal bleeding K50.811
                - specified complication NEC K50.818
          - rectal bleeding K50.011
          - specified complication NEC K50.018
  - rotaviral A08.0
  - Salmonella, salmonellosis (arizonae) (choleraesuis) (enteritidis) (typhimurium) A02.0
  - segmental —*see* Enteritis, regional
  - septic A09
  - Shigella —*see* Infection, Shigella
  - small round structured NEC A08.19
  - spasmodic, spastic —*see* Syndrome, irritable bowel
  - staphylococcal A04.8
    - due to food A05.0
  - torovirus A08.39
  - toxic NEC K52.1
    - ~~due to Clostridium difficile~~
      - ~~not specified as recurrent A04.72~~
      - ~~recurrent A04.71~~
    - ▶due to
      - ▶Clostridioides difficile
        - ▶not specified as recurrent A04.72
        - ▶recurrent A04.71
      - ▶Clostridium difficile
        - ▶not specified as recurrent A04.72
        - ▶recurrent A04.71
  - trichomonal A07.8
  - tuberculous A18.32
  - typhosa A01.00
  - ulcerative (chronic) —*see* Colitis, ulcerative
  - viral A08.4
    - adenovirus A08.2
    - enterovirus A08.39
    - Rotavirus A08.0
    - small round structured NEC A08.19
    - specified NEC A08.39
    - virus specified NEC A08.39
- **Enterobiasis** B80
- **Enterobius vermicularis** (infection) (infestation) B80
- **Enterocele** —*see also* Hernia, abdomen
  - pelvic, pelvis (acquired) (congenital) N81.5
  - vagina, vaginal (acquired) (congenital) NEC N81.5
- **Enterocolitis** —*see also* Enteritis K52.9
  - ~~due to Clostridium difficile~~
    - ~~not specified as recurrent A04.72~~
    - ~~recurrent A04.71~~
  - ▶due to
    - ▶Clostridioides difficile
      - ▶not specified as recurrent A04.72
      - ▶recurrent A04.71
    - ▶Clostridium difficile
      - ▶not specified as recurrent A04.72
      - ▶recurrent A04.71
- **Enterocolitis** *(Continued)*
  - fulminant ischemic —*see also* Ischemia, intestine, acute K55.059
  - granulomatous —*see* Enteritis, regional
  - hemorrhagic (acute) —*see also* Ischemia, intestine, acute K55.059
    - chronic K55.1
  - infectious NEC A09
  - ischemic K55.9
  - necrotizing K55.30
    - with
      - perforation K55.33
      - pneumatosis K55.32
        - and perforation K55.33
      - ~~due to Clostridium difficile~~
        - ~~not specified as recurrent A04.72~~
        - ~~recurrent A04.71~~
    - ▶due to
      - ▶Clostridioides difficile
        - ▶not specified as recurrent A04.72
        - ▶recurrent A04.71
      - ▶Clostridium difficile
        - ▶not specified as recurrent A04.72
        - ▶recurrent A04.71
    - in non-newborn K55.30
      - stage 1 (without pneumatosis, without perforation) K55.31
      - stage 2 (with pneumatosis, without perforation) K55.32
      - stage 3 (with pneumatosis, with perforation) K55.33
    - in newborn P77.9
      - stage 1 (without pneumatosis, without perforation) P77.1
      - stage 2 (with pneumatosis, without perforation) P77.2
      - stage 3 (with pneumatosis, with perforation) P77.3
    - without pneumatosis or perforation K55.31
  - noninfectious K52.9
    - newborn —*see* Enterocolitis, necrotizing, in newborn
  - pseudomembranous (newborn)
    - not specified as recurrent A04.72
    - recurrent A04.71
  - radiation K52.0
    - newborn —*see* Enterocolitis, necrotizing, in newborn
  - ulcerative (chronic) —*see* Pancolitis, ulcerative (chronic)
- **Enterogastritis** —*see* Enteritis
- **Enteropathy** K63.9
  - celiac-gluten-sensitive K90.0
    - non-celiac K90.41
  - food protein-induced K52.22
  - hemorrhagic, terminal —*see also* Ischemia, intestine, acute K55.059
  - protein-losing K90.49
- **Enteroperitonitis** —*see* Peritonitis
- **Enteroptosis** K63.4
- **Enterorrhagia** K92.2
- **Enterospasm** —*see also* Syndrome, irritable, bowel
  - psychogenic F45.8
- **Enterostenosis** —*see also* Obstruction, intestine, specified NEC K56.699
- **Enterostomy**
  - complication —*see* Complication, enterostomy
  - status Z93.4
- **Enterovirus, as cause of disease classified elsewhere** B97.10
  - coxsackievirus B97.11
  - echovirus B97.12
  - other specified B97.19
- **Enthesopathy** (peripheral) M77.5-●
  - Achilles tendinitis —*see* Tendinitis, Achilles
  - ankle and tarsus M77.9
    - specified type NEC —*see* Enthesopathy, foot, specified type NEC
  - anterior tibial syndrome M76.81-●
  - calcaneal spur —*see* Spur, bone, calcaneal
  - elbow region M77.8
    - lateral epicondylitis —*see* Epicondylitis, lateral
    - medial epicondylitis —*see* Epicondylitis, medial
  - foot NEC M77.8
    - metatarsalgia —*see* Metatarsalgia
    - specified type NEC M77.5-●
  - forearm M77.8
  - gluteal tendinitis —*see* Tendinitis, gluteal
  - hand M77.8
  - hip —*see* Enthesopathy, lower limb, specified type NEC
- **Enthesopathy** *(Continued)*
  - iliac crest spur —*see* Spur, bone, iliac crest
  - iliotibial band syndrome —*see* Syndrome, iliotibial band
  - knee —*see* Enthesopathy, lower limb, lower leg, specified type NEC
  - lateral epicondylitis —*see* Epicondylitis, lateral
  - lower limb (excluding foot) M76.9
    - Achilles tendinitis —*see* Tendinitis, Achilles
    - ankle and tarsus M77.5-
      - specified type NEC - *see* Enthesopathy, foot, specified type NEC
    - anterior tibial syndrome M76.81-●
    - gluteal tendinitis —*see* Tendinitis, gluteal
    - iliac crest spur —*see* Spur, bone, iliac crest
    - iliotibial band syndrome —*see* Syndrome, iliotibial band
    - patellar tendinitis —*see* Tendinitis, patellar
    - pelvic region —*see* Enthesopathy, lower limb, specified type NEC
    - peroneal tendinitis —*see* Tendinitis, peroneal
    - posterior tibial syndrome M76.82-●
    - psoas tendinitis —*see* Tendinitis, psoas
    - specified type NEC M76.89-●
    - tibial collateral bursitis —*see* Bursitis, tibial collateral
  - medial epicondylitis —*see* Epicondylitis, medial
  - multiple sites M77.8
  - patellar tendinitis —*see* Tendinitis, patellar
  - pelvis M77.8
  - periarthritis of wrist —*see* Periarthritis, wrist
  - peroneal tendinitis —*see* Tendinitis, peroneal
  - posterior tibial syndrome M76.82-●
  - psoas tendinitis —*see* Tendinitis, psoas
  - shoulder M77.8
  - shoulder region —*see* Lesion, shoulder
  - specified type NEC M77.8
  - spinal M46.00
    - cervical region M46.02
    - cervicothoracic region M46.03
    - lumbar region M46.06
    - lumbosacral region M46.07
    - multiple sites M46.09
    - occipito-atlanto-axial region M46.01
    - sacrococcygeal region M46.08
    - thoracic region M46.04
    - thoracolumbar region M46.05
  - tibial collateral bursitis —*see* Bursitis, tibial collateral
  - upper arm M77.8
  - wrist and carpus NEC M77.8
    - calcaneal spur —*see* Spur, bone, calcaneal
    - periarthritis of wrist —*see* Periarthritis, wrist
- **Entomophobia** F40.218
- **Entomophthoromycosis** B46.8
- **Entrance, air into vein** —*see* Embolism, air
- **Entrapment, nerve** —*see also* Neuropathy, entrapment
  - muscle
    - eye
      - extraocular H50.68-●
      - oblique
        - inferior H50.62-●
        - superior H50.66-●
      - rectus
        - inferior H50.63-●
        - lateral H50.64-●
        - medial H50.65-●
        - superior H50.67-●
- **Entropion** (eyelid) (paralytic) H02.009
  - cicatricial H02.019
    - left H02.016
      - lower H02.015
      - upper H02.014
    - right H02.013
      - lower H02.012
      - upper H02.011
  - congenital Q10.2
  - left H02.006
    - lower H02.005
    - upper H02.004
  - mechanical H02.029
    - left H02.026
      - lower H02.025
      - upper H02.024
    - right H02.023
      - lower H02.022
      - upper H02.021
  - right H02.003
    - lower H02.002
    - upper H02.001

Entropion *(Continued)*
 senile H02.039
 left H02.036
 lower H02.035
 upper H02.034
 right H02.033
 lower H02.032
 upper H02.031
 spastic H02.049
 left H02.046
 lower H02.045
 upper H02.044
 right H02.043
 lower H02.042
 upper H02.041
Enucleated eye (traumatic, current) S05.7-•
Enuresis R32
 functional F98.0
 habit disturbance F98.0
 nocturnal N39.44
 psychogenic F98.0
 nonorganic origin F98.0
 psychogenic F98.0
Eosinopenia —*see* Agranulocytosis
Eosinophilia (allergic) (idiopathic) (secondary)
 D72.10
 with
 angiolymphoid hyperplasia (ALHE) D18.01
 familial D72.19
 hereditary D72.19
 in disease classified elsewhere D72.18
 infiltrative —*see* Eosinophilia, pulmonary
 Löffler's J82.89
 peritoneal —*see* Peritonitis, eosinophilic
 pulmonary NEC J82.89
 acute J82.82
 asthmatic J82.83
 chronic J82.81
 specified NEC D72.19
 tropical (pulmonary) J82.89
Eosinophilia-myalgia syndrome M35.89
Ependymitis (acute) (cerebral) (chronic)
 (granular) —*see* Encephalomyelitis
Ependymoblastoma
 specified site —*see* Neoplasm, malignant, by
 site
 unspecified site C71.9
Ependymoma (epithelial) (malignant)
 anaplastic
 specified site —*see* Neoplasm, malignant, by
 site
 unspecified site C71.9
 benign
 specified site —*see* Neoplasm, benign, by site
 unspecified site D33.2
 myxopapillary D43.2
 specified site —*see* Neoplasm, uncertain
 behavior, by site
 unspecified site D43.2
 papillary D43.2
 specified site —*see* Neoplasm, uncertain
 behavior, by site
 unspecified site D43.2
 specified site —*see* Neoplasm, malignant, by site
 unspecified site C71.9
Ependymopathy G93.89
Ephelis, ephelides L81.2
Epiblepharon (congenital) Q10.3
Epicanthus, epicanthic fold (eyelid) (congenital)
 Q10.3
Epicondylitis (elbow)
 lateral M77.1-•
 medial M77.0-•
Epicystitis —*see* Cystitis
Epidemic —*see* condition
Epidermidalization, cervix —*see* Dysplasia, cervix
Epidermis, epidermal —*see* condition
Epidermodysplasia verruciformis B07.8
Epidermolysis
 bullosa (congenital) Q81.9
 acquired L12.30
 drug-induced L12.31
 specified cause NEC L12.35
 dystrophica Q81.2
 letalis Q81.1
 simplex Q81.0
 specified NEC Q81.8
 necroticans combustiformis L51.2
 due to drug —*see* Table of Drugs and
 Chemicals, by drug
Epidermophytid —*see* Dermatophytosis

Epidermophytosis (infected) —*see*
 Dermatophytosis
Epididymis —*see* condition
Epididymitis (acute) (nonvenereal) (recurrent)
 (residual) N45.1
 with orchitis N45.3
 blennorrhagic (gonococcal) A54.23
 caseous (tuberculous) A18.15
 chlamydial A56.19
 filarial —*see also* Infestation, filarial B74.9 [N51]
 gonococcal A54.23
 syphilitic A52.76
 tuberculous A18.15
Epididymo-orchitis —*see also* Epididymitis N45.3
Epidural —*see* condition
Epigastrium, epigastric —*see* condition
Epigastrocele —*see* Hernia, ventral
Epiglottis —*see* condition
Epiglottitis, epiglottiditis (acute) J05.10
 with obstruction J05.11
 chronic J37.0
Epignathus Q89.4
Epilepsia partialis continua —*see also*
 Kozhevnikof's epilepsy G40.1-•
Epilepsy, epileptic, epilepsia (attack) (cerebral)
 (convulsion) (fit) (seizure) G40.909

> Note: the following terms are to be considered
> equivalent to intractable: pharmacoresistant
> (pharmacologically resistant), treatment
> resistant, refractory (medically) and poorly
> controlled

 with
 complex partial seizures —*see* Epilepsy,
 localization-related, symptomatic, with
 complex partial seizures
 grand mal seizures on awakening —
 see Epilepsy, generalized, specified NEC
 myoclonic absences —*see* Epilepsy,
 generalized, specified NEC
 myoclonic-astatic seizures —*see* Epilepsy,
 generalized, specified NEC
 simple partial seizures —*see* Epilepsy,
 localization-related, symptomatic, with
 simple partial seizures
 akinetic —*see* Epilepsy, generalized, specified
 NEC
 benign childhood with centrotemporal EEG
 spikes —*see* Epilepsy, localization-related,
 idiopathic
 benign myoclonic in infancy G40.80-•
 Bravais-jacksonian —*see* Epilepsy, localization-
 related, symptomatic,
 with simple partial seizures
 childhood
 with occipital EEG paroxysms —*see* Epilepsy,
 localization-related, idiopathic
 absence G40.A09
 intractable G40.A19
 with status epilepticus G40.A11
 without status epilepticus G40.A19
 not intractable G40.A09
 with status epilepticus G40.A01
 without status epilepticus G40.A09
 climacteric —*see* Epilepsy, specified NEC
 cysticercosis B69.0
 deterioration (mental) F06.8
 due to syphilis A52.19
 focal —*see* Epilepsy, localization-related,
 symptomatic, with simple partial
 seizures
 generalized
 idiopathic G40.309
 intractable G40.319
 with status epilepticus G40.311
 without status epilepticus G40.319
 not intractable G40.309
 with status epilepticus G40.301
 without status epilepticus G40.309
 specified NEC G40.409
 intractable G40.419
 with status epilepticus G40.411
 without status epilepticus G40.419
 not intractable G40.409
 with status epilepticus G40.401
 without status epilepticus G40.409
 impulsive petit mal —*see* Epilepsy, juvenile
 myoclonic

Epilepsy, epileptic, epilepsia *(Continued)*
 intractable G40.919
 with status epilepticus G40.911
 without status epilepticus G40.919
 juvenile absence G40.A09
 intractable G40.A19
 with status epilepticus G40.A11
 without status epilepticus G40.A19
 not intractable G40.A09
 with status epilepticus G40.A01
 without status epilepticus G40.A09
 juvenile myoclonic G40.B11
 intractable G40.B19
 with status epilepticus G40.B11
 without status epilepticus G40.B19
 not intractable G40.B09
 with status epilepticus G40.B01
 without status epilepticus G40.B09
▶KCNQ2-related G40.842
 ▶intractable G40.844
 ▶with status epilepticus G40.843
 ▶without status epilepticus G40.844
 ▶not intractable G40.842
 ▶with status epilepticus G40.841
 ▶without status epilepticus G40.842
 Lafora progressive myoclonus (*see also* Epilepsy,
 progressive, Lafora) G40.C09
 localization-related (focal) (partial)
 idiopathic G40.009
 with seizures of localized onset G40.009
 intractable G40.019
 with status epilepticus G40.011
 without status epilepticus G40.019
 not intractable G40.009
 with status epilepticus G40.001
 without status epilepticus G40.009
 symptomatic
 with complex partial seizures G40.209
 intractable G40.219
 with status epilepticus G40.211
 without status epilepticus G40.219
 not intractable G40.209
 with status epilepticus G40.201
 without status epilepticus G40.209
 with simple partial seizures G40.109
 intractable G40.119
 with status epilepticus G40.111
 without status epilepticus G40.119
 not intractable G40.109
 with status epilepticus G40.101
 without status epilepticus G40.109
 myoclonus, myoclonic —*see also* Epilepsy,
 generalized, specified NEC
 progressive —*see also* Epilepsy, generalized,
 idiopathic
 Lafora G40.C09
 intractable G40.C19
 with status epilepticus G40.C11
 without status epilepticus G40.C19
 not intractable G40.C09
 with status epilepticus G40.C01
 without status epilepticus G40.C09
 type 1 - see Epilepsy, generalized,
 idiopathic
 type 2 - see Epilepsy, myoclonus,
 progressive, Lafora
 severe, in infancy (SMEI) G40.83-•
 not intractable G40.909
 with status epilepticus G40.901
 without status epilepticus G40.909
 on awakening —*see* Epilepsy, generalized,
 specified NEC
 parasitic NOS B71.9 [*G94*]
 partial —*see* Epilepsy, localization-related,
 symptomatic, with simple partial seizures
 partialis continua —*see also* Kozhevnikof's
 epilepsy G40.1-•
 peripheral —*see* Epilepsy, specified NEC
 polymorphic, in infancy (PMEI) G40.83-•
 procursiva —*see* Epilepsy, localization-related,
 symptomatic, with simple partial seizures
 progressive (familial) myoclonic —*see* Epilepsy,
 myoclonus, progressive
 Lafora (*see also* Epilepsy, progressive, Lafora)
 G40.C09
 reflex —*see* Epilepsy, specified NEC
 related to
 alcohol G40.509
 not intractable G40.509
 with status epilepticus G40.501
 without status epilepticus G40.509

E

Epilepsy, epileptic, epilepsia *(Continued)*
 related to *(Continued)*
 drugs G40.509
 not intractable G40.509
 with status epliepticus G40.501
 without status epliepticus G40.509
 external causes G40.509
 not intractable G40.509
 with status epliepticus G40.501
 without status epliepticus G40.509
 hormonal changes G40.509
 not intractable G40.509
 with status epliepticus G40.501
 without status epliepticus G40.509
 sleep deprivation G40.509
 not intractable G40.509
 with status epliepticus G40.501
 without status epliepticus G40.509
 stress G40.509
 not intractable G40.509
 with status epliepticus G40.501
 without status epliepticus G40.509
 somatomotor —*see* Epilepsy, localization-related, symptomatic, with simple partial seizures
 somatosensory —*see* Epilepsy, localization-related, symptomatic, with simple partial seizures
 spasms G40.822
 intractable G40.824
 with status epilepticus G40.823
 without status epilepticus G40.824
 not intractable G40.822
 with status epilepticus G40.821
 without status epilepticus G40.822
 specified NEC G40.802
 intractable G40.804
 with status epilepticus G40.803
 without status epilepticus G40.804
 not intractable G40.802
 with status epilepticus G40.801
 without status epilepticus G40.802
 syndromes
 generalized
 idiopathic G40.309
 intractable G40.319
 with status epilepticus G40.311
 without status epilepticus G40.319
 not intractable G40.309
 with status epilepticus G40.301
 without status epilepticus G40.309
 specified NEC G40.409
 intractable G40.419
 with status epilepticus G40.411
 without status epilepticus G40.419
 not intractable G40.409
 with status epilepticus G40.401
 without status epilepticus G40.409
 localization-related (focal) (partial)
 idiopathic G40.009
 with seizures of localized onset G40.009
 intractable G40.019
 with status epilepticus G40.011
 without status epilepticus G40.019
 not intractable G40.009
 with status epilepticus G40.001
 without status epilepticus G40.009
 symptomatic
 with complex partial seizures G40.209
 intractable G40.219
 with status epilepticus G40.211
 without status epilepticus G40.219
 not intractable G40.209
 with status epilepticus G40.201
 without status epilepticus G40.209
 with simple partial seizures G40.109
 intractable G40.119
 with status epilepticus G40.111
 without status epilepticus G40.119
 not intractable G40.109
 with status epilepticus G40.101
 without status epilepticus G40.109
 specified NEC G40.802
 intractable G40.804
 with status epilepticus G40.803
 without status epilepticus G40.804
 not intractable G40.802
 with status epilepticus G40.801
 without status epilepticus G40.802
 tonic (-clonic) —*see* Epilepsy, generalized, specified NEC
 twilight F05

Epilepsy, epileptic, epilepsia *(Continued)*
 uncinate (gyrus) —*see* Epilepsy, localization-related, symptomatic, with complex partial seizures
 Unverricht (-Lundborg) (familial myoclonic) —*see* Epilepsy, generalized, idiopathic
 visceral —*see* Epilepsy, specified NEC
 visual —*see* Epilepsy, specified NEC
Epiloia Q85.1
Epimenorrhea N92.0
Epipharyngitis —*see* Nasopharyngitis
Epiphora H04.20-●
 due to
 excess lacrimation H04.21-●
 insufficient drainage H04.22-●
Epiphyseal arrest —*see* Arrest, epiphyseal
Epiphyseolysis, epiphysiolysis —*see* Osteochondropathy
Epiphysitis —*see also* Osteochondropathy
 juvenile M92.9
 syphilitic (congenital) A50.02
Epiplocele —*see* Hernia, abdomen
Epiploitis —*see* Peritonitis
Epiplosarcomphalocele —*see* Hernia, umbilicus
Episcleritis (suppurative) H15.10-●
 in (due to)
 syphilis A52.71
 tuberculosis A18.51
 nodular H15.12-●
 periodica fugax H15.11-●
 angioneurotic —*see* Edema, angioneurotic
 syphilitic (late) A52.71
 tuberculous A18.51
Episode
 affective, mixed F39
 depersonalization (in neurotic state) F48.1
 depressive F32.A
 major F32.9
 mild F32.0
 moderate F32.1
 severe (without psychotic symptoms) F32.2
 with psychotic symptoms F32.3
 recurrent F33.9
 brief F33.8
 specified NEC F32.89
 hypomanic F30.8
 manic F30.9
 with
 psychotic symptoms F30.2
 remission (full) F30.4
 partial F30.3
 without psychotic symptoms F30.10
 mild F30.11
 moderate F30.12
 severe (without psychotic symptoms) F30.13
 with psychotic symptoms F30.2
 other specified F30.8
 recurrent F31.89
 psychotic F23
 organic F06.8
 schizophrenic (acute) NEC, brief F23
Epispadias (female) (male) Q64.0
Episplenitis D73.89
Epistaxis (multiple) R04.0
 hereditary I78.0
 vicarious menstruation N94.89
Epithelioma (malignant) —*see also* Neoplasm, malignant, by site
 adenoides cysticum —*see* Neoplasm, skin, benign
 basal cell —*see* Neoplasm, skin, malignant
 benign —*see* Neoplasm, benign, by site
 Bowen's —*see* Neoplasm, skin, in situ
 calcifying, of Malherbe —*see* Neoplasm, skin, benign
 external site —*see* Neoplasm, skin, malignant
 intraepidermal, Jadassohn —*see* Neoplasm, skin, benign
 squamous cell —*see* Neoplasm, malignant, by site
Epitheliomatosis pigmented Q82.1
Epitheliopathy, multifocal placoid pigment H30.14-●
Epithelium, epithelial —*see* condition
Epituberculosis (with atelectasis) (allergic) A15.7
Eponychia Q84.6
Epstein's
 nephrosis or syndrome —*see* Nephrosis
 pearl K09.8
Epulis (gingiva) (fibrous) (giant cell) K06.8

Equinia A24.0
Equinovarus (congenital) (talipes) Q66.0-●
 acquired —*see* Deformity, limb, clubfoot
Equivalent
 convulsive (abdominal) —*see* Epilepsy, specified NEC
 epileptic (psychic) —*see* Epilepsy, localization-related, symptomatic, with complex partial seizures
Erb (-Duchenne) paralysis (birth injury) (newborn) P14.0
Erb's
 disease G71.02
 palsy, paralysis (brachial) (birth) (newborn) P14.0
 spinal (spastic) syphilitic A52.17
 pseudohypertrophic muscular dystrophy G71.02
Erb-Goldflam disease or syndrome G70.00
 with exacerbation (acute) G70.01
 in crisis G70.01
Erdheim's syndrome (acromegalic macrospondylitis) E22.0
Erection, painful (persistent) —*see* Priapism
Ergosterol deficiency (vitamin D) E55.9
 with
 adult osteomalacia M83.8
 rickets —*see* Rickets
Ergotism —*see also* Poisoning, food, noxious, plant
 from ergot used as drug (migraine therapy) —*see* Table of Drugs and Chemicals
Erosio interdigitalis blastomycetica B37.2
Erosion
 artery I77.2
 without rupture I77.89
 bone —*see* Disorder, bone, density and structure, specified NEC
 bronchus J98.09
 cameron —*see* Ulcer, stomach
 cartilage (joint) —*see* Disorder, cartilage, specified type NEC
 cervix (uteri) (acquired) (chronic) (congenital) N86
 with cervicitis N72
 cornea (nontraumatic) —*see* Ulcer, cornea
 recurrent H18.83-●
 traumatic —*see* Abrasion, cornea
 dental (idiopathic) (occupational) (due to diet, drugs or vomiting) K03.2
 duodenum, postpyloric —*see* Ulcer, duodenum
 esophagus K22.10
 with bleeding K22.11
 gastric —*see* Ulcer, stomach
 gastrojejunal —*see* Ulcer, gastrojejunal
 implanted mesh —*see* Complications, prosthetic device or implant, mesh
 intestine K63.3
 lymphatic vessel I89.8
 pylorus, pyloric (ulcer) —*see* Ulcer, stomach
 spine, aneurysmal A52.09
 stomach —*see* Ulcer, stomach
 subcutaneous device pocket
 nervous system prosthetic device, implant, or graft T85.890
 other internal prosthetic device, implant, or graft T85.898
 teeth (idiopathic) (occupational) (due to diet, drugs or vomiting) K03.2
 urethra N36.8
 uterus N85.8
Erotomania F52.8
Error
 metabolism, inborn —*see* Disorder, metabolism
 refractive —*see* Disorder, refraction
Eructation R14.2
 nervous or psychogenic F45.8
Eruption
 creeping B76.9
 drug (generalized) (taken internally) L27.0
 fixed L27.1
 in contact with skin —*see* Dermatitis, due to drugs
 localized L27.1
 Hutchinson, summer L56.4
 Kaposi's varicelliform B00.0
 napkin L22
 polymorphous light (sun) L56.4
 recalcitrant pustular L13.8
 ringed R23.8

E

Examination *(Continued)*
- dental Z01.20
  - with abnormal findings Z01.21
- developmental —*see* Examination, child
- donor (potential) Z00.5
- ear Z01.10
  - with abnormal findings NEC Z01.118
- eye Z01.00
  - with abnormal findings Z01.01
  - following failed vision screening Z01.020
    - with abnormal findings Z01.021
- following
  - accident NEC Z04.3
    - transport Z04.1
    - work Z04.2
  - assault, alleged, ruled out
    - adult Z04.71
    - child Z04.72
  - motor vehicle accident Z04.1
  - treatment (for) Z09
    - combined NEC Z09
      - fracture Z09
      - malignant neoplasm Z08
    - malignant neoplasm Z08
    - mental disorder Z09
    - specified condition NEC Z09
- follow-up (routine) (following) Z09
  - chemotherapy NEC Z09
    - malignant neoplasm Z08
  - fracture Z09
  - malignant neoplasm Z08
  - postpartum Z39.2
  - psychotherapy Z09
  - radiotherapy NEC Z09
    - malignant neoplasm Z08
  - surgery NEC Z09
    - malignant neoplasm Z08
- forced sexual exploitation Z04.81
- forced labor exploitation Z04.82
- gynecological Z01.419
  - with abnormal findings Z01.411
  - for contraceptive maintenance Z30.8
- health —*see* Examination, medical
- hearing Z01.10
  - with abnormal findings NEC Z01.118
  - infant or child (over 28 days old) Z00.129
    - with abnormal findings Z00.121
  - following failed hearing screening Z01.110
- immunity status testing Z01.84
- laboratory (as part of a general medical examination) Z00.00
  - with abnormal findings Z00.01
  - preprocedural Z01.812
- lactating mother Z39.1
- medical (adult) (for) (of) Z00.00
  - with abnormal findings Z00.01
  - administrative purpose only Z02.9
    - specified NEC Z02.89
  - admission to
    - armed forces Z02.3
    - old age home Z02.2
    - prison Z02.89
    - residential institution Z02.2
    - school Z02.0
      - following illness or medical treatment Z02.0
    - summer camp Z02.89
  - adoption Z02.82
  - blood alcohol or drug level Z02.83
  - camp (summer) Z02.89
  - clinical research, normal subject (control) (participant) Z00.6
  - control subject in clinical research (normal comparison) (participant) Z00.6
  - donor (potential) Z00.5
  - driving license Z02.4
  - general (adult) Z00.00
    - with abnormal findings Z00.01
  - immigration Z02.89
  - insurance purposes Z02.6
  - marriage Z02.89
  - medicolegal reasons NEC Z04.89
  - naturalization Z02.89
  - participation in sport Z02.5
  - paternity testing Z02.81
  - population survey Z00.8
  - pre-employment Z02.1
  - pre-operative —*see* Examination, pre-procedural

Examination *(Continued)*
- medical *(Continued)*
  - pre-procedural
    - cardiovascular Z01.810
    - respiratory Z01.811
    - specified NEC Z01.818
  - preschool children
    - for admission to school Z02.0
  - prisoners
    - for entrance into prison Z02.89
  - recruitment for armed forces Z02.3
  - specified NEC Z00.8
  - sport competition Z02.5
- medicolegal reason NEC Z04.89
  - forced sexual exploitation Z04.81
  - forced labor exploitation Z04.82
- newborn —*see* Newborn, examination
- pelvic (annual) (periodic) Z01.419
  - with abnormal findings Z01.411
- period of rapid growth in childhood Z00.2
- periodic (adult) (annual) (routine) Z00.00
  - with abnormal findings Z00.01
- physical (adult) —*see also* Examination, medical Z00.00
  - sports Z02.5
- postpartum
  - immediately after delivery Z39.0
  - routine follow-up Z39.2
- pre-chemotherapy (antineoplastic) Z01.818
- prenatal (normal pregnancy) —*see also* Pregnancy, normal Z34.9- ●
- pre-procedural (pre-operative)
  - cardiovascular Z01.810
  - laboratory Z01.812
  - respiratory Z01.811
  - specified NEC Z01.818
- prior to chemotherapy (antineoplastic) Z01.818
- psychiatric NEC Z00.8
  - follow-up not needing further care Z09
  - requested by authority Z04.6
- radiological (as part of a general medical examination) Z00.00
  - with abnormal findings Z00.01
- repeat cervical smear to confirm findings of recent normal smear following initial abnormal smear Z01.42
- skin (hypersensitivity) Z01.82
- special —*see also* Examination, by type Z01.89
  - specified type NEC Z01.89
- specified type or reason NEC Z04.89
- teeth Z01.20
  - with abnormal findings Z01.21
- urine —*see* Examination, laboratory
- vision Z01.00
  - with abnormal findings Z01.01
  - following failed vision screening Z01.020
    - with abnormal findings Z01.021
  - infant or child (over 28 days old) Z00.129
    - with abnormal findings Z00.121

Exanthem, exanthema —*see also* Rash
- with enteroviral vesicular stomatitis B08.4
- Boston A88.0
- epidemic with meningitis A88.0 *[G02]*
- subitum B08.20
  - due to human herpesvirus 6 B08.21
  - due to human herpesvirus 7 B08.22
- viral, virus B09
  - specified type NEC B08.8

Excess, excessive, excessively
- alcohol level in blood R78.0
- androgen (ovarian) E28.1
- attrition, tooth, teeth K03.0
- carotene, carotin (dietary) E67.1
- cold, effects of T69.9
  - specified effect NEC T69.8
- convergence H51.12
- crying
  - in child, adolescent, or adult R45.83
  - in infant R68.11
- development, breast N62
- divergence H51.8
- drinking (alcohol) NEC (without dependence) F10.10
  - habitual (continual) (without remission) F10.20
- eating R63.2
- estrogen E28.0
- fat —*see also* Obesity
  - in heart —*see* Degeneration, myocardial
  - localized E65
- foreskin N47.8

Excess, excessive, excessively *(Continued)*
- gas R14.0
- glucagon E16.3
- heat —*see* Heat
- intermaxillary vertical dimension of fully erupted teeth M26.37
- interocclusal distance of fully erupted teeth M26.37
- kalium E87.5
- large
  - colon K59.39
    - congenital Q43.8
  - infant P08.0
  - organ or site, congenital NEC —*see* Anomaly, by site
- long
  - organ or site, congenital NEC —*see* Anomaly, by site
- menstruation (with regular cycle) N92.0
  - with irregular cycle N92.1
- napping Z72.821
- natrium E87.0
- number of teeth K00.1
- nutrient (dietary) NEC R63.2
- potassium (K) E87.5
- salivation K11.7
- secretion —*see also* Hypersecretion
  - milk O92.6
  - sputum R09.3
  - sweat R61
- sexual drive F52.8
- short
  - organ or site, congenital NEC —*see* Anomaly, by site
  - umbilical cord in labor or delivery O69.3
- skin L98.7
  - and subcutaneous tissue L98.7
  - eyelid (acquired) —*see* Blepharochalasis
    - congenital Q10.3
- sodium (Na) E87.0
- spacing of fully erupted teeth M26.32
- sputum R09.3
- sweating R61
- thirst R63.1
  - due to deprivation of water T73.1
- transportation time Z59.82
- tuberosity of jaw M26.07
- vitamin
  - A (dietary) E67.0
    - administered as drug (prolonged intake) —*see* Table of Drugs and Chemicals, vitamins, adverse effect
    - overdose or wrong substance given or taken —*see* Table of Drugs and Chemicals, vitamins, poisoning
  - D (dietary) E67.3
    - administered as drug (prolonged intake) —*see* Table of Drugs and Chemicals, vitamins, adverse effect
    - overdose or wrong substance given or taken —*see* Table of Drugs and Chemicals, vitamins, poisoning
- weight
  - gain R63.5
  - loss R63.4

Excitability, abnormal, under minor stress (personality disorder) F60.3

Excitation
- anomalous atrioventricular I45.6
- psychogenic F30.8
- reactive (from emotional stress, psychological trauma) F30.8

Excitement
- hypomanic F30.8
- manic F30.9
- mental, reactive (from emotional stress, psychological trauma) F30.8
- state, reactive (from emotional stress, psychological trauma) F30.8

Excoriation (traumatic) —*see also* Abrasion
- neurotic L98.1
- skin picking disorder F42.4

Exfoliation
- due to erythematous conditions according to extent of body surface involved L49.0
- 10-19 percent of body surface L49.1
- 20-29 percent of body surface L49.2
- 30-39 percent of body surface L49.3
- 40-49 percent of body surface L49.4
- 50-59 percent of body surface L49.5

E

F

- **Failure, failed** *(Continued)*
  - renal N19
    - with
      - tubular necrosis (acute) N17.0
    - acute N17.9
      - with
        - cortical necrosis N17.1
        - medullary necrosis N17.2
        - tubular necrosis N17.0
      - specified NEC N17.8
    - chronic N18.9
      - hypertensive —*see* Hypertension, kidney
    - congenital P96.0
    - end stage (chronic) N18.6
      - due to hypertension I12.0
    - following
      - abortion —*see* Abortion by type complicated by specified condition NEC
      - crushing T79.5
      - ectopic or molar pregnancy O08.4
      - labor and delivery (acute) O90.49
    - hypertensive —*see* Hypertension, kidney
    - postprocedural N99.0
  - respiration, respiratory J96.90
    - with
      - hypercapnia J96.92
      - hypercarbia J96.02
      - hypoxia J96.91
    - acute J96.00
      - with
        - hypercapnia J96.02
        - hypercarbia J96.92
        - hypoxia J96.01
    - acute and (on) chronic J96.20
      - with
        - hypercapnia J96.22
        - hypercarbia J96.22
        - hypoxia J96.21
    - center G93.89
    - chronic J96.10
      - with
        - hypercapnia J96.12
        - hypercarbia J96.12
        - hypoxia J96.11
    - newborn P28.5
    - postprocedural (acute) J95.821
      - acute and chronic J95.822
  - rotation
    - cecum Q43.3
    - colon Q43.3
    - intestine Q43.3
    - kidney Q63.2
  - sedation (conscious) (moderate) during procedure T88.52
    - history of Z92.83
  - segmentation —*see also* Fusion
    - fingers —*see* Syndactylism, complex, fingers
    - vertebra Q76.49
      - with scoliosis Q76.3
  - seminiferous tubule, adult E29.1
  - senile (general) R54
  - sexual arousal (male) F52.21
    - female F52.22
  - testicular endocrine function E29.1
  - to thrive (child over 28 days old) R62.51
    - adult R62.7
    - newborn P92.6
  - transplant T86.92
    - bone T86.831
      - marrow T86.02
    - cornea T86.841-●
    - heart T86.22
      - with lung(s) T86.32
    - intestine T86.851
    - kidney T86.12
    - liver T86.42
    - lung(s) T86.811
      - with heart T86.32
    - pancreas T86.891
    - skin (allograft) (autograft) T86.821
    - specified organ or tissue NEC T86.891
    - stem cell (peripheral blood) (umbilical cord) T86.5
  - trial of labor (with subsequent cesarean delivery) O66.40
    - following previous cesarean delivery O66.41
  - tubal ligation N99.89
  - urinary —*see* Disease, kidney, chronic
  - vacuum extraction NOS (with subsequent cesarean delivery) O66.5

- **Failure, failed** *(Continued)*
  - vasectomy N99.89
  - ventouse NOS (with subsequent cesarean delivery) O66.5
  - ventricular —*see also* Failure, heart I50.9
    - left —*see also* Failure, heart, left I50.1
      - with rheumatic fever (conditions in I00)
        - active I01.8
          - with chorea I02.0
        - inactive or quiescent (with chorea) I09.81
      - rheumatic (chronic) (inactive) (with chorea) I09.81
        - active or acute I01.8
          - with chorea I02.0
    - right —*see* Failure, heart, right
  - vital centers, newborn P91.88
- **Fainting** (fit) R55
- **Fallen arches** —*see* Deformity, limb, flat foot
- **Falling, falls** (repeated) R29.6
  - any organ or part —*see* Prolapse
- **Fallopian**
  - insufflation Z31.41
  - tube —*see* condition
- **Fallot's**
  - pentalogy Q21.8
  - tetrad or tetralogy Q21.3
  - triad or trilogy Q22.3
- **False** —*see also* condition
  - croup J38.5
  - joint —*see* Nonunion, fracture
  - labor (pains) O47.9
    - at or after 37 completed weeks of gestation O47.1
    - before 37 completed weeks of gestation O47.0-●
  - passage, urethra (prostatic) N36.5
  - pregnancy F45.8
- **Family, familial** —*see also* condition
  - disruption Z63.8
    - involving divorce or separation Z63.5
  - Li-Fraumeni (syndrome) Z15.01
  - planning advice Z30.09
  - problem Z63.9
    - specified NEC Z63.8
  - retinoblastoma C69.2-●
- **Famine** (effects of) T73.0
  - edema —*see* Malnutrition, severe
- **Fanconi** (-de Toni)(-Debré) **syndrome** E72.09
  - with cystinosis E72.04
- ~~Fanconi's anemia (congenital pancytopenia) D61.09~~
- ▶ **Fanconi('s) anemia** D61.03
- ▶ **Fanconi hypoplastic anemia** D61.03
- ▶ **Fanconi panmyelopathy** D61.03
- **Farber's disease or syndrome** E75.29
- **Farcy** A24.0
- **Farmer's**
  - lung J67.0
  - skin L57.8
- **Farsightedness** —*see* Hypermetropia
- **Fascia** —*see* condition
- **Fasciculation** R25.3
- **Fasciitis** M72.9
  - diffuse (eosinophilic) M35.4
  - infective M72.8
    - necrotizing M72.6
  - necrotizing M72.6
  - nodular M72.4
  - perirenal (with ureteral obstruction) N13.5
    - with infection N13.6
  - plantar M72.2
  - specified NEC M72.8
  - traumatic (old) M72.8
    - current - code by site under Sprain
- **Fascioliasis** B66.3
- **Fasciolopsis, fasciolopsiasis** (intestinal) B66.5
- **Fascioscapulohumeral myopathy** G71.02
- **Fast pulse** R00.0
- **Fat**
  - embolism —*see* Embolism, fat
  - excessive —*see also* Obesity
    - in heart —*see* Degeneration, myocardial
  - in stool R19.5
  - localized (pad) E65
    - heart —*see* Degeneration, myocardial
    - knee M79.4
    - retropatellar M79.4

- **Fat** *(Continued)*
  - necrosis
    - breast N64.1
    - mesentery K65.4
    - omentum K65.4
  - pad E65
    - knee M79.4
- **Fatigue** R53.83
  - auditory deafness —*see* Deafness
  - chronic R53.82
  - combat F43.0
  - general R53.83
    - psychogenic F48.8
  - heat (transient) T67.6
  - muscle M62.89
  - myocardium —*see* Failure, heart
  - neoplasm-related R53.0
  - nervous, neurosis F48.8
  - operational F48.8
  - psychogenic (general) F48.8
  - senile R54
  - voice R49.8
- **Fatness** —*see* Obesity
- **Fatty** —*see also* condition
  - apron E65
  - degeneration —*see* Degeneration, fatty
  - heart (enlarged) —*see* Degeneration, myocardial
  - liver NEC K76.0
    - alcoholic K70.0
    - nonalcoholic K76.0
  - necrosis —*see* Degeneration, fatty
- **Fauces** —*see* condition
- **Fauchard's disease** (periodontitis) —*see* Periodontitis
- **Faucitis** J02.9
- **Favism** (anemia) D55.0
- **Favus** —*see* Dermatophytosis
- **Fazio-Londe disease or syndrome** G12.1
- **Fear complex or reaction** F40.9
- **Fear of** —*see* Phobia
- **Feared complaint unfounded** Z71.1
- **Febris, febrile** —*see also* Fever
  - flava —*see also* Fever, yellow A95.9
  - melitensis A23.0
  - pestis —*see* Plague
  - recurrens —*see* Fever, relapsing
  - rubra A38.9
- **Fecal**
  - incontinence R15.9
  - smearing R15.1
  - soiling R15.1
  - urgency R15.2
- **Fecalith** (impaction) K56.41
  - appendix K38.1
  - congenital P76.8
- **Fede's disease** K14.0
- **Feeble rapid pulse due to shock following injury** T79.4
- **Feeble-minded** F70
- **Feeding**
  - difficulties R63.30
  - problem (elderly) (infant) R63.39
    - newborn P92.9
      - specified NEC P92.8
    - nonorganic (adult) —*see* Disorder, eating
- **Feeling** (of)
  - foreign body in throat R09.A2
- **Feer's disease** —*see* Poisoning, mercury
- **Feet** —*see* condition
- **Feigned illness** Z76.5
- **Feil-Klippel syndrome** (brevicollis) Q76.1
- **Feinmesser's** (hidrotic) **ectodermal dysplasia** Q82.4
- **Felinophobia** F40.218
- **Felon** —*see also* Cellulitis, digit
  - with lymphangitis —*see* Lymphangitis, acute, digit
- **Felty's syndrome** M05.00
  - ankle M05.07-●
  - elbow M05.02-●
  - foot joint M05.07-●
  - hand joint M05.04-●
  - hip M05.05-●
  - knee M05.06-●
  - multiple site M05.09
  - shoulder M05.01-●
  - vertebra —*see* Spondylitis, ankylosing
  - wrist M05.03-●

F

▶ New ▶ Revised ~~deleted~~ Deleted ● Use Additional Character(s)

F

Findings, abnormal, inconclusive, without diagnosis —*(Continued)*
- hemoglobinuria R82.3
- human papillomavirus (HPV) DNA test positive
  - cervix
    - high risk R87.810
    - low risk R87.820
  - vagina
    - high risk R87.811
    - low risk R87.821
- in blood (of substance not normally found in blood) R78.9
  - addictive drug NEC R78.4
  - alcohol (excessive level) R78.0
  - cocaine R78.2
  - hallucinogen R78.3
  - heavy metals (abnormal level) R78.79
  - lead R78.71
  - lithium (abnormal level) R78.89
  - opiate drug R78.1
  - psychotropic drug R78.5
  - specified substance NEC R78.89
  - steroid agent R78.6
- indoleacetic acid, elevated R82.5
- ketonuria R82.4
- lactic acid dehydrogenase (LDH) R74.02
- liver function test (*see also* Elevated, liver function, test) R79.89
- mammogram NEC R92.8
  - calcification (calculus) R92.1
  - inconclusive result R92.2
  - microcalcification R92.0
- mediastinal shift R93.89
- melanin, urine R82.998
- myoglobinuria R82.1
- neonatal screening —*see* Abnormal, neonatal screening
- newborn screens, state mandated —*see* Abnormal, neonatal screening
- nonvisualization of gallbladder R93.2
- odor of urine NOS R82.90
- Papanicolaou cervix R87.619
  - non-atypical endometrial cells R87.618
- pneumoencephalogram R93.0
- poikilocytosis R71.8
- potassium (deficiency) E87.6
  - excess E87.5
- PPD R76.11
- radiologic (X-ray) R93.89
  - abdomen R93.5
  - biliary tract R93.2
  - breast R92.8
  - gastrointestinal tract R93.3
  - genitourinary organs R93.89
  - head R93.0
  - inconclusive due to excess body fat of patient R93.9
  - intrathoracic organs NEC R93.1
  - musculoskeletal
    - limbs R93.6
    - other than limb R93.7
  - placenta R93.89
  - retroperitoneum R93.5
  - skin R93.89
  - skull R93.0
  - subcutaneous tissue R93.89
  - testis R93.81-●
- red blood cell (count) (morphology) (sickling) (volume) R71.8
- scan NEC R94.8
  - bladder R94.8
  - bone R94.8
  - kidney R94.4
  - liver R93.2
  - lung R94.2
  - pancreas R94.8
  - placental R94.8
  - spleen R94.8
  - thyroid R94.6
- sedimentation rate, elevated R70.0
- SGOT R74.01
- SGPT R74.01
- sodium (deficiency) E87.1
  - excess E87.0
- specified body fluid NEC R88.8
- stress test R94.39
- thyroid (function) (metabolic rate) (scan) (uptake) R94.6
- transaminase (level) R74.01

Findings, abnormal, inconclusive, without diagnosis —*(Continued)*
- triglycerides E78.9
  - high E78.1
    - with high cholesterol E78.2
- tuberculin skin test (without active tuberculosis) R76.11
- urine R82.90
  - acetone R82.4
  - bacteria R82.71
  - bile R82.2
  - casts or cells R82.998
  - chyle R82.0
  - culture positive R82.79
  - glucose R81
  - hemoglobin R82.3
  - ketone R82.4
  - sugar R81
- vanillylmandelic acid (VMA), elevated R82.5
- vectorcardiogram (VCG) R94.39
- ventriculogram R93.0
- white blood cell (count) (differential) (morphology) D72.9
- xerography R92.8

Finger —*see* condition

Fire, Saint Anthony's —*see* Erysipelas

Fire-setting
- pathological (compulsive) F63.1

Fish hook stomach K31.89

Fishmeal-worker's lung J67.8

Fissure, fissured
- anus, anal K60.2
  - acute K60.0
  - chronic K60.1
  - congenital Q43.8
- ear, lobule, congenital Q17.8
- epiglottis (congenital) Q31.8
- larynx J38.7
  - congenital Q31.8
- lip K13.0
  - congenital —*see* Cleft, lip
- nipple N64.0
  - associated with
    - lactation O92.13
    - pregnancy O92.11-●
    - puerperium O92.12
- nose Q30.2
- palate (congenital) —*see* Cleft, palate
- skin R23.4
- spine (congenital) —*see also* Spina bifida
  - with hydrocephalus —*see* Spina bifida, by site, with hydrocephalus
- tongue (acquired) K14.5
  - congenital Q38.3

Fistula (cutaneous) L98.8
- abdomen (wall) K63.2
  - bladder N32.2
  - intestine NEC K63.2
  - ureter N28.89
  - uterus N82.5
- abdominorectal K63.2
- abdominosigmoidal K63.2
- abdominothoracic J86.0
- abdominouterine N82.5
  - congenital Q51.7
- abdominovesical N32.2
- accessory sinuses —*see* Sinusitis
- actinomycotic —*see* Actinomycosis
- alveolar antrum —*see* Sinusitis, maxillary
- alveolar process K04.6
- ➡anorectal (infectional) K60.50
  - ▶complex K60.529
    - ▶chronic K60.522
    - ▶initial K60.521
    - ▶new K60.521
    - ▶occurring following complete healing K60.523
    - ▶persistent K60.522
    - ▶recurrent K60.523
  - ▶extrasphincteric K60.52-●
  - ▶high intersphincteric K60.52-●
  - ▶low intersphincteric K60.51-●
  - ▶simple K60.519
    - ▶chronic K60.512
    - ▶initial K60.511
    - ▶new K60.511
    - ▶occurring following complete healing K60.513
    - ▶persistent K60.512
    - ▶recurrent K60.513
  - ▶superficial K60.51-●

Fistula *(Continued)*
- anorectal *(Continued)*
  - ▶suprasphincteric K60.52-●
  - ▶transsphincteric K60.52-●
- antrobuccal —*see* Sinusitis, maxillary
- antrum —*see* Sinusitis, maxillary
- ➡anus, anal (recurrent) (infectional) K60.30
  - ▶complex K60.329
    - ▶chronic K60.322
    - ▶initial K60.321
    - ▶new K60.321
    - ▶occurring following complete healing K60.323
    - ▶persistent K60.322
    - ▶recurrent K60.323
  - ▶extrasphincteric K60.32-●
  - ▶high intersphincteric K60.32-●
  - ▶low intersphincteric K60.31-●
  - ▶simple K60.319
    - ▶chronic K60.312
    - ▶initial K60.311
    - ▶new K60.311
    - ▶occurring following complete healing K60.313
    - ▶persistent K60.312
    - ▶recurrent K60.313
  - ▶superficial K60.31-●
  - ▶suprasphincteric K60.32-●
  - ▶transsphincteric K60.32-●
  - congenital Q43.6
    - with absence, atresia and stenosis Q42.2
  - tuberculous A18.32
- aorta-duodenal I77.2
- appendix, appendicular K38.3
- arteriovenous (acquired) (nonruptured) I77.0
  - brain I67.1
    - congenital Q28.2
      - ruptured —*see* Fistula, arteriovenous, brain, ruptured
    - ruptured I60.8
      - intracerebral I61.8
      - intraparenchymal I61.8
      - intraventricular I61.5
      - subarachnoid I60.8
  - cerebral —*see* Fistula, arteriovenous, brain
  - congenital (peripheral) —*see also* Malformation, arteriovenous
    - brain Q28.2
      - ruptured —*see* Fistula, arteriovenous, brain, ruptured
    - coronary Q24.5
    - pulmonary Q25.72
  - coronary I25.41
    - congenital Q24.5
  - pulmonary I28.0
    - congenital Q25.72
  - surgically created (for dialysis) Z99.2
    - complication —*see* Complication, arteriovenous, fistula, surgically created
  - traumatic —*see* Injury, blood vessel
- artery I77.2
- aural (mastoid) —*see* Mastoiditis, chronic
- auricle —*see also* Disorder, pinna, specified type NEC
  - congenital Q18.1
- Bartholin's gland N82.8
- bile duct (common) (hepatic) K83.3
  - with calculus, stones —*see also* Calculus, bile duct K83.3
- biliary (tract) —*see* Fistula, bile duct
- bladder (sphincter) NEC —*see also* Fistula, vesico- N32.2
  - into seminal vesicle N32.2
- bone —*see also* Disorder, bone, specified type NEC
  - with osteomyelitis, chronic —*see* Osteomyelitis, chronic, with draining sinus
- brain G93.89
  - arteriovenous (acquired) (*see* Fistula, arteriovenous, brain) I67.1
    - congenital Q28.2
- branchial (cleft) Q18.0
- branchiogenous Q18.0
- breast N61.0
  - puerperal, postpartum or gestational, due to mastitis (purulent) —*see* Mastitis, obstetric, purulent
- bronchial J86.0

F

F

F

- **Fracture, pathological** *(Continued)*
  - due to *(Continued)*
    - specified disease NEC M84.60
      - ankle M84.67-●
      - carpus M84.64-●
      - clavicle M84.61-●
      - femur M84.65-●
      - fibula M84.66-●
      - finger M84.64-●
      - hip M84.65-●
      - humerus M84.62-●
      - ilium M84.650
      - ischium M84.650
      - metacarpus M84.64-●
      - metatarsus M84.67-●
      - neck M84.68
      - radius M84.63-●
      - rib M84.68
      - scapula M84.61-●
      - skull M84.68
      - tarsus M84.67-●
      - tibia M84.66-●
      - toe M84.67-●
      - ulna M84.63-●
      - vertebra M84.68
  - femur M84.45-●
  - fibula M84.46-●
  - finger M84.44-●
  - hip M84.459
  - humerus M84.42-●
  - ilium M84.454
  - ischium M84.454
  - joint prosthesis —*see* Complications, joint prosthesis, mechanical, breakdown, by site
    - periprosthetic —*see* Fracture, pathological, periprosthetic
  - metacarpus M84.44-●
  - metatarsus M84.47-●
  - neck M84.48
  - pelvis M84.454
  - periprosthetic M97.9
    - ankle M97.2-●
    - elbow M97.4-●
    - finger M97.8
    - hip M97.0-●
    - knee M97.1-●
    - other specified joint M97.8
    - shoulder M97.3-●
    - spinal joint M97.8
    - toe joint M97.8
    - wrist joint M97.8
  - radius M84.43-●
  - restorative material (dental) K08.539
    - with loss of material K08.531
    - without loss of material K08.530
  - rib M84.48
  - scapula M84.41-●
  - skull M84.48
  - tarsus M84.47-●
  - tibia M84.46-●
  - toe M84.47-●
  - ulna M84.43-●
  - vertebra M84.48
- **Fracture, traumatic** (abduction) (adduction) (separation) —*see also* Fracture, pathological T14.8
  - associated with chest compression and cardiopulmonary resuscitation M96.A9
  - acetabulum S32.40-●
    - column
      - anterior (displaced) (iliopubic) S32.43-●
        - nondisplaced S32.436
      - posterior (displaced) (ilioischial) S32.443
        - nondisplaced S32.44-●
    - dome (displaced) S32.48-●
      - nondisplaced S32.48
    - specified NEC S32.49-●
    - transverse (displaced) S32.45-●
      - with associated posterior wall fracture (displaced) S32.46-●
        - nondisplaced S32.46-●
      - nondisplaced S32.45-●
    - wall
      - anterior (displaced) S32.41-●
        - nondisplaced S32.41-●
      - medial (displaced) S32.47-●
        - nondisplaced S32.47-●
      - posterior (displaced) S32.42-●
        - with associated transverse fracture (displaced) S32.46-●
          - nondisplaced S32.46-●
        - nondisplaced S32.42-●

- **Fracture, traumatic** *(Continued)*
  - acromion —*see* Fracture, scapula, acromial process
  - ankle S82.899
    - bimalleolar (displaced) S82.84-●
      - nondisplaced S82.84-●
    - lateral malleolus only (displaced) S82.6-●
      - nondisplaced S82.6-●
    - medial malleolus (displaced) S82.5-●
      - associated with Maisonneuve's fracture —*see* Fracture, Maisonneuve's
      - nondisplaced S82.5-●
    - talus —*see* Fracture, tarsal, talus
    - trimalleolar (displaced) S82.85-●
      - nondisplaced S82.85-●
  - arm (upper) —*see also* Fracture, humerus, shaft
    - humerus —*see* Fracture, humerus
    - radius —*see* Fracture, radius
    - ulna —*see* Fracture, ulna
  - astragalus —*see* Fracture, tarsal, talus
  - atlas —*see* Fracture, neck, cervical vertebra, first
  - axis —*see* Fracture, neck, cervical vertebra, second
  - back —*see* Fracture, vertebra
  - Barton's —*see* Barton's fracture
  - base of skull —*see* Fracture, skull, base
  - basicervical (basal) (femoral) S72.0
  - Bennett's —*see* Bennett's fracture
  - bimalleolar —*see* Fracture, ankle, bimalleolar
  - blow-out S02.3-●
  - bone NEC T14.8
    - birth injury P13.9
    - following insertion of orthopedic implant, joint prosthesis or bone plate —*see* Fracture, following insertion of orthopedic implant, joint prosthesis or bone plate
    - in (due to) neoplastic disease NEC —*see* Fracture, pathological, due to, neoplastic disease
    - pathological (cause unknown) —*see* Fracture, pathological
  - breast bone —*see* Fracture, sternum
  - buckle —*see* Fracture, by site, torus
  - bucket handle (semilunar cartilage) —*see* Tear, meniscus
  - burst —*see* Fracture, traumatic, by site
  - calcaneus —*see* Fracture, tarsal, calcaneus
  - carpal bone(s) S62.10-●
    - capitate (displaced) S62.13-●
      - nondisplaced S62.13-●
    - cuneiform —*see* Fracture, carpal bone, triquetrum
    - hamate (body) (displaced) S62.143
      - hook process (displaced) S62.15-●
        - nondisplaced S62.15-●
      - nondisplaced S62.14-●
    - larger multangular —*see* Fracture, carpal bones, trapezium
    - lunate (displaced) S62.12-●
      - nondisplaced S62.12-●
    - navicular S62.00-●
      - distal pole (displaced) S62.01-●
        - nondisplaced S62.01-●
      - middle third (displaced) S62.02-●
        - nondisplaced S62.02-●
      - proximal third (displaced) S62.03-●
        - nondisplaced S62.03-●
      - volar tuberosity —*see* Fracture, carpal bones, navicular, distal pole
    - os magnum —*see* Fracture, carpal bones, capitate
    - pisiform (displaced) S62.16-●
      - nondisplaced S62.16-●
    - semilunar —*see* Fracture, carpal bones, lunate
    - smaller multangular —*see* Fracture, carpal bones, trapezoid
    - trapezium (displaced) S62.17-●
      - nondisplaced S62.17-●
    - trapezoid (displaced) S62.18-●
      - nondisplaced S62.18-●
    - triquetrum (displaced) S62.11-●
      - nondisplaced S62.11-●
    - unciform —*see* Fracture, carpal bones, hamate
  - cervical —*see* Fracture, vertebra, cervical
  - clavicle S42.00-●
    - acromial end (displaced) S42.03-●
      - nondisplaced S42.03-●
    - birth injury P13.4
    - lateral end —*see* Fracture, clavicle, acromial end

- **Fracture, traumatic** *(Continued)*
  - clavicle *(Continued)*
    - shaft (displaced) S42.02-●
      - nondisplaced S42.02-●
    - sternal end (anterior) (displaced) S42.01-●
      - nondisplaced S42.01-●
      - posterior S42.01-●
  - coccyx S32.2
  - collapsed —*see* Collapse, vertebra
  - collar bone —*see* Fracture, clavicle
  - Colles' —*see* Colles' fracture
  - coronoid process —*see* Fracture, ulna, upper end, coronoid process
  - corpus cavernosum penis S39.840
  - costochondral cartilage S23.41
  - costochondral, costosternal junction —*see* Fracture, rib
  - cranium —*see* Fracture, skull
  - cricoid cartilage S12.8
  - cuboid (ankle) —*see* Fracture, tarsal, cuboid
  - cuneiform
    - foot —*see* Fracture, tarsal, cuneiform
    - wrist —*see* Fracture, carpal, triquetrum
  - delayed union —*see* Delay, union, fracture
  - dental restorative material K08.539
    - with loss of material K08.531
    - without loss of material K08.530
  - due to
    - birth injury —*see* Birth, injury, fracture
    - osteoporosis —*see* Osteoporosis, with fracture
  - Dupuytren's —*see* Fracture, ankle, lateral malleolus
  - elbow S42.40-●
  - ethmoid (bone) (sinus) —*see* Fracture, skull, base
  - face bone S02.92
  - fatigue —*see also* Fracture, stress
    - vertebra M48.40
      - cervical region M48.42
      - cervicothoracic region M48.43
      - lumbar region M48.46
      - lumbosacral region M48.47
      - occipito-atlanto-axial region M48.41
      - sacrococcygeal region M48.48
      - thoracic region M48.44
      - thoracolumbar region M48.45
  - femur, femoral S72.9-●
    - basicervical (basal) S72.0
    - birth injury P13.2
    - capital epiphyseal S79.01-●
    - condyles, epicondyles —*see* Fracture, femur, lower end
    - distal end —*see* Fracture, femur, lower end
    - epiphysis
      - head —*see* Fracture, femur, upper end, epiphysis
      - lower —*see* Fracture, femur, lower end, epiphysis
      - upper —*see* Fracture, femur, upper end, epiphysis
    - following insertion of implant, prosthesis or plate M96.66-●
    - head —*see* Fracture, femur, upper end, head
    - intertrochanteric —*see* Fracture, femur, trochanteric
    - intratrochanteric —*see* Fracture, femur, trochanteric
    - lower end S72.40-●
      - condyle (displaced) S72.41-●
        - lateral (displaced) S72.42-●
          - nondisplaced S72.42-●
        - medial (displaced) S72.43-●
          - nondisplaced S72.43-●
        - nondisplaced S72.41-●
      - epiphysis (displaced) S72.44-●
        - nondisplaced S72.44-●
      - physeal S79.10-●
        - Salter-Harris
          - Type I S79.11-●
          - Type II S79.12-●
          - Type III S79.13-●
          - Type IV S79.14-●
        - specified NEC S79.19-●
      - specified NEC S72.49-●
      - supracondylar (displaced) S72.45-●
        - with intracondylar extension (displaced) S72.46-●
          - nondisplaced S72.46-●
        - nondisplaced S72.45-●
      - torus S72.47-●
    - neck —*see* Fracture, femur, upper end, neck
    - pertrochanteric —*see* Fracture, femur, trochanteric

F

F

F

▶ New ➡ Revised ~~deleted~~ Deleted • Use Additional Character(s)

F

G

G

▶ New ➠ Revised ~~deleted~~ Deleted ● Use Additional Character(s)

Gerhardt's
- disease (erythromelalgia) I73.81
- syndrome (vocal cord paralysis) J38.ØØ
  - bilateral J38.Ø2
  - unilateral J38.Ø1

German measles *—see also* Rubella
- exposure to Z2Ø.4

Germinoblastoma (diffuse) C85.9-●
- follicular C82.9-●

Germinoma *—see* Neoplasm, malignant, by site

Gerontoxon *—see* Degeneration, cornea, senile

Gerstmann-Sträussler-Scheinker syndrome (GSS) A81.82

Gerstmann's syndrome R48.8
- developmental F81.2

Gestation (period) *—see also* Pregnancy
- ectopic *—see* Pregnancy, by site
- multiple O3Ø.9-●
  - greater than quadruplets *—see* Pregnancy, multiple (gestation), specified NEC
  - specified NEC *—see* Pregnancy, multiple (gestation), specified NEC

Gestational
- mammary abscess O91.11-●
- purulent mastitis O91.11-●
- subareolar abscess O91.11-●

Ghon tubercle, primary infection A15.7

Ghost
- teeth KØØ.4
- vessels (cornea) H16.41-●

Ghoul hand A66.3

Gianotti-Crosti disease L44.4

Giant
- cell
  - epulis KØ6.8
  - peripheral granuloma KØ6.8
- esophagus, congenital Q39.5
- kidney, congenital Q63.3
- urticaria T78.3
  - hereditary D84.1

Giardiasis AØ7.1

Gibert's disease or pityriasis L42

Giddiness R42
- hysterical F44.89
- psychogenic F45.8

Gierke's disease (glycogenosis I) E74.Ø1

Gigantism (cerebral) (hypophyseal) (pituitary) E22.Ø
- constitutional E34.4

Gilbert's disease or syndrome E8Ø.4

Gilchrist's disease B4Ø.9

Gilford-Hutchinson disease E34.8

Gilles de la Tourette's disease or syndrome (motor-verbal tic) F95.2

Gingivitis KØ5.1Ø
- acute (catarrhal) KØ5.ØØ
  - necrotizing A69.1
  - nonplaque induced KØ5.Ø1
  - plaque induced KØ5.ØØ
- chronic (desquamative) (hyperplastic) (simple marginal) (pregnancy associated) (ulcerative) KØ5.1Ø
  - nonplaque induced KØ5.11
  - plaque induced KØ5.1Ø
- expulsiva *—see* Periodontitis
- necrotizing ulcerative (acute) A69.1
- pellagrous E52
  - acute necrotizing A69.1
- Vincent's A69.1

Gingivoglossitis K14.Ø

Gingivopericementitis *—see* Periodontitis

Gingivosis *—see* Gingivitis, chronic

Gingivostomatitis KØ5.1Ø
- herpesviral BØØ.2
- necrotizing ulcerative (acute) A69.1

Gland, glandular *—see* condition

Glanders A24.Ø

Glanzmann (-Naegeli) disease or thrombasthenia D69.1

Glasgow coma scale
- total score
  - 3-8 R4Ø.243
  - 9-12 R4Ø.242
  - 13-15 R4Ø.241

Glass-blower's disease (cataract) *—see* Cataract, specified NEC

Glaucoma H4Ø.9
- with
  - increased episcleral venous pressure H4Ø.81-●
  - pseudoexfoliation of lens *—see* Glaucoma, open angle, primary, capsular

Glaucoma *(Continued)*
- absolute H44.51-●
- angle-closure (primary) H4Ø.2Ø-●
  - acute (attack) (crisis) H4Ø.21-●
  - chronic H4Ø.22-●
  - intermittent H4Ø.23-●
  - residual stage H4Ø.24-●
- borderline H4Ø.ØØ-●
- capsular (with pseudoexfoliation of lens) *—see* Glaucoma, open angle, primary, capsular
- childhood Q15.Ø
- closed angle *—see* Glaucoma, angle-closure
- congenital Q15.Ø
- corticosteroid-induced *—see* Glaucoma, secondary, drugs
- hypersecretion H4Ø.82-●
- in (due to)
  - amyloidosis E85.4 *[H42]*
  - aniridia Q13.1 *[H42]*
  - concussion of globe *—see* Glaucoma, secondary, trauma
  - dislocation of lens *—see* Glaucoma, secondary
  - disorder of lens NEC *—see* Glaucoma, secondary
  - drugs *—see* Glaucoma, secondary, drugs
  - endocrine disease NOS E34.9 *[H42]*
  - eye
    - inflammation *—see* Glaucoma, secondary, inflammation
    - trauma *—see* Glaucoma, secondary, trauma
  - hypermature cataract *—see* Glaucoma, secondary
  - iridocyclitis *—see* Glaucoma, secondary, inflammation
  - lens disorder *—see* Glaucoma, secondary,
  - Lowe's syndrome E72.Ø3 *[H42]*
  - metabolic disease NOS E88.9 *[H42]*
  - ocular disorders NEC *—see* Glaucoma, secondary
  - onchocerciasis B73.Ø2
  - pupillary block *—see* Glaucoma, secondary
  - retinal vein occlusion *—see* Glaucoma, secondary
  - ~~Rieger's anomaly Q13.81 [H42]~~
  - ▶ Rieger anomaly Q13.81 *[H42]*
  - rubeosis of iris *—see* Glaucoma, secondary
  - tumor of globe *—see* Glaucoma, secondary
- infantile Q15.Ø
- low tension *—see* Glaucoma, open angle, primary, low-tension
- malignant H4Ø.83-●
- narrow angle *—see* Glaucoma, angle-closure
- newborn Q15.Ø
- noncongestive (chronic) *—see* Glaucoma, open angle
- nonobstructive *—see* Glaucoma, open angle
- obstructive *—see also* Glaucoma, angle-closure
  - due to lens changes *—see* Glaucoma, secondary
- open angle H4Ø.1Ø-●
  - primary H4Ø.11-●
    - capsular (with pseudoexfoliation of lens) H4Ø.14-●
    - low-tension H4Ø.12-●
    - pigmentary H4Ø.13-●
    - residual stage H4Ø.15-●
- phacolytic *—see* Glaucoma, secondary
- pigmentary *—see* Glaucoma, open angle, primary, pigmentary
- postinfectious *—see* Glaucoma, secondary, inflammation
- secondary (to) H4Ø.5-●
  - drugs H4Ø.6-●
  - inflammation H4Ø.4-●
  - trauma H4Ø.3-●
- simple (chronic) H4Ø.11-●
- simplex H4Ø.11-●
- specified type NEC H4Ø.89
- suspect H4Ø.ØØ-●
- syphilitic A52.71
- traumatic *—see also* Glaucoma, secondary, trauma
  - newborn (birth injury) P15.3
- tuberculous A18.59

Glaucomatous flecks (subcapsular) *—see* Cataract, complicated

Glazed tongue K14.4

Gleet (gonococcal) A54.Ø1

Glénard's disease K63.4

Glioblastoma (multiforme)
- with sarcomatous component
  - specified site *—see* Neoplasm, malignant, by site
  - unspecified site C71.9
- giant cell
  - specified site *—see* Neoplasm, malignant, by site
  - unspecified site C71.9
- specified site *—see* Neoplasm, malignant, by site
- unspecified site C71.9

Glioma (malignant)
- astrocytic
  - specified site *—see* Neoplasm, malignant, by site
  - unspecified site C71.9
- mixed
  - specified site *—see* Neoplasm, malignant, by site
  - unspecified site C71.9
- nose Q3Ø.8
- specified site NEC *—see* Neoplasm, malignant, by site
- subependymal D43.2
  - specified site *—see* Neoplasm, uncertain behavior, by site
  - unspecified site D43.2
- unspecified site C71.9

Gliomatosis cerebri C71.Ø

Glioneuroma *—see* Neoplasm, uncertain behavior, by site

Gliosarcoma
- specified site *—see* Neoplasm, malignant, by site
- unspecified site C71.9

Gliosis (cerebral) G93.89
- spinal G95.89

Glisson's disease *—see* Rickets

Globinuria R82.3

Globus (hystericus) F45.8

Glomangioma D18.ØØ
- intra-abdominal D18.Ø3
- intracranial D18.Ø2
- skin D18.Ø1
- specified site NEC D18.Ø9

Glomangiomyoma D18.ØØ
- intra-abdominal D18.Ø3
- intracranial D18.Ø2
- skin D18.Ø1
- specified site NEC D18.Ø9

Glomangiosarcoma *—see* Neoplasm, connective tissue, malignant

Glomerular
- disease in syphilis A52.75
- nephritis *—see* Glomerulonephritis

Glomerulitis *—see* Glomerulonephritis

Glomerulonephritis *—see also* Nephritis NØ5.9
- with
  - C3
    - glomerulonephritis NØ5.A
    - glomerulopathy NØ5.A
      - with dense deposit disease NØ5.6
  - edema *—see* Nephrosis
  - minimal change NØ5.Ø
  - minor glomerular abnormality NØ5.Ø
- acute NØØ.9
- chronic NØ3.9
- crescentic (diffuse) NEC *—see also* NØØ-NØ7 with fourth character .7 NØ5.7
- dense deposit *—see also* NØØ-NØ7 with fourth character .6 NØ5.6
- diffuse
  - crescentic *—see also* NØØ-NØ7 with fourth character .7 NØ5.7
  - endocapillary proliferative *—see also* NØØNØ7 with fourth character .4 NØ5.4
  - membranous *—see also* NØØ-NØ7 with fourth character .2 NØ5.2
  - mesangial proliferative *—see also* NØØ-NØ7 with fourth character .3 NØ5.3
  - mesangiocapillary *—see also* NØØ-NØ7 with fourth character .5 NØ5.5
  - sclerosing N18.9
- endocapillary proliferative (diffuse) NEC *—see also* NØØ-NØ7 with fourth character .4 NØ5.4
- extracapillary NEC *—see also* NØØ-NØ7 with fourth character .7 NØ5.7
- focal (and segmental) *—see also* NØØ-NØ7 with fourth character .1 NØ5.1
- hypocomplementemic *—see* Glomerulonephritis, membranoproliferative
- IgA *—see* Nephropathy, IgA

▶ New ➡ Revised ~~deleted~~ Deleted ● Use Additional Character(s)

H

H

- Hallucinosis *(Continued)*
  - drug-induced *(Continued)*
    - in *(Continued)*
      - dependence *(Continued)*
        - sedative, anxiolytic or hypnotic F13.251
        - stimulant NEC F15.251
    - inhalant F18.951
    - opioid F11.951
    - sedative, anxiolytic or hypnotic F13.951
    - stimulant NEC F15.951
  - organic FØ6.Ø
- Hallux
  - deformity (acquired) NEC M2Ø.5X-●
  - limitus M2Ø.5X-●
  - malleus (acquired) NEC M2Ø.3-●
  - rigidus (acquired) M2Ø.2-●
    - congenital Q74.2
    - sequelae (late effect) of rickets E64.3
  - valgus (acquired) M2Ø.1-●
    - congenital Q66.6
  - varus (acquired) M2Ø.3-●
    - congenital Q66.3-●
- Halo, visual H53.19
- Hamartoma, hamartoblastoma Q85.9
  - epithelial (gingival), odontogenic, central or peripheral —*see* Cyst, calcifying odontogenic
- Hamartosis Q85.9
- Hamman-Rich syndrome J84.114
- Hammer toe (acquired) NEC —*see also* Deformity, toe, hammer toe
  - congenital Q66.89
  - sequelae (late effect) of rickets E64.3
- Hand —*see* condition
- Hand-foot syndrome L27.1
- Handicap, handicapped
  - educational Z55.9
    - specified NEC Z55.8
- Hand-Schüller-Christian disease or syndrome C96.5
- Hanging (asphyxia) (strangulation) (suffocation) —*see* Asphyxia, traumatic, due to mechanical threat
- Hangnail —*see also* Cellulitis, digit
  - with lymphangitis —*see* Lymphangitis, acute, digit
- Hangover (alcohol) F1Ø.129
- Hanhart's syndrome Q87.Ø
- Hanot-Chauffard (-Troisier) syndrome E83.19
- Hanot's cirrhosis or disease K74.3
- Hansen's disease —*see* Leprosy
- Hantaan virus disease (Korean hemorrhagic fever) A98.5
- Hantavirus disease (with renal manifestations) (Dobrava) (Puumala) (Seoul) A98.5
  - with pulmonary manifestations (Andes) (Bayou) (Bermejo) (Black Creek Canal) (Choclo) (Juquitiba) (Laguna negra) (Lechiguanas) (New York) (Oran) (Sin nombre) B33.4
- Happy puppet syndrome Q93.59
- Harada's disease or syndrome H3Ø.81-●
- Hardening
  - artery —*see* Arteriosclerosis
  - brain G93.89
- Harelip (complete) (incomplete) —*see* Cleft, lip
- Harlequin (newborn) Q8Ø.4
- Harley's disease D59.6
- Harmful use (of)
  - alcohol F1Ø.1Ø
  - anxiolytics —*see* Abuse, drug, sedative
  - cannabinoids —*see* Abuse, drug, cannabis
  - cocaine —*see* Abuse, drug, cocaine
  - drug —*see* Abuse, drug
  - hallucinogens —*see* Abuse, drug, hallucinogen
  - hypnotics —*see* Abuse, drug, sedative -
    - opioids —*see* Abuse, drug, opioid
  - PCP (phencyclidine) —*see* Abuse, drug, hallucinogen
  - sedatives —*see* Abuse, drug, sedative
  - stimulants NEC —*see* Abuse, drug, stimulant
- Harris' lines —*see* Arrest, epiphyseal
- Hardship, material, due to limited financial resources, specified NEC Z59.87
- Hartnup's disease E72.Ø2
- Harvester's lung J67.Ø
- Harvesting ovum for in vitro fertilization Z31.83
- Hashimoto's disease or thyroiditis EØ6.3
- Hashitoxicosis (transient) EØ6.3
- Hassal-Henle bodies or warts (cornea) H18.49
- Haut mal —*see* Epilepsy, generalized, specified NEC
- Haverhill fever A25.1
- Hay fever —*see also* Fever, hay J3Ø.1
- Hayem-Widal syndrome D59.8
- Haygarth's nodes M15.8
- Haymaker's lung J67.Ø
- Hb (abnormal)
  - Bart's disease D56.Ø
  - disease —*see* Disease, hemoglobin
  - trait —*see* Trait
- Head —*see* condition
- Headache R51.9
  - with
    - orthostatic component NEC R51.Ø
    - positional component NEC R51.Ø
  - allergic NEC G44.89
  - associated with sexual activity G44.82
  - cervicogenic G44.86
  - chronic daily R51.9
  - cluster G44.ØØ9
    - chronic G44.Ø29
      - intractable G44.Ø21
      - not intractable G44.Ø29
    - episodic G44.Ø19
      - intractable G44.Ø11
      - not intractable G44.Ø19
    - intractable G44.ØØ1
    - not intractable G44.ØØ9
  - cough (primary) G44.83
  - daily chronic R51.9
  - drug-induced NEC G44.4Ø
    - intractable G44.41
    - not intractable G44.4Ø
  - exertional (primary) G44.84
  - histamine G44.ØØ9
    - intractable G44.ØØ1
    - not intractable G44.ØØ9
  - hypnic G44.81
  - lumbar puncture G97.1
  - medication overuse G44.4Ø
    - intractable G44.41
    - not intractable G44.4Ø
  - menstrual —*see* Migraine, menstrual
  - migraine (type) —*see also* Migraine G43.9Ø9
  - nasal septum R51.9
  - neuralgiform, short lasting unilateral, with conjunctival injection and tearing (SUNCT) G44.Ø59
    - intractable G44.Ø51
    - not intractable G44.Ø59
  - new daily persistent (NDPH) G44.52
  - orgasmic G44.82
  - periodic syndromes in adults and children G43.CØ
    - with refractory migraine G43.C1
    - intractable G43.C1
    - not intractable G43.CØ
    - without refractory migraine G43.CØ
  - postspinal puncture G97.1
  - post-traumatic G44.3Ø9
    - acute G44.319
      - intractable G44.311
      - not intractable G44.319
    - chronic G44.329
      - intractable G44.321
      - not intractable G44.329
    - intractable G44.3Ø1
    - not intractable G44.3Ø9
  - pre-menstrual —*see* Migraine, menstrual
  - preorgasmic G44.82
  - primary
    - cough G44.83
    - exertional G44.84
    - stabbing G44.85
    - thunderclap G44.53
  - rebound G44.4Ø
    - intractable G44.41
    - not intractable G44.4Ø
  - short lasting unilateral neuralgiform, with conjunctival injection and tearing (SUNCT) G44.Ø59
    - intractable G44.Ø51
    - not intractable G44.Ø59
  - specified syndrome NEC G44.89
  - spinal and epidural anesthesia - induced T88.59
    - in labor and delivery O74.5
    - in pregnancy O29.4-●
    - postpartum, puerperal O89.4
  - spinal fluid loss (from puncture) G97.1
  - stabbing (primary) G44.85
- Headache *(Continued)*
  - tension (-type) G44.2Ø9
    - chronic G44.229
      - intractable G44.221
      - not intractable G44.229
    - episodic G44.219
      - intractable G44.211
      - not intractable G44.219
    - intractable G44.2Ø1
    - not intractable G44.2Ø9
  - thunderclap (primary) G44.53
  - vascular NEC G44.1
- Healthy
  - infant
    - accompanying sick mother Z76.3
    - receiving care Z76.2
  - person accompanying sick person Z76.3
- Hearing examination ZØ1.1Ø
  - with abnormal findings NEC ZØ1.118
  - infant or child (over 28 days old) ZØØ.129
    - with abnormal findings ZØØ.121
  - following failed hearing screening ZØ1.11Ø
  - for hearing conservation and treatment ZØ1.12
- Heart —*see* condition
  - ▶carcinoid - see Syndrome, carcinoid, heart
- Heart beat
  - abnormality RØØ.9
    - specified NEC RØØ.8
  - awareness RØØ.2
  - rapid RØØ.Ø
  - slow RØØ.1
- Heartburn R12
  - psychogenic F45.8
- Heartland virus disease A93.8
- Heat (effects) T67.9
  - apoplexy T67.Ø1
  - burn —*see also* Burn L55.9
  - collapse T67.1
  - cramps T67.2
  - dermatitis or eczema L59.Ø
  - edema T67.7
  - erythema - code by site under Burn, first degree
  - excessive T67.9
    - specified effect NEC T67.8
  - exhaustion T67.5
    - anhydrotic T67.3
    - due to
      - salt (and water) depletion T67.4
      - water depletion T67.3
        - with salt depletion T67.4
  - fatigue (transient) T67.6
  - fever T67.Ø1
  - hyperpyrexia T67.Ø1
  - prickly L74.Ø
  - prostration —*see* Heat, exhaustion
  - pyrexia T67.Ø1
  - rash L74.Ø
  - specified effect NEC T67.8
  - stroke T67.Ø1
    - exertional T67.Ø2
    - specified NEC T67.Ø9
  - sunburn —*see* Sunburn
  - syncope T67.1
- Heavy-for-dates NEC (infant) (4ØØØg to 4499g) PØ8.1
  - exceptionally (45ØØg or more) PØ8.Ø
- Hebephrenia, hebephrenic (schizophrenia) F2Ø.1
- Heberden's disease or nodes (with arthropathy) M15.1
- Hebra's
  - pityriasis L26
  - prurigo L28.2
- Heel —*see* condition
- Heerfordt's disease D86.89
- Hegglin's anomaly or syndrome D72.Ø
- Heilmeyer-Schoner disease D45
- Heine-Medin disease A8Ø.9
- Heinz body anemia, congenital D58.2
- Heliophobia F4Ø.228
- Heller's disease or syndrome F84.3
- HELLP syndrome (hemolysis, elevated liver enzymes and low platelet count) O14.2-●
  - complicating
    - childbirth O14.24
    - puerperium O14.25
- Helminthiasis —*see also* Infestation, helminth
  - Ancylostoma B76.Ø
  - intestinal B82.Ø
    - mixed types (types classifiable to more than one of the titles B65.Ø-B81.3 and B81.8) B81.4
    - specified type NEC B81.8

H

▶ New ➡ Revised ~~deleted~~ Deleted ● Use Additional Character(s)

H

Hemorrhage, hemorrhagic *(Continued)*
- joint (nontraumatic) —*see* Hemarthrosis
- kidney N28.89
- knee (joint) (nontraumatic) —*see* Hemarthrosis, knee
- labyrinth —*see* subcategory H83.8
- lenticular striate artery I61.0
- ligature, vessel —*see* Hemorrhage, postoperative
- liver K76.89
- lung R04.89
  - newborn P26.9
    - massive P26.1
    - specified NEC P26.8
  - tuberculous —*see* Tuberculosis, pulmonary
- massive umbilical, newborn P51.0
- mediastinum —*see* Hemorrhage, lung
- medulla I61.3
- membrane (brain) I60.8
  - spinal cord —*see* Hemorrhage, spinal cord
- meninges, meningeal (brain) (middle) I60.8
  - spinal cord —*see* Hemorrhage, spinal cord
- mesentery K66.1
- metritis —*see* Endometritis
- mouth K13.79
- mucous membrane NEC R58
  - newborn P54.8
- muscle M62.89
- nail (subungual) L60.8
- nasal turbinate R04.0
  - newborn P54.8
- navel, newborn P51.9
- newborn P54.9
  - specified NEC P54.8
- nipple N64.59
- nose R04.0
  - newborn P54.8
- omentum K66.1
- optic nerve (sheath) H47.02-●
- orbit, orbital H05.23-●
- ovary NEC N83.8
- oviduct N83.6
- pancreas K86.89
- parathyroid (gland) (spontaneous) E21.4
- parturition —*see* Hemorrhage, complicating, delivery
- penis N48.89
- pericardium, pericarditis I31.2
- peritoneum, peritoneal K66.1
- peritonsillar tissue J35.8
  - due to infection J36
- petechial R23.3
  - due to autosensitivity, erythrocyte D69.2
- pituitary (gland) E23.6
- pleura —*see* Hemorrhage, lung
- polioencephalitis, superior E51.2
- polymyositis —*see* Polymyositis
- pons, pontine I61.3
- posterior fossa (nontraumatic) I61.8
  - newborn P52.6
- postmenopausal N95.0
- postnasal R04.0
- postoperative —*see* Complications, postprocedural, hemorrhage, by site
- postpartum NEC (following delivery of placenta) O72.1
  - delayed or secondary O72.2
  - retained placenta O72.0
  - third stage O72.0
- pregnancy —*see* Hemorrhage, antepartum
- preretinal —*see* Hemorrhage, retina
- prostate N42.1
- puerperal —*see* Hemorrhage, postpartum
  - delayed or secondary O72.2
- pulmonary R04.89
  - newborn P26.9
    - massive P26.1
    - specified NEC P26.8
  - tuberculous —*see* Tuberculosis, pulmonary
- purpura (primary) D69.3
- rectum (sphincter) K62.5
  - newborn P54.2
- recurring, following initial hemorrhage at time of injury T79.2
- renal N28.89
- respiratory passage or tract R04.9
  - specified NEC R04.89
- retina, retinal (vessels) H35.6-●
  - diabetic —*see* Microaneurysm, retinal, diabetic
- retroperitoneal K68.3
- scalp R58
- scrotum N50.1

Hemorrhage, hemorrhagic *(Continued)*
- secondary (nontraumatic) R58
  - following initial hemorrhage at time of injury T79.2
- seminal vesicle N50.1
- skin R23.3
  - newborn P54.5
- slipped umbilical ligature P51.8
- spermatic cord N50.1
- spinal (cord) G95.19
  - newborn (birth injury) P11.5
- spleen D73.5
  - intraoperative —*see* Complications, intraoperative, hemorrhage, spleen
  - postprocedural —*see* Complications, postprocedural, hemorrhage, spleen
- stomach K92.2
  - newborn P54.3
  - ulcer —*see* Ulcer, stomach, with hemorrhage
- subarachnoid (nontraumatic) —*see* Hemorrhage, intracranial, subarachnoid
- subconjunctival —*see also* Hemorrhage, conjunctiva
  - birth injury P15.3
- subcortical (brain) I61.0
- subcutaneous R23.3
- subdiaphragmatic R58
- subdural (acute) (nontraumatic) —*see* Hemorrhage, intracranial, subdural
- subependymal
  - newborn P52.0
    - with intraventricular extension P52.1
      - and intracerebral extension P52.22
- subgaleal P12.2
- subhyaloid —*see* Hemorrhage, retina
- subperiosteal —*see* Disorder, bone, specified type NEC
- subretinal —*see* Hemorrhage, retina
- subtentorial —*see* Hemorrhage, intracranial, subdural
- subungual L60.8
- suprarenal (capsule) (gland) E27.49
  - newborn P54.4
- tentorium (traumatic) NEC —*see* Hemorrhage, brain
  - newborn (birth injury) P10.4
- testis N50.1
- third stage (postpartum) O72.0
- thorax —*see* Hemorrhage, lung
- throat R04.1
- thymus (gland) E32.8
- thyroid (cyst) (gland) E07.89
- tongue K14.8
- tonsil J35.8
- trachea —*see* Hemorrhage, lung
- tracheobronchial R04.89
  - newborn P26.0
- traumatic — code to specific injury
  - cerebellar —*see* Hemorrhage, brain
  - intracranial —*see* Hemorrhage, brain
  - recurring or secondary (following initial hemorrhage at time of injury) T79.2
- tuberculous NEC —*see also* Tuberculosis, pulmonary A15.0
- tunica vaginalis N50.1
- ulcer - code by site under Ulcer, with hemorrhage K27.4
- umbilicus, umbilical
  - cord
    - after birth, newborn P51.9
    - complicating delivery O69.5
  - newborn P51.9
    - massive P51.0
    - slipped ligature P51.8
  - stump P51.9
- urethra (idiopathic) N36.8
- uterus, uterine (abnormal) N93.9
  - climacteric N92.4
  - complicating delivery —*see* Hemorrhage, complicating, delivery
  - dysfunctional or functional N93.8
  - intermenstrual (regular) N92.3
    - irregular N92.1
  - postmenopausal N95.0
  - postpartum —*see* Hemorrhage, postpartum
  - preclimacteric or premenopausal N92.4
  - prepubertal N93.8
  - pubertal N92.2
- vagina (abnormal) N93.9
  - newborn P54.6
- vas deferens N50.1
- vasa previa O69.4

Hemorrhage, hemorrhagic *(Continued)*
- ventricular I61.5
- vesical N32.89
- viscera NEC R58
  - newborn P54.8
- vitreous (humor) (intraocular) H43.1-●
- vulva N90.89

Hemorrhoids (bleeding) (without mention of degree) K64.9
- 1st degree (grade/stage I) (without prolapse outside of anal canal) K64.0
- 2nd degree (grade/stage II) (that prolapse with straining but retract spontaneously) K64.1
- 3rd degree (grade/stage III) (that prolapse with straining and require manual replacement back inside anal canal) K64.2
- 4th degree (grade/stage IV) (with prolapsed tissue that cannot be manually replaced) K64.3
- complicating
  - pregnancy O22.4
  - puerperium O87.2
- external K64.4
  - with
    - thrombosis K64.5
- internal (without mention of degree) K64.8
- prolapsed K64.8
- skin tags
  - anus K64.4
  - residual K64.4
- specified NEC K64.8
- strangulated —*see also* Hemorrhoids, by degree K64.8
- thrombosed —*see also* Hemorrhoids, by degree K64.5
- ulcerated —*see also* Hemorrhoids, by degree K64.8

Hemosalpinx N83.6
- with
  - hematocolpos N89.7
  - hematometra N85.7
    - with hematocolpos N89.7

Hemosiderosis (dietary) E83.19
- pulmonary, idiopathic E83.1 *[J84.03]*
- transfusion T80.89

Hemothorax (bacterial) (nontuberculous) J94.2
- newborn P54.8
- traumatic S27.1
  - with pneumothorax S27.2
- tuberculous NEC A15.6

Henoch (-Schönlein) disease or syndrome (purpura) D69.0

Henpue, henpuye A66.6

Hepar lobatum (syphilitic) A52.74

Hepatalgia K76.89

Hepatitis K75.9
- ▶A —*see* Hepatitis, viral, type, A
- acute B17.9
  - with coma K72.01
  - with hepatic failure —*see* Failure, hepatic
  - alcoholic —*see* Hepatitis, alcoholic
  - infectious B15.9
  - non-viral K72.0
  - ➡viral (*see also,* Hepatitis, viral) B17.9
- alcoholic (acute) (chronic) K70.10
  - with ascites K70.11
- amebic —*see* Abscess, liver, amebic
- anicteric (viral) —*see* Hepatitis, viral
- antigen-associated (HAA) —*see* Hepatitis, B
- Australia-antigen (positive) —*see* Hepatitis, B
- autoimmune K75.4
- B B19.10
  - ~~with hepatic coma B19.11~~
  - ▶with
    - ▶delta (agent) —*see* Hepatitis, D
    - ▶hepatic coma B19.11
  - acute B16.9
    - with
      - delta-agent (coinfection) (without hepatic coma) B16.1
        - with hepatic coma B16.0
      - hepatic coma (without delta-agent coinfection) B16.2
  - chronic B18.1
    - with delta-agent B18.0
- bacterial NEC K75.89
- C (viral) B19.20
  - with hepatic coma B19.21
  - acute B17.10
    - with hepatic coma B17.11
  - chronic B18.2
- catarrhal (acute) B15.9
  - with hepatic coma B15.0

▶ New ➡ Revised ~~deleted~~ Deleted ● Use Additional Character(s)

Hepatitis *(Continued)*
cholangiolitic K75.89
cholestatic K75.89
chronic K73.9
active NEC K73.2
▶toxic —*see* Disease, liver, toxic, with, hepatitis, chronic, active
lobular NEC K73.1
persistent NEC K73.Ø
specified NEC K73.8
▶toxic —*see* Disease, liver, toxic, with, hepatitis, chronic
▶viral —*see* Hepatitis, viral, chronic
cytomegaloviral B25.1
▶D B16.1
▶acute B16.1
▶with hepatic coma B16.Ø
▶in hepatitis B carrier B17.Ø
▶chronic B18.Ø
▶delta (agent) —*see* Hepatitis, D
due to ethanol (acute) (chronic) —*see* Hepatitis, alcoholic
epidemic B15.9
with hepatic coma B15.Ø
fulminant NEC (viral) —*see* Hepatitis, viral
granulomatous NEC K75.3
herpesviral BØØ.81
history of
B Z86.19
C Z86.19
homologous serum —*see* Hepatitis, viral, type B
in (due to)
mumps B26.81
toxoplasmosis (acquired) B58.1
congenital (active) P37.1 *[K77]*
infectious, infective B15.9
acute (subacute) B17.9
chronic B18.9
inoculation —*see* Hepatitis, viral, type B
interstitial (chronic) K74.69
ischemia, ischemic K72.ØØ
lupoid NEC K75.2
malignant NEC (with hepatic failure) K72.9Ø
with coma K72.91
neonatal giant cell P59.29
neonatal (idiopathic) (toxic) P59.29
newborn P59.29
postimmunization —*see* Hepatitis, viral, type B
post-transfusion —*see* Hepatitis, viral, type B
reactive, nonspecific K75.2
serum —*see* Hepatitis, viral, type B
shock K72.ØØ
specified type NEC
with hepatic failure —*see* Failure, hepatic
syphilitic (late) A52.74
congenital (early) A5Ø.Ø8 *[K77]*
late A5Ø.59 *[K77]*
secondary A51.45
toxic —*see also* Disease, liver, toxic K71.6
tuberculous A18.83
viral, virus B19.9
with hepatic coma B19.Ø
acute B17.9
chronic B18.9
specified NEC B18.8
type
B B18.1
with delta-agent B18.Ø
C B18.2
▶D B18.Ø
congenital P35.3
coxsackie B33.8 *[K77]*
cytomegalic inclusion B25.1
in remission, any type — code to Hepatitis, chronic, by type
non-A, non-B B17.8
specified type NEC (with or without coma) B17.8
type
A B15.9
with hepatic coma B15.Ø
B B19.1Ø
with hepatic coma B19.11
acute B16.9
with
delta-agent (coinfection) (without hepatic coma) B16.1
with hepatic coma B16.Ø
hepatic coma (without delta-agent coinfection) B16.2
chronic B18.1
with delta-agent B18.Ø

Hepatitis *(Continued)*
viral, virus *(Continued)*
type *(Continued)*
C B19.2Ø
with hepatic coma B19.21
acute B17.1Ø
with hepatic coma B17.11
chronic B18.2
▶D B16.1
▶acute B16.1
▶with hepatic coma B16.Ø
▶in hepatitis B carrier B17.Ø
▶chronic B18.Ø
▶delta (agent) —*see* Hepatitis, viral, type, D
E B17.2
non-A, non-B B17.8
Hepatization lung (acute) —*see* Pneumonia, lobar
Hepatoblastoma C22.2
Hepatocarcinoma C22.Ø
Hepatocholangiocarcinoma C22.Ø
Hepatocholangioma, benign D13.4
Hepatocholangitis K75.89
Hepatolenticular degeneration E83.Ø1
Hepatoma (malignant) C22.Ø
benign D13.4
embryonal C22.Ø
Hepatomegaly —*see also* Hypertrophy, liver
with splenomegaly R16.2
congenital Q44.79
in mononucleosis
gammaherpesviral B27.Ø9
infectious specified NEC B27.89
Hepatoptosis K76.89
Hepatorenal syndrome following labor and delivery O9Ø.41
Hepatosis K76.89
Hepatosplenomegaly R16.2
hyperlipemic (Bürger-Grütz type) E78.3 *[K77]*
Hereditary —*see* condition
Hereditary alpha tryptasemia (syndrome) D89.44
Heredodegeneration, macular —*see* Dystrophy, retina
Heredopathia atactica polyneuritiformis G6Ø.1
Heredosyphilis —*see* Syphilis, congenital
Herlitz' syndrome Q81.1
Hermansky-Pudlak syndrome E7Ø.331
Hermaphrodite, hermaphroditism (true) Q56.Ø
46,XX with streak gonads Q99.1
46,XX/46,XY Q99.Ø
46,XY with streak gonads Q99.1
chimera 46,XX/46,XY Q99.Ø
Hernia, hernial (acquired) (recurrent) K46.9
with
gangrene —*see* Hernia, by site, with, gangrene
incarceration —*see* Hernia, by site, with, obstruction
irreducible —*see* Hernia, by site, with, obstruction
obstruction —*see* Hernia, by site, with, obstruction
strangulation —*see* Hernia, by site, with, obstruction
abdomen, abdominal K46.9
with
gangrene (and obstruction) K46.1
obstruction K46.Ø
femoral —*see* Hernia, femoral
incisional —*see* Hernia, incisional
inguinal —*see* Hernia, inguinal
specified site NEC K45.8
with
gangrene (and obstruction) K45.1
obstruction K45.Ø
umbilical —*see* Hernia, umbilical
wall —*see* Hernia, ventral
appendix —*see* Hernia, abdomen
bladder (mucosa) (sphincter)
congenital (female) (male) Q79.51
female —*see* Cystocele
male N32.89
brain, congenital —*see* Encephalocele
cartilage, vertebra —*see* Displacement, intervertebral disc
cerebral, congenital —*see also* Encephalocele
endaural QØ1.8
ciliary body (traumatic) SØ5.2-●
colon —*see* Hernia, abdomen
Cooper's —*see* Hernia, abdomen, specified site NEC
crural —*see* Hernia, femoral

Hernia, hernial *(Continued)*
diaphragm, diaphragmatic K44.9
with
gangrene (and obstruction) K44.1
obstruction K44.Ø
congenital Q79.Ø
direct (inguinal) —*see* Hernia, inguinal
diverticulum, intestine —*see* Hernia, abdomen
double (inguinal) —*see* Hernia, inguinal, bilateral
due to adhesions (with obstruction) K56.5Ø
epigastric —*see also* Hernia, ventral K43.9
esophageal hiatus —*see* Hernia, hiatal
external (inguinal) —*see* Hernia, inguinal
fallopian tube N83.4-●
fascia M62.89
femoral K41.9Ø
with
gangrene (and obstruction) K41.4Ø
not specified as recurrent K41.4Ø
recurrent K41.41
obstruction K41.3Ø
not specified as recurrent K41.3Ø
recurrent K41.31
bilateral K41.2Ø
with
gangrene (and obstruction) K41.1Ø
not specified as recurrent K41.1Ø
recurrent K41.11
obstruction K41.ØØ
not specified as recurrent K41.ØØ
recurrent K41.Ø1
not specified as recurrent K41.2Ø
recurrent K41.21
not specified as recurrent K41.9Ø
recurrent K41.91
unilateral K41.9Ø
with
gangrene (and obstruction) K41.4Ø
not specified as recurrent K41.4Ø
recurrent K41.41
obstruction K41.3Ø
not specified as recurrent K41.3Ø
recurrent K41.31
not specified as recurrent K41.9Ø
recurrent K41.91
foramen magnum G93.5
congenital QØ1.8
funicular (umbilical) —*see also* Hernia, umbilicus
spermatic (cord) —*see* Hernia, inguinal
gastrointestinal tract —*see* Hernia, abdomen
Hesselbach's —*see* Hernia, femoral, specified site NEC
hiatal (esophageal) (sliding) K44.9
with
gangrene (and obstruction) K44.1
obstruction K44.Ø
congenital Q4Ø.1
hypogastric —*see* Hernia, ventral
incarcerated —*see also* Hernia, by site, with obstruction
with gangrene —*see* Hernia, by site, with gangrene
incisional K43.2
with
gangrene (and obstruction) K43.1
obstruction K43.Ø
indirect (inguinal) —*see* Hernia, inguinal
inguinal (direct) (external) (funicular) (indirect) (internal) (oblique) (scrotal) (sliding) K4Ø.9Ø
with
gangrene (and obstruction) K4Ø.4Ø
not specified as recurrent K4Ø.4Ø
recurrent K4Ø.41
obstruction K4Ø.3Ø
not specified as recurrent K4Ø.3Ø
recurrent K4Ø.31
bilateral K4Ø.2Ø
with
gangrene (and obstruction) K4Ø.1Ø
not specified as recurrent K4Ø.1Ø
recurrent K4Ø.11
obstruction K4Ø.ØØ
not specified as recurrent K4Ø.ØØ
recurrent K4Ø.Ø1
not specified as recurrent K4Ø.2Ø
recurrent K4Ø.21
not specified as recurrent K4Ø.9Ø
recurrent K4Ø.91

H

Hernia, hernial *(Continued)*
inguinal *(Continued)*
unilateral K40.90
with
gangrene (and obstruction) K40.40
not specified as recurrent K40.40
recurrent K40.41
obstruction K40.30
not specified as recurrent K40.30
recurrent K40.31
not specified as recurrent K40.90
recurrent K40.91
internal —*see also* Hernia, abdomen
inguinal —*see* Hernia, inguinal
interstitial —*see* Hernia, abdomen
intervertebral cartilage or disc —*see* Displacement, intervertebral disc
intestine, intestinal —*see* Hernia, by site
intra-abdominal —*see* Hernia, abdomen
iris (traumatic) S05.2- ●
irreducible —*see also* Hernia, by site, with obstruction
with gangrene —*see* Hernia, by site, with gangrene
ischiatic —*see* Hernia, abdomen, specified site NEC
ischiorectal —*see* Hernia, abdomen, specified site NEC
lens (traumatic) S05.2- ●
linea (alba) (semilunaris) —*see* Hernia, ventral
Littre's —*see* Hernia, abdomen
lumbar —*see* Hernia, abdomen, specified site NEC
lung (subcutaneous) J98.4
mediastinum J98.59
mesenteric (internal) —*see* Hernia, abdomen
midline —*see* Hernia, ventral
muscle (sheath) M62.89
nucleus pulposus —*see* Displacement, intervertebral disc
oblique (inguinal) —*see* Hernia, inguinal
obstructive —*see also* Hernia, by site, with obstruction
with gangrene —*see* Hernia, by site, with gangrene
obturator —*see* Hernia, abdomen, specified site NEC
omental —*see* Hernia, abdomen
ovary N83.4- ●
oviduct N83.4- ●
paraesophageal —*see also* Hernia, diaphragm
congenital Q40.1
parastomal K43.5
with
gangrene (and obstruction) K43.4
obstruction K43.3
paraumbilical —*see* Hernia, umbilicus
perineal —*see* Hernia, abdomen, specified site NEC
Petit's —*see* Hernia, abdomen, specified site NEC
postoperative —*see* Hernia, incisional
pregnant uterus —*see* Abnormal, uterus in pregnancy or childbirth
prevesical N32.89
properitoneal —*see* Hernia, abdomen, specified site NEC
pudendal —*see* Hernia, abdomen, specified site NEC
rectovaginal N81.6
retroperitoneal —*see* Hernia, abdomen, specified site NEC
Richter's —*see* Hernia, abdomen, with obstruction
Rieux's, Riex's —*see* Hernia, abdomen, specified site NEC
sac condition (adhesion) (dropsy) (inflammation) (laceration) (suppuration) - code by site under Hernia
sciatic —*see* Hernia, abdomen, specified site NEC
scrotum, scrotal —*see* Hernia, inguinal
sliding (inguinal) —*see also* Hernia, inguinal
hiatus —*see* Hernia, hiatal
spigelian —*see* Hernia, ventral
spinal —*see* Spina bifida
strangulated —*see also* Hernia, by site, with obstruction
with gangrene —*see* Hernia, by site, with gangrene
subxiphoid —*see* Hernia, ventral

Hernia, hernial *(Continued)*
supra-umbilicus —*see* Hernia, ventral
tendon —*see* Disorder, tendon, specified type NEC
Treitz's (fossa) —*see* Hernia, abdomen, specified site NEC
tunica vaginalis Q55.29
umbilicus, umbilical K42.9
with
gangrene (and obstruction) K42.1
obstruction K42.0
ureter N28.89
urethra, congenital Q64.79
urinary meatus, congenital Q64.79
uterus N81.4
pregnant —*see* Abnormal, uterus in pregnancy or childbirth
vaginal (anterior) (wall) —*see* Cystocele
Velpeau's —*see* Hernia, femoral
ventral K43.9
with
gangrene (and obstruction) K43.7
obstruction K43.6
incisional K43.2
with
gangrene (and obstruction) K43.1
obstruction K43.0
recurrent —*see* Hernia, incisional
specified NEC K43.9
with
gangrene (and obstruction) K43.7
obstruction K43.6
vesical
congenital (female) (male) Q79.51
female —*see* Cystocele
male N32.89
vitreous (into wound) S05.2- ●
into anterior chamber —*see* Prolapse, vitreous
Herniation —*see also* Hernia
brain (stem) G93.5
nontraumatic G93.5
traumatic S06.A1
cerebellar S06.A1
subfalcine (cingulate) S06.A1
tonsillar S06.A1
transtentorial (central) (upward cerebellar) S06.A1
uncal S06.A1
cerebral G93.5
nontraumatic G93.5
traumatic S06.A1
mediastinum J98.59
nucleus pulposus —*see* Displacement, intervertebral disc
Herpangina B08.5
Herpes, herpesvirus, herpetic B00.9
anogenital A60.9
perianal skin A60.1
rectum A60.1
urogenital tract A60.00
cervix A60.03
male genital organ NEC A60.02
penis A60.01
specified site NEC A60.09
vagina A60.04
vulva A60.04
blepharitis (zoster) B02.39
simplex B00.59
circinatus B35.4
bullosus L12.0
conjunctivitis (simplex) B00.53
zoster B02.31
cornea B02.33
encephalitis B00.4
due to herpesvirus 6 B10.01
due to herpesvirus 7 B10.09
specified NEC B10.09
eye (zoster) B02.30
simplex B00.50
eyelid (zoster) B02.39
simplex B00.59
facialis B00.1
febrilis B00.1
geniculate ganglionitis B02.21
genital, genitalis A60.00
female A60.09
male A60.02
gestational, gestationis O26.4- ●
gingivostomatitis B00.2

Herpes, herpesvirus, herpetic *(Continued)*
human B00.9
1 —*see* Herpes, simplex
2 —*see* Herpes, simplex
3 —*see* Varicella
4 —*see* Mononucleosis, Epstein-Barr (virus)
5 —*see* Disease, cytomegalic inclusion (generalized)
6
encephalitis B10.01
specified NEC B10.81
7
encephalitis B10.09
specified NEC B10.82
8 B10.89
infection NEC B10.89
Kaposi's sarcoma associated B10.89
iridocyclitis (simplex) B00.51
zoster B02.32
iris (vesicular erythema multiforme) L51.9
iritis (simplex) B00.51
Kaposi's sarcoma associated B10.89
keratitis (simplex) (dendritic) (disciform) (interstitial) B00.52
zoster (interstitial) B02.33
keratoconjunctivitis (simplex) B00.52
zoster B02.33
labialis B00.1
lip B00.1
meningitis (simplex) B00.3
zoster B02.1
ophthalmicus (zoster) NEC B02.30
simplex B00.50
penis A60.01
perianal skin A60.1
pharyngitis, pharyngotonsillitis B00.2
rectum A60.1
scrotum A60.02
sepsis B00.7
simplex B00.9
complicated NEC B00.89
congenital P35.2
conjunctivitis B00.53
external ear B00.1
eyelid B00.59
hepatitis B00.81
keratitis (interstitial) B00.52
~~myelitis B00.82~~
▶ myelitis B00.82
specified complication NEC B00.89
visceral B00.89
stomatitis B00.2
tonsurans B35.0
visceral B00.89
vulva A60.04
whitlow B00.89
zoster —*see also* condition B02.9
auricularis B02.21
complicated NEC B02.8
conjunctivitis B02.31
disseminated B02.7
encephalitis B02.0
eye(lid) B02.39
geniculate ganglionitis B02.21
keratitis (interstitial) B02.33
meningitis B02.1
myelitis B02.24
neuritis, neuralgia B02.29
ophthalmicus NEC B02.30
oticus B02.21
polyneuropathy B02.23
specified complication NEC B02.8
trigeminal neuralgia B02.22
Herpesvirus (human) —*see* Herpes
Herpetophobia F40.218
Herrick's anemia —*see* Disease, sickle-cell
Hers' disease E74.09
Herter-Gee syndrome K90.0
Herxheimer's reaction R68.89
Hesitancy
of micturition R39.11
urinary R39.11
Hesselbach's hernia —*see* Hernia, femoral, specified site NEC
Heterochromia (congenital) Q13.2
cataract —*see* Cataract, complicated
cyclitis (Fuchs) —*see* Cyclitis, Fuchs' heterochromic
hair L67.1
iritis —*see* Cyclitis, Fuchs' heterochromic

H

- **Heterochromia** *(Continued)*
  - retained metallic foreign body (nonmagnetic) —*see* Foreign body, intraocular, old, retained
    - magnetic —*see* Foreign body, intraocular, old, retained, magnetic
  - uveitis —*see* Cyclitis, Fuchs' heterochromic
- **Heterophoria** —*see* Strabismus, heterophoria
- **Heterophyes, heterophyiasis** (small intestine) B66.8
- **Heterotopia, heterotopic** —*see also* Malposition, congenital
  - cerebralis Q04.8
- **Heterotropia** —*see* Strabismus
- **Heubner-Herter disease** K90.0
- **Hexadactylism** Q69.9
- **HGSIL** (cytology finding) (high grade squamous intraepithelial lesion on cytologic smear) (Pap smear finding)
  - anus R85.613
  - cervix R87.613
    - biopsy (histology) finding — *see* Neoplasia, intraepithelial, cervix, grade II or grade III
  - vagina R87.623
    - biopsy (histology) finding — *see* Neoplasia, intraepithelial, vagina, grade II or grade III
- **Hibernoma** —*see* Lipoma
- **Hiccup, hiccough** R06.6
  - epidemic B33.0
  - psychogenic F45.8
- **Hidden penis** (congenital) Q55.64
  - acquired N48.83
- **Hidradenitis** (axillaris) (suppurative) L73.2
- **Hidradenoma** (nodular) —*see also* Neoplasm, skin, benign
  - clear cell —*see* Neoplasm, skin, benign
  - papillary —*see* Neoplasm, skin, benign
- **Hidrocystoma** —*see* Neoplasm, skin, benign
- **High**
  - altitude effects T70.20
    - anoxia T70.29
    - on
      - ears T70.0
      - sinuses T70.1
    - polycythemia D75.1
  - arch
    - foot Q66.7- •
    - palate, congenital Q38.5
  - arterial tension —*see* Hypertension
  - basal metabolic rate R94.8
  - blood pressure —*see also* Hypertension
    - borderline R03.0
    - reading (incidental) (isolated) (nonspecific), without diagnosis of hypertension R03.0
  - cholesterol E78.00
    - with high triglycerides E78.2
  - diaphragm (congenital) Q79.1
  - expressed emotional level within family Z63.8
  - head at term O32.4
  - palate, congenital Q38.5
  - risk
    - infant NEC Z76.2
    - sexual behavior (heterosexual) Z72.51
      - bisexual Z72.53
      - homosexual Z72.52
  - scrotal testis, testes
    - bilateral Q53.23
    - unilateral Q53.13
  - temperature (of unknown origin) R50.9
  - thoracic rib Q76.6
  - triglycerides E78.1
    - with high cholesterol E78.2
- **Hildenbrand's disease** A75.0
- **Hilum** —*see* condition
- **Hip** —*see* condition
- **Hippel's disease** Q85.83
- **Hippophobia** F40.218
- **Hippus** H57.09
- **Hirschsprung's disease or megacolon** Q43.1
- **Hirsutism, hirsuties** L68.0
- **Hirudiniasis**
  - external B88.3
  - internal B83.4
- **Hiss-Russell dysentery** A03.1
- **Histidinemia, histidinuria** E70.41
- **Histiocytoma** —*see also* Neoplasm, skin, benign
  - fibrous —*see also* Neoplasm, skin, benign
    - atypical —*see* Neoplasm, connective tissue, uncertain behavior
    - malignant —*see* Neoplasm, connective tissue, malignant
- **Histiocytosis** D76.3
  - acute differentiated progressive C96.0
  - Langerhans' cell NEC C96.6
    - multifocal X
      - multisystemic (disseminated) C96.0
      - unisystemic C96.5
    - pulmonary, adult (adult PLCH) J84.82
    - unifocal (X) C96.6
  - lipid, lipoid D76.3
    - essential E75.29
  - malignant C96.A
  - mononuclear phagocytes NEC D76.1
    - Langerhans' cells C96.6
  - non-Langerhans cell D76.3
  - polyostotic sclerosing D76.3
  - sinus, with massive lymphadenopathy D76.3
  - syndrome NEC D76.3
  - X NEC C96.6
    - acute (progressive) C96.0
    - chronic C96.6
    - multifocal C96.5
    - multisystemic C96.0
    - unifocal C96.6
- **Histoplasmosis** B39.9
  - with pneumonia NEC B39.2
  - African B39.5
  - American —*see* Histoplasmosis, capsulati
  - capsulati B39.4
    - disseminated B39.3
    - generalized B39.3
    - pulmonary B39.2
      - acute B39.0
      - chronic B39.1
  - Darling's B39.4
  - duboisii B39.5
  - lung NEC B39.2
- **History**
  - family (of) —*see also* History, personal (of)
    - ▶ adenomatous polyposis Z83.72
    - alcohol abuse Z81.1
    - allergy NEC Z84.89
    - anemia Z83.2
    - arthritis Z82.61
    - asthma Z82.5
    - blindness Z82.1
    - cardiac death (sudden) Z82.41
    - carrier of genetic disease Z84.81
    - chromosomal anomaly Z82.79
    - chronic
      - disabling disease NEC Z82.8
      - lower respiratory disease Z82.5
    - colonic polyps Z83.719
      - adenomatous and serrated Z83.710
      - hyperplastic Z83.711
      - inflammatory Z83.718
      - specified, NEC Z83.718
      - tubular adenoma Z83.710
      - tubulovillous adenoma Z83.710
      - villous adenoma Z83.710
    - congenital malformations and deformations Z82.79
      - polycystic kidney Z82.71
    - consanguinity Z84.3
    - deafness Z82.2
    - diabetes mellitus Z83.3
    - disability NEC Z82.8
    - disease or disorder (of)
      - allergic NEC Z84.89
      - behavioral NEC Z81.8
      - blood and blood-forming organs Z83.2
      - cardiovascular NEC Z82.49
      - chronic disabling NEC Z82.8
      - digestive Z83.79
      - ear NEC Z83.52
      - elevated lipoprotein (a) (Lp(a)) Z83.430
      - endocrine NEC Z83.49
      - eye NEC Z83.518
        - glaucoma Z83.511
      - familial hypercholesterolemia Z83.42
      - genitourinary NEC Z84.2
      - glaucoma Z83.511
      - hematological Z83.2
      - immune mechanism Z83.2
      - infectious NEC Z83.1
- **History** *(Continued)*
  - family *(Continued)*
    - disease or disorder *(Continued)*
      - ischemic heart Z82.49
      - kidney Z84.1
      - lipoprotein metabolism Z83.438
      - mental NEC Z81.8
      - metabolic Z83.49
      - musculoskeletal NEC Z82.69
      - neurological NEC Z82.0
      - nutritional Z83.49
      - parasitic NEC Z83.1
      - psychiatric NEC Z81.8
      - respiratory NEC Z83.6
      - skin and subcutaneous tissue NEC Z84.0
      - specified NEC Z84.89
    - drug abuse NEC Z81.3
    - elevated lipoprotein(a) (Lp (a)) Z83.430
    - epilepsy Z82.0
    - familial hypercholesterolemia Z83.42
    - genetic disease carrier Z84.81
    - glaucoma Z83.511
    - hearing loss Z82.2
    - human immunodeficiency virus (HIV) infection Z83.0
    - Huntington's chorea Z82.0
    - hyperlipidemia, familial combined Z83.438
    - intellectual disability Z81.0
    - leukemia Z80.6
    - lipidemia NEC Z83.438
    - malignant neoplasm (of) NOS Z80.9
      - bladder Z80.52
      - breast Z80.3
      - bronchus Z80.1
      - digestive organ Z80.0
      - gastrointestinal tract Z80.0
      - genital organ Z80.49
        - ovary Z80.41
        - prostate Z80.42
        - specified organ NEC Z80.49
        - testis Z80.43
      - hematopoietic NEC Z80.7
      - intrathoracic organ NEC Z80.2
      - kidney Z80.51
      - lung Z80.1
      - lymphatic NEC Z80.7
      - ovary Z80.41
      - prostate Z80.42
      - respiratory organ NEC Z80.2
      - specified site NEC Z80.8
      - testis Z80.43
      - trachea Z80.1
      - urinary organ or tract Z80.59
        - bladder Z80.52
        - kidney Z80.51
    - mental
      - disorder NEC Z81.8
    - multiple endocrine neoplasia (MEN) syndrome Z83.41
    - osteoporosis Z82.62
    - polycystic kidney Z82.71
    - ▶ polyposis, adenomatous Z83.72
    - polyps (colon) (*see also* History, family, colonic polyps) Z83.719
    - psychiatric disorder Z81.8
    - psychoactive substance abuse NEC Z81.3
    - respiratory condition NEC Z83.6
      - asthma and other lower respiratory conditions Z82.5
    - self-harmful behavior Z81.8
    - SIDS (sudden infant death syndrome) Z84.82
    - skin condition Z84.0
    - specified condition NEC Z84.89
    - stroke (cerebrovascular) Z82.3
    - substance abuse NEC Z81.4
      - alcohol Z81.1
      - drug NEC Z81.3
      - psychoactive NEC Z81.3
      - tobacco Z81.2
    - sudden
      - cardiac death Z82.41
      - infant death syndrome (SIDS) Z84.82
    - tobacco abuse Z81.2
    - violence, violent behavior Z81.8
    - visual loss Z82.1

▶ New ➡ Revised ~~deleted~~ Deleted • Use Additional Character(s)

- **History** *(Continued)*
  - personal *(Continued)*
    - malignant neoplasm *(Continued)*
      - breast Z85.3
      - bronchus NEC Z85.118
        - carcinoid Z85.110
      - carcinoid —*see* History, personal (of), malignant neoplasm, by site, carcinoid
      - cervix Z85.41
      - colon NEC Z85.038
        - carcinoid Z85.030
      - digestive organ Z85.00
        - specified NEC Z85.09
      - endocrine gland NEC Z85.858
      - epididymis Z85.48
      - esophagus Z85.01
      - eye Z85.840
      - gastrointestinal tract —*see* History, malignant neoplasm, digestive organ
      - genital organ
        - female Z85.40
          - specified NEC Z85.44
        - male Z85.45
          - specified NEC Z85.49
      - hematopoietic NEC Z85.79
      - intrathoracic organ Z85.20-●
      - kidney NEC Z85.528
        - carcinoid Z85.520
      - large intestine NEC Z85.038
        - carcinoid Z85.030
      - larynx Z85.21
      - liver Z85.05
      - lung NEC Z85.118
        - carcinoid Z85.110
      - mediastinum Z85.29
      - Merkel cell Z85.821
      - middle ear Z85.22
      - nasal cavities Z85.22
      - nervous system NEC Z85.848
        - oral cavity Z85.819
        - specified site NEC Z85.818
      - ovary Z85.43
      - pancreas Z85.07
      - pelvis Z85.53
      - pharynx Z85.819
        - specified site NEC Z85.818
      - pleura Z85.29
      - prostate Z85.46
      - rectosigmoid junction NEC Z85.048
        - carcinoid Z85.040
      - rectum NEC Z85.048
        - carcinoid Z85.040
      - respiratory organ Z85.20
      - sinuses, accessory Z85.22
      - skin NEC Z85.828
        - melanoma Z85.820
        - Merkel cell Z85.821
      - small intestine NEC Z85.068
        - carcinoid Z85.060
      - soft tissue Z85.831
      - specified site NEC Z85.89
      - stomach NEC Z85.028
        - carcinoid Z85.020
      - testis Z85.47
      - thymus NEC Z85.238
        - carcinoid Z85.230
      - thyroid Z85.850
      - tongue Z85.810
      - trachea Z85.12
      - ureter Z85.54
      - urinary organ or tract Z85.50
        - specified NEC Z85.59
      - uterus Z85.42
    - maltreatment Z91.89
    - medical treatment NEC Z92.89
    - melanoma Z85.820
      - in situ Z86.06
      - malignant (skin) Z85.820
    - meningitis Z86.61
    - mental disorder Z86.59
    - Merkel cell carcinoma (skin) Z85.821
    - Methicillin resistant Staphylococcus aureus (MRSA) Z86.14
    - military deployment Z91.82
    - military service Z91.85
    - military war, peacekeeping and humanitarian deployment (current or past conflict) Z91.82
    - myocardial infarction (old) I25.2
    - neglect (in)
      - adult Z91.412
      - childhood Z62.812
    - neoplasia
      - anal intraepithelial, III [AIN III] Z86.004
      - high-grade prostatic intraepithelial, III [HGPIN III] Z86.002
      - vaginal intraepithelial, III [VAIN III] Z86.002
      - vulvar intraepithelial, III [VIN III] Z86.002
    - neoplasm
      - benign Z86.018
        - brain Z86.011
        - colon polyp Z86.0100
          - ►adenomatous (sessile) Z86.0101
          - ►hyperplastic Z86.0102
          - ►serrated (sessile) Z86.0101
          - ►specified NEC Z86.0109
          - ►traditional serrated adenoma Z86.0101
          - ►tubular adenoma Z86.0101
          - ►tubulovillous adenoma Z86.0101
          - ►villous adenoma Z86.0101
      - in situ
        - breast Z86.000
        - cervix uteri Z86.001
        - digestive organs, specified NEC Z86.004
        - esophagus Z86.003
        - genital organs, specified NEC Z86.002
        - melanoma Z86.006
        - middle ear Z86.005
        - oral cavity Z86.003
        - respiratory system Z86.005
        - skin Z86.007
        - specified NEC Z86.008
        - stomach Z86.003
      - malignant —*see* History of, malignant neoplasm
      - uncertain behavior Z86.03
    - nephrotic syndrome Z87.441
    - nicotine dependence Z87.891
    - noncompliance with medical treatment or regimen —*see* Noncompliance
    - nutritional deficiency Z86.39
    - obstetric complications Z87.59
      - childbirth Z87.59
      - pregnancy Z87.59
      - pre-term labor Z87.51
      - puerperium Z87.59
    - osteoporosis fractures Z87.31
    - parasuicide (attempt) Z91.51
    - physical trauma NEC Z87.828
      - self-harm or suicide attempt Z91.51
    - pneumonia (recurrent) Z87.01
    - poisoning NEC Z91.89
      - self-harm or suicide attempt Z91.51
    - poor personal hygiene Z91.89
    - preterm labor Z87.51
    - procedure during pregnancy Z98.870
    - procedure while a fetus Z98.871
    - prolonged reversible ischemic neurologic deficit (PRINO) Z86.73
    - prostatic dysplasia Z87.430
    - psychiatric disorder NEC Z87.89
    - psychological
      - abuse
        - adult Z91.411
        - child Z62.811
      - trauma, specified NEC Z91.49
    - radiation therapy Z92.3
    - removal
      - implant
        - breast Z98.86
    - renal calculi Z87.442
    - respiratory condition NEC Z87.09
    - retained foreign body fully removed Z87.821
    - risk factors NEC Z91.89
    - SARS-CoV-2 infection Z86.16
    - self-harm
      - nonsuicidal Z91.52
      - suicidal Z91.51
    - self-inflicted injury without suicidal intent Z91.52
    - self-injury
      - nonsuicidal Z91.52
    - self-mutilation Z91.52
    - self-poisoning attempt Z91.51
      - suicidal behavior Z91.51
    - sex reassignment Z87.890
    - sleep-wake cycle problem Z72.821
    - specified NEC Z87.898
    - steroid therapy (systemic) Z92.241
      - inhaled Z92.240
    - stroke without residual deficits Z86.73
    - substance abuse NEC F10-F19
    - sudden cardiac arrest Z86.74
    - sudden cardiac death successfully resuscitated Z86.74
    - suicide attempt Z91.51
    - surgery NEC Z98.890
      - with uterine scar Z98.891
      - sex reassignment Z87.890
      - transplant —*see* Transplant
    - thrombophlebitis Z86.72
    - thrombosis (venous) Z86.718
      - pulmonary Z86.711
    - tobacco dependence Z87.891
    - transient ischemic attack (TIA) without residual deficits Z86.73
    - trauma (physical) NEC Z87.828
      - psychological NEC Z91.49
      - self-harm Z91.51
    - traumatic brain injury Z87.820
    - tuberculosis, latent infection Z86.15
    - unhealthy sleep-wake cycle Z72.821
    - unintended awareness under general anesthesia Z92.84
    - urinary (recurrent) (tract) infection(s) Z87.440
    - urinary calculi Z87.42
    - uterine scar from previous surgery Z98.891
    - vaginal dysplasia Z87.411
    - venous thrombosis or embolism Z86.718
      - pulmonary Z86.711
    - vulvar dysplasia Z87.412
- **His-Werner disease** A79.0
- **HIV** —*see also* Human, immunodeficiency virus B20
  - laboratory evidence (nonconclusive) R75
  - nonconclusive test (in infants) R75
  - positive, seropositive Z21
- **Hives** (bold) —*see* Urticaria
- **Hoarseness** R49.0
- **Hobo** Z59.00
- **Hodgkin** disease —*see* Lymphoma, Hodgkin
- **Hodgson's** (*see also* Aneurysm, aorta, thorax) I71.20
  - ruptured (*see also* Aneurysm, aorta, thorax, ruptured) I71.10
- **Hoffa-Kastert disease** E88.89
- **Hoffa's disease** E88.89
- **Hoffmann-Bouveret syndrome** I47.9
- **Hoffmann's syndrome** E03.9 *[G73.7]*
- **Hole** (round)
  - macula H35.34-●
  - retina (without detachment) —*see* Break, retina, round hole
    - with detachment —*see* Detachment, retina, with retinal, break
- **Holiday relief care** Z75.5
- **Hollenhorst's plaque** —*see* Occlusion, artery, retina
- **Hollow foot** (congenital) Q66.7-●
  - acquired —*see* Deformity, limb, foot, specified NEC
- **Holoprosencephaly** Q04.2
- **Holt-Oram syndrome** Q87.2
- **Homelessness** Z59.00
  - sheltered Z59.01
  - unsheltered Z59.02
- **Homesickness** —*see* Disorder, adjustment
- **Homocysteinemia** R79.83
- **Homocystinemia** R79.83
- **Homocystinuria** E72.11
- **Homogentisate 1,2-dioxygenase deficiency** E70.29
- **Homologous serum hepatitis** (prophylactic) (therapeutic) —*see* Hepatitis, viral, type B
- **Honeycomb lung** J98.4
  - congenital Q33.0
- **Hooded**
  - clitoris Q52.6
  - penis Q55.69
- **Hookworm** (disease) (infection) (infestation) B76.9
  - with anemia B76.9 *[D63.8]*
  - specified NEC B76.8
- **Hordeolum** (eyelid) (externum) (recurrent) H00.019
  - internum H00.029
    - left H00.026
      - lower H00.025
      - upper H00.024

- **Hordeolum** *(Continued)*
  - internum *(Continued)*
    - right HØØ.Ø23
      - lower HØØ.Ø22
      - upper HØØ.Ø21
  - left HØØ.Ø16
    - lower HØØ.Ø15
    - upper HØØ.Ø14
  - right HØØ.Ø13
    - lower HØØ.Ø12
    - upper HØØ.Ø11
- **Horn**
  - cutaneous L85.8
  - nail L6Ø.2
    - congenital Q84.6
- **Horner** (-Claude Bernard) syndrome G9Ø.2
  - traumatic —*see* Injury, nerve, cervical sympathetic
- **Horseshoe kidney** (congenital) Q63.1
- **Horton's headache or neuralgia** G44.Ø99
  - intractable G44.Ø91
  - not intractable G44.Ø99
- **Hospital hopper syndrome** —*see* Disorder, factitious
- **Hospitalism in children** —*see* Disorder, adjustment
- **Hostility** R45.5
  - towards child Z62.3
- **Hot flashes**
  - menopausal N95.1
- **Hourglass** (contracture) —*see also* Contraction, hourglass
  - stomach K31.89
    - congenital Q4Ø.2
    - stricture K31.2
- **Household, housing circumstance affecting care** Z59.9
  - specified NEC Z59.89
- **Housemaid's knee** —*see* Bursitis, prepatellar
- **HSCT-TMA (hematopoietic stem cell transplantation-associated thrombotic microangiopathy)** M31.11
- **Hudson** (-Stähli) line (cornea) —*see* Pigmentation, cornea, anterior
- **Human**
  - bite (open wound) —*see also* Bite
    - intact skin surface —*see* Bite, superficial
  - herpesvirus —*see* Herpes
  - immunodeficiency virus (HIV) disease (infection) B2Ø
    - asymptomatic status Z21
    - contact Z2Ø.6
    - counseling Z71.7
    - dementia (*see also* Dementia, in, diseases specified elsewhere) B2Ø *[FØ2.8Ø]*
      - with behavioral disturbance (*see also* Dementia, in, diseases specified elsewhere) B2Ø *[FØ2.81-●]*
    - exposure to Z2Ø.6
    - laboratory evidence R75
    - type-2 (HIV 2) as cause of disease classified elsewhere B97.35
  - papillomavirus (HPV)
    - DNA test positive
      - high risk
        - cervix R87.81Ø
        - vagina R87.811
      - low risk
        - cervix R87.82Ø
        - vagina R87.821
    - screening for Z11.51
  - T-cell lymphotropic virus
    - type-1 (HTLV-I) infection B33.3
      - as cause of disease classified elsewhere B97.33
      - carrier Z22.6
    - type-2 (HTLV-II) as cause of disease classified elsewhere B97.34
- **Humidifier lung or pneumonitis** J67.7
- **Humiliation** (experience) in childhood Z62.898
- **Humpback** (acquired) —*see* Kyphosis
- **Hunchback** (acquired) —*see* Kyphosis
- **Hunger** T73.Ø
  - air, psychogenic F45.8
- **Hungry bone syndrome** E83.81
- **Hunner's ulcer** —*see* Cystitis, chronic, interstitial
- **Hunter's**
  - glossitis D51.Ø
  - syndrome E76.1
- **Huntington's disease or chorea** G1Ø
  - with dementia (*see also* Dementia, in, diseases specified elsewhere) G1Ø *[FØ2.8Ø]*
    - with behavioral disturbance (*see also* Dementia, in, diseases specified elsewhere) G1Ø *[FØ2.81-●]*
- **Hunt's**
  - disease or syndrome (herpetic geniculate ganglionitis) BØ2.21
    - dyssynergia cerebellaris myoclonica G11.19
  - neuralgia BØ2.21
- **Hurler** (-Scheie) **disease or syndrome** E76.Ø2
- **Hurst's disease** G36.1
- **Hurthle cell**
  - adenocarcinoma C73
  - adenoma D34
  - carcinoma C73
  - tumor D34
- **Hutchinson-Boeck disease or syndrome** —*see* Sarcoidosis
- **Hutchinson-Gilford disease or syndrome** E34.8
- **Hutchinson's**
  - disease, meaning
    - angioma serpiginosum L81.7
    - pompholyx (cheiropompholyx) L3Ø.1
    - prurigo estivalis L56.4
    - summer eruption or summer prurigo L56.4
  - melanotic freckle —*see* Melanoma, in situ
    - malignant melanoma in —*see* Melanoma
  - teeth or incisors (congenital syphilis) A5Ø.52
  - triad (congenital syphilis) A5Ø.53
- **Hyalin plaque, sclera, senile** H15.89
- **Hyaline membrane** (disease) (lung) (pulmonary) (newborn) P22.Ø
- **Hyalinosis**
  - cutis (et mucosae) E78.89
  - focal and segmental (glomerular) —*see also* NØØ-NØ7 with fourth character .1 NØ5.1
- **Hyalitis, hyalosis, asteroid** —*see also* Deposit, crystalline
  - syphilitic (late) A52.71
- **Hydatid**
  - cyst or tumor —*see* Echinococcus
  - mole —*see* Hydatidiform mole
  - Morgagni
    - female Q5Ø.5
    - male (epididymal) Q55.4
      - testicular Q55.29
- **Hydatidiform mole** (benign) (complicating pregnancy) (delivered) (undelivered) OØ1.9
  - classical OØ1.Ø
  - complete OØ1.Ø
  - incomplete OØ1.1
  - invasive D39.2
  - malignant D39.2
  - partial OØ1.1
- **Hydatidosis** —*see* Echinococcus
- **Hydradenitis** (axillaris) (suppurative) L73.2
- **Hydradenoma** —*see* Hidradenoma
- **Hydramnios** O4Ø.-●
- **Hydrancephaly, hydranencephaly** QØ4.3
  - with spina bifida —*see* Spina bifida, with hydrocephalus
- **Hydrargyrism NEC** —*see* Poisoning, mercury
- **Hydrarthrosis** —*see also* Effusion, joint
  - gonococcal A54.42
  - intermittent M12.4Ø
    - ankle M12.47-●
    - elbow M12.42-●
    - foot joint M12.47-●
    - hand joint M12.44-●
    - hip M12.45-●
    - knee M12.46-●
    - multiple site M12.49
    - shoulder M12.41-●
    - specified joint NEC M12.48
    - wrist M12.43-●
  - of yaws (early) (late) —*see also* subcategory M14.8-● A66.6
  - syphilitic (late) A52.77
    - congenital A5Ø.55 *[M12.8Ø]*
- **Hydremia** D64.89
- **Hydrencephalocele** (congenital) —*see* Encephalocele
- **Hydrencephalomeningocele** (congenital) —*see* Encephalocele
- **Hydroa** R23.8
  - aestivale L56.4
  - vacciniforme L56.4
- **Hydroadenitis** (axillaris) (suppurative) L73.2
- **Hydrocalycosis** —*see* Hydronephrosis
- **Hydrocele** (spermatic cord) (testis) (tunica vaginalis) N43.3
  - canal of Nuck N94.89
  - communicating N43.2
    - congenital P83.5
  - congenital P83.5
  - encysted N43.Ø
- **Hydrocele** *(Continued)*
  - female NEC N94.89
  - infected N43.1
  - newborn P83.5
  - round ligament N94.89
  - specified NEC N43.2
  - spinalis —*see* Spina bifida
  - vulva N9Ø.89
- **Hydrocephalus** (acquired) (external) (internal) (malignant) (recurrent) G91.9
  - aqueduct Sylvius stricture QØ3.Ø
  - causing disproportion O33.6
    - with obstructed labor O66.3
  - communicating G91.Ø
  - congenital (external) (internal) QØ3.9
    - with spina bifida QØ5.4
      - cervical QØ5.Ø
      - dorsal QØ5.1
      - lumbar QØ5.2
      - lumbosacral QØ5.2
      - sacral QØ5.3
      - thoracic QØ5.1
      - thoracolumbar QØ5.1
    - specified NEC QØ3.8
  - due to toxoplasmosis (congenital) P37.1
  - foramen Magendie block (acquired) G91.1
    - congenital —*see also* Hydrocephalus, congenital QØ3.1
  - in (due to)
    - infectious disease NEC B89 *[G91.4]*
    - neoplastic disease NEC (*see also* Neoplasm) G91.4
    - parasitic disease B89 *[G91.4]*
  - newborn QØ3.9
    - with spina bifida —*see* Spina bifida, with hydrocephalus
  - noncommunicating G91.1
  - normal pressure G91.2
    - secondary G91.Ø
  - obstructive G91.1
  - otitic G93.2
  - post-traumatic NEC G91.3
  - secondary G91.4
    - post-traumatic G91.3
  - specified NEC G91.8
  - syphilitic, congenital A5Ø.49
- **Hydrocolpos** (congenital) N89.8
- **Hydrocystoma** —*see* Neoplasm, skin, benign
- **Hydroencephalocele** (congenital) —*see* Encephalocele
- **Hydroencephalomeningocele** (congenital) —*see* Encephalocele
- **Hydrohematopneumothorax** —*see* Hemothorax
- **Hydromeningitis** —*see* Meningitis
- **Hydromeningocele** (spinal) —*see also* Spina bifida
  - cranial —*see* Encephalocele
- **Hydrometra** N85.8
- **Hydrometrocolpos** N89.8
- **Hydromicrocephaly** QØ2
- **Hydromphalos** (since birth) Q45.8
- **Hydromyelia** QØ6.4
- **Hydromyelocele** —*see* Spina bifida
- **Hydronephrosis** (atrophic) (early) (functionless) (intermittent) (primary) (secondary) NEC N13.3Ø
  - with
    - infection N13.6
    - obstruction (by) (of)
      - renal calculus N13.2
        - with infection N13.6
      - ureteral NEC N13.1
        - with infection N13.6
        - calculus N13.2
          - with infection N13.6
      - ureteropelvic junction (congenital) Q62.11
        - acquired N13.Ø
          - with infection N13.6
    - ureteral stricture NEC N13.1
      - with infection N13.6
  - congenital Q62.Ø
    - due to acquired occlusion of ureteropelvic junction N13.Ø
  - specified type NEC N13.39
  - tuberculous A18.11
- **Hydropericarditis** —*see* Pericarditis
- **Hydropericardium** —*see* Pericarditis
- **Hydroperitoneum** R18.8
- **Hydrophobia** —*see* Rabies
- **Hydrophthalmos** Q15.Ø
- **Hydropneumohemothorax** —*see* Hemothorax
- **Hydropneumopericarditis** —*see* Pericarditis

H

H

- **Hypersecretion** *(Continued)*
  - gastric K31.89
    - psychogenic F45.8
  - gastrin E16.4
  - glucagon E16.3
  - hormone(s)
    - ACTH (not associated with Cushing's syndrome) E27.0
      - pituitary E24.0
    - antidiuretic E22.2
    - growth E22.0
    - intestinal NEC E34.1
    - ovarian androgen E28.1
    - pituitary E22.9
    - testicular E29.0
    - thyroid stimulating E05.80
      - with thyroid storm E05.81
  - insulin —*see* Hyperinsulinism
  - lacrimal glands —*see* Epiphora
  - medulloadrenal E27.5
  - milk O92.6
  - ovarian androgens E28.1
  - salivary gland (any) K11.7
  - thyrocalcitonin E07.0
  - upper respiratory J39.8
- **Hypersegmentation, leukocytic, hereditary** D72.0
- **Hypersensitive, hypersensitiveness, hypersensitivity** —*see also* Allergy
  - carotid sinus G90.01
  - colon —*see* Irritable, colon
  - drug T88.7
  - gastrointestinal K52.29
    - immediate K52.29
    - psychogenic F45.8
  - labyrinth —*see* subcategory H83.2
  - pain R20.8
  - pneumonitis —*see* Pneumonitis, allergic
  - reaction T78.40
    - upper respiratory tract NEC J39.3
- **Hypersomnia** (organic) G47.10
  - due to
    - alcohol
      - abuse F10.182
      - dependence F10.282
      - use F10.982
    - amphetamines
      - abuse F15.182
      - dependence F15.282
      - use F15.982
    - caffeine
      - abuse F15.182
      - dependence F15.282
      - use F15.982
    - cocaine
      - abuse F14.182
      - dependence F14.282
      - use F14.982
    - drug NEC
      - abuse F19.182
      - dependence F19.282
      - use F19.982
    - medical condition G47.14
    - mental disorder F51.13
    - opioid
      - abuse F11.182
      - dependence F11.282
      - use F11.982
    - psychoactive substance NEC
      - abuse F19.182
      - dependence F19.282
      - use F19.982
    - sedative, hypnotic, or anxiolytic
      - abuse F13.182
      - dependence F13.282
      - use F13.982
    - stimulant NEC
      - abuse F15.182
      - dependence F15.282
      - use F15.982
  - idiopathic G47.11
    - with long sleep time G47.11
    - without long sleep time G47.12
  - menstrual related G47.13
  - nonorganic origin F51.11
    - specified NEC F51.19
  - not due to a substance or known physiological condition F51.11
    - specified NEC F51.19
  - primary F51.11
  - recurrent G47.13
  - specified NEC G47.19
- **Hypersplenia, hypersplenism** D73.1
- **Hyperstimulation, ovaries** (associated with induced ovulation) N98.1
- **Hypersusceptibility** —*see* Allergy
- **Hypertelorism** (ocular) (orbital) Q75.2
- **Hypertension, hypertensive** (accelerated) (benign) (essential) (idiopathic) (malignant) (systemic) I10
  - with
    - heart failure (congestive) I11.0
    - heart involvement (conditions in I50.- or I51.4-I51.7, I51.89, I51.9, due to hypertension) —*see* Hypertension, heart
    - kidney involvement —*see* Hypertension, kidney
  - benign, intracranial G93.2
  - borderline R03.0
  - cardiorenal (disease) I13.10
    - with heart failure I13.0
      - with stage 1 through stage 4 chronic kidney disease I13.0
      - with stage 5 or end stage renal disease I13.2
    - without heart failure I13.10
      - with stage 1 through stage 4 chronic kidney disease I13.10
      - with stage 5 or end stage renal disease I13.11
  - cardiovascular
    - disease (arteriosclerotic) (sclerotic) —*see* Hypertension, heart
    - renal (disease) —*see* Hypertension, cardiorenal
  - chronic venous —*see* Hypertension, venous (chronic)
  - complicating
    - childbirth (labor) O16.4
      - pre-existing O10.92
        - with
          - heart disease O10.12
            - with renal disease O10.32
          - pre-eclampsia O11.4
          - renal disease O10.22
            - with heart disease O10.32
        - essential O10.02
        - secondary O10.42
    - pregnancy O16.-●
      - with edema —*see also* Pre-eclampsia O14.9-●
      - gestational (pregnancy induced) (without proteinuria) O13.-●
        - with proteinuria O14.9-●
          - mild pre-eclampsia O14.0-●
          - moderate pre-eclampsia O14.0-●
          - severe pre-eclampsia O14.1-●
            - with hemolysis, elevated liver enzymes and low platelet count (HELLP) O14.2-●
      - pre-existing O10.91-●
        - with
          - heart disease O10.11-●
            - with renal disease O10.31-●
          - pre-eclampsia —*see* category O11
          - renal disease O10.21-●
            - with heart disease O10.31-●
        - essential O10.01-●
        - secondary O10.41-●
      - transient O13.-●
    - puerperium pre-existing O16.5
      - pre-existing
        - with
          - heart disease O10.13
            - with renal disease O10.33
          - pre-eclampsia O11.5
          - renal disease O10.23
            - with heart disease O10.33
        - essential O10.03
      - pregnancy-induced O13.9
      - secondary O10.43
  - crisis I16.9
  - due to
    - endocrine disorders I15.2
    - ➡ pheochromocytoma (*see also* Pheochromocytoma, by type) I15.2
    - renal disorders NEC I15.1
      - arterial I15.0
    - renovascular disorders I15.0
    - specified disease NEC I15.8
  - emergency I16.1
  - encephalopathy I67.4
  - gestational (without significant proteinuria) (pregnancy-induced) (transient) O13.-●
    - with significant proteinuria —*see* Pre-eclampsia
- **Hypertension, hypertensive** *(Continued)*
  - gestational *(Continued)*
    - complicating
      - delivery O13.4
      - puerperium O13.5
  - Goldblatt's I70.1
  - heart (disease) (conditions in I51.4-I51.9 due to hypertension) I11.9
    - with
      - heart failure (congestive) I11.0
      - kidney disease (chronic) —*see* Hypertension, cardiorenal
  - intracranial, benign G93.2
  - kidney I12.9
    - with
      - heart disease —*see* Hypertension, cardiorenal
      - stage 1 through stage 4 chronic kidney disease I12.9
      - stage 5 chronic kidney disease (CKD) or end stage renal disease (ESRD) I12.0
  - lesser circulation I27.0
    - maternal O16.-●
  - newborn P29.2
    - pulmonary (persistent) P29.30
  - ocular H40.05-●
  - pancreatic duct — code to underlying condition
    - with chronic pancreatitis K86.1
  - portal (due to chronic liver disease) (idiopathic) K76.6
    - gastropathy K31.89
    - in (due to) schistosomiasis (bilharziasis) B65.9 *[K77]*
  - postoperative I97.3
  - psychogenic F45.8
  - pulmonary NEC I27.20
    - with
      - cor pulmonale (chronic) I27.29
        - acute I26.09
      - right heart ventricular strain/failure I27.29
        - acute I26.09
      - right to left shunt related to congenital heart disease I27.83
      - unclear multifactorial mechanisms I27.29
    - arterial (associated) (drug-induced) (toxin-induced) I27.21
    - chronic thromboembolic I27.24
    - due to
      - hematologic disorders I27.29
      - kyphoscoliotic heart disease I27.1
      - left heart disease I27.22
      - lung diseases and hypoxia I27.23
      - metabolic disorders I27.29
      - specified systemic disorders NEC I27.29
    - group 1 (associated) (drug-induced) (toxin-induced) I27.21
    - group 2 I27.22
    - group 3 I27.23
    - group 4 I27.24
    - group 5 I27.29
    - of newborn (persistent) P29.30
    - secondary
      - arterial I27.21
      - specified NEC I27.29
    - primary (idiopathic) I27.0
  - renal —*see* Hypertension, kidney
  - renovascular I15.0
  - resistant (apparent treatment) (treatment) (true) I1A.0
  - secondary NEC I15.9
    - due to
      - endocrine disorders I15.2
      - ➡ pheochromocytoma (*see also* Pheochromocytoma, by type) I15.2
      - renal disorders NEC I15.1
        - arterial I15.0
      - renovascular disorders I15.0
    - specified NEC I15.8
  - transient R03.0
    - of pregnancy O13.●
  - urgency I16.0
  - venous (chronic)
    - due to
      - deep vein thrombosis —*see* Syndrome, postthrombotic
    - idiopathic I87.309
      - with
        - inflammation I87.32-●
          - with ulcer I87.33-●
        - specified complication NEC I87.39-●
        - ulcer I87.31-●
          - with inflammation I87.33-●
      - asymptomatic I87.30-●

H

H

H

- **Hypoplasia, hypoplastic** *(Continued)*
  - endocrine (gland) NEC Q89.2
  - endometrium N85.8
  - epididymis (congenital) Q55.4
  - epiglottis Q31.2
  - erythroid, congenital D61.Ø1
  - esophagus (congenital) Q39.8
  - eustachian tube Q17.8
  - eye Q11.2
  - eyelid (congenital) Q1Ø.3
  - face Q18.8
    - bone(s) Q75.8
  - femur (congenital) —*see* Defect, reduction, lower limb, specified type NEC
  - fibula (congenital) —*see* Defect, reduction, lower limb, specified type NEC
  - finger (congenital) —*see* Defect, reduction, upper limb, specified type NEC
  - focal dermal Q82.8
  - foot —*see* Defect, reduction, lower limb, specified type NEC
  - gallbladder Q44.Ø
  - genitalia, genital organ(s)
    - female, congenital Q52.8
      - external Q52.79
      - internal NEC Q52.8
    - in adiposogenital dystrophy E23.6
  - glottis Q31.2
  - hair Q84.2
  - hand (congenital) —*see* Defect, reduction, upper limb, specified type NEC
  - heart Q24.8
  - humerus (congenital) —*see* Defect, reduction, upper limb, specified type NEC
  - intestine (small) Q41.9
    - large Q42.9
      - specified NEC Q42.8
  - jaw M26.Ø9
    - alveolar M26.79
    - lower M26.Ø4
      - alveolar M26.74
    - upper M26.Ø2
      - alveolar M26.73
  - kidney(s) Q6Ø.5
    - bilateral Q6Ø.4
    - unilateral Q6Ø.3
  - labium (majus) (minus), congenital Q52.79
  - larynx Q31.2
  - left heart syndrome Q23.4
  - leg (congenital) —*see* Defect, reduction, lower limb
  - limb Q73.8
    - lower (congenital) —*see* Defect, reduction, lower limb
    - upper (congenital) —*see* Defect, reduction, upper limb
  - liver Q44.79
  - lung (lobe) (not associated with short gestation) Q33.6
    - associated with immaturity, low birth weight, prematurity, or short gestation P28.Ø
  - mammary (areola), congenital Q83.8
  - mandible, mandibular M26.Ø4
    - alveolar M26.74
    - unilateral condylar M27.8
  - maxillary M26.Ø2
    - alveolar M26.73
  - medullary D61.9
  - megakaryocytic D69.49
  - metacarpus —*see* Defect, reduction, upper limb, specified type NEC
  - metatarsus —*see* Defect, reduction, lower limb, specified type NEC
  - muscle Q79.8
  - nail(s) Q84.6
  - nose, nasal Q3Ø.1
  - optic nerve H47.Ø3- ●
  - osseous meatus (ear) Q17.8
  - ovary, congenital Q5Ø.39
  - pancreas Q45.Ø
  - parathyroid (gland) Q89.2
  - parotid gland Q38.4
  - patella Q74.1
  - pelvis, pelvic girdle Q74.2
  - penis (congenital) Q55.62
  - peripheral vascular system Q27.8
    - digestive system Q27.8
    - lower limb Q27.8
    - specified site NEC Q27.8
    - upper limb Q27.8
  - pituitary (gland) (congenital) Q89.2
  - pulmonary (not associated with short gestation) Q33.6
    - artery, functional J43.Ø
    - associated with short gestation P28.Ø
  - radioulnar —*see* Defect, reduction, upper limb, specified type NEC
  - radius —*see* Defect, reduction, upper limb
  - rectum Q42.1
    - with fistula Q42.Ø
  - respiratory system NEC Q34.8
  - rib Q76.6
  - right heart syndrome Q22.6
  - sacrum Q76.49
  - scapula Q74.Ø
  - scrotum Q55.1
  - shoulder girdle Q74.Ø
  - skin Q82.8
  - skull (bone) Q75.8
    - with
      - anencephaly QØØ.Ø
      - encephalocele —*see* Encephalocele
      - hydrocephalus QØ3.9
        - with spina bifida —*see* Spina bifida, by site, with hydrocephalus
      - microcephaly QØ2
  - spinal (cord) (ventral horn cell) QØ6.1
  - spine Q76.49
  - sternum Q76.7
  - tarsus —*see* Defect, reduction, lower limb, specified type NEC
  - testis Q55.1
  - thymic, with immunodeficiency D82.1
  - thymus (gland) Q89.2
    - with immunodeficiency D82.1
  - thyroid (gland) EØ3.1
    - cartilage Q31.2
  - tibiofibular (congenital) —*see* Defect, reduction, lower limb, specified type NEC
  - toe —*see* Defect, reduction, lower limb, specified type NEC
  - tongue Q38.3
  - Turner's KØØ.4
  - ulna (congenital) —*see* Defect, reduction, upper limb
  - umbilical artery Q27.Ø
  - unilateral condylar M27.8
  - ureter Q62.8
  - uterus, congenital Q51.811
  - vagina Q52.4
  - vascular NEC peripheral Q27.8
    - brain Q28.3
    - digestive system Q27.8
    - lower limb Q27.8
    - specified site NEC Q27.8
    - upper limb Q27.8
  - vein(s) (peripheral) Q27.8
    - brain Q28.3
    - digestive system Q27.8
    - great Q26.8
    - lower limb Q27.8
    - specified site NEC Q27.8
    - upper limb Q27.8
  - vena cava (inferior) (superior) Q26.8
  - vertebra Q76.49
  - vulva, congenital Q52.79
  - zonule (ciliary) Q12.8
- **Hypoplasminogenemia** E88.Ø2
- **Hypopnea, obstructive sleep apnea** G47.33
- **Hypopotassemia** E87.6
- **Hypoproconvertinemia, congenital** (hereditary) D68.2
- **Hypoproteinemia** E77.8
- **Hypoprothrombinemia** (congenital) (hereditary) (idiopathic) D68.2
  - acquired D68.4
  - newborn, transient P61.6
- **Hypoptyalism** K11.7
- **Hypopyon** (eye) (anterior chamber) —*see* Iridocyclitis, acute, hypopyon
- **Hypopyrexia** R68.Ø
- **Hyporeflexia** R29.2
- **Hyposecretion**
  - ACTH E23.Ø
  - antidiuretic hormone E23.2
  - ovary E28.39
  - salivary gland (any) K11.7
  - vasopressin E23.2
- **Hyposegmentation, leukocytic, hereditary** D72.Ø
- **Hyposiderinemia** D5Ø.9
- **Hypospadias** Q54.9
  - balanic Q54.Ø
  - coronal Q54.Ø
  - glandular Q54.Ø
  - penile Q54.1
  - penoscrotal Q54.2
  - perineal Q54.3
  - specified NEC Q54.8
- **Hypospermatogenesis** —*see* Oligospermia
- **Hyposplenism** D73.Ø
- **Hypostasis pulmonary, passive** —*see* Edema, lung
- **Hypostatic** —*see* condition
- **Hyposthenuria** N28.89
- **Hypotension** (arterial) (constitutional) I95.9
  - chronic I95.89
  - drug-induced I95.2
  - due to (of) hemodialysis I95.3
  - iatrogenic I95.89
  - idiopathic (permanent) I95.Ø
  - intracranial G96.81Ø
    - following
      - lumbar cerebrospinal fluid shunting G97.83
      - specified procedure NEC G97.84
      - ventricular shunting (ventriculostomy) G97.2
    - specified NEC G96.819
    - spontaneous G96.811
- **Hypothermia** (accidental) T68
  - intra-dialytic I95.3
  - maternal, syndrome (following labor and delivery) O26.5- ●
  - neurogenic, orthostatic G9Ø.3
  - orthostatic (chronic) I95.1
    - due to drugs I95.2
    - neurogenic G9Ø.3
  - postoperative I95.81
  - postural I95.1
  - specified NEC I95.89
  - due to anesthesia, anesthetic T88.51
  - low environmental temperature T68
  - neonatal P8Ø.9
    - environmental (mild) NEC P8Ø.8
    - mild P8Ø.8
    - severe (chronic) (cold injury syndrome) P8Ø.Ø
    - specified NEC P8Ø.8
  - not associated with low environmental temperature R68.Ø
- **Hypothyroidism** (acquired) EØ3.9
  - autoimmune —*see* Thyroiditis, autoimmune
  - congenital (without goiter) EØ3.1
    - with goiter (diffuse) EØ3.Ø
  - due to
    - exogenous substance NEC EØ3.2
    - iodine-deficiency, acquired EØ1.8
      - subclinical EØ2
    - irradiation therapy E89.Ø
    - medicament NEC EØ3.2
    - P-aminosalicylic acid (PAS) EØ3.2
    - phenylbutazone EØ3.2
    - resorcinol EØ3.2
    - sulfonamide EØ3.2
    - surgery E89.Ø
    - thiourea group drugs EØ3.2
  - iatrogenic NEC EØ3.2
  - iodine-deficiency (acquired) EØ1.8
    - congenital —*see* Syndrome, iodine-deficiency, congenital
    - subclinical EØ2
  - neonatal, transitory P72.2
  - postinfectious EØ3.3
  - postirradiation E89.Ø
  - postprocedural E89.Ø
  - postsurgical E89.Ø
  - specified NEC EØ3.8
  - subclinical, iodine-deficiency related EØ2
- **Hypotonia, hypotonicity, hypotony**
  - bladder N31.2
  - congenital (benign) P94.2
  - eye —*see* Disorder, globe, hypotony
- **Hypotrichosis** —*see* Alopecia
- **Hypotropia** H5Ø.2- ●
- **Hypoventilation** RØ6.89
  - congenital central alveolar G47.35
  - sleep related
    - idiopathic nonobstructive alveolar G47.34
    - in conditions classified elsewhere G47.36
- **Hypovitaminosis** —*see* Deficiency, vitamin
- **Hypovolemia** E86.1
  - surgical shock T81.19
  - traumatic (shock) T79.4

Hypoxemia R09.Ø2
- newborn P84
- sleep related, in conditions classified elsewhere G47.36

Hypoxia —*see also* Anoxia R09.Ø2
- cerebral, during a procedure NEC G97.81
  - postprocedural NEC G97.82
- intrauterine P84
- myocardial —*see* Insufficiency, coronary
- newborn P84
- sleep-related G47.34

~~Hypsarhythmia —see Epilepsy, generalized, specified NEC~~

▶ **Hypsarrhythmia** —*see* Epilepsy, generalized, specified NEC

Hysteralgia, pregnant uterus O26.89-●

Hysteria, hysterical (conversion) (dissociative state) F44.9
- anxiety F41.8
- convulsions F44.5
- psychosis, acute F44.9

Hysteroepilepsy F44.5

I

IBDU (colonic inflammatory bowel dissease unclassified) K52.3

ICANS (immune effector cell-associated neurotoxicity syndrome) —see Syndrome, immune effector cell-associated neurotoxicity

Ichthyoparasitism due to Vandellia cirrhosa B88.8

Ichthyosis (congenital) Q8Ø.9
- acquired L85.Ø
- fetalis Q8Ø.4
- hystrix Q8Ø.8
- lamellar Q8Ø.2
- lingual K13.29
- palmaris and plantaris Q82.8
- simplex Q8Ø.Ø
- vera Q8Ø.8
- vulgaris Q8Ø.Ø
- X-linked Q8Ø.1

Ichthyotoxism —*see* Poisoning, fish
- bacterial —*see* Intoxication, foodborne

Icteroanemia, hemolytic (acquired) D59.9
- congenital —*see* Spherocytosis

Icterus —*see also* Jaundice
- conjunctiva R17
- gravis, newborn P55.Ø
- hematogenous (acquired) D59.9
- hemolytic (acquired) D59.9
  - congenital —*see* Spherocytosis
- hemorrhagic (acute) (leptospiral) (spirochetal) A27.Ø
  - newborn P53
- infectious B15.9
  - with hepatic coma B15.Ø
  - leptospiral A27.Ø
  - spirochetal A27.Ø
- neonatorum —*see* Jaundice, newborn
- newborn P59.9
- spirochetal A27.Ø

Ictus solaris, solis T67.Ø1

Ideation
- homicidal R45.85Ø
- suicidal R45.851

Identity disorder (child) F64.9
- gender role F64.2
- psychosexual F64.2

Idioglossia F8Ø.Ø

Idiopathic —*see* condition

Idiot, idiocy (congenital) F73
- amaurotic (Bielschowsky(-Jansky)) (family) (infantile (late)) (juvenile (late)) (Vogt-Spielmeyer) E75.4
- microcephalic QØ2

Id reaction (due to bacteria) L3Ø.2

IgE asthma J45.909

IIAC (idiopathic infantile arterial calcification) Q28.8

Ileitis (chronic) (noninfectious) —*see also* Enteritis K52.9
- backwash —*see* Pancolitis, ulcerative (chronic)
- infectious AØ9
- regional (ulcerative) —*see* Enteritis, regional, small intestine
- segmental —*see* Enteritis, regional
- terminal (ulcerative) —*see* Enteritis, regional, small intestine

Ileocolitis —*see also* Enteritis K52.9
- infectious AØ9
- regional —*see* Enteritis, regional
- ulcerative K51.Ø-●

Ileostomy
- attention to Z43.2
- malfunctioning K94.13
- ➡ status (ileal pouch) (Kock pouch) Z93.2
  - with complication —*see* Complications, enterostomy

Ileotyphus —*see* Typhoid

Ileum —*see* condition

Ileus (bowel) (colon) (inhibitory) (intestine) K56.7
- adynamic K56.Ø
- due to gallstone (in intestine) K56.3
- duodenal (chronic) K31.5
- gallstone K56.3
- mechanical NEC —*see also* Obstruction, intestine, specified K56.699
- meconium P76.Ø
  - in cystic fibrosis E84.11
  - meaning meconium plug (without cystic fibrosis) P76.Ø
- myxedema K59.89
- neurogenic K56.Ø
  - Hirschsprung's disease or megacolon Q43.1
- newborn
  - due to meconium P76.Ø
    - in cystic fibrosis E84.11
    - meaning meconium plug (without cystic fibrosis) P76.Ø
  - transitory P76.1
- obstructive —*see also* Obstruction, intestine, specified K56.699
- paralytic K56.Ø
- postoperative K91.89

Iliac —*see* condition

Iliotibial band syndrome M76.3-●

Illiteracy Z55.Ø
- health Z55.6

Illness—*see also* Disease R69
- manic-depressive —*see* Disorder, bipolar

Imbalance R26.89
- ➡ autonomic G9Ø.89
- constituents of food intake E63.1
- electrolyte E87.8
  - with
    - abortion —*see* Abortion by type, complicated by, electrolyte imbalance
    - molar pregnancy OØ8.5
  - due to hyperemesis gravidarum O21.1
  - following ectopic or molar pregnancy OØ8.5
  - neonatal, transitory NEC P74.49
    - potassium
      - hyperkalemia P74.31
      - hypokalemia P74.32
    - sodium
      - hypernatremia P74.21
      - hyponatremia P74.22
- endocrine E34.9
- eye muscle NOS H5Ø.9
- hormone E34.9
- hysterical F44.4
- labyrinth —*see* subcategory H83.2
- posture R29.3
- protein-energy —*see* Malnutrition
- ➡ sympathetic G9Ø.89

Imbecile, imbecility (I.Q. 35-49) F71

Imbedding, intrauterine device T83.39

Imbibition, cholesterol (gallbladder) K82.4

Imbrication, teeth, fully erupted M26.3Ø

Imerslund (-Gräsbeck) **syndrome** D51.1

Immature —*see also* Immaturity
- birth (less than 37 completed weeks) —*see* Preterm, newborn
  - extremely (less than 28 completed weeks) —*see* Immaturity, extreme
- personality F6Ø.89

Immaturity (less than 37 completed weeks) —*see also* Preterm, newborn
- extreme of newborn (less than 28 completed weeks of gestation) (less than 196 completed days of gestation) (unspecified weeks of gestation) PØ7.2Ø
  - gestational age
    - 23 completed weeks (23 weeks, Ø days through 23 weeks, 6 days) PØ7.22
    - 24 completed weeks (24 weeks, Ø days through 24 weeks, 6 days) PØ7.23
    - 25 completed weeks (25 weeks, Ø days through 25 weeks, 6 days) PØ7.24
    - 26 completed weeks (26 weeks, Ø days through 26 weeks, 6 days) PØ7.25
    - 27 completed weeks (27 weeks, Ø days through 27 weeks, 6 days) PØ7.26
    - less than 23 completed weeks PØ7.21
- fetus or infant light-for-dates —*see* Light-for-dates
- lung, newborn P28.Ø
- organ or site NEC —*see* Hypoplasia
- pulmonary, newborn P28.Ø
- reaction F6Ø.89
- sexual (female) (male), after puberty E3Ø.Ø

Immersion T75.1
- foot T69.Ø2-●
- hand T69.Ø1-●

Immobile, immobility
- complete, due to severe physical disability or frailty R53.2
- intestine K59.89
- syndrome (paraplegic) M62.3

Immune reconstitution (inflammatory) **syndrome [IRIS]** D89.3

Immunization —*see also* Vaccination
- ABO —*see* Incompatibility, ABO
  - in newborn P55.1
- appropriate for age
  - child (over 28 days old) ZØØ.129
    - with abnormal findings ZØØ.121
- complication —*see* Complications, vaccination
- encounter for Z23
- not done (not carried out) Z28.9
  - because (of)
    - acute illness of patient Z28.Ø1
    - allergy to vaccine (or component) Z28.Ø4
    - caregiver refusal Z28.82
    - chronic illness of patient Z28.Ø2
    - contraindication NEC Z28.Ø9
    - delay in delivery of vaccine Z28.83
    - group pressure Z28.1
    - guardian refusal Z28.82
    - immune compromised state of patient Z28.Ø3
    - lack of availability of vaccine Z28.83
    - manufacturer delay of vaccine Z28.83
    - parent refusal Z28.82
    - patient's belief Z28.1
    - patient had disease being vaccinated against Z28.81
    - patient refusal Z28.21
    - religious beliefs of patient Z28.1
    - specified reason NEC Z28.89
      - of patient Z28.29
    - unavailability of vaccine Z28.83
    - unspecified patient reason Z28.2Ø
- Rh factor
  - affecting management of pregnancy NEC O36.Ø9-●
    - anti-D antibody O36.Ø1-●
  - from transfusion —*see* Complication(s), transfusion, incompatibility reaction, Rh (factor)

Immunocompromised NOS D84.9

Immunocytoma C83.Ø-●

New Revised ~~deleted~~ Deleted • Use Additional Character(s)

Implantation *(Continued)*
- cyst *(Continued)*
  - vagina N89.8
  - vulva N9Ø.7
- dermoid (cyst) —*see* Implantation, cyst

Impotence (sexual) N52.9
- counseling Z7Ø.1
- organic origin —*see also* Dysfunction, sexual, male, erectile N52.9
- psychogenic F52.21

Impression, basilar Q75.8

Imprisonment, anxiety concerning Z65.1

Improper care (child) (newborn) —*see* Maltreatment

Improperly tied umbilical cord (causing hemorrhage) P51.8

Impulsiveness (impulsive) R45.87

Inability to
- comply with dietary regimen Z91.118
- swallow - see Aphagia

Inaccessible, inaccessibility
- health care NEC Z75.3
  - due to
    - waiting period Z75.2
      - for admission to facility elsewhere Z75.1
- other helping agencies Z75.4
- transportation Z59.82

Inactive —*see* condition

Inadequate, inadequacy
- aesthetics of dental restoration KØ8.56
- biologic, constitutional, functional, or social F6Ø.7
- development
  - child R62.5Ø
  - genitalia
    - after puberty NEC E3Ø.Ø
    - congenital
      - female Q52.8
        - external Q52.79
        - internal Q52.8
      - male Q55.8
  - lungs Q33.6
    - associated with short gestation P28.Ø
  - organ or site not listed —*see* Anomaly, by site
- diet (causing nutritional deficiency) E63.9
- drinking-water supply Z58.6
- eating habits Z72.4
- environment, household Z59.11
- family support Z63.8
- food (supply) NEC Z59.48
  - hunger effects T73.Ø
- functional F6Ø.7
- household care, due to
  - family member
    - handicapped or ill Z74.2
    - on vacation Z75.5
    - temporarily away from home Z74.2
  - technical defects in home Z59.19
  - temporary absence from home of person rendering care Z74.2
- housing Z59.1Ø
- environmental temperature Z59.11
- heating Z59.11
- space Z59.19
- specified NEC Z59.19
- utilities Z59.12
- income (financial) Z59.6
- intrafamilial communication Z63.8
- material resources due to limited financial resources, specified NEC Z59.87
- mental —*see* Disability, intellectual
- parental supervision or control of child Z62.Ø
- personality F6Ø.7
- pulmonary
  - function RØ6.89
    - newborn P28.5
  - ventilation, newborn P28.5
- sample of cytologic smear
  - anus R85.615
  - cervix R87.615
  - vagina R87.625
- social F6Ø.7
  - insurance Z59.71
  - skills NEC Z73.4
- social support Z6Ø.8
- supervision of child by parent Z62.Ø
- teaching affecting education Z55.8
- transportation Z59.82
- welfare support Z59.72

Inanition R64
- with edema —*see* Malnutrition, severe
- due to
  - deprivation of food T73.Ø
  - malnutrition —*see* Malnutrition
- fever R5Ø.9

Inappropriate
- change in quantitative human chorionic gonadotropin (hCG) in early pregnancy OØ2.81
- diet or eating habits Z72.4
- level of quantitative human chorionic gonadotropin (hCG) for gestational age in early pregnancy OØ2.81
- secretion
  - antidiuretic hormone (ADH) (excessive) E22.2
    - deficiency E23.2
  - pituitary (posterior) E22.2
- sinus tachycardia, so stated (IST) I47.11

Inattention at or after birth —*see* Neglect

Incarceration, incarcerated
- enterocele K46.Ø
  - gangrenous K46.1
- epiplocele K46.Ø
  - gangrenous K46.1
- exomphalos K42.Ø
  - gangrenous K42.1
- hernia —*see also* Hernia, by site, with obstruction
  - with gangrene —*see* Hernia, by site, with gangrene
- iris, in wound —*see* Injury, eye, laceration, with prolapse
- lens, in wound —*see* Injury, eye, laceration, with prolapse
- omphalocele K42.Ø
- prison, anxiety concerning Z65.1
- rupture —*see* Hernia, by site
- sarcoepiplocele K46.Ø
  - gangrenous K46.1
- sarcoepiplomphalocele K42.Ø
  - with gangrene K42.1
- uterus N85.8
  - gravid O34.51-●
    - causing obstructed labor O65.5

Incised wound
- external —*see* Laceration
- internal organs —*see* Injury, by site

Incision, incisional
- hernia K43.2
  - with
    - gangrene (and obstruction) K43.1
    - obstruction K43.Ø
- surgical, complication —*see* Complications, surgical procedure
- traumatic
  - external —*see* Laceration
  - internal organs —*see* Injury, by site

Inclusion
- azurophilic leukocytic D72.Ø
- blennorrhea (neonatal) (newborn) P39.1
- gallbladder in liver (congenital) Q44.1

Incompatibility
- ABO
  - affecting management of pregnancy O36.11-●
    - anti-A sensitization O36.11-●
    - anti-B sensitization O36.19-●
    - specified NEC O36.19-●
  - infusion or transfusion reaction —*see* Complication(s), transfusion, incompatibility reaction, ABO
  - newborn P55.1
- blood (group) (Duffy) (K) (Kell) (Kidd) (Lewis) (M) (S) NEC
  - affecting management of pregnancy O36.11-●
    - anti-A sensitization O36.11-●
    - anti-B sensitization O36.19-●
  - infusion or transfusion reaction T8Ø.89
  - newborn P55.8
- divorce or estrangement Z63.5
- Rh (blood group) (factor) Z31.82
  - affecting management of pregnancy NEC O36.Ø9-●
    - anti-D antibody O36.Ø1-●
  - infusion or transfusion reaction —*see* Complication(s), transfusion, incompatibility reaction, Rh (factor)
  - newborn P55.Ø
- rhesus —*see* Incompatibility, Rh

Incompetency, incompetent, incompetence
- annular
  - aortic (valve) —*see* Insufficiency, aortic
  - mitral (valve) I34.Ø
  - pulmonary valve (heart) I37.1
- aortic (valve) —*see* Insufficiency, aortic
- cardiac valve —*see* Endocarditis
- cervix, cervical (os) N88.3
  - in pregnancy O34.3-●
- chronotropic I45.89
  - with
    - autonomic dysfunction G9Ø.89
    - ischemic heart disease I25.89
    - left ventricular dysfunction I51.89
    - sinus node dysfunction I49.8
- esophagogastric (junction) (sphincter) K22.Ø
- mitral (valve) —*see* Insufficiency, mitral
- pelvic fundus N81.89
- pubocervical tissue N81.82
- pulmonary valve (heart) I37.1
  - congenital Q22.3
- rectovaginal tissue N81.83
- tricuspid (annular) (valve) —*see* Insufficiency, tricuspid
- valvular —*see* Endocarditis
  - congenital Q24.8
- vein, venous (saphenous) (varicose) —*see* Varix, leg

Incomplete —*see also* condition
- atrioventricular
  - canal Q21.21
  - septal defect Q21.21
- bladder, emptying R33.9
- defecation R15.Ø
- endocardial cushion defect Q21.21
- expansion lungs (newborn) NEC —*see* Atelectasis
- rotation, intestine Q43.3

Inconclusive
- diagnostic imaging due to excess body fat of patient R93.9
- findings on diagnostic imaging of breast NEC R92.8
- mammogram R92.2

Incontinence R32
- anal sphincter R15.9
- coital N39.491
- feces R15.9
  - nonorganic origin F98.1
- insensible (urinary) N39.42
- overflow N39.49Ø
- postural (urinary) N39.492
- psychogenic F45.8
- rectal R15.9
- reflex N39.498
- stress (female) (male) N39.3
  - and urge N39.46
- urethral sphincter R32
- urge N39.41
  - and stress (female) (male) N39.46
- urine (urinary) R32
  - continuous N39.45
  - due to cognitive impairment, or severe physical disability or immobility R39.81
  - functional R39.81
  - insensible N39.42
  - mixed (stress and urge) N39.46
  - nocturnal N39.44
  - nonorganic origin F98.Ø
  - overflow N39.49Ø
  - post dribbling N39.43
  - postural N39.492
  - reflex N39.498
  - specified NEC N39.498
  - stress (female) (male) N39.3
    - and urge N39.46
  - total N39.498
  - unaware N39.42
  - urge N39.41
    - and stress (female) (male) N39.46

Incontinentia pigmenti Q82.3

Incoordinate, incoordination
- esophageal-pharyngeal (newborn) —*see* Dysphagia
- muscular R27.8
- uterus (action) (contractions) (complicating delivery) O62.4

Increase, increased
- abnormal, in development R63.8
- androgens (ovarian) E28.1

▶ New ➡ Revised ~~deleted~~ Deleted ● Use Additional Character(s)

- Injury *(Continued)*
  - genital organ(s) *(Continued)*
    - internal *(Continued)*
      - prostate —*see* Injury, prostate
      - seminal vesicle —*see* Injury, pelvis, organ, specified site NEC
      - uterus —*see* Injury, uterus
      - vas deferens —*see* Injury, pelvis, organ, specified site NEC
    - obstetrical trauma O71.9
  - gland
    - lacrimal laceration —*see* Injury, eye, specified site NEC
    - salivary SØ9.93
    - thyroid NEC S19.84
  - globe (eye) SØ5.9Ø
    - specified NEC SØ5.8X- •
  - groin —*see* Injury, abdomen
  - gum SØ9.9Ø
  - hand S69.9- •
    - blood vessel —*see* Injury, blood vessel, hand
    - contusion —*see* Contusion, hand
    - fracture —*see* Fracture, hand
    - muscle —*see* Injury, muscle, hand
    - nerve —*see* Injury, nerve, hand
    - open —*see* Wound, open, hand
    - specified NEC S69.8- •
    - sprain —*see* Sprain, hand
    - superficial —*see* Injury, superficial, hand
  - head SØ9.9Ø
    - with loss of consciousness SØ6.9- •
    - specified NEC SØ9.8- •
  - heart (traumatic) S26.9Ø
    - with hemopericardium S26.ØØ
      - contusion S26.Ø1
      - laceration (mild) S26.Ø2Ø
        - major S26.Ø22
        - moderate S26.Ø21
      - specified type NEC S26.Ø9
    - without hemopericardium S26.1Ø
      - contusion S26.11
      - laceration S26.12
      - specified type NEC S26.19
    - contusion S26.91
    - laceration S26.92
    - non-traumatic (acute) (chronic) (non-ischemic) I5A
    - specified type NEC S26.99
  - heel —*see* Injury, foot
  - hepatic
    - artery —*see* Injury, blood vessel, celiac artery, branch
    - duct —*see* Injury, liver
    - vein —*see* Injury, vena cava, inferior
  - hip S79.91- •
    - blood vessel —*see* Injury, blood vessel, hip
    - contusion —*see* Contusion, hip
    - dislocation —*see* Dislocation, hip
    - fracture —*see* Fracture, femur, neck
    - muscle —*see* Injury, muscle, hip
    - nerve —*see* Injury, nerve, hip
    - open —*see* Wound, open, hip
    - specified NEC S79.81- •
    - sprain —*see* Sprain, hip
    - superficial —*see* Injury, superficial, hip
  - hymen S39.94
  - hypogastric
    - blood vessel —*see* Injury, blood vessel, iliac
    - plexus —*see* Injury, nerve, lumbosacral, sympathetic
  - ileum —*see* Injury, intestine, small
  - iliac region S39.91
  - instrumental (during surgery) —*see* Laceration, accidental complicating surgery
    - birth injury —*see* Birth, injury
    - nonsurgical —*see* Injury, by site
    - obstetrical O71.9
      - bladder O71.5
      - cervix O71.3
      - high vaginal O71.4
      - perineal NOS O7Ø.9
      - urethra O71.5
      - uterus O71.5
        - with rupture or perforation O71.1
  - internal T14.8
    - aorta —*see* Injury, aorta
    - bladder (sphincter) —*see* Injury, bladder
      - with
        - ectopic or molar pregnancy OØ8.6
      - following ectopic or molar pregnancy OØ8.6
      - obstetrical trauma O71.5

- Injury *(Continued)*
  - internal *(Continued)*
    - bronchus, bronchi —*see* Injury, intrathoracic, bronchus
    - cecum —*see* Injury, intestine, large
    - cervix (uteri) —*see also* Injury, uterus
      - with ectopic or molar pregnancy OØ8.6
      - following ectopic or molar pregnancy OØ8.6
      - obstetrical trauma O71.3
    - chest —*see* Injury, intrathoracic
    - gastrointestinal tract —*see* Injury, intra-abdominal
    - heart —*see* Injury, heart
    - intestine NEC —*see* Injury, intestine
    - intrauterine —*see* Injury, uterus
    - mesentery —*see* Injury, intra-abdominal, specified, site NEC
    - pelvis, pelvic (organ) S37.9Ø
      - following ectopic or molar pregnancy (subsequent episode) OØ8.6
      - obstetrical trauma NEC O71.5
        - rupture or perforation O71.1
      - specified NEC S39.83
    - rectum —*see* Injury, intestine, large, rectum
    - stomach —*see* Injury, stomach
    - ureter —*see* Injury, ureter
    - urethra (sphincter) following ectopic or molar pregnancy OØ8.6
    - uterus —*see* Injury, uterus
  - interscapular area —*see* Injury, thorax
  - intestine
    - large S36.5Ø9
      - ascending (right) S36.5ØØ
        - blast injury (primary) S36.51Ø
          - secondary S36.59Ø
        - contusion S36.52Ø
        - laceration S36.53Ø
        - specified type NEC S36.59Ø
      - blast injury (primary) S36.519
        - ascending (right) S36.51Ø
        - descending (left) S36.512
        - rectum S36.61
        - sigmoid S36.513
        - specified site NEC S36.518
        - transverse S36.511
      - contusion S36.529
        - ascending (right) S36.52Ø
        - descending (left) S36.522
        - rectum S36.62
        - sigmoid S36.523
        - specified site NEC S36.528
        - transverse S36.521
      - descending (left) S36.5Ø2
        - blast injury (primary) S36.512
          - secondary S36.592
        - contusion S36.522
        - laceration S36.532
        - specified type NEC S36.592
      - laceration S36.539
        - ascending (right) S36.53Ø
        - descending (left) S36.532
        - rectum S36.63
        - sigmoid S36.533
        - specified site NEC S36.538
        - transverse S36.531
      - rectum S36.6Ø
        - blast injury (primary) S36.61
          - secondary S36.69
        - contusion S36.62
        - laceration S36.63
        - specified type NEC S36.69
      - sigmoid S36.5Ø3
        - blast injury (primary) S36.513
          - secondary S36.593
        - contusion S36.523
        - laceration S36.533
        - specified type NEC S36.593
      - specified
        - site NEC S36.5Ø8
          - blast injury (primary) S36.518
            - secondary S36.598
          - contusion S36.528
          - laceration S36.538
          - specified type NEC S36.598
        - type NEC S36.599
          - ascending (right) S36.59Ø
          - descending (left) S36.592
          - rectum S36.69
          - sigmoid S36.593

- Injury *(Continued)*
  - intestine *(Continued)*
    - large *(Continued)*
      - specified *(Continued)*
        - type *(Continued)*
          - specified site NEC S36.598
          - transverse S36.591
      - transverse S36.5Ø1
        - blast injury (primary) S36.511
          - secondary S36.591
        - contusion S36.521
        - laceration S36.531
        - specified type NEC S36.591
    - small S36.4Ø9
      - blast injury (primary) S36.419
        - duodenum S36.41Ø
        - secondary S36.499
          - duodenum S36.49Ø
          - specified site NEC S36.498
        - specified site NEC S36.418
      - contusion S36.429
        - duodenum S36.42Ø
        - specified site NEC S36.428
      - duodenum S36.4ØØ
        - blast injury (primary) S36.41Ø
          - secondary S36.49Ø
        - contusion S36.42Ø
        - laceration S36.43Ø
        - specified NEC S36.49Ø
      - laceration S36.439
        - duodenum S36.43Ø
        - specified site NEC S36.438
      - specified
        - site NEC S36.4Ø8
        - type NEC S36.499
          - duodenum S36.49Ø
          - specified site NEC S36.498
  - intra-abdominal S36.9Ø
    - adrenal gland —*see* Injury, adrenal gland
    - bladder —*see* Injury, bladder
    - colon —*see* Injury, intestine, large
    - contusion S36.92
    - fallopian tube —*see* Injury, fallopian tube
    - gallbladder —*see* Injury, gallbladder
    - intestine —*see* Injury, intestine
    - kidney —*see* Injury, kidney
    - laceration S36.93
    - liver —*see* Injury, liver
    - ovary —*see* Injury, ovary
    - pancreas —*see* Injury, pancreas
    - pelvic NOS S37.9Ø
    - peritoneum —*see* Injury, intra-abdominal, specified, site NEC
    - prostate —*see* Injury, prostate
    - rectum —*see* Injury, intestine, large, rectum
    - retroperitoneum —*see* Injury, intra-abdominal, specified, site NEC
    - seminal vesicle —*see* Injury, pelvis, organ, specified site NEC
    - small intestine —*see* Injury, intestine, small
    - specified
      - pelvic S37.9Ø
        - specified
          - site NEC S37.899
            - specified type NEC S37.898
          - type NEC S37.99
      - site NEC S36.899
        - contusion S36.892
        - laceration S36.893
        - specified type NEC S36.898
      - type NEC S36.99
    - spleen —*see* Injury, spleen
    - stomach —*see* Injury, stomach
    - ureter —*see* Injury, ureter
    - urethra —*see* Injury, urethra
    - uterus —*see* Injury, uterus
    - vas deferens —*see* Injury, pelvis, organ, specified site NEC
  - intracranial (traumatic) (*see also*, if applicable, Compression, brain, traumatic) SØ6.9- •
    - cerebellar hemorrhage, traumatic —*see* Injury, intracranial, focal
    - cerebral edema, traumatic SØ6.1X- •
      - diffuse SØ6.1X- •
      - focal SØ6.1X- •
    - diffuse (axonal) SØ6.2X- •
    - epidural hemorrhage (traumatic) SØ6.4X- •
    - focal brain injury SØ6.3Ø- •
      - contusion —*see* Contusion, cerebral
      - laceration —*see* Laceration, cerebral

- Injury *(Continued)*
  - nerve NEC T14.8
    - abdomen S34.9
      - peripheral S34.6
      - specified site NEC S34.8
    - abducens S04.4-●
      - contusion S04.4-●
      - laceration S04.4-●
      - specified type NEC S04.4-●
    - abducent —*see* Injury, nerve, abducens
    - accessory S04.7-●
      - contusion S04.7-●
      - laceration S04.7-●
      - specified type NEC S04.7-●
    - acoustic S04.6-●
      - contusion S04.6-●
      - laceration S04.6-●
      - specified type NEC S04.6-●
    - ankle S94.9-●
      - cutaneous sensory S94.3-●
      - specified site NEC —*see* subcategory S94.8
    - anterior crural, femoral —*see* Injury, nerve, femoral
    - arm (upper) S44.9-●
      - axillary —*see* Injury, nerve, axillary
      - cutaneous —*see* Injury, nerve, cutaneous, arm
      - median —*see* Injury, nerve, median, upper arm
      - musculocutaneous —*see* Injury, nerve, musculocutaneous
      - radial —*see* Injury, nerve, radial, upper arm
      - specified site NEC —*see* subcategory S44.8
      - ulnar —*see* Injury, nerve, ulnar, arm
    - auditory —*see* Injury, nerve, acoustic
    - axillary S44.3-●
    - brachial plexus —*see* Injury, brachial plexus
    - cervical sympathetic S14.5
    - cranial S04.9
      - contusion S04.9
      - eighth (acoustic or auditory) —*see* Injury, nerve, acoustic
      - eleventh (accessory) —*see* Injury, nerve, accessory
      - fifth (trigeminal) —*see* Injury, nerve, trigeminal
      - first (olfactory) —*see* Injury, nerve, olfactory
      - fourth (trochlear) —*see* Injury, nerve, trochlear
      - laceration S04.9
      - ninth (glossopharyngeal) —*see* Injury, nerve, glossopharyngeal
      - second (optic) —*see* Injury, nerve, optic
      - seventh (facial) —*see* Injury, nerve, facial
      - sixth (abducent) —*see* Injury, nerve, abducens
      - specified
        - nerve NEC S04.89-●
          - contusion S04.89-●
          - laceration S04.89-●
          - specified type NEC S04.89-●
        - type NEC S04.9
      - tenth (pneumogastric or vagus) —*see* Injury, nerve, vagus
      - third (oculomotor) —*see* Injury, nerve, oculomotor
      - twelfth (hypoglossal) —*see* Injury, nerve, hypoglossal
    - cutaneous sensory
      - ankle (level) S94.3-●
      - arm (upper) (level) S44.5-●
      - foot (level) —*see* Injury, nerve, cutaneous sensory, ankle
      - forearm (level) S54.3-●
      - hip (level) S74.2-●
      - leg (lower level) S84.2-●
      - shoulder (level) —*see* Injury, nerve, cutaneous sensory, arm
      - thigh (level) —*see* Injury, nerve, cutaneous sensory, hip
    - deep peroneal —*see* Injury, nerve, peroneal, foot
    - digital
      - finger S64.4-●
        - index S64.49-●
        - little S64.49-●
        - middle S64.49-●
        - ring S64.49-●
      - thumb S64.3-●
      - toe —*see* Injury, nerve, ankle, specified site NEC

- Injury *(Continued)*
  - nerve NEC *(Continued)*
    - eighth cranial (acoustic or auditory) —*see* Injury, nerve, acoustic
    - eleventh cranial (accessory) —*see* Injury, nerve, accessory
    - facial S04.5-●
      - contusion S04.5-●
      - laceration S04.5-●
      - newborn P11.3
      - specified type NEC S04.5-●
    - femoral (hip level) (thigh level) S74.1-●
    - fifth cranial (trigeminal) —*see* Injury, nerve, trigeminal
    - finger (digital) —*see* Injury, nerve, digital, finger
    - first cranial (olfactory) —*see* Injury, nerve, olfactory
    - foot S94.9-●
      - cutaneous sensory S94.3-●
      - deep peroneal S94.2-●
      - lateral plantar S94.Ø-●
      - medial plantar S94.1-●
      - specified site NEC —*see* subcategory S94.8
    - forearm (level) S54.9-●
      - cutaneous sensory —*see* Injury, nerve, cutaneous sensory, forearm
      - median —*see* Injury, nerve, median
      - radial —*see* Injury, nerve, radial
      - specified site NEC —*see* subcategory S54.8
      - ulnar —*see* Injury, nerve, ulnar
    - fourth cranial (trochlear) —*see* Injury, nerve, trochlear
    - glossopharyngeal S04.89-●
      - specified type NEC S04.89-●
    - hand S64.9-●
      - median —*see* Injury, nerve, median, hand
      - radial —*see* Injury, nerve, radial, hand
      - specified NEC —*see* subcategory S64.8
      - ulnar —*see* Injury, nerve, ulnar, hand
    - hip (level) S74.9-●
      - cutaneous sensory —*see* Injury, nerve, cutaneous sensory, hip
      - femoral —*see* Injury, nerve, femoral
      - sciatic —*see* Injury, nerve, sciatic
      - specified site NEC —*see* subcategory S74.8
    - hypoglossal S04.89-●
      - specified type NEC S04.89-●
    - lateral plantar S94.Ø-●
    - leg (lower) S84.9-●
      - cutaneous sensory —*see* Injury, nerve, cutaneous sensory, leg
      - peroneal —*see* Injury, nerve, peroneal
      - specified site NEC —*see* subcategory S84.8
      - tibial —*see* Injury, nerve, tibial
      - upper —*see* Injury, nerve, thigh
    - lower
      - back —*see* Injury, nerve, abdomen, specified site NEC
        - peripheral —*see* Injury, nerve, abdomen, peripheral
      - limb —*see* Injury, nerve, leg
    - lumbar plexus —*see* Injury, nerve, lumbosacral, sympathetic
    - lumbar spinal —*see* Injury, spinal, lumbar
    - peripheral S34.6
      - root S34.21
      - sympathetic S34.5
    - lumbosacral
      - plexus —*see* Injury, nerve, lumbosacral, sympathetic
      - sympathetic S34.5
    - medial plantar S94.1-●
    - median (forearm level) S54.1-●
      - hand (level) S64.1-●
      - upper arm (level) S44.1-●
      - wrist (level) —*see* Injury, nerve, median, hand
    - musculocutaneous S44.4-●
    - musculospiral (upper arm level) —*see* Injury, nerve, radial, upper arm
    - neck S14.9
      - peripheral S14.4
      - specified site NEC S14.8
      - sympathetic S14.5
    - ninth cranial (glossopharyngeal) —*see* Injury, nerve, glossopharyngeal
    - oculomotor S04.1-●
      - contusion S04.1-●
      - laceration S04.1-●
      - specified type NEC S04.1-●

- Injury *(Continued)*
  - nerve *(Continued)*
    - olfactory S04.81-●
      - specified type NEC S04.81-●
    - optic S04.Ø1-●
      - contusion S04.Ø1-●
      - laceration S04.Ø1-●
      - specified type NEC S04.Ø1-●
    - pelvic girdle —*see* Injury, nerve, hip
    - pelvis —*see* Injury, nerve, abdomen, specified site NEC
      - peripheral —*see* Injury, nerve, abdomen, peripheral
    - peripheral NEC T14.8
      - abdomen —*see* Injury, nerve, abdomen, peripheral
      - lower back —*see* Injury, nerve, abdomen, peripheral
      - neck —*see* Injury, nerve, neck, peripheral
      - pelvis —*see* Injury, nerve, abdomen, peripheral
      - specified NEC T14.8
    - peroneal (lower leg level) S84.1-●
      - foot S94.2-●
    - plexus
      - brachial —*see* Injury, brachial plexus
      - celiac, coeliac —*see* Injury, nerve, lumbosacral, sympathetic
      - mesenteric, inferior —*see* Injury, nerve, lumbosacral, sympathetic
      - sacral —*see* Injury, lumbosacral plexus
      - spinal
        - brachial —*see* Injury, brachial plexus
        - lumbosacral —*see* Injury, lumbosacral plexus
    - pneumogastric —*see* Injury, nerve, vagus
    - radial (forearm level) S54.2-●
      - hand (level) S64.2-●
      - upper arm (level) S44.2-●
      - wrist (level) —*see* Injury, nerve, radial, hand
    - root —*see* Injury, nerve, spinal, root
    - sacral plexus —*see* Injury, lumbosacral plexus
    - sacral spinal —*see* Injury, spinal, sacral
    - peripheral S34.6
      - root S34.22
      - sympathetic S34.5
    - sciatic (hip level) (thigh level) S74.Ø-●
    - second cranial (optic) —*see* Injury, nerve, optic
    - self-inflicted, without suicidal intent R45.88
    - seventh cranial (facial) —*see* Injury, nerve, facial
    - shoulder —*see* Injury, nerve, arm
    - sixth cranial (abducent) —*see* Injury, nerve, abducens
    - spinal
      - plexus —*see* Injury, nerve, plexus, spinal
      - root
        - cervical S14.2
        - dorsal S24.2
        - lumbar S34.21
        - sacral S34.22
        - thoracic —*see* Injury, nerve, spinal, root, dorsal
    - splanchnic —*see* Injury, nerve, lumbosacral, sympathetic
    - sympathetic NEC —*see* Injury, nerve, lumbosacral, sympathetic
      - cervical —*see* Injury, nerve, cervical sympathetic
    - tenth cranial (pneumogastric or vagus) —*see* Injury, nerve, vagus
    - thigh (level) —*see* Injury, nerve, hip
      - cutaneous sensory —*see* Injury, nerve, cutaneous sensory, hip
      - femoral —*see* Injury, nerve, femoral
      - sciatic —*see* Injury, nerve, sciatic
      - specified NEC —*see* Injury, nerve, hip
    - third cranial (oculomotor) —*see* Injury, nerve, oculomotor
    - thorax S24.9
      - peripheral S24.3
      - specified site NEC S24.8
      - sympathetic S24.4
    - thumb, digital —*see* Injury, nerve, digital, thumb
    - tibial (lower leg level) (posterior) S84.Ø-●
    - toe —*see* Injury, nerve, ankle
    - trigeminal S04.3-●
      - contusion S04.3-●
      - laceration S04.3-●
      - specified type NEC S04.3-●

Injury (Continued)
superficial (Continued)
head (Continued)
oral cavity S00.502
scalp S00.00
specified site NEC S00.80
heel —see Injury, superficial, foot
hip S70.91- •
abrasion —see Abrasion, hip
bite —see Bite, superficial, hip
blister —see Blister, hip
contusion —see Contusion, hip
external constriction —see Constriction, external, hip
foreign body —see Foreign body, superficial, hip
iliac region —see Injury, superficial, abdomen
inguinal region —see Injury, superficial, abdomen
insect bite —see Bite, by site, superficial, insect
interscapular region —see Injury, superficial, thorax, back
jaw —see Injury, superficial, head, specified NEC
knee S80.91- •
abrasion —see Abrasion, knee
bite —see Bite, superficial, knee
blister —see Blister, knee
contusion —see Contusion, knee
external constriction —see Constriction, external, knee
foreign body —see Foreign body, superficial, knee
labium (majus) (minus) S30.95
lacrimal (apparatus) (gland) (sac) —see Injury, eye, specified site NEC
larynx —see Injury, superficial, throat
leg (lower) S80.92- •
abrasion —see Abrasion, leg
bite —see Bite, superficial, leg
contusion —see Contusion, leg
external constriction —see Constriction, external, leg
foreign body —see Foreign body, superficial, leg
knee —see Injury, superficial, knee
limb NEC T14.8
lip S00.501
lower back S30.91
lumbar region S30.91
malar region —see Injury, superficial, head, specified NEC
mammary —see Injury, superficial, breast
mastoid region —see Injury, superficial, head, specified NEC
mouth —see Injury, superficial, oral cavity
muscle NEC T14.8
nail NEC T14.8
finger —see Injury, superficial, finger
toe —see Injury, superficial, toe
nasal (septum) —see Injury, superficial, nose
neck S10.90
specified site NEC S10.80
nose (septum) S00.30
occipital region —see Injury, superficial, scalp
oral cavity S00.502
orbital region —see Injury, superficial, periocular area
palate —see Injury, superficial, oral cavity
palm —see Injury, superficial, hand
parietal region —see Injury, superficial, scalp
pelvis S30.91
girdle —see Injury, superficial, hip
penis S30.93
perineum
female S30.95
male S30.91
periocular area S00.20- •
abrasion —see Abrasion, eyelid
bite —see Bite, superficial, eyelid
contusion —see Contusion, eyelid
external constriction —see Constriction, external, eyelid
foreign body —see Foreign body, superficial, eyelid
phalanges
finger —see Injury, superficial, finger
toe —see Injury, superficial, toe
pharynx —see Injury, superficial, throat
pinna —see Injury, superficial, ear

Injury (Continued)
superficial (Continued)
popliteal space —see Injury, superficial, knee
prepuce S30.93
pubic region S30.91
pudendum
female S30.97
male S30.96
sacral region S30.91
scalp S00.00
scapular region —see Injury, superficial, shoulder
sclera —see Injury, eye, specified site NEC
scrotum S30.94
shin —see Injury, superficial, leg
shoulder S40.91- •
abrasion —see Abrasion, shoulder
bite —see Bite, superficial, shoulder
blister —see Blister, shoulder
contusion —see Contusion, shoulder
external constriction —see Constriction, external, shoulder
foreign body —see Foreign body, superficial, shoulder
skin NEC T14.8
sternal region —see Injury, superficial, thorax, front
subconjunctival —see Injury, eye, specified site NEC
subcutaneous NEC T14.8
submaxillary region —see Injury, superficial, head, specified NEC
submental region —see Injury, superficial, head, specified NEC
subungual
finger(s) —see Injury, superficial, finger
toe(s) —see Injury, superficial, toe
supraclavicular fossa —see Injury, superficial, neck
supraorbital —see Injury, superficial, head, specified NEC
temple —see Injury, superficial, head, specified NEC
temporal region —see Injury, superficial, head, specified NEC
testis S30.94
thigh S70.92- •
abrasion —see Abrasion, thigh
bite —see Bite, superficial, thigh
blister —see Blister, thigh
contusion —see Contusion, thigh
external constriction —see Constriction, external, thigh
foreign body —see Foreign body, superficial, thigh
thorax, thoracic (wall) S20.90
abrasion —see Abrasion, thorax
back S20.40- •
bite —see Bite, thorax, superficial
blister —see Blister, thorax
contusion —see Contusion, thorax
external constriction —see Constriction, external, thorax
foreign body —see Foreign body, superficial, thorax
front S20.30- •
throat S10.10
abrasion S10.11
bite S10.17
insect S10.16
blister S10.12
contusion S10.0
external constriction S10.14
foreign body S10.15
thumb S60.93- •
abrasion —see Abrasion, thumb
bite —see Bite, superficial, thumb
blister —see Blister, thumb
contusion —see Contusion, thumb
external constriction —see Constriction, external, thumb
foreign body —see Foreign body, superficial, thumb
insect bite —see Bite, by site, superficial, insect
specified type NEC S60.39- •
toe(s) S90.93- •
abrasion —see Abrasion, toe
bite —see Bite, toe
blister —see Blister, toe
contusion —see Contusion, toe

Injury (Continued)
superficial (Continued)
toe(s) (Continued)
external constriction —see Constriction, external, toe
foreign body —see Foreign body, superficial, toe
great S90.93- •
tongue —see Injury, superficial, oral cavity
tooth, teeth —see Injury, superficial, oral cavity
trachea S10.10
tunica vaginalis S30.94
tympanum, tympanic membrane —see Injury, superficial, ear
uvula —see Injury, superficial, oral cavity
vagina S30.95
vocal cords —see Injury, superficial, throat
vulva S30.95
wrist S60.91- •
supraclavicular region —see Injury, neck
supraorbital S09.93
suprarenal gland (multiple) —see Injury, adrenal
surgical complication (external or internal site) —see Laceration, accidental complicating surgery
temple S09.90
temporal region S09.90
tendon —see also Injury, muscle, by site
abdomen —see Injury, muscle, abdomen
Achilles —see Injury, Achilles tendon
lower back —see Injury, muscle, lower back
pelvic organs —see Injury, muscle, pelvis
tenth cranial nerve (pneumogastric or vagus) —see Injury, nerve, vagus
testis S39.94
thigh S79.92- •
blood vessel —see Injury, blood vessel, hip
contusion —see Contusion, thigh
fracture —see Fracture, femur
muscle —see Injury, muscle, thigh
nerve —see Injury, nerve, thigh
open —see Wound, open, thigh
specified NEC S79.82- •
superficial —see Injury, superficial, thigh
third cranial nerve (oculomotor) —see Injury, nerve, oculomotor
thorax, thoracic S29.9
blood vessel —see Injury, blood vessel, thorax
cavity —see Injury, intrathoracic
dislocation —see Dislocation, thorax
external (wall) S29.9
contusion —see Contusion, thorax
nerve —see Injury, nerve, thorax
open —see Wound, open, thorax
specified NEC S29.8
sprain —see Sprain, thorax
superficial —see Injury, superficial, thorax
fracture —see Fracture, thorax
internal —see Injury, intrathoracic
intrathoracic organ —see Injury, intrathoracic
sympathetic ganglion —see Injury, nerve, thorax, sympathetic
throat —see also Injury, neck S19.9
thumb S69.9- •
blood vessel —see Injury, blood vessel, thumb
contusion —see Contusion, thumb
dislocation —see Dislocation, thumb
fracture —see Fracture, thumb
muscle —see Injury, muscle, thumb
nerve —see Injury, nerve, digital, thumb
open —see Wound, open, thumb
specified NEC S69.8- •
sprain —see Sprain, thumb
superficial —see Injury, superficial, thumb
thymus (gland) —see Injury, intrathoracic, specified organ NEC
thyroid (gland) NEC S19.84
toe S99.92- •
contusion —see Contusion, toe
dislocation —see Dislocation, toe
fracture —see Fracture, toe
muscle —see Injury, muscle, toe
open —see Wound, open, toe
specified type NEC S99.82- •
sprain —see Sprain, toe
superficial —see Injury, superficial, toe
tongue S09.93
tonsil S09.93
tooth S09.93

▶ New ➡ Revised ~~deleted~~ Deleted • Use Additional Character(s)

Injury *(Continued)*
trachea (cervical) NEC S19.82
thoracic —*see* Injury, intrathoracic, trachea, thoracic
transfusion-related acute lung (TRALI) J95.84
tunica vaginalis S39.94
twelfth cranial nerve (hypoglossal) —*see* Injury, nerve, hypoglossal
ureter S37.10
contusion S37.12
laceration S37.13
specified type NEC S37.19
urethra (sphincter) S37.30
at delivery O71.5
contusion S37.32
laceration S37.33
specified type NEC S37.38
urinary organ S37.899
contusion S37.92
laceration S37.93
specified
site NEC S37.899
contusion S37.892
laceration S37.893
specified type NEC S37.898
type NEC S37.99
uterus, uterine S37.60
with ectopic or molar pregnancy O08.6
blood vessel —*see* Injury, blood vessel, iliac
contusion S37.62
laceration S37.63
cervix at delivery O71.3
rupture associated with obstetrics —*see* Rupture, uterus
specified type NEC S37.69
uvula S09.93
vagina S39.93
abrasion S30.814
bite S31.45
insect S30.864
superficial NEC S30.874
contusion S30.23
crush S38.03
during delivery —*see* Laceration, vagina, during delivery
external constriction S30.844
insect bite S30.864
laceration S31.41
with foreign body S31.42
open wound S31.40
puncture S31.43
with foreign body S31.44
superficial S30.95
foreign body S30.854
vas deferens —*see* Injury, pelvic organ, specified site NEC
vascular NEC T14.8
vein —*see* Injury, blood vessel
vena cava (superior) S25.20
inferior S35.10
laceration (minor) (superficial) S35.11
major S35.12
specified type NEC S35.19
laceration (minor) (superficial) S25.21
major S25.22
specified type NEC S25.29
vesical (sphincter) —*see* Injury, bladder
visual cortex S04.04- ●
vitreous (humor) S05.90
specified NEC S05.8X- ●
vocal cord NEC S19.83
vulva S39.94
abrasion S30.814
bite S31.45
insect S30.864
superficial NEC S30.874
contusion S30.23
crush S38.03
during delivery —*see* Laceration, perineum, female, during delivery
external constriction S30.844
insect bite S30.864
laceration S31.41
with foreign body S31.42
open wound S31.40
puncture S31.43
with foreign body S31.44
superficial S30.95
foreign body S30.854
whiplash (cervical spine) S13.4

Injury *(Continued)*
wrist S69.9- ●
blood vessel —*see* Injury, blood vessel, hand
contusion —*see* Contusion, wrist
dislocation —*see* Dislocation, wrist
fracture —*see* Fracture, wrist
muscle —*see* Injury, muscle, hand
nerve —*see* Injury, nerve, hand
open —*see* Wound, open, wrist
specified NEC S69.8- ●
sprain —*see* Sprain, wrist
superficial —*see* Injury, superficial, wrist
Inoculation —*see also* Vaccination
complication or reaction —*see* Complications, vaccination
Insanity, insane —*see also* Psychosis
adolescent —*see* Schizophrenia
confusional F28
acute or subacute F05
delusional F22
senile F03
Insect
bite —*see* Bite, by site, superficial, insect
venomous, poisoning NEC (by) —*see* Venom, arthropod
Insecurity
financial Z59.86
food Z59.41
transportation Z59.82
Insensitivity
adrenocorticotropin hormone (ACTH) E27.49
androgen E34.50
complete E34.51
partial E34.52
Insertion
cord (umbilical) lateral or velamentous O43.12- ●
intrauterine contraceptive device (encounter for) —*see* Intrauterine contraceptive device
Insolation (sunstroke) T67.01
Insomnia (organic) G47.00
without objective findings F51.02
adjustment F51.02
adjustment disorder F51.02
behavioral, of childhood Z73.819
combined type Z73.812
limit setting type Z73.811
sleep-onset association type Z73.810
childhood Z73.819
chronic F51.04
somatized tension F51.04
conditioned F51.04
due to
alcohol
abuse F10.182
dependence F10.282
use F10.982
amphetamines
abuse F15.182
dependence F15.282
use F15.982
anxiety disorder F51.05
caffeine
abuse F15.182
dependence F15.282
use F15.982
cocaine
abuse F14.182
dependence F14.282
use F14.982
depression F51.05
drug NEC
abuse F19.182
dependence F19.282
use F19.982
medical condition G47.01
mental disorder NEC F51.05
opioid
abuse F11.182
dependence F11.282
use F11.982
psychoactive substance NEC
abuse F19.182
dependence F19.282
use F19.982
sedative, hypnotic, or anxiolytic
abuse F13.182
dependence F13.282
use F13.982

Insomnia *(Continued)*
due to *(Continued)*
stimulant NEC
abuse F15.182
dependence F15.282
use F15.982
fatal familial (FFI) A81.83
idiopathic F51.01
learned F51.3
nonorganic origin F51.01
not due to a substance or known physiological condition F51.01
specified NEC F51.09
paradoxical F51.03
primary F51.01
psychiatric F51.05
psychophysiologic F51.04
related to psychopathology F51.05
short-term F51.02
specified NEC G47.09
stress-related F51.02
transient F51.02
Inspiration
food or foreign body —*see* Foreign body, by site
mucus —*see* Asphyxia, mucus
Inspissated bile syndrome (newborn) P59.1
Instability
emotional (excessive) F60.3
housing
housed Z59.819
with risk of homelessness Z59.811
homelessness in past 12 months Z59.812
joint (post-traumatic) M25.30
ankle M25.37- ●
due to old ligament injury —*see* Disorder, ligament
elbow M25.32- ●
flail —*see* Flail, joint
foot M25.37- ●
hand M25.34- ●
hip M25.35- ●
knee M25.36- ●
lumbosacral —*see* subcategory M53.2
prosthesis —*see* Complications, joint prosthesis, mechanical, displacement, by site
sacroiliac —*see* subcategory M53.2
secondary to
old ligament injury —*see* Disorder, ligament
removal of joint prosthesis M96.89
shoulder (region) M25.31- ●
specified site NEC M25.39
spine —*see* subcategory M53.2
wrist M25.33- ●
knee (chronic) M23.5- ●
lumbosacral —*see* subcategory M53.2
nervous F48.8
personality (emotional) F60.3
spine —*see* Instability, joint, spine
vasomotor R55
Institutional syndrome (childhood) F94.2
Institutionalization, affecting child Z62.22
disinhibited attachment F94.2
Insufficiency, insufficient
accommodation, old age H52.4
adrenal (gland) E27.40
primary E27.1
adrenocortical E27.40
drug-induced E27.3
iatrogenic E27.3
primary E27.1
anatomic crown height K08.89
anterior (occlusal) guidance M26.54
anus K62.89
aortic (valve) I35.1
with
mitral (valve) disease I08.0
with tricuspid (valve) disease I08.3
stenosis I35.2
tricuspid (valve) disease I08.2
with mitral (valve) disease I08.3
congenital Q23.1
rheumatic I06.1
with
mitral (valve) disease I08.0
with tricuspid (valve) disease I08.3
stenosis I06.2
with mitral (valve) disease I08.0
with tricuspid (valve) disease I08.3

INDEX TO DISEASES AND INJURIES / Insufficiency, insufficient

Insufficiency, insufficient *(Continued)*
  aortic *(Continued)*
    rheumatic *(Continued)*
      with *(Continued)*
        tricuspid (valve) disease I08.2
          with mitral (valve) disease I08.3
    specified cause NEC I35.1
    syphilitic A52.03
  arterial I77.1
    basilar G45.0
    carotid (hemispheric) G45.1
    cerebral I67.81
    coronary (acute or subacute) I24.89
    mesenteric K55.1
    peripheral I73.9
    precerebral (multiple) (bilateral) G45.2
    vertebral G45.0
  arteriovenous I99.8
  biliary K83.8
  cardiac —*see also* Insufficiency, myocardial
    due to presence of (cardiac) prosthesis I97.11-•
    postprocedural I97.11-•
  cardiorenal, hypertensive I13.2
  cardiovascular —*see* Disease, cardiovascular
  cerebrovascular (acute) I67.81
    with transient focal neurological signs and symptoms G45.8
  circulatory NEC I99.8
    newborn P29.89
  clinical crown length K08.89
  convergence H51.11
  coronary (acute or subacute) I24.89
    chronic or with a stated duration of over 4 weeks I25.89
  corticoadrenal E27.40
    primary E27.1
  dietary E63.9
  divergence H51.8
  food T73.0
  gastroesophageal K22.89
  gonadal
    ovary E28.39
    testis E29.1
  ▶health insurance coverage Z59.71
  heart —*see also* Insufficiency, myocardial
    newborn P29.0
    valve —*see* Endocarditis
  hepatic —*see* Failure, hepatic
  idiopathic autonomic G90.09
  interocclusal distance of fully erupted teeth (ridge) M26.36
  kidney N28.9
    acute N28.9
    chronic N18.9
  lacrimal (secretion) H04.12-•
    passages —*see* Stenosis, lacrimal
  liver —*see* Failure, hepatic
  lung —*see* Insufficiency, pulmonary
  mental (congenital) —*see* Disability, intellectual
  mesenteric K55.1
  mitral (valve) I34.0
    with
      aortic valve disease I08.0
        with tricuspid (valve) disease I08.3
      obstruction or stenosis I05.2
        with aortic valve disease I08.0
      tricuspid (valve) disease I08.1
        with aortic (valve) disease I08.3
    congenital Q23.3
    rheumatic I05.1
      with
        aortic valve disease I08.0
          with tricuspid (valve) disease I08.3
        obstruction or stenosis I05.2
          with aortic valve disease I08.0
            with tricuspid (valve) disease I08.3
        tricuspid (valve) disease I08.1
          with aortic (valve) disease I08.3
      active or acute I01.1
        with chorea, rheumatic (Sydenham's) I02.0
    specified cause, except rheumatic I34.0
  muscle —*see also* Disease, muscle
    heart —*see* Insufficiency, myocardial
    ocular NEC H50.9
  myocardial, myocardium (with arteriosclerosis) —*see also* Failure, heart I50.9

Insufficiency, insufficient *(Continued)*
  myocardial, myocardium *(Continued)*
    with
      rheumatic fever (conditions in I00) I09.0
        active, acute or subacute I01.2
          with chorea I02.0
        inactive or quiescent (with chorea) I09.0
    congenital Q24.8
    hypertensive —*see* Hypertension, heart
    newborn P29.0
    rheumatic I09.0
      active, acute, or subacute I01.2
    syphilitic A52.06
  nourishment (*see also* Nutrition deficient) T73.0
  pancreatic K86.89
    exocrine K86.81
  parathyroid (gland) E20.9
  peripheral vascular (arterial) I73.9
  pituitary E23.0
  placental (mother) O36.51-•
  platelets D69.6
  prenatal care affecting management of pregnancy O09.3-•
  progressive pluriglandular E31.0
  pulmonary J98.4
    acute, following surgery (nonthoracic) J95.2
      thoracic J95.1
    chronic, following surgery J95.3
    following
      shock J98.4
      trauma J98.4
    newborn P28.89
    valve I37.1
      with stenosis I37.2
      congenital Q22.2
      rheumatic I09.89
        with aortic, mitral or tricuspid (valve) disease I08.8
  pyloric K31.89
  renal (acute) N28.9
    chronic N18.9
  respiratory R06.89
    newborn P28.5
  rotation —*see* Malrotation
  sleep syndrome F51.12
  ➡social insurance Z59.71
  suprarenal E27.40
    primary E27.1
  tarso-orbital fascia, congenital Q10.3
  testis E29.1
  thyroid (gland) (acquired) E03.9
    congenital E03.1
  tricuspid (valve) (rheumatic) I07.1
    with
      aortic (valve) disease I08.2
        with mitral (valve) disease I08.3
      mitral (valve) disease I08.1
        with aortic (valve) disease I08.3
      obstruction or stenosis I07.2
        with aortic (valve) disease I08.2
          with mitral (valve) disease I08.3
    congenital Q22.8
    nonrheumatic I36.1
      with stenosis I36.2
  urethral sphincter R32
  valve, valvular (heart) I38
    aortic —*see* Insufficiency, aortic (valve)
    mitral —*see* Insufficiency, mitral (valve)
    pulmonary —*see* Insufficiency, pulmonary, valve
    tricuspid —*see* Insufficiency, tricuspid (valve)
    congenital Q24.8
  vascular I99.8
    intestine K55.9
      acute —*see also* Ischemia, intestine, acute K55.059
    mesenteric K55.1
    peripheral I73.9
    renal —*see* Hypertension, kidney
  velopharyngeal
    acquired K13.79
    congenital Q38.8
  venous (chronic) (peripheral) I87.2
  ventricular —*see* Insufficiency, myocardial
  ➡welfare support Z59.72
Insufflation, fallopian Z31.41
Insular —*see* condition
Insulinoma
  pancreas
    benign D13.7
    malignant C25.4
    uncertain behavior D37.8

Insulinoma *(Continued)*
  specified site
    benign —*see* Neoplasm, by site, benign
    malignant —*see* Neoplasm, by site, malignant
    uncertain behavior —*see* Neoplasm, by site, uncertain behavior
  unspecified site
    benign D13.7
    malignant C25.4
    uncertain behavior D37.8
Insuloma —*see* Insulinoma
Interference
  balancing side M26.56
  non-working side M26.56
Intermenstrual —*see* condition
Intermittent —*see* condition
Internal —*see* condition
Interrogation
  cardiac defibrillator (automatic) (implantable) Z45.02
  cardiac pacemaker Z45.018
  cardiac (event) (loop) recorder Z45.09
  infusion pump (implanted) (intrathecal) Z45.1
  neurostimulator Z46.2
Interruption
  aortic arch Q25.21
  phase-shift, sleep cycle —*see* Disorder, sleep, circadian rhythm
  sleep phase-shift, or 24 hour sleep-wake cycle —*see* Disorder, sleep, circadian rhythm
Interstitial —*see* condition
Intertrigo L30.4
  labialis K13.0
Intervertebral disc —*see* condition
Intestine, intestinal —*see* condition
Intolerance
  carbohydrate K90.49
  disaccharide, hereditary E73.0
  fat NEC K90.49
    pancreatic K90.3
  food K90.49
    dietary counseling and surveillance Z71.3
  fructose E74.10
    hereditary E74.12
  glucose(-galactose) E74.39
  gluten K90.01
  lactose E73.9
    specified NEC E73.8
  lysine E72.3
  milk NEC K90.49
    lactose E73.9
  orthostatic, chronic G90.A
  protein K90.49
  starch NEC K90.49
  sucrose (-isomaltose) E74.31
Intoxicated NEC (without dependence) —*see* Alcohol, intoxication
Intoxication
  acid (*see also* Acidosis) E87.29
  alcoholic (acute) (without dependence) —*see* Alcohol, intoxication
  alimentary canal K52.1
  amphetamine (without dependence) —*see also* Abuse, drug, stimulant, with intoxication
    stimulant NEC F15.10
      with
        anxiety disorder F15.180
        intoxication F15.129
          with
            delirium F15.121
            perceptual disturbance F15.122
    with dependence —*see* Dependence, drug, stimulant, with intoxication
  anxiolytic (acute) (without dependence) —*see* Abuse, drug, sedative, with intoxication
    with dependence —*see* Dependence, drug, sedative, with intoxication
  caffeine F15.929
    with dependence —*see* Dependence, drug, stimulant, with intoxication
  cannabinoids (acute) (without dependence) —*see* Use, cannabis, with intoxication
    with
      abuse —*see* Abuse, drug, cannabis, with intoxication
      dependence —*see* Dependence, drug, cannabis, with intoxication
  chemical —*see* Table of Drugs and Chemicals
    via placenta or breast milk —*see* Absorption, chemical, through placenta

▶ New ➠ Revised ~~deleted~~ Deleted ● Use Additional Character(s)

- **Irritable, irritability** R45.4
  - bladder N32.89
  - bowel (syndrome) K58.9
    - with
      - constipation K58.1
      - diarrhea K58.0
    - mixed K58.2
    - psychogenic F45.8
    - specified NEC K58.8
  - bronchial —*see* Bronchitis
  - cerebral, in newborn P91.3
  - colon —*see also* Irritable, bowel K58.9
    - with diarrhea K58.0
    - psychogenic F45.8
  - duodenum K59.89
  - heart (psychogenic) F45.8
  - hip —*see* Derangement, joint, specified type NEC, hip
  - ileum K59.89
  - infant R68.12
  - jejunum K59.89
  - rectum K59.89
  - stomach K31.89
    - psychogenic F45.8
  - ➡sympathetic G90.89
  - urethra N36.8
  - ▶without diarrhea K58.9
- **Irritation**
  - anus K62.89
  - axillary nerve G54.0
  - bladder N32.89
  - brachial plexus G54.0
  - bronchial —*see* Bronchitis
  - cervical plexus G54.2
  - cervix —*see* Cervicitis
  - choroid, sympathetic —*see* Endophthalmitis
  - cranial nerve —*see* Disorder, nerve, cranial
  - gastric K31.89
    - psychogenic F45.8
  - globe, sympathetic —*see* Uveitis, sympathetic
  - labyrinth —*see* subcategory H83.2
  - lumbosacral plexus G54.1
  - meninges (traumatic) —*see* Injury, intracranial
    - nontraumatic —*see* Meningismus
  - nerve —*see* Disorder, nerve
  - nervous R45.0
  - penis N48.89
  - perineum NEC L29.3
  - ➡peripheral autonomic nervous system G90.89
  - peritoneum —*see* Peritonitis
  - pharynx J39.2
  - plantar nerve —*see* Lesion, nerve, plantar
  - spinal (cord) (traumatic) —*see also* Injury, spinal cord, by region
    - nerve G58.9
      - root NEC —*see* Radiculopathy
    - nontraumatic —*see* Myelopathy
  - stomach K31.89
    - psychogenic F45.8
  - ➡sympathetic nerve NEC G90.89
  - ulnar nerve —*see* Lesion, nerve, ulnar
  - vagina N89.8
- **Ischemia, ischemic** I99.8
  - bowel (transient)
    - acute —*see also* Ischemia, intestine, acute K55.059
    - chronic K55.1
      - due to mesenteric artery insufficiency K55.1
  - brain —*see* Ischemia, cerebral
  - cardiac (*see* Disease, heart, ischemic)
  - cardiomyopathy I25.5
  - cerebral (chronic) (generalized) I67.82
    - arteriosclerotic I67.2
    - intermittent G45.9
    - newborn P91.0
    - recurrent focal G45.8
    - transient G45.9
  - colon chronic (due to mesenteric artery insufficiency) K55.1
  - coronary —*see* Disease, heart, ischemic
  - demand (coronary) —*see also* Angina I24.89
    - with myocardial infarction I21.A1
      - resulting in myocardial infarction I21.A1
  - heart (chronic or with a stated duration of over 4 weeks) I25.9
    - acute or with a stated duration of 4 weeks or less I24.9
    - subacute I24.9
- **Ischemia, ischemic** *(Continued)*
  - infarction, muscle —*see* Infarct, muscle
  - intestine (large) (small) (transient) K55.9
    - acute K55.059
      - diffuse K55.052
      - focal K55.051
      - large K55.039
        - diffuse K55.032
        - focal K55.031
      - small K55.019
        - diffuse K55.012
        - focal K55.011
    - chronic K55.1
    - due to mesenteric artery insufficiency K55.1
  - IST (inappropriate sinus tachycardia, so stated) I47.11
  - kidney N28.0
  - limb, critical —*see* Arteriosclerosis, with critical limb ischemia
  - limb-threatening, chronic —*see* Arteriosclerosis, with critical limb ischemia
  - mesenteric, acute —*see also* Ischemia, intestine, acute K55.059
  - muscle, traumatic T79.6
  - myocardium, myocardial (chronic or with a stated duration of over 4 weeks) I25.9
    - acute, without myocardial infarction I51.3
    - silent (asymptomatic) I25.6
    - transient of newborn P29.4
  - renal N28.0
  - retina, retinal —*see* Occlusion, artery, retina
  - small bowel
    - acute K55.019
      - diffuse K55.012
      - focal K55.011
    - chronic K55.1
    - due to mesenteric artery insufficiency K55.1
  - spinal cord G95.11
  - subendocardial —*see* Insufficiency, coronary
  - supply (coronary) —*see also* Angina I25.9
    - due to vasospasm I20.1
- **Ischial spine** —*see* condition
- **Ischialgia** —*see* Sciatica
- **Ischiopagus** Q89.4
- **Ischium, ischial** —*see* condition
- **Ischuria** R34
- **Iselin's disease or osteochondrosis** —*see* Osteochondrosis, juvenile, metatarsus
- **Islands of**
  - parotid tissue in
    - lymph nodes Q38.6
    - neck structures Q38.6
  - submaxillary glands in
    - fascia Q38.6
    - lymph nodes Q38.6
    - neck muscles Q38.6
- **Islet cell tumor, pancreas** D13.7
- **Isoimmunization NEC** —*see also* Incompatibility
  - affecting management of pregnancy (ABO) (with hydrops fetalis) O36.11-●
    - anti-A sensitization O36.11-●
    - anti-B sensitization O36.19-●
    - anti-c sensitization O36.09-●
    - anti-C sensitization O36.09-●
    - anti-e sensitization O36.09-●
    - anti-E sensitization O36.09-●
    - Rh NEC O36.09-●
      - anti-D antibody O36.01-●
    - specified NEC O36.19-●
  - newborn P55.9
    - with
      - hydrops fetalis P56.0
      - kernicterus P57.0
    - ABO (blood groups) P55.1
    - Rhesus (Rh) factor P55.0
    - specified type NEC P55.8
- **Isolation, isolated**
  - dwelling Z59.89
  - family Z63.79
  - social Z60.4
- **Isoleucinosis** E71.19
- **Isomerism atrial appendages** (with asplenia or polysplenia) Q20.6
- **Isosporiasis, isosporosis** A07.3
- **Isovaleric acidemia** E71.110
- **Issue of**
  - medical certificate Z02.79
    - for disability determination Z02.71
  - repeat prescription (appliance) (glasses) (medicinal substance, medicament, medicine) Z76.0
    - contraception —*see* Contraception
- **Itch, itching** —*see also* Pruritus
  - baker's L23.6
  - barber's B35.0
  - bricklayer's L24.5
  - cheese B88.0
  - clam digger's B65.3
  - coolie B76.9
  - copra B88.0
  - dew B76.9
  - dhobi B35.6
  - filarial —*see* Infestation, filarial
  - grain B88.0
  - grocer's B88.0
  - ground B76.9
  - harvest B88.0
  - jock B35.6
  - Malabar B35.5
    - beard B35.0
    - foot B35.3
    - scalp B35.0
  - meaning scabies B86
  - Norwegian B86
  - perianal L29.0
  - poultrymen's B88.0
  - sarcoptic B86
  - scabies B86
  - scrub B88.0
  - straw B88.0
  - swimmer's B65.3
  - water B76.9
  - ➡winter L29.89
- **Ivemark's syndrome** (asplenia with congenital heart disease) Q89.01
- **Ivory bones** Q78.2
- **Ixodiasis NEC** B88.8

J

- **Jaccoud's syndrome** —*see* Arthropathy, postrheumatic, chronic
- **Jackson's**
  - membrane Q43.3
  - paralysis or syndrome G83.89
  - veil Q43.3
- **Jacquet's dermatitis** (diaper dermatitis) L22
- **Jadassohn-Pellizari's disease or anetoderma** L90.2
- **Jadassohn's**
  - blue nevus —*see* Nevus
  - intraepidermal epithelioma —*see* Neoplasm, skin, benign
- **Jaffe-Lichtenstein (-Uehlinger) syndrome** —*see* Dysplasia, fibrous, bone NEC
- **Jakob-Creutzfeldt disease or syndrome** —*see* Creutzfeldt-Jakob disease or syndrome
- **Jaksch-Luzet disease** D64.89
- **Jamaican**
  - neuropathy G92.8
  - paraplegic tropical ataxic-spastic syndrome G92.8
- **Janet's disease** F48.8
- **Janiceps** Q89.4
- **Jansky-Bielschowsky amaurotic idiocy** E75.4
- **Japanese**
  - B-type encephalitis A83.0
  - river fever A75.3
- **Jaundice** (yellow) R17
  - acholuric (familial) (splenomegalic) —*see also* Spherocytosis
    - acquired D59.8
  - breast-milk (inhibitor) P59.3
  - catarrhal (acute) B15.9
    - with hepatic coma B15.0
  - cholestatic (benign) R17

▶ New ➡ Revised ~~deleted~~ Deleted ● Use Additional Character(s)

K

L

L

Laceration *(Continued)*
- penis S31.21
  - with foreign body S31.22
- perineum
  - female S31.41
    - with
      - ectopic or molar pregnancy OØ8.6
      - foreign body S31.42
    - during delivery O7Ø.9
      - first degree O7Ø.Ø
      - fourth degree O7Ø.3
      - second degree O7Ø.1
      - third degree —*see also* Delivery, complicated, by, laceration, perineum, third degree O7Ø.2Ø
    - old (postpartal) N81.89
    - postpartal N81.89
    - secondary (postpartal) O9Ø.1
  - male S31.119
    - with foreign body S31.129
- periocular area (with or without lacrimal passages) —*see* Laceration, eyelid
- peritoneum S36.893
- periumbilic region —*see* Laceration, abdomen, wall, periumbilic
- periurethral tissue —*see* Laceration, urethra
- phalanges
  - finger —*see* Laceration, finger
  - toe —*see* Laceration, toe
- pharynx S11.21
  - with foreign body S11.22
- pinna —*see* Laceration, ear
- popliteal space —*see* Laceration, knee
- prepuce —*see* Laceration, penis
- prostate S37.823
- pubic region S31.119
  - with foreign body S31.129
- pudendum —*see* Laceration, genital organs, external
- rectovaginal septum —*see* Laceration, vagina
- rectum S36.63
- retroperitoneum S36.893
- round ligament S37.893
- sacral region —*see* Laceration, back, lower
- sacroiliac region —*see* Laceration, back, lower
- salivary gland —*see* Laceration, oral cavity
- scalp SØ1.Ø1
  - with foreign body SØ1.Ø2
- scapular region —*see* Laceration, shoulder
- scrotum S31.31
  - with foreign body S31.32
- seminal vesicle S37.893
- shin —*see* Laceration, leg
- shoulder S41.Ø19
  - with foreign body S41.Ø29
  - left S41.Ø12
    - with foreign body S41.Ø22
  - right S41.Ø11
    - with foreign body S41.Ø21
- small intestine —*see* Laceration, intestine, small
- spermatic cord —*see* Laceration, testis
- spinal cord (meninges) —*see also* Injury, spinal cord, by region
  - due to injury at birth P11.5
  - newborn (birth injury) P11.5
- spleen S36.Ø39
  - major (massive) (stellate) S36.Ø32
  - moderate S36.Ø31
  - superficial (minor) S36.Ø3Ø
- sternal region —*see* Laceration, thorax, front
- stomach S36.33
- submaxillary region —*see* Laceration, head, specified site NEC
- submental region —*see* Laceration, head, specified site NEC
- subungual
  - finger(s) —*see* Laceration, finger, with damage to nail
  - toe(s) —*see* Laceration, toe, with damage to nail
- suprarenal gland —*see* Laceration, adrenal gland
- temple, temporal region —*see* Laceration, head, specified site NEC
- temporomandibular area —*see* Laceration, cheek
- tendon —*see* Injury, muscle, by site, laceration
  - Achilles S86.Ø2-•
- tentorium cerebelli —*see* Injury, intracranial, diffuse

Laceration *(Continued)*
- testis S31.31
  - with foreign body S31.32
- thigh S71.11-•
  - with foreign body S71.12-•
- thorax, thoracic (wall) S21.91
  - with foreign body S21.92
    - back S21.22-•
      - with penetration into thoracic cavity S21.42-•
    - front S21.12-•
      - with penetration into thoracic cavity S21.32-•
  - back S21.21-•
    - with
      - foreign body S21.22-•
        - with penetration into thoracic cavity S21.42-•
      - penetration into thoracic cavity S21.41-•
  - breast —*see* Laceration, breast
  - front S21.11-•
    - with
      - foreign body S21.12-•
        - with penetration into thoracic cavity S21.32-•
      - penetration into thoracic cavity S21.31-•
- thumb S61.Ø19
  - with
    - damage to nail S61.119
      - with
        - foreign body S61.129
    - foreign body S61.Ø29
  - left S61.Ø12
    - with
      - damage to nail S61.112
        - with
          - foreign body S61.122
      - foreign body S61.Ø22
  - right S61.Ø11
    - with
      - damage to nail S61.111
        - with
          - foreign body S61.121
      - foreign body S61.Ø21
- thyroid gland S11.11
  - with foreign body S11.12
- toe(s) S91.119
  - with
    - damage to nail S91.219
      - with
        - foreign body S91.229
    - foreign body S91.129
  - great S91.113
    - with
      - damage to nail S91.213
        - with
          - foreign body S91.223
      - foreign body S91.123
    - left S91.112
      - with
        - damage to nail S91.212
          - with
            - foreign body S91.222
        - foreign body S91.122
    - right S91.111
      - with
        - damage to nail S91.211
          - with
            - foreign body S91.221
        - foreign body S91.121
  - lesser S91.116
    - with
      - damage to nail S91.216
        - with
          - foreign body S91.226
      - foreign body S91.126
    - left S91.115
      - with
        - damage to nail S91.215
          - with
            - foreign body S91.225
        - foreign body S91.125
    - right S91.114
      - with
        - damage to nail S91.214
          - with
            - foreign body S91.224
        - foreign body S91.124
- tongue —*see* Laceration, oral cavity
- trachea S11.Ø21
  - with foreign body S11.Ø22

Laceration *(Continued)*
- tunica vaginalis —*see* Laceration, testis
- tympanum, tympanic membrane —*see* Laceration, ear, drum
- umbilical region S31.115
  - with foreign body S31.125
- ureter S37.13
- urethra S37.33
  - with or following ectopic or molar pregnancy OØ8.6
  - obstetrical trauma O71.5
- urinary organ NEC S37.893
- uterus S37.63
  - with ectopic or molar pregnancy OØ8.6
  - following ectopic or molar pregnancy OØ8.6
  - nonpuerperal, nontraumatic N85.8
  - obstetrical trauma NEC O71.81
  - old (postpartal) N85.8
- uvula —*see* Laceration, oral cavity
- vagina S31.41
  - with
    - ectopic or molar pregnancy OØ8.6
    - foreign body S31.42
  - during delivery O71.4
    - with perineal laceration —*see* Laceration, perineum, female, during delivery
  - following ectopic or molar pregnancy OØ8.6
  - nonpuerperal, nontraumatic N89.8
  - old (postpartal) N89.8
- vas deferens S37.893
- vesical —*see* Laceration, bladder
- vocal cords S11.Ø31
  - with foreign body S11.Ø32
- vulva S31.41
  - with
    - ectopic or molar pregnancy OØ8.6
    - foreign body S31.42
  - complicating delivery O7Ø.Ø
  - following ectopic or molar pregnancy OØ8.6
  - nonpuerperal, nontraumatic N9Ø.89
  - old (postpartal) N9Ø.89
- wrist S61.519
  - with
    - foreign body S61.529
  - left S61.512
    - with
      - foreign body S61.522
  - right S61.511
    - with
      - foreign body S61.521

Lack of
- achievement in school Z55.3
- adequate
  - food Z59.48
  - intermaxillary vertical dimension of fully erupted teeth M26.36
  - sleep Z72.82Ø
- air conditioning Z59.11
- appetite (*see* Anorexia) R63.Ø
- awareness R41.9
- basic services in physical environment Z58.81
- care
  - in home Z74.2
  - of infant (at or after birth) T76.Ø2
    - confirmed T74.Ø2
- cognitive functions R41.9
- coordination R27.9
  - ataxia R27.Ø
  - specified type NEC R27.8
- development (physiological) R62.5Ø
  - failure to thrive (child over 28 days old) R62.51
    - adult R62.7
    - newborn P92.6
  - short stature R62.52
  - specified type NEC R62.59
- electricity services Z59.12
- emotional support Z6Ø.8
- energy R53.83
- financial resources Z59.6
- food Z59.48
- gas services Z59.12
- growth R62.52
- heating Z59.11
- housing (permanent) (temporary) Z59.ØØ
  - adequate Z59.1Ø
- learning experiences in childhood Z62.898
- leisure time (affecting life-style) Z73.2
- material resources due to limited financial resources, specified NEC Z59.87

Lack of *(Continued)*
memory —*see also* Amnesia
mild, following organic brain damage F06.8
oil services Z59.12
ovulation N97.0
parental supervision or control of child Z62.0
person able to render necessary care Z74.2
physical exercise Z72.3
play experience in childhood Z62.898
posterior occlusal support M26.57
relaxation (affecting life-style) Z73.2
safe drinking water Z58.6
sexual
desire F52.0
enjoyment F52.1
shelter Z59.02
sleep (adequate) Z72.820
supervision of child by parent Z62.0
support, posterior occlusal M26.57
transportation Z59.82
water T73.1
safe drinking Z58.6
services Z59.12
Lacrimal —*see* condition
Lacrimation, abnormal —*see* Epiphora
Lacrimonasal duct —*see* condition
Lactate, elevated —*see* Acidosis, lactic
Lactation, lactating (breast) (puerperal, postpartum)
associated
cracked nipple O92.13
retracted nipple O92.03
defective O92.4
disorder NEC O92.79
excessive O92.6
failed (complete) O92.3
partial O92.4
mastitis NEC —*see* Mastitis, obstetric
mother (care and/or examination) Z39.1
nonpuerperal N64.3
Lacticemia, excessive (*see also* Acidosis) E87.20
Lacunar skull Q75.8
Laennec's cirrhosis K70.30
with ascites K70.31
nonalcoholic K74.69
Lafora disease (see also Epilepsy, progressive, Lafora) G40.C09
Lag, lid (nervous) —*see* Retraction, lid
Lagophthalmos (eyelid) (nervous) H02.209
bilateral, upper and lower eyelids H02.20C
cicatricial H02.219
bilateral, upper and lower eyelids H02.21C
left H02.216
lower H02.215
upper H02.214
upper and lower eyelids H02.21B
right H02.213
lower H02.212
upper H02.211
upper and lower eyelids H02.21A
keratoconjunctivitis —*see* Keratoconjunctivitis
left H02.206
lower H02.205
upper H02.204
upper and lower eyelids H02.20B
mechanical H02.229
bilateral, upper and lower eyelids H02.22C
left H02.226
lower H02.225
upper H02.224
upper and lower eyelids H02.22B
right H02.223
lower H02.222
upper H02.221
upper and lower eyelids H02.22A
paralytic H02.239
bilateral, upper and lower eyelids H02.23C
left H02.236
lower H02.235
upper H02.234
upper and lower eyelids H02.23B
right H02.233
lower H02.232
upper H02.231
upper and lower eyelids H02.23A
right H02.203
lower H02.202
upper H02.201
upper and lower eyelids H02.20A
Laki-Lorand factor deficiency —*see* Defect, coagulation, specified type NEC
Lalling F80.0
Lambert-Eaton syndrome —*see* Syndrome, Lambert-Eaton
Lambliasis, lambliosis A07.1
Landau-Kleffner syndrome —*see* Epilepsy, specified NEC
Landouzy-Déjérine dystrophy or facioscapulohumeral atrophy G71.02
Landouzy's disease (icterohemorrhagic leptospirosis) A27.0
Landry-Guillain-Barré, syndrome or paralysis G61.0
Landry's disease or paralysis G61.0
Lane's
band Q43.3
kink —*see* Obstruction, intestine
syndrome K90.2
Langdon Down's syndrome —*see* Trisomy, 21
Lapsed immunization schedule status Z28.3
Large
baby (regardless of gestational age) (4000g to 4499g) P08.1
ear, congenital Q17.1
physiological cup Q14.2
stature R68.89
Large-for-dates NEC (infant) (4000g to 4499g) P08.1
affecting management of pregnancy O36.6-●
exceptionally (4500g or more) P08.0
➠ **Larsen-Johansson disease or osteochondrosis** — *see* Osteochondrosis, juvenile, patella
Larsen's syndrome (flattened facies and multiple congenital dislocations) Q74.8
Larva migrans
cutaneous B76.9
Ancylostoma B76.0
visceral B83.0
Laryngeal —*see* condition
Laryngismus (stridulus) J38.5
congenital P28.89
diphtheritic A36.2
Laryngitis (acute) (edematous) (fibrinous) (infective) (infiltrative) (malignant) (membranous) (phlegmonous) (pneumococcal) (pseudomembranous) (septic) (subglottic) (suppurative) (ulcerative) J04.0
with
influenza, flu, or grippe —*see* Influenza, with, laryngitis
tracheitis (acute) —*see* Laryngotracheitis
atrophic J37.0
catarrhal J37.0
chronic J37.0
with tracheitis (chronic) J37.1
diphtheritic A36.2
due to external agent —*see* Inflammation, respiratory, upper, due to
Hemophilus influenzae J04.0
H. influenzae J04.0
hypertrophic J37.0
influenzal —*see* Influenza, with, respiratory manifestations NEC
obstructive J05.0
sicca J37.0
spasmodic J05.0
acute J04.0
streptococcal J04.0
stridulous J05.0
syphilitic (late) A52.73
congenital A50.59 *[J99]*
early A50.03 *[J99]*
tuberculous A15.5
Vincent's A69.1
Laryngocele (congenital) (ventricular) Q31.3
Laryngofissure J38.7
congenital Q31.8
Laryngomalacia (congenital) Q31.5
Laryngopharyngitis (acute) J06.0
chronic J37.0
due to external agent —*see* Inflammation, respiratory, upper, due to
Laryngoplegia J38.00
bilateral J38.02
unilateral J38.01
Laryngoptosis J38.7
Laryngospasm J38.5
Laryngostenosis J38.6
Laryngotracheitis (acute) (Infectional) (infective) (viral) J04.2
atrophic J37.1
catarrhal J37.1
chronic J37.1
Laryngotracheitis *(Continued)*
diphtheritic A36.2
due to external agent —*see* Inflammation, respiratory, upper, due to
Hemophilus influenzae J04.2
hypertrophic J37.1
influenzal —*see* Influenza, with, respiratory manifestations NEC
pachydermic J38.7
sicca J37.1
spasmodic J38.5
acute J05.0
streptococcal J04.2
stridulous J38.5
syphilitic (late) A52.73
congenital A50.59 *[J99]*
early A50.03 *[J99]*
tuberculous A15.5
Vincent's A69.1
Laryngotracheobronchitis —*see* Bronchitis
Larynx, laryngeal —*see* condition
Lassa fever A96.2
Lassitude —*see* Weakness
Late
talker R62.0
walker R62.0
Late effect(s) —*see* Sequelae
Latent —*see* condition
Laterocession —*see* Lateroversion
Lateroflexion —*see* Lateroversion
Lateroversion
cervix —*see* Lateroversion, uterus
uterus, uterine (cervix) (postinfectional) (postpartal, old) N85.4
congenital Q51.818
in pregnancy or childbirth O34.59-●
Lathyrism —*see* Poisoning, food, noxious, plant
Launois' syndrome (pituitary gigantism) E22.0
Launois-Bensaude adenolipomatosis E88.89
Laurence-Moon syndrome Q87.84
Lax, laxity —*see also* Relaxation
ligament (ous) —*see also* Disorder, ligament
familial M35.7
knee —*see* Derangement, knee
skin (acquired) L57.4
congenital Q82.8
Laxative habit F55.2
Lazy leukocyte syndrome D70.8
Lead miner's lung J63.6
Leak, leakage
air NEC J93.82
postprocedural J95.812
amniotic fluid —*see* Rupture, membranes, premature
blood (microscopic), fetal, into maternal circulation affecting management of pregnancy —*see* Pregnancy, complicated by
cerebrospinal fluid G96.00
cranial
postoperative G96.08
specified NEC G96.08
spontaneous G96.01
traumatic G96.08
from spinal (lumbar) puncture G97.0
spinal
postoperative G96.09
post-traumatic G96.09
specified NEC G96.09
spontaneous G96.02
spontaneous
from
skull base G96.01
spine G96.02
CSF —*see* Leak, cerebrospinal fluid
device, implant or graft —*see also* Complications, by site and type, mechanical
arterial graft NEC —*see* Complication, vascular, graft, mechanical, leakage T82.838
breast (implant) T85.43
catheter NEC T85.638
dialysis (renal) T82.43
intraperitoneal T85.631
infusion NEC T82.534
spinal (epidural) (subdural) T85.630
urinary T83.038
cystostomy T83.030
Hopkins T83.038
ileostomy T83.038
indwelling T83.031

▶ New ➠ Revised ~~deleted~~ Deleted ● Use Additional Character(s)

Leukopenia D72.819
- basophilic D72.818
- chemotherapy (cancer) induced D70.1
- congenital D70.0
- cyclic D70.0
- drug induced NEC D70.2
  - due to cytoreductive cancer chemotherapy D70.1
- eosinophilic D72.818
- familial D70.0
- infantile genetic D70.0
- malignant D70.9
- periodic D70.0
- transitory neonatal P61.5

Leukopenic —*see* condition

Leukoplakia
- anus K62.89
- bladder (postinfectional) N32.89
- buccal K13.21
- cervix (uteri) N88.0
- esophagus K22.89
- gingiva K13.21
- hairy (oral mucosa) (tongue) K13.3
- kidney (pelvis) N28.89
- larynx J38.7
- lip K13.21
- mouth K13.21
- oral epithelium, including tongue (mucosa) K13.21
- palate K13.21
- pelvis (kidney) N28.89
- penis (infectional) N48.0
- rectum K62.89
- syphilitic (late) A52.79
- tongue K13.21
- ureter (postinfectional) N28.89
- urethra (postinfectional) N36.8
- uterus N85.8
- vagina N89.4
- vocal cord J38.3
- vulva N90.4

Leukorrhea N89.8
- due to Trichomonas (vaginalis) A59.00
- trichomonal A59.00

Leukosarcoma C85.9

Levocardia (isolated) Q24.1
- with situs inversus Q89.3

Levotransposition Q20.5

Lev's disease or syndrome (acquired complete heart block) I44.2

Levulosuria —*see* Fructosuria

Levurid L30.2

Lewy body (ies) (disease) G31.83

Leyden-Möbius dystrophy —*see* Dystrophy, Leyden-Möbius

Leydig cell
- carcinoma
  - specified site —*see* Neoplasm, malignant, by site
  - unspecified site
    - female C56.9-●
    - male C62.9-●
- tumor
  - benign
    - specified site —*see* Neoplasm, benign, by site
    - unspecified site
      - female D27.-●
      - male D29.2-●
  - malignant
    - specified site —*see* Neoplasm, malignant, by site
    - unspecified site
      - female C56.-●
      - male C62.9-●
  - specified site —*see* Neoplasm, uncertain behavior, by site
  - unspecified site
    - female D39.1-●
    - male D40.1-●

Leydig-Sertoli cell tumor
- specified site —*see* Neoplasm, benign, by site
- unspecified site
  - female D27.-●
  - male D29.2-●

LGMD —*see* Dystrophy, muscular, limb-girdle

LGSIL (Low grade squamous intraepithelial lesion on cytologic smear of)
- anus R85.612
- cervix R87.612
- vagina R87.622

Liar, pathologic F60.2

Libido
- decreased R68.82

Libman-Sacks disease M32.11

Lice (infestation) B85.2
- body (Pediculus corporis) B85.1
- crab B85.3
- head (Pediculus capitis) B85.0
- mixed (classifiable to more than one of the titles B85.0-B85.3) B85.4
- pubic (Phthirus pubis) B85.3

Lichen L28.0
- albus L90.0
  - penis N48.0
  - vulva N90.4
- amyloidosis E85.4 *[L99]*
- atrophicus L90.0
  - penis N48.0
  - vulva N90.4
- congenital Q82.8
- myxedematosus L98.5
- nitidus L44.1
- pilaris Q82.8
  - acquired L85.8
- ➡ planopilaris L66.10
  - ▶ classic L66.11
  - ▶ follicular L66.11
  - ▶ specified NEC L66.19
- planus (chronicus) L43.9
  - annularis L43.8
  - bullous L43.1
  - ➡ follicular L66.11
  - hypertrophic L43.0
  - moniliformis L44.3
  - of Wilson L43.9
  - specified NEC L43.8
  - subacute (active) L43.3
  - tropicus L43.3
- ruber
  - acuminatus L44.0
  - moniliformis L44.3
  - planus L43.9
- sclerosus (et atrophicus) L90.0
  - penis N48.0
  - vulva N90.4
- scrofulosus (primary) (tuberculous) A18.4
- simplex (chronicus) (circumscriptus) L28.0
- striatus L44.2
- urticatus L28.2

Lichenification L28.0

Lichenoid keratosis —*see* Keratosis, lichenoid

Lichenoides tuberculosis (primary) A18.4

Lichtheim's disease or syndrome D51.0

Lien migrans D73.89

Ligament —*see* condition

Light
- for gestational age —*see* Light for dates
- headedness R42

Light-for-dates (infant) P05.00
- with weight of
  - 499 grams or less P05.01
  - 500-749 grams P05.02
  - 750-999 grams P05.03
  - 1000-1249 grams P05.04
  - 1250-1499 grams P05.05
  - 1500-1749 grams P05.06
  - 1750-1999 grams P05.07
  - 2000-2499 grams P05.08
  - 2500 grams and over P05.09
- affecting management of pregnancy O36.59-●
- and small-for-dates —*see* Small for dates
- specified NEC P05.09

Lightning (effects) (stroke) (struck by) T75.00
- burn —*see* Burn
- foot E53.8
- shock T75.01
- specified effect NEC T75.09

Lightwood-Albright syndrome N25.89

Lightwood's disease or syndrome (renal tubular acidosis) N25.89

Lignac (-de Toni) (-Fanconi) (-Debré) disease or syndrome E72.09
- with cystinosis E72.04

Ligneous thyroiditis E06.5

Likoff's syndrome I20.89

Limb —*see* condition

Limbic epilepsy personality syndrome F07.0

Limitation, limited
- activities due to disability Z73.6
- cardiac reserve —*see* Disease, heart

Limitation, limited *(Continued)*
- eye muscle duction, traumatic —*see* Strabismus, mechanical
- mandibular range of motion M26.52

Lindau (-von Hippel) **disease** Q85.83

Line(s)
- Beau's L60.4
- Harris' —*see* Arrest, epiphyseal
- Hudson's (cornea) —*see* Pigmentation, cornea, anterior
- Stähli's (cornea) —*see* Pigmentation, cornea, anterior

Linea corneae senilis —*see* Change, cornea, senile

Lingua
- geographica K14.1
- nigra (villosa) K14.3
- plicata K14.5
- tylosis K13.29

Lingual —*see* condition

Linguatulosis B88.8

Linitis (gastric) **plastica** C16.9

Lip —*see* condition

Lipedema —*see* Edema

Lipemia —*see also* Hyperlipidemia
- retina, retinalis E78.3

Lipidosis E75.6
- cerebral (infantile) (juvenile) (late) E75.4
- cerebroretinal E75.4
- cerebroside E75.22
- cholesterol (cerebral) E75.5
- glycolipid E75.21
- hepatosplenomegalic E78.3
- sphingomyelin —*see* Niemann-Pick disease or syndrome
- sulfatide E75.29

Lipoadenoma —*see* Neoplasm, benign, by site

Lipoblastoma —*see* Lipoma

Lipoblastomatosis —*see* Lipoma

Lipochondrodystrophy E76.01

Lipochrome histiocytosis (familial) D71

Lipodermatosclerosis —(*see also* Insufficiency, venous) M79.3
- with
  - varicose veins - see Varix, leg, with, inflammation
  - ulcerated - see Varix, leg, with, ulcer, with inflammation by site
- ulcerated —*see* Ulcer, by site

Lipodystrophia progressiva E88.1

Lipodystrophy (progressive) E88.1
- insulin E88.1
- intestinal K90.81
- mesenteric K65.4

Lipofibroma —*see* Lipoma

Lipofuscinosis, neuronal (with ceroidosis) E75.4

Lipogranuloma, sclerosing L92.8

Lipogranulomatosis E78.89

Lipoid —*see also* condition
- histiocytosis D76.3
  - essential E75.29
- nephrosis N04.9
- proteinosis of Urbach E78.89

Lipoidemia —*see* Hyperlipidemia

Lipoidosis —*see* Lipidosis

Lipoma D17.9
- fetal D17.9
  - fat cell D17.9
- infiltrating D17.9
- intramuscular D17.9
- pleomorphic D17.9
- site classification
  - arms (skin) (subcutaneous) D17.2-●
  - connective tissue D17.30
    - intra-abdominal D17.5
    - intrathoracic D17.4
    - peritoneum D17.79
    - retroperitoneum D17.79
    - specified site NEC D17.39
    - spermatic cord D17.6
  - face (skin) (subcutaneous) D17.0
  - genitourinary organ NEC D17.72
  - head (skin) (subcutaneous) D17.0
  - intra-abdominal D17.5
  - intrathoracic D17.4
  - kidney D17.71
  - legs (skin) (subcutaneous) D17.2-●
  - neck (skin) (subcutaneous) D17.0
  - peritoneum D17.79
  - retroperitoneum D17.79
  - skin D17.30
    - specified site NEC D17.39

L

L

- **Lymphoma** *(Continued)*
  - Hodgkin C81.9-•
    - lymphocyte-rich (classical) C81.4-•
    - lymphocyte depleted (classical) C81.3-•
    - mixed cellularity (classical) C81.2-•
    - nodular sclerosis (classical) C81.1-•
    - specified NEC (classical) C81.7-•
    - lymphocyte-rich classical C81.4-•
    - lymphocyte depleted classical C81.3-•
    - mixed cellularity classical C81.2-•
    - nodular
      - lymphocyte predominant C81.0-•
      - sclerosis (classical) C81.1-•
  - intravascular large B-cell C83.8-•
  - Lennert's C84.4-•
  - lymphoblastic (diffuse) C83.5-•
  - lymphoblastic B-cell C83.5-•
  - lymphoblastic T-cell C83.5-•
  - lymphoepithelioid C84.4-•
  - lymphoplasmacytic C83.0-•
    - ➡with IgM-production C88.0-•
  - ➡MALT C88.4-•
  - mantle cell C83.1-•
  - mature T-cell NEC C84.4-•
  - mature T/NK-cell C84.9-•
    - specified NEC C84.Z-•
  - mediastinal (thymic) large B-cell C85.2-•
  - ➡Mediterranean C88.3-•
  - ▶meninges, primary —*see* Lymphoma, primary central nervous system
  - ➡mucosa-associated lymphoid tissue [MALT-lymphoma] C88.4-•
  - NK/T cell C84.9-•
  - nodal marginal zone C83.0-•
  - non-follicular (diffuse) C83.9-•
    - specified NEC C83.8-•
  - non-Hodgkin —*see also* Lymphoma, by type C85.9-•
    - specified NEC C85.8-•
  - non-leukemic variant of B-CLL C83.0-•
  - peripheral T-cell NEC C84.4-•
  - ▶primary central nervous system (brain) (meninges) (PCNSL) (spinal cord) C83.390
    - ▶Burkitt C83.79
    - ▶diffuse large B-cell C83.390
    - ▶lymphoblastic C83.59
    - ▶peripheral T-cell C84.49
  - primary cutaneous
    - ➡anaplastic large cell C86.6-•
    - ➡CD30-positive large T-cell C86.6-•
  - primary effusion B-cell C83.8-•
  - ➡SALT C88.4-•
  - ➡skin-associated lymphoid tissue [SALT-lymphoma] C88.4-•
  - small cell B-cell C83.0-•
  - ▶spinal cord, primary —*see* Lymphoma, primary central nervous system
  - splenic marginal zone C83.0-•
  - ➡subcutaneous panniculitis-like T-cell C86.3-•
  - T-precursor C83.5-•
  - true histiocytic C96.A
- **Lymphomatosis** —*see* Lymphoma
- **Lymphopathia venereum, veneris** A55
- **Lymphopenia** D72.810
- **Lymphoplasmacytic leukemia** —*see* Leukemia, chronic lymphocytic, B-cell type
- **Lymphoproliferation, X-linked disease** D82.3
- **Lymphoreticulosis, benign** (of inoculation) A28.1
- **Lymphorrhea** I89.8
- **Lymphosarcoma** (diffuse) —*see also* Lymphoma C85.9-•
- **Lymphostasis** I89.8
- **Lypemania** —*see* Melancholia
- **Lysine and hydroxylysine metabolism disorder** E72.3
- **Lyssa** —*see* Rabies

M

- **Macacus ear** Q17.3
- **Maceration, wet feet, tropical** (syndrome) T69.02-•
- **MacLeod's syndrome** J43.0
- **Macrocephalia, macrocephaly** Q75.3
- **Macrocheilia, macrochilia** (congenital)Q18.6
- **Macrocolon** —*see also* Megacolon Q43.1
- **Macrocornea** Q15.8
  - with glaucoma Q15.0
- **Macrocytic** —*see* condition
- **Macrocytosis** D75.89
- **Macrodactylia, macrodactylism** (fingers) (thumbs) Q74.0
  - toes Q74.2
- **Macrodontia** K00.2
- **Macrogenia** M26.05
- **Macrogenitosomia** (adrenal) (male) (praecox) E25.9
  - congenital E25.0
- ➡**Macroglobulinemia** (idiopathic) (primary) C88.0-•
  - monoclonal (essential) D47.2
  - ➡Waldenström C88.0-•
- **Macroglossia** (congenital) Q38.2
  - acquired K14.8
- **Macrognathia, macrognathism** (congenital) (mandibular) (maxillary) M26.09
- **Macrogyria** (congenital) Q04.8
- **Macrohydrocephalus** —*see* Hydrocephalus
- **Macromastia** —*see* Hypertrophy, breast
- **Macrophthalmos** Q11.3
  - in congenital glaucoma Q15.0
- **Macropsia** H53.15
- **Macrosigmoid** K59.39
  - congenital Q43.2
- **Macrospondylitis, acromegalic** E22.0
- **Macrostomia** (congenital) Q18.4
- **Macrotia** (external ear) (congenital) Q17.1
- **Macula**
  - cornea, corneal —*see* Opacity, cornea
  - degeneration (atrophic) (exudative) (senile) —*see also* Degeneration, macula
    - hereditary —*see* Dystrophy, retina
- **Maculae ceruleae** — B85.1
- **Maculopathy, toxic** —*see* Degeneration, macula, toxic
- **Madarosis** (eyelid) H02.729
  - left H02.726
    - lower H02.725
    - upper H02.724
  - right H02.723
    - lower H02.722
    - upper H02.721
- **Madelung's**
  - deformity (radius) Q74.0
  - disease
    - radial deformity Q74.0
    - symmetrical lipomas, neck E88.89
- **Madness** —*see* Psychosis
- **Madura**
  - foot B47.9
    - actinomycotic B47.1
    - mycotic B47.0
- **Maduromycosis** B47.0
- **Maffucci's syndrome** Q78.4
- **Magnesium metabolism disorder** —*see* Disorder, metabolism, magnesium
- **Main en griffe** (acquired) —*see also* Deformity, limb, clawhand
  - congenital Q68.1
- **Maintenance** (encounter for)
  - antineoplastic chemotherapy Z51.11
  - antineoplastic radiation therapy Z51.0
  - methadone F11.20
- **Majocchi's**
  - disease L81.7
  - granuloma B35.8
- **Major** —*see* condition
- **Malabar itch** (any site) B35.5
- **Malabsorption** K90.9
  - calcium K90.89
  - carbohydrate K90.49
  - disaccharide E73.9
  - fat K90.49
  - galactose E74.20
  - glucose(-galactose) E74.39
  - intestinal K90.9
    - specified NEC K90.89
  - isomaltose E74.31
  - lactose E73.9
  - methionine E72.19
  - monosaccharide E74.39
  - postgastrectomy K91.2
  - postsurgical K91.2
  - protein K90.49
  - starch K90.49
  - sucrose E74.39
  - syndrome K90.9
    - postsurgical K91.2
- **Malacia, bone** (adult) M83.9
  - juvenile —*see* Rickets
- **Malacoplakia**
  - bladder N32.89
  - pelvis (kidney) N28.89
  - ureter N28.89
  - urethra N36.8
- **Malacosteon, juvenile** —*see* Rickets
- **Maladaptation** —*see* Maladjustment
- **Maladie de Roger** Q21.0
- **Maladjustment**
  - conjugal Z63.0
    - involving divorce or estrangement Z63.5
  - educational Z55.4
  - family Z63.9
  - marital Z63.0
    - involving divorce or estrangement Z63.5
  - occupational NEC Z56.89
  - simple, adult —*see* Disorder, adjustment
  - situational —*see* Disorder, adjustment
  - social Z60.9
    - due to
      - acculturation difficulty Z60.3
      - discrimination and persecution (perceived) Z60.5
      - exclusion and isolation Z60.4
      - life-cycle (phase of life) transition Z60.0
      - rejection Z60.4
      - specified reason NEC Z60.8
- **Malaise** R53.81
- **Malakoplakia** —*see* Malacoplakia
- **Malaria, malarial** (fever) B54
  - with
    - blackwater fever B50.8
      - hemoglobinuric (bilious) B50.8
    - hemoglobinuria B50.8
  - accidentally induced (therapeutically) - code by type under Malaria
  - algid B50.9
  - cerebral B50.0 *[G94]*
  - clinically diagnosed (without parasitological confirmation) B54
  - congenital NEC P37.4
    - falciparum P37.3
  - congestion, congestive B54
  - continued (fever) B50.9
  - estivo-autumnal B50.9
  - falciparum B50.9
    - with complications NEC B50.8
      - cerebral B50.0 *[G94]*
    - severe B50.8
  - hemorrhagic B54
  - malariae B52.9
    - with
      - complications NEC B52.8
      - glomerular disorder B52.0
  - malignant (tertian) —*see* Malaria, falciparum
  - mixed infections — code to first listed type in B50-B53
  - ovale B53.0
  - parasitologically confirmed NEC B53.8
  - pernicious, acute —*see* Malaria, falciparum
  - Plasmodium (P.)
    - falciparum NEC —*see* Malaria, falciparum
    - malariae NEC B52.9
      - with Plasmodium
        - falciparum (and or vivax) —*see* Malaria, falciparum
        - vivax —*see also* Malaria, vivax
          - and falciparum —*see* Malaria, falciparum
    - ovale B53.0
      - with Plasmodium malariae —*see also* Malaria, malariae
        - and vivax —*see also* Malaria, vivax
          - and falciparum —*see* Malaria, falciparum
    - simian B53.1
      - with Plasmodium malariae —*see also* Malaria, malariae
        - and vivax —*see also* Malaria, vivax
          - and falciparum —*see* Malaria, falciparum
    - vivax NEC B51.9
      - with Plasmodium falciparum —*see* Malaria, falciparum
  - quartan —*see* Malaria, malariae
  - quotidian —*see* Malaria, falciparum
  - recurrent B54
  - remittent B54
  - specified type NEC (parasitologically confirmed) B53.8
  - spleen B54

Malformation *(Continued)*
- thyroid gland Q89.2
- tongue (congenital) Q38.3
  - hypertrophy Q38.2
  - tie Q38.1
- trachea Q32.1
- tricuspid valve Q22.9
  - specified type NEC Q22.8
- umbilical cord NEC (complicating delivery) O69.89
- umbilicus Q89.9
- ureter Q62.8
  - agenesis Q62.4
  - duplication Q62.5
  - malposition —*see* Malposition, congenital, ureter
  - obstructive defect —*see* Defect, obstructive, ureter
  - vesico-uretero-renal reflux Q62.7
- urethra Q64.79
  - aplasia Q64.5
  - duplication Q64.74
  - posterior valves Q64.2
  - prolapse Q64.71
  - stricture Q64.32
- urinary system Q64.9
- uterus Q51.9
  - specified type NEC Q51.818
- vagina Q52.4
- vascular system, peripheral Q27.9
- vas deferens Q55.4
  - atresia Q55.3
- venous —*see* Anomaly, vein(s)
- vulva Q52.70

Malfunction —*see also* Dysfunction
- cardiac electronic device T82.119
  - electrode T82.11Ø
  - pulse generator T82.111
  - specified type NEC T82.118
- catheter device NEC T85.618
  - cystostomy T83.Ø1Ø
  - dialysis (renal) (vascular) T82.41
    - intraperitoneal T85.611
  - infusion NEC T82.514
    - cranial (*see also* Complication(s), catheter, cranial infusion, mechanical) T85.69Ø
    - epidural (*see also* Complication(s), catheter, cranial infusion, mechanical) T85.69Ø
    - intrathecal (*see also* Complication(s), catheter, cranial infusion, mechanical) T85.69Ø
    - spinal (*see also* Complication(s), catheter, cranial infusion, mechanical) T85.69Ø
    - subarachnoid (*see also* Complication(s), catheter, cranial infusion, mechanical) T85.69Ø
    - subdural (*see also* Complication(s), catheter, cranial infusion, mechanical) T85.69Ø
  - urinary —*see also* Breakdown, device, catheter T83.Ø18
- colostomy K94.Ø3
  - valve K94.Ø3
- cystostomy (stoma) N99.512
  - catheter T83.Ø1Ø
- enteric stoma K94.13
- enterostomy K94.13
- esophagostomy K94.33
- gastroenteric K31.89
- gastrostomy K94.23
- ileostomy K94.13
  - valve K94.13
- intrathecal infusion pump T85.615
- jejunostomy K94.13
- nervous system device, implant or graft, specified NEC T85.615
- pacemaker —*see* Malfunction, cardiac electronic device
- prosthetic device, internal —*see* Complications, prosthetic device, by site, mechanical
- tracheostomy J95.Ø3
- urinary device NEC —*see* Complication, genitourinary, device, urinary, mechanical
- valve
  - colostomy K94.Ø3
  - heart T82.Ø9
  - ileostomy K94.13
- vascular graft or shunt NEC —*see* Complication, cardiovascular device, mechanical, vascular
- ventricular (communicating shunt) T85.Ø1

Malherbe's tumor —*see* Neoplasm, skin, benign

Malibu disease L98.8-●

Malignancy —*see also* Neoplasm, malignant, by site
- unspecified site (primary) C8Ø.1

Malignant —*see* condition

Malingerer, malingering Z76.5

Mallet finger (acquired) —*see* Deformity, finger, mallet finger
- congenital Q74.Ø
- sequelae of rickets E64.3

Malleus A24.Ø

Mallory's bodies R89.7

Mallory-Weiss syndrome K22.6

Malnutrition E46
- degree
  - first E44.1
  - mild (protein) E44.1
  - moderate (protein) E44.Ø
  - second E44.Ø
  - severe (protein-energy) E43
    - ▶with
      - ▶kwashiorkor E4Ø
      - ▶marasmus E41
    - intermediate form E42
      - with
        - kwashiorkor E42
        - ~~marasmus E41~~
  - third E43
- following gastrointestinal surgery K91.2
- intrauterine
  - light-for-dates —*see* Light for dates
  - small-for-dates —*see* Small for dates
- lack of care, or neglect (child) (infant) T76.Ø2
  - confirmed T74.Ø2
- malignant E4Ø
- protein E46
  - calorie E46
    - mild E44.1
    - moderate E44.Ø
    - severe E43
      - ▶with
        - ▶kwashiorkor E4Ø
        - ▶marasmus E41
      - intermediate form E42
        - with
          - kwashiorkor (and marasmus) E42
          - ~~marasmus E41~~
  - energy E46
    - mild E44.1
    - moderate E44.Ø
    - severe E43
      - ▶with
        - ▶kwashiorkor E4Ø
        - ▶marasmus E41
      - intermediate form E42
        - with
          - kwashiorkor (and marasmus) E42
          - ~~marasmus E41~~
- severe (protein-energy) E43
  - with
    - ➡kwashiorkor E4Ø
      - ▶with marasmus E42
    - ~~marasmus E41~~
  - ▶intermediate form E42
    - ▶with
      - ▶kwashiorkor (and marasmus) E42
    - ▶marasmus E41

Malocclusion (teeth) M26.4
- Angle's M26.219
  - class I M26.211
  - class II M26.212
  - class III M26.213
- due to
  - abnormal swallowing M26.59
  - mouth breathing M26.59
  - tongue, lip or finger habits M26.59
- temporomandibular (joint) M26.69

Malposition
- cervix —*see* Malposition, uterus
- congenital
  - adrenal (gland) Q89.1
  - alimentary tract Q45.8
    - lower Q43.8
    - upper Q4Ø.8
  - aorta Q25.49
  - appendix Q43.8
  - arterial trunk Q2Ø.Ø
  - artery (peripheral) Q27.8
    - coronary Q24.5
    - digestive system Q27.8
    - lower limb Q27.8

Malposition *(Continued)*
- congenital *(Continued)*
  - artery *(Continued)*
    - pulmonary Q25.79
    - specified site NEC Q27.8
    - upper limb Q27.8
  - auditory canal Q17.8
    - causing impairment of hearing Q16.9
  - auricle (ear) Q17.4
    - causing impairment of hearing Q16.9
    - cervical Q18.2
  - biliary duct or passage Q44.5
  - bladder (mucosa) —*see* Exstrophy, bladder
  - brachial plexus QØ7.8
  - brain tissue QØ4.8
  - breast Q83.8
  - bronchus Q32.4
  - cecum Q43.8
  - clavicle Q74.Ø
  - colon Q43.8
  - digestive organ or tract NEC Q45.8
    - lower Q43.8
    - upper Q4Ø.8
  - ear (auricle) (external) Q17.4
    - ossicles Q16.3
  - endocrine (gland) NEC Q89.2
  - epiglottis Q31.8
  - eustachian tube Q17.8
  - eye Q15.8
  - facial features Q18.8
  - fallopian tube Q5Ø.6
  - finger(s) Q68.1
    - supernumerary Q69.Ø
  - foot Q66.9-●
  - gallbladder Q44.1
  - gastrointestinal tract Q45.8
  - genitalia, genital organ(s) or tract
    - female Q52.8
      - external Q52.79
      - internal NEC Q52.8
    - male Q55.8
  - glottis Q31.8
  - hand Q68.1
  - heart Q24.8
    - dextrocardia Q24.Ø
      - with complete transposition of viscera Q89.3
  - hepatic duct Q44.5
  - hip (joint) Q65.89
  - intestine (large) (small) Q43.8
    - with anomalous adhesions, fixation or malrotation Q43.3
  - joint NEC Q68.8
  - kidney Q63.2
  - larynx Q31.8
  - limb Q68.8
    - lower Q68.8
    - upper Q68.8
  - liver Q44.79
  - lung (lobe) Q33.8
  - nail(s) Q84.6
  - nerve QØ7.8
  - nervous system NEC QØ7.8
  - nose, nasal (septum) Q3Ø.8
  - organ or site not listed —*see* Anomaly, by site
  - ovary Q5Ø.39
  - pancreas Q45.3
  - parathyroid (gland) Q89.2
  - patella Q74.1
  - peripheral vascular system Q27.8
  - pituitary (gland) Q89.2
  - respiratory organ or system NEC Q34.8
  - rib (cage) Q76.6
    - supernumerary in cervical region Q76.5
  - scapula Q74.Ø
  - shoulder Q74.Ø
  - spinal cord QØ6.8
  - spleen Q89.Ø9
  - sternum NEC Q76.7
  - stomach Q4Ø.2
  - symphysis pubis Q74.2
  - thymus (gland) Q89.2
  - thyroid (gland) (tissue) Q89.2
    - cartilage Q31.8
  - toe(s) Q66.9-●
    - supernumerary Q69.2
  - tongue Q38.3
  - trachea Q32.1
  - ureter Q62.6Ø
    - deviation Q62.61
    - displacement Q62.62

M

M

M

- **Meige's syndrome** Q82.Ø
- **Melalgia, nutritional** E53.8
- **Melancholia** F32.A
  - climacteric (single episode) F32.89
    - recurrent episode F33.8
  - hypochondriac F45.29
  - intermittent (single episode) F32.89
    - recurrent episode F33.8
  - involutional (single episode) F32.89
    - recurrent episode F33.8
  - menopausal (single episode) F32.89
    - recurrent episode F33.8
  - puerperal F32.89
  - reactive (emotional stress or trauma) F32.3
  - recurrent F33.9
  - senile FØ3
  - stuporous (single episode) F32.89
    - recurrent episode F33.8
- **Melanemia** R79.89
- **Melanoameloblastoma** —*see* Neoplasm, bone, benign
- **Melanoblastoma** —*see* Melanoma
- **Melanocarcinoma** —*see* Melanoma
- **Melanocytoma, eyeball** D31.9-●
- **Melanocytosis, neurocutaneous** Q82.8
- **Melanoderma, melanodermia** L81.4
- **Melanodontia, infantile** KØ3.89
- **Melanodontoclasia** KØ3.89
- **Melanoepithelioma** —*see* Melanoma
- **Melanoma (malignant)** C43.9
  - acral lentiginous, malignant —*see* Melanoma, skin, by site
  - amelanotic —*see* Melanoma, skin, by site
  - balloon cell —*see* Melanoma, skin, by site
  - benign —*see* Nevus
  - desmoplastic, malignant —*see* Melanoma, skin, by site
  - epithelioid cell —*see* Melanoma, skin, by site
    - with spindle cell, mixed —*see* Melanoma, skin, by site
  - in
    - giant pigmented nevus —*see* Melanoma, skin, by site
    - Hutchinson's melanotic freckle —*see* Melanoma, skin, by site
    - junctional nevus —*see* Melanoma, skin, by site
    - precancerous melanosis —*see* Melanoma, skin, by site
  - in situ DØ3.9
    - abdominal wall DØ3.59
    - ala nasi DØ3.39
    - ankle DØ3.7-●
    - anus, anal (margin) (skin) DØ3.51
    - arm DØ3.6-●
    - auditory canal DØ3.2-●
    - auricle (ear) DØ3.2-●
    - auricular canal (external) DØ3.2-●
    - axilla, axillary fold DØ3.59
    - back DØ3.59
    - breast DØ3.52
    - brow DØ3.39
    - buttock DØ3.59
    - canthus (eye) DØ3.1-●
    - cheek (external) DØ3.39
    - chest wall DØ3.59
    - chin DØ3.39
    - choroid DØ3.8
    - conjunctiva DØ3.8
    - ear (external) DØ3.2-●
    - external meatus (ear) DØ3.2-●
    - eye DØ3.8
    - eyebrow DØ3.39
    - eyelid (lower) (upper) DØ3.1-●
    - face DØ3.3Ø
      - specified NEC DØ3.39
    - female genital organ (external) NEC DØ3.8
    - finger DØ3.6-●
    - flank DØ3.59
    - foot DØ3.7-●
    - forearm DØ3.6-●
    - forehead DØ3.39
    - foreskin DØ3.8
    - gluteal region DØ3.59
    - groin DØ3.59
    - hand DØ3.6-●
    - heel DØ3.7-●
    - helix DØ3.2-●
    - hip DØ3.7-●
    - interscapular region DØ3.59
    - iris DØ3.8
    - jaw DØ3.39

Melanoma *(Continued)*
  - in situ *(Continued)*
    - knee DØ3.7-●
    - labium (majus) (minus) DØ3.8
    - lacrimal gland DØ3.8
    - leg DØ3.7-●
    - lip (lower) (upper) DØ3.Ø
    - lower limb NEC DØ3.7-●
    - male genital organ (external) NEC DØ3.8
    - nail DØ3.9
      - finger DØ3.6-●
      - toe DØ3.7-●
    - neck DØ3.4
    - nose (external) DØ3.39
    - orbit DØ3.8
    - penis DØ3.8
    - perianal skin DØ3.51
    - perineum DØ3.51
    - pinna DØ3.2-●
    - popliteal fossa or space DØ3.7-●
    - prepuce DØ3.8
    - pudendum DØ3.8
    - retina DØ3.8
    - retrobulbar DØ3.8
    - scalp DØ3.4
    - scrotum DØ3.8
    - shoulder DØ3.6-●
    - specified site NEC DØ3.8
    - submammary fold DØ3.52
    - temple DØ3.39
    - thigh DØ3.7-●
    - toe DØ3.7-●
    - trunk NEC DØ3.59
    - umbilicus DØ3.59
    - upper limb NEC DØ3.6-●
    - vulva DØ3.8
  - juvenile —*see* Nevus
  - malignant, of soft parts except skin —*see* Neoplasm, connective tissue, malignant
  - metastatic
    - breast C79.81
    - genital organ C79.82
    - specified site NEC C79.89
  - neurotropic, malignant —*see* Melanoma, skin, by site
  - nodular —*see* Melanoma, skin, by site
  - regressing, malignant —*see* Melanoma, skin, by site
  - skin C43.9
    - abdominal wall C43.59
    - ala nasi C43.31
    - ankle C43.7-●
    - anus, anal (skin) C43.51
    - arm C43.6-●
    - auditory canal (external) C43.2-●
    - auricle (ear) C43.2-●
    - auricular canal (external) C43.2-●
    - axilla, axillary fold C43.59
    - back C43.59
    - breast (female) (male) C43.52
    - brow C43.39
    - buttock C43.59
    - canthus (eye) C43.1-●
    - cheek (external) C43.39
    - chest wall C43.59
    - chin C43.39
    - ear (external) C43.2-●
    - elbow C43.6-●
    - external meatus (ear) C43.2-●
    - eyebrow C43.39
    - eyelid (lower) (upper) C43.1-●
    - face C43.3Ø
      - specified NEC C43.39
    - female genital organ (external) NEC C51.9
    - finger C43.6-●
    - flank C43.59
    - foot C43.7-●
    - forearm C43.6-●
    - forehead C43.39
    - foreskin C6Ø.Ø
    - glabella C43.39
    - gluteal region C43.59
    - groin C43.59
    - hand C43.6-●
    - heel C43.7-●
    - helix C43.2-●
    - hip C43.7-●
    - interscapular region C43.59
    - jaw (external) C43.39
    - knee C43.7-●

Melanoma *(Continued)*
  - skin *(Continued)*
    - labium C51.9
      - majus C51.Ø
      - minus C51.1
    - leg C43.7-●
    - lip (lower) (upper) C43.Ø
    - lower limb NEC C43.7-●
    - male genital organ (external) NEC C63.9
    - nail
      - finger C43.6-●
      - toe C43.7-●
    - nasolabial groove C43.39
    - nates C43.59
    - neck C43.4
    - nose (external) C43.31
    - overlapping site C43.8
    - palpebra C43.1-●
    - penis C6Ø.9
    - perianal skin C43.51
    - perineum C43.51
    - pinna C43.2-●
    - popliteal fossa or space C43.7-●
    - prepuce C6Ø.Ø
    - pudendum C51.9
    - scalp C43.4
    - scrotum C63.2
    - shoulder C43.6-●
    - skin NEC C43.9
    - submammary fold C43.52
    - temple C43.39
    - thigh C43.7-●
    - toe C43.7-●
    - trunk NEC C43.59
    - umbilicus C43.59
    - upper limb NEC C43.6-●
    - vulva C51.9
      - overlapping sites C51.8
  - spindle cell
    - with epithelioid, mixed —*see* Melanoma, skin, by site
    - type A C69.4-●
    - type B C69.4-●
  - superficial spreading —*see* Melanoma, skin, by site
- **Melanosarcoma** —*see also* Melanoma
  - epithelioid cell —*see* Melanoma
- **Melanosis** L81.4
  - addisonian E27.1
    - tuberculous A18.7
  - adrenal E27.1
  - colon K63.89
  - conjunctiva —*see* Pigmentation, conjunctiva
    - congenital Q13.89
  - cornea (presenile) (senile) —*see also* Pigmentation, cornea
    - congenital Q13.4
  - eye NEC H57.89
    - congenital Q15.8
  - lenticularis progressiva Q82.1
  - liver K76.89
  - precancerous —*see also* Melanoma, in situ
    - malignant melanoma in —*see* Melanoma
  - Riehl's L81.4
  - sclera H15.89
    - congenital Q13.89
  - suprarenal E27.1
  - tar L81.4
  - toxic L81.4
- **Melanuria** R82.998
- **MELAS syndrome** E88.41
- **Melasma** L81.1
  - adrenal (gland) E27.1
  - suprarenal (gland) E27.1
- **Melena** K92.1
  - with ulcer - code by site under Ulcer, with hemorrhage K27.4
  - due to swallowed maternal blood P78.2
  - newborn, neonatal P54.1
    - due to swallowed maternal blood P78.2
- **Meleney's**
  - gangrene (cutaneous) —*see* Ulcer, skin
  - ulcer (chronic undermining) —*see* Ulcer, skin
- **Melioidosis** A24.9
  - acute A24.1
  - chronic A24.2
  - fulminating A24.1
  - pneumonia A24.1
  - pulmonary (chronic) A24.2
    - acute A24.1
    - subacute A24.2

M

M

M

M

M

M

▶ New ➡ Revised ~~deleted~~ Deleted ● Use Additional Character(s)

M

Myositis *(Continued)*
interstitial *(Continued)*
lower leg M60.16-●
multiple sites M60.19
shoulder region M60.11-●
specified site NEC M60.18
thigh M60.15-●
upper arm M60.12-●
mycotic B49 *[M63.8-●]*
ossificans or ossifying (circumscripta) —*see also* Ossification, muscle, specified NEC
in (due to)
burns M61.30
ankle M61.37-●
foot M61.37-●
forearm M61.33-●
hand M61.34-●
lower leg M61.36-●
multiple sites M61.39
pelvic region M61.35-●
shoulder region M61.31-●
specified site NEC M61.38
thigh M61.35-●
upper arm M61.32-●
quadriplegia or paraplegia M61.20
ankle M61.27-●
foot M61.27-●
forearm M61.23-●
hand M61.24-●
lower leg M61.26-●
multiple sites M61.29
pelvic region M61.25-●
shoulder region M61.21-●
specified site NEC M61.28
thigh M61.25-●
upper arm M61.22-●
progressiva M61.10
ankle M61.17-●
finger M61.14-●
foot M61.17-●
forearm M61.13-●
hand M61.14-●
lower leg M61.16-●
multiple sites M61.19
pelvic region M61.15-●
shoulder region M61.11-●
specified site NEC M61.18
thigh M61.15-●
toe M61.17-●
upper arm M61.12-●
traumatica M61.00
ankle M61.07-●
foot M61.07-●
forearm M61.03-●
hand M61.04-●
lower leg M61.06-●
multiple sites M61.09
pelvic region M61.05-●
shoulder region M61.01-●
specified site NEC M61.08
thigh M61.05-●
upper arm M61.02-●
purulent —*see* Myositis, infective
specified type NEC M60.80
ankle M60.87-●
foot M60.87-●
forearm M60.83-●
hand M60.84-●
lower leg M60.86-●
multiple sites M60.89
pelvic region M60.85-●
shoulder region M60.81-●
specified site NEC M60.88
thigh M60.85-●
upper arm M60.82-●
suppurative —*see* Myositis, infective
traumatic (old) —*see* Myositis, specified type NEC
Myospasia impulsiva F95.2
Myotonia (acquisita) (intermittens) M62.89
atrophica G71.11
chondrodystrophic G71.13
congenita (acetazolamide responsive) (dominant) (recessive) G71.12
drug-induced G71.14
dystrophica G71.11
fluctuans G71.19
levior G71.12
permanens G71.19
symptomatic G71.19
Myotonic pupil —*see* Anomaly, pupil, function, tonic pupil
Myriapodiasis B88.2
Myringitis H73.2-●
with otitis media —*see* Otitis, media
acute H73.00-●
bullous H73.01-●
specified NEC H73.09-●
bullous —*see* Myringitis, acute, bullous
chronic H73.1-●
Mysophobia F40.228
Mytilotoxism —*see* Poisoning, fish
Myxadenitis labialis K13.0
Myxedema (adult) (idiocy) (infantile) (juvenile) —*see also* Hypothyroidism E03.9
circumscribed E05.90
with storm E05.91
coma E03.5
congenital E00.1
cutis L98.5
localized (pretibial) E05.90
with storm E05.91
papular L98.5
Myxochondrosarcoma —*see* Neoplasm, cartilage, malignant
Myxofibroma —*see* Neoplasm, connective tissue, benign
odontogenic —*see* Cyst, calcifying odontogenic
Myxofibrosarcoma —*see* Neoplasm, connective tissue, malignant
Myxolipoma D17.9
Myxoliposarcoma —*see* Neoplasm, connective tissue, malignant
Myxoma —*see also* Neoplasm, connective tissue, benign
nerve sheath —*see* Neoplasm, nerve, benign
odontogenic —*see* Cyst, calcifying odontogenic
Myxosarcoma —*see* Neoplasm, connective tissue, malignant

N

Naegeli's
disease Q82.8
leukemia, monocytic C93.1-●
Naegleriasis (with meningoencephalitis) B60.2
Naffziger's syndrome G54.0
Naga sore —*see* Ulcer, skin
Nägele's pelvis M95.5
with disproportion (fetopelvic) O33.0
causing obstructed labor O65.0
Nail —*see also* condition
biting F98.8
patella syndrome Q87.2
Nanism, nanosomia —*see* Dwarfism
Nanophyetiasis B66.8
Nanukayami A27.89
Napkin rash L22
Narcolepsy G47.419
with cataplexy G47.411
in conditions classified elsewhere G47.429
with cataplexy G47.421
Narcosis R06.89
Narcotism —*see* Dependence
NARP (Neuropathy, Ataxia and Retinitis pigmentosa) syndrome E88.49
Narrow
anterior chamber angle H40.03-●
gingival width (of periodontal soft tissue) K05.5
pelvis —*see* Contraction, pelvis
Narrowing —*see also* Stenosis
artery I77.1
auditory, internal I65.8
basilar —*see* Occlusion, artery, basilar
carotid —*see* Occlusion, artery, carotid
▶caudal septum, fixed, lower lateral cartilage, alar rim and nasal sill J34.8211
cerebellar —*see* Occlusion, artery, cerebellar
cerebral —*see* Occlusion artery, cerebral
choroidal —*see* Occlusion, artery, precerebral, specified NEC
communicating posterior —*see* Occlusion, artery, precerebral, specified NEC
coronary —*see also* Disease, heart, ischemic, atherosclerotic
congenital Q24.5
syphilitic A50.54 *[I52]*
due to syphilis NEC A52.06

Narrowing *(Continued)*
artery *(Continued)*
hypophyseal —*see* Occlusion, artery, precerebral, specified NEC
pontine —*see* Occlusion, artery, precerebral, specified NEC
precerebral —*see* Occlusion, artery, precerebral
vertebral —*see* Occlusion, artery, vertebral
auditory canal (external) —*see* Stenosis, external ear canal
eustachian tube —*see* Obstruction, eustachian tube
eyelid —*see* Disorder, eyelid function
larynx J38.6
mesenteric artery —*see also* Ischemia, intestine, acute K55.059
palate M26.89
palpebral fissure —*see* Disorder, eyelid function
ureter N13.5
with infection N13.6
urethra —*see* Stricture, urethra
Narrowness, abnormal, eyelid Q10.3
Nasal —*see* condition
Nasolachrymal, nasolacrimal —*see* condition
Nasopharyngeal —*see also* condition
pituitary gland Q89.2
torticollis M43.6
Nasopharyngitis (acute) (infective) (streptococcal) (subacute) J00
chronic (suppurative) (ulcerative) J31.1
Nasopharynx, nasopharyngeal —*see* condition
Natal tooth, teeth K00.6
Nausea (without vomiting) R11.0
with vomiting R11.2
gravidarum —*see* Hyperemesis, gravidarum
marina T75.3
navalis T75.3
Navel —*see* condition
Neapolitan fever —*see* Brucellosis
Near drowning T75.1
Nearsightedness —*see* Myopia
Near-syncope R55
Nebula, cornea —*see* Opacity, cornea
Necator americanus infestation B76.1
Necatoriasis B76.1
Neck —*see* condition
Necrobiosis R68.89
lipoidica NEC L92.1
with diabetes —*see* E08-E13 with .620
Necrolysis, toxic epidermal L51.2
due to drug
correct substance properly administered —*see* Table of Drugs and Chemicals, by drug, adverse effect
overdose or wrong substance given or taken —*see* Table of Drugs and Chemicals, by drug, poisoning
Necrophilia F65.89
Necrosis, necrotic (ischemic) —*see also* Gangrene
adrenal (capsule) (gland) E27.49
amputation stump (surgical) (late) T87.50
arm T87.5-●
leg T87.5-●
antrum J32.0
aorta (hyaline) —*see also* Aneurysm, aorta
cystic medial —*see* Dissection, aorta
artery I77.5
bladder (aseptic) (sphincter) N32.89
bone —*see also* Osteonecrosis M87.9
aseptic or avascular —*see* Osteonecrosis
idiopathic M87.00
ethmoid J32.2
jaw M27.2
tuberculous —*see* Tuberculosis, bone
brain I67.89
breast (aseptic) (fat) (segmental) N64.1
bronchus J98.09
central nervous system NEC I67.89
cerebellar I67.89
cerebral I67.89
colon —*see also* Infarct, intestine K55.049
cornea H18.89-●
cortical (acute) (renal) N17.1
cystic medial (aorta) —*see* Dissection, aorta
dental pulp K04.1
esophagus K22.89
ethmoid (bone) J32.2
eyelid —*see* Disorder, eyelid, degenerative
fat, fatty (generalized) —*see also* Disorder, soft tissue, specified type NEC
abdominal wall K65.4
breast (aseptic) (segmental) N64.1

N

▶ New ➠ Revised ~~deleted~~ Deleted ● Use Additional Character(s)

Nephritis, nephritic *(Continued)*
  chronic NØ3.9
    with
      C3
        glomerulonephritis NØ3.A
        glomerulopathy NØ3.A
          with dense deposit disease NØ3.6
      dense deposit disease NØ3.6
      diffuse
        crescentic glomerulonephritis NØ3.7
        endocapillary proliferative glomerulonephritis NØ3.4
        membranous glomerulonephritis NØ3.2
        mesangial proliferative glomerulonephritis NØ3.3
        mesangiocapillary glomerulonephritis NØ3.5
      focal and segmental glomerular lesions NØ3.1
      minor glomerular abnormality NØ3.Ø
      specified morphological changes NEC NØ3.8
    arteriosclerotic *—see* Hypertension, kidney
  cirrhotic N26.9
  complicating pregnancy O26.83-●
  croupous NØØ.9
  degenerative *—see* Nephrosis
  diffuse sclerosing NØ5.8
  due to
    diabetes mellitus *—see* EØ8-E13 with .21
    subacute bacterial endocarditis I33.Ø
    systemic lupus erythematosus (chronic) M32.14
    typhoid fever AØ1.Ø9
  gonococcal (acute) (chronic) A54.21
  hypocomplementemic *—see* Nephritis, membranoproliferative
  IgA *—see* Nephropathy, IgA
  immune complex (circulating) NEC NØ5.8
  infective *—see* Nephritis, tubulo-interstitial
  interstitial *—see* Nephritis, tubulo-interstitial
  lead N14.3
  membranoproliferative (diffuse) (type 1 or 3) *—see also* NØØ-NØ7 with fourth character .5 NØ5.5
    type 2 *—see also* NØØ-NØ7 with fourth character .6 NØ5.6
  minimal change NØ5.Ø
  necrotic, necrotizing NEC *—see also* NØØ-NØ7 with fourth character .8 NØ5.8
  nephrotic *—see* Nephrosis
  nodular *—see* Nephritis, membranoproliferative
  polycystic Q61.3
    adult type Q61.2
    autosomal
      dominant Q61.2
      recessive NEC Q61.19
    childhood type NEC Q61.19
    infantile type NEC Q61.19
  poststreptococcal NØ5.9
    acute NØØ.9
    chronic NØ3.9
    rapidly progressive NØ1.9
  proliferative NEC *—see also* NØØ-NØ7 with fourth character .8 NØ5.8
  purulent *—see* Nephritis, tubulo-interstitial
  rapidly progressive NØ1.9
    with
      C3
        glomerulonephritis NØ1.A
        glomerulopathy NØ1.A
          with dense deposit disease NØ1.6
      dense deposit disease NØ1.6
      diffuse
        crescentic glomerulonephritis NØ1.7
        endocapillary proliferative glomerulonephritis NØ1.4
        membranous glomerulonephritis NØ1.2
        mesangial proliferative glomerulonephritis NØ1.3
        mesangiocapillary glomerulonephritis NØ1.5
      focal and segmental glomerular lesions NØ1.1
      minor glomerular abnormality NØ1.Ø
      specified morphological changes NEC NØ1.8
  salt losing or wasting NEC N28.89
  saturnine N14.3

Nephritis, nephritic *(Continued)*
  sclerosing, diffuse NØ5.8
  septic *—see* Nephritis, tubulo-interstitial
  specified pathology NEC *—see also* NØØ-NØ7 with fourth character .8 NØ5.8
  subacute NØ1.9
  suppurative *—see* Nephritis, tubulo-interstitial
  syphilitic (late) A52.75
    congenital A5Ø.59 *[NØ8]*
    early (secondary) A51.44
  toxic *—see* Nephropathy, toxic
  tubal, tubular *—see* Nephritis, tubulo-interstitial
  tuberculous A18.11
  tubulo-interstitial (in) N12
    acute (infectious) N1Ø
    chronic (infectious) N11.9
      nonobstructive N11.8
        reflux-associated N11.Ø
      obstructive N11.1
      specified NEC N11.8
    due to
      brucellosis A23.9 *[N16]*
      cryoglobulinemia D89.1 *[N16]*
      glycogen storage disease E74.ØØ *[N16]*
    Sjögren's syndrome M35.Ø4
  vascular *—see* Hypertension, kidney
  war NØØ.9
Nephroblastoma (epithelial) (mesenchymal) C64-●
Nephrocalcinosis E83.59 *[N29]*
Nephrocystitis, pustular *—see* Nephritis, tubulo-interstitial
Nephrolithiasis (congenital) (pelvis) (recurrent) *—see also* Calculus, kidney
Nephroma C64-●
  mesoblastic D41.Ø-●
Nephronephritis *—see* Nephrosis
Nephronophthisis Q61.5
Nephropathia epidemica A98.5
Nephropathy *—see also* Nephritis N28.9
  with
    edema *—see* Nephrosis
    glomerular lesion *—see* Glomerulonephritis
  amyloid, hereditary E85.Ø
  analgesic N14.Ø
    with medullary necrosis, acute N17.2
  Balkan (endemic) N15.Ø
  chemical *—see* Nephropathy, toxic
  contrast-induced N14.11
  contrast medium, radiography N14.11
  diabetic *—see* EØ8-E13 with .21
  drug-induced N14.2
    contrast-induced N14.11
    specified NEC N14.19
  focal and segmental hyalinosis or sclerosis NØ2.1
  heavy metal-induced N14.3
  hereditary NEC NØ7.9
    with
      C3
        glomerulonephritis NØ7.A
        glomerulopathy NØ7.A
          with dense deposit disease NØ7.6
      dense deposit disease NØ7.6
      diffuse
        crescentic glomerulonephritis NØ7.7
        endocapillary proliferative glomerulonephritis NØ7.4
        membranous glomerulonephritis NØ7.2
        mesangial proliferative glomerulonephritis NØ7.3
        mesangiocapillary glomerulonephritis NØ7.5
      focal and segmental glomerular lesions NØ7.1
      minor glomerular abnormality NØ7.Ø
      specified morphological changes NEC NØ7.8
  hypercalcemic N25.89
  hypertensive *—see* Hypertension, kidney
  hypokalemic (vacuolar) N25.89
  IgA IgA NØ2.B-●
    with glomerular lesion NØ2.B1
      focal and segmental hyalinosis or sclerosis NØ2.B2
      membranoproliferative (diffuse) NØ2.B3
      membranous (diffuse) NØ2.B4
      mesangial proliferative (diffuse) NØ2.B5
      mesangiocapillary (diffuse) NØ2.B6
      proliferative NEC NØ2.B9
      specified pathology NEC NØ2.B9
  lead N14.3
  membranoproliferative (diffuse) NØ2.5

Nephropathy *(Continued)*
  membranous (diffuse) NØ2.2Ø
    with
      nephrotic syndrome NØ4.2Ø
        primary NØ4.21
        secondary NØ4.22
    idiopathic, with nephrotic syndrome NØ4.21
    primary NØ6.21
      with nephrotic syndrome NØ4.21
    secondary NØ6.22
      with nephrotic syndrome NØ4.22
  mesangial (IgA/IgG) *—see* Nephropathy, IgA
    proliferative (diffuse) NØ2.3
  mesangiocapillary (diffuse) NØ2.5
  obstructive N13.8
  phenacetin N17.2
  phosphate-losing N25.Ø
  potassium depletion N25.89
  pregnancy-related O26.83-●
  proliferative NEC (*see also* NØØ-NØ7 with fourth character .8) NØ5.8
  protein-losing N25.89
  saturnine N14.3
  sickle-cell D57.-● *[NØ8]*
  toxic NEC N14.4
    due to
      drugs N14.2
        analgesic N14.Ø
        specified NEC N14.19
      heavy metals N14.3
  vasomotor N17.Ø
  water-losing N25.89
Nephroptosis N28.83
Nephropyosis *—see* Abscess, kidney
Nephrorrhagia N28.89
Nephrosclerosis (arteriolar) (arteriosclerotic) (chronic) (hyaline) *—see also* Hypertension, kidney
  hyperplastic *—see* Hypertension, kidney
  senile N26.9
Nephrosis, nephrotic (Epstein's) (syndrome) (congenital) NØ4.9
  with
    foot process disease NØ4.9
    glomerular lesion NØ4.1
    hypocomplementemic NØ4.5
  acute NØ4.9
  anoxic *—see* Nephrosis, tubular
  chemical *—see* Nephrosis, tubular
  cholemic K76.7
  diabetic *—see* EØ8-E13 with .21
  Finnish type (congenital) Q89.8
  hemoglobin N1Ø
  hemoglobinuric *—see* Nephrosis, tubular
  in
    amyloidosis E85.4 *[NØ8]*
    diabetes mellitus *—see* EØ8-E13 with .21
    epidemic hemorrhagic fever A98.5
    malaria (malariae) B52.Ø
  ischemic *—see* Nephrosis, tubular
  lipoid NØ4.9
  lower nephron *—see* Nephrosis, tubular
  malarial (malariae) B52.Ø
  minimal change NØ4.Ø
  myoglobin N1Ø
  necrotizing *—see* Nephrosis, tubular
  osmotic (sucrose) N25.89
  radiation NØ4.9
  syphilitic (late) A52.75
  toxic *—see* Nephrosis, tubular
  tubular (acute) N17.Ø
    postprocedural N99.Ø
    radiation NØ4.9
Nephrosonephritis, hemorrhagic (endemic) A98.5
Nephrostomy
  attention to Z43.6
  status Z93.6
Nerve *—see also* condition
  injury *—see* Injury, nerve, by body site
Nerves R45.Ø
Nervous *—see also* condition R45.Ø
  heart F45.8
  stomach F45.8
  tension R45.Ø
Nervousness R45.Ø
Nesidioblastoma
  pancreas D13.7
  specified site NEC *—see* Neoplasm, benign, by site
  unspecified site D13.7

328 ▶ New ➠ Revised ~~deleted~~ Deleted ● Use Additional Character(s)

N

- **Nettleship's syndrome** —*see* Urticaria pigmentosa
- **Neumann's disease or syndrome** L1Ø.1
- **Neuralgia, neuralgic** (acute) M79.2
  - accessory (nerve) G52.8
  - acoustic (nerve) —*see* subcategory H93.3
  - auditory (nerve) —*see* subcategory H93.3
  - ciliary G44.ØØ9
    - intractable G44.ØØ1
    - not intractable G44.ØØ9
  - cranial
    - nerve —*see also* Disorder, nerve, cranial
      - fifth or trigeminal —*see* Neuralgia, trigeminal
    - postherpetic, postzoster BØ2.29
  - ear —*see* subcategory H92.Ø
  - facialis vera G51.1
  - Fothergill's —*see* Neuralgia, trigeminal
  - glossopharyngeal (nerve) G52.1
  - Horton's G44.Ø99
    - intractable G44.Ø91
    - not intractable G44.Ø99
  - Hunt's BØ2.21
  - hypoglossal (nerve) G52.3
  - infraorbital —*see* Neuralgia, trigeminal
  - malarial —*see* Malaria
  - migrainous G44.ØØ9
    - intractable G44.ØØ1
    - not intractable G44.ØØ9
  - Morton's G57.6-●
  - nerve, cranial —*see* Disorder, nerve, cranial
  - nose G52.Ø
  - occipital M54.81
  - olfactory G52.Ø
  - penis N48.9
  - perineum R1Ø.2
  - postherpetic NEC BØ2.29
    - trigeminal BØ2.22
  - pubic region R1Ø.2
  - scrotum R1Ø.2
  - Sluder's G44.89
  - specified nerve NEC G58.8
  - spermatic cord R1Ø.2
  - sphenopalatine (ganglion) G9Ø.Ø9
  - trifacial —*see* Neuralgia, trigeminal
  - trigeminal G5Ø.Ø
    - postherpetic, postzoster BØ2.22
  - vagus (nerve) G52.2
  - writer's F48.8
    - organic G25.89
- **Neurapraxia** —*see* Injury, nerve
- **Neurasthenia** F48.8
  - cardiac F45.8
  - gastric F45.8
  - heart F45.8
- **Neurilemmoma** —*see also* Neoplasm, nerve, benign
  - acoustic (nerve) D33.3
  - malignant —*see also* Neoplasm, nerve, malignant
    - acoustic (nerve) C72.4
- **Neurilemmosarcoma** —*see* Neoplasm, nerve, malignant
- **Neurinoma** —*see* Neoplasm, nerve, benign
- **Neurinomatosis** —*see* Neoplasm, nerve, uncertain behavior
- **Neuritis** (rheumatoid) M79.2
  - abducens (nerve) —*see* Strabismus, paralytic, sixth nerve
  - accessory (nerve) G52.8
  - acoustic (nerve) —*see also* subcategory H93.3
    - in (due to)
      - infectious disease NEC B99 *[H94.Ø-●]*
      - parasitic disease NEC B89 *[H94.Ø-●]*
    - syphilitic A52.15
  - alcoholic G62.1
    - with psychosis —*see* Psychosis, alcoholic
  - amyloid, any site E85.4 *[G63]*
  - auditory (nerve) —*see* subcategory H93.3
  - brachial —*see* Radiculopathy
    - due to displacement, intervertebral disc —*see* Disorder, disc, cervical, with neuritis
  - cranial nerve
    - due to Lyme disease A69.22
    - eighth or acoustic or auditory —*see* subcategory H93.3
    - eleventh or accessory G52.8
    - fifth or trigeminal G5Ø.-●
    - first or olfactory G52.Ø
    - fourth or trochlear —*see* Strabismus, paralytic, fourth nerve
    - second or optic —*see* Neuritis, optic
    - seventh or facial G51.8
      - newborn (birth injury) P11.3

- **Neuritis** *(Continued)*
  - cranial nerve *(Continued)*
    - sixth or abducent —*see* Strabismus, paralytic, sixth nerve
    - tenth or vagus G52.2
    - third or oculomotor —*see* Strabismus, paralytic, third nerve
    - twelfth or hypoglossal G52.3
  - Déjérine-Sottas G6Ø.Ø
  - diabetic (mononeuropathy) —*see* EØ8-E13 with .41
    - polyneuropathy —*see* EØ8-E13 with .42
  - due to
    - beriberi E51.11
    - displacement, prolapse or rupture, intervertebral disc —*see* Disorder, disc, with, radiculopathy
    - herniation, nucleus pulposus M51.9 *[G55]*
  - endemic E51.11
  - facial G51.8
    - newborn (birth injury) P11.3
  - general —*see* Polyneuropathy
  - geniculate ganglion G51.1
    - due to herpes (zoster) BØ2.21
  - gouty —*see also* Gout, by type M1Ø.9 *[G63]*
  - hypoglossal (nerve) G52.3
  - ilioinguinal (nerve) G57.9-●
  - infectious (multiple) NEC G61.Ø
  - interstitial hypertrophic progressive G6Ø.Ø
  - lumbar M54.16
  - lumbosacral M54.17
  - multiple —*see also* Polyneuropathy
    - endemic E51.11
    - infective, acute G61.Ø
  - multiplex endemica E51.11
  - nerve root —*see* Radiculopathy
  - oculomotor (nerve) —*see* Strabismus, paralytic, third nerve
  - olfactory nerve G52.Ø
  - optic (nerve) (hereditary) (sympathetic) H46.9
    - with demyelination G36.Ø
    - in myelitis G36.Ø
    - nutritional H46.2
    - papillitis —*see* Papillitis, optic
    - retrobulbar H46.1-●
    - specified type NEC H46.8
    - toxic H46.3
  - peripheral (nerve) G62.9
    - multiple —*see* Polyneuropathy
    - single —*see* Mononeuritis
  - pneumogastric (nerve) G52.2
  - postherpetic, postzoster BØ2.29
  - progressive hypertrophic interstitial G6Ø.Ø
  - retrobulbar —*see also* Neuritis, optic, retrobulbar
    - in (due to)
      - late syphilis A52.15
      - meningococcal infection A39.82
    - meningococcal A39.82
    - syphilitic A52.15
  - sciatic (nerve) —*see also* Sciatica
    - due to displacement of intervertebral disc —*see* Disorder, disc, with, radiculopathy
  - serum —*see also* Reaction, serum T8Ø.69
  - shoulder-girdle G54.5
  - specified nerve NEC G58.8
  - spinal (nerve) root —*see* Radiculopathy
  - syphilitic A52.15
  - thenar (median) G56.1-●
  - thoracic M54.14
  - toxic NEC G62.2
  - trochlear (nerve) —*see* Strabismus, paralytic, fourth nerve
  - vagus (nerve) G52.2
- **Neuroastrocytoma** —*see* Neoplasm, uncertain behavior, by site
- **Neuroavitaminosis** E56.9 *[G99.8]*
- **Neuroblastoma**
  - olfactory C3Ø.Ø
  - specified site —*see* Neoplasm, malignant, by site
  - unspecified site C74.9Ø
- **Neurochorioretinitis** —*see* Chorioretinitis
- **Neurocirculatory asthenia** F45.8
- **Neurocysticercosis** B69.Ø
- **Neurocytoma** —*see* Neoplasm, benign, by site
- **Neurodermatitis** (circumscribed) (circumscripta) (local) L28.Ø
  - atopic L2Ø.81
  - diffuse (Brocq) L2Ø.81
  - disseminated L2Ø.81
- **Neuroencephalomyelopathy, optic** G36.Ø

- **Neuroepithelioma** —*see also* Neoplasm, malignant, by site
  - olfactory C3Ø.Ø
- **Neurofibroma** —*see also* Neoplasm, nerve, benign
  - melanotic —*see* Neoplasm, nerve, benign
  - multiple —*see* Neurofibromatosis
  - plexiform —*see* Neoplasm, nerve, benign
- **Neurofibromatosis** (multiple) (nonmalignant) Q85.ØØ
  - acoustic Q85.Ø2
  - malignant —*see* Neoplasm, nerve, malignant
  - specified NEC Q85.Ø9
  - type 1 (von Recklinghausen) Q85.Ø1
  - type 2 Q85.Ø2
- **Neurofibrosarcoma** —*see* Neoplasm, nerve, malignant
- **Neurogenic** —*see also* condition
  - bladder —*see also* Dysfunction, bladder, neuromuscular N31.9
    - cauda equina syndrome G83.4
  - bowel NEC K59.2
  - heart F45.8
- **Neuroglioma** —*see* Neoplasm, uncertain behavior, by site
- **Neurolabyrinthitis** (of Dix and Hallpike) —*see* Neuronitis, vestibular
- **Neurolathyrism** —*see* Poisoning, food, noxious, plant
- **Neuroleprosy** A3Ø.9
- **Neuroma** —*see also* Neoplasm, nerve, benign
  - acoustic (nerve) D33.3
  - amputation (stump) (traumatic) (surgical complication) (late) T87.3-●
    - arm T87.3-●
    - leg T87.3-●
  - digital (toe) G57.6-●
  - interdigital G58.8
    - lower limb toe G57.8-●
    - upper limb G56.8-●
  - intermetatarsal G57.8-●
  - Morton's G57.6-●
  - nonneoplastic
    - arm G56.9-●
    - leg G57.9-●
    - lower extremity G57.9-●
    - upper extremity G56.9-●
  - optic (nerve) D33.3
  - plantar G57.6-●
  - plexiform —*see* Neoplasm, nerve, benign
  - surgical (nonneoplastic)
    - arm G56.9-●
    - leg G57.9-●
    - lower extremity G57.9-●
    - upper extremity G56.9-●
- **Neuromyalgia** —*see* Neuralgia
- **Neuromyasthenia** (epidemic) (postinfectious) G93.39
- **Neuromyelitis** G36.9
  - ascending G61.Ø
  - optica G36.Ø
- **Neuromyopathy** G7Ø.9
  - paraneoplastic (*see also*, Neoplasm, by site, if known) D49.9 *[G13.Ø]*
- **Neuromyotonia** (Isaacs) G71.19
- **Neuronevus** —*see* Nevus
- **Neuronitis** G58.9
  - ascending (acute) G57.2-●
  - vestibular H81.2-●
- **Neuroparalytic** —*see* condition
- **Neuropathy, neuropathic** G62.9
  - acute motor G62.81
  - alcoholic G62.1
    - with psychosis —*see* Psychosis, alcoholic
  - arm G56.9-●
  - autonomic, peripheral —*see* Neuropathy, peripheral, autonomic
  - axillary G56.9-●
  - bladder N31.9
    - atonic (motor) (sensory) N31.2
    - autonomous N31.2
    - flaccid N31.2
    - nonreflex N31.2
    - reflex N31.1
    - uninhibited N31.Ø
  - brachial plexus G54.Ø
  - cervical plexus G54.2
  - chronic
    - progressive segmentally demyelinating G62.89
    - relapsing demyelinating G62.89

Neuropathy, neuropathic *(Continued)*
- Déjérine-Sottas G6Ø.Ø
- diabetic —*see* EØ8-E13 with .4Ø
  - mononeuropathy —*see* EØ8-E13 with .41
  - polyneuropathy —*see* EØ8-E13 with .42
- entrapment G58.9
  - iliohypogastric nerve G57.8-●
  - ilioinguinal nerve G57.8-●
  - lateral cutaneous nerve of thigh G57.1-●
  - median nerve G56.Ø-●
  - obturator nerve G57.8-●
  - peroneal nerve G57.3-●
  - posterior tibial nerve G57.5-●
  - saphenous nerve G57.8-●
  - ulnar nerve G56.2-●
- facial nerve G51.9
- hereditary G6Ø.9
  - motor and sensory (types I-IV) G6Ø.Ø
  - sensory G6Ø.8
  - specified NEC G6Ø.8
- hypertrophic G6Ø.Ø
  - Charcot-Marie-Tooth G6Ø.Ø
  - Déjérine-Sottas G6Ø.Ø
  - interstitial progressive G6Ø.Ø
  - of infancy G6Ø.Ø
  - Refsum G6Ø.1
- idiopathic G6Ø.9
  - progressive G6Ø.3
  - specified NEC G6Ø.8
- in association with hereditary ataxia G6Ø.2
- intercostal G58.Ø
- ischemic —*see* Disorder, nerve
- Jamaica (ginger) G62.2
- leg NEC G57.9-●
- lower extremity G57.9-●
- lumbar plexus G54.1
- median nerve G56.1-●
- motor and sensory —*see also* Polyneuropathy
  - hereditary (types I-IV) G6Ø.Ø
- multifocal motor (MMN) G61.82
- multiple (acute) (chronic) —*see* Polyneuropathy
- optic (nerve) —*see also* Neuritis, optic
  - ischemic H47.Ø1-●
- paraneoplastic (sensorial) (Denny Brown) (*see also*, Neoplasm, by site, if known) D49.9 *[G13.Ø]*
- peripheral (nerve) —*see also* Polyneuropathy G62.9
  - autonomic G9Ø.9
    - idiopathic G9Ø.Ø9
    - in (due to)
      - amyloidosis E85.4 *[G99.Ø]*
      - diabetes mellitus —*see* EØ8-E13 with .43
      - endocrine disease NEC E34.9 *[G99.Ø]*
      - gout M1Ø.ØØ *[G99.Ø]*
      - hyperthyroidism EØ5.9Ø *[G99.Ø]*
        - with thyroid storm EØ5.91 *[G99.Ø]*
      - metabolic disease NEC E88.9 *[G99.Ø]*
  - idiopathic G6Ø.9
    - progressive G6Ø.3
  - in (due to)
    - antitetanus serum G62.Ø
    - arsenic G62.2
    - drugs NEC G62.Ø
    - lead G62.2
    - organophosphate compounds G62.2
    - toxic agent NEC G62.2
- plantar nerves G57.6-●
- progressive
  - hypertrophic interstitial G6Ø.Ø
  - inflammatory G62.81
- radicular NEC —*see* Radiculopathy
- sacral plexus G54.1
- sciatic G57.Ø-●
- serum G61.1
- toxic NEC G62.2
- trigeminal sensory G5Ø.8
- ulnar nerve G56.2-●
- uremic N18.9 *[G63]*
- vitamin B12 E53.8 *[G63]*
  - with anemia (pernicious) D51.Ø *[G63]*
    - due to dietary deficiency D51.3 *[G63]*

Neurophthisis —*see also* Disorder, nerve
- peripheral, diabetic —*see* EØ8-E13 with .42

Neuroretinitis —*see* Chorioretinitis

Neuroretinopathy, hereditary optic H47.22

Neurosarcoma —*see* Neoplasm, nerve, malignant

Neurosclerosis —*see* Disorder, nerve

Neurosis, neurotic F48.9
- anankastic F42.8
- anxiety (state) F41.1
  - panic type F41.Ø
- asthenic F48.8
- bladder F45.8
- cardiac (reflex) F45.8
- cardiovascular F45.8
- character F6Ø.9
- colon F45.8
- compensation F68.1Ø
- compulsive, compulsion F42.8
- conversion F44.9
- craft F48.8
- cutaneous F45.8
- depersonalization F48.1
- depressive (reaction) (type) F34.1
- environmental F48.8
- excoriation L98.1
- fatigue F48.8
- functional —*see* Disorder, somatoform
- gastric F45.8
- gastrointestinal F45.8
- heart F45.8
- hypochondriacal F45.21
- hysterical F44.9
- incoordination F45.8
  - larynx F45.8
  - vocal cord F45.8
- intestine F45.8
- larynx (sensory) F45.8
  - hysterical F44.4
- mixed NEC F48.8
- musculoskeletal F45.8
- obsessional F42.8
- obsessive-compulsive F42.8
- occupational F48.8
- ocular NEC F45.8
- organ —*see* Disorder, somatoform
- pharynx F45.8
- phobic F4Ø.9
- posttraumatic (situational) F43.1Ø
  - acute F43.11
  - chronic F43.12
- psychasthenic (type) F48.8
- railroad F48.8
- rectum F45.8
- respiratory F45.8
- rumination F45.8
- sexual F65.9
- situational F48.8
- social F4Ø.1Ø
  - generalized F4Ø.11
- specified type NEC F48.8
- state F48.9
  - with depersonalization episode F48.1
- stomach F45.8
- traumatic F43.1Ø
  - acute F43.11
  - chronic F43.12
- vasomotor F45.8
- visceral F45.8
- war F48.8

Neurospongioblastosis diffusa Q85.1

Neurosyphilis (arrested) (early) (gumma) (late) (latent) (recurrent) (relapse) A52.3
- with ataxia (cerebellar) (locomotor) (spastic) (spinal) A52.19
- aneurysm (cerebral) A52.Ø5
- arachnoid (adhesive) A52.13
- arteritis (any artery) (cerebral) A52.Ø4
- asymptomatic A52.2
- congenital A5Ø.4Ø
- dura (mater) A52.13
- general paresis A52.17
- hemorrhagic A52.Ø5
- juvenile (asymptomatic) (meningeal) A5Ø.4Ø
- leptomeninges (aseptic) A52.13
- meningeal, meninges (adhesive) A52.13
- meningitis A52.13
- meningovascular (diffuse) A52.13
- optic atrophy A52.15
- parenchymatous (degenerative) A52.19
- paresis, paretic A52.17
  - juvenile A5Ø.45
- remission in (sustained) A52.3
- serological (without symptoms) A52.2
- specified nature or site NEC A52.19
- tabes, tabetic (dorsalis) A52.11
  - juvenile A5Ø.45

Neurosyphilis *(Continued)*
- ➡ taboparesis (taboparetic) A52.17
  - juvenile A5Ø.45
- thrombosis (cerebral) A52.Ø5
- vascular (cerebral) NEC A52.Ø5

Neurothekeoma —*see* Neoplasm, nerve, benign

Neurotic —*see* Neurosis

Neurotoxemia —*see* Toxemia

Neutroclusion M26.211

Neutropenia, neutropenic (chronic) (genetic) (idiopathic) (immune) (infantile) (malignant) (pernicious) (splenic) D7Ø.9
- ▶ benign ethnic —*see* Phenotype, Duffy, null
- congenital (primary) D7Ø.Ø
- cyclic D7Ø.4
- cytoreductive cancer chemotherapy sequela D7Ø.1
- drug-induced D7Ø.2
  - due to cytoreductive cancer chemotherapy D7Ø.1
- due to infection D7Ø.3
- fever D7Ø.9
- neonatal, transitory (isoimmune) (maternal transfer) P61.5
- periodic D7Ø.4
- secondary (cyclic) (periodic) (splenic) D7Ø.4
  - drug-induced D7Ø.2
    - due to cytoreductive cancer chemotherapy D7Ø.1
- specified NEC D7Ø.8
- toxic D7Ø.8

Neutrophilia, hereditary giant D72.Ø

Nevocarcinoma —*see* Melanoma

Nevus D22.9
- achromic —*see* Neoplasm, skin, benign
- amelanotic —*see* Neoplasm, skin, benign
- angiomatous D18.ØØ
  - intra-abdominal D18.Ø3
  - intracranial D18.Ø2
  - skin D18.Ø1
  - specified site NEC D18.Ø9
- araneus I78.1
- balloon cell —*see* Neoplasm, skin, benign
- bathing trunk D48.5
- blue —*see* Neoplasm, skin, benign
  - cellular —*see* Neoplasm, skin, benign
  - giant —*see* Neoplasm, skin, benign
  - Jadassohn's —*see* Neoplasm, skin, benign
  - malignant —*see* Melanoma
- capillary D18.ØØ
  - intra-abdominal D18.Ø3
  - intracranial D18.Ø2
  - skin D18.Ø1
  - specified site NEC D18.Ø9
- cavernous D18.ØØ
  - intra-abdominal D18.Ø3
  - intracranial D18.Ø2
  - skin D18.Ø1
  - specified site NEC D18.Ø9
- cellular —*see* Neoplasm, skin, benign
  - blue —*see* Neoplasm, skin, benign
- choroid D31.3-●
- comedonicus Q82.5
- conjunctiva D31.Ø-●
- dermal —*see* Neoplasm, skin, benign
  - with epidermal nevus —*see* Neoplasm, skin, benign
- dysplastic —*see* Neoplasm, skin, benign
- eye D31.9-●
- flammeus Q82.5
- hemangiomatous D18.ØØ
  - intra-abdominal D18.Ø3
  - intracranial D18.Ø2
  - skin D18.Ø1
  - specified site NEC D18.Ø9
- iris D31.4-●
- lacrimal gland D31.5-●
- lymphatic D18.1
- magnocellular
  - specified site —*see* Neoplasm, benign, by site
  - unspecified site D31.4Ø
- malignant —*see* Melanoma
- meaning hemangioma D18.ØØ
  - intra-abdominal D18.Ø3
  - intracranial D18.Ø2
  - skin D18.Ø1
  - specified site NEC D18.Ø9
- mouth (mucosa) D1Ø.3Ø
  - specified site NEC D1Ø.39
  - white sponge Q38.6
- multiplex Q85.1

Newborn *(Continued)*
affected by *(Continued)*
placenta previa P02.0
placental
abnormality (functional) (morphological) P02.20
specified NEC P02.29
dysfunction P02.29
infarction P02.29
insufficiency P02.29
separation NEC P02.1
transfusion syndromes P02.3
placentitis P02.78
precipitate delivery P03.5
prolapsed cord P02.4
respiratory arrest P28.81
slow intrauterine growth P05.9
tobacco P04.2
twin to twin transplacental transfusion P02.3
umbilical cord (tightly) around neck P02.5
umbilical cord condition P02.60
short cord P02.69
specified NEC P02.69
uterine contractions (abnormal) P03.6
vasa previa P02.69
from intrauterine blood loss P50.0
apnea (*see also* Apnea, newborn) P28.40
obstructive P28.42
primary (*see also* Apnea, newborn, sleep, primary) P28.30
sleep (central) (obstructive) (primary) (*see also* Apnea, newborn, sleep, primary) P28.30
born in hospital Z38.00
by cesarean Z38.01
born outside hospital Z38.1
breast buds P96.89
breast engorgement P83.4
check-up —*see* Newborn, examination
convulsion P90
dehydration P74.1
examination
8 to 28 days old Z00.111
under 8 days old Z00.110
fever P81.9
environmentally-induced P81.0
hyperbilirubinemia P59.9
of prematurity P59.0
hypernatremia P74.21
hyponatremia P74.22
infection P39.9
candidal P37.5
specified NEC P39.8
urinary tract P39.3
jaundice P59.9
due to
breast milk inhibitor P59.3
hepatocellular damage P59.20
specified NEC P59.29
preterm delivery P59.0
of prematurity P59.0
specified NEC P59.8
late metabolic acidosis P74.0
mastitis P39.0
infective P39.0
noninfective P83.4
multiple born NEC Z38.8
born in hospital Z38.68
by cesarean Z38.69
born outside hospital Z38.7
omphalitis P38.9
with mild hemorrhage P38.1
without hemorrhage P38.9
post-term P08.21
prolonged gestation (over 42 completed weeks) P08.22
quadruplet Z38.8
born in hospital Z38.63
by cesarean Z38.64
born outside hospital Z38.7
quintuplet Z38.8
born in hospital Z38.65
by cesarean Z38.66
born outside hospital Z38.7
seizure P90
sepsis (congenital) P36.9
due to
anaerobes NEC P36.5
Escherichia coli P36.4
Staphylococcus P36.30
aureus P36.2
specified NEC P36.39

Newborn *(Continued)*
sepsis *(Continued)*
due to *(Continued)*
Streptococcus P36.10
group B P36.0
specified NEC P36.19
specified NEC P36.8
triplet Z38.8
born in hospital Z38.61
by cesarean Z38.62
born outside hospital Z38.7
twin Z38.5
born in hospital Z38.30
by cesarean Z38.31
born outside hospital Z38.4
vomiting P92.09
bilious P92.01
weight check Z00.111
Newcastle conjunctivitis or disease B30.8
Nezelof's syndrome (pure alymphocytosis) D81.4
Niacin (amide) **deficiency** E52
Nicolas (-Durand)-Favre disease A55
Nicotine —*see* Tobacco
Nicotinic acid deficiency E52
Niemann-Pick disease or syndrome E75.249
specified NEC E75.248
type
A E75.240
A/B E75.244
B E75.241
C E75.242
D E75.243
Night
blindness —*see* Blindness, night
sweats R61
terrors (child) F51.4
Nightmares (REM sleep type) F51.5
NIHSS (National Institutes of Health Stroke Scale) score R29.7-●
Nipple —*see* condition
Nisbet's chancre A57
Nishimoto (-Takeuchi) disease I67.5
Nitritoid crisis or reaction —*see* Crisis, nitritoid
Nitrosohemoglobinemia D74.8
Njovera A65
~~No general equivalence degree (GED) Z55.5~~
▶**No**
▶general equivalence degree (GED) Z55.5
▶health insurance coverage Z59.71
Nocardiosis, nocardiasis A43.9
cutaneous A43.1
lung A43.0
pneumonia A43.0
pulmonary A43.0
specified site NEC A43.8
Nocturia R35.1
psychogenic F45.8
Nocturnal —*see* condition
Nodal rhythm I49.8
Node(s) —*see also* Nodule
Bouchard's (with arthropathy) M15.2
Haygarth's M15.8
Heberden's (with arthropathy) M15.1
larynx J38.7
lymph —*see* condition
milker's B08.03
Osler's I33.0
Schmorl's —*see* Schmorl's disease
singer's J38.2
teacher's J38.2
tuberculous —*see* Tuberculosis, lymph gland
vocal cord J38.2
Nodule(s), nodular
actinomycotic —*see* Actinomycosis
breast NEC —*see also* Lump, breast N63.0
colloid (cystic), thyroid E04.1
cutaneous —*see* Swelling, localized
endometrial (stromal) D26.1
Haygarth's M15.8
inflammatory —*see* Inflammation
juxta-articular
syphilitic A52.77
yaws A66.7
larynx J38.7
lung, solitary (subsegmental branch of the bronchial tree) R91.1
multiple R91.8
milker's B08.03
prostate N40.2
with lower urinary tract symptoms (LUTS) N40.3
without lower urinary tract symptoms (LUTS) N40.2

Nodule(s), nodular *(Continued)*
pulmonary, solitary (subsegmental branch of the bronchial tree) R91.1
retrocardiac R09.89
rheumatoid M06.30
ankle M06.37-●
elbow M06.32-●
foot joint M06.37-●
hand joint M06.34-●
hip M06.35-●
knee M06.36-●
multiple site M06.39
shoulder M06.31-●
vertebra M06.38
wrist M06.33-●
scrotum (inflammatory) N49.2
singer's J38.2
solitary, lung (subsegmental branch of the bronchial tree) R91.1
multiple R91.8
subcutaneous —*see* Swelling, localized
teacher's J38.2
thyroid (cold) (gland) (nontoxic) E04.1
with thyrotoxicosis E05.20
with thyroid storm E05.21
toxic or with hyperthyroidism E05.20
with thyroid storm E05.21
vocal cord J38.2
Noma (gangrenous) (hospital) (infective) A69.0
auricle I96
mouth A69.0
pudendi N76.89
vulvae N76.89
Nomad, nomadism Z59.00
NOMID (neonatal onset multisystemic inflammatory disorder) M04.2
Nonadherence to medical treatment, specified NEC Z91.199
due to
financial hardship Z91.190
specified reason NEC Z91.198
Nonautoimmune hemolytic anemia D59.4
drug-induced D59.2
Nonclosure —*see also* Imperfect, closure
ductus arteriosus (Botallo's) Q25.0
foramen
botalli Q21.12
ovale Q21.12
Noncompliance Z91.199
with
caregiver
with patient's
dietary regimen
due to
financial hardship Z91.A10
specified reason NEC Z91.A18
medical treatment and regimen
financial hardship Z91.A91
specified reason NEC Z91.A98
medication regimen
due to financial hardship Z91.A41
specified reason NEC Z91.A48
renal dialysis
financial hardship Z91.A51
specified reason NEC Z91.A58
dialysis Z91.158
due to financial hardship Z91.151
dietary regimen Z91.119
due to
financial hardship Z91.110
specified reason NEC Z91.118
medical treatment, specified NEC Z91.199
due to
financial hardship Z91.190
specified reason NEC Z91.198
medication regimen Z91.148
due to financial hardship Z91.151
underdosing —*see also* Table of Drugs and Chemicals, categories T36-T50, with final character 6 Z91.148
intentional NEC Z91.128
by caregiver
due to
financial hardship Z91.A20
specified reason NEC Z91.A28
due to financial hardship of patient Z91.120
unintentional NEC Z91.138
by caregiver Z91.A3
renal dialysis Z91.158
due to financial hardship Z91.151

N

O

O

- **Obstruction, obstructed, obstructive** *(Continued)*
  - valvular *—see* Endocarditis
  - vein, venous I87.1
    - caval (inferior) (superior) I87.1
    - thrombotic *—see* Thrombosis
  - vena cava (inferior) (superior) I87.1
  - vesical NEC N32.Ø
  - vesicourethral orifice N32.Ø
    - congenital Q64.31
  - vessel NEC I99.8
    - stent *—see* Restenosis, stent
- **Obturator** *—see* condition
- **Occlusal wear, teeth** KØ3.Ø
- **Occlusio pupillae** *—see* Membrane, pupillary
- **Occlusion, occluded**
  - anus K62.4
    - congenital Q42.3
      - with fistula Q42.2
  - aortoiliac (chronic) I74.Ø9
  - aqueduct of Sylvius G91.1
    - congenital QØ3.Ø
      - with spina bifida *—see* Spina bifida, by site, with hydrocephalus
  - artery *—see also* Atherosclerosis, artery I7Ø.9
    - auditory, internal I65.8
    - basilar I65.1
      - with
        - infarction I63.22
          - due to
            - embolism I63.12
            - thrombosis I63.Ø2
    - brain or cerebral I66.9
      - with infarction (due to) I63.5-●
        - embolism I63.4-●
        - thrombosis I63.3-●
    - carotid I65.2-●
      - with
        - infarction I63.23-●
          - due to
            - embolism I63.13-●
            - thrombosis I63.Ø3-●
    - cerebellar (anterior inferior) (posterior inferior) (superior) I66.3
      - with infarction I63.54-●
        - due to
          - embolism I63.44-●
          - thrombosis I63.34-●
    - cerebral I66.9
      - with infarction I63.5Ø
        - due to
          - embolism I63.4Ø
            - specified NEC I63.49
          - thrombosis I63.3Ø
            - specified NEC I63.39
      - anterior I66.1-●
        - with infarction I63.52-●
          - due to
            - embolism I63.42-●
            - thrombosis I63.32-●
      - middle I66.Ø-●
        - with infarction I63.51-●
          - due to
            - embolism I63.41-●
            - thrombosis I63.31-●
      - posterior I66.2-●
        - with infarction I63.53-●
          - due to
            - embolism I63.43-●
            - thrombosis I63.33-●
      - specified NEC I66.8
        - with infarction I63.59
          - due to
            - embolism I63.4-●
            - thrombosis I63.3-●
    - choroidal (anterior) *—see* Occlusion, artery, cerebral, specified NEC
    - communicating posterior *—see* Occlusion, artery, precerebral, specified NEC
    - complete
      - coronary I25.82
      - extremities I7Ø.92
    - coronary (acute) (thrombotic) (without myocardial infarction) I24.Ø
      - with myocardial infarction *—see* Infarction, myocardium
      - chronic total I25.82
      - complete I25.82
      - healed or old I25.2
      - total (chronic) I25.82
    - hypophyseal *—see* Occlusion, artery, precerebral, specified NEC
    - iliac I74.5

- **Occlusion, occluded** *(Continued)*
  - artery *(Continued)*
    - lower extremities due to stenosis or stricture I77.1
    - mesenteric (embolic) (thrombotic) *—see also* Infarct, intestine K55.Ø69
    - perforating *—see* Occlusion, artery, cerebral, specified NEC
    - peripheral I77.9
      - thrombotic or embolic I74.4
    - pontine *—see* Occlusion, artery, precerebral, specified NEC
    - precerebral I65.9
      - with infarction I63.2Ø
        - due to
          - embolism I63.1Ø
            - specified NEC I63.19
          - thrombosis I63.ØØ
            - specified NEC I63.Ø9
        - specified NEC I63.29
      - basilar *—see* Occlusion, artery, basilar
      - carotid *—see* Occlusion, artery, carotid
      - puerperal O88.23
      - specified NEC I65.8
        - with infarction I63.29
          - due to
            - embolism I63.19
            - thrombosis I63.Ø9
      - vertebral *—see* Occlusion, artery, vertebral
    - renal N28.Ø
    - retinal
      - branch H34.23-●
      - central H34.1-●
      - partial H34.21-●
      - transient H34.Ø-●
    - spinal *—see* Occlusion, artery, precerebral, vertebral
    - total (chronic)
      - coronary I25.82
      - extremities I7Ø.92
    - vertebral I65.Ø-●
      - with
        - infarction I63.21-●
          - due to
            - embolism I63.11-●
            - thrombosis I63.Ø1-●
  - basilar artery *—see* Occlusion, artery, basilar
  - bile duct (common) (hepatic) (noncalculous) K83.1
  - bowel *—see* Obstruction, intestine
  - carotid (artery) (common) (internal) *—see* Occlusion, artery, carotid
  - centric (of teeth) M26.59
    - maximum intercuspation discrepancy M26.55
  - cerebellar (artery) *—see* Occlusion, artery, cerebellar
  - cerebral (artery) *—see* Occlusion, artery, cerebral
  - cerebrovascular *—see also* Occlusion, artery, cerebral
    - with infarction I63.5-●
  - cervical canal *—see* Stricture, cervix
  - cervix (uteri) *—see* Stricture, cervix
  - choanal Q3Ø.Ø
  - choroidal (artery) *—see* Occlusion, artery, precerebral, specified NEC
  - colon *—see* Obstruction, intestine
  - communicating posterior artery *—see* Occlusion, artery, precerebral, specified NEC
  - coronary (artery) (vein) (thrombotic) *—see also* Infarct, myocardium
    - chronic total I25.82
    - healed or old I25.2
    - not resulting in infarction I24.Ø
    - total (chronic) I25.82
  - cystic duct *—see* Obstruction, gallbladder
  - embolic *—see* Embolism
  - fallopian tube N97.1
    - congenital Q5Ø.6
  - gallbladder *—see also* Obstruction, gallbladder
    - congenital (causing jaundice) Q44.1
  - gingiva, traumatic KØ6.2
  - hymen N89.6
    - congenital Q52.3
  - hypophyseal (artery) *—see* Occlusion, artery, precerebral, specified NEC
  - iliac artery I74.5
  - intestine *—see* Obstruction, intestine
  - lacrimal passages *—see* Obstruction, lacrimal
  - lung J98.4
  - lymph or lymphatic channel I89.Ø
  - mammary duct N64.89

- **Occlusion, occluded** *(Continued)*
  - mesenteric artery (embolic) (thrombotic) *—see also* Infarct, intestine K55.Ø69
  - nose J34.89
    - congenital Q3Ø.Ø
  - organ or site, congenital NEC *—see* Atresia, by site
  - oviduct N97.1
    - congenital Q5Ø.6
  - peripheral arteries
    - due to stricture or stenosis I77.1
    - upper extremity I74.2
  - pontine (artery) *—see* Occlusion, artery, precerebral, specified NEC
  - posterior lingual, of mandibular teeth M26.29
  - precerebral artery *—see* Occlusion, artery, precerebral
  - punctum lacrimale *—see* Obstruction, lacrimal
  - pupil *—see* Membrane, pupillary
  - pylorus, adult *—see also* Stricture, pylorus K31.1
  - renal artery N28.Ø
  - retina, retinal
    - artery *—see* Occlusion, artery, retinal
    - vein (central) H34.81-●
      - engorgement H34.82-●
      - tributary H34.83-●
    - vessels H34.9
  - spinal artery *—see* Occlusion, artery, precerebral, vertebral
  - teeth (mandibular) (posterior lingual) M26.29
  - thoracic duct I89.Ø
  - thrombotic *—see* Thrombosis, artery
  - traumatic
    - edentulous (alveolar) ridge KØ6.2
    - gingiva KØ6.2
    - periodontal KØ5.5
  - tubal N97.1
  - ureter (complete) (partial) N13.5
    - congenital Q62.1Ø
  - ureteropelvic junction N13.5
    - congenital Q62.11
  - ureterovesical orifice N13.5
    - congenital Q62.12
  - urethra *—see* Stricture, urethra
  - uterus N85.8
  - vagina N89.5
  - vascular NEC I99.8
  - vein *—see* Thrombosis
    - retinal *—see* Occlusion, retinal, vein
  - vena cava (inferior) (superior) *—see* Embolism, vena cava
  - ventricle (brain) NEC G91.1
  - vertebral (artery) *—see* Occlusion, artery, vertebral
  - vessel (blood) I99.8
  - vulva N9Ø.5
- **Occult**
  - blood in feces (stools) R19.5
- **Occupational**
  - problems NEC Z56.89
- **Ochlophobia** *—see* Agoraphobia
- **Ochronosis (endogenous)** E7Ø.29
- **Ocular muscle** *—see* condition
- **Oculogyric crisis or disturbance** H51.8
  - psychogenic F45.8
- **Oculomotor syndrome** H51.9
- **Oculopathy**
  - syphilitic NEC A52.71
    - congenital
      - early A5Ø.Ø1
      - late A5Ø.3Ø
    - early (secondary) A51.43
    - late A52.71
- **Oddi's sphincter spasm** K83.4
- **Odontalgia** KØ8.89
- **Odontoameloblastoma** *—see* Cyst, calcifying odontogenic
- **Odontoclasia** KØ3.89
- **Odontodysplasia, regional** KØØ.4
- **Odontogenesis imperfecta** KØØ.5
- **Odontoma (ameloblastic) (complex) (compound) (fibroameloblastic)** *—see* Cyst, calcifying odontogenic
- **Odontomyelitis (closed) (open)** KØ4.Ø1
  - irreversible KØ4.Ø2
  - reversible KØ4.Ø1
- **Odontorrhagia** KØ8.89
- **Odontosarcoma, ameloblastic** C41.1
  - upper jaw (bone) C41.Ø
- **Oestriasis** *—see* Myiasis
- **Oguchi's disease** H53.63
- **Ohara's disease** *—see* Tularemia

▶ New ➡ Revised ~~deleted~~ Deleted ● Use Additional Character(s)

Osteochondrosis *(Continued)*
Sinding-Larsen —*see* Osteochondrosis, juvenile, patella
adult M42.10
cervical region M42.12
cervicothoracic region M42.13
lumbar region M42.16
lumbosacral region M42.17
multiple sites M42.19
occipito-atlanto-axial region M42.11
sacrococcygeal region M42.18
thoracic region M42.14
thoracolumbar region M42.15
juvenile —*see* Osteochondrosis, juvenile, spine
symphysis pubis (juvenile) M91.0
syphilitic (congenital) A50.02
talus (juvenile) —*see* Osteochondrosis, juvenile, tarsus
tarsus (navicular) (juvenile) —*see* Osteochondrosis, juvenile, tarsus
tibia (proximal) (tubercle) (juvenile) —*see* Osteochondrosis, juvenile, tibia
tuberculous —*see* Tuberculosis, bone
ulna (lower) (juvenile) —*see* Osteochondrosis, juvenile, ulna
van Neck's M91.0
vertebral —*see* Osteochondrosis, spine
Osteoclastoma D48.0
malignant —*see* Neoplasm, bone, malignant
Osteodynia —*see* Disorder, bone, specified type NEC
Osteodystrophy Q78.9
azotemic N25.0
congenital Q78.9
parathyroid, secondary E21.1
renal N25.0
Osteofibroma —*see* Neoplasm, bone, benign
Osteofibrosarcoma —*see* Neoplasm, bone, malignant
Osteogenesis imperfecta Q78.0
Osteogenic —*see* condition
Osteolysis M89.50
carpus M89.54-●
clavicle M89.51-●
femur M89.55-●
fibula M89.56-●
finger M89.54-●
humerus M89.52-●
ilium M89.58
ischium M89.58
joint prosthesis (periprosthetic) —*see* Complications, joint prosthesis, mechanical, periprosthetic, osteolysis, by site
metacarpus M89.54-●
metatarsus M89.57-●
multiple sites M89.59
neck M89.58
periprosthetic —*see* Complications, joint prosthesis, mechanical, periprosthetic, osteolysis, by site
pubic ramus M89.58
radius M89.53-●
rib M89.58
scapula M89.51-●
skull M89.58
tarsus M89.57-●
tibia M89.56-●
toe M89.57-●
ulna M89.53-●
vertebra M89.58
Osteoma —*see also* Neoplasm, bone, benign
osteoid —*see also* Neoplasm, bone, benign
giant —*see* Neoplasm, bone, benign
Osteomalacia M83.9
adult M83.9
drug-induced NEC M83.5
due to
malabsorption (postsurgical) M83.2
malnutrition M83.3
specified NEC M83.8
aluminium-induced M83.4
infantile —*see* Rickets
juvenile —*see* Rickets
oncogenic E83.89
pelvis M83.8
puerperal M83.0
senile M83.1
vitamin-D-resistant in adults E83.31 *[M90.8-●]*
carpus E83.31 *[M90.84-●]*
clavicle E83.31 *[M90.81-●]*
femur E83.31 *[M90.85-●]*

Osteomalacia *(Continued)*
vitamin-D-resistant in adults *(Continued)*
fibula E83.31 *[M90.86-●]*
finger E83.31 *[M90.84-●]*
humerus E83.31 *[M90.82-●]*
ilium E83.31 *[M90.88]*
ischium E83.31 *[M90.88]*
metacarpus E83.31 *[M90.84-●]*
metatarsus E83.31 *[M90.87-●]*
multiple sites E83.31 *[M90.89]*
neck E83.31 *[M90.88]*
pubic ramus E83.31 *[M90.88]*
radius E83.31 *[M90.83-●]*
rib E83.31 *[M90.88]*
scapula E83.31 *[M90.819]*
skull E83.31 *[M90.88]*
tarsus E83.31 *[M90.879]*
tibia E83.31 *[M90.869]*
toe E83.31 *[M90.879]*
ulna E83.31 *[M90.839]*
vertebra E83.31 *[M90.88]*
Osteomyelitis (general) (infective) (localized) (neonatal) (purulent) (septic) (staphylococcal) (streptococcal) (suppurative) (with periostitis) M86.9
acute M86.10
carpus M86.14-●
clavicle M86.11-●
femur M86.15-●
fibula M86.16-●
finger M86.14-●
hematogenous M86.00
carpus M86.04-●
clavicle M86.01-●
femur M86.05-●
fibula M86.06-●
finger M86.04-●
humerus M86.02-●
ilium M86.08
ischium M86.08
mandible M27.2
metacarpus M86.04-●
metatarsus M86.07-●
multiple sites M86.09
neck M86.08
orbit H05.02-●
petrous bone —*see* Petrositis
radius M86.03-●
rib M86.08
scapula M86.01-●
skull M86.08
tarsus M86.07-●
tibia M86.06-●
toe M86.07-●
ulna M86.03-●
vertebra —*see* Osteomyelitis, vertebra
humerus M86.12-●
ilium M86.18
ischium M86.18
mandible M27.2
metacarpus M86.14-●
metatarsus M86.17-●
multiple sites M86.19
neck M86.18
orbit H05.02-●
petrous bone —*see* Petrositis
radius M86.13-●
rib M86.18
scapula M86.11-●
skull M86.18
tarsus M86.17-●
tibia M86.16-●
toe M86.17-●
ulna M86.13-●
vertebra —*see* Osteomyelitis, vertebra
chronic (or old) M86.60
with draining sinus M86.40
carpus M86.44-●
clavicle M86.41-●
femur M86.45-●
fibula M86.46-●
finger M86.44-●
humerus M86.42-●
ilium M86.48
ischium M86.48
mandible M27.2
metacarpus M86.44-●
metatarsus M86.47-●
multiple sites M86.49
neck M86.48
orbit H05.02-●

Osteomyelitis *(Continued)*
chronic *(Continued)*
with draining sinus *(Continued)*
petrous bone —*see* Petrositis
pubic ramus M86.48
radius M86.43-●
rib M86.48
scapula M86.41-●
skull M86.48
tarsus M86.47-●
tibia M86.46-●
toe M86.47-●
ulna M86.43-●
vertebra —*see* Osteomyelitis, vertebra
carpus M86.64-●
clavicle M86.61-●
femur M86.65-●
fibula M86.66-●
finger M86.64-●
hematogenous NEC M86.50
carpus M86.54-●
clavicle M86.51-●
femur M86.55-●
fibula M86.56-●
finger M86.54-●
humerus M86.52-●
ilium M86.58
ischium M86.58
mandible M27.2
metacarpus M86.54-●
metatarsus M86.57-●
multifocal M86.30
carpus M86.34-●
clavicle M86.31-●
femur M86.35-●
fibula M86.36-●
finger M86.34-●
humerus M86.32-●
ilium M86.38
ischium M86.38
metacarpus M86.34-●
metatarsus M86.37-●
multiple sites M86.39
neck M86.38
pubic ramus M86.38
radius M86.33-●
rib M86.38
scapula M86.31-●
skull M86.38
tarsus M86.37-●
tibia M86.36-●
toe M86.37-●
ulna M86.33-●
vertebra —*see* Osteomyelitis, vertebra
multiple sites M86.59
neck M86.58
orbit H05.02-●
petrous bone —*see* Petrositis
pubic ramus M86.58
radius M86.53-●
rib M86.58
scapula M86.51-●
skull M86.58
tarsus M86.57-●
tibia M86.56-●
toe M86.57-●
ulna M86.53-●
vertebra —*see* Osteomyelitis, vertebra
humerus M86.62-●
ilium M86.659
ischium M86.659
mandible M27.2
metacarpus M86.64-●
metatarsus M86.67-●
multifocal —*see* Osteomyelitis, chronic, hematogenous, multifocal
multiple sites M86.69
neck M86.68
orbit H05.02-●
petrous bone —*see* Petrositis
radius M86.63-●
rib M86.68
scapula M86.61-●
skull M86.68
tarsus M86.67-●
tibia M86.66-●
toe M86.67-●
ulna M86.63-●
vertebra —*see* Osteomyelitis, vertebra
echinococcal B67.2
Garr's —*see* Osteomyelitis, specified type NEC

▶ New ➡ Revised ~~deleted~~ Deleted ● Use Additional Character(s)

- **Osteophyte** M25.7Ø
  - ankle M25.77-●
  - elbow M25.72-●
  - foot joint M25.77-●
  - hand joint M25.74-●
  - hip M25.75-●
  - knee M25.76-●
  - shoulder M25.71-●
  - spine M25.78
  - vertebrae M25.78
  - wrist M25.73-●
- **Osteopoikilosis** Q78.8
- **Osteoporosis** (female) (male) M81.Ø
  - with current pathological fracture M8Ø.ØØ
  - age-related M81.Ø
    - with current pathologic fracture M8Ø.ØØ
      - carpus M8Ø.Ø4-●
      - clavicle M8Ø.Ø1-●
      - femur M8Ø.Ø5-●
      - fibula M8Ø.Ø6-●
      - finger M8Ø.Ø4-●
      - hip M8Ø.Ø5-●
      - humerus M8Ø.Ø2-●
      - ilium M8Ø.ØA
      - ischium M8Ø.ØA
      - metacarpus M8Ø.Ø4-●
      - metatarsus M8Ø.Ø7-●
      - pelvis M8Ø.ØB
      - pubis ramus M8Ø.ØA
      - radius M8Ø.Ø3-●
      - rib(s) M8Ø.ØA
      - scapula M8Ø.Ø1-●
      - site specified NEC M8Ø.ØA
      - specified site NEC M8Ø.ØA
      - tarsus M8Ø.Ø7-●
      - tibia M8Ø.Ø6-●
      - toe M8Ø.Ø7-●
      - ulna M8Ø.Ø3-●
      - vertebra M8Ø.Ø8
  - disuse M81.8
    - with current pathological fracture M8Ø.8Ø
      - carpus M8Ø.84-●
      - clavicle M8Ø.81-●
      - fibula M8Ø.86-●
      - finger M8Ø.84-●
      - humerus M8Ø.82-●
      - ilium M8Ø.8A
      - ischium M8Ø.8A
      - metacarpus M8Ø.84-●
      - metatarsus M8Ø.87-●
      - pelvis M8Ø.8B
      - pubis ramus M8Ø.8A
      - radius M8Ø.83-●
      - scapula M8Ø.81-●
      - site specified NEC M8Ø.8A
      - tarsus M8Ø.87-●
      - tibia M8Ø.86-●
      - toe M8Ø.87-●
      - ulna M8Ø.83-●
      - vertebra M8Ø.88
  - drug-induced —*see* Osteoporosis, specified type NEC
  - idiopathic —*see* Osteoporosis, specified type NEC
  - involutional —*see* Osteoporosis, age-related
  - Lequesne M81.6
  - localized M81.6
  - postmenopausal M81.Ø
    - with pathological fracture M8Ø.ØØ
      - carpus M8Ø.Ø4-●
      - clavicle M8Ø.Ø1-●
      - femur M8Ø.85-●
      - fibula M8Ø.Ø6-●
      - finger M8Ø.Ø4-●
      - hip M8Ø.85-●
      - humerus M8Ø.Ø2-●
      - ilium M8Ø.ØA
      - ischium M8Ø.ØA
      - metacarpus M8Ø.Ø4-●
      - metatarsus M8Ø.Ø7-●
      - pelvis M8Ø.ØB
      - pubis ramus M8Ø.ØA
      - radius M8Ø.Ø3-●
      - scapula M8Ø.Ø1-●
      - site specified NEC M8Ø.ØA
      - tarsus M8Ø.Ø7-●
      - tibia M8Ø.Ø6-●
      - toe M8Ø.Ø7-●
      - ulna M8Ø.Ø3-●
      - vertebra M8Ø.Ø8

- **Osteoporosis** *(Continued)*
  - postoophorectomy —*see* Osteoporosis, specified type NEC
  - postsurgical malabsorption —*see* Osteoporosis, specified type NEC
  - post-traumatic —*see* Osteoporosis, specified type NEC
  - senile —*see* Osteoporosis, age-related
  - specified type NEC M81.8
    - with pathological fracture M8Ø.8Ø
      - carpus M8Ø.84-●
      - clavicle M8Ø.81-●
      - femur M8Ø.85-●
      - fibula M8Ø.86-●
      - finger M8Ø.84-●
      - hip M8Ø.85-●
      - humerus M8Ø.82-●
      - ilium M8Ø.8A
      - ischium M8Ø.8A
      - metacarpus M8Ø.84-●
      - metatarsus M8Ø.87-●
      - pelvis M8Ø.8B
      - radius M8Ø.83-●
      - pubis ramus M8Ø.8A
      - scapula M8Ø.81-●
      - site specified NEC M8Ø.8A
      - tarsus M8Ø.87-●
      - tibia M8Ø.86-●
      - toe M8Ø.87-●
      - ulna M8Ø.83-●
      - vertebra M8Ø.88
- **Osteopsathyrosis** (idiopathica) Q78.Ø
- **Osteoradionecrosis, jaw** (acute) (chronic) (lower) (suppurative) (upper) M27.2
- **Osteosarcoma** (any form) —*see* Neoplasm, bone, malignant
- **Osteosclerosis** Q78.2
  - acquired M85.8-●
  - congenita Q77.4
  - fragilitas (generalisata) Q78.2
  - myelofibrosis D75.81
- **Osteosclerotic anemia** D64.89
- **Osteosis**
  - cutis L94.2
  - renal fibrocystic N25.Ø
- **Österreicher-Turner syndrome** Q87.2
- **Ostium**
  - atrioventriculare commune Q21.23
  - primum (arteriosum) (defect) (persistent) Q21.2Ø
  - secundum (arteriosum) (defect) (patent) (persistent) Q21.11
- **Ostrum-Furst syndrome** Q75.8
- **Otalgia** —*see* subcategory H92.Ø
- **Otitis** (acute) H66.9Ø
  - with effusion —*see also* Otitis, media, nonsuppurative
    - purulent —*see* Otitis, media, suppurative
  - adhesive —*see* subcategory H74.1
  - chronic —*see also* Otitis, media, chronic
    - with effusion —*see also* Otitis, media, nonsuppurative, chronic
  - externa H6Ø.9-●
    - abscess —*see* Abscess, ear, external
    - acute (noninfective) H6Ø.5Ø-●
      - actinic H6Ø.51-●
      - chemical H6Ø.52-●
      - contact H6Ø.53-●
      - eczematoid H6Ø.54-●
      - infective —*see* Otitis, externa, infective
      - reactive H6Ø.55-●
      - specified NEC H6Ø.59-●
    - cellulitis —*see* Cellulitis, ear
    - chronic H6Ø.6-●
    - diffuse —*see* Otitis, externa, infective, diffuse
    - hemorrhagic —*see* Otitis, externa, infective, hemorrhagic
    - in (due to)
      - aspergillosis B44.89
      - candidiasis B37.84
      - erysipelas A46 *[H62.4Ø]*
      - herpes (simplex) virus infection BØØ.1
        - zoster BØ2.8
      - impetigo LØ1.ØØ *[H62.4Ø]*
      - infectious disease NEC B99 *[H62.4-●]*
      - mycosis NEC B36.9 *[H62.4Ø]*
      - parasitic disease NEC B89 *[H62.4Ø]*
      - viral disease NEC B34.9 *[H62.4Ø]*
      - zoster BØ2.8
    - infective NEC H6Ø.39-●
      - abscess —*see* Abscess, ear, external
      - cellulitis —*see* Cellulitis, ear

- **Otitis** *(Continued)*
  - externa *(Continued)*
    - infective *(Continued)*
      - diffuse H6Ø.31-●
      - hemorrhagic H6Ø.32-●
      - swimmer's ear —*see* Swimmer's, ear
    - malignant H6Ø.2-●
    - mycotic NEC B36.9 *[H62.4Ø]*
      - in
        - aspergillosis B44.89
        - candidiasis B37.84
        - moniliasis B37.84
    - necrotizing —*see* Otitis, externa, malignant
    - Pseudomonas aeruginosa —*see* Otitis, externa, malignant
    - reactive —*see* Otitis, externa, acute, reactive
    - specified NEC —*see* subcategory H6Ø.8
    - tropical NEC B36.9 *[H62.4Ø]*
      - in
        - aspergillosis B44.89
        - candidiasis B37.84
        - moniliasis B37.84
  - insidiosa —*see* Otosclerosis
  - interna —*see* subcategory H83.Ø
  - media (hemorrhagic) (staphylococcal) (streptococcal) H66.9-●
    - with effusion (nonpurulent) —*see* Otitis, media, nonsuppurative
    - acute, subacute H66.9Ø
      - allergic —*see* Otitis, media, nonsuppurative, acute, allergic
      - exudative —*see* Otitis, media, suppurative, acute
      - mucoid —*see* Otitis, media, nonsuppurative, acute
      - necrotizing —*see also* Otitis, media, suppurative, acute
        - in
          - measles BØ5.3
          - scarlet fever A38.Ø
      - nonsuppurative NEC —*see* Otitis, media, nonsuppurative, acute
      - purulent —*see* Otitis, media, suppurative, acute
      - sanguinous —*see* Otitis, media, nonsuppurative, acute
      - secretory —*see* Otitis, media, nonsuppurative, acute, serous
      - seromucinous —*see* Otitis, media, nonsuppurative, acute
      - serous —*see* Otitis, media, nonsuppurative, acute, serous
      - suppurative —*see* Otitis, media, suppurative, acute
    - allergic —*see* Otitis, media, nonsuppurative
    - catarrhal —*see* Otitis, media, nonsuppurative
    - chronic H66.9Ø
      - with effusion (nonpurulent) —*see* Otitis, media, nonsuppurative, chronic
      - allergic —*see* Otitis, media, nonsuppurative, chronic, allergic
      - benign suppurative —*see* Otitis, media, suppurative, chronic, tubotympanic
      - catarrhal —*see* Otitis, media, nonsuppurative, chronic, serous
      - exudative —*see* Otitis, media, suppurative, chronic
      - mucinous —*see* Otitis, media, nonsuppurative, chronic, mucoid
      - mucoid —*see* Otitis, media, nonsuppurative, chronic, mucoid
      - nonsuppurative NEC —*see* Otitis, media, nonsuppurative, chronic
      - purulent —*see* Otitis, media, suppurative, chronic
      - secretory —*see* Otitis, media, nonsuppurative, chronic, mucoid
      - seromucinous —*see* Otitis, media, nonsuppurative, chronic
      - serous —*see* Otitis, media, nonsuppurative, chronic, serous
      - suppurative —*see* Otitis, media, suppurative, chronic
      - transudative —*see* Otitis, media, nonsuppurative, chronic, mucoid
    - exudative —*see* Otitis, media, nonsuppurative

P

▶ New ➠ Revised ~~deleted~~ Deleted ● Use Additional Character(s)

Paralysis, paralytic *(Continued)*
- lung J98.4
- median nerve G56.1-●
- medullary (tegmental) G83.89
- mesencephalic NEC G83.89
  - tegmental G83.89
- middle alternating G83.89
- Millard-Gubler-Foville G46.3
- monoplegic —*see* Monoplegia
- motor G83.9
- muscle, muscular NEC G72.89
  - due to nerve lesion G58.9
  - eye (extrinsic) H49.9
    - intrinsic —*see* Paresis, of accommodation
    - oblique —*see* Strabismus, paralytic, fourth nerve
  - iris sphincter H21.9
  - ischemic (Volkmann's) (complicating trauma) T79.6
  - progressive G12.21
  - progressive, spinal G12.25
  - pseudohypertrophic G71.02
  - spinal progressive G12.25
- musculocutaneous nerve G56.9-●
- musculospiral G56.9-●
- nerve —*see also* Disorder, nerve
  - abducent —*see* Strabismus, paralytic, sixth nerve
  - accessory G52.8
  - auditory (except Deafness) —*see* subcategory H93.3
  - birth injury P14.9
  - cranial or cerebral G52.9
  - facial G51.0
    - birth injury P11.3
    - congenital P11.3
    - newborn (birth injury) P11.3
  - fourth or trochlear —*see* Strabismus, paralytic, fourth nerve
  - newborn (birth injury) P14.9
  - oculomotor —*see* Strabismus, paralytic, third nerve
  - phrenic (birth injury) P14.2
  - radial G56.3-●
  - seventh or facial G51.0
    - newborn (birth injury) P11.3
  - sixth or abducent —*see* Strabismus, paralytic, sixth nerve
  - syphilitic A52.15
  - third or oculomotor —*see* Strabismus, paralytic, third nerve
  - trigeminal G50.9
  - trochlear —*see* Strabismus, paralytic, fourth nerve
  - ulnar G56.2-●
- normokalemic periodic G72.3
- ocular H49.9
  - alternating G83.89
- oculofacial, congenital (Moebius) Q87.0
- oculomotor (external bilateral) (nerve) —*see* Strabismus, paralytic, third nerve
- palate (soft) K13.79
- paratrigeminal G50.9
- periodic (familial) (hyperkalemic) (hypokalemic) (myotonic) (normokalemic) (potassium sensitive) (secondary) G72.3
- peripheral autonomic nervous system —*see* Neuropathy, peripheral, autonomic
- peroneal (nerve) G57.3-●
- pharynx J39.2
- phrenic nerve G56.8-●
- plantar nerve(s) G57.6-●
- pneumogastric nerve G52.2
- poliomyelitis (current) —*see* Poliomyelitis, paralytic
- popliteal nerve G57.3-●
- postepileptic transitory G83.84
- progressive (atrophic) (bulbar) (spinal) G12.22
  - general A52.17
  - infantile acute —*see* Poliomyelitis, paralytic
  - supranuclear G23.1
- pseudobulbar G12.29
- pseudohypertrophic (muscle) (*see also* Dystrophy, muscular, by type, if applicable) G71.09
- psychogenic F44.4
- quadriceps G57.9-●
- quadriplegic —*see* Tetraplegia
- radial nerve G56.3-●
- rectus muscle (eye) H49.9
- recurrent isolated sleep G47.53

Paralysis, paralytic *(Continued)*
- respiratory (muscle) (system) (tract) R06.81
  - center NEC G93.89
  - congenital P28.89
  - newborn P28.89
- right side —*see* Hemiplegia
- saturnine —*see* subcategory T56.0
- sciatic nerve G57.0-●
- senile G83.9
- shaking —*see* Parkinsonism
- shoulder G56.9-●
- sleep, recurrent isolated G47.53
- spastic G83.9
  - cerebral —*see* Palsy, cerebral, spastic
  - congenital (cerebral) —*see* Palsy, cerebral, spastic
  - familial G11.4
  - hereditary G11.4
  - quadriplegic G80.0
  - syphilitic (spinal) A52.17
- sphincter, bladder —*see* Paralysis, bladder
- spinal (cord) G83.9
  - accessory nerve G52.8
  - acute —*see* Poliomyelitis, paralytic
  - ascending acute G61.0
  - atrophic (acute) —*see also* Poliomyelitis, paralytic
    - spastic, syphilitic A52.17
  - congenital NEC —*see* Palsy, cerebral
  - hereditary G95.89
  - infantile —*see* Poliomyelitis, paralytic
  - progressive G12.21
  - muscle G12.25
  - sequelae NEC G83.89
- sternomastoid G52.8
- stomach K31.84
  - diabetic —*see* Diabetes, by type, with gastroparesis
  - nerve G52.2
    - diabetic —*see* Diabetes, by type, with gastroparesis
- stroke —*see* Infarct, brain
- ~~subcapsularis G56.8-●~~
- ▶ subscapularis G56.8-●
- supranuclear (progressive) G23.1
- ➠ sympathetic G90.89
  - cervical G90.09
  - nervous system —*see* Neuropathy, peripheral, autonomic
- syndrome G83.9
  - specified NEC G83.89
- syphilitic spastic spinal (Erb's) A52.17
- thigh G57.9-●
- throat J39.2
  - diphtheritic A36.0
  - muscle J39.2
- thrombotic (current episode) I63.3-●
- thumb G56.9-●
- tick —*see* Toxicity, venom, arthropod, specified NEC
- Todd's (postepileptic transitory paralysis) G83.84
- toe G57.6-●
- tongue K14.8
- transient R29.5
  - arm or leg NEC R29.818
  - traumatic NEC —*see* Injury, nerve
- trapezius G52.8
- traumatic, transient NEC —*see* Injury, nerve
- trembling —*see* Parkinsonism
- triceps brachii G56.9-●
- trigeminal nerve G50.9
- trochlear (nerve) —*see* Strabismus, paralytic, fourth nerve
- ulnar nerve G56.2-●
- upper limb —*see* Monoplegia, upper limb
- uremic N18.9 *[G99.8]*
- uveoparotitic D86.89
- uvula K13.79
  - postdiphtheritic A36.0
- vagus nerve G52.2
- ➠ vasomotor NEC G90.89
- velum palati K13.79
- vesical —*see* Paralysis, bladder
- vestibular nerve (except Vertigo) —*see* subcategory H93.3
- vocal cords J38.00
  - bilateral J38.02
  - unilateral J38.01
- Volkmann's (complicating trauma) T79.6
- wasting G12.29
- Weber's G46.3
- wrist G56.9-●

Paramedial urethrovesical orifice Q64.79

Paramenia N92.6

Parametritis —*see also* Disease, pelvis, inflammatory N73.2
- acute N73.0
- complicating abortion —*see* Abortion, by type, complicated by, parametritis

Parametrium, parametric —*see* condition

Paramnesia —*see* Amnesia

Paramolar K00.1

Paramyloidosis E85.89

Paramyoclonus multiplex G25.3

Paramyotonia (congenita) G71.19

Parangi —*see* Yaws

Paranoia (querulans) F22
- senile F03

Paranoid
- dementia (senile) F03
  - praecox —*see* Schizophrenia
- personality F60.0
- psychosis (climacteric) (involutional) (menopausal) F22
  - psychogenic (acute) F23
  - senile F03
- reaction (acute) F23
  - chronic F22
- schizophrenia F20.0
- state (climacteric) (involutional) (menopausal) (simple) F22
  - senile F03
- tendencies F60.0
- traits F60.0
- trends F60.0
- type, psychopathic personality F60.0

Paraparesis —*see* Paraplegia

Paraphasia R47.02

Paraphilia F65.9

Paraphimosis (congenital) N47.2
- chancroidal A57

Paraphrenia, paraphrenic (late) F22
- schizophrenia F20.0

Paraplegia (lower) G82.20
- ataxic —*see* Degeneration, combined, spinal cord
- complete G82.21
- congenital (cerebral) G80.8
  - spastic G80.1
- familial spastic G11.4
- functional (hysterical) F44.4
- hereditary, spastic G11.4
- hysterical F44.4
- incomplete G82.22
- Pott's A18.01
- psychogenic F44.4
- spastic
  - Erb's spinal, syphilitic A52.17
  - hereditary G11.4
  - tropical G04.1
- syphilitic (spastic) A52.17
- traumatic
  - current injury - code to injury with seventh character A
  - sequela of previous injury - code to injury with seventh character S
- tropical spastic G04.1

Parapoxvirus B08.60
- specified NEC B08.69

Paraproteinemia D89.2
- benign (familial) D89.2
- monoclonal D47.2
- secondary to malignant disease D47.2

Parapsoriasis L41.9
- en plaques L41.4
- guttata L41.1
- large plaque L41.4
- retiform, retiformis L41.5
- small plaque L41.3
- specified NEC L41.8
- varioliformis (acuta) L41.0

Parasitic —*see also* condition
- disease NEC B89
- stomatitis B37.0
- sycosis (beard) (scalp) B35.0
- twin Q89.4

Parasitism B89
- intestinal B82.9
- skin B88.9
- specified —*see* Infestation

Parasitophobia F40.218

Parasomnia G47.5Ø
due to
alcohol
abuse F1Ø.182
dependence F1Ø.282
use F1Ø.982
amphetamines
abuse F15.182
dependence F15.282
use F15.982
caffeine
abuse F15.182
dependence F15.282
use F15.982
cocaine
abuse F14.182
dependence F14.282
use F14.982
drug NEC
abuse F19.182
dependence F19.282
use F19.982
opioid
abuse F11.182
dependence F11.282
use F11.982
psychoactive substance NEC
abuse F19.182
dependence F19.282
use F19.982
sedative, hypnotic, or anxiolytic
abuse F13.182
dependence F13.282
use F13.982
stimulant NEC
abuse F15.182
dependence F15.282
use F15.982
in conditions classified elsewhere G47.54
nonorganic origin F51.8
organic G47.5Ø
specified NEC G47.59
Paraspadias Q54.9
Paraspasmus facialis G51.8
Parasuicide (attempt)
history of (personal) Z91.51
in family Z81.8
Parathyroid gland —*see* condition
Parathyroid tetany E2Ø.9
Paratrachoma A74.Ø
Paratyphilitis —*see* Appendicitis
Paratyphoid (fever) —*see* Fever, paratyphoid
Paratyphus —*see* Fever, paratyphoid
Paraurethral duct Q64.79
Paraurethritis —*see also* Urethritis
gonococcal (acute) (chronic) (with abscess) A54.1
Paravaccinia NEC BØ8.Ø4
Paravaginitis —*see* Vaginitis
Parencephalitis —*see also* Encephalitis
sequelae GØ9
Parent-child conflict —*see* Conflict, parent-child
estrangement NEC Z62.89Ø
Paresis —*see also* Paralysis
accommodation —*see* Paresis, of accommodation
Bernhardt's G57.1- ●
bladder (sphincter) —*see also* Paralysis, bladder
tabetic A52.17
bowel, colon or intestine K56.Ø
extrinsic muscle, eye H49.9
general (progressive) (syphilitic) A52.17
juvenile A5Ø.45
heart —*see* Failure, heart
insane (syphilitic) A52.17
juvenile (general) A5Ø.45
of accommodation H52.52- ●
peripheral progressive (idiopathic) G6Ø.3
pseudohypertrophic (*see also* Dystrophy, muscular, by type, if applicable) G71.Ø9
senile G83.9
syphilitic (general) A52.17
congenital A5Ø.45
vesical NEC N31.2
Paresthesia —*see also* Disturbance, sensation, skin R2Ø.2
Bernhardt G57.1- ●
Paretic —*see* condition
Parinaud's
conjunctivitis H1Ø.89
oculoglandular syndrome H1Ø.89
ophthalmoplegia H49.88
Parkinsonism (idiopathic) (primary) G2Ø.C
with neurogenic orthostatic hypotension (symptomatic) G9Ø.3
arteriosclerotic G21.4
dementia (*see also* Dementia, in, diseases specified elsewhere) G2Ø.C *[FØ2.8Ø]*
with behavioral disturbance (*see also* Dementia, in, diseases specified elsewhere) G2Ø.C *[FØ2.81- ●]*
due to
drugs NEC G21.19
neuroleptic G21.11
medication-induced NEC G21.19
neuroleptic induced G21.11
postencephalitic G21.3
secondary G21.9
due to
arteriosclerosis G21.4
drugs NEC G21.19
neuroleptic G21.11
encephalitis G21.3
external agents NEC G21.2
syphilis A52.19
specified NEC G21.8
syphilitic A52.19
treatment-induced NEC G21.19
vascular G21.4
Parkinson's disease, syndrome or tremor —*see* Parkinsonism
Parodontitis —*see* Periodontitis
Parodontosis KØ5.4
Paronychia —*see also* Cellulitis, digit
with lymphangitis —*see* Lymphangitis, acute, digit
candidal (chronic) B37.2
tuberculous (primary) A18.4
Parorexia (psychogenic) F5Ø.89
Parosmia R43.1
psychogenic F45.8
Parotid gland —*see* condition
Parotitis, parotiditis (allergic) (nonspecific toxic) (purulent) (septic) (suppurative) —*see also* Sialoadenitis
epidemic —*see* Mumps
infectious —*see* Mumps
postoperative K91.89
surgical K91.89
Parrot fever A7Ø
Parrot's disease (early congenital syphilitic pseudoparalysis) A5Ø.Ø2
Parry-Romberg syndrome G51.8
Parry's disease or syndrome EØ5.ØØ
with thyroid storm EØ5.Ø1
Pars planitis —*see* Cyclitis
Parsonage (-Aldren)-Turner syndrome G54.5
Parson's disease (exophthalmic goiter) EØ5.ØØ
with thyroid storm EØ5.Ø1
Particolored infant Q82.8
Parturition —*see* Delivery
Parulis KØ4.7
with sinus KØ4.6
Parvovirus, as cause of disease classified elsewhere B97.6
Pasini and Pierini's atrophoderma L9Ø.3
Passage
false, urethra N36.5
meconium (newborn) during delivery PØ3.82
of sounds or bougies —*see* Attention to, artificial, opening
Passive —*see* condition
smoking Z77.22
Past due on rent or mortgage Z59.81- ●
Pasteurella septica A28.Ø
Pasteurellosis —*see* Infection, Pasteurella
PAT (paroxysmal atrial tachycardia) I47.19
Patau's syndrome —*see* Trisomy, 13
Patches
mucous (syphilitic) A51.39
congenital A5Ø.Ø7
smokers' (mouth) K13.24
Patellar —*see* condition
Patent —*see also* Imperfect, closure
canal of Nuck Q52.4
cervix N88.3
ductus arteriosus or Botallo's Q25.Ø
foramen
botalli Q21.12
ovale Q21.12
interauricular septum Q21.1Ø
interventricular septum Q21.Ø
omphalomesenteric duct Q43.Ø
Patent *(Continued)*
os (uteri) —*see* Patent, cervix
ostium secundum (type II) Q21.11
urachus Q64.4
vitelline duct Q43.Ø
Paterson (-Brown)(-Kelly) syndrome or web D5Ø.1
Pathologic, pathological —*see also* condition
asphyxia RØ9.Ø1
fire-setting F63.1
gambling F63.Ø
ovum OØ2.Ø
resorption, tooth KØ3.3
stealing F63.2
Pathology (of) —*see* Disease
periradicular, associated with previous endodontic treatment NEC M27.59
Pattern, sleep-wake, irregular G47.23
Patulous —*see also* Imperfect, closure (congenital)
alimentary tract Q45.8
lower Q43.8
upper Q4Ø.8
eustachian tube H69.Ø- ●
Pause, sinoatrial I49.5
Paxton's disease B36.2
Pearl(s)
enamel KØØ.2
Epstein's KØ9.8
Pearl-worker's disease —*see* Osteomyelitis, specified type NEC
Pectenosis K62.4
Pectoral —*see* condition
Pectus
carinatum (congenital) Q67.7
acquired M95.4
rachitic sequelae (late effect) E64.3
excavatum (congenital) Q67.6
acquired M95.4
rachitic sequelae (late effect) E64.3
recurvatum (congenital) Q67.6
Pedatrophia E41
Pederosis F65.4
Pediatric inflammatory multisystem syndrome M35.81
Pediculosis (infestation) B85.2
capitis (head-louse) (any site) B85.Ø
corporis (body-louse) (any site) B85.1
eyelid B85.Ø
mixed (classifiable to more than one of the titles B85.Ø-B85.3) B85.4
pubis (pubic louse) (any site) B85.3
vestimenti B85.1
vulvae B85.3
Pediculus (infestation) —*see* Pediculosis
Pedophilia F65.4
Peg-shaped teeth KØØ.2
Pelade —*see* Alopecia, areata
Pelger-Huët anomaly or syndrome D72.Ø
Peliosis (rheumatica) D69.Ø
hepatis K76.4
with toxic liver disease K71.8
Pelizaeus-Merzbacher disease E75.27
Pellagra (alcoholic) E52
with
polyneuropathy E52 [G63]
Pellagra-cerebellar-ataxia-renal aminoaciduria syndrome E72.Ø2
Pellegrini (-Stieda) disease or syndrome —*see* Bursitis, tibial collateral
Pellizzi's syndrome E34.8
Pel's crisis A52.11
Pelvic —*see also* condition
examination (periodic) (routine) ZØ1.419
with abnormal findings ZØ1.411
kidney, congenital Q63.2
Pelviolithiasis —*see* Calculus, kidney
Pelviperitonitis —*see also* Peritonitis, pelvic
gonococcal A54.24
puerperal O85
Pelvis —*see* condition or type
Pemphigoid L12.9
benign, mucous membrane L12.1
bullous L12.Ø
cicatricial L12.1
juvenile L12.2
ocular L12.1
specified NEC L12.8
Pemphigus L1Ø.9
benign familial (chronic) Q82.8
Brazilian L1Ø.3
circinatus L13.Ø
conjunctiva L12.1

P

P

▶ New ➡ Revised ~~deleted~~ Deleted ● Use Additional Character(s)

Perforation, perforated *(Continued)*
- urethra *(Continued)*
  - obstetrical trauma O71.5
  - traumatic S37.39
    - at delivery O71.5
- uterus
  - with ectopic or molar pregnancy OØ8.6
  - by intrauterine contraceptive device T83.39
  - following ectopic or molar pregnancy OØ8.6
  - obstetrical trauma O71.1
  - traumatic S37.69
    - obstetric O71.1
- uvula K13.79
  - syphilitic A52.79
- vagina
  - obstetrical trauma O71.4
  - other trauma - *see* Puncture, vagina

Periadenitis mucosa necrotica recurrens K12.Ø

Periappendicitis (acute) *—see* Appendicitis

Periarteritis nodosa (disseminated) (infectious) (necrotizing) M3Ø.Ø

Periarthritis (joint) *—see also* Enthesopathy
- Duplay's M75.Ø-●
- gonococcal A54.42
- humeroscapularis *—see* Capsulitis, adhesive
- scapulohumeral *—see* Capsulitis, adhesive
- shoulder *—see* Capsulitis, adhesive
- wrist M77.2-●

Periarthrosis (angioneural) *—see* Enthesopathy

Pericapsulitis, adhesive (shoulder) *—see* Capsulitis, adhesive

Pericarditis (with decompensation) (with effusion) I31.9
- with rheumatic fever (conditions in IØØ)
  - active *—see* Pericarditis, rheumatic
  - inactive or quiescent IØ9.2
- acute (hemorrhagic) (nonrheumatic) (Sicca) I3Ø.9
  - with chorea (acute) (rheumatic) (Sydenham's) IØ2.Ø
  - benign I3Ø.8
  - nonspecific I3Ø.Ø
  - rheumatic IØ1.Ø
    - with chorea (acute) (Sydenham's) IØ2.Ø
- adhesive or adherent (chronic) (external) (internal) I31.Ø
  - acute *—see* Pericarditis, acute
  - rheumatic IØ9.2
- bacterial (acute) (subacute) (with serous or seropurulent effusion) I3Ø.1
- calcareous I31.1
- cholesterol (chronic) I31.8
  - acute I3Ø.9
- chronic (nonrheumatic) I31.9
  - rheumatic IØ9.2
- constrictive (chronic) I31.1
- coxsackie B33.23
- fibrinocaseous (tuberculous) A18.84
- fibrinopurulent I3Ø.1
- fibrinous I3Ø.8
- fibrous I31.Ø
- gonococcal A54.83
- idiopathic I3Ø.Ø
- in systemic lupus erythematosus M32.12
- infective I3Ø.1
- meningococcal A39.53
- neoplastic (chronic) I31.8
  - acute I3Ø.9
- obliterans, obliterating I31.Ø
- plastic I31.Ø
- pneumococcal I3Ø.1
- postinfarction I24.1
- purulent I3Ø.1
- rheumatic (active) (acute) (with effusion) (with pneumonia) IØ1.Ø
  - with chorea (acute) (rheumatic) (Sydenham's) IØ2.Ø
  - chronic or inactive (with chorea) IØ9.2
- rheumatoid *—see* Rheumatoid, carditis
- septic I3Ø.1
- serofibrinous I3Ø.8
- staphylococcal I3Ø.1
- streptococcal I3Ø.1
- suppurative I3Ø.1
- syphilitic A52.Ø6
- tuberculous A18.84
- uremic N18.9 *[I32]*
- viral I3Ø.1

Pericardium, pericardial *—see* condition

Pericellulitis *—see* Cellulitis

Pericementitis (chronic) (suppurative) *—see also* Periodontitis
- acute KØ5.2Ø
  - generalized *—see* Periodontitis, aggressive, generalized
  - localized *—see* Periodontitis, aggressive, localized

Perichondritis
- auricle *—see* Perichondritis, ear
- bronchus J98.Ø9
- ear (external) H61.ØØ-●
  - acute H61.Ø1-●
  - chronic H61.Ø2-●
- external auditory canal *—see* Perichondritis, ear
- larynx J38.7
  - syphilitic A52.73
  - typhoid AØ1.Ø9
- nose J34.89
- pinna *—see* Perichondritis, ear
- trachea J39.8

Periclasia KØ5.4

Pericoronitis *—see* Periodontitis

Pericystitis N3Ø.9Ø
- with hematuria N3Ø.91

Peridiverticulitis (intestine) K57.92
- cecum *—see* Diverticulitis, intestine, large
- colon *—see* Diverticulitis, intestine, large
- duodenum *—see* Diverticulitis, intestine, small
- intestine *—see* Diverticulitis, intestine
- jejunum *—see* Diverticulitis, intestine, small
- rectosigmoid *—see* Diverticulitis, intestine, large
- rectum *—see* Diverticulitis, intestine, large
- sigmoid *—see* Diverticulitis, intestine, large

Periendocarditis *—see* Endocarditis

Periepididymitis N45.1

Perifolliculitis LØ1.Ø2
- abscedens, caput, scalp L66.3
- capitis, abscedens (et suffodiens) L66.3
- superficial pustular LØ1.Ø2

Perihepatitis K65.8

Perilabyrinthitis (acute) *—see* subcategory H83.Ø

Perimeningitis *—see* Meningitis

Perimetritis *—see* Endometritis

Perimetrosalpingitis *—see* Salpingo-oophoritis

Perineocele N81.81

Perinephric, perinephritic *—see* condition

Perinephritis *—see also* Infection, kidney
- purulent *—see* Abscess, kidney

Perineum, perineal *—see* condition

Perineuritis NEC *—see* Neuralgia

Periodic *—see* condition

Periodontitis (chronic) (complex) (compound) (local) (simplex) KØ5.3Ø
- acute KØ5.2Ø
  - generalized KØ5.229
    - moderate KØ5.222
    - severe KØ5.223
    - slight KØ5.221
  - localized KØ5.219
    - moderate KØ5.212
    - severe KØ5.213
    - slight KØ5.211
- aggressive KØ5.2Ø
  - generalized KØ5.229
    - moderate KØ5.222
    - severe KØ5.223
    - slight KØ5.221
  - localized KØ5.219
    - moderate KØ5.212
    - severe KØ5.213
    - slight KØ5.211
- apical KØ4.5
  - acute (pulpal origin) KØ4.4
- generalized KØ5.329
  - moderate KØ5.322
  - severe KØ5.323
  - slight KØ5.321
- localized KØ5.319
  - moderate KØ5.312
  - severe KØ5.313
  - slight KØ5.311

Periodontoclasia KØ5.4

Periodontosis (juvenile) KØ5.4

Periods *—see also* Menstruation
- heavy N92.Ø
- irregular N92.6
- shortened intervals (irregular) N92.1

Perionychia *—see also* Cellulitis, digit
- with lymphangitis *—see* Lymphangitis, acute, digit

Perioophoritis *—see* Salpingo-oophoritis

Periorchitis N45.2

Periosteum, periosteal *—see* condition

Periostitis (albuminosa) (circumscribed) (diffuse) (infective) (monomelic) *—see also* Osteomyelitis
- alveolar M27.3
- alveolodental M27.3
- dental M27.3
- gonorrheal A54.43
- jaw (lower) (upper) M27.2
- orbit HØ5.Ø3-●
- syphilitic A52.77
  - congenital (early) A5Ø.Ø2 *[M9Ø.8Ø]*
  - secondary A51.46
- tuberculous *—see* Tuberculosis, bone
- yaws (hypertrophic) (early) (late) A66.6 *[M9Ø.8Ø]*

Periostosis (hyperplastic) *—see also* Disorder, bone, specified type NEC
- with osteomyelitis *—see* Osteomyelitis, specified type NEC

Peripartum
- cardiomyopathy O9Ø.3

Periphlebitis *—see* Phlebitis

Periproctitis K62.89

Periprostatitis *—see* Prostatitis

Perirectal *—see* condition

Perirenal *—see* condition

Perisalpingitis *—see* Salpingo-oophoritis

Perisplenitis (infectional) D73.89

Peristalsis, visible or reversed R19.2

Peritendinitis *—see* Enthesopathy

Peritoneum, peritoneal *—see* condition

Peritonitis (adhesive) (bacterial) (fibrinous) (hemorrhagic) (idiopathic) (localized) (perforative) (primary) (with adhesions) (with effusion) K65.9
- with or following
  - abscess K65.1
  - appendicitis
    - with perforation or rupture K35.32
    - generalized (*see also* Appendicitis) K35.2Ø9
    - localized (*see also* Appendicitis) K35.3Ø
  - diverticular disease (intestine) K57.8Ø
    - with bleeding K57.81
    - ectopic or molar pregnancy OØ8.Ø
    - large intestine K57.2Ø
      - with
        - bleeding K57.21
        - small intestine K57.4Ø
          - with bleeding K57.41
    - small intestine K57.ØØ
      - with
        - bleeding K57.Ø1
        - large intestine K57.4Ø
          - with bleeding K57.41
- acute (generalized) K65.Ø
- aseptic T81.61
- bile, biliary K65.3
- chemical T81.61
- chlamydial A74.81
- chronic proliferative K65.8
- complicating abortion *—see* Abortion, by type, complicated by, pelvic peritonitis
- congenital P78.1
- diaphragmatic K65.Ø
- diffuse K65.Ø
- diphtheritic A36.89
- disseminated K65.Ø
- due to
  - bile K65.3
  - foreign
    - body or object accidentally left during a procedure (instrument) (sponge) (swab) T81.599
    - substance accidentally left during a procedure (chemical) (powder) (talc) T81.61
  - talc T81.61
  - urine K65.8
- eosinophilic K65.8
  - acute K65.Ø
- fibrocaseous (tuberculous) A18.31
- fibropurulent K65.Ø
- following ectopic or molar pregnancy OØ8.Ø
- general (ized) K65.Ø
- gonococcal A54.85
- meconium (newborn) P78.Ø
- neonatal P78.1
  - meconium P78.Ø
- pancreatic K65.Ø

P

Peritonitis *(Continued)*
- paroxysmal, familial E85.Ø
  - benign E85.Ø
- pelvic
  - female N73.5
    - acute N73.3
    - chronic N73.4
      - with adhesions N73.6
  - male K65.Ø
- periodic, familial E85.Ø
- proliferative, chronic K65.8
- puerperal, postpartum, childbirth O85
- purulent K65.Ø
- septic K65.Ø
- specified NEC K65.8
- spontaneous bacterial K65.2
- subdiaphragmatic K65.Ø
- subphrenic K65.Ø
- suppurative K65.Ø
- syphilitic A52.74
  - congenital (early) A5Ø.Ø8 *[K67]*
- talc T81.61
- tuberculous A18.31
- urine K65.8

Peritonsillar —*see* condition
Peritonsillitis J36
Perityphlitis (*see also* Cecitis) K37
Periureteritis N28.89
Periurethral —*see* condition
Periurethritis (gangrenous) —*see* Urethritis
Periuterine —*see* condition
Perivaginitis —*see* Vaginitis
Perivasculitis, retinal H35.Ø6- ●
Perivasitis (chronic) N49.1
Perivesiculitis (seminal) —*see* Vesiculitis
Perlèche NEC K13.Ø
- due to
  - candidiasis B37.83
  - moniliasis B37.83
  - riboflavin deficiency E53.Ø
  - vitamin B2 (riboflavin) deficiency E53.Ø

Pernicious —*see* condition
Pernio, perniosis T69.1
Perpetrator (of abuse) —*see* Index to External Causes of Injury, Perpetrator
Persecution
- delusion F22
- social Z6Ø.5

Perseveration (tonic) R48.8
Persistence, persistent (congenital)
- anal membrane Q42.3
  - with fistula Q42.2
- arteria stapedia Q16.3
- atrioventricular canal Q21.2Ø
- branchial cleft NOS Q18.2
  - cyst Q18.Ø
  - fistula Q18.Ø
  - sinus Q18.Ø
- bulbus cordis in left ventricle Q21.8
- canal of Cloquet Q14.Ø
- capsule (opaque) Q12.8
- cilioretinal artery or vein Q14.8
- cloaca Q43.7
- communication —*see* Fistula, congenital
- convolutions
  - aortic arch Q25.46
  - fallopian tube Q5Ø.6
  - oviduct Q5Ø.6
  - uterine tube Q5Ø.6
- double aortic arch Q25.45
- ductus arteriosus (Botalli) Q25.Ø
- fetal
  - circulation P29.38
  - form of cervix (uteri) Q51.828
  - hemoglobin, hereditary (HPFH) D56.4
- foramen
  - Botalli Q21.12
  - ovale Q21.12
- Gartner's duct Q52.4
- hemoglobin, fetal (hereditary) (HPFH) D56.4
- hyaloid
  - artery (generally incomplete) Q14.Ø
  - system Q14.8
- hymen, in pregnancy or childbirth —*see* Pregnancy, complicated by, abnormal, vulva
- lanugo Q84.2
- left
  - posterior cardinal vein Q26.8
  - root with right arch of aorta Q25.49
  - superior vena cava Q26.1

Persistence, persistent *(Continued)*
- Meckel's diverticulum Q43.Ø
  - malignant —*see* Table of Neoplasms, small intestine, malignant
- mucosal disease (middle ear) —*see* Otitis, media, suppurative, chronic, tubotympanic
- nail(s), anomalous Q84.6
- omphalomesenteric duct Q43.Ø
- organ or site not listed —*see* Anomaly, by site
- ostium
  - atrioventriculare commune Q21.23
  - primum Q21.2Ø
  - secundum Q21.11
- ovarian rests in fallopian tube Q5Ø.6
- pancreatic tissue in intestinal tract Q43.8
- primary (deciduous)
  - teeth KØØ.6
  - vitreous hyperplasia Q14.Ø
- pupillary membrane Q13.89
- rhesus (Rh)titer —*see* Complication(s), transfusion, incompatibility reaction, Rh (factor)
- right aortic arch Q25.47
- sinus
  - urogenitalis
    - female Q52.8
    - male Q55.8
  - venosus with imperfect incorporation in right auricle Q26.8
- thymus (gland) (hyperplasia) E32.Ø
- thyroglossal duct Q89.2
- thyrolingual duct Q89.2
- truncus arteriosus or communis Q2Ø.Ø
- tunica vasculosa lentis Q12.2
- umbilical sinus Q64.4
- urachus Q64.4
- vitelline duct Q43.Ø

Person (with)
- admitted for clinical research, as a control subject (normal comparison) (participant) ZØØ.6
- awaiting admission to adequate facility elsewhere Z75.1
- concern (normal) about sick person in family Z63.6
- consulting on behalf of another Z71.Ø
- feigning illness Z76.5
- living (in)
  - without
    - adequate housing (heating) (space) Z59.1Ø
    - air conditioning Z59.11
    - environmental temperature Z59.11
    - heating Z59.11
    - space Z59.19
    - housing (permanent) (temporary) Z59.ØØ
    - person able to render necessary care Z74.2
    - shelter Z59.Ø2
  - alone Z6Ø.2
  - boarding school Z59.3
  - residential institution Z59.3
- on waiting list Z75.1
- sick or handicapped in family Z63.6

Personality (disorder) F6Ø.9
- accentuation of traits (type A pattern) Z73.1
- affective F34.Ø
- aggressive F6Ø.3
- amoral F6Ø.2
- anacastic, anankastic F6Ø.5
- antisocial F6Ø.2
- anxious F6Ø.6
- asocial F6Ø.2
- asthenic F6Ø.7
- avoidant F6Ø.6
- borderline F6Ø.3
- change due to organic condition (enduring) FØ7.Ø
- compulsive F6Ø.5
- cycloid F34.Ø
- cyclothymic F34.Ø
- dependent F6Ø.7
- depressive F34.1
- dissocial F6Ø.2
- dual F44.81
- eccentric F6Ø.89
- emotionally unstable F6Ø.3
- expansive paranoid F6Ø.Ø
- explosive F6Ø.3
- fanatic F6Ø.Ø
- haltlose type F6Ø.89
- histrionic F6Ø.4
- hyperthymic F34.Ø
- hypothymic F34.1

Personality *(Continued)*
- hysterical F6Ø.4
- immature F6Ø.89
- inadequate F6Ø.7
- labile (emotional) F6Ø.3
- mixed (nonspecific) F6Ø.89
- morally defective F6Ø.2
- multiple F44.81
- narcissistic F6Ø.81
- obsessional F6Ø.5
- obsessive (-compulsive) F6Ø.5
- organic FØ7.Ø
- overconscientious F6Ø.5
- paranoid F6Ø.Ø
- passive (-dependent) F6Ø.7
- passive-aggressive F6Ø.89
- pathologic F6Ø.9
- pattern defect or disturbance F6Ø.9
- pseudopsychopathic (organic) FØ7.Ø
- pseudoretarded (organic) FØ7.Ø
- psychoinfantile F6Ø.4
- psychoneurotic NEC F6Ø.89
- psychopathic F6Ø.2
- querulant F6Ø.Ø
- sadistic F6Ø.89
- schizoid F6Ø.1
- self-defeating F6Ø.89
- sensitive paranoid F6Ø.Ø
- sociopathic (amoral) (antisocial) (asocial) (dissocial) F6Ø.2
- specified NEC F6Ø.89
- type A Z73.1
- unstable (emotional) F6Ø.3

Perthes' disease —*see* Legg-Calvé-Perthes disease
Pertussis (*see also* Whooping cough) A37.9Ø
Perversion, perverted
- appetite F5Ø.89
  - psychogenic F5Ø.89
- function
  - pituitary gland E23.2
    - posterior lobe E22.2
- sense of smell and taste R43.8
  - psychogenic F45.8
- sexual —*see* Deviation, sexual

Pervious, congenital —*see also* Imperfect, closure
- ductus arteriosus Q25.Ø

Pes (congenital) —*see also* Talipes
- acquired —*see also* Deformity, limb, foot, specified NEC
  - planus —*see* Deformity, limb, flat foot
- adductus Q66.89
- cavus Q66.7- ●
- deformity NEC, acquired —*see* Deformity, limb, foot, specified NEC
- planus (acquired) (any degree) —*see also* Deformity, limb, flat foot
  - rachitic sequelae (late effect) E64.3
- valgus Q66.6

Pest, pestis —*see* Plague
Petechia, petechiae R23.3
- newborn P54.5

Petechial typhus A75.9
Peter's anomaly Q13.4
Petit mal seizure —*see* Epilepsy, childhood, absence
Petit's hernia —*see* Hernia, abdomen, specified site NEC
Petrellidosis B48.2
Petrositis H7Ø.2Ø- ●
- acute H7Ø.21- ●
- chronic H7Ø.22- ●

Peutz-Jeghers disease or syndrome Q85.89
Peyronie's disease N48.6
PFAPA (periodic fever, aphthous stomatitis, pharyngitis, and adenopathy syndrome) MØ4.8
Pfeiffer's disease —*see* Mononucleosis, infectious
Phagedena (dry) (moist) (sloughing) —*see also* Gangrene
- geometric L88
- penis N48.29
- tropical —*see* Ulcer, skin
- vulva N76.6

Phagedenic —*see* condition
Phakoma H35.89
Phakomatosis —*see also* specific eponymous syndromes Q85.9
- Bourneville's Q85.1
- specified NEC Q85.89

Phantom limb syndrome (without pain) G54.7
- with pain G54.6

P

P

Pick's *(Continued)*
disease or syndrome (brain) (*see also* Dementia, in, diseases specified elsewhere) G31.Ø1 *[FØ2.8Ø]*
with behavioral disturbance (*see also* Dementia, in, diseases specified elsewhere) G31.Ø1 *[FØ2.81-●]*
brain (*see also* Dementia, in, diseases specified elsewhere) G31.Ø1 *[FØ2.8Ø]*
with behavioral disturbance (*see also* Dementia, in, diseases specified elsewhere) G31.Ø1 *[FØ2.81-●]*
pericardium (pericardial pseudocirrhosis of liver) I31.1
syndrome
brain (*see also* Dementia, in, diseases specified elsewhere) G31.Ø1 *[FØ2.8Ø]*
with behavioral disturbance (*see also* Dementia, in, diseases specified elsewhere) G31.Ø1 *[FØ2.81-●]*
of heart (pericardial pseudocirrhosis of liver) I31.1
Pickwickian syndrome E66.2
Piebaldism E7Ø.39
Piedra (beard) (scalp) B36.8
black B36.3
white B36.2
Pierre Robin deformity or syndrome Q87.Ø
Pierson's disease or osteochondrosis M91.Ø
Pig-bel AØ5.2
Pigeon
breast or chest (acquired) M95.4
congenital Q67.7
rachitic sequelae (late effect) E64.3
breeder's disease or lung J67.2
fancier's disease or lung J67.2
toe —*see* Deformity, toe, specified NEC
Pigmentation (abnormal) (anomaly) L81.9
conjunctiva H11.13-●
cornea (anterior) H18.Ø1-●
posterior H18.Ø5-●
stromal H18.Ø6-●
diminished melanin formation NEC L81.6
iron L81.8
lids, congenital Q82.8
limbus corneae —*see* Pigmentation, cornea
metals L81.8
optic papilla, congenital Q14.2
retina, congenital (grouped) (nevoid) Q14.1
scrotum, congenital Q82.8
tattoo L81.8
Piles —*see also* Hemorrhoids K64.9
Pili
annulati or torti (congenital) Q84.1
incarnati L73.1
Pill roller hand (intrinsic) —*see* Parkinsonism
Pilomatrixoma —*see* Neoplasm, skin, benign
malignant —*see* Neoplasm, skin, malignant
Pilonidal —*see* condition
Pimple R23.8
PIMS M35.81
PIN —*see* Neoplasia, intraepithelial, prostate
Pinched nerve —*see* Neuropathy, entrapment
Pindborg tumor —*see* Cyst, calcifying odontogenic
Pineal body or gland —*see* condition
Pinealoblastoma C75.3
Pinealoma D44.5
malignant C75.3
Pineoblastoma C75.3
Pineocytoma D44.5
Pinguecula H11.15-●
Pingueculitis H1Ø.81-●
Pinhole meatus —*see also* Stricture, urethra N35.919
Pink
disease —*see* subcategory T56.1
eye —*see* Conjunctivitis, acute, mucopurulent
Pinkus' disease (lichen nitidus) L44.1
Pinpoint
meatus —*see* Stricture, urethra
os (uteri) —*see* Stricture, cervix
Pins and needles R2Ø.2
Pinta A67.9
cardiovascular lesions A67.2
chancre (primary) A67.Ø
erythematous plaques A67.1
hyperchromic lesions A67.1
hyperkeratosis A67.1
lesions A67.9
cardiovascular A67.2
hyperchromic A67.1
Pinta *(Continued)*
lesions *(Continued)*
intermediate A67.1
late A67.2
mixed A67.3
primary A67.Ø
skin (achromic) (cicatricial) (dyschromic) A67.2
hyperchromic A67.1
mixed (achromic and hyperchromic) A67.3
papule (primary) A67.Ø
skin lesions (achromic) (cicatricial) (dyschromic) A67.2
hyperchromic A67.1
mixed (achromic and hyperchromic) A67.3
vitiligo A67.2
Pintids A67.1
Pinworm (disease) (infection) (infestation) B8Ø
Piroplasmosis (*see also* Babesiosis) B6Ø.ØØ
specified NEC B6Ø.Ø9
Pistol wound —*see* Gunshot wound
Pitchers' elbow —*see* Derangement, joint, specified type NEC, elbow
Pithecoid pelvis Q74.2
with disproportion (fetopelvic) O33.Ø
causing obstructed labor O65.Ø
Pithiatism F48.8
Pitted —*see* Pitting
Pitting —*see also* Edema R6Ø.9
lip R6Ø.Ø
nail L6Ø.8
teeth KØØ.4
Pituitary gland —*see* condition
Pituitary-snuff-taker's disease J67.8
Pityriasis (capitis) L21.Ø
alba L3Ø.5
circinata (et maculata) L42
furfuracea L21.Ø
Hebra's L26
lichenoides L41.Ø
chronica L41.1
et varioliformis (acuta) L41.Ø
maculata (et circinata) L3Ø.5
nigra B36.1
pilaris, Hebra's L44.Ø
rosea L42
rotunda L44.8
rubra (Hebra) pilaris L44.Ø
simplex L3Ø.5
specified type NEC L3Ø.5
streptogenes L3Ø.5
versicolor (scrotal) B36.Ø
Placenta, placental —*see* Pregnancy, complicated by (care of) (management affected by), specified condition
Placentitis O41.14-●
Plagiocephaly Q67.3
non-deformational
anterior Q75.Ø21
posterior Q75.Ø4-●
Plague A2Ø.9
abortive A2Ø.8
ambulatory A2Ø.8
asymptomatic A2Ø.8
bubonic A2Ø.Ø
cellulocutaneous A2Ø.1
cutaneobubonic A2Ø.1
lymphatic gland A2Ø.Ø
meningitis A2Ø.3
pharyngeal A2Ø.8
pneumonic (primary) (secondary) A2Ø.2
pulmonary, pulmonic A2Ø.2
septicemic A2Ø.7
tonsillar A2Ø.8
septicemic A2Ø.7
Planning, family
contraception Z3Ø.9
procreation Z31.69
Plaque(s)
artery, arterial —*see* Arteriosclerosis
calcareous —*see* Calcification
coronary, lipid rich I25.83
epicardial I31.8
erythematous, of pinta A67.1
Hollenhorst's —*see* Occlusion, artery, retina
lipid rich, coronary I25.83
pleural (without asbestos) J92.9
with asbestos J92.Ø
tongue K13.29
Plasmacytoma C9Ø.3-●
extramedullary C9Ø.2-●
medullary C9Ø.Ø-●
solitary C9Ø.3-●
Plasmacytopenia D72.818
Plasmacytosis D72.822
Plaster ulcer —*see* Ulcer, pressure, by site
Plateau iris syndrome (post-iridectomy) (postprocedural) (without glaucoma)H21.82
with glaucoma H4Ø.22-●
Platybasia Q75.8
Platyonychia (congenital) Q84.6
acquired L6Ø.8
Platypelloid pelvis M95.5
with disproportion (fetopelvic) O33.Ø
causing obstructed labor O65.Ø
congenital Q74.2
Platyspondylisis Q76.49
Plaut (-Vincent) disease —*see also* Vincent's A69.1
Plethora R23.2
newborn P61.1
Pleura, pleural —*see* condition
Pleuralgia RØ7.81
Pleurisy (acute) (adhesive) (chronic) (costal) (diaphragmatic) (double) (dry) (fibrinous) (fibrous) (interlobar) (latent) (plastic) (primary) (residual) (sicca) (sterile) (subacute) (unresolved) RØ9.1
with
adherent pleura J86.Ø
effusion J9Ø
chylous, chyliform J94.Ø
tuberculous (non primary) A15.6
primary (progressive) A15.7
tuberculosis —*see* Pleurisy, tuberculous (non primary)
encysted —*see* Pleurisy, with effusion
exudative —*see* Pleurisy, with effusion
fibrinopurulent, fibropurulent —*see* Pyothorax
hemorrhagic —*see* Hemothorax
pneumococcal J9Ø
purulent —*see* Pyothorax
septic —*see* Pyothorax
serofibrinous —*see* Pleurisy, with effusion
seropurulent —*see* Pyothorax
serous —*see* Pleurisy, with effusion
staphylococcal J86.9
streptococcal J9Ø
suppurative —*see* Pyothorax
traumatic (post) (current) —*see* Injury, intrathoracic, pleura
tuberculous (with effusion) (non primary) A15.6
primary (progressive) A15.7
Pleuritis sicca —*see* Pleurisy
Pleurobronchopneumonia —*see* Pneumonia, broncho
Pleurodynia RØ7.81
epidemic B33.Ø
viral B33.Ø
Pleuropericarditis —*see also* Pericarditis
acute I3Ø.9
Pleuropneumonia (acute) (bilateral) (double) (septic) —*see also* Pneumonia J18.8
chronic —*see* Fibrosis, lung
Pleuro-pneumonia-like-organism (PPLO), as cause of disease classified elsewhere B96.Ø
Pleurorrhea —*see* Pleurisy, with effusion
Plexitis, brachial G54.Ø
Plica
polonica B85.Ø
syndrome, knee M67.5
tonsil J35.8
Plicated tongue K14.5
Plug
bronchus NEC J98.Ø9
meconium (newborn) NEC syndrome P76.Ø
mucus —*see* Asphyxia, mucus
Plumbism —*see* subcategory T56.Ø
Plummer's disease EØ5.2Ø
with thyroid storm EØ5.21
Plummer-Vinson syndrome D5Ø.1
Pluricarential syndrome of infancy E4Ø
Plus (and minus) **hand** (intrinsic) —*see* Deformity, limb, specified type NEC, forearm
PMEI (polymorphic epilepsy in infancy) G4Ø.83-●
Pneumathemia —*see* Air, embolism
Pneumatic hammer (drill) **syndrome** T75.21
Pneumatocele (lung) J98.4
intracranial G93.89
tension J98.8

352
▶ New ➡ Revised ~~deleted~~ Deleted ● Use Additional Character(s)

- **Pneumatosis**
  - cystoides intestinalis K63.89
  - intestinalis K63.89
  - peritonei K66.8
- **Pneumaturia** R39.89
- **Pneumoblastoma** —*see* Neoplasm, lung, malignant
- **Pneumocephalus** G93.89
- **Pneumococcemia** A4Ø.3
- **Pneumococcus, pneumococcal** —*see* condition
- **Pneumoconiosis** (due to) (inhalation of) J64
  - with tuberculosis (any type in A15) J65
  - aluminum J63.Ø
  - asbestos J61
  - bagasse, bagassosis J67.1
  - bauxite J63.1
  - beryllium J63.2
  - coal miners' (simple) J6Ø
  - coalworkers' (simple) J6Ø
  - collier's J6Ø
  - cotton dust J66.Ø
  - diatomite (diatomaceous earth) J62.8
  - dust
    - inorganic NEC J63.6
    - lime J62.8
    - marble J62.8
    - organic NEC J66.8
  - fumes or vapors (from silo) J68.9
  - graphite J63.3
  - grinder's J62.8
  - kaolin J62.8
  - mica J62.8
  - millstone maker's J62.8
  - mineral fibers NEC J61
  - miner's J6Ø
  - moldy hay J67.Ø
  - potter's J62.8
  - rheumatoid —*see* Rheumatoid, lung
  - sandblaster's J62.8
  - silica, silicate NEC J62.8
    - with carbon J6Ø
  - stonemason's J62.8
  - talc (dust) J62.Ø
- **Pneumocystis carinii pneumonia** B59
- **Pneumocystis jiroveci** (pneumonia) B59
- **Pneumocystosis** (with pneumonia) B59
- **Pneumohemopericardium** I31.2
- **Pneumohemothorax** J94.2
  - traumatic S27.2
- **Pneumohydropericardium** —*see* Pericarditis
- **Pneumohydrothorax** —*see* Hydrothorax
- **Pneumomediastinum** J98.2
  - congenital or perinatal P25.2
- **Pneumomycosis** B49 *[J99]*
- **Pneumonia** (acute) (double) (migratory) (purulent) (septic) (unresolved) J18.9
  - with
    - influenza —*see* Influenza, with, pneumonia
    - lung abscess J85.1
      - due to specified organism —*see* Pneumonia, in (due to)
  - 2Ø19 (novel) coronavirus J12.82
  - adenoviral J12.Ø
  - adynamic J18.2
  - alba A5Ø.Ø4
  - allergic (*see also* Pneumonitis, hypersensitivity) J82.89
  - alveolar —*see* Pneumonia, lobar
  - anaerobes J15.8
  - anthrax A22.1
  - apex, apical —*see* Pneumonia, lobar
  - Ascaris B77.81
  - aspiration J69.Ø
    - due to
      - aspiration of microorganisms
        - bacterial J15.9
        - viral J12.9
      - food (regurgitated) J69.Ø
      - gastric secretions J69.Ø
      - milk (regurgitated) J69.Ø
      - oils, essences J69.1
      - solids, liquids NEC J69.8
      - vomitus J69.Ø
    - newborn P24.81
      - amniotic fluid (clear) P24.11
      - blood P24.21
      - food (regurgitated) P24.31
      - liquor (amnii) P24.11
      - meconium P24.Ø1
      - milk P24.31

Pneumonia *(Continued)*
  - aspiration *(Continued)*
    - newborn *(Continued)*
      - mucus P24.11
      - specified NEC P24.81
      - stomach contents P24.31
    - postprocedural J95.4
  - atypical NEC J18.9
  - bacillus J15.9
    - specified NEC J15.8
  - bacterial J15.9
    - specified NEC J15.8
  - Bacteroides (fragilis) (oralis) (melaninogenicus) J15.8
  - basal, basic, basilar —*see* Pneumonia, by type
  - bronchiolitis obliterans organized (BOOP) J84.89
  - broncho-, bronchial (confluent) (croupous) (diffuse) (disseminated) (hemorrhagic) (involving lobes) (lobar) (terminal) J18.Ø
    - allergic (*see also* Pneumonitis, hypersensitivity) J82.89
    - aspiration —*see* Pneumonia, aspiration
    - bacterial J15.9
      - specified NEC J15.8
    - chronic —*see* Fibrosis, lung
    - diplococcal J13
    - Eaton's agent J15.7
    - Escherichia coli (E. coli) J15.5
    - Friedländer's bacillus J15.Ø
    - Hemophilus influenzae J14
    - hypostatic J18.2
    - inhalation —*see also* Pneumonia, aspiration
      - due to fumes or vapors (chemical) J68.Ø
      - of oils or essences J69.1
    - Klebsiella (pneumoniae) J15.Ø
    - lipid, lipoid J69.1
      - endogenous J84.89
    - Mycoplasma (pneumoniae) J15.7
    - pleuro-pneumonia-like-organisms (PPLO) J15.7
    - pneumococcal J13
    - Proteus J15.69
    - Pseudomonas J15.1
    - Serratia marcescens J15.69
    - specified organism NEC J16.8
    - staphylococcal —*see* Pneumonia, staphylococcal
    - streptococcal NEC J15.4
      - group B J15.3
      - pneumoniae J13
    - viral, virus —*see* Pneumonia, viral
  - Butyrivibrio (fibriosolvens) J15.8
  - Candida B37.1
  - caseous —*see* Tuberculosis, pulmonary
  - catarrhal —*see* Pneumonia, broncho
  - chlamydial J16.Ø
    - congenital P23.1
  - cholesterol J84.89
  - cirrhotic (chronic) —*see* Fibrosis, lung
  - Clostridium (haemolyticum) (novyi) J15.8
  - confluent —*see* Pneumonia, broncho
  - congenital (infective) P23.9
    - due to
      - bacterium NEC P23.6
      - Chlamydia P23.1
      - Escherichia coli P23.4
      - Haemophilus influenzae P23.6
      - infective organism NEC P23.8
      - Klebsiella pneumoniae P23.6
      - Mycoplasma P23.6
      - Pseudomonas P23.5
      - Staphylococcus P23.2
      - Streptococcus (except group B) P23.6
        - group B P23.3
      - viral agent P23.Ø
    - specified NEC P23.8
  - coronavirus (novel) (disease) 2Ø19 J12.82
  - COVID-19 J12.82
  - croupous —*see* Pneumonia, lobar
  - cryptogenic organizing J84.116
  - cytomegalic inclusion B25.Ø
  - cytomegaloviral B25.Ø
  - deglutition —*see* Pneumonia, aspiration
  - desquamative interstitial J84.117
  - diffuse —*see* Pneumonia, broncho
  - diplococcal, diplococcus (broncho-) (lobar) J13
  - disseminated (focal) —*see* Pneumonia, broncho
  - Eaton's agent J15.7
  - embolic, embolism —*see* Embolism, pulmonary
  - Enterobacter J15.69

Pneumonia *(Continued)*
  - eosinophilic J82.81
    - acute J82.82
    - chronic J82.81
  - Escherichia coli (E. coli) J15.5
  - Eubacterium J15.8
  - fibrinous —*see* Pneumonia, lobar
  - fibroid, fibrous (chronic) —*see* Fibrosis, lung
  - Friedländer's bacillus J15.Ø
  - Fusobacterium (nucleatum) J15.8
  - gangrenous J85.Ø
  - giant cell (measles) BØ5.2
  - gonococcal A54.84
  - gram-negative bacteria NEC J15.69
    - anaerobic J15.8
  - Hemophilus influenzae (broncho) (lobar) J14
  - human metapneumovirus J12.3
  - hypostatic (broncho) (lobar) J18.2
  - in (due to)
    - Acinetobacter baumannii J15.61
    - actinomycosis A42.Ø
    - adenovirus J12.Ø
    - anthrax A22.1
    - ascariasis B77.81
    - aspergillosis B44.9
    - Bacillus anthracis A22.1
    - Bacterium anitratum J15.69
    - candidiasis B37.1
    - chickenpox BØ1.2
    - Chlamydia J16.Ø
      - neonatal P23.1
    - coccidioidomycosis B38.2
      - acute B38.Ø
      - chronic B38.1
    - cytomegalovirus disease B25.Ø
    - Diplococcus (pneumoniae) J13
    - Eaton's agent J15.7
    - Enterobacter J15.69
    - Escherichia coli (E. coli) J15.5
    - Friedländer's bacillus J15.Ø
    - fumes and vapors (chemical) (inhalation) J68.Ø
    - gonorrhea A54.84
    - Hemophilus influenzae (H. influenzae) J14
    - Herellea J15.69
    - histoplasmosis B39.2
      - acute B39.Ø
      - chronic B39.1
    - human metapneumovirus J12.3
    - Klebsiella (pneumoniae) J15.Ø
    - measles BØ5.2
    - Mycoplasma (pneumoniae) J15.7
    - nocardiosis, nocardiasis A43.Ø
    - ornithosis A7Ø
    - parainfluenza virus J12.2
    - pleuro-pneumonia-like-organism (PPLO) J15.7
    - pneumococcus J13
    - pneumocystosis (Pneumocystis carinii) (Pneumocystis jiroveci) B59
    - Proteus J15.69
    - Pseudomonas NEC J15.1
      - pseudomallei A24.1
    - psittacosis A7Ø
    - Q fever A78
    - respiratory syncytial virus (RSV) J12.1
    - rheumatic fever IØØ *[J17]*
    - rubella BØ6.81
    - Salmonella (infection) AØ2.22
      - typhi AØ1.Ø3
    - schistosomiasis B65.9 *[J17]*
    - Serratia marcescens J15.69
    - specified
      - bacterium NEC J15.8
      - organism NEC J16.8
    - spirochetal NEC A69.8
    - Staphylococcus J15.2Ø
      - aureus (methicillin susceptible) (MSSA) J15.211
        - methicillin resistant (MRSA) J15.212
      - specified NEC J15.29
    - Streptococcus J15.4
      - group B J15.3
      - pneumoniae J13
      - specified NEC J15.4
    - toxoplasmosis B58.3
    - tularemia A21.2
    - typhoid (fever) AØ1.Ø3
    - varicella BØ1.2
    - virus —*see* Pneumonia, viral

Pneumonia *(Continued)*
- in (due to) *(Continued)*
  - whooping cough A37.91
    - due to
      - Bordetella parapertussis A37.11
      - Bordetella pertussis A37.Ø1
      - specified NEC A37.81
  - Yersinia pestis A2Ø.2
- inhalation of food or vomit *—see* Pneumonia, aspiration
- interstitial J84.9
  - chronic J84.111
  - desquamative J84.117
  - due to
    - collagen vascular disease J84.178
    - known underlying cause J84.178
  - idiopathic NOS J84.111
  - in disease classified elsewhere J84.178
  - lymphocytic (due to collagen vascular disease) (in diseases classified elsewhere) J84.178
  - lymphoid J84.2
  - non-specific J84.89
    - due to
      - collagen vascular disease J84.178
      - known underlying cause J84.178
    - idiopathic J84.113
    - in diseases classified elsewhere J84.178
  - plasma cell B59
  - pseudomonas J15.1
  - usual J84.112
    - due to collagen vascular disease J84.178
    - idiopathic J84.112
    - in diseases classified elsewhere J84.178
- Klebsiella (pneumoniae) J15.Ø
- lipid, lipoid (exogenous) J69.1
  - endogenous J84.89
- lobar (disseminated) (double) (interstitial) J18.1
  - bacterial J15.9
    - specified NEC J15.8
  - chronic *—see* Fibrosis, lung
  - Escherichia coli (E. coli) J15.5
  - Friedländer's bacillus J15.Ø
  - Hemophilus influenzae J14
  - hypostatic J18.2
  - Klebsiella (pneumoniae) J15.Ø
  - pneumococcal J13
  - Proteus J15.69
  - Pseudomonas J15.1
  - specified organism NEC J16.8
  - staphylococcal *—see* Pneumonia, staphylococcal
  - streptococcal NEC J15.4
  - Streptococcus pneumoniae J13
  - viral, virus *—see* Pneumonia, viral
- lobular *—see* Pneumonia, broncho
- Löffler's J82.89
- lymphoid interstitial J84.2
- massive *—see* Pneumonia, lobar
- meconium P24.Ø1
- MRSA (Methicillin resistant Staphylococcus aureus) J15.212
- MSSA (methicillin susceptible Staphylococcus aureus) J15.211
- multilobar *—see* Pneumonia, by type
- Mycoplasma (pneumoniae) J15.7
- necrotic J85.Ø
- neonatal P23.9
  - aspiration *—see* Aspiration, by substance, with pneumonia
- nitrogen dioxide J68.Ø
- organizing J84.89
  - due to
    - collagen vascular disease J84.178
    - known underlying cause J84.178
  - in diseases classified elsewhere J84.178
- orthostatic J18.2
- parainfluenza virus J12.2
- parenchymatous *—see* Fibrosis, lung
- passive J18.2
- patchy *—see* Pneumonia, broncho
- Peptococcus J15.8
- Peptostreptococcus J15.8
- plasma cell (of infants) B59
- pleurolobar *—see* Pneumonia, lobar
- pleuro-pneumonia-like organism (PPLO) J15.7
- pneumococcal (broncho) (lobar) J13
- Pneumocystis (carinii) (jiroveci) B59
- postinfectional NEC B99 *[J17]*
- postmeasles BØ5.2
- Proteus J15.69
- Pseudomonas J15.1
- psittacosis A7Ø
- radiation J7Ø.Ø
  - respiratory syncytial virus (RSV) J12.1
- resulting from a procedure J95.89
- rheumatic IØØ *[J17]*
- Salmonella (arizonae) (cholerae-suis) (enteritidis) (typhimurium) AØ2.22
  - typhi AØ1.Ø3
  - typhoid fever AØ1.Ø3
- SARS-associated coronavirus J12.81
- SARS-CoV-2 J12.82
- segmented, segmental *—see* Pneumonia, broncho-●
- Serratia marcescens J15.69
- specified NEC J18.8
  - bacterium NEC J15.8
  - organism NEC J16.8
  - virus NEC J12.89
- spirochetal NEC A69.8
- staphylococcal (broncho) (lobar) J15.2Ø
  - aureus (methicillin susceptible) (MSSA) J15.211
    - methicillin resistant (MRSA) J15.212
  - specified NEC J15.29
- static, stasis J18.2
- streptococcal NEC (broncho) (lobar) J15.4
  - group
    - A J15.4
    - B J15.3
    - specified NEC J15.4
- Streptococcus pneumoniae J13
- syphilitic, congenital (early) A5Ø.Ø4
- traumatic (complication) (early) (secondary) T79.8
- tuberculous (any) *—see* Tuberculosis, pulmonary
- tularemic A21.2
- varicella BØ1.2
- Veillonella J15.8
- ventilator associated J95.851
- viral, virus (broncho) (interstitial) (lobar) J12.9
  - adenoviral J12.Ø
  - congenital P23.Ø
  - human metapneumovirus J12.3
  - parainfluenza J12.2
  - respiratory syncytial (RSV) J12.1
  - SARS-associated coronavirus J12.81
  - specified NEC J12.89
- white (congenital) A5Ø.Ø4

Pneumonic *—see* condition

Pneumonitis (acute) (primary) (*see also* Pneumonia) J98.4
- air-conditioner J67.7
- allergic (due to) J67.9
  - organic dust NEC J67.8
  - red cedar dust J67.8
  - sequoiosis J67.8
  - wood dust J67.8
- aspiration J69.Ø
  - due to
    - anesthesia J95.4
      - during
        - labor and delivery O74.Ø
        - pregnancy O29.Ø1-●
        - puerperium O89.Ø1
    - fumes or gases J68.Ø
  - obstetric O74.Ø
- chemical (due to gases, fumes or vapors) (inhalation) J68.Ø
  - due to anesthesia J95.4
- cholesterol J84.89
- chronic *—see* Fibrosis, lung
- congenital rubella P35.Ø
- crack (cocaine) J68.Ø
- due to
  - beryllium J68.Ø
  - cadmium J68.Ø
  - crack (cocaine) J68.Ø
  - detergent J69.8
  - fluorocarbon-polymer J68.Ø
  - food, vomit (aspiration) J69.Ø
  - fumes or vapors J68.Ø
  - gases, fumes or vapors (inhalation) J68.Ø
  - inhalation
    - blood J69.8
    - essences J69.1
    - food (regurgitated), milk, vomit J69.Ø
    - oils, essences J69.1
    - saliva J69.Ø
    - solids, liquids NEC J69.8

Pneumonitis *(Continued)*
- due to *(Continued)*
  - manganese J68.Ø
  - nitrogen dioxide J68.Ø
  - oils, essences J69.1
  - solids, liquids NEC J69.8
  - toxoplasmosis (acquired) B58.3
    - congenital P37.1
  - vanadium J68.Ø
  - ventilator J95.851
- eosinophilic J82.81
  - acute J82.82
  - chronic J82.81
- hypersensitivity J67.9
  - air conditioner lung J67.7
  - bagassosis J67.1
  - bird fancier's lung J67.2
  - farmer's lung J67.Ø
  - maltworker's lung J67.4
  - maple bark-stripper's lung J67.6
  - mushroom worker's lung J67.5
  - specified organic dust NEC J67.8
  - suberosis J67.3
- interstitial (chronic) J84.89
  - acute J84.114
  - lymphoid J84.2
  - non-specific J84.89
    - idiopathic J84.113
- lymphoid, interstitial J84.2
- meconium P24.Ø1
- noninfectious J98.4
- postanesthetic J95.4
  - correct substance properly administered *—see* Table of Drugs and Chemcials, by drug, adverse effect
  - in labor and delivery O74.Ø
  - in pregnancy O29.Ø1-●
  - obstetric O74.Ø
  - overdose or wrong substance given or taken (by accident) *—see* Table of Drugs and Chemicals, by drug, poisoning
  - postpartum, puerperal O89.Ø1
- postoperative J95.4
  - obstetric O74.Ø
- radiation J7Ø.Ø
- rubella, congenital P35.Ø
- specified NEC J98.4
- ventilation (air-conditioning) J67.7
- ventilator associated J95.851
- wood-dust J67.8

Pneumonoconiosis *—see* Pneumoconiosis

Pneumoparotid K11.8

Pneumopathy NEC J98.4
- alveolar J84.Ø9
- due to organic dust NEC J66.8
- parietoalveolar J84.Ø9

Pneumopericarditis *—see also* Pericarditis
- acute I3Ø.9

Pneumopericardium *—see also* Pericarditis
- congenital P25.3
- newborn P25.3
- traumatic (post) *—see* Injury, heart

Pneumophagia (psychogenic) F45.8

Pneumopleurisy, pneumopleuritis *—see also* Pneumonia J18.8

Pneumopyopericardium I3Ø.1

Pneumopyothorax *—see* Pyopneumothorax
- with fistula J86.Ø

Pneumorrhagia *—see also* Hemorrhage, lung
- tuberculous *—see* Tuberculosis, pulmonary

Pneumothorax NOS J93.9
- acute J93.83
- chronic J93.81
- congenital P25.1
- perinatal period P25.1
- postprocedural J95.811
- specified NEC J93.83
- spontaneous NOS J93.83
  - newborn P25.1
  - primary J93.11
  - secondary J93.12
  - tension J93.Ø
- tense valvular, infectional J93.Ø
- tension (spontaneous) J93.Ø
- traumatic S27.Ø
  - with hemothorax S27.2
- tuberculous *—see* Tuberculosis, pulmonary

Podagra *—see also* Gout M1Ø.9

Podencephalus QØ1.9

Poikilocytosis R71.8

Poikiloderma L81.6
Civatte's L57.3
congenital Q82.8
vasculare atrophicans L94.5
Poikilodermatomyositis M33.10
with
myopathy M33.12
respiratory involvement M33.11
specified organ involvement NEC M33.19
amyopathic M33.13
without myopathy M33.13
Pointed ear (congenital) Q17.3
Poison ivy, oak, sumac or other plant dermatitis (allergic) (contact) L23.7
Poisoning (acute) —*see also* Table of Drugs and Chemicals
algae and toxins T65.82-●
Bacillus B (aertrycke) (cholerae (suis)) (paratyphosus) (suipestifer) A02.9
botulinus A05.1
bacterial toxins A05.9
berries, noxious —*see* Poisoning, food, noxious, berries
botulism A05.1
ciguatera fish T61.0-●
Clostridium botulinum A05.1
death-cap (Amanita phalloides) (Amanita verna) —*see* Poisoning, food, noxious, mushrooms
drug —*see* Table of Drugs and Chemicals, by drug, poisoning
epidemic, fish (noxious) —*see* Poisoning, seafood
bacterial A05.9
fava bean D55.0
fish (noxious) T61.9-●
bacterial —*see* Intoxication, foodborne, by agent
ciguatera fish —*see* Poisoning, ciguatera fish
scombroid fish —*see* Poisoning, scombroid fish
specified type NEC T61.77-●
food NEC A05.9
bacterial —*see* Intoxication, foodborne, by agent
due to
Bacillus (aertrycke) (choleraesuis) (paratyphosus) (suipestifer) A02.9
botulinus A05.1
Clostridium (perfringens) (Welchii) A05.2
salmonella (aertrycke) (choleraesuis) (enteritidis) (gallinarum) (paratyphi) (suipestifer) A02.9
with
gastroenteritis A02.0
sepsis A02.1
staphylococcus A05.0
Vibrio
parahaemolyticus A05.3
vulnificus A05.5
noxious or naturally toxic T62.9-●
berries —*see* subcategory T62.1-●
fish —*see* Poisoning, seafood
mushrooms —*see* subcategory T62.0X-●
plants NEC —*see* subcategory T62.2X-●
seafood —*see* Poisoning, seafood
specified NEC —*see* subcategory T62.8X-●
ichthyotoxism —*see* Poisoning, seafood
kreotoxism, food A05.9
latex T65.81-●
lead T56.0-●
mushroom —*see* Poisoning, food, noxious, mushroom
mussels —*see also* Poisoning, shellfish
bacterial —*see* Intoxication, foodborne, by agent
nicotine (tobacco) T65.2-●
noxious foodstuffs —*see* Poisoning, food, noxious
plants, noxious —*see* Poisoning, food, noxious, plants NEC
ptomaine —*see* Poisoning, food
radiation J70.0
Salmonella (arizonae) (cholerae-suis) (enteritidis) (typhimurium) A02.9
scombroid fish T61.1-●
seafood (noxious) T61.9-●
bacterial —*see* Intoxication, foodborne, by agent
fish —*see* Poisoning, fish
Poisoning *(Continued)*
seafood *(Continued)*
shellfish —*see* Poisoning, shellfish
specified NEC —*see* subcategory T61.8X-●
shellfish (amnesic) (azaspiracid) (diarrheic) (neurotoxic) (noxious) (paralytic) T61.78-●
bacterial —*see* Intoxication, foodborne, by agent
ciguatera mollusk —*see* Poisoning, ciguatera fish
specified substance NEC T65.891
Staphylococcus, food A05.0
tobacco (nicotine) T65.2-●
water E87.79
Poker spine —*see* Spondylitis, ankylosing
Poland syndrome Q79.8
Polioencephalitis (acute) (bulbar) A80.9
inferior G12.22
influenzal —*see* Influenza, with, encephalopathy
superior hemorrhagic (acute) (Wernicke's) E51.2
Wernicke's E51.2
Polioencephalomyelitis (acute) (anterior) A80.9
with beriberi E51.2
Polioencephalopathy, superior hemorrhagic E51.2
with
beriberi E51.11
pellagra E52
Poliomeningoencephalitis —*see* Meningoencephalitis
Poliomyelitis (acute) (anterior) (epidemic) A80.9
with paralysis (bulbar) —*see* Poliomyelitis, paralytic
abortive A80.4
ascending (progressive) —*see* Poliomyelitis, paralytic
bulbar (paralytic) —*see* Poliomyelitis, paralytic
congenital P35.8
nonepidemic A80.9
nonparalytic A80.4
paralytic A80.30
specified NEC A80.39
vaccine-associated A80.0
wild virus
imported A80.1
indigenous A80.2
spinal, acute A80.9
Poliosis (eyebrow) (eyelashes) L67.1
circumscripta, acquired L67.1
Pollakiuria R35.0
Pollinosis J30.1
Pollitzer's disease L73.2
Polyadenitis —*see also* Lymphadenitis
malignant A20.0
Polyalgia M79.89
Polyangiitis M30.0
microscopic M31.7
overlap syndrome M30.8
Polyarteritis
microscopic M31.7
nodosa M30.0
with lung involvement M30.1
juvenile M30.2
related condition NEC M30.8
Polyarthralgia —*see* Pain, joint
Polyarthritis, polyarthropathy —*see also* Arthritis M13.0
due to or associated with other specified conditions —*see* Arthritis
epidemic (Australian) (with exanthema) B33.1
infective —*see* Arthritis, pyogenic or pyemic
inflammatory M06.4
juvenile (chronic) (seronegative) M08.3
migratory M13.8-●
rheumatic, acute —*see* Fever, rheumatic
Polyarthrosis M15.9
post-traumatic M15.3
primary M15.0
specified NEC M15.8
Polycarential syndrome of infancy E40
Polychondritis (atrophic) (chronic) —*see also* Disorder, cartilage, specified type NEC
relapsing M94.1
Polycoria Q13.2
Polycystic (disease)
degeneration, kidney Q61.3
autosomal dominant (adult type) Q61.2
autosomal recessive (infantile type) NEC Q61.19
Polycystic *(Continued)*
kidney Q61.3
autosomal
dominant Q61.2
recessive NEC Q61.19
autosomal dominant (adult type) Q61.2
autosomal recessive (childhood type) NEC Q61.19
infantile type NEC Q61.19
liver Q44.6
lung J98.4
congenital Q33.0
ovary, ovaries E28.2
spleen Q89.09
Polycythemia (secondary) D75.1
acquired D75.1
benign (familial) D75.0
due to
donor twin P61.1
erythropoietin D75.1
fall in plasma volume D75.1
high altitude D75.1
maternal-fetal transfusion P61.1
stress D75.1
emotional D75.1
erythropoietin D75.1
familial (benign) D75.0
Gaisböck's (hypertonica) D75.1
high altitude D75.1
hypertonica D75.1
hypoxemic D75.1
neonatorum P61.1
nephrogenous D75.1
relative D75.1
secondary D75.1
spurious D75.1
stress D75.1
vera D45
Polycytosis cryptogenica D75.1
Polydactylism, polydactyly Q69.9
toes Q69.2
Polydipsia R63.1
Polydystrophy, pseudo-Hurler E77.0
Polyembryoma —*see* Neoplasm, malignant, by site
Polyglandular
deficiency E31.0
dyscrasia E31.9
dysfunction E31.9
syndrome E31.8
Polyhydramnios O40.-●
Polymastia Q83.1
Polymenorrhea N92.0
Polymyalgia M35.3
arteritica, giant cell M31.5
rheumatica M35.3
with giant cell arteritis M31.5
Polymyositis (acute) (chronic) (hemorrhagic) M33.20
with
myopathy M33.22
respiratory involvement M33.21
skin involvement —*see* Dermatopolymyositis
specified organ involvement NEC M33.29
ossificans (generalisata) (progressiva) —*see* Myositis, ossificans, progressiva
Polyneuritis, polyneuritic —*see also* Polyneuropathy
acute (post-)infective G61.0
alcoholic G62.1
cranialis G52.7
demyelinating, chronic inflammatory (CIDP) G61.81
diabetic —*see* Diabetes, polyneuropathy
diphtheritic A36.83
due to lack of vitamin NEC E56.9 *[G63]*
endemic E51.11
erythredema —*see* subcategory T56.1
febrile, acute G61.0
hereditary ataxic G60.1
idiopathic, acute G61.0
infective (acute) G61.0
inflammatory, chronic demyelinating (CIDP) G61.81
nutritional E63.9 *[G63]*
postinfective (acute) G61.0
specified NEC G62.89
Polyneuropathy (peripheral) G62.9
alcoholic G62.1
amyloid (Portuguese) E85.1 *[G63]*
transthyretin-related (ATTR) familial E85.1

Polyneuropathy *(Continued)*
- arsenical E85.1 *[G63]*
- critical illness G62.81
- demyelinating, chronic inflammatory (CIDP) G61.81
- diabetic *—see* Diabetes, polyneuropathy
- drug-induced G62.Ø
- hereditary G6Ø.9
  - specified NEC G6Ø.8
- idiopathic G6Ø.9
  - progressive G6Ø.3
- in (due to)
  - alcohol G62.1
    - sequelae G65.2
  - amyloidosis, familial (Portuguese) E85.1 *[G63]*
  - antitetanus serum G61.1
  - arsenic G62.2
    - sequelae G65.2
  - avitaminosis NEC E56.9 *[G63]*
  - beriberi E51.11
  - collagen vascular disease NEC M35.9 *[G63]*
  - deficiency (of)
    - B (-complex) vitamins E53.9 *[G63]*
    - vitamin B6 E53.1 *[G63]*
  - diabetes *—see* Diabetes, polyneuropathy
  - diphtheria A36.83
  - drug or medicament G62.Ø
    - correct substance properly administered *—see* Table of Drugs and Chemicals, by drug, adverse effect
    - overdose or wrong substance given or taken *—see* Table of Drugs and Chemicals, by drug, poisoning
  - endocrine disease NEC E34.9 *[G63]*
  - herpes zoster BØ2.23
  - hypoglycemia E16.2 *[G63]*
  - infectious
    - disease NEC B99 *[G63]*
    - mononucleosis B27.91
  - lack of vitamin NEC E56.9 *[G63]*
  - lead G62.2
    - sequelae G65.2
  - leprosy A3Ø.9 *[G63]*
  - Lyme disease A69.22
  - metabolic disease NEC E88.9 *[G63]*
  - microscopic polyangiitis M31.7 *[G63]*
  - mumps B26.84
  - neoplastic disease *—see also* Neoplasm D49.9 *[G63]*
  - nutritional deficiency NEC E63.9 *[G63]*
  - organophosphate compounds G62.2
    - sequelae G65.2
  - parasitic disease NEC B89 *[G63]*
  - pellagra E52 *[G63]*
  - polyarteritis nodosa M3Ø.Ø
  - porphyria E8Ø.2Ø *[G63]*
  - radiation G62.82
  - rheumatoid arthritis *—see* Rheumatoid, polyneuropathy
  - sarcoidosis D86.89
  - serum G61.1
  - syphilis (late) A52.15
    - congenital A5Ø.43
  - systemic
    - connective tissue disorder M35.9 *[G63]*
    - lupus erythematosus M32.19
  - toxic agent NEC G62.2
    - sequelae G65.2
  - transthyretin-related (ATTR) familial amyloid E85.1
  - triorthocresyl phosphate G62.2
    - sequelae G65.2
  - tuberculosis A17.89
  - uremia N18.9 [G63]
  - vitamin B12 deficiency E53.8 [G63]
    - with anemia (pernicious) D51.Ø [G63]
      - due to dietary deficiency D51.3 [G63]
  - zoster BØ2.23
- inflammatory G61.9
  - chronic demyelinating (CIDP) G61.81
  - sequelae G65.1
  - specified NEC G61.89
- lead G62.2
  - sequelae G65.2
- nutritional NEC E63.9 *[G63]*
- postherpetic (zoster) BØ2.23
- progressive G6Ø.3
- radiation-induced G62.82
- sensory (hereditary) (idiopathic) G6Ø.8
- specified NEC G62.89
- syphilitic (late) A52.15
  - congenital A5Ø.43

Polyopia H53.8

Polyorchism, polyorchidism Q55.21

Polyosteoarthritis *—see also* Osteoarthritis, generalized M15.9-●
- post-traumatic M15.3
- specified NEC M15.8

Polyostotic fibrous dysplasia Q78.1

Polyotia Q17.Ø

Polyp, polypus
- accessory sinus J33.8
- adenocarcinoma in *—see* Neoplasm, malignant, by site
- adenocarcinoma in situ in *—see* Neoplasm, in situ, by site
- adenoid tissue J33.Ø
- adenomatous *—see also* Neoplasm, benign, by site
  - adenocarcinoma in *—see* Neoplasm, malignant, by site
  - adenocarcinoma in situ in *—see* Neoplasm, in situ, by site
  - carcinoma in *—see* Neoplasm, malignant, by site
  - carcinoma in situ in *—see* Neoplasm, in situ, by site
  - multiple *—see* Neoplasm, benign
    - adenocarcinoma in *—see* Neoplasm, malignant, by site
    - adenocarcinoma in situ in *—see* Neoplasm, in situ, by site
- antrum J33.8
- anus, anal (canal) K62.Ø
- Bartholin's gland N84.3
- bladder D41.4
- carcinoma in *—see* Neoplasm, malignant, by site
- carcinoma in situ in *—see* Neoplasm, in situ, by site
- cecum D12.Ø
- cervix (uteri) N84.1
  - in pregnancy or childbirth *—see* Pregnancy, complicated by, abnormal, cervix
  - mucous N84.1
  - nonneoplastic N84.1
- choanal J33.Ø
- cholesterol K82.4
- clitoris N84.3
- colon K63.5
  - adenomatous D12.6
    - ascending D12.6
    - cecum D12.Ø
    - descending D12.4
  - ascending K63.5
    - sigmoid D12.5
    - transverse D12.3
  - cecum K63.5
  - descending K63.5
  - inflammatory K51.4Ø
    - with
      - abscess K51.414
      - complication K51.419
        - specified NEC K51.418
      - fistula K51.413
      - intestinal obstruction K51.412
      - rectal bleeding K51.411
  - sigmoid D12.5
  - transverse D12.3
- corpus uteri N84.Ø
- dental KØ4.Ø1
  - irreversible KØ4.Ø2
  - reversible KØ4.Ø1
- duodenum K31.7
- ear (middle) H74.4-●
- endometrium N84.Ø
- esophageal K22.81
- esophagogastric junction K22.82
- ethmoidal (sinus) J33.8
- fallopian tube N84.8
- female genital tract N84.9
  - specified NEC N84.8
- frontal (sinus) J33.8
- gallbladder K82.4
- gingiva, gum KØ6.8
- hyperplastic, (any site) K63.5
- labia, labium (majus) (minus) N84.3
- larynx (mucous) J38.1
  - adenomatous D14.1
- malignant *—see* Neoplasm, malignant, by site
- maxillary (sinus) J33.8
- middle ear *—see* Polyp, ear (middle)
- myometrium N84.Ø

Polyp, polypus *(Continued)*
- nares
  - anterior J33.9
  - posterior J33.Ø
- nasal (mucous) J33.9
  - cavity J33.Ø
  - septum J33.Ø
- nasopharyngeal J33.Ø
- nose (mucous) J33.9
- oviduct N84.8
- pharynx J39.2
- placenta O9Ø.89
- prostate *—see* Enlargement, enlarged, prostate
- pudenda, pudendum N84.3
- pulpal (dental) KØ4.Ø1
  - irreversible KØ4.Ø2
  - reversible KØ4.Ø1
- rectum (nonadenomatous) K62.1
  - adenomatous *—see* Polyp, adenomatous
- septum (nasal) J33.Ø
- sinus (accessory) (ethmoidal) (frontal) (maxillary) (sphenoidal) J33.8
- sphenoidal (sinus) J33.8
- stomach K31.7
  - adenomatous D13.1
- tube, fallopian N84.8
- turbinate, mucous membrane J33.8
- umbilical, newborn P83.6
- ureter N28.89
- urethra N36.2
- uterus (body) (corpus) (mucous) N84.Ø
  - cervix N84.1
  - in pregnancy or childbirth *—see* Pregnancy, complicated by, tumor, uterus
- vagina N84.2
- vocal cord (mucous) J38.1
- vulva N84.3

Polyphagia R63.2

Polyploidy Q92.7

Polypoid *—see* condition

Polyposis *—see also* Polyp
- adenomatous D13.91
- coli (adenomatous) D12.6
  - adenocarcinoma in C18.9
  - adenocarcinoma in situ in *—see* Neoplasm, in situ, by site
  - carcinoma in C18.9
- colon (adenomatous) D12.6
- familial D12.6
  - adenocarcinoma in situ in *—see* Neoplasm, in situ, by site
- intestinal D12.6
  - adenomatous D13.91
- malignant lymphomatous C83.1
- multiple, adenomatous *—see also* Neoplasm, benign D36.9

Polyradiculitis *—see* Polyneuropathy

Polyradiculoneuropathy (acute) (postinfective) (segmentally demyelinating) G61.Ø

Polyserositis
- due to pericarditis I31.1
- pericardial I31.1
- periodic, familial E85.Ø
- tuberculous A19.9
  - acute A19.1
  - chronic A19.8

Polysplenia syndrome Q89.Ø9

Polysyndactyly *—see also* Syndactylism, syndactyly Q7Ø.4

Polytrichia L68.3

Polyunguia Q84.6

Polyuria R35.89
- nocturnal R35.81
- psychogenic F45.8
- specified NEC R35.89

Pompe's disease (glycogen storage) E74.Ø2

Pompholyx L3Ø.1

Poncet's disease (tuberculous rheumatism) A18.Ø9

Pond fracture *—see* Fracture, skull

Ponos B55.Ø

Pons, pontine *—see* condition

Poor
- aesthetic of existing restoration of tooth KØ8.56
- contractions, labor O62.2
- gingival margin to tooth restoration KØ8.51
- personal hygiene R46.Ø
- prenatal care, affecting management of pregnancy *—see* Pregnancy, complicated by, insufficient, prenatal care
- sucking reflex (newborn) R29.2
- urinary stream R39.12
- vision NEC H54.7

Poradenitis, nostras inguinalis or venerea A55
Porencephaly (congenital) (developmental) (true) Q04.6
  acquired G93.Ø
  nondevelopmental G93.Ø
  traumatic (post) FØ7.89
Porocephaliasis B88.8
Porokeratosis Q82.8
Poroma, eccrine —*see* Neoplasm, skin, benign
Porphyria (South African) E8Ø.2Ø
  acquired E8Ø.2Ø
  acute intermittent (hepatic) (Swedish) E8Ø.21
  cutanea tarda (hereditary) (symptomatic) E8Ø.1
  due to drugs E8Ø.2Ø
    correct substance properly administered —*see* Table of Drugs and Chemicals, by drug, adverse effect
    overdose or wrong substance given or taken —*see* Table of Drugs and Chemicals, by drug, poisoning
  erythropoietic (congenital) (hereditary) E8Ø.Ø
  hepatocutaneous type E8Ø.1
  secondary E8Ø.2Ø
  toxic NEC E8Ø.2Ø
  variegata E8Ø.2Ø
Porphyrinuria —*see* Porphyria
Porphyruria —*see* Porphyria
Portal —*see* condition
Port wine nevus, mark, or stain Q82.5
Posadas-Wernicke disease B38.9
Positive
  culture (nonspecific)
    blood R78.81
    bronchial washings R84.5
    cerebrospinal fluid R83.5
    cervix uteri R87.5
    nasal secretions R84.5
    nipple discharge R89.5
    nose R84.5
      staphylococcus (Methicillin susceptible) Z22.321
        Methicillin resistant Z22.322
    peritoneal fluid R85.5
    pleural fluid R84.5
    prostatic secretions R86.5
    saliva R85.5
    seminal fluid R86.5
    sputum R84.5
    synovial fluid R89.5
    throat scrapings R84.5
    urine R82.79
    vagina R87.5
    vulva R87.5
    wound secretions R89.5
  PPD (skin test) R76.11
  serology for syphilis A53.Ø
    with signs or symptoms - code as Syphilis, by site and stage
    false R76.8
  skin test, tuberculin (without active tuberculosis) R76.11
  test, human immunodeficiency virus (HIV) R75
  VDRL A53.Ø
    with signs or symptoms - code by site and stage under Syphilis A53.9
  Wassermann reaction A53.Ø
Post COVID-19 condition, unspecified UØ9.9
Postcardiotomy syndrome I97.Ø
Postcaval ureter Q62.62
Postcholecystectomy syndrome K91.5
Postclimacteric bleeding N95.Ø
Postcommissurotomy syndrome I97.Ø
Postconcussional syndrome FØ7.81
Postcontusional syndrome FØ7.81
Postcricoid region —*see* condition
Post-dates (40-42 weeks) (pregnancy) (mother) O48.Ø
  more than 42 weeks gestation O48.1
Postencephalitic syndrome FØ7.89
Posterior —*see* condition
Posterolateral sclerosis (spinal cord) —*see* Degeneration, combined
Postexanthematous —*see* condition
Postfebrile —*see* condition
Postgastrectomy dumping syndrome K91.1
Posthemiplegic chorea —*see* Monoplegia
Posthemorrhagic anemia (chronic) D5Ø.Ø
  acute D62
  newborn P61.3
Postherpetic neuralgia (zoster) BØ2.29
  trigeminal BØ2.22
Posthitis N47.7
Postimmunization complication or reaction —*see* Complications, vaccination
Postinfectious —*see* condition
Postlaminectomy syndrome NEC M96.1
Postleukotomy syndrome FØ7.Ø
Postmastectomy lymphedema (syndrome) I97.2
Postmaturity, postmature (over 42 weeks)
  maternal (over 42 weeks gestation) O48.1
  newborn PØ8.22
Postmeasles complication NEC —*see also* condition BØ5.89
Postmenopausal
  endometrium (atrophic) N95.8
    suppurative —*see also* Endometritis N71.9
  osteoporosis —*see* Osteoporosis, postmenopausal
Postnasal drip RØ9.82
  due to
    allergic rhinitis —*see* Rhinitis, allergic
    common cold JØØ
    gastroesophageal reflux —*see* Reflux, gastroesophageal
    nasopharyngitis —*see* Nasopharyngitis
    other know condition — code to condition
    sinusitis —*see* Sinusitis
Postnatal —*see* condition
Postoperative (postprocedural) —*see also* Complication, postoperative
  pneumothorax, therapeutic Z98.3
  state NEC Z98.89Ø
  visit - *see* Aftercare
  wound check - *see* Aftercare
Postpancreatectomy hyperglycemia E89.1
Postpartum —*see* Puerperal
Postphlebitic syndrome —*see* Syndrome, postthrombotic
Postpolio (myelitic) syndrome G14
Postpoliomyelitic —*see also* condition
  osteopathy —*see* Osteopathy, after poliomyelitis
Postprocedural —*see also* Postoperative
  hypoinsulinemia E89.1
Postschizophrenic depression F32.89
Postsurgery status —*see also* Status (post)
  pneumothorax, therapeutic Z98.3
Post-term (40-42 weeks) (pregnancy) (mother) O48.Ø
  infant PØ8.21
  more than 42 weeks gestation (mother) O48.1
Post-traumatic brain syndrome, nonpsychotic FØ7.81
Post-typhoid abscess AØ1.Ø9
Postures, hysterical F44.2
Postvaccinal reaction or complication —*see* Complications, vaccination
Postvalvulotomy syndrome I97.Ø
Potain's
  disease (pulmonary edema) —*see* Edema, lung
  syndrome (gastrectasis with dyspepsia) K31.Ø
POTS (postural orthostatic tachycardia syndrome) G9Ø.A
Potter's
  asthma J62.8
  facies Q6Ø.6
  lung J62.8
  syndrome (with renal agenesis) Q6Ø.6
Pott's
  curvature (spinal) A18.Ø1
  disease or paraplegia A18.Ø1
  spinal curvature A18.Ø1
  tumor, puffy —*see* Osteomyelitis, specified type NEC
Pouch
  bronchus Q32.4
  Douglas' —*see* condition
  esophagus, esophageal, congenital Q39.6
    acquired K22.5
  gastric K31.4
  Hartmann's K82.8
  pharynx, pharyngeal (congenital) Q38.7
Pouchitis K91.85Ø
Poultrymen's itch B88.Ø
Poverty NEC Z59.6
  extreme Z59.5
Poxvirus NEC BØ8.8
Prader-Willi syndrome Q87.11
Prader-Willi-like syndrome Q87.11
Preauricular appendage or tag Q17.Ø
Prebetalipoproteinemia (acquired) (essential) (familial) (hereditary) (primary) (secondary) E78.1
  with chylomicronemia E78.3
Precipitate labor or delivery O62.3
Preclimacteric bleeding (menorrhagia) N92.4
Precocious
  adrenarche E3Ø.1
  menarche E3Ø.1
  menstruation E3Ø.1
  pubarche E3Ø.1
  puberty E3Ø.1
    central E22.8
  sexual development NEC E3Ø.1
  thelarche E3Ø.8
Precocity, sexual (constitutional) (cryptogenic) (female) (idiopathic) (male) E3Ø.1
  with adrenal hyperplasia E25.9
    congenital E25.Ø
Precordial pain RØ7.2
Predeciduous teeth KØØ.2
Prediabetes, prediabetic R73.Ø3
  complicating
    pregnancy —*see* Pregnancy, complicated by, diseases of, specified type or system NEC
    puerperium O99.893
Predislocation status of hip at birth Q65.6
Pre-eclampsia O14.9- ●
  with pre-existing hypertension —*see* Hypertension, complicating pregnancy, pre-existing, with, pre-eclampsia
  complicating
    childbirth O14.94
    puerperium O14.95
  mild O14.Ø- ●
    complicating
      childbirth O14.Ø4
      puerperium O14.Ø5
  moderate O14.Ø- ●
    complicating
      childbirth O14.Ø4
      puerperium O14.Ø5
  severe O14.1- ●
    with hemolysis, elevated liver enzymes and low platelet count (HELLP) O14.2- ●
      complicating
        childbirth O14.24
        puerperium O14.25
    complicating
      childbirth O14.14
      puerperium O14.15
Pre-eruptive color change, teeth, tooth KØØ.8
Pre-excitation atrioventricular conduction I45.6
Preglaucoma H4Ø.ØØ- ●
Pregnancy (single) (uterine) —*see also* Delivery and Puerperal Z33.1

Note: The Tabular must be reviewed for assignment of the appropriate character indicating the trimester of the pregnancy

Note: The Tabular must be reviewed for assignment of appropriate seventh character for multiple gestation codes in Chapter 15

  abdominal (ectopic) OØØ.ØØ
    with intrauterine pregnancy OØØ.Ø1
    with viable fetus O36.7- ●
  ampullar OØØ.1Ø- ●
    with intrauterine pregnancy OØØ.11- ●
  biochemical OØ2.81
  broad ligament OØØ.8Ø
    with intrauterine pregnancy OØØ.81
  cervical OØØ.8Ø
    with intrauterine pregnancy OØØ.81
  chemical OØ2.81
  complicated NOS O26.9- ●
  complicated by (care of) (management affected by)
    abnormal, abnormality
      cervix O34.4- ●
        causing obstructed labor O65.5
      cord (umbilical) O69.9
      fetal heart rate or rhythm O36.83- ●
      findings on antenatal screening of mother O28.9
        biochemical O28.1
        chromosomal O28.5
        cytological O28.2
        genetic O28.5
        hematological O28.Ø
        radiological O28.4
        specified NEC O28.8
        ultrasonic O28.3
      glucose (tolerance) NEC O99.81Ø

P

P

P

- **Presence** *(Continued)*
  - cardioverter-defibrillator (ICD) Z95.81Ø
  - cerebrospinal fluid drainage device Z98.2
  - cochlear implant (functional) Z96.21
  - contact lens (es) Z97.3
  - coronary artery graft or prosthesis Z95.5
  - CRT-D (cardiac resynchronization therapy defibrillator) Z95.81Ø
  - CRT-P (cardiac resynchronization therapy pacemaker) Z95.Ø
  - cardioverter-defribrillator (ICD) Z95.81Ø
  - CSF shunt Z98.2
  - dental prosthesis device Z97.2
  - dentures Z97.2
  - device (external) NEC Z97.8
    - cardiac NEC Z95.818
    - heart assist Z95.811
    - implanted (functional) Z96.9
      - specified NEC Z96.89
    - prosthetic Z97.8
  - ear implant Z96.2Ø
    - cochlear implant Z96.21
    - myringotomy tube Z96.22
    - specified type NEC Z96.29
  - elbow-joint implant (functional) (prosthesis) Z96.62-•
  - endocrine implant (functional) NEC Z96.49
  - eustachian tube stent or device (functional) Z96.29
  - external hearing-aid or device Z97.4
  - finger-joint implant (functional) (prosthetic) Z96.69-•
  - functional implant Z96.9
    - specified NEC Z96.89
  - graft
    - cardiac NEC Z95.818
    - vascular NEC Z95.828
  - hearing-aid or device (external) Z97.4
    - implant (bone) (cochlear) (functional) Z96.21
  - heart assist device Z95.811
  - heart valve implant (functional) Z95.2
    - prosthetic Z95.2
    - specified type NEC Z95.4
    - xenogenic Z95.3
  - hip-joint implant (functional) (prosthesis) Z96.64-•
  - ICD (cardioverter-defibrillator) Z95.81Ø
  - implanted device (artificial) (functional) (prosthetic) Z96.9
    - automatic cardiac defibrillator (with synchronous cardiac pacemaker)Z95.81Ø
    - cardiac pacemaker Z95.Ø
    - cochlear Z96.21
    - dental Z96.5
    - heart Z95.812
    - heart valve Z95.2
      - prosthetic Z95.2
      - specified NEC Z95.4
      - xenogenic Z95.3
    - insulin pump Z96.41
    - intraocular lens Z96.1
    - joint Z96.6Ø
      - ankle Z96.66-•
      - elbow Z96.62-•
      - finger Z96.69-•
      - hip Z96.64-•
      - Pknee Z96.65-•
      - shoulder Z96.61-•
      - specified NEC Z96.698
      - wrist Z96.63-•
    - larynx Z96.3
    - myringotomy tube Z96.22
    - otological Z96.2Ø
      - cochlear Z96.21
      - eustachian stent Z96.29
      - myringotomy Z96.22
      - specified NEC Z96.29
      - stapes Z96.29
    - skin Z96.81
    - skull plate Z96.7
    - specified NEC Z96.89
    - urogenital Z96.Ø
  - insulin pump (functional) Z96.41
  - intestinal bypass or anastomosis Z98.Ø
  - intraocular lens (functional) Z96.1
  - intrauterine contraceptive device (IUD) Z97.5
  - intravascular implant (functional) (prosthetic) NEC Z95.9
    - coronary artery Z95.5
    - defibrillator (with synchronous cardiac pacemaker) Z95.81Ø
    - peripheral vessel (with angioplasty) Z95.82Ø
- **Presence** *(Continued)*
  - joint implant (prosthetic) (any) Z96.6Ø
    - ankle *—see* Presence, ankle joint implant
    - elbow *—see* Presence, elbow joint implant
    - finger *—see* Presence, finger joint implant
    - hip *—see* Presence, hip joint implant
    - knee *—see* Presence, knee joint implant
    - shoulder *—see* Presence, shoulder joint implant
    - specified joint NEC Z96.698
    - wrist *—see* Presence, wrist joint implant
  - knee-joint implant (functional) (prosthesis) Z96.65-•
  - laryngeal implant (functional) Z96.3
  - mandibular implant (dental) Z96.5
  - myringotomy tube(s) Z96.22
  - neurostimulator (brain) (gastric) (peripheral nerve) (sacral nerve) (spinal cord) (vagus nerve) Z96.82
  - orthopedic-joint implant (prosthetic) (any) *—see* Presence, joint implant
  - otological implant (functional) Z96.29
  - shoulder-joint implant (functional) (prosthesis) Z96.61-•
  - skull-plate implant Z96.7
  - spectacles Z97.3
  - stapes implant (functional) Z96.29
  - systemic lupus erythematosus [SLE] inhibitor D68.62
  - tendon implant (functional) (graft) Z96.7
  - tooth root(s) implant Z96.5
  - ureteral stent Z96.Ø
  - urethral stent Z96.Ø
  - urogenital implant (functional) Z96.Ø
  - vascular implant or device Z95.9
    - access port device Z95.828
    - specified type NEC Z95.828
  - wrist-joint implant (functional) (prosthesis) Z96.63-•
- **Presenile** *—see also* condition
  - dementia FØ3
  - premature aging E34.8
- **Presentation, fetal** *—see* Delivery, complicated by, malposition
- **Prespondylolisthesis** (congenital) Q76.2
- **Pressure**
  - area, skin *—see* Ulcer, pressure, by site
  - brachial plexus G54.Ø
  - brain G93.5
    - injury at birth NEC P11.1
  - cerebral *—see* Pressure, brain
  - chest RØ7.89
  - cone, tentorial G93.5
  - hyposystolic *—see also* Hypotension
    - incidental reading, without diagnosis of hypotension RØ3.1
  - increased
    - intracranial, benign G93.2
      - injury at birth P11.Ø
    - intraocular H4Ø.Ø5-•
  - injury *—see* Ulcer, pressure, by site
  - lumbosacral plexus G54.1
  - mediastinum J98.59
  - necrosis (chronic) *—see* Ulcer, pressure, by site
  - parental, inappropriate (excessive) Z62.6
  - sore (chronic) *—see* Ulcer, pressure, by site
  - spinal cord G95.2Ø
  - ulcer (chronic) *—see* Ulcer, pressure, by site
  - venous, increased I87.8
- **Pre-syncope** R55
- **Preterm**
  - delivery (*see also* Pregnancy, complicated by, preterm labor) O6Ø.1Ø
  - labor *—see* Pregnancy, complicated by, preterm labor
  - newborn (infant) PØ7.3Ø
    - gestational age
      - 28 completed weeks (28 weeks, Ø days through 28 weeks, 6 days) PØ7.31
      - 29 completed weeks (29 weeks, Ø days through 29 weeks, 6 days) PØ7.32
      - 3Ø completed weeks (3Ø weeks, Ø days through 3Ø weeks, 6 days) PØ7.33
      - 31 completed weeks (31 weeks, Ø days through 31 weeks, 6 days) PØ7.34
      - 32 completed weeks (32 weeks, Ø days through 32 weeks, 6 days) PØ7.35
      - 33 completed weeks (33 weeks, Ø days through 33 weeks, 6 days) PØ7.36
      - 34 completed weeks (34 weeks, Ø days through 34 weeks, 6 days) PØ7.37
- **Preterm** *(Continued)*
  - newborn *(Continued)*
    - gestational age *(Continued)*
      - 35 completed weeks (35 weeks, Ø days through 35 weeks, 6 days) PØ7.38
      - 36 completed weeks (36 weeks, Ø days through 36 weeks, 6 days) PØ7.39
- **Previa**
  - placenta (total) (without hemorrhage) O44.Ø-•
    - with hemorrhage O44.1-•
    - complete O44.Ø-•
      - with hemorrhage O44.1-•
    - low *—see also* Delivery, complicated, by, placenta, low O44.4-•
      - with hemorrhage O44.5-•
    - marginal O44.2-•
      - with hemorrhage O44.3-•
    - partial O44.2-•
      - with hemorrhage O44.3-•
  - vasa O69.4
- **Priapism** N48.3Ø
  - due to
    - disease classified elsewhere N48.32
    - drug N48.33
    - specified cause NEC N48.39
    - trauma N48.31
- **Prickling sensation** (skin) R2Ø.2
- **Prickly heat** L74.Ø
- **Primary** *—see* condition
- **Primigravida**
  - elderly, affecting management of pregnancy, labor and delivery (supervision only) *—see* Pregnancy, complicated by, elderly, primigravida
  - older, affecting management of pregnancy, labor and delivery (supervision only) *—see* Pregnancy, complicated by, elderly, primigravida
  - very young, affecting management of pregnancy, labor and delivery (supervision only) *—see* Pregnancy, complicated by, young mother, primigravida
- **Primipara**
  - elderly, affecting management of pregnancy, labor and delivery (supervision only) *—see* Pregnancy, complicated by, elderly, primigravida
  - older, affecting management of pregnancy, labor and delivery (supervision only) *—see* Pregnancy, complicated by, elderly, primigravida
  - very young, affecting management of pregnancy, labor and delivery (supervision only) *—see* Pregnancy, complicated by, young mother, primigravida
- **Primus varus** (bilateral) Q66.21-•
- **PRIND** (Prolonged reversible ischemic neurologic deficit) I63.9
- **Pringle's disease** (tuberous sclerosis)Q85.1
- **Prinzmetal angina** I2Ø.1
- **Prizefighter ear** *—see* Cauliflower ear
- **Problem** (with) (related to)
  - academic Z55.8
  - acculturation Z6Ø.3
  - adjustment (to)
    - change of job Z56.1
    - life-cycle transition Z6Ø.Ø
    - pension Z6Ø.Ø
    - retirement Z6Ø.Ø
  - adopted child Z62.821
  - alcoholism in family Z63.72
  - atypical parenting situation Z62.9
  - bankruptcy Z59.89
  - behavioral (adult) F69
    - drug seeking Z76.5
  - birth of sibling affecting child Z62.898
  - care (of)
    - provider dependency Z74.9
      - specified NEC Z74.8
    - sick or handicapped person in family or household Z63.6
  - child
    - abuse (affecting the child) *—see* Maltreatment, child
    - custody or support proceedings Z65.3
    - in
      - care of non-parental family member Z62.23
      - custody of
        - grandparent Z62.23
        - non-parental relative Z62.23
        - non-relative guardian Z62.24

P

P

P

Protrusion, protrusio *(Continued)*
- device, implant or graft *(Continued)*
  - genital NEC T83.498
    - intrauterine contraceptive device T83.39
    - ➠penile prosthesis (cylinder) (implanted) (pump) (reservoir) T83.490
    - testicular prosthesis T83.491
  - heart NEC —*see* Complication, cardiovascular device, mechanical
  - joint prosthesis —*see* Complications, joint prosthesis, mechanical, specified NEC, by site
  - ocular NEC —*see* Complications, prosthetic device, mechanical, ocular device
  - orthopedic NEC —*see* Complication, orthopedic, device, mechanical
  - specified NEC T85.628
  - urinary NEC —*see also* Complication, genitourinary, device, urinary, mechanical
    - graft T83.29
  - vascular NEC —*see* Complication, cardiovascular device, mechanical
  - ventricular intracranial shunt T85.09
- intervertebral disc —*see* Displacement, intervertebral disc
- joint prosthesis —*see* Complications, joint prosthesis, mechanical, specified NEC, by site
- nucleus pulposus —*see* Displacement, intervertebral disc

Prune belly (syndrome) Q79.4
Prurigo (ferox) (gravis) (Hebrae) (Hebra's) (mitis) (simplex) L28.2
- Besnier's L20.0
- estivalis L56.4
- nodularis L28.1
- psychogenic F45.8

Pruritus, pruritic (essential) L29.9
- ani, anus L29.0
  - psychogenic F45.8
- anogenital L29.3
  - psychogenic F45.8
- ▶cholestatic L29.81
- due to onchocerca volvulus B73.1
- gravidarum —*see* Pregnancy, complicated by, specified pregnancy-related condition NEC
- ➠hiemalis L29.89
- neurogenic (any site) F45.8
- perianal L29.0
- psychogenic (any site) F45.8
- scroti, scrotum L29.1
  - psychogenic F45.8
- ➠senile, senilis L29.89
- ➠specified NEC L29.89
  - psychogenic F45.8
- Trichomonas A59.9
- vulva, vulvae L29.2
  - psychogenic F45.8

Pseudarthrosis, pseudoarthrosis (bone) —*see* Nonunion, fracture
- clavicle, congenital Q74.0
- joint, following fusion or arthrodesis M96.0

Pseudoaneurysm —*see* Aneurysm
Pseudoangina (pectoris) —*see* Angina
Pseudoangioma I81
Pseudoarteriosus Q28.8
Pseudoarthrosis —*see* Pseudarthrosis
Pseudobulbar affect (PBA) F48.2
Pseudochromhidrosis L67.8
Pseudocirrhosis, liver, pericardial I31.1
Pseudocowpox B08.03
Pseudocoxalgia M91.3-●
Pseudocroup J38.5
Pseudo-Cushing's syndrome, alcohol-induced E24.4
Pseudocyesis F45.8
Pseudocyst
- lung J98.4
- pancreas K86.3
- retina —*see* Cyst, retina

Pseudoelephantiasis neuroarthritica Q82.0
Pseudoexfoliation, capsule (lens) —*see* Cataract, specified NEC
Pseudofolliculitis barbae L73.1
Pseudoglioma H44.89
Pseudohemophilia (Bernuth's) (hereditary) (type B) —*see* Disease, von Willebrand
- Type A D69.8
- vascular D69.8

Pseudohermaphroditism Q56.3
- adrenal E25.8
- female (*see also* Disorder, adrenogenital) Q56.2
  - with adrenocortical disorder E25.8
  - without adrenocortical disorder Q56.2
  - adrenal (congenital) E25.0
- male (*see also* Disorder, adrenogenital) Q56.1
  - with
    - adrenocortical disorder E25.8
    - androgen resistance E34.51
    - cleft scrotum Q56.1
    - feminizing testis E34.51
    - 5-alpha-reductase deficiency E29.1
  - without gonadal disorder Q56.1
  - adrenal E25.8

Pseudo-Hurler's polydystrophy E77.0
Pseudohydrocephalus G93.2
Pseudohypertrophic muscular dystrophy (Erb's) G71.02
Pseudohypertrophy, muscle (*see also* Dystrophy, muscular, by type, if applicable) G71.09
Pseudohypoparathyroidism E20.1
Pseudoinsomnia F51.03
Pseudoleukemia, infantile D64.89
Pseudomembranous —*see* condition
Pseudomeningocele (cerebral) (infective) (post-traumatic) G96.198
- postprocedural (spinal) G97.82

Pseudomenses (newborn) P54.6
Pseudomenstruation (newborn) P54.6
Pseudomonas
- aeruginosa, as cause of disease classified elsewhere B96.5
- mallei infection A24.0
  - as cause of disease classified elsewhere B96.5
- pseudomallei, as cause of disease classified elsewhere B96.5

Pseudomyotonia G71.19
Pseudomyxoma peritonei C78.6
Pseudoneuritis, optic (nerve) (disc) (papilla), **congenital** Q14.2
Pseudo-obstruction intestine (acute) (chronic) (idiopathic) (intermittent secondary) (primary) K59.89
- colonic K59.81

Pseudopapilledema H47.33-●
- congenital Q14.2

Pseudoparalysis
- arm or leg R29.818
- atonic, congenital P94.2

Pseudopelade L66.0
Pseudophakia Z96.1
Pseudopolyarthritis, rhizomelic M35.3
Pseudopolycythemia D75.1
Pseudopseudohypoparathyroidism E20.1
Pseudopterygium H11.81-●
Pseudoptosis (eyelid) —*see* Blepharochalasis
Pseudopuberty, precocious
- female heterosexual E25.8
- male isosexual E25.8

Pseudorickets (renal) N25.0
Pseudorubella B08.20
Pseudosclerema, newborn P83.88
Pseudosclerosis (brain)
- Jakob's —*see* Creutzfeldt-Jakob disease or syndrome
- of Westphal (Strüümpell) E83.01
- spastic —*see* Creutzfeldt-Jakob disease or syndrome

Pseudotetanus —*see* Convulsions
Pseudotetany R29.0
- hysterical F44.5

Pseudotruncus arteriosus Q25.49
Pseudotuberculosis A28.2
- enterocolitis A04.8
- pasteurella (infection) A28.0

Pseudotumor G93.2
- cerebri G93.2
- orbital H05.11-●

Pseudoxanthoma elasticum Q82.8
Psilosis (sprue) (tropical) K90.1
- nontropical K90.0

Psittacosis A70
Psoitis M60.88
Psoriasis L40.9
- arthropathic L40.50
  - arthritis mutilans L40.52
  - distal interphalangeal L40.51
  - juvenile L40.54
  - other specified L40.59
  - spondylitis L40.53

Psoriasis *(Continued)*
- buccal K13.29
- flexural L40.8
- guttate L40.4
- mouth K13.29
- nummular L40.0
- plaque L40.0
- psychogenic F54
- pustular (generalized) L40.1
  - palmaris et plantaris L40.3
- specified NEC L40.8
- vulgaris L40.0

Psychasthenia F48.8
Psychiatric disorder or problem F99
Psychogenic —*see also* condition
- factors associated with physical conditions F54

Psychological and behavioral factors affecting medical condition F59
Psychoneurosis, psychoneurotic —*see also* Neurosis
- anxiety (state) F41.1
- depersonalization F48.1
- hypochondriacal F45.21
- hysteria F44.9
- neurasthenic F48.8
- personality NEC F60.89

Psychopathy, psychopathic
- affectionless F94.2
- autistic F84.5
- constitution, post-traumatic F07.81
- personality —*see* Disorder, personality
- sexual —*see* Deviation, sexual
- state F60.2

Psychosexual identity disorder of childhood F64.2
Psychosis, psychotic F29
- acute (transient) F23
  - hysterical F44.9
- affective —*see* Disorder, mood
- alcoholic F10.959
  - with
    - abuse F10.159
    - anxiety disorder F10.980
      - with
        - abuse F10.180
        - dependence F10.280
    - delirium tremens F10.231
    - delusions F10.950
      - with
        - abuse F10.150
        - dependence F10.250
    - dementia F10.97
      - with dependence F10.27
    - dependence F10.259
    - hallucinosis F10.951
      - with
        - abuse F10.151
        - dependence F10.251
    - mood disorder F10.94
      - with
        - abuse F10.14
        - dependence F10.24
    - paranoia F10.950
      - with
        - abuse F10.150
        - dependence F10.250
    - persisting amnesia F10.96
      - with dependence F10.26
  - amnestic confabulatory F10.96
    - with dependence F10.26
  - delirium tremens F10.231
  - Korsakoff's, Korsakov's, Korsakow's F10.26
  - paranoid type F10.950
    - with
      - abuse F10.150
      - dependence F10.250
- anergastic —*see* Psychosis, organic
- arteriosclerotic (simple type) (uncomplicated) (*see also* Dementia, vascular) F01.50
  - with behavioral disturbance —*see* Dementia, vascular
- childhood F84.0
  - atypical F84.8
- climacteric —*see* Psychosis, involutional
- confusional F29
  - acute or subacute F05
  - reactive F23
- cycloid F23
- depressive —*see* Disorder, depressive
- disintegrative (childhood) F84.3
- drug-induced —*see* F11-F19 with .x59
  - paranoid and hallucinatory states —*see* F11-F19 with .x50 or .x51

P

- **Psychosis, psychotic** *(Continued)*
  - due to or associated with
    - addiction, drug —*see* F11-F19 with .X59
    - dependence
      - alcohol F10.259
      - drug —*see* F11-F19 with .x59
    - epilepsy F06.8
    - Huntington's chorea F06.8
    - ischemia, cerebrovascular (generalized) F06.8
    - multiple sclerosis F06.8
    - physical disease F06.8
    - presenile dementia F03
    - senile dementia F03
    - vascular disease (arteriosclerotic) (cerebral) (*see also* Dementia, vascular) F01.50
      - with behavioral disturbance —*see* Dementia, vascular
  - epileptic F06.8
  - episode F23
    - due to or associated with physical condition F06.8
  - exhaustive F43.0
  - hallucinatory, chronic F28
  - hypomanic F30.8
  - hysterical (acute) F44.9
  - induced F24
  - infantile F84.0
    - atypical F84.8
  - infective (acute) (subacute) F05
  - involutional F28
    - depressive —*see* Disorder, depressive
    - melancholic —*see* Disorder, depressive
    - paranoid (state) F22
  - Korsakoff's, Korsakov's, Korsakow's (nonalcoholic) F04
    - alcoholic F10.96
      - in dependence F10.26
    - induced by other psychoactive substance —*see* categories F11-F19 with .x5x
  - mania, manic (single episode) F30.2
    - recurrent type F31.89
  - manic-depressive —*see* Disorder, bipolar
  - menopausal —*see* Psychosis, involutional
  - mixed schizophrenic and affective F25.8
  - multi-infarct (cerebrovascular) (*see also* Dementia, vascular) F01.50
    - with behavioral disturbance —*see* Dementia, vascular
  - nonorganic F29
    - specified NEC F28
  - organic F09
    - due to or associated with
      - arteriosclerosis (cerebral) —*see* Psychosis, arteriosclerotic
      - cerebrovascular disease, arteriosclerotic —*see* Psychosis, arteriosclerotic
      - childbirth —*see* Psychosis, puerperal
      - Creutzfeldt-Jakob disease or syndrome —*see* Creutzfeldt-Jakob disease or syndrome
      - dependence, alcohol F10.259
      - disease
        - alcoholic liver F10.259
        - brain, arteriosclerotic —*see* Psychosis, arteriosclerotic
        - cerebrovascular (*see also* Dementia, vascular) F01.50
          - with behavioral disturbance —*see* Dementia, vascular
        - Creutzfeldt-Jakob —*see* Creutzfeldt-Jakob disease or syndrome
        - endocrine or metabolic F06.8
          - acute or subacute F05
        - liver, alcoholic F10.259
      - epilepsy transient (acute) F05
      - infection
        - brain (intracranial) F06.8
          - acute or subacute F05
      - intoxication
        - alcoholic (acute) F10.259
        - drug F11-F19 with .x59
      - ischemia, cerebrovascular (generalized) —*see* Psychosis, arteriosclerotic
      - puerperium —*see* Psychosis, puerperal
      - trauma, brain (birth) (from electric current) (surgical) F06.8
        - acute or subacute F05
    - infective F06.8
      - acute or subacute F05
    - post-traumatic F06.8
      - acute or subacute F05
- **Psychosis, psychotic** *(Continued)*
  - paranoiac F22
  - paranoid (climacteric) (involutional) (menopausal) F22
    - psychogenic (acute) F23
    - schizophrenic F20.0
    - senile F03
  - postpartum F53.1
  - presbyophrenic (type) F03
  - presenile F03
  - psychogenic (paranoid) F23
    - depressive F32.3
  - puerperal F53.1
    - specified type —*see* Psychosis, by type
  - reactive (brief) (transient) (emotional stress) (psychological trauma) F23
    - depressive F32.3
      - recurrent F33.3
    - excitative type F30.8
  - schizoaffective F25.9
    - depressive type F25.1
    - manic type F25.0
  - schizophrenia, schizophrenic —*see* Schizophrenia
  - schizophrenia-like, in epilepsy F06.2
  - schizophreniform F20.81
    - affective type F25.9
    - brief F23
    - confusional type F23
    - mixed type F25.0
  - senile NEC F03
    - depressed or paranoid type F03
    - simple deterioration F03
    - specified type — code to condition
  - shared F24
  - situational (reactive) F23
  - symbiotic (childhood) F84.3
  - symptomatic F09
- **Psychosomatic** —*see* Disorder, psychosomatic
- **Psychosyndrome, organic** F07.9
- **Psychotic episode due to or associated with physical condition** F06.8
- **Pterygium** (eye) H11.00-•
  - amyloid H11.01-•
  - central H11.02-•
  - colli Q18.3
  - double H11.03-•
  - peripheral
    - progressive H11.05-•
    - stationary H11.04-•
  - recurrent H11.06-•
- **Ptilosis** (eyelid) —*see* Madarosis
- **Ptomaine** (poisoning) —*see* Poisoning, food
- **Ptosis** —*see also* Blepharoptosis
  - adiposa (false) —*see* Blepharoptosis
  - breast N64.81
  - brow H57.81-•
  - cecum K63.4
  - colon K63.4
  - congenital (eyelid) Q10.0
    - specified site NEC —*see* Anomaly, by site
  - eyebrow H57.81-•
  - eyelid —*see* Blepharoptosis
    - congenital Q10.0
  - gastric K31.89
  - intestine K63.4
  - kidney N28.83
  - liver K76.89
  - renal N28.83
  - splanchnic K63.4
  - spleen D73.89
  - stomach K31.89
  - viscera K63.4
- **PTP** D69.51
- **Ptyalism** (periodic) K11.7
  - hysterical F45.8
  - pregnancy —*see* Pregnancy, complicated by, specified pregnancy-related condition NEC
  - psychogenic F45.8
- **Ptyalolithiasis** K11.5
- **Pubarche, precocious** E30.1
- **Pubertas praecox** E30.1
- **Puberty** (development state) Z00.3
  - bleeding (excessive) N92.2
  - delayed E30.0
  - precocious (constitutional) (cryptogenic) (idiopathic) E30.1
    - central E22.8
    - due to
      - ovarian hyperfunction E28.1
        - estrogen E28.0
      - testicular hyperfunction E29.0
- **Puberty** *(Continued)*
  - premature E30.1
    - due to
      - adrenal cortical hyperfunction E25.8
      - pineal tumor E34.8
      - pituitary (anterior) hyperfunction E22.8
- **Puckering, macula** —*see* Degeneration, macula, puckering
- **Pudenda, pudendum** —*see* condition
- **Puente's disease** (simple glandular cheilitis) K13.0
- **Puerperal, puerperium** (complicated by, complications)
  - abnormal glucose (tolerance test) O99.815
  - abscess
    - areola O91.02
      - associated with lactation O91.03
    - Bartholin's gland O86.19
    - breast O91.12
      - associated with lactation O91.13
    - cervix (uteri) O86.11
    - genital organ NEC O86.19
    - kidney O86.21
    - mammary O91.12
      - associated with lactation O91.13
    - nipple O91.02
      - associated with lactation O91.03
    - peritoneum O85
    - subareolar O91.12
      - associated with lactation O91.13
    - urinary tract —*see* Puerperal, infection, urinary
    - uterus O86.12
    - vagina (wall) O86.13
    - vaginorectal O86.13
    - vulvovaginal gland O86.13
  - adnexitis O86.19
  - afibrinogenemia, or other coagulation defect O72.3
  - albuminuria (acute) (subacute) —*see* Proteinuria, gestational
  - alcohol use O99.315
  - anemia O90.81
    - pre-existing (pre-pregnancy) O99.03
  - anesthetic death O89.8
  - apoplexy O99.43
  - bariatric surgery status O99.845
  - blood disorder NEC O99.13
  - blood dyscrasia O72.3
  - cardiomyopathy O90.3
  - cerebrovascular disorder (conditions in I60-I69) O99.43
  - cervicitis O86.11
  - circulatory system disorder O99.43
  - coagulopathy (any) O99.13
    - with hemorrhage O72.3
  - complications O90.9
    - specified NEC O90.89
  - convulsions —*see* Eclampsia
  - cystitis O86.22
  - cystopyelitis O86.29
  - delirium NEC F05
  - diabetes O24.93
    - gestational —*see* Puerperal, gestational diabetes
    - pre-existing O24.33
      - specified NEC O24.83
      - type 1 O24.03
      - type 2 O24.13
  - digestive system disorder O99.63
  - disease O90.9
    - breast NEC O92.29
    - cerebrovascular (acute) O99.43
    - nonobstetric NEC O99.893
    - tubo-ovarian O86.19
    - Valsuani's O99.03
  - disorder O90.9
    - biliary tract O26.63
    - lactation O92.70
    - liver O26.63
    - nonobstetric NEC O99.893
  - disruption
    - cesarean wound O90.0
    - episiotomy wound O90.1
    - perineal laceration wound O90.1
  - drug use O99.325
  - eclampsia (with pre-existing hypertension) O15.2
  - embolism (pulmonary) (blood clot) —*see* Embolism, obstetric, puerperal
  - endocrine, nutritional or metabolic disease NEC O99.285
  - endophlebitis —*see* Puerperal, phlebitis

P

Puncture *(Continued)*
- accidental, complicating surgery —*see* Complication, accidental puncture or laceration
- alveolar (process) —*see* Puncture, oral cavity
- ankle S91.039
  - with
    - foreign body S91.049
  - left S91.032
    - with
      - foreign body S91.042
  - right S91.031
    - with
      - foreign body S91.041
- anus S31.833
  - with foreign body S31.834
- arm (upper) S41.139
  - with foreign body S41.149
  - left S41.132
    - with foreign body S41.142
  - lower —*see* Puncture, forearm
  - right S41.131
    - with foreign body S41.141
- auditory canal (external) (meatus) —*see* Puncture, ear
- auricle, ear —*see* Puncture, ear
- axilla —*see* Puncture, arm
- back —*see also* Puncture, thorax, back
  - lower S31.030
    - with
      - foreign body S31.040
        - with penetration into retroperitoneal space S31.041
      - penetration into retroperitoneal space S31.031
- bladder (traumatic) S37.29
  - nontraumatic N32.89
- breast S21.039
  - with foreign body S21.049
  - left S21.032
    - with foreign body S21.042
  - right S21.031
    - with foreign body S21.041
- buttock S31.803
  - with foreign body S31.804
  - left S31.823
    - with foreign body S31.824
  - right S31.813
    - with foreign body S31.814
- by
  - device, implant or graft —*see* Complications, by site and type, mechanical
  - foreign body left accidentally in operative wound T81.539
  - instrument (any) during a procedure, accidental —*see* Puncture, accidental complicating surgery
- calf —*see* Puncture, leg
- canaliculus lacrimalis —*see* Puncture, eyelid
- canthus, eye —*see* Puncture, eyelid
- cervical esophagus S11.23
  - with foreign body S11.24
- cheek (external) S01.439
  - with foreign body S01.449
  - internal —*see* Puncture, oral cavity
  - left S01.432
    - with foreign body S01.442
  - right S01.431
    - with foreign body S01.441
- chest wall —*see* Puncture, thorax
- chin —*see* Puncture, head, specified site NEC
- clitoris —*see* Puncture, vulva
- costal region —*see* Puncture, thorax
- digit(s)
  - foot —*see* Puncture, toe
  - hand —*see* Puncture, finger
- ear (canal) (external) S01.339
  - with foreign body S01.349
  - drum S09.2-●
  - left S01.332
    - with foreign body S01.342
  - right S01.331
    - with foreign body S01.341
- elbow S51.039
  - with
    - foreign body S51.049
  - left S51.032
    - with
      - foreign body S51.042

Puncture *(Continued)*
- elbow *(Continued)*
  - right S51.031
    - with
      - foreign body S51.041
- epididymis —*see* Puncture, testis
- epigastric region —*see* Puncture, abdomen, wall, epigastric
- epiglottis S11.83
  - with foreign body S11.84
- esophagus
  - cervical S11.23
    - with foreign body S11.24
  - thoracic S27.818
- eyeball S05.6-●
  - with foreign body S05.5-●
- eyebrow —*see* Puncture, eyelid
- eyelid S01.13-●
  - with foreign body S01.14-●
  - left S01.132
    - with foreign body S01.142
  - right S01.131
    - with foreign body S01.141
- face NEC —*see* Puncture, head, specified site NEC
- finger(s) S61.239
  - with
    - damage to nail S61.339
      - with
        - foreign body S61.349
    - foreign body S61.249
  - index S61.238
    - with
      - damage to nail S61.338
        - with
          - foreign body S61.348
      - foreign body S61.248
    - left S61.231
      - with
        - damage to nail S61.331
          - with
            - foreign body S61.341
        - foreign body S61.241
    - right S61.230
      - with
        - damage to nail S61.330
          - with
            - foreign body S61.340
        - foreign body S61.240
  - little S61.238
    - with
      - damage to nail S61.338
        - with
          - foreign body S61.348
      - foreign body S61.248
    - left S61.237
      - with
        - damage to nail S61.337
          - with
            - foreign body S61.347
        - foreign body S61.247
    - right S61.236
      - with
        - damage to nail S61.336
          - with
            - foreign body S61.346
        - foreign body S61.246
  - middle S61.238
    - with
      - damage to nail S61.338
        - with
          - foreign body S61.348
      - foreign body S61.248
    - left S61.233
      - with
        - damage to nail S61.333
          - with
            - foreign body S61.343
        - foreign body S61.243
    - right S61.232
      - with
        - damage to nail S61.332
          - with
            - foreign body S61.342
        - foreign body S61.242
  - ring S61.238
    - with
      - damage to nail S61.338
        - with
          - foreign body S61.348
      - foreign body S61.248

Puncture *(Continued)*
- finger(s) *(Continued)*
  - ring *(Continued)*
    - left S61.235
      - with
        - damage to nail S61.335
          - with
            - foreign body S61.345
        - foreign body S61.245
    - right S61.234
      - with
        - damage to nail S61.334
          - with
            - foreign body S61.344
        - foreign body S61.244
- flank S31.139
  - with foreign body S31.149
- foot (except toe(s) alone) S91.339
  - with foreign body S91.349
  - left S91.332
    - with foreign body S91.342
  - right S91.331
    - with foreign body S91.341
  - toe —*see* Puncture, toe
- forearm S51.839
  - with
    - foreign body S51.849
  - elbow only —*see* Puncture, elbow
  - left S51.832
    - with
      - foreign body S51.842
  - right S51.831
    - with
      - foreign body S51.841
- forehead —*see* Puncture, head, specified site NEC
- genital organs, external
  - female S31.532
    - with foreign body S31.542
    - vagina —*see* Puncture, vagina
    - vulva —*see* Puncture, vulva
  - male S31.531
    - with foreign body S31.541
    - penis —*see* Puncture, penis
    - scrotum —*see* Puncture, scrotum
    - testis —*see* Puncture, testis
- groin —*see* Puncture, abdomen, wall
- gum —*see* Puncture, oral cavity
- hand S61.439
  - with
    - foreign body S61.449
  - finger —*see* Puncture, finger
  - left S61.432
    - with
      - foreign body S61.442
  - right S61.431
    - with
      - foreign body S61.441
  - thumb —*see* Puncture, thumb
- head S01.93
  - with foreign body S01.94
  - cheek —*see* Puncture, cheek
  - ear —*see* Puncture, ear
  - eyelid —*see* Puncture, eyelid
  - lip —*see* Puncture, oral cavity
  - nose —*see* Puncture, nose
  - oral cavity —*see* Puncture, oral cavity
  - scalp S01.03
    - with foreign body S01.04
  - specified site NEC S01.83
    - with foreign body S01.84
  - temporomandibular area —*see* Puncture, cheek
- heart S26.99
  - with hemopericardium S26.09
  - without hemopericardium S26.19
- heel —*see* Puncture, foot
- hip S71.039
  - with foreign body S71.049
  - left S71.032
    - with foreign body S71.042
  - right S71.031
    - with foreign body S71.041
- hymen —*see* Puncture, vagina
- hypochondrium —*see* Puncture, abdomen, wall
- hypogastric region —*see* Puncture, abdomen, wall
- inguinal region —*see* Puncture, abdomen, wall
- instep —*see* Puncture, foot
- internal organs —*see* Injury, by site
- interscapular region —*see* Puncture, thorax, back

Q

R

▶ New ➠ Revised ~~deleted~~ Deleted ● Use Additional Character(s)

R

R

Retardation *(Continued)*
- reading (specific) F81.0
- spelling (specific) (without reading disorder) F81.81

Retching —*see* Vomiting
Retention —*see also* Retained
- bladder —*see* Retention, urine
- carbon dioxide E87.29
- cholelithiasis following cholecystectomy K91.86
- cyst —*see* Cyst
- dead
  - fetus (at or near term) (mother) O36.4
    - early fetal death O02.1
  - ovum O02.0
- decidua (fragments) (following delivery) (with hemorrhage) O72.2
  - without hemorrhage O73.1
- deciduous tooth K00.6
- dental root K08.3
- fecal —*see* Constipation
- fetus
  - dead O36.4
    - early O02.1
- fluid R60.9
- foreign body —*see also* Foreign body, retained
  - current trauma - code as Foreign body, by site or type
- gallstones, following cholecystectomy K91.86
- gastric K31.89
- intrauterine contraceptive device, in pregnancy —*see* Pregnancy, complicated by, retention, intrauterine device
- membranes (complicating delivery) (with hemorrhage) O72.2
  - with abortion —*see* Abortion, by type
  - without hemorrhage O73.1
- meniscus —*see* Derangement, meniscus
- menses N94.89
- milk (puerperal, postpartum) O92.79
- nitrogen, extrarenal R39.2
- ovary syndrome N99.83
- placenta (total) (with hemorrhage) O72.0
  - without hemorrhage O73.0
  - portions or fragments (with hemorrhage) O72.2
    - without hemorrhage O73.1
- products of conception
  - early pregnancy (dead fetus) O02.1
  - following
    - delivery (with hemorrhage) O72.2
      - without hemorrhage O73.1
- secundines (following delivery) (with hemorrhage) O72.0
  - without hemorrhage O73.0
  - complicating puerperium (delayed hemorrhage) O72.2
  - partial O72.2
    - without hemorrhage O73.1
- smegma, clitoris N90.89
- urine R33.9
  - drug-induced R33.0
  - due to hyperplasia (hypertrophy) of prostate —*see* Hyperplasia, prostate
  - organic R33.8
    - drug-induced R33.0
  - psychogenic F45.8
  - specified NEC R33.8
- water (in tissues) —*see* Edema

Reticular erythematous mucinosis L98.5
Reticulation, dust —*see* Pneumoconiosis
Reticulocytosis R70.1
Reticuloendotheliosis
- acute infantile C96.0
- leukemic C91.4-•
- nonlipid C96.0

Reticulohistiocytoma (giant-cell) D76.3
Reticuloid, actinic L57.1
Reticulosis (skin)
- acute of infancy C96.0
- hemophagocytic, familial D76.1
- histiocytic medullary C96.A
- lipomelanotic I89.8
- ➡malignant (midline) C86.0-•
- ➡polymorphic C86.0-•
- Sézary —*see* Sézary disease

Retina, retinal —*see also* condition
- dark area D49.81

Retinitis —*see also* Inflammation, chorioretinal
- albuminurica N18.9 *[H32]*
- diabetic —*see* Diabetes, retinitis
- disciformis —*see* Degeneration, macula

Retinitis *(Continued)*
- focal —*see* Inflammation, chorioretinal, focal
- gravidarum —*see* Pregnancy, complicated by, specified pregnancy-related condition NEC
- juxtapapillaris —*see* Inflammation, chorioretinal, focal, juxtapapillary
- luetic —*see* Retinitis, syphilitic
- pigmentosa H35.52
- proliferans —*see* Disorder, globe, degenerative, specified type NEC
- proliferating —*see* Disorder, globe, degenerative, specified type NEC
- renal N18.9 *[H32]*
- syphilitic (early) (secondary) A51.43
  - central, recurrent A52.71
  - congenital (early) A50.01 *[H32]*
  - late A52.71
- tuberculous A18.53

Retinoblastoma C69.2-•
- differentiated C69.2-•
- undifferentiated C69.2-•

Retinochoroiditis —*see also* Inflammation, chorioretinal
- disseminated —*see* Inflammation, chorioretinal, disseminated
  - syphilitic A52.71
- focal —*see* Inflammation, chorioretinal
- juxtapapillaris —*see* Inflammation, chorioretinal, focal, juxtapapillary

Retinopathy (background) H35.00
- arteriosclerotic I70.8 *[H35.0-•]*
- atherosclerotic I70.8 *[H35.0-•]*
- central serous —*see* Chorioretinopathy, central serous
- Coats H35.02-•
- diabetic —*see* Diabetes, retinopathy
- exudative H35.02-•
- hypertensive H35.03-•
- in (due to)
  - diabetes —*see* Diabetes, retinopathy
- sickle-cell disorders
  - nonproliferative D57.-• [H36.81-•]
  - proliferative D57.-• [H36.82-•]
- of prematurity H35.10-•
  - stage 0 H35.11-•
  - stage 1 H35.12-•
  - stage 2 H35.13-•
  - stage 3 H35.14-•
  - stage 4 H35.15-•
  - stage 5 H35.16-•
- pigmentary, congenital —*see* Dystrophy, retina
- proliferative NEC H35.2-•
  - diabetic —*see* Diabetes, retinopathy, proliferative
  - sickle-cell D57.-• *[H36.82-•]*
  - ~~thaslassemia H35.2~~
  - ▶thalassemia H35.2
- solar H31.02-•

Retinoschisis H33.10-•
- congenital Q14.1
- specified type NEC H33.19-•

Retortamoniasis A07.8
Retractile testis Q55.22
Retraction
- cervix —*see* Retroversion, uterus
- drum (membrane) —*see* Disorder, tympanic membrane, specified NEC
- finger —*see* Deformity, finger
- lid H02.539
  - left H02.536
    - lower H02.535
    - upper H02.534
  - right H02.533
    - lower H02.532
    - upper H02.531
- lung J98.4
- mediastinum J98.59
- nipple N64.53
  - associated with
    - lactation O92.03
    - pregnancy O92.01-•
    - puerperium O92.02
  - congenital Q83.8
- palmar fascia M72.0
- pleura —*see* Pleurisy
- ring, uterus (Bandl's) (pathological) O62.4
- sternum (congenital) Q76.7
  - acquired M95.4
- uterus —*see* Retroversion, uterus
- valve (heart) —*see* Endocarditis

Retrobulbar —*see* condition
Retrocecal —*see* condition
Retrocession —*see* Retroversion
Retrodisplacement —*see* Retroversion
Retroflection, retroflexion —*see* Retroversion
Retrognathia, retrognathism (mandibular) (maxillary) M26.19
Retrograde menstruation N92.5
Retroperineal —*see* condition
Retroperitoneal —*see* condition
Retroperitonitis K68.9
Retropharyngeal —*see* condition
Retroplacental —*see* condition
Retroposition —*see* Retroversion
Retroprosthetic membrane T85.398
Retrosternal thyroid (congenital) Q89.2
Retroversion, retroverted
- cervix —*see* Retroversion, uterus
- female NEC —*see* Retroversion, uterus
- iris H21.89
- testis (congenital) Q55.29
- uterus (acquired) (acute) (any degree) (asymptomatic) (cervix) (postinfectional) (postpartal, old) N85.4
  - congenital Q51.818
  - in pregnancy O34.53-•

Retrovirus, as cause of disease classified elsewhere B97.30
- human
  - immunodeficiency, type 2 (HIV 2) B97.35
  - T-cell lymphotropic
    - type I (HTLV-I) B97.33
    - type II (HTLV-II) B97.34
- lentivirus B97.31
- oncovirus B97.32
- specified NEC B97.39

Retrusion, premaxilla (developmental) M26.09
Rett's disease or syndrome F84.2
Reverse peristalsis R19.2
Reye's syndrome G93.7
Rh (factor)
- hemolytic disease (newborn) P55.0
- incompatibility, immunization or sensitization
  - affecting management of pregnancy NEC O36.09-•
    - anti-D antibody O36.01-•
  - newborn P55.0
  - transfusion reaction —*see* Complication(s), transfusion, incompatibility reaction, Rh (factor)
- negative mother affecting newborn P55.0
- titer elevated —*see* Complication(s), transfusion, incompatibility reaction, Rh (factor)
- transfusion reaction —*see* Complication(s), transfusion, incompatibility reaction, Rh (factor)

Rhabdomyolysis (idiopathic) NEC M62.82
- traumatic T79.6

Rhabdomyoma —*see also* Neoplasm, connective tissue, benign
- adult —*see* Neoplasm, connective tissue, benign
- fetal —*see* Neoplasm, connective tissue, benign
- glycogenic —*see* Neoplasm, connective tissue, benign

Rhabdomyosarcoma (any type) —*see* Neoplasm, connective tissue, malignant
Rhabdosarcoma —*see* Rhabdomyosarcoma
Rhesus (factor) **incompatibility** —*see* Rh, incompatibility
Rheumatic (acute) (subacute)
- adherent pericardium I09.2
- chronic I09.89
- coronary arteritis I01.8
- degeneration, myocardium I09.0
- fever (acute) —*see* Fever, rheumatic
- heart —*see* Disease, heart, rheumatic
- myocardial degeneration —*see* Degeneration, myocardium
- myocarditis (chronic) (inactive) (with chorea) I09.0
  - with chorea (acute) (rheumatic) (Sydenham's) I02.0
  - active or acute I01.2
- pancarditis, acute I01.8
  - with chorea (acute rheumatic) Sydenham's) I02.0
- pericarditis (active) (acute) (with effusion) (with pneumonia) I01.0
  - with chorea (acute) (rheumatic) (Sydenham's) I02.0
  - chronic or inactive I09.2
- pneumonia I00 *[J17]*

R

Rheumatic *(Continued)*
torticollis M43.6
typhoid fever A01.09
Rheumatism (articular) (neuralgic) (nonarticular) M79.0
gout —*see* Arthritis, rheumatoid
intercostal, meaning Tietze's disease M94.0
palindromic (any site) M12.30
ankle M12.37-●
elbow M12.32-●
foot joint M12.37-●
hand joint M12.34-●
hip M12.35-●
knee M12.36-●
multiple site M12.39
shoulder M12.31-●
specified joint NEC M12.38
vertebrae M12.38
wrist M12.33-●
sciatic M54.4-●
Rheumatoid —*see also* condition
arthritis —*see also* Arthritis, rheumatoid
with involvement of organs NEC M05.60
ankle M05.67-●
elbow M05.62-●
foot joint M05.67-●
hand joint M05.64-●
hip M05.65-●
knee M05.66-●
multiple site M05.69
shoulder M05.61-●
vertebra —*see* Spondylitis, ankylosing
wrist M05.63-●
seronegative —*see* Arthritis, rheumatoid, seronegative
seropositive —*see* Arthritis, rheumatoid, seropositive
carditis M05.30
ankle M05.37-●
elbow M05.32-●
foot joint M05.37-●
hand joint M05.34-●
hip M05.35-●
knee M05.36-●
multiple site M05.39
shoulder M05.31-●
vertebra —*see* Spondylitis, ankylosing
wrist M05.33-●
endocarditis —*see* Rheumatoid, carditis
lung (disease) M05.10
ankle M05.17-●
elbow M05.12-●
foot joint M05.17-●
hand joint M05.14-●
hip M05.15-●
knee M05.16-●
multiple site M05.19
shoulder M05.11-●
vertebra —*see* Spondylitis, ankylosing
wrist M05.13-●
myocarditis —*see* Rheumatoid, carditis
myopathy M05.40
ankle M05.47-●
elbow M05.42-●
foot joint M05.47-●
hand joint M05.44-●
hip M05.45-●
knee M05.46-●
multiple site M05.49
shoulder M05.41-●
vertebra —*see* Spondylitis, ankylosing
wrist M05.43-●
pericarditis —*see* Rheumatoid, carditis
polyarthritis —*see* Arthritis, rheumatoid
polyneuropathy M05.50
ankle M05.57-●
elbow M05.52-●
foot joint M05.57-●
hand joint M05.54-●
hip M05.55-●
knee M05.56-●
multiple site M05.59
shoulder M05.51-●
vertebra —*see* Spondylitis, ankylosing
wrist M05.53-●
vasculitis M05.20
ankle M05.27-●
elbow M05.22-●
foot joint M05.27-●
hand joint M05.24-●
hip M05.25-●

Rheumatoid *(Continued)*
vasculitis *(Continued)*
knee M05.26-●
multiple site M05.29
shoulder M05.21-●
vertebra —*see* Spondylitis, ankylosing
wrist M05.23-●
Rhinitis (atrophic) (catarrhal) (chronic) (croupous) (fibrinous) (granulomatous) (hyperplastic) (hypertrophic) (membranous) (obstructive) (purulent) (suppurative) (ulcerative) J31.0
with
sore throat —*see* Nasopharyngitis
acute J00
allergic J30.9
with asthma J45.909
with
exacerbation (acute) J45.901
status asthmaticus J45.902
due to
food J30.5
pollen J30.1
nonseasonal J30.89
perennial J30.89
seasonal NEC J30.2
specified NEC J30.89
infective J00
pneumococcal J00
syphilitic A52.73
congenital A50.05 *[J99]*
tuberculous A15.8
vasomotor J30.0
Rhinoantritis (chronic) —*see* Sinusitis, maxillary
Rhinodacryolith —*see* Dacryolith
Rhinolith (nasal sinus) J34.89
Rhinomegaly J34.89
Rhinopharyngitis (acute) (subacute) —*see also* Nasopharyngitis
chronic J31.1
destructive ulcerating A66.5
mutilans A66.5
Rhinophyma L71.1
Rhinorrhea J34.89
cerebrospinal (fluid) G96.01
postoperative G96.08
specified NEC G96.08
spontaneous G96.01
traumatic G96.08
paroxysmal —*see* Rhinitis, allergic
spasmodic —*see* Rhinitis, allergic
Rhinosalpingitis —*see* Salpingitis, eustachian
Rhinoscleroma A48.8
Rhinosinusitis —*see* Sinusitis
Rhinosporidiosis B48.1
Rhinovirus infection NEC B34.8
Rhizomelic chondrodysplasia punctata E71.540
Rhythm
atrioventricular nodal I49.8
disorder I49.9
coronary sinus I49.8
ectopic I49.8
nodal I49.8
escape I49.9
heart, abnormal I49.9
idioventricular I44.2
nodal I49.8
sleep, inversion G47.2-●
nonorganic origin —*see* Disorder, sleep, circadian rhythm, psychogenic
Rhytidosis facialis L98.8
Rib —*see also* condition
cervical Q76.5
Riboflavin deficiency E53.0
Rice bodies —*see also* Loose, body, joint
knee M23.4-●
Richter syndrome —*see* Leukemia, chronic lymphocytic, B-cell type
Richter's hernia —*see* Hernia, abdomen, with obstruction
Ricinism —*see* Poisoning, food, noxious, plant
Rickets (active) (acute) (adolescent) (chest wall) (congenital) (current) (infantile) (intestinal) E55.0
adult —*see* Osteomalacia
celiac K90.0
hypophosphatemic with nephrotic-glycosuric dwarfism E72.09
inactive E64.3
kidney N25.0
renal N25.0
sequelae, any E64.3
vitamin-D-resistant E83.31 *[M90.80]*

Rickettsia 364D/R. philipii (Pacific Coast tick fever) A77.8
Rickettsial disease A79.9
specified type NEC A79.89
Rickettsialpox (Rickettsia akari) A79.1
Rickettsiosis A79.9
due to
Ehrlichia sennetsu A79.81
Neorickettsia sennetsu A79.81
Rickettsia akari (rickettsialpox) A79.1
specified type NEC A79.89
tick-borne A77.9
vesicular A79.1
Rider's bone —*see* Ossification, muscle, specified NEC
Ridge, alveolus —*see also* condition
flabby K06.8
Ridged ear, congenital Q17.3
Riedel's
lobe, liver Q44.79
struma, thyroiditis or disease E06.5
~~Rieger's anomaly or syndrome Q13.81~~
▶ **Rieger anomaly or syndrome** Q13.81
Riehl's melanosis L81.4
Rietti-Greppi-Micheli anemia D56.9
Rieux's hernia —*see* Hernia, abdomen, specified site NEC
Riga (-Fede) disease K14.0
Riggs' disease —*see* Periodontitis
Right aortic arch Q25.47
Right middle lobe syndrome J98.11
Rigid, rigidity —*see also* condition
abdominal R19.30
with severe abdominal pain R10.0
epigastric R19.36
generalized R19.37
left lower quadrant R19.34
left upper quadrant R19.32
periumbilic R19.35
right lower quadrant R19.33
right upper quadrant R19.31
articular, multiple, congenital Q68.8
cervix (uteri) in pregnancy —*see* Pregnancy, complicated by, abnormal, cervix
hymen (acquired) (congenital) N89.6
nuchal R29.1
pelvic floor in pregnancy —*see* Pregnancy, complicated by, abnormal, pelvic organs or tissues NEC
perineum or vulva in pregnancy —*see* Pregnancy, complicated by, abnormal, vulva
spine —*see* Dorsopathy, specified NEC
vagina in pregnancy —*see* Pregnancy, complicated by, abnormal, vagina
Rigors R68.89
with fever R50.9
Riley-Day syndrome G90.1
RIND (reversible ischemic neurologic deficit) I63.9
Ring(s)
aorta (vascular) Q25.45
Bandl's O62.4
contraction, complicating delivery O62.4
esophageal, lower (muscular) K22.2
Fleischer's (cornea) H18.04-●
hymenal, tight (acquired) (congenital) N89.6
Kayser-Fleischer (cornea) H18.04-●
retraction, uterus, pathological O62.4
Schatzki's (esophagus) (lower) K22.2
congenital Q39.3
Soemmerring's —*see* Cataract, secondary
vascular (congenital) Q25.8
aorta Q25.45
Ringed hair (congenital) Q84.1
Ringworm B35.9
beard B35.0
black dot B35.0
body B35.4
Burmese B35.5
corporeal B35.4
foot B35.3
groin B35.6
hand B35.2
honeycomb B35.0
nails B35.1
perianal (area) B35.6
scalp B35.0
specified NEC B35.8
Tokelau B35.5
Rise, venous pressure I87.8

R

Rising, PSA following treatment for malignant neoplasm of prostate R97.21
Risk
- for
  - dental caries Z91.849
    - high Z91.843
    - low Z91.841
    - moderate Z91.842
  - homelessness, imminent Z59.811
- suffocation (smothering) under another while sleeping Z72.823
- suicidal
  - meaning personal history of attempted suicide Z91.51
  - meaning suicidal ideation —*see* Ideation, suicidal

Ritter's disease L00
Rivalry, sibling Z62.891
Rivalta's disease A42.2
River blindness B73.01
Robert's pelvis Q74.2
- with disproportion (fetopelvic) O33.0
  - causing obstructed labor O65.0

Robin (-Pierre) syndrome Q87.0
~~Robinow-Silvermann-Smith syndrome Q87.19~~
▶ **Robinow-Silverman-Smith syndrome** Q87.19
Robinson's (hidrotic) ectodermal dysplasia or syndrome Q82.4
Robles' disease B73.01
Rocky Mountain (spotted) fever A77.0
Roetheln —*see* Rubella
Roger's disease Q21.0
Rokitansky-Aschoff sinuses (gallbladder) K82.8
Rolando's fracture (displaced) S62.22-●
- nondisplaced S62.22-●

Romano-Ward (prolonged QT interval) **syndrome** I45.81
Romberg's disease or syndrome G51.8
Roof, mouth —*see* condition
Rosacea L71.9
- acne L71.9
- keratitis L71.8
- specified NEC L71.8

Rosary, rachitic E55.0
Rose
- cold J30.1
- fever J30.1
- rash R21
  - epidemic B06.9

Rosenbach's erysipeloid A26.0
Rosenthal's disease or syndrome D68.1
Roseola B09
- infantum B08.20
  - due to human herpesvirus 6 B08.21
  - due to human herpesvirus 7 B08.22

Ross River disease or fever B33.1
Rossbach's disease K31.89
- psychogenic F45.8

Rostan's asthma (cardiac) —*see* Failure, ventricular, left
Rotation
- anomalous, incomplete or insufficient, intestine Q43.3
- cecum (congenital) Q43.3
- colon (congenital) Q43.3
- spine, incomplete or insufficient —*see* Dorsopathy, deforming, specified NEC
- tooth, teeth, fully erupted M26.35
- vertebra, incomplete or insufficient —*see* Dorsopathy, deforming, specified NEC

Rotes Quérol disease or syndrome —*see* Hyperostosis, ankylosing
Roth (-Bernhardt) disease or syndrome —*see* Meralgia paraesthetica
Rothmund (-Thomson) syndrome Q82.8
Rotor's disease or syndrome E80.6
Round
- back (with wedging of vertebrae) —*see* Kyphosis
  - sequelae (late effect) of rickets E64.3
- worms (large) (infestation) NEC B82.0
  - Ascariasis —*see also* Ascariasis B77.9

Roussy-Lévy syndrome G60.0
Rubella (German measles) B06.9
- complication NEC B06.09
  - neurological B06.00
- congenital P35.0
- contact Z20.4
- exposure to Z20.4
- maternal
  - care for (suspected) damage to fetus O35.3
  - manifest rubella in infant P35.0
  - suspected damage to fetus affecting management of pregnancy O35.3
- specified complications NEC B06.89

Rubeola (meaning measles) —*see* Measles
- meaning rubella —*see* Rubella

Rubeosis, iris —*see* Disorder, iris, vascular
Rubinstein-Taybi syndrome Q87.2
Rudimentary (congenital) —*see also* Agenesis
- arm —*see* Defect, reduction, upper limb
- bone Q79.9
- cervix uteri Q51.828
- eye Q11.2
- lobule of ear Q17.3
- patella Q74.1
- respiratory organs in thoracopagus Q89.4
- tracheal bronchus Q32.4
- uterus Q51.818
  - in male Q56.1
- vagina Q52.0

Ruled out condition —*see* Observation, suspected
Rumination R11.10
- with nausea R11.2
- ~~disorder of infancy F98.21~~
- ▶ disorder of infancy or childhood (in remission) F98.21
  - ▶ in adults (in remission) F50.84
- neurotic F42.8
- newborn P92.1
- obsessional F42.8
- psychogenic F42.8

Runaway [from current living environment] Z62.892
Runeberg's disease D51.0
Runny nose R09.89
Running out of money Z59.86
Rupia (syphilitic) A51.39
- congenital A50.06
- tertiary A52.79

Rupture, ruptured
- abscess (spontaneous) - code by site under Abscess
- aneurysm —*see* Aneurysm
- anus (sphincter) —*see* Laceration, anus
- aorta, aortic I71.8
  - abdominal I71.30
    - infrarenal I71.33
    - juxtarenal I71.32
    - pararenal I71.31
  - arch I71.12
  - ascending I71.11
  - descending I71.8
    - abdominal I71.30
    - thoracic I71.13
  - syphilitic A52.01
  - thoracoabdominal I71.50
    - paravisceral I71.52
    - supraceliac I71.51
  - thorax, thoracic I71.10
  - transverse I71.12
  - traumatic —*see* Injury, aorta, laceration, major
  - valve or cusp —*see also* Endocarditis, aortic I35.8
- appendix (with peritonitis) (*see also* Appendicitis) K35.32
  - with localized peritonitis (*see also* Appendicitis) K35.32
- arteriovenous fistula, brain —*see* Fistula, arteriovenous, brain, ruptured
- artery I77.2
  - brain —*see* Hemorrhage, intracranial, intracerebral
  - coronary —*see* Infarct, myocardium
  - heart —*see* Infarct, myocardium
  - pulmonary I28.8
  - traumatic (complication) —*see* Injury, blood vessel
- bile duct (common) (hepatic) K83.2
  - cystic K82.2
- bladder (sphincter) (nontraumatic) (spontaneous) N32.89
  - following ectopic or molar pregnancy O08.6
  - obstetrical trauma O71.5
  - traumatic S37.29
- blood vessel —*see also* Hemorrhage
  - brain —*see* Hemorrhage, intracranial, intracerebral
  - heart —*see* Infarct, myocardium
  - traumatic (complication) —*see* Injury, blood vessel, laceration, major, by site
- bone —*see* Fracture
- bowel (nontraumatic) K63.1
- brain
  - aneurysm (congenital) —*see also* Hemorrhage, intracranial, subarachnoid
    - syphilitic A52.05
  - hemorrhagic —*see* Hemorrhage, intracranial, intracerebral
- capillaries I78.8
- cardiac (auricle) (ventricle) (wall) I23.3
  - with hemopericardium I23.0
  - infectional I40.9
  - traumatic —*see* Injury, heart
- cartilage (articular) (current) —*see also* Sprain
  - knee S83.3-●
  - semilunar —*see* Tear, meniscus
- cecum (with peritonitis) K65.0
  - with peritoneal abscess K35.33
  - traumatic S36.598
- celiac artery, traumatic —*see* Injury, blood vessel, celiac artery, laceration, major
- cerebral aneurysm (congenital) (*see* Hemorrhage, intracranial, subarachnoid)
- cervix (uteri)
  - with ectopic or molar pregnancy O08.6
  - following ectopic or molar pregnancy O08.6
  - obstetrical trauma O71.3
  - traumatic S37.69
- chordae tendineae NEC I51.1
  - concurrent with acute myocardial infarction —*see* Infarct, myocardium
  - following acute myocardial infarction (current complication) I23.4
- choroid (direct) (indirect) (traumatic) H31.32-●
- circle of Willis I60.6
- colon (nontraumatic) K63.1
  - traumatic —*see* Injury, intestine, large
- cornea (traumatic) —*see* Injury, eye, laceration
- coronary (artery) (thrombotic) —*see* Infarct, myocardium
- corpus luteum (infected) (ovary) N83.1-●
- cyst —*see* Cyst
- cystic duct K82.2
- Descemet's membrane —*see* Change, corneal membrane, Descemet's, rupture
  - traumatic —*see* Injury, eye, laceration
- diaphragm, traumatic —*see* Injury, intrathoracic, diaphragm
- disc —*see* Rupture, intervertebral disc
- diverticulum (intestine) K57.80
  - with bleeding K57.81
  - bladder N32.3
  - large intestine K57.20
    - with
      - bleeding K57.21
      - small intestine K57.40
        - with bleeding K57.41
  - small intestine K57.00
    - with
      - bleeding K57.01
      - large intestine K57.40
        - with bleeding K57.41
- duodenal stump K31.89
- ear drum (nontraumatic) —*see also* Perforation, tympanum
  - traumatic S09.2-●
    - due to blast injury —*see* Injury, blast, ear
- esophagus K22.3
- eye (without prolapse or loss of intraocular tissue) —*see* Injury, eye, laceration
- fallopian tube NEC (nonobstetric) (nontraumatic) N83.8
  - due to pregnancy O00.10-●
    - with intrauterine pregnancy O00.11-●
- fontanel P13.1
- gallbladder K82.2
  - traumatic S36.128
- gastric —*see also* Rupture, stomach
  - vessel K92.2
- globe (eye) (traumatic) —*see* Injury, eye, laceration
  - ▶ nontraumatic (*see also* Disorder, globe) H44.89
- graafian follicle (hematoma) N83.0-●
- heart —*see* Rupture, cardiac
- hymen (nontraumatic) (nonintentional) N89.8
- internal organ, traumatic —*see* Injury, by site

▶ New ➡ Revised ~~deleted~~ Deleted ● Use Additional Character(s)

Rupture, ruptured *(Continued)*
- intervertebral disc —*see* Displacement, intervertebral disc
  - traumatic —*see* Rupture, traumatic, intervertebral disc
- intestine NEC (nontraumatic) K63.1
  - traumatic —*see* Injury, intestine
- iris —*see also* Abnormality, pupillary
  - traumatic —*see* Injury, eye, laceration
- joint capsule, traumatic —*see* Sprain
- kidney (traumatic) S37.06- ●
  - birth injury P15.8
  - nontraumatic N28.89
- lacrimal duct (traumatic) —*see* Injury, eye, specified site NEC
- lens (cataract) (traumatic) —*see* Cataract, traumatic
- ligament, traumatic —*see* Rupture, traumatic, ligament, by site
- liver S36.116
  - birth injury P15.0
- lymphatic vessel I89.8
- marginal sinus (placental) (with hemorrhage) —*see* Hemorrhage, antepartum, specified cause NEC
- membrana tympani (nontraumatic) —*see* Perforation, tympanum
- membranes (spontaneous)
  - artificial
    - delayed delivery following O75.5
  - delayed delivery following —*see* Pregnancy, complicated by, premature rupture of membranes
- meningeal artery I60.8
- meniscus (knee) —*see also* Tear, meniscus
  - old —*see* Derangement, meniscus
  - site other than knee - code as Sprain
- mesenteric artery, traumatic —*see* Injury, mesenteric, artery, laceration, major
- mesentery (nontraumatic) K66.8
  - traumatic —*see* Injury, intra-abdominal, specified, site NEC
- mitral (valve) I34.89
- muscle (traumatic) —*see also* Strain
  - diastasis —*see* Diastasis, muscle
  - nontraumatic M62.10
    - ankle M62.17- ●
    - foot M62.17- ●
    - forearm M62.13- ●
    - hand M62.14- ●
    - lower leg M62.16- ●
    - pelvic region M62.15- ●
    - shoulder region M62.11- ●
    - specified site NEC M62.18
    - thigh M62.15- ●
    - upper arm M62.12- ●
  - traumatic —*see* Strain, by site
- musculotendinous junction NEC, nontraumatic —*see* Rupture, tendon, spontaneous
- mycotic aneurysm causing cerebral hemorrhage —*see* Hemorrhage, intracranial, subarachnoid
- myocardium, myocardial —*see* Rupture, cardiac
  - traumatic —*see* Injury, heart
- nontraumatic, meaning hernia —*see* Hernia
- obstructed —*see* Hernia, by site, obstructed
- operation wound —*see* Disruption, wound, operation
- ovary, ovarian N83.8
  - corpus luteum cyst N83.1- ●
  - follicle (graafian) N83.0- ●
- oviduct (nonobstetric) (nontraumatic) N83.8
  - due to pregnancy O00.10- ●
    - with intrauterine pregnancy O00.11- ●
- pancreas (nontraumatic) K86.89
  - traumatic S36.299
- papillary muscle NEC I51.2
  - following acute myocardial infarction (current complication) I23.5
- pelvic
  - floor, complicating delivery O70.1
  - organ NEC, obstetrical trauma O71.5
- perineum (nonobstetric) (nontraumatic) N90.89
  - complicating delivery —*see* Delivery, complicated, by, laceration, anus (sphincter)
- postoperative wound —*see* Disruption, wound, operation
- prostate (traumatic) S37.828
- pulmonary
  - artery I28.8
  - valve (heart) I37.8
  - vein I28.8
  - vessel I28.8
- pus tube —*see* Salpingitis
- pyosalpinx —*see* Salpingitis
- rectum (nontraumatic) K63.1
  - traumatic S36.69
- retina, retinal (traumatic) (without detachment) —*see also* Break, retina
  - with detachment —*see* Detachment, retina, with retinal, break
- rotator cuff (nontraumatic) M75.10- ●
  - complete M75.12- ●
  - incomplete M75.11- ●
- sclera —*see* Injury, eye, laceration
- sigmoid (nontraumatic) K63.1
  - traumatic S36.593
- spinal cord —*see also* Injury, spinal cord, by region
  - due to injury at birth P11.5
  - newborn (birth injury) P11.5
- spleen (traumatic) S36.09
  - birth injury P15.1
  - congenital (birth injury) P15.1
  - due to P. vivax malaria B51.0
  - nontraumatic D73.5
  - spontaneous D73.5
- splenic vein R58
  - traumatic —*see* Injury, blood vessel, splenic vein
- stomach (nontraumatic) (spontaneous) K31.89
  - traumatic S36.39
- supraspinatus (complete) (incomplete) (nontraumatic) —*see* Tear, rotator cuff
- symphysis pubis
  - obstetric O71.6
  - traumatic S33.4
- synovium (cyst) M66.10
  - ankle M66.17- ●
  - elbow M66.12- ●
  - finger M66.14- ●
  - foot M66.17- ●
  - forearm M66.13- ●
  - hand M66.14- ●
  - pelvic region M66.15- ●
  - shoulder region M66.11- ●
  - specified site NEC M66.18
  - thigh M66.15- ●
  - toe M66.17- ●
  - upper arm M66.12- ●
  - wrist M66.13- ●
- tendon (traumatic) —*see* Strain
  - nontraumatic (spontaneous) M66.9
    - ankle M66.87- ●
    - extensor M66.20
      - ankle M66.27- ●
      - foot M66.27- ●
      - forearm M66.23- ●
      - hand M66.24- ●
      - lower leg M66.26- ●
      - multiple sites M66.29
      - pelvic region M66.25- ●
      - shoulder region M66.21- ●
      - specified site NEC M66.28
      - thigh M66.25- ●
      - upper arm M66.22- ●
    - flexor M66.30
      - ankle M66.37- ●
      - foot M66.37- ●
      - forearm M66.33- ●
      - hand M66.34- ●
      - lower leg M66.36- ●
      - multiple sites M66.39
      - pelvic region M66.35- ●
      - shoulder region M66.31- ●
      - specified site NEC M66.38
      - thigh M66.35- ●
      - upper arm M66.32- ●
    - foot M66.87- ●
    - forearm M66.83- ●
    - hand M66.84- ●
    - lower leg M66.86- ●
    - multiple sites M66.89
    - pelvic region M66.85- ●
    - shoulder region M66.81- ●
    - specified
      - site NEC M66.88
      - tendon M66.80

Rupture, ruptured *(Continued)*
- tendon *(Continued)*
  - nontraumatic *(Continued)*
    - thigh M66.85- ●
    - upper arm M66.82- ●
- thoracic duct I89.8
- tonsil J35.8
- traumatic
  - aorta —*see* Injury, aorta, laceration, major
  - diaphragm —*see* Injury, intrathoracic, diaphragm
  - external site —*see* Wound, open, by site
  - eye —*see* Injury, eye, laceration
  - internal organ —*see* Injury, by site
  - intervertebral disc
    - cervical S13.0
    - lumbar S33.0
    - thoracic S23.0
  - kidney S37.06- ●
  - ligament —*see also* Sprain
    - ankle —*see* Sprain, ankle
    - carpus —*see* Rupture, traumatic, ligament, wrist
    - collateral (hand) —*see* Rupture, traumatic, ligament, finger, collateral
    - finger (metacarpophalangeal) (interphalangeal) S63.40- ●
      - collateral S63.41- ●
        - index S63.41- ●
        - little S63.41- ●
        - middle S63.41- ●
        - ring S63.41- ●
      - index S63.40- ●
      - little S63.40- ●
      - middle S63.40- ●
      - palmar S63.42- ●
        - index S63.42- ●
        - little S63.42- ●
        - middle S63.42- ●
        - ring S63.42- ●
      - ring S63.40- ●
      - specified site NEC S63.499
        - index S63.49- ●
        - little S63.49- ●
        - middle S63.49- ●
        - ring S63.49- ●
      - volar plate S63.43- ●
        - index S63.43- ●
        - little S63.43- ●
        - middle S63.43- ●
        - ring S63.43- ●
    - foot —*see* Sprain, foot
    - radial collateral S53.2- ●
    - radiocarpal —*see* Rupture, traumatic, ligament, wrist, radiocarpal
    - ulnar collateral S53.3- ●
    - ulnocarpal —*see* Rupture, traumatic, ligament, wrist, ulnocarpal
    - wrist S63.30- ●
      - collateral S63.31- ●
      - radiocarpal S63.32- ●
      - specified site NEC S63.39- ●
      - ulnocarpal (palmar) S63.33- ●
  - liver S36.116
  - membrana tympani —*see* Rupture, ear drum, traumatic
  - muscle or tendon —*see* Strain
  - myocardium —*see* Injury, heart
  - pancreas S36.299
  - rectum S36.69
  - sigmoid S36.593
  - spleen S36.09
  - stomach S36.39
  - symphysis pubis S33.4
  - tympanum, tympanic (membrane) —*see* Rupture, ear drum, traumatic
  - ureter S37.19
  - uterus S37.69
  - vagina —*see* Injury, vagina
  - vena cava —*see* Injury, vena cava, laceration, major
- tricuspid (heart) (valve) I07.8
- tube, tubal (nonobstetric) (nontraumatic) N83.8
  - abscess —*see* Salpingitis
  - due to pregnancy O00.10- ●
    - with intrauterine pregnancy O00.11- ●
- tympanum, tympanic (membrane) (nontraumatic) —*see also* Perforation, tympanic membrane H72.9- ●
  - traumatic —*see* Rupture, ear drum, traumatic
- umbilical cord, complicating delivery O69.89

Rupture, ruptured *(Continued)*
- ureter (traumatic) S37.19
  - nontraumatic N28.89
- urethra (nontraumatic) N36.8
  - with ectopic or molar pregnancy O08.6
  - following ectopic or molar pregnancy O08.6
  - obstetrical trauma O71.5
  - traumatic S37.39
- uterosacral ligament (nonobstetric) (nontraumatic) N83.8
- uterus (traumatic) S37.69
  - before labor O71.0-●
  - during or after labor O71.1
  - nonpuerperal, nontraumatic N85.8
  - pregnant (during labor) O71.1
    - before labor O71.0-●
- vagina *—see* Injury, vagina
- valve, valvular (heart) *—see* Endocarditis
- varicose vein *—see* Varix
- varix *—see* Varix
- vena cava R58
  - traumatic *—see* Injury, vena cava, laceration, major
- vesical (urinary) N32.89
- vessel (blood) R58
  - pulmonary I28.8
  - traumatic *—see* Injury, blood vessel
- viscus R19.8
- vulva complicating delivery O70.0

Russell-Silver syndrome Q87.19

Russian spring-summer type encephalitis A84.0

Rust's disease (tuberculous cervical spondylitis) A18.01

Ruvalcaba-Myhre-Smith syndrome E71.440

Rytand-Lipsitch syndrome I44.2

S

Saber, sabre shin or tibia (syphilitic) A50.56 *[M90.8-●]*

Sac lacrimal *—see* condition

Saccharomyces infection B37.9

Saccharopinuria E72.3

Saccular *—see* condition

Sacculation
- aorta (nonsyphilitic) *—see* Aneurysm, aorta
- bladder N32.3
- intralaryngeal (congenital) (ventricular) Q31.3
- larynx (congenital) (ventricular) Q31.3
- organ or site, congenital *—see* Distortion
- pregnant uterus *—see* Pregnancy, complicated by, abnormal, uterus
- ureter N28.89
- urethra N36.1
- vesical N32.3

Sachs' amaurotic familial idiocy or disease E75.02

Sachs-Tay disease E75.02

Sacks-Libman disease M32.11

Sacralgia M53.3

Sacralization Q76.49

Sacrodynia M53.3

Sacroiliac joint *—see* condition

Sacroiliitis NEC M46.1

Sacrum *—see* condition

Saddle
- back *—see* Lordosis
- embolus
  - abdominal aorta I74.01
  - pulmonary artery I26.92
    - with acute cor pulmonale I26.02
- injury — code to condition
- nose M95.0
  - due to syphilis A50.57

Sadism (sexual) F65.52

Sadness, postpartal O90.6

Sadomasochism F65.50

Saemisch's ulcer (cornea) *—see* Ulcer, cornea, central

Sagging
- skin and subcutaneous tissue (following bariatric surgery weight loss) (following dietary weight loss) L98.7

Sahib disease B55.0

Sailors' skin L57.8

Saint
- Anthony's fire *—see* Erysipelas
- triad *—see* Hernia, diaphragm
- Vitus' dance *—see* Chorea, Sydenham's

Salaam
- attack(s) *—see* Epilepsy, spasms
- tic R25.8

Salicylism
- abuse F55.8
- overdose or wrong substance given *—see* Table of Drugs and Chemicals, by drug, poisoning

Salivary duct or gland *—see* condition

Salivation, excessive K11.7

Salmonella *—see* Infection, Salmonella

Salmonellosis A02.0

Salpingitis (catarrhal) (fallopian tube) (nodular) (pseudofollicular) (purulent) (septic) N70.91
- with oophoritis N70.93
- acute N70.01
  - with oophoritis N70.03
- chlamydial A56.11
- chronic N70.11
  - with oophoritis N70.13
- complicating abortion *—see* Abortion, by type, complicated by, salpingitis
- ear *—see* Salpingitis, eustachian
- eustachian (tube) H68.00-●
  - acute H68.01-●
  - chronic H68.02-●
- follicularis N70.11
  - with oophoritis N70.13
- gonococcal (acute) (chronic) A54.24
- interstitial, chronic N70.11
  - with oophoritis N70.13
- isthmica nodosa N70.11
  - with oophoritis N70.13
- specific (gonococcal) (acute) (chronic) A54.24
- tuberculous (acute) (chronic) A18.17
- venereal (gonococcal) (acute) (chronic) A54.24

Salpingocele N83.4-●

Salpingo-oophoritis (catarrhal) (purulent) (ruptured) (septic) (suppurative) N70.93
- acute N70.03
  - with ectopic or molar pregnancy O08.0
  - following ectopic or molar pregnancy O08.0
  - gonococcal A54.24
- chronic N70.13
- following ectopic or molar pregnancy O08.0
- gonococcal (acute) (chronic) A54.24
- puerperal O86.19
- specific (gonococcal) (acute) (chronic) A54.24
- subacute N70.03
- tuberculous (acute) (chronic) A18.17
- venereal (gonococcal) (acute) (chronic) A54.24

Salpingo-ovaritis *—see* Salpingo-oophoritis

Salpingoperitonitis *—see* Salpingo-oophoritis

Salzmann's nodular dystrophy *—see* Degeneration, cornea, nodular

Sampson's cyst or tumor N80.10-●

San Joaquin (Valley) **fever** B38.0

Sandblaster's asthma, lung or pneumoconiosis J62.8

Sander's disease (paranoia) F22

Sandfly fever A93.1

Sandhoff's disease E75.01

Sanfilippo (Type B) (Type C) (Type D) **syndrome** E76.22

Sanger-Brown ataxia G11.2

Sao Paulo fever or typhus A77.0

Saponification, mesenteric K65.8

Sarcocele (benign)
- syphilitic A52.76
  - congenital A50.59

Sarcocystosis A07.8

Sarcoepiplocele *—see* Hernia

Sarcoepiplomphalocele Q79.2

Sarcoglycanopathy G71.0340
- alpha G71.0341
- beta G71.0342
- delta G71.0349
- gamma G71.0349

Sarcoid *—see also* Sarcoidosis
- arthropathy D86.86
- Boeck's D86.9
- Darier-Roussy D86.3
- iridocyclitis D86.83
- meningitis D86.81
- myocarditis D86.85
- myositis D86.87
- pyelonephritis D86.84
- Spiegler-Fendt L08.89

Sarcoidosis D86.9
- with
  - cranial nerve palsies D86.82
  - hepatic granuloma D86.89
  - polyarthritis D86.86
  - tubulo-interstitial nephropathy D86.84
- combined sites NEC D86.89
- lung D86.0
  - and lymph nodes D86.2
- lymph nodes D86.1
  - and lung D86.2
- meninges D86.81
- skin D86.3
- specified type NEC D86.89

Sarcoma (of) *—see also* Neoplasm, connective tissue, malignant
- alveolar soft part *—see* Neoplasm, connective tissue, malignant
- ameloblastic C41.1
  - upper jaw (bone) C41.0
- botryoid *—see* Neoplasm, connective tissue, malignant
- botryoides *—see* Neoplasm, connective tissue, malignant
- cerebellar C71.6
  - circumscribed (arachnoidal) C71.6
- circumscribed (arachnoidal) cerebellar C71.6
- clear cell *—see also* Neoplasm, connective tissue, malignant
  - kidney C64.-●
- dendritic cells (accessory cells) C96.4
- embryonal *—see* Neoplasm, connective tissue, malignant
- endometrial (stromal) C54.1
  - isthmus C54.0
- epithelioid (cell) *—see* Neoplasm, connective tissue, malignant
- Ewing's *—see* Neoplasm, bone, malignant
- follicular dendritic cell C96.4
- germinoblastic (diffuse) *—see* Lymphoma, diffuse, large cell
  - follicular *—see* Lymphoma, follicular, specified NEC
- giant cell (except of bone) *—see also* Neoplasm, connective tissue, malignant
  - bone *—see* Neoplasm, bone, malignant
- glomoid *—see* Neoplasm, connective tissue, malignant
- granulocytic C92.3-●
- hemangioendothelial *—see* Neoplasm, connective tissue, malignant
- hemorrhagic, multiple *—see* Sarcoma, Kaposi's
- histiocytic C96.A
- Hodgkin *—see* Lymphoma, Hodgkin
- immunoblastic (diffuse) *—see* Lymphoma, diffuse large cell
- interdigitating dendritic cell C96.4
- Kaposi's
  - colon C46.4
  - connective tissue C46.1
  - gastrointestinal organ C46.4
  - lung C46.5-●
  - lymph node(s) C46.3
  - palate (hard) (soft) C46.2
  - rectum C46.4
  - skin C46.0
  - specified site NEC C46.7
  - stomach C46.4
  - unspecified site C46.9
- Kupffer cell C22.3
- Langerhans cell C96.4
- leptomeningeal *—see* Neoplasm, meninges, malignant
- liver NEC C22.4
- lymphangioendothelial *—see* Neoplasm, connective tissue, malignant
- lymphoblastic *—see* Lymphoma, lymphoblastic (diffuse)
- lymphocytic *—see* Lymphoma, small cell B-cell
- mast cell C96.22
- melanotic *—see* Melanoma
- meningeal *—see* Neoplasm, meninges, malignant
- meningothelial *—see* Neoplasm, meninges, malignant
- mesenchymal *—see also* Neoplasm, connective tissue, malignant
  - mixed *—see* Neoplasm, connective tissue, malignant
- mesothelial *—see* Mesothelioma

Sarcoma *(Continued)*
monstrocellular
specified site —*see* Neoplasm, malignant, by site
unspecified site C71.9
myeloid C92.3-●
neurogenic —*see* Neoplasm, nerve, malignant
odontogenic C41.1
upper jaw (bone) C41.Ø
osteoblastic —*see* Neoplasm, bone, malignant
osteogenic —*see also* Neoplasm, bone, malignant
juxtacortical —*see* Neoplasm, bone, malignant
periosteal —*see* Neoplasm, bone, malignant
periosteal —*see also* Neoplasm, bone, malignant
osteogenic —*see* Neoplasm, bone, malignant
pleomorphic cell —*see* Neoplasm, connective tissue, malignant
reticulum cell (diffuse) —*see* Lymphoma, diffuse large cell
nodular —*see* Lymphoma, follicular
pleomorphic cell type —*see* Lymphoma, diffuse large cell
rhabdoid —*see* Neoplasm, malignant, by site
round cell —*see* Neoplasm, connective tissue, malignant
small cell —*see* Neoplasm, connective tissue, malignant
soft tissue —*see* Neoplasm, connective tissue, malignant
spindle cell —*see* Neoplasm, connective tissue, malignant
stromal (endometrial) C54.1
isthmus C54.Ø
synovial —*see also* Neoplasm, connective tissue, malignant
biphasic —*see* Neoplasm, connective tissue, malignant
epithelioid cell —*see* Neoplasm, connective tissue, malignant
spindle cell —*see* Neoplasm, connective tissue, malignant
Sarcomatosis
meningeal —*see* Neoplasm, meninges, malignant
specified site NEC —*see* Neoplasm, connective tissue, malignant
unspecified site C8Ø.1
Sarcopenia (age-related) M62.84
Sarcosinemia E72.59
Sarcosporidiosis (intestinal) AØ7.8
SARS-CoV-2 —*see also* COVID-19
sequelae (post acute) UØ9.9
Satiety, early R68.81
Saturnine —*see* condition
Saturnism
overdose or wrong substance given or taken —*see* Table of Drugs and Chemicals, by drug, poisoning
Satyriasis F52.8
Sauriasis —*see* Ichthyosis
SBE (subacute bacterial endocarditis) I33.Ø
Scabies (any site) B86
Scabs R23.4
Scaglietti-Dagnini syndrome E22.Ø
Scald —*see* Burn
Scalenus anticus (anterior) **syndrome** G54.Ø
Scales R23.4
Scaling, skin R23.4
Scalp —*see* condition
Scapegoating affecting child Z62.3
Scaphocephaly, non-deformational Q75.Ø1
Scapulalgia M89.8X1
Scapulohumeral myopathy G71.Ø2
Scar, scarring —*see also* Cicatrix L9Ø.5
adherent L9Ø.5
atrophic L9Ø.5
cervix
in pregnancy or childbirth —*see* Pregnancy, complicated by, abnormal cervix
cheloid L91.Ø
chorioretinal H31.ØØ-●
posterior pole macula H31.Ø1-●
postsurgical H59.81-●
solar retinopathy H31.Ø2-●
specified type NEC H31.Ø9-●
choroid —*see* Scar, chorioretinal
conjunctiva H11.24-●
cornea H17.9
xerophthalmic —*see also* Opacity, cornea
vitamin A deficiency E5Ø.6
defect (isthmocele) O34.22
duodenum, obstructive K31.5

Scar, scarring *(Continued)*
hypertrophic L91.Ø
keloid L91.Ø
labia N9Ø.89
lung (base) J98.4
macula —*see* Scar, chorioretinal, posterior pole
muscle M62.89
myocardium, myocardial I25.2
painful L9Ø.5
posterior pole (eye) —*see* Scar, chorioretinal, posterior pole
retina —*see* Scar, chorioretinal
trachea J39.8
transmural uterine, in pregnancy O34.29
uterus N85.8
in pregnancy O34.29
vagina N89.8
postoperative N99.2
vulva N9Ø.89
Scarabiasis B88.2
Scarlatina (anginosa) (maligna) A38.9
myocarditis (acute) A38.1
old —*see* Myocarditis
otitis media A38.Ø
ulcerosa A38.8
Scarlet fever (albuminuria) (angina) A38.9
Schamberg's disease (progressive pigmentary dermatosis) L81.7
Schatzki's ring (acquired) (esophagus) (lower) K22.2
congenital Q39.3
Schaufenster krankheit I2Ø.89
Schaumann's
benign lymphogranulomatosis D86.1
disease or syndrome —*see* Sarcoidosis
Scheie's syndrome E76.Ø3
Schenck's disease B42.1
Scheuermann's disease or osteochondrosis —*see* Osteochondrosis, juvenile, spine
Schilder (-Flatau) **disease** G37.Ø
Schilling-type monocytic leukemia C93.Ø-●
Schimmelbusch's disease, cystic mastitis, or hyperplasia —*see* Mastopathy, cystic
Schistosoma infestation —*see* Infestation, Schistosoma
Schistosomiasis B65.9
with muscle disorder B65.9 *[M63.8Ø]*
ankle B65.9 *[M63.87-●]*
foot B65.9 *[M63.87-●]*
forearm B65.9 *[M63.83-●]*
hand B65.9 *[M63.84-●]*
lower leg B65.9 *[M63.86-●]*
multiple sites B65.9 *[M63.89]*
pelvic region B65.9 *[M63.85-●]*
shoulder region B65.9 *[M63.81-●]*
specified site NEC B65.9 *[M63.88]*
thigh B65.9 *[M63.85-●]*
upper arm B65.9 *[M63.82-●]*
Asiatic B65.2
bladder B65.Ø
chestermani B65.8
colon B65.1
cutaneous B65.3
due to
S. haematobium B65.Ø
S. japonicum B65.2
S. mansoni B65.1
S. mattheii B65.8
Eastern B65.2
genitourinary tract B65.Ø
intestinal B65.1
lung NEC B65.9 *[J99]*
pneumonia B65.9 *[J17]*
Manson's (intestinal) B65.1
oriental B65.2
pulmonary NEC B65.9 *[J99]*
pneumonia B65.9
Schistosoma
haematobium B65.Ø
japonicum B65.2
mansoni B65.1
specified type NEC B65.8
urinary B65.Ø
vesical B65.Ø
Schizencephaly QØ4.6
Schizoaffective psychosis F25.9
Schizodontia KØØ.2
Schizoid personality F6Ø.1
Schizophrenia, schizophrenic F2Ø.9
acute (brief) (undifferentiated) F23
atypical (form) F2Ø.3

Schizophrenia, schizophrenic *(Continued)*
borderline F21
catalepsy F2Ø.2
catatonic (type) (excited) (withdrawn) F2Ø.2
cenesthopathic, cenesthesiopathic F2Ø.89
childhood type F2Ø.9
chronic undifferentiated F2Ø.9
cyclic F25.Ø
disorganized (type) F2Ø.1
flexibilitas cerea F2Ø.2
hebephrenic (type) F2Ø.1
incipient F21
latent F21
negative type F2Ø.5
paranoid (type) F2Ø.Ø
paraphrenic F2Ø.Ø
post-psychotic depression F32.89
prepsychotic F21
prodromal F21
pseudoneurotic F21
pseudopsychopathic F21
reaction F23
residual (state) (type) F2Ø.5
restzustand F2Ø.5
schizoaffective (type) —*see* Psychosis, schizoaffective
simple (type) F2Ø.89
simplex F2Ø.89
specified type NEC F2Ø.89
spectrum and other psychotic disorder F29
specified NEC F28
stupor F2Ø.2
syndrome of childhood F84.5
undifferentiated (type) F2Ø.3
chronic F2Ø.5
Schizothymia (persistent) F6Ø.1
Schlatter-Osgood disease or osteochondrosis M92.52-●
Schlatter's tibia —*see* Osteochondrosis, juvenile, tibia
Schmidt's syndrome (polyglandular, autoimmune) E31.Ø
Schmincke's carcinoma or tumor —*see* Neoplasm, nasopharynx, malignant
Schmitz (-Stutzer) **dysentery** AØ3.Ø
Schmorl's disease or nodes
lumbar region M51.46
lumbosacral region M51.47
sacrococcygeal region M53.3
thoracic region M51.44
thoracolumbar region M51.45
Schneiderian
papilloma —*see* Neoplasm, nasopharynx benign
specified site —*see* Neoplasm, benign, by site
unspecified site D14.Ø
specified site —*see* Neoplasm, malignant, by site
unspecified site C3Ø.Ø
Scholte's syndrome (malignant carcinoid) E34.Ø9
Scholz (-Bielchowsky-Henneberg) **disease or syndrome** E75.25
Schönlein (-Henoch) **disease or purpura** (primary) (rheumatic) D69.Ø
Schottmuller's disease AØ1.4
Schroeder's syndrome (endocrine hypertensive) E27.Ø
Schüller-Christian disease or syndrome C96.5
Schultze's type acroparesthesia, simple I73.89
Schultz's disease or syndrome —*see* Agranulocytosis
Schwalbe-Ziehen-Oppenheim disease G24.1
Schwannoma —*see also* Neoplasm, nerve, benign
malignant —*see also* Neoplasm, nerve, malignant
with rhabdomyoblastic differentiation —*see* Neoplasm, nerve, malignant
melanocytic —*see* Neoplasm, nerve, benign
pigmented —*see* Neoplasm, nerve, benign
Schwannomatosis Q85.Ø3
Schwartz (-Jampel) **syndrome** G71.13
Schwartz-Bartter syndrome E22.2
~~Schweniger-Buzzi anetoderma L9Ø.1~~
Schweninger-Buzzi anetoderma L9Ø.1
Sciatic —*see* condition
Sciatica (infective) M54.3-●
with lumbago M54.4-●
due to intervertebral disc disorder —*see* Disorder, disc, with, radiculopathy
due to displacement of intervertebral disc (with lumbago) —*see* Disorder, disc, with, radiculopathy
wallet M54.3-●

S

- **Scimitar syndrome** Q26.8
- **Sclera** —*see* condition
- **Sclerectasia** H15.84-●
- **Scleredema**
  - adultorum —*see* Sclerosis, systemic
  - Buschke's —*see* Sclerosis, systemic
  - newborn P83.Ø
- **Sclerema** (adiposum) (edematosum) (neonatorum) (newborn) P83.Ø
  - adultorum —*see* Sclerosis, systemic
- **Scleriasis** —*see* Scleroderma
- **Scleritis** H15.ØØ-●
  - with corneal involvement H15.Ø4-●
  - anterior H15.Ø1-●
  - brawny H15.Ø2-●
  - in (due to) zoster BØ2.34
  - posterior H15.Ø3-●
  - specified type NEC H15.Ø9-●
  - syphilitic A52.71
  - tuberculous (nodular) A18.51
- **Sclerochoroiditis** H31.8
- **Scleroconjunctivitis** —*see* Scleritis
- **Sclerocystic ovary syndrome** E28.2
- **Sclerodactyly, sclerodactylia** L94.3
- **Scleroderma, sclerodermia** (acrosclerotic) (diffuse) (generalized) (progressive) (pulmonary) —*see also* Sclerosis, systemic M34.9-●
  - circumscribed L94.Ø
  - linear L94.1
  - localized L94.Ø
  - newborn P83.88
  - systemic M34.9
- **Sclerokeratitis** H16.8
  - tuberculous A18.52
- **Scleroma nasi** A48.8
- **Scleromalacia** (perforans) H15.Ø5-●
- **Scleromyxedema** L98.5
- **Sclérose en plaques** G35
- **Sclerosis, sclerotic**
  - adrenal (gland) E27.8
  - Alzheimer's —*see* Disease, Alzheimer's
  - amyotrophic (lateral) G12.21
  - aorta, aortic I7Ø.Ø
    - valve —*see* Endocarditis, aortic
  - artery, arterial, arteriolar, arteriovascular —*see* Arteriosclerosis
  - ascending multiple G35
  - brain (generalized) (lobular) G37.9
    - artery, arterial I67.2
    - diffuse G37.Ø
    - disseminated G35
    - insular G35
    - Krabbe's E75.23
    - miliary G35
    - multiple G35
    - presenile (Alzheimer's) —*see* Disease, Alzheimer's, early onset
    - senile (arteriosclerotic) I67.2
    - stem, multiple G35
    - tuberous Q85.1
  - bulbar, multiple G35
  - bundle of His I44.39
  - cardiac —*see* Disease, heart, ischemic, atherosclerotic
  - cardiorenal —*see* Hypertension, cardiorenal
  - cardiovascular —*see also* Disease, cardiovascular
    - renal —*see* Hypertension, cardiorenal
  - cerebellar —*see* Sclerosis, brain
  - cerebral —*see* Sclerosis, brain
  - cerebrospinal (disseminated) (multiple) G35
  - cerebrovascular I67.2
  - choroid —*see* Degeneration, choroid
  - combined (spinal cord) —*see also* Degeneration, combined
    - multiple G35
  - concentric (Balo) G37.5
  - cornea —*see* Opacity, cornea
  - coronary (artery) I25.1Ø
    - with angina pectoris —*see* Arteriosclerosis, coronary (artery),
  - corpus cavernosum
    - female N9Ø.89
    - male N48.6
  - diffuse (brain) (spinal cord) G37.Ø
  - disseminated G35
  - dorsal G35
  - dorsolateral (spinal cord) —*see* Degeneration, combined
  - endometrium N85.5
  - extrapyramidal G25.9

Sclerosis, sclerotic *(Continued)*

  - eye, nuclear (senile) —*see* Cataract, senile, nuclear
  - focal and segmental (glomerular) —*see also* NØØ-NØ7 with fourth character .1 NØ5.1
  - Friedreich's (spinal cord) G11.11
  - funicular (spermatic cord) N5Ø.89
  - general (vascular) —*see* Arteriosclerosis
  - gland (lymphatic) I89.8
  - hepatic K74.1
    - alcoholic K7Ø.2
  - hereditary
    - cerebellar G11.9
    - spinal (Friedreich's ataxia) G11.11
  - hippocampal G93.81
  - insular G35
  - kidney —*see* Sclerosis, renal
  - larynx J38.7
  - lateral (amyotrophic) (descending) (spinal) G12.21
    - primary G12.23
  - lens, senile nuclear —*see* Cataract, senile, nuclear
  - liver K74.1
    - with fibrosis K74.2
      - alcoholic K7Ø.2
    - alcoholic K7Ø.2
    - cardiac K76.1
  - lung —*see* Fibrosis, lung
  - mastoid —*see* Mastoiditis, chronic
  - mesial temporal G93.81
  - mitral IØ5.8
  - Mönckeberg's (medial) —*see* Arteriosclerosis, extremities
  - multiple (brain stem) (cerebral) (generalized) (spinal cord) G35
  - myocardium, myocardial —*see* Disease, heart, ischemic, atherosclerotic
  - nuclear (senile), eye —*see* Cataract, senile, nuclear
  - ovary N83.8
  - pancreas K86.89
  - penis N48.6
  - peripheral arteries —*see* Arteriosclerosis, extremities
  - plaques G35
  - pluriglandular E31.8
  - polyglandular E31.8
  - posterolateral (spinal cord) —*see* Degeneration, combined
  - presenile (Alzheimer's) —*see* Disease, Alzheimer's, early onset
  - primary, lateral G12.23
  - progressive, systemic M34.Ø
  - pulmonary —*see* Fibrosis, lung
    - artery I27.Ø
    - valve (heart) —*see* Endocarditis, pulmonary
  - renal N26.9
    - with
      - cystine storage disease E72.Ø9
      - hypertensive heart disease (conditions in I11) —*see* Hypertension, cardiorenal
    - arteriolar (hyaline) (hyperplastic) —*see* Hypertension, kidney
  - retina (senile) (vascular) H35.ØØ
  - senile (vascular) —*see* Arteriosclerosis
  - spinal (cord) (progressive) G95.89
    - ascending G61.Ø
    - combined —*see also* Degeneration, combined
      - multiple G35
      - syphilitic A52.11
    - disseminated G35
    - dorsolateral —*see* Degeneration, combined
    - hereditary (Friedreich's) (mixed form) G11.11
    - lateral (amyotrophic) G12.21
      - progressive G12.23
    - multiple G35
    - posterior (syphilitic) A52.11
  - stomach K31.89
  - subendocardial, congenital I42.4
  - systemic M34.9
    - with
      - lung involvement M34.81
      - myopathy M34.82
      - polyneuropathy M34.83
    - drug-induced M34.2
    - due to chemicals NEC M34.2
    - progressive M34.Ø
    - specified NEC M34.89
  - temporal (mesial) G93.81
  - tricuspid (heart) (valve) IØ7.8
  - tuberous (brain) Q85.1

Sclerosis, sclerotic *(Continued)*

  - tympanic membrane —*see* Disorder, tympanic membrane, specified NEC
  - valve, valvular (heart) —*see* Endocarditis
  - vascular —*see* Arteriosclerosis
  - vein I87.8
- **Scoliosis** (acquired) (postural) M41.9
  - adolescent (idiopathic) —*see* Scoliosis, idiopathic, adolescent
  - congenital Q67.5
    - due to bony malformation Q76.3
    - failure of segmentation (hemivertebra) Q76.3
    - hemivertebra fusion Q76.3
    - postural Q67.5
  - degenerative M41.5-●
  - idiopathic M41.2Ø
    - adolescent M41.129
      - cervical region M41.122
      - cervicothoracic region M41.123
      - lumbar region M41.126
      - lumbosacral region M41.127
      - thoracic region M41.124
      - thoracolumbar region M41.125
    - cervical region M41.22
    - cervicothoracic region M41.23
    - infantile M41.ØØ
      - cervical region M41.Ø2
      - cervicothoracic region M41.Ø3
      - lumbar region M41.Ø6
      - lumbosacral region M41.Ø7
      - sacrococcygeal region M41.Ø8
      - thoracic region M41.Ø4
      - thoracolumbar region M41.Ø5
    - juvenile M41.119
      - cervical region M41.112
      - cervicothoracic region M41.113
      - lumbar region M41.116
      - lumbosacral region M41.117
      - thoracic region M41.114
      - thoracolumbar region M41.115
    - lumbar region M41.26
    - lumbosacral region M41.27
    - thoracic region M41.24
    - thoracolumbar region M41.25
  - infantile —*see* Scoliosis, idiopathic, infantile
  - neuromuscular M41.4Ø
    - cervical region M41.42
    - cervicothoracic region M41.43
    - lumbar region M41.46
    - lumbosacral region M41.47
    - occipito-atlanto-axial region M41.41
    - thoracic region M41.44
    - thoracolumbar region M41.45
  - paralytic —*see* Scoliosis, neuromuscular
  - postprocedural M96.89
  - postradiation therapy M96.5
  - rachitic (late effect or sequelae) E64.3 *[M49.8Ø]*
    - cervical region E64.3 *[M49.82]*
    - cervicothoracic region E64.3 *[M49.83]*
    - lumbar region E64.3 *[M49.86]*
    - lumbosacral region E64.3 *[M49.87]*
    - multiple sites E64.3 *[M49.89]*
    - occipito-atlanto-axial region E64.3 *[M49.81]*
    - sacrococcygeal region E64.3 *[M49.88]*
    - thoracic region E64.3 *[M49.84]*
    - thoracolumbar region E64.3 *[M49.85]*
  - sciatic M54.4-●
  - secondary (to) NEC M41.5Ø
    - cerebral palsy, Friedreich's ataxia, poliomyelitis, neuromuscular disorders —*see* Scoliosis, neuromuscular
    - cervical region M41.52
    - cervicothoracic region M41.53
    - lumbar region M41.56
    - lumbosacral region M41.57
    - thoracic region M41.54
    - thoracolumbar region M41.55
  - specified form NEC M41.8Ø
    - cervical region M41.82
    - cervicothoracic region M41.83
    - lumbar region M41.86
    - lumbosacral region M41.87
    - thoracic region M41.84
    - thoracolumbar region M41.85
  - thoracogenic M41.3Ø
    - thoracic region M41.34
    - thoracolumbar region M41.35
  - tuberculous A18.Ø1

S

New   Revised   ~~deleted~~ Deleted   ● Use Additional Character(s)

S

Sequelae *(Continued)*
- hemorrhage *(Continued)*
  - intracranial, nontraumatic *(Continued)*
    - hemiplegia I69.25-•
    - language deficit NEC I69.228
    - monoplegia
      - lower limb I69.24-•
      - upper limb I69.23-•
    - paralytic syndrome I69.26-•
    - specified effect NEC I69.298
    - speech deficit NEC I69.228
  - subarachnoid I69.00
    - alteration of sensation I69.098
    - aphasia I69.020
    - apraxia I69.090
    - ataxia I69.093
    - cognitive deficits —*see* subcategory I69.01-•
    - disturbance of vision I69.098
    - dysarthria I69.022
    - dysphagia I69.091
    - dysphasia I69.021
    - facial droop I69.092
    - facial weakness I69.092
    - fluency disorder I69.023
    - hemiplegia I69.05-•
    - language deficit NEC I69.028
    - monoplegia
      - lower limb I69.04-•
      - upper limb I69.03-•
    - paralytic syndrome I69.06-•
    - specified effect NEC I69.098
    - speech deficit NEC I69.028
- hepatitis, viral B94.2
- hyperalimentation E68
- infarction
  - cerebral I69.30
    - alteration of sensation I69.398
    - aphasia I69.320
    - apraxia I69.390
    - ataxia I69.393
    - cognitive deficits I69.31
    - disturbance of vision I69.398
    - dysarthria I69.322
    - dysphagia I69.391
    - dysphasia I69.321
    - facial droop I69.392
    - facial weakness I69.392
    - fluency disorder I69.323
    - hemiplegia I69.35-•
    - language deficit NEC I69.328
    - monoplegia
      - lower limb I69.34-•
      - upper limb I69.33-•
    - paralytic syndrome I69.36-•
    - specified effect NEC I69.398
    - speech deficit NEC I69.328
- infection, pyogenic, intracranial or intraspinal G09
- infectious disease B94.9
  - specified NEC B94.8
- injury — code to injury with seventh character S
- leprosy B92
- meningitis
  - bacterial (conditions in G00) G09
  - other or unspecified cause (conditions in G03) G09
- muscle (and tendon) injury — code to injury with seventh character S
- myelitis —*see* Sequelae, encephalitis
- niacin deficiency E64.8
- nutritional deficiency E64.9
  - specified NEC E64.8
- obstetrical condition O94
- parasitic disease B94.9
- phlebitis or thrombophlebitis of intracranial or intraspinal venous sinuses and veins (conditions in G08) G09
- poisoning — code to poisoning with seventh character S
  - nonmedicinal substance —*see* Sequelae, toxic effect, nonmedicinal substance
- poliomyelitis (acute) B91
- pregnancy O94
- protein-energy malnutrition E64.0
- puerperium O94
- rickets E64.3
- SARS-CoV-2 (post acute) U09.9
- selenium deficiency E64.8
- sprain and strain — code to injury with seventh character S

Sequelae *(Continued)*
- stroke NOS I69.30
  - alteration in sensation I69.398
  - aphasia I69.320
  - apraxia I69.390
  - ataxia I69.393
  - cognitive deficits I69.31
  - disturbance of vision I69.398
  - dysarthria I69.322
  - dysphagia I69.391
  - dysphasia I69.321
  - facial droop I69.392
  - facial weakness I69.392
  - hemiplegia I69.35-•
  - language deficit NEC I69.328
  - monoplegia
    - lower limb I69.34-•
    - upper limb I69.33-•
  - paralytic syndrome I69.36-•
  - specified effect NEC I69.398
  - speech deficit NEC I69.328
- tendon and muscle injury — code to injury with seventh character S
- thiamine deficiency E64.8
- trachoma B94.0
- tuberculosis B90.9
  - bones and joints B90.2
  - central nervous system B90.0
  - genitourinary B90.1
  - pulmonary (respiratory) B90.9
  - specified organs NEC B90.8
- viral
  - encephalitis B94.1
  - hepatitis B94.2
- vitamin deficiency NEC E64.8
  - A E64.1
  - B E64.8
  - C E64.2
- wound, open — code to injury with seventh character S

Sequestration —*see also* Sequestrum
- disc —*see* Displacement, intervertebral disc
- lung, congenital Q33.2

Sequestrum
- bone —*see* Osteomyelitis, chronic
- dental M27.2
- jaw bone M27.2
- orbit —*see* Osteomyelitis, orbit
- sinus (accessory) (nasal) —*see* Sinusitis

Sequoiosis lung or pneumonitis J67.8

Serology for syphilis
- doubtful
  - with signs or symptoms - code by site and stage under Syphilis
  - follow-up of latent syphilis —*see* Syphilis, latent
- negative, with signs or symptoms — code by site and stage under Syphilis
- positive A53.0
  - with signs or symptoms - code by site and stage under Syphilis
- reactivated A53.0

Seroma —*see also* Hematoma
- postprocedural —*see* Complication, postprocedural, seroma
- traumatic, secondary and recurrent T79.2

Seropurulent —*see* condition

Serositis, multiple K65.8
- pericardial I31.1
- peritoneal K65.8

Serous —*see* condition

Sertoli cell
- adenoma
  - specified site —*see* Neoplasm, benign, by site
  - unspecified site
    - female D27.9
    - male D29.20
- carcinoma
  - specified site —*see* Neoplasm, malignant, by site
  - unspecified site (male) C62.9-•
    - female C56.9
- tumor
  - with lipid storage
    - specified site —*see* Neoplasm, benign, by site
    - unspecified site
      - female D27.9
      - male D29.20
  - specified site —*see* Neoplasm, benign, by site
  - unspecified site
    - female D27.9
    - male D29.20

Sertoli-Leydig cell tumor —*see* Neoplasm, benign, by site
- specified site —*see* Neoplasm, benign, by site
- unspecified site
  - female D27.9
  - male D29.20

Serum
- allergy, allergic reaction —*see also* Reaction, serum T80.69
  - shock —*see also* Shock, anaphylactic T80.59
- arthritis —*see also* Reaction, serum T80.69
- complication or reaction NEC —*see also* Reaction, serum T80.69
- disease NEC —*see also* Reaction, serum T80.69
- hepatitis —*see also* Hepatitis, viral, type B carrier (suspected) of B18.1
- intoxication —*see also* Reaction, serum T80.69
- neuritis —*see also* Reaction, serum T80.69
- neuropathy G61.1
- poisoning NEC —*see also* Reaction, serum T80.69
- rash NEC —*see also* Reaction, serum T80.69
- reaction NEC —*see also* Reaction, serum T80.69
- sickness NEC —*see also* Reaction, serum T80.69
- urticaria —*see also* Reaction, serum T80.69

Sesamoiditis M25.8-•

Sever's disease or osteochondrosis —*see* Osteochondrosis, juvenile, tarsus

Severe sepsis R65.20
- with septic shock R65.21

Sex
- chromosome mosaics Q97.8
  - lines with various numbers of X chromosomes Q97.2
- education Z70.8
- reassignment surgery status Z87.890

Sextuplet pregnancy —*see* Pregnancy, sextuplet

Sexual
- function, disorder of (psychogenic) F52.9
- immaturity (female) (male) E30.0
- impotence (psychogenic) organic origin NEC —*see* Dysfunction, sexual, male
- precocity (constitutional) (cryptogenic) (female) (idiopathic) (male) E30.1

Sexuality, pathologic —*see* Deviation, sexual

Sézary disease C84.1-•

Shadow, lung R91.8

Shaking palsy or paralysis —*see* Parkinsonism

Shallowness, acetabulum —*see* Derangement, joint, specified type NEC, hip

Shaver's disease J63.1

Sheath (tendon) —*see* condition

Sheathing, retinal vessels H35.01-•

Shedding
- nail L60.8
- premature, primary (deciduous) teeth K00.6

Sheehan's disease or syndrome E23.0

Shelf, rectal K62.89

Shell teeth K00.5

Shellshock (current) F43.0
- lasting state —*see* Disorder, post-traumatic stress

Shield kidney Q63.1

Shift
- auditory threshold (temporary) H93.24-•
- mediastinal R93.89

Shifting sleep-work schedule (affecting sleep) G47.26

Shiga (-Kruse) dysentery A03.0

Shiga's bacillus A03.0

Shigella (dysentery) —*see* Dysentery, bacillary

Shigellosis A03.9
- Group A A03.0
- Group B A03.1
- Group C A03.2
- Group D A03.3

Shin splints S86.89

Shingles —*see* Herpes, zoster

Shipyard disease or eye B30.0

Shirodkar suture, in pregnancy —*see* Pregnancy, complicated by, incompetent cervix

Shock R57.9
- with ectopic or molar pregnancy O08.3
- adrenal (cortical) (Addisonian) E27.2
- adverse food reaction (anaphylactic) —*see* Shock, anaphylactic, due to food
- allergic —*see* Shock, anaphylactic

S

S

S

Spondylosis *(Continued)*
  with *(Continued)*
    radiculopathy M47.2Ø
      cervical region M47.22
      cervicothoracic region M47.23
      lumbar region M47.26
      lumbosacral region M47.27
      occipito-atlanto-axial region M47.21
      sacrococcygeal region M47.28
      thoracic region M47.24
      thoracolumbar region M47.25
  without myelopathy or radiculopathy M47.819
    cervical region M47.812
    cervicothoracic region M47.813
    lumbar region M47.816
    lumbosacral region M47.817
    occipito-atlanto-axial region M47.811
    sacrococcygeal region M47.818
    thoracic region M47.814
    thoracolumbar region M47.815
  specified NEC M47.899
    cervical region M47.892
    cervicothoracic region M47.893
    facet joint M47.819
    lumbar region M47.896
    lumbosacral region M47.897
    occipito-atlanto-axial region M47.891
    sacrococcygeal region M47.898
    thoracic region M47.894
    thoracolumbar region M47.895
  traumatic —*see* Spondylopathy, traumatic
Sponge
  inadvertently left in operation wound —*see* Foreign body, accidentally left during a procedure
  kidney (medullary) Q61.5
Sponge-diver's disease —*see* Toxicity, venom, marine animal, sea anemone
Spongioblastoma (any type) —*see* Neoplasm, malignant, by site
  specified site —*see* Neoplasm, malignant, by site
  unspecified site C71.9
Spongioneuroblastoma —*see* Neoplasm, malignant, by site
Spontaneous —*see also* condition
  fracture (cause unknown) —*see* Fracture, pathological
Spoon nail L6Ø.3
  congenital Q84.6
Sporadic —*see* condition
Sporothrix schenckii infection —*see* Sporotrichosis
Sporotrichosis B42.9
  arthritis B42.82
  disseminated B42.7
  generalized B42.7
  lymphocutaneous (fixed) (progressive) B42.1
  pulmonary B42.Ø
  specified NEC B42.89
Spots, spotting (in) (of)
  Bitot's —*see also* Pigmentation, conjunctiva
    in the young child E5Ø.1
    vitamin A deficiency E5Ø.1
  café, au lait L81.3
  Cayenne pepper I78.1
  cotton wool, retina —*see* Occlusion, artery, retina
  de Morgan's (senile angiomas) I78.1
  Fuchs' black (myopic) —*see also* Myopia, degenerative H44.2-●
  intermenstrual (regular) N92.Ø
    irregular N92.1
  Koplik's BØ5.9
  liver L81.4
  pregnancy O26.85-●
  purpuric R23.3
  ruby I78.1
Spotted fever —*see* Fever, spotted A77.9
Sprain (joint) (ligament)
  acromioclavicular joint or ligament S43.5-●
  ankle S93.4Ø-●
    calcaneofibular ligament S93.41-●
    deltoid ligament S93.42-●
    internal collateral ligament —*see* Sprain, ankle, specified ligament NEC
    specified ligament NEC S93.49-●
    talofibular ligament —*see* Sprain, ankle, specified ligament NEC
    tibiofibular ligament S93.43-●
  anterior longitudinal, cervical S13.4
  atlas, atlanto-axial, atlanto-occipital S13.4
  breast bone —*see* Sprain, sternum
  calcaneofibular —*see* Sprain, ankle

Sprain *(Continued)*
  carpal —*see* Sprain, wrist
  carpometacarpal —*see* Sprain, hand, specified site NEC
  cartilage
    costal S23.41
    semilunar (knee) —*see* Sprain, knee, specified site NEC
      with current tear —*see* Tear, meniscus
    thyroid region S13.5
    xiphoid —*see* Sprain, sternum
  cervical, cervicodorsal, cervicothoracic S13.4
  chondrosternal S23.421
  coracoclavicular S43.8-●
  coracohumeral S43.41-●
  coronary, knee —*see* Sprain, knee, specified site NEC
  costal cartilage S23.41
  cricoarytenoid articulation or ligament S13.5
  cricothyroid articulation S13.5
  cruciate, knee —*see* Sprain, knee, cruciate
  deltoid, ankle —*see* Sprain, ankle
  dorsal (spine) S23.3
  elbow S53.4Ø-●
    radial collateral ligament S53.43-●
    radiohumeral S53.41-●
    rupture
      radial collateral ligament —*see* Rupture, traumatic, ligament, radial collateral
      ulnar collateral ligament —*see* Rupture, traumatic, ligament, ulnar collateral
    specified type NEC S53.49-●
    ulnar collateral ligament S53.44-●
    ulnohumeral S53.42-●
  femur, head —*see* Sprain, hip
  fibular collateral, knee —*see* Sprain, knee, collateral
  fibulocalcaneal —*see* Sprain, ankle
  finger(s) S63.61-●
    index S63.61-●
    interphalangeal (joint) S63.63-●
      index S63.63-●
      little S63.63-●
      middle S63.63-●
      ring S63.63-●
    little S63.61-●
    metacarpophalangeal (joint) S63.65-●
    middle S63.61-●
    ring S63.61-●
    specified site NEC S63.69-●
      index S63.69-●
      little S63.69-●
      middle S63.69-●
      ring S63.69-●
  foot S93.6Ø-●
    specified ligament NEC S93.69-●
    tarsal ligament S93.61-●
    tarsometatarsal ligament S93.62-●
    toe —*see* Sprain, toe
  hand S63.9-●
    finger —*see* Sprain, finger
    specified site NEC —*see* subcategory S63.8
    thumb —*see* Sprain, thumb
  head SØ3.9
  hip S73.1Ø-●
    iliofemoral ligament S73.11-●
    ischiocapsular (ligament) S73.12-●
    specified NEC S73.19-●
  iliofemoral —*see* Sprain, hip
  innominate
    acetabulum —*see* Sprain, hip
    sacral junction S33.6
  internal
    collateral, ankle —*see* Sprain, ankle
    semilunar cartilage —*see* Sprain, knee, specified site NEC
  interphalangeal
    finger —*see* Sprain, finger, interphalangeal (joint)
    toe —*see* Sprain, toe, interphalangeal joint
  ischiocapsular —*see* Sprain, hip
  ischiofemoral —*see* Sprain, hip
  jaw (articular disc) (cartilage) (meniscus) SØ3.4-●
    old M26.69
  knee S83.9-●
    collateral ligament S83.4Ø-●
      lateral (fibular) S83.42-●
      medial (tibial) S83.41-●
    cruciate ligament S83.5Ø-●
      anterior S83.51-●
      posterior S83.52-●

Sprain *(Continued)*
  knee *(Continued)*
    lateral (fibular) collateral ligament S83.42-●
    medial (tibial) collateral ligament S83.41-●
    patellar ligament S76.11-●
    specified site NEC S83.8X-●
    superior tibiofibular joint (ligament) S83.6-●
  lateral collateral, knee —*see* Sprain, knee, collateral
  lumbar (spine) S33.5
  lumbosacral S33.9
  mandible (articular disc) SØ3.4-●
    old M26.69
  medial collateral, knee —*see* Sprain, knee, collateral
  meniscus
    jaw SØ3.4-●
      old M26.69
    knee —*see* Sprain, knee, specified site NEC
      with current tear —*see* Tear, meniscus
        old —*see* Derangement, knee, meniscus, due to old tear
    mandible SØ3.4-●
      old M26.69
  metacarpal (distal) (proximal) —*see* Sprain, hand, specified site NEC
  metacarpophalangeal —*see* Sprain, finger, metacarpophalangeal (joint)
  metatarsophalangeal —*see* Sprain, toe, metatarsophalangeal joint
  midcarpal —*see* Sprain, hand, specified site NEC
  midtarsal —*see* Sprain, foot, specified site NEC
  neck S13.9
    anterior longitudinal cervical ligament S13.4
    atlanto-axial joint S13.4
    atlanto-occipital joint S13.4
    cervical spine S13.4
    cricoarytenoid ligament S13.5
    cricothyroid ligament S13.5
    specified site NEC S13.8
    thyroid region (cartilage) S13.5
  nose SØ3.8
  orbicular, hip —*see* Sprain, hip
  patella —*see* Sprain, knee, specified site NEC
  patellar ligament S76.11-●
  pelvis NEC S33.8
  phalanx
    finger —*see* Sprain, finger
    toe —*see* Sprain, toe
  pubofemoral —*see* Sprain, hip
  radiocarpal —*see* Sprain, wrist
  radiohumeral —*see* Sprain, elbow
  radius, collateral —*see* Rupture, traumatic, ligament, radial collateral
  rib (cage) S23.41
  rotator cuff (capsule) S43.42-●
  sacroiliac (region)
    chronic or old —*see* subcategory M53.2
    joint S33.6
  scaphoid (hand) —*see* Sprain, hand, specified site NEC
  scapula (r) —*see* Sprain, shoulder girdle, specified site NEC
  semilunar cartilage (knee) —*see* Sprain, knee, specified site NEC
    with current tear —*see* Tear, meniscus
      old —*see* Derangement, knee, meniscus, due to old tear
  shoulder joint S43.4Ø-●
    acromioclavicular joint (ligament) —*see* Sprain, acromioclavicular joint
    blade —*see* Sprain, shoulder, girdle, specified site NEC
    coracoclavicular joint (ligament) —*see* Sprain, coracoclavicular joint
    coracohumeral ligament —*see* Sprain, coracohumeral joint
    girdle S43.9-●
      specified site NEC S43.8-●
    rotator cuff —*see* Sprain, rotator cuff
    specified site NEC S43.49-●
    sternoclavicular joint (ligament) —*see* Sprain, sternoclavicular joint
  spine
    cervical S13.4
    lumbar S33.5
    thoracic S23.3
  sternoclavicular joint S43.6-●
  sternum S23.429
    chondrosternal joint S23.421
    specified site NEC S23.428
    sternoclavicular (joint) (ligament) S43.6-●

S

Status *(Continued)*
  asthmaticus —*see* Asthma, by type, with status asthmaticus
  awaiting organ transplant Z76.82
  bariatric surgery Z98.84
  bed confinement Z74.Ø1
  bleb, filtering (vitreous), after glaucoma surgery Z98.83
  breast implant Z98.82
    removal Z98.86
  cataract extraction Z98.4-●
  cholecystectomy Z9Ø.49
  clitorectomy N9Ø.811
    with excision of labia minora N9Ø.812
  colectomy (complete) (partial) Z9Ø.49
  colonization —*see* Carrier (suspected) of
  colostomy Z93.3
  ▶combined receptor
    ▶negative
      ▶hormone receptor negative with human epidermal growth factor receptor 2 negative Z17.421
      ▶hormone receptor negative with human epidermal growth factor receptor 2 positive Z17.42Ø
    ▶positive
      ▶hormone receptor positive with human epidermal growth factor receptor 2 negative Z17.411
      ▶hormone receptor positive with human epidermal growth factor receptor 2 positive Z17.41Ø
  convulsivus idiopathicus —*see* Epilepsy, by type, with status epilepticus
  coronary artery angioplasty —*see* Status, angioplasty, coronary artery
  coronary artery bypass graft Z95.1
  cystectomy (urinary bladder) Z9Ø.6
  cystostomy Z93.5Ø
    appendico-vesicostomy Z93.52
    cutaneous Z93.51
    specified NEC Z93.59
  delinquent immunization Z28.3
  dental Z98.818
    crown Z98.811
    fillings Z98.811
    restoration Z98.811
    sealant Z98.81Ø
    specified NEC Z98.818
  deployment (current) (military) Z56.82
  dialysis (hemodialysis) (peritoneal) Z99.2
  do not resuscitate (DNR) Z66
  donor —*see* Donor
  embedded fragments —*see* Retained, foreign body fragments (type of)
  embedded splinter —*see* Retained, foreign body fragments (type of)
  enterostomy Z93.4
  epileptic, epilepticus —*see also* Epilepsy, by type, with status epilepticus G4Ø.9Ø1
  estrogen receptor
    negative Z17.1
    positive Z17.Ø
  female genital cutting —*see* Female genital mutilation status
  female genital mutilation —*see* Female genital mutilation status
  filtering (vitreous) bleb after glaucoma surgery Z98.83
  gastrectomy (complete) (partial) Z9Ø.3
  gastric banding Z98.84
  gastric bypass for obesity Z98.84
  gastrostomy Z93.1
  ▶human epidermal growth factor 2 receptor
    ▶negative Z17.32
    ▶positive Z17.31
  human immunodeficiency virus (HIV) infection, asymptomatic Z21
  ➡hysterectomy (complete) (total) Z9Ø.71Ø
    partial (with remaining cervical stump) Z9Ø.711
  ➡ileostomy (ileal pouch) (Kock pouch) Z93.2
  implant
    breast Z98.82
  infibulation N9Ø.813
  intestinal bypass Z98.Ø
  jejunostomy Z93.4
  lapsed immunization schedule Z28.3
  laryngectomy Z9Ø.Ø2
  lymphaticus E32.8

Status *(Continued)*
  malignancy
    castrate resistant prostate Z19.2
    hormone resistant Z19.2
    hormone sensitive Z19.1
  marmoratus G8Ø.3
  mastectomy (unilateral) (bilateral) Z9Ø.1-●
  military deployment status (current) Z56.82
    in theater or in support of military war, peacekeeping and humanitarian operations Z56.82
  nephrectomy (unilateral) (bilateral) Z9Ø.5
  nephrostomy Z93.6
  obesity surgery Z98.84
  oophorectomy
    bilateral Z9Ø.722
    unilateral Z9Ø.721
  organ replacement
    by artificial or mechanical device or prosthesis of
      artery Z95.828
      bladder Z96.Ø
      blood vessel Z95.828
      breast Z97.8
      eye globe Z97.Ø
      heart Z95.812
        valve Z95.2
      intestine Z97.8
      joint Z96.6Ø
        hip —*see* Presence, hip joint implant
        knee —*see* Presence, knee joint implant
        specified site NEC Z96.698
      kidney Z97.8
      larynx Z96.3
      lens Z96.1
      limbs —*see* Presence, artificial, limb
      liver Z97.8
      lung Z97.8
      pancreas Z97.8
    by organ transplant (heterologous) (homologous) —*see* Transplant
  pacemaker
    brain Z96.89
    cardiac Z95.Ø
    specified NEC Z96.89
  pancreatectomy Z9Ø.41Ø
    complete Z9Ø.41Ø
    partial Z9Ø.411
    total Z9Ø.41Ø
  pneumonectomy (complete) (partial) Z9Ø.2
  pneumothorax, therapeutic Z98.3
  postcommotio cerebri FØ7.81
  postoperative (postprocedural) NEC Z98.89Ø
    breast implant Z98.82
    dental Z98.818
      crown Z98.811
      fillings Z98.811
      restoration Z98.811
      sealant Z98.81Ø
      specified NEC Z98.818
    pneumothorax, therapeutic Z98.3
    uterine scar Z98.891
  postpartum (routine follow-up) Z39.2
    care immediately after delivery Z39.Ø
  postsurgical (postprocedural) NEC Z98.89Ø
    pneumothorax, therapeutic Z98.3
  pregnancy, incidental Z33.1
  ▶progesterone receptor
    ▶negative Z17.22
    ▶positive Z17.21
  prosthesis coronary angioplasty Z95.5
  pseudophakia Z96.1
  renal dialysis (hemodialysis) (peritoneal) Z99.2
  retained foreign body —*see* Retained, foreign body fragments (type of)
  reversed jejunal transposition (for bypass Z98.Ø
  salpingo-oophorectomy
    bilateral Z9Ø.722
    unilateral Z9Ø.721
  sex reassignment surgery status Z87.89Ø
  shunt
    arteriovenous (for dialysis) Z99.2
    cerebrospinal fluid Z98.2
    ventricular (communicating) (for drainage) Z98.2
  splenectomy Z9Ø.81
  thymicolymphaticus E32.8

Status *(Continued)*
  thymicus E32.8
  thymolymphaticus E32.8
  thyroidectomy (hypothyroidism) E89.Ø
  tooth (teeth) extraction —*see also* Absence, teeth, acquired KØ8.4Ø9
  tPA (rtPA) administration in a different facility within the last 24 hours prior to admission to current facility Z92.82
  tracheostomy Z93.Ø
  transplant —*see* Transplant
    organ removed Z98.85
  tubal ligation Z98.51
  underimmunization Z28.3
  ureterostomy Z93.6
  urethrostomy Z93.6
  vagina, artificial Z93.8
  vasectomy Z98.52
  wheelchair confinement Z99.3
Stealing
  child problem F91.8
    in company with others Z72.81Ø
  pathological (compulsive) F63.2
Steam burn —*see* Burn
Steatocystoma multiplex L72.2
Steatohepatitis (nonalcoholic) (NASH) K75.81
Steatoma L72.3
  eyelid (cystic) —*see* Dermatosis, eyelid
    infected —*see* Hordeolum
Steatorrhea (chronic) K9Ø.9
  with lacteal obstruction K9Ø.2
  idiopathic (adult) (infantile) K9Ø.9
  pancreatic K9Ø.3
  primary K9Ø.Ø
  tropical K9Ø.1
Steatosis E88.89
  heart —*see* Degeneration, myocardial
  kidney N28.89
  liver NEC K76.Ø
Steele-Richardson-Olszewski disease or syndrome G23.1
➡**Steinbrocker's syndrome** G9Ø.89
Steinert's disease G71.11
Stein-Leventhal syndrome E28.2
Stein's syndrome E28.2
STEMI —*see also* Infarct, myocardium, ST elevation I21.3
Stenocardia I2Ø.89
Stenocephaly Q75.8
Stenosis, stenotic (cicatricial) —*see also* Stricture
  ampulla of Vater K83.1
  anus, anal (canal) (sphincter) K62.4
    and rectum K62.4
    congenital Q42.3
      with fistula Q42.2
  aorta (ascending) (supraventricular) (congenital) Q25.1
    arteriosclerotic I7Ø.Ø
    calcified I7Ø.Ø
    supravalvular Q25.3
  aortic (valve) I35.Ø
    with insufficiency I35.2
    congenital Q23.Ø
    rheumatic IØ6.Ø
      with
        incompetency, insufficiency or regurgitation IØ6.2
          with mitral (valve) disease IØ8.Ø
            with tricuspid (valve) disease IØ8.3
        mitral (valve) disease IØ8.Ø
          with tricuspid (valve) disease IØ8.3
        tricuspid (valve) disease IØ8.2
          with mitral (valve) disease IØ8.3
    specified cause NEC I35.Ø
    syphilitic A52.Ø3
  aqueduct of Sylvius (congenital) QØ3.Ø
    with spina bifida —*see* Spina bifida, by site, with hydrocephalus
    acquired G91.1
  artery NEC —*see also* Arteriosclerosis I77.1
    ➡celiac (compression) I77.4
      ▶arteriosclerotic I7Ø.8
      ▶atherosclerosis I7Ø.8
    cerebral —*see* Occlusion, artery, cerebral
    extremities —*see* Arteriosclerosis, extremities
    precerebral —*see* Occlusion, artery, precerebral
    pulmonary (congenital) Q25.6
      acquired I28.8
    renal I7Ø.1

S

Stenosis, stenotic *(Continued)*
  pulmonary *(Continued)*
    valve I37.0
      with insufficiency I37.2
      congenital Q22.1
      rheumatic I09.89
        with aortic, mitral or tricuspid (valve) disease I08.8
    vein, acquired I28.8
    vessel NEC I28.8
  pulmonic (congenital) Q22.1
    infundibular Q24.3
    subvalvular Q24.3
  pylorus (hypertrophic) (acquired) K31.1
    adult K31.1
    congenital Q40.0
    infantile Q40.0
  rectum (sphincter) —*see* Stricture, rectum
  renal artery I70.1
    congenital Q27.1
  salivary duct (any) K11.8
  sphincter of Oddi K83.1
  spinal M48.00
    cervical region M48.02
    cervicothoracic region M48.03
    lumbar region (NOS) (without neurogenic claudication) M48.061
      with neurogenic claudication M48.062
    lumbosacral region M48.07
    occipito-atlanto-axial region M48.01
    sacrococcygeal region M48.08
    thoracic region M48.04
    thoracolumbar region M48.05
  stent
    vascular
      end stent
        adjacent to stent —*see* Arteriosclerosis
        within the stent
          coronary T82.855
          peripheral T82.856
      in stent
        coronary vessel T82.855
        peripheral vessel T82.856
  stomach, hourglass K31.2
  subaortic (congenital) Q24.4
    hypertrophic (idiopathic) I42.1
  subglottic J38.6
    congenital Q31.1
    postprocedural J95.5
  trachea J39.8
    congenital Q32.1
    syphilitic A52.73
    tuberculous NEC A15.5
  tracheostomy J95.03
  tricuspid (valve) I07.0
    with
      aortic (valve) disease I08.2
      incompetency, insufficiency or regurgitation I07.2
        with aortic (valve) disease I08.2
          with mitral (valve) disease I08.3
      mitral (valve) disease I08.1
        with aortic (valve) disease I08.3
    congenital Q22.4
    nonrheumatic I36.0
      with insufficiency I36.2
  tubal N97.1
  ureter —*see* Atresia, ureter
  ureteropelvic junction, congenital Q62.11
  ureterovesical orifice, congenital Q62.12
  urethra (valve) —*see also* Stricture, urethra
    congenital Q64.32
  urinary meatus, congenital Q64.33
  vagina N89.5
    congenital Q52.4
    in pregnancy —*see* Pregnancy, complicated by, abnormal vagina
      causing obstructed labor O65.5
  valve (cardiac) (heart) —*see also* Endocarditis I38
    congenital Q24.8
      aortic Q23.0
      mitral Q23.2
      pulmonary Q22.1
      tricuspid Q22.4
  vena cava (inferior) (superior) I87.1
    congenital Q26.0
  vesicourethral orifice Q64.31
  vulva N90.5
Stent jail T82.897
Stercolith (impaction) K56.41
  appendix K38.1
Stercoraceous, stercoral ulcer K63.3
  anus or rectum K62.6
Stereotypies NEC F98.4
Sterility —*see* Infertility
Sterilization —*see* Encounter (for), sterilization
Sternalgia —*see* Angina
Sternopagus Q89.4
Sternum bifidum Q76.7
Steroid
  effects (adverse) (adrenocortical) (iatrogenic)
    cushingoid E24.2
      correct substance properly administered —*see* Table of Drugs and Chemicals, by drug, adverse effect
      overdose or wrong substance given or taken —*see* Table of Drugs and Chemicals, by drug, poisoning
    diabetes —*see* category E09
      correct substance properly administered —*see* Table of Drugs and Chemicals, by drug, adverse effect
      overdose or wrong substance given or taken —*see* Table of Drugs and Chemicals, by drug, poisoning
    fever R50.2
    insufficiency E27.3
      correct substance properly administered —*see* Table of Drugs and Chemicals, by drug, adverse effect
      overdose or wrong substance given or taken —*see* Table of Drugs and Chemicals, by drug, poisoning
  responder H40.04- ●
Stevens-Johnson disease or syndrome L51.1
  toxic epidermal necrolysis overlap L51.3
Stewart-Morel syndrome M85.2
Sticker's disease B08.3
Sticky eye —*see* Conjunctivitis, acute, mucopurulent
Stieda's disease —*see* Bursitis, tibial collateral
Stiff neck —*see* Torticollis
Stiff-man syndrome G25.82
Stiffness, joint NEC M25.60- ●
  ankle M25.67- ●
  ankylosis —*see* Ankylosis, joint
  contracture —*see* Contraction, joint
  elbow M25.62- ●
  foot M25.67- ●
  hand M25.64- ●
  hip M25.65- ●
  knee M25.66- ●
  shoulder M25.61- ●
  specified site NEC M25.69
  wrist M25.63- ●
Stigmata congenital syphilis A50.59
Stillbirth P95
Still-Felty syndrome —*see* Felty's syndrome
Still's disease or syndrome (juvenile) M08.20
  adult-onset M06.1
  ankle M08.27- ●
  elbow M08.22- ●
  foot joint M08.27- ●
  hand joint M08.24- ●
  hip M08.25- ●
  knee M08.26- ●
  multiple site M08.29
  shoulder M08.21- ●
  specified site NEC M08.2A
  vertebra M08.28
  wrist M08.23- ●
Stimulation, ovary E28.1
Sting (venomous) (with allergic or anaphylactic shock) —*see* Table of Drugs and Chemicals, by animal or substance, poisoning
Stippled epiphyses Q78.8
Stitch
  abscess T81.41
  burst (in operation wound) —*see* Disruption, wound, operation
Stokes-Adams disease or syndrome I45.9
Stokes' disease E05.00
  with thyroid storm E05.01
Stokvis (-Talma) disease D74.8
Stoma malfunction
  colostomy K94.03
  enterostomy K94.13
  gastrostomy K94.23
  ileostomy K94.13
  tracheostomy J95.03
Stomach —*see* condition
Stomatitis (denture) (ulcerative) K12.1
  angular K13.0
    due to dietary or vitamin deficiency E53.0
  aphthous K12.0
  bovine B08.61
  candidal B37.0
  catarrhal K12.1
  diphtheritic A36.89
  due to
    dietary deficiency E53.0
    thrush B37.0
    vitamin deficiency
      B group NEC E53.9
      B2 (riboflavin) E53.0
  epidemic B08.8
  epizootic B08.8
  follicular K12.1
  gangrenous A69.0
  Geotrichum B48.3
  herpesviral, herpetic B00.2
  herpetiformis K12.0
  malignant K12.1
  membranous acute K12.1
  monilial B37.0
  mycotic B37.0
  necrotizing ulcerative A69.0
  parasitic B37.0
  septic K12.1
  spirochetal A69.1
  suppurative (acute) K12.2
  ulceromembranous A69.1
  vesicular K12.1
    with exanthem (enteroviral) B08.4
    virus disease A93.8
  Vincent's A69.1
Stomatocytosis D58.8
Stomatomycosis B37.0
Stomatorrhagia K13.79
Stone(s) —*see also* Calculus
  bladder (diverticulum) N21.0
  cystine E72.09
  heart syndrome I50.1
  kidney N20.0
  prostate N42.0
  pulpal (dental) K04.2
  renal N20.0
  salivary gland or duct (any) K11.5
  urethra (impacted) N21.1
  urinary (duct) (impacted) (passage) N20.9
    bladder (diverticulum) N21.0
    lower tract N21.9
    specified NEC N21.8
  xanthine E79.82 *[N22]*
Stonecutter's lung J62.8
Stonemason's asthma, disease, lung or pneumoconiosis J62.8
Stoppage
  heart —*see* Arrest, cardiac
  urine —*see* Retention, urine
Storm, thyroid —*see* Thyrotoxicosis
Strabismus (congenital) (nonparalytic) H50.9
  concomitant H50.40
    convergent —*see* Strabismus, convergent concomitant
    divergent —*see* Strabismus, divergent concomitant
  convergent concomitant H50.00
    accommodative component H50.43
    alternating H50.05
      with
        A pattern H50.06
        specified nonconcomitances NEC H50.08
        V pattern H50.07
    monocular H50.01- ●
      with
        A pattern H50.02- ●
        specified nonconcomitances NEC H50.04- ●
        V pattern H50.03- ●
    intermittent H50.31- ●
      alternating H50.32
  cyclotropia H50.41
  divergent concomitant H50.10
    alternating H50.15
      with
        A pattern H50.16
        specified noncomitances NEC H50.18
        V pattern H50.17

- **Strabismus** *(Continued)*
  - divergent concomitant *(Continued)*
    - monocular H50.11-●
      - with
        - A pattern H50.12-●
        - specified noncomitances NEC H50.14-●
        - V pattern H50.13-●
      - intermittent H50.33-●
        - alternating H50.34
  - Duane's syndrome H50.81-●
  - due to adhesions, scars H50.69
  - heterophoria H50.50
    - alternating H50.55
    - cyclophoria H50.54
    - esophoria H50.51
    - exophoria H50.52
    - vertical H50.53
  - heterotropia H50.40
    - intermittent H50.30
  - hypertropia H50.2-●
  - hypotropia —*see* Hypertropia
  - latent H50.50
  - mechanical H50.60
    - Brown's sheath syndrome H50.61-●
    - specified type NEC H50.69
  - monofixation syndrome H50.42
  - paralytic H49.9
    - abducens nerve H49.2-●
    - fourth nerve H49.1-●
    - Kearns-Sayre syndrome H49.81-●
    - ophthalmoplegia (external)
      - progressive H49.4-●
        - with pigmentary retinopathy H49.81-●
      - total H49.3-●
    - sixth nerve H49.2-●
    - specified type NEC H49.88-●
    - third nerve H49.0-●
    - trochlear nerve H49.1-●
  - specified type NEC H50.89
  - vertical H50.2-●
- **Strain**
  - back S39.012
  - cervical S16.1
  - eye NEC —*see* Disturbance, vision, subjective
  - heart —*see* Disease, heart
  - low back S39.012
  - mental NOS Z73.3
    - work-related Z56.6
  - muscle (tendon) —*see* Injury, muscle, by site, strain
  - neck S16.1
  - physical NOS Z73.3
    - work-related Z56.6
  - postural —*see also* Disorder, soft tissue, due to use
  - psychological NEC Z73.3
  - tendon —*see* Injury, muscle, by site, strain
- **Straining,** on urination R39.16
- **Strand, vitreous** —*see* Opacity, vitreous, membranes and strands
- **Strangulation, strangulated** —*see also* Asphyxia, traumatic
  - appendix K38.8
  - bladder-neck N32.0
  - bowel or colon K56.2
  - food or foreign body —*see* Foreign body, by site
  - hemorrhoids —*see* Hemorrhoids, with complication
  - hernia —*see also* Hernia, by site, with obstruction
    - with gangrene —*see* Hernia, by site, with gangrene
  - intestine (large) (small) K56.2
    - with hernia —*see also* Hernia, by site, with obstruction
      - with gangrene —*see* Hernia, by site, with gangrene
  - mesentery K56.2
  - mucus —*see* Asphyxia, mucus
  - omentum K56.2
  - organ or site, congenital NEC —*see* Atresia, by site
  - ovary —*see* Torsion, ovary
  - penis N48.89
    - foreign body T19.4
  - rupture —*see* Hernia, by site, with obstruction
  - stomach due to hernia —*see also* Hernia, by site, with obstruction
    - with gangrene —*see* Hernia, by site, with gangrene
  - vesicourethral orifice N32.0
- **Strangury** R30.0
- **Straw itch** B88.0
- **Strawberry**
  - gallbladder K82.4
  - mark Q82.5
  - tongue (red) (white) K14.3
- **Streak(s)**
  - macula, angioid H35.33
  - ovarian Q50.32
- **Strephosymbolia** F81.0
  - secondary to organic lesion R48.8
- **Streptobacillary fever** A25.1
- **Streptobacillosis** A25.1
- **Streptobacillus moniliformis** A25.1
- **Streptococcus, streptococcal** —*see also* condition
  - as cause of disease classified elsewhere B95.5
  - group
    - A, as cause of disease classified elsewhere B95.0
    - B, as cause of disease classified elsewhere B95.1
    - D, as cause of disease classified elsewhere B95.2
  - pneumoniae, as cause of disease classified elsewhere B95.3
  - specified NEC, as cause of disease classified elsewhere B95.4
- **Streptomycosis** B47.1
- **Streptotrichosis** A48.8
- **Stress** F43.9
  - family —*see* Disruption, family
  - fetal P84
    - complicating pregnancy O77.9
      - due to drug administration O77.1
  - mental NEC Z73.3
    - work-related Z56.6
  - physical NEC Z73.3
    - work-related Z56.6
  - polycythemia D75.1
  - reaction —*see also* Reaction, stress F43.9
  - work schedule Z56.3
- **Stretching, nerve** —*see* Injury, nerve
- **Striae albicantes, atrophicae or distensae** (cutis) L90.6
- **Stricture** —*see also* Stenosis
  - ampulla of Vater K83.1
  - anus (sphincter) K62.4
    - congenital Q42.3
      - with fistula Q42.2
    - infantile Q42.3
      - with fistula Q42.2
  - aorta (ascending) (congenital) Q25.1
    - arteriosclerotic I70.0
    - calcified I70.0
    - supravalvular, congenital Q25.3
  - aortic (valve) —*see* Stenosis, aortic
  - aqueduct of Sylvius (congenital) Q03.0
    - with spina bifida —*see* Spina bifida, by site, with hydrocephalus
    - acquired G91.1
  - artery I77.1
    - basilar —*see* Occlusion, artery, basilar
    - carotid —*see* Occlusion, artery, carotid
    - celiac (compression) I77.4
      - ▶arteriosclerotic I70.8
      - ▶atherosclerosis I70.8
    - congenital (peripheral) Q27.8
      - cerebral Q28.3
      - coronary Q24.5
      - digestive system Q27.8
      - lower limb Q27.8
      - retinal Q14.1
      - specified site NEC Q27.8
      - umbilical Q27.0
      - upper limb Q27.8
    - coronary —*see* Disease, heart, ischemic, atherosclerotic
      - congenital Q24.5
    - precerebral —*see* Occlusion, artery, precerebral
    - pulmonary (congenital) Q25.6
      - acquired I28.8
    - renal I70.1
    - vertebral —*see* Occlusion, artery, vertebral
  - auditory canal (external) (congenital)
    - acquired —*see* Stenosis, external ear canal
  - bile duct (common) (hepatic) K83.1
    - congenital Q44.3
    - postoperative K91.89
  - bladder N32.89
    - neck N32.0
  - bowel —*see* Obstruction, intestine
  - brain G93.89
- **Stricture** *(Continued)*
  - bronchus J98.09
    - congenital Q32.3
    - syphilitic A52.72
  - cardia (stomach) K22.2
    - congenital Q39.3
  - cardiac —*see also* Disease, heart
    - orifice (stomach) K22.2
  - cecum —*see* Obstruction, intestine
  - cervix, cervical (canal) N88.2
    - congenital Q51.828
    - in pregnancy —*see* Pregnancy, complicated by, abnormal cervix
      - causing obstructed labor O65.5
  - colon —*see also* Obstruction, intestine
    - congenital Q42.9
      - specified NEC Q42.8
  - colostomy K94.03
  - common (bile) duct K83.1
  - coronary (artery) —*see* Disease, heart, ischemic, atherosclerotic
  - cystic duct —*see* Obstruction, gallbladder
  - digestive organs NEC, congenital Q45.8
  - duodenum K31.5
    - congenital Q41.0
  - ear canal (external) (congenital) Q16.1
    - acquired —*see* Stricture, auditory canal, acquired
  - ejaculatory duct N50.89
  - enterostomy K94.13
  - esophagus K22.2
    - congenital Q39.3
    - syphilitic A52.79
      - congenital A50.59 *[K23]*
  - eustachian tube —*see also* Obstruction, eustachian tube
    - congenital Q17.8
  - fallopian tube N97.1
    - gonococcal A54.24
    - tuberculous A18.17
  - gallbladder —*see* Obstruction, gallbladder
  - glottis J38.6
  - heart —*see also* Disease, heart
    - valve (*see also* Endocarditis) I38
      - aortic Q23.0
      - mitral Q23.2
      - pulmonary Q22.1
      - tricuspid Q22.4
  - hepatic duct K83.1
  - hourglass, of stomach K31.2
  - hymen N89.6
  - hypopharynx J39.2
  - ileum —*see also* Obstruction, intestine, specified NEC K56.699
    - congenital Q41.2
  - intestine —*see also* Obstruction, intestine
    - congenital (small) Q41.9
      - large Q42.9
        - specified NEC Q42.8
      - specified NEC Q41.8
    - ischemic K55.1
  - jejunum —*see also* Obstruction, intestine, specified NEC K56.699
    - congenital Q41.1
  - lacrimal passages —*see also* Stenosis, lacrimal
    - congenital Q10.5
  - larynx J38.6
    - congenital NEC Q31.8
      - subglottic Q31.1
    - syphilitic A52.73
      - congenital A50.59 *[J99]*
  - meatus
    - ear (congenital) Q16.1
      - acquired —*see* Stricture, auditory canal, acquired
    - osseous (ear) (congenital) Q16.1
      - acquired —*see* Stricture, auditory canal, acquired
    - urinarius —*see also* Stricture, urethra
      - congenital Q64.33
  - mitral (valve) —*see* Stenosis, mitral
  - myocardium, myocardial I51.5
    - hypertrophic subaortic (idiopathic) I42.1
  - nares (anterior) (posterior) J34.89
    - congenital Q30.0
  - nasal duct —*see also* Stenosis, lacrimal, duct
    - congenital Q10.5
  - nasolacrimal duct —*see also* Stenosis, lacrimal, duct
    - congenital Q10.5

S

Subcortical —*see* condition
Subcostal syndrome, nerve compression —*see* Mononeuropathy, upper limb, specified site NEC
Subcutaneous, subcuticular —*see* condition
Subdural —*see* condition
Subendocardium —*see* condition
Subependymoma
specified site —*see* Neoplasm, uncertain behavior, by site
unspecified site D43.2
Suberosis J67.3
Subglossitis —*see* Glossitis
Subhemophilia D66
Subinvolution
breast (postlactational) (postpuerperal) N64.89
puerperal O90.89
uterus (chronic) (nonpuerperal) N85.3
puerperal O90.89
Sublingual —*see* condition
Sublinguitis —*see* Sialoadenitis
Subluxatable hip Q65.6
Subluxation —*see also* Dislocation
acromioclavicular S43.11-•
ankle S93.0-•
atlantoaxial, recurrent M43.4
with myelopathy M43.3
carpometacarpal (joint) NEC S63.05-•
thumb S63.04-•
complex, vertebral —*see* Complex, subluxation
congenital —*see also* Malposition, congenital
hip —*see* Dislocation, hip, congenital, partial
joint (excluding hip)
lower limb Q68.8
shoulder Q68.8
upper limb Q68.8
elbow (traumatic) S53.10-•
anterior S53.11-•
lateral S53.14-•
medial S53.13-•
posterior S53.12-•
specified type NEC S53.19-•
finger S63.20-•
index S63.20-•
interphalangeal S63.22-•
distal S63.24-•
index S63.24-•
little S63.24-•
middle S63.24-•
ring S63.24-•
index S63.22-•
little S63.22-•
middle S63.22-•
proximal S63.23-•
index S63.23-•
little S63.23-•
middle S63.23-•
ring S63.23-•
ring S63.22-•
little S63.20-•
metacarpophalangeal S63.21-•
index S63.21-•
little S63.21-•
middle S63.21-•
ring S63.21-•
middle S63.20-•
ring S63.20-•
foot S93.30-•
specified site NEC S93.33-•
tarsal joint S93.31-•
tarsometatarsal joint S93.32-•
toe —*see* Subluxation, toe
hip S73.00-•
anterior S73.03-•
obturator S73.02-•
central S73.04-•
posterior S73.01-•
interphalangeal (joint)
finger S63.22-•
distal joint S63.24-•
index S63.24-•
little S63.24-•
middle S63.24-•
ring S63.24-•
index S63.22-•
little S63.22-•
middle S63.22-•
proximal joint S63.23-•
index S63.23-•
little S63.23-•

Subluxation *(Continued)*
interphalangeal *(Continued)*
finger *(Continued)*
proximal joint *(Continued)*
middle S63.23-•
ring S63.23-•
ring S63.22-•
thumb S63.12-•
toe S93.13-•
great S93.13-•
lesser S93.13-•
joint prosthesis —*see* Complications, joint prosthesis, mechanical, displacement, by site
knee S83.10-•
cap —*see* Subluxation, patella
patella —*see* Subluxation, patella
proximal tibia
anteriorly S83.11-•
laterally S83.14-•
medially S83.13-•
posteriorly S83.12-•
specified type NEC S83.19-•
lens —*see* Dislocation, lens, partial
ligament, traumatic —*see* Sprain, by site
metacarpal (bone)
proximal end S63.06-•
metacarpophalangeal (joint)
finger S63.21-•
index S63.21-•
little S63.21-•
middle S63.21-•
ring S63.21-•
thumb S63.11-•
metatarsophalangeal joint S93.14-•
great toe S93.14-•
lesser toe S93.14-•
midcarpal (joint) S63.03-•
patella S83.00-•
lateral S83.01-•
recurrent (nontraumatic) —*see* Dislocation, patella, recurrent, incomplete
specified type NEC S83.09-•
pathological —*see* Dislocation, pathological
radial head S53.00-•
anterior S53.01-•
nursemaid's elbow S53.03-•
posterior S53.02-•
specified type NEC S53.09-•
radiocarpal (joint) S63.02-•
radioulnar (joint)
distal S63.01-•
proximal —*see* Subluxation, elbow
shoulder
congenital Q68.8
girdle S43.30-•
scapula S43.31-•
specified site NEC S43.39-•
traumatic S43.00-•
anterior S43.01-•
inferior S43.03-•
posterior S43.02-•
specified type NEC S43.08-•
sternoclavicular (joint) S43.20-•
anterior S43.21-•
posterior S43.22-•
symphysis (pubis) —*see also* Dislocation, symphysis pubis
thumb S63.103
interphalangeal joint —*see* Subluxation, interphalangeal (joint), thumb
metacarpophalangeal joint —*see* Subluxation, metacarpophalangeal (joint), thumb
toe(s) S93.10-•
great S93.10-•
interphalangeal joint S93.13-•
metatarsophalangeal joint S93.14-•
interphalangeal joint S93.13-•
lesser S93.10-•
interphalangeal joint S93.13-•
metatarsophalangeal joint S93.14-•
metatarsophalangeal joint S93.149
ulnohumeral joint —*see* Subluxation, elbow
vertebral
recurrent NEC —*see* subcategory M43.5
traumatic
cervical S13.100
atlantoaxial joint S13.120
atlantooccipital joint S13.110
atloidooccipital joint S13.110

Subluxation *(Continued)*
vertebral *(Continued)*
traumatic *(Continued)*
cervical *(Continued)*
joint between
C0 and C1 S13.110
C1 and C2 S13.120
C2 and C3 S13.130
C3 and C4 S13.140
C4 and C5 S13.150
C5 and C6 S13.160
C6 and C7 S13.170
C7 and T1 S13.180
occipitoatloid joint S13.110
lumbar S33.100
joint between
L1 and L2 S33.110
L2 and L3 S33.120
L3 and L4 S33.130
L4 and L5 S33.140
thoracic S23.100
joint between
T1 and T2 S23.110
T2 and T3 S23.120
T3 and T4 S23.122
T4 and T5 S23.130
T5 and T6 S23.132
T6 and T7 S23.140
T7 and T8 S23.142
T8 and T9 S23.150
T9 and T10 S23.152
T10 and T11 S23.160
T11 and T12 S23.162
T12 and L1 S23.170
ulna
distal end S63.07-•
proximal end —*see* Subluxation, elbow
wrist (carpal bone) S63.00-•
carpometacarpal joint —*see* Subluxation, carpometacarpal (joint)
distal radioulnar joint —*see* Subluxation, radioulnar (joint), distal
metacarpal bone, proximal —*see* Subluxation, metacarpal (bone), proximal end
midcarpal —*see* Subluxation, midcarpal (joint)
radiocarpal joint —*see* Subluxation, radiocarpal (joint)
recurrent —*see* Dislocation, recurrent, wrist
specified site NEC S63.09-•
ulna —*see* Subluxation, ulna, distal end
Submaxillary —*see* condition
Submersion (fatal) (nonfatal) T75.1
Submucous —*see* condition
Subnormal, subnormality
accommodation (old age) H52.4
mental —*see* Disability, intellectual
temperature (accidental) T68
Subphrenic —*see* condition
Subscapular nerve —*see* condition
Subseptus uterus Q51.28
Subsiding appendicitis K36
Substance (other psychoactive) -induced
anxiety disorder F19.980
bipolar and related disorder F19.94
delirium F19.921
depressive disorder F19.94
major neurocognitive disorder F19.97
mild neurocognitive disorder F19.988
obsessive-compulsive and related disorder F19.988
psychotic disorder F19.959
sexual dysfunction F19.981
sleep disorder F19.982
Substernal thyroid E04.9
congenital Q89.2
Substitution disorder F44.9
Subtentorial —*see* condition
Subthyroidism (acquired) —*see also* Hypothyroidism
congenital E03.1
Succenturiate placenta O43.19-•
Sucking thumb, child (excessive) F98.8
Sudamen, sudamina L74.1
Sudanese kala-azar B55.0
Sudden
hearing loss —*see* Deafness, sudden
heart failure —*see* Failure, heart
Sudeck's atrophy, disease, or syndrome —*see* Algoneurodystrophy
Suffocation —*see* Asphyxia, traumatic

Sugar
blood
high (transient) R73.9
low (transient) E16.2
in urine R81
Suicide, suicidal (attempted) T14.91
by poisoning —*see* Table of Drugs and Chemicals
history of (personal) Z91.51
in family Z81.8
ideation —*see* Ideation, suicidal
risk
meaning personal history of attempted suicide Z91.51
meaning suicidal ideation —*see* Ideation, suicidal
tendencies
meaning personal history of attempted suicide Z91.51
meaning suicidal ideation —*see* Ideation, suicidal
trauma —*see* nature of injury by site
Suipestifer infection —*see* Infection, salmonella
Sulfhemoglobinemia, sulphemoglobinemia (acquired) (with methemoglobinemia) D74.8
Sumatran mite fever A75.3
Summer —*see* condition
Sunburn L55.9
due to
tanning bed (acute) L56.8
chronic L57.8
ultraviolet radiation (acute) L56.8
chronic L57.8
first degree L55.0
second degree L55.1
third degree L55.2
SUNCT (short lasting unilateral neuralgiform headache with conjunctival injection and tearing) G44.059
intractable G44.051
not intractable G44.059
Sundowning F05
Sunken acetabulum —*see* Derangement, joint, specified type NEC, hip
Sunstroke T67.01
specified NEC T67.09
Superfecundation —*see* Pregnancy, multiple
Superfetation —*see* Pregnancy, multiple
Superinvolution (uterus) N85.8
Supernumerary (congenital)
aortic cusps Q23.88
auditory ossicles Q16.3
bone Q79.8
breast Q83.1
carpal bones Q74.0
cusps, heart valve NEC Q24.8
aortic Q23.88
mitral Q23.2
pulmonary Q22.3
digit(s) Q69.9
ear (lobule) Q17.0
fallopian tube Q50.6
finger Q69.0
hymen Q52.4
kidney Q63.0
lacrimonasal duct Q10.6
lobule (ear) Q17.0
mitral cusps Q23.2
muscle Q79.8
nipple(s) Q83.3
organ or site not listed —*see* Accessory
ossicles, auditory Q16.3
ovary Q50.31
oviduct Q50.6
pulmonary, pulmonic cusps Q22.3
rib Q76.6
cervical or first (syndrome) Q76.5
roots (of teeth) K00.2
spleen Q89.09
tarsal bones Q74.2
teeth K00.1
testis Q55.29
thumb Q69.1
toe Q69.2
uterus Q51.28
vagina Q52.1
vertebra Q76.49
Supervision (of)
contraceptive —*see* Prescription, contraceptives
dietary (for) Z71.3
allergy (food) Z71.3
colitis Z71.3
Supervision *(Continued)*
dietary *(Continued)*
diabetes mellitus Z71.3
food allergy or intolerance Z71.3
gastritis Z71.3
hypercholesterolemia Z71.3
hypoglycemia Z71.3
intolerance (food) Z71.3
obesity Z71.3
specified NEC Z71.3
healthy infant or child Z76.2
foundling Z76.1
high-risk pregnancy —*see* Pregnancy, supervision of, high, risk
lactation Z39.1
pregnancy —*see* Pregnancy, supervision of
Supplemental teeth K00.1
Suppression
binocular vision H53.34
lactation O92.5
menstruation N94.89
ovarian secretion E28.39
renal N28.9
urine, urinary secretion R34
Suppuration, suppurative —*see also* condition
accessory sinus (chronic) —*see* Sinusitis
adrenal gland
antrum (chronic) —*see* Sinusitis, maxillary
bladder —*see* Cystitis
brain G06.0
sequelae G09
breast N61.1
puerperal, postpartum or gestational —*see* Mastitis, obstetric, purulent
dental periosteum M27.3
ear (middle) —*see also* Otitis, media
external NEC —*see* Otitis, externa, infective
internal —*see* subcategory H83.0
ethmoidal (chronic) (sinus) —*see* Sinusitis, ethmoidal
fallopian tube —*see* Salpingo-oophoritis
frontal (chronic) (sinus) —*see* Sinusitis, frontal
gallbladder (acute) K81.0
gum K05.20
generalized —*see* Periodontitis, aggressive, generalized
localized —*see* Periodontitis, aggressive, localized
intracranial G06.0
joint —*see* Arthritis, pyogenic or pyemic
labyrinthine —*see* subcategory H83.0
lung —*see* Abscess, lung
mammary gland N61.1
puerperal, postpartum O91.12
associated with lactation O91.13
maxilla, maxillary M27.2
sinus (chronic) —*see* Sinusitis, maxillary
muscle —*see* Myositis, infective
nasal sinus (chronic) —*see* Sinusitis
pancreas, acute —*see also* Pancreatitis, acute K85.80
parotid gland —*see* Sialoadenitis
pelvis, pelvic
female —*see* Disease, pelvis, inflammatory
male K65.0
pericranial —*see* Osteomyelitis
salivary duct or gland (any) —*see* Sialoadenitis
sinus (accessory) (chronic) (nasal) —*see* Sinusitis
sphenoidal sinus (chronic) —*see* Sinusitis, sphenoidal
thymus (gland) E32.1
thyroid (gland) E06.0
tonsil —*see* Tonsillitis
uterus —*see* Endometritis
Supraeruption of tooth (teeth) M26.34
Supraglottitis J04.30
with obstruction J04.31
Suprarenal (gland) —*see* condition
Suprascapular nerve —*see* condition
Suprasellar —*see* condition
Surfer's knots or nodules S89.8-●
Surgical
emphysema T81.82
procedures, complication or misadventure —*see* Complications, surgical procedures
shock T81.10
Surveillance (of) (for) —*see also* Observation
alcohol abuse Z71.41
contraceptive —*see* Prescription, contraceptives
dietary Z71.3
drug abuse Z71.51
neoplasm —*see* Screening, neoplasm
Susceptibility to disease, genetic Z15.89
malignant neoplasm Z15.09
breast Z15.01
endometrium Z15.04
ovary Z15.02
prostate Z15.03
specified NEC Z15.09
multiple endocrine neoplasia Z15.81
Suspected condition, ruled out —*see also* Observation, suspected
amniotic cavity and membrane Z03.71
cervical shortening Z03.75
fetal anomaly Z03.73
fetal growth Z03.74
maternal and fetal conditions NEC Z03.79
newborn —*see also* Observation, newborn, suspected condition ruled out Z05.9
oligohydramnios Z03.71
placental problem Z03.72
polyhydramnios Z03.71
Suspended uterus
in pregnancy or childbirth —*see* Pregnancy, complicated by, abnormal uterus
Sutton's nevus D22.9
Suture
burst (in operation wound) T81.31
external operation wound T81.31
internal operation wound T81.329
inadvertently left in operation wound —*see* Foreign body, accidentally left during a procedure
removal Z48.02
Swab inadvertently left in operation wound —*see* Foreign body, accidentally left during a procedure
Swallowed, swallowing
difficulty —*see* Dysphagia
foreign body —*see* Foreign body, alimentary tract
Swan-neck deformity (finger) —*see* Deformity, finger, swan-neck
Swearing, compulsive F42.8
in Gilles de la Tourette's syndrome F95.2
Sweat, sweats
fetid L75.0
night R61
Sweating, excessive R61
Sweeley-Klionsky disease E75.21
Sweet's disease or dermatosis L98.2
Swelling (of) R60.9
abdomen, abdominal (not referable to any particular organ) —*see* Mass, abdominal
ankle —*see* Effusion, joint, ankle
arm M79.89
forearm M79.89
breast —*see also* Lump, breast N63.0
Calabar B74.3
cervical gland R59.0
chest, localized R22.2
ear H93.8-●
extremity (lower) (upper) —*see* Disorder, soft tissue, specified type NEC
finger M79.89
foot M79.89
glands R59.9
generalized R59.1
localized R59.0
hand M79.89
head (localized) R22.0
inflammatory —*see* Inflammation
intra-abdominal —*see* Mass, abdominal
joint —*see* Effusion, joint
leg M79.89
lower M79.89
limb —*see* Disorder, soft tissue, specified type NEC
localized (skin) R22.9
chest R22.2
head R22.0
limb
lower —*see* Mass, localized, limb, lower
upper —*see* Mass, localized, limb, upper
neck R22.1
trunk R22.2
neck (localized) R22.1
pelvic —*see* Mass, abdominal
scrotum N50.89
splenic —*see* Splenomegaly
testis N50.89
toe M79.89
umbilical R19.09

Swelling *(Continued)*
wandering, due to Gnathostoma (spinigerum) B83.1
white —*see* Tuberculosis, arthritis
Swift (-Feer) disease
overdose or wrong substance given or taken —*see* Table of Drugs and Chemicals, by drug, poisoning
Swimmer's
cramp T75.1
ear H60.33-●
itch B65.3
Swimming in the head R42
Swollen —*see* Swelling
Swyer syndrome Q99.1
Sycosis L73.8
barbae (not parasitic) L73.8
contagiosa (mycotic) B35.0
lupoides L73.8
mycotic B35.0
parasitic B35.0
vulgaris L73.8
Sydenham's chorea —*see* Chorea, Sydenham's
Sylvatic yellow fever A95.0
Sylvest's disease B33.0
Symblepharon H11.23-●
congenital Q10.3
Symond's syndrome G93.2
Sympathetic —*see* condition
Sympatheticotonia G90.89
Sympathicoblastoma
specified site —*see* Neoplasm, malignant, by site
unspecified site C74.90
Sympathogonioma —*see* Sympathicoblastoma
Symphalangy (fingers) (toes) Q70.9
Symptoms NEC R68.89
breast NEC N64.59
cold J00
development NEC R63.8
factitious, self-induced —*see* Disorder, factitious
genital organs, female R10.2
involving
abdomen NEC R19.8
appearance NEC R46.89
awareness R41.9
altered mental status R41.82
amnesia —*see* Amnesia
borderline intellectual functioning R41.83
coma —*see* Coma
disorientation R41.0
neurologic neglect syndrome R41.4
senile cognitive decline R41.81
specified symptom NEC R41.89
behavior NEC R46.89
cardiovascular system NEC R09.89
chest NEC R09.89
circulatory system NEC R09.89
cognitive functions R41.9
altered mental status R41.82
amnesia —*see* Amnesia
borderline intellectual functioning R41.83
coma —*see* Coma
disorientation R41.0
neurologic neglect syndrome R41.4
senile cognitive decline R41.81
specified symptom NEC R41.89
development NEC R62.50
digestive system NEC R19.8
emotional state NEC R45.89
emotional lability R45.86
food and fluid intake R63.8
general perceptions and sensations R44.9
specified NEC R44.8
musculoskeletal system R29.91
specified NEC R29.898
nervous system R29.90
specified NEC R29.818
pelvis NEC R19.8
respiratory system NEC R09.89
skin and integument R23.9
urinary system R39.9
menopausal N95.1
metabolism NEC R63.8
neurotic F48.8
of infancy R68.19
pelvis NEC, female R10.2
skin and integument NEC R23.9
subcutaneous tissue NEC R23.9
viral cold J00
Sympus Q74.2
Syncephalus Q89.4
Synchondrosis
abnormal (congenital) Q78.8
ischiopubic M91.0
Synchysis (scintillans) (senile) (vitreous body) H43.89
Syncope (near) (pre-) R55
anginosa I20.89
bradycardia R00.1
cardiac R55
carotid sinus G90.01
due to spinal (lumbar) puncture G97.1
heart R55
heat T67.1
laryngeal R05.4
psychogenic F48.8
tussive R05.8
vasoconstriction R55
vasodepressor R55
vasomotor R55
vasovagal R55
Syndactylism, syndactyly Q70.9
complex (with synostosis)
fingers Q70.0-●
toes Q70.2-●
simple (without synostosis)
fingers Q70.1-●
toes Q70.3-●
Syndrome —*see also* Disease
22q13.3 deletion Q93.52
4H G11.5
48,XXXX Q97.1
49,XXXXX Q97.1
5q minus NOS D46.C
abdominal
acute R10.0
muscle deficiency Q79.4
abnormal innervation H02.519
left H02.516
lower H02.515
upper H02.514
right H02.513
lower H02.512
upper H02.511
abstinence, neonatal P96.1
acid pulmonary aspiration, obstetric O74.0
acquired immunodeficiency —*see* Human, immunodeficiency virus (HIV) disease
activated phosphoinositide 3-kinase delta syndrome [APDS] D81.82
acute abdominal R10.0
acute respiratory distress (adult) (child) J80
idiopathic J84.114
Adair-Dighton Q78.0
Adams-Stokes (-Morgagni) I45.9
adiposogenital E23.6
adrenal
hemorrhage (meningococcal) A39.1
meningococcic A39.1
adrenocortical —*see* Cushing's, syndrome
adrenogenital E25.9
congenital, associated with enzyme deficiency E25.0
afferent loop NEC K91.89
Aicardi-Goutières E79.81
Alagille (-Watson) Q44.71
alcohol withdrawal (without convulsions) —*see* Dependence, alcohol, with, withdrawal
Alder's D72.0
Aldrich (-Wiskott) D82.0
alien hand R41.4
Alport Q87.81
alveolar hypoventilation E66.2
alveolocapillary block J84.10
amnesic, amnestic (confabulatory) (due to) —*see* Disorder, amnesic
amyostatic (Wilson's disease) E83.01
androgen insensitivity E34.50
complete E34.51
partial E34.52
androgen resistance (*see also* Syndrome, androgen insensitivity) E34.50
Angelman Q93.51
anginal —*see* Angina
ankyloglossia superior Q38.1
anterior
chest wall R07.89
cord G83.82
spinal artery G95.19
compression M47.019
cervical region M47.012
cervicothoracic region M47.013
Syndrome *(Continued)*
anterior *(Continued)*
spinal artery *(Continued)*
compression *(Continued)*
lumbar region M47.016
occipito-atlanto-axial region M47.011
thoracic region M47.014
thoracolumbar region M47.015
tibial M76.81-●
antibody deficiency D80.9
agammaglobulinemic D80.1
hereditary D80.0
congenital D80.0
hypogammaglobulinemic D80.1
hereditary D80.0
anticardiolipin (-antibody) D68.61
antidepressant discontinuation T43.205
antiphospholipid (-antibody) D68.61
aortic
arch M31.4
bifurcation I74.09
aortomesenteric duodenum occlusion K31.5
apical ballooning (transient left ventricular) I51.81
arcuate ligament I77.4
argentaffin, argintaffinoma E34.09
Arnold-Chiari —*see* Arnold-Chiari disease
Arrillaga-Ayerza I27.0
arterial tortuosity Q87.82
arteriovenous steal T82.898-●
Asherman's N85.6
aspiration, of newborn —*see* Aspiration, by substance, with pneumonia
meconium P24.01
ataxia-telangiectasia G11.3
auriculotemporal G50.8
autoerythrocyte sensitization (Gardner-Diamond) D69.2
autoimmune lymphoproliferative [ALPS] D89.82
autoimmune polyglandular E31.0
autoinflammatory M04.9
specified type NEC M04.8
autosomal —*see* Abnormal, autosomes
Avellis' G46.8
Axenfeld-Rieger Q13.81
Ayerza (-Arrillaga) I27.0
Babinski-Nageotte G83.89
Bakwin-Krida Q78.5
Bardet-Biedl Q87.83
bare lymphocyte D81.6
Barré-Guillain G61.0
Barré-Liéou M53.0
Barrett's —*see* Barrett's, esophagus
Barsony-Polgar K22.4
Barsony-Teschendorf K22.4
Barth E78.71
Bartter's E26.81
basal cell nevus Q87.89
Basedow's E05.00
with thyroid storm E05.01
basilar artery G45.0
Batten-Steinert G71.11
battered
baby or child —*see* Maltreatment, child, physical abuse
spouse —*see* Maltreatment, adult, physical abuse
Beals Q87.40
Beau's I51.5
Beck's I65.8
Benedikt's G46.3
Béquez César (-Steinbrinck-Chédiak-Higashi) D70.330
Bernhardt-Roth —*see* Meralgia paresthetica
Bernheim's —*see* Failure, heart, right
big spleen D73.1
bilateral polycystic ovarian E28.2
Bing-Horton's —*see* Horton's headache
Birt-Hogg-Dube syndrome Q87.89
Björck (-Thorsen) E34.09
black
lung J60
widow spider bite —*see* Toxicity, venom, spider, black widow
Blackfan-Diamond D61.01
Blau M04.8
blind loop K90.2
congenital Q43.8
postsurgical K91.2
blue sclera Q78.0
blue toe I75.02-●

S

New Revised ~~deleted~~ Deleted ● Use Additional Character(s)

Syndrome *(Continued)*
- Boder-Sedgewick G11.3
- Boerhaave's K22.3
- Borjeson Forssman Lehmann Q89.8
- Bouillaud's I01.9
- Bourneville (-Pringle) Q85.1
- Bouveret (-Hoffman) I47.9
- brachial plexus G54.0
- bradycardia-tachycardia I49.5
- brain (nonpsychotic) F09
  - with psychosis, psychotic reaction F09
  - acute or subacute —*see* Delirium
  - congenital —*see* Disability, intellectual
  - organic F09
    - post-traumatic (nonpsychotic) F07.81
      - psychotic F09
  - personality change F07.0
  - postcontusional F07.81
  - post-traumatic, nonpsychotic F07.81
  - psycho-organic F09
  - psychotic F06.8
- brain stem stroke G46.3
- Brandt's (acrodermatitis enteropathica) E83.2
- broad ligament laceration N83.8
- Brock's J98.11
- bronchiolitis obliterans (*see also* Bronchiolitis, obliterative) J44.81
- bronze baby P83.88
- Brown-Sequard G83.81
- Brugada I49.8
- bubbly lung P27.0
- Buchem's M85.2
- Budd-Chiari I82.0
- bulbar (progressive) G12.22
- Bürger-Grütz E78.3
- Burke's K86.89
- Burnett's (milk-alkali) E83.52
- burning feet E53.9
- Bywaters' T79.5
- Call-Fleming I67.841
- carbohydrate-deficient glycoprotein (CDGS) E77.8
- carcinogenic thrombophlebitis I82.1
- ➡ carcinoid E34.00
  - ▶ heart E34.01
  - ▶ specified NEC E34.09
- cardiac asthma I50.1
- cardiacos negros I27.0
- cardiofaciocutaneous Q87.89
- cardiopulmonary-obesity E66.2
- cardiorenal —*see* Hypertension, cardiorenal
- cardiorespiratory distress (idiopathic), newborn P22.0
- cardiovascular renal —*see* Hypertension, cardiorenal
- carotid
  - artery (hemispheric) (internal) G45.1
  - body G90.01
  - sinus G90.01
- carpal tunnel G56.0- ●
- ➡ Cassidy (-Scholte) E34.09
- cat-cry Q93.4
- cat eye Q92.8
- cauda equina G83.4
- causalgia —*see* Causalgia
- celiac K90.0
  - artery compression I77.4
  - axis I77.4
- central pain G89.0
- cerebellar
  - hereditary G11.9
  - stroke G46.4
- cerebellomedullary malformation —*see* Spina bifida
- cerebral
  - artery
    - anterior G46.1
    - middle G46.0
    - posterior G46.2
  - gigantism E22.0
- cervical (root) M53.1
  - disc —*see* Disorder, disc, cervical, with neuritis
  - fusion Q76.1
  - posterior, sympathicus M53.0
  - rib Q76.5
  - sympathetic paralysis G90.2
- cervicobrachial (diffuse) M53.1
- cervicocranial M53.0
- cervicodorsal outlet G54.2
- ➡ cervicothoracic outlet (*see also* Syndrome, thoracic outlet) G54.0
- Céstan (-Raymond) I65.8
- Charcot's (angina cruris) (intermittent claudication) I73.9
- Charcot-Weiss-Baker G90.09
- CHARGE Q89.8
- Chédiak-Higashi (-Steinbrinck) E70.330
- chest wall R07.1
- Chiari's (hepatic vein thrombosis) I82.0
- Chilaiditi's Q43.3
- child maltreatment —*see* Maltreatment, child
- chondrocostal junction M94.0
- chondroectodermal dysplasia Q77.6
- chromosome 4 short arm deletion Q93.3
- chromosome 5 short arm deletion Q93.4
- chronic
  - infantile neurological, cutaneous and articular (CINCA) M04.2
  - pain G89.4
    - personality F68.8
- Churg-Strauss M30.1
- Clarke-Hadfield K86.89
- Clerambault's automatism G93.89
- Clouston's (hidrotic ectodermal dysplasia) Q82.4
- clumsiness, clumsy child F82
- cluster headache G44.009
  - intractable G44.001
  - not intractable G44.009
- Coffin-Lowry Q89.8
- cold injury (newborn) P80.0
- combined immunity deficiency D81.9
- compartment (deep) (posterior) (traumatic) T79.A0
  - abdomen T79.A3
  - lower extremity (hip, buttock, thigh, leg, foot, toes) T79.A2
  - nontraumatic
    - abdomen M79.A3
    - lower extremity (hip, buttock, thigh, leg, foot, toes) M79.A2- ●
    - specified site NEC M79.A9
    - upper extremity (shoulder, arm, forearm, wrist, hand, fingers) M79.A1- ●
  - postprocedural —*see* Syndrome compartment, nontraumatic
  - specified site NEC T79.A9
  - upper extremity (shoulder, arm, forearm, wrist, hand, fingers) T79.A1
- complex regional pain —*see* Syndrome, pain, complex regional
- compression T79.5
  - anterior spinal —*see* Syndrome, anterior, spinal artery, compression
  - cauda equina G83.4
  - celiac artery I77.4
  - vertebral artery M47.029
    - cervical region M47.022
    - occipito-atlanto-axial region M47.021
- concussion F07.81
- congenital
  - affecting multiple systems NEC Q87.89
  - central alveolar hypoventilation G47.35
  - facial diplegia Q87.0
  - muscular hypertrophy-cerebral Q87.89
  - oculo-auriculovertebral Q87.0
  - oculofacial diplegia (Moebius) Q87.0
  - rubella (manifest) P35.0
- congestion-fibrosis (pelvic), female N94.89
- congestive dysmenorrhea N94.6
- Conn's E26.01
- connective tissue M35.9
  - overlap NEC M35.1
- conus medullaris G95.81
- cord
  - anterior G83.82
  - posterior G83.83
- coronary
  - acute NEC I24.9
  - insufficiency or intermediate I20.0
  - slow flow I20.89
- Costen's (complex) M26.69
- costochondral junction M94.0
- costoclavicular G54.0
- costovertebral E22.0
- Cowden
  - PTEN related Q85.81
  - specified NEC Q85.82
- craniovertebral M53.0
- Creutzfeldt-Jakob —*see* Creutzfeldt-Jakob disease or syndrome
- cri-du-chat Q93.4
- crib death R99
- cricopharyngeal —*see* Dysphagia
- croup J05.0
- CRPS I —*see* Syndrome, pain, complex regional I
- crush T79.5
- cubital tunnel —*see* Lesion, nerve, ulnar
- Curschmann (-Batten) (-Steinert) G71.11
- Cushing's E24.9
  - alcohol-induced E24.4
  - drug-induced E24.2
  - due to
    - alcohol
    - drugs E24.2
    - ectopic ACTH E24.3
    - overproduction of pituitary ACTH E24.0
  - overdose or wrong substance given or taken —*see* Table of Drugs and Chemicals, by drug, poisoning
  - pituitary-dependent E24.0
  - specified type NEC E24.8
- cryopyrin-associated periodic M04.2
- cryptophthalmos Q87.0
- cystic duct stump K91.5
- cytokine release D89.839
  - grade 1 D89.831
  - grade 2 D89.832
  - grade 3 D89.833
  - grade 4 D89.834
  - grade 5 D89.835
- Dana-Putnam D51.0
- Danbolt (-Cross) (acrodermatitis enteropathica) E83.2
- Dandy-Walker Q03.1
  - with spina bifida Q07.01
- Danlos' (*see also* Syndrome, Ehlers-Danlos) Q79.60
- defibrination —*see also* Fibrinolysis
  - with
    - antepartum hemorrhage —*see* Hemorrhage, antepartum, with coagulation defect
    - intrapartum hemorrhage —*see* Hemorrhage, complicating, delivery
  - newborn P60
  - postpartum O72.3
- Degos' I77.8
- Déjérine-Roussy G89.0
- delayed sleep phase G47.21
- demyelinating G37.9
- dependence —*see* F10-F19 with fourth character .2
- depersonalization (-derealization) F48.1
- De Quervain E34.51
- de Toni-Fanconi (-Debré) E72.09
  - with cystinosis E72.04
- de Vivo syndrome E74.810
- diabetes mellitus-hypertension-nephrosis —*see* Diabetes, nephrosis
- diabetes mellitus in newborn infant P70.2
- diabetes-nephrosis —*see* Diabetes, nephrosis
- diabetic amyotrophy —*see* Diabetes, amyotrophy
- dialysis associated steal T82.898- ●
- Diamond-Blackfan D61.01
- Diamond-Gardener D69.2
- DIC (diffuse or disseminated intravascular coagulopathy) D65
- di George's D82.1
- Dighton's Q78.0
- disequilibrium E87.8
- Döhle body-panmyelopathic D72.0
- dorsolateral medullary G46.4
- double athetosis G80.3
- Down (*see also* Down syndrome) Q90.9
- Dravet (intractable) G40.834
  - with status epilepticus G40.833
  - without status epilepticus G40.834
- Dresbach's (elliptocytosis) D58.1
- DRESS (drug rash with eosinophilia and systemic symptoms) D72.12
- Dressler's (postmyocardial infarction) I24.1
  - postcardiotomy I97.0
- drug rash with eosinophilia and systemic symptoms (DRESS) D72.12
- drug withdrawal, infant of dependent mother P96.1
- dry eye H04.12- ●
- due to abnormality
  - chromosomal Q99.9
    - sex
      - female phenotype Q97.9
      - male phenotype Q98.9
    - specified NEC Q99.8

Syndrome *(Continued)*
  dumping (postgastrectomy) K91.1
    nonsurgical K31.89
  Dupré's (meningism) R29.1
  dysmetabolic X E88.81Ø
  dyspraxia, developmental F82
  Eagle-Barrett Q79.4
  Eaton-Lambert —*see* Syndrome, Lambert-Eaton
  Ebstein's Q22.5
  ectopic ACTH E24.3
  eczema-thrombocytopenia D82.Ø
  Eddowes' Q78.Ø
  effort (psychogenic) F45.8
  Ehlers-Danlos Q79.6Ø
    classical (cEDS) (classical EDS) Q79.61
    hypermobile (hEDS) (hypermobile EDS) Q79.62
    specified NEC Q79.69
    vascular (vascular EDS) (vEDS) Q79.63
  Eisenmenger's I27.83
  Ekman's Q78.Ø
  electric feet E53.8
  Ellis-van Creveld Q77.6
  empty nest Z6Ø.Ø
  endocrine-hypertensive E27.Ø
  entrapment —*see* Neuropathy, entrapment
  eosinophilia-myalgia M35.89
  epileptic —*see also* Epilepsy, by type
    absence G4Ø.AØ9
      intractable G4Ø.A19
        with status epilepticus G4Ø.A11
        without status epilepticus G4Ø.A19
      not intractable G4Ø.AØ9
        with status epilepticus G4Ø.AØ1
        without status epilepticus G4Ø.AØ9
  Erdheim-Chester (ECD) E88.89
  Erdheim's E22.Ø
  erythrocyte fragmentation D59.4
  Evans D69.41
  exhaustion F48.8
  extrapyramidal G25.9
    specified NEC G25.89
  eye retraction —*see* Strabismus
  eyelid-malar-mandible Q87.Ø
  Faber's D5Ø.9
  facet M47.89- ●
  facet joint (*see also* Spondylosis) M47.819
  facial pain, paroxysmal G5Ø.Ø
  Fallot's Q21.3
  familial cold autoinflammatory MØ4.2
  familial eczema-thrombocytopenia (Wiskott-Aldrich) D82.Ø
  Fanconi (-de Toni) (-Debré) E72.Ø9
    with cystinosis E72.Ø4
  ~~Fanconi's (anemia) (congenital pancytopenia) D61.Ø9~~
  fatigue
    chronic G93.32
    postviral G93.31
    psychogenic F48.8
  faulty bowel habit K59.39
  Feil-Klippel (brevicollis) Q76.1
  Felty's —*see* Felty's syndrome
  fertile eunuch E23.Ø
  fetal
    alcohol (dysmorphic) Q86.Ø
    hydantoin Q86.1
  Fiedler's I4Ø.1
  first arch Q87.Ø
  fish odor E72.89
  Fisher's G61.Ø
  Fitzhugh-Curtis
    due to
      Chlamydia trachomatis A74.81
      ~~Neisseria gonorrhorea (gonococcal peritonitis) A54.85~~
      ▶ Neisseria gonorrhea (gonococcal peritonitis) A54.85
  Fitz's —*see also* Pancreatitis, acute K85.8Ø
  Flajani (-Basedow) EØ5.ØØ
    with thyroid storm EØ5.Ø1
  flatback —*see* Flatback syndrome
  floppy
    baby P94.2
    iris (intraoeprative) (IFIS) H21.81
    mitral valve I34.1
  ➡ flush E34.Ø9
  Foix-Alajouanine G95.19
  Fong's Q87.2
  food protein-induced enterocolitis (FPIES) K52.21
  foramen magnum G93.5

Syndrome *(Continued)*
  Foster-Kennedy H47.14- ●
  Foville's (peduncular) G46.3
  fragile X Q99.2
  Franceschetti Q75.4
  Frey's
    auriculotemporal G5Ø.8
    hyperhidrosis L74.52
  Friderichsen-Waterhouse A39.1
  Froin's G95.89
  frontal lobe FØ7.Ø
  Fukuhara E88.49
  functional
    bowel K59.9
    prepubertal castrate E29.1
  Gaisböck's D75.1
  ganglion (basal ganglia brain) G25.9
    geniculi G51.1
  Gardner-Diamond D69.2
  gastroesophageal
    junction K22.Ø
    laceration-hemorrhage K22.6
  gastrojejunal loop obstruction K91.89
  Gee-Herter-Heubner K9Ø.Ø
  Gelineau's G47.419
    with cataplexy G47.411
  genito-anorectal A55
  Gerstmann-Sträussler-Scheinker (GSS) A81.82
  Gianotti-Crosti L44.4
  giant platelet (Bernard-Soulier) D69.1
  Gilles de la Tourette's F95.2
  Glass Q87.89
  Gleich's D72.118
  goiter-deafness EØ7.1
  Goldberg Q89.8
  Goldberg-Maxwell E34.51
  Good's D83.8
  Gopalan' (burning feet) E53.8
  Gorlin's Q87.89
  Gougerot-Blum L81.7
  Gouley's I31.1
  Gower's R55
  gray or grey (newborn) P93.Ø
    platelet D69.1
  Gubler-Millard G46.3
  Guillain-Barré (-Strohl) G61.Ø
  gustatory sweating G5Ø.8
  Hadfield-Clarke K86.89
  hair tourniquet —*see* Constriction, external, by site
  Hamman's J98.19
  hand-foot L27.1
  ➡ hand-shoulder G9Ø.89
  hantavirus (cardio)-pulmonary (HPS) (HCPS) B33.4
  happy puppet Q93.51
  Harada's H3Ø.81- ●
  Hayem-Faber D5Ø.9
  headache NEC G44.89
    complicated NEC G44.59
  Heberden's I2Ø.89
  ➡ Hedinger's E34.Ø1
  Hegglin's D72.Ø
  HELLP (hemolysis, elevated liver enzymes and low platelet count) O14.2- ●
    complicating
      childbirth O14.24
        puerperium O14.25
  hemolytic-uremic D59.3Ø
    atypical D59.39
      genetic D59.32
      hereditary D59.32
      infection-associated D59.31
      secondary D59.39
      specified NEC D59.39
    due to genetic disorder D59.32
    familial D59.32
    hereditary D59.32
    infection-associated D59.31
    secondary D59.39
    Shiga toxin-producing E. coli [STEC] related D59.31
    specified NEC D59.39
    typical D59.31
  hemophagocytic, infection-associated D76.2
  Henoch-Schönlein D69.Ø
  hepatic flexure K59.89
  hepatopulmonary K76.81
  hepatorenal K76.7
    following delivery O9Ø.41
    postoperative or postprocedural K91.83
    postpartum, puerperal O9Ø.41

Syndrome *(Continued)*
  hepatourologic K76.7
  hereditary alpha tryptasemia D89.44
  Herter (-Gee) (nontropical sprue) K9Ø.Ø
  Heubner-Herter K9Ø.Ø
  Heyd's K76.7
  Hilger's G9Ø.Ø9
  histamine-like (fish poisoning) —*see* Poisoning, fish
  histiocytic D76.3
  histiocytosis NEC D76.3
  HIV infection, acute B2Ø
  Hoffmann-Werdnig G12.Ø
  Hollander-Simons E88.1
  Hoppe-Goldflam G7Ø.ØØ
    with exacerbation (acute) G7Ø.Ø1
    in crisis G7Ø.Ø1
  Horner's G9Ø.2
  hungry bone E83.81
  hunterian glossitis D51.Ø
  Hunt's (herpetic geniculate ganglionitis) (neuralgia) BØ2.21
    dyssynergia cerebellaris myoclonica G11.19
  Hutchinson's triad A5Ø.53
  hyperabduction G54.Ø
  hyperammonemia-hyperornithinemia-homocitrullinemia E72.4
  hypereosinophilic (HES) D72.119
    idiopathic (IHES) D72.11Ø
    lymphocytic variant (LHES) D72.111
    myeloid D72.118
    specified NEC D72.118
  hyperimmunoglobulin D MØ4.1
  hyperimmunoglobulin E (IgE) D82.4
  hyperkalemic E87.5
  hyperkinetic —*see* Hyperkinesia
  hypermobility M35.7
  hypernatremia E87.Ø
  hyperosmolarity (*see also*, Diabetes, by type, with hyperosmolarity) E87.Ø
  hyperperfusion G97.82
  hypersplenic D73.1
  hypertransfusion, newborn P61.1
  hyperventilation F45.8
  hyperviscosity (of serum)
    polycythemic D75.1
    sclerothymic D58.8
  hypoglycemic (familial) (neonatal) E16.2
  hypokalemic E87.6
  hyponatremic E87.1
  hypopituitarism E23.Ø
  hypoplastic left-heart Q23.4
  hypopotassemia E87.6
  hyposmolality E87.1
  hypotension, maternal O26.5- ●
  hypothenar hammer I73.89
  hypoventilation, obesity (OHS) E66.2
  ICF (intravascular coagulation-fibrinolysis) D65
  idiopathic
    cardiorespiratory distress, newborn P22.Ø
    nephrotic (infantile) NØ4.9
  iliotibial band M76.3- ●
  immobility, immobilization (paraplegic) M62.3
  immune effector cell-associated neurotoxicity (ICANS) G92.ØØ
    grade
      1 G92.Ø1
      2 G92.Ø2
      3 G92.Ø3
      4 G92.Ø4
      5 G92.Ø5
      unspecified G92.ØØ
  immune reconstitution D89.3
  immune reconstitution inflammatory [IRIS] D89.3
  immunity deficiency, combined D81.9
  immunodeficiency
    acquired —*see* Human, immunodeficiency virus (HIV) disease
    combined D81.9
  impending coronary I2Ø.Ø
  impingement, shoulder M75.4- ●
  inappropriate secretion of antidiuretic hormone E22.2
  infant
    gestational diabetes P7Ø.Ø
    of diabetic mother P7Ø.1
  infantilism (pituitary) E23.Ø
  inferior vena cava I87.1
  inspissated bile (newborn) P59.1
  institutional (childhood) F94.2
  insufficient sleep F51.12

Syndrome *(Continued)*
- insulin resistance
  - type A E88.811
  - type B E88.818
- intermediate coronary (artery) I20.0
- interspinous ligament —*see* Spondylopathy, specified NEC
- intestinal
  - ➡carcinoid E34.09
  - knot K56.2
- intravascular coagulation-fibrinolysis (ICF) D65
- iodine-deficiency, congenital E00.9
  - type
    - mixed E00.2
    - myxedematous E00.1
    - neurological E00.0
- IRDS (idiopathic respiratory distress, newborn) P22.0
- irritable
  - bowel K58.9
    - with
      - constipation K58.1
      - diarrhea K58.0
    - mixed K58.2
    - psychogenic F45.8
    - specified NEC K58.8
  - heart (psychogenic) F45.8
  - weakness F48.8
- ischemic
  - bowel (transient) K55.9
    - chronic K55.1
    - due to mesenteric artery insufficiency K55.1
  - steal T82.898
- IVC (intravascular coagulopathy) D65
- Ivemark's Q89.01
- Jaccoud's —*see* Arthropathy, postrheumatic, chronic
- Jackson's G83.89
- Jakob-Creutzfeldt —*see* Creutzfeldt-Jakob disease or syndrome
- jaw-winking Q07.8
- Jervell-Lange-Nielsen I45.81
- jet lag G47.25
- Job's D71
- Joseph-Diamond-Blackfan D61.01
- jugular foramen G52.7
- Kabuki Q89.8
- Kanner's (autism) F84.0
- Kartagener's Q89.3
- Kelly's D50.1
- Kimmelstiel-Wilson —*see* Diabetes, specified type, with Kimmelstiel-Wilson disease
- ▶Kleefstra Q87.86
- Klein (e)-Levine G47.13
- Klippel-Feil (brevicollis) Q76.1
- ~~Köhler-Pellegrini-Steida —*see* Bursitis, tibial collateral~~
- ▶Köhler-Pellegrini-Stieda —*see* Bursitis, tibial collateral
- König's K59.89
- Korsakoff (-Wernicke) (nonalcoholic) F04
  - alcoholic F10.26
- Kostmann's D70.0
- Krabbe's congenital muscle hypoplasia Q79.8
- labyrinthine —*see* subcategory H83.2
- lacunar NEC G46.7
- Lambert-Eaton G70.80
  - in
    - neoplastic disease G73.1
    - specified disease NEC G70.81
- Landau-Kleffner —*see* Epilepsy, specified NEC
- Larsen's Q74.8
- ▶Lassueur Graham-Little Piccardi L66.19
- lateral
  - cutaneous nerve of thigh G57.1-●
  - medullary G46.4
- Launois' E22.0
- Laurence-Moon Q87.84
- lazy
  - leukocyte D70.8
  - posture M62.3
- ~~Lemiere I80.8~~
- ▶Lemierre I80.8
- Lennox-Gastaut G40.812
  - intractable G40.814
    - with status epilepticus G40.813
    - without status epilepticus G40.814
  - not intractable G40.812
    - with status epilepticus G40.811
    - without status epilepticus G40.812
- lenticular, progressive E83.01
- Leopold-Levi's E05.90

Syndrome *(Continued)*
- Lev's I44.2
- Li-Fraumeni Z15.01
- Lichtheim's D51.0
- Lightwood's N25.89
- Lignac (de Toni) (-Fanconi) (-Debré) E72.09
  - with cystinosis E72.04
- Likoff's I20.89
- limbic epilepsy personality F07.0
- liver-kidney K76.7
- lobotomy F07.0
- Löffler's J82.89
- long arm 18 or 21 deletion Q93.89
- long QT I45.81
- Louis-Barré G11.3
- low
  - atmospheric pressure T70.29
  - back M54.50
  - output (cardiac) I50.9
- lower radicular, newborn (birth injury) P14.8
- Luetscher's (dehydration) E86.0
- Lupus anticoagulant D68.62
- Lutembacher's Q21.19
- macrophage activation D76.1
  - due to infection D76.2
- magnesium-deficiency R29.0
- Majeed M04.8
- Mal de Debarquement R42
- malabsorption K90.9
  - postsurgical K91.2
- malformation, congenital, due to
  - alcohol Q86.0
  - exogenous cause NEC Q86.8
  - hydantoin Q86.1
  - warfarin Q86.2
- malignant
  - ➡carcinoid E34.00
  - neuroleptic G21.0
- Mallory-Weiss K22.6
- mandibulofacial dysostosis Q75.4
- manic-depressive —*see* Disorder, bipolar
- maple-syrup-urine E71.0
- Marable's I77.4
- Marfan Q87.40
  - with
    - cardiovascular manifestations Q87.418
      - aortic dilation Q87.410
    - ocular manifestations Q87.42
    - skeletal manifestations Q87.43
- Marie's (acromegaly) E22.0
- mast cell activation —*see* Activation, mast cell
- maternal hypotension —*see* Syndrome, hypotension, maternal
- May (-Hegglin) D72.0
- McArdle (-Schmidt) (-Pearson) E74.04
- McQuarrie's E16.2
- meconium plug (newborn) P76.0
- MED13L (mediator complex subunit 13L) Q87.85
- median arcuate ligament I77.4
- mediator complex subunit 13L (MED13L) Q87.85
- Meekeren-Ehlers-Danlos Q79.6
- megavitamin-B6 E67.2
- Meige G24.4
- MELAS E88.41
- Mendelson's O74.0
- MERRF (myoclonic epilepsy associated with ragged-red fibers) E88.42
- mesenteric
  - artery (superior) K55.1
  - vascular insufficiency K55.1
- metabolic E88.810
- ➡metastatic carcinoid E34.00
- micrognathia-glossoptosis Q87.0
- midbrain NEC G93.89
- middle lobe (lung) J98.19
- middle radicular G54.0
- migraine —*see also* Migraine G43.909-●
- Mikulicz' K11.8
- milk-alkali E83.52
- Millard-Gubler G46.3
- Miller-Dieker Q93.88
- Miller-Fisher G61.0
- Minkowski-Chauffard D58.0
- Mirizzi's K83.1
- MNGIE (Mitochondrial Neurogastrointestinal Encephalopathy) E88.49
- Möbius, ophthalmoplegic migraine —*see* Migraine, ophthalmoplegic
- monofixation H50.42
- Morel-Moore M85.2
- Morel-Morgagni M85.2
- Morgagni (-Morel) (-Stewart) M85.2

Syndrome *(Continued)*
- Morgagni-Adams-Stokes I45.9
- Mounier-Kuhn Q32.4
  - with bronchiectasis J47.9
    - with
      - exacerbation (acute) J47.1
      - lower respiratory infection J47.0
  - acquired J98.09
    - with bronchiectasis J47.9
      - with
        - exacerbation (acute) J47.1
        - lower respiratory infection J47.0
- Muckle-Wells M04.2
- mucocutaneous lymph node (acute febrile) (MCLS) M30.3
- multiple endocrine neoplasia (MEN) —*see* Neoplasia, endocrine, multiple (MEN)
- multiple operations —*see* Disorder, factitious
- multisystem inflammatory (in adults) (in children) M35.81
- myasthenic G70.9
  - in
    - diabetes mellitus —*see* Diabetes, amyotrophy
    - endocrine disease NEC E34.9 *[G73.3]*
    - neoplastic disease —*see also* Neoplasm D49.9 *[G73.3]*
    - thyrotoxicosis (hyperthyroidism) E05.90 *[G73.3]*
      - with thyroid storm E05.91 *[G73.3]*
- myelodysplastic D46.9
  - with
    - 5q deletion D46.C
    - isolated del (5q) chromosomal abnormality D46.C
    - multilineage dysplasia D46.A
      - with ringed sideroblasts D46.B
  - lesions, low grade D46.20
  - specified NEC D46.Z
- myeloid hypereosinophilic D72.118
- myelopathic pain G89.0
- myeloproliferative (chronic) D47.1
- myofascial pain M79.18
- Naffziger's G54.0
- nail patella Q87.2
- NARP (Neuropathy, Ataxia and Retinitis pigmentosa) E88.49
- neonatal abstinence P96.1
- nephritic —*see also* Nephritis
  - with edema —*see* Nephrosis
  - acute N00.9
  - chronic N03.9
  - rapidly progressive N01.9
- nephrotic (congenital) —*see also* Nephrosis N04.9
  - with
    - C3
      - glomerulonephritis N04.A
      - glomerulopathy N04.A
        - with dense deposit disease N04.6
    - dense deposit disease N04.6
    - diffuse
      - crescentic glomerulonephritis N04.7
      - endocapillary proliferative glomerulonephritis N04.4
      - membranous glomerulonephritis N04.20
      - mesangial proliferative glomerulonephritis N04.3
      - mesangiocapillary glomerulonephritis N04.5
    - focal and segmental glomerular lesions N04.1
    - minor glomerular abnormality N04.0
    - specified morphological changes NEC N04.8
  - diabetic —*see* Diabetes, nephrosis
  - specified type NEC with diffuse membranous glomerulonephritis N04.29
- neurologic neglect R41.4
- Nezelof's D81.4
- Nonne-Milroy-Meige Q82.0
- Nothnagel's vasomotor acroparesthesia I73.89
- obesity hypoventilation (OHS) E66.2
- obliterans
  - bronchiolitis (see also Bronchiolitis, obliterative) J44.81
- oculomotor H51.9
- Ogilvie K59.81
- Oliver-McFarlane Q87.89
- ophthalmoplegia-cerebellar ataxia —*see* Strabismus, paralytic, third nerve
- oral allergy T78.1
- oral-facial-digital Q87.0

▶ New ➡ Revised ~~deleted~~ Deleted ● Use Additional Character(s)

Syndrome *(Continued)*
- organic
  - affective FØ6.3Ø
  - amnesic (not alcohol- or drug-induced) FØ4
  - brain FØ9
  - depressive FØ6.31
  - hallucinosis FØ6.Ø
  - personality FØ7.Ø
- Ormond's N13.5
- oro-facial-digital Q87.Ø
- os trigonum Q68.8
- Osler-Weber-Rendu I78.Ø
- osteoporosis-osteomalacia M83.8
- Osterreicher-Turner Q87.2
- otolith *—see* subcategory H81.8
- oto-palatal-digital Q87.Ø
- ➠ outlet (thoracic) (*see also* Syndrome, thoracic outlet) G54.Ø
- ovary
  - polycystic E28.2
  - resistant E28.39
  - sclerocystic E28.2
- Owren's D68.2
- Paget-Schroetter I82.89Ø
- pain *—see also* Pain
  - complex regional I G9Ø.5Ø
    - lower limb G9Ø.52-●
    - specified site NEC G9Ø.59
    - upper limb G9Ø.51-●
  - complex regional II *—see* Causalgia
- painful
  - bruising D69.2
  - feet E53.8
  - prostate N42.81
- paralysis agitans *—see* Parkinsonism
- paralytic G83.9
  - specified NEC G83.89
- Parinaud's H51.Ø
- parkinsonian *—see* Parkinsonism
- Parkinson's *—see* Parkinsonism
- paroxysmal facial pain G5Ø.Ø
- Parry's EØ5.ØØ
  - with thyroid storm EØ5.Ø1
- Parsonage (-Aldren)-Turner G54.5
- patella clunk M25.86-●
- Paterson (-Brown) (-Kelly) D5Ø.1
- pectoral girdle I77.89
- pectoralis minor I77.89
- pediatric autoimmune neuropsychiatric disorders associated with streptococcal infections (PANDAS) D89.89
- pediatric inflammatory multisystem M35.81
- Pelger-Huet D72.Ø
- pellagra-cerebellar ataxia-renal aminoaciduria E72.Ø2
- pellagroid E52
- Pellegrini-Stieda *—see* Bursitis, tibial collateral
- pelvic congestion-fibrosis, female N94.89
- penta X Q97.1
- peptic ulcer *—see* Ulcer, peptic
- perabduction I77.89
- periodic fever MØ4.1
- periodic fever, aphthous stomatitis, pharyngitis, and adenopathy [PFAPA] MØ4.8
- periodic headache, in adults and children *—see* Headache, periodic syndromes in adults and children
- periurethral fibrosis N13.5
- Peutz-Jeghers Q85.89
- phantom limb (without pain) G54.7
  - with pain G54.6
- pharyngeal pouch D82.1
- Phelan-McDermid Q93.52
- Pick's *—see* Disease, Pick's
- Pickwickian E66.2
- PIE (pulmonary infiltration with eosinophilia) J82.89
- pigmentary pallidal degeneration (progressive) G23.Ø
- pineal E34.8
- pituitary E22.Ø
- placental transfusion *—see* Pregnancy, complicated by, placental transfusion syndromes
- plantar fascia M72.2
- plateau iris (post-iridectomy) (postprocedural) H21.82
- Plummer-Vinson D5Ø.1
- pluricarential of infancy E4Ø
- plurideficiency E4Ø
- pluriglandular (compensatory) E31.8
  - autoimmune E31.Ø
- pneumatic hammer T75.21

Syndrome *(Continued)*
- polyangiitis overlap M3Ø.8
- polycarential of infancy E4Ø
- polyglandular E31.8
  - autoimmune E31.Ø
- polysplenia Q89.Ø9
- pontine NEC G93.89
- popliteal
  - artery entrapment I77.89
  - web Q87.89
- postbacterial fatigue G93.39
- postcardiac injury
  - postcardiotomy I97.Ø
  - postmyocardial infarction I24.1
- postcardiotomy I97.Ø
- post chemoembolization — code to associated conditions
- postcholecystectomy K91.5
- postcommissurotomy I97.Ø
- postconcussional FØ7.81
- postcontusional FØ7.81
- post-COVID (-19) UØ9.9
- postencephalitic FØ7.89
- post endometrial ablation N99.85
- posterior
  - cervical sympathetic M53.Ø
  - cord G83.83
  - fossa compression G93.5
  - reversible encephalopathy (PRES) I67.83
- postgastrectomy (dumping) K91.1
- postgastric surgery K91.1
- postinfarction I24.1
- postinfectious fatigue G93.39
- postlaminectomy NEC M96.1
- postleukotomy FØ7.Ø
- postmastectomy lymphedema I97.2
- postmyocardial infarction I24.1
- postoperative NEC T81.9
  - blind loop K9Ø.2
- postpartum panhypopituitary (Sheehan) E23.Ø
- postpolio (myelitic) G14
- postthrombotic I87.ØØ9
  - with
    - inflammation I87.Ø2-●
      - with ulcer I87.Ø3-●
    - specified complication NEC I87.Ø9-●
    - ulcer I87.Ø1-●
      - with inflammation I87.Ø3-●
  - asymptomatic I87.ØØ-●
- postural
  - orthostatic tachycardia [POTS] G9Ø.A
  - tachycardia G9Ø.A
- postvagotomy K91.1
- postvalvulotomy I97.Ø
- postviral NEC G93.31
  - fatigue G93.31
- Potain's K31.Ø
- potassium intoxication E87.5
- Prader-Willi Q87.11
- Prader-Willi-like Q87.19
- precerebral artery (multiple) (bilateral) G45.2
- preinfarction I2Ø.Ø
- preleukemic D46.9
- premature senility E34.8
- premenstrual dysphoric F32.81
- premenstrual tension N94.3
- Prinzmetal-Massumi RØ7.1
- prune belly Q79.4
- pseudocarpal tunnel (sublimis) *—see* Syndrome, carpal tunnel
- pseudoparalytica G7Ø.ØØ
  - with exacerbation (acute) G7Ø.Ø1
  - in crisis G7Ø.Ø1
- pseudo-Turner's Q87.19
- psycho-organic (nonpsychotic severity) FØ7.9
  - acute or subacute FØ5
  - depressive type FØ6.31
  - hallucinatory type FØ6.Ø
  - nonpsychotic severity FØ7.Ø
  - specified NEC FØ7.89
- PTEN (hamartoma) tumor Q85.81
- pulmonary
  - arteriosclerosis I27.Ø
  - dysmaturity (Wilson-Mikity) P27.Ø
  - hypoperfusion (idiopathic) P22.Ø
  - renal (hemorrhagic) (Goodpasture's) M31.Ø
- pure
  - motor lacunar G46.5
  - sensory lacunar G46.6

Syndrome *(Continued)*
- Putnam-Dana D51.Ø
- pyogenic arthritis, pyoderma gangrenosum, and acne [PAPA] MØ4.8
- pyramidopallidonigral G2Ø.C
- pyriformis *—see* Lesion, nerve, sciatic
- QT interval prolongation I45.81
- radicular NEC *—see* Radiculopathy
  - upper limbs, newborn (birth injury) P14.3
- rapid time-zone change G47.25
- Rasmussen GØ4.81
- Raymond (-Céstan) I65.8
- Raynaud's I73.ØØ
  - with gangrene I73.Ø1
- RDS (respiratory distress syndrome, newborn) P22.Ø
- reactive airways dysfunction J68.3
- Refsum's G6Ø.1
- Reifenstein E34.52
- renal glomerulohyalinosis-diabetic *—see* Diabetes, nephrosis
- Rendu-Osler-Weber I78.Ø
- residual ovary N99.83
- resistant ovary E28.39
- respiratory
  - distress
    - acute J8Ø
      - adult J8Ø
      - child J8Ø
      - idiopathic J84.114
    - newborn (idiopathic) (type I) P22.Ø
      - type II P22.1
- restless legs G25.81
- restrictive allograft J4A.Ø
- retinoblastoma (familial) C69.2
- retroperitoneal fibrosis K68.2
- retroviral seroconversion (acute) Z21
- Reye's G93.7
- Richter *—see* Leukemia, chronic lymphocytic, B-cell type
- Ridley's I5Ø.1
- right
  - heart, hypoplastic Q22.6
  - ventricular obstruction *—see* Failure, heart, right
- Romano-Ward (prolonged QT interval) I45.81
- rotator cuff, shoulder *—see also* Tear, rotator cuff M75.1Ø-●
- Rotes Quérol *—see* Hyperostosis, ankylosing
- Roth *—see* Meralgia paresthetica
- rubella (congenital) P35.Ø
- Ruvalcaba-Myhre-Smith E71.44Ø
- Rytand-Lipsitch I44.2
- salt
  - depletion E87.1
    - due to heat NEC T67.8
      - causing heat exhaustion or prostration T67.4
  - low E87.1
- salt-losing N28.89
- SATB2-associated Q87.89
- Scaglietti-Dagnini E22.Ø
- scalenus anticus (anterior) G54.Ø
- scapulocostal *—see* Mononeuropathy, upper limb, specified site NEC
- scapuloperoneal G71.Ø9
- schizophrenic, of childhood NEC F2Ø.9
- Schnitzler D47.2
- ➠ Scholte's E34.Ø9
- Schroeder's E27.Ø
- Schüller-Christian C96.5
- Schwachman (-Diamond) D61.Ø2
- Schwartz (-Jampel) G71.13
- Schwartz-Bartter E22.2
- scimitar Q26.8
- sclerocystic ovary E28.2
- Seitelberger's G31.89
- septicemic adrenal hemorrhage A39.1
- seroconversion, retroviral (acute) Z21
- ▶ serotonin G9Ø.81
- serous meningitis G93.2
- severe acute respiratory (SARS) J12.81
- coronavirus 2 *-see also* COVID-19 UØ7.1
  - pneumonia J12.82
- shaken infant T74.4
- shock (traumatic) T79.4
  - kidney N17.Ø
    - following crush injury T79.5
  - toxic A48.3
- shock-lung J8Ø
- Shone's — code to specific anomalies

Synovial sarcoma —*see* Neoplasm, connective tissue, malignant
Synovioma (malignant) —*see also* Neoplasm, connective tissue, malignant
benign —*see* Neoplasm, connective tissue, benign
Synoviosarcoma —*see* Neoplasm, connective tissue, malignant
Synovitis —*see also* Tenosynovitis M65.9Ø
ankle and foot M65.97-●
arm, upper M65.92-●
crepitant
hand M7Ø.Ø-●
wrist M7Ø.Ø3-●
forearm M65.93-●
gonococcal A54.49
gouty —*see* Gout
hand M65.94-●
in (due to)
crystals M65.8-●
gonorrhea A54.49
syphilis (late) A52.78
use, overuse, pressure —*see* Disorder, soft tissue, due to use
infective NEC —*see* Tenosynovitis, infective NEC
leg, lower M65.96-●
multiple sites, unspecified type M65.99
shoulder M65.91-●
specified NEC —*see* Tenosynovitis, specified type NEC
specified site, unspecified type M65.98
syphilitic A52.78
congenital (early) A5Ø.Ø2
thigh M65.95-●
toxic —*see* Synovitis, transient
transient M67.3-●
ankle M67.37-●
elbow M67.32-●
foot joint M67.37-●
hand joint M67.34-●
hip M67.35-●
knee M67.36-●
multiple site M67.39
pelvic region M67.35-●
shoulder M67.31-●
specified joint NEC M67.38
wrist M67.33-●
traumatic, current —*see* Sprain
tuberculous —*see* Tuberculosis, synovitis
villonodular (pigmented) M12.2-●
ankle M12.27-●
elbow M12.22-●
foot joint M12.27-●
hand joint M12.24-●
hip M12.25-●
knee M12.26-●
multiple site M12.29
pelvic region M12.25-●
shoulder M12.21-●
specified joint NEC M12.28
vertebrae M12.28
wrist M12.23-●
Syphilid A51.39
congenital A5Ø.Ø6
newborn A5Ø.Ø6
tubercular (late) A52.79
Syphilis, syphilitic (acquired) A53.9
abdomen (late) A52.79
acoustic nerve A52.15
adenopathy (secondary) A51.49
adrenal (gland) (with cortical hypofunction) A52.79
age under 2 years NOS —*see also* Syphilis, congenital, early
acquired A51.9
alopecia (secondary) A51.32
anemia (late) A52.79 *[D63.8]*
aneurysm (aorta) (ruptured) A52.Ø1
central nervous system A52.Ø5
congenital A5Ø.54 *[I79.Ø]*
anus (late) A52.74
primary A51.1
secondary A51.39
aorta (arch) (abdominal) (thoracic) A52.Ø2
aneurysm A52.Ø1
aortic (insufficiency) (regurgitation) (stenosis)A52.Ø3
aneurysm A52.Ø1
arachnoid (adhesive) (cerebral) (spinal) A52.13
asymptomatic —*see* Syphilis, latent
ataxia (locomotor) A52.11
atrophoderma maculatum A51.39
auricular fibrillation A52.Ø6
bladder (late) A52.76

Syphilis, syphilitic *(Continued)*
bone A52.77
secondary A51.46
brain A52.17
breast (late) A52.79
bronchus (late) A52.72
bubo (primary) A51.Ø
bulbar palsy A52.19
bursa (late) A52.78
cardiac decompensation A52.Ø6
cardiovascular A52.ØØ
central nervous system (late) (recurrent) (relapse) (tertiary) A52.3
with
ataxia A52.11
general paralysis A52.17
juvenile A5Ø.45
paresis (general) A52.17
juvenile A5Ø.45
tabes (dorsalis) A52.11
juvenile A5Ø.45
taboparesis A52.17
juvenile A5Ø.45
aneurysm A52.Ø5
congenital A5Ø.4Ø
juvenile A5Ø.4Ø
remission in (sustained) A52.3
serology doubtful, negative, or positive A52.3
specified nature or site NEC A52.19
vascular A52.Ø5
cerebral A52.17
meningovascular A52.13
nerves (multiple palsies) A52.15
sclerosis A52.17
thrombosis A52.Ø5
cerebrospinal (tabetic type) A52.12
cerebrovascular A52.Ø5
cervix (late) A52.76
chancre (multiple) A51.Ø
extragenital A51.2
Rollet's A51.Ø
Charcot's joint A52.16
chorioretinitis A51.43
congenital A5Ø.Ø1
late A52.71
prenatal A5Ø.Ø1
choroiditis —*see* Syphilitic chorioretinitis
choroidoretinitis —*see* Syphilitic chorioretinitis
ciliary body (secondary) A51.43
late A52.71
colon (late) A52.74
combined spinal sclerosis A52.11
condyloma (latum) A51.31
congenital A5Ø.9
with
paresis (general) A5Ø.45
tabes (dorsalis) A5Ø.45
taboparesis A5Ø.45
chorioretinitis, choroiditis A5Ø.Ø1 *[H32]*
early, or less than 2 years after birth NEC A5Ø.2
with manifestations —*see* Syphilis, congenital, early, symptomatic
latent (without manifestations) A5Ø.1
negative spinal fluid test A5Ø.1
serology positive A5Ø.1
symptomatic A5Ø.Ø9
cutaneous A5Ø.Ø6
mucocutaneous A5Ø.Ø7
oculopathy A5Ø.Ø1
osteochondropathy A5Ø.Ø2
pharyngitis A5Ø.Ø3
pneumonia A5Ø.Ø4
rhinitis A5Ø.Ø5
visceral A5Ø.Ø8
interstitial keratitis A5Ø.31
juvenile neurosyphilis A5Ø.45
late, or 2 years or more after birth NEC A5Ø.7
chorioretinitis, choroiditis A5Ø.32
interstitial keratitis A5Ø.31
juvenile neurosyphilis A5Ø.45
latent (without manifestations) A5Ø.6
negative spinal fluid test A5Ø.6
serology positive A5Ø.6
symptomatic or with manifestations NEC A5Ø.59
arthropathy A5Ø.55
cardiovascular A5Ø.54
Clutton's joints A5Ø.51
Hutchinson's teeth A5Ø.52
Hutchinson's triad A5Ø.53
osteochondropathy A5Ø.56
saddle nose A5Ø.57

Syphilis, syphilitic *(Continued)*
conjugal A53.9
tabes A52.11
conjunctiva (late) A52.71
contact Z2Ø.2
cord bladder A52.19
cornea, late A52.71
coronary (artery) (sclerosis) A52.Ø6
coryza, congenital A5Ø.Ø5
cranial nerve A52.15
multiple palsies A52.15
cutaneous —*see* Syphilis, skin
dacryocystitis (late) A52.71
degeneration, spinal cord A52.12
dementia paralytica A52.17
juvenilis A5Ø.45
destruction of bone A52.77
dilatation, aorta A52.Ø1
due to blood transfusion A53.9
dura mater A52.13
ear A52.79
inner A52.79
nerve (eighth) A52.15
neurorecurrence A52.15
early A51.9
cardiovascular A52.ØØ
central nervous system A52.3
latent (without manifestations) (less than 2 years after infection) A51.5
negative spinal fluid test A51.5
serological relapse after treatment A51.5
serology positive A51.5
relapse (treated, untreated) A51.9
skin A51.39
symptomatic A51.9
extragenital chancre A51.2
primary, except extragenital chancre A51.Ø
secondary —*see also* Syphilis, secondary A51.39
relapse (treated, untreated) A51.49
ulcer A51.39
eighth nerve (neuritis) A52.15
endemic A65
endocarditis A52.Ø3
aortic A52.Ø3
pulmonary A52.Ø3
epididymis (late) A52.76
epiglottis (late) A52.73
epiphysitis (congenital) (early) A5Ø.Ø2
episcleritis (late) A52.71
esophagus A52.79
eustachian tube A52.73
exposure to Z2Ø.2
eye A52.71
eyelid (late) (with gumma) A52.71
fallopian tube (late) A52.76
fracture A52.77
gallbladder (late) A52.74
gastric (polyposis) (late) A52.74
general A53.9
paralysis A52.17
juvenile A5Ø.45
genital (primary) A51.Ø
glaucoma A52.71
gumma NEC A52.79
cardiovascular system A52.ØØ
central nervous system A52.3
congenital A5Ø.59
heart (block) (decompensation) (disease) (failure) A52.Ø6 *[I52]*
valve NEC A52.Ø3
hemianesthesia A52.19
hemianopsia A52.71
hemiparesis A52.17
hemiplegia A52.17
hepatic artery A52.Ø9
hepatis A52.74
hepatomegaly, congenital A5Ø.Ø8
hereditaria tarda —*see* Syphilis, congenital, late
hereditary —*see* Syphilis, congenital
Hutchinson's teeth A5Ø.52
hyalitis A52.71
inactive —*see* Syphilis, latent
infantum —*see* Syphilis, congenital
inherited —*see* Syphilis, congenital
internal ear A52.79
intestine (late) A52.74
iris, iritis (secondary) A51.43
late A52.71
joint (late) A52.77
keratitis (congenital) (interstitial) (late) A5Ø.31
kidney (late) A52.75

S

Syphilis, syphilitic *(Continued)*
- lacrimal passages (late) A52.71
- larynx (late) A52.73
- late A52.9
  - cardiovascular A52.00
  - central nervous system A52.3
  - kidney A52.75
  - latent or 2 years or more after infection (without manifestations) A52.8
    - negative spinal fluid test A52.8
    - serology positive A52.8
  - paresis A52.17
  - specified site NEC A52.79
  - symptomatic or with manifestations A52.79
  - tabes A52.11
- latent A53.0
  - with signs or symptoms - code by site and stage under Syphilis
  - central nervous system A52.2
  - date of infection unspecified A53.0
  - early, or less than 2 years after infection A51.5
  - follow-up of latent syphilis A53.0
    - date of infection unspecified A53.0
    - late, or 2 years or more after infection A52.8
  - late, or 2 years or more after infection A52.8
  - positive serology (only finding) A53.0
    - date of infection unspecified A53.0
    - early, or less than 2 years after infection A51.5
    - late, or 2 years or more after infection A52.8
- lens (late) A52.71
- leukoderma A51.39
  - late A52.79
- lienitis A52.79
- lip A51.39
  - chancre (primary) A51.2
  - late A52.79
- Lissauer's paralysis A52.17
- liver A52.74
- locomotor ataxia A52.11
- lung A52.72
- lymph gland (early) (secondary) A51.49
  - late A52.79
- lymphadenitis (secondary) A51.49
- macular atrophy of skin A51.39
  - striated A52.79
- mediastinum (late) A52.73
- meninges (adhesive) (brain) (spinal cord) A52.13
- meningitis A52.13
  - acute (secondary) A51.41
  - congenital A50.41
- meningoencephalitis A52.14
- meningovascular A52.13
  - congenital A50.41
- mesarteritis A52.09
  - brain A52.04
- middle ear A52.77
- mitral stenosis A52.03
- monoplegia A52.17
- mouth (secondary) A51.39
  - late A52.79
- mucocutaneous (secondary) A51.39
  - late A52.79
- mucous
  - membrane (secondary) A51.39
    - late A52.79
  - patches A51.39
    - congenital A50.07
- mulberry molars A50.52
- muscle A52.78
- myocardium A52.06
- nasal sinus (late) A52.73
- neonatorum —*see* Syphilis, congenital
- nephrotic syndrome (secondary) A51.44
- nerve palsy (any cranial nerve) A52.15
  - multiple A52.15
- nervous system, central A52.3
- neuritis A52.15
  - acoustic A52.15
- neurorecidive of retina A52.19
- neuroretinitis A52.19
- newborn —*see* Syphilis, congenital
- nodular superficial (late) A52.79
- nonvenereal A65
- nose (late) A52.73
  - saddle back deformity A50.57
- occlusive arterial disease A52.09
- oculopathy A52.71
- ophthalmic (late) A52.71
- optic nerve (atrophy) (neuritis) (papilla) A52.15
- orbit (late) A52.71
- organic A53.9
- osseous (late) A52.77

Syphilis, syphilitic *(Continued)*
- osteochondritis (congenital) (early) A50.02 *[M90.80]*
- osteoporosis A52.77
- ovary (late) A52.76
- oviduct (late) A52.76
- palate (late) A52.79
- pancreas (late) A52.74
- paralysis A52.17
  - general A52.17
    - juvenile A50.45
- paresis (general) A52.17
  - juvenile A50.45
- paresthesia A52.19
- Parkinson's disease or syndrome A52.19
- paroxysmal tachycardia A52.06
- pemphigus (congenital) A50.06
- penis (chancre) A51.0
  - late A52.76
- pericardium A52.06
- perichondritis, larynx (late) A52.73
- periosteum (late) A52.77
  - congenital (early) A50.02 *[M90.80]*
  - early (secondary) A51.46
- peripheral nerve A52.79
- petrous bone (late) A52.77
- pharynx (late) A52.73
  - secondary A51.39
- pituitary (gland) A52.79
- pleura (late) A52.73
- pneumonia, white A50.04
- pontine lesion A52.17
- portal vein A52.09
- primary A51.0
  - anal A51.1
  - and secondary —*see* Syphilis, secondary
  - central nervous system A52.3
  - extragenital chancre NEC A51.2
  - fingers A51.2
  - genital A51.0
  - lip A51.2
  - specified site NEC A51.2
  - tonsils A51.2
- prostate (late) A52.76
- ptosis (eyelid) A52.71
- pulmonary (late) A52.72
  - artery A52.09
- pyelonephritis (late) A52.75
- recently acquired, symptomatic A51.9
- rectum (late) A52.74
- respiratory tract (late) A52.73
- retina, late A52.71
- retrobulbar neuritis A52.15
- salpingitis A52.76
- sclera (late) A52.71
- sclerosis
  - cerebral A52.17
  - coronary A52.06
  - multiple A52.11
- scotoma (central) A52.71
- scrotum (late) A52.76
- secondary (and primary) A51.49
  - adenopathy A51.49
  - anus A51.39
  - bone A51.46
  - chorioretinitis, choroiditis A51.43
  - hepatitis A51.45
  - liver A51.45
  - lymphadenitis A51.49
  - meningitis (acute) A51.41
  - mouth A51.39
  - mucous membranes A51.39
  - periosteum, periostitis A51.46
  - pharynx A51.39
  - relapse (treated, untreated) A51.49
  - skin A51.39
  - specified form NEC A51.49
  - tonsil A51.39
  - ulcer A51.39
  - viscera NEC A51.49
  - vulva A51.39
- seminal vesicle (late) A52.76
- seronegative with signs or symptoms - code by site and stage under Syphilis
- seropositive
  - with signs or symptoms - code by site and stage under Syphilis
  - follow-up of latent syphilis —*see* Syphilis, latent
  - only finding —*see* Syphilis, latent
- seventh nerve (paralysis) A52.15
- sinus, sinusitis (late) A52.73

Syphilis, syphilitic *(Continued)*
- skeletal system A52.77
- skin (with ulceration) (early) (secondary) A51.39
  - late or tertiary A52.79
- small intestine A52.74
- spastic spinal paralysis A52.17
- spermatic cord (late) A52.76
- spinal (cord) A52.12
- spleen A52.79
- splenomegaly A52.79
- spondylitis A52.77
- staphyloma A52.71
- stigmata (congenital) A50.59
- stomach A52.74
- synovium A52.78
- tabes dorsalis (late) A52.11
  - juvenile A50.45
- tabetic type A52.11
  - juvenile A50.45
- taboparesis A52.17
  - juvenile A50.45
- tachycardia A52.06
- tendon (late) A52.78
- tertiary A52.9
  - with symptoms NEC A52.79
  - cardiovascular A52.00
  - central nervous system A52.3
  - multiple NEC A52.79
  - specified site NEC A52.79
- testis A52.76
- thorax A52.73
- throat A52.73
- thymus (gland) (late) A52.79
- thyroid (late) A52.79
- tongue (late) A52.79
- tonsil (lingual) (late) A52.73
  - primary A51.2
  - secondary A51.39
- trachea (late) A52.73
- tunica vaginalis (late) A52.76
- ulcer (any site) (early) (secondary) A51.39
  - late A52.79
  - perforating A52.79
    - foot A52.11
- urethra (late) A52.76
- urogenital (late) A52.76
- uterus (late) A52.76
- uveal tract (secondary) A51.43
  - late A52.71
- uveitis (secondary) A51.43
  - late A52.71
- uvula (late) (perforated) A52.79
- vagina A51.0
  - late A52.76
- valvulitis NEC A52.03
- vascular A52.00
  - brain (cerebral) A52.05
- ventriculi A52.74
- vesicae urinariae (late) A52.76
- viscera (abdominal) (late) A52.74
  - secondary A51.49
- vitreous (opacities) (late) A52.71
  - hemorrhage A52.71
- vulva A51.0
  - late A52.76
  - secondary A51.39

Syphiloma A52.79
- cardiovascular system A52.00
- central nervous system A52.3
- circulatory system A52.00
- congenital A50.59

Syphilophobia F45.29

Syringadenoma —*see also* Neoplasm, skin, benign
- papillary —*see* Neoplasm, skin, benign

Syringobulbia G95.0

Syringocystadenoma —*see* Neoplasm, skin, benign
- papillary —*see* Neoplasm, skin, benign

Syringoma —*see also* Neoplasm, skin, benign
- chondroid —*see* Neoplasm, skin, benign

Syringomyelia G95.0

Syringomyelitis —*see* Encephalitis

Syringomyelocele —*see* Spina bifida

Syringopontia G95.0

System, systemic —*see also* condition
- disease, combined —*see* Degeneration, combined
- inflammatory response syndrome (SIRS) of non-infectious origin (without organ dysfunction) R65.10
  - with acute organ dysfunction R65.11
- lupus erythematosus M32.9
  - inhibitor present D68.62

Systemic exertion intolerance disease [SEID] G93.32

S

T

Tabacism, tabacosis, tabagism —*see also* Poisoning, tobacco
- meaning dependence (without remission) F17.200
  - with
    - disorder F17.299
      - in remission F17.211
      - specified disorder NEC F17.298
      - withdrawal F17.203

Tabardillo A75.9
- flea-borne A75.2
- louse-borne A75.0

Tabes, tabetic A52.10
- with
  - central nervous system syphilis A52.10
  - Charcot's joint A52.16
  - cord bladder A52.19
  - crisis, viscera (any) A52.19
  - paralysis, general A52.17
  - paresis (general) A52.17
  - perforating ulcer (foot) A52.19
- arthropathy (Charcot) A52.16
- bladder A52.19
- bone A52.11
- cerebrospinal A52.12
- congenital A50.45
- conjugal A52.10
- dorsalis A52.11
  - juvenile A50.49
- juvenile A50.49
- latent A52.19
- mesenterica A18.39
- paralysis, insane, general A52.17
- spasmodic A52.17
- syphilis (cerebrospinal) A52.12

Taboparalysis A52.17

Taboparesis (remission) A52.17
- juvenile A50.45

TAC (trigeminal autonomic cephalgia) NEC G44.099
- intractable G44.091
- not intractable G44.099

Tache noir S60.22-●

Tachyalimentation K91.2

Tachyarrhythmia, tachyrhythmia —*see* Tachycardia

Tachycardia R00.0
- atrial (paroxysmal) I47.19
- auricular I47.19
- AV nodal re-entry (re-entrant) I47.19
- junctional (paroxysmal) I47.19
- newborn P29.11
- nodal (paroxysmal) I47.19
- non-paroxysmal AV nodal I45.89
- paroxysmal (sustained) (nonsustained) I47.9
  - with sinus bradycardia I49.5
  - atrial (PAT) I47.19
  - atrioventricular (AV) (re-entrant) I47.19
    - psychogenic F54
  - junctional I47.19
    - ectopic I47.19
  - nodal I47.19
  - psychogenic (atrial) (supraventricular) (ventricular) F54
  - supraventricular (sustained) I47.10
    - psychogenic F54
  - ventricular I47.20
    - psychogenic F54
    - specified type NEC I47.29
- psychogenic F45.8
- sick sinus I49.5
- sinoauricular NOS R00.0
  - Inappropriate, so stated (IST) I47.11
  - paroxysmal I47.19
- sinus [sinusal] NOS R00.0
  - paroxysmal I47.19
- supraventricular I47.10
- ventricular (paroxysmal) (sustained) I47.20
  - psychogenic F54
  - specified type NEC I47.29

Tachygastria K31.89

Tachypnea R06.82
- hysterical F45.8
- newborn (idiopathic) (transitory) P22.1
- psychogenic F45.8
- transitory, of newborn P22.1

TACO (transfusion associated circulatory overload) E87.71

TAD (transfusion-associated dyspnea) J95.87

Taenia (infection) (infestation) B68.9
- diminuta B71.0
- echinococcal infestation B67.90
- mediocanellata B68.1
- nana B71.0
- saginata B68.1
- solium (intestinal form) B68.0
  - larval form —*see* Cysticercosis

Taeniasis (intestine) —*see* Taenia

Tag (hypertrophied skin) (infected) L91.8
- adenoid J35.8
- anus K64.4
- hemorrhoidal K64.4
- hymen N89.8
- perineal N90.89
- preauricular Q17.0
- sentinel K64.4
- skin L91.8
  - accessory (congenital) Q82.8
  - anus K64.4
  - congenital Q82.8
  - preauricular Q17.0
- tonsil J35.8
- urethra, urethral N36.8
- vulva N90.89

Tahyna fever B33.8

Takahara's disease E80.3

Takayasu's disease or syndrome M31.4

Talaromycosis B48.4

Talcosis (pulmonary) J62.0

Talipes (congenital) Q66.89
- acquired, planus —*see* Deformity, limb, flat foot
- asymmetric Q66.89
- calcaneovalgus Q66.4-●
- calcaneovarus Q66.1-●
- calcaneus Q66.89
- cavus Q66.7-●
- equinovalgus Q66.6
- equinovarus Q66.0-●
- equinus Q66.89
- percavus Q66.7-●
- planovalgus Q66.6
- planus (acquired) (any degree) —*see also* Deformity, limb, flat foot
  - congenital Q66.5-●
  - due to rickets (sequelae) E64.3
- valgus Q66.6
- varus Q66.3-●

Tall stature, constitutional E34.4

Talma's disease M62.89

Talon noir S90.3-●
- hand S60.22-●
- heel S90.3-●
- toe S90.1-●

Tamponade, heart I31.4

Tanapox (virus disease) B08.71

Tangier disease E78.6

Tantrum, child problem F91.8

Tapeworm (infection) (infestation) —*see* Infestation, tapeworm

Tapia's syndrome G52.7

TAR (thrombocytopenia with absent radius) syndrome Q87.2

Tarral-Besnier disease L44.0

Tarsal tunnel syndrome —*see* Syndrome, tarsal tunnel

Tarsalgia —*see* Pain, limb, lower

Tarsitis (eyelid) H01.8
- syphilitic A52.71
- tuberculous A18.4

Tartar (teeth) (dental calculus) K03.6

Tattoo (mark) L81.8

Tauri's disease E74.09

Taurodontism K00.2

Taussig-Bing syndrome Q20.1

Taybi's syndrome Q87.2

Tay-Sachs amaurotic familial idiocy or disease E75.02

TBI (traumatic brain injury) S06.9

Teacher's node or nodule J38.2

Tear, torn (traumatic) —*see also* Laceration
- with abortion —*see* Abortion
- annular fibrosis M51.35
- anus, anal (sphincter) S31.831
  - complicating delivery
    - with third degree perineal laceration —*see also* Delivery, complicated, by, laceration, perineum, third degree O70.20
      - with mucosa O70.3
    - without third degree perineal laceration O70.4
  - nontraumatic (healed) (old) K62.81
- articular cartilage, old —*see* Derangement, joint, articular cartilage, by site
- bladder
  - with ectopic or molar pregnancy O08.6
  - following ectopic or molar pregnancy O08.6
  - obstetrical O71.5
  - traumatic —*see* Injury, bladder
- bowel
  - with ectopic or molar pregnancy O08.6
  - following ectopic or molar pregnancy O08.6
  - obstetrical trauma O71.5
- broad ligament
  - with ectopic or molar pregnancy O08.6
  - following ectopic or molar pregnancy O08.6
  - obstetrical trauma O71.6
- bucket handle (knee) (meniscus) —*see* Tear, meniscus
- capsule, joint —*see* Sprain
- cartilage —*see also* Sprain
  - articular, old —*see* Derangement, joint, articular cartilage, by site
- cervix
  - with ectopic or molar pregnancy O08.6
  - following ectopic or molar pregnancy O08.6
  - obstetrical trauma (current) O71.3
  - old N88.1
  - traumatic —*see* Injury, uterus
- dural G97.41
  - nontraumatic G96.11
- internal organ —*see* Injury, by site
- knee cartilage
  - articular (current) S83.3-●
  - old —*see* Derangement, knee, meniscus, due to old tear
- ligament —*see* Sprain
- meniscus (knee) (current injury) S83.209
  - bucket-handle S83.20-●
  - lateral
    - bucket-handle S83.25-●
    - complex S83.27-●
    - peripheral S83.26-●
    - specified type NEC S83.28-●
  - medial
    - bucket-handle S83.21-●
    - complex S83.23-●
    - peripheral S83.22-●
    - specified type NEC S83.24-●
  - old —*see* Derangement, knee, meniscus, due to old tear
  - site other than knee - code as Sprain
  - specified type NEC S83.20-●
- muscle —*see* Strain
- pelvic
  - floor, complicating delivery O70.1
  - organ NEC, obstetrical trauma O71.5
    - with ectopic or molar pregnancy O08.6
    - following ectopic or molar pregnancy O08.6
- perineal, secondary O90.1
- periurethral tissue, obstetrical trauma O71.82
  - with ectopic or molar pregnancy O08.6
  - following ectopic or molar pregnancy O08.6
- rectovaginal septum —*see* Laceration, vagina
- retina, retinal (without detachment) (horseshoe) —*see also* Break, retina, horseshoe
  - with detachment —*see* Detachment, retina, with retinal, break
- rotator cuff (nontraumatic) M75.10-●
  - complete M75.12-●
  - incomplete M75.11-●
  - traumatic S46.01-●
    - capsule S43.42-●
- semilunar cartilage, knee —*see* Tear, meniscus
- supraspinatus (complete) (incomplete) (nontraumatic) —*see also* Tear, rotator cuff M75.10-●
- tendon —*see* Strain
- tentorial, at birth P10.4
- umbilical cord
  - complicating delivery O69.89
- urethra
  - with ectopic or molar pregnancy O08.6
  - following ectopic or molar pregnancy O08.6
  - obstetrical trauma O71.5
- uterus —*see* Injury, uterus
- vagina —*see* Laceration, vagina
- vessel, from catheter —*see* Puncture, accidental complicating surgery
- vulva, complicating delivery O70.0

Tear-stone —*see* Dacryolith

Teeth —*see also* condition
  grinding
    psychogenic F45.8
    sleep related G47.63
Teething (syndrome) K00.7
Telangiectasia, telangiectasis (verrucous) I78.1
  ataxic (cerebellar) (Louis-Bar) G11.3
  familial I78.0
  hemorrhagic, hereditary (congenital) (senile) I78.0
  hereditary, hemorrhagic (congenital) (senile) I78.0
  juxtafoveal H35.07-●
  macular H35.07-●
  macularis eruptiva perstans D47.01
  parafoveal H35.07-●
  retinal (idiopathic) (juxtafoveal) (macular) (parafoveal) H35.07-●
  spider I78.1
Telephone scatologia F65.89
Telescoped bowel or intestine K56.1
  congenital Q43.8
Temperature
  body, high (of unknown origin) R50.9
  cold, trauma from T69.9
    newborn P80.0
    specified effect NEC T69.8
Temple —*see* condition
Temporal —*see* condition
Temporomandibular joint pain-dysfunction syndrome M26.62-●
Temporosphenoidal —*see* condition
Tendency
  bleeding —*see* Defect, coagulation
  suicide
    meaning personal history of attempted suicide Z91.51
    meaning suicidal ideation —*see* Ideation, suicidal
  to fall R29.6
Tenderness, abdominal R10.819
  epigastric R10.816
  generalized R10.817
  left lower quadrant R10.814
  left upper quadrant R10.812
  periumbilic R10.815
  rebound R10.829
    epigastric R10.826
    generalized R10.827
    left lower quadrant R10.824
    left upper quadrant R10.822
    periumbilic R10.825
    right lower quadrant R10.823
    right upper quadrant R10.821
  right lower quadrant R10.813
  right upper quadrant R10.811
Tendinitis, tendonitis —*see also* Enthesopathy
  Achilles M76.6-●
  adhesive —*see* Tenosynovitis, specified type NEC
    shoulder —*see* Capsulitis, adhesive
  bicipital M75.2-●
  calcific M65.2-●
    ankle M65.27-●
    foot M65.27-●
    forearm M65.23-●
    hand M65.24-●
    lower leg M65.26-●
    multiple sites M65.29
    pelvic region M65.25-●
    shoulder M75.3-●
    specified site NEC M65.28
    thigh M65.25-●
    upper arm M65.22-●
  due to use, overuse, pressure —*see also* Disorder, soft tissue, due to use
    specified NEC —*see* Disorder, soft tissue, due to use, specified NEC
  gluteal M76.0-●
  patellar M76.5-●
  peroneal M76.7-●
  psoas M76.1-●
  tibial (posterior) M76.82-●
    anterior M76.81-●
  trochanteric —*see* Bursitis, hip, trochanteric
Tendon —*see* condition
Tendosynovitis —*see* Tenosynovitis
Tenesmus (rectal) R19.8
  vesical R30.1
Tennis elbow —*see* Epicondylitis, lateral
Tenonitis —*see also* Tenosynovitis
  eye (capsule) H05.04-●
Tenontosynovitis —*see* Tenosynovitis
Tenontothecitis —*see* Tenosynovitis
Tenophyte —*see* Disorder, synovium, specified type NEC
Tenosynovitis —*see also* Synovitis M65.90
  adhesive —*see* Tenosynovitis, specified type NEC
    shoulder —*see* Capsulitis, adhesive
  bicipital (calcifying) —*see* Tendinitis, bicipital
  gonococcal A54.49
  in (due to)
    crystals M65.8-●
    gonorrhea A54.49
    syphilis (late) A52.78
    use, overuse, pressure —*see also* Disorder, soft tissue, due to use
      specified NEC —*see* Disorder, soft tissue, due to use, specified NEC
  infective NEC M65.1-●
    ankle M65.17-●
    foot M65.17-●
    forearm M65.13-●
    hand M65.14-●
    lower leg M65.16-●
    multiple sites M65.19
    pelvic region M65.15-●
    shoulder region M65.11-●
    specified site NEC M65.18
    thigh M65.15-●
    upper arm M65.12-●
  radial styloid M65.4
  shoulder region M65.81-●
    adhesive —*see* Capsulitis, adhesive
  specified type NEC M65.88-●
    ankle M65.87-●
    foot M65.87-●
    forearm M65.83-●
    hand M65.84-●
    lower leg M65.86-●
    multiple sites M65.89
    pelvic region M65.85-●
    shoulder region M65.81-●
    specified site NEC M65.88
    thigh M65.85-●
    upper arm M65.82-●
  tuberculous —*see* Tuberculosis, tenosynovitis
Tenovaginitis —*see* Tenosynovitis
Tension
  arterial, high —*see also* Hypertension
    without diagnosis of hypertension R03.0
  headache G44.209
    intractable G44.201
    not intractable G44.209
  nervous R45.0
  pneumothorax J93.0
  premenstrual N94.3
  state (mental) F48.9
Tentorium —*see* condition
Tentatencephalus Q89.8
Teratism Q89.7
Teratoblastoma (malignant) —*see* Neoplasm, malignant, by site
Teratocarcinoma —*see also* Neoplasm, malignant, by site
  liver C22.7
Teratoma (solid) —*see also* Neoplasm, uncertain behavior, by site
  with embryonal carcinoma, mixed —*see* Neoplasm, malignant, by site
  with malignant transformation —*see* Neoplasm, malignant, by site
  adult (cystic) —*see* Neoplasm, benign, by site
  benign —*see* Neoplasm, benign, by site
  combined with choriocarcinoma —*see* Neoplasm, malignant, by site
  cystic (adult) —*see* Neoplasm, benign, by site
  differentiated —*see* Neoplasm, benign, by site
  embryonal —*see also* Neoplasm, malignant, by site
    liver C22.7
  immature —*see* Neoplasm, malignant, by site
  liver C22.7
    adult, benign, cystic, differentiated type or mature D13.4
  malignant —*see also* Neoplasm, malignant, by site
    anaplastic —*see* Neoplasm, malignant, by site
    intermediate —*see* Neoplasm, malignant, by site
      specified site —*see* Neoplasm, malignant, by site
      unspecified site C62.90
    undifferentiated —*see* Neoplasm, malignant, by site
Teratoma *(Continued)*
  mature —*see* Neoplasm, uncertain behavior, by site
    malignant —*see* Neoplasm, by site, malignant, by site
  ovary D27.-●
    embryonal, immature or malignant C56-●
  solid —*see* Neoplasm, uncertain behavior, by site
  testis C62.9-●
    adult, benign, cystic, differentiated type or mature D29.2-●
    scrotal C62.1-●
    undescended C62.0-●
Termination
  anomalous —*see also* Malposition, congenital
    right pulmonary vein Q26.3
  pregnancy, elective Z33.2
Ternidens diminutus infestation B81.8
Ternidensiasis B81.8
Terror(s) night (child) F51.4
Terrorism, victim of Z65.4
Terry's syndrome —*see also* Myopia, degenerative H44.2-●
Tertiary —*see* condition
Test, tests, testing (for)
  adequacy (for dialysis)
    hemodialysis Z49.31
    peritoneal Z49.32
  blood pressure Z01.30
    abnormal reading —*see* Blood, pressure
  blood typing Z01.83
    Rh typing Z01.83
  blood-alcohol Z02.83
    positive —*see* Findings, abnormal, in blood
  blood-drug Z02.83
    positive —*see* Findings, abnormal, in blood
  cardiac pulse generator (battery) Z45.010
  fertility Z31.41
  genetic
    disease carrier status for procreative management
      female Z31.430
      male Z31.440
    male partner of patient with recurrent pregnancy loss Z31.441
    procreative management NEC
      female Z31.438
      male Z31.448
  hearing Z01.10
    with abnormal findings NEC Z01.118
    infant or child (over 28 days old) Z00.129
      with abnormal findings Z00.121
  HIV (human immunodeficiency virus)
    nonconclusive (in infants) R75
    positive Z21
    seropositive Z21
  immunity status Z01.84
  intelligence NEC Z01.89
  laboratory (as part of a general medical examination) Z00.00
    with abnormal finding Z00.01
    for medicolegal reason NEC Z04.89
  male partner of patient with recurrent pregnancy loss Z31.441
  Mantoux (for tuberculosis) Z11.1
    abnormal result R76.11
  pregnancy, positive first pregnancy —*see* Pregnancy, normal, first
  procreative Z31.49
    fertility Z31.41
  skin, diagnostic
    allergy Z01.82
      special screening examination —*see* Screening, by name of disease
    Mantoux Z11.1
    tuberculin Z11.1
  specified NEC Z01.89
  tuberculin Z11.1
    abnormal result R76.11
  vision Z01.00
    with abnormal findings Z01.01
    following failed vision screening Z01.020
      with abnormal findings Z01.021
    infant or child (over 28 days old) Z00.129
      with abnormal findings Z00.121
  Wassermann Z11.3
    positive —*see* Serology for syphilis, positive
Testicle, testicular, testis —*see also* condition
  feminization syndrome —*see also* Syndrome, androgen insensitivity E34.51
  migrans Q55.29

T

- **Tetanus, tetanic** (cephalic) (convulsions) A35
  - with
    - abortion A34
    - ectopic or molar pregnancy O08.0
  - following ectopic or molar pregnancy O08.0
  - inoculation reaction (due to serum) —*see* Complications, vaccination
  - neonatorum A33
  - obstetrical A34
  - puerperal, postpartum, childbirth A34
- **Tetany** (due to) R29.0
  - alkalosis E87.3
  - associated with rickets E55.0
  - convulsions R29.0
    - hysterical F44.5
  - functional (hysterical) F44.5
  - hyperkinetic R29.0
    - hysterical F44.5
  - hyperpnea R06.4
    - hysterical F44.5
    - psychogenic F45.8
  - hyperventilation —*see also* Hyperventilation R06.4
    - hysterical F44.5
  - neonatal (without calcium or magnesium deficiency) P71.3
  - parathyroid (gland) E20.9
  - parathyroprival E89.2
  - post- (para)thyroidectomy E89.2
  - postoperative E89.2
  - pseudotetany R29.0
  - psychogenic (conversion reaction) F44.5
- **Tetralogy of Fallot** Q21.3
- **Tetraplegia** (chronic) —*see also* Quadriplegia G82.50-●
- **Thailand hemorrhagic fever** A91
- **Thalassanemia** —*see* Thalassemia
- **Thalassemia** (anemia) (disease) D56.9
  - with other hemoglobinopathy D56.8
  - alpha (major) (severe) (triple gene defect) D56.0
    - minor D56.3
    - silent carrier D56.3
    - trait D56.3
  - beta (severe) D56.1
    - homozygous D56.1
    - major D56.1
    - minor D56.3
    - trait D56.3
  - delta-beta (homozygous) D56.2
    - minor D56.3
    - trait D56.3
  - dominant D56.8
  - hemoglobin
    - C D56.8
    - E-beta D56.5
  - intermedia D56.1
  - major D56.1
  - minor D56.3
  - mixed D56.8
  - sickle-cell —*see* Disease, sickle-cell, thalassemia
  - specified type NEC D56.8
  - trait D56.3
  - variants D56.8
- **Thanatophoric dwarfism or short stature** Q77.1
- **Thaysen-Gee disease** (nontropical sprue) K90.0
- **Thaysen's disease** K90.0
- **Thecoma** D27-●
  - luteinized D27-●
  - malignant C56-●
- **Thelarche, premature** E30.8
- **Thelaziasis** B83.8
- **Thelitis** N61.0
  - puerperal, postpartum or gestational —*see* Infection, nipple
- **Therapeutic** —*see* condition
- **Therapy**
  - drug, long-term (current) (prophylactic)
    - agents affecting estrogen receptors and estrogen levels NEC Z79.818
    - anastrozole (Arimidex) Z79.811
    - antibiotics Z79.2
      - short-term use - omit code
    - anticoagulants Z79.01
    - anti-inflammatory Z79.1
    - antiplatelet Z79.02
    - antithrombotics Z79.02
    - aromatase inhibitors Z79.811
    - aspirin Z79.82
    - birth control pill or patch Z79.3
    - bisphosphonates Z79.83
    - contraceptive, oral Z79.3
    - drug, specified NEC Z79.899
    - estrogen receptor downregulators Z79.818

- **Therapy** *(Continued)*
  - drug, long-term *(Continued)*
    - Evista Z79.810
    - exemestane (Aromasin) Z79.811
    - Fareston Z79.810
    - fulvestrant (Faslodex) Z79.818
    - gonadotropin-releasing hormone (GnRH) agonist Z79.818
    - goserelin acetate (Zoladex) Z79.818
    - hormone replacement Z79.890
    - insulin Z79.4
    - letrozole (Femara) Z79.811
    - leuprolide acetate (leuprorelin) (Lupron) Z79.818
    - megestrol acetate (Megace) Z79.818
    - methadone
      - for pain management Z79.891
      - maintenance therapy F11.20
    - Nolvadex Z79.810
    - opiate analgesic Z79.891
    - oral antidiabetic Z79.84
    - oral contraceptive Z79.3
    - oral hypoglycemic Z79.84
    - raloxifene (Evista) Z79.810
    - selective estrogen receptor modulators (SERMs) Z79.810
    - short term - omit code
    - steroids
      - inhaled Z79.51
      - systemic Z79.52
    - tamoxifen (Nolvadex) Z79.810
    - toremifene (Fareston) Z79.810
- **Thermic** —*see* condition
- **Thermography** (abnormal) —*see also* Abnormal, diagnostic imaging R93.89
  - breast R92.8
- **Thermoplegia** T67.01
- **Thesaurismosis, glycogen** —*see* Disease, glycogen storage
- **Thiamin deficiency** E51.9
  - specified NEC E51.8
- **Thiaminic deficiency with beriberi** E51.11
- **Thibierge-Weissenbach syndrome** —*see* Sclerosis, systemic
- **Thickening**
  - bone —*see* Hypertrophy, bone
  - breast N64.59
  - endometrium R93.89
  - epidermal L85.9
    - specified NEC L85.8
  - hymen N89.6
  - larynx J38.7
  - nail L60.2
    - congenital Q84.5
  - periosteal —*see* Hypertrophy, bone
  - pleura J92.9
    - with asbestos J92.0
  - skin R23.4
  - subepiglottic J38.7
  - tongue K14.8
  - valve, heart —*see* Endocarditis
- **Thigh** —*see* condition
- **Thinning vertebra** —*see* Spondylopathy, specified NEC
- **Thirst, excessive** R63.1
  - due to deprivation of water T73.1
- **Thomsen disease** G71.12
- **Thoracic** —*see also* condition
  - kidney Q63.2
  - ➡outlet syndrome (*see also* Syndrome, thoracic outlet) G54.0
- **Thoracogastroschisis** (congenital) Q79.8
- **Thoracopagus** Q89.4
- **Thorax** —*see* condition
- **Thorn's syndrome** N28.89
- ➡**Thorson-Björck syndrome** E34.09
- **Threadworm** (infection) (infestation) B80
- **Threatened**
  - abortion O20.0
    - with subsequent abortion O03.9
  - ➡abuse (harm)
    - ▶adult —*see* Maltreatment, adult, threatened abuse
    - ▶child —*see* Maltreatment, child, threatened abuse
  - job loss, anxiety concerning Z56.2
  - labor (without delivery) O47.9
    - at or after 37 completed weeks of gestation O47.1
    - before 37 completed weeks of gestation O47.0-●

- **Threatened** *(Continued)*
  - loss of job, anxiety concerning Z56.2
  - miscarriage O20.0
  - unemployment, anxiety concerning Z56.2
- **Three-day fever** A93.1
- **Threshers' lung** J67.0
- **Thrix annulata** (congenital) Q84.1
- **Throat** —*see* condition
- **Thrombasthenia** (Glanzmann) (hemorrhagic) (hereditary) D69.1
- **Thromboangiitis I73.1**
  - obliterans (general) I73.1
    - cerebral I67.89
    - vessels
      - brain I67.89
      - spinal cord I67.89
- **Thromboarteritis** —*see* Arteritis
- **Thromboasthenia** (Glanzmann) (hemorrhagic) (hereditary) D69.1
- **Thrombocytasthenia** (Glanzmann) D69.1
- **Thrombocythemia** (hemorrhagic) (see also Thrombocytosis) D75.839
  - essential D47.3
  - idiopathic D47.3
  - primary D47.3
- **Thrombocytopathy** (dystrophic) (granulopenic) D69.1
- **Thrombocytopenia, thrombocytopenic** D69.6
  - with absent radius (TAR) Q87.2
  - congenital D69.42
  - dilutional D69.59
  - due to
    - drugs D69.59
    - extracorporeal circulation of blood D69.59
    - (massive)blood transfusion D69.59
    - platelet alloimmunization D69.59
  - essential D69.3
  - heparin-associated D75.821
  - heparin induced (HIT) D75.829
  - delayed-onset D75.828
  - immune-mediated D75.822
  - non-immune D75.821
  - persisting D75.828
  - syndrome
    - autoimmune D75.828
    - specified NEC D75.828
    - spontaneous (without heparin exposure) D75.84
  - type 1 D75.821
  - type 2 D75.822
  - hereditary D69.42
  - idiopathic D69.3
  - neonatal, transitory P61.0
    - due to
      - exchange transfusion P61.0
      - idiopathic maternal thrombocytopenia P61.0
      - isoimmunization P61.0
  - primary NEC D69.49
    - idiopathic D69.3
  - puerperal, postpartum O72.3
  - secondary D69.59
  - transient neonatal P61.0
  - vaccine-induced thrombotic D75.84
- **Thrombocytosis** D75.839
  - essential D47.3
  - idiopathic D47.3
  - primary D47.3
  - reactive D75.838
  - secondary D75.838
  - specified NEC D75.838
- **Thromboembolism** —*see* Embolism
- **Thrombopathy** (Bernard-Soulier) D69.1
  - constitutional —*see* Disease, von Willebrand
  - Willebrand-Jurgens —*see* Disease, von Willebrand
- **Thrombopenia** —*see* Thrombocytopenia
- **Thrombophilia** D68.59
  - primary NEC D68.59
  - secondary NEC D68.69
  - specified NEC D68.69
- **Thrombophlebitis** I80.9
  - antepartum O22.2-●
    - deep O22.3-●
    - superficial O22.2-●
  - calf muscular vein (NOS) I80.25-●
  - cavernous (venous) sinus G08
    - complicating pregnancy O22.5-●
    - nonpyogenic I67.6
  - cerebral (sinus) (vein) G08
    - nonpyogenic I67.6
    - sequelae G09

T

- **Thrombophlebitis** *(Continued)*
  - due to implanted device —*see* Complications, by site and type, specified NEC
  - during or resulting from a procedure NEC T81.72
  - femoral vein (superficial) I8Ø.1-●
  - femoropopliteal vein I8Ø.Ø-●
  - gastrocnemial vein I8Ø.25-●
  - hepatic (vein) I8Ø.8
  - idiopathic, recurrent I82.1
  - iliac vein (common) (external) (internal) I8Ø.21-●
  - iliofemoral I8Ø.1-●
  - intracranial venous sinus (any) GØ8
    - nonpyogenic I67.6
    - sequelae GØ9
  - intraspinal venous sinuses and veins GØ8
    - nonpyogenic G95.19
  - lateral (venous) sinus GØ8
    - nonpyogenic I67.6
  - leg I8Ø.3
    - superficial I8Ø.Ø-●
  - longitudinal (venous) sinus GØ8
    - nonpyogenic I67.6
  - lower extremity I8Ø.299
  - migrans, migrating I82.1
  - pelvic
    - with ectopic or molar pregnancy OØ8.Ø
    - following ectopic or molar pregnancy OØ8.Ø
    - puerperal O87.1
  - peroneal vein I8Ø.24-●
  - popliteal vein —*see* Phlebitis, leg, deep, popliteal
  - portal (vein) K75.1
  - postoperative T81.72
  - pregnancy —*see* Thrombophlebitis, antepartum
  - puerperal, postpartum, childbirth O87.Ø
    - deep O87.1
    - pelvic O87.1
    - septic O86.81
    - superficial O87.Ø
  - saphenous (greater) (lesser) I8Ø.Ø-●
  - sinus (intracranial) GØ8
    - nonpyogenic I67.6
  - soleal vein I8Ø.25-●
  - specified site NEC I8Ø.8
  - tibial vein (anterior) (posterior) I8Ø.23-●
- **Thrombosis, thrombotic** (bland) (multiple) (progressive) (silent) (vessel) I82.9Ø
  - anal K64.5
  - antepartum —*see* Thrombophlebitis, antepartum
  - aorta, aortic I74.1Ø
    - abdominal I74.Ø9
      - saddle I74.Ø1
    - bifurcation I74.Ø9
    - saddle I74.Ø1
    - specified site NEC I74.19
    - terminal I74.Ø9
    - thoracic I74.11
    - valve —*see* Endocarditis, aortic
  - apoplexy I63.3-●
  - artery, arteries (postinfectional) I74.9
    - auditory, internal —*see* Occlusion, artery, precerebral, specified NEC
    - basilar —*see* Occlusion, artery, basilar
    - carotid (common) (internal) —*see* Occlusion, artery, carotid
    - cerebellar (anterior inferior) (posterior inferior) (superior) —*see* Occlusion, artery, cerebellar
    - cerebral —*see* Occlusion, artery, cerebral
    - choroidal (anterior) —*see* Occlusion, artery, precerebral, specified NEC
    - communicating, posterior —*see* Occlusion, artery, precerebral, specified NEC
    - coronary —*see also* Infarct, myocardium
      - not resulting in infarction I24.Ø
    - hepatic I74.8
    - hypophyseal —*see* Occlusion, artery, precerebral, specified NEC
    - iliac I74.5
    - limb I74.4
      - lower I74.3
      - upper I74.2
    - meningeal, anterior or posterior —*see* Occlusion, artery, cerebral, specified NEC
    - mesenteric (with gangrene) —*see also* Infarct, intestine K55.Ø69
    - ophthalmic —*see* Occlusion, artery, retina
    - pontine —*see* Occlusion, artery, precerebral, specified NEC
    - precerebral —*see* Occlusion, artery, precerebral

- **Thrombosis, thrombotic** *(Continued)*
  - artery, arteries *(Continued)*
    - pulmonary (iatrogenic) —*see* Embolism, pulmonary
    - renal N28.Ø
    - retinal —*see* Occlusion, artery, retina
    - spinal, anterior or posterior G95.11
    - traumatic NEC T14.8
    - vertebral —*see* Occlusion, artery, vertebral
  - atrium, auricular —*see also* Infarct, myocardium
    - following acute myocardial infarction (current complication) I23.6
    - not resulting in infarction I51.3
    - old I51.3
  - basilar (artery) —*see* Occlusion, artery, basilar
  - brain (artery) (stem) —*see also* Occlusion, artery, cerebral
    - due to syphilis A52.Ø5
    - puerperal O99.43
    - ➡sinus —*see* Thrombosis, intracranial, venous sinus
  - capillary I78.8
  - cardiac —*see also* Infarct, myocardium
    - not resulting in infarction I51.3
    - valve —*see* Endocarditis
    - old I51.3
  - carotid (artery) (common) (internal) —*see* Occlusion, artery, carotid
  - ➡cavernous (venous) sinus —*see* Thrombosis, intracranial, venous sinus
  - cerebellar artery (anterior inferior) (posterior inferior) (superior) I66.3
  - cerebral (artery) —*see* Occlusion, artery, cerebral
  - ➡cerebrovenous sinus —*see also* Thrombosis, intracranial, venous sinus
    - puerperium O87.3
  - chronic I82.91
  - coronary (artery) (vein) —*see also* Infarct, myocardium
    - not resulting in infarction I24.Ø
  - corpus cavernosum N48.89
  - cortical I66.9
  - deep —*see* Embolism, vein, lower extremity
  - due to device, implant or graft —*see also* Complications, by site and type, specified NEC T85.868
    - arterial graft NEC T82.868
    - breast (implant) T85.868
    - catheter NEC T85.868
      - dialysis (renal) T82.868
        - intraperitoneal T85.868
      - infusion NEC T82.868
        - spinal (epidural) (subdural) T85.86Ø
      - urinary (indwelling) T83.86
    - electronic (electrode) (pulse generator) (stimulator)
      - bone T84.86
      - cardiac T82.867
      - nervous system (brain) (peripheral nerve) (spinal) T85.86Ø
      - urinary T83.86
    - fixation, internal (orthopedic) NEC T84.86
    - gastrointestinal (bile duct) (esophagus) T85.868
    - genital NEC T83.86
    - heart T82.867
    - joint prosthesis T84.86
    - ocular (corneal graft) (orbital implant) NEC T85.868
    - orthopedic NEC T84.86
    - specified NEC T85.868
    - urinary NEC T83.86
    - vascular NEC T82.868
    - ventricular intracranial shunt T85.86Ø
  - during the puerperium —*see* Thrombosis, puerperal
  - endocardial —*see also* Infarct, myocardium
    - not resulting in infarction I51.3
  - eye —*see* Occlusion, retina
  - genital organ
    - female NEC N94.89
      - pregnancy —*see* Thrombophlebitis, antepartum
    - male N5Ø.1
  - gestational —*see* Phlebopathy, gestational
  - heart (chamber) —*see also* Infarct, myocardium
    - not resulting in infarction I51.3
    - old I51.3
  - hepatic (vein) I82.Ø
    - artery I74.8

- **Thrombosis, thrombotic** *(Continued)*
  - history (of) Z86.718
  - intestine (with gangrene) —*see also* Infarct, intestine K55.Ø69
  - intracardiac NEC (apical) (atrial) (auricular) (ventricular) (old) I51.3
  - intracranial (arterial) I66.9
    - venous sinus (any) GØ8
      - ▶nonpyogenic I67.6
      - nonpyogenic origin I67.6
      - puerperium O87.3
  - intramural —*see also* Infarct, myocardium
    - not resulting in infarction I51.3
    - old I51.3
  - intraspinal venous sinuses and veins GØ8
    - nonpyogenic G95.19
  - kidney (artery) N28.Ø
  - ➡lateral (venous) sinus —*see* Thrombosis, intracranial, venous sinus
  - leg —*see* Thrombosis, vein, lower extremity
    - arterial I74.3
  - liver (venous) I82.Ø
    - artery I74.8
    - portal vein I81
  - ➡longitudinal (venous) sinus —*see* Thrombosis, intracranial, venous sinus
  - lower limb —*see* Thrombosis, vein, lower extremity
  - lung (iatrogenic) (postoperative) —*see* Embolism, pulmonary
  - meninges (brain) (arterial) I66.8
  - mesenteric (artery) (with gangrene) —*see also* Infarct, intestine K55.Ø69
    - vein (inferior) (superior) K55.Ø-●
  - mitral I34.89
  - mural —*see also* Infarct, myocardium
    - due to syphilis A52.Ø6
    - not resulting in infarction I51.3
    - old I51.3
  - omentum (with gangrene) —*see also* Infarct, intestine K55.Ø69
  - ophthalmic —*see* Occlusion, retina
  - pampiniform plexus (male) N5Ø.1
  - parietal —*see also* Infarct, myocardium
    - not resulting in infarction I24.Ø
  - penis, superficial vein N48.81
  - perianal venous K64.5
  - peripheral arteries I74.4
    - upper I74.2
  - personal history (of) Z86.718
  - portal I81
    - due to syphilis A52.Ø9
  - precerebral artery —*see* Occlusion, artery, precerebral
  - puerperal, postpartum O87.Ø
    - brain (artery) O99.43
      - venous (sinus) O87.3
    - cardiac O99.43
    - cerebral (artery) O99.43
      - venous (sinus) O87.3
    - superficial O87.Ø
  - pulmonary (artery) (iatrogenic) (postoperative) (vein) —*see* Embolism, pulmonary
  - renal (artery) N28.Ø
    - vein I82.3
  - resulting from presence of device, implant or graft —*see* Complications, by site and type, specified NEC
  - retina, retinal —*see* Occlusion, retina
  - scrotum N5Ø.1
  - seminal vesicle N5Ø.1
  - sigmoid (venous) sinus —*see* Thrombosis, intracranial venous sinus
  - ➡sinus, intracranial (any) —*see* Thrombosis, intracranial, venous sinus
  - specified site NEC I82.89Ø
    - chronic I82.891
  - spermatic cord N5Ø.1
  - spinal cord (arterial) G95.11
    - due to syphilis A52.Ø9
    - pyogenic origin GØ6.1
  - spleen, splenic D73.5
    - artery I74.8
  - testis N5Ø.1
  - traumatic NEC T14.8
  - tricuspid IØ7.8
  - tumor —*see* Neoplasm, by site
  - tunica vaginalis N5Ø.1
  - umbilical cord (vessels), complicating delivery O69.5
  - vas deferens N5Ø.1

- **Thrombosis, thrombotic** *(Continued)*
  - vein (acute) I82.9Ø
    - antecubital I82.61-●
      - chronic I82.71-●
    - axillary I82.A1-●
      - chronic I82.A2-●
    - basilic I82.61-●
      - chronic I82.71-●
    - brachial I82.62-●
      - chronic I82.72-●
    - brachiocephalic (innominate) I82.29Ø
      - chronic I82.291
    - calf muscular I82.46-●
      - chronic I82.56-●
    - cerebral, nonpyogenic I67.6
    - cephalic I82.61-●
      - chronic I82.71-●
    - chronic I82.91
    - deep (DVT) I82.4Ø-●
      - calf I82.4Z-●
        - chronic I82.5Z-●
      - lower leg I82.4Z-●
        - chronic I82.5Z-●
      - thigh I82.4Y-●
        - chronic I82.5Y-●
      - upper leg I82.4Y●
        - chronic I82.5Y-●
    - femoral I82.41-●
      - chronic I82.51-●
    - iliac (iliofemoral) I82.42-●
      - chronic I82.52-●
    - innominate I82.29Ø
      - chronic I82.291
    - internal jugular I82.C1-●
      - chronic I82.C2-●
    - lower extremity
      - deep I82.4Ø-●
        - chronic I82.5Ø-●
        - specified NEC I82.49-●
          - chronic NEC I82.59-●
      - distal
        - deep I82.4Z-●
      - proximal
        - deep I82.4Y-●
          - chronic I82.5Y-●
      - superficial I82.81-●
    - perianal K64.5
    - peroneal I82.45-●
      - chronic I82.55-●
    - popliteal I82.43-●
      - chronic I82.53-●
    - radial I82.62-●
      - chronic I82.72-●
    - renal I82.3
    - saphenous (greater) (lesser) I82.81-●
    - specified NEC I82.89Ø
      - chronic NEC I82.891
    - subclavian I82.B1-●
      - chronic I82.B2-●
    - thoracic NEC I82.29Ø
      - chronic I82.291
    - tibial I82.44-●
      - chronic I82.54-●
    - ulnar I82.62-●
      - chronic I82.72-●
    - upper extremity I82.6Ø-●
      - chronic I82.7Ø-●
      - deep I82.62-●
        - chronic I82.72-●
      - superficial I82.61-●
        - chronic I82.71-●
  - vena cava
    - inferior I82.22Ø
      - chronic I82.221
    - superior I82.21Ø
      - chronic I82.211
  - venous, perianal K64.5
  - ventricle —*see also* Infarct, myocardium
    - following acute myocardial infarction (current complication) I23.6
    - not resulting in infarction I24.Ø
    - old I51.3
- **Thrombus** —*see* Thrombosis
- **Thrush** —*see also* Candidiasis
  - newborn P37.5
  - oral B37.Ø
  - vaginal (acute) B37.31
    - chronic (recurrent) B37.32
- **Thumb** —*see also* condition
  - sucking (child problem) F98.8
- **Thymitis** E32.8
- **Thymoma** —*see* also Neoplasm, thymus, by type
  - malignant C37
  - metaplastic C37
  - microscopic D15.Ø
  - sclerosing C37
  - type A C37
  - type AB C37
  - type B1 C37
  - type B2 C37
  - type B3 C37
- **Thymus, thymic (gland)** —*see* condition
- **Thyrocele** —*see* Goiter
- **Thyroglossal** —*see also* condition
  - cyst Q89.2
  - duct, persistent Q89.2
- **Thyroid** (gland) (body) —*see also* condition
  - hormone resistance E07.89
  - lingual Q89.2
  - nodule (cystic) (nontoxic) (single) E04.1
- **Thyroiditis** E06.9
  - acute (nonsuppurative) (pyogenic) (suppurative) E06.Ø
  - autoimmune E06.3
  - chronic (nonspecific) (sclerosing) E06.5
    - with thyrotoxicosis, transient E06.2
    - fibrous E06.5
    - lymphadenoid E06.3
    - lymphocytic E06.3
    - lymphoid E06.3
  - de Quervain's E06.1
  - drug-induced E06.4
  - fibrous (chronic) E06.5
  - giant-cell (follicular) E06.1
  - granulomatous (de Quervain) (subacute) E06.1
  - Hashimoto's (struma lymphomatosa) E06.3
  - iatrogenic E06.4
  - ligneous E06.5
  - lymphocytic (chronic) E06.3
  - lymphoid E06.3
  - lymphomatous E06.3
  - nonsuppurative E06.1
  - postpartum, puerperal O90.5
  - pseudotuberculous E06.1
  - pyogenic E06.Ø
  - radiation E06.4
  - Riedel's E06.5
  - subacute (granulomatous) E06.1
  - suppurative E06.Ø
  - tuberculous A18.81
  - viral E06.1
  - woody E06.5
- **Thyrolingual duct, persistent** Q89.2
- **Thyromegaly** E01.Ø
- **Thyrotoxic**
  - crisis —*see* Thyrotoxicosis
  - heart disease or failure —*see also* Thyrotoxicosis E05.9Ø *[I43]*
    - with thyroid storm E05.91 *[I43]*
  - storm —*see* Thyrotoxicosis
- **Thyrotoxicosis** (recurrent) E05.9Ø
  - with
    - goiter (diffuse) E05.ØØ
      - with thyroid storm E05.Ø1
      - adenomatous uninodular E05.1Ø
        - with thyroid storm E05.11
      - multinodular E05.2Ø
        - with thyroid storm E05.21
      - nodular E05.2Ø
        - with thyroid storm E05.21
      - uninodular E05.1Ø
        - with thyroid storm E05.11
    - infiltrative
      - dermopathy E05.ØØ
        - with thyroid storm E05.Ø1
      - ophthalmopathy E05.ØØ
        - with thyroid storm E05.Ø1
    - single thyroid nodule E05.1Ø
      - with thyroid storm E05.11
    - thyroid storm E05.91
  - due to
    - ectopic thyroid nodule or tissue E05.3Ø
      - with thyroid storm E05.31
    - ingestion of (excessive) thyroid material E05.4Ø
      - with thyroid storm E05.41
    - overproduction of thyroid-stimulating hormone E05.8Ø
      - with thyroid storm E05.81
    - specified cause NEC E05.8Ø
      - with thyroid storm E05.81
- **Thyrotoxicosis** *(Continued)*
  - factitia E05.4Ø
    - with thyroid storm E05.41
  - heart —*see also* Failure, heart, high-output E05.9Ø *[I43]*
    - with thyroid storm —*see also* Failure, heart, high-output E05.91 *[I43]*
    - failure —*see also* Failure, heart, high-output E05.9Ø *[I43]*
  - neonatal (transient) P72.1
  - transient with chronic thyroiditis E06.2
- **Tibia vara** M92.51-●
- **Tic** (disorder) F95.9
  - breathing F95.8
  - child problem F95.Ø
  - compulsive F95.1
  - de la Tourette F95.2
  - degenerative (generalized) (localized) G25.69
    - facial G25.69
  - disorder
    - chronic
      - motor F95.1
      - vocal F95.1
    - combined vocal and multiple motor F95.2
    - transient F95.Ø
  - douloureux G5Ø.Ø
    - atypical G5Ø.1
    - postherpetic, postzoster B02.22
  - drug-induced G25.61
  - eyelid F95.8
  - habit F95.9
    - chronic F95.1
    - transient of childhood F95.Ø
  - lid, transient of childhood F95.Ø
  - motor-verbal F95.2
  - occupational F48.8
  - orbicularis F95.8
    - transient of childhood F95.Ø
  - organic origin G25.69
  - postchoreic G25.69
  - provisional F95.Ø
  - psychogenic, compulsive F95.1
  - salaam R25.8
  - spasm (motor or vocal) F95.9
    - chronic F95.1
    - transient of childhood F95.Ø
  - specified NEC F95.8
- **Tick-borne** —*see* condition
- **Tietze's disease or syndrome** M94.Ø
- **Tight, tightness**
  - anus K62.89
  - chest R07.89
  - fascia (lata) M62.89
  - foreskin (congenital) N47.1
  - hymen, hymenal ring N89.6
  - introitus (acquired) (congenital) N89.6
  - rectal sphincter K62.89
  - tendon —*see* Short, tendon
  - urethral sphincter N35.919
- **Tilting vertebra** —*see* Dorsopathy, deforming, specified NEC
- **Timidity, child** F93.8
- **Tin-miner's lung** J63.5
- **Tinea** (intersecta) (tarsi) B35.9
  - amiantacea L44.8
  - asbestina B35.Ø
  - barbae B35.Ø
  - beard B35.Ø
  - black dot B35.Ø
  - blanca B36.2
  - capitis B35.Ø
  - corporis B35.4
  - cruris B35.6
  - flava B36.Ø
  - foot B35.3
  - furfuracea B36.Ø
  - imbricata (Tokelau) B35.5
  - kerion B35.Ø
  - manuum B35.2
  - microsporic —*see* Dermatophytosis
  - nigra B36.1
  - nodosa —*see* Piedra
  - pedis B35.3
  - scalp B35.Ø
  - specified NEC B35.8
  - sycosis B35.Ø
  - tonsurans B35.Ø
  - trichophytic —*see* Dermatophytosis
  - unguium B35.1
  - versicolor B36.Ø
- **Tingling sensation** (skin) R2Ø.2

- **Tinnitus NOS** H93.1-●
  - audible H93.1-●
  - aurium H93.1-●
  - pulsatile H93.A-●
  - subjective H93.1-●
- **Tipped tooth** (teeth) M26.33
- **Tipping**
  - pelvis M95.5
    - with disproportion (fetopelvic) O33.0
      - causing obstructed labor O65.0
  - tooth (teeth), fully erupted M26.33
- **Tiredness** R53.83
- **Tissue** —*see* condition
- **Tobacco** (nicotine)
  - abuse —*see* Tobacco, use
  - dependence —*see* Dependence, drug, nicotine
  - harmful use Z72.0
  - heart —*see* Tobacco, toxic effect
  - maternal use, affecting newborn P04.2
  - toxic effect —*see* Table of Drugs and Chemicals, by substance, poisoning
    - chewing tobacco —*see* Table of Drugs and Chemicals, by substance, poisoning
    - cigarettes —*see* Table of Drugs and Chemicals, by substance, poisoning
  - use Z72.0
    - complicating
      - childbirth O99.334
      - pregnancy O99.33-●
      - puerperium O99.335
    - counseling and surveillance Z71.6
    - history Z87.891
  - withdrawal state —*see also* Dependence, drug, nicotine F17.203
- **Tocopherol deficiency** E56.0
- **Todd's**
  - cirrhosis K74.3
  - paralysis (postepileptic) (transitory) G83.84
- **Toe** —*see* condition
- **Toilet, artificial opening** —*see* Attention to, artificial, opening
- **Tokelau** (ringworm) B35.5
- **Tollwut** —*see* Rabies
- **Tommaselli's disease** R31.9
  - correct substance properly administered —*see* Table of Drugs and Chemicals, by drug, adverse effect
  - overdose or wrong substance given or taken —*see* Table of Drugs and Chemicals, by drug, poisoning
- **Tongue** —*see also* condition
  - tie Q38.1
- **Tonic pupil** —*see* Anomaly, pupil, function, tonic pupil
- **Toni-Fanconi syndrome** (cystinosis) E72.09
  - with cystinosis E72.04
- **Tonsil** —*see* condition
- **Tonsillitis** (acute) (catarrhal) (croupous) (follicular) (gangrenous) (infective) (lacunar) (lingual) (malignant) (membranous) (parenchymatous) (phlegmonous) (pseudomembranous) (purulent) (septic) (subacute) (suppurative) (toxic) (ulcerative) (vesicular) (viral) J03.90
  - chronic J35.01
    - with adenoiditis J35.03
  - diphtheritic A36.0
  - hypertrophic J35.01
    - with adenoiditis J35.03
  - recurrent J03.91
  - specified organism NEC J03.80
    - recurrent J03.81
  - staphylococcal J03.80
    - recurrent J03.81
  - streptococcal J03.00
    - recurrent J03.01
  - tuberculous A15.8
  - Vincent's A69.1
- **Tooth, teeth** —*see* condition
- **Toothache** K08.89
- **Topagnosis** R20.8
- **Tophi** —*see* Gout, chronic
- **TORCH infection** —*see* Infection, congenital
  - without active infection P00.2
- **Torn** —*see* Tear
- **Tornwaldt's cyst or disease** J39.2
- **Torsades de pointes** I47.21
- **Torsion**
  - accessory tube —*see* Torsion, fallopian tube
  - adnexa (female) —*see* Torsion, fallopian tube
  - aorta, acquired I77.1
  - appendix epididymis N44.04
  - appendix testis N44.03
  - bile duct (common) (hepatic) K83.8
    - congenital Q44.5
  - bowel, colon or intestine K56.2
  - cervix —*see* Malposition, uterus
  - cystic duct K82.8
  - dystonia —*see* Dystonia, torsion
  - epididymis (appendix) N44.04
  - fallopian tube N83.52-●
    - with ovary N83.53
  - gallbladder K82.8
    - congenital Q44.1
  - hydatid of Morgagni
    - female N83.52-●
    - male N44.03
  - kidney (pedicle) (leading to infarction) N28.0
  - Meckel's diverticulum (congenital) Q43.0
    - malignant —*see* Table of Neoplasms, small intestine, malignant
  - mesentery K56.2
  - omentum K56.2
  - organ or site, congenital NEC —*see* Anomaly, by site
  - ovary (pedicle) N83.51-●
    - with fallopian tube N83.53
    - congenital Q50.2
  - oviduct —*see* Torsion, fallopian tube
  - penis (acquired) N48.82
    - congenital Q55.63
  - spasm —*see* Dystonia, torsion
  - spermatic cord N44.02
    - extravaginal N44.01
    - intravaginal N44.02
  - spleen D73.5
  - testis, testicle N44.00
    - appendix N44.03
  - tibia —*see* Deformity, limb, specified type NEC, lower leg
  - uterus —*see* Malposition, uterus
- **Torticollis** (intermittent) (spastic) M43.6
  - congenital (sternomastoid) Q68.0
  - due to birth injury P15.8
  - hysterical F44.4
  - ocular R29.891
  - psychogenic F45.8
    - conversion reaction F44.4
  - rheumatic M43.6
  - rheumatoid M06.88
  - spasmodic G24.3
  - traumatic, current S13.4
- **Tortipelvis** G24.1
- **Tortuous**
  - aortic arch Q25.46
  - artery I77.1
  - organ or site, congenital NEC —*see* Distortion
  - retinal vessel, congenital Q14.1
  - ureter N13.8
  - urethra N36.8
  - vein —*see* Varix
- **Torture, victim of** Z65.4
- **Torula, torular** (histolytica) (infection) —*see* Cryptococcosis
- **Torulosis** —*see* Cryptococcosis
- **Torus** (mandibularis) (palatinus) M27.0
  - fracture —*see* Fracture, by site, torus
- **Touraine's syndrome** Q79.8
- **Tourette's syndrome** F95.2
- **Tourniquet syndrome** —*see* Constriction, external, by site
- **Tower skull** Q75.009
  - with exophthalmos Q87.0
- **Toxemia** R68.89
  - bacterial —*see* Sepsis
  - burn —*see* Burn
  - eclamptic (with pre-existing hypertension) —*see* Eclampsia
  - erysipelatous —*see* Erysipelas
  - fatigue R68.89
  - food —*see* Poisoning, food
  - gastrointestinal K52.1
  - intestinal K52.1
  - kidney —*see* Uremia
  - malarial —*see* Malaria
  - myocardial —*see* Myocarditis, toxic
  - of pregnancy —*see* Pre-eclampsia
  - pre-eclamptic —*see* Pre-eclampsia
  - small intestine K52.1
  - staphylococcal, due to food A05.0
  - stasis R68.89
  - uremic —*see* Uremia
  - urinary —*see* Uremia
- **Toxemica cerebropathia psychica** (nonalcoholic) F04
  - alcoholic —*see* Alcohol, amnestic disorder
- **Toxic** (poisoning) —*see also* condition T65.91
  - effect —*see* Table of Drugs and Chemicals, by substance, poisoning
  - shock syndrome A48.3
  - thyroid (gland) —*see* Thyrotoxicosis
- **Toxicemia** —*see* Toxemia
- **Toxicity** —*see* Table of Drugs and Chemicals, by substance, poisoning
  - fava bean D55.0
  - food, noxious —*see* Poisoning, food
  - from drug or nonmedicinal substance —*see* Table of Drugs and Chemicals, by drug
- **Toxicosis** —*see also* Toxemia
  - capillary, hemorrhagic D69.0
- **Toxinfection, gastrointestinal** K52.1
- **Toxocariasis** B83.0
- **Toxoplasma, toxoplasmosis** (acquired) B58.9
  - with
    - hepatitis B58.1
    - meningoencephalitis B58.2
    - ocular involvement B58.00
    - other organ involvement B58.89
    - pneumonia, pneumonitis B58.3
  - congenital (acute) (subacute) (chronic) P37.1
  - maternal, manifest toxoplasmosis in infant (acute) (subacute) (chronic) P37.1
- **tPA** (rtPA) administation in a different facility within the last 24 hours prior to admission to current facility Z92.82
- **Trabeculation, bladder** N32.89
- **Trachea** —*see* condition
- **Tracheitis** (catarrhal) (infantile) (membranous) (plastic) (septal) (suppurative) (viral) J04.10
  - with
    - bronchitis (15 years of age and above) J40
      - acute or subacute —*see* Bronchitis, acute
      - chronic J42
      - tuberculous NEC A15.5
      - under 15 years of age J20.9
    - laryngitis (acute) J04.2
      - chronic J37.1
      - tuberculous NEC A15.5
  - acute J04.10
    - with obstruction J04.11
  - chronic J42
    - with
      - bronchitis (chronic) J42
      - laryngitis (chronic) J37.1
  - diphtheritic (membranous) A36.89
  - due to external agent —*see* Inflammation, respiratory, upper, due to
  - syphilitic A52.73
  - tuberculous A15.5
- **Trachelitis** (nonvenereal) —*see* Cervicitis
- **Tracheobronchial** —*see* condition
- **Tracheobronchitis** (15 years of age and above) —*see also* Bronchitis
  - due to
    - Bordetella bronchiseptica A37.80
      - with pneumonia A37.81
    - Francisella tularensis A21.8
- **Tracheobronchomegaly** Q32.4
  - with bronchiectasis J47.9
    - with
      - exacerbation (acute) J47.1
      - lower respiratory infection J47.0
  - acquired J98.09
    - with bronchiectasis J47.9
      - with
        - exacerbation (acute) J47.1
        - lower respiratory infection J47.0
- **Tracheobronchopneumonitis** —*see* Pneumonia, broncho-●
- **Tracheocele** (external) (internal) J39.8
  - congenital Q32.1
- **Tracheomalacia** J39.8
  - congenital Q32.0
- **Tracheopharyngitis** (acute) J06.9
  - chronic J42
  - due to external agent —*see* Inflammation, respiratory, upper, due to
- **Tracheostenosis** J39.8

T

Trichomycosis
  axillaris A48.8
  nodosa, nodularis B36.8
Trichonodosis L67.8
Trichophytid, trichophyton infection —*see* Dermatophytosis
Trichophytobezoar T18.9
  intestine T18.3
  stomach T18.2
Trichophytosis —*see* Dermatophytosis
Trichoptilosis L67.8
Trichorrhexis (nodosa) (invaginata) L67.Ø
Trichosis axillaris A48.8
Trichosporosis nodosa B36.2
Trichostasis spinulosa (congenital) Q84.1
Trichostrongyliasis, trichostrongylosis (small intestine) B81.2
Trichostrongylus infection B81.2
Trichotillomania F63.3
Trichromat, trichromatopsia, anomalous (congenital) H53.55
Trichuriasis B79
Trichuris trichiura (infection) (infestation) (any site) B79
Tricuspid (valve) —*see* condition
Trifid —*see also* Accessory
  kidney (pelvis) Q63.8
  tongue Q38.3
Trigeminal neuralgia —*see* Neuralgia, trigeminal
Trigeminy RØØ.8
Trigger finger (acquired) M65.3Ø
  congenital Q74.Ø
  index finger M65.32- •
  little finger M65.35- •
  middle finger M65.33- •
  ring finger M65.34- •
  thumb M65.31- •
Trigonitis (bladder) (chronic) (pseudomembranous) N3Ø.3Ø
  with hematuria N3Ø.31
Trigonocephaly Q75.Ø3
Trilocular heart —*see* Cor triloculare
Trimethylaminuria E72.52
Tripartite placenta O43.19- •
Triphalangeal thumb Q74.Ø
Triple —*see also* Accessory
  kidneys Q63.Ø
  ▶ negative breast cancer (TNBC) Z17.421
  uteri Q51.818
  X, female Q97.Ø
Triple I O41.12- •
Triplegia G83.89
  congenital G8Ø.8
Triplet (newborn) —*see also* Newborn, triplet
  complicating pregnancy —*see* Pregnancy, triplet
Triplication —*see* Accessory
Triploidy Q92.7
Trismus R25.2
  neonatorum A33
  newborn A33
Trisomy (syndrome) Q92.9
  13 (partial) Q91.7
    meiotic nondisjunction Q91.4
    mitotic nondisjunction Q91.5
    mosaicism Q91.5
    translocation Q91.6
  18 (partial) Q91.3
    meiotic nondisjunction Q91.Ø
    mitotic nondisjunction Q91.1
    mosaicism Q91.1
    translocation Q91.2
  2Ø Q92.8
  21 (partial) Q9Ø.9
    meiotic nondisjunction Q9Ø.Ø
    mitotic nondisjunction Q9Ø.1
    mosaicism Q9Ø.1
    translocation Q9Ø.2
  22 Q92.8
  autosomes Q92.9
  chromosome specified NEC Q92.8
    partial Q92.2
      due to unbalanced translocation Q92.5
    specified NEC Q92.8
    whole (nonsex chromosome)
      meiotic nondisjunction Q92.Ø
      mitotic nondisjunction Q92.1
      mosaicism Q92.1
  due to
    dicentrics —*see* Extra, marker chromosomes
    extra rings —*see* Extra, marker chromosomes
    isochromosomes —*see* Extra, marker chromosomes

Trisomy *(Continued)*
  specified NEC Q92.8
  whole chromosome Q92.9
    meiotic nondisjunction Q92.Ø
    mitotic nondisjunction Q92.1
    mosaicism Q92.1
    partial Q92.9
    specified NEC Q92.8
Tritanomaly, tritanopia H53.55
Trombiculosis, trombiculiasis, trombidiosis B88.Ø
Trophedema (congenital) (hereditary) Q82.Ø
Trophoblastic disease —*see also* Mole, hydatidiform OØ1.9
Tropholymphedema Q82.Ø
Trophoneurosis NEC G96.89
  disseminated M34.9
Tropical —*see* condition
Trouble —*see also* Disease
  heart —*see* Disease, heart
  kidney —*see* Disease, renal
  nervous R45.Ø
  sinus —*see* Sinusitis
Trousseau's syndrome (thrombophlebitis migrans) I82.1
Truancy, childhood
  from school Z72.81Ø
Truncus
  arteriosus (persistent) Q2Ø.Ø
  communis Q2Ø.Ø
Trunk —*see* condition
Trypanosomiasis
  African B56.9
    by Trypanosoma brucei
      gambiense B56.Ø
      rhodesiense B56.1
  American —*see* Chagas' disease
  Brazilian —*see* Chagas' disease
  by Trypanosoma
    brucei gambiense B56.Ø
    brucei rhodesiense B56.1
    cruzi —*see* Chagas' disease
  gambiensis, Gambian B56.Ø
  rhodesiensis, Rhodesian B56.1
  South American —*see* Chagas' disease
  where
    African trypanosomiasis is prevalent B56.9
    Chagas' disease is prevalent B57.2
Tryptasemia, hereditary alpha D89.44
T-shaped incisors KØØ.2
Tsutsugamushi (disease) (fever) A75.3
Tube, tubal, tubular —*see* condition
Tubercle —*see also* Tuberculosis
  brain, solitary A17.81
  Darwin's Q17.8
  Ghon, primary infection A15.7
Tuberculid, tuberculide (indurating, subcutaneous) (lichenoid) (miliary) (papulonecrotic) (primary) (skin) A18.4
Tuberculoma —*see also* Tuberculosis
  brain A17.81
  meninges (cerebral) (spinal) A17.1
  spinal cord A17.81
Tuberculosis, tubercular, tuberculous (calcification) (calcified) (caseous) (chromogenic acid-fast bacilli) (degeneration) (fibrocaseous) (fistula) (interstitial) (isolated circumscribed lesions) (necrosis) (parenchymatous) (ulcerative) A15.9
  with pneumoconiosis (any condition in J6Ø-J64) J65
  abdomen (lymph gland) A18.39
  abscess (respiratory) A15.9
    bone A18.Ø3
      hip A18.Ø2
      knee A18.Ø2
      sacrum A18.Ø1
      specified site NEC A18.Ø3
      spinal A18.Ø1
      vertebra A18.Ø1
    brain A17.81
    breast A18.89
    Cowper's gland A18.15
    dura (mater) (cerebral) (spinal) A17.81
    epidural (cerebral) (spinal) A17.81
    female pelvis A18.17
    frontal sinus A15.8
    genital organs NEC A18.1Ø
    genitourinary A18.1Ø
    gland (lymphatic) —*see* Tuberculosis, lymph gland
    hip A18.Ø2
    intestine A18.32

Tuberculosis, tubercular, tuberculous *(Continued)*
  abscess *(Continued)*
    ischiorectal A18.32
    joint NEC A18.Ø2
      hip A18.Ø2
      knee A18.Ø2
      specified NEC A18.Ø2
      vertebral A18.Ø1
    kidney A18.11
    knee A18.Ø2
    latent Z22.7
    lumbar (spine) A18.Ø1
    lung —*see* Tuberculosis, pulmonary
    meninges (cerebral) (spinal) A17.Ø
    muscle A18.Ø9
    perianal (fistula) A18.32
    perinephritic A18.11
    perirectal A18.32
    rectum A18.32
    retropharyngeal A15.8
    sacrum A18.Ø1
    scrofulous A18.2
    scrotum A18.15
    skin (primary) A18.4
    spinal cord A17.81
    spine or vertebra (column) A18.Ø1
    subdiaphragmatic A18.31
    testis A18.15
    urinary A18.13
    uterus A18.17
  accessory sinus —*see* Tuberculosis, sinus
  Addison's disease A18.7
  adenitis —*see* Tuberculosis, lymph gland
  adenoids A15.8
  adenopathy —*see* Tuberculosis, lymph gland
  adherent pericardium A18.84
  adnexa (uteri) A18.17
  adrenal (capsule) (gland) A18.7
  alimentary canal A18.32
  anemia A18.89
  ankle (joint) (bone) A18.Ø2
  anus A18.32
  apex, apical —*see* Tuberculosis, pulmonary
  appendicitis, appendix A18.32
  arachnoid A17.Ø
  artery, arteritis A18.89
    cerebral A18.89
  arthritis (chronic) (synovial) A18.Ø2
    spine or vertebra (column) A18.Ø1
  articular —*see* Tuberculosis, joint
  ascites A18.31
  asthma —*see* Tuberculosis, pulmonary
  axilla, axillary (gland) A18.2
  bladder A18.12
  bone A18.Ø3
    hip A18.Ø2
    knee A18.Ø2
    limb NEC A18.Ø3
    sacrum A18.Ø1
    spine or vertebral column A18.Ø1
  bowel (miliary) A18.32
  brain A17.81
  breast A18.89
  broad ligament A18.17
  bronchi, bronchial, bronchus A15.5
    ectasia, ectasis (bronchiectasis) —*see* Tuberculosis, pulmonary
    fistula A15.5
      primary (progressive) A15.7
    gland or node A15.4
      primary (progressive) A15.7
    lymph gland or node A15.4
      primary (progressive) A15.7
  bronchiectasis —*see* Tuberculosis, pulmonary
  bronchitis A15.5
  bronchopleural A15.6
  bronchopneumonia, bronchopneumonic —*see* Tuberculosis, pulmonary
  bronchorrhagia A15.5
  bronchotracheal A15.5
  bronze disease A18.7
  buccal cavity A18.83
  bulbourethral gland A18.15
  bursa A18.Ø9
  cachexia A15.9
  cardiomyopathy A18.84
  caries —*see* Tuberculosis, bone
  cartilage A18.Ø2
    intervertebral A18.Ø1
  catarrhal —*see* Tuberculosis, respiratory
  cecum A18.32
  cellulitis (primary) A18.4

T

T

- **Tumor** *(Continued)*
  - stromal *(Continued)*
    - gastrointestinal *(Continued)*
      - malignant *(Continued)*
        - small intestine C49.A3
        - specified site NEC C49.A9
        - stomach C49.A2
      - rectum C49.A5
      - small intestine C49.A3
      - specified site NEC C49.A9
      - stomach C49.A2
      - uncertain behavior D48.19
    - intestine
      - benign D21.4
      - malignant
        - large C49.A4
        - small C49.A3
      - uncertain behavior D48.19
    - ovarian D39.1- ●
    - stomach C49.A2
      - benign D21.4
      - malignant C49.A2
      - uncertain behavior D48.19
  - sweat gland —*see also* Neoplasm, skin, uncertain behavior
    - benign —*see* Neoplasm, skin, benign
    - malignant —*see* Neoplasm, skin, malignant
  - syphilitic, brain A52.17
  - testicular D40.10
  - testicular stromal D40.1- ●
  - theca cell D27.- ●
  - theca cell-granulosa cell D39.1- ●
  - Triton, malignant —*see* Neoplasm, nerve, malignant
  - trophoblastic, placental site D39.2
  - turban D23.4
  - uterus (body), in pregnancy or childbirth —*see* Pregnancy, complicated by, tumor, uterus
  - vagina, in pregnancy or childbirth —*see* Pregnancy, complicated by
  - varicose —*see* Varix
  - von Recklinghausen's —*see* Neurofibromatosis
  - vulva or perineum, in pregnancy or childbirth —*see* Pregnancy, complicated by
    - causing obstructed labor O65.5
  - ➡ Warthin's —*see* Neoplasm, salivary gland or duct, benign
  - Wilms' C64- ●
  - yolk sac —*see* Neoplasm, malignant, by site
    - specified site —*see* Neoplasm, malignant, by site
    - unspecified site
      - female C56.9
      - male C62.90
- **Tumor lysis syndrome** (following antineoplastic chemotherapy) (spontaneous) NEC E88.3
- **Tumorlet**—*see* Neoplasm, uncertain behavior, by site
- **Tungiasis** B88.1
- **Tunica vasculosa lentis** Q12.2
- **Turban tumor** D23.4
- **Türck's trachoma** J37.0
- **Turner-Kieser syndrome** Q87.2
- **Turner-like syndrome** Q87.19
- **Turner's**
  - hypoplasia (tooth) K00.4
  - syndrome Q96.9
    - specified NEC Q96.8
  - tooth K00.4
- **Turner-Ullrich syndrome** Q96.9
- **Tussis convulsiva**—*see* Whooping cough
- **Twiddler's syndrome** (due to)
  - automatic implantable defibrillator T82.198
  - cardiac pacemaker T82.198
- **Twilight state**
  - epileptic F05
  - psychogenic F44.89
- **Twin** (newborn) —*see also* Newborn, twin
  - conjoined Q89.4
  - pregnancy —*see* Pregnancy, twin
- **Twinning, teeth** K00.2
- **Twist, twisted**
  - bowel, colon or intestine K56.2
  - hair (congenital) Q84.1
  - mesentery K56.2
  - omentum K56.2
  - organ or site, congenital NEC —*see* Anomaly, by site
  - ovarian pedicle —*see* Torsion, ovary
- **Twitching** R25.3
- **Tylosis** (acquired) L84
  - buccalis K13.29
  - linguae K13.29
  - palmaris et plantaris (congenital) (inherited) Q82.8
    - acquired L85.1
- **Tympanism** R14.0
- **Tympanites** (abdominal) (intestinal) R14.0
- **Tympanitis**—*see* Myringitis
- **Tympanosclerosis**—*see* subcategory H74.0
- **Tympanum**—*see* condition
- **Tympany**
  - abdomen R14.0
  - chest R09.89
- **Type A behavior pattern** Z73.1
- **Typhlitis**—*see* Cecitis
- **Typhoenteritis**—*see* Typhoid
- **Typhoid** (abortive) (ambulant) (any site) (clinical) (fever) (hemorrhagic) (infection) (intermittent) (malignant) (rheumatic) (Widal negative) A01.00
  - with pneumonia A01.03
  - abdominal A01.09
  - arthritis A01.04
  - carrier (suspected) of Z22.0
  - cholecystitis (current) A01.09
  - endocarditis A01.02
  - heart involvement A01.02
  - inoculation reaction —*see* Complications, vaccination
  - meningitis A01.01
  - mesenteric lymph nodes A01.09
  - myocarditis A01.02
  - Orientia Tsutsugamushi (scrub typhus) A75.3
  - osteomyelitis A01.05
  - perichondritis, larynx A01.09
  - pneumonia A01.03
  - specified NEC A01.09
  - spine A01.05
  - ulcer (perforating) A01.09
- **Typhomalaria** (fever) —*see* Malaria
- **Typhomania** A01.00
- **Typhoperitonitis** A01.09
- **Typhus** (fever) A75.9
  - abdominal, abdominalis —*see* Typhoid
  - African tick A77.1
  - amarillic A95.9
  - brain A75.9 *[G94]*
  - cerebral A75.9 *[G94]*
  - classical A75.0
  - due to Rickettsia
    - prowazekii A75.0
      - recrudescent A75.1
    - tsutsugamushi A75.3
    - typhi A75.2
  - endemic (flea-borne) A75.2
  - epidemic (louse-borne) A75.0
  - exanthematic NEC A75.0
  - exanthematicus SAI A75.0
    - brillii SAI A75.1
    - mexicanus SAI A75.2
    - typhus murinus A75.2
  - flea-borne A75.2
  - India tick A77.1
  - Kenya (tick) A77.1
  - louse-borne A75.0
  - Mexican A75.2
  - mite-borne A75.3
  - murine A75.2
  - North Asian tick-borne A77.2
  - petechial A75.9
  - Queensland tick A77.3
  - rat A75.2
  - recrudescent A75.1
  - recurrens —*see* Fever, relapsing
  - Sao Paulo A77.0
  - scrub (China) (India) (Malaysia) (New Guinea) A75.3
  - shop (of Malaysia) A75.2
  - Siberian tick A77.2
  - tick-borne A77.9
  - tropical (mite-borne) A75.3
- **Tyrosinemia** E70.21
  - newborn, transitory P74.5
- **Tyrosinosis** E70.21
- **Tyrosinuria** E70.29

U

- **Uhl's anomaly or disease** Q24.8
- **Ulcer, ulcerated, ulcerating, ulceration, ulcerative**
  - alveolar process M27.3
  - amebic (intestine) A06.1
    - skin A06.7
  - anastomotic —*see* Ulcer, gastrojejunal
  - anorectal K62.6
  - antral —*see* Ulcer, stomach
  - anus (sphincter) (solitary) K62.6
  - aorta —*see* Aneurysm
  - aphthous (oral) (recurrent) K12.0
    - genital organ(s)
      - female N76.6
      - male N50.89
  - artery I77.2
  - atrophic —*see* Ulcer, skin
    - decubitus —*see* Ulcer, pressure, by site
  - back L98.429
    - with
      - bone involvement without evidence of necrosis L98.426
      - bone necrosis L98.424
      - exposed fat layer L98.422
      - muscle involvement without evidence of necrosis L98.425
      - muscle necrosis L98.423
      - skin breakdown only L98.421
      - specified severity NEC L98.428
  - Barrett's (esophagus) K22.10
    - with bleeding K22.11
  - bile duct (common) (hepatic) K83.8
  - bladder (solitary) (sphincter) NEC N32.89
    - bilharzial B65.9 *[N33]*
    - in schistosomiasis (bilharzial) B65.9 *[N33]*
    - submucosal —*see* Cystitis, interstitial
    - tuberculous A18.12
  - bleeding K27.4
  - bone —*see* Osteomyelitis, specified type NEC
  - bowel —*see* Ulcer, intestine
  - breast N61.1
  - bronchus J98.09
  - buccal (cavity) (traumatic) K12.1
  - Buruli A31.1
  - buttock L98.419
    - with
      - bone involvement without evidence of necrosis L98.416
      - bone necrosis L98.414
      - exposed fat layer L98.412
      - muscle involvement without evidence of necrosis L98.415
      - muscle necrosis L98.413
      - skin breakdown only L98.411
      - specified severity NEC L98.418
  - cameron - see Ulcer, stomach
  - cancerous —*see* Neoplasm, malignant, by site
  - cardia K22.10
    - with bleeding K22.11
  - cardioesophageal (peptic) K22.10
    - with bleeding K22.11
  - cecum —*see* Ulcer, intestine
  - cervix (uteri) (decubitus) (trophic) N86
    - with cervicitis N72
  - chancroidal A57
  - chiclero B55.1
  - chronic (cause unknown) —*see* Ulcer, skin
  - Cochin-China B55.1
  - colon —*see* Ulcer, intestine
  - conjunctiva H10.89
  - cornea H16.00- ●
    - with hypopyon H16.03- ●
    - central H16.01- ●
    - dendritic (herpes simplex) B00.52
    - marginal H16.04- ●
    - Mooren's H16.05- ●
    - mycotic H16.06- ●
    - perforated H16.07- ●
    - ring H16.02- ●
    - tuberculous (phlyctenular) A18.52
  - corpus cavernosum (chronic) N48.5
  - crural —*see* Ulcer, lower limb
  - Curling's —*see* Ulcer, peptic, acute
  - Cushing's —*see* Ulcer, peptic, acute
  - cystic duct K82.8
  - cystitis (interstitial) —*see* Cystitis, interstitial
  - decubitus —*see* Ulcer, pressure, by site
  - dendritic, cornea (herpes simplex) B00.52
  - diabetes, diabetic —*see* Diabetes, ulcer

U

- **Urticaria** *(Continued)*
  - serum —*see also* Reaction, serum T8Ø.69
  - solar L56.3
  - specified type NEC L5Ø.8
  - thermal (cold) (heat) L5Ø.2
  - vibratory L5Ø.4
  - xanthelasmoidea —*see* Urticaria pigmentosa
- Use (of)
  - ▶alcohol (*see also* Alcohol, alcoholic, by disorder) F1Ø.9Ø
    - with
      - ▶anxiety disorder F1Ø.98Ø
      - intoxication F1Ø.929
      - sleep disorder F1Ø.982
      - withdrawal F1Ø.939
        - with
          - perceptual disturbance F1Ø.932
        - delirium F1Ø.931
        - uncomplicated F1Ø.93Ø
    - harmful —*see* Abuse, alcohol
    - in remission F1Ø.91
  - amphetamines —*see* Use, stimulant NEC
  - caffeine —*see* Use, stimulant NEC
  - cannabis F12.9Ø
    - with
      - anxiety disorder F12.98Ø
      - intoxication F12.929
        - with
          - delirium F12.921
          - perceptual disturbance F12.922
        - uncomplicated F12.92Ø
      - other specified disorder F12.988
      - psychosis F12.959
        - delusions F12.95Ø
        - hallucinations F12.951
      - unspecified disorder F12.99
      - withdrawal F12.93
    - in remission F12.91
  - cocaine F14.9Ø
    - with
      - anxiety disorder F14.98Ø
      - intoxication F14.929
        - with
          - delirium F14.921
          - perceptual disturbance F14.922
        - uncomplicated F14.92Ø
      - other specified disorder F14.988
      - psychosis F14.959
        - delusions F14.95Ø
        - hallucinations F14.951
      - sexual dysfunction F14.981
      - sleep disorder F14.982
      - unspecified disorder F14.99
      - withdrawal F14.93
    - harmful —*see* Abuse, drug, cocaine
    - in remission F14.91
  - drug(s) NEC F19.9Ø
    - with sleep disorder F19.982
    - harmful —*see* Abuse, drug, by type
  - hallucinogen NEC F16.9Ø
    - with
      - anxiety disorder F16.98Ø
      - intoxication F16.929
        - with
          - delirium F16.921
        - uncomplicated F16.92Ø
      - mood disorder F16.94
      - other specified disorder F16.988
      - perception disorder (flashbacks) F16.983
      - psychosis F16.959
        - delusions F16.95Ø
        - hallucinations F16.951
      - unspecified disorder F16.99
    - harmful —*see* Abuse, drug, hallucinogen NEC
    - in remission F16.91
  - inhalants F18.9Ø
    - with
      - anxiety disorder F18.98Ø
      - intoxication F18.929
        - with delirium F18.921
        - uncomplicated F18.92Ø
      - mood disorder F18.94
      - other specified disorder F18.988
      - persisting dementia F18.97
      - psychosis F18.959
        - delusions F18.95Ø
        - hallucinations F18.951
      - unspecified disorder F18.99
    - harmful —*see* Abuse, drug, inhalant
    - in remission F18.91

- Use *(Continued)*
  - methadone —*see* Use, opioid
  - nonprescribed drugs F19.9Ø
    - harmful —*see* Abuse, non-psychoactive substance
  - opioid F11.9Ø
    - with
      - disorder F11.99
        - mood F11.94
        - sleep F11.982
        - specified type NEC F11.988
      - intoxication F11.929
        - with
          - delirium F11.921
          - perceptual disturbance F11.922
        - uncomplicated F11.92Ø
      - opioid-associated amnestic syndrome F11.988
      - withdrawal F11.93
    - harmful —*see* Abuse, drug, opioid
    - in remission F11.91
  - patent medicines F19.9Ø
    - harmful —*see* Abuse, non-psychoactive substance
  - psychoactive drug NEC F19.9Ø
    - with
      - anxiety disorder F19.98Ø
      - intoxication F19.929
        - with
          - delirium F19.921
          - perceptual disturbance F19.922
        - uncomplicated F19.92Ø
      - mood disorder F19.94
      - other specified disorder F19.988
      - persisting
        - amnestic disorder F19.96
        - dementia F19.97
      - psychosis F19.959
        - delusions F19.95Ø
        - hallucinations F19.951
      - sexual dysfunction F19.981
      - sleep disorder F19.982
      - unspecified disorder F19.99
      - withdrawal F19.939
        - with
          - delirium F19.931
          - perceptual disturbance F19.932
        - uncomplicated F19.93Ø
    - harmful —*see* Abuse, drug NEC, psychoactive NEC
    - in remission F19.91
  - sedative, hypnotic, or anxiolytic F13.9Ø
    - with
      - anxiety disorder F13.98Ø
      - intoxication F13.929
        - with
          - delirium F13.921
        - uncomplicated F13.92Ø
      - other specified disorder F13.988
      - persisting
        - amnestic disorder F13.96
        - dementia F13.97
      - psychosis F13.959
        - delusions F13.95Ø
        - hallucinations F13.951
      - sexual dysfunction F13.981
      - sleep disorder F13.982
      - unspecified disorder F13.99
    - harmful —*see* Abuse, drug, sedative, hypnotic, or anxiolytic
    - in remission F13.91
  - stimulant NEC F15.9Ø
    - with
      - anxiety disorder F15.98Ø
      - intoxication F15.929
        - with
          - delirium F15.921
          - perceptual disturbance F15.922
        - uncomplicated F15.92Ø
      - mood disorder F15.94
      - other specified disorder F15.988
      - psychosis F15.959
        - delusions F15.95Ø
        - hallucinations F15.951
      - sexual dysfunction F15.981
      - sleep disorder F15.982
      - unspecified disorder F15.99
      - withdrawal F15.93
    - harmful —*see* Abuse, drug, stimulant NEC
    - in remission F15.91

- Use *(Continued)*
  - tobacco Z72.Ø
    - with dependence —*see* Dependence, drug, nicotine
  - volatile solvents —*see also* Use, inhalant F18.9Ø
    - harmful —*see* Abuse, drug, inhalant
- **Usher-Senear disease or syndrome** L1Ø.4
- **Uta** B55.1
- **Uteromegaly** N85.2
- **Uterovaginal** —*see* condition
- **Uterovesical** —*see* condition
- **Uveal** —*see* condition
- **Uveitis** (anterior) —*see also* Iridocyclitis
  - acute —*see* Iridocyclitis, acute
  - chronic —*see* Iridocyclitis, chronic
  - due to toxoplasmosis (acquired) B58.Ø9
    - congenital P37.1
  - granulomatous —*see* Iridocyclitis, chronic
  - heterochromic —*see* Cyclitis, Fuchs' heterochromic
  - lens-induced —*see* Iridocyclitis, lens-induced
  - posterior —*see* Chorioretinitis
  - sympathetic H44.13-●
  - syphilitic (secondary) A51.43
    - congenital (early) A5Ø.Ø1
    - late A52.71
  - tuberculous A18.54
- **Uveoencephalitis** —*see* Inflammation, chorioretinal
- **Uveokeratitis** —*see* Iridocyclitis
- **Uveoparotitis** D86.89
- **Uvula** —*see* condition
- **Uvulitis** (acute) (catarrhal) (chronic) (membranous) (suppurative) (ulcerative) K12.2

V

- **Vaccination** (prophylactic)
  - complication or reaction —*see* Complications, vaccination
  - delayed Z28.9
  - encounter for Z23
  - not done —*see* Immunization, not done, because (of)
- **Vaccinia** (generalized) (localized) T88.1
  - without vaccination BØ8.Ø11
  - congenital P35.8
- **Vacuum, in sinus** (accessory) (nasal) J34.89
- **Vagabond, vagabondage** Z59.ØØ
- **Vagabond's disease** B85.1
- **Vagina, vaginal** —*see* condition
- **Vaginalitis** (tunica) (testis) N49.1
- **Vaginismus** (reflex) N94.2
  - functional F52.5
  - nonorganic F52.5
  - psychogenic F52.5
  - secondary N94.2
- **Vaginitis** (acute) (circumscribed) (diffuse) (emphysematous) (nonvenereal) (ulcerative) N76.Ø
  - with ectopic or molar pregnancy OØ8.Ø
  - amebic AØ6.82
  - atrophic, postmenopausal N95.2
  - bacterial N76.Ø
  - blennorrhagic (gonococcal) A54.Ø2
  - candidal (acute) B37.31
  - chronic (recurrent) B37.32
  - chlamydial A56.Ø2
  - chronic N76.1
  - due to Trichomonas (vaginalis) A59.Ø1
  - following ectopic or molar pregnancy OØ8.Ø
  - gonococcal A54.Ø2
    - with abscess (accessory gland) (periurethral) A54.1
  - granuloma A58
  - in (due to)
    - candidiasis (acute) B37.31
    - chronic (recurrent) B37.32
    - herpesviral (herpes simplex) infection A6Ø.Ø4
    - pinworm infection B8Ø *[N77.1]*
  - monilial (acute) B37.31
    - chronic (recurrent) B37.32
  - mycotic (candidal) (acute) B37.31
    - chronic (recurrent) B37.32
  - postmenopausal atrophic N95.2
  - puerperal (postpartum) O86.13
  - senile (atrophic) N95.2
  - subacute or chronic N76.1

- **Vasospasm** (vasoconstriction) (*see also* Angiospasm) I73.9
  - cerebral (cerebrovascular) (artery) I67.848
    - reversible I67.841
  - coronary I2Ø.1
  - nerve
    - arm —*see* Mononeuropathy, upper limb
    - brachial plexus G54.Ø
    - cervical plexus G54.2
    - leg —*see* Mononeuropathy, lower limb
  - peripheral NOS I73.9
  - retina (artery) —*see* Occlusion, artery, retina
- **Vasospastic** —*see* condition
- **Vasovagal attack** (paroxysmal) R55
  - psychogenic F45.8
- **VATER syndrome** Q87.2
- **Vater's ampulla** —*see* condition
- **Vegetation, vegetative**
  - adenoid (nasal fossa) J35.8
  - endocarditis (acute) (any valve) (subacute) I33.Ø
  - heart (mycotic) (valve) I33.Ø
- **Veil**
  - Jackson's Q43.3
- **Vein, venous** —*see* condition
- **Veldt sore** —*see* Ulcer, skin
- **Velpeau's hernia** —*see* Hernia, femoral
- **Venereal**
  - bubo A55
  - disease A64
  - granuloma inguinale A58
  - lymphogranuloma (Durand-Nicolas-Favre) A55
- **Venofibrosis** I87.8
- **Venom, venomous** —*see* Table of Drugs and Chemicals, by animal or substance, poisoning
- **Venous** —*see* condition
- **Ventilator lung, newborn** P27.8
- **Ventral** —*see* condition
- **Ventricle, ventricular** —*see also* condition
  - escape I49.3
  - inversion Q2Ø.5
- **Ventriculitis** (cerebral) —*see also* Encephalitis G04.90
- **Ventriculostomy status** Z98.2
- **Vernet's syndrome** G52.7
- **Verneuil's disease** (syphilitic bursitis) A52.78
- **Verruca** (due to HPV) (filiformis) (simplex) (viral) (vulgaris) BØ7.9
  - acuminata A63.Ø
  - necrogenica (primary) (tuberculosa) A18.4
  - plana BØ7.8
  - plantaris BØ7.Ø
  - seborrheica L82.1
    - inflamed L82.Ø
  - senile (seborrheic) L82.1
    - inflamed L82.Ø
  - tuberculosa (primary) A18.4
  - venereal A63.Ø
- **Verrucosities** —*see* Verruca
- **Verruga peruana, peruviana** A44.1
- **Version**
  - cervix —*see* Malposition, uterus
  - uterus (postinfectional) (postpartal, old) —*see* Malposition, uterus
- **Vertebra, vertebral** —*see* condition
- **Vertical talus** (congenital) Q66.8Ø
  - left foot Q66.82
  - right foot Q66.81
- **Vertigo** R42
  - auditory —*see* Vertigo, aural
  - aural H81.31- ●
  - benign paroxysmal (positional) H81.1- ●
  - central (origin) H81.4
  - cerebral H81.4
  - Dix and Hallpike (epidemic) —*see* Neuronitis, vestibular
  - due to infrasound T75.23
  - epidemic A88.1
    - Dix and Hallpike —*see* Neuronitis, vestibular
    - Pedersen's —*see* Neuronitis, vestibular
    - vestibular neuronitis —*see* Neuronitis, vestibular
  - hysterical F44.89
  - infrasound T75.23
  - labyrinthine —*see* subcategory H81.Ø
  - laryngeal RØ5.4
  - malignant positional H81.4
  - Ménière's —*see* subcategory H81.4Ø
  - menopausal N95.11
  - otogenic —*see* Vertigo, aural
  - paroxysmal positional, benign —*see* Vertigo, benign paroxysmal

Vertigo *(Continued)*
  - Pedersen's (epidemic) —*see* Neuronitis, vestibular
  - peripheral NEC H81.39- ●
  - positional
    - benign paroxysmal —*see* Vertigo, benign paroxysmal
    - malignant H81.4
- **Very-low-density-lipoprotein-type (VLDL) hyperlipoproteinemia** E78.1
- **Vesania** —*see* Psychosis
- **Vesical** —*see* condition
- **Vesicle**
  - cutaneous R23.8
  - seminal —*see* condition
  - skin R23.8
- **Vesicocolic** —*see* condition
- **Vesicoperineal** —*see* condition
- **Vesicorectal** —*see* condition
- **Vesicourethrorectal** —*see* condition
- **Vesicovaginal** —*see* condition
- **Vesicular** —*see* condition
- **Vesiculitis** (seminal) N49.Ø
  - amebic AØ6.82
  - gonorrheal (acute) (chronic) A54.23
  - trichomonal A59.Ø9
  - tuberculous A18.15
- **Vestibulitis** (ear) —*see also* subcategory H83.Ø
  - nose (external) J34.89
  - vulvar N94.81Ø
- **Vestibulopathy, acute peripheral** (recurrent) —*see* Neuronitis, vestibular
- **Vestige, vestigial** —*see also* Persistence
  - branchial Q18.Ø
  - structures in vitreous Q14.Ø
- **Vibration**
  - adverse effects T75.2Ø
    - pneumatic hammer syndrome T75.21
    - specified effect NEC T75.29
    - vasospastic syndrome T75.22
    - vertigo from infrasound T75.23
  - exposure (occupational) Z57.7
  - vertigo T75.23
- **Vibriosis** A28.9
- **Victim** (of)
  - crime Z65.4
  - disaster Z65.5
  - terrorism Z65.4
  - torture Z65.4
  - war Z65.5
- **Vidal's disease** L28.Ø
- **Villaret's syndrome** G52.7
- **Villous** —*see* condition
- **VIN** —*see* Neoplasia, intraepithelial, vulva
- **Vincent's infection** (angina) (gingivitis) A69.1
  - stomatitis NEC A69.1
- **Vinson-Plummer syndrome** D5Ø.1
- **Violence, physical** R45.6
- **Viosterol deficiency** —*see* Deficiency, calciferol
- **Vipoma** —*see* Neoplasm, malignant, by site
- **Viremia** B34.9
- **Virilism** (adrenal) E25.9
  - congenital E25.Ø
- **Virilization** (female) (suprarenal) E25.9
  - congenital E25.Ø
  - isosexual E28.2
- **Virulent bubo** A57
- **Virus, viral** —*see also* condition
  - as cause of disease classified elsewhere B97.89
    - respiratory syncytial virus (RSV) —*see* Virus, infection, respiratory syncytial (RSV)
  - cytomegalovirus B25.9
  - human immunodeficiency (HIV) —*see* Human, immunodeficiency virus (HIV) disease
  - infection —*see* Infection, virus
  - respiratory syncytial (RSV)
    - as cause of disease classified elsewhere B97.4
    - bronchiolitis J21.Ø
    - bronchitis J2Ø.5
    - bronchopneumonia J12.1
    - otitis media H65- ● *[B97.4]*
    - pneumonia J12.1
    - upper respiratory infection JØ6.9 *[B97.4]*
  - specified NEC B34.8
  - swine influenza (viruses that normally cause infections in pigs) —*see also* Influenza, due to, identified novel influenza A virus JØ9.X2

Virus, viral *(Continued)*
  - West Nile (fever) A92.3Ø
    - with
      - complications NEC A92.39
      - cranial nerve disorders A92.32
      - encephalitis A92.31
      - encephalomyelitis A92.31
      - neurologic manifestation NEC A92.32
      - optic neuritis A92.32
      - polyradiculitis A92.32
- **Viscera, visceral** —*see* condition
- **Visceroptosis** K63.4
- **Visible peristalsis** R19.2
- **Vision, visual**
  - binocular, suppression H53.34
  - blurred, blurring H53.8
    - hysterical F44.6
  - defect, defective NEC H54.7
  - disorientation (syndrome) H53.8
  - disturbance H53.9
    - hysterical F44.6
  - double H53.2
  - examination ZØ1.ØØ
    - with abnormal findings ZØ1.Ø1
    - following failed vision screening ZØ1.Ø2Ø
      - with abnormal findings ZØ1.Ø21
  - field, limitation (defect) —*see* Defect, visual field
  - hallucinations R44.1
  - halos H53.19
  - loss —*see* Loss, vision
    - sudden —*see* Disturbance, vision, subjective, loss, sudden
  - low (both eyes) —*see* Low, vision
  - perception, simultaneous without fusion H53.33
- **Vitality, lack or want of** R53.83
  - newborn P96.89
- **Vitamin deficiency** —*see* Deficiency, vitamin
- **Vitelline duct, persistent** Q43.Ø
- **Vitiligo** L8Ø
  - eyelid HØ2.739
    - left HØ2.736
      - lower HØ2.735
      - upper HØ2.734
    - right HØ2.733
      - lower HØ2.732
      - upper HØ2.731
  - pinta A67.2
  - vulva N9Ø.89
- **Vitreal corneal syndrome** H59.Ø1- ●
- **Vitreoretinopathy, proliferative** —*see also* Retinopathy, proliferative
  - with retinal detachment —*see* Detachment, retina, traction
- **Vitreous** —*see also* condition
  - touch syndrome —*see* Complication, postprocedural, following cataract surgery
- **Vocal cord** —*see* condition
- **Vogt-Koyanagi syndrome** H2Ø.82- ●
- **Vogt's disease or syndrome** G8Ø.3
- **Vogt-Spielmeyer amaurotic idiocy or disease** E75.4
- **Voice**
  - change R49.9
    - specified NEC R49.8
  - loss —*see* Aphonia
- **Volhynian fever** A79.Ø
- **Volkmann's ischemic contracture or paralysis** (complicating trauma) T79.6
- **Volvulus** (bowel) (colon) (intestine) K56.2
  - with perforation K56.2
  - congenital Q43.8
  - duodenum K31.5
  - fallopian tube —*see* Torsion, fallopian tube
  - oviduct —*see* Torsion, fallopian tube
  - stomach (due to absence of gastrocolic ligament) K31.89
- **Vomiting** R11.1Ø
  - with nausea R11.2
  - without nausea R11.11
  - asphyxia —*see* Foreign body, by site, causing asphyxia, gastric contents
  - bilious (cause unknown) R11.14
    - following gastro-intestinal surgery K91.Ø
    - in newborn P92.Ø1
  - blood —*see* Hematemesis
  - causing asphyxia, choking, or suffocation —*see* Foreign body, by site
  - cyclical, in migraine G43.AØ
    - with refractory migraine G43.A1
    - intractable G43.A1
    - not intractable G43.AØ

V

W

W

W

X

Y

Z

TON

ICD-10-CM Table of Neoplasms

The list below gives the code numbers for neoplasms by anatomical site. For each site there are six possible code numbers according to whether the neoplasm in question is malignant, benign, in situ, of uncertain behavior, or of unspecified nature. The description of the neoplasm will often indicate which of the six columns is appropriate; e.g., malignant melanoma of skin, benign fibroadenoma of breast, carcinoma in situ of cervix uteri.

Where such descriptors are not present, the remainder of the Index should be consulted where guidance is given to the appropriate column for each morphological (histological) variety listed; e.g., Mesonephroma—*see Neoplasm, malignant;* Embryoma—*see also Neoplasm, uncertain behavior;* Disease, Bowen's—*see Neoplasm, skin, in situ.* However, the guidance in the Index can be overridden if one of the descriptors mentioned above is present; e.g., malignant adenoma of colon is coded to C18.9 and not to D12.6 as the adjective "Malignant" overrides the Index entry 'Adenoma—*see also Neoplasm, benign.*'

Codes listed with a dash -, following the code have a required additional character for laterality. The Tablular must be reviewed for the complete code.

	Malignant Primary	Malignant Secondary	Ca in situ	Benign	Uncertain Behavior	Unspecified Behavior
Neoplasm, neoplastic	C80.1	C79.9	D09.9	D36.9	D48.9	D49.9
abdomen, abdominal	C76.2	C79.8-•	D09.8	D36.7	D48.7	D49.89
cavity	C76.2	C79.8-•	D09.8	D36.7	D48.7	D49.89
organ	C76.2	C79.8-•	D09.8	D36.7	D48.7	D49.89
viscera	C76.2	C79.8-•	D09.8	D36.7	D48.7	D49.89
wall—*see also Neoplasm, abdomen, wall, skin*	C44.509	C79.2-•	D04.5	D23.5	D48.5	D49.2
connective tissue	C49.4	C79.8-•	—	D21.4	D48.1	D49.2
skin	C44.509					
basal cell carcinoma	C44.519	—	—	—	—	—
specified type NEC	C44.599	—	—	—	—	—
squamous cell carcinoma	C44.529	—	—	—	—	—
abdominopelvic	C76.8	C79.8-•	—	D36.7	D48.7	D49.89
accessory sinus—*see Neoplasm, sinus*						
acoustic nerve	C72.4-•	C79.49	—	D33.3	D43.3	D49.7
adenoid (pharynx) (tissue)	C11.1	C79.89	D00.08	D10.6	D37.05	D49.0
adipose tissue—*see also Neoplasm, connective tissue*	C49.4	C79.89	—	D21.9	D48.1	D49.2
adnexa (uterine)	C57.4	C79.89	D07.39	D28.7	D39.8	D49.59
adrenal	C74.9-•	C79.7-•	D09.3	D35.0-•	D44.1-•	D49.7
capsule	C74.9-•	C79.7-•	D09.3	D35.0-•	D44.1-•	D49.7
cortex	C74.0-•	C79.7-•	D09.3	D35.0-•	D44.1-•	D49.7
gland	C74.9-•	C79.7-•	D09.3	D35.0-•	D44.1-•	D49.7
medulla	C74.1-•	C79.7-•	D09.3	D35.0-•	D44.1-•	D49.7
ala nasi (external)—*see also Neoplasm, skin, nose*	C44.301	C79.2	D04.39	D23.39	D48.5	D49.2
alimentary canal or tract NEC	C26.9	C78.80	D01.9	D13.99	D37.9	D49.0
alveolar	C03.9	C79.89	D00.03	D10.39	D37.09	D49.0
mucosa	C03.9	C79.89	D00.03	D10.39	D37.09	D49.0
lower	C03.1	C79.89	D00.03	D10.39	D37.09	D49.0
upper	C03.0	C79.89	D00.03	D10.39	D37.09	D49.0
ridge or process	C41.1	C79.51	—	D16.5-•	D48.0	D49.2
carcinoma	C03.9	C79.8-•	—	—	—	—
lower	C03.1	C79.8-•	—	—	—	—
upper	C03.0	C79.8-•	—	—	—	—
lower	C41.1	C79.51	—	D16.5-•	D48.0	D49.2
mucosa	C03.9	C79.89	D00.03	D10.39	D37.09	D49.0
lower	C03.1	C79.89	D00.03	D10.39	D37.09	D49.0
upper	C03.0	C79.89	D00.03	D10.39	D37.09	D49.0
upper	C41.0	C79.51	—	D16.4-•	D48.0	D49.2
sulcus	C06.1	C79.89	D00.02	D10.39	D37.09	D49.0
alveolus	C03.9	C79.89	D00.03	D10.39	D37.09	D49.0
lower	C03.1	C79.89	D00.03	D10.39	D37.09	D49.0
upper	C03.0	C79.89	D00.03	D10.39	D37.09	D49.0
ampulla of Vater	C24.1	C78.89	D01.5	D13.5	D37.6	D49.0
ankle NEC	C76.5-•	C79.89	D04.7-•	D36.7	D48.7	D49.89
anorectum, anorectal (junction)	C21.8	C78.5	D01.3	D12.9	D37.8	D49.0
antecubital fossa or space	C76.4-•	C79.89	D04.6-•	D36.7	D48.7	D49.89
antrum (Highmore) (maxillary)	C31.0	C78.39	D02.3	D14.0	D38.5	D49.1
pyloric	C16.3	C78.89	D00.2	D13.1	D37.1	D49.0
tympanicum	C30.1	C78.39	D02.3	D14.0	D38.5	D49.1
anus, anal	C21.0	C78.5	D01.3	D12.9	D37.8	D49.0
canal	C21.1	C78.5	D01.3	D12.9	D37.8	D49.0
cloacogenic zone	C21.2	C78.5	D01.3	D12.9	D37.8	D49.0
margin—*see also Neoplasm, anus, skin*	C44.500	C79.2	D04.5	D23.5	D48.5	D49.2
overlapping lesion with rectosigmoid junction or rectum	C21.8	—	—	—	—	—
skin	C44.500	C79.2	D04.5	D23.5	D48.5	D49.2
basal cell carcinoma	C44.510	—	—	—	—	—
specified type NEC	C44.590	—	—	—	—	—
squamous cell carcinoma	C44.520	—	—	—	—	—
sphincter	C21.1	C78.5	D01.3	D12.9	D37.8	D49.0
aorta (thoracic)	C49.3	C79.89	—	D21.3	D48.1	D49.2
abdominal	C49.4	C79.89	—	D21.4	D48.1	D49.2
aortic body	C75.5	C79.89	—	D35.6	D44.7	D49.7
aponeurosis	C49.9	C79.89	—	D21.9	D48.1	D49.2
palmar	C49.1-•	C79.89	—	D21.1-•	D48.1	D49.2
plantar	C49.2-•	C79.89	—	D21.2-•	D48.1	D49.2

TABLE OF NEOPLASMS

	Malignant Primary	Malignant Secondary	Ca in situ	Benign	Uncertain Behavior	Unspecified Behavior
appendix	C18.1	C78.5	DØ1.Ø	D12.1	D37.3	D49.Ø
arachnoid	C7Ø.9	C79.49	—	D32.9	D42.9	D49.7
cerebral	C7Ø.Ø	C79.32	—	D32.Ø	D42.Ø	D49.7
spinal	C7Ø.1	C79.49	—	D32.1	D42.1	D49.7
areola	C5Ø.Ø-●	C79.81	DØ5.-●	D24.-●	D48.6-●	D49.3
arm NEC	C76.4-●	C79.89	DØ4.6-●	D36.7	D48.7	D49.89
artery — *see Neoplasm, connective tissue*						
aryepiglottic fold	C13.1	C79.89	DØØ.Ø8	D1Ø.7	D37.Ø5	D49.Ø
hypopharyngeal aspect	C13.1	C79.89	DØØ.Ø8	D1Ø.7	D37.Ø5	D49.Ø
laryngeal aspect	C32.1	C78.39	DØ2.Ø	D14.1	D38.Ø	D49.1
marginal zone	C13.1	C79.89	DØØ.Ø8	D1Ø.7	D37.Ø5	D49.Ø
arytenoid (cartilage)	C32.3	C78.39	DØ2.Ø	D14.1	D38.Ø	D49.1
fold — *see Neoplasm, aryepiglottic*						
associated with transplanted organ	C8Ø.2	—	—	—	—	—
atlas	C41.2	C79.51	—	D16.6	D48.Ø	D49.2
atrium, cardiac	C38.Ø	C79.89	—	D15.1	D48.7	D49.89
auditory						
canal (external) (skin)	C44.2Ø-●	C79.2	DØ4.2-●	D23.2-●	D48.5	D49.2
internal	C3Ø.1	C78.39	DØ2.3	D14.Ø	D38.5	D49.1
nerve	C72.4-●	C79.49	—	D33.3	D43.3	D49.7
tube	C3Ø.1	C78.39	DØ2.3	D14.Ø	D38.5	D49.1
opening	C11.2	C79.89	DØØ.Ø8	D1Ø.6	D37.Ø5	D49.Ø
auricle, ear — *see also Neoplasm, skin, ear*	C44.2Ø-●	C79.2	DØ4.2-●	D23.2-●	D48.5	D49.2
auricular canal (external) — *see also Neoplasm, skin, ear*	C44.2Ø-●	C79.2	DØ4.2-●	D23.2-●	D48.5	D49.2
internal	C3Ø.1	C78.39	DØ2.3	D14.Ø	D38.5	D49.2
autonomic nerve or nervous system NEC *(see Neoplasm, nerve, peripheral)*						
axilla, axillary	C76.1	C79.89	DØ9.8	D36.7	D48.7	D49.89
fold — *see also Neoplasm, skin, trunk*	C44.5Ø9	C79.2	DØ4.5	D23.5	D48.5	D49.2
back NEC	C76.8	C79.89	DØ4.5	D36.7	D48.7	D49.89
Bartholin's gland	C51.Ø	C79.82	DØ7.1	D28.Ø	D39.8	D49.59
basal ganglia	C71.Ø	C79.31	—	D33.Ø	D43.Ø	D49.6
basis pedunculi	C71.7	C79.31	—	D33.1	D43.1	D49.6
bile or biliary (tract)	C24.9	C78.89	DØ1.5	D13.5	D37.6	D49.Ø
canaliculi (biliferi) (intrahepatic)	C22.1	C78.7	DØ1.5	D13.4	D37.6	D49.Ø
canals, interlobular	C22.1	C78.89	DØ1.5	D13.4	D37.6	D49.Ø
bile or biliary *(Continued)*						
duct or passage (common) (cystic) (extrahepatic)	C24.Ø	C78.89	DØ1.5	D13.5	D37.6	D49.Ø
interlobular	C22.1	C78.89	DØ1.5	D13.4	D37.6	D49.Ø
intrahepatic	C22.1	C78.7	DØ1.5	D13.4	D37.6	D49.Ø
and extrahepatic	C24.8	C78.89	DØ1.5	D13.5	D37.6	D49.Ø
bladder (urinary)	C67.9	C79.11	DØ9.Ø	D3Ø.3	D41.4	D49.4
dome	C67.1	C79.11	DØ9.Ø	D3Ø.3	D41.4	D49.4
neck	C67.5	C79.11	DØ9.Ø	D3Ø.3	D41.4	D49.4
orifice	C67.9	C79.11	DØ9.Ø	D3Ø.3	D41.4	D49.4
ureteric	C67.6	C79.11	DØ9.Ø	D3Ø.3	D41.4	D49.4
urethral	C67.5	C79.11	DØ9.Ø	D3Ø.3	D41.4	D49.4
overlapping lesion	C67.8	—	—	—	—	—
sphincter	C67.8	C79.11	DØ9.Ø	D3Ø.3	D41.4	D49.4
trigone	C67.Ø	C79.11	DØ9.Ø	D3Ø.3	D41.4	D49.4
urachus	C67.7	C79.11	DØ9.Ø	D3Ø.3	D41.4	D49.4
wall	C67.9	C79.11	DØ9.Ø	D3Ø.3	D41.4	D49.4
anterior	C67.3	C79.11	DØ9.Ø	D3Ø.3	D41.4	D49.4
lateral	C67.2	C79.11	DØ9.Ø	D3Ø.3	D41.4	D49.4
posterior	C67.4	C79.11	DØ9.Ø	D3Ø.3	D41.4	D49.4
blood vessel — *see Neoplasm, connective tissue*						
bone (periosteum)	C41.9	C79.51	—	D16.9-●	D48.Ø	D49.2
acetabulum	C41.4	C79.51	—	D16.8-●	D48.Ø	D49.2
ankle	C4Ø.3-●	C79.51	—	D16.3-●	—	—
arm NEC	C4Ø.Ø-●	C79.51	—	D16.Ø-●	—	—
astragalus	C4Ø.3-●	C79.51	—	D16.3-●	—	—
atlas	C41.2	C79.51	—	D16.6-●	D48.Ø	D49.2
axis	C41.2	C79.51	—	D16.6-●	D48.Ø	D49.2
back NEC	C41.2	C79.51	—	D16.6-●	D48.Ø	D49.2
calcaneus	C4Ø.3-●	C79.51	—	D16.3-●	—	—
calvarium	C41.Ø	C79.51	—	D16.4-●	D48.Ø	D49.2
carpus (any)	C4Ø.1-●	C79.51	—	D16.1-●	—	—
cartilage NEC	C41.9	C79.51	—	D16.9-●	D48.Ø	D49.2
clavicle	C41.3	C79.51	—	D16.7-●	D48.Ø	D49.2
clivus	C41.Ø	C79.51	—	D16.4-●	D48.Ø	D49.2
coccygeal vertebra	C41.4	C79.51	—	D16.8-●	D48.Ø	D49.2
coccyx	C41.4	C79.51	—	D16.8-●	D48.Ø	D49.2
costal cartilage	C41.3	C79.51	—	D16.7-●	D48.Ø	D49.2
costovertebral joint	C41.3	C79.51	—	D16.7-●	D48.Ø	D49.2
cranial	C41.Ø	C79.51	—	D16.4-●	D48.Ø	D49.2
cuboid	C4Ø.3-●	C79.51	—	D16.3-●	—	—
cuneiform	C41.9	C79.51	—	D16.9-●	D48.Ø	D49.2
elbow	C4Ø.Ø-●	C79.51	—	D16.Ø-●	—	—

TABLE OF NEOPLASMS

◀ New ◀ Revised ~~deleted~~ Deleted ● Use Additional Character(s)

	Malignant Primary	Malignant Secondary	Ca in situ	Benign	Uncertain Behavior	Unspecified Behavior
bone *(Continued)*						
ethmoid (labyrinth)	C41.0	C79.51	—	D16.4-	D48.0	D49.2
face	C41.0	C79.51	—	D16.4-	D48.0	D49.2
femur (any part)	C40.2-	C79.51	—	D16.2-	—	—
fibula (any part)	C40.2-	C79.51	—	D16.2-	—	—
finger (any)	C40.1-	C79.51	—	D16.1-	—	—
foot	C40.3-	C79.51	—	D16.3-	—	—
forearm	C40.0-	C79.51	—	D16.0-	—	—
frontal	C41.0	C79.51	—	D16.4-	D48.0	D49.2
hand	C40.1-	C79.51	—	D16.1-	—	—
heel	C40.3-	C79.51	—	D16.3-	—	—
hip	C41.4	C79.51	—	D16.8-	D48.0	D49.2
humerus (any part)	C40.0-	C79.51	—	D16.0-	—	—
hyoid	C41.0	C79.51	—	D16.4-	D48.0	D49.2
ilium	C41.4	C79.51	—	D16.8-	D48.0	D49.2
innominate	C41.4	C79.51	—	D16.8-	D48.0	D49.2
intervertebral cartilage or disc	C41.2	C79.51	—	D16.6-	D48.0	D49.2
ischium	C41.4	C79.51	—	D16.8-	D48.0	D49.2
jaw (lower)	C41.1	C79.51	—	D16.5-	D48.0	D49.2
knee	C40.2-	C79.51	—	D16.2-	—	—
leg NEC	C40.2-	C79.51	—	D16.2-	—	—
limb NEC	C40.9-	C79.51	—	D16.9-	—	—
lower (long bones)	C40.2-	C79.51	—	D16.2-	—	—
short bones	C40.3-	C79.51	—	D16.3-	—	—
upper (long bones)	C40.0-	C79.51	—	D16.0-	—	—
short bones	C40.1-	C79.51	—	D16.1-	—	—
malar	C41.0	C79.51	—	D16.4-	D48.0	D49.2
mandible	C41.1	C79.51	—	D16.5-	D48.0	D49.2
marrow NEC (any bone)	C96.9	C79.52	—	—	D47.9	D49.89
mastoid	C41.0	C79.51	—	D16.4-	D48.0	D49.2
maxilla, maxillary (superior)	C41.0	C79.51	—	D16.4-	D48.0	D49.2
inferior	C41.1	C79.51	—	D16.5-	D48.0	D49.2
metacarpus (any)	C40.1-	C79.51	—	D16.1-	—	—
metatarsus (any)	C40.3-	C79.51	—	D16.3-	—	—
overlapping sites	C40.8-	—	—	—	—	—
navicular						
ankle	C40.3-	C79.51	—	—	—	—
hand	C40.1-	C79.51	—	—	—	—
nose, nasal	C41.0	C79.51	—	D16.4-	D48.0	D49.2
occipital	C41.0	C79.51	—	D16.4-	D48.0	D49.2
orbit	C41.0	C79.51	—	D16.4-	D48.0	D49.2
parietal	C41.0	C79.51	—	D16.4-	D48.0	D49.2
patella	C40.2-	C79.51	—	—	—	—
pelvic	C41.4	C79.51	—	D16.8	D48.0	D49.2
bone *(Continued)*						
phalanges						
foot	C40.3-	C79.51	—	—	—	—
hand	C40.1-	C79.51	—	—	—	—
pubic	C41.4	C79.51	—	D16.8	D48.0	D49.2
radius (any part)	C40.0-	C79.51	—	D16.0-	—	—
rib	C41.3	C79.51	—	D16.7	D48.0	D49.2
sacral vertebra	C41.4	C79.51	—	D16.8	D48.0	D49.2
sacrum	C41.4	C79.51	—	D16.8	D48.0	D49.2
scaphoid	—	—	—		—	—
of ankle	C40.3-	C79.51	—	—	—	—
of hand	C40.1-	C79.51	—	—	—	—
scapula (any part)	C40.0-	C79.51	—	D16.0-	—	—
sella turcica	C41.0	C79.51	—	D16.4-	D48.0	D49.2
shoulder	C40.0-	C79.51	—	D16.0-	—	—
skull	C41.0	C79.51	—	D16.4-	D48.0	D49.2
sphenoid	C41.0	C79.51	—	D16.4-	D48.0	D49.2
spine, spinal (column)	C41.2	C79.51	—	D16.6	D48.0	D49.2
coccyx	C41.4	C79.51	—	D16.8	D48.0	D49.2
sacrum	C41.4	C79.51	—	D16.8	D48.0	D49.2
sternum	C41.3	C79.51	—	D16.7	D48.0	D49.2
tarsus (any)	C40.3-	C79.51	—	—	—	—
temporal	C41.0	C79.51	—	D16.4-	D48.0	D49.2
thumb	C40.1-	C79.51	—	—	—	—
tibia (any part)	C40.2-	C79.51	—	—	—	—
toe (any)	C40.3-	C79.51	—	—	—	—
trapezium	C40.1-	C79.51	—	—	—	—
trapezoid	C40.1-	C79.51	—	—	—	—
turbinate	C41.0	C79.51	—	D16.4-	D48.0	D49.2
ulna (any part)	C40.0-	C79.51	—	D16.0-	—	—
unciform	C40.1-	C79.51	—	—	—	—
vertebra (column)	C41.2	C79.51	—	D16.6	D48.0	D49.2
coccyx	C41.4	C79.51	—	D16.8	D48.0	D49.2
sacrum	C41.4	C79.51	—	D16.8	D48.0	D49.2
vomer	C41.0	C79.51	—	D16.4-	D48.0	D49.2
wrist	C40.1-	C79.51	—	—	—	—
xiphoid process	C41.3	C79.51	—	D16.7	D48.0	D49.2
zygomatic	C41.0	C79.51	—	D16.4-	D48.0	D49.2
book-leaf (mouth)	C06.89	C79.89	D00.00	D10.39	D37.09	D49.0
bowel—*see Neoplasm, intestine*						
brachial plexus	C47.1-	C79.89	—	D36.12	D48.2	D49.2
brain NEC	C71.9	C79.31	—	D33.2	D43.2	D49.6
basal ganglia	C71.0	C79.31	—	D33.0	D43.0	D49.6
cerebellopontine angle	C71.6	C79.31	—	D33.1	D43.1	D49.6

TABLE OF NEOPLASMS

	Malignant Primary	Malignant Secondary	Ca in situ	Benign	Uncertain Behavior	Unspecified Behavior
brain NEC *(Continued)*						
cerebellum NOS	C71.6	C79.31	—	D33.1	D43.1	D49.6
cerebrum	C71.Ø	C79.31	—	D33.Ø	D43.Ø	D49.6
choroid plexus	C71.7	C79.31	—	D33.1	D43.1	D49.6
corpus callosum	C71.8	C79.31	—	D33.2	D43.2	D49.6
corpus striatum	C71.Ø	C79.31	—	D33.Ø	D43.Ø	D49.6
cortex (cerebral)	C71.Ø	C79.31	—	D33.Ø	D43.Ø	D49.6
frontal lobe	C71.1	C79.31	—	D33.Ø	D43.Ø	D49.6
globus pallidus	C71.Ø	C79.31	—	D33.Ø	D43.Ø	D49.6
hippocampus	C71.2	C79.31	—	D33.Ø	D43.Ø	D49.6
hypothalamus	C71.Ø	C79.31	—	D33.Ø	D43.Ø	D49.6
internal capsule	C71.Ø	C79.31	—	D33.Ø	D43.Ø	D49.6
medulla oblongata	C71.7	C79.31	—	D33.1	D43.1	D49.6
meninges	C7Ø.Ø	C79.32	—	D32.Ø	D42.Ø	D49.7
midbrain	C71.7	C79.31	—	D33.1	D43.1	D49.6
occipital lobe	C71.4	C79.31	—	D33.Ø	D43.Ø	D49.6
overlapping lesion	C71.8	C79.31	—	—	—	—
parietal lobe	C71.3	C79.31	—	D33.Ø	D43.Ø	D49.6
peduncle	C71.7	C79.31	—	D33.1	D43.1	D49.6
pons	C71.7	C79.31	—	D33.1	D43.1	D49.6
stem	C71.7	C79.31	—	D33.1	D43.1	D49.6
tapetum	C71.8	C79.31	—	D33.2	D43.2	D49.6
temporal lobe	C71.2	C79.31	—	D33.Ø	D43.Ø	D49.6
thalamus	C71.Ø	C79.31	—	D33.Ø	D43.Ø	D49.6
uncus	C71.2	C79.31	—	D33.Ø	D43.Ø	D49.6
ventricle (floor)	C71.5	C79.31	—	D33.Ø	D43.Ø	D49.6
fourth	C71.7	C79.31	—	D33.1	D43.1	D49.6
branchial (cleft) (cyst) (vestiges)	C1Ø.4	C79.89	DØØ.Ø8	D1Ø.5	D37.Ø5	D49.Ø
breast (connective tissue) (glandular tissue) (soft parts)	C5Ø.9-●	C79.81	DØ5.-●	D24.-●	D48.6-●	D49.3
areola	C5Ø.Ø-●	C79.81	DØ5.-●	D24.-●	D48.6-●	D49.3
axillary tail	C5Ø.6-●	C79.81	DØ5.-●	D24.-●	D48.6-●	D49.3
central portion	C5Ø.1-●	C79.81	DØ5.-●	D24.-●	D48.6-●	D49.3
inner	C5Ø.8-●	C79.81	DØ5.-●	D24.-●	D48.6-●	D49.3
lower	C5Ø.8-●	C79.81	DØ5.-●	D24.-●	D48.6-●	D49.3
lower-inner quadrant	C5Ø.3-●	C79.81	DØ5.-●	D24.-●	D48.6-●	D49.3
lower-outer quadrant	C5Ø.5-●	C79.81	DØ5.-●	D24.-●	D48.6-●	D49.3
mastectomy site (skin)—*see also Neoplasm, breast, skin*	C44.5Ø1	C79.2	—	—	—	—
specified as breast tissue	C5Ø.8-●	C79.81	—	—	—	—
midline	C5Ø.8-●	C79.81	DØ5.-●	D24.-●	D48.6-●	D49.3
nipple	C5Ø.Ø-●	C79.81	DØ5.-●	D24.-●	D48.6-●	D49.3
outer	C5Ø.8-●	C79.81	DØ5.-●	D24.-●	D48.6-●	D49.3
overlapping lesion	C5Ø.8-●	—	—	—	—	—

	Malignant Primary	Malignant Secondary	Ca in situ	Benign	Uncertain Behavior	Unspecified Behavior
breast *(Continued)*						
skin	C44.5Ø1	C79.2	DØ4.5	D23.5	D48.5	D49.2
basal cell carcinoma	C44.511	—	—	—	—	—
specified type NEC	C44.591	—	—	—	—	—
squamous cell carcinoma	C44.521	—	—	—	—	—
tail (axillary)	C5Ø.6-●	C79.81	DØ5.-●	D24.-●	D48.6-●	D49.3
upper	C5Ø.8-●	C79.81	DØ5.-●	D24.-●	D48.6-●	D49.3
upper-inner quadrant	C5Ø.2-●	C79.81	DØ5.-●	D24.-●	D48.6-●	D49.3
upper-outer quadrant	C5Ø.4-●	C79.81	DØ5.-●	D24.-●	D48.6-●	D49.3
broad ligament	C57.1	C79.82	DØ7.39	D28.2	D39.8	D49.59
bronchiogenic, bronchogenic (lung)	C34.9-●	C78.Ø-●	DØ2.2-●	D14.3-●	D38.1	D49.1
bronchiole	C34.9-●	C78.Ø-●	DØ2.2-●	D14.3-●	D38.1	D49.1
bronchus	C34.9-●	C78.Ø-●	DØ2.2-●	D14.3-●	D38.1	D49.1
carina	C34.Ø-●	C78.Ø-●	DØ2.2-●	D14.3-●	D38.1	D49.1
lower lobe of lung	C34.3-●	C78.Ø-●	DØ2.2-●	D14.3-●	D38.1	D49.1
main	C34.Ø-●	C78.Ø-●	DØ2.2-●	D14.3-●	D38.1	D49.1
middle lobe of lung	C34.2	C78.Ø-●	DØ2.21	D14.31	D38.1	D49.1
overlapping lesion	C34.8-●	—	—	—	—	—
upper lobe of lung	C34.1-●	C78.Ø-●	DØ2.2-●	D14.3-●	D38.1	D49.1
brow	C44.3Ø9	C79.2	DØ4.39	D23.39	D48.5	D49.2
basal cell carcinoma	C44.319	—	—	—	—	—
specified type NEC	C44.399	—	—	—	—	—
squamous cell carcinoma	C44.329	—	—	—	—	—
buccal (cavity)	CØ6.9	C79.89	DØØ.ØØ	D1Ø.39	D37.Ø9	D49.Ø
commissure	CØ6.Ø	C79.89	DØØ.Ø2	D1Ø.39	D37.Ø9	D49.Ø
groove (lower) (upper)	CØ6.1	C79.89	DØØ.Ø2	D1Ø.39	D37.Ø9	D49.Ø
mucosa	CØ6.Ø	C79.89	DØØ.Ø2	D1Ø.39	D37.Ø9	D49.Ø
sulcus (lower) (upper)	CØ6.1	C79.89	DØØ.Ø2	D1Ø.39	D37.Ø9	D49.Ø
bulbourethral gland	C68.Ø	C79.19	DØ9.19	D3Ø.4	D41.3	D49.59
bursa—*see Neoplasm, connective tissue*						
buttock NEC	C76.3	C79.89	DØ4.5	D36.7	D48.7	D49.89
calf	C76.5-●	C79.89	DØ4.7-●	D36.7	D48.7	D49.89
calvarium	C41.Ø	C79.51	—	D16.4-●	D48.Ø	D49.2
calyx, renal	C65.-●	C79.Ø-●	DØ9.19	D3Ø.1-●	D41.1-●	D49.51-●
canal						
anal	C21.1	C78.5	DØ1.3	D12.9	D37.8	D49.Ø
auditory (external)—*see also Neoplasm, skin, ear*	C44.2Ø-●	C79.2	DØ4.2-●	D23.2-●	D48.5	D49.2
auricular (external)—*see also Neoplasm, skin, ear*	C44.2Ø-●	C79.2	DØ4.2-●	D23.2-●	D48.5	D49.2
canaliculi, biliary (biliferi) (intrahepatic)	C22.1	C78.7	DØ1.5	D13.4	D37.6	D49.Ø

◀ New ▮ Revised ~~deleted~~ Deleted ● Use Additional Character(s)

	Malignant Primary	Malignant Secondary	Ca in situ	Benign	Uncertain Behavior	Unspecified Behavior
canthus (eye) (inner) (outer)	C44.1Ø-●	C79.2	DØ4.1-●	D23.1-●	D48.5	D49.2
basal cell carcinoma	C44.11-●	—	—	—	—	—
sebaceous cell	C44.13-●	—	—	—	—	—
specified type NEC	C44.19-●	—	—	—	—	—
squamous cell carcinoma	C44.12-●	—	—	—	—	—
capillary — *see Neoplasm, connective tissue*						
caput coli	C18.Ø	C78.5	DØ1.Ø	D12.Ø	D37.4	D49.Ø
carcinoid — *see Tumor, carcinoid*						
cardia (gastric)	C16.Ø	C78.89	DØØ.2	D13.1	D37.1	D49.Ø
cardiac orifice (stomach)	C16.Ø	C78.89	DØØ.2	D13.1	D37.1	D49.Ø
cardio-esophageal junction	C16.Ø	C78.89	DØØ.2	D13.1	D37.1	D49.Ø
cardio-esophagus	C16.Ø	C78.89	DØØ.2	D13.1	D37.1	D49.Ø
carina (bronchus)	C34.Ø-●	C78.Ø-●	DØ2.2-●	D14.3-●	D38.1	D49.1
carotid (artery)	C49.Ø	C79.89	—	D21.Ø	D48.1	D49.2
body	C75.4	C79.89	—	D35.5	D44.6	D49.7
carpus (any bone)	C4Ø.1-●	C79.51	—	D16.1-●	—	—
cartilage (articular) (joint) NEC — *see also Neoplasm, bone*	C41.9	C79.51	—	D16.9-●	D48.Ø	D49.2
arytenoid	C32.3	C78.39	DØ2.Ø	D14.1	D38.Ø	D49.1
auricular	C49.Ø	C79.89	—	D21.Ø	D48.1	D49.2
bronchi	C34.Ø-●	C78.39	—	D14.3-●	D38.1	D49.1
costal	C41.3	C79.51	—	D16.7	D48.Ø	D49.2
cricoid	C32.3	C78.39	DØ2.Ø	D14.1	D38.Ø	D49.1
cuneiform	C32.3	C78.39	DØ2.Ø	D14.1	D38.Ø	D49.1
ear (external)	C49.Ø	C79.89	—	D21.Ø	D48.1	D49.2
ensiform	C41.3	C79.51	—	D16.7	D48.Ø	D49.2
epiglottis	C32.1	C78.39	DØ2.Ø	D14.1	D38.Ø	D49.1
anterior surface	C1Ø.1	C79.89	DØØ.Ø8	D1Ø.5	D37.Ø5	D49.Ø
eyelid	C49.Ø	C79.89	—	D21.Ø	D48.1	D49.2
intervertebral	C41.2	C79.51	—	D16.6	D48.Ø	D49.2
larynx, laryngeal	C32.3	C78.39	DØ2.Ø	D14.1	D38.Ø	D49.1
nose, nasal	C3Ø.Ø	C78.39	DØ2.3	D14.Ø	D38.5	D49.1
pinna	C49.Ø	C79.89	—	D21.Ø	D48.1	D49.2
rib	C41.3	C79.51	—	D16.7	D48.Ø	D49.2
semilunar (knee)	C4Ø.2-●	C79.51	—	D16.2-●	D48.Ø	D49.2
thyroid	C32.3	C78.39	DØ2.Ø	D14.1	D38.Ø	D49.1
trachea	C33	C78.39	DØ2.1	D14.2	D38.1	D49.1
cauda equina	C72.1	C79.49	—	D33.4	D43.4	D49.7
cavity						
buccal	CØ6.9	C79.89	DØØ.ØØ	D1Ø.3Ø	D37.Ø9	D49.Ø
nasal	C3Ø.Ø	C78.39	DØ2.3	D14.Ø	D38.5	D49.1
oral	CØ6.9	C79.89	DØØ.ØØ	D1Ø.3Ø	D37.Ø9	D49.Ø

	Malignant Primary	Malignant Secondary	Ca in situ	Benign	Uncertain Behavior	Unspecified Behavior
cavity *(Continued)*						
peritoneal	C48.2	C78.6	—	D2Ø.1	D48.4	D49.Ø
tympanic	C3Ø.1	C78.39	DØ2.3	D14.Ø	D38.5	D49.1
cecum	C18.Ø	C78.5	DØ1.Ø	D12.Ø	D37.4	D49.Ø
central nervous system	C72.9	C79.4Ø	—	—	—	—
cerebellopontine (angle)	C71.6	C79.31	—	D33.1	D43.1	D49.6
cerebellum, cerebellar	C71.6	C79.31	—	D33.1	D43.1	D49.6
cerebrum, cerebra (cortex) (hemisphere) (white matter)	C71.Ø	C79.31	—	D33.Ø	D43.Ø	D49.6
meninges	C7Ø.Ø	C79.32	—	D32.Ø	D42.Ø	D49.7
peduncle	C71.7	C79.31	—	D33.1	D43.1	D49.6
ventricle	C71.5	C79.31	—	D33.Ø	D43.Ø	D49.6
fourth	C71.7	C79.31	—	D33.1	D43.1	D49.6
cervical region	C76.Ø	C79.89	DØ9.8	D36.7	D48.7	D49.89
cervix (cervical) (uteri) (uterus)	C53.9	C79.82	DØ6.9	D26.Ø	D39.Ø	D49.59
canal	C53.Ø	C79.82	DØ6.Ø	D26.Ø	D39.Ø	D49.59
endocervix (canal) (gland)	C53.Ø	C79.82	DØ6.Ø	D26.Ø	D39.Ø	D49.59
exocervix	C53.1	C79.82	DØ6.1	D26.Ø	D39.Ø	D49.59
external os	C53.1	C79.82	DØ6.1	D26.Ø	D39.Ø	D49.59
internal os	C53.Ø	C79.82	DØ6.Ø	D26.Ø	D39.Ø	D49.59
nabothian gland	C53.Ø	C79.82	DØ6.Ø	D26.Ø	D39.Ø	D49.59
overlapping lesion	C53.8	—	—	—	—	—
squamocolumnar junction	C53.8	C79.82	DØ6.7	D26.Ø	D39.Ø	D49.59
stump	C53.8	C79.82	DØ6.7	D26.Ø	D39.Ø	D49.59
cheek	C76.Ø	C79.89	DØ9.8	D36.7	D48.7	D49.89
external	C44.3Ø9	C79.2	DØ4.39	D23.39	D48.5	D49.2
basal cell carcinoma	C44.319	—	—	—	—	—
specified type NEC	C44.399	—	—	—	—	—
squamous cell carcinoma	C44.329	—	—	—	—	—
inner aspect	CØ6.Ø	C79.89	DØØ.Ø2	D1Ø.39	D37.Ø9	D49.Ø
internal	CØ6.Ø	C79.89	DØØ.Ø2	D1Ø.39	D37.Ø9	D49.Ø
mucosa	CØ6.Ø	C79.89	DØØ.Ø2	D1Ø.39	D37.Ø9	D49.Ø
chest (wall) NEC	C76.1	C79.89	DØ9.8	D36.7	D48.7	D49.89
chiasma opticum	C72.3-●	C79.49	—	D33.3	D43.3	D49.7
chin	C44.3Ø9	C79.2	DØ4.39	D23.39	D48.5	D49.2
basal cell carcinoma	C44.319	—	—	—	—	—
specified type NEC	C44.399	—	—	—	—	—
squamous cell carcinoma	C44.329	—	—	—	—	—
choana	C11.3	C79.89	DØØ.Ø8	D1Ø.6	D37.Ø5	D49.Ø
cholangiole	C22.1	C78.89	DØ1.5	D13.4	D37.6	D49.Ø
choledochal duct	C24.Ø	C78.89	DØ1.5	D13.5	D37.6	D49.Ø
choroid	C69.3-●	C79.49	DØ9.2-●	D31.3-●	D48.7	D49.81
plexus	C71.5	C79.31	—	D33.Ø	D43.Ø	D49.6
ciliary body	C69.4-●	C79.49	DØ9.2-●	D31.4-●	D48.7	D49.89

	Malignant Primary	Malignant Secondary	Ca in situ	Benign	Uncertain Behavior	Unspecified Behavior
clavicle	C41.3	C79.51	—	D16.7	D48.0	D49.2
clitoris	C51.2	C79.82	D07.1	D28.0	D39.8	D49.59
clivus	C41.0	C79.51	—	D16.4-●	D48.0	D49.2
cloacogenic zone	C21.2	C78.5	D01.3	D12.9	D37.8	D49.0
coccygeal						
body or glomus	C49.5	C79.89	—	D21.5	D48.1	D49.2
vertebra	C41.4	C79.51	—	D16.8	D48.0	D49.2
coccyx	C41.4	C79.51	—	D16.8	D48.0	D49.2
colon — *see also Neoplasm, intestine, large*	C18.9	C78.5	—	—	—	—
with rectum	C19	C78.5	D01.1	D12.7	D37.5	D49.0
column, spinal — *see Neoplasm, spine*						
columnella — *see also Neoplasm, skin, face*	C44.390	C79.2	D04.39	D23.39	D48.5	D49.2
commissure						
labial, lip	C00.6	C79.89	D00.01	D10.39	D37.01	D49.0
laryngeal	C32.0	C78.39	D02.0	D14.1	D38.0	D49.1
common (bile) duct	C24.0	C78.89	D01.5	D13.5	D37.6	D49.0
concha — *see also Neoplasm, skin, ear*	C44.20-●	C79.2	D04.2-●	D23.2-●	D48.5	D49.2
nose	C30.0	C78.39	D02.3	D14.0	D38.5	D49.1
conjunctiva	C69.0-●	C79.49	D09.2-●	D31.0-●	D48.7	D49.89
connective tissue NEC	C49.9	C79.89	—	D21.9	D48.1	D49.2

Note: For neoplasms of connective tissue (blood vessel, bursa, fascia, ligament, muscle, peripheral nerves, sympathetic and parasympathetic nerves and ganglia, synovia, tendon, etc.) or of morphological types that indicate connective tissue, code according to the list under "Neoplasm, connective tissue." For sites that do not appear in this list, code to neoplasm of that site; e.g., fibrosarcoma, pancreas (C25.9)

Note: Morphological types that indicate connective tissue appear in their proper place in the alphabetic index with the instruction "*see Neoplasm, connective tissue ....*"

	Malignant Primary	Malignant Secondary	Ca in situ	Benign	Uncertain Behavior	Unspecified Behavior
connective tissue NEC *(Continued)*						
abdomen	C49.4	C79.89	—	D21.4	D48.1	D49.2
abdominal wall	C49.4	C79.89	—	D21.4	D48.1	D49.2
ankle	C49.2-●	C79.89	—	D21.2-●	D48.1	D49.2
antecubital fossa or space	C49.1-●	C79.89	—	D21.1-●	D48.1	D49.2
arm	C49.1-●	C79.89	—	D21.1-●	D48.1	D49.2
auricle (ear)	C49.0	C79.89	—	D21.0	D48.1	D49.2
axilla	C49.3	C79.89	—	D21.3	D48.1	D49.2
back	C49.6	C79.89	—	D21.6	D48.1	D49.2
breast — *see Neoplasm, breast*						
buttock	C49.5	C79.89	—	D21.5	D48.1	D49.2
calf	C49.2-●	C79.89	—	D21.2-●	D48.1	D49.2
cervical region	C49.0	C79.89	—	D21.0	D48.1	D49.2
cheek	C49.0	C79.89	—	D21.0	D48.1	D49.2
chest (wall)	C49.3	C79.89	—	D21.3	D48.1	D49.2
chin	C49.0	C79.89	—	D21.0	D48.1	D49.2
diaphragm	C49.3	C79.89	—	D21.3	D48.1	D49.2
ear (external)	C49.0	C79.89	—	D21.0	D48.1	D49.2
elbow	C49.1-●	C79.89	—	D21.1-●	D48.1	D49.2
extrarectal	C49.5	C79.89	—	D21.5	D48.1	D49.2
extremity	C49.9	C79.89	—	D21.9	D48.1	D49.2
lower	C49.2-●	C79.89	—	D21.2-●	D48.1	D49.2
upper	C49.1-●	C79.89	—	D21.1-●	D48.1	D49.2
eyelid	C49.0	C79.89	—	D21.0	D48.1	D49.2
face	C49.0	C79.89	—	D21.0	D48.1	D49.2
finger	C49.1-●	C79.89	—	D21.1-●	D48.1	D49.2
flank	C49.6	C79.89	—	D21.6	D48.1	D49.2
foot	C49.2-●	C79.89	—	D21.2-●	D48.1	D49.2
forearm	C49.1-●	C79.89	—	D21.1-●	D48.1	D49.2
forehead	C49.0	C79.89	—	D21.0	D48.1	D49.2
gastric	C49.4	C79.89	—	D21.4	D48.1	D49.2
gastrointestinal	C49.4	C79.89	—	D21.4	D48.1	D49.2
gluteal region	C49.5	C79.89	—	D21.5	D48.1	D49.2
great vessels NEC	C49.3	C79.89	—	D21.3	D48.1	D49.2
groin	C49.5	C79.89	—	D21.5	D48.1	D49.2
hand	C49.1-●	C79.89	—	D21.1-●	D48.1	D49.2
head	C49.0	C79.89	—	D21.0	D48.1	D49.2
heel	C49.2-●	C79.89	—	D21.2-●	D48.1	D49.2
hip	C49.2-●	C79.89	—	D21.2-●	D48.1	D49.2
hypochondrium	C49.4	C79.89	—	D21.4	D48.1	D49.2
iliopsoas muscle	C49.5	C79.89	—	D21.5	D48.1	D49.2
infraclavicular region	C49.3	C79.89	—	D21.3	D48.1	D49.2
inguinal (canal) (region)	C49.5	C79.89	—	D21.5	D48.1	D49.2
intestinal	C49.4	C79.89	—	D21.4	D48.1	D49.2
intrathoracic	C49.3	C79.89	—	D21.3	D48.1	D49.2
ischiorectal fossa	C49.5	C79.89	—	D21.5	D48.1	D49.2
jaw	C03.9	C79.89	D00.03	D10.39	D48.1	D49.0
knee	C49.2-●	C79.89	—	D21.2-●	D48.1	D49.2
leg	C49.2-●	C79.89	—	D21.2-●	D48.1	D49.2
limb NEC	C49.9	C79.89	—	D21.9	D48.1	D49.2
lower	C49.2-●	C79.89	—	D21.2-●	D48.1	D49.2
upper	C49.1-●	C79.89	—	D21.1-●	D48.1	D49.2
nates	C49.5	C79.89	—	D21.5	D48.1	D49.2
neck	C49.0	C79.89	—	D21.0	D48.1	D49.2
orbit	C69.6-●	C79.49	D09.2-●	D31.6-●	D48.1	D49.89
overlapping lesion	C49.8	—	—	—	—	—

TABLE OF NEOPLASMS

◄ New ◄ Revised ~~deleted~~ Deleted ● Use Additional Character(s)

	Malignant Primary	Malignant Secondary	Ca in situ	Benign	Uncertain Behavior	Unspecified Behavior
connective tissue NEC *(Continued)*						
pararectal	C49.5	C79.89	—	D21.5	D48.1	D49.2
para-urethral	C49.5	C79.89	—	D21.5	D48.1	D49.2
paravaginal	C49.5	C79.89	—	D21.5	D48.1	D49.2
pelvis (floor)	C49.5	C79.89	—	D21.5	D48.1	D49.2
pelvo-abdominal	C49.8	C79.89	—	D21.6	D48.1	D49.2
perineum	C49.5	C79.89	—	D21.5	D48.1	D49.2
perirectal (tissue)	C49.5	C79.89	—	D21.5	D48.1	D49.2
periurethral (tissue)	C49.5	C79.89	—	D21.5	D48.1	D49.2
popliteal fossa or space	C49.2-●	C79.89	—	D21.2-●	D48.1	D49.2
presacral	C49.5	C79.89	—	D21.5	D48.1	D49.2
psoas muscle	C49.4	C79.89	—	D21.4	D48.1	D49.2
pterygoid fossa	C49.Ø	C79.89	—	D21.Ø	D48.1	D49.2
rectovaginal septum or wall	C49.5	C79.89	—	D21.5	D48.1	D49.2
rectovesical	C49.5	C79.89	—	D21.5	D48.1	D49.2
retroperitoneum	C48.Ø	C78.6	—	D2Ø.Ø	D48.3	D49.Ø
sacrococcygeal region	C49.5	C79.89	—	D21.5	D48.1	D49.2
scalp	C49.Ø	C79.89	—	D21.Ø	D48.1	D49.2
scapular region	C49.3	C79.89	—	D21.3	D48.1	D49.2
shoulder	C49.1-●	C79.89	—	D21.1-●	D48.1	D49.2
skin (dermis) NEC—*see also Neoplasm, skin, by site*	C44.9Ø	C79.2	DØ4.9	D23.9	D48.5	D49.2
stomach	C49.4	C79.89	—	D21.4	D48.1	D49.2
submental	C49.Ø	C79.89	—	D21.Ø	D48.1	D49.2
supraclavicular region	C49.Ø	C79.89	—	D21.Ø	D48.1	D49.2
temple	C49.Ø	C79.89	—	D21.Ø	D48.1	D49.2
temporal region	C49.Ø	C79.89	—	D21.Ø	D48.1	D49.2
thigh	C49.2-●	C79.89	—	D21.2-●	D48.1	D49.2
thoracic (duct) (wall)	C49.3	C79.89	—	D21.3	D48.1	D49.2
thorax	C49.3	C79.89	—	D21.3	D48.1	D49.2
thumb	C49.1-●	C79.89	—	D21.1-●	D48.1	D49.2
toe	C49.2-●	C79.89	—	D21.2-●	D48.1	D49.2
trunk	C49.6	C79.89	—	D21.6	D48.1	D49.2
umbilicus	C49.4	C79.89	—	D21.4	D48.1	D49.2
vesicorectal	C49.5	C79.89	—	D21.5	D48.1	D49.2
wrist	C49.1-●	C79.89	—	D21.1-●	D48.1	D49.2
conus medullaris	C72.Ø	C79.49	—	D33.4	D43.4	D49.7
cord (true) (vocal)	C32.Ø	C78.39	DØ2.Ø	D14.1	D38.Ø	D49.1
false	C32.1	C78.39	DØ2.Ø	D14.1	D38.Ø	D49.1
spermatic	C63.1-●	C79.82	DØ7.69	D29.8	D4Ø.8	D49.59
spinal (cervical) (lumbar) (thoracic)	C72.Ø	C79.49	—	D33.4	D43.4	D49.7
cornea (limbus)	C69.1-●	C79.49	DØ9.2-●	D31.1-●	D48.7	D49.89
corpus						

	Malignant Primary	Malignant Secondary	Ca in situ	Benign	Uncertain Behavior	Unspecified Behavior
corpus *(Continued)*						
albicans	C56.-●	C79.6-●	DØ7.39	D27.-●	D39.1-●	D49.59
callosum, brain	C71.Ø	C79.31	—	D33.2	D43.2	D49.6
cavernosum	C6Ø.2	C79.82	DØ7.4	D29.Ø	D4Ø.8	D49.59
gastric	C16.2	C78.89	DØØ.2	D13.1	D37.1	D49.Ø
overlapping sites	C54.8	—	—	—	—	—
penis	C6Ø.2	C79.82	DØ7.4	D29.Ø	D4Ø.8	D49.59
striatum, cerebrum	C71.Ø	C79.31	—	D33.Ø	D43.Ø	D49.6
uteri	C54.9	C79.82	DØ7.Ø	D26.1	D39.Ø	D49.59
isthmus	C54.Ø	C79.82	DØ7.Ø	D26.1	D39.Ø	D49.59
cortex						
adrenal	C74.Ø-●	C79.7-●	DØ9.3	D35.Ø-●	D44.1-●	D49.7
cerebral	C71.Ø	C79.31	—	D33.Ø	D43.Ø	D49.6
costal cartilage	C41.3	C79.51	—	D16.7	D48.Ø	D49.2
costovertebral joint	C41.3	C79.51	—	D16.7	D48.Ø	D49.2
Cowper's gland	C68.Ø	C79.19	DØ9.19	D3Ø.4	D41.3	D49.59
cranial (fossa, any)	C71.9	C79.31	—	D33.2	D43.2	D49.6
meninges	C7Ø.Ø	C79.32	—	D32.Ø	D42.Ø	D49.7
nerve	C72.5Ø	C79.49	—	D33.3	D43.3	D49.7
specified NEC	C72.59	C79.49	—	D33.3	D43.3	D49.7
craniobuccal pouch	C75.2	C79.89	DØ9.3	D35.2	D44.3	D49.7
craniopharyngeal (duct) (pouch)	C75.2	C79.89	DØ9.3	D35.3	D44.4	D49.7
cricoid	C13.Ø	C79.89	DØØ.Ø8	D1Ø.7	D37.Ø5	D49.Ø
cartilage	C32.3	C78.39	DØ2.Ø	D14.1	D38.Ø	D49.1
cricopharynx	C13.Ø	C79.89	DØØ.Ø8	D1Ø.7	D37.Ø5	D49.Ø
crypt of Morgagni	C21.8	C78.5	DØ1.3	D12.9	D37.8	D49.Ø
crystalline lens	C69.4-●	C79.49	DØ9.2-●	D31.4-●	D48.7	D49.89
cul-de-sac (Douglas')	C48.1	C78.6	—	D2Ø.1	D48.4	D49.Ø
cuneiform cartilage	C32.3	C78.39	DØ2.Ø	D14.1	D38.Ø	D49.1
cutaneous—*see Neoplasm, skin*						
cutis—*see Neoplasm, skin*						
cystic (bile) duct (common)	C24.Ø	C78.89	DØ1.5	D13.5	D37.6	D49.Ø
dermis—*see Neoplasm, skin*						
diaphragm	C49.3	C79.89	—	D21.3	D48.1	D49.2
digestive organs, system, tube, or tract NEC	C26.9	C78.89	DØ1.9	D13.99	D37.9	D49.Ø
disc, intervertebral	C41.2	C79.51	—	D16.6	D48.Ø	D49.2
disease, generalized	C8Ø.Ø	—	—	—	—	—
disseminated	C8Ø.Ø	—	—	—	—	—
Douglas' cul-de-sac or pouch	C48.1	C78.6	—	D2Ø.1	D48.4	D49.Ø
duodenojejunal junction	C17.8	C78.4	DØ1.49	D13.39	D37.2	D49.Ø
duodenum	C17.Ø	C78.4	DØ1.49	D13.2	D37.2	D49.Ø

TABLE OF NEOPLASMS

	Malignant Primary	Malignant Secondary	Ca in situ	Benign	Uncertain Behavior	Unspecified Behavior
dura (cranial) (mater)	C70.9	C79.49	—	D32.9	D42.9	D49.7
cerebral	C70.0	C79.32	—	D32.0	D42.0	D49.7
spinal	C70.1	C79.49	—	D32.1	D42.1	D49.7
ear (external) — *see also Neoplasm, skin, ear*	C44.20•	C79.2	D04.2•	D23.2•	D48.5	D49.2
auricle or auris — *see also Neoplasm, skin, ear*	C44.20•	C79.2	D04.2•	D23.2•	D48.5	D49.2
canal, external — *see also Neoplasm, skin, ear*	C44.20•	C79.2	D04.2•	D23.2•	D48.5	D49.2
cartilage	C49.0	C79.89	—	D21.0	D48.1	D49.2
external meatus — *see also Neoplasm, skin, ear*	C44.20•	C79.2	D04.2•	D23.2•	D48.5	D49.2
inner	C30.1	C78.39	D02.3	D14.0	D38.5	D49.1
lobule — *see also Neoplasm, skin, ear*	C44.20•	C79.2	D04.2•	D23.2•	D48.5	D49.2
middle	C30.1	C78.39	D02.3	D14.0	D38.5	D49.1
overlapping lesion with accessory sinuses	C31.8	—	—	—	—	—
skin	C44.20•	C79.2	D04.2•	D23.2•	D48.5	D49.2
basal cell carcinoma	C44.21•	—	—	—	—	—
specified type NEC	C44.29•	—	—	—	—	—
squamous cell carcinoma	C44.22•	—	—	—	—	—
earlobe	C44.20•	C79.2	D04.2•	D23.2•	D48.5	D49.2
basal cell carcinoma	C44.21•	—	—	—	—	—
specified type NEC	C44.29•	—	—	—	—	—
squamous cell carcinoma	C44.22•	—	—	—	—	—
ejaculatory duct	C63.7	C79.82	D07.69	D29.8	D40.8	D49.59
elbow NEC	C76.4•	C79.89	D04.6•	D36.7	D48.7	D49.89
endocardium	C38.0	C79.89	—	D15.1	D48.7	D49.89
endocervix (canal) (gland)	C53.0	C79.82	D06.0	D26.0	D39.0	D49.59
endocrine gland NEC	C75.9	C79.89	D09.3	D35.9	D44.9	D49.7
pluriglandular	C75.8	C79.89	D09.3	D35.7	D44.9	D49.7
endometrium (gland) (stroma)	C54.1	C79.82	D07.0	D26.1	D39.0	D49.59
ensiform cartilage	C41.3	C79.51	—	D16.7	D48.0	D49.2
enteric — *see Neoplasm, intestine*						
ependyma (brain)	C71.5	C79.31	—	D33.0	D43.0	D49.6
fourth ventricle	C71.7	C79.31	—	D33.1	D43.1	D49.6
epicardium	C38.0	C79.89	—	D15.1	D48.7	D49.89
epididymis	C63.0•	C79.82	D07.69	D29.3•	D40.8	D49.59
epidural	C72.9	C79.49	—	D33.9	D43.9	D49.7
epiglottis	C32.1	C78.39	D02.0	D14.1	D38.0	D49.1
anterior aspect or surface	C10.1	C79.89	D00.08	D10.5	D37.05	D49.0
cartilage	C32.3	C78.39	D02.0	D14.1	D38.0	D49.1
free border (margin)	C10.1	C79.89	D00.08	D10.5	D37.05	D49.0
junctional region	C10.8	C79.89	D00.08	D10.5	D37.05	D49.0
posterior (laryngeal) surface	C32.1	C78.39	D02.0	D14.1	D38.0	D49.1
suprahyoid portion	C32.1	C78.39	D02.0	D14.1	D38.0	D49.1
esophagogastric junction	C16.0	C78.89	D00.2	D13.1	D37.1	D49.0
esophagus	C15.9	C78.89	D00.1	D13.0	D37.8	D49.0
abdominal	C15.5	C78.89	D00.1	D13.0	D37.8	D49.0
cervical	C15.3	C78.89	D00.1	D13.0	D37.8	D49.0
distal (third)	C15.5	C78.89	D00.1	D13.0	D37.8	D49.0
lower (third)	C15.5	C78.89	D00.1	D13.0	D37.8	D49.0
middle (third)	C15.4	C78.89	D00.1	D13.0	D37.8	D49.0
overlapping lesion	C15.8	—	—	—	—	—
proximal (third)	C15.3	C78.89	D00.1	D13.0	D37.8	D49.0
thoracic	C15.4	C78.89	D00.1	D13.0	D37.8	D49.0
upper (third)	C15.3	C78.89	D00.1	D13.0	D37.8	D49.0
ethmoid (sinus)	C31.1	C78.39	D02.3	D14.0	D38.5	D49.1
bone or labyrinth	C41.0	C79.51	—	D16.4•	D48.0	D49.2
eustachian tube	C30.1	C78.39	D02.3	D14.0	D38.5	D49.1
exocervix	C53.1	C79.82	D06.1	D26.0	D39.0	D49.59
external						
meatus (ear) — *see also Neoplasm, skin, ear*	C44.20•	C79.2	D04.2•	D23.2•	D48.5	D49.2
os, cervix uteri	C53.1	C79.82	D06.1	D26.0	D39.0	D49.59
extradural	C72.9	C79.49	—	D33.9	D43.9	D49.7
extrahepatic (bile) duct	C24.0	C78.89	D01.5	D13.5	D37.6	D49.0
overlapping lesion with gallbladder	C24.8	—	—	—	—	—
extraocular muscle	C69.6•	C79.49	D09.2•	D31.6•	D48.7	D49.89
extrarectal	C76.3	C79.89	D09.8	D36.7	D48.7	D49.89
extremity	C76.8	C79.89	D04.8	D36.7	D48.7	D49.89
lower	C76.5•	C79.89	D04.7•	D36.7	D48.7	D49.89
upper	C76.4•	C79.89	D04.6•	D36.7	D48.7	D49.89
eye NEC	C69.9•	C79.49	D09.2	D31.9	D48.7	D49.89
overlapping sites	C69.8	—	—	—	—	—
eyeball	C69.9•	C79.49	D09.2•	D31.9•	D48.7	D49.89
eyebrow	C44.309	C79.2	D04.39	D23.39	D48.5	D49.2
basal cell carcinoma	C44.319	—	—	—	—	—
specified type NEC	C44.399	—	—	—	—	—
squamous cell carcinoma	C44.329	—	—	—	—	—
eyelid (lower) (skin) (upper)	C44.10•	—	—	—	—	—
basal cell carcinoma	C44.11•	—	—	—	—	—
cartilage	C49.0	C79.89	—	D21.0	D48.1	D49.2
sebaceous cell	C44.13•	—	—	—	—	—
specified type NEC	C44.19•	—	—	—	—	—
squamous cell carcinoma	C44.12•	—	—	—	—	—

New   Revised   ~~deleted~~ Deleted   • Use Additional Character(s)

	Malignant Primary	Malignant Secondary	Ca in situ	Benign	Uncertain Behavior	Unspecified Behavior
face NEC	C76.0	C79.89	D04.39	D36.7	D48.7	D49.89
fallopian tube (accessory)	C57.0•	C79.82	D07.39	D28.2	D39.8	D49.59
falx (cerebella) (cerebri)	C70.0	C79.32	—	D32.0	D42.0	D49.7
fascia — *see also Neoplasm, connective tissue*						
palmar	C49.1•	C79.89	—	D21.1•	D48.1	D49.2
plantar	C49.2•	C79.89	—	D21.2•	D48.1	D49.2
fatty tissue — *see Neoplasm, connective tissue*						
fauces, faucial NEC	C10.9	C79.89	D00.08	D10.5	D37.05	D49.0
pillars	C09.1	C79.89	D00.08	D10.5	D37.05	D49.0
tonsil	C09.9	C79.89	D00.08	D10.4	D37.05	D49.0
femur (any part)	C40.2•	—	—	D16.2•	—	—
fetal membrane	C58	C79.82	D07.0	D26.7	D39.2	D49.59
fibrous tissue — *see Neoplasm, connective tissue*						
fibula (any part)	C40.2•	C79.51	—	D16.2•	—	—
filum terminale	C72.0	C79.49	—	D33.4	D43.4	D49.7
finger NEC	C76.4•	C79.89	D04.6•	D36.7	D48.7	D49.89
flank NEC	C76.8	C79.89	D04.5	D36.7	D48.7	D49.89
follicle, nabothian	C53.0	C79.82	D06.0	D26.0	D39.0	D49.59
foot NEC	C76.5•	C79.89	D04.7•	D36.7	D48.7	D49.89
forearm NEC	C76.4•	C79.89	D04.6•	D36.7	D48.7	D49.89
forehead (skin)	C44.309	C79.2	D04.39	D23.39	D48.5	D49.2
basal cell carcinoma	C44.319	—	—	—	—	—
specified type NEC	C44.399	—	—	—	—	—
squamous cell carcinoma	C44.329	—	—	—	—	—
foreskin	C60.0	C79.82	D07.4	D29.0	D40.8	D49.59
fornix						
pharyngeal	C11.3	C79.89	D00.08	D10.6	D37.05	D49.0
vagina	C52	C79.82	D07.2	D28.1	D39.8	D49.59
fossa (of)						
anterior (cranial)	C71.9	C79.31	—	D33.2	D43.2	D49.6
cranial	C71.9	C79.31	—	D33.2	D43.2	D49.6
ischiorectal	C76.3	C79.89	D09.8	D36.7	D48.7	D49.89
middle (cranial)	C71.9	C79.31	—	D33.2	D43.2	D49.6
piriform	C12	C79.89	D00.08	D10.7	D37.05	D49.0
pituitary	C75.1	C79.89	D09.3	D35.2	D44.3	D49.7
posterior (cranial)	C71.9	C79.31	—	D33.2	D43.2	D49.6
pterygoid	C49.0	C79.89	—	D21.0	D48.1	D49.2
pyriform	C12	C79.89	D00.08	D10.7	D37.05	D49.0
Rosenmuller	C11.2	C79.89	D00.08	D10.6	D37.05	D49.0
tonsillar	C09.0	C79.89	D00.08	D10.5	D37.05	D49.0
fourchette	C51.9	C79.82	D07.1	D28.0	D39.8	D49.59
frenulum						
labii — *see Neoplasm, lip, internal*						
linguae	C02.2	C79.89	D00.07	D10.1	D37.02	D49.0
frontal						
bone	C41.0	C79.51	—	D16.4•	D48.0	D49.2
lobe, brain	C71.1	C79.31	—	D33.0	D43.0	D49.6
pole	C71.1	C79.31	—	D33.0	D43.0	D49.6
sinus	C31.2	C78.39	D02.3	D14.0	D38.5	D49.1
fundus						
stomach	C16.1	C78.89	D00.2	D13.1	D37.1	D49.0
uterus	C54.3	C79.82	D07.0	D26.1	D39.0	D49.59
gall duct (extrahepatic)	C24.0	C78.89	D01.5	D13.5	D37.6	D49.0
intrahepatic	C22.1	C78.7	D01.5	D13.4	D37.6	D49.0
gallbladder	C23	C78.89	D01.5	D13.5	D37.6	D49.0
overlapping lesion with extrahepatic bile ducts	C24.8	—	—	—	—	—
ganglia — *see also Neoplasm, nerve, peripheral*	C47.9	C79.89	—	D36.10	D48.2	D49.2
basal	C71.0	C79.31	—	D33.0	D43.0	D49.6
cranial nerve	C72.50	C79.49	—	D33.3	D43.3	D49.7
Gartner's duct	C52	C79.82	D07.2	D28.1	D39.8	D49.59
gastric — *see Neoplasm, stomach*						
gastrocolic	C26.9	C78.89	D01.9	D13.99	D37.9	D49.0
gastroesophageal junction	C16.0	C78.89	D00.2	D13.1	D37.1	D49.0
gastrointestinal (tract) NEC	C26.9	C78.89	D01.9	D13.99	D37.9	D49.0
generalized	C80.0	—	—	—	—	—
genital organ or tract						
female NEC	C57.9	C79.82	D07.30	D28.9	D39.9	D49.59
overlapping lesion	C57.8	—	—	—	—	—
specified site NEC	C57.7	C79.82	D07.39	D28.7	D39.8	D49.59
male NEC	C63.9	C79.82	D07.60	D29.9	D40.9	D49.59
overlapping lesion	C63.8	—	—	—	—	—
specified site NEC	C63.7	C79.82	D07.69	D29.8	D40.8	D49.59
genitourinary tract						
female	C57.9	C79.82	D07.30	D28.9	D39.9	D49.59
male	C63.9	C79.82	D07.60	D29.9	D40.9	D49.59
gingiva (alveolar) (marginal)	C03.9	C79.89	D00.03	D10.39	D37.09	D49.0
lower	C03.1	C79.89	D00.03	D10.39	D37.09	D49.0
mandibular	C03.1	C79.89	D00.03	D10.39	D37.09	D49.0
maxillary	C03.0	C79.89	D00.03	D10.39	D37.09	D49.0
upper	C03.0	C79.89	D00.03	D10.39	D37.09	D49.0

	Malignant Primary	Malignant Secondary	Ca in situ	Benign	Uncertain Behavior	Unspecified Behavior
gland, glandular (lymphatic) (system) — *see also Neoplasm, lymph gland*						
endocrine NEC	C75.9	C79.89	DØ9.3	D35.9	D44.9	D49.7
salivary — *see Neoplasm, salivary gland*						
glans penis	C6Ø.1	C79.82	DØ7.4	D29.Ø	D4Ø.8	D49.59
globus pallidus	C71.Ø	C79.31	—	D33.Ø	D43.Ø	D49.6
glomus						
coccygeal	C49.5	C79.89	—	D21.5	D48.1	D49.2
jugularis	C75.5	C79.89	—	D35.6	D44.7	D49.7
glosso-epiglottic fold(s)	C1Ø.1	C79.89	DØØ.Ø8	D1Ø.5	D37.Ø5	D49.Ø
glossopalatine fold	CØ9.1	C79.89	DØØ.Ø8	D1Ø.5	D37.Ø5	D49.Ø
glossopharyngeal sulcus	CØ9.Ø	C79.89	DØØ.Ø8	D1Ø.5	D37.Ø5	D49.Ø
glottis	C32.Ø	C78.39	DØ2.Ø	D14.1	D38.Ø	D49.1
gluteal region	C76.3	C79.89	DØ4.5	D36.7	D48.7	D49.89
great vessels NEC	C49.3	C79.89	—	D21.3	D48.1	D49.2
groin NEC	C76.3	C79.89	DØ4.5	D36.7	D48.7	D49.89
gum	CØ3.9	C79.89	DØØ.Ø3	D1Ø.39	D37.Ø9	D49.Ø
lower	CØ3.1	C79.89	DØØ.Ø3	D1Ø.39	D37.Ø9	D49.Ø
upper	CØ3.Ø	C79.89	DØØ.Ø3	D1Ø.39	D37.Ø9	D49.Ø
hand NEC	C76.4-●	C79.89	DØ4.6-●	D36.7	D48.7	D49.89
head NEC	C76.Ø	C79.89	DØ4.4	D36.7	D48.7	D49.89
heart	C38.Ø	C79.89	—	D15.1	D48.7	D49.89
heel NEC	C76.5-●	C79.89	DØ4.7-●	D36.7	D48.7	D49.89
helix — *see also Neoplasm, skin, ear*	C44.2Ø-●	C79.2	DØ4.2-●	D23.2-●	D48.5	D49.2
hematopoietic, hemopoietic tissue NEC	C96.9	—	—	—	—	—
specified NEC	C96.Z	—	—	—	—	—
hemisphere, cerebral	C71.Ø	C79.31	—	D33.Ø	D43.Ø	D49.6
hemorrhoidal zone	C21.1	C78.5	DØ1.3	D12.9	D37.8	D49.Ø
hepatic — *see also Index to disease, by histology*	C22.9	C78.7	DØ1.5	D13.4	D37.6	D49.Ø
duct (bile)	C24.Ø	C78.89	DØ1.5	D13.5	D37.6	D49.Ø
flexure (colon)	C18.3	C78.5	DØ1.Ø	D12.3	D37.4	D49.Ø
primary	C22.8	C78.7	DØ1.5	D13.4	D37.6	D49.Ø
hepatobiliary	C24.9	C79.89	DØ1.5	D13.5	D37.6	D49.Ø
hepatoblastoma	C22.2	C78.7	DØ1.5	D13.4	D37.6	D49.Ø
hepatoma	C22.Ø	C78.7	DØ1.5	D13.4	D37.6	D49.Ø
hilus of lung	C34.Ø-●	C78.Ø-●	DØ2.2-●	D14.3-●	D38.1	D49.1
hip NEC	C76.5-●	C79.89	DØ4.7-●	D36.7	D48.7	D49.89
hippocampus, brain	C71.2	C79.31	—	D33.Ø	D43.Ø	D49.6
humerus (any part)	C4Ø.Ø-●	C79.51	—	D16.Ø-●	—	—
hymen	C52	C79.82	DØ7.2	D28.1	D39.8	D49.59

	Malignant Primary	Malignant Secondary	Ca in situ	Benign	Uncertain Behavior	Unspecified Behavior
hypopharynx, hypopharyngeal NEC	C13.9	C79.89	DØØ.Ø8	D1Ø.7	D37.Ø5	D49.Ø
overlapping lesion	C13.8	—	—	—	—	—
postcricoid region	C13.Ø	C79.89	DØØ.Ø8	D1Ø.7	D37.Ø5	D49.Ø
posterior wall	C13.2	C79.89	DØØ.Ø8	D1Ø.7	D37.Ø5	D49.Ø
pyriform fossa (sinus)	C12	C79.89	DØØ.Ø8	D1Ø.7	D37.Ø5	D49.Ø
hypophysis	C75.1	C79.89	DØ9.3	D35.2	D44.3	D49.7
hypothalamus	C71.Ø	C79.31	—	D33.Ø	D43.Ø	D49.6
ileocecum, ileocecal (coil) (junction) (valve)	C18.Ø	C78.5	DØ1.Ø	D12.Ø	D37.4	D49.Ø
ileum	C17.2	C78.4	DØ1.49	D13.39	D37.2	D49.Ø
ilium	C41.4	C79.51	—	D16.8	D48.Ø	D49.2
immunoproliferative NEC	C88.9	—	—	—	—	—
infraclavicular (region)	C76.1	C79.89	DØ4.5	D36.7	D48.7	D49.89
inguinal (region)	C76.3	C79.89	DØ4.5	D36.7	D48.7	D49.89
insula	C71.Ø	C79.31	—	D33.Ø	D43.Ø	D49.6
insular tissue (pancreas)	C25.4	C78.89	DØ1.7	D13.7	D37.8	D49.Ø
brain	C71.Ø	C79.31	—	D33.Ø	D43.Ø	D49.6
interarytenoid fold	C13.1	C79.89	DØØ.Ø8	D1Ø.7	D37.Ø5	D49.Ø
hypopharyngeal aspect	C13.1	C79.89	DØØ.Ø8	D1Ø.7	D37.Ø5	D49.Ø
laryngeal aspect	C32.1	C78.39	DØ2.Ø	D14.1	D38.Ø	D49.1
marginal zone	C13.1	C79.89	DØØ.Ø8	D1Ø.7	D37.Ø5	D49.Ø
interdental papillae	CØ3.9	C79.89	DØØ.Ø3	D1Ø.39	D37.Ø9	D49.Ø
lower	CØ3.1	C79.89	DØØ.Ø3	D1Ø.39	D37.Ø9	D49.Ø
upper	CØ3.Ø	C79.89	DØØ.Ø3	D1Ø.39	D37.Ø9	D49.Ø
internal						
capsule	C71.Ø	C79.31	—	D33.Ø	D43.Ø	D49.6
os (cervix)	C53.Ø	C79.82	DØ6.Ø	D26.Ø	D39.Ø	D49.59
intervertebral cartilage or disc	C41.2	C79.51	—	D16.6	D48.Ø	D49.2
intestine, intestinal	C26.Ø	C78.8Ø	DØ1.4Ø	D13.99	D37.8	D49.Ø
large	C18.9	C78.5	DØ1.Ø	D12.6	D37.4	D49.Ø
appendix	C18.1	C78.5	DØ1.Ø	D12.1	D37.3	D49.Ø
caput coli	C18.Ø	C78.5	DØ1.Ø	D12.Ø	D37.4	D49.Ø
cecum	C18.Ø	C78.5	DØ1.Ø	D12.Ø	D37.4	D49.Ø
colon	C18.9	C78.5	DØ1.Ø	D12.6	D37.4	D49.Ø
and rectum	C19	C78.5	DØ1.1	D12.7	D37.5	D49.Ø
ascending	C18.2	C78.5	DØ1.Ø	D12.2	D37.4	D49.Ø
caput	C18.Ø	C78.5	DØ1.Ø	D12.Ø	D37.4	D49.Ø
descending	C18.6	C78.5	DØ1.Ø	D12.4	D37.4	D49.Ø
distal	C18.6	C78.5	DØ1.Ø	D12.4	D37.4	D49.Ø
left	C18.6	C78.5	DØ1.Ø	D12.4	D37.4	D49.Ø
overlapping lesion	C18.8	—	—	—	—	—
pelvic	C18.7	C78.5	DØ1.Ø	D12.5	D37.4	D49.Ø
right	C18.2	C78.5	DØ1.Ø	D12.2	D37.4	D49.Ø

◄ New ◄ Revised ~~deleted~~ Deleted ● Use Additional Character(s)

	Malignant Primary	Malignant Secondary	Ca in situ	Benign	Uncertain Behavior	Unspecified Behavior
intestine, intestinal *(Continued)*						
large *(Continued)*						
colon *(Continued)*						
sigmoid (flexure)	C18.7	C78.5	D01.0	D12.5	D37.4	D49.0
transverse	C18.4	C78.5	D01.0	D12.3	D37.4	D49.0
hepatic flexure	C18.3	C78.5	D01.0	D12.3	D37.4	D49.0
ileocecum, ileocecal (coil) (valve)	C18.0	C78.5	D01.0	D12.0	D37.4	D49.0
overlapping lesion	C18.8	—	—	—	—	—
sigmoid flexure (lower) (upper)	C18.7	C78.5	D01.0	D12.5	D37.4	D49.0
splenic flexure	C18.5	C78.5	D01.0	D12.3	D37.4	D49.0
small	C17.9	C78.4	D01.40	D13.30	D37.2	D49.0
duodenum	C17.0	C78.4	D01.49	D13.2	D37.2	D49.0
ileum	C17.2	C78.4	D01.49	D13.39	D37.2	D49.0
jejunum	C17.1	C78.4	D01.49	D13.39	D37.2	D49.0
overlapping lesion	C17.8	—	—	—	—	—
tract NEC	C26.0	C78.89	D01.40	D13.99	D37.8	D49.0
intra-abdominal	C76.2	C79.89	D09.8	D36.7	D48.7	D49.89
intracranial NEC	C71.9	C79.31	—	D33.2	D43.2	D49.6
intrahepatic (bile) duct	C22.1	C78.7	D01.5	D13.4	D37.6	D49.0
intraocular	C69.9-•	C79.49	D09.2-•	D31.9-•	D48.7	D49.89
intraorbital	C69.6-•	C79.49	D09.2-•	D31.6-•	D48.7	D49.89
intrasellar	C75.1	C79.89	D09.3	D35.2	D44.3	D49.7
intrathoracic (cavity) (organs)	C76.1	C79.89	D09.8	D15.9	D48.7	D49.89
specified NEC	C76.1	C79.89	D09.8	D15.7	—	—
iris	C69.4-•	C79.49	D09.2-•	D31.4-•	D48.7	D49.89
ischiorectal (fossa)	C76.3	C79.89	D09.8	D36.7	D48.7	D49.89
ischium	C41.4	C79.51	—	D16.8	D48.0	D49.2
island of Reil	C71.0	C79.31	—	D33.0	D43.0	D49.6
islands or islets of Langerhans	C25.4	C78.89	D01.7	D13.7	D37.8	D49.0
isthmus uteri	C54.0	C79.82	D07.0	D26.1	D39.0	D49.59
jaw	C76.0	C79.89	D09.8	D36.7	D48.7	D49.89
bone	C41.1	C79.51	—	D16.5-•	D48.0	D49.2
lower	C41.1	C79.51	—	D16.5-•	—	—
upper	C41.0	C79.51	—	D16.4-•	—	—
carcinoma (any type) (lower) (upper)	C76.0	C79.89	—	—	—	—
skin—*see also Neoplasm, skin, face*	C44.309	C79.2	D04.39	D23.39	D48.5	D49.2
soft tissues	C03.9	C79.89	D00.03	D10.39	D37.09	D49.0
lower	C03.1	C79.89	D00.03	D10.39	D37.09	D49.0
upper	C03.0	C79.89	D00.03	D10.39	D37.09	D49.0
jejunum	C17.1	C78.4	D01.49	D13.39	D37.2	D49.0

	Malignant Primary	Malignant Secondary	Ca in situ	Benign	Uncertain Behavior	Unspecified Behavior
joint NEC—*see also Neoplasm, bone*	C41.9	C79.51	—	D16.9-•	D48.0	D49.2
acromioclavicular	C40.0-•	C79.51	—	D16.0-•	—	—
bursa or synovial membrane—*see Neoplasm, connective tissue*						
costovertebral	C41.3	C79.51	—	D16.7	D48.0	D49.2
sternocostal	C41.3	C79.51	—	D16.7	D48.0	D49.2
temporomandibular	C41.1	C79.51	—	D16.5-•	D48.0	D49.2
junction						
anorectal	C21.8	C78.5	D01.3	D12.9	D37.8	D49.0
cardioesophageal	C16.0	C78.89	D00.2	D13.1	D37.1	D49.0
esophagogastric	C16.0	C78.89	D00.2	D13.1	D37.1	D49.0
gastroesophageal	C16.0	C78.89	D00.2	D13.1	D37.1	D49.0
hard and soft palate	C05.9	C79.89	D00.00	D10.39	D37.09	D49.0
ileocecal	C18.0	C78.5	D01.0	D12.0	D37.4	D49.0
pelvirectal	C19	C78.5	D01.1	D12.7	D37.5	D49.0
pelviureteric	C65.-•	C79.0-•	D09.19	D30.1-•	D41.1-•	D49.59
rectosigmoid	C19	C78.5	D01.1	D12.7	D37.5	D49.0
squamocolumnar, of cervix	C53.8	C79.82	D06.7	D26.0	D39.0	D49.59
Kaposi's sarcoma—*see Kaposi's, sarcoma*						
kidney (parenchymal)	C64.-•	C79.0-•	D09.19	D30.0-•	D41.0-•	D49.51-•
calyx	C65.-•	C79.0-•	D09.19	D30.1-•	D41.1-•	D49.51-•
hilus	C65.-•	C79.0-•	D09.19	D30.1-•	D41.1-•	D49.51-•
pelvis	C65.-•	C79.0-•	D09.19	D30.1-•	D41.1-•	D49.51-•
knee NEC	C76.5-•	C79.89	D04.7-•	D36.7	D48.7	D49.89
labia (skin)	C51.9	C79.82	D07.1	D28.0	D39.8	D49.59
majora	C51.0	C79.82	D07.1	D28.0	D39.8	D49.59
minora	C51.1	C79.82	D07.1	D28.0	D39.8	D49.59
labial—*see also Neoplasm, lip*	C00.9	C79.89	D00.01	D10.0	D37.01	D49.0
sulcus (lower) (upper)	C06.1	C79.89	D00.02	D10.39	D37.09	D49.0
labium (skin)	C51.9	C79.82	D07.1	D28.0	D39.8	D49.59
majus	C51.0	C79.82	D07.1	D28.0	D39.8	D49.59
minus	C51.1	C79.82	D07.1	D28.0	D39.8	D49.59
lacrimal						
canaliculi	C69.5-•	C79.49	D09.2-•	D31.5-•	D48.7	D49.89
duct (nasal)	C69.5-•	C79.49	D09.2-•	D31.5-•	D48.7	D49.89
gland	C69.5-•	C79.49	D09.2-•	D31.5-•	D48.7	D49.89
punctum	C69.5-•	C79.49	D09.2-•	D31.5-•	D48.7	D49.89
sac	C69.5-•	C79.49	D09.2-•	D31.5-•	D48.7	D49.89
Langerhans, islands or islets	C25.4	C78.89	D01.7	D13.7	D37.8	D49.0
laryngopharynx	C13.9	C79.89	D00.08	D10.7	D37.05	D49.0

	Malignant Primary	Malignant Secondary	Ca in situ	Benign	Uncertain Behavior	Unspecified Behavior
larynx, laryngeal NEC	C32.9	C78.39	D02.Ø	D14.1	D38.Ø	D49.1
aryepiglottic fold	C32.1	C78.39	D02.Ø	D14.1	D38.Ø	D49.1
cartilage (arytenoid) (cricoid) (cuneiform) (thyroid)	C32.3	C78.39	D02.Ø	D14.1	D38.Ø	D49.1
commissure (anterior) (posterior)	C32.Ø	C78.39	D02.Ø	D14.1	D38.Ø	D49.1
extrinsic NEC	C32.1	C78.39	D02.Ø	D14.1	D38.Ø	D49.1
meaning hypopharynx	C13.9	C79.89	DØØ.Ø8	D1Ø.7	D37.Ø5	D49.Ø
interarytenoid fold	C32.1	C78.39	D02.Ø	D14.1	D38.Ø	D49.1
intrinsic	C32.Ø	C78.39	D02.Ø	D14.1	D38.Ø	D49.1
overlapping lesion	C32.8	—	—	—	—	—
ventricular band	C32.1	C78.39	D02.Ø	D14.1	D38.Ø	D49.1
leg NEC	C76.5-•	C79.89	D04.7-•	D36.7	D48.7	D49.89
lens, crystalline	C69.4-•	C79.49	D09.2-•	D31.4-•	D48.7	D49.89
lid (lower) (upper)	C44.1Ø-•	C79.2	D04.1-•	D23.1-•	D48.5	D49.2
basal cell carcinoma	C44.11-•	—	—	—	—	—
sebaceous cell	C44.13-•	—	—	—	—	—
specified type NEC	C44.19-•	—	—	—	—	—
squamous cell carcinoma	C44.12-•	—	—	—	—	—
ligament — *see also Neoplasm, connective tissue*						
broad	C57.1	C79.82	D07.39	D28.2	D39.8	D49.59
Mackenrodt's	C57.7	C79.82	D07.39	D28.7	D39.8	D49.59
non-uterine — *see Neoplasm, connective tissue*						
round	C57.2	C79.82	—	D28.2	D39.8	D49.59
sacro-uterine	C57.3	C79.82	—	D28.2	D39.8	D49.59
uterine	C57.3	C79.82	—	D28.2	D39.8	D49.59
utero-ovarian	C57.7	C79.82	D07.39	D28.2	D39.8	D49.59
uterosacral	C57.3	C79.82	—	D28.2	D39.8	D49.59
limb	C76.8	C79.89	D04.8	D36.7	D48.7	D49.89
lower	C76.5-•	C79.89	D04.7-•	D36.7	D48.7	D49.89
upper	C76.4-•	C79.89	D04.6-•	D36.7	D48.7	D49.89
limbus of cornea	C69.1-•	C79.49	D09.2-•	D31.1-•	D48.7	D49.89
lingual NEC — *see also Neoplasm, tongue*	CØ2.9	C79.89	DØØ.Ø7	D1Ø.1	D37.Ø2	D49.Ø
lingula, lung	C34.1-•	C78.Ø-•	DØ2.2-•	D14.3-•	D38.1	D49.1
lip	CØØ.9	C79.89	DØØ.Ø1	D1Ø.Ø	D37.Ø1	D49.Ø
buccal aspect — *see Neoplasm, lip, internal*						
commissure	CØØ.6	C79.89	DØØ.Ø1	D1Ø.Ø	D37.Ø1	D49.Ø
external	CØØ.2	C79.89	DØØ.Ø1	D1Ø.Ø	D37.Ø1	D49.Ø
lower	CØØ.1	C79.89	DØØ.Ø1	D1Ø.Ø	D37.Ø1	D49.Ø
upper	CØØ.Ø	C79.89	DØØ.Ø1	D1Ø.Ø	D37.Ø1	D49.Ø
frenulum — *see Neoplasm, lip, internal*						
lip *(Continued)*						
inner aspect — *see Neoplasm, lip, internal*						
internal	CØØ.5	C79.89	DØØ.Ø1	D1Ø.Ø	D37.Ø1	D49.Ø
lower	CØØ.4	C79.89	DØØ.Ø1	D1Ø.Ø	D37.Ø1	D49.Ø
upper	CØØ.3	C79.89	DØØ.Ø1	D1Ø.Ø	D37.Ø1	D49.Ø
lipstick area	CØØ.2	C79.89	DØØ.Ø1	D1Ø.Ø	D37.Ø1	D49.Ø
lower	CØØ.1	C79.89	DØØ.Ø1	D1Ø.Ø	D37.Ø1	D49.Ø
upper	CØØ.Ø	C79.89	DØØ.Ø1	D1Ø.Ø	D37.Ø1	D49.Ø
lower	CØØ.1	C79.89	DØØ.Ø1	D1Ø.Ø	D37.Ø1	D49.Ø
internal	CØØ.4	C79.89	DØØ.Ø1	D1Ø.Ø	D37.Ø1	D49.Ø
mucosa — *see Neoplasm, lip, internal*						
oral aspect — *see Neoplasm, lip, internal*						
overlapping lesion	CØØ.8	—	—	—	—	—
with oral cavity or pharynx	C14.8	—	—	—	—	—
skin (commissure) (lower) (upper)	C44.ØØ	C79.2	DØ4.Ø	D23.Ø	D48.5	D49.2
basal cell carcinoma	C44.Ø1	—	—	—	—	—
specified type NEC	C44.Ø9	—	—	—	—	—
squamous cell carcinoma	C44.Ø2	—	—	—	—	—
upper	CØØ.Ø	C79.89	DØØ.Ø1	D1Ø.Ø	D37.Ø1	D49.Ø
internal	CØØ.3	C79.89	DØØ.Ø1	D1Ø.Ø	D37.Ø1	D49.Ø
vermilion border	CØØ.2	C79.89	DØØ.Ø1	D1Ø.Ø	D37.Ø1	D49.Ø
lower	CØØ.1	C79.89	DØØ.Ø1	D1Ø.Ø	D37.Ø1	D49.Ø
upper	CØØ.Ø	C79.89	DØØ.Ø1	D1Ø.Ø	D37.Ø1	D49.Ø
lipomatous — *see Lipoma, by site*						
liver — *see also Index to disease, by histology*	C22.9	C78.7	DØ1.5	D13.4	D37.6	D49.Ø
primary	C22.8	C78.7	DØ1.5	D13.4	D37.6	D49.Ø
lumbosacral plexus	C47.5	C79.89	—	D36.16	D48.2	D49.2
lung	C34.9-•	C78.Ø-•	DØ2.2-•	D14.3-•	D38.1	D49.1
azygos lobe	C34.1-•	C78.Ø-•	DØ2.2-•	D14.3-•	D38.1	D49.1
carina	C34.Ø-•	C78.Ø-•	DØ2.2-•	D14.3-•	D38.1	D49.1
hilus	C34.Ø-•	C78.Ø-•	DØ2.2-•	D14.3-•	D38.1	D49.1
linqula	C34.1-•	C78.Ø-•	DØ2.2-•	D14.3-•	D38.1	D49.1
lobe NEC	C34.9-•	C78.Ø-•	DØ2.2-•	D14.3-•	D38.1	D49.1
lower lobe	C34.3-•	C78.Ø-•	DØ2.2-•	D14.3-•	D38.1	D49.1
main bronchus	C34.Ø-•	C78.Ø-•	DØ2.2-•	D14.3-•	D38.1	D49.1
mesothelioma — *see Mesothelioma*						
middle lobe	C34.2	C78.Ø-•	DØ2.21	D14.31	D38.1	D49.1
overlapping lesion	C34.8-•	—	—	—	—	—
upper lobe	C34.1-•	C78.Ø-•	DØ2.2-•	D14.3-•	D38.1	D49.1

◄ New ▐ Revised ~~deleted~~ Deleted • Use Additional Character(s)

	Malignant Primary	Malignant Secondary	Ca in situ	Benign	Uncertain Behavior	Unspecified Behavior
lymph, lymphatic channel NEC	C49.9	C79.89	—	D21.9	D48.1	D49.2
gland (secondary)	—	C77.9	—	D36.0	D48.7	D49.89
abdominal	—	C77.2	—	D36.0	D48.7	D49.89
aortic	—	C77.2	—	D36.0	D48.7	D49.89
arm	—	C77.3	—	D36.0	D48.7	D49.89
auricular (anterior) (posterior)	—	C77.0	—	D36.0	D48.7	D49.89
axilla, axillary	—	C77.3	—	D36.0	D48.7	D49.89
brachial	—	C77.3	—	D36.0	D48.7	D49.89
bronchial	—	C77.1	—	D36.0	D48.7	D49.89
bronchopulmonary	—	C77.1	—	D36.0	D48.7	D49.89
celiac	—	C77.2	—	D36.0	D48.7	D49.89
cervical	—	C77.0	—	D36.0	D48.7	D49.89
cervicofacial	—	C77.0	—	D36.0	D48.7	D49.89
Cloquet	—	C77.4	—	D36.0	D48.7	D49.89
colic	—	C77.2	—	D36.0	D48.7	D49.89
common duct	—	C77.2	—	D36.0	D48.7	D49.89
cubital	—	C77.3	—	D36.0	D48.7	D49.89
diaphragmatic	—	C77.1	—	D36.0	D48.7	D49.89
epigastric, inferior	—	C77.1	—	D36.0	D48.7	D49.89
epitrochlear	—	C77.3	—	D36.0	D48.7	D49.89
esophageal	—	C77.1	—	D36.0	D48.7	D49.89
face	—	C77.0	—	D36.0	D48.7	D49.89
femoral	—	C77.4	—	D36.0	D48.7	D49.89
gastric	—	C77.2	—	D36.0	D48.7	D49.89
groin	—	C77.4	—	D36.0	D48.7	D49.89
head	—	C77.0	—	D36.0	D48.7	D49.89
hepatic	—	C77.2	—	D36.0	D48.7	D49.89
hilar (pulmonary)	—	C77.1	—	D36.0	D48.7	D49.89
splenic	—	C77.2	—	D36.0	D48.7	D49.89
hypogastric	—	C77.5	—	D36.0	D48.7	D49.89
ileocolic	—	C77.2	—	D36.0	D48.7	D49.89
iliac	—	C77.5	—	D36.0	D48.7	D49.89
infraclavicular	—	C77.3	—	D36.0	D48.7	D49.89
inguina, inguinal	—	C77.4	—	D36.0	D48.7	D49.89
innominate	—	C77.1	—	D36.0	D48.7	D49.89
intercostal	—	C77.1	—	D36.0	D48.7	D49.89
intestinal	—	C77.2	—	D36.0	D48.7	D49.89
intrabdominal	—	C77.2	—	D36.0	D48.7	D49.89
intrapelvic	—	C77.5	—	D36.0	D48.7	D49.89
intrathoracic	—	C77.1	—	D36.0	D48.7	D49.89
jugular	—	C77.0	—	D36.0	D48.7	D49.89
leg	—	C77.4	—	D36.0	D48.7	D49.89
limb						
lower	—	C77.4	—	D36.0	D48.7	D49.89
upper	—	C77.3	—	D36.0	D48.7	D49.89

	Malignant Primary	Malignant Secondary	Ca in situ	Benign	Uncertain Behavior	Unspecified Behavior
lymph, lymphatic channel NEC *(Continued)*						
gland *(Continued)*						
lower limb	—	C77.4	—	D36.0	D48.7	D49.89
lumbar	—	C77.2	—	D36.0	D48.7	D49.89
mandibular	—	C77.0	—	D36.0	D48.7	D49.89
mediastinal	—	C77.1	—	D36.0	D48.7	D49.89
mesenteric (inferior) (superior)	—	C77.2	—	D36.0	D48.7	D49.89
midcolic	—	C77.2	—	D36.0	D48.7	D49.89
multiple sites in categories C77.0 - C77.5	—	C77.8	—	D36.0	D48.7	D49.89
neck	—	C77.0	—	D36.0	D48.7	D49.89
obturator	—	C77.5	—	D36.0	D48.7	D49.89
occipital	—	C77.0	—	D36.0	D48.7	D49.89
pancreatic	—	C77.2	—	D36.0	D48.7	D49.89
para-aortic	—	C77.2	—	D36.0	D48.7	D49.89
paracervical	—	C77.5	—	D36.0	D48.7	D49.89
parametrial	—	C77.5	—	D36.0	D48.7	D49.89
parasternal	—	C77.1	—	D36.0	D48.7	D49.89
parotid	—	C77.0	—	D36.0	D48.7	D49.89
pectoral	—	C77.3	—	D36.0	D48.7	D49.89
pelvic	—	C77.5	—	D36.0	D48.7	D49.89
peri-aortic	—	C77.2	—	D36.0	D48.7	D49.89
peripancreatic	—	C77.2	—	D36.0	D48.7	D49.89
popliteal	—	C77.4	—	D36.0	D48.7	D49.89
porta hepatis	—	C77.2	—	D36.0	D48.7	D49.89
portal	—	C77.2	—	D36.0	D48.7	D49.89
preauricular	—	C77.0	—	D36.0	D48.7	D49.89
prelaryngeal	—	C77.0	—	D36.0	D48.7	D49.89
presymphysial	—	C77.5	—	D36.0	D48.7	D49.89
pretracheal	—	C77.0	—	D36.0	D48.7	D49.89
primary (any site) NEC	C96.9	—	—	—	—	—
pulmonary (hiler)	—	C77.1	—	D36.0	D48.7	D49.89
pyloric	—	C77.2	—	D36.0	D48.7	D49.89
retroperitoneal	—	C77.2	—	D36.0	D48.7	D49.89
retropharyngeal	—	C77.0	—	D36.0	D48.7	D49.89
Rosenmuller's	—	C77.4	—	D36.0	D48.7	D49.89
sacral	—	C77.5	—	D36.0	D48.7	D49.89
scalene	—	C77.0	—	D36.0	D48.7	D49.89
site NEC	—	C77.9	—	D36.0	D48.7	D49.89
splenic (hilar)	—	C77.2	—	D36.0	D48.7	D49.89
subclavicular	—	C77.3	—	D36.0	D48.7	D49.89
subinguinal	—	C77.4	—	D36.0	D48.7	D49.89

TABLE OF NEOPLASMS

◄ New   Revised   ~~deleted~~ Deleted   • Use Additional Character(s)

	Malignant Primary	Malignant Secondary	Ca in situ	Benign	Uncertain Behavior	Unspecified Behavior
lymph, lymphatic channel NEC *(Continued)*						
gland *(Continued)*						
sublingual	—	C77.0	—	D36.0	D48.7	D49.89
submandibular	—	C77.0	—	D36.0	D48.7	D49.89
submaxillary	—	C77.0	—	D36.0	D48.7	D49.89
submental	—	C77.0	—	D36.0	D48.7	D49.89
subscapular	—	C77.3	—	D36.0	D48.7	D49.89
supraclavicular	—	C77.0	—	D36.0	D48.7	D49.89
thoracic	—	C77.1	—	D36.0	D48.7	D49.89
tibial	—	C77.4	—	D36.0	D48.7	D49.89
tracheal	—	C77.1	—	D36.0	D48.7	D49.89
tracheobronchial	—	C77.1	—	D36.0	D48.7	D49.89
upper limb	—	C77.3	—	D36.0	D48.7	D49.89
Virchow's	—	C77.0	—	D36.0	D48.7	D49.89
node — *see also Neoplasm, lymph gland*						
primary NEC	C96.9	—	—	—	—	—
vessel — *see also Neoplasm, connective tissue*	C49.9	C79.89	—	D21.9	D48.1	D49.2
Mackenrodt's ligament	C57.7	C79.82	D07.39	D28.7	D39.8	D49.59
malar	C41.0	C79.51	—	D16.4-●	D48.0	D49.2
region — *see Neoplasm, cheek*						
mammary gland — *see Neoplasm, breast*						
mandible	C41.1	C79.51	—	D16.5-●	D48.0	D49.2
alveolar						
mucosa (carcinoma)	C03.1	C79.89	D00.03	D10.39	D37.09	D49.0
ridge or process	C41.1	C79.51	—	D16.5-●	D48.0	D49.2
marrow (bone) NEC	C96.9	C79.52	—	—	D47.9	D49.89
mastectomy site (skin) — *see also Neoplasm, breast, skin*	C44.501	C79.2	—	—	—	—
specified as breast tissue	C50.8-●	C79.81	—	—	—	—
mastoid (air cells) (antrum) (cavity)	C30.1	C78.39	D02.3	D14.0	D38.5	D49.1
bone or process	C41.0	C79.51	—	D16.4-●	D48.0	D49.2
maxilla, maxillary (superior)	C41.0	C79.51	—	D16.4-●	D48.0	D49.2
alveolar						
mucosa	C03.0	C79.89	D00.03	D10.39	D37.09	D49.0
ridge or process (carcinoma)	C41.0	C79.51	—	D16.4-●	D48.0	D49.2
antrum	C31.0	C78.39	D02.3	D14.0	D38.5	D49.1
carcinoma	C03.0	C79.51	—	—	—	—
inferior — *see Neoplasm, mandible*						
sinus	C31.0	C78.39	D02.3	D14.0	D38.5	D49.1
meatus external (ear) — *see also Neoplasm, skin, ear*	C44.20-●	C79.2	D04.2-●	D23.2-●	D48.5	D49.2
Meckel diverticulum, malignant	C17.3	C78.4	D01.49	D13.39	D37.2	D49.0
mediastinum, mediastinal	C38.3	C78.1	—	D15.2	D38.3	D49.89
anterior	C38.1	C78.1	—	D15.2	D38.3	D49.89
posterior	C38.2	C78.1	—	D15.2	D38.3	D49.89
medulla						
adrenal	C74.1-●	C79.7-●	D09.3	D35.0-●	D44.1-●	D49.7
oblongata	C71.7	C79.31	—	D33.1	D43.1	D49.6
meibomian gland	C44.10-●	C79.2	D04.1-●	D23.1-●	D48.5	D49.2
basal cell carcinoma	C44.11-●	—	—	—	—	—
sebaceous cell	C44.13-●	—	—	—	—	—
specified type NEC	C44.19-●	—	—	—	—	—
squamous cell carcinoma	C44.12-●	—	—	—	—	—
melanoma — *see Melanoma*						
meninges	C70.9	C79.49	—	D32.9	D42.9	D49.7
brain	C70.0	C79.32	—	D32.0	D42.0	D49.7
cerebral	C70.0	C79.32	—	D32.0	D42.0	D49.7
crainial	C70.0	C79.32	—	D32.0	D42.0	D49.7
intracranial	C70.0	C79.32	—	D32.0	D42.0	D49.7
spinal (cord)	C70.1	C79.49	—	D32.1	D42.1	D49.7
meniscus, knee joint (lateral) (medial)	C40.2-●	C79.51	—	D16.2-●	D48.0	D49.2
Merkel cell — *see Carcinoma, Merkel cell*						
mesentery, mesenteric	C48.1	C78.6	—	D20.1	D48.4	D49.0
mesoappendix	C48.1	C78.6	—	D20.1	D48.4	D49.0
mesocolon	C48.1	C78.6	—	D20.1	D48.4	D49.0
mesopharynx — *see Neoplasm, oropharynx*						
mesosalpinx	C57.1	C79.82	D07.39	D28.2	D39.8	D49.59
mesothelial tissue — *see Mesothelioma*						
mesothelioma — *see Mesothelioma*						
mesovarium	C57.1	C79.82	D07.39	D28.2	D39.8	D49.59
metacarpus (any bone)	C40.1-●	C79.51	—	D16.1-●	—	—
metastatic NEC — *see also Neoplasm, by site, secondary*	—	C79.9	—	—	—	—
metatarsus (any bone)	C40.3-●	C79.51	—	D16.3-●	—	—
midbrain	C71.7	C79.31	—	D33.1	D43.1	D49.6
milk duct — *see Neoplasm, breast*						
mons						
pubis	C51.9	C79.82	D07.1	D28.0	D39.8	D49.59
veneris	C51.9	C79.82	D07.1	D28.0	D39.8	D49.59

TABLE OF NEOPLASMS

◄ New ▒ Revised ~~deleted~~ Deleted ● Use Additional Character(s)

	Malignant Primary	Malignant Secondary	Ca in situ	Benign	Uncertain Behavior	Unspecified Behavior
motor tract	C72.9	C79.49	—	D33.9	D43.9	D49.7
brain	C71.9	C79.31	—	D33.2	D43.2	D49.6
cauda equina	C72.1	C79.49	—	D33.4	D43.4	D49.7
spinal	C72.0	C79.49	—	D33.4	D43.4	D49.7
mouth	C06.9	C79.89	D00.00	D10.30	D37.09	D49.0
book-leaf	C06.89	C79.89	—	—	—	—
floor	C04.9	C79.89	D00.06	D10.2	D37.09	D49.0
anterior portion	C04.0	C79.89	D00.06	D10.2	D37.09	D49.0
lateral portion	C04.1	C79.89	D00.06	D10.2	D37.09	D49.0
overlapping lesion	C04.8	—	—	—	—	—
overlapping NEC	C06.80	—	—	—	—	—
roof	C05.9	C79.89	D00.00	D10.39	D37.09	D49.0
specified part NEC	C06.89	C79.89	D00.00	D10.39	D37.09	D49.0
vestibule	C06.1	C79.89	D00.00	D10.39	D37.09	D49.0
mucosa						
alveolar (ridge or process)	C03.9	C79.89	D00.03	D10.39	D37.09	D49.0
lower	C03.1	C79.89	D00.03	D10.39	D37.09	D49.0
upper	C03.0	C79.89	D00.03	D10.39	D37.09	D49.0
buccal	C06.0	C79.89	D00.02	D10.39	D37.09	D49.0
cheek	C06.0	C79.89	D00.02	D10.39	D37.09	D49.0
lip — *see Neoplasm, lip, internal*						
nasal	C30.0	C78.39	D02.3	D14.0	D38.5	D49.1
oral	C06.0	C79.89	D00.02	D10.39	D37.09	D49.0
Mullerian duct						
female	C57.7	C79.82	D07.39	D28.7	D39.8	D49.59
male	C63.7	C79.82	D07.69	D29.8	D40.8	D49.59
muscle — *see also Neoplasm, connective tissue*						
extraocular	C69.6-•	C79.49	D09.2-•	D31.6-•	D48.7	D49.89
myocardium	C38.0	C79.89	—	D15.1	D48.7	D49.89
myometrium	C54.2	C79.82	D07.0	D26.1	D39.0	D49.59
myopericardium	C38.0	C79.89	—	D15.1	D48.7	D49.89
nabothian gland (follicle)	C53.0	C79.82	D06.0	D26.0	D39.0	D49.59
nail — *see also Neoplasm, skin, limb*	C44.90	C79.2	D04.9	D23.9	D48.5	D49.2
finger — *see also Neoplasm, skin, limb, upper*	C44.60-•	C79.2	D04.6-•	D23.6-•	D48.5	D49.2
toe — *see also Neoplasm, skin, limb, lower*	C44.70-•	C79.2	D04.7-•	D23.7-•	D48.5	D49.2
nares, naris (anterior) (posterior)	C30.0	C78.39	D02.3	D14.0	D38.5	D49.1
nasal — *see Neoplasm, nose*						
nasolabial groove — *see also Neoplasm, skin, face*	C44.309	C79.2	D04.39	D23.39	D48.5	D49.2
nasolacrimal duct	C69.5-•	C79.49	D09.2-•	D31.5-•	D48.7	D49.89

	Malignant Primary	Malignant Secondary	Ca in situ	Benign	Uncertain Behavior	Unspecified Behavior
nasopharynx, nasopharyngeal	C11.9	C79.89	D00.08	D10.6	D37.05	D49.0
floor	C11.3	C79.89	D00.08	D10.6	D37.05	D49.0
overlapping lesion	C11.8	—	—	—	—	—
roof	C11.0	C79.89	D00.08	D10.6	D37.05	D49.0
wall	C11.9	C79.89	D00.08	D10.6	D37.05	D49.0
anterior	C11.3	C79.89	D00.08	D10.6	D37.05	D49.0
lateral	C11.2	C79.89	D00.08	D10.6	D37.05	D49.0
posterior	C11.1	C79.89	D00.08	D10.6	D37.05	D49.0
superior	C11.0	C79.89	D00.08	D10.6	D37.05	D49.0
nates — *see also Neoplasm, skin, trunk*	C44.509	C79.2	D04.5	D23.5	D48.5	D49.2
neck NEC	C76.0	C79.89	D09.8	D36.7	D48.7	D49.89
skin	C44.40	—	—	—	—	—
basal cell carcinoma	C44.41	—	—	—	—	—
specified type NEC	C44.49	—	—	—	—	—
squamous cell carcinoma	C44.42	—	—	—	—	—
nerve (ganglion)	C47.9	C79.89	—	D36.10	D48.2	D49.2
abducens	C72.59	C79.49	—	D33.3	D43.3	D49.7
accessory (spinal)	C72.59	C79.49	—	D33.3	D43.3	D49.7
acoustic	C72.4-•	C79.49	—	D33.3	D43.3	D49.7
auditory	C72.4-•	C79.49	—	D33.3	D43.3	D49.7
autonomic NEC — *see also Neoplasm, nerve, peripheral*	C47.9	C79.89	—	D36.10	D48.2	D49.2
brachial	C47.1-•	C79.89	—	D36.12	D48.2	D49.2
cranial	C72.50	C79.49	—	D33.3	D43.3	D49.7
specified NEC	C72.59	C79.49	—	D33.3	D43.3	D49.7
facial	C72.59	C79.49	—	D33.3	D43.3	D49.7
femoral	C47.2-•	C79.89	—	D36.13	D48.2	D49.2
ganglion NEC — *see also Neoplasm, nerve, peripheral*	C47.9	C79.89	—	D36.10	D48.2	D49.2
glossopharyngeal	C72.59	C79.49	—	D33.3	D43.3	D49.7
hypoglossal	C72.59	C79.49	—	D33.3	D43.3	D49.7
intercostal	C47.3	C79.89	—	D36.14	D48.2	D49.2
lumbar	C47.6	C79.89	—	D36.17	D48.2	D49.2
median	C47.1-•	C79.89	—	D36.12	D48.2	D49.2
obturator	C47.2-•	C79.89	—	D36.13	D48.2	D49.2
oculomotor	C72.59	C79.49	—	D33.3	D43.3	D49.7
olfactory	C47.2-•	C79.49	—	D33.3	D43.3	D49.7
optic	C72.3-•	C79.49	—	D33.3	D43.3	D49.7
parasympathetic NEC	C47.9	C79.89	—	D36.10	D48.2	D49.2
peripheral NEC	C47.9	C79.89	—	D36.10	D48.2	D49.2
abdomen	C47.4	C79.89	—	D36.15	D48.2	D49.2
abdominal wall	C47.4	C79.89	—	D36.15	D48.2	D49.2

	Malignant Primary	Malignant Secondary	Ca in situ	Benign	Uncertain Behavior	Unspecified Behavior
nerve *(Continued)*						
peripheral NEC *(Continued)*						
ankle	C47.2●	C79.89	—	D36.13	D48.2	D49.2
antecubital fossa or space	C47.1●	C79.89	—	D36.12	D48.2	D49.2
arm	C47.1●	C79.89	—	D36.12	D48.2	D49.2
auricle (ear)	C47.0	C79.89	—	D36.11	D48.2	D49.2
axilla	C47.3	C79.89	—	D36.12	D48.2	D49.2
back	C47.6	C79.89	—	D36.17	D48.2	D49.2
buttock	C47.5	C79.89	—	D36.16	D48.2	D49.2
calf	C47.2●	C79.89	—	D36.13	D48.2	D49.2
cervical region	C47.0	C79.89	—	D36.11	D48.2	D49.2
cheek	C47.0	C79.89	—	D36.11	D48.2	D49.2
chest (wall)	C47.3	C79.89	—	D36.14	D48.2	D49.2
chin	C47.0	C79.89	—	D36.11	D48.2	D49.2
ear (external)	C47.0	C79.89	—	D36.11	D48.2	D49.2
elbow	C47.1●	C79.89	—	D36.12	D48.2	D49.2
extrarectal	C47.5	C79.89	—	D36.16	D48.2	D49.2
extremity	C47.9	C79.89	—	D36.10	D48.2	D49.2
lower	C47.2●	C79.89	—	D36.13	D48.2	D49.2
upper	C47.1●	C79.89	—	D36.12	D48.2	D49.2
eyelid	C47.0	C79.89	—	D36.11	D48.2	D49.2
face	C47.0	C79.89	—	D36.11	D48.2	D49.2
finger	C47.1●	C79.89	—	D36.12	D48.2	D49.2
flank	C47.6	C79.89	—	D36.17	D48.2	D49.2
foot	C47.2●	C79.89	—	D36.13	D48.2	D49.2
forearm	C47.1●	C79.89	—	D36.12	D48.2	D49.2
forehead	C47.0	C79.89	—	D36.11	D48.2	D49.2
gluteal region	C47.5	C79.89	—	D36.16	D48.2	D49.2
groin	C47.5	C79.89	—	D36.16	D48.2	D49.2
hand	C47.1●	C79.89	—	D36.12	D48.2	D49.2
head	C47.0	C79.89	—	D36.11	D48.2	D49.2
heel	C47.2●	C79.89	—	D36.13	D48.2	D49.2
hip	C47.2●	C79.89	—	D36.13	D48.2	D49.2
infraclavicular region	C47.3	C79.89	—	D36.14	D48.2	D49.2
inguinal (canal) (region)	C47.5	C79.89	—	D36.16	D48.2	D49.2
intrathoracic	C47.3	C79.89	—	D36.14	D48.2	D49.2
ischiorectal fossa	C47.5	C79.89	—	D36.16	D48.2	D49.2
knee	C47.2●	C79.89	—	D36.13	D48.2	D49.2
leg	C47.2●	C79.89	—	D36.13	D48.2	D49.2
limb NEC	C47.9	C79.89	—	D36.10	D48.2	D49.2
lower	C47.2●	C79.89	—	D36.13	D48.2	D49.2
upper	C47.1●	C79.89	—	D36.12	D48.2	D49.2
nates	C47.5	C79.89	—	D36.16	D48.2	D49.2
neck	C47.0	C79.89	—	D36.11	D48.2	D49.2
nerve *(Continued)*						
peripheral NEC *(Continued)*						
orbit	C69.6●	C79.49	—	D31.6●	D48.7	D49.2
pararectal	C47.5	C79.89	—	D36.16	D48.2	D49.2
paraurethral	C47.5	C79.89	—	D36.16	D48.2	D49.2
paravaginal	C47.5	C79.89	—	D36.16	D48.2	D49.2
pelvis (floor)	C47.5	C79.89	—	D36.16	D48.2	D49.2
pelvoabdominal	C47.8	C79.89	—	D36.17	D48.2	D49.2
perineum	C47.5	C79.89	—	D36.16	D48.2	D49.2
perirectal (tissue)	C47.5	C79.89	—	D36.16	D48.2	D49.2
periurethral (tissue)	C47.5	C79.89	—	D36.16	D48.2	D49.2
popliteal fossa or space	C47.2●	C79.89	—	D36.13	D48.2	D49.2
presacral	C47.5	C79.89	—	D36.16	D48.2	D49.2
pterygoid fossa	C47.0	C79.89	—	D36.11	D48.2	D49.2
rectovaginal septum or wall	C47.5	C79.89	—	D36.16	D48.2	D49.2
rectovesical	C47.5	C79.89	—	D36.16	D48.2	D49.2
sacrococcygeal region	C47.5	C79.89	—	D36.16	D48.2	D49.2
scalp	C47.0	C79.89	—	D36.11	D48.2	D49.2
scapular region	C47.3	C79.89	—	D36.14	D48.2	D49.2
shoulder	C47.1●	C79.89	—	D36.12	D48.2	D49.2
submental	C47.0	C79.89	—	D36.11	D48.2	D49.2
supraclavicular region	C47.0	C79.89	—	D36.11	D48.2	D49.2
temple	C47.0	C79.89	—	D36.11	D48.2	D49.2
temporal region	C47.0	C79.89	—	D36.11	D48.2	D49.2
thigh	C47.2●	C79.89	—	D36.13	D48.2	D49.2
thoracic (duct) (wall)	C47.3	C79.89	—	D36.14	D48.2	D49.2
thorax	C47.3	C79.89	—	D36.14	D48.2	D49.2
thumb	C47.1●	C79.89	—	D36.12	D48.2	D49.2
toe	C47.2●	C79.89	—	D36.13	D48.2	D49.2
trunk	C47.6	C79.89	—	D36.17	D48.2	D49.2
umbilicus	C47.4	C79.89	—	D36.15	D48.2	D49.2
vesicorectal	C47.5	C79.89	—	D36.16	D48.2	D49.2
wrist	C47.1●	C79.89	—	D36.12	D48.2	D49.2
radial	C47.1●	C79.89	—	D36.12	D48.2	D49.2
sacral	C47.5	C79.89	—	D36.16	D48.2	D49.2
sciatic	C47.2●	C79.89	—	D36.13	D48.2	D49.2
spinal NEC	C47.9	C79.89	—	D36.10	D48.2	D49.2
accessory	C72.59	C79.49	—	D33.3	D43.3	D49.7
sympathetic NEC — *see also Neoplasm, nerve, peripheral*	C47.9	C79.89	—	D36.10	D48.2	D49.2
trigeminal	C72.59	C79.49	—	D33.3	D43.3	D49.7
trochlear	C72.59	C79.49	—	D33.3	D43.3	D49.7
ulnar	C47.1●	C79.89	—	D36.12	D48.2	D49.2
vagus	C72.59	C79.49	—	D33.3	D43.3	D49.7

New   Revised   ~~deleted~~ Deleted   ● Use Additional Character(s)

	Malignant Primary	Malignant Secondary	Ca in situ	Benign	Uncertain Behavior	Unspecified Behavior
nervous system (central)	C72.9	C79.40	—	D33.9	D43.9	D49.7
autonomic — *see Neoplasm, nerve, peripheral*						
parasympathetic — *see Neoplasm, nerve, peripheral*						
specified site NEC	—	C79.49	—	D33.7	D43.8	—
sympathetic — *see Neoplasm, nerve, peripheral*						
nevus — *see Nevus*						
nipple	C50.0•	C79.81	D05.•	D24.•	—	—
nose, nasal	C76.0	C79.89	D09.8	D36.7	D48.7	D49.89
ala (external) (nasi) — *see also Neoplasm, nose, skin*	C44.301	C79.2	D04.39	D23.39	D48.5	D49.2
bone	C41.0	C79.51	—	D16.4•	D48.0	D49.2
cartilage	C30.0	C78.39	D02.3	D14.0	D38.5	D49.1
cavity	C30.0	C78.39	D02.3	D14.0	D38.5	D49.1
choana	C11.3	C79.89	D00.08	D10.6	D37.05	D49.0
external (skin) — *see also Neoplasm, nose, skin*	C44.301	C79.2	D04.39	D23.39	D48.5	D49.2
fossa	C30.0	C78.39	D02.3	D14.0	D38.5	D49.1
internal	C30.0	C78.39	D02.3	D14.0	D38.5	D49.1
mucosa	C30.0	C78.39	D02.3	D14.0	D38.5	D49.1
septum	C30.0	C78.39	D02.3	D14.0	D38.5	D49.1
posterior margin	C11.3	C79.89	D00.08	D10.6	D37.05	D49.0
sinus — *see Neoplasm, sinus*						
skin	C44.301	C79.2	D04.39	D23.39	D48.5	D49.2
basal cell carcinoma	C44.311	—	—	—	—	—
specified type NEC	C44.391	—	—	—	—	—
squamous cell carcinoma	C44.321	—	—	—	—	—
turbinate (mucosa)	C30.0	C78.39	D02.3	D14.0	D38.5	D49.1
bone	C41.0	C79.51	—	D16.4•	D48.0	D49.2
vestibule	C30.0	C78.39	D02.3	D14.0	D38.5	D49.1
nostril	C30.0	C78.39	D02.3	D14.0	D38.5	D49.1
nucleus pulposus	C41.2	C79.51	—	D16.6	D48.0	D49.2
occipital						
bone	C41.0	C79.51	—	D16.4•	D48.0	D49.2
lobe or pole, brain	C71.4	C79.31	—	D33.0	D43.0	D49.6
odontogenic — *see Neoplasm, jaw, bone*						
olfactory nerve or bulb	C72.2•	C79.49	—	D33.3	D43.3	D49.7
olive (brain)	C71.7	C79.31	—	D33.1	D43.1	D49.6
omentum	C48.1	C78.6	—	D20.1	D48.4	D49.0
operculum (brain)	C71.0	C79.31	—	D33.0	D43.0	D49.6
optic nerve, chiasm, or tract	C72.3•	C79.49	—	D33.3	D43.3	D49.7
oral (cavity)	C06.9	C79.89	D00.00	D10.30	D37.09	D49.0
ill-defined	C14.8	C79.89	D00.00	D10.30	D37.09	D49.0
mucosa	C06.0	C79.89	D00.02	D10.39	D37.09	D49.0
orbit	C69.6•	C79.49	D09.2•	D31.6•	D48.7	D49.89
autonomic nerve	C69.6•	C79.49	—	D31.6•	D48.7	D49.2
bone	C41.0	C79.51	—	D16.4•	D48.0	D49.2
eye	C69.6•	C79.49	D09.2•	D31.6•	D48.7	D49.89
peripheral nerves	C69.6•	C79.49	—	D31.6•	D48.7	D49.2
soft parts	C69.6•	C79.49	D09.2•	D31.6•	D48.7	D49.89
organ of Zuckerkandl	C75.5	C79.89	—	D35.6	D44.7	D49.7
oropharynx	C10.9	C79.89	D00.08	D10.5	D37.05	D49.0
branchial cleft (vestige)	C10.4	C79.89	D00.08	D10.5	D37.05	D49.0
junctional region	C10.8	C79.89	D00.08	D10.5	D37.05	D49.0
lateral wall	C10.2	C79.89	D00.08	D10.5	D37.05	D49.0
overlapping lesion	C10.8	—	—	—	—	—
pillars or fauces	C09.1	C79.89	D00.08	D10.5	D37.05	D49.0
posterior wall	C10.3	C79.89	D00.08	D10.5	D37.05	D49.0
vallecula	C10.0	C79.89	D00.08	D10.5	D37.05	D49.0
os						
external	C53.1	C79.82	D06.1	D26.0	D39.0	D49.59
internal	C53.0	C79.82	D06.0	D26.0	D39.0	D49.59
ovary	C56.•	C79.6•	D07.39	D27.•	D39.1•	D49.59
oviduct	C57.0•	C79.82	D07.39	D28.2	D39.8	D49.59
palate	C05.9	C79.89	D00.00	D10.39	D37.09	D49.0
hard	C05.0	C79.89	D00.05	D10.39	D37.09	D49.0
junction of hard and soft palate	C05.9	C79.89	D00.00	D10.39	D37.09	D49.0
overlapping lesions	C05.8	—	—	—	—	—
soft	C05.1	C79.89	D00.04	D10.39	D37.09	D49.0
nasopharyngeal surface	C11.3	C79.89	D00.08	D10.6	D37.05	D49.0
posterior surface	C11.3	C79.89	D00.08	D10.6	D37.05	D49.0
superior surface	C11.3	C79.89	D00.08	D10.6	D37.05	D49.0
palatoglossal arch	C09.1	C79.89	D00.00	D10.5	D37.09	D49.0
palatopharyngeal arch	C09.1	C79.89	D00.00	D10.5	D37.09	D49.0
pallium	C71.0	C79.31	—	D33.0	D43.0	D49.6
palpebra	C44.10•	C79.2	D04.1•	D23.1•	D48.5	D49.2
basal cell carcinoma	C44.11•	—	—	—	—	—
sebaceous cell	C44.13•	—	—	—	—	—
specified type NEC	C44.19•	—	—	—	—	—
squamous cell carcinoma	C44.12•	—	—	—	—	—
pancreas	C25.9	C78.89	D01.7	D13.6	D37.8	D49.0
body	C25.1	C78.89	D01.7	D13.6	D37.8	D49.0
duct (of Santorini) (of Wirsung)	C25.3	C78.89	D01.7	D13.6	D37.8	D49.0
ectopic tissue	C25.7	C78.89	—	D13.6	D37.8	D49.0
head	C25.0	C78.89	D01.7	D13.6	D37.8	D49.0

TABLE OF NEOPLASMS

	Malignant Primary	Malignant Secondary	Ca in situ	Benign	Uncertain Behavior	Unspecified Behavior
pancreas *(Continued)*						
islet cells	C25.4	C78.89	D01.7	D13.7	D37.8	D49.0
neck	C25.7	C78.89	D01.7	D13.6	D37.8	D49.0
overlapping lesion	C25.8	—	—	—	—	—
tail	C25.2	C78.89	D01.7	D13.6	D37.8	D49.0
para-aortic body	C75.5	C79.89	—	D35.6	D44.7	D49.7
paraganglion NEC	C75.5	C79.89	—	D35.6	D44.7	D49.7
parametrium	C57.3	C79.82	—	D28.2	D39.8	D49.59
paranephric	C48.0	C78.6	—	D20.0	D48.3	D49.0
pararectal	C76.3	C79.89	—	D36.7	D48.7	D49.89
parasagittal (region)	C76.0	C79.89	D09.8	D36.7	D48.7	D49.89
parasellar	C72.9	C79.49	—	D33.9	D43.8	D49.7
parathyroid (gland)	C75.0	C79.89	D09.3	D35.1	D44.2	D49.7
paraurethral	C76.3	C79.89	—	D36.7	D48.7	D49.89
gland	C68.1	C79.19	D09.19	D30.8	D41.8	D49.59
paravaginal	C76.3	C79.89	—	D36.7	D48.7	D49.89
parenchyma, kidney	C64.-•	C79.0-•	D09.19	D30.0-•	D41.0-•	D49.51-•
parietal						
bone	C41.0	C79.51	—	D16.4-•	D48.0	D49.2
lobe, brain	C71.3	C79.31	—	D33.0	D43.0	D49.6
paroophoron	C57.1	C79.82	D07.39	D28.2	D39.8	D49.59
parotid (duct) (gland)	C07	C79.89	D00.00	D11.0	D37.030	D49.0
parovarium	C57.1	C79.82	D07.39	D28.2	D39.8	D49.59
patella	C40.20	C79.51	—	—	—	—
peduncle, cerebral	C71.7	C79.31	—	D33.1	D43.1	D49.6
pelvirectal junction	C19	C78.5	D01.1	D12.7	D37.5	D49.0
pelvis, pelvic	C76.3	C79.89	D09.8	D36.7	D48.7	D49.89
bone	C41.4	C79.51	—	D16.8	D48.0	D49.2
floor	C76.3	C79.89	D09.8	D36.7	D48.7	D49.89
renal	C65.-•	C79.0-•	D09.19	D30.1-•	D41.1-•	D49.51-•
viscera	C76.3	C79.89	D09.8	D36.7	D48.7	D49.89
wall	C76.3	C79.89	D09.8	D36.7	D48.7	D49.89
pelvo-abdominal	C76.8	C79.89	D09.8	D36.7	D48.7	D49.89
penis	C60.9	C79.82	D07.4	D29.0	D40.8	D49.59
body	C60.2	C79.82	D07.4	D29.0	D40.8	D49.59
corpus (cavernosum)	C60.2	C79.82	D07.4	D29.0	D40.8	D49.59
glans	C60.1	C79.82	D07.4	D29.0	D40.8	D49.59
overlapping sites	C60.8	—	—	—	—	—
skin NEC	C60.9	C79.82	D07.4	D29.0	D40.8	D49.59
periadrenal (tissue)	C48.0	C78.6	—	D20.0	D48.3	D49.0
perianal (skin) — *see also Neoplasm, anus, skin*	C44.500	C79.2	D04.5	D23.5	D48.5	D49.2
pericardium	C38.0	C79.89	—	D15.1	D48.7	D49.89
perinephric	C48.0	C78.6	—	D20.0	D48.3	D49.0
perineum	C76.3	C79.89	D09.8	D36.7	D48.7	D49.89
periodontal tissue NEC	C03.9	C79.89	D00.03	D10.39	D37.09	D49.0
periosteum — *see Neoplasm, bone*						
peripancreatic	C48.0	C78.6	—	D20.0	D48.3	D49.0
peripheral nerve NEC	C47.9	C79.89	—	D36.10	D48.2	D49.2
perirectal (tissue)	C76.3	C79.89	—	D36.7	D48.7	D49.89
perirenal (tissue)	C48.0	C78.6	—	D20.0	D48.3	D49.0
peritoneum, peritoneal (cavity)	C48.2	C78.6	—	D20.1	D48.4	D49.0
benign mesothelial tissue — *see Mesothelioma, benign*						
overlapping lesion	C48.8	—	—	—	—	—
with digestive organs	C26.9	—	—	—	—	—
parietal	C48.1	C78.6	—	D20.1	D48.4	D49.0
pelvic	C48.1	C78.6	—	D20.1	D48.4	D49.0
specified part NEC	C48.1	C78.6	—	D20.1	D48.4	D49.0
peritonsillar (tissue)	C76.0	C79.89	D09.8	D36.7	D48.7	D49.89
periurethral tissue	C76.3	C79.89	—	D36.7	D48.7	D49.89
phalanges						
foot	C40.3-•	C79.51	—	D16.3-•	—	—
hand	C40.1-•	C79.51	—	D16.1-•	—	—
pharynx, pharyngeal	C14.0	C79.89	D00.08	D10.9	D37.05	D49.0
bursa	C11.1	C79.89	D00.08	D10.6	D37.05	D49.0
fornix	C11.3	C79.89	D00.08	D10.6	D37.05	D49.0
recess	C11.2	C79.89	D00.08	D10.6	D37.05	D49.0
region	C14.0	C79.89	D00.08	D10.9	D37.05	D49.0
tonsil	C11.1	C79.89	D00.08	D10.6	D37.05	D49.0
wall (lateral) (posterior)	C14.0	C79.89	D00.08	D10.9	D37.05	D49.0
pia mater	C70.9	C79.40	—	D32.9	D42.9	D49.7
cerebral	C70.0	C79.32	—	D32.0	D42.0	D49.7
cranial	C70.0	C79.32	—	D32.0	D42.0	D49.7
spinal	C70.1	C79.49	—	D32.1	D42.1	D49.7
pillars of fauces	C09.1	C79.89	D00.08	D10.5	D37.05	D49.0
pineal (body) (gland)	C75.3	C79.89	D09.3	D35.4	D44.5	D49.7
pinna (ear) NEC — *see also Neoplasm, skin, ear*	C44.20-•	C79.2	D04.2-•	D23.2-•	D48.5	D49.2
piriform fossa or sinus	C12	C79.89	D00.08	D10.7	D37.05	D49.0
pituitary (body) (fossa) (gland) (lobe)	C75.1	C79.89	D09.3	D35.2	D44.3	D49.7
placenta	C58	C79.82	D07.0	D26.7	D39.2	D49.59
pleura, pleural (cavity)	C38.4	C78.2	—	D19.0	D38.2	D49.1
overlapping lesion with heart or mediastinum	C38.8	—	—	—	—	—
parietal	C38.4	C78.2	—	D19.0	D38.2	D49.1
visceral	C38.4	C78.2	—	D19.0	D38.2	D49.1

◄ New ▪ Revised ~~deleted~~ Deleted • Use Additional Character(s)

	Malignant Primary	Malignant Secondary	Ca in situ	Benign	Uncertain Behavior	Unspecified Behavior
plexus						
brachial	C47.1-•	C79.89	—	D36.12	D48.2	D49.2
cervical	C47.0	C79.89	—	D36.11	D48.2	D49.2
choroid	C71.5	C79.31	—	D33.0	D43.0	D49.6
lumbosacral	C47.5	C79.89	—	D36.16	D48.2	D49.2
sacral	C47.5	C79.89	—	D36.16	D48.2	D49.2
pluriendocrine	C75.8	C79.89	D09.3	D35.7	D44.9	D49.7
pole						
frontal	C71.1	C79.31	—	D33.0	D43.0	D49.6
occipital	C71.4	C79.31	—	D33.0	D43.0	D49.6
pons (varolii)	C71.7	C79.31	—	D33.1	D43.1	D49.6
popliteal fossa or space	C76.5-•	C79.89	D04.7-•	D36.7	D48.7	D49.89
postcricoid (region)	C13.0	C79.89	D00.08	D10.7	D37.05	D49.0
posterior fossa (cranial)	C71.9	C79.31	—	D33.2	D43.2	D49.6
postnasal space	C11.9	C79.89	D00.08	D10.6	D37.05	D49.0
prepuce	C60.0	C79.82	D07.4	D29.0	D40.8	D49.59
prepylorus	C16.4	C78.89	D00.2	D13.1	D37.1	D49.0
presacral (region)	C76.3	C79.89	—	D36.7	D48.7	D49.89
prostate (gland)	C61	C79.82	D07.5	D29.1	D40.0	D49.59
utricle	C68.0	C79.19	D09.19	D30.4	D41.3	D49.59
pterygoid fossa	C49.0	C79.89	—	D21.0	D48.1	D49.2
pubic bone	C41.4	C79.51	—	D16.8	D48.0	D49.2
pudenda, pudendum (femaie)	C51.9	C79.82	D07.1	D28.0	D39.8	D49.59
pulmonary — *see also Neoplasm, lung*	C34.9-•	C78.0-•	D02.2-•	D14.3-•	D38.1	D49.1
putamen	C71.0	C79.31	—	D33.0	D43.0	D49.6
pyloric						
antrum	C16.3	C78.89	D00.2	D13.1	D37.1	D49.0
canal	C16.4	C78.89	D00.2	D13.1	D37.1	D49.0
pylorus	C16.4	C78.89	D00.2	D13.1	D37.1	D49.0
pyramid (brain)	C71.7	C79.31	—	D33.1	D43.1	D49.6
pyriform fossa or sinus	C12	C79.89	D00.08	D10.7	D37.05	D49.0
radius (any part)	C40.0-•	C79.51	—	D16.0-•	—	—
Rathke's pouch	C75.1	C79.89	D09.3	D35.2	D44.3	D49.7
rectosigmoid (junction)	C19	C78.5	D01.1	D12.7	D37.5	D49.0
overlapping lesion with anus or rectum	C21.8	—	—	—	—	—
rectouterine pouch	C48.1	C78.6	—	D20.1	D48.4	D49.0
rectovaginal septum or wall	C76.3	C79.89	D09.8	D36.7	D48.7	D49.89
rectovesical septum	C76.3	C79.89	D09.8	D36.7	D48.7	D49.89
rectum (ampulla)	C20	C78.5	D01.2	D12.8	D37.5	D49.0
and colon	C19	C78.5	D01.1	D12.7	D37.5	D49.0
overlapping lesion with anus or rectosigmoid junction	C21.8	—	—	—	—	—
renal	C64.-•	C79.0-•	D09.19	D30.0-•	D41.0-•	D49.51-•
calyx	C65.-•	C79.0-•	D09.19	D30.1-•	D41.1-•	D49.51-•
hilus	C65.-•	C79.0-•	D09.19	D30.1-•	D41.1-•	D49.51-•
parenchyma	C64.-•	C79.0-•	D09.19	D30.0-•	D41.0-•	D49.51-•
pelvis	C65.-•	C79.0-•	D09.19	D30.1-•	D41.1-•	D49.51-•
respiratory						
organs or system NEC	C39.9	C78.30	D02.4	D14.4	D38.6	D49.1
tract NEC	C39.9	C78.30	D02.4	D14.4	D38.5	D49.1
upper	C39.0	C78.30	D02.4	D14.4	D38.5	D49.1
retina	C69.2-•	C79.49	D09.2-•	D31.2-•	D48.7	D49.81
retrobulbar	C69.6-•	C79.49	—	D31.6-•	D48.7	D49.89
retrocecal	C48.0	C78.6	—	D20.0	D48.3	D49.0
retromolar (area) (triangle) (trigone)	C06.2	C79.89	D00.00	D10.39	D37.09	D49.0
retro-orbital	C76.0	C79.89	D09.8	D36.7	D48.7	D49.89
retroperitoneal (space) (tissue)	C48.0	C78.6	—	D20.0	D48.3	D49.0
retroperitoneum	C48.0	C78.6	—	D20.0	D48.3	D49.0
retropharyngeal	C14.0	C79.89	D00.08	D10.9	D37.05	D49.0
retrovesical (septum)	C76.3	C79.89	D09.8	D36.7	D48.7	D49.89
rhinencephalon	C71.0	C79.31	—	D33.0	D43.0	D49.6
rib	C41.3	C79.51	—	D16.7	D48.0	D49.2
Rosenmuller's fossa	C11.2	C79.89	D00.08	D10.6	D37.05	D49.0
round ligament	C57.2	C79.82	—	D28.2	D39.8	D49.59
sacrococcyx, sacrococcygeal	C41.4	C79.51	—	D16.8	D48.0	D49.2
region	C76.3	C79.89	D09.8	D36.7	D48.7	D49.89
sacrouterine ligament	C57.3	C79.82	—	D28.2	D39.8	D49.59
sacrum, sacral (vertebra)	C41.4	C79.51	—	D16.8	D48.0	D49.2
salivary gland or duct (major)	C08.9	C79.89	D00.00	D11.9	D37.039	D49.0
minor NEC	C06.9	C79.89	D00.00	D10.39	D37.04	D49.0
overlapping lesion	C08.9	—	—	—	—	—
parotid	C07	C79.89	D00.00	D11.0	D37.030	D49.0
pluriglandular	C08.9	C79.89	D00.00	D11.9	D37.039	D49.0
sublingual	C08.1	C79.89	D00.00	D11.7	D37.031	D49.0
submandibular	C08.0	C79.89	D00.00	D11.7	D37.032	D49.0
submaxillary	C08.0	C79.89	D00.00	D11.7	D37.032	D49.0
salpinx (uterine)	C57.0-•	C79.82	D07.39	D28.2	D39.8	D49.59
Santorini's duct	C25.3	C78.89	D01.7	D13.6	D37.8	D49.0
scalp	C44.40	C79.2	D04.4	D23.4	D48.5	D49.2
basal cell carcinoma	C44.41	—	—	—	—	—
specified type NEC	C44.49	—	—	—	—	—
squamous cell carcinoma	C44.42	—	—	—	—	—
scapula (any part)	C40.0-•	C79.51	—	D16.0-•	—	—
scapular region	C76.1	C79.89	D09.8	D36.7	D48.7	D49.89

	Malignant Primary	Malignant Secondary	Ca in situ	Benign	Uncertain Behavior	Unspecified Behavior
scar NEC — *see also Neoplasm, skin, by site*	C44.90	C79.2	D04.9	D23.9	D48.5	D49.2
sciatic nerve	C47.2-●	C79.89	—	D36.13	D48.2	D49.2
sclera	C69.4-●	C79.49	D09.2-●	D31.4-●	D48.7	D49.89
scrotum (skin)	C63.2	C79.82	D07.61	D29.4	D40.8	D49.59
sebaceous gland — *see Neoplasm, skin*						
sella turcica	C75.1	C79.89	D09.3	D35.2	D44.3	D49.7
bone	C41.0	C79.51	—	D16.4-●	D48.0	D49.2
semilunar cartilage (knee)	C40.2-●	C79.51	—	D16.2-●	D48.0	D49.2
seminal vesicle	C63.7	C79.82	D07.69	D29.8	D40.8	D49.59
septum						
nasal	C30.0	C78.39	D02.3	D14.0	D38.5	D49.1
posterior margin	C11.3	C79.89	D00.08	D10.6	D37.05	D49.0
rectovaginal	C76.3	C79.89	D09.8	D36.7	D48.7	D49.89
rectovesical	C76.3	C79.89	D09.8	D36.7	D48.7	D49.89
urethrovaginal	C57.9	C79.82	D07.30	D28.9	D39.9	D49.59
vesicovaginal	C57.9	C79.82	D07.30	D28.9	D39.9	D49.59
shoulder NEC	C76.4-●	C79.89	D04.6-●	D36.7	D48.7	D49.89
sigmoid flexure (lower) (upper)	C18.7	C78.5	D01.0	D12.5	D37.4	D49.0
sinus (accessory)	C31.9	C78.39	D02.3	D14.0	D38.5	D49.1
bone (any)	C41.0	C79.51	—	D16.4-●	D48.0	D49.2
ethmoidal	C31.1	C78.39	D02.3	D14.0	D38.5	D49.1
frontal	C31.2	C78.39	D02.3	D14.0	D38.5	D49.1
maxillary	C31.0	C78.39	D02.3	D14.0	D38.5	D49.1
nasal, paranasal NEC	C31.9	C78.39	D02.3	D14.0	D38.5	D49.1
overlapping lesion	C31.8	—	—	—	—	—
pyriform	C12	C79.89	D00.08	D10.7	D37.05	D49.0
sphenoid	C31.3	C78.39	D02.3	D14.0	D38.5	D49.1
skeleton, skeletal NEC	C41.9	C79.51	—	D16.9-●	D48.0	D49.2
Skene's gland	C68.1	C79.19	D09.19	D30.8	D41.8	D49.59
skin NOS	C44.90	C79.2	D04.9	D23.9	D48.5	D49.2
abdominal wall	C44.509	C79.2	D04.5	D23.5	D48.5	D49.2
basal cell carcinoma	C44.519	—	—	—	—	—
specified type NEC	C44.599	—	—	—	—	—
squamous cell carcinoma	C44.529	—	—	—	—	—
ala nasi — *see also Neoplasm, nose, skin*	C44.301	C79.2	D04.39	D23.39	D48.5	D49.2
ankle — *see also Neoplasm, skin, limb, lower*	C44.70-●	C79.2	D04.7-●	D23.7-●	D48.5	D49.2
antecubital space — *see also Neoplasm, skin, limb, upper*	C44.60-●	C79.2	D04.6-●	D23.6-●	D48.5	D49.2
skin NOS *(Continued)*						
anus	C44.500	C79.2	D04.5	D23.5	D48.5	D49.2
basal cell carcinoma	C44.510	—	—	—	—	—
specified type NEC	C44.590	—	—	—	—	—
squamous cell carcinoma	C44.520	—	—	—	—	—
arm — *see also Neoplasm, skin, limb, upper*	C44.60-●	C79.2	D04.6-●	D23.6-●	D48.5	D49.2
auditory canal (external) — *see also Neoplasm, skin, ear*	C44.20-●	C79.2	D04.2-●	D23.2-●	D48.5	D49.2
auricle (ear) — *see also Neoplasm, skin, ear*	C44.20-●	C79.2	D04.2-●	D23.2-●	D48.5	D49.2
auricular canal (external) — *see also Neoplasm, skin, ear*	C44.20-●	C79.2	D04.2-●	D23.2-●	D48.5	D49.2
axilla, axillary fold — *see also Neoplasm, skin, trunk*	C44.509	C79.2	D04.5	D23.5	D48.5	D49.2
back — *see also Neoplasm, skin, trunk*	C44.509	C79.2	D04.5	D23.5	D48.5	D49.2
basal cell carcinoma	C44.91					
breast	C44.501	C79.2	D04.5	D23.5	D48.5	D49.2
basal cell carcinoma	C44.511	—	—	—	—	—
specified type NEC	C44.591	—	—	—	—	—
squamous cell carcinoma	C44.521	—	—	—	—	—
brow — *see also Neoplasm, skin, face*	C44.309	C79.2	D04.39	D23.39	D48.5	D49.2
buttock — *see also Neoplasm, skin, trunk*	C44.509	C79.2	D04.5	D23.5	D48.5	D49.2
calf — *see also Neoplasm, skin, limb, lower*	C44.70-●	C79.2	D04.7-●	D23.7-●	D48.5	D49.2
canthus (eye) (inner) (outer)	C44.10-●	C79.2	D04.1-●	D23.1-●	D48.5	D49.2
basal cell carcinoma	C44.11-●	—	—	—	—	—
sebaceous cell	C44.13-●	—	—	—	—	—
specified type NEC	C44.19-●	—	—	—	—	—
squamous cell carcinoma	C44.12-●	—	—	—	—	—
cervical region — *see also Neoplasm, skin, neck*	C44.40	C79.2	D04.4	D23.4	D48.5	D49.2
cheek (external) — *see also Neoplasm, skin, face*	C44.309	C79.2	D04.39	D23.39	D48.5	D49.2
chest (wall) — *see also Neoplasm, skin, trunk*	C44.509	C79.2	D04.5	D23.5	D48.5	D49.2
chin — *see also Neoplasm, skin, face*	C44.309	C79.2	D04.39	D23.39	D48.5	D49.2
clavicular area — *see also Neoplasm, skin, trunk*	C44.509	C79.2	D04.5	D23.5	D48.5	D49.2
clitoris	C51.2	C79.82	D07.1	D28.0	D39.8	D49.59

TABLE OF NEOPLASMS

◀ New ⬅ Revised ~~deleted~~ Deleted ● Use Additional Character(s)

	Malignant Primary	Malignant Secondary	Ca in situ	Benign	Uncertain Behavior	Unspecified Behavior
skin NOS *(Continued)*						
columnella — *see also Neoplasm, skin, face*	C44.309	C79.2	D04.39	D23.39	D48.5	D49.2
concha — *see also Neoplasm, skin, ear*	C44.20-●	C79.2	D04.2-●	D23.2-●	D48.5	D49.2
ear (external)	C44.20-●	C79.2	D04.2-●	D23.2-●	D48.5	D49.2
basal cell carcinoma	C44.21-●	—	—	—	—	—
specified type NEC	C44.29-●	—	—	—	—	—
squamous cell carcinoma	C44.22-●	—	—	—	—	—
elbow — *see also Neoplasm, skin, limb, upper*	C44.60-●	C79.2	D04.6-●	D23.6-●	D48.5	D49.2
eyebrow — *see also Neoplasm, skin, face*	C44.309	C79.2	D04.39	D23.39	D48.5	D49.2
eyelid	C44.10-●	C79.2	D04.1-●	D23.1-●	D48.5	D49.2
basal cell carcinoma	C44.11-●	—	—	—	—	—
sebaceous cell	C44.13-●	—	—	—	—	—
specified type NEC	C44.19-●	—	—	—	—	—
squamous cell carcinoma	C44.12-●	—	—	—	—	—
face NOS	C44.300	C79.2	D04.30	D23.30	D48.5	D49.2
basal cell carcinoma	C44.310	—	—	—	—	—
specified type NEC	C44.390	—	—	—	—	—
squamous cell carcinoma	C44.320	—	—	—	—	—
female genital organs (external)	C51.9	C79.82	D07.1	D28.0	D39.8	D49.59
clitoris	C51.2	C79.82	D07.1	D28.0	D39.8	D49.59
labium NEC	C51.9	C79.82	D07.1	D28.0	D39.8	D49.59
majus	C51.0	C79.82	D07.1	D28.0	D39.8	D49.59
minus	C51.1	C79.82	D07.1	D28.0	D39.8	D49.59
pudendum	C51.9	C79.82	D07.1	D28.0	D39.8	D49.59
vulva	C51.9	C79.82	D07.1	D28.0	D39.8	D49.59
finger — *see also Neoplasm, skin, limb, upper*	C44.60-●	C79.2	D04.6-●	D23.6-●	D48.5	D49.2
flank — *see also Neoplasm, skin, trunk*	C44.509	C79.2	D04.5	D23.5	D48.5	D49.2
foot — *see also Neoplasm, skin, limb, lower*	C44.70-●	C79.2	D04.7-●	D23.7-●	D48.5	D49.2
forearm — *see also Neoplasm, skin, limb, upper*	C44.60-●	C79.2	D04.6-●	D23.6-●	D48.5	D49.2
forehead — *see also Neoplasm, skin, face*	C44.309	C79.2	D04.39	D23.39	D48.5	D49.2
glabella — *see also Neoplasm, skin, face*	C44.309	C79.2	D04.39	D23.39	D48.5	D49.2
gluteal region — *see also Neoplasm, skin, trunk*	C44.509	C79.2	D04.5	D23.5	D48.5	D49.2
groin — *see also Neoplasm, skin, trunk*	C44.509	C79.2	D04.5	D23.5	D48.5	D49.2

	Malignant Primary	Malignant Secondary	Ca in situ	Benign	Uncertain Behavior	Unspecified Behavior
skin NOS *(Continued)*						
hand — *see also Neoplasm, skin, limb, upper*	C44.60-●	C79.2	D04.6-●	D23.6-●	D48.5	D49.2
head NEC — *see also Neoplasm, skin, scalp*	C44.40	C79.2	D04.4	D23.4	D48.5	D49.2
heel — *see also Neoplasm, skin, limb, lower*	C44.70-●	C79.2	D04.7-●	D23.7-●	D48.5	D49.2
helix — *see also Neoplasm, skin, ear*	C44.20-●	C79.2	D04.2-●	D23.2-●	D48.5	D49.2
hip — *see also Neoplasm, skin, limb, lower*	C44.70-●	C79.2	D04.7-●	D23.7-●	D48.5	D49.2
infraclavicular region — *see also Neoplasm, skin, trunk*	C44.509	C79.2	D04.5	D23.5	D48.5	D49.2
inguinal region — *see also Neoplasm, skin, trunk*	C44.509	C79.2	D04.5	D23.5	D48.5	D49.2
jaw — *see also Neoplasm, skin, face*	C44.309	C79.2	D04.39	D23.39	D48.5	D49.2
Kaposi's sarcoma — *see Kaposi's, sarcoma, skin*						
knee — *see also Neoplasm, skin, limb, lower*	C44.70-●	C79.2	D04.7-●	D23.7-●	D48.5	D49.2
labia						
majora	C51.0	C79.82	D07.1	D28.0	D39.8	D49.59
minora	C51.1	C79.82	D07.1	D28.0	D39.8	D49.59
leg — *see also Neoplasm, skin, limb, lower*	C44.70-●	C79.2	D04.7-●	D23.7-●	D48.5	D49.2
lid (lower) (upper)	C44.10-●	C79.2	D04.1-●	D23.1-●	D48.5	D49.2
basal cell carcinoma	C44.11-●	—	—	—	—	—
sebaceous cell	C44.13-●	—	—	—	—	—
specified type NEC	C44.19-●	—	—	—	—	—
squamous cell carcinoma	C44.12-●	—	—	—	—	—
limb NEC	C44.90	C79.2	D04.9	D23.9	D48.5	D49.2
basal cell carcinoma	C44.91					
lower	C44.70-●	C79.2	D04.7-●	D23.7-●	D48.5	D49.2
basal cell carcinoma	C44.71-●	—	—	—	—	—
specified type NEC	C44.79-●	—	—	—	—	—
squamous cell carcinoma	C44.72-●	—	—	—	—	—
upper	C44.60-●	C79.2	D04.6-●	D23.6-●	D48.5	D49.2
basal cell carcinoma	C44.61-●	—	—	—	—	—
specified type NEC	C44.69-●	—	—	—	—	—
squamous cell carcinoma	C44.62-●	—	—	—	—	—
lip (lower) (upper)	C44.00	C79.2	D04.0	D23.0	D48.5	D49.2
basal cell carcinoma	C44.01	—	—	—	—	—
specified type NEC	C44.09	—	—	—	—	—
squamous cell carcinoma	C44.02	—	—	—	—	—

TABLE OF NEOPLASMS

	Malignant Primary	Malignant Secondary	Ca in situ	Benign	Uncertain Behavior	Unspecified Behavior
skin NOS *(Continued)*						
male genital organs	C63.9	C79.82	D07.60	D29.9	D40.8	D49.59
penis	C60.9	C79.82	D07.4	D29.0	D40.8	D49.59
prepuce	C60.0	C79.82	D07.4	D29.0	D40.8	D49.59
scrotum	C63.2	C79.82	D07.61	D29.4	D40.8	D49.59
mastectomy site (skin) — *see also Neoplasm, skin, breast*	C44.501	C79.2	—	—	—	—
specified as breast tissue	C50.8-•	C79.81	—	—	—	—
meatus, acoustic (external) — *see also Neoplasm, skin, ear*	C44.20-•	C79.2	D04.2-•	D23.2-•	D48.5	D49.2
melanotic — *see Melanoma*						
Merkel cell — *see Carcinoma, Merkel cell*						
nates — *see also Neoplasm, skin, trunk*	C44.509	C79.2	D04.5	D23.5	D48.5	D49.2
neck	C44.40	C79.2	D04.4	D23.4	D48.5	D49.2
basal cell carcinoma	C44.41	—	—	—	—	—
specified type NEC	C44.49	—	—	—	—	—
squamous cell carcinoma	C44.42	—	—	—	—	—
nevus — *see Nevus, skin*						
nose (external) — *see also Neoplasm, nose, skin*	C44.301	C79.2	D04.39	D23.39	D48.5	D49.2
overlapping lesion	C44.80	—	—	—	—	—
basal cell carcinoma	C44.81	—	—	—	—	—
specified type NEC	C44.89	—	—	—	—	—
squamous cell carcinoma	C44.82	—	—	—	—	—
palm — *see also Neoplasm, skin, limb, upper*	C44.60-•	C79.2	D04.6-•	D23.6-•	D48.5	D49.2
palpebra	C44.10-•	C79.2	D04.1-•	D23.1-•	D48.5	D49.2
basal cell carcinoma	C44.11-•	—	—	—	—	—
sebaceous cell	C44.13-•	—	—	—	—	—
specified type NEC	C44.19-•	—	—	—	—	—
squamous cell carcinoma	C44.12-•	—	—	—	—	—
penis NEC	C60.9	C79.82	D07.4	D29.0	D40.8	D49.59
perianal — *see also Neoplasm, skin, anus*	C44.500	C79.2	D04.5	D23.5	D48.5	D49.2
perineum — *see also Neoplasm, skin, anus*	C44.500	C79.2	D04.5	D23.5	D48.5	D49.2
pinna — *see also Neoplasm, skin, ear*	C44.20-•	C79.2	D04.2-•	D23.2-•	D48.5	D49.2
plantar — *see also Neoplasm, skin, limb, lower*	C44.70-•	C79.2	D04.7-•	D23.7-•	D48.5	D49.2
popliteal fossa or space — *see also Neoplasm, skin, limb, lower*	C44.70-•	C79.2	D04.7-•	D23.7-•	D48.5	D49.2
skin NOS *(Continued)*						
prepuce	C60.0	C79.82	D07.4	D29.0	D40.8	D49.59
pubes — *see also Neoplasm, skin, trunk*	C44.509	C79.2	D04.5	D23.5	D48.5	D49.2
sacrococcygeal region — *see also Neoplasm, skin, trunk*	C44.509	C79.2	D04.5	D23.5	D48.5	D49.2
scalp	C44.40	C79.2	D04.4	D23.4	D48.5	D49.2
basal cell carcinoma	C44.41	—	—	—	—	—
specified type NEC	C44.49	—	—	—	—	—
squamous cell carcinoma	C44.42	—	—	—	—	—
scapular region — *see also Neoplasm, skin, trunk*	C44.509	C79.2	D04.5	D23.5	D48.5	D49.2
scrotum	C63.2	C79.82	D07.61	D29.4	D40.8	D49.59
shoulder — *see also Neoplasm, skin, limb, upper*	C44.60-•	C79.2	D04.6-•	D23.6-•	D48.5	D49.2
sole (foot) — *see also Neoplasm, skin, limb, lower*	C44.70-•	C79.2	D04.7-•	D23.7-•	D48.5	D49.2
specified sites NEC	C44.80	C79.2	D04.8	D23.9	D48.5	D49.2
basal cell carcinoma	C44.81	—	—	—	—	—
specified type NEC	C44.89	—	—	—	—	—
squamous cell carcinoma	C44.82	—	—	—	—	—
specified type NEC	C44.99	—	—	—	—	—
squamous cell carcinoma	C44.92	—	—	—	—	—
submammary fold — *see also Neoplasm, skin, trunk*	C44.509	C79.2	D04.5	D23.5	D48.5	D49.2
supraclavicular region — *see also Neoplasm, skin, neck*	C44.40	C79.2	D04.4	D23.4	D48.5	D49.2
temple — *see also Neoplasm, skin, face*	C44.309	C79.2	D04.39	D23.39	D48.5	D49.2
thigh — *see also Neoplasm, skin, limb, lower*	C44.70-•	C79.2	D04.7-•	D23.7-•	D48.5	D49.2
thoracic wall — *see also Neoplasm, skin, trunk*	C44.509	C79.2	D04.5	D23.5	D48.5	D49.2
thumb — *see also Neoplasm, skin, limb, upper*	C44.60-•	C79.2	D04.6-•	D23.6-•	D48.5	D49.2
toe — *see also Neoplasm, skin, limb, lower*	C44.70-•	C79.2	D04.7-•	D23.7-•	D48.5	D49.2
tragus — *see also Neoplasm, skin, ear*	C44.20-•	C79.2	D04.2-•	D23.2-•	D48.5	D49.2
trunk	C44.509	C79.2	D04.5	D23.5	D48.5	D49.2
basal cell carcinoma	C44.519	—	—	—	—	—
specified type NEC	C44.599	—	—	—	—	—
squamous cell carcinoma	C44.529	—	—	—	—	—
umbilicus — *see also Neoplasm, skin, trunk*	C44.509	C79.2	D04.5	D23.5	D48.5	D49.2

◀ New ▮ Revised ~~deleted~~ Deleted • Use Additional Character(s)

	Malignant Primary	Malignant Secondary	Ca in situ	Benign	Uncertain Behavior	Unspecified Behavior
skin NOS *(Continued)*						
vulva	C51.9	C79.82	DØ7.1	D28.Ø	D39.8	D49.59
overlapping lesion	C51.8	—	—	—	—	—
wrist—*see also Neoplasm, skin, limb, upper*	C44.6Ø-●	C79.2	DØ4.6-●	D23.6-●	D48.5	D49.2
skull	C41.Ø	C79.51	—	D16.4-●	D48.Ø	D49.2
soft parts or tissues—*see Neoplasm, connective tissue*						
specified site NEC	C76.8	C79.89	DØ9.8	D36.7	D48.7	D49.89
spermatic cord	C63.1-●	C79.82	DØ7.69	D29.8	D4Ø.8	D49.59
sphenoid	C31.3	C78.39	DØ2.3	D14.Ø	D38.5	D49.1
bone	C41.Ø	C79.51	—	D16.4-●	D48.Ø	D49.2
sinus	C31.3	C78.39	DØ2.3	D14.Ø	D38.5	D49.1
sphincter						
anal	C21.1	C78.5	DØ1.3	D12.9	D37.8	D49.Ø
of Oddi	C24.Ø	C78.89	DØ1.5	D13.5	D37.6	D49.Ø
spine, spinal (column)	C41.2	C79.51	—	D16.6	D48.Ø	D49.2
bulb	C71.7	C79.31	—	D33.1	D43.1	D49.6
coccyx	C41.4	C79.51	—	D16.8	D48.Ø	D49.2
cord (cervical) (lumbar) (sacral) (thoracic)	C72.Ø	C79.49	—	D33.4	D43.4	D49.7
dura mater	C7Ø.1	C79.49	—	D32.1	D42.1	D49.7
lumbosacral	C41.2	C79.51	—	D16.6	D48.Ø	D49.2
marrow NEC	C96.9	C79.52	—	—	D47.9	D49.89
membrane	C7Ø.1	C79.49	—	D32.1	D42.1	D49.7
meninges	C7Ø.1	C79.49	—	D32.1	D42.1	D49.7
nerve (root)	C47.9	C79.89	—	D36.1Ø	D48.2	D49.2
pia mater	C7Ø.1	C79.49	—	D32.1	D42.1	D49.7
root	C47.9	C79.89	—	D36.1Ø	D48.2	D49.2
sacrum	C41.4	C79.51	—	D16.8	D48.Ø	D49.2
spleen, splenic NEC	C26.1	C78.89	DØ1.7	D13.99	D37.8	D49.Ø
flexure (colon)	C18.5	C78.5	DØ1.Ø	D12.3	D37.4	D49.Ø
stem, brain	C71.7	C79.31	—	D33.1	D43.1	D49.6
Stensen's duct	CØ7	C79.89	DØØ.ØØ	D11.Ø	D37.Ø3Ø	D49.Ø
sternum	C41.3	C79.51	—	D16.7	D48.Ø	D49.2
stomach	C16.9	C78.89	DØØ.2	D13.1	D37.1	D49.Ø
antrum (pyloric)	C16.3	C78.89	DØØ.2	D13.1	D37.1	D49.Ø
body	C16.2	C78.89	DØØ.2	D13.1	D37.1	D49.Ø
cardia	C16.Ø	C78.89	DØØ.2	D13.1	D37.1	D49.Ø
cardiac orifice	C16.Ø	C78.89	DØØ.2	D13.1	D37.1	D49.Ø
corpus	C16.2	C78.89	DØØ.2	D13.1	D37.1	D49.Ø
fundus	C16.1	C78.89	DØØ.2	D13.1	D37.1	D49.Ø
greater curvature NEC	C16.6	C78.89	DØØ.2	D13.1	D37.1	D49.Ø
lesser curvature NEC	C16.5	C78.89	DØØ.2	D13.1	D37.1	D49.Ø
stomach *(Continued)*						
overlapping lesion	C16.8	—	—	—	—	—
prepylorus	C16.4	C78.89	DØØ.2	D13.1	D37.1	D49.Ø
pylorus	C16.4	C78.89	DØØ.2	D13.1	D37.1	D49.Ø
wall NEC	C16.9	C78.89	DØØ.2	D13.1	D37.1	D49.Ø
anterior NEC	C16.8	C78.89	DØØ.2	D13.1	D37.1	D49.Ø
posterior NEC	C16.8	C78.89	DØØ.2	D13.1	D37.1	D49.Ø
stroma, endometrial	C54.1	C79.82	DØ7.Ø	D26.1	D39.Ø	D49.59
stump, cervical	C53.8	C79.82	DØ6.7	D26.Ø	D39.Ø	D49.59
subcutaneous (nodule) (tissue) NEC—*see Neoplasm, connective tissue*						
subdural	C7Ø.9	C79.32	—	D32.9	D42.9	D49.7
subglottis, subglottic	C32.2	C78.39	DØ2.Ø	D14.1	D38.Ø	D49.1
sublingual	CØ4.9	C79.89	DØØ.Ø6	D1Ø.2	D37.Ø9	D49.Ø
gland or duct	CØ8.1	C79.89	DØØ.ØØ	D11.7	D37.Ø31	D49.Ø
submandibular gland	CØ8.Ø	C79.89	DØØ.ØØ	D11.7	D37.Ø32	D49.Ø
submaxillary gland or duct	CØ8.Ø	C79.89	DØØ.ØØ	D11.7	D37.Ø32	D49.Ø
submental	C76.Ø	C79.89	DØ9.8	D36.7	D48.7	D49.89
subpleural	C34.9-●	C78.Ø-●	DØ2.2-●	D14.3-●	D38.1	D49.1
substernal	C38.1	C78.1	—	D15.2	D38.3	D49.89
sudoriferous, sudoriparous gland, site unspecified	C44.9Ø	C79.2	DØ4.9	D23.9	D48.5	D49.2
specified site—*see Neoplasm, skin*						
supraclavicular region	C76.Ø	C79.89	DØ9.8	D36.7	D48.7	D49.89
supraglottis	C32.1	C78.39	DØ2.Ø	D14.1	D38.Ø	D49.1
suprarenal	C74.9-●	C79.7-●	DØ9.3	D35.Ø-●	D44.1-●	D49.7
capsule	C74.9-●	C79.7-●	DØ9.3	D35.Ø-●	D44.1-●	D49.7
cortex	C74.Ø-●	C79.7-●	DØ9.3	D35.Ø-●	D44.1-●	D49.7
gland	C74.9-●	C79.7-●	DØ9.3	D35.Ø-●	D44.1-●	D49.7
medulla	C74.1-●	C79.7-●	DØ9.3	D35.Ø-●	D44.1-●	D49.7
suprasellar (region)	C71.9	C79.31	—	D33.2	D43.2	D49.6
supratentorial (brain) NEC	C71.Ø	C79.31	—	D33.Ø	D43.Ø	D49.6
sweat gland (apocrine) (eccrine), site unspecified	C44.9Ø	C79.2	DØ4.9	D23.9	D48.5	D49.2
specified site—*see Neoplasm, skin*						
sympathetic nerve or nervous system NEC	C47.9	C79.89	—	D36.1Ø	D48.2	D49.2
symphysis pubis	C41.4	C79.51	—	D16.8	D48.Ø	D49.2
synovial membrane—*see Neoplasm, connective tissue*						
tapetum, brain	C71.8	C79.31	—	D33.2	D43.2	D49.6

TABLE OF NEOPLASMS

	Malignant Primary	Malignant Secondary	Ca in situ	Benign	Uncertain Behavior	Unspecified Behavior
tarsus (any bone)	C40.3•	C79.51	—	D16.3•	—	—
temple (skin)—*see also Neoplasm, skin, face*	C44.309	C79.2	D04.39	D23.39	D48.5	D49.2
temporal						
bone	C41.0	C79.51	—	D16.4•	D48.0	D49.2
lobe or pole	C71.2	C79.31	—	D33.0	D43.0	D49.6
region	C76.0	C79.89	D09.8	D36.7	D48.7	D49.89
skin—*see also Neoplasm, skin, face*	C44.309	C79.2	D04.39	D23.39	D48.5	D49.2
tendon (sheath)—*see Neoplasm, connective tissue*						
tentorium (cerebelli)	C70.0	C79.32	—	D32.0	D42.0	D49.7
testis, testes	C62.9•	C79.82	D07.69	D29.2•	D40.1•	D49.59
descended	C62.1•	C79.82	D07.69	D29.2•	D40.1•	D49.59
ectopic	C62.0•	C79.82	D07.69	D29.2•	D40.1•	D49.59
retained	C62.0•	C79.82	D07.69	D29.2•	D40.1•	D49.59
scrotal	C62.1•	C79.82	D07.69	D29.2•	D40.1•	D49.59
undescended	C62.0•	C79.82	D07.69	D29.2•	D40.1•	D49.59
unspecified whether descended or undescended	C62.9•	C79.82	D07.69	D29.2•	D40.1•	D49.59
thalamus	C71.0	C79.31	—	D33.0	D43.0	D49.6
thigh NEC	C76.5•	C79.89	D04.7•	D36.7	D48.7	D49.89
thorax, thoracic (cavity) (organs NEC)	C76.1	C79.89	D09.8	D36.7	D48.7	D49.89
duct	C49.3	C79.89	—	D21.3	D48.1	D49.2
wall NEC	C76.1	C79.89	D09.8	D36.7	D48.7	D49.89
throat	C14.0	C79.89	D00.08	D10.9	D37.05	D49.0
thumb NEC	C76.4•	C79.89	D04.6•	D36.7	D48.7	D49.89
thymus (gland)	C37	C79.89	D09.3	D15.0	D38.4	D49.89
thyroglossal duct	C73	C79.89	D09.3	D34	D44.0	D49.7
thyroid (gland)	C73	C79.89	D09.3	D34	D44.0	D49.7
cartilage	C32.3	C78.39	D02.0	D14.1	D38.0	D49.1
tibia (any part)	C40.2•	C79.51	—	D16.2•	—	—
toe NEC	C76.5•	C79.89	D04.7•	D36.7	D48.7	D49.89
tongue	C02.9	C79.89	D00.07	D10.1	D37.02	D49.0
anterior (two-thirds) NEC	C02.3	C79.89	D00.07	D10.1	D37.02	D49.0
dorsal surface	C02.0	C79.89	D00.07	D10.1	D37.02	D49.0
ventral surface	C02.2	C79.89	D00.07	D10.1	D37.02	D49.0
base (dorsal surface)	C01	C79.89	D00.07	D10.1	D37.02	D49.0
border (lateral)	C02.1	C79.89	D00.07	D10.1	D37.02	D49.0
dorsal surface NEC	C02.0	C79.89	D00.07	D10.1	D37.02	D49.0
fixed part NEC	C01	C79.89	D00.07	D10.1	D37.02	D49.0
foreamen cecum	C02.0	C79.89	D00.07	D10.1	D37.02	D49.0
frenulum linguae	C02.2	C79.89	D00.07	D10.1	D37.02	D49.0

	Malignant Primary	Malignant Secondary	Ca in situ	Benign	Uncertain Behavior	Unspecified Behavior
tongue *(Continued)*						
junctional zone	C02.8	C79.89	D00.07	D10.1	D37.02	D49.0
margin (lateral)	C02.1	C79.89	D00.07	D10.1	D37.02	D49.0
midline NEC	C02.0	C79.89	D00.07	D10.1	D37.02	D49.0
mobile part NEC	C02.3	C79.89	D00.07	D10.1	D37.02	D49.0
overlapping lesion	C02.8	—	—	—	—	—
posterior (third)	C01	C79.89	D00.07	D10.1	D37.02	D49.0
root	C01	C79.89	D00.07	D10.1	D37.02	D49.0
surface (dorsal)	C02.0	C79.89	D00.07	D10.1	D37.02	D49.0
base	C01	C79.89	D00.07	D10.1	D37.02	D49.0
ventral	C02.2	C79.89	D00.07	D10.1	D37.02	D49.0
tip	C02.1	C79.89	D00.07	D10.1	D37.02	D49.0
tonsil	C02.4	C79.89	D00.07	D10.1	D37.02	D49.0
tonsil	C09.9	C79.89	D00.08	D10.4	D37.05	D49.0
fauces, faucial	C09.9	C79.89	D00.08	D10.4	D37.05	D49.0
lingual	C02.4	C79.89	D00.07	D10.1	D37.02	D49.0
overlapping sites	C09.8	—	—	—	—	—
palatine	C09.9	C79.89	D00.08	D10.4	D37.05	D49.0
pharyngeal	C11.1	C79.89	D00.08	D10.6	D37.05	D49.0
pillar (anterior) (posterior)	C09.1	C79.89	D00.08	D10.5	D37.05	D49.0
tonsillar fossa	C09.0	C79.89	D00.08	D10.5	D37.05	D49.0
tooth socket NEC	C03.9	C79.89	D00.03	D10.39	D37.09	D49.0
trachea (cartilage) (mucosa)	C33	C78.39	D02.1	D14.2	D38.1	D49.1
overlapping lesion with bronchus or lung	C34.8•	—	—	—	—	—
tracheobronchial	C34.8•	C78.39	D02.1	D14.2	D38.1	D49.1
overlapping lesion with lung	C34.8•	—	—	—	—	—
tragus—*see also Neoplasm, skin, ear*	C44.20•	C79.2	D04.2•	D23.2•	D48.5	D49.2
trunk NEC	C76.8	C79.89	D04.5	D36.7	D48.7	D49.89
tubo-ovarian	C57.8	C79.82	D07.39	D28.7	D39.8	D49.59
tunica vaginalis	C63.7	C79.82	D07.69	D29.8	D40.8	D49.59
turbinate (bone)	C41.0	C79.51	—	D16.4•	D48.0	D49.2
nasal	C30.0	C78.39	D02.3	D14.0	D38.5	D49.1
tympanic cavity	C30.1	C78.39	D02.3	D14.0	D38.5	D49.1
ulna (any part)	C40.0•	C79.51	—	D16.0•	—	—
umbilicus, umbilical—*see also Neoplasm, skin, trunk*	C44.509	C79.2	D04.5	D23.5	D48.5	D49.2
uncus, brain	C71.2	C79.31	—	D33.0	D43.0	D49.6
unknown site or unspecified	C80.1	C79.9	D09.9	D36.9	D48.9	D49.9
urachus	C67.7	C79.11	D09.0	D30.3	D41.4	D49.4
ureter, ureteral	C66.•	C79.19	D09.19	D30.2•	D41.2•	D49.59
orifice (bladder)	C67.6	C79.11	D09.0	D30.3	D41.4	D49.4
ureter-bladder (junction)	C67.6	C79.11	D09.0	D30.3	D41.4	D49.4

TABLE OF NEOPLASMS

◄ New ◄ Revised ~~deleted~~ Deleted • Use Additional Character(s)

	Malignant Primary	Malignant Secondary	Ca in situ	Benign	Uncertain Behavior	Unspecified Behavior
urethra, urethral (gland)	C68.0	C79.19	D09.19	D30.4	D41.3	D49.59
orifice, internal	C67.5	C79.11	D09.0	D30.3	D41.4	D49.4
urethrovaginal (septum)	C57.9	C79.82	D07.30	D28.9	D39.8	D49.59
urinary organ or system	C68.9	C79.10	D09.10	D30.9	D41.9	D49.59
bladder — *see Neoplasm, bladder*						
overlapping lesion	C68.8	—	—	—	—	—
specified sites NEC	C68.8	C79.19	D09.19	D30.8	D41.8	D49.59
utero-ovarian	C57.8	C79.82	D07.39	D28.7	D39.8	D49.59
ligament	C57.1	C79.82	D07.39	D28.2	D39.8	D49.59
uterosacral ligament	C57.3	C79.82	—	D28.2	D39.8	D49.59
uterus, uteri, uterine	C55	C79.82	D07.0	D26.9	D39.0	D49.59
adnexa NEC	C57.4	C79.82	D07.39	D28.7	D39.8	D49.59
body	C54.9	C79.82	D07.0	D26.1	D39.0	D49.59
cervix	C53.9	C79.82	D06.9	D26.0	D39.0	D49.59
cornu	C54.9	C79.82	D07.0	D26.1	D39.0	D49.59
corpus	C54.9	C79.82	D07.0	D26.1	D39.0	D49.59
endocervix (canal) (gland)	C53.0	C79.82	D06.0	D26.0	D39.0	D49.59
endometrium	C54.1	C79.82	D07.0	D26.1	D39.0	D49.59
exocervix	C53.1	C79.82	D06.1	D26.0	D39.0	D49.59
external os	C53.1	C79.82	D06.1	D26.0	D39.0	D49.59
fundus	C54.3	C79.82	D07.0	D26.1	D39.0	D49.59
internal os	C53.0	C79.82	D06.0	D26.0	D39.0	D49.59
isthmus	C54.0	C79.82	D07.0	D26.1	D39.0	D49.59
ligament	C57.3	C79.82	—	D28.2	D39.8	D49.59
broad	C57.1	C79.82	D07.39	D28.2	D39.8	D49.59
round	C57.2	C79.82	—	D28.2	D39.8	D49.59
lower segment	C54.0	C79.82	D07.0	D26.1	D39.0	D49.59
myometrium	C54.2	C79.82	D07.0	D26.1	D39.0	D49.59
overlapping sites	C54.8	—	—	—	—	—
squamocolumnar junction	C53.8	C79.82	D06.7	D26.0	D39.0	D49.59
tube	C57.0	C79.82	D07.39	D28.2	D39.8	D49.59
utricle, prostatic	C68.0	C79.19	D09.19	D30.4	D41.3	D49.59
uveal tract	C69.4	C79.49	D09.2	D31.4	D48.7	D49.89
uvula	C05.2	C79.89	D00.04	D10.39	D37.09	D49.0
vagina, vaginal (fornix) (vault) (wall)	C52	C79.82	D07.2	D28.1	D39.8	D49.59
vaginovesical	C57.9	C79.82	D07.30	D28.9	D39.9	D49.59
septum	C57.9	C79.82	D07.30	D28.9	D39.9	D49.59
vallecula (epiglottis)	C10.0	C79.89	D00.08	D10.5	D37.05	D49.0
vas deferens	C63.1	C79.82	D07.69	D29.8	D40.8	D49.59
vascular — *see Neoplasm, connective tissue*						
Vater's ampulla	C24.1	C78.89	D01.5	D13.5	D37.6	D49.0
vein, venous — *see Neoplasm, connective tissue*						
vena cava (abdominal) (inferior)	C49.4	C79.89	—	D21.4	D48.1	D49.2
superior	C49.3	C79.89	—	D21.3	D48.1	D49.2
ventricle (cerebral) (floor) (lateral) (third)	C71.5	C79.31	—	D33.0	D43.0	D49.6
cardiac (left) (right)	C38.0	C79.89	—	D15.1	D48.7	D49.89
fourth	C71.7	C79.31	—	D33.1	D43.1	D49.6
ventricular band of larynx	C32.1	C78.39	D02.0	D14.1	D38.0	D49.1
ventriculus — *see Neoplasm, stomach*						
vermillion border — *see Neoplasm, lip*						
vermis, cerebellum	C71.6	C79.31	—	D33.1	D43.1	D49.6
vertebra (column)	C41.2	C79.51	—	D16.6	D48.0	D49.2
coccyx	C41.4	C79.51	—	D16.8	D48.0	D49.2
marrow NEC	C96.9	C79.52	—	—	D47.9	D49.89
sacrum	C41.4	C79.51	—	D16.8	D48.0	D49.2
vesical — *see Neoplasm, bladder*						
vesicle, seminal	C63.7	C79.82	D07.69	D29.8	D40.8	D49.59
vesicocervical tissue	C57.9	C79.82	D07.30	D28.9	D39.9	D49.59
vesicorectal	C76.3	C79.82	D09.8	D36.7	D48.7	D49.89
vesicovaginal	C57.9	C79.82	D07.30	D28.9	D39.9	D49.59
septum	C57.9	C79.82	D07.30	D28.9	D39.8	D49.59
vessel (blood) — *see Neoplasm, connective tissue*						
vestibular gland, greater	C51.0	C79.82	D07.1	D28.0	D39.8	D49.59
vestibule						
mouth	C06.1	C79.89	D00.00	D10.39	D37.09	D49.0
nose	C30.0	C78.39	D02.3	D14.0	D38.5	D49.1
Virchow's gland	C77.0	C77.0	—	D36.0	D48.7	D49.89
viscera NEC	C76.8	C79.89	D09.8	D36.7	D48.7	D49.89
vocal cords (true)	C32.0	C78.39	D02.0	D14.1	D38.0	D49.1
false	C32.1	C78.39	D02.0	D14.1	D38.0	D49.1
vomer	C41.0	C79.51	—	D16.4	D48.0	D49.2
vulva	C51.9	C79.82	D07.1	D28.0	D39.8	D49.59
vulvovaginal gland	C51.0	C79.82	D07.1	D28.0	D39.8	D49.59
Waldeyer's ring	C14.2	C79.89	D00.08	D10.9	D37.05	D49.0
Wharton's duct	C08.0	C79.89	D00.00	D11.7	D37.032	D49.0
white matter (central) (cerebral)	C71.0	C79.31	—	D33.0	D43.0	D49.6
windpipe	C33	C78.39	D02.1	D14.2	D38.1	D49.1

	Malignant Primary	Malignant Secondary	Ca in situ	Benign	Uncertain Behavior	Unspecified Behavior
Wirsung's duct	C25.3	C78.89	DØ1.7	D13.6	D37.8	D49.Ø
wolffian (body) (duct)						
female	C57.7	C79.82	DØ7.39	D28.7	D39.8	D49.59
male	C63.7	C79.82	DØ7.69	D29.8	D4Ø.8	D49.59

	Malignant Primary	Malignant Secondary	Ca in situ	Benign	Uncertain Behavior	Unspecified Behavior
womb — *see Neoplasm, uterus*						
wrist NEC	C76.4-•	C79.89	DØ4.6-•	D36.7	D48.7	D49.89
xiphoid process	C41.3	C79.51	—	D16.7	D48.Ø	D49.2
Zuckerkandl organ	C75.5	C79.89	—	D35.6	D44.7	D49.7

TABLE OF NEOPLASMS

New Revised ~~deleted~~ Deleted • Use Additional Character(s)

TOD

ICD-10-CM Table of Drugs and Chemicals

Substance	External Cause (T-Code) Poisoning, Accidental (Unintentional)	Poisoning, Intentional Self-Harm	Poisoning, Assault	Poisoning, Undetermined	Adverse Effect	Underdosing
#						
1-propanol	T51.3X1	T51.3X2	T51.3X3	T51.3X4	—	—
2-propanol	T51.2X1	T51.2X2	T51.2X3	T51.2X4	—	—
2,4-D (dichlorophen-oxyacetic acid)	T60.3X1	T60.3X2	T60.3X3	T60.3X4	—	—
2,4-toluene diisocyanate	T65.0X1	T65.0X2	T65.0X3	T65.0X4	—	—
2,4,5-T (trichloro-phenoxyacetic acid)	T60.1X1	T60.1X2	T60.1X3	T60.1X4	—	—
3,4-methylenedioxy-methamphetamine	T43.641	T43.642	T43.643	T43.644	—	—
14-hydroxydihydro-morphinone	T40.2X1	T40.2X2	T40.2X3	T40.2X4	T40.2X5	T40.2X6
A						
ABOB	T37.5X1	T37.5X2	T37.5X3	T37.5X4	T37.5X5	T37.5X6
Abrine	T62.2X1	T62.2X2	T62.2X3	T62.2X4	—	—
Abrus (seed)	T62.2X1	T62.2X2	T62.2X3	T62.2X4	—	—
Absinthe	T51.0X1	T51.0X2	T51.0X3	T51.0X4	—	—
beverage	T51.0X1	T51.0X2	T51.0X3	T51.0X4	—	—
Acaricide	T60.8X1	T60.8X2	T60.8X3	T60.8X4	—	—
Acebutolol	T44.7X1	T44.7X2	T44.7X3	T44.7X4	T44.7X5	T44.7X6
Acecarbromal	T42.6X1	T42.6X2	T42.6X3	T42.6X4	T42.6X5	T42.6X6
Aceclidine	T44.1X1	T44.1X2	T44.1X3	T44.1X4	T44.1X5	T44.1X6
Acedapsone	T37.0X1	T37.0X2	T37.0X3	T37.0X4	T37.0X5	T37.0X6
Acefylline piperazine	T48.6X1	T48.6X2	T48.6X3	T48.6X4	T48.6X5	T48.6X6
Acemorphan	T40.2X1	T40.2X2	T40.2X3	T40.2X4	T40.2X5	T40.2X6
Acenocoumarin	T45.511	T45.512	T45.513	T45.514	T45.515	T45.516
Acenocoumarol	T45.511	T45.512	T45.513	T45.514	T45.515	T45.516
Acepifylline	T48.6X1	T48.6X2	T48.6X3	T48.6X4	T48.6X5	T48.6X6
Acepromazine	T43.3X1	T43.3X2	T43.3X3	T43.3X4	T43.3X5	T43.3X6
Acesulfamethoxypyridazine	T37.0X1	T37.0X2	T37.0X3	T37.0X4	T37.0X5	T37.0X6
Acetal	T52.8X1	T52.8X2	T52.8X3	T52.8X4	—	—
Acetaldehyde (vapor)	T52.8X1	T52.8X2	T52.8X3	T52.8X4	—	—
liquid	T65.891	T65.892	T65.893	T65.894	—	—
P-Acetamidophenol	T39.1X1	T39.1X2	T39.1X3	T39.1X4	T39.1X5	T39.1X6
Acetaminophen	T39.1X1	T39.1X2	T39.1X3	T39.1X4	T39.1X5	T39.1X6
Acetaminosalol	T39.1X1	T39.1X2	T39.1X3	T39.1X4	T39.1X5	T39.1X6
Acetanilide	T39.1X1	T39.1X2	T39.1X3	T39.1X4	T39.1X5	T39.1X6
Acetarsol	T37.3X1	T37.3X2	T37.3X3	T37.3X4	T37.3X5	T37.3X6
Acetazolamide	T50.2X1	T50.2X2	T50.2X3	T50.2X4	T50.2X5	T50.2X6
Acetiamine	T45.2X1	T45.2X2	T45.2X3	T45.2X4	T45.2X5	T45.2X6
Acetic						
acid	T54.2X1	T54.2X2	T54.2X3	T54.2X4	—	—
with sodium acetate (ointment)	T49.3X1	T49.3X2	T49.3X3	T49.3X4	T49.3X5	T49.3X6
Acetic *(Continued)*						
acid *(Continued)*						
ester (solvent) (vapor)	T52.8X1	T52.8X2	T52.8X3	T52.8X4	—	—
irrigating solution	T50.3X1	T50.3X2	T50.3X3	T50.3X4	T50.3X5	T50.3X6
medicinal (lotion)	T49.2X1	T49.2X2	T49.2X3	T49.2X4	T49.2X5	T49.2X6
anhydride	T65.891	T65.892	T65.893	T65.894	—	—
ether (vapor)	T52.8X1	T52.8X2	T52.8X3	T52.8X4	—	—
Acetohexamide	T38.3X1	T38.3X2	T38.3X3	T38.3X4	T38.3X5	T38.3X6
Acetohydroxamic acid	T50.991	T50.992	T50.993	T50.994	T50.995	T50.996
Acetomenaphthone	T45.7X1	T45.7X2	T45.7X3	T45.7X4	T45.7X5	T45.7X6
Acetomorphine	T40.1X1	T40.1X2	T40.1X3	T40.1X4	—	—
Acetone (oils)	T52.4X1	T52.4X2	T52.4X3	T52.4X4	—	—
chlorinated	T52.4X1	T52.4X2	T52.4X3	T52.4X4	—	—
vapor	T52.4X1	T52.4X2	T52.4X3	T52.4X4	—	—
Acetonitrile	T52.8X1	T52.8X2	T52.8X3	T52.8X4	—	—
Acetophenazine	T43.3X1	T43.3X2	T43.3X3	T43.3X4	T43.3X5	T43.3X6
Acetophenetedin	T39.1X1	T39.1X2	T39.1X3	T39.1X4	T39.1X5	T39.1X6
Acetophenone	T52.4X1	T52.4X2	T52.4X3	T52.4X4	—	—
Acetorphine	T40.2X1	T40.2X2	T40.2X3	T40.2X4	—	—
Acetosulfone (sodium)	T37.1X1	T37.1X2	T37.1X3	T37.1X4	T37.1X5	T37.1X6
Acetrizoate (sodium)	T50.8X1	T50.8X2	T50.8X3	T50.8X4	T50.8X5	T50.8X6
Acetylcarbromal	T42.6X1	T42.6X2	T42.6X3	T42.6X4	T42.6X5	T42.6X6
Acetrizoic acid	T50.8X1	T50.8X2	T50.8X3	T50.8X4	T50.8X5	T50.8X6
Acetyl						
bromide	T53.6X1	T53.6X2	T53.6X3	T53.6X4	—	—
chloride	T53.6X1	T53.6X2	T53.6X3	T53.6X4	—	—
Acetylcholine						
chloride	T44.1X1	T44.1X2	T44.1X3	T44.1X4	T44.1X5	T44.1X6
derivative	T44.1X1	T44.1X2	T44.1X3	T44.1X4	T44.1X5	T44.1X6
Acetylcysteine	T48.4X1	T48.4X2	T48.4X3	T48.4X4	T48.4X5	T48.4X6
Acetyldigitoxin	T46.0X1	T46.0X2	T46.0X3	T46.0X4	T46.0X5	T46.0X6
Acetyldigoxin	T46.0X1	T46.0X2	T46.0X3	T46.0X4	T46.0X5	T46.0X6
Acetyldihydrocodeine	T40.2X1	T40.2X2	T40.2X3	T40.2X4	—	—
Acetyldihydrocodeinone	T40.2X1	T40.2X2	T40.2X3	T40.2X4	—	—
Acetylene (gas)	T59.891	T59.892	T59.893	T59.894	—	—
dichloride	T53.6X1	T53.6X2	T53.6X3	T53.6X4	—	—
incomplete combustion of	T58.11	T58.12	T58.13	T58.14	—	—
industrial	T59.891	T59.892	T59.893	T59.894	—	—
tetrachloride	T53.6X1	T53.6X2	T53.6X3	T53.6X4	—	—
vapor	T53.6X1	T53.6X2	T53.6X3	T53.6X4	—	—
Acetylphenylhydrazine	T39.8X1	T39.8X2	T39.8X3	T39.8X4	T39.8X5	T39.8X6
Acetylpheneturide	T42.6X1	T42.6X2	T42.6X3	T42.6X4	T42.6X5	T42.6X6

◀ New ◀ Revised ~~deleted~~ Deleted

Substance	External Cause (T-Code) Poisoning, Accidental (Unintentional)	Poisoning, Intentional Self-Harm	Poisoning, Assault	Poisoning, Undetermined	Adverse Effect	Underdosing
Acetylsalicylic acid (salts)	T39.011	T39.012	T39.013	T39.014	T39.015	T39.016
enteric coated	T39.011	T39.012	T39.013	T39.014	T39.015	T39.016
Acetylsulfamethoxypyridazine	T37.0X1	T37.0X2	T37.0X3	T37.0X4	T37.0X5	T37.0X6
Achromycin	T36.4X1	T36.4X2	T36.4X3	T36.4X4	T36.4X5	T36.4X6
ophthalmic preparation	T49.5X1	T49.5X2	T49.5X3	T49.5X4	T49.5X5	T49.5X6
topical NEC	T49.0X1	T49.0X2	T49.0X3	T49.0X4	T49.0X5	T49.0X6
Aciclovir	T37.5X1	T37.5X2	T37.5X3	T37.5X4	T37.5X5	T37.5X6
Acid (corrosive) NEC	T54.2X1	T54.2X2	T54.2X3	T54.2X4	—	—
Acidifying agent NEC	T50.901	T50.902	T50.903	T50.904	T50.905	T50.906
Acipimox	T46.6X1	T46.6X2	T46.6X3	T46.6X4	T46.6X5	T46.6X6
Acitretin	T50.991	T50.992	T50.993	T50.994	T50.995	T50.996
Aclarubicin	T45.1X1	T45.1X2	T45.1X3	T45.1X4	T45.1X5	T45.1X6
Aclatonium napadisilate	T48.1X1	T48.1X2	T48.1X3	T48.1X4	T48.1X5	T48.1X6
Aconite (wild)	T46.991	T46.992	T46.993	T46.994	T46.995	T46.996
Aconitine	T46.991	T46.992	T46.993	T46.994	T46.995	T46.996
Aconitum ferox	T46.991	T46.992	T46.993	T46.994	T46.995	T46.996
Acridine	T65.6X1	T65.6X2	T65.6X3	T65.6X4	—	—
vapor	T59.891	T59.892	T59.893	T59.894	—	—
Acriflavine	T37.91	T37.92	T37.93	T37.94	T37.95	T37.96
Acriflavinium chloride	T49.0X1	T49.0X2	T49.0X3	T49.0X4	T49.0X5	T49.0X6
Acrinol	T49.0X1	T49.0X2	T49.0X3	T49.0X4	T49.0X5	T49.0X6
Acrisorcin	T49.0X1	T49.0X2	T49.0X3	T49.0X4	T49.0X5	T49.0X6
Acrivastine	T45.0X1	T45.0X2	T45.0X3	T45.0X4	T45.0X5	T45.0X6
Acrolein (gas)	T59.891	T59.892	T59.893	T59.894	—	—
liquid	T54.1X1	T54.1X2	T54.1X3	T54.1X4	—	—
Acrylamide	T65.891	T65.892	T65.893	T65.894	—	—
Acrylic resin	T49.3X1	T49.3X2	T49.3X3	T49.3X4	T49.3X5	T49.3X6
Acrylonitrile	T65.891	T65.892	T65.893	T65.894	—	—
Actaea spicata	T62.2X1	T62.2X2	T62.2X3	T62.2X4	—	—
berry	T62.1X1	T62.1X2	T62.1X3	T62.1X4	—	—
Acterol	T37.3X1	T37.3X2	T37.3X3	T37.3X4	T37.3X5	T37.3X6
ACTH	T38.811	T38.812	T38.813	T38.814	T38.815	T38.816
Actinomycin C	T45.1X1	T45.1X2	T45.1X3	T45.1X4	T45.1X5	T45.1X6
Actinomycin D	T45.1X1	T45.1X2	T45.1X3	T45.1X4	T45.1X5	T45.1X6
Activated charcoal — *see also Charcoal, medicinal*	T47.6X1	T47.6X2	T47.6X3	T47.6X4	T47.6X5	T47.6X6
Acyclovir	T37.5X1	T37.5X2	T37.5X3	T37.5X4	T37.5X5	T37.5X6
Adenine	T45.2X1	T45.2X2	T45.2X3	T45.2X4	T45.2X5	T45.2X6
arabinoside	T37.5X1	T37.5X2	T37.5X3	T37.5X4	T37.5X5	T37.5X6
Adenosine (phosphate)	T46.2X1	T46.2X2	T46.2X3	T46.2X4	T46.2X5	T46.2X6
ADH	T38.891	T38.892	T38.893	T38.894	T38.895	T38.896
Adhesive NEC	T65.891	T65.892	T65.893	T65.894	—	—

Substance	External Cause (T-Code) Poisoning, Accidental (Unintentional)	Poisoning, Intentional Self-Harm	Poisoning, Assault	Poisoning, Undetermined	Adverse Effect	Underdosing
Adicillin	T36.0X1	T36.0X2	T36.0X3	T36.0X4	T36.0X5	T36.0X6
Adiphenine	T44.3X1	T44.3X2	T44.3X3	T44.3X4	T44.3X5	T44.3X6
Adipiodone	T50.8X1	T50.8X2	T50.8X3	T50.8X4	T50.8X5	T50.8X6
Adjunct, pharmaceutical	T50.901	T50.902	T50.903	T50.904	T50.905	T50.906
Adrenal (extract, cortex or medulla) (glucocorticoids) (hormones) (mineralo corticoids)	T38.0X1	T38.0X2	T38.0X3	T38.0X4	T38.0X5	T38.0X6
ENT agent	T49.6X1	T49.6X2	T49.6X3	T49.6X4	T49.6X5	T49.6X6
ophthalmic preparation	T49.5X1	T49.5X2	T49.5X3	T49.5X4	T49.5X5	T49.5X6
topical NEC	T49.0X1	T49.0X2	T49.0X3	T49.0X4	T49.0X5	T49.0X6
Adrenaline	T44.5X1	T44.5X2	T44.5X3	T44.5X4	T44.5X5	T44.5X6
Adrenalin — *see Adrenaline*						
Adrenergic NEC	T44.901	T44.902	T44.903	T44.904	T44.905	T44.906
blocking agent NEC	T44.8X1	T44.8X2	T44.8X3	T44.8X4	T44.8X5	T44.8X6
beta, heart	T44.7X1	T44.7X2	T44.7X3	T44.7X4	T44.7X5	T44.7X6
specified NEC	T44.991	T44.992	T44.993	T44.994	T44.995	T44.996
Adrenochrome						
(mono) semicarbazone	T46.991	T46.992	T46.993	T46.994	T46.995	T46.996
derivative	T46.991	T46.992	T46.993	T46.994	T46.995	T46.996
Adrenocorticotrophic hormone	T38.811	T38.812	T38.813	T38.814	T38.815	T38.816
Adrenocorticotrophin	T38.811	T38.812	T38.813	T38.814	T38.815	T38.816
Adriamycin	T45.1X1	T45.1X2	T45.1X3	T45.1X4	T45.1X5	T45.1X6
Aerosol spray NEC	T65.91	T65.92	T65.93	T65.94	—	—
Aerosporin	T36.8X1	T36.8X2	T36.8X3	T36.8X4	T36.8X5	T36.8X6
ENT agent	T49.6X1	T49.6X2	T49.6X3	T49.6X4	T49.6X5	T49.6X6
ophthalmic preparation	T49.5X1	T49.5X2	T49.5X3	T49.5X4	T49.5X5	T49.5X6
topical NEC	T49.0X1	T49.0X2	T49.0X3	T49.0X4	T49.0X5	T49.0X6
Aethusa cynapium	T62.2X1	T62.2X2	T62.2X3	T62.2X4	—	—
Afghanistan black	T40.711	T40.712	T40.713	T40.714	T40.715	T40.716
Aflatoxin	T64.01	T64.02	T64.03	T64.04	—	—
Afloqualone	T42.8X1	T42.8X2	T42.8X3	T42.8X4	T42.8X5	T42.8X6
African boxwood	T62.2X1	T62.2X2	T62.2X3	T62.2X4	—	—
Agar	T47.4X1	T47.4X2	T47.4X3	T47.4X4	T47.4X5	T47.4X6
Agonist						
predominantly						
alpha-adrenoreceptor	T44.4X1	T44.4X2	T44.4X3	T44.4X4	T44.4X5	T44.4X6
beta-adrenoreceptor	T44.5X1	T44.5X2	T44.5X3	T44.5X4	T44.5X5	T44.5X6
Agricultural agent NEC	T65.91	T65.92	T65.93	T65.94	—	—
Agrypnal	T42.3X1	T42.3X2	T42.3X3	T42.3X4	T42.3X5	T42.3X6
AHLG	T50.Z11	T50.Z12	T50.Z13	T50.Z14	T50.Z15	T50.Z16
Air contaminant(s), source/type NOS	T65.91	T65.92	T65.93	T65.94	—	—

Substance	External Cause (T-Code) Poisoning, Accidental (Unintentional)	Poisoning, Intentional Self-Harm	Poisoning, Assault	Poisoning, Undetermined	Adverse Effect	Underdosing
Ajmaline	T46.2X1	T46.2X2	T46.2X3	T46.2X4	T46.2X5	T46.2X6
Akritoin	T37.8X1	T37.8X2	T37.8X3	T37.8X4	T37.8X5	T37.8X6
Akee	T62.1X1	T62.1X2	T62.1X3	T62.1X4	—	—
Akrinol	T49.ØX1	T49.ØX2	T49.ØX3	T49.ØX4	T49.ØX5	T49.ØX6
Alacepril	T46.4X1	T46.4X2	T46.4X3	T46.4X4	T46.4X5	T46.4X6
Alantolactone	T37.4X1	T37.4X2	T37.4X3	T37.4X4	T37.4X5	T37.4X6
Albamycin	T36.8X1	T36.8X2	T36.8X3	T36.8X4	T36.8X5	T36.8X6
Albendazole	T37.4X1	T37.4X2	T37.4X3	T37.4X4	T37.4X5	T37.4X6
Albumin						
bovine	T45.8X1	T45.8X2	T45.8X3	T45.8X4	T45.8X5	T45.8X6
human serum	T45.8X1	T45.8X2	T45.8X3	T45.8X4	T45.8X5	T45.8X6
salt-poor	T45.8X1	T45.8X2	T45.8X3	T45.8X4	T45.8X5	T45.8X6
normal human serum	T45.8X1	T45.8X2	T45.8X3	T45.8X4	T45.8X5	T45.8X6
Albuterol	T48.6X1	T48.6X2	T48.6X3	T48.6X4	T48.6X5	T48.6X6
Albutoin	T42.ØX1	T42.ØX2	T42.ØX3	T42.ØX4	T42.ØX5	T42.ØX6
Alclometasone	T49.ØX1	T49.ØX2	T49.ØX3	T49.ØX4	T49.ØX5	T49.ØX6
Alcohol	T51.91	T51.92	T51.93	T51.94	—	—
absolute	T51.ØX1	T51.ØX2	T51.ØX3	T51.ØX4	—	—
beverage	T51.ØX1	T51.ØX2	T51.ØX3	T51.ØX4	—	—
allyl	T51.8X1	T51.8X2	T51.8X3	T51.8X4	—	—
amyl	T51.3X1	T51.3X2	T51.3X3	T51.3X4	—	—
antifreeze	T51.1X1	T51.1X2	T51.1X3	T51.1X4	—	—
beverage	T51.ØX1	T51.ØX2	T51.ØX3	T51.ØX4	—	—
butyl	T51.3X1	T51.3X2	T51.3X3	T51.3X4	—	—
dehydrated	T51.ØX1	T51.ØX2	T51.ØX3	T51.ØX4	—	—
beverage	T51.ØX1	T51.ØX2	T51.ØX3	T51.ØX4	—	—
denatured	T51.ØX1	T51.ØX2	T51.ØX3	T51.ØX4	—	—
deterrent NEC	T5Ø.6X1	T5Ø.6X2	T5Ø.6X3	T5Ø.6X4	T5Ø.6X5	T5Ø.6X6
diagnostic (gastric function)	T5Ø.8X1	T5Ø.8X2	T5Ø.8X3	T5Ø.8X4	T5Ø.8X5	T5Ø.8X6
ethyl	T51.ØX1	T51.ØX2	T51.ØX3	T51.ØX4	—	—
beverage	T51.ØX1	T51.ØX2	T51.ØX3	T51.ØX4	—	—
grain	T51.ØX1	T51.ØX2	T51.ØX3	T51.ØX4	—	—
beverage	T51.ØX1	T51.ØX2	T51.ØX3	T51.ØX4	—	—
industrial	T51.ØX1	T51.ØX2	T51.ØX3	T51.ØX4	—	—
isopropyl	T51.2X1	T51.2X2	T51.2X3	T51.2X4	—	—
methyl	T51.1X1	T51.1X2	T51.1X3	T51.1X4	—	—
preparation for consumption	T51.ØX1	T51.ØX2	T51.ØX3	T51.ØX4	—	—
propyl	T51.3X1	T51.3X2	T51.3X3	T51.3X4	—	—
secondary	T51.2X1	T51.2X2	T51.2X3	T51.2X4	—	—
radiator	T51.1X1	T51.1X2	T51.1X3	T51.1X4	—	—
rubbing	T51.2X1	T51.2X2	T51.2X3	T51.2X4	—	—
specified type NEC	T51.8X1	T51.8X2	T51.8X3	T51.8X4	—	—

Substance	External Cause (T-Code) Poisoning, Accidental (Unintentional)	Poisoning, Intentional Self-Harm	Poisoning, Assault	Poisoning, Undetermined	Adverse Effect	Underdosing
Alcohol *(Continued)*						
surgical	T51.ØX1	T51.ØX2	T51.ØX3	T51.ØX4	—	—
vapor (from any type of Alcohol)	T59.891	T59.892	T59.893	T59.894	—	—
wood	T51.1X1	T51.1X2	T51.1X3	T51.1X4	—	—
Alcuronium (chloride)	T48.1X1	T48.1X2	T48.1X3	T48.1X4	T48.1X5	T48.1X6
Aldactone	T5Ø.ØX1	T5Ø.ØX2	T5Ø.ØX3	T5Ø.ØX4	T5Ø.ØX5	T5Ø.ØX6
Aldesulfone sodium	T37.1X1	T37.1X2	T37.1X3	T37.1X4	T37.1X5	T37.1X6
Aldicarb	T6Ø.ØX1	T6Ø.ØX2	T6Ø.ØX3	T6Ø.ØX4	—	—
Aldomet	T46.5X1	T46.5X2	T46.5X3	T46.5X4	T46.5X5	T46.5X6
Aldosterone	T5Ø.ØX1	T5Ø.ØX2	T5Ø.ØX3	T5Ø.ØX4	T5Ø.ØX5	T5Ø.ØX6
Aldrin (dust)	T6Ø.1X1	T6Ø.1X2	T6Ø.1X3	T6Ø.1X4	—	—
Aleve — *see Naproxen*						
Alexitol sodium	T47.1X1	T47.1X2	T47.1X3	T47.1X4	T47.1X5	T47.1X6
Alfacalcidol	T45.2X1	T45.2X2	T45.2X3	T45.2X4	T45.2X5	T45.2X6
Alfadolone	T41.1X1	T41.1X2	T41.1X3	T41.1X4	T41.1X5	T41.1X6
Alfaxalone	T41.1X1	T41.1X2	T41.1X3	T41.1X4	T41.1X5	T41.1X6
Alfentanil	T4Ø.411	T4Ø.412	T4Ø.413	T4Ø.414	T4Ø.415	T4Ø.416
Alfuzosin (hydrochloride)	T44.8X1	T44.8X2	T44.8X3	T44.8X4	T44.8X5	T44.8X6
Algae (harmful) (toxin)	T65.821	T65.822	T65.823	T65.824	—	—
Algeldrate	T47.1X1	T47.1X2	T47.1X3	T47.1X4	T47.1X5	T47.1X6
Algin	T47.8X1	T47.8X2	T47.8X3	T47.8X4	T47.8X5	T47.8X6
Alglucerase	T45.3X1	T45.3X2	T45.3X3	T45.3X4	T45.3X5	T45.3X6
Alidase	T45.3X1	T45.3X2	T45.3X3	T45.3X4	T45.3X5	T45.3X6
Alimemazine	T43.3X1	T43.3X2	T43.3X3	T43.3X4	T43.3X5	T43.3X6
Aliphatic thiocyanates	T65.ØX1	T65.ØX2	T65.ØX3	T65.ØX4	—	—
Alizapride	T45.ØX1	T45.ØX2	T45.ØX3	T45.ØX4	T45.ØX5	T45.ØX6
Alkali (caustic)	T54.3X1	T54.3X2	T54.3X3	T54.3X4	—	—
Alkalizing agent NEC	T5Ø.9Ø1	T5Ø.9Ø2	T5Ø.9Ø3	T5Ø.9Ø4	T5Ø.9Ø5	T5Ø.9Ø6
Alkaline antiseptic solution (aromatic)	T49.6X1	T49.6X2	T49.6X3	T49.6X4	T49.6X5	T49.6X6
Alkalinizing agents (medicinal)	T5Ø.9Ø1	T5Ø.9Ø2	T5Ø.9Ø3	T5Ø.9Ø4	T5Ø.9Ø5	T5Ø.9Ø6
Alka-seltzer	T39.Ø11	T39.Ø12	T39.Ø13	T39.Ø14	T39.Ø15	T39.Ø16
Alkavervir	T46.5X1	T46.5X2	T46.5X3	T46.5X4	T46.5X5	T46.5X6
Alkonium (bromide)	T49.ØX1	T49.ØX2	T49.ØX3	T49.ØX4	T49.ØX5	T49.ØX6
Alkylating drug NEC	T45.1X1	T45.1X2	T45.1X3	T45.1X4	T45.1X5	T45.1X6
antimyeloproliferative	T45.1X1	T45.1X2	T45.1X3	T45.1X4	T45.1X5	T45.1X6
lymphatic	T45.1X1	T45.1X2	T45.1X3	T45.1X4	T45.1X5	T45.1X6
Alkylisocyanate	T65.ØX1	T65.ØX2	T65.ØX3	T65.ØX4	—	—
Allantoin	T49.411	T49.412	T49.413	T49.414	T49.415	T49.416
Allegron	T43.ØX1	T43.ØX2	T43.ØX3	T43.ØX4	T43.ØX5	T43.ØX6
Allethrin	T49.ØX1	T49.ØX2	T49.ØX3	T49.ØX4	T49.ØX5	T49.ØX6
Allobarbital	T42.3X1	T42.3X2	T42.3X3	T42.3X4	T42.3X5	T42.3X6

	External Cause (T-Code)					
Substance	Poisoning, Accidental (Unintentional)	Poisoning, Intentional Self-Harm	Poisoning, Assault	Poisoning, Undetermined	Adverse Effect	Underdosing
Allopurinol	T5Ø.4X1	T5Ø.4X2	T5Ø.4X3	T5Ø.4X4	T5Ø.4X5	T5Ø.4X6
Allyl						
alcohol	T51.8X1	T51.8X2	T51.8X3	T51.8X4	—	—
disulfide	T46.6X1	T46.6X2	T46.6X3	T46.6X4	T46.6X5	T46.6X6
Allylestrenol	T38.5X1	T38.5X2	T38.5X3	T38.5X4	T38.5X5	T38.5X6
Allylisopropylacetylurea	T42.6X1	T42.6X2	T42.6X3	T42.6X4	T42.6X5	T42.6X6
Allylisopropylmalonylurea	T42.3X1	T42.3X2	T42.3X3	T42.3X4	T42.3X5	T42.3X6
Allylthiourea	T49.3X1	T49.3X2	T49.3X3	T49.3X4	T49.3X5	T49.3X6
Allyltribromide	T42.6X1	T42.6X2	T42.6X3	T42.6X4	T42.6X5	T42.6X6
Allypropymal	T42.3X1	T42.3X2	T42.3X3	T42.3X4	T42.3X5	T42.3X6
Almagate	T47.1X1	T47.1X2	T47.1X3	T47.1X4	T47.1X5	T47.1X6
Almasilate	T47.1X1	T47.1X2	T47.1X3	T47.1X4	T47.1X5	T47.1X6
Almitrine	T5Ø.7X1	T5Ø.7X2	T5Ø.7X3	T5Ø.7X4	T5Ø.7X5	T5Ø.7X6
Aloes	T47.2X1	T47.2X2	T47.2X3	T47.2X4	T47.2X5	T47.2X6
Aloglutamol	T47.1X1	T47.1X2	T47.1X3	T47.1X4	T47.1X5	T47.1X6
Aloin	T47.2X1	T47.2X2	T47.2X3	T47.2X4	T47.2X5	T47.2X6
Aloxidone	T42.2X1	T42.2X2	T42.2X3	T42.2X4	T42.2X5	T42.2X6
Alpha						
acetyldigoxin	T46.ØX1	T46.ØX2	T46.ØX3	T46.ØX4	T46.ØX5	T46.ØX6
adrenergic blocking drug	T44.6X1	T44.6X2	T44.6X3	T44.6X4	T44.6X5	T44.6X6
amylase	T45.3X1	T45.3X2	T45.3X3	T45.3X4	T45.3X5	T45.3X6
tocoferol (acetate)	T45.2X1	T45.2X2	T45.2X3	T45.2X4	T45.2X5	T45.2X6
tocopherol	T45.2X1	T45.2X2	T45.2X3	T45.2X4	T45.2X5	T45.2X6
Alphadolone	T41.1X1	T41.1X2	T41.1X3	T41.1X4	T41.1X5	T41.1X6
Alphaprodine	T4Ø.491	T4Ø.492	T4Ø.493	T4Ø.494	T4Ø.495	T4Ø.496
Alphaxalone	T41.1X1	T41.1X2	T41.1X3	T41.1X4	T41.1X5	T41.1X6
Alprazolam	T42.4X1	T42.4X2	T42.4X3	T42.4X4	T42.4X5	T42.4X6
Alprenolol	T44.7X1	T44.7X2	T44.7X3	T44.7X4	T44.7X5	T44.7X6
Alprostadil	T46.7X1	T46.7X2	T46.7X3	T46.7X4	T46.7X5	T46.7X6
Alsactide	T38.811	T38.812	T38.813	T38.814	T38.815	T38.816
Alseroxylon	T46.5X1	T46.5X2	T46.5X3	T46.5X4	T46.5X5	T46.5X6
Alteplase	T45.611	T45.612	T45.613	T45.614	T45.615	T45.616
Altizide	T5Ø.2X1	T5Ø.2X2	T5Ø.2X3	T5Ø.2X4	T5Ø.2X5	T5Ø.2X6
Altretamine	T45.1X1	T45.1X2	T45.1X3	T45.1X4	T45.1X5	T45.1X6
Alum (medicinal)	T49.4X1	T49.4X2	T49.4X3	T49.4X4	T49.4X5	T49.4X6
nonmedicinal (ammonium) (potassium)	T56.891	T56.892	T56.893	T56.894	—	—
Aluminium, aluminum						
acetate	T49.2X1	T49.2X2	T49.2X3	T49.2X4	T49.2X5	T49.2X6
solution	T49.ØX1	T49.ØX2	T49.ØX3	T49.ØX4	T49.ØX5	T49.ØX6
aspirin	T39.Ø11	T39.Ø12	T39.Ø13	T39.Ø14	T39.Ø15	T39.Ø16
bis (acetylsalicylate)	T39.Ø11	T39.Ø12	T39.Ø13	T39.Ø14	T39.Ø15	T39.Ø16
Aluminium, aluminum *(Continued)*						
carbonate (gel, basic)	T47.1X1	T47.1X2	T47.1X3	T47.1X4	T47.1X5	T47.1X6
chlorhydroxide-complex	T47.1X1	T47.1X2	T47.1X3	T47.1X4	T47.1X5	T47.1X6
chloride	T49.2X1	T49.2X2	T49.2X3	T49.2X4	T49.2X5	T49.2X6
clofibrate	T46.6X1	T46.6X2	T46.6X3	T46.6X4	T46.6X5	T46.6X6
diacetate	T49.2X1	T49.2X2	T49.2X3	T49.2X4	T49.2X5	T49.2X6
glycinate	T47.1X1	T47.1X2	T47.1X3	T47.1X4	T47.1X5	T47.1X6
hydroxide (gel)	T47.1X1	T47.1X2	T47.1X3	T47.1X4	T47.1X5	T47.1X6
hydroxide-magnesium carb. gel	T47.1X1	T47.1X2	T47.1X3	T47.1X4	T47.1X5	T47.1X6
magnesium silicate	T47.1X1	T47.1X2	T47.1X3	T47.1X4	T47.1X5	T47.1X6
nicotinate	T46.7X1	T46.7X2	T46.7X3	T46.7X4	T46.7X5	T46.7X6
ointment (surgical) (topical)	T49.3X1	T49.3X2	T49.3X3	T49.3X4	T49.3X5	T49.3X6
phosphate	T47.1X1	T47.1X2	T47.1X3	T47.1X4	T47.1X5	T47.1X6
salicylate	T39.Ø91	T39.Ø92	T39.Ø93	T39.Ø94	T39.Ø95	T39.Ø96
silicate	T47.1X1	T47.1X2	T47.1X3	T47.1X4	T47.1X5	T47.1X6
sodium silicate	T47.1X1	T47.1X2	T47.1X3	T47.1X4	T47.1X5	T47.1X6
subacetate	T49.2X1	T49.2X2	T49.2X3	T49.2X4	T49.2X5	T49.2X6
sulfate	T49.ØX1	T49.ØX2	T49.ØX3	T49.ØX4	T49.ØX5	T49.ØX6
tannate	T47.6X1	T47.6X2	T47.6X3	T47.6X4	T47.6X5	T47.6X6
topical NEC	T49.3X1	T49.3X2	T49.3X3	T49.3X4	T49.3X5	T49.3X6
Alurate	T42.3X1	T42.3X2	T42.3X3	T42.3X4	T42.3X5	T42.3X6
Alverine	T44.3X1	T44.3X2	T44.3X3	T44.3X4	T44.3X5	T44.3X6
Alvodine	T4Ø.2X1	T4Ø.2X2	T4Ø.2X3	T4Ø.2X4	T4Ø.2X5	T4Ø.2X6
Amanita phalloides	T62.ØX1	T62.ØX2	T62.ØX3	T62.ØX4	—	—
Amanitine	T62.ØX1	T62.ØX2	T62.ØX3	T62.ØX4	—	—
Amantadine	T42.8X1	T42.8X2	T42.8X3	T42.8X4	T42.8X5	T42.8X6
Ambazone	T49.6X1	T49.6X2	T49.6X3	T49.6X4	T49.6X5	T49.6X6
Ambenonium (chloride)	T44.ØX1	T44.ØX2	T44.ØX3	T44.ØX4	T44.ØX5	T44.ØX6
Ambroxol	T48.4X1	T48.4X2	T48.4X3	T48.4X4	T48.4X5	T48.4X6
Ambuphylline	T48.6X1	T48.6X2	T48.6X3	T48.6X4	T48.6X5	T48.6X6
Ambutonium bromide	T44.3X1	T44.3X2	T44.3X3	T44.3X4	T44.3X5	T44.3X6
Amcinonide	T49.ØX1	T49.ØX2	T49.ØX3	T49.ØX4	T49.ØX5	T49.ØX6
Amdinocilline	T36.ØX1	T36.ØX2	T36.ØX3	T36.ØX4	T36.ØX5	T36.ØX6
Ametazole	T5Ø.8X1	T5Ø.8X2	T5Ø.8X3	T5Ø.8X4	T5Ø.8X5	T5Ø.8X6
Amethocaine	T41.3X1	T41.3X2	T41.3X3	T41.3X4	T41.3X5	T41.3X6
regional	T41.3X1	T41.3X2	T41.3X3	T41.3X4	T41.3X5	T41.3X6
spinal	T41.3X1	T41.3X2	T41.3X3	T41.3X4	T41.3X5	T41.3X6
Amethopterin	T45.1X1	T45.1X2	T45.1X3	T45.1X4	T45.1X5	T45.1X6
Amezinium metilsulfate	T44.991	T44.992	T44.993	T44.994	T44.995	T44.996
Amfebutamone	T43.291	T43.292	T43.293	T43.294	T43.295	T43.296
Amfepramone	T5Ø.5X1	T5Ø.5X2	T5Ø.5X3	T5Ø.5X4	T5Ø.5X5	T5Ø.5X6

New Revised ~~deleted~~ Deleted

Substance	Poisoning, Accidental (Unintentional)	Poisoning, Intentional Self-Harm	Poisoning, Assault	Poisoning, Undetermined	Adverse Effect	Underdosing
	External Cause (T-Code)					
Amfetamine	T43.621	T43.622	T43.623	T43.624	T43.625	T43.626
Amfetaminil	T43.621	T43.622	T43.623	T43.624	T43.625	T43.626
Amfomycin	T36.8X1	T36.8X2	T36.8X3	T36.8X4	T36.8X5	T36.8X6
Amidefrine mesilate	T48.5X1	T48.5X2	T48.5X3	T48.5X4	T48.5X5	T48.5X6
Amidone	T40.3X1	T40.3X2	T40.3X3	T40.3X4	T40.3X5	T40.3X6
Amidopyrine	T39.2X1	T39.2X2	T39.2X3	T39.2X4	T39.2X5	T39.2X6
Amidotrizoate	T50.8X1	T50.8X2	T50.8X3	T50.8X4	T50.8X5	T50.8X6
Amiflamine	T43.1X1	T43.1X2	T43.1X3	T43.1X4	T43.1X5	T43.1X6
Amikacin	T36.5X1	T36.5X2	T36.5X3	T36.5X4	T36.5X5	T36.5X6
Amikhelline	T46.3X1	T46.3X2	T46.3X3	T46.3X4	T46.3X5	T46.3X6
Amiloride	T50.2X1	T50.2X2	T50.2X3	T50.2X4	T50.2X5	T50.2X6
Aminacrine	T49.0X1	T49.0X2	T49.0X3	T49.0X4	T49.0X5	T49.0X6
Amineptine	T43.011	T43.012	T43.013	T43.014	T43.015	T43.016
Aminitrozole	T37.3X1	T37.3X2	T37.3X3	T37.3X4	T37.3X5	T37.3X6
Aminoacetic acid (derivatives)	T50.3X1	T50.3X2	T50.3X3	T50.3X4	T50.3X5	T50.3X6
Amino acids	T50.3X1	T50.3X2	T50.3X3	T50.3X4	T50.3X5	T50.3X6
Aminoacridine	T49.0X1	T49.0X2	T49.0X3	T49.0X4	T49.0X5	T49.0X6
Aminobenzoic acid (-p)	T49.3X1	T49.3X2	T49.3X3	T49.3X4	T49.3X5	T49.3X6
4-Aminobutyric acid	T43.8X1	T43.8X2	T43.8X3	T43.8X4	T43.8X5	T43.8X6
Aminocaproic acid	T45.621	T45.622	T45.623	T45.624	T45.625	T45.626
Aminofenazone	T39.2X1	T39.2X2	T39.2X3	T39.2X4	T39.2X5	T39.2X6
Aminoethylisothiourium	T45.8X1	T45.8X2	T45.8X3	T45.8X4	T45.8X5	T45.8X6
Aminoglutethimide	T45.1X1	T45.1X2	T45.1X3	T45.1X4	T45.1X5	T45.1X6
Aminohippuric acid	T50.8X1	T50.8X2	T50.8X3	T50.8X4	T50.8X5	T50.8X6
Aminomethylbenzoic acid	T45.691	T45.692	T45.693	T45.694	T45.695	T45.696
Aminometradine	T50.2X1	T50.2X2	T50.2X3	T50.2X4	T50.2X5	T50.2X6
Aminopentamide	T44.3X1	T44.3X2	T44.3X3	T44.3X4	T44.3X5	T44.3X6
Aminophenazone	T39.2X1	T39.2X2	T39.2X3	T39.2X4	T39.2X5	T39.2X6
Aminophenol	T54.0X1	T54.0X2	T54.0X3	T54.0X4	—	—
4-Aminophenol derivatives	T39.1X1	T39.1X2	T39.1X3	T39.1X4	T39.1X5	T39.1X6
Aminophenylpyridone	T43.591	T43.592	T43.593	T43.594	T43.595	T43.596
Aminophylline	T48.6X1	T48.6X2	T48.6X3	T48.6X4	T48.6X5	T48.6X6
Aminopterin sodium	T45.1X1	T45.1X2	T45.1X3	T45.1X4	T45.1X5	T45.1X6
Aminopyrine	T39.2X1	T39.2X2	T39.2X3	T39.2X4	T39.2X5	T39.2X6
8-Aminoquinoline drugs	T37.2X1	T37.2X2	T37.2X3	T37.2X4	T37.2X5	T37.2X6
Aminorex	T50.5X1	T50.5X2	T50.5X3	T50.5X4	T50.5X5	T50.5X6
Aminosalicylic acid	T37.1X1	T37.1X2	T37.1X3	T37.1X4	T37.1X5	T37.1X6
Aminosalylum	T37.1X1	T37.1X2	T37.1X3	T37.1X4	T37.1X5	T37.1X6
Amiodarone	T46.2X1	T46.2X2	T46.2X3	T46.2X4	T46.2X5	T46.2X6
Amiphenazole	T50.7X1	T50.7X2	T50.7X3	T50.7X4	T50.7X5	T50.7X6
Amiquinsin	T46.5X1	T46.5X2	T46.5X3	T46.5X4	T46.5X5	T46.5X6
Amisometradine	T50.2X1	T50.2X2	T50.2X3	T50.2X4	T50.2X5	T50.2X6

Substance	Poisoning, Accidental (Unintentional)	Poisoning, Intentional Self-Harm	Poisoning, Assault	Poisoning, Undetermined	Adverse Effect	Underdosing
	External Cause (T-Code)					
Amisulpride	T43.591	T43.592	T43.593	T43.594	T43.595	T43.596
Amitriptyline	T43.021	T43.022	T43.023	T43.024	T43.025	T43.026
Amitriptylinoxide	T43.021	T43.022	T43.023	T43.024	T43.025	T43.026
Amlexanox	T48.6X1	T48.6X2	T48.6X3	T48.6X4	T48.6X5	T48.6X6
Ammonia (fumes) (gas) (vapor)	T59.891	T59.892	T59.893	T59.894	—	—
aromatic spirit	T48.991	T48.992	T48.993	T48.994	T48.995	T48.996
liquid (household)	T54.3X1	T54.3X2	T54.3X3	T54.3X4	—	—
Ammoniated mercury	T49.0X1	T49.0X2	T49.0X3	T49.0X4	T49.0X5	T49.0X6
Ammonium						
acid tartrate	T49.5X1	T49.5X2	T49.5X3	T49.5X4	T49.5X5	T49.5X6
bromide	T42.6X1	T42.6X2	T42.6X3	T42.6X4	T42.6X5	T42.6X6
carbonate	T54.3X1	T54.3X2	T54.3X3	T54.3X4	—	—
chloride	T50.991	T50.992	T50.993	T50.994	T50.995	T50.996
expectorant	T48.4X1	T48.4X2	T48.4X3	T48.4X4	T48.4X5	T48.4X6
compounds (household) NEC	T54.3X1	T54.3X2	T54.3X3	T54.3X4	—	—
fumes (any usage)	T59.891	T59.892	T59.893	T59.894	—	—
industrial	T54.3X1	T54.3X2	T54.3X3	T54.3X4	—	—
ichthyosulronate	T49.4X1	T49.4X2	T49.4X3	T49.4X4	T49.4X5	T49.4X6
mandelate	T37.91	T37.92	T37.93	T37.94	T37.95	T37.96
sulfamate	T60.3X1	T60.3X2	T60.3X3	T60.3X4	—	—
sulfonate resin	T47.8X1	T47.8X2	T47.8X3	T47.8X4	T47.8X5	T47.8X6
Amobarbital (sodium)	T42.3X1	T42.3X2	T42.3X3	T42.3X4	T42.3X5	T42.3X6
Amodiaquine	T37.2X1	T37.2X2	T37.2X3	T37.2X4	T37.2X5	T37.2X6
Amopyroquin(e)	T37.2X1	T37.2X2	T37.2X3	T37.2X4	T37.2X5	T37.2X6
Amoxapine	T43.011	T43.012	T43.013	T43.014	T43.015	T43.016
Amoxicillin	T36.0X1	T36.0X2	T36.0X3	T36.0X4	T36.0X5	T36.0X6
Amperozide	T43.591	T43.592	T43.593	T43.594	T43.595	T43.596
Amphenidone	T43.591	T43.592	T43.593	T43.594	T43.595	T43.596
Amphetamine NEC	T43.621	T43.622	T43.623	T43.624	T43.625	T43.626
Amphomycin	T36.8X1	T36.8X2	T36.8X3	T36.8X4	T36.8X5	T36.8X6
Amphotalide	T37.4X1	T37.4X2	T37.4X3	T37.4X4	T37.4X5	T37.4X6
Amphotericin B	T36.7X1	T36.7X2	T36.7X3	T36.7X4	T36.7X5	T36.7X6
topical	T49.0X1	T49.0X2	T49.0X3	T49.0X4	T49.0X5	T49.0X6
Ampicillin	T36.0X1	T36.0X2	T36.0X3	T36.0X4	T36.0X5	T36.0X6
Amprotropine	T44.3X1	T44.3X2	T44.3X3	T44.3X4	T44.3X5	T44.3X6
Amsacrine	T45.1X1	T45.1X2	T45.1X3	T45.1X4	T45.1X5	T45.1X6
Amygdaline	T62.2X1	T62.2X2	T62.2X3	T62.2X4	—	—
Amyl						
acetate	T52.8X1	T52.8X2	T52.8X3	T52.8X4	—	—
vapor	T59.891	T59.892	T59.893	T59.894	—	—
alcohol	T51.3X1	T51.3X2	T51.3X3	T51.3X4	—	—
chloride	T53.6X1	T53.6X2	T53.6X3	T53.6X4	—	—

		External Cause (T-Code)				
Substance	**Poisoning, Accidental (Unintentional)**	**Poisoning, Intentional Self-Harm**	**Poisoning, Assault**	**Poisoning, Undetermined**	**Adverse Effect**	**Underdosing**
Amyl *(Continued)*						
formate	T52.8X1	T52.8X2	T52.8X3	T52.8X4	—	—
nitrite	T46.3X1	T46.3X2	T46.3X3	T46.3X4	T46.3X5	T46.3X6
propionate	T65.891	T65.892	T65.893	T65.894	—	—
Amylase	T47.5X1	T47.5X2	T47.5X3	T47.5X4	T47.5X5	T47.5X6
Amyleine, regional	T41.3X1	T41.3X2	T41.3X3	T41.3X4	T41.3X5	T41.3X6
Amylene						
dichloride	T53.6X1	T53.6X2	T53.6X3	T53.6X4	—	—
hydrate	T51.3X1	T51.3X2	T51.3X3	T51.3X4	—	—
Amylmetacresol	T49.6X1	T49.6X2	T49.6X3	T49.6X4	T49.6X5	T49.6X6
Amylobarbitone	T42.3X1	T42.3X2	T42.3X3	T42.3X4	T42.3X5	T42.3X6
Amylocaine, regional	T41.3X1	T41.3X2	T41.3X3	T41.3X4	T41.3X5	T41.3X6
infiltration (subcutaneous)	T41.3X1	T41.3X2	T41.3X3	T41.3X4	T41.3X5	T41.3X6
nerve block (peripheral) (plexus)	T41.3X1	T41.3X2	T41.3X3	T41.3X4	T41.3X5	T41.3X6
spinal	T41.3X1	T41.3X2	T41.3X3	T41.3X4	T41.3X5	T41.3X6
topical (surface)	T41.3X1	T41.3X2	T41.3X3	T41.3X4	T41.3X5	T41.3X6
Amylopectin	T47.6X1	T47.6X2	T47.6X3	T47.6X4	T47.6X5	T47.6X6
Amytal (sodium)	T42.3X1	T42.3X2	T42.3X3	T42.3X4	T42.3X5	T42.3X6
Anabolic steroid	T38.7X1	T38.7X2	T38.7X3	T38.7X4	T38.7X5	T38.7X6
Analeptic NEC	T50.7X1	T50.7X2	T50.7X3	T50.7X4	T50.7X5	T50.7X6
Analgesic	T39.91	T39.92	T39.93	T39.94	T39.95	T39.96
anti-inflammatory NEC	T39.91	T39.92	T39.93	T39.94	T39.95	T39.96
propionic acid derivative	T39.311	T39.312	T39.313	T39.314	T39.315	T39.316
antirheumatic NEC	T39.4X1	T39.4X2	T39.4X3	T39.4X4	T39.4X5	T39.4X6
aromatic NEC	T39.1X1	T39.1X2	T39.1X3	T39.1X4	T39.1X5	T39.1X6
narcotic NEC	T40.601	T40.602	T40.603	T40.604	T40.605	T40.606
combination	T40.601	T40.602	T40.603	T40.604	T40.605	T40.606
obstetric	T40.601	T40.602	T40.603	T40.604	T40.605	T40.606
non-narcotic NEC	T39.91	T39.92	T39.93	T39.94	T39.95	T39.96
combination	T39.91	T39.92	T39.93	T39.94	T39.95	T39.96
pyrazole	T39.2X1	T39.2X2	T39.2X3	T39.2X4	T39.2X5	T39.2X6
specified NEC	T39.8X1	T39.8X2	T39.8X3	T39.8X4	T39.8X5	T39.8X6
Analgin	T39.2X1	T39.2X2	T39.2X3	T39.2X4	T39.2X5	T39.2X6
Anamirta cocculus	T62.1X1	T62.1X2	T62.1X3	T62.1X4	—	—
Ancillin	T36.0X1	T36.0X2	T36.0X3	T36.0X4	T36.0X5	T36.0X6
Ancrod	T45.691	T45.692	T45.693	T45.694	T45.695	T45.696
Androgen	T38.7X1	T38.7X2	T38.7X3	T38.7X4	T38.7X5	T38.7X6
Androgen-estrogen mixture	T38.7X1	T38.7X2	T38.7X3	T38.7X4	T38.7X5	T38.7X6
Androstalone	T38.7X1	T38.7X2	T38.7X3	T38.7X4	T38.7X5	T38.7X6
Androstanolone	T38.7X1	T38.7X2	T38.7X3	T38.7X4	T38.7X5	T38.7X6
Androsterone	T38.7X1	T38.7X2	T38.7X3	T38.7X4	T38.7X5	T38.7X6
Anemone pulsatilla	T62.2X1	T62.2X2	T62.2X3	T62.2X4	—	—
Anesthesia						
caudal	T41.3X1	T41.3X2	T41.3X3	T41.3X4	T41.3X5	T41.3X6
endotracheal	T41.0X1	T41.0X2	T41.0X3	T41.0X4	T41.0X5	T41.0X6
epidural	T41.3X1	T41.3X2	T41.3X3	T41.3X4	T41.3X5	T41.3X6
inhalation	T41.0X1	T41.0X2	T41.0X3	T41.0X4	T41.0X5	T41.0X6
local	T41.3X1	T41.3X2	T41.3X3	T41.3X4	T41.3X5	T41.3X6
mucosal	T41.3X1	T41.3X2	T41.3X3	T41.3X4	T41.3X5	T41.3X6
muscle relaxation	T48.1X1	T48.1X2	T48.1X3	T48.1X4	T48.1X5	T48.1X6
nerve blocking	T41.3X1	T41.3X2	T41.3X3	T41.3X4	T41.3X5	T41.3X6
plexus blocking	T41.3X1	T41.3X2	T41.3X3	T41.3X4	T41.3X5	T41.3X6
potentiated	T41.201	T41.202	T41.203	T41.204	T41.205	T41.206
rectal	T41.201	T41.202	T41.203	T41.204	T41.205	T41.206
general	T41.201	T41.202	T41.203	T41.204	T41.205	T41.206
local	T41.3X1	T41.3X2	T41.3X3	T41.3X4	T41.3X5	T41.3X6
regional	T41.3X1	T41.3X2	T41.3X3	T41.3X4	T41.3X5	T41.3X6
surface	T41.3X1	T41.3X2	T41.3X3	T41.3X4	T41.3X5	T41.3X6
Anesthetic NEC—*see also Anesthesia*	T41.41	T41.42	T41.43	T41.44	T41.45	T41.46
with muscle relaxant	T41.201	T41.202	T41.203	T41.204	T41.205	T41.206
general	T41.201	T41.202	T41.203	T41.204	T41.205	T41.206
local	T41.3X1	T41.3X2	T41.3X3	T41.3X4	T41.3X5	T41.3X6
gaseous NEC	T41.0X1	T41.0X2	T41.0X3	T41.0X4	T41.0X5	T41.0X6
general NEC	T41.201	T41.202	T41.203	T41.204	T41.205	T41.206
halogenated hydrocarbon derivatives NEC	T41.0X1	T41.0X2	T41.0X3	T41.0X4	T41.0X5	T41.0X6
infiltration NEC	T41.3X1	T41.3X2	T41.3X3	T41.3X4	T41.3X5	T41.3X6
intravenous NEC	T41.1X1	T41.1X2	T41.1X3	T41.1X4	T41.1X5	T41.1X6
local NEC	T41.3X1	T41.3X2	T41.3X3	T41.3X4	T41.3X5	T41.3X6
rectal	T41.201	T41.202	T41.203	T41.204	T41.205	T41.206
general	T41.201	T41.202	T41.203	T41.204	T41.205	T41.206
local	T41.3X1	T41.3X2	T41.3X3	T41.3X4	T41.3X5	T41.3X6
regional NEC	T41.3X1	T41.3X2	T41.3X3	T41.3X4	T41.3X5	T41.3X6
spinal NEC	T41.3X1	T41.3X2	T41.3X3	T41.3X4	T41.3X5	T41.3X6
thiobarbiturate	T41.1X1	T41.1X2	T41.1X3	T41.1X4	T41.1X5	T41.1X6
topical	T41.3X1	T41.3X2	T41.3X3	T41.3X4	T41.3X5	T41.3X6
Aneurine	T45.2X1	T45.2X2	T45.2X3	T45.2X4	T45.2X5	T45.2X6
Angio-Conray	T50.8X1	T50.8X2	T50.8X3	T50.8X4	T50.8X5	T50.8X6
Angiotensin	T44.5X1	T44.5X2	T44.5X3	T44.5X4	T44.5X5	T44.5X6
Angiotensinamide	T44.991	T44.992	T44.993	T44.994	T44.995	T44.996
Anhydrohydroxy-progesterone	T38.5X1	T38.5X2	T38.5X3	T38.5X4	T38.5X5	T38.5X6
Anhydron	T50.2X1	T50.2X2	T50.2X3	T50.2X4	T50.2X5	T50.2X6
Anileridine	T40.491	T40.492	T40.493	T40.494	T40.495	T40.496

Substance	External Cause (T-Code) Poisoning, Accidental (Unintentional)	Poisoning, Intentional Self-Harm	Poisoning, Assault	Poisoning, Undetermined	Adverse Effect	Underdosing
Aniline (dye) (liquid)	T65.3X1	T65.3X2	T65.3X3	T65.3X4	—	—
analgesic	T39.1X1	T39.1X2	T39.1X3	T39.1X4	T39.1X5	T39.1X6
derivatives, therapeutic NEC	T39.1X1	T39.1X2	T39.1X3	T39.1X4	T39.1X5	T39.1X6
vapor	T65.3X1	T65.3X2	T65.3X3	T65.3X4	—	—
Anise oil	T47.5X1	T47.5X2	T47.5X3	T47.5X4	T47.5X5	T47.5X6
Aniscoropine	T44.3X1	T44.3X2	T44.3X3	T44.3X4	T44.3X5	T44.3X6
Anisidine	T65.3X1	T65.3X2	T65.3X3	T65.3X4	—	—
Anisindione	T45.511	T45.512	T45.513	T45.514	T45.515	T45.516
Anisotropine methyl-bromide	T44.3X1	T44.3X2	T44.3X3	T44.3X4	T44.3X5	T44.3X6
Anistreplase	T45.611	T45.612	T45.613	T45.614	T45.615	T45.616
Anorexiant (central)	T5Ø.5X1	T5Ø.5X2	T5Ø.5X3	T5Ø.5X4	T5Ø.5X5	T5Ø.5X6
Anorexic agents	T5Ø.5X1	T5Ø.5X2	T5Ø.5X3	T5Ø.5X4	T5Ø.5X5	T5Ø.5X6
Ansamycin	T36.6X1	T36.6X2	T36.6X3	T36.6X4	T36.6X5	T36.6X6
Ant (bite) (sting)	T63.421	T63.422	T63.423	T63.424	—	—
Antabuse	T5Ø.6X1	T5Ø.6X2	T5Ø.6X3	T5Ø.6X4	T5Ø.6X5	T5Ø.6X6
Ant poison — *see Insecticide*						
Antacid NEC	T47.1X1	T47.1X2	T47.1X3	T47.1X4	T47.1X5	T47.1X6
Antagonist						
Aldosterone	T5Ø.ØX1	T5Ø.ØX2	T5Ø.ØX3	T5Ø.ØX4	T5Ø.ØX5	T5Ø.ØX6
alpha-adrenoreceptor	T44.6X1	T44.6X2	T44.6X3	T44.6X4	T44.6X5	T44.6X6
anticoagulant	T45.7X1	T45.7X2	T45.7X3	T45.7X4	T45.7X5	T45.7X6
beta-adrenoreceptor	T44.7X1	T44.7X2	T44.7X3	T44.7X4	T44.7X5	T44.7X6
extrapyramidal NEC	T44.3X1	T44.3X2	T44.3X3	T44.3X4	T44.3X5	T44.3X6
folic acid	T45.1X1	T45.1X2	T45.1X3	T45.1X4	T45.1X5	T45.1X6
H2 receptor	T47.ØX1	T47.ØX2	T47.ØX3	T47.ØX4	T47.ØX5	T47.ØX6
heavy metal	T45.8X1	T45.8X2	T45.8X3	T45.8X4	T45.8X5	T45.8X6
narcotic analgesic	T5Ø.7X1	T5Ø.7X2	T5Ø.7X3	T5Ø.7X4	T5Ø.7X5	T5Ø.7X6
opiate	T5Ø.7X1	T5Ø.7X2	T5Ø.7X3	T5Ø.7X4	T5Ø.7X5	T5Ø.7X6
pyrimidine	T45.1X1	T45.1X2	T45.1X3	T45.1X4	T45.1X5	T45.1X6
serotonin	T46.5X1	T46.5X2	T46.5X3	T46.5X4	T46.5X5	T46.5X6
Antazolin(e)	T45.ØX1	T45.ØX2	T45.ØX3	T45.ØX4	T45.ØX5	T45.ØX6
Anterior pituitary hormone NEC	T38.811	T38.812	T38.813	T38.814	T38.815	T38.816
Anthelmintic NEC	T37.4X1	T37.4X2	T37.4X3	T37.4X4	T37.4X5	T37.4X6
Anthiolimine	T37.4X1	T37.4X2	T37.4X3	T37.4X4	T37.4X5	T37.4X6
Anthralin	T49.4X1	T49.4X2	T49.4X3	T49.4X4	T49.4X5	T49.4X6
Anthramycin	T45.1X1	T45.1X2	T45.1X3	T45.1X4	T45.1X5	T45.1X6
Antiadrenergic NEC	T44.8X1	T44.8X2	T44.8X3	T44.8X4	T44.8X5	T44.8X6
Antiallergic NEC	T45.ØX1	T45.ØX2	T45.ØX3	T45.ØX4	T45.ØX5	T45.ØX6
Anti-anemic (drug) (preparation)	T45.8X1	T45.8X2	T45.8X3	T45.8X4	T45.8X5	T45.8X6
Antiandrogen NEC	T38.6X1	T38.6X2	T38.6X3	T38.6X4	T38.6X5	T38.6X6
Antianxiety drug NEC	T43.5Ø1	T43.5Ø2	T43.5Ø3	T43.5Ø4	T43.5Ø5	T43.5Ø6
Antiaris toxicaria	T65.891	T65.892	T65.893	T65.894	—	—

Substance	External Cause (T-Code) Poisoning, Accidental (Unintentional)	Poisoning, Intentional Self-Harm	Poisoning, Assault	Poisoning, Undetermined	Adverse Effect	Underdosing
Antiarteriosclerotic drug	T46.6X1	T46.6X2	T46.6X3	T46.6X4	T46.6X5	T46.6X6
Antiasthmatic drug NEC	T48.6X1	T48.6X2	T48.6X3	T48.6X4	T48.6X5	T48.6X6
Antibiotic NEC	T36.91	T36.92	T36.93	T36.94	T36.95	T36.96
aminoglycoside	T36.5X1	T36.5X2	T36.5X3	T36.5X4	T36.5X5	T36.5X6
anticancer	T45.1X1	T45.1X2	T45.1X3	T45.1X4	T45.1X5	T45.1X6
antifungal	T36.7X1	T36.7X2	T36.7X3	T36.7X4	T36.7X5	T36.7X6
antimycobacterial	T36.5X1	T36.5X2	T36.5X3	T36.5X4	T36.5X5	T36.5X6
antineoplastic	T45.1X1	T45.1X2	T45.1X3	T45.1X4	T45.1X5	T45.1X6
cephalosporin (group)	T36.1X1	T36.1X2	T36.1X3	T36.1X4	T36.1X5	T36.1X6
chloramphenicol (group)	T36.2X1	T36.2X2	T36.2X3	T36.2X4	T36.2X5	T36.2X6
ENT	T49.6X1	T49.6X2	T49.6X3	T49.6X4	T49.6X5	T49.6X6
eye	T49.5X1	T49.5X2	T49.5X3	T49.5X4	T49.5X5	T49.5X6
fungicidal (local)	T49.ØX1	T49.ØX2	T49.ØX3	T49.ØX4	T49.ØX5	T49.ØX6
intestinal	T36.8X1	T36.8X2	T36.8X3	T36.8X4	T36.8X5	T36.8X6
b-lactam NEC	T36.1X1	T36.1X2	T36.1X3	T36.1X4	T36.1X5	T36.1X6
local	T49.ØX1	T49.ØX2	T49.ØX3	T49.ØX4	T49.ØX5	T49.ØX6
macrolides	T36.3X1	T36.3X2	T36.3X3	T36.3X4	T36.3X5	T36.3X6
polypeptide	T36.8X1	T36.8X2	T36.8X3	T36.8X4	T36.8X5	T36.8X6
specified NEC	T36.8X1	T36.8X2	T36.8X3	T36.8X4	T36.8X5	T36.8X6
tetracycline (group)	T36.4X1	T36.4X2	T36.4X3	T36.4X4	T36.4X5	T36.4X6
throat	T49.6X1	T49.6X2	T49.6X3	T49.6X4	T49.6X5	T49.6X6
Anticancer agents NEC	T45.1X1	T45.1X2	T45.1X3	T45.1X4	T45.1X5	T45.1X6
Anticholesterolemic drug NEC	T46.6X1	T46.6X2	T46.6X3	T46.6X4	T46.6X5	T46.6X6
Anticholinergic NEC	T44.3X1	T44.3X2	T44.3X3	T44.3X4	T44.3X5	T44.3X6
Anticholinesterase	T44.ØX1	T44.ØX2	T44.ØX3	T44.ØX4	T44.ØX5	T44.ØX6
organophosphorus	T44.ØX1	T44.ØX2	T44.ØX3	T44.ØX4	T44.ØX5	T44.ØX6
insecticide	T6Ø.ØX1	T6Ø.ØX2	T6Ø.ØX3	T6Ø.ØX4	—	—
nerve gas	T59.891	T59.892	T59.893	T59.894	—	—
reversible	T44.ØX1	T44.ØX2	T44.ØX3	T44.ØX4	T44.ØX5	T44.ØX6
ophthalmological	T49.5X1	T49.5X2	T49.5X3	T49.5X4	T49.5X5	T49.5X6
Anticoagulant NEC	T45.511	T45.512	T45.513	T45.514	T45.515	T45.516
Antagonist	T45.7X1	T45.7X2	T45.7X3	T45.7X4	T45.7X5	T45.7X6
Anti-common-cold drug NEC	T48.5X1	T48.5X2	T48.5X3	T48.5X4	T48.5X5	T48.5X6
Anticonvulsant	T42.71	T42.72	T42.73	T42.74	T42.75	T42.76
barbiturate	T42.3X1	T42.3X2	T42.3X3	T42.3X4	T42.3X5	T42.3X6
combination (with barbiturate)	T42.3X1	T42.3X2	T42.3X3	T42.3X4	T42.3X5	T42.3X6
hydantoin	T42.ØX1	T42.ØX2	T42.ØX3	T42.ØX4	T42.ØX5	T42.ØX6
hypnotic NEC	T42.6X1	T42.6X2	T42.6X3	T42.6X4	T42.6X5	T42.6X6
oxazolidinedione	T42.2X1	T42.2X2	T42.2X3	T42.2X4	T42.2X5	T42.2X6
pyrimidinedione	T42.6X1	T42.6X2	T42.6X3	T42.6X4	T42.6X5	T42.6X6
specified NEC	T42.6X1	T42.6X2	T42.6X3	T42.6X4	T42.6X5	T42.6X6
succinimide	T42.2X1	T42.2X2	T42.2X3	T42.2X4	T42.2X5	T42.2X6

Substance	External Cause (T-Code)					
	Poisoning, Accidental (Unintentional)	Poisoning, Intentional Self-Harm	Poisoning, Assault	Poisoning, Undetermined	Adverse Effect	Underdosing
Anti-D immunoglobulin (human)	T50.Z11	T50.Z12	T50.Z13	T50.Z14	T50.Z15	T50.Z16
Antidepressant NEC	T43.201	T43.202	T43.203	T43.204	T43.205	T43.206
monoamine oxidase inhibitor	T43.1X1	T43.1X2	T43.1X3	T43.1X4	T43.1X5	T43.1X6
selective serotonin norepinephrine reuptake inhibitor	T43.211	T43.212	T43.213	T43.214	T43.215	T43.216
selective serotonin reuptake inhibitor	T43.221	T43.222	T43.223	T43.224	T43.225	T43.226
specified NEC	T43.291	T43.292	T43.293	T43.294	T43.295	T43.296
tetracyclic	T43.021	T43.022	T43.023	T43.024	T43.025	T43.026
triazolopyridine	T43.221	T43.222	T43.223	T43.224	T43.225	T43.226
tricyclic	T43.011	T43.012	T43.013	T43.014	T43.015	T43.016
Antidiabetic NEC	T38.3X1	T38.3X2	T38.3X3	T38.3X4	T38.3X5	T38.3X6
biguanide	T38.3X1	T38.3X2	T38.3X3	T38.3X4	T38.3X5	T38.3X6
and sulfonyl combined	T38.3X1	T38.3X2	T38.3X3	T38.3X4	T38.3X5	T38.3X6
combined	T38.3X1	T38.3X2	T38.3X3	T38.3X4	T38.3X5	T38.3X6
sulfonylurea	T38.3X1	T38.3X2	T38.3X3	T38.3X4	T38.3X5	T38.3X6
Antidiarrheal drug NEC	T47.6X1	T47.6X2	T47.6X3	T47.6X4	T47.6X5	T47.6X6
absorbent	T47.6X1	T47.6X2	T47.6X3	T47.6X4	T47.6X5	T47.6X6
Antidiphtheria serum	T50.Z11	T50.Z12	T50.Z13	T50.Z14	T50.Z15	T50.Z16
Antidiuretic hormone	T38.891	T38.892	T38.893	T38.894	T38.895	T38.896
Antidote NEC	T50.6X1	T50.6X2	T50.6X3	T50.6X4	T50.6X5	T50.6X6
heavy metal	T45.8X1	T45.8X2	T45.8X3	T45.8X4	T45.8X5	T45.8X6
Antidysrhythmic NEC	T46.2X1	T46.2X2	T46.2X3	T46.2X4	T46.2X5	T46.2X6
Antiemetic drug	T45.0X1	T45.0X2	T45.0X3	T45.0X4	T45.0X5	T45.0X6
Antiepilepsy agent	T42.71	T42.72	T42.73	T42.74	T42.75	T42.76
combination	T42.5X1	T42.5X2	T42.5X3	T42.5X4	T42.5X5	T42.5X6
mixed	T42.5X1	T42.5X2	T42.5X3	T42.5X4	T42.5X5	T42.5X6
specified, NEC	T42.6X1	T42.6X2	T42.6X3	T42.6X4	T42.6X5	T42.6X6
Antiestrogen NEC	T38.6X1	T38.6X2	T38.6X3	T38.6X4	T38.6X5	T38.6X6
Antifertility pill	T38.4X1	T38.4X2	T38.4X3	T38.4X4	T38.4X5	T38.4X6
Antifibrinolytic drug	T45.621	T45.622	T45.623	T45.624	T45.625	T45.626
Antifilarial drug	T37.4X1	T37.4X2	T37.4X3	T37.4X4	T37.4X5	T37.4X6
Antiflatulent	T47.5X1	T47.5X2	T47.5X3	T47.5X4	T47.5X5	T47.5X6
Antifreeze	T65.91	T65.92	T65.93	T65.94	—	—
alcohol	T51.1X1	T51.1X2	T51.1X3	T51.1X4	—	—
ethylene glycol	T51.8X1	T51.8X2	T51.8X3	T51.8X4	—	—
Antifungal						
antibiotic (systemic)	T36.7X1	T36.7X2	T36.7X3	T36.7X4	T36.7X5	T36.7X6
anti-infective NEC	T37.91	T37.92	T37.93	T37.94	T37.95	T37.96
disinfectant, local	T49.0X1	T49.0X2	T49.0X3	T49.0X4	T49.0X5	T49.0X6
nonmedicinal (spray)	T60.3X1	T60.3X2	T60.3X3	T60.3X4	—	—
topical	T49.0X1	T49.0X2	T49.0X3	T49.0X4	T49.0X5	T49.0X6

Substance	External Cause (T-Code)					
	Poisoning, Accidental (Unintentional)	Poisoning, Intentional Self-Harm	Poisoning, Assault	Poisoning, Undetermined	Adverse Effect	Underdosing
Anti-gastric-secretion drug NEC	T47.1X1	T47.1X2	T47.1X3	T47.1X4	T47.1X5	T47.1X6
Antigonadotrophin NEC	T38.6X1	T38.6X2	T38.6X3	T38.6X4	T38.6X5	T38.6X6
Antihallucinogen	T43.501	T43.502	T43.503	T43.504	T43.505	T43.506
Antihelmintics	T37.4X1	T37.4X2	T37.4X3	T37.4X4	T37.4X5	T37.4X6
Antihemophilic						
factor	T45.8X1	T45.8X2	T45.8X3	T45.8X4	T45.8X5	T45.8X6
fraction	T45.8X1	T45.8X2	T45.8X3	T45.8X4	T45.8X5	T45.8X6
globulin concentrate	T45.7X1	T45.7X2	T45.7X3	T45.7X4	T45.7X5	T45.7X6
human plasma	T45.8X1	T45.8X2	T45.8X3	T45.8X4	T45.8X5	T45.8X6
plasma, dried	T45.7X1	T45.7X2	T45.7X3	T45.7X4	T45.7X5	T45.7X6
Antihemorrhoidal preparation	T49.2X1	T49.2X2	T49.2X3	T49.2X4	T49.2X5	T49.2X6
Antiheparin drug	T45.7X1	T45.7X2	T45.7X3	T45.7X4	T45.7X5	T45.7X6
Antihistamine	T45.0X1	T45.0X2	T45.0X3	T45.0X4	T45.0X5	T45.0X6
Antihookworm drug	T37.4X1	T37.4X2	T37.4X3	T37.4X4	T37.4X5	T37.4X6
Anti-human lymphocytic globulin	T50.Z11	T50.Z12	T50.Z13	T50.Z14	T50.Z15	T50.Z16
Antihyperlipidemic drug	T46.6X1	T46.6X2	T46.6X3	T46.6X4	T46.6X5	T46.6X6
Antihypertensive drug NEC	T46.5X1	T46.5X2	T46.5X3	T46.5X4	T46.5X5	T46.5X6
Anti-infective NEC	T37.91	T37.92	T37.93	T37.94	T37.95	T37.96
anthelmintic	T37.4X1	T37.4X2	T37.4X3	T37.4X4	T37.4X5	T37.4X6
antibiotics	T36.91	T36.92	T36.93	T36.94	T36.95	T36.96
specified NEC	T36.8X1	T36.8X2	T36.8X3	T36.8X4	T36.8X5	T36.8X6
antimalarial	T37.2X1	T37.2X2	T37.2X3	T37.2X4	T37.2X5	T37.2X6
antimycobacterial NEC	T37.1X1	T37.1X2	T37.1X3	T37.1X4	T37.1X5	T37.1X6
antibiotics	T36.5X1	T36.5X2	T36.5X3	T36.5X4	T36.5X5	T36.5X6
antiprotozoal NEC	T37.3X1	T37.3X2	T37.3X3	T37.3X4	T37.3X5	T37.3X6
blood	T37.2X1	T37.2X2	T37.2X3	T37.2X4	T37.2X5	T37.2X6
antiviral	T37.5X1	T37.5X2	T37.5X3	T37.5X4	T37.5X5	T37.5X6
arsenical	T37.8X1	T37.8X2	T37.8X3	T37.8X4	T37.8X5	T37.8X6
bismuth, local	T49.0X1	T49.0X2	T49.0X3	T49.0X4	T49.0X5	T49.0X6
ENT	T49.6X1	T49.6X2	T49.6X3	T49.6X4	T49.6X5	T49.6X6
eye NEC	T49.5X1	T49.5X2	T49.5X3	T49.5X4	T49.5X5	T49.5X6
heavy metals NEC	T37.8X1	T37.8X2	T37.8X3	T37.8X4	T37.8X5	T37.8X6
local NEC	T49.0X1	T49.0X2	T49.0X3	T49.0X4	T49.0X5	T49.0X6
specified NEC	T49.0X1	T49.0X2	T49.0X3	T49.0X4	T49.0X5	T49.0X6
mixed	T37.91	T37.92	T37.93	T37.94	T37.95	T37.96
ophthalmic preparation	T49.5X1	T49.5X2	T49.5X3	T49.5X4	T49.5X5	T49.5X6
topical NEC	T49.0X1	T49.0X2	T49.0X3	T49.0X4	T49.0X5	T49.0X6
Anti-inflammatory drug NEC	T49.0X1	T49.0X2	T49.0X3	T49.0X4	T49.0X5	T49.0X6
local	T49.0X1	T49.0X2	T49.0X3	T49.0X4	T49.0X5	T49.0X6
nonsteroidal NEC	T39.391	T39.392	T39.393	T39.394	T39.395	T39.396
propionic acid derivative	T39.311	T39.312	T39.313	T39.314	T39.315	T39.316
specified NEC	T39.391	T39.392	T39.393	T39.394	T39.395	T39.396

◀ New ◀ Revised ~~deleted~~ Deleted

Substance	External Cause (T-Code)					
	Poisoning, Accidental (Unintentional)	Poisoning, Intentional Self-Harm	Poisoning, Assault	Poisoning, Undetermined	Adverse Effect	Underdosing
Antikaluretic	T5Ø.3X1	T5Ø.3X2	T5Ø.3X3	T5Ø.3X4	T5Ø.3X5	T5Ø.3X6
Antiknock (tetraethyl lead)	T56.ØX1	T56.ØX2	T56.ØX3	T56.ØX4	—	—
Antilipemic drug NEC	T46.6X1	T46.6X2	T46.6X3	T46.6X4	T46.6X5	T46.6X6
Antimalarial	T37.2X1	T37.2X2	T37.2X3	T37.2X4	T37.2X5	T37.2X6
prophylactic NEC	T37.2X1	T37.2X2	T37.2X3	T37.2X4	T37.2X5	T37.2X6
pyrimidine derivative	T37.2X1	T37.2X2	T37.2X3	T37.2X4	T37.2X5	T37.2X6
Antimetabolite	T45.1X1	T45.1X2	T45.1X3	T45.1X4	T45.1X5	T45.1X6
Antimitotic agent	T45.1X1	T45.1X2	T45.1X3	T45.1X4	T45.1X5	T45.1X6
Antimony (compounds) (vapor) NEC	T56.891	T56.892	T56.893	T56.894	—	—
anti-infectives	T37.8X1	T37.8X2	T37.8X3	T37.8X4	T37.8X5	T37.8X6
dimercaptosuccinate	T37.3X1	T37.3X2	T37.3X3	T37.3X4	T37.3X5	T37.3X6
hydride	T56.891	T56.892	T56.893	T56.894	—	—
pesticide (vapor)	T6Ø.8X1	T6Ø.8X2	T6Ø.8X3	T6Ø.8X4	—	—
potassium (sodium) tartrate	T37.8X1	T37.8X2	T37.8X3	T37.8X4	T37.8X5	T37.8X6
sodium dimercaptosuccinate	T37.3X1	T37.3X2	T37.3X3	T37.3X4	T37.3X5	T37.3X6
tartrated	T37.8X1	T37.8X2	T37.8X3	T37.8X4	T37.8X5	T37.8X6
Antimuscarinic NEC	T44.3X1	T44.3X2	T44.3X3	T44.3X4	T44.3X5	T44.3X6
Antimycobacterial drug NEC	T37.1X1	T37.1X2	T37.1X3	T37.1X4	T37.1X5	T37.1X6
antibiotics	T36.5X1	T36.5X2	T36.5X3	T36.5X4	T36.5X5	T36.5X6
combination	T37.1X1	T37.1X2	T37.1X3	T37.1X4	T37.1X5	T37.1X6
Antinausea drug	T45.ØX1	T45.ØX2	T45.ØX3	T45.ØX4	T45.ØX5	T45.ØX6
Antinematode drug	T37.4X1	T37.4X2	T37.4X3	T37.4X4	T37.4X5	T37.4X6
Antineoplastic NEC	T45.1X1	T45.1X2	T45.1X3	T45.1X4	T45.1X5	T45.1X6
alkaloidal	T45.1X1	T45.1X2	T45.1X3	T45.1X4	T45.1X5	T45.1X6
antibiotics	T45.1X1	T45.1X2	T45.1X3	T45.1X4	T45.1X5	T45.1X6
combination	T45.1X1	T45.1X2	T45.1X3	T45.1X4	T45.1X5	T45.1X6
estrogen	T38.5X1	T38.5X2	T38.5X3	T38.5X4	T38.5X5	T38.5X6
steroid	T38.7X1	T38.7X2	T38.7X3	T38.7X4	T38.7X5	T38.7X6
Antiparasitic drug (systemic)	T37.91	T37.92	T37.93	T37.94	T37.95	T37.96
local	T49.ØX1	T49.ØX2	T49.ØX3	T49.ØX4	T49.ØX5	T49.ØX6
specified NEC	T37.8X1	T37.8X2	T37.8X3	T37.8X4	T37.8X5	T37.8X6
Antiparkinsonism drug NEC	T42.8X1	T42.8X2	T42.8X3	T42.8X4	T42.8X5	T42.8X6
Antiperspirant NEC	T49.2X1	T49.2X2	T49.2X3	T49.2X4	T49.2X5	T49.2X6
Antiphlogistic NEC	T39.4X1	T39.4X2	T39.4X3	T39.4X4	T39.4X5	T39.4X6
Antiplatyhelmintic drug	T37.4X1	T37.4X2	T37.4X3	T37.4X4	T37.4X5	T37.4X6
Antiprotozoal drug NEC	T37.3X1	T37.3X2	T37.3X3	T37.3X4	T37.3X5	T37.3X6
blood	T37.2X1	T37.2X2	T37.2X3	T37.2X4	T37.2X5	T37.2X6
local	T49.ØX1	T49.ØX2	T49.ØX3	T49.ØX4	T49.ØX5	T49.ØX6
Antipruritic drug NEC	T49.1X1	T49.1X2	T49.1X3	T49.1X4	T49.1X5	T49.1X6
Antipsychotic drug	T43.5Ø1	T43.5Ø2	T43.5Ø3	T43.5Ø4	T43.5Ø5	T43.5Ø6
specified NEC	T43.591	T43.592	T43.593	T43.594	T43.595	T43.596
Antipyretic	T39.91	T39.92	T39.93	T39.94	T39.95	T39.96
specified NEC	T39.8X1	T39.8X2	T39.8X3	T39.8X4	T39.8X5	T39.8X6
Antipyrine	T39.2X1	T39.2X2	T39.2X3	T39.2X4	T39.2X5	T39.2X6
Antirabies hyperimmune serum	T5Ø.Z11	T5Ø.Z12	T5Ø.Z13	T5Ø.Z14	T5Ø.Z15	T5Ø.Z16
Antirheumatic NEC	T39.4X1	T39.4X2	T39.4X3	T39.4X4	T39.4X5	T39.4X6
Antirigidity drug NEC	T42.8X1	T42.8X2	T42.8X3	T42.8X4	T42.8X5	T42.8X6
Antischistosomal drug	T37.4X1	T37.4X2	T37.4X3	T37.4X4	T37.4X5	T37.4X6
Antiscorpion sera	T5Ø.Z11	T5Ø.Z12	T5Ø.Z13	T5Ø.Z14	T5Ø.Z15	T5Ø.Z16
Antiseborrheics	T49.4X1	T49.4X2	T49.4X3	T49.4X4	T49.4X5	T49.4X6
Antiseptics (external) (medicinal)	T49.ØX1	T49.ØX2	T49.ØX3	T49.ØX4	T49.ØX5	T49.ØX6
Antistine	T45.ØX1	T45.ØX2	T45.ØX3	T45.ØX4	T45.ØX5	T45.ØX6
Antitapeworm drug	T37.4X1	T37.4X2	T37.4X3	T37.4X4	T37.4X5	T37.4X6
Antitetanus immunoglobulin	T5Ø.Z11	T5Ø.Z12	T5Ø.Z13	T5Ø.Z14	T5Ø.Z15	T5Ø.Z16
Antithrombotic	T45.521	T45.522	T45.523	T45.524	T45.525	T45.526
Antithyroid drug NEC	T38.2X1	T38.2X2	T38.2X3	T38.2X4	T38.2X5	T38.2X6
Antitoxin	T5Ø.Z11	T5Ø.Z12	T5Ø.Z13	T5Ø.Z14	T5Ø.Z15	T5Ø.Z16
diphtheria	T5Ø.Z11	T5Ø.Z12	T5Ø.Z13	T5Ø.Z14	T5Ø.Z15	T5Ø.Z16
gas gangrene	T5Ø.Z11	T5Ø.Z12	T5Ø.Z13	T5Ø.Z14	T5Ø.Z15	T5Ø.Z16
tetanus	T5Ø.Z11	T5Ø.Z12	T5Ø.Z13	T5Ø.Z14	T5Ø.Z15	T5Ø.Z16
Antitoxin, any	T5Ø.9Ø1	T5Ø.9Ø2	T5Ø.9Ø3	T5Ø.9Ø4	T5Ø.9Ø5	T5Ø.9Ø6
Antitrichomonal drug	T37.3X1	T37.3X2	T37.3X3	T37.3X4	T37.3X5	T37.3X6
Antituberculars	T37.1X1	T37.1X2	T37.1X3	T37.1X4	T37.1X5	T37.1X6
antibiotics	T36.5X1	T36.5X2	T36.5X3	T36.5X4	T36.5X5	T36.5X6
Antitussive NEC	T48.3X1	T48.3X2	T48.3X3	T48.3X4	T48.3X5	T48.3X6
codeine mixture	T4Ø.2X1	T4Ø.2X2	T4Ø.2X3	T4Ø.2X4	T4Ø.2X5	T4Ø.2X6
opiate	T4Ø.2X1	T4Ø.2X2	T4Ø.2X3	T4Ø.2X4	T4Ø.2X5	T4Ø.2X6
Antivaricose drug	T46.8X1	T46.8X2	T46.8X3	T46.8X4	T46.8X5	T46.8X6
Antivenin, antivenom (sera)	T5Ø.Z11	T5Ø.Z12	T5Ø.Z13	T5Ø.Z14	T5Ø.Z15	T5Ø.Z16
crotaline	T5Ø.Z11	T5Ø.Z12	T5Ø.Z13	T5Ø.Z14	T5Ø.Z15	T5Ø.Z16
spider bite	T5Ø.Z11	T5Ø.Z12	T5Ø.Z13	T5Ø.Z14	T5Ø.Z15	T5Ø.Z16
Antivertigo drug	T45.ØX1	T45.ØX2	T45.ØX3	T45.ØX4	T45.ØX5	T45.ØX6
Antiviral drug NEC	T37.5X1	T37.5X2	T37.5X3	T37.5X4	T37.5X5	T37.5X6
eye	T49.5X1	T49.5X2	T49.5X3	T49.5X4	T49.5X5	T49.5X6
Antiwhipworm drug	T37.4X1	T37.4X2	T37.4X3	T37.4X4	T37.4X5	T37.4X6
Ant poisons — *see Pesticides*						
Antrol — *see also by specific chemical substance*	T6Ø.91	T6Ø.92	T6Ø.93	T6Ø.94	—	—
fungicide	T6Ø.91	T6Ø.92	T6Ø.93	T6Ø.94	—	—
ANTU (alpha naphthylthiourea)	T6Ø.4X1	T6Ø.4X2	T6Ø.4X3	T6Ø.4X4	—	—
Apalcillin	T36.ØX1	T36.ØX2	T36.ØX3	T36.ØX4	T36.ØX5	T36.ØX6
APC	T48.5X1	T48.5X2	T48.5X3	T48.5X4	T48.5X5	T48.5X6
Aplonidine	T44.4X1	T44.4X2	T44.4X3	T44.4X4	T44.4X5	T44.4X6
Apomorphine	T47.7X1	T47.7X2	T47.7X3	T47.7X4	T47.7X5	T47.7X6

Substance	External Cause (T-Code)					
	Poisoning, Accidental (Unintentional)	Poisoning, Intentional Self-Harm	Poisoning, Assault	Poisoning, Undetermined	Adverse Effect	Underdosing
Appetite depressants, central	T5Ø.5X1	T5Ø.5X2	T5Ø.5X3	T5Ø.5X4	T5Ø.5X5	T5Ø.5X6
Apraclonidine (hydrochloride)	T44.4X1	T44.4X2	T44.4X3	T44.4X4	T44.4X5	T44.4X6
Apresoline	T46.5X1	T46.5X2	T46.5X3	T46.5X4	T46.5X5	T46.5X6
Aprindine	T46.2X1	T46.2X2	T46.2X3	T46.2X4	T46.2X5	T46.2X6
Aprobarbital	T42.3X1	T42.3X2	T42.3X3	T42.3X4	T42.3X5	T42.3X6
Apronalide	T42.6X1	T42.6X2	T42.6X3	T42.6X4	T42.6X5	T42.6X6
Aprotinin	T45.621	T45.622	T45.623	T45.624	T45.625	T45.626
Aptocaine	T41.3X1	T41.3X2	T41.3X3	T41.3X4	T41.3X5	T41.3X6
Aqua fortis	T54.2X1	T54.2X2	T54.2X3	T54.2X4	—	—
Ara-A	T37.5X1	T37.5X2	T37.5X3	T37.5X4	T37.5X5	T37.5X6
Ara-C	T45.1X1	T45.1X2	T45.1X3	T45.1X4	T45.1X5	T45.1X6
Arachis oil	T49.3X1	T49.3X2	T49.3X3	T49.3X4	T49.3X5	T49.3X6
cathartic	T47.4X1	T47.4X2	T47.4X3	T47.4X4	T47.4X5	T47.4X6
Aralen	T37.2X1	T37.2X2	T37.2X3	T37.2X4	T37.2X5	T37.2X6
Arecoline	T44.1X1	T44.1X2	T44.1X3	T44.1X4	T44.1X5	T44.1X6
Arginine	T5Ø.991	T5Ø.992	T5Ø.993	T5Ø.994	T5Ø.995	T5Ø.996
glutamate	T5Ø.991	T5Ø.992	T5Ø.993	T5Ø.994	T5Ø.995	T5Ø.996
Argyrol	T49.ØX1	T49.ØX2	T49.ØX3	T49.ØX4	T49.ØX5	T49.ØX6
ENT agent	T49.6X1	T49.6X2	T49.6X3	T49.6X4	T49.6X5	T49.6X6
ophthalmic preparation	T49.5X1	T49.5X2	T49.5X3	T49.5X4	T49.5X5	T49.5X6
Aristocort	T38.ØX1	T38.ØX2	T38.ØX3	T38.ØX4	T38.ØX5	T38.ØX6
ENT agent	T49.6X1	T49.6X2	T49.6X3	T49.6X4	T49.6X5	T49.6X6
ophthalmic preparation	T49.5X1	T49.5X2	T49.5X3	T49.5X4	T49.5X5	T49.5X6
topical NEC	T49.ØX1	T49.ØX2	T49.ØX3	T49.ØX4	T49.ØX5	T49.ØX6
Aromatics, corrosive	T54.1X1	T54.1X2	T54.1X3	T54.1X4	—	—
disinfectants	T54.1X1	T54.1X2	T54.1X3	T54.1X4	—	—
Arsenate of lead	T57.ØX1	T57.ØX2	T57.ØX3	T57.ØX4	—	—
herbicide	T57.ØX1	T57.ØX2	T57.ØX3	T57.ØX4	—	—
Arsenic, arsenicals (compounds) (dust) (vapor) NEC	T57.ØX1	T57.ØX2	T57.ØX3	T57.ØX4	—	—
anti-infectives	T37.8X1	T37.8X2	T37.8X3	T37.8X4	T37.8X5	T37.8X6
pesticide (dust) (fumes)	T57.ØX1	T57.ØX2	T57.ØX3	T57.ØX4	—	—
Arsine (gas)	T57.ØX1	T57.ØX2	T57.ØX3	T57.ØX4	—	—
Arsphenamine (silver)	T37.8X1	T37.8X2	T37.8X3	T37.8X4	T37.8X5	T37.8X6
Arsthinol	T37.3X1	T37.3X2	T37.3X3	T37.3X4	T37.3X5	T37.3X6
Artane	T44.3X1	T44.3X2	T44.3X3	T44.3X4	T44.3X5	T44.3X6
Arthropod (venomous) NEC	T63.481	T63.482	T63.483	T63.484	—	—
Articaine	T41.3X1	T41.3X2	T41.3X3	T41.3X4	T41.3X5	T41.3X6
Asbestos	T57.8X1	T57.8X2	T57.8X3	T57.8X4	—	—
Ascaridole	T37.4X1	T37.4X2	T37.4X3	T37.4X4	T37.4X5	T37.4X6
Ascorbic acid	T45.2X1	T45.2X2	T45.2X3	T45.2X4	T45.2X5	T45.2X6
Asiaticoside	T49.ØX1	T49.ØX2	T49.ØX3	T49.ØX4	T49.ØX5	T49.ØX6

Substance	External Cause (T-Code)					
	Poisoning, Accidental (Unintentional)	Poisoning, Intentional Self-Harm	Poisoning, Assault	Poisoning, Undetermined	Adverse Effect	Underdosing
Asparaginase	T45.1X1	T45.1X2	T45.1X3	T45.1X4	T45.1X5	T45.1X6
Aspidium (oleoresin)	T37.4X1	T37.4X2	T37.4X3	T37.4X4	T37.4X5	T37.4X6
Aspirin (aluminum) (soluble)	T39.Ø11	T39.Ø12	T39.Ø13	T39.Ø14	T39.Ø15	T39.Ø16
Aspoxicillin	T36.ØX1	T36.ØX2	T36.ØX3	T36.ØX4	T36.ØX5	T36.ØX6
Astemizole	T45.ØX1	T45.ØX2	T45.ØX3	T45.ØX4	T45.ØX5	T45.ØX6
Astringent (local)	T49.2X1	T49.2X2	T49.2X3	T49.2X4	T49.2X5	T49.2X6
specified NEC	T49.2X1	T49.2X2	T49.2X3	T49.2X4	T49.2X5	T49.2X6
Astromicin	T36.5X1	T36.5X2	T36.5X3	T36.5X4	T36.5X5	T36.5X6
Ataractic drug NEC	T43.5Ø1	T43.5Ø2	T43.5Ø3	T43.5Ø4	T43.5Ø5	T43.5Ø6
Atenolol	T44.7X1	T44.7X2	T44.7X3	T44.7X4	T44.7X5	T44.7X6
Atonia drug, intestinal	T47.4X1	T47.4X2	T47.4X3	T47.4X4	T47.4X5	T47.4X6
Atophan	T5Ø.4X1	T5Ø.4X2	T5Ø.4X3	T5Ø.4X4	T5Ø.4X5	T5Ø.4X6
Atracurium besilate	T48.1X1	T48.1X2	T48.1X3	T48.1X4	T48.1X5	T48.1X6
Atropine	T44.3X1	T44.3X2	T44.3X3	T44.3X4	T44.3X5	T44.3X6
derivative	T44.3X1	T44.3X2	T44.3X3	T44.3X4	T44.3X5	T44.3X6
methonitrate	T44.3X1	T44.3X2	T44.3X3	T44.3X4	T44.3X5	T44.3X6
Attapulgite	T47.6X1	T47.6X2	T47.6X3	T47.6X4	T47.6X5	T47.6X6
Attenuvax	T5Ø.991	T5Ø.992	T5Ø.993	T5Ø.994	T5Ø.995	T5Ø.996
Auramine	T65.891	T65.892	T65.893	T65.894	—	—
dye	T65.6X1	T65.6X2	T65.6X3	T65.6X4	—	—
fungicide	T6Ø.3X1	T6Ø.3X2	T6Ø.3X3	T6Ø.3X4	—	—
Auranofin	T39.4X1	T39.4X2	T39.4X3	T39.4X4	T39.4X5	T39.4X6
Aurantiin	T46.991	T46.992	T46.993	T46.994	T46.995	T46.996
Aureomycin	T36.4X1	T36.4X2	T36.4X3	T36.4X4	T36.4X5	T36.4X6
ophthalmic preparation	T49.5X1	T49.5X2	T49.5X3	T49.5X4	T49.5X5	T49.5X6
topical NEC	T49.ØX1	T49.ØX2	T49.ØX3	T49.ØX4	T49.ØX5	T49.ØX6
Aurothioglucose	T39.4X1	T39.4X2	T39.4X3	T39.4X4	T39.4X5	T39.4X6
Aurothioglycanide	T39.4X1	T39.4X2	T39.4X3	T39.4X4	T39.4X5	T39.4X6
Aurothiomalate sodium	T39.4X1	T39.4X2	T39.4X3	T39.4X4	T39.4X5	T39.4X6
Aurotioprol	T39.4X1	T39.4X2	T39.4X3	T39.4X4	T39.4X5	T39.4X6
Automobile fuel	T52.ØX1	T52.ØX2	T52.ØX3	T52.ØX4	—	—
Autonomic nervous system agent NEC	T44.9Ø1	T44.9Ø2	T44.9Ø3	T44.9Ø4	T44.9Ø5	T44.9Ø6
Avlosulfon	T37.1X1	T37.1X2	T37.1X3	T37.1X4	T37.1X5	T37.1X6
Avomine	T42.6X1	T42.6X2	T42.6X3	T42.6X4	T42.6X5	T42.6X6
Axerophthol	T45.2X1	T45.2X2	T45.2X3	T45.2X4	T45.2X5	T45.2X6
Azacitidine	T45.1X1	T45.1X2	T45.1X3	T45.1X4	T45.1X5	T45.1X6
Azacyclonol	T43.591	T43.592	T43.593	T43.594	T43.595	T43.596
Azadirachta	T6Ø.2X1	T6Ø.2X2	T6Ø.2X3	T6Ø.2X4	—	—
Azanidazole	T37.3X1	T37.3X2	T37.3X3	T37.3X4	T37.3X5	T37.3X6
Azapetine	T46.7X1	T46.7X2	T46.7X3	T46.7X4	T46.7X5	T46.7X6
Azapropazone	T39.2X1	T39.2X2	T39.2X3	T39.2X4	T39.2X5	T39.2X6

Substance	External Cause (T-Code)					
	Poisoning, Accidental (Unintentional)	Poisoning, Intentional Self-Harm	Poisoning, Assault	Poisoning, Undetermined	Adverse Effect	Underdosing
Azaribine	T45.1X1	T45.1X2	T45.1X3	T45.1X4	T45.1X5	T45.1X6
Azaserine	T45.1X1	T45.1X2	T45.1X3	T45.1X4	T45.1X5	T45.1X6
Azatadine	T45.0X1	T45.0X2	T45.0X3	T45.0X4	T45.0X5	T45.0X6
Azatepa	T45.1X1	T45.1X2	T45.1X3	T45.1X4	T45.1X5	T45.1X6
Azathioprine	T45.1X1	T45.1X2	T45.1X3	T45.1X4	T45.1X5	T45.1X6
Azelaic acid	T49.0X1	T49.0X2	T49.0X3	T49.0X4	T49.0X5	T49.0X6
Azelastine	T45.0X1	T45.0X2	T45.0X3	T45.0X4	T45.0X5	T45.0X6
Azidocillin	T36.0X1	T36.0X2	T36.0X3	T36.0X4	T36.0X5	T36.0X6
Azidothymidine	T37.5X1	T37.5X2	T37.5X3	T37.5X4	T37.5X5	T37.5X6
Azinphos (ethyl) (methyl)	T60.0X1	T60.0X2	T60.0X3	T60.0X4	—	—
Aziridine (chelating)	T54.1X1	T54.1X2	T54.1X3	T54.1X4	—	—
Azithromycin	T36.3X1	T36.3X2	T36.3X3	T36.3X4	T36.3X5	T36.3X6
Azlocillin	T36.01	T36.02	T36.03	T36.04	T36.05	T36.06
Azobenzene smoke	T65.3X1	T65.3X2	T65.3X3	T65.3X4	—	—
acaricide	T60.8X1	T60.8X2	T60.8X3	T60.8X4	—	—
Azosulfamide	T37.0X1	T37.0X2	T37.0X3	T37.0X4	T37.0X5	T37.0X6
AZT	T37.5X1	T37.5X2	T37.5X3	T37.5X4	T37.5X5	T37.5X6
Aztreonam	T36.1X1	T36.1X2	T36.1X3	T36.1X4	T36.1X5	T36.1X6
Azulfidine	T37.0X1	T37.0X2	T37.0X3	T37.0X4	T37.0X5	T37.0X6
Azuresin	T50.8X1	T50.8X2	T50.8X3	T50.8X4	T50.8X5	T50.8X6
B						
Bacampicillin	T36.0X1	T36.0X2	T36.0X3	T36.0X4	T36.0X5	T36.0X6
Bacillus						
lactobacillus	T47.8X1	T47.8X2	T47.8X3	T47.8X4	T47.8X5	T47.8X6
subtilis	T47.6X1	T47.6X2	T47.6X3	T47.6X4	T47.6X5	T47.6X6
Bacimycin	T49.0X1	T49.0X2	T49.0X3	T49.0X4	T49.0X5	T49.0X6
ophthalmic preparation	T49.5X1	T49.5X2	T49.5X3	T49.5X4	T49.5X5	T49.5X6
Bacitracin zinc	T49.0X1	T49.0X2	T49.0X3	T49.0X4	T49.0X5	T49.0X6
with neomycin	T49.0X1	T49.0X2	T49.0X3	T49.0X4	T49.0X5	T49.0X6
ENT agent	T49.6X1	T49.6X2	T49.6X3	T49.6X4	T49.6X5	T49.6X6
ophthalmic preparation	T49.5X1	T49.5X2	T49.5X3	T49.5X4	T49.5X5	T49.5X6
topical NEC	T49.0X1	T49.0X2	T49.0X3	T49.0X4	T49.0X5	T49.0X6
Baclofen	T42.8X1	T42.8X2	T42.8X3	T42.8X4	T42.8X5	T42.8X6
Baking soda	T50.991	T50.992	T50.993	T50.994	T50.995	T50.996
BAL	T45.8X1	T45.8X2	T45.8X3	T45.8X4	T45.8X5	T45.8X6
Bambuterol	T48.6X1	T48.6X2	T48.6X3	T48.6X4	T48.6X5	T48.6X6
Bamethan (sulfate)	T46.7X1	T46.7X2	T46.7X3	T46.7X4	T46.7X5	T46.7X6
Bamifylline	T48.6X1	T48.6X2	T48.6X3	T48.6X4	T48.6X5	T48.6X6
Bamipine	T45.0X1	T45.0X2	T45.0X3	T45.0X4	T45.0X5	T45.0X6
Baneberry — *see Actaea spicata*						
Banewort — *see Belladonna*						

Substance	External Cause (T-Code)					
	Poisoning, Accidental (Unintentional)	Poisoning, Intentional Self-Harm	Poisoning, Assault	Poisoning, Undetermined	Adverse Effect	Underdosing
Barbenyl	T42.3X1	T42.3X2	T42.3X3	T42.3X4	T42.3X5	T42.3X6
Barbexaclone	T42.6X1	T42.6X2	T42.6X3	T42.6X4	T42.6X5	T42.6X6
Barbital	T42.3X1	T42.3X2	T42.3X3	T42.3X4	T42.3X5	T42.3X6
sodium	T42.3X1	T42.3X2	T42.3X3	T42.3X4	T42.3X5	T42.3X6
Barbitone	T42.3X1	T42.3X2	T42.3X3	T42.3X4	T42.3X5	T42.3X6
Barbiturate NEC	T42.3X1	T42.3X2	T42.3X3	T42.3X4	T42.3X5	T42.3X6
with tranquilizer	T42.3X1	T42.3X2	T42.3X3	T42.3X4	T42.3X5	T42.3X6
anesthetic (intravenous)	T41.1X1	T41.1X2	T41.1X3	T41.1X4	T41.1X5	T41.1X6
Barium (carbonate) (chloride) (sulfite)	T57.8X1	T57.8X2	T57.8X3	T57.8X4	—	—
diagnostic agent	T50.8X1	T50.8X2	T50.8X3	T50.8X4	T50.8X5	T50.8X6
pesticide	T60.4X1	T60.4X2	T60.4X3	T60.4X4	—	—
rodenticide	T60.4X1	T60.4X2	T60.4X3	T60.4X4	—	—
sulfate (medicinal)	T50.8X1	T50.8X2	T50.8X3	T50.8X4	T50.8X5	T50.8X6
Barrier cream	T49.3X1	T49.3X2	T49.3X3	T49.3X4	T49.3X5	T49.3X6
Basic fuchsin	T49.0X1	T49.0X2	T49.0X3	T49.0X4	T49.0X5	T49.0X6
Battery acid or fluid	T54.2X1	T54.2X2	T54.2X3	T54.2X4	—	—
Bay rum	T51.8X1	T51.8X2	T51.8X3	T51.8X4	—	—
BCG (vaccine)	T50.A91	T50.A92	T50.A93	T50.A94	T50.A95	T50.A96
BCNU	T45.1X1	T45.1X2	T45.1X3	T45.1X4	T45.1X5	T45.1X6
Bearsfoot	T62.2X1	T62.2X2	T62.2X3	T62.2X4	—	—
Beclamide	T42.6X1	T42.6X2	T42.6X3	T42.6X4	T42.6X5	T42.6X6
Beclomethasone	T44.5X1	T44.5X2	T44.5X3	T44.5X4	T44.5X5	T44.5X6
Bee (sting) (venom)	T63.441	T63.442	T63.443	T63.444	—	—
Befunolol	T49.5X1	T49.5X2	T49.5X3	T49.5X4	T49.5X5	T49.5X6
Bekanamycin	T36.5X1	T36.5X2	T36.5X3	T36.5X4	T36.5X5	T36.5X6
Belladonna — *see also Nightshade*						
alkaloids	T44.3X1	T44.3X2	T44.3X3	T44.3X4	T44.3X5	T44.3X6
extract	T44.3X1	T44.3X2	T44.3X3	T44.3X4	T44.3X5	T44.3X6
herb	T44.3X1	T44.3X2	T44.3X3	T44.3X4	T44.3X5	T44.3X6
Bemegride	T50.7X1	T50.7X2	T50.7X3	T50.7X4	T50.7X5	T50.7X6
Benactyzine	T44.3X1	T44.3X2	T44.3X3	T44.3X4	T44.3X5	T44.3X6
Benadryl	T45.0X1	T45.0X2	T45.0X3	T45.0X4	T45.0X5	T45.0X6
Benaprizine	T44.3X1	T44.3X2	T44.3X3	T44.3X4	T44.3X5	T44.3X6
Benazepril	T46.4X1	T46.4X2	T46.4X3	T46.4X4	T46.4X5	T46.4X6
Bencyclane	T46.7X1	T46.7X2	T46.7X3	T46.7X4	T46.7X5	T46.7X6
Bendazol	T46.3X1	T46.3X2	T46.3X3	T46.3X4	T46.3X5	T46.3X6
Bendrofluazide	T50.2X1	T50.2X2	T50.2X3	T50.2X4	T50.2X5	T50.2X6
Bendroflumethiazide	T50.2X1	T50.2X2	T50.2X3	T50.2X4	T50.2X5	T50.2X6
Benemid	T50.4X1	T50.4X2	T50.4X3	T50.4X4	T50.4X5	T50.4X6
Benethamine penicillin	T36.0X1	T36.0X2	T36.0X3	T36.0X4	T36.0X5	T36.0X6
Benisone	T49.0X1	T49.0X2	T49.0X3	T49.0X4	T49.0X5	T49.0X6

Substance	External Cause (T-Code)					
	Poisoning, Accidental (Unintentional)	Poisoning, Intentional Self-Harm	Poisoning, Assault	Poisoning, Undetermined	Adverse Effect	Underdosing
Benexate	T47.1X1	T47.1X2	T47.1X3	T47.1X4	T47.1X5	T47.1X6
Benfluorex	T46.6X1	T46.6X2	T46.6X3	T46.6X4	T46.6X5	T46.6X6
Benfotiamine	T45.2X1	T45.2X2	T45.2X3	T45.2X4	T45.2X5	T45.2X6
Benomyl	T6Ø.ØX1	T6Ø.ØX2	T6Ø.ØX3	T6Ø.ØX4	—	—
Benoquin	T49.8X1	T49.8X2	T49.8X3	T49.8X4	T49.8X5	T49.8X6
Benoxinate	T41.3X1	T41.3X2	T41.3X3	T41.3X4	T41.3X5	T41.3X6
Benperidol	T43.4X1	T43.4X2	T43.4X3	T43.4X4	T43.4X5	T43.4X6
Benproperine	T48.3X1	T48.3X2	T48.3X3	T48.3X4	T48.3X5	T48.3X6
Benserazide	T42.8X1	T42.8X2	T42.8X3	T42.8X4	T42.8X5	T42.8X6
Bentazepam	T42.4X1	T42.4X2	T42.4X3	T42.4X4	T42.4X5	T42.4X6
Bentiromide	T5Ø.8X1	T5Ø.8X2	T5Ø.8X3	T5Ø.8X4	T5Ø.8X5	T5Ø.8X6
Bentonite	T49.3X1	T49.3X2	T49.3X3	T49.3X4	T49.3X5	T49.3X6
Benzalbutyramide	T46.6X1	T46.6X2	T46.6X3	T46.6X4	T46.6X5	T46.6X6
Benzalkonium (chloride)	T49.ØX1	T49.ØX2	T49.ØX3	T49.ØX4	T49.ØX5	T49.ØX6
ophthalmic preparation	T49.5X1	T49.5X2	T49.5X3	T49.5X4	T49.5X5	T49.5X6
Benzamine	T41.3X1	T41.3X2	T41.3X3	T41.3X4	T41.3X5	T41.3X6
lactate	T49.1X1	T49.1X2	T49.1X3	T49.1X4	T49.1X5	T49.1X6
Benzamidosalicylate (calcium)	T37.1X1	T37.1X2	T37.1X3	T37.1X4	T37.1X5	T37.1X6
Benzamphetamine	T5Ø.5X1	T5Ø.5X2	T5Ø.5X3	T5Ø.5X4	T5Ø.5X5	T5Ø.5X6
Benzapril hydrochloride	T46.5X1	T46.5X2	T46.5X3	T46.5X4	T46.5X5	T46.5X6
Benzathine benzylpenicillin	T36.ØX1	T36.ØX2	T36.ØX3	T36.ØX4	T36.ØX5	T36.ØX6
Benzathine penicillin	T36.ØX1	T36.ØX2	T36.ØX3	T36.ØX4	T36.ØX5	T36.ØX6
Benzatropine	T42.8X1	T42.8X2	T42.8X3	T42.8X4	T42.8X5	T42.8X6
Benzbromarone	T5Ø.4X1	T5Ø.4X2	T5Ø.4X3	T5Ø.4X4	T5Ø.4X5	T5Ø.4X6
Benzcarbimine	T45.1X1	T45.1X2	T45.1X3	T45.1X4	T45.1X5	T45.1X6
Benzedrex	T44.991	T44.992	T44.993	T44.994	T44.995	T44.996
Benzedrine (amphetamine)	T43.621	T43.622	T43.623	T43.624	T43.625	T43.626
Benzenamine	T65.3X1	T65.3X2	T65.3X3	T65.3X4	—	—
Benzene	T52.1X1	T52.1X2	T52.1X3	T52.1X4	—	—
homologues (acetyl) (dimethyl) (methyl) (solvent)	T52.2X1	T52.2X2	T52.2X3	T52.2X4	—	—
Benzethonium (chloride)	T49.ØX1	T49.ØX2	T49.ØX3	T49.ØX4	T49.ØX5	T49.ØX6
Benzfetamine	T5Ø.5X1	T5Ø.5X2	T5Ø.5X3	T5Ø.5X4	T5Ø.5X5	T5Ø.5X6
Benzhexol	T44.3X1	T44.3X2	T44.3X3	T44.3X4	T44.3X5	T44.3X6
Benzhydramine (chloride)	T45.ØX1	T45.ØX2	T45.ØX3	T45.ØX4	T45.ØX5	T45.ØX6
Benzidine	T65.891	T65.892	T65.893	T65.894	—	—
Benzilonium bromide	T44.3X1	T44.3X2	T44.3X3	T44.3X4	T44.3X5	T44.3X6
Benzimidazole	T6Ø.3X1	T6Ø.3X2	T6Ø.3X3	T6Ø.3X4	—	—
Benzin(e) — *see Ligroin*						
Benziodarone	T46.3X1	T46.3X2	T46.3X3	T46.3X4	T46.3X5	T46.3X6
Benznidazole	T37.3X1	T37.3X2	T37.3X3	T37.3X4	T37.3X5	T37.3X6
Benzocaine	T41.3X1	T41.3X2	T41.3X3	T41.3X4	T41.3X5	T41.3X6
Benzoctamine	T43.ØX1	T43.ØX2	T43.ØX3	T43.ØX4	T43.ØX5	T43.ØX6
Benzodiapin	T42.4X1	T42.4X2	T42.4X3	T42.4X4	T42.4X5	T42.4X6
Benzodiazepine NEC	T42.4X1	T42.4X2	T42.4X3	T42.4X4	T42.4X5	T42.4X6
Benzoic acid	T49.ØX1	T49.ØX2	T49.ØX3	T49.ØX4	T49.ØX5	T49.ØX6
with salicylic acid	T49.ØX1	T49.ØX2	T49.ØX3	T49.ØX4	T49.ØX5	T49.ØX6
Benzoin (tincture)	T48.5X1	T48.5X2	T48.5X3	T48.5X4	T48.5X5	T48.5X6
Benzol (benzene)	T52.1X1	T52.1X2	T52.1X3	T52.1X4	—	—
vapor	T52.ØX1	T52.ØX2	T52.ØX3	T52.ØX4	—	—
Benzomorphan	T4Ø.2X1	T4Ø.2X2	T4Ø.2X3	T4Ø.2X4	T4Ø.2X5	T4Ø.2X6
Benzonatate	T48.3X1	T48.3X2	T48.3X3	T48.3X4	T48.3X5	T48.3X6
Benzophenones	T49.3X1	T49.3X2	T49.3X3	T49.3X4	T49.3X5	T49.3X6
Benzopyrone	T46.991	T46.992	T46.993	T46.994	T46.995	T46.996
Benzothiadiazides	T5Ø.2X1	T5Ø.2X2	T5Ø.2X3	T5Ø.2X4	T5Ø.2X5	T5Ø.2X6
Benzoxonium chloride	T49.ØX1	T49.ØX2	T49.ØX3	T49.ØX4	T49.ØX5	T49.ØX6
Benzoyl peroxide	T49.ØX1	T49.ØX2	T49.ØX3	T49.ØX4	T49.ØX5	T49.ØX6
Benzoylpas calcium	T37.1X1	T37.1X2	T37.1X3	T37.1X4	T37.1X5	T37.1X6
Benzperidin	T43.591	T43.592	T43.593	T43.594	T43.595	T43.596
Benzperidol	T43.591	T43.592	T43.593	T43.594	T43.595	T43.596
Benzphetamine	T5Ø.5X1	T5Ø.5X2	T5Ø.5X3	T5Ø.5X4	T5Ø.5X5	T5Ø.5X6
Benzpyrinium bromide	T44.1X1	T44.1X2	T44.1X3	T44.1X4	T44.1X5	T44.1X6
Benzquinamide	T45.ØX1	T45.ØX2	T45.ØX3	T45.ØX4	T45.ØX5	T45.ØX6
Benzthiazide	T5Ø.2X1	T5Ø.2X2	T5Ø.2X3	T5Ø.2X4	T5Ø.2X5	T5Ø.2X6
Benztropine						
anticholinergic	T44.3X1	T44.3X2	T44.3X3	T44.3X4	T44.3X5	T44.3X6
antiparkinson	T42.8X1	T42.8X2	T42.8X3	T42.8X4	T42.8X5	T42.8X6
Benzydamine	T49.ØX1	T49.ØX2	T49.ØX3	T49.ØX4	T49.ØX5	T49.ØX6
Benzyl						
acetate	T52.8X1	T52.8X2	T52.8X3	T52.8X4	—	—
alcohol	T49.ØX1	T49.ØX2	T49.ØX3	T49.ØX4	T49.ØX5	T49.ØX6
benzoate	T49.ØX1	T49.ØX2	T49.ØX3	T49.ØX4	T49.ØX5	T49.ØX6
Benzoic acid	T49.ØX1	T49.ØX2	T49.ØX3	T49.ØX4	T49.ØX5	T49.ØX6
morphine	T4Ø.2X1	T4Ø.2X2	T4Ø.2X3	T4Ø.2X4	—	—
nicotinate	T46.6X1	T46.6X2	T46.6X3	T46.6X4	T46.6X5	T46.6X6
penicillin	T36.ØX1	T36.ØX2	T36.ØX3	T36.ØX4	T36.ØX5	T36.ØX6
Benzylhydrochlorthia-zide	T5Ø.2X1	T5Ø.2X2	T5Ø.2X3	T5Ø.2X4	T5Ø.2X5	T5Ø.2X6
Benzylpenicillin	T36.ØX1	T36.ØX2	T36.ØX3	T36.ØX4	T36.ØX5	T36.ØX6
Benzylthiouracil	T38.2X1	T38.2X2	T38.2X3	T38.2X4	T38.2X5	T38.2X6
Bephenium hydroxy-naphthoate	T37.4X1	T37.4X2	T37.4X3	T37.4X4	T37.4X5	T37.4X6
Bepridil	T46.1X1	T46.1X2	T46.1X3	T46.1X4	T46.1X5	T46.1X6
Bergamot oil	T65.891	T65.892	T65.893	T65.894	—	—
Bergapten	T5Ø.991	T5Ø.992	T5Ø.993	T5Ø.994	T5Ø.995	T5Ø.996
Berries, poisonous	T62.1X1	T62.1X2	T62.1X3	T62.1X4	—	—

◄ New ◄ Revised ~~deleted~~ Deleted

Substance	External Cause (T-Code) Poisoning, Accidental (Unintentional)	Poisoning, Intentional Self-Harm	Poisoning, Assault	Poisoning, Undetermined	Adverse Effect	Underdosing
Beryllium (compounds)	T56.7X1	T56.7X2	T56.7X3	T56.7X4	—	—
b-acetyldigoxin	T46.ØX1	T46.ØX2	T46.ØX3	T46.ØX4	T46.ØX5	T46.ØX6
beta adrenergic blocking agent, heart	T44.7X1	T44.7X2	T44.7X3	T44.7X4	T44.7X5	T44.7X6
b-benzalbutyramide	T46.6X1	T46.6X2	T46.6X3	T46.6X4	T46.6X5	T46.6X6
Betacarotene	T45.2X1	T45.2X2	T45.2X3	T45.2X4	T45.2X5	T45.2X6
b-eucaine	T49.1X1	T49.1X2	T49.1X3	T49.1X4	T49.1X5	T49.1X6
Beta-Chlor	T42.6X1	T42.6X2	T42.6X3	T42.6X4	T42.6X5	T42.6X6
b-galactosidase	T47.5X1	T47.5X2	T47.5X3	T47.5X4	T47.5X5	T47.5X6
Betahistine	T46.7X1	T46.7X2	T46.7X3	T46.7X4	T46.7X5	T46.7X6
Betaine	T47.5X1	T47.5X2	T47.5X3	T47.5X4	T47.5X5	T47.5X6
Betamethasone	T49.ØX1	T49.ØX2	T49.ØX3	T49.ØX4	T49.ØX5	T49.ØX6
topical	T49.ØX1	T49.ØX2	T49.ØX3	T49.ØX4	T49.ØX5	T49.ØX6
Betamicin	T36.8X1	T36.8X2	T36.8X3	T36.8X4	T36.8X5	T36.8X6
Betanidine	T46.5X1	T46.5X2	T46.5X3	T46.5X4	T46.5X5	T46.5X6
b-sitosterol(s)	T46.6X1	T46.6X2	T46.6X3	T46.6X4	T46.6X5	T46.6X6
Betaxolol	T44.7X1	T44.7X2	T44.7X3	T44.7X4	T44.7X5	T44.7X6
Betazole	T5Ø.8X1	T5Ø.8X2	T5Ø.8X3	T5Ø.8X4	T5Ø.8X5	T5Ø.8X6
Bethanechol	T44.1X1	T44.1X2	T44.1X3	T44.1X4	T44.1X5	T44.1X6
chloride	T44.1X1	T44.1X2	T44.1X3	T44.1X4	T44.1X5	T44.1X6
Bethanidine	T46.5X1	T46.5X2	T46.5X3	T46.5X4	T46.5X5	T46.5X6
Betoxycaine	T41.3X1	T41.3X2	T41.3X3	T41.3X4	T41.3X5	T41.3X6
Betula oil	T49.3X1	T49.3X2	T49.3X3	T49.3X4	T49.3X5	T49.3X6
Bevantolol	T44.7X1	T44.7X2	T44.7X3	T44.7X4	T44.7X5	T44.7X6
Bevonium metilsulfate	T44.3X1	T44.3X2	T44.3X3	T44.3X4	T44.3X5	T44.3X6
Bezafibrate	T46.6X1	T46.6X2	T46.6X3	T46.6X4	T46.6X5	T46.6X6
Bezitramide	T4Ø.491	T4Ø.492	T4Ø.493	T4Ø.494	T4Ø.495	T4Ø.496
BHA	T5Ø.991	T5Ø.992	T5Ø.993	T5Ø.994	T5Ø.995	T5Ø.996
Bhang	T4Ø.711	T4Ø.712	T4Ø.713	T4Ø.714	T4Ø.715	T4Ø.716
BHC (medicinal)	T49.ØX1	T49.ØX2	T49.ØX3	T49.ØX4	T49.ØX5	T49.ØX6
nonmedicinal (vapor)	T53.6X1	T53.6X2	T53.6X3	T53.6X4	—	—
Bialamicol	T37.3X1	T37.3X2	T37.3X3	T37.3X4	T37.3X5	T37.3X6
Bibenzonium bromide	T48.3X1	T48.3X2	T48.3X3	T48.3X4	T48.3X5	T48.3X6
Bibrocathol	T49.5X1	T49.5X2	T49.5X3	T49.5X4	T49.5X5	T49.5X6
Bichloride of mercury — *see Mercury, chloride*						
Bichromates (calcium) (potassium) (sodium) (crystals)	T57.8X1	T57.8X2	T57.8X3	T57.8X4	—	—
fumes	T56.2X1	T56.2X2	T56.2X3	T56.2X4	—	—
Biclotymol	T49.6X1	T49.6X2	T49.6X3	T49.6X4	T49.6X5	T49.6X6
Bicuculline	T5Ø.7X1	T5Ø.7X2	T5Ø.7X3	T5Ø.7X4	T5Ø.7X5	T5Ø.7X6
Bifemelane	T43.291	T43.292	T43.293	T43.294	T43.295	T43.296
Biguanide derivatives, oral	T38.3X1	T38.3X2	T38.3X3	T38.3X4	T38.3X5	T38.3X6

Substance	External Cause (T-Code) Poisoning, Accidental (Unintentional)	Poisoning, Intentional Self-Harm	Poisoning, Assault	Poisoning, Undetermined	Adverse Effect	Underdosing
Biligrafin	T5Ø.8X1	T5Ø.8X2	T5Ø.8X3	T5Ø.8X4	T5Ø.8X5	T5Ø.8X6
Bile salts	T47.5X1	T47.5X2	T47.5X3	T47.5X4	T47.5X5	T47.5X6
Bilopaque	T5Ø.8X1	T5Ø.8X2	T5Ø.8X3	T5Ø.8X4	T5Ø.8X5	T5Ø.8X6
Binifibrate	T46.6X1	T46.6X2	T46.6X3	T46.6X4	T46.6X5	T46.6X6
Binitrobenzol	T65.3X1	T65.3X2	T65.3X3	T65.3X4	—	—
Bioflavonoid(s)	T46.991	T46.992	T46.993	T46.994	T46.995	T46.996
Biological substance NEC	T5Ø.9Ø1	T5Ø.9Ø2	T5Ø.9Ø3	T5Ø.9Ø4	T5Ø.9Ø5	T5Ø.9Ø6
Biotin	T45.2X1	T45.2X2	T45.2X3	T45.2X4	T45.2X5	T45.2X6
Biperiden	T44.3X1	T44.3X2	T44.3X3	T44.3X4	T44.3X5	T44.3X6
Bisacodyl	T47.2X1	T47.2X2	T47.2X3	T47.2X4	T47.2X5	T47.2X6
Bisbentiamine	T45.2X1	T45.2X2	T45.2X3	T45.2X4	T45.2X5	T45.2X6
Bisbutiamine	T45.2X1	T45.2X2	T45.2X3	T45.2X4	T45.2X5	T45.2X6
Bisdequalinium (salts) (diacetate)	T49.6X1	T49.6X2	T49.6X3	T49.6X4	T49.6X5	T49.6X6
Bishydroxycoumarin	T45.511	T45.512	T45.513	T45.514	T45.515	T45.516
Bismarsen	T37.8X1	T37.8X2	T37.8X3	T37.8X4	T37.8X5	T37.8X6
Bismuth salts	T47.6X1	T47.6X2	T47.6X3	T47.6X4	T47.6X5	T47.6X6
aluminate	T47.1X1	T47.1X2	T47.1X3	T47.1X4	T47.1X5	T47.1X6
anti-infectives	T37.8X1	T37.8X2	T37.8X3	T37.8X4	T37.8X5	T37.8X6
formic iodide	T49.ØX1	T49.ØX2	T49.ØX3	T49.ØX4	T49.ØX5	T49.ØX6
glycolylarsenate	T49.ØX1	T49.ØX2	T49.ØX3	T49.ØX4	T49.ØX5	T49.ØX6
nonmedicinal (compounds) NEC	T65.91	T65.92	T65.93	T65.94	—	—
subcarbonate	T47.6X1	T47.6X2	T47.6X3	T47.6X4	T47.6X5	T47.6X6
subsalicylate	T37.8X1	T37.8X2	T37.8X3	T37.8X4	T37.8X5	T37.8X6
sulfarsphenamine	T37.8X1	T37.8X2	T37.8X3	T37.8X4	T37.8X5	T37.8X6
Bisoprolol	T44.7X1	T44.7X2	T44.7X3	T44.7X4	T44.7X5	T44.7X6
Bisoxatin	T47.2X1	T47.2X2	T47.2X3	T47.2X4	T47.2X5	T47.2X6
Bisulepin (hydrochloride)	T45.ØX1	T45.ØX2	T45.ØX3	T45.ØX4	T45.ØX5	T45.ØX6
Bithionol	T37.8X1	T37.8X2	T37.8X3	T37.8X4	T37.8X5	T37.8X6
anthelminthic	T37.4X1	T37.4X2	T37.4X3	T37.4X4	T37.4X5	T37.4X6
Bitolterol	T48.6X1	T48.6X2	T48.6X3	T48.6X4	T48.6X5	T48.6X6
Bitoscanate	T37.4X1	T37.4X2	T37.4X3	T37.4X4	T37.4X5	T37.4X6
Bitter almond oil	T62.8X1	T62.8X2	T62.8X3	T62.8X4	—	—
Bittersweet	T62.2X1	T62.2X2	T62.2X3	T62.2X4	—	—
Black						
flag	T6Ø.91	T6Ø.92	T6Ø.93	T6Ø.94	—	—
henbane	T62.2X1	T62.2X2	T62.2X3	T62.2X4	—	—
leaf (4Ø)	T6Ø.91	T6Ø.92	T6Ø.93	T6Ø.94	—	—
widow spider (bite)	T63.311	T63.312	T63.313	T63.314	—	—
antivenin	T5Ø.Z11	T5Ø.Z12	T5Ø.Z13	T5Ø.Z14	T5Ø.Z15	T5Ø.Z16
Blast furnace gas (carbon monoxide from)	T58.8X1	T58.8X2	T58.8X3	T58.8X4	—	—
Bleach	T54.91	T54.92	T54.93	T54.94	—	—

TABLE OF DRUGS AND CHEMICALS

New Revised ~~deleted~~ Deleted

Substance	External Cause (T-Code)					
	Poisoning, Accidental (Unintentional)	Poisoning, Intentional Self-Harm	Poisoning, Assault	Poisoning, Undetermined	Adverse Effect	Underdosing
Bleaching agent (medicinal)	T49.4X1	T49.4X2	T49.4X3	T49.4X4	T49.4X5	T49.4X6
Bleomycin	T45.1X1	T45.1X2	T45.1X3	T45.1X4	T45.1X5	T45.1X6
Blockain	T41.3X1	T41.3X2	T41.3X3	T41.3X4	T41.3X5	T41.3X6
infiltration (subcutaneous)	T41.3X1	T41.3X2	T41.3X3	T41.3X4	T41.3X5	T41.3X6
nerve block (peripheral) (plexus)	T41.3X1	T41.3X2	T41.3X3	T41.3X4	T41.3X5	T41.3X6
topical (surface)	T41.3X1	T41.3X2	T41.3X3	T41.3X4	T41.3X5	T41.3X6
Blockers, calcium channel	T46.1X1	T46.1X2	T46.1X3	T46.1X4	T46.1X5	T46.1X6
Blood (derivatives) (natural) (plasma) (whole)	T45.8X1	T45.8X2	T45.8X3	T45.8X4	T45.8X5	T45.8X6
dried	T45.8X1	T45.8X2	T45.8X3	T45.8X4	T45.8X5	T45.8X6
drug affecting NEC	T45.91	T45.92	T45.93	T45.94	T45.95	T45.96
expander NEC	T45.8X1	T45.8X2	T45.8X3	T45.8X4	T45.8X5	T45.8X6
fraction NEC	T45.8X1	T45.8X2	T45.8X3	T45.8X4	T45.8X5	T45.8X6
substitute (macromolecular)	T45.8X1	T45.8X2	T45.8X3	T45.8X4	T45.8X5	T45.8X6
Blue velvet	T4Ø.2X1	T4Ø.2X2	T4Ø.2X3	T4Ø.2X4	—	—
Bone meal	T62.8X1	T62.8X2	T62.8X3	T62.8X4	—	—
Bonine	T45.ØX1	T45.ØX2	T45.ØX3	T45.ØX4	T45.ØX5	T45.ØX6
Bopindolol	T44.7X1	T44.7X2	T44.7X3	T44.7X4	T44.7X5	T44.7X6
Boracic acid	T49.ØX1	T49.ØX2	T49.ØX3	T49.ØX4	T49.ØX5	T49.ØX6
ENT agent	T49.6X1	T49.6X2	T49.6X3	T49.6X4	T49.6X5	T49.6X6
ophthalmic preparation	T49.5X1	T49.5X2	T49.5X3	T49.5X4	T49.5X5	T49.5X6
Borane complex	T57.8X1	T57.8X2	T57.8X3	T57.8X4	—	—
Borate(s)	T57.8X1	T57.8X2	T57.8X3	T57.8X4	—	—
buffer	T5Ø.991	T5Ø.992	T5Ø.993	T5Ø.994	T5Ø.995	T5Ø.996
cleanser	T54.91	T54.92	T54.93	T54.94	—	—
sodium	T57.8X1	T57.8X2	T57.8X3	T57.8X4	—	—
Borax (cleanser)	T54.91	T54.92	T54.93	T54.94	—	—
Bordeaux mixture	T6Ø.3X1	T6Ø.3X2	T6Ø.3X3	T6Ø.3X4	—	—
Boric acid	T49.ØX1	T49.ØX2	T49.ØX3	T49.ØX4	T49.ØX5	T49.ØX6
ENT agent	T49.6X1	T49.6X2	T49.6X3	T49.6X4	T49.6X5	T49.6X6
ophthalmic preparation	T49.5X1	T49.5X2	T49.5X3	T49.5X4	T49.5X5	T49.5X6
Bornaprine	T44.3X1	T44.3X2	T44.3X3	T44.3X4	T44.3X5	T44.3X6
Boron	T57.8X1	T57.8X2	T57.8X3	T57.8X4	—	—
hydride NEC	T57.8X1	T57.8X2	T57.8X3	T57.8X4	—	—
fumes or gas	T57.8X1	T57.8X2	T57.8X3	T57.8X4	—	—
trifluoride	T59.891	T59.892	T59.893	T59.894	—	—
Botox	T48.291	T48.292	T48.293	T48.294	T48.295	T48.296
Botulinus anti-toxin (type A, B)	T5Ø.Z11	T5Ø.Z12	T5Ø.Z13	T5Ø.Z14	T5Ø.Z15	T5Ø.Z16
Brake fluid vapor	T59.891	T59.892	T59.893	T59.894	—	—
Brallobarbital	T42.3X1	T42.3X2	T42.3X3	T42.3X4	T42.3X5	T42.3X6
Bran (wheat)	T47.4X1	T47.4X2	T47.4X3	T47.4X4	T47.4X5	T47.4X6
Brass (fumes)	T56.891	T56.892	T56.893	T56.894	—	—
Brasso	T52.ØX1	T52.ØX2	T52.ØX3	T52.ØX4	—	—
Bretylium tosilate	T46.2X1	T46.2X2	T46.2X3	T46.2X4	T46.2X5	T46.2X6
Brevital (sodium)	T41.1X1	T41.1X2	T41.1X3	T41.1X4	T41.1X5	T41.1X6
Brinase	T45.3X1	T45.3X2	T45.3X3	T45.3X4	T45.3X5	T45.3X6
British antilewisite	T45.8X1	T45.8X2	T45.8X3	T45.8X4	T45.8X5	T45.8X6
Brodifacoum	T6Ø.4X1	T6Ø.4X2	T6Ø.4X3	T6Ø.4X4	—	—
Bromal (hydrate)	T42.6X1	T42.6X2	T42.6X3	T42.6X4	T42.6X5	T42.6X6
Bromazepam	T42.4X1	T42.4X2	T42.4X3	T42.4X4	T42.4X5	T42.4X6
Bromazine	T45.ØX1	T45.ØX2	T45.ØX3	T45.ØX4	T45.ØX5	T45.ØX6
Brombenzylcyanide	T59.3X1	T59.3X2	T59.3X3	T59.3X4	—	—
Bromelains	T45.3X1	T45.3X2	T45.3X3	T45.3X4	T45.3X5	T45.3X6
Bromethalin	T6Ø.4X1	T6Ø.4X2	T6Ø.4X3	T6Ø.4X4	—	—
Bromhexine	T48.4X1	T48.4X2	T48.4X3	T48.4X4	T48.4X5	T48.4X6
Bromide salts	T42.6X1	T42.6X2	T42.6X3	T42.6X4	T42.6X5	T42.6X6
Bromindione	T45.511	T45.512	T45.513	T45.514	T45.515	T45.516
Bromine						
compounds (medicinal)	T42.6X1	T42.6X2	T42.6X3	T42.6X4	T42.6X5	T42.6X6
sedative	T42.6X1	T42.6X2	T42.6X3	T42.6X4	T42.6X5	T42.6X6
vapor	T59.891	T59.892	T59.893	T59.894	—	—
Bromisovalum	T42.6X1	T42.6X2	T42.6X3	T42.6X4	T42.6X5	T42.6X6
Bromisoval	T42.6X1	T42.6X2	T42.6X3	T42.6X4	T42.6X5	T42.6X6
Bromobenzylcyanide	T59.3X1	T59.3X2	T59.3X3	T59.3X4	—	—
Bromochlorosalicylani-lide	T49.ØX1	T49.ØX2	T49.ØX3	T49.ØX4	T49.ØX5	T49.ØX6
Bromocriptine	T42.8X1	T42.8X2	T42.8X3	T42.8X4	T42.8X5	T42.8X6
Bromodiphenhydramine	T45.ØX1	T45.ØX2	T45.ØX3	T45.ØX4	T45.ØX5	T45.ØX6
Bromoform	T42.6X1	T42.6X2	T42.6X3	T42.6X4	T42.6X5	T42.6X6
Bromophenol blue reagent	T5Ø.991	T5Ø.992	T5Ø.993	T5Ø.994	T5Ø.995	T5Ø.996
Bromopride	T47.8X1	T47.8X2	T47.8X3	T47.8X4	T47.8X5	T47.8X6
Bromosalicylchloranitide	T49.ØX1	T49.ØX2	T49.ØX3	T49.ØX4	T49.ØX5	T49.ØX6
Bromosalicylhydroxamic acid	T37.1X1	T37.1X2	T37.1X3	T37.1X4	T37.1X5	T37.1X6
Bromo-seltzer	T39.1X1	T39.1X2	T39.1X3	T39.1X4	T39.1X5	T39.1X6
Bromoxynil	T6Ø.3X1	T6Ø.3X2	T6Ø.3X3	T6Ø.3X4	—	—
Bromperidol	T43.4X1	T43.4X2	T43.4X3	T43.4X4	T43.4X5	T43.4X6
Brompheniramine	T45.ØX1	T45.ØX2	T45.ØX3	T45.ØX4	T45.ØX5	T45.ØX6
Bromsulfophthalein	T5Ø.8X1	T5Ø.8X2	T5Ø.8X3	T5Ø.8X4	T5Ø.8X5	T5Ø.8X6
Bromural	T42.6X1	T42.6X2	T42.6X3	T42.6X4	T42.6X5	T42.6X6
Bromvaletone	T42.6X1	T42.6X2	T42.6X3	T42.6X4	T42.6X5	T42.6X6
Bronchodilator NEC	T48.6X1	T48.6X2	T48.6X3	T48.6X4	T48.6X5	T48.6X6
Brotizolam	T42.4X1	T42.4X2	T42.4X3	T42.4X4	T42.4X5	T42.4X6
Brovincamine	T46.7X1	T46.7X2	T46.7X3	T46.7X4	T46.7X5	T46.7X6
Brown spider (bite) (venom)	T63.391	T63.392	T63.393	T63.394	—	—

Substance	External Cause (T-Code)					
	Poisoning, Accidental (Unintentional)	Poisoning, Intentional Self-Harm	Poisoning, Assault	Poisoning, Undetermined	Adverse Effect	Underdosing
Brown recluse spider (bite) (venom)	T63.331	T63.332	T63.333	T63.334	—	—
Broxaterol	T48.6X1	T48.6X2	T48.6X3	T48.6X4	T48.6X5	T48.6X6
Broxuridine	T45.1X1	T45.1X2	T45.1X3	T45.1X4	T45.1X5	T45.1X6
Broxyquinoline	T37.8X1	T37.8X2	T37.8X3	T37.8X4	T37.8X5	T37.8X6
Bruceine	T48.291	T48.292	T48.293	T48.294	T48.295	T48.296
Brucia	T62.2X1	T62.2X2	T62.2X3	T62.2X4	—	—
Brucine	T65.1X1	T65.1X2	T65.1X3	T65.1X4	—	—
Brunswick green — *see Copper*						
Bruten — *see Ibuprofen*						
Bryonia	T47.2X1	T47.2X2	T47.2X3	T47.2X4	T47.2X5	T47.2X6
Buclizine	T45.0X1	T45.0X2	T45.0X3	T45.0X4	T45.0X5	T45.0X6
Buclosamide	T49.0X1	T49.0X2	T49.0X3	T49.0X4	T49.0X5	T49.0X6
Budesonide	T44.5X1	T44.5X2	T44.5X3	T44.5X4	T44.5X5	T44.5X6
Budralazine	T46.5X1	T46.5X2	T46.5X3	T46.5X4	T46.5X5	T46.5X6
Bufferin	T39.011	T39.012	T39.013	T39.014	T39.015	T39.016
Buflomedil	T46.7X1	T46.7X2	T46.7X3	T46.7X4	T46.7X5	T46.7X6
Buformin	T38.3X1	T38.3X2	T38.3X3	T38.3X4	T38.3X5	T38.3X6
Bufotenine	T40.991	T40.992	T40.993	T40.994	—	—
Bufrolin	T48.6X1	T48.6X2	T48.6X3	T48.6X4	T48.6X5	T48.6X6
Bufylline	T48.6X1	T48.6X2	T48.6X3	T48.6X4	T48.6X5	T48.6X6
Bulk filler	T50.5X1	T50.5X2	T50.5X3	T50.5X4	T50.5X5	T50.5X6
cathartic	T47.4X1	T47.4X2	T47.4X3	T47.4X4	T47.4X5	T47.4X6
Bumetanide	T50.1X1	T50.1X2	T50.1X3	T50.1X4	T50.1X5	T50.1X6
Bunaftine	T46.2X1	T46.2X2	T46.2X3	T46.2X4	T46.2X5	T46.2X6
Bunamiodyl	T50.8X1	T50.8X2	T50.8X3	T50.8X4	T50.8X5	T50.8X6
Bunazosin	T44.6X1	T44.6X2	T44.6X3	T44.6X4	T44.6X5	T44.6X6
Bunitrolol	T44.7X1	T44.7X2	T44.7X3	T44.7X4	T44.7X5	T44.7X6
Buphenine	T46.7X1	T46.7X2	T46.7X3	T46.7X4	T46.7X5	T46.7X6
Bupivacaine	T41.3X1	T41.3X2	T41.3X3	T41.3X4	T41.3X5	T41.3X6
infiltration (subcutaneous)	T41.3X1	T41.3X2	T41.3X3	T41.3X4	T41.3X5	T41.3X6
nerve block (peripheral) (plexus)	T41.3X1	T41.3X2	T41.3X3	T41.3X4	T41.3X5	T41.3X6
spinal	T41.3X1	T41.3X2	T41.3X3	T41.3X4	T41.3X5	T41.3X6
Bupranolol	T44.7X1	T44.7X2	T44.7X3	T44.7X4	T44.7X5	T44.7X6
Buprenorphine	T40.491	T40.492	T40.493	T40.494	T40.495	T40.496
Bupropion	T43.291	T43.292	T43.293	T43.294	T43.295	T43.296
Burimamide	T47.1X1	T47.1X2	T47.1X3	T47.1X4	T47.1X5	T47.1X6
Buserelin	T38.891	T38.892	T38.893	T38.894	T38.895	T38.896
Buspirone	T43.591	T43.592	T43.593	T43.594	T43.595	T43.596
Busulfan, busulphan	T45.1X1	T45.1X2	T45.1X3	T45.1X4	T45.1X5	T45.1X6
Butabarbital (sodium)	T42.3X1	T42.3X2	T42.3X3	T42.3X4	T42.3X5	T42.3X6
Butabarbitone	T42.3X1	T42.3X2	T42.3X3	T42.3X4	T42.3X5	T42.3X6

Substance	External Cause (T-Code)					
	Poisoning, Accidental (Unintentional)	Poisoning, Intentional Self-Harm	Poisoning, Assault	Poisoning, Undetermined	Adverse Effect	Underdosing
Butabarpal	T42.3X1	T42.3X2	T42.3X3	T42.3X4	T42.3X5	T42.3X6
Butacaine	T41.3X1	T41.3X2	T41.3X3	T41.3X4	T41.3X5	T41.3X6
Butalamine	T46.7X1	T46.7X2	T46.7X3	T46.7X4	T46.7X5	T46.7X6
Butalbital	T42.3X1	T42.3X2	T42.3X3	T42.3X4	T42.3X5	T42.3X6
Butallylonal	T42.3X1	T42.3X2	T42.3X3	T42.3X4	T42.3X5	T42.3X6
Butamben	T41.3X1	T41.3X2	T41.3X3	T41.3X4	T41.3X5	T41.3X6
Butamirate	T48.3X1	T48.3X2	T48.3X3	T48.3X4	T48.3X5	T48.3X6
Butane (distributed in mobile container)	T59.891	T59.892	T59.893	T59.894	—	—
distributed through pipes	T59.891	T59.892	T59.893	T59.894	—	—
incomplete combustion	T58.11	T58.12	T58.13	T58.14	—	—
Butanilicaine	T41.3X1	T41.3X2	T41.3X3	T41.3X4	T41.3X5	T41.3X6
Butanol	T51.3X1	T51.3X2	T51.3X3	T51.3X4	—	—
Butanone, 2-butanone	T52.4X1	T52.4X2	T52.4X3	T52.4X4	—	—
Butantrone	T49.4X1	T49.4X2	T49.4X3	T49.4X4	T49.4X5	T49.4X6
Butaperazine	T43.3X1	T43.3X2	T43.3X3	T43.3X4	T43.3X5	T43.3X6
Butazolidin	T39.2X1	T39.2X2	T39.2X3	T39.2X4	T39.2X5	T39.2X6
Butetamate	T48.6X1	T48.6X2	T48.6X3	T48.6X4	T48.6X5	T48.6X6
Butethal	T42.3X1	T42.3X2	T42.3X3	T42.3X4	T42.3X5	T42.3X6
Butethamate	T44.3X1	T44.3X2	T44.3X3	T44.3X4	T44.3X5	T44.3X6
Buthalitone (sodium)	T41.1X1	T41.1X2	T41.1X3	T41.1X4	T41.1X5	T41.1X6
Butisol (sodium)	T42.3X1	T42.3X2	T42.3X3	T42.3X4	T42.3X5	T42.3X6
Butizide	T50.2X1	T50.2X2	T50.2X3	T50.2X4	T50.2X5	T50.2X6
Butobarbital	T42.3X1	T42.3X2	T42.3X3	T42.3X4	T42.3X5	T42.3X6
sodium	T42.3X1	T42.3X2	T42.3X3	T42.3X4	T42.3X5	T42.3X6
Butobarbitone	T42.3X1	T42.3X2	T42.3X3	T42.3X4	T42.3X5	T42.3X6
Butoconazole (nitrate)	T49.0X1	T49.0X2	T49.0X3	T49.0X4	T49.0X5	T49.0X6
Butorphanol	T40.491	T40.492	T40.493	T40.494	T40.495	T40.496
Butriptyline	T43.011	T43.012	T43.013	T43.014	T43.015	T43.016
Butropium bromide	T44.3X1	T44.3X2	T44.3X3	T44.3X4	T44.3X5	T44.3X6
Buttercups	T62.2X1	T62.2X2	T62.2X3	T62.2X4	—	—
Butter of antimony — *see Antimony*						
Butyl						
acetate (secondary)	T52.8X1	T52.8X2	T52.8X3	T52.8X4	—	—
alcohol	T51.3X1	T51.3X2	T51.3X3	T51.3X4	—	—
aminobenzoate	T41.3X1	T41.3X2	T41.3X3	T41.3X4	T41.3X5	T41.3X6
butyrate	T52.8X1	T52.8X2	T52.8X3	T52.8X4	—	—
carbinol	T51.3X1	T51.3X2	T51.3X3	T51.3X4	—	—
carbitol	T52.3X1	T52.3X2	T52.3X3	T52.3X4	—	—
cellosolve	T52.3X1	T52.3X2	T52.3X3	T52.3X4	—	—
chloral (hydrate)	T42.6X1	T42.6X2	T42.6X3	T42.6X4	T42.6X5	T42.6X6
formate	T52.8X1	T52.8X2	T52.8X3	T52.8X4	—	—

	External Cause (T-Code)					
Substance	Poisoning, Accidental (Unintentional)	Poisoning, Intentional Self-Harm	Poisoning, Assault	Poisoning, Undetermined	Adverse Effect	Underdosing
Butyl *(Continued)*						
lactate	T52.8X1	T52.8X2	T52.8X3	T52.8X4	—	—
propionate	T52.8X1	T52.8X2	T52.8X3	T52.8X4	—	—
scopolamine bromide	T44.3X1	T44.3X2	T44.3X3	T44.3X4	T44.3X5	T44.3X6
thiobarbital sodium	T41.1X1	T41.1X2	T41.1X3	T41.1X4	T41.1X5	T41.1X6
Butylated hydroxy-anisole	T5Ø.991	T5Ø.992	T5Ø.993	T5Ø.994	T5Ø.995	T5Ø.996
Butylchloral hydrate	T42.6X1	T42.6X2	T42.6X3	T42.6X4	T42.6X5	T42.6X6
Butyltoluene	T52.2X1	T52.2X2	T52.2X3	T52.2X4	—	—
Butyn	T41.3X1	T41.3X2	T41.3X3	T41.3X4	T41.3X5	T41.3X6
Butyrophenone (-based tranquilizers)	T43.4X1	T43.4X2	T43.4X3	T43.4X4	T43.4X5	T43.4X6
C						
Cabergoline	T42.8X1	T42.8X2	T42.8X3	T42.8X4	T42.8X5	T42.8X6
Cacodyl, cacodylic acid	T57.ØX1	T57.ØX2	T57.ØX3	T57.ØX4	—	—
Cactinomycin	T45.1X1	T45.1X2	T45.1X3	T45.1X4	T45.1X5	T45.1X6
Cade oil	T49.4X1	T49.4X2	T49.4X3	T49.4X4	T49.4X5	T49.4X6
Cadexomer iodine	T49.ØX1	T49.ØX2	T49.ØX3	T49.ØX4	T49.ØX5	T49.ØX6
Cadmium (chloride) (fumes) (oxide)	T56.3X1	T56.3X2	T56.3X3	T56.3X4	—	—
sulfide (medicinal) NEC	T49.4X1	T49.4X2	T49.4X3	T49.4X4	T49.4X5	T49.4X6
Cadralazine	T46.5X1	T46.5X2	T46.5X3	T46.5X4	T46.5X5	T46.5X6
Caffeine	T43.611	T43.612	T43.613	T43.614	T43.615	T43.616
Calabar bean	T62.2X1	T62.2X2	T62.2X3	T62.2X4	—	—
Caladium seguinum	T62.2X1	T62.2X2	T62.2X3	T62.2X4	—	—
Calamine (lotion)	T49.3X1	T49.3X2	T49.3X3	T49.3X4	T49.3X5	T49.3X6
Calcifediol	T45.2X1	T45.2X2	T45.2X3	T45.2X4	T45.2X5	T45.2X6
Calciferol	T45.2X1	T45.2X2	T45.2X3	T45.2X4	T45.2X5	T45.2X6
Calcitonin	T5Ø.991	T5Ø.992	T5Ø.993	T5Ø.994	T5Ø.995	T5Ø.996
Calcitriol	T45.2X1	T45.2X2	T45.2X3	T45.2X4	T45.2X5	T45.2X6
Calcium	T5Ø.3X1	T5Ø.3X2	T5Ø.3X3	T5Ø.3X4	T5Ø.3X5	T5Ø.3X6
actylsalicylate	T39.Ø11	T39.Ø12	T39.Ø13	T39.Ø14	T39.Ø15	T39.Ø16
benzamidosalicylate	T37.1X1	T37.1X2	T37.1X3	T37.1X4	T37.1X5	T37.1X6
bromide	T42.6X1	T42.6X2	T42.6X3	T42.6X4	T42.6X5	T42.6X6
bromolactobionate	T42.6X1	T42.6X2	T42.6X3	T42.6X4	T42.6X5	T42.6X6
carbaspirin	T39.Ø11	T39.Ø12	T39.Ø13	T39.Ø14	T39.Ø15	T39.Ø16
carbimide	T5Ø.6X1	T5Ø.6X2	T5Ø.6X3	T5Ø.6X4	T5Ø.6X5	T5Ø.6X6
carbonate	T47.1X1	T47.1X2	T47.1X3	T47.1X4	T47.1X5	T47.1X6
chloride	T5Ø.991	T5Ø.992	T5Ø.993	T5Ø.994	T5Ø.995	T5Ø.996
anhydrous	T5Ø.991	T5Ø.992	T5Ø.993	T5Ø.994	T5Ø.995	T5Ø.996
cyanide	T57.8X1	T57.8X2	T57.8X3	T57.8X4	—	—
dioctyl sulfosuccinate	T47.4X1	T47.4X2	T47.4X3	T47.4X4	T47.4X5	T47.4X6
disodium edathamil	T45.8X1	T45.8X2	T45.8X3	T45.8X4	T45.8X5	T45.8X6

	External Cause (T-Code)					
Substance	Poisoning, Accidental (Unintentional)	Poisoning, Intentional Self-Harm	Poisoning, Assault	Poisoning, Undetermined	Adverse Effect	Underdosing
Calcium *(Continued)*						
disodium edetate	T45.8X1	T45.8X2	T45.8X3	T45.8X4	T45.8X5	T45.8X6
dobesilate	T46.991	T46.992	T46.993	T46.994	T46.995	T46.996
EDTA	T45.8X1	T45.8X2	T45.8X3	T45.8X4	T45.8X5	T45.8X6
ferrous citrate	T45.4X1	T45.4X2	T45.4X3	T45.4X4	T45.4X5	T45.4X6
folinate	T45.8X1	T45.8X2	T45.8X3	T45.8X4	T45.8X5	T45.8X6
glubionate	T5Ø.3X1	T5Ø.3X2	T5Ø.3X3	T5Ø.3X4	T5Ø.3X5	T5Ø.3X6
gluconate	T5Ø.3X1	T5Ø.3X2	T5Ø.3X3	T5Ø.3X4	T5Ø.3X5	T5Ø.3X6
gluconogalactogluconate	T5Ø.3X1	T5Ø.3X2	T5Ø.3X3	T5Ø.3X4	T5Ø.3X5	T5Ø.3X6
hydrate, hydroxide	T54.3X1	T54.3X2	T54.3X3	T54.3X4	—	—
hypochlorite	T54.3X1	T54.3X2	T54.3X3	T54.3X4	—	—
iodide	T48.4X1	T48.4X2	T48.4X3	T48.4X4	T48.4X5	T48.4X6
ipodate	T5Ø.8X1	T5Ø.8X2	T5Ø.8X3	T5Ø.8X4	T5Ø.8X5	T5Ø.8X6
lactate	T5Ø.3X1	T5Ø.3X2	T5Ø.3X3	T5Ø.3X4	T5Ø.3X5	T5Ø.3X6
leucovorin	T45.8X1	T45.8X2	T45.8X3	T45.8X4	T45.8X5	T45.8X6
mandelate	T37.91	T37.92	T37.93	T37.94	T37.95	T37.96
oxide	T54.3X1	T54.3X2	T54.3X3	T54.3X4	—	—
pantothenate	T45.2X1	T45.2X2	T45.2X3	T45.2X4	T45.2X5	T45.2X6
phosphate	T5Ø.3X1	T5Ø.3X2	T5Ø.3X3	T5Ø.3X4	T5Ø.3X5	T5Ø.3X6
salicylate	T39.Ø91	T39.Ø92	T39.Ø93	T39.Ø94	T39.Ø95	T39.Ø96
salts	T5Ø.3X1	T5Ø.3X2	T5Ø.3X3	T5Ø.3X4	T5Ø.3X5	T5Ø.3X6
Calculus-dissolving drug	T5Ø.991	T5Ø.992	T5Ø.993	T5Ø.994	T5Ø.995	T5Ø.996
Calomel	T49.ØX1	T49.ØX2	T49.ØX3	T49.ØX4	T49.ØX5	T49.ØX6
Caloric agent	T5Ø.3X1	T5Ø.3X2	T5Ø.3X3	T5Ø.3X4	T5Ø.3X5	T5Ø.3X6
Calusterone	T38.7X1	T38.7X2	T38.7X3	T38.7X4	T38.7X5	T38.7X6
Camazepam	T42.4X1	T42.4X2	T42.4X3	T42.4X4	T42.4X5	T42.4X6
Camomile	T49.ØX1	T49.ØX2	T49.ØX3	T49.ØX4	T49.ØX5	T49.ØX6
Camoquin	T37.2X1	T37.2X2	T37.2X3	T37.2X4	T37.2X5	T37.2X6
Camphor						
insecticide	T6Ø.2X1	T6Ø.2X2	T6Ø.2X3	T6Ø.2X4	—	—
medicinal	T49.8X1	T49.8X2	T49.8X3	T49.8X4	T49.8X5	T49.8X6
Camylofin	T44.3X1	T44.3X2	T44.3X3	T44.3X4	T44.3X5	T44.3X6
Cancer chemotherapy drug regimen	T45.1X1	T45.1X2	T45.1X3	T45.1X4	T45.1X5	T45.1X6
Candeptin	T49.ØX1	T49.ØX2	T49.ØX3	T49.ØX4	T49.ØX5	T49.ØX6
Candicidin	T49.ØX1	T49.ØX2	T49.ØX3	T49.ØX4	T49.ØX5	T49.ØX6
Cannabinoids, synthetic	T4Ø.721	T4Ø.722	T4Ø.723	T4Ø.724	T4Ø.725	T4Ø.726
Cannabinol	T4Ø.711	T4Ø.712	T4Ø.713	T4Ø.714	T4Ø.715	T4Ø.716
Cannabis (derivatives)	T4Ø.711	T4Ø.712	T4Ø.713	T4Ø.714	T4Ø.715	T4Ø.716
Canned heat	T51.1X1	T51.1X2	T51.1X3	T51.1X4	—	—
Canrenoic acid	T5Ø.ØX1	T5Ø.ØX2	T5Ø.ØX3	T5Ø.ØX4	T5Ø.ØX5	T5Ø.ØX6
Canrenone	T5Ø.ØX1	T5Ø.ØX2	T5Ø.ØX3	T5Ø.ØX4	T5Ø.ØX5	T5Ø.ØX6

New Revised ~~deleted~~ Deleted

Substance	Poisoning, Accidental (Unintentional)	Poisoning, Intentional Self-Harm	Poisoning, Assault	Poisoning, Undetermined	Adverse Effect	Underdosing
Cantharides, cantharidin, cantharis	T49.8X1	T49.8X2	T49.8X3	T49.8X4	T49.8X5	T49.8X6
Canthaxanthin	T50.991	T50.992	T50.993	T50.994	T50.995	T50.996
Capillary-active drug NEC	T46.901	T46.902	T46.903	T46.904	T46.905	T46.906
Capreomycin	T36.8X1	T36.8X2	T36.8X3	T36.8X4	T36.8X5	T36.8X6
Capsicum	T49.4X1	T49.4X2	T49.4X3	T49.4X4	T49.4X5	T49.4X6
Captafol	T60.3X1	T60.3X2	T60.3X3	T60.3X4	—	—
Captan	T60.3X1	T60.3X2	T60.3X3	T60.3X4	—	—
Captodiame, captodiamine	T43.591	T43.592	T43.593	T43.594	T43.595	T43.596
Captopril	T46.4X1	T46.4X2	T46.4X3	T46.4X4	T46.4X5	T46.4X6
Caramiphen	T44.3X1	T44.3X2	T44.3X3	T44.3X4	T44.3X5	T44.3X6
Carazolol	T44.7X1	T44.7X2	T44.7X3	T44.7X4	T44.7X5	T44.7X6
Carbachol	T44.1X1	T44.1X2	T44.1X3	T44.1X4	T44.1X5	T44.1X6
Carbacrylamine (resin)	T50.3X1	T50.3X2	T50.3X3	T50.3X4	T50.3X5	T50.3X6
Carbamate (insecticide)	T60.0X1	T60.0X2	T60.0X3	T60.0X4	—	—
Carbamate (sedative)	T42.6X1	T42.6X2	T42.6X3	T42.6X4	T42.6X5	T42.6X6
herbicide	T60.0X1	T60.0X2	T60.0X3	T60.0X4	—	—
insecticide	T60.0X1	T60.0X2	T60.0X3	T60.0X4	—	—
Carbamazepine	T42.1X1	T42.1X2	T42.1X3	T42.1X4	T42.1X5	T42.1X6
Carbamide	T47.3X1	T47.3X2	T47.3X3	T47.3X4	T47.3X5	T47.3X6
peroxide	T49.0X1	T49.0X2	T49.0X3	T49.0X4	T49.0X5	T49.0X6
topical	T49.8X1	T49.8X2	T49.8X3	T49.8X4	T49.8X5	T49.8X6
Carbamylcholine chloride	T44.1X1	T44.1X2	T44.1X3	T44.1X4	T44.1X5	T44.1X6
Carbaril	T60.0X1	T60.0X2	T60.0X3	T60.0X4	—	—
Carbarsone	T37.3X1	T37.3X2	T37.3X3	T37.3X4	T37.3X5	T37.3X6
Carbaryl	T60.0X1	T60.0X2	T60.0X3	T60.0X4	—	—
Carbaspirin	T39.011	T39.012	T39.013	T39.014	T39.015	T39.016
Carbazochrome (salicylate) (sodium sulfonate)	T49.4X1	T49.4X2	T49.4X3	T49.4X4	T49.4X5	T49.4X6
Carbenicillin	T36.0X1	T36.0X2	T36.0X3	T36.0X4	T36.0X5	T36.0X6
Carbenoxolone	T47.1X1	T47.1X2	T47.1X3	T47.1X4	T47.1X5	T47.1X6
Carbetapentane	T48.3X1	T48.3X2	T48.3X3	T48.3X4	T48.3X5	T48.3X6
Carbethyl salicylate	T39.091	T39.092	T39.093	T39.094	T39.095	T39.096
Carbidopa (with levodopa)	T42.8X1	T42.8X2	T42.8X3	T42.8X4	T42.8X5	T42.8X6
Carbimazole	T38.2X1	T38.2X2	T38.2X3	T38.2X4	T38.2X5	T38.2X6
Carbinol	T51.1X1	T51.1X2	T51.1X3	T51.1X4	—	—
Carbinoxamine	T45.0X1	T45.0X2	T45.0X3	T45.0X4	T45.0X5	T45.0X6
Carbiphene	T39.8X1	T39.8X2	T39.8X3	T39.8X4	T39.8X5	T39.8X6
Carbitol	T52.3X1	T52.3X2	T52.3X3	T52.3X4	—	—
Carbocaine	T41.3X1	T41.3X2	T41.3X3	T41.3X4	T41.3X5	T41.3X6
infiltration (subcutaneous)	T41.3X1	T41.3X2	T41.3X3	T41.3X4	T41.3X5	T41.3X6
nerve block (peripheral) (plexus)	T41.3X1	T41.3X2	T41.3X3	T41.3X4	T41.3X5	T41.3X6
topical (surface)	T41.3X1	T41.3X2	T41.3X3	T41.3X4	T41.3X5	T41.3X6

Substance	Poisoning, Accidental (Unintentional)	Poisoning, Intentional Self-Harm	Poisoning, Assault	Poisoning, Undetermined	Adverse Effect	Underdosing
Carbo medicinalis	T47.6X1	T47.6X2	T47.6X3	T47.6X4	T47.6X5	T47.6X6
Carbomycin	T36.8X1	T36.8X2	T36.8X3	T36.8X4	T36.8X5	T36.8X6
Carbocisteine	T48.4X1	T48.4X2	T48.4X3	T48.4X4	T48.4X5	T48.4X6
Carbocromen	T46.3X1	T46.3X2	T46.3X3	T46.3X4	T46.3X5	T46.3X6
Carbol fuchsin	T49.0X1	T49.0X2	T49.0X3	T49.0X4	T49.0X5	T49.0X6
Carbolic acid—*see also Phenol*	T54.0X1	T54.0X2	T54.0X3	T54.0X4	—	—
Carbolonium (bromide)	T48.1X1	T48.1X2	T48.1X3	T48.1X4	T48.1X5	T48.1X6
Carbon						
bisulfide (liquid)	T65.4X1	T65.4X2	T65.4X3	T65.4X4	—	—
vapor	T65.4X1	T65.4X2	T65.4X3	T65.4X4	—	—
dioxide (gas)	T59.7X1	T59.7X2	T59.7X3	T59.7X4	—	—
medicinal	T41.5X1	T41.5X2	T41.5X3	T41.5X4	T41.5X5	T41.5X6
nonmedicinal	T59.7X1	T59.7X2	T59.7X3	T59.7X4	—	—
snow	T49.4X1	T49.4X2	T49.4X3	T49.4X4	T49.4X5	T49.4X6
disulfide (liquid)	T65.4X1	T65.4X2	T65.4X3	T65.4X4	—	—
vapor	T65.4X1	T65.4X2	T65.4X3	T65.4X4	—	—
monoxide (from incomplete combustion)	T58.91	T58.92	T58.93	T58.94	—	—
blast furnace gas	T58.8X1	T58.8X2	T58.8X3	T58.8X4	—	—
butane (distributed in mobile container)	T58.11	T58.12	T58.13	T58.14	—	—
distributed through pipes	T58.11	T58.12	T58.13	T58.14	—	—
charcoal fumes	T58.2X1	T58.2X2	T58.2X3	T58.2X4	—	—
coal	T58.2X1	T58.2X2	T58.2X3	T58.2X4		
coke (in domestic stoves, fireplaces)	T58.2X1	T58.2X2	T58.2X3	T58.2X4	—	—
gas (piped)	T58.11	T58.12	T58.13	T58.14	—	—
solid (in domestic stoves, fireplaces)	T58.2X1	T58.2X2	T58.2X3	T58.2X4	—	—
exhaust gas (motor) not in transit	T58.01	T58.02	T58.03	T58.04	—	—
combustion engine, any not in watercraft	T58.01	T58.02	T58.03	T58.04	—	—
farm tractor, not in transit	T58.01	T58.02	T58.03	T58.04	—	—
gas engine	T58.01	T58.02	T58.03	T58.04	—	—
motor pump	T58.01	T58.02	T58.03	T58.04	—	—
motor vehicle, not in transit	T58.01	T58.02	T58.03	T58.04	—	—
fuel (in domestic use)	T58.2X1	T58.2X2	T58.2X3	T58.2X4	—	—
gas (piped)	T58.11	T58.12	T58.13	T58.14	—	—
in mobile container	T58.11	T58.12	T58.13	T58.14	—	—
utility	T58.11	T58.12	T58.13	T58.14	—	—
in mobile container	T58.11	T58.12	T58.13	T58.14	—	—
piped (natural)	T58.11	T58.12	T58.13	T58.14	—	—

Substance	External Cause (T-Code) Poisoning, Accidental (Unintentional)	Poisoning, Intentional Self-Harm	Poisoning, Assault	Poisoning, Undetermined	Adverse Effect	Underdosing
Carbon *(Continued)*						
monoxide *(Continued)*						
illuminating gas	T58.11	T58.12	T58.13	T58.14	—	—
industrial fuels or gases, any	T58.8X1	T58.8X2	T58.8X3	T58.8X4	—	—
kerosene (in domestic stoves, fireplaces)	T58.2X1	T58.2X2	T58.2X3	T58.2X4	—	—
kiln gas or vapor	T58.8X1	T58.8X2	T58.8X3	T58.8X4	—	—
motor exhaust gas, not in transit	T58.01	T58.02	T58.03	T58.04	—	—
piped gas (manufactured) (natural)	T58.11	T58.12	T58.13	T58.14	—	—
producer gas	T58.8X1	T58.8X2	T58.8X3	T58.8X4	—	—
propane (distributed in mobile container)	T58.11	T58.12	T58.13	T58.14	—	—
distributed through pipes	T58.11	T58.12	T58.13	T58.14	—	—
specified source NEC	T58.8X1	T58.8X2	T58.8X3	T58.8X4	—	—
stove gas	T58.11	T58.12	T58.13	T58.14	—	—
piped	T58.11	T58.12	T58.13	T58.14	—	—
utility gas	T58.11	T58.12	T58.13	T58.14	—	—
piped	T58.11	T58.12	T58.13	T58.14	—	—
water gas	T58.11	T58.12	T58.13	T58.14	—	—
wood (in domestic stoves, fireplaces)	T58.2X1	T58.2X2	T58.2X3	T58.2X4	—	—
tetrachloride (vapor) NEC	T53.0X1	T53.0X2	T53.0X3	T53.0X4	—	—
liquid (cleansing agent) NEC	T53.0X1	T53.0X2	T53.0X3	T53.0X4	—	—
solvent	T53.0X1	T53.0X2	T53.0X3	T53.0X4	—	—
Carbonic acid gas	T59.7X1	T59.7X2	T59.7X3	T59.7X4	—	—
anhydrase inhibitor NEC	T50.2X1	T50.2X2	T50.2X3	T50.2X4	T50.2X5	T50.2X6
Carbophenothion	T60.0X1	T60.0X2	T60.0X3	T60.0X4	—	—
Carboplatin	T45.1X1	T45.1X2	T45.1X3	T45.1X4	T45.1X5	T45.1X6
Carboprost	T48.0X1	T48.0X2	T48.0X3	T48.0X4	T48.0X5	T48.0X6
Carboquone	T45.1X1	T45.1X2	T45.1X3	T45.1X4	T45.1X5	T45.1X6
Carbowax	T49.3X1	T49.3X2	T49.3X3	T49.3X4	T49.3X5	T49.3X6
Carboxymethyl-cellulose	T47.4X1	T47.4X2	T47.4X3	T47.4X4	T47.4X5	T47.4X6
S-Carboxymethyl-cysteine	T48.4X1	T48.4X2	T48.4X3	T48.4X4	T48.4X5	T48.4X6
Carbrital	T42.3X1	T42.3X2	T42.3X3	T42.3X4	T42.3X5	T42.3X6
Carbromal	T42.6X1	T42.6X2	T42.6X3	T42.6X4	T42.6X5	T42.6X6
Carbutamide	T38.3X1	T38.3X2	T38.3X3	T38.3X4	T38.3X5	T38.3X6
Carbuterol	T48.6X1	T48.6X2	T48.6X3	T48.6X4	T48.6X5	T48.6X6
Cardiac						
depressants	T46.2X1	T46.2X2	T46.2X3	T46.2X4	T46.2X5	T46.2X6
rhythm regulator	T46.2X1	T46.2X2	T46.2X3	T46.2X4	T46.2X5	T46.2X6
specified NEC	T46.2X1	T46.2X2	T46.2X3	T46.2X4	T46.2X5	T46.2X6
Cardiografin	T50.8X1	T50.8X2	T50.8X3	T50.8X4	T50.8X5	T50.8X6
Cardio-green	T50.8X1	T50.8X2	T50.8X3	T50.8X4	T50.8X5	T50.8X6
Cardiotonic (glycoside) NEC	T46.0X1	T46.0X2	T46.0X3	T46.0X4	T46.0X5	T46.0X6
Cardiovascular drug NEC	T46.901	T46.902	T46.903	T46.904	T46.905	T46.906
Cardrase	T50.2X1	T50.2X2	T50.2X3	T50.2X4	T50.2X5	T50.2X6
Carfusin	T49.0X1	T49.0X2	T49.0X3	T49.0X4	T49.0X5	T49.0X6
Carfecillin	T36.0X1	T36.0X2	T36.0X3	T36.0X4	T36.0X5	T36.0X6
Carfenazine	T43.3X1	T43.3X2	T43.3X3	T43.3X4	T43.3X5	T43.3X6
Carindacillin	T36.0X1	T36.0X2	T36.0X3	T36.0X4	T36.0X5	T36.0X6
Carisoprodol	T42.8X1	T42.8X2	T42.8X3	T42.8X4	T42.8X5	T42.8X6
Carmellose	T47.4X1	T47.4X2	T47.4X3	T47.4X4	T47.4X5	T47.4X6
Carminative	T47.5X1	T47.5X2	T47.5X3	T47.5X4	T47.5X5	T47.5X6
Carmofur	T45.1X1	T45.1X2	T45.1X3	T45.1X4	T45.1X5	T45.1X6
Carmustine	T45.1X1	T45.1X2	T45.1X3	T45.1X4	T45.1X5	T45.1X6
Carotene	T45.2X1	T45.2X2	T45.2X3	T45.2X4	T45.2X5	T45.2X6
Carphenazine	T43.3X1	T43.3X2	T43.3X3	T43.3X4	T43.3X5	T43.3X6
Carpipramine	T42.4X1	T42.4X2	T42.4X3	T42.4X4	T42.4X5	T42.4X6
Carprofen	T39.311	T39.312	T39.313	T39.314	T39.315	T39.316
Carpronium chloride	T44.3X1	T44.3X2	T44.3X3	T44.3X4	T44.3X5	T44.3X6
Carrageenan	T47.8X1	T47.8X2	T47.8X3	T47.8X4	T47.8X5	T47.8X6
Carteolol	T44.7X1	T44.7X2	T44.7X3	T44.7X4	T44.7X5	T44.7X6
Carter's Little Pills	T47.2X1	T47.2X2	T47.2X3	T47.2X4	T47.2X5	T47.2X6
Cascara (sagrada)	T47.2X1	T47.2X2	T47.2X3	T47.2X4	T47.2X5	T47.2X6
Cassava	T62.2X1	T62.2X2	T62.2X3	T62.2X4	—	—
Castellani's paint	T49.0X1	T49.0X2	T49.0X3	T49.0X4	T49.0X5	T49.0X6
Castor						
bean	T62.2X1	T62.2X2	T62.2X3	T62.2X4	—	—
oil	T47.2X1	T47.2X2	T47.2X3	T47.2X4	T47.2X5	T47.2X6
Catalase	T45.3X1	T45.3X2	T45.3X3	T45.3X4	T45.3X5	T45.3X6
Caterpillar (sting)	T63.431	T63.432	T63.433	T63.434	—	—
Catha (edulis) (tea)	T43.691	T43.692	T43.693	T43.694	—	—
Cathartic NEC	T47.4X1	T47.4X2	T47.4X3	T47.4X4	T47.4X5	T47.4X6
anthacene derivative	T47.2X1	T47.2X2	T47.2X3	T47.2X4	T47.2X5	T47.2X6
bulk	T47.4X1	T47.4X2	T47.4X3	T47.4X4	T47.4X5	T47.4X6
contact	T47.2X1	T47.2X2	T47.2X3	T47.2X4	T47.2X5	T47.2X6
emollient NEC	T47.4X1	T47.4X2	T47.4X3	T47.4X4	T47.4X5	T47.4X6
irritant NEC	T47.2X1	T47.2X2	T47.2X3	T47.2X4	T47.2X5	T47.2X6
mucilage	T47.4X1	T47.4X2	T47.4X3	T47.4X4	T47.4X5	T47.4X6
saline	T47.3X1	T47.3X2	T47.3X3	T47.3X4	T47.3X5	T47.3X6
vegetable	T47.2X1	T47.2X2	T47.2X3	T47.2X4	T47.2X5	T47.2X6
Cathine	T50.5X1	T50.5X2	T50.5X3	T50.5X4	T50.5X5	T50.5X6
Cathomycin	T36.8X1	T36.8X2	T36.8X3	T36.8X4	T36.8X5	T36.8X6

New Revised ~~deleted~~ Deleted

TABLE OF DRUGS AND CHEMICALS

Substance	External Cause (T-Code) Poisoning, Accidental (Unintentional)	Poisoning, Intentional Self-Harm	Poisoning, Assault	Poisoning, Undetermined	Adverse Effect	Underdosing
Cation exchange resin	T50.3X1	T50.3X2	T50.3X3	T50.3X4	T50.3X5	T50.3X6
Caustic(s) NEC	T54.91	T54.92	T54.93	T54.94	—	—
alkali	T54.3X1	T54.3X2	T54.3X3	T54.3X4	—	—
hydroxide	T54.3X1	T54.3X2	T54.3X3	T54.3X4	—	—
potash	T54.3X1	T54.3X2	T54.3X3	T54.3X4	—	—
soda	T54.3X1	T54.3X2	T54.3X3	T54.3X4	—	—
specified NEC	T54.91	T54.92	T54.93	T54.94	—	—
Ceepryn	T49.0X1	T49.0X2	T49.0X3	T49.0X4	T49.0X5	T49.0X6
ENT agent	T49.6X1	T49.6X2	T49.6X3	T49.6X4	T49.6X5	T49.6X6
lozenges	T49.6X1	T49.6X2	T49.6X3	T49.6X4	T49.6X5	T49.6X6
Cefacetrile	T36.1X1	T36.1X2	T36.1X3	T36.1X4	T36.1X5	T36.1X6
Cefaclor	T36.1X1	T36.1X2	T36.1X3	T36.1X4	T36.1X5	T36.1X6
Cefadroxil	T36.1X1	T36.1X2	T36.1X3	T36.1X4	T36.1X5	T36.1X6
Cefalexin	T36.1X1	T36.1X2	T36.1X3	T36.1X4	T36.1X5	T36.1X6
Cefaloglycin	T36.1X1	T36.1X2	T36.1X3	T36.1X4	T36.1X5	T36.1X6
Cefaloridine	T36.1X1	T36.1X2	T36.1X3	T36.1X4	T36.1X5	T36.1X6
Cefalosporins	T36.1X1	T36.1X2	T36.1X3	T36.1X4	T36.1X5	T36.1X6
Cefalotin	T36.1X1	T36.1X2	T36.1X3	T36.1X4	T36.1X5	T36.1X6
Cefamandole	T36.1X1	T36.1X2	T36.1X3	T36.1X4	T36.1X5	T36.1X6
Cefamycin antibiotic	T36.1X1	T36.1X2	T36.1X3	T36.1X4	T36.1X5	T36.1X6
Cefapirin	T36.1X1	T36.1X2	T36.1X3	T36.1X4	T36.1X5	T36.1X6
Cefatrizine	T36.1X1	T36.1X2	T36.1X3	T36.1X4	T36.1X5	T36.1X6
Cefazedone	T36.1X1	T36.1X2	T36.1X3	T36.1X4	T36.1X5	T36.1X6
Cefazolin	T36.1X1	T36.1X2	T36.1X3	T36.1X4	T36.1X5	T36.1X6
Cefbuperazone	T36.1X1	T36.1X2	T36.1X3	T36.1X4	T36.1X5	T36.1X6
Cefetamet	T36.1X1	T36.1X2	T36.1X3	T36.1X4	T36.1X5	T36.1X6
Cefixime	T36.1X1	T36.1X2	T36.1X3	T36.1X4	T36.1X5	T36.1X6
Cefmenoxime	T36.1X1	T36.1X2	T36.1X3	T36.1X4	T36.1X5	T36.1X6
Cefmetazole	T36.1X1	T36.1X2	T36.1X3	T36.1X4	T36.1X5	T36.1X6
Cefminox	T36.1X1	T36.1X2	T36.1X3	T36.1X4	T36.1X5	T36.1X6
Cefonicid	T36.1X1	T36.1X2	T36.1X3	T36.1X4	T36.1X5	T36.1X6
Cefoperazone	T36.1X1	T36.1X2	T36.1X3	T36.1X4	T36.1X5	T36.1X6
Ceforanide	T36.1X1	T36.1X2	T36.1X3	T36.1X4	T36.1X5	T36.1X6
Cefotaxime	T36.1X1	T36.1X2	T36.1X3	T36.1X4	T36.1X5	T36.1X6
Cefotetan	T36.1X1	T36.1X2	T36.1X3	T36.1X4	T36.1X5	T36.1X6
Cefotiam	T36.1X1	T36.1X2	T36.1X3	T36.1X4	T36.1X5	T36.1X6
Cefoxitin	T36.1X1	T36.1X2	T36.1X3	T36.1X4	T36.1X5	T36.1X6
Cefpimizole	T36.1X1	T36.1X2	T36.1X3	T36.1X4	T36.1X5	T36.1X6
Cefpiramide	T36.1X1	T36.1X2	T36.1X3	T36.1X4	T36.1X5	T36.1X6
Cefradine	T36.1X1	T36.1X2	T36.1X3	T36.1X4	T36.1X5	T36.1X6
Cefroxadine	T36.1X1	T36.1X2	T36.1X3	T36.1X4	T36.1X5	T36.1X6
Cefsulodin	T36.1X1	T36.1X2	T36.1X3	T36.1X4	T36.1X5	T36.1X6

Substance	External Cause (T-Code) Poisoning, Accidental (Unintentional)	Poisoning, Intentional Self-Harm	Poisoning, Assault	Poisoning, Undetermined	Adverse Effect	Underdosing
Ceftazidime	T36.1X1	T36.1X2	T36.1X3	T36.1X4	T36.1X5	T36.1X6
Cefteram	T36.1X1	T36.1X2	T36.1X3	T36.1X4	T36.1X5	T36.1X6
Ceftezole	T36.1X1	T36.1X2	T36.1X3	T36.1X4	T36.1X5	T36.1X6
Ceftizoxime	T36.1X1	T36.1X2	T36.1X3	T36.1X4	T36.1X5	T36.1X6
Ceftriaxone	T36.1X1	T36.1X2	T36.1X3	T36.1X4	T36.1X5	T36.1X6
Cefuroxime	T36.1X1	T36.1X2	T36.1X3	T36.1X4	T36.1X5	T36.1X6
Cefuzonam	T36.1X1	T36.1X2	T36.1X3	T36.1X4	T36.1X5	T36.1X6
Celestone	T38.0X1	T38.0X2	T38.0X3	T38.0X4	T38.0X5	T38.0X6
topical	T49.0X1	T49.0X2	T49.0X3	T49.0X4	T49.0X5	T49.0X6
Celiprolol	T44.7X1	T44.7X2	T44.7X3	T44.7X4	T44.7X5	T44.7X6
Cellosolve	T52.91	T52.92	T52.93	T52.94	—	—
Cell stimulants and proliferants	T49.8X1	T49.8X2	T49.8X3	T49.8X4	T49.8X5	T49.8X6
Cellulose						
cathartic	T47.4X1	T47.4X2	T47.4X3	T47.4X4	T47.4X5	T47.4X6
hydroxyethyl	T47.4X1	T47.4X2	T47.4X3	T47.4X4	T47.4X5	T47.4X6
nitrates (topical)	T49.3X1	T49.3X2	T49.3X3	T49.3X4	T49.3X5	T49.3X6
oxidized	T49.4X1	T49.4X2	T49.4X3	T49.4X4	T49.4X5	T49.4X6
Centipede (bite)	T63.411	T63.412	T63.413	T63.414	—	—
Central nervous system						
depressants	T42.71	T42.72	T42.73	T42.74	T42.75	T42.76
anesthetic (general) NEC	T41.201	T41.202	T41.203	T41.204	T41.205	T41.206
gases NEC	T41.0X1	T41.0X2	T41.0X3	T41.0X4	T41.0X5	T41.0X6
intravenous	T41.1X1	T41.1X2	T41.1X3	T41.1X4	T41.1X5	T41.1X6
barbiturates	T42.3X1	T42.3X2	T42.3X3	T42.3X4	T42.3X5	T42.3X6
benzodiazepines	T42.4X1	T42.4X2	T42.4X3	T42.4X4	T42.4X5	T42.4X6
bromides	T42.6X1	T42.6X2	T42.6X3	T42.6X4	T42.6X5	T42.6X6
cannabis sativa	T40.711	T40.712	T40.713	T40.714	T40.715	T40.716
chloral hydrate	T42.6X1	T42.6X2	T42.6X3	T42.6X4	T42.6X5	T42.6X6
ethanol	T51.0X1	T51.0X2	T51.0X3	T51.0X4	—	—
hallucinogenics	T40.901	T40.902	T40.903	T40.904	T40.905	T40.906
hypnotics	T42.71	T42.72	T42.73	T42.74	T42.75	T42.76
specified NEC	T42.6X1	T42.6X2	T42.6X3	T42.6X4	T42.6X5	T42.6X6
muscle relaxants	T42.8X1	T42.8X2	T42.8X3	T42.8X4	T42.8X5	T42.8X6
paraldehyde	T42.6X1	T42.6X2	T42.6X3	T42.6X4	T42.6X5	T42.6X6
sedatives; sedative-hypnotics	T42.71	T42.72	T42.73	T42.74	T42.75	T42.76
mixed NEC	T42.6X1	T42.6X2	T42.6X3	T42.6X4	T42.6X5	T42.6X6
specified NEC	T42.6X1	T42.6X2	T42.6X3	T42.6X4	T42.6X5	T42.6X6
muscle-tone depressants	T42.8X1	T42.8X2	T42.8X3	T42.8X4	T42.8X5	T42.8X6
stimulants	T43.601	T43.602	T43.603	T43.604	T43.605	T43.606
amphetamines	T43.621	T43.622	T43.623	T43.624	T43.625	T43.626
analeptics	T50.7X1	T50.7X2	T50.7X3	T50.7X4	T50.7X5	T50.7X6

TABLE OF DRUGS AND CHEMICALS

Substance	External Cause (T-Code)					
	Poisoning, Accidental (Unintentional)	Poisoning, Intentional Self-Harm	Poisoning, Assault	Poisoning, Undetermined	Adverse Effect	Underdosing
Central nervous system *(Continued)*						
stimulants *(Continued)*						
antidepressants	T43.201	T43.202	T43.203	T43.204	T43.205	T43.206
opiate antagonists	T50.7X1	T50.7X2	T50.7X3	T50.7X4	T50.7X5	T50.7X6
specified NEC	T43.691	T43.692	T43.693	T43.694	T43.695	T43.696
Cephalexin	T36.1X1	T36.1X2	T36.1X3	T36.1X4	T36.1X5	T36.1X6
Cephaloglycin	T36.1X1	T36.1X2	T36.1X3	T36.1X4	T36.1X5	T36.1X6
Cephaloridine	T36.1X1	T36.1X2	T36.1X3	T36.1X4	T36.1X5	T36.1X6
Cephalosporins	T36.1X1	T36.1X2	T36.1X3	T36.1X4	T36.1X5	T36.1X6
N (adicillin)	T36.0X1	T36.0X2	T36.0X3	T36.0X4	T36.0X5	T36.0X6
Cephalothin	T36.1X1	T36.1X2	T36.1X3	T36.1X4	T36.1X5	T36.1X6
Cephalotin	T36.1X1	T36.1X2	T36.1X3	T36.1X4	T36.1X5	T36.1X6
Cephradine	T36.1X1	T36.1X2	T36.1X3	T36.1X4	T36.1X5	T36.1X6
Cerbera (odallam)	T62.2X1	T62.2X2	T62.2X3	T62.2X4	—	—
Cerberin	T46.0X1	T46.0X2	T46.0X3	T46.0X4	T46.0X5	T46.0X6
Cerebral stimulants	T43.601	T43.602	T43.603	T43.604	T43.605	T43.606
psychotherapeutic	T43.601	T43.602	T43.603	T43.604	T43.605	T43.606
specified NEC	T43.691	T43.692	T43.693	T43.694	T43.695	T43.696
Cerium oxalate	T45.0X1	T45.0X2	T45.0X3	T45.0X4	T45.0X5	T45.0X6
Cerous oxalate	T45.0X1	T45.0X2	T45.0X3	T45.0X4	T45.0X5	T45.0X6
Ceruletide	T50.8X1	T50.8X2	T50.8X3	T50.8X4	T50.8X5	T50.8X6
Cetalkonium (chloride)	T49.0X1	T49.0X2	T49.0X3	T49.0X4	T49.0X5	T49.0X6
Cethexonium chloride	T49.0X1	T49.0X2	T49.0X3	T49.0X4	T49.0X5	T49.0X6
Cetiedil	T46.7X1	T46.7X2	T46.7X3	T46.7X4	T46.7X5	T46.7X6
Cetirizine	T45.0X1	T45.0X2	T45.0X3	T45.0X4	T45.0X5	T45.0X6
Cetomacrogol	T50.991	T50.992	T50.993	T50.994	T50.995	T50.996
Cetotiamine	T45.2X1	T45.2X2	T45.2X3	T45.2X4	T45.2X5	T45.2X6
Cetoxime	T45.0X1	T45.0X2	T45.0X3	T45.0X4	T45.0X5	T45.0X6
Cetraxate	T47.1X1	T47.1X2	T47.1X3	T47.1X4	T47.1X5	T47.1X6
Cetrimide	T49.0X1	T49.0X2	T49.0X3	T49.0X4	T49.0X5	T49.0X6
Cetrimonium (bromide)	T49.0X1	T49.0X2	T49.0X3	T49.0X4	T49.0X5	T49.0X6
Cetylpyridinium chloride	T49.0X1	T49.0X2	T49.0X3	T49.0X4	T49.0X5	T49.0X6
ENT agent	T49.6X1	T49.6X2	T49.6X3	T49.6X4	T49.6X5	T49.6X6
lozenges	T49.6X1	T49.6X2	T49.6X3	T49.6X4	T49.6X5	T49.6X6
Cevadillasee Sabadilla						
Cevitamic acid	T45.2X1	T45.2X2	T45.2X3	T45.2X4	T45.2X5	T45.2X6
Chalk, precipitated	T47.1X1	T47.1X2	T47.1X3	T47.1X4	T47.1X5	T47.1X6
Chamomile	T49.0X1	T49.0X2	T49.0X3	T49.0X4	T49.0X5	T49.0X6
Ch'an su	T46.0X1	T46.0X2	T46.0X3	T46.0X4	T46.0X5	T46.0X6
Charcoal	T47.6X1	T47.6X2	T47.6X3	T47.6X4	T47.6X5	T47.6X6
activated—*see also Charcoal, medicinal*	T47.6X1	T47.6X2	T47.6X3	T47.6X4	T47.6X5	T47.6X6
Charcoal *(Continued)*						
fumes (Carbon monoxide)	T58.2X1	T58.2X2	T58.2X3	T58.2X4	—	—
industrial	T58.8X1	T58.8X2	T58.8X3	T58.8X4	—	—
medicinal (activated)	T47.6X1	T47.6X2	T47.6X3	T47.6X4	T47.6X5	T47.6X6
antidiarrheal	T47.6X1	T47.6X2	T47.6X3	T47.6X4	T47.6X5	T47.6X6
poison control	T47.8X1	T47.8X2	T47.8X3	T47.8X4	T47.8X5	T47.8X6
specified use other than for diarrhea	T47.8X1	T47.8X2	T47.8X3	T47.8X4	T47.8X5	T47.8X6
topical	T49.8X1	T49.8X2	T49.8X3	T49.8X4	T49.8X5	T49.8X6
Chaulmosulfone	T37.1X1	T37.1X2	T37.1X3	T37.1X4	T37.1X5	T37.1X6
Chelating agent NEC	T50.6X1	T50.6X2	T50.6X3	T50.6X4	T50.6X5	T50.6X6
Chelidonium majus	T62.2X1	T62.2X2	T62.2X3	T62.2X4	—	—
Chemical substance NEC	T65.91	T65.92	T65.93	T65.94	—	—
Chenodeoxycholic acid	T47.5X1	T47.5X2	T47.5X3	T47.5X4	T47.5X5	T47.5X6
Chenodiol	T47.5X1	T47.5X2	T47.5X3	T47.5X4	T47.5X5	T47.5X6
Chenopodium	T37.4X1	T37.4X2	T37.4X3	T37.4X4	T37.4X5	T37.4X6
Cherry laurel	T62.2X1	T62.2X2	T62.2X3	T62.2X4	—	—
Chinidin(e)	T46.2X1	T46.2X2	T46.2X3	T46.2X4	T46.2X5	T46.2X6
Chiniofon	T37.8X1	T37.8X2	T37.8X3	T37.8X4	T37.8X5	T37.8X6
Chlophedianol	T48.3X1	T48.3X2	T48.3X3	T48.3X4	T48.3X5	T48.3X6
Chloral	T42.6X1	T42.6X2	T42.6X3	T42.6X4	T42.6X5	T42.6X6
derivative	T42.6X1	T42.6X2	T42.6X3	T42.6X4	T42.6X5	T42.6X6
hydrate	T42.6X1	T42.6X2	T42.6X3	T42.6X4	T42.6X5	T42.6X6
Chloralamide	T42.6X1	T42.6X2	T42.6X3	T42.6X4	T42.6X5	T42.6X6
Chloralodol	T42.6X1	T42.6X2	T42.6X3	T42.6X4	T42.6X5	T42.6X6
Chloralose	T60.4X1	T60.4X2	T60.4X3	T60.4X4	—	—
Chlorambucil	T45.1X1	T45.1X2	T45.1X3	T45.1X4	T45.1X5	T45.1X6
Chloramine	T57.8X1	T57.8X2	T57.8X3	T57.8X4	—	—
T	T49.0X1	T49.0X2	T49.0X3	T49.0X4	T49.0X5	T49.0X6
topical	T49.0X1	T49.0X2	T49.0X3	T49.0X4	T49.0X5	T49.0X6
Chloramphenicol	T36.2X1	T36.2X2	T36.2X3	T36.2X4	T36.2X5	T36.2X6
ENT agent	T49.6X1	T49.6X2	T49.6X3	T49.6X4	T49.6X5	T49.6X6
ophthalmic preparation	T49.5X1	T49.5X2	T49.5X3	T49.5X4	T49.5X5	T49.5X6
topical NEC	T49.0X1	T49.0X2	T49.0X3	T49.0X4	T49.0X5	T49.0X6
Chlorate (potassium) (sodium) NEC	T60.3X1	T60.3X2	T60.3X3	T60.3X4	—	—
herbicide	T60.3X1	T60.3X2	T60.3X3	T60.3X4	—	—
Chlorazanil	T50.2X1	T50.2X2	T50.2X3	T50.2X4	T50.2X5	T50.2X6
Chlorbenzene, chlorbenzol	T53.7X1	T53.7X2	T53.7X3	T53.7X4	—	—
Chlorbenzoxamine	T44.3X1	T44.3X2	T44.3X3	T44.3X4	T44.3X5	T44.3X6
Chlorbutol	T42.6X1	T42.6X2	T42.6X3	T42.6X4	T42.6X5	T42.6X6
Chlorcyclizine	T45.0X1	T45.0X2	T45.0X3	T45.0X4	T45.0X5	T45.0X6

◀ New ◀ Revised ~~deleted~~ Deleted

Substance	External Cause (T-Code) Poisoning, Accidental (Unintentional)	Poisoning, Intentional Self-Harm	Poisoning, Assault	Poisoning, Undetermined	Adverse Effect	Underdosing
Chlordan(e) (dust)	T60.1X1	T60.1X2	T60.1X3	T60.1X4	—	—
Chlordantoin	T49.0X1	T49.0X2	T49.0X3	T49.0X4	T49.0X5	T49.0X6
Chlordiazepoxide	T42.4X1	T42.4X2	T42.4X3	T42.4X4	T42.4X5	T42.4X6
Chlordiethyl benzamide	T49.3X1	T49.3X2	T49.3X3	T49.3X4	T49.3X5	T49.3X6
Chloresium	T49.8X1	T49.8X2	T49.8X3	T49.8X4	T49.8X5	T49.8X6
Chlorethiazol	T42.6X1	T42.6X2	T42.6X3	T42.6X4	T42.6X5	T42.6X6
Chlorethyl — *see Ethyl, chloride*						
Chloretone	T42.6X1	T42.6X2	T42.6X3	T42.6X4	T42.6X5	T42.6X6
Chlorex	T53.6X1	T53.6X2	T53.6X3	T53.6X4	—	—
insecticide	T60.1X1	T60.1X2	T60.1X3	T60.1X4	—	—
Chlorfenvinphos	T60.0X1	T60.0X2	T60.0X3	T60.0X4	—	—
Chlorhexadol	T42.6X1	T42.6X2	T42.6X3	T42.6X4	T42.6X5	T42.6X6
Chlorhexamide	T45.1X1	T45.1X2	T45.1X3	T45.1X4	T45.1X5	T45.1X6
Chlorhexidine	T49.0X1	T49.0X2	T49.0X3	T49.0X4	T49.0X5	T49.0X6
Chlorhydroxyquinolin	T49.0X1	T49.0X2	T49.0X3	T49.0X4	T49.0X5	T49.0X6
Chloride of lime (bleach)	T54.3X1	T54.3X2	T54.3X3	T54.3X4	—	—
Chlorimipramine	T43.011	T43.012	T43.013	T43.014	T43.015	T43.016
Chlorinated						
camphene	T53.6X1	T53.6X2	T53.6X3	T53.6X4	—	—
diphenyl	T53.7X1	T53.7X2	T53.7X3	T53.7X4	—	—
hydrocarbons NEC	T53.91	T53.92	T53.93	T53.94	—	—
solvents	T53.91	T53.92	T53.93	T53.94	—	—
lime (bleach)	T54.3X1	T54.3X2	T54.3X3	T54.3X4	—	—
and boric acid solution	T49.0X1	T49.0X2	T49.0X3	T49.0X4	T49.0X5	T49.0X6
naphthalene (insecticide)	T60.1X1	T60.1X2	T60.1X3	T60.1X4	—	—
industrial (non-pesticide)	T53.7X1	T53.7X2	T53.7X3	T53.7X4	—	—
pesticide NEC	T60.8X1	T60.8X2	T60.8X3	T60.8X4	—	—
soda — *see also Sodium hypochlorite*						
solution	T49.0X1	T49.0X2	T49.0X3	T49.0X4	T49.0X5	T49.0X6
Chlorine (fumes) (gas)	T59.4X1	T59.4X2	T59.4X3	T59.4X4	—	—
bleach	T54.3X1	T54.3X2	T54.3X3	T54.3X4	—	—
compound gas NEC	T59.4X1	T59.4X2	T59.4X3	T59.4X4	—	—
disinfectant	T59.4X1	T59.4X2	T59.4X3	T59.4X4	—	—
releasing agents NEC	T59.4X1	T59.4X2	T59.4X3	T59.4X4	—	—
Chlorisondamine chloride	T46.991	T46.992	T46.993	T46.994	T46.995	T46.996
Chlormadinone	T38.5X1	T38.5X2	T38.5X3	T38.5X4	T38.5X5	T38.5X6
Chlormephos	T60.0X1	T60.0X2	T60.0X3	T60.0X4	—	—
Chlormerodrin	T50.2X1	T50.2X2	T50.2X3	T50.2X4	T50.2X5	T50.2X6
Chlormethiazole	T42.6X1	T42.6X2	T42.6X3	T42.6X4	T42.6X5	T42.6X6
Chlormethine	T45.1X1	T45.1X2	T45.1X3	T45.1X4	T45.1X5	T45.1X6
Chlormethylenecycline	T36.4X1	T36.4X2	T36.4X3	T36.4X4	T36.4X5	T36.4X6

Substance	External Cause (T-Code) Poisoning, Accidental (Unintentional)	Poisoning, Intentional Self-Harm	Poisoning, Assault	Poisoning, Undetermined	Adverse Effect	Underdosing
Chlormezanone	T42.6X1	T42.6X2	T42.6X3	T42.6X4	T42.6X5	T42.6X6
Chloroacetic acid	T60.3X1	T60.3X2	T60.3X3	T60.3X4	—	—
Chloroacetone	T59.3X1	T59.3X2	T59.3X3	T59.3X4	—	—
Chloroacetophenone	T59.3X1	T59.3X2	T59.3X3	T59.3X4	—	—
Chloroaniline	T53.7X1	T53.7X2	T53.7X3	T53.7X4	—	—
Chlorobenzene, chlorobenzol	T53.7X1	T53.7X2	T53.7X3	T53.7X4	—	—
Chlorobromomethane (fire extinguisher)	T53.6X1	T53.6X2	T53.6X3	T53.6X4	—	—
Chlorobutanol	T49.0X1	T49.0X2	T49.0X3	T49.0X4	T49.0X5	T49.0X6
Chlorocresol	T49.0X1	T49.0X2	T49.0X3	T49.0X4	T49.0X5	T49.0X6
Chlorodehydro-methyltestosterone	T38.7X1	T38.7X2	T38.7X3	T38.7X4	T38.7X5	T38.7X6
Chlorodinitrobenzene	T53.7X1	T53.7X2	T53.7X3	T53.7X4	—	—
dust or vapor	T53.7X1	T53.7X2	T53.7X3	T53.7X4	—	—
Chlorodiphenyl	T53.7X1	T53.7X2	T53.7X3	T53.7X4	—	—
Chloroethane — *see Ethyl, chloride*						
Chloroethylene	T53.6X1	T53.6X2	T53.6X3	T53.6X4	—	—
Chlorofluorocarbons	T53.5X1	T53.5X2	T53.5X3	T53.5X4	—	—
Chloroform (fumes) (vapor)	T53.1X1	T53.1X2	T53.1X3	T53.1X4	—	—
anesthetic	T41.0X1	T41.0X2	T41.0X3	T41.0X4	T41.0X5	T41.0X6
solvent	T53.1X1	T53.1X2	T53.1X3	T53.1X4	—	—
water, concentrated	T41.0X1	T41.0X2	T41.0X3	T41.0X4	T41.0X5	T41.0X6
Chloroguanide	T37.2X1	T37.2X2	T37.2X3	T37.2X4	T37.2X5	T37.2X6
Chloromycetin	T36.2X1	T36.2X2	T36.2X3	T36.2X4	T36.2X5	T36.2X6
ENT agent	T49.6X1	T49.6X2	T49.6X3	T49.6X4	T49.6X5	T49.6X6
ophthalmic preparation	T49.5X1	T49.5X2	T49.5X3	T49.5X4	T49.5X5	T49.5X6
otic solution	T49.6X1	T49.6X2	T49.6X3	T49.6X4	T49.6X5	T49.6X6
topical NEC	T49.0X1	T49.0X2	T49.0X3	T49.0X4	T49.0X5	T49.0X6
Chloronitrobenzene	T53.7X1	T53.7X2	T53.7X3	T53.7X4	—	—
dust or vapor	T53.7X1	T53.7X2	T53.7X3	T53.7X4	—	—
Chlorophacinone	T60.4X1	T60.4X2	T60.4X3	T60.4X4	—	—
Chlorophenol	T53.7X1	T53.7X2	T53.7X3	T53.7X4	—	—
Chlorophenothane	T60.1X1	T60.1X2	T60.1X3	T60.1X4	—	—
Chlorophyll	T50.991	T50.992	T50.993	T50.994	T50.995	T50.996
Chloropicrin (fumes)	T53.6X1	T53.6X2	T53.6X3	T53.6X4	—	—
fumigant	T60.8X1	T60.8X2	T60.8X3	T60.8X4	—	—
fungicide	T60.3X1	T60.3X2	T60.3X3	T60.3X4	—	—
pesticide	T60.8X1	T60.8X2	T60.8X3	T60.8X4	—	—
Chloroprocaine	T41.3X1	T41.3X2	T41.3X3	T41.3X4	T41.3X5	T41.3X6
infiltration (subcutaneous)	T41.3X1	T41.3X2	T41.3X3	T41.3X4	T41.3X5	T41.3X6
nerve block (peripheral) (plexus)	T41.3X1	T41.3X2	T41.3X3	T41.3X4	T41.3X5	T41.3X6
spinal	T41.3X1	T41.3X2	T41.3X3	T41.3X4	T41.3X5	T41.3X6

TABLE OF DRUGS AND CHEMICALS

Substance	External Cause (T-Code) Poisoning, Accidental (Unintentional)	Poisoning, Intentional Self-Harm	Poisoning, Assault	Poisoning, Undetermined	Adverse Effect	Underdosing
Chloroptic	T49.5X1	T49.5X2	T49.5X3	T49.5X4	T49.5X5	T49.5X6
Chloropurine	T45.1X1	T45.1X2	T45.1X3	T45.1X4	T45.1X5	T45.1X6
Chloropyramine	T45.0X1	T45.0X2	T45.0X3	T45.0X4	T45.0X5	T45.0X6
Chloropyrifos	T60.0X1	T60.0X2	T60.0X3	T60.0X4	—	—
Chloropyrilene	T45.0X1	T45.0X2	T45.0X3	T45.0X4	T45.0X5	T45.0X6
Chloroquine	T37.2X1	T37.2X2	T37.2X3	T37.2X4	T37.2X5	T37.2X6
Chlorothalonil	T60.3X1	T60.3X2	T60.3X3	T60.3X4	—	—
Chlorothen	T45.0X1	T45.0X2	T45.0X3	T45.0X4	T45.0X5	T45.0X6
Chlorothiazide	T50.2X1	T50.2X2	T50.2X3	T50.2X4	T50.2X5	T50.2X6
Chlorothymol	T49.4X1	T49.4X2	T49.4X3	T49.4X4	T49.4X5	T49.4X6
Chlorotrianisene	T38.5X1	T38.5X2	T38.5X3	T38.5X4	T38.5X5	T38.5X6
Chlorovinyldichloro-arsine, not in war	T57.0X1	T57.0X2	T57.0X3	T57.0X4	—	—
Chloroxine	T49.4X1	T49.4X2	T49.4X3	T49.4X4	T49.4X5	T49.4X6
Chloroxylenol	T49.0X1	T49.0X2	T49.0X3	T49.0X4	T49.0X5	T49.0X6
Chlorphenamine	T45.0X1	T45.0X2	T45.0X3	T45.0X4	T45.0X5	T45.0X6
Chlorphenesin	T42.8X1	T42.8X2	T42.8X3	T42.8X4	T42.8X5	T42.8X6
topical (antifungal)	T49.0X1	T49.0X2	T49.0X3	T49.0X4	T49.0X5	T49.0X6
Chlorpheniramine	T45.0X1	T45.0X2	T45.0X3	T45.0X4	T45.0X5	T45.0X6
Chlorphenoxamine	T45.0X1	T45.0X2	T45.0X3	T45.0X4	T45.0X5	T45.0X6
Chlorphentermine	T50.5X1	T50.5X2	T50.5X3	T50.5X4	T50.5X5	T50.5X6
Chlorprocaine—*see Chloroprocaine*						
Chlorproguanil	T37.2X1	T37.2X2	T37.2X3	T37.2X4	T37.2X5	T37.2X6
Chlorpromazine	T43.3X1	T43.3X2	T43.3X3	T43.3X4	T43.3X5	T43.3X6
Chlorpropamide	T38.3X1	T38.3X2	T38.3X3	T38.3X4	T38.3X5	T38.3X6
Chlorprothixene	T43.4X1	T43.4X2	T43.4X3	T43.4X4	T43.4X5	T43.4X6
Chlorquinaldol	T49.0X1	T49.0X2	T49.0X3	T49.0X4	T49.0X5	T49.0X6
Chlorquinol	T49.0X1	T49.0X2	T49.0X3	T49.0X4	T49.0X5	T49.0X6
Chlortalidone	T50.2X1	T50.2X2	T50.2X3	T50.2X4	T50.2X5	T50.2X6
Chlortetracycline	T36.4X1	T36.4X2	T36.4X3	T36.4X4	T36.4X5	T36.4X6
Chlorthalidone	T50.2X1	T50.2X2	T50.2X3	T50.2X4	T50.2X5	T50.2X6
Chlorthiophos	T60.0X1	T60.0X2	T60.0X3	T60.0X4	—	—
Chlorotrianisene	T38.5X1	T38.5X2	T38.5X3	T38.5X4	T38.5X5	T38.5X6
Chlor-Trimeton	T45.0X1	T45.0X2	T45.0X3	T45.0X4	T45.0X5	T45.0X6
Chlorthion	T60.0X1	T60.0X2	T60.0X3	T60.0X4	—	—
Chlorzoxazone	T42.8X1	T42.8X2	T42.8X3	T42.8X4	T42.8X5	T42.8X6
Choke damp	T59.7X1	T59.7X2	T59.7X3	T59.7X4	—	—
Cholagogues	T47.5X1	T47.5X2	T47.5X3	T47.5X4	T47.5X5	T47.5X6
Cholebrine	T50.8X1	T50.8X2	T50.8X3	T50.8X4	T50.8X5	T50.8X6
Cholecalciferol	T45.2X1	T45.2X2	T45.2X3	T45.2X4	T45.2X5	T45.2X6
Cholecystokinin	T50.8X1	T50.8X2	T50.8X3	T50.8X4	T50.8X5	T50.8X6
Cholera vaccine	T50.A91	T50.A92	T50.A93	T50.A94	T50.A95	T50.A96
Choleretic	T47.5X1	T47.5X2	T47.5X3	T47.5X4	T47.5X5	T47.5X6
Cholesterol-lowering agents	T46.6X1	T46.6X2	T46.6X3	T46.6X4	T46.6X5	T46.6X6
Cholestyramine (resin)	T46.6X1	T46.6X2	T46.6X3	T46.6X4	T46.6X5	T46.6X6
Cholic acid	T47.5X1	T47.5X2	T47.5X3	T47.5X4	T47.5X5	T47.5X6
Choline	T48.6X1	T48.6X2	T48.6X3	T48.6X4	T48.6X5	T48.6X6
chloride	T50.991	T50.992	T50.993	T50.994	T50.995	T50.996
dihydrogen citrate	T50.991	T50.992	T50.993	T50.994	T50.995	T50.996
salicylate	T39.091	T39.092	T39.093	T39.094	T39.095	T39.096
theophyllinate	T48.6X1	T48.6X2	T48.6X3	T48.6X4	T48.6X5	T48.6X6
Cholinergic (drug) NEC	T44.1X1	T44.1X2	T44.1X3	T44.1X4	T44.1X5	T44.1X6
muscle tone enhancer	T44.1X1	T44.1X2	T44.1X3	T44.1X4	T44.1X5	T44.1X6
organophosphorus	T44.0X1	T44.0X2	T44.0X3	T44.0X4	T44.0X5	T44.0X6
insecticide	T60.0X1	T60.0X2	T60.0X3	T60.0X4	—	—
nerve gas	T59.891	T59.892	T59.893	T59.894	—	—
trimethyl ammonium propanediol	T44.1X1	T44.1X2	T44.1X3	T44.1X4	T44.1X5	T44.1X6
Cholinesterase reactivator	T50.6X1	T50.6X2	T50.6X3	T50.6X4	T50.6X5	T50.6X6
Chlolografin	T50.8X1	T50.8X2	T50.8X3	T50.8X4	T50.8X5	T50.8X6
Chorionic gonadotropin	T38.891	T38.892	T38.893	T38.894	T38.895	T38.896
Chromate	T56.2X1	T56.2X2	T56.2X3	T56.2X4	—	—
dust or mist	T56.2X1	T56.2X2	T56.2X3	T56.2X4	—	—
lead—*see also Lead*	T56.0X1	T56.0X2	T56.0X3	T56.0X4	—	—
paint	T56.0X1	T56.0X2	T56.0X3	T56.0X4	—	—
Chromic						
acid	T56.2X1	T56.2X2	T56.2X3	T56.2X4	—	—
dust or mist	T56.2X1	T56.2X2	T56.2X3	T56.2X4	—	—
phosphate 32P	T45.1X1	T45.1X2	T45.1X3	T45.1X4	T45.1X5	T45.1X6
Chromium	T56.2X1	T56.2X2	T56.2X3	T56.2X4	—	—
compounds—*see Chromate*						
sesquioxide	T50.8X1	T50.8X2	T50.8X3	T50.8X4	T50.8X5	T50.8X6
Chromomycin A3	T45.1X1	T45.1X2	T45.1X3	T45.1X4	T45.1X5	T45.1X6
Chromonar	T46.3X1	T46.3X2	T46.3X3	T46.3X4	T46.3X5	T46.3X6
Chromyl chloride	T56.2X1	T56.2X2	T56.2X3	T56.2X4	—	—
Chrysarobin	T49.4X1	T49.4X2	T49.4X3	T49.4X4	T49.4X5	T49.4X6
Chrysazin	T47.2X1	T47.2X2	T47.2X3	T47.2X4	T47.2X5	T47.2X6
Chymar	T45.3X1	T45.3X2	T45.3X3	T45.3X4	T45.3X5	T45.3X6
ophthalmic preparation	T49.5X1	T49.5X2	T49.5X3	T49.5X4	T49.5X5	T49.5X6
Chymopapain	T45.3X1	T45.3X2	T45.3X3	T45.3X4	T45.3X5	T45.3X6
Chymotrypsin	T45.3X1	T45.3X2	T45.3X3	T45.3X4	T45.3X5	T45.3X6
ophthalmic preparation	T49.5X1	T49.5X2	T49.5X3	T49.5X4	T49.5X5	T49.5X6
Cianidanol	T50.991	T50.992	T50.993	T50.994	T50.995	T50.996
Cianopramine	T43.011	T43.012	T43.013	T43.014	T43.015	T43.016
Cibenzoline	T46.2X1	T46.2X2	T46.2X3	T46.2X4	T46.2X5	T46.2X6

Substance	External Cause (T-Code) Poisoning, Accidental (Unintentional)	Poisoning, Intentional Self-Harm	Poisoning, Assault	Poisoning, Undetermined	Adverse Effect	Underdosing
Ciclacillin	T36.ØX1	T36.ØX2	T36.ØX3	T36.ØX4	T36.ØX5	T36.ØX6
Ciclobarbital — *see Hexobarbital*						
Ciclonicate	T46.7X1	T46.7X2	T46.7X3	T46.7X4	T46.7X5	T46.7X6
Ciclopirox (olamine)	T49.ØX1	T49.ØX2	T49.ØX3	T49.ØX4	T49.ØX5	T49.ØX6
Ciclosporin	T45.1X1	T45.1X2	T45.1X3	T45.1X4	T45.1X5	T45.1X6
Cicuta maculata or virosa	T62.2X1	T62.2X2	T62.2X3	T62.2X4	—	—
Cicutoxin	T62.2X1	T62.2X2	T62.2X3	T62.2X4	—	—
Cigarette lighter fluid	T52.ØX1	T52.ØX2	T52.ØX3	T52.ØX4	—	—
Cigarettes (tobacco)	T65.221	T65.222	T65.223	T65.224	—	—
Ciguatoxin	T61.Ø1	T61.Ø2	T61.Ø3	T61.Ø4	—	—
Cilazapril	T46.4X1	T46.4X2	T46.4X3	T46.4X4	T46.4X5	T46.4X6
Cimetidine	T47.ØX1	T47.ØX2	T47.ØX3	T47.ØX4	T47.ØX5	T47.ØX6
Cimetropium bromide	T44.3X1	T44.3X2	T44.3X3	T44.3X4	T44.3X5	T44.3X6
Cinchocaine	T41.3X1	T41.3X2	T41.3X3	T41.3X4	T41.3X5	T41.3X6
topical (surface)	T41.3X1	T41.3X2	T41.3X3	T41.3X4	T41.3X5	T41.3X6
Cinchona	T37.2X1	T37.2X2	T37.2X3	T37.2X4	T37.2X5	T37.2X6
Cinchonine alkaloids	T37.2X1	T37.2X2	T37.2X3	T37.2X4	T37.2X5	T37.2X6
Cinchophen	T5Ø.4X1	T5Ø.4X2	T5Ø.4X3	T5Ø.4X4	T5Ø.4X5	T5Ø.4X6
Cinepazide	T46.7X1	T46.7X2	T46.7X3	T46.7X4	T46.7X5	T46.7X6
Cinnamedrine	T48.5X1	T48.5X2	T48.5X3	T48.5X4	T48.5X5	T48.5X6
Cinnarizine	T45.ØX1	T45.ØX2	T45.ØX3	T45.ØX4	T45.ØX5	T45.ØX6
Cinoxacin	T37.8X1	T37.8X2	T37.8X3	T37.8X4	T37.8X5	T37.8X6
Ciprofibrate	T46.6X1	T46.6X2	T46.6X3	T46.6X4	T46.6X5	T46.6X6
Ciprofloxacin	T36.8X1	T36.8X2	T36.8X3	T36.8X4	T36.8X5	T36.8X6
Cisapride	T47.8X1	T47.8X2	T47.8X3	T47.8X4	T47.8X5	T47.8X6
Cisplatin	T45.1X1	T45.1X2	T45.1X3	T45.1X4	T45.1X5	T45.1X6
Citalopram	T43.221	T43.222	T43.223	T43.224	T43.225	T43.226
Citanest	T41.3X1	T41.3X2	T41.3X3	T41.3X4	T41.3X5	T41.3X6
infiltration (subcutaneous)	T41.3X1	T41.3X2	T41.3X3	T41.3X4	T41.3X5	T41.3X6
nerve block (peripheral) (plexus)	T41.3X1	T41.3X2	T41.3X3	T41.3X4	T41.3X5	T41.3X6
Citric acid	T47.5X1	T47.5X2	T47.5X3	T47.5X4	T47.5X5	T47.5X6
Citrovorum (factor)	T45.8X1	T45.8X2	T45.8X3	T45.8X4	T45.8X5	T45.8X6
Claviceps purpurea	T62.2X1	T62.2X2	T62.2X3	T62.2X4	—	—
Clavulanic acid	T36.1X1	T36.1X2	T36.1X3	T36.1X4	T36.1X5	T36.1X6
Cleaner, cleansing agent, type not specified	T65.891	T65.892	T65.893	T65.894	—	—
of paint or varnish	T52.91	T52.92	T52.93	T52.94	—	—
specified type NEC	T65.891	T65.892	T65.893	T65.894	—	—
Clebopride	T47.8X1	T47.8X2	T47.8X3	T47.8X4	T47.8X5	T47.8X6
Clefamide	T37.3X1	T37.3X2	T37.3X3	T37.3X4	T37.3X5	T37.3X6
Clemastine	T45.ØX1	T45.ØX2	T45.ØX3	T45.ØX4	T45.ØX5	T45.ØX6
Clematis vitalba	T62.2X1	T62.2X2	T62.2X3	T62.2X4		
Clemizole	T45.ØX1	T45.ØX2	T45.ØX3	T45.ØX4	T45.ØX5	T45.ØX6
penicillin	T36.ØX1	T36.ØX2	T36.ØX3	T36.ØX4	T36.ØX5	T36.ØX6
Clenbuterol	T48.6X1	T48.6X2	T48.6X3	T48.6X4	T48.6X5	T48.6X6
Clidinium bromide	T44.3X1	T44.3X2	T44.3X3	T44.3X4	T44.3X5	T44.3X6
Clindamycin	T36.8X1	T36.8X2	T36.8X3	T36.8X4	T36.8X5	T36.8X6
Clinofibrate	T46.6X1	T46.6X2	T46.6X3	T46.6X4	T46.6X5	T46.6X6
Clioquinol	T37.8X1	T37.8X2	T37.8X3	T37.8X4	T37.8X5	T37.8X6
Cliradon	T40.2X1	T40.2X2	T40.2X3	T40.2X4	—	—
Clobazam	T42.4X1	T42.4X2	T42.4X3	T42.4X4	T42.4X5	T42.4X6
Clobenzorex	T5Ø.5X1	T5Ø.5X2	T5Ø.5X3	T5Ø.5X4	T5Ø.5X5	T5Ø.5X6
Clobetasol	T49.ØX1	T49.ØX2	T49.ØX3	T49.ØX4	T49.ØX5	T49.ØX6
Clobetasone	T49.ØX1	T49.ØX2	T49.ØX3	T49.ØX4	T49.ØX5	T49.ØX6
Clobutinol	T48.3X1	T48.3X2	T48.3X3	T48.3X4	T48.3X5	T48.3X6
Clocapramine	T43.ØX1	T43.ØX2	T43.ØX3	T43.ØX4	T43.ØX5	T43.ØX6
Clocortolone	T38.ØX1	T38.ØX2	T38.ØX3	T38.ØX4	T38.ØX5	T38.ØX6
Clodantoin	T49.ØX1	T49.ØX2	T49.ØX3	T49.ØX4	T49.ØX5	T49.ØX6
Clodronic acid	T5Ø.991	T5Ø.992	T5Ø.993	T5Ø.994	T5Ø.995	T5Ø.996
Clofazimine	T37.1X1	T37.1X2	T37.1X3	T37.1X4	T37.1X5	T37.1X6
Clofedanol	T48.3X1	T48.3X2	T48.3X3	T48.3X4	T48.3X5	T48.3X6
Clofenamide	T5Ø.2X1	T5Ø.2X2	T5Ø.2X3	T5Ø.2X4	T5Ø.2X5	T5Ø.2X6
Clofenotane	T49.ØX1	T49.ØX2	T49.ØX3	T49.ØX4	T49.ØX5	T49.ØX6
Clofezone	T39.2X1	T39.2X2	T39.2X3	T39.2X4	T39.2X5	T39.2X6
Clofibrate	T46.6X1	T46.6X2	T46.6X3	T46.6X4	T46.6X5	T46.6X6
Clofibride	T46.6X1	T46.6X2	T46.6X3	T46.6X4	T46.6X5	T46.6X6
Cloforex	T5Ø.5X1	T5Ø.5X2	T5Ø.5X3	T5Ø.5X4	T5Ø.5X5	T5Ø.5X6
Clomacran	T43.ØX1	T43.ØX2	T43.ØX3	T43.ØX4	T43.ØX5	T43.ØX6
Clomethiazole	T42.6X1	T42.6X2	T42.6X3	T42.6X4	T42.6X5	T42.6X6
Clometocillin	T36.ØX1	T36.ØX2	T36.ØX3	T36.ØX4	T36.ØX5	T36.ØX6
Clomifene	T38.5X1	T38.5X2	T38.5X3	T38.5X4	T38.5X5	T38.5X6
Clomiphene	T38.5X1	T38.5X2	T38.5X3	T38.5X4	T38.5X5	T38.5X6
Clomipramine	T43.Ø11	T43.Ø12	T43.Ø13	T43.Ø14	T43.Ø15	T43.Ø16
Clomocycline	T36.4X1	T36.4X2	T36.4X3	T36.4X4	T36.4X5	T36.4X6
Clonazepam	T42.4X1	T42.4X2	T42.4X3	T42.4X4	T42.4X5	T42.4X6
Clonidine	T46.5X1	T46.5X2	T46.5X3	T46.5X4	T46.5X5	T46.5X6
Clonixin	T39.8X1	T39.8X2	T39.8X3	T39.8X4	T39.8X5	T39.8X6
Clopamide	T5Ø.2X1	T5Ø.2X2	T5Ø.2X3	T5Ø.2X4	T5Ø.2X5	T5Ø.2X6
Clopenthixol	T43.4X1	T43.4X2	T43.4X3	T43.4X4	T43.4X5	T43.4X6
Cloperastine	T48.3X1	T48.3X2	T48.3X3	T48.3X4	T48.3X5	T48.3X6
Clophedianol	T48.3X1	T48.3X2	T48.3X3	T48.3X4	T48.3X5	T48.3X6
Cloponone	T36.2X1	T36.2X2	T36.2X3	T36.2X4	T36.2X5	T36.2X6
Cloprednol	T38.ØX1	T38.ØX2	T38.ØX3	T38.ØX4	T38.ØX5	T38.ØX6
Cloral betaine	T42.6X1	T42.6X2	T42.6X3	T42.6X4	T42.6X5	T42.6X6

TABLE OF DRUGS AND CHEMICALS

◀ New ⇐ Revised ~~deleted~~ Deleted

	External Cause (T-Code)					
Substance	Poisoning, Accidental (Unintentional)	Poisoning, Intentional Self-Harm	Poisoning, Assault	Poisoning, Undetermined	Adverse Effect	Underdosing
Cloramfenicol	T36.2X1	T36.2X2	T36.2X3	T36.2X4	T36.2X5	T36.2X6
Clorazepate (dipotassium)	T42.4X1	T42.4X2	T42.4X3	T42.4X4	T42.4X5	T42.4X6
Clorexolone	T50.2X1	T50.2X2	T50.2X3	T50.2X4	T50.2X5	T50.2X6
Clorox (bleach)	T54.91	T54.92	T54.93	T54.94	—	—
Clorfenamine	T45.0X1	T45.0X2	T45.0X3	T45.0X4	T45.0X5	T45.0X6
Clorgiline	T43.1X1	T43.1X2	T43.1X3	T43.1X4	T43.1X5	T43.1X6
Clorotepine	T44.3X1	T44.3X2	T44.3X3	T44.3X4	T44.3X5	T44.3X6
Clorprenaline	T48.6X1	T48.6X2	T48.6X3	T48.6X4	T48.6X5	T48.6X6
Clortermine	T50.5X1	T50.5X2	T50.5X3	T50.5X4	T50.5X5	T50.5X6
Clotiapine	T43.591	T43.592	T43.593	T43.594	T43.595	T43.596
Clotiazepam	T42.4X1	T42.4X2	T42.4X3	T42.4X4	T42.4X5	T42.4X6
Clotibric acid	T46.6X1	T46.6X2	T46.6X3	T46.6X4	T46.6X5	T46.6X6
Clotrimazole	T49.0X1	T49.0X2	T49.0X3	T49.0X4	T49.0X5	T49.0X6
Cloxacillin	T36.0X1	T36.0X2	T36.0X3	T36.0X4	T36.0X5	T36.0X6
Cloxazolam	T42.4X1	T42.4X2	T42.4X3	T42.4X4	T42.4X5	T42.4X6
Cloxiquine	T49.0X1	T49.0X2	T49.0X3	T49.0X4	T49.0X5	T49.0X6
Clozapine	T42.4X1	T42.4X2	T42.4X3	T42.4X4	T42.4X5	T42.4X6
Coagulant NEC	T45.7X1	T45.7X2	T45.7X3	T45.7X4	T45.7X5	T45.7X6
Coal (carbon monoxide from) — *see also Carbon, monoxide, coal*	T58.2X1	T58.2X2	T58.2X3	T58.2X4	—	—
oil — *see Kerosene*						
tar	T49.1X1	T49.1X2	T49.1X3	T49.1X4	T49.1X5	T49.1X6
fumes	T59.891	T59.892	T59.893	T59.894	—	—
medicinal (ointment)	T49.4X1	T49.4X2	T49.4X3	T49.4X4	T49.4X5	T49.4X6
analgesics NEC	T39.2X1	T39.2X2	T39.2X3	T39.2X4	T39.2X5	T39.2X6
naphtha (solvent)	T52.0X1	T52.0X2	T52.0X3	T52.0X4		
Cobalamine	T45.2X1	T45.2X2	T45.2X3	T45.2X4	T45.2X5	T45.2X6
Cobalt (nonmedicinal) (fumes) (industrial)	T56.891	T56.892	T56.893	T56.894		
medicinal (trace) (chloride)	T45.8X1	T45.8X2	T45.8X3	T45.8X4	T45.8X5	T45.8X6
Cobra (venom)	T63.041	T63.042	T63.043	T63.044		
Coca (leaf)	T40.5X1	T40.5X2	T40.5X3	T40.5X4	T40.5X5	T40.5X6
Cocaine	T40.5X1	T40.5X2	T40.5X3	T40.5X4	T40.5X5	T40.5X6
topical anesthetic	T41.3X1	T41.3X2	T41.3X3	T41.3X4	T41.3X5	T41.3X6
Cocarboxylase	T45.3X1	T45.3X2	T45.3X3	T45.3X4	T45.3X5	T45.3X6
Coccidioidin	T50.8X1	T50.8X2	T50.8X3	T50.8X4	T50.8X5	T50.8X6
Cocculus indicus	T62.1X1	T62.1X2	T62.1X3	T62.1X4		
Cochineal	T65.6X1	T65.6X2	T65.6X3	T65.6X4		
medicinal products	T50.991	T50.992	T50.993	T50.994	T50.995	T50.996
Codeine	T40.2X1	T40.2X2	T40.2X3	T40.2X4	T40.2X5	T40.2X6
Cod-liver oil	T45.2X1	T45.2X2	T45.2X3	T45.2X4	T45.2X5	T45.2X6

	External Cause (T-Code)					
Substance	Poisoning, Accidental (Unintentional)	Poisoning, Intentional Self-Harm	Poisoning, Assault	Poisoning, Undetermined	Adverse Effect	Underdosing
Coenzyme A	T50.991	T50.992	T50.993	T50.994	T50.995	T50.996
Coffee	T62.8X1	T62.8X2	T62.8X3	T62.8X4	—	—
Cogalactoisomerase	T50.991	T50.992	T50.993	T50.994	T50.995	T50.996
Cogentin	T44.3X1	T44.3X2	T44.3X3	T44.3X4	T44.3X5	T44.3X6
Coke fumes or gas (carbon monoxide)	T58.2X1	T58.2X2	T58.2X3	T58.2X4	—	—
industrial use	T58.8X1	T58.8X2	T58.8X3	T58.8X4	—	—
Colace	T47.4X1	T47.4X2	T47.4X3	T47.4X4	T47.4X5	T47.4X6
Colaspase	T45.1X1	T45.1X2	T45.1X3	T45.1X4	T45.1X5	T45.1X6
Colchicine	T50.4X1	T50.4X2	T50.4X3	T50.4X4	T50.4X5	T50.4X6
Colchicum	T62.2X1	T62.2X2	T62.2X3	T62.2X4	—	—
Cold cream	T49.3X1	T49.3X2	T49.3X3	T49.3X4	T49.3X5	T49.3X6
Colecalciferol	T45.2X1	T45.2X2	T45.2X3	T45.2X4	T45.2X5	T45.2X6
Colestipol	T46.6X1	T46.6X2	T46.6X3	T46.6X4	T46.6X5	T46.6X6
Colestyramine	T46.6X1	T46.6X2	T46.6X3	T46.6X4	T46.6X5	T46.6X6
Colimycin	T36.8X1	T36.8X2	T36.8X3	T36.8X4	T36.8X5	T36.8X6
Colistimethate	T36.8X1	T36.8X2	T36.8X3	T36.8X4	T36.8X5	T36.8X6
Colistin	T36.8X1	T36.8X2	T36.8X3	T36.8X4	T36.8X5	T36.8X6
sulfate (eye preparation)	T49.5X1	T49.5X2	T49.5X3	T49.5X4	T49.5X5	T49.5X6
Collagen	T50.991	T50.992	T50.993	T50.994	T50.995	T50.996
Collagenase	T49.4X1	T49.4X2	T49.4X3	T49.4X4	T49.4X5	T49.4X6
Collodion	T49.3X1	T49.3X2	T49.3X3	T49.3X4	T49.3X5	T49.3X6
Colocynth	T47.2X1	T47.2X2	T47.2X3	T47.2X4	T47.2X5	T47.2X6
Colophony adhesive	T49.3X1	T49.3X2	T49.3X3	T49.3X4	T49.3X5	T49.3X6
Colorant — *see also Dye*	T50.991	T50.992	T50.993	T50.994	T50.995	T50.996
Coloring matter — *see Dye(s)*						
Combustion gas (after combustion) — *see Carbon, monoxide*						
prior to combustion	T59.891	T59.892	T59.893	T59.894	—	—
Compazine	T43.3X1	T43.3X2	T43.3X3	T43.3X4	T43.3X5	T43.3X6
Compound						
42 (warfarin)	T60.4X1	T60.4X2	T60.4X3	T60.4X4	—	—
269 (endrin)	T60.1X1	T60.1X2	T60.1X3	T60.1X4	—	—
497 (dieldrin)	T60.1X1	T60.1X2	T60.1X3	T60.1X4	—	—
1080 (sodium fluoroacetate)	T60.4X1	T60.4X2	T60.4X3	T60.4X4	—	—
3422 (parathion)	T60.0X1	T60.0X2	T60.0X3	T60.0X4	—	—
3911 (phorate)	T60.0X1	T60.0X2	T60.0X3	T60.0X4	—	—
3956 (toxaphene)	T60.1X1	T60.1X2	T60.1X3	T60.1X4	—	—
4049 (malathion)	T60.0X1	T60.0X2	T60.0X3	T60.0X4	—	—
4069 (malathion)	T60.0X1	T60.0X2	T60.0X3	T60.0X4	—	—
4124 (dicapthon)	T60.0X1	T60.0X2	T60.0X3	T60.0X4	—	—

Substance	External Cause (T-Code)					
	Poisoning, Accidental (Unintentional)	Poisoning, Intentional Self-Harm	Poisoning, Assault	Poisoning, Undetermined	Adverse Effect	Underdosing
Compound *(Continued)*						
E (cortisone)	T38.ØX1	T38.ØX2	T38.ØX3	T38.ØX4	T38.ØX5	T38.ØX6
F (hydrocortisone)	T38.ØX1	T38.ØX2	T38.ØX3	T38.ØX4	T38.ØX5	T38.ØX6
Congener, anabolic	T38.7X1	T38.7X2	T38.7X3	T38.7X4	T38.7X5	T38.7X6
Congo red	T5Ø.8X1	T5Ø.8X2	T5Ø.8X3	T5Ø.8X4	T5Ø.8X5	T5Ø.8X6
Coniine, conine	T62.2X1	T62.2X2	T62.2X3	T62.2X4	—	—
Conium (maculatum)	T62.2X1	T62.2X2	T62.2X3	T62.2X4	—	—
Conjugated estrogenic substances	T38.5X1	T38.5X2	T38.5X3	T38.5X4	T38.5X5	T38.5X6
Contac	T48.5X1	T48.5X2	T48.5X3	T48.5X4	T48.5X5	T48.5X6
Contact lens solution	T49.5X1	T49.5X2	T49.5X3	T49.5X4	T49.5X5	T49.5X6
Contraceptive (oral)	T38.4X1	T38.4X2	T38.4X3	T38.4X4	T38.4X5	T38.4X6
vaginal	T49.8X1	T49.8X2	T49.8X3	T49.8X4	T49.8X5	T49.8X6
Contrast medium, radiography	T5Ø.8X1	T5Ø.8X2	T5Ø.8X3	T5Ø.8X4	T5Ø.8X5	T5Ø.8X6
Convallaria glycosides	T46.ØX1	T46.ØX2	T46.ØX3	T46.ØX4	T46.ØX5	T46.ØX6
Convallaria majalis	T62.2X1	T62.2X2	T62.2X3	T62.2X4	—	—
berry	T62.1X1	T62.1X2	T62.1X3	T62.1X4	—	—
Copper (dust) (fumes) (nonmedicinal) NEC	T56.4X1	T56.4X2	T56.4X3	T56.4X4	—	—
arsenate, arsenite	T57.ØX1	T57.ØX2	T57.ØX3	T57.ØX4	—	—
insecticide	T6Ø.2X1	T6Ø.2X2	T6Ø.2X3	T6Ø.2X4	—	—
emetic	T47.7X1	T47.7X2	T47.7X3	T47.7X4	T47.7X5	T47.7X6
fungicide	T6Ø.3X1	T6Ø.3X2	T6Ø.3X3	T6Ø.3X4	—	—
gluconate	T49.ØX1	T49.ØX2	T49.ØX3	T49.ØX4	T49.ØX5	T49.ØX6
insecticide	T6Ø.2X1	T6Ø.2X2	T6Ø.2X3	T6Ø.2X4	—	—
medicinal (trace)	T45.8X1	T45.8X2	T45.8X3	T45.8X4	T45.8X5	T45.8X6
oleate	T49.ØX1	T49.ØX2	T49.ØX3	T49.ØX4	T49.ØX5	T49.ØX6
sulfate	T56.4X1	T56.4X2	T56.4X3	T56.4X4	—	—
cupric	T56.4X1	T56.4X2	T56.4X3	T56.4X4	—	—
fungicide	T6Ø.3X1	T6Ø.3X2	T6Ø.3X3	T6Ø.3X4	—	—
medicinal						
ear	T49.6X1	T49.6X2	T49.6X3	T49.6X4	T49.6X5	T49.6X6
emetic	T47.7X1	T47.7X2	T47.7X3	T47.7X4	T47.7X5	T47.7X6
eye	T49.5X1	T49.5X2	T49.5X3	T49.5X4	T49.5X5	T49.5X6
cuprous	T56.4X1	T56.4X2	T56.4X3	T56.4X4	—	—
fungicide	T6Ø.3X1	T6Ø.3X2	T6Ø.3X3	T6Ø.3X4	—	—
medicinal						
ear	T49.6X1	T49.6X2	T49.6X3	T49.6X4	T49.6X5	T49.6X6
emetic	T47.7X1	T47.7X2	T47.7X3	T47.7X4	T47.7X5	T47.7X6
eye	T49.5X1	T49.5X2	T49.5X3	T49.5X4	T49.5X5	T49.5X6
Copperhead snake (bite) (venom)	T63.Ø61	T63.Ø62	T63.Ø63	T63.Ø64	—	—
Coral (sting)	T63.691	T63.692	T63.693	T63.694	—	—
snake (bite) (venom)	T63.Ø21	T63.Ø22	T63.Ø23	T63.Ø24	—	—

Substance	External Cause (T-Code)					
	Poisoning, Accidental (Unintentional)	Poisoning, Intentional Self-Harm	Poisoning, Assault	Poisoning, Undetermined	Adverse Effect	Underdosing
Corbadrine	T49.6X1	T49.6X2	T49.6X3	T49.6X4	T49.6X5	T49.6X6
Cordran	T49.ØX1	T49.ØX2	T49.ØX3	T49.ØX4	T49.ØX5	T49.ØX6
Cordite	T65.891	T65.892	T65.893	T65.894	—	—
vapor	T59.891	T59.892	T59.893	T59.894	—	—
Corn cures	T49.4X1	T49.4X2	T49.4X3	T49.4X4	T49.4X5	T49.4X6
Cornhusker's lotion	T49.3X1	T49.3X2	T49.3X3	T49.3X4	T49.3X5	T49.3X6
Corn starch	T49.3X1	T49.3X2	T49.3X3	T49.3X4	T49.3X5	T49.3X6
Coronary vasodilator NEC	T46.3X1	T46.3X2	T46.3X3	T46.3X4	T46.3X5	T46.3X6
Corrosive NEC	T54.91	T54.92	T54.93	T54.94	—	—
acid NEC	T54.2X1	T54.2X2	T54.2X3	T54.2X4	—	—
aromatics	T54.1X1	T54.1X2	T54.1X3	T54.1X4	—	—
disinfectant	T54.1X1	T54.1X2	T54.1X3	T54.1X4	—	—
fumes NEC	T54.91	T54.92	T54.93	T54.94	—	—
specified NEC	T54.91	T54.92	T54.93	T54.94	—	—
sublimate	T56.1X1	T56.1X2	T56.1X3	T56.1X4	—	—
Cortate	T38.ØX1	T38.ØX2	T38.ØX3	T38.ØX4	T38.ØX5	T38.ØX6
Cort-Dome	T38.ØX1	T38.ØX2	T38.ØX3	T38.ØX4	T38.ØX5	T38.ØX6
ENT agent	T49.6X1	T49.6X2	T49.6X3	T49.6X4	T49.6X5	T49.6X6
ophthalmic preparation	T49.5X1	T49.5X2	T49.5X3	T49.5X4	T49.5X5	T49.5X6
topical NEC	T49.ØX1	T49.ØX2	T49.ØX3	T49.ØX4	T49.ØX5	T49.ØX6
Cortef	T38.ØX1	T38.ØX2	T38.ØX3	T38.ØX4	T38.ØX5	T38.ØX6
ENT agent	T49.6X1	T49.6X2	T49.6X3	T49.6X4	T49.6X5	T49.6X6
ophthalmic preparation	T49.5X1	T49.5X2	T49.5X3	T49.5X4	T49.5X5	T49.5X6
topical NEC	T49.ØX1	T49.ØX2	T49.ØX3	T49.ØX4	T49.ØX5	T49.ØX6
Corticosteroid	T38.ØX1	T38.ØX2	T38.ØX3	T38.ØX4	T38.ØX5	T38.ØX6
ENT agent	T49.6X1	T49.6X2	T49.6X3	T49.6X4	T49.6X5	T49.6X6
mineral	T5Ø.ØX1	T5Ø.ØX2	T5Ø.ØX3	T5Ø.ØX4	T5Ø.ØX5	T5Ø.ØX6
ophthalmic	T49.5X1	T49.5X2	T49.5X3	T49.5X4	T49.5X5	T49.5X6
topical NEC	T49.ØX1	T49.ØX2	T49.ØX3	T49.ØX4	T49.ØX5	T49.ØX6
Corticotropin	T38.811	T38.812	T38.813	T38.814	T38.815	T38.816
Cortisol	T49.ØX1	T49.ØX2	T49.ØX3	T49.ØX4	T49.ØX5	T49.ØX6
ENT agent	T49.6X1	T49.6X2	T49.6X3	T49.6X4	T49.6X5	T49.6X6
ophthalmic preparation	T49.5X1	T49.5X2	T49.5X3	T49.5X4	T49.5X5	T49.5X6
topical NEC	T49.ØX1	T49.ØX2	T49.ØX3	T49.ØX4	T49.ØX5	T49.ØX6
Cortisone (acetate)	T38.ØX1	T38.ØX2	T38.ØX3	T38.ØX4	T38.ØX5	T38.ØX6
ENT agent	T49.6X1	T49.6X2	T49.6X3	T49.6X4	T49.6X5	T49.6X6
ophthalmic preparation	T49.5X1	T49.5X2	T49.5X3	T49.5X4	T49.5X5	T49.5X6
topical NEC	T49.ØX1	T49.ØX2	T49.ØX3	T49.ØX4	T49.ØX5	T49.ØX6
Cortivazol	T38.ØX1	T38.ØX2	T38.ØX3	T38.ØX4	T38.ØX5	T38.ØX6
Cortogen	T38.ØX1	T38.ØX2	T38.ØX3	T38.ØX4	T38.ØX5	T38.ØX6
ENT agent	T49.6X1	T49.6X2	T49.6X3	T49.6X4	T49.6X5	T49.6X6
ophthalmic preparation	T49.5X1	T49.5X2	T49.5X3	T49.5X4	T49.5X5	T49.5X6

Substance	External Cause (T-Code)					
	Poisoning, Accidental (Unintentional)	Poisoning, Intentional Self-Harm	Poisoning, Assault	Poisoning, Undetermined	Adverse Effect	Underdosing
Cortone	T38.ØX1	T38.ØX2	T38.ØX3	T38.ØX4	T38.ØX5	T38.ØX6
ENT agent	T49.6X1	T49.6X2	T49.6X3	T49.6X4	T49.6X5	T49.6X6
ophthalmic preparation	T49.5X1	T49.5X2	T49.5X3	T49.5X4	T49.5X5	T49.5X6
Cortril	T38.ØX1	T38.ØX2	T38.ØX3	T38.ØX4	T38.ØX5	T38.ØX6
ENT agent	T49.6X1	T49.6X2	T49.6X3	T49.6X4	T49.6X5	T49.6X6
ophthalmic preparation	T49.5X1	T49.5X2	T49.5X3	T49.5X4	T49.5X5	T49.5X6
topical NEC	T49.ØX1	T49.ØX2	T49.ØX3	T49.ØX4	T49.ØX5	T49.ØX6
Corynebacterium parvum	T45.1X1	T45.1X2	T45.1X3	T45.1X4	T45.1X5	T45.1X6
Cosmetic preparation	T49.8X1	T49.8X2	T49.8X3	T49.8X4	T49.8X5	T49.8X6
Cosmetics	T49.8X1	T49.8X2	T49.8X3	T49.8X4	T49.8X5	T49.8X6
Cosyntropin	T38.811	T38.812	T38.813	T38.814	T38.815	T38.816
Cotarnine	T45.7X1	T45.7X2	T45.7X3	T45.7X4	T45.7X5	T45.7X6
Co-trimoxazole	T36.8X1	T36.8X2	T36.8X3	T36.8X4	T36.8X5	T36.8X6
Cottonseed oil	T49.3X1	T49.3X2	T49.3X3	T49.3X4	T49.3X5	T49.3X6
Cough mixture (syrup)	T48.4X1	T48.4X2	T48.4X3	T48.4X4	T48.4X5	T48.4X6
containing opiates	T40.2X1	T40.2X2	T40.2X3	T40.2X4	T40.2X5	T40.2X6
expectorants	T48.4X1	T48.4X2	T48.4X3	T48.4X4	T48.4X5	T48.4X6
Coumadin	T45.511	T45.512	T45.513	T45.514	T45.515	T45.516
rodenticide	T60.4X1	T60.4X2	T60.4X3	T60.4X4	—	—
Coumaphos	T60.ØX1	T60.ØX2	T60.ØX3	T60.ØX4	—	—
Coumarin	T45.511	T45.512	T45.513	T45.514	T45.515	T45.516
Coumetarol	T45.511	T45.512	T45.513	T45.514	T45.515	T45.516
Cowbane	T62.2X1	T62.2X2	T62.2X3	T62.2X4	—	—
Cozyme	T45.2X1	T45.2X2	T45.2X3	T45.2X4	T45.2X5	T45.2X6
Crack	T40.5X1	T40.5X2	T40.5X3	T40.5X4	—	—
Crataegus extract	T46.ØX1	T46.ØX2	T46.ØX3	T46.ØX4	T46.ØX5	T46.ØX6
Creolin	T54.1X1	T54.1X2	T54.1X3	T54.1X4	—	—
disinfectant	T54.1X1	T54.1X2	T54.1X3	T54.1X4	—	—
Creosol (compound)	T49.ØX1	T49.ØX2	T49.ØX3	T49.ØX4	T49.ØX5	T49.ØX6
Creosote (coal tar) (beechwood)	T49.ØX1	T49.ØX2	T49.ØX3	T49.ØX4	T49.ØX5	T49.ØX6
medicinal (expectorant)	T48.4X1	T48.4X2	T48.4X3	T48.4X4	T48.4X5	T48.4X6
syrup	T48.4X1	T48.4X2	T48.4X3	T48.4X4	T48.4X5	T48.4X6
Cresol(s)	T49.ØX1	T49.ØX2	T49.ØX3	T49.ØX4	T49.ØX5	T49.ØX6
and soap solution	T49.ØX1	T49.ØX2	T49.ØX3	T49.ØX4	T49.ØX5	T49.ØX6
Cresyl acetate	T49.ØX1	T49.ØX2	T49.ØX3	T49.ØX4	T49.ØX5	T49.ØX6
Cresylic acid	T49.ØX1	T49.ØX2	T49.ØX3	T49.ØX4	T49.ØX5	T49.ØX6
Crimidine	T60.4X1	T60.4X2	T60.4X3	T60.4X4	—	—
Croconazole	T37.8X1	T37.8X2	T37.8X3	T37.8X4	T37.8X5	T37.8X6
Cromoglicic acid	T48.6X1	T48.6X2	T48.6X3	T48.6X4	T48.6X5	T48.6X6
Cromolyn	T48.6X1	T48.6X2	T48.6X3	T48.6X4	T48.6X5	T48.6X6
Cromonar	T46.3X1	T46.3X2	T46.3X3	T46.3X4	T46.3X5	T46.3X6
Cropropamide	T39.8X1	T39.8X2	T39.8X3	T39.8X4	T39.8X5	T39.8X6
with crotethamide	T50.7X1	T50.7X2	T50.7X3	T50.7X4	T50.7X5	T50.7X6
Crotamiton	T49.ØX1	T49.ØX2	T49.ØX3	T49.ØX4	T49.ØX5	T49.ØX6
Crotethamide	T39.8X1	T39.8X2	T39.8X3	T39.8X4	T39.8X5	T39.8X6
with cropropamide	T50.7X1	T50.7X2	T50.7X3	T50.7X4	T50.7X5	T50.7X6
Croton (oil)	T47.2X1	T47.2X2	T47.2X3	T47.2X4	T47.2X5	T47.2X6
chloral	T42.6X1	T42.6X2	T42.6X3	T42.6X4	T42.6X5	T42.6X6
Crude oil	T52.ØX1	T52.ØX2	T52.ØX3	T52.ØX4	—	—
Cryogenine	T39.8X1	T39.8X2	T39.8X3	T39.8X4	T39.8X5	T39.8X6
Cryolite (vapor)	T60.1X1	T60.1X2	T60.1X3	T60.1X4	—	—
insecticide	T60.1X1	T60.1X2	T60.1X3	T60.1X4	—	—
Cryptenamine (tannates)	T46.5X1	T46.5X2	T46.5X3	T46.5X4	T46.5X5	T46.5X6
Crystal violet	T49.ØX1	T49.ØX2	T49.ØX3	T49.ØX4	T49.ØX5	T49.ØX6
Cuckoopint	T62.2X1	T62.2X2	T62.2X3	T62.2X4	—	—
Cumetharol	T45.511	T45.512	T45.513	T45.514	T45.515	T45.516
Cupric						
acetate	T60.3X1	T60.3X2	T60.3X3	T60.3X4	—	—
acetoarsenite	T57.ØX1	T57.ØX2	T57.ØX3	T57.ØX4	—	—
arsenate	T57.ØX1	T57.ØX2	T57.ØX3	T57.ØX4	—	—
gluconate	T49.ØX1	T49.ØX2	T49.ØX3	T49.ØX4	T49.ØX5	T49.ØX6
oleate	T49.ØX1	T49.ØX2	T49.ØX3	T49.ØX4	T49.ØX5	T49.ØX6
sulfate	T56.4X1	T56.4X2	T56.4X3	T56.4X4	—	—
Cuprous sulfate — *see also Copper, sulfate*	T56.4X1	T56.4X2	T56.4X3	T56.4X4	—	—
Curare, curarine	T48.1X1	T48.1X2	T48.1X3	T48.1X4	T48.1X5	T48.1X6
Cyamemazine	T43.3X1	T43.3X2	T43.3X3	T43.3X4	T43.3X5	T43.3X6
Cyamopsis tetragono-loba	T46.6X1	T46.6X2	T46.6X3	T46.6X4	T46.6X5	T46.6X6
Cyanacetyl hydrazide	T37.1X1	T37.1X2	T37.1X3	T37.1X4	T37.1X5	T37.1X6
Cyanic acid (gas)	T59.891	T59.892	T59.893	T59.894	—	—
Cyanide(s) (compounds) (potassium) (sodium) NEC	T65.ØX1	T65.ØX2	T65.ØX3	T65.ØX4	—	—
dust or gas (inhalation) NEC	T57.3X1	T57.3X2	T57.3X3	T57.3X4	—	—
fumigant	T65.ØX1	T65.ØX2	T65.ØX3	T65.ØX4	—	—
hydrogen	T57.3X1	T57.3X2	T57.3X3	T57.3X4	—	—
mercuric — *see Mercury*						
pesticide (dust) (fumes)	T65.ØX1	T65.ØX2	T65.ØX3	T65.ØX4	—	—
Cyanoacrylate adhesive	T49.3X1	T49.3X2	T49.3X3	T49.3X4	T49.3X5	T49.3X6
Cyanocobalamin	T45.8X1	T45.8X2	T45.8X3	T45.8X4	T45.8X5	T45.8X6
Cyanogen (chloride) (gas) NEC	T59.891	T59.892	T59.893	T59.894	—	—
Cyclacillin	T36.ØX1	T36.ØX2	T36.ØX3	T36.ØX4	T36.ØX5	T36.ØX6
Cyclaine	T41.3X1	T41.3X2	T41.3X3	T41.3X4	T41.3X5	T41.3X6
Cyclamate	T50.991	T50.992	T50.993	T50.994	T50.995	T50.996

Substance	External Cause (T-Code)					
	Poisoning, Accidental (Unintentional)	Poisoning, Intentional Self-Harm	Poisoning, Assault	Poisoning, Undetermined	Adverse Effect	Underdosing
Cyclamen europaeum	T62.2X1	T62.2X2	T62.2X3	T62.2X4	—	—
Cyclandelate	T46.7X1	T46.7X2	T46.7X3	T46.7X4	T46.7X5	T46.7X6
Cyclazocine	T50.7X1	T50.7X2	T50.7X3	T50.7X4	T50.7X5	T50.7X6
Cyclizine	T45.0X1	T45.0X2	T45.0X3	T45.0X4	T45.0X5	T45.0X6
Cyclobarbital	T42.3X1	T42.3X2	T42.3X3	T42.3X4	T42.3X5	T42.3X6
Cyclobarbitone	T42.3X1	T42.3X2	T42.3X3	T42.3X4	T42.3X5	T42.3X6
Cyclobenzaprine	T48.1X1	T48.1X2	T48.1X3	T48.1X4	T48.1X5	T48.1X6
Cyclodrine	T44.3X1	T44.3X2	T44.3X3	T44.3X4	T44.3X5	T44.3X6
Cycloguanil embonate	T37.2X1	T37.2X2	T37.2X3	T37.2X4	T37.2X5	T37.2X6
Cycloheptadiene	T43.291	T43.292	T43.293	T43.294	T43.295	T43.296
Cyclohexane	T52.8X1	T52.8X2	T52.8X3	T52.8X4	—	—
Cyclohexanol	T51.8X1	T51.8X2	T51.8X3	T51.8X4	—	—
Cyclohexanone	T52.4X1	T52.4X2	T52.4X3	T52.4X4	—	—
Cycloheximide	T60.3X1	T60.3X2	T60.3X3	T60.3X4	—	—
Cyclohexyl acetate	T52.8X1	T52.8X2	T52.8X3	T52.8X4	—	—
Cycloleucin	T45.1X1	T45.1X2	T45.1X3	T45.1X4	T45.1X5	T45.1X6
Cyclomethycaine	T41.3X1	T41.3X2	T41.3X3	T41.3X4	T41.3X5	T41.3X6
Cyclopentamine	T44.4X1	T44.4X2	T44.4X3	T44.4X4	T44.4X5	T44.4X6
Cyclopenthiazide	T50.2X1	T50.2X2	T50.2X3	T50.2X4	T50.2X5	T50.2X6
Cyclopentolate	T44.3X1	T44.3X2	T44.3X3	T44.3X4	T44.3X5	T44.3X6
Cyclophosphamide	T45.1X1	T45.1X2	T45.1X3	T45.1X4	T45.1X5	T45.1X6
Cycloplegic drug	T49.5X1	T49.5X2	T49.5X3	T49.5X4	T49.5X5	T49.5X6
Cyclopropane	T41.291	T41.292	T41.293	T41.294	T41.295	T41.296
Cyclopyrabital	T39.8X1	T39.8X2	T39.8X3	T39.8X4	T39.8X5	T39.8X6
Cycloserine	T37.1X1	T37.1X2	T37.1X3	T37.1X4	T37.1X5	T37.1X6
Cyclosporin	T45.1X1	T45.1X2	T45.1X3	T45.1X4	T45.1X5	T45.1X6
Cyclothiazide	T50.2X1	T50.2X2	T50.2X3	T50.2X4	T50.2X5	T50.2X6
Cycrimine	T44.3X1	T44.3X2	T44.3X3	T44.3X4	T44.3X5	T44.3X6
Cyhalothrin	T60.1X1	T60.1X2	T60.1X3	T60.1X4	—	—
Cymarin	T46.0X1	T46.0X2	T46.0X3	T46.0X4	T46.0X5	T46.0X6
Cypermethrin	T60.1X1	T60.1X2	T60.1X3	T60.1X4	—	—
Cyphenothrin	T60.2X1	T60.2X2	T60.2X3	T60.2X4	—	—
Cyproheptadine	T45.0X1	T45.0X2	T45.0X3	T45.0X4	T45.0X5	T45.0X6
Cyprolidol	T43.291	T43.292	T43.293	T43.294	T43.295	T43.296
Cyproterone	T38.6X1	T38.6X2	T38.6X3	T38.6X4	T38.6X5	T38.6X6
Cysteamine	T50.6X1	T50.6X2	T50.6X3	T50.6X4	T50.6X5	T50.6X6
Cytarabine	T45.1X1	T45.1X2	T45.1X3	T45.1X4	T45.1X5	T45.1X6
Cytisus						
laburnum	T62.2X1	T62.2X2	T62.2X3	T62.2X4	—	—
scoparius	T62.2X1	T62.2X2	T62.2X3	T62.2X4	—	—
Cytochrome C	T47.5X1	T47.5X2	T47.5X3	T47.5X4	T47.5X5	T47.5X6
Cytomel	T38.1X1	T38.1X2	T38.1X3	T38.1X4	T38.1X5	T38.1X6
Cytosine arabinoside	T45.1X1	T45.1X2	T45.1X3	T45.1X4	T45.1X5	T45.1X6
Cytoxan	T45.1X1	T45.1X2	T45.1X3	T45.1X4	T45.1X5	T45.1X6
Cytozyme	T45.7X1	T45.7X2	T45.7X3	T45.7X4	T45.7X5	T45.7X6
2,4-D	T60.3X1	T60.3X2	T60.3X3	T60.3X4	—	—
D						
Dacarbazine	T45.1X1	T45.1X2	T45.1X3	T45.1X4	T45.1X5	T45.1X6
Dactinomycin	T45.1X1	T45.1X2	T45.1X3	T45.1X4	T45.1X5	T45.1X6
DADPS	T37.1X1	T37.1X2	T37.1X3	T37.1X4	T37.1X5	T37.1X6
Dakin's solution	T49.0X1	T49.0X2	T49.0X3	T49.0X4	T49.0X5	T49.0X6
Dalapon (sodium)	T60.3X1	T60.3X2	T60.3X3	T60.3X4	—	—
Dalmane	T42.4X1	T42.4X2	T42.4X3	T42.4X4	T42.4X5	T42.4X6
Danazol	T38.6X1	T38.6X2	T38.6X3	T38.6X4	T38.6X5	T38.6X6
Danilone	T45.511	T45.512	T45.513	T45.514	T45.515	T45.516
Danthron	T47.2X1	T47.2X2	T47.2X3	T47.2X4	T47.2X5	T47.2X6
Dantrolene	T42.8X1	T42.8X2	T42.8X3	T42.8X4	T42.8X5	T42.8X6
Dantron	T47.2X1	T47.2X2	T47.2X3	T47.2X4	T47.2X5	T47.2X6
Daphne (gnidium) (mezereum)	T62.2X1	T62.2X2	T62.2X3	T62.2X4	—	—
berry	T62.1X1	T62.1X2	T62.1X3	T62.1X4	—	—
Dapsone	T37.1X1	T37.1X2	T37.1X3	T37.1X4	T37.1X5	T37.1X6
Daraprim	T37.2X1	T37.2X2	T37.2X3	T37.2X4	T37.2X5	T37.2X6
Darnel	T62.2X1	T62.2X2	T62.2X3	T62.2X4	—	—
Darvon	T39.8X1	T39.8X2	T39.8X3	T39.8X4	T39.8X5	T39.8X6
Daunomycin	T45.1X1	T45.1X2	T45.1X3	T45.1X4	T45.1X5	T45.1X6
Daunorubicin	T45.1X1	T45.1X2	T45.1X3	T45.1X4	T45.1X5	T45.1X6
DBI	T38.3X1	T38.3X2	T38.3X3	T38.3X4	T38.3X5	T38.3X6
D-Con	T60.91	T60.92	T60.93	T60.94	—	—
insecticide	T60.2X1	T60.2X2	T60.2X3	T60.2X4	—	—
rodenticide	T60.4X1	T60.4X2	T60.4X3	T60.4X4	—	—
DDAVP	T38.891	T38.892	T38.893	T38.894	T38.895	T38.896
DDE (bis(chlorophenyl)-dichloroethylene)	T60.2X1	T60.2X2	T60.2X3	T60.2X4	—	—
DDS	T37.1X1	T37.1X2	T37.1X3	T37.1X4	T37.1X5	T37.1X6
DDT (dust)	T60.1X1	T60.1X2	T60.1X3	T60.1X4	—	—
Deadly nightshade — *see also Belladonna*	T62.2X1	T62.2X2	T62.2X3	T62.2X4	—	—
berry	T62.1X1	T62.1X2	T62.1X3	T62.1X4	—	—
Deamino-D-arginine vasopressin	T38.891	T38.892	T38.893	T38.894	T38.895	T38.896
Deanol (aceglumate)	T50.991	T50.992	T50.993	T50.994	T50.995	T50.996
Debrisoquine	T46.5X1	T46.5X2	T46.5X3	T46.5X4	T46.5X5	T46.5X6
Decaborane	T57.8X1	T57.8X2	T57.8X3	T57.8X4	—	—
fumes	T59.891	T59.892	T59.893	T59.894	—	—

Substance	External Cause (T-Code) Poisoning, Accidental (Unintentional)	Poisoning, Intentional Self-Harm	Poisoning, Assault	Poisoning, Undetermined	Adverse Effect	Underdosing
Decadron	T38.0X1	T38.0X2	T38.0X3	T38.0X4	T38.0X5	T38.0X6
ENT agent	T49.6X1	T49.6X2	T49.6X3	T49.6X4	T49.6X5	T49.6X6
ophthalmic preparation	T49.5X1	T49.5X2	T49.5X3	T49.5X4	T49.5X5	T49.5X6
topical NEC	T49.0X1	T49.0X2	T49.0X3	T49.0X4	T49.0X5	T49.0X6
Decahydronaphthalene	T52.8X1	T52.8X2	T52.8X3	T52.8X4	—	—
Decalin	T52.8X1	T52.8X2	T52.8X3	T52.8X4	—	—
Decamethonium (bromide)	T48.1X1	T48.1X2	T48.1X3	T48.1X4	T48.1X5	T48.1X6
Decholin	T47.5X1	T47.5X2	T47.5X3	T47.5X4	T47.5X5	T47.5X6
Declomycin	T36.4X1	T36.4X2	T36.4X3	T36.4X4	T36.4X5	T36.4X6
Decongestant, nasal (mucosa)	T48.5X1	T48.5X2	T48.5X3	T48.5X4	T48.5X5	T48.5X6
combination	T48.5X1	T48.5X2	T48.5X3	T48.5X4	T48.5X5	T48.5X6
Deet	T60.8X1	T60.8X2	T60.8X3	T60.8X4	—	—
Deferoxamine	T45.8X1	T45.8X2	T45.8X3	T45.8X4	T45.8X5	T45.8X6
Deflazacort	T38.0X1	T38.0X2	T38.0X3	T38.0X4	T38.0X5	T38.0X6
Deglycyrrhizinized extract of licorice	T48.4X1	T48.4X2	T48.4X3	T48.4X4	T48.4X5	T48.4X6
Dehydrocholic acid	T47.5X1	T47.5X2	T47.5X3	T47.5X4	T47.5X5	T47.5X6
Dehydroemetine	T37.3X1	T37.3X2	T37.3X3	T37.3X4	T37.3X5	T37.3X6
Dekalin	T52.8X1	T52.8X2	T52.8X3	T52.8X4	—	—
Delalutin	T38.5X1	T38.5X2	T38.5X3	T38.5X4	T38.5X5	T38.5X6
Delphinium	T62.2X1	T62.2X2	T62.2X3	T62.2X4	—	—
Deltasone	T38.0X1	T38.0X2	T38.0X3	T38.0X4	T38.0X5	T38.0X6
Deltra	T38.0X1	T38.0X2	T38.0X3	T38.0X4	T38.0X5	T38.0X6
Delvinal	T42.3X1	T42.3X2	T42.3X3	T42.3X4	T42.3X5	T42.3X6
Delorazepam	T42.4X1	T42.4X2	T42.4X3	T42.4X4	T42.4X5	T42.4X6
Deltamethrin	T60.1X1	T60.1X2	T60.1X3	T60.1X4	—	—
Demecarium (bromide)	T49.5X1	T49.5X2	T49.5X3	T49.5X4	T49.5X5	T49.5X6
Demeclocycline	T36.4X1	T36.4X2	T36.4X3	T36.4X4	T36.4X5	T36.4X6
Demecolcine	T45.1X1	T45.1X2	T45.1X3	T45.1X4	T45.1X5	T45.1X6
Demegestone	T38.5X1	T38.5X2	T38.5X3	T38.5X4	T38.5X5	T38.5X6
Demelanizing agents	T49.8X1	T49.8X2	T49.8X3	T49.8X4	T49.8X5	T49.8X6
Demephion -O and -S	T60.0X1	T60.0X2	T60.0X3	T60.0X4	—	—
Demerol	T40.2X1	T40.2X2	T40.2X3	T40.2X4	T40.2X5	T40.2X6
Demethylchlortetracycline	T36.4X1	T36.4X2	T36.4X3	T36.4X4	T36.4X5	T36.4X6
Demethyltetracycline	T36.4X1	T36.4X2	T36.4X3	T36.4X4	T36.4X5	T36.4X6
Demeton -O and -S	T60.0X1	T60.0X2	T60.0X3	T60.0X4	—	—
Demulcent (external)	T49.3X1	T49.3X2	T49.3X3	T49.3X4	T49.3X5	T49.3X6
specified NEC	T49.3X1	T49.3X2	T49.3X3	T49.3X4	T49.3X5	T49.3X6
Demulen	T38.4X1	T38.4X2	T38.4X3	T38.4X4	T38.4X5	T38.4X6
Denatured alcohol	T51.0X1	T51.0X2	T51.0X3	T51.0X4	—	—
Dendrid	T49.5X1	T49.5X2	T49.5X3	T49.5X4	T49.5X5	T49.5X6
Dental drug, topical application NEC	T49.7X1	T49.7X2	T49.7X3	T49.7X4	T49.7X5	T49.7X6

Substance	External Cause (T-Code) Poisoning, Accidental (Unintentional)	Poisoning, Intentional Self-Harm	Poisoning, Assault	Poisoning, Undetermined	Adverse Effect	Underdosing
Dentifrice	T49.7X1	T49.7X2	T49.7X3	T49.7X4	T49.7X5	T49.7X6
Deodorant spray (feminine hygiene)	T49.8X1	T49.8X2	T49.8X3	T49.8X4	T49.8X5	T49.8X6
Deoxycortone	T50.0X1	T50.0X2	T50.0X3	T50.0X4	T50.0X5	T50.0X6
2-Deoxy-5-fluorouridine	T45.1X1	T45.1X2	T45.1X3	T45.1X4	T45.1X5	T45.1X6
5-Deoxy-5-fluorouridine	T45.1X1	T45.1X2	T45.1X3	T45.1X4	T45.1X5	T45.1X6
Deoxyribonuclease (pancreatic)	T45.3X1	T45.3X2	T45.3X3	T45.3X4	T45.3X5	T45.3X6
Depilatory	T49.4X1	T49.4X2	T49.4X3	T49.4X4	T49.4X5	T49.4X6
Deprenalin	T42.8X1	T42.8X2	T42.8X3	T42.8X4	T42.8X5	T42.8X6
Deprenyl	T42.8X1	T42.8X2	T42.8X3	T42.8X4	T42.8X5	T42.8X6
Depressant, appetite	T50.5X1	T50.5X2	T50.5X3	T50.5X4	T50.5X5	T50.5X6
Depressant						
appetite, central	T50.5X1	T50.5X2	T50.5X3	T50.5X4	T50.5X5	T50.5X6
cardiac	T46.2X1	T46.2X2	T46.2X3	T46.2X4	T46.2X5	T46.2X6
central nervous system (anesthetic) — *see also Central nervous system, depressants*	T42.71	T42.72	T42.73	T42.74	T42.75	T42.76
general anesthetic	T41.201	T41.202	T41.203	T41.204	T41.205	T41.206
muscle tone	T42.8X1	T42.8X2	T42.8X3	T42.8X4	T42.8X5	T42.8X6
muscle tone, central	T42.8X1	T42.8X2	T42.8X3	T42.8X4	T42.8X5	T42.8X6
psychotherapeutic	T43.501	T43.502	T43.503	T43.504	T43.505	T43.506
Deptropine	T45.0X1	T45.0X2	T45.0X3	T45.0X4	T45.0X5	T45.0X6
Dequalinium (chloride)	T49.0X1	T49.0X2	T49.0X3	T49.0X4	T49.0X5	T49.0X6
Derris root	T60.2X1	T60.2X2	T60.2X3	T60.2X4	—	—
Deserpidine	T43.011	T43.012	T43.013	T43.014	T43.015	T43.016
Desferrioxamine	T45.8X1	T45.8X2	T45.8X3	T45.8X4	T45.8X5	T45.8X6
Desipramine	T43.0X1	T43.0X2	T43.0X3	T43.0X4	T43.0X5	T43.0X6
Deslanoside	T46.0X1	T46.0X2	T46.0X3	T46.0X4	T46.0X5	T46.0X6
Desloughing agent	T49.4X1	T49.4X2	T49.4X3	T49.4X4	T49.4X5	T49.4X6
Desmethylimipramine	T43.011	T43.012	T43.013	T43.014	T43.015	T43.016
Desmopressin	T38.891	T38.892	T38.893	T38.894	T38.895	T38.896
Desocodeine	T40.2X1	T40.2X2	T40.2X3	T40.2X4	T40.2X5	T40.2X6
Desogestrel	T38.5X1	T38.5X2	T38.5X3	T38.5X4	T38.5X5	T38.5X6
Desomorphine	T40.2X1	T40.2X2	T40.2X3	T40.2X4	—	—
Desonide	T49.0X1	T49.0X2	T49.0X3	T49.0X4	T49.0X5	T49.0X6
Desoximetasone	T49.0X1	T49.0X2	T49.0X3	T49.0X4	T49.0X5	T49.0X6
Desoxycorticosteroid	T50.0X1	T50.0X2	T50.0X3	T50.0X4	T50.0X5	T50.0X6
Desoxycortone	T50.0X1	T50.0X2	T50.0X3	T50.0X4	T50.0X5	T50.0X6
Desoxyephedrine	T43.651	T43.652	T43.653	T43.654	T43.655	T43.656
Detaxtran	T46.6X1	T46.6X2	T46.6X3	T46.6X4	T46.6X5	T46.6X6
Detergent	T49.2X1	T49.2X2	T49.2X3	T49.2X4	T49.2X5	T49.2X6
external medication	T49.2X1	T49.2X2	T49.2X3	T49.2X4	T49.2X5	T49.2X6
local	T49.2X1	T49.2X2	T49.2X3	T49.2X4	T49.2X5	T49.2X6

	External Cause (T-Code)					
Substance	Poisoning, Accidental (Unintentional)	Poisoning, Intentional Self-Harm	Poisoning, Assault	Poisoning, Undetermined	Adverse Effect	Underdosing
Detergent *(Continued)*						
medicinal	T49.2X1	T49.2X2	T49.2X3	T49.2X4	T49.2X5	T49.2X6
nonmedicinal	T55.1X1	T55.1X2	T55.1X3	T55.1X4	—	—
specified NEC	T55.1X1	T55.1X2	T55.1X3	T55.1X4	T55.1X5	T55.1X6
Deterrent, alcohol	T50.6X1	T50.6X2	T50.6X3	T50.6X4	T50.6X5	T50.6X6
Detoxifying agent	T50.6X1	T50.6X2	T50.6X3	T50.6X4	T50.6X5	T50.6X6
Detrothyronine	T38.1X1	T38.1X2	T38.1X3	T38.1X4	T38.1X5	T38.1X6
Dettol (external medication)	T49.0X1	T49.0X2	T49.0X3	T49.0X4	T49.0X5	T49.0X6
Dexamethasone	T38.0X1	T38.0X2	T38.0X3	T38.0X4	T38.0X5	T38.0X6
ENT agent	T49.6X1	T49.6X2	T49.6X3	T49.6X4	T49.6X5	T49.6X6
ophthalmic preparation	T49.5X1	T49.5X2	T49.5X3	T49.5X4	T49.5X5	T49.5X6
topical NEC	T49.0X1	T49.0X2	T49.0X3	T49.0X4	T49.0X5	T49.0X6
Dexamfetamine	T43.621	T43.622	T43.623	T43.624	T43.625	T43.626
Dexamphetamine	T43.621	T43.622	T43.623	T43.624	T43.625	T43.626
Dexbrompheniramine	T45.0X1	T45.0X2	T45.0X3	T45.0X4	T45.0X5	T45.0X6
Dexchlorpheniramine	T45.0X1	T45.0X2	T45.0X3	T45.0X4	T45.0X5	T45.0X6
Dexedrine	T43.621	T43.622	T43.623	T43.624	T43.625	T43.626
Dexetimide	T44.3X1	T44.3X2	T44.3X3	T44.3X4	T44.3X5	T44.3X6
Dexfenfluramine	T50.5X1	T50.5X2	T50.5X3	T50.5X4	T50.5X5	T50.5X6
Dexpanthenol	T45.2X1	T45.2X2	T45.2X3	T45.2X4	T45.2X5	T45.2X6
Dextran (40) (70) (150)	T45.8X1	T45.8X2	T45.8X3	T45.8X4	T45.8X5	T45.8X6
Dextriferron	T45.4X1	T45.4X2	T45.4X3	T45.4X4	T45.4X5	T45.4X6
Dextroamphetamine	T43.621	T43.622	T43.623	T43.624	T43.625	T43.626
Dextro calcium pantothenate	T45.2X1	T45.2X2	T45.2X3	T45.2X4	T45.2X5	T45.2X6
Dextromethorphan	T48.3X1	T48.3X2	T48.3X3	T48.3X4	T48.3X5	T48.3X6
Dextromoramide	T40.491	T40.492	T40.493	T40.494	—	—
topical	T49.8X1	T49.8X2	T49.8X3	T49.8X4	T49.8X5	T49.8X6
Dextro pantothenyl alcohol	T45.2X1	T45.2X2	T45.2X3	T45.2X4	T45.2X5	T45.2X6
Dextropropoxyphene	T40.491	T40.492	T40.493	T40.494	T40.495	T40.496
Dextrorphan	T40.2X1	T40.2X2	T40.2X3	T40.2X4	T40.2X5	T40.2X6
Dextrose	T50.3X1	T50.3X2	T50.3X3	T50.3X4	T50.3X5	T50.3X6
concentrated solution, intravenous	T46.8X1	T46.8X2	T46.8X3	T46.8X4	T46.8X5	T46.8X6
Dextrothyroxin	T38.1X1	T38.1X2	T38.1X3	T38.1X4	T38.1X5	T38.1X6
Dextrothyroxine sodium	T38.1X1	T38.1X2	T38.1X3	T38.1X4	T38.1X5	T38.1X6
DFP	T44.0X1	T44.0X2	T44.0X3	T44.0X4	T44.0X5	T44.0X6
DHE	T37.3X1	T37.3X2	T37.3X3	T37.3X4	T37.3X5	T37.3X6
45	T46.5X1	T46.5X2	T46.5X3	T46.5X4	T46.5X5	T46.5X6
Diabinese	T38.3X1	T38.3X2	T38.3X3	T38.3X4	T38.3X5	T38.3X6
Diacetone alcohol	T52.4X1	T52.4X2	T52.4X3	T52.4X4	—	—
Diacetyl monoxime	T50.991	T50.992	T50.993	T50.994	—	—
Diacetylmorphine	T40.1X1	T40.1X2	T40.1X3	T40.1X4	—	—

	External Cause (T-Code)					
Substance	Poisoning, Accidental (Unintentional)	Poisoning, Intentional Self-Harm	Poisoning, Assault	Poisoning, Undetermined	Adverse Effect	Underdosing
Diachylon plaster	T49.4X1	T49.4X2	T49.4X3	T49.4X4	T49.4X5	T49.4X6
Diaethylstilboestrolum	T38.5X1	T38.5X2	T38.5X3	T38.5X4	T38.5X5	T38.5X6
Diagnostic agent NEC	T50.8X1	T50.8X2	T50.8X3	T50.8X4	T50.8X5	T50.8X6
Dial (soap)	T49.2X1	T49.2X2	T49.2X3	T49.2X4	T49.2X5	T49.2X6
sedative	T42.3X1	T42.3X2	T42.3X3	T42.3X4	T42.3X5	T42.3X6
Dialkyl carbonate	T52.91	T52.92	T52.93	T52.94	—	—
Diallylbarbituric acid	T42.3X1	T42.3X2	T42.3X3	T42.3X4	T42.3X5	T42.3X6
Diallymal	T42.3X1	T42.3X2	T42.3X3	T42.3X4	T42.3X5	T42.3X6
Dialysis solution (intraperitoneal)	T50.3X1	T50.3X2	T50.3X3	T50.3X4	T50.3X5	T50.3X6
Diaminodiphenylsulfone	T37.1X1	T37.1X2	T37.1X3	T37.1X4	T37.1X5	T37.1X6
Diamorphine	T40.1X1	T40.1X2	T40.1X3	T40.1X4	—	—
Diamox	T50.2X1	T50.2X2	T50.2X3	T50.2X4	T50.2X5	T50.2X6
Diamthazole	T49.0X1	T49.0X2	T49.0X3	T49.0X4	T49.0X5	T49.0X6
Dianthone	T47.2X1	T47.2X2	T47.2X3	T47.2X4	T47.2X5	T47.2X6
Diaphenylsulfone	T37.0X1	T37.0X2	T37.0X3	T37.0X4	T37.0X5	T37.0X6
Diasone (sodium)	T37.1X1	T37.1X2	T37.1X3	T37.1X4	T37.1X5	T37.1X6
Diastase	T47.5X1	T47.5X2	T47.5X3	T47.5X4	T47.5X5	T47.5X6
Diatrizoate	T50.8X1	T50.8X2	T50.8X3	T50.8X4	T50.8X5	T50.8X6
Diazepam	T42.4X1	T42.4X2	T42.4X3	T42.4X4	T42.4X5	T42.4X6
Diazinon	T60.0X1	T60.0X2	T60.0X3	T60.0X4	—	—
Diazomethane (gas)	T59.891	T59.892	T59.893	T59.894	—	—
Diazoxide	T46.5X1	T46.5X2	T46.5X3	T46.5X4	T46.5X5	T46.5X6
Dibekacin	T36.5X1	T36.5X2	T36.5X3	T36.5X4	T36.5X5	T36.5X6
Dibenamine	T44.6X1	T44.6X2	T44.6X3	T44.6X4	T44.6X5	T44.6X6
Dibenzepin	T43.011	T43.012	T43.013	T43.014	T43.015	T43.016
Dibenzheptropine	T45.0X1	T45.0X2	T45.0X3	T45.0X4	T45.0X5	T45.0X6
Dibenzyline	T44.6X1	T44.6X2	T44.6X3	T44.6X4	T44.6X5	T44.6X6
Diborane (gas)	T59.891	T59.892	T59.893	T59.894	—	—
Dibromochloropropane	T60.8X1	T60.8X2	T60.8X3	T60.8X4	—	—
Dibromodulcitol	T45.1X1	T45.1X2	T45.1X3	T45.1X4	T45.1X5	T45.1X6
Dibromoethane	T53.6X1	T53.6X2	T53.6X3	T53.6X4	—	—
Dibromomannitol	T45.1X1	T45.1X2	T45.1X3	T45.1X4	T45.1X5	T45.1X6
Dibromopropamidine isethionate	T49.0X1	T49.0X2	T49.0X3	T49.0X4	T49.0X5	T49.0X6
Dibrompropamidine	T49.0X1	T49.0X2	T49.0X3	T49.0X4	T49.0X5	T49.0X6
Dibucaine	T41.3X1	T41.3X2	T41.3X3	T41.3X4	T41.3X5	T41.3X6
topical (surface)	T41.3X1	T41.3X2	T41.3X3	T41.3X4	T41.3X5	T41.3X6
Dibunate sodium	T48.3X1	T48.3X2	T48.3X3	T48.3X4	T48.3X5	T48.3X6
Dibutoline sulfate	T44.3X1	T44.3X2	T44.3X3	T44.3X4	T44.3X5	T44.3X6
Dicamba	T60.3X1	T60.3X2	T60.3X3	T60.3X4	—	—
Dicapthon	T60.0X1	T60.0X2	T60.0X3	T60.0X4	—	—
Dichlobenil	T60.3X1	T60.3X2	T60.3X3	T60.3X4	—	—
Dichlone	T60.3X1	T60.3X2	T60.3X3	T60.3X4	—	—

Substance	Poisoning, Accidental (Unintentional)	Poisoning, Intentional Self-Harm	Poisoning, Assault	Poisoning, Undetermined	Adverse Effect	Underdosing
	External Cause (T-Code)					
Dichloralphenozone	T42.6X1	T42.6X2	T42.6X3	T42.6X4	T42.6X5	T42.6X6
Dichlorbenzidine	T65.3X1	T65.3X2	T65.3X3	T65.3X4	—	—
Dichlorhydrin	T52.8X1	T52.8X2	T52.8X3	T52.8X4	—	—
Dichlorhydroxyquinoline	T37.8X1	T37.8X2	T37.8X3	T37.8X4	T37.8X5	T37.8X6
Dichlorobenzene	T53.7X1	T53.7X2	T53.7X3	T53.7X4	—	—
Dichlorobenzyl alcohol	T49.6X1	T49.6X2	T49.6X3	T49.6X4	T49.6X5	T49.6X6
Dichlorodifluoromethane	T53.5X1	T53.5X2	T53.5X3	T53.5X4	—	—
Dichloroethane	T52.8X1	T52.8X2	T52.8X3	T52.8X4	—	—
Sym-Dichloroethyl ether	T53.6X1	T53.6X2	T53.6X3	T53.6X4	—	—
Dichloroethyl sulfide, not in war	T59.891	T59.892	T59.893	T59.894	—	—
Dichloroethylene	T53.6X1	T53.6X2	T53.6X3	T53.6X4	—	—
Dichloroformoxine, not in war	T59.891	T59.892	T59.893	T59.894	—	—
Dichlorohydrin, alpha-dichlorohydrin	T52.8X1	T52.8X2	T52.8X3	T52.8X4	—	—
Dichloromethane (solvent)	T53.4X1	T53.4X2	T53.4X3	T53.4X4	—	—
vapor	T53.4X1	T53.4X2	T53.4X3	T53.4X4	—	—
Dichloronaphthoquinone	T60.3X1	T60.3X2	T60.3X3	T60.3X4	—	—
Dichlorophen	T37.4X1	T37.4X2	T37.4X3	T37.4X4	T37.4X5	T37.4X6
2,4-Dichlorophenoxy-acetic acid	T60.3X1	T60.3X2	T60.3X3	T60.3X4	—	—
Dichloropropene	T60.3X1	T60.3X2	T60.3X3	T60.3X4	—	—
Dichloropropionic acid	T60.3X1	T60.3X2	T60.3X3	T60.3X4	—	—
Dichlorphenamide	T50.2X1	T50.2X2	T50.2X3	T50.2X4	T50.2X5	T50.2X6
Dichlorvos	T60.0X1	T60.0X2	T60.0X3	T60.0X4	—	—
Diclofenac	T39.391	T39.392	T39.393	T39.394	T39.395	T39.396
Diclofenamide	T50.2X1	T50.2X2	T50.2X3	T50.2X4	T50.2X5	T50.2X6
Diclofensine	T43.291	T43.292	T43.293	T43.294	T43.295	T43.296
Diclonixine	T39.8X1	T39.8X2	T39.8X3	T39.8X4	T39.8X5	T39.8X6
Dicloxacillin	T36.0X1	T36.0X2	T36.0X3	T36.0X4	T36.0X5	T36.0X6
Dicophane	T49.0X1	T49.0X2	T49.0X3	T49.0X4	T49.0X5	T49.0X6
Dicoumarol, dicoumarin, dicumarol	T45.511	T45.512	T45.513	T45.514	T45.515	T45.516
Dicrotophos	T60.0X1	T60.0X2	T60.0X3	T60.0X4	—	—
Dicyanogen (gas)	T65.0X1	T65.0X2	T65.0X3	T65.0X4	—	—
Dicyclomine	T44.3X1	T44.3X2	T44.3X3	T44.3X4	T44.3X5	T44.3X6
Dicycloverine	T44.3X1	T44.3X2	T44.3X3	T44.3X4	T44.3X5	T44.3X6
Dideoxycytidine	T37.5X1	T37.5X2	T37.5X3	T37.5X4	T37.5X5	T37.5X6
Dideoxyinosine	T37.5X1	T37.5X2	T37.5X3	T37.5X4	T37.5X5	T37.5X6
Dieldrin (vapor)	T60.1X1	T60.1X2	T60.1X3	T60.1X4	—	—
Diemal	T42.3X1	T42.3X2	T42.3X3	T42.3X4	T42.3X5	T42.3X6
Dienestrol	T38.5X1	T38.5X2	T38.5X3	T38.5X4	T38.5X5	T38.5X6
Dienoestrol	T38.5X1	T38.5X2	T38.5X3	T38.5X4	T38.5X5	T38.5X6
Dietetic drug NEC	T50.901	T50.902	T50.903	T50.904	T50.905	T50.906
Diethazine	T42.8X1	T42.8X2	T42.8X3	T42.8X4	T42.8X5	T42.8X6
Diethyl						
barbituric acid	T42.3X1	T42.3X2	T42.3X3	T42.3X4	T42.3X5	T42.3X6
carbamazine	T37.4X1	T37.4X2	T37.4X3	T37.4X4	T37.4X5	T37.4X6
carbinol	T51.3X1	T51.3X2	T51.3X3	T51.3X4	—	—
carbonate	T52.8X1	T52.8X2	T52.8X3	T52.8X4	—	—
ether (vapor) — *see also Ether*	T41.0X1	T41.0X2	T41.0X3	T41.0X4	T41.0X5	T41.0X6
oxide	T52.8X1	T52.8X2	T52.8X3	T52.8X4	—	—
propion	T50.5X1	T50.5X2	T50.5X3	T50.5X4	T50.5X5	T50.5X6
stilbestrol	T38.5X1	T38.5X2	T38.5X3	T38.5X4	T38.5X5	T38.5X6
toluamide (nonmedicinal)	T60.8X1	T60.8X2	T60.8X3	T60.8X4	—	—
medicinal	T49.3X1	T49.3X2	T49.3X3	T49.3X4	T49.3X5	T49.3X6
Diethylcarbamazine	T37.4X1	T37.4X2	T37.4X3	T37.4X4	T37.4X5	T37.4X6
Diethylene						
dioxide	T52.8X1	T52.8X2	T52.8X3	T52.8X4	—	—
glycol (monoacetate) (monobutyl ether) (monoethyl ether)	T52.3X1	T52.3X2	T52.3X3	T52.3X4	—	—
Diethylhexylphthalate	T65.891	T65.892	T65.893	T65.894	—	—
Diethylpropion	T50.5X1	T50.5X2	T50.5X3	T50.5X4	T50.5X5	T50.5X6
Diethylstilbestrol	T38.5X1	T38.5X2	T38.5X3	T38.5X4	T38.5X5	T38.5X6
Diethylstilboestrol	T38.5X1	T38.5X2	T38.5X3	T38.5X4	T38.5X5	T38.5X6
Diethylsulfone-diethylmethane	T42.6X1	T42.6X2	T42.6X3	T42.6X4	T42.6X5	T42.6X6
Diethyltoluamide	T49.0X1	T49.0X2	T49.0X3	T49.0X4	T49.0X5	T49.0X6
Diethyltryptamine (DET)	T40.991	T40.992	T40.993	T40.994	—	—
Difebarbamate	T42.3X1	T42.3X2	T42.3X3	T42.3X4	T42.3X5	T42.3X6
Difencloxazine	T40.2X1	T40.2X2	T40.2X3	T40.2X4	T40.2X5	T40.2X6
Difenidol	T45.0X1	T45.0X2	T45.0X3	T45.0X4	T45.0X5	T45.0X6
Difenoxin	T47.6X1	T47.6X2	T47.6X3	T47.6X4	T47.6X5	T47.6X6
Difetarsone	T37.3X1	T37.3X2	T37.3X3	T37.3X4	T37.3X5	T37.3X6
Diffusin	T45.3X1	T45.3X2	T45.3X3	T45.3X4	T45.3X5	T45.3X6
Diflorasone	T49.0X1	T49.0X2	T49.0X3	T49.0X4	T49.0X5	T49.0X6
Diflubenzuron	T60.1X1	T60.1X2	T60.1X3	T60.1X4	—	—
Diflos	T44.0X1	T44.0X2	T44.0X3	T44.0X4	T44.0X5	T44.0X6
Diflucortolone	T49.0X1	T49.0X2	T49.0X3	T49.0X4	T49.0X5	T49.0X6
Diflunisal	T39.091	T39.092	T39.093	T39.094	T39.095	T39.096
Difluoromethyldopa	T42.8X1	T42.8X2	T42.8X3	T42.8X4	T42.8X5	T42.8X6
Difluorophate	T44.0X1	T44.0X2	T44.0X3	T44.0X4	T44.0X5	T44.0X6
Digestant NEC	T47.5X1	T47.5X2	T47.5X3	T47.5X4	T47.5X5	T47.5X6
Digitalin(e)	T46.0X1	T46.0X2	T46.0X3	T46.0X4	T46.0X5	T46.0X6
Digitalis (leaf) (glycoside)	T46.0X1	T46.0X2	T46.0X3	T46.0X4	T46.0X5	T46.0X6
lanata	T46.0X1	T46.0X2	T46.0X3	T46.0X4	T46.0X5	T46.0X6
purpurea	T46.0X1	T46.0X2	T46.0X3	T46.0X4	T46.0X5	T46.0X6
Digitoxin	T46.0X1	T46.0X2	T46.0X3	T46.0X4	T46.0X5	T46.0X6

New Revised ~~deleted~~ Deleted

Substance	External Cause (T-Code) Poisoning, Accidental (Unintentional)	Poisoning, Intentional Self-Harm	Poisoning, Assault	Poisoning, Undetermined	Adverse Effect	Underdosing
Digitoxose	T46.0X1	T46.0X2	T46.0X3	T46.0X4	T46.0X5	T46.0X6
Digoxin	T46.0X1	T46.0X2	T46.0X3	T46.0X4	T46.0X5	T46.0X6
Digoxine	T46.0X1	T46.0X2	T46.0X3	T46.0X4	T46.0X5	T46.0X6
Dihydralazine	T46.5X1	T46.5X2	T46.5X3	T46.5X4	T46.5X5	T46.5X6
Dihydrazine	T46.5X1	T46.5X2	T46.5X3	T46.5X4	T46.5X5	T46.5X6
Dihydrocodeinone	T40.2X1	T40.2X2	T40.2X3	T40.2X4	T40.2X5	T40.2X6
Dihydroergocornine	T46.7X1	T46.7X2	T46.7X3	T46.7X4	T46.7X5	T46.7X6
Dihydroergocristine (mesilate)	T46.7X1	T46.7X2	T46.7X3	T46.7X4	T46.7X5	T46.7X6
Dihydroergokryptine	T46.7X1	T46.7X2	T46.7X3	T46.7X4	T46.7X5	T46.7X6
Dihydroergotamine	T46.5X1	T46.5X2	T46.5X3	T46.5X4	T46.5X5	T46.5X6
Dihydroergotoxine	T46.7X1	T46.7X2	T46.7X3	T46.7X4	T46.7X5	T46.7X6
mesilate	T46.7X1	T46.7X2	T46.7X3	T46.7X4	T46.7X5	T46.7X6
Dihydrohydroxycodein-one	T40.2X1	T40.2X2	T40.2X3	T40.2X4	T40.2X5	T40.2X6
Dihydrohydroxymorphinone	T40.2X1	T40.2X2	T40.2X3	T40.2X4	T40.2X5	T40.2X6
Dihydroisocodeine	T40.2X1	T40.2X2	T40.2X3	T40.2X4	T40.2X5	T40.2X6
Dihydromorphine	T40.2X1	T40.2X2	T40.2X3	T40.2X4	—	—
Dihydromorphinone	T40.2X1	T40.2X2	T40.2X3	T40.2X4	T40.2X5	T40.2X6
Dihydrostreptomycin	T36.5X1	T36.5X2	T36.5X3	T36.5X4	T36.5X5	T36.5X6
Dihydrotachysterol	T45.2X1	T45.2X2	T45.2X3	T45.2X4	T45.2X5	T45.2X6
Dihydroxyaluminum aminoacetate	T47.1X1	T47.1X2	T47.1X3	T47.1X4	T47.1X5	T47.1X6
Dihydroxyaluminum sodium carbonate	T47.1X1	T47.1X2	T47.1X3	T47.1X4	T47.1X5	T47.1X6
Dihydroxyanthraquinone	T47.2X1	T47.2X2	T47.2X3	T47.2X4	T47.2X5	T47.2X6
Dihydroxycodeinone	T40.2X1	T40.2X2	T40.2X3	T40.2X4	T40.2X5	T40.2X6
Dihydroxypropyl theophylline	T50.2X1	T50.2X2	T50.2X3	T50.2X4	T50.2X5	T50.2X6
Diiodohydroxyquin	T37.8X1	T37.8X2	T37.8X3	T37.8X4	T37.8X5	T37.8X6
topical	T49.0X1	T49.0X2	T49.0X3	T49.0X4	T49.0X5	T49.0X6
Diiodohydroxyquinoline	T37.8X1	T37.8X2	T37.8X3	T37.8X4	T37.8X5	T37.8X6
Diiodotyrosine	T38.2X1	T38.2X2	T38.2X3	T38.2X4	T38.2X5	T38.2X6
Diisopromine	T44.3X1	T44.3X2	T44.3X3	T44.3X4	T44.3X5	T44.3X6
Diisopropylamine	T46.3X1	T46.3X2	T46.3X3	T46.3X4	T46.3X5	T46.3X6
Diisopropylfluorophosphonate	T44.0X1	T44.0X2	T44.0X3	T44.0X4	T44.0X5	T44.0X6
Dilantin	T42.0X1	T42.0X2	T42.0X3	T42.0X4	T42.0X5	T42.0X6
Dilaudid	T40.2X1	T40.2X2	T40.2X3	T40.2X4	T40.2X5	T40.2X6
Dilazep	T46.3X1	T46.3X2	T46.3X3	T46.3X4	T46.3X5	T46.3X6
Dill	T47.5X1	T47.5X2	T47.5X3	T47.5X4	T47.5X5	T47.5X6
Diloxanide	T37.3X1	T37.3X2	T37.3X3	T37.3X4	T37.3X5	T37.3X6
Diltiazem	T46.1X1	T46.1X2	T46.1X3	T46.1X4	T46.1X5	T46.1X6
Dimazole	T49.0X1	T49.0X2	T49.0X3	T49.0X4	T49.0X5	T49.0X6
Dimefline	T50.7X1	T50.7X2	T50.7X3	T50.7X4	T50.7X5	T50.7X6
Dimefox	T60.0X1	T60.0X2	T60.0X3	T60.0X4	—	—

Substance	External Cause (T-Code) Poisoning, Accidental (Unintentional)	Poisoning, Intentional Self-Harm	Poisoning, Assault	Poisoning, Undetermined	Adverse Effect	Underdosing
Dimemorfan	T48.3X1	T48.3X2	T48.3X3	T48.3X4	T48.3X5	T48.3X6
Dimenhydrinate	T45.0X1	T45.0X2	T45.0X3	T45.0X4	T45.0X5	T45.0X6
Dimercaprol (British anti-lewisite)	T45.8X1	T45.8X2	T45.8X3	T45.8X4	T45.8X5	T45.8X6
Dimercaptopropanol	T45.8X1	T45.8X2	T45.8X3	T45.8X4	T45.8X5	T45.8X6
Dimestrol	T38.5X1	T38.5X2	T38.5X3	T38.5X4	T38.5X5	T38.5X6
Dimetane	T45.0X1	T45.0X2	T45.0X3	T45.0X4	T45.0X5	T45.0X6
Dimethicone	T47.1X1	T47.1X2	T47.1X3	T47.1X4	T47.1X5	T47.1X6
Dimethindene	T45.0X1	T45.0X2	T45.0X3	T45.0X4	T45.0X5	T45.0X6
Dimethisoquin	T49.1X1	T49.1X2	T49.1X3	T49.1X4	T49.1X5	T49.1X6
Dimethisterone	T38.5X1	T38.5X2	T38.5X3	T38.5X4	T38.5X5	T38.5X6
Dimethoate	T60.0X1	T60.0X2	T60.0X3	T60.0X4	—	—
Dimethocaine	T41.3X1	T41.3X2	T41.3X3	T41.3X4	T41.3X5	T41.3X6
Dimethoxanate	T48.3X1	T48.3X2	T48.3X3	T48.3X4	T48.3X5	T48.3X6
Dimethyl						
arsine, arsinic acid	T57.0X1	T57.0X2	T57.0X3	T57.0X4	—	—
carbinol	T51.2X1	T51.2X2	T51.2X3	T51.2X4	—	—
carbonate	T52.8X1	T52.8X2	T52.8X3	T52.8X4	—	—
diguanide	T38.3X1	T38.3X2	T38.3X3	T38.3X4	T38.3X5	T38.3X6
ketone	T52.4X1	T52.4X2	T52.4X3	T52.4X4	—	—
vapor	T52.4X1	T52.4X2	T52.4X3	T52.4X4	—	—
meperidine	T40.2X1	T40.2X2	T40.2X3	T40.2X4	T40.2X5	T40.2X6
parathion	T60.0X1	T60.0X2	T60.0X3	T60.0X4	—	—
phthlate	T49.3X1	T49.3X2	T49.3X3	T49.3X4	T49.3X5	T49.3X6
polysiloxane	T47.8X1	T47.8X2	T47.8X3	T47.8X4	T47.8X5	T47.8X6
sulfate (fumes)	T59.891	T59.892	T59.893	T59.894	—	—
liquid	T65.891	T65.892	T65.893	T65.894	—	—
sulfoxide (nonmedicinal)	T52.8X1	T52.8X2	T52.8X3	T52.8X4	—	—
medicinal	T49.4X1	T49.4X2	T49.4X3	T49.4X4	T49.4X5	T49.4X6
tryptamine	T40.991	T40.992	T40.993	T40.994	—	—
tubocurarine	T48.1X1	T48.1X2	T48.1X3	T48.1X4	T48.1X5	T48.1X6
Dimethylamine sulfate	T49.4X1	T49.4X2	T49.4X3	T49.4X4	T49.4X5	T49.4X6
Dimethylformamide	T52.8X1	T52.8X2	T52.8X3	T52.8X4	—	—
Dimethyltubocurarinium chloride	T48.1X1	T48.1X2	T48.1X3	T48.1X4	T48.1X5	T48.1X6
Dimeticone	T47.1X1	T47.1X2	T47.1X3	T47.1X4	T47.1X5	T47.1X6
Dimetilan	T60.0X1	T60.0X2	T60.0X3	T60.0X4	—	—
Dimetindene	T45.0X1	T45.0X2	T45.0X3	T45.0X4	T45.0X5	T45.0X6
Dimetotiazine	T43.3X1	T43.3X2	T43.3X3	T43.3X4	T43.3X5	T43.3X6
Dimorpholamine	T50.7X1	T50.7X2	T50.7X3	T50.7X4	T50.7X5	T50.7X6
Dimoxyline	T46.3X1	T46.3X2	T46.3X3	T46.3X4	T46.3X5	T46.3X6
Dinitrobenzene	T65.3X1	T65.3X2	T65.3X3	T65.3X4	—	—
vapor	T59.891	T59.892	T59.893	T59.894	—	—

Substance	Poisoning, Accidental (Unintentional)	Poisoning, Intentional Self-Harm	Poisoning, Assault	Poisoning, Undetermined	Adverse Effect	Underdosing
	External Cause (T-Code)					
Dinitrobenzol	T65.3X1	T65.3X2	T65.3X3	T65.3X4	—	—
vapor	T59.891	T59.892	T59.893	T59.894	—	—
Dinitrobutylphenol	T65.3X1	T65.3X2	T65.3X3	T65.3X4	—	—
Dinitro (-ortho-)cresol (pesticide) (spray)	T65.3X1	T65.3X2	T65.3X3	T65.3X4	—	—
Dinitrocyclohexylphenol	T65.3X1	T65.3X2	T65.3X3	T65.3X4	—	—
Dinitrophenol	T65.3X1	T65.3X2	T65.3X3	T65.3X4	—	—
Dinoprost	T48.ØX1	T48.ØX2	T48.ØX3	T48.ØX4	T48.ØX5	T48.ØX6
Dinoprostone	T48.ØX1	T48.ØX2	T48.ØX3	T48.ØX4	T48.ØX5	T48.ØX6
Dinoseb	T6Ø.3X1	T6Ø.3X2	T6Ø.3X3	T6Ø.3X4	—	—
Dioctyl sulfosuccinate (calcium) (sodium)	T47.4X1	T47.4X2	T47.4X3	T47.4X4	T47.4X5	T47.4X6
Diodone	T5Ø.8X1	T5Ø.8X2	T5Ø.8X3	T5Ø.8X4	T5Ø.8X5	T5Ø.8X6
Diodoquin	T37.8X1	T37.8X2	T37.8X3	T37.8X4	T37.8X5	T37.8X6
Dionin	T4Ø.2X1	T4Ø.2X2	T4Ø.2X3	T4Ø.2X4	T4Ø.2X5	T4Ø.2X6
Diosmin	T46.991	T46.992	T46.993	T46.994	T46.995	T46.996
Dioxane	T52.8X1	T52.8X2	T52.8X3	T52.8X4	—	—
Dioxathion	T6Ø.ØX1	T6Ø.ØX2	T6Ø.ØX3	T6Ø.ØX4	—	—
Dioxin	T53.7X1	T53.7X2	T53.7X3	T53.7X4	—	—
Dioxopromethazine	T43.3X1	T43.3X2	T43.3X3	T43.3X4	T43.3X5	T43.3X6
Dioxyline	T46.3X1	T46.3X2	T46.3X3	T46.3X4	T46.3X5	T46.3X6
Dipentene	T52.8X1	T52.8X2	T52.8X3	T52.8X4	—	—
Diperodon	T41.3X1	T41.3X2	T41.3X3	T41.3X4	T41.3X5	T41.3X6
Diphacinone	T6Ø.4X1	T6Ø.4X2	T6Ø.4X3	T6Ø.4X4	—	—
Diphemanil	T44.3X1	T44.3X2	T44.3X3	T44.3X4	T44.3X5	T44.3X6
metilsulfate	T44.3X1	T44.3X2	T44.3X3	T44.3X4	T44.3X5	T44.3X6
Diphenadione	T45.511	T45.512	T45.513	T45.514	T45.515	T45.516
rodenticide	T6Ø.4X1	T6Ø.4X2	T6Ø.4X3	T6Ø.4X4	—	—
Diphenhydramine	T45.ØX1	T45.ØX2	T45.ØX3	T45.ØX4	T45.ØX5	T45.ØX6
Diphenidol	T45.ØX1	T45.ØX2	T45.ØX3	T45.ØX4	T45.ØX5	T45.ØX6
Diphenoxylate	T47.6X1	T47.6X2	T47.6X3	T47.6X4	T47.6X5	T47.6X6
Diphenylamine	T65.3X1	T65.3X2	T65.3X3	T65.3X4	—	—
Diphenylbutazone	T39.2X1	T39.2X2	T39.2X3	T39.2X4	T39.2X5	T39.2X6
Diphenylchloroarsine, not in war	T57.ØX1	T57.ØX2	T57.ØX3	T57.ØX4	—	—
Diphenylhydantoin	T42.ØX1	T42.ØX2	T42.ØX3	T42.ØX4	T42.ØX5	T42.ØX6
Diphenylmethane dye	T52.1X1	T52.1X2	T52.1X3	T52.1X4	—	—
Diphenylpyraline	T45.ØX1	T45.ØX2	T45.ØX3	T45.ØX4	T45.ØX5	T45.ØX6
Diphtheria						
antitoxin	T5Ø.Z11	T5Ø.Z12	T5Ø.Z13	T5Ø.Z14	T5Ø.Z15	T5Ø.Z16
toxoid	T5Ø.A91	T5Ø.A92	T5Ø.A93	T5Ø.A94	T5Ø.A95	T5Ø.A96
with tetanus toxoid	T5Ø.A21	T5Ø.A22	T5Ø.A23	T5Ø.A24	T5Ø.A25	T5Ø.A26
with pertussis component	T5Ø.A11	T5Ø.A12	T5Ø.A13	T5Ø.A14	T5Ø.A15	T5Ø.A16

Substance	Poisoning, Accidental (Unintentional)	Poisoning, Intentional Self-Harm	Poisoning, Assault	Poisoning, Undetermined	Adverse Effect	Underdosing
	External Cause (T-Code)					
Diphtheria *(Continued)*						
vaccine (combination)	T5Ø.A91	T5Ø.A92	T5Ø.A93	T5Ø.A94	T5Ø.A95	T5Ø.A96
combination						
including pertussis	T5Ø.A11	T5Ø.A12	T5Ø.A13	T5Ø.A14	T5Ø.A15	T5Ø.A16
without pertussis	T5Ø.A21	T5Ø.A22	T5Ø.A23	T5Ø.A24	T5Ø.A25	T5Ø.A26
Diphylline	T5Ø.2X1	T5Ø.2X2	T5Ø.2X3	T5Ø.2X4	T5Ø.2X5	T5Ø.2X6
Dipipanone	T4Ø.491	T4Ø.492	T4Ø.493	T4Ø.494	—	—
Dipivefrine	T49.5X1	T49.5X2	T49.5X3	T49.5X4	T49.5X5	T49.5X6
Diplovax	T5Ø.B91	T5Ø.B92	T5Ø.B93	T5Ø.B94	T5Ø.B95	T5Ø.B96
Diprophylline	T5Ø.2X1	T5Ø.2X2	T5Ø.2X3	T5Ø.2X4	T5Ø.2X5	T5Ø.2X6
Dipropyline	T48.291	T48.292	T48.293	T48.294	T48.295	T48.296
Dipyridamole	T46.3X1	T46.3X2	T46.3X3	T46.3X4	T46.3X5	T46.3X6
Dipyrone	T39.2X1	T39.2X2	T39.2X3	T39.2X4	T39.2X5	T39.2X6
Diquat (dibromide)	T6Ø.3X1	T6Ø.3X2	T6Ø.3X3	T6Ø.3X4	—	—
Disinfectant	T65.891	T65.892	T65.893	T65.894	—	—
alkaline	T54.3X1	T54.3X2	T54.3X3	T54.3X4	—	—
aromatic	T54.1X1	T54.1X2	T54.1X3	T54.1X4	—	—
intestinal	T37.8X1	T37.8X2	T37.8X3	T37.8X4	T37.8X5	T37.8X6
Disipal	T42.8X1	T42.8X2	T42.8X3	T42.8X4	T42.8X5	T42.8X6
Disodium edetate	T5Ø.6X1	T5Ø.6X2	T5Ø.6X3	T5Ø.6X4	T5Ø.6X5	T5Ø.6X6
Disoprofol	T41.291	T41.292	T41.293	T41.294	T41.295	T41.296
Disopyramide	T46.2X1	T46.2X2	T46.2X3	T46.2X4	T46.2X5	T46.2X6
Distigmine (bromide)	T44.ØX1	T44.ØX2	T44.ØX3	T44.ØX4	T44.ØX5	T44.ØX6
Disulfamide	T5Ø.2X1	T5Ø.2X2	T5Ø.2X3	T5Ø.2X4	T5Ø.2X5	T5Ø.2X6
Disulfanilamide	T37.ØX1	T37.ØX2	T37.ØX3	T37.ØX4	T37.ØX5	T37.ØX6
Disulfiram	T5Ø.6X1	T5Ø.6X2	T5Ø.6X3	T5Ø.6X4	T5Ø.6X5	T5Ø.6X6
Disulfoton	T6Ø.ØX1	T6Ø.ØX2	T6Ø.ØX3	T6Ø.ØX4	—	—
Dithiazanine iodide	T37.4X1	T37.4X2	T37.4X3	T37.4X4	T37.4X5	T37.4X6
Dithiocarbamate	T6Ø.ØX1	T6Ø.ØX2	T6Ø.ØX3	T6Ø.ØX4	—	—
Dithranol	T49.4X1	T49.4X2	T49.4X3	T49.4X4	T49.4X5	T49.4X6
Diucardin	T5Ø.2X1	T5Ø.2X2	T5Ø.2X3	T5Ø.2X4	T5Ø.2X5	T5Ø.2X6
Diupres	T5Ø.2X1	T5Ø.2X2	T5Ø.2X3	T5Ø.2X4	T5Ø.2X5	T5Ø.2X6
Diuretic NEC	T5Ø.2X1	T5Ø.2X2	T5Ø.2X3	T5Ø.2X4	T5Ø.2X5	T5Ø.2X6
benzothiadiazine	T5Ø.2X1	T5Ø.2X2	T5Ø.2X3	T5Ø.2X4	T5Ø.2X5	T5Ø.2X6
carbonic acid anhydrase inhibitors	T5Ø.2X1	T5Ø.2X2	T5Ø.2X3	T5Ø.2X4	T5Ø.2X5	T5Ø.2X6
furfuryl NEC	T5Ø.2X1	T5Ø.2X2	T5Ø.2X3	T5Ø.2X4	T5Ø.2X5	T5Ø.2X6
loop (high-ceiling)	T5Ø.1X1	T5Ø.1X2	T5Ø.1X3	T5Ø.1X4	T5Ø.1X5	T5Ø.1X6
mercurial NEC	T5Ø.2X1	T5Ø.2X2	T5Ø.2X3	T5Ø.2X4	T5Ø.2X5	T5Ø.2X6
osmotic	T5Ø.2X1	T5Ø.2X2	T5Ø.2X3	T5Ø.2X4	T5Ø.2X5	T5Ø.2X6
purine NEC	T5Ø.2X1	T5Ø.2X2	T5Ø.2X3	T5Ø.2X4	T5Ø.2X5	T5Ø.2X6
saluretic NEC	T5Ø.2X1	T5Ø.2X2	T5Ø.2X3	T5Ø.2X4	T5Ø.2X5	T5Ø.2X6

Substance	External Cause (T-Code)					
	Poisoning, Accidental (Unintentional)	Poisoning, Intentional Self-Harm	Poisoning, Assault	Poisoning, Undetermined	Adverse Effect	Underdosing
Diuretic NEC *(Continued)*						
sulfonamide	T5Ø.2X1	T5Ø.2X2	T5Ø.2X3	T5Ø.2X4	T5Ø.2X5	T5Ø.2X6
thiazide NEC	T5Ø.2X1	T5Ø.2X2	T5Ø.2X3	T5Ø.2X4	T5Ø.2X5	T5Ø.2X6
xanthine	T5Ø.2X1	T5Ø.2X2	T5Ø.2X3	T5Ø.2X4	T5Ø.2X5	T5Ø.2X6
Diurgin	T5Ø.2X1	T5Ø.2X2	T5Ø.2X3	T5Ø.2X4	T5Ø.2X5	T5Ø.2X6
Diuril	T5Ø.2X1	T5Ø.2X2	T5Ø.2X3	T5Ø.2X4	T5Ø.2X5	T5Ø.2X6
Diuron	T6Ø.3X1	T6Ø.3X2	T6Ø.3X3	T6Ø.3X4	—	—
Divalproex	T42.6X1	T42.6X2	T42.6X3	T42.6X4	T42.6X5	T42.6X6
Divinyl ether	T41.ØX1	T41.ØX2	T41.ØX3	T41.ØX4	T41.ØX5	T41.ØX6
Dixanthogen	T49.ØX1	T49.ØX2	T49.ØX3	T49.ØX4	T49.ØX5	T49.ØX6
Dixyrazine	T43.3X1	T43.3X2	T43.3X3	T43.3X4	T43.3X5	T43.3X6
D-lysergic acid diethylamide	T4Ø.8X1	T4Ø.8X2	T4Ø.8X3	T4Ø.8X4	—	—
DMCT	T36.4X1	T36.4X2	T36.4X3	T36.4X4	T36.4X5	T36.4X6
DMSO — *see Dimethyl, sulfoxide*						
DNBP	T6Ø.3X1	T6Ø.3X2	T6Ø.3X3	T6Ø.3X4	—	—
DNOC	T65.3X1	T65.3X2	T65.3X3	T65.3X4	—	—
DOCA	T38.ØX1	T38.ØX2	T38.ØX3	T38.ØX4	T38.ØX5	T38.ØX6
Dobutamine	T44.5X1	T44.5X2	T44.5X3	T44.5X4	T44.5X5	T44.5X6
Docusate sodium	T47.4X1	T47.4X2	T47.4X3	T47.4X4	T47.4X5	T47.4X6
Dodicin	T49.ØX1	T49.ØX2	T49.ØX3	T49.ØX4	T49.ØX5	T49.ØX6
Dofamium chloride	T49.ØX1	T49.ØX2	T49.ØX3	T49.ØX4	T49.ØX5	T49.ØX6
Dolophine	T4Ø.3X1	T4Ø.3X2	T4Ø.3X3	T4Ø.3X4	T4Ø.3X5	T4Ø.3X6
Doloxene	T39.8X1	T39.8X2	T39.8X3	T39.8X4	T39.8X5	T39.8X6
Domestic gas (after combustion) — *see Gas, utility*						
prior to combustion	T59.891	T59.892	T59.893	T59.894	—	—
Domiodol	T48.4X1	T48.4X2	T48.4X3	T48.4X4	T48.4X5	T48.4X6
Domiphen (bromide)	T49.ØX1	T49.ØX2	T49.ØX3	T49.ØX4	T49.ØX5	T49.ØX6
Domperidone	T45.ØX1	T45.ØX2	T45.ØX3	T45.ØX4	T45.ØX5	T45.ØX6
Dopa	T42.8X1	T42.8X2	T42.8X3	T42.8X4	T42.8X5	T42.8X6
Dopamine	T44.991	T44.992	T44.993	T44.994	T44.995	T44.996
Doriden	T42.6X1	T42.6X2	T42.6X3	T42.6X4	T42.6X5	T42.6X6
Dormiral	T42.3X1	T42.3X2	T42.3X3	T42.3X4	T42.3X5	T42.3X6
Dormison	T42.6X1	T42.6X2	T42.6X3	T42.6X4	T42.6X5	T42.6X6
Dornase	T48.4X1	T48.4X2	T48.4X3	T48.4X4	T48.4X5	T48.4X6
Dorsacaine	T41.3X1	T41.3X2	T41.3X3	T41.3X4	T41.3X5	T41.3X6
Dosulepin	T43.Ø11	T43.Ø12	T43.Ø13	T43.Ø14	T43.Ø15	T43.Ø16
Dothiepin	T43.Ø11	T43.Ø12	T43.Ø13	T43.Ø14	T43.Ø15	T43.Ø16
Doxantrazole	T48.6X1	T48.6X2	T48.6X3	T48.6X4	T48.6X5	T48.6X6
Doxapram	T5Ø.7X1	T5Ø.7X2	T5Ø.7X3	T5Ø.7X4	T5Ø.7X5	T5Ø.7X6
Doxazosin	T44.6X1	T44.6X2	T44.6X3	T44.6X4	T44.6X5	T44.6X6
Doxepin	T43.Ø11	T43.Ø12	T43.Ø13	T43.Ø14	T43.Ø15	T43.Ø16
Doxifluridine	T45.1X1	T45.1X2	T45.1X3	T45.1X4	T45.1X5	T45.1X6
Doxorubicin	T45.1X1	T45.1X2	T45.1X3	T45.1X4	T45.1X5	T45.1X6
Doxycycline	T36.4X1	T36.4X2	T36.4X3	T36.4X4	T36.4X5	T36.4X6
Doxylamine	T45.ØX1	T45.ØX2	T45.ØX3	T45.ØX4	T45.ØX5	T45.ØX6
Dramamine	T45.ØX1	T45.ØX2	T45.ØX3	T45.ØX4	T45.ØX5	T45.ØX6
Drano (drain cleaner)	T54.3X1	T54.3X2	T54.3X3	T54.3X4	—	—
Dressing, live pulp	T49.7X1	T49.7X2	T49.7X3	T49.7X4	T49.7X5	T49.7X6
Drocode	T4Ø.2X1	T4Ø.2X2	T4Ø.2X3	T4Ø.2X4	T4Ø.2X5	T4Ø.2X6
Dromoran	T4Ø.2X1	T4Ø.2X2	T4Ø.2X3	T4Ø.2X4	T4Ø.2X5	T4Ø.2X6
Dromostanolone	T38.7X1	T38.7X2	T38.7X3	T38.7X4	T38.7X5	T38.7X6
Dronabinol	T4Ø.711	T4Ø.712	T4Ø.713	T4Ø.714	T4Ø.715	T4Ø.716
Droperidol	T43.591	T43.592	T43.593	T43.594	T43.595	T43.596
Dropropizine	T48.3X1	T48.3X2	T48.3X3	T48.3X4	T48.3X5	T48.3X6
Drostanolone	T38.7X1	T38.7X2	T38.7X3	T38.7X4	T38.7X5	T38.7X6
Drotaverine	T44.3X1	T44.3X2	T44.3X3	T44.3X4	T44.3X5	T44.3X6
Drotrecogin alfa	T45.511	T45.512	T45.513	T45.514	T45.515	T45.516
Drug NEC	T5Ø.9Ø1	T5Ø.9Ø2	T5Ø.9Ø3	T5Ø.9Ø4	T5Ø.9Ø5	T5Ø.9Ø6
specified NEC	T5Ø.991	T5Ø.992	T5Ø.993	T5Ø.994	T5Ø.995	T5Ø.996
DTIC	T45.1X1	T45.1X2	T45.1X3	T45.1X4	T45.1X5	T45.1X6
Duboisine	T44.3X1	T44.3X2	T44.3X3	T44.3X4	T44.3X5	T44.3X6
Dulcolax	T47.2X1	T47.2X2	T47.2X3	T47.2X4	T47.2X5	T47.2X6
Duponol (C) (EP)	T49.2X1	T49.2X2	T49.2X3	T49.2X4	T49.2X5	T49.2X6
Durabolin	T38.7X1	T38.7X2	T38.7X3	T38.7X4	T38.7X5	T38.7X6
Dyclone	T41.3X1	T41.3X2	T41.3X3	T41.3X4	T41.3X5	T41.3X6
Dyclonine	T41.3X1	T41.3X2	T41.3X3	T41.3X4	T41.3X5	T41.3X6
Dydrogesterone	T38.5X1	T38.5X2	T38.5X3	T38.5X4	T38.5X5	T38.5X6
Dye NEC	T65.6X1	T65.6X2	T65.6X3	T65.6X4	—	—
antiseptic	T49.ØX1	T49.ØX2	T49.ØX3	T49.ØX4	T49.ØX5	T49.ØX6
diagnostic agents	T5Ø.8X1	T5Ø.8X2	T5Ø.8X3	T5Ø.8X4	T5Ø.8X5	T5Ø.8X6
pharmaceutical NEC	T5Ø.9Ø1	T5Ø.9Ø2	T5Ø.9Ø3	T5Ø.9Ø4	T5Ø.9Ø5	T5Ø.9Ø6
Dyflos	T44.ØX1	T44.ØX2	T44.ØX3	T44.ØX4	T44.ØX5	T44.ØX6
Dymelor	T38.3X1	T38.3X2	T38.3X3	T38.3X4	T38.3X5	T38.3X6
Dynamite	T65.3X1	T65.3X2	T65.3X3	T65.3X4	—	—
fumes	T59.891	T59.892	T59.893	T59.894	—	—
Dyphylline	T44.3X1	T44.3X2	T44.3X3	T44.3X4	T44.3X5	T44.3X6
E						
Ear drug NEC	T49.6X1	T49.6X2	T49.6X3	T49.6X4	T49.6X5	T49.6X6
Ear preparations	T49.6X1	T49.6X2	T49.6X3	T49.6X4	T49.6X5	T49.6X6
Econazole	T49.ØX1	T49.ØX2	T49.ØX3	T49.ØX4	T49.ØX5	T49.ØX6
Ecothiopate iodide	T49.5X1	T49.5X2	T49.5X3	T49.5X4	T49.5X5	T49.5X6
Echothiophate, echothiopate, ecothiopate	T49.5X1	T49.5X2	T49.5X3	T49.5X4	T49.5X5	T49.5X6

Substance	External Cause (T-Code)					
	Poisoning, Accidental (Unintentional)	Poisoning, Intentional Self-Harm	Poisoning, Assault	Poisoning, Undetermined	Adverse Effect	Underdosing
Ecstasy	T43.641	T43.642	T43.643	T43.644	—	—
Ectylurea	T42.6X1	T42.6X2	T42.6X3	T42.6X4	T42.6X5	T42.6X6
Edathamil disodium	T45.8X1	T45.8X2	T45.8X3	T45.8X4	T45.8X5	T45.8X6
Edecrin	T50.1X1	T50.1X2	T50.1X3	T50.1X4	T50.1X5	T50.1X6
Edetate, disodium (calcium)	T45.8X1	T45.8X2	T45.8X3	T45.8X4	T45.8X5	T45.8X6
Edoxudine	T49.5X1	T49.5X2	T49.5X3	T49.5X4	T49.5X5	T49.5X6
Edrophonium	T44.0X1	T44.0X2	T44.0X3	T44.0X4	T44.0X5	T44.0X6
chloride	T44.0X1	T44.0X2	T44.0X3	T44.0X4	T44.0X5	T44.0X6
EDTA	T50.6X1	T50.6X2	T50.6X3	T50.6X4	T50.6X5	T50.6X6
Eflornithine	T37.2X1	T37.2X2	T37.2X3	T37.2X4	T37.2X5	T37.2X6
Efloxate	T46.3X1	T46.3X2	T46.3X3	T46.3X4	T46.3X5	T46.3X6
Elase	T49.8X1	T49.8X2	T49.8X3	T49.8X4	T49.8X5	T49.8X6
Elastase	T47.5X1	T47.5X2	T47.5X3	T47.5X4	T47.5X5	T47.5X6
Elaterium	T47.2X1	T47.2X2	T47.2X3	T47.2X4	T47.2X5	T47.2X6
Elcatonin	T50.991	T50.992	T50.993	T50.994	T50.995	T50.996
Elder	T62.2X1	T62.2X2	T62.2X3	T62.2X4	—	—
berry (unripe)	T62.1X1	T62.1X2	T62.1X3	T62.1X4	—	—
Electrolyte balance drug	T50.3X1	T50.3X2	T50.3X3	T50.3X4	T50.3X5	T50.3X6
Electrolytes NEC	T50.3X1	T50.3X2	T50.3X3	T50.3X4	T50.3X5	T50.3X6
Electrolytic agent NEC	T50.3X1	T50.3X2	T50.3X3	T50.3X4	T50.3X5	T50.3X6
Elemental diet	T50.901	T50.902	T50.903	T50.904	T50.905	T50.906
Elliptinium acetate	T45.1X1	T45.1X2	T45.1X3	T45.1X4	T45.1X5	T45.1X6
Embramine	T45.0X1	T45.0X2	T45.0X3	T45.0X4	T45.0X5	T45.0X6
Emepronium (salts)	T44.3X1	T44.3X2	T44.3X3	T44.3X4	T44.3X5	T44.3X6
bromide	T44.3X1	T44.3X2	T44.3X3	T44.3X4	T44.3X5	T44.3X6
Emetic NEC	T47.7X1	T47.7X2	T47.7X3	T47.7X4	T47.7X5	T47.7X6
Emetine	T37.3X1	T37.3X2	T37.3X3	T37.3X4	T37.3X5	T37.3X6
Emollient NEC	T49.3X1	T49.3X2	T49.3X3	T49.3X4	T49.3X5	T49.3X6
Emorfazone	T39.8X1	T39.8X2	T39.8X3	T39.8X4	T39.8X5	T39.8X6
Emylcamate	T43.591	T43.592	T43.593	T43.594	T43.595	T43.596
Enalapril	T46.4X1	T46.4X2	T46.4X3	T46.4X4	T46.4X5	T46.4X6
Enalaprilat	T46.4X1	T46.4X2	T46.4X3	T46.4X4	T46.4X5	T46.4X6
Encainide	T46.2X1	T46.2X2	T46.2X3	T46.2X4	T46.2X5	T46.2X6
Endocaine	T41.3X1	T41.3X2	T41.3X3	T41.3X4	T41.3X5	T41.3X6
Endosulfan	T60.2X1	T60.2X2	T60.2X3	T60.2X4	—	—
Endothall	T60.3X1	T60.3X2	T60.3X3	T60.3X4	—	—
Endralazine	T46.5X1	T46.5X2	T46.5X3	T46.5X4	T46.5X5	T46.5X6
Endrin	T60.1X1	T60.1X2	T60.1X3	T60.1X4	—	—
Enflurane	T41.0X1	T41.0X2	T41.0X3	T41.0X4	T41.0X5	T41.0X6
Enhexymal	T42.3X1	T42.3X2	T42.3X3	T42.3X4	T42.3X5	T42.3X6
Enocitabine	T45.1X1	T45.1X2	T45.1X3	T45.1X4	T45.1X5	T45.1X6
Enovid	T38.4X1	T38.4X2	T38.4X3	T38.4X4	T38.4X5	T38.4X6

Substance	External Cause (T-Code)					
	Poisoning, Accidental (Unintentional)	Poisoning, Intentional Self-Harm	Poisoning, Assault	Poisoning, Undetermined	Adverse Effect	Underdosing
Enoxacin	T36.8X1	T36.8X2	T36.8X3	T36.8X4	T36.8X5	T36.8X6
Enoxaparin (sodium)	T45.511	T45.512	T45.513	T45.514	T45.515	T45.516
Enpiprazole	T43.591	T43.592	T43.593	T43.594	T43.595	T43.596
Enprofylline	T48.6X1	T48.6X2	T48.6X3	T48.6X4	T48.6X5	T48.6X6
Enprostil	T47.1X1	T47.1X2	T47.1X3	T47.1X4	T47.1X5	T47.1X6
ENT preparations (anti-infectives)	T49.6X1	T49.6X2	T49.6X3	T49.6X4	T49.6X5	T49.6X6
Enviomycin	T36.8X1	T36.8X2	T36.8X3	T36.8X4	T36.8X5	T36.8X6
Enzodase	T45.3X1	T45.3X2	T45.3X3	T45.3X4	T45.3X5	T45.3X6
Enzyme NEC	T45.3X1	T45.3X2	T45.3X3	T45.3X4	T45.3X5	T45.3X6
depolymerizing	T49.8X1	T49.8X2	T49.8X3	T49.8X4	T49.8X5	T49.8X6
fibrolytic	T45.3X1	T45.3X2	T45.3X3	T45.3X4	T45.3X5	T45.3X6
gastric	T47.5X1	T47.5X2	T47.5X3	T47.5X4	T47.5X5	T47.5X6
intestinal	T47.5X1	T47.5X2	T47.5X3	T47.5X4	T47.5X5	T47.5X6
local action	T49.4X1	T49.4X2	T49.4X3	T49.4X4	T49.4X5	T49.4X6
proteolytic	T49.4X1	T49.4X2	T49.4X3	T49.4X4	T49.4X5	T49.4X6
thrombolytic	T45.3X1	T45.3X2	T45.3X3	T45.3X4	T45.3X5	T45.3X6
EPAB	T41.3X1	T41.3X2	T41.3X3	T41.3X4	T41.3X5	T41.3X6
Epanutin	T42.0X1	T42.0X2	T42.0X3	T42.0X4	T42.0X5	T42.0X6
Ephedra	T44.991	T44.992	T44.993	T44.994	T44.995	T44.996
Ephedrine	T44.991	T44.992	T44.993	T44.994	T44.995	T44.996
Epichlorhydrin, epichlorohydrin	T52.8X1	T52.8X2	T52.8X3	T52.8X4	—	—
Epicillin	T36.0X1	T36.0X2	T36.0X3	T36.0X4	T36.0X5	T36.0X6
Epiestriol	T38.5X1	T38.5X2	T38.5X3	T38.5X4	T38.5X5	T38.5X6
Epilim — *see Sodium, valproate*						
Epimestrol	T38.5X1	T38.5X2	T38.5X3	T38.5X4	T38.5X5	T38.5X6
Epinephrine	T44.5X1	T44.5X2	T44.5X3	T44.5X4	T44.5X5	T44.5X6
Epirubicin	T45.1X1	T45.1X2	T45.1X3	T45.1X4	T45.1X5	T45.1X6
Epitiostanol	T38.7X1	T38.7X2	T38.7X3	T38.7X4	T38.7X5	T38.7X6
Epitizide	T50.2X1	T50.2X2	T50.2X3	T50.2X4	T50.2X5	T50.2X6
EPN	T60.0X1	T60.0X2	T60.0X3	T60.0X4	—	—
EPO	T45.8X1	T45.8X2	T45.8X3	T45.8X4	T45.8X5	T45.8X6
Epoetin alpha	T45.8X1	T45.8X2	T45.8X3	T45.8X4	T45.8X5	T45.8X6
Epomediol	T50.991	T50.992	T50.993	T50.994	T50.995	T50.996
Epoprostenol	T45.521	T45.522	T45.523	T45.524	T45.525	T45.526
Epoxy resin	T65.891	T65.892	T65.893	T65.894	—	—
Eprazinone	T48.4X1	T48.4X2	T48.4X3	T48.4X4	T48.4X5	T48.4X6
Epsilon amino-caproic acid	T45.621	T45.622	T45.623	T45.624	T45.625	T45.626
Epsom salt	T47.3X1	T47.3X2	T47.3X3	T47.3X4	T47.3X5	T47.3X6
Eptazocine	T40.491	T40.492	T40.493	T40.494	T40.495	T40.496
Equanil	T43.591	T43.592	T43.593	T43.594	T43.595	T43.596
Equisetum	T62.2X1	T62.2X2	T62.2X3	T62.2X4	—	—
diuretic	T50.2X1	T50.2X2	T50.2X3	T50.2X4	T50.2X5	T50.2X6

◀ New ⇐ Revised ~~deleted~~ Deleted

Substance	Poisoning, Accidental (Unintentional)	Poisoning, Intentional Self-Harm	Poisoning, Assault	Poisoning, Undetermined	Adverse Effect	Underdosing
	External Cause (T-Code)					
Ergobasine	T48.ØX1	T48.ØX2	T48.ØX3	T48.ØX4	T48.ØX5	T48.ØX6
Ergocalciferol	T45.2X1	T45.2X2	T45.2X3	T45.2X4	T45.2X5	T45.2X6
Ergoloid mesylates	T46.7X1	T46.7X2	T46.7X3	T46.7X4	T46.7X5	T46.7X6
Ergometrine	T48.ØX1	T48.ØX2	T48.ØX3	T48.ØX4	T48.ØX5	T48.ØX6
Ergonovine	T48.ØX1	T48.ØX2	T48.ØX3	T48.ØX4	T48.ØX5	T48.ØX6
Ergot NEC	T64.81	T64.82	T64.83	T64.84	—	—
derivative	T48.ØX1	T48.ØX2	T48.ØX3	T48.ØX4	T48.ØX5	T48.ØX6
medicinal (alkaloids)	T48.ØX1	T48.ØX2	T48.ØX3	T48.ØX4	T48.ØX5	T48.ØX6
prepared	T48.ØX1	T48.ØX2	T48.ØX3	T48.ØX4	T48.ØX5	T48.ØX6
Ergotamine	T46.5X1	T46.5X2	T46.5X3	T46.5X4	T46.5X5	T46.5X6
Ergotocine	T48.ØX1	T48.ØX2	T48.ØX3	T48.ØX4	T48.ØX5	T48.ØX6
Ergotrate	T48.ØX1	T48.ØX2	T48.ØX3	T48.ØX4	T48.ØX5	T48.ØX6
Eritrityl tetranitrate	T46.3X1	T46.3X2	T46.3X3	T46.3X4	T46.3X5	T46.3X6
Erythrityl tetranitrate	T46.3X1	T46.3X2	T46.3X3	T46.3X4	T46.3X5	T46.3X6
Erythrol tetranitrate	T46.3X1	T46.3X2	T46.3X3	T46.3X4	T46.3X5	T46.3X6
Erythromycin (salts)	T36.3X1	T36.3X2	T36.3X3	T36.3X4	T36.3X5	T36.3X6
ophthalmic preparation	T49.5X1	T49.5X2	T49.5X3	T49.5X4	T49.5X5	T49.5X6
topical NEC	T49.ØX1	T49.ØX2	T49.ØX3	T49.ØX4	T49.ØX5	T49.ØX6
Erythropoietin	T45.8X1	T45.8X2	T45.8X3	T45.8X4	T45.8X5	T45.8X6
human	T45.8X1	T45.8X2	T45.8X3	T45.8X4	T45.8X5	T45.8X6
Escin	T46.991	T46.992	T46.993	T46.994	T46.995	T46.996
Esculin	T45.2X1	T45.2X2	T45.2X3	T45.2X4	T45.2X5	T45.2X6
Esculoside	T45.2X1	T45.2X2	T45.2X3	T45.2X4	T45.2X5	T45.2X6
ESDT (ether-soluble tar distillate)	T49.1X1	T49.1X2	T49.1X3	T49.1X4	T49.1X5	T49.1X6
Eserine	T49.5X1	T49.5X2	T49.5X3	T49.5X4	T49.5X5	T49.5X6
Esflurbiprofen	T39.311	T39.312	T39.313	T39.314	T39.315	T39.316
Eskabarb	T42.3X1	T42.3X2	T42.3X3	T42.3X4	T42.3X5	T42.3X6
Eskalith	T43.8X1	T43.8X2	T43.8X3	T43.8X4	T43.8X5	T43.8X6
Esmolol	T44.7X1	T44.7X2	T44.7X3	T44.7X4	T44.7X5	T44.7X6
Estanozolol	T38.7X1	T38.7X2	T38.7X3	T38.7X4	T38.7X5	T38.7X6
Estazolam	T42.4X1	T42.4X2	T42.4X3	T42.4X4	T42.4X5	T42.4X6
Estradiol	T38.5X1	T38.5X2	T38.5X3	T38.5X4	T38.5X5	T38.5X6
with testosterone	T38.7X1	T38.7X2	T38.7X3	T38.7X4	T38.7X5	T38.7X6
benzoate	T38.5X1	T38.5X2	T38.5X3	T38.5X4	T38.5X5	T38.5X6
Estramustine	T45.1X1	T45.1X2	T45.1X3	T45.1X4	T45.1X5	T45.1X6
Estriol	T38.5X1	T38.5X2	T38.5X3	T38.5X4	T38.5X5	T38.5X6
Estrogen	T38.5X1	T38.5X2	T38.5X3	T38.5X4	T38.5X5	T38.5X6
with progesterone	T38.5X1	T38.5X2	T38.5X3	T38.5X4	T38.5X5	T38.5X6
conjugated	T38.5X1	T38.5X2	T38.5X3	T38.5X4	T38.5X5	T38.5X6
Estrone	T38.5X1	T38.5X2	T38.5X3	T38.5X4	T38.5X5	T38.5X6
Estropipate	T38.5X1	T38.5X2	T38.5X3	T38.5X4	T38.5X5	T38.5X6

Substance	Poisoning, Accidental (Unintentional)	Poisoning, Intentional Self-Harm	Poisoning, Assault	Poisoning, Undetermined	Adverse Effect	Underdosing
	External Cause (T-Code)					
Etacrynate sodium	T5Ø.1X1	T5Ø.1X2	T5Ø.1X3	T5Ø.1X4	T5Ø.1X5	T5Ø.1X6
Etacrynic acid	T5Ø.1X1	T5Ø.1X2	T5Ø.1X3	T5Ø.1X4	T5Ø.1X5	T5Ø.1X6
Etafedrine	T48.6X1	T48.6X2	T48.6X3	T48.6X4	T48.6X5	T48.6X6
Etafenone	T46.3X1	T46.3X2	T46.3X3	T46.3X4	T46.3X5	T46.3X6
Etambutol	T37.1X1	T37.1X2	T37.1X3	T37.1X4	T37.1X5	T37.1X6
Etamiphyllin	T48.6X1	T48.6X2	T48.6X3	T48.6X4	T48.6X5	T48.6X6
Etamivan	T5Ø.7X1	T5Ø.7X2	T5Ø.7X3	T5Ø.7X4	T5Ø.7X5	T5Ø.7X6
Etamsylate	T45.7X1	T45.7X2	T45.7X3	T45.7X4	T45.7X5	T45.7X6
Etebenecid	T5Ø.4X1	T5Ø.4X2	T5Ø.4X3	T5Ø.4X4	T5Ø.4X5	T5Ø.4X6
Ethacridine	T49.ØX1	T49.ØX2	T49.ØX3	T49.ØX4	T49.ØX5	T49.ØX6
Ethacrynic acid	T5Ø.1X1	T5Ø.1X2	T5Ø.1X3	T5Ø.1X4	T5Ø.1X5	T5Ø.1X6
Ethadione	T42.2X1	T42.2X2	T42.2X3	T42.2X4	T42.2X5	T42.2X6
Ethambutol	T37.1X1	T37.1X2	T37.1X3	T37.1X4	T37.1X5	T37.1X6
Ethamide	T5Ø.2X1	T5Ø.2X2	T5Ø.2X3	T5Ø.2X4	T5Ø.2X5	T5Ø.2X6
Ethamivan	T5Ø.7X1	T5Ø.7X2	T5Ø.7X3	T5Ø.7X4	T5Ø.7X5	T5Ø.7X6
Ethamsylate	T45.7X1	T45.7X2	T45.7X3	T45.7X4	T45.7X5	T45.7X6
Ethanol	T51.ØX1	T51.ØX2	T51.ØX3	T51.ØX4	—	—
beverage	T51.ØX1	T51.ØX2	T51.ØX3	T51.ØX4	—	—
Ethanolamine oleate	T46.8X1	T46.8X2	T46.8X3	T46.8X4	T46.8X5	T46.8X6
Ethaverine	T44.3X1	T44.3X2	T44.3X3	T44.3X4	T44.3X5	T44.3X6
Ethchlorvynol	T42.6X1	T42.6X2	T42.6X3	T42.6X4	T42.6X5	T42.6X6
Ethebenecid	T5Ø.4X1	T5Ø.4X2	T5Ø.4X3	T5Ø.4X4	T5Ø.4X5	T5Ø.4X6
Ether (vapor)	T41.ØX1	T41.ØX2	T41.ØX3	T41.ØX4	T41.ØX5	T41.ØX6
anesthetic	T41.ØX1	T41.ØX2	T41.ØX3	T41.ØX4	T41.ØX5	T41.ØX6
divinyl	T41.ØX1	T41.ØX2	T41.ØX3	T41.ØX4	T41.ØX5	T41.ØX6
ethyl (medicinal)	T41.ØX1	T41.ØX2	T41.ØX3	T41.ØX4	T41.ØX5	T41.ØX6
nonmedicinal	T52.8X1	T52.8X2	T52.8X3	T52.8X4	—	—
petroleum — *see Ligroin*						
solvent	T52.8X1	T52.8X2	T52.8X3	T52.8X4	—	—
Ethiazide	T5Ø.2X1	T5Ø.2X2	T5Ø.2X3	T5Ø.2X4	T5Ø.2X5	T5Ø.2X6
Ethidium chloride (vapor)	T59.891	T59.892	T59.893	T59.894	—	—
Ethinamate	T42.6X1	T42.6X2	T42.6X3	T42.6X4	T42.6X5	T42.6X6
Ethinylestradiol, ethinyloestradiol	T38.5X1	T38.5X2	T38.5X3	T38.5X4	T38.5X5	T38.5X6
with						
levonorgestrel	T38.4X1	T38.4X2	T38.4X3	T38.4X4	T38.4X5	T38.4X6
norethisterone	T38.4X1	T38.4X2	T38.4X3	T38.4X4	T38.4X5	T38.4X6
Ethiodized oil (131 I)	T5Ø.8X1	T5Ø.8X2	T5Ø.8X3	T5Ø.8X4	T5Ø.8X5	T5Ø.8X6
Ethion	T6Ø.ØX1	T6Ø.ØX2	T6Ø.ØX3	T6Ø.ØX4	—	—
Ethionamide	T37.1X1	T37.1X2	T37.1X3	T37.1X4	T37.1X5	T37.1X6
Ethioniamide	T37.1X1	T37.1X2	T37.1X3	T37.1X4	T37.1X5	T37.1X6
Ethisterone	T38.5X1	T38.5X2	T38.5X3	T38.5X4	T38.5X5	T38.5X6
Ethobral	T42.3X1	T42.3X2	T42.3X3	T42.3X4	T42.3X5	T42.3X6

	External Cause (T-Code)					
Substance	Poisoning, Accidental (Unintentional)	Poisoning, Intentional Self-Harm	Poisoning, Assault	Poisoning, Undetermined	Adverse Effect	Underdosing
Ethocaine (infiltration) (topical)	T41.3X1	T41.3X2	T41.3X3	T41.3X4	T41.3X5	T41.3X6
nerve block (peripheral) (plexus)	T41.3X1	T41.3X2	T41.3X3	T41.3X4	T41.3X5	T41.3X6
spinal	T41.3X1	T41.3X2	T41.3X3	T41.3X4	T41.3X5	T41.3X6
Ethoheptazine	T4Ø.491	T4Ø.492	T4Ø.493	T4Ø.494	T4Ø.495	T4Ø.496
Ethopropazine	T44.3X1	T44.3X2	T44.3X3	T44.3X4	T44.3X5	T44.3X6
Ethosuximide	T42.2X1	T42.2X2	T42.2X3	T42.2X4	T42.2X5	T42.2X6
Ethotoin	T42.ØX1	T42.ØX2	T42.ØX3	T42.ØX4	T42.ØX5	T42.ØX6
Ethoxazene	T37.91	T37.92	T37.93	T37.94	T37.95	T37.96
Ethoxazorutoside	T46.991	T46.992	T46.993	T46.994	T46.995	T46.996
2-Ethoxyethanol	T52.3X1	T52.3X2	T52.3X3	T52.3X4	—	—
Ethoxzolamide	T5Ø.2X1	T5Ø.2X2	T5Ø.2X3	T5Ø.2X4	T5Ø.2X5	T5Ø.2X6
Ethyl						
acetate	T52.8X1	T52.8X2	T52.8X3	T52.8X4	—	—
alcohol	T51.ØX1	T51.ØX2	T51.ØX3	T51.ØX4	—	—
beverage	T51.ØX1	T51.ØX2	T51.ØX3	T51.ØX4	—	—
aldehyde (vapor)	T59.891	T59.892	T59.893	T59.894	—	—
liquid	T52.8X1	T52.8X2	T52.8X3	T52.8X4	—	—
aminobenzoate	T41.3X1	T41.3X2	T41.3X3	T41.3X4	T41.3X5	T41.3X6
aminophenothiazine	T43.3X1	T43.3X2	T43.3X3	T43.3X4	T43.3X5	T43.3X6
benzoate	T52.8X1	T52.8X2	T52.8X3	T52.8X4	—	—
biscoumacetate	T45.511	T45.512	T45.513	T45.514	T45.515	T45.516
bromide (anesthetic)	T41.ØX1	T41.ØX2	T41.ØX3	T41.ØX4	T41.ØX5	T41.ØX6
carbamate	T45.1X1	T45.1X2	T45.1X3	T45.1X4	T45.1X5	T45.1X6
carbinol	T51.3X1	T51.3X2	T51.3X3	T51.3X4	—	—
carbonate	T52.8X1	T52.8X2	T52.8X3	T52.8X4	—	—
chaulmoograte	T37.1X1	T37.1X2	T37.1X3	T37.1X4	T37.1X5	T37.1X6
chloride (anesthetic)	T41.ØX1	T41.ØX2	T41.ØX3	T41.ØX4	T41.ØX5	T41.ØX6
anesthetic (local)	T41.3X1	T41.3X2	T41.3X3	T41.3X4	T41.3X5	T41.3X6
inhaled	T41.ØX1	T41.ØX2	T41.ØX3	T41.ØX4	T41.ØX5	T41.ØX6
local	T49.4X1	T49.4X2	T49.4X3	T49.4X4	T49.4X5	T49.4X6
solvent	T53.6X1	T53.6X2	T53.6X3	T53.6X4	—	—
dibunate	T48.3X1	T48.3X2	T48.3X3	T48.3X4	T48.3X5	T48.3X6
dichloroarsine (vapor)	T57.ØX1	T57.ØX2	T57.ØX3	T57.ØX4	—	—
estranol	T38.7X1	T38.7X2	T38.7X3	T38.7X4	T38.7X5	T38.7X6
ether — *see also Ether*	T52.8X1	T52.8X2	T52.8X3	T52.8X4	—	—
formate NEC (solvent)	T52.ØX1	T52.ØX2	T52.ØX3	T52.ØX4	—	—
fumarate	T49.4X1	T49.4X2	T49.4X3	T49.4X4	T49.4X5	T49.4X6
hydroxyisobutyrate NEC (solvent)	T52.8X1	T52.8X2	T52.8X3	T52.8X4	—	—
iodoacetate	T59.3X1	T59.3X2	T59.3X3	T59.3X4	—	—
lactate NEC (solvent)	T52.8X1	T52.8X2	T52.8X3	T52.8X4	—	—
loflazepate	T42.4X1	T42.4X2	T42.4X3	T42.4X4	T42.4X5	T42.4X6
Ethyl *(Continued)*						
mercuric chloride	T56.1X1	T56.1X2	T56.1X3	T56.1X4	—	—
methylcarbinol	T51.8X1	T51.8X2	T51.8X3	T51.8X4	—	—
morphine	T4Ø.2X1	T4Ø.2X2	T4Ø.2X3	T4Ø.2X4	T4Ø.2X5	T4Ø.2X6
noradrenaline	T48.6X1	T48.6X2	T48.6X3	T48.6X4	T48.6X5	T48.6X6
oxybutyrate NEC (solvent)	T52.8X1	T52.8X2	T52.8X3	T52.8X4	—	—
Ethylene (gas)	T59.891	T59.892	T59.893	T59.894	—	—
anesthetic (general)	T41.ØX1	T41.ØX2	T41.ØX3	T41.ØX4	T41.ØX5	T41.ØX6
chlorohydrin	T52.8X1	T52.8X2	T52.8X3	T52.8X4	—	—
vapor	T53.6X1	T53.6X2	T53.6X3	T53.6X4	—	—
dichloride	T52.8X1	T52.8X2	T52.8X3	T52.8X4	—	—
vapor	T53.6X1	T53.6X2	T53.6X3	T53.6X4	—	—
dinitrate	T52.3X1	T52.3X2	T52.3X3	T52.3X4	—	—
glycol(s)	T52.8X1	T52.8X2	T52.8X3	T52.8X4	—	—
dinitrate	T52.3X1	T52.3X2	T52.3X3	T52.3X4	—	—
monobutyl ether	T52.3X1	T52.3X2	T52.3X3	T52.3X4	—	—
imine	T54.1X1	T54.1X2	T54.1X3	T54.1X4	—	—
oxide (fumigant) (nonmedicinal)	T59.891	T59.892	T59.893	T59.894	—	—
medicinal	T49.ØX1	T49.ØX2	T49.ØX3	T49.ØX4	T49.ØX5	T49.ØX6
Ethylenediamine theophylline	T48.6X1	T48.6X2	T48.6X3	T48.6X4	T48.6X5	T48.6X6
Ethylenediaminetetra-acetic acid	T5Ø.6X1	T5Ø.6X2	T5Ø.6X3	T5Ø.6X4	T5Ø.6X5	T5Ø.6X6
Ethylenedinitrilotetra-acetate	T5Ø.6X1	T5Ø.6X2	T5Ø.6X3	T5Ø.6X4	T5Ø.6X5	T5Ø.6X6
Ethylestrenol	T38.7X1	T38.7X2	T38.7X3	T38.7X4	T38.7X5	T38.7X6
Ethylhydroxycellulose	T47.4X1	T47.4X2	T47.4X3	T47.4X4	T47.4X5	T47.4X6
Ethylidene						
chloride NEC	T53.6X1	T53.6X2	T53.6X3	T53.6X4	—	—
diacetate	T6Ø.3X1	T6Ø.3X2	T6Ø.3X3	T6Ø.3X4	—	—
dicoumarin	T45.511	T45.512	T45.513	T45.514	T45.515	T45.516
dicoumarol	T45.511	T45.512	T45.513	T45.514	T45.515	T45.516
diethyl ether	T52.ØX1	T52.ØX2	T52.ØX3	T52.ØX4	—	—
Ethylmorphine	T4Ø.2X1	T4Ø.2X2	T4Ø.2X3	T4Ø.2X4	T4Ø.2X5	T4Ø.2X6
Ethylnorepinephrine	T48.6X1	T48.6X2	T48.6X3	T48.6X4	T48.6X5	T48.6X6
Ethylparachlorophen-oxyisobutyrate	T46.6X1	T46.6X2	T46.6X3	T46.6X4	T46.6X5	T46.6X6
Ethynodiol	T38.4X1	T38.4X2	T38.4X3	T38.4X4	T38.4X5	T38.4X6
with mestranol diacetate	T38.4X1	T38.4X2	T38.4X3	T38.4X4	T38.4X5	T38.4X6
Etidocaine	T41.3X1	T41.3X2	T41.3X3	T41.3X4	T41.3X5	T41.3X6
infiltration (subcutaneous)	T41.3X1	T41.3X2	T41.3X3	T41.3X4	T41.3X5	T41.3X6
nerve (peripheral) (plexus)	T41.3X1	T41.3X2	T41.3X3	T41.3X4	T41.3X5	T41.3X6
Etidronate	T5Ø.991	T5Ø.992	T5Ø.993	T5Ø.994	T5Ø.995	T5Ø.996
Etidronic acid (disodium salt)	T5Ø.991	T5Ø.992	T5Ø.993	T5Ø.994	T5Ø.995	T5Ø.996
Etifoxine	T42.6X1	T42.6X2	T42.6X3	T42.6X4	T42.6X5	T42.6X6

New Revised ~~deleted~~ Deleted

Substance	External Cause (T-Code) Poisoning, Accidental (Unintentional)	Poisoning, Intentional Self-Harm	Poisoning, Assault	Poisoning, Undetermined	Adverse Effect	Underdosing
Etilefrine	T44.4X1	T44.4X2	T44.4X3	T44.4X4	T44.4X5	T44.4X6
Etilfen	T42.3X1	T42.3X2	T42.3X3	T42.3X4	T42.3X5	T42.3X6
Etinodiol	T38.4X1	T38.4X2	T38.4X3	T38.4X4	T38.4X5	T38.4X6
Etiroxate	T46.6X1	T46.6X2	T46.6X3	T46.6X4	T46.6X5	T46.6X6
Etizolam	T42.4X1	T42.4X2	T42.4X3	T42.4X4	T42.4X5	T42.4X6
Etodolac	T39.391	T39.392	T39.393	T39.394	T39.395	T39.396
Etofamide	T37.3X1	T37.3X2	T37.3X3	T37.3X4	T37.3X5	T37.3X6
Etofibrate	T46.6X1	T46.6X2	T46.6X3	T46.6X4	T46.6X5	T46.6X6
Etofylline	T46.7X1	T46.7X2	T46.7X3	T46.7X4	T46.7X5	T46.7X6
clofibrate	T46.6X1	T46.6X2	T46.6X3	T46.6X4	T46.6X5	T46.6X6
Etoglucid	T45.1X1	T45.1X2	T45.1X3	T45.1X4	T45.1X5	T45.1X6
Etomidate	T41.1X1	T41.1X2	T41.1X3	T41.1X4	T41.1X5	T41.1X6
Etomide	T39.8X1	T39.8X2	T39.8X3	T39.8X4	T39.8X5	T39.8X6
Etomidoline	T44.3X1	T44.3X2	T44.3X3	T44.3X4	T44.3X5	T44.3X6
Etoposide	T45.1X1	T45.1X2	T45.1X3	T45.1X4	T45.1X5	T45.1X6
Etorphine	T40.2X1	T40.2X2	T40.2X3	T40.2X4	T40.2X5	T40.2X6
Etoval	T42.3X1	T42.3X2	T42.3X3	T42.3X4	T42.3X5	T42.3X6
Etozolin	T50.1X1	T50.1X2	T50.1X3	T50.1X4	T50.1X5	T50.1X6
Etretinate	T50.991	T50.992	T50.993	T50.994	T50.995	T50.996
Etryptamine	T43.691	T43.692	T43.693	T43.694	T43.695	T43.696
Etybenzatropine	T44.3X1	T44.3X2	T44.3X3	T44.3X4	T44.3X5	T44.3X6
Etynodiol	T38.4X1	T38.4X2	T38.4X3	T38.4X4	T38.4X5	T38.4X6
Eucaine	T41.3X1	T41.3X2	T41.3X3	T41.3X4	T41.3X5	T41.3X6
Eucalyptus oil	T49.7X1	T49.7X2	T49.7X3	T49.7X4	T49.7X5	T49.7X6
Eucatropine	T49.5X1	T49.5X2	T49.5X3	T49.5X4	T49.5X5	T49.5X6
Eucodal	T40.2X1	T40.2X2	T40.2X3	T40.2X4	T40.2X5	T40.2X6
Euneryl	T42.3X1	T42.3X2	T42.3X3	T42.3X4	T42.3X5	T42.3X6
Euphthalmine	T44.3X1	T44.3X2	T44.3X3	T44.3X4	T44.3X5	T44.3X6
Eurax	T49.0X1	T49.0X2	T49.0X3	T49.0X4	T49.0X5	T49.0X6
Euresol	T49.4X1	T49.4X2	T49.4X3	T49.4X4	T49.4X5	T49.4X6
Euthroid	T38.1X1	T38.1X2	T38.1X3	T38.1X4	T38.1X5	T38.1X6
Evans blue	T50.8X1	T50.8X2	T50.8X3	T50.8X4	T50.8X5	T50.8X6
Evipal	T42.3X1	T42.3X2	T42.3X3	T42.3X4	T42.3X5	T42.3X6
sodium	T41.1X1	T41.1X2	T41.1X3	T41.1X4	T41.1X5	T41.1X6
Evipan	T42.3X1	T42.3X2	T42.3X3	T42.3X4	T42.3X5	T42.3X6
sodium	T41.1X1	T41.1X2	T41.1X3	T41.1X4	T41.1X5	T41.1X6
Exalamide	T49.0X1	T49.0X2	T49.0X3	T49.0X4	T49.0X5	T49.0X6
Exalgin	T39.1X1	T39.1X2	T39.1X3	T39.1X4	T39.1X5	T39.1X6
Excipients, pharmaceutical	T50.901	T50.902	T50.903	T50.904	T50.905	T50.906
Exhaust gas (engine) (motor vehicle)	T58.01	T58.02	T58.03	T58.04	—	—
Ex-Lax (phenolphthalein)	T47.2X1	T47.2X2	T47.2X3	T47.2X4	T47.2X5	T47.2X6
Expectorant NEC	T48.4X1	T48.4X2	T48.4X3	T48.4X4	T48.4X5	T48.4X6

Substance	External Cause (T-Code) Poisoning, Accidental (Unintentional)	Poisoning, Intentional Self-Harm	Poisoning, Assault	Poisoning, Undetermined	Adverse Effect	Underdosing
Extended insulin zinc suspension	T38.3X1	T38.3X2	T38.3X3	T38.3X4	T38.3X5	T38.3X6
External medications (skin) (mucous membrane)	T49.91	T49.92	T49.93	T49.94	T49.95	T49.96
dental agent	T49.7X1	T49.7X2	T49.7X3	T49.7X4	T49.7X5	T49.7X6
ENT agent	T49.6X1	T49.6X2	T49.6X3	T49.6X4	T49.6X5	T49.6X6
ophthalmic preparation	T49.5X1	T49.5X2	T49.5X3	T49.5X4	T49.5X5	T49.5X6
specified NEC	T49.8X1	T49.8X2	T49.8X3	T49.8X4	T49.8X5	T49.8X6
Extrapyramidal antagonist NEC	T44.3X1	T44.3X2	T44.3X3	T44.3X4	T44.3X5	T44.3X6
Eye agents (anti-infective)	T49.5X1	T49.5X2	T49.5X3	T49.5X4	T49.5X5	T49.5X6
Eye drug NEC	T49.5X1	T49.5X2	T49.5X3	T49.5X4	T49.5X5	T49.5X6
F						
FAC (fluorouracil + doxorubicin + cyclophosphamide)	T45.1X1	T45.1X2	T45.1X3	T45.1X4	T45.1X5	T45.1X6
Factor						
I (fibrinogen)	T45.8X1	T45.8X2	T45.8X3	T45.8X4	T45.8X5	T45.8X6
III (thromboplastin)	T45.8X1	T45.8X2	T45.8X3	T45.8X4	T45.8X5	T45.8X6
VIII (antihemophilic Factor) (Concentrate)	T45.8X1	T45.8X2	T45.8X3	T45.8X4	T45.8X5	T45.8X6
IX complex	T45.7X1	T45.7X2	T45.7X3	T45.7X4	T45.7X5	T45.7X6
human	T45.8X1	T45.8X2	T45.8X3	T45.8X4	T45.8X5	T45.8X6
Famotidine	T47.0X1	T47.0X2	T47.0X3	T47.0X4	T47.0X5	T47.0X6
Fat suspension, intravenous	T50.991	T50.992	T50.993	T50.994	T50.995	T50.996
Fazadinium bromide	T48.1X1	T48.1X2	T48.1X3	T48.1X4	T48.1X5	T48.1X6
Febarbamate	T42.3X1	T42.3X2	T42.3X3	T42.3X4	T42.3X5	T42.3X6
Fecal softener	T47.4X1	T47.4X2	T47.4X3	T47.4X4	T47.4X5	T47.4X6
Fedrilate	T48.3X1	T48.3X2	T48.3X3	T48.3X4	T48.3X5	T48.3X6
Felodipine	T46.1X1	T46.1X2	T46.1X3	T46.1X4	T46.1X5	T46.1X6
Felypressin	T38.891	T38.892	T38.893	T38.894	T38.895	T38.896
Femoxetine	T43.221	T43.222	T43.223	T43.224	T43.225	T43.226
Fenalcomine	T46.3X1	T46.3X2	T46.3X3	T46.3X4	T46.3X5	T46.3X6
Fenamisal	T37.1X1	T37.1X2	T37.1X3	T37.1X4	T37.1X5	T37.1X6
Fenazone	T39.2X1	T39.2X2	T39.2X3	T39.2X4	T39.2X5	T39.2X6
Fenbendazole	T37.4X1	T37.4X2	T37.4X3	T37.4X4	T37.4X5	T37.4X6
Fenbutrazate	T50.5X1	T50.5X2	T50.5X3	T50.5X4	T50.5X5	T50.5X6
Fencamfamine	T43.691	T43.692	T43.693	T43.694	T43.695	T43.696
Fendiline	T46.1X1	T46.1X2	T46.1X3	T46.1X4	T46.1X5	T46.1X6
Fenetylline	T43.691	T43.692	T43.693	T43.694	T43.695	T43.696
Fenflumizole	T39.391	T39.392	T39.393	T39.394	T39.395	T39.396
Fenfluramine	T50.5X1	T50.5X2	T50.5X3	T50.5X4	T50.5X5	T50.5X6
Fenobarbital	T42.3X1	T42.3X2	T42.3X3	T42.3X4	T42.3X5	T42.3X6
Fenofibrate	T46.6X1	T46.6X2	T46.6X3	T46.6X4	T46.6X5	T46.6X6
Fenoprofen	T39.311	T39.312	T39.313	T39.314	T39.315	T39.316
Fenoterol	T48.6X1	T48.6X2	T48.6X3	T48.6X4	T48.6X5	T48.6X6

Substance	External Cause (T-Code)					
	Poisoning, Accidental (Unintentional)	Poisoning, Intentional Self-Harm	Poisoning, Assault	Poisoning, Undetermined	Adverse Effect	Underdosing
Fenoverine	T44.3X1	T44.3X2	T44.3X3	T44.3X4	T44.3X5	T44.3X6
Fenoxazoline	T48.5X1	T48.5X2	T48.5X3	T48.5X4	T48.5X5	T48.5X6
Fenproporex	T5Ø.5X1	T5Ø.5X2	T5Ø.5X3	T5Ø.5X4	T5Ø.5X5	T5Ø.5X6
Fenquizone	T5Ø.2X1	T5Ø.2X2	T5Ø.2X3	T5Ø.2X4	T5Ø.2X5	T5Ø.2X6
Fentanyl (analogs)	T4Ø.411	T4Ø.412	T4Ø.413	T4Ø.414	T4Ø.415	T4Ø.416
Fentazin	T43.3X1	T43.3X2	T43.3X3	T43.3X4	T43.3X5	T43.3X6
Fenthion	T6Ø.ØX1	T6Ø.ØX2	T6Ø.ØX3	T6Ø.ØX4	—	—
Fenticlor	T49.ØX1	T49.ØX2	T49.ØX3	T49.ØX4	T49.ØX5	T49.ØX6
Fenylbutazone	T39.2X1	T39.2X2	T39.2X3	T39.2X4	T39.2X5	T39.2X6
Feprazone	T39.2X1	T39.2X2	T39.2X3	T39.2X4	T39.2X5	T39.2X6
Fer de lance (bite) (venom)	T63.Ø61	T63.Ø62	T63.Ø63	T63.Ø64	—	—
Ferric—*see also* *Iron*						
chloride	T45.4X1	T45.4X2	T45.4X3	T45.4X4	T45.4X5	T45.4X6
citrate	T45.4X1	T45.4X2	T45.4X3	T45.4X4	T45.4X5	T45.4X6
hydroxide						
colloidal	T45.4X1	T45.4X2	T45.4X3	T45.4X4	T45.4X5	T45.4X6
polymaltose	T45.4X1	T45.4X2	T45.4X3	T45.4X4	T45.4X5	T45.4X6
pyrophosphate	T45.4X1	T45.4X2	T45.4X3	T45.4X4	T45.4X5	T45.4X6
Ferritin	T45.4X1	T45.4X2	T45.4X3	T45.4X4	T45.4X5	T45.4X6
Ferrocholinate	T45.4X1	T45.4X2	T45.4X3	T45.4X4	T45.4X5	T45.4X6
Ferrodextrane	T45.4X1	T45.4X2	T45.4X3	T45.4X4	T45.4X5	T45.4X6
Ferropolimaler	T45.4X1	T45.4X2	T45.4X3	T45.4X4	T45.4X5	T45.4X6
Ferrous—*see also* *Iron*						
phosphate	T45.4X1	T45.4X2	T45.4X3	T45.4X4	T45.4X5	T45.4X6
salt	T45.4X1	T45.4X2	T45.4X3	T45.4X4	T45.4X5	T45.4X6
with folic acid	T45.4X1	T45.4X2	T45.4X3	T45.4X4	T45.4X5	T45.4X6
Ferrous fumerate, gluconate, lactate, salt NEC, sulfate (medicinal)	T45.4X1	T45.4X2	T45.4X3	T45.4X4	T45.4X5	T45.4X6
Ferrovanadium (fumes)	T59.891	T59.892	T59.893	T59.894	—	—
Ferrum—*see* *Iron*						
Fertilizers NEC	T65.891	T65.892	T65.893	T65.894	—	—
with herbicide mixture	T6Ø.3X1	T6Ø.3X2	T6Ø.3X3	T6Ø.3X4	—	—
Fetoxilate	T47.6X1	T47.6X2	T47.6X3	T47.6X4	T47.6X5	T47.6X6
Fiber, dietary	T47.4X1	T47.4X2	T47.4X3	T47.4X4	T47.4X5	T47.4X6
Fibrinogen (human)	T45.8X1	T45.8X2	T45.8X3	T45.8X4	T45.8X5	T45.8X6
Fibrinolysin (human)	T45.691	T45.692	T45.693	T45.694	T45.695	T45.696
Fibrinolysis						
affecting drug	T45.6Ø1	T45.6Ø2	T45.6Ø3	T45.6Ø4	T45.6Ø5	T45.6Ø6
inhibitor NEC	T45.621	T45.622	T45.623	T45.624	T45.625	T45.626
Fibrinolytic drug	T45.611	T45.612	T45.613	T45.614	T45.615	T45.616
Filix mas	T37.4X1	T37.4X2	T37.4X3	T37.4X4	T37.4X5	T37.4X6
Filtering cream	T49.3X1	T49.3X2	T49.3X3	T49.3X4	T49.3X5	T49.3X6

Substance	External Cause (T-Code)					
	Poisoning, Accidental (Unintentional)	Poisoning, Intentional Self-Harm	Poisoning, Assault	Poisoning, Undetermined	Adverse Effect	Underdosing
Fiorinal	T39.Ø11	T39.Ø12	T39.Ø13	T39.Ø14	T39.Ø15	T39.Ø16
Firedamp	T59.891	T59.892	T59.893	T59.894	—	—
Fish, noxious, nonbacterial	T61.91	T61.92	T61.93	T61.94	—	—
ciguatera	T61.Ø1	T61.Ø2	T61.Ø3	T61.Ø4	—	—
scombroid	T61.11	T61.12	T61.13	T61.14	—	—
shell	T61.781	T61.782	T61.783	T61.784	—	—
specified NEC	T61.771	T61.772	T61.773	T61.774	—	—
Flagyl	T37.3X1	T37.3X2	T37.3X3	T37.3X4	T37.3X5	T37.3X6
Flavine adenine dinucleotide	T45.2X1	T45.2X2	T45.2X3	T45.2X4	T45.2X5	T45.2X6
Flavodic acid	T46.991	T46.992	T46.993	T46.994	T46.995	T46.996
Flavoxate	T44.3X1	T44.3X2	T44.3X3	T44.3X4	T44.3X5	T44.3X6
Flaxedil	T48.1X1	T48.1X2	T48.1X3	T48.1X4	T48.1X5	T48.1X6
Flaxseed (medicinal)	T49.3X1	T49.3X2	T49.3X3	T49.3X4	T49.3X5	T49.3X6
Flecainide	T46.2X1	T46.2X2	T46.2X3	T46.2X4	T46.2X5	T46.2X6
Fleroxacin	T36.8X1	T36.8X2	T36.8X3	T36.8X4	T36.8X5	T36.8X6
Floctafenine	T39.8X1	T39.8X2	T39.8X3	T39.8X4	T39.8X5	T39.8X6
Flomax	T44.6X1	T44.6X2	T44.6X3	T44.6X4	T44.6X5	T44.6X6
Flomoxef	T36.1X1	T36.1X2	T36.1X3	T36.1X4	T36.1X5	T36.1X6
Flopropione	T44.3X1	T44.3X2	T44.3X3	T44.3X4	T44.3X5	T44.3X6
Florantyrone	T47.5X1	T47.5X2	T47.5X3	T47.5X4	T47.5X5	T47.5X6
Floraquin	T37.8X1	T37.8X2	T37.8X3	T37.8X4	T37.8X5	T37.8X6
Florinef	T38.ØX1	T38.ØX2	T38.ØX3	T38.ØX4	T38.ØX5	T38.ØX6
ENT agent	T49.6X1	T49.6X2	T49.6X3	T49.6X4	T49.6X5	T49.6X6
ophthalmic preparation	T49.5X1	T49.5X2	T49.5X3	T49.5X4	T49.5X5	T49.5X6
topical NEC	T49.ØX1	T49.ØX2	T49.ØX3	T49.ØX4	T49.ØX5	T49.ØX6
Flowers of sulfur	T49.4X1	T49.4X2	T49.4X3	T49.4X4	T49.4X5	T49.4X6
Floxuridine	T45.1X1	T45.1X2	T45.1X3	T45.1X4	T45.1X5	T45.1X6
Fluanisone	T43.4X1	T43.4X2	T43.4X3	T43.4X4	T43.4X5	T43.4X6
Flubendazole	T37.4X1	T37.4X2	T37.4X3	T37.4X4	T37.4X5	T37.4X6
Fluclorolone acetonide	T49.ØX1	T49.ØX2	T49.ØX3	T49.ØX4	T49.ØX5	T49.ØX6
Flucloxacillin	T36.ØX1	T36.ØX2	T36.ØX3	T36.ØX4	T36.ØX5	T36.ØX6
Fluconazole	T37.8X1	T37.8X2	T37.8X3	T37.8X4	T37.8X5	T37.8X6
Flucytosine	T37.8X1	T37.8X2	T37.8X3	T37.8X4	T37.8X5	T37.8X6
Fludeoxyglucose (18F)	T5Ø.8X1	T5Ø.8X2	T5Ø.8X3	T5Ø.8X4	T5Ø.8X5	T5Ø.8X6
Fludiazepam	T42.4X1	T42.4X2	T42.4X3	T42.4X4	T42.4X5	T42.4X6
Fludrocortisone	T5Ø.ØX1	T5Ø.ØX2	T5Ø.ØX3	T5Ø.ØX4	T5Ø.ØX5	T5Ø.ØX6
ENT agent	T49.6X1	T49.6X2	T49.6X3	T49.6X4	T49.6X5	T49.6X6
ophthalmic preparation	T49.5X1	T49.5X2	T49.5X3	T49.5X4	T49.5X5	T49.5X6
topical NEC	T49.ØX1	T49.ØX2	T49.ØX3	T49.ØX4	T49.ØX5	T49.ØX6
Fludroxycortide	T49.ØX1	T49.ØX2	T49.ØX3	T49.ØX4	T49.ØX5	T49.ØX6
Flufenamic acid	T39.391	T39.392	T39.393	T39.394	T39.395	T39.396
Fluindione	T45.511	T45.512	T45.513	T45.514	T45.515	T45.516

Substance	External Cause (T-Code)					
	Poisoning, Accidental (Unintentional)	Poisoning, Intentional Self-Harm	Poisoning, Assault	Poisoning, Undetermined	Adverse Effect	Underdosing
Flumequine	T37.8X1	T37.8X2	T37.8X3	T37.8X4	T37.8X5	T37.8X6
Flumethasone	T49.0X1	T49.0X2	T49.0X3	T49.0X4	T49.0X5	T49.0X6
Flumethiazide	T50.2X1	T50.2X2	T50.2X3	T50.2X4	T50.2X5	T50.2X6
Flumidin	T37.5X1	T37.5X2	T37.5X3	T37.5X4	T37.5X5	T37.5X6
Flunarizine	T46.7X1	T46.7X2	T46.7X3	T46.7X4	T46.7X5	T46.7X6
Flunidazole	T37.8X1	T37.8X2	T37.8X3	T37.8X4	T37.8X5	T37.8X6
Flunisolide	T48.6X1	T48.6X2	T48.6X3	T48.6X4	T48.6X5	T48.6X6
Flunitrazepam	T42.4X1	T42.4X2	T42.4X3	T42.4X4	T42.4X5	T42.4X6
Fluocinolone (acetonide)	T49.0X1	T49.0X2	T49.0X3	T49.0X4	T49.0X5	T49.0X6
Fluocinonide	T49.0X1	T49.0X2	T49.0X3	T49.0X4	T49.0X5	T49.0X6
Fluocortin (butyl)	T49.0X1	T49.0X2	T49.0X3	T49.0X4	T49.0X5	T49.0X6
Fluocortolone	T49.0X1	T49.0X2	T49.0X3	T49.0X4	T49.0X5	T49.0X6
Fluohydrocortisone	T38.0X1	T38.0X2	T38.0X3	T38.0X4	T38.0X5	T38.0X6
ENT agent	T49.6X1	T49.6X2	T49.6X3	T49.6X4	T49.6X5	T49.6X6
ophthalmic preparation	T49.5X1	T49.5X2	T49.5X3	T49.5X4	T49.5X5	T49.5X6
topical NEC	T49.0X1	T49.0X2	T49.0X3	T49.0X4	T49.0X5	T49.0X6
Fluonid	T49.0X1	T49.0X2	T49.0X3	T49.0X4	T49.0X5	T49.0X6
Fluopromazine	T43.3X1	T43.3X2	T43.3X3	T43.3X4	T43.3X5	T43.3X6
Fluoroacetate	T60.8X1	T60.8X2	T60.8X3	T60.8X4	—	—
Fluorescein	T50.8X1	T50.8X2	T50.8X3	T50.8X4	T50.8X5	T50.8X6
Fluorhydrocortisone	T50.0X1	T50.0X2	T50.0X3	T50.0X4	T50.0X5	T50.0X6
Fluoride (nonmedicinal) (pesticide) (sodium) NEC	T60.8X1	T60.8X2	T60.8X3	T60.8X4	—	—
hydrogen — *see Hydrofluoric acid*						
medicinal NEC	T50.991	T50.992	T50.993	T50.994	T50.995	T50.996
dental use	T49.7X1	T49.7X2	T49.7X3	T49.7X4	T49.7X5	T49.7X6
not pesticide NEC	T54.91	T54.92	T54.93	T54.94	—	—
stannous	T49.7X1	T49.7X2	T49.7X3	T49.7X4	T49.7X5	T49.7X6
Fluorinated corticosteroids	T38.0X1	T38.0X2	T38.0X3	T38.0X4	T38.0X5	T38.0X6
Fluorine (gas)	T59.5X1	T59.5X2	T59.5X3	T59.5X4	—	—
salt — *see Fluoride(s)*						
Fluoristan	T49.7X1	T49.7X2	T49.7X3	T49.7X4	T49.7X5	T49.7X6
Fluormetholone	T49.0X1	T49.0X2	T49.0X3	T49.0X4	T49.0X5	T49.0X6
Fluoroacetate	T60.8X1	T60.8X2	T60.8X3	T60.8X4	—	—
Fluorocarbon monomer	T53.6X1	T53.6X2	T53.6X3	T53.6X4	—	—
Fluorocytosine	T37.8X1	T37.8X2	T37.8X3	T37.8X4	T37.8X5	T37.8X6
Fluorodeoxyuridine	T45.1X1	T45.1X2	T45.1X3	T45.1X4	T45.1X5	T45.1X6
Fluorometholone	T49.0X1	T49.0X2	T49.0X3	T49.0X4	T49.0X5	T49.0X6
ophthalmic preparation	T49.5X1	T49.5X2	T49.5X3	T49.5X4	T49.5X5	T49.5X6
Fluorophosphate insecticide	T60.0X1	T60.0X2	T60.0X3	T60.0X4	—	—
Fluorosol	T46.3X1	T46.3X2	T46.3X3	T46.3X4	T46.3X5	T46.3X6
Fluorouracil	T45.1X1	T45.1X2	T45.1X3	T45.1X4	T45.1X5	T45.1X6

Substance	External Cause (T-Code)					
	Poisoning, Accidental (Unintentional)	Poisoning, Intentional Self-Harm	Poisoning, Assault	Poisoning, Undetermined	Adverse Effect	Underdosing
Fluorphenylalanine	T49.5X1	T49.5X2	T49.5X3	T49.5X4	T49.5X5	T49.5X6
Fluothane	T41.0X1	T41.0X2	T41.0X3	T41.0X4	T41.0X5	T41.0X6
Fluoxetine	T43.221	T43.222	T43.223	T43.224	T43.225	T43.226
Fluoxymesterone	T38.7X1	T38.7X2	T38.7X3	T38.7X4	T38.7X5	T38.7X6
Flupenthixol	T43.4X1	T43.4X2	T43.4X3	T43.4X4	T43.4X5	T43.4X6
Flupentixol	T43.4X1	T43.4X2	T43.4X3	T43.4X4	T43.4X5	T43.4X6
Fluphenazine	T43.3X1	T43.3X2	T43.3X3	T43.3X4	T43.3X5	T43.3X6
Fluprednidene	T49.0X1	T49.0X2	T49.0X3	T49.0X4	T49.0X5	T49.0X6
Fluprednisolone	T38.0X1	T38.0X2	T38.0X3	T38.0X4	T38.0X5	T38.0X6
Fluradoline	T39.8X1	T39.8X2	T39.8X3	T39.8X4	T39.8X5	T39.8X6
Flurandrenolide	T49.0X1	T49.0X2	T49.0X3	T49.0X4	T49.0X5	T49.0X6
Flurandrenolone	T49.0X1	T49.0X2	T49.0X3	T49.0X4	T49.0X5	T49.0X6
Flurazepam	T42.4X1	T42.4X2	T42.4X3	T42.4X4	T42.4X5	T42.4X6
Flurbiprofen	T39.311	T39.312	T39.313	T39.314	T39.315	T39.316
Flurobate	T49.0X1	T49.0X2	T49.0X3	T49.0X4	T49.0X5	T49.0X6
Flurotyl	T43.291	T43.292	T43.293	T43.294	T43.295	T43.296
Fluroxene	T41.0X1	T41.0X2	T41.0X3	T41.0X4	T41.0X5	T41.0X6
Fluspirilene	T43.591	T43.592	T43.593	T43.594	T43.595	T43.596
Flutamide	T38.6X1	T38.6X2	T38.6X3	T38.6X4	T38.6X5	T38.6X6
Flutazolam	T42.4X1	T42.4X2	T42.4X3	T42.4X4	T42.4X5	T42.4X6
Fluticasone propionate	T38.0X1	T38.0X2	T38.0X3	T38.0X4	T38.0X5	T38.0X6
Flutoprazepam	T42.4X1	T42.4X2	T42.4X3	T42.4X4	T42.4X5	T42.4X6
Flutropium bromide	T48.6X1	T48.6X2	T48.6X3	T48.6X4	T48.6X5	T48.6X6
Fluvoxamine	T43.221	T43.222	T43.223	T43.224	T43.225	T43.226
Folacin	T45.8X1	T45.8X2	T45.8X3	T45.8X4	T45.8X5	T45.8X6
Folic acid	T45.8X1	T45.8X2	T45.8X3	T45.8X4	T45.8X5	T45.8X6
with ferrous salt	T45.2X1	T45.2X2	T45.2X3	T45.2X4	T45.2X5	T45.2X6
antagonist	T45.1X1	T45.1X2	T45.1X3	T45.1X4	T45.1X5	T45.1X6
Folinic acid	T45.8X1	T45.8X2	T45.8X3	T45.8X4	T45.8X5	T45.8X6
Folium stramoniae	T48.6X1	T48.6X2	T48.6X3	T48.6X4	T48.6X5	T48.6X6
Follicle-stimulating hormone, human	T38.811	T38.812	T38.813	T38.814	T38.815	T38.816
Folpet	T60.3X1	T60.3X2	T60.3X3	T60.3X4	—	—
Fominoben	T48.3X1	T48.3X2	T48.3X3	T48.3X4	T48.3X5	T48.3X6
Food, foodstuffs, noxious, nonbacterial, NEC	T62.91	T62.92	T62.93	T62.94	—	—
berries	T62.1X1	T62.1X2	T62.1X3	T62.1X4	—	—
fish — *see also Fish*	T61.91	T61.92	T61.93	T61.94	—	—
mushrooms	T62.0X1	T62.0X2	T62.0X3	T62.0X4	—	—
plants	T62.2X1	T62.2X2	T62.2X3	T62.2X4	—	—
seafood	T61.91	T61.92	T61.93	T61.94	—	—
specified NEC	T61.8X1	T61.8X2	T61.8X3	T61.8X4	—	—
seeds	T62.2X1	T62.2X2	T62.2X3	T62.2X4	—	—

Substance	Poisoning, Accidental (Unintentional)	Poisoning, Intentional Self-Harm	Poisoning, Assault	Poisoning, Undetermined	Adverse Effect	Underdosing
	External Cause (T-Code)					
Food, foodstuffs, noxious, nonbacterial, NEC *(Continued)*						
shellfish	T61.781	T61.782	T61.783	T61.784	—	—
specified NEC	T62.8X1	T62.8X2	T62.8X3	T62.8X4	—	—
Fool's parsley	T62.2X1	T62.2X2	T62.2X3	T62.2X4	—	—
Formaldehyde (solution), gas or vapor	T59.2X1	T59.2X2	T59.2X3	T59.2X4	—	—
fungicide	T6Ø.3X1	T6Ø.3X2	T6Ø.3X3	T6Ø.3X4	—	—
Formalin	T59.2X1	T59.2X2	T59.2X3	T59.2X4	—	—
fungicide	T6Ø.3X1	T6Ø.3X2	T6Ø.3X3	T6Ø.3X4	—	—
vapor	T59.2X1	T59.2X2	T59.2X3	T59.2X4	—	—
Formic acid	T54.2X1	T54.2X2	T54.2X3	T54.2X4	—	—
vapor	T59.891	T59.892	T59.893	T59.894	—	—
Foscarnet sodium	T37.5X1	T37.5X2	T37.5X3	T37.5X4	T37.5X5	T37.5X6
Fosfestrol	T38.5X1	T38.5X2	T38.5X3	T38.5X4	T38.5X5	T38.5X6
Fosfomycin	T36.8X1	T36.8X2	T36.8X3	T36.8X4	T36.8X5	T36.8X6
Fosfonet sodium	T37.5X1	T37.5X2	T37.5X3	T37.5X4	T37.5X5	T37.5X6
Fosinopril	T46.4X1	T46.4X2	T46.4X3	T46.4X4	T46.4X5	T46.4X6
sodium	T46.4X1	T46.4X2	T46.4X3	T46.4X4	T46.4X5	T46.4X6
Fowler's solution	T57.ØX1	T57.ØX2	T57.ØX3	T57.ØX4	—	—
Foxglove	T62.2X1	T62.2X2	T62.2X3	T62.2X4	—	—
Framycetin	T36.5X1	T36.5X2	T36.5X3	T36.5X4	T36.5X5	T36.5X6
Frangula	T47.2X1	T47.2X2	T47.2X3	T47.2X4	T47.2X5	T47.2X6
extract	T47.2X1	T47.2X2	T47.2X3	T47.2X4	T47.2X5	T47.2X6
Frei antigen	T5Ø.8X1	T5Ø.8X2	T5Ø.8X3	T5Ø.8X4	T5Ø.8X5	T5Ø.8X6
Freon	T53.5X1	T53.5X2	T53.5X3	T53.5X4	—	—
Fructose	T5Ø.3X1	T5Ø.3X2	T5Ø.3X3	T5Ø.3X4	T5Ø.3X5	T5Ø.3X6
Frusemide	T5Ø.1X1	T5Ø.1X2	T5Ø.1X3	T5Ø.1X4	T5Ø.1X5	T5Ø.1X6
FSH	T38.811	T38.812	T38.813	T38.814	T38.815	T38.816
Ftorafur	T45.1X1	T45.1X2	T45.1X3	T45.1X4	T45.1X5	T45.1X6
Fuel						
automobile	T52.ØX1	T52.ØX2	T52.ØX3	T52.ØX4	—	—
exhaust gas, not in transit	T58.Ø1	T58.Ø2	T58.Ø3	T58.Ø4	—	—
vapor NEC	T52.ØX1	T52.ØX2	T52.ØX3	T52.ØX4	—	—
gas (domestic use) — *see also Carbon, monoxide, fuel, utility*	T59.891	T59.892	T59.893	T59.894	—	—
utility	T59.891	T59.892	T59.893	T59.894	—	—
in mobile container	T59.891	T59.892	T59.893	T59.894	—	—
incomplete combustion of — *see Carbon, monoxide, fuel, utility*						
piped (natural)	T59.891	T59.892	T59.893	T59.894	—	—
industrial, incomplete combustion	T58.8X1	T58.8X2	T58.8X3	T58.8X4	—	—

Substance	Poisoning, Accidental (Unintentional)	Poisoning, Intentional Self-Harm	Poisoning, Assault	Poisoning, Undetermined	Adverse Effect	Underdosing
	External Cause (T-Code)					
Fugillin	T36.8X1	T36.8X2	T36.8X3	T36.8X4	T36.8X5	T36.8X6
Fulminate of mercury	T56.1X1	T56.1X2	T56.1X3	T56.1X4	—	—
Fulvicin	T36.7X1	T36.7X2	T36.7X3	T36.7X4	T36.7X5	T36.7X6
Fumadil	T36.8X1	T36.8X2	T36.8X3	T36.8X4	T36.8X5	T36.8X6
Fumagillin	T36.8X1	T36.8X2	T36.8X3	T36.8X4	T36.8X5	T36.8X6
Fumaric acid	T49.4X1	T49.4X2	T49.4X3	T49.4X4	T49.4X5	T49.4X6
Fumes (from)	T59.91	T59.92	T59.93	T59.94	—	—
carbon monoxide — *see Carbon, monoxide*						
charcoal (domestic use) — *see Charcoal, fumes*						
chloroform — *see Chloroform*						
coke (in domestic stoves, fireplaces) — *see Coke, fumes*						
corrosive NEC	T54.91	T54.92	T54.93	T54.94	—	—
ether — *see Ether*						
freons	T53.5X1	T53.5X2	T53.5X3	T53.5X4	—	—
hydrocarbons	T59.891	T59.892	T59.893	T59.894	—	—
petroleum (liquefied)	T59.891	T59.892	T59.893	T59.894	—	—
distributed through pipes (pure or mixed with air)	T59.891	T59.892	T59.893	T59.894	—	—
lead — *see Lead*						
metal — *see Metals, or the specified metal*						
nitrogen dioxide	T59.ØX1	T59.ØX2	T59.ØX3	T59.ØX4	—	—
pesticides — *see Pesticide*						
petroleum (liquefied)	T59.891	T59.892	T59.893	T59.894	—	—
distributed through pipes (pure or mixed with air)	T59.891	T59.892	T59.893	T59.894	—	—
polyester	T59.891	T59.892	T59.893	T59.894	—	—
specified source NEC — *see also substance specified*	T59.891	T59.892	T59.893	T59.894	—	—
sulfur dioxide	T59.1X1	T59.1X2	T59.1X3	T59.1X4	—	—
Fumigant NEC	T6Ø.91	T6Ø.92	T6Ø.93	T6Ø.94	—	—
Fungi, noxious, used as food	T62.ØX1	T62.ØX2	T62.ØX3	T62.ØX4	—	—
Fungicide NEC (nonmedicinal)	T6Ø.3X1	T6Ø.3X2	T6Ø.3X3	T6Ø.3X4	—	—
Fungizone	T36.7X1	T36.7X2	T36.7X3	T36.7X4	T36.7X5	T36.7X6
topical	T49.ØX1	T49.ØX2	T49.ØX3	T49.ØX4	T49.ØX5	T49.ØX6
Furacin	T49.ØX1	T49.ØX2	T49.ØX3	T49.ØX4	T49.ØX5	T49.ØX6
Furadantin	T37.91	T37.92	T37.93	T37.94	T37.95	T37.96
Furazolidone	T37.8X1	T37.8X2	T37.8X3	T37.8X4	T37.8X5	T37.8X6
Furazolium chloride	T49.ØX1	T49.ØX2	T49.ØX3	T49.ØX4	T49.ØX5	T49.ØX6
Furfural	T52.8X1	T52.8X2	T52.8X3	T52.8X4	—	—

◀ New ◀ Revised ~~deleted~~ Deleted

	External Cause (T-Code)					
Substance	**Poisoning, Accidental (Unintentional)**	**Poisoning, Intentional Self-Harm**	**Poisoning, Assault**	**Poisoning, Undetermined**	**Adverse Effect**	**Underdosing**
Furnace (coal burning) (domestic), gas from industrial	T58.2X1	T58.2X2	T58.2X3	T58.2X4	—	—
industrial	T58.8X1	T58.8X2	T58.8X3	T58.8X4	—	—
Furniture polish	T65.891	T65.892	T65.893	T65.894	—	—
Furosemide	T5Ø.1X1	T5Ø.1X2	T5Ø.1X3	T5Ø.1X4	T5Ø.1X5	T5Ø.1X6
Furoxone	T37.91	T37.92	T37.93	T37.94	T37.95	T37.96
Fursultiamine	T45.2X1	T45.2X2	T45.2X3	T45.2X4	T45.2X5	T45.2X6
Fusafungine	T36.8X1	T36.8X2	T36.8X3	T36.8X4	T36.8X5	T36.8X6
Fusel oil (any) (amyl) (butyl) (propyl), vapor	T51.3X1	T51.3X2	T51.3X3	T51.3X4	—	—
Fusidate (ethanolamine) (sodium)	T36.8X1	T36.8X2	T36.8X3	T36.8X4	T36.8X5	T36.8X6
Fusidic acid	T36.8X1	T36.8X2	T36.8X3	T36.8X4	T36.8X5	T36.8X6
Fytic acid, nonasodium	T5Ø.6X1	T5Ø.6X2	T5Ø.6X3	T5Ø.6X4	T5Ø.6X5	T5Ø.6X6
G						
GABA	T43.8X1	T43.8X2	T43.8X3	T43.8X4	T43.8X5	T43.8X6
Gadolinium	T56.821	T56.822	T56.823	T56.824	T56.825	—
Gadopentetic acid	T5Ø.8X1	T5Ø.8X2	T5Ø.8X3	T5Ø.8X4	T5Ø.8X5	T5Ø.8X6
Galactose	T5Ø.3X1	T5Ø.3X2	T5Ø.3X3	T5Ø.3X4	T5Ø.3X5	T5Ø.3X6
b-Galactosidase	T47.5X1	T47.5X2	T47.5X3	T47.5X4	T47.5X5	T47.5X6
Galantamine	T44.ØX1	T44.ØX2	T44.ØX3	T44.ØX4	T44.ØX5	T44.ØX6
Gallamine (triethiodide)	T48.1X1	T48.1X2	T48.1X3	T48.1X4	T48.1X5	T48.1X6
Gallium citrate	T5Ø.991	T5Ø.992	T5Ø.993	T5Ø.994	T5Ø.995	T5Ø.996
Gallopamil	T46.1X1	T46.1X2	T46.1X3	T46.1X4	T46.1X5	T46.1X6
Gamboge	T47.2X1	T47.2X2	T47.2X3	T47.2X4	T47.2X5	T47.2X6
Gamimune	T5Ø.Z11	T5Ø.Z12	T5Ø.Z13	T5Ø.Z14	T5Ø.Z15	T5Ø.Z16
Gamma-aminobutyric acid	T43.8X1	T43.8X2	T43.8X3	T43.8X4	T43.8X5	T43.8X6
Gamma-benzene hexachloride (medicinal)	T49.ØX1	T49.ØX2	T49.ØX3	T49.ØX4	T49.ØX5	T49.ØX6
nonmedicinal, vapor	T53.6X1	T53.6X2	T53.6X3	T53.6X4	—	—
Gamma-BHC (medicinal) — *see also Gamma-benzene hexachloride*	T49.ØX1	T49.ØX2	T49.ØX3	T49.ØX4	T49.ØX5	T49.ØX6
Gamma globulin	T5Ø.Z11	T5Ø.Z12	T5Ø.Z13	T5Ø.Z14	T5Ø.Z15	T5Ø.Z16
Gamulin	T5Ø.Z11	T5Ø.Z12	T5Ø.Z13	T5Ø.Z14	T5Ø.Z15	T5Ø.Z16
Ganciclovir (sodium)	T37.5X1	T37.5X2	T37.5X3	T37.5X4	T37.5X5	T37.5X6
Ganglionic blocking drug NEC	T44.2X1	T44.2X2	T44.2X3	T44.2X4	T44.2X5	T44.2X6
specified NEC	T44.2X1	T44.2X2	T44.2X3	T44.2X4	T44.2X5	T44.2X6
Ganja	T4Ø.711	T4Ø.712	T4Ø.713	T4Ø.714	T4Ø.715	T4Ø.716
Garamycin	T36.5X1	T36.5X2	T36.5X3	T36.5X4	T36.5X5	T36.5X6
ophthalmic preparation	T49.5X1	T49.5X2	T49.5X3	T49.5X4	T49.5X5	T49.5X6
topical NEC	T49.ØX1	T49.ØX2	T49.ØX3	T49.ØX4	T49.ØX5	T49.ØX6
Gardenal	T42.3X1	T42.3X2	T42.3X3	T42.3X4	T42.3X5	T42.3X6

	External Cause (T-Code)					
Substance	**Poisoning, Accidental (Unintentional)**	**Poisoning, Intentional Self-Harm**	**Poisoning, Assault**	**Poisoning, Undetermined**	**Adverse Effect**	**Underdosing**
Gardepanyl	T42.3X1	T42.3X2	T42.3X3	T42.3X4	T42.3X5	T42.3X6
Gas NEC	T59.91	T59.92	T59.93	T59.94	—	—
acetylene	T59.891	T59.892	T59.893	T59.894	—	—
incomplete combustion of	T58.11	T58.12	T58.13	T58.14	—	—
air contaminants, source or type not specified	T59.91	T59.92	T59.93	T59.94	—	—
anesthetic	T41.ØX1	T41.ØX2	T41.ØX3	T41.ØX4	T41.ØX5	T41.ØX6
blast furnace	T58.8X1	T58.8X2	T58.8X3	T58.8X4	—	—
butane — see Butane						
carbon monoxide — see Carbon, monoxide						
chlorine	T59.4X1	T59.4X2	T59.4X3	T59.4X4	—	—
coal	T58.2X1	T58.2X2	T58.2X3	T58.2X4	—	—
cyanide	T57.3X1	T57.3X2	T57.3X3	T57.3X4	—	—
dicyanogen	T65.ØX1	T65.ØX2	T65.ØX3	T65.ØX4	—	—
domestic — see Domestic gas	T57.91	T57.92	T57.93	T57.94	—	—
exhaust	T57.91	T57.92	T57.93	T57.94	—	—
from utility (for cooking, heating, or lighting) (after combustion) — see Carbon, monoxide, fuel, utility						
prior to combustion	T59.891	T59.892	T59.893	T59.894	—	—
from wood or coal-burning stove or fireplace	T57.91	T57.92	T57.93	T57.94	—	—
fuel (domestic use) (after combustion) — see also Carbon, monoxide, fuel	T57.91	T57.92	T57.93	T57.94	—	—
industrial use	T58.8X1	T58.8X2	T58.8X3	T58.8X4	—	—
prior to combustion	T59.891	T59.892	T59.893	T59.894	—	—
utility	T59.891	T59.892	T59.893	T59.894	—	—
in mobile container	T59.891	T59.892	T59.893	T59.894	—	—
incomplete combustion of — see Carbon, monoxide, fuel, utility						
piped (natural)	T59.891	T59.892	T59.893	T59.894	—	—
garage	T58.Ø1	T58.Ø2	T58.Ø3	T58.Ø4	—	—
hydrocarbon NEC	T59.891	T59.892	T59.893	T59.894	—	—
incomplete combustion of — see Carbon, monoxide, fuel, utility						
liquefied — see Butane						
piped	T59.891	T59.892	T59.893	T59.894	—	—
hydrocyanic acid	T65.ØX1	T65.ØX2	T65.ØX3	T65.ØX4	—	—

Substance	External Cause (T-Code) Poisoning, Accidental (Unintentional)	Poisoning, Intentional Self-Harm	Poisoning, Assault	Poisoning, Undetermined	Adverse Effect	Underdosing
Gas NEC *(Continued)*						
illuminating (after combustion)	T58.11	T58.12	T58.13	T58.14	—	—
prior to combustion	T59.891	T59.892	T59.893	T59.894	—	—
incomplete combustion, any—see Carbon, monoxide						
kiln	T58.8X1	T58.8X2	T58.8X3	T58.8X4	—	—
lacrimogenic	T59.3X1	T59.3X2	T59.3X3	T59.3X4	—	—
liquefied petroleum—see Butane						
marsh	T59.891	T59.892	T59.893	T59.894	—	—
motor exhaust, not in transit	T58.Ø1	T58.Ø2	T58.Ø3	T58.Ø4	—	—
mustard, not in war	T59.891	T59.892	T59.893	T59.894	—	—
natural	T59.891	T59.892	T59.893	T59.894	—	—
nerve, not in war	T59.91	T59.92	T59.93	T59.94	—	—
oil	T52.ØX1	T52.ØX2	T52.ØX3	T52.ØX4	—	—
petroleum (liquefied) (distributed in mobile containers)	T59.891	T59.892	T59.893	T59.894	—	—
piped (pure or mixed with air)	T59.891	T59.892	T59.893	T59.894	—	—
piped (manufactured) (natural) NEC	T59.891	T59.892	T59.893	T59.894	—	—
producer	T58.8X1	T58.8X2	T58.8X3	T58.8X4	—	—
propane—see Propane						
refrigerant (chlorofluoro-carbon)	T53.5X1	T53.5X2	T53.5X3	T53.5X4	—	—
not chlorofluoro-carbon	T59.891	T59.892	T59.893	T59.894	—	—
sewer	T59.91	T59.92	T59.93	T59.94	—	—
specified source NEC	T59.91	T59.92	T59.93	T59.94	—	—
stove (after combustion)	T58.11	T58.12	T58.13	T58.14	—	—
tear	T59.3X1	T59.3X2	T59.3X3	T59.3X4	—	—
therapeutic	T41.5X1	T41.5X2	T41.5X3	T41.5X4	T41.5X5	T41.5X6
utility (for cooking, heating, or lighting) (piped) NEC	T59.891	T59.892	T59.893	T59.894	—	—
in mobile container	T59.891	T59.892	T59.893	T59.894	—	—
incomplete combustion of—see Carbon, monoxide, fuel, utility						
piped (natural)	T59.891	T59.892	T59.893	T59.894	—	—
water	T58.11	T58.12	T58.13	T58.14	—	—
incomplete combustion of—see Carbon, monoxide, fuel, utility						

Substance	External Cause (T-Code) Poisoning, Accidental (Unintentional)	Poisoning, Intentional Self-Harm	Poisoning, Assault	Poisoning, Undetermined	Adverse Effect	Underdosing
Gaseous substance—*see Gas*						
Gasoline	T52.ØX1	T52.ØX2	T52.ØX3	T52.ØX4	—	—
vapor	T52.ØX1	T52.ØX2	T52.ØX3	T52.ØX4	—	—
Gastric enzymes	T47.5X1	T47.5X2	T47.5X3	T47.5X4	T47.5X5	T47.5X6
Gastrografin	T5Ø.8X1	T5Ø.8X2	T5Ø.8X3	T5Ø.8X4	T5Ø.8X5	T5Ø.8X6
Gastrointestinal drug	T47.91	T47.92	T47.93	T47.94	T47.95	T47.96
biological	T47.8X1	T47.8X2	T47.8X3	T47.8X4	T47.8X5	T47.8X6
specified NEC	T47.8X1	T47.8X2	T47.8X3	T47.8X4	T47.8X5	T47.8X6
Gaultheria procumbens	T62.2X1	T62.2X2	T62.2X3	T62.2X4	—	—
Gelatin (intravenous)	T45.8X1	T45.8X2	T45.8X3	T45.8X4	T45.8X5	T45.8X6
absorbable (sponge)	T45.7X1	T45.7X2	T45.7X3	T45.7X4	T45.7X5	T45.7X6
Gefarnate	T44.3X1	T44.3X2	T44.3X3	T44.3X4	T44.3X5	T44.3X6
Gelfilm	T49.8X1	T49.8X2	T49.8X3	T49.8X4	T49.8X5	T49.8X6
Gelfoam	T45.7X1	T45.7X2	T45.7X3	T45.7X4	T45.7X5	T45.7X6
Gelsemine	T5Ø.991	T5Ø.992	T5Ø.993	T5Ø.994	T5Ø.995	T5Ø.996
Gelsemium (sempervirens)	T62.2X1	T62.2X2	T62.2X3	T62.2X4	—	—
Gemeprost	T48.ØX1	T48.ØX2	T48.ØX3	T48.ØX4	T48.ØX5	T48.ØX6
Gemfibrozil	T46.6X1	T46.6X2	T46.6X3	T46.6X4	T46.6X5	T46.6X6
Gemonil	T42.3X1	T42.3X2	T42.3X3	T42.3X4	T42.3X5	T42.3X6
Gentamicin	T36.5X1	T36.5X2	T36.5X3	T36.5X4	T36.5X5	T36.5X6
ophthalmic preparation	T49.5X1	T49.5X2	T49.5X3	T49.5X4	T49.5X5	T49.5X6
topical NEC	T49.ØX1	T49.ØX2	T49.ØX3	T49.ØX4	T49.ØX5	T49.ØX6
Gentian	T47.5X1	T47.5X2	T47.5X3	T47.5X4	T47.5X5	T47.5X6
violet	T49.ØX1	T49.ØX2	T49.ØX3	T49.ØX4	T49.ØX5	T49.ØX6
Gepefrine	T44.4X1	T44.4X2	T44.4X3	T44.4X4	T44.4X5	T44.4X6
Gestonorone caproate	T38.5X1	T38.5X2	T38.5X3	T38.5X4	T38.5X5	T38.5X6
Gexane	T49.ØX1	T49.ØX2	T49.ØX3	T49.ØX4	T49.ØX5	T49.ØX6
Gila monster (venom)	T63.111	T63.112	T63.113	T63.114	—	—
Ginger	T47.5X1	T47.5X2	T47.5X3	T47.5X4	T47.5X5	T47.5X6
Jamaica—*see Jamaica, ginger*						
Gitalin	T46.ØX1	T46.ØX2	T46.ØX3	T46.ØX4	T46.ØX5	T46.ØX6
amorphous	T46.ØX1	T46.ØX2	T46.ØX3	T46.ØX4	T46.ØX5	T46.ØX6
Gitaloxin	T46.ØX1	T46.ØX2	T46.ØX3	T46.ØX4	T46.ØX5	T46.ØX6
Gitoxin	T46.ØX1	T46.ØX2	T46.ØX3	T46.ØX4	T46.ØX5	T46.ØX6
Glafenine	T39.8X1	T39.8X2	T39.8X3	T39.8X4	T39.8X5	T39.8X6
Glandular extract (medicinal) NEC	T5Ø.Z91	T5Ø.Z92	T5Ø.Z93	T5Ø.Z94	T5Ø.Z95	T5Ø.Z96
Glaucarubin	T37.3X1	T37.3X2	T37.3X3	T37.3X4	T37.3X5	T37.3X6
Glibenclamide	T38.3X1	T38.3X2	T38.3X3	T38.3X4	T38.3X5	T38.3X6
Glibornuride	T38.3X1	T38.3X2	T38.3X3	T38.3X4	T38.3X5	T38.3X6
Gliclazide	T38.3X1	T38.3X2	T38.3X3	T38.3X4	T38.3X5	T38.3X6
Glimidine	T38.3X1	T38.3X2	T38.3X3	T38.3X4	T38.3X5	T38.3X6

◀ New ◀ Revised ~~deleted~~ Deleted

Substance	External Cause (T-Code)					
	Poisoning, Accidental (Unintentional)	Poisoning, Intentional Self-Harm	Poisoning, Assault	Poisoning, Undetermined	Adverse Effect	Underdosing
Glipizide	T38.3X1	T38.3X2	T38.3X3	T38.3X4	T38.3X5	T38.3X6
Gliquidone	T38.3X1	T38.3X2	T38.3X3	T38.3X4	T38.3X5	T38.3X6
Glisolamide	T38.3X1	T38.3X2	T38.3X3	T38.3X4	T38.3X5	T38.3X6
Glisoxepide	T38.3X1	T38.3X2	T38.3X3	T38.3X4	T38.3X5	T38.3X6
Globin zinc insulin	T38.3X1	T38.3X2	T38.3X3	T38.3X4	T38.3X5	T38.3X6
Globulin						
antilymphocytic	T5Ø.Z11	T5Ø.Z12	T5Ø.Z13	T5Ø.Z14	T5Ø.Z15	T5Ø.Z16
antirhesus	T5Ø.Z11	T5Ø.Z12	T5Ø.Z13	T5Ø.Z14	T5Ø.Z15	T5Ø.Z16
antivenin	T5Ø.Z11	T5Ø.Z12	T5Ø.Z13	T5Ø.Z14	T5Ø.Z15	T5Ø.Z16
antiviral	T5Ø.Z11	T5Ø.Z12	T5Ø.Z13	T5Ø.Z14	T5Ø.Z15	T5Ø.Z16
Glucagon	T38.3X1	T38.3X2	T38.3X3	T38.3X4	T38.3X5	T38.3X6
Glucocorticoids	T38.ØX1	T38.ØX2	T38.ØX3	T38.ØX4	T38.ØX5	T38.ØX6
Glucocorticosteroid	T38.ØX1	T38.ØX2	T38.ØX3	T38.ØX4	T38.ØX5	T38.ØX6
Gluconic acid	T5Ø.991	T5Ø.992	T5Ø.993	T5Ø.994	T5Ø.995	T5Ø.996
Glucosamine sulfate	T39.4X1	T39.4X2	T39.4X3	T39.4X4	T39.4X5	T39.4X6
Glucose	T5Ø.3X1	T5Ø.3X2	T5Ø.3X3	T5Ø.3X4	T5Ø.3X5	T5Ø.3X6
with sodium chloride	T5Ø.3X1	T5Ø.3X2	T5Ø.3X3	T5Ø.3X4	T5Ø.3X5	T5Ø.3X6
Glucosulfone sodium	T37.1X1	T37.1X2	T37.1X3	T37.1X4	T37.1X5	T37.1X6
Glucurolactone	T47.8X1	T47.8X2	T47.8X3	T47.8X4	T47.8X5	T47.8X6
Glue NEC	T52.8X1	T52.8X2	T52.8X3	T52.8X4	—	—
Glutamic acid	T47.5X1	T47.5X2	T47.5X3	T47.5X4	T47.5X5	T47.5X6
Glutaral (medicinal)	T49.ØX1	T49.ØX2	T49.ØX3	T49.ØX4	T49.ØX5	T49.ØX6
nonmedicinal	T65.891	T65.892	T65.893	T65.894	—	—
Glutaraldehyde (nonmedicinal)	T65.891	T65.892	T65.893	T65.894	—	—
medicinal	T49.ØX1	T49.ØX2	T49.ØX3	T49.ØX4	T49.ØX5	T49.ØX6
Glutathione	T5Ø.6X1	T5Ø.6X2	T5Ø.6X3	T5Ø.6X4	T5Ø.6X5	T5Ø.6X6
Glutethimide	T42.6X1	T42.6X2	T42.6X3	T42.6X4	T42.6X5	T42.6X6
Glyburide	T38.3X1	T38.3X2	T38.3X3	T38.3X4	T38.3X5	T38.3X6
Glycerin	T47.4X1	T47.4X2	T47.4X3	T47.4X4	T47.4X5	T47.4X6
Glycerol	T47.4X1	T47.4X2	T47.4X3	T47.4X4	T47.4X5	T47.4X6
borax	T49.6X1	T49.6X2	T49.6X3	T49.6X4	T49.6X5	T49.6X6
intravenous	T5Ø.3X1	T5Ø.3X2	T5Ø.3X3	T5Ø.3X4	T5Ø.3X5	T5Ø.3X6
iodinated	T48.4X1	T48.4X2	T48.4X3	T48.4X4	T48.4X5	T48.4X6
Glycerophosphate	T5Ø.991	T5Ø.992	T5Ø.993	T5Ø.994	T5Ø.995	T5Ø.996
Glyceryl						
gualacolate	T48.4X1	T48.4X2	T48.4X3	T48.4X4	T48.4X5	T48.4X6
nitrate	T46.3X1	T46.3X2	T46.3X3	T46.3X4	T46.3X5	T46.3X6
triacetate (topical)	T49.ØX1	T49.ØX2	T49.ØX3	T49.ØX4	T49.ØX5	T49.ØX6
trinitrate	T46.3X1	T46.3X2	T46.3X3	T46.3X4	T46.3X5	T46.3X6
Glycine	T5Ø.3X1	T5Ø.3X2	T5Ø.3X3	T5Ø.3X4	T5Ø.3X5	T5Ø.3X6
Glyclopyramide	T38.3X1	T38.3X2	T38.3X3	T38.3X4	T38.3X5	T38.3X6
Glycobiarsol	T37.3X1	T37.3X2	T37.3X3	T37.3X4	T37.3X5	T37.3X6

Substance	External Cause (T-Code)					
	Poisoning, Accidental (Unintentional)	Poisoning, Intentional Self-Harm	Poisoning, Assault	Poisoning, Undetermined	Adverse Effect	Underdosing
Glycols (ether)	T52.3X1	T52.3X2	T52.3X3	T52.3X4	—	—
Glyconiazide	T37.1X1	T37.1X2	T37.1X3	T37.1X4	T37.1X5	T37.1X6
Glycopyrrolate	T44.3X1	T44.3X2	T44.3X3	T44.3X4	T44.3X5	T44.3X6
Glycopyrronium	T44.3X1	T44.3X2	T44.3X3	T44.3X4	T44.3X5	T44.3X6
bromide	T44.3X1	T44.3X2	T44.3X3	T44.3X4	T44.3X5	T44.3X6
Glycoside, cardiac (stimulant)	T46.ØX1	T46.ØX2	T46.ØX3	T46.ØX4	T46.ØX5	T46.ØX6
Glycyclamide	T38.3X1	T38.3X2	T38.3X3	T38.3X4	T38.3X5	T38.3X6
Glycyrrhiza extract	T48.4X1	T48.4X2	T48.4X3	T48.4X4	T48.4X5	T48.4X6
Glycyrrhizic acid	T48.4X1	T48.4X2	T48.4X3	T48.4X4	T48.4X5	T48.4X6
Glycyrrhizinate potassium	T48.4X1	T48.4X2	T48.4X3	T48.4X4	T48.4X5	T48.4X6
Glymidine sodium	T38.3X1	T38.3X2	T38.3X3	T38.3X4	T38.3X5	T38.3X6
Glyphosate	T6Ø.3X1	T6Ø.3X2	T6Ø.3X3	T6Ø.3X4	—	—
Glyphylline	T48.6X1	T48.6X2	T48.6X3	T48.6X4	T48.6X5	T48.6X6
Gold						
colloidal (l98Au)	T45.1X1	T45.1X2	T45.1X3	T45.1X4	T45.1X5	T45.1X6
salts	T39.4X1	T39.4X2	T39.4X3	T39.4X4	T39.4X5	T39.4X6
Golden sulfide of antimony	T56.891	T56.892	T56.893	T56.894	—	—
Goldylocks	T62.2X1	T62.2X2	T62.2X3	T62.2X4	—	—
Gonadal tissue extract	T38.9Ø1	T38.9Ø2	T38.9Ø3	T38.9Ø4	T38.9Ø5	T38.9Ø6
female	T38.5X1	T38.5X2	T38.5X3	T38.5X4	T38.5X5	T38.5X6
male	T38.7X1	T38.7X2	T38.7X3	T38.7X4	T38.7X5	T38.7X6
Gonadorelin	T38.891	T38.892	T38.893	T38.894	T38.895	T38.896
Gonadotropin	T38.891	T38.892	T38.893	T38.894	T38.895	T38.896
chorionic	T38.891	T38.892	T38.893	T38.894	T38.895	T38.896
pituitary	T38.811	T38.812	T38.813	T38.814	T38.815	T38.816
Goserelin	T45.1X1	T45.1X2	T45.1X3	T45.1X4	T45.1X5	T45.1X6
Grain alcohol	T51.ØX1	T51.ØX2	T51.ØX3	T51.ØX4	—	—
Gramicidin	T49.ØX1	T49.ØX2	T49.ØX3	T49.ØX4	T49.ØX5	T49.ØX6
Granisetron	T45.ØX1	T45.ØX2	T45.ØX3	T45.ØX4	T45.ØX5	T45.ØX6
Gratiola officinalis	T62.2X1	T62.2X2	T62.2X3	T62.2X4	—	—
Grease	T65.891	T65.892	T65.893	T65.894	—	—
Green hellebore	T62.2X1	T62.2X2	T62.2X3	T62.2X4	—	—
Green soap	T49.2X1	T49.2X2	T49.2X3	T49.2X4	T49.2X5	T49.2X6
Grifulvin	T36.7X1	T36.7X2	T36.7X3	T36.7X4	T36.7X5	T36.7X6
Griseofulvin	T36.7X1	T36.7X2	T36.7X3	T36.7X4	T36.7X5	T36.7X6
Growth hormone	T38.811	T38.812	T38.813	T38.814	T38.815	T38.816
Guaiacol derivatives	T48.4X1	T48.4X2	T48.4X3	T48.4X4	T48.4X5	T48.4X6
Guaiac reagent	T5Ø.991	T5Ø.992	T5Ø.993	T5Ø.994	T5Ø.995	T5Ø.996
Guaifenesin	T48.4X1	T48.4X2	T48.4X3	T48.4X4	T48.4X5	T48.4X6
Guaimesal	T48.4X1	T48.4X2	T48.4X3	T48.4X4	T48.4X5	T48.4X6
Guaiphenesin	T48.4X1	T48.4X2	T48.4X3	T48.4X4	T48.4X5	T48.4X6
Guamecycline	T36.4X1	T36.4X2	T36.4X3	T36.4X4	T36.4X5	T36.4X6

TABLE OF DRUGS AND CHEMICALS

	External Cause (T-Code)					
Substance	Poisoning, Accidental (Unintentional)	Poisoning, Intentional Self-Harm	Poisoning, Assault	Poisoning, Undetermined	Adverse Effect	Underdosing
Guanabenz	T46.5X1	T46.5X2	T46.5X3	T46.5X4	T46.5X5	T46.5X6
Guanacline	T46.5X1	T46.5X2	T46.5X3	T46.5X4	T46.5X5	T46.5X6
Guanadrel	T46.5X1	T46.5X2	T46.5X3	T46.5X4	T46.5X5	T46.5X6
Guanatol	T37.2X1	T37.2X2	T37.2X3	T37.2X4	T37.2X5	T37.2X6
Guanethidine	T46.5X1	T46.5X2	T46.5X3	T46.5X4	T46.5X5	T46.5X6
Guanfacine	T46.5X1	T46.5X2	T46.5X3	T46.5X4	T46.5X5	T46.5X6
Guano	T65.891	T65.892	T65.893	T65.894	—	—
Guanochlor	T46.5X1	T46.5X2	T46.5X3	T46.5X4	T46.5X5	T46.5X6
Guanoclor	T46.5X1	T46.5X2	T46.5X3	T46.5X4	T46.5X5	T46.5X6
Guanoctine	T46.5X1	T46.5X2	T46.5X3	T46.5X4	T46.5X5	T46.5X6
Guanoxabenz	T46.5X1	T46.5X2	T46.5X3	T46.5X4	T46.5X5	T46.5X6
Guanoxan	T46.5X1	T46.5X2	T46.5X3	T46.5X4	T46.5X5	T46.5X6
Guar gum (medicinal)	T46.6X1	T46.6X2	T46.6X3	T46.6X4	T46.6X5	T46.6X6
H						
Hachimycin	T36.7X1	T36.7X2	T36.7X3	T36.7X4	T36.7X5	T36.7X6
Hair						
dye	T49.4X1	T49.4X2	T49.4X3	T49.4X4	T49.4X5	T49.4X6
preparation NEC	T49.4X1	T49.4X2	T49.4X3	T49.4X4	T49.4X5	T49.4X6
Halazepam	T42.4X1	T42.4X2	T42.4X3	T42.4X4	T42.4X5	T42.4X6
Halcinolone	T49.0X1	T49.0X2	T49.0X3	T49.0X4	T49.0X5	T49.0X6
Halcinonide	T49.0X1	T49.0X2	T49.0X3	T49.0X4	T49.0X5	T49.0X6
Halethazole	T49.0X1	T49.0X2	T49.0X3	T49.0X4	T49.0X5	T49.0X6
Hallucinogen NOS	T40.901	T40.902	T40.903	T40.904	T40.905	T40.906
specified NEC	T40.991	T40.992	T40.993	T40.994	T40.995	T40.996
Halofantrine	T37.2X1	T37.2X2	T37.2X3	T37.2X4	T37.2X5	T37.2X6
Halofenate	T46.6X1	T46.6X2	T46.6X3	T46.6X4	T46.6X5	T46.6X6
Halometasone	T49.0X1	T49.0X2	T49.0X3	T49.0X4	T49.0X5	T49.0X6
Haloperidol	T43.4X1	T43.4X2	T43.4X3	T43.4X4	T43.4X5	T43.4X6
Haloprogin	T49.0X1	T49.0X2	T49.0X3	T49.0X4	T49.0X5	T49.0X6
Halotex	T49.0X1	T49.0X2	T49.0X3	T49.0X4	T49.0X5	T49.0X6
Halothane	T41.0X1	T41.0X2	T41.0X3	T41.0X4	T41.0X5	T41.0X6
Haloxazolam	T42.4X1	T42.4X2	T42.4X3	T42.4X4	T42.4X5	T42.4X6
Halquinols	T49.0X1	T49.0X2	T49.0X3	T49.0X4	T49.0X5	T49.0X6
Hamamelis	T49.2X1	T49.2X2	T49.2X3	T49.2X4	T49.2X5	T49.2X6
Haptendextran	T45.8X1	T45.8X2	T45.8X3	T45.8X4	T45.8X5	T45.8X6
Harmonyl	T46.5X1	T46.5X2	T46.5X3	T46.5X4	T46.5X5	T46.5X6
Hartmann's solution	T50.3X1	T50.3X2	T50.3X3	T50.3X4	T50.3X5	T50.3X6
Hashish	T40.711	T40.712	T40.713	T40.714	T40.715	T40.716
Hawaiian Woodrose seeds	T40.991	T40.992	T40.993	T40.994	—	—
HCB	T60.3X1	T60.3X2	T60.3X3	T60.3X4	—	—
HCH	T53.6X1	T53.6X2	T53.6X3	T53.6X4	—	—
medicinal	T49.0X1	T49.0X2	T49.0X3	T49.0X4	T49.0X5	T49.0X6
HCN	T57.3X1	T57.3X2	T57.3X3	T57.3X4	—	—
Headache cures, drugs, powders NEC	T50.901	T50.902	T50.903	T50.904	T50.905	T50.906
Heavenly Blue (morning glory)	T40.991	T40.992	T40.993	T40.994	—	—
Heavy metal antidote	T45.8X1	T45.8X2	T45.8X3	T45.8X4	T45.8X5	T45.8X6
Hedaquinium	T49.0X1	T49.0X2	T49.0X3	T49.0X4	T49.0X5	T49.0X6
Hedge hyssop	T62.2X1	T62.2X2	T62.2X3	T62.2X4	—	—
Heet	T49.8X1	T49.8X2	T49.8X3	T49.8X4	T49.8X5	T49.8X6
Helium	T48.991	T48.992	T48.993	T48.994	T48.995	T48.996
Helenin	T37.4X1	T37.4X2	T37.4X3	T37.4X4	T37.4X5	T37.4X6
Hellebore (black) (green) (white)	T62.2X1	T62.2X2	T62.2X3	T62.2X4	—	—
Helium (nonmedicinal) NEC	T59.891	T59.892	T59.893	T59.894	—	—
medicinal	T48.991	T48.992	T48.993	T48.994	T48.995	T48.996
Hematin	T45.8X1	T45.8X2	T45.8X3	T45.8X4	T45.8X5	T45.8X6
Hematinic preparation	T45.8X1	T45.8X2	T45.8X3	T45.8X4	T45.8X5	T45.8X6
Hemlock	T62.2X1	T62.2X2	T62.2X3	T62.2X4	—	—
Hemostatic	T45.621	T45.622	T45.623	T45.624	T45.625	T45.626
drug, systemic	T45.621	T45.622	T45.623	T45.624	T45.625	T45.626
Hemostyptic	T49.4X1	T49.4X2	T49.4X3	T49.4X4	T49.4X5	T49.4X6
Henbane	T62.2X1	T62.2X2	T62.2X3	T62.2X4	—	—
Heparin (sodium)	T45.511	T45.512	T45.513	T45.514	T45.515	T45.516
action reverser	T45.7X1	T45.7X2	T45.7X3	T45.7X4	T45.7X5	T45.7X6
Heparin-fraction	T45.511	T45.512	T45.513	T45.514	T45.515	T45.516
Heparinoid (systemic)	T45.511	T45.512	T45.513	T45.514	T45.515	T45.516
Hepatic secretion stimulant	T47.8X1	T47.8X2	T47.8X3	T47.8X4	T47.8X5	T47.8X6
Hepatitis B						
immune globulin	T50.Z11	T50.Z12	T50.Z13	T50.Z14	T50.Z15	T50.Z16
vaccine	T50.B91	T50.B92	T50.B93	T50.B94	T50.B95	T50.B96
Hepronicate	T46.7X1	T46.7X2	T46.7X3	T46.7X4	T46.7X5	T46.7X6
Heptabarb	T42.3X1	T42.3X2	T42.3X3	T42.3X4	T42.3X5	T42.3X6
Heptabarbitone	T42.3X1	T42.3X2	T42.3X3	T42.3X4	T42.3X5	T42.3X6
Heptabarbital	T42.3X1	T42.3X2	T42.3X3	T42.3X4	T42.3X5	T42.3X6
Heptachlor	T60.1X1	T60.1X2	T60.1X3	T60.1X4	—	—
Heptalgin	T40.2X1	T40.2X2	T40.2X3	T40.2X4	T40.2X5	T40.2X6
Heptaminol	T46.3X1	T46.3X2	T46.3X3	T46.3X4	T46.3X5	T46.3X6
Herbicide NEC	T60.3X1	T60.3X2	T60.3X3	T60.3X4	—	—
Heroin	T40.1X1	T40.1X2	T40.1X3	T40.1X4	—	—
Herplex	T49.5X1	T49.5X2	T49.5X3	T49.5X4	T49.5X5	T49.5X6
HES	T45.8X1	T45.8X2	T45.8X3	T45.8X4	T45.8X5	T45.8X6
Hesperidin	T46.991	T46.992	T46.993	T46.994	T46.995	T46.996
Hetacillin	T36.0X1	T36.0X2	T36.0X3	T36.0X4	T36.0X5	T36.0X6

Substance	External Cause (T-Code)					
	Poisoning, Accidental (Unintentional)	Poisoning, Intentional Self-Harm	Poisoning, Assault	Poisoning, Undetermined	Adverse Effect	Underdosing
Hetastarch	T45.8X1	T45.8X2	T45.8X3	T45.8X4	T45.8X5	T45.8X6
HETP	T60.0X1	T60.0X2	T60.0X3	T60.0X4	—	—
Hexachlorobenzene (vapor)	T60.3X1	T60.3X2	T60.3X3	T60.3X4	—	—
Hexachlorocyclohexane	T53.6X1	T53.6X2	T53.6X3	T53.6X4	—	—
Hexachlorophene	T49.0X1	T49.0X2	T49.0X3	T49.0X4	T49.0X5	T49.0X6
Hexadiline	T46.3X1	T46.3X2	T46.3X3	T46.3X4	T46.3X5	T46.3X6
Hexadimethrine (bromide)	T45.7X1	T45.7X2	T45.7X3	T45.7X4	T45.7X5	T45.7X6
Hexadylamine	T46.3X1	T46.3X2	T46.3X3	T46.3X4	T46.3X5	T46.3X6
Hexaethyl tetraphosphate	T60.0X1	T60.0X2	T60.0X3	T60.0X4	—	—
Hexafluorenium bromide	T48.1X1	T48.1X2	T48.1X3	T48.1X4	T48.1X5	T48.1X6
Hexafluorodiethyl ether	T43.291	T43.292	T43.293	T43.294	T43.295	T43.296
Hexafluronium (bromide)	T48.1X1	T48.1X2	T48.1X3	T48.1X4	T48.1X5	T48.1X6
Hexahydrobenzol	T52.8X1	T52.8X2	T52.8X3	T52.8X4	—	—
Hexahydrocresol(s)	T51.8X1	T51.8X2	T51.8X3	T51.8X4	—	—
arsenide	T57.0X1	T57.0X2	T57.0X3	T57.0X4	—	—
arseniurated	T57.0X1	T57.0X2	T57.0X3	T57.0X4	—	—
cyanide	T57.3X1	T57.3X2	T57.3X3	T57.3X4	—	—
gas	T59.891	T59.892	T59.893	T59.894	—	—
Fluoride (liquid)	T57.8X1	T57.8X2	T57.8X3	T57.8X4	—	—
vapor	T59.891	T59.892	T59.893	T59.894	—	—
phohorated	T60.0X1	T60.0X2	T60.0X3	T60.0X4	—	—
sulfate	T57.8X1	T57.8X2	T57.8X3	T57.8X4	—	—
sulfide (gas)	T59.6X1	T59.6X2	T59.6X3	T59.6X4	—	—
arseniurated	T57.0X1	T57.0X2	T57.0X3	T57.0X4	—	—
sulfurated	T57.8X1	T57.8X2	T57.8X3	T57.8X4	—	—
Hexahydrophenol	T51.8X1	T51.8X2	T51.8X3	T51.8X4	—	—
Hexa-germ	T49.2X1	T49.2X2	T49.2X3	T49.2X4	T49.2X5	T49.2X6
Hexalen	T51.8X1	T51.8X2	T51.8X3	T51.8X4	—	—
Hexamethonium bromide	T44.2X1	T44.2X2	T44.2X3	T44.2X4	T44.2X5	T44.2X6
Hexamethylene	T52.8X1	T52.8X2	T52.8X3	T52.8X4	—	—
Hexamethylmelamine	T45.1X1	T45.1X2	T45.1X3	T45.1X4	T45.1X5	T45.1X6
Hexamidine	T49.0X1	T49.0X2	T49.0X3	T49.0X4	T49.0X5	T49.0X6
Hexamine (mandelate)	T37.8X1	T37.8X2	T37.8X3	T37.8X4	T37.8X5	T37.8X6
Hexanone, 2-hexanone	T52.4X1	T52.4X2	T52.4X3	T52.4X4	—	—
Hexanuorenium	T48.1X1	T48.1X2	T48.1X3	T48.1X4	T48.1X5	T48.1X6
Hexapropymate	T42.6X1	T42.6X2	T42.6X3	T42.6X4	T42.6X5	T42.6X6
Hexasonium iodide	T44.3X1	T44.3X2	T44.3X3	T44.3X4	T44.3X5	T44.3X6
Hexcarbacholine bromide	T48.1X1	T48.1X2	T48.1X3	T48.1X4	T48.1X5	T48.1X6
Hexemal	T42.3X1	T42.3X2	T42.3X3	T42.3X4	T42.3X5	T42.3X6
Hexestrol	T38.5X1	T38.5X2	T38.5X3	T38.5X4	T38.5X5	T38.5X6
Hexethal (sodium)	T42.3X1	T42.3X2	T42.3X3	T42.3X4	T42.3X5	T42.3X6
Hexetidine	T37.8X1	T37.8X2	T37.8X3	T37.8X4	T37.8X5	T37.8X6
Hexobarbital	T42.3X1	T42.3X2	T42.3X3	T42.3X4	T42.3X5	T42.3X6
rectal	T41.291	T41.292	T41.293	T41.294	T41.295	T41.296
sodium	T41.1X1	T41.1X2	T41.1X3	T41.1X4	T41.1X5	T41.1X6
Hexobendine	T46.3X1	T46.3X2	T46.3X3	T46.3X4	T46.3X5	T46.3X6
Hexocyclium	T44.3X1	T44.3X2	T44.3X3	T44.3X4	T44.3X5	T44.3X6
metilsulfate	T44.3X1	T44.3X2	T44.3X3	T44.3X4	T44.3X5	T44.3X6
Hexoestrol	T38.5X1	T38.5X2	T38.5X3	T38.5X4	T38.5X5	T38.5X6
Hexone	T52.4X1	T52.4X2	T52.4X3	T52.4X4	—	—
Hexoprenaline	T48.6X1	T48.6X2	T48.6X3	T48.6X4	T48.6X5	T48.6X6
Hexylcaine	T41.3X1	T41.3X2	T41.3X3	T41.3X4	T41.3X5	T41.3X6
Hexylresorcinol	T52.2X1	T52.2X2	T52.2X3	T52.2X4	—	—
HGH (human growth hormone)	T38.811	T38.812	T38.813	T38.814	T38.815	T38.816
Hinkle's pills	T47.2X1	T47.2X2	T47.2X3	T47.2X4	T47.2X5	T47.2X6
Histalog	T50.8X1	T50.8X2	T50.8X3	T50.8X4	T50.8X5	T50.8X6
Histamine (phosphate)	T50.8X1	T50.8X2	T50.8X3	T50.8X4	T50.8X5	T50.8X6
Histoplasmin	T50.8X1	T50.8X2	T50.8X3	T50.8X4	T50.8X5	T50.8X6
Holly berries	T62.2X1	T62.2X2	T62.2X3	T62.2X4	—	—
Homatropine	T44.3X1	T44.3X2	T44.3X3	T44.3X4	T44.3X5	T44.3X6
methylbromide	T44.3X1	T44.3X2	T44.3X3	T44.3X4	T44.3X5	T44.3X6
Homochlorcyclizine	T45.0X1	T45.0X2	T45.0X3	T45.0X4	T45.0X5	T45.0X6
Homosalate	T49.3X1	T49.3X2	T49.3X3	T49.3X4	T49.3X5	T49.3X6
Homo-tet	T50.Z11	T50.Z12	T50.Z13	T50.Z14	T50.Z15	T50.Z16
Hormone	T38.801	T38.802	T38.803	T38.804	T38.805	T38.806
adrenal cortical steroids	T38.0X1	T38.0X2	T38.0X3	T38.0X4	T38.0X5	T38.0X6
androgenic	T38.7X1	T38.7X2	T38.7X3	T38.7X4	T38.7X5	T38.7X6
anterior pituitary NEC	T38.811	T38.812	T38.813	T38.814	T38.815	T38.816
antidiabetic agents	T38.3X1	T38.3X2	T38.3X3	T38.3X4	T38.3X5	T38.3X6
antidiuretic	T38.891	T38.892	T38.893	T38.894	T38.895	T38.896
cancer therapy	T45.1X1	T45.1X2	T45.1X3	T45.1X4	T45.1X5	T45.1X6
follicle stimulating	T38.811	T38.812	T38.813	T38.814	T38.815	T38.816
gonadotropic	T38.891	T38.892	T38.893	T38.894	T38.895	T38.896
pituitary	T38.811	T38.812	T38.813	T38.814	T38.815	T38.816
growth	T38.811	T38.812	T38.813	T38.814	T38.815	T38.816
luteinizing	T38.811	T38.812	T38.813	T38.814	T38.815	T38.816
ovarian	T38.5X1	T38.5X2	T38.5X3	T38.5X4	T38.5X5	T38.5X6
oxytocic	T48.0X1	T48.0X2	T48.0X3	T48.0X4	T48.0X5	T48.0X6
parathyroid (derivatives)	T50.991	T50.992	T50.993	T50.994	T50.995	T50.996
pituitary (posterior) NEC	T38.891	T38.892	T38.893	T38.894	T38.895	T38.896
anterior	T38.811	T38.812	T38.813	T38.814	T38.815	T38.816
specified, NEC	T38.891	T38.892	T38.893	T38.894	T38.895	T38.896
thyroid	T38.1X1	T38.1X2	T38.1X3	T38.1X4	T38.1X5	T38.1X6
Hornet (sting)	T63.451	T63.452	T63.453	T63.454	—	—

Substance	External Cause (T-Code) Poisoning, Accidental (Unintentional)	Poisoning, Intentional Self-Harm	Poisoning, Assault	Poisoning, Undetermined	Adverse Effect	Underdosing
Horse anti-human lymphocytic serum	T5Ø.Z11	T5Ø.Z12	T5Ø.Z13	T5Ø.Z14	T5Ø.Z15	T5Ø.Z16
Horticulture agent NEC	T65.91	T65.92	T65.93	T65.94	—	—
with pesticide	T6Ø.91	T6Ø.92	T6Ø.93	T6Ø.94	—	—
Human						
albumin	T45.8X1	T45.8X2	T45.8X3	T45.8X4	T45.8X5	T45.8X6
growth hormone (HGH)	T38.811	T38.812	T38.813	T38.814	T38.815	T38.816
immune serum	T5Ø.Z11	T5Ø.Z12	T5Ø.Z13	T5Ø.Z14	T5Ø.Z15	T5Ø.Z16
Hyaluronidase	T45.3X1	T45.3X2	T45.3X3	T45.3X4	T45.3X5	T45.3X6
Hyazyme	T45.3X1	T45.3X2	T45.3X3	T45.3X4	T45.3X5	T45.3X6
Hycodan	T4Ø.2X1	T4Ø.2X2	T4Ø.2X3	T4Ø.2X4	T4Ø.2X5	T4Ø.2X6
Hydantoin derivative NEC	T42.ØX1	T42.ØX2	T42.ØX3	T42.ØX4	T42.ØX5	T42.ØX6
Hydeltra	T38.ØX1	T38.ØX2	T38.ØX3	T38.ØX4	T38.ØX5	T38.ØX6
Hydergine	T44.6X1	T44.6X2	T44.6X3	T44.6X4	T44.6X5	T44.6X6
Hydrabamine penicillin	T36.ØX1	T36.ØX2	T36.ØX3	T36.ØX4	T36.ØX5	T36.ØX6
Hydralazine	T46.5X1	T46.5X2	T46.5X3	T46.5X4	T46.5X5	T46.5X6
Hydrargaphen	T49.ØX1	T49.ØX2	T49.ØX3	T49.ØX4	T49.ØX5	T49.ØX6
Hydrargyri amino-chloridum	T49.ØX1	T49.ØX2	T49.ØX3	T49.ØX4	T49.ØX5	T49.ØX6
Hydrastine	T48.291	T48.292	T48.293	T48.294	T48.295	T48.296
Hydrazine	T54.1X1	T54.1X2	T54.1X3	T54.1X4	—	—
monoamine oxidase inhibitors	T43.1X1	T43.1X2	T43.1X3	T43.1X4	T43.1X5	T43.1X6
Hydrazoic acid, azides	T54.2X1	T54.2X2	T54.2X3	T54.2X4	—	—
Hydriodic acid	T48.4X1	T48.4X2	T48.4X3	T48.4X4	T48.4X5	T48.4X6
Hydrocarbon gas	T59.891	T59.892	T59.893	T59.894	—	—
incomplete combustion of—*see Carbon, monoxide, fuel, utility*						
liquefied (mobile container)	T59.891	T59.892	T59.893	T59.894	—	—
piped (natural)	T59.891	T59.892	T59.893	T59.894	—	—
Hydrochloric acid (liquid)	T54.2X1	T54.2X2	T54.2X3	T54.2X4	—	—
medicinal (digestant)	T47.5X1	T47.5X2	T47.5X3	T47.5X4	T47.5X5	T47.5X6
vapor	T59.891	T59.892	T59.893	T59.894	—	—
Hydrochlorothiazide	T5Ø.2X1	T5Ø.2X2	T5Ø.2X3	T5Ø.2X4	T5Ø.2X5	T5Ø.2X6
Hydrocodone	T4Ø.2X1	T4Ø.2X2	T4Ø.2X3	T4Ø.2X4	T4Ø.2X5	T4Ø.2X6
Hydrocortisone (derivatives)	T38.ØX1	T38.ØX2	T38.ØX3	T38.ØX4	T38.ØX5	T38.ØX6
aceponate	T49.ØX1	T49.ØX2	T49.ØX3	T49.ØX4	T49.ØX5	T49.ØX6
ENT agent	T49.6X1	T49.6X2	T49.6X3	T49.6X4	T49.6X5	T49.6X6
ophthalmic preparation	T49.5X1	T49.5X2	T49.5X3	T49.5X4	T49.5X5	T49.5X6
topical NEC	T49.ØX1	T49.ØX2	T49.ØX3	T49.ØX4	T49.ØX5	T49.ØX6
Hydrocortone	T38.ØX1	T38.ØX2	T38.ØX3	T38.ØX4	T38.ØX5	T38.ØX6
ENT agent	T49.6X1	T49.6X2	T49.6X3	T49.6X4	T49.6X5	T49.6X6
ophthalmic preparation	T49.5X1	T49.5X2	T49.5X3	T49.5X4	T49.5X5	T49.5X6
topical NEC	T49.ØX1	T49.ØX2	T49.ØX3	T49.ØX4	T49.ØX5	T49.ØX6

Substance	External Cause (T-Code) Poisoning, Accidental (Unintentional)	Poisoning, Intentional Self-Harm	Poisoning, Assault	Poisoning, Undetermined	Adverse Effect	Underdosing
Hydrocyanic acid (liquid)	T57.3X1	T57.3X2	T57.3X3	T57.3X4	—	—
gas	T65.ØX1	T65.ØX2	T65.ØX3	T65.ØX4	—	—
Hydroflumethiazide	T5Ø.2X1	T5Ø.2X2	T5Ø.2X3	T5Ø.2X4	T5Ø.2X5	T5Ø.2X6
Hydrofluoric acid (liquid)	T54.2X1	T54.2X2	T54.2X3	T54.2X4	—	—
vapor	T59.891	T59.892	T59.893	T59.894	—	—
Hydrogen	T59.891	T59.892	T59.893	T59.894	—	—
arsenide	T57.ØX1	T57.ØX2	T57.ØX3	T57.ØX4	—	—
arseniureted	T57.ØX1	T57.ØX2	T57.ØX3	T57.ØX4	—	—
chloride	T57.8X1	T57.8X2	T57.8X3	T57.8X4	—	—
cyanide (salts)	T57.3X1	T57.3X2	T57.3X3	T57.3X4	—	—
gas	T57.3X1	T57.3X2	T57.3X3	T57.3X4	—	—
Fluoride	T59.5X1	T59.5X2	T59.5X3	T59.5X4	—	—
vapor	T59.5X1	T59.5X2	T59.5X3	T59.5X4	—	—
peroxide	T49.ØX1	T49.ØX2	T49.ØX3	T49.ØX4	T49.ØX5	T49.ØX6
phosphureted	T57.1X1	T57.1X2	T57.1X3	T57.1X4	—	—
sulfide	T59.6X1	T59.6X2	T59.6X3	T59.6X4	—	—
arseniureted	T57.ØX1	T57.ØX2	T57.ØX3	T57.ØX4	—	—
sulfureted	T59.6X1	T59.6X2	T59.6X3	T59.6X4	—	—
Hydromethylpyridine	T46.7X1	T46.7X2	T46.7X3	T46.7X4	T46.7X5	T46.7X6
Hydromorphinol	T4Ø.2X1	T4Ø.2X2	T4Ø.2X3	T4Ø.2X4	—	—
Hydromorphinone	T4Ø.2X1	T4Ø.2X2	T4Ø.2X3	T4Ø.2X4	T4Ø.2X5	T4Ø.2X6
Hydromorphone	T4Ø.2X1	T4Ø.2X2	T4Ø.2X3	T4Ø.2X4	T4Ø.2X5	T4Ø.2X6
Hydromox	T5Ø.2X1	T5Ø.2X2	T5Ø.2X3	T5Ø.2X4	T5Ø.2X5	T5Ø.2X6
Hydrophilic lotion	T49.3X1	T49.3X2	T49.3X3	T49.3X4	T49.3X5	T49.3X6
Hydroquinidine	T46.2X1	T46.2X2	T46.2X3	T46.2X4	T46.2X5	T46.2X6
Hydroquinone	T52.2X1	T52.2X2	T52.2X3	T52.2X4	—	—
vapor	T59.891	T59.892	T59.893	T59.894	—	—
Hydrosulfuric acid (gas)	T59.6X1	T59.6X2	T59.6X3	T59.6X4	—	—
Hydrotalcite	T47.1X1	T47.1X2	T47.1X3	T47.1X4	T47.1X5	T47.1X6
Hydrous wool fat	T49.3X1	T49.3X2	T49.3X3	T49.3X4	T49.3X5	T49.3X6
Hydroxide, caustic	T54.3X1	T54.3X2	T54.3X3	T54.3X4	—	—
Hydroxocobalamin	T45.8X1	T45.8X2	T45.8X3	T45.8X4	T45.8X5	T45.8X6
Hydroxyamphetamine	T49.5X1	T49.5X2	T49.5X3	T49.5X4	T49.5X5	T49.5X6
Hydroxycarbamide	T45.1X1	T45.1X2	T45.1X3	T45.1X4	T45.1X5	T45.1X6
Hydroxychloroquine	T37.8X1	T37.8X2	T37.8X3	T37.8X4	T37.8X5	T37.8X6
Hydroxydihydrocodeinone	T4Ø.2X1	T4Ø.2X2	T4Ø.2X3	T4Ø.2X4	T4Ø.2X5	T4Ø.2X6
Hydroxyestrone	T38.5X1	T38.5X2	T38.5X3	T38.5X4	T38.5X5	T38.5X6
Hydroxyethyl starch	T45.8X1	T45.8X2	T45.8X3	T45.8X4	T45.8X5	T45.8X6
Hydroxymethylpentanone	T52.4X1	T52.4X2	T52.4X3	T52.4X4	—	—
Hydroxyphenamate	T43.591	T43.592	T43.593	T43.594	T43.595	T43.596
Hydroxyphenylbutazone	T39.2X1	T39.2X2	T39.2X3	T39.2X4	T39.2X5	T39.2X6

Substance	External Cause (T-Code)					
	Poisoning, Accidental (Unintentional)	Poisoning, Intentional Self-Harm	Poisoning, Assault	Poisoning, Undetermined	Adverse Effect	Underdosing
Hydroxyprogesterone	T38.5X1	T38.5X2	T38.5X3	T38.5X4	T38.5X5	T38.5X6
caproate	T38.5X1	T38.5X2	T38.5X3	T38.5X4	T38.5X5	T38.5X6
Hydroxyquinoline (derivatives) NEC	T37.8X1	T37.8X2	T37.8X3	T37.8X4	T37.8X5	T37.8X6
Hydroxystilbamidine	T37.3X1	T37.3X2	T37.3X3	T37.3X4	T37.3X5	T37.3X6
Hydroxytoluene (nonmedicinal)	T54.ØX1	T54.ØX2	T54.ØX3	T54.ØX4	—	—
medicinal	T49.ØX1	T49.ØX2	T49.ØX3	T49.ØX4	T49.ØX5	T49.ØX6
Hydroxyurea	T45.1X1	T45.1X2	T45.1X3	T45.1X4	T45.1X5	T45.1X6
Hydroxyzine	T43.591	T43.592	T43.593	T43.594	T43.595	T43.596
antiallergic	T45.ØX1	T45.ØX2	T45.ØX3	T45.ØX4	T45.ØX5	T45.ØX6
Hyoscine	T44.3X1	T44.3X2	T44.3X3	T44.3X4	T44.3X5	T44.3X6
Hyoscyamine	T44.3X1	T44.3X2	T44.3X3	T44.3X4	T44.3X5	T44.3X6
Hyoscyamus	T44.3X1	T44.3X2	T44.3X3	T44.3X4	T44.3X5	T44.3X6
dry extract	T44.3X1	T44.3X2	T44.3X3	T44.3X4	T44.3X5	T44.3X6
Hypaque	T5Ø.8X1	T5Ø.8X2	T5Ø.8X3	T5Ø.8X4	T5Ø.8X5	T5Ø.8X6
Hypertussis	T5Ø.Z11	T5Ø.Z12	T5Ø.Z13	T5Ø.Z14	T5Ø.Z15	T5Ø.Z16
Hypnotic	T42.71	T42.72	T42.73	T42.74	T42.75	T42.76
anticonvulsant	T42.71	T42.72	T42.73	T42.74	T42.75	T42.76
specified NEC	T42.6X1	T42.6X2	T42.6X3	T42.6X4	T42.6X5	T42.6X6
Hypochlorite	T49.ØX1	T49.ØX2	T49.ØX3	T49.ØX4	T49.ØX5	T49.ØX6
Hypophysis, posterior	T38.891	T38.892	T38.893	T38.894	T38.895	T38.896
Hypotensive NEC	T46.5X1	T46.5X2	T46.5X3	T46.5X4	T46.5X5	T46.5X6
Hypromellose	T49.5X1	T49.5X2	T49.5X3	T49.5X4	T49.5X5	T49.5X6
I						
Ibacitabine	T37.5X1	T37.5X2	T37.5X3	T37.5X4	T37.5X5	T37.5X6
Ibopamine	T44.991	T44.992	T44.993	T44.994	T44.995	T44.996
Ibufenac	T39.311	T39.312	T39.313	T39.314	T39.315	T39.316
Ibuprofen	T39.311	T39.312	T39.313	T39.314	T39.315	T39.316
Ibuproxam	T39.311	T39.312	T39.313	T39.314	T39.315	T39.316
Ibuterol	T48.6X1	T48.6X2	T48.6X3	T48.6X4	T48.6X5	T48.6X6
Ichthammol	T49.ØX1	T49.ØX2	T49.ØX3	T49.ØX4	T49.ØX5	T49.ØX6
Ichthyol	T49.4X1	T49.4X2	T49.4X3	T49.4X4	T49.4X5	T49.4X6
Idarubicin	T45.1X1	T45.1X2	T45.1X3	T45.1X4	T45.1X5	T45.1X6
Idrocilamide	T42.8X1	T42.8X2	T42.8X3	T42.8X4	T42.8X5	T42.8X6
Ifenprodil	T46.7X1	T46.7X2	T46.7X3	T46.7X4	T46.7X5	T46.7X6
Ifosfamide	T45.1X1	T45.1X2	T45.1X3	T45.1X4	T45.1X5	T45.1X6
Iletin	T38.3X1	T38.3X2	T38.3X3	T38.3X4	T38.3X5	T38.3X6
Ilex	T62.2X1	T62.2X2	T62.2X3	T62.2X4	—	—
Illuminating gas (after combustion)	T58.11	T58.12	T58.13	T58.14	—	—
prior to combustion	T59.891	T59.892	T59.893	T59.894	—	—
Ilopan	T45.2X1	T45.2X2	T45.2X3	T45.2X4	T45.2X5	T45.2X6

Substance	External Cause (T-Code)					
	Poisoning, Accidental (Unintentional)	Poisoning, Intentional Self-Harm	Poisoning, Assault	Poisoning, Undetermined	Adverse Effect	Underdosing
Iloprost	T46.7X1	T46.7X2	T46.7X3	T46.7X4	T46.7X5	T46.7X6
Ilotycin	T36.3X1	T36.3X2	T36.3X3	T36.3X4	T36.3X5	T36.3X6
ophthalmic preparation	T49.5X1	T49.5X2	T49.5X3	T49.5X4	T49.5X5	T49.5X6
topical NEC	T49.ØX1	T49.ØX2	T49.ØX3	T49.ØX4	T49.ØX5	T49.ØX6
Imidazole-4-carboxamide	T45.1X1	T45.1X2	T45.1X3	T45.1X4	T45.1X5	T45.1X6
Imipenem	T36.ØX1	T36.ØX2	T36.ØX3	T36.ØX4	T36.ØX5	T36.ØX6
Imipramine	T43.Ø11	T43.Ø12	T43.Ø13	T43.Ø14	T43.Ø15	T43.Ø16
Iminostilbene	T42.1X1	T42.1X2	T42.1X3	T42.1X4	T42.1X5	T42.1X6
Immu-G	T5Ø.Z11	T5Ø.Z12	T5Ø.Z13	T5Ø.Z14	T5Ø.Z15	T5Ø.Z16
Immuglobin	T5Ø.Z11	T5Ø.Z12	T5Ø.Z13	T5Ø.Z14	T5Ø.Z15	T5Ø.Z16
Immune						
checkpoint inhibitors	T45.AX1	T45.AX2	T45.AX3	T45.AX4	T45.AX5	T45.AX6
globulin	T5Ø.Z11	T5Ø.Z12	T5Ø.Z13	T5Ø.Z14	T5Ø.Z15	T5Ø.Z16
serum globulin	T5Ø.Z11	T5Ø.Z12	T5Ø.Z13	T5Ø.Z14	T5Ø.Z15	T5Ø.Z16
Immunoglobin human (intravenous) (normal)	T5Ø.Z11	T5Ø.Z12	T5Ø.Z13	T5Ø.Z14	T5Ø.Z15	T5Ø.Z16
unmodified	T5Ø.Z11	T5Ø.Z12	T5Ø.Z13	T5Ø.Z14	T5Ø.Z15	T5Ø.Z16
Immunostimulant drug	T45.AX1	T45.AX2	T45.AX3	T45.AX4	T45.AX5	T45.AX6
Immunosuppressive drug	T45.1X1	T45.1X2	T45.1X3	T45.1X4	T45.1X5	T45.1X6
Immu-tetanus	T5Ø.Z11	T5Ø.Z12	T5Ø.Z13	T5Ø.Z14	T5Ø.Z15	T5Ø.Z16
Indalpine	T43.221	T43.222	T43.223	T43.224	T43.225	T43.226
Indanazoline	T48.5X1	T48.5X2	T48.5X3	T48.5X4	T48.5X5	T48.5X6
Indandione (derivatives)	T45.511	T45.512	T45.513	T45.514	T45.515	T45.516
Indapamide	T46.5X1	T46.5X2	T46.5X3	T46.5X4	T46.5X5	T46.5X6
Indendione (derivatives)	T45.511	T45.512	T45.513	T45.514	T45.515	T45.516
Indenolol	T44.7X1	T44.7X2	T44.7X3	T44.7X4	T44.7X5	T44.7X6
Inderal	T44.7X1	T44.7X2	T44.7X3	T44.7X4	T44.7X5	T44.7X6
Indian						
hemp	T4Ø.711	T4Ø.712	T4Ø.713	T4Ø.714	T4Ø.715	T4Ø.716
tobacco	T62.2X1	T62.2X2	T62.2X3	T62.2X4	—	—
Indigo carmine	T5Ø.8X1	T5Ø.8X2	T5Ø.8X3	T5Ø.8X4	T5Ø.8X5	T5Ø.8X6
Indobufen	T45.521	T45.522	T45.523	T45.524	T45.525	T45.526
Indocin	T39.2X1	T39.2X2	T39.2X3	T39.2X4	T39.2X5	T39.2X6
Indocyanine green	T5Ø.8X1	T5Ø.8X2	T5Ø.8X3	T5Ø.8X4	T5Ø.8X5	T5Ø.8X6
Indometacin	T39.391	T39.392	T39.393	T39.394	T39.395	T39.396
Indomethacin	T39.391	T39.392	T39.393	T39.394	T39.395	T39.396
farnesil	T39.4X1	T39.4X2	T39.4X3	T39.4X4	T39.4X5	T39.4X6
Indoramin	T44.6X1	T44.6X2	T44.6X3	T44.6X4	T44.6X5	T44.6X6
Industrial						
alcohol	T51.ØX1	T51.ØX2	T51.ØX3	T51.ØX4	—	—
fumes	T59.891	T59.892	T59.893	T59.894	—	—
solvents (fumes) (vapors)	T52.91	T52.92	T52.93	T52.94	—	—
Influenza vaccine	T5Ø.B91	T5Ø.B92	T5Ø.B93	T5Ø.B94	T5Ø.B95	T5Ø.B96

◄ New   Revised   ~~deleted~~ Deleted

	External Cause (T-Code)					
Substance	**Poisoning, Accidental (Unintentional)**	**Poisoning, Intentional Self-Harm**	**Poisoning, Assault**	**Poisoning, Undetermined**	**Adverse Effect**	**Underdosing**
Ingested substance NEC	T65.91	T65.92	T65.93	T65.94	—	—
INH	T37.1X1	T37.1X2	T37.1X3	T37.1X4	T37.1X5	T37.1X6
Inhalation, gas (noxious)—*see Gas*						
Inhibitor						
angiotensin-converting enzyme	T46.4X1	T46.4X2	T46.4X3	T46.4X4	T46.4X5	T46.4X6
carbonic anhydrase	T50.2X1	T50.2X2	T50.2X3	T50.2X4	T50.2X5	T50.2X6
fibrinolysis	T45.621	T45.622	T45.623	T45.624	T45.625	T45.626
monoamine oxidase NEC	T43.1X1	T43.1X2	T43.1X3	T43.1X4	T43.1X5	T43.1X6
hydrazine	T43.1X1	T43.1X2	T43.1X3	T43.1X4	T43.1X5	T43.1X6
postsynaptic	T43.8X1	T43.8X2	T43.8X3	T43.8X4	T43.8X5	T43.8X6
prothrombin synthesis	T45.511	T45.512	T45.513	T45.514	T45.515	T45.516
Ink	T65.891	T65.892	T65.893	T65.894	—	—
Inorganic substance NEC	T57.91	T57.92	T57.93	T57.94	—	—
Inosine pranobex	T37.5X1	T37.5X2	T37.5X3	T37.5X4	T37.5X5	T37.5X6
Inositol	T50.991	T50.992	T50.993	T50.994	T50.995	T50.996
nicotinate	T46.7X1	T46.7X2	T46.7X3	T46.7X4	T46.7X5	T46.7X6
Inproquone	T45.1X1	T45.1X2	T45.1X3	T45.1X4	T45.1X5	T45.1X6
Insect (sting), venomous	T63.481	T63.482	T63.483	T63.484	—	—
ant	T63.421	T63.422	T63.423	T63.424	—	—
bee	T63.441	T63.442	T63.443	T63.444	—	—
caterpillar	T63.431	T63.432	T63.433	T63.434	—	—
hornet	T63.451	T63.452	T63.453	T63.454	—	—
wasp	T63.461	T63.462	T63.463	T63.464	—	—
Insecticide NEC	T60.91	T60.92	T60.93	T60.94	—	—
carbamate	T60.0X1	T60.0X2	T60.0X3	T60.0X4	—	—
chlorinated	T60.1X1	T60.1X2	T60.1X3	T60.1X4	—	—
mixed	T60.91	T60.92	T60.93	T60.94	—	—
organochlorine	T60.1X1	T60.1X2	T60.1X3	T60.1X4	—	—
organophosphorus	T60.0X1	T60.0X2	T60.0X3	T60.0X4	—	—
Insular tissue extract	T38.3X1	T38.3X2	T38.3X3	T38.3X4	T38.3X5	T38.3X6
Insulin (amorphous) (globin) (isophane) (Lente) (NPH) (Semilente) (Ultralente)	T38.3X1	T38.3X2	T38.3X3	T38.3X4	T38.3X5	T38.3X6
defalan	T38.3X1	T38.3X2	T38.3X3	T38.3X4	T38.3X5	T38.3X6
human	T38.3X1	T38.3X2	T38.3X3	T38.3X4	T38.3X5	T38.3X6
injection, soluble	T38.3X1	T38.3X2	T38.3X3	T38.3X4	T38.3X5	T38.3X6
biphasic	T38.3X1	T38.3X2	T38.3X3	T38.3X4	T38.3X5	T38.3X6
intermediate acting	T38.3X1	T38.3X2	T38.3X3	T38.3X4	T38.3X5	T38.3X6
protamine zinc	T38.3X1	T38.3X2	T38.3X3	T38.3X4	T38.3X5	T38.3X6
slow acting	T38.3X1	T38.3X2	T38.3X3	T38.3X4	T38.3X5	T38.3X6
zinc						
protamine injection	T38.3X1	T38.3X2	T38.3X3	T38.3X4	T38.3X5	T38.3X6
suspension (amorphous) (crystalline)	T38.3X1	T38.3X2	T38.3X3	T38.3X4	T38.3X5	T38.3X6
Interferon (alpha) (beta) (gamma)	T37.5X1	T37.5X2	T37.5X3	T37.5X4	T37.5X5	T37.5X6
Intestinal motility control drug	T47.6X1	T47.6X2	T47.6X3	T47.6X4	T47.6X5	T47.6X6
biological	T47.8X1	T47.8X2	T47.8X3	T47.8X4	T47.8X5	T47.8X6
Intranarcon	T41.1X1	T41.1X2	T41.1X3	T41.1X4	T41.1X5	T41.1X6
Intravenous						
amino acids	T50.991	T50.992	T50.993	T50.994	T50.995	T50.996
fat suspension	T50.991	T50.992	T50.993	T50.994	T50.995	T50.996
Inulin	T50.8X1	T50.8X2	T50.8X3	T50.8X4	T50.8X5	T50.8X6
Invert sugar	T50.3X1	T50.3X2	T50.3X3	T50.3X4	T50.3X5	T50.3X6
Inza—*see Naproxen*						
Iobenzamic acid	T50.8X1	T50.8X2	T50.8X3	T50.8X4	T50.8X5	T50.8X6
Iocarmic acid	T50.8X1	T50.8X2	T50.8X3	T50.8X4	T50.8X5	T50.8X6
Iocetamic acid	T50.8X1	T50.8X2	T50.8X3	T50.8X4	T50.8X5	T50.8X6
Iodamide	T50.8X1	T50.8X2	T50.8X3	T50.8X4	T50.8X5	T50.8X6
Iodide NEC—*see also Iodine*	T49.0X1	T49.0X2	T49.0X3	T49.0X4	T49.0X5	T49.0X6
mercury (ointment)	T49.0X1	T49.0X2	T49.0X3	T49.0X4	T49.0X5	T49.0X6
methylate	T49.0X1	T49.0X2	T49.0X3	T49.0X4	T49.0X5	T49.0X6
potassium (expectorant) NEC	T48.4X1	T48.4X2	T48.4X3	T48.4X4	T48.4X5	T48.4X6
Iodinated						
contrast medium	T50.8X1	T50.8X2	T50.8X3	T50.8X4	T50.8X5	T50.8X6
glycerol	T48.4X1	T48.4X2	T48.4X3	T48.4X4	T48.4X5	T48.4X6
human serum albumin (131I)	T50.8X1	T50.8X2	T50.8X3	T50.8X4	T50.8X5	T50.8X6
Iodine (antiseptic, external) (tincture) NEC	T49.0X1	T49.0X2	T49.0X3	T49.0X4	T49.0X5	T49.0X6
125—*see also Radiation sickness, and Exposure to radioactive isotopes*						
therapeutic	T50.991	T50.992	T50.993	T50.994	T50.995	T50.996
131—*see also Radiation sickness, and Exposure to radioactive isotopes*						
therapeutic	T38.2X1	T38.2X2	T38.2X3	T38.2X4	T38.2X5	T38.2X6
diagnostic	T50.8X1	T50.8X2	T50.8X3	T50.8X4	T50.8X5	T50.8X6
for thyroid conditions (antithyroid)	T38.2X1	T38.2X2	T38.2X3	T38.2X4	T38.2X5	T38.2X6
solution	T49.0X1	T49.0X2	T49.0X3	T49.0X4	T49.0X5	T49.0X6
vapor	T59.891	T59.892	T59.893	T59.894	—	—
Iodipamide	T50.8X1	T50.8X2	T50.8X3	T50.8X4	T50.8X5	T50.8X6
Iodized (poppy seed) oil	T50.8X1	T50.8X2	T50.8X3	T50.8X4	T50.8X5	T50.8X6
Iodobismitol	T37.8X1	T37.8X2	T37.8X3	T37.8X4	T37.8X5	T37.8X6

New Revised ~~deleted~~ Deleted

	External Cause (T-Code)					
Substance	Poisoning, Accidental (Unintentional)	Poisoning, Intentional Self-Harm	Poisoning, Assault	Poisoning, Undetermined	Adverse Effect	Underdosing
Iodochlorhydroxyquin	T37.8X1	T37.8X2	T37.8X3	T37.8X4	T37.8X5	T37.8X6
topical	T49.ØX1	T49.ØX2	T49.ØX3	T49.ØX4	T49.ØX5	T49.ØX6
Iodochlorhydroxyquino-line	T37.8X1	T37.8X2	T37.8X3	T37.8X4	T37.8X5	T37.8X6
Iodocholesterol (131I)	T5Ø.8X1	T5Ø.8X2	T5Ø.8X3	T5Ø.8X4	T5Ø.8X5	T5Ø.8X6
Iodoform	T49.ØX1	T49.ØX2	T49.ØX3	T49.ØX4	T49.ØX5	T49.ØX6
Iodohippuric acid	T5Ø.8X1	T5Ø.8X2	T5Ø.8X3	T5Ø.8X4	T5Ø.8X5	T5Ø.8X6
Iodopanoic acid	T5Ø.8X1	T5Ø.8X2	T5Ø.8X3	T5Ø.8X4	T5Ø.8X5	T5Ø.8X6
Iodophthalein (sodium)	T5Ø.8X1	T5Ø.8X2	T5Ø.8X3	T5Ø.8X4	T5Ø.8X5	T5Ø.8X6
Iodopyracet	T5Ø.8X1	T5Ø.8X2	T5Ø.8X3	T5Ø.8X4	T5Ø.8X5	T5Ø.8X6
Iodoquinol	T37.8X1	T37.8X2	T37.8X3	T37.8X4	T37.8X5	T37.8X6
Iodoxamic acid	T5Ø.8X1	T5Ø.8X2	T5Ø.8X3	T5Ø.8X4	T5Ø.8X5	T5Ø.8X6
Iofendylate	T5Ø.8X1	T5Ø.8X2	T5Ø.8X3	T5Ø.8X4	T5Ø.8X5	T5Ø.8X6
Ioglycamic acid	T5Ø.8X1	T5Ø.8X2	T5Ø.8X3	T5Ø.8X4	T5Ø.8X5	T5Ø.8X6
Iohexol	T5Ø.8X1	T5Ø.8X2	T5Ø.8X3	T5Ø.8X4	T5Ø.8X5	T5Ø.8X6
Ion exchange resin						
anion	T47.8X1	T47.8X2	T47.8X3	T47.8X4	T47.8X5	T47.8X6
cation	T5Ø.3X1	T5Ø.3X2	T5Ø.3X3	T5Ø.3X4	T5Ø.3X5	T5Ø.3X6
cholestyramine	T46.6X1	T46.6X2	T46.6X3	T46.6X4	T46.6X5	T46.6X6
intestinal	T47.8X1	T47.8X2	T47.8X3	T47.8X4	T47.8X5	T47.8X6
Iopamidol	T5Ø.8X1	T5Ø.8X2	T5Ø.8X3	T5Ø.8X4	T5Ø.8X5	T5Ø.8X6
Iopanoic acid	T5Ø.8X1	T5Ø.8X2	T5Ø.8X3	T5Ø.8X4	T5Ø.8X5	T5Ø.8X6
Iophenoic acid	T5Ø.8X1	T5Ø.8X2	T5Ø.8X3	T5Ø.8X4	T5Ø.8X5	T5Ø.8X6
Iopodate, sodium	T5Ø.8X1	T5Ø.8X2	T5Ø.8X3	T5Ø.8X4	T5Ø.8X5	T5Ø.8X6
Iopodic acid	T5Ø.8X1	T5Ø.8X2	T5Ø.8X3	T5Ø.8X4	T5Ø.8X5	T5Ø.8X6
Iopromide	T5Ø.8X1	T5Ø.8X2	T5Ø.8X3	T5Ø.8X4	T5Ø.8X5	T5Ø.8X6
Iopydol	T5Ø.8X1	T5Ø.8X2	T5Ø.8X3	T5Ø.8X4	T5Ø.8X5	T5Ø.8X6
Iotalamic acid	T5Ø.8X1	T5Ø.8X2	T5Ø.8X3	T5Ø.8X4	T5Ø.8X5	T5Ø.8X6
Iothalamate	T5Ø.8X1	T5Ø.8X2	T5Ø.8X3	T5Ø.8X4	T5Ø.8X5	T5Ø.8X6
Iothiouracil	T38.2X1	T38.2X2	T38.2X3	T38.2X4	T38.2X5	T38.2X6
Iotrol	T5Ø.8X1	T5Ø.8X2	T5Ø.8X3	T5Ø.8X4	T5Ø.8X5	T5Ø.8X6
Iotrolan	T5Ø.8X1	T5Ø.8X2	T5Ø.8X3	T5Ø.8X4	T5Ø.8X5	T5Ø.8X6
Iotroxate	T5Ø.8X1	T5Ø.8X2	T5Ø.8X3	T5Ø.8X4	T5Ø.8X5	T5Ø.8X6
Iotroxic acid	T5Ø.8X1	T5Ø.8X2	T5Ø.8X3	T5Ø.8X4	T5Ø.8X5	T5Ø.8X6
Ioversol	T5Ø.8X1	T5Ø.8X2	T5Ø.8X3	T5Ø.8X4	T5Ø.8X5	T5Ø.8X6
Ioxaglate	T5Ø.8X1	T5Ø.8X2	T5Ø.8X3	T5Ø.8X4	T5Ø.8X5	T5Ø.8X6
Ioxaglic acid	T5Ø.8X1	T5Ø.8X2	T5Ø.8X3	T5Ø.8X4	T5Ø.8X5	T5Ø.8X6
Ioxitalamic acid	T5Ø.8X1	T5Ø.8X2	T5Ø.8X3	T5Ø.8X4	T5Ø.8X5	T5Ø.8X6
Ipecac	T47.7X1	T47.7X2	T47.7X3	T47.7X4	T47.7X5	T47.7X6
Ipecacuanha	T48.4X1	T48.4X2	T48.4X3	T48.4X4	T48.4X5	T48.4X6
Ipodate, calcium	T5Ø.8X1	T5Ø.8X2	T5Ø.8X3	T5Ø.8X4	T5Ø.8X5	T5Ø.8X6
Ipral	T42.3X1	T42.3X2	T42.3X3	T42.3X4	T42.3X5	T42.3X6
Ipratropium (bromide)	T48.6X1	T48.6X2	T48.6X3	T48.6X4	T48.6X5	T48.6X6

	External Cause (T-Code)					
Substance	Poisoning, Accidental (Unintentional)	Poisoning, Intentional Self-Harm	Poisoning, Assault	Poisoning, Undetermined	Adverse Effect	Underdosing
Ipriflavone	T46.3X1	T46.3X2	T46.3X3	T46.3X4	T46.3X5	T46.3X6
Iprindole	T43.Ø11	T43.Ø12	T43.Ø13	T43.Ø14	T43.Ø15	T43.Ø16
Iproclozide	T43.1X1	T43.1X2	T43.1X3	T43.1X4	T43.1X5	T43.1X6
Iprofenin	T5Ø.8X1	T5Ø.8X2	T5Ø.8X3	T5Ø.8X4	T5Ø.8X5	T5Ø.8X6
Iproheptine	T49.2X1	T49.2X2	T49.2X3	T49.2X4	T49.2X5	T49.2X6
Iproniazid	T43.1X1	T43.1X2	T43.1X3	T43.1X4	T43.1X5	T43.1X6
Iproplatin	T45.1X1	T45.1X2	T45.1X3	T45.1X4	T45.1X5	T45.1X6
Iproveratril	T46.1X1	T46.1X2	T46.1X3	T46.1X4	T46.1X5	T46.1X6
Iron (compounds) (medicinal) NEC	T45.4X1	T45.4X2	T45.4X3	T45.4X4	T45.4X5	T45.4X6
ammonium	T45.4X1	T45.4X2	T45.4X3	T45.4X4	T45.4X5	T45.4X6
dextran injection	T45.4X1	T45.4X2	T45.4X3	T45.4X4	T45.4X5	T45.4X6
nonmedicinal	T56.891	T56.892	T56.893	T56.894	—	—
salts	T45.4X1	T45.4X2	T45.4X3	T45.4X4	T45.4X5	T45.4X6
sorbitex	T45.4X1	T45.4X2	T45.4X3	T45.4X4	T45.4X5	T45.4X6
sorbitol citric acid complex	T45.4X1	T45.4X2	T45.4X3	T45.4X4	T45.4X5	T45.4X6
Irrigating fluid (vaginal)	T49.8X1	T49.8X2	T49.8X3	T49.8X4	T49.8X5	T49.8X6
eye	T49.5X1	T49.5X2	T49.5X3	T49.5X4	T49.5X5	T49.5X6
Isepamicin	T36.5X1	T36.5X2	T36.5X3	T36.5X4	T36.5X5	T36.5X6
Isoaminile (citrate)	T48.3X1	T48.3X2	T48.3X3	T48.3X4	T48.3X5	T48.3X6
Isoamyl nitrite	T46.3X1	T46.3X2	T46.3X3	T46.3X4	T46.3X5	T46.3X6
Isobenzan	T6Ø.1X1	T6Ø.1X2	T6Ø.1X3	T6Ø.1X4	—	—
Isobutyl acetate	T52.8X1	T52.8X2	T52.8X3	T52.8X4	—	—
Isocarboxazid	T43.1X1	T43.1X2	T43.1X3	T43.1X4	T43.1X5	T43.1X6
Isoconazole	T49.ØX1	T49.ØX2	T49.ØX3	T49.ØX4	T49.ØX5	T49.ØX6
Isocyanate	T65.ØX1	T65.ØX2	T65.ØX3	T65.ØX4	—	—
Isoephedrine	T44.991	T44.992	T44.993	T44.994	T44.995	T44.996
Isoetarine	T48.6X1	T48.6X2	T48.6X3	T48.6X4	T48.6X5	T48.6X6
Isoethadione	T42.2X1	T42.2X2	T42.2X3	T42.2X4	T42.2X5	T42.2X6
Isoetharine	T44.5X1	T44.5X2	T44.5X3	T44.5X4	T44.5X5	T44.5X6
Isoflurane	T41.ØX1	T41.ØX2	T41.ØX3	T41.ØX4	T41.ØX5	T41.ØX6
Isoflurophate	T44.ØX1	T44.ØX2	T44.ØX3	T44.ØX4	T44.ØX5	T44.ØX6
Isomaltose, ferric complex	T45.4X1	T45.4X2	T45.4X3	T45.4X4	T45.4X5	T45.4X6
Isometheptene	T44.3X1	T44.3X2	T44.3X3	T44.3X4	T44.3X5	T44.3X6
Isoniazid	T37.1X1	T37.1X2	T37.1X3	T37.1X4	T37.1X5	T37.1X6
with						
rifampicin	T36.6X1	T36.6X2	T36.6X3	T36.6X4	T36.6X5	T36.6X6
thioacetazone	T37.1X1	T37.1X2	T37.1X3	T37.1X4	T37.1X5	T37.1X6
Isonicotinic acid hydrazide	T37.1X1	T37.1X2	T37.1X3	T37.1X4	T37.1X5	T37.1X6
Isonipecaine	T4Ø.491	T4Ø.492	T4Ø.493	T4Ø.494	T4Ø.495	T4Ø.496
Isopentaquine	T37.2X1	T37.2X2	T37.2X3	T37.2X4	T37.2X5	T37.2X6
Isophane insulin	T38.3X1	T38.3X2	T38.3X3	T38.3X4	T38.3X5	T38.3X6
Isophorone	T65.891	T65.892	T65.893	T65.894	—	—

Substance	External Cause (T-Code): Poisoning, Accidental (Unintentional)	Poisoning, Intentional Self-Harm	Poisoning, Assault	Poisoning, Undetermined	Adverse Effect	Underdosing
Isophosphamide	T45.1X1	T45.1X2	T45.1X3	T45.1X4	T45.1X5	T45.1X6
Isopregnenone	T38.5X1	T38.5X2	T38.5X3	T38.5X4	T38.5X5	T38.5X6
Isoprenaline	T48.6X1	T48.6X2	T48.6X3	T48.6X4	T48.6X5	T48.6X6
Isopromethazine	T43.3X1	T43.3X2	T43.3X3	T43.3X4	T43.3X5	T43.3X6
Isopropamide	T44.3X1	T44.3X2	T44.3X3	T44.3X4	T44.3X5	T44.3X6
iodide	T44.3X1	T44.3X2	T44.3X3	T44.3X4	T44.3X5	T44.3X6
Isopropanol	T51.2X1	T51.2X2	T51.2X3	T51.2X4	—	—
Isopropyl						
acetate	T52.8X1	T52.8X2	T52.8X3	T52.8X4	—	—
alcohol	T51.2X1	T51.2X2	T51.2X3	T51.2X4	—	—
medicinal	T49.4X1	T49.4X2	T49.4X3	T49.4X4	T49.4X5	T49.4X6
ether	T52.8X1	T52.8X2	T52.8X3	T52.8X4	—	—
Isopropylaminophena-zone	T39.2X1	T39.2X2	T39.2X3	T39.2X4	T39.2X5	T39.2X6
Isoproterenol	T48.6X1	T48.6X2	T48.6X3	T48.6X4	T48.6X5	T48.6X6
Isosorbide dinitrate	T46.3X1	T46.3X2	T46.3X3	T46.3X4	T46.3X5	T46.3X6
Isothipendyl	T45.0X1	T45.0X2	T45.0X3	T45.0X4	T45.0X5	T45.0X6
Isotretinoin	T50.991	T50.992	T50.993	T50.994	T50.995	T50.996
Isoxazolyl penicillin	T36.0X1	T36.0X2	T36.0X3	T36.0X4	T36.0X5	T36.0X6
Isoxicam	T39.391	T39.392	T39.393	T39.394	T39.395	T39.396
Isoxsuprine	T46.7X1	T46.7X2	T46.7X3	T46.7X4	T46.7X5	T46.7X6
Ispagula	T47.4X1	T47.4X2	T47.4X3	T47.4X4	T47.4X5	T47.4X6
husk	T47.4X1	T47.4X2	T47.4X3	T47.4X4	T47.4X5	T47.4X6
Isradipine	T46.1X1	T46.1X2	T46.1X3	T46.1X4	T46.1X5	T46.1X6
I-thyroxine sodium	T38.1X1	T38.1X2	T38.1X3	T38.1X4	T38.1X5	T38.1X6
Itraconazole	T37.8X1	T37.8X2	T37.8X3	T37.8X4	T37.8X5	T37.8X6
Itramin tosilate	T46.3X1	T46.3X2	T46.3X3	T46.3X4	T46.3X5	T46.3X6
Ivermectin	T37.4X1	T37.4X2	T37.4X3	T37.4X4	T37.4X5	T37.4X6
Izoniazid	T37.1X1	T37.1X2	T37.1X3	T37.1X4	T37.1X5	T37.1X6
with thioacetazone	T37.1X1	T37.1X2	T37.1X3	T37.1X4	T37.1X5	T37.1X6
J						
Jalap	T47.2X1	T47.2X2	T47.2X3	T47.2X4	T47.2X5	T47.2X6
Jamaica						
dogwood (bark)	T39.8X1	T39.8X2	T39.8X3	T39.8X4	T39.8X5	T39.8X6
ginger	T65.891	T65.892	T65.893	T65.894	—	—
root	T62.2X1	T62.2X2	T62.2X3	T62.2X4	—	—
Jatropha	T62.2X1	T62.2X2	T62.2X3	T62.2X4	—	—
curcas	T62.2X1	T62.2X2	T62.2X3	T62.2X4	—	—
Jectofer	T45.4X1	T45.4X2	T45.4X3	T45.4X4	T45.4X5	T45.4X6
Jellyfish (sting)	T63.621	T63.622	T63.623	T63.624	—	—
Jequirity (bean)	T62.2X1	T62.2X2	T62.2X3	T62.2X4	—	—
Jimson weed (stramonium)	T62.2X1	T62.2X2	T62.2X3	T62.2X4	—	—
seeds	T62.2X1	T62.2X2	T62.2X3	T62.2X4	—	—
Josamycin	T36.3X1	T36.3X2	T36.3X3	T36.3X4	T36.3X5	T36.3X6
Juniper tar	T49.1X1	T49.1X2	T49.1X3	T49.1X4	T49.1X5	T49.1X6
K						
Kallidinogenase	T46.7X1	T46.7X2	T46.7X3	T46.7X4	T46.7X5	T46.7X6
Kallikrein	T46.7X1	T46.7X2	T46.7X3	T46.7X4	T46.7X5	T46.7X6
Kanamycin	T36.5X1	T36.5X2	T36.5X3	T36.5X4	T36.5X5	T36.5X6
Kantrex	T36.5X1	T36.5X2	T36.5X3	T36.5X4	T36.5X5	T36.5X6
Kaolin	T47.6X1	T47.6X2	T47.6X3	T47.6X4	T47.6X5	T47.6X6
light	T47.6X1	T47.6X2	T47.6X3	T47.6X4	T47.6X5	T47.6X6
Karaya (gum)	T47.4X1	T47.4X2	T47.4X3	T47.4X4	T47.4X5	T47.4X6
Kebuzone	T39.2X1	T39.2X2	T39.2X3	T39.2X4	T39.2X5	T39.2X6
Kelevan	T60.1X1	T60.1X2	T60.1X3	T60.1X4	—	—
Kemithal	T41.1X1	T41.1X2	T41.1X3	T41.1X4	T41.1X5	T41.1X6
Kenacort	T38.0X1	T38.0X2	T38.0X3	T38.0X4	T38.0X5	T38.0X6
Keratolytic drug NEC	T49.4X1	T49.4X2	T49.4X3	T49.4X4	T49.4X5	T49.4X6
anthracene	T49.4X1	T49.4X2	T49.4X3	T49.4X4	T49.4X5	T49.4X6
Keratoplastic NEC	T49.4X1	T49.4X2	T49.4X3	T49.4X4	T49.4X5	T49.4X6
Kerosene, kerosine (fuel) (solvent) NEC	T52.0X1	T52.0X2	T52.0X3	T52.0X4	—	—
insecticide	T52.0X1	T52.0X2	T52.0X3	T52.0X4	—	—
vapor	T52.0X1	T52.0X2	T52.0X3	T52.0X4	—	—
Ketamine	T41.291	T41.292	T41.293	T41.294	T41.295	T41.296
Ketazolam	T42.4X1	T42.4X2	T42.4X3	T42.4X4	T42.4X5	T42.4X6
Ketazon	T39.2X1	T39.2X2	T39.2X3	T39.2X4	T39.2X5	T39.2X6
Ketobemidone	T40.491	T40.492	T40.493	T40.494	—	—
Ketoconazole	T49.0X1	T49.0X2	T49.0X3	T49.0X4	T49.0X5	T49.0X6
Ketols	T52.4X1	T52.4X2	T52.4X3	T52.4X4	—	—
Ketone oils	T52.4X1	T52.4X2	T52.4X3	T52.4X4	—	—
Ketoprofen	T39.311	T39.312	T39.313	T39.314	T39.315	T39.316
Ketorolac	T39.8X1	T39.8X2	T39.8X3	T39.8X4	T39.8X5	T39.8X6
Ketotifen	T45.0X1	T45.0X2	T45.0X3	T45.0X4	T45.0X5	T45.0X6
Khat	T43.691	T43.692	T43.693	T43.694	—	—
Khellin	T46.3X1	T46.3X2	T46.3X3	T46.3X4	T46.3X5	T46.3X6
Khelloside	T46.3X1	T46.3X2	T46.3X3	T46.3X4	T46.3X5	T46.3X6
Kiln gas or vapor (carbon monoxide)	T58.8X1	T58.8X2	T58.8X3	T58.8X4	—	—
Kitasamycin	T36.3X1	T36.3X2	T36.3X3	T36.3X4	T36.3X5	T36.3X6
Konsyl	T47.4X1	T47.4X2	T47.4X3	T47.4X4	T47.4X5	T47.4X6
Kosam seed	T62.2X1	T62.2X2	T62.2X3	T62.2X4	—	—
Krait (venom)	T63.091	T63.092	T63.093	T63.094	—	—
Kwell (insecticide)	T60.1X1	T60.1X2	T60.1X3	T60.1X4	—	—
anti-infective (topical)	T49.0X1	T49.0X2	T49.0X3	T49.0X4	T49.0X5	T49.0X6

New Revised ~~deleted~~ Deleted

	External Cause (T-Code)					
Substance	Poisoning, Accidental (Unintentional)	Poisoning, Intentional Self-Harm	Poisoning, Assault	Poisoning, Undetermined	Adverse Effect	Underdosing
L						
Labetalol	T44.8X1	T44.8X2	T44.8X3	T44.8X4	T44.8X5	T44.8X6
Laburnum (seeds)	T62.2X1	T62.2X2	T62.2X3	T62.2X4	—	—
leaves	T62.2X1	T62.2X2	T62.2X3	T62.2X4	—	—
Lachesine	T49.5X1	T49.5X2	T49.5X3	T49.5X4	T49.5X5	T49.5X6
Lacidipine	T46.5X1	T46.5X2	T46.5X3	T46.5X4	T46.5X5	T46.5X6
Lacquer	T65.6X1	T65.6X2	T65.6X3	T65.6X4	—	—
Lacrimogenic gas	T59.3X1	T59.3X2	T59.3X3	T59.3X4	—	—
Lactated potassic saline	T50.3X1	T50.3X2	T50.3X3	T50.3X4	T50.3X5	T50.3X6
Lactic acid	T49.8X1	T49.8X2	T49.8X3	T49.8X4	T49.8X5	T49.8X6
Lactobacillus						
acidophilus	T47.6X1	T47.6X2	T47.6X3	T47.6X4	T47.6X5	T47.6X6
compound	T47.6X1	T47.6X2	T47.6X3	T47.6X4	T47.6X5	T47.6X6
bifidus, lyophilized	T47.6X1	T47.6X2	T47.6X3	T47.6X4	T47.6X5	T47.6X6
bulgaricus	T47.6X1	T47.6X2	T47.6X3	T47.6X4	T47.6X5	T47.6X6
sporogenes	T47.6X1	T47.6X2	T47.6X3	T47.6X4	T47.6X5	T47.6X6
Lactoflavin	T45.2X1	T45.2X2	T45.2X3	T45.2X4	T45.2X5	T45.2X6
Lactose (as excipient)	T50.901	T50.902	T50.903	T50.904	T50.905	T50.906
Lactuca (virosa) (extract)	T42.6X1	T42.6X2	T42.6X3	T42.6X4	T42.6X5	T42.6X6
Lactucarium	T42.6X1	T42.6X2	T42.6X3	T42.6X4	T42.6X5	T42.6X6
Lactulose	T47.3X1	T47.3X2	T47.3X3	T47.3X4	T47.3X5	T47.3X6
Laevo — *see Levo-*						
Lanatosides	T46.0X1	T46.0X2	T46.0X3	T46.0X4	T46.0X5	T46.0X6
Lanolin	T49.3X1	T49.3X2	T49.3X3	T49.3X4	T49.3X5	T49.3X6
Largactil	T43.3X1	T43.3X2	T43.3X3	T43.3X4	T43.3X5	T43.3X6
Larkspur	T62.2X1	T62.2X2	T62.2X3	T62.2X4	—	—
Laroxyl	T43.011	T43.012	T43.013	T43.014	T43.015	T43.016
Lassar's paste	T49.4X1	T49.4X2	T49.4X3	T49.4X4	T49.4X5	T49.4X6
Lasix	T50.1X1	T50.1X2	T50.1X3	T50.1X4	T50.1X5	T50.1X6
Latamoxef	T36.1X1	T36.1X2	T36.1X3	T36.1X4	T36.1X5	T36.1X6
Latex	T65.811	T65.812	T65.813	T65.814	—	—
Lathyrus (seed)	T62.2X1	T62.2X2	T62.2X3	T62.2X4	—	—
Laudanum	T40.0X1	T40.0X2	T40.0X3	T40.0X4	T40.0X5	T40.0X6
Laudexium	T48.1X1	T48.1X2	T48.1X3	T48.1X4	T48.1X5	T48.1X6
Laughing gas	T41.0X1	T41.0X2	T41.0X3	T41.0X4	T41.0X5	T41.0X6
Laurel, black or cherry	T62.2X1	T62.2X2	T62.2X3	T62.2X4	—	—
Laurolinium	T49.0X1	T49.0X2	T49.0X3	T49.0X4	T49.0X5	T49.0X6
Lauryl sulfoacetate	T49.2X1	T49.2X2	T49.2X3	T49.2X4	T49.2X5	T49.2X6
Laxative NEC	T47.4X1	T47.4X2	T47.4X3	T47.4X4	T47.4X5	T47.4X6
osmotic	T47.3X1	T47.3X2	T47.3X3	T47.3X4	T47.3X5	T47.3X6
saline	T47.3X1	T47.3X2	T47.3X3	T47.3X4	T47.3X5	T47.3X6
stimulant	T47.2X1	T47.2X2	T47.2X3	T47.2X4	T47.2X5	T47.2X6
L-dopa	T42.8X1	T42.8X2	T42.8X3	T42.8X4	T42.8X5	T42.8X6
Lead (dust) (fumes) (vapor) NEC	T56.0X1	T56.0X2	T56.0X3	T56.0X4	—	—
acetate	T49.2X1	T49.2X2	T49.2X3	T49.2X4	T49.2X5	T49.2X6
alkyl (fuel additive)	T56.0X1	T56.0X2	T56.0X3	T56.0X4	—	—
anti-infectives	T37.8X1	T37.8X2	T37.8X3	T37.8X4	T37.8X5	T37.8X6
antiknock compound (tetraethyl)	T56.0X1	T56.0X2	T56.0X3	T56.0X4	—	—
arsenate, arsenite (dust) (herbicide) (insecticide) (vapor)	T57.0X1	T57.0X2	T57.0X3	T57.0X4	—	—
carbonate	T56.0X1	T56.0X2	T56.0X3	T56.0X4	—	—
paint	T56.0X1	T56.0X2	T56.0X3	T56.0X4	—	—
chromate	T56.0X1	T56.0X2	T56.0X3	T56.0X4	—	—
paint	T56.0X1	T56.0X2	T56.0X3	T56.0X4	—	—
dioxide	T56.0X1	T56.0X2	T56.0X3	T56.0X4	—	—
inorganic	T56.0X1	T56.0X2	T56.0X3	T56.0X4	—	—
iodide	T56.0X1	T56.0X2	T56.0X3	T56.0X4	—	—
pigment (paint)	T56.0X1	T56.0X2	T56.0X3	T56.0X4	—	—
monoxide (dust)	T56.0X1	T56.0X2	T56.0X3	T56.0X4	—	—
paint	T56.0X1	T56.0X2	T56.0X3	T56.0X4	—	—
organic	T56.0X1	T56.0X2	T56.0X3	T56.0X4	—	—
oxide	T56.0X1	T56.0X2	T56.0X3	T56.0X4	—	—
paint	T56.0X1	T56.0X2	T56.0X3	T56.0X4	—	—
paint	T56.0X1	T56.0X2	T56.0X3	T56.0X4	—	—
salts	T56.0X1	T56.0X2	T56.0X3	T56.0X4	—	—
specified compound NEC	T56.0X1	T56.0X2	T56.0X3	T56.0X4	—	—
tetra-ethyl	T56.0X1	T56.0X2	T56.0X3	T56.0X4	—	—
Lebanese red	T40.711	T40.712	T40.713	T40.714	T40.715	T40.716
Lefetamine	T39.8X1	T39.8X2	T39.8X3	T39.8X4	T39.8X5	T39.8X6
Lenperone	T43.4X1	T43.4X2	T43.4X3	T43.4X4	T43.4X5	T43.4X6
Lente lietin (insulin)	T38.3X1	T38.3X2	T38.3X3	T38.3X4	T38.3X5	T38.3X6
Leptazol	T50.7X1	T50.7X2	T50.7X3	T50.7X4	T50.7X5	T50.7X6
Leptophos	T60.0X1	T60.0X2	T60.0X3	T60.0X4	—	—
Leritine	T40.2X1	T40.2X2	T40.2X3	T40.2X4	T40.2X5	T40.2X6
Letosteine	T48.4X1	T48.4X2	T48.4X3	T48.4X4	T48.4X5	T48.4X6
Letter	T38.1X1	T38.1X2	T38.1X3	T38.1X4	T38.1X5	T38.1X6
Lettuce opium	T42.6X1	T42.6X2	T42.6X3	T42.6X4	T42.6X5	T42.6X6
Leucinocaine	T41.3X1	T41.3X2	T41.3X3	T41.3X4	T41.3X5	T41.3X6

Substance	External Cause (T-Code)					
	Poisoning, Accidental (Unintentional)	Poisoning, Intentional Self-Harm	Poisoning, Assault	Poisoning, Undetermined	Adverse Effect	Underdosing
Leucocianidol	T46.991	T46.992	T46.993	T46.994	T46.995	T46.996
Leucovorin (factor)	T45.8X1	T45.8X2	T45.8X3	T45.8X4	T45.8X5	T45.8X6
Leukeran	T45.1X1	T45.1X2	T45.1X3	T45.1X4	T45.1X5	T45.1X6
Leuprolide	T38.891	T38.892	T38.893	T38.894	T38.895	T38.896
Levalbuterol	T48.6X1	T48.6X2	T48.6X3	T48.6X4	T48.6X5	T48.6X6
Levallorphan	T50.7X1	T50.7X2	T50.7X3	T50.7X4	T50.7X5	T50.7X6
Levamisole	T37.4X1	T37.4X2	T37.4X3	T37.4X4	T37.4X5	T37.4X6
Levanil	T42.6X1	T42.6X2	T42.6X3	T42.6X4	T42.6X5	T42.6X6
Levarterenol	T44.4X1	T44.4X2	T44.4X3	T44.4X4	T44.4X5	T44.4X6
Levdropropizine	T48.3X1	T48.3X2	T48.3X3	T48.3X4	T48.3X5	T48.3X6
Levobunolol	T49.5X1	T49.5X2	T49.5X3	T49.5X4	T49.5X5	T49.5X6
Levocabastine (hydrochloride)	T45.0X1	T45.0X2	T45.0X3	T45.0X4	T45.0X5	T45.0X6
Levocarnitine	T50.991	T50.992	T50.993	T50.994	T50.995	T50.996
Levodopa	T42.8X1	T42.8X2	T42.8X3	T42.8X4	T42.8X5	T42.8X6
with carbidopa	T42.8X1	T42.8X2	T42.8X3	T42.8X4	T42.8X5	T42.8X6
Levo-dromoran	T40.2X1	T40.2X2	T40.2X3	T40.2X4	T40.2X5	T40.2X6
Levoglutamide	T50.991	T50.992	T50.993	T50.994	T50.995	T50.996
Levoid	T38.1X1	T38.1X2	T38.1X3	T38.1X4	T38.1X5	T38.1X6
Levo-iso-methadone	T40.3X1	T40.3X2	T40.3X3	T40.3X4	T40.3X5	T40.3X6
Levomepromazine	T43.3X1	T43.3X2	T43.3X3	T43.3X4	T43.3X5	T43.3X6
Levonordefrin	T49.6X1	T49.6X2	T49.6X3	T49.6X4	T49.6X5	T49.6X6
Levonorgestrel	T38.4X1	T38.4X2	T38.4X3	T38.4X4	T38.4X5	T38.4X6
with ethinylestradiol	T38.5X1	T38.5X2	T38.5X3	T38.5X4	T38.5X5	T38.5X6
Levopromazine	T43.3X1	T43.3X2	T43.3X3	T43.3X4	T43.3X5	T43.3X6
Levoprome	T42.6X1	T42.6X2	T42.6X3	T42.6X4	T42.6X5	T42.6X6
Levopropoxyphene	T40.491	T40.492	T40.493	T40.494	T40.495	T40.496
Levopropylhexedrine	T50.5X1	T50.5X2	T50.5X3	T50.5X4	T50.5X5	T50.5X6
Levoproxyphylline	T48.6X1	T48.6X2	T48.6X3	T48.6X4	T48.6X5	T48.6X6
Levorphanol	T40.491	T40.492	T40.493	T40.494	T40.495	T40.496
Levothyroxine	T38.1X1	T38.1X2	T38.1X3	T38.1X4	T38.1X5	T38.1X6
sodium	T38.1X1	T38.1X2	T38.1X3	T38.1X4	T38.1X5	T38.1X6
Levsin	T44.3X1	T44.3X2	T44.3X3	T44.3X4	T44.3X5	T44.3X6
Levulose	T50.3X1	T50.3X2	T50.3X3	T50.3X4	T50.3X5	T50.3X6
Lewisite (gas), not in war	T57.0X1	T57.0X2	T57.0X3	T57.0X4	—	—
Librium	T42.4X1	T42.4X2	T42.4X3	T42.4X4	T42.4X5	T42.4X6
Lidex	T49.0X1	T49.0X2	T49.0X3	T49.0X4	T49.0X5	T49.0X6
Lidocaine	T41.3X1	T41.3X2	T41.3X3	T41.3X4	T41.3X5	T41.3X6
regional	T41.3X1	T41.3X2	T41.3X3	T41.3X4	T41.3X5	T41.3X6
spinal	T41.3X1	T41.3X2	T41.3X3	T41.3X4	T41.3X5	T41.3X6
Lidofenin	T50.8X1	T50.8X2	T50.8X3	T50.8X4	T50.8X5	T50.8X6
Lidoflazine	T46.1X1	T46.1X2	T46.1X3	T46.1X4	T46.1X5	T46.1X6
Lighter fluid	T52.0X1	T52.0X2	T52.0X3	T52.0X4	—	—
Lignin hemicellulose	T47.6X1	T47.6X2	T47.6X3	T47.6X4	T47.6X5	T47.6X6
Lignocaine	T41.3X1	T41.3X2	T41.3X3	T41.3X4	T41.3X5	T41.3X6
regional	T41.3X1	T41.3X2	T41.3X3	T41.3X4	T41.3X5	T41.3X6
spinal	T41.3X1	T41.3X2	T41.3X3	T41.3X4	T41.3X5	T41.3X6
Ligroin(e) (solvent)	T52.0X1	T52.0X2	T52.0X3	T52.0X4	—	—
vapor	T59.891	T59.892	T59.893	T59.894	—	—
Ligustrum vulgare	T62.2X1	T62.2X2	T62.2X3	T62.2X4	—	—
Lily of the valley	T62.2X1	T62.2X2	T62.2X3	T62.2X4	—	—
Lime (chloride)	T54.3X1	T54.3X2	T54.3X3	T54.3X4	—	—
Limonene	T52.8X1	T52.8X2	T52.8X3	T52.8X4	—	—
Lincomycin	T36.8X1	T36.8X2	T36.8X3	T36.8X4	T36.8X5	T36.8X6
Lindane (insecticide) (nonmedicinal) (vapor)	T53.6X1	T53.6X2	T53.6X3	T53.6X4	—	—
medicinal	T49.0X1	T49.0X2	T49.0X3	T49.0X4	T49.0X5	T49.0X6
Liniments NEC	T49.91	T49.92	T49.93	T49.94	T49.95	T49.96
Linoleic acid	T46.6X1	T46.6X2	T46.6X3	T46.6X4	T46.6X5	T46.6X6
Linolenic acid	T46.6X1	T46.6X2	T46.6X3	T46.6X4	T46.6X5	T46.6X6
Linseed	T47.4X1	T47.4X2	T47.4X3	T47.4X4	T47.4X5	T47.4X6
Liothyronine	T38.1X1	T38.1X2	T38.1X3	T38.1X4	T38.1X5	T38.1X6
Liotrix	T38.1X1	T38.1X2	T38.1X3	T38.1X4	T38.1X5	T38.1X6
Lipancreatin	T47.5X1	T47.5X2	T47.5X3	T47.5X4	T47.5X5	T47.5X6
Lipo-alprostadil	T46.7X1	T46.7X2	T46.7X3	T46.7X4	T46.7X5	T46.7X6
Lipo-Lutin	T38.5X1	T38.5X2	T38.5X3	T38.5X4	T38.5X5	T38.5X6
Lipotropic drug NEC	T50.901	T50.902	T50.903	T50.904	T50.905	T50.906
Liquefied petroleum gases	T59.891	T59.892	T59.893	T59.894	—	—
piped (pure or mixed with air)	T59.891	T59.892	T59.893	T59.894	—	—
Liquid						
paraffin	T47.4X1	T47.4X2	T47.4X3	T47.4X4	T47.4X5	T47.4X6
petrolatum	T47.4X1	T47.4X2	T47.4X3	T47.4X4	T47.4X5	T47.4X6
topical	T49.3X1	T49.3X2	T49.3X3	T49.3X4	T49.3X5	T49.3X6
specified NEC	T65.891	T65.892	T65.893	T65.894	—	—
substance	T65.91	T65.92	T65.93	T65.94	—	—
Liquor creosolis compositus	T65.891	T65.892	T65.893	T65.894	—	—
Liquorice	T48.4X1	T48.4X2	T48.4X3	T48.4X4	T48.4X5	T48.4X6
extract	T47.8X1	T47.8X2	T47.8X3	T47.8X4	T47.8X5	T47.8X6
Lirugen	T50.991	T50.992	T50.993	T50.994	T50.995	T50.996
Lisinopril	T46.4X1	T46.4X2	T46.4X3	T46.4X4	T46.4X5	T46.4X6
Lisuride	T42.8X1	T42.8X2	T42.8X3	T42.8X4	T42.8X5	T42.8X6
Lithane	T43.8X1	T43.8X2	T43.8X3	T43.8X4	T43.8X5	T43.8X6
Lithium	T56.891	T56.892	T56.893	T56.894	—	—
gluconate	T43.591	T43.592	T43.593	T43.594	T43.595	T43.596
salts (carbonate)	T43.591	T43.592	T43.593	T43.594	T43.595	T43.596

◀ New ◀ Revised ~~deleted~~ Deleted

Substance	External Cause (T-Code) Poisoning, Accidental (Unintentional)	Poisoning, Intentional Self-Harm	Poisoning, Assault	Poisoning, Undetermined	Adverse Effect	Underdosing
Lithonate	T43.8X1	T43.8X2	T43.8X3	T43.8X4	T43.8X5	T43.8X6
Liver						
extract	T45.8X1	T45.8X2	T45.8X3	T45.8X4	T45.8X5	T45.8X6
for parenteral use	T45.8X1	T45.8X2	T45.8X3	T45.8X4	T45.8X5	T45.8X6
fraction 1	T45.8X1	T45.8X2	T45.8X3	T45.8X4	T45.8X5	T45.8X6
hydrolysate	T45.8X1	T45.8X2	T45.8X3	T45.8X4	T45.8X5	T45.8X6
Lizard (bite) (venom)	T63.121	T63.122	T63.123	T63.124	—	—
LMD	T45.8X1	T45.8X2	T45.8X3	T45.8X4	T45.8X5	T45.8X6
Lobelia	T62.2X1	T62.2X2	T62.2X3	T62.2X4	—	—
Lobeline	T5Ø.7X1	T5Ø.7X2	T5Ø.7X3	T5Ø.7X4	T5Ø.7X5	T5Ø.7X6
Local action drug NEC	T49.8X1	T49.8X2	T49.8X3	T49.8X4	T49.8X5	T49.8X6
Locorten	T49.ØX1	T49.ØX2	T49.ØX3	T49.ØX4	T49.ØX5	T49.ØX6
Lofepramine	T43.Ø11	T43.Ø12	T43.Ø13	T43.Ø14	T43.Ø15	T43.Ø16
Lolium temulentum	T62.2X1	T62.2X2	T62.2X3	T62.2X4	—	—
Lomotil	T47.6X1	T47.6X2	T47.6X3	T47.6X4	T47.6X5	T47.6X6
Lomustine	T45.1X1	T45.1X2	T45.1X3	T45.1X4	T45.1X5	T45.1X6
Lonidamine	T45.1X1	T45.1X2	T45.1X3	T45.1X4	T45.1X5	T45.1X6
Loperamide	T47.6X1	T47.6X2	T47.6X3	T47.6X4	T47.6X5	T47.6X6
Loprazolam	T42.4X1	T42.4X2	T42.4X3	T42.4X4	T42.4X5	T42.4X6
Lorajmine	T46.2X1	T46.2X2	T46.2X3	T46.2X4	T46.2X5	T46.2X6
Loratidine	T45.ØX1	T45.ØX2	T45.ØX3	T45.ØX4	T45.ØX5	T45.ØX6
Lorazepam	T42.4X1	T42.4X2	T42.4X3	T42.4X4	T42.4X5	T42.4X6
Lorcainide	T46.2X1	T46.2X2	T46.2X3	T46.2X4	T46.2X5	T46.2X6
Lormetazepam	T42.4X1	T42.4X2	T42.4X3	T42.4X4	T42.4X5	T42.4X6
Lotions NEC	T49.91	T49.92	T49.93	T49.94	T49.95	T49.96
Lotusate	T42.3X1	T42.3X2	T42.3X3	T42.3X4	T42.3X5	T42.3X6
Lovastatin	T46.6X1	T46.6X2	T46.6X3	T46.6X4	T46.6X5	T46.6X6
Loxapine	T43.591	T43.592	T43.593	T43.594	T43.595	T43.596
Lowila	T49.2X1	T49.2X2	T49.2X3	T49.2X4	T49.2X5	T49.2X6
Lozenges (throat)	T49.6X1	T49.6X2	T49.6X3	T49.6X4	T49.6X5	T49.6X6
LSD	T4Ø.8X1	T4Ø.8X2	T4Ø.8X3	T4Ø.8X4	—	—
L-Tryptophan — *see Amino acid*						
Lubricant, eye	T49.5X1	T49.5X2	T49.5X3	T49.5X4	T49.5X5	T49.5X6
Lubricating oil NEC	T52.ØX1	T52.ØX2	T52.ØX3	T52.ØX4	—	—
Lucanthone	T37.4X1	T37.4X2	T37.4X3	T37.4X4	T37.4X5	T37.4X6
Luminal	T42.3X1	T42.3X2	T42.3X3	T42.3X4	T42.3X5	T42.3X6
Lung irritant (gas) NEC	T59.91	T59.92	T59.93	T59.94	—	—
Luteinizing hormone	T38.811	T38.812	T38.813	T38.814	T38.815	T38.816
Lutocylol	T38.5X1	T38.5X2	T38.5X3	T38.5X4	T38.5X5	T38.5X6
Lutromone	T38.5X1	T38.5X2	T38.5X3	T38.5X4	T38.5X5	T38.5X6
Lututrin	T48.291	T48.292	T48.293	T48.294	T48.295	T48.296
Lye (Concentrated)	T54.3X1	T54.3X2	T54.3X3	T54.3X4	—	
Lygranum (skin test)	T5Ø.8X1	T5Ø.8X2	T5Ø.8X3	T5Ø.8X4	T5Ø.8X5	T5Ø.8X6
Lymecycline	T36.4X1	T36.4X2	T36.4X3	T36.4X4	T36.4X5	T36.4X6
Lymphogranuloma venereum antigen	T5Ø.8X1	T5Ø.8X2	T5Ø.8X3	T5Ø.8X4	T5Ø.8X5	T5Ø.8X6
Lynestrenol	T38.4X1	T38.4X2	T38.4X3	T38.4X4	T38.4X5	T38.4X6
Lypressin	T38.891	T38.892	T38.893	T38.894	T38.895	T38.896
Lyovac Sodium Edecrin	T5Ø.1X1	T5Ø.1X2	T5Ø.1X3	T5Ø.1X4	T5Ø.1X5	T5Ø.1X6
Lysergic acid diethylamide	T4Ø.8X1	T4Ø.8X2	T4Ø.8X3	T4Ø.8X4	—	—
Lysergide	T4Ø.8X1	T4Ø.8X2	T4Ø.8X3	T4Ø.8X4	—	—
Lysine vasopressin	T38.891	T38.892	T38.893	T38.894	T38.895	T38.896
Lysol	T54.1X1	T54.1X2	T54.1X3	T54.1X4	—	—
Lysozyme	T49.ØX1	T49.ØX2	T49.ØX3	T49.ØX4	T49.ØX5	T49.ØX6
Lytta (vitatta)	T49.8X1	T49.8X2	T49.8X3	T49.8X4	T49.8X5	T49.8X6

M

Substance	External Cause (T-Code) Poisoning, Accidental (Unintentional)	Poisoning, Intentional Self-Harm	Poisoning, Assault	Poisoning, Undetermined	Adverse Effect	Underdosing
Mace	T59.3X1	T59.3X2	T59.3X3	T59.3X4	—	—
Macrogol	T5Ø.991	T5Ø.992	T5Ø.993	T5Ø.994	T5Ø.995	T5Ø.996
Macrolide						
anabolic drug	T38.7X1	T38.7X2	T38.7X3	T38.7X4	T38.7X5	T38.7X6
antibiotic	T36.3X1	T36.3X2	T36.3X3	T36.3X4	T36.3X5	T36.3X6
Mafenide	T49.ØX1	T49.ØX2	T49.ØX3	T49.ØX4	T49.ØX5	T49.ØX6
Magaldrate	T47.1X1	T47.1X2	T47.1X3	T47.1X4	T47.1X5	T47.1X6
Magic mushroom	T4Ø.991	T4Ø.992	T4Ø.993	T4Ø.994	—	—
Magnamycin	T36.8X1	T36.8X2	T36.8X3	T36.8X4	T36.8X5	T36.8X6
Magnesia magma	T47.1X1	T47.1X2	T47.1X3	T47.1X4	T47.1X5	T47.1X6
Magnesium NEC	T56.891	T56.892	T56.893	T56.894	—	—
carbonate	T47.1X1	T47.1X2	T47.1X3	T47.1X4	T47.1X5	T47.1X6
citrate	T47.4X1	T47.4X2	T47.4X3	T47.4X4	T47.4X5	T47.4X6
hydroxide	T47.1X1	T47.1X2	T47.1X3	T47.1X4	T47.1X5	T47.1X6
oxide	T47.1X1	T47.1X2	T47.1X3	T47.1X4	T47.1X5	T47.1X6
peroxide	T49.ØX1	T49.ØX2	T49.ØX3	T49.ØX4	T49.ØX5	T49.ØX6
salicylate	T39.Ø91	T39.Ø92	T39.Ø93	T39.Ø94	T39.Ø95	T39.Ø96
silicofluoride	T5Ø.3X1	T5Ø.3X2	T5Ø.3X3	T5Ø.3X4	T5Ø.3X5	T5Ø.3X6
sulfate	T47.4X1	T47.4X2	T47.4X3	T47.4X4	T47.4X5	T47.4X6
thiosulfate	T45.ØX1	T45.ØX2	T45.ØX3	T45.ØX4	T45.ØX5	T45.ØX6
trisilicate	T47.1X1	T47.1X2	T47.1X3	T47.1X4	T47.1X5	T47.1X6
Malathion (medicinal)	T49.ØX1	T49.ØX2	T49.ØX3	T49.ØX4	T49.ØX5	T49.ØX6
insecticide	T6Ø.ØX1	T6Ø.ØX2	T6Ø.ØX3	T6Ø.ØX4	—	—
Male fern extract	T37.4X1	T37.4X2	T37.4X3	T37.4X4	T37.4X5	T37.4X6
M-AMSA	T45.1X1	T45.1X2	T45.1X3	T45.1X4	T45.1X5	T45.1X6
Mandelic acid	T37.8X1	T37.8X2	T37.8X3	T37.8X4	T37.8X5	T37.8X6
Manganese (dioxide) (salts)	T57.2X1	T57.2X2	T57.2X3	T57.2X4	—	—
medicinal	T5Ø.991	T5Ø.992	T5Ø.993	T5Ø.994	T5Ø.995	T5Ø.996

TABLE OF DRUGS AND CHEMICALS

Substance	External Cause (T-Code) Poisoning, Accidental (Unintentional)	Poisoning, Intentional Self-Harm	Poisoning, Assault	Poisoning, Undetermined	Adverse Effect	Underdosing
Mannitol	T47.3X1	T47.3X2	T47.3X3	T47.3X4	T47.3X5	T47.3X6
hexanitrate	T46.3X1	T46.3X2	T46.3X3	T46.3X4	T46.3X5	T46.3X6
Mannomustine	T45.1X1	T45.1X2	T45.1X3	T45.1X4	T45.1X5	T45.1X6
MAO inhibitors	T43.1X1	T43.1X2	T43.1X3	T43.1X4	T43.1X5	T43.1X6
Mapharsen	T37.8X1	T37.8X2	T37.8X3	T37.8X4	T37.8X5	T37.8X6
Maphenide	T49.0X1	T49.0X2	T49.0X3	T49.0X4	T49.0X5	T49.0X6
Maprotiline	T43.021	T43.022	T43.023	T43.024	T43.025	T43.026
Marcaine	T41.3X1	T41.3X2	T41.3X3	T41.3X4	T41.3X5	T41.3X6
infiltration (subcutaneous)	T41.3X1	T41.3X2	T41.3X3	T41.3X4	T41.3X5	T41.3X6
nerve block (peripheral) (plexus)	T41.3X1	T41.3X2	T41.3X3	T41.3X4	T41.3X5	T41.3X6
Marezine	T45.0X1	T45.0X2	T45.0X3	T45.0X4	T45.0X5	T45.0X6
Marihuana	T40.711	T40.712	T40.713	T40.714	T40.715	T40.716
Marijuana	T40.711	T40.712	T40.713	T40.714	T40.715	T40.716
Marine (sting)	T63.691	T63.692	T63.693	T63.694	—	—
animals (sting)	T63.691	T63.692	T63.693	T63.694	—	—
plants (sting)	T63.711	T63.712	T63.713	T63.714	—	—
Marplan	T43.1X1	T43.1X2	T43.1X3	T43.1X4	T43.1X5	T43.1X6
Marsh gas	T59.891	T59.892	T59.893	T59.894	—	—
Marsilid	T43.1X1	T43.1X2	T43.1X3	T43.1X4	T43.1X5	T43.1X6
Matulane	T45.1X1	T45.1X2	T45.1X3	T45.1X4	T45.1X5	T45.1X6
Mazindol	T50.5X1	T50.5X2	T50.5X3	T50.5X4	T50.5X5	T50.5X6
MCPA	T60.3X1	T60.3X2	T60.3X3	T60.3X4	—	—
MDMA	T43.641	T43.642	T43.643	T43.644	—	—
Meadow saffron	T62.2X1	T62.2X2	T62.2X3	T62.2X4	—	—
Measles virus vaccine (attenuated)	T50.B91	T50.B92	T50.B93	T50.B94	T50.B95	T50.B96
Meat, noxious	T62.8X1	T62.8X2	T62.8X3	T62.8X4	—	—
Meballymal	T42.3X1	T42.3X2	T42.3X3	T42.3X4	T42.3X5	T42.3X6
Mebanazine	T43.1X1	T43.1X2	T43.1X3	T43.1X4	T43.1X5	T43.1X6
Mebaral	T42.3X1	T42.3X2	T42.3X3	T42.3X4	T42.3X5	T42.3X6
Mebendazole	T37.4X1	T37.4X2	T37.4X3	T37.4X4	T37.4X5	T37.4X6
Mebeverine	T44.3X1	T44.3X2	T44.3X3	T44.3X4	T44.3X5	T44.3X6
Mebhydrolin	T45.0X1	T45.0X2	T45.0X3	T45.0X4	T45.0X5	T45.0X6
Mebumal	T42.3X1	T42.3X2	T42.3X3	T42.3X4	T42.3X5	T42.3X6
Mebutamate	T43.591	T43.592	T43.593	T43.594	T43.595	T43.596
Mecamylamine	T44.2X1	T44.2X2	T44.2X3	T44.2X4	T44.2X5	T44.2X6
Mechlorethamine	T45.1X1	T45.1X2	T45.1X3	T45.1X4	T45.1X5	T45.1X6
Mecillinam	T36.0X1	T36.0X2	T36.0X3	T36.0X4	T36.0X5	T36.0X6
Meclizine (hydrochloride)	T45.0X1	T45.0X2	T45.0X3	T45.0X4	T45.0X5	T45.0X6
Meclocycline	T36.4X1	T36.4X2	T36.4X3	T36.4X4	T36.4X5	T36.4X6
Meclofenamate	T39.391	T39.392	T39.393	T39.394	T39.395	T39.396
Meclofenamic acid	T39.391	T39.392	T39.393	T39.394	T39.395	T39.396

Substance	External Cause (T-Code) Poisoning, Accidental (Unintentional)	Poisoning, Intentional Self-Harm	Poisoning, Assault	Poisoning, Undetermined	Adverse Effect	Underdosing
Meclofenoxate	T43.691	T43.692	T43.693	T43.694	T43.695	T43.696
Meclozine	T45.0X1	T45.0X2	T45.0X3	T45.0X4	T45.0X5	T45.0X6
Mecobalamin	T45.8X1	T45.8X2	T45.8X3	T45.8X4	T45.8X5	T45.8X6
Mecoprop	T60.3X1	T60.3X2	T60.3X3	T60.3X4	—	—
Mecrilate	T49.3X1	T49.3X2	T49.3X3	T49.3X4	T49.3X5	T49.3X6
Mecysteine	T48.4X1	T48.4X2	T48.4X3	T48.4X4	T48.4X5	T48.4X6
Medazepam	T42.4X1	T42.4X2	T42.4X3	T42.4X4	T42.4X5	T42.4X6
Medicament NEC	T50.901	T50.902	T50.903	T50.904	T50.905	T50.906
Medinal	T42.3X1	T42.3X2	T42.3X3	T42.3X4	T42.3X5	T42.3X6
Medomin	T42.3X1	T42.3X2	T42.3X3	T42.3X4	T42.3X5	T42.3X6
Medrogestone	T38.5X1	T38.5X2	T38.5X3	T38.5X4	T38.5X5	T38.5X6
Medroxalol	T44.8X1	T44.8X2	T44.8X3	T44.8X4	T44.8X5	T44.8X6
Medroxyprogesterone acetate (depot)	T38.5X1	T38.5X2	T38.5X3	T38.5X4	T38.5X5	T38.5X6
Medrysone	T49.0X1	T49.0X2	T49.0X3	T49.0X4	T49.0X5	T49.0X6
Mefenamic acid	T39.391	T39.392	T39.393	T39.394	T39.395	T39.396
Mefenorex	T50.5X1	T50.5X2	T50.5X3	T50.5X4	T50.5X5	T50.5X6
Mefloquine	T37.2X1	T37.2X2	T37.2X3	T37.2X4	T37.2X5	T37.2X6
Mefruside	T50.2X1	T50.2X2	T50.2X3	T50.2X4	T50.2X5	T50.2X6
Megahallucinogen	T40.901	T40.902	T40.903	T40.904	T40.905	T40.906
Megestrol	T38.5X1	T38.5X2	T38.5X3	T38.5X4	T38.5X5	T38.5X6
Meglumine						
antimoniate	T37.8X1	T37.8X2	T37.8X3	T37.8X4	T37.8X5	T37.8X6
diatrizoate	T50.8X1	T50.8X2	T50.8X3	T50.8X4	T50.8X5	T50.8X6
iodipamide	T50.8X1	T50.8X2	T50.8X3	T50.8X4	T50.8X5	T50.8X6
iotroxate	T50.8X1	T50.8X2	T50.8X3	T50.8X4	T50.8X5	T50.8X6
MEK (methyl ethyl ketone)	T52.4X1	T52.4X2	T52.4X3	T52.4X4	—	—
Meladrazine	T44.3X1	T44.3X2	T44.3X3	T44.3X4	T44.3X5	T44.3X6
Meladinin	T49.3X1	T49.3X2	T49.3X3	T49.3X4	T49.3X5	T49.3X6
Melaleuca alternifolia oil	T49.0X1	T49.0X2	T49.0X3	T49.0X4	T49.0X5	T49.0X6
Melanizing agents	T49.3X1	T49.3X2	T49.3X3	T49.3X4	T49.3X5	T49.3X6
Melanocyte-stimulating hormone	T38.891	T38.892	T38.893	T38.894	T38.895	T38.896
Melarsonyl potassium	T37.3X1	T37.3X2	T37.3X3	T37.3X4	T37.3X5	T37.3X6
Melarsoprol	T37.3X1	T37.3X2	T37.3X3	T37.3X4	T37.3X5	T37.3X6
Melia azedarach	T62.2X1	T62.2X2	T62.2X3	T62.2X4	—	—
Melitracen	T43.011	T43.012	T43.013	T43.014	T43.015	T43.016
Mellaril	T43.3X1	T43.3X2	T43.3X3	T43.3X4	T43.3X5	T43.3X6
Meloxine	T49.3X1	T49.3X2	T49.3X3	T49.3X4	T49.3X5	T49.3X6
Melperone	T43.4X1	T43.4X2	T43.4X3	T43.4X4	T43.4X5	T43.4X6
Melphalan	T45.1X1	T45.1X2	T45.1X3	T45.1X4	T45.1X5	T45.1X6
Memantine	T43.8X1	T43.8X2	T43.8X3	T43.8X4	T43.8X5	T43.8X6

New Revised ~~deleted~~ Deleted

Substance	Poisoning, Accidental (Unintentional)	Poisoning, Intentional Self-Harm	Poisoning, Assault	Poisoning, Undetermined	Adverse Effect	Underdosing
	External Cause (T-Code)					
Menadiol	T45.7X1	T45.7X2	T45.7X3	T45.7X4	T45.7X5	T45.7X6
sodium sulfate	T45.7X1	T45.7X2	T45.7X3	T45.7X4	T45.7X5	T45.7X6
Menadione	T45.7X1	T45.7X2	T45.7X3	T45.7X4	T45.7X5	T45.7X6
sodium bisulfite	T45.7X1	T45.7X2	T45.7X3	T45.7X4	T45.7X5	T45.7X6
Menaphthone	T45.7X1	T45.7X2	T45.7X3	T45.7X4	T45.7X5	T45.7X6
Menaquinone	T45.7X1	T45.7X2	T45.7X3	T45.7X4	T45.7X5	T45.7X6
Menatetrenone	T45.7X1	T45.7X2	T45.7X3	T45.7X4	T45.7X5	T45.7X6
Meningococcal vaccine	T50.A91	T50.A92	T50.A93	T50.A94	T50.A95	T50.A96
Menningovax (-AC) (-C)	T50.A91	T50.A92	T50.A93	T50.A94	T50.A95	T50.A96
Menotropins	T38.811	T38.812	T38.813	T38.814	T38.815	T38.816
Menthol	T48.5X1	T48.5X2	T48.5X3	T48.5X4	T48.5X5	T48.5X6
Mepacrine	T37.2X1	T37.2X2	T37.2X3	T37.2X4	T37.2X5	T37.2X6
Meparfynol	T42.6X1	T42.6X2	T42.6X3	T42.6X4	T42.6X5	T42.6X6
Mepartricin	T36.7X1	T36.7X2	T36.7X3	T36.7X4	T36.7X5	T36.7X6
Mepazine	T43.3X1	T43.3X2	T43.3X3	T43.3X4	T43.3X5	T43.3X6
Mepenzolate	T44.3X1	T44.3X2	T44.3X3	T44.3X4	T44.3X5	T44.3X6
bromide	T44.3X1	T44.3X2	T44.3X3	T44.3X4	T44.3X5	T44.3X6
Meperidine	T40.491	T40.492	T40.493	T40.494	T40.495	T40.496
Mephebarbital	T42.3X1	T42.3X2	T42.3X3	T42.3X4	T42.3X5	T42.3X6
Mephenamin(e)	T42.8X1	T42.8X2	T42.8X3	T42.8X4	T42.8X5	T42.8X6
Mephenesin	T42.8X1	T42.8X2	T42.8X3	T42.8X4	T42.8X5	T42.8X6
Mephenhydramine	T45.0X1	T45.0X2	T45.0X3	T45.0X4	T45.0X5	T45.0X6
Mephenoxalone	T42.8X1	T42.8X2	T42.8X3	T42.8X4	T42.8X5	T42.8X6
Mephentermine	T44.991	T44.992	T44.993	T44.994	T44.995	T44.996
Mephenytoin	T42.0X1	T42.0X2	T42.0X3	T42.0X4	T42.0X5	T42.0X6
with phenobarbital	T42.3X1	T42.3X2	T42.3X3	T42.3X4	T42.3X5	T42.3X6
Mephobarbital	T42.3X1	T42.3X2	T42.3X3	T42.3X4	T42.3X5	T42.3X6
Mephosfolan	T60.0X1	T60.0X2	T60.0X3	T60.0X4	—	—
Mepindolol	T44.7X1	T44.7X2	T44.7X3	T44.7X4	T44.7X5	T44.7X6
Mepiperphenidol	T44.3X1	T44.3X2	T44.3X3	T44.3X4	T44.3X5	T44.3X6
Mepitiostane	T38.7X1	T38.7X2	T38.7X3	T38.7X4	T38.7X5	T38.7X6
Mepivacaine	T41.3X1	T41.3X2	T41.3X3	T41.3X4	T41.3X5	T41.3X6
epidural	T41.3X1	T41.3X2	T41.3X3	T41.3X4	T41.3X5	T41.3X6
Meprednisone	T38.0X1	T38.0X2	T38.0X3	T38.0X4	T38.0X5	T38.0X6
Meprobam	T43.591	T43.592	T43.593	T43.594	T43.595	T43.596
Meprobamate	T43.591	T43.592	T43.593	T43.594	T43.595	T43.596
Meproscillarin	T46.0X1	T46.0X2	T46.0X3	T46.0X4	T46.0X5	T46.0X6
Meprylcaine	T41.3X1	T41.3X2	T41.3X3	T41.3X4	T41.3X5	T41.3X6
Meptazinol	T39.8X1	T39.8X2	T39.8X3	T39.8X4	T39.8X5	T39.8X6
Mepyramine	T45.0X1	T45.0X2	T45.0X3	T45.0X4	T45.0X5	T45.0X6
Mequitazine	T43.3X1	T43.3X2	T43.3X3	T43.3X4	T43.3X5	T43.3X6
Meralluride	T50.2X1	T50.2X2	T50.2X3	T50.2X4	T50.2X5	T50.2X6
Merbaphen	T50.2X1	T50.2X2	T50.2X3	T50.2X4	T50.2X5	T50.2X6
Merbromin	T49.0X1	T49.0X2	T49.0X3	T49.0X4	T49.0X5	T49.0X6
Mercaptobenzothiazole salts	T49.0X1	T49.0X2	T49.0X3	T49.0X4	T49.0X5	T49.0X6
Mercaptomerin	T50.2X1	T50.2X2	T50.2X3	T50.2X4	T50.2X5	T50.2X6
Mercaptopurine	T45.1X1	T45.1X2	T45.1X3	T45.1X4	T45.1X5	T45.1X6
Mercumatilin	T50.2X1	T50.2X2	T50.2X3	T50.2X4	T50.2X5	T50.2X6
Mercuramide	T50.2X1	T50.2X2	T50.2X3	T50.2X4	T50.2X5	T50.2X6
Mercurochrome	T49.0X1	T49.0X2	T49.0X3	T49.0X4	T49.0X5	T49.0X6
Mercurophylline	T50.2X1	T50.2X2	T50.2X3	T50.2X4	T50.2X5	T50.2X6
Mercury, mercurial, mercuric, mercurous (compounds) (cyanide) (fumes) (nonmedicinal) (vapor) NEC	T56.1X1	T56.1X2	T56.1X3	T56.1X4	—	—
ammoniated	T49.0X1	T49.0X2	T49.0X3	T49.0X4	T49.0X5	T49.0X6
anti-infective						
local	T49.0X1	T49.0X2	T49.0X3	T49.0X4	T49.0X5	T49.0X6
systemic	T37.8X1	T37.8X2	T37.8X3	T37.8X4	T37.8X5	T37.8X6
topical	T49.0X1	T49.0X2	T49.0X3	T49.0X4	T49.0X5	T49.0X6
chloride (ammoniated)	T49.0X1	T49.0X2	T49.0X3	T49.0X4	T49.0X5	T49.0X6
fungicide	T56.1X1	T56.1X2	T56.1X3	T56.1X4	—	—
diuretic NEC	T50.2X1	T50.2X2	T50.2X3	T50.2X4	T50.2X5	T50.2X6
fungicide	T56.1X1	T56.1X2	T56.1X3	T56.1X4	—	—
organic (fungicide)	T56.1X1	T56.1X2	T56.1X3	T56.1X4	—	—
oxide, yellow	T49.0X1	T49.0X2	T49.0X3	T49.0X4	T49.0X5	T49.0X6
Mersalyl	T50.2X1	T50.2X2	T50.2X3	T50.2X4	T50.2X5	T50.2X6
Merthiolate	T49.0X1	T49.0X2	T49.0X3	T49.0X4	T49.0X5	T49.0X6
ophthalmic preparation	T49.5X1	T49.5X2	T49.5X3	T49.5X4	T49.5X5	T49.5X6
Meruvax	T50.B91	T50.B92	T50.B93	T50.B94	T50.B95	T50.B96
Mesalazine	T47.8X1	T47.8X2	T47.8X3	T47.8X4	T47.8X5	T47.8X6
Mescal buttons	T40.991	T40.992	T40.993	T40.994	—	—
Mescaline	T40.991	T40.992	T40.993	T40.994	—	—
Mesna	T48.4X1	T48.4X2	T48.4X3	T48.4X4	T48.4X5	T48.4X6
Mesoglycan	T46.6X1	T46.6X2	T46.6X3	T46.6X4	T46.6X5	T46.6X6
Mesoridazine	T43.3X1	T43.3X2	T43.3X3	T43.3X4	T43.3X5	T43.3X6
Mestanolone	T38.7X1	T38.7X2	T38.7X3	T38.7X4	T38.7X5	T38.7X6
Mesterolone	T38.7X1	T38.7X2	T38.7X3	T38.7X4	T38.7X5	T38.7X6
Mestranol	T38.5X1	T38.5X2	T38.5X3	T38.5X4	T38.5X5	T38.5X6
Mesulergine	T42.8X1	T42.8X2	T42.8X3	T42.8X4	T42.8X5	T42.8X6
Mesulfen	T49.0X1	T49.0X2	T49.0X3	T49.0X4	T49.0X5	T49.0X6
Mesuximide	T42.2X1	T42.2X2	T42.2X3	T42.2X4	T42.2X5	T42.2X6
Metabutethamine	T41.3X1	T41.3X2	T41.3X3	T41.3X4	T41.3X5	T41.3X6
Metactesylacetate	T49.0X1	T49.0X2	T49.0X3	T49.0X4	T49.0X5	T49.0X6
Metacycline	T36.4X1	T36.4X2	T36.4X3	T36.4X4	T36.4X5	T36.4X6

Substance	External Cause (T-Code)					
	Poisoning, Accidental (Unintentional)	Poisoning, Intentional Self-Harm	Poisoning, Assault	Poisoning, Undetermined	Adverse Effect	Underdosing
Metaldehyde (snail killer) NEC	T60.8X1	T60.8X2	T60.8X3	T60.8X4	—	—
Metals (heavy) (nonmedicinal)	T56.91	T56.92	T56.93	T56.94	—	—
dust, fumes, or vapor NEC	T56.91	T56.92	T56.93	T56.94	—	—
gadolinium	T56.821	T56.822	T56.823	T56.824	T56.825	—
light NEC	T56.91	T56.92	T56.93	T56.94	—	—
dust, fumes, or vapor NEC	T56.91	T56.92	T56.93	T56.94	—	—
specified NEC	T56.891	T56.892	T56.893	T56.894	—	—
thallium	T56.811	T56.812	T56.813	T56.814	—	—
Metamfetamine	T43.651	T43.652	T43.652	T43.654	T43.655	T43.656
Metamizole sodium	T39.2X1	T39.2X2	T39.2X3	T39.2X4	T39.2X5	T39.2X6
Metampicillin	T36.0X1	T36.0X2	T36.0X3	T36.0X4	T36.0X5	T36.0X6
Metamucil	T47.4X1	T47.4X2	T47.4X3	T47.4X4	T47.4X5	T47.4X6
Metaphen	T49.0X1	T49.0X2	T49.0X3	T49.0X4	T49.0X5	T49.0X6
Metandienone	T38.7X1	T38.7X2	T38.7X3	T38.7X4	T38.7X5	T38.7X6
Metandrostenolone	T38.7X1	T38.7X2	T38.7X3	T38.7X4	T38.7X5	T38.7X6
Metaphos	T60.0X1	T60.0X2	T60.0X3	T60.0X4	—	—
Metapramine	T43.011	T43.012	T43.013	T43.014	T43.015	T43.016
Metaproterenol	T48.291	T48.292	T48.293	T48.294	T48.295	T48.296
Metaraminol	T44.4X1	T44.4X2	T44.4X3	T44.4X4	T44.4X5	T44.4X6
Metaxalone	T42.8X1	T42.8X2	T42.8X3	T42.8X4	T42.8X5	T42.8X6
Metenolone	T38.7X1	T38.7X2	T38.7X3	T38.7X4	T38.7X5	T38.7X6
Metergoline	T42.8X1	T42.8X2	T42.8X3	T42.8X4	T42.8X5	T42.8X6
Metescufylline	T46.991	T46.992	T46.993	T46.994	T46.995	T46.996
Metetoin	T42.0X1	T42.0X2	T42.0X3	T42.0X4	T42.0X5	T42.0X6
Metformin	T38.3X1	T38.3X2	T38.3X3	T38.3X4	T38.3X5	T38.3X6
Methacholine	T44.1X1	T44.1X2	T44.1X3	T44.1X4	T44.1X5	T44.1X6
Methacycline	T36.4X1	T36.4X2	T36.4X3	T36.4X4	T36.4X5	T36.4X6
Methadone	T40.3X1	T40.3X2	T40.3X3	T40.3X4	T40.3X5	T40.3X6
Methallenestril	T38.5X1	T38.5X2	T38.5X3	T38.5X4	T38.5X5	T38.5X6
Methallenoestril	T38.5X1	T38.5X2	T38.5X3	T38.5X4	T38.5X5	T38.5X6
Methamphetamine	T43.651	T43.652	T43.652	T43.654	T43.655	T43.656
Methampyrone	T39.2X1	T39.2X2	T39.2X3	T39.2X4	T39.2X5	T39.2X6
Methandienone	T38.7X1	T38.7X2	T38.7X3	T38.7X4	T38.7X5	T38.7X6
Methandriol	T38.7X1	T38.7X2	T38.7X3	T38.7X4	T38.7X5	T38.7X6
Methandrostenolone	T38.7X1	T38.7X2	T38.7X3	T38.7X4	T38.7X5	T38.7X6
Methane	T59.891	T59.892	T59.893	T59.894	—	—
Methanethiol	T59.891	T59.892	T59.893	T59.894	—	—
Methaniazide	T37.1X1	T37.1X2	T37.1X3	T37.1X4	T37.1X5	T37.1X6
Methanol (vapor)	T51.1X1	T51.1X2	T51.1X3	T51.1X4	—	—
Methantheline	T44.3X1	T44.3X2	T44.3X3	T44.3X4	T44.3X5	T44.3X6
Methanthelinium bromide	T44.3X1	T44.3X2	T44.3X3	T44.3X4	T44.3X5	T44.3X6
Methaphenilene	T45.0X1	T45.0X2	T45.0X3	T45.0X4	T45.0X5	T45.0X6
Methapyrilene	T45.0X1	T45.0X2	T45.0X3	T45.0X4	T45.0X5	T45.0X6
Methaqualone (compound)	T42.6X1	T42.6X2	T42.6X3	T42.6X4	T42.6X5	T42.6X6
Metharbital	T42.3X1	T42.3X2	T42.3X3	T42.3X4	T42.3X5	T42.3X6
Methazolamide	T50.2X1	T50.2X2	T50.2X3	T50.2X4	T50.2X5	T50.2X6
Methdilazine	T43.3X1	T43.3X2	T43.3X3	T43.3X4	T43.3X5	T43.3X6
Methedrine	T43.651	T43.652	T43.652	T43.654	T43.655	T43.656
Methenamine (mandelate)	T37.8X1	T37.8X2	T37.8X3	T37.8X4	T37.8X5	T37.8X6
Methenolone	T38.7X1	T38.7X2	T38.7X3	T38.7X4	T38.7X5	T38.7X6
Methergine	T48.0X1	T48.0X2	T48.0X3	T48.0X4	T48.0X5	T48.0X6
Methetoin	T42.0X1	T42.0X2	T42.0X3	T42.0X4	T42.0X5	T42.0X6
Methiacil	T38.2X1	T38.2X2	T38.2X3	T38.2X4	T38.2X5	T38.2X6
Methicillin	T36.0X1	T36.0X2	T36.0X3	T36.0X4	T36.0X5	T36.0X6
Methimazole	T38.2X1	T38.2X2	T38.2X3	T38.2X4	T38.2X5	T38.2X6
Methiodal sodium	T50.8X1	T50.8X2	T50.8X3	T50.8X4	T50.8X5	T50.8X6
Methionine	T50.991	T50.992	T50.993	T50.994	T50.995	T50.996
Methisazone	T37.5X1	T37.5X2	T37.5X3	T37.5X4	T37.5X5	T37.5X6
Methisoprinol	T37.5X1	T37.5X2	T37.5X3	T37.5X4	T37.5X5	T37.5X6
Methitural	T42.3X1	T42.3X2	T42.3X3	T42.3X4	T42.3X5	T42.3X6
Methixene	T44.3X1	T44.3X2	T44.3X3	T44.3X4	T44.3X5	T44.3X6
Methobarbital, methobarbitone	T42.3X1	T42.3X2	T42.3X3	T42.3X4	T42.3X5	T42.3X6
Methocarbamol	T42.8X1	T42.8X2	T42.8X3	T42.8X4	T42.8X5	T42.8X6
skeletal muscle relaxant	T48.1X1	T48.1X2	T48.1X3	T48.1X4	T48.1X5	T48.1X6
Methohexital	T41.1X1	T41.1X2	T41.1X3	T41.1X4	T41.1X5	T41.1X6
Methohexitone	T41.1X1	T41.1X2	T41.1X3	T41.1X4	T41.1X5	T41.1X6
Methoin	T42.0X1	T42.0X2	T42.0X3	T42.0X4	T42.0X5	T42.0X6
Methopholine	T39.8X1	T39.8X2	T39.8X3	T39.8X4	T39.8X5	T39.8X6
Methopromazine	T43.3X1	T43.3X2	T43.3X3	T43.3X4	T43.3X5	T43.3X6
Methorate	T48.3X1	T48.3X2	T48.3X3	T48.3X4	T48.3X5	T48.3X6
Methoserpidine	T46.5X1	T46.5X2	T46.5X3	T46.5X4	T46.5X5	T46.5X6
Methotrexate	T45.1X1	T45.1X2	T45.1X3	T45.1X4	T45.1X5	T45.1X6
Methotrimeprazine	T43.3X1	T43.3X2	T43.3X3	T43.3X4	T43.3X5	T43.3X6
Methoxa-Dome	T49.3X1	T49.3X2	T49.3X3	T49.3X4	T49.3X5	T49.3X6
Methoxamine	T44.4X1	T44.4X2	T44.4X3	T44.4X4	T44.4X5	T44.4X6
Methoxsalen	T50.991	T50.992	T50.993	T50.994	T50.995	T50.996
Methoxyaniline	T65.3X1	T65.3X2	T65.3X3	T65.3X4	—	—
Methoxybenzyl penicillin	T36.0X1	T36.0X2	T36.0X3	T36.0X4	T36.0X5	T36.0X6
Methoxychlor	T53.7X1	T53.7X2	T53.7X3	T53.7X4	—	—
Methoxy-DDT	T53.7X1	T53.7X2	T53.7X3	T53.7X4	—	—
2-Methoxyethanol	T52.3X1	T52.3X2	T52.3X3	T52.3X4	—	—
Methoxyflurane	T41.0X1	T41.0X2	T41.0X3	T41.0X4	T41.0X5	T41.0X6
Methoxyphenamine	T48.6X1	T48.6X2	T48.6X3	T48.6X4	T48.6X5	T48.6X6
Methoxypromazine	T43.3X1	T43.3X2	T43.3X3	T43.3X4	T43.3X5	T43.3X6

New Revised ~~deleted~~ Deleted

Substance	External Cause (T-Code) Poisoning, Accidental (Unintentional)	Poisoning, Intentional Self-Harm	Poisoning, Assault	Poisoning, Undetermined	Adverse Effect	Underdosing
5-Methoxypsoralen (5-MOP)	T5Ø.991	T5Ø.992	T5Ø.993	T5Ø.994	T5Ø.995	T5Ø.996
8-Methoxypsoralen (8-MOP)	T5Ø.991	T5Ø.992	T5Ø.993	T5Ø.994	T5Ø.995	T5Ø.996
Methscopolamine bromide	T44.3X1	T44.3X2	T44.3X3	T44.3X4	T44.3X5	T44.3X6
Methsuximide	T42.2X1	T42.2X2	T42.2X3	T42.2X4	T42.2X5	T42.2X6
Methyclothiazide	T5Ø.2X1	T5Ø.2X2	T5Ø.2X3	T5Ø.2X4	T5Ø.2X5	T5Ø.2X6
Methyl						
acetate	T52.4X1	T52.4X2	T52.4X3	T52.4X4	—	—
acetone	T52.4X1	T52.4X2	T52.4X3	T52.4X4	—	—
acrylate	T65.891	T65.892	T65.893	T65.894	—	—
alcohol	T51.1X1	T51.1X2	T51.1X3	T51.1X4	—	—
aminophenol	T65.3X1	T65.3X2	T65.3X3	T65.3X4	—	—
amphetamine	T43.651	T43.652	T43.652	T43.654	T43.655	T43.656
androstanolone	T38.7X1	T38.7X2	T38.7X3	T38.7X4	T38.7X5	T38.7X6
atropine	T44.3X1	T44.3X2	T44.3X3	T44.3X4	T44.3X5	T44.3X6
benzene	T52.2X1	T52.2X2	T52.2X3	T52.2X4	—	—
benzoate	T52.8X1	T52.8X2	T52.8X3	T52.8X4	—	—
benzol	T52.2X1	T52.2X2	T52.2X3	T52.2X4	—	—
bromide (gas)	T59.891	T59.892	T59.893	T59.894	—	—
fumigant	T6Ø.8X1	T6Ø.8X2	T6Ø.8X3	T6Ø.8X4	—	—
butanol	T51.3X1	T51.3X2	T51.3X3	T51.3X4	—	—
carbinol	T51.1X1	T51.1X2	T51.1X3	T51.1X4	—	—
carbonate	T52.8X1	T52.8X2	T52.8X3	T52.8X4	—	—
CCNU	T45.1X1	T45.1X2	T45.1X3	T45.1X4	T45.1X5	T45.1X6
cellosolve	T52.91	T52.92	T52.93	T52.94	—	—
cellulose	T47.4X1	T47.4X2	T47.4X3	T47.4X4	T47.4X5	T47.4X6
chloride (gas)	T59.891	T59.892	T59.893	T59.894	—	—
chloroformate	T59.3X1	T59.3X2	T59.3X3	T59.3X4	—	—
cyclohexane	T52.8X1	T52.8X2	T52.8X3	T52.8X4	—	—
cyclohexanol	T51.8X1	T51.8X2	T51.8X3	T51.8X4	—	—
cyclohexanone	T52.8X1	T52.8X2	T52.8X3	T52.8X4	—	—
cyclohexyl acetate	T52.8X1	T52.8X2	T52.8X3	T52.8X4	—	—
demeton	T6Ø.ØX1	T6Ø.ØX2	T6Ø.ØX3	T6Ø.ØX4	—	—
dihydromorphinone	T4Ø.2X1	T4Ø.2X2	T4Ø.2X3	T4Ø.2X4	T4Ø.2X5	T4Ø.2X6
ergometrine	T48.ØX1	T48.ØX2	T48.ØX3	T48.ØX4	T48.ØX5	T48.ØX6
ergonovine	T48.ØX1	T48.ØX2	T48.ØX3	T48.ØX4	T48.ØX5	T48.ØX6
ethyl ketone	T52.4X1	T52.4X2	T52.4X3	T52.4X4	—	—
glucamine antimonate	T37.8X1	T37.8X2	T37.8X3	T37.8X4	T37.8X5	T37.8X6
hydrazine	T65.891	T65.892	T65.893	T65.894	—	—
iodide	T65.891	T65.892	T65.893	T65.894	—	—
isobutyl ketone	T52.4X1	T52.4X2	T52.4X3	T52.4X4	—	—
isothiocyanate	T6Ø.3X1	T6Ø.3X2	T6Ø.3X3	T6Ø.3X4	—	—
mercaptan	T59.891	T59.892	T59.893	T59.894	—	—
Methyl *(Continued)*						
morphine NEC	T4Ø.2X1	T4Ø.2X2	T4Ø.2X3	T4Ø.2X4	T4Ø.2X5	T4Ø.2X6
nicotinate	T49.4X1	T49.4X2	T49.4X3	T49.4X4	T49.4X5	T49.4X6
paraben	T49.ØX1	T49.ØX2	T49.ØX3	T49.ØX4	T49.ØX5	T49.ØX6
parafynol	T42.6X1	T42.6X2	T42.6X3	T42.6X4	T42.6X5	T42.6X6
parathion	T6Ø.ØX1	T6Ø.ØX2	T6Ø.ØX3	T6Ø.ØX4	—	—
peridol	T43.4X1	T43.4X2	T43.4X3	T43.4X4	T43.4X5	T43.4X6
phenidate	T43.631	T43.632	T43.633	T43.634	T43.635	T43.636
prednisolone	T38.ØX1	T38.ØX2	T38.ØX3	T38.ØX4	T38.ØX5	T38.ØX6
ENT agent	T49.6X1	T49.6X2	T49.6X3	T49.6X4	T49.6X5	T49.6X6
ophthalmic preparation	T49.5X1	T49.5X2	T49.5X3	T49.5X4	T49.5X5	T49.5X6
topical NEC	T49.ØX1	T49.ØX2	T49.ØX3	T49.ØX4	T49.ØX5	T49.ØX6
propylcarbinol	T51.3X1	T51.3X2	T51.3X3	T51.3X4	—	—
rosaniline NEC	T49.ØX1	T49.ØX2	T49.ØX3	T49.ØX4	T49.ØX5	T49.ØX6
salicylate	T49.2X1	T49.2X2	T49.2X3	T49.2X4	T49.2X5	T49.2X6
sulfate (fumes)	T59.891	T59.892	T59.893	T59.894	—	—
liquid	T52.8X1	T52.8X2	T52.8X3	T52.8X4	—	—
sulfonal	T42.6X1	T42.6X2	T42.6X3	T42.6X4	T42.6X5	T42.6X6
testosterone	T38.7X1	T38.7X2	T38.7X3	T38.7X4	T38.7X5	T38.7X6
thiouracil	T38.2X1	T38.2X2	T38.2X3	T38.2X4	T38.2X5	T38.2X6
Methylamphetamine	T43.651	T43.652	T43.652	T43.654	T43.655	T43.656
Methylated spirit	T51.1X1	T51.1X2	T51.1X3	T51.1X4	—	—
Methylatropine nitrate	T44.3X1	T44.3X2	T44.3X3	T44.3X4	T44.3X5	T44.3X6
Methylbenactyzium bromide	T44.3X1	T44.3X2	T44.3X3	T44.3X4	T44.3X5	T44.3X6
Methylbenzethonium chloride	T49.ØX1	T49.ØX2	T49.ØX3	T49.ØX4	T49.ØX5	T49.ØX6
Methylcellulose	T47.4X1	T47.4X2	T47.4X3	T47.4X4	T47.4X5	T47.4X6
laxative	T47.4X1	T47.4X2	T47.4X3	T47.4X4	T47.4X5	T47.4X6
Methylchlorophenoxy-acetic acid	T6Ø.3X1	T6Ø.3X2	T6Ø.3X3	T6Ø.3X4	—	—
Methyldopa	T46.5X1	T46.5X2	T46.5X3	T46.5X4	T46.5X5	T46.5X6
Methyldopate	T46.5X1	T46.5X2	T46.5X3	T46.5X4	T46.5X5	T46.5X6
Methylene						
blue	T5Ø.6X1	T5Ø.6X2	T5Ø.6X3	T5Ø.6X4	T5Ø.6X5	T5Ø.6X6
chloride or dichloride (solvent) NEC	T53.4X1	T53.4X2	T53.4X3	T53.4X4	—	—
Methylenedioxyamphet-amine	T43.621	T43.622	T43.623	T43.624	T43.625	T43.626
Methylenedioxymethamphetamine	T43.641	T43.642	T43.643	T43.644	—	—
Methylergometrine	T48.ØX1	T48.ØX2	T48.ØX3	T48.ØX4	T48.ØX5	T48.ØX6
Methylergonovine	T48.ØX1	T48.ØX2	T48.ØX3	T48.ØX4	T48.ØX5	T48.ØX6
Methylestrenolone	T38.5X1	T38.5X2	T38.5X3	T38.5X4	T38.5X5	T38.5X6
Methylethyl cellulose	T5Ø.991	T5Ø.992	T5Ø.993	T5Ø.994	T5Ø.995	T5Ø.996
Methylhexabital	T42.3X1	T42.3X2	T42.3X3	T42.3X4	T42.3X5	T42.3X6
Methylmorphine	T4Ø.2X1	T4Ø.2X2	T4Ø.2X3	T4Ø.2X4	T4Ø.2X5	T4Ø.2X6

Substance	External Cause (T-Code) Poisoning, Accidental (Unintentional)	Poisoning, Intentional Self-Harm	Poisoning, Assault	Poisoning, Undetermined	Adverse Effect	Underdosing
Methylparaben (ophthalmic)	T49.5X1	T49.5X2	T49.5X3	T49.5X4	T49.5X5	T49.5X6
Methylparafynol	T42.6X1	T42.6X2	T42.6X3	T42.6X4	T42.6X5	T42.6X6
Methylpentynol, methylpenthynol	T42.6X1	T42.6X2	T42.6X3	T42.6X4	T42.6X5	T42.6X6
Methylphenidate	T43.631	T43.632	T43.633	T43.634	T43.635	T43.636
Methylphenobarbital	T42.3X1	T42.3X2	T42.3X3	T42.3X4	T42.3X5	T42.3X6
Methylpolysiloxane	T47.1X1	T47.1X2	T47.1X3	T47.1X4	T47.1X5	T47.1X6
Methylprednisolone — *see Methyl, prednisolone*						
Methylrosaniline	T49.0X1	T49.0X2	T49.0X3	T49.0X4	T49.0X5	T49.0X6
Methylrosanilinium chloride	T49.0X1	T49.0X2	T49.0X3	T49.0X4	T49.0X5	T49.0X6
Methyltestosterone	T38.7X1	T38.7X2	T38.7X3	T38.7X4	T38.7X5	T38.7X6
Methylthionine chloride	T50.6X1	T50.6X2	T50.6X3	T50.6X4	T50.6X5	T50.6X6
Methylthioninium chloride	T50.6X1	T50.6X2	T50.6X3	T50.6X4	T50.6X5	T50.6X6
Methylthiouracil	T38.2X1	T38.2X2	T38.2X3	T38.2X4	T38.2X5	T38.2X6
Methyprylon	T42.6X1	T42.6X2	T42.6X3	T42.6X4	T42.6X5	T42.6X6
Methysergide	T46.5X1	T46.5X2	T46.5X3	T46.5X4	T46.5X5	T46.5X6
Metiamide	T47.1X1	T47.1X2	T47.1X3	T47.1X4	T47.1X5	T47.1X6
Meticillin	T36.0X1	T36.0X2	T36.0X3	T36.0X4	T36.0X5	T36.0X6
Meticrane	T50.2X1	T50.2X2	T50.2X3	T50.2X4	T50.2X5	T50.2X6
Metildigoxin	T46.0X1	T46.0X2	T46.0X3	T46.0X4	T46.0X5	T46.0X6
Metipranolol	T49.5X1	T49.5X2	T49.5X3	T49.5X4	T49.5X5	T49.5X6
Metirosine	T46.5X1	T46.5X2	T46.5X3	T46.5X4	T46.5X5	T46.5X6
Metisazone	T37.5X1	T37.5X2	T37.5X3	T37.5X4	T37.5X5	T37.5X6
Metixene	T44.3X1	T44.3X2	T44.3X3	T44.3X4	T44.3X5	T44.3X6
Metizoline	T48.5X1	T48.5X2	T48.5X3	T48.5X4	T48.5X5	T48.5X6
Metoclopramide	T45.0X1	T45.0X2	T45.0X3	T45.0X4	T45.0X5	T45.0X6
Metofenazate	T43.3X1	T43.3X2	T43.3X3	T43.3X4	T43.3X5	T43.3X6
Metofoline	T39.8X1	T39.8X2	T39.8X3	T39.8X4	T39.8X5	T39.8X6
Metolazone	T50.2X1	T50.2X2	T50.2X3	T50.2X4	T50.2X5	T50.2X6
Metopon	T40.2X1	T40.2X2	T40.2X3	T40.2X4	T40.2X5	T40.2X6
Metoprine	T45.1X1	T45.1X2	T45.1X3	T45.1X4	T45.1X5	T45.1X6
Metoprolol	T44.7X1	T44.7X2	T44.7X3	T44.7X4	T44.7X5	T44.7X6
Metrifonate	T60.0X1	T60.0X2	T60.0X3	T60.0X4	—	—
Metrizamide	T50.8X1	T50.8X2	T50.8X3	T50.8X4	T50.8X5	T50.8X6
Metrizoic acid	T50.8X1	T50.8X2	T50.8X3	T50.8X4	T50.8X5	T50.8X6
Metronidazole	T37.8X1	T37.8X2	T37.8X3	T37.8X4	T37.8X5	T37.8X6
Metycaine	T41.3X1	T41.3X2	T41.3X3	T41.3X4	T41.3X5	T41.3X6
infiltration (subcutaneous)	T41.3X1	T41.3X2	T41.3X3	T41.3X4	T41.3X5	T41.3X6
nerve block (peripheral) (plexus)	T41.3X1	T41.3X2	T41.3X3	T41.3X4	T41.3X5	T41.3X6
topical (surface)	T41.3X1	T41.3X2	T41.3X3	T41.3X4	T41.3X5	T41.3X6
Metyrapone	T50.8X1	T50.8X2	T50.8X3	T50.8X4	T50.8X5	T50.8X6
Mevinphos	T60.0X1	T60.0X2	T60.0X3	T60.0X4	—	—

Substance	External Cause (T-Code) Poisoning, Accidental (Unintentional)	Poisoning, Intentional Self-Harm	Poisoning, Assault	Poisoning, Undetermined	Adverse Effect	Underdosing
Mexazolam	T42.4X1	T42.4X2	T42.4X3	T42.4X4	T42.4X5	T42.4X6
Mexenone	T49.3X1	T49.3X2	T49.3X3	T49.3X4	T49.3X5	T49.3X6
Mexiletine	T46.2X1	T46.2X2	T46.2X3	T46.2X4	T46.2X5	T46.2X6
Mezereon	T62.2X1	T62.2X2	T62.2X3	T62.2X4	—	—
berries	T62.1X1	T62.1X2	T62.1X3	T62.1X4	—	—
Mezlocillin	T36.0X1	T36.0X2	T36.0X3	T36.0X4	T36.0X5	T36.0X6
Mianserin	T43.021	T43.022	T43.023	T43.024	T43.025	T43.026
Micatin	T49.0X1	T49.0X2	T49.0X3	T49.0X4	T49.0X5	T49.0X6
Miconazole	T49.0X1	T49.0X2	T49.0X3	T49.0X4	T49.0X5	T49.0X6
Micronomicin	T36.5X1	T36.5X2	T36.5X3	T36.5X4	T36.5X5	T36.5X6
Midazolam	T42.4X1	T42.4X2	T42.4X3	T42.4X4	T42.4X5	T42.4X6
Midecamycin	T36.3X1	T36.3X2	T36.3X3	T36.3X4	T36.3X5	T36.3X6
Mifepristone	T38.6X1	T38.6X2	T38.6X3	T38.6X4	T38.6X5	T38.6X6
Milk of magnesia	T47.1X1	T47.1X2	T47.1X3	T47.1X4	T47.1X5	T47.1X6
Millipede (tropical) (venomous)	T63.411	T63.412	T63.413	T63.414	—	—
Miltown	T43.591	T43.592	T43.593	T43.594	T43.595	T43.596
Milverine	T44.3X1	T44.3X2	T44.3X3	T44.3X4	T44.3X5	T44.3X6
Minaprine	T43.291	T43.292	T43.293	T43.294	T43.295	T43.296
Minaxolone	T41.291	T41.292	T41.293	T41.294	T41.295	T41.296
Mineral						
acids	T54.2X1	T54.2X2	T54.2X3	T54.2X4	—	—
oil (laxative) (medicinal)	T47.4X1	T47.4X2	T47.4X3	T47.4X4	T47.4X5	T47.4X6
emulsion	T47.2X1	T47.2X2	T47.2X3	T47.2X4	T47.2X5	T47.2X6
nonmedicinal	T52.0X1	T52.0X2	T52.0X3	T52.0X4	—	—
topical	T49.3X1	T49.3X2	T49.3X3	T49.3X4	T49.3X5	T49.3X6
salt NEC	T50.3X1	T50.3X2	T50.3X3	T50.3X4	T50.3X5	T50.3X6
spirits	T52.0X1	T52.0X2	T52.0X3	T52.0X4	—	—
Mineralocorticosteroid	T50.0X1	T50.0X2	T50.0X3	T50.0X4	T50.0X5	T50.0X6
Minocycline	T36.4X1	T36.4X2	T36.4X3	T36.4X4	T36.4X5	T36.4X6
Minoxidil	T46.7X1	T46.7X2	T46.7X3	T46.7X4	T46.7X5	T46.7X6
Miokamycin	T36.3X1	T36.3X2	T36.3X3	T36.3X4	T36.3X5	T36.3X6
Miotic drug	T49.5X1	T49.5X2	T49.5X3	T49.5X4	T49.5X5	T49.5X6
Mipafox	T60.0X1	T60.0X2	T60.0X3	T60.0X4	—	—
Mirex	T60.1X1	T60.1X2	T60.1X3	T60.1X4	—	—
Mirtazapine	T43.021	T43.022	T43.023	T43.024	T43.025	T43.026
Misonidazole	T37.3X1	T37.3X2	T37.3X3	T37.3X4	T37.3X5	T37.3X6
Misoprostol	T47.1X1	T47.1X2	T47.1X3	T47.1X4	T47.1X5	T47.1X6
Mithramycin	T45.1X1	T45.1X2	T45.1X3	T45.1X4	T45.1X5	T45.1X6
Mitobronitol	T45.1X1	T45.1X2	T45.1X3	T45.1X4	T45.1X5	T45.1X6
Mitoguazone	T45.1X1	T45.1X2	T45.1X3	T45.1X4	T45.1X5	T45.1X6
Mitolactol	T45.1X1	T45.1X2	T45.1X3	T45.1X4	T45.1X5	T45.1X6
Mitomycin	T45.1X1	T45.1X2	T45.1X3	T45.1X4	T45.1X5	T45.1X6

New Revised ~~deleted~~ Deleted

Substance	External Cause (T-Code) Poisoning, Accidental (Unintentional)	Poisoning, Intentional Self-Harm	Poisoning, Assault	Poisoning, Undetermined	Adverse Effect	Underdosing
Mitopodozide	T45.1X1	T45.1X2	T45.1X3	T45.1X4	T45.1X5	T45.1X6
Mitotane	T45.1X1	T45.1X2	T45.1X3	T45.1X4	T45.1X5	T45.1X6
Mitoxantrone	T45.1X1	T45.1X2	T45.1X3	T45.1X4	T45.1X5	T45.1X6
Mivacurium chloride	T48.1X1	T48.1X2	T48.1X3	T48.1X4	T48.1X5	T48.1X6
Miyari bacteria	T47.6X1	T47.6X2	T47.6X3	T47.6X4	T47.6X5	T47.6X6
Moclobemide	T43.1X1	T43.1X2	T43.1X3	T43.1X4	T43.1X5	T43.1X6
Moderil	T46.5X1	T46.5X2	T46.5X3	T46.5X4	T46.5X5	T46.5X6
Mofebutazone	T39.2X1	T39.2X2	T39.2X3	T39.2X4	T39.2X5	T39.2X6
Mogadon — *see Nitrazepam*						
Molindone	T43.591	T43.592	T43.593	T43.594	T43.595	T43.596
Molsidomine	T46.3X1	T46.3X2	T46.3X3	T46.3X4	T46.3X5	T46.3X6
Mometasone	T49.ØX1	T49.ØX2	T49.ØX3	T49.ØX4	T49.ØX5	T49.ØX6
Monistat	T49.ØX1	T49.ØX2	T49.ØX3	T49.ØX4	T49.ØX5	T49.ØX6
Monkshood	T62.2X1	T62.2X2	T62.2X3	T62.2X4	—	—
Monoamine oxidase inhibitor NEC	T43.1X1	T43.1X2	T43.1X3	T43.1X4	T43.1X5	T43.1X6
hydrazine	T43.1X1	T43.1X2	T43.1X3	T43.1X4	T43.1X5	T43.1X6
Monobenzone	T49.4X1	T49.4X2	T49.4X3	T49.4X4	T49.4X5	T49.4X6
Monochloroacetic acid	T6Ø.3X1	T6Ø.3X2	T6Ø.3X3	T6Ø.3X4	—	—
Monochlorobenzene	T53.7X1	T53.7X2	T53.7X3	T53.7X4	—	—
Monoethanolamine	T46.8X1	T46.8X2	T46.8X3	T46.8X4	T46.8X5	T46.8X6
oleate	T46.8X1	T46.8X2	T46.8X3	T46.8X4	T46.8X5	T46.8X6
Monooctanoin	T5Ø.991	T5Ø.992	T5Ø.993	T5Ø.994	T5Ø.995	T5Ø.996
Monophenylbutazone	T39.2X1	T39.2X2	T39.2X3	T39.2X4	T39.2X5	T39.2X6
Monosodium glutamate	T65.891	T65.892	T65.893	T65.894	—	—
Monosulfiram	T49.ØX1	T49.ØX2	T49.ØX3	T49.ØX4	T49.ØX5	T49.ØX6
Monoxide, carbon — *see Carbon, monoxide*	T57.91	T57.92	T57.93	T57.94	—	—
Monoxidine hydrochloride	T46.1X1	T46.1X2	T46.1X3	T46.1X4	T46.1X5	T46.1X6
Monuron	T6Ø.3X1	T6Ø.3X2	T6Ø.3X3	T6Ø.3X4	—	—
Moperone	T43.4X1	T43.4X2	T43.4X3	T43.4X4	T43.4X5	T43.4X6
Mopidamol	T45.1X1	T45.1X2	T45.1X3	T45.1X4	T45.1X5	T45.1X6
MOPP (mechlorethamine + vincristine + prednisone + procarbazine)	T45.1X1	T45.1X2	T45.1X3	T45.1X4	T45.1X5	T45.1X6
Morfin	T4Ø.2X1	T4Ø.2X2	T4Ø.2X3	T4Ø.2X4	T4Ø.2X5	T4Ø.2X6
Morinamide	T37.1X1	T37.1X2	T37.1X3	T37.1X4	T37.1X5	T37.1X6
Morning glory seeds	T4Ø.991	T4Ø.992	T4Ø.993	T4Ø.994	—	—
Moroxydine	T37.5X1	T37.5X2	T37.5X3	T37.5X4	T37.5X5	T37.5X6
Morphazinamide	T37.1X1	T37.1X2	T37.1X3	T37.1X4	T37.1X5	T37.1X6
Morphine	T4Ø.2X1	T4Ø.2X2	T4Ø.2X3	T4Ø.2X4	T4Ø.2X5	T4Ø.2X6
antagonist	T5Ø.7X1	T5Ø.7X2	T5Ø.7X3	T5Ø.7X4	T5Ø.7X5	T5Ø.7X6
Morpholinylethylmorphine	T4Ø.2X1	T4Ø.2X2	T4Ø.2X3	T4Ø.2X4	—	—
Morsuximide	T42.2X1	T42.2X2	T42.2X3	T42.2X4	T42.2X5	T42.2X6
Mosapramine	T43.591	T43.592	T43.593	T43.594	T43.595	T43.596
Moth balls — *see also Pesticide*	T6Ø.2X1	T6Ø.2X2	T6Ø.2X3	T6Ø.2X4	—	—
naphthalene	T6Ø.2X1	T6Ø.2X2	T6Ø.2X3	T6Ø.2X4	—	—
paradichlorobenzene	T6Ø.1X1	T6Ø.1X2	T6Ø.1X3	T6Ø.1X4	—	—
Motor exhaust gas	T58.Ø1	T58.Ø2	T58.Ø3	T58.Ø4	—	—
Mouthwash (antiseptic) (zinc chloride)	T49.6X1	T49.6X2	T49.6X3	T49.6X4	T49.6X5	T49.6X6
Moxastine	T45.ØX1	T45.ØX2	T45.ØX3	T45.ØX4	T45.ØX5	T45.ØX6
Moxaverine	T44.3X1	T44.3X2	T44.3X3	T44.3X4	T44.3X5	T44.3X6
Moxifensine	T43.291	T43.292	T43.293	T43.294	T43.295	T43.296
Moxisylyte	T46.7X1	T46.7X2	T46.7X3	T46.7X4	T46.7X5	T46.7X6
Mucilage, plant	T47.4X1	T47.4X2	T47.4X3	T47.4X4	T47.4X5	T47.4X6
Mucolytic drug	T48.4X1	T48.4X2	T48.4X3	T48.4X4	T48.4X5	T48.4X6
Mucomyst	T48.4X1	T48.4X2	T48.4X3	T48.4X4	T48.4X5	T48.4X6
Mucous membrane agents (external)	T49.91	T49.92	T49.93	T49.94	T49.95	T49.96
specified NEC	T49.8X1	T49.8X2	T49.8X3	T49.8X4	T49.8X5	T49.8X6
Multiple unspecified drugs, medicaments and biological substances	T5Ø.911	T5Ø.912	T5Ø.913	T5Ø.914	T5Ø.915	T5Ø.916
Mumps						
immune globulin (human)	T5Ø.Z11	T5Ø.Z12	T5Ø.Z13	T5Ø.Z14	T5Ø.Z15	T5Ø.Z16
skin test antigen	T5Ø.8X1	T5Ø.8X2	T5Ø.8X3	T5Ø.8X4	T5Ø.8X5	T5Ø.8X6
vaccine	T5Ø.B91	T5Ø.B92	T5Ø.B93	T5Ø.B94	T5Ø.B95	T5Ø.B96
Mumpsvax	T5Ø.B91	T5Ø.B92	T5Ø.B93	T5Ø.B94	T5Ø.B95	T5Ø.B96
Mupirocin	T49.ØX1	T49.ØX2	T49.ØX3	T49.ØX4	T49.ØX5	T49.ØX6
Muriatic acid — *see Hydrochloric acid*						
Muromonab-CD3	T45.1X1	T45.1X2	T45.1X3	T45.1X4	T45.1X5	T45.1X6
Muscle relaxant — *see Relaxant, muscle*						
Muscle-action drug NEC	T48.2Ø1	T48.2Ø2	T48.2Ø3	T48.2Ø4	T48.2Ø5	T48.2Ø6
Muscle affecting agents NEC	T48.2Ø1	T48.2Ø2	T48.2Ø3	T48.2Ø4	T48.2Ø5	T48.2Ø6
oxytocic	T48.ØX1	T48.ØX2	T48.ØX3	T48.ØX4	T48.ØX5	T48.ØX6
relaxants	T48.2Ø1	T48.2Ø2	T48.2Ø3	T48.2Ø4	T48.2Ø5	T48.2Ø6
central nervous system	T42.8X1	T42.8X2	T42.8X3	T42.8X4	T42.8X5	T42.8X6
skeletal	T48.1X1	T48.1X2	T48.1X3	T48.1X4	T48.1X5	T48.1X6
smooth	T44.3X1	T44.3X2	T44.3X3	T44.3X4	T44.3X5	T44.3X6
Muscle-tone depressant, central NEC	T42.8X1	T42.8X2	T42.8X3	T42.8X4	T42.8X5	T42.8X6
specified NEC	T42.8X1	T42.8X2	T42.8X3	T42.8X4	T42.8X5	T42.8X6
Mushroom, noxious	T62.ØX1	T62.ØX2	T62.ØX3	T62.ØX4	—	—
Mussel, noxious	T61.781	T61.782	T61.783	T61.784	—	—

	External Cause (T-Code)					
Substance	Poisoning, Accidental (Unintentional)	Poisoning, Intentional Self-Harm	Poisoning, Assault	Poisoning, Undetermined	Adverse Effect	Underdosing
Mustard (emetic)	T47.7X1	T47.7X2	T47.7X3	T47.7X4	T47.7X5	T47.7X6
black	T47.7X1	T47.7X2	T47.7X3	T47.7X4	T47.7X5	T47.7X6
gas, not in war	T59.91	T59.92	T59.93	T59.94	—	—
nitrogen	T45.1X1	T45.1X2	T45.1X3	T45.1X4	T45.1X5	T45.1X6
Mustine	T45.1X1	T45.1X2	T45.1X3	T45.1X4	T45.1X5	T45.1X6
M-vac	T45.1X1	T45.1X2	T45.1X3	T45.1X4	T45.1X5	T45.1X6
Mycifradin	T36.5X1	T36.5X2	T36.5X3	T36.5X4	T36.5X5	T36.5X6
topical	T49.0X1	T49.0X2	T49.0X3	T49.0X4	T49.0X5	T49.0X6
Mycitracin	T36.8X1	T36.8X2	T36.8X3	T36.8X4	T36.8X5	T36.8X6
ophthalmic preparation	T49.5X1	T49.5X2	T49.5X3	T49.5X4	T49.5X5	T49.5X6
Mycostatin	T36.7X1	T36.7X2	T36.7X3	T36.7X4	T36.7X5	T36.7X6
topical	T49.0X1	T49.0X2	T49.0X3	T49.0X4	T49.0X5	T49.0X6
Mycotoxins	T64.81	T64.82	T64.83	T64.84	—	—
aflatoxin	T64.01	T64.02	T64.03	T64.04	—	—
specified NEC	T64.81	T64.82	T64.83	T64.84	—	—
Mydriacyl	T44.3X1	T44.3X2	T44.3X3	T44.3X4	T44.3X5	T44.3X6
Mydriatic drug	T49.5X1	T49.5X2	T49.5X3	T49.5X4	T49.5X5	T49.5X6
Myelobromal	T45.1X1	T45.1X2	T45.1X3	T45.1X4	T45.1X5	T45.1X6
Myleran	T45.1X1	T45.1X2	T45.1X3	T45.1X4	T45.1X5	T45.1X6
Myochrysin(e)	T39.2X1	T39.2X2	T39.2X3	T39.2X4	T39.2X5	T39.2X6
Myoneural blocking agents	T48.1X1	T48.1X2	T48.1X3	T48.1X4	T48.1X5	T48.1X6
Myralact	T49.0X1	T49.0X2	T49.0X3	T49.0X4	T49.0X5	T49.0X6
Myristica fragrans	T62.2X1	T62.2X2	T62.2X3	T62.2X4	—	—
Myristicin	T65.891	T65.892	T65.893	T65.894	—	—
Mysoline	T42.3X1	T42.3X2	T42.3X3	T42.3X4	T42.3X5	T42.3X6
N						
Nabilone	T40.711	T40.712	T40.713	T40.714	T40.715	T40.716
Nabumetone	T39.391	T39.392	T39.393	T39.394	T39.395	T39.396
Nadolol	T44.7X1	T44.7X2	T44.7X3	T44.7X4	T44.7X5	T44.7X6
Nafcillin	T36.0X1	T36.0X2	T36.0X3	T36.0X4	T36.0X5	T36.0X6
Nafoxidine	T38.6X1	T38.6X2	T38.6X3	T38.6X4	T38.6X5	T38.6X6
Naftazone	T46.991	T46.992	T46.993	T46.994	T46.995	T46.996
Naftidrofuryl (oxalate)	T46.7X1	T46.7X2	T46.7X3	T46.7X4	T46.7X5	T46.7X6
Naftifine	T49.0X1	T49.0X2	T49.0X3	T49.0X4	T49.0X5	T49.0X6
Nail polish remover	T52.91	T52.92	T52.93	T52.94	—	—
Nalbuphine	T40.491	T40.492	T40.493	T40.494	T40.495	T40.496
Naled	T60.0X1	T60.0X2	T60.0X3	T60.0X4	—	—
Nalidixic acid	T37.8X1	T37.8X2	T37.8X3	T37.8X4	T37.8X5	T37.8X6
Nalorphine	T50.7X1	T50.7X2	T50.7X3	T50.7X4	T50.7X5	T50.7X6
Naloxone	T50.7X1	T50.7X2	T50.7X3	T50.7X4	T50.7X5	T50.7X6
Naltrexone	T50.7X1	T50.7X2	T50.7X3	T50.7X4	T50.7X5	T50.7X6
Namenda	T43.8X1	T43.8X2	T43.8X3	T43.8X4	T43.8X5	T43.8X6

	External Cause (T-Code)					
Substance	Poisoning, Accidental (Unintentional)	Poisoning, Intentional Self-Harm	Poisoning, Assault	Poisoning, Undetermined	Adverse Effect	Underdosing
Nandrolone	T38.7X1	T38.7X2	T38.7X3	T38.7X4	T38.7X5	T38.7X6
Naphazoline	T48.5X1	T48.5X2	T48.5X3	T48.5X4	T48.5X5	T48.5X6
Naphtha (painters') (petroleum)	T52.0X1	T52.0X2	T52.0X3	T52.0X4	—	—
solvent	T52.0X1	T52.0X2	T52.0X3	T52.0X4	—	—
vapor	T52.0X1	T52.0X2	T52.0X3	T52.0X4	—	—
Naphthalene (non-chlorinated)	T60.2X1	T60.2X2	T60.2X3	T60.2X4	—	—
chlorinated	T60.1X1	T60.1X2	T60.1X3	T60.1X4	—	—
vapor	T60.1X1	T60.1X2	T60.1X3	T60.1X4	—	—
insecticide or moth repellent	T60.2X1	T60.2X2	T60.2X3	T60.2X4	—	—
chlorinated	T60.1X1	T60.1X2	T60.1X3	T60.1X4	—	—
vapor	T60.2X1	T60.2X2	T60.2X3	T60.2X4	—	—
chlorinated	T60.1X1	T60.1X2	T60.1X3	T60.1X4	—	—
Naphthol	T65.891	T65.892	T65.893	T65.894	—	—
Naphthylamine	T65.891	T65.892	T65.893	T65.894	—	—
Naphthylthiourea (ANTU)	T60.4X1	T60.4X2	T60.4X3	T60.4X4	—	—
Naprosyn — *see Naproxen*						
Naproxen	T39.311	T39.312	T39.313	T39.314	T39.315	T39.316
Narcotic (drug)	T40.601	T40.602	T40.603	T40.604	T40.605	T40.606
analgesic NEC	T40.601	T40.602	T40.603	T40.604	T40.605	T40.606
antagonist	T50.7X1	T50.7X2	T50.7X3	T50.7X4	T50.7X5	T50.7X6
specified NEC	T40.691	T40.692	T40.693	T40.694	T40.695	T40.696
synthetic	T40.491	T40.492	T40.493	T40.494	T40.495	T40.496
Narcotine	T48.3X1	T48.3X2	T48.3X3	T48.3X4	T48.3X5	T48.3X6
Nardil	T43.1X1	T43.1X2	T43.1X3	T43.1X4	T43.1X5	T43.1X6
Nasal drug NEC	T49.6X1	T49.6X2	T49.6X3	T49.6X4	T49.6X5	T49.6X6
Natamycin	T49.0X1	T49.0X2	T49.0X3	T49.0X4	T49.0X5	T49.0X6
Natrium cyanide — *see Cyanide(s)*						
Natural gas	T59.891	T59.892	T59.893	T59.894	—	—
incomplete combustion	T57.91	T57.92	T57.93	T57.94	—	—
Natural						
blood (product)	T45.8X1	T45.8X2	T45.8X3	T45.8X4	T45.8X5	T45.8X6
gas (piped)	T59.891	T59.892	T59.893	T59.894	—	—
incomplete combustion	T58.11	T58.12	T58.13	T58.14	—	—
Nealbarbital	T42.3X1	T42.3X2	T42.3X3	T42.3X4	T42.3X5	T42.3X6
Nectadon	T48.3X1	T48.3X2	T48.3X3	T48.3X4	T48.3X5	T48.3X6
Nedocromil	T48.6X1	T48.6X2	T48.6X3	T48.6X4	T48.6X5	T48.6X6
Nefopam	T39.8X1	T39.8X2	T39.8X3	T39.8X4	T39.8X5	T39.8X6
Nematocyst (sting)	T63.691	T63.692	T63.693	T63.694	—	—
Nembutal	T42.3X1	T42.3X2	T42.3X3	T42.3X4	T42.3X5	T42.3X6
Nemonapride	T43.591	T43.592	T43.593	T43.594	T43.595	T43.596
Neoarsphenamine	T37.8X1	T37.8X2	T37.8X3	T37.8X4	T37.8X5	T37.8X6

Substance	External Cause (T-Code)					
	Poisoning, Accidental (Unintentional)	Poisoning, Intentional Self-Harm	Poisoning, Assault	Poisoning, Undetermined	Adverse Effect	Underdosing
Neocinchophen	T50.4X1	T50.4X2	T50.4X3	T50.4X4	T50.4X5	T50.4X6
Neomycin (derivatives)	T36.5X1	T36.5X2	T36.5X3	T36.5X4	T36.5X5	T36.5X6
with						
bacitracin	T49.0X1	T49.0X2	T49.0X3	T49.0X4	T49.0X5	T49.0X6
neostigmine	T44.0X1	T44.0X2	T44.0X3	T44.0X4	T44.0X5	T44.0X6
ENT agent	T49.6X1	T49.6X2	T49.6X3	T49.6X4	T49.6X5	T49.6X6
ophthalmic preparation	T49.5X1	T49.5X2	T49.5X3	T49.5X4	T49.5X5	T49.5X6
topical NEC	T49.0X1	T49.0X2	T49.0X3	T49.0X4	T49.0X5	T49.0X6
Neonal	T42.3X1	T42.3X2	T42.3X3	T42.3X4	T42.3X5	T42.3X6
Neoprontosil	T37.0X1	T37.0X2	T37.0X3	T37.0X4	T37.0X5	T37.0X6
Neosalvarsan	T37.8X1	T37.8X2	T37.8X3	T37.8X4	T37.8X5	T37.8X6
Neosilversalvarsan	T37.8X1	T37.8X2	T37.8X3	T37.8X4	T37.8X5	T37.8X6
Neosporin	T36.8X1	T36.8X2	T36.8X3	T36.8X4	T36.8X5	T36.8X6
ENT agent	T49.6X1	T49.6X2	T49.6X3	T49.6X4	T49.6X5	T49.6X6
opthalmic preparation	T49.5X1	T49.5X2	T49.5X3	T49.5X4	T49.5X5	T49.5X6
topical NEC	T49.0X1	T49.0X2	T49.0X3	T49.0X4	T49.0X5	T49.0X6
Neostigmine bromide	T44.0X1	T44.0X2	T44.0X3	T44.0X4	T44.0X5	T44.0X6
Neraval	T42.3X1	T42.3X2	T42.3X3	T42.3X4	T42.3X5	T42.3X6
Neravan	T42.3X1	T42.3X2	T42.3X3	T42.3X4	T42.3X5	T42.3X6
Nerium oleander	T62.2X1	T62.2X2	T62.2X3	T62.2X4	—	—
Nerve gas, not in war	T59.91	T59.92	T59.93	T59.94	—	—
Nesacaine	T41.3X1	T41.3X2	T41.3X3	T41.3X4	T41.3X5	T41.3X6
infiltration (subcutaneous)	T41.3X1	T41.3X2	T41.3X3	T41.3X4	T41.3X5	T41.3X6
nerve block (peripheral) (plexus)	T41.3X1	T41.3X2	T41.3X3	T41.3X4	T41.3X5	T41.3X6
Netilmicin	T36.5X1	T36.5X2	T36.5X3	T36.5X4	T36.5X5	T36.5X6
Neurobarb	T42.3X1	T42.3X2	T42.3X3	T42.3X4	T42.3X5	T42.3X6
Neuroleptic drug NEC	T43.501	T43.502	T43.503	T43.504	T43.505	T43.506
Neuromuscular blocking drug	T48.1X1	T48.1X2	T48.1X3	T48.1X4	T48.1X5	T48.1X6
Neutral insulin injection	T38.3X1	T38.3X2	T38.3X3	T38.3X4	T38.3X5	T38.3X6
Neutral spirits	T51.0X1	T51.0X2	T51.0X3	T51.0X4	—	—
beverage	T51.0X1	T51.0X2	T51.0X3	T51.0X4	—	—
Niacin	T46.7X1	T46.7X2	T46.7X3	T46.7X4	T46.7X5	T46.7X6
Niacinamide	T45.2X1	T45.2X2	T45.2X3	T45.2X4	T45.2X5	T45.2X6
Nialamide	T43.1X1	T43.1X2	T43.1X3	T43.1X4	T43.1X5	T43.1X6
Niaprazine	T42.6X1	T42.6X2	T42.6X3	T42.6X4	T42.6X5	T42.6X6
Nicametate	T46.7X1	T46.7X2	T46.7X3	T46.7X4	T46.7X5	T46.7X6
Nicardipine	T46.1X1	T46.1X2	T46.1X3	T46.1X4	T46.1X5	T46.1X6
Nicergoline	T46.7X1	T46.7X2	T46.7X3	T46.7X4	T46.7X5	T46.7X6
Nickel (carbonyl) (tetra-carbonyl) (fumes) (vapor)	T56.891	T56.892	T56.893	T56.894	—	—
Nickelocene	T56.891	T56.892	T56.893	T56.894	—	—
Niclosamide	T37.4X1	T37.4X2	T37.4X3	T37.4X4	T37.4X5	T37.4X6
Nicofuranose	T46.7X1	T46.7X2	T46.7X3	T46.7X4	T46.7X5	T46.7X6
Nicomorphine	T40.2X1	T40.2X2	T40.2X3	T40.2X4	—	—
Nicorandil	T46.3X1	T46.3X2	T46.3X3	T46.3X4	T46.3X5	T46.3X6
Nicotiana (plant)	T62.2X1	T62.2X2	T62.2X3	T62.2X4	—	—
Nicotinamide	T45.2X1	T45.2X2	T45.2X3	T45.2X4	T45.2X5	T45.2X6
Nicotine (insecticide) (spray) (sulfate) NEC	T60.2X1	T60.2X2	T60.2X3	T60.2X4	—	—
from tobacco	T65.291	T65.292	T65.293	T65.294	—	—
cigarettes	T65.221	T65.222	T65.223	T65.224	—	—
not insecticide	T65.291	T65.292	T65.293	T65.294	—	—
Nicotinic acid	T46.7X1	T46.7X2	T46.7X3	T46.7X4	T46.7X5	T46.7X6
Nicotinyl alcohol	T46.7X1	T46.7X2	T46.7X3	T46.7X4	T46.7X5	T46.7X6
Nicoumalone	T45.511	T45.512	T45.513	T45.514	T45.515	T45.516
Nifedipine	T46.1X1	T46.1X2	T46.1X3	T46.1X4	T46.1X5	T46.1X6
Nifenazone	T39.2X1	T39.2X2	T39.2X3	T39.2X4	T39.2X5	T39.2X6
Nifuraldezone	T37.91	T37.92	T37.93	T37.94	T37.95	T37.96
Nifuratel	T37.8X1	T37.8X2	T37.8X3	T37.8X4	T37.8X5	T37.8X6
Nifurtimox	T37.3X1	T37.3X2	T37.3X3	T37.3X4	T37.3X5	T37.3X6
Nifurtoinol	T37.8X1	T37.8X2	T37.8X3	T37.8X4	T37.8X5	T37.8X6
Nightshade, deadly (solanum)—*see also Belladonna*	T62.2X1	T62.2X2	T62.2X3	T62.2X4	—	—
berry	T62.1X1	T62.1X2	T62.1X3	T62.1X4	—	—
Nikethamide	T50.7X1	T50.7X2	T50.7X3	T50.7X4	T50.7X5	T50.7X6
Nilstat	T36.7X1	T36.7X2	T36.7X3	T36.7X4	T36.7X5	T36.7X6
topical	T49.0X1	T49.0X2	T49.0X3	T49.0X4	T49.0X5	T49.0X6
Nilutamide	T38.6X1	T38.6X2	T38.6X3	T38.6X4	T38.6X5	T38.6X6
Nimesulide	T39.391	T39.392	T39.393	T39.394	T39.395	T39.396
Nimetazepam	T42.4X1	T42.4X2	T42.4X3	T42.4X4	T42.4X5	T42.4X6
Nimodipine	T46.1X1	T46.1X2	T46.1X3	T46.1X4	T46.1X5	T46.1X6
Nimorazole	T37.3X1	T37.3X2	T37.3X3	T37.3X4	T37.3X5	T37.3X6
Nimustine	T45.1X1	T45.1X2	T45.1X3	T45.1X4	T45.1X5	T45.1X6
Niridazole	T37.4X1	T37.4X2	T37.4X3	T37.4X4	T37.4X5	T37.4X6
Nisentil	T40.2X1	T40.2X2	T40.2X3	T40.2X4	T40.2X5	T40.2X6
Nisoldipine	T46.1X1	T46.1X2	T46.1X3	T46.1X4	T46.1X5	T46.1X6
Nitramine	T65.3X1	T65.3X2	T65.3X3	T65.3X4	—	—
Nitrate, organic	T46.3X1	T46.3X2	T46.3X3	T46.3X4	T46.3X5	T46.3X6
Nitrazepam	T42.4X1	T42.4X2	T42.4X3	T42.4X4	T42.4X5	T42.4X6
Nitrefazole	T50.6X1	T50.6X2	T50.6X3	T50.6X4	T50.6X5	T50.6X6
Nitrendipine	T46.1X1	T46.1X2	T46.1X3	T46.1X4	T46.1X5	T46.1X6

Substance	External Cause (T-Code) Poisoning, Accidental (Unintentional)	Poisoning, Intentional Self-Harm	Poisoning, Assault	Poisoning, Undetermined	Adverse Effect	Underdosing
Nitric						
acid (liquid)	T54.2X1	T54.2X2	T54.2X3	T54.2X4	—	—
vapor	T59.891	T59.892	T59.893	T59.894	—	—
oxide (gas)	T59.0X1	T59.0X2	T59.0X3	T59.0X4	—	—
Nitrimidazine	T37.3X1	T37.3X2	T37.3X3	T37.3X4	T37.3X5	T37.3X6
Nitrite, amyl (medicinal) (vapor)	T46.3X1	T46.3X2	T46.3X3	T46.3X4	T46.3X5	T46.3X6
Nitroaniline	T65.3X1	T65.3X2	T65.3X3	T65.3X4	—	—
vapor	T59.891	T59.892	T59.893	T59.894	—	—
Nitrobenzene, nitrobenzol	T65.3X1	T65.3X2	T65.3X3	T65.3X4	—	—
vapor	T65.3X1	T65.3X2	T65.3X3	T65.3X4	—	—
Nitrocellulose	T65.891	T65.892	T65.893	T65.894	—	—
lacquer	T65.891	T65.892	T65.893	T65.894	—	—
Nitrodiphenyl	T65.3X1	T65.3X2	T65.3X3	T65.3X4	—	—
Nitrofural	T49.0X1	T49.0X2	T49.0X3	T49.0X4	T49.0X5	T49.0X6
Nitrofurantoin	T37.8X1	T37.8X2	T37.8X3	T37.8X4	T37.8X5	T37.8X6
Nitrofurazone	T49.0X1	T49.0X2	T49.0X3	T49.0X4	T49.0X5	T49.0X6
Nitrogen	T59.0X1	T59.0X2	T59.0X3	T59.0X4	—	—
mustard	T45.1X1	T45.1X2	T45.1X3	T45.1X4	T45.1X5	T45.1X6
Nitroglycerin, nitro-glycerol (medicinal)	T46.3X1	T46.3X2	T46.3X3	T46.3X4	T46.3X5	T46.3X6
nonmedicinal	T65.5X1	T65.5X2	T65.5X3	T65.5X4	—	—
fumes	T65.5X1	T65.5X2	T65.5X3	T65.5X4	—	—
Nitroglycol	T52.3X1	T52.3X2	T52.3X3	T52.3X4	—	—
Nitrohydrochloric acid	T54.2X1	T54.2X2	T54.2X3	T54.2X4	—	—
Nitromersol	T49.0X1	T49.0X2	T49.0X3	T49.0X4	T49.0X5	T49.0X6
Nitronaphthalene	T65.891	T65.892	T65.893	T65.894	—	—
Nitrophenol	T54.0X1	T54.0X2	T54.0X3	T54.0X4	—	—
Nitropropane	T52.8X1	T52.8X2	T52.8X3	T52.8X4	—	—
Nitroprusside	T46.5X1	T46.5X2	T46.5X3	T46.5X4	T46.5X5	T46.5X6
Nitrosodimethylamine	T65.3X1	T65.3X2	T65.3X3	T65.3X4	—	—
Nitrothiazol	T37.4X1	T37.4X2	T37.4X3	T37.4X4	T37.4X5	T37.4X6
Nitrotoluene, nitrotoluol	T65.3X1	T65.3X2	T65.3X3	T65.3X4	—	—
vapor	T65.3X1	T65.3X2	T65.3X3	T65.3X4	—	—
Nitrous						
acid (liquid)	T54.2X1	T54.2X2	T54.2X3	T54.2X4	—	—
fumes	T59.891	T59.892	T59.893	T59.894	—	—
ether spirit	T46.3X1	T46.3X2	T46.3X3	T46.3X4	T46.3X5	T46.3X6
oxide	T41.0X1	T41.0X2	T41.0X3	T41.0X4	T41.0X5	T41.0X6
Nitroxoline	T37.8X1	T37.8X2	T37.8X3	T37.8X4	T37.8X5	T37.8X6
Nitrozone	T49.0X1	T49.0X2	T49.0X3	T49.0X4	T49.0X5	T49.0X6
Nizatidine	T47.0X1	T47.0X2	T47.0X3	T47.0X4	T47.0X5	T47.0X6

Substance	External Cause (T-Code) Poisoning, Accidental (Unintentional)	Poisoning, Intentional Self-Harm	Poisoning, Assault	Poisoning, Undetermined	Adverse Effect	Underdosing
Nizofenone	T43.8X1	T43.8X2	T43.8X3	T43.8X4	T43.8X5	T43.8X6
Noctec	T42.6X1	T42.6X2	T42.6X3	T42.6X4	T42.6X5	T42.6X6
Noludar	T42.6X1	T42.6X2	T42.6X3	T42.6X4	T42.6X5	T42.6X6
Noptil	T42.3X1	T42.3X2	T42.3X3	T42.3X4	T42.3X5	T42.3X6
Nomegestrol	T38.5X1	T38.5X2	T38.5X3	T38.5X4	T38.5X5	T38.5X6
Nomifensine	T43.291	T43.292	T43.293	T43.294	T43.295	T43.296
Nonoxinol	T49.8X1	T49.8X2	T49.8X3	T49.8X4	T49.8X5	T49.8X6
Nonylphenoxy (polyethoxy-ethanol)	T49.8X1	T49.8X2	T49.8X3	T49.8X4	T49.8X5	T49.8X6
Noptil	T42.3X1	T42.3X2	T42.3X3	T42.3X4	T42.3X5	T42.3X6
Noradrenaline	T44.4X1	T44.4X2	T44.4X3	T44.4X4	T44.4X5	T44.4X6
Noramidopyrine	T39.2X1	T39.2X2	T39.2X3	T39.2X4	T39.2X5	T39.2X6
methanesulfonate sodium	T39.2X1	T39.2X2	T39.2X3	T39.2X4	T39.2X5	T39.2X6
Norbormide	T60.4X1	T60.4X2	T60.4X3	T60.4X4	—	—
Nordazepam	T42.4X1	T42.4X2	T42.4X3	T42.4X4	T42.4X5	T42.4X6
Norepinephrine	T44.4X1	T44.4X2	T44.4X3	T44.4X4	T44.4X5	T44.4X6
Norethandrolone	T38.7X1	T38.7X2	T38.7X3	T38.7X4	T38.7X5	T38.7X6
Norethindrone	T38.4X1	T38.4X2	T38.4X3	T38.4X4	T38.4X5	T38.4X6
Norethisterone (acetate) (enantate)	T38.4X1	T38.4X2	T38.4X3	T38.4X4	T38.4X5	T38.4X6
with ethinylestradiol	T38.5X1	T38.5X2	T38.5X3	T38.5X4	T38.5X5	T38.5X6
Noretynodrel	T38.5X1	T38.5X2	T38.5X3	T38.5X4	T38.5X5	T38.5X6
Norfenefrine	T44.4X1	T44.4X2	T44.4X3	T44.4X4	T44.4X5	T44.4X6
Norfloxacin	T36.8X1	T36.8X2	T36.8X3	T36.8X4	T36.8X5	T36.8X6
Norgestrel	T38.4X1	T38.4X2	T38.4X3	T38.4X4	T38.4X5	T38.4X6
Norgestrienone	T38.4X1	T38.4X2	T38.4X3	T38.4X4	T38.4X5	T38.4X6
Norlestrin	T38.4X1	T38.4X2	T38.4X3	T38.4X4	T38.4X5	T38.4X6
Norlutin	T38.4X1	T38.4X2	T38.4X3	T38.4X4	T38.4X5	T38.4X6
Normal serum albumin (human), salt-poor	T45.8X1	T45.8X2	T45.8X3	T45.8X4	T45.8X5	T45.8X6
Normethandrone	T38.5X1	T38.5X2	T38.5X3	T38.5X4	T38.5X5	T38.5X6
Normison—*see Benzodiazepines*						
Normorphine	T40.2X1	T40.2X2	T40.2X3	T40.2X4	—	—
Norpseudoephedrine	T50.5X1	T50.5X2	T50.5X3	T50.5X4	T50.5X5	T50.5X6
Nortestosterone (furanpropionate)	T38.7X1	T38.7X2	T38.7X3	T38.7X4	T38.7X5	T38.7X6
Nortriptyline	T43.011	T43.012	T43.013	T43.014	T43.015	T43.016
Noscapine	T48.3X1	T48.3X2	T48.3X3	T48.3X4	T48.3X5	T48.3X6
Nose preparations	T49.6X1	T49.6X2	T49.6X3	T49.6X4	T49.6X5	T49.6X6
Novobiocin	T36.5X1	T36.5X2	T36.5X3	T36.5X4	T36.5X5	T36.5X6
Novocain (infiltration) (topical)	T41.3X1	T41.3X2	T41.3X3	T41.3X4	T41.3X5	T41.3X6
nerve block (peripheral) (plexus)	T41.3X1	T41.3X2	T41.3X3	T41.3X4	T41.3X5	T41.3X6
spinal	T41.3X1	T41.3X2	T41.3X3	T41.3X4	T41.3X5	T41.3X6

New Revised ~~deleted~~ Deleted

Substance	External Cause (T-Code) Poisoning, Accidental (Unintentional)	Poisoning, Intentional Self-Harm	Poisoning, Assault	Poisoning, Undetermined	Adverse Effect	Underdosing
Noxious foodstuff	T62.91	T62.92	T62.93	T62.94	—	—
specified NEC	T62.8X1	T62.8X2	T62.8X3	T62.8X4	—	—
Noxiptiline	T43.011	T43.012	T43.013	T43.014	T43.015	T43.016
Noxytiolin	T49.0X1	T49.0X2	T49.0X3	T49.0X4	T49.0X5	T49.0X6
NPH Iletin (insulin)	T38.3X1	T38.3X2	T38.3X3	T38.3X4	T38.3X5	T38.3X6
Numorphan	T40.2X1	T40.2X2	T40.2X3	T40.2X4	T40.2X5	T40.2X6
Nunol	T42.3X1	T42.3X2	T42.3X3	T42.3X4	T42.3X5	T42.3X6
Nupercaine (spinal anesthetic)	T41.3X1	T41.3X2	T41.3X3	T41.3X4	T41.3X5	T41.3X6
topical (surface)	T41.3X1	T41.3X2	T41.3X3	T41.3X4	T41.3X5	T41.3X6
Nutmeg oil (liniment)	T49.3X1	T49.3X2	T49.3X3	T49.3X4	T49.3X5	T49.3X6
Nutritional supplement	T50.901	T50.902	T50.903	T50.904	T50.905	T50.906
Nux vomica	T65.1X1	T65.1X2	T65.1X3	T65.1X4	—	—
Nydrazid	T37.1X1	T37.1X2	T37.1X3	T37.1X4	T37.1X5	T37.1X6
Nylidrin	T46.7X1	T46.7X2	T46.7X3	T46.7X4	T46.7X5	T46.7X6
Nystatin	T36.7X1	T36.7X2	T36.7X3	T36.7X4	T36.7X5	T36.7X6
topical	T49.0X1	T49.0X2	T49.0X3	T49.0X4	T49.0X5	T49.0X6
Nytol	T45.0X1	T45.0X2	T45.0X3	T45.0X4	T45.0X5	T45.0X6
O						
Obidoxime chloride	T50.6X1	T50.6X2	T50.6X3	T50.6X4	T50.6X5	T50.6X6
Octafonium (chloride)	T49.3X1	T49.3X2	T49.3X3	T49.3X4	T49.3X5	T49.3X6
Octamethyl pyrophosphoramide	T60.0X1	T60.0X2	T60.0X3	T60.0X4	—	—
Octanoin	T50.991	T50.992	T50.993	T50.994	T50.995	T50.996
Octatropine methylbromide	T44.3X1	T44.3X2	T44.3X3	T44.3X4	T44.3X5	T44.3X6
Octotiamine	T45.2X1	T45.2X2	T45.2X3	T45.2X4	T45.2X5	T45.2X6
Octoxinol (9)	T49.8X1	T49.8X2	T49.8X3	T49.8X4	T49.8X5	T49.8X6
Octreotide	T38.991	T38.992	T38.993	T38.994	T38.995	T38.996
Octyl nitrite	T46.3X1	T46.3X2	T46.3X3	T46.3X4	T46.3X5	T46.3X6
Oestradiol	T38.5X1	T38.5X2	T38.5X3	T38.5X4	T38.5X5	T38.5X6
Oestriol	T38.5X1	T38.5X2	T38.5X3	T38.5X4	T38.5X5	T38.5X6
Oestrogen	T38.5X1	T38.5X2	T38.5X3	T38.5X4	T38.5X5	T38.5X6
Oestrone	T38.5X1	T38.5X2	T38.5X3	T38.5X4	T38.5X5	T38.5X6
Ofloxacin	T36.8X1	T36.8X2	T36.8X3	T36.8X4	T36.8X5	T36.8X6
Oil (of)	T65.891	T65.892	T65.893	T65.894	—	—
bitter almond	T62.8X1	T62.8X2	T62.8X3	T62.8X4	—	—
cloves	T49.7X1	T49.7X2	T49.7X3	T49.7X4	T49.7X5	T49.7X6
colors	T65.6X1	T65.6X2	T65.6X3	T65.6X4	—	—
fumes	T59.891	T59.892	T59.893	T59.894	—	—
lubricating	T52.0X1	T52.0X2	T52.0X3	T52.0X4	—	—
Niobe	T52.0X1	T52.8X2	T52.8X3	T52.8X4	—	—

Substance	External Cause (T-Code) Poisoning, Accidental (Unintentional)	Poisoning, Intentional Self-Harm	Poisoning, Assault	Poisoning, Undetermined	Adverse Effect	Underdosing
Oil (of) *(Continued)*						
vitriol (liquid)	T54.2X1	T54.2X2	T54.2X3	T54.2X4	—	—
fumes	T54.2X1	T54.2X2	T54.2X3	T54.2X4	—	—
wintergreen (bitter) NEC	T49.3X1	T49.3X2	T49.3X3	T49.3X4	T49.3X5	T49.3X6
Oily preparation (for skin)	T49.3X1	T49.3X2	T49.3X3	T49.3X4	T49.3X5	T49.3X6
Ointment NEC	T49.3X1	T49.3X2	T49.3X3	T49.3X4	T49.3X5	T49.3X6
Olanzapine	T43.591	T43.592	T43.593	T43.594	T43.595	T43.596
Oleander	T62.2X1	T62.2X2	T62.2X3	T62.2X4	—	—
Oleandomycin	T36.3X1	T36.3X2	T36.3X3	T36.3X4	T36.3X5	T36.3X6
Oleandrin	T46.0X1	T46.0X2	T46.0X3	T46.0X4	T46.0X5	T46.0X6
Oleic acid	T46.6X1	T46.6X2	T46.6X3	T46.6X4	T46.6X5	T46.6X6
Oleovitamin A	T45.2X1	T45.2X2	T45.2X3	T45.2X4	T45.2X5	T45.2X6
Oleum ricini	T47.2X1	T47.2X2	T47.2X3	T47.2X4	T47.2X5	T47.2X6
Olive oil (medicinal) NEC	T47.4X1	T47.4X2	T47.4X3	T47.4X4	T47.4X5	T47.4X6
Olivomycin	T45.1X1	T45.1X2	T45.1X3	T45.1X4	T45.1X5	T45.1X6
Olsalazine	T47.8X1	T47.8X2	T47.8X3	T47.8X4	T47.8X5	T47.8X6
Omeprazole	T47.1X1	T47.1X2	T47.1X3	T47.1X4	T47.1X5	T47.1X6
OMPA	T60.0X1	T60.0X2	T60.0X3	T60.0X4	—	—
Ondansetron	T45.0X1	T45.0X2	T45.0X3	T45.0X4	T45.0X5	T45.0X6
Oncovin	T45.1X1	T45.1X2	T45.1X3	T45.1X4	T45.1X5	T45.1X6
Ophthaine	T41.3X1	T41.3X2	T41.3X3	T41.3X4	T41.3X5	T41.3X6
Ophthetic	T41.3X1	T41.3X2	T41.3X3	T41.3X4	T41.3X5	T41.3X6
Opiate NEC	T40.601	T40.602	T40.603	T40.604	T40.605	T40.606
antagonists	T50.7X1	T50.7X2	T50.7X3	T50.7X4	T50.7X5	T50.7X6
Opioid NEC	T40.2X1	T40.2X2	T40.2X3	T40.2X4	T40.2X5	T40.2X6
Opipramol	T43.011	T43.012	T43.013	T43.014	T43.015	T43.016
Opium alkaloids (total)	T40.0X1	T40.0X2	T40.0X3	T40.0X4	T40.0X5	T40.0X6
standardized powdered	T40.0X1	T40.0X2	T40.0X3	T40.0X4	T40.0X5	T40.0X6
tincture (camphorated)	T40.0X1	T40.0X2	T40.0X3	T40.0X4	T40.0X5	T40.0X6
Oracon	T38.4X1	T38.4X2	T38.4X3	T38.4X4	T38.4X5	T38.4X6
Oragrafin	T50.8X1	T50.8X2	T50.8X3	T50.8X4	T50.8X5	T50.8X6
Oral contraceptives	T38.4X1	T38.4X2	T38.4X3	T38.4X4	T38.4X5	T38.4X6
Oral rehydration salts	T50.3X1	T50.3X2	T50.3X3	T50.3X4	T50.3X5	T50.3X6
Orazamide	T50.991	T50.992	T50.993	T50.994	T50.995	T50.996
Orciprenaline	T48.291	T48.292	T48.293	T48.294	T48.295	T48.296
Organidin	T48.4X1	T48.4X2	T48.4X3	T48.4X4	T48.4X5	T48.4X6
Organonitrate NEC	T46.3X1	T46.3X2	T46.3X3	T46.3X4	T46.3X5	T46.3X6
Organophosphates	T60.0X1	T60.0X2	T60.0X3	T60.0X4	—	—
Orimune	T50.B91	T50.B92	T50.B93	T50.B94	T50.B95	T50.B96
Orinase	T38.3X1	T38.3X2	T38.3X3	T38.3X4	T38.3X5	T38.3X6
Ormeloxifene	T38.6X1	T38.6X2	T38.6X3	T38.6X4	T38.6X5	T38.6X6

Substance	External Cause (T-Code) Poisoning, Accidental (Unintentional)	Poisoning, Intentional Self-Harm	Poisoning, Assault	Poisoning, Undetermined	Adverse Effect	Underdosing
Ornidazole	T37.3X1	T37.3X2	T37.3X3	T37.3X4	T37.3X5	T37.3X6
Ornithine aspartate	T5Ø.991	T5Ø.992	T5Ø.993	T5Ø.994	T5Ø.995	T5Ø.996
Ornoprostil	T47.1X1	T47.1X2	T47.1X3	T47.1X4	T47.1X5	T47.1X6
Orphenadrine (hydrochloride)	T42.8X1	T42.8X2	T42.8X3	T42.8X4	T42.8X5	T42.8X6
Ortal (sodium)	T42.3X1	T42.3X2	T42.3X3	T42.3X4	T42.3X5	T42.3X6
Orthoboric acid	T49.ØX1	T49.ØX2	T49.ØX3	T49.ØX4	T49.ØX5	T49.ØX6
ENT agent	T49.6X1	T49.6X2	T49.6X3	T49.6X4	T49.6X5	T49.6X6
ophthalmic preparation	T49.5X1	T49.5X2	T49.5X3	T49.5X4	T49.5X5	T49.5X6
Orthocaine	T41.3X1	T41.3X2	T41.3X3	T41.3X4	T41.3X5	T41.3X6
Orthodichlorobenzene	T53.7X1	T53.7X2	T53.7X3	T53.7X4	—	—
Ortho-Novum	T38.4X1	T38.4X2	T38.4X3	T38.4X4	T38.4X5	T38.4X6
Orthotolidine (reagent)	T54.2X1	T54.2X2	T54.2X3	T54.2X4	—	—
Osmic acid (liquid)	T54.2X1	T54.2X2	T54.2X3	T54.2X4	—	—
fumes	T54.2X1	T54.2X2	T54.2X3	T54.2X4	—	—
Osmotic diuretics	T5Ø.2X1	T5Ø.2X2	T5Ø.2X3	T5Ø.2X4	T5Ø.2X5	T5Ø.2X6
Otilonium bromide	T44.3X1	T44.3X2	T44.3X3	T44.3X4	T44.3X5	T44.3X6
Otorhinolaryngological drug NEC	T49.6X1	T49.6X2	T49.6X3	T49.6X4	T49.6X5	T49.6X6
Ouabain(e)	T46.ØX1	T46.ØX2	T46.ØX3	T46.ØX4	T46.ØX5	T46.ØX6
Ovarian						
hormone	T38.5X1	T38.5X2	T38.5X3	T38.5X4	T38.5X5	T38.5X6
stimulant	T38.5X1	T38.5X2	T38.5X3	T38.5X4	T38.5X5	T38.5X6
Ovral	T38.4X1	T38.4X2	T38.4X3	T38.4X4	T38.4X5	T38.4X6
Ovulen	T38.4X1	T38.4X2	T38.4X3	T38.4X4	T38.4X5	T38.4X6
Oxacillin	T36.ØX1	T36.ØX2	T36.ØX3	T36.ØX4	T36.ØX5	T36.ØX6
Oxalic acid	T54.2X1	T54.2X2	T54.2X3	T54.2X4	—	—
ammonium salt	T5Ø.991	T5Ø.992	T5Ø.993	T5Ø.994	T5Ø.995	T5Ø.996
Oxamniquine	T37.4X1	T37.4X2	T37.4X3	T37.4X4	T37.4X5	T37.4X6
Oxanamide	T43.591	T43.592	T43.593	T43.594	T43.595	T43.596
Oxandrolone	T38.7X1	T38.7X2	T38.7X3	T38.7X4	T38.7X5	T38.7X6
Oxantel	T37.4X1	T37.4X2	T37.4X3	T37.4X4	T37.4X5	T37.4X6
Oxapium iodide	T44.3X1	T44.3X2	T44.3X3	T44.3X4	T44.3X5	T44.3X6
Oxaprotiline	T43.Ø21	T43.Ø22	T43.Ø23	T43.Ø24	T43.Ø25	T43.Ø26
Oxaprozin	T39.311	T39.312	T39.313	T39.314	T39.315	T39.316
Oxatomide	T45.ØX1	T45.ØX2	T45.ØX3	T45.ØX4	T45.ØX5	T45.ØX6
Oxazepam	T42.4X1	T42.4X2	T42.4X3	T42.4X4	T42.4X5	T42.4X6
Oxazimedrine	T5Ø.5X1	T5Ø.5X2	T5Ø.5X3	T5Ø.5X4	T5Ø.5X5	T5Ø.5X6
Oxazolam	T42.4X1	T42.4X2	T42.4X3	T42.4X4	T42.4X5	T42.4X6
Oxazolidine derivatives	T42.2X1	T42.2X2	T42.2X3	T42.2X4	T42.2X5	T42.2X6
Oxazolidinedione (derivative)	T42.2X1	T42.2X2	T42.2X3	T42.2X4	T42.2X5	T42.2X6
Ox bile extract	T47.5X1	T47.5X2	T47.5X3	T47.5X4	T47.5X5	T47.5X6
Oxcarbazepine	T42.1X1	T42.1X2	T42.1X3	T42.1X4	T42.1X5	T42.1X6
Oxedrine	T44.4X1	T44.4X2	T44.4X3	T44.4X4	T44.4X5	T44.4X6

Substance	External Cause (T-Code) Poisoning, Accidental (Unintentional)	Poisoning, Intentional Self-Harm	Poisoning, Assault	Poisoning, Undetermined	Adverse Effect	Underdosing
Oxeladin (citrate)	T48.3X1	T48.3X2	T48.3X3	T48.3X4	T48.3X5	T48.3X6
Oxendolone	T38.5X1	T38.5X2	T38.5X3	T38.5X4	T38.5X5	T38.5X6
Oxetacaine	T41.3X1	T41.3X2	T41.3X3	T41.3X4	T41.3X5	T41.3X6
Oxethazine	T41.3X1	T41.3X2	T41.3X3	T41.3X4	T41.3X5	T41.3X6
Oxetorone	T39.8X1	T39.8X2	T39.8X3	T39.8X4	T39.8X5	T39.8X6
Oxiconazole	T49.ØX1	T49.ØX2	T49.ØX3	T49.ØX4	T49.ØX5	T49.ØX6
Oxidizing agent NEC	T54.91	T54.92	T54.93	T54.94	—	—
Oxipurinol	T5Ø.4X1	T5Ø.4X2	T5Ø.4X3	T5Ø.4X4	T5Ø.4X5	T5Ø.4X6
Oxitriptan	T43.291	T43.292	T43.293	T43.294	T43.295	T43.296
Oxitropium bromide	T48.6X1	T48.6X2	T48.6X3	T48.6X4	T48.6X5	T48.6X6
Oxodipine	T46.1X1	T46.1X2	T46.1X3	T46.1X4	T46.1X5	T46.1X6
Oxolamine	T48.3X1	T48.3X2	T48.3X3	T48.3X4	T48.3X5	T48.3X6
Oxolinic acid	T37.8X1	T37.8X2	T37.8X3	T37.8X4	T37.8X5	T37.8X6
Oxomemazine	T43.3X1	T43.3X2	T43.3X3	T43.3X4	T43.3X5	T43.3X6
Oxophenarsine	T37.3X1	T37.3X2	T37.3X3	T37.3X4	T37.3X5	T37.3X6
Oxprenolol	T44.7X1	T44.7X2	T44.7X3	T44.7X4	T44.7X5	T44.7X6
Oxsoralen	T49.3X1	T49.3X2	T49.3X3	T49.3X4	T49.3X5	T49.3X6
Oxtriphylline	T48.6X1	T48.6X2	T48.6X3	T48.6X4	T48.6X5	T48.6X6
Oxybate sodium	T41.291	T41.292	T41.293	T41.294	T41.295	T41.296
Oxybuprocaine	T41.3X1	T41.3X2	T41.3X3	T41.3X4	T41.3X5	T41.3X6
Oxybutynin	T44.3X1	T44.3X2	T44.3X3	T44.3X4	T44.3X5	T44.3X6
Oxychlorosene	T49.ØX1	T49.ØX2	T49.ØX3	T49.ØX4	T49.ØX5	T49.ØX6
Oxycodone	T4Ø.2X1	T4Ø.2X2	T4Ø.2X3	T4Ø.2X4	T4Ø.2X5	T4Ø.2X6
Oxyfedrine	T46.3X1	T46.3X2	T46.3X3	T46.3X4	T46.3X5	T46.3X6
Oxygen	T41.5X1	T41.5X2	T41.5X3	T41.5X4	T41.5X5	T41.5X6
Oxylone	T49.ØX1	T49.ØX2	T49.ØX3	T49.ØX4	T49.ØX5	T49.ØX6
ophthalmic preparation	T49.5X1	T49.5X2	T49.5X3	T49.5X4	T49.5X5	T49.5X6
Oxymesterone	T38.7X1	T38.7X2	T38.7X3	T38.7X4	T38.7X5	T38.7X6
Oxymetazoline	T48.5X1	T48.5X2	T48.5X3	T48.5X4	T48.5X5	T48.5X6
Oxymetholone	T38.7X1	T38.7X2	T38.7X3	T38.7X4	T38.7X5	T38.7X6
Oxymorphone	T4Ø.2X1	T4Ø.2X2	T4Ø.2X3	T4Ø.2X4	T4Ø.2X5	T4Ø.2X6
Oxypertine	T43.591	T43.592	T43.593	T43.594	T43.595	T43.596
Oxyphenbutazone	T39.2X1	T39.2X2	T39.2X3	T39.2X4	T39.2X5	T39.2X6
Oxyphencyclimine	T44.3X1	T44.3X2	T44.3X3	T44.3X4	T44.3X5	T44.3X6
Oxyphenisatine	T47.2X1	T47.2X2	T47.2X3	T47.2X4	T47.2X5	T47.2X6
Oxyphenonium bromide	T44.3X1	T44.3X2	T44.3X3	T44.3X4	T44.3X5	T44.3X6
Oxypolygelatin	T45.8X1	T45.8X2	T45.8X3	T45.8X4	T45.8X5	T45.8X6
Oxyquinoline (derivatives)	T37.8X1	T37.8X2	T37.8X3	T37.8X4	T37.8X5	T37.8X6
Oxytetracycline	T36.4X1	T36.4X2	T36.4X3	T36.4X4	T36.4X5	T36.4X6
Oxytocic drug NEC	T48.ØX1	T48.ØX2	T48.ØX3	T48.ØX4	T48.ØX5	T48.ØX6
Oxytocin (synthetic)	T48.ØX1	T48.ØX2	T48.ØX3	T48.ØX4	T48.ØX5	T48.ØX6
Ozone	T59.891	T59.892	T59.893	T59.894	—	—

Substance	External Cause (T-Code)					
	Poisoning, Accidental (Unintentional)	Poisoning, Intentional Self-Harm	Poisoning, Assault	Poisoning, Undetermined	Adverse Effect	Underdosing
P						
PABA	T49.3X1	T49.3X2	T49.3X3	T49.3X4	T49.3X5	T49.3X6
Packed red cells	T45.8X1	T45.8X2	T45.8X3	T45.8X4	T45.8X5	T45.8X6
Padimate	T49.3X1	T49.3X2	T49.3X3	T49.3X4	T49.3X5	T49.3X6
Paint NEC	T65.6X1	T65.6X2	T65.6X3	T65.6X4	—	—
cleaner	T52.91	T52.92	T52.93	T52.94	—	—
fumes NEC	T59.891	T59.892	T59.893	T59.894	—	—
lead (fumes)	T56.ØX1	T56.ØX2	T56.ØX3	T56.ØX4	—	—
solvent NEC	T52.8X1	T52.8X2	T52.8X3	T52.8X4	—	—
stripper	T52.8X1	T52.8X2	T52.8X3	T52.8X4	—	—
Palfium	T40.2X1	T40.2X2	T40.2X3	T40.2X4	—	—
Palm kernel oil	T5Ø.991	T5Ø.992	T5Ø.993	T5Ø.994	T5Ø.995	T5Ø.996
Paludrine	T37.2X1	T37.2X2	T37.2X3	T37.2X4	T37.2X5	T37.2X6
PAM (pralidoxime)	T5Ø.6X1	T5Ø.6X2	T5Ø.6X3	T5Ø.6X4	T5Ø.6X5	T5Ø.6X6
Pamaquine (naphthoute)	T37.2X1	T37.2X2	T37.2X3	T37.2X4	T37.2X5	T37.2X6
Panadol	T39.1X1	T39.1X2	T39.1X3	T39.1X4	T39.1X5	T39.1X6
Pancreatic						
digestive secretion stimulant	T47.8X1	T47.8X2	T47.8X3	T47.8X4	T47.8X5	T47.8X6
dornase	T45.3X1	T45.3X2	T45.3X3	T45.3X4	T45.3X5	T45.3X6
Pancreatin	T47.5X1	T47.5X2	T47.5X3	T47.5X4	T47.5X5	T47.5X6
Pancrelipase	T47.5X1	T47.5X2	T47.5X3	T47.5X4	T47.5X5	T47.5X6
Pancuronium (bromide)	T48.1X1	T48.1X2	T48.1X3	T48.1X4	T48.1X5	T48.1X6
Pangamic acid	T45.2X1	T45.2X2	T45.2X3	T45.2X4	T45.2X5	T45.2X6
Panthenol	T45.2X1	T45.2X2	T45.2X3	T45.2X4	T45.2X5	T45.2X6
topical	T49.8X1	T49.8X2	T49.8X3	T49.8X4	T49.8X5	T49.8X6
Pantopon	T40.ØX1	T40.ØX2	T40.ØX3	T40.ØX4	T40.ØX5	T40.ØX6
Pantothenic acid	T45.2X1	T45.2X2	T45.2X3	T45.2X4	T45.2X5	T45.2X6
Panwarfin	T45.511	T45.512	T45.513	T45.514	T45.515	T45.516
Papain	T47.5X1	T47.5X2	T47.5X3	T47.5X4	T47.5X5	T47.5X6
digestant	T47.5X1	T47.5X2	T47.5X3	T47.5X4	T47.5X5	T47.5X6
Papaveretum	T40.ØX1	T40.ØX2	T40.ØX3	T40.ØX4	T40.ØX5	T40.ØX6
Papaverine	T44.3X1	T44.3X2	T44.3X3	T44.3X4	T44.3X5	T44.3X6
Para-acetamidophenol	T39.1X1	T39.1X2	T39.1X3	T39.1X4	T39.1X5	T39.1X6
Para-aminobenzoic acid	T49.3X1	T49.3X2	T49.3X3	T49.3X4	T49.3X5	T49.3X6
Para-aminophenol derivatives	T39.1X1	T39.1X2	T39.1X3	T39.1X4	T39.1X5	T39.1X6
Para-aminosalicylic acid	T37.1X1	T37.1X2	T37.1X3	T37.1X4	T37.1X5	T37.1X6
Paracetaldehyde	T42.6X1	T42.6X2	T42.6X3	T42.6X4	T42.6X5	T42.6X6
Paracetamol	T39.1X1	T39.1X2	T39.1X3	T39.1X4	T39.1X5	T39.1X6
Parachlorophenol (camphorated)	T49.ØX1	T49.ØX2	T49.ØX3	T49.ØX4	T49.ØX5	T49.ØX6
Paracodin	T40.2X1	T40.2X2	T40.2X3	T40.2X4	T40.2X5	T40.2X6
Paradione	T42.2X1	T42.2X2	T42.2X3	T42.2X4	T42.2X5	T42.2X6

Substance	External Cause (T-Code)					
	Poisoning, Accidental (Unintentional)	Poisoning, Intentional Self-Harm	Poisoning, Assault	Poisoning, Undetermined	Adverse Effect	Underdosing
Paraffin(s) (wax)	T52.ØX1	T52.ØX2	T52.ØX3	T52.ØX4	—	—
liquid (medicinal)	T47.4X1	T47.4X2	T47.4X3	T47.4X4	T47.4X5	T47.4X6
nonmedicinal	T52.ØX1	T52.ØX2	T52.ØX3	T52.ØX4	—	—
Paraformaldehyde	T6Ø.3X1	T6Ø.3X2	T6Ø.3X3	T6Ø.3X4	—	—
Paraldehyde	T42.6X1	T42.6X2	T42.6X3	T42.6X4	T42.6X5	T42.6X6
Paramethadione	T42.2X1	T42.2X2	T42.2X3	T42.2X4	T42.2X5	T42.2X6
Paramethasone	T38.ØX1	T38.ØX2	T38.ØX3	T38.ØX4	T38.ØX5	T38.ØX6
acetate	T49.ØX1	T49.ØX2	T49.ØX3	T49.ØX4	T49.ØX5	T49.ØX6
Paraoxon	T6Ø.ØX1	T6Ø.ØX2	T6Ø.ØX3	T6Ø.ØX4	—	—
Paraquat	T6Ø.3X1	T6Ø.3X2	T6Ø.3X3	T6Ø.3X4	—	—
Parasympatholytic NEC	T44.3X1	T44.3X2	T44.3X3	T44.3X4	T44.3X5	T44.3X6
Parasympathomimetic drug NEC	T44.1X1	T44.1X2	T44.1X3	T44.1X4	T44.1X5	T44.1X6
Parathion	T6Ø.ØX1	T6Ø.ØX2	T6Ø.ØX3	T6Ø.ØX4	—	—
Parathormone	T5Ø.991	T5Ø.992	T5Ø.993	T5Ø.994	T5Ø.995	T5Ø.996
Parathyroid extract	T5Ø.991	T5Ø.992	T5Ø.993	T5Ø.994	T5Ø.995	T5Ø.996
Paratyphoid vaccine	T5Ø.A91	T5Ø.A92	T5Ø.A93	T5Ø.A94	T5Ø.A95	T5Ø.A96
Paredrine	T44.4X1	T44.4X2	T44.4X3	T44.4X4	T44.4X5	T44.4X6
Paregoric	T40.ØX1	T40.ØX2	T40.ØX3	T40.ØX4	T40.ØX5	T40.ØX6
Pargyline	T46.5X1	T46.5X2	T46.5X3	T46.5X4	T46.5X5	T46.5X6
Paris green	T57.ØX1	T57.ØX2	T57.ØX3	T57.ØX4	—	—
insecticide	T57.ØX1	T57.ØX2	T57.ØX3	T57.ØX4	—	—
Parnate	T43.1X1	T43.1X2	T43.1X3	T43.1X4	T43.1X5	T43.1X6
Paromomycin	T36.5X1	T36.5X2	T36.5X3	T36.5X4	T36.5X5	T36.5X6
Paroxypropione	T45.1X1	T45.1X2	T45.1X3	T45.1X4	T45.1X5	T45.1X6
Parzone	T40.2X1	T40.2X2	T40.2X3	T40.2X4	T40.2X5	T40.2X6
PAS	T37.1X1	T37.1X2	T37.1X3	T37.1X4	T37.1X5	T37.1X6
Pasiniazid	T37.1X1	T37.1X2	T37.1X3	T37.1X4	T37.1X5	T37.1X6
PBB (polybrominated biphenyls)	T65.891	T65.892	T65.893	T65.894	—	—
PCB	T65.891	T65.892	T65.893	T65.894	—	—
PCP						
meaning pentachlorophenol	T6Ø.1X1	T6Ø.1X2	T6Ø.1X3	T6Ø.1X4	—	—
fungicide	T6Ø.3X1	T6Ø.3X2	T6Ø.3X3	T6Ø.3X4	—	—
herbicide	T6Ø.3X1	T6Ø.3X2	T6Ø.3X3	T6Ø.3X4	—	—
insecticide	T6Ø.1X1	T6Ø.1X2	T6Ø.1X3	T6Ø.1X4	—	—
meaning phencyclidine	T40.991	T40.992	T40.993	T40.994	—	—
Peach kernel oil (emulsion)	T47.4X1	T47.4X2	T47.4X3	T47.4X4	T47.4X5	T47.4X6
Peanut oil (emulsion) NEC	T47.4X1	T47.4X2	T47.4X3	T47.4X4	T47.4X5	T47.4X6
topical	T49.3X1	T49.3X2	T49.3X3	T49.3X4	T49.3X5	T49.3X6
Pearly Gates (morning glory seeds)	T40.991	T40.992	T40.993	T40.994	—	—
Pecazine	T43.3X1	T43.3X2	T43.3X3	T43.3X4	T43.3X5	T43.3X6
Pectin	T47.6X1	T47.6X2	T47.6X3	T47.6X4	T47.6X5	T47.6X6

Substance	External Cause (T-Code) Poisoning, Accidental (Unintentional)	Poisoning, Intentional Self-Harm	Poisoning, Assault	Poisoning, Undetermined	Adverse Effect	Underdosing
Pefloxacin	T37.8X1	T37.8X2	T37.8X3	T37.8X4	T37.8X5	T37.8X6
Pegademase, bovine	T50.Z91	T50.Z92	T50.Z93	T50.Z94	T50.Z95	T50.Z96
Pelletierine tannate	T37.4X1	T37.4X2	T37.4X3	T37.4X4	T37.4X5	T37.4X6
Pemirolast (potassium)	T48.6X1	T48.6X2	T48.6X3	T48.6X4	T48.6X5	T48.6X6
Pemoline	T50.7X1	T50.7X2	T50.7X3	T50.7X4	T50.7X5	T50.7X6
Pempidine	T44.2X1	T44.2X2	T44.2X3	T44.2X4	T44.2X5	T44.2X6
Penamecillin	T36.0X1	T36.0X2	T36.0X3	T36.0X4	T36.0X5	T36.0X6
Penbutolol	T44.7X1	T44.7X2	T44.7X3	T44.7X4	T44.7X5	T44.7X6
Penethamate	T36.0X1	T36.0X2	T36.0X3	T36.0X4	T36.0X5	T36.0X6
Penfluridol	T43.591	T43.592	T43.593	T43.594	T43.595	T43.596
Penflutizide	T50.2X1	T50.2X2	T50.2X3	T50.2X4	T50.2X5	T50.2X6
Pengitoxin	T46.0X1	T46.0X2	T46.0X3	T46.0X4	T46.0X5	T46.0X6
Penicillamine	T50.6X1	T50.6X2	T50.6X3	T50.6X4	T50.6X5	T50.6X6
Penicillin (any)	T36.0X1	T36.0X2	T36.0X3	T36.0X4	T36.0X5	T36.0X6
Penicillinase	T45.3X1	T45.3X2	T45.3X3	T45.3X4	T45.3X5	T45.3X6
Penicilloyl polylysine	T50.8X1	T50.8X2	T50.8X3	T50.8X4	T50.8X5	T50.8X6
Penimepicycline	T36.4X1	T36.4X2	T36.4X3	T36.4X4	T36.4X5	T36.4X6
Pentachloroethane	T53.6X1	T53.6X2	T53.6X3	T53.6X4	—	—
Pentachloronaphthalene	T53.7X1	T53.7X2	T53.7X3	T53.7X4	—	—
Pentachlorophenol (pesticide)	T60.1X1	T60.1X2	T60.1X3	T60.1X4	—	—
fungicide	T60.3X1	T60.3X2	T60.3X3	T60.3X4	—	—
herbicide	T60.3X1	T60.3X2	T60.3X3	T60.3X4	—	—
insecticide	T60.1X1	T60.1X2	T60.1X3	T60.1X4	—	—
Pentaerythritol tetranitrate	T46.3X1	T46.3X2	T46.3X3	T46.3X4	T46.3X5	T46.3X6
Pentaerythritol	T46.3X1	T46.3X2	T46.3X3	T46.3X4	T46.3X5	T46.3X6
chloral	T42.6X1	T42.6X2	T42.6X3	T42.6X4	T42.6X5	T42.6X6
tetranitrate NEC	T46.3X1	T46.3X2	T46.3X3	T46.3X4	T46.3X5	T46.3X6
Pentagastrin	T50.8X1	T50.8X2	T50.8X3	T50.8X4	T50.8X5	T50.8X6
Pentalin	T53.6X1	T53.6X2	T53.6X3	T53.6X4	—	—
Pentamethonium bromide	T44.2X1	T44.2X2	T44.2X3	T44.2X4	T44.2X5	T44.2X6
Pentamidine	T37.3X1	T37.3X2	T37.3X3	T37.3X4	T37.3X5	T37.3X6
Pentanol	T51.3X1	T51.3X2	T51.3X3	T51.3X4	—	—
Pentapyrrolinium (bitartrate)	T44.2X1	T44.2X2	T44.2X3	T44.2X4	T44.2X5	T44.2X6
Pentaquine	T37.2X1	T37.2X2	T37.2X3	T37.2X4	T37.2X5	T37.2X6
Pentazocine	T40.491	T40.492	T40.493	T40.494	T40.495	T40.496
Pentetrazole	T50.7X1	T50.7X2	T50.7X3	T50.7X4	T50.7X5	T50.7X6
Penthienate bromide	T44.3X1	T44.3X2	T44.3X3	T44.3X4	T44.3X5	T44.3X6
Pentifylline	T46.7X1	T46.7X2	T46.7X3	T46.7X4	T46.7X5	T46.7X6
Pentobarbital	T42.3X1	T42.3X2	T42.3X3	T42.3X4	T42.3X5	T42.3X6
sodium	T42.3X1	T42.3X2	T42.3X3	T42.3X4	T42.3X5	T42.3X6
Pentobarbitone	T42.3X1	T42.3X2	T42.3X3	T42.3X4	T42.3X5	T42.3X6
Pentolonium tartrate	T44.2X1	T44.2X2	T44.2X3	T44.2X4	T44.2X5	T44.2X6

Substance	External Cause (T-Code) Poisoning, Accidental (Unintentional)	Poisoning, Intentional Self-Harm	Poisoning, Assault	Poisoning, Undetermined	Adverse Effect	Underdosing
Pentosan polysulfate (sodium)	T39.8X1	T39.8X2	T39.8X3	T39.8X4	T39.8X5	T39.8X6
Pentostatin	T45.1X1	T45.1X2	T45.1X3	T45.1X4	T45.1X5	T45.1X6
Pentothal	T41.1X1	T41.1X2	T41.1X3	T41.1X4	T41.1X5	T41.1X6
Pentoxifylline	T46.7X1	T46.7X2	T46.7X3	T46.7X4	T46.7X5	T46.7X6
Pentoxyverine	T48.3X1	T48.3X2	T48.3X3	T48.3X4	T48.3X5	T48.3X6
Pentrinat	T46.3X1	T46.3X2	T46.3X3	T46.3X4	T46.3X5	T46.3X6
Pentylenetetrazole	T50.7X1	T50.7X2	T50.7X3	T50.7X4	T50.7X5	T50.7X6
Pentylsalicylamide	T37.1X1	T37.1X2	T37.1X3	T37.1X4	T37.1X5	T37.1X6
Pentymal	T42.3X1	T42.3X2	T42.3X3	T42.3X4	T42.3X5	T42.3X6
Peplomycin	T45.1X1	T45.1X2	T45.1X3	T45.1X4	T45.1X5	T45.1X6
Peppermint (oil)	T47.5X1	T47.5X2	T47.5X3	T47.5X4	T47.5X5	T47.5X6
Pepsin	T47.5X1	T47.5X2	T47.5X3	T47.5X4	T47.5X5	T47.5X6
digestant	T47.5X1	T47.5X2	T47.5X3	T47.5X4	T47.5X5	T47.5X6
Pepstatin	T47.1X1	T47.1X2	T47.1X3	T47.1X4	T47.1X5	T47.1X6
Peptavlon	T50.8X1	T50.8X2	T50.8X3	T50.8X4	T50.8X5	T50.8X6
Perazine	T43.3X1	T43.3X2	T43.3X3	T43.3X4	T43.3X5	T43.3X6
Percaine (spinal)	T41.3X1	T41.3X2	T41.3X3	T41.3X4	T41.3X5	T41.3X6
topical (surface)	T41.3X1	T41.3X2	T41.3X3	T41.3X4	T41.3X5	T41.3X6
Perchloroethylene	T53.3X1	T53.3X2	T53.3X3	T53.3X4	—	—
medicinal	T37.4X1	T37.4X2	T37.4X3	T37.4X4	T37.4X5	T37.4X6
vapor	T53.3X1	T53.3X2	T53.3X3	T53.3X4	—	—
Percodan	T40.2X1	T40.2X2	T40.2X3	T40.2X4	T40.2X5	T40.2X6
Percogesic — *see also Acetaminophen*	T45.0X1	T45.0X2	T45.0X3	T45.0X4	T45.0X5	T45.0X6
Percorten	T38.0X1	T38.0X2	T38.0X3	T38.0X4	T38.0X5	T38.0X6
Pergolide	T42.8X1	T42.8X2	T42.8X3	T42.8X4	T42.8X5	T42.8X6
Pergonal	T38.811	T38.812	T38.813	T38.814	T38.815	T38.816
Perhexilene	T46.3X1	T46.3X2	T46.3X3	T46.3X4	T46.3X5	T46.3X6
Perhexiline (maleate)	T46.3X1	T46.3X2	T46.3X3	T46.3X4	T46.3X5	T46.3X6
Periactin	T45.0X1	T45.0X2	T45.0X3	T45.0X4	T45.0X5	T45.0X6
Periciazine	T43.3X1	T43.3X2	T43.3X3	T43.3X4	T43.3X5	T43.3X6
Periclor	T42.6X1	T42.6X2	T42.6X3	T42.6X4	T42.6X5	T42.6X6
Perindopril	T46.4X1	T46.4X2	T46.4X3	T46.4X4	T46.4X5	T46.4X6
Perisoxal	T39.8X1	T39.8X2	T39.8X3	T39.8X4	T39.8X5	T39.8X6
Peritrate	T46.3X1	T46.3X2	T46.3X3	T46.3X4	T46.3X5	T46.3X6
Peritoneal dialysis solution	T50.3X1	T50.3X2	T50.3X3	T50.3X4	T50.3X5	T50.3X6
Perlapine	T42.4X1	T42.4X2	T42.4X3	T42.4X4	T42.4X5	T42.4X6
Permanganate	T65.891	T65.892	T65.893	T65.894	—	—
Permethrin	T60.1X1	T60.1X2	T60.1X3	T60.1X4	—	—
Pernocton	T42.3X1	T42.3X2	T42.3X3	T42.3X4	T42.3X5	T42.3X6
Pernoston	T42.3X1	T42.3X2	T42.3X3	T42.3X4	T42.3X5	T42.3X6
Peronine	T40.2X1	T40.2X2	T40.2X3	T40.2X4	—	—
Perphenazine	T43.3X1	T43.3X2	T43.3X3	T43.3X4	T43.3X5	T43.3X6

Substance	External Cause (T-Code)					
	Poisoning, Accidental (Unintentional)	Poisoning, Intentional Self-Harm	Poisoning, Assault	Poisoning, Undetermined	Adverse Effect	Underdosing
Pertofrane	T43.Ø11	T43.Ø12	T43.Ø13	T43.Ø14	T43.Ø15	T43.Ø16
Pertussis						
immune serum (human)	T5Ø.Z11	T5Ø.Z12	T5Ø.Z13	T5Ø.Z14	T5Ø.Z15	T5Ø.Z16
vaccine (with diphtheria toxoid) (with tetanus toxoid)	T5Ø.A11	T5Ø.A12	T5Ø.A13	T5Ø.A14	T5Ø.A15	T5Ø.A16
Peruvian balsam	T49.ØX1	T49.ØX2	T49.ØX3	T49.ØX4	T49.ØX5	T49.ØX6
Peruvoside	T46.ØX1	T46.ØX2	T46.ØX3	T46.ØX4	T46.ØX5	T46.ØX6
Pesticide (dust) (fumes) (vapor) NEC	T6Ø.91	T6Ø.92	T6Ø.93	T6Ø.94	—	—
arsenic	T57.ØX1	T57.ØX2	T57.ØX3	T57.ØX4	—	—
chlorinated	T6Ø.1X1	T6Ø.1X2	T6Ø.1X3	T6Ø.1X4	—	—
cyanide	T65.ØX1	T65.ØX2	T65.ØX3	T65.ØX4	—	—
kerosene	T52.ØX1	T52.ØX2	T52.ØX3	T52.ØX4	—	—
mixture (of compounds)	T6Ø.91	T6Ø.92	T6Ø.93	T6Ø.94	—	—
naphthalene	T6Ø.2X1	T6Ø.2X2	T6Ø.2X3	T6Ø.2X4	—	—
organochlorine (compounds)	T6Ø.1X1	T6Ø.1X2	T6Ø.1X3	T6Ø.1X4	—	—
petroleum (distillate) (products) NEC	T6Ø.8X1	T6Ø.8X2	T6Ø.8X3	T6Ø.8X4	—	—
specified ingredient NEC	T6Ø.8X1	T6Ø.8X2	T6Ø.8X3	T6Ø.8X4	—	—
strychnine	T65.1X1	T65.1X2	T65.1X3	T65.1X4	—	—
thallium	T6Ø.4X1	T6Ø.4X2	T6Ø.4X3	T6Ø.4X4	—	—
Pethidine	T4Ø.491	T4Ø.492	T4Ø.493	T4Ø.494	T4Ø.495	T4Ø.496
Petrichloral	T42.6X1	T42.6X2	T42.6X3	T42.6X4	T42.6X5	T42.6X6
Petrol	T52.ØX1	T52.ØX2	T52.ØX3	T52.ØX4	—	—
vapor	T52.ØX1	T52.ØX2	T52.ØX3	T52.ØX4	—	—
Petrolatum	T49.3X1	T49.3X2	T49.3X3	T49.3X4	T49.3X5	T49.3X6
hydrophilic	T49.3X1	T49.3X2	T49.3X3	T49.3X4	T49.3X5	T49.3X6
liquid	T47.4X1	T47.4X2	T47.4X3	T47.4X4	T47.4X5	T47.4X6
topical	T49.3X1	T49.3X2	T49.3X3	T49.3X4	T49.3X5	T49.3X6
nonmedicinal	T52.ØX1	T52.ØX2	T52.ØX3	T52.ØX4	—	—
red veterinary	T49.3X1	T49.3X2	T49.3X3	T49.3X4	T49.3X5	T49.3X6
white	T49.3X1	T49.3X2	T49.3X3	T49.3X4	T49.3X5	T49.3X6
Petroleum (products) NEC	T52.ØX1	T52.ØX2	T52.ØX3	T52.ØX4	—	—
benzine(s) — *see Ligroin*						
ether — *see Ligroin*						
jelly — *see Petrolatum*						
naphtha — *see Ligroin*						
pesticide	T6Ø.8X1	T6Ø.8X2	T6Ø.8X3	T6Ø.8X4	—	—
solids	T52.ØX1	T52.ØX2	T52.ØX3	T52.ØX4	—	—
solvents	T52.ØX1	T52.ØX2	T52.ØX3	T52.ØX4	—	—
vapor	T52.ØX1	T52.ØX2	T52.ØX3	T52.ØX4	—	—
Peyote	T4Ø.991	T4Ø.992	T4Ø.993	T4Ø.994	—	—
Phanodorm, phanodorn	T42.3X1	T42.3X2	T42.3X3	T42.3X4	T42.3X5	T42.3X6
Phanquinone	T37.3X1	T37.3X2	T37.3X3	T37.3X4	T37.3X5	T37.3X6
Phanquone	T37.3X1	T37.3X2	T37.3X3	T37.3X4	T37.3X5	T37.3X6
Pharmaceutical						
adjunct NEC	T5Ø.9Ø1	T5Ø.9Ø2	T5Ø.9Ø3	T5Ø.9Ø4	T5Ø.9Ø5	T5Ø.9Ø6
excipient NEC	T5Ø.9Ø1	T5Ø.9Ø2	T5Ø.9Ø3	T5Ø.9Ø4	T5Ø.9Ø5	T5Ø.9Ø6
sweetener	T5Ø.9Ø1	T5Ø.9Ø2	T5Ø.9Ø3	T5Ø.9Ø4	T5Ø.9Ø5	T5Ø.9Ø6
viscous agent	T5Ø.9Ø1	T5Ø.9Ø2	T5Ø.9Ø3	T5Ø.9Ø4	T5Ø.9Ø5	T5Ø.9Ø6
Phemitone	T42.3X1	T42.3X2	T42.3X3	T42.3X4	T42.3X5	T42.3X6
Phenacaine	T41.3X1	T41.3X2	T41.3X3	T41.3X4	T41.3X5	T41.3X6
Phenacemide	T42.6X1	T42.6X2	T42.6X3	T42.6X4	T42.6X5	T42.6X6
Phenacetin	T39.1X1	T39.1X2	T39.1X3	T39.1X4	T39.1X5	T39.1X6
Phenadoxone	T4Ø.2X1	T4Ø.2X2	T4Ø.2X3	T4Ø.2X4	—	—
Phenaglycodol	T43.591	T43.592	T43.593	T43.594	T43.595	T43.596
Phenantoin	T42.ØX1	T42.ØX2	T42.ØX3	T42.ØX4	T42.ØX5	T42.ØX6
Phenaphthazine reagent	T5Ø.991	T5Ø.992	T5Ø.993	T5Ø.994	T5Ø.995	T5Ø.996
Phenazocine	T4Ø.491	T4Ø.492	T4Ø.493	T4Ø.494	T4Ø.495	T4Ø.496
Phenazone	T39.2X1	T39.2X2	T39.2X3	T39.2X4	T39.2X5	T39.2X6
Phenazopyridine	T39.8X1	T39.8X2	T39.8X3	T39.8X4	T39.8X5	T39.8X6
Phenbenicillin	T36.ØX1	T36.ØX2	T36.ØX3	T36.ØX4	T36.ØX5	T36.ØX6
Phenbutrazate	T5Ø.5X1	T5Ø.5X2	T5Ø.5X3	T5Ø.5X4	T5Ø.5X5	T5Ø.5X6
Phencyclidine	T4Ø.991	T4Ø.992	T4Ø.993	T4Ø.994	T4Ø.995	T4Ø.996
Phendimetrazine	T5Ø.5X1	T5Ø.5X2	T5Ø.5X3	T5Ø.5X4	T5Ø.5X5	T5Ø.5X6
Phenelzine	T43.1X1	T43.1X2	T43.1X3	T43.1X4	T43.1X5	T43.1X6
Phenemal	T42.3X1	T42.3X2	T42.3X3	T42.3X4	T42.3X5	T42.3X6
Phenergan	T42.6X1	T42.6X2	T42.6X3	T42.6X4	T42.6X5	T42.6X6
Pheneticillin	T36.ØX1	T36.ØX2	T36.ØX3	T36.ØX4	T36.ØX5	T36.ØX6
Pheneturide	T42.6X1	T42.6X2	T42.6X3	T42.6X4	T42.6X5	T42.6X6
Phenformin	T38.3X1	T38.3X2	T38.3X3	T38.3X4	T38.3X5	T38.3X6
Phenglutarimide	T44.3X1	T44.3X2	T44.3X3	T44.3X4	T44.3X5	T44.3X6
Phenicarbazide	T39.8X1	T39.8X2	T39.8X3	T39.8X4	T39.8X5	T39.8X6
Phenindamine	T45.ØX1	T45.ØX2	T45.ØX3	T45.ØX4	T45.ØX5	T45.ØX6
Phenindione	T45.511	T45.512	T45.513	T45.514	T45.515	T45.516
Pheniprazine	T43.1X1	T43.1X2	T43.1X3	T43.1X4	T43.1X5	T43.1X6
Pheniramine	T45.ØX1	T45.ØX2	T45.ØX3	T45.ØX4	T45.ØX5	T45.ØX6
Phenisatin	T47.2X1	T47.2X2	T47.2X3	T47.2X4	T47.2X5	T47.2X6
Phenmetrazine	T5Ø.5X1	T5Ø.5X2	T5Ø.5X3	T5Ø.5X4	T5Ø.5X5	T5Ø.5X6
Phenobal	T42.3X1	T42.3X2	T42.3X3	T42.3X4	T42.3X5	T42.3X6
Phenobarbital	T42.3X1	T42.3X2	T42.3X3	T42.3X4	T42.3X5	T42.3X6
with						
mephenytoin	T42.3X1	T42.3X2	T42.3X3	T42.3X4	T42.3X5	T42.3X6
phenytoin	T42.3X1	T42.3X2	T42.3X3	T42.3X4	T42.3X5	T42.3X6
sodium	T42.3X1	T42.3X2	T42.3X3	T42.3X4	T42.3X5	T42.3X6

TABLE OF DRUGS AND CHEMICALS

Substance	External Cause (T-Code) Poisoning, Accidental (Unintentional)	Poisoning, Intentional Self-Harm	Poisoning, Assault	Poisoning, Undetermined	Adverse Effect	Underdosing
Phenobarbitone	T42.3X1	T42.3X2	T42.3X3	T42.3X4	T42.3X5	T42.3X6
Phenobutiodil	T5Ø.8X1	T5Ø.8X2	T5Ø.8X3	T5Ø.8X4	T5Ø.8X5	T5Ø.8X6
Phenoctide	T49.ØX1	T49.ØX2	T49.ØX3	T49.ØX4	T49.ØX5	T49.ØX6
Phenol	T49.ØX1	T49.ØX2	T49.ØX3	T49.ØX4	T49.ØX5	T49.ØX6
disinfectant	T54.ØX1	T54.ØX2	T54.ØX3	T54.ØX4	—	—
in oil injection	T46.8X1	T46.8X2	T46.8X3	T46.8X4	T46.8X5	T46.8X6
medicinal	T49.1X1	T49.1X2	T49.1X3	T49.1X4	T49.1X5	T49.1X6
nonmedicinal NEC	T54.ØX1	T54.ØX2	T54.ØX3	T54.ØX4	—	—
pesticide	T6Ø.8X1	T6Ø.8X2	T6Ø.8X3	T6Ø.8X4	—	—
red	T5Ø.8X1	T5Ø.8X2	T5Ø.8X3	T5Ø.8X4	T5Ø.8X5	T5Ø.8X6
Phenolic preparation	T49.1X1	T49.1X2	T49.1X3	T49.1X4	T49.1X5	T49.1X6
Phenolphthalein	T47.2X1	T47.2X2	T47.2X3	T47.2X4	T47.2X5	T47.2X6
Phenolsulfonphthalein	T5Ø.8X1	T5Ø.8X2	T5Ø.8X3	T5Ø.8X4	T5Ø.8X5	T5Ø.8X6
Phenomorphan	T4Ø.2X1	T4Ø.2X2	T4Ø.2X3	T4Ø.2X4	—	—
Phenonyl	T42.3X1	T42.3X2	T42.3X3	T42.3X4	T42.3X5	T42.3X6
Phenoperidine	T4Ø.491	T4Ø.492	T4Ø.493	T4Ø.494	—	—
Phenopyrazone	T46.991	T46.992	T46.993	T46.994	T46.995	T46.996
Phenoquin	T5Ø.4X1	T5Ø.4X2	T5Ø.4X3	T5Ø.4X4	T5Ø.4X5	T5Ø.4X6
Phenothiazine (psychotropic) NEC	T43.3X1	T43.3X2	T43.3X3	T43.3X4	T43.3X5	T43.3X6
insecticide	T6Ø.2X1	T6Ø.2X2	T6Ø.2X3	T6Ø.2X4	—	—
Phenothrin	T49.ØX1	T49.ØX2	T49.ØX3	T49.ØX4	T49.ØX5	T49.ØX6
Phenoxybenzamine	T46.7X1	T46.7X2	T46.7X3	T46.7X4	T46.7X5	T46.7X6
Phenoxyethanol	T49.ØX1	T49.ØX2	T49.ØX3	T49.ØX4	T49.ØX5	T49.ØX6
Phenoxymethyl penicillin	T36.ØX1	T36.ØX2	T36.ØX3	T36.ØX4	T36.ØX5	T36.ØX6
Phenprobamate	T42.8X1	T42.8X2	T42.8X3	T42.8X4	T42.8X5	T42.8X6
Phenprocoumon	T45.511	T45.512	T45.513	T45.514	T45.515	T45.516
Phensuximide	T42.2X1	T42.2X2	T42.2X3	T42.2X4	T42.2X5	T42.2X6
Phentermine	T5Ø.5X1	T5Ø.5X2	T5Ø.5X3	T5Ø.5X4	T5Ø.5X5	T5Ø.5X6
Phenthicillin	T36.ØX1	T36.ØX2	T36.ØX3	T36.ØX4	T36.ØX5	T36.ØX6
Phentolamine	T46.7X1	T46.7X2	T46.7X3	T46.7X4	T46.7X5	T46.7X6
Phenyl						
butazone	T39.2X1	T39.2X2	T39.2X3	T39.2X4	T39.2X5	T39.2X6
enediamine	T65.3X1	T65.3X2	T65.3X3	T65.3X4	—	—
hydrazine	T65.3X1	T65.3X2	T65.3X3	T65.3X4	—	—
antineoplastic	T45.1X1	T45.1X2	T45.1X3	T45.1X4	T45.1X5	T45.1X6
mercuric compounds — *see* *Mercury*						
salicylate	T49.3X1	T49.3X2	T49.3X3	T49.3X4	T49.3X5	T49.3X6
Phenylalanine mustard	T45.1X1	T45.1X2	T45.1X3	T45.1X4	T45.1X5	T45.1X6
Phenylbutazone	T39.2X1	T39.2X2	T39.2X3	T39.2X4	T39.2X5	T39.2X6
Phenylenediamine	T65.3X1	T65.3X2	T65.3X3	T65.3X4	—	—
Phenylephrine	T44.4X1	T44.4X2	T44.4X3	T44.4X4	T44.4X5	T44.4X6
Phenylethylbiguanide	T38.3X1	T38.3X2	T38.3X3	T38.3X4	T38.3X5	T38.3X6
Phenylmercuric						
acetate	T49.ØX1	T49.ØX2	T49.ØX3	T49.ØX4	T49.ØX5	T49.ØX6
borate	T49.ØX1	T49.ØX2	T49.ØX3	T49.ØX4	T49.ØX5	T49.ØX6
nitrate	T49.ØX1	T49.ØX2	T49.ØX3	T49.ØX4	T49.ØX5	T49.ØX6
Phenylmethylbarbitone	T42.3X1	T42.3X2	T42.3X3	T42.3X4	T42.3X5	T42.3X6
Phenylpropanol	T47.5X1	T47.5X2	T47.5X3	T47.5X4	T47.5X5	T47.5X6
Phenylpropanolamine	T44.991	T44.992	T44.993	T44.994	T44.995	T44.996
Phenylsulfthion	T6Ø.ØX1	T6Ø.ØX2	T6Ø.ØX3	T6Ø.ØX4	—	—
Phenyltoloxamine	T45.ØX1	T45.ØX2	T45.ØX3	T45.ØX4	T45.ØX5	T45.ØX6
Phenyramidol, phenyramidon	T39.8X1	T39.8X2	T39.8X3	T39.8X4	T39.8X5	T39.8X6
Phenytoin	T42.ØX1	T42.ØX2	T42.ØX3	T42.ØX4	T42.ØX5	T42.ØX6
with Phenobarbital	T42.3X1	T42.3X2	T42.3X3	T42.3X4	T42.3X5	T42.3X6
pHisoHex	T49.2X1	T49.2X2	T49.2X3	T49.2X4	T49.2X5	T49.2X6
Pholcodine	T48.3X1	T48.3X2	T48.3X3	T48.3X4	T48.3X5	T48.3X6
Pholedrine	T46.991	T46.992	T46.993	T46.994	T46.995	T46.996
Phorate	T6Ø.ØX1	T6Ø.ØX2	T6Ø.ØX3	T6Ø.ØX4	—	—
Phosdrin	T6Ø.ØX1	T6Ø.ØX2	T6Ø.ØX3	T6Ø.ØX4	—	—
Phosfolan	T6Ø.ØX1	T6Ø.ØX2	T6Ø.ØX3	T6Ø.ØX4	—	—
Phosgene (gas)	T59.891	T59.892	T59.893	T59.894	—	—
Phosphamidon	T6Ø.ØX1	T6Ø.ØX2	T6Ø.ØX3	T6Ø.ØX4	—	—
Phosphate	T65.891	T65.892	T65.893	T65.894	—	—
laxative	T47.4X1	T47.4X2	T47.4X3	T47.4X4	T47.4X5	T47.4X6
organic	T6Ø.ØX1	T6Ø.ØX2	T6Ø.ØX3	T6Ø.ØX4	—	—
solvent	T52.91	T52.92	T52.93	T52.94	—	—
tricresyl	T65.891	T65.892	T65.893	T65.894	—	—
Phosphine	T57.1X1	T57.1X2	T57.1X3	T57.1X4	—	—
fumigant	T57.1X1	T57.1X2	T57.1X3	T57.1X4	—	—
Phospholine	T49.5X1	T49.5X2	T49.5X3	T49.5X4	T49.5X5	T49.5X6
Phosphoric acid	T54.2X1	T54.2X2	T54.2X3	T54.2X4	—	—
Phosphorus (compound) NEC	T57.1X1	T57.1X2	T57.1X3	T57.1X4	—	—
pesticide	T6Ø.ØX1	T6Ø.ØX2	T6Ø.ØX3	T6Ø.ØX4	—	—
Phthalates	T65.891	T65.892	T65.893	T65.894	—	—
Phthalic anhydride	T65.891	T65.892	T65.893	T65.894	—	—
Phthalimidoglutarimide	T42.6X1	T42.6X2	T42.6X3	T42.6X4	T42.6X5	T42.6X6
Phthalylsulfathiazole	T37.ØX1	T37.ØX2	T37.ØX3	T37.ØX4	T37.ØX5	T37.ØX6
Phylloquinone	T45.7X1	T45.7X2	T45.7X3	T45.7X4	T45.7X5	T45.7X6
Physeptone	T4Ø.3X1	T4Ø.3X2	T4Ø.3X3	T4Ø.3X4	T4Ø.3X5	T4Ø.3X6
Physostigma venenosum	T62.2X1	T62.2X2	T62.2X3	T62.2X4	—	—
Physostigmine	T49.5X1	T49.5X2	T49.5X3	T49.5X4	T49.5X5	T49.5X6
Phytolacca decandra	T62.2X1	T62.2X2	T62.2X3	T62.2X4	—	—
berries	T62.1X1	T62.1X2	T62.1X3	T62.1X4	—	—

Substance	External Cause (T-Code)					
	Poisoning, Accidental (Unintentional)	Poisoning, Intentional Self-Harm	Poisoning, Assault	Poisoning, Undetermined	Adverse Effect	Underdosing
Phytomenadione	T45.7X1	T45.7X2	T45.7X3	T45.7X4	T45.7X5	T45.7X6
Phytonadione	T45.7X1	T45.7X2	T45.7X3	T45.7X4	T45.7X5	T45.7X6
Picoperine	T48.3X1	T48.3X2	T48.3X3	T48.3X4	T48.3X5	T48.3X6
Picosulfate (sodium)	T47.2X1	T47.2X2	T47.2X3	T47.2X4	T47.2X5	T47.2X6
Picric (acid)	T54.2X1	T54.2X2	T54.2X3	T54.2X4	—	—
Picrotoxin	T5Ø.7X1	T5Ø.7X2	T5Ø.7X3	T5Ø.7X4	T5Ø.7X5	T5Ø.7X6
Piketoprofen	T49.ØX1	T49.ØX2	T49.ØX3	T49.ØX4	T49.ØX5	T49.ØX6
Pilocarpine	T44.1X1	T44.1X2	T44.1X3	T44.1X4	T44.1X5	T44.1X6
Pilocarpus (jaborandi) extract	T44.1X1	T44.1X2	T44.1X3	T44.1X4	T44.1X5	T44.1X6
Pilsicainide (hydrochloride)	T46.2X1	T46.2X2	T46.2X3	T46.2X4	T46.2X5	T46.2X6
Pimaricin	T36.7X1	T36.7X2	T36.7X3	T36.7X4	T36.7X5	T36.7X6
Pimeclone	T5Ø.7X1	T5Ø.7X2	T5Ø.7X3	T5Ø.7X4	T5Ø.7X5	T5Ø.7X6
Pimelic ketone	T52.8X1	T52.8X2	T52.8X3	T52.8X4	—	—
Pimethixene	T45.ØX1	T45.ØX2	T45.ØX3	T45.ØX4	T45.ØX5	T45.ØX6
Piminodine	T4Ø.2X1	T4Ø.2X2	T4Ø.2X3	T4Ø.2X4	T4Ø.2X5	T4Ø.2X6
Pimozide	T43.591	T43.592	T43.593	T43.594	T43.595	T43.596
Pinacidil	T46.5X1	T46.5X2	T46.5X3	T46.5X4	T46.5X5	T46.5X6
Pinaverium bromide	T44.3X1	T44.3X2	T44.3X3	T44.3X4	T44.3X5	T44.3X6
Pinazepam	T42.4X1	T42.4X2	T42.4X3	T42.4X4	T42.4X5	T42.4X6
Pindolol	T44.7X1	T44.7X2	T44.7X3	T44.7X4	T44.7X5	T44.7X6
Pindone	T6Ø.4X1	T6Ø.4X2	T6Ø.4X3	T6Ø.4X4	—	—
Pine oil (disinfectant)	T65.891	T65.892	T65.893	T65.894	—	—
Pinkroot	T37.4X1	T37.4X2	T37.4X3	T37.4X4	T37.4X5	T37.4X6
Pipadone	T4Ø.2X1	T4Ø.2X2	T4Ø.2X3	T4Ø.2X4	—	—
Pipamazine	T45.ØX1	T45.ØX2	T45.ØX3	T45.ØX4	T45.ØX5	T45.ØX6
Pipamperone	T43.4X1	T43.4X2	T43.4X3	T43.4X4	T43.4X5	T43.4X6
Pipazetate	T48.3X1	T48.3X2	T48.3X3	T48.3X4	T48.3X5	T48.3X6
Pipemidic acid	T37.8X1	T37.8X2	T37.8X3	T37.8X4	T37.8X5	T37.8X6
Pipenzolate bromide	T44.3X1	T44.3X2	T44.3X3	T44.3X4	T44.3X5	T44.3X6
Piperacetazine	T43.3X1	T43.3X2	T43.3X3	T43.3X4	T43.3X5	T43.3X6
Piperacillin	T36.ØX1	T36.ØX2	T36.ØX3	T36.ØX4	T36.ØX5	T36.ØX6
Piperazine	T37.4X1	T37.4X2	T37.4X3	T37.4X4	T37.4X5	T37.4X6
estrone sulfate	T38.5X1	T38.5X2	T38.5X3	T38.5X4	T38.5X5	T38.5X6
Piper cubeba	T62.2X1	T62.2X2	T62.2X3	T62.2X4	—	—
Piperidione	T48.3X1	T48.3X2	T48.3X3	T48.3X4	—	—
Piperidolate	T44.3X1	T44.3X2	T44.3X3	T44.3X4	T44.3X5	T44.3X6
Piperocaine	T41.3X1	T41.3X2	T41.3X3	T41.3X4	T41.3X5	T41.3X6
infiltration (subcutaneous)	T41.3X1	T41.3X2	T41.3X3	T41.3X4	T41.3X5	T41.3X6
nerve block (peripheral) (plexus)	T41.3X1	T41.3X2	T41.3X3	T41.3X4	T41.3X5	T41.3X6
topical (surface)	T41.3X1	T41.3X2	T41.3X3	T41.3X4	T41.3X5	T41.3X6
Piperonyl butoxide	T6Ø.8X1	T6Ø.8X2	T6Ø.8X3	T6Ø.8X4	—	—
Pipethanate	T44.3X1	T44.3X2	T44.3X3	T44.3X4	T44.3X5	T44.3X6

Substance	External Cause (T-Code)					
	Poisoning, Accidental (Unintentional)	Poisoning, Intentional Self-Harm	Poisoning, Assault	Poisoning, Undetermined	Adverse Effect	Underdosing
Pipobroman	T45.1X1	T45.1X2	T45.1X3	T45.1X4	T45.1X5	T45.1X6
Pipofezine	T43.ØX1	T43.ØX2	T43.ØX3	T43.ØX4	T43.ØX5	T43.ØX6
Pipotiazine	T43.3X1	T43.3X2	T43.3X3	T43.3X4	T43.3X5	T43.3X6
Pipoxizine	T45.ØX1	T45.ØX2	T45.ØX3	T45.ØX4	T45.ØX5	T45.ØX6
Pipradrol	T43.691	T43.692	T43.693	T43.694	T43.695	T43.696
Piprinhydrinate	T45.ØX1	T45.ØX2	T45.ØX3	T45.ØX4	T45.ØX5	T45.ØX6
Pirarubicin	T45.1X1	T45.1X2	T45.1X3	T45.1X4	T45.1X5	T45.1X6
Pirazinamide	T37.1X1	T37.1X2	T37.1X3	T37.1X4	T37.1X5	T37.1X6
Pirbuterol	T48.6X1	T48.6X2	T48.6X3	T48.6X4	T48.6X5	T48.6X6
Pirenzepine	T47.1X1	T47.1X2	T47.1X3	T47.1X4	T47.1X5	T47.1X6
Piretanide	T5Ø.1X1	T5Ø.1X2	T5Ø.1X3	T5Ø.1X4	T5Ø.1X5	T5Ø.1X6
Piribedil	T42.8X1	T42.8X2	T42.8X3	T42.8X4	T42.8X5	T42.8X6
Piridoxilate	T46.3X1	T46.3X2	T46.3X3	T46.3X4	T46.3X5	T46.3X6
Piritramide	T4Ø.491	T4Ø.492	T4Ø.493	T4Ø.494	—	—
Pirlindole	T43.ØX1	T43.ØX2	T43.ØX3	T43.ØX4	T43.ØX5	T43.ØX6
Piromidic acid	T37.8X1	T37.8X2	T37.8X3	T37.8X4	T37.8X5	T37.8X6
Piroxicam	T39.391	T39.392	T39.393	T39.394	T39.395	T39.396
beta-cyclodextrin complex	T39.8X1	T39.8X2	T39.8X3	T39.8X4	T39.8X5	T39.8X6
Pirozadil	T46.6X1	T46.6X2	T46.6X3	T46.6X4	T46.6X5	T46.6X6
Piscidia (bark) (erythrina)	T39.8X1	T39.8X2	T39.8X3	T39.8X4	T39.8X5	T39.8X6
Pitch	T65.891	T65.892	T65.893	T65.894	—	—
Pitkin's solution	T41.3X1	T41.3X2	T41.3X3	T41.3X4	T41.3X5	T41.3X6
Pitocin	T48.ØX1	T48.ØX2	T48.ØX3	T48.ØX4	T48.ØX5	T48.ØX6
Pitressin (tannate)	T38.891	T38.892	T38.893	T38.894	T38.895	T38.896
Pituitary extracts (posterior)	T38.891	T38.892	T38.893	T38.894	T38.895	T38.896
anterior	T38.811	T38.812	T38.813	T38.814	T38.815	T38.816
Pituitrin	T38.891	T38.892	T38.893	T38.894	T38.895	T38.896
Pivampicillin	T36.ØX1	T36.ØX2	T36.ØX3	T36.ØX4	T36.ØX5	T36.ØX6
Pivmecillinam	T36.ØX1	T36.ØX2	T36.ØX3	T36.ØX4	T36.ØX5	T36.ØX6
Placental hormone	T38.891	T38.892	T38.893	T38.894	T38.895	T38.896
Placidyl	T42.6X1	T42.6X2	T42.6X3	T42.6X4	T42.6X5	T42.6X6
Plague vaccine	T5Ø.A91	T5Ø.A92	T5Ø.A93	T5Ø.A94	T5Ø.A95	T5Ø.A96
Plant						
food or fertilizer NEC	T65.891	T65.892	T65.893	T65.894	—	—
containing herbicide	T6Ø.3X1	T6Ø.3X2	T6Ø.3X3	T6Ø.3X4	—	—
noxious, used as food	T62.2X1	T62.2X2	T62.2X3	T62.2X4	—	—
berries	T62.1X1	T62.1X2	T62.1X3	T62.1X4	—	—
seeds	T62.2X1	T62.2X2	T62.2X3	T62.2X4	—	—
specified type NEC	T62.2X1	T62.2X2	T62.2X3	T62.2X4	—	—
Plasma	T45.8X1	T45.8X2	T45.8X3	T45.8X4	T45.8X5	T45.8X6
expander NEC	T45.8X1	T45.8X2	T45.8X3	T45.8X4	T45.8X5	T45.8X6
protein fraction (human)	T45.8X1	T45.8X2	T45.8X3	T45.8X4	T45.8X5	T45.8X6

TABLE OF DRUGS AND CHEMICALS

New Revised ~~deleted~~ Deleted

Substance	Poisoning, Accidental (Unintentional)	Poisoning, Intentional Self-Harm	Poisoning, Assault	Poisoning, Undetermined	Adverse Effect	Underdosing
Plasmanate	T45.8X1	T45.8X2	T45.8X3	T45.8X4	T45.8X5	T45.8X6
Plasminogen (tissue) activator	T45.611	T45.612	T45.613	T45.614	T45.615	T45.616
Plaster dressing	T49.3X1	T49.3X2	T49.3X3	T49.3X4	T49.3X5	T49.3X6
Plastic dressing	T49.3X1	T49.3X2	T49.3X3	T49.3X4	T49.3X5	T49.3X6
Plegicil	T43.3X1	T43.3X2	T43.3X3	T43.3X4	T43.3X5	T43.3X6
Plicamycin	T45.1X1	T45.1X2	T45.1X3	T45.1X4	T45.1X5	T45.1X6
Podophyllotoxin	T49.8X1	T49.8X2	T49.8X3	T49.8X4	T49.8X5	T49.8X6
Podophyllum (resin)	T49.4X1	T49.4X2	T49.4X3	T49.4X4	T49.4X5	T49.4X6
Poison NEC	T65.91	T65.92	T65.93	T65.94	—	—
Poisonous berries	T62.1X1	T62.1X2	T62.1X3	T62.1X4	—	—
Pokeweed (any part)	T62.2X1	T62.2X2	T62.2X3	T62.2X4	—	—
Poldine metilsulfate	T44.3X1	T44.3X2	T44.3X3	T44.3X4	T44.3X5	T44.3X6
Polidexide (sulfate)	T46.6X1	T46.6X2	T46.6X3	T46.6X4	T46.6X5	T46.6X6
Polidocanol	T46.8X1	T46.8X2	T46.8X3	T46.8X4	T46.8X5	T46.8X6
Poliomyelitis vaccine	T50.B91	T50.B92	T50.B93	T50.B94	T50.B95	T50.B96
Polish (car) (floor) (furniture) (metal) (porcelain) (silver)	T65.891	T65.892	T65.893	T65.894	—	—
abrasive	T65.891	T65.892	T65.893	T65.894	—	—
porcelain	T65.891	T65.892	T65.893	T65.894	—	—
Poloxalkol	T47.4X1	T47.4X2	T47.4X3	T47.4X4	T47.4X5	T47.4X6
Poloxamer	T47.4X1	T47.4X2	T47.4X3	T47.4X4	T47.4X5	T47.4X6
Polyaminostyrene resins	T50.3X1	T50.3X2	T50.3X3	T50.3X4	T50.3X5	T50.3X6
Polycarbophil	T47.4X1	T47.4X2	T47.4X3	T47.4X4	T47.4X5	T47.4X6
Polychlorinated biphenyl	T65.891	T65.892	T65.893	T65.894	—	—
Polycycline	T36.4X1	T36.4X2	T36.4X3	T36.4X4	T36.4X5	T36.4X6
Polyester fumes	T59.891	T59.892	T59.893	T59.894	—	—
Polyester resin hardener	T52.91	T52.92	T52.93	T52.94	—	—
fumes	T59.891	T59.892	T59.893	T59.894	—	—
Polyestradiol phosphate	T38.5X1	T38.5X2	T38.5X3	T38.5X4	T38.5X5	T38.5X6
Polyethanolamine alkyl sulfate	T49.2X1	T49.2X2	T49.2X3	T49.2X4	T49.2X5	T49.2X6
Polyethylene adhesive	T49.3X1	T49.3X2	T49.3X3	T49.3X4	T49.3X5	T49.3X6
Polyferose	T45.4X1	T45.4X2	T45.4X3	T45.4X4	T45.4X5	T45.4X6
Polygeline	T45.8X1	T45.8X2	T45.8X3	T45.8X4	T45.8X5	T45.8X6
Polymyxin	T36.8X1	T36.8X2	T36.8X3	T36.8X4	T36.8X5	T36.8X6
B	T36.8X1	T36.8X2	T36.8X3	T36.8X4	T36.8X5	T36.8X6
ENT agent	T49.6X1	T49.6X2	T49.6X3	T49.6X4	T49.6X5	T49.6X6
ophthalmic preparation	T49.5X1	T49.5X2	T49.5X3	T49.5X4	T49.5X5	T49.5X6
topical NEC	T49.0X1	T49.0X2	T49.0X3	T49.0X4	T49.0X5	T49.0X6
E sulfate (eye preparation)	T49.5X1	T49.5X2	T49.5X3	T49.5X4	T49.5X5	T49.5X6
Polynoxylin	T49.0X1	T49.0X2	T49.0X3	T49.0X4	T49.0X5	T49.0X6
Polyoestradiol phosphate	T38.5X1	T38.5X2	T38.5X3	T38.5X4	T38.5X5	T38.5X6
Polyoxymethyleneurea	T49.0X1	T49.0X2	T49.0X3	T49.0X4	T49.0X5	T49.0X6
Polysilane	T47.8X1	T47.8X2	T47.8X3	T47.8X4	T47.8X5	T47.8X6
Polytetrafluoroethylene (inhaled)	T59.891	T59.892	T59.893	T59.894	—	—
Polythiazide	T50.2X1	T50.2X2	T50.2X3	T50.2X4	T50.2X5	T50.2X6
Polyvidone	T45.8X1	T45.8X2	T45.8X3	T45.8X4	T45.8X5	T45.8X6
Polyvinylpyrrolidone	T45.8X1	T45.8X2	T45.8X3	T45.8X4	T45.8X5	T45.8X6
Pontocaine (hydrochloride) (infiltration) (topical)	T41.3X1	T41.3X2	T41.3X3	T41.3X4	T41.3X5	T41.3X6
nerve block (peripheral) (plexus)	T41.3X1	T41.3X2	T41.3X3	T41.3X4	T41.3X5	T41.3X6
spinal	T41.3X1	T41.3X2	T41.3X3	T41.3X4	T41.3X5	T41.3X6
Porfiromycin	T45.1X1	T45.1X2	T45.1X3	T45.1X4	T45.1X5	T45.1X6
Posterior pituitary hormone NEC	T38.891	T38.892	T38.893	T38.894	T38.895	T38.896
Pot	T40.711	T40.712	T40.713	T40.714	T40.715	T40.716
Potash (caustic)	T54.3X1	T54.3X2	T54.3X3	T54.3X4	—	—
Potassic saline injection (lactated)	T50.3X1	T50.3X2	T50.3X3	T50.3X4	T50.3X5	T50.3X6
Potassium (salts) NEC	T50.3X1	T50.3X2	T50.3X3	T50.3X4	T50.3X5	T50.3X6
aminobenzoate	T45.8X1	T45.8X2	T45.8X3	T45.8X4	T45.8X5	T45.8X6
aminosalicylate	T37.1X1	T37.1X2	T37.1X3	T37.1X4	T37.1X5	T37.1X6
antimony 'tartrate'	T37.8X1	T37.8X2	T37.8X3	T37.8X4	T37.8X5	T37.8X6
arsenite (solution)	T57.0X1	T57.0X2	T57.0X3	T57.0X4	—	—
bichromate	T56.2X1	T56.2X2	T56.2X3	T56.2X4	—	—
bisulfate	T47.3X1	T47.3X2	T47.3X3	T47.3X4	T47.3X5	T47.3X6
bromide	T42.6X1	T42.6X2	T42.6X3	T42.6X4	T42.6X5	T42.6X6
canrenoate	T50.0X1	T50.0X2	T50.0X3	T50.0X4	T50.0X5	T50.0X6
carbonate	T54.3X1	T54.3X2	T54.3X3	T54.3X4	—	—
chlorate NEC	T65.891	T65.892	T65.893	T65.894	—	—
chloride	T50.3X1	T50.3X2	T50.3X3	T50.3X4	T50.3X5	T50.3X6
citrate	T50.991	T50.992	T50.993	T50.994	T50.995	T50.996
cyanide	T65.0X1	T65.0X2	T65.0X3	T65.0X4	—	—
ferric hexacyanoferrate (medicinal)	T50.6X1	T50.6X2	T50.6X3	T50.6X4	T50.6X5	T50.6X6
nonmedicinal	T65.891	T65.892	T65.893	T65.894	—	—
Fluoride	T57.8X1	T57.8X2	T57.8X3	T57.8X4	—	—
glucaldrate	T47.1X1	T47.1X2	T47.1X3	T47.1X4	T47.1X5	T47.1X6
hydroxide	T54.3X1	T54.3X2	T54.3X3	T54.3X4	—	—
iodate	T49.0X1	T49.0X2	T49.0X3	T49.0X4	T49.0X5	T49.0X6
iodide	T48.4X1	T48.4X2	T48.4X3	T48.4X4	T48.4X5	T48.4X6
nitrate	T57.8X1	T57.8X2	T57.8X3	T57.8X4	—	—
oxalate	T65.891	T65.892	T65.893	T65.894	—	—
perchlorate (nonmedicinal) NEC	T65.891	T65.892	T65.893	T65.894	—	—
antithyroid	T38.2X1	T38.2X2	T38.2X3	T38.2X4	T38.2X5	T38.2X6
medicinal	T38.2X1	T38.2X2	T38.2X3	T38.2X4	T38.2X5	T38.2X6

New Revised ~~deleted~~ Deleted

Substance	External Cause (T-Code)					
	Poisoning, Accidental (Unintentional)	Poisoning, Intentional Self-Harm	Poisoning, Assault	Poisoning, Undetermined	Adverse Effect	Underdosing
Permanganate (nonmedicinal)	T65.891	T65.892	T65.893	T65.894	—	—
medicinal	T49.ØX1	T49.ØX2	T49.ØX3	T49.ØX4	T49.ØX5	T49.ØX6
sulfate	T47.2X1	T47.2X2	T47.2X3	T47.2X4	T47.2X5	T47.2X6
Potassium-removing resin	T5Ø.3X1	T5Ø.3X2	T5Ø.3X3	T5Ø.3X4	T5Ø.3X5	T5Ø.3X6
Potassium-retaining drug	T5Ø.3X1	T5Ø.3X2	T5Ø.3X3	T5Ø.3X4	T5Ø.3X5	T5Ø.3X6
Povidone	T45.8X1	T45.8X2	T45.8X3	T45.8X4	T45.8X5	T45.8X6
iodine	T49.ØX1	T49.ØX2	T49.ØX3	T49.ØX4	T49.ØX5	T49.ØX6
Practolol	T44.7X1	T44.7X2	T44.7X3	T44.7X4	T44.7X5	T44.7X6
Prajmalium bitartrate	T46.2X1	T46.2X2	T46.2X3	T46.2X4	T46.2X5	T46.2X6
Pralidoxime (iodide)	T5Ø.6X1	T5Ø.6X2	T5Ø.6X3	T5Ø.6X4	T5Ø.6X5	T5Ø.6X6
chloride	T5Ø.6X1	T5Ø.6X2	T5Ø.6X3	T5Ø.6X4	T5Ø.6X5	T5Ø.6X6
Pramiverine	T44.3X1	T44.3X2	T44.3X3	T44.3X4	T44.3X5	T44.3X6
Pramocaine	T49.1X1	T49.1X2	T49.1X3	T49.1X4	T49.1X5	T49.1X6
Pramoxine	T49.1X1	T49.1X2	T49.1X3	T49.1X4	T49.1X5	T49.1X6
Prasterone	T38.7X1	T38.7X2	T38.7X3	T38.7X4	T38.7X5	T38.7X6
Pravastatin	T46.6X1	T46.6X2	T46.6X3	T46.6X4	T46.6X5	T46.6X6
Prazepam	T42.4X1	T42.4X2	T42.4X3	T42.4X4	T42.4X5	T42.4X6
Praziquantel	T37.4X1	T37.4X2	T37.4X3	T37.4X4	T37.4X5	T37.4X6
Prazitone	T43.291	T43.292	T43.293	T43.294	T43.295	T43.296
Prazosin	T44.6X1	T44.6X2	T44.6X3	T44.6X4	T44.6X5	T44.6X6
Prednicarbate	T49.ØX1	T49.ØX2	T49.ØX3	T49.ØX4	T49.ØX5	T49.ØX6
Prednimustine	T45.1X1	T45.1X2	T45.1X3	T45.1X4	T45.1X5	T45.1X6
Prednisolone	T38.ØX1	T38.ØX2	T38.ØX3	T38.ØX4	T38.ØX5	T38.ØX6
ENT agent	T49.6X1	T49.6X2	T49.6X3	T49.6X4	T49.6X5	T49.6X6
ophthalmic preparation	T49.5X1	T49.5X2	T49.5X3	T49.5X4	T49.5X5	T49.5X6
steaglate	T49.ØX1	T49.ØX2	T49.ØX3	T49.ØX4	T49.ØX5	T49.ØX6
topical NEC	T49.ØX1	T49.ØX2	T49.ØX3	T49.ØX4	T49.ØX5	T49.ØX6
Prednisone	T38.ØX1	T38.ØX2	T38.ØX3	T38.ØX4	T38.ØX5	T38.ØX6
Prednylidene	T38.ØX1	T38.ØX2	T38.ØX3	T38.ØX4	T38.ØX5	T38.ØX6
Pregnandiol	T38.5X1	T38.5X2	T38.5X3	T38.5X4	T38.5X5	T38.5X6
Pregneninolone	T38.5X1	T38.5X2	T38.5X3	T38.5X4	T38.5X5	T38.5X6
Preludin	T43.691	T43.692	T43.693	T43.694	T43.695	T43.696
Premarin	T38.5X1	T38.5X2	T38.5X3	T38.5X4	T38.5X5	T38.5X6
Premedication anesthetic	T41.2Ø1	T41.2Ø2	T41.2Ø3	T41.2Ø4	T41.2Ø5	T41.2Ø6
Prenalterol	T44.5X1	T44.5X2	T44.5X3	T44.5X4	T44.5X5	T44.5X6
Prenoxdiazine	T48.3X1	T48.3X2	T48.3X3	T48.3X4	T48.3X5	T48.3X6
Prenylamine	T46.3X1	T46.3X2	T46.3X3	T46.3X4	T46.3X5	T46.3X6
Preparation, local	T49.4X1	T49.4X2	T49.4X3	T49.4X4	T49.4X5	T49.4X6
Preparation H	T49.8X1	T49.8X2	T49.8X3	T49.8X4	T49.8X5	T49.8X6
Preservative (nonmedicinal)	T65.891	T65.892	T65.893	T65.894	—	—
medicinal	T5Ø.9Ø1	T5Ø.9Ø2	T5Ø.9Ø3	T5Ø.9Ø4	T5Ø.9Ø5	T5Ø.9Ø6
wood	T6Ø.91	T6Ø.92	T6Ø.93	T6Ø.94	—	—
Prethcamide	T5Ø.7X1	T5Ø.7X2	T5Ø.7X3	T5Ø.7X4	T5Ø.7X5	T5Ø.7X6
Pride of China	T62.2X1	T62.2X2	T62.2X3	T62.2X4	—	—
Pridinol	T44.3X1	T44.3X2	T44.3X3	T44.3X4	T44.3X5	T44.3X6
Prifinium bromide	T44.3X1	T44.3X2	T44.3X3	T44.3X4	T44.3X5	T44.3X6
Prilocaine	T41.3X1	T41.3X2	T41.3X3	T41.3X4	T41.3X5	T41.3X6
infiltration (subcutaneous)	T41.3X1	T41.3X2	T41.3X3	T41.3X4	T41.3X5	T41.3X6
nerve block (peripheral) (plexus)	T41.3X1	T41.3X2	T41.3X3	T41.3X4	T41.3X5	T41.3X6
regional	T41.3X1	T41.3X2	T41.3X3	T41.3X4	T41.3X5	T41.3X6
Primaquine	T37.2X1	T37.2X2	T37.2X3	T37.2X4	T37.2X5	T37.2X6
Primidone	T42.6X1	T42.6X2	T42.6X3	T42.6X4	T42.6X5	T42.6X6
Primula (veris)	T62.2X1	T62.2X2	T62.2X3	T62.2X4	—	—
Prinadol	T4Ø.2X1	T4Ø.2X2	T4Ø.2X3	T4Ø.2X4	T4Ø.2X5	T4Ø.2X6
Priscol, Priscoline	T44.6X1	T44.6X2	T44.6X3	T44.6X4	T44.6X5	T44.6X6
Pristinamycin	T36.3X1	T36.3X2	T36.3X3	T36.3X4	T36.3X5	T36.3X6
Privet	T62.2X1	T62.2X2	T62.2X3	T62.2X4	—	—
berries	T62.1X1	T62.1X2	T62.1X3	T62.1X4	—	—
Privine	T44.4X1	T44.4X2	T44.4X3	T44.4X4	T44.4X5	T44.4X6
Pro-Banthine	T44.3X1	T44.3X2	T44.3X3	T44.3X4	T44.3X5	T44.3X6
Probarbital	T42.3X1	T42.3X2	T42.3X3	T42.3X4	T42.3X5	T42.3X6
Probenecid	T5Ø.4X1	T5Ø.4X2	T5Ø.4X3	T5Ø.4X4	T5Ø.4X5	T5Ø.4X6
Probucol	T46.6X1	T46.6X2	T46.6X3	T46.6X4	T46.6X5	T46.6X6
Procainamide	T46.2X1	T46.2X2	T46.2X3	T46.2X4	T46.2X5	T46.2X6
Procaine	T41.3X1	T41.3X2	T41.3X3	T41.3X4	T41.3X5	T41.3X6
benzylpenicillin	T36.ØX1	T36.ØX2	T36.ØX3	T36.ØX4	T36.ØX5	T36.ØX6
nerve block (periphreal) (plexus)	T41.3X1	T41.3X2	T41.3X3	T41.3X4	T41.3X5	T41.3X6
penicillin G	T36.ØX1	T36.ØX2	T36.ØX3	T36.ØX4	T36.ØX5	T36.ØX6
regional	T41.3X1	T41.3X2	T41.3X3	T41.3X4	T41.3X5	T41.3X6
spinal	T41.3X1	T41.3X2	T41.3X3	T41.3X4	T41.3X5	T41.3X6
Procalmidol	T43.591	T43.592	T43.593	T43.594	T43.595	T43.596
Procarbazine	T45.1X1	T45.1X2	T45.1X3	T45.1X4	T45.1X5	T45.1X6
Procaterol	T44.5X1	T44.5X2	T44.5X3	T44.5X4	T44.5X5	T44.5X6
Prochlorperazine	T43.3X1	T43.3X2	T43.3X3	T43.3X4	T43.3X5	T43.3X6
Procyclidine	T44.3X1	T44.3X2	T44.3X3	T44.3X4	T44.3X5	T44.3X6
Producer gas	T58.8X1	T58.8X2	T58.8X3	T58.8X4	—	—
Profadol	T4Ø.491	T4Ø.492	T4Ø.493	T4Ø.494	T4Ø.495	T4Ø.496
Profenamine	T44.3X1	T44.3X2	T44.3X3	T44.3X4	T44.3X5	T44.3X6
Profenil	T44.3X1	T44.3X2	T44.3X3	T44.3X4	T44.3X5	T44.3X6
Proflavine	T49.ØX1	T49.ØX2	T49.ØX3	T49.ØX4	T49.ØX5	T49.ØX6
Progabide	T42.6X1	T42.6X2	T42.6X3	T42.6X4	T42.6X5	T42.6X6
Progestin	T38.5X1	T38.5X2	T38.5X3	T38.5X4	T38.5X5	T38.5X6
oral contraceptive	T38.4X1	T38.4X2	T38.4X3	T38.4X4	T38.4X5	T38.4X6

TABLE OF DRUGS AND CHEMICALS

	External Cause (T-Code)					
Substance	Poisoning, Accidental (Unintentional)	Poisoning, Intentional Self-Harm	Poisoning, Assault	Poisoning, Undetermined	Adverse Effect	Underdosing
Progesterone	T38.5X1	T38.5X2	T38.5X3	T38.5X4	T38.5X5	T38.5X6
Progestogen NEC	T38.5X1	T38.5X2	T38.5X3	T38.5X4	T38.5X5	T38.5X6
Progestone	T38.5X1	T38.5X2	T38.5X3	T38.5X4	T38.5X5	T38.5X6
Proglumide	T47.1X1	T47.1X2	T47.1X3	T47.1X4	T47.1X5	T47.1X6
Proguanil	T37.2X1	T37.2X2	T37.2X3	T37.2X4	T37.2X5	T37.2X6
Prolactin	T38.811	T38.812	T38.813	T38.814	T38.815	T38.816
Prolintane	T43.691	T43.692	T43.693	T43.694	T43.695	T43.696
Proloid	T38.1X1	T38.1X2	T38.1X3	T38.1X4	T38.1X5	T38.1X6
Proluton	T38.5X1	T38.5X2	T38.5X3	T38.5X4	T38.5X5	T38.5X6
Promacetin	T37.1X1	T37.1X2	T37.1X3	T37.1X4	T37.1X5	T37.1X6
Promazine	T43.3X1	T43.3X2	T43.3X3	T43.3X4	T43.3X5	T43.3X6
Promedol	T40.2X1	T40.2X2	T40.2X3	T40.2X4	—	—
Promegestone	T38.5X1	T38.5X2	T38.5X3	T38.5X4	T38.5X5	T38.5X6
Promethazine (teoclate)	T43.3X1	T43.3X2	T43.3X3	T43.3X4	T43.3X5	T43.3X6
Promin	T37.1X1	T37.1X2	T37.1X3	T37.1X4	T37.1X5	T37.1X6
Pronase	T45.3X1	T45.3X2	T45.3X3	T45.3X4	T45.3X5	T45.3X6
Pronestyl (hydrochloride)	T46.2X1	T46.2X2	T46.2X3	T46.2X4	T46.2X5	T46.2X6
Pronetalol	T44.7X1	T44.7X2	T44.7X3	T44.7X4	T44.7X5	T44.7X6
Prontosil	T37.0X1	T37.0X2	T37.0X3	T37.0X4	T37.0X5	T37.0X6
Propachlor	T60.3X1	T60.3X2	T60.3X3	T60.3X4	—	—
Propafenone	T46.2X1	T46.2X2	T46.2X3	T46.2X4	T46.2X5	T46.2X6
Propallylonal	T42.3X1	T42.3X2	T42.3X3	T42.3X4	T42.3X5	T42.3X6
Propamidine	T49.0X1	T49.0X2	T49.0X3	T49.0X4	T49.0X5	T49.0X6
Propane (distributed in mobile container)	T59.891	T59.892	T59.893	T59.894	—	—
distributed through pipes	T59.891	T59.892	T59.893	T59.894	—	—
incomplete combustion	T57.11	T57.12	T57.13	T57.14	—	—
Propanidid	T41.291	T41.292	T41.293	T41.294	T41.295	T41.296
Propanil	T60.3X1	T60.3X2	T60.3X3	T60.3X4	—	—
1-Propanol	T51.3X1	T51.3X2	T51.3X3	T51.3X4	—	—
2-Propanol	T51.2X1	T51.2X2	T51.2X3	T51.2X4	—	—
Propantheline	T44.3X1	T44.3X2	T44.3X3	T44.3X4	T44.3X5	T44.3X6
bromide	T44.3X1	T44.3X2	T44.3X3	T44.3X4	T44.3X5	T44.3X6
Proparacaine	T41.3X1	T41.3X2	T41.3X3	T41.3X4	T41.3X5	T41.3X6
Propatylnitrate	T46.3X1	T46.3X2	T46.3X3	T46.3X4	T46.3X5	T46.3X6
Propicillin	T36.0X1	T36.0X2	T36.0X3	T36.0X4	T36.0X5	T36.0X6
Propiolactone	T49.0X1	T49.0X2	T49.0X3	T49.0X4	T49.0X5	T49.0X6
Propiomazine	T45.0X1	T45.0X2	T45.0X3	T45.0X4	T45.0X5	T45.0X6
Propionaldehyde (medicinal)	T42.6X1	T42.6X2	T42.6X3	T42.6X4	T42.6X5	T42.6X6
Propionate (calcium) (sodium)	T49.0X1	T49.0X2	T49.0X3	T49.0X4	T49.0X5	T49.0X6
Propion gel	T49.0X1	T49.0X2	T49.0X3	T49.0X4	T49.0X5	T49.0X6
Propitocaine	T41.3X1	T41.3X2	T41.3X3	T41.3X4	T41.3X5	T41.3X6
infiltration (subcutaneous)	T41.3X1	T41.3X2	T41.3X3	T41.3X4	T41.3X5	T41.3X6
nerve block (peripheral) (plexus)	T41.3X1	T41.3X2	T41.3X3	T41.3X4	T41.3X5	T41.3X6
Propofol	T41.291	T41.292	T41.293	T41.294	T41.295	T41.296
Propoxur	T60.0X1	T60.0X2	T60.0X3	T60.0X4	—	—
Propoxycaine	T41.3X1	T41.3X2	T41.3X3	T41.3X4	T41.3X5	T41.3X6
infiltration (subcutaneous)	T41.3X1	T41.3X2	T41.3X3	T41.3X4	T41.3X5	T41.3X6
nerve block (peripheral) (plexus)	T41.3X1	T41.3X2	T41.3X3	T41.3X4	T41.3X5	T41.3X6
topical (surface)	T41.3X1	T41.3X2	T41.3X3	T41.3X4	T41.3X5	T41.3X6
Propoxyphene	T40.491	T40.492	T40.493	T40.494	T40.495	T40.496
Propranolol	T44.7X1	T44.7X2	T44.7X3	T44.7X4	T44.7X5	T44.7X6
Propyl						
alcohol	T51.3X1	T51.3X2	T51.3X3	T51.3X4	—	—
carbinol	T51.3X1	T51.3X2	T51.3X3	T51.3X4	—	—
hexadrine	T44.4X1	T44.4X2	T44.4X3	T44.4X4	T44.4X5	T44.4X6
iodone	T50.8X1	T50.8X2	T50.8X3	T50.8X4	T50.8X5	T50.8X6
thiouracil	T38.2X1	T38.2X2	T38.2X3	T38.2X4	T38.2X5	T38.2X6
Propylaminophenothiazine	T43.3X1	T43.3X2	T43.3X3	T43.3X4	T43.3X5	T43.3X6
Propylene	T59.891	T59.892	T59.893	T59.894	—	—
Propylhexedrine	T48.5X1	T48.5X2	T48.5X3	T48.5X4	T48.5X5	T48.5X6
Propyliodone	T50.8X1	T50.8X2	T50.8X3	T50.8X4	T50.8X5	T50.8X6
Propylthiouracil	T38.2X1	T38.2X2	T38.2X3	T38.2X4	T38.2X5	T38.2X6
Propylparaben (ophthalmic)	T49.5X1	T49.5X2	T49.5X3	T49.5X4	T49.5X5	T49.5X6
Propyphenazone	T39.2X1	T39.2X2	T39.2X3	T39.2X4	T39.2X5	T39.2X6
Proquazone	T39.391	T39.392	T39.393	T39.394	T39.395	T39.396
Proscillaridin	T46.0X1	T46.0X2	T46.0X3	T46.0X4	T46.0X5	T46.0X6
Prostacyclin	T45.521	T45.522	T45.523	T45.524	T45.525	T45.526
Prostaglandin (I2)	T45.521	T45.522	T45.523	T45.524	T45.525	T45.526
E1	T46.7X1	T46.7X2	T46.7X3	T46.7X4	T46.7X5	T46.7X6
E2	T48.0X1	T48.0X2	T48.0X3	T48.0X4	T48.0X5	T48.0X6
F2 alpha	T48.0X1	T48.0X2	T48.0X3	T48.0X4	T48.0X5	T48.0X6
Prostigmin	T44.0X1	T44.0X2	T44.0X3	T44.0X4	T44.0X5	T44.0X6
Prosultiamine	T45.2X1	T45.2X2	T45.2X3	T45.2X4	T45.2X5	T45.2X6
Protamine sulfate	T45.7X1	T45.7X2	T45.7X3	T45.7X4	T45.7X5	T45.7X6
zinc insulin	T38.3X1	T38.3X2	T38.3X3	T38.3X4	T38.3X5	T38.3X6
Protease	T47.5X1	T47.5X2	T47.5X3	T47.5X4	T47.5X5	T47.5X6
Protectant, skin NEC	T49.3X1	T49.3X2	T49.3X3	T49.3X4	T49.3X5	T49.3X6
Protein hydrolysate	T50.991	T50.992	T50.993	T50.994	T50.995	T50.996
Prothiaden — *see Dothiepin hydrochloride*						
Prothionamide	T37.1X1	T37.1X2	T37.1X3	T37.1X4	T37.1X5	T37.1X6

New Revised ~~deleted~~ Deleted

Substance	Poisoning, Accidental (Unintentional)	Poisoning, Intentional Self-Harm	Poisoning, Assault	Poisoning, Undetermined	Adverse Effect	Underdosing
	External Cause (T-Code)					
Prothipendyl	T43.591	T43.592	T43.593	T43.594	T43.595	T43.596
Prothoate	T60.0X1	T60.0X2	T60.0X3	T60.0X4	—	—
Prothrombin						
activator	T45.7X1	T45.7X2	T45.7X3	T45.7X4	T45.7X5	T45.7X6
synthesis inhibitor	T45.511	T45.512	T45.513	T45.514	T45.515	T45.516
Protionamide	T37.1X1	T37.1X2	T37.1X3	T37.1X4	T37.1X5	T37.1X6
Protirelin	T38.891	T38.892	T38.893	T38.894	T38.895	T38.896
Protokylol	T48.6X1	T48.6X2	T48.6X3	T48.6X4	T48.6X5	T48.6X6
Protopam	T50.6X1	T50.6X2	T50.6X3	T50.6X4	T50.6X5	T50.6X6
Protoveratrine(s) (A) (B)	T46.5X1	T46.5X2	T46.5X3	T46.5X4	T46.5X5	T46.5X6
Protriptyline	T43.011	T43.012	T43.013	T43.014	T43.015	T43.016
Provera	T38.5X1	T38.5X2	T38.5X3	T38.5X4	T38.5X5	T38.5X6
Provitamin A	T45.2X1	T45.2X2	T45.2X3	T45.2X4	T45.2X5	T45.2X6
Proxibarbal	T42.3X1	T42.3X2	T42.3X3	T42.3X4	T42.3X5	T42.3X6
Proxymetacaine	T41.3X1	T41.3X2	T41.3X3	T41.3X4	T41.3X5	T41.3X6
Proxyphylline	T48.6X1	T48.6X2	T48.6X3	T48.6X4	T48.6X5	T48.6X6
Prozac — *see Fluoxetine hydrochloride*						
Prunus						
laurocerasus	T62.2X1	T62.2X2	T62.2X3	T62.2X4	—	—
virginiana	T62.2X1	T62.2X2	T62.2X3	T62.2X4	—	—
Prussian blue						
commercial	T65.891	T65.892	T65.893	T65.894	—	—
therapeutic	T50.6X1	T50.6X2	T50.6X3	T50.6X4	T50.6X5	T50.6X6
Prussic acid	T65.0X1	T65.0X2	T65.0X3	T65.0X4	—	—
vapor	T57.3X1	T57.3X2	T57.3X3	T57.3X4	—	—
Pseudoephedrine	T44.991	T44.992	T44.993	T44.994	T44.995	T44.996
Psilocin	T40.991	T40.992	T40.993	T40.994	—	—
Psilocybin	T40.991	T40.992	T40.993	T40.994	—	—
Psilocybine	T40.991	T40.992	T40.993	T40.994	—	—
Psoralene (nonmedicinal)	T65.891	T65.892	T65.893	T65.894	—	—
Psoralens (medicinal)	T50.991	T50.992	T50.993	T50.994	T50.995	T50.996
PSP (phenolsulfonphthalein)	T50.8X1	T50.8X2	T50.8X3	T50.8X4	T50.8X5	T50.8X6
Psychodysleptic drug NOS	T40.901	T40.902	T40.903	T40.904	T40.905	T40.906
specified NEC	T40.991	T40.992	T40.993	T40.994	T40.995	T40.996
Psychostimulant	T43.601	T43.602	T43.603	T43.604	T43.605	T43.606
amphetamine	T43.621	T43.622	T43.623	T43.624	T43.625	T43.626
caffeine	T43.611	T43.612	T43.613	T43.614	T43.615	T43.616
methylphenidate	T43.631	T43.632	T43.633	T43.634	T43.635	T43.636
specified NEC	T43.691	T43.692	T43.693	T43.694	T43.695	T43.696
Psychotherapeutic drug NEC	T43.91	T43.92	T43.93	T43.94	T43.95	T43.96
antidepressants — *see also Antidepressant*	T43.201	T43.202	T43.203	T43.204	T43.205	T43.206

Substance	Poisoning, Accidental (Unintentional)	Poisoning, Intentional Self-Harm	Poisoning, Assault	Poisoning, Undetermined	Adverse Effect	Underdosing
	External Cause (T-Code)					
Psychotherapeutic drug NEC *(Continued)*						
specified NEC	T43.8X1	T43.8X2	T43.8X3	T43.8X4	T43.8X5	T43.8X6
tranquilizers NEC	T43.501	T43.502	T43.503	T43.504	T43.505	T43.506
Psychotomimetic agents	T40.901	T40.902	T40.903	T40.904	T40.905	T40.906
Psychotropic drug NEC	T43.91	T43.92	T43.93	T43.94	T43.95	T43.96
specified NEC	T43.8X1	T43.8X2	T43.8X3	T43.8X4	T43.8X5	T43.8X6
Psyllium hydrophilic mucilloid	T47.4X1	T47.4X2	T47.4X3	T47.4X4	T47.4X5	T47.4X6
Pteroylglutamic acid	T45.8X1	T45.8X2	T45.8X3	T45.8X4	T45.8X5	T45.8X6
Pteroyltriglutamate	T45.1X1	T45.1X2	T45.1X3	T45.1X4	T45.1X5	T45.1X6
PTFE — *see Polytetrafluoroethylene*						
Pulp						
devitalizing paste	T49.7X1	T49.7X2	T49.7X3	T49.7X4	T49.7X5	T49.7X6
dressing	T49.7X1	T49.7X2	T49.7X3	T49.7X4	T49.7X5	T49.7X6
Pulsatilla	T62.2X1	T62.2X2	T62.2X3	T62.2X4	—	—
Pumpkin seed extract	T37.4X1	T37.4X2	T37.4X3	T37.4X4	T37.4X5	T37.4X6
Purex (bleach)	T54.91	T54.92	T54.93	T54.94	—	—
Purgative NEC — *see also Cathartic*	T47.4X1	T47.4X2	T47.4X3	T47.4X4	T47.4X5	T47.4X6
Purine analogue (antineoplastic)	T45.1X1	T45.1X2	T45.1X3	T45.1X4	T45.1X5	T45.1X6
Purine diuretics	T50.2X1	T50.2X2	T50.2X3	T50.2X4	T50.2X5	T50.2X6
Purinethol	T45.1X1	T45.1X2	T45.1X3	T45.1X4	T45.1X5	T45.1X6
PVP	T45.8X1	T45.8X2	T45.8X3	T45.8X4	T45.8X5	T45.8X6
Pyrabital	T39.8X1	T39.8X2	T39.8X3	T39.8X4	T39.8X5	T39.8X6
Pyramidon	T39.2X1	T39.2X2	T39.2X3	T39.2X4	T39.2X5	T39.2X6
Pyrantel	T37.4X1	T37.4X2	T37.4X3	T37.4X4	T37.4X5	T37.4X6
Pyrathiazine	T45.0X1	T45.0X2	T45.0X3	T45.0X4	T45.0X5	T45.0X6
Pyrazinamide	T37.1X1	T37.1X2	T37.1X3	T37.1X4	T37.1X5	T37.1X6
Pyrazinoic acid (amide)	T37.1X1	T37.1X2	T37.1X3	T37.1X4	T37.1X5	T37.1X6
Pyrazole (derivatives)	T39.2X1	T39.2X2	T39.2X3	T39.2X4	T39.2X5	T39.2X6
Pyrazolone analgesic NEC	T39.2X1	T39.2X2	T39.2X3	T39.2X4	T39.2X5	T39.2X6
Pyrethrin, pyrethrum (nonmedicinal)	T60.2X1	T60.2X2	T60.2X3	T60.2X4	—	—
Pyrethrum extract	T49.0X1	T49.0X2	T49.0X3	T49.0X4	T49.0X5	T49.0X6
Pyribenzamine	T45.0X1	T45.0X2	T45.0X3	T45.0X4	T45.0X5	T45.0X6
Pyridine	T52.8X1	T52.8X2	T52.8X3	T52.8X4	—	—
aldoxime methiodide	T50.6X1	T50.6X2	T50.6X3	T50.6X4	T50.6X5	T50.6X6
aldoxime methyl chloride	T50.6X1	T50.6X2	T50.6X3	T50.6X4	T50.6X5	T50.6X6
vapor	T59.891	T59.892	T59.893	T59.894	—	—
Pyridium	T39.8X1	T39.8X2	T39.8X3	T39.8X4	T39.8X5	T39.8X6
Pyridostigmine bromide	T44.0X1	T44.0X2	T44.0X3	T44.0X4	T44.0X5	T44.0X6
Pyridoxal phosphate	T45.2X1	T45.2X2	T45.2X3	T45.2X4	T45.2X5	T45.2X6

	External Cause (T-Code)					
Substance	Poisoning, Accidental (Unintentional)	Poisoning, Intentional Self-Harm	Poisoning, Assault	Poisoning, Undetermined	Adverse Effect	Underdosing
Pyridoxine	T45.2X1	T45.2X2	T45.2X3	T45.2X4	T45.2X5	T45.2X6
Pyrilamine	T45.0X1	T45.0X2	T45.0X3	T45.0X4	T45.0X5	T45.0X6
Pyrimethamine	T37.2X1	T37.2X2	T37.2X3	T37.2X4	T37.2X5	T37.2X6
with sulfadoxine	T37.2X1	T37.2X2	T37.2X3	T37.2X4	T37.2X5	T37.2X6
Pyrimidine antagonist	T45.1X1	T45.1X2	T45.1X3	T45.1X4	T45.1X5	T45.1X6
Pyriminil	T60.4X1	T60.4X2	T60.4X3	T60.4X4	—	—
Pyrithione zinc	T49.4X1	T49.4X2	T49.4X3	T49.4X4	T49.4X5	T49.4X6
Pyrithyldione	T42.6X1	T42.6X2	T42.6X3	T42.6X4	T42.6X5	T42.6X6
Pyrogallic acid	T49.0X1	T49.0X2	T49.0X3	T49.0X4	T49.0X5	T49.0X6
Pyrogallol	T49.0X1	T49.0X2	T49.0X3	T49.0X4	T49.0X5	T49.0X6
Pyroxylin	T49.3X1	T49.3X2	T49.3X3	T49.3X4	T49.3X5	T49.3X6
Pyrrobutamine	T45.0X1	T45.0X2	T45.0X3	T45.0X4	T45.0X5	T45.0X6
Pyrrolizidine alkaloids	T62.8X1	T62.8X2	T62.8X3	T62.8X4	—	—
Pyrvinium chloride	T37.4X1	T37.4X2	T37.4X3	T37.4X4	T37.4X5	T37.4X6
PZI	T38.3X1	T38.3X2	T38.3X3	T38.3X4	T38.3X5	T38.3X6
Q						
Quaalude	T42.6X1	T42.6X2	T42.6X3	T42.6X4	T42.6X5	T42.6X6
Quarternary ammonium						
anti-infective	T49.0X1	T49.0X2	T49.0X3	T49.0X4	T49.0X5	T49.0X6
ganglion blocking	T44.2X1	T44.2X2	T44.2X3	T44.2X4	T44.2X5	T44.2X6
parasympatholytic	T44.3X1	T44.3X2	T44.3X3	T44.3X4	T44.3X5	T44.3X6
Quazepam	T42.4X1	T42.4X2	T42.4X3	T42.4X4	T42.4X5	T42.4X6
Quicklime	T54.3X1	T54.3X2	T54.3X3	T54.3X4	—	—
Quillaja extract	T48.4X1	T48.4X2	T48.4X3	T48.4X4	T48.4X5	T48.4X6
Quinacrine	T37.2X1	T37.2X2	T37.2X3	T37.2X4	T37.2X5	T37.2X6
Quinaglute	T46.2X1	T46.2X2	T46.2X3	T46.2X4	T46.2X5	T46.2X6
Quinalbarbital	T42.3X1	T42.3X2	T42.3X3	T42.3X4	T42.3X5	T42.3X6
Quinalbarbitone sodium	T42.3X1	T42.3X2	T42.3X3	T42.3X4	T42.3X5	T42.3X6
Quinalphos	T60.0X1	T60.0X2	T60.0X3	T60.0X4	—	—
Quinapril	T46.4X1	T46.4X2	T46.4X3	T46.4X4	T46.4X5	T46.4X6
Quinestradiol	T38.5X1	T38.5X2	T38.5X3	T38.5X4	T38.5X5	T38.5X6
Quinestradol	T38.5X1	T38.5X2	T38.5X3	T38.5X4	T38.5X5	T38.5X6
Quinestrol	T38.5X1	T38.5X2	T38.5X3	T38.5X4	T38.5X5	T38.5X6
Quinethazone	T50.2X1	T50.2X2	T50.2X3	T50.2X4	T50.2X5	T50.2X6
Quingestanol	T38.4X1	T38.4X2	T38.4X3	T38.4X4	T38.4X5	T38.4X6
Quinidine	T46.2X1	T46.2X2	T46.2X3	T46.2X4	T46.2X5	T46.2X6
Quinine	T37.2X1	T37.2X2	T37.2X3	T37.2X4	T37.2X5	T37.2X6
Quiniobine	T37.8X1	T37.8X2	T37.8X3	T37.8X4	T37.8X5	T37.8X6
Quinisocaine	T49.1X1	T49.1X2	T49.1X3	T49.1X4	T49.1X5	T49.1X6
Quinocide	T37.2X1	T37.2X2	T37.2X3	T37.2X4	T37.2X5	T37.2X6
Quinoline (derivatives) NEC	T37.8X1	T37.8X2	T37.8X3	T37.8X4	T37.8X5	T37.8X6
Quinupramine	T43.011	T43.012	T43.013	T43.014	T43.015	T43.016
Quotane	T41.3X1	T41.3X2	T41.3X3	T41.3X4	T41.3X5	T41.3X6
R						
Rabies						
immune globulin (human)	T50.Z11	T50.Z12	T50.Z13	T50.Z14	T50.Z15	T50.Z16
vaccine	T50.B91	T50.B92	T50.B93	T50.B94	T50.B95	T50.B96
Racemoramide	T40.2X1	T40.2X2	T40.2X3	T40.2X4	—	—
Racemorphan	T40.2X1	T40.2X2	T40.2X3	T40.2X4	T40.2X5	T40.2X6
Racepinefrin	T44.5X1	T44.5X2	T44.5X3	T44.5X4	T44.5X5	T44.5X6
Raclopride	T43.591	T43.592	T43.593	T43.594	T43.595	T43.596
Radiator alcohol	T51.1X1	T51.1X2	T51.1X3	T51.1X4	—	—
Radioactive drug NEC	T50.8X1	T50.8X2	T50.8X3	T50.8X4	T50.8X5	T50.8X6
Radio-opaque (drugs) (materials)	T50.8X1	T50.8X2	T50.8X3	T50.8X4	T50.8X5	T50.8X6
Ramifenazone	T39.2X1	T39.2X2	T39.2X3	T39.2X4	T39.2X5	T39.2X6
Ramipril	T46.4X1	T46.4X2	T46.4X3	T46.4X4	T46.4X5	T46.4X6
Ranitidine	T47.0X1	T47.0X2	T47.0X3	T47.0X4	T47.0X5	T47.0X6
Ranunculus	T62.2X1	T62.2X2	T62.2X3	T62.2X4	—	—
Rat poison NEC	T60.4X1	T60.4X2	T60.4X3	T60.4X4	—	—
Rattlesnake (venom)	T63.011	T63.012	T63.013	T63.014	—	—
Raubasine	T46.7X1	T46.7X2	T46.7X3	T46.7X4	T46.7X5	T46.7X6
Raudixin	T46.5X1	T46.5X2	T46.5X3	T46.5X4	T46.5X5	T46.5X6
Rautensin	T46.5X1	T46.5X2	T46.5X3	T46.5X4	T46.5X5	T46.5X6
Rautina	T46.5X1	T46.5X2	T46.5X3	T46.5X4	T46.5X5	T46.5X6
Rautotal	T46.5X1	T46.5X2	T46.5X3	T46.5X4	T46.5X5	T46.5X6
Rauwiloid	T46.5X1	T46.5X2	T46.5X3	T46.5X4	T46.5X5	T46.5X6
Rauwoldin	T46.5X1	T46.5X2	T46.5X3	T46.5X4	T46.5X5	T46.5X6
Rauwolfia (alkaloids)	T46.5X1	T46.5X2	T46.5X3	T46.5X4	T46.5X5	T46.5X6
Razoxane	T45.1X1	T45.1X2	T45.1X3	T45.1X4	T45.1X5	T45.1X6
Realgar	T57.0X1	T57.0X2	T57.0X3	T57.0X4	—	—
Recombinant (R) — *see specific protein*						
Red blood cells, packed	T45.8X1	T45.8X2	T45.8X3	T45.8X4	T45.8X5	T45.8X6
Red squill (scilliroside)	T60.4X1	T60.4X2	T60.4X3	T60.4X4	—	—
Reducing agent, industrial NEC	T65.891	T65.892	T65.893	T65.894	—	—
Refrigerant gas (chlorofluoro-carbon)	T53.5X1	T53.5X2	T53.5X3	T53.5X4	—	—
not chlorofluoro-carbon	T59.891	T59.892	T59.893	T59.894	—	—
Regroton	T50.2X1	T50.2X2	T50.2X3	T50.2X4	T50.2X5	T50.2X6
Rehydration salts (oral)	T50.3X1	T50.3X2	T50.3X3	T50.3X4	T50.3X5	T50.3X6
Rela	T42.8X1	T42.8X2	T42.8X3	T42.8X4	T42.8X5	T42.8X6

◀ New ◀ Revised ~~deleted~~ Deleted

	External Cause (T-Code)					
Substance	**Poisoning, Accidental (Unintentional)**	**Poisoning, Intentional Self-Harm**	**Poisoning, Assault**	**Poisoning, Undetermined**	**Adverse Effect**	**Underdosing**
Relaxant, muscle						
anesthetic	T48.1X1	T48.1X2	T48.1X3	T48.1X4	T48.1X5	T48.1X6
central nervous system	T42.8X1	T42.8X2	T42.8X3	T42.8X4	T42.8X5	T42.8X6
skeletal NEC	T48.1X1	T48.1X2	T48.1X3	T48.1X4	T48.1X5	T48.1X6
smooth NEC	T44.3X1	T44.3X2	T44.3X3	T44.3X4	T44.3X5	T44.3X6
Remoxipride	T43.591	T43.592	T43.593	T43.594	T43.595	T43.596
Renese	T5Ø.2X1	T5Ø.2X2	T5Ø.2X3	T5Ø.2X4	T5Ø.2X5	T5Ø.2X6
Renografin	T5Ø.8X1	T5Ø.8X2	T5Ø.8X3	T5Ø.8X4	T5Ø.8X5	T5Ø.8X6
Replacement solution	T5Ø.3X1	T5Ø.3X2	T5Ø.3X3	T5Ø.3X4	T5Ø.3X5	T5Ø.3X6
Reproterol	T48.6X1	T48.6X2	T48.6X3	T48.6X4	T48.6X5	T48.6X6
Rescinnamine	T46.5X1	T46.5X2	T46.5X3	T46.5X4	T46.5X5	T46.5X6
Reserpin(e)	T46.5X1	T46.5X2	T46.5X3	T46.5X4	T46.5X5	T46.5X6
Resorcin, resorcinol (nonmedicinal)	T65.891	T65.892	T65.893	T65.894	—	—
medicinal	T49.4X1	T49.4X2	T49.4X3	T49.4X4	T49.4X5	T49.4X6
Respaire	T48.4X1	T48.4X2	T48.4X3	T48.4X4	T48.4X5	T48.4X6
Respiratory drug NEC	T48.9Ø1	T48.9Ø2	T48.9Ø3	T48.9Ø4	T48.9Ø5	T48.9Ø6
antiasthmatic NEC	T48.6X1	T48.6X2	T48.6X3	T48.6X4	T48.6X5	T48.6X6
anti-common-cold NEC	T48.5X1	T48.5X2	T48.5X3	T48.5X4	T48.5X5	T48.5X6
expectorant NEC	T48.4X1	T48.4X2	T48.4X3	T48.4X4	T48.4X5	T48.4X6
stimulant	T48.9Ø1	T48.9Ø2	T48.9Ø3	T48.9Ø4	T48.9Ø5	T48.9Ø6
Retinoic acid	T49.ØX1	T49.ØX2	T49.ØX3	T49.ØX4	T49.ØX5	T49.ØX6
Retinol	T45.2X1	T45.2X2	T45.2X3	T45.2X4	T45.2X5	T45.2X6
Rh (D) immune globulin (human)	T5Ø.Z11	T5Ø.Z12	T5Ø.Z13	T5Ø.Z14	T5Ø.Z15	T5Ø.Z16
Rhodine	T39.Ø11	T39.Ø12	T39.Ø13	T39.Ø14	T39.Ø15	T39.Ø16
RhoGAM	T5Ø.Z11	T5Ø.Z12	T5Ø.Z13	T5Ø.Z14	T5Ø.Z15	T5Ø.Z16
Rhubarb						
dry extract	T47.2X1	T47.2X2	T47.2X3	T47.2X4	T47.2X5	T47.2X6
tincture, compound	T47.2X1	T47.2X2	T47.2X3	T47.2X4	T47.2X5	T47.2X6
Ribavirin	T37.5X1	T37.5X2	T37.5X3	T37.5X4	T37.5X5	T37.5X6
Riboflavin	T45.2X1	T45.2X2	T45.2X3	T45.2X4	T45.2X5	T45.2X6
Ribostamycin	T36.5X1	T36.5X2	T36.5X3	T36.5X4	T36.5X5	T36.5X6
Ricin	T62.2X1	T62.2X2	T62.2X3	T62.2X4	—	—
Ricinus communis	T62.2X1	T62.2X2	T62.2X3	T62.2X4	—	—
Rickettsial vaccine NEC	T5Ø.A91	T5Ø.A92	T5Ø.A93	T5Ø.A94	T5Ø.A95	T5Ø.A96
Rifabutin	T36.6X1	T36.6X2	T36.6X3	T36.6X4	T36.6X5	T36.6X6
Rifamide	T36.6X1	T36.6X2	T36.6X3	T36.6X4	T36.6X5	T36.6X6
Rifampicin	T36.6X1	T36.6X2	T36.6X3	T36.6X4	T36.6X5	T36.6X6
with isoniazid	T37.1X1	T37.1X2	T37.1X3	T37.1X4	T37.1X5	T37.1X6
Rifampin	T36.6X1	T36.6X2	T36.6X3	T36.6X4	T36.6X5	T36.6X6
Rifamycin	T36.6X1	T36.6X2	T36.6X3	T36.6X4	T36.6X5	T36.6X6
Rifaximin	T36.6X1	T36.6X2	T36.6X3	T36.6X4	T36.6X5	T36.6X6

	External Cause (T-Code)					
Substance	**Poisoning, Accidental (Unintentional)**	**Poisoning, Intentional Self-Harm**	**Poisoning, Assault**	**Poisoning, Undetermined**	**Adverse Effect**	**Underdosing**
Rimantadine	T37.5X1	T37.5X2	T37.5X3	T37.5X4	T37.5X5	T37.5X6
Rimazolium metilsulfate	T39.8X1	T39.8X2	T39.8X3	T39.8X4	T39.8X5	T39.8X6
Rimifon	T37.1X1	T37.1X2	T37.1X3	T37.1X4	T37.1X5	T37.1X6
Rimiterol	T48.6X1	T48.6X2	T48.6X3	T48.6X4	T48.6X5	T48.6X6
Ringer (lactate) solution	T5Ø.3X1	T5Ø.3X2	T5Ø.3X3	T5Ø.3X4	T5Ø.3X5	T5Ø.3X6
Ristocetin	T36.8X1	T36.8X2	T36.8X3	T36.8X4	T36.8X5	T36.8X6
Ritalin	T43.631	T43.632	T43.633	T43.634	T43.635	T43.636
Ritodrine	T44.5X1	T44.5X2	T44.5X3	T44.5X4	T44.5X5	T44.5X6
Roach killer — *see Insecticide*						
Rociverine	T44.3X1	T44.3X2	T44.3X3	T44.3X4	T44.3X5	T44.3X6
Rocky Mountain spotted fever vaccine	T5Ø.A91	T5Ø.A92	T5Ø.A93	T5Ø.A94	T5Ø.A95	T5Ø.A96
Rodenticide NEC	T6Ø.4X1	T6Ø.4X2	T6Ø.4X3	T6Ø.4X4	—	—
Rohypnol	T42.4X1	T42.4X2	T42.4X3	T42.4X4	T42.4X5	T42.4X6
Rokitamycin	T36.3X1	T36.3X2	T36.3X3	T36.3X4	T36.3X5	T36.3X6
Rolaids	T47.1X1	T47.1X2	T47.1X3	T47.1X4	T47.1X5	T47.1X6
Rolitetracycline	T36.4X1	T36.4X2	T36.4X3	T36.4X4	T36.4X5	T36.4X6
Romilar	T48.3X1	T48.3X2	T48.3X3	T48.3X4	T48.3X5	T48.3X6
Ronifibrate	T46.6X1	T46.6X2	T46.6X3	T46.6X4	T46.6X5	T46.6X6
Rosaprostol	T47.1X1	T47.1X2	T47.1X3	T47.1X4	T47.1X5	T47.1X6
Rose bengal sodium (131I)	T5Ø.8X1	T5Ø.8X2	T5Ø.8X3	T5Ø.8X4	T5Ø.8X5	T5Ø.8X6
Rose water ointment	T49.3X1	T49.3X2	T49.3X3	T49.3X4	T49.3X5	T49.3X6
Rosoxacin	T37.8X1	T37.8X2	T37.8X3	T37.8X4	T37.8X5	T37.8X6
Rotenone	T6Ø.2X1	T6Ø.2X2	T6Ø.2X3	T6Ø.2X4	—	—
Rotoxamine	T45.ØX1	T45.ØX2	T45.ØX3	T45.ØX4	T45.ØX5	T45.ØX6
Rough-on-rats	T6Ø.4X1	T6Ø.4X2	T6Ø.4X3	T6Ø.4X4	—	—
Roxatidine	T47.ØX1	T47.ØX2	T47.ØX3	T47.ØX4	T47.ØX5	T47.ØX6
Roxithromycin	T36.3X1	T36.3X2	T36.3X3	T36.3X4	T36.3X5	T36.3X6
Rt-PA	T45.611	T45.612	T45.613	T45.614	T45.615	T45.616
Rubbing alcohol	T51.2X1	T51.2X2	T51.2X3	T51.2X4	—	—
Rubefacient	T49.4X1	T49.4X2	T49.4X3	T49.4X4	T49.4X5	T49.4X6
Rubella vaccine	T5Ø.B91	T5Ø.B92	T5Ø.B93	T5Ø.B94	T5Ø.B95	T5Ø.B96
Rubelogen	T5Ø.B91	T5Ø.B92	T5Ø.B93	T5Ø.B94	T5Ø.B95	T5Ø.B96
Rubeovax	T5Ø.991	T5Ø.992	T5Ø.993	T5Ø.994	T5Ø.995	T5Ø.996
Rubidium chloride Rb82	T5Ø.8X1	T5Ø.8X2	T5Ø.8X3	T5Ø.8X4	T5Ø.8X5	T5Ø.8X6
Rubidomycin	T45.1X1	T45.1X2	T45.1X3	T45.1X4	T45.1X5	T45.1X6
Rue	T62.2X1	T62.2X2	T62.2X3	T62.2X4	—	—
Rufocromomycin	T45.1X1	T45.1X2	T45.1X3	T45.1X4	T45.1X5	T45.1X6
Russel's viper venin	T45.7X1	T45.7X2	T45.7X3	T45.7X4	T45.7X5	T45.7X6
Ruta (graveolens)	T62.2X1	T62.2X2	T62.2X3	T62.2X4	—	—
Rutinum	T46.991	T46.992	T46.993	T46.994	T46.995	T46.996
Rutoside	T46.991	T46.992	T46.993	T46.994	T46.995	T46.996

Substance	External Cause (T-Code)					
	Poisoning, Accidental (Unintentional)	Poisoning, Intentional Self-Harm	Poisoning, Assault	Poisoning, Undetermined	Adverse Effect	Underdosing
S						
Sabadilla (plant)	T62.2X1	T62.2X2	T62.2X3	T62.2X4	—	—
pesticide	T60.2X1	T60.2X2	T60.2X3	T60.2X4	—	—
Saccharated iron oxide	T45.8X1	T45.8X2	T45.8X3	T45.8X4	T45.8X5	T45.8X6
Saccharin	T50.901	T50.902	T50.903	T50.904	T50.905	T50.906
Saccharomyces boulardii	T47.6X1	T47.6X2	T47.6X3	T47.6X4	T47.6X5	T47.6X6
Safflower oil	T46.6X1	T46.6X2	T46.6X3	T46.6X4	T46.6X5	T46.6X6
Safrazine	T43.1X1	T43.1X2	T43.1X3	T43.1X4	T43.1X5	T43.1X6
Salazosulfapyridine	T37.0X1	T37.0X2	T37.0X3	T37.0X4	T37.0X5	T37.0X6
Salbutamol	T48.6X1	T48.6X2	T48.6X3	T48.6X4	T48.6X5	T48.6X6
Salicylamide	T39.091	T39.092	T39.093	T39.094	T39.095	T39.096
Salicylate NEC	T39.091	T39.092	T39.093	T39.094	T39.095	T39.096
methyl	T49.3X1	T49.3X2	T49.3X3	T49.3X4	T49.3X5	T49.3X6
theobromine calcium	T50.2X1	T50.2X2	T50.2X3	T50.2X4	T50.2X5	T50.2X6
Salicylazosulfapyridine	T37.0X1	T37.0X2	T37.0X3	T37.0X4	T37.0X5	T37.0X6
Salicylhydroxamic acid	T49.0X1	T49.0X2	T49.0X3	T49.0X4	T49.0X5	T49.0X6
Salicylic acid	T49.4X1	T49.4X2	T49.4X3	T49.4X4	T49.4X5	T49.4X6
with benzoic acid	T49.4X1	T49.4X2	T49.4X3	T49.4X4	T49.4X5	T49.4X6
congeners	T39.091	T39.092	T39.093	T39.094	T39.095	T39.096
derivative	T39.091	T39.092	T39.093	T39.094	T39.095	T39.096
salts	T39.091	T39.092	T39.093	T39.094	T39.095	T39.096
Salinazid	T37.1X1	T37.1X2	T37.1X3	T37.1X4	T37.1X5	T37.1X6
Salmeterol	T48.6X1	T48.6X2	T48.6X3	T48.6X4	T48.6X5	T48.6X6
Salol	T49.3X1	T49.3X2	T49.3X3	T49.3X4	T49.3X5	T49.3X6
Salsalate	T39.091	T39.092	T39.093	T39.094	T39.095	T39.096
Salt substitute	T50.901	T50.902	T50.903	T50.904	T50.905	T50.906
Salt-replacing drug	T50.901	T50.902	T50.903	T50.904	T50.905	T50.906
Salt-retaining mineralocorticoid	T50.0X1	T50.0X2	T50.0X3	T50.0X4	T50.0X5	T50.0X6
Saluretic NEC	T50.2X1	T50.2X2	T50.2X3	T50.2X4	T50.2X5	T50.2X6
Saluron	T50.2X1	T50.2X2	T50.2X3	T50.2X4	T50.2X5	T50.2X6
Salvarsan 606 (neosilver) (silver)	T37.8X1	T37.8X2	T37.8X3	T37.8X4	T37.8X5	T37.8X6
Sambucus canadensis	T62.2X1	T62.2X2	T62.2X3	T62.2X4	—	—
berry	T62.1X1	T62.1X2	T62.1X3	T62.1X4	—	—
Sandril	T46.5X1	T46.5X2	T46.5X3	T46.5X4	T46.5X5	T46.5X6
Sanguinaria canadensis	T62.2X1	T62.2X2	T62.2X3	T62.2X4	—	—
Saniflush (cleaner)	T54.2X1	T54.2X2	T54.2X3	T54.2X4	—	—
Santonin	T37.4X1	T37.4X2	T37.4X3	T37.4X4	T37.4X5	T37.4X6
Santyl	T49.8X1	T49.8X2	T49.8X3	T49.8X4	T49.8X5	T49.8X6
Saralasin	T46.5X1	T46.5X2	T46.5X3	T46.5X4	T46.5X5	T46.5X6
Sarcolysin	T45.1X1	T45.1X2	T45.1X3	T45.1X4	T45.1X5	T45.1X6
Sarkomycin	T45.1X1	T45.1X2	T45.1X3	T45.1X4	T45.1X5	T45.1X6
Saroten	T43.011	T43.012	T43.013	T43.014	T43.015	T43.016
Saturnine — *see Lead*						
Savin (oil)	T49.4X1	T49.4X2	T49.4X3	T49.4X4	T49.4X5	T49.4X6
Scammony	T47.2X1	T47.2X2	T47.2X3	T47.2X4	T47.2X5	T47.2X6
Scarlet red	T49.8X1	T49.8X2	T49.8X3	T49.8X4	T49.8X5	T49.8X6
Scheele's green	T57.0X1	T57.0X2	T57.0X3	T57.0X4	—	—
insecticide	T57.0X1	T57.0X2	T57.0X3	T57.0X4	—	—
Schizontozide (blood) (tissue)	T37.2X1	T37.2X2	T37.2X3	T37.2X4	T37.2X5	T37.2X6
Schradan	T60.0X1	T60.0X2	T60.0X3	T60.0X4	—	—
Schweinfurth green	T57.0X1	T57.0X2	T57.0X3	T57.0X4	—	—
insecticide	T57.0X1	T57.0X2	T57.0X3	T57.0X4	—	—
Scilla, rat poison	T60.4X1	T60.4X2	T60.4X3	T60.4X4	—	—
Scillaren	T60.4X1	T60.4X2	T60.4X3	T60.4X4	—	—
Sclerosing agent	T46.8X1	T46.8X2	T46.8X3	T46.8X4	T46.8X5	T46.8X6
Scombrotoxin	T61.11	T61.12	T61.13	T61.14	—	—
Scopolamine	T44.3X1	T44.3X2	T44.3X3	T44.3X4	T44.3X5	T44.3X6
Scopolia extract	T44.3X1	T44.3X2	T44.3X3	T44.3X4	T44.3X5	T44.3X6
Scouring powder	T65.891	T65.892	T65.893	T65.894	—	—
Sea						
anemone (sting)	T63.631	T63.632	T63.633	T63.634	—	—
cucumber (sting)	T63.691	T63.692	T63.693	T63.694	—	—
snake (bite) (venom)	T63.091	T63.092	T63.093	T63.094	—	—
urchin spine (puncture)	T63.691	T63.692	T63.693	T63.694	—	—
Seafood	T61.91	T61.92	T61.93	T61.94	—	—
specified NEC	T61.8X1	T61.8X2	T61.8X3	T61.8X4	—	—
Secbutabarbital	T42.3X1	T42.3X2	T42.3X3	T42.3X4	T42.3X5	T42.3X6
Secbutabarbitone	T42.3X1	T42.3X2	T42.3X3	T42.3X4	T42.3X5	T42.3X6
Secnidazole	T37.3X1	T37.3X2	T37.3X3	T37.3X4	T37.3X5	T37.3X6
Secobarbital	T42.3X1	T42.3X2	T42.3X3	T42.3X4	T42.3X5	T42.3X6
Seconal	T42.3X1	T42.3X2	T42.3X3	T42.3X4	T42.3X5	T42.3X6
Secretin	T50.8X1	T50.8X2	T50.8X3	T50.8X4	T50.8X5	T50.8X6
Sedative NEC	T42.71	T42.72	T42.73	T42.74	T42.75	T42.76
mixed NEC	T42.6X1	T42.6X2	T42.6X3	T42.6X4	T42.6X5	T42.6X6
Sedormid	T42.6X1	T42.6X2	T42.6X3	T42.6X4	T42.6X5	T42.6X6
Seed disinfectant or dressing	T60.8X1	T60.8X2	T60.8X3	T60.8X4	—	—
Seeds (poisonous)	T62.2X1	T62.2X2	T62.2X3	T62.2X4	—	—
Selegiline	T42.8X1	T42.8X2	T42.8X3	T42.8X4	T42.8X5	T42.8X6
Selenium NEC	T56.891	T56.892	T56.893	T56.894	—	—
disulfide or sulfide	T49.4X1	T49.4X2	T49.4X3	T49.4X4	T49.4X5	T49.4X6
fumes	T59.891	T59.892	T59.893	T59.894	—	—
sulfide	T49.4X1	T49.4X2	T49.4X3	T49.4X4	T49.4X5	T49.4X6
Selenomethionine (75Se)	T50.8X1	T50.8X2	T50.8X3	T50.8X4	T50.8X5	T50.8X6
Selsun	T49.4X1	T49.4X2	T49.4X3	T49.4X4	T49.4X5	T49.4X6

◀ New ◀ Revised ~~deleted~~ Deleted

Substance	External Cause (T-Code)					
	Poisoning, Accidental (Unintentional)	Poisoning, Intentional Self-Harm	Poisoning, Assault	Poisoning, Undetermined	Adverse Effect	Underdosing
Semustine	T45.1X1	T45.1X2	T45.1X3	T45.1X4	T45.1X5	T45.1X6
Senega syrup	T48.4X1	T48.4X2	T48.4X3	T48.4X4	T48.4X5	T48.4X6
Senna	T47.2X1	T47.2X2	T47.2X3	T47.2X4	T47.2X5	T47.2X6
Sennoside A+B	T47.2X1	T47.2X2	T47.2X3	T47.2X4	T47.2X5	T47.2X6
Septisol	T49.2X1	T49.2X2	T49.2X3	T49.2X4	T49.2X5	T49.2X6
Seractide	T38.811	T38.812	T38.813	T38.814	T38.815	T38.816
Serax	T42.4X1	T42.4X2	T42.4X3	T42.4X4	T42.4X5	T42.4X6
Serenesil	T42.6X1	T42.6X2	T42.6X3	T42.6X4	T42.6X5	T42.6X6
Serenium (hydrochloride)	T37.91	T37.92	T37.93	T37.94	T37.95	T37.96
Serepax — *see Oxazepam*						
Sermorelin	T38.891	T38.892	T38.893	T38.894	T38.895	T38.896
Sernyl	T41.1X1	T41.1X2	T41.1X3	T41.1X4	T41.1X5	T41.1X6
Serotonin	T5Ø.991	T5Ø.992	T5Ø.993	T5Ø.994	T5Ø.995	T5Ø.996
Serpasil	T46.5X1	T46.5X2	T46.5X3	T46.5X4	T46.5X5	T46.5X6
Serrapeptase	T45.3X1	T45.3X2	T45.3X3	T45.3X4	T45.3X5	T45.3X6
Serum						
antibotulinus	T5Ø.Z11	T5Ø.Z12	T5Ø.Z13	T5Ø.Z14	T5Ø.Z15	T5Ø.Z16
anticytotoxic	T5Ø.Z11	T5Ø.Z12	T5Ø.Z13	T5Ø.Z14	T5Ø.Z15	T5Ø.Z16
antidiphtheria	T5Ø.Z11	T5Ø.Z12	T5Ø.Z13	T5Ø.Z14	T5Ø.Z15	T5Ø.Z16
antimeningococcus	T5Ø.Z11	T5Ø.Z12	T5Ø.Z13	T5Ø.Z14	T5Ø.Z15	T5Ø.Z16
anti-Rh	T5Ø.Z11	T5Ø.Z12	T5Ø.Z13	T5Ø.Z14	T5Ø.Z15	T5Ø.Z16
anti-snake-bite	T5Ø.Z11	T5Ø.Z12	T5Ø.Z13	T5Ø.Z14	T5Ø.Z15	T5Ø.Z16
antitetanic	T5Ø.Z11	T5Ø.Z12	T5Ø.Z13	T5Ø.Z14	T5Ø.Z15	T5Ø.Z16
antitoxic	T5Ø.Z11	T5Ø.Z12	T5Ø.Z13	T5Ø.Z14	T5Ø.Z15	T5Ø.Z16
complement (inhibitor)	T45.8X1	T45.8X2	T45.8X3	T45.8X4	T45.8X5	T45.8X6
convalescent	T5Ø.Z11	T5Ø.Z12	T5Ø.Z13	T5Ø.Z14	T5Ø.Z15	T5Ø.Z16
hemolytic complement	T45.8X1	T45.8X2	T45.8X3	T45.8X4	T45.8X5	T45.8X6
immune (human)	T5Ø.Z11	T5Ø.Z12	T5Ø.Z13	T5Ø.Z14	T5Ø.Z15	T5Ø.Z16
protective NEC	T5Ø.Z11	T5Ø.Z12	T5Ø.Z13	T5Ø.Z14	T5Ø.Z15	T5Ø.Z16
Setastine	T45.ØX1	T45.ØX2	T45.ØX3	T45.ØX4	T45.ØX5	T45.ØX6
Setoperone	T43.591	T43.592	T43.593	T43.594	T43.595	T43.596
Sewer gas	T59.91	T59.92	T59.93	T59.94	—	—
Shampoo	T55.ØX1	T55.ØX2	T55.ØX3	T55.ØX4	—	—
Shellfish, noxious, nonbacterial	T61.781	T61.782	T61.783	T61.784	—	—
Sildenafil	T46.7X1	T46.7X2	T46.7X3	T46.7X4	T46.7X5	T46.7X6
Silibinin	T5Ø.991	T5Ø.992	T5Ø.993	T5Ø.994	T5Ø.995	T5Ø.996
Silicone NEC	T65.891	T65.892	T65.893	T65.894	—	—
medicinal	T49.3X1	T49.3X2	T49.3X3	T49.3X4	T49.3X5	T49.3X6
Silvadene	T49.ØX1	T49.ØX2	T49.ØX3	T49.ØX4	T49.ØX5	T49.ØX6
Silver	T49.ØX1	T49.ØX2	T49.ØX3	T49.ØX4	T49.ØX5	T49.ØX6
anti-infectives	T49.ØX1	T49.ØX2	T49.ØX3	T49.ØX4	T49.ØX5	T49.ØX6
arsphenamine	T37.8X1	T37.8X2	T37.8X3	T37.8X4	T37.8X5	T37.8X6

Substance	External Cause (T-Code)					
	Poisoning, Accidental (Unintentional)	Poisoning, Intentional Self-Harm	Poisoning, Assault	Poisoning, Undetermined	Adverse Effect	Underdosing
Silver *(Continued)*						
colloidal	T49.ØX1	T49.ØX2	T49.ØX3	T49.ØX4	T49.ØX5	T49.ØX6
nitrate	T49.ØX1	T49.ØX2	T49.ØX3	T49.ØX4	T49.ØX5	T49.ØX6
ophthalmic preparation	T49.5X1	T49.5X2	T49.5X3	T49.5X4	T49.5X5	T49.5X6
toughened (keratolytic)	T49.4X1	T49.4X2	T49.4X3	T49.4X4	T49.4X5	T49.4X6
nonmedicinal (dust)	T56.891	T56.892	T56.893	T56.894	—	—
protein	T49.5X1	T49.5X2	T49.5X3	T49.5X4	T49.5X5	T49.5X6
salvarsan	T37.8X1	T37.8X2	T37.8X3	T37.8X4	T37.8X5	T37.8X6
sulfadiazine	T49.4X1	T49.4X2	T49.4X3	T49.4X4	T49.4X5	T49.4X6
Silymarin	T5Ø.991	T5Ø.992	T5Ø.993	T5Ø.994	T5Ø.995	T5Ø.996
Simaldrate	T47.1X1	T47.1X2	T47.1X3	T47.1X4	T47.1X5	T47.1X6
Simazine	T6Ø.3X1	T6Ø.3X2	T6Ø.3X3	T6Ø.3X4	—	—
Simethicone	T47.1X1	T47.1X2	T47.1X3	T47.1X4	T47.1X5	T47.1X6
Simfibrate	T46.6X1	T46.6X2	T46.6X3	T46.6X4	T46.6X5	T46.6X6
Simvastatin	T46.6X1	T46.6X2	T46.6X3	T46.6X4	T46.6X5	T46.6X6
Sincalide	T5Ø.8X1	T5Ø.8X2	T5Ø.8X3	T5Ø.8X4	T5Ø.8X5	T5Ø.8X6
Sinequan	T43.Ø11	T43.Ø12	T43.Ø13	T43.Ø14	T43.Ø15	T43.Ø16
Singoserp	T46.5X1	T46.5X2	T46.5X3	T46.5X4	T46.5X5	T46.5X6
Sintrom	T45.511	T45.512	T45.513	T45.514	T45.515	T45.516
Sisomicin	T36.5X1	T36.5X2	T36.5X3	T36.5X4	T36.5X5	T36.5X6
Sitosterols	T46.6X1	T46.6X2	T46.6X3	T46.6X4	T46.6X5	T46.6X6
Skeletal muscle relaxants	T48.1X1	T48.1X2	T48.1X3	T48.1X4	T48.1X5	T48.1X6
Skin						
agents (external)	T49.91	T49.92	T49.93	T49.94	T49.95	T49.96
specified NEC	T49.8X1	T49.8X2	T49.8X3	T49.8X4	T49.8X5	T49.8X6
test antigen	T5Ø.8X1	T5Ø.8X2	T5Ø.8X3	T5Ø.8X4	T5Ø.8X5	T5Ø.8X6
Sleep-eze	T45.ØX1	T45.ØX2	T45.ØX3	T45.ØX4	T45.ØX5	T45.ØX6
Sleeping draught, pill	T42.71	T42.72	T42.73	T42.74	T42.75	T42.76
Smallpox vaccine	T5Ø.B11	T5Ø.B12	T5Ø.B13	T5Ø.B14	T5Ø.B15	T5Ø.B16
Smelter fumes NEC	T56.91	T56.92	T56.93	T56.94	—	—
Smog	T59.1X1	T59.1X2	T59.1X3	T59.1X4	—	—
Smoke NEC	T59.811	T59.812	T59.813	T59.814	—	—
Smooth muscle relaxant	T44.3X1	T44.3X2	T44.3X3	T44.3X4	T44.3X5	T44.3X6
Snail killer NEC	T6Ø.8X1	T6Ø.8X2	T6Ø.8X3	T6Ø.8X4	—	—
Snake venom or bite	T63.ØØ1	T63.ØØ2	T63.ØØ3	T63.ØØ4	—	—
hemocoagulase	T45.7X1	T45.7X2	T45.7X3	T45.7X4	T45.7X5	T45.7X6
Snuff	T65.211	T65.212	T65.213	T65.214	—	—
Soap (powder) (product)	T55.ØX1	T55.ØX2	T55.ØX3	T55.ØX4	—	—
enema	T47.4X1	T47.4X2	T47.4X3	T47.4X4	T47.4X5	T47.4X6
medicinal, soft	T49.2X1	T49.2X2	T49.2X3	T49.2X4	T49.2X5	T49.2X6
superfatted	T49.2X1	T49.2X2	T49.2X3	T49.2X4	T49.2X5	T49.2X6
Sobrerol	T48.4X1	T48.4X2	T48.4X3	T48.4X4	T48.4X5	T48.4X6

TABLE OF DRUGS AND CHEMICALS

New Revised ~~deleted~~ Deleted

Substance	External Cause (T-Code)					
	Poisoning, Accidental (Unintentional)	Poisoning, Intentional Self-Harm	Poisoning, Assault	Poisoning, Undetermined	Adverse Effect	Underdosing
Soda (caustic)	T54.3X1	T54.3X2	T54.3X3	T54.3X4	—	—
bicarb	T47.1X1	T47.1X2	T47.1X3	T47.1X4	T47.1X5	T47.1X6
chlorinated — *see Sodium, hypochlorite*						
Sodium						
acetosulfone	T37.1X1	T37.1X2	T37.1X3	T37.1X4	T37.1X5	T37.1X6
acetrizoate	T50.8X1	T50.8X2	T50.8X3	T50.8X4	T50.8X5	T50.8X6
acid phosphate	T50.3X1	T50.3X2	T50.3X3	T50.3X4	T50.3X5	T50.3X6
alginate	T47.8X1	T47.8X2	T47.8X3	T47.8X4	T47.8X5	T47.8X6
amidotrizoate	T50.8X1	T50.8X2	T50.8X3	T50.8X4	T50.8X5	T50.8X6
aminopterin	T45.1X1	T45.1X2	T45.1X3	T45.1X4	T45.1X5	T45.1X6
amylosulfate	T47.8X1	T47.8X2	T47.8X3	T47.8X4	T47.8X5	T47.8X6
amytal	T42.3X1	T42.3X2	T42.3X3	T42.3X4	T42.3X5	T42.3X6
antimony gluconate	T37.3X1	T37.3X2	T37.3X3	T37.3X4	T37.3X5	T37.3X6
arsenate	T57.0X1	T57.0X2	T57.0X3	T57.0X4	—	—
aurothiomalate	T39.4X1	T39.4X2	T39.4X3	T39.4X4	T39.4X5	T39.4X6
aurothiosulfate	T39.4X1	T39.4X2	T39.4X3	T39.4X4	T39.4X5	T39.4X6
barbiturate	T42.3X1	T42.3X2	T42.3X3	T42.3X4	T42.3X5	T42.3X6
basic phosphate	T47.4X1	T47.4X2	T47.4X3	T47.4X4	T47.4X5	T47.4X6
bicarbonate	T47.1X1	T47.1X2	T47.1X3	T47.1X4	T47.1X5	T47.1X6
bichromate	T57.8X1	T57.8X2	T57.8X3	T57.8X4	—	—
biphosphate	T50.3X1	T50.3X2	T50.3X3	T50.3X4	T50.3X5	T50.3X6
bisulfate	T65.891	T65.892	T65.893	T65.894	—	—
borate						
cleanser	T57.8X1	T57.8X2	T57.8X3	T57.8X4	—	—
eye	T49.5X1	T49.5X2	T49.5X3	T49.5X4	T49.5X5	T49.5X6
therapeutic	T49.8X1	T49.8X2	T49.8X3	T49.8X4	T49.8X5	T49.8X6
bromide	T42.6X1	T42.6X2	T42.6X3	T42.6X4	T42.6X5	T42.6X6
cacodylate (nonmedicinal) NEC	T50.8X1	T50.8X2	T50.8X3	T50.8X4	T50.8X5	T50.8X6
anti-infective	T37.8X1	T37.8X2	T37.8X3	T37.8X4	T37.8X5	T37.8X6
herbicide	T60.3X1	T60.3X2	T60.3X3	T60.3X4	—	—
calcium edetate	T45.8X1	T45.8X2	T45.8X3	T45.8X4	T45.8X5	T45.8X6
carbonate NEC	T54.3X1	T54.3X2	T54.3X3	T54.3X4	—	—
chlorate NEC	T65.891	T65.892	T65.893	T65.894	—	—
herbicide	T54.91	T54.92	T54.93	T54.94	—	—
chloride	T50.3X1	T50.3X2	T50.3X3	T50.3X4	T50.3X5	T50.3X6
with glucose	T50.3X1	T50.3X2	T50.3X3	T50.3X4	T50.3X5	T50.3X6
chromate	T65.891	T65.892	T65.893	T65.894	—	—
citrate	T50.991	T50.992	T50.993	T50.994	T50.995	T50.996
cromoglicate	T48.6X1	T48.6X2	T48.6X3	T48.6X4	T48.6X5	T48.6X6
cyanide	T65.0X1	T65.0X2	T65.0X3	T65.0X4	—	—
cyclamate	T50.3X1	T50.3X2	T50.3X3	T50.3X4	T50.3X5	T50.3X6

Substance	External Cause (T-Code)					
	Poisoning, Accidental (Unintentional)	Poisoning, Intentional Self-Harm	Poisoning, Assault	Poisoning, Undetermined	Adverse Effect	Underdosing
Sodium *(Continued)*						
dehydrocholate	T45.8X1	T45.8X2	T45.8X3	T45.8X4	T45.8X5	T45.8X6
diatrizoate	T50.8X1	T50.8X2	T50.8X3	T50.8X4	T50.8X5	T50.8X6
dibunate	T48.4X1	T48.4X2	T48.4X3	T48.4X4	T48.4X5	T48.4X6
dioctyl sulfosuccinate	T47.4X1	T47.4X2	T47.4X3	T47.4X4	T47.4X5	T47.4X6
dipantoyl ferrate	T45.8X1	T45.8X2	T45.8X3	T45.8X4	T45.8X5	T45.8X6
edetate	T45.8X1	T45.8X2	T45.8X3	T45.8X4	T45.8X5	T45.8X6
ethacrynate	T50.1X1	T50.1X2	T50.1X3	T50.1X4	T50.1X5	T50.1X6
feredetate	T45.8X1	T45.8X2	T45.8X3	T45.8X4	T45.8X5	T45.8X6
Fluoride — *see Fluoride*						
fluoroacetate (dust) (pesticide)	T60.4X1	T60.4X2	T60.4X3	T60.4X4	—	—
free salt	T50.3X1	T50.3X2	T50.3X3	T50.3X4	T50.3X5	T50.3X6
fusidate	T36.8X1	T36.8X2	T36.8X3	T36.8X4	T36.8X5	T36.8X6
glucaldrate	T47.1X1	T47.1X2	T47.1X3	T47.1X4	T47.1X5	T47.1X6
glucosulfone	T37.1X1	T37.1X2	T37.1X3	T37.1X4	T37.1X5	T37.1X6
glutamate	T45.8X1	T45.8X2	T45.8X3	T45.8X4	T45.8X5	T45.8X6
hydrogen carbonate	T50.3X1	T50.3X2	T50.3X3	T50.3X4	T50.3X5	T50.3X6
hydroxide	T54.3X1	T54.3X2	T54.3X3	T54.3X4	—	—
hypochlorite (bleach) NEC	T54.3X1	T54.3X2	T54.3X3	T54.3X4	—	—
disinfectant	T54.3X1	T54.3X2	T54.3X3	T54.3X4	—	—
medicinal (anti-infective) (external)	T49.0X1	T49.0X2	T49.0X3	T49.0X4	T49.0X5	T49.0X6
vapor	T54.3X1	T54.3X2	T54.3X3	T54.3X4	—	—
hyposulfite	T49.0X1	T49.0X2	T49.0X3	T49.0X4	T49.0X5	T49.0X6
indigotin disulfonate	T50.8X1	T50.8X2	T50.8X3	T50.8X4	T50.8X5	T50.8X6
iodide	T50.991	T50.992	T50.993	T50.994	T50.995	T50.996
I-131	T50.8X1	T50.8X2	T50.8X3	T50.8X4	T50.8X5	T50.8X6
therapeutic	T38.2X1	T38.2X2	T38.2X3	T38.2X4	T38.2X5	T38.2X6
iodohippurate (131I)	T50.8X1	T50.8X2	T50.8X3	T50.8X4	T50.8X5	T50.8X6
iopodate	T50.8X1	T50.8X2	T50.8X3	T50.8X4	T50.8X5	T50.8X6
iothalamate	T50.8X1	T50.8X2	T50.8X3	T50.8X4	T50.8X5	T50.8X6
iron edetate	T45.4X1	T45.4X2	T45.4X3	T45.4X4	T45.4X5	T45.4X6
lactate (compound solution)	T45.8X1	T45.8X2	T45.8X3	T45.8X4	T45.8X5	T45.8X6
lauryl (sulfate)	T49.2X1	T49.2X2	T49.2X3	T49.2X4	T49.2X5	T49.2X6
(L)-triiodothyronine	T38.1X1	T38.1X2	T38.1X3	T38.1X4	T38.1X5	T38.1X6
magnesium citrate	T50.991	T50.992	T50.993	T50.994	T50.995	T50.996
mersalate	T50.2X1	T50.2X2	T50.2X3	T50.2X4	T50.2X5	T50.2X6
metasilicate	T65.891	T65.892	T65.893	T65.894	—	—
metrizoate	T50.8X1	T50.8X2	T50.8X3	T50.8X4	T50.8X5	T50.8X6
monofluoroacetate (pesticide)	T60.1X1	T60.1X2	T60.1X3	T60.1X4	—	—
morrhuate	T46.8X1	T46.8X2	T46.8X3	T46.8X4	T46.8X5	T46.8X6
nafcillin	T36.0X1	T36.0X2	T36.0X3	T36.0X4	T36.0X5	T36.0X6

Substance	Poisoning, Accidental (Unintentional)	Poisoning, Intentional Self-Harm	Poisoning, Assault	Poisoning, Undetermined	Adverse Effect	Underdosing
	External Cause (T-Code)					
Sodium *(Continued)*						
nitrate (oxidizing agent)	T65.891	T65.892	T65.893	T65.894	—	—
nitrite	T50.6X1	T50.6X2	T50.6X3	T50.6X4	T50.6X5	T50.6X6
nitroferricyanide	T46.5X1	T46.5X2	T46.5X3	T46.5X4	T46.5X5	T46.5X6
nitroprusside	T46.5X1	T46.5X2	T46.5X3	T46.5X4	T46.5X5	T46.5X6
oxalate	T65.891	T65.892	T65.893	T65.894	—	—
oxide/peroxide	T65.891	T65.892	T65.893	T65.894	—	—
oxybate	T41.291	T41.292	T41.293	T41.294	T41.295	T41.296
para-aminohippurate	T50.8X1	T50.8X2	T50.8X3	T50.8X4	T50.8X5	T50.8X6
perborate (nonmedicinal) NEC	T65.891	T65.892	T65.893	T65.894	—	—
medicinal	T49.0X1	T49.0X2	T49.0X3	T49.0X4	T49.0X5	T49.0X6
soap	T55.0X1	T55.0X2	T55.0X3	T55.0X4	—	—
percarbonate — *see Sodium, perborate*						
pertechnetate Tc99m	T50.8X1	T50.8X2	T50.8X3	T50.8X4	T50.8X5	T50.8X6
phosphate						
cellulose	T45.8X1	T45.8X2	T45.8X3	T45.8X4	T45.8X5	T45.8X6
dibasic	T47.2X1	T47.2X2	T47.2X3	T47.2X4	T47.2X5	T47.2X6
monobasic	T47.2X1	T47.2X2	T47.2X3	T47.2X4	T47.2X5	T47.2X6
phytate	T50.6X1	T50.6X2	T50.6X3	T50.6X4	T50.6X5	T50.6X6
picosulfate	T47.2X1	T47.2X2	T47.2X3	T47.2X4	T47.2X5	T47.2X6
polyhydroxyaluminium monocarbonate	T47.1X1	T47.1X2	T47.1X3	T47.1X4	T47.1X5	T47.1X6
polystyrene sulfonate	T50.3X1	T50.3X2	T50.3X3	T50.3X4	T50.3X5	T50.3X6
propionate	T49.0X1	T49.0X2	T49.0X3	T49.0X4	T49.0X5	T49.0X6
propyl hydroxybenzoate	T50.991	T50.992	T50.993	T50.994	T50.995	T50.996
psylliate	T46.8X1	T46.8X2	T46.8X3	T46.8X4	T46.8X5	T46.8X6
removing resins	T50.3X1	T50.3X2	T50.3X3	T50.3X4	T50.3X5	T50.3X6
salicylate	T39.091	T39.092	T39.093	T39.094	T39.095	T39.096
salt NEC	T50.3X1	T50.3X2	T50.3X3	T50.3X4	T50.3X5	T50.3X6
selenate	T60.2X1	T60.2X2	T60.2X3	T60.2X4	—	—
stibogluconate	T37.3X1	T37.3X2	T37.3X3	T37.3X4	T37.3X5	T37.3X6
sulfate	T47.4X1	T47.4X2	T47.4X3	T47.4X4	T47.4X5	T47.4X6
sulfoxone	T37.1X1	T37.1X2	T37.1X3	T37.1X4	T37.1X5	T37.1X6
tetradecyl sulfate	T46.8X1	T46.8X2	T46.8X3	T46.8X4	T46.8X5	T46.8X6
thiopental	T41.1X1	T41.1X2	T41.1X3	T41.1X4	T41.1X5	T41.1X6
thiosalicylate	T39.091	T39.092	T39.093	T39.094	T39.095	T39.096
thiosulfate	T50.6X1	T50.6X2	T50.6X3	T50.6X4	T50.6X5	T50.6X6
tolbutamide	T38.3X1	T38.3X2	T38.3X3	T38.3X4	T38.3X5	T38.3X6
l-triiodothyronine	T38.1X1	T38.1X2	T38.1X3	T38.1X4	T38.1X5	T38.1X6
tyropanoate	T50.8X1	T50.8X2	T50.8X3	T50.8X4	T50.8X5	T50.8X6
valproate	T42.6X1	T42.6X2	T42.6X3	T42.6X4	T42.6X5	T42.6X6
versenate	T50.6X1	T50.6X2	T50.6X3	T50.6X4	T50.6X5	T50.6X6

Substance	Poisoning, Accidental (Unintentional)	Poisoning, Intentional Self-Harm	Poisoning, Assault	Poisoning, Undetermined	Adverse Effect	Underdosing
	External Cause (T-Code)					
Sodium-free salt	T50.901	T50.902	T50.903	T50.904	T50.905	T50.906
Sodium-removing resin	T50.3X1	T50.3X2	T50.3X3	T50.3X4	T50.3X5	T50.3X6
Soft soap	T55.0X1	T55.0X2	T55.0X3	T55.0X4	—	—
Solanine	T62.2X1	T62.2X2	T62.2X3	T62.2X4	—	—
berries	T62.1X1	T62.1X2	T62.1X3	T62.1X4	—	—
Solanum dulcamara	T62.2X1	T62.2X2	T62.2X3	T62.2X4	—	—
berries	T62.1X1	T62.1X2	T62.1X3	T62.1X4	—	—
Solapsone	T37.1X1	T37.1X2	T37.1X3	T37.1X4	T37.1X5	T37.1X6
Solar lotion	T49.3X1	T49.3X2	T49.3X3	T49.3X4	T49.3X5	T49.3X6
Solasulfone	T37.1X1	T37.1X2	T37.1X3	T37.1X4	T37.1X5	T37.1X6
Soldering fluid	T65.891	T65.892	T65.893	T65.894	—	—
Solid substance	T65.91	T65.92	T65.93	T65.94	—	—
specified NEC	T65.891	T65.892	T65.893	T65.894	—	—
Solvent, industrial NEC	T52.91	T52.92	T52.93	T52.94	—	—
naphtha	T52.0X1	T52.0X2	T52.0X3	T52.0X4	—	—
petroleum	T52.0X1	T52.0X2	T52.0X3	T52.0X4	—	—
specified NEC	T52.8X1	T52.8X2	T52.8X3	T52.8X4	—	—
Soma	T42.8X1	T42.8X2	T42.8X3	T42.8X4	T42.8X5	T42.8X6
Somatorelin	T38.891	T38.892	T38.893	T38.894	T38.895	T38.896
Somatostatin	T38.991	T38.992	T38.993	T38.994	T38.995	T38.996
Somatotropin	T38.811	T38.812	T38.813	T38.814	T38.815	T38.816
Somatrem	T38.811	T38.812	T38.813	T38.814	T38.815	T38.816
Somatropin	T38.811	T38.812	T38.813	T38.814	T38.815	T38.816
Sominex	T45.0X1	T45.0X2	T45.0X3	T45.0X4	T45.0X5	T45.0X6
Somnos	T42.6X1	T42.6X2	T42.6X3	T42.6X4	T42.6X5	T42.6X6
Somonal	T42.3X1	T42.3X2	T42.3X3	T42.3X4	T42.3X5	T42.3X6
Soneryl	T42.3X1	T42.3X2	T42.3X3	T42.3X4	T42.3X5	T42.3X6
Soothing syrup	T50.901	T50.902	T50.903	T50.904	T50.905	T50.906
Sopor	T42.6X1	T42.6X2	T42.6X3	T42.6X4	T42.6X5	T42.6X6
Soporific	T42.71	T42.72	T42.73	T42.74	T42.75	T42.76
Soporific drug	T42.71	T42.72	T42.73	T42.74	T42.75	T42.76
specified type NEC	T42.6X1	T42.6X2	T42.6X3	T42.6X4	T42.6X5	T42.6X6
Sorbide nitrate	T46.3X1	T46.3X2	T46.3X3	T46.3X4	T46.3X5	T46.3X6
Sorbitol	T47.4X1	T47.4X2	T47.4X3	T47.4X4	T47.4X5	T47.4X6
Sotalol	T44.7X1	T44.7X2	T44.7X3	T44.7X4	T44.7X5	T44.7X6
Sotradecol	T46.8X1	T46.8X2	T46.8X3	T46.8X4	T46.8X5	T46.8X6
Soysterol	T46.6X1	T46.6X2	T46.6X3	T46.6X4	T46.6X5	T46.6X6
Spacoline	T44.3X1	T44.3X2	T44.3X3	T44.3X4	T44.3X5	T44.3X6
Spanish fly	T49.8X1	T49.8X2	T49.8X3	T49.8X4	T49.8X5	T49.8X6
Sparine	T43.3X1	T43.3X2	T43.3X3	T43.3X4	T43.3X5	T43.3X6
Sparteine	T48.0X1	T48.0X2	T48.0X3	T48.0X4	T48.0X5	T48.0X6

TABLE OF DRUGS AND CHEMICALS

New Revised ~~deleted~~ Deleted

Substance	External Cause (T-Code)					
	Poisoning, Accidental (Unintentional)	Poisoning, Intentional Self-Harm	Poisoning, Assault	Poisoning, Undetermined	Adverse Effect	Underdosing
Spasmolytic						
anticholinergics	T44.3X1	T44.3X2	T44.3X3	T44.3X4	T44.3X5	T44.3X6
autonomic	T44.3X1	T44.3X2	T44.3X3	T44.3X4	T44.3X5	T44.3X6
bronchial NEC	T48.6X1	T48.6X2	T48.6X3	T48.6X4	T48.6X5	T48.6X6
quaternary ammonium	T44.3X1	T44.3X2	T44.3X3	T44.3X4	T44.3X5	T44.3X6
skeletal muscle NEC	T48.1X1	T48.1X2	T48.1X3	T48.1X4	T48.1X5	T48.1X6
Spectinomycin	T36.5X1	T36.5X2	T36.5X3	T36.5X4	T36.5X5	T36.5X6
Speed	T43.651	T43.652	T43.652	T43.654	T43.655	T43.656
Spermicide	T49.8X1	T49.8X2	T49.8X3	T49.8X4	T49.8X5	T49.8X6
Spider (bite) (venom)	T63.391	T63.392	T63.393	T63.394	—	—
antivenin	T50.Z11	T50.Z12	T50.Z13	T50.Z14	T50.Z15	T50.Z16
Spigelia (root)	T37.4X1	T37.4X2	T37.4X3	T37.4X4	T37.4X5	T37.4X6
Spindle inactivator	T50.4X1	T50.4X2	T50.4X3	T50.4X4	T50.4X5	T50.4X6
Spiperone	T43.4X1	T43.4X2	T43.4X3	T43.4X4	T43.4X5	T43.4X6
Spiramycin	T36.3X1	T36.3X2	T36.3X3	T36.3X4	T36.3X5	T36.3X6
Spirapril	T46.4X1	T46.4X2	T46.4X3	T46.4X4	T46.4X5	T46.4X6
Spirilene	T43.591	T43.592	T43.593	T43.594	T43.595	T43.596
Spirit(s) (neutral) NEC	T51.ØX1	T51.ØX2	T51.ØX3	T51.ØX4	—	—
beverage	T51.ØX1	T51.ØX2	T51.ØX3	T51.ØX4	—	—
industrial	T51.ØX1	T51.ØX2	T51.ØX3	T51.ØX4	—	—
mineral	T52.ØX1	T52.ØX2	T52.ØX3	T52.ØX4	—	—
of salt — *see Hydrochloric acid*						
surgical	T51.ØX1	T51.ØX2	T51.ØX3	T51.ØX4	—	—
Spironolactone	T50.ØX1	T50.ØX2	T50.ØX3	T50.ØX4	T50.ØX5	T50.ØX6
Spiroperidol	T43.4X1	T43.4X2	T43.4X3	T43.4X4	T43.4X5	T43.4X6
Sponge, absorbable (gelatin)	T45.7X1	T45.7X2	T45.7X3	T45.7X4	T45.7X5	T45.7X6
Sporostacin	T49.ØX1	T49.ØX2	T49.ØX3	T49.ØX4	T49.ØX5	T49.ØX6
Spray (aerosol)	T65.91	T65.92	T65.93	T65.94	—	—
cosmetic	T65.891	T65.892	T65.893	T65.894	—	—
medicinal NEC	T50.901	T50.902	T50.903	T50.904	T50.905	T50.906
pesticides — *see Pesticide*						
specified content — *see specific substance*						
Spurge flax	T62.2X1	T62.2X2	T62.2X3	T62.2X4	—	—
Spurges	T62.2X1	T62.2X2	T62.2X3	T62.2X4	—	—
Sputum viscosity-lowering drug	T48.4X1	T48.4X2	T48.4X3	T48.4X4	T48.4X5	T48.4X6
Squill	T46.ØX1	T46.ØX2	T46.ØX3	T46.ØX4	T46.ØX5	T46.ØX6
rat poison	T60.4X1	T60.4X2	T60.4X3	T60.4X4	—	—
Squirting cucumber (cathartic)	T47.2X1	T47.2X2	T47.2X3	T47.2X4	T47.2X5	T47.2X6
Stains	T65.6X1	T65.6X2	T65.6X3	T65.6X4	—	—
Stannous fluoride	T49.7X1	T49.7X2	T49.7X3	T49.7X4	T49.7X5	T49.7X6
Stanolone	T38.7X1	T38.7X2	T38.7X3	T38.7X4	T38.7X5	T38.7X6
Stanozolol	T38.7X1	T38.7X2	T38.7X3	T38.7X4	T38.7X5	T38.7X6
Staphisagria or stavesacre (pediculicide)	T49.ØX1	T49.ØX2	T49.ØX3	T49.ØX4	T49.ØX5	T49.ØX6
Starch	T50.901	T50.902	T50.903	T50.904	T50.905	T50.906
Stelazine	T43.3X1	T43.3X2	T43.3X3	T43.3X4	T43.3X5	T43.3X6
Stemetil	T43.3X1	T43.3X2	T43.3X3	T43.3X4	T43.3X5	T43.3X6
Stepronin	T48.4X1	T48.4X2	T48.4X3	T48.4X4	T48.4X5	T48.4X6
Sterculia	T47.4X1	T47.4X2	T47.4X3	T47.4X4	T47.4X5	T47.4X6
Sternutator gas	T59.891	T59.892	T59.893	T59.894	—	—
Steroid	T38.ØX1	T38.ØX2	T38.ØX3	T38.ØX4	T38.ØX5	T38.ØX6
anabolic	T38.7X1	T38.7X2	T38.7X3	T38.7X4	T38.7X5	T38.7X6
androgenic	T38.7X1	T38.7X2	T38.7X3	T38.7X4	T38.7X5	T38.7X6
antineoplastic, hormone	T38.7X1	T38.7X2	T38.7X3	T38.7X4	T38.7X5	T38.7X6
estrogen	T38.5X1	T38.5X2	T38.5X3	T38.5X4	T38.5X5	T38.5X6
ENT agent	T49.6X1	T49.6X2	T49.6X3	T49.6X4	T49.6X5	T49.6X6
ophthalmic preparation	T49.5X1	T49.5X2	T49.5X3	T49.5X4	T49.5X5	T49.5X6
topical NEC	T49.ØX1	T49.ØX2	T49.ØX3	T49.ØX4	T49.ØX5	T49.ØX6
Stibine	T56.891	T56.892	T56.893	T56.894	—	—
Stibogluconate	T37.3X1	T37.3X2	T37.3X3	T37.3X4	T37.3X5	T37.3X6
Stibophen	T37.4X1	T37.4X2	T37.4X3	T37.4X4	T37.4X5	T37.4X6
Stilbamidine (isetionate)	T37.3X1	T37.3X2	T37.3X3	T37.3X4	T37.3X5	T37.3X6
Stilbestrol	T38.5X1	T38.5X2	T38.5X3	T38.5X4	T38.5X5	T38.5X6
Stilboestrol	T38.5X1	T38.5X2	T38.5X3	T38.5X4	T38.5X5	T38.5X6
Stimulant						
central nervous system — *see also Psychostimulant*	T43.601	T43.602	T43.603	T43.604	T43.605	T43.606
analeptics	T50.7X1	T50.7X2	T50.7X3	T50.7X4	T50.7X5	T50.7X6
opiate antagonist	T50.7X1	T50.7X2	T50.7X3	T50.7X4	T50.7X5	T50.7X6
psychotherapeutic NEC — *see also Psychotherapeutic drug*	T43.601	T43.602	T43.603	T43.604	T43.605	T43.606
specified NEC	T43.691	T43.692	T43.693	T43.694	T43.695	T43.696
respiratory	T48.901	T48.902	T48.903	T48.904	T48.905	T48.906
Stone-dissolving drug	T50.901	T50.902	T50.903	T50.904	T50.905	T50.906
Storage battery (cells) (acid)	T54.2X1	T54.2X2	T54.2X3	T54.2X4	—	—
Stovaine	T41.3X1	T41.3X2	T41.3X3	T41.3X4	T41.3X5	T41.3X6
infiltration (subcutaneous)	T41.3X1	T41.3X2	T41.3X3	T41.3X4	T41.3X5	T41.3X6
nerve block (peripheral) (plexus)	T41.3X1	T41.3X2	T41.3X3	T41.3X4	T41.3X5	T41.3X6
spinal	T41.3X1	T41.3X2	T41.3X3	T41.3X4	T41.3X5	T41.3X6
topical (surface)	T41.3X1	T41.3X2	T41.3X3	T41.3X4	T41.3X5	T41.3X6
Stovarsal	T37.8X1	T37.8X2	T37.8X3	T37.8X4	T37.8X5	T37.8X6
Stove gas — *see Gas, stove*	T57.91	T57.92	T57.93	T57.94	—	—

◀ New ◀ Revised ~~deleted~~ Deleted

Substance	External Cause (T-Code) Poisoning, Accidental (Unintentional)	Poisoning, Intentional Self-Harm	Poisoning, Assault	Poisoning, Undetermined	Adverse Effect	Underdosing
Stoxil	T49.5X1	T49.5X2	T49.5X3	T49.5X4	T49.5X5	T49.5X6
Stramonium	T48.6X1	T48.6X2	T48.6X3	T48.6X4	T48.6X5	T48.6X6
natural state	T62.2X1	T62.2X2	T62.2X3	T62.2X4	—	—
Streptodornase	T45.3X1	T45.3X2	T45.3X3	T45.3X4	T45.3X5	T45.3X6
Streptoduocin	T36.5X1	T36.5X2	T36.5X3	T36.5X4	T36.5X5	T36.5X6
Streptokinase	T45.611	T45.612	T45.613	T45.614	T45.615	T45.616
Streptomycin (derivative)	T36.5X1	T36.5X2	T36.5X3	T36.5X4	T36.5X5	T36.5X6
Streptonivicin	T36.5X1	T36.5X2	T36.5X3	T36.5X4	T36.5X5	T36.5X6
Streptovarycin	T36.5X1	T36.5X2	T36.5X3	T36.5X4	T36.5X5	T36.5X6
Streptozocin	T45.1X1	T45.1X2	T45.1X3	T45.1X4	T45.1X5	T45.1X6
Streptozotocin	T45.1X1	T45.1X2	T45.1X3	T45.1X4	T45.1X5	T45.1X6
Stripper (paint) (solvent)	T52.8X1	T52.8X2	T52.8X3	T52.8X4	—	—
Strobane	T60.1X1	T60.1X2	T60.1X3	T60.1X4	—	—
Strofantina	T46.0X1	T46.0X2	T46.0X3	T46.0X4	T46.0X5	T46.0X6
Strophanthin (g) (k)	T46.0X1	T46.0X2	T46.0X3	T46.0X4	T46.0X5	T46.0X6
Strophanthus	T46.0X1	T46.0X2	T46.0X3	T46.0X4	T46.0X5	T46.0X6
Strophantin	T46.0X1	T46.0X2	T46.0X3	T46.0X4	T46.0X5	T46.0X6
Strophantin-g	T46.0X1	T46.0X2	T46.0X3	T46.0X4	T46.0X5	T46.0X6
Strychnine (nonmedicinal) (pesticide) (salts)	T65.1X1	T65.1X2	T65.1X3	T65.1X4	—	—
medicinal	T48.291	T48.292	T48.293	T48.294	T48.295	T48.296
Strychnos (ignatii) — *see Strychnine*						
Styramate	T42.8X1	T42.8X2	T42.8X3	T42.8X4	T42.8X5	T42.8X6
Styrene	T65.891	T65.892	T65.893	T65.894	—	—
Succinimide, antiepileptic or anticonvulsant	T42.2X1	T42.2X2	T42.2X3	T42.2X4	T42.2X5	T42.2X6
mercuric — *see Mercury*						
Succinylcholine	T48.1X1	T48.1X2	T48.1X3	T48.1X4	T48.1X5	T48.1X6
Succinylsulfathiazole	T37.0X1	T37.0X2	T37.0X3	T37.0X4	T37.0X5	T37.0X6
Sucralfate	T47.1X1	T47.1X2	T47.1X3	T47.1X4	T47.1X5	T47.1X6
Sucrose	T50.3X1	T50.3X2	T50.3X3	T50.3X4	T50.3X5	T50.3X6
Sufentanil	T40.411	T40.412	T40.413	T40.414	T40.415	T40.416
Sulbactam	T36.0X1	T36.0X2	T36.0X3	T36.0X4	T36.0X5	T36.0X6
Sulbenicillin	T36.0X1	T36.0X2	T36.0X3	T36.0X4	T36.0X5	T36.0X6
Sulbentine	T49.0X1	T49.0X2	T49.0X3	T49.0X4	T49.0X5	T49.0X6
Sulfacetamide	T49.0X1	T49.0X2	T49.0X3	T49.0X4	T49.0X5	T49.0X6
ophthalmic preparation	T49.5X1	T49.5X2	T49.5X3	T49.5X4	T49.5X5	T49.5X6
Sulfachlorpyridazine	T37.0X1	T37.0X2	T37.0X3	T37.0X4	T37.0X5	T37.0X6
Sulfacitine	T37.0X1	T37.0X2	T37.0X3	T37.0X4	T37.0X5	T37.0X6
Sulfadiasulfone sodium	T37.0X1	T37.0X2	T37.0X3	T37.0X4	T37.0X5	T37.0X6
Sulfadiazine	T37.0X1	T37.0X2	T37.0X3	T37.0X4	T37.0X5	T37.0X6
silver (topical)	T49.0X1	T49.0X2	T49.0X3	T49.0X4	T49.0X5	T49.0X6

Substance	External Cause (T-Code) Poisoning, Accidental (Unintentional)	Poisoning, Intentional Self-Harm	Poisoning, Assault	Poisoning, Undetermined	Adverse Effect	Underdosing
Sulfadimethoxine	T37.0X1	T37.0X2	T37.0X3	T37.0X4	T37.0X5	T37.0X6
Sulfadimidine	T37.0X1	T37.0X2	T37.0X3	T37.0X4	T37.0X5	T37.0X6
Sulfadoxine	T37.0X1	T37.0X2	T37.0X3	T37.0X4	T37.0X5	T37.0X6
with pyrimethamine	T37.2X1	T37.2X2	T37.2X3	T37.2X4	T37.2X5	T37.2X6
Sulfaethidole	T37.0X1	T37.0X2	T37.0X3	T37.0X4	T37.0X5	T37.0X6
Sulfafurazole	T37.0X1	T37.0X2	T37.0X3	T37.0X4	T37.0X5	T37.0X6
Sulfaguanidine	T37.0X1	T37.0X2	T37.0X3	T37.0X4	T37.0X5	T37.0X6
Sulfalene	T37.0X1	T37.0X2	T37.0X3	T37.0X4	T37.0X5	T37.0X6
Sulfaloxate	T37.0X1	T37.0X2	T37.0X3	T37.0X4	T37.0X5	T37.0X6
Sulfaloxic acid	T37.0X1	T37.0X2	T37.0X3	T37.0X4	T37.0X5	T37.0X6
Sulfamazone	T39.2X1	T39.2X2	T39.2X3	T39.2X4	T39.2X5	T39.2X6
Sulfamerazine	T37.0X1	T37.0X2	T37.0X3	T37.0X4	T37.0X5	T37.0X6
Sulfameter	T37.0X1	T37.0X2	T37.0X3	T37.0X4	T37.0X5	T37.0X6
Sulfamethazine	T37.0X1	T37.0X2	T37.0X3	T37.0X4	T37.0X5	T37.0X6
Sulfamethizole	T37.0X1	T37.0X2	T37.0X3	T37.0X4	T37.0X5	T37.0X6
Sulfamethoxazole	T37.0X1	T37.0X2	T37.0X3	T37.0X4	T37.0X5	T37.0X6
with trimethoprim	T36.8X1	T36.8X2	T36.8X3	T36.8X4	T36.8X5	T36.8X6
Sulfamethoxydiazine	T37.0X1	T37.0X2	T37.0X3	T37.0X4	T37.0X5	T37.0X6
Sulfamethoxypyridazine	T37.0X1	T37.0X2	T37.0X3	T37.0X4	T37.0X5	T37.0X6
Sulfamethylthiazole	T37.0X1	T37.0X2	T37.0X3	T37.0X4	T37.0X5	T37.0X6
Sulfametoxydiazine	T37.0X1	T37.0X2	T37.0X3	T37.0X4	T37.0X5	T37.0X6
Sulfamidopyrine	T39.2X1	T39.2X2	T39.2X3	T39.2X4	T39.2X5	T39.2X6
Sulfamonomethoxine	T37.0X1	T37.0X2	T37.0X3	T37.0X4	T37.0X5	T37.0X6
Sulfamoxole	T37.0X1	T37.0X2	T37.0X3	T37.0X4	T37.0X5	T37.0X6
Sulfamylon	T49.0X1	T49.0X2	T49.0X3	T49.0X4	T49.0X5	T49.0X6
Sulfan blue (diagnostic dye)	T50.8X1	T50.8X2	T50.8X3	T50.8X4	T50.8X5	T50.8X6
Sulfanilamide	T37.0X1	T37.0X2	T37.0X3	T37.0X4	T37.0X5	T37.0X6
Sulfanilylguanidine	T37.0X1	T37.0X2	T37.0X3	T37.0X4	T37.0X5	T37.0X6
Sulfaperin	T37.0X1	T37.0X2	T37.0X3	T37.0X4	T37.0X5	T37.0X6
Sulfaphenazole	T37.0X1	T37.0X2	T37.0X3	T37.0X4	T37.0X5	T37.0X6
Sulfaphenylthiazole	T37.0X1	T37.0X2	T37.0X3	T37.0X4	T37.0X5	T37.0X6
Sulfaproxyline	T37.0X1	T37.0X2	T37.0X3	T37.0X4	T37.0X5	T37.0X6
Sulfapyridine	T37.0X1	T37.0X2	T37.0X3	T37.0X4	T37.0X5	T37.0X6
Sulfapyrimidine	T37.0X1	T37.0X2	T37.0X3	T37.0X4	T37.0X5	T37.0X6
Sulfarsphenamine	T37.8X1	T37.8X2	T37.8X3	T37.8X4	T37.8X5	T37.8X6
Sulfasalazine	T37.0X1	T37.0X2	T37.0X3	T37.0X4	T37.0X5	T37.0X6
Sulfasuxidine	T37.0X1	T37.0X2	T37.0X3	T37.0X4	T37.0X5	T37.0X6
Sulfasymazine	T37.0X1	T37.0X2	T37.0X3	T37.0X4	T37.0X5	T37.0X6
Sulfated amylopectin	T47.8X1	T47.8X2	T47.8X3	T47.8X4	T47.8X5	T47.8X6
Sulfathiazole	T37.0X1	T37.0X2	T37.0X3	T37.0X4	T37.0X5	T37.0X6
Sulfatostearate	T49.2X1	T49.2X2	T49.2X3	T49.2X4	T49.2X5	T49.2X6
Sulfinpyrazone	T50.1X1	T50.4X2	T50.4X3	T50.4X4	T50.4X5	T50.4X6

◀ New ⇐ Revised ~~deleted~~ Deleted

Substance	External Cause (T-Code)					
	Poisoning, Accidental (Unintentional)	Poisoning, Intentional Self-Harm	Poisoning, Assault	Poisoning, Undetermined	Adverse Effect	Underdosing
Sulfiram	T49.ØX1	T49.ØX2	T49.ØX3	T49.ØX4	T49.ØX5	T49.ØX6
Sulfisomidine	T37.ØX1	T37.ØX2	T37.ØX3	T37.ØX4	T37.ØX5	T37.ØX6
Sulfisoxazole	T37.ØX1	T37.ØX2	T37.ØX3	T37.ØX4	T37.ØX5	T37.ØX6
ophthalmic preparation	T49.5X1	T49.5X2	T49.5X3	T49.5X4	T49.5X5	T49.5X6
Sulfobromophthalein (sodium)	T5Ø.8X1	T5Ø.8X2	T5Ø.8X3	T5Ø.8X4	T5Ø.8X5	T5Ø.8X6
Sulfobromphthalein	T5Ø.8X1	T5Ø.8X2	T5Ø.8X3	T5Ø.8X4	T5Ø.8X5	T5Ø.8X6
Sulfogaiacol	T48.4X1	T48.4X2	T48.4X3	T48.4X4	T48.4X5	T48.4X6
Sulfomyxin	T36.8X1	T36.8X2	T36.8X3	T36.8X4	T36.8X5	T36.8X6
Sulfonal	T42.6X1	T42.6X2	T42.6X3	T42.6X4	T42.6X5	T42.6X6
Sulfonamide NEC	T37.ØX1	T37.ØX2	T37.ØX3	T37.ØX4	T37.ØX5	T37.ØX6
eye	T49.5X1	T49.5X2	T49.5X3	T49.5X4	T49.5X5	T49.5X6
Sulfonazide	T37.1X1	T37.1X2	T37.1X3	T37.1X4	T37.1X5	T37.1X6
Sulfones	T37.1X1	T37.1X2	T37.1X3	T37.1X4	T37.1X5	T37.1X6
Sulfonethylmethane	T42.6X1	T42.6X2	T42.6X3	T42.6X4	T42.6X5	T42.6X6
Sulfonmethane	T42.6X1	T42.6X2	T42.6X3	T42.6X4	T42.6X5	T42.6X6
Sulfonphthal, sulfonphthol	T5Ø.8X1	T5Ø.8X2	T5Ø.8X3	T5Ø.8X4	T5Ø.8X5	T5Ø.8X6
Sulfonylurea derivatives, oral	T38.3X1	T38.3X2	T38.3X3	T38.3X4	T38.3X5	T38.3X6
Sulforidazine	T43.3X1	T43.3X2	T43.3X3	T43.3X4	T43.3X5	T43.3X6
Sulfoxone	T37.1X1	T37.1X2	T37.1X3	T37.1X4	T37.1X5	T37.1X6
Sulfur, sulfurated, sulfuric, sulfurous, sulfuryl (compounds NEC) (medicinal)	T49.4X1	T49.4X2	T49.4X3	T49.4X4	T49.4X5	T49.4X6
acid	T54.2X1	T54.2X2	T54.2X3	T54.2X4	—	—
dioxide (gas)	T59.1X1	T59.1X2	T59.1X3	T59.1X4	—	—
ether — *see Ether(s)*						
hydrogen	T59.6X1	T59.6X2	T59.6X3	T59.6X4	—	—
medicinal (keratolytic) (ointment) NEC	T49.4X1	T49.4X2	T49.4X3	T49.4X4	T49.4X5	T49.4X6
ointment	T49.ØX1	T49.ØX2	T49.ØX3	T49.ØX4	T49.ØX5	T49.ØX6
pesticide (vapor)	T6Ø.91	T6Ø.92	T6Ø.93	T6Ø.94	—	—
vapor NEC	T59.891	T59.892	T59.893	T59.894	—	—
Sulfuric acid	T54.2X1	T54.2X2	T54.2X3	T54.2X4	—	—
Sulglicotide	T47.1X1	T47.1X2	T47.1X3	T47.1X4	T47.1X5	T47.1X6
Sulindac	T39.391	T39.392	T39.393	T39.394	T39.395	T39.396
Sulisatin	T47.2X1	T47.2X2	T47.2X3	T47.2X4	T47.2X5	T47.2X6
Sulisobenzone	T49.3X1	T49.3X2	T49.3X3	T49.3X4	T49.3X5	T49.3X6
Sulkowitch's reagent	T5Ø.8X1	T5Ø.8X2	T5Ø.8X3	T5Ø.8X4	T5Ø.8X5	T5Ø.8X6
Sulmetozine	T44.3X1	T44.3X2	T44.3X3	T44.3X4	T44.3X5	T44.3X6
Suloctidil	T46.7X1	T46.7X2	T46.7X3	T46.7X4	T46.7X5	T46.7X6
Sulph — *see also Sulf-*						
Sulphadiazine	T37.ØX1	T37.ØX2	T37.ØX3	T37.ØX4	T37.ØX5	T37.ØX6
Sulphadimethoxine	T37.ØX1	T37.ØX2	T37.ØX3	T37.ØX4	T37.ØX5	T37.ØX6
Sulphadimidine	T37.ØX1	T37.ØX2	T37.ØX3	T37.ØX4	T37.ØX5	T37.ØX6
Sulphadione	T37.1X1	T37.1X2	T37.1X3	T37.1X4	T37.1X5	T37.1X6
Sulphafurazole	T37.ØX1	T37.ØX2	T37.ØX3	T37.ØX4	T37.ØX5	T37.ØX6
Sulphamethizole	T37.ØX1	T37.ØX2	T37.ØX3	T37.ØX4	T37.ØX5	T37.ØX6
Sulphamethoxazole	T37.ØX1	T37.ØX2	T37.ØX3	T37.ØX4	T37.ØX5	T37.ØX6
Sulphan blue	T5Ø.8X1	T5Ø.8X2	T5Ø.8X3	T5Ø.8X4	T5Ø.8X5	T5Ø.8X6
Sulphaphenazole	T37.ØX1	T37.ØX2	T37.ØX3	T37.ØX4	T37.ØX5	T37.ØX6
Sulphapyridine	T37.ØX1	T37.ØX2	T37.ØX3	T37.ØX4	T37.ØX5	T37.ØX6
Sulphasalazine	T37.ØX1	T37.ØX2	T37.ØX3	T37.ØX4	T37.ØX5	T37.ØX6
Sulphinpyrazone	T5Ø.4X1	T5Ø.4X2	T5Ø.4X3	T5Ø.4X4	T5Ø.4X5	T5Ø.4X6
Sulpiride	T43.591	T43.592	T43.593	T43.594	T43.595	T43.596
Sulprostone	T48.ØX1	T48.ØX2	T48.ØX3	T48.ØX4	T48.ØX5	T48.ØX6
Sulpyrine	T39.2X1	T39.2X2	T39.2X3	T39.2X4	T39.2X5	T39.2X6
Sultamicillin	T36.ØX1	T36.ØX2	T36.ØX3	T36.ØX4	T36.ØX5	T36.ØX6
Sulthiame	T42.6X1	T42.6X2	T42.6X3	T42.6X4	T42.6X5	T42.6X6
Sultiame	T42.6X1	T42.6X2	T42.6X3	T42.6X4	T42.6X5	T42.6X6
Sultopride	T43.591	T43.592	T43.593	T43.594	T43.595	T43.596
Sumatriptan	T39.8X1	T39.8X2	T39.8X3	T39.8X4	T39.8X5	T39.8X6
Sunflower seed oil	T46.6X1	T46.6X2	T46.6X3	T46.6X4	T46.6X5	T46.6X6
Superinone	T48.4X1	T48.4X2	T48.4X3	T48.4X4	T48.4X5	T48.4X6
Suprofen	T39.311	T39.312	T39.313	T39.314	T39.315	T39.316
Suramin (sodium)	T37.4X1	T37.4X2	T37.4X3	T37.4X4	T37.4X5	T37.4X6
Surfacaine	T41.3X1	T41.3X2	T41.3X3	T41.3X4	T41.3X5	T41.3X6
Surital	T41.1X1	T41.1X2	T41.1X3	T41.1X4	T41.1X5	T41.1X6
Sutilains	T45.3X1	T45.3X2	T45.3X3	T45.3X4	T45.3X5	T45.3X6
Suxamethonium (chloride)	T48.1X1	T48.1X2	T48.1X3	T48.1X4	T48.1X5	T48.1X6
Suxethonium (chloride)	T48.1X1	T48.1X2	T48.1X3	T48.1X4	T48.1X5	T48.1X6
Suxibuzone	T39.2X1	T39.2X2	T39.2X3	T39.2X4	T39.2X5	T39.2X6
Sweet oil (birch)	T49.3X1	T49.3X2	T49.3X3	T49.3X4	T49.3X5	T49.3X6
Sweet niter spirit	T46.3X1	T46.3X2	T46.3X3	T46.3X4	T46.3X5	T46.3X6
Sweetener	T5Ø.9Ø1	T5Ø.9Ø2	T5Ø.9Ø3	T5Ø.9Ø4	T5Ø.9Ø5	T5Ø.9Ø6
Sym-dichloroethyl ether	T53.6X1	T53.6X2	T53.6X3	T53.6X4	—	—
Sympatholytic NEC	T44.8X1	T44.8X2	T44.8X3	T44.8X4	T44.8X5	T44.8X6
haloalkylamine	T44.8X1	T44.8X2	T44.8X3	T44.8X4	T44.8X5	T44.8X6
Sympathomimetic NEC	T44.9Ø1	T44.9Ø2	T44.9Ø3	T44.9Ø4	T44.9Ø5	T44.9Ø6
anti-common-cold	T48.5X1	T48.5X2	T48.5X3	T48.5X4	T48.5X5	T48.5X6
bronchodilator	T48.6X1	T48.6X2	T48.6X3	T48.6X4	T48.6X5	T48.6X6
specified NEC	T44.991	T44.992	T44.993	T44.994	T44.995	T44.996
Synagis	T5Ø.B91	T5Ø.B92	T5Ø.B93	T5Ø.B94	T5Ø.B95	T5Ø.B96
Synalar	T49.ØX1	T49.ØX2	T49.ØX3	T49.ØX4	T49.ØX5	T49.ØX6
Synthetic cannabinoids	T4Ø.721	T4Ø.722	T4Ø.723	T4Ø.724	T4Ø.725	T4Ø.726
Synthroid	T38.1X1	T38.1X2	T38.1X3	T38.1X4	T38.1X5	T38.1X6

Substance	Poisoning, Accidental (Unintentional)	Poisoning, Intentional Self-Harm	Poisoning, Assault	Poisoning, Undetermined	Adverse Effect	Underdosing
Syntocinon	T48.ØX1	T48.ØX2	T48.ØX3	T48.ØX4	T48.ØX5	T48.ØX6
Syrosingopine	T46.5X1	T46.5X2	T46.5X3	T46.5X4	T46.5X5	T46.5X6
Systemic drug	T45.91	T45.92	T45.93	T45.94	T45.95	T45.96
specified NEC	T45.8X1	T45.8X2	T45.8X3	T45.8X4	T45.8X5	T45.8X6
2,4,5-T	T6Ø.3X1	T6Ø.3X2	T6Ø.3X3	T6Ø.3X4	—	—
T						
Tablets — *see also specified substance*	T5Ø.9Ø1	T5Ø.9Ø2	T5Ø.9Ø3	T5Ø.9Ø4	T5Ø.9Ø5	T5Ø.9Ø6
Tace	T38.5X1	T38.5X2	T38.5X3	T38.5X4	T38.5X5	T38.5X6
Tacrine	T44.ØX1	T44.ØX2	T44.ØX3	T44.ØX4	T44.ØX5	T44.ØX6
Tadalafil	T46.7X1	T46.7X2	T46.7X3	T46.7X4	T46.7X5	T46.7X6
Talampicillin	T36.ØX1	T36.ØX2	T36.ØX3	T36.ØX4	T36.ØX5	T36.ØX6
Talbutal	T42.3X1	T42.3X2	T42.3X3	T42.3X4	T42.3X5	T42.3X6
Talc powder	T49.3X1	T49.3X2	T49.3X3	T49.3X4	T49.3X5	T49.3X6
Talcum	T49.3X1	T49.3X2	T49.3X3	T49.3X4	T49.3X5	T49.3X6
Taleranol	T38.6X1	T38.6X2	T38.6X3	T38.6X4	T38.6X5	T38.6X6
Tamoxifen	T38.6X1	T38.6X2	T38.6X3	T38.6X4	T38.6X5	T38.6X6
Tamsulosin	T44.6X1	T44.6X2	T44.6X3	T44.6X4	T44.6X5	T44.6X6
Tandearil, tanderil	T39.2X1	T39.2X2	T39.2X3	T39.2X4	T39.2X5	T39.2X6
Tannic acid	T49.2X1	T49.2X2	T49.2X3	T49.2X4	T49.2X5	T49.2X6
medicinal (astringent)	T49.2X1	T49.2X2	T49.2X3	T49.2X4	T49.2X5	T49.2X6
Tannin — *see Tannic acid*						
Tansy	T62.2X1	T62.2X2	T62.2X3	T62.2X4	—	—
TAO	T36.3X1	T36.3X2	T36.3X3	T36.3X4	T36.3X5	T36.3X6
Tapazole	T38.2X1	T38.2X2	T38.2X3	T38.2X4	T38.2X5	T38.2X6
Tar NEC	T52.ØX1	T52.ØX2	T52.ØX3	T52.ØX4	—	—
camphor	T6Ø.1X1	T6Ø.1X2	T6Ø.1X3	T6Ø.1X4	—	—
distillate	T49.1X1	T49.1X2	T49.1X3	T49.1X4	T49.1X5	T49.1X6
fumes	T59.891	T59.892	T59.893	T59.894	—	—
medicinal	T49.1X1	T49.1X2	T49.1X3	T49.1X4	T49.1X5	T49.1X6
ointment	T49.1X1	T49.1X2	T49.1X3	T49.1X4	T49.1X5	T49.1X6
Taractan	T43.591	T43.592	T43.593	T43.594	T43.595	T43.596
Tarantula (venomous)	T63.321	T63.322	T63.323	T63.324	—	—
Tartar emetic	T37.8X1	T37.8X2	T37.8X3	T37.8X4	T37.8X5	T37.8X6
Tartaric acid	T65.891	T65.892	T65.893	T65.894	—	—
Tartrated antimony (anti-infective)	T37.8X1	T37.8X2	T37.8X3	T37.8X4	T37.8X5	T37.8X6
Tartrate, laxative	T47.4X1	T47.4X2	T47.4X3	T47.4X4	T47.4X5	T47.4X6
Tauromustine	T45.1X1	T45.1X2	T45.1X3	T45.1X4	T45.1X5	T45.1X6
TCA — *see Trichloroacetic acid*						
TCDD	T53.7X1	T53.7X2	T53.7X3	T53.7X4	—	—
TDI (vapor)	T65.ØX1	T65.ØX2	T65.ØX3	T65.ØX4	—	—

Substance	Poisoning, Accidental (Unintentional)	Poisoning, Intentional Self-Harm	Poisoning, Assault	Poisoning, Undetermined	Adverse Effect	Underdosing
Tear						
gas	T59.3X1	T59.3X2	T59.3X3	T59.3X4	—	—
solution	T49.5X1	T49.5X2	T49.5X3	T49.5X4	T49.5X5	T49.5X6
Teclothiazide	T5Ø.2X1	T5Ø.2X2	T5Ø.2X3	T5Ø.2X4	T5Ø.2X5	T5Ø.2X6
Teclozan	T37.3X1	T37.3X2	T37.3X3	T37.3X4	T37.3X5	T37.3X6
Tegafur	T45.1X1	T45.1X2	T45.1X3	T45.1X4	T45.1X5	T45.1X6
Tegretol	T42.1X1	T42.1X2	T42.1X3	T42.1X4	T42.1X5	T42.1X6
Teicoplanin	T36.8X1	T36.8X2	T36.8X3	T36.8X4	T36.8X5	T36.8X6
Telepaque	T5Ø.8X1	T5Ø.8X2	T5Ø.8X3	T5Ø.8X4	T5Ø.8X5	T5Ø.8X6
Tellurium	T56.891	T56.892	T56.893	T56.894	—	—
fumes	T56.891	T56.892	T56.893	T56.894	—	—
TEM	T45.1X1	T45.1X2	T45.1X3	T45.1X4	T45.1X5	T45.1X6
Temazepam	T42.4X1	T42.4X2	T42.4X3	T42.4X4	T42.4X5	T42.4X6
Temocillin	T36.ØX1	T36.ØX2	T36.ØX3	T36.ØX4	T36.ØX5	T36.ØX6
Tenamfetamine	T43.621	T43.622	T43.623	T43.624	T43.625	T43.626
Teniposide	T45.1X1	T45.1X2	T45.1X3	T45.1X4	T45.1X5	T45.1X6
Tenitramine	T46.3X1	T46.3X2	T46.3X3	T46.3X4	T46.3X5	T46.3X6
Tenoglicin	T48.4X1	T48.4X2	T48.4X3	T48.4X4	T48.4X5	T48.4X6
Tenonitrozole	T37.3X1	T37.3X2	T37.3X3	T37.3X4	T37.3X5	T37.3X6
Tenoxicam	T39.391	T39.392	T39.393	T39.394	T39.395	T39.396
TEPA	T45.1X1	T45.1X2	T45.1X3	T45.1X4	T45.1X5	T45.1X6
TEPP	T6Ø.ØX1	T6Ø.ØX2	T6Ø.ØX3	T6Ø.ØX4	—	—
Teprotide	T46.5X1	T46.5X2	T46.5X3	T46.5X4	T46.5X5	T46.5X6
Terazosin	T44.6X1	T44.6X2	T44.6X3	T44.6X4	T44.6X5	T44.6X6
Terbufos	T6Ø.ØX1	T6Ø.ØX2	T6Ø.ØX3	T6Ø.ØX4	—	—
Terbutaline	T48.6X1	T48.6X2	T48.6X3	T48.6X4	T48.6X5	T48.6X6
Terconazole	T49.ØX1	T49.ØX2	T49.ØX3	T49.ØX4	T49.ØX5	T49.ØX6
Terfenadine	T45.ØX1	T45.ØX2	T45.ØX3	T45.ØX4	T45.ØX5	T45.ØX6
Teriparatide (acetate)	T5Ø.991	T5Ø.992	T5Ø.993	T5Ø.994	T5Ø.995	T5Ø.996
Terizidone	T37.1X1	T37.1X2	T37.1X3	T37.1X4	T37.1X5	T37.1X6
Terlipressin	T38.891	T38.892	T38.893	T38.894	T38.895	T38.896
Terodiline	T46.3X1	T46.3X2	T46.3X3	T46.3X4	T46.3X5	T46.3X6
Teroxalene	T37.4X1	T37.4X2	T37.4X3	T37.4X4	T37.4X5	T37.4X6
Terpin(cis) hydrate	T48.4X1	T48.4X2	T48.4X3	T48.4X4	T48.4X5	T48.4X6
Terramycin	T36.4X1	T36.4X2	T36.4X3	T36.4X4	T36.4X5	T36.4X6
Tertatolol	T44.7X1	T44.7X2	T44.7X3	T44.7X4	T44.7X5	T44.7X6
Tessalon	T48.3X1	T48.3X2	T48.3X3	T48.3X4	T48.3X5	T48.3X6
Testolactone	T38.7X1	T38.7X2	T38.7X3	T38.7X4	T38.7X5	T38.7X6
Testosterone	T38.7X1	T38.7X2	T38.7X3	T38.7X4	T38.7X5	T38.7X6
Tetanus toxoid or vaccine	T5Ø.A91	T5Ø.A92	T5Ø.A93	T5Ø.A94	T5Ø.A95	T5Ø.A96
antitoxin	T5Ø.Z11	T5Ø.Z12	T5Ø.Z13	T5Ø.Z14	T5Ø.Z15	T5Ø.Z16
immune globulin (human)	T5Ø.Z11	T5Ø.Z12	T5Ø.Z13	T5Ø.Z14	T5Ø.Z15	T5Ø.Z16

Substance	Poisoning, Accidental (Unintentional)	Poisoning, Intentional Self-Harm	Poisoning, Assault	Poisoning, Undetermined	Adverse Effect	Underdosing
	External Cause (T-Code)					
Tetanus toxoid or vaccine *(Continued)*						
toxoid	T5Ø.A91	T5Ø.A92	T5Ø.A93	T5Ø.A94	T5Ø.A95	T5Ø.A96
with diphtheria toxoid	T5Ø.A21	T5Ø.A22	T5Ø.A23	T5Ø.A24	T5Ø.A25	T5Ø.A26
with pertussis	T5Ø.A11	T5Ø.A12	T5Ø.A13	T5Ø.A14	T5Ø.A15	T5Ø.A16
Tetrabenazine	T43.591	T43.592	T43.593	T43.594	T43.595	T43.596
Tetracaine	T41.3X1	T41.3X2	T41.3X3	T41.3X4	T41.3X5	T41.3X6
nerve block (peripheral) (plexus)	T41.3X1	T41.3X2	T41.3X3	T41.3X4	T41.3X5	T41.3X6
regional	T41.3X1	T41.3X2	T41.3X3	T41.3X4	T41.3X5	T41.3X6
spinal	T41.3X1	T41.3X2	T41.3X3	T41.3X4	T41.3X5	T41.3X6
Tetrachlorethylene — *see Tetrachloroethylene*						
Tetrachlormethiazide	T5Ø.2X1	T5Ø.2X2	T5Ø.2X3	T5Ø.2X4	T5Ø.2X5	T5Ø.2X6
2,3,7,8-Tetrachlorodibenzo-p-dioxin	T53.7X1	T53.7X2	T53.7X3	T53.7X4	—	—
Tetrachloroethane	T53.6X1	T53.6X2	T53.6X3	T53.6X4	—	—
vapor	T53.6X1	T53.6X2	T53.6X3	T53.6X4	—	—
paint or varnish	T53.6X1	T53.6X2	T53.6X3	T53.6X4	—	—
Tetrachloroethylene (liquid)	T53.3X1	T53.3X2	T53.3X3	T53.3X4	—	—
medicinal	T37.4X1	T37.4X2	T37.4X3	T37.4X4	T37.4X5	T37.4X6
vapor	T53.3X1	T53.3X2	T53.3X3	T53.3X4	—	—
Tetrachloromethane — *see Carbon tetrachloride*						
Tetracosactide	T38.811	T38.812	T38.813	T38.814	T38.815	T38.816
Tetracosactrin	T38.811	T38.812	T38.813	T38.814	T38.815	T38.816
Tetracycline	T36.4X1	T36.4X2	T36.4X3	T36.4X4	T36.4X5	T36.4X6
ophthalmic preparation	T49.5X1	T49.5X2	T49.5X3	T49.5X4	T49.5X5	T49.5X6
topical NEC	T49.ØX1	T49.ØX2	T49.ØX3	T49.ØX4	T49.ØX5	T49.ØX6
Tetradifon	T6Ø.8X1	T6Ø.8X2	T6Ø.8X3	T6Ø.8X4	—	—
Tetradotoxin	T61.771	T61.772	T61.773	T61.774	—	—
Tetraethyl						
lead	T56.ØX1	T56.ØX2	T56.ØX3	T56.ØX4	—	—
pyrophosphate	T6Ø.ØX1	T6Ø.ØX2	T6Ø.ØX3	T6Ø.ØX4	—	—
Tetraethylammonium chloride	T44.2X1	T44.2X2	T44.2X3	T44.2X4	T44.2X5	T44.2X6
Tetraethylthiuram disulfide	T5Ø.6X1	T5Ø.6X2	T5Ø.6X3	T5Ø.6X4	T5Ø.6X5	T5Ø.6X6
Tetrahydroaminoacridine	T44.ØX1	T44.ØX2	T44.ØX3	T44.ØX4	T44.ØX5	T44.ØX6
Tetrahydrocannabinol	T4Ø.711	T4Ø.712	T4Ø.713	T4Ø.714	T4Ø.715	T4Ø.716
Tetrahydrofuran	T52.8X1	T52.8X2	T52.8X3	T52.8X4	—	—
Tetrahydronaphthalene	T52.8X1	T52.8X2	T52.8X3	T52.8X4	—	—
Tetrahydrozoline	T49.5X1	T49.5X2	T49.5X3	T49.5X4	T49.5X5	T49.5X6
Tetralin	T52.8X1	T52.8X2	T52.8X3	T52.8X4	—	—
Tetramethrin	T6Ø.2X1	T6Ø.2X2	T6Ø.2X3	T6Ø.2X4	—	—
Tetramethylthiuram (disulfide) NEC	T6Ø.3X1	T6Ø.3X2	T6Ø.3X3	T6Ø.3X4	—	—
medicinal	T49.ØX1	T49.ØX2	T49.ØX3	T49.ØX4	T49.ØX5	T49.ØX6
Tetramisole	T37.4X1	T37.4X2	T37.4X3	T37.4X4	T37.4X5	T37.4X6
Tetranicotinoyl fructose	T46.7X1	T46.7X2	T46.7X3	T46.7X4	T46.7X5	T46.7X6
Tetronal	T42.6X1	T42.6X2	T42.6X3	T42.6X4	T42.6X5	T42.6X6
Tetrazepam	T42.4X1	T42.4X2	T42.4X3	T42.4X4	T42.4X5	T42.4X6
Tetryl	T65.3X1	T65.3X2	T65.3X3	T65.3X4	—	—
Tetrylammonium chloride	T44.2X1	T44.2X2	T44.2X3	T44.2X4	T44.2X5	T44.2X6
Tetryzoline	T49.5X1	T49.5X2	T49.5X3	T49.5X4	T49.5X5	T49.5X6
Thalidomide	T45.1X1	T45.1X2	T45.1X3	T45.1X4	T45.1X5	T45.1X6
Thallium (compounds) (dust) NEC	T56.811	T56.812	T56.813	T56.814	—	—
pesticide	T6Ø.4X1	T6Ø.4X2	T6Ø.4X3	T6Ø.4X4	—	—
THC	T4Ø.711	T4Ø.712	T4Ø.713	T4Ø.714	T4Ø.715	T4Ø.716
Thebacon	T48.3X1	T48.3X2	T48.3X3	T48.3X4	T48.3X5	T48.3X6
Thebaine	T4Ø.2X1	T4Ø.2X2	T4Ø.2X3	T4Ø.2X4	T4Ø.2X5	T4Ø.2X6
Thenoic acid	T49.6X1	T49.6X2	T49.6X3	T49.6X4	T49.6X5	T49.6X6
Thenyldiamine	T45.ØX1	T45.ØX2	T45.ØX3	T45.ØX4	T45.ØX5	T45.ØX6
Theobromine (calcium salicylate)	T48.6X1	T48.6X2	T48.6X3	T48.6X4	T48.6X5	T48.6X6
sodium salicylate	T48.6X1	T48.6X2	T48.6X3	T48.6X4	T48.6X5	T48.6X6
Theophyllamine	T48.6X1	T48.6X2	T48.6X3	T48.6X4	T48.6X5	T48.6X6
Theophylline	T48.6X1	T48.6X2	T48.6X3	T48.6X4	T48.6X5	T48.6X6
aminobenzoic acid	T48.6X1	T48.6X2	T48.6X3	T48.6X4	T48.6X5	T48.6X6
ethylenediamine	T48.6X1	T48.6X2	T48.6X3	T48.6X4	T48.6X5	T48.6X6
piperazine p-amino-benzoate	T48.6X1	T48.6X2	T48.6X3	T48.6X4	T48.6X5	T48.6X6
Thiabendazole	T37.4X1	T37.4X2	T37.4X3	T37.4X4	T37.4X5	T37.4X6
Thialbarbital	T41.1X1	T41.1X2	T41.1X3	T41.1X4	T41.1X5	T41.1X6
Thiamazole	T38.2X1	T38.2X2	T38.2X3	T38.2X4	T38.2X5	T38.2X6
Thiambutosine	T37.1X1	T37.1X2	T37.1X3	T37.1X4	T37.1X5	T37.1X6
Thiamine	T45.2X1	T45.2X2	T45.2X3	T45.2X4	T45.2X5	T45.2X6
Thiamphenicol	T36.2X1	T36.2X2	T36.2X3	T36.2X4	T36.2X5	T36.2X6
Thiamylal	T41.1X1	T41.1X2	T41.1X3	T41.1X4	T41.1X5	T41.1X6
sodium	T41.1X1	T41.1X2	T41.1X3	T41.1X4	T41.1X5	T41.1X6
Thiazesim	T43.291	T43.292	T43.293	T43.294	T43.295	T43.296
Thiazides (diuretics)	T5Ø.2X1	T5Ø.2X2	T5Ø.2X3	T5Ø.2X4	T5Ø.2X5	T5Ø.2X6
Thiazinamium metilsulfate	T43.3X1	T43.3X2	T43.3X3	T43.3X4	T43.3X5	T43.3X6
Thiethylperazine	T43.3X1	T43.3X2	T43.3X3	T43.3X4	T43.3X5	T43.3X6
Thimerosal	T49.ØX1	T49.ØX2	T49.ØX3	T49.ØX4	T49.ØX5	T49.ØX6
ophthalmic preparation	T49.5X1	T49.5X2	T49.5X3	T49.5X4	T49.5X5	T49.5X6
Thioacetazone	T37.1X1	T37.1X2	T37.1X3	T37.1X4	T37.1X5	T37.1X6
with isoniazid	T37.1X1	T37.1X2	T37.1X3	T37.1X4	T37.1X5	T37.1X6
Thiobarbital sodium	T41.1X1	T41.1X2	T41.1X3	T41.1X4	T41.1X5	T41.1X6

Substance	External Cause (T-Code)					
	Poisoning, Accidental (Unintentional)	Poisoning, Intentional Self-Harm	Poisoning, Assault	Poisoning, Undetermined	Adverse Effect	Underdosing
Thiobarbiturate anesthetic	T41.1X1	T41.1X2	T41.1X3	T41.1X4	T41.1X5	T41.1X6
Thiobismol	T37.8X1	T37.8X2	T37.8X3	T37.8X4	T37.8X5	T37.8X6
Thiobutabarbital sodium	T41.1X1	T41.1X2	T41.1X3	T41.1X4	T41.1X5	T41.1X6
Thiocarbamate (insecticide)	T60.0X1	T60.0X2	T60.0X3	T60.0X4	—	—
Thiocarbamide	T38.2X1	T38.2X2	T38.2X3	T38.2X4	T38.2X5	T38.2X6
Thiocarbarsone	T37.8X1	T37.8X2	T37.8X3	T37.8X4	T37.8X5	T37.8X6
Thiocarlide	T37.1X1	T37.1X2	T37.1X3	T37.1X4	T37.1X5	T37.1X6
Thioctamide	T50.991	T50.992	T50.993	T50.994	T50.995	T50.996
Thioctic acid	T50.991	T50.992	T50.993	T50.994	T50.995	T50.996
Thiofos	T60.0X1	T60.0X2	T60.0X3	T60.0X4	—	—
Thioglycolate	T49.4X1	T49.4X2	T49.4X3	T49.4X4	T49.4X5	T49.4X6
Thioglycolic acid	T65.891	T65.892	T65.893	T65.894	—	—
Thioguanine	T45.1X1	T45.1X2	T45.1X3	T45.1X4	T45.1X5	T45.1X6
Thiomercaptomerin	T50.2X1	T50.2X2	T50.2X3	T50.2X4	T50.2X5	T50.2X6
Thiomerin	T50.2X1	T50.2X2	T50.2X3	T50.2X4	T50.2X5	T50.2X6
Thiomersal	T49.0X1	T49.0X2	T49.0X3	T49.0X4	T49.0X5	T49.0X6
Thionazin	T60.0X1	T60.0X2	T60.0X3	T60.0X4	—	—
Thiopental (sodium)	T41.1X1	T41.1X2	T41.1X3	T41.1X4	T41.1X5	T41.1X6
Thiopentone (sodium)	T41.1X1	T41.1X2	T41.1X3	T41.1X4	T41.1X5	T41.1X6
Thiopropazate	T43.3X1	T43.3X2	T43.3X3	T43.3X4	T43.3X5	T43.3X6
Thioproperazine	T43.3X1	T43.3X2	T43.3X3	T43.3X4	T43.3X5	T43.3X6
Thioridazine	T43.3X1	T43.3X2	T43.3X3	T43.3X4	T43.3X5	T43.3X6
Thiosinamine	T49.3X1	T49.3X2	T49.3X3	T49.3X4	T49.3X5	T49.3X6
Thiotepa	T45.1X1	T45.1X2	T45.1X3	T45.1X4	T45.1X5	T45.1X6
Thiothixene	T43.4X1	T43.4X2	T43.4X3	T43.4X4	T43.4X5	T43.4X6
Thiouracil (benzyl) (methyl) (propyl)	T38.2X1	T38.2X2	T38.2X3	T38.2X4	T38.2X5	T38.2X6
Thiourea	T38.2X1	T38.2X2	T38.2X3	T38.2X4	T38.2X5	T38.2X6
Thiphenamil	T44.3X1	T44.3X2	T44.3X3	T44.3X4	T44.3X5	T44.3X6
Thiram	T60.3X1	T60.3X2	T60.3X3	T60.3X4	—	—
medicinal	T49.2X1	T49.2X2	T49.2X3	T49.2X4	T49.2X5	T49.2X6
Thonzylamine (systemic)	T45.0X1	T45.0X2	T45.0X3	T45.0X4	T45.0X5	T45.0X6
mucosal decongestant	T48.5X1	T48.5X2	T48.5X3	T48.5X4	T48.5X5	T48.5X6
Thorazine	T43.3X1	T43.3X2	T43.3X3	T43.3X4	T43.3X5	T43.3X6
Thorium dioxide suspension	T50.8X1	T50.8X2	T50.8X3	T50.8X4	T50.8X5	T50.8X6
Thornapple	T62.2X1	T62.2X2	T62.2X3	T62.2X4	—	—
Throat drug NEC	T49.6X1	T49.6X2	T49.6X3	T49.6X4	T49.6X5	T49.6X6
Thrombin	T45.7X1	T45.7X2	T45.7X3	T45.7X4	T45.7X5	T45.7X6
Thrombolysin	T45.611	T45.612	T45.613	T45.614	T45.615	T45.616
Thromboplastin	T45.7X1	T45.7X2	T45.7X3	T45.7X4	T45.7X5	T45.7X6
Thurfyl nicotinate	T46.7X1	T46.7X2	T46.7X3	T46.7X4	T46.7X5	T46.7X6
Thymol	T49.0X1	T49.0X2	T49.0X3	T49.0X4	T49.0X5	T49.0X6
Thymopentin	T37.5X1	T37.5X2	T37.5X3	T37.5X4	T37.5X5	T37.5X6
Thymoxamine	T46.7X1	T46.7X2	T46.7X3	T46.7X4	T46.7X5	T46.7X6
Thymus extract	T38.891	T38.892	T38.893	T38.894	T38.895	T38.896
Thyreotrophic hormone	T38.811	T38.812	T38.813	T38.814	T38.815	T38.816
Thyroglobulin	T38.1X1	T38.1X2	T38.1X3	T38.1X4	T38.1X5	T38.1X6
Thyroid (hormone)	T38.1X1	T38.1X2	T38.1X3	T38.1X4	T38.1X5	T38.1X6
Thyrolar	T38.1X1	T38.1X2	T38.1X3	T38.1X4	T38.1X5	T38.1X6
Thyrotrophin	T38.811	T38.812	T38.813	T38.814	T38.815	T38.816
Thyrotropic hormone	T38.811	T38.812	T38.813	T38.814	T38.815	T38.816
Thyroxine	T38.1X1	T38.1X2	T38.1X3	T38.1X4	T38.1X5	T38.1X6
Tiabendazole	T37.4X1	T37.4X2	T37.4X3	T37.4X4	T37.4X5	T37.4X6
Tiamizide	T50.2X1	T50.2X2	T50.2X3	T50.2X4	T50.2X5	T50.2X6
Tianeptine	T43.291	T43.292	T43.293	T43.294	T43.295	T43.296
Tiapamil	T46.1X1	T46.1X2	T46.1X3	T46.1X4	T46.1X5	T46.1X6
Tiapride	T43.591	T43.592	T43.593	T43.594	T43.595	T43.596
Tiaprofenic acid	T39.311	T39.312	T39.313	T39.314	T39.315	T39.316
Tiaramide	T39.8X1	T39.8X2	T39.8X3	T39.8X4	T39.8X5	T39.8X6
Ticarcillin	T36.0X1	T36.0X2	T36.0X3	T36.0X4	T36.0X5	T36.0X6
Ticlatone	T49.0X1	T49.0X2	T49.0X3	T49.0X4	T49.0X5	T49.0X6
Ticlopidine	T45.521	T45.522	T45.523	T45.524	T45.525	T45.526
Ticrynafen	T50.1X1	T50.1X2	T50.1X3	T50.1X4	T50.1X5	T50.1X6
Tidiacic	T50.991	T50.992	T50.993	T50.994	T50.995	T50.996
Tiemonium	T44.3X1	T44.3X2	T44.3X3	T44.3X4	T44.3X5	T44.3X6
iodide	T44.3X1	T44.3X2	T44.3X3	T44.3X4	T44.3X5	T44.3X6
Tienilic acid	T50.1X1	T50.1X2	T50.1X3	T50.1X4	T50.1X5	T50.1X6
Tifenamil	T44.3X1	T44.3X2	T44.3X3	T44.3X4	T44.3X5	T44.3X6
Tigan	T45.0X1	T45.0X2	T45.0X3	T45.0X4	T45.0X5	T45.0X6
Tigloidine	T44.3X1	T44.3X2	T44.3X3	T44.3X4	T44.3X5	T44.3X6
Tilactase	T47.5X1	T47.5X2	T47.5X3	T47.5X4	T47.5X5	T47.5X6
Tiletamine	T41.291	T41.292	T41.293	T41.294	T41.295	T41.296
Tilidine	T40.441	T40.442	T40.443	T40.444	—	—
Timepidium bromide	T44.3X1	T44.3X2	T44.3X3	T44.3X4	T44.3X5	T44.3X6
Timiperone	T43.4X1	T43.4X2	T43.4X3	T43.4X4	T43.4X5	T43.4X6
Timolol	T44.7X1	T44.7X2	T44.7X3	T44.7X4	T44.7X5	T44.7X6
Tin (chloride) (dust) (oxide) NEC	T56.6X1	T56.6X2	T56.6X3	T56.6X4	—	—
anti-infectives	T37.8X1	T37.8X2	T37.8X3	T37.8X4	T37.8X5	T37.8X6
Tincture, iodine — *see Iodine*						
Tindal	T43.3X1	T43.3X2	T43.3X3	T43.3X4	T43.3X5	T43.3X6
Tinidazole	T37.3X1	T37.3X2	T37.3X3	T37.3X4	T37.3X5	T37.3X6
Tinoridine	T39.8X1	T39.8X2	T39.8X3	T39.8X4	T39.8X5	T39.8X6
Tiocarlide	T37.1X1	T37.1X2	T37.1X3	T37.1X4	T37.1X5	T37.1X6
Tioclomarol	T45.511	T45.512	T45.513	T45.514	T45.515	T45.516

Substance	External Cause (T-Code): Poisoning, Accidental (Unintentional)	Poisoning, Intentional Self-Harm	Poisoning, Assault	Poisoning, Undetermined	Adverse Effect	Underdosing
Tioconazole	T49.ØX1	T49.ØX2	T49.ØX3	T49.ØX4	T49.ØX5	T49.ØX6
Tioguanine	T45.1X1	T45.1X2	T45.1X3	T45.1X4	T45.1X5	T45.1X6
Tiopronin	T5Ø.991	T5Ø.992	T5Ø.993	T5Ø.994	T5Ø.995	T5Ø.996
Tiotixene	T43.4X1	T43.4X2	T43.4X3	T43.4X4	T43.4X5	T43.4X6
Tioxolone	T49.4X1	T49.4X2	T49.4X3	T49.4X4	T49.4X5	T49.4X6
Tipepidine	T48.3X1	T48.3X2	T48.3X3	T48.3X4	T48.3X5	T48.3X6
Tiquizium bromide	T44.3X1	T44.3X2	T44.3X3	T44.3X4	T44.3X5	T44.3X6
Tiratricol	T38.1X1	T38.1X2	T38.1X3	T38.1X4	T38.1X5	T38.1X6
Tisopurine	T5Ø.4X1	T5Ø.4X2	T5Ø.4X3	T5Ø.4X4	T5Ø.4X5	T5Ø.4X6
Titanium (compounds) (vapor)	T56.891	T56.892	T56.893	T56.894	—	—
dioxide	T49.3X1	T49.3X2	T49.3X3	T49.3X4	T49.3X5	T49.3X6
ointment	T49.3X1	T49.3X2	T49.3X3	T49.3X4	T49.3X5	T49.3X6
oxide	T49.3X1	T49.3X2	T49.3X3	T49.3X4	T49.3X5	T49.3X6
tetrachloride	T56.891	T56.892	T56.893	T56.894	—	—
Titanocene	T56.891	T56.892	T56.893	T56.894	—	—
Titroid	T38.1X1	T38.1X2	T38.1X3	T38.1X4	T38.1X5	T38.1X6
Tizanidine	T42.8X1	T42.8X2	T42.8X3	T42.8X4	T42.8X5	T42.8X6
TMTD	T6Ø.3X1	T6Ø.3X2	T6Ø.3X3	T6Ø.3X4	—	—
TNT (fumes)	T65.3X1	T65.3X2	T65.3X3	T65.3X4	—	—
Toadstool	T62.ØX1	T62.ØX2	T62.ØX3	T62.ØX4	—	—
Tobacco NEC	T65.291	T65.292	T65.293	T65.294	—	—
cigarettes	T65.221	T65.222	T65.223	T65.224	—	—
Indian	T62.2X1	T62.2X2	T62.2X3	T62.2X4	—	—
smoke, second-hand	T65.221	T65.222	T65.223	T65.224	—	—
Tobramycin	T36.5X1	T36.5X2	T36.5X3	T36.5X4	T36.5X5	T36.5X6
Tocainide	T46.2X1	T46.2X2	T46.2X3	T46.2X4	T46.2X5	T46.2X6
Tocoferol	T45.2X1	T45.2X2	T45.2X3	T45.2X4	T45.2X5	T45.2X6
Tocopherol	T45.2X1	T45.2X2	T45.2X3	T45.2X4	T45.2X5	T45.2X6
acetate	T45.2X1	T45.2X2	T45.2X3	T45.2X4	T45.2X5	T45.2X6
Tocosamine	T48.ØX1	T48.ØX2	T48.ØX3	T48.ØX4	T48.ØX5	T48.ØX6
Todralazine	T46.5X1	T46.5X2	T46.5X3	T46.5X4	T46.5X5	T46.5X6
Tofisopam	T42.4X1	T42.4X2	T42.4X3	T42.4X4	T42.4X5	T42.4X6
Tofranil	T43.Ø11	T43.Ø12	T43.Ø13	T43.Ø14	T43.Ø15	T43.Ø16
Toilet deodorizer	T65.891	T65.892	T65.893	T65.894	—	—
Tolamolol	T44.7X1	T44.7X2	T44.7X3	T44.7X4	T44.7X5	T44.7X6
Tolazamide	T38.3X1	T38.3X2	T38.3X3	T38.3X4	T38.3X5	T38.3X6
Tolazoline	T46.7X1	T46.7X2	T46.7X3	T46.7X4	T46.7X5	T46.7X6
Tolbutamide (sodium)	T38.3X1	T38.3X2	T38.3X3	T38.3X4	T38.3X5	T38.3X6
Tolciclate	T49.ØX1	T49.ØX2	T49.ØX3	T49.ØX4	T49.ØX5	T49.ØX6
Tolmetin	T39.391	T39.392	T39.393	T39.394	T39.395	T39.396
Tolnaftate	T49.ØX1	T49.ØX2	T49.ØX3	T49.ØX4	T49.ØX5	T49.ØX6
Tolonidine	T46.5X1	T46.5X2	T46.5X3	T46.5X4	T46.5X5	T46.5X6

Substance	External Cause (T-Code): Poisoning, Accidental (Unintentional)	Poisoning, Intentional Self-Harm	Poisoning, Assault	Poisoning, Undetermined	Adverse Effect	Underdosing
Toloxatone	T42.6X1	T42.6X2	T42.6X3	T42.6X4	T42.6X5	T42.6X6
Tolperisone	T44.3X1	T44.3X2	T44.3X3	T44.3X4	T44.3X5	T44.3X6
Tolserol	T42.8X1	T42.8X2	T42.8X3	T42.8X4	T42.8X5	T42.8X6
Toluene (liquid)	T52.2X1	T52.2X2	T52.2X3	T52.2X4	—	—
diisocyanate	T65.ØX1	T65.ØX2	T65.ØX3	T65.ØX4	—	—
Toluidine	T65.891	T65.892	T65.893	T65.894	—	—
vapor	T59.891	T59.892	T59.893	T59.894	—	—
Toluol (liquid)	T52.2X1	T52.2X2	T52.2X3	T52.2X4	—	—
vapor	T52.2X1	T52.2X2	T52.2X3	T52.2X4	—	—
Toluylenediamine	T65.3X1	T65.3X2	T65.3X3	T65.3X4	—	—
Tolylene-2,4-diisocyanate	T65.ØX1	T65.ØX2	T65.ØX3	T65.ØX4	—	—
Tonic NEC	T5Ø.9Ø1	T5Ø.9Ø2	T5Ø.9Ø3	T5Ø.9Ø4	T5Ø.9Ø5	T5Ø.9Ø6
Topical action drug NEC	T49.91	T49.92	T49.93	T49.94	T49.95	T49.96
ear, nose or throat	T49.6X1	T49.6X2	T49.6X3	T49.6X4	T49.6X5	T49.6X6
eye	T49.5X1	T49.5X2	T49.5X3	T49.5X4	T49.5X5	T49.5X6
skin	T49.91	T49.92	T49.93	T49.94	T49.95	T49.96
specified NEC	T49.8X1	T49.8X2	T49.8X3	T49.8X4	T49.8X5	T49.8X6
Toquizine	T44.3X1	T44.3X2	T44.3X3	T44.3X4	T44.3X5	T44.3X6
Toremifene	T38.6X1	T38.6X2	T38.6X3	T38.6X4	T38.6X5	T38.6X6
Tosylchloramide sodium	T49.8X1	T49.8X2	T49.8X3	T49.8X4	T49.8X5	T49.8X6
Toxaphene (dust) (spray)	T6Ø.1X1	T6Ø.1X2	T6Ø.1X3	T6Ø.1X4	—	—
Toxin, diphtheria (Schick Test)	T5Ø.8X1	T5Ø.8X2	T5Ø.8X3	T5Ø.8X4	T5Ø.8X5	T5Ø.8X6
Toxoid						
combined	T5Ø.A21	T5Ø.A22	T5Ø.A23	T5Ø.A24	T5Ø.A25	T5Ø.A26
diphtheria	T5Ø.A91	T5Ø.A92	T5Ø.A93	T5Ø.A94	T5Ø.A95	T5Ø.A96
tetanus	T5Ø.A91	T5Ø.A92	T5Ø.A93	T5Ø.A94	T5Ø.A95	T5Ø.A96
Trace element NEC	T45.8X1	T45.8X2	T45.8X3	T45.8X4	T45.8X5	T45.8X6
Tractor fuel NEC	T52.ØX1	T52.ØX2	T52.ØX3	T52.ØX4	—	—
Tragacanth	T5Ø.991	T5Ø.992	T5Ø.993	T5Ø.994	T5Ø.995	T5Ø.996
Tramadol	T4Ø.421	T4Ø.422	T4Ø.423	T4Ø.424	T4Ø.425	T4Ø.426
Tramazoline	T48.5X1	T48.5X2	T48.5X3	T48.5X4	T48.5X5	T48.5X6
Tranexamic acid	T45.621	T45.622	T45.623	T45.624	T45.625	T45.626
Tranilast	T45.ØX1	T45.ØX2	T45.ØX3	T45.ØX4	T45.ØX5	T45.ØX6
Tranquilizer NEC	T43.5Ø1	T43.5Ø2	T43.5Ø3	T43.5Ø4	T43.5Ø5	T43.5Ø6
with hypnotic or sedative	T42.6X1	T42.6X2	T42.6X3	T42.6X4	T42.6X5	T42.6X6
benzodiazepine NEC	T42.4X1	T42.4X2	T42.4X3	T42.4X4	T42.4X5	T42.4X6
butyrophenone NEC	T43.4X1	T43.4X2	T43.4X3	T43.4X4	T43.4X5	T43.4X6
carbamate	T43.591	T43.592	T43.593	T43.594	T43.595	T43.596
dimethylamine	T43.3X1	T43.3X2	T43.3X3	T43.3X4	T43.3X5	T43.3X6
ethylamine	T43.3X1	T43.3X2	T43.3X3	T43.3X4	T43.3X5	T43.3X6
hydroxyzine	T43.591	T43.592	T43.593	T43.594	T43.595	T43.596
major NEC	T43.5Ø1	T43.5Ø2	T43.5Ø3	T43.5Ø4	T43.5Ø5	T43.5Ø6

Substance	External Cause (T-Code) Poisoning, Accidental (Unintentional)	Poisoning, Intentional Self-Harm	Poisoning, Assault	Poisoning, Undetermined	Adverse Effect	Underdosing
Tranquilizer NEC *(Continued)*						
penothiazine NEC	T43.3X1	T43.3X2	T43.3X3	T43.3X4	T43.3X5	T43.3X6
phenothiazine-based	T43.3X1	T43.3X2	T43.3X3	T43.3X4	T43.3X5	T43.3X6
piperazine NEC	T43.3X1	T43.3X2	T43.3X3	T43.3X4	T43.3X5	T43.3X6
piperidine	T43.3X1	T43.3X2	T43.3X3	T43.3X4	T43.3X5	T43.3X6
propylamine	T43.3X1	T43.3X2	T43.3X3	T43.3X4	T43.3X5	T43.3X6
specified NEC	T43.591	T43.592	T43.593	T43.594	T43.595	T43.596
thioxanthene NEC	T43.591	T43.592	T43.593	T43.594	T43.595	T43.596
Tranxene	T42.4X1	T42.4X2	T42.4X3	T42.4X4	T42.4X5	T42.4X6
Tranylcypromine	T43.1X1	T43.1X2	T43.1X3	T43.1X4	T43.1X5	T43.1X6
Trapidil	T46.3X1	T46.3X2	T46.3X3	T46.3X4	T46.3X5	T46.3X6
Trasentine	T44.3X1	T44.3X2	T44.3X3	T44.3X4	T44.3X5	T44.3X6
Travert	T50.3X1	T50.3X2	T50.3X3	T50.3X4	T50.3X5	T50.3X6
Trazodone	T43.211	T43.212	T43.213	T43.214	T43.215	T43.216
Trecator	T37.1X1	T37.1X2	T37.1X3	T37.1X4	T37.1X5	T37.1X6
Treosulfan	T45.1X1	T45.1X2	T45.1X3	T45.1X4	T45.1X5	T45.1X6
Tretamine	T45.1X1	T45.1X2	T45.1X3	T45.1X4	T45.1X5	T45.1X6
Tretinoin	T49.0X1	T49.0X2	T49.0X3	T49.0X4	T49.0X5	T49.0X6
Tretoquinol	T48.6X1	T48.6X2	T48.6X3	T48.6X4	T48.6X5	T48.6X6
Triacetin	T49.0X1	T49.0X2	T49.0X3	T49.0X4	T49.0X5	T49.0X6
Triacetoxyanthracene	T49.4X1	T49.4X2	T49.4X3	T49.4X4	T49.4X5	T49.4X6
Triacetyloleandomycin	T36.3X1	T36.3X2	T36.3X3	T36.3X4	T36.3X5	T36.3X6
Triamcinolone	T38.0X1	T38.0X2	T38.0X3	T38.0X4	T38.0X5	T38.0X6
ENT agent	T49.6X1	T49.6X2	T49.6X3	T49.6X4	T49.6X5	T49.6X6
hexacetonide	T49.0X1	T49.0X2	T49.0X3	T49.0X4	T49.0X5	T49.0X6
ophthalmic preparation	T49.5X1	T49.5X2	T49.5X3	T49.5X4	T49.5X5	T49.5X6
topical NEC	T49.0X1	T49.0X2	T49.0X3	T49.0X4	T49.0X5	T49.0X6
Triampyzine	T44.3X1	T44.3X2	T44.3X3	T44.3X4	T44.3X5	T44.3X6
Triamterene	T50.2X1	T50.2X2	T50.2X3	T50.2X4	T50.2X5	T50.2X6
Triazine (herbicide)	T60.3X1	T60.3X2	T60.3X3	T60.3X4	—	—
Triaziquone	T45.1X1	T45.1X2	T45.1X3	T45.1X4	T45.1X5	T45.1X6
Triazolam	T42.4X1	T42.4X2	T42.4X3	T42.4X4	T42.4X5	T42.4X6
Triazole (herbicide)	T60.3X1	T60.3X2	T60.3X3	T60.3X4	—	—
Tribenoside	T46.991	T46.992	T46.993	T46.994	T46.995	T46.996
Tribromacetaldehyde	T42.6X1	T42.6X2	T42.6X3	T42.6X4	T42.6X5	T42.6X6
Tribromoethanol, rectal	T41.291	T41.292	T41.293	T41.294	T41.295	T41.296
Tribromomethane	T42.6X1	T42.6X2	T42.6X3	T42.6X4	T42.6X5	T42.6X6
Trichlorethane	T53.2X1	T53.2X2	T53.2X3	T53.2X4	—	—
Trichlorethylene	T53.2X1	T53.2X2	T53.2X3	T53.2X4	—	—
Trichlorfon	T60.0X1	T60.0X2	T60.0X3	T60.0X4	—	—
Trichlormethiazide	T50.2X1	T50.2X2	T50.2X3	T50.2X4	T50.2X5	T50.2X6
Trichlormethine	T45.1X1	T45.1X2	T45.1X3	T45.1X4	T45.1X5	T45.1X6
Trichloroacetic acid, Trichloracetic acid	T54.2X1	T54.2X2	T54.2X3	T54.2X4	—	—
medicinal	T49.4X1	T49.4X2	T49.4X3	T49.4X4	T49.4X5	T49.4X6
Trichloroethane	T53.2X1	T53.2X2	T53.2X3	T53.2X4	—	—
Trichloroethanol	T42.6X1	T42.6X2	T42.6X3	T42.6X4	T42.6X5	T42.6X6
Trichloroethylene (liquid) (vapor)	T53.2X1	T53.2X2	T53.2X3	T53.2X4	—	—
anesthetic (gas)	T41.0X1	T41.0X2	T41.0X3	T41.0X4	T41.0X5	T41.0X6
vapor NEC	T53.2X1	T53.2X2	T53.2X3	T53.2X4	—	—
Trichloroethyl phosphate	T42.6X1	T42.6X2	T42.6X3	T42.6X4	T42.6X5	T42.6X6
Trichlorofluoromethane NEC	T53.5X1	T53.5X2	T53.5X3	T53.5X4	—	—
Trichloronate	T60.0X1	T60.0X2	T60.0X3	T60.0X4	—	—
2,4,5-Trichlorophen-oxyacetic acid	T60.3X1	T60.3X2	T60.3X3	T60.3X4	—	—
Trichloropropane	T53.6X1	T53.6X2	T53.6X3	T53.6X4	—	—
Trichlorotriethylamine	T45.1X1	T45.1X2	T45.1X3	T45.1X4	T45.1X5	T45.1X6
Trichomonacides NEC	T37.3X1	T37.3X2	T37.3X3	T37.3X4	T37.3X5	T37.3X6
Trichomycin	T36.7X1	T36.7X2	T36.7X3	T36.7X4	T36.7X5	T36.7X6
Triclobisonium chloride	T49.0X1	T49.0X2	T49.0X3	T49.0X4	T49.0X5	T49.0X6
Triclocarban	T49.0X1	T49.0X2	T49.0X3	T49.0X4	T49.0X5	T49.0X6
Triclofos	T42.6X1	T42.6X2	T42.6X3	T42.6X4	T42.6X5	T42.6X6
Triclosan	T49.0X1	T49.0X2	T49.0X3	T49.0X4	T49.0X5	T49.0X6
Tricresyl phosphate	T65.891	T65.892	T65.893	T65.894	—	—
solvent	T52.91	T52.92	T52.93	T52.94	—	—
Tricyclamol chloride	T44.3X1	T44.3X2	T44.3X3	T44.3X4	T44.3X5	T44.3X6
Tridesilon	T49.0X1	T49.0X2	T49.0X3	T49.0X4	T49.0X5	T49.0X6
Tridihexethyl iodide	T44.3X1	T44.3X2	T44.3X3	T44.3X4	T44.3X5	T44.3X6
Tridione	T42.2X1	T42.2X2	T42.2X3	T42.2X4	T42.2X5	T42.2X6
Trientine	T45.8X1	T45.8X2	T45.8X3	T45.8X4	T45.8X5	T45.8X6
Triethanolamine NEC	T54.3X1	T54.3X2	T54.3X3	T54.3X4	—	—
detergent	T54.3X1	T54.3X2	T54.3X3	T54.3X4	—	—
trinitrate (biphosphate)	T46.3X1	T46.3X2	T46.3X3	T46.3X4	T46.3X5	T46.3X6
Triethanomelamine	T45.1X1	T45.1X2	T45.1X3	T45.1X4	T45.1X5	T45.1X6
Triethylenemelamine	T45.1X1	T45.1X2	T45.1X3	T45.1X4	T45.1X5	T45.1X6
Triethylenephosphoramide	T45.1X1	T45.1X2	T45.1X3	T45.1X4	T45.1X5	T45.1X6
Triethylenethiophosphoramide	T45.1X1	T45.1X2	T45.1X3	T45.1X4	T45.1X5	T45.1X6
Trifluoperazine	T43.3X1	T43.3X2	T43.3X3	T43.3X4	T43.3X5	T43.3X6
Trifluoroethyl vinyl ether	T41.0X1	T41.0X2	T41.0X3	T41.0X4	T41.0X5	T41.0X6
Trifluperidol	T43.4X1	T43.4X2	T43.4X3	T43.4X4	T43.4X5	T43.4X6
Triflupromazine	T43.3X1	T43.3X2	T43.3X3	T43.3X4	T43.3X5	T43.3X6
Trifluridine	T37.5X1	T37.5X2	T37.5X3	T37.5X4	T37.5X5	T37.5X6
Triflusal	T45.521	T45.522	T45.523	T45.524	T45.525	T45.526
Trihexyphenidyl	T44.3X1	T44.3X2	T44.3X3	T44.3X4	T44.3X5	T44.3X6
Triiodothyronine	T38.1X1	T38.1X2	T38.1X3	T38.1X4	T38.1X5	T38.1X6

TABLE OF DRUGS AND CHEMICALS

Substance	External Cause (T-Code)					
	Poisoning, Accidental (Unintentional)	Poisoning, Intentional Self-Harm	Poisoning, Assault	Poisoning, Undetermined	Adverse Effect	Underdosing
Trilene	T41.0X1	T41.0X2	T41.0X3	T41.0X4	T41.0X5	T41.0X6
Trilostane	T38.991	T38.992	T38.993	T38.994	T38.995	T38.996
Trimebutine	T44.3X1	T44.3X2	T44.3X3	T44.3X4	T44.3X5	T44.3X6
Trimecaine	T41.3X1	T41.3X2	T41.3X3	T41.3X4	T41.3X5	T41.3X6
Trimeprazine (tartrate)	T44.3X1	T44.3X2	T44.3X3	T44.3X4	T44.3X5	T44.3X6
Trimetaphan camsilate	T44.2X1	T44.2X2	T44.2X3	T44.2X4	T44.2X5	T44.2X6
Trimetazidine	T46.7X1	T46.7X2	T46.7X3	T46.7X4	T46.7X5	T46.7X6
Trimethadione	T42.2X1	T42.2X2	T42.2X3	T42.2X4	T42.2X5	T42.2X6
Trimethaphan	T44.2X1	T44.2X2	T44.2X3	T44.2X4	T44.2X5	T44.2X6
Trimethidinium	T44.2X1	T44.2X2	T44.2X3	T44.2X4	T44.2X5	T44.2X6
Trimethobenzamide	T45.0X1	T45.0X2	T45.0X3	T45.0X4	T45.0X5	T45.0X6
Trimethoprim	T37.8X1	T37.8X2	T37.8X3	T37.8X4	T37.8X5	T37.8X6
with sulfamethoxazole	T36.8X1	T36.8X2	T36.8X3	T36.8X4	T36.8X5	T36.8X6
Trimethylcarbinol	T51.3X1	T51.3X2	T51.3X3	T51.3X4	—	—
Trimethylpsoralen	T49.3X1	T49.3X2	T49.3X3	T49.3X4	T49.3X5	T49.3X6
Trimeton	T45.0X1	T45.0X2	T45.0X3	T45.0X4	T45.0X5	T45.0X6
Trimetrexate	T45.1X1	T45.1X2	T45.1X3	T45.1X4	T45.1X5	T45.1X6
Trimipramine	T43.011	T43.012	T43.013	T43.014	T43.015	T43.016
Trimustine	T45.1X1	T45.1X2	T45.1X3	T45.1X4	T45.1X5	T45.1X6
Trinitrine	T46.3X1	T46.3X2	T46.3X3	T46.3X4	T46.3X5	T46.3X6
Trinitrobenzol	T65.3X1	T65.3X2	T65.3X3	T65.3X4	—	—
Trinitrophenol	T65.3X1	T65.3X2	T65.3X3	T65.3X4	—	—
Trinitrotoluene (fumes)	T65.3X1	T65.3X2	T65.3X3	T65.3X4	—	—
Trional	T42.6X1	T42.6X2	T42.6X3	T42.6X4	T42.6X5	T42.6X6
Triorthocresyl phosphate	T65.891	T65.892	T65.893	T65.894	—	—
Trioxide of arsenic	T57.0X1	T57.0X2	T57.0X3	T57.0X4	—	—
Trioxysalen	T49.4X1	T49.4X2	T49.4X3	T49.4X4	T49.4X5	T49.4X6
Tripamide	T50.2X1	T50.2X2	T50.2X3	T50.2X4	T50.2X5	T50.2X6
Triparanol	T46.6X1	T46.6X2	T46.6X3	T46.6X4	T46.6X5	T46.6X6
Tripelennamine	T45.0X1	T45.0X2	T45.0X3	T45.0X4	T45.0X5	T45.0X6
Triperiden	T44.3X1	T44.3X2	T44.3X3	T44.3X4	T44.3X5	T44.3X6
Triperidol	T43.4X1	T43.4X2	T43.4X3	T43.4X4	T43.4X5	T43.4X6
Triphenylphosphate	T65.891	T65.892	T65.893	T65.894	—	—
Triple						
bromides	T42.6X1	T42.6X2	T42.6X3	T42.6X4	T42.6X5	T42.6X6
carbonate	T47.1X1	T47.1X2	T47.1X3	T47.1X4	T47.1X5	T47.1X6
vaccine						
DPT	T50.A11	T50.A12	T50.A13	T50.A14	T50.A15	T50.A16
including pertussis	T50.A11	T50.A12	T50.A13	T50.A14	T50.A15	T50.A16
MMR	T50.B91	T50.B92	—	—	—	—
Triprolidine	T45.0X1	T45.0X2	T45.0X3	T45.0X4	T45.0X5	T45.0X6
Trisodium hydrogen edetate	T50.6X1	T50.6X2	T50.6X3	T50.6X4	T50.6X5	T50.6X6
Trisoralen	T49.3X1	T49.3X2	T49.3X3	T49.3X4	T49.3X5	T49.3X6
Trisulfapyrimidines	T37.0X1	T37.0X2	T37.0X3	T37.0X4	T37.0X5	T37.0X6
Trithiozine	T44.3X1	T44.3X2	T44.3X3	T44.3X4	T44.3X5	T44.3X6
Tritiozine	T44.3X1	T44.3X2	T44.3X3	T44.3X4	T44.3X5	T44.3X6
Tritoqualine	T45.0X1	T45.0X2	T45.0X3	T45.0X4	T45.0X5	T45.0X6
Trofosfamide	T45.1X1	T45.1X2	T45.1X3	T45.1X4	T45.1X5	T45.1X6
Troleandomycin	T36.3X1	T36.3X2	T36.3X3	T36.3X4	T36.3X5	T36.3X6
Trolnitrate (phosphate)	T46.3X1	T46.3X2	T46.3X3	T46.3X4	T46.3X5	T46.3X6
Tromantadine	T37.5X1	T37.5X2	T37.5X3	T37.5X4	T37.5X5	T37.5X6
Trometamol	T50.2X1	T50.2X2	T50.2X3	T50.2X4	T50.2X5	T50.2X6
Tromethamine	T50.2X1	T50.2X2	T50.2X3	T50.2X4	T50.2X5	T50.2X6
Tronothane	T41.3X1	T41.3X2	T41.3X3	T41.3X4	T41.3X5	T41.3X6
Tropacine	T44.3X1	T44.3X2	T44.3X3	T44.3X4	T44.3X5	T44.3X6
Tropatepine	T44.3X1	T44.3X2	T44.3X3	T44.3X4	T44.3X5	T44.3X6
Tropicamide	T44.3X1	T44.3X2	T44.3X3	T44.3X4	T44.3X5	T44.3X6
Trospium chloride	T44.3X1	T44.3X2	T44.3X3	T44.3X4	T44.3X5	T44.3X6
Troxerutin	T46.991	T46.992	T46.993	T46.994	T46.995	T46.996
Troxidone	T42.2X1	T42.2X2	T42.2X3	T42.2X4	T42.2X5	T42.2X6
Tryparsamide	T37.3X1	T37.3X2	T37.3X3	T37.3X4	T37.3X5	T37.3X6
Trypsin	T45.3X1	T45.3X2	T45.3X3	T45.3X4	T45.3X5	T45.3X6
Tryptizol	T43.011	T43.012	T43.013	T43.014	T43.015	T43.016
TSH	T38.811	T38.812	T38.813	T38.814	T38.815	T38.816
Tuaminoheptane	T48.5X1	T48.5X2	T48.5X3	T48.5X4	T48.5X5	T48.5X6
Tuberculin, purified protein derivative (PPD)	T50.8X1	T50.8X2	T50.8X3	T50.8X4	T50.8X5	T50.8X6
Tubocurare	T48.1X1	T48.1X2	T48.1X3	T48.1X4	T48.1X5	T48.1X6
Tubocurarine (chloride)	T48.1X1	T48.1X2	T48.1X3	T48.1X4	T48.1X5	T48.1X6
Tulobuterol	T48.6X1	T48.6X2	T48.6X3	T48.6X4	T48.6X5	T48.6X6
Turpentine (spirits of)	T52.8X1	T52.8X2	T52.8X3	T52.8X4	—	—
vapor	T52.8X1	T52.8X2	T52.8X3	T52.8X4	—	—
Tybamate	T43.591	T43.592	T43.593	T43.594	T43.595	T43.596
Tyloxapol	T48.4X1	T48.4X2	T48.4X3	T48.4X4	T48.4X5	T48.4X6
Tymazoline	T48.5X1	T48.5X2	T48.5X3	T48.5X4	T48.5X5	T48.5X6
Typhoid-paratyphoid vaccine	T50.A91	T50.A92	T50.A93	T50.A94	T50.A95	T50.A96
Typhus vaccine	T50.A91	T50.A92	T50.A93	T50.A94	T50.A95	T50.A96
Tyropanoate	T50.8X1	T50.8X2	T50.8X3	T50.8X4	T50.8X5	T50.8X6
Tyrothricin	T49.6X1	T49.6X2	T49.6X3	T49.6X4	T49.6X5	T49.6X6
ENT agent	T49.6X1	T49.6X2	T49.6X3	T49.6X4	T49.6X5	T49.6X6
ophthalmic preparation	T49.5X1	T49.5X2	T49.5X3	T49.5X4	T49.5X5	T49.5X6
U						
Ufenamate	T39.391	T39.392	T39.393	T39.394	T39.395	T39.396
Ultraviolet light protectant	T49.3X1	T49.3X2	T49.3X3	T49.3X4	T49.3X5	T49.3X6

Substance	External Cause (T-Code)					
	Poisoning, Accidental (Unintentional)	Poisoning, Intentional Self-Harm	Poisoning, Assault	Poisoning, Undetermined	Adverse Effect	Underdosing
Undecenoic acid	T49.0X1	T49.0X2	T49.0X3	T49.0X4	T49.0X5	T49.0X6
Undecoylium	T49.0X1	T49.0X2	T49.0X3	T49.0X4	T49.0X5	T49.0X6
Undecylenic acid (derivatives)	T49.0X1	T49.0X2	T49.0X3	T49.0X4	T49.0X5	T49.0X6
Unna's boot	T49.3X1	T49.3X2	T49.3X3	T49.3X4	T49.3X5	T49.3X6
Unsaturated fatty acid	T46.6X1	T46.6X2	T46.6X3	T46.6X4	T46.6X5	T46.6X6
Uracil mustard	T45.1X1	T45.1X2	T45.1X3	T45.1X4	T45.1X5	T45.1X6
Uramustine	T45.1X1	T45.1X2	T45.1X3	T45.1X4	T45.1X5	T45.1X6
Urapidil	T46.5X1	T46.5X2	T46.5X3	T46.5X4	T46.5X5	T46.5X6
Urari	T48.1X1	T48.1X2	T48.1X3	T48.1X4	T48.1X5	T48.1X6
Urate oxidase	T50.4X1	T50.4X2	T50.4X3	T50.4X4	T50.4X5	T50.4X6
Urea	T47.3X1	T47.3X2	T47.3X3	T47.3X4	T47.3X5	T47.3X6
peroxide	T49.0X1	T49.0X2	T49.0X3	T49.0X4	T49.0X5	T49.0X6
stibamine	T37.4X1	T37.4X2	T37.4X3	T37.4X4	T37.4X5	T37.4X6
topical	T49.8X1	T49.8X2	T49.8X3	T49.8X4	T49.8X5	T49.8X6
Urethane	T45.1X1	T45.1X2	T45.1X3	T45.1X4	T45.1X5	T45.1X6
Urginea (maritima) (scilla) — *see Squill*						
Uric acid metabolism drug NEC	T50.4X1	T50.4X2	T50.4X3	T50.4X4	T50.4X5	T50.4X6
Uricosuric agent	T50.4X1	T50.4X2	T50.4X3	T50.4X4	T50.4X5	T50.4X6
Urinary anti-infective	T37.8X1	T37.8X2	T37.8X3	T37.8X4	T37.8X5	T37.8X6
Urofollitropin	T38.811	T38.812	T38.813	T38.814	T38.815	T38.816
Urokinase	T45.611	T45.612	T45.613	T45.614	T45.615	T45.616
Urokon	T50.8X1	T50.8X2	T50.8X3	T50.8X4	T50.8X5	T50.8X6
Ursodeoxycholic acid	T50.991	T50.992	T50.993	T50.994	T50.995	T50.996
Ursodiol	T50.991	T50.992	T50.993	T50.994	T50.995	T50.996
Urtica	T62.2X1	T62.2X2	T62.2X3	T62.2X4	—	—
Utility gas — *see Gas, utility*						
V						
Vaccine NEC	T50.Z91	T50.Z92	T50.Z93	T50.Z94	T50.Z95	T50.Z96
antineoplastic	T50.Z91	T50.Z92	T50.Z93	T50.Z94	T50.Z95	T50.Z96
bacterial NEC	T50.A91	T50.A92	T50.A93	T50.A94	T50.A95	T50.A96
with						
other bacterial component	T50.A91	T50.A92	T50.A93	T50.A94	T50.A95	T50.A96
pertussis component	T50.A91	T50.A92	T50.A93	T50.A94	T50.A95	T50.A96
viral-rickettsial component	T50.A91	T50.A92	T50.A93	T50.A94	T50.A95	T50.A96
mixed NEC	T50.A91	T50.A92	T50.A93	T50.A94	T50.A95	T50.A96
BCG	T50.A91	T50.A92	T50.A93	T50.A94	T50.A95	T50.A96
cholera	T50.A91	T50.A92	T50.A93	T50.A94	T50.A95	T50.A96
diphtheria	T50.A91	T50.A92	T50.A93	T50.A94	T50.A95	T50.A96
with tetanus	T50.A21	T50.A22	T50.A23	T50.A24	T50.A25	T50.A26
and pertussis	T50.A11	T50.A12	T50.A13	T50.A14	T50.A15	T50.A16
Vaccine NEC *(Continued)*						
influenza	T50.B91	T50.B92	T50.B93	T50.B94	T50.B95	T50.B96
measles	T50.B91	T50.B92	T50.B93	T50.B94	T50.B95	T50.B96
with mumps and rubella	T50.B91	T50.B92	T50.B93	T50.B94	T50.B95	T50.B96
meningococcal	T50.A91	T50.A92	T50.A93	T50.A94	T50.A95	T50.A96
mumps	T50.B91	T50.B92	T50.B93	T50.B94	T50.B95	T50.B96
paratyphoid	T50.A91	T50.A92	T50.A93	T50.A94	T50.A95	T50.A96
pertussis	T50.A11	T50.A12	T50.A13	T50.A14	T50.A15	T50.A16
with diphtheria	T50.A11	T50.A12	T50.A13	T50.A14	T50.A15	T50.A16
and tetanus	T50.A11	T50.A12	T50.A13	T50.A14	T50.A15	T50.A16
plague	T50.A91	T50.A92	T50.A93	T50.A94	T50.A95	T50.A96
poliomyelitis	T50.B91	T50.B92	T50.B93	T50.B94	T50.B95	T50.B96
poliovirus	T50.B91	T50.B92	T50.B93	T50.B94	T50.B95	T50.B96
rabies	T50.B91	T50.B92	T50.B93	T50.B94	T50.B95	T50.B96
respiratory syncytial virus	T50.B91	T50.B92	T50.B93	T50.B94	T50.B95	T50.B96
rickettsial NEC	T50.A91	T50.A92	T50.A93	T50.A94	T50.A95	T50.A96
with						
bacterial component	T50.A21	T50.A22	T50.A23	T50.A24	T50.A25	T50.A26
Rocky Mountain spotted fever	T50.A91	T50.A92	T50.A93	T50.A94	T50.A95	T50.A96
rubella	T50.B91	T50.B92	T50.B93	T50.B94	T50.B95	T50.B96
sabin oral	T50.B91	T50.B92	T50.B93	T50.B94	T50.B95	T50.B96
smallpox	T50.B11	T50.B12	T50.B13	T50.B14	T50.B15	T50.B16
TAB	T50.A91	T50.A92	T50.A93	T50.A94	T50.A95	T50.A96
tetanus	T50.A91	T50.A92	T50.A93	T50.A94	T50.A95	T50.A96
typhoid	T50.A91	T50.A92	T50.A93	T50.A94	T50.A95	T50.A96
typhus	T50.A91	T50.A92	T50.A93	T50.A94	T50.A95	T50.A96
viral NEC	T50.B91	T50.B92	T50.B93	T50.B94	T50.B95	T50.B96
yellow fever	T50.B91	T50.B92	T50.B93	T50.B94	T50.B95	T50.B96
Vaccinia immune globulin	T50.Z11	T50.Z12	T50.Z13	T50.Z14	T50.Z15	T50.Z16
Vaginal contraceptives	T49.8X1	T49.8X2	T49.8X3	T49.8X4	T49.8X5	T49.8X6
Valerian						
root	T42.6X1	T42.6X2	T42.6X3	T42.6X4	T42.6X5	T42.6X6
tincture	T42.6X1	T42.6X2	T42.6X3	T42.6X4	T42.6X5	T42.6X6
Valethamate bromide	T44.3X1	T44.3X2	T44.3X3	T44.3X4	T44.3X5	T44.3X6
Valisone	T49.0X1	T49.0X2	T49.0X3	T49.0X4	T49.0X5	T49.0X6
Valium	T42.4X1	T42.4X2	T42.4X3	T42.4X4	T42.4X5	T42.4X6
Valmid	T42.6X1	T42.6X2	T42.6X3	T42.6X4	T42.6X5	T42.6X6
Valnoctamide	T42.6X1	T42.6X2	T42.6X3	T42.6X4	T42.6X5	T42.6X6
Valproate (sodium)	T42.6X1	T42.6X2	T42.6X3	T42.6X4	T42.6X5	T42.6X6
Valproic acid	T42.6X1	T42.6X2	T42.6X3	T42.6X4	T42.6X5	T42.6X6
Valpromide	T42.6X1	T42.6X2	T42.6X3	T42.6X4	T42.6X5	T42.6X6
Vanadium	T56.891	T56.892	T56.893	T56.894	—	—

Substance	External Cause (T-Code) Poisoning, Accidental (Unintentional)	Poisoning, Intentional Self-Harm	Poisoning, Assault	Poisoning, Undetermined	Adverse Effect	Underdosing
Vancomycin	T36.8X1	T36.8X2	T36.8X3	T36.8X4	T36.8X5	T36.8X6
Vapor — *see also Gas*	T59.91	T59.92	T59.93	T59.94	—	—
kiln (carbon monoxide)	T58.8X1	T58.8X2	T58.8X3	T58.8X4	—	—
lead — *see Lead*						
specified source NEC	T59.891	T59.892	T59.893	T59.894	—	—
Vardenafil	T46.7X1	T46.7X2	T46.7X3	T46.7X4	T46.7X5	T46.7X6
Varicose reduction drug	T46.8X1	T46.8X2	T46.8X3	T46.8X4	T46.8X5	T46.8X6
Varnish	T65.4X1	T65.4X2	T65.4X3	T65.4X4	—	—
cleaner	T52.91	T52.92	T52.93	T52.94	—	—
Vaseline	T49.3X1	T49.3X2	T49.3X3	T49.3X4	T49.3X5	T49.3X6
Vasodilan	T46.7X1	T46.7X2	T46.7X3	T46.7X4	T46.7X5	T46.7X6
Vasodilator						
coronary NEC	T46.3X1	T46.3X2	T46.3X3	T46.3X4	T46.3X5	T46.3X6
peripheral NEC	T46.7X1	T46.7X2	T46.7X3	T46.7X4	T46.7X5	T46.7X6
Vasopressin	T38.891	T38.892	T38.893	T38.894	T38.895	T38.896
Vasopressor drugs	T38.891	T38.892	T38.893	T38.894	T38.895	T38.896
Vecuronium bromide	T48.1X1	T48.1X2	T48.1X3	T48.1X4	T48.1X5	T48.1X6
Vegetable extract, astringent	T49.2X1	T49.2X2	T49.2X3	T49.2X4	T49.2X5	T49.2X6
Venlafaxine	T43.211	T43.212	T43.213	T43.214	T43.215	T43.216
Venom, venomous (bite) (sting)	T63.91	T63.92	T63.93	T63.94	—	—
amphibian NEC	T63.831	T63.832	T63.833	T63.834	—	—
animal NEC	T63.891	T63.892	T63.893	T63.894	—	—
ant	T63.421	T63.422	T63.423	T63.424	—	—
arthropod NEC	T63.481	T63.482	T63.483	T63.484	—	—
bee	T63.441	T63.442	T63.443	T63.444	—	—
centipede	T63.411	T63.412	T63.413	T63.414	—	—
fish	T63.591	T63.592	T63.593	T63.594	—	—
frog	T63.811	T63.812	T63.813	T63.814	—	—
hornet	T63.451	T63.452	T63.453	T63.454	—	—
insect NEC	T63.481	T63.482	T63.483	T63.484	—	—
lizard	T63.121	T63.122	T63.123	T63.124	—	—
marine						
animals	T63.691	T63.692	T63.693	T63.694	—	—
bluebottle	T63.611	T63.612	T63.613	T63.614	—	—
jellyfish NEC	T63.621	T63.622	T63.623	T63.624	—	—
Portuguese Man-o-war	T63.611	T63.612	T63.613	T63.614	—	—
sea anemone	T63.631	T63.632	T63.633	T63.634	—	—
specified NEC	T63.691	T63.692	T63.693	T63.694	—	—
fish	T63.591	T63.592	T63.593	T63.594	—	—
plants	T63.711	T63.712	T63.713	T63.714	—	—
sting ray	T63.511	T63.512	T63.513	T63.514	—	—
Venom, venomous *(Continued)*						
millipede (tropical)	T63.411	T63.412	T63.413	T63.414	—	—
plant NEC	T63.791	T63.792	T63.793	T63.794	—	—
marine	T63.711	T63.712	T63.713	T63.714	—	—
reptile	T63.191	T63.192	T63.193	T63.194	—	—
gila monster	T63.111	T63.112	T63.113	T63.114	—	—
lizard NEC	T63.121	T63.122	T63.123	T63.124	—	—
scorpion	T63.2X1	T63.2X2	T63.2X3	T63.2X4	—	—
snake	T63.001	T63.002	T63.003	T63.004	—	—
African NEC	T63.081	T63.082	T63.083	T63.084	—	—
American (North) (South) NEC	T63.061	T63.062	T63.063	T63.064	—	—
Asian	T63.081	T63.082	T63.083	T63.084	—	—
Australian	T63.071	T63.072	T63.073	T63.074	—	—
cobra	T63.041	T63.042	T63.043	T63.044	—	—
coral snake	T63.021	T63.022	T63.023	T63.024	—	—
rattlesnake	T63.011	T63.012	T63.013	T63.014	—	—
specified NEC	T63.091	T63.092	T63.093	T63.094	—	—
taipan	T63.031	T63.032	T63.033	T63.034	—	—
specified NEC	T63.891	T63.892	T63.893	T63.894	—	—
spider	T63.301	T63.302	T63.303	T63.304	—	—
black widow	T63.311	T63.312	T63.313	T63.314	—	—
brown recluse	T63.331	T63.332	T63.333	T63.334	—	—
specified NEC	T63.391	T63.392	T63.393	T63.394	—	—
tarantula	T63.321	T63.322	T63.323	T63.324	—	—
sting ray	T63.511	T63.512	T63.513	T63.514	—	—
toad	T63.821	T63.822	T63.823	T63.824	—	—
wasp	T63.461	T63.462	T63.463	T63.464	—	—
Venous sclerosing drug NEC	T46.8X1	T46.8X2	T46.8X3	T46.8X4	T46.8X5	T46.8X6
Ventolin — *see Albuterol*						
Verapamil	T46.1X1	T46.1X2	T46.1X3	T46.1X4	T46.1X5	T46.1X6
Veramon	T42.3X1	T42.3X2	T42.3X3	T42.3X4	T42.3X5	T42.3X6
Veratrine	T46.5X1	T46.5X2	T46.5X3	T46.5X4	T46.5X5	T46.5X6
Veratrum						
album	T62.2X1	T62.2X2	T62.2X3	T62.2X4	—	—
alkaloids	T46.5X1	T46.5X2	T46.5X3	T46.5X4	T46.5X5	T46.5X6
viride	T62.2X1	T62.2X2	T62.2X3	T62.2X4	—	—
Verdigris	T60.3X1	T60.3X2	T60.3X3	T60.3X4	—	—
Veronal	T42.3X1	T42.3X2	T42.3X3	T42.3X4	T42.3X5	T42.3X6
Veroxil	T37.4X1	T37.4X2	T37.4X3	T37.4X4	T37.4X5	T37.4X6
Versenate	T50.6X1	T50.6X2	T50.6X3	T50.6X4	T50.6X5	T50.6X6

Substance	External Cause (T-Code) Poisoning, Accidental (Unintentional)	Poisoning, Intentional Self-Harm	Poisoning, Assault	Poisoning, Undetermined	Adverse Effect	Underdosing
Versidyne	T39.8X1	T39.8X2	T39.8X3	T39.8X4	T39.8X5	T39.8X6
Vetrabutine	T48.0X1	T48.0X2	T48.0X3	T48.0X4	T48.0X5	T48.0X6
Vidarabine	T37.5X1	T37.5X2	T37.5X3	T37.5X4	T37.5X5	T37.5X6
Vienna						
green	T57.0X1	T57.0X2	T57.0X3	T57.0X4	—	—
insecticide	T60.2X1	T60.2X2	T60.2X3	T60.2X4	—	—
red	T57.0X1	T57.0X2	T57.0X3	T57.0X4	—	—
pharmaceutical dye	T50.991	T50.992	T50.993	T50.994	T50.995	T50.996
Vigabatrin	T42.6X1	T42.6X2	T42.6X3	T42.6X4	T42.6X5	T42.6X6
Viloxazine	T43.291	T43.292	T43.293	T43.294	T43.295	T43.296
Viminol	T39.8X1	T39.8X2	T39.8X3	T39.8X4	T39.8X5	T39.8X6
Vinbarbital, vinbarbitone	T42.3X1	T42.3X2	T42.3X3	T42.3X4	T42.3X5	T42.3X6
Vinblastine	T45.1X1	T45.1X2	T45.1X3	T45.1X4	T45.1X5	T45.1X6
Vinburnine	T46.7X1	T46.7X2	T46.7X3	T46.7X4	T46.7X5	T46.7X6
Vincamine	T45.1X1	T45.1X2	T45.1X3	T45.1X4	T45.1X5	T45.1X6
Vincristine	T45.1X1	T45.1X2	T45.1X3	T45.1X4	T45.1X5	T45.1X6
Vindesine	T45.1X1	T45.1X2	T45.1X3	T45.1X4	T45.1X5	T45.1X6
Vinesthene, vinethene	T41.0X1	T41.0X2	T41.0X3	T41.0X4	T41.0X5	T41.0X6
Vinorelbine tartrate	T45.1X1	T45.1X2	T45.1X3	T45.1X4	T45.1X5	T45.1X6
Vinpocetine	T46.7X1	T46.7X2	T46.7X3	T46.7X4	T46.7X5	T46.7X6
Vinyl						
acetate	T65.891	T65.892	T65.893	T65.894	—	—
bital	T42.3X1	T42.3X2	T42.3X3	T42.3X4	T42.3X5	T42.3X6
bromide	T65.891	T65.892	T65.893	T65.894	—	—
chloride	T59.891	T59.892	T59.893	T59.894	—	—
ether	T41.0X1	T41.0X2	T41.0X3	T41.0X4	T41.0X5	T41.0X6
Vinylbital	T42.3X1	T42.3X2	T42.3X3	T42.3X4	T42.3X5	T42.3X6
Vinylidene chloride	T65.891	T65.892	T65.893	T65.894	—	—
Vioform	T37.8X1	T37.8X2	T37.8X3	T37.8X4	T37.8X5	T37.8X6
topical	T49.0X1	T49.0X2	T49.0X3	T49.0X4	T49.0X5	T49.0X6
Viomycin	T36.8X1	T36.8X2	T36.8X3	T36.8X4	T36.8X5	T36.8X6
Viosterol	T45.2X1	T45.2X2	T45.2X3	T45.2X4	T45.2X5	T45.2X6
Viper (venom)	T63.091	T63.092	T63.093	T63.094	—	—
Viprynium	T37.4X1	T37.4X2	T37.4X3	T37.4X4	T37.4X5	T37.4X6
Viquidil	T46.7X1	T46.7X2	T46.7X3	T46.7X4	T46.7X5	T46.7X6
Viral vaccine NEC	T50.B91	T50.B92	T50.B93	T50.B94	T50.B95	T50.B96
Virginiamycin	T36.8X1	T36.8X2	T36.8X3	T36.8X4	T36.8X5	T36.8X6
Virugon	T37.5X1	T37.5X2	T37.5X3	T37.5X4	T37.5X5	T37.5X6
Viscous agent	T50.901	T50.902	T50.903	T50.904	T50.905	T50.906
Visine	T49.5X1	T49.5X2	T49.5X3	T49.5X4	T49.5X5	T49.5X6
Visnadine	T46.3X1	T46.3X2	T46.3X3	T46.3X4	T46.3X5	T46.3X6

Substance	External Cause (T-Code) Poisoning, Accidental (Unintentional)	Poisoning, Intentional Self-Harm	Poisoning, Assault	Poisoning, Undetermined	Adverse Effect	Underdosing
Vitamin NEC	T45.2X1	T45.2X2	T45.2X3	T45.2X4	T45.2X5	T45.2X6
A	T45.2X1	T45.2X2	T45.2X3	T45.2X4	T45.2X5	T45.2X6
B NEC	T45.2X1	T45.2X2	T45.2X3	T45.2X4	T45.2X5	T45.2X6
nicotinic acid	T46.7X1	T46.7X2	T46.7X3	T46.7X4	T46.7X5	T46.7X6
B1	T45.2X1	T45.2X2	T45.2X3	T45.2X4	T45.2X5	T45.2X6
B2	T45.2X1	T45.2X2	T45.2X3	T45.2X4	T45.2X5	T45.2X6
B6	T45.2X1	T45.2X2	T45.2X3	T45.2X4	T45.2X5	T45.2X6
B12	T45.2X1	T45.2X2	T45.2X3	T45.2X4	T45.2X5	T45.2X6
B15	T45.2X1	T45.2X2	T45.2X3	T45.2X4	T45.2X5	T45.2X6
C	T45.2X1	T45.2X2	T45.2X3	T45.2X4	T45.2X5	T45.2X6
D	T45.2X1	T45.2X2	T45.2X3	T45.2X4	T45.2X5	T45.2X6
D2	T45.2X1	T45.2X2	T45.2X3	T45.2X4	T45.2X5	T45.2X6
D3	T45.2X1	T45.2X2	T45.2X3	T45.2X4	T45.2X5	T45.2X6
E	T45.2X1	T45.2X2	T45.2X3	T45.2X4	T45.2X5	T45.2X6
E acetate	T45.2X1	T45.2X2	T45.2X3	T45.2X4	T45.2X5	T45.2X6
hematopoietic	T45.8X1	T45.8X2	T45.8X3	T45.8X4	T45.8X5	T45.8X6
K NEC	T45.7X1	T45.7X2	T45.7X3	T45.7X4	T45.7X5	T45.7X6
K1	T45.7X1	T45.7X2	T45.7X3	T45.7X4	T45.7X5	T45.7X6
K2	T45.7X1	T45.7X2	T45.7X3	T45.7X4	T45.7X5	T45.7X6
PP	T45.2X1	T45.2X2	T45.2X3	T45.2X4	T45.2X5	T45.2X6
ulceroprotectant	T47.1X1	T47.1X2	T47.1X3	T47.1X4	T47.1X5	T47.1X6
Vleminckx's solution	T49.4X1	T49.4X2	T49.4X3	T49.4X4	T49.4X5	T49.4X6
Voltaren — *see Diclofenac sodium*						

W

Substance	Poisoning, Accidental (Unintentional)	Poisoning, Intentional Self-Harm	Poisoning, Assault	Poisoning, Undetermined	Adverse Effect	Underdosing
Warfarin	T45.511	T45.512	T45.513	T45.514	T45.515	T45.516
rodenticide	T60.4X1	T60.4X2	T60.4X3	T60.4X4	—	—
sodium	T45.511	T45.512	T45.513	T45.514	T45.515	T45.516
Wasp (sting)	T63.461	T63.462	T63.463	T63.464	—	—
Water						
balance drug	T50.3X1	T50.3X2	T50.3X3	T50.3X4	T50.3X5	T50.3X6
distilled	T50.3X1	T50.3X2	T50.3X3	T50.3X4	T50.3X5	T50.3X6
gas — *see Gas, water*						
incomplete combustion of — *see Carbon, monoxide, fuel, utility*						
hemlock	T62.2X1	T62.2X2	T62.2X3	T62.2X4	—	—
moccasin (venom)	T63.061	T63.062	T63.063	T63.064	—	—
purified	T50.3X1	T50.3X2	T50.3X3	T50.3X4	T50.3X5	T50.3X6
Wax (paraffin) (petroleum)	T52.0X1	T52.0X2	T52.0X3	T52.0X4	—	—
automobile	T65.891	T65.892	T65.893	T65.894	—	—
floor	T52.0X1	T52.0X2	T52.0X3	T52.0X4	—	—

Substance	Poisoning, Accidental (Unintentional)	Poisoning, Intentional Self-Harm	Poisoning, Assault	Poisoning, Undetermined	Adverse Effect	Underdosing
	External Cause (T-Code)					
Weed killers NEC	T60.3X1	T60.3X2	T60.3X3	T60.3X4	—	—
Welldorm	T42.6X1	T42.6X2	T42.6X3	T42.6X4	T42.6X5	T42.6X6
White						
arsenic	T57.0X1	T57.0X2	T57.0X3	T57.0X4	—	—
hellebore	T62.2X1	T62.2X2	T62.2X3	T62.2X4	—	—
lotion (keratolytic)	T49.4X1	T49.4X2	T49.4X3	T49.4X4	T49.4X5	T49.4X6
spirit	T52.0X1	T52.0X2	T52.0X3	T52.0X4	—	—
Whitewash	T65.891	T65.892	T65.893	T65.894	—	—
Whole blood (human)	T45.8X1	T45.8X2	T45.8X3	T45.8X4	T45.8X5	T45.8X6
Wild						
black cherry	T62.2X1	T62.2X2	T62.2X3	T62.2X4	—	—
poisonous plants NEC	T62.2X1	T62.2X2	T62.2X3	T62.2X4	—	—
Window cleaning fluid	T65.891	T65.892	T65.893	T65.894	—	—
Wintergreen (oil)	T49.3X1	T49.3X2	T49.3X3	T49.3X4	T49.3X5	T49.3X6
Wisterine	T62.2X1	T62.2X2	T62.2X3	T62.2X4	—	—
Witch hazel	T49.2X1	T49.2X2	T49.2X3	T49.2X4	T49.2X5	T49.2X6
Wood alcohol or spirit	T51.1X1	T51.1X2	T51.1X3	T51.1X4	—	—
Wool fat (hydrous)	T49.3X1	T49.3X2	T49.3X3	T49.3X4	T49.3X5	T49.3X6
Woorali	T48.1X1	T48.1X2	T48.1X3	T48.1X4	T48.1X5	T48.1X6
Wormseed, American	T37.4X1	T37.4X2	T37.4X3	T37.4X4	T37.4X5	T37.4X6
X						
Xamoterol	T44.5X1	T44.5X2	T44.5X3	T44.5X4	T44.5X5	T44.5X6
Xanthine diuretics	T50.2X1	T50.2X2	T50.2X3	T50.2X4	T50.2X5	T50.2X6
Xanthinol nicotinate	T46.7X1	T46.7X2	T46.7X3	T46.7X4	T46.7X5	T46.7X6
Xanthotoxin	T49.3X1	T49.3X2	T49.3X3	T49.3X4	T49.3X5	T49.3X6
Xantinol nicotinate	T46.7X1	T46.7X2	T46.7X3	T46.7X4	T46.7X5	T46.7X6
Xantocillin	T36.0X1	T36.0X2	T36.0X3	T36.0X4	T36.0X5	T36.0X6
Xenon (127Xe) (133Xe)	T50.8X1	T50.8X2	T50.8X3	T50.8X4	T50.8X5	T50.8X6
Xenysalate	T49.4X1	T49.4X2	T49.4X3	T49.4X4	T49.4X5	T49.4X6
Xibornol	T37.8X1	T37.8X2	T37.8X3	T37.8X4	T37.8X5	T37.8X6
Xigris	T45.511	T45.512	T45.513	T45.514	T45.515	T45.516
Xipamide	T50.2X1	T50.2X2	T50.2X3	T50.2X4	T50.2X5	T50.2X6
Xylene (vapor)	T52.2X1	T52.2X2	T52.2X3	T52.2X4	—	—
Xylocaine (infiltration) (topical)	T41.3X1	T41.3X2	T41.3X3	T41.3X4	T41.3X5	T41.3X6
nerve block (peripheral) (plexus)	T41.3X1	T41.3X2	T41.3X3	T41.3X4	T41.3X5	T41.3X6
spinal	T41.3X1	T41.3X2	T41.3X3	T41.3X4	T41.3X5	T41.3X6
Xylol (vapor)	T52.2X1	T52.2X2	T52.2X3	T52.2X4	—	—
Xylometazoline	T48.5X1	T48.5X2	T48.5X3	T48.5X4	T48.5X5	T48.5X6

Substance	Poisoning, Accidental (Unintentional)	Poisoning, Intentional Self-Harm	Poisoning, Assault	Poisoning, Undetermined	Adverse Effect	Underdosing
	External Cause (T-Code)					
Y						
Yeast	T45.2X1	T45.2X2	T45.2X3	T45.2X4	T45.2X5	T45.2X6
dried	T45.2X1	T45.2X2	T45.2X3	T45.2X4	T45.2X5	T45.2X6
Yellow						
fever vaccine	T50.B91	T50.B92	T50.B93	T50.B94	T50.B95	T50.B96
jasmine	T62.2X1	T62.2X2	T62.2X3	T62.2X4	—	—
phenolphthalein	T47.2X1	T47.2X2	T47.2X3	T47.2X4	T47.2X5	T47.2X6
Yew	T62.2X1	T62.2X2	T62.2X3	T62.2X4	—	—
Yohimbic acid	T40.991	T40.992	T40.993	T40.994	T40.995	T40.996
Z						
Zactane	T39.8X1	T39.8X2	T39.8X3	T39.8X4	T39.8X5	T39.8X6
Zalcitabine	T37.5X1	T37.5X2	T37.5X3	T37.5X4	T37.5X5	T37.5X6
Zaroxolyn	T50.2X1	T50.2X2	T50.2X3	T50.2X4	T50.2X5	T50.2X6
Zephiran (topical)	T49.0X1	T49.0X2	T49.0X3	T49.0X4	T49.0X5	T49.0X6
ophthalmic preparation	T49.5X1	T49.5X2	T49.5X3	T49.5X4	T49.5X5	T49.5X6
Zeranol	T38.7X1	T38.7X2	T38.7X3	T38.7X4	T38.7X5	T38.7X6
Zerone	T51.1X1	T51.1X2	T51.1X3	T51.1X4	—	—
Zidovudine	T37.5X1	T37.5X2	T37.5X3	T37.5X4	T37.5X5	T37.5X6
Zimeldine	T43.221	T43.222	T43.223	T43.224	T43.225	T43.226
Zinc (compounds) (fumes) (vapor) NEC	T56.5X1	T56.5X2	T56.5X3	T56.5X4	—	—
anti-infectives	T49.0X1	T49.0X2	T49.0X3	T49.0X4	T49.0X5	T49.0X6
antivaricose	T46.8X1	T46.8X2	T46.8X3	T46.8X4	T46.8X5	T46.8X6
bacitracin	T49.0X1	T49.0X2	T49.0X3	T49.0X4	T49.0X5	T49.0X6
chloride (mouthwash)	T49.6X1	T49.6X2	T49.6X3	T49.6X4	T49.6X5	T49.6X6
chromate	T56.5X1	T56.5X2	T56.5X3	T56.5X4	—	—
gelatin	T49.3X1	T49.3X2	T49.3X3	T49.3X4	T49.3X5	T49.3X6
oxide	T49.3X1	T49.3X2	T49.3X3	T49.3X4	T49.3X5	T49.3X6
plaster	T49.3X1	T49.3X2	T49.3X3	T49.3X4	T49.3X5	T49.3X6
peroxide	T49.0X1	T49.0X2	T49.0X3	T49.0X4	T49.0X5	T49.0X6
pesticides	T56.5X1	T56.5X2	T56.5X3	T56.5X4	—	—
phosphide	T60.4X1	T60.4X2	T60.4X3	T60.4X4	—	—
pyrithionate	T49.4X1	T49.4X2	T49.4X3	T49.4X4	T49.4X5	T49.4X6
stearate	T49.3X1	T49.3X2	T49.3X3	T49.3X4	T49.3X5	T49.3X6
sulfate	T49.5X1	T49.5X2	T49.5X3	T49.5X4	T49.5X5	T49.5X6
ENT agent	T49.6X1	T49.6X2	T49.6X3	T49.6X4	T49.6X5	T49.6X6
ophthalmic solution	T49.5X1	T49.5X2	T49.5X3	T49.5X4	T49.5X5	T49.5X6
topical NEC	T49.0X1	T49.0X2	T49.0X3	T49.0X4	T49.0X5	T49.0X6
undecylenate	T49.0X1	T49.0X2	T49.0X3	T49.0X4	T49.0X5	T49.0X6

◀ New ◀ Revised ~~deleted~~ Deleted

Substance	External Cause (T-Code)					
	Poisoning, Accidental (Unintentional)	Poisoning, Intentional Self-Harm	Poisoning, Assault	Poisoning, Undetermined	Adverse Effect	Underdosing
Zineb	T60.0X1	T60.0X2	T60.0X3	T60.0X4	—	—
Zinostatin	T45.1X1	T45.1X2	T45.1X3	T45.1X4	T45.1X5	T45.1X6
Zipeprol	T48.3X1	T48.3X2	T48.3X3	T48.3X4	T48.3X5	T48.3X6
Zofenopril	T46.4X1	T46.4X2	T46.4X3	T46.4X4	T46.4X5	T46.4X6
Zolpidem	T42.6X1	T42.6X2	T42.6X3	T42.6X4	T42.6X5	T42.6X6
Zomepirac	T39.391	T39.392	T39.393	T39.394	T39.395	T39.396
Zopiclone	T42.6X1	T42.6X2	T42.6X3	T42.6X4	T42.6X5	T42.6X6
Zorubicin	T45.1X1	T45.1X2	T45.1X3	T45.1X4	T45.1X5	T45.1X6
Zotepine	T43.591	T43.592	T43.593	T43.594	T43.595	T43.596
Zovant	T45.511	T45.512	T45.513	T45.514	T45.515	T45.516
Zoxazolamine	T42.8X1	T42.8X2	T42.8X3	T42.8X4	T42.8X5	T42.8X6
Zuclopenthixol	T43.4X1	T43.4X2	T43.4X3	T43.4X4	T43.4X5	T43.4X6
Zygadenus (venenosus)	T62.2X1	T62.2X2	T62.2X3	T62.2X4	—	—
Zyprexa	T43.591	T43.592	T43.593	T43.594	T43.595	T43.596

ECI

External Cause of Injuries Index

ICD-10-CM EXTERNAL CAUSE OF INJURIES INDEX

A

- **Abandonment** (causing exposure to weather conditions) (with intent to injure or kill) NEC X58
- **Abuse** (adult) (child) (mental) (physical) (sexual) X58
- **Accident** (to) X58
  - aircraft (in transit) (powered) —*see also* Accident, transport, aircraft
    - due to, caused by cataclysm —*see* Forces of nature, by type
  - animal-drawn vehicle —*see* Accident, transport, animal-drawn vehicle occupant
  - animal-rider —*see* Accident, transport, animal-rider
  - automobile —*see* Accident, transport, car occupant
  - bare foot water skiier V94.4
  - boat, boating —*see also* Accident, watercraft
    - striking swimmer
      - powered V94.11
      - unpowered V94.12
  - bus —*see* Accident, transport, bus occupant
  - cable car, not on rails V98.0
    - on rails —*see* Accident, transport, streetcar occupant
  - car —*see* Accident, transport, car occupant
  - caused by, due to
    - animal NEC W64
    - chain hoist W24.0
    - cold (excessive) —*see* Exposure, cold
    - corrosive liquid, substance —*see* Table of Drugs and Chemicals
    - cutting or piercing instrument —*see* Contact, with, by type of instrument
    - drive belt W24.0
    - electric
      - current —*see* Exposure, electric current
      - motor —*see also* Contact, with, by type of machine W31.3
        - current (of) W86.8
    - environmental factor NEC X58
    - explosive material —*see* Explosion
    - fire, flames —*see* Exposure, fire
    - firearm missile —*see* Discharge, firearm by type
    - heat (excessive) —*see* Heat
    - hot —*see* Contact, with, hot
    - ignition —*see* Ignition
    - lifting device W24.0
    - lightning —*see* subcategory T75.0
      - causing fire —*see* Exposure, fire
    - machine, machinery —*see* Contact, with, by type of machine
    - natural factor NEC X58
    - pulley (block) W24.0
    - radiation —*see* Radiation
    - steam X13.1
      - inhalation X13.0
      - pipe X16
    - thunderbolt —*see* subcategory T75.0
      - causing fire —*see* Exposure, fire
    - transmission device W24.1
  - coach —*see* Accident, transport, bus occupant
  - coal car —*see* Accident, transport, industrial vehicle occupant
  - diving —*see also* Fall, into, water
    - with
      - drowning or submersion —*see* Drowning
  - forklift —*see* Accident, transport, industrial vehicle occupant
  - heavy transport vehicle NOS —*see* Accident, transport, truck occupant
  - ice yacht V98.2
  - in
    - medical, surgical procedure
      - as, or due to misadventure —*see* Misadventure
      - causing an abnormal reaction or later complication without mention of misadventure —*see also* Complication of or following, by type of procedure Y84.9
  - land yacht V98.1
  - late effect of —*see* W00-X58 with 7th character S
  - logging car —*see* Accident, transport, industrial vehicle occupant

- **Accident** *(Continued)*
  - machine, machinery —*see also* Contact, with, by type of machine
    - on board watercraft V93.69
      - explosion —*see* Explosion, in, watercraft
      - fire —*see* Burn, on board watercraft
      - powered craft V93.63
        - ferry boat V93.61
        - fishing boat V93.62
        - jet ski V93.63
        - liner V93.61
        - merchant ship V93.60
        - passenger ship V93.61
        - sailboat V93.64
  - mine tram —*see* Accident, transport, industrial vehicle occupant
  - mobility scooter (motorized) —*see* Accident, transport, pedestrian, conveyance, specified type NEC
  - motor scooter —*see* Accident, transport, motorcycle
  - motor vehicle NOS (traffic) —*see also* Accident, transport V89.2
    - nontraffic V89.0
    - three-wheeled NOS —*see* Accident, transport, three-wheeled motor vehicle occupant
  - motorcycle NOS —*see* Accident, transport, motorcycle
  - nonmotor vehicle NOS (nontraffic) —*see also* Accident, transport V89.1
    - traffic NOS V89.3
  - nontraffic (victim's mode of transport NOS) V88.9
    - collision (between) V88.7
      - bus and truck V88.5
      - car and:
        - bus V88.3
        - pickup V88.2
        - three-wheeled motor vehicle V88.0
        - train V88.6
        - truck V88.4
        - two-wheeled motor vehicle V88.0
        - van V88.2
      - specified vehicle NEC and:
        - three-wheeled motor vehicle V88.1
        - two-wheeled motor vehicle V88.1
    - known mode of transport —*see* Accident, transport, by type of vehicle
    - noncollision V88.8
  - on board watercraft V93.89
    - powered craft V93.83
      - ferry boat V93.81
      - fishing boat V93.82
      - jet ski V93.83
      - liner V93.81
      - merchant ship V93.80
      - passenger ship V93.81
    - unpowered craft V93.88
      - canoe V93.85
      - inflatable V93.86
        - in tow
          - recreational V94.31
          - specified NEC V94.32
      - kayak V93.85
      - sailboat V93.84
      - surf-board V93.88
      - water skis V93.87
      - windsurfer V93.88
  - parachutist V97.29
    - entangled in object V97.21
    - injured on landing V97.22
  - pedal cycle —*see* Accident, transport, pedal cyclist
  - pedestrian (on foot)
    - with
      - another pedestrian W51
        - with fall W03
          - due to ice or snow W00.0
        - on pedestrian conveyance NEC V00.09
      - rider of
        - hoverboard V00.038
        - Segway V00.038
        - standing
          - electric scooter V00.031
          - micro-mobility pedestrian conveyance NEC V00.038
      - roller skater (in-line) V00.01
      - skate boarder V00.02
      - transport vehicle —*see* Accident, transport
    - on pedestrian conveyance —*see* Accident, transport, pedestrian, conveyance

- **Accident** *(Continued)*
  - pick-up truck or van —*see* Accident, transport, pickup truck occupant
  - quarry truck —*see* Accident, transport, industrial vehicle occupant
  - railway vehicle (any) (in motion) —*see* Accident, transport, railway vehicle occupant
    - due to cataclysm —*see* Forces of nature, by type
  - scooter (non-motorized) —*see* Accident, transport, pedestrian, conveyance, scooter
  - sequelae of —*see* W00-X58 with 7th character S
  - skateboard —*see* Accident, transport, pedestrian, conveyance, skateboard
  - ski (ing) —*see* Accident, transport, pedestrian, conveyance
    - lift V98.3
  - specified cause NEC X58
  - streetcar —*see* Accident, transport, streetcar occupant
  - traffic (victim's mode of transport NOS) V87.9
    - collision (between) V87.7
      - bus and truck V87.5
      - car and:
        - bus V87.3
        - pickup V87.2
        - three-wheeled motor vehicle V87.0
        - train V87.6
        - truck V87.4
        - two-wheeled motor vehicle V87.0
        - van V87.2
      - specified vehicle NEC V86.39
        - and
          - three-wheeled motor vehicle V87.1
          - two-wheeled motor vehicle V87.1
        - driver V86.09
        - person on outside V86.29
        - passenger V86.19
        - while boarding or alighting V86.49
    - known mode of transport —*see* Accident, transport, by type of vehicle
    - noncollision V87.8
  - transport (involving injury to) V99
    - 18 wheeler —*see* Accident, transport, truck occupant
    - agricultural vehicle occupant (nontraffic) V84.9
      - driver V84.5
      - hanger-on V84.7
      - passenger V84.6
      - traffic V84.3
        - driver V84.0
        - hanger-on V84.2
        - passenger V84.1
      - while boarding or alighting V84.4
    - aircraft NEC V97.89
      - military NEC V97.818
        - with civilian aircraft V97.810
        - civilian injured by V97.811
      - occupant injured (in)
        - nonpowered craft accident V96.9
          - balloon V96.00
            - collision V96.03
            - crash V96.01
            - explosion V96.05
            - fire V96.04
            - forced landing V96.02
            - specified type NEC V96.09
          - glider V96.20
            - collision V96.23
            - crash V96.21
            - explosion V96.25
            - fire V96.24
            - forced landing V96.22
            - specified type NEC V96.29
          - hang glider V96.10
            - collision V96.13
            - crash V96.11
            - explosion V96.15
            - fire V96.14
            - forced landing V96.12
            - specified type NEC V96.19
          - specified craft NEC V96.8
        - powered craft accident V95.9
          - fixed wing NEC
            - commercial V95.30
              - collision V95.33
              - crash V95.31

A

A

- **Accident** *(Continued)*
  - transport *(Continued)*
    - bus occupant *(Continued)*
      - hanger-on *(Continued)*
        - collision *(Continued)*
          - two wheeled motor vehicle (traffic) V72.7
            - nontraffic V72.2
          - van (traffic) V73.7
            - nontraffic V73.2
        - noncollision accident (traffic) V78.7
          - nontraffic V78.2
      - noncollision accident (traffic) V78.9
        - nontraffic V78.3
        - while boarding or alighting V78.4
      - nontraffic V79.3
      - passenger
        - collision (with)
          - animal (traffic) V7Ø.6
            - being ridden (traffic) V76.6
              - nontraffic V76.1
            - nontraffic V7Ø.1
          - animal-drawn vehicle (traffic) V76.6
            - nontraffic V76.1
          - bus (traffic) V74.6
            - nontraffic V74.1
          - car (traffic) V73.6
            - nontraffic V73.1
          - motor vehicle NOS (traffic) V79.5Ø
            - nontraffic V79.1Ø
            - specified type NEC (traffic) V79.59
              - nontraffic V79.19
          - pedal cycle (traffic) V71.6
            - nontraffic V71.1
          - pickup truck (traffic) V73.6
            - nontraffic V73.1
          - railway vehicle (traffic) V75.6
            - nontraffic V75.1
          - specified vehicle NEC (traffic) V76.6
            - nontraffic V76.1
          - stationary object (traffic) V77.6
            - nontraffic V77.1
          - streetcar (traffic) V76.6
            - nontraffic V76.1
          - three wheeled motor vehicle (traffic) V72.6
            - nontraffic V72.1
          - truck (traffic) V74.6
            - nontraffic V74.1
          - two wheeled motor vehicle (traffic) V72.6
            - nontraffic V72.1
          - van (traffic) V73.6
            - nontraffic V73.1
        - noncollision accident (traffic) V78.6
          - nontraffic V78.1
      - specified type NEC V79.88
        - military vehicle V79.81
    - cable car, not on rails V98.Ø
      - on rails —*see* Accident, transport, streetcar occupant
    - car occupant V49.9
      - ambulance occupant —*see* Accident, transport, ambulance occupant
      - collision (with)
        - animal (traffic) V4Ø.9
          - being ridden (traffic) V46.9
            - nontraffic V46.3
            - while boarding or alighting V46.4
          - nontraffic V4Ø.3
          - while boarding or alighting V4Ø.4
        - animal-drawn vehicle (traffic) V46.9
          - nontraffic V46.3
          - while boarding or alighting V46.4
        - bus (traffic) V44.9
          - nontraffic V44.3
          - while boarding or alighting V44.4
        - car (traffic) V43.92
          - nontraffic V43.32
          - while boarding or alighting V43.42
        - motor vehicle NOS (traffic) V49.6Ø
          - nontraffic V49.2Ø
          - specified type NEC (traffic) V49.69
            - nontraffic V49.29
        - pedal cycle (traffic) V41.9
          - nontraffic V41.3
          - while boarding or alighting V41.4
        - pickup truck (traffic) V43.93
          - nontraffic V43.33
          - while boarding or alighting V43.43

- **Accident** *(Continued)*
  - transport *(Continued)*
    - car occupant *(Continued)*
      - collision *(Continued)*
        - railway vehicle (traffic) V45.9
          - nontraffic V45.3
          - while boarding or alighting V45.4
        - specified vehicle NEC (traffic) V46.9
          - nontraffic V46.3
          - while boarding or alighting V46.4
        - sport utility vehicle (traffic) V43.91
          - nontraffic V43.31
          - while boarding or alighting V43.41
        - stationary object (traffic) V47.9
          - nontraffic V47.3
          - while boarding or alighting V47.4
        - streetcar (traffic) V46.9
          - nontraffic V46.3
          - while boarding or alighting V46.4
        - three wheeled motor vehicle (traffic) V42.9
          - nontraffic V42.3
          - while boarding or alighting V42.4
        - truck (traffic) V44.9
          - nontraffic V44.3
          - while boarding or alighting V44.4
        - two wheeled motor vehicle (traffic) V42.9
          - nontraffic V42.3
          - while boarding or alighting V42.4
        - van (traffic) V43.94
          - nontraffic V43.34
          - while boarding or alighting V43.44
      - driver
        - collision (with)
          - animal (traffic) V4Ø.5
            - being ridden (traffic) V46.5
              - nontraffic V46.Ø
            - nontraffic V4Ø.Ø
          - animal-drawn vehicle (traffic) V46.5
            - nontraffic V46.Ø
          - bus (traffic) V44.5
            - nontraffic V44.Ø
          - car (traffic) V43.52
            - nontraffic V43.Ø2
          - motor vehicle NOS (traffic) V49.4Ø
            - nontraffic V49.ØØ
            - specified type NEC (traffic) V49.49
              - nontraffic V49.Ø9
          - pedal cycle (traffic) V41.5
            - nontraffic V41.Ø
          - pickup truck (traffic) V43.53
            - nontraffic V43.Ø3
          - railway vehicle (traffic) V45.5
            - nontraffic V45.Ø
          - specified vehicle NEC (traffic) V46.5
            - nontraffic V46.Ø
          - sport utility vehicle (traffic) V43.51
            - nontraffic V43.Ø1
          - stationary object (traffic) V47.5
            - nontraffic V47.Ø
          - streetcar (traffic) V46.5
            - nontraffic V46.Ø
          - three wheeled motor vehicle (traffic) V42.5
            - nontraffic V42.Ø
          - truck (traffic) V44.5
            - nontraffic V44.Ø
          - two wheeled motor vehicle (traffic) V42.5
            - nontraffic V42.Ø
          - van (traffic) V43.54
            - nontraffic V43.Ø4
        - noncollision accident (traffic) V48.5
          - nontraffic V48.Ø
      - hanger-on
        - collision (with)
          - animal (traffic) V4Ø.7
            - being ridden (traffic) V46.7
              - nontraffic V46.2
            - nontraffic V4Ø.2
          - animal-drawn vehicle (traffic) V46.7
            - nontraffic V46.2
          - bus (traffic) V44.7
            - nontraffic V44.2
          - car (traffic) V43.72
            - nontraffic V43.22
          - pedal cycle (traffic) V41.7
            - nontraffic V41.2
          - pickup truck (traffic) V43.73
            - nontraffic V43.23

- **Accident** *(Continued)*
  - transport *(Continued)*
    - car occupant *(Continued)*
      - hanger-on *(Continued)*
        - collision *(Continued)*
          - railway vehicle (traffic) V45.7
            - nontraffic V45.2
          - specified vehicle NEC (traffic) V46.7
            - nontraffic V46.2
          - sport utility vehicle (traffic) V43.71
            - nontraffic V43.21
          - stationary object (traffic) V47.7
            - nontraffic V47.2
          - streetcar (traffic) V46.7
            - nontraffic V46.2
          - three wheeled motor vehicle (traffic) V42.7
            - nontraffic V42.2
          - truck (traffic) V44.7
            - nontraffic V44.2
          - two wheeled motor vehicle (traffic) V42.7
            - nontraffic V42.2
          - van (traffic) V43.74
            - nontraffic V43.24
        - noncollision accident (traffic) V48.7
          - nontraffic V48.2
      - noncollision accident (traffic) V48.9
        - nontraffic V48.3
        - while boarding or alighting V48.4
      - nontraffic V49.3
      - passenger
        - collision (with)
          - animal (traffic) V4Ø.6
            - being ridden (traffic) V46.6
              - nontraffic V46.1
            - nontraffic V4Ø.1
          - animal-drawn vehicle (traffic) V46.6
            - nontraffic V46.1
          - bus (traffic) V44.6
            - nontraffic V44.1
          - car (traffic) V43.62
            - nontraffic V43.12
          - motor vehicle NOS (traffic) V49.5Ø
            - nontraffic V49.1Ø
            - specified type NEC (traffic) V49.59
              - nontraffic V49.19
          - pedal cycle (traffic) V41.6
            - nontraffic V41.1
          - pickup truck (traffic) V43.63
            - nontraffic V43.13
          - railway vehicle (traffic) V45.6
            - nontraffic V45.1
          - specified vehicle NEC (traffic) V46.6
            - nontraffic V46.1
          - sport utility vehicle (traffic) V43.61
            - nontraffic V43.11
          - stationary object (traffic) V47.6
            - nontraffic V47.1
          - streetcar (traffic) V46.6
            - nontraffic V46.1
          - three wheeled motor vehicle (traffic) V42.6
            - nontraffic V42.1
          - truck (traffic) V44.6
            - nontraffic V44.1
          - two wheeled motor vehicle (traffic) V42.6
            - nontraffic V42.1
          - van (traffic) V43.64
            - nontraffic V43.14
        - noncollision accident (traffic) V48.6
          - nontraffic V48.1
      - specified type NEC V49.88
        - military vehicle V49.81
    - coal car —*see* Accident, transport, industrial vehicle occupant
    - construction vehicle occupant (nontraffic) V85.9
      - driver V85.5
      - hanger-on V85.7
      - passenger V85.6
      - traffic V85.3
        - driver V85.Ø
        - hanger-on V85.2
        - passenger V85.1
      - while boarding or alighting V85.4
    - dirt bike rider (nontraffic) V86.96
      - driver V86.56
      - hanger-on V86.76
      - passenger V86.66

A

A

A

- **Accident** *(Continued)*
  - transport *(Continued)*
    - pedestrian *(Continued)*
      - conveyance *(Continued)*
        - roller skates *(Continued)*
          - collision *(Continued)*
            - car V03.91
              - nontraffic V03.01
              - traffic V03.11
            - pedal cycle V01.91
              - nontraffic V01.01
              - traffic V01.11
            - pick-up truck or van V03.91
              - nontraffic V03.01
              - traffic V03.11
            - railway (train) (vehicle) V05.91
              - nontraffic V05.01
              - traffic V05.11
            - stationary object V00.122
            - streetcar V06.91
              - nontraffic V06.01
              - traffic V06.11
            - two- or three-wheeled motor vehicle V02.91
              - nontraffic V02.01
              - traffic V02.11
            - vehicle V09.9
              - animal-drawn V06.91
                - nontraffic V06.01
                - traffic V06.11
              - motor
                - nontraffic V09.00
                - traffic V09.20
          - fall V00.121
          - in-line V00.118
            - collision —*see also* Accident, transport, pedestrian, conveyance occupant, roller skates, collision
              - with stationary object V00.112
            - fall V00.111
            - nontraffic V09.1
              - involving motor vehicle NEC V09.00
            - traffic V09.3
              - involving motor vehicle NEC V09.20
        - rolling shoes V00.158
          - colliding with stationary object V00.152
          - fall V00.151
        - rolling type NEC V00.188
          - collision (with) V09.9
            - animal being ridden or animal drawn vehicle V06.99
              - nontraffic V06.09
              - traffic V06.19
            - bus or heavy transport V04.99
              - nontraffic V04.09
              - traffic V04.19
            - car V03.99
              - nontraffic V03.09
              - traffic V03.19
            - pedal cycle V01.99
              - nontraffic V01.09
              - traffic V01.19
            - pick-up truck or van V03.99
              - nontraffic V03.09
              - traffic V03.19
            - railway (train) (vehicle) V05.99
              - nontraffic V05.09
              - traffic V05.19
            - stationary object V00.182
            - streetcar V06.99
              - nontraffic V06.09
              - traffic V06.19
            - two- or three-wheeled motor vehicle V02.99
              - nontraffic V02.09
              - traffic V02.19
            - vehicle V09.9
              - animal-drawn V06.99
                - nontraffic V06.09
                - traffic V06.19
              - motor
                - nontraffic V09.00
                - traffic V09.20

- **Accident** *(Continued)*
  - transport *(Continued)*
    - pedestrian *(Continued)*
      - conveyance *(Continued)*
        - rolling type *(Continued)*
          - fall V00.181
          - in-line roller skate —*see* Accident, transport, pedestrian, conveyance, roller skate, in-line
          - nontraffic V09.1
            - involving motor vehicle NEC V09.00
          - roller skate —*see* Accident, transport, pedestrian, conveyance, roller skate
          - scooter (non-motorized) —*see* Accident, transport, pedestrian, conveyance, scooter
          - skateboard —*see* Accident, transport, pedestrian, conveyance, skateboard
          - traffic V09.3
            - involving motor vehicle NEC V09.20
        - scooter (non-motorized) V00.148
          - collision (with) V09.9
            - animal being ridden or animal drawn vehicle V06.99
              - nontraffic V06.09
              - traffic V06.19
            - bus or heavy transport V04.99
              - nontraffic V04.09
              - traffic V04.19
            - car V03.99
              - nontraffic V03.09
              - traffic V03.19
            - pedal cycle V01.99
              - nontraffic V01.09
              - traffic V01.19
            - pick-up truck or van V03.99
              - nontraffic V03.09
              - traffic V03.19
            - railway (train) (vehicle) V05.99
              - nontraffic V05.09
              - traffic V05.19
            - stationary object V00.142
            - streetcar V06.99
              - nontraffic V06.09
              - traffic V06.19
            - two- or three-wheeled motor vehicle V02.99
              - nontraffic V02.09
              - traffic V02.19
            - vehicle V09.9
              - animal-drawn V06.99
                - nontraffic V06.09
                - traffic V06.19
              - motor
                - nontraffic V09.00
                - traffic V09.20
          - fall V00.141
          - nontraffic V09.1
            - involving motor vehicle NEC V09.00
          - traffic V09.3
            - involving motor vehicle NEC V09.20
        - skateboard V00.138
          - collision (with) V09.9
            - animal being ridden or animal drawn vehicle V06.92
              - nontraffic V06.02
              - traffic V06.12
            - bus or heavy transport V04.92
              - nontraffic V04.02
              - traffic V04.12
            - car V03.92
              - nontraffic V03.02
              - traffic V03.12
            - pedal cycle V01.92
              - nontraffic V01.02
              - traffic V01.12
            - pick-up truck or van V03.92
              - nontraffic V03.02
              - traffic V03.12
            - railway (train) (vehicle) V05.92
              - nontraffic V05.02
              - traffic V05.12

- **Accident** *(Continued)*
  - transport *(Continued)*
    - pedestrian *(Continued)*
      - conveyance *(Continued)*
        - skateboard *(Continued)*
          - collision *(Continued)*
            - stationary object V00.132
            - streetcar V06.92
              - nontraffic V06.02
              - traffic V06.12
            - two- or three-wheeled motor vehicle V02.92
              - nontraffic V02.02
              - traffic V02.12
            - vehicle V09.9
              - animal-drawn V06.92
                - nontraffic V06.02
                - traffic V06.12
              - motor
                - nontraffic V09.00
                - traffic V09.20
          - fall V00.131
          - nontraffic V09.1
            - involving motor vehicle NEC V09.00
          - traffic V09.3
            - involving motor vehicle NEC V09.20
        - skis (snow) V00.328
          - collision (with) V09.9
            - animal being ridden or animal drawn vehicle V06.99
              - nontraffic V06.09
              - traffic V06.19
            - bus or heavy transport V04.99
              - nontraffic V04.09
              - traffic V04.19
            - car V03.99
              - nontraffic V03.09
              - traffic V03.19
            - pedal cycle V01.99
              - nontraffic V01.09
              - traffic V01.19
            - pick-up truck or van V03.99
              - nontraffic V03.09
              - traffic V03.19
            - railway (train) (vehicle) V05.99
              - nontraffic V05.09
              - traffic V05.19
            - stationary object V00.322
            - streetcar V06.99
              - nontraffic V06.09
              - traffic V06.19
            - two- or three-wheeled motor vehicle V02.99
              - nontraffic V02.09
              - traffic V02.19
            - vehicle V09.9
              - animal-drawn V06.99
                - nontraffic V06.09
                - traffic V06.19
              - motor
                - nontraffic V09.00
                - traffic V09.20
          - fall V00.321
          - nontraffic V09.1
            - involving motor vehicle NEC V09.00
          - traffic V09.3
            - involving motor vehicle NEC V09.20
        - sled V00.228
          - collision (with) V09.9
            - animal being ridden or animal drawn vehicle V06.99
              - nontraffic V06.09
              - traffic V06.19
            - bus or heavy transport V04.99
              - nontraffic V04.09
              - traffic V04.19
            - car V03.99
              - nontraffic V03.09
              - traffic V03.19
            - pedal cycle V01.99
              - nontraffic V01.09
              - traffic V01.19
            - pick-up truck or van V03.99
              - nontraffic V03.09
              - traffic V03.19
            - railway (train) (vehicle) V05.99
              - nontraffic V05.09
              - traffic V05.19

A

A

- **Accident** *(Continued)*
  - transport *(Continued)*
    - three-wheeled motor vehicle occupant—*(Continued)*
      - collision *(Continued)*
        - truck (traffic) V34.9
          - nontraffic V34.3
          - while boarding or alighting V34.4
        - two wheeled motor vehicle (traffic) V32.9
          - nontraffic V32.3
          - while boarding or alighting V32.4
        - van (traffic) V33.9
          - nontraffic V33.3
          - while boarding or alighting V33.4
      - driver
        - collision (with)
          - animal (traffic) V3Ø.5
            - being ridden (traffic) V36.5
              - nontraffic V36.Ø
            - nontraffic V3Ø.Ø
          - animal-drawn vehicle (traffic) V36.5
            - nontraffic V36.Ø
          - bus (traffic) V34.5
            - nontraffic V34.Ø
          - car (traffic) V33.5
            - nontraffic V33.Ø
          - motor vehicle NOS (traffic) V39.4Ø
            - nontraffic V39.ØØ
            - specified type NEC (traffic) V39.49
              - nontraffic V39.Ø9
          - pedal cycle (traffic) V31.5
            - nontraffic V31.Ø
          - pickup truck (traffic) V33.5
            - nontraffic V33.Ø
          - railway vehicle (traffic) V35.5
            - nontraffic V35.Ø
          - specified vehicle NEC (traffic) V36.5
            - nontraffic V36.Ø
          - stationary object (traffic) V37.5
            - nontraffic V37.Ø
          - streetcar (traffic) V36.5
            - nontraffic V36.Ø
          - three wheeled motor vehicle (traffic) V32.5
            - nontraffic V32.Ø
          - truck (traffic) V34.5
            - nontraffic V34.Ø
          - two wheeled motor vehicle (traffic) V32.5
            - nontraffic V32.Ø
          - van (traffic) V33.5
            - nontraffic V33.Ø
        - noncollision accident (traffic) V38.5
          - nontraffic V38.Ø
      - hanger-on
        - collision (with)
          - animal (traffic) V3Ø.7
            - being ridden (traffic) V36.7
              - nontraffic V36.2
            - nontraffic V3Ø.2
          - animal-drawn vehicle (traffic) V36.7
            - nontraffic V36.2
          - bus (traffic) V34.7
            - nontraffic V34.2
          - car (traffic) V33.7
            - nontraffic V33.2
          - pedal cycle (traffic) V31.7
            - nontraffic V31.2
          - pickup truck (traffic) V33.7
            - nontraffic V33.2
          - railway vehicle (traffic) V35.7
            - nontraffic V35.2
          - specified vehicle NEC (traffic) V36.7
            - nontraffic V36.2
          - stationary object (traffic) V37.7
            - nontraffic V37.2
          - streetcar (traffic) V36.7
            - nontraffic V36.2
          - three wheeled motor vehicle (traffic) V32.7
            - nontraffic V32.2
          - truck (traffic) V34.7
            - nontraffic V34.2
          - two wheeled motor vehicle (traffic) V32.7
            - nontraffic V32.2
          - van (traffic) V33.7
            - nontraffic V33.2
        - noncollision accident (traffic) V38.7
          - nontraffic V38.2

- **Accident** *(Continued)*
  - transport *(Continued)*
    - three-wheeled motor vehicle occupant—*(Continued)*
      - noncollision accident (traffic) V38.9
        - nontraffic V38.3
        - while boarding or alighting V38.4
      - nontraffic V39.3
      - passenger
        - collision (with)
          - animal (traffic) V3Ø.6
            - being ridden (traffic) V36.6
              - nontraffic V36.1
            - nontraffic V3Ø.1
          - animal-drawn vehicle (traffic) V36.6
            - nontraffic V36.1
          - bus (traffic) V34.6
            - nontraffic V34.1
          - car (traffic) V33.6
            - nontraffic V33.1
          - motor vehicle NOS (traffic) V39.5Ø
            - nontraffic V39.1Ø
            - specified type NEC (traffic) V39.59
              - nontraffic V39.19
          - pedal cycle (traffic) V31.6
            - nontraffic V31.1
          - pickup truck (traffic) V33.6
            - nontraffic V33.1
          - railway vehicle (traffic) V35.6
            - nontraffic V35.1
          - specified vehicle NEC (traffic) V36.6
            - nontraffic V36.1
          - stationary object (traffic) V37.6
            - nontraffic V37.1
          - streetcar (traffic) V36.6
            - nontraffic V36.1
          - three wheeled motor vehicle (traffic) V32.6
            - nontraffic V32.1
          - truck (traffic) V34.6
            - nontraffic V34.1
          - two wheeled motor vehicle (traffic) V32.6
            - nontraffic V32.1
          - van (traffic) V33.6
            - nontraffic V33.1
        - noncollision accident (traffic) V38.6
          - nontraffic V38.1
      - specified type NEC V39.89
        - military vehicle V39.81
    - tractor (farm) (and trailer) —*see* Accident, transport, agricultural vehicle occupant
    - tram —*see* Accident, transport, streetcar
      - in mine or quarry —*see* Accident, transport, industrial vehicle occupant
    - trolley —*see* Accident, transport, streetcar
      - in mine or quarry —*see* Accident, transport, industrial vehicle occupant
    - truck (heavy) occupant V69.9
      - collision (with)
        - animal (traffic) V6Ø.9
          - being ridden (traffic) V66.9
            - nontraffic V66.3
            - while boarding or alighting V66.4
          - nontraffic V6Ø.3
          - while boarding or alighting V6Ø.4
        - animal-drawn vehicle (traffic) V66.9
          - nontraffic V66.3
          - while boarding or alighting V66.4
        - bus (traffic) V64.9
          - nontraffic V64.3
          - while boarding or alighting V64.4
        - car (traffic) V63.9
          - nontraffic V63.3
          - while boarding or alighting V63.4
        - motor vehicle NOS (traffic) V69.6Ø
          - nontraffic V69.2Ø
          - specified type NEC (traffic) V69.69
            - nontraffic V69.29
        - pedal cycle (traffic) V61.9
          - nontraffic V61.3
          - while boarding or alighting V61.4
        - pickup truck (traffic) V63.9
          - nontraffic V63.3
          - while boarding or alighting V63.4
        - railway vehicle (traffic) V65.9
          - nontraffic V65.3
          - while boarding or alighting V65.4
        - specified vehicle NEC (traffic) V66.9
          - nontraffic V66.3
          - while boarding or alighting V66.4

- **Accident** *(Continued)*
  - transport *(Continued)*
    - truck (heavy) occupant *(Continued)*
      - collision *(Continued)*
        - stationary object (traffic) V67.9
          - nontraffic V67.3
          - while boarding or alighting V67.4
        - streetcar (traffic) V66.9
          - nontraffic V66.3
          - while boarding or alighting V66.4
        - three wheeled motor vehicle (traffic) V62.9
          - nontraffic V62.3
          - while boarding or alighting V62.4
        - truck (traffic) V64.9
          - nontraffic V64.3
          - while boarding or alighting V64.4
        - two wheeled motor vehicle (traffic) V62.9
          - nontraffic V62.3
          - while boarding or alighting V62.4
        - van (traffic) V63.9
          - nontraffic V63.3
          - while boarding or alighting V63.4
      - driver
        - collision (with)
          - animal (traffic) V6Ø.5
            - being ridden (traffic) V66.5
              - nontraffic V66.Ø
            - nontraffic V6Ø.Ø
          - animal-drawn vehicle (traffic) V66.5
            - nontraffic V66.Ø
          - bus (traffic) V64.5
            - nontraffic V64.Ø
          - car (traffic) V63.5
            - nontraffic V63.Ø
          - motor vehicle NOS (traffic) V69.4Ø
            - nontraffic V69.ØØ
            - specified type NEC (traffic) V69.49
              - nontraffic V69.Ø9
          - pedal cycle (traffic) V61.5
            - nontraffic V61.Ø
          - pickup truck (traffic) V63.5
            - nontraffic V63.Ø
          - railway vehicle (traffic) V65.5
            - nontraffic V65.Ø
          - specified vehicle NEC (traffic) V66.5
            - nontraffic V66.Ø
          - stationary object (traffic) V67.5
            - nontraffic V67.Ø
          - streetcar (traffic) V66.5
            - nontraffic V66.Ø
          - three wheeled motor vehicle (traffic) V62.5
            - nontraffic V62.Ø
          - truck (traffic) V64.5
            - nontraffic V64.Ø
          - two wheeled motor vehicle (traffic) V62.5
            - nontraffic V62.Ø
          - van (traffic) V63.5
            - nontraffic V63.Ø
        - noncollision accident (traffic) V68.5
          - nontraffic V68.Ø
      - dump —*see* Accident, transport, construction vehicle occupant
      - hanger-on
        - collision (with)
          - animal (traffic) V6Ø.7
            - being ridden (traffic) V66.7
              - nontraffic V66.2
            - nontraffic V6Ø.2
          - animal-drawn vehicle (traffic) V66.7
            - nontraffic V66.2
          - bus (traffic) V64.7
            - nontraffic V64.2
          - car (traffic) V63.7
            - nontraffic V63.2
          - pedal cycle (traffic) V61.7
            - nontraffic V61.2
          - pickup truck (traffic) V63.7
            - nontraffic V63.2
          - railway vehicle (traffic) V65.7
            - nontraffic V65.2
          - specified vehicle NEC (traffic) V66.7
            - nontraffic V66.2
          - stationary object (traffic) V67.7
            - nontraffic V67.2
          - streetcar (traffic) V66.7
            - nontraffic V66.2

A

Accident *(Continued)*
  transport *(Continued)*
    truck (heavy) occupant *(Continued)*
      hanger-on *(Continued)*
        collision *(Continued)*
          three wheeled motor vehicle (traffic) V62.7
            nontraffic V62.2
          truck (traffic) V64.7
            nontraffic V64.2
          two wheeled motor vehicle (traffic) V62.7
            nontraffic V62.2
          van (traffic) V63.7
            nontraffic V63.2
        noncollision accident (traffic) V68.7
          nontraffic V68.2
      noncollision accident (traffic) V68.9
        nontraffic V68.3
        while boarding or alighting V68.4
      nontraffic V69.3
      passenger
        collision (with)
          animal (traffic) V6Ø.6
            being ridden (traffic) V66.6
              nontraffic V66.1
            nontraffic V6Ø.1
          animal-drawn vehicle (traffic) V66.6
            nontraffic V66.1
          bus (traffic) V64.6
            nontraffic V64.1
          car (traffic) V63.6
            nontraffic V63.1
          motor vehicle NOS (traffic) V69.5Ø
            nontraffic V69.1Ø
            specified type NEC (traffic) V69.59
              nontraffic V69.19
          pedal cycle (traffic) V61.6
            nontraffic V61.1
          pickup truck (traffic) V63.6
            nontraffic V63.1
          railway vehicle (traffic) V65.6
            nontraffic V65.1
          specified vehicle NEC (traffic) V66.6
            nontraffic V66.1
          stationary object (traffic) V67.6
            nontraffic V67.1
          streetcar (traffic) V66.6
            nontraffic V66.1
          three wheeled motor vehicle (traffic) V62.6
            nontraffic V62.1
          truck (traffic) V64.6
            nontraffic V64.1
          two wheeled motor vehicle (traffic) V62.6
            nontraffic V62.1
          van (traffic) V63.6
            nontraffic V63.1
        noncollision accident (traffic) V68.6
          nontraffic V68.1
      pickup —*see* Accident, transport, pickup truck occupant
      specified type NEC V69.88
        military vehicle V69.81
    van occupant V59.9
      collision (with)
        animal (traffic) V5Ø.9
          being ridden (traffic) V56.9
            nontraffic V56.3
            while boarding or alighting V56.4
          nontraffic V5Ø.3
          while boarding or alighting V5Ø.4
        animal-drawn vehicle (traffic) V56.9
          nontraffic V56.3
          while boarding or alighting V56.4
        bus (traffic) V54.9
          nontraffic V54.3
          while boarding or alighting V54.4
        car (traffic) V53.9
          nontraffic V53.3
          while boarding or alighting V53.4
        motor vehicle NOS (traffic) V59.6Ø
          nontraffic V59.2Ø
          specified type NEC (traffic) V59.69
            nontraffic V59.29
        pedal cycle (traffic) V51.9
          nontraffic V51.3
          while boarding or alighting V51.4

Accident *(Continued)*
  transport *(Continued)*
    van occupant *(Continued)*
      collision *(Continued)*
        pickup truck (traffic) V53.9
          nontraffic V53.3
          while boarding or alighting V53.4
        railway vehicle (traffic) V55.9
          nontraffic V55.3
          while boarding or alighting V55.4
        specified vehicle NEC (traffic) V56.9
          nontraffic V56.3
          while boarding or alighting V56.4
        stationary object (traffic) V57.9
          nontraffic V57.3
          while boarding or alighting V57.4
        streetcar (traffic) V56.9
          nontraffic V56.3
          while boarding or alighting V56.4
        three wheeled motor vehicle (traffic) V52.9
          nontraffic V52.3
          while boarding or alighting V52.4
        truck (traffic) V54.9
          nontraffic V54.3
          while boarding or alighting V54.4
        two wheeled motor vehicle (traffic) V52.9
          nontraffic V52.3
          while boarding or alighting V52.4
        van (traffic) V53.9
          nontraffic V53.3
          while boarding or alighting V53.4
      driver
        collision (with)
          animal (traffic) V5Ø.5
            being ridden (traffic) V56.5
              nontraffic V56.Ø
            nontraffic V5Ø.Ø
          animal-drawn vehicle (traffic) V56.5
            nontraffic V56.Ø
          bus (traffic) V54.5
            nontraffic V54.Ø
          car (traffic) V53.5
            nontraffic V53.Ø
          motor vehicle NOS (traffic) V59.4Ø
            nontraffic V59.ØØ
            specified type NEC (traffic) V59.49
              nontraffic V59.Ø9
          pedal cycle (traffic) V51.5
            nontraffic V51.Ø
          pickup truck (traffic) V53.5
            nontraffic V53.Ø
          railway vehicle (traffic) V55.5
            nontraffic V55.Ø
          specified vehicle NEC (traffic) V56.5
            nontraffic V56.Ø
          stationary object (traffic) V57.5
            nontraffic V57.Ø
          streetcar (traffic) V56.5
            nontraffic V56.Ø
          three wheeled motor vehicle (traffic) V52.5
            nontraffic V52.Ø
          truck (traffic) V54.5
            nontraffic V54.Ø
          two wheeled motor vehicle (traffic) V52.5
            nontraffic V52.Ø
          van (traffic) V53.5
            nontraffic V53.Ø
        noncollision accident (traffic) V58.5
          nontraffic V58.Ø
      hanger-on
        collision (with)
          animal (traffic) V5Ø.7
            being ridden (traffic) V56.7
              nontraffic V56.2
            nontraffic V5Ø.2
          animal-drawn vehicle (traffic) V56.7
            nontraffic V56.2
          bus (traffic) V54.7
            nontraffic V54.2
          car (traffic) V53.7
            nontraffic V53.2
          pedal cycle (traffic) V51.7
            nontraffic V51.2
          pickup truck (traffic) V53.7
            nontraffic V53.2
          railway vehicle (traffic) V55.7
            nontraffic V55.2

Accident *(Continued)*
  transport *(Continued)*
    van occupant *(Continued)*
      hanger-on *(Continued)*
        collision *(Continued)*
          specified vehicle NEC (traffic) V56.7
            nontraffic V56.2
          stationary object (traffic) V57.7
            nontraffic V57.2
          streetcar (traffic) V56.7
            nontraffic V56.2
          three wheeled motor vehicle (traffic) V52.7
            nontraffic V52.2
          truck (traffic) V54.7
            nontraffic V54.2
          two wheeled motor vehicle (traffic) V52.7
            nontraffic V52.2
          van (traffic) V53.7
            nontraffic V53.2
        noncollision accident (traffic) V58.7
          nontraffic V58.2
      noncollision accident (traffic) V58.9
        nontraffic V58.3
        while boarding or alighting V58.4
      nontraffic V59.3
      passenger
        collision (with)
          animal (traffic) V5Ø.6
            being ridden (traffic) V56.6
              nontraffic V56.1
            nontraffic V5Ø.1
          animal-drawn vehicle (traffic) V56.6
            nontraffic V56.1
          bus (traffic) V54.6
            nontraffic V54.1
          car (traffic) V53.6
            nontraffic V53.1
          motor vehicle NOS (traffic) V59.5Ø
            nontraffic V59.1Ø
            specified type NEC (traffic) V59.59
              nontraffic V59.19
          pedal cycle (traffic) V51.6
            nontraffic V51.1
          pickup truck (traffic) V53.6
            nontraffic V53.1
          railway vehicle (traffic) V55.6
            nontraffic V55.1
          specified vehicle NEC (traffic) V56.6
            nontraffic V56.1
          stationary object (traffic) V57.6
            nontraffic V57.1
          streetcar (traffic) V56.6
            nontraffic V56.1
          three wheeled motor vehicle (traffic) V52.6
            nontraffic V52.1
          truck (traffic) V54.6
            nontraffic V54.1
          two wheeled motor vehicle (traffic) V52.6
            nontraffic V52.1
          van (traffic) V53.6
            nontraffic V53.1
        noncollision accident (traffic) V58.6
          nontraffic V58.1
      specified type NEC V59.88
        military vehicle V59.81
    watercraft occupant —*see* Accident, watercraft
  vehicle NEC V89.9
    animal-drawn NEC —*see* Accident, transport, animal-drawn vehicle occupant
    special
      agricultural —*see* Accident, transport, agricultural vehicle occupant
      construction —*see* Accident, transport, construction vehicle occupant
      industrial —*see* Accident, transport, industrial vehicle occupant
    three-wheeled NEC (motorized) —*see* Accident, transport, three-wheeled motor vehicle occupant
  watercraft V94.9
    causing
      drowning —*see* Drowning, due to, accident to, watercraft
      injury NEC V91.89
        crushed between craft and object V91.19
          powered craft V91.13
            ferry boat V91.11
            fishing boat V91.12

A

- **Accident** *(Continued)*
  - watercraft *(Continued)*
    - causing *(Continued)*
      - injury *(Continued)*
        - crushed between craft and object— *(Continued)*
          - powered craft *(Continued)*
            - jet ski V91.13
            - liner V91.11
            - merchant ship V91.10
            - passenger ship V91.11
          - unpowered craft V91.18
            - canoe V91.15
            - inflatable V91.16
            - kayak V91.15
            - sailboat V91.14
            - surf-board V91.18
            - windsurfer V91.18
        - fall on board V91.29
          - powered craft V91.23
            - ferry boat V91.21
            - fishing boat V91.22
            - jet ski V91.23
            - liner V91.21
            - merchant ship V91.20
            - passenger ship V91.21
          - unpowered craft
            - canoe V91.25
            - inflatable V91.26
            - kayak V91.25
            - sailboat V91.24
        - fire on board causing burn V91.09
          - powered craft V91.03
            - ferry boat V91.01
            - fishing boat V91.02
            - jet ski V91.03
            - liner V91.01
            - merchant ship V91.00
            - passenger ship V91.01
          - unpowered craft V91.08
            - canoe V91.05
            - inflatable V91.06
            - kayak V91.05
            - sailboat V91.04
            - surf-board V91.08
            - water skis V91.07
            - windsurfer V91.08
        - hit by falling object V91.39
          - powered craft V91.33
            - ferry boat V91.31
            - fishing boat V91.32
            - jet skis V91.33
            - liner V91.31
            - merchant ship V91.30
            - passenger ship V91.31
          - unpowered craft V91.38
            - canoe V91.35
            - inflatable V91.36
            - kayak V91.35
            - sailboat V91.34
            - surf-board V91.38
            - water skis V91.37
            - windsurfer V91.38
        - specified type NEC V91.89
          - powered craft V91.83
            - ferry boat V91.81
            - fishing boat V91.82
            - jet ski V91.83
            - liner V91.81
            - merchant ship V91.80
            - passenger ship V91.81
          - unpowered craft V91.88
            - canoe V91.85
            - inflatable V91.86
            - kayak V91.85
            - sailboat V91.84
            - surf-board V91.88
            - water skis V91.87
            - windsurfer V91.88
    - due to, caused by cataclysm —*see* Forces of nature, by type
    - military NEC V94.818
      - with civilian watercraft V94.810
      - civilian in water injured by V94.811
    - nonpowered, struck by
      - nonpowered vessel V94.22
      - powered vessel V94.21
    - specified type NEC V94.89
    - striking swimmer
      - powered V94.11
      - unpowered V94.12

- **Acid throwing** (assault) Y08.89
- **Activity** (involving) (of victim at time of event) Y93.9
  - aerobic and step exercise (class) Y93.A3
  - alpine skiing Y93.23
  - animal care NEC Y93.K9
  - arts and handcrafts NEC Y93.D9
  - athletics NEC Y93.79
  - athletics played as a team or group NEC Y93.69
  - athletics played individually NEC Y93.59
  - baking Y93.G3
  - ballet Y93.41
  - barbells Y93.B3
  - BASE (Building, Antenna, Span, Earth) jumping Y93.33
  - baseball Y93.64
  - basketball Y93.67
  - bathing (personal) Y93.E1
  - beach volleyball Y93.68
  - bike riding Y93.55
  - blackout game Y93.85
  - boogie boarding Y93.18
  - bowling Y93.54
  - boxing Y93.71
  - brass instrument playing Y93.J4
  - building construction Y93.H3
  - bungee jumping Y93.34
  - calisthenics Y93.A2
  - canoeing (in calm and turbulent water) Y93.16
  - capture the flag Y93.6A
  - cardiorespiratory exercise NEC Y93.A9
  - caregiving (providing) NEC Y93.F9
    - bathing Y93.F1
    - lifting Y93.F2
  - cellular
    - communication device Y93.C2
    - telephone Y93.C2
  - challenge course Y93.A5
  - cheerleading Y93.45
  - choking game Y93.85
  - circuit training Y93.A4
  - cleaning
    - floor Y93.E5
  - climbing NEC Y93.39
    - mountain Y93.31
    - rock Y93.31
    - wall Y93.31
  - clothing care and maintenance NEC Y93.E9
  - combatives Y93.75
  - computer
    - keyboarding Y93.C1
    - technology NEC Y93.C9
  - confidence course Y93.A5
  - construction (building) Y93.H3
  - cooking and baking Y93.G3
  - cool down exercises Y93.A2
  - cricket Y93.69
  - crocheting Y93.D1
  - cross country skiing Y93.24
  - dancing (all types) Y93.41
  - digging
    - dirt Y93.H1
  - dirt digging Y93.H1
  - dishwashing Y93.G1
  - diving (platform) (springboard) Y93.12
    - underwater Y93.15
  - dodge ball Y93.6A
  - downhill skiing Y93.23
  - drum playing Y93.J2
  - dumbbells Y93.B3
  - electronic
    - devices NEC Y93.C9
      - hand held interactive Y93.C2
    - game playing (using) (with)
      - interactive device Y93.C2
      - keyboard or other stationary device Y93.C1
  - elliptical machine Y93.A1
  - exercise(s)
    - machines ((primarily) for)
      - cardiorespiratory conditioning Y93.A1
      - muscle strengthening Y93.B1
    - muscle strengthening (non-machine) NEC Y93.B9
  - external motion NEC Y93.I9
    - rollercoaster Y93.I1
  - fainting game Y93.85
  - field hockey Y93.65
  - figure skating (pairs) (singles) Y93.21
  - flag football Y93.62
  - floor mopping and cleaning Y93.E5
  - food preparation and clean up Y93.G1

- **Activity** *(Continued)*
  - football (American) NOS Y93.61
    - flag Y93.62
    - tackle Y93.61
    - touch Y93.62
  - four square Y93.6A
  - free weights Y93.B3
  - frisbee (ultimate) Y93.74
  - furniture
    - building Y93.D3
    - finishing Y93.D3
    - repair Y93.D3
  - game playing (electronic)
    - using interactive device Y93.C2
    - using keyboard or other stationary device Y93.C1
  - gardening Y93.H2
  - golf Y93.53
  - grass drills Y93.A6
  - grilling and smoking food Y93.G2
  - grooming and shearing an animal Y93.K3
  - guerilla drills Y93.A6
  - gymnastics (rhythmic) Y93.43
  - hand held interactive electronic device Y93.C2
  - handball Y93.73
  - handcrafts NEC Y93.D9
  - hang gliding Y93.35
  - hiking (on level or elevated terrain) Y93.01
  - hockey (ice) Y93.22
    - field Y93.65
  - horseback riding Y93.52
  - household (interior) maintenance NEC Y93.E9
  - ice NEC Y93.29
    - dancing Y93.21
    - hockey Y93.22
    - skating Y93.21
  - inline roller skating Y93.51
  - ironing Y93.E4
  - judo Y93.75
  - jumping (off) NEC Y93.39
    - BASE (Building, Antenna, Span, Earth) Y93.33
    - bungee Y93.34
    - jacks Y93.A2
    - rope Y93.56
  - jumping jacks Y93.A2
  - jumping rope Y93.56
  - karate Y93.75
  - kayaking (in calm and turbulent water) Y93.16
  - keyboarding (computer) Y93.C1
  - kickball Y93.6A
  - knitting Y93.D1
  - lacrosse Y93.65
  - land maintenance NEC Y93.H9
  - landscaping Y93.H2
  - laundry Y93.E2
  - machines (exercise)
    - primarily for cardiorespiratory conditioning Y93.A1
    - primarily for muscle strengthening Y93.B1
  - maintenance
    - exterior building NEC Y93.H9
    - household (interior) NEC Y93.E9
    - land Y93.H9
    - property Y93.H9
  - marching (on level or elevated terrain) Y93.01
  - martial arts Y93.75
  - microwave oven Y93.G3
  - milking an animal Y93.K2
  - mopping (floor) Y93.E5
  - mountain climbing Y93.31
  - muscle strengthening
    - exercises (non-machine) NEC Y93.B9
    - machines Y93.B1
  - musical keyboard (electronic) playing Y93.J1
  - nordic skiing Y93.24
  - obstacle course Y93.A5
  - oven (microwave) Y93.G3
  - packing up and unpacking in moving to a new residence Y93.E6
  - parasailing Y93.19
  - pass out game Y93.85
  - percussion instrument playing NEC Y93.J2
  - personal
    - bathing and showering Y93.E1
    - hygiene NEC Y93.E8
    - showering Y93.E1
  - physical games generally associated with school recess, summer camp and children Y93.6A
  - physical training NEC Y93.A9
  - piano playing Y93.J1
  - pilates Y93.B4

A

A

Assault *(Continued)*
- steam X98.0
- striking against
  - other person Y04.2
  - sports equipment Y08.09
    - baseball bat Y08.02
    - hockey stick Y08.01
- struck by
  - sports equipment Y08.09
    - baseball bat Y08.02
    - hockey stick Y08.01
- submersion —*see* Assault, drowning
- violence Y09
- weapon Y09
  - blunt Y00
  - cutting or piercing —*see* Assault, cutting or piercing instrument
  - firearm —*see* Assault, firearm
- wound Y09
  - cutting —*see* Assault, cutting or piercing instrument
  - gunshot —*see* Assault, firearm
  - knife X99.1
  - piercing —*see* Assault, cutting or piercing instrument
  - puncture —*see* Assault, cutting or piercing instrument
  - stab —*see* Assault, cutting or piercing instrument

Attack by mammals NEC W55.89

Avalanche —*see* Landslide

Aviator's disease —*see* Air, pressure

B

Barotitis, barodontalgia, barosinusitis, barotrauma (otitic) (sinus) —*see* Air, pressure

Battered (baby) (child) (person) (syndrome) X58

Bayonet wound W26.1
- in
  - legal intervention —*see* Legal, intervention, sharp object, bayonet
  - war operations —*see* War operations, combat
- stated as undetermined whether accidental or intentional Y28.8
- suicide (attempt) X78.2

Bean in nose —*see* categories T17 and T18

Bed set on fire NEC —*see* Exposure, fire, uncontrolled, building, bed

Beheading (by guillotine)
- homicide X99.9
- legal execution —*see* Legal, intervention

Bending, injury in (prolonged) (static) X50.1

Bends —*see* Air, pressure, change

Bite, bitten by
- alligator W58.01
- arthropod (nonvenomous) NEC W57
- bull W55.21
- cat W55.01
- cow W55.21
- crocodile W58.11
- dog W54.0
- goat W55.31
- hoof stock NEC W55.31
- horse W55.11
- human being (accidentally) W50.3
  - with intent to injure or kill Y04.1
  - as, or caused by, a crowd or human stampede (with fall) W52
  - assault Y04.1
  - homicide (attempt) Y04.1
  - in
    - fight Y04.1
- insect (nonvenomous) W57
- lizard (nonvenomous) W59.01
- mammal NEC W55.81
  - marine W56.31
- marine animal (nonvenomous) W56.81
- millipede W57
- moray eel W56.51
- mouse W53.01
- person(s) (accidentally) W50.3
  - with intent to injure or kill Y04.1
  - as, or caused by, a crowd or human stampede (with fall) W52
  - assault Y04.1

Bite, bitten by *(Continued)*
- person(s) *(Continued)*
  - homicide (attempt) Y04.1
  - in
    - fight Y04.1
- pig W55.41
- raccoon W55.51
- rat W53.11
- reptile W59.81
  - lizard W59.01
  - snake W59.11
  - turtle W59.21
    - terrestrial W59.81
- rodent W53.81
  - mouse W53.01
  - rat W53.11
  - specified NEC W53.81
  - squirrel W53.21
- shark W56.41
- sheep W55.31
- snake (nonvenomous) W59.11
- spider (nonvenomous) W57
- squirrel W53.21

Blast (air) **in war operations** —*see* War operations, blast

Blizzard X37.2

Blood alcohol level Y90.9
- 20-39mg/100ml Y90.1
- 40-59mg/100ml Y90.2
- 60-79mg/100ml Y90.3
- 80-99mg/100ml Y90.4
- 100-119mg/100ml Y90.5
- 120-199mg/100ml Y90.6
- 200-239mg/100ml Y90.7
- less than 20mg/100ml Y90.0
- presence in blood, level not specified Y90.9

Blow X58
- by law-enforcing agent, police (on duty) —*see* Legal, intervention, manhandling
  - blunt object —*see* Legal, intervention, blunt object

Blowing up —*see* Explosion

Brawl (hand) (fists) (foot) Y04.0

Breakage (accidental) (part of)
- ladder (causing fall) W11
- scaffolding (causing fall) W12

Broken
- glass, contact with —*see* Contact, with, glass
- power line (causing electric shock) W85

Bumping against, into (accidentally)
- object NEC W22.8
  - with fall —*see* Fall, due to, bumping against, object
  - caused by crowd or human stampede (with fall) W52
  - sports equipment W21.9
- person(s) W51
  - with fall W03
    - due to ice or snow W00.0
  - assault Y04.2
  - caused by, a crowd or human stampede (with fall) W52
  - homicide (attempt) Y04.2
- sports equipment W21.9

Burn, burned, burning (accidental) (by) (from) (on)
- acid NEC —*see* Table of Drugs and Chemicals
- bed linen —*see* Exposure, fire, uncontrolled, in building, bed
- blowtorch X08.8
  - with ignition of clothing NEC X06.2
    - nightwear X05
- bonfire, campfire (controlled) —*see also* Exposure, fire, controlled, not in building
  - uncontrolled —*see* Exposure, fire, uncontrolled, not in building
- candle X08.8
  - with ignition of clothing NEC X06.2
    - nightwear X05
- caustic liquid, substance (external) (internal) NEC —*see* Table of Drugs and Chemicals
- chemical (external) (internal) —*see also* Table of Drugs and Chemicals
  - in war operations —*see* War operations, fire
- cigar(s) or cigarette(s) X08.8
  - with ignition of clothing NEC X06.2
    - nightwear X05

Burn, burned, burning *(Continued)*
- clothes, clothing NEC (from controlled fire) X06.2
  - with conflagration —*see* Exposure, fire, uncontrolled, building
    - not in building or structure —*see* Exposure, fire, uncontrolled, not in building
- cooker (hot) X15.8
  - stated as undetermined whether accidental or intentional Y27.3
  - suicide (attempt) X77.3
- electric blanket X16
- engine (hot) X17
- fire, flames —*see* Exposure, fire
- flare, Very pistol —*see* Discharge, firearm NEC
- heat
  - from appliance (electrical) (household) X15.8
    - cooker X15.8
    - hotplate X15.2
    - kettle X15.8
    - light bulb X15.8
    - saucepan X15.3
    - skillet X15.3
    - stated as undetermined whether accidental or intentional Y27.3
    - stove X15.0
    - suicide (attempt) X77.3
    - toaster X15.1
  - in local application or packing during medical or surgical procedure Y63.5
- heating
  - appliance, radiator or pipe X16
- homicide (attempt) —*see* Assault, burning
- hot
  - air X14.1
  - cooker X15.8
  - drink X10.0
  - engine X17
  - fat X10.2
  - fluid NEC X12
  - food X10.1
  - gases X14.1
  - heating appliance X16
  - household appliance NEC X15.8
  - kettle X15.8
  - liquid NEC X12
  - machinery X17
  - metal (molten) (liquid) NEC X18
  - object (not producing fire or flames) NEC X19
  - oil (cooking) X10.2
  - pipe(s) X16
  - radiator X16
  - saucepan (glass) (metal) X15.3
  - stove (kitchen) X15.0
  - substance NEC X19
    - caustic or corrosive NEC —*see* Table of Drugs and Chemicals
  - toaster X15.1
  - tool X17
  - vapor X13.1
  - water (tap) —*see* Contact, with, hot, tap water
- hotplate X15.2
  - suicide (attempt) X77.3
- ignition —*see* Ignition
- in war operations —*see* War operations, fire
- inflicted by other person X97
  - by hot objects, hot vapor, and steam —*see* Assault, burning, hot object
- internal, from swallowed caustic, corrosive liquid, substance —*see* Table of Drugs and Chemicals
- iron (hot) X15.8
  - stated as undetermined whether accidental or intentional Y27.3
  - suicide (attempt) X77.3
- kettle (hot) X15.8
  - stated as undetermined whether accidental or intentional Y27.3
  - suicide (attempt) X77.3
- lamp (flame) X08.8
  - with ignition of clothing NEC X06.2
    - nightwear X05
- lighter (cigar) (cigarette) X08.8
  - with ignition of clothing NEC X06.2
    - nightwear X05
- lightning —*see* subcategory T75.0
  - causing fire —*see* Exposure, fire
- liquid (boiling) (hot) NEC X12
  - stated as undetermined whether accidental or intentional Y27.2
  - suicide (attempt) X77.2

A & B

C

C

- **Contact** *(Continued)*
  - with *(Continued)*
    - sewing-machine (electric) (powered) W29.2
      - not powered W27.8
    - shaft (hoist) (lift) (transmission) NEC W24.Ø
      - agricultural W3Ø.89
    - shark W56.49
      - bite W56.41
      - strike W56.42
    - sharp object(s) W26.9
      - specified NEC W26.8
    - shears (hand) W27.2
      - powered (industrial) W31.1
        - domestic W29.2
    - sheep W55.39
      - bite W55.31
      - strike W55.32
    - shovel W27.8
      - steam —*see* Accident, transport, construction vehicle
    - snake (nonvenomous) W59.19
      - bite W59.11
      - crushing W59.13
      - strike W59.12
    - spade W27.1
    - spider (venomous) X58
    - spin-drier W29.2
    - spinning machine W31.89
    - splinter W45.8
    - sports equipment W21.9
    - staple gun (powered) W29.8
    - steam X13.1
      - engine W31.3
      - inhalation X13.Ø
      - pipe X16
      - shovel W31.89
    - stove (hot) (kitchen) X15.Ø
    - substance, hot NEC X19
      - molten (metal) X18
    - sword W26.1
      - assault X99.2
      - stated as undetermined whether accidental or intentional Y28.2
      - suicide (attempt) X78.2
    - tarantula X58
    - thresher W3Ø.Ø
    - tin can lid W26.8
    - toad W62.1
    - toaster (hot) X15.1
    - tool W27.8
      - hand (not powered) W27.8
        - auger W27.Ø
        - axe W27.Ø
        - can opener W27.4
        - chisel W27.Ø
        - fork W27.4
        - garden W27.1
        - handsaw W27.Ø
        - hoe W27.1
        - ice-pick W27.4
        - kitchen utensil W27.4
        - manual
          - lawn mower W27.1
          - sewing machine W27.8
        - meat grinder W27.4
        - needle (sewing) W27.3
          - hypodermic W46.Ø
            - contaminated W46.1
        - paper cutter W27.5
        - pitchfork W27.1
        - rake W27.1
        - scissors W27.2
        - screwdriver W27.Ø
        - specified NEC W27.8
        - workbench W27.Ø
      - hot X17
      - powered W29.8
        - blender W29.Ø
          - commercial W31.82
        - can opener W29.Ø
          - commercial W31.82
        - chainsaw W29.3
        - clothes dryer W29.2
          - commercial W31.82
        - dishwasher W29.2
          - commercial W31.82
        - edger W29.3
        - electric fan W29.2
          - commercial W31.82
        - electric knife W29.1

- **Contact** *(Continued)*
  - with *(Continued)*
    - tool *(Continued)*
      - powered *(Continued)*
        - food processor W29.Ø
          - commercial W31.82
        - garbage disposal W29.Ø
          - commercial W31.82
        - garden tool W29.3
        - hedge trimmer W29.3
        - ice maker W29.Ø
          - commercial W31.82
        - kitchen appliance W29.Ø
          - commercial W31.82
        - lawn mower W28
        - meat grinder W29.Ø
          - commercial W31.82
        - mixer W29.Ø
          - commercial W31.82
        - rototiller W29.3
        - sewing machine W29.2
          - commercial W31.82
        - washing machine W29.2
          - commercial W31.82
    - transmission device (belt, cable, chain, gear, pinion, shaft) W24.1
      - agricultural operations W3Ø.89
    - turbine (gas) (water-driven) W31.3
    - turkey W61.49
      - peck W61.43
      - strike W61.42
    - turtle (nonvenomous) W59.29
      - bite W59.21
      - strike W59.22
      - terrestrial W59.89
        - bite W59.81
        - crushing W59.83
        - strike W59.82
    - under-cutter W31.Ø
    - urine —*see* Contact, with, by type of animal
    - vehicle
      - agricultural use (transport) —*see* Accident, transport, agricultural vehicle
        - not on public highway W3Ø.81
      - industrial use (transport) —*see* Accident, transport, industrial vehicle
        - not on public highway W31.83
      - off-road use (transport) —*see* Accident, transport, all-terrain or off-road vehicle
        - not on public highway W31.83
      - special construction use (transport) —*see* Accident, transport, construction vehicle
        - not on public highway W31.83
    - venomous
      - animal X58
      - arthropods X58
      - lizard X58
      - marine animal NEC X58
      - marine plant NEC X58
      - millipedes (tropical) X58
      - plant(s) X58
      - snake X58
      - spider X58
    - viper X58
    - washing-machine (powered) W29.2
    - wasp X58
    - weaving-machine W31.89
    - winch W24.Ø
      - agricultural operations W3Ø.89
    - wire NEC W24.Ø
      - agricultural operations W3Ø.89
    - wood slivers W45.8
    - yellow jacket X58
    - zebra —*see* Contact, with, hoof stock NEC
  - pressure X5Ø.9
  - stress X5Ø.9
- **Coup de soleil** X32
- **Crash**
  - aircraft (in transit) (powered) V95.9
    - balloon V96.Ø1
    - fixed wing NEC (private) V95.21
      - commercial V95.31
    - glider V96.21
      - hang V96.11
      - powered V95.11
    - helicopter V95.Ø1
    - in war operations —*see* War operations, destruction of aircraft
    - microlight V95.11

- **Crash** *(Continued)*
  - aircraft *(Continued)*
    - nonpowered V96.9
      - specified NEC V96.8
    - powered NEC V95.8
    - stated as
      - homicide (attempt) YØ8.81
      - suicide (attempt) X83.Ø
    - ultralight V95.11
  - spacecraft V95.41
  - transport vehicle NEC —*see also* Accident, transport V89.9
    - homicide (attempt) YØ3.8
    - motor NEC (traffic) V89.2
      - homicide (attempt) YØ3.8
      - suicide (attempt) —*see* Suicide, collision
- **Cruelty** (mental) (physical) (sexual) X58
- **Crushed** (accidentally) X58
  - between objects (moving) (stationary and moving) W23.Ø
    - stationary W23.1
  - by
    - alligator W58.Ø3
    - avalanche NEC —*see* Landslide
    - cave-in W2Ø.Ø
      - caused by cataclysmic earth surface movement —*see* Landslide
    - crocodile W58.13
    - crowd or human stampede W52
    - falling
      - aircraft V97.39
        - in war operations —*see* War operations, destruction of aircraft
      - earth, material W2Ø.Ø
        - caused by cataclysmic earth surface movement —*see* Landslide
      - object NEC W2Ø.8
    - landslide NEC —*see* Landslide
    - lizard (nonvenomous) W59.Ø9
    - machinery —*see* Contact, with, by type of machine
    - reptile NEC W59.89
    - snake (nonvenomous) W59.13
  - in
    - machinery —*see* Contact, with, by type of machine
- **Cut, cutting** (any part of body) (accidental) —*see also* Contact, with, by object or machine
  - during medical or surgical treatment as misadventure —*see* Index to Diseases and Injuries, Complications
  - homicide (attempt) —*see* Assault, cutting or piercing instrument
  - inflicted by other person —*see* Assault, cutting or piercing instrument
  - legal
    - execution —*see* Legal, intervention
    - intervention —*see* Legal, intervention, sharp object
  - machine NEC —*see also* Contact, with, by type of machine W31.9
  - self-inflicted —*see* Suicide, cutting or piercing instrument
  - suicide (attempt) —*see* Suicide, cutting or piercing instrument
- **Cyclone** (any injury) X37.1

D

- **Decapitation** (accidental circumstances) NEC X58
  - homicide X99.9
  - legal execution —*see* Legal, intervention
- **Dehydration from lack of water** X58
- **Deprivation** X58
- **Derailment** (accidental)
  - railway (rolling stock) (train) (vehicle) (without antecedent collision) V81.7
    - with antecedent collision —*see* Accident, transport, railway vehicle occupant
  - streetcar (without antecedent collision) V82.7
    - with antecedent collision —*see* Accident, transport, streetcar occupant
- **Descent**
  - parachute (voluntary) (without accident to aircraft) V97.29
    - due to accident to aircraft —*see* Accident, transport, aircraft
- **Desertion** X58

C & D

- **Destitution** X58
- **Disability, late effect or sequela of injury** —*see* Sequelae
- **Discharge** (accidental)
  - airgun W34.010
    - assault X95.01
    - homicide (attempt) X95.01
    - stated as undetermined whether accidental or intentional Y24.0
    - suicide (attempt) X74.01
  - BB gun —*see* Discharge, airgun
  - firearm (accidental) W34.00
    - assault X95.9
    - handgun (pistol) (revolver) W32.0
      - assault X93
      - homicide (attempt) X93
      - legal intervention —*see* Legal, intervention, firearm, handgun
      - stated as undetermined whether accidental or intentional Y22
      - suicide (attempt) X72
    - homicide (attempt) X95.9
    - hunting rifle W33.02
      - assault X94.1
      - homicide (attempt) X94.1
      - legal intervention
        - injuring
          - bystander Y35.032
          - law enforcement personnel Y35.031
          - suspect Y35.033
          - unspecified person Y35.039
      - stated as undetermined whether accidental or intentional Y23.1
      - suicide (attempt) X73.1
    - larger W33.00
      - assault X94.9
      - homicide (attempt) X94.9
      - hunting rifle —*see* Discharge, firearm, hunting rifle
      - legal intervention —*see* Legal, intervention, firearm by type of firearm
      - machine gun —*see* Discharge, firearm, machine gun
      - shotgun —*see* Discharge, firearm, shotgun
      - specified NEC W33.09
        - assault X94.8
        - homicide (attempt) X94.8
        - legal intervention
          - injuring
            - bystander Y35.092
            - law enforcement personnel Y35.091
            - suspect Y35.093
            - unspecified person Y35.099
        - stated as undetermined whether accidental or intentional Y23.8
        - suicide (attempt) X73.8
      - stated as undetermined whether accidental or intentional Y23.9
      - suicide (attempt) X73.9
    - legal intervention
      - injuring
        - bystander Y35.002
        - law enforcement personnel Y35.001
        - suspect Y35.03
        - unspecified person Y35.009
      - using rubber bullet
        - injuring
          - bystander Y35.042
          - law enforcement personnel Y35.041
          - suspect Y35.043
          - unspecified person Y35.049
    - machine gun W33.03
      - assault X94.2
      - homicide (attempt) X94.2
      - legal intervention —*see* Legal, intervention, firearm, machine gun
      - stated as undetermined whether accidental or intentional Y23.3
      - suicide (attempt) X73.2
    - pellet gun —*see* Discharge, airgun
    - shotgun W33.01
      - assault X94.0
      - homicide (attempt) X94.0
      - legal intervention —*see* Legal, intervention, firearm, specified NEC
      - stated as undetermined whether accidental or intentional Y23.0
      - suicide (attempt) X73.0
    - specified NEC W34.09
      - assault X95.8
      - homicide (attempt) X95.8

- **Discharge** *(Continued)*
  - firearm *(Continued)*
    - specified *(Continued)*
      - legal intervention —*see* Legal, intervention, firearm, specified NEC
      - stated as undetermined whether accidental or intentional Y24.8
      - suicide (attempt) X74.8
    - stated as undetermined whether accidental or intentional Y24.9
    - suicide (attempt) X74.9
    - Very pistol W34.09
      - assault X95.8
      - homicide (attempt) X95.8
      - stated as undetermined whether accidental or intentional Y24.8
      - suicide (attempt) X74.8
  - firework(s) W39
    - stated as undetermined whether accidental or intentional Y25
  - gas-operated gun NEC W34.018
    - airgun —*see* Discharge, airgun
    - assault X95.09
    - homicide (attempt) X95.09
    - paintball gun —*see* Discharge, paintball gun
    - stated as undetermined whether accidental or intentional Y24.8
    - suicide (attempt) X74.09
  - gun NEC —*see also* Discharge, firearm NEC
    - air —*see* Discharge, airgun
    - BB —*see* Discharge, airgun
    - for single hand use —*see* Discharge, firearm, handgun
    - hand —*see* Discharge, firearm, handgun
    - machine —*see* Discharge, firearm, machine gun
    - other specified —*see* Discharge, firearm NEC
    - paintball —*see* Discharge, paintball gun
    - pellet —*see* Discharge, airgun
  - handgun —*see* Discharge, firearm, handgun
  - machine gun —*see* Discharge, firearm, machine gun
  - paintball gun W34.011
    - assault X95.02
    - homicide (attempt) X95.02
    - stated as undetermined whether accidental or intentional Y24.8
    - suicide (attempt) X74.02
  - pistol —*see* Discharge, firearm, handgun
    - flare —*see* Discharge, firearm, Very pistol
    - pellet —*see* Discharge, airgun
    - Very —*see* Discharge, firearm, Very pistol
  - revolver —*see* Discharge, firearm, handgun
  - rifle (hunting) —*see* Discharge, firearm, hunting rifle
  - shotgun —*see* Discharge, firearm, shotgun
  - spring-operated gun NEC W34.018
    - assault X95.09
    - homicide (attempt) X95.09
    - stated as undetermined whether accidental or intentional Y24.8
    - suicide (attempt) X74.09
- **Disease**
  - Andes W94.11
  - aviator's —*see* Air, pressure
  - range W94.11
- **Diver's disease, palsy, paralysis, squeeze** —*see* Air, pressure
- **Diving** (into water) —*see* Accident, diving
- **Dog bite** W54.0
- **Dragged by transport vehicle NEC** —*see also* Accident, transport V09.9
- **Drinking poison** (accidental) —*see* Table of Drugs and Chemicals
- **Dropped** (accidentally) **while being carried or supported by other person** W04
- **Drowning** (accidental) W74
  - assault X92.9
  - due to
    - accident (to)
      - machinery —*see* Contact, with, by type of machine
      - watercraft V90.89
        - burning V90.29
          - powered V90.23
            - fishing boat V90.22
            - jet ski V90.23
            - merchant ship V90.20
            - passenger ship V90.21
          - unpowered V90.28
            - canoe V90.25
            - inflatable V90.26

- **Drowning** *(Continued)*
  - due to *(Continued)*
    - accident *(Continued)*
      - watercraft *(Continued)*
        - burning *(Continued)*
          - unpowered *(Continued)*
            - kayak V90.25
            - sailboat V90.24
            - water skis V90.27
        - crushed V90.39
          - powered V90.33
            - fishing boat V90.32
            - jet ski V90.33
            - merchant ship V90.30
            - passenger ship V90.31
          - unpowered V90.38
            - canoe V90.35
            - inflatable V90.36
            - kayak V90.35
            - sailboat V90.34
            - water skis V90.37
        - overturning V90.09
          - powered V90.03
            - fishing boat V90.02
            - jet ski V90.03
            - merchant ship V90.00
            - passenger ship V90.01
          - unpowered V90.08
            - canoe V90.05
            - inflatable V90.06
            - kayak V90.05
            - sailboat V90.04
        - sinking V90.19
          - powered V90.13
            - fishing boat V90.12
            - jet ski V90.13
            - merchant ship V90.10
            - passenger ship V90.11
          - unpowered V90.18
            - canoe V90.15
            - inflatable V90.16
            - kayak V90.15
            - sailboat V90.14
        - specified type NEC V90.89
          - powered V90.83
            - fishing boat V90.82
            - jet ski V90.83
            - merchant ship V90.80
            - passenger ship V90.81
          - unpowered V90.88
            - canoe V90.85
            - inflatable V90.86
            - kayak V90.85
            - sailboat V90.84
            - water skis V90.87
    - avalanche —*see* Landslide
    - cataclysmic
      - earth surface movement NEC —*see* Forces of nature, earth movement
      - storm —*see* Forces of nature, cataclysmic storm
    - cloudburst X37.8
    - cyclone X37.1
    - fall overboard (from) V92.09
      - powered craft V92.03
        - ferry boat V92.01
        - fishing boat V92.02
        - jet ski V92.03
        - liner V92.01
        - merchant ship V92.00
        - passenger ship V92.01
      - resulting from
        - accident to watercraft —*see* Drowning, due to, accident to, watercraft
        - being washed overboard (from) V92.29
          - powered craft V92.23
            - ferry boat V92.21
            - fishing boat V92.22
            - jet ski V92.23
            - liner V92.21
            - merchant ship V92.20
            - passenger ship V92.21
          - unpowered craft V92.28
            - canoe V92.25
            - inflatable V92.26
            - kayak V92.25
            - sailboat V92.24
            - surf-board V92.28
            - water skis V92.27
            - windsurfer V92.28

D

- **Drowning** *(Continued)*
  - due to *(Continued)*
    - fall overboard *(Continued)*
      - resulting from *(Continued)*
        - motion of watercraft V92.19
          - powered craft V92.13
            - ferry boat V92.11
            - fishing boat V92.12
            - jet ski V92.13
            - liner V92.11
            - merchant ship V92.10
            - passenger ship V92.11
          - unpowered craft
            - canoe V92.15
            - inflatable V92.16
            - kayak V92.15
            - sailboat V92.14
      - unpowered craft V92.08
        - canoe V92.05
        - inflatable V92.06
        - kayak V92.05
        - sailboat V92.04
        - surf-board V92.08
        - water skis V92.07
        - windsurfer V92.08
    - hurricane X37.0
    - jumping into water from watercraft (involved in accident) —*see also* Drowning, due to, accident to, watercraft
      - without accident to or on watercraft W16.711
    - tidal wave NEC —*see* Forces of nature, tidal wave
    - torrential rain X37.8
  - following
    - fall
      - into
        - bathtub W16.211
        - bucket W16.221
        - fountain —*see* Drowning, following, fall, into, water, specified NEC
        - quarry —*see* Drowning, following, fall, into, water, specified NEC
        - reservoir —*see* Drowning, following, fall, into, water, specified NEC
        - swimming-pool W16.011
          - stated as undetermined whether accidental or intentional Y21.3
          - striking
            - bottom W16.021
            - wall W16.031
          - suicide (attempt) X71.2
        - water NOS W16.41
          - natural (lake) (open sea) (river) (stream) (pond) W16.111
            - striking
              - bottom W16.121
              - side W16.131
          - specified NEC W16.311
            - striking
              - bottom W16.321
              - wall W16.331
      - overboard NEC —*see* Drowning, due to, fall overboard
    - jump or dive
      - from boat W16.711
        - striking bottom W16.721
      - into
        - fountain —*see* Drowning, following, jump or dive, into, water, specified NEC
        - quarry —*see* Drowning, following, jump or dive, into, water, specified NEC
        - reservoir —*see* Drowning, following, jump or dive, into, water, specified NEC
        - swimming-pool W16.511
          - striking
            - bottom W16.521
            - wall W16.531
          - suicide (attempt) X71.2
        - water NOS W16.91
          - natural (lake) (open sea) (river) (stream) (pond) W16.611
          - specified NEC W16.811
            - striking
              - bottom W16.821
              - wall W16.831
          - striking bottom W16.621
  - homicide (attempt) X92.9
- **Drowning** *(Continued)*
  - in
    - bathtub (accidental) W65
      - assault X92.0
      - following fall W16.211
        - stated as undetermined whether accidental or intentional Y21.1
      - stated as undetermined whether accidental or intentional Y21.0
      - suicide (attempt) X71.0
    - lake —*see* Drowning, in, natural water
    - natural water (lake) (open sea) (river) (stream) (pond) W69
      - assault X92.3
      - following
        - dive or jump W16.611
          - striking bottom W16.621
        - fall W16.111
          - striking
            - bottom W16.121
            - side W16.131
      - stated as undetermined whether accidental or intentional Y21.4
      - suicide (attempt) X71.3
    - quarry —*see* Drowning, in, specified place NEC
    - quenching tank —*see* Drowning, in, specified place NEC
    - reservoir —*see* Drowning, in, specified place NEC
    - river —*see* Drowning, in, natural water
    - sea —*see* Drowning, in, natural water
    - specified place NEC W73
      - assault X92.8
      - following
        - dive or jump W16.811
          - striking
            - bottom W16.821
            - wall W16.831
        - fall W16.311
          - striking
            - bottom W16.321
            - wall W16.331
      - stated as undetermined whether accidental or intentional Y21.8
      - suicide (attempt) X71.8
    - stream —*see* Drowning, in, natural water
    - swimming-pool W67
      - assault X92.1
        - following fall X92.2
      - following
        - dive or jump W16.511
          - striking
            - bottom W16.521
            - wall W16.531
        - fall W16.011
          - striking
            - bottom W16.021
            - wall W16.031
      - stated as undetermined whether accidental or intentional Y21.2
        - following fall Y21.3
      - suicide (attempt) X71.1
        - following fall X71.2
    - war operations —*see* War operations, restriction of airway
  - resulting from accident to watercraft —*see* Drowning, due to, accident, watercraft
  - self-inflicted X71.9
  - stated as undetermined whether accidental or intentional Y21.9
  - suicide (attempt) X71.9

E

- **Earth** (surface) movement NEC —*see* Forces of nature, earth movement
- **Earth falling** (on) W20.0
  - caused by cataclysmic earth surface movement or eruption —*see* Landslide
- **Earthquake** (any injury) X34
- **Effect(s)** (adverse) of
  - air pressure (any) —*see* Air, pressure
  - cold, excessive (exposure to) —*see* Exposure, cold
  - heat (excessive) —*see* Heat
  - hot place (weather) —*see* Heat
- **Effect** *(Continued)*
  - insolation X30
  - late —*see* Sequelae
  - motion —*see* Motion
  - nuclear explosion or weapon in war operations —*see* War operations, nuclear weapon
  - radiation —*see* Radiation
  - travel —*see* Travel
- **Electric shock** (accidental) (by) (in) —*see* Exposure, electric current
- **Electrocution** (accidental) —*see* Exposure, electric current
- **Endotracheal tube wrongly placed during anesthetic procedure** Y65.3
- **Entanglement**
  - in
    - bed linen, causing suffocation —*see* category T71
    - wheel of pedal cycle V19.88
- **Entry of foreign body or material** —*see* Foreign body
- **Environmental pollution related condition** —*see* Z57
- **Execution, legal** (any method) —*see* Legal, intervention
- **Exhaustion**
  - cold —*see* Exposure, cold
  - due to excessive exertion —*see also* Overexertion X50.9
  - heat —*see* Heat
- **Explosion** (accidental) (of) (with secondary fire) W40.9
  - acetylene W40.1
  - aerosol can W36.1
  - air tank (compressed) (in machinery) W36.2
  - aircraft (in transit) (powered) NEC V95.9
    - balloon V96.05
    - fixed wing NEC (private) V95.25
      - commercial V95.35
    - glider V96.25
      - hang V96.15
      - powered V95.15
    - helicopter V95.05
    - in war operations —*see* War operations, destruction of aircraft
    - microlight V95.15
    - nonpowered V96.9
      - specified NEC V96.8
    - powered NEC V95.8
    - stated as
      - ➡homicide (attempt) Y08.81
      - suicide (attempt) X83.0
    - ultralight V95.15
  - anesthetic gas in operating room W40.1
  - antipersonnel bomb W40.8
    - assault X96.0
    - homicide (attempt) X96.0
    - suicide (attempt) X75
  - assault X96.9
  - bicycle tire W37.0
  - blasting (cap) (materials) W40.0
  - boiler (machinery), not on transport vehicle W35
    - on watercraft —*see* Explosion, in, watercraft
  - butane W40.1
  - caused by other person X96.9
  - coal gas W40.1
  - detonator W40.0
  - dump (munitions) W40.8
  - dynamite W40.0
    - in
      - assault X96.8
      - homicide (attempt) X96.8
      - legal intervention
        - injuring
          - bystander Y35.112
          - law enforcement personnel Y35.111
          - suspect Y35.113
          - unspecified person Y35.119
      - suicide (attempt) X75
  - explosive (material) W40.9
    - gas W40.1
    - in blasting operation W40.0
    - specified NEC W40.8
      - in
        - assault X96.8
        - homicide (attempt) X96.8
        - legal intervention
          - injuring
            - bystander Y35.192
            - law enforcement personnel Y35.191

E

- **Exposure** *(Continued)*
  - fire, flames *(Continued)*
    - in, of, on, starting in *(Continued)*
      - war operations —*see also* War operations, fire
        - from nuclear explosion —*see* War operations, nuclear weapons
      - watercraft (in transit) (not in transit) V91.09
        - localized —*see* Burn, on board watercraft, due to, fire on board
        - powered craft V91.03
          - ferry boat V91.01
          - fishing boat V91.02
          - jet skis V91.03
          - liner V91.01
          - merchant ship V91.00
          - passenger ship V91.01
        - unpowered craft V91.08
          - canoe V91.05
          - inflatable V91.06
          - kayak V91.05
          - sailboat V91.04
          - surf-board V91.08
          - waterskis V91.07
          - windsurfer V91.08
    - lumber (uncontrolled) —*see* Exposure, fire, uncontrolled, not in building
    - mine (uncontrolled) —*see* Exposure, fire, uncontrolled, not in building
    - prairie (uncontrolled) —*see* Exposure, fire, uncontrolled, not in building
    - resulting from
      - explosion —*see* Explosion
      - lightning X08.8
    - self-inflicted X76
    - specified NEC X08.8
    - started by other person X97
    - stated as undetermined whether accidental or intentional Y26
    - stove —*see* Exposure, fire, controlled, building
    - suicide (attempt) X76
    - tunnel (uncontrolled) —*see* Exposure, fire, uncontrolled, not in building
    - uncontrolled
      - in building or structure X00.0
        - with
          - fall from building X00.3
          - injury due to building collapse X00.2
          - jump from building X00.5
          - smoke inhalation X00.1
        - bed X08.00
          - due to
            - cigarette X08.01
            - specified material NEC X08.09
        - furniture NEC X08.20
          - due to
            - cigarette X08.21
            - specified material NEC X08.29
        - hit by object from building X00.4
        - sofa X08.10
          - due to
            - cigarette X08.11
            - specified material NEC X08.19
        - specified mode of injury NEC X00.8
      - not in building or structure (any) X01.0
        - with
          - fall X01.3
          - smoke inhalation X01.1
        - hit by object X01.4
        - specified mode of injury NEC X01.8
    - undetermined whether accidental or intentional Y26
  - forces of nature NEC —*see* Forces of nature
  - G-forces (abnormal) W49.9
  - gravitational forces (abnormal) W49.9
  - heat (natural) NEC —*see* Heat
  - high-pressure jet (hydraulic) (pneumatic) W49.9
  - hydraulic jet W49.9
  - inanimate mechanical force W49.9
  - jet, high-pressure (hydraulic) (pneumatic) W49.9
  - lightning —*see* subcategory T75.0
    - causing fire —*see* Exposure, fire
  - mechanical forces NEC W49.9
    - animate NEC W64
    - inanimate NEC W49.9
  - noise W42.9
    - supersonic W42.0
  - noxious substance —*see* Table of Drugs and Chemicals
  - pneumatic jet W49.9

- **Exposure** *(Continued)*
  - prolonged in deep-freeze unit or refrigerator W93.2
  - radiation —*see* Radiation
  - smoke —*see also* Exposure, fire
    - tobacco, second hand Z77.22
  - specified factors NEC X58
  - sunlight X32
    - man-made (sun lamp) W89.8
      - tanning bed W89.1
  - supersonic waves W42.0
  - transmission line(s), electric W85
  - vibration W49.9
  - waves
    - infrasound W49.9
    - sound W42.9
    - supersonic W42.0
  - weather NEC —*see* Forces of nature
- **External cause status** Y99.9
  - child assisting in compensated work for family Y99.8
  - civilian activity done for financial or other compensation Y99.0
  - civilian activity done for income or pay Y99.0
  - family member assisting in compensated work for other family member Y99.8
  - hobby not done for income Y99.8
  - leisure activity Y99.8
  - military activity Y99.1
  - off-duty activity of military personnel Y99.8
  - recreation or sport not for income or while a student Y99.8
  - specified NEC Y99.8
  - student activity Y99.8
  - volunteer activity Y99.2

F

- **Factors, supplemental**
  - alcohol
    - blood level
      - less than 20mg/100ml Y90.0
      - presence in blood, level not specified Y90.9
      - 20-39mg/100ml Y90.1
      - 40-59mg/100ml Y90.2
      - 60-79mg/100ml Y90.3
      - 80-99mg/100ml Y90.4
      - 100-119mg/100ml Y90.5
      - 120-199mg/100ml Y90.6
      - 200-239mg/100ml Y90.7
      - 240mg/100ml or more Y90.8
    - presence in blood, but level not specified Y90.9
  - environmental-pollution-related condition —*see* Z57
  - nosocomial condition Y95
  - work-related condition Y99.0
- **Failure**
  - in suture or ligature during surgical procedure Y65.2
  - mechanical, of instrument or apparatus (any) (during any medical or surgical procedure) Y65.8
  - sterile precautions (during medical and surgical care) —*see* Misadventure, failure, sterile precautions, by type of procedure
  - to
    - introduce tube or instrument Y65.4
      - endotracheal tube during anesthesia Y65.3
    - make curve (transport vehicle) NEC —*see* Accident, transport
    - remove tube or instrument Y65.4
- **Fall, falling** (accidental) W19
  - building W20.1
    - burning (uncontrolled fire) X00.3
  - down
    - embankment W17.81
    - escalator W10.0
    - hill W17.81
    - ladder W11
    - ramp W10.2
    - stairs, steps W10.9
  - due to
    - bumping against
      - object W18.00
        - sharp glass W18.02
        - specified NEC W18.09
        - sports equipment W18.01

- **Fall, falling** *(Continued)*
  - due to *(Continued)*
    - bumping against *(Continued)*
      - person W03
        - due to ice or snow W00.0
        - on pedestrian conveyance —*see* Accident, transport, pedestrian, conveyance
    - collision with another person W03
      - due to ice or snow W00.0
      - involving pedestrian conveyance —*see* Accident, transport, pedestrian, conveyance
    - grocery cart tipping over W17.82
    - ice or snow W00.9
      - from one level to another W00.2
        - on stairs or steps W00.1
      - involving pedestrian conveyance —*see* Accident, transport, pedestrian, conveyance
      - on same level W00.0
    - slipping (on moving sidewalk) W01.0
      - with subsequent striking against object W01.10
        - furniture W01.190
        - sharp object W01.119
          - glass W01.110
          - power tool or machine W01.111
          - specified NEC W01.118
        - specified NEC W01.198
    - striking against
      - object W18.00
        - sharp glass W18.02
        - specified NEC W18.09
        - sports equipment W18.01
      - person W03
        - due to ice or snow W00.0
        - on pedestrian conveyance —*see* Accident, transport, pedestrian, conveyance
  - earth (with asphyxia or suffocation (by pressure)) —*see* Earth, falling
  - from, off, out of
    - aircraft NEC (with accident to aircraft NEC) V97.0
      - while boarding or alighting V97.1
    - balcony W13.0
    - bed W06
    - boat, ship, watercraft NEC (with drowning or submersion) —*see* Drowning, due to, fall overboard
      - with hitting bottom or object V94.0
    - bridge W13.1
    - building W13.9
      - burning (uncontrolled fire) X00.3
    - cavity W17.2
    - chair W07
    - cherry picker W17.89
    - cliff W15
    - dock W17.4
    - embankment W17.81
    - escalator W10.0
    - flagpole W13.8
    - furniture NEC W08
    - grocery cart W17.82
    - haystack W17.89
    - high place NEC W17.89
      - stated as undetermined whether accidental or intentional Y30
    - hole W17.2
    - incline W10.2
    - ladder W11
    - lifting device W17.89
    - machine, machinery —*see also* Contact, with, by type of machine
      - not in operation W17.89
    - manhole W17.1
    - mobile elevated work platform [MEWP] W17.89
    - motorized mobility scooter W05.2
    - one level to another NEC W17.89
      - intentional, purposeful, suicide (attempt) X80
      - stated as undetermined whether accidental or intentional Y30
    - pit W17.2
    - playground equipment W09.8
      - jungle gym W09.2
      - slide W09.0
      - swing W09.1
    - quarry W17.89
    - railing W13.9
    - ramp W10.2
    - roof W13.2
    - scaffolding W12

E & F

Firearm discharge —*see* Discharge, firearm
Fireball effects from nuclear explosion in war operations —*see* War operations, nuclear weapons
Fireworks (explosion) W39
Flash burns from explosion —*see* Explosion
Flood (any injury) (caused by) X38
  collapse of man-made structure causing earth movement X36.Ø
  tidal wave —*see* Forces of nature, tidal wave
Food (any type) in
  air passages (with asphyxia, obstruction, or suffocation) —*see* categories T17 and T18
  alimentary tract causing asphyxia (due to compression of trachea) —*see* categories T17 and T18
Forces of nature X39.8
  avalanche X36.1
    causing transport accident —*see* Accident, transport, by type of vehicle
  blizzard X37.2
  cataclysmic storm X37.9
    with flood X38
    blizzard X37.2
    cloudburst X37.8
    cyclone X37.1
    dust storm X37.3
    hurricane X37.Ø
    specified storm NEC X37.8
    storm surge X37.Ø
    tornado X37.1
    twister X37.1
    typhoon X37.Ø
  cloudburst X37.8
  cold (natural) X31
  cyclone X37.1
  dam collapse causing earth movement X36.Ø
  dust storm X37.3
  earth movement X36.1
    caused by dam or structure collapse X36.Ø
    earthquake X34
  earthquake X34
  flood (caused by) X38
    dam collapse X36.Ø
    tidal wave —*see* Forces of nature, tidal wave
  heat (natural) X3Ø
  hurricane X37.Ø
  landslide X36.1
    causing transport accident —*see* Accident, transport, by type of vehicle
  lightning —*see* subcategory T75.Ø
    causing fire —*see* Exposure, fire
  mudslide X36.1
    causing transport accident —*see* Accident, transport, by type of vehicle
  radiation (natural) X39.Ø8
    radon X39.Ø1
  radon X39.Ø1
  specified force NEC X39.8
  storm surge X37.Ø
  structure collapse causing earth movement X36.Ø
  sunlight X32
  tidal wave X37.41
    due to
      earthquake X37.41
      landslide X37.43
      storm X37.42
      volcanic eruption X37.41
  tornado X37.1
  tsunami X37.41
  twister X37.1
  typhoon X37.Ø
  volcanic eruption X35
Foreign body
  aspiration —*see* Index to Diseases and Injuries, Foreign body, respitory tract
  embedded in skin W45
  entering through
    natural orifice W44.9
      audio device W44.G1
      battery W44.AØ
        button W44.A1
        cylindrical W44.A9
        other specified NEC W44.A9
    bezoar W44.F1
      bottle cap W44.E9
      can lid W44.E9
      combination metal and plastic
        jewelry W44.G3
        toy and toy part W44.G2
      dagger W44.H2
      dart W44.H1

Foreign body *(Continued)*
  entering through *(Continued)*
    bezoar *(Continued)*
      ear buds W44.G1
      food W44.F3
      glass W44.CØ
        intact W44.C2
          bottle W44.C2
        shard W44.C1
        sharp W44.C1
      hearing aids W44.G1
      insect W44.F4
      knife W44.H2
      magnetic metal W44.DØ
        bead W44.D1
        coin W44.D2
        jewelry W44.D4
        object specified NEC W44.D9
        toy W44.D3
      needle (hypodermic) (sewing) W44.H1
      non-magnetic metal W44.EØ
        bead W44.E1
        coin W44.E2
        jewelry W44.E4
        object specified NEC W44.E9
        toy W44.E3
      objects of natural or organic material W44.FØ
        specified NEC W44.F9
      other
        non-organic objects W44.GØ
          specified NEC W44.G9
        sharp object unspecified W44.HØ
      plastic
        bead W44.B1
        bottle W44.B5
        coin W44.B2
        jewelry W44.B4
        object W44.BØ
          specified NEC W44.B9
        toy and toy part W44.B3
      pull tab W44.E9
      rubber band W44.F2
      safety pin W44.H1
      specified NEC W44.8
      sword W44.H2
    skin W45.8
      can lid W26.8
      nail W45.Ø
      paper W26.2
      specified NEC W45.8
      splinter W45.8
Forest fire (exposure to) —*see* Exposure, fire, uncontrolled, not in building
Found injured X58
  from exposure (to) —*see* Exposure
  on
    highway, road(way), street V89.9
    railway right of way V81.9
Fracture (circumstances unknown or unspecified) X58
  due to specified cause NEC X58
Freezing —*see* Exposure, cold
Frostbite X31
  due to man-made conditions —*see* Exposure, cold, man-made
Frozen —*see* Exposure, cold

G

Gored by bull W55.22
Gunshot wound W34.ØØ

H

Hailstones, injured by X39.8
Hanged herself or himself —*see* Hanging, self-inflicted
Hanging (accidental) —*see also* category T71
  legal execution —*see* Legal, intervention, specified means NEC
Heat (effects of) (excessive) X3Ø
  due to
    man-made conditions W92
      on board watercraft V93.29
        fishing boat V93.22
        merchant ship V93.2Ø

Heat *(Continued)*
  due to *(Continued)*
    man-made conditions *(Continued)*
      on board watercraft *(Continued)*
        passenger ship V93.21
        sailboat V93.24
        specified powered craft NEC V93.23
    weather (conditions) X3Ø
  from
    electric heating apparatus causing burning X16
    nuclear explosion in war operations —*see* War operations, nuclear weapons
  inappropriate in local application or packing in medical or surgical procedure Y63.5
Hemorrhage
  delayed following medical or surgical treatment without mention of misadventure —*see* Index to Diseases and Injuries, Complication(s)
  during medical or surgical treatment as misadventure —*see* Index to Diseases and Injuries, Complication(s)
High
  altitude (effects) —*see* Air, pressure, low
  level of radioactivity, effects —*see* Radiation
  pressure (effects) —*see* Air, pressure, high
  temperature, effects —*see* Heat
Hit, hitting (accidental) by —*see* Struck by
Hitting against —*see* Striking against
Homicide (attempt) (justifiable) —*see* Assault
Hot
  place, effects —*see also* Heat
  weather, effects X3Ø
House fire (uncontrolled) —*see* Exposure, fire, uncontrolled, building
Humidity, causing problem X39.8
Hunger X58
Hurricane (any injury) X37.Ø
Hypobarism, hypobaropathy —*see* Air, pressure, low

I

Ictus
  caloris —*see also* Heat
  solaris X3Ø
Ignition (accidental) —*see also* Exposure, fire XØ8.8
  anesthetic gas in operating room W4Ø.1
  apparel XØ6.2
    from highly flammable material XØ4
    nightwear XØ5
  bed linen (sheets) (spreads) (pillows) (mattress) —*see* Exposure, fire, uncontrolled, building, bed
  benzine XØ4
  clothes, clothing NEC (from controlled fire) XØ6.2
    from
      highly flammable material XØ4
  ether XØ4
    in operating room W4Ø.1
  explosive material —*see* Explosion
  gasoline XØ4
  jewelry (plastic) (any) XØ6.Ø
  kerosene XØ4
  material
    explosive —*see* Explosion
    highly flammable with secondary explosion XØ4
  nightwear XØ5
  paraffin XØ4
  petrol XØ4
Immersion (accidental) —*see also* Drowning
  hand or foot due to cold (excessive) X31
Implantation of quills of porcupine W55.89
Inanition (from) (hunger) X58
  thirst X58.8
Inappropriate operation performed
  correct operation on wrong side or body part (wrong side) (wrong site) Y65.53
  operation intended for another patient done on wrong patient Y65.52
  wrong operation performed on correct patient Y65.51
Inattention after, at birth (homicidal intent) (infanticidal intent) X58

▶ New ➡ Revised ~~deleted~~ Deleted • Use Additional Character(s)

- **Incident, adverse**
  - device
    - anesthesiology Y7Ø.8
      - accessory Y7Ø.2
      - diagnostic Y7Ø.Ø
      - miscellaneous Y7Ø.8
      - monitoring Y7Ø.Ø
      - prosthetic Y7Ø.2
      - rehabilitative Y7Ø.1
      - surgical Y7Ø.3
      - therapeutic Y7Ø.1
    - cardiovascular Y71.8
      - accessory Y71.2
      - diagnostic Y71.Ø
      - miscellaneous Y71.8
      - monitoring Y71.Ø
      - prosthetic Y71.2
      - rehabilitative Y71.1
      - surgical Y71.3
      - therapeutic Y71.1
    - gastroenterology Y73.8
      - accessory Y73.2
      - diagnostic Y73.Ø
      - miscellaneous Y73.8
      - monitoring Y73.Ø
      - prosthetic Y73.2
      - rehabilitative Y73.1
      - surgical Y73.3
      - therapeutic Y73.1
    - general
      - hospital Y74.8
        - accessory Y74.2
        - diagnostic Y74.Ø
        - miscellaneous Y74.8
        - monitoring Y74.Ø
        - prosthetic Y74.2
        - rehabilitative Y74.1
        - surgical Y74.3
        - therapeutic Y74.1
      - surgical Y81.8
        - accessory Y81.2
        - diagnostic Y81.Ø
        - miscellaneous Y81.8
        - monitoring Y81.Ø
        - prosthetic Y81.2
        - rehabilitative Y81.1
        - surgical Y81.3
        - therapeutic Y81.1
    - gynecological Y76.8
      - accessory Y76.2
      - diagnostic Y76.Ø
      - miscellaneous Y76.8
      - monitoring Y76.Ø
      - prosthetic Y76.2
      - rehabilitative Y76.1
      - surgical Y76.3
      - therapeutic Y76.1
    - medical Y82.9
      - specified type NEC Y82.8
    - neurological Y75.8
      - accessory Y75.2
      - diagnostic Y75.Ø
      - miscellaneous Y75.8
      - monitoring Y75.Ø
      - prosthetic Y75.2
      - rehabilitative Y75.1
      - surgical Y75.3
      - therapeutic Y75.1
    - obstetrical Y76.8
      - accessory Y76.2
      - diagnostic Y76.Ø
      - miscellaneous Y76.8
      - monitoring Y76.Ø
      - prosthetic Y76.2
      - rehabilitative Y76.1
      - surgical Y76.3
      - therapeutic Y76.1
    - ophthalmic Y77.8
      - accessory Y77.2
      - contact lens (rigid gas permeable) (soft) (hydrophilic)) Y77.11
      - diagnostic Y77.Ø
      - miscellaneous Y77.8
      - monitoring Y77.Ø
      - prosthetic Y77.2
      - rehabilitative Y77.19
      - surgical Y77.3
      - therapeutic Y77.19
    - orthopedic Y79.8
      - accessory Y79.2
      - diagnostic Y79.Ø
      - miscellaneous Y79.8

- **Incident, adverse** *(Continued)*
  - device *(Continued)*
    - orthopedic *(Continued)*
      - monitoring Y79.Ø
      - prosthetic Y79.2
      - rehabilitative Y79.1
      - surgical Y79.3
      - therapeutic Y79.1
    - otorhinolaryngological Y72.8
      - accessory Y72.2
      - diagnostic Y72.Ø
      - miscellaneous Y72.8
      - monitoring Y72.Ø
      - prosthetic Y72.2
      - rehabilitative Y72.1
      - surgical Y72.3
      - therapeutic Y72.1
    - personal use Y74.8
      - accessory Y74.2
      - diagnostic Y74.Ø
      - miscellaneous Y74.8
      - monitoring Y74.Ø
      - prosthetic Y74.2
      - rehabilitative Y74.1
      - surgical Y74.3
      - therapeutic Y74.1
    - physical medicine Y8Ø.8
      - accessory Y8Ø.2
      - diagnostic Y8Ø.Ø
      - miscellaneous Y8Ø.8
      - monitoring Y8Ø.Ø
      - prosthetic Y8Ø.2
      - rehabilitative Y8Ø.1
      - surgical Y8Ø.3
      - therapeutic Y8Ø.1
    - plastic surgical Y81.8
      - accessory Y81.2
      - diagnostic Y81.Ø
      - miscellaneous Y81.8
      - monitoring Y81.Ø
      - prosthetic Y81.2
      - rehabilitative Y81.1
      - surgical Y81.3
      - therapeutic Y81.1
    - radiological Y78.8
      - accessory Y78.2
      - diagnostic Y78.Ø
      - miscellaneous Y78.8
      - monitoring Y78.Ø
      - prosthetic Y78.2
      - rehabilitative Y78.1
      - surgical Y78.3
      - therapeutic Y78.1
    - urology Y73.8
      - accessory Y73.2
      - diagnostic Y73.Ø
      - miscellaneous Y73.8
      - monitoring Y73.Ø
      - prosthetic Y73.2
      - rehabilitative Y73.1
      - surgical Y73.3
      - therapeutic Y73.1
- **Incineration** (accidental) —*see* Exposure, fire
- **Infanticide** —*see* Assault
- **Infrasound waves** (causing injury) W49.9
- **Ingestion**
  - foreign body (causing injury) (with obstruction) —*see* Foreign body, alimentary canal
  - poisonous
    - plant(s) X58
    - substance NEC —*see* Table of Drugs and Chemicals
- **Inhalation**
  - excessively cold substance, man-made —*see* Exposure, cold, man-made
  - food (any type) (into respiratory tract) (with asphyxia, obstruction respiratory tract, suffocation) —*see* categories T17 and T18
  - foreign body —*see* Foreign body, aspiration
  - gastric contents (with asphyxia, obstruction respiratory passage, suffocation) T17.81-●
  - hot air or gases X14.Ø
  - liquid air, hydrogen, nitrogen W93.12
    - suicide (attempt) X83.2
  - steam X13.Ø
    - assault X98.Ø
    - stated as undetermined whether accidental or intentional Y27.Ø
    - suicide (attempt) X77.Ø

- **Inhalation** *(Continued)*
  - toxic gas —*see* Table of Drugs and Chemicals
  - vomitus (with asphyxia, obstruction respiratory passage, suffocation) T17.81-●
- **Injury, injured** (accidental(ly)) **NOS** X58
  - by, caused by, from
    - assault —*see* Assault
    - law-enforcing agent, police, in course of legal intervention —*see* Legal intervention
    - suicide (attempt) X83.8
  - due to, in
    - civil insurrection —*see* War operations
    - fight —*see also* Assault, fight YØ4.Ø
    - war operations —*see* War operations
  - homicide —*see also* Assault YØ9
  - inflicted (by)
    - in course of arrest (attempted), suppression of disturbance, maintenance of order, by law-enforcing agents —*see* Legal intervention
    - other person
      - stated as
        - accidental X58
        - intentional, homicide (attempt) —*see* Assault
        - undetermined whether accidental or intentional Y33
  - purposely (inflicted) by other person(s) —*see* Assault
  - self-inflicted X83.8
    - stated as accidental X58
  - specified cause NEC X58
  - undetermined whether accidental or intentional Y33
- **Insolation, effects** X3Ø
- **Insufficient nourishment** X58
- **Interruption of respiration** (by)
  - food (lodged in esophagus) —*see* categories T17 and T18
  - vomitus (lodged in esophagus) T17.81-●
- **Intervention, legal** —*see* Legal intervention
- **Intoxication**
  - drug —*see* Table of Drugs and Chemicals
  - poison —*see* Table of Drugs and Chemicals

J

- **Jammed** (accidentally)
  - between objects (moving) (stationary and moving) W23.Ø
    - stationary W23.1
- **Jumped, jumping**
  - before moving object NEC X81.8
    - motor vehicle X81.Ø
    - subway train X81.1
    - train X81.1
    - undetermined whether accidental or intentional Y31
  - from
    - boat (into water) voluntarily, without accident (to or on boat) W16.712
      - with
        - accident to or on boat —*see* Accident, watercraft
        - drowning or submersion W16.711
          - suicide (attempt) X71.3
      - striking bottom W16.722
        - causing drowning W16.721
    - building —*see also* Jumped, from, high place W13.9
      - burning (uncontrolled fire) XØØ.5
    - high place NEC W17.89
      - suicide (attempt) X8Ø
      - undetermined whether accidental or intentional Y3Ø
    - structure —*see also* Jumped, from, high place W13.9
      - burning (uncontrolled fire) XØØ.5
  - into water W16.92
    - causing drowning W16.91
    - from, off watercraft —*see* Jumped, from, boat
    - in
      - natural body W16.612
        - causing drowning W16.611
        - striking bottom W16.622
          - causing drowning W16.621

I & J

- **Jumped, jumping** *(Continued)*
  - into water *(Continued)*
    - in *(Continued)*
      - specified place NEC W16.812
        - causing drowning W16.811
        - striking
          - bottom W16.822
            - causing drowning W16.821
          - wall W16.832
            - causing drowning W16.831
      - swimming pool W16.512
        - causing drowning W16.511
        - striking
          - bottom W16.522
            - causing drowning W16.521
          - wall W16.532
            - causing drowning W16.531
    - suicide (attempt) X71.3

K

- **Kicked by**
  - animal NEC W55.82
  - person(s) (accidentally) W5Ø.1
    - with intent to injure or kill YØ4.Ø
    - as, or caused by, a crowd or human stampede (with fall) W52
    - assault YØ4.Ø
    - homicide (attempt) YØ4.Ø
    - in
      - fight YØ4.Ø
      - legal intervention
        - injuring
          - bystander Y35.812
          - law enforcement personnel Y35.811
          - suspect Y35.813
          - unspecified person Y35.819
- **Kicking**
  - against
    - object W22.8
      - sports equipment W21.9
      - stationary W22.Ø9
        - sports equipment W21.89
    - person *—see* Striking against, person
    - sports equipment W21.9
  - carpet stretcher with knee X5Ø.3
- **Killed, killing** (accidentally) **NOS** *—see also* Injury X58
  - in
    - action *—see* War operations
    - brawl, fight (hand) (fists) (foot) YØ4.Ø
      - by weapon *—see also* Assault
        - cutting, piercing *—see* Assault, cutting or piercing instrument
        - firearm *—see* Discharge, firearm, by type, homicide
  - self
    - stated as
      - accident NOS X58
      - suicide *—see* Suicide
      - undetermined whether accidental or intentional Y33
- **Kneeling** (prolonged) (static) X5Ø.1
- **Knocked down** (accidentally) (by) **NOS** X58
  - animal (not being ridden) NEC *—see also* Struck by, by type of animal
  - crowd or human stampede W52
  - person W51
    - in brawl, fight YØ4.Ø
  - transport vehicle NEC *—see also* Accident, transport VØ9.9

L

- **Laceration NEC** *—see* Injury
- **Lack of**
  - care (helpless person) (infant) (newborn) X58
  - food except as result of abandonment or neglect X58
    - due to abandonment or neglect X58
  - water except as result of transport accident X58
    - due to transport accident *—see* Accident, transport, by type
    - helpless person, infant, newborn X58
- **Landslide** (falling on transport vehicle) X36.1
  - caused by collapse of man-made structure X36.Ø
- **Late effect** *—see* Sequelae
- **Legal**
  - execution (any method) *—see* Legal, intervention
  - intervention (by)
    - baton *—see* Legal, intervention, blunt object, baton
    - bayonet *—see* Legal, intervention, sharp object, bayonet
    - blow *—see* Legal, intervention, manhandling
    - blunt object
      - baton
        - injuring
          - bystander Y35.312
          - law enforcement personnel Y35.311
          - suspect Y35.313
          - unspecified person Y35.319
      - injuring
        - bystander Y35.3Ø2
        - law enforcement personnel Y35.3Ø1
        - suspect Y35.3Ø3
        - unspecified person Y35.3Ø9
      - specified NEC
        - injuring
          - bystander Y35.392
          - law enforcement personnel Y35.391
          - suspect Y35.393
          - unspecified person Y35.399
      - stave
        - injuring
          - bystander Y35.392
          - law enforcement personnel Y35.391
          - suspect Y35.393
          - unspecified person Y35.399
    - bomb *—see* Legal, intervention, explosive
    - conducted energy device
      - injuring
        - bystander Y35.832
        - law enforcement personnel Y35.831
        - suspect Y35.833
        - unspecified person Y35.839
    - cutting or piercing instrument *—see* Legal, intervention, sharp object
    - dynamite *—see* Legal, intervention, explosive, dynamite
    - electroshock device (taser)
      - injuring
        - bystander Y35.832
        - law enforcement personnel Y35.831
        - suspect Y35.833
        - unspecified person Y35.839
    - explosive(s)
      - dynamite
        - injuring
          - bystander Y35.112
          - law enforcement personnel Y35.111
          - suspect Y35.113
          - unspecified person Y35.119
      - grenade
        - injuring
          - bystander Y35.192
          - law enforcement personnel Y35.191
          - suspect Y35.193
          - unspecified person Y35.199
      - injuring
        - bystander Y35.1Ø2
        - law enforcement personnel Y35.1Ø1
        - suspect Y35.1Ø3
        - unspecified person Y35.1Ø9
      - mortar bomb
        - injuring
          - bystander Y35.192
          - law enforcement personnel Y35.191
          - suspect Y35.193
          - unspecified person Y35.199
      - shell
        - injuring
          - bystander Y35.122
          - law enforcement personnel Y35.121
          - suspect Y35.123
          - unspecified person Y35.129
      - specified NEC
        - injuring
          - bystander Y35.192
          - law enforcement personnel Y35.191
          - suspect Y35.193
          - unspecified person Y35.199
- **Legal** *(Continued)*
  - intervention (by) *(Continued)*
    - firearm(s) (discharge)
      - handgun
        - injuring
          - bystander Y35.Ø22
          - law enforcement personnel Y35.Ø21
          - suspect Y35.Ø23
          - unspecified person Y35.Ø29
      - injuring
        - bystander Y35.ØØ2
        - law enforcement personnel Y35.ØØ1
        - suspect Y35.ØØ3
        - unspecified person Y35.ØØ9
      - machine gun
        - injuring
          - bystander Y35.Ø12
          - law enforcement personnel Y35.Ø11
          - suspect Y35.Ø13
          - unspecified person Y35.Ø19
      - rifle pellet
        - injuring
          - bystander Y35.Ø32
          - law enforcement personnel Y35.Ø31
          - suspect Y35.Ø33
          - unspecified person Y35.Ø39
      - rubber bullet
        - injuring
          - bystander Y35.Ø42
          - law enforcement personnel Y35.Ø41
          - suspect Y35.Ø43
          - unspecified person Y35.Ø49
      - shotgun *—see* Legal, intervention, firearm, specified NEC
      - specified NEC
        - injuring
          - bystander Y35.Ø92
          - law enforcement personnel Y35.Ø91
          - suspect Y35.Ø93
          - unspecified person Y35.Ø99
    - gas (asphyxiation) (poisoning)
      - injuring
        - bystander Y35.2Ø2
        - law enforcement personnel Y35.2Ø1
        - suspect Y35.2Ø3
        - unspecified person Y35.2Ø9
      - specified NEC
        - injuring
          - bystander Y35.292
          - law enforcement personnel Y35.291
          - suspect Y35.293
          - unspecified person Y35.299
      - tear gas
        - injuring
          - bystander Y35.212
          - law enforcement personnel Y35.211
          - suspect Y35.213
          - unspecified person Y35.219
    - grenade *—see* Legal, intervention, explosive, grenade
    - injuring
      - bystander Y35.92
      - law enforcement personnel Y35.91
      - suspect Y35.93
      - unspecified person Y35.99
    - late effect (of) *—see* with 7th character S Y35
    - manhandling
      - injuring
        - bystander Y35.812
        - law enforcement personnel Y35.811
        - suspect Y35.813
        - unspecified person Y35.819
    - sequelae (of) *—see* with 7th character S Y35
    - sharp objects
      - bayonet
        - injuring
          - bystander Y35.412
          - law enforcement personnel Y35.411
          - suspect Y35.413
          - unspecified person Y35.419
      - injuring
        - bystander Y35.4Ø2
        - law enforcement personnel Y35.4Ø1
        - suspect Y35.4Ø3
        - unspecified person Y35.4Ø9
      - specified NEC
        - injuring
          - bystander Y35.492
          - law enforcement personnel Y35.491

J, K, & L

L & M

N

O

P

M, N, O, & P

P

- **Place of occurrence** *(Continued)*
  - residence *(Continued)*
    - institutional *(Continued)*
      - orphanage *(Continued)*
        - specified NEC Y92.118
        - swimming pool Y92.115
        - yard Y92.116
      - prison Y92.149
        - bathroom Y92.142
        - cell Y92.143
        - courtyard Y92.147
        - dining room Y92.141
        - kitchen Y92.140
        - specified NEC Y92.148
        - swimming pool Y92.146
      - reform school Y92.159
        - bathroom Y92.152
        - bedroom Y92.153
        - dining room Y92.151
        - driveway Y92.154
        - garage Y92.155
        - garden Y92.157
        - kitchen Y92.150
        - specified NEC Y92.158
        - swimming pool Y92.156
        - yard Y92.157
      - school dormitory Y92.169
        - bathroom Y92.162
        - bedroom Y92.163
        - dining room Y92.161
        - kitchen Y92.160
        - specified NEC Y92.168
      - specified NEC Y92.199
        - bathroom Y92.192
        - bedroom Y92.193
        - dining room Y92.191
        - driveway Y92.194
        - garage Y92.195
        - garden Y92.197
        - kitchen Y92.190
        - specified NEC Y92.198
        - swimming pool Y92.196
        - yard Y92.197
    - kitchen Y92.000
    - mobile home Y92.029
      - bathroom Y92.022
      - bedroom Y92.023
      - dining room Y92.021
      - driveway Y92.024
      - garage Y92.025
      - garden Y92.027
      - kitchen Y92.020
      - specified NEC Y92.028
      - swimming pool Y92.026
      - yard Y92.027
    - specified place in residence NEC Y92.008
    - specified residence type NEC Y92.099
      - bathroom Y92.091
      - bedroom Y92.092
      - driveway Y92.093
      - garage Y92.094
      - garden Y92.096
      - kitchen Y92.090
      - specified NEC Y92.098
      - swimming pool Y92.095
      - yard Y92.096
  - restaurant Y92.511
  - riding school Y92.39
  - river Y92.828
  - road Y92.410
  - rodeo ring Y92.39
  - rugby field Y92.328
  - same day surgery center Y92.530
  - sand pit Y92.64
  - school (private) (public) (state) Y92.219
    - college Y92.214
    - daycare center Y92.210
    - elementary school Y92.211
    - high school Y92.213
    - kindergarten Y92.211
    - middle school Y92.212
    - specified NEC Y92.218
    - trace school Y92.215
    - university Y92.214
    - vocational school Y92.215
  - sea (shore) Y92.832
  - senior citizen center Y92.29
  - service area
    - airport Y92.520
    - bus station Y92.521
    - gas station Y92.524

- **Place of occurrence** *(Continued)*
  - service area *(Continued)*
    - highway rest stop Y92.523
    - railway station Y92.522
  - shipyard Y92.62
  - shop(commercial) Y92.513
  - sidewalk Y92.480
  - silo Y92.79
  - skating rink (roller) Y92.331
    - ice Y92.330
  - slaughter house Y92.86
  - soccer field Y92.322
  - specified place NEC Y92.89
  - sports area Y92.39
    - athletic
      - court Y92.318
        - basketball Y92.310
        - specified NEC Y92.318
        - squash Y92.311
        - tennis Y92.312
      - field Y92.328
        - baseball Y92.320
        - cricket ground Y92.328
        - football Y92.321
        - hockey Y92.328
        - soccer Y92.322
        - specified NEC Y92.328
    - golf course Y92.39
    - gymnasium Y92.39
    - riding school Y92.39
    - skating rink (roller) Y92.331
      - ice Y92.330
    - stadium Y92.39
    - swimming pool Y92.34
  - squash court Y92.311
  - stadium Y92.39
  - steeplechasing course Y92.39
  - store Y92.512
  - stream Y92.828
  - street and highway Y92.410
    - bike path Y92.482
    - freeway Y92.411
    - highway ramp Y92.415
    - interstate highway Y92.411
    - local residential or business street Y92.414
    - motorway Y92.411
    - parking lot Y92.481
    - parkway Y92.412
    - sidewalk Y92.480
    - specified NEC Y92.488
    - state road Y92.413
  - subway car Y92.816
  - supermarket Y92.512
  - swamp Y92.828
  - swimming pool (public) Y92.34
    - private (at) Y92.095
      - boarding house Y92.045
      - military base Y92.136
      - mobile home Y92.026
      - nursing home Y92.125
      - orphanage Y92.115
      - prison Y92.146
      - reform school Y92.156
      - single family residence Y92.016
  - synagogue Y92.22
  - tavern
  - television station Y92.59
  - tennis court Y92.312
  - theater Y92.254
  - trade area Y92.59
    - bank Y92.510
    - cafe Y92.511
    - casino Y92.59
    - garage Y92.59
    - hotel Y92.59
    - market Y92.512
    - office building Y92.59
    - radio station Y92.59
    - restaurant Y92.511
    - shop Y92.513
    - shopping mall Y92.59
    - store Y92.512
    - supermarket Y92.512
    - television station Y92.59
    - warehouse Y92.59
  - trailer park, residential *—see* Place of occurrence, residence, mobile home
  - trailer site NOS Y92.89
  - train Y92.815
    - station Y92.522
  - truck Y92.812

- **Place of occurrence** *(Continued)*
  - tunnel under construction Y92. 69
  - university Y92.214
  - urgent (health) care center Y92.532
  - vehicle (transport) Y92.818
    - airplane Y92.813
    - boat Y92.814
    - bus Y92.811
    - car Y92.810
    - specified NEC Y92.818
    - subway car Y92.816
    - train Y92.815
    - truck Y92.812
  - warehouse Y92.59
  - water reservoir Y92.89
  - wilderness area Y92.828
    - desert Y92.820
    - forest Y92.821
    - marsh Y92.828
    - mountain Y92.828
    - prairie Y92.828
    - specified NEC Y92.828
    - swamp Y92.828
  - workshop Y92.69
  - yard, private Y92.096
    - boarding house Y92.046
    - mobile home Y92.027
    - single family house Y92.017
  - youth center Y92.29
  - zoo (zoological garden) Y92.834
- **Plumbism** *—see* Table of Drugs and Chemicals, lead
- **Poisoning** (accidental) (by) *—see also* Table of Drugs and Chemicals
  - by plant, thorns, spines, sharp leaves or other mechanisms NEC X58
  - carbon monoxide
    - generated by
      - motor vehicle *—see* Accident, transport
      - watercraft (in transit) (not in transit) V93.89
        - ferry boat V93.81
        - fishing boat V93.82
        - jet skis V93.83
        - liner V93.81
        - merchant ship V93.80
        - passenger ship V93.81
        - powered craft NEC V93.83
  - caused by injection of poisons into skin by plant thorns, spines, sharp leaves X58
    - marine or sea plants (venomous) X58
  - exhaust gas
    - generated by
      - motor vehicle *—see* Accident, transport
      - watercraft (in transit) (not in transit) V93.89
        - ferry boat V93.81
        - fishing boat V93.82
        - jet skis V93.83
        - liner V93.81
        - merchant ship V93.80
        - passenger ship V93.81
        - powered craft NEC V93.83
  - fumes or smoke due to
    - explosion *—see also* Explosion W40.9
    - fire *—see* Exposure, fire
    - ignition *—see* Ignition
  - gas
    - in legal intervention *—see* Legal, intervention, gas
    - legal execution *—see* Legal, intervention, gas
  - in war operations *—see* War operations
  - legal
  - execution *—see* Legal, intervention, gas
    - intervention
      - by gas *—see* Legal, intervention, gas
      - other specified means *—see* Legal, intervention, specified means NEC
- **Powder burn** (by) (from)
  - airgun W34.110
  - BB gun W34.110
  - firearm NEC W34.19
  - gas, air or spring-operated gun NEC W34.118
  - handgun W32.1
  - hunting rifle W33.12
  - larger firearm W33.10
    - specified NEC W33.19
  - machine gun W33.13
  - paintball gun W34.111
  - pellet gun W34.110
  - shotgun W33.11
  - Very pistol [flare] W34.19

P

- **Premature cessation** (of) **surgical and medical care** Y66
- **Privation** (food) (water) X58
- **Procedure** (operation)
  - correct, on wrong side or body part (wrong side) (wrong site) Y65.53
  - intended for another patient done on wrong patient Y65.52
  - performed on patient not scheduled for surgery Y65.52
  - performed on wrong patient Y65.52
  - wrong, performed on correct patient Y65.51
- **Prolonged**
  - sitting in transport vehicle —*see* Sitting
  - stay in
    - high altitude as cause of anoxia, barodontalgia, barotitis or hypoxia W94.11
    - weightless environment X52
- **Pulling, excessive** —*see also* Overexertion X50.9
- **Puncture, puncturing** —*see also* Contact, with, by type of object or machine
  - by
    - plant thorns, spines, sharp leaves or other mechanisms NEC W60
  - during medical or surgical treatment as misadventure —*see* Index to Diseases and Injuries, Complication(s)
- **Pushed, pushing** (accidental) (injury in)
  - by other person(s) (accidental) W51
    - with fall W03
      - due to ice or snow W00.0
    - as, or caused by, a crowd or human stampede (with fall) W52
    - before moving object NEC Y02.8
      - motor vehicle Y02.0
      - subway train Y02.1
      - train Y02.1
    - from
      - high place NEC
        - in accidental circumstances W17.89
        - stated as
          - intentional, homicide (attempt) Y01
          - undetermined whether accidental or intentional Y30
      - transport vehicle NEC —*see also* Accident, transport V89.9
        - stated as
          - intentional, homicide (attempt) Y08.89
      - overexertion X50.9

R

- **Radiation** (exposure to)
  - arc lamps W89.0
  - atomic power plant (malfunction) NEC W88.1
  - complication of or abnormal reaction to medical radiotherapy Y84.2
  - electromagnetic, ionizing W88.0
  - gamma rays W88.1
  - in
    - war operations (from or following nuclear explosion) —*see also* War operations
  - inadvertent exposure of patient (receiving test or therapy) Y63.3
  - infrared (heaters and lamps) W90.1
    - excessive heat from W92
  - ionized, ionizing (particles, artificially accelerated)
    - radioisotopes W88.1
    - specified NEC W88.8
    - x-rays W88.0
  - isotopes, radioactive —*see* Radiation, radioactive isotopes
  - laser(s) W90.2
    - in war operations —*see* War operations
    - misadventure in medical care Y63.2
  - light sources (man-made visible and ultraviolet) W89.9
    - natural X32
    - specified NEC W89.8
    - tanning bed W89.1
    - welding light W89.0
  - man-made visible light W89.9
    - specified NEC W89.8
    - tanning bed W89.1
    - welding light W89.0
  - microwave W90.8
  - misadventure in medical or surgical procedure Y63.2
  - natural NEC X39.08
    - radon X39.01
  - overdose (in medical or surgical procedure) Y63.2
  - radar W90.0
  - radioactive isotopes (any) W88.1
    - atomic power plant malfunction W88.1
    - misadventure in medical or surgical treatment Y63.2
  - radiofrequency W90.0
  - radium NEC W88.1
  - sun X32
  - ultraviolet (light) (man-made) W89.9
    - natural X32
    - specified NEC W89.8
    - tanning bed W89.1
    - welding light W89.0
  - welding arc, torch, or light W89.0
    - excessive heat from W92
  - x-rays (hard) (soft) W88.0
- **Range disease** W94.11
- ➡ **Rape** (attempted) (confirmed) T74.2-●
  - ▶ suspected T76.2-●
- **Rat bite** W53.11
- **Reaching** (prolonged) (static) X50.1
- **Reaction, abnormal to medical procedure** —*see also* Complication of or following, by type of procedure Y84.9
  - with misadventure —*see* Misadventure
  - biologicals —*see* Table of Drugs and Chemicals
  - drugs —*see* Table of Drugs and Chemicals
  - vaccine —*see* Table of Drugs and Chemicals
- **Recoil**
  - airgun W34.110
  - BB gun W34.110
  - firearm NEC W34.19
  - gas, air or spring-operated gun NEC W34.118
  - handgun W32.1
  - hunting rifle W33.12
  - larger firearm W33.10
    - specified NEC W33.19
  - machine gun W33.13
  - paintball gun W34.111
  - pellet W34.110
  - shotgun W33.11
  - Very pistol [flare] W34.19
- **Reduction in**
  - atmospheric pressure —*see* Air, pressure, change
- **Rock falling on or hitting** (accidentally) (person) W20.8
  - in cave-in W20.0
- **Run over** (accidentally) (by)
  - animal (not being ridden) NEC W55.89
  - machinery —*see* Contact, with, by specified type of machine
  - transport vehicle NEC —*see also* Accident, transport V09.9
    - intentional homicide (attempt) Y03.0
    - motor NEC V09.20
      - intentional homicide (attempt) Y03.0
- **Running**
  - before moving object X81.8
    - motor vehicle X81.0
- **Running off, away**
  - animal (being ridden) —*see also* Accident, transport V80.918
    - not being ridden W55.89
  - animal-drawn vehicle NEC —*see also* Accident, transport V80.928
  - highway, road(way), street
    - transport vehicle NEC —*see also* Accident, transport V89.9
- **Rupture pressurized devices** —*see* Explosion, by type of device

S

- **Saturnism** —*see* Table of Drugs and Chemicals, lead
- **Scald, scalding** (accidental) (by) (from) (in) X19
  - air (hot) X14.1
  - gases (hot) X14.1
  - homicide (attempt) —*see* Assault, burning, hot object
  - inflicted by other person
    - stated as intentional, homicide (attempt) —*see* Assault, burning, hot object
  - liquid (boiling) (hot) NEC X12
    - stated as undetermined whether accidental or intentional Y27.2
    - suicide (attempt) X77.2
  - local application of externally applied substance in medical or surgical care Y63.5
  - metal (molten) (liquid) (hot) NEC X18
  - self-inflicted X77.9
  - stated as undetermined whether accidental or intentional Y27.8
  - steam X13.1
    - assault X98.0
    - stated as undetermined whether accidental or intentional Y27.0
    - suicide (attempt) X77.0
  - suicide (attempt) X77.9
  - vapor (hot) X13.1
    - assault X98.0
    - stated as undetermined whether accidental or intentional Y27.0
    - suicide (attempt) X77.0
- **Scratched by**
  - cat W55.03
  - person(s) (accidentally) W50.4
    - with intent to injure or kill Y04.0
    - as, or caused by, a crowd or human stampede (with fall) W52
    - assault Y04.0
    - homicide (attempt) Y04.0
    - in
      - fight Y04.0
      - legal intervention
        - injuring
          - bystander Y35.892
          - law enforcement personnel Y35.891
          - suspect Y35.893
          - unspecified person Y35.899
- **Seasickness** T75.3
- **Self-harm NEC** —*see also* External cause by type, undetermined whether accidental or intentional
  - intentional —*see* Suicide
  - poisoning NEC —*see* Table of drugs and biologicals, accident
- **Self-inflicted** (injury) **NEC** —*see also* External cause by type, undetermined whether accidental or intentional
  - intentional —*see* Suicide
  - poisoning NEC —*see* Table of drugs and biologicals, accident
- **Sequelae** (of)
  - accident NEC —*see* W00-X58 with 7th character S
  - assault (homicidal) (any means) —*see* X92-Y08 with 7th character S
  - homicide, attempt (any means) —*see* X92-Y08 with 7th character S
  - injury undetermined whether accidentally or purposely inflicted —*see* Y21-Y33 with 7th character S
  - intentional self-harm (classifiable to X71-X83) —*see* X71-X83 with 7th character S
  - legal intervention (*see* with 7th character S Y35)
  - motor vehicle accident —*see* V00-V99 with 7th character S
  - suicide, attempt (any means) —*see* X71-X83 with 7th character S
  - transport accident —*see* V00-V99 with 7th character S
  - war operations —*see* War operations
- **Shock**
  - electric —*see* Exposure, electric current
  - from electric appliance (any) (faulty) W86.8
    - domestic W86.0
    - suicide (attempt) X83.1
- **Shooting, shot** (accidental (ly)) —*see also* Discharge, firearm, by type
  - herself or himself —*see* Discharge, firearm by type, self-inflicted
  - homicide (attempt) —*see* Discharge, firearm by type, homicide
  - in war operations —*see* War operations
  - inflicted by other person —*see* Discharge, firearm by type, homicide
    - accidental —*see* Discharge, firearm, by type of firearm

Shooting, shot *(Continued)*
legal
execution —*see* Legal, intervention, firearm
intervention —*see* Legal, intervention, firearm
self-inflicted —*see* Discharge, firearm by type, suicide
accidental —*see* Discharge, firearm, by type of firearm
suicide (attempt) —*see* Discharge, firearm by type, suicide
Shoving (accidentally) **by other person** —*see* Pushed, by other person
Sickness
alpine W94.11
motion —*see* Motion
mountain W94.11
Sinking (accidental)
watercraft (causing drowning, submersion) —*see also* Drowning, due to, accident to, watercraft, sinking
causing injury except drowning or submersion —*see* Accident, watercraft, causing, injury NEC
Siriasis X32
Sitting (prolonged) (static) X50.1
Slashed wrists —*see* Cut, self-inflicted
Slipping (accidental) (on same level) (with fall) W01.0
without fall W18.40
due to
specified NEC W18.49
stepping from one level to another W18.43
stepping into hole or opening W18.42
stepping on object W18.41
on
ice W00.0
with skates —*see* Accident, transport, pedestrian, conveyance
mud W01.0
oil W01.0
snow W00.0
with skis —*see* Accident, transport, pedestrian, conveyance
surface (slippery) (wet) NEC W01.0
Sliver, wood, contact with W45.8
Smoldering (due to fire) —*see* Exposure, fire
Sodomy (attempted) **by force** T74.2-•
Sound waves (causing injury) W42.9
supersonic W42.0
Splinter, contact with W45.8
Stab, stabbing —*see* Cut
Standing (prolonged) (static) X50.1
Starvation X58
Status of external cause Y99.9
child assisting in compensated work for family Y99.8
civilian activity done for financial or other compensation Y99.0
civilian activity done for income or pay Y99.0
family member assisting in compensated work for other family member Y99.8
hobby not done for income Y99.8
leisure activity Y99.8
military activity Y99.1
off-duty activity of military personnel Y99.8
recreation or sport not for income or while a student Y99.8
specified NEC Y99.8
student activity Y99.8
volunteer activity Y99.2
Stepped on
by
animal (not being ridden) NEC W55.89
crowd or human stampede W52
person W50.0
Stepping on
object W22.8
with fall W18.31
sports equipment W21.9
stationary W22.09
sports equipment W21.89
person W51
by crowd or human stampede W52
sports equipment W21.9
Sting
arthropod, nonvenomous W57
insect, nonvenomous W57
Storm (cataclysmic) —*see* Forces of nature, cataclysmic storm
Straining, excessive —*see also* Overexertion X50.9
Strangling —*see* Strangulation
Strangulation (accidental) —*see* category T71
Strenuous movements —*see also* Overexertion X50.9
Striking against
airbag (automobile) W22.10
driver side W22.11
front passenger side W22.12
specified NEC W22.19
bottom when
diving or jumping into water (in) W16.822
causing drowning W16.821
from boat W16.722
causing drowning W16.721
natural body W16.622
causing drowning W16.821
swimming pool W16.522
causing drowning W16.521
falling into water (in) W16.322
causing drowning W16.321
fountain —*see* Striking against, bottom when, falling into water, specified NEC
natural body W16.122
causing drowning W16.121
reservoir —*see* Striking against, bottom when, falling into water, specified NEC
specified NEC W16.322
causing drowning W16.321
swimming pool W16.022
causing drowning W16.021
diving board (swimming-pool) W21.4
object W22.8
with
drowning or submersion —*see* Drowning
fall —*see* Fall, due to, bumping against, object
caused by crowd or human stampede (with fall) W52
furniture W22.03
lamppost W22.02
sports equipment W21.9
stationary W22.09
sports equipment W21.89
wall W22.01
person(s) W51
with fall W03
due to ice or snow W00.0
as, or caused by, a crowd or human stampede (with fall) W52
assault Y04.2
homicide (attempt) Y04.2
sports equipment W21.9
wall (when) W22.01
diving or jumping into water (in) W16.832
causing drowning W16.831
swimming pool W16.532
causing drowning W16.531
falling into water (in) W16.332
causing drowning W16.331
fountain —*see* Striking against, wall when, falling into water, specified NEC
natural body W16.132
causing drowning W16.131
reservoir —*see* Striking against, wall when, falling into water, specified NEC
specified NEC W16.332
causing drowning W16.331
swimming pool W16.032
causing drowning W16.031
swimming pool (when) W22.042
causing drowning W22.041
diving or jumping into water W16.532
causing drowning W16.531
falling into water W16.032
causing drowning W16.031
Struck (accidentally) **by**
airbag (automobile) W22.10
driver side W22.11
front passenger side W22.12
specified NEC W22.19
alligator W58.02
animal (not being ridden) NEC W55.89
avalanche —*see* Landslide
ball (hit) (thrown) W21.00
assault Y08.09
baseball W21.03
Struck *(Continued)*
ball *(Continued)*
basketball W21.05
football W21.01
golf ball W21.04
football W21.01
soccer W21.02
softball W21.07
specified NEC W21.09
volleyball W21.06
bat or racquet
baseball bat W21.11
assault Y08.02
golf club W21.13
assault Y08.09
specified NEC W21.19
assault Y08.09
tennis racquet W21.12
assault Y08.09
bullet —*see also* Discharge, firearm by type
in war operations —*see* War operations
crocodile W58.12
dog W54.1
flare, Very pistol —*see* Discharge, firearm NEC
hailstones X39.8
hockey (ice)
field
puck W21.221
stick W21.211
puck W21.220
stick W21.210
assault Y08.01
landslide —*see* Landslide
law-enforcement agent (on duty) —*see* Legal, intervention, manhandling
with blunt object —*see* Legal, intervention, blunt object
lightning —*see* subcategory T75.0
causing fire —*see* Exposure, fire
machine —*see* Contact, with, by type of machine
mammal NEC W55.89
marine W56.32
marine animal W56.82
missile
firearm —*see* Discharge, firearm by type
in war operations —*see* War operations, missile
object W22.8
blunt W22.8
assault Y00
suicide (attempt) X79
undetermined whether accidental or intentional Y29
falling W20.8
from, in, on
building W20.1
burning (uncontrolled fire) X00.4
cataclysmic
earth surface movement NEC —*see* Landslide
storm —*see* Forces of nature, cataclysmic storm
cave-in W20.0
earthquake X34
machine (in operation) —*see* Contact, with, by type of machine
structure W20.1
burning X00.4
transport vehicle (in motion) —*see* Accident, transport, by type of vehicle
watercraft V93.49
due to
accident to craft V91.39
powered craft V91.33
ferry boat V91.31
fishing boat V91.32
jet ski V91.33
liner V91.31
merchant ship V91.30
passenger ship V91.31
unpowered craft V91.38
canoe V91.35
inflatable V91.36
kayak V91.35
sailboat V91.34
surf-board V91.38
windsurfer V91.38

S

- **Struck** *(Continued)*
  - object *(Continued)*
    - falling *(Continued)*
      - from, in *(Continued)*
        - watercraft *(Continued)*
          - powered craft V93.43
            - ferry boat V93.41
            - fishing boat V93.42
            - jet ski V93.43
            - liner V93.41
            - merchant ship V93.4Ø
            - passenger ship V93.41
          - unpowered craft V93.48
            - sailboat V93.44
            - surf-board V93.48
            - windsurfer V93.48
    - moving NEC W2Ø.8
    - projected W2Ø.8
      - assault YØØ
      - in sports W21.9
        - assault YØ8.Ø9
        - ball W21.ØØ
          - baseball W21.Ø3
          - basketball W21.Ø5
          - football W21.Ø1
          - golf ball W21.Ø4
          - soccer W21.Ø2
          - softball W21.Ø7
          - specified NEC W21.Ø9
          - volleyball W21.Ø6
        - bat or racquet
          - baseball bat W21.11
            - assault YØ8.Ø2
          - golf club W21.13
            - assault YØ8.Ø9-●
          - specified NEC W21.19
            - assault YØ8.Ø9
          - tennis racquet W21.12
            - assault YØ8.Ø9
        - hockey (ice)
          - field
            - puck W21.221
            - stick W21.211
          - puck W21.22Ø
          - stick W21.21Ø
            - assault YØ8.Ø1
        - specified NEC W21.89
    - set in motion by explosion —*see* Explosion
    - thrown W2Ø.8
      - assault YØØ
      - in sports W21.9
        - assault YØ8.Ø9
        - ball W21.ØØ
          - baseball W21.Ø3
          - basketball W21.Ø5
          - football W21.Ø1
          - golf ball W21.Ø4
          - soccer W21.Ø2
          - soft ball W21.Ø7
          - specified NEC W21.Ø9
          - volleyball W21.Ø6
        - bat or racquet
          - baseball bat W21.11
            - assault YØ8.Ø2
          - golf club W21.13
            - assault YØ8.Ø9
          - specified NEC W21.19
            - assault YØ8.Ø9
          - tennis racquet W21.12
            - assault YØ8.Ø9
        - hockey (ice)
          - field
            - puck W21.221
            - stick W21.211
          - puck W21.22Ø
          - stick W21.21Ø
            - assault YØ8.Ø1
        - specified NEC W21.89
  - other person(s) W5Ø.Ø
    - with
      - blunt object W22.8
        - intentional, homicide (attempt) YØØ
        - sports equipment W21.9
        - undetermined whether accidental or intentional Y29
      - fall WØ3
        - due to ice or snow WØØ.Ø
    - as, or caused by, a crowd or human stampede (with fall) W52
    - assault YØ4.2
    - homicide (attempt) YØ4.2
    - in legal intervention
      - injuring
        - bystander Y35.812
        - law enforcement personnel Y35.811
        - suspect Y35.813
        - unspecified person Y35.819
    - sports equipment W21.9
  - police (on duty) —*see* Legal, intervention, manhandling
    - with blunt object —*see* Legal, intervention, blunt object
  - sports equipment W21.9
    - assault YØ8.Ø9
    - ball W21.ØØ
      - baseball W21.Ø3
      - basketball W21.Ø5
      - football W21.Ø1
      - golf ball W21.Ø4
      - soccer W21.Ø2
      - soft ball W21.Ø7
      - specified NEC W21.Ø9
      - volleyball W21.Ø6
    - bat or racquet
      - baseball bat W21.11
        - assault YØ8.Ø2
      - golf club W21.13
        - assault YØ8.Ø9
      - specified NEC W21.19
      - tennis racquet W21.12
        - assault YØ8.Ø9
    - cleats (shoe) W21.31
    - foot wear NEC W21.39
    - football helmet W21.81
    - hockey (ice)
      - field
        - puck W21.221
        - stick W21.211
      - puck W21.22Ø
      - stick W21.21Ø
        - assault YØ8.Ø1
    - skate blades W21.32
    - specified NEC W21.89
      - assault YØ8.Ø9
  - thunderbolt —*see* subcategory T75.Ø
    - causing fire —*see* Exposure, fire
  - transport vehicle NEC —*see also* Accident, transport VØ9.9
    - intentional, homicide (attempt) YØ3.Ø
    - motor NEC —*see also* Accident, transport VØ9.2Ø
      - homicide YØ3.Ø
  - vehicle (transport) NEC —*see* Accident, transport, by type of vehicle
    - stationary (falling from jack, hydraulic lift, ramp) W2Ø.8
- **Stumbling**
  - without fall W18.4Ø
    - due to
      - specified NEC W18.49
      - stepping from one level to another W18.43
      - stepping into hole or opening W18.42
      - stepping on object W18.41
  - over
    - animal NEC WØ1.Ø
      - with fall W18.Ø9
    - carpet, rug or (small) object W22.8
      - with fall W18.Ø9
    - person W51
      - with fall WØ3
        - due to ice or snow WØØ.Ø
- **Submersion** (accidental) —*see* Drowning
- **Suffocation** (accidental) (by external means) (by pressure) (mechanical) —*see also* category T71
  - due to, by
    - avalanche —*see* Landslide
    - explosion —*see* Explosion
    - fire —*see* Exposure, fire
    - food, any type (aspiration) (ingestion) (inhalation) —*see* categories T17 and T18
    - ignition —*see* Ignition
    - landslide —*see* Landslide
    - machine (ry) —*see* Contact, with, by type of machine
    - vomitus (aspiration) (inhalation) T17.81-●
  - in
    - burning building XØØ.8
- **Suicide, suicidal** (attempted) (by) X83.8
  - blunt object X79
  - burning, burns X76
    - hot object X77.9
      - fluid NEC X77.2
      - household appliance X77.3
      - specified NEC X77.8
      - steam X77.Ø
      - tap water X77.1
      - vapors X77.Ø
  - caustic substance —*see* Table of Drugs and Chemicals
  - cold, extreme X83.2
  - collision of motor vehicle with
    - motor vehicle X82.Ø
    - specified NEC X82.8
    - train X82.1
    - tree X82.2
  - crashing of aircraft X83.Ø
  - cut (any part of body) X78.9
  - cutting or piercing instrument X78.9
    - dagger X78.2
    - glass X78.Ø
    - knife X78.1
    - specified NEC X78.8
    - sword X78.2
  - drowning (in) X71.9
    - bathtub X71.Ø
    - natural water X71.3
    - specified NEC X71.8
    - swimming pool X71.1
      - following fall X71.2
  - electrocution X83.1
  - explosive(s) (material) X75
  - fire, flames X76
  - firearm X74.9
    - airgun X74.Ø1
    - handgun X72
    - hunting rifle X73.1
    - larger X73.9
      - specified NEC X73.8
    - machine gun X73.2
    - shotgun X73.Ø
    - specified NEC X74.8
  - hanging X83.8
  - hot object —*see* Suicide, burning, hot object
  - jumping
    - before moving object X81.8
      - motor vehicle X81.Ø
      - subway train X81.1
      - train X81.1
    - from high place X8Ø
  - late effect of attempt —*see* X71-X83 with 7th character S
  - lying before moving object, train, vehicle X81.8
  - poisoning —*see* Table of Drugs and Chemicals
  - puncture (any part of body) —*see* Suicide, cutting or piercing instrument
  - scald —*see* Suicide, burning, hot object
  - sequelae of attempt —*see* X71-X83 with 7th character S
  - sharp object (any) —*see* Suicide, cutting or piercing instrument
  - shooting —*see* Suicide, firearm
  - specified means NEC X83.8
  - stab (any part of body) —*see* Suicide, cutting or piercing instrument
  - steam, hot vapors X77.Ø
  - strangulation X83.8
  - submersion —*see* Suicide, drowning
  - suffocation X83.8
  - wound NEC X83.8
- **Sunstroke** X32
- **Supersonic waves** (causing injury) W42.Ø
- **Surgical procedure, complication of** (delayed or as an abnormal reaction without mention of misadventure) —*see also* Complication of or following, by type of procedure
  - due to or as a result of misadventure —*see* Misadventure

S

- **Swallowed, swallowing**
  - foreign body —*see* Foreign body, alimentary canal
  - poison —*see* Table of Drugs and Chemicals
  - substance
    - caustic or corrosive —*see* Table of Drugs and Chemicals
    - poisonous —*see* Table of Drugs and Chemicals

T

- **Tackle in sport** WØ3
- **Terrorism** (involving) Y38.8Ø
  - biological weapons Y38.6X-•
  - chemical weapons Y38.7X-•
  - conflagration Y38.3X-•
  - drowning and submersion Y38.89-•
  - explosion Y38.2X-•
    - destruction of aircraft Y38.1X-•
    - marine weapons Y38.ØX-•
  - fire Y38.3X-•
  - firearms Y38.4X-•
  - hot substances Y38.3X-•
  - lasers Y38.89-•
  - nuclear weapons Y38.5X-•
  - piercing or stabbing instruments Y38.89-•
  - secondary effects Y38.9X-•
  - specified method NEC Y38.89-•
  - suicide bomber Y38.81-•
- **Thirst** X58
- **Threat to breathing**
  - aspiration —*see* Aspiration
  - due to cave-in, falling earth or substance NEC —*see* category T71
- **Thrown** (accidentally)
  - against part (any) of or object in transport vehicle (in motion) NEC —*see also* Accident, transport
  - from
    - high place, homicide (attempt) YØ1
    - machinery —*see* Contact, with, by type of machine
    - transport vehicle NEC —*see also* Accident, transport V89.9
  - off —*see* Thrown, from
- **Thunderbolt** —*see* subcategory T75.Ø
  - causing fire —*see* Exposure, fire
- **Tidal wave** (any injury) **NEC** —*see* Forces of nature, tidal wave
- **Took**
  - overdose (drug) —*see* Table of Drugs and Chemicals
  - poison —*see* Table of Drugs and Chemicals
- **Tornado** (any injury) X37.1
- **Torrential rain** (any injury) X37.8
- **Torture** X58
- **Trampled by animal NEC** W55.89
- **Trapped** (accidentally)
  - between objects (moving) (stationary and moving) —*see* Caught
  - by part (any) of
    - electric (assisted) bicycle V29.881
    - motorcycle V29.888
    - pedal cycle V19.88
    - transport vehicle NEC —*see also* Accident, transport V89.9
- **Travel** (effects) (sickness) T75.3
- **Tree falling on or hitting** (accidentally) (person) W2Ø.8
- **Tripping**
  - without fall W18.4Ø
    - due to
      - specified NEC W18.49
      - stepping from one level to another W18.43
      - stepping into hole or opening W18.42
      - stepping on object W18.41
  - over
    - animal WØ1.Ø
      - with fall WØ1.Ø
    - carpet, rug or (small) object W22.8
      - with fall W18.Ø9
    - person W51
      - with fall WØ3
        - due to ice or snow WØØ.Ø
- **Twisted by person**(s) (accidentally) W5Ø.2
  - with intent to injure or kill YØ4.Ø
  - as, or caused by, a crowd or human stampede (with fall) W52
  - assault YØ4.Ø
  - homicide (attempt) YØ4.Ø
  - in
    - fight YØ4.Ø
    - legal intervention —*see* Legal, intervention, manhandling
- **Twisting** (prolonged) (static) X5Ø.1

U

- **Underdosing of necessary drugs, medicaments or biological substances** Y63.6
- **Undetermined intent** (contact) (exposure)
  - automobile collision Y32
  - blunt object Y29
  - drowning (submersion) (in) Y21.9
    - bathtub Y21.Ø
      - after fall Y21.1
    - natural water (lake) (ocean) (pond) (river) (stream) Y21.4
    - specified place NEC Y21.8
    - swimming pool Y21.2
      - after fall Y21.3
  - explosive material Y25
  - fall, jump or push from high place Y3Ø
  - falling, lying or running before moving object Y31
  - fire Y26
  - firearm discharge Y24.9
    - airgun (BB) (pellet) Y24.Ø
    - handgun (pistol) (revolver) Y22
    - hunting rifle Y23.1
    - larger Y23.9
      - hunting rifle Y23.1
      - machine gun Y23.3
      - military Y23.2
      - shotgun Y23.Ø
      - specified type NEC Y23.8
    - machine gun Y23.3
    - military Y23.2
    - shotgun Y23.Ø
    - specified type NEC Y24.8
    - Very pistol Y24.8
  - hot object Y27.9
    - fluid NEC Y27.2
    - household appliance Y27.3
    - specified object NEC Y27.8
    - steam Y27.Ø
    - tap water Y27.1
    - vapor Y27.Ø
  - jump, fall or push from high place Y3Ø
  - lying, falling or running before moving object Y31
  - motor vehicle crash Y32
  - push, fall or jump from high place Y3Ø
  - running, falling or lying before moving object Y31
  - sharp object Y28.9
    - dagger Y28.2
    - glass Y28.Ø
    - knife Y28.1
    - specified object NEC Y28.8
    - sword Y28.2
  - smoke Y26
  - specified event NEC Y33
- **Use of hand as hammer** X5Ø.3

V

- **Vibration** (causing injury) W49.9
- **Victim** (of)
  - avalanche —*see* Landslide
  - earth movements NEC —*see* Forces of nature, earth movement
  - earthquake X34
  - flood —*see* Flood
  - landslide —*see* Landslide
  - lightning —*see* subcategory T75.Ø
    - causing fire —*see* Exposure, fire
  - storm (cataclysmic) NEC —*see* Forces of nature, cataclysmic storm
  - volcanic eruption X35
- **Volcanic eruption** (any injury) X35
- **Vomitus, gastric contents in air passages** (with asphyxia, obstruction or suffocation) T17.81-•

W

- **Walked into stationary object** (any) W22.Ø9
  - furniture W22.Ø3
  - lamppost W22.Ø2
  - wall W22.Ø1
- **War operations** (injuries to military personnel and civilians during war, civil insurrection and peacekeeping missions) (by) (from) (involving) Y36.9Ø-•
  - after cessation of hostilities Y36.89-•
    - explosion (of)
      - bomb placed during war operations Y36.82-•
      - mine placed during war operations Y36.81-•
    - specified NEC Y36.88-•
  - air blast Y36.2Ø-•
  - aircraft
    - destruction —*see* War operations, destruction of aircraft
  - airway restriction —*see* War operations, restriction of airways
  - asphyxiation —*see* War operations, restriction of airways
  - biological weapons Y36.6X-•
  - blast Y36.2Ø-•
  - blast fragments Y36.2Ø-•
  - blast wave Y36.2Ø-•
  - blast wind Y36.2Ø-•
  - bomb Y36.2Ø-•
    - dirty Y36.5Ø-•
    - gasoline Y36.31-•
    - incendiary Y36.31-•
    - petrol Y36.31-•
  - bullet Y36.43-•
    - incendiary Y36.32-•
    - rubber Y36.41-•
  - chemical weapons Y36.7X-•
  - combat
    - hand to hand (unarmed) combat Y36.44-•
    - using blunt or piercing object Y36.45-•
  - conflagration —*see* War operations, fire
  - conventional warfare NEC Y36.49-•
  - depth-charge Y36.Ø1-•
  - destruction of aircraft Y36.1Ø-•
    - due to
      - air to air missile Y36.11-•
      - collision with other aircraft Y36.12-•
      - detonation (accidental) of onboard munitions and explosives Y36.14-•
      - enemy fire or explosives Y36.11-•
      - explosive placed on aircraft Y36.11-•
      - onboard fire Y36.13-•
      - rocket propelled grenade [RPG] Y36.11-•
      - small arms fire Y36.11-•
      - surface to air missile Y36.11-•
    - specified NEC Y36.19-•
  - detonation (accidental) of
    - onboard marine weapons Y36.Ø5-•
    - own munitions or munitions launch device Y36.24-•
  - dirty bomb Y36.5Ø-•
  - explosion (of) Y36.2Ø-•
    - aerial bomb Y36.21-•
    - after cessation of hostilities
      - bomb placed during war operations Y36.82-•
      - mine placed during war operations Y36.81-•
    - bomb NOS —*see also* War operations, bomb(s) Y36.2Ø-•
    - fragments Y36.2Ø-•
    - grenade Y36.29-•

S, T, U, V, & W

War operations *(Continued)*
explosion *(Continued)*
guided missile Y36.22-●
improvised explosive device [IED] (person-borne) (roadside) (vehicle-borne) Y36.23-●
land mine Y36.29-●
marine mine (at sea) (in harbor) Y36.02-●
marine weapon Y36.00-●
specified NEC Y36.09-●
own munitions or munitions launch device (accidental) Y36.24-●
sea-based artillery shell Y36.03-●
specified NEC Y36.29-●
torpedo Y36.04-●
fire Y36.30-●
specified NEC Y36.39-●
firearms
discharge Y36.43-●
pellets Y36.42-●
flamethrower Y36.33-●
fragments (from) (of)
improvised explosive device [IED] (person-borne) (roadside) (vehicle-borne) Y36.26-●
munitions Y36.25-●
specified NEC Y36.29-●
weapons Y36.27-●
friendly fire Y36.92
hand to hand (unarmed) combat Y36.44-●
hot substances —*see* War operations, fire
incendiary bullet Y36.32-●
nuclear weapon (effects of) Y36.50-●
acute radiation exposure Y36.54-●
blast pressure Y36.51-●

War operations *(Continued)*
nuclear weapon *(Continued)*
direct blast Y36.51-●
direct heat Y36.53-●
fallout exposure Y36.54-●
fireball Y36.53-●
indirect blast (struck or crushed by blast debris) (being thrown by blast) Y36.52-●
ionizing radiation (immediate exposure) Y36.54-●
nuclear radiation Y36.54-●
radiation
ionizing (immediate exposure) Y36.54-●
nuclear Y36.54-●
thermal Y36.53-●
secondary effects Y36.54-●
specified NEC Y36.59-●
thermal radiation Y36.53-●
restriction of air (airway)
intentional Y36.46-●
unintentional Y36.47-●
rubber bullets Y36.41-●
shrapnel NOS Y36.29-●
suffocation —*see* War operations, restriction of airways
unconventional warfare NEC Y36.7X-●
underwater blast NOS Y36.00-●
warfare
conventional NEC Y36.49-●
unconventional NEC Y36.7X-●
weapon of mass destruction [WMD] Y36.91
weapons
biological weapons Y36.6X-●
chemical Y36.7X-●

War operations *(Continued)*
weapons *(Continued)*
nuclear (effects of) Y36.50-●
acute radiation exposure Y36.54-●
blast pressure Y36.51-●
direct blast Y36.51-●
direct heat Y36.53-●
fallout exposure Y36.54-●
fireball Y36.53-●
radiation
ionizing (immediate exposure) Y36.54-●
nuclear Y36.54-●
thermal Y36.53-●
secondary effects Y36.54-●
specified NEC Y36.59-●
of mass destruction [WMD] Y36.91-●
Washed
away by flood —*see* Flood
off road by storm (transport vehicle) —*see* Forces of nature, cataclysmic storm
Weather exposure NEC —*see* Forces of nature
Weightlessness (causing injury) (effects of) (in spacecraft, real or simulated) X52
Work related condition Y99.0
Wound (accidental) NEC —*see also* Injury X58
battle —*see also* War operations Y36.90
gunshot —*see* Discharge, firearm by type
Wreck transport vehicle NEC —*see also* Accident, transport V89.9
Wrong
device implanted into correct surgical site Y65.51
fluid in infusion Y65.1
patient, procedure performed on Y65.52
procedure (operation) on correct patient Y65.51

W

PART III

ICD-10-CM Tabular List of Diseases and Injuries

CHAPTER 1

CERTAIN INFECTIOUS AND PARASITIC DISEASES (AØØ-B99)

OGCR Chapter-Specific Coding Guidelines

1. **Chapter 1: Certain Infectious and Parasitic Diseases (AØØ-B99)**

a. **Human Immunodeficiency Virus (HIV) Infections**

1) **Code only confirmed cases**

Code only confirmed cases of HIV infection/illness. This is an exception to the hospital inpatient guideline Section II, H.

In this context, "confirmation" does not require documentation of positive serology or culture for HIV; the provider's diagnostic statement that the patient is HIV positive, or has an HIV-related illness is sufficient.

2) **Selection and sequencing of HIV codes**

(a) **Patient admitted for HIV-related condition**

If a patient is admitted for an HIV-related condition, the principal diagnosis should be B2Ø, Human immunodeficiency virus [HIV] disease followed by additional diagnosis codes for all reported HIV-related conditions.

(b) **Patient with HIV disease admitted for unrelated condition**

If a patient with HIV disease is admitted for an unrelated condition (such as a traumatic injury), the code for the unrelated condition (e.g., the nature of injury code) should be the principal diagnosis. Other diagnoses would be B2Ø followed by additional diagnosis codes for all reported HIV-related conditions.

(c) **Whether the patient is newly diagnosed**

Whether the patient is newly diagnosed or has had previous admissions/encounters for HIV conditions is irrelevant to the sequencing decision.

(d) **Asymptomatic human immunodeficiency virus**

Z21, Asymptomatic human immunodeficiency virus [HIV] infection status, is to be applied when the patient without any documentation of symptoms is listed as being "HIV positive," "known HIV," "HIV test positive," or similar terminology. Do not use this code if the term "AIDS" is used or if the patient is treated for any HIV-related illness or is described as having any condition(s) resulting from his/her HIV positive status; use B2Ø in these cases.

(e) **Patients with inconclusive HIV serology**

Patients with inconclusive HIV serology, but no definitive diagnosis or manifestations of the illness, may be assigned code R75, Inconclusive laboratory evidence of human immunodeficiency virus [HIV].

(f) **Previously diagnosed HIV-related illness**

Patients with any known prior diagnosis of an HIV-related illness should be coded to B2Ø. Once a patient has developed an HIV-related illness, the patient should always be assigned code B2Ø on every subsequent admission/encounter. Patients previously diagnosed with any HIV illness (B2Ø) should never be assigned to R75 or Z21, Asymptomatic human immunodeficiency virus [HIV] infection status.

(g) **HIV Infection in Pregnancy, Childbirth and the Puerperium**

During pregnancy, childbirth or the puerperium, a patient admitted (or presenting for a health care encounter) because of an HIV-related illness should receive a principal diagnosis code of O98.7-, Human immunodeficiency [HIV] disease complicating pregnancy, childbirth and the puerperium, followed by B2Ø and the code(s) for the HIV-related illness(es). Codes from Chapter 15 always take sequencing priority.

Patients with asymptomatic HIV infection status admitted (or presenting for a health care encounter) during pregnancy, childbirth, or the puerperium should receive codes of O98.7- and Z21.

(h) **Encounters for testing for HIV**

If a patient is being seen to determine his/her HIV status, use code Z11.4, Encounter for screening for human immunodeficiency virus [HIV]. Use additional codes for any associated high-risk behavior.

If a patient with signs or symptoms is being seen for HIV testing, code the signs and symptoms. An additional counseling code Z71.7, Human immunodeficiency virus [HIV] counseling, may be used if counseling is provided during the encounter for the test.

When a patient returns to be informed of his/her HIV test results and the test result is negative, use code Z71.7, Human immunodeficiency virus [HIV] counseling.

If the results are positive, see previous guidelines and assign codes as appropriate.

b. **Infectious agents as the cause of diseases classified to other chapters**

Certain infections are classified in chapters other than Chapter 1 and no organism is identified as part of the infection code. In these instances, it is necessary to use an additional code from Chapter 1 to identify the organism. A code from category B95, Streptococcus, Staphylococcus, and Enterococcus as the cause of diseases classified to other chapters, B96, Other bacterial agents as the cause of diseases classified to other chapters, or B97, Viral agents as the cause of diseases classified to other chapters, is to be used as an additional code to identify the organism. An instructional note will be found at the infection code advising that an additional organism code is required.

c. **Infections resistant to antibiotics**

Many bacterial infections are resistant to current antibiotics. It is necessary to identify all infections documented as antibiotic resistant. Assign a code from category Z16, Resistance to antimicrobial drugs, following the infection code only if the infection code does not identify drug resistance.

d. **Sepsis, Severe Sepsis, and Septic Shock**

1) **Coding of Sepsis and Severe Sepsis**

(a) **Sepsis**

For a diagnosis of sepsis, assign the appropriate code for the underlying systemic infection. If the type of infection or causal organism is not further specified, assign code A41.9, Sepsis, unspecified organism.

A code from subcategory R65.2, Severe sepsis, should not be assigned unless severe sepsis or an associated acute organ dysfunction is documented.

(i) Negative or inconclusive blood cultures and sepsis
Negative or inconclusive blood cultures do not preclude a diagnosis of sepsis in patients with clinical evidence of the condition, however, the provider should be queried.

(ii) Urosepsis
The term urosepsis is a nonspecific term. It is not to be considered synonymous with sepsis. It has no default code in the Alphabetic Index. Should a provider use this term, he/she must be queried for clarification.

(iii) Sepsis with organ dysfunction
If a patient has sepsis and associated acute organ dysfunction or multiple organ dysfunction (MOD), follow the instructions for coding severe sepsis.

(iv) Acute organ dysfunction that is not clearly associated with the sepsis
If a patient has sepsis and an acute organ dysfunction, but the medical record documentation indicates that the acute organ dysfunction is related to a medical condition other than the sepsis, do not assign a code from subcategory R65.2, Severe sepsis. An acute organ dysfunction must be associated with the sepsis in order to assign the severe sepsis code. If the documentation is not clear as to whether an acute organ dysfunction is related to the sepsis or another medical condition, query the provider.

(b) **Severe sepsis**

The coding of severe sepsis requires a minimum of 2 codes: first a code for the underlying systemic infection, followed by a code from subcategory R65.2, Severe sepsis. If the causal organism is not documented, assign code A41.9, Sepsis, unspecified organism, for the infection. Additional code(s) for the associated acute organ dysfunction are also required.

Due to the complex nature of severe sepsis, some cases may require querying the provider prior to assignment of the codes.

2) **Septic shock**

(a) Septic shock generally refers to circulatory failure associated with severe sepsis, and therefore, it represents a type of acute organ dysfunction.

For all cases of septic shock, the code for the systemic infection should be sequenced first, followed by code R65.21, Severe sepsis with septic shock or code T81.12, Postprocedural septic shock.

Any additional codes for the other acute organ dysfunctions should also be assigned. As noted in the sequencing instructions in the Tabular List, the code for septic shock cannot be assigned as a principal diagnosis.

3) Sequencing of severe sepsis

If severe sepsis is present on admission, and meets the definition of principal diagnosis, the underlying systemic infection should be assigned as principal diagnosis followed by the appropriate code from subcategory R65.2 as required by the sequencing rules in the Tabular List. A code from subcategory R65.2 can never be assigned as a principal diagnosis.

When severe sepsis develops during an encounter (it was not present on admission) the underlying systemic infection and the appropriate code from subcategory R65.2 should be assigned as secondary diagnoses.

Severe sepsis may be present on admission but the diagnosis may not be confirmed until sometime after admission. If the documentation is not clear whether severe sepsis was present on admission, the provider should be queried.

4) Sepsis and severe sepsis with a localized infection

If the reason for admission is both sepsis or severe sepsis and a localized infection, such as pneumonia or cellulitis, a code(s) for the underlying systemic infection should be assigned first and the code for the localized infection should be assigned as a secondary diagnosis. If the patient has severe sepsis, a code from subcategory R65.2 should also be assigned as a secondary diagnosis. If the patient is admitted with a localized infection, such as pneumonia, and sepsis/severe sepsis doesn't develop until after admission, the localized infection should be assigned first, followed by the appropriate sepsis/severe sepsis codes.

5) Sepsis due to a postprocedural infection

(a) Documentation of causal relationship

As with all postprocedural complications, code assignment is based on the provider's documentation of the relationship between the infection and the procedure.

(b) Sepsis due to a postprocedural infection

For infections following a procedure, a code from T81.4Ø, to T81.43. Infection following a procedure, or O86.ØØ to O86.Ø3, Infection of obstetric surgical wound, that identifies the site of the infection should be coded first, if known. Assign an additional code for sepsis following a procedure (T81.44) or sepsis following an obstetrical procedure (O86.Ø4). Use an additional code to identify the infectious agent. If the patient has severe sepsis the appropriate code from subcategory R65.2 should also be assigned with the additional code(s) for any acute organ dysfunction.

For infections following infusion, transfusion, therapeutic injection, or immunization, a code from subcategory T8Ø.2, Infections following infusion, transfusion, and therapeutic injection, or code T88.Ø-, Infection following immunization, should be coded first, followed by the code for the specific infection. If the patient has severe sepsis, the appropriate code from subcategory R65.2 should also be assigned, with the additional codes(s) for any acute organ dysfunction.

(c) Postprocedural infection and postprocedural septic shock

If a postprocedural infection has resulted in postprocedural septic shock, assign the codes indicated above for sepsis due to a postprocedural infection, followed by code T81.12-, Postprocedural septic shock. Do not assign code R65.21, Severe sepsis with septic shock. Additional code(s) should be assigned for any acute organ dysfunction.

6) Sepsis and severe sepsis associated with a noninfectious process (condition)

In some cases a noninfectious process (condition), such as trauma, may lead to an infection which can result in sepsis or severe sepsis. If sepsis or severe sepsis is documented as associated with a noninfectious condition, such as a burn or serious injury, and this condition meets the definition for principal diagnosis, the code for the noninfectious condition should be sequenced first, followed by the code for the resulting infection. If severe sepsis is present, a code from subcategory R65.2 should also be assigned with any associated organ dysfunction(s) codes. It is not necessary to assign a code from subcategory R65.1, Systemic inflammatory response syndrome (SIRS) of noninfectious origin, for these cases.

If the infection meets the definition of principal diagnosis it should be sequenced before the noninfectious condition. When both the associated noninfectious condition and the infection meet the definition of principal diagnosis either may be assigned as principal diagnosis.

Only one code from category R65, Symptoms and signs specifically associated with systemic inflammation and infection, should be assigned. Therefore, when a noninfectious condition leads to an infection resulting in severe sepsis, assign the appropriate code from subcategory R65.2, Severe sepsis. Do not additionally assign a code from subcategory R65.1, Systemic inflammatory response syndrome (SIRS) of noninfectious origin.

See Section I.C.18. SIRS due to non-infectious process

7) Sepsis and septic shock complicating abortion, pregnancy, childbirth, and the puerperium

See Section I.C.15. Sepsis and septic shock complicating abortion, pregnancy, childbirth and the puerperium

8) Newborn sepsis

See Section I.C.16. f. Bacterial sepsis of Newborn

e. Methicillin Resistant Staphylococcus aureus (MRSA) Conditions

1) Selection and sequencing of MRSA codes

(a) Combination codes for MRSA infection

When a patient is diagnosed with an infection that is due to methicillin resistant *Staphylococcus aureus* (MRSA), and that infection has a combination code that includes the causal organism (e.g., sepsis, pneumonia) assign the appropriate combination code for the condition (e.g., code A41.Ø2, Sepsis due to Methicillin resistant Staphylococcus aureus or code J15.212, Pneumonia due to Methicillin resistant Staphylococcus aureus). Do not assign code B95.62, Methicillin resistant Staphylococcus aureus infection as the cause of diseases classified elsewhere, as an additional code because the combination code includes the type of infection and the MRSA organism. Do not assign a code from subcategory Z16.11, Resistance to penicillins, as an additional diagnosis.

See Section C.1. for instructions on coding and sequencing of sepsis and severe sepsis.

(b) Other codes for MRSA infection

When there is documentation of a current infection (e.g., wound infection, stitch abscess, urinary tract infection) due to MRSA, and that infection does not have a combination code that includes the causal organism, assign the appropriate code to identify the condition along with code B95.62, Methicillin resistant Staphylococcus aureus infection as the cause of diseases classified elsewhere for the MRSA infection. Do not assign a code from subcategory Z16.11, Resistance to penicillins.

(c) Methicillin susceptible Staphylococcus aureus (MSSA) and MRSA colonization

The condition or state of being colonized or carrying MSSA or MRSA is called colonization or carriage, while an individual person is described as being colonized or being a carrier. Colonization means that MSSA or MSRA is present on or in the body without necessarily causing illness. A positive MRSA colonization test might be documented by the provider as "MRSA screen positive" or "MRSA nasal swab positive".

Assign code Z22.322, Carrier or suspected carrier of Methicillin resistant Staphylococcus aureus, for patients documented as having MRSA colonization. Assign code Z22.321, Carrier or suspected carrier of Methicillin susceptible Staphylococcus aureus, for patient documented as having MSSA colonization. Colonization is not necessarily indicative of a disease process or as the cause of a specific condition the patient may have unless documented as such by the provider.

(d) MRSA colonization and infection

If a patient is documented as having both MRSA colonization and infection during a hospital admission, code Z22.322, Carrier or suspected carrier of Methicillin resistant Staphylococcus aureus, and a code for the MRSA infection may both be assigned.

f. Zika virus infections

1) Code only confirmed cases

Code only a confirmed diagnosis of Zika virus (A92.5, Zika virus disease) as documented by the provider. This is an exception to the hospital inpatient guideline Section II, H.

In this context, "confirmation" does not require documentation of the type of test performed; the physician's diagnostic statement that the condition is confirmed is sufficient. This code should be assigned regardless of the stated mode of transmission.

If the provider documents "suspected", "possible" or "probable" Zika, do not assign code A92.5. Assign a code(s) explaining the reason for encounter (such as fever, rash, or joint pain) or Z2Ø.821, Contact with and (suspected) exposure to Zika virus.

CHAPTER 1

CERTAIN INFECTIOUS AND PARASITIC DISEASES (A00-B99)

Includes diseases generally recognized as communicable or transmissible

Use additional code to identify resistance to antimicrobial drugs (Z16.-)

Excludes1 certain localized infections - see body system-related chapters

Excludes2 carrier or suspected carrier of infectious disease (Z22.-)
infectious and parasitic diseases complicating pregnancy, childbirth and the puerperium (O98.-)
infectious and parasitic diseases specific to the perinatal period (P35-P39)
influenza and other acute respiratory infections (J00-J22)

This chapter contains the following blocks:

A00-A09	Intestinal infectious diseases
A15-A19	Tuberculosis
A20-A28	Certain zoonotic bacterial diseases
A30-A49	Other bacterial diseases
A50-A64	Infections with a predominantly sexual mode of transmission
A65-A69	Other spirochetal diseases
A70-A74	Other diseases caused by chlamydiae
A75-A79	Rickettsioses
A80-A89	Viral and prion infections of the central nervous system
A90-A99	Arthropod-borne viral fevers and viral hemorrhagic fevers
B00-B09	Viral infections characterized by skin and mucous membrane lesions
B10	Other human herpesviruses
B15-B19	Viral hepatitis
B20	Human immunodeficiency virus [HIV] disease
B25-B34	Other viral diseases
B35-B49	Mycoses
B50-B64	Protozoal diseases
B65-B83	Helminthiases
B85-B89	Pediculosis, acariasis and other infestations
B90-B94	Sequelae of infectious and parasitic diseases
B95-B97	Bacterial and viral infectious agents
B99	Other infectious diseases

INTESTINAL INFECTIOUS DISEASES (A00-A09)

● **A00 Cholera** Ex PDX 2
A serious, often deadly, infectious disease of the small intestine

A00.0 Cholera due to Vibrio cholerae 01, biovar cholerae
Classical cholera

A00.1 Cholera due to Vibrio cholerae 01, biovar eltor
Cholera eltor

A00.9 Cholera, unspecified

● **A01 Typhoid and paratyphoid fevers** Ex PDX 3
Caused by Salmonella typhi and Salmonella paratyphi A, B, and C bacteria

● **A01.0 Typhoid fever**
Infection due to Salmonella typhi

A01.00 Typhoid fever, unspecified

A01.01 Typhoid meningitis

A01.02 Typhoid fever with heart involvement
Typhoid endocarditis
Typhoid myocarditis

A01.03 Typhoid pneumonia

A01.04 Typhoid arthritis

A01.05 Typhoid osteomyelitis

A01.09 Typhoid fever with other complications

A01.1 Paratyphoid fever A

A01.2 Paratyphoid fever B

A01.3 Paratyphoid fever C

A01.4 Paratyphoid fever, unspecified
Infection due to Salmonella paratyphi NOS

● **A02 Other salmonella infections**

Includes infection or foodborne intoxication due to any Salmonella species other than S. typhi and S. paratyphi

A02.0 Salmonella enteritis Ex PDX 4
Salmonellosis

A02.1 Salmonella sepsis Ex PDX 5

● **A02.2 Localized salmonella infections**

A02.20 Localized salmonella infection, unspecified
Specified in the documentation as localized, but unspecified as to type

A02.21 Salmonella meningitis Ex PDX 6
Specified as localized in the meninges

A02.22 Salmonella pneumonia Ex PDX 7
Specified as localized in the lungs

A02.23 Salmonella arthritis Ex PDX 8
Specified as localized in the joints

A02.24 Salmonella osteomyelitis Ex PDX 9
Specified as localized in bone

A02.25 Salmonella pyelonephritis Ex PDX 10
Salmonella tubulo-interstitial nephropathy

A02.29 Salmonella with other localized infection Ex PDX 10
Specified as localized (because it is still under localized heading) but does not assign into any of the above codes

A02.8 Other specified salmonella infections Ex PDX 11
Any specified salmonella infection which does NOT assign into any of the above codes (not specified as localized)

A02.9 Salmonella infection, unspecified Ex PDX 12
Unspecified in the documentation as to specific type of salmonella

● **A03 Shigellosis**
An infectious disease caused by bacteria (Shigella)

A03.0 Shigellosis due to Shigella dysenteriae Ex PDX 13
Group A shigellosis [Shiga-Kruse dysentery]

A03.1 Shigellosis due to Shigella flexneri
Group B shigellosis

A03.2 Shigellosis due to Shigella boydii
Group C shigellosis

A03.3 Shigellosis due to Shigella sonnei
Group D shigellosis

A03.8 Other shigellosis

A03.9 Shigellosis, unspecified
Bacillary dysentery NOS

● **A04 Other bacterial intestinal infections** Ex PDX 14

Excludes1 bacterial foodborne intoxications, NEC (A05.-)
tuberculous enteritis (A18.32)

A04.0 Enteropathogenic Escherichia coli infection
Pertaining to or producing intestinal disease

A04.1 Enterotoxigenic Escherichia coli infection
Producing or containing intestinal toxin

Item 1–1 Salmonella is a bacterium that lives in the intestines of fowl and mammals and can spread to humans through improper food preparation and cooking. Salmonellosis is an infection with the bacterium. Symptoms include diarrhea, fever, and abdominal cramps 12 to 72 hours after infection. The illness usually lasts 4 to 7 days, and most persons recover without treatment. The diarrhea may be so severe that the patient needs to be hospitalized. Patients with immunocompromised systems in chronic, ill health are more likely to have the infection invade their bloodstream with life-threatening results. For example, patients with sickle cell disease are more prone to salmonella osteomyelitis than others.

A04.2 Enteroinvasive Escherichia coli infection
Capable of penetrating and spreading through intestinal mucosal epithelium

A04.3 Enterohemorrhagic Escherichia coli infection
Causing bloody diarrhea, resulting from microorganisms

A04.4 Other intestinal Escherichia coli infections
Escherichia coli enteritis NOS

A04.5 Campylobacter enteritis (Ex) PDX 15
Spiral shaped bacterium

A04.6 Enteritis due to Yersinia enterocolitica (Ex) PDX 15
Excludes1 extraintestinal yersiniosis (A28.2)
Transmitted by infected food/water and person-to-person contact, affecting intestinal tract

● A04.7 Enterocolitis due to Clostridium difficile
▶Clostridioides difficile colitis
Foodborne intoxication by Clostridium difficile
Pseudomembraneous colitis
Marked by fibrinous deposit (false membrane) with enmeshed necrotic cells

A04.71 Enterocolitis due to Clostridium difficile, recurrent (Ex) PDX 15
Coding Clinic: 2020, Q1, P18

A04.72 Enterocolitis due to Clostridium difficile, not specified as recurrent (Ex) PDX 15

A04.8 Other specified bacterial intestinal infections (Ex) PDX 15

A04.9 Bacterial intestinal infection, unspecified (Ex) PDX 16
Bacterial enteritis NOS

● A05 Other bacterial foodborne intoxications, not elsewhere classified
Excludes1 Clostridium difficile foodborne intoxication and infection (A04.7-)
Escherichia coli infection (A04.0-A04.4)
listeriosis (A32.-)
salmonella foodborne intoxication and infection (A02.-)
toxic effect of noxious foodstuffs (T61-T62)

A05.0 Foodborne staphylococcal intoxication (Ex) PDX 17

A05.1 Botulism food poisoning (Ex) PDX 18
Botulism NOS
Classical foodborne intoxication due to Clostridium botulinum
Excludes1 infant botulism (A48.51)
wound botulism (A48.52)

A05.2 Foodborne Clostridium perfringens [Clostridium welchii] intoxication (Ex) PDX 19
Type A causes gas gangrene and necrotizing colitis; major cause of food poisoning in humans
Enteritis necroticans
Pig-bel

A05.3 Foodborne Vibrio parahaemolyticus intoxication (Ex) PDX 17
Organism that survives only in high salt environment (halophilic), major cause of gastroenteritis due to consumption of raw or improperly cooked fish/seafood

A05.4 Foodborne Bacillus cereus intoxication (Ex) PDX 17
Spore-forming species commonly found in soil, causes food poisoning from formation of intestinal toxins in contaminated foods

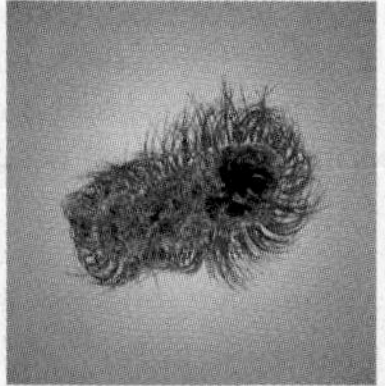

Figure 1-1 Electron micrograph of escherichia coli (E. coli) expressing P fimbriae. (Getty Image)

Item 1-2 ***Escherichia coli [E. coli]*** is a Gram-negative bacterium found in the intestinal tracts of humans and animals and is usually nonpathogenic. Pathogenic strains can cause diarrhea or pyogenic (pus-producing) infections. Can be a threat to food safety.

A05.5 Foodborne Vibrio vulnificus intoxication (Ex) PDX 17
Species that survives in high salt environment (halophilic) with infection by eating raw seafood causes septicemia and cellulitis

A05.8 Other specified bacterial foodborne intoxications (Ex) PDX 17

A05.9 Bacterial foodborne intoxication, unspecified

● A06 Amebiasis
An intestinal illness caused by the microscopic parasite Entamoeba histolytica
Includes infection due to Entamoeba histolytica
Excludes1 other protozoal intestinal diseases (A07.-)
Excludes2 acanthamebiasis (B60.1-)
Naegleriasis (B60.2)

A06.0 Acute amebic dysentery (Ex) PDX 20
Acute amebiasis
Intestinal amebiasis NOS

A06.1 Chronic intestinal amebiasis (Ex) PDX 20

A06.2 Amebic nondysenteric colitis (Ex) PDX 21
Pertaining to single cell microorganism

A06.3 Ameboma of intestine (Ex) PDX 22
Tumorlike mass produced by localized inflammation often in intestine
Ameboma NOS

A06.4 Amebic liver abscess (Ex) PDX 23
Hepatic amebiasis

A06.5 Amebic lung abscess (Ex) PDX 24
Amebic abscess of lung (and liver)

A06.6 Amebic brain abscess (Ex) PDX 25
Amebic abscess of brain (and liver) (and lung)

A06.7 Cutaneous amebiasis

● A06.8 Amebic infection of other sites (Ex) PDX 22

A06.81 Amebic cystitis

A06.82 Other amebic genitourinary infections
Amebic balanitis
Amebic vesiculitis
Amebic vulvovaginitis

A06.89 Other amebic infections
Amebic appendicitis
Amebic splenic abscess

A06.9 Amebiasis, unspecified

● A07 Other protozoal intestinal diseases

A07.0 Balantidiasis
Balantidial dysentery
Infection by protozoa that may cause diarrhea and dysentery, with ulceration of colonic mucous membranes

A07.1 Giardiasis [lambliasis] (Ex) PDX 26
Common infection in small intestine spread by contaminated food, water, or direct person-to-person contact

A07.2 Cryptosporidiosis (Ex) PDX 26
Human infection with protozoa usually seen as self-limited diarrhea in those who work with cattle

A07.3 Isosporiasis (Ex) PDX 26
Human intestinal disease caused by protozoa
Infection due to Isospora belli and Isospora hominis
Intestinal coccidiosis
Isosporosis

A07.4 Cyclosporiasis (Ex) PDX 27
Infection by protozoa with most common species infecting humans being C cayetanensis

A07.8 Other specified protozoal intestinal diseases (Ex) PDX 26
Intestinal microsporidiosis
Intestinal trichomoniasis
Sarcocystosis
Sarcosporidiosis

A07.9 **Protozoal intestinal disease, unspecified** (Ex) PDX 26
Flagellate diarrhea
Protozoal colitis
Protozoal diarrhea
Protozoal dysentery

● **A08 Viral and other specified intestinal infections** (Ex) PDX 28
Excludes1 influenza with involvement of gastrointestinal tract (J09.X3, J10.2, J11.2)

A08.0 **Rotaviral enteritis**

● A08.1 **Acute gastroenteropathy due to Norwalk agent and other small round viruses**

A08.11 **Acute gastroenteropathy due to Norwalk agent**
Acute gastroenteropathy due to Norovirus
Acute gastroenteropathy due to Norwalk-like agent

A08.19 **Acute gastroenteropathy due to other small round viruses**
Acute gastroenteropathy due to small round virus [SRV] NOS

A08.2 **Adenoviral enteritis**

● A08.3 **Other viral enteritis**

A08.31 **Calicivirus enteritis**

A08.32 **Astrovirus enteritis**

A08.39 **Other viral enteritis**
Coxsackie virus enteritis
Echovirus enteritis
Enterovirus enteritis NEC
Torovirus enteritis

A08.4 **Viral intestinal infection, unspecified**
Viral enteritis NOS
Viral gastroenteritis NOS
Viral gastroenteropathy NOS
Coding Clinic: 2016, Q3, P12

A08.8 **Other specified intestinal infections**

A09 Infectious gastroenteritis and colitis, unspecified (Ex) PDX 17
Infectious colitis NOS
Infectious enteritis NOS
Infectious gastroenteritis NOS
Excludes1 colitis NOS (K52.9)
diarrhea NOS (R19.7)
enteritis NOS (K52.9)
gastroenteritis NOS (K52.9)
noninfective gastroenteritis and colitis, unspecified (K52.9)

TUBERCULOSIS (A15-A19)

Includes infections due to Mycobacterium tuberculosis and Mycobacterium bovis
Excludes1 congenital tuberculosis (P37.0)
nonspecific reaction to test for tuberculosis without active tuberculosis (R76.1-)
pneumoconiosis associated with tuberculosis, any type in A15 (J65)
positive PPD (R76.11)
positive tuberculin skin test without active tuberculosis (R76.11)
sequelae of tuberculosis (B90.-)
silicotuberculosis (J65)

● **A15 Respiratory tuberculosis** (Ex) PDX 29

A15.0 **Tuberculosis of lung**
Tuberculous bronchiectasis
Chronic dilatation of bronchi
Tuberculous fibrosis of lung
Tuberculous pneumonia
Tuberculous pneumothorax

A15.4 **Tuberculosis of intrathoracic lymph nodes**
Tuberculosis of hilar lymph nodes
Tuberculosis of mediastinal lymph nodes
Tuberculosis of tracheobronchial lymph nodes
Excludes1 tuberculosis specified as primary (A15.7)

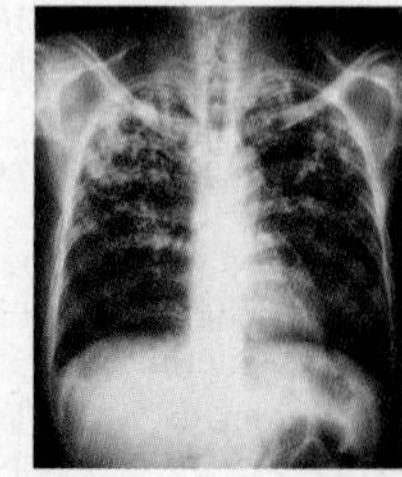

Figure 1-2 Far advanced bilateral pulmonary tuberculosis before and after 8 months of treatment with streptomycin, PAS, and isoniazid. (Getty Image)

A15.5 **Tuberculosis of larynx, trachea and bronchus**
Tuberculosis of bronchus
Tuberculosis of glottis
Tuberculosis of larynx
Tuberculosis of trachea

A15.6 **Tuberculous pleurisy**
Tuberculosis of pleura
Tuberculous empyema
Excludes1 primary respiratory tuberculosis (A15.7)

A15.7 **Primary respiratory tuberculosis** (Ex) PDX 30

A15.8 **Other respiratory tuberculosis** (Ex) PDX 31
Mediastinal tuberculosis
Nasopharyngeal tuberculosis
Tuberculosis of nose
Tuberculosis of sinus [any nasal]

A15.9 **Respiratory tuberculosis unspecified** (Ex) PDX 31

● **A17 Tuberculosis of nervous system**

A17.0 **Tuberculous meningitis** (Ex) PDX 32
Tuberculosis of meninges (cerebral) (spinal)
Tuberculous leptomeningitis
Excludes1 tuberculous meningoencephalitis (A17.82)

A17.1 **Meningeal tuberculoma** (Ex) PDX 32
Tuberculoma of meninges (cerebral) (spinal)
Excludes2 tuberculoma of brain and spinal cord (A17.81)

● A17.8 **Other tuberculosis of nervous system**

A17.81 **Tuberculoma of brain and spinal cord** (Ex) PDX 33
Tuberculous abscess of brain and spinal cord

A17.82 **Tuberculous meningoencephalitis** (Ex) PDX 33
Inflammation of brain and meninges; AKA cerebromeningitis and encephalomeningitis
Tuberculous myelitis

A17.83 **Tuberculous neuritis** (Ex) PDX 34
Tuberculous mononeuropathy

A17.89 **Other tuberculosis of nervous system** (Ex) PDX 35
Tuberculous polyneuropathy

A17.9 **Tuberculosis of nervous system, unspecified** (Ex) PDX 36

Item 1-3 Tuberculosis is a common and deadly infectious disease caused by the *Mycobacterium tuberculosis* organism. The first tuberculosis infection is called the **primary infection** and most commonly attacks the lungs but can affect the central nervous system, lymphatic system, circulatory system, genitourinary system, bones, joints, and even the skin. A **Ghon** lesion is the **initial lesion.** A **secondary lesion** occurs when the tubercle bacilli are carried to other areas.

Item 1-4 Although it primarily affects the lungs, the bacteria ***Mycobacterium tuberculosis*** can travel from the pulmonary circulation to virtually any organ in the body, much as a cancer metastasizes to a secondary site. If the immune system becomes compromised by age or disease, what would otherwise be a self-limiting primary tuberculosis in the lungs will develop in other organs. These are known as extrapulmonary sites.

CHAPTER 1 (A00-B99)

● A18 Tuberculosis of other organs

● A18.0 Tuberculosis of bones and joints

A18.01 Tuberculosis of spine (Ex) PDX 37
Pott's disease or curvature of spine
Tuberculous arthritis
Tuberculous osteomyelitis of spine
Tuberculous spondylitis

A18.02 Tuberculous arthritis of other joints (Ex) PDX 38
Tuberculosis of hip (joint)
Tuberculosis of knee (joint)

A18.03 Tuberculosis of other bones (Ex) PDX 39
Tuberculous mastoiditis
Tuberculous osteomyelitis

A18.09 Other musculoskeletal tuberculosis (Ex) PDX 40
Tuberculous myositis
Tuberculous synovitis
Tuberculous tenosynovitis

● A18.1 Tuberculosis of genitourinary system

A18.10 Tuberculosis of genitourinary system, unspecified (Ex) PDX 41

A18.11 Tuberculosis of kidney and ureter (Ex) PDX 42

A18.12 Tuberculosis of bladder (Ex) PDX 42

A18.13 Tuberculosis of other urinary organs (Ex) PDX 42
Tuberculous urethritis

A18.14 Tuberculosis of prostate (Ex) PDX 43 A

A18.15 Tuberculosis of other male genital organs (Ex) PDX 43

A18.16 Tuberculosis of cervix (Ex) PDX 44

A18.17 Tuberculous female pelvic inflammatory disease (Ex) PDX 44
Tuberculous endometritis
Tuberculous oophoritis and salpingitis
Oophoritis = inflammation of ovary
Salpingitis = inflammation of fallopian tube

A18.18 Tuberculosis of other female genital organs (Ex) PDX 44
Tuberculous ulceration of vulva

A18.2 Tuberculous peripheral lymphadenopathy (Ex) PDX 45
Tuberculous adenitis

Excludes2 tuberculosis of bronchial and mediastinal lymph nodes (A15.4)
tuberculosis of mesenteric and retroperitoneal lymph nodes (A18.39)
tuberculous tracheobronchial adenopathy (A15.4)

● A18.3 Tuberculosis of intestines, peritoneum and mesenteric glands (Ex) PDX 46

A18.31 Tuberculous peritonitis
Tuberculous ascites

A18.32 Tuberculous enteritis
Tuberculosis of anus and rectum
Tuberculosis of intestine (large) (small)

A18.39 Retroperitoneal tuberculosis
Tuberculosis of mesenteric glands
Tuberculosis of retroperitoneal (lymph glands)

A18.4 Tuberculosis of skin and subcutaneous tissue (Ex) PDX 30
Erythema induratum, tuberculous
Lupus exedens
Lupus vulgaris NOS
Lupus vulgaris of eyelid
Cutaneous tuberculosis characterized by reddish brown plaque on skin surrounded by papules and nodules
Scrofuloderma
Type of cutaneous tuberculosis, with direct extension of tuberculosis into skin from underlying structures; AKA tuberculosis colliquativa
Tuberculosis of external ear

Excludes2 lupus erythematosus (L93.-)
systemic lupus erythematosus (M32.-)

● A18.5 Tuberculosis of eye (Ex) PDX 47

Excludes2 lupus vulgaris of eyelid (A18.4)

A18.50 Tuberculosis of eye, unspecified

A18.51 Tuberculous episcleritis
Inflammation of episclera and adjacent tissues

A18.52 Tuberculous keratitis
Tuberculous interstitial keratitis
Tuberculous keratoconjunctivitis (interstitial) (phlyctenular)
Inflammation of cornea and conjunctiva

A18.53 Tuberculous chorioretinitis
Inflammation of choroid and retina; retinochoroiditis

A18.54 Tuberculous iridocyclitis
Inflammation of iris and ciliary body

A18.59 Other tuberculosis of eye
Tuberculous conjunctivitis

A18.6 Tuberculosis of (inner) (middle) ear (Ex) PDX 48
Tuberculous otitis media

Excludes2 tuberculosis of external ear (A18.4)
tuberculous mastoiditis (A18.03)

A18.7 Tuberculosis of adrenal glands (Ex) PDX 49
Tuberculous Addison's disease

● A18.8 Tuberculosis of other specified organs

A18.81 Tuberculosis of thyroid gland (Ex) PDX 50

A18.82 Tuberculosis of other endocrine glands (Ex) PDX 36
Tuberculosis of pituitary gland
Tuberculosis of thymus gland

A18.83 Tuberculosis of digestive tract organs, not elsewhere classified (Ex) PDX 46

Excludes1 tuberculosis of intestine (A18.32)

A18.84 Tuberculosis of heart (Ex) PDX 36
Tuberculous cardiomyopathy
Tuberculous endocarditis
Tuberculous myocarditis
Tuberculous pericarditis

A18.85 Tuberculosis of spleen (Ex) PDX 51

A18.89 Tuberculosis of other sites (Ex) PDX 36
Tuberculosis of muscle
Tuberculous cerebral arteritis

● A19 Miliary tuberculosis (Ex) PDX 52

Includes disseminated tuberculosis
generalized tuberculosis
tuberculous polyserositis

A19.0 Acute miliary tuberculosis of a single specified site

A19.1 Acute miliary tuberculosis of multiple sites

A19.2 Acute miliary tuberculosis, unspecified

A19.8 Other miliary tuberculosis

A19.9 Miliary tuberculosis, unspecified

Item 1-5 Miliary tuberculosis can be a life-threatening condition. If a tuberculous lesion enters a blood vessel, immense dissemination of tuberculous organisms can occur if the immune system is weak. High-risk populations—children under 4 years of age, the elderly, or the immunocompromised—are particularly prone to this type of infection. The lesions will have a millet seedlike appearance on chest x-ray. Bronchial washings and biopsy may aid in diagnosis.

CERTAIN ZOONOTIC BACTERIAL DISEASES (A20-A28)

● A20 Plague
Infectious disease caused by a Yersinia pestis bacterium, transmitted by a rodent flea bite or handling of infected animal
Includes infection due to Yersinia pestis

A20.0 **Bubonic** plague (Ex) PDX 53
A20.1 **Cellulocutaneous** plague (Ex) PDX 53
Skin and subcutaneous tissue plague
A20.2 **Pneumonic** plague (Ex) PDX 54
A20.3 Plague **meningitis** (Ex) PDX 55
A20.7 **Septicemic** plague (Ex) PDX 56
A20.8 **Other** forms of plague (Ex) PDX 55
Abortive plague
Asymptomatic plague
Pestis minor
Systemic bacterial disease
A20.9 Plague, **unspecified** (Ex) PDX 57

● A21 Tularemia
Caused by Francisella tularensis bacterium found in rodents, rabbits, and hares and transmitted to humans by contact with infected animal tissues or by ticks, biting flies, or mosquitoes
Includes deer-fly fever
infection due to Francisella tularensis
rabbit fever

Coding Clinic: 2016, Q4, P25

A21.0 **Ulceroglandular** tularemia (Ex) PDX 58
Most common form of tularemia in humans is painful, swollen, erythematous papule at point of inoculation that ruptures to form shallow ulcer
A21.1 **Oculoglandular** tularemia (Ex) PDX 59
Primary site of entry is conjunctival sac, results in granulomatous corneal lesions
Ophthalmic tularemia
A21.2 **Pulmonary** tularemia (Ex) PDX 60
A21.3 **Gastrointestinal** tularemia (Ex) PDX 61
Abdominal tularemia
A21.7 **Generalized** tularemia (Ex) PDX 62
A21.8 **Other** forms of tularemia (Ex) PDX 62
A21.9 Tularemia, **unspecified** (Ex) PDX 62

● A22 Anthrax
An acute infectious disease caused by the spore-forming Bacillus anthracis; occurs in humans exposed to infected animals or tissue from infected animals
Includes infection due to Bacillus anthracis

A22.0 **Cutaneous** anthrax (Ex) PDX 63
Malignant carbuncle
Malignant pustule
A22.1 **Pulmonary** anthrax (Ex) PDX 64
Inhalation anthrax
Ragpicker's disease
Woolsorter's disease
A22.2 **Gastrointestinal** anthrax (Ex) PDX 65
A22.7 Anthrax **sepsis** (Ex) PDX 5
Infectious bacterial disease
MCC when PDx is its own MCC
A22.8 **Other** forms of anthrax (Ex) PDX 66
Anthrax meningitis
A22.9 Anthrax, **unspecified** (Ex) PDX 67

● A23 Brucellosis
Includes Malta fever
Mediterranean fever
undulant fever

A23.0 Brucellosis due to Brucella **melitensis**
Resulting in flu-like symptoms that may lead to chronic symptoms that include recurrent fevers, joint pain, and fatigue
A23.1 Brucellosis due to Brucella **abortus**
Most common cause of brucellosis in humans; AKA Bang bacillus

Item 1-6 Brucellosis: An infectious disease caused by the bacterium Brucella. Humans are infected by contact with contaminated animals or animal products. In humans brucellosis symptoms that are similar to the flu include fever, sweats, headaches, back pains, and physical weakness. Severe infections of the central nervous system or lining of the heart may occur. Brucellosis can also cause chronic symptoms that include recurrent fevers, joint pain, and fatigue.

A23.2 Brucellosis due to Brucella **suis**
Species found primarily in pigs, rabbits, and reindeer
A23.3 Brucellosis due to Brucella **canis**
Species that causes respiratory tract infection in humans
A23.8 Other brucellosis (Ex) PDX 68
A23.9 Brucellosis, **unspecified** (Ex) PDX 68

● A24 Glanders and melioidosis
Infection, usually of rodents, which spreads to other animals and humans, caused by Burkholderia pseudomallei *through break in skin contaminated with infested soil or water*

A24.0 **Glanders** (Ex) PDX 69
Infection due to Pseudomonas mallei
Malleus
A24.1 **Acute and fulminating** melioidosis (Ex) PDX 70
Melioidosis pneumonia
Melioidosis sepsis
A24.2 **Subacute and chronic** melioidosis (Ex) PDX 70
A24.3 **Other** melioidosis (Ex) PDX 70
A24.9 Melioidosis, **unspecified** (Ex) PDX 70
Infection due to Pseudomonas pseudomallei NOS
Whitmore's disease

● A25 Rat-bite fevers (Ex) PDX 71
RBF, infectious disease caused by Streptobacillus moniliformis or Spirillum minus.

A25.0 Spirillosis
Any disease condition caused by spirilla
Sodoku
A25.1 Streptobacillosis
Acute, febrile human illness caused by bacteria transmitted by rats in most cases, passed from rodent to human via rodent's urine or mucous secretions; AKA rat fever
Epidemic arthritic erythema
Haverhill fever
Streptobacillary rat-bite fever
A25.9 Rat-bite fever, **unspecified**

● A26 Erysipeloid
Infection with Erysipelothrix rhusiopathiae, *occurring often as occupational disease resulting from handling infected fish, shellfish, meat, or poultry*

A26.0 **Cutaneous** erysipeloid
Erythema migrans
A26.7 Erysipelothrix **sepsis** (Ex) PDX 72
MCC when PDx is its own MCC
A26.8 **Other** forms of erysipeloid
A26.9 Erysipeloid, **unspecified**

● A27 Leptospirosis
Occurs most commonly in the tropics

A27.0 Leptospirosis **icterohemorrhagica** (Ex) PDX 73
Leptospiral or spirochetal jaundice (hemorrhagic)
Weil's disease
● A27.8 Other forms of leptospirosis
A27.81 **Aseptic meningitis** in leptospirosis (Ex) PDX 74
A27.89 **Other** forms of leptospirosis (Ex) PDX 73
A27.9 Leptospirosis, **unspecified** (Ex) PDX 73

● A28 Other zoonotic bacterial diseases, not elsewhere classified

A28.0 Pasteurellosis (Ex) PDX 75
Infection of humans or other animals by species of Pasteurella
A28.1 Cat-scratch disease (Ex) PDX 76
Cat-scratch fever

A28.2 **Extraintestinal yersiniosis** (Ex) PDX 75
Infection from Yersinia enterocolitica; *AKA enteric yersiniosis, intestinal yersiniosis, Yersinia enteritis*
Excludes1 enteritis due to Yersinia enterocolitica (A04.6)
plague (A20.-)

A28.8 **Other specified zoonotic bacterial diseases, not elsewhere classified** (Ex) PDX 75

A28.9 **Zoonotic bacterial disease, unspecified** (Ex) PDX 75

OTHER BACTERIAL DISEASES (A30-A49)

● A30 Leprosy [Hansen's disease]
Chronic infectious disease attacking the skin, peripheral nerves, and mucous membranes
Includes infection due to Mycobacterium leprae
Excludes1 sequelae of leprosy (B92)

A30.0 **Indeterminate leprosy** (Ex) PDX 77
I leprosy

A30.1 **Tuberculoid leprosy** (Ex) PDX 78
TT leprosy

A30.2 **Borderline tuberculoid leprosy** (Ex) PDX 79
BT leprosy

A30.3 **Borderline leprosy** (Ex) PDX 79
BB leprosy

A30.4 **Borderline lepromatous leprosy** (Ex) PDX 79
BL leprosy

A30.5 **Lepromatous leprosy** (Ex) PDX 80
LL leprosy

A30.8 **Other forms of leprosy** (Ex) PDX 81

A30.9 **Leprosy, unspecified** (Ex) PDX 82

● A31 **Infection due to other mycobacteria** (Ex) PDX 84
Excludes2 leprosy (A30.-)
tuberculosis (A15-A19)

A31.0 **Pulmonary mycobacterial infection** (Ex) PDX 83
Infection due to Mycobacterium avium
Infection due to Mycobacterium intracellulare [Battey bacillus]
Infection due to Mycobacterium kansasii

A31.1 **Cutaneous mycobacterial infection**
Buruli ulcer
Infection due to Mycobacterium marinum
Infection due to Mycobacterium ulcerans

A31.2 **Disseminated mycobacterium avium-intracellulare complex (DMAC)**
MAC sepsis

A31.8 **Other mycobacterial infections**

A31.9 **Mycobacterial infection, unspecified**
Atypical mycobacterial infection NOS
Mycobacteriosis NOS

● A32 Listeriosis
Infection caused by Listeria monocytogenes
Includes listerial foodborne infection
Excludes1 neonatal (disseminated) listeriosis (P37.2)

A32.0 **Cutaneous listeriosis** (Ex) PDX 75

● A32.1 **Listerial meningitis and meningoencephalitis**

A32.11 **Listerial meningitis** (Ex) PDX 75

A32.12 **Listerial meningoencephalitis** (Ex) PDX 75

A32.7 **Listerial sepsis** (Ex) PDX 72
MCC when PDx is its own MCC

● A32.8 **Other forms of listeriosis** (Ex) PDX 75

A32.81 **Oculoglandular listeriosis**
Primary infection site is conjunctival sac, which if untreated may result in perforation of cornea and optic atrophy

A32.82 **Listerial endocarditis**
Exudative and proliferative inflammatory condition of endocardium caused by listeria bacteria

A32.89 **Other forms of listeriosis**
Listerial cerebral arteritis

A32.9 **Listeriosis, unspecified** (Ex) PDX 75

A33 **Tetanus neonatorum** (Ex) PDX 85 N
Neonate = newborn

A34 **Obstetrical tetanus** (Ex) PDX 86 M

A35 **Other tetanus** (Ex) PDX 87
Tetanus NOS
Excludes1 tetanus neonatorum (A33)
obstetrical tetanus (A34)

● A36 **Diphtheria** (Ex) PDX 88

A36.0 **Pharyngeal diphtheria**
Diphtheritic membranous angina
Tonsillar diphtheria

A36.1 **Nasopharyngeal diphtheria**

A36.2 **Laryngeal diphtheria**
Diphtheritic laryngotracheitis

A36.3 **Cutaneous diphtheria**
Excludes2 erythrasma (L08.1)

● A36.8 **Other diphtheria**

A36.81 **Diphtheritic cardiomyopathy** (Ex) PDX 89
Diphtheritic myocarditis

A36.82 **Diphtheritic radiculomyelitis**

A36.83 **Diphtheritic polyneuritis**

A36.84 **Diphtheritic tubulo-interstitial nephropathy**

A36.85 **Diphtheritic cystitis**

A36.86 **Diphtheritic conjunctivitis**

A36.89 **Other diphtheritic complications**
Diphtheritic peritonitis

A36.9 **Diphtheria, unspecified**

● A37 **Whooping cough**
Pertussis is a highly contagious disease caused by the bacterium Bordetella pertussis and results in a whooping sounding cough.

● A37.0 **Whooping cough due to Bordetella pertussis**

A37.00 **Whooping cough due to Bordetella pertussis without pneumonia** (Ex) PDX 90
Paroxysmal cough due to Bordetella pertussis without pneumonia

A37.01 **Whooping cough due to Bordetella pertussis with pneumonia** (Ex) PDX 91
Paroxysmal cough due to Bordetella pertussis without pneumonia
MCC when PDx is its own MCC

● A37.1 **Whooping cough due to Bordetella parapertussis**

A37.10 **Whooping cough due to Bordetella parapertussis without pneumonia** (Ex) PDX 90

A37.11 **Whooping cough due to Bordetella parapertussis with pneumonia** (Ex) PDX 91
MCC when PDx is its own MCC

● A37.8 **Whooping cough due to other Bordetella species**

A37.80 **Whooping cough due to other Bordetella species without pneumonia** (Ex) PDX 90

A37.81 **Whooping cough due to other Bordetella species with pneumonia** (Ex) PDX 91
MCC when PDx is its own MCC

Item 1-7 Diphtheria: A highly contagious bacterial disease that results in the formation of an adherent membrane in the throat that may lead to suffocation. In its most poisonous form, it attacks the heart and lungs. It is spread by direct physical contact or breathing the aerosolized secretions of infected individuals. The exact location is specified in the codes.

CHAPTER 1 (A00-B99)

● **A37.9 Whooping cough, unspecified species**

A37.90 Whooping cough, unspecified species without pneumonia (Ex:) PDX 90

A37.91 Whooping cough, unspecified species with pneumonia (Ex:) PDX 91

MCC when PDx is its own MCC

● **A38 Scarlet fever** (Ex:) PDX 92

Most commonly caused by the bacteria Streptococcus pneumoniae and Neisseria meningitides

Includes scarlatina

Excludes2 streptococcal sore throat (J02.0)

A38.0 Scarlet fever with otitis media

A38.1 Scarlet fever with myocarditis

A38.8 Scarlet fever with other complications

A38.9 Scarlet fever, uncomplicated

Scarlet fever, NOS

● **A39 Meningococcal infection**

Most commonly caused by the bacteria Streptococcus pneumoniae and Neisseria meningitides

A39.0 Meningococcal meningitis (Ex:) PDX 93

A39.1 Waterhouse-Friderichsen syndrome (Ex:) PDX 94

Fulminating complication of meningococcemia

Meningococcal hemorrhagic adrenalitis

Meningococcic adrenal syndrome

A39.2 Acute meningococcemia (Ex:) PDX 95

A39.3 Chronic meningococcemia (Ex:) PDX 95

A39.4 Meningococcemia, unspecified (Ex:) PDX 95

● **A39.5 Meningococcal heart disease**

A39.50 Meningococcal carditis, unspecified (Ex:) PDX 96

A39.51 Meningococcal endocarditis (Ex:) PDX 97

A39.52 Meningococcal myocarditis (Ex:) PDX 98

A39.53 Meningococcal pericarditis (Ex:) PDX 99

● **A39.8 Other meningococcal infections**

A39.81 Meningococcal encephalitis (Ex:) PDX 100

A39.82 Meningococcal retrobulbar neuritis (Ex:) PDX 101

Optic neuritis in portion of optic nerve posterior to eyeball; AKA postocular optic neuritis

A39.83 Meningococcal arthritis (Ex:) PDX 102

A39.84 Postmeningococcal arthritis (Ex:) PDX 102

A39.89 Other meningococcal infections (Ex:) PDX 103

Meningococcal conjunctivitis

A39.9 Meningococcal infection, unspecified (Ex:) PDX 103

Meningococcal disease NOS

● **A40 Streptococcal sepsis** (Ex:) PDX 72

Code first

, if applicable, postprocedural sepsis (T81.44-)
sepsis due to central venous catheter (T80.211-)
streptococcal sepsis during labor (O75.3)
streptococcal sepsis following abortion or ectopic or molar pregnancy (O03.37, O03.87, O04.87, O07.37, O08.82)
streptococcal sepsis following immunization (T88.0-)
streptococcal sepsis following infusion, transfusion or therapeutic injection (T80.22-, T80.29-)

Excludes1 neonatal (P36.0-P36.1)
puerperal sepsis (O85)
sepsis due to Streptococcus, group D (A41.81)

A40.0 Sepsis due to streptococcus, group A

A40.1 Sepsis due to streptococcus, group B

Coding Clinic: 2019, Q1, P14

A40.3 Sepsis due to Streptococcus pneumoniae (Ex:) PDX 104

Pneumococcal sepsis

A40.8 Other streptococcal sepsis

A40.9 Streptococcal sepsis, unspecified

● **A41 Other sepsis** (Ex:) PDX 72

Code first

, if applicable, postprocedural sepsis (T81.44-)
sepsis due to central venous catheter (T80.211-)
sepsis during labor (O75.3)
sepsis following abortion, ectopic or molar pregnancy (O03.37, O03.87, O04.87, O07.37, O08.82)
sepsis following immunization (T88.0-)
sepsis following infusion, transfusion or therapeutic injection (T80.22-, T80.29-)

Excludes1 bacteremia NOS (R78.81)
neonatal (P36.-)
puerperal sepsis (O85)
streptococcal sepsis (A40.-)

Excludes2 sepsis (due to) (in) actinomycotic (A42.7)
sepsis (due to) (in) anthrax (A22.7)
sepsis (due to) (in) candidal (B37.7)
sepsis (due to) (in) Erysipelothrix (A26.7)
sepsis (due to) (in) extraintestinal yersiniosis (A28.2)
sepsis (due to) (in) gonococcal (A54.86)
sepsis (due to) (in) herpesviral (B00.7)
sepsis (due to) (in) listerial (A32.7)
sepsis (due to) (in) melioidosis (A24.1)
sepsis (due to) (in) meningococcal (A39.2-A39.4)
sepsis (due to) (in) plague (A20.7)
sepsis (due to) (in) tularemia (A21.7)
toxic shock syndrome (A48.3)

Coding Clinic: 2022, Q1, P35; 2016, Q1, P39

● **A41.0 Sepsis due to Staphylococcus aureus**

A41.01 Sepsis due to Methicillin susceptible Staphylococcus aureus

MSSA sepsis

Staphylococcus aureus sepsis NOS

A41.02 Sepsis due to Methicillin resistant Staphylococcus aureus

A41.1 Sepsis due to other specified staphylococcus

Coagulase negative staphylococcus sepsis

Coding Clinic: 2024, Q1, P19

A41.2 Sepsis due to unspecified staphylococcus

A41.3 Sepsis due to Hemophilus influenzae

A41.4 Sepsis due to anaerobes

Excludes1 gas gangrene (A48.0)

● **A41.5 Sepsis due to other Gram-negative organisms**

A41.50 Gram-negative sepsis, unspecified

Gram-negative sepsis NOS

A41.51 Sepsis due to Escherichia coli [E. coli]

Coding Clinic: 2018, Q1, P16

A41.52 Sepsis due to Pseudomonas

Pseudomonas aeruginosa

A41.53 Sepsis due to Serratia

A41.54 Sepsis due to Acinetobacter baumannii (Ex:) PDX 105

A41.59 Other Gram-negative sepsis

Coding Clinic: 2019, Q1, P13

● **A41.8 Other specified sepsis**

A41.81 Sepsis due to Enterococcus

A41.89 Other specified sepsis

Coding Clinic: 2021, Q1, P33; 2016, Q3, P8-14

A41.9 Sepsis, unspecified organism

Septicemia NOS

Coding Clinic: 2022, Q2, P5; Q1, P30; 2018, Q4, P18

● **A42 Actinomycosis**

Excludes1 actinomycetoma (B47.1)

A42.0 Pulmonary actinomycosis (Ex:) PDX 106

A42.1 Abdominal actinomycosis (Ex:) PDX 107

A42.2 Cervicofacial actinomycosis (Ex:) PDX 108

A42.7 Actinomycotic sepsis (Ex:) PDX 72

● A42.8 Other forms of actinomycosis (Ex) PDX 109
 A42.81 Actinomycotic meningitis
 A42.82 Actinomycotic encephalitis
 A42.89 Other forms of actinomycosis
A42.9 Actinomycosis, unspecified (Ex) PDX 109

● A43 Nocardiosis
A43.0 Pulmonary nocardiosis (Ex) PDX 106
A43.1 Cutaneous nocardiosis (Ex) PDX 110
A43.8 Other forms of nocardiosis (Ex) PDX 109
A43.9 Nocardiosis, unspecified (Ex) PDX 109

● A44 Bartonellosis (Ex) PDX 111
A44.0 Systemic bartonellosis
 Oroya fever
A44.1 Cutaneous and mucocutaneous bartonellosis
 Verruga peruana
A44.8 Other forms of bartonellosis
A44.9 Bartonellosis, unspecified

A46 Erysipelas
Excludes1 postpartum or puerperal erysipelas (O86.89)

● A48 Other bacterial diseases, not elsewhere classified
Excludes1 actinomycetoma (B47.1)
A48.0 Gas gangrene (Ex) PDX 112
 Clostridial cellulitis
 Clostridial myonecrosis
 Coding Clinic: 2017, Q4, P102
A48.1 Legionnaires' disease (Ex) PDX 113
A48.2 Nonpneumonic Legionnaires' disease [Pontiac fever]
A48.3 Toxic shock syndrome (Ex) PDX 114
 Use additional code to identify the organism (B95, B96)
 Excludes1 endotoxic shock NOS (R57.8)
 sepsis NOS (A41.9)
 Coding Clinic: 2022, Q1, P35
A48.4 Brazilian purpuric fever
 Systemic Hemophilus aegyptius infection
● A48.5 Other specified botulism (Ex) PDX 18
 Non-foodborne intoxication due to toxins of Clostridium botulinum [C. botulinum]
 Excludes1 food poisoning due to toxins of Clostridium botulinum (A05.1)
 A48.51 Infant botulism P
 A48.52 Wound botulism
 Non-foodborne botulism NOS
 Use additional code for associated wound
A48.8 Other specified bacterial diseases

● A49 Bacterial infection of unspecified site
Excludes1 bacterial agents as the cause of diseases classified elsewhere (B95-B96)
chlamydial infection NOS (A74.9)
meningococcal infection NOS (A39.9)
rickettsial infection NOS (A79.9)
spirochetal infection NOS (A69.9)

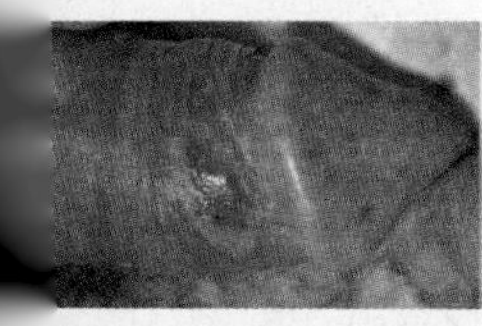

Figure 1-3 Chancre of primary syphilis. (From James WD, Berger TG, Elston DM: Andrews' Diseases of the Skin: Clinical Dermatology, Philadelphia, Saunders Elsevier, 2006)

Item 1-8 Gas gangrene is a necrotizing subcutaneous infection that will cause tissue death. Patients with poor circulation (e.g., diabetes, peripheral nephropathy) will have low oxygen content in their tissues (hypoxia), which allows the Clostridium bacteria to flourish. Gas gangrene often occurs at the site of a surgical wound or trauma. Onset is sudden and dramatic. Treatment can include debridement, amputation, and/or hyperbaric oxygen treatments.

Item 1-9 Syphilis, also known as lues, is the most serious of the venereal diseases caused by *Treponema pallidum*. The **primary** stage is characterized by an ulceration known as **chancre,** which usually appears on the genitals but can also develop on the anus, lips, tonsils, breasts, or fingers. Syphilis is easy to cure in its early stages. A single intramuscular injection of penicillin will usually cure a person who has had syphilis for less than a year.

The **secondary** stage is characterized by a rash that can affect any area of the body. **Latent** syphilis is divided into **early,** which is diagnosed within two years of infection, and **late,** which is diagnosed two years or more after infection. Additional doses of penicillin or another antibiotic are needed to treat someone who has had syphilis for longer than a year. For those allergic to penicillin, there are other antibiotic treatments. **Congenital** syphilis is also labeled **early** or **late** based on the time of diagnosis.

● A49.0 Staphylococcal infection, unspecified site
 A49.01 Methicillin susceptible Staphylococcus aureus infection, unspecified site
 Methicillin susceptible Staphylococcus aureus (MSSA) infection
 Staphylococcus aureus infection NOS
 A49.02 Methicillin resistant Staphylococcus aureus infection, unspecified site
 Methicillin resistant Staphylococcus aureus (MRSA) infection
A49.1 Streptococcal infection, unspecified site
A49.2 Hemophilus influenzae infection, unspecified site
 Any of seven bacterium of genus Haemophilus
A49.3 Mycoplasma infection, unspecified site
 Bacterium of class Mollicutes, unusual group of bacteria distinguished by absence of cell wall
A49.8 Other bacterial infections of unspecified site
A49.9 Bacterial infection, unspecified
 Excludes1 bacteremia NOS (R78.81)

INFECTIONS WITH A PREDOMINANTLY SEXUAL MODE OF TRANSMISSION (A50-A64)

Excludes1 nonspecific and nongonococcal urethritis (N34.1)
Reiter's disease (M02.3-)
Excludes2 human immunodeficiency virus [HIV] disease (B20)

● A50 Congenital syphilis
● A50.0 Early congenital syphilis, symptomatic (Ex) PDX 115
 Any congenital syphilitic condition specified as early or manifest less than two years after birth
 A50.01 Early congenital syphilitic oculopathy
 A50.02 Early congenital syphilitic osteochondropathy
 A50.03 Early congenital syphilitic pharyngitis
 Early congenital syphilitic laryngitis
 A50.04 Early congenital syphilitic pneumonia
 A50.05 Early congenital syphilitic rhinitis
 A50.06 Early cutaneous congenital syphilis
 A50.07 Early mucocutaneous congenital syphilis
 A50.08 Early visceral congenital syphilis
 A50.09 Other early congenital syphilis, symptomatic
A50.1 Early congenital syphilis, latent
 Congenital syphilis without clinical manifestations, with positive serological reaction and negative spinal fluid test, less than two years after birth
A50.2 Early congenital syphilis, unspecified (Ex) PDX 116
 Congenital syphilis NOS less than two years after birth
● A50.3 Late congenital syphilitic oculopathy (Ex) PDX 115
 Excludes1 Hutchinson's triad (A50.53)
 A50.30 Late congenital syphilitic oculopathy, unspecified
 A50.31 Late congenital syphilitic interstitial keratitis
 A50.32 Late congenital syphilitic chorioretinitis
 A50.39 Other late congenital syphilitic oculopathy

● A50.4 Late congenital neurosyphilis [juvenile neurosyphilis] (Ex) PDX 117
Use additional code to identify any associated mental disorder
Excludes1 Hutchinson's triad (A50.53)
- A50.40 Late congenital neurosyphilis, unspecified
  - Juvenile neurosyphilis NOS
- A50.41 Late congenital syphilitic meningitis (Ex) PDX 118
- A50.42 Late congenital syphilitic encephalitis
- A50.43 Late congenital syphilitic polyneuropathy
- A50.44 Late congenital syphilitic optic nerve atrophy (Ex) PDX 115
- A50.45 Juvenile general paresis
  - Dementia paralytica juvenilis
  - Juvenile taboparetic neurosyphilis
- A50.49 Other late congenital neurosyphilis
  - Juvenile tabes dorsalis

● A50.5 Other late congenital syphilis, symptomatic (Ex) PDX 115
Any congenital syphilitic condition specified as late or manifest two years or more after birth
- A50.51 Clutton's joints
- A50.52 Hutchinson's teeth
- A50.53 Hutchinson's triad
- A50.54 Late congenital cardiovascular syphilis
- A50.55 Late congenital syphilitic arthropathy
- A50.56 Late congenital syphilitic osteochondropathy
- A50.57 Syphilitic saddle nose
- A50.59 Other late congenital syphilis, symptomatic

A50.6 Late congenital syphilis, latent
Congenital syphilis without clinical manifestations, with positive serological reaction and negative spinal fluid test, two years or more after birth.

A50.7 Late congenital syphilis, unspecified
Congenital syphilis NOS two years or more after birth.

A50.9 Congenital syphilis, unspecified

● A51 Early syphilis

A51.0 Primary genital syphilis
Syphilitic chancre NOS

A51.1 Primary anal syphilis

A51.2 Primary syphilis of other sites

● A51.3 Secondary syphilis of skin and mucous membranes
- A51.31 Condyloma latum (Ex) PDX 115
- A51.32 Syphilitic alopecia (Ex) PDX 119
- A51.39 Other secondary syphilis of skin (Ex) PDX 15
  - Syphilitic leukoderma
  - Syphilitic mucous patch
  - **Excludes1** late syphilitic leukoderma (A52.79)

● A51.4 Other secondary syphilis
- A51.41 Secondary syphilitic meningitis (Ex) PDX 120
- A51.42 Secondary syphilitic female pelvic disease (Ex) PDX 116
- A51.43 Secondary syphilitic oculopathy (Ex) PDX 115
  - Secondary syphilitic chorioretinitis
  - Secondary syphilitic iridocyclitis, iritis
  - Secondary syphilitic uveitis
- A51.44 Secondary syphilitic nephritis (Ex) PDX 116
- A51.45 Secondary syphilitic hepatitis (Ex) PDX 121
- A51.46 Secondary syphilitic osteopathy (Ex) PDX 122
- A51.49 Other secondary syphilitic conditions (Ex) PDX 123
  - Secondary syphilitic lymphadenopathy
  - Secondary syphilitic myositis

A51.5 Early syphilis, latent
Syphilis (acquired) without clinical manifestations, with positive serological reaction and negative spinal fluid test, less than two years after infection.

A51.9 Early syphilis, unspecified

● A52 Late syphilis

● A52.0 Cardiovascular and cerebrovascular syphilis (Ex) PDX 117
- A52.00 Cardiovascular syphilis, unspecified
- A52.01 Syphilitic aneurysm of aorta
- A52.02 Syphilitic aortitis
- A52.03 Syphilitic endocarditis
  - Syphilitic aortic valve incompetence or stenosis
  - Syphilitic mitral valve stenosis
  - Syphilitic pulmonary valve regurgitation
- A52.04 Syphilitic cerebral arteritis
- A52.05 Other cerebrovascular syphilis
  - Syphilitic cerebral aneurysm (ruptured) (non-ruptured)
  - Syphilitic cerebral thrombosis
- A52.06 Other syphilitic heart involvement
  - Syphilitic coronary artery disease
  - Syphilitic myocarditis
  - Syphilitic pericarditis
- A52.09 Other cardiovascular syphilis

● A52.1 Symptomatic neurosyphilis (Ex) PDX 117
- A52.10 Symptomatic neurosyphilis, unspecified
- A52.11 Tabes dorsalis
  - *Cognitive decline with progressive degeneration of posterior columns, roots, and ganglia of spinal cord, occur 15-20 years after initial infection of syphilis; AKA Duchenne disease*
  - Locomotor ataxia (progressive)
  - Tabetic neurosyphilis
- A52.12 Other cerebrospinal syphilis
- A52.13 Late syphilitic meningitis (Ex) PDX 118
- A52.14 Late syphilitic encephalitis
- A52.15 Late syphilitic neuropathy
  - Late syphilitic acoustic neuritis
  - Late syphilitic optic (nerve) atrophy
  - Late syphilitic polyneuropathy
  - Late syphilitic retrobulbar neuritis
- A52.16 Charcôt's arthropathy (tabetic)
  - *Progressive musculoskeletal condition characterized by joint dislocation, fractures, and deformities, results in progressive destruction of bone and soft tissue of weight-bearing joints*
- A52.17 General paresis
  - *Chronic meningoencephalitis results in loss of cortical function, or progressive dementia and generalized paralysis, occurring 10-20 years after initial infection of syphilis; AKA Bayle disease, dementia paralytica, paralytic dementiaparetic neurosyphilis, syphilitic meningoencephalitis*
  - Dementia paralytica
- A52.19 Other symptomatic neurosyphilis
  - Syphilitic parkinsonism

A52.2 Asymptomatic neurosyphilis (Ex) PDX 117

A52.3 Neurosyphilis, unspecified (Ex) PDX 117
Gumma (syphilitic)
Destructive lesions of syphilis
Syphilis (late)
Syphiloma
Coding Clinic: 2021, Q2, P6

● A52.7 Other symptomatic late syphilis (Ex) PDX 119
- A52.71 Late syphilitic oculopathy (Ex) PDX 124
  - Late syphilitic chorioretinitis
  - Late syphilitic episcleritis
- A52.72 Syphilis of lung and bronchus
- A52.73 Symptomatic late syphilis of other respiratory organs

A52.74 **Syphilis of liver and other viscera**
Late syphilitic peritonitis

A52.75 **Syphilis of kidney and ureter**
Syphilitic glomerular disease

A52.76 **Other genitourinary symptomatic late syphilis**
Late syphilitic female pelvic inflammatory disease

A52.77 **Syphilis of bone and joint**

A52.78 **Syphilis of other musculoskeletal tissue**
Late syphilitic bursitis
Syphilis [stage unspecified] of bursa
Syphilis [stage unspecified] of muscle
Syphilis [stage unspecified] of synovium
Syphilis [stage unspecified] of tendon

A52.79 **Other symptomatic late syphilis**
Late syphilitic leukoderma
Syphilis of adrenal gland
Syphilis of pituitary gland
Syphilis of thyroid gland
Syphilitic splenomegaly
Excludes1 syphilitic leukoderma (secondary) (A51.39)

A52.8 **Late syphilis, latent**
Syphilis (acquired) without clinical manifestations, with positive serological reaction and negative spinal fluid test, two years or more after infection

A52.9 **Late syphilis, unspecified**

● A53 **Other and unspecified syphilis**

A53.Ø **Latent syphilis, unspecified as early or late**
Latent syphilis NOS
Positive serological reaction for syphilis

A53.9 **Syphilis, unspecified**
Infection due to Treponema pallidum NOS
Syphilis (acquired) NOS
Excludes1 syphilis NOS under two years of age (A5Ø.2)

● A54 **Gonococcal infection**

● A54.Ø **Gonococcal infection of lower genitourinary tract without periurethral or accessory gland abscess** (Ex) PDX 125
Excludes1 gonococcal infection with genitourinary gland abscess (A54.1)
gonococcal infection with periurethral abscess (A54.1)

A54.ØØ **Gonococcal infection of lower genitourinary tract, unspecified**

A54.Ø1 **Gonococcal cystitis and urethritis, unspecified**

A54.Ø2 **Gonococcal vulvovaginitis, unspecified**

A54.Ø3 **Gonococcal cervicitis, unspecified**

A54.Ø9 **Other gonococcal infection of lower genitourinary tract**

A54.1 **Gonococcal infection of lower genitourinary tract with periurethral and accessory gland abscess** (Ex) PDX 125
Gonococcal Bartholin's gland abscess

● A54.2 **Gonococcal pelviperitonitis and other gonococcal genitourinary infection** (Ex) PDX 125

A54.21 **Gonococcal infection of kidney and ureter**

A54.22 **Gonococcal prostatitis**

A54.23 **Gonococcal infection of other male genital organs**
Gonococcal epididymitis
Gonococcal orchitis

A54.24 **Gonococcal female pelvic inflammatory disease**
Gonococcal pelviperitonitis
Excludes1 gonococcal peritonitis (A54.85)

A54.29 **Other gonococcal genitourinary infections**

Item 1-10 An STD (sexually transmitted disease) caused by **Neisseria gonorrhoeae** that flourishes in the warm, moist areas of the reproductive tract. Untreated gonorrhea spreads to other parts of the body, causing inflammation of the testes or prostate or pelvic inflammatory disease (PID).

● A54.3 **Gonococcal infection of eye** (Ex) PDX 119

A54.3Ø **Gonococcal infection of eye, unspecified**

A54.31 **Gonococcal conjunctivitis**
Form of bacterial conjunctivitis contracted by newborns during delivery; AKA neonatal conjunctivitis
Ophthalmia neonatorum due to gonococcus

A54.32 **Gonococcal iridocyclitis**
Inflammation of iris and of ciliary body due to gonococcal infection

A54.33 **Gonococcal keratitis**
Inflammation of cornea due to gonococcal infection; AKA keratoconjunctivitis, keratopathy

A54.39 **Other gonococcal eye infection**
Gonococcal endophthalmia

● A54.4 **Gonococcal infection of musculoskeletal system** (Ex) PDX 126

A54.4Ø **Gonococcal infection of musculoskeletal system, unspecified**

A54.41 **Gonococcal spondylopathy**
Disorder of vertebrae due to gonococcal infection; AKA rachiopathy

A54.42 **Gonococcal arthritis**
Excludes2 gonococcal infection of spine (A54.41)

A54.43 **Gonococcal osteomyelitis**
Excludes2 gonococcal infection of spine (A54.41)

A54.49 **Gonococcal infection of other musculoskeletal tissue**
Gonococcal bursitis
Gonococcal myositis
Gonococcal synovitis
Gonococcal tenosynovitis

A54.5 **Gonococcal pharyngitis**

A54.6 **Gonococcal infection of anus and rectum**

● A54.8 **Other gonococcal infections**

A54.81 **Gonococcal meningitis** (Ex) PDX 120

A54.82 **Gonococcal brain abscess** (Ex) PDX 127

A54.83 **Gonococcal heart infection** (Ex) PDX 128
Gonococcal endocarditis
Gonococcal myocarditis
Gonococcal pericarditis

A54.84 **Gonococcal pneumonia** (Ex) PDX 127

A54.85 **Gonococcal peritonitis** (Ex) PDX 129
Excludes1 gonococcal pelviperitonitis (A54.24)

A54.86 **Gonococcal sepsis** (Ex) PDX 72
MCC when PDx is its own MCC

A54.89 **Other gonococcal infections** (Ex) PDX 127
Gonococcal keratoderma
Gonococcal lymphadenitis

A54.9 **Gonococcal infection, unspecified** (Ex) PDX 127

A55 **Chlamydial lymphogranuloma (venereum)**
Climatic or tropical bubo
Durand-Nicolas-Favre disease
Esthiomene
Lymphogranuloma inguinale

● A56 **Other sexually transmitted chlamydial diseases**
Includes sexually transmitted diseases due to Chlamydia trachomatis
Excludes1 neonatal chlamydial conjunctivitis (P39.1)
neonatal chlamydial pneumonia (P23.1)
Excludes2 chlamydial lymphogranuloma (A55)
conditions classified to A74.-

CHAPTER 1 (AØØ-B99)

● A56.0 **Chlamydial infection of lower genitourinary tract**

A56.00 **Chlamydial infection of lower genitourinary tract, unspecified**

A56.01 **Chlamydial cystitis and urethritis**

A56.02 **Chlamydial vulvovaginitis**

A56.09 **Other chlamydial infection of lower genitourinary tract**
Chlamydial cervicitis

● A56.1 **Chlamydial infection of pelviperitoneum and other genitourinary organs**

A56.11 **Chlamydial female pelvic inflammatory disease**

A56.19 **Other chlamydial genitourinary infection**
Chlamydial epididymitis
Chlamydial orchitis

A56.2 **Chlamydial infection of genitourinary tract, unspecified**

A56.3 **Chlamydial infection of anus and rectum**

A56.4 **Chlamydial infection of pharynx**

A56.8 **Sexually transmitted chlamydial infection of other sites**

A57 **Chancroid**
Ulcus molle
Sexually transmitted infection caused by bacteria, Haemophilus ducreyi

A58 **Granuloma inguinale**
Chronic, progressive, ulcerative granulomatous disease
Donovanosis

● A59 **Trichomoniasis**
Excludes2 intestinal trichomoniasis (AØ7.8)
A common STD caused by a parasite, Trichomonas vaginalis

● A59.0 **Urogenital trichomoniasis**

A59.00 **Urogenital trichomoniasis, unspecified**
Fluor (vaginalis) due to Trichomonas
Leukorrhea (vaginalis) due to Trichomonas

A59.01 **Trichomonal vulvovaginitis**

A59.02 **Trichomonal prostatitis**

A59.03 **Trichomonal cystitis and urethritis**

A59.09 **Other urogenital trichomoniasis**
Common sexually transmitted disease (STD) caused by single-celled protozoan parasite; AKA trich
Trichomonas cervicitis

A59.8 **Trichomoniasis of other sites**

A59.9 **Trichomoniasis, unspecified**

● A60 **Anogenital herpesviral [herpes simplex] infections**

● A60.0 **Herpesviral infection of genitalia and urogenital tract**

A60.00 **Herpesviral infection of urogenital system, unspecified**

A60.01 **Herpesviral infection of penis**

A60.02 **Herpesviral infection of other male genital organs**

A60.03 **Herpesviral cervicitis**

A60.04 **Herpesviral vulvovaginitis**
Herpesviral [herpes simplex] ulceration
Herpesviral [herpes simplex] vaginitis
Herpesviral [herpes simplex] vulvitis

A60.09 **Herpesviral infection of other urogenital tract**
Coding Clinic: 2020, Q1, P20

A60.1 **Herpesviral infection of perianal skin and rectum**

A60.9 **Anogenital herpesviral infection, unspecified**

● A63 **Other predominantly sexually transmitted diseases, not elsewhere classified**
Excludes2 molluscum contagiosum (BØ8.1)
papilloma of cervix (D26.Ø)

A63.0 **Anogenital (venereal) warts**
Anogenital warts due to (human) papillomavirus [HPV]
Condyloma acuminatum

A63.8 **Other specified predominantly sexually transmitted diseases**

A64 **Unspecified sexually transmitted disease**

OTHER SPIROCHETAL DISEASES (A65-A69)

Excludes2 leptospirosis (A27.-)
syphilis (A5Ø-A53)

A65 **Nonvenereal syphilis**
Bejel
Endemic syphilis
Njovera

● A66 **Yaws**
Endemic, infectious, tropical disease caused by spirochete, spread by direct contact; AKA frambesia, framboesia, frambesia tropica
Includes bouba
frambesia (tropica)
pian

A66.0 **Initial lesions of yaws**
Chancre of yaws
Frambesia, initial or primary
Initial frambesial ulcer
Mother yaw

A66.1 **Multiple papillomata and wet crab yaws**
Frambesioma
Pianoma
Plantar or palmar papilloma of yaws

A66.2 **Other early skin lesions of yaws**
Cutaneous yaws, less than five years after infection
Early yaws (cutaneous)(macular)(maculopapular)(micropapular)(papular)
Frambeside of early yaws

A66.3 **Hyperkeratosis of yaws**
Hypertrophy of stratum corneum of skin in which there are small, hard, verrucous scales
Ghoul hand
Hyperkeratosis, palmar or plantar (early) (late) due to yaws
Worm-eaten soles

A66.4 **Gummata and ulcers of yaws**
Small, rubbery granuloma with necrotic center and inflamed characteristic of advanced stage of syphilis; AKA syphiloma
Gummatous frambeside
Nodular late yaws (ulcerated)

A66.5 **Gangosa**
Manifestation of yaws that develops in the soft palate and spreads eroding bone, cartilage, and soft tissue
Rhinopharyngitis mutilans

A66.6 **Bone and joint lesions of yaws**
Yaws ganglion
Yaws goundou
Yaws gumma, bone
Yaws gummatous osteitis or periostitis
Yaws hydrarthrosis
Yaws osteitis
Yaws periostitis (hypertrophic)

A66.7 **Other manifestations of yaws**
Juxta-articular nodules of yaws
Mucosal yaws

A66.8 **Latent yaws**
Yaws without clinical manifestations, with positive serology

A66.9 **Yaws, unspecified**

CHAPTER 1 (AØØ-B99)

Item 1-11 Cancrum oris, also known as **noma** or **gangrenous stomatitis,** begins as an ulcer of the gingiva and results in a progressive gangrenous process.

● **A67 Pinta [carate]**
Group of nonvenereal diseases caused by Treponema species
A67.0 Primary lesions of pinta
Chancre (primary) of pinta
Papule (primary) of pinta
A67.1 Intermediate lesions of pinta
Erythematous plaques of pinta
Hyperchromic lesions of pinta
Hyperkeratosis of pinta
Pintids
A67.2 Late lesions of pinta
Achromic skin lesions of pinta
Cicatricial skin lesions of pinta
Dyschromic skin lesions of pinta
A67.3 Mixed lesions of pinta
Achromic with hyperchromic skin lesions of pinta [carate]
A67.9 Pinta, unspecified

● **A68 Relapsing fevers** (Ex) PDX 111
Includes recurrent fever
Excludes2 Lyme disease (A69.2-)
A68.0 Louse-borne relapsing fever
Relapsing fever due to Borrelia recurrentis
A68.1 Tick-borne relapsing fever
Relapsing fever due to any Borrelia species other than Borrelia recurrentis
A68.9 Relapsing fever, unspecified

● **A69 Other spirochetal infections**
A69.0 Necrotizing ulcerative stomatitis
Cancrum oris
Fusospirochetal gangrene
Noma
Stomatitis gangrenosa
A69.1 Other Vincent's infections (Ex) PDX 130
Fusospirochetal pharyngitis
Necrotizing ulcerative (acute) gingivitis
Necrotizing ulcerative (acute) gingivostomatitis
Spirochetal stomatitis
Trench mouth
Vincent's angina
Vincent's gingivitis
● **A69.2 Lyme disease** (Ex) PDX 111
Erythema chronicum migrans due to Borrelia burgdorferi
A69.20 Lyme disease, unspecified
Coding Clinic: 2021, Q4, P5
A69.21 Meningitis due to Lyme disease
A69.22 Other neurologic disorders in Lyme disease
Cranial neuritis
Meningoencephalitis
Polyneuropathy
A69.23 Arthritis due to Lyme disease
A69.29 Other conditions associated with Lyme disease
Myopericarditis due to Lyme disease
Coding Clinic: 2016, Q3, P12
A69.8 Other specified spirochetal infections
A69.9 Spirochetal infection, unspecified

OTHER DISEASES CAUSED BY CHLAMYDIAE (A70-A74)

Excludes1 sexually transmitted chlamydial diseases (A55-A56)

A70 Chlamydia psittaci infections (Ex) PDX 131
Ornithosis
Parrot fever
Psittacosis

Item 1-12 Rickettsioses are diseases spread from ticks, lice, fleas, or mites to humans.
Typhus is spread to humans chiefly by the fleas of rats.
Endemic identifies a disease as being present in low numbers of humans at all times, whereas **epidemic** identifies a disease as being present in high numbers of humans at a specific time. Morbidity (death) is higher in epidemic diseases.
Brill's disease, also known as **Brill-Zinsser disease,** is spread from human to human by body lice and also from the lice of flying squirrels. **Scrub typhus** is spread in the same ways as Brill's disease.
Malaria is spread to humans by mosquitoes.

● **A71 Trachoma**
Excludes1 sequelae of trachoma (B94.0)
A71.0 Initial stage of trachoma
Trachoma dubium
A71.1 Active stage of trachoma
Granular conjunctivitis (trachomatous)
Trachomatous follicular conjunctivitis
Trachomatous pannus
A71.9 Trachoma, unspecified

● **A74 Other diseases caused by chlamydiae**
Excludes1 neonatal chlamydial conjunctivitis (P39.1)
neonatal chlamydial pneumonia (P23.1)
Reiter's disease (M02.3-)
sexually transmitted chlamydial diseases (A55-A56)
Excludes2 chlamydial pneumonia (J16.0)
A74.0 Chlamydial conjunctivitis
Paratrachoma
● **A74.8 Other chlamydial diseases**
A74.81 Chlamydial peritonitis
A74.89 Other chlamydial diseases
A74.9 Chlamydial infection, unspecified
Chlamydiosis NOS

RICKETTSIOSES (A75-A79)

● **A75 Typhus fever** (Ex) PDX 111
Excludes1 rickettsiosis due to Ehrlichia sennetsu (A79.81)
A75.0 Epidemic louse-borne typhus fever due to Rickettsia prowazekii
Organisms transmitted between humans via louse
Classical typhus (fever)
Epidemic (louse-borne) typhus
A75.1 Recrudescent typhus [Brill's disease]
Brill-Zinsser disease
A75.2 Typhus fever due to Rickettsia typhi
Murine (flea-borne) typhus
A75.3 Typhus fever due to Rickettsia tsutsugamushi
Scrub (mite-borne) typhus
Tsutsugamushi fever
Typhus fever due to Orientia Tsutsugamushi (scrub typhus)
A75.9 Typhus fever, unspecified (Ex) PDX 132
Typhus (fever) NOS

● **A77 Spotted fever [tick-borne rickettsioses]** (Ex) PDX 111
A77.0 Spotted fever due to Rickettsia rickettsii
Rocky Mountain spotted fever
Sao Paulo fever
A77.1 Spotted fever due to Rickettsia conorii
African tick typhus
Boutonneuse fever
India tick typhus
Kenya tick typhus
Marseilles fever
Mediterranean tick fever
A77.2 Spotted fever due to Rickettsia siberica
North Asian tick fever
Siberian tick typhus
A77.3 Spotted fever due to Rickettsia australis
Queensland tick typhus

● A77.4 **Ehrlichiosis** (Ex:) PDX 133
Type of tick-borne fever caused by bacteria infection
Excludes1 anaplasmosis [A. phagocytophilum] (A79.82)
rickettsiosis due to Ehrlichia sennetsu (A79.81)
Coding Clinic: 2021, Q4, P5

A77.40 **Ehrlichiosis, unspecified**
Coding Clinic: 2021, Q4, P5

A77.41 **Ehrlichiosis chaffeensis [E. chaffeensis]**

A77.49 **Other ehrlichiosis**
Ehrlichiosis due to E. ewingii
Ehrlichiosis due to E. muris euclairensis

A77.8 **Other spotted fevers** (Ex:) PDX 111
Rickettsia 364D/R. philipii (Pacific Coast tick fever)
Spotted fever due to Rickettsia africae (African tick bite fever)
Spotted fever due to Rickettsia parkeri]

A77.9 **Spotted fever, unspecified** (Ex:) PDX 111
Tick-borne typhus NOS

A78 **Q fever** (Ex:) PDX 111
Infection due to Coxiella burnetii
Nine Mile fever
Quadrilateral fever

● A79 **Other rickettsioses**

A79.0 **Trench fever** (Ex:) PDX 111
Quintan fever
Wolhynian fever

A79.1 **Rickettsialpox due to Rickettsia akari** (Ex:) PDX 134
Kew Garden fever
Vesicular rickettsiosis

● A79.8 **Other specified rickettsioses**

A79.81 **Rickettsiosis due to Ehrlichia sennetsu** (Ex:) PDX 135
Rickettsiosis due to Neorickettsia sennetsu

A79.82 **Anaplasmosis [A. phagocytophilum]** (Ex:) PDX 136
Transfusion transmitted A. phagocytophilum
Coding Clinic: 2021, Q4, P5

A79.89 **Other specified rickettsioses** (Ex:) PDX 134

A79.9 **Rickettsiosis, unspecified** (Ex:) PDX 134
Rickettsial infection NOS

VIRAL AND PRION INFECTIONS OF THE CENTRAL NERVOUS SYSTEM (A80-A89)

Excludes1 postpolio syndrome (G14)
sequelae of poliomyelitis (B91)
sequelae of viral encephalitis (B94.1)

● A80 **Acute poliomyelitis** (Ex:) PDX 137
Excludes1 acute flaccid myelitis (G04.82)

A80.0 **Acute paralytic poliomyelitis, vaccine-associated**

A80.1 **Acute paralytic poliomyelitis, wild virus, imported**

A80.2 **Acute paralytic poliomyelitis, wild virus, indigenous**

● A80.3 **Acute paralytic poliomyelitis, other and unspecified**

A80.30 **Acute paralytic poliomyelitis, unspecified**

A80.39 **Other acute paralytic poliomyelitis**

A80.4 **Acute nonparalytic poliomyelitis**

A80.9 **Acute poliomyelitis, unspecified**

● A81 **Atypical virus infections of central nervous system**
Includes diseases of the central nervous system caused by prions
Use additional, if applicable, code to identify:
dementia with anxiety (F02.84, F02.A4, F02.B4, F02.C4)
dementia with behavioral disturbance (F02.81-, F02.A1-, F02.B1-, F02.C1-)
dementia with mood disturbance (F02.83, F02.A3, F02.B3, F02.C3)
dementia with psychotic disturbance (F02.82, F02.A2, F02.B2, F02.C2)
dementia without behavioral disturbance (F02.80, F02.A0, F02.B0, F02.C0)
mild neurocognitive disorder due to known physiological condition (F06.7-)

Item 1-13 Acute Poliomyelitis: Also called infantile paralysis and is caused by the poliovirus, which enters the body orally and infects the intestinal wall and then enters the blood stream and central nervous system, causing muscle weakness and paralysis. This disease has been nearly eradicated with the polio vaccine.

● A81.0 **Creutzfeldt-Jakob disease** (Ex:) PDX 138

A81.00 **Creutzfeldt-Jakob disease, unspecified**
Jakob-Creutzfeldt disease, unspecified

A81.01 **Variant Creutzfeldt-Jakob disease**
vCJD

A81.09 **Other Creutzfeldt-Jakob disease**
CJD
Familial Creutzfeldt-Jakob disease
Iatrogenic Creutzfeldt-Jakob disease
Sporadic Creutzfeldt-Jakob disease
Subacute spongiform encephalopathy (with dementia)

A81.1 **Subacute sclerosing panencephalitis** (Ex:) PDX 139
Type of viral encephalitis that causes parenchymatous lesions in gray and white matter of brain
Dawson's inclusion body encephalitis
Van Bogaert's sclerosing leukoencephalopathy

A81.2 **Progressive multifocal leukoencephalopathy** (Ex:) PDX 140
Group of diseases affecting white matter of brain
Multifocal leukoencephalopathy NOS

● A81.8 **Other atypical virus infections of central nervous system** (Ex:) PDX 142

A81.81 **Kuru** (Ex:) PDX 141

A81.82 **Gerstmann-Sträussler-Scheinker syndrome**
GSS syndrome

A81.83 **Fatal familial insomnia**
FFI

A81.89 **Other atypical virus infections of central nervous system**

A81.9 **Atypical virus infection of central nervous system, unspecified** (Ex:) PDX 141
Prion diseases of the central nervous system NOS

● A82 **Rabies** (Ex:) PDX 143
Viral disease affecting the central nervous system and transmitted from infected mammals to man

A82.0 **Sylvatic rabies**

A82.1 **Urban rabies**

A82.9 **Rabies, unspecified**

● A83 **Mosquito-borne viral encephalitis** (Ex:) PDX 144
Inflammation of the brain caused most commonly by Herpes Simplex virus
Includes mosquito-borne viral meningoencephalitis
Excludes2 Venezuelan equine encephalitis (A92.2)
West Nile fever (A92.3-)
West Nile virus (A92.3-)

A83.0 **Japanese encephalitis**

A83.1 **Western equine encephalitis**

A83.2 **Eastern equine encephalitis**

A83.3 **St. Louis encephalitis**

A83.4 **Australian encephalitis**
Kunjin virus disease

A83.5 **California encephalitis**
California meningoencephalitis
La Crosse encephalitis

A83.6 **Rocio virus disease**
Mosquito-borne virus

A83.8 **Other mosquito-borne viral encephalitis**

A83.9 **Mosquito-borne viral encephalitis, unspecified**

Item 1-14 Encephalitis is an inflammation of the brain most often caused by a virus but may also be caused by a bacteria and most commonly transmitted by a mosquito. **Myelitis** is an inflammation of the spinal cord that may disrupt CNS function. Untreated myelitis may rapidly lead to permanent damage to the spinal cord. **Encephalomyelitis** is a general term for an inflammation of the brain and spinal cord.

● **A84 Tick-borne viral encephalitis** (Ex) PDX 144
 Includes tick-borne viral meningoencephalitis
 A84.0 Far Eastern tick-borne encephalitis [Russian spring-summer encephalitis]
 A84.1 Central European tick-borne encephalitis
 A84.8 Other tick-borne viral encephalitis
  A84.81 Powassan virus disease (Ex) PDX 145
  A84.89 Other tick-borne viral encephalitis (Ex) PDX 146
   Louping ill
   Code first, if applicable, transfusion related infection (T80.22-)
 A84.9 Tick-borne viral encephalitis, unspecified

● **A85 Other viral encephalitis, not elsewhere classified** (Ex) PDX 147
 Includes specified viral encephalomyelitis NEC
  specified viral meningoencephalitis NEC
 Excludes1 encephalitis due to cytomegalovirus (B25.8)
  encephalitis due to herpesvirus NEC (B10.0-)
  encephalitis due to herpesvirus [herpes simplex] (B00.4)
  encephalitis due to measles virus (B05.0)
  encephalitis due to mumps virus (B26.2)
  encephalitis due to poliomyelitis virus (A80.-)
  encephalitis due to zoster (B02.0)
  lymphocytic choriomeningitis (A87.2)
  myalgic encephalomyelitis (G93.32)
 A85.0 Enteroviral encephalitis
  Enteroviral encephalomyelitis
 A85.1 Adenoviral encephalitis
  Adenoviral meningoencephalitis
 A85.2 Arthropod-borne viral encephalitis, unspecified (Ex) PDX 144
  Excludes1 West nile virus with encephalitis (A92.31)
 A85.8 Other specified viral encephalitis
  Encephalitis lethargica
  Von Economo-Cruchet disease

A86 Unspecified viral encephalitis (Ex) PDX 148
 Viral encephalomyelitis NOS
 Viral meningoencephalitis NOS

● **A87 Viral meningitis** (Ex) PDX 149
 Excludes1 meningitis due to herpesvirus [herpes simplex] (B00.3)
  meningitis due to measles virus (B05.1)
  meningitis due to mumps virus (B26.1)
  meningitis due to poliomyelitis virus (A80.-)
  meningitis due to zoster (B02.1)
 A87.0 Enteroviral meningitis
  Group of common viruses responsible for the majority of viral meningitis
  Coxsackievirus meningitis
  Echovirus meningitis
 A87.1 Adenoviral meningitis
 A87.2 Lymphocytic choriomeningitis (Ex) PDX 150
  Lymphocytic meningoencephalitis
 A87.8 Other viral meningitis
 A87.9 Viral meningitis, unspecified

● **A88 Other viral infections of central nervous system, not elsewhere classified**
 Excludes1 viral encephalitis NOS (A86)
  viral meningitis NOS (A87.9)
 A88.0 Enteroviral exanthematous fever [Boston exanthem] (Ex) PDX 144
  Infectious skin eruption
 A88.1 Epidemic vertigo
 A88.8 Other specified viral infections of central nervous system (Ex) PDX 147

A89 Unspecified viral infection of central nervous system (Ex) PDX 148

OGCR Section I. C.1.f.

Certain Infectious and Parasitic Diseases (A00-B99)

Zika virus infections

Code only confirmed cases

Code only a confirmed diagnosis of Zika virus (A92.5, Zika virus disease) as documented by the provider. This is an exception to the hospital inpatient guideline Section II, H.

In this context, "confirmation" does not require documentation of the type of test performed; the physician's diagnostic statement that the condition is confirmed is sufficient. This code should be assigned regardless of the stated mode of transmission.

If the provider documents "suspected", "possible" or "probable" Zika, do not assign code A92.5. Assign a code(s) explaining the reason for encounter (such as fever, rash, or joint pain) or Z20.828, Contact with and (suspected) exposure to other viral communicable diseases.

ARTHROPOD-BORNE VIRAL FEVERS AND VIRAL HEMORRHAGIC FEVERS (A90-A99)

A90 Dengue fever [classical dengue] (Ex) PDX 151
 Acute, self-limited disease, characterized by fever, prostration, severe muscle pains, headache, rash, lymphadenopathy, and leukopenia, caused by dengue virus; AKA breakbone, dandy
 Excludes1 dengue hemorrhagic fever (A91)
 Coding Clinic: 2016, Q3, P13

A91 Dengue hemorrhagic fever (Ex) PDX 152
 Serious follow-up to regular dengue, with symptoms of hemorrhage

● **A92 Other mosquito-borne viral fevers**
 Excludes1 Ross River disease (B33.1)
 A92.0 Chikungunya virus disease (Ex) PDX 152
  Transmitted by mosquitoes
  Chikungunya (hemorrhagic) fever
 A92.1 O'nyong-nyong fever (Ex) PDX 153
  Acute, nonfatal febrile disease transmitted by mosquitoes, which clinically resembles dengue and chikungunya
 A92.2 Venezuelan equine fever (Ex) PDX 153
  Venezuelan equine encephalitis
  Venezuelan equine encephalomyelitis virus disease
 ● **A92.3 West Nile virus infection**
  West Nile fever
  A92.30 West Nile virus infection, unspecified (Ex) PDX 154
   West Nile fever NOS
   West Nile fever without complications
   West Nile virus NOS
  A92.31 West Nile virus infection with encephalitis (Ex) PDX 155
   West Nile encephalitis
   West Nile encephalomyelitis
   Coding Clinic: 2016, Q3, P13
  A92.32 West Nile virus infection with other neurologic manifestation (Ex) PDX 156
   Use additional code to specify the neurologic manifestation
  A92.39 West Nile virus infection with other complications (Ex) PDX 157
   Use additional code to specify the other conditions
 A92.4 Rift Valley fever (Ex) PDX 153

A92.5 **Zika virus disease** (Ex) PDX 153
Zika virus fever
Zika virus infection
Zika NOS
Excludes1 congenital Zika virus disease (P35.4)
Coding Clinic: 2016, Q4, P4-7, 121

A92.8 **Other specified mosquito-borne viral fevers** (Ex) PDX 153

A92.9 **Mosquito-borne viral fever, unspecified** (Ex) PDX 152

● A93 **Other arthropod-borne viral fevers, not elsewhere classified** (Ex) PDX 152

A93.0 **Oropouche virus disease** (Ex) PDX 153
Tropical viral infection
Oropouche fever

A93.1 **Sandfly fever**
Pappataci fever
Phlebotomus fever

A93.2 **Colorado tick fever**

A93.8 **Other specified arthropod-borne viral fevers**
Piry virus disease
Vesicular stomatitis virus disease [Indiana fever]

A94 **Unspecified arthropod-borne viral fever** (Ex) PDX 152
Arboviral fever NOS
Arbovirus infection NOS

● A95 **Yellow fever** (Ex) PDX 158
Acute infectious disease transmitted by mosquitoes

A95.0 **Sylvatic yellow fever**
Jungle yellow fever

A95.1 **Urban yellow fever**

A95.9 **Yellow fever, unspecified**

● A96 **Arenaviral hemorrhagic fever** (Ex) PDX 159
Virus that causes various hemorrhagic fevers

A96.0 **Junin hemorrhagic fever**
Argentinian hemorrhagic fever

A96.1 **Machupo hemorrhagic fever**
Transmitted by contact with infected rodents
Bolivian hemorrhagic fever

A96.2 **Lassa fever**
Acute type of hemorrhagic fever caused by contact with disease carrying mouse or person

A96.8 **Other arenaviral hemorrhagic fevers**

A96.9 **Arenaviral hemorrhagic fever, unspecified**

● A98 **Other viral hemorrhagic fevers, not elsewhere classified** (Ex) PDX 152
Excludes1 chikungunya hemorrhagic fever (A92.0)
dengue hemorrhagic fever (A91)

A98.0 **Crimean-Congo hemorrhagic fever**
Virus transmitted by ticks and contact with blood, secretions, or fluids from infected humans or animals
Central Asian hemorrhagic fever

A98.1 **Omsk hemorrhagic fever**
Transmitted to humans by bites of infected ticks or contact with infected muskrats

A98.2 **Kyasanur Forest disease**
Transmitted via infected monkeys, voles, ticks

A98.3 **Marburg virus disease**
Rare, acute, often fatal type of hemorrhagic fever

A98.4 **Ebola virus disease**

A98.5 **Hemorrhagic fever with renal syndrome** (Ex) PDX 160
Epidemic hemorrhagic fever
Korean hemorrhagic fever
Russian hemorrhagic fever
Hantaan virus disease
Hantavirus disease with renal manifestations
Nephropathia epidemica
Songo fever
Excludes1 hantavirus (cardio)-pulmonary syndrome (B33.4)

A98.8 **Other specified viral hemorrhagic fevers**

A99 **Unspecified viral hemorrhagic fever** (Ex) PDX 152

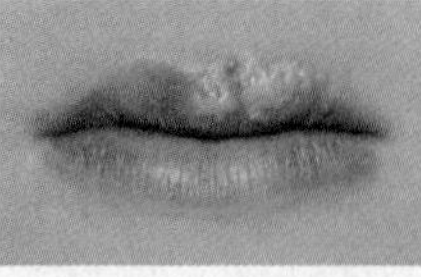

Figure 1-4 Primary herpes simplex in and around the mouth. The infection is usually acquired from siblings or parents and is readily transmitted to other direct contacts. (Getty Image)

Item 1-15 **Herpes** is a viral disease for which there is no cure. There are two types of the herpes simplex virus: **Type I** causes **cold sores** or **fever blisters,** and **Type II** causes **genital herpes.** The virus can be spread from a sore on the lips to the genitals or from the genitals to the lips.

VIRAL INFECTIONS CHARACTERIZED BY SKIN AND MUCOUS MEMBRANE LESIONS (B00-B09)

● B00 **Herpesviral [herpes simplex] infections**
Excludes1 congenital herpesviral infections (P35.2)
Excludes2 anogenital herpesviral infection (A60.-)
gammaherpesviral mononucleosis (B27.0-)
herpangina (B08.5)

B00.0 **Eczema herpeticum**
Cutaneous eruption caused by herpes simplex virus (HSV) type 1, HSV-2, coxsackievirus A16, or vaccinia virus
Kaposi's varicelliform eruption

B00.1 **Herpesviral vesicular dermatitis**
Vesicle formation; characteristics include formation of blisters and scabs on feet and legs
Herpes simplex facialis
Herpes simplex labialis
Herpes simplex otitis externa
Vesicular dermatitis of ear
Vesicular dermatitis of lip

B00.2 **Herpesviral gingivostomatitis and pharyngotonsillitis** (Ex) PDX 161
Inflammation involving both gingivae and oral mucosa
Herpesviral pharyngitis
Inflammation of pharynx and tonsils; AKA tonsillopharyngitis

B00.3 **Herpesviral meningitis** (Ex) PDX 162

B00.4 **Herpesviral encephalitis** (Ex) PDX 163
Herpesviral meningoencephalitis
Simian B disease
Excludes1 herpesviral encephalitis due to herpesvirus 6 and 7 (B10.01, B10.09)
non-simplex herpesviral encephalitis (B10.0-)

● B00.5 **Herpesviral ocular disease** (Ex) PDX 164

B00.50 **Herpesviral ocular disease, unspecified**

B00.51 **Herpesviral iridocyclitis**
Herpesviral iritis
Herpesviral uveitis, anterior

B00.52 **Herpesviral keratitis**
Herpesviral keratoconjunctivitis

B00.53 **Herpesviral conjunctivitis**

B00.59 **Other herpesviral disease of eye**
Herpesviral dermatitis of eyelid

B00.7 **Disseminated herpesviral disease** (Ex) PDX 165
Herpesviral sepsis

● B00.8 **Other forms of herpesviral infections**

B00.81 **Herpesviral hepatitis** (Ex) PDX 166

B00.82 **Herpes simplex myelitis** (Ex) PDX 167

B00.89 **Other herpesviral infection** (Ex) PDX 168
Herpesviral whitlow

B00.9 **Herpesviral infection, unspecified**
Herpes simplex infection NOS

● **B01 Varicella [chickenpox]**
Very contagious disease caused by the varicella zoster virus that results in an itchy outbreak of skin blisters (varicella). The same virus causes shingles (zoster).

B01.0 Varicella meningitis (Ex) PDX 169
● **B01.1** Varicella encephalitis, myelitis and encephalomyelitis
Postchickenpox encephalitis, myelitis and encephalomyelitis
B01.11 Varicella encephalitis and encephalomyelitis (Ex) PDX 170
Postchickenpox encephalitis and encephalomyelitis
B01.12 Varicella myelitis (Ex) PDX 171
Postchickenpox myelitis
B01.2 Varicella pneumonia (Ex) PDX 172
● **B01.8** Varicella with other complications (Ex) PDX 169
B01.81 Varicella keratitis
B01.89 Other varicella complications
B01.9 Varicella without complication (Ex) PDX 169
Varicella NOS

● **B02 Zoster [herpes zoster]**
Includes shingles
zona
B02.0 Zoster encephalitis (Ex) PDX 173
Zoster meningoencephalitis
B02.1 Zoster meningitis (Ex) PDX 174
● **B02.2** Zoster with other nervous system involvement (Ex) PDX 173
Coding Clinic: 2019, Q1, P18
B02.21 Postherpetic geniculate ganglionitis
B02.22 Postherpetic trigeminal neuralgia
B02.23 Postherpetic polyneuropathy
B02.24 Postherpetic myelitis (Ex) PDX 175
Herpes zoster myelitis
B02.29 Other postherpetic nervous system involvement
Postherpetic radiculopathy
● **B02.3** Zoster ocular disease (Ex) PDX 176
B02.30 Zoster ocular disease, unspecified
B02.31 Zoster conjunctivitis
B02.32 Zoster iridocyclitis
B02.33 Zoster keratitis
Herpes zoster keratoconjunctivitis
B02.34 Zoster scleritis
B02.39 Other herpes zoster eye disease
Zoster blepharitis
B02.7 Disseminated zoster (Ex) PDX 177
B02.8 Zoster with other complications (Ex) PDX 177
Herpes zoster otitis externa
B02.9 Zoster without complications
Zoster NOS

B03 Smallpox (Ex) PDX 178
Note: In 1980 the 33rd World Health Assembly declared that smallpox had been eradicated. The classification is maintained for surveillance purposes.

B04 Monkeypox (Ex) PDX 179
▶**Mpox**
Disease occurring in captive monkeys and other mammals that may be transmitted to humans, clinically similar to smallpox
Coding Clinic: 2022, Q3, P3

Item 1-16 Zoster: Also known as ***shingles*** and is caused by the same virus as chickenpox. After exposure, the virus lies dormant in nerve tissue and is activated by factors including aging, stress, suppression of the immune system, and certain medication. It begins as a unilateral rash that leads to blisters and sores on the skin. It may involve the nerve pathways of the eye, forehead, nose, and eyelids and may be very painful with long-term systemic effects.

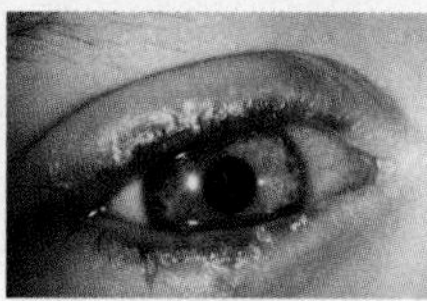

Figure 1-5 Photograph of eyelids with marginal blepharitis. (From Hoyt CS, Taylor D: Pediatric Ophthalmology and Strabismus, London, Elsevier Saunders, 2005)

Item 1-17 Blepharitis is a common condition in which the eyelid is swollen and yellow scaling and conjunctivitis develop. Usually the hair on the scalp and brow is involved.

● **B05 Measles**
Includes morbilli
Excludes1 subacute sclerosing panencephalitis (A81.1)
B05.0 Measles complicated by encephalitis (Ex) PDX 180
Postmeasles encephalitis
B05.1 Measles complicated by meningitis (Ex) PDX 181
Postmeasles meningitis
B05.2 Measles complicated by pneumonia (Ex) PDX 182
Postmeasles pneumonia
B05.3 Measles complicated by otitis media
Postmeasles otitis media
B05.4 Measles with intestinal complications (Ex) PDX 179
● **B05.8** Measles with other complications
B05.81 Measles keratitis and keratoconjunctivitis (Ex) PDX 183
B05.89 Other measles complications (Ex) PDX 181
B05.9 Measles without complication
Measles NOS

● **B06 Rubella [German measles]** (Ex) PDX 184
Excludes1 congenital rubella (P35.0)
● **B06.0** Rubella with neurological complications
B06.00 Rubella with neurological complication, unspecified
B06.01 Rubella encephalitis
Rubella meningoencephalitis
B06.02 Rubella meningitis
B06.09 Other neurological complications of rubella
● **B06.8** Rubella with other complications
B06.81 Rubella pneumonia
B06.82 Rubella arthritis (Ex) PDX 185
B06.89 Other rubella complications
B06.9 Rubella without complication
Rubella NOS

● **B07 Viral warts**
Includes verruca simplex
verruca vulgaris
viral warts due to human papillomavirus
Excludes2 anogenital (venereal) warts (A63.0)
papilloma of bladder (D41.4)
papilloma of cervix (D26.0)
papilloma larynx (D14.1)
B07.0 Plantar wart
Verruca plantaris
B07.8 Other viral warts
Common wart
Flat wart
Verruca plana
B07.9 Viral wart, unspecified

B08 Other viral infections characterized by skin and mucous membrane lesions, not elsewhere classified
Excludes1 vesicular stomatitis virus disease (A93.8)

B08.0 Other orthopoxvirus infections
Excludes2 monkeypox (B04)

B08.01 Cowpox and vaccinia not from vaccine

B08.010 Cowpox

B08.011 Vaccinia not from vaccine
Excludes1 vaccinia (from vaccination) (generalized) (T88.1)

B08.02 Orf virus disease
Contagious pustular dermatitis
Ecthyma contagiosum

B08.03 Pseudocowpox [milker's node]

B08.04 Paravaccinia, unspecified

B08.09 Other orthopoxvirus infections
Orthopoxvirus infection NOS

B08.1 Molluscum contagiosum
Various skin diseases characterized by soft, rounded, cutaneous lesions

B08.2 Exanthema subitum [sixth disease] Roseola infantum
Acute, short-lived high fever in infants and young children followed by a rash mainly on the trunk, caused by human herpesvirus 6

B08.20 Exanthema subitum [sixth disease], unspecified Roseola infantum, unspecified P

B08.21 Exanthema subitum [sixth disease] due to human herpesvirus 6 Roseola infantum due to human herpesvirus 6 P
Virus results in sudden rash; infection results in lifelong persistence

B08.22 Exanthema subitum [sixth disease] due to human herpesvirus 7 Roseola infantum due to human herpesvirus 7 P

B08.3 Erythema infectiosum [fifth disease] PDX 186
Moderately contagious, epidemic disease in children caused by B19 virus; onset of rash that begins as redness of cheeks, later there is rash on trunk and limbs; when this fades, there may be central clearing that leaves lacelike pattern

B08.4 Enteroviral vesicular stomatitis with exanthem
Hand, foot and mouth disease
Check your documentation—this code is HAND, foot, and mouth disease. Code B08.8 is foot and mouth disease.

B08.5 Enteroviral vesicular pharyngitis
Herpangina

B08.6 Parapoxvirus infections

B08.60 Parapoxvirus infection, unspecified

B08.61 Bovine stomatitis

B08.62 Sealpox

B08.69 Other parapoxvirus infections

B08.7 Yatapoxvirus infections

B08.70 Yatapoxvirus infection, unspecified

B08.71 Tanapox virus disease PDX 179

B08.72 Yaba pox virus disease
Yaba monkey tumor disease

B08.79 Other yatapoxvirus infections

B08.8 Other specified viral infections characterized by skin and mucous membrane lesions
Enteroviral lymphonodular pharyngitis
Foot-and-mouth disease
Check your documentation. Code B08.4 is for HAND, foot, and mouth disease.
Poxvirus NEC

B09 Unspecified viral infection characterized by skin and mucous membrane lesions
Viral enanthema NOS
Viral exanthema NOS

OTHER HUMAN HERPESVIRUSES (B10)

B10 Other human herpesviruses
Excludes2 cytomegalovirus (B25.9)
Epstein-Barr virus (B27.0-)
herpes NOS (B00.9)
herpes simplex (B00.-)
herpes zoster (B02.-)
human herpesvirus NOS (B00.-)
human herpesvirus 1 and 2 (B00.-)
human herpesvirus 3 (B01.-, B02.-)
human herpesvirus 4 (B27.0-)
human herpesvirus 5 (B25.-)
varicella (B01.-)
zoster (B02.-)
Coding Clinic: 2024, Q2, P21

B10.0 Other human herpesvirus encephalitis PDX 163
Excludes2 herpes encephalitis NOS (B00.4)
herpes simplex encephalitis (B00.4)
human herpesvirus encephalitis (B00.4)
simian B herpes virus encephalitis (B00.4)

B10.01 Human herpesvirus 6 encephalitis
Sudden rash or roseola

B10.09 Other human herpesvirus encephalitis
Human herpesvirus 7 encephalitis
Virus closely related to human herpesvirus 6, but not known to cause any disease
Coding Clinic: 2024, Q2, P21

B10.8 Other human herpesvirus infection

B10.81 Human herpesvirus 6 infection
Causative agent of exanthema subitum that results in sudden rash

B10.82 Human herpesvirus 7 infection
Closely related to human herpesvirus 6, but not known cause any disease

B10.89 Other human herpesvirus infection
Human herpesvirus 8 infection
May be the cause of Kaposi sarcoma, a malignant tumor
Kaposi's sarcoma-associated herpesvirus infection

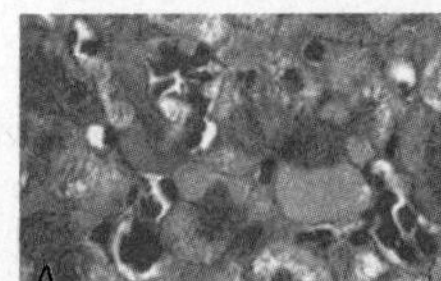

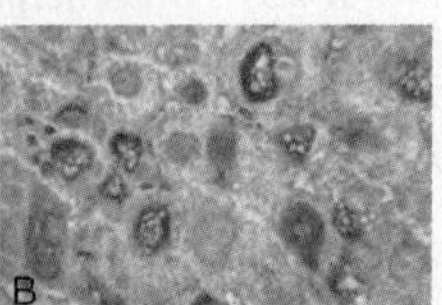

Figure 1-6 Hepatitis B viral infection. **A.** Liver parenchyma showing hepatocytes with diffuse granular cytoplasm, so-called ground glass hepatocytes (H&E). **B.** Immunoperoxidase stains from the same case, showing cytoplasmic inclusions of viral particles. (From Kumar: Robbins and Cotran: Pathologic Basis of Disease, ed 8, Saunders, An Imprint of Elsevier, 2009)

Item 1-18 Hepatitis A (HAV) was formerly called epidemic, infectious, short-incubation, or acute catarrhal jaundice hepatitis. The primary transmission mode is the oral–fecal route. **Hepatitis B (HBV)** was formerly called long-incubation period, serum, or homologous serum hepatitis. Transmission modes are through blood from infected persons and from body fluids of infected mother to neonate. **Hepatitis C (HCV),** caused by the hepatitis C virus, is primarily transfusion associated. **Hepatitis D (HDV),** also called delta hepatitis, is caused by the hepatitis D virus in patients formerly or currently infected with hepatitis B. **Hepatitis E (HEV)** is also called enterically transmitted non-A, non-B hepatitis. The primary transmission mode is the oral–fecal route, usually through contaminated water.

VIRAL HEPATITIS (B15-B19)

Excludes1 sequelae of viral hepatitis (B94.2)
Excludes2 cytomegaloviral hepatitis (B25.1)
herpesviral [herpes simplex] hepatitis (BØØ.81)

● **B15 Acute hepatitis A** Ex PDX 187
B15.Ø Hepatitis A with hepatic coma
B15.9 Hepatitis A without hepatic coma
Hepatitis A (acute) (viral) NOS

● **B16 Acute hepatitis B** Ex PDX 187
B16.Ø Acute hepatitis B with delta-agent with hepatic coma
B16.1 Acute hepatitis B with delta-agent without hepatic coma
B16.2 Acute hepatitis B without delta-agent with hepatic coma
B16.9 Acute hepatitis B without delta-agent and without hepatic coma
Hepatitis B (acute) (viral) NOS
Coding Clinic: 2016, Q3, P13

● **B17 Other acute viral hepatitis** Ex PDX 187
B17.Ø Acute delta-(super) infection of hepatitis B carrier
● **B17.1 Acute hepatitis C**
B17.1Ø Acute hepatitis C without hepatic coma
Acute hepatitis C NOS
B17.11 Acute hepatitis C with hepatic coma
B17.2 Acute hepatitis E
B17.8 Other specified acute viral hepatitis
Hepatitis non-A non-B (acute) (viral) NEC
B17.9 Acute viral hepatitis, unspecified
Acute hepatitis NOS
Acute infectious hepatitis NOS

● **B18 Chronic viral hepatitis** Ex PDX 187
Includes Carrier of viral hepatitis
B18.Ø Chronic viral hepatitis B with delta-agent
B18.1 Chronic viral hepatitis B without delta-agent
Carrier of viral hepatitis B
Chronic (viral) hepatitis B
B18.2 Chronic viral hepatitis C
Carrier of viral hepatitis C
Coding Clinic: 2018, Q1, P4; 2017, Q1, P41
B18.8 Other chronic viral hepatitis
Carrier of other viral hepatitis
B18.9 Chronic viral hepatitis, unspecified
Carrier of unspecified viral hepatitis

● **B19 Unspecified viral hepatitis** Ex PDX 187
B19.Ø Unspecified viral hepatitis with hepatic coma
● **B19.1 Unspecified viral hepatitis B**
B19.1Ø Unspecified viral hepatitis B without hepatic coma
Unspecified viral hepatitis B NOS
B19.11 Unspecified viral hepatitis B with hepatic coma
● **B19.2 Unspecified viral hepatitis C**
B19.2Ø Unspecified viral hepatitis C without hepatic coma
Viral hepatitis C NOS
B19.21 Unspecified viral hepatitis C with hepatic coma
B19.9 Unspecified viral hepatitis without hepatic coma
Viral hepatitis NOS

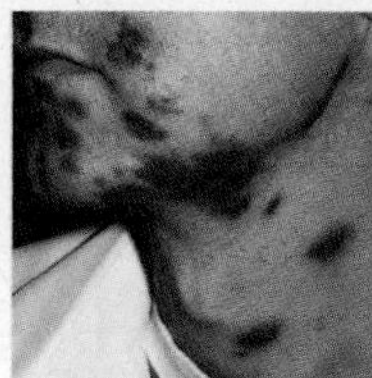

Figure 1-7 Kaposi's sarcoma. There are large confluent hyperpigmented patch-stage lesions with lymphedema. (From Kanski, JJ: Clinical Diagnosis in Ophthalmology, London, Elsevier Mosby, 2006)

Item 1-19 AIDS (acquired immune deficiency syndrome) is caused by **HIV** (human immunodeficiency virus). HIV affects certain white blood cells (T-4 lymphocytes) and destroys the ability of the cells to fight infections, making patients susceptible to a host of infectious diseases (e.g., ***Pneumocystis carinii pneumonia [PCP], Kaposi's sarcoma,*** and ***lymphoma***). ***AIDS-related complex (ARC)*** is an early stage of AIDS in which tests for HIV are positive but the symptoms are mild.

OGCR Section I. C.1.a.

Certain Infectious and Parasitic Diseases (AØØ-B99)
a. Human Immunodeficiency Virus (HIV) Infections
1) Code only confirmed cases
Code only confirmed cases of HIV infection illness. This is an exception to the hospital inpatient guideline Section II, H.
In this context, "confirmation" does not require documentation of positive serology or culture for HIV; the provider's diagnostic statement that the patient is HIV positive or has an HIV-related illness is sufficient.

HUMAN IMMUNODEFICIENCY VIRUS [HIV] DISEASE (B2Ø)

B2Ø Human immunodeficiency virus [HIV] disease Ex PDX 188
Includes acquired immune deficiency syndrome [AIDS]
AIDS-related complex [ARC]
HIV infection, symptomatic
Code first Human immunodeficiency virus [HIV] disease complicating pregnancy, childbirth and the puerperium, if applicable (O98.7-)
Use additional code(s) to identify all manifestations of HIV infection
Excludes1 asymptomatic human immunodeficiency virus [HIV] infection status (Z21)
exposure to HIV virus (Z2Ø.6)
inconclusive serologic evidence of HIV (R75)
Coding Clinic: 2022, Q1, P36; 2021, Q2, P6; 2019, Q1, P9-11

OTHER VIRAL DISEASES (B25-B34)

● **B25 Cytomegaloviral disease**
AKA: HCMV or Human Herpesvirus 5 (HHV-5)
Excludes1 congenital cytomegalovirus infection (P35.1)
cytomegaloviral mononucleosis (B27.1-)
B25.Ø Cytomegaloviral pneumonitis Ex PDX 113
MCC when PDx is its own MCC
B25.1 Cytomegaloviral hepatitis Ex PDX 189
CC when PDx is its own CC
B25.2 Cytomegaloviral pancreatitis Ex PDX 190
MCC when PDx is its own MCC
B25.8 Other cytomegaloviral diseases Ex PDX 191
Cytomegaloviral encephalitis
B25.9 Cytomegaloviral disease, unspecified Ex PDX 191

● **B26 Mumps**
Includes epidemic parotitis
infectious parotitis
Acute, contagious, viral disease
B26.Ø Mumps orchitis Ex PDX 192
B26.1 Mumps meningitis Ex PDX 193
B26.2 Mumps encephalitis Ex PDX 194
B26.3 Mumps pancreatitis Ex PDX 195

CHAPTER 1 (AØØ-B99)

- B26.8 Mumps with other complications
  - B26.81 Mumps hepatitis (Ex) PDX 196
  - B26.82 Mumps myocarditis (Ex) PDX 197
  - B26.83 Mumps nephritis (Ex) PDX 197
  - B26.84 Mumps polyneuropathy (Ex) PDX 198
  - B26.85 Mumps arthritis (Ex) PDX 197
  - B26.89 Other mumps complications (Ex) PDX 197
- B26.9 Mumps without complication
  Mumps NOS
  Mumps parotitis NOS

B27 Infectious mononucleosis

Includes glandular fever
monocytic angina
Pfeiffer's disease

- **B27.0 Gammaherpesviral mononucleosis**
  AKA: Pfeiffer's disease, infective mononucleosis
  Mononucleosis due to Epstein-Barr virus
  - B27.00 Gammaherpesviral mononucleosis without complication
    Infective mononucleosis
  - B27.01 Gammaherpesviral mononucleosis with polyneuropathy
  - B27.02 Gammaherpesviral mononucleosis with meningitis
  - B27.09 Gammaherpesviral mononucleosis with other complications
    Hepatomegaly in gammaherpesviral mononucleosis
    Coding Clinic: 2024, Q2, P21,22
- **B27.1 Cytomegaloviral mononucleosis**
  Infectious disease resembling infectious mononucleosis
  - B27.10 Cytomegaloviral mononucleosis without complications
  - B27.11 Cytomegaloviral mononucleosis with polyneuropathy
  - B27.12 Cytomegaloviral mononucleosis with meningitis
  - B27.19 Cytomegaloviral mononucleosis with other complication
    Hepatomegaly in cytomegaloviral mononucleosis
- **B27.8 Other infectious mononucleosis**
  - B27.80 Other infectious mononucleosis without complication
  - B27.81 Other infectious mononucleosis with polyneuropathy
  - B27.82 Other infectious mononucleosis with meningitis
  - B27.89 Other infectious mononucleosis with other complication
    Hepatomegaly in other infectious mononucleosis
- **B27.9 Infectious mononucleosis, unspecified**
  - B27.90 Infectious mononucleosis, unspecified without complication
  - B27.91 Infectious mononucleosis, unspecified with polyneuropathy
  - B27.92 Infectious mononucleosis, unspecified with meningitis
  - B27.99 Infectious mononucleosis, unspecified with other complication
    Hepatomegaly in unspecified infectious mononucleosis

B30 Viral conjunctivitis

Excludes1 herpesviral [herpes simplex] ocular disease (B00.5)
ocular zoster (B02.3)

- B30.0 Keratoconjunctivitis due to adenovirus
  Epidemic keratoconjunctivitis
  Shipyard eye
- B30.1 Conjunctivitis due to adenovirus
  Acute adenoviral follicular conjunctivitis
  Swimming-pool conjunctivitis
- B30.2 Viral pharyngoconjunctivitis
- B30.3 Acute epidemic hemorrhagic conjunctivitis (enteroviral)
  Conjunctivitis due to coxsackievirus 24
  Conjunctivitis due to enterovirus 70
  Hemorrhagic conjunctivitis (acute)(epidemic)
- B30.8 Other viral conjunctivitis
  Newcastle conjunctivitis
- B30.9 Viral conjunctivitis, unspecified

B33 Other viral diseases, not elsewhere classified

- B33.0 Epidemic myalgia
  Acute infectious disease, caused by group A coxsackie viruses or other enteroviruses with symptoms that include sudden pain in chest or upper abdomen with fever
  Bornholm disease
- B33.1 Ross River disease (Ex) PDX 163
  Epidemic polyarthritis and exanthema
  Ross River fever
- **B33.2 Viral carditis**
  Coxsackie (virus) carditis
  - B33.20 Viral carditis, unspecified (Ex) PDX 199
  - B33.21 Viral endocarditis (Ex) PDX 200
  - B33.22 Viral myocarditis (Ex) PDX 199
  - B33.23 Viral pericarditis (Ex) PDX 201
  - B33.24 Viral cardiomyopathy
- B33.3 Retrovirus infections, not elsewhere classified
  Retrovirus infection NOS
- B33.4 Hantavirus (cardio)-pulmonary syndrome [HPS] [HCPS] (Ex) PDX 202
  Hantavirus disease with pulmonary manifestations
  Sin nombre virus disease
  Use additional code to identify any associated acute kidney failure (N17.9)
  Excludes1 hantavirus disease with renal manifestations (A98.5)
  hemorrhagic fever with renal manifestations (A98.5)
- B33.8 Other specified viral diseases
  Excludes1 anogenital human papillomavirus infection (A63.0)
  viral warts due to human papillomavirus infection (B07)

B34 Viral infection of unspecified site

Excludes1 anogenital human papillomavirus infection (A63.0)
cytomegaloviral disease NOS (B25.9)
herpesvirus [herpes simplex] infection NOS (B00.9)
retrovirus infection NOS (B33.3)
viral agents as the cause of diseases classified elsewhere (B97.-)
viral warts due to human papillomavirus infection (B07)

- B34.0 Adenovirus infection, unspecified
- B34.1 Enterovirus infection, unspecified
  Intestinal tract infection
  Coxsackievirus infection NOS
  Echovirus infection NOS

CHAPTER 1 (A00-B99)

B34.2 Coronavirus infection, unspecified
Excludes1 COVID-19 (U07.1)
pneumonia due to SARS-associated coronavirus (J12.81)
B34.3 Parvovirus infection, unspecified (Ex) PDX 186
B34.4 Papovavirus infection, unspecified
B34.8 Other viral infections of unspecified site
B34.9 Viral infection, unspecified
Viremia NOS
Coding Clinic: 2016, Q3, P10

MYCOSES (B35-B49)

Excludes2 hypersensitivity pneumonitis due to organic dust (J67.-)
mycosis fungoides (C84.0-)

● B35 Dermatophytosis
AKA tinea or ringworm
Includes favus
infections due to species of Epidermophyton, Micro-sporum and Trichophyton
tinea, any type except those in B36.-
B35.0 Tinea barbae and tinea capitis
Beard ringworm
Kerion
Scalp ringworm
Sycosis, mycotic
B35.1 Tinea unguium
White patches or pits on surface or edges of nails, followed by infection under nail plate
Dermatophytic onychia
Dermatophytosis of nail
Onychomycosis
Ringworm of nails
B35.2 Tinea manuum
Tinea of hands
Dermatophytosis of hand
Hand ringworm
B35.3 Tinea pedis
Tinea affecting feet
Athlete's foot
Dermatophytosis of foot
Foot ringworm
B35.4 Tinea corporis
Infecting skin areas other than hands
Ringworm of the body
B35.5 Tinea imbricata
Chronic tropical tinea corporis; AKA Oriental ringworm, tinea inguinalis, tinea cruris
Tokelau
B35.6 Tinea cruris
In groin or perineal area, spreading to adjacent regions; AKA jock itch, eczema marginatum, ringworm of groin, or tinea inguinalis
Dhobi itch
Groin ringworm
Jock itch
B35.8 Other dermatophytoses
Disseminated dermatophytosis
Granulomatous dermatophytosis
B35.9 Dermatophytosis, unspecified
Ringworm NOS

● B36 Other superficial mycoses
B36.0 Pityriasis versicolor
Common, chronic, symptomless disorder that includes macular patches of various sizes and shapes; AKA liver spots
Tinea flava
Tinea versicolor
B36.1 Tinea nigra
Minor fungal infection, with dark lesions, usually on skin of hands
Keratomycosis nigricans palmaris
Microsporosis nigra
Pityriasis nigra
B36.2 White piedra
White to light brown nodules on hair of beard, axilla, or groin; AKA trichosporosis
Tinea blanca
B36.3 Black piedra
Characterized by small black or brown nodules on shafts of scalp hair
B36.8 Other specified superficial mycoses
B36.9 Superficial mycosis, unspecified

● B37 Candidiasis
Includes candidosis
moniliasis
Excludes1 neonatal candidiasis (P37.5)
B37.0 Candidal stomatitis (Ex) PDX 203
Oral thrush
B37.1 Pulmonary candidiasis (Ex) PDX 203
Candidal bronchitis
Candidal pneumonia
B37.2 Candidiasis of skin and nail
Candidal onychia
Candidal paronychia
Excludes2 diaper dermatitis (L22)
B37.3 Candidiasis of vulva and vagina
Candidal vulvovaginitis
Monilial vulvovaginitis
Vaginal thrush
B37.31 Acute candidiasis of vulva and vagina
Candidiasis of vulva and vagina NOS
B37.32 Chronic candidiasis of vulva and vagina
Recurrent candidiasis of vulva and vagina
● B37.4 Candidiasis of other urogenital sites
B37.41 Candidal cystitis and urethritis (Ex) PDX 204
B37.42 Candidal balanitis
Male condition only
B37.49 Other urogenital candidiasis (Ex) PDX 204
Candidal pyelonephritis
B37.5 Candidal meningitis (Ex) PDX 205
B37.6 Candidal endocarditis (Ex) PDX 203
B37.7 Candidal sepsis (Ex) PDX 206
Disseminated candidiasis systemic candidiasis
MCC when PDx is its own MCC
● B37.8 Candidiasis of other sites (Ex) PDX 203
B37.81 Candidal esophagitis
B37.82 Candidal enteritis
Candidal proctitis
B37.83 Candidal cheilitis
Inflammation affecting lip
B37.84 Candidal otitis externa
Inflammation of external auditory canal
B37.89 Other sites of candidiasis (Ex) PDX 207
Infection manifested by invasive candidiasis
Candidal osteomyelitis
B37.9 Candidiasis, unspecified
Thrush NOS

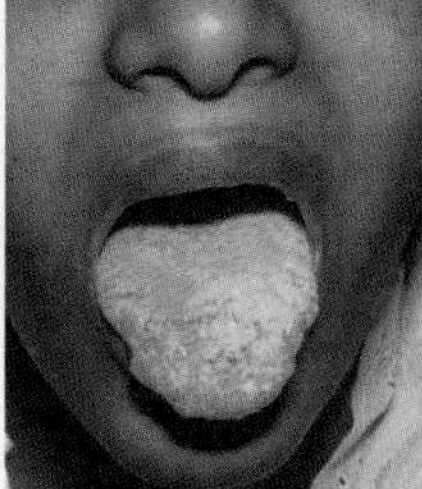

Figure 1-8 Oral candidiasis (thrush). (From James WD, Berger T, Elston D: Andrews' Diseases of the Skin: Clinical Dermatology, 11e, Saunders, 2011)

Item 1-20 Candidiasis, also called oidiomycosis or moniliasis, is a fungal infection. It most often appears on moist cutaneous areas of the body but can also be responsible for a variety of systemic infections such as endocarditis, meningitis, arthritis, and myositis. Antifungal medications cure most yeast infections.

Item 1–21 Bird and bat droppings that fall into the soil give rise to a fungus that can spread airborne spores. When inhaled into the lungs, these spores divide and multiply into lesions. Histoplasmosis capsulatum takes three forms: primary (lodged in the lungs only), chronic (resembles TB), and disseminated (infection has moved to other organs). This is an opportunistic infection in immunosuppressed patients.

● **B38 Coccidioidomycosis**
Fungal disease; AKA coccidioidosis, coccidioidal granuloma, Posadas, or Posadas-Wernicke disease

- **B38.0** Acute pulmonary coccidioidomycosis (Ex) PDX 208
- **B38.1** Chronic pulmonary coccidioidomycosis (Ex) PDX 209
- **B38.2** Pulmonary coccidioidomycosis, unspecified (Ex) PDX 209
- **B38.3** Cutaneous coccidioidomycosis (Ex) PDX 210
- **B38.4** Coccidioidomycosis meningitis (Ex) PDX 211
- **B38.7** Disseminated coccidioidomycosis (Ex) PDX 212
  Generalized coccidioidomycosis
- ● **B38.8** Other forms of coccidioidomycosis
  - **B38.81** Prostatic coccidioidomycosis (Ex) PDX 210
  - **B38.89** Other forms of coccidioidomycosis (Ex) PDX 212
- **B38.9** Coccidioidomycosis, unspecified (Ex) PDX 212

● **B39 Histoplasmosis**
Infection resulting from inhalation or ingestion of spores; AKA Darling disease

Code first associated AIDS (B20)

Use additional code for any associated manifestations, such as:
endocarditis (I39)
meningitis (G02)
pericarditis (I32)
retinitis (H32)

- **B39.0** Acute pulmonary histoplasmosis capsulati (Ex) PDX 213
- **B39.1** Chronic pulmonary histoplasmosis capsulati (Ex) PDX 213
- **B39.2** Pulmonary histoplasmosis capsulati, unspecified (Ex) PDX 213
- **B39.3** Disseminated histoplasmosis capsulati (Ex) PDX 214
  Generalized histoplasmosis capsulati
- **B39.4** Histoplasmosis capsulati, unspecified
  American histoplasmosis
- **B39.5** Histoplasmosis duboisii
  African histoplasmosis
- **B39.9** Histoplasmosis, unspecified

● **B40 Blastomycosis** (Ex) PDX 215
Rare and potentially fatal infection caused by inhaling fungus found in moist soil in temperate climates.

Excludes1 Brazilian blastomycosis (B41.-)
keloidal blastomycosis (B48.0)

- **B40.0** Acute pulmonary blastomycosis
- **B40.1** Chronic pulmonary blastomycosis
- **B40.2** Pulmonary blastomycosis, unspecified
- **B40.3** Cutaneous blastomycosis
- **B40.7** Disseminated blastomycosis
  Generalized blastomycosis
- ● **B40.8** Other forms of blastomycosis
  - **B40.81** Blastomycotic meningoencephalitis
    Meningomyelitis due to blastomycosis
  - **B40.89** Other forms of blastomycosis
- **B40.9** Blastomycosis, unspecified

● **B41 Paracoccidioidomycosis** (Ex) PDX 216
Fungal infection usually chronic that begins in lungs, spreads to mucocutaneous areas which may extend to skin, tonsils, gastrointestinal lymphatics, liver, and spleen; AKA Almeida or Lutz-Splendore-Almeida disease, Brazilian or South American blastomycosis, or paracoccidioidal granuloma

Includes Brazilian blastomycosis
Lutz' disease

- **B41.0** Pulmonary paracoccidioidomycosis
- **B41.7** Disseminated paracoccidioidomycosis
  Generalized paracoccidioidomycosis
- **B41.8** Other forms of paracoccidioidomycosis
- **B41.9** Paracoccidioidomycosis, unspecified

● **B42 Sporotrichosis**
Chronic fungal infection with nodular lesions

- **B42.0** Pulmonary sporotrichosis
- **B42.1** Lymphocutaneous sporotrichosis
- **B42.7** Disseminated sporotrichosis
  Generalized sporotrichosis
- ● **B42.8** Other forms of sporotrichosis
  - **B42.81** Cerebral sporotrichosis
    Meningitis due to sporotrichosis
  - **B42.82** Sporotrichosis arthritis
  - **B42.89** Other forms of sporotrichosis
- **B42.9** Sporotrichosis, unspecified

● **B43 Chromomycosis and pheomycotic abscess**
Chronic fungal infection of skin, initiated at site of puncture affecting lower limb or foot (mossy foot)

- **B43.0** Cutaneous chromomycosis
  Dermatitis verrucosa
- **B43.1** Pheomycotic brain abscess
  Cerebral chromomycosis
- **B43.2** Subcutaneous pheomycotic abscess and cyst
- **B43.8** Other forms of chromomycosis
- **B43.9** Chromomycosis, unspecified

● **B44 Aspergillosis** (Ex) PDX 217
Infection marked by inflammatory lesions in skin, ear, orbit, nasal sinuses, lungs, and occasionally bones and meninges

Includes aspergilloma

- **B44.0** Invasive pulmonary aspergillosis (Ex) PDX 113
  MCC when PDx is its own MCC
- **B44.1** Other pulmonary aspergillosis
- **B44.2** Tonsillar aspergillosis
- **B44.7** Disseminated aspergillosis
  Generalized aspergillosis
- ● **B44.8** Other forms of aspergillosis
  - **B44.81** Allergic bronchopulmonary a spergillosis (Ex) PDX 218
  - **B44.89** Other forms of aspergillosis
- **B44.9** Aspergillosis, unspecified

● **B45 Cryptococcosis** (Ex) PDX 219
Infection in the immunocompromised and fatal if left untreated; AKA torulosis, Buschke, or Busse-Buschke disease

- **B45.0** Pulmonary cryptococcosis
- **B45.1** Cerebral cryptococcosis (Ex) PDX 221
  Cryptococcal meningitis
  Cryptococcosis meningocerebralis
  MCC when PDx is its own MCC
- **B45.2** Cutaneous cryptococcosis
- **B45.3** Osseous cryptococcosis
- **B45.7** Disseminated cryptococcosis
  Generalized cryptococcosis
- **B45.8** Other forms of cryptococcosis
- **B45.9** Cryptococcosis, unspecified

CHAPTER 1 (A00-B99)

New | Revised | ~~deleted~~ Deleted | Excludes 1 | Excludes 2 | Includes | Use additional | Code first | Code also | Key words
OGCR Official Guidelines | ● Unacceptable Principal Diagnosis | X Assign placeholder X | ● Use Additional Character(s) | Manifestation Code | Coding Clinic

B46 Zygomycosis (Ex) PDX 221
Fungal infections including subcutaneous lesions and infection of sinuses, brain, or lungs

B46.0 Pulmonary mucormycosis
Fungal infection affecting lung

B46.1 Rhinocerebral mucormycosis

B46.2 Gastrointestinal mucormycosis

B46.3 Cutaneous mucormycosis
Subcutaneous mucormycosis

B46.4 Disseminated mucormycosis
Generalized mucormycosis

B46.5 Mucormycosis, unspecified

B46.8 Other zygomycoses
Entomophthoromycosis

B46.9 Zygomycosis, unspecified
Phycomycosis NOS

B47 Mycetoma
Slow progressive, destructive fungal infection of cutaneous and subcutaneous tissues, fascia, and bone, primarily seen in foot (Madura foot) or leg

B47.0 Eumycetoma (Ex) PDX 222
Madura foot, mycotic Maduromycosis

B47.1 Actinomycetoma (Ex) PDX 109

B47.9 Mycetoma, unspecified (Ex) PDX 223
Madura foot NOS

B48 Other mycoses, not elsewhere classified

B48.0 Lobomycosis
Infection with symptoms of red, smooth, hard cutaneous nodules resembling keloids
Keloidal blastomycosis
Lobo's disease

B48.1 Rhinosporidiosis
Chronic, localized granulomatous fungal infection, affecting mucocutaneous tissues, usually of nose characterized by polyps, papillomas, and wartlike lesions

B48.2 Allescheriasis (Ex) PDX 224
Fungal infection
Infection due to Pseudallescheria boydii
Excludes1 eumycetoma (B47.0)

B48.3 Geotrichosis (Ex) PDX 225
Fungal infection usually of bronchi, lungs, mouth, or intestinal tract
Geotrichum stomatitis

B48.4 Penicillosis (Ex) PDX 217
Fungal infection
Talaromycosis

B48.8 Other specified mycoses (Ex) PDX 226
Adiaspiromycosis
Infection of tissue and organs by Alternaria
Infection of tissue and organs by Drechslera
Infection of tissue and organs by Fusarium
Infection of tissue and organs by saprophytic fungi NEC

B49 Unspecified mycosis (Ex) PDX 225
Fungemia NOS

PROTOZOAL DISEASES (B50-B64)

Excludes1 amebiasis (A06.-)
other protozoal intestinal diseases (A07.-)

B50 Plasmodium falciparum malaria (Ex) PDX 227
Severe form of malaria that can be fatal
Includes mixed infections of Plasmodium falciparum with any other Plasmodium species

B50.0 Plasmodium falciparum malaria with cerebral complications
Cerebral malaria NOS

B50.8 Other severe and complicated Plasmodium falciparum malaria
Severe or complicated Plasmodium falciparum malaria NOS

B50.9 Plasmodium falciparum malaria, unspecified

B51 Plasmodium vivax malaria (Ex) PDX 227
Includes mixed infections of Plasmodium vivax with other Plasmodium species, except Plasmodium falciparum
Excludes1 plasmodium vivax with Plasmodium falciparum (B50.-)

B51.0 Plasmodium vivax malaria with rupture of spleen

B51.8 Plasmodium vivax malaria with other complications

B51.9 Plasmodium vivax malaria without complication (Ex) PDX 228
Plasmodium vivax malaria NOS

B52 Plasmodium malariae malaria
Causes fever that recurs at approximately three-day intervals (quartan fever), longer than two-day (tertian) intervals of other malarial parasites
Includes mixed infections of Plasmodium malariae with other Plasmodium species, except Plasmodium falciparum and Plasmodium vivax
Excludes1 plasmodium falciparum (B50.-)
plasmodium vivax (B51.-)

B52.0 Plasmodium malariae malaria with nephropathy (Ex) PDX 229
CC when PDx is its own CC

B52.8 Plasmodium malariae malaria with other complications (Ex) PDX 227

B52.9 Plasmodium malariae malaria without complication (Ex) PDX 227
Plasmodium malariae malaria NOS

B53 Other specified malaria (Ex) PDX 227

B53.0 Plasmodium ovale malaria
Least diagnosed type of malaria spread by female mosquitoes of rare species
Excludes1 plasmodium ovale with Plasmodium falciparum (B50.-)
plasmodium ovale with Plasmodium malariae (B52.-)
plasmodium ovale with Plasmodium vivax (B51.-)

B53.1 Malaria due to simian plasmodia
Malaria-like disease (parasite infection)
Excludes1 malaria due to simian plasmodia with Plasmodium falciparum (B50.-)
malaria due to simian plasmodia with Plasmodium malariae (B52.-)
malaria due to simian plasmodia with Plasmodium ovale (B53.0)
malaria due to simian plasmodia with Plasmodium vivax (B51.-)

B53.8 Other malaria, not elsewhere classified

B54 Unspecified malaria (Ex) PDX 227

B55 Leishmaniasis (Ex) PDX 230
Protozoal infection

B55.0 Visceral leishmaniasis
Kala-azar
Post-kala-azar dermal leishmaniasis

B55.1 Cutaneous leishmaniasis

B55.2 Mucocutaneous leishmaniasis

B55.9 Leishmaniasis, unspecified

● **B56 African trypanosomiasis** (Ex) PDX 230
Human African trypanosomiasis (HAT) is transmitted by fly bites

B56.0 Gambiense trypanosomiasis
Infection due to Trypanosoma brucei gambiense
West African sleeping sickness

B56.1 Rhodesiense trypanosomiasis
East African sleeping sickness
Infection due to Trypanosoma brucei rhodesiense

B56.9 African trypanosomiasis, unspecified
Sleeping sickness NOS

● **B57 Chagas' disease** (Ex) PDX 230
Tropical parasitic disease

Includes American trypanosomiasis
infection due to Trypanosoma cruzi

B57.0 Acute Chagas' disease with heart involvement (Ex) PDX 231
Acute Chagas' disease with myocarditis

B57.1 Acute Chagas' disease without heart involvement
Acute Chagas' disease NOS

B57.2 Chagas' disease (chronic) with heart involvement (Ex) PDX 231
American trypanosomiasis NOS
Chagas' disease (chronic) NOS
Chagas' disease (chronic) with myocarditis
Trypanosomiasis NOS

● **B57.3 Chagas' disease (chronic) with digestive system involvement**

B57.30 Chagas' disease with digestive system involvement, unspecified

B57.31 Megaesophagus in Chagas' disease

B57.32 Megacolon in Chagas' disease

B57.39 Other digestive system involvement in Chagas' disease

● **B57.4 Chagas' disease (chronic) with nervous system involvement**

B57.40 Chagas' disease with nervous system involvement, unspecified

B57.41 Meningitis in Chagas' disease

B57.42 Meningoencephalitis in Chagas' disease

B57.49 Other nervous system involvement in Chagas' disease

B57.5 Chagas' disease (chronic) with other organ involvement

● **B58 Toxoplasmosis**
Infection by protozoon transmitted in cysts in feces of cats

Includes infection due to Toxoplasma gondii

Excludes1 congenital toxoplasmosis (P37.1)

● **B58.0 Toxoplasma oculopathy**

B58.00 Toxoplasma oculopathy, unspecified (Ex) PDX 232

B58.01 Toxoplasma chorioretinitis (Ex) PDX 233

B58.09 Other toxoplasma oculopathy (Ex) PDX 234
Toxoplasma uveitis

B58.1 Toxoplasma hepatitis (Ex) PDX 235

B58.2 Toxoplasma meningoencephalitis (Ex) PDX 236

B58.3 Pulmonary toxoplasmosis (Ex) PDX 237

Item 1–22 Toxoplasmosis is caused by the protozoa **Toxoplasma gondii,** of which the house cat can be a host. Human infection occurs when contact is made with materials containing the pathogen, such as feces, contaminated soil, or ingestion of infected lamb, goat, or pork. Of the infected, very few have symptoms because a healthy person's immune system keeps the parasite from causing illness. When the immune system is compromised, symptoms may occur. Clinical symptoms include flu-like symptoms, but the disease progresses to include the eyes and the brain in babies.

● **B58.8 Toxoplasmosis with other organ involvement**

B58.81 Toxoplasma myocarditis (Ex) PDX 238

B58.82 Toxoplasma myositis (Ex) PDX 232

B58.83 Toxoplasma tubulo-interstitial nephropathy (Ex) PDX 232
Toxoplasma pyelonephritis

B58.89 Toxoplasmosis with other organ involvement (Ex) PDX 232

B58.9 Toxoplasmosis, unspecified (Ex) PDX 239

B59 Pneumocystosis (Ex) PDX 240
Caused by fungus
Pneumonia due to Pneumocystis carinii
Pneumonia due to Pneumocystis jiroveci

● **B60 Other protozoal diseases, not elsewhere classified**

Excludes1 cryptosporidiosis (A07.2)
intestinal microsporidiosis (A07.8)
isosporiasis (A07.3)

B60.0 Babesiosis (Ex) PDX 241
Tickborne disease caused by microscopic organisms

B60.00 Babesiosis, unspecified
Babesiosis due to unspecified Babesia species
Piroplasmosis, unspecified

B60.01 Babesiosis due to Babesia microti
Infection due to B. microti

B60.02 Babesiosis due to Babesia duncani
Infection due to B. duncani and B. duncani-type species

B60.03 Babesiosis due to Babesia divergens
Babesiosis due to Babesia MO-1
Infection due to B. divergens and B. divergens-like strains

B60.09 Other babesiosis
Babesiosis due to Babesia KO-1
Babesiosis due to Babesia venatorum
Infection due to other Babesia species
Infection due to other protozoa of the order Piroplasmida
Other piroplasmosis

● **B60.1 Acanthamebiasis** (Ex) PDX 242

B60.10 Acanthamebiasis, unspecified

B60.11 Meningoencephalitis due to Acanthamoeba (culbertsoni)

B60.12 Conjunctivitis due to Acanthamoeba

B60.13 Keratoconjunctivitis due to Acanthamoeba

B60.19 Other acanthamebic disease

B60.2 Naegleriasis
Infection with microscopic organisms
Primary amebic meningoencephalitis

B60.8 Other specified protozoal diseases
Microsporidiosis

B64 Unspecified protozoal disease

HELMINTHIASES (B65-B83)

Diseases or infestations caused by parasitic worms

● **B65 Schistosomiasis [bilharziasis]** (Ex) PDX 243
Infection with flukes (flat parasitic worms)

Includes snail fever

B65.0 Schistosomiasis due to Schistosoma haematobium [urinary schistosomiasis]

B65.1 Schistosomiasis due to Schistosoma mansoni [intestinal schistosomiasis]

B65.2 Schistosomiasis due to Schistosoma japonicum
Asiatic schistosomiasis

B65.3 Cercarial dermatitis
Swimmer's itch

B65.8 Other schistosomiasis
Infection due to Schistosoma intercalatum
Infection due to Schistosoma mattheei
Infection due to Schistosoma mekongi

B65.9 Schistosomiasis, unspecified

B66 Other fluke infections (Ex) PDX 244
Trematode (parasitic worms)

B66.0 Opisthorchiasis
Infection due to cat liver fluke
Infection due to Opisthorchis (felineus)(viverrini)

B66.1 Clonorchiasis
Chinese liver fluke disease
Infection due to Clonorchis sinensis
Oriental liver fluke disease

B66.2 Dicroceliasis
Liver fluke
Infection due to Dicrocoelium dendriticum
Lancet fluke infection

B66.3 Fascioliasis
Infection due to Fasciola gigantica
Infection due to Fasciola hepatica
Infection due to Fasciola indica
Sheep liver fluke disease

B66.4 Paragonimiasis
Infection due to Paragonimus species
Lung fluke disease
Pulmonary distomiasis

B66.5 Fasciolopsiasis
Largest intestinal fluke in humans
Infection due to Fasciolopsis buski
Intestinal distomiasis

B66.8 Other specified fluke infections
Echinostomiasis
Heterophyiasis
Metagonimiasis
Nanophyetiasis
Watsoniasis

B66.9 Fluke infection, unspecified

B67 Echinococcosis
Larval forms of tapeworms usually of liver or lungs
Includes hydatidosis

B67.0 Echinococcus granulosus infection of liver (Ex) PDX 245

B67.1 Echinococcus granulosus infection of lung (Ex) PDX 246

B67.2 Echinococcus granulosus infection of bone (Ex) PDX 247

B67.3 Echinococcus granulosus infection, other and multiple sites

B67.31 Echinococcus granulosus infection, thyroid gland (Ex) PDX 248

B67.32 Echinococcus granulosus infection, multiple sites (Ex) PDX 247

B67.39 Echinococcus granulosus infection, other sites (Ex) PDX 247

B67.4 Echinococcus granulosus infection, unspecified (Ex) PDX 249
Dog tapeworm (infection)

B67.5 Echinococcus multilocularis infection of liver (Ex) PDX 250

B67.6 Echinococcus multilocularis infection, other and multiple sites (Ex) PDX 251

B67.61 Echinococcus multilocularis infection, multiple sites

B67.69 Echinococcus multilocularis infection, other sites

B67.7 Echinococcus multilocularis infection, unspecified (Ex) PDX 252

B67.8 Echinococcosis, unspecified, of liver (Ex) PDX 253

B67.9 Echinococcosis, other and unspecified (Ex) PDX 253

B67.90 Echinococcosis, unspecified
Echinococcosis NOS

B67.99 Other echinococcosis

Item 1-23 Echinococcosis: Also known as hydatid disease; is caused by Echinococcus granulosus, E. multilocularis, and E. vogeli tapeworms; and is contracted from infected food. Found in southern South America, the Mediterranean, the Middle East, central Asia, and Africa and uncommon in the United States but has been reported in California, New Mexico, Arizona and Utah. The disease is treated with medication over a long course, as it is resistive.

B68 Taeniasis
Intestinal tapeworm (cestode) infection from raw or undercooked meat of infected animal
Excludes1 cysticercosis (B69.-)

B68.0 Taenia solium taeniasis (Ex) PDX 254
Pork tapeworm (infection)

B68.1 Taenia saginata taeniasis (Ex) PDX 255
Beef tapeworm (infection)
Infection due to adult tapeworm Taenia saginata

B68.9 Taeniasis, unspecified (Ex) PDX 255

B69 Cysticercosis (Ex) PDX 255
Systemic illness caused by the larvae of pork tapeworm
Includes cysticerciasis infection due to larval form of Taenia solium

B69.0 Cysticercosis of central nervous system

B69.1 Cysticercosis of eye

B69.8 Cysticercosis of other sites

B69.81 Myositis in cysticercosis

B69.89 Cysticercosis of other sites

B69.9 Cysticercosis, unspecified

B70 Diphyllobothriasis and sparganosis (Ex) PDX 255
Infection with tapeworms seen most often from inadequately cooked fish

B70.0 Diphyllobothriasis
Diphyllobothrium (adult) (latum) (pacificum) infection
Fish tapeworm (infection)
Excludes2 larval diphyllobothriasis (B70.1)

B70.1 Sparganosis
Infection with migrating tapeworm larvae, which invade subcutaneous tissues, causing inflammation and fibrosis that resembles cellulitis
Infection due to Sparganum (mansoni) (proliferum)
Infection due to Spirometra larva
Larval diphyllobothriasis
Spirometrosis

B71 Other cestode infections (Ex) PDX 255

B71.0 Hymenolepiasis
Intestinal infestation with tapeworms
Dwarf tapeworm infection
Rat tapeworm (infection)

B71.1 Dipylidiasis
Infection with tapeworm common to dogs and cats and seen in children having close contact with infected pets

B71.8 Other specified cestode infections
Infection by the larval stage of a tapeworm, usually through fruit or vegetables
Coenurosis

B71.9 Cestode infection, unspecified
Tapeworm (infection) NOS

B72 Dracunculiasis (Ex) PDX 256
Infection with roundworms
Includes guinea worm infection
infection due to Dracunculus medinensis

CHAPTER 1 (A00-B99)

B73 Onchocerciasis PDX 256
Infection with parasitic worm
Includes onchocerca volvulus infection
onchocercosis
river blindness

B73.0 Onchocerciasis with eye disease
B73.00 Onchocerciasis with eye involvement, unspecified
B73.01 Onchocerciasis with endophthalmitis
B73.02 Onchocerciasis with glaucoma
B73.09 Onchocerciasis with other eye involvement
Infestation of eyelid due to onchocerciasis
B73.1 Onchocerciasis without eye disease

B74 Filariasis PDX 256
Infestation with slender threadlike worms
Excludes2 onchocerciasis (B73)
tropical (pulmonary) eosinophilia NOS (J82.89)

B74.0 Filariasis due to Wuchereria bancrofti
Bancroftian elephantiasis
Bancroftian filariasis
B74.1 Filariasis due to Brugia malayi
B74.2 Filariasis due to Brugia timori
B74.3 Loiasis
Infection with round worms growing in subcutaneous connective tissue
Calabar swelling
Eyeworm disease of Africa
Loa loa infection
B74.4 Mansonelliasis
Infection with filarial parasite
Infection due to Mansonella ozzardi
Infection due to Mansonella perstans
Infection due to Mansonella streptocerca
B74.8 Other filariases
Dirofilariasis
B74.9 Filariasis, unspecified

B75 Trichinellosis PDX 257
Infestation with parasitic roundworms ingested in undercooked contaminated meat
Includes infection due to Trichinella species trichiniasis

B76 Hookworm diseases PDX 258
Occurs in hot, humid parts of world where larvae are soil borne, enter digestive tract through skin of feet/legs or in contaminated food/water; AKA ground itch
Includes uncinariasis

B76.0 Ancylostomiasis
Infection due to Ancylostoma species
B76.1 Necatoriasis
Infection due to Necator americanus
B76.8 Other hookworm diseases
B76.9 Hookworm disease, unspecified
Cutaneous larva migrans NOS

B77 Ascariasis
Infection by roundworm in small intestine
Includes ascaridiasis
roundworm infection

B77.0 Ascariasis with intestinal complications PDX 259
B77.8 Ascariasis with other complications
B77.81 Ascariasis pneumonia PDX 260
MCC when PDx is its own MCC
B77.89 Ascariasis with other complications PDX 259
B77.9 Ascariasis, unspecified PDX 259

B78 Strongyloidiasis PDX 259
Infection with adult female roundworms
Excludes1 trichostrongyliasis (B81.2)

B78.0 Intestinal strongyloidiasis
B78.1 Cutaneous strongyloidiasis
B78.7 Disseminated strongyloidiasis
B78.9 Strongyloidiasis, unspecified

B79 Trichuriasis PDX 259
Intestinal infection with roundworms
Includes trichocephaliasis
whipworm (disease)(infection)

B80 Enterobiasis PDX 259
Intestinal infection with pinworms
Includes oxyuriasis
pinworm infection
threadworm infection

B81 Other intestinal helminthiases, not elsewhere classified
Diseases or infestations caused by parasitic worms
Excludes1 angiostrongyliasis due to:
Angiostrongylus cantonensis (B83.2)
Parastrongylus cantonensis (B83.2)

B81.0 Anisakiasis PDX 259
Roundworm infection via contaminated undercooked infected fish or marine mammals
Infection due to Anisakis larva
B81.1 Intestinal capillariasis PDX 259
Infestation with of parasites (nematodes)
Capillariasis NOS
Infection due to Capillaria philippinensis
Excludes2 hepatic capillariasis (B83.8)
B81.2 Trichostrongyliasis PDX 259
B81.3 Intestinal angiostrongyliasis PDX 261
Angiostrongyliasis due to:
Angiostrongylus costaricensis (B83.2)
Parastrongylus costaricensis (B83.2)
B81.4 Mixed intestinal helminthiases PDX 261
Infection due to intestinal helminths classified to more than one of the categories B65.0-B81.3 and B81.8
Mixed helminthiasis NOS
B81.8 Other specified intestinal helminthiases PDX 261
Infection due to Oesophagostomum species [esophagostomiasis]
Infection due to Ternidens diminutus [ternidensiasis]

B82 Unspecified intestinal parasitism
B82.0 Intestinal helminthiasis, unspecified PDX 261
Infected with worms
B82.9 Intestinal parasitism, unspecified

B83 Other helminthiases
Caused by parasitic worms
Excludes1 capillariasis NOS (B81.1)
Excludes2 intestinal capillariasis (B81.1)

B83.0 Visceral larva migrans
Prolonged migration of nematode larvae
Toxocariasis
B83.1 Gnathostomiasis
Infection with nematode occurring from ingested undercooked fish contaminated with larvae; larvae migrate to subcutaneous tissue or deeper tissues, results are abscesses
Wandering swelling
B83.2 Angiostrongyliasis due to Parastrongylus cantonensis
Nematode infection caused by eating contaminated raw snails, slugs, or paratenic hosts such as prawns or crabs; larval worms migrate to central nervous system resulting in eosinophilic meningitis
Eosinophilic meningoencephalitis due to Parastrongylus cantonensis
Excludes2 intestinal angiostrongyliasis (B81.3)

B83.3 Syngamiasis
Infestation with gapeworm from turkey, pheasant, guinea fowl, goose, and wild birds
Syngamosis

B83.4 Internal hirudiniasis
Infestation by leeches
Excludes2 external hirudiniasis (B88.3)

B83.8 Other specified helminthiases
Parasitic worm infestation
Acanthocephaliasis
Gongylonemiasis
Hepatic capillariasis
Metastrongyliasis
Thelaziasis

B83.9 Helminthiasis, unspecified
Worms NOS
Excludes1 intestinal helminthiasis NOS (B82.0)

PEDICULOSIS, ACARIASIS AND OTHER INFESTATIONS (B85-B89)

B85 Pediculosis and phthiriasis
Infestation of lice

B85.0 Pediculosis due to Pediculus humanus capitis
Head-louse infestation

B85.1 Pediculosis due to Pediculus humanus corporis
Body-louse infestation

B85.2 Pediculosis, unspecified

B85.3 Phthiriasis
Crab or pubic lice
Infestation by crab-louse
Infestation by Phthirus pubis

B85.4 Mixed pediculosis and phthiriasis
Infestation classifiable to more than one of the categories B85.0-B85.3

B86 Scabies
Contagious dermatitis caused by mites
Sarcoptic itch

B87 Myiasis
Infestation by fly maggots
Includes infestation by larva of flies

B87.0 Cutaneous myiasis
Creeping myiasis

B87.1 Wound myiasis
Traumatic myiasis

B87.2 Ocular myiasis

B87.3 Nasopharyngeal myiasis
Laryngeal myiasis

B87.4 Aural myiasis

B87.8 Myiasis of other sites

B87.81 Genitourinary myiasis

B87.82 Intestinal myiasis

B87.89 Myiasis of other sites

B87.9 Myiasis, unspecified

B88 Other infestations

B88.0 Other acariasis
Acarine dermatitis
Dermatitis due to Demodex species
Dermatitis due to Dermanyssus gallinae
Dermatitis due to Liponyssoides sanguineus
Trombiculosis
Excludes2 scabies (B86)

B88.1 Tungiasis [sandflea infestation]
Inflammatory skin disease caused by infestation of fleas

B88.2 Other arthropod infestations
Scarabiasis

B88.3 External hirudiniasis
Leech infestation NOS
Excludes2 internal hirudiniasis (B83.4)

B88.8 Other specified infestations
Infection of topical fresh water fish parasite
Ichthyoparasitism due to Vandellia cirrhosa
Linguatulosis
Porocephaliasis

B88.9 Infestation, unspecified
Infestation (skin) NOS
Infestation by mites NOS
Skin parasites NOS

B89 Unspecified parasitic disease

SEQUELAE OF INFECTIOUS AND PARASITIC DISEASES (B90-B94)

Note: Categories B90-B94 are to be used to indicate conditions in categories A00-B89 as the cause of sequelae, which are themselves classified elsewhere. The 'sequelae' include conditions specified as such; they also include residuals of diseases classifiable to the above categories if there is evidence that the disease itself is no longer present. Codes from these categories are not to be used for chronic infections. Code chronic current infections to active infectious disease as appropriate.

Code first condition resulting from (sequela) the infectious or parasitic disease

B90 Sequelae of tuberculosis
Condition resulting from tuberculosis

B90.0 Sequelae of central nervous system tuberculosis

B90.1 Sequelae of genitourinary tuberculosis

B90.2 Sequelae of tuberculosis of bones and joints

B90.8 Sequelae of tuberculosis of other organs
Excludes2 sequelae of respiratory tuberculosis (B90.9)

B90.9 Sequelae of respiratory and unspecified tuberculosis
Sequelae of tuberculosis NOS

B91 Sequelae of poliomyelitis
Excludes1 postpolio syndrome (G14)

B92 Sequelae of leprosy

B94 Sequelae of other and unspecified infectious and parasitic diseases

B94.0 Sequelae of trachoma

B94.1 Sequelae of viral encephalitis

B94.2 Sequelae of viral hepatitis

B94.8 Sequelae of other specified infectious and parasitic diseases
Coding Clinic: 2021, Q4, P102-106; 2021, Q1, P34,37,41,44,46,48

B94.9 Sequelae of unspecified infectious and parasitic disease
Excludes2 post COVID-19 condition (U09.9)
Coding Clinic: 2017, Q4, P109

OGCR Section I.C.1.b.

Certain infectious and parasitic diseases

Infectious agents as the cause of diseases classified to other chapters

Certain infections are classified in chapters other than Chapter 1 and no organism is identified as part of the infection code. In these instances, it is necessary to use an additional code from Chapter 1 to identify the organism. A code from category B95, Streptococcus, Staphylococcus, and Enterococcus as the cause of diseases classified to other chapters, B96, Other bacterial agents as the cause of diseases classified to other chapters, or B97, Viral agents as the cause of diseases classified to other chapters, is to be used as an additional code to identify the organism. An instructional note will be found at the infection code advising that an additional organism code is required.

BACTERIAL AND VIRAL INFECTIOUS AGENTS (B95-B97)

Note: These categories are provided for use as supplementary or additional codes to identify the infectious agent(s) in diseases classified elsewhere.

Code the disease first, then the bacterium. Do not report codes from B95-B97 for sepsis.

B95 Streptococcus, Staphylococcus, and Enterococcus as the cause of diseases classified elsewhere

- **B95.0 Streptococcus, group A, as the cause of diseases classified elsewhere**
- **B95.1 Streptococcus, group B, as the cause of diseases classified elsewhere**
  Coding Clinic: 2020, Q1, P10; 2019, Q2, P9-10; 2018, Q4, P23
- **B95.2 Enterococcus as the cause of diseases classified elsewhere**
- **B95.3 Streptococcus pneumoniae as the cause of diseases classified elsewhere**
- **B95.4 Other streptococcus as the cause of diseases classified elsewhere**
- **B95.5 Unspecified streptococcus as the cause of diseases classified elsewhere**
- **B95.6 Staphylococcus aureus as the cause of diseases classified elsewhere**
  - **B95.61 Methicillin susceptible Staphylococcus aureus infection as the cause of diseases classified elsewhere**
    Methicillin susceptible Staphylococcus aureus (MSSA) infection as the cause of diseases classified elsewhere
    Staphylococcus aureus infection NOS as the cause of diseases classified elsewhere
  - **B95.62 Methicillin resistant Staphylococcus aureus infection as the cause of diseases classified elsewhere**
    Methicillin resistant staphylococcus aureus (MRSA) infection as the cause of diseases classified elsewhere
    Coding Clinic: 2016, Q1, P13
- **B95.7 Other staphylococcus as the cause of diseases classified elsewhere**
- **B95.8 Unspecified staphylococcus as the cause of diseases classified elsewhere**

B96 Other bacterial agents as the cause of diseases classified elsewhere

- **B96.0 Mycoplasma pneumoniae [M. pneumoniae] as the cause of diseases classified elsewhere**
  Pleuro-pneumonia-like-organism [PPLO]
- **B96.1 Klebsiella pneumoniae [K. pneumoniae] as the cause of diseases classified elsewhere**
- **B96.2 Escherichia coli [E. coli] as the cause of diseases classified elsewhere**
  - **B96.20 Unspecified Escherichia coli [E. coli] as the cause of diseases classified elsewhere**
    Escherichia coli [E. coli] NOS
    Coding Clinic: 2022, Q1, P31; 2018, Q4, P34; 2018, Q1, P16
  - **B96.21 Shiga toxin-producing Escherichia coli [E. coli] [STEC] O157 as the cause of diseases classified elsewhere**
    E. coli O157:H- (nonmotile) with confirmation of Shiga toxin
    E. coli O157 with confirmation of Shiga toxin when H antigen is unknown, or is not H7
    O157:H7 Escherichia coli [E.coli] with or without confirmation of Shiga toxin-production
    Shiga toxin-producing Escherichia coli [E.coli] O157:H7 with or without confirmation of Shiga toxin-production
    STEC O157:H7 with or without confirmation of Shiga toxin-production
  - **B96.22 Other specified Shiga toxin-producing Escherichia coli [E. coli] [STEC] as the cause of diseases classified elsewhere**
    Non-O157 Shiga toxin-producing Escherichia coli [E.coli]
    Non-O157 Shiga toxin-producing Escherichia coli [E.coli] with known O group
  - **B96.23 Unspecified Shiga toxin-producing Escherichia coli [E. coli] [STEC] as the cause of diseases classified elsewhere**
    Shiga toxin-producing Escherichia coli [E. coli] with unspecified O group
    STEC NOS
  - **B96.29 Other Escherichia coli [E. coli] as the cause of diseases classified elsewhere**
    Non-Shiga toxin-producing E. coli
- **B96.3 Hemophilus influenzae [H. influenzae] as the cause of diseases classified elsewhere**
- **B96.4 Proteus (mirabilis) (morganii) as the cause of diseases classified elsewhere**
- **B96.5 Pseudomonas (aeruginosa) (mallei) (pseudomallei) as the cause of diseases classified elsewhere**
  Coding Clinic: 2015, Q1, P18
- **B96.6 Bacteroides fragilis [B. fragilis] as the cause of diseases classified elsewhere**
- **B96.7 Clostridium perfringens [C. perfringens] as the cause of diseases classified elsewhere**
- **B96.8 Other specified bacterial agents as the cause of diseases classified elsewhere**
  - **B96.81 Helicobacter pylori [H. pylori] as the cause of diseases classified elsewhere**
  - **B96.82 Vibrio vulnificus as the cause of diseases classified elsewhere**
  - **B96.83 Acinetobacter baumannii as the cause of diseases classified elsewhere**
  - **B96.89 Other specified bacterial agents as the cause of diseases classified elsewhere**

B97 Viral agents as the cause of diseases classified elsewhere

- **B97.0 Adenovirus as the cause of diseases classified elsewhere**
- **B97.1 Enterovirus as the cause of diseases classified elsewhere**
  - **B97.10 Unspecified enterovirus as the cause of diseases classified elsewhere**
  - **B97.11 Coxsackievirus as the cause of diseases classified elsewhere**
  - **B97.12 Echovirus as the cause of diseases classified elsewhere**
  - **B97.19 Other enterovirus as the cause of diseases classified elsewhere**
- **B97.2 Coronavirus as the cause of diseases classified elsewhere**
  - **B97.21 SARS-associated coronavirus as the cause of diseases classified elsewhere** PDX 262
    Excludes1 pneumonia due to SARS-associated coronavirus (J12.81)
  - **B97.29 Other coronavirus as the cause of diseases classified elsewhere**

Item 1–24 Retrovirus develops by copying its RNA, genetic materials, into the DNA, which then produces new virus particles. It is from the Retroviridae virus family. **Human T-cell lymphotropic virus, Type I (HTLV-I),** is also called human T-cell leukemia virus, Type I, and is a retrovirus thought to cause T-cell leukemia/lymphoma. **Human T-cell lymphotropic virus, Type II (HTLV-II),** is also called human T-cell leukemia virus, Type II, and is a retrovirus associated with hematologic disorders.

HIV-2 is one of the serotypes of HIV and is usually confined to West Africa, whereas **HIV-1** is found worldwide.

● **B97.3 Retrovirus as the cause of diseases classified elsewhere**
  Excludes1 human immunodeficiency virus [HIV] disease (B2Ø)
- ● **B97.3Ø Unspecified retrovirus as the cause of diseases classified elsewhere**
- ● **B97.31 Lentivirus as the cause of diseases classified elsewhere**
- ● **B97.32 Oncovirus as the cause of diseases classified elsewhere**
- ● **B97.33 Human T-cell lymphotrophic virus, type I [HTLV-I] as the cause of diseases classified elsewhere** Ex: PDX 263
- ● **B97.34 Human T-cell lymphotrophic virus, type II [HTLV-II] as the cause of diseases classified elsewhere** Ex: PDX 263
- ● **B97.35 Human immunodeficiency virus, type 2 [HIV 2] as the cause of diseases classified elsewhere** Ex: PDX 264
- ● B97.39 Other retrovirus as the cause of diseases classified elsewhere

● **B97.4 Respiratory syncytial virus as the cause of diseases classified elsewhere**
  RSV as the cause of diseases classified elsewhere
  Code first related disorders, such as:
  otitis media (H65.-)
  upper respiratory infection (JØ6.9)
  Excludes1 acute bronchiolitis due to respiratory syncytial virus (RSV) (J21.Ø)
  acute bronchitis due to respiratory syncytial virus (RSV) (J2Ø.5)
  respiratory syncytial virus (RSV) pneumonia (J12.1)

● **B97.5 Reovirus as the cause of diseases classified elsewhere**

● **B97.6 Parvovirus as the cause of diseases classified elsewhere**

● **B97.7 Papillomavirus as the cause of diseases classified elsewhere**

● **B97.8 Other viral agents as the cause of diseases classified elsewhere**
- ● **B97.81 Human metapneumovirus as the cause of diseases classified elsewhere**
- ● **B97.89 Other viral agents as the cause of diseases classified elsewhere**
  Coding Clinic: 2Ø16, Q3, P8-1Ø, 14

OTHER INFECTIOUS DISEASES (B99)

● B99 Other and unspecified infectious diseases
- B99.8 Other infectious disease
- B99.9 Unspecified infectious disease

CHAPTER 2

NEOPLASMS (CØØ-D49)

OGCR Chapter-Specific Coding Guidelines

2. **Chapter 2: Neoplasms (CØØ-D49)**
General guidelines
Chapter 2 of the ICD-10-CM contains the codes for most benign and all malignant neoplasms. Certain benign neoplasms, such as prostatic adenomas, may be found in the specific body system chapters. To properly code a neoplasm it is necessary to determine from the record if the neoplasm is benign, in-situ, malignant, or of uncertain histologic behavior. If malignant, any secondary (metastatic) sites should also be determined.

Primary malignant neoplasms overlapping site boundaries

A primary malignant neoplasm that overlaps two or more contiguous (next to each other) sites should be classified to the subcategory/code .8 ('overlapping lesion'), unless the combination is specifically indexed elsewhere. For multiple neoplasms of the same site that are not contiguous such as tumors in different quadrants of the same breast, codes for each site should be assigned.

Malignant neoplasm of ectopic tissue

Malignant neoplasms of ectopic tissue are to be coded to the site of origin mentioned, e.g., ectopic pancreatic malignant neoplasms involving the stomach are coded to malignant neoplasm of pancreas, unspecified (C25.9).

The neoplasm table in the Alphabetic Index should be referenced first. However, if the histological term is documented, that term should be referenced first, rather than going immediately to the Neoplasm Table, in order to determine which column in the Neoplasm Table is appropriate. For example, if the documentation indicates "adenoma," refer to the term in the Alphabetic Index to review the entries under this term and the instructional note to "see also neoplasm, by site, benign." The table provides the proper code based on the type of neoplasm and the site. It is important to select the proper column in the table that corresponds to the type of neoplasm. The Tabular List should then be referenced to verify that the correct code has been selected from the table and that a more specific site code does not exist.

See Section I.C.21. Factors influencing health status and contact with health services, Status, for information regarding Z15.Ø, codes for genetic susceptibility to cancer.

a. Treatment directed at the malignancy
If the treatment is directed at the malignancy, designate the malignancy as the principal diagnosis.

The only exception to this guideline is if a patient admission/encounter is solely for the administration of chemotherapy, immunotherapy or external beam radiation therapy, assign the appropriate Z51.— code as the first-listed or principal diagnosis, and the diagnosis or problem for which the service is being performed as a secondary diagnosis.

b. Treatment of secondary site
When a patient is admitted because of a primary neoplasm with metastasis and treatment is directed toward the secondary site only, the secondary neoplasm is designated as the principal diagnosis even though the primary malignancy is still present.

c. Coding and sequencing of complications
Coding and sequencing of complications associated with the malignancies or with the therapy thereof are subject to the following guidelines:

1) Anemia associated with malignancy
When admission/encounter is for management of an anemia associated with the malignancy, and the treatment is only for anemia, the appropriate code for the malignancy is sequenced as the principal or first-listed diagnosis followed by the appropriate code for the anemia (such as code D63.Ø, Anemia in neoplastic disease).

2) Anemia associated with chemotherapy, immunotherapy and radiation therapy
When the admission/encounter is for management of an anemia associated with an adverse effect of the administration of chemotherapy or immunotherapy and the only treatment is for the anemia, the anemia code is sequenced first followed by the appropriate codes for the neoplasm and the adverse effect (T45.1X5, Adverse effect of antineoplastic and immunosuppressive drugs).

When the admission/encounter is for management of an anemia associated with an adverse effect of radiotherapy, the anemia code should be sequenced first, followed by the appropriate neoplasm code and code Y84.2, Radiological procedure and radiotherapy as the cause of abnormal reaction of the patient, or of later complication, without mention of misadventure at the time of the procedure.

3) Management of dehydration due to the malignancy
When the admission/encounter is for management of dehydration due to the malignancy and only the dehydration is being treated (intravenous rehydration), the dehydration is sequenced first, followed by the code(s) for the malignancy.

4) Treatment of a complication resulting from a surgical procedure
When the admission/encounter is for treatment of a complication resulting from a surgical procedure, designate the complication as the principal or first-listed diagnosis if treatment is directed at resolving the complication.

d. Primary malignancy previously excised
When a primary malignancy has been previously excised or eradicated from its site and there is no further treatment directed to that site and there is no evidence of any existing primary malignancy at that site, a code from category Z85, Personal history of malignant neoplasm, should be used to indicate the former site of the malignancy. Any mention of extension, invasion, or metastasis to another site is coded as a secondary malignant neoplasm to that site. The secondary site may be the principal or first-listed with the Z85 code used as a secondary code.

e. Admissions/Encounters involving chemotherapy, immunotherapy and radiation therapy

1) Episode of care involves surgical removal of neoplasm
When an episode of care involves the surgical removal of a neoplasm, primary or secondary site, followed by adjunct chemotherapy or radiation treatment during the same episode of care, the code for the neoplasm should be assigned as principal or first-listed diagnosis.

2) Patient admission/encounter solely for administration of chemotherapy, immunotherapy and radiation therapy
If a patient admission/encounter is solely for the administration of chemotherapy, immunotherapy or external beam radiation therapy assign code Z51.Ø, Encounter for antineoplastic radiation therapy, or Z51.11, Encounter for antineoplastic chemotherapy, or Z51.12, Encounter for antineoplastic immunotherapy as the first-listed or principal diagnosis. If a patient receives more than one of these therapies during the same admission more than one of these codes may be assigned, in any sequence.

The malignancy for which the therapy is being administered should be assigned as a secondary diagnosis.

If a patient admission/encounter is for the insertion or implantation of radioactive elements (e.g., brachytherapy) the appropriate code for the malignancy is sequenced as the principal or first-listed diagnosis. Code Z51.Ø should not be assigned.

3) Patient admitted for radiation therapy, chemotherapy or immunotherapy and develops complications
When a patient is admitted for the purpose of external beam radiotherapy, immunotherapy or chemotherapy and develops complications such as uncontrolled nausea and vomiting or dehydration, the principal or first-listed diagnosis is Z51.Ø, Encounter for antineoplastic radiation therapy, or Z51.11, Encounter for antineoplastic chemotherapy, or Z51.12, Encounter for antineoplastic immunotherapy followed by any codes for the complications.

When a patient is admitted for the purpose of insertion or implantation of radioactive elements (e.g., brachytherapy) and develops complications such as uncontrolled nausea and vomiting or dehydration, the principal or first-listed diagnosis is the appropriate code for the malignancy followed by any codes for the complications.

f. Admission/encounter to determine extent of malignancy
When the reason for admission/encounter is to determine the extent of the malignancy, or for a procedure such as paracentesis

or thoracentesis, the primary malignancy or appropriate metastatic site is designated as the principal or first-listed diagnosis, even though chemotherapy or radiotherapy is administered.

g. Symptoms, signs, and abnormal findings listed in Chapter 18 associated with neoplasms

Symptoms, signs, and ill-defined conditions listed in Chapter 18 characteristic of, or associated with, an existing primary or secondary site malignancy cannot be used to replace the malignancy as principal or first-listed diagnosis, regardless of the number of admissions or encounters for treatment and care of the neoplasm.

See Section I.C.21. Factors influencing health status and contact with health services, Encounter for prophylactic organ removal.

h. Admission/encounter for pain control/management

See Section I.C.6. for information on coding admission/encounter for pain control/management.

i. Malignancy in two or more noncontiguous sites

A patient may have more than one malignant tumor in the same organ. These tumors may represent different primaries or metastatic disease, depending on the site. Should the documentation be unclear, the provider should be queried as to the status of each tumor so that the correct codes can be assigned.

j. Disseminated malignant neoplasm, unspecified

Code C80.0, Disseminated malignant neoplasm, unspecified, is for use only in those cases where the patient has advanced metastatic disease and no known primary or secondary sites are specified. It should not be used in place of assigning codes for the primary site and all known secondary sites.

k. Malignant neoplasm without specification of site

Code C80.1, Malignant (primary) neoplasm, unspecified, equates to Cancer, unspecified. This code should only be used when no determination can be made as to the primary site of a malignancy. This code should rarely be used in the inpatient setting.

l. Sequencing of neoplasm codes

1) Encounter for treatment of primary malignancy

If the reason for the encounter is for treatment of a primary malignancy, assign the malignancy as the principal/first-listed diagnosis. The primary site is to be sequenced first, followed by any metastatic sites.

2) Encounter for treatment of secondary malignancy

When an encounter is for a primary malignancy with metastasis and treatment is directed toward the metastatic (secondary) site(s) only, the metastatic site(s) is designated as the principal/first-listed diagnosis. The primary malignancy is coded as an additional code.

3) Malignant neoplasm in a pregnant patient

When a pregnant woman has a malignant neoplasm, a code from subcategory O9A.1-, Malignant neoplasm complicating pregnancy, childbirth, and the puerperium, should be sequenced first, followed by the appropriate code from Chapter 2 to indicate the type of neoplasm.

4) Encounter for complication associated with a neoplasm

When an encounter is for management of a complication associated with a neoplasm, such as dehydration, and the treatment is only for the complication, the complication is coded first, followed by the appropriate code(s) for the neoplasm.

The exception to this guideline is anemia. When the admission/encounter is for management of an anemia associated with the malignancy, and the treatment is only for anemia, the appropriate code for the malignancy is sequenced as the principal or first-listed diagnosis followed by code D63.0, Anemia in neoplastic disease.

5) Complication from surgical procedure for treatment of a neoplasm

When an encounter is for treatment of a complication resulting from a surgical procedure performed for the treatment of the neoplasm, designate the complication as the principal/first-listed diagnosis. See guideline regarding the coding of a current malignancy versus personal history to determine if the code for the neoplasm should also be assigned.

6) Pathologic fracture due to a neoplasm

When an encounter is for a pathological fracture due to a neoplasm, and the focus of treatment is the fracture, a code from subcategory M84.5, Pathological fracture in neoplastic disease, should be sequenced first, followed by the code for the neoplasm.

If the focus of treatment is the neoplasm with an associated pathological fracture, the neoplasm code should be sequenced first, followed by a code from M84.5 for the pathological fracture.

m. Current malignancy versus personal history of malignancy

When a primary malignancy has been excised but further treatment, such as an additional surgery for the malignancy, radiation therapy or chemotherapy is directed to that site, the primary malignancy code should be used until treatment is completed.

When a primary malignancy has been previously excised or eradicated from its site, there is no further treatment (of the malignancy) directed to that site, and there is no evidence of any existing primary malignancy at that site, a code from category Z85, Personal history of malignant neoplasm, should be used to indicate the former site of the malignancy.

Subcategories Z85.0–Z85.7 should only be assigned for the former site of a primary malignancy, not the site of a secondary malignancy. Codes from subcategory Z85.8-, may be assigned for the former site(s) of either a primary or secondary malignancy included in this subcategory.

See Section I.C.21. Factors influencing health status and contact with health services, History (of)

n. Leukemia, Multiple Myeloma, and Malignant Plasma Cell Neoplasms in remission versus personal history

The categories for leukemia, and category C90, Multiple myeloma and malignant plasma cell neoplasms, have codes indicating whether or not the leukemia has achieved remission. There are also codes Z85.6, Personal history of leukemia, and Z85.79, Personal history of other malignant neoplasms of lymphoid, hematopoietic and related tissues. If the documentation is unclear, as to whether the leukemia has achieved remission, the provider should be queried.

See Section I.C.21. Factors influencing health status and contact with health services, History (of)

o. Aftercare following surgery for neoplasm

See Section I.C.21. Factors influencing health status and contact with health services, Aftercare

p. Follow-up care for completed treatment of a malignancy

See Section I.C.21. Factors influencing health status and contact with health services, Follow-up

q. Prophylactic organ removal for prevention of malignancy

See Section I.C. 21, Factors influencing health status and contact with health services, Prophylactic organ removal

r. Malignant neoplasm associated with transplanted organ

A malignant neoplasm of a transplanted organ should be coded as a transplant complication. Assign first the appropriate code from category T86.-, Complications of transplanted organs and tissue, followed by code C80.2, Malignant neoplasm associated with transplanted organ. Use an additional code for the specific malignancy.

Item 2-1 Neoplasm: Neo = new, plasm = growth, development, formation. This new growth (mass, tumor) can be malignant or benign, which is confirmed by the pathology report. Do not assign a code to a neoplasm until you review the pathology report. Certain CPT codes will specify benign or malignant lesion, so be certain the diagnosis code supports the procedure code.

CHAPTER 2

NEOPLASMS (C00-D49)

This chapter contains the following blocks:

C00-C14	Malignant neoplasms of lip, oral cavity and pharynx
C15-C26	Malignant neoplasms of digestive organs
C30-C39	Malignant neoplasms of respiratory and intrathoracic organs
C40-C41	Malignant neoplasms of bone and articular cartilage
C43-C44	Melanoma and other malignant neoplasms of skin
C45-C49	Malignant neoplasms of mesothelial and soft tissue
C50	Malignant neoplasms of breast
C51-C58	Malignant neoplasms of female genital organs
C60-C63	Malignant neoplasms of male genital organs
C64-C68	Malignant neoplasms of urinary tract
C69-C72	Malignant neoplasms of eye, brain and other parts of central nervous system
C73-C75	Malignant neoplasms of thyroid and other endocrine glands
C7A	Malignant neuroendocrine tumors
C7B	Secondary neuroendocrine tumors
C76-C80	Malignant neoplasms of ill-defined, other secondary and unspecified sites
C81-C96	Malignant neoplasms of lymphoid, hematopoietic and related tissue
D00-D09	In situ neoplasms
D10-D36	Benign neoplasms, except benign neuroendocrine tumors
D3A	Benign neuroendocrine tumors
D37-D48	Neoplasms of uncertain behavior, polycythemia vera and myelodysplastic syndromes
D49	Neoplasms of unspecified behavior

Notes: Functional activity

All neoplasms are classified in this chapter, whether they are functionally active or not. An additional code from Chapter 4 may be used, to identify functional activity associated with any neoplasm.

Morphology [Histology]

Chapter 2 classifies neoplasms primarily by site (topography), with broad groupings for behavior, malignant, in situ, benign, etc. The Table of Neoplasms should be used to identify the correct topography code. In a few cases, such as for malignant melanoma and certain neuroendocrine tumors, the morphology (histologic type) is included in the category and codes.

Primary malignant neoplasms overlapping site boundaries

A primary malignant neoplasm that overlaps two or more contiguous (next to each other) sites should be classified to the subcategory/code .8 ("overlapping lesion"), unless the combination is specifically indexed elsewhere. For multiple neoplasms of the same site that are not contiguous, such as tumors in different quadrants of the same breast, codes for each site should be assigned.

Malignant neoplasm of ectopic tissue

Malignant neoplasms of ectopic tissue are to be coded to the site mentioned, e.g., ectopic pancreatic malignant neoplasms are coded to pancreas, unspecified (C25.9).

MALIGNANT NEOPLASMS (C00-C96)

MALIGNANT NEOPLASMS, STATED OR PRESUMED TO BE PRIMARY (OF SPECIFIED SITES), AND CERTAIN SPECIFIED HISTOLOGIES, EXCEPT NEUROENDOCRINE, AND OF LYMPHOID, HEMATOPOIETIC AND RELATED TISSUE (C00-C75)

MALIGNANT NEOPLASMS OF LIP, ORAL CAVITY AND PHARYNX (C00-C14)

● **C00 Malignant neoplasm of lip**

Use additional code to identify:
- alcohol abuse and dependence (F10.-)
- history of tobacco dependence (Z87.891)
- tobacco dependence (F17.-)
- tobacco use (Z72.0)

Excludes1 malignant melanoma of lip (C43.0)
Merkel cell carcinoma of lip (C4A.0)
other and unspecified malignant neoplasm of skin of lip (C44.0-)

C00.0 Malignant neoplasm of external upper lip
Malignant neoplasm of lipstick area of upper lip
Malignant neoplasm of upper lip NOS
Malignant neoplasm of vermilion border of upper lip

C00.1 Malignant neoplasm of external lower lip
Malignant neoplasm of lower lip NOS
Malignant neoplasm of lipstick area of lower lip
Malignant neoplasm of vermilion border of lower lip

C00.2 Malignant neoplasm of external lip, unspecified
Malignant neoplasm of vermilion border of lip NOS

C00.3 Malignant neoplasm of upper lip, inner aspect
Malignant neoplasm of buccal aspect of upper lip
Malignant neoplasm of frenulum of upper lip
Malignant neoplasm of mucosa of upper lip
Malignant neoplasm of oral aspect of upper lip

C00.4 Malignant neoplasm of lower lip, inner aspect
Malignant neoplasm of buccal aspect of lower lip
Malignant neoplasm of frenulum of lower lip
Malignant neoplasm of mucosa of lower lip
Malignant neoplasm of oral aspect of lower lip

C00.5 Malignant neoplasm of lip, unspecified, inner aspect
Malignant neoplasm of buccal aspect of lip, unspecified
Malignant neoplasm of frenulum of lip, unspecified
Malignant neoplasm of mucosa of lip, unspecified
Malignant neoplasm of oral aspect of lip, unspecified

C00.6 Malignant neoplasm of commissure of lip, unspecified
Commissure: Site of union of corresponding parts

C00.8 Malignant neoplasm of overlapping sites of lip

C00.9 Malignant neoplasm of lip, unspecified

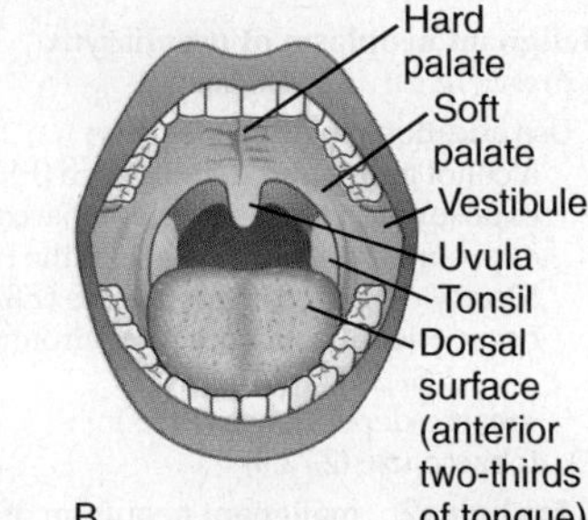

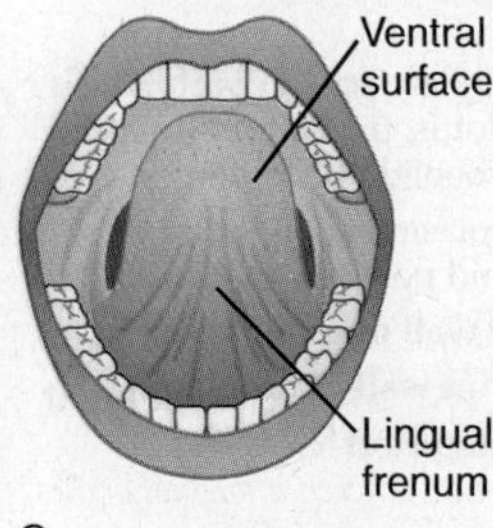

Figure 2-1 Anatomical structures of the mouth and lips. **A.** Transitional or vermilion borders. Lips are connected to the gums by frenulum. **B.** Dorsal surface. **C.** Ventral surface.

C01 Malignant neoplasm of base of tongue
Malignant neoplasm of dorsal surface of base of tongue
Malignant neoplasm of fixed part of tongue NOS
Malignant neoplasm of posterior third of tongue
Use additional code to identify:
alcohol abuse and dependence (F10.-)
history of tobacco dependence (Z87.891)
tobacco dependence (F17.-)
tobacco use (Z72.0)

● **C02 Malignant neoplasm of other and unspecified parts of tongue**
Use additional code to identify:
alcohol abuse and dependence (F10.-)
history of tobacco dependence (Z87.891)
tobacco dependence (F17.-)
tobacco use (Z72.0)

C02.0 Malignant neoplasm of dorsal surface of tongue
Malignant neoplasm of anterior two-thirds of tongue, dorsal surface
Excludes2 malignant neoplasm of dorsal surface of base of tongue (C01)

C02.1 Malignant neoplasm of border of tongue
Malignant neoplasm of tip of tongue

C02.2 Malignant neoplasm of ventral surface of tongue
Malignant neoplasm of anterior two-thirds of tongue, ventral surface
Malignant neoplasm of frenulum linguae

C02.3 Malignant neoplasm of anterior two-thirds of tongue, part unspecified
Malignant neoplasm of middle third of tongue NOS
Malignant neoplasm of mobile part of tongue NOS

C02.4 Malignant neoplasm of lingual tonsil
Lingual tonsil: Aggregation of lymph follicles at root of tongue
Excludes2 malignant neoplasm of tonsil NOS (C09.9)

C02.8 Malignant neoplasm of overlapping sites of tongue
Malignant neoplasm of two or more contiguous sites of tongue

C02.9 Malignant neoplasm of tongue, unspecified

● **C03 Malignant neoplasm of gum**
Includes malignant neoplasm of alveolar (ridge) mucosa
malignant neoplasm of gingiva
Use additional code to identify:
alcohol abuse and dependence (F10.-)
history of tobacco dependence (Z87.891)
tobacco dependence (F17.-)
tobacco use (Z72.0)
Excludes2 malignant odontogenic neoplasms (C41.0-C41.1)

C03.0 Malignant neoplasm of upper gum

C03.1 Malignant neoplasm of lower gum

C03.9 Malignant neoplasm of gum, unspecified

● **C04 Malignant neoplasm of floor of mouth**
Use additional code to identify:
alcohol abuse and dependence (F10.-)
history of tobacco dependence (Z87.891)
tobacco dependence (F17.-)
tobacco use (Z72.0)

C04.0 Malignant neoplasm of anterior floor of mouth
Malignant neoplasm of anterior to the premolar-canine junction

C04.1 Malignant neoplasm of lateral floor of mouth

C04.8 Malignant neoplasm of overlapping sites of floor of mouth

C04.9 Malignant neoplasm of floor of mouth, unspecified

● **C05 Malignant neoplasm of palate**
Use additional code to identify:
alcohol abuse and dependence (F10.-)
history of tobacco dependence (Z87.891)
tobacco dependence (F17.-)
tobacco use (Z72.0)
Excludes1 Kaposi's sarcoma of palate (C46.2)

C05.0 Malignant neoplasm of hard palate

C05.1 Malignant neoplasm of soft palate
Excludes2 malignant neoplasm of nasopharyngeal surface of soft palate (C11.3)

C05.2 Malignant neoplasm of uvula

C05.8 Malignant neoplasm of overlapping sites of palate

C05.9 Malignant neoplasm of palate, unspecified
Malignant neoplasm of roof of mouth

● **C06 Malignant neoplasm of other and unspecified parts of mouth**
Use additional code to identify:
alcohol abuse and dependence (F10.-)
history of tobacco dependence (Z87.891)
tobacco dependence (F17.-)
tobacco use (Z72.0)

C06.0 Malignant neoplasm of cheek mucosa
Malignant neoplasm of buccal mucosa NOS
Malignant neoplasm of internal cheek

C06.1 Malignant neoplasm of vestibule of mouth
Malignant neoplasm of buccal sulcus (upper) (lower)
Malignant neoplasm of labial sulcus (upper) (lower)

C06.2 Malignant neoplasm of retromolar area

● **C06.8 Malignant neoplasm of overlapping sites of other and unspecified parts of mouth**

C06.80 Malignant neoplasm of overlapping sites of unspecified parts of mouth

C06.89 Malignant neoplasm of overlapping sites of other parts of mouth
'book leaf' neoplasm [ventral surface of tongue and floor of mouth]

C06.9 Malignant neoplasm of mouth, unspecified
Malignant neoplasm of minor salivary gland, unspecified site
Malignant neoplasm of oral cavity NOS

CHAPTER 2 (C00-D49)

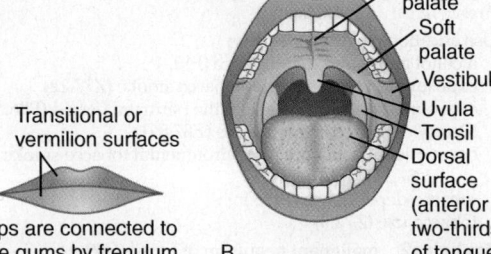

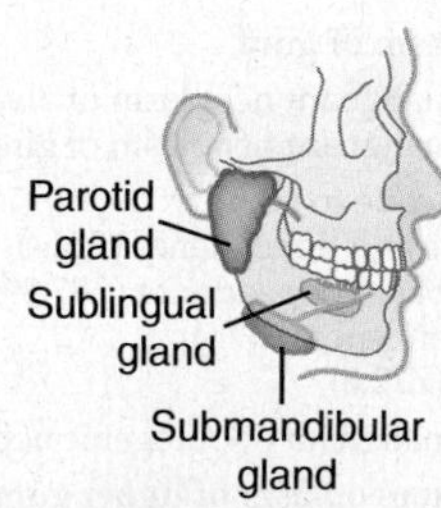

Figure 2-2 Major salivary glands.

C07 Malignant neoplasm of parotid gland
Use additional code to identify:
alcohol abuse and dependence (F10.-)
exposure to environmental tobacco smoke (Z77.22)
exposure to tobacco smoke in the perinatal period (P96.81)
history of tobacco dependence (Z87.891)
occupational exposure to environmental tobacco smoke (Z57.31)
tobacco dependence (F17.-)
tobacco use (Z72.0)

C08 Malignant neoplasm of other and unspecified major salivary glands
Includes malignant neoplasm of salivary ducts
Use additional code to identify:
alcohol abuse and dependence (F10.-)
exposure to environmental tobacco smoke (Z77.22)
exposure to tobacco smoke in the perinatal period (P96.81)
history of tobacco dependence (Z87.891)
occupational exposure to environmental tobacco smoke (Z57.31)
tobacco dependence (F17.-)
tobacco use (Z72.0)
Excludes1 malignant neoplasms of specified minor salivary glands which are classified according to their anatomical location
Excludes2 malignant neoplasms of minor salivary glands NOS (C06.9)
malignant neoplasm of parotid gland (C07)

C08.0 Malignant neoplasm of submandibular gland
Malignant neoplasm of submaxillary gland

C08.1 Malignant neoplasm of sublingual gland

C08.9 Malignant neoplasm of major salivary gland, unspecified
Malignant neoplasm of salivary gland (major) NOS

★**(See Plate 28 of the Anatomy Illustrations.)**

C09 Malignant neoplasm of tonsil
Use additional code to identify:
alcohol abuse and dependence (F10.-)
exposure to environmental tobacco smoke (Z77.22)
exposure to tobacco smoke in the perinatal period (P96.81)
history of tobacco dependence (Z87.891)
occupational exposure to environmental tobacco smoke (Z57.31)
tobacco dependence (F17.-)
tobacco use (Z72.0)
Excludes2 malignant neoplasm of lingual tonsil (C02.4)
malignant neoplasm of pharyngeal tonsil (C11.1)

C09.0 Malignant neoplasm of tonsillar fossa
Surface of palatine (two masses of lymphatic tissue on sides of throat) tonsils

C09.1 Malignant neoplasm of tonsillar pillar (anterior) (posterior)
Extension from palatine (two masses of lymphatic tissue on sides of throat) tonsils

C09.8 Malignant neoplasm of overlapping sites of tonsil

C09.9 Malignant neoplasm of tonsil, unspecified
Malignant neoplasm of tonsil NOS
Malignant neoplasm of faucial tonsils
Malignant neoplasm of palatine tonsils

C10 Malignant neoplasm of oropharynx
Area of throat at back of mouth
Use additional code to identify:
alcohol abuse and dependence (F10.-)
exposure to environmental tobacco smoke (Z77.22)
exposure to tobacco smoke in the perinatal period (P96.81)
history of tobacco dependence (Z87.891)
occupational exposure to environmental tobacco smoke (Z57.31)
tobacco dependence (F17.-)
tobacco use (Z72.0)
Excludes2 malignant neoplasm of tonsil (C09.-)

C10.0 Malignant neoplasm of vallecula
Vallecula, depression or furrow

C10.1 Malignant neoplasm of anterior surface of epiglottis
Malignant neoplasm of epiglottis, free border [margin]
Malignant neoplasm of glossoepiglottic fold(s)
Excludes2 malignant neoplasm of epiglottis (suprahyoid portion) NOS (C32.1)

C10.2 Malignant neoplasm of lateral wall of oropharynx

C10.3 Malignant neoplasm of posterior wall of oropharynx

C10.4 Malignant neoplasm of branchial cleft
Congenital slitlike openings formed between branchial arches pharyngeal groove
Malignant neoplasm of branchial cyst [site of neoplasm]

C10.8 Malignant neoplasm of overlapping sites of oropharynx
Malignant neoplasm of junctional region of oropharynx

C10.9 Malignant neoplasm of oropharynx, unspecified

C11 Malignant neoplasm of nasopharynx
Use additional code to identify:
exposure to environmental tobacco smoke (Z77.22)
exposure to tobacco smoke in the perinatal period (P96.81)
history of tobacco dependence (Z87.891)
occupational exposure to environmental tobacco smoke (Z57.31)
tobacco dependence (F17.-)
tobacco use (Z72.0)

C11.0 Malignant neoplasm of superior wall of nasopharynx
Part of pharynx that lies above soft palate
Malignant neoplasm of roof of nasopharynx

C11.1 Malignant neoplasm of posterior wall of nasopharynx
Malignant neoplasm of adenoid
Malignant neoplasm of pharyngeal tonsil

C11.2 Malignant neoplasm of lateral wall of nasopharynx
Malignant neoplasm of fossa of Rosenmüller
Malignant neoplasm of opening of auditory tube
Malignant neoplasm of pharyngeal recess

C11.3 Malignant neoplasm of anterior wall of nasopharynx
Malignant neoplasm of floor of nasopharynx
Malignant neoplasm of nasopharyngeal (anterior) (posterior) surface of soft palate
Malignant neoplasm of posterior margin of nasal choana
Malignant neoplasm of posterior margin of nasal septum

C11.8 Malignant neoplasm of overlapping sites of nasopharynx

C11.9 Malignant neoplasm of nasopharynx, unspecified
Malignant neoplasm of nasopharyngeal wall NOS

C12 Malignant neoplasm of pyriform sinus
Malignant neoplasm of pyriform fossa
Use additional code to identify:
exposure to environmental tobacco smoke (Z77.22)
exposure to tobacco smoke in the perinatal period (P96.81)
history of tobacco dependence (Z87.891)
occupational exposure to environmental tobacco smoke (Z57.31)
tobacco dependence (F17.-)
tobacco use (Z72.0)

C13 Malignant neoplasm of hypopharynx
Use additional code to identify:
exposure to environmental tobacco smoke (Z77.22)
exposure to tobacco smoke in the perinatal period (P96.81)
history of tobacco dependence (Z87.891)
occupational exposure to environmental tobacco smoke (Z57.31)
tobacco dependence (F17.-)
tobacco use (Z72.Ø)
Excludes2 malignant neoplasm of pyriform sinus (C12)

C13.Ø Malignant neoplasm of postcricoid region
Behind the cricoid cartilage of neck

C13.1 Malignant neoplasm of aryepiglottic fold, hypopharyngeal aspect
Arytenoepiglottic fold, triangular opening between side of epiglottis and apex of arytenoid cartilage
Malignant neoplasm of aryepiglottic fold, marginal zone
Malignant neoplasm of aryepiglottic fold NOS
Malignant neoplasm of interarytenoid fold, marginal zone
Malignant neoplasm of interarytenoid fold NOS
Excludes2 malignant neoplasm of aryepiglottic fold or interarytenoid fold, laryngeal aspect (C32.1)

C13.2 Malignant neoplasm of posterior wall of hypopharynx

C13.8 Malignant neoplasm of overlapping sites of hypopharynx

C13.9 Malignant neoplasm of hypopharynx, unspecified
Malignant neoplasm of hypopharyngeal wall NOS

C14 Malignant neoplasm of other and ill-defined sites in the lip, oral cavity and pharynx
Use additional code to identify:
alcohol abuse and dependence (F1Ø.-)
exposure to environmental tobacco smoke (Z77.22)
exposure to tobacco smoke in the perinatal period (P96.81)
history of tobacco dependence (Z87.891)
occupational exposure to environmental tobacco smoke (Z57.31)
tobacco dependence (F17.-)
tobacco use (Z72.Ø)
Excludes1 malignant neoplasm of oral cavity NOS (CØ6.9)

C14.Ø Malignant neoplasm of pharynx, unspecified

C14.2 Malignant neoplasm of Waldeyer's ring

C14.8 Malignant neoplasm of overlapping sites of lip, oral cavity and pharynx
Primary malignant neoplasm of two or more contiguous sites of lip, oral cavity and pharynx
Excludes1 'book leaf' neoplasm [ventral surface of tongue and floor of mouth] (CØ6.89)

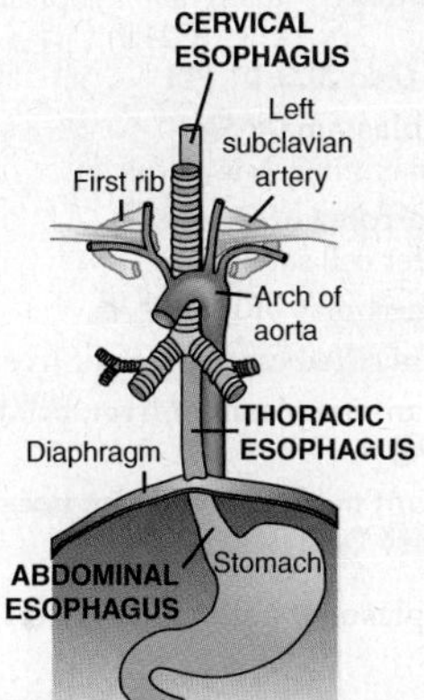

Figure 2-3 The esophagus is the muscular tube that connects the pharynx and the stomach. The 1Ø inch (25 cm) long esophagus is divided into three parts: **cervical, thoracic,** and **abdominal.**

MALIGNANT NEOPLASM OF DIGESTIVE ORGANS (C15-C26)

Excludes1 Kaposi's sarcoma of gastrointestinal sites (C46.4)
Excludes2 gastrointestinal stromal tumors (C49.A-)

C15 Malignant neoplasms of esophagus PDX 265
Use additional code to identify:
alcohol abuse and dependence (F1Ø.-)

C15.3 Malignant neoplasm of upper third of esophagus

C15.4 Malignant neoplasm of middle third of esophagus

C15.5 Malignant neoplasm of lower third of esophagus
Excludes1 malignant neoplasm of cardio-esophageal junction (C16.Ø)
Coding Clinic: 2022, Q3, P1Ø

C15.8 Malignant neoplasm of overlapping sites of esophagus

C15.9 Malignant neoplasm of esophagus, unspecified

C16 Malignant neoplasm of stomach PDX 266
Use additional code to identify:
alcohol abuse and dependence (F1Ø.-)
Excludes2 malignant carcinoid tumor of the stomach (C7A.Ø92)

C16.Ø Malignant neoplasm of cardia
Malignant neoplasm of cardiac orifice
Malignant neoplasm of cardio-esophageal junction
Malignant neoplasm of esophagus and stomach
Malignant neoplasm of gastro-esophageal junction

C16.1 Malignant neoplasm of fundus of stomach

C16.2 Malignant neoplasm of body of stomach

C16.3 Malignant neoplasm of pyloric antrum
Malignant neoplasm of gastric antrum

C16.4 Malignant neoplasm of pylorus
Malignant neoplasm of prepylorus
Malignant neoplasm of pyloric canal

C16.5 Malignant neoplasm of lesser curvature of stomach, unspecified
Malignant neoplasm of lesser curvature of stomach, not classifiable to C16.1-C16.4

C16.6 Malignant neoplasm of greater curvature of stomach, unspecified
Malignant neoplasm of greater curvature of stomach, not classifiable to C16.Ø-C16.4

C16.8 Malignant neoplasm of overlapping sites of stomach

C16.9 Malignant neoplasm of stomach, unspecified
Gastric cancer NOS

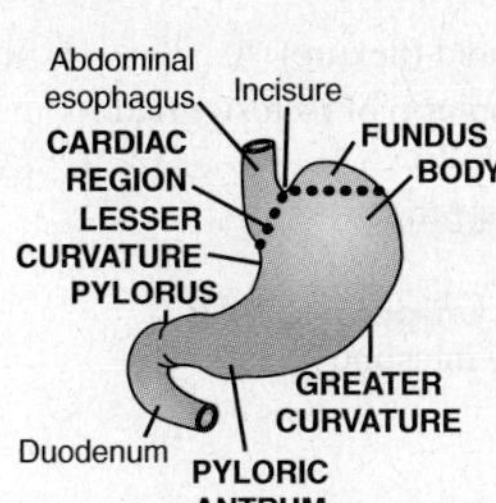

Figure 2-4 Parts of the stomach.

Item 2-2 The esophagus opens into the stomach through the **cardiac orifice,** also called the **cardioesophageal junction.** The **cardia** is adjacent to the cardiac orifice. The stomach widens into the **greater** and **lesser curvatures.** The **pyloric antrum** precedes the **pylorus,** which opens to the duodenum.

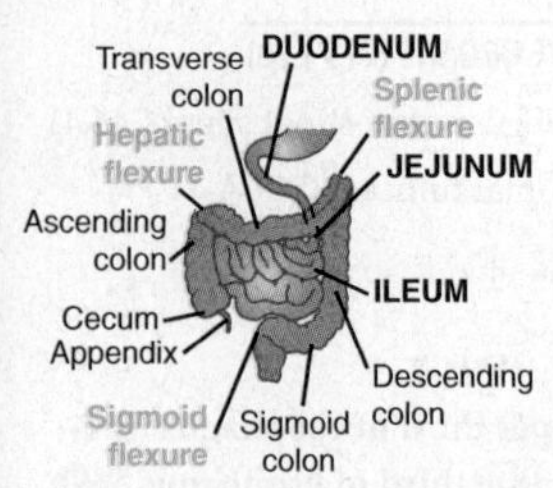

Figure 2-5 Small intestine and colon.

● **C17 Malignant neoplasm of small intestine**
Excludes1 malignant carcinoid tumor of the small intestine (C7A.Ø1)

C17.Ø Malignant neoplasm of duodenum Ex PDX 267
First or proximal portion of small intestine, extending from pylorus to jejunum

C17.1 Malignant neoplasm of jejunum Ex PDX 268
Second section of small intestine, extending from duodenum to ileum

C17.2 Malignant neoplasm of ileum Ex PDX 269
Distal and longest portion of small intestine, extending from jejunum to cecum
Excludes1 malignant neoplasm of ileocecal valve (C18.Ø)

C17.3 Meckel's diverticulum, malignant Ex PDX 270
Appendage of ileum
Excludes1 Meckel's diverticulum, congenital (Q43.Ø)

C17.8 Malignant neoplasm of overlapping sites of small intestine Ex PDX 271

C17.9 Malignant neoplasm of small intestine, unspecified Ex PDX 271

● **C18 Malignant neoplasm of colon**
Excludes1 malignant carcinoid tumors of the colon (C7A.Ø2)

C18.Ø Malignant neoplasm of cecum Ex PDX 272
First section of large intestine
Malignant neoplasm of ileocecal valve

C18.1 Malignant neoplasm of appendix Ex PDX 273
Blind ended tube connected to the cecum; AKA vermiform appendix

C18.2 Malignant neoplasm of ascending colon Ex PDX 274
Ascending colon is between cecum and right colic flexure

C18.3 Malignant neoplasm of hepatic flexure Ex PDX 275
A flexure is a bending in a structure or organ. Note the three flexures illustrated in Figure 2–5.

C18.4 Malignant neoplasm of transverse colon Ex PDX 276
Portion of colon that runs transversely across upper part of abdomen, between right and left colic flexures

C18.5 Malignant neoplasm of splenic flexure Ex PDX 277
Bend at junction of transverse and descending colon

C18.6 Malignant neoplasm of descending colon Ex PDX 278
Portion between left colic flexure and sigmoid colon at pelvic brim; AKA iliac colon

C18.7 Malignant neoplasm of sigmoid colon Ex PDX 279
S-shaped part of colon extending from pelvic brim to third segment of sacrum
Malignant neoplasm of sigmoid (flexure)
Excludes1 malignant neoplasm of rectosigmoid junction (C19)

C18.8 Malignant neoplasm of overlapping sites of colon Ex PDX 280

C18.9 Malignant neoplasm of colon, unspecified
Malignant neoplasm of large intestine NOS
Ex PDX 280

C19 Malignant neoplasm of rectosigmoid junction Ex PDX 281
Malignant neoplasm of colon with rectum
Malignant neoplasm of rectosigmoid (colon)
Excludes1 malignant carcinoid tumors of the colon (C7A.Ø2-)

C2Ø Malignant neoplasm of rectum Ex PDX 282
Malignant neoplasm of rectal ampulla
Excludes1 malignant carcinoid tumor of the rectum (C7A.Ø26)

● **C21 Malignant neoplasm of anus and anal canal**
Excludes2 malignant carcinoid tumors of the colon (C7A.Ø2-)
malignant melanoma of anal margin (C43.51)
malignant melanoma of anal skin (C43.51)
malignant melanoma of perianal skin (C43.51)
other and unspecified malignant neoplasm of anal margin (C44.5ØØ, C44.51Ø, C44.52Ø, C44.59Ø)
other and unspecified malignant neoplasm of anal skin (C44.5ØØ, C44.51Ø, C44.52Ø, C44.59Ø)
other and unspecified malignant neoplasm of perianal skin (C44.5ØØ, C44.51Ø, C44.52Ø, C44.59Ø)

C21.Ø Malignant neoplasm of anus, unspecified Ex PDX 283

C21.1 Malignant neoplasm of anal canal Ex PDX 283
Terminal part of large intestine
Malignant neoplasm of anal sphincter

C21.2 Malignant neoplasm of cloacogenic zone Ex PDX 284

C21.8 Malignant neoplasm of overlapping sites of rectum, anus and anal canal Ex PDX 284
Malignant neoplasm of anorectal junction
Malignant neoplasm of anorectum
Primary malignant neoplasm of two or more contiguous sites of rectum, anus and anal canal

● **C22 Malignant neoplasm of liver and intrahepatic bile ducts** Ex PDX 285
Intrahepatic: Within liver
Use additional code to identify:
alcohol abuse and dependence (F1Ø.-)
hepatitis B (B16.-, B18.Ø-B18.1) hepatitis C (B17.1-, B18.2)
Excludes1 malignant neoplasm of biliary tract NOS (C24.9)
secondary malignant neoplasm of liver and intrahepatic bile duct (C78.7)

C22.Ø Liver cell carcinoma
Hepatocellular carcinoma
Hepatoma

C22.1 Intrahepatic bile duct carcinoma
Cholangiocarcinoma
Adenocarcinoma (cancer that originates in glandular tissue) arising from epithelium of intrahepatic bile ducts
Excludes1 malignant neoplasm of hepatic duct (C24.Ø)
Coding Clinic: 2Ø23, Q1, P24

C22.2 Hepatoblastoma
Malignant intrahepatic tumor

C22.3 Angiosarcoma of liver
Kupffer cell sarcoma

C22.4 Other sarcomas of liver

C22.7 Other specified carcinomas of liver

C22.8 Malignant neoplasm of liver, primary, unspecified as to type

C22.9 Malignant neoplasm of liver, not specified as primary or secondary

C23 Malignant neoplasm of gallbladder Ex PDX 286

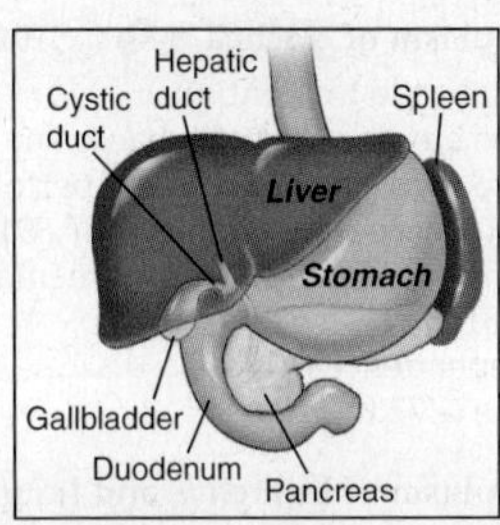

Figure 2-6 Diagram of liver, gallbladder, hepatic duct, pancreas, and spleen. (From Thibodeau and Patton: Anatomy and Physiology, ed 7, Mosby, 2010)

● C24 Malignant neoplasm of other and unspecified parts of biliary tract

Excludes1 malignant neoplasm of intrahepatic bile duct (C22.1)

C24.0 Malignant neoplasm of extrahepatic bile duct (Ex) PDX 287

Extrahepatic = outside the liver

Malignant neoplasm of biliary duct or passage NOS
Malignant neoplasm of common bile duct
Malignant neoplasm of cystic duct
Malignant neoplasm of hepatic duct

C24.1 Malignant neoplasm of ampulla of Vater (Ex) PDX 288

Union of pancreatic duct and common bile duct

C24.8 Malignant neoplasm of overlapping sites of biliary tract (Ex) PDX 289

Malignant neoplasm involving both intrahepatic and extrahepatic bile ducts
Primary malignant neoplasm of two or more contiguous sites of biliary tract

C24.9 Malignant neoplasm of biliary tract, unspecified (Ex) PDX 289

● C25 Malignant neoplasm of pancreas (Ex) PDX 290

Check documentation for specific site.

Code also if applicable exocrine pancreatic insufficiency (K86.81)

Use additional code to identify:
alcohol abuse and dependence (F10.-)

C25.0 Malignant neoplasm of head of pancreas

C25.1 Malignant neoplasm of body of pancreas

Coding Clinic: 2018, Q4, P40

C25.2 Malignant neoplasm of tail of pancreas

C25.3 Malignant neoplasm of pancreatic duct

C25.4 Malignant neoplasm of endocrine pancreas

Malignant neoplasm of islets of Langerhans

That part of the pancreas that acts as endocrine gland and consists of islets of Langerhans

Use additional code to identify any functional activity.

C25.7 Malignant neoplasm of other parts of pancreas

Malignant neoplasm of neck of pancreas

C25.8 Malignant neoplasm of overlapping sites of pancreas

C25.9 Malignant neoplasm of pancreas, unspecified

Item 2-3 Islets of Langerhans (endocrine producing cells comprising 1% to 2% of the pancreatic mass) make and secrete hormones that regulate the body's production of insulin, glucagon, and stomach acid. Breakdown of the insulin-producing cells can cause diabetes mellitus. Islet cell tumors can be benign or malignant and include glucagonomas, insulinomas, gastrinomas, and neuroendocrine tumor. The neoplasm table must be consulted for the correct neoplasm code.

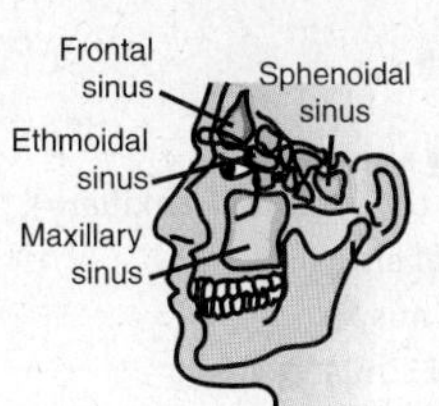

Figure 2-7 Paranasal sinuses. (From Buck CJ: Step-by-Step Medical Coding, ed 2016, St. Louis, Elsevier, 2016)

● C26 Malignant neoplasm of other and ill-defined digestive organs

Excludes1 malignant neoplasm of peritoneum and retroperitoneum (C48.-)

C26.0 Malignant neoplasm of intestinal tract, part unspecified

Malignant neoplasm of intestine NOS

C26.1 Malignant neoplasm of spleen

Excludes1 Hodgkin lymphoma (C81.-)
non-Hodgkin lymphoma (C82-C85)

C26.9 Malignant neoplasm of ill-defined sites within the digestive system

Malignant neoplasm of alimentary canal or tract NOS
Malignant neoplasm of gastrointestinal tract NOS

Excludes1 malignant neoplasm of abdominal NOS (C76.2)
malignant neoplasm of intra-abdominal NOS (C76.2)

MALIGNANT NEOPLASMS OF RESPIRATORY AND INTRATHORACIC ORGANS (C30-C39)

Includes malignant neoplasm of middle ear

Excludes1 mesothelioma (C45.-)

● C30 Malignant neoplasm of nasal cavity and middle ear

C30.0 Malignant neoplasm of nasal cavity

Malignant neoplasm of cartilage of nose
Malignant neoplasm of nasal concha
Malignant neoplasm of internal nose
Malignant neoplasm of septum of nose
Malignant neoplasm of vestibule of nose

Anterior part of nasal cavity

Excludes1 malignant neoplasm of nasal bone (C41.0)
malignant neoplasm of nose NOS (C76.0)
malignant neoplasm of olfactory bulb (C72.2-)
malignant neoplasm of posterior margin of nasal septum and choana (C11.3)
malignant melanoma of skin of nose (C43.31)
malignant neoplasm of turbinates (C41.0)
other and unspecified malignant neoplasm of skin of nose (C44.301, C44.311, C44.321, C44.391)

C30.1 Malignant neoplasm of middle ear

Malignant neoplasm of antrum tympanicum

Boney cavity or chamber

Malignant neoplasm of auditory tube
Malignant neoplasm of eustachian tube
Malignant neoplasm of inner ear
Malignant neoplasm of mastoid air cells
Malignant neoplasm of tympanic cavity

Excludes1 malignant neoplasm of auricular canal (external) (C43.2-, C44.2-)
malignant neoplasm of bone of ear (meatus) (C41.0)
malignant neoplasm of cartilage of ear (C49.0)
malignant melanoma of skin of (external) ear (C43.2-)
other and unspecified malignant neoplasm of skin of (external) ear (C44.2-)

CHAPTER 2 (C00-D49)

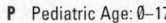

C31 Malignant neoplasm of accessory sinuses
Paired sinuses in bones of face
C31.Ø Malignant neoplasm of maxillary sinus
Malignant neoplasm of antrum (Highmore) (maxillary)
C31.1 Malignant neoplasm of ethmoidal sinus
C31.2 Malignant neoplasm of frontal sinus
C31.3 Malignant neoplasm of sphenoid sinus
C31.8 Malignant neoplasm of overlapping sites of accessory sinuses
C31.9 Malignant neoplasm of accessory sinus, unspecified

C32 Malignant neoplasm of larynx
Use additional code to identify:
alcohol abuse and dependence (F1Ø.-)
exposure to environmental tobacco smoke (Z77.22)
exposure to tobacco smoke in the perinatal period (P96.81)
history of tobacco dependence (Z87.891)
occupational exposure to environmental tobacco smoke (Z57.31)
tobacco dependence (F17.-)
tobacco use (Z72.Ø)
C32.Ø Malignant neoplasm of glottis
Vocal apparatus of larynx, consisting of true vocal cords (plicae vocales) and opening between them (rima glottidis)
Malignant neoplasm of intrinsic larynx
Malignant neoplasm of laryngeal commissure (anterior) (posterior)
Malignant neoplasm of vocal cord (true) NOS
True vocal cords ("lower vocal folds") produce vocalization when air from the lungs passes between them. Check your documentation. Code C32.1 is for malignant neoplasm of the false vocal cords.
C32.1 Malignant neoplasm of supraglottis
Area of pharynx above glottis
Malignant neoplasm of aryepiglottic fold or interarytenoid fold, laryngeal aspect
Malignant neoplasm of epiglottis (suprahyoid portion) NOS
Malignant neoplasm of extrinsic larynx
Malignant neoplasm of false vocal cord
False vocal cords ("upper vocal folds") are not involved in vocalization. Check your documentation. Code C32.Ø is for true vocal cords.
Malignant neoplasm of posterior (laryngeal) surface of epiglottis
Malignant neoplasm of ventricular bands
Excludes2 malignant neoplasm of anterior surface of epiglottis (C1Ø.1)
malignant neoplasm of aryepiglottic fold or interarytenoid fold, hypopharyngeal aspect (C13.1)
malignant neoplasm of aryepiglottic fold or interarytenoid fold, marginal zone (C13.1)
malignant neoplasm of aryepiglottic fold or interarytenoid fold NOS (C13.1)
C32.2 Malignant neoplasm of subglottis
Lowest part of larynx from just below vocal cords down to top of trachea
C32.3 Malignant neoplasm of laryngeal cartilage
Cartilages of larynx, including cricoid, thyroid, and epiglottic, and two each of arytenoid, corniculate, and cuneiform
C32.8 Malignant neoplasm of overlapping sites of larynx
C32.9 Malignant neoplasm of larynx, unspecified

C33 Malignant neoplasm of trachea PDX 291
Use additional code to identify:
exposure to environmental tobacco smoke (Z77.22)
exposure to tobacco smoke in the perinatal period (P96.81)
history of tobacco dependence (Z87.891)
occupational exposure to environmental tobacco smoke (Z57.31)
tobacco dependence (F17.-)
tobacco use (Z72.Ø)

C34 Malignant neoplasm of bronchus and lung
Use additional code to identify:
exposure to environmental tobacco smoke (Z77.22)
exposure to tobacco smoke in the perinatal period (P96.81)
history of tobacco dependence (Z87.891)
occupational exposure to environmental tobacco smoke (Z57.31)
tobacco dependence (F17.-)
tobacco use (Z72.Ø)
Excludes1 Kaposi's sarcoma of lung (C46.5-)
malignant carcinoid tumor of the bronchus and lung (C7A.Ø9Ø)
Coding Clinic: 2Ø23, Q1, P2Ø
C34.Ø Malignant neoplasm of main bronchus PDX 292
Malignant neoplasm of carina
Ridgelike structure
Malignant neoplasm of hilus (of lung)
Anatomic depression or pit
C34.ØØ Malignant neoplasm of unspecified main bronchus
C34.Ø1 Malignant neoplasm of right main bronchus
C34.Ø2 Malignant neoplasm of left main bronchus
C34.1 Malignant neoplasm of upper lobe, bronchus or lung PDX 293
C34.1Ø Malignant neoplasm of unspecified bronchus or lung
C34.11 Malignant neoplasm of upper lobe, right bronchus or lung
C34.12 Malignant neoplasm of upper lobe, left bronchus or lung
C34.2 Malignant neoplasm of middle lobe, bronchus or lung PDX 294
C34.3 Malignant neoplasm of lower lobe, bronchus or lung PDX 295
C34.3Ø Malignant neoplasm of lower lobe, unspecified bronchus or lung
C34.31 Malignant neoplasm of lower lobe, right bronchus or lung
C34.32 Malignant neoplasm of lower lobe, left bronchus or lung
C34.8 Malignant neoplasm of overlapping sites of bronchus and lung PDX 296
C34.8Ø Malignant neoplasm of overlapping sites of unspecified bronchus and lung
C34.81 Malignant neoplasm of overlapping sites of right bronchus and lung
C34.82 Malignant neoplasm of overlapping sites of left bronchus and lung
C34.9 Malignant neoplasm of unspecified part of bronchus or lung PDX 296
C34.9Ø Malignant neoplasm of unspecified part of unspecified bronchus or lung
Lung cancer NOS
Coding Clinic: 2Ø22, Q4, P23
C34.91 Malignant neoplasm of unspecified part of right bronchus or lung
C34.92 Malignant neoplasm of unspecified part of left bronchus or lung

C37 Malignant neoplasm of thymus PDX 297
Excludes1 malignant carcinoid tumor of the thymus (C7A.Ø91)

C38 Malignant neoplasm of heart, mediastinum and pleura Ex PDX 299
Excludes1 mesothelioma (C45.-)
C38.0 **Malignant neoplasm of heart** Ex PDX 298
Malignant neoplasm of pericardium
Excludes1 malignant neoplasm of great vessels (C49.3)
C38.1 **Malignant neoplasm of anterior mediastinum**
C38.2 **Malignant neoplasm of posterior mediastinum**
C38.3 **Malignant neoplasm of mediastinum, part unspecified**
C38.4 **Malignant neoplasm of pleura** Ex PDX 300
C38.8 **Malignant neoplasm of overlapping sites of heart, mediastinum and pleura**
Pleura are comprised of serous membrane that lines the thoracic cavity (parietal) and covers the lungs (visceral).

C39 Malignant neoplasm of other and ill-defined sites in the respiratory system and intrathoracic organs
Intrathoracic: within thorax/chest
Use additional code to identify:
exposure to environmental tobacco smoke (Z77.22)
exposure to tobacco smoke in the perinatal period (P96.81)
history of tobacco dependence (Z87.891)
occupational exposure to environmental tobacco smoke (Z57.31)
tobacco dependence (F17.-)
tobacco use (Z72.0)
Excludes1 intrathoracic malignant neoplasm NOS (C76.1)
thoracic malignant neoplasm NOS (C76.1)
C39.0 **Malignant neoplasm of upper respiratory tract, part unspecified**
C39.9 **Malignant neoplasm of lower respiratory tract, part unspecified**
Malignant neoplasm of respiratory tract NOS

MALIGNANT NEOPLASMS OF BONE AND ARTICULAR CARTILAGE (C40-C41)

Includes malignant neoplasm of cartilage (articular) (joint)
malignant neoplasm of periosteum
Excludes1 malignant neoplasm of bone marrow NOS (C96.9)
malignant neoplasm of synovia (C49.-)

C40 Malignant neoplasm of bone and articular cartilage of limbs
Use additional code to identify major osseous defect, if applicable (M89.7-)
C40.0 Malignant neoplasm of scapula and long bones of upper limb Ex PDX 301
C40.00 **Malignant neoplasm of scapula and long bones of unspecified upper limb**
C40.01 **Malignant neoplasm of scapula and long bones of right upper limb**
C40.02 **Malignant neoplasm of scapula and long bones of left upper limb**
C40.1 Malignant neoplasm of short bones of upper limb Ex PDX 302
C40.10 **Malignant neoplasm of short bones of unspecified upper limb**
C40.11 **Malignant neoplasm of short bones of right upper limb**
C40.12 **Malignant neoplasm of short bones of left upper limb**

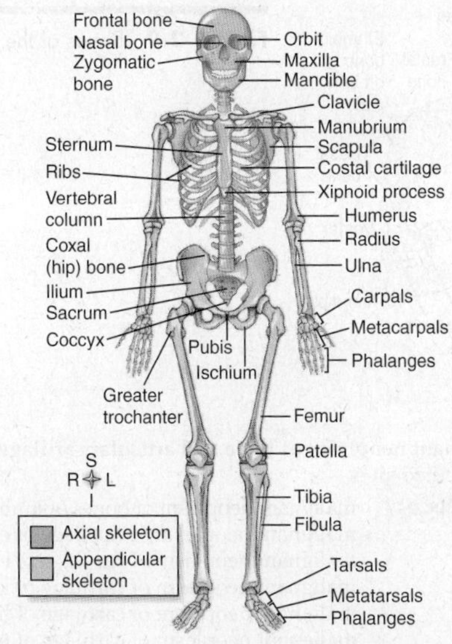

Figure 2-8 Diagram of skeleton of trunk and limbs with bones labeled. (From Thibodeau and Patton: Anatomy and Physiology, ed 7, Mosby, 2010)

C40.2 Malignant neoplasm of long bones of lower limb Ex PDX 303
C40.20 **Malignant neoplasm of long bones of unspecified lower limb**
C40.21 **Malignant neoplasm of long bones of right lower limb**
C40.22 **Malignant neoplasm of long bones of left lower limb**
C40.3 Malignant neoplasm of short bones of lower limb Ex PDX 304
C40.30 **Malignant neoplasm of short bones of unspecified lower limb**
C40.31 **Malignant neoplasm of short bones of right lower limb**
C40.32 **Malignant neoplasm of short bones of left lower limb**
C40.8 Malignant neoplasm of overlapping sites of bone and articular cartilage of limb Ex PDX 305
C40.80 **Malignant neoplasm of overlapping sites of bone and articular cartilage of unspecified limb**
C40.81 **Malignant neoplasm of overlapping sites of bone and articular cartilage of right limb**
C40.82 **Malignant neoplasm of overlapping sites of bone and articular cartilage of left limb**
C40.9 Malignant neoplasm of unspecified bones and articular cartilage of limb Ex PDX 305
C40.90 **Malignant neoplasm of unspecified bones and articular cartilage of unspecified limb**
C40.91 **Malignant neoplasm of unspecified bones and articular cartilage of right limb**
C40.92 **Malignant neoplasm of unspecified bones and articular cartilage of left limb**

CHAPTER 2 (C00-D49)

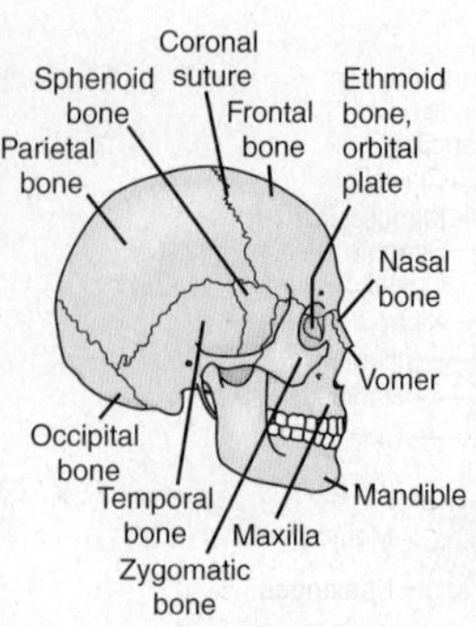

Figure 2-9 Bones of the skull.

● **C41 Malignant neoplasm of bone and articular cartilage of other and unspecified sites**

Excludes1 malignant neoplasm of bones of limbs (C40.-)
malignant neoplasm of cartilage of ear (C49.0)
malignant neoplasm of cartilage of eyelid (C49.0)
malignant neoplasm of cartilage of larynx (C32.3)
malignant neoplasm of cartilage of limbs (C40.-)
malignant neoplasm of cartilage of nose (C30.0)

C41.0 **Malignant neoplasm of bones of skull and face** (Ex) PDX 306
Malignant neoplasm of maxilla (superior)
Malignant neoplasm of orbital bone
Excludes2 carcinoma, any type except intraosseous or odontogenic of:
maxillary sinus (C31.0)
upper jaw (C03.0)
malignant neoplasm of jaw bone (lower) (C41.1)

C41.1 **Malignant neoplasm of mandible** (Ex) PDX 307
Malignant neoplasm of inferior maxilla
Malignant neoplasm of lower jaw bone
Excludes2 carcinoma, any type except intraosseous or odontogenic of:
jaw NOS (C03.9)
lower (C03.1)
malignant neoplasm of upper jaw bone (C41.0)

C41.2 **Malignant neoplasm of vertebral column** (Ex) PDX 308
Excludes1 malignant neoplasm of sacrum and coccyx (C41.4)

C41.3 **Malignant neoplasm of ribs, sternum and clavicle** (Ex) PDX 309

C41.4 **Malignant neoplasm of pelvic bones, sacrum and coccyx** (Ex) PDX 310

C41.9 **Malignant neoplasm of bone and articular cartilage, unspecified** (Ex) PDX 305

MELANOMA AND OTHER MALIGNANT NEOPLASMS OF SKIN (C43-C44)

● **C43 Malignant melanoma of skin**

Excludes1 melanoma in situ (D03.-)
Excludes2 malignant melanoma of skin of genital organs (C51-C52, C60.-, C63.-)
Merkel cell carcinoma (C4A.-)
sites other than skin-code to malignant neoplasm of the site

C43.0 **Malignant melanoma of lip**
Excludes1 malignant neoplasm of vermilion border of lip (C00.0-C00.2)

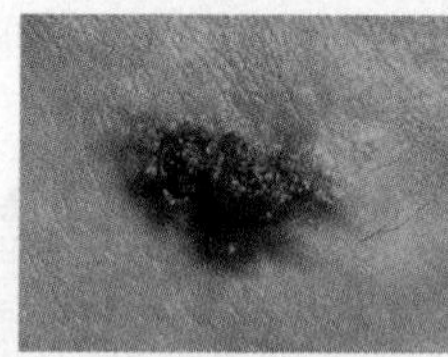

Figure 2-10 Malignant melanoma of skin. (Getty Image)

Item 2-4 Malignant melanoma is a serious form of skin cancer that affects the melanocytes (pigment-forming cells) and is caused by ultraviolet (UV) rays from the sun that damage skin. It is most commonly seen in the 40- to 60-year-olds with fair skin, blue or green eyes, and red or blond hair who sunburn easily.

Melanoma can spread very rapidly and is the most deadly form of skin cancer. It is less common than other types of skin cancer. The rate of melanoma is increasing and currently is the leading cause of death from skin disease.

● C43.1 **Malignant melanoma of eyelid, including canthus**
Canthus: Either corner of eye where upper and lower eyelids meet
C43.10 **Malignant melanoma of unspecified eyelid, including canthus**
● C43.11 **Malignant melanoma of right eyelid, including canthus**
C43.111 **Malignant melanoma of right upper eyelid, including canthus**
C43.112 **Malignant melanoma of right lower eyelid, including canthus**
● C43.12 **Malignant melanoma of left eyelid, including canthus**
C43.121 **Malignant melanoma of left upper eyelid, including canthus**
C43.122 **Malignant melanoma of left lower eyelid, including canthus**

● C43.2 **Malignant melanoma of ear and external auricular canal**
C43.20 **Malignant melanoma of unspecified ear and external auricular canal**
C43.21 **Malignant melanoma of right ear and external auricular canal**
C43.22 **Malignant melanoma of left ear and external auricular canal**

● C43.3 **Malignant melanoma of other and unspecified parts of face**
C43.30 **Malignant melanoma of unspecified part of face**
C43.31 **Malignant melanoma of nose**
C43.39 **Malignant melanoma of other parts of face**

C43.4 **Malignant melanoma of scalp and neck**

● C43.5 **Malignant melanoma of trunk**
Excludes2 malignant neoplasm of anus NOS (C21.0)
malignant neoplasm of scrotum (C63.2)
C43.51 **Malignant melanoma of anal skin**
Malignant melanoma of anal margin
Malignant melanoma of perianal skin
C43.52 **Malignant melanoma of skin of breast**
C43.59 **Malignant melanoma of other part of trunk**

● C43.6 **Malignant melanoma of upper limb, including shoulder**
C43.60 **Malignant melanoma of upper limb, including shoulder, unspecified side**
C43.61 **Malignant melanoma of right upper limb, including shoulder**
C43.62 **Malignant melanoma of left upper limb, including shoulder**

- **C43.7 Malignant melanoma of lower limb, including hip**
  - **C43.70 Malignant melanoma of unspecified lower limb, including hip**
  - **C43.71 Malignant melanoma of right lower limb, including hip**
  - **C43.72 Malignant melanoma of left lower limb, including hip**
- **C43.8 Malignant melanoma of overlapping sites of skin**
- **C43.9 Malignant melanoma of skin, unspecified**
  - Malignant melanoma of unspecified site of skin
  - Melanoma (malignant) NOS

C44 Other and unspecified malignant neoplasm of skin

Includes malignant neoplasm of sebaceous glands
malignant neoplasm of sweat glands

Excludes1 Kaposi's sarcoma of skin (C46.Ø)
malignant melanoma of skin (C43.-)
malignant neoplasm of skin of genital organs (C51-C52, C6Ø.-, C63.2)
Merkel cell carcinoma (C4A.-)

- **C44.Ø Other and unspecified malignant neoplasm of skin of lip**
  - **Excludes1** malignant neoplasm of lip (CØØ.-)
  - **C44.ØØ Unspecified malignant neoplasm of skin of lip**
  - **C44.Ø1 Basal cell carcinoma of skin of lip**
  - **C44.Ø2 Squamous cell carcinoma of skin of lip**
  - **C44.Ø9 Other specified malignant neoplasm of skin of lip**
- **C44.1 Other and unspecified malignant neoplasm of skin of eyelid, including canthus**
  - **Excludes1** connective tissue of eyelid (C49.Ø)
  - **C44.1Ø Unspecified malignant neoplasm of skin of eyelid, including canthus**
    - **C44.1Ø1 Unspecified malignant neoplasm of skin of unspecified eyelid, including canthus**
    - **C44.1Ø2 Unspecified malignant neoplasm of skin of right eyelid, including canthus**
      - **C44.1Ø21 Unspecified malignant neoplasm of skin of right upper eyelid, including canthus**
      - **C44.1Ø22 Unspecified malignant neoplasm of skin of right lower eyelid, including canthus**
    - **C44.1Ø9 Unspecified malignant neoplasm of skin of left eyelid, including canthus**
      - **C44.1Ø91 Unspecified malignant neoplasm of skin of left upper eyelid, including canthus**
      - **C44.1Ø92 Unspecified malignant neoplasm of skin of left lower eyelid, including canthus**
  - **C44.11 Basal cell carcinoma of skin of eyelid, including canthus**
    - **C44.111 Basal cell carcinoma of skin of unspecified eyelid, including canthus**
    - **C44.112 Basal cell carcinoma of skin of right eyelid, including canthus**
      - **C44.1121 Basal cell carcinoma of skin of right upper eyelid, including canthus**
      - **C44.1122 Basal cell carcinoma of skin of right lower eyelid, including canthus**
    - **C44.119 Basal cell carcinoma of skin of left eyelid, including canthus**
      - **C44.1191 Basal cell carcinoma of skin of left upper eyelid, including canthus**
      - **C44.1192 Basal cell carcinoma of skin of left lower eyelid, including canthus**
  - **C44.12 Squamous cell carcinoma of skin of eyelid, including canthus**
    - **C44.121 Squamous cell carcinoma of skin of unspecified eyelid, including canthus**
    - **C44.122 Squamous cell carcinoma of skin of right eyelid, including canthus**
      - **C44.1221 Squamous cell carcinoma of skin of right upper eyelid, including canthus**
      - **C44.1222 Squamous cell carcinoma of skin of right lower eyelid, including canthus**
    - **C44.129 Squamous cell carcinoma of skin of left eyelid, including canthus**
      - **C44.1291 Squamous cell carcinoma of skin of left upper eyelid, including canthus**
      - **C44.1292 Squamous cell carcinoma of skin of left lower eyelid, including canthus**
  - **C44.13 Sebaceous cell carcinoma of skin of eyelid, including canthus**
    - **C44.131 Sebaceous cell carcinoma of skin of unspecified eyelid, including canthus**
    - **C44.132 Sebaceous cell carcinoma of skin of right eyelid, including canthus**
      - **C44.1321 Sebaceous cell carcinoma of skin of right upper eyelid, including canthus**
      - **C44.1322 Sebaceous cell carcinoma of skin of right lower eyelid, including canthus**
    - **C44.139 Sebaceous cell carcinoma of skin of left eyelid, including canthus**
      - **C44.1391 Sebaceous cell carcinoma of skin of left upper eyelid, including canthus**
      - **C44.1392 Sebaceous cell carcinoma of skin of left lower eyelid, including canthus**
  - **C44.19 Other specified malignant neoplasm of skin of eyelid, including canthus**
    - **C44.191 Other specified malignant neoplasm of skin of unspecified eyelid, including canthus**
    - **C44.192 Other specified malignant neoplasm of skin of right eyelid, including canthus**
      - **C44.1921 Other specified malignant neoplasm of skin of right upper eyelid, including canthus**
      - **C44.1922 Other specified malignant neoplasm of skin of right lower eyelid, including canthus**

CHAPTER 2 (CØØ-D49)

- C44.199 **Other specified malignant neoplasm of skin of left eyelid, including canthus**
  - C44.1991 **Other specified malignant neoplasm of skin of left upper eyelid, including canthus**
  - C44.1992 **Other specified malignant neoplasm of skin of left lower eyelid, including canthus**
- C44.2 **Other and unspecified malignant neoplasm of skin of ear and external auricular canal**
  - **Excludes1** connective tissue of ear (C49.Ø)
  - C44.2Ø **Unspecified malignant neoplasm of skin of ear and external auricular canal**
    - C44.2Ø1 **Unspecified malignant neoplasm of skin of unspecified ear and external auricular canal**
    - C44.2Ø2 **Unspecified malignant neoplasm of skin of right ear and external auricular canal**
    - C44.2Ø9 **Unspecified malignant neoplasm of skin of left ear and external auricular canal**
  - C44.21 **Basal cell carcinoma of skin of ear and external auricular canal**
    - C44.211 **Basal cell carcinoma of skin of unspecified ear and external auricular canal**
    - C44.212 **Basal cell carcinoma of skin of right ear and external auricular canal**
    - C44.219 **Basal cell carcinoma of skin of left ear and external auricular canal**
  - C44.22 **Squamous cell carcinoma of skin of ear and external auricular canal**
    - C44.221 **Squamous cell carcinoma of skin of unspecified ear and external auricular canal**
    - C44.222 **Squamous cell carcinoma of skin of right ear and external auricular canal**
    - C44.229 **Squamous cell carcinoma of skin of left ear and external auricular canal**
  - C44.29 **Other specified malignant neoplasm of skin of ear and external auricular canal**
    - C44.291 **Other specified malignant neoplasm of skin of unspecified ear and external auricular canal**
    - C44.292 **Other specified malignant neoplasm of skin of right ear and external auricular canal**
    - C44.299 **Other specified malignant neoplasm of skin of left ear and external auricular canal**
- C44.3 **Other and unspecified malignant neoplasm of skin of other and unspecified parts of face**
  - C44.3Ø **Unspecified malignant neoplasm of skin of other and unspecified parts of face**
    - C44.3ØØ **Unspecified malignant neoplasm of skin of unspecified part of face**
    - C44.3Ø1 **Unspecified malignant neoplasm of skin of nose**
    - C44.3Ø9 **Unspecified malignant neoplasm of skin of other parts of face**
  - C44.31 **Basal cell carcinoma of skin of other and unspecified parts of face**
    - C44.31Ø **Basal cell carcinoma of skin of unspecified parts of face**
    - C44.311 **Basal cell carcinoma of skin of nose**
    - C44.319 **Basal cell carcinoma of skin of other parts of face**
      - Coding Clinic: 2017, Q1, P4
  - C44.32 **Squamous cell carcinoma of skin of other and unspecified parts of face**
    - C44.32Ø **Squamous cell carcinoma of skin of unspecified parts of face**
    - C44.321 **Squamous cell carcinoma of skin of nose**
    - C44.329 **Squamous cell carcinoma of skin of other parts of face**
  - C44.39 **Other specified malignant neoplasm of skin of other and unspecified parts of face**
    - C44.39Ø **Other specified malignant neoplasm of skin of unspecified parts of face**
    - C44.391 **Other specified malignant neoplasm of skin of nose**
    - C44.399 **Other specified malignant neoplasm of skin of other parts of face**
- C44.4 **Other and unspecified malignant neoplasm of skin of scalp and neck**
  - C44.4Ø **Unspecified malignant neoplasm of skin of scalp and neck**
  - C44.41 **Basal cell carcinoma of skin of scalp and neck**
  - C44.42 **Squamous cell carcinoma of skin of scalp and neck**
  - C44.49 **Other specified malignant neoplasm of skin of scalp and neck**
- C44.5 **Other and unspecified malignant neoplasm of skin of trunk**
  - **Excludes1** anus NOS (C21.Ø)
    scrotum (C63.2)
  - C44.5Ø **Unspecified malignant neoplasm of skin of trunk**
    - C44.5ØØ **Unspecified malignant neoplasm of anal skin**
      - Unspecified malignant neoplasm of anal margin
      - Unspecified malignant neoplasm of perianal skin
    - C44.5Ø1 **Unspecified malignant neoplasm of skin of breast**
    - C44.5Ø9 **Unspecified malignant neoplasm of skin of other part of trunk**
  - C44.51 **Basal cell carcinoma of skin of trunk**
    - C44.51Ø **Basal cell carcinoma of anal skin**
      - Basal cell carcinoma of anal margin
      - Basal cell carcinoma of perianal skin
    - C44.511 **Basal cell carcinoma of skin of breast**
    - C44.519 **Basal cell carcinoma of skin of other part of trunk**
  - C44.52 **Squamous cell carcinoma of skin of trunk**
    - C44.52Ø **Squamous cell carcinoma of anal skin**
      - Squamous cell carcinoma of anal margin
      - Squamous cell carcinoma of perianal skin
    - C44.521 **Squamous cell carcinoma of skin of breast**
    - C44.529 **Squamous cell carcinoma of skin of other part of trunk**
  - C44.59 **Other specified malignant neoplasm of skin of trunk**
    - C44.59Ø **Other specified malignant neoplasm of anal skin**
      - Other specified malignant neoplasm of anal margin
      - Other specified malignant neoplasm of perianal skin
    - C44.591 **Other specified malignant neoplasm of skin of breast**
    - C44.599 **Other specified malignant neoplasm of skin of other part of trunk**

● C44.6 Other and unspecified malignant neoplasm of skin of upper limb, including shoulder
● C44.60 Unspecified malignant neoplasm of skin of upper limb, including shoulder
C44.601 Unspecified malignant neoplasm of skin of unspecified upper limb, including shoulder
C44.602 Unspecified malignant neoplasm of skin of right upper limb, including shoulder
C44.609 Unspecified malignant neoplasm of skin of left upper limb, including shoulder
● C44.61 Basal cell carcinoma of skin of upper limb, including shoulder
C44.611 Basal cell carcinoma of skin of unspecified upper limb, including shoulder
C44.612 Basal cell carcinoma of skin of right upper limb, including shoulder
C44.619 Basal cell carcinoma of skin of left upper limb, including shoulder
● C44.62 Squamous cell carcinoma of skin of upper limb, including shoulder
C44.621 Squamous cell carcinoma of skin of unspecified upper limb, including shoulder
C44.622 Squamous cell carcinoma of skin of right upper limb, including shoulder
C44.629 Squamous cell carcinoma of skin of left upper limb, including shoulder
● C44.69 Other specified malignant neoplasm of skin of upper limb, including shoulder
C44.691 Other specified malignant neoplasm of skin of unspecified upper limb, including shoulder
C44.692 Other specified malignant neoplasm of skin of right upper limb, including shoulder
C44.699 Other specified malignant neoplasm of skin of left upper limb, including shoulder
● C44.7 Other and unspecified malignant neoplasm of skin of lower limb, including hip
● C44.70 Unspecified malignant neoplasm of skin of lower limb, including hip
C44.701 Unspecified malignant neoplasm of skin of unspecified lower limb, including hip
C44.702 Unspecified malignant neoplasm of skin of right lower limb, including hip
C44.709 Unspecified malignant neoplasm of skin of left lower limb, including hip
● C44.71 Basal cell carcinoma of skin of lower limb, including hip
C44.711 Basal cell carcinoma of skin of unspecified lower limb, including hip
C44.712 Basal cell carcinoma of skin of right lower limb, including hip
C44.719 Basal cell carcinoma of skin of left lower limb, including hip
● C44.72 Squamous cell carcinoma of skin of lower limb, including hip
C44.721 Squamous cell carcinoma of skin of unspecified lower limb, including hip
C44.722 Squamous cell carcinoma of skin of right lower limb, including hip
C44.729 Squamous cell carcinoma of skin of left lower limb, including hip
● C44.79 Other specified malignant neoplasm of skin of lower limb, including hip
C44.791 Other specified malignant neoplasm of skin of unspecified lower limb, including hip
C44.792 Other specified malignant neoplasm of skin of right lower limb, including hip
C44.799 Other specified malignant neoplasm of skin of left lower limb, including hip
● C44.8 Other and unspecified malignant neoplasm of overlapping sites of skin
C44.80 Unspecified malignant neoplasm of overlapping sites of skin
C44.81 Basal cell carcinoma of overlapping sites of skin
C44.82 Squamous cell carcinoma of overlapping sites of skin
C44.89 Other specified malignant neoplasm of overlapping sites of skin
● C44.9 Other and unspecified malignant neoplasm of skin, unspecified
C44.90 Unspecified malignant neoplasm of skin, unspecified
Malignant neoplasm of unspecified site of skin
C44.91 Basal cell carcinoma of skin, unspecified
C44.92 Squamous cell carcinoma of skin, unspecified
C44.99 Other specified malignant neoplasm of skin, unspecified

MALIGNANT NEOPLASMS OF MESOTHELIAL AND SOFT TISSUE (C45-C49)

● C45 Mesothelioma
Malignant cells develop in protective lining that covers internal organs (mesothelium) caused by exposure to asbestos
C45.0 Mesothelioma of pleura (Ex) PDX 300
Excludes1 other malignant neoplasm of pleura (C38.4)
Coding Clinic: 2017, Q2, P11
C45.1 Mesothelioma of peritoneum (Ex) PDX 311
Mesothelioma of cul-de-sac
Mesothelioma of mesentery
Mesothelioma of mesocolon
Mesothelioma of omentum
Mesothelioma of peritoneum (parietal) (pelvic)
Excludes1 other malignant neoplasm of soft tissue of peritoneum (C48.-)
C45.2 Mesothelioma of pericardium (Ex) PDX 298
Excludes1 other malignant neoplasm of pericardium (C38.0)
C45.7 Mesothelioma of other sites
C45.9 Mesothelioma, unspecified
● C46 Kaposi's sarcoma
Code first any human immunodeficiency virus [HIV] disease (B20)
C46.0 Kaposi's sarcoma of skin (Ex) PDX 312
C46.1 Kaposi's sarcoma of soft tissue (Ex) PDX 313
Kaposi's sarcoma of blood vessel
Kaposi's sarcoma of connective tissue
Kaposi's sarcoma of fascia
Kaposi's sarcoma of ligament
Kaposi's sarcoma of lymphatic(s) NEC
Kaposi's sarcoma of muscle
Excludes2 Kaposi's sarcoma of lymph glands and nodes (C46.3)
C46.2 Kaposi's sarcoma of palate (Ex) PDX 314
C46.3 Kaposi's sarcoma of lymph nodes (Ex) PDX 315
C46.4 Kaposi's sarcoma of gastrointestinal sites (Ex) PDX 316

CHAPTER 2 (C00-D49)

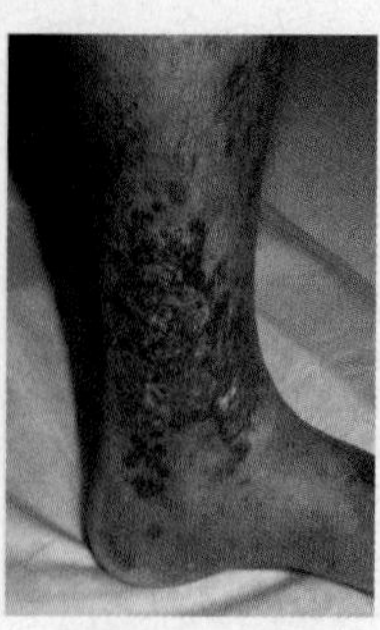

Figure 2-11 Kaposi's sarcoma. There are large confluent hyperpigmented patch-stage lesions with lymphedema. (From Goldman L, Ausiello D, Arend W, Armitage J, Clemmons D, Drazen J, Griggs R, et al: Cecil Medicine: Expert Consult, 23e, Saunders, 2007)

Item 2–5 Kaposi's sarcoma is a cancer that causes patches of abnormal tissue to grow under the skin; in the lining of the mouth, nose, and throat; or in other organs, often beginning and spreading to other organs. Patients who have had organ transplants or patients with AIDS are at high risk for this malignancy.

C46.5 Kaposi's sarcoma of lung Ex PDX 296

- **C46.50 Kaposi's sarcoma of unspecified lung**
- **C46.51 Kaposi's sarcoma of right lung**
- **C46.52 Kaposi's sarcoma of left lung**

C46.7 Kaposi's sarcoma of other sites Ex PDX 317

C46.9 Kaposi's sarcoma, unspecified Ex PDX 318
Kaposi's sarcoma of unspecified site

C47 Malignant neoplasm of peripheral nerves and autonomic nervous system

Includes malignant neoplasm of sympathetic and parasympathetic nerves and ganglia

Excludes1 Kaposi's sarcoma of soft tissue (C46.1)

C47.0 Malignant neoplasm of peripheral nerves of head, face and neck Ex PDX 319

Excludes1 malignant neoplasm of peripheral nerves of orbit (C69.6-)

C47.1 Malignant neoplasm of peripheral nerves of upper limb, including shoulder

- **C47.10 Malignant neoplasm of peripheral nerves of unspecified upper limb, including shoulder** Ex PDX 320
- **C47.11 Malignant neoplasm of peripheral nerves of right upper limb, including shoulder** Ex PDX 321
- **C47.12 Malignant neoplasm of peripheral nerves of left upper limb, including shoulder** Ex PDX 322

C47.2 Malignant neoplasm of peripheral nerves of lower limb, including hip

- **C47.20 Malignant neoplasm of peripheral nerves of unspecified lower limb, including hip** Ex PDX 323
- **C47.21 Malignant neoplasm of peripheral nerves of right lower limb, including hip** Ex PDX 324
- **C47.22 Malignant neoplasm of peripheral nerves of left lower limb, including hip** Ex PDX 325

C47.3 Malignant neoplasm of peripheral nerves of thorax Ex PDX 326

C47.4 Malignant neoplasm of peripheral nerves of abdomen Ex PDX 327

C47.5 Malignant neoplasm of peripheral nerves of pelvis Ex PDX 328

C47.6 Malignant neoplasm of peripheral nerves of trunk, unspecified Ex PDX 329
Malignant neoplasm of peripheral nerves of unspecified part of trunk

C47.8 Malignant neoplasm of overlapping sites of peripheral nerves and autonomic nervous system Ex PDX 330

C47.9 Malignant neoplasm of peripheral nerves and autonomic nervous system, unspecified Ex PDX 331
Malignant neoplasm of unspecified site of peripheral nerves and autonomic nervous system

C48 Malignant neoplasm of retroperitoneum and peritoneum

Excludes1 Kaposi's sarcoma of connective tissue (C46.1)
mesothelioma (C45.-)

C48.0 Malignant neoplasm of retroperitoneum Ex PDX 332
Behind/outside of peritoneum

C48.1 Malignant neoplasm of specified parts of peritoneum Ex PDX 311
Serous membrane lining abdominopelvic walls and covering viscera
Malignant neoplasm of cul-de-sac
Malignant neoplasm of mesentery
Malignant neoplasm of mesocolon
Malignant neoplasm of omentum
Malignant neoplasm of parietal peritoneum
Malignant neoplasm of pelvic peritoneum

C48.2 Malignant neoplasm of peritoneum, unspecified Ex PDX 311

C48.8 Malignant neoplasm of overlapping sites of retroperitoneum and peritoneum Ex PDX 311

C49 Malignant neoplasm of other connective and soft tissue

Includes malignant neoplasm of blood vessel
malignant neoplasm of bursa
malignant neoplasm of cartilage
malignant neoplasm of fascia
malignant neoplasm of fat
malignant neoplasm of ligament, except uterine
malignant neoplasm of lymphatic vessel
malignant neoplasm of muscle
malignant neoplasm of synovia
malignant neoplasm of tendon (sheath)

Excludes1 malignant neoplasm of cartilage (of):
articular (C40-C41)
larynx (C32.3)
nose (C30.0)
malignant neoplasm of connective tissue of breast (C50.-)

Excludes2 Kaposi's sarcoma of soft tissue (C46.1)
malignant neoplasm of heart (C38.0)
malignant neoplasm of peripheral nerves and autonomic nervous system (C47.-)
malignant neoplasm of peritoneum (C48.2)
malignant neoplasm of retroperitoneum (C48.0)
malignant neoplasm of uterine ligament (C57.3)
mesothelioma (C45.-)

C49.0 Malignant neoplasm of connective and soft tissue of head, face and neck Ex PDX 333
Malignant neoplasm of connective tissue of ear
Malignant neoplasm of connective tissue of eyelid

Excludes1 connective tissue of orbit (C69.6-)

C49.1 Malignant neoplasm of connective and soft tissue of upper limb, including shoulder

- **C49.10 Malignant neoplasm of connective and soft tissue of unspecified upper limb, including shoulder** Ex PDX 334
- **C49.11 Malignant neoplasm of connective and soft tissue of right upper limb, including shoulder** Ex PDX 335
- **C49.12 Malignant neoplasm of connective and soft tissue of left upper limb, including shoulder** Ex PDX 336

C49.2 Malignant neoplasm of connective and soft tissue of lower limb, including hip

- **C49.20 Malignant neoplasm of connective and soft tissue of unspecified lower limb, including hip** Ex PDX 337
- **C49.21 Malignant neoplasm of connective and soft tissue of right lower limb, including hip** Ex PDX 338
- **C49.22 Malignant neoplasm of connective and soft tissue of left lower limb, including hip** Ex PDX 339

C49.3 Malignant neoplasm of connective and soft tissue of thorax (Ex) PDX 340
Malignant neoplasm of axilla
Malignant neoplasm of diaphragm
Malignant neoplasm of great vessels
Excludes1 malignant neoplasm of breast (C50.-)
malignant neoplasm of heart (C38.0)
malignant neoplasm of mediastinum (C38.1-C38.3)
malignant neoplasm of thymus (C37)
Coding Clinic: 2015, Q3, P19

C49.4 Malignant neoplasm of connective and soft tissue of abdomen (Ex) PDX 341
Malignant neoplasm of abdominal wall
Malignant neoplasm of hypochondrium
Coding Clinic: 2019, Q4, P44

C49.5 Malignant neoplasm of connective and soft tissue of pelvis (Ex) PDX 342
Malignant neoplasm of buttock
Malignant neoplasm of groin
Malignant neoplasm of perineum

C49.6 Malignant neoplasm of connective and soft tissue of trunk, unspecified (Ex) PDX 343
Malignant neoplasm of back NOS

C49.8 Malignant neoplasm of overlapping sites of connective and soft tissue (Ex) PDX 344
Primary malignant neoplasm of two or more contiguous sites of connective and soft tissue

C49.9 Malignant neoplasm of connective and soft tissue, unspecified (Ex) PDX 345

● **C49.A Gastrointestinal stromal tumor**
Coding Clinic: 2016, Q4, P8

C49.A0 Gastrointestinal stromal tumor, unspecified site (Ex) PDX 346

C49.A1 Gastrointestinal stromal tumor of esophagus (Ex) PDX 347

C49.A2 Gastrointestinal stromal tumor of stomach (Ex) PDX 266

C49.A3 Gastrointestinal stromal tumor of small intestine (Ex) PDX 348

C49.A4 Gastrointestinal stromal tumor of large intestine (Ex) PDX 349

C49.A5 Gastrointestinal stromal tumor of rectum (Ex) PDX 350

C49.A9 Gastrointestinal stromal tumor of other sites (Ex) PDX 351

● **C4A Merkel cell carcinoma**

C4A.0 Merkel cell carcinoma of lip
Excludes1 malignant neoplasm of vermilion border of lip (C00.0-C00.2)

● **C4A.1 Merkel cell carcinoma of eyelid, including canthus**

C4A.10 Merkel cell carcinoma of unspecified eyelid, including canthus

● **C4A.11 Merkel cell carcinoma of right eyelid, including canthus**

C4A.111 Merkel cell carcinoma of right upper eyelid, including canthus

C4A.112 Merkel cell carcinoma of right lower eyelid, including canthus

● **C4A.12 Merkel cell carcinoma of left eyelid, including canthus**

C4A.121 Merkel cell carcinoma of left upper eyelid, including canthus

C4A.122 Merkel cell carcinoma of left lower eyelid, including canthus

● **C4A.2 Merkel cell carcinoma of ear and external auricular canal**

C4A.20 Merkel cell carcinoma of unspecified ear and external auricular canal

C4A.21 Merkel cell carcinoma of right ear and external auricular canal

C4A.22 Merkel cell carcinoma of left ear and external auricular canal

● **C4A.3 Merkel cell carcinoma of other and unspecified parts of face**

C4A.30 Merkel cell carcinoma of unspecified part of face

C4A.31 Merkel cell carcinoma of nose

C4A.39 Merkel cell carcinoma of other parts of face

C4A.4 Merkel cell carcinoma of scalp and neck

● **C4A.5 Merkel cell carcinoma of trunk**
Excludes2 malignant neoplasm of anus NOS (C21.0)
malignant neoplasm of scrotum (C63.2)

C4A.51 Merkel cell carcinoma of anal skin
Merkel cell carcinoma of anal margin
Merkel cell carcinoma of perianal skin

C4A.52 Merkel cell carcinoma of skin of breast

C4A.59 Merkel cell carcinoma of other part of trunk

● **C4A.6 Merkel cell carcinoma of upper limb, including shoulder**

C4A.60 Merkel cell carcinoma of unspecified upper limb, including shoulder

C4A.61 Merkel cell carcinoma of right upper limb, including shoulder

C4A.62 Merkel cell carcinoma of left upper limb, including shoulder

● **C4A.7 Merkel cell carcinoma of lower limb, including hip**

C4A.70 Merkel cell carcinoma of unspecified lower limb, including hip

C4A.71 Merkel cell carcinoma of right lower limb, including hip

C4A.72 Merkel cell carcinoma of left lower limb, including hip

C4A.8 Merkel cell carcinoma of overlapping sites

C4A.9 Merkel cell carcinoma, unspecified
Merkel cell carcinoma of unspecified site
Merkel cell carcinoma NOS

MALIGNANT NEOPLASMS OF BREAST (C50)

● **C50 Malignant neoplasm of breast**
Includes connective tissue of breast
Paget's disease of breast
Paget's disease of nipple
Intraductal carcinoma of breast characterized by eczema-like inflammatory skin changes
Use additional code to identify estrogen, and other hormones and factors receptor status (Z17.0, Z17.1)
Excludes1 skin of breast (C44.501, C44.511, C44.521, C44.591)

● **C50.0 Malignant neoplasm of nipple and areola**

● **C50.01 Malignant neoplasm of nipple and areola, female**

C50.011 Malignant neoplasm of nipple and areola, right female breast

C50.012 Malignant neoplasm of nipple and areola, left female breast

C50.019 Malignant neoplasm of nipple and areola, unspecified female breast

CHAPTER 2 (C00-D49)

- ● C50.02 Malignant neoplasm of nipple and areola, male
  - C50.021 Malignant neoplasm of nipple and areola, right male breast
  - C50.022 Malignant neoplasm of nipple and areola, left male breast
  - C50.029 Malignant neoplasm of nipple and areola, unspecified male breast
- ● C50.1 Malignant neoplasm of central portion of breast
  - ● C50.11 Malignant neoplasm of central portion of breast, female
    - C50.111 Malignant neoplasm of central portion of right female breast
    - C50.112 Malignant neoplasm of central portion of left female breast
    - C50.119 Malignant neoplasm of central portion of unspecified female breast
  - ● C50.12 Malignant neoplasm of central portion of breast, male
    - C50.121 Malignant neoplasm of central portion of right male breast
    - C50.122 Malignant neoplasm of central portion of left male breast
    - C50.129 Malignant neoplasm of central portion of unspecified male breast
- ● C50.2 Malignant neoplasm of upper-inner quadrant of breast
  - ● C50.21 Malignant neoplasm of upper-inner quadrant of breast, female
    - C50.211 Malignant neoplasm of upper-inner quadrant of right female breast
    - C50.212 Malignant neoplasm of upper-inner quadrant of left female breast
    - C50.219 Malignant neoplasm of upper-inner quadrant of unspecified female breast
  - ● C50.22 Malignant neoplasm of upper-inner quadrant of breast, male
    - C50.221 Malignant neoplasm of upper-inner quadrant of right male breast
    - C50.222 Malignant neoplasm of upper-inner quadrant of left male breast
    - C50.229 Malignant neoplasm of upper-inner quadrant of unspecified male breast
- ● C50.3 Malignant neoplasm of lower-inner quadrant of breast
  - ● C50.31 Malignant neoplasm of lower-inner quadrant of breast, female
    - C50.311 Malignant neoplasm of lower-inner quadrant of right female breast
    - C50.312 Malignant neoplasm of lower-inner quadrant of left female breast
    - C50.319 Malignant neoplasm of lower-inner quadrant of unspecified female breast

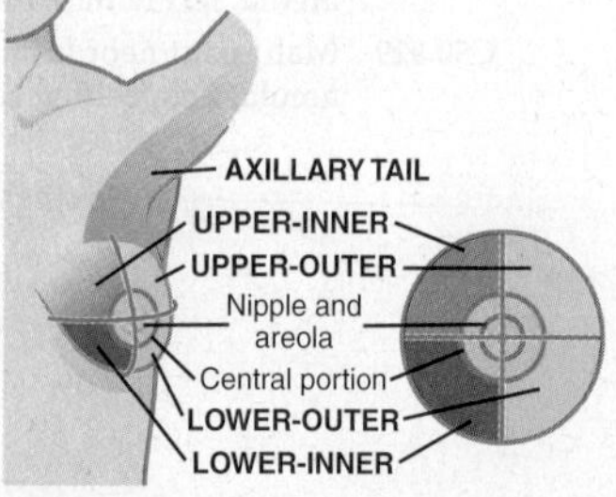

Figure 2-12 Female breast quadrants and axillary tail.

  - ● C50.32 Malignant neoplasm of lower-inner quadrant of breast, male
    - C50.321 Malignant neoplasm of lower-inner quadrant of right male breast
    - C50.322 Malignant neoplasm of lower-inner quadrant of left male breast
    - C50.329 Malignant neoplasm of lower-inner quadrant of unspecified male breast
- ● C50.4 Malignant neoplasm of upper-outer quadrant of breast
  - ● C50.41 Malignant neoplasm of upper-outer quadrant of breast, female
    - C50.411 Malignant neoplasm of upper-outer quadrant of right female breast
    - C50.412 Malignant neoplasm of upper-outer quadrant of left female breast
    - C50.419 Malignant neoplasm of upper-outer quadrant of unspecified female breast
  - ● C50.42 Malignant neoplasm of upper-outer quadrant of breast, male
    - C50.421 Malignant neoplasm of upper-outer quadrant of right male breast
    - C50.422 Malignant neoplasm of upper-outer quadrant of left male breast
    - C50.429 Malignant neoplasm of upper-outer quadrant of unspecified male breast
- ● C50.5 Malignant neoplasm of lower-outer quadrant of breast
  - ● C50.51 Malignant neoplasm of lower-outer quadrant of breast, female
    - C50.511 Malignant neoplasm of lower-outer quadrant of right female breast
    - C50.512 Malignant neoplasm of lower-outer quadrant of left female breast
    - C50.519 Malignant neoplasm of lower-outer quadrant of unspecified female breast
  - ● C50.52 Malignant neoplasm of lower-outer quadrant of breast, male
    - C50.521 Malignant neoplasm of lower-outer quadrant of right male breast
    - C50.522 Malignant neoplasm of lower-outer quadrant of left male breast
    - C50.529 Malignant neoplasm of lower-outer quadrant of unspecified male breast
- ● C50.6 Malignant neoplasm of axillary tail of breast
  - ● C50.61 Malignant neoplasm of axillary tail of breast, female
    - C50.611 Malignant neoplasm of axillary tail of right female breast
    - C50.612 Malignant neoplasm of axillary tail of left female breast
    - C50.619 Malignant neoplasm of axillary tail of unspecified female breast
  - ● C50.62 Malignant neoplasm of axillary tail of breast, male
    - C50.621 Malignant neoplasm of axillary tail of right male breast
    - C50.622 Malignant neoplasm of axillary tail of left male breast
    - C50.629 Malignant neoplasm of axillary tail of unspecified male breast

C50.8 Malignant neoplasm of overlapping sites of breast

C50.81 Malignant neoplasm of overlapping sites of breast, female

C50.811 Malignant neoplasm of overlapping sites of right female breast

C50.812 Malignant neoplasm of overlapping sites of left female breast

C50.819 Malignant neoplasm of overlapping sites of unspecified female breast

C50.82 Malignant neoplasm of overlapping sites of breast, male

C50.821 Malignant neoplasm of overlapping sites of right male breast

C50.822 Malignant neoplasm of overlapping sites of left male breast

C50.829 Malignant neoplasm of overlapping sites of unspecified male breast

C50.9 Malignant neoplasm of breast of unspecified site

C50.91 Malignant neoplasm of breast of unspecified site, female

C50.911 Malignant neoplasm of unspecified site of right female breast

C50.912 Malignant neoplasm of unspecified site of left female breast

Coding Clinic: 2022, Q3, P11,15

C50.919 Malignant neoplasm of unspecified site of unspecified female breast

C50.92 Malignant neoplasm of breast of unspecified site, male

C50.921 Malignant neoplasm of unspecified site of right male breast

C50.922 Malignant neoplasm of unspecified site of left male breast

C50.929 Malignant neoplasm of unspecified site of unspecified male breast

MALIGNANT NEOPLASMS OF FEMALE GENITAL ORGANS (C51-C58)

Includes malignant neoplasm of skin of female genital organs

C51 Malignant neoplasm of vulva

Excludes1 carcinoma in situ of vulva (D07.1)

C51.0 Malignant neoplasm of labium majus

Outer folds of skin external female genitalia

Malignant neoplasm of Bartholin's [greater vestibular] gland

C51.1 Malignant neoplasm of labium minus

Two inner folds surrounding vulva in female genitalia

C51.2 Malignant neoplasm of clitoris

C51.8 Malignant neoplasm of overlapping sites of vulva

C51.9 Malignant neoplasm of vulva, unspecified

Malignant neoplasm of external female genitalia NOS

Malignant neoplasm of pudendum

C52 Malignant neoplasm of vagina

Excludes1 carcinoma in situ of vagina (D07.2)

C53 Malignant neoplasm of cervix uteri

Excludes1 carcinoma in situ of cervix uteri (D06.-)

C53.0 Malignant neoplasm of endocervix

Inside the cervix

C53.1 Malignant neoplasm of exocervix

Outside the cervix

C53.8 Malignant neoplasm of overlapping sites of cervix uteri

C53.9 Malignant neoplasm of cervix uteri, unspecified

Coding Clinic: 2017, Q4, P103

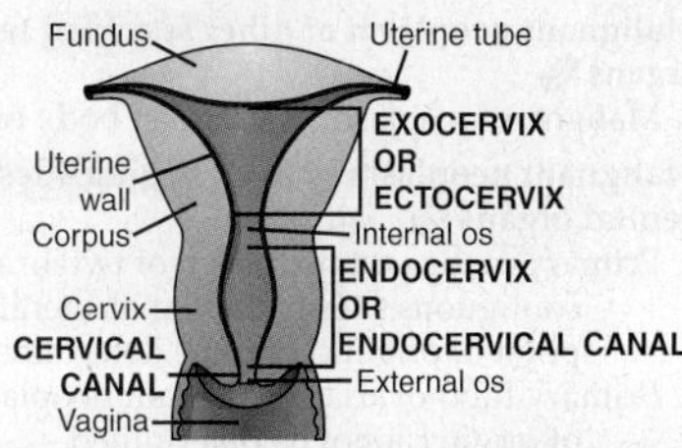

Figure 2-13 Cervix uteri.

C54 Malignant neoplasm of corpus uteri

C54.0 Malignant neoplasm of isthmus uteri

Constricted part of uterus between cervix and body

Malignant neoplasm of lower uterine segment

C54.1 Malignant neoplasm of endometrium

Lining of uterus

C54.2 Malignant neoplasm of myometrium

Middle layer of uterine wall consisting of smooth muscle supporting stromal and vascular tissue

C54.3 Malignant neoplasm of fundus uteri

Top rounded portion of uterus

C54.8 Malignant neoplasm of overlapping sites of corpus uteri ♀

Main body of uterus

Coding Clinic: 2023, Q3, P15

C54.9 Malignant neoplasm of corpus uteri, unspecified

C55 Malignant neoplasm of uterus, part unspecified

C56 Malignant neoplasm of ovary (Ex) PDX 352

Use additional code to identify any functional activity

C56.1 Malignant neoplasm of right ovary

C56.2 Malignant neoplasm of left ovary

C56.3 Malignant neoplasm of bilateral ovaries (Ex) PDX 353

C56.9 Malignant neoplasm of unspecified ovary

C57 Malignant neoplasm of other and unspecified female genital organs

C57.0 Malignant neoplasm of fallopian tube

Malignant neoplasm of oviduct

Malignant neoplasm of uterine tube

C57.00 Malignant neoplasm of unspecified fallopian tube

C57.01 Malignant neoplasm of right fallopian tube

C57.02 Malignant neoplasm of left fallopian tube

C57.1 Malignant neoplasm of broad ligament

C57.10 Malignant neoplasm of unspecified broad ligament

C57.11 Malignant neoplasm of right broad ligament

C57.12 Malignant neoplasm of left broad ligament

C57.2 Malignant neoplasm of round ligament

C57.20 Malignant neoplasm of unspecified round ligament

C57.21 Malignant neoplasm of right round ligament

C57.22 Malignant neoplasm of left round ligament

C57.3 Malignant neoplasm of parametrium

Malignant neoplasm of uterine ligament NOS

C57.4 Malignant neoplasm of uterine adnexa, unspecified ♀

C57.7 **Malignant neoplasm of other specified female genital organs**
Malignant neoplasm of wolffian body or duct

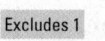

C57.8 **Malignant neoplasm of overlapping sites of female genital organs**
Primary malignant neoplasm of two or more contiguous sites of the female genital organs whose point of origin cannot be determined
Primary tubo-ovarian malignant neoplasm whose point of origin cannot be determined
Primary utero-ovarian malignant neoplasm whose point of origin cannot be determined

C57.9 **Malignant neoplasm of female genital organ, unspecified**
Malignant neoplasm of female genitourinary tract NOS

C58 **Malignant neoplasm of placenta** M
Includes choriocarcinoma NOS
chorionepithelioma NOS
Excludes1 chorioadenoma (destruens) (D39.2)
hydatidiform mole NOS (O01.9)
invasive hydatidiform mole (D39.2)
male choriocarcinoma NOS (C62.9-)
malignant hydatidiform mole (D39.2)

MALIGNANT NEOPLASMS OF MALE GENITAL ORGANS (C60-C63)

Includes malignant neoplasm of skin of male genital organs

● C60 **Malignant neoplasm of penis**

C60.0 **Malignant neoplasm of prepuce**
Malignant neoplasm of foreskin

C60.1 **Malignant neoplasm of glans penis**

C60.2 **Malignant neoplasm of body of penis**
Malignant neoplasm of corpus cavernosum

C60.8 **Malignant neoplasm of overlapping sites of penis**

C60.9 **Malignant neoplasm of penis, unspecified**
Malignant neoplasm of skin of penis NOS

C61 **Malignant neoplasm of prostate**
Use additional, if applicable, code to identify:
hormone sensitivity status (Z19.1-Z19.2)
rising PSA following treatment for malignant neoplasm of prostate (R97.21)
Excludes1 malignant neoplasm of seminal vesicle (C63.7)

● C62 **Malignant neoplasm of testis**
Use additional code to identify any functional activity.

● C62.0 **Malignant neoplasm of undescended testis**
Malignant neoplasm of ectopic testis
Malignant neoplasm of retained testis

C62.00 **Malignant neoplasm of unspecified undescended testis**

C62.01 **Malignant neoplasm of undescended right testis**

C62.02 **Malignant neoplasm of undescended left testis**

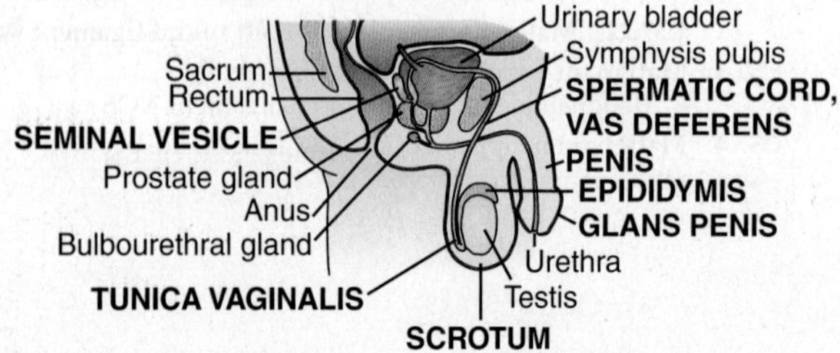

Figure 2-14 Penis and other male genital organs.

● C62.1 **Malignant neoplasm of descended testis**
Malignant neoplasm of scrotal testis

C62.10 **Malignant neoplasm of unspecified descended testis, unspecified side**

C62.11 **Malignant neoplasm of descended right testis**

C62.12 **Malignant neoplasm of descended left testis**

● C62.9 **Malignant neoplasm of testis, unspecified whether descended or undescended**

C62.90 **Malignant neoplasm of unspecified testis, unspecified whether descended or undescended**
Malignant neoplasm of testis NOS

C62.91 **Malignant neoplasm of right testis, unspecified whether descended or undescended**

C62.92 **Malignant neoplasm of left testis, unspecified whether descended or undescended**

● C63 **Malignant neoplasm of other and unspecified male genital organs**

● C63.0 **Malignant neoplasm of epididymis**

C63.00 **Malignant neoplasm of unspecified epididymis**

C63.01 **Malignant neoplasm of right epididymis**

C63.02 **Malignant neoplasm of left epididymis**

● C63.1 **Malignant neoplasm of spermatic cord**

C63.10 **Malignant neoplasm of unspecified spermatic cord**

C63.11 **Malignant neoplasm of right spermatic cord**

C63.12 **Malignant neoplasm of left spermatic cord**

C63.2 **Malignant neoplasm of scrotum**
Malignant neoplasm of skin of scrotum

C63.7 **Malignant neoplasm of other specified male genital organs**
Malignant neoplasm of seminal vesicle
Malignant neoplasm of tunica vaginalis

C63.8 **Malignant neoplasm of overlapping sites of male genital organs**
Primary malignant neoplasm of two or more contiguous sites of male genital organs whose point of origin cannot be determined

C63.9 **Malignant neoplasm of male genital organ, unspecified**
Malignant neoplasm of male genitourinary tract NOS

MALIGNANT NEOPLASMS OF URINARY TRACT (C64-C68)

● C64 **Malignant neoplasm of kidney, except renal pelvis** (Ex) PDX 354
Excludes1 malignant carcinoid tumor of the kidney (C7A.093)
malignant neoplasm of renal calyces (C65.-)
malignant neoplasm of renal pelvis (C65.-)

C64.1 **Malignant neoplasm of right kidney, except renal pelvis**

C64.2 **Malignant neoplasm of left kidney, except renal pelvis**

C64.9 **Malignant neoplasm of unspecified kidney, except renal pelvis**

● C65 **Malignant neoplasm of renal pelvis** (Ex) PDX 354
Includes malignant neoplasm of pelviureteric junction
malignant neoplasm of renal calyces

C65.1 **Malignant neoplasm of right renal pelvis**

C65.2 **Malignant neoplasm of left renal pelvis**

C65.9 **Malignant neoplasm of unspecified renal pelvis**

C66 Malignant neoplasm of ureter PDX 355

Excludes1 malignant neoplasm of ureteric orifice of bladder (C67.6)

C66.1 Malignant neoplasm of right ureter

C66.2 Malignant neoplasm of left ureter

C66.9 Malignant neoplasm of unspecified ureter

C67 Malignant neoplasm of bladder

C67.0 Malignant neoplasm of trigone of bladder

Triangular area formed by three openings in the floor of urinary bladder

C67.1 Malignant neoplasm of dome of bladder

Vaulted roof

Coding Clinic: 2023, Q3, P16

C67.2 Malignant neoplasm of lateral wall of bladder

Side walls

Coding Clinic: 2023, Q3, P16

C67.3 Malignant neoplasm of anterior wall of bladder

Front wall

Coding Clinic: 2023, Q3, P16

C67.4 Malignant neoplasm of posterior wall of bladder

Back wall

C67.5 Malignant neoplasm of bladder neck

Joining of bladder and urethra

Malignant neoplasm of internal urethral orifice

Coding Clinic: 2023, Q3, P16

C67.6 Malignant neoplasm of ureteric orifice

Opening from bladder to ureters

C67.7 Malignant neoplasm of urachus

Embryonic canal that connects the urinary bladder with the structure that forms the umbilical cord (allantois)

C67.8 Malignant neoplasm of overlapping sites of bladder

C67.9 Malignant neoplasm of bladder, unspecified

Coding Clinic: 2017, Q1, P6; 2016, Q1, P19

C68 Malignant neoplasm of other and unspecified urinary organs

Excludes1 malignant neoplasm of female genitourinary tract NOS (C57.9)
malignant neoplasm of male genitourinary tract NOS (C63.9)

C68.0 Malignant neoplasm of urethra PDX 356

Excludes1 malignant neoplasm of urethral orifice of bladder (C67.5)

C68.1 Malignant neoplasm of paraurethral glands PDX 356

Group of glands of female urethra drained by paraurethral ducts; AKA Skene glands, female prostate

C68.8 Malignant neoplasm of overlapping sites of urinary organs PDX 357

Primary malignant neoplasm of two or more contiguous sites of urinary organs whose point of origin cannot be determined

C68.9 Malignant neoplasm of urinary organ, unspecified PDX 357

Malignant neoplasm of urinary system NOS

MALIGNANT NEOPLASMS OF EYE, BRAIN AND OTHER PARTS OF CENTRAL NERVOUS SYSTEM (C69-C72)

C69 Malignant neoplasm of eye and adnexa

Excludes1 malignant neoplasm of connective tissue of eyelid (C49.0)
malignant neoplasm of eyelid (skin) (C43.1-, C44.1-)
malignant neoplasm of optic nerve (C72.3-)

C69.0 Malignant neoplasm of conjunctiva

C69.00 Malignant neoplasm of unspecified conjunctiva

C69.01 Malignant neoplasm of right conjunctiva

C69.02 Malignant neoplasm of left conjunctiva

C69.1 Malignant neoplasm of cornea

C69.10 Malignant neoplasm of unspecified cornea

C69.11 Malignant neoplasm of right cornea

C69.12 Malignant neoplasm of left cornea

C69.2 Malignant neoplasm of retina

Excludes1 dark area on retina (D49.81)
neoplasm of unspecified behavior of retina and choroid (D49.81)
retinal freckle (D49.81)

C69.20 Malignant neoplasm of unspecified retina

C69.21 Malignant neoplasm of right retina

C69.22 Malignant neoplasm of left retina

C69.3 Malignant neoplasm of choroid

C69.30 Malignant neoplasm of unspecified choroid

C69.31 Malignant neoplasm of right choroid

C69.32 Malignant neoplasm of left choroid

C69.4 Malignant neoplasm of ciliary body

C69.40 Malignant neoplasm of unspecified ciliary body

C69.41 Malignant neoplasm of right ciliary body

C69.42 Malignant neoplasm of left ciliary body

C69.5 Malignant neoplasm of lacrimal gland and duct

Malignant neoplasm of lacrimal sac
Malignant neoplasm of nasolacrimal duct

C69.50 Malignant neoplasm of unspecified lacrimal gland and duct

C69.51 Malignant neoplasm of right lacrimal gland and duct

C69.52 Malignant neoplasm of left lacrimal gland and duct

C69.6 Malignant neoplasm of orbit

Malignant neoplasm of connective tissue of orbit
Malignant neoplasm of extraocular muscle
Malignant neoplasm of peripheral nerves of orbit
Malignant neoplasm of retrobulbar tissue
Malignant neoplasm of retro-ocular tissue

Excludes1 malignant neoplasm of orbital bone (C41.0)

C69.60 Malignant neoplasm of unspecified orbit

C69.61 Malignant neoplasm of right orbit

C69.62 Malignant neoplasm of left orbit

C69.8 Malignant neoplasm of overlapping sites of eye and adnexa

C69.80 Malignant neoplasm of overlapping sites of unspecified eye and adnexa

C69.81 Malignant neoplasm of overlapping sites of right eye and adnexa

C69.82 Malignant neoplasm of overlapping sites of left eye and adnexa

C69.9 Malignant neoplasm of unspecified site of eye

Malignant neoplasm of eyeball

C69.90 Malignant neoplasm of unspecified site of unspecified eye

C69.91 Malignant neoplasm of unspecified site of right eye

C69.92 Malignant neoplasm of unspecified site of left eye

C70 Malignant neoplasm of meninges

C70.0 Malignant neoplasm of cerebral meninges PDX 358

C70.1 Malignant neoplasm of spinal meninges PDX 359

C70.9 Malignant neoplasm of meninges, unspecified PDX 358

CHAPTER 2 (C00-D49)

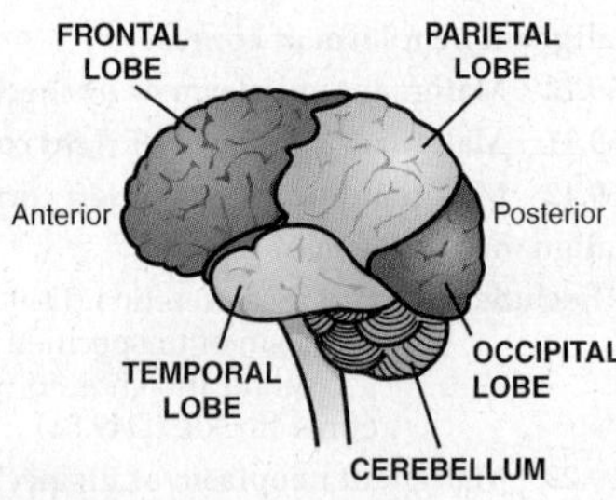

Figure 2-15 The brain.

● **C71 Malignant neoplasm of brain** Ex: PDX 360

Excludes1 malignant neoplasm of cranial nerves (C72.2-C72.5)
retrobulbar malignant neoplasm (C69.6-)

C71.0 **Malignant neoplasm of cerebrum, except lobes and ventricles**
Malignant neoplasm of supratentorial NOS

C71.1 **Malignant neoplasm of frontal lobe**

C71.2 **Malignant neoplasm of temporal lobe**

C71.3 **Malignant neoplasm of parietal lobe**

C71.4 **Malignant neoplasm of occipital lobe**

C71.5 **Malignant neoplasm of cerebral ventricle**

Excludes1 malignant neoplasm of fourth cerebral ventricle (C71.7)

C71.6 **Malignant neoplasm of cerebellum**

C71.7 **Malignant neoplasm of brain stem**
Malignant neoplasm of fourth cerebral ventricle
Infratentorial malignant neoplasm NOS

C71.8 **Malignant neoplasm of overlapping sites of brain**

C71.9 **Malignant neoplasm of brain, unspecified**

● **C72 Malignant neoplasm of spinal cord, cranial nerves and other parts of central nervous system** Ex: PDX 361

Excludes1 malignant neoplasm of meninges (C70.-)
malignant neoplasm of peripheral nerves and autonomic nervous system (C47.-)

C72.0 **Malignant neoplasm of spinal cord**

C72.1 **Malignant neoplasm of cauda equina**
Lower end of spinal column

● C72.2 **Malignant neoplasm of olfactory nerve** Ex: PDX 362
Malignant neoplasm of olfactory bulb

C72.20 **Malignant neoplasm of unspecified olfactory nerve**

C72.21 **Malignant neoplasm of right olfactory nerve**

C72.22 **Malignant neoplasm of left olfactory nerve**

● C72.3 **Malignant neoplasm of optic nerve** Ex: PDX 362

C72.30 **Malignant neoplasm of unspecified optic nerve**

C72.31 **Malignant neoplasm of right optic nerve**

C72.32 **Malignant neoplasm of left optic nerve**

● C72.4 **Malignant neoplasm of acoustic nerve** Ex: PDX 362

C72.40 **Malignant neoplasm of unspecified acoustic nerve**

C72.41 **Malignant neoplasm of right acoustic nerve**

C72.42 **Malignant neoplasm of left acoustic nerve**

● C72.5 **Malignant neoplasm of other and unspecified cranial nerves** Ex: PDX 362

C72.50 **Malignant neoplasm of unspecified cranial nerve**
Malignant neoplasm of cranial nerve NOS

C72.59 **Malignant neoplasm of other cranial nerves**

C72.9 **Malignant neoplasm of central nervous system, unspecified** Ex: PDX 363
Malignant neoplasm of unspecified site of central nervous system
Malignant neoplasm of nervous system NOS

MALIGNANT NEOPLASMS OF THYROID AND OTHER ENDOCRINE GLANDS (C73-C75)

C73 Malignant neoplasm of thyroid gland
Use additional code to identify any functional activity

● **C74 Malignant neoplasm of adrenal gland** Ex: PDX 364

● C74.0 **Malignant neoplasm of cortex of adrenal gland**

C74.00 **Malignant neoplasm of cortex of unspecified adrenal gland**

C74.01 **Malignant neoplasm of cortex of right adrenal gland**

C74.02 **Malignant neoplasm of cortex of left adrenal gland**

● C74.1 **Malignant neoplasm of medulla of adrenal gland**
Pair of glands situated on top of or above each kidney ("suprarenal")

C74.10 **Malignant neoplasm of medulla of unspecified adrenal gland**

C74.11 **Malignant neoplasm of medulla of right adrenal gland**

C74.12 **Malignant neoplasm of medulla of left adrenal gland**

● C74.9 **Malignant neoplasm of unspecified part of adrenal gland**

C74.90 **Malignant neoplasm of unspecified part of unspecified adrenal gland**

C74.91 **Malignant neoplasm of unspecified part of right adrenal gland**

C74.92 **Malignant neoplasm of unspecified part of left adrenal gland**

● **C75 Malignant neoplasm of other endocrine glands and related structures**

Excludes1 malignant carcinoid tumors (C7A.0-)
malignant neoplasm of adrenal gland (C74.-)
malignant neoplasm of endocrine pancreas (C25.4)
malignant neoplasm of islets of Langerhans (C25.4)
malignant neoplasm of ovary (C56.-)
malignant neoplasm of testis (C62.-)
malignant neoplasm of thymus (C37)
malignant neoplasm of thyroid gland (C73)
malignant neuroendocrine tumors (C7A.-)

C75.0 **Malignant neoplasm of parathyroid gland** Ex: PDX 365

C75.1 **Malignant neoplasm of pituitary gland** Ex: PDX 366

C75.2 **Malignant neoplasm of craniopharyngeal duct** Ex: PDX 366

C75.3 **Malignant neoplasm of pineal gland** Ex: PDX 367

C75.4 **Malignant neoplasm of carotid body** Ex: PDX 368

C75.5 **Malignant neoplasm of aortic body and other paraganglia** Ex: PDX 369

C75.8 **Malignant neoplasm with pluriglandular involvement, unspecified** Ex: PDX 370

C75.9 **Malignant neoplasm of endocrine gland, unspecified** Ex: PDX 370

CHAPTER 2 (C00-D49)

MALIGNANT NEOPLASMS OF ILL-DEFINED, OTHER SECONDARY AND UNSPECIFIED SITES (C76-C8Ø)

C76 Malignant neoplasm of other and ill-defined sites

Excludes1 malignant neoplasm of female genitourinary tract NOS (C57.9)
malignant neoplasm of male genitourinary tract NOS (C63.9)
malignant neoplasm of lymphoid, hematopoietic and related tissue (C81-C96)
malignant neoplasm of skin (C44.-)
malignant neoplasm of unspecified site NOS (C8Ø.1)

C76.Ø Malignant neoplasm of head, face and neck
Malignant neoplasm of cheek NOS
Malignant neoplasm of nose NOS

C76.1 Malignant neoplasm of thorax
Intrathoracic malignant neoplasm NOS
Malignant neoplasm of axilla NOS
Thoracic malignant neoplasm NOS

C76.2 Malignant neoplasm of abdomen

C76.3 Malignant neoplasm of pelvis
Malignant neoplasm of groin NOS
Malignant neoplasm of sites overlapping systems within the pelvis
Rectovaginal (septum) malignant neoplasm
Between rectum and vagina
Rectovesical (septum) malignant neoplasm
Between rectum and urinary bladder; AKA vesicorectal

C76.4 Malignant neoplasm of upper limb

C76.4Ø Malignant neoplasm of unspecified upper limb

C76.41 Malignant neoplasm of right upper limb

C76.42 Malignant neoplasm of left upper limb

C76.5 Malignant neoplasm of lower limb

C76.5Ø Malignant neoplasm of unspecified lower limb

C76.51 Malignant neoplasm of right lower limb

C76.52 Malignant neoplasm of left lower limb

C76.8 Malignant neoplasm of other specified ill-defined sites
Malignant neoplasm of overlapping ill-defined sites

C77 Secondary and unspecified malignant neoplasm of lymph nodes (Ex) PDX 315

Excludes1 malignant neoplasm of lymph nodes, specified as primary (C81-C86, C88, C96.-)
mesentary metastasis of carcinoid tumor (C7B.Ø4)
secondary carcinoid tumors of distant lymph nodes (C7B.Ø1)

C77.Ø Secondary and unspecified malignant neoplasm of lymph nodes of head, face and neck
Secondary and unspecified malignant neoplasm of supraclavicular lymph nodes
Coding Clinic: 2Ø22, Q3, P15

C77.1 Secondary and unspecified malignant neoplasm of intrathoracic lymph nodes

C77.2 Secondary and unspecified malignant neoplasm of intra-abdominal lymph nodes

C77.3 Secondary and unspecified malignant neoplasm of axilla and upper limb lymph nodes
Secondary and unspecified malignant neoplasm of pectoral lymph nodes

C77.4 Secondary and unspecified malignant neoplasm of inguinal and lower limb lymph nodes

C77.5 Secondary and unspecified malignant neoplasm of intrapelvic lymph nodes

C77.8 Secondary and unspecified malignant neoplasm of lymph nodes of multiple regions

C77.9 Secondary and unspecified malignant neoplasm of lymph node, unspecified

Item 2-6 The adrenal glands are a pair of glands situated on top of or above each kidney ("suprarenal") and chiefly responsible for regulating the stress response through the synthesis of corticosteroids and catecholamines, including cortisol and adrenaline.

C78 Secondary malignant neoplasm of respiratory and digestive organs

Excludes1 secondary carcinoid tumors of liver (C7B.Ø2)
secondary carcinoid tumors of peritoneum (C7B.Ø4)

Excludes2 lymph node metastases (C77.Ø)

Coding Clinic: 2Ø23, Q1, P22

C78.Ø Secondary malignant neoplasm of lung (Ex) PDX 371

C78.ØØ Secondary malignant neoplasm of unspecified lung
Coding Clinic: 2Ø22, Q3, P9

C78.Ø1 Secondary malignant neoplasm of right lung
Coding Clinic: 2Ø24, Q2, P11; 2Ø23, Q3, P15

C78.Ø2 Secondary malignant neoplasm of left lung
Coding Clinic: 2Ø23, Q3, P15

C78.1 Secondary malignant neoplasm of mediastinum (Ex) PDX 372
Thoracic cavity between pleural cavities

C78.2 Secondary malignant neoplasm of pleura (Ex) PDX 373
Serous membrane covering lungs and lining thoracic cavity

C78.3 Secondary malignant neoplasm of other and unspecified respiratory organs (Ex) PDX 374

C78.3Ø Secondary malignant neoplasm of unspecified respiratory organ

C78.39 Secondary malignant neoplasm of other respiratory organs

C78.4 Secondary malignant neoplasm of small intestine (Ex) PDX 375

C78.5 Secondary malignant neoplasm of large intestine and rectum (Ex) PDX 376

C78.6 Secondary malignant neoplasm of retroperitoneum and peritoneum (Ex) PDX 377
Coding Clinic: 2Ø17, Q2, P12

C78.7 Secondary malignant neoplasm of liver and intrahepatic bile duct (Ex) PDX 378
Coding Clinic: 2Ø24, Q1, P25; 2Ø22, Q3, P15

C78.8 Secondary malignant neoplasm of other and unspecified digestive organs (Ex) PDX 379

C78.8Ø Secondary malignant neoplasm of unspecified digestive organ

C78.89 Secondary malignant neoplasm of other digestive organs
Code also exocrine pancreatic insufficiency (K86.81)

C79 Secondary malignant neoplasm of other and unspecified sites

Excludes1 secondary carcinoid tumors (C7B.-)
secondary neuroendocrine tumors (C7B.-)

Coding Clinic: 2Ø23, Q1, P22

C79.Ø Secondary malignant neoplasm of kidney and renal pelvis (Ex) PDX 380

C79.ØØ Secondary malignant neoplasm of unspecified kidney and renal pelvis

C79.Ø1 Secondary malignant neoplasm of right kidney and renal pelvis

C79.Ø2 Secondary malignant neoplasm of left kidney and renal pelvis

C79.1 Secondary malignant neoplasm of bladder and other and unspecified urinary organs (Ex) PDX 380

C79.1Ø Secondary malignant neoplasm of unspecified urinary organs

C79.11 Secondary malignant neoplasm of bladder

Excludes2 lymph node metastases (C77.Ø)

C79.19 Secondary malignant neoplasm of other urinary organs

CHAPTER 2 (CØØ-D49)

C79.2 Secondary malignant neoplasm of skin PDX 381
Excludes1 secondary Merkel cell carcinoma (C7B.1)

● **C79.3** Secondary malignant neoplasm of brain and cerebral meninges
C79.31 Secondary malignant neoplasm of brain PDX 382
Coding Clinic: 2022, Q3, P9,11
C79.32 Secondary malignant neoplasm of cerebral meninges PDX 383
Coding Clinic: 2020, Q1, P13

● **C79.4** Secondary malignant neoplasm of other and unspecified parts of nervous system PDX 383
C79.40 Secondary malignant neoplasm of unspecified part of nervous system
C79.49 Secondary malignant neoplasm of other parts of nervous system

● **C79.5** Secondary malignant neoplasm of bone and bone marrow PDX 384
Excludes1 secondary carcinoid tumors of bone (C7B.03)
C79.51 Secondary malignant neoplasm of bone
Coding Clinic: 2022, Q3, P15
C79.52 Secondary malignant neoplasm of bone marrow

● **C79.6** Secondary malignant neoplasm of ovary PDX 385
C79.60 Secondary malignant neoplasm of unspecified ovary
C79.61 Secondary malignant neoplasm of right ovary
C79.62 Secondary malignant neoplasm of left ovary
C79.63 Secondary malignant neoplasm of bilateral ovaries PDX 386

● **C79.7** Secondary malignant neoplasm of adrenal gland PDX 387
C79.70 Secondary malignant neoplasm of unspecified adrenal gland
C79.71 Secondary malignant neoplasm of right adrenal gland
C79.72 Secondary malignant neoplasm of left adrenal gland

● **C79.8** Secondary malignant neoplasm of other specified sites
C79.81 Secondary malignant neoplasm of breast PDX 388
C79.82 Secondary malignant neoplasm of genital organs PDX 389
Coding Clinic: 2023, Q3, P15
C79.89 Secondary malignant neoplasm of other specified sites PDX 390
Coding Clinic: 2017, Q2, P11

C79.9 Secondary malignant neoplasm of unspecified site PDX 390
Metastatic cancer NOS
Metastatic disease NOS
Excludes1 carcinomatosis NOS (C80.0)
generalized cancer NOS (C80.0)
malignant (primary) neoplasm of unspecified site (C80.1)
Coding Clinic: 2023, Q2, P5

MALIGNANT NEUROENDOCRINE TUMORS (C7A)

● **C7A** Malignant neuroendocrine tumors
Code also any associated multiple endocrine neoplasia [MEN] syndromes (E31.2-)
Use additional code to identify any associated endocrine syndrome, such as:
carcinoid syndrome (E34.00)
Excludes2 malignant pancreatic islet cell tumors (C25.4)
Merkel cell carcinoma (C4A.-)

● **C7A.0** Malignant carcinoid tumors
C7A.00 Malignant carcinoid tumor of unspecified site PDX 391

● **C7A.01** Malignant carcinoid tumors of the small intestine
C7A.010 Malignant carcinoid tumor of the duodenum PDX 392
C7A.011 Malignant carcinoid tumor of the jejunum PDX 393
C7A.012 Malignant carcinoid tumor of the ileum PDX 394
C7A.019 Malignant carcinoid tumor of the small intestine, unspecified portion PDX 395

● **C7A.02** Malignant carcinoid tumors of the appendix, large intestine, and rectum
C7A.020 Malignant carcinoid tumor of the appendix PDX 396
C7A.021 Malignant carcinoid tumor of the cecum PDX 397
C7A.022 Malignant carcinoid tumor of the ascending colon PDX 398
C7A.023 Malignant carcinoid tumor of the transverse colon PDX 399
C7A.024 Malignant carcinoid tumor of the descending colon PDX 400
C7A.025 Malignant carcinoid tumor of the sigmoid colon PDX 401
C7A.026 Malignant carcinoid tumor of the rectum PDX 402
C7A.029 Malignant carcinoid tumor of the large intestine, unspecified portion PDX 403
Malignant carcinoid tumor of the colon NOS

● **C7A.09** Malignant carcinoid tumors of other sites
C7A.090 Malignant carcinoid tumor of the bronchus and lung PDX 404
C7A.091 Malignant carcinoid tumor of the thymus PDX 405
C7A.092 Malignant carcinoid tumor of the stomach PDX 406
C7A.093 Malignant carcinoid tumor of the kidney PDX 407
C7A.094 Malignant carcinoid tumor of the foregut, unspecified PDX 406
C7A.095 Malignant carcinoid tumor of the midgut, unspecified PDX 406
C7A.096 Malignant carcinoid tumor of the hindgut, unspecified PDX 406
C7A.098 Malignant carcinoid tumors of other sites PDX 391

C7A.1 Malignant poorly differentiated neuroendocrine tumors PDX 391
Malignant poorly differentiated neuroendocrine tumor NOS
Malignant poorly differentiated neuroendocrine carcinoma, any site
High grade neuroendocrine carcinoma, any site
Coding Clinic: 2023, Q1, P21-22

C7A.8 Other malignant neuroendocrine tumors PDX 391
Secondary neuroendocrine tumors (C7B)
Coding Clinic: 2019, Q3, P7

SECONDARY NEUROENDOCRINE TUMORS (C7B)

C7B Secondary neuroendocrine tumors
Use additional code to identify any functional activity

C7B.0 Secondary carcinoid tumors
- C7B.00 Secondary carcinoid tumors, unspecified site
- C7B.01 Secondary carcinoid tumors of distant lymph nodes (Ex) PDX 408
- C7B.02 Secondary carcinoid tumors of liver (Ex) PDX 409
- C7B.03 Secondary carcinoid tumors of bone (Ex) PDX 410
- C7B.04 Secondary carcinoid tumors of peritoneum (Ex) PDX 411
  Mesentary metastasis of carcinoid tumor
- C7B.09 Secondary carcinoid tumors of other sites (Ex) PDX 412

C7B.1 Secondary Merkel cell carcinoma
Merkel cell carcinoma nodal presentation
Merkel cell carcinoma visceral metastatic presentation

C7B.8 Other secondary neuroendocrine tumors (Ex) PDX 412
Coding Clinic: 2024, Q2, P10; 2023, Q1, P21; 2019, Q3, P7

OGCR Section I.C.2.j and k

Disseminated malignant neoplasm, unspecified

j. Code C80.0, Disseminated malignant neoplasm, unspecified, is for use only in those cases where the patient has advanced metastatic disease and no known primary or secondary sites are specified. It should not be used in place of assigning codes for the primary site and all known secondary sites.

Malignant neoplasm without specification of site

k. Code C80.1, Malignant (primary) neoplasm, unspecified, equates to Cancer, unspecified. This code should only be used when no determination can be made as to the primary site of a malignancy. This code should rarely be used in the inpatient setting.

C80 Malignant neoplasm without specification of site
Excludes1 malignant carcinoid tumor of unspecified site (C7A.00)
malignant neoplasm of specified multiple sites- code to each site

C80.0 Disseminated malignant neoplasm, unspecified (Ex) PDX 390
Carcinomatosis NOS
Generalized cancer, unspecified site (primary) (secondary)
Generalized malignancy, unspecified site (primary) (secondary)

C80.1 Malignant (primary) neoplasm, unspecified
Cancer NOS
Cancer unspecified site (primary)
Carcinoma unspecified site (primary)
Malignancy unspecified site (primary)
Excludes1 secondary malignant neoplasm of unspecified site (C79.9)

C80.2 Malignant neoplasm associated with transplanted organ (Ex) PDX 390
Code first complication of transplanted organ (T86.-)
Use additional code to identify the specific malignancy

★**(See Plate 1 of the Anatomy Illustrations.)**

MALIGNANT NEOPLASMS OF LYMPHOID, HEMATOPOIETIC AND RELATED TISSUE (C81-C96)

Excludes2 Kaposi's sarcoma of lymph nodes (C46.3)
secondary and unspecified neoplasm of lymph nodes (C77.-)
secondary neoplasm of bone marrow (C79.52)
secondary neoplasm of spleen (C78.89)

C81 Hodgkin lymphoma
Form of malignant lymphoma with four types, nodular sclerosis, mixed cellularity, lymphocyte depleted, and lymphocyte predominant
Excludes1 personal history of Hodgkin lymphoma (Z85.71)

C81.0 Nodular lymphocyte predominant Hodgkin lymphoma
Least aggressive, least common, typically no symptoms
Lymphocytic-histiocytic predominance Hodgkin's disease
- C81.00 Nodular lymphocyte predominant Hodgkin lymphoma, unspecified site (Ex) PDX 413
- C81.01 Nodular lymphocyte predominant Hodgkin lymphoma, lymph nodes of head, face, and neck (Ex) PDX 414
- C81.02 Nodular lymphocyte predominant Hodgkin lymphoma, intrathoracic lymph nodes (Ex) PDX 415
- C81.03 Nodular lymphocyte predominant Hodgkin lymphoma, intra-abdominal lymph nodes (Ex) PDX 416
- C81.04 Nodular lymphocyte predominant Hodgkin lymphoma, lymph nodes of axilla and upper limb (Ex) PDX 417
- C81.05 Nodular lymphocyte predominant Hodgkin lymphoma, lymph nodes of inguinal region and lower limb (Ex) PDX 418
- C81.06 Nodular lymphocyte predominant Hodgkin lymphoma, intrapelvic lymph nodes (Ex) PDX 419
- C81.07 Nodular lymphocyte predominant Hodgkin lymphoma, spleen (Ex) PDX 420
- C81.08 Nodular lymphocyte predominant Hodgkin lymphoma, lymph nodes of multiple sites (Ex) PDX 413
- C81.09 Nodular lymphocyte predominant Hodgkin lymphoma, extranodal and solid organ sites (Ex) PDX 413
- ▶C81.0A Nodular lymphocyte predominant Hodgkin lymphoma, in remission (Ex) PDX 413

C81.1 Nodular sclerosis Hodgkin lymphoma
Nodular sclerosis classical Hodgkin lymphoma
Moderately aggressive; most common in young adults
- C81.10 Nodular sclerosis Hodgkin lymphoma, unspecified site (Ex) PDX 421
- C81.11 Nodular sclerosis Hodgkin lymphoma, lymph nodes of head, face, and neck (Ex) PDX 422
- C81.12 Nodular sclerosis Hodgkin lymphoma, intrathoracic lymph nodes (Ex) PDX 423
- C81.13 Nodular sclerosis Hodgkin lymphoma, intra-abdominal lymph nodes (Ex) PDX 424
- C81.14 Nodular sclerosis Hodgkin lymphoma, lymph nodes of axilla and upper limb (Ex) PDX 425
- C81.15 Nodular sclerosis Hodgkin lymphoma, lymph nodes of inguinal region and lower limb (Ex) PDX 426
- C81.16 Nodular sclerosis Hodgkin lymphoma, intrapelvic lymph nodes (Ex) PDX 427
- C81.17 Nodular sclerosis Hodgkin lymphoma, spleen (Ex) PDX 428
- C81.18 Nodular sclerosis Hodgkin lymphoma, lymph nodes of multiple sites (Ex) PDX 421
- C81.19 Nodular sclerosis Hodgkin lymphoma, extranodal and solid organ sites (Ex) PDX 421
- ▶C81.1A Nodular sclerosis Hodgkin lymphoma, in remission (Ex) PDX 421

C81.2 Mixed cellularity Hodgkin lymphoma
Mixed cellularity classical Hodgkin lymphoma
A type of Hodgkin's that is moderately aggressive with mixed cell types
- C81.20 Mixed cellularity Hodgkin lymphoma, unspecified site (Ex) PDX 429
- C81.21 Mixed cellularity Hodgkin lymphoma, lymph nodes of head, face, and neck (Ex) PDX 430

CHAPTER 2 (C00-D49)

C81.22 Mixed cellularity Hodgkin lymphoma, intrathoracic lymph nodes PDX 431

C81.23 Mixed cellularity Hodgkin lymphoma, intra-abdominal lymph nodes PDX 432

C81.24 Mixed cellularity Hodgkin lymphoma, lymph nodes of axilla and upper limb PDX 433

C81.25 Mixed cellularity Hodgkin lymphoma, lymph nodes of inguinal region and lower limb PDX 434

C81.26 Mixed cellularity Hodgkin lymphoma, intrapelvic lymph nodes PDX 435

C81.27 Mixed cellularity Hodgkin lymphoma, spleen PDX 429

C81.28 Mixed cellularity Hodgkin lymphoma, lymph nodes of multiple sites PDX 429

C81.29 Mixed cellularity Hodgkin lymphoma, extranodal and solid organ sites PDX 429

C81.2A Mixed cellularity Hodgkin lymphoma, in remission PDX 429

C81.3 Lymphocyte depleted Hodgkin lymphoma

Lymphocyte depleted classical Hodgkin lymphoma

Most aggressive type with poor prognosis

C81.30 Lymphocyte depleted Hodgkin lymphoma, unspecified site PDX 437

C81.31 Lymphocyte depleted Hodgkin lymphoma, lymph nodes of head, face, and neck PDX 438

C81.32 Lymphocyte depleted Hodgkin lymphoma, intrathoracic lymph nodes PDX 439

C81.33 Lymphocyte depleted Hodgkin lymphoma, intra-abdominal lymph nodes PDX 440

C81.34 Lymphocyte depleted Hodgkin lymphoma, lymph nodes of axilla and upper limb PDX 441

C81.35 Lymphocyte depleted Hodgkin lymphoma, lymph nodes of inguinal region and lower limb PDX 442

C81.36 Lymphocyte depleted Hodgkin lymphoma, intrapelvic lymph nodes PDX 443

C81.37 Lymphocyte depleted Hodgkin lymphoma, spleen PDX 444

C81.38 Lymphocyte depleted Hodgkin lymphoma, lymph nodes of multiple sites PDX 445

C81.39 Lymphocyte depleted Hodgkin lymphoma, extranodal and solid organ sites PDX 437

C81.3A Lymphocyte depleted Hodgkin lymphoma, in remission PDX 437

C81.4 Lymphocyte-rich Hodgkin lymphoma

Lymphocyte-rich classical Hodgkin lymphoma

Excludes1 nodular lymphocyte predominant Hodgkin lymphoma (C81.0-)

C81.40 Lymphocyte-rich Hodgkin lymphoma, unspecified site PDX 413

C81.41 Lymphocyte-rich Hodgkin lymphoma, lymph nodes of head, face, and neck PDX 414

C81.42 Lymphocyte-rich Hodgkin lymphoma, intrathoracic lymph nodes PDX 415

C81.43 Lymphocyte-rich Hodgkin lymphoma, intra-abdominal lymph nodes PDX 416

C81.44 Lymphocyte-rich Hodgkin lymphoma, lymph nodes of axilla and upper limb PDX 417

C81.45 Lymphocyte-rich Hodgkin lymphoma, lymph nodes of inguinal region and lower limb PDX 418

C81.46 Lymphocyte-rich Hodgkin lymphoma, intrapelvic lymph nodes PDX 419

C81.47 Lymphocyte-rich Hodgkin lymphoma, spleen PDX 420

C81.48 Lymphocyte-rich Hodgkin lymphoma, lymph nodes of multiple sites PDX 413

C81.49 Lymphocyte-rich Hodgkin lymphoma, extranodal and solid organ sites PDX 413

C81.4A Lymphocyte-rich Hodgkin lymphoma, in remission PDX 413

C81.7 Other Hodgkin lymphoma

Classical Hodgkin lymphoma NOS

Other classical Hodgkin lymphoma

C81.70 Other Hodgkin lymphoma, unspecified site PDX 446

C81.71 Other Hodgkin lymphoma, lymph nodes of head, face, and neck PDX 447

C81.72 Other Hodgkin lymphoma, intrathoracic lymph nodes PDX 448

C81.73 Other Hodgkin lymphoma, intra-abdominal lymph nodes PDX 449

C81.74 Other Hodgkin lymphoma, lymph nodes of axilla and upper limb PDX 450

C81.75 Other Hodgkin lymphoma, lymph nodes of inguinal region and lower limb PDX 451

C81.76 Other Hodgkin lymphoma, intrapelvic lymph nodes PDX 452

C81.77 Other Hodgkin lymphoma, spleen PDX 453

C81.78 Other Hodgkin lymphoma, lymph nodes of multiple sites PDX 446

C81.79 Other Hodgkin lymphoma, extranodal and solid organ sites PDX 446

C81.7A Other Hodgkin lymphoma, in remission PDX 446

C81.9 Hodgkin lymphoma, unspecified

C81.90 Hodgkin lymphoma, unspecified, unspecified site PDX 454

C81.91 Hodgkin lymphoma, unspecified, lymph nodes of head, face, and neck PDX 455

C81.92 Hodgkin lymphoma, unspecified, intrathoracic lymph nodes PDX 456

C81.93 Hodgkin lymphoma, unspecified, intra-abdominal lymph nodes PDX 457

C81.94 Hodgkin lymphoma, unspecified, lymph nodes of axilla and upper limb PDX 458

C81.95 Hodgkin lymphoma, unspecified, lymph nodes of inguinal region and lower limb PDX 459

C81.96 Hodgkin lymphoma, unspecified, intrapelvic lymph nodes PDX 460

C81.97 Hodgkin lymphoma, unspecified, spleen PDX 461

C81.98 Hodgkin lymphoma, unspecified, lymph nodes of multiple sites PDX 454

C81.99 Hodgkin lymphoma, unspecified, extranodal and solid organ sites PDX 462

C81.9A Hodgkin lymphoma, unspecified, in remission PDX 454

C82 Follicular lymphoma

Group of malignant lymphomas

Includes follicular lymphoma with or without diffuse areas

Excludes1 mature T/NK-cell lymphomas (C84.-)
personal history of non-Hodgkin lymphoma (Z85.72)

C82.0 Follicular lymphoma grade I

C82.00 Follicular lymphoma grade I, unspecified site PDX 463

C82.01 Follicular lymphoma grade I, lymph nodes of head, face, and neck PDX 464

C82.02 Follicular lymphoma grade I, intrathoracic lymph nodes PDX 465

C82.03 Follicular lymphoma grade I, intra-abdominal lymph nodes PDX 466

C82.04 Follicular lymphoma grade I, lymph nodes of axilla and upper limb PDX 467

C82.05 Follicular lymphoma grade I, lymph nodes of inguinal region and lower limb (Ex) PDX 468

C82.06 Follicular lymphoma grade I, intrapelvic lymph nodes (Ex) PDX 469

C82.07 Follicular lymphoma grade I, spleen (Ex) PDX 470

C82.08 Follicular lymphoma grade I, lymph nodes of multiple sites (Ex) PDX 471

C82.09 Follicular lymphoma grade I, extranodal and solid organ sites (Ex) PDX 463

C82.0A Follicular lymphoma grade I, in remission (Ex) PDX 463

C82.1 Follicular lymphoma grade II

C82.10 Follicular lymphoma grade II, unspecified site (Ex) PDX 463

C82.11 Follicular lymphoma grade II, lymph nodes of head, face, and neck (Ex) PDX 464

C82.12 Follicular lymphoma grade II, intrathoracic lymph nodes (Ex) PDX 465

C82.13 Follicular lymphoma grade II, intra-abdominal lymph nodes (Ex) PDX 466

C82.14 Follicular lymphoma grade II, lymph nodes of axilla and upper limb (Ex) PDX 467

C82.15 Follicular lymphoma grade II, lymph nodes of inguinal region and lower limb (Ex) PDX 468

C82.16 Follicular lymphoma grade II, intrapelvic lymph nodes (Ex) PDX 469

C82.17 Follicular lymphoma grade II, spleen (Ex) PDX 470

C82.18 Follicular lymphoma grade II, lymph nodes of multiple sites (Ex) PDX 471

C82.19 Follicular lymphoma grade II, extranodal and solid organ sites (Ex) PDX 463

C82.1A Follicular lymphoma grade II, in remission (Ex) PDX 463

C82.2 Follicular lymphoma grade III, unspecified

C82.20 Follicular lymphoma grade III, unspecified, unspecified site (Ex) PDX 463

C82.21 Follicular lymphoma grade III, unspecified, lymph nodes of head, face, and neck (Ex) PDX 464

C82.22 Follicular lymphoma grade III, unspecified, intrathoracic lymph nodes (Ex) PDX 465

C82.23 Follicular lymphoma grade III, unspecified, intra-abdominal lymph nodes (Ex) PDX 466

C82.24 Follicular lymphoma grade III, unspecified, lymph nodes of axilla and upper limb (Ex) PDX 467

C82.25 Follicular lymphoma grade III, unspecified, lymph nodes of inguinal region and lower limb (Ex) PDX 468

C82.26 Follicular lymphoma grade III, unspecified, intrapelvic lymph nodes (Ex) PDX 469

C82.27 Follicular lymphoma grade III, unspecified, spleen (Ex) PDX 470

C82.28 Follicular lymphoma grade III, unspecified, lymph nodes of multiple sites (Ex) PDX 471

C82.29 Follicular lymphoma grade III, unspecified, extranodal and solid organ sites (Ex) PDX 463

C82.2A Follicular lymphoma grade III, unspecified, in remission (Ex) PDX 463

C82.3 Follicular lymphoma grade IIIa

C82.30 Follicular lymphoma grade IIIa, unspecified site (Ex) PDX 463

C82.31 Follicular lymphoma grade IIIa, lymph nodes of head, face, and neck (Ex) PDX 464

C82.32 Follicular lymphoma grade IIIa, intrathoracic lymph nodes (Ex) PDX 465

C82.33 Follicular lymphoma grade IIIa, intra-abdominal lymph nodes (Ex) PDX 466

C82.34 Follicular lymphoma grade IIIa, lymph nodes of axilla and upper limb (Ex) PDX 467

C82.35 Follicular lymphoma grade IIIa, lymph nodes of inguinal region and lower limb (Ex) PDX 468

C82.36 Follicular lymphoma grade IIIa, intrapelvic lymph nodes (Ex) PDX 469

C82.37 Follicular lymphoma grade IIIa, spleen (Ex) PDX 470

C82.38 Follicular lymphoma grade IIIa, lymph nodes of multiple sites (Ex) PDX 471

C82.39 Follicular lymphoma grade IIIa, extranodal and solid organ sites (Ex) PDX 463

C82.3A Follicular lymphoma grade IIIa, in remission (Ex) PDX 463

C82.4 Follicular lymphoma grade IIIb

C82.40 Follicular lymphoma grade IIIb, unspecified site (Ex) PDX 463

C82.41 Follicular lymphoma grade IIIb, lymph nodes of head, face, and neck (Ex) PDX 464

C82.42 Follicular lymphoma grade IIIb, intrathoracic lymph nodes (Ex) PDX 465

C82.43 Follicular lymphoma grade IIIb, intra-abdominal lymph nodes (Ex) PDX 466

C82.44 Follicular lymphoma grade IIIb, lymph nodes of axilla and upper limb (Ex) PDX 467

C82.45 Follicular lymphoma grade IIIb, lymph nodes of inguinal region and lower limb (Ex) PDX 468

C82.46 Follicular lymphoma grade IIIb, intrapelvic lymph nodes (Ex) PDX 469

C82.47 Follicular lymphoma grade IIIb, spleen (Ex) PDX 470

C82.48 Follicular lymphoma grade IIIb, lymph nodes of multiple sites (Ex) PDX 471

C82.49 Follicular lymphoma grade IIIb, extranodal and solid organ sites (Ex) PDX 463

C82.4A Follicular lymphoma grade IIIb, in remission (Ex) PDX 463

C82.5 Diffuse follicle center lymphoma

C82.50 Diffuse follicle center lymphoma, unspecified site (Ex) PDX 472

C82.51 Diffuse follicle center lymphoma, lymph nodes of head, face, and neck (Ex) PDX 473

C82.52 Diffuse follicle center lymphoma, intrathoracic lymph nodes (Ex) PDX 474

C82.53 Diffuse follicle center lymphoma, intra-abdominal lymph nodes (Ex) PDX 475

C82.54 Diffuse follicle center lymphoma, lymph nodes of axilla and upper limb (Ex) PDX 476

C82.55 Diffuse follicle center lymphoma, lymph nodes of inguinal region and lower limb (Ex) PDX 477

C82.56 Diffuse follicle center lymphoma, intrapelvic lymph nodes (Ex) PDX 478

C82.57 Diffuse follicle center lymphoma, spleen (Ex) PDX 479

C82.58 Diffuse follicle center lymphoma, lymph nodes of multiple sites (Ex) PDX 480

C82.59 Diffuse follicle center lymphoma, extranodal and solid organ sites (Ex) PDX 472

C82.5A Diffuse follicle center lymphoma, in remission (Ex) PDX 472

C82.6 Cutaneous follicle center lymphoma

C82.60 Cutaneous follicle center lymphoma, unspecified site (Ex) PDX 463

C82.61 Cutaneous follicle center lymphoma, lymph nodes of head, face, and neck (Ex) PDX 464

C82.62 Cutaneous follicle center lymphoma, intrathoracic lymph nodes (Ex) PDX 465

CHAPTER 2 (C00-D49)

C82.63 Cutaneous follicle center lymphoma, intra-abdominal lymph nodes (Ex:) PDX 466
C82.64 Cutaneous follicle center lymphoma, lymph nodes of axilla and upper limb (Ex:) PDX 467
C82.65 Cutaneous follicle center lymphoma, lymph nodes of inguinal region and lower limb (Ex:) PDX 468
C82.66 Cutaneous follicle center lymphoma, intrapelvic lymph nodes (Ex:) PDX 469
C82.67 Cutaneous follicle center lymphoma, spleen (Ex:) PDX 470
C82.68 Cutaneous follicle center lymphoma, lymph nodes of multiple sites (Ex:) PDX 471
C82.69 Cutaneous follicle center lymphoma, extranodal and solid organ sites (Ex:) PDX 463
▶C82.6A Cutaneous follicle center lymphoma, in remission (Ex:) PDX 463

●C82.8 Other types of follicular lymphoma
C82.80 Other types of follicular lymphoma, unspecified site (Ex:) PDX 463
C82.81 Other types of follicular lymphoma, lymph nodes of head, face, and neck (Ex:) PDX 464
C82.82 Other types of follicular lymphoma, intrathoracic lymph nodes (Ex:) PDX 465
C82.83 Other types of follicular lymphoma, intra-abdominal lymph nodes (Ex:) PDX 466
C82.84 Other types of follicular lymphoma, lymph nodes of axilla and upper limb (Ex:) PDX 467
C82.85 Other types of follicular lymphoma, lymph nodes of inguinal region and lower limb (Ex:) PDX 468
C82.86 Other types of follicular lymphoma, intra pelvic lymph nodes (Ex:) PDX 469
C82.87 Other types of follicular lymphoma, spleen (Ex:) PDX 470
C82.88 Other types of follicular lymphoma, lymph nodes of multiple sites (Ex:) PDX 471
C82.89 Other types of follicular lymphoma, extranodal and solid organ sites (Ex:) PDX 463
▶C82.8A Other types of follicular lymphoma, in remission (Ex:) PDX 463

●C82.9 Follicular lymphoma, unspecified
C82.90 Follicular lymphoma, unspecified, unspecified site (Ex:) PDX 463
C82.91 Follicular lymphoma, unspecified, lymph nodes of head, face, and neck (Ex:) PDX 464
C82.92 Follicular lymphoma, unspecified, intrathoracic lymph nodes (Ex:) PDX 465
C82.93 Follicular lymphoma, unspecified, intra-abdominal lymph nodes (Ex:) PDX 466
C82.94 Follicular lymphoma, unspecified, lymph nodes of axilla and upper limb (Ex:) PDX 467
C82.95 Follicular lymphoma, unspecified, lymph nodes of inguinal region and lower limb (Ex:) PDX 468
C82.96 Follicular lymphoma, unspecified, intra pelvic lymph nodes (Ex:) PDX 469
C82.97 Follicular lymphoma, unspecified, spleen (Ex:) PDX 470
C82.98 Follicular lymphoma, unspecified, lymph nodes of multiple sites (Ex:) PDX 471
C82.99 Follicular lymphoma, unspecified, extranodal and solid organ sites (Ex:) PDX 463
▶C82.9A Follicular lymphoma, unspecified, in remission (Ex:) PDX 463

●C83 Non-follicular lymphoma
Excludes1 personal history of non-Hodgkin lymphoma (Z85.72)

●C83.0 Small cell B-cell lymphoma
Lymphoplasmacytic lymphoma
Nodal marginal zone lymphoma
Non-leukemic variant of B-CLL
Splenic marginal zone lymphoma
Excludes1 chronic lymphocytic leukemia (C91.1)
mature T/NK-cell lymphomas (C84.-)
➡Waldenström macroglobulinemia (C88.00)
Coding Clinic: 2023, Q1, P18-19
C83.00 Small cell B-cell lymphoma, unspecified site (Ex:) PDX 481
C83.01 Small cell B-cell lymphoma, lymph nodes of head, face, and neck (Ex:) PDX 482
C83.02 Small cell B-cell lymphoma, intrathoracic lymph nodes (Ex:) PDX 483
C83.03 Small cell B-cell lymphoma, intra-abdominal lymph nodes (Ex:) PDX 484
C83.04 Small cell B-cell lymphoma, lymph nodes of axilla and upper limb (Ex:) PDX 485
C83.05 Small cell B-cell lymphoma, lymph nodes of inguinal region and lower limb (Ex:) PDX 476
C83.06 Small cell B-cell lymphoma, intrapelvic lymph nodes (Ex:) PDX 487
C83.07 Small cell B-cell lymphoma, spleen (Ex:) PDX 488
C83.08 Small cell B-cell lymphoma, lymph nodes of multiple sites (Ex:) PDX 481
C83.09 Small cell B-cell lymphoma, extranodal and solid organ sites (Ex:) PDX 481
▶C83.0A Small cell B-cell lymphoma, in remission (Ex:) PDX 481

●C83.1 Mantle cell lymphoma
Centrocytic lymphoma
Malignant lymphomatous polyposis
C83.10 Mantle cell lymphoma, unspecified site (Ex:) PDX 472
Coding Clinic: 2024, Q1, P24
C83.11 Mantle cell lymphoma, lymph nodes of head, face, and neck (Ex:) PDX 473
C83.12 Mantle cell lymphoma, intrathoracic lymph nodes (Ex:) PDX 474
C83.13 Mantle cell lymphoma, intra-abdominal lymph nodes (Ex:) PDX 475
C83.14 Mantle cell lymphoma, lymph nodes of axilla and upper limb (Ex:) PDX 476
C83.15 Mantle cell lymphoma, lymph nodes of inguinal region and lower limb (Ex:) PDX 477
C83.16 Mantle cell lymphoma, intrapelvic lymph nodes (Ex:) PDX 478
C83.17 Mantle cell lymphoma, spleen (Ex:) PDX 479
C83.18 Mantle cell lymphoma, lymph nodes of multiple sites (Ex:) PDX 480
C83.19 Mantle cell lymphoma, extranodal and solid organ sites (Ex:) PDX 472
▶C83.1A Mantle cell lymphoma, in remission (Ex:) PDX 472
▶Centrocytic lymphoma, in remission

●C83.3 Diffuse large B-cell lymphoma
Anaplastic diffuse large B-cell lymphoma
CD30-positive diffuse large B-cell lymphoma
Centroblastic diffuse large B-cell lymphoma
~~Diffuse large B-cell lymphoma, subtype not specified~~
Immunoblastic diffuse large B-cell lymphoma
Plasmablastic diffuse large B-cell lymphoma
Diffuse large B-cell lymphoma, subtype not specified
T-cell rich diffuse large B-cell lymphoma
Excludes1 mediastinal (thymic) large B-cell lymphoma (C85.2-)
mature T/NK-cell lymphomas (C84.-)

C83.30 Diffuse large B-cell lymphoma, unspecified site (Ex) PDX 489
C83.31 Diffuse large B-cell lymphoma, lymph nodes of head, face, and neck (Ex) PDX 490
C83.32 Diffuse large B-cell lymphoma, intrathoracic lymph nodes (Ex) PDX 491
C83.33 Diffuse large B-cell lymphoma, intra-abdominal lymph nodes (Ex) PDX 492
C83.34 Diffuse large B-cell lymphoma, lymph nodes of axilla and upper limb (Ex) PDX 493
C83.35 Diffuse large B-cell lymphoma, lymph nodes of inguinal region and lower limb (Ex) PDX 494
C83.36 Diffuse large B-cell lymphoma, intrapelvic lymph nodes (Ex) PDX 495
C83.37 Diffuse large B-cell lymphoma, spleen (Ex) PDX 496
C83.38 Diffuse large B-cell lymphoma, lymph nodes of multiple sites (Ex) PDX 489
Coding Clinic: 2023, Q1, P22
C83.39 Diffuse large B-cell lymphoma, extranodal and solid organ sites (Ex) PDX 489
Coding Clinic: 2023, Q1, P22
▶C83.390 Primary central nervous system lymphoma
▶PCNSL of brain
▶PCNSL of meninges
▶PCNSL of spinal cord
▶PCNSL NOS
▶ **Excludes1** Primary central nervous system lymphoma, Burkitt (C83.79)
▶Primary central nervous system lymphoma, lymphoblastic (C83.59)
▶Primary central nervous system lymphoma, other (C83.89)
▶Primary central nervous system lymphoma, peripheral T-cell (C84.49)
▶C83.398 Diffuse large B-cell lymphoma of other extranodal and solid organ sites
▶C83.3A Diffuse large B-cell lymphoma, in remission (Ex) PDX 489

● C83.5 Lymphoblastic (diffuse) lymphoma
Highly malignant type of non-Hodgkin lymphoma with diffuse infiltration
B-precursor lymphoma
Lymphoblastic B-cell lymphoma
Lymphoblastic lymphoma NOS
Lymphoblastic T-cell lymphoma
T-precursor lymphoma
C83.50 Lymphoblastic (diffuse) lymphoma, unspecified site (Ex) PDX 497
C83.51 Lymphoblastic (diffuse) lymphoma, lymph nodes of head, face, and neck (Ex) PDX 498
C83.52 Lymphoblastic (diffuse) lymphoma, intrathoracic lymph nodes (Ex) PDX 499
C83.53 Lymphoblastic (diffuse) lymphoma, intra-abdominal lymph nodes (Ex) PDX 500
C83.54 Lymphoblastic (diffuse) lymphoma, lymph nodes of axilla and upper limb (Ex) PDX 501
C83.55 Lymphoblastic (diffuse) lymphoma, lymph nodes of inguinal region and lower limb (Ex) PDX 502
C83.56 Lymphoblastic (diffuse) lymphoma, intrapelvic lymph nodes (Ex) PDX 503
C83.57 Lymphoblastic (diffuse) lymphoma, spleen (Ex) PDX 504
C83.58 Lymphoblastic (diffuse) lymphoma, lymph nodes of multiple sites (Ex) PDX 497
C83.59 Lymphoblastic (diffuse) lymphoma, extranodal and solid organ sites (Ex) PDX 497
▶C83.5A Lymphoblastic (diffuse) lymphoma, in remission (Ex) PDX 497

● C83.7 Burkitt lymphoma
Form of small cell lymphoma
Atypical Burkitt lymphoma
Burkitt-like lymphoma
Excludes1 mature B-cell leukemia Burkitt type (C91.A-)
C83.70 Burkitt lymphoma, unspecified site (Ex) PDX 505
C83.71 Burkitt lymphoma, lymph nodes of head, face, and neck (Ex) PDX 506
C83.72 Burkitt lymphoma, intrathoracic lymph nodes (Ex) PDX 507
C83.73 Burkitt lymphoma, intra-abdominal lymph nodes (Ex) PDX 508
C83.74 Burkitt lymphoma, lymph nodes of axilla and upper limb (Ex) PDX 509
C83.75 Burkitt lymphoma, lymph nodes of inguinal region and lower limb (Ex) PDX 510
C83.76 Burkitt lymphoma, intrapelvic lymph nodes (Ex) PDX 511
C83.77 Burkitt lymphoma, spleen (Ex) PDX 512
C83.78 Burkitt lymphoma, lymph nodes of multiple sites (Ex) PDX 505
C83.79 Burkitt lymphoma, extranodal and solid organ sites (Ex) PDX 505
▶C83.7A Burkitt lymphoma, in remission (Ex) PDX 505

● C83.8 Other non-follicular lymphoma
Intravascular large B-cell lymphoma
Lymphoid granulomatosis
Primary effusion B-cell lymphoma
Excludes1 mediastinal (thymic) large B-cell lymphoma (C85.2-)
T-cell rich B-cell lymphoma (C83.3-)
C83.80 Other non-follicular lymphoma, unspecified site (Ex) PDX 481
C83.81 Other non-follicular lymphoma, lymph nodes of head, face, and neck (Ex) PDX 482
C83.82 Other non-follicular lymphoma, intrathoracic lymph nodes (Ex) PDX 483
C83.83 Other non-follicular lymphoma, intra-abdominal lymph nodes (Ex) PDX 484
C83.84 Other non-follicular lymphoma, lymph nodes of axilla and upper limb (Ex) PDX 485
C83.85 Other non-follicular lymphoma, lymph nodes of inguinal region and lower limb (Ex) PDX 486
C83.86 Other non-follicular lymphoma, intrapelvic lymph nodes (Ex) PDX 487
C83.87 Other non-follicular lymphoma, spleen (Ex) PDX 488
C83.88 Other non-follicular lymphoma, lymph nodes of multiple sites (Ex) PDX 481
C83.89 Other non-follicular lymphoma, extranodal and solid organ sites (Ex) PDX 481
▶C83.8A Other non-follicular lymphoma, in remission (Ex) PDX 481

● C83.9 Non-follicular (diffuse) lymphoma, unspecified
C83.90 Non-follicular (diffuse) lymphoma, unspecified, unspecified site (Ex) PDX 481
C83.91 Non-follicular (diffuse) lymphoma, unspecified, lymph nodes of head, face, and neck (Ex) PDX 482
C83.92 Non-follicular (diffuse) lymphoma, unspecified, intrathoracic lymph nodes (Ex) PDX 483
C83.93 Non-follicular (diffuse) lymphoma, unspecified, intra-abdominal lymph nodes (Ex) PDX 484

C83.94 **Non-follicular (diffuse) lymphoma, unspecified, lymph nodes of axilla and upper limb** PDX 485

C83.95 **Non-follicular (diffuse) lymphoma, unspecified, lymph nodes of inguinal region and lower limb** PDX 486

C83.96 **Non-follicular (diffuse) lymphoma, unspecified, intrapelvic lymph nodes** PDX 487

C83.97 **Non-follicular (diffuse) lymphoma, unspecified, spleen** PDX 488

C83.98 **Non-follicular (diffuse) lymphoma, unspecified, lymph nodes of multiple sites** PDX 481

C83.99 **Non-follicular (diffuse) lymphoma, unspecified, extranodal and solid organ sites** PDX 481

▶C83.9A **Non-follicular (diffuse) lymphoma, unspecified, in remission** PDX 481

C84 Mature T/NK-cell lymphomas

Excludes1 personal history of non-Hodgkin lymphoma (Z85.72)

C84.Ø Mycosis fungoides

Chronic or rapidly progressive form of cutaneous T-cell lymphoma; AKA granuloma fungoides

Excludes1 peripheral T-cell lymphoma, not elsewhere classified (C84.4-)

C84.ØØ **Mycosis fungoides, unspecified site** PDX 513

C84.Ø1 **Mycosis fungoides, lymph nodes of head, face, and neck** PDX 514

C84.Ø2 **Mycosis fungoides, intrathoracic lymph nodes** PDX 515

C84.Ø3 **Mycosis fungoides, intra-abdominal lymph nodes** PDX 516

C84.Ø4 **Mycosis fungoides, lymph nodes of axilla and upper limb** PDX 517

C84.Ø5 **Mycosis fungoides, lymph nodes of inguinal region and lower limb** PDX 518

C84.Ø6 **Mycosis fungoides, intrapelvic lymph nodes** PDX 519

C84.Ø7 **Mycosis fungoides, spleen** PDX 520

C84.Ø8 **Mycosis fungoides, lymph nodes of multiple sites** PDX 521

C84.Ø9 **Mycosis fungoides, extranodal and solid organ sites** PDX 513

▶C84.ØA **Mycosis fungoides, in remission** PDX 513

C84.1 Sézary disease

Type of cutaneous lymphoma affecting T-cells

C84.1Ø **Sézary disease, unspecified site** PDX 522

C84.11 **Sézary disease, lymph nodes of head, face, and neck** PDX 523

C84.12 **Sézary disease, intrathoracic lymph nodes** PDX 524

C84.13 **Sézary disease, intra-abdominal lymph nodes** PDX 525

C84.14 **Sézary disease, lymph nodes of axilla and upper limb** PDX 526

C84.15 **Sézary disease, lymph nodes of inguinal region and lower limb** PDX 527

C84.16 **Sézary disease, intrapelvic lymph nodes** PDX 528

C84.17 **Sézary disease, spleen** PDX 529

C84.18 **Sézary disease, lymph nodes of multiple sites** PDX 530

C84.19 **Sézary disease, extranodal and solid organ sites** PDX 522

▶C84.1A **Sézary disease, in remission** PDX 522

C84.4 Peripheral T-cell lymphoma, not elsewhere classified

Diverse group of blood carcinomas originating from T-cells, requiring aggressive chemotherapy

Lennert's lymphoma
Lymphoepithelioid lymphoma
Mature T-cell lymphoma, not elsewhere classified

C84.4Ø **Peripheral T-cell lymphoma, not elsewhere classified, unspecified site** PDX 472

C84.41 **Peripheral T-cell lymphoma, not elsewhere classified, lymph nodes of head, face, and neck** PDX 473

C84.42 **Peripheral T-cell lymphoma, not elsewhere classified, intrathoracic lymph nodes** PDX 474

C84.43 **Peripheral T-cell lymphoma, not elsewhere classified, intra-abdominal lymph nodes** PDX 475

C84.44 **Peripheral T-cell lymphoma, not elsewhere classified, lymph nodes of axilla and upper limb** PDX 476

C84.45 **Peripheral T-cell lymphoma, not elsewhere classified, lymph nodes of inguinal region and lower limb** PDX 477

C84.46 **Peripheral T-cell lymphoma, not elsewhere classified, intrapelvic lymph nodes** PDX 478

C84.47 **Peripheral T-cell lymphoma, not elsewhere classified, spleen** PDX 479

C84.48 **Peripheral T-cell lymphoma, not elsewhere classified, lymph nodes of multiple sites** PDX 480

C84.49 **Peripheral T-cell lymphoma, not elsewhere classified, extranodal and solid organ sites** PDX 472

▶C84.4A **Peripheral T-cell lymphoma, not elsewhere classified, in remission** PDX 472

C84.6 Anaplastic large cell lymphoma, ALK-positive

Anaplastic large cell lymphoma, CD3Ø-positive

C84.6Ø **Anaplastic large cell lymphoma, ALK-positive, unspecified site** PDX 472

C84.61 **Anaplastic large cell lymphoma, ALK-positive, lymph nodes of head, face, and neck** PDX 473

C84.62 **Anaplastic large cell lymphoma, ALK-positive, intrathoracic lymph nodes** PDX 474

C84.63 **Anaplastic large cell lymphoma, ALK-positive, intra-abdominal lymph nodes** PDX 475

C84.64 **Anaplastic large cell lymphoma, ALK-positive, lymph nodes of axilla and upper limb** PDX 476

C84.65 **Anaplastic large cell lymphoma, ALK-positive, lymph nodes of inguinal region and lower limb** PDX 477

C84.66 **Anaplastic large cell lymphoma, ALK-positive, intrapelvic lymph nodes** PDX 478

C84.67 **Anaplastic large cell lymphoma, ALK-positive, spleen** PDX 479

C84.68 **Anaplastic large cell lymphoma, ALK-positive, lymph nodes of multiple sites** PDX 480

C84.69 **Anaplastic large cell lymphoma, ALK-positive, extranodal and solid organ sites** PDX 472

▶C84.6A **Anaplastic large cell lymphoma, ALK-positive, in remission** PDX 472

Item 2–7 Lymphosarcoma, also known as malignant lymphoma, is a cancer of the lymph system exhibiting abnormal cells encompassing an entire lymph node creating a diffuse pattern without any definite organization. Diffuse pattern lymphoma has a more unfavorable survival outlook than those with a follicular or nodular pattern. Reticulosarcoma is the most common aggressive form of non-Hodgkin lymphoma.

C84.7 Anaplastic large cell lymphoma, ALK-negative
Excludes1 primary cutaneous CD3Ø-positive T-cell proliferations (C86.6-)

C84.7Ø Anaplastic large cell lymphoma, ALK-negative, unspecified site PDX 472
C84.71 Anaplastic large cell lymphoma, ALK-negative, lymph nodes of head, face, and neck PDX 473
C84.72 Anaplastic large cell lymphoma, ALK-negative, intrathoracic lymph nodes PDX 474
C84.73 Anaplastic large cell lymphoma, ALK-negative, intra-abdominal lymph nodes PDX 475
C84.74 Anaplastic large cell lymphoma, ALK-negative, lymph nodes of axilla and upper limb PDX 476
C84.75 Anaplastic large cell lymphoma, ALK-negative, lymph nodes of inguinal region and lower limb PDX 477
C84.76 Anaplastic large cell lymphoma, ALK-negative, intrapelvic lymph nodes PDX 478
C84.77 Anaplastic large cell lymphoma, ALK-negative, spleen PDX 479
C84.78 Anaplastic large cell lymphoma, ALK-negative, lymph nodes of multiple sites PDX 480
C84.79 Anaplastic large cell lymphoma, ALK-negative, extranodal and solid organ sites PDX 472
C84.7A Anaplastic large cell lymphoma, ALK-negative, breast PDX 531
Breast implant associated anaplastic large cell lymphoma (BIA-ALCL)
Use additional code to identify:
breast implant status (Z98.82)
personal history of breast implant removal (Z98.86)
C84.7B Anaplastic large cell lymphoma, ALK-negative, in remission PDX 472

C84.9 Mature T/NK-cell lymphomas, unspecified
NK/T cell lymphoma NOS
Excludes1 mature T-cell lymphoma, not elsewhere classified (C84.4-)

C84.9Ø Mature T/NK-cell lymphomas, unspecified, unspecified site PDX 472
C84.91 Mature T/NK-cell lymphomas, unspecified, lymph nodes of head, face, and neck PDX 473
C84.92 Mature T/NK-cell lymphomas, unspecified, intrathoracic lymph nodes PDX 474
C84.93 Mature T/NK-cell lymphomas, unspecified, intra-abdominal lymph nodes PDX 475
C84.94 Mature T/NK-cell lymphomas, unspecified, lymph nodes of axilla and upper limb PDX 476
C84.95 Mature T/NK-cell lymphomas, unspecified, lymph nodes of inguinal region and lower limb PDX 477
C84.96 Mature T/NK-cell lymphomas, unspecified, intrapelvic lymph nodes PDX 478
C84.97 Mature T/NK-cell lymphomas, unspecified, spleen PDX 479
C84.98 Mature T/NK-cell lymphomas, unspecified, lymph nodes of multiple sites PDX 480
C84.99 Mature T/NK-cell lymphomas, unspecified, extranodal and solid organ sites PDX 472
C84.9A Mature T/NK-cell lymphomas, unspecified, in remission PDX 472

C84.A Cutaneous T-cell lymphoma, unspecified

C84.AØ Cutaneous T-cell lymphoma, unspecified, unspecified site PDX 472
C84.A1 Cutaneous T-cell lymphoma, unspecified lymph nodes of head, face, and neck PDX 473
C84.A2 Cutaneous T-cell lymphoma, unspecified, intrathoracic lymph nodes PDX 474
C84.A3 Cutaneous T-cell lymphoma, unspecified, intra-abdominal lymph nodes PDX 475
C84.A4 Cutaneous T-cell lymphoma, unspecified, lymph nodes of axilla and upper limb PDX 476
C84.A5 Cutaneous T-cell lymphoma, unspecified, lymph nodes of inguinal region and lower limb PDX 477
C84.A6 Cutaneous T-cell lymphoma, unspecified, intrapelvic lymph nodes PDX 478
C84.A7 Cutaneous T-cell lymphoma, unspecified, spleen PDX 479
Coding Clinic: 2Ø21, Q2, P7
C84.A8 Cutaneous T-cell lymphoma, unspecified, lymph nodes of multiple sites PDX 480
Coding Clinic: 2Ø21, Q2, P7
C84.A9 Cutaneous T-cell lymphoma, unspecified, extranodal and solid organ sites PDX 472
C84.AA Cutaneous T-cell lymphoma, unspecified, in remission PDX 472

C84.Z Other mature T/NK-cell lymphomas
Note: If T-cell lineage or involvement is mentioned in conjunction with a specific lymphoma, code to the more specific description.
Excludes1 angioimmunoblastic T-cell lymphoma (C86.5Ø)
blastic NK-cell lymphoma (C86.4Ø)
enteropathy-type T-cell lymphoma (C86.2Ø)
extranodal NK-cell lymphoma, nasal type (C86.ØØ)
hepatosplenic T-cell lymphoma (C86.1Ø)
primary cutaneous CD3Ø-positive T-cell proliferations (C86.6Ø)
subcutaneous panniculitis-like T-cell lymphoma (C86.3Ø)
T-cell leukemia (C91.1-)

C84.ZØ Other mature T/NK-cell lymphomas, unspecified site PDX 472
C84.Z1 Other mature T/NK-cell lymphomas, lymph nodes of head, face, and neck PDX 473
C84.Z2 Other mature T/NK-cell lymphomas, intrathoracic lymph nodes PDX 474
C84.Z3 Other mature T/NK-cell lymphomas, intra-abdominal lymph nodes PDX 475
C84.Z4 Other mature T/NK-cell lymphomas, lymph nodes of axilla and upper limb PDX 476
C84.Z5 Other mature T/NK-cell lymphomas, lymph nodes of inguinal region and lower limb PDX 477
C84.Z6 Other mature T/NK-cell lymphomas, intrapelvic lymph nodes PDX 478
C84.Z7 Other mature T/NK-cell lymphomas, spleen PDX 479
C84.Z8 Other mature T/NK-cell lymphomas, lymph nodes of multiple sites PDX 480
C84.Z9 Other mature T/NK-cell lymphomas, extranodal and solid organ sites PDX 472
C84.ZA Other mature T/NK-cell lymphomas, in remission PDX 472

CHAPTER 2 (CØØ-D49)

● C85 Other specified and unspecified types of non-Hodgkin lymphoma
Excludes1 other specified types of T/NK-cell lymphoma (C86.-)
personal history of non-Hodgkin lymphoma (Z85.72)

● C85.1 Unspecified B-cell lymphoma
Note: If B-cell lineage or involvement is mentioned in conjunction with a specific lymphoma, code to the more specific description.
C85.10 Unspecified B-cell lymphoma, unspecified site PDX 472
C85.11 Unspecified B-cell lymphoma, lymph nodes of head, face, and neck PDX 473
C85.12 Unspecified B-cell lymphoma, intrathoracic lymph nodes PDX 474
C85.13 Unspecified B-cell lymphoma, intra-abdominal lymph nodes PDX 475
C85.14 Unspecified B-cell lymphoma, lymph nodes of axilla and upper limb PDX 476
C85.15 Unspecified B-cell lymphoma, lymph nodes of inguinal region and lower limb PDX 477
C85.16 Unspecified B-cell lymphoma, intrapelvic lymph nodes PDX 478
C85.17 Unspecified B-cell lymphoma, spleen PDX 479
C85.18 Unspecified B-cell lymphoma, lymph nodes of multiple sites PDX 480
C85.19 Unspecified B-cell lymphoma, extranodal and solid organ sites PDX 472
▶ C85.1A Unspecified B-cell lymphoma, in remission PDX 472

● C85.2 Mediastinal (thymic) large B-cell lymphoma
C85.20 Mediastinal (thymic) large B-cell lymphoma, unspecified site PDX 472
C85.21 Mediastinal (thymic) large B-cell lymphoma, lymph nodes of head, face, and neck PDX 473
C85.22 Mediastinal (thymic) large B-cell lymphoma, intrathoracic lymph nodes PDX 474
C85.23 Mediastinal (thymic) large B-cell lymphoma, intra-abdominal lymph nodes PDX 475
C85.24 Mediastinal (thymic) large B-cell lymphoma, lymph nodes of axilla and upper limb PDX 476
C85.25 Mediastinal (thymic) large B-cell lymphoma, lymph nodes of inguinal region and lower limb PDX 477
C85.26 Mediastinal (thymic) large B-cell lymphoma, intrapelvic lymph nodes PDX 478
C85.27 Mediastinal (thymic) large B-cell lymphoma, spleen PDX 479
C85.28 Mediastinal (thymic) large B-cell lymphoma, lymph nodes of multiple sites PDX 480
C85.29 Mediastinal (thymic) large B-cell lymphoma, extranodal and solid organ sites PDX 472
▶ C85.2A Mediastinal (thymic) large B-cell lymphoma, in remission PDX 472

● C85.8 Other specified types of non-Hodgkin lymphoma
C85.80 Other specified types of non-Hodgkin lymphoma, unspecified site PDX 472
C85.81 Other specified types of non-Hodgkin lymphoma, lymph nodes of head, face, and neck PDX 473
C85.82 Other specified types of non-Hodgkin lymphoma, intrathoracic lymph nodes PDX 474
C85.83 Other specified types of non-Hodgkin lymphoma, intra-abdominal lymph nodes PDX 475
C85.84 Other specified types of non-Hodgkin lymphoma, lymph nodes of axilla and upper limb PDX 476
C85.85 Other specified types of non-Hodgkin lymphoma, lymph nodes of inguinal region and lower limb PDX 477
C85.86 Other specified types of non-Hodgkin lymphoma, intrapelvic lymph nodes PDX 478
C85.87 Other specified types of non-Hodgkin lymphoma, spleen PDX 479
C85.88 Other specified types of non-Hodgkin lymphoma, lymph nodes of multiple sites PDX 480
C85.89 Other specified types of non-Hodgkin lymphoma, extranodal and solid organ sites PDX 472
▶ C85.8A Other specified types of non-Hodgkin lymphoma, in remission PDX 472

● C85.9 Non-Hodgkin lymphoma, unspecified
Lymphoma NOS
Malignant lymphoma NOS
Non-Hodgkin lymphoma NOS
C85.90 Non-Hodgkin lymphoma, unspecified, unspecified site PDX 472
C85.91 Non-Hodgkin lymphoma, unspecified, lymph nodes of head, face, and neck PDX 473
C85.92 Non-Hodgkin lymphoma, unspecified, intrathoracic lymph nodes PDX 474
C85.93 Non-Hodgkin lymphoma, unspecified, intra-abdominal lymph nodes PDX 475
C85.94 Non-Hodgkin lymphoma, unspecified, lymph nodes of axilla and upper limb PDX 476
C85.95 Non-Hodgkin lymphoma, unspecified, lymph nodes of inguinal region and lower limb PDX 477
C85.96 Non-Hodgkin lymphoma, unspecified, intrapelvic lymph nodes PDX 478
C85.97 Non-Hodgkin lymphoma, unspecified, spleen PDX 479
C85.98 Non-Hodgkin lymphoma, unspecified, lymph nodes of multiple sites PDX 480
C85.99 Non-Hodgkin lymphoma, unspecified, extranodal and solid organ sites PDX 472
▶ C85.9A Non-Hodgkin lymphoma, unspecified, in remission PDX 472

● C86 Other specified types of T/NK-cell lymphoma
Excludes1 anaplastic large cell lymphoma, ALK negative (C84.7-)
anaplastic large cell lymphoma, ALK positive (C84.6-)
mature T/NK-cell lymphomas (C84.-)
other specified types of non-Hodgkin lymphoma (C85.8-)

C86.0 Extranodal NK/T-cell lymphoma, nasal type PDX 473
▶ C86.00 Extranodal NK/T-cell lymphoma, nasal type not having achieved remission
▶ Extranodal NK/T-cell lymphoma, nasal type NOS
▶ Extranodal NK/T-cell lymphoma, nasal type with failed remission
▶ C86.01 Extranodal NK/T-cell lymphoma, nasal type, in remission

C86.1 Hepatosplenic T-cell lymphoma PDX 479
Alpha-beta and gamma delta types
▶ C86.10 Hepatosplenic T-cell lymphoma not having achieved remission
▶ Hepatosplenic T-cell lymphoma NOS
▶ Hepatosplenic T-cell lymphoma with failed remission
▶ C86.11 Hepatosplenic T-cell lymphoma, in remission

C86.2 Enteropathy-type (intestinal) T-cell lymphoma PDX 475
Enteropathy associated T-cell lymphoma

▶C86.2Ø **Enteropathy-type (intestinal) T-cell lymphoma not having achieved remission**
▶Enteropathy associated T-cell lymphoma NOS
▶Enteropathy associated T-cell lymphoma not having achieved remission
▶Enteropathy associated T-cell lymphoma with failed remission
▶Enteropathy-type (intestinal) T-cell lymphoma NOS
▶Enteropathy-type (intestinal) T-cell lymphoma with failed remission

▶C86.21 **Enteropathy-type (intestinal) T-cell lymphoma, in remission**
▶Enteropathy associated T-cell lymphoma, in remission

C86.3 **Subcutaneous panniculitis-like T-cell lymphoma** (Ex) PDX 475

▶C86.3Ø **Subcutaneous panniculitis-like T-cell lymphoma not having achieved remission**
▶Subcutaneous panniculitis-like T-cell lymphoma NOS
▶Subcutaneous panniculitis-like T-cell lymphoma with failed remission

▶C86.3 **Subcutaneous panniculitis-like T-cell lymphoma, in remission**

C86.4 **Blastic NK-cell lymphoma** (Ex) PDX 472
Blastic plasmacytoid dendritic cell neoplasm (BPDCN)

▶C86.4Ø **Blastic NK-cell lymphoma not having achieved remission**
▶Blastic NK-cell lymphoma NOS
▶Blastic NK-cell lymphoma with failed remission
▶Blastic plasmacytoid dendritic cell neoplasm (BPDCN) NOS
▶Blastic plasmacytoid dendritic cell neoplasm (BPDCN) not having achieved remission
▶Blastic plasmacytoid dendritic cell neoplasm (BPDCN) with failed remission

▶C86.41 **Blastic NK-cell lymphoma, in remission**
Blastic plasmacytoid dendritic cell neoplasm (BPDCN), in remission

C86.5 **Angioimmunoblastic T-cell lymphoma** (Ex) PDX 481
Angioimmunoblastic lymphadenopathy with dysproteinemia (AILD)

▶C86.5Ø **Angioimmunoblastic T-cell lymphoma not having achieved remission**
▶Angioimmunoblastic lymphadenopathy with dysproteinemia (AILD) NOS
▶Angioimmunoblastic lymphadenopathy with dysproteinemia (AILD) not having achieved remission
▶Angioimmunoblastic lymphadenopathy with dysproteinemia (AILD) with failed remission
▶Angioimmunoblastic T-cell lymphoma NOS
▶Angioimmunoblastic T-cell lymphoma with failed remission

▶C86.51 **Angioimmunoblastic T-cell lymphoma, in remission**
▶Angioimmunoblastic lymphadenopathy with dysproteinemia (AILD), in remission

C86.6 **Primary cutaneous CD3Ø-positive T-cell proliferations** (Ex) PDX 481
Lymphomatoid papulosis
Primary cutaneous anaplastic large cell lymphoma
Primary cutaneous CD3Ø-positive large T-cell lymphoma

▶C86.6Ø **Primary cutaneous CD3Ø-positive T-cell proliferations not having achievedremission**
▶Lymphomatoid papulosis NOS
▶Lymphomatoid papulosis not having achieved remission
▶Lymphomatoid papulosis with failed remission
▶Primary cutaneous anaplastic large cell lymphoma NOS
▶Primary cutaneous anaplastic large cell lymphoma not having achieved remission
▶Primary cutaneous anaplastic large cell lymphoma with failed remission
▶Primary cutaneous CD3Ø-positive large T-cell lymphoma NOS
▶Primary cutaneous CD3Ø-positive large T-cell lymphoma not having achieved remission
▶Primary cutaneous CD3Ø-positive large T-cell lymphoma with failed remission
▶Primary cutaneous CD3Ø-positive T-cell proliferations NOS
▶Primary cutaneous CD3Ø-positive T-cell proliferations with failed remission

▶C86.61 **Primary cutaneous CD3Ø-positive T-cell proliferations, in remission**

● C88 **Malignant immunoproliferative diseases and certain other B-cell lymphomas**
Diseases involving immune system
Excludes1 B-cell lymphoma, unspecified (C85.1-)
personal history of other malignant neoplasms of lymphoid, hematopoietic and related tissues (Z85.79)

C88.Ø **Waldenström's macroglobulinemia**
Lymphoplasmacytic lymphoma with IgM-production
Macroglobulinemia (idiopathic) (primary)
Excludes1 small cell B-cell lymphoma (C83.Ø)

▶C88.ØØ **Waldenström macroglobulinemia not having achieved remission**
▶Lymphoplasmacytic lymphoma with IgM-production, NOS
▶Lymphoplasmacytic lymphoma with IgM-production not having achieved remission
▶Lymphoplasmacytic lymphoma with IgM-production with failed remission
▶Macroglobulinemia (idiopathic) (primary) NOS
▶Macroglobulinemia (idiopathic) (primary) not having achieved remission
▶Macroglobulinemia (idiopathic) (primary) with failed remission
▶Waldenström macroglobulinemia NOS
▶Waldenström macroglobulinemia with failed remission

▶C88.Ø1 **Waldenström macroglobulinemia, in remission**

C88.2 **Heavy chain disease** (Ex) PDX 532
Franklin disease
Gamma heavy chain disease
Mu heavy chain disease

▶C88.20 **Heavy chain disease not having achieved remission**
▶Franklin disease NOS
Franklin disease not having achieved remission
▶Franklin disease with failed remission
▶Gamma heavy chain disease NOS
▶Gamma heavy chain disease not having achieved remission
▶Gamma heavy chain disease with failed remission
▶Heavy chain disease NOS
▶Heavy chain disease with failed remissionMu heavy chain disease not having achieved remission
▶Mu heavy chain disease NOS
▶Mu heavy chain disease not having achieved remission
▶Mu heavy chain disease with failed remission

▶C88.21 **Heavy chain disease, in remission**

C88.3 **Immunoproliferative small intestinal disease** (Ex) PDX 532
Alpha heavy chain disease
Mediterranean lymphoma

▶C88.30 **Immunoproliferative small intestinal disease not having achieved remission**
▶Alpha heavy chain disease NOS
▶Alpha heavy chain disease not having achieved remission
▶Alpha heavy chain disease with failed remission
▶Immunoproliferative small intestinal disease NOS
▶Immunoproliferative small intestinal disease with failed remission
▶Mediterranean lymphoma NOS
▶Mediterranean lymphoma not having achieved remission
▶Mediterranean lymphoma with failed remission

▶C88.31 **Immunoproliferative small intestinal disease, in remission**

C88.4 **Extranodal marginal zone B-cell lymphoma of mucosa-associated lymphoid tissue [MALT-lymphoma]** (Ex) PDX 472
Lymphoma of skin-associated lymphoid tissue [SALT-lymphoma]
Lymphoma of bronchial-associated lymphoid tissue [BALT-lymphoma]
Excludes1 high malignant (diffuse large B-cell) lymphoma (C83.3-)

▶C88.40 **Extranodal marginal zone B-cell lymphoma of mucosa-associated lymphoid tissue[MALT-lymphoma] not having achieved remission**
▶Extranodal marginal zone B-cell lymphoma of mucosa-associated lymphoid tissue [MALT-lymphoma] NOS
▶Extranodal marginal zone B-cell lymphoma of mucosa-associated lymphoid tissue [MALT-lymphoma] with failed remission
▶Lymphoma of bronchial-associated lymphoid tissue [BALT-lymphoma] NOS
▶Lymphoma of bronchial-associated lymphoid tissue [BALT-lymphoma] not having achieved remission
▶Lymphoma of bronchial-associated lymphoid tissue [BALT-lymphoma] with failed remission
▶Lymphoma of skin-associated lymphoid tissue [SALT-lymphoma] NOS
▶Lymphoma of skin-associated lymphoid tissue [SALT-lymphoma] not having achieved remission
▶Lymphoma of skin-associated lymphoid tissue [SALT-lymphoma] with failed remission

▶C88.41 **Extranodal marginal zone B-cell**

Item 2-8 Multiple myeloma is a cancer of a plasma cell (a type of white blood cell) and is an incurable but treatable disease. Immunoproliferative neoplasm is a term for diseases (mostly cancers) in which the immune system cells proliferate.

C88.8 **Other malignant immunoproliferative diseases** (Ex) PDX 533

▶C88.80 **Other malignant immunoproliferative diseases not having achieved remission**
▶Other malignant immunoproliferative diseases NOS
▶Other malignant immunoproliferative diseases with failed remission

▶C88.81 **Other malignant immunoproliferative diseases, in remission**

C88.9 **Malignant immunoproliferative disease, unspecified**
Immunoproliferative disease NOS

▶C88.90 **Malignant immunoproliferative disease, unspecified not having achieved remission**
▶Immunoproliferative disease NOS
▶Immunoproliferative disease NOS not having achieved remission
▶Immunoproliferative disease NOS with failed remission
▶Malignant immunoproliferative disease, unspecified NOS
▶Malignant immunoproliferative disease, unspecified with failed remission

▶C88.91 **Malignant immunoproliferative disease, unspecified, in remission**

● C90 **Multiple myeloma and malignant plasma cell neoplasms** (Ex) PDX 532
Excludes1 personal history of other malignant neoplasms of lymphoid, hematopoietic and related tissues (Z85.79)

● C90.0 **Multiple myeloma**
Kahler's disease
Medullary plasmacytoma
Myelomatosis
Plasma cell myeloma
Excludes1 solitary myeloma (C90.3-)
solitary plasmacytoma (C90.3-)

C90.00 **Multiple myeloma not having achieved remission**
Multiple myeloma with failed remission
Multiple myeloma NOS

C90.01 **Multiple myeloma in remission**

C90.02 **Multiple myeloma in relapse**

● C90.1 **Plasma cell leukemia**
Rare type of acute leukemia
Plasmacytic leukemia
Coding Clinic: 2019, Q2, P30

C90.10 **Plasma cell leukemia not having achieved remission**
Plasma cell leukemia with failed remission
Plasma cell leukemia NOS
Coding Clinic: 2019, Q2, P30

C90.11 **Plasma cell leukemia in remission**

C90.12 **Plasma cell leukemia in relapse**

● C90.2 **Extramedullary plasmacytoma**
Malignant monoclonal plasma cell tumor growing in soft tissue; AKA plasma cell dyscrasias

C90.20 **Extramedullary plasmacytoma not having achieved remission**
Extramedullary plasmacytoma with failed remission
Extramedullary plasmacytoma NOS

C90.21 **Extramedullary plasmacytoma in remission**

C90.22 **Extramedullary plasmacytoma in relapse**

C90.3 Solitary plasmacytoma (Ex) PDX 532
Localized malignant plasma cell tumor NOS
Plasmacytoma NOS
Solitary myeloma

C90.30 Solitary plasmacytoma not having achieved remission
Solitary plasmacytoma with failed remission
Solitary plasmacytoma NOS

C90.31 Solitary plasmacytoma in remission

C90.32 Solitary plasmacytoma in relapse

C91 Lymphoid leukemia
Type of leukemia affecting circulating cells of lymphoid origin
Excludes1 personal history of leukemia (Z85.6)

C91.0 Acute lymphoblastic leukemia [ALL] (Ex) PDX 532
Note: Codes in subcategory C91.0 should only be used for T-cell and B-cell precusor leukemia

C91.00 Acute lymphoblastic leukemia not having achieved remission
Acute lymphoblastic leukemia with failed remission
Acute lymphoblastic leukemia NOS
Coding Clinic: 2022, Q1, P16

C91.01 Acute lymphoblastic leukemia, in remission

C91.02 Acute lymphoblastic leukemia, in relapse

C91.1 Chronic lymphocytic leukemia of B-cell type (Ex) PDX 532
Lymphoplasmacytic leukemia
Richter syndrome
Excludes1 lymphoplasmacytic lymphoma (C83.0-)
Coding Clinic: 2023, Q1, P18

C91.10 Chronic lymphocytic leukemia of B-cell type not having achieved remission
Chronic lymphocytic leukemia of B-cell type with failed remission
Chronic lymphocytic leukemia of B-cell type NOS

C91.11 Chronic lymphocytic leukemia of B-cell type in remission

C91.12 Chronic lymphocytic leukemia of B-cell type in relapse
Coding Clinic: 2023, Q1, P18

C91.3 Prolymphocytic leukemia of B-cell type (Ex) PDX 532
Chronic leukemia with symptoms of large number of circulating lymphocytes

C91.30 Prolymphocytic leukemia of B-cell type not having achieved remission
Prolymphocytic leukemia of B-cell type with failed remission
Prolymphocytic leukemia of B-cell type NOS

C91.31 Prolymphocytic leukemia of B-cell type, in remission

C91.32 Prolymphocytic leukemia of B-cell type, in relapse

Item 2-9 Leukemia is a cancer (acute or chronic) of the blood-forming tissues of the bone marrow. Blood cells all start out as stem cells. They mature and become red cells, white cells, or platelets. There are three main types of leukocytes (white cells that fight infection): monocytes, lymphocytes, and granulocytes. **Acute monocytic leukemia** (AML) affects monocytes. **Acute lymphoid leukemia** (ALL) affects lymphocytes, and **acute myeloid leukemia** (AML) affects cells that typically develop into white blood cells (not lymphocytes), though it may develop in other blood cells.

C91.4 Hairy cell leukemia (Ex) PDX 532
Chronic leukemia with splenomegaly and excessive number of abnormal large mononuclear cells covered by hairlike villi
Leukemic reticuloendotheliosis

C91.40 Hairy cell leukemia not having achieved remission
Hairy cell leukemia with failed remission
Hairy cell leukemia NOS

C91.41 Hairy cell leukemia, in remission

C91.42 Hairy cell leukemia, in relapse

C91.5 Adult T-cell lymphoma/leukemia (HTLV-1-associated) (Ex) PDX 532
Acute variant of adult T-cell lymphoma/leukemia (HTLV-1-associated)
Chronic variant of adult T-cell lymphoma/leukemia (HTLV-1-associated)
Lymphomatoid variant of adult T-cell lymphoma/leukemia (HTLV-1-associated)
Smouldering variant of adult T-cell lymphoma/leukemia (HTLV-1-associated)

C91.50 Adult T-cell lymphoma/leukemia (HTLV-1-associated) not having achieved remission A
Adult T-cell lymphoma/leukemia (HTLV-1-associated) with failed remission
Adult T-cell lymphoma/leukemia (HTLV-1-associated) NOS

C91.51 Adult T-cell lymphoma/leukemia (HTLV-1-associated), in remission A

C91.52 Adult T-cell lymphoma/leukemia (HTLV-1-associated), in relapse A

C91.6 Prolymphocytic leukemia of T-cell type (Ex) PDX 532

C91.60 Prolymphocytic leukemia of T-cell type not having achieved remission
Prolymphocytic leukemia of T-cell type with failed remission
Prolymphocytic leukemia of T-cell type NOS

C91.61 Prolymphocytic leukemia of T-cell type, in remission

C91.62 Prolymphocytic leukemia of T-cell type, in relapse

C91.9 Lymphoid leukemia, unspecified (Ex) PDX 532

C91.90 Lymphoid leukemia, unspecified not having achieved remission
Lymphoid leukemia with failed remission
Lymphoid leukemia NOS

C91.91 Lymphoid leukemia, unspecified, in remission

C91.92 Lymphoid leukemia, unspecified, in relapse

C91.A Mature B-cell leukemia Burkitt-type (Ex) PDX 532
Excludes1 Burkitt lymphoma (C83.7-)

C91.A0 Mature B-cell leukemia Burkitt-type not having achieved remission
Mature B-cell leukemia Burkitt-type with failed remission
Mature B-cell leukemia Burkitt-type NOS

C91.A1 Mature B-cell leukemia Burkitt-type, in remission

C91.A2 Mature B-cell leukemia Burkitt-type, in relapse

C91.Z Other lymphoid leukemia (Ex) PDX 532
T-cell large granular lymphocytic leukemia (associated with rheumatoid arthritis)

C91.Z0 Other lymphoid leukemia not having achieved remission
Other lymphoid leukemia with failed remission
Other lymphoid leukemia NOS
Coding Clinic: 2019, Q2, P25

C91.Z1 Other lymphoid leukemia, in remission

C91.Z2 Other lymphoid leukemia, in relapse

CHAPTER 2 (C00-D49)

C92 Myeloid leukemia Ex: PDX 532
Code also, if applicable, pancytopenia (acquired) (D61.818)
Includes granulocytic leukemia
myelogenous leukemia
Excludes1 personal history of leukemia (Z85.6)
Coding Clinic: 2019, Q1, P16

C92.0 Acute myeloblastic leukemia
Acute myeloblastic leukemia, minimal differentiation
Acute myeloblastic leukemia (with maturation)
Acute myeloblastic leukemia 1/ETO
Acute myeloblastic leukemia M0
Acute myeloblastic leukemia M1
Acute myeloblastic leukemia M2
Acute myeloblastic leukemia with t(8;21)
Acute myeloblastic leukemia (without a FAB classification) NOS
Refractory anemia with excess blasts in transformation [RAEB T]
Excludes1 acute exacerbation of chronic myeloid leukemia (C92.10)
refractory anemia with excess of blasts not in transformation (D46.2-)
Coding Clinic: 2018, Q4, P87

C92.00 Acute myeloblastic leukemia, not having achieved remission
Acute myeloblastic leukemia with failed remission
Acute myeloblastic leukemia NOS

C92.01 Acute myeloblastic leukemia, in remission
Coding Clinic: 2021, Q3, P4

C92.02 Acute myeloblastic leukemia, in relapse
Coding Clinic: 2023, Q1, P23

C92.1 Chronic myeloid leukemia, BCR/ABL-positive
Chronic myelogenous leukemia, Philadelphia chromosome (Ph1) positive
Chronic myelogenous leukemia, t(9;22) (q34;q11)
Chronic myelogenous leukemia with crisis of blast cells
Excludes1 atypical chronic myeloid leukemia BCR/ABL-negative (C92.2-)
chronic myelomonocytic leukemia (C93.1-)
chronic myeloproliferative disease (D47.1)

C92.10 Chronic myeloid leukemia, BCR/ABL-positive, not having achieved remission
Chronic myeloid leukemia, BCR/ABL-positive with failed remission
Chronic myeloid leukemia, BCR/ABL-positive NOS
Coding Clinic: 2017, Q1, P7

C92.11 Chronic myeloid leukemia, BCR/ABL-positive, in remission

C92.12 Chronic myeloid leukemia, BCR/ABL-positive, in relapse

C92.2 Atypical chronic myeloid leukemia, BCR/ABL-negative

C92.20 Atypical chronic myeloid leukemia, BCR/ABL-negative, not having achieved remission
Atypical chronic myeloid leukemia, BCR/ABL-negative with failed remission
Atypical chronic myeloid leukemia, BCR/ABL-negative NOS

C92.21 Atypical chronic myeloid leukemia, BCR/ABL-negative, in remission

C92.22 Atypical chronic myeloid leukemia, BCR/ABL-negative, in relapse

C92.3 Myeloid sarcoma
A malignant tumor of immature myeloid cells
Chloroma
Granulocytic sarcoma

C92.30 Myeloid sarcoma, not having achieved remission
Myeloid sarcoma with failed remission
Myeloid sarcoma NOS

C92.31 Myeloid sarcoma, in remission

C92.32 Myeloid sarcoma, in relapse

C92.4 Acute promyelocytic leukemia
AML M3
AML Me with t(15;17) and variants

C92.40 Acute promyelocytic leukemia, not having achieved remission
Acute promyelocytic leukemia with failed remission
Acute promyelocytic leukemia NOS

C92.41 Acute promyelocytic leukemia, in remission

C92.42 Acute promyelocytic leukemia, in relapse

C92.5 Acute myelomonocytic leukemia
AML M4
AML M4 Eo with inv(16) or t(16;16)

C92.50 Acute myelomonocytic leukemia, not having achieved remission
Acute myelomonocytic leukemia with failed remission
Acute myelomonocytic leukemia NOS

C92.51 Acute myelomonocytic leukemia, in remission

C92.52 Acute myelomonocytic leukemia, in relapse

C92.6 Acute myeloid leukemia with 11q23-abnormality
Acute myeloid leukemia with variation of MLL-gene

C92.60 Acute myeloid leukemia with 11q23-abnormality not having achieved remission
Acute myeloid leukemia with 11q23-abnormality with failed remission
Acute myeloid leukemia with 11q23-abnormality NOS

C92.61 Acute myeloid leukemia with 11q23-abnormality in remission

C92.62 Acute myeloid leukemia with 11q23-abnormality in relapse

C92.9 Myeloid leukemia, unspecified

C92.90 Myeloid leukemia, unspecified, not having achieved remission
Myeloid leukemia, unspecified with failed remission
Myeloid leukemia, unspecified NOS

C92.91 Myeloid leukemia, unspecified in remission

C92.92 Myeloid leukemia, unspecified in relapse

C92.A Acute myeloid leukemia with multilineage dysplasia
Acute myeloid leukemia with dysplasia of remaining hematopoesis and/or myelodysplastic disease in its history

C92.A0 Acute myeloid leukemia with multilineage dysplasia, not having achieved remission
Acute myeloid leukemia with multilineage dysplasia with failed remission
Acute myeloid leukemia with multilineage dysplasia NOS

C92.A1 Acute myeloid leukemia with multilineage dysplasia, in remission

C92.A2 Acute myeloid leukemia with multilineage dysplasia, in relapse

CHAPTER 2 (C00-D49)

C92.Z Other myeloid leukemia PDX 532

C92.Z0 Other myeloid leukemia not having achieved remission
Myeloid leukemia NEC with failed remission
Myeloid leukemia NEC

C92.Z1 Other myeloid leukemia, in remission

C92.Z2 Other myeloid leukemia, in relapse

C93 Monocytic leukemia PDX 532
Includes monocytoid leukemia
Excludes1 personal history of leukemia (Z85.6)

C93.0 Acute monoblastic/monocytic leukemia
AML M5
AML M5a
AML M5b

C93.00 Acute monoblastic/monocytic leukemia, not having achieved remission
Acute monoblastic/monocytic leukemia with failed remission
Acute monoblastic/monocytic leukemia NOS

C93.01 Acute monoblastic/monocytic leukemia, in remission

C93.02 Acute monoblastic/monocytic leukemia, in relapse

C93.1 Chronic myelomonocytic leukemia
Chronic monocytic leukemia
CMML-1
CMML-2
CMML with eosinophilia
Code also, if applicable, eosinophilia (D72.18)

C93.10 Chronic myelomonocytic leukemia not having achieved remission
Chronic myelomonocytic leukemia with failed remission
Chronic myelomonocytic leukemia NOS

C93.11 Chronic myelomonocytic leukemia, in remission

C93.12 Chronic myelomonocytic leukemia, in relapse

C93.3 Juvenile myelomonocytic leukemia

C93.30 Juvenile myelomonocytic leukemia, not having achieved remission P
Juvenile myelomonocytic leukemia with failed remission
Juvenile myelomonocytic leukemia NOS

C93.31 Juvenile myelomonocytic leukemia, in remission P

C93.32 Juvenile myelomonocytic leukemia, in relapse P

C93.9 Monocytic leukemia, unspecified

C93.90 Monocytic leukemia, unspecified, not having achieved remission
Monocytic leukemia, unspecified with failed remission
Monocytic leukemia, unspecified NOS

C93.91 Monocytic leukemia, unspecified in remission

C93.92 Monocytic leukemia, unspecified in relapse

C93.Z Other monocytic leukemia

C93.Z0 Other monocytic leukemia, not having achieved remission
Other monocytic leukemia NOS

C93.Z1 Other monocytic leukemia, in remission

C93.Z2 Other monocytic leukemia, in relapse

C94 Other leukemias of specified cell type
Excludes1 leukemic reticuloendotheliosis (C91.4-)
myelodysplastic syndromes (D46.-)
personal history of leukemia (Z85.6)
plasma cell leukemia (C90.1-)

C94.0 Acute erythroid leukemia PDX 532
Acute myeloid leukemia M6(a)(b)
Erythroleukemia

C94.00 Acute erythroid leukemia, not having achieved remission
Acute erythroid leukemia with failed remission
Acute erythroid leukemia NOS

C94.01 Acute erythroid leukemia, in remission

C94.02 Acute erythroid leukemia, in relapse

C94.2 Acute megakaryoblastic leukemia PDX 532
Acute myeloid leukemia M7
Acute megakaryocytic leukemia

C94.20 Acute megakaryoblastic leukemia not having achieved remission
Acute megakaryoblastic leukemia with failed remission
Acute megakaryoblastic leukemia NOS

C94.21 Acute megakaryoblastic leukemia, in remission

C94.22 Acute megakaryoblastic leukemia, in relapse

C94.3 Mast cell leukemia PDX 532

C94.30 Mast cell leukemia not having achieved remission
Mast cell leukemia with failed remission
Mast cell leukemia NOS

C94.31 Mast cell leukemia, in remission

C94.32 Mast cell leukemia, in relapse

C94.4 Acute panmyelosis with myelofibrosis PDX 532
Acute myelofibrosis
Excludes1 myelofibrosis NOS (D75.81)
secondary myelofibrosis NOS (D75.81)

C94.40 Acute panmyelosis with myelofibrosis not having achieved remission
Acute myelofibrosis NOS
Acute panmyelosis with myelofibrosis with failed remission
Acute panmyelosis NOS

C94.41 Acute panmyelosis with myelofibrosis, in remission

C94.42 Acute panmyelosis with myelofibrosis, in relapse

C94.6 Myelodysplastic disease, not elsewhere classified PDX 532
Myelodysplastic/myeloproliferative neoplasm, unclassifiable
Myeloproliferative disease, not elsewhere classified

C94.8 Other specified leukemias PDX 532
Aggressive NK-cell leukemia
Acute basophilic leukemia
Code also, if applicable, eosinophilia (D72.18)

C94.80 Other specified leukemias not having achieved remission
Other specified leukemia with failed remission
Other specified leukemias NOS

C94.81 Other specified leukemias, in remission

C94.82 Other specified leukemias, in relapse

CHAPTER 2 (C00-D49)

C95 Leukemia of unspecified cell type PDX 532

Excludes1 personal history of leukemia (Z85.6)

C95.Ø Acute leukemia of unspecified cell type

Acute bilineal leukemia
Acute mixed lineage leukemia
Biphenotypic acute leukemia
Stem cell leukemia of unclear lineage

Excludes1 acute exacerbation of unspecified chronic leukemia (C95.1Ø)

C95.ØØ Acute leukemia of unspecified cell type not having achieved remission

Acute leukemia of unspecified cell type with failed remission
Acute leukemia NOS

C95.Ø1 Acute leukemia of unspecified cell type, in remission

C95.Ø2 Acute leukemia of unspecified cell type, in relapse

C95.1 Chronic leukemia of unspecified cell type

C95.1Ø Chronic leukemia of unspecified cell type not having achieved remission

Chronic leukemia of unspecified cell type with failed remission
Chronic leukemia NOS

C95.11 Chronic leukemia of unspecified cell type, in remission

C95.12 Chronic leukemia of unspecified cell type, in relapse

C95.9 Leukemia, unspecified

C95.9Ø Leukemia, unspecified not having achieved remission

Leukemia, unspecified with failed remission
Leukemia NOS

C95.91 Leukemia, unspecified, in remission

C95.92 Leukemia, unspecified, in relapse

C96 Other and unspecified malignant neoplasms of lymphoid, hematopoietic and related tissue

Excludes1 personal history of other malignant neoplasms of lymphoid, hematopoietic and related tissues (Z85.79)

C96.Ø Multifocal and multisystemic (disseminated) Langerhans-cell histiocytosis PDX 536

Histiocytosis X, multisystemic
Letterer-Siwe disease

Excludes1 adult pulmonary Langerhans cell histiocytosis (J84.82)
multifocal and unisystemic Langerhans-cell histiocytosis (C96.5)
unifocal Langerhans-cell histiocytosis (C96.6)

C96.2 Malignant mast cell neoplasm PDX 537

Excludes1 indolent mastocytosis (D47.Ø2)
mast cell leukemia (C94.3Ø)
mastocytosis (congenital) (cutaneous) (Q82.2)

C96.2Ø Malignant mast cell neoplasm, unspecified

C96.21 Aggressive systemic mastocytosis

C96.22 Mast cell sarcoma

C96.29 Other malignant mast cell neoplasm

C96.4 Sarcoma of dendritic cells (accessory cells) PDX 538

Follicular dendritic cell sarcoma
Interdigitating dendritic cell sarcoma
Langerhans cell sarcoma

C96.5 Multifocal and unisystemic Langerhans-cell histiocytosis PDX 539

Hand-Schüller-Christian disease
Histiocytosis X, multifocal

Excludes1 multifocal and multisystemic (disseminated) Langerhans-cell histiocytosis (C96.Ø)
unifocal Langerhans-cell histiocytosis (C96.6)

C96.6 Unifocal Langerhans-cell histiocytosis PDX 540

Eosinophilic granuloma
Histiocytosis X, unifocal
Histiocytosis X NOS
Langerhans-cell histiocytosis NOS

Excludes1 multifocal and multisysemic (disseminated) Langerhans-cell histiocytosis (C96.Ø)
multifocal and unisystemic Langerhans-cell histiocytosis (C96.5)

C96.9 Malignant neoplasm of lymphoid, hematopoietic and related tissue, unspecified PDX 538

C96.A Histiocytic sarcoma PDX 541

Malignant histiocytosis

C96.Z Other specified malignant neoplasms of lymphoid, hematopoietic and related tissue PDX 538

IN SITU NEOPLASMS (DØØ-DØ9)

In situ is carcinoma involving cells in localized tissues that has not spread to nearby tissues

Includes Bowen's disease
erythroplasia
grade III intraepithelial neoplasia
Queyrat's erythroplasia

DØØ Carcinoma in situ of oral cavity, esophagus and stomach

Excludes1 melanoma in situ (DØ3.-)

DØØ.Ø Carcinoma in situ of lip, oral cavity and pharynx

Use additional code to identify:
exposure to environmental tobacco smoke (Z77.22)
exposure to tobacco smoke in the perinatal period (P96.81)
history of tobacco dependence (Z87.891)
occupational exposure to environmental tobacco smoke (Z57.31)
tobacco dependence (F17.-)
tobacco use (Z72.Ø)

Excludes1 carcinoma in situ of aryepiglottic fold or interarytenoid fold, laryngeal aspect (DØ2.Ø)
carcinoma in situ of epiglottis NOS (DØ2.Ø)
carcinoma in situ of epiglottis suprahyoid portion (DØ2.Ø)
carcinoma in situ of skin of lip (DØ3.Ø, DØ4.Ø)

DØØ.ØØ Carcinoma in situ of oral cavity, unspecified site

DØØ.Ø1 Carcinoma in situ of labial mucosa and vermilion border

DØØ.Ø2 Carcinoma in situ of buccal mucosa

DØØ.Ø3 Carcinoma in situ of gingiva and edentulous alveolar ridge

DØØ.Ø4 Carcinoma in situ of soft palate

DØØ.Ø5 Carcinoma in situ of hard palate

DØØ.Ø6 Carcinoma in situ of floor of mouth

DØØ.Ø7 Carcinoma in situ of tongue

DØØ.Ø8 Carcinoma in situ of pharynx

Carcinoma in situ of aryepiglottic fold NOS
Carcinoma in situ of hypopharyngeal aspect of aryepiglottic fold
Carcinoma in situ of marginal zone of aryepiglottic fold

DØØ.1 Carcinoma in situ of esophagus

DØØ.2 Carcinoma in situ of stomach

D01 Carcinoma in situ of other and unspecified digestive organs
Excludes1 melanoma in situ (D03.-)
D01.0 Carcinoma in situ of colon
Excludes1 carcinoma in situ of rectosigmoid junction (D01.1)
D01.1 Carcinoma in situ of rectosigmoid junction
D01.2 Carcinoma in situ of rectum
D01.3 Carcinoma in situ of anus and anal canal
Anal intraepithelial neoplasia III [AIN III]
Severe dysplasia of anus
Excludes1 anal intraepithelial neoplasia I and II [AIN I and AIN II] (K62.82)
carcinoma in situ of anal margin (D04.5)
carcinoma in situ of anal skin (D04.5)
carcinoma in situ of perianal skin (D04.5)
D01.4 Carcinoma in situ of other and unspecified parts of intestine
Excludes1 carcinoma in situ of ampulla of Vater (D01.5)
D01.40 Carcinoma in situ of unspecified part of intestine
D01.49 Carcinoma in situ of other parts of intestine
D01.5 Carcinoma in situ of liver, gallbladder and bile ducts
Carcinoma in situ of ampulla of Vater
D01.7 Carcinoma in situ of other specified digestive organs
Carcinoma in situ of pancreas
D01.9 Carcinoma in situ of digestive organ, unspecified

D02 Carcinoma in situ of middle ear and respiratory system
Use additional code to identify:
exposure to environmental tobacco smoke (Z77.22)
exposure to tobacco smoke in the perinatal period (P96.81)
history of tobacco dependence (Z87.891)
occupational exposure to environmental tobacco smoke (Z57.31)
tobacco dependence (F17.-)
tobacco use (Z72.0)
Excludes1 melanoma in situ (D03.-)
D02.0 Carcinoma in situ of larynx
Carcinoma in situ of aryepiglottic fold or interarytenoid fold, laryngeal aspect
Carcinoma in situ of epiglottis (suprahyoid portion)
Excludes1 carcinoma in situ of aryepiglottic fold or interarytenoid fold NOS (D00.08)
carcinoma in situ of hypopharyngeal aspect (D00.08)
carcinoma in situ of marginal zone (D00.08)
D02.1 Carcinoma in situ of trachea
D02.2 Carcinoma in situ of bronchus and lung
D02.20 Carcinoma in situ of unspecified bronchus and lung
D02.21 Carcinoma in situ of right bronchus and lung
D02.22 Carcinoma in situ of left bronchus and lung
D02.3 Carcinoma in situ of other parts of respiratory system
Carcinoma in situ of accessory sinuses
Carcinoma in situ of middle ear
Carcinoma in situ of nasal cavities
Excludes1 carcinoma in situ of ear (external) (skin) (D04.2-)
carcinoma in situ of nose NOS (D09.8)
carcinoma in situ of skin of nose (D04.3)
D02.4 Carcinoma in situ of respiratory system, unspecified

D03 Melanoma in situ
D03.0 Melanoma in situ of lip
D03.1 Melanoma in situ of eyelid, including canthus
D03.10 Melanoma in situ of unspecified eyelid, including canthus
D03.11 Melanoma in situ of right eyelid, including canthus
D03.111 Melanoma in situ of right upper eyelid, including canthus
D03.112 Melanoma in situ of right lower eyelid, including canthus
D03.12 Melanoma in situ of left eyelid, including canthus
D03.121 Melanoma in situ of left upper eyelid, including canthus
D03.122 Melanoma in situ of left lower eyelid, including canthus
D03.2 Melanoma in situ of ear and external auricular canal
D03.20 Melanoma in situ of unspecified ear and external auricular canal
D03.21 Melanoma in situ of right ear and external auricular canal
D03.22 Melanoma in situ of left ear and external auricular canal
D03.3 Melanoma in situ of other and unspecified parts of face
D03.30 Melanoma in situ of unspecified part of face
D03.39 Melanoma in situ of other parts of face
D03.4 Melanoma in situ of scalp and neck
D03.5 Melanoma in situ of trunk
D03.51 Melanoma in situ of anal skin
Melanoma in situ of anal margin
Melanoma in situ of perianal skin
D03.52 Melanoma in situ of breast (skin) (soft tissue)
D03.59 Melanoma in situ of other part of trunk
D03.6 Melanoma in situ of upper limb, including shoulder
D03.60 Melanoma in situ of unspecified upper limb, including shoulder
D03.61 Melanoma in situ of right upper limb, including shoulder
D03.62 Melanoma in situ of left upper limb, including shoulder
D03.7 Melanoma in situ of lower limb, including hip
D03.70 Melanoma in situ of unspecified lower limb, including hip
D03.71 Melanoma in situ of right lower limb, including hip
D03.72 Melanoma in situ of left lower limb, including hip
D03.8 Melanoma in situ of other sites
Melanoma in situ of scrotum
Excludes1 carcinoma in situ of scrotum (D07.61)
D03.9 Melanoma in situ, unspecified

D04 Carcinoma in situ of skin
Excludes1 erythroplasia of Queyrat (penis) NOS (D07.4)
melanoma in situ (D03.-)
D04.0 Carcinoma in situ of skin of lip
Excludes2 carcinoma in situ of vermilion border of lip (D00.01)
D04.1 Carcinoma in situ of skin of eyelid, including canthus
D04.10 Carcinoma in situ of skin of unspecified eyelid, including canthus
D04.11 Carcinoma in situ of skin of right eyelid, including canthus
D04.111 Carcinoma in situ of skin of right upper eyelid, including canthus
D04.112 Carcinoma in situ of skin of right lower eyelid, including canthus
D04.12 Carcinoma in situ of skin of left eyelid, including canthus
D04.121 Carcinoma in situ of skin of left upper eyelid, including canthus
D04.122 Carcinoma in situ of skin of left lower eyelid, including canthus

CHAPTER 2 (C00-D49)

- **D04.2 Carcinoma in situ of skin of ear and external auricular canal**
  - **D04.20** Carcinoma in situ of skin of unspecified ear and external auricular canal
  - **D04.21** Carcinoma in situ of skin of right ear and external auricular canal
  - **D04.22** Carcinoma in situ of skin of left ear and external auricular canal
- **D04.3 Carcinoma in situ of skin of other and unspecified parts of face**
  - **D04.30** Carcinoma in situ of skin of unspecified part of face
  - **D04.39** Carcinoma in situ of skin of other parts of face
- **D04.4** Carcinoma in situ of skin of scalp and neck
- **D04.5** Carcinoma in situ of skin of trunk
  - Carcinoma in situ of anal margin
  - Carcinoma in situ of anal skin
  - Carcinoma in situ of perianal skin
  - Carcinoma in situ of skin of breast
  - **Excludes1** carcinoma in situ of anus NOS (D01.3)
    carcinoma in situ of scrotum (D07.61)
    carcinoma in situ of skin of genital organs (D07.-)
- **D04.6 Carcinoma in situ of skin of upper limb, including shoulder**
  - **D04.60** Carcinoma in situ of skin of unspecified upper limb, including shoulder
  - **D04.61** Carcinoma in situ of skin of right upper limb, including shoulder
  - **D04.62** Carcinoma in situ of skin of left upper limb, including shoulder
- **D04.7 Carcinoma in situ of skin of lower limb, including hip**
  - **D04.70** Carcinoma in situ of skin of unspecified lower limb, including hip
  - **D04.71** Carcinoma in situ of skin of right lower limb, including hip
  - **D04.72** Carcinoma in situ of skin of left lower limb, including hip
- **D04.8** Carcinoma in situ of skin of other sites
- **D04.9** Carcinoma in situ of skin, unspecified

D05 Carcinoma in situ of breast

- **Excludes1** carcinoma in situ of skin of breast (D04.5)
  melanoma in situ of breast (skin) (D03.5)
  Paget's disease of breast or nipple (C50.-)
- **Excludes2** malignant neoplasm of breast (C50.-)
- **D05.0 Lobular carcinoma in situ of breast**
  - **D05.00** Lobular carcinoma in situ of unspecified breast
  - **D05.01** Lobular carcinoma in situ of right breast
  - **D05.02** Lobular carcinoma in situ of left breast
- **D05.1 Intraductal carcinoma in situ of breast**
  - **D05.10** Intraductal carcinoma in situ of unspecified breast
  - **D05.11** Intraductal carcinoma in situ of right breast
  - **D05.12** Intraductal carcinoma in situ of left breast
- **D05.8 Other specified type of carcinoma in situ of breast**
  - **D05.80** Other specified type of carcinoma in situ of unspecified breast
  - **D05.81** Other specified type of carcinoma in situ of right breast
  - **D05.82** Other specified type of carcinoma in situ of left breast
- **D05.9 Unspecified type of carcinoma in situ of breast**
  - **D05.90** Unspecified type of carcinoma in situ of unspecified breast
  - **D05.91** Unspecified type of carcinoma in situ of right breast
  - **D05.92** Unspecified type of carcinoma in situ of left breast

D06 Carcinoma in situ of cervix uteri

- **Includes** cervical adenocarcinoma in situ
  cervical intraepithelial glandular neoplasia
  cervical intraepithelial neoplasia III [CIN III]
  severe dysplasia of cervix uteri
- **Excludes1** cervical intraepithelial neoplasia II [CIN II] (N87.1)
  cytologic evidence of malignancy of cervix without histologic confirmation (R87.614)
  high grade squamous intraepithelial lesion (HGSIL) of cervix (R87.613)
  melanoma in situ of cervix (D03.5)
  moderate cervical dysplasia (N87.1)
- **D06.0** Carcinoma in situ of endocervix
- **D06.1** Carcinoma in situ of exocervix
- **D06.7** Carcinoma in situ of other parts of cervix
- **D06.9** Carcinoma in situ of cervix, unspecified

D07 Carcinoma in situ of other and unspecified genital organs

- **Excludes1** melanoma in situ of trunk (D03.5)
- **D07.0** Carcinoma in situ of endometrium
- **D07.1** Carcinoma in situ of vulva
  - Severe dysplasia of vulva
  - Vulvar intraepithelial neoplasia III [VIN III]
  - **Excludes1** moderate dysplasia of vulva (N90.1)
    vulvar intraepithelial neoplasia II [VIN II] (N90.1)
- **D07.2** Carcinoma in situ of vagina
  - Severe dysplasia of vagina
  - Vaginal intraepithelial neoplasia III [VIN III]
  - **Excludes1** moderate dysplasia of vagina (N89.1)
    vaginal intraepithelial neoplasia II [VIN II] (N89.1)
- **D07.3 Carcinoma in situ of other and unspecified female genital organs**
  - **D07.30** Carcinoma in situ of unspecified female genital organs
  - **D07.39** Carcinoma in situ of other female genital organs
- **D07.4** Carcinoma in situ of penis
  - Erythroplasia of Queyrat NOS
- **D07.5** Carcinoma in situ of prostate
  - Prostatic intraepithelial neoplasia III (PIN III)
  - Severe dysplasia of prostate
  - **Excludes1** dysplasia (mild) (moderate) of prostate (N42.3-)
    prostatic intraepithelial neoplasia II [PIN II] (N42.3-)
- **D07.6 Carcinoma in situ of other and unspecified male genital organs**
  - **D07.60** Carcinoma in situ of unspecified male genital organs
  - **D07.61** Carcinoma in situ of scrotum
  - **D07.69** Carcinoma in situ of other male genital organs

D09 Carcinoma in situ of other and unspecified sites

- **Excludes1** melanoma in situ (D03.-)
- **D09.0** Carcinoma in situ of bladder
- **D09.1 Carcinoma in situ of other and unspecified urinary organs**
  - **D09.10** Carcinoma in situ of unspecified urinary organ
  - **D09.19** Carcinoma in situ of other urinary organs
- **D09.2 Carcinoma in situ of eye**
  - **Excludes1** carcinoma in situ of skin of eyelid (D04.1-)
  - **D09.20** Carcinoma in situ of unspecified eye
  - **D09.21** Carcinoma in situ of right eye
  - **D09.22** Carcinoma in situ of left eye

D09.3 Carcinoma in situ of **thyroid and other endocrine glands**
Excludes1 carcinoma in situ of endocrine pancreas (D01.7)
carcinoma in situ of ovary (D07.39)
carcinoma in situ of testis (D07.69)

D09.8 Carcinoma in situ of **other specified sites**

D09.9 Carcinoma in situ, **unspecified**

BENIGN NEOPLASMS, EXCEPT BENIGN NEUROENDOCRINE TUMORS (D10-D36)

● **D10 Benign neoplasm of mouth and pharynx**

D10.0 Benign neoplasm of **lip**
Benign neoplasm of lip (frenulum) (inner aspect) (mucosa) (vermilion border)
Excludes1 benign neoplasm of skin of lip (D22.0, D23.0)

D10.1 Benign neoplasm of **tongue**
Benign neoplasm of lingual tonsil

D10.2 Benign neoplasm of **floor of mouth**

● D10.3 Benign neoplasm of **other and unspecified** parts of mouth

D10.30 Benign neoplasm of **unspecified** part of mouth

D10.39 Benign neoplasm of **other** parts of mouth
Benign neoplasm of minor salivary gland NOS
Excludes1 benign odontogenic neoplasms (D16.4-D16.5)
benign neoplasm of mucosa of lip (D10.0)
benign neoplasm of nasopharyngeal surface of soft palate (D10.6)

D10.4 Benign neoplasm of **tonsil**
Benign neoplasm of tonsil (faucial) (palatine)
Excludes1 benign neoplasm of lingual tonsil (D10.1)
benign neoplasm of pharyngeal tonsil (D10.6)
benign neoplasm of tonsillar fossa (D10.5)
benign neoplasm of tonsillar pillars (D10.5)

D10.5 Benign neoplasm of **other parts of oropharynx**
Division of pharynx lying between soft palate and upper edge of epiglottis
Benign neoplasm of epiglottis, anterior aspect
Benign neoplasm of tonsillar fossa
Benign neoplasm of tonsillar pillars
Benign neoplasm of vallecula
Excludes1 benign neoplasm of epiglottis NOS (D14.1)
benign neoplasm of epiglottis, suprahyoid portion (D14.1)

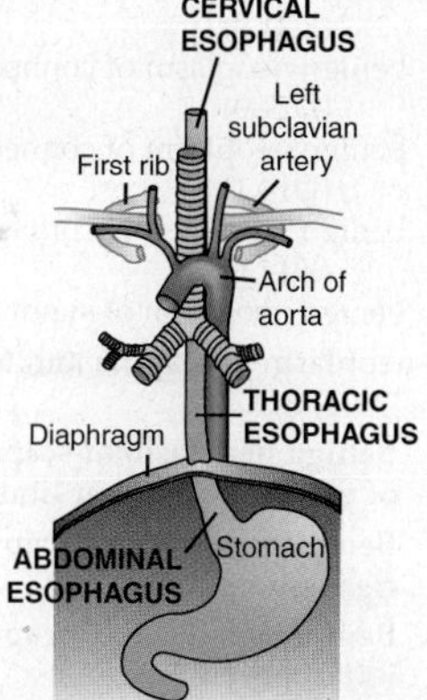

Figure 2-16 The esophagus is the muscular tube that connects the pharynx and the stomach. The 10 inch (25 cm) long esophagus is divided into three parts: **cervical, thoracic,** and **abdominal.**

D10.6 Benign neoplasm of **nasopharynx**
Segment of pharynx that lies above soft palate
Benign neoplasm of pharyngeal tonsil
Benign neoplasm of posterior margin of septum and choanae

D10.7 Benign neoplasm of **hypopharynx**
Segment of pharynx that lies below upper edge of epiglottis and opens into larynx and esophagus

D10.9 Benign neoplasm of **pharynx, unspecified**

● **D11 Benign neoplasm of major salivary glands**
Excludes1 benign neoplasms of specified minor salivary glands which are classified according to their anatomical location
benign neoplasms of minor salivary glands NOS (D10.39)

D11.0 Benign neoplasm of **parotid gland**

D11.7 Benign neoplasm of **other** major salivary glands
Benign neoplasm of sublingual salivary gland
Benign neoplasm of submandibular salivary gland

D11.9 Benign neoplasm of major salivary gland, **unspecified**

● **D12 Benign neoplasm of colon, rectum, anus and anal canal**
Excludes2 benign carcinoid tumors of the large intestine and rectum (D3A.02-)
polyp of colon NOS (K63.5)
Coding Clinic: 2017, Q1, P15; 2015, Q2, P14

D12.0 Benign neoplasm of **cecum**
Benign neoplasm of ileocecal valve

D12.1 Benign neoplasm of **appendix**
Excludes1 benign carcinoid tumor of the appendix (D3A.020)

D12.2 Benign neoplasm of **ascending** colon
Coding Clinic: 2018, Q2, P14; 2017, Q1, P15

D12.3 Benign neoplasm of **transverse** colon
Benign neoplasm of hepatic flexure
Benign neoplasm of splenic flexure
Flexure is a bending in a structure or organ. Note the three flexures illustrated in Figure 2–17. Hepatic = liver, sigmoid = colon, splenic = spleen.
Coding Clinic: 2017, Q1, P16

D12.4 Benign neoplasm of **descending** colon
Coding Clinic: 2015, Q2, P14

D12.5 Benign neoplasm of **sigmoid** colon

D12.6 Benign neoplasm of colon, **unspecified**
Adenomatosis of colon
Benign neoplasm of large intestine NOS
Polyposis (hereditary) of colon
Excludes1 inflammatory polyp of colon (K51.4-)
Coding Clinic: 2017, Q1, P8-9

D12.7 Benign neoplasm of **rectosigmoid junction**
Angle where sigmoid colon becomes rectum

D12.8 Benign neoplasm of **rectum**
Excludes1 benign carcinoid tumor of the rectum (D3A.026)
Coding Clinic: 2018, Q1, P7

D12.9 Benign neoplasm of **anus and anal canal**
Benign neoplasm of anus NOS
Excludes1 benign neoplasm of anal margin (D22.5, D23.5)
benign neoplasm of anal skin (D22.5, D23.5)
benign neoplasm of perianal skin (D22.5, D23.5)

CHAPTER 2 (C00-D49)

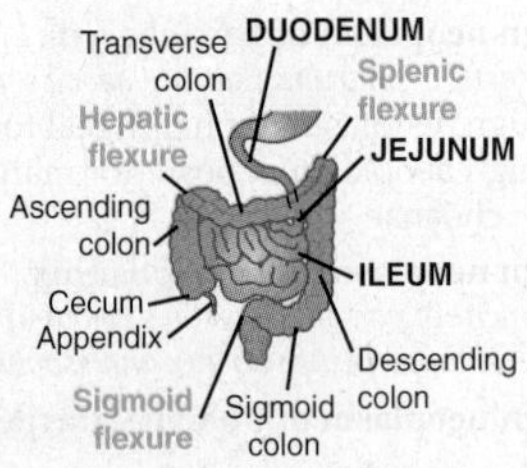

Figure 2-17 Small intestine and colon.

● **D13 Benign neoplasm of other and ill-defined parts of digestive system**

Excludes1 benign stromal tumors of digestive system (D21.4)

D13.0 Benign neoplasm of esophagus

D13.1 Benign neoplasm of stomach

Excludes1 benign carcinoid tumor of the stomach (D3A.092)

D13.2 Benign neoplasm of duodenum

Excludes1 benign carcinoid tumor of the duodenum (D3A.010)

● **D13.3 Benign neoplasm of other and unspecified parts of small intestine**

Excludes1 benign carcinoid tumors of the small intestine (D3A.01-)
benign neoplasm of ileocecal valve (D12.0)

D13.30 Benign neoplasm of unspecified part of small intestine

D13.39 Benign neoplasm of other parts of small intestine

D13.4 Benign neoplasm of liver

Benign neoplasm of intrahepatic bile ducts

D13.5 Benign neoplasm of extrahepatic bile ducts

Extensions of common hepatic bile duct (tube that collects bile from liver)

D13.6 Benign neoplasm of pancreas

Excludes1 benign neoplasm of endocrine pancreas (D13.7)

D13.7 Benign neoplasm of endocrine pancreas

Pancreatic islets: Cells scattered throughout pancreas

Islet cell tumor

Benign neoplasm of islets of Langerhans

Use additional code to identify any functional activity.

D13.9 Benign neoplasm of ill-defined sites within the digestive system

D13.91 Familial adenomatous polyposis

Code also associated conditions, such as:
benign neoplasm of colon (D12.6)
malignant neoplasm of colon (C18.-)

D13.99 Benign neoplasm of ill-defined sites within the digestive system

Benign neoplasm of digestive system NOS

Benign neoplasm of intestine NOS

Benign neoplasm of spleen

● **D14 Benign neoplasm of middle ear and respiratory system**

D14.0 Benign neoplasm of middle ear, nasal cavity and accessory sinuses

Benign neoplasm of cartilage of nose

Excludes1 benign neoplasm of auricular canal (external) (D22.2-, D23.2-)
benign neoplasm of bone of ear (D16.4)
benign neoplasm of bone of nose (D16.4)
benign neoplasm of cartilage of ear (D21.0)
benign neoplasm of ear (external) (skin) (D22.2-, D23.2-)
benign neoplasm of nose NOS (D36.7)
benign neoplasm of skin of nose (D22.39, D23.39)
benign neoplasm of olfactory bulb (D33.3)
benign neoplasm of posterior margin of septum and choanae (D10.6)
polyp of accessory sinus (J33.8)
polyp of ear (middle) (H74.4)
polyp of nasal (cavity) (J33.-)

D14.1 Benign neoplasm of larynx

Adenomatous polyp of larynx

Benign neoplasm of epiglottis (suprahyoid portion)

Horseshoe-shaped bone in anterior midline of neck between chin and thyroid cartilage

Excludes1 benign neoplasm of epiglottis, anterior aspect (D10.5)
polyp (nonadenomatous) of vocal cord or larynx (J38.1)

D14.2 Benign neoplasm of trachea

● **D14.3 Benign neoplasm of bronchus and lung**

Excludes1 benign carcinoid tumor of the bronchus and lung (D3A.090)

D14.30 Benign neoplasm of unspecified bronchus and lung

D14.31 Benign neoplasm of right bronchus and lung

D14.32 Benign neoplasm of left bronchus and lung

D14.4 Benign neoplasm of respiratory system, unspecified

● **D15 Benign neoplasm of other and unspecified intrathoracic organs**

Excludes1 benign neoplasm of mesothelial tissue (D19.-)

D15.0 Benign neoplasm of thymus

Excludes1 benign carcinoid tumor of the thymus (D3A.091)

D15.1 Benign neoplasm of heart

Excludes1 benign neoplasm of great vessels (D21.3)

D15.2 Benign neoplasm of mediastinum

D15.7 Benign neoplasm of other specified intrathoracic organs

D15.9 Benign neoplasm of intrathoracic organ, unspecified

● **D16 Benign neoplasm of bone and articular cartilage**

Excludes1 benign neoplasm of connective tissue of ear (D21.0)
benign neoplasm of connective tissue of eyelid (D21.0)
benign neoplasm of connective tissue of larynx (D14.1)
benign neoplasm of connective tissue of nose (D14.0)
benign neoplasm of synovia (D21.-)

● **D16.0 Benign neoplasm of scapula and long bones of upper limb**

D16.00 Benign neoplasm of scapula and long bones of unspecified upper limb

D16.01 Benign neoplasm of scapula and long bones of right upper limb

D16.02 Benign neoplasm of scapula and long bones of left upper limb

● **D16.1 Benign neoplasm of short bones of upper limb**
- **D16.10 Benign neoplasm of short bones of unspecified upper limb**
- **D16.11 Benign neoplasm of short bones of right upper limb**
- **D16.12 Benign neoplasm of short bones of left upper limb**

● **D16.2 Benign neoplasm of long bones of lower limb**
- **D16.20 Benign neoplasm of long bones of unspecified lower limb**
- **D16.21 Benign neoplasm of long bones of right lower limb**
- **D16.22 Benign neoplasm of long bones of left lower limb**

● **D16.3 Benign neoplasm of short bones of lower limb**
- **D16.30 Benign neoplasm of short bones of unspecified lower limb**
- **D16.31 Benign neoplasm of short bones of right lower limb**
- **D16.32 Benign neoplasm of short bones of left lower limb**

D16.4 Benign neoplasm of bones of skull and face
Benign neoplasm of maxilla (superior)
Benign neoplasm of orbital bone
Cavity or socket of skull in which eye and its appendages are located
Keratocyst of maxilla
Keratocystic odontogenic tumor of maxilla
Excludes2 benign neoplasm of lower jaw bone (D16.5)

D16.5 Benign neoplasm of lower jaw bone
Keratocyst of mandible
Keratocystic odontogenic tumor of mandible

D16.6 Benign neoplasm of vertebral column
Excludes1 benign neoplasm of sacrum and coccyx (D16.8)

D16.7 Benign neoplasm of ribs, sternum and clavicle

D16.8 Benign neoplasm of pelvic bones, sacrum and coccyx

D16.9 Benign neoplasm of bone and articular cartilage, unspecified

● **D17 Benign lipomatous neoplasm**
Slow-growing benign tumors (rubbery masses) of mature fat cells enclosed in a thin fibrous capsule

D17.0 Benign lipomatous neoplasm of skin and subcutaneous tissue of head, face and neck

D17.1 Benign lipomatous neoplasm of skin and subcutaneous tissue of trunk

● **D17.2 Benign lipomatous neoplasm of skin and subcutaneous tissue of limb**
- **D17.20 Benign lipomatous neoplasm of skin and subcutaneous tissue of unspecified limb**
- **D17.21 Benign lipomatous neoplasm of skin and subcutaneous tissue of right arm**
- **D17.22 Benign lipomatous neoplasm of skin and subcutaneous tissue of left arm**
- **D17.23 Benign lipomatous neoplasm of skin and subcutaneous tissue of right leg**
- **D17.24 Benign lipomatous neoplasm of skin and subcutaneous tissue of left leg**

● **D17.3 Benign lipomatous neoplasm of skin and subcutaneous tissue of other and unspecified sites**
- **D17.30 Benign lipomatous neoplasm of skin and subcutaneous tissue of unspecified sites**
- **D17.39 Benign lipomatous neoplasm of skin and subcutaneous tissue of other sites**

D17.4 Benign lipomatous neoplasm of intrathoracic organs

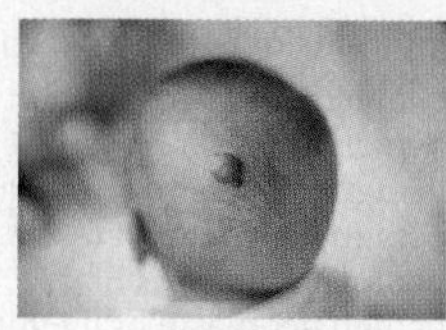

Figure 2-18 Hemangioma of skin and subcutaneous tissue. (Getty Image)

Item 2-10 Hemangiomas are abnormally dense collections of dilated capillaries that occur on the skin or in internal organs. Hemangiomas are both deep and superficial and undergo a rapid growth phase when the size increases rapidly, followed by a rest phase, in which the tumor changes very little, followed by an involutional phase in which the tumor begins to and can disappear altogether. **Lymphangiomas** or cystic hygroma are benign collections of overgrown lymph vessels and, although rare, may occur anywhere but most commonly on the head and neck of children and infants. Visceral organs, lungs, and gastrointestinal tract may also be involved.

D17.5 Benign lipomatous neoplasm of intra-abdominal organs
Excludes1 benign lipomatous neoplasm of peritoneum and retroperitoneum (D17.79)

D17.6 Benign lipomatous neoplasm of spermatic cord

● **D17.7 Benign lipomatous neoplasm of other sites**
- **D17.71 Benign lipomatous neoplasm of kidney**
- **D17.72 Benign lipomatous neoplasm of other genitourinary organ**
- **D17.79 Benign lipomatous neoplasm of other sites**
  Benign lipomatous neoplasm of peritoneum
  Benign lipomatous neoplasm of retroperitoneum

D17.9 Benign lipomatous neoplasm, unspecified
Lipoma NOS

● **D18 Hemangioma and lymphangioma, any site**
Excludes1 benign neoplasm of glomus jugulare (D35.6)
blue or pigmented nevus (D22.-)
nevus NOS (D22.-)
vascular nevus (Q82.5)

● **D18.0 Hemangioma**
Common type of vascular malformation
Angioma NOS
Cavernous nevus
- **D18.00 Hemangioma unspecified site**
- **D18.01 Hemangioma of skin and subcutaneous tissue**
- **D18.02 Hemangioma of intracranial structures** HCC
- **D18.03 Hemangioma of intra-abdominal structures**
- **D18.09 Hemangioma of other sites**

D18.1 Lymphangioma, any site
Coding Clinic: 2018, Q2, P13

● **D19 Benign neoplasm of mesothelial tissue**
Mesothelial tissue is the membrane lining several body cavities

D19.0 Benign neoplasm of mesothelial tissue of pleura

D19.1 Benign neoplasm of mesothelial tissue of peritoneum

D19.7 Benign neoplasm of mesothelial tissue of other sites

D19.9 Benign neoplasm of mesothelial tissue, unspecified
Benign mesothelioma NOS

● **D20 Benign neoplasm of soft tissue of retroperitoneum and peritoneum**
Excludes1 benign lipomatous neoplasm of peritoneum and retroperitoneum (D17.79)
benign neoplasm of mesothelial tissue (D19.-)

D20.0 Benign neoplasm of soft tissue of retroperitoneum

D20.1 Benign neoplasm of soft tissue of peritoneum

CHAPTER 2 (C00-D49)

● **D21 Other benign neoplasms of connective and other soft tissue**

Includes benign neoplasm of blood vessel
benign neoplasm of bursa
benign neoplasm of cartilage
benign neoplasm of fascia
benign neoplasm of fat
benign neoplasm of ligament, except uterine
benign neoplasm of lymphatic channel
benign neoplasm of muscle
benign neoplasm of synovia
benign neoplasm of tendon (sheath)
benign stromal tumors

Excludes1 benign neoplasm of articular cartilage (D16.-)
benign neoplasm of cartilage of larynx (D14.1)
benign neoplasm of cartilage of nose (D14.0)
benign neoplasm of connective tissue of breast (D24.-)
benign neoplasm of peripheral nerves and autonomic nervous system (D36.1-)
benign neoplasm of peritoneum (D20.1)
benign neoplasm of retroperitoneum (D20.0)
benign neoplasm of uterine ligament, any (D28.2)
benign neoplasm of vascular tissue (D18.-)
hemangioma (D18.0-)
lipomatous neoplasm (D17.-)
lymphangioma (D18.1)
uterine leiomyoma (D25.-)

D21.0 Benign neoplasm of connective and other soft tissue of head, face and neck
Benign neoplasm of connective tissue of ear
Benign neoplasm of connective tissue of eyelid
Excludes1 benign neoplasm of connective tissue of orbit (D31.6-)

● **D21.1 Benign neoplasm of connective and other soft tissue of upper limb, including shoulder**
D21.10 Benign neoplasm of connective and other soft tissue of unspecified upper limb, including shoulder
D21.11 Benign neoplasm of connective and other soft tissue of right upper limb, including shoulder
D21.12 Benign neoplasm of connective and other soft tissue of left upper limb, including shoulder

● **D21.2 Benign neoplasm of connective and other soft tissue of lower limb, including hip**
D21.20 Benign neoplasm of connective and other soft tissue of unspecified lower limb, including hip
D21.21 Benign neoplasm of connective and other soft tissue of right lower limb, including hip
D21.22 Benign neoplasm of connective and other soft tissue of left lower limb, including hip

D21.3 Benign neoplasm of connective and other soft tissue of thorax
Benign neoplasm of axilla
Benign neoplasm of diaphragm
Benign neoplasm of great vessels
Excludes1 benign neoplasm of heart (D15.1)
benign neoplasm of mediastinum (D15.2)
benign neoplasm of thymus (D15.0)

D21.4 Benign neoplasm of connective and other soft tissue of abdomen
Benign stromal tumors of abdomen

D21.5 Benign neoplasm of connective and other soft tissue of pelvis
Excludes1 benign neoplasm of any uterine ligament (D28.2)
uterine leiomyoma (D25.-)

D21.6 Benign neoplasm of connective and other soft tissue of trunk, unspecified
Benign neoplasm of connective and other soft tissue of back NOS

D21.9 Benign neoplasm of connective and other soft tissue, unspecified

● **D22 Melanocytic nevi**

Includes atypical nevus
blue hairy pigmented nevus
nevus NOS

D22.0 Melanocytic nevi of lip
Skin lesions composed of nests of nevus cells with macules/papules

● **D22.1 Melanocytic nevi of eyelid, including canthus**
D22.10 Melanocytic nevi of unspecified eyelid, including canthus
● **D22.11 Melanocytic nevi of right eyelid, including canthus**
D22.111 Melanocytic nevi of right upper eyelid, including canthus
D22.112 Melanocytic nevi of right lower eyelid, including canthus
● **D22.12 Melanocytic nevi of left eyelid, including canthus**
D22.121 Melanocytic nevi of left upper eyelid, including canthus
D22.122 Melanocytic nevi of left lower eyelid, including canthus

● **D22.2 Melanocytic nevi of ear and external auricular canal**
D22.20 Melanocytic nevi of unspecified ear and external auricular canal
D22.21 Melanocytic nevi of right ear and external auricular canal
D22.22 Melanocytic nevi of left ear and external auricular canal

● **D22.3 Melanocytic nevi of other and unspecified parts of face**
D22.30 Melanocytic nevi of unspecified part of face
D22.39 Melanocytic nevi of other parts of face

D22.4 Melanocytic nevi of scalp and neck

D22.5 Melanocytic nevi of trunk
Melanocytic nevi of anal margin
Melanocytic nevi of anal skin
Melanocytic nevi of perianal skin
Melanocytic nevi of skin of breast

● **D22.6 Melanocytic nevi of upper limb, including shoulder**
D22.60 Melanocytic nevi of unspecified upper limb, including shoulder
D22.61 Melanocytic nevi of right upper limb, including shoulder
D22.62 Melanocytic nevi of left upper limb, including shoulder

● **D22.7 Melanocytic nevi of lower limb, including hip**
D22.70 Melanocytic nevi of unspecified lower limb, including hip
D22.71 Melanocytic nevi of right lower limb, including hip
D22.72 Melanocytic nevi of left lower limb, including hip

D22.9 Melanocytic nevi, unspecified

● **D23 Other benign neoplasms of skin**

Includes benign neoplasm of hair follicles
benign neoplasm of sebaceous glands
benign neoplasm of sweat glands

Excludes1 benign lipomatous neoplasms of skin (D17.0-D17.3)

Excludes2 melanocytic nevi (D22.-)

D23.0 Other benign neoplasm of skin of lip
Excludes1 benign neoplasm of vermilion border of lip (D10.0)

● **D23.1 Other benign neoplasm of skin of eyelid, including canthus**
D23.10 Other benign neoplasm of skin unspecified of eyelid, including canthus

- **D23.11 Other benign neoplasm of skin of right eyelid, including canthus**
  - **D23.111 Other benign neoplasm of skin of right upper eyelid, including canthus**
  - **D23.112 Other benign neoplasm of skin of right lower eyelid, including canthus**
- **D23.12 Other benign neoplasm of skin of left eyelid, including canthus**
  - **D23.121 Other benign neoplasm of skin of left upper eyelid, including canthus**
  - **D23.122 Other benign neoplasm of skin of left lower eyelid, including canthus**

D23.2 Other benign neoplasm of skin of ear and external auricular canal
- **D23.20 Other benign neoplasm of skin of unspecified ear and external auricular canal**
- **D23.21 Other benign neoplasm of skin of right ear and external auricular canal**
- **D23.22 Other benign neoplasm of skin of left ear and external auricular canal**

D23.3 Other benign neoplasm of skin of other and unspecified parts of face
- **D23.30 Other benign neoplasm of skin of unspecified part of face**
- **D23.39 Other benign neoplasm of skin of other parts of face**

D23.4 Other benign neoplasm of skin of scalp and neck

D23.5 Other benign neoplasm of skin of trunk
Other benign neoplasm of anal margin
Other benign neoplasm of anal skin
Other benign neoplasm of perianal skin
Other benign neoplasm of skin of breast
Excludes1 benign neoplasm of anus NOS (D12.9)

D23.6 Other benign neoplasm of skin of upper limb, including shoulder
- **D23.60 Other benign neoplasm of skin of unspecified upper limb, including shoulder**
- **D23.61 Other benign neoplasm of skin of right upper limb, including shoulder**
- **D23.62 Other benign neoplasm of skin of left upper limb, including shoulder**

D23.7 Other benign neoplasm of skin of lower limb, including hip
- **D23.70 Other benign neoplasm of skin of unspecified lower limb, including hip**
- **D23.71 Other benign neoplasm of skin of right lower limb, including hip**
- **D23.72 Other benign neoplasm of skin of left lower limb, including hip**

D23.9 Other benign neoplasm of skin, unspecified

D24 Benign neoplasm of breast
Includes benign neoplasm of connective tissue of breast
benign neoplasm of soft parts of breast
fibroadenoma of breast
Excludes2 adenofibrosis of breast (N60.2)
benign cyst of breast (N60.-)
benign mammary dysplasia (N60.-)
benign neoplasm of skin of breast (D22.5, D23.5)
fibrocystic disease of breast (N60.-)

- **D24.1 Benign neoplasm of right breast**
  Coding Clinic: 2017, Q1, P5
- **D24.2 Benign neoplasm of left breast**
- **D24.9 Benign neoplasm of unspecified breast**

Item 2-11 Teratoma: terat = monster, oma = mass, tumor. Alternate terms: dermoid cyst of the ovary, ovarian teratoma. Teratomas are neoplasms and arise from germ cells (ovaries in female and testes in male) and can be benign or malignant. Teratomas have been known to contain hair, nails, and teeth, giving them a bizarre ("monster") appearance.

D25 Leiomyoma of uterus
Benign tumors or nodules of the uterine wall
Includes uterine fibroid
uterine fibromyoma
uterine myoma
- **D25.0 Submucous leiomyoma of uterus**
- **D25.1 Intramural leiomyoma of uterus**
  Interstitial leiomyoma of uterus
- **D25.2 Subserosal leiomyoma of uterus**
  Subperitoneal leiomyoma of uterus
- **D25.9 Leiomyoma of uterus, unspecified**

D26 Other benign neoplasms of uterus
- **D26.0 Other benign neoplasm of cervix uteri**
- **D26.1 Other benign neoplasm of corpus uteri**
- **D26.7 Other benign neoplasm of other parts of uterus**
- **D26.9 Other benign neoplasm of uterus, unspecified**

D27 Benign neoplasm of ovary
Use additional code to identify any functional activity.
Excludes2 corpus albicans cyst (N83.2-)
corpus luteum cyst (N83.1-)
endometrial cyst (N80.1-)
follicular (atretic) cyst (N83.0-)
graafian follicle cyst (N83.0-)
ovarian cyst NEC (N83.2-)
ovarian retention cyst (N83.2-)
- **D27.0 Benign neoplasm of right ovary**
- **D27.1 Benign neoplasm of left ovary**
- **D27.9 Benign neoplasm of unspecified ovary**
  Ovarian teratoma

D28 Benign neoplasm of other and unspecified female genital organs
Includes adenomatous polyp
benign neoplasm of skin of female genital organs
benign teratoma
Excludes1 epoophoron cyst (Q50.5)
fimbrial cyst (Q50.4)
Gartner's duct cyst (Q52.4)
parovarian cyst (Q50.5)
- **D28.0 Benign neoplasm of vulva**
- **D28.1 Benign neoplasm of vagina**
- **D28.2 Benign neoplasm of uterine tubes and ligaments**
  Benign neoplasm of fallopian tube
  Benign neoplasm of uterine ligament (broad) (round)
- **D28.7 Benign neoplasm of other specified female genital organs**
- **D28.9 Benign neoplasm of female genital organ, unspecified**

D29 Benign neoplasm of male genital organs
Includes benign neoplasm of skin of male genital organs
- **D29.0 Benign neoplasm of penis**
- **D29.1 Benign neoplasm of prostate**
  Excludes1 enlarged prostate (N40.-)
- **D29.2 Benign neoplasm of testis**
  Use additional code to identify any functional activity.
  - **D29.20 Benign neoplasm of unspecified testis**
  - **D29.21 Benign neoplasm of right testis**
  - **D29.22 Benign neoplasm of left testis**
- **D29.3 Benign neoplasm of epididymis**
  - **D29.30 Benign neoplasm of unspecified epididymis**
  - **D29.31 Benign neoplasm of right epididymis**
  - **D29.32 Benign neoplasm of left epididymis**

CHAPTER 2 (C00-D49)

D29.4 Benign neoplasm of scrotum
Benign neoplasm of skin of scrotum

D29.8 Benign neoplasm of other specified male genital organs
Benign neoplasm of seminal vesicle
Benign neoplasm of spermatic cord
Benign neoplasm of tunica vaginalis

D29.9 Benign neoplasm of male genital organ, unspecified

● **D30 Benign neoplasm of urinary organs**

● **D30.0 Benign neoplasm of kidney**

Excludes1 benign carcinoid tumor of the kidney (D3A.093)
benign neoplasm of renal calyces (D30.1-)
benign neoplasm of renal pelvis (D30.1-)

D30.00 Benign neoplasm of unspecified kidney
D30.01 Benign neoplasm of right kidney
D30.02 Benign neoplasm of left kidney

● **D30.1 Benign neoplasm of renal pelvis**
D30.10 Benign neoplasm of unspecified renal pelvis
D30.11 Benign neoplasm of right renal pelvis
D30.12 Benign neoplasm of left renal pelvis

● **D30.2 Benign neoplasm of ureter**

Excludes1 benign neoplasm of ureteric orifice of bladder (D30.3)

D30.20 Benign neoplasm of unspecified ureter
D30.21 Benign neoplasm of right ureter
D30.22 Benign neoplasm of left ureter

D30.3 Benign neoplasm of bladder
Benign neoplasm of ureteric orifice of bladder
Benign neoplasm of urethral orifice of bladder

D30.4 Benign neoplasm of urethra

Excludes1 benign neoplasm of urethral orifice of bladder (D30.3)

D30.8 Benign neoplasm of other specified urinary organs
Benign neoplasm of paraurethral glands

D30.9 Benign neoplasm of urinary organ, unspecified
Benign neoplasm of urinary system NOS

● **D31 Benign neoplasm of eye and adnexa**

Excludes1 benign neoplasm of connective tissue of eyelid (D21.0)
benign neoplasm of optic nerve (D33.3)
benign neoplasm of skin of eyelid (D22.1-, D23.1-)

● **D31.0 Benign neoplasm of conjunctiva**
D31.00 Benign neoplasm of unspecified conjunctiva
D31.01 Benign neoplasm of right conjunctiva
D31.02 Benign neoplasm of left conjunctiva

● **D31.1 Benign neoplasm of cornea**
D31.10 Benign neoplasm of unspecified cornea
D31.11 Benign neoplasm of right cornea
D31.12 Benign neoplasm of left cornea

● **D31.2 Benign neoplasm of retina**

Excludes1 dark area on retina (D49.81)
hemangioma of retina (D49.81)
neoplasm of unspecified behavior of retina and choroid (D49.81)
retinal freckle (D49.81)

D31.20 Benign neoplasm of unspecified retina
D31.21 Benign neoplasm of right retina
D31.22 Benign neoplasm of left retina

● **D31.3 Benign neoplasm of choroid**
D31.30 Benign neoplasm of unspecified choroid
D31.31 Benign neoplasm of right choroid
D31.32 Benign neoplasm of left choroid

● **D31.4 Benign neoplasm of ciliary body**
D31.40 Benign neoplasm of unspecified ciliary body
D31.41 Benign neoplasm of right ciliary body
D31.42 Benign neoplasm of left ciliary body

● **D31.5 Benign neoplasm of lacrimal gland and duct**
Benign neoplasm of lacrimal sac
Benign neoplasm of nasolacrimal duct

D31.50 Benign neoplasm of unspecified lacrimal gland and duct
D31.51 Benign neoplasm of right lacrimal gland and duct
D31.52 Benign neoplasm of left lacrimal gland and duct

● **D31.6 Benign neoplasm of unspecified site of orbit**
Benign neoplasm of connective tissue of orbit
Benign neoplasm of extraocular muscle
Benign neoplasm of peripheral nerves of orbit
Benign neoplasm of retrobulbar tissue
Benign neoplasm of retro-ocular tissue

Excludes1 benign neoplasm of orbital bone (D16.4)

D31.60 Benign neoplasm of unspecified site of unspecified orbit
D31.61 Benign neoplasm of unspecified site of right orbit
D31.62 Benign neoplasm of unspecified site of left orbit

● **D31.9 Benign neoplasm of unspecified part of eye**
Benign neoplasm of eyeball

D31.90 Benign neoplasm of unspecified part of unspecified eye
D31.91 Benign neoplasm of unspecified part of right eye
D31.92 Benign neoplasm of unspecified part of left eye

● **D32 Benign neoplasm of meninges**
D32.0 Benign neoplasm of cerebral meninges
D32.1 Benign neoplasm of spinal meninges
D32.9 Benign neoplasm of meninges, unspecified
Meningioma NOS

● **D33 Benign neoplasm of brain and other parts of central nervous system**

Excludes1 angioma (D18.0-)
benign neoplasm of meninges (D32.-)
benign neoplasm of peripheral nerves and autonomic nervous system (D36.1-)
hemangioma (D18.0-)
neurofibromatosis (Q85.0-)
retro-ocular benign neoplasm (D31.6-)

D33.0 Benign neoplasm of brain, supratentorial
Benign neoplasm of cerebral ventricle
Benign neoplasm of cerebrum
Benign neoplasm of frontal lobe
Benign neoplasm of occipital lobe
Benign neoplasm of parietal lobe
Benign neoplasm of temporal lobe

Excludes1 benign neoplasm of fourth ventricle (D33.1)

D33.1 Benign neoplasm of brain, infratentorial
Benign neoplasm of brain stem
Benign neoplasm of cerebellum
Benign neoplasm of fourth ventricle

D33.2 Benign neoplasm of brain, unspecified
D33.3 Benign neoplasm of cranial nerves
Benign neoplasm of olfactory bulb

D33.4 Benign neoplasm of spinal cord
D33.7 Benign neoplasm of other specified parts of central nervous system
D33.9 Benign neoplasm of central nervous system, unspecified
Benign neoplasm of nervous system (central) NOS

D34 Benign neoplasm of thyroid gland
Use additional code to identify any functional activity.

CHAPTER 2 (C00-D49)

D35 Benign neoplasm of other and unspecified endocrine glands
Use additional code to identify any functional activity.
Excludes1 benign neoplasm of endocrine pancreas (D13.7)
benign neoplasm of ovary (D27.-)
benign neoplasm of testis (D29.2.-)
benign neoplasm of thymus (D15.0)

D35.0 Benign neoplasm of adrenal gland
D35.00 Benign neoplasm of unspecified adrenal gland
D35.01 Benign neoplasm of right adrenal gland
D35.02 Benign neoplasm of left adrenal gland
D35.1 Benign neoplasm of parathyroid gland
D35.2 Benign neoplasm of pituitary gland
D35.3 Benign neoplasm of craniopharyngeal duct
D35.4 Benign neoplasm of pineal gland
D35.5 Benign neoplasm of carotid body
D35.6 Benign neoplasm of aortic body and other paraganglia
Benign tumor of glomus jugulare
D35.7 Benign neoplasm of other specified endocrine glands
D35.9 Benign neoplasm of endocrine gland, unspecified
Benign neoplasm of unspecified endocrine gland

D36 Benign neoplasm of other and unspecified sites
D36.0 Benign neoplasm of lymph nodes
Excludes1 lymphangioma (D18.1)
D36.1 Benign neoplasm of peripheral nerves and autonomic nervous system
Excludes1 benign neoplasm of peripheral nerves of orbit (D31.6-)
neurofibromatosis (Q85.0-)
D36.10 Benign neoplasm of peripheral nerves and autonomic nervous system, unspecified
D36.11 Benign neoplasm of peripheral nerves and autonomic nervous system of face, head, and neck
D36.12 Benign neoplasm of peripheral nerves and autonomic nervous system, upper limb, including shoulder
D36.13 Benign neoplasm of peripheral nerves and autonomic nervous system of lower limb, including hip
D36.14 Benign neoplasm of peripheral nerves and autonomic nervous system of thorax
D36.15 Benign neoplasm of peripheral nerves and autonomic nervous system of abdomen
D36.16 Benign neoplasm of peripheral nerves and autonomic nervous system of pelvis
D36.17 Benign neoplasm of peripheral nerves and autonomic nervous system of trunk, unspecified
D36.7 Benign neoplasm of other specified sites
Benign neoplasm of nose NOS
Benign neoplasm of back NOS
D36.9 Benign neoplasm, unspecified site

NEOPLASMS OF UNCERTAIN BEHAVIOR, POLYCYTHEMIA VERA AND MYELODYSPLASTIC SYNDROMES (D37-D48)

Note: Categories D37-D44, and D48 classify by site neoplasms of uncertain behavior, i.e., histologic confirmation whether the neoplasm is malignant or benign cannot be made.
Excludes1 neoplasms of unspecified behavior (D49.-)

D37 Neoplasm of uncertain behavior of oral cavity and digestive organs
Excludes1 stromal tumors of uncertain behavior of digestive system (D48.1-)
D37.0 Neoplasm of uncertain behavior of lip, oral cavity and pharynx
Excludes1 neoplasm of uncertain behavior of aryepiglottic fold or interarytenoid fold, laryngeal aspect (D38.0)
neoplasm of uncertain behavior of epiglottis NOS (D38.0)
neoplasm of uncertain behavior of skin of lip (D48.5)
neoplasm of uncertain behavior of suprahyoid portion of epiglottis (D38.0)
D37.01 Neoplasm of uncertain behavior of lip
Neoplasm of uncertain behavior of vermilion border of lip
D37.02 Neoplasm of uncertain behavior of tongue
D37.03 Neoplasm of uncertain behavior of the major salivary glands
D37.030 Neoplasm of uncertain behavior of the parotid salivary glands
D37.031 Neoplasm of uncertain behavior of the sublingual salivary glands
D37.032 Neoplasm of uncertain behavior of the submandibular salivary glands
D37.039 Neoplasm of uncertain behavior of the major salivary glands, unspecified
D37.04 Neoplasm of uncertain behavior of the minor salivary glands
Neoplasm of uncertain behavior of submucosal salivary glands of lip
Neoplasm of uncertain behavior of submucosal salivary glands of cheek
Neoplasm of uncertain behavior of submucosal salivary glands of hard palate
Neoplasm of uncertain behavior of submucosal salivary glands of soft palate
D37.05 Neoplasm of uncertain behavior of pharynx
Neoplasm of uncertain behavior of aryepiglottic fold of pharynx NOS
Neoplasm of uncertain behavior of hypopharyngeal aspect of aryepiglottic fold of pharynx
Neoplasm of uncertain behavior of marginal zone of aryepiglottic fold of pharynx
D37.09 Neoplasm of uncertain behavior of other specified sites of the oral cavity
D37.1 Neoplasm of uncertain behavior of stomach
D37.2 Neoplasm of uncertain behavior of small intestine
D37.3 Neoplasm of uncertain behavior of appendix
D37.4 Neoplasm of uncertain behavior of colon
D37.5 Neoplasm of uncertain behavior of rectum
Neoplasm of uncertain behavior of rectosigmoid junction
Rectosigmoid junction: Angle where sigmoid colon becomes rectum
D37.6 Neoplasm of uncertain behavior of liver, gallbladder and bile ducts
Neoplasm of uncertain behavior of ampulla of Vater
Ampulla of Vater: Enlarged segment of ducts from liver and pancreas at entry point to small intestine

CHAPTER 2 (C00-D49)

D37.8 Neoplasm of uncertain behavior of other specified digestive organs
Neoplasm of uncertain behavior of anal canal
Neoplasm of uncertain behavior of anal sphincter
Neoplasm of uncertain behavior of anus NOS
Neoplasm of uncertain behavior of esophagus
Neoplasm of uncertain behavior of intestine NOS
Neoplasm of uncertain behavior of pancreas
Excludes1 neoplasm of uncertain behavior of anal margin (D48.5)
neoplasm of uncertain behavior of anal skin (D48.5)
neoplasm of uncertain behavior of perianal skin (D48.5)

D37.9 Neoplasm of uncertain behavior of digestive organ, unspecified

● **D38 Neoplasm of uncertain behavior of middle ear and respiratory and intrathoracic organs**
Excludes1 neoplasm of uncertain behavior of heart (D48.7)

D38.0 Neoplasm of uncertain behavior of larynx
Neoplasm of uncertain behavior of aryepiglottic fold or interarytenoid fold, laryngeal aspect
Neoplasm of uncertain behavior of epiglottis (suprahyoid portion)
Excludes1 neoplasm of uncertain behavior of aryepiglottic fold or interarytenoid fold NOS (D37.05)
neoplasm of uncertain behavior of hypopharyngeal aspect of aryepiglottic fold (D37.05)
neoplasm of uncertain behavior of marginal zone of aryepiglottic fold (D37.05)

D38.1 Neoplasm of uncertain behavior of trachea, bronchus and lung
D38.2 Neoplasm of uncertain behavior of pleura
D38.3 Neoplasm of uncertain behavior of mediastinum
D38.4 Neoplasm of uncertain behavior of thymus
D38.5 Neoplasm of uncertain behavior of other respiratory organs
Neoplasm of uncertain behavior of accessory sinuses
Neoplasm of uncertain behavior of cartilage of nose
Neoplasm of uncertain behavior of middle ear
Neoplasm of uncertain behavior of nasal cavities
Excludes1 neoplasm of uncertain behavior of ear (external) (skin) (D48.5)
neoplasm of uncertain behavior of nose NOS (D48.7)
neoplasm of uncertain behavior of skin of nose (D48.5)

D38.6 Neoplasm of uncertain behavior of respiratory organ, unspecified

● **D39 Neoplasm of uncertain behavior of female genital organs**

D39.0 Neoplasm of uncertain behavior of uterus

● **D39.1 Neoplasm of uncertain behavior of ovary**
Use additional code to identify any functional activity.
D39.10 Neoplasm of uncertain behavior of unspecified ovary
D39.11 Neoplasm of uncertain behavior of right ovary
D39.12 Neoplasm of uncertain behavior of left ovary

D39.2 Neoplasm of uncertain behavior of placentaM
Chorioadenoma destruens
Invasive hydatidiform mole
Malignant hydatidiform mole
Excludes1 hydatidiform mole NOS (O01.9)
Coding Clinic: 2023, Q3, P15

D39.8 Neoplasm of uncertain behavior of other specified female genital organs
Neoplasm of uncertain behavior of skin of female genital organs

D39.9 Neoplasm of uncertain behavior of female genital organ, unspecified

BENIGN NEUROENDOCRINE TUMORS (D3A)

● **D3A Benign neuroendocrine tumors**
Code also any associated multiple endocrine neoplasia [MEN] syndromes (E31.2-)
Use additional code to identify any associated endocrine syndrome, such as:
carcinoid syndrome (E34.00)
Excludes2 benign pancreatic islet cell tumors (D13.7)

● **D3A.0 Benign carcinoid tumors**
D3A.00 Benign carcinoid tumor of unspecified site
Carcinoid tumor NOS

● **D3A.01 Benign carcinoid tumors of the small intestine**
D3A.010 Benign carcinoid tumor of the duodenum
D3A.011 Benign carcinoid tumor of the jejunum
D3A.012 Benign carcinoid tumor of the ileum
D3A.019 Benign carcinoid tumor of the small intestine, unspecified portion

● **D3A.02 Benign carcinoid tumors of the appendix, large intestine, and rectum**
D3A.020 Benign carcinoid tumor of the appendix
D3A.021 Benign carcinoid tumor of the cecum
D3A.022 Benign carcinoid tumor of the ascending colon
D3A.023 Benign carcinoid tumor of the transverse colon
D3A.024 Benign carcinoid tumor of the descending colon
D3A.025 Benign carcinoid tumor of the sigmoid colon
D3A.026 Benign carcinoid tumor of the rectum
D3A.029 Benign carcinoid tumor of the large intestine, unspecified portion
Benign carcinoid tumor of the colon NOS

● **D3A.09 Benign carcinoid tumors of other sites**
D3A.090 Benign carcinoid tumor of the bronchus and lung
D3A.091 Benign carcinoid tumor of the thymus
D3A.092 Benign carcinoid tumor of the stomach
D3A.093 Benign carcinoid tumor of the kidney
D3A.094 Benign carcinoid tumor of the foregut, unspecified
D3A.095 Benign carcinoid tumor of the midgut, unspecified
D3A.096 Benign carcinoid tumor of the hindgut, unspecified
D3A.098 Benign carcinoid tumors of other sites

D3A.8 Other benign neuroendocrine tumors
Neuroendocrine tumor NOS

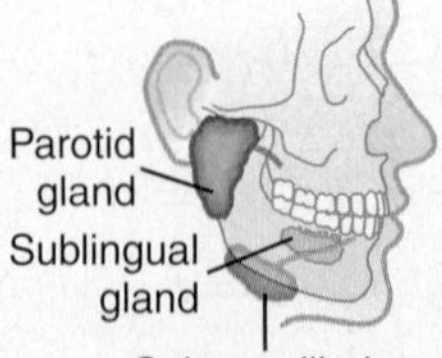

Figure 2-19 Major salivary glands.

D40 Neoplasm of uncertain behavior of male genital organs

D40.0 Neoplasm of uncertain behavior of prostate

D40.1 Neoplasm of uncertain behavior of testis

D40.10 Neoplasm of uncertain behavior of unspecified testis

D40.11 Neoplasm of uncertain behavior of right testis

D40.12 Neoplasm of uncertain behavior of left testis

D40.8 Neoplasm of uncertain behavior of other specified male genital organs

Neoplasm of uncertain behavior of skin of male genital organs

D40.9 Neoplasm of uncertain behavior of male genital organ, unspecified

D41 Neoplasm of uncertain behavior of urinary organs

D41.0 Neoplasm of uncertain behavior of kidney

Excludes1 neoplasm of uncertain behavior of renal pelvis (D41.1-)

D41.00 Neoplasm of uncertain behavior of unspecified kidney

D41.01 Neoplasm of uncertain behavior of right kidney

D41.02 Neoplasm of uncertain behavior of left kidney

D41.1 Neoplasm of uncertain behavior of renal pelvis

D41.10 Neoplasm of uncertain behavior of unspecified renal pelvis

D41.11 Neoplasm of uncertain behavior of right renal pelvis

D41.12 Neoplasm of uncertain behavior of left renal pelvis

D41.2 Neoplasm of uncertain behavior of ureter

D41.20 Neoplasm of uncertain behavior of unspecified ureter

D41.21 Neoplasm of uncertain behavior of right ureter

D41.22 Neoplasm of uncertain behavior of left ureter

D41.3 Neoplasm of uncertain behavior of urethra

D41.4 Neoplasm of uncertain behavior of bladder

D41.8 Neoplasm of uncertain behavior of other specified urinary organs

D41.9 Neoplasm of uncertain behavior of unspecified urinary organ

D42 Neoplasm of uncertain behavior of meninges

D42.0 Neoplasm of uncertain behavior of cerebral meninges

D42.1 Neoplasm of uncertain behavior of spinal meninges

D42.9 Neoplasm of uncertain behavior of meninges, unspecified

D43 Neoplasm of uncertain behavior of brain and central nervous system

Excludes1 neoplasm of uncertain behavior of peripheral nerves and autonomic nervous system (D48.2)

D43.0 Neoplasm of uncertain behavior of brain, supratentorial

Superior to tentorium of cerebellum

Neoplasm of uncertain behavior of cerebral ventricle
Neoplasm of uncertain behavior of cerebrum
Neoplasm of uncertain behavior of frontal lobe
Neoplasm of uncertain behavior of occipital lobe
Neoplasm of uncertain behavior of parietal lobe
Neoplasm of uncertain behavior of temporal lobe

Excludes1 neoplasm of uncertain behavior of fourth ventricle (D43.1)

D43.1 Neoplasm of uncertain behavior of brain, infratentorial

Beneath the tentorium of cerebellum

Neoplasm of uncertain behavior of brain stem
Neoplasm of uncertain behavior of cerebellum
Neoplasm of uncertain behavior of fourth ventricle

Coding Clinic: 2023, Q2, P16

D43.2 Neoplasm of uncertain behavior of brain, unspecified

D43.3 Neoplasm of uncertain behavior of cranial nerves

D43.4 Neoplasm of uncertain behavior of spinal cord

D43.8 Neoplasm of uncertain behavior of other specified parts of central nervous system

D43.9 Neoplasm of uncertain behavior of central nervous system, unspecified

Neoplasm of uncertain behavior of nervous system (central) NOS

D44 Neoplasm of uncertain behavior of endocrine glands

Excludes1 multiple endocrine adenomatosis (E31.2-)
multiple endocrine neoplasia (E31.2-)
neoplasm of uncertain behavior of endocrine pancreas (D37.8)
neoplasm of uncertain behavior of ovary (D39.1-)
neoplasm of uncertain behavior of testis (D40.1-)
neoplasm of uncertain behavior of thymus (D38.4)

D44.0 Neoplasm of uncertain behavior of thyroid gland

D44.1 Neoplasm of uncertain behavior of adrenal gland

Use additional code to identify any functional activity.

D44.10 Neoplasm of uncertain behavior of unspecified adrenal gland

D44.11 Neoplasm of uncertain behavior of right adrenal gland

D44.12 Neoplasm of uncertain behavior of left adrenal gland

D44.2 Neoplasm of uncertain behavior of parathyroid gland

D44.3 Neoplasm of uncertain behavior of pituitary gland

Use additional code to identify any functional activity.

D44.4 Neoplasm of uncertain behavior of craniopharyngeal duct

D44.5 Neoplasm of uncertain behavior of pineal gland

D44.6 Neoplasm of uncertain behavior of carotid body

D44.7 Neoplasm of uncertain behavior of aortic body and other paraganglia

Coding Clinic: 2016, Q4, P26

D44.9 Neoplasm of uncertain behavior of unspecified endocrine gland

D45 Polycythemia vera

Excludes1 familial polycythemia (D75.0)
secondary polycythemia (D75.1)

Primary polycythemia. Secondary polycythemia is D75.1. Check your documentation. Polycythemia is caused by too many red blood cells, which increase the thickness of blood (viscosity). This can cause engorgement of the spleen (splenomegaly) with extra RBCs and potential clot formation.

D46 Myelodysplastic syndromes

Use additional code for adverse effect, if applicable, to identify drug (T36-T50 with fifth or sixth character 5)

Excludes2 drug-induced aplastic anemia (D61.1)

D46.0 Refractory anemia without ring sideroblasts, so stated

Refractory anemia without sideroblasts, without excess of blasts

D46.1 Refractory anemia with ring sideroblasts RARS

D46.2 Refractory anemia with excess of blasts [RAEB]

Form of myelodysplasia with increased immature white blood cells (blasts) in bone marrow

D46.20 Refractory anemia with excess of blasts, unspecified RAEB NOS

D46.21 Refractory anemia with excess of blasts 1 RAEB 1

Bone marrow disease which results in insufficient RBCs (anemia) in which level of blasts is less than 10%

D46.22 Refractory anemia with excess of blasts 2 RAEB 2 Ex: PDX 535

Bone marrow disease manifested by insufficient numbers of RBCs (anemia) with level of blasts 10-20%

D46.A Refractory cytopenia with multilineage dysplasia

D46.B Refractory cytopenia with multilineage dysplasia and ring sideroblasts
RCMD RS

D46.C Myelodysplastic syndrome with isolated del(5q) chromosomal abnormality PDX 535
Myelodysplastic syndrome with 5q deletion
5q minus syndrome NOS

D46.4 Refractory anemia, unspecified

D46.Z Other myelodysplastic syndromes
Excludes1 chronic myelomonocytic leukemia (C93.1-)

D46.9 Myelodysplastic syndrome, unspecified
Myelodysplasia NOS

D47 Other neoplasms of uncertain behavior of lymphoid, hematopoietic and related tissue

D47.Ø Mast cell neoplasms of uncertain behavior PDX 542
Excludes1 congenital cutaneous mastocytosis (Q82.2)
histiocytic neoplasms of uncertain behavior (D47.Z9)
malignant mast cell neoplasm (C96.2-)

D47.Ø1 Cutaneous mastocytosis
Diffuse cutaneous mastocytosis
Maculopapular cutaneous mastocytosis
Solitary mastocytoma
Telangiectasia macularis eruptiva perstans
Urticaria pigmentosa
Excludes1 congenital (diffuse) (maculopapular) cutaneous mastocytosis (Q82.2)
congenital urticaria pigmentosa (Q82.2)
extracutaneous mastocytoma (D47.Ø9)

D47.Ø2 Systemic mastocytosis
Indolent systemic mastocytosis
Isolated bone marrow mastocytosis
Smoldering systemic mastocytosis
Systemic mastocytosis, with an associated hematological non-mast cell lineage disease (SM-AHNMD)
Code also if applicable, any associated hematological non-mast cell lineage disease, such as:
acute myeloid leukemia (C92.6-, C92.A-)
chronic myelomonocytic leukemia (C93.1-)
essential thrombocytosis (D47.3)
hypereosinophilic syndrome (D72.1)
myelodysplastic syndrome (D46.9)
myeloproliferative syndrome (D47.1)
non-Hodgkin lymphoma (C82-C85)
plasma cell myeloma (C90.0-)
polycythemia vera (D45)
Excludes1 aggressive systemic mastocytosis (C96.21)
mast cell leukemia (C94.3-)

D47.Ø9 Other mast cell neoplasms of uncertain behavior
Extracutaneous mastocytoma
Mast cell tumor NOS
Mastocytoma NOS
Mastocytosis NOS

D47.1 Chronic myeloproliferative disease PDX 535
Chronic neutrophilic leukemia
Myeloproliferative disease, unspecified
Excludes1 atypical chronic myeloid leukemia BCR/ABL-negative (C92.2-)
chronic myeloid leukemia BCR/ABL-positive (C92.1-)
myelofibrosis NOS (D75.81)
myelophthisic anemia (D61.82)
myelophthisis (D61.82)
secondary myelofibrosis NOS (D75.81)

D47.2 Monoclonal gammopathy
Monoclonal gammopathy of undetermined significance [MGUS]
Coding Clinic: 2Ø21, Q3, P5

D47.3 Essential (hemorrhagic) thrombocythemia
Essential thrombocytosis
Idiopathic hemorrhagic thrombocythemia
Primary thrombocytosis
Excludes2 reactive thrombocytosis (D75.838)
secondary thrombocytosis (D75.838)
thrombocythemia NOS (D75.839)
thrombocytosis NOS (D75.839)

D47.4 Osteomyelofibrosis
Chronic idiopathic myelofibrosis
Myelofibrosis (idiopathic) (with myeloid metaplasia)
Myelosclerosis (megakaryocytic) with myeloid metaplasia
Secondary myelofibrosis in myeloproliferative disease
Excludes1 acute myelofibrosis (C94.4-)

D47.9 Neoplasm of uncertain behavior of lymphoid, hematopoietic and related tissue, unspecified PDX 535
Lymphoproliferative disease NOS

D47.Z Other specified neoplasms of uncertain behavior of lymphoid, hematopoietic and related tissue

D47.Z1 Post-transplant lymphoproliferative disorder (PTLD) PDX 542
Code first complications of transplanted organs and tissue (T86.-)

D47.Z2 Castleman disease PDX 535
Code also if applicable, human herpesvirus 8 infection (B10.89)
Excludes2 Kaposi's sarcoma (C46.-)
Coding Clinic: 2Ø16, Q4, P8

D47.Z9 Other specified neoplasms of uncertain behavior of lymphoid, hematopoietic and related tissue PDX 535
Histiocytic tumors of uncertain behavior

D48 Neoplasm of uncertain behavior of other and unspecified sites
Excludes1 neurofibromatosis (nonmalignant) (Q85.Ø-)

D48.Ø Neoplasm of uncertain behavior of bone and articular cartilage
Excludes1 neoplasm of uncertain behavior of cartilage of ear (D48.1-)
neoplasm of uncertain behavior of cartilage of larynx (D38.Ø)
neoplasm of uncertain behavior of cartilage of nose (D38.5)
neoplasm of uncertain behavior of connective tissue of eyelid (D48.1-)
neoplasm of uncertain behavior of synovia (D48.1-)

D48.1 Neoplasm of uncertain behavior of connective and other soft tissue
Neoplasm of uncertain behavior of connective tissue of ear
Neoplasm of uncertain behavior of connective tissue of eyelid
Stromal tumors of uncertain behavior of digestive system
Excludes1 neoplasm of uncertain behavior of articular cartilage (D48.Ø)
neoplasm of uncertain behavior of cartilage of larynx (D38.Ø)
neoplasm of uncertain behavior of cartilage of nose (D38.5)
neoplasm of uncertain behavior of connective tissue of breast (D48.6-)

D48.11 Desmoid tumor
D48.11Ø Desmoid tumor of head and neck
D48.111 Desmoid tumor of chest wall
D48.112 Desmoid tumor, intrathoracic
D48.113 Desmoid tumor of abdominal wall

D48.114 **Desmoid tumor, intraabdomin**
Desmoid tumor of pelvic cavity
Desmoid tumor, peritoneal, retroperitoneal

D48.115 **Desmoid tumor of upper extremity and shoulder girdle**

D48.116 **Desmoid tumor of lower extremity and pelvic girdle**
Desmoid tumor of buttock

D48.117 **Desmoid tumor of back**

D48.118 **Desmoid tumor of other site**

D48.119 **Desmoid tumor of unspecified site**

D48.19 **Other specified neoplasm of uncertain behavior of connective and other soft tissue**

D48.2 **Neoplasm of uncertain behavior of peripheral nerves and autonomic nervous system**
Excludes1 neoplasm of uncertain behavior of peripheral nerves of orbit (D48.7)

D48.3 **Neoplasm of uncertain behavior of retroperitoneum**

D48.4 **Neoplasm of uncertain behavior of peritoneum**

D48.5 **Neoplasm of uncertain behavior of skin**
Neoplasm of uncertain behavior of anal margin
Neoplasm of uncertain behavior of anal skin
Neoplasm of uncertain behavior of perianal skin
Neoplasm of uncertain behavior of skin of breast
Excludes1 neoplasm of uncertain behavior of anus NOS (D37.8)
neoplasm of uncertain behavior of skin of genital organs (D39.8, D4Ø.8)
neoplasm of uncertain behavior of vermilion border of lip (D37.Ø)

● D48.6 **Neoplasm of uncertain behavior of breast**
Neoplasm of uncertain behavior of connective tissue of breast
Cystosarcoma phyllodes
Excludes1 neoplasm of uncertain behavior of skin of breast (D48.5)

D48.6Ø **Neoplasm of uncertain behavior of unspecified breast**

D48.61 **Neoplasm of uncertain behavior of right breast**

D48.62 **Neoplasm of uncertain behavior of left breast**

D48.7 **Neoplasm of uncertain behavior of other specified sites**
Neoplasm of uncertain behavior of eye
Neoplasm of uncertain behavior of heart
Neoplasm of uncertain behavior of peripheral nerves of orbit
Excludes1 neoplasm of uncertain behavior of connective tissue (D48.1-)
neoplasm of uncertain behavior of skin of eyelid (D48.5)

D48.9 **Neoplasm of uncertain behavior, unspecified**

● D49 **Neoplasms of unspecified behavior**

Note: Category D49 classifies by site neoplasms of unspecified morphology and behavior. The term "mass," unless otherwise stated, is not to be regarded as a neoplastic growth.

Includes 'growth' NOS
neoplasm NOS
new growth NOS
tumor NOS

Excludes1 neoplasms of uncertain behavior (D37-D44, D48)

D49.Ø **Neoplasm of unspecified behavior of digestive system**
Excludes1 neoplasm of unspecified behavior of margin of anus (D49.2)
neoplasm of unspecified behavior of perianal skin (D49.2)
neoplasm of unspecified behavior of skin of anus (D49.2)

D49.1 **Neoplasm of unspecified behavior of respiratory system**

D49.2 **Neoplasm of unspecified behavior of bone, soft tissue, and skin**
Excludes1 neoplasm of unspecified behavior of anal canal (D49.Ø)
neoplasm of unspecified behavior of anus NOS (D49.Ø)
neoplasm of unspecified behavior of bone marrow (D49.89)
neoplasm of unspecified behavior of cartilage of larynx (D49.1)
neoplasm of unspecified behavior of cartilage of nose (D49.1)
neoplasm of unspecified behavior of connective tissue of breast (D49.3)
neoplasm of unspecified behavior of skin of genital organs (D49.59)
neoplasm of unspecified behavior of vermilion border of lip (D49.Ø)

D49.3 **Neoplasm of unspecified behavior of breast**
Excludes1 neoplasm of unspecified behavior of skin of breast (D49.2)

D49.4 **Neoplasm of unspecified behavior of bladder**

● D49.5 **Neoplasm of unspecified behavior of other genitourinary organs**

● D49.51 **Neoplasm of unspecified behavior of kidney**

D49.511 **Neoplasm of unspecified behavior of right kidney**
Coding Clinic: 2Ø16, Q4, P9

D49.512 **Neoplasm of unspecified behavior of left kidney**
Coding Clinic: 2Ø16, Q4, P9

D49.519 **Neoplasm of unspecified behavior of unspecified kidney**
Coding Clinic: 2Ø16, Q4, P9

D49.59 **Neoplasm of unspecified behavior of other genitourinary organ**
Coding Clinic: 2Ø16, Q4, P9

D49.6 **Neoplasm of unspecified behavior of brain**
Excludes1 neoplasm of unspecified behavior of cerebral meninges (D49.7)
neoplasm of unspecified behavior of cranial nerves (D49.7)

D49.7 **Neoplasm of unspecified behavior of endocrine glands and other parts of nervous system**
Excludes1 neoplasm of unspecified behavior of peripheral, sympathetic, and parasympathetic nerves and ganglia (D49.2)

● D49.8 **Neoplasm of unspecified behavior of other specified sites**
Excludes1 neoplasm of unspecified behavior of eyelid (skin) (D49.2)
neoplasm of unspecified behavior of eyelid cartilage (D49.2)
neoplasm of unspecified behavior of great vessels (D49.2)
neoplasm of unspecified behavior of optic nerve (D49.7)

D49.81 **Neoplasm of unspecified behavior of retina and choroid**
Dark area on retina
Retinal freckle

D49.89 **Neoplasm of unspecified behavior of other specified sites**

D49.9 **Neoplasm of unspecified behavior of unspecified site**

CHAPTER 2 (CØØ-D49)

OGCR Chapter-Specific Coding Guidelines

3. Chapter 3: Disease of the blood and blood-forming organs and certain disorders involving the immune mechanism (D50-D89)
Reserved for future guideline expansion

CHAPTER 3

DISEASES OF THE BLOOD AND BLOOD-FORMING ORGANS AND CERTAIN DISORDERS INVOLVING THE IMMUNE MECHANISM (D50-D89)

Excludes2 autoimmune disease (systemic) NOS (M35.9)
certain conditions originating in the perinatal period (P00-P96)
complications of pregnancy, childbirth and the puerperium (O00-O9A)
congenital malformations, deformations and chromosomal abnormalities (Q00-Q99)
endocrine, nutritional and metabolic diseases (E00-E88)
human immunodeficiency virus [HIV] disease (B20)
injury, poisoning and certain other consequences of external causes (S00-T88)
neoplasms (C00-D49)
symptoms, signs and abnormal clinical and laboratory findings, not elsewhere classified (R00-R94)

This chapter contains the following blocks:

D50-D53	Nutritional anemias
D55-D59	Hemolytic anemias
D60-D64	Aplastic and other anemias and other bone marrow failure syndromes
D65-D69	Coagulation defects, purpura and other hemorrhagic conditions
D70-D77	Other disorders of blood and blood-forming organs
D78	Intraoperative and postprocedural complications of the spleen
D80-D89	Certain disorders involving the immune mechanism

NUTRITIONAL ANEMIAS (D50-D53)

● **D50 Iron deficiency anemia**
A disease characterized by a decrease in the number of red cells (hemoglobin) in the blood.
Includes asiderotic anemia
hypochromic anemia

D50.0 Iron deficiency anemia secondary to blood loss (chronic)
Posthemorrhagic anemia (chronic)
Excludes1 acute posthemorrhagic anemia (D62)
congenital anemia from fetal blood loss (P61.3)
Coding Clinic: 2019, Q3, P17

D50.1 Sideropenic dysphagia
Weblike growth of membranes in throat that makes swallowing difficult
Kelly-Paterson syndrome
Plummer-Vinson syndrome

D50.8 Other iron deficiency anemias
Iron deficiency anemia due to inadequate dietary iron intake

D50.9 Iron deficiency anemia, unspecified

● **D51 Vitamin B12 deficiency anemia**
Excludes1 vitamin B12 deficiency (E53.8)

D51.0 Vitamin B12 deficiency anemia due to intrinsic factor deficiency
Addison anemia
Biermer anemia
Pernicious (congenital) anemia
Congenital intrinsic factor deficiency

D51.1 Vitamin B12 deficiency anemia due to selective vitamin B12 malabsorption with proteinuria
Imerslund (Gräsbeck) syndrome
Megaloblastic hereditary anemia

D51.2 Transcobalamin II deficiency

D51.3 Other dietary vitamin B12 deficiency anemia
Vegan anemia

D51.8 Other vitamin B12 deficiency anemias

D51.9 Vitamin B12 deficiency anemia, unspecified

● **D52 Folate deficiency anemia**
Excludes1 folate deficiency without anemia (E53.8)

D52.0 Dietary folate deficiency anemia
Nutritional megaloblastic anemia

D52.1 Drug-induced folate deficiency anemia
Use additional code for adverse effect, if applicable, to identify drug (T36-T50 with fifth or sixth character 5)

D52.8 Other folate deficiency anemias

D52.9 Folate deficiency anemia, unspecified
Folic acid deficiency anemia NOS

● **D53 Other nutritional anemias**
Includes megaloblastic anemia unresponsive to vitamin B12 or folate therapy

D53.0 Protein deficiency anemia
Amino-acid deficiency anemia
Orotaciduric anemia
Excludes1 Lesch-Nyhan syndrome (E79.1)

D53.1 Other megaloblastic anemias, not elsewhere classified
Megaloblastic anemia NOS
Excludes1 Di Guglielmo's disease (C94.0)

D53.2 Scorbutic anemia
Anemia resulting from deficiency of ascorbic acid (vitamin C)
Excludes1 scurvy (E54)

D53.8 Other specified nutritional anemias
Anemia associated with deficiency of copper
Anemia associated with deficiency of molybdenum
Anemia associated with deficiency of zinc
Excludes1 nutritional deficiencies without anemia, such as:
copper deficiency NOS (E61.0)
molybdenum deficiency NOS (E61.5)
zinc deficiency NOS (E60)

D53.9 Nutritional anemia, unspecified
Simple chronic anemia
Excludes1 anemia NOS (D64.9)
Coding Clinic: 2018, Q4, P88

HEMOLYTIC ANEMIAS (D55-D59)

● **D55 Anemia due to enzyme disorders**
Excludes1 drug-induced enzyme deficiency anemia (D59.2)

D55.0 Anemia due to glucose-6-phosphate dehydrogenase [G6PD] deficiency
Favism
G6PD deficiency anemia
Excludes1 glucose-6-phosphate dehydrogenase (G6PD) deficiency without anemia (D75.A)

D55.1 Anemia due to other disorders of glutathione metabolism
Anemia (due to) enzyme deficiencies, except G6PD, related to the hexose monophosphate [HMP] shunt pathway
Anemia (due to) hemolytic nonspherocytic (hereditary), type I

● **D55.2 Anemia due to disorders of glycolytic enzymes**

D55.21 Anemia due to pyruvate kinase deficiency
PK deficiency anemia
Pyruvate kinase deficiency anemia

D55.29 Anemia due to other disorders of glycolytic enzymes
Hexokinase deficiency anemia
Triose-phosphate isomerase deficiency anemia
Excludes1 disorders of glycolysis not associated with anemia (E74.81-)

D55.3 Anemia due to disorders of nucleotide metabolism

D55.8 Other anemias due to enzyme disorders

D55.9 Anemia due to enzyme disorder, unspecified

● **D56 Thalassemia**
Hereditary disorders characterized by low production of hemoglobin or excessive destruction of red blood cells
Excludes1 sickle-cell thalassemia (D57.4-)

D56.0 Alpha thalassemia
Alpha thalassemia major
Hemoglobin H Constant Spring
Hemoglobin H disease
Hydrops fetalis due to alpha thalassemia
Severe alpha thalassemia
Triple gene defect alpha thalassemia
Use additional code, if applicable, for hydrops fetalis due to alpha thalassemia (P56.99)
Excludes1 alpha thalassemia trait or minor (D56.3)
asymptomatic alpha thalassemia (D56.3)
hydrops fetalis due to isoimmunization (P56.0)
hydrops fetalis not due to immune hemolysis (P83.2)

D56.1 Beta thalassemia
Beta thalassemia major
Cooley's anemia
Homozygous beta thalassemia
Severe beta thalassemia
Thalassemia intermedia
Thalassemia major
Excludes1 beta thalassemia minor (D56.3)
beta thalassemia trait (D56.3)
delta-beta thalassemia (D56.2)
hemoglobin E-beta thalassemia (D56.5)
sickle-cell beta thalassemia (D57.4-)

D56.2 Delta-beta thalassemia
Homozygous delta-beta thalassemia
Excludes1 delta-beta thalassemia minor (D56.3)
delta-beta thalassemia trait (D56.3)

D56.3 Thalassemia minor
Genetic disorders that have in common defective production of hemoglobin
Alpha thalassemia minor
Alpha thalassemia silent carrier
Alpha thalassemia trait
Beta thalassemia minor
Beta thalassemia trait
Delta-beta thalassemia minor
Delta-beta thalassemia trait
Thalassemia trait NOS
Excludes1 alpha thalassemia (D56.0)
beta thalassemia (D56.1)
delta-beta thalassemia (D56.2)
hemoglobin E-beta thalassemia (D56.5)
sickle-cell trait (D57.3)

D56.4 Hereditary persistence of fetal hemoglobin [HPFH]
Persistent production of hemoglobin

D56.5 Hemoglobin E-beta thalassemia
Excludes1 beta thalassemia (D56.1)
beta thalassemia minor (D56.3)
beta thalassemia trait (D56.3)
delta-beta thalassemia (D56.2)
delta-beta thalassemia trait (D56.3)
hemoglobin E disease (D58.2)
other hemoglobinopathies (D58.2)
sickle-cell beta thalassemia (D57.4-)

D56.8 Other thalassemias
Dominant thalassemia
Hemoglobin C thalassemia
Mixed thalassemia
Thalassemia with other hemoglobinopathy
Excludes1 hemoglobin C disease (D58.2)
hemoglobin E disease (D58.2)
other hemoglobinopathies (D58.2)
sickle cell anemia (D57.-)
sickle-cell thalassemia (D57.4-)

D56.9 Thalassemia, unspecified
Mediterranean anemia (with other hemoglobinopathy)

● **D57 Sickle-cell disorders**
Inherited disease in which red blood cells, normally disc-shaped, become crescent shaped
Use additional code for any associated fever (R50.81)
Excludes1 other hemoglobinopathies (D58.-)
Coding Clinic: 2022, Q2, P29

● **D57.0 Hb-SS disease with crisis**
Sickle-cell disease with crisis
Hb-SS disease with (vaso-occlusive) pain

D57.00 Hb-SS disease with crisis, unspecified (Ex) PDX 544
Hb-SS disease with (painful) crisis NOS
Hb-SS disease with (vaso-occlusive) pain NOS

D57.01 Hb-SS disease with acute chest syndrome (Ex) PDX 544

D57.02 Hb-SS disease with splenic sequestration (Ex) PDX 544

D57.03 Hb-SS disease with cerebral vascular involvement (Ex) PDX 545
Code also, if applicable, cerebral infarction (I63.-)

D57.04 Hb-SS disease with dactylitis (Ex) PDX 545
Coding Clinic: 2023, Q4, P7

D57.09 Hb-SS disease with crisis with other specified complication (Ex) PDX 545
Use additional code to identify complications, such as:
cholelithiasis (K80.-)
priapism (N48.32)

D57.1 Sickle-cell disease without crisis Hb-SS disease without crisis
Sickle-cell anemia NOS
Sickle-cell disease NOS
Sickle-cell disorder NOS

● **D57.2 Sickle-cell/Hb-C disease**
Hb-SC disease
Hb-S/Hb-C disease

D57.20 Sickle-cell/Hb-C disease without crisis

● **D57.21 Sickle-cell/Hb-C disease with crisis**

D57.211 Sickle-cell/Hb-C disease with acute chest syndrome (Ex) PDX 544
CC when PDX is its own CC

D57.212 Sickle-cell/Hb-C disease with splenic sequestration (Ex) PDX 544

D57.213 Sickle-cell/Hb-C disease with cerebral vascular involvement (Ex) PDX 545
Code also, if applicable, cerebral infarction (I63.-)

D57.214 Sickle-cell/Hb-C disease with dactylitis (Ex) PDX 545

D57.218 Sickle-cell/Hb-C disease with crisis with other specified complication (Ex) PDX 545
Use additional code to identify complications, such as:
cholelithiasis (K80.-)
priapism (N48.32)

CHAPTER 3 (D50-D89)

D57.219 Sickle-cell/Hb-C disease with crisis, unspecified Ex: PDX 544
Sickle-cell/Hb-C disease with crisis NOS
Sickle-cell/Hb-C disease with (vaso-occlusive) pain NOS

D57.3 Sickle-cell trait
Hb-S trait
Heterozygous hemoglobin S

● **D57.4 Sickle-cell thalassemia**
Sickle-cell beta thalassemia
Thalassemia Hb-S disease

D57.40 Sickle-cell thalassemia without crisis
Microdrepanocytosis
Sickle-cell thalassemia NOS

● **D57.41 Sickle-cell thalassemia, unspecified, with crisis**
Sickle-cell "crisis" is precipitated when abnormally crescent-shaped red blood cells form clots and interrupt blood flow to major organs, causing severe pain and organ damage.
Sickle-cell thalassemia with (painful) crisis NOS
Sickle-cell thalassemia with (vaso-occlusive) pain NOS

D57.411 Sickle-cell thalassemia, unspecified, with acute chest syndrome Ex: PDX 544
CC when PDX is its own CC

D57.412 Sickle-cell thalassemia with, unspecified, splenic sequestration Ex: PDX 544

D57.413 Sickle-cell thalassemia, unspecified, with cerebral vascular involvement Ex: PDX 546
Code also, if applicable cerebral infarction (I63.-)

D57.414 Sickle-cell thalassemia, unspecified, with dactylitis Ex: PDX 546

D57.418 Sickle-cell thalassemia, unspecified, with crisis with other specified complication Ex: PDX 546
Use additional code to identify complications, such as:
cholelithiasis (K80.-)
priapism (N48.32)

D57.419 Sickle-cell thalassemia with, unspecified, crisis Ex: PDX 544
Sickle-cell thalassemia with (painful) crisis NOS
Sickle-cell thalassemia with (vaso-occlusive) pain NOS

D57.42 Sickle-cell thalassemia beta zero without crisis
HbS-beta zero without crisis
Sickle-cell beta zero without crisis

● **D57.43 Sickle-cell thalassemia beta zero with crisis** Ex: PDX 547
HbS-beta zero with crisis
Sickle-cell beta zero with crisis

D57.431 Sickle-cell thalassemia beta zero with acute chest syndrome
HbS-beta zero with acute chest syndrome
Sickle-cell beta zero with acute chest syndrome

D57.432 Sickle-cell thalassemia beta zero with splenic sequestration
HbS-beta zero with splenic sequestration
Sickle-cell beta zero with splenic sequestration

D57.433 Sickle-cell thalassemia beta zero with cerebral vascular involvement
HbS-beta zero with cerebral vascular involvement
Sickle-cell beta zero with cerebral vascular involvement
Code also, if applicable cerebral infarction (I63.-)

D57.434 Sickle-cell thalassemia beta zero with dactylitis

D57.438 Sickle-cell thalassemia beta zero with crisis with other specified complication
HbS-beta zero with other specified complication
Sickle-cell beta zero with other specified complication
Use additional code to identify complications, such as:
cholelithiasis (K80.-)
priapism (N48.32)

D57.439 Sickle-cell thalassemia beta zero with crisis, unspecified
HbS-beta zero with other specified complication
Sickle-cell beta zero with crisis unspecified
Sickle-cell thalassemia beta zero with (painful) crisis NOS
Sickle-cell thalassemia beta zero with (vaso-occlusive) pain NOS

D57.44 Sickle-cell thalassemia beta plus without crisis
HbS-beta plus without crisis
Sickle-cell beta plus without crisis

● **D57.45 Sickle-cell thalassemia beta plus with crisis** Ex: PDX 547
HbS-beta plus with crisis
Sickle-cell beta plus with crisis

D57.451 Sickle-cell thalassemia beta plus with acute chest syndrome
HbS-beta plus with acute chest syndrome
Sickle-cell beta plus with acute chest syndrome

D57.452 Sickle-cell thalassemia beta plus with splenic sequestration
HbS-beta plus with splenic sequestration
Sickle-cell beta plus with splenic sequestration

D57.453 Sickle-cell thalassemia beta plus with cerebral vascular involvement
HbS-beta plus with cerebral vascular involvement
Sickle-cell beta plus with cerebral vascular involvement
Code also, if applicable cerebral infarction (I63.-)

D57.454 Sickle-cell thalassemia beta plus with dactylitis

D57.458 Sickle-cell thalassemia beta plus with crisis with other specified complication
HbS-beta plus with crisis with other specified complication
Sickle-cell beta plus with crisis with other specified complication
Use additional code to identify complications, such as:
cholelithiasis (K80.-)
priapism (N48.32)

D57.459 **Sickle-cell thalassemia beta plus with crisis, unspecified** PDX 547
HbS-beta plus with crisis with unspecified complication
Sickle-cell beta plus with crisis with unspecified complication
Sickle-cell thalassemia beta plus with (painful) crisis NOS
Sickle-cell thalassemia beta plus with (vaso-occlusive) pain NOS

● **D57.8 Other sickle-cell disorders**
Hb-SD disease
Hb-SE disease

D57.80 Other sickle-cell disorders without crisis

● **D57.81 Other sickle-cell disorders with crisis**

D57.811 Other sickle-cell disorders with acute chest syndrome PDX 544

D57.812 Other sickle-cell disorders with splenic sequestration PDX 544

D57.813 Other sickle-cell disorders with cerebral vascular involvement PDX 548
Code also, if applicable: cerebral infarction (I63.-)

D57.814 Other sickle-cell disorders with dactylitis PDX 548

D57.818 Other sickle-cell disorders with crisis with other specified complication PDX 548
Use additional code to identify complications, such as:
cholelithiasis (K80.-)
priapism (N48.32)

D57.819 Other sickle-cell disorders with crisis, unspecified PDX 544
Other sickle-cell disorders with crisis NOS
Other sickle-cell disorders with (vaso-occlusive) pain NOS

● **D58 Other hereditary hemolytic anemias**
Genetic condition in which bone marrow is unable to compensate for premature destruction of red blood cells
Excludes1 hemolytic anemia of the newborn (P55.-)

D58.0 Hereditary spherocytosis
Presence of spherocytes (spherically shaped red blood cells)
Acholuric (familial) jaundice
Congenital (spherocytic) hemolytic icterus
Minkowski-Chauffard syndrome

D58.1 Hereditary elliptocytosis
Presence of large numbers of elliptocytes in blood
Elliptocytosis (congenital)
Ovalocytosis (congenital) (hereditary)

D58.2 Other hemoglobinopathies
Abnormal hemoglobin NOS
Congenital Heinz body anemia
Hb-C disease
Hb-D disease
Hb-E disease
Hemoglobinopathy NOS
Unstable hemoglobin hemolytic disease
Excludes1 familial polycythemia (D75.0)
Hb-M disease (D74.0)
hemoglobin E-beta thalassemia (D56.5)
hereditary persistence of fetal hemoglobin [HPFH] (D56.4)
high-altitude polycythemia (D75.1)
methemoglobinemia (D74.-)
other hemoglobinopathies with thalassemia (D56.8)

D58.8 Other specified hereditary hemolytic anemias PDX 549
Stomatocytosis

D58.9 Hereditary hemolytic anemia, unspecified PDX 549

● **D59 Acquired hemolytic anemia**

D59.0 Drug-induced autoimmune hemolytic anemia PDX 550
Use additional code for adverse effect, if applicable, to identify drug (T36-T50 with fifth or sixth character 5)

D59.1 Other autoimmune hemolytic anemias PDX 551
Excludes2 Evans syndrome (D69.41)
hemolytic disease of newborn (P55.-)
paroxysmal cold hemoglobinuria (D59.6)

D59.10 Autoimmune hemolytic anemia, unspecified

D59.11 Warm autoimmune hemolytic anemia
Warm type (primary) (secondary) (symptomatic) autoimmune hemolytic anemia
Warm type autoimmune hemolytic disease

D59.12 Cold autoimmune hemolytic anemia
Chronic cold hemagglutinin disease
Cold agglutinin disease
Cold agglutinin hemoglobinuria
Cold type (primary) (secondary) (symptomatic) autoimmune hemolytic anemia
Cold type autoimmune hemolytic disease

D59.13 Mixed type autoimmune hemolytic anemia
Mixed type autoimmune hemolytic disease
Mixed type, cold and warm, (primary) (secondary) (symptomatic) autoimmune hemolyticanemia

D59.19 Other autoimmune hemolytic anemia

D59.2 Drug-induced nonautoimmune hemolytic anemia PDX 550
Drug-induced enzyme deficiency anemia
Use additional code for adverse effect, if applicable, to identify drug (T36-T50 with fifth or sixth character 5)

D59.3 Hemolytic-uremic syndrome PDX 552
Code also, if applicable, any associated:
acute kidney failure (N17.-)
chronic kidney disease (N18.-)

D59.30 Hemolytic-uremic syndrome, unspecified
Hemolytic-uremic syndrome NOS

D59.31 Infection-associated hemolytic-uremic syndrome
Shiga toxin-producing E. coli [STEC] related hemolytic uremic syndrome
Typical hemolytic uremic syndrome
Use Additional code to identify associated infection, such as:
E. coli infection (B96.2-)
Human immunodeficiency virus [HIV] disease (B20)
Pneumococcal meningitis (G00.1)
Pneumococcal pneumonia (J13)
Sepsis due to Streptococcus pneumoniae (A40.3)
Shigella dysenteriae (A03.9)
Streptococcus pneumoniae as the cause of diseases classified elsewhere (B95.3)

D59.32 Hereditary hemolytic-uremic syndrome
Atypical hemolytic uremic syndrome with an identified genetic cause
Code also, if applicable:
defects in the complement system (D84.1)
methylmalonic acidemia (E71.120)

D59.39 Other hemolytic-uremic syndrome (Ex) PDX 552
Atypical (nongenetic) hemolytic uremic syndrome
Secondary hemolytic-uremic syndrome
Code first, if applicable, any associated:
COVID-19 (U07.1)
complications of kidney transplant (T86.1-)
complications of heart transplant (T86.2-)
complications of liver transplant (T86.4-)
Code also, if applicable, any associated condition, such as:
hypertensive emergency (I16.1)
malignant neoplasm (C00-C96)
systemic lupus erythematosus (M32.-)
Use Additional code, if applicable, for adverse effect to identify drug (T36-T50 with fifth or sixth character 5)
Coding Clinic: 2022, Q4, P6

D59.4 Other nonautoimmune hemolytic anemias (Ex) PDX 552
Mechanical hemolytic anemia
Microangiopathic hemolytic anemia
Toxic hemolytic anemia

D59.5 Paroxysmal nocturnal hemoglobinuria [Marchiafava-Micheli]
Excludes1 hemoglobinuria NOS (R82.3)

D59.6 Hemoglobinuria due to hemolysis from other external causes
Hemoglobinuria from exertion
March hemoglobinuria
Paroxysmal cold hemoglobinuria
Use additional code (Chapter 20) to identify external cause
Excludes1 hemoglobinuria NOS (R82.3)

D59.8 Other acquired hemolytic anemias

D59.9 Acquired hemolytic anemia, unspecified (Ex) PDX 552
Idiopathic hemolytic anemia, chronic

APLASTIC AND OTHER ANEMIAS AND OTHER BONE MARROW FAILURE SYNDROMES (D60-D64)

● **D60 Acquired pure red cell aplasia [erythroblastopenia]** (Ex) PDX 552
Deficiency of erythroblasts
Includes red cell aplasia (acquired) (adult) (with thymoma)
Excludes1 congenital red cell aplasia (D61.01)

D60.0 Chronic acquired pure red cell aplasia
Lack of development of blood cell

D60.1 Transient acquired pure red cell aplasia

D60.8 Other acquired pure red cell aplasias

D60.9 Acquired pure red cell aplasia, unspecified

● **D61 Other aplastic anemias and other bone marrow failure syndromes**
Excludes2 neutropenia (D70.-)

● **D61.0 Constitutional aplastic anemia**
Condition where bone marrow is unable to produce blood cells

D61.01 Constitutional (pure) red blood cell aplasia (Ex) PDX 553
Blackfan-Diamond syndrome
Congenital (pure) red cell aplasia
Familial hypoplastic anemia
Primary (pure) red cell aplasia
Red cell (pure) aplasia of infants
Excludes1 acquired red cell aplasia (D60.9)

D61.02 Shwachman-Diamond syndrome (Ex) PDX 554
Code also, if applicable, associated conditions such as:
acute myeloblastic leukemia (C92.0-)
exocrine pancreatic insufficiency (K86.81)
myelodysplastic syndrome (D46.-)
Use additional code, if applicable, for genetic susceptibility to other malignant neoplasm(Z15.09)

▶ **D61.03 Fanconi anemia** (Ex) PDX 555
▶ Fanconi pancytopenia
▶ Fanconi's anemia
▶ **Excludes1** Fanconi syndrome (E72.0-)

D61.09 Other constitutional aplastic anemia (Ex) PDX 555
~~Fanconi's anemia~~
Pancytopenia with malformations

D61.1 Drug-induced aplastic anemia (Ex) PDX 552
Use additional code for adverse effect, if applicable, to identify drug (T36-T50 with fifth or sixth character 5)

D61.2 Aplastic anemia due to other external agents (Ex) PDX 552
Code first, if applicable, toxic effects of substances chiefly nonmedicinal as to source (T51-T65)

D61.3 Idiopathic aplastic anemia (Ex) PDX 552

● **D61.8 Other specified aplastic anemias and other bone marrow failure syndromes**

● **D61.81 Pancytopenia** (Ex) PDX 556
Marked deficiency of all the blood elements: Red blood cells (erythrocytes), white blood cells (leukocytes), and platelets (thrombocytes). Check laboratory results.
Excludes1 pancytopenia (due to) (with) aplastic anemia (D61.9)
pancytopenia (due to) (with) bone marrow infiltration (D61.82)
pancytopenia (due to) (with) congenital (pure) red cell aplasia (D61.01)
pancytopenia (due to) (with) hairy cell leukemia (C91.4-)
pancytopenia (due to) (with) human immunodeficiency virus disease (B20.-)
pancytopenia (due to) (with) leukoerythroblastic anemia (D61.82)
pancytopenia (due to) (with) myeloproliferative disease (D47.1)
Excludes2 pancytopenia (due to) (with) myelodysplastic syndromes (D46.-)

D61.810 Antineoplastic chemotherapy induced pancytopenia
Excludes2 aplastic anemia due to antineoplastic chemotherapy (D61.1)

D61.811 Other drug-induced pancytopenia
Excludes2 aplastic anemia due to drugs (D61.1)

D61.818 Other pancytopenia
Coding Clinic: 2023, Q1, P23; 2019, Q1, P16

D61.82 Myelophthisis (Ex:) PDX 556
Leukoerythroblastic anemia
Myelophthisic anemia
Panmyelophthisis
Code also the underlying disorder, such as:
malignant neoplasm of breast (C50.-)
tuberculosis (A15.-)
Excludes1 idiopathic myelofibrosis (D47.1)
myelofibrosis NOS (D75.81)
myelofibrosis with myeloid metaplasia (D47.4)
primary myelofibrosis (D47.1)
secondary myelofibrosis (D75.81)

D61.89 Other specified aplastic anemias and other bone marrow failure syndromes (Ex:) PDX 552

D61.9 Aplastic anemia, unspecified (Ex:) PDX 552
Hypoplastic anemia NOS
Medullary hypoplasia

D62 Acute posthemorrhagic anemia (Ex:) PDX 557
Excludes1 anemia due to chronic blood loss (D50.0)
blood loss anemia NOS (D50.0)
congenital anemia from fetal blood loss (P61.3)
Coding Clinic: 2019, Q3, P13,17

D63 Anemia in chronic diseases classified elsewhere

D63.0 Anemia in neoplastic disease
Code first neoplasm (C00-D49)
Excludes1 aplastic anemia due to antineoplastic chemotherapy (D61.1)
Excludes2 anemia due to antineoplastic chemotherapy (D64.81)
OGCR Section I.C.2.e.2.
2) Anemia associated with chemotherapy, immunotherapy and radiation therapy
When the admission/encounter is for management of an anemia associated with an adverse effect of the administration of chemotherapy or immunotherapy and the only treatment is for the anemia, the anemia code is sequenced first followed by the appropriate codes for the neoplasm and the adverse effect (T45.1X5, Adverse effect of antineoplastic and immunosuppressive drugs).

D63.1 Anemia in chronic kidney disease
Erythropoietin resistant anemia (EPO resistant anemia)
Code first underlying chronic kidney disease (CKD) (N18.-)

D63.8 Anemia in other chronic diseases classified elsewhere
Code first underlying disease, such as:
diphyllobothriasis (B70.0)
hookworm disease (B76.0-B76.9)
hypothyroidism (E00.0-E03.9)
malaria (B50.0-B54)
symptomatic late syphilis (A52.79)
tuberculosis (A18.89)

D64 Other anemias
Excludes1 refractory anemia (D46.-)
refractory anemia with excess blasts in transformation [RAEB T] (C92.0-)

D64.0 Hereditary sideroblastic anemia
Abnormal production RBCs (erythrocytes)
Sex-linked hypochromic sideroblastic anemia

D64.1 Secondary sideroblastic anemia due to disease
Code first underlying disease

D64.2 Secondary sideroblastic anemia due to drugs and toxins
Code first poisoning due to drug or toxin, if applicable (T36-T65 with fifth or sixth character 1-4)
Use additional code for adverse effect, if applicable, to identify drug (T36-T50 with fifth or sixth character 5)

D64.3 Other sideroblastic anemias
Sideroblastic anemia NOS
Pyridoxine-responsive sideroblastic anemia NEC

D64.4 Congenital dyserythropoietic anemia
Any of several rare hereditary anemias, mostly types of macrocytic anemia
Dyshematopoietic anemia (congenital)
Excludes1 Blackfan-Diamond syndrome (D61.01)
Di Guglielmo's disease (C94.0)

D64.8 Other specified anemias

D64.81 Anemia due to antineoplastic chemotherapy
Antineoplastic chemotherapy induced anemia
aplastic anemia due to antineoplastic chemotherapy (D61.1)
Excludes2 anemia in neoplastic disease (D63.0)
Coding Clinic: 2023, Q3, P4; 2023, Q2, P18; 2021, Q3, P4

D64.89 Other specified anemias
Infantile pseudoleukemia

D64.9 Anemia, unspecified
Coding Clinic: 2018, Q4, P88; 2017, Q1, P7

COAGULATION DEFECTS, PURPURA AND OTHER HEMORRHAGIC CONDITIONS (D65-D69)

D65 Disseminated intravascular coagulation [defibrination syndrome] (Ex:) PDX 558
Blood clots form and consume all coagulation proteins and platelets and disrupt normal coagulation, resulting in abnormal bleeding
Afibrinogenemia, acquired
Consumption coagulopathy
COVID-19 associated diffuse or disseminated intravascular coagulopathy
Diffuse or disseminated intravascular coagulation [DIC]
Fibrinolytic hemorrhage, acquired
Fibrinolytic purpura
Purpura fulminans
Code also, if applicable, associated condition
Excludes1 disseminated intravascular coagulation (complicating):
abortion or ectopic or molar pregnancy (O00-O07, O08.1)
in newborn (P60)
pregnancy, childbirth and the puerperium (O45.0, O46.0, O67.0, O72.3)
Coding Clinic: 2022, Q4, P9; 2021, Q1, P39; 2019, Q2, P25

D66 Hereditary factor VIII deficiency (Ex:) PDX 558
Inherited coagulation disorder carried by females but most often affecting males
Classical hemophilia
Deficiency factor VIII (with functional defect)
Hemophilia NOS
Hemophilia A
Excludes1 factor VIII deficiency with vascular defect (D68.0-)

D67 Hereditary factor IX deficiency (Ex:) PDX 558
Christmas disease
Factor IX deficiency (with functional defect)
Hemophilia B
Plasma thromboplastin component [PTC] deficiency

D68 Other coagulation defects
Excludes1 abnormal coagulation profile NOS (R79.1)
Excludes2 coagulation defects complicating abortion or ectopic or molar pregnancy (O00-O07, O08.1)
coagulation defects complicating pregnancy, childbirth and the puerperium (O45.0, O46.0, O67.0, O72.3)
Coding Clinic: 2016, Q1, P14

D68.0 Von Willebrand disease (Ex:) PDX 559
Congenital bleeding disorder
Excludes1 capillary fragility (hereditary) (D69.8)
factor VIII deficiency NOS (D66)
factor VIII deficiency with functional defect (D66)

D68.00 Von Willebrand disease, unspecified

D68.01 Von Willebrand disease, type 1
Partial quantitative deficiency of von Willebrand factor
Type 1C von Willebrand disease
Coding Clinic: 2022, Q4, P9

D68.02 Von Willebrand disease, type 2 PDX 559
Qualitative defects of von Willebrand factor

D68.020 Von Willebrand disease, type 2A
Qualitative defects of von Willebrand factor with decreased platelet adhesion and selective deficiency of high-molecular-weight multimers

D68.021 Von Willebrand disease, type 2B
Qualitative defects of von Willebrand factor with high-molecular-weight von Willebrand factor loss
Qualitative defects of von Willebrand factor with hyper-adhesive forms
Qualitative defects of von Willebrand factor with increased affinity for platelet glycoprotein lb

D68.022 Von Willebrand disease, type 2M
Qualitative defects of von Willebrand factor with defective platelet adhesion with anormal size distribution of von Willebrand factor multimers

D68.023 Von Willebrand disease, type 2N
Qualitative defects of von Willebrand factor with defective von Willebrand factor to factor VIII binding
Qualitative defects of von Willebrand factor with markedly decreased affinity for factor VIII

D68.029 Von Willebrand disease, type 2, unspecified
Qualitative defect in von Willebrand factor function, with no further subtyping

D68.03 Von Willebrand disease, type 3
(Near) complete absence of von Willebrand factor
Total quantitative deficiency of von Willebrand factor

D68.04 Acquired von Willebrand disease
Acquired von Willebrand syndrome

D68.09 Other von Willebrand disease
Platelet-type von Willebrand disease
Pseudo-von Willebrand disease
Code also, if applicable, qualitative platelet defects (D69.1)

D68.1 Hereditary factor XI deficiency PDX 558
Deficiency of blood coagulation resulting in systemic blood-clotting defect
Hemophilia C
Plasma thromboplastin antecedent [PTA] deficiency
Rosenthal's disease

D68.2 Hereditary deficiency of other clotting factors PDX 558
Blood clotting disorders caused by hereditary deficiencies of one or more clotting factors
AC globulin deficiency
Congenital afibrinogenemia
Deficiency of factor I [fibrinogen]
Deficiency of factor II [prothrombin]
Deficiency of factor V [labile]
Deficiency of factor VII [stable]
Deficiency of factor X [Stuart-Prower]
Deficiency of factor XII [Hageman]
Deficiency of factor XIII [fibrin stabilizing]
Dysfibrinogenemia (congenital)
Hypoproconvertinemia
Owren's disease
Proaccelerin deficiency

D68.3 Hemorrhagic disorder due to circulating anticoagulants
Blood clotting disorders caused by anticoagulants (warfarin and heparin)

D68.31 Hemorrhagic disorder due to intrinsic circulating anticoagulants, antibodies, or inhibitors

D68.311 Acquired hemophilia PDX 558
Autoimmune hemophilia
Autoimmune inhibitors to clotting factors
Secondary hemophilia

D68.312 Antiphospholipid antibody with hemorrhagic disorder PDX 560
Lupus anticoagulant (LAC) with hemorrhagic disorder
Systemic lupus erythematosus [SLE] inhibitor with hemorrhagic disorder

Excludes1 antiphospholipid antibody, finding without diagnosis (R76.0)
antiphospholipid antibody syndrome (D68.61)
antiphospholipid antibody with hypercoagulable state (D68.61)
lupus anticoagulant (LAC) finding without diagnosis (R76.0)
lupus anticoagulant (LAC) with hypercoagulable state (D68.62)
systemic lupus erythematosus [SLE] inhibitor finding without diagnosis (R76.0)
systemic lupus erythematosus [SLE] inhibitor with hypercoagulable state (D68.62)

CHAPTER 3 (D50-D89)

D68.318 Other hemorrhagic disorder due to intrinsic circulating anticoagulants, antibodies, or inhibitors (Ex) PDX 558
Antithromboplastinemia
Antithromboplastinogenemia
Hemorrhagic disorder due to intrinsic increase in antithrombin
Hemorrhagic disorder due to intrinsic increase in anti-VIIIa
Hemorrhagic disorder due to intrinsic increase in anti-IXa
Hemorrhagic disorder due to intrinsic increase in anti-XIa

D68.32 Hemorrhagic disorder due to extrinsic circulating anticoagulants (Ex) PDX 558
Drug-induced hemorrhagic disorder
Hemorrhagic disorder due to increase in anti-IIa
Hemorrhagic disorder due to increase in anti-Xa
Hyperheparinemia
Use additional code for adverse effect, if applicable, to identify drug (T45.515, T45.525)
Coding Clinic: 2021, Q1, P5; 2016, Q1, P14-15

D68.4 Acquired coagulation factor deficiency (Ex) PDX 558
Deficiency of coagulation factor due to liver disease
Deficiency of coagulation factor due to vitamin K deficiency
Excludes1 vitamin K deficiency of newborn (P53)

● **D68.5 Primary thrombophilia**
AKA idiopathic thrombocytopenia, may be acquired or congenital and is a common cause of coagulation disorders.
Primary hypercoagulable states
Excludes1 antiphospholipid syndrome (D68.61)
lupus anticoagulant (D68.62)
secondary activated protein C resistance (D68.69)
secondary antiphospholipid antibody syndrome (D68.69)
secondary lupus anticoagulant with hypercoagulable state (D68.69)
secondary systemic lupus erythematosus [SLE] inhibitor with hypercoagulable state (D68.69)
systemic lupus erythematosus [SLE] inhibitor finding without diagnosis (R76.Ø)
systemic lupus erythematosus [SLE] inhibitor with hemorrhagic disorder (D68.312)
thrombotic thrombocytopenic purpura (M31.19)

D68.51 Activated protein C resistance (Ex) PDX 561
Factor V Leiden mutation

D68.52 Prothrombin gene mutation (Ex) PDX 561

D68.59 Other primary thrombophilia (Ex) PDX 562
Antithrombin III deficiency
Hypercoagulable state NOS
Primary hypercoagulable state NEC
Primary thrombophilia NEC
Protein C deficiency
Protein S deficiency
Thrombophilia NOS
Coding Clinic: 2021, Q2, P8-9

● **D68.6 Other thrombophilia**
Other hypercoagulable states
Excludes1 diffuse or disseminated intravascular coagulation [DIC] (D65)
heparin induced thrombocytopenia (HIT) (D75.82-)
hyperhomocysteinemia (E72.11)

D68.61 Antiphospholipid syndrome (Ex) PDX 561
Anticardiolipin syndrome
Antiphospholipid antibody syndrome
Excludes1 anti-phospholipid antibody, finding without diagnosis (R76.Ø)
anti-phospholipid antibody with hemorrhagic disorder (D68.312)
lupus anticoagulant syndrome (D68.62)

D68.62 Lupus anticoagulant syndrome (Ex) PDX 561
Lupus anticoagulant
Presence of systemic lupus erythematosus [SLE] inhibitor
Excludes1 anticardiolipin syndrome (D68.61)
antiphospholipid syndrome (D68.61)
lupus anticoagulant (LAC) finding without diagnosis (R76.Ø)
lupus anticoagulant (LAC) with hemorrhagic disorder (D68.312)

D68.69 Other thrombophilia (Ex) PDX 562
COVID-19 associated hypercoagulability
Hypercoagulable states NEC
Secondary hypercoagulable state NOS
Code also, if applicable, associated condition
Coding Clinic: 2021, Q2, P8

D68.8 Other specified coagulation defects (Ex) PDX 558
COVID-19 associated coagulopathy
Code also, if applicable, associated condition
Excludes1 hemorrhagic disease of newborn (P53)
Coding Clinic: 2021, Q1, P39-40

D68.9 Coagulation defect, unspecified (Ex) PDX 558

● **D69 Purpura and other hemorrhagic conditions**
Group of conditions characterized by small hemorrhages in skin, mucous membranes, or serosal surfaces
Excludes1 benign hypergammaglobulinemic purpura (D89.Ø)
cryoglobulinemic purpura (D89.1)
essential (hemorrhagic) thrombocythemia (D47.3)
hemorrhagic thrombocythemia (D47.3)
purpura fulminans (D65)
thrombotic thrombocytopenic purpura (M31.19)
Waldenström hypergammaglobulinemic purpura (D89.Ø)

D69.Ø Allergic purpura (Ex) PDX 558
Allergic vasculitis
Nonthrombocytopenic hemorrhagic purpura
Nonthrombocytopenic idiopathic purpura
Purpura anaphylactoid
Purpura Henoch(-Schönlein)
Purpura rheumatica
Vascular purpura
Excludes1 thrombocytopenic hemorrhagic purpura (D69.3)

D69.1 Qualitative platelet defects
Bernard-Soulier [giant platelet] syndrome
Glanzmann's disease
Grey platelet syndrome
Thromboasthenia (hemorrhagic) (hereditary)
Thrombocytopathy
Excludes1 hemolytic-uremic syndrome (D59.3-)
Excludes2 von Willebrand disease (D68.Ø-)

CHAPTER 3 (D5Ø-D89)

D69.2 Other nonthrombocytopenic purpura
Purpura NOS
Purpura simplex
Senile purpura

D69.3 Immune thrombocytopenic purpura PDX 563
Hemorrhagic (thrombocytopenic) purpura
Idiopathic thrombocytopenic purpura
Tidal platelet dysgenesis

D69.4 Other primary thrombocytopenia
Excludes1 transient neonatal thrombocytopenia (P61.0)
Wiskott-Aldrich syndrome (D82.0)

D69.41 Evans syndrome PDX 563
Acquired hemolytic anemia and thrombocytopenia

D69.42 Congenital and hereditary thrombocytopenia purpura PDX 563
Congenital thrombocytopenia
Hereditary thrombocytopenia
Code first congential or hereditary disorder, such as:
thrombocytopenia with absent radius (TAR syndrome) (Q87.2)

D69.49 Other primary thrombocytopenia
Megakaryocytic hypoplasia
Primary thrombocytopenia NOS

D69.5 Secondary thrombocytopenia
Acquired reduction of number of platelets required for blood clotting
Excludes1 heparin induced thrombocytopenia (HIT) (D75.82-)
transient thrombocytopenia of newborn (P61.0)

D69.51 Posttransfusion purpura
Posttransfusion purpura from whole blood (fresh) or blood products PTP

D69.59 Other secondary thrombocytopenia

D69.6 Thrombocytopenia, unspecified

D69.8 Other specified hemorrhagic conditions
Capillary fragility (hereditary)
Vascular pseudohemophilia

D69.9 Hemorrhagic condition, unspecified

OTHER DISORDERS OF BLOOD AND BLOOD-FORMING ORGANS (D70-D77)

D70 Neutropenia
Code also, if applicable, mucositis (J34.81, K12.3-, K92.81, N76.81)
Decrease in number of neutrophils (type of white blood cell)
Includes agranulocytosis
decreased absolute neurophile count (ANC)
Excludes1 neutropenic splenomegaly (D73.81)
transient neonatal neutropenia (P61.5)

D70.0 Congenital agranulocytosis
Reduced numbers of neutrophils (type of white blood cell)
Congenital neutropenia
Infantile genetic agranulocytosis
Kostmann's disease

D70.1 Agranulocytosis secondary to cancer chemotherapy
Decreased numbers of granulocytes (type of white blood cell)
Code also *underlying neoplasm*
Use additional code for adverse effect, if applicable, to identify drug (T45.1X5)

D70.2 Other drug-induced agranulocytosis
Use additional code for adverse effect, if applicable, to identify drug (T36-T50 with fifth or sixth character 5)

D70.3 Neutropenia due to infection

D70.4 Cyclic neutropenia
Chronic neutropenia (low number of type of white blood cell)
Cyclic hematopoiesis
Periodic neutropenia

D70.8 Other neutropenia

D70.9 Neutropenia, unspecified
Coding Clinic: 2019, Q2, P25

D71 Functional disorders of polymorphonuclear neutrophils
Polymorphonuclear: varying shapes of nucleus; AKA PMNs
Cell membrane receptor complex [CR3] defect
Chronic (childhood) granulomatous disease
Congenital dysphagocytosis
Progressive septic granulomatosis

D72 Other disorders of white blood cells
Excludes1 basophilia (D72.824)
immunity disorders (D80-D89)
neutropenia (D70)
preleukemia (syndrome) (D46.9)

D72.0 Genetic anomalies of leukocytes
Alder (granulation) (granulocyte) anomaly
Alder syndrome
Hereditary leukocytic hypersegmentation
Hereditary leukocytic hyposegmentation
Hereditary leukomelanopathy
May-Hegglin (granulation) (granulocyte) anomaly
May-Hegglin syndrome
Pelger-Huët (granulation) (granulocyte) anomaly
Pelger-Huët syndrome
Excludes1 Chédiak (-Steinbrinck)-Higashi syndrome (E70.330)

D72.1 Eosinophilia
Formation and accumulation of high number of white cells in blood/tissue
Excludes2 Löffler's syndrome (J82.89)
pulmonary eosinophilia (J82.-)

D72.10 Eosinophilia, unspecified

D72.11 Hypereosinophilic syndrome [HES]

D72.110 Idiopathic hypereosinophilic syndrome [IHES]

D72.111 Lymphocytic Variant Hypereosinophilic Syndrome [LHES]
Lymphocyte variant hypereosinophilia
Code also, if applicable, any associated lymphocytic neoplastic disorder

D72.118 Other hypereosinophilic syndrome
Episodic angioedema with eosinophilia
Gleich's syndrome

D72.119 Hypereosinophilic syndrome [HES], unspecified

D72.12 Drug rash with eosinophilia and systemic symptoms syndrome
DRESS syndrome
Use additional code for adverse effect, if applicable, to identify drug (T36-T50 with fifth or sixth character 5)

D72.18 Eosinophilia in diseases classified elsewhere
Code first underlying disease, such as:
chronic myelomonocytic leukemia (C93.1-)

D72.19 Other eosinophilia
Familial eosinophilia
Hereditary eosinophilia

D72.8 Other specified disorders of white blood cells
Excludes1 leukemia (C91-C95)

D72.81 Decreased white blood cell count
Excludes1 neutropenia (D70.-)

D72.810 Lymphocytopenia
Decreased lymphocytes
Reduction in number of lympho cytes in blood

D72.818 Other decreased white blood cell count
Basophilic leukopenia
Eosinophilic leukopenia
Monocytopenia
Other decreased leukocytes
Plasmacytopenia

D72.819 Decreased white blood cell count, unspecified
Decreased leukocytes, unspecified
Leukocytopenia, unspecified
Leukopenia
Excludes1 malignant leukopenia (D7Ø.9)

D72.82 Elevated white blood cell count
Excludes1 eosinophilia (D72.1)

D72.82Ø Lymphocytosis (symptomatic)
Elevated lymphocytes
Excess of normal lymphocytes

D72.821 Monocytosis (symptomatic)
Excludes1 infectious mononucleosis (B27.-)

D72.822 Plasmacytosis
Presence of excess plasma cells

D72.823 Leukemoid reaction
Basophilic leukemoid reaction
Leukemoid reaction NOS
Lymphocytic leukemoid reaction
Monocytic leukemoid reaction
Myelocytic leukemoid reaction
Neutrophilic leukemoid reaction

D72.824 Basophilia
Increase of basophils in blood

D72.825 Bandemia
Bandemia without diagnosis of specific infection
Excess number of band cells (immature white blood cells) released by bone marrow
Excludes1 confirmed infection -code to infection
leukemia (C91.-, C92.-, C93.-, C94.-, C95.-)

D72.828 Other elevated white blood cell count

D72.829 Elevated white blood cell count, unspecified
Elevated leukocytes, unspecified
Leukocytosis, unspecified

D72.89 Other specified disorders of white blood cells
Abnormality of white blood cells NEC

D72.9 Disorder of white blood cells, unspecified
Abnormal leukocyte differential NOS

D73 Diseases of spleen

D73.Ø Hyposplenism
Diminished functioning of spleen
Atrophy of spleen
Excludes1 asplenia (congenital) (Q89.Ø1)
postsurgical absence of spleen (Z9Ø.81)

D73.1 Hypersplenism
Accelerated function of spleen
Excludes1 neutropenic splenomegaly (D73.81)
primary splenic neutropenia (D73.81)
splenitis, splenomegaly in late syphilis (A52.79)
splenitis, splenomegaly in tuberculosis (A18.85)
splenomegaly NOS (R16.1)
splenomegaly congenital (Q89.Ø)

D73.2 Chronic congestive splenomegaly
Enlargement of spleen

D73.3 Abscess of spleen

D73.4 Cyst of spleen

D73.5 Infarction of spleen
Splenic rupture, nontraumatic
Torsion of spleen
Excludes1 rupture of spleen due to Plasmodium vivax malaria (B51.Ø)
traumatic rupture of spleen (S36.Ø3-)

D73.8 Other diseases of spleen

D73.81 Neutropenic splenomegaly
Werner-Schultz disease
Enlarged spleen responding to inadequate number of neutrophils

D73.89 Other diseases of spleen
Fibrosis of spleen NOS
Perisplenitis
Splenitis NOS

D73.9 Disease of spleen, unspecified

D74 Methemoglobinemia (Ex) PDX 564
Excessive methemoglobin (form of hemoglobin)

D74.Ø Congenital methemoglobinemia
Congenital NADH-methemoglobin reductase deficiency
Hemoglobin-M [Hb-M] disease
Methemoglobinemia, hereditary

D74.8 Other methemoglobinemias
Acquired methemoglobinemia (with sulfhemoglobinemia)
Toxic methemoglobinemia

D74.9 Methemoglobinemia, unspecified

D75 Other and unspecified diseases of blood and blood-forming organs
Excludes2 acute lymphadenitis (LØ4.-)
chronic lymphadenitis (I88.1)
enlarged lymph nodes (R59.-)
hypergammaglobulinemia NOS (D89.2)
lymphadenitis NOS (I88.9)
mesenteric lymphadenitis (acute) (chronic) (I88.Ø)

D75.Ø Familial erythrocytosis
Genetic mutation of gene that results in increased circulating RBCs
Benign polycythemia
Familial polycythemia
Excludes1 hereditary ovalocytosis (D58.1)

D75.1 Secondary polycythemia
Increase in total red cell mass
Acquired polycythemia
Emotional polycythemia
Erythrocytosis NOS
Hypoxemic polycythemia
Nephrogenous polycythemia
Polycythemia due to erythropoietin
Polycythemia due to fall in plasma volume
Polycythemia due to high altitude
Polycythemia due to stress
Polycythemia NOS
Relative polycythemia
Excludes1 polycythemia neonatorum (P61.1)
polycythemia vera (D45)

CHAPTER 3 (D5Ø-D89)

D75.8 Other specified diseases of blood and blood-forming organs

D75.81 Myelofibrosis PDX 535
Replacing bone marrow by fibrous tissue
Myelofibrosis NOS
Secondary myelofibrosis NOS
Code first the underlying disorder, such as:
malignant neoplasm of breast (C5Ø.-)
Use additional code, if applicable, for associated therapy-related myelodysplastic syndrome (D46.-)
Use additional code for adverse effect, if applicable, to identify drug (T45.1X5)
Excludes1 acute myelofibrosis (C94.4-)
idiopathic myelofibrosis (D47.1)
leukoerythroblastic anemia (D61.82)
myelofibrosis with myeloid metaplasia (D47.4)
myelophthisic anemia (D61.82)
myelophthisis (D61.82)
primary myelofibrosis (D47.1)

D75.82 Heparin induced thrombocytopenia (HIT)
Use Additional code, if applicable, for adverse effect of heparin (T45.515-)

D75.821 Non-immune heparin-induced thrombocytopenia
Non-immune HIT
Type 1 heparin-induced thrombocytopenia

D75.822 Immune-mediated heparin-induced thrombocytopenia
Immune-mediated HIT
Type 2 heparin-induced thrombocytopenia

D75.828 Other heparin-induced thrombocytopenia syndrome
Autoimmune heparin-induced thrombocytopenia syndrome
Delayed-onset heparin-induced thrombocytopenia
Persisting heparin-induced thrombocytopenia

D75.829 Heparin-induced thrombocytopenia, unspecified

D75.83 Thrombocytosis
Excludes2 essential thrombocythemia (D47.3)

D75.838 Other thrombocytosis
Reactive thrombocytosis
Secondary thrombocytosis
Code also, underlying condition, if known and applicable

D75.839 Thrombocytosis, unspecified
Thrombocythemia NOS
Thrombocytosis NOS

D75.84 Other platelet-activating anti-PF4 disorders
Spontaneous heparin-induced thrombocytopenia syndrome (without heparin exposure)
Thrombosis with thrombocytopenia syndrome
Vaccine-induced thrombotic thrombocytopenia
Use Additional code, if applicable, for adverse effect of other viral vaccine (T50.B95-)

D75.89 Other specified diseases of blood and blood-forming organs

D75.9 Disease of blood and blood-forming organs, unspecified

D75.A Glucose-6-phosphate dehydrogenase (G6PD) deficiency without anemia
Excludes1 glucose-6-phosphate dehydrogenase (G6PD) deficiency with anemia (D55.Ø)

D76 Other specified diseases with participation of lymphoreticular and reticulohistiocytic tissue
Excludes1 (Abt-) Letterer-Siwe disease (C96.Ø)
eosinophilic granuloma (C96.6)
Hand-Schüller-Christian disease (C96.5)
histiocytic medullary reticulosis (C96.9)
histiocytic sarcoma (C96.A)
histiocytosis X, multifocal (C96.5)
histiocytosis X, unifocal (C96.6)
Langerhans-cell histiocytosis, multifocal (C96.5)
Langerhans-cell histiocytosis NOS (C96.6)
Langerhans-cell histiocytosis, unifocal (C96.6)
leukemic reticuloendotheliosis (C91.4-)
lipomelanotic reticulosis (I89.8)
malignant histiocytosis (C96.A)
malignant reticulosis (C86.Ø)
nonlipid reticuloendotheliosis (C96.Ø)

D76.1 Hemophagocytic lymphohistiocytosis PDX 565
Familial hemophagocytic reticulosis
Histiocytoses of mononuclear phagocytes

D76.2 Hemophagocytic syndrome, infection-associated PDX 566
Use additional code to identify infectious agent or disease.

D76.3 Other histiocytosis syndromes PDX 567
Reticulohistiocytoma (giant-cell)
Sinus histiocytosis with massive lymphadenopathy
Xanthogranuloma

D77 Other disorders of blood and blood-forming organs in diseases classified elsewhere
Code first underlying disease, such as:
amyloidosis (E85.-)
congenital early syphilis (A5Ø.Ø-)
echinococcosis (B67.Ø-B67.9)
malaria (B5Ø.Ø-B54)
schistosomiasis [bilharziasis] (B65.Ø-B65.9)
vitamin C deficiency (E54)
Excludes1 rupture of spleen due to Plasmodium vivax malaria (B51.Ø)
splenitis, splenomegaly in late syphilis (A52.79)
splenitis, splenomegaly in tuberculosis (A18.85)

INTRAOPERATIVE AND POSTPROCEDURAL COMPLICATIONS OF THE SPLEEN (D78)

D78 Intraoperative and postprocedural complications of the spleen
Coding Clinic: 2016, Q4, P9

D78.Ø Intraoperative hemorrhage and hematoma of the spleen complicating a procedure PDX 568
Excludes1 intraoperative hemorrhage and hematoma of the spleen due to accidental puncture or laceration during a procedure (D78.1-)

D78.Ø1 Intraoperative hemorrhage and hematoma of the spleen complicating a procedure on the spleen

D78.Ø2 Intraoperative hemorrhage and hematoma of the spleen complicating other procedure

D78.1 Accidental puncture and laceration of the spleen during a procedure PDX 569

D78.11 Accidental puncture and laceration of the spleen during a procedure on the spleen

D78.12 Accidental puncture and laceration of the spleen during other procedure
Coding Clinic: 2022, Q1, P22-23

D78.2 Postprocedural hemorrhage of the spleen following a procedure PDX 568

D78.21 Postprocedural hemorrhage of the spleen following a procedure on the spleen

D78.22 Postprocedural hemorrhage of the spleen following other procedure

● **D78.3 Postprocedural hematoma and seroma of the spleen following a procedure** PDX 568
- **D78.31 Postprocedural hematoma of the spleen following a procedure on the spleen**
- **D78.32 Postprocedural hematoma of the spleen following other procedure**
- **D78.33 Postprocedural seroma of the spleen following a procedure on the spleen**
- **D78.34 Postprocedural seroma of the spleen following other procedure**

● **D78.8 Other intraoperative and postprocedural complications of the spleen**
Use additional code, if applicable, to further specify disorder
- **D78.81 Other intraoperative complications of the spleen**
- **D78.89 Other postprocedural complications of the spleen**

CERTAIN DISORDERS INVOLVING THE IMMUNE MECHANISM (D80-D89)

Includes defects in the complement system
immunodeficiency disorders, except human immunodeficiency virus [HIV] disease
sarcoidosis

Excludes1 autoimmune disease (systemic) NOS (M35.9)
functional disorders of polymorphonuclear neutrophils (D71)
human immunodeficiency virus [HIV] disease (B20)

● **D80 Immunodeficiency with predominantly antibody defects** PDX 571
- **D80.0 Hereditary hypogammaglobulinemia**
  Autosomal recessive agammaglobulinemia (Swiss type)
  X-linked agammaglobulinemia [Bruton] (with growth hormone deficiency)
- **D80.1 Nonfamilial hypogammaglobulinemia** PDX 572
  Abnormally low levels of all classes of immunoglobulins
  Agammaglobulinemia with immunoglobulin-bearing B-lymphocytes
  Common variable agammaglobulinemia [CVAgamma]
  Hypogammaglobulinemia NOS
- **D80.2 Selective deficiency of immunoglobulin A [IgA]** PDX 572
- **D80.3 Selective deficiency of immunoglobulin G [IgG] subclasses**
- **D80.4 Selective deficiency of immunoglobulin M [IgM]**
- **D80.5 Immunodeficiency with increased immunoglobulin M [IgM]**
- **D80.6 Antibody deficiency with near-normal immunoglobulins or with hyperimmunoglobulinemia**
  Abnormally high levels of immunoglobulins in serum
- **D80.7 Transient hypogammaglobulinemia of infancy**
- **D80.8 Other immunodeficiencies with predominantly antibody defects**
  Kappa light chain deficiency
- **D80.9 Immunodeficiency with predominantly antibody defects, unspecified**

● **D81 Combined immunodeficiencies** PDX 571
Excludes1 autosomal recessive agammaglobulinemia (Swiss type) (D80.0)
- **D81.0 Severe combined immunodeficiency [SCID] with reticular dysgenesis**
- **D81.1 Severe combined immunodeficiency [SCID] with low T- and B-cell numbers**
- **D81.2 Severe combined immunodeficiency [SCID] with low or normal B-cell numbers**

● **D81.3 Adenosine deaminase [ADA] deficiency** PDX 573
- **D81.30 Adenosine deaminase deficiency, unspecified**
  ADA deficiency NOS
- **D81.31 Severe combined immunodeficiency due to adenosine deaminase deficiency**
  ADA deficiency with SCID
  Adenosine deaminase [ADA] deficiency with severe combined immunodeficiency
- **D81.32 Adenosine deaminase 2 deficiency**
  ADA2 deficiency
  Adenosine deaminase deficiency type 2
  Code also, if applicable, any associated manifestations, such as:
  polyarteritis nodosa (M30.0)
  stroke (I63.-)
- **D81.39 Other adenosine deaminase deficiency**
  Adenosine deaminase [ADA] deficiency type 1, NOS
  Adenosine deaminase [ADA] deficiency type 1, without SCID
  Adenosine deaminase [ADA] deficiency type 1, without severe combined immunodeficiency
  Partial ADA deficiency (type 1)
  Partial adenosine deaminase deficiency (type 1)

D81.4 Nezelof's syndrome PDX 571

D81.5 Purine nucleoside phosphorylase [PNP] deficiency PDX 573

D81.6 Major histocompatibility complex class I deficiency PDX 571
Bare lymphocyte syndrome

D81.7 Major histocompatibility complex class II deficiency PDX 571

● **D81.8 Other combined immunodeficiencies**

● **D81.81 Biotin-dependent carboxylase deficiency**
Multiple carboxylase deficiency
Excludes1 biotin-dependent carboxylase deficiency due to dietary deficiency of biotin (E53.8)
- **D81.810 Biotinidase deficiency**
- **D81.818 Other biotin-dependent carboxylase deficiency**
  Holocarboxylase synthetase deficiency
  Other multiple carboxylase deficiency
- **D81.819 Biotin-dependent carboxylase deficiency, unspecified**
  Multiple carboxylase deficiency, unspecified

D81.82 Activated Phosphoinositide 3-kinase Delta Syndrome [APDS] PDX 571
p110d-activating mutation causing senescent T cells, lymphadenopathy, and immunodeficiency [PASLI] disease
Code also, if applicable, any associated manifestations, such as:
bronchiectasis (J47.-)
herpes virus infections (B00.-)
other acute respiratory tract infections (J00-J06; J20-J22)
other infections (A00-B99)
pneumonia (J12-J18)

D81.89 Other combined immunodeficiencies PDX 571

D81.9 Combined immunodeficiency, unspecified PDX 571
Severe combined immunodeficiency disorder [SCID] NOS

CHAPTER 3 (D50-D89)

D82 Immunodeficiency associated with other major defects (Ex) PDX 571
Excludes1 ataxia telangiectasia [Louis-Bar] (G11.3)
D82.0 Wiskott-Aldrich syndrome
X-linked immunodeficiency
Immunodeficiency with thrombocytopenia and eczema
D82.1 Di George's syndrome
Congenital disorder with defective development of third and fourth pharyngeal pouches
Pharyngeal pouch syndrome
Thymic alymphoplasia
Thymic aplasia or hypoplasia with immunodeficiency
Coding Clinic: 2019, Q3, P14
D82.2 Immunodeficiency with short-limbed stature
D82.3 Immunodeficiency following hereditary defective response to Epstein-Barr virus
X-linked lymphoproliferative disease
D82.4 Hyperimmunoglobulin E [IgE] syndrome
Suspected genetic defect that produces high levels of antibody immunoglobulin (IgE) that causes skin and lung infections and eczema
D82.8 Immunodeficiency associated with other specified major defects
D82.9 Immunodeficiency associated with major defect, unspecified

D83 Common variable immunodeficiency (Ex) PDX 571
D83.0 Common variable immunodeficiency with predominant abnormalities of B-cell numbers and function
D83.1 Common variable immunodeficiency with predominant immunoregulatory T-cell disorders
D83.2 Common variable immunodeficiency with autoantibodies to B- or T-cells
D83.8 Other common variable immunodeficiencies
D83.9 Common variable immunodeficiency, unspecified

D84 Other immunodeficiencies (Ex) PDX 571
D84.0 Lymphocyte function antigen-1 [LFA-1] defect
D84.1 Defects in the complement system
C1 esterase inhibitor [C1-INH] deficiency
D84.8 Other specified immunodeficiencies
D84.81 Immunodeficiency due to conditions classified elsewhere
Code first underlying condition, such as:
chromosomal abnormalities (Q90-Q99)
diabetes mellitus (E08-E13)
malignant neoplasms (C00-C96)
Excludes1 *certain disorders involving the immune mechanism (D80-D83, D84.0, D84.1, D84.9)*
human immunodeficiency virus [HIV] disease (B20)
D84.82 Immunodeficiency due to drugs and external causes
D84.821 Immunodeficiency due to drugs
Immunodeficiency due to (current or past) medication
Use additional code for adverse effect if applicable, to identify adverse effect of drug (T36-T50 with fifth or six character 5)
Use additional code, if applicable, for associated long term (current) drug therapy drug or medication such as:
long term (current) drug therapy systemic steroids (Z79.52)
other long term (current) drug therapy (Z79.899)
D84.822 Immunodeficiency due to external causes
Code also, if applicable, radiological procedure and radiotherapy (Y84.2)
Use additional code for external cause such as:
exposure to ionizing radiation (W88)
D84.89 Other immunodeficiencies
D84.9 Immunodeficiency, unspecified
Immunocompromised NOS
Immunodeficient NOS
Immunosuppressed NOS

D86 Sarcoidosis
D86.0 Sarcoidosis of lung
D86.1 Sarcoidosis of lymph nodes
D86.2 Sarcoidosis of lung with sarcoidosis of lymph nodes
D86.3 Sarcoidosis of skin
D86.8 Sarcoidosis of other sites
D86.81 Sarcoid meningitis
D86.82 Multiple cranial nerve palsies in sarcoidosis
D86.83 Sarcoid iridocyclitis
Rare large tumor with irregular surface of iris
D86.84 Sarcoid pyelonephritis
Systemic disease of unknown etiology characterized by chronic granulomatous inflammation with tissue destruction of pelvis kidney
Tubulo-interstitial nephropathy in sarcoidosis
D86.85 Sarcoid myocarditis
D86.86 Sarcoid arthropathy
Polyarthritis in sarcoidosis
D86.87 Sarcoid myositis
Granumloma of muscle
D86.89 Sarcoidosis of other sites
Hepatic granuloma
Uveoparotid fever [Heerfordt]
D86.9 Sarcoidosis, unspecified

D89 Other disorders involving the immune mechanism, not elsewhere classified
Excludes1 hyperglobulinemia NOS (R77.1)
monoclonal gammopathy (of undetermined significance) (D47.2)
Excludes2 transplant failure and rejection (T86.-)
D89.0 Polyclonal hypergammaglobulinemia
Benign hypergammaglobulinemic purpura
Polyclonal gammopathy NOS
D89.1 Cryoglobulinemia
Cryoglobulin (proteins) in blood that precipitate temperatures below 98.6° F; usually symptomatic of underlying disease
Cryoglobulinemic purpura
Cryoglobulinemic vasculitis
Essential cryoglobulinemia
Idiopathic cryoglobulinemia
Mixed cryoglobulinemia
Primary cryoglobulinemia
Secondary cryoglobulinemia
D89.2 Hypergammaglobulinemia, unspecified
D89.3 Immune reconstitution syndrome
Immune reconstitution inflammatory syndrome [IRIS]
Use additional code for adverse effect, if applicable, to identify drug (T36-T50 with fifth or sixth character 5)

Item 3-1 Sarcoidosis: A symptom of an inflammation producing tiny lumps of cells (granulomas) in various organs, most commonly the lungs and lymph nodes, that affect organ function. Cause is unknown occurring primarily in 20- to 40-year-olds, African-American, especially women, and those of Asian, German, Irish, Scandinavian, and Puerto Rican heritage.

CHAPTER 3 (D50-D89)

D89.4 Mast cell activation syndrome and related disorders

Excludes1 aggressive systemic mastocytosis (C96.21)
congenital cutaneous mastocytosis (Q82.2)
(non-congenital) cutaneous mastocytosis (D47.Ø1)
(indolent) systemic mastocytosis (D47.Ø2)
malignant mast cell neoplasm (C96.2-)
malignant mastocytoma (C96.29)
mast cell leukemia (C94.3-)
mast cell sarcoma (C96.22)
mastocytoma NOS (D47.Ø9)
other mast cell neoplasms of uncertain behavior (D47.Ø9)
systemic mastocytosis associated with a clonal hematologic non-mast cell lineage disease (SM-AHNMD) (D47.Ø2)

Coding Clinic: 2Ø16, Q4, P11

D89.4Ø Mast cell activation, unspecified
Mast cell activation disorder, unspecified
Mast cell activation syndrome, NOS

D89.41 Monoclonal mast cell activation syndrome
Coding Clinic: 2Ø16, Q4, P11

D89.42 Idiopathic mast cell activation syndrome
Coding Clinic: 2Ø16, Q4, P11

D89.44 Hereditary alpha tryptasemia
Use additional code, if applicable, for:
allergy status, other than to drugs and biological substances (Z91.Ø-)
personal history of anaphylaxis (Z87.892)

D89.43 Secondary mast cell activation
Secondary mast cell activation syndrome
Code also underlying etiology, if known
Coding Clinic: 2Ø16, Q4, P11

D89.49 Other mast cell activation disorder
Other mast cell activation syndrome
Coding Clinic: 2Ø16, Q4, P11

D89.8 Other specified disorders involving the immune mechanism, not elsewhere classified

D89.81 Graft-versus-host disease Ex: PDX 574
Code first underlying cause, such as:
complications of transplanted organs and tissue (T86.-)
complications of blood transfusion (T8Ø.89)
Use additional code to identify associated manifestations, such as:
desquamative dermatitis (L3Ø.8)
diarrhea (R19.7)
elevated bilirubin (R17)
hair loss (L65.9)

D89.81Ø Acute graft-versus-host disease

D89.811 Chronic graft-versus-host disease
Coding Clinic: 2Ø23, Q3, P2Ø

D89.812 Acute on chronic graft-versus-host disease

D89.813 Graft-versus-host disease, unspecified

D89.82 Autoimmune lymphoproliferative syndrome [ALPS]

D89.84 IgG4-related disease
Immunoglobulin G4-related disease

D89.83 Cytokine release syndrome No Exclusions
Code first underlying cause, such as:
complications following infusion, transfusion and therapeutic injection (T8Ø.89-)
complications of transplanted organs and tissue (T86.-)
Use additional code to identify associated manifestations
code for adverse effect, if applicable, to identify immune checkpointinhibitors and immunostimulant drugs (T45.AX5)

D89.831 Cytokine release syndrome, grade 1

D89.832 Cytokine release syndrome, grade 2

D89.833 Cytokine release syndrome, grade 3

D89.834 Cytokine release syndrome, grade 4

D89.835 Cytokine release syndrome, grade 5

D89.839 Cytokine release syndrome, grade unspecified

D89.89 Other specified disorders involving the immune mechanism, not elsewhere classified
Excludes1 human immunodeficiency virus disease (B2Ø)
Coding Clinic: 2Ø17, Q4, P1Ø9

D89.9 Disorder involving the immune mechanism, unspecified
Immune disease NOS
Coding Clinic: 2Ø15, Q3, P22

CHAPTER 4

ENDOCRINE, NUTRITIONAL AND METABOLIC DISEASES (EØØ-E89)

OGCR Chapter-Specific Coding Guidelines

4. **Chapter 4: Endocrine, Nutritional, and Metabolic Diseases (EØØ-E89)**

a. Diabetes mellitus

The diabetes mellitus codes are combination codes that include the type of diabetes mellitus, the body system affected, and the complications affecting that body system. As many codes within a particular category as are necessary to describe all of the complications of the disease may be used. They should be sequenced based on the reason for a particular encounter. Assign as many codes from categories EØ8 – E13 as needed to identify all of the associated conditions that the patient has.

1) Type of diabetes

The age of a patient is not the sole determining factor, though most type 1 diabetics develop the condition before reaching puberty. For this reason type 1 diabetes mellitus is also referred to as juvenile diabetes.

2) Type of diabetes mellitus not documented

If the type of diabetes mellitus is not documented in the medical record the default is E11.-, Type 2 diabetes mellitus.

3) Diabetes mellitus and the use of insulin oral hypoglycemics

If the documentation in a medical record does not indicate the type of diabetes but does indicate that the patient uses insulin, code E11, Type 2 diabetes mellitus, should be assigned. An additional code should be assigned from category Z79 to identify the long-term (current) use of insulin or oral hypoglycemic drugs. If the patient is treated with both oral medications and insulin, only the code for long-term (current) use of insulin should be assigned. Code Z79.4 should not be assigned if insulin is given temporarily to bring a type 2 patient's blood sugar under control during an encounter.

4) Diabetes mellitus in pregnancy and gestational diabetes

See Section I.C.15. Diabetes mellitus in pregnancy.
See Section I.C.15. Gestational (pregnancy induced) diabetes

5) Complications due to insulin pump malfunction

(a) Underdose of insulin due to insulin pump failure

An underdose of insulin due to an insulin pump failure should be assigned to a code from subcategory T85.6, Mechanical complication of other specified internal and external prosthetic devices, implants and grafts, that specifies the type of pump malfunction, as the principal or first-listed code, followed by code T38.3X6-, Underdosing of insulin and oral hypoglycemic [antidiabetic] drugs. Additional codes for the type of diabetes mellitus and any associated complications due to the underdosing should also be assigned.

(b) Overdose of insulin due to insulin pump failure

The principal or first-listed code for an encounter due to an insulin pump malfunction resulting in an overdose of insulin, should also be T85.6-, Mechanical complication of other specified internal and external prosthetic devices, implants and grafts, followed by code T38.3X1-, Poisoning by insulin and oral hypoglycemic [antidiabetic] drugs, accidental (unintentional).

6) Secondary diabetes mellitus

Codes under categories EØ8, Diabetes mellitus due to underlying condition, EØ9, Drug or chemical induced diabetes mellitus and E13, Other specified diabetes mellitus, identify complications/manifestations associated with secondary diabetes mellitus. Secondary diabetes is always caused by another condition or event (e.g., cystic fibrosis, malignant neoplasm of pancreas, pancreatectomy, adverse effect of drug, or poisoning).

(a) Secondary diabetes mellitus and the use of insulin or hypoglycemic drugs

For patients with secondary diabetes mellitus who routinely use insulin or oral hypoglycemic drugs, an additional code from category Z79 should be assigned to identify the long-term (current) use of insulin or oral hypoglycemic drugs. If the patient is treated with both oral medications and insulin, only the code for long-term (current) use of insulin should be assigned. Code Z79.4 should not be assigned if insulin is given temporarily to bring a type 2 patient's blood sugar under control during an encounter.

(b) Assigning and sequencing secondary diabetes codes and its causes

The sequencing of the secondary diabetes codes in relationship to codes for the cause of the diabetes is based on the Tabular List instructions for categories EØ8, EØ9 and E13.

(i) **Secondary diabetes mellitus due to pancreatectomy** For postpancreatectomy diabetes mellitus (lack of insulin due to the surgical removal of all or part of the pancreas), assign code E89.1, Postprocedural hypoinsulinemia. Assign a code from category E13 and a code from subcategory Z90.41-, Acquired absence of pancreas, as additional codes.

(ii) **Secondary diabetes due to drugs** Secondary diabetes may be caused by an adverse effect of correctly administered medications, poisoning or sequela of poisoning.

See Section I.C.19.e for coding of adverse effects and poisoning, and Section I.C.2Ø for external cause code reporting.

CHAPTER 4 (EØØ-E89)

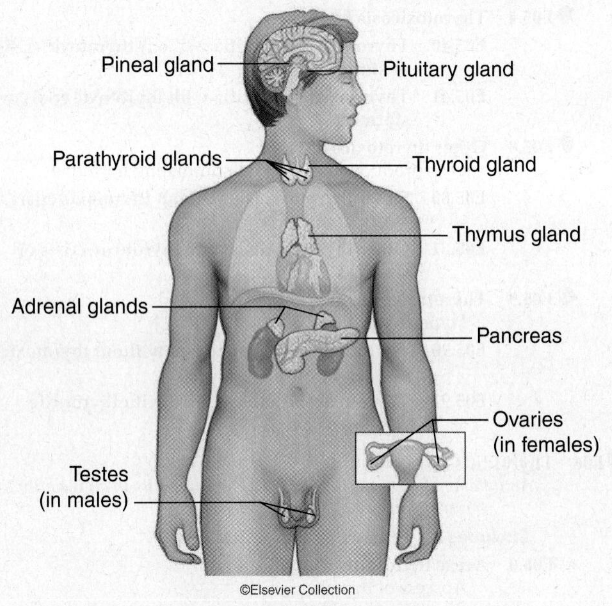

Figure 4-1 The endocrine system. ©Elsevier Collection.

CHAPTER 4

ENDOCRINE, NUTRITIONAL AND METABOLIC DISEASES (E00-E89)

All neoplasms, whether functionally active or not, are classified in Chapter 2. Appropriate codes in this chapter (i.e., E05.8, E07.0, E16-E31, E34.-) may be used as additional codes to indicate either functional activity by neoplasms and ectopic endocrine tissue or hyperfunction and hypofunction of endocrine glands associated with neoplasms and other conditions classified elsewhere.

Excludes1 transitory endocrine and metabolic disorders specific to newborn (P70-P74)

This chapter contains the following blocks:

E00-E07	Disorders of thyroid gland
E08-E13	Diabetes mellitus
E15-E16	Other disorders of glucose regulation and pancreatic internal secretion
E20-E35	Disorders of other endocrine glands
E36	Intraoperative complications of endocrine system
E40-E46	Malnutrition
E50-E64	Other nutritional deficiencies
E65-E68	Overweight, obesity and other hyperalimentation
E70-E88	Metabolic disorders
E89	Postprocedural endocrine and metabolic complications and disorders, not elsewhere classified

DISORDERS OF THYROID GLAND (E00-E07)

● **E00 Congenital iodine-deficiency syndrome**

Use additional code (F70-F79) to identify associated intellectual disabilities.

Excludes1 subclinical iodine-deficiency hypothyroidism (E02)

E00.0 Congenital iodine-deficiency syndrome, neurological type

Endemic cretinism, neurological type

E00.1 Congenital iodine-deficiency syndrome, myxedematous type

Dry, waxy type of swelling (nonpitting edema) with abnormal deposits of mucin in skin (mucinosis) and other tissues

Endemic hypothyroid cretinism

Endemic cretinism, myxedematous type

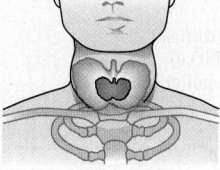

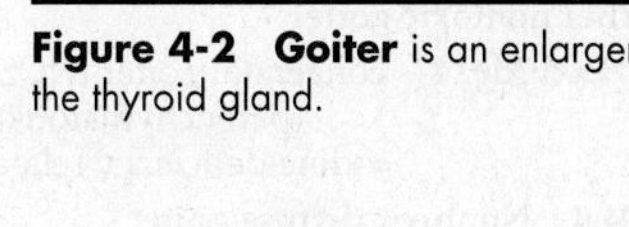

Figure 4-2 Goiter is an enlargement of the thyroid gland.

Item 4–1 Simple goiter indicates no nodules are present. The most common type of goiter is a **diffuse colloidal,** also called a **nontoxic** or **endemic** goiter.

E00.2 Congenital iodine-deficiency syndrome, mixed type

Endemic cretinism, mixed type

E00.9 Congenital iodine-deficiency syndrome, unspecified

Congenital iodine-deficiency hypothyroidism NOS

Endemic cretinism NOS

● **E01 Iodine-deficiency related thyroid disorders and allied conditions**

Excludes1 congenital iodine-deficiency syndrome (E00.-)
subclinical iodine-deficiency hypothyroidism (E02)

E01.0 Iodine-deficiency related diffuse (endemic) goiter

Thyroid gland is enlarged

E01.1 Iodine-deficiency related multinodular (endemic) goiter

Iodine-deficiency related nodular goiter

E01.2 Iodine-deficiency related (endemic) goiter, unspecified

Endemic goiter NOS

E01.8 Other iodine-deficiency related thyroid disorders and allied conditions

Acquired iodine-deficiency hypothyroidism NOS

E02 Subclinical iodine-deficiency hypothyroidism

Coding Clinic: 2021, Q1, P8-9

● **E03 Other hypothyroidism**

Excludes1 iodine-deficiency related hypothyroidism (E00-E02)
postprocedural hypothyroidism (E89.0)

E03.0 Congenital hypothyroidism with diffuse goiter

Congenital parenchymatous goiter (nontoxic)

Congenital goiter (nontoxic) NOS

Excludes1 transitory congenital goiter with normal function (P72.0)

E03.1 Congenital hypothyroidism without goiter

Aplasia of thyroid (with myxedema)

Congenital atrophy of thyroid

Congenital hypothyroidism NOS

E03.2 Hypothyroidism due to medicaments and other exogenous substances

Code first poisoning due to drug or toxin, if applicable (T36-T65 with fifth or sixth character 1-4)

Use additional code for adverse effect, if applicable, to identify drug (T36-T50 with fifth or sixth character 5)

E03.3 Postinfectious hypothyroidism

E03.4 Atrophy of thyroid (acquired)

Excludes1 congenital atrophy of thyroid (E03.1)

E03.5 Myxedema coma (Ex) PDX 575

Often fatal complication of long-term hypothyroidism

E03.8 Other specified hypothyroidism

E03.9 Hypothyroidism, unspecified

Myxedema NOS

Coding Clinic: 2021, Q1, P9

Item 4–2 Hypothyroidism is a condition in which there are insufficient levels of thyroxine. **Cretinism** is congenital hypothyroidism, which can result in mental and physical retardation.

CHAPTER 4 (E00-E89)

E04 Other nontoxic goiter
Excludes1 congenital goiter (NOS) (diffuse) (parenchymatous) (E03.0)
iodine-deficiency related goiter (E00-E02)

E04.0 Nontoxic diffuse goiter
Thyroid gland is enlarged
Diffuse (colloid) nontoxic goiter
Simple nontoxic goiter

E04.1 Nontoxic single thyroid nodule
Colloid nodule (cystic) (thyroid)
Nontoxic uninodular goiter
Thyroid (cystic) nodule NOS

E04.2 Nontoxic multinodular goiter
Enlarged thyroid gland with multiple nodules
Cystic goiter NOS
Multinodular (cystic) goiter NOS

E04.8 Other specified nontoxic goiter

E04.9 Nontoxic goiter, unspecified
Goiter NOS
Nodular goiter (nontoxic) NOS

E05 Thyrotoxicosis [hyperthyroidism] (Ex) PDX 576
Enlarged thyroid gland with multiple nodules
Excludes1 chronic thyroiditis with transient thyrotoxicosis (E06.2)
neonatal thyrotoxicosis (P72.1)

E05.0 Thyrotoxicosis with diffuse goiter
Exophthalmic or toxic goiter NOS
Graves' disease
Toxic diffuse goiter

E05.00 Thyrotoxicosis with diffuse goiter without thyrotoxic crisis or storm

E05.01 Thyrotoxicosis with diffuse goiter with thyrotoxic crisis or storm

E05.1 Thyrotoxicosis with toxic single thyroid nodule
Thyrotoxicosis with toxic uninodular goiter

E05.10 Thyrotoxicosis with toxic single thyroid nodule without thyrotoxic crisis or storm

E05.11 Thyrotoxicosis with toxic single thyroid nodule with thyrotoxic crisis or storm

E05.2 Thyrotoxicosis with toxic multinodular goiter
Toxic nodular goiter NOS

E05.20 Thyrotoxicosis with toxic multinodular goiter without thyrotoxic crisis or storm

E05.21 Thyrotoxicosis with toxic multinodular goiter with thyrotoxic crisis or storm

E05.3 Thyrotoxicosis from ectopic thyroid tissue

E05.30 Thyrotoxicosis from ectopic thyroid tissue without thyrotoxic crisis or storm

E05.31 Thyrotoxicosis from ectopic thyroid tissue with thyrotoxic crisis or storm

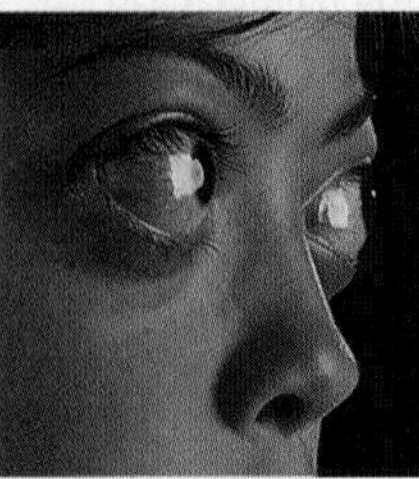

Figure 4-3 Graves' disease. In Graves' disease, exophthalmos often looks more pronounced than it actually is because of the extreme lid retraction that may occur. This patient, for instance, had minimal proptosis of the left eye but marked lid retraction. (From Lissauer T, Clayden G, and Craft A: Illustrated Textbook of Paediatrics, Edinburgh, Mosby, 2015)

Item 4-3 Thyrotoxicosis is a condition caused by excessive amounts of the thyroid hormone thyroxine production or hyperthyroidism. **Graves' disease is associated with hyperthyroidism** (known as **Basedow's disease** in Europe).

E05.4 Thyrotoxicosis factitia

E05.40 Thyrotoxicosis factitia without thyrotoxic crisis or storm

E05.41 Thyrotoxicosis factitia with thyrotoxic crisis or storm

E05.8 Other thyrotoxicosis
Overproduction of thyroid-stimulating hormone

E05.80 Other thyrotoxicosis without thyrotoxic crisis or storm

E05.81 Other thyrotoxicosis with thyrotoxic crisis or storm

E05.9 Thyrotoxicosis, unspecified
Hyperthyroidism NOS

E05.90 Thyrotoxicosis, unspecified without thyrotoxic crisis or storm

E05.91 Thyrotoxicosis, unspecified with thyrotoxic crisis or storm

E06 Thyroiditis
An inflammation of the thyroid gland which results in an inability to convert iodine into thyroid hormone
Excludes1 postpartum thyroiditis (O90.5)

E06.0 Acute thyroiditis (Ex) PDX 577
Abscess of thyroid
Pyogenic thyroiditis
Suppurative thyroiditis
Use additional code (B95-B97) to identify infectious agent.

E06.1 Subacute thyroiditis
Inflammation of thyroid gland following viral upper respiratory infection
de Quervain thyroiditis
Giant-cell thyroiditis
Granulomatous thyroiditis
Nonsuppurative thyroiditis
Viral thyroiditis
Excludes1 autoimmune thyroiditis (E06.3)

E06.2 Chronic thyroiditis with transient thyrotoxicosis
Chronic inflammation of thyroid gland with intermittent overproduction of thyroid hormone
Excludes1 autoimmune thyroiditis (E06.3)

E06.3 Autoimmune thyroiditis
Hashimoto's thyroiditis
Hashitoxicosis (transient)
Lymphadenoid goiter
Lymphocytic thyroiditis
Struma lymphomatosa
Coding Clinic: 2024, Q1, P14

E06.4 Drug-induced thyroiditis
Use additional code for adverse effect, if applicable, to identify drug (T36-T50 with fifth or sixth character 5)

E06.5 Other chronic thyroiditis
Chronic fibrous thyroiditis
Chronic thyroiditis NOS
Ligneous thyroiditis
Riedel thyroiditis

E06.9 Thyroiditis, unspecified

E07 Other disorders of thyroid

E07.0 Hypersecretion of calcitonin
C-cell hyperplasia of thyroid
Hypersecretion of thyrocalcitonin

E07.1 Dyshormogenetic goiter
Group of several types of goiter resulting from enzyme defects in hormone synthesis
▶Dyshormonogenetic goiter
Familial dyshormogenetic goiter
Pendred's syndrome
Excludes1 transitory congenital goiter with normal function (P72.0)

● **E07.8 Other specified disorders of thyroid**

E07.81 Sick-euthyroid syndrome
Euthyroid sick-syndrome

E07.89 Other specified disorders of thyroid
Abnormality of thyroid-binding globulin
Hemorrhage of thyroid
Infarction of thyroid

E07.9 Disorder of thyroid, unspecified

OGCR Section I.C.4.a.

Diabetes mellitus

The diabetes mellitus codes are combination codes that include the type of diabetes mellitus, body system affected, and the complications affecting that body system. As many codes within a particular category as are necessary to describe all of the complications of the disease may be used. They should be sequenced based on the reason for a particular visit. Assign as many codes from categories E08–E13 as needed to identify all of the associated conditions that the patient has.

DIABETES MELLITUS (E08-E13)

A metabolic disease that results in persistent hyperglycemia

Coding Clinic: 2016, Q4, P142

● **E08 Diabetes mellitus due to underlying condition**

Code first the underlying condition, such as:
congenital rubella (P35.0)
Cushing's syndrome (E24.-)
cystic fibrosis (E84.-)
malignant neoplasm (C00-C96)
malnutrition (E40-E46)
pancreatitis and other diseases of the pancreas (K85-K86.-)

Use additional code to identify control using:
▶injectable non-insulin antidiabetic drugs (Z79.85)
insulin (Z79.4)
oral antidiabetic drugs (Z79.84)
oral hypoglycemic drugs (Z79.84)

Excludes1 drug or chemical induced diabetes mellitus (E09.-)
gestational diabetes (O24.4-)
neonatal diabetes mellitus (P70.2)
postpancreatectomy diabetes mellitus (E13.-)
postprocedural diabetes mellitus (E13.-)
secondary diabetes mellitus NEC (E13.-)
type 1 diabetes mellitus (E10.-)
type 2 diabetes mellitus (E11.-)

● **E08.0 Diabetes mellitus due to underlying condition with hyperosmolarity** (Ex) PDX 578

E08.00 Diabetes mellitus due to underlying condition with hyperosmolarity without nonketotic hyperglycemic-hyperosmolar coma (NKHHC)

E08.01 Diabetes mellitus due to underlying condition with hyperosmolarity with coma

● **E08.1 Diabetes mellitus due to underlying condition with ketoacidosis** (Ex) PDX 578

E08.10 Diabetes mellitus due to underlying condition with ketoacidosis without coma

E08.11 Diabetes mellitus due to underlying condition with ketoacidosis with coma

● **E08.2 Diabetes mellitus due to underlying condition with kidney complications**

E08.21 Diabetes mellitus due to underlying condition with diabetic nephropathy
Diabetes mellitus due to underlying condition with intercapillary glomerulosclerosis
Diabetes mellitus due to underlying condition with intracapillary glomerulonephrosis
Diabetes mellitus due to underlying condition with Kimmelstiel-Wilson disease

E08.22 Diabetes mellitus due to underlying condition with diabetic chronic kidney disease
Use additional code to identify stage of chronic kidney disease (N18.1-N18.6)

E08.29 Diabetes mellitus due to underlying condition with other diabetic kidney complication
Renal tubular degeneration in diabetes mellitus due to underlying condition

● **E08.3 Diabetes mellitus due to underlying condition with ophthalmic complications**

Changes in blood vessels of retina in which blood vessels swell and leak fluid into retinal surface.

Coding Clinic: 2016, Q4, P11

● **E08.31 Diabetes mellitus due to underlying condition with unspecified diabetic retinopathy**

E08.311 Diabetes mellitus due to underlying condition with unspecified diabetic retinopathy with macular edema

E08.319 Diabetes mellitus due to underlying condition with unspecified diabetic retinopathy without macular edema

● **E08.32 Diabetes mellitus due to underlying condition with mild nonproliferative diabetic retinopathy**
Diabetes mellitus due to underlying condition with nonproliferative diabetic retinopathy NOS

One of the following 7th characters is to be assigned to codes in subcategory E08.32 to designate laterality of the disease:

1	right eye
2	left eye
3	bilateral
9	unspecified eye

E08.321 Diabetes mellitus due to underlying condition with mild nonproliferative diabetic retinopathy with macular edema

E08.329 Diabetes mellitus due to underlying condition with mild nonproliferative diabetic retinopathy without macular edema

● **E08.33 Diabetes mellitus due to underlying condition with moderate nonproliferative diabetic retinopathy**

One of the following 7th characters is to be assigned to codes in subcategory E08.33 to designate laterality of the disease:

1	right eye
2	left eye
3	bilateral
9	unspecified eye

E08.331 Diabetes mellitus due to underlying condition with moderate nonproliferative diabetic retinopathy with macular edema

E08.339 Diabetes mellitus due to underlying condition with moderate nonproliferative diabetic retinopathy without macular edema

CHAPTER 4 (E00-E89)

E08.34 Diabetes mellitus due to underlying condition with severe nonproliferative diabetic retinopathy

One of the following 7th characters is to be assigned to codes in subcategory E08.34 to designate laterality of the disease:

1	right eye
2	left eye
3	bilateral
9	unspecified eye

E08.341 Diabetes mellitus due to underlying condition with severe nonproliferative diabetic retinopathy with macular edema

E08.349 Diabetes mellitus due to underlying condition with severe nonproliferative diabetic retinopathy without macular edema

E08.35 Diabetes mellitus due to underlying condition with proliferative diabetic retinopathy

One of the following 7th characters is to be assigned to codes in subcategory E08.35 to designate laterality of the disease:

1	right eye
2	left eye
3	bilateral
9	unspecified eye

E08.351 Diabetes mellitus due to underlying condition with proliferative diabetic retinopathy with macular edema

E08.352 Diabetes mellitus due to underlying condition with proliferative diabetic retinopathy with traction retinal detachment involving the macula

E08.353 Diabetes mellitus due to underlying condition with proliferative diabetic retinopathy with traction retinal detachment not involving the macula

E08.354 Diabetes mellitus due to underlying condition with proliferative diabetic retinopathy with combined traction retinal detachment and rhegmatogenous retinal detachment

E08.355 Diabetes mellitus due to underlying condition with stable proliferative diabetic retinopathy

E08.359 Diabetes mellitus due to underlying condition with proliferative diabetic retinopathy without macular edema

E08.36 Diabetes mellitus due to underlying condition with diabetic cataract

X *E08.37 Diabetes mellitus due to underlying condition with diabetic macular edema, resolved following treatment*

One of the following 7th characters is to be assigned to code E08.37 to designate laterality of the disease:

1	right eye
2	left eye
3	bilateral
9	unspecified eye

E08.39 Diabetes mellitus due to underlying condition with other diabetic ophthalmic complication

Use additional code to identify manifestation, such as:
diabetic glaucoma (H40-H42)

E08.4 Diabetes mellitus due to underlying condition with neurological complications

E08.40 Diabetes mellitus due to underlying condition with diabetic neuropathy, unspecified

E08.41 Diabetes mellitus due to underlying condition with diabetic mononeuropathy

E08.42 Diabetes mellitus due to underlying condition with diabetic polyneuropathy

Diabetes mellitus due to underlying condition with diabetic neuralgia

E08.43 Diabetes mellitus due to underlying condition with diabetic autonomic (poly)neuropathy

Diabetes mellitus due to underlying condition with diabetic gastroparesis

E08.44 Diabetes mellitus due to underlying condition with diabetic amyotrophy

E08.49 Diabetes mellitus due to underlying condition with other diabetic neurological complication

E08.5 Diabetes mellitus due to underlying condition with circulatory complications

E08.51 Diabetes mellitus due to underlying condition with diabetic peripheral angiopathy without gangrene

E08.52 Diabetes mellitus due to underlying condition with diabetic peripheral angiopathy with gangrene (Ex) PDX 579

Diabetes mellitus due to underlying condition with diabetic gangrene

CC when PDx is its own CC

E08.59 Diabetes mellitus due to underlying condition with other circulatory complications

E08.6 Diabetes mellitus due to underlying condition with other specified complications

E08.61 Diabetes mellitus due to underlying condition with diabetic arthropathy

E08.610 Diabetes mellitus due to underlying condition with diabetic neuropathic arthropathy

Diabetes mellitus due to underlying condition with Charcôt's joints

E08.618 Diabetes mellitus due to underlying condition with other diabetic arthropathy

E08.62 Diabetes mellitus due to underlying condition with skin complications

E08.620 Diabetes mellitus due to underlying condition with diabetic dermatitis

Diabetes mellitus due to underlying condition with diabetic necrobiosis lipoidica

E08.621 Diabetes mellitus due to underlying condition with foot ulcer

Use additional code to identify site of ulcer (L97.4-, L97.5-)

E08.622 Diabetes mellitus due to underlying condition with other skin ulcer

Use additional code to identify site of ulcer (L97.1-L97.9, L98.41-L98.49)

E08.628 Diabetes mellitus due to underlying condition with other skin complications

E08.63 Diabetes mellitus due to underlying condition with oral complications

E08.630 Diabetes mellitus due to underlying condition with periodontal disease

E08.638 Diabetes mellitus due to underlying condition with other oral complications

E08.64 Diabetes mellitus due to underlying condition with hypoglycemia
Use additional code for hypoglycemia level, if applicable (E16.A-)

E08.641 Diabetes mellitus due to underlying condition with hypoglycemia with coma (Ex) PDX 578

E08.649 Diabetes mellitus due to underlying condition with hypoglycemia without coma

E08.65 Diabetes mellitus due to underlying condition with hyperglycemia

E08.69 Diabetes mellitus due to underlying condition with other specified complication
Use additional code to identify complication

E08.8 Diabetes mellitus due to underlying condition with unspecified complications

E08.9 Diabetes mellitus due to underlying condition without complications

E09 Drug or chemical induced diabetes mellitus
Code first poisoning due to drug or toxin, if applicable (T36-T65 with fifth or sixth character 1-4)
Use additional code for adverse effect, if applicable, to identify drug (T36-T50 with fifth or sixth character 5)
Use additional code to identify control using:
injectable non-insulin antidiabetic drugs (Z79.85)
insulin (Z79.4)
oral antidiabetic drugs (Z79.84)
oral hypoglycemic drugs (Z79.84)

Excludes1 diabetes mellitus due to underlying condition (E08.-)
gestational diabetes (O24.4-)
neonatal diabetes mellitus (P70.2)
postpancreatectomy diabetes mellitus (E13.-)
postprocedural diabetes mellitus (E13.-)
secondary diabetes mellitus NEC (E13.-)
type 1 diabetes mellitus (E10.-)
type 2 diabetes mellitus (E11.-)

E09.0 Drug or chemical induced diabetes mellitus with hyperosmolarity (Ex) PDX 578

E09.00 Drug or chemical induced diabetes mellitus with hyperosmolarity without nonketotic hyperglycemic-hyperosmolar coma (NKHHC)

E09.01 Drug or chemical induced diabetes mellitus with hyperosmolarity with coma

E09.1 Drug or chemical induced diabetes mellitus with ketoacidosis (Ex) PDX 578

E09.10 Drug or chemical induced diabetes mellitus with ketoacidosis without coma

E09.11 Drug or chemical induced diabetes mellitus with ketoacidosis with coma

E09.2 Drug or chemical induced diabetes mellitus with kidney complications

E09.21 Drug or chemical induced diabetes mellitus with diabetic nephropathy
Drug or chemical induced diabetes mellitus with intercapillary glomerulosclerosis
Drug or chemical induced diabetes mellitus with intracapillary glomerulonephrosis
Drug or chemical induced diabetes mellitus with Kimmelstiel-Wilson disease

E09.22 Drug or chemical induced diabetes mellitus with diabetic chronic kidney disease
Use additional code to identify stage of chronic kidney disease (N18.1-N18.6)

E09.29 Drug or chemical induced diabetes mellitus with other diabetic kidney complication
Drug or chemical induced diabetes mellitus with renal tubular degeneration

E09.3 Drug or chemical induced diabetes mellitus with ophthalmic complications
Coding Clinic: 2016, Q4, P11

E09.31 Drug or chemical induced diabetes mellitus with unspecified diabetic retinopathy

E09.311 Drug or chemical induced diabetes mellitus with unspecified diabetic retinopathy with macular edema

E09.319 Drug or chemical induced diabetes mellitus with unspecified diabetic retinopathy without macular edema

E09.32 Drug or chemical induced diabetes mellitus with mild nonproliferative diabetic retinopathy
Drug or chemical induced diabetes mellitus with nonproliferative diabetic retinopathy NOS
One of the following 7th characters is to be assigned to codes in subcategory E09.32 to designate laterality of the disease:

1	right eye
2	left eye
3	bilateral
9	unspecified eye

E09.321 Drug or chemical induced diabetes mellitus with mild nonproliferative diabetic retinopathy with macular edema

E09.329 Drug or chemical induced diabetes mellitus with mild nonproliferative diabetic retinopathy without macular edema

E09.33 Drug or chemical induced diabetes mellitus with moderate nonproliferative diabetic retinopathy
One of the following 7th characters is to be assigned to codes in subcategory E09.33 to designate laterality of the disease:

1	right eye
2	left eye
3	bilateral
9	unspecified eye

E09.331 Drug or chemical induced diabetes mellitus with moderate nonproliferative diabetic retinopathy with macular edema

E09.339 Drug or chemical induced diabetes mellitus with moderate nonproliferative diabetic retinopathy without macular edema

E09.34 Drug or chemical induced diabetes mellitus with severe nonproliferative diabetic retinopathy
One of the following 7th characters is to be assigned to codes in subcategory E09.34 to designate laterality of the disease:

1	right eye
2	left eye
3	bilateral
9	unspecified eye

E09.341 Drug or chemical induced diabetes mellitus with severe nonproliferative diabetic retinopathy with macular edema

E09.349 Drug or chemical induced diabetes mellitus with severe nonproliferative diabetic retinopathy without macular edema

● E09.35 Drug or chemical induced diabetes mellitus with proliferative diabetic retinopathy

One of the following 7th characters is to be assigned to codes in subcategory E09.35 to designate laterality of the disease:

1 right eye
2 left eye
3 bilateral
9 unspecified eye

● E09.351 Drug or chemical induced diabetes mellitus with proliferative diabetic retinopathy with macular edema

● E09.352 Drug or chemical induced diabetes mellitus with proliferative diabetic retinopathy with traction retinal detachment involving the macula

● E09.353 Drug or chemical induced diabetes mellitus with proliferative diabetic retinopathy with traction retinal detachment not involving the macula

● E09.354 Drug or chemical induced diabetes mellitus with proliferative diabetic retinopathy with combined traction retinal detachment and rhegmatogenous retinal detachment

● E09.355 Drug or chemical induced diabetes mellitus with stable proliferative diabetic retinopathy

● E09.359 Drug or chemical induced diabetes mellitus with proliferative diabetic retinopathy without macular edema

E09.36 Drug or chemical induced diabetes mellitus with diabetic cataract

X● E09.37 Drug or chemical induced diabetes mellitus with diabetic macular edema, resolved following treatment

One of the following 7th characters is to be assigned to code E09.37 to designate laterality of the disease:

1 right eye
2 left eye
3 bilateral
9 unspecified eye

E09.39 Drug or chemical induced diabetes mellitus with other diabetic ophthalmic complication

Use additional code to identify manifestation, such as:
diabetic glaucoma (H40-H42)

● E09.4 Drug or chemical induced diabetes mellitus with neurological complications

E09.40 Drug or chemical induced diabetes mellitus with neurological complications with diabetic neuropathy, unspecified

E09.41 Drug or chemical induced diabetes mellitus with neurological complications with diabetic mononeuropathy

E09.42 Drug or chemical induced diabetes mellitus with neurological complications with diabetic polyneuropathy

Drug or chemical induced diabetes mellitus with diabetic neuralgia

E09.43 Drug or chemical induced diabetes mellitus with neurological complications with diabetic autonomic (poly)neuropathy

Drug or chemical induced diabetes mellitus with diabetic gastroparesis

E09.44 Drug or chemical induced diabetes mellitus with neurological complications with diabetic amyotrophy

E09.49 Drug or chemical induced diabetes mellitus with neurological complications with other diabetic neurological complication

● E09.5 Drug or chemical induced diabetes mellitus with circulatory complications

E09.51 Drug or chemical induced diabetes mellitus with diabetic peripheral angiopathy without gangrene

E09.52 Drug or chemical induced diabetes mellitus with diabetic peripheral angiopathy with gangrene (Ex) PDX 580

Drug or chemical induced diabetes mellitus with diabetic gangrene

CC when PDx is its own CC

E09.59 Drug or chemical induced diabetes mellitus with other circulatory complications

● E09.6 Drug or chemical induced diabetes mellitus with other specified complications

● E09.61 Drug or chemical induced diabetes mellitus with diabetic arthropathy

E09.610 Drug or chemical induced diabetes mellitus with diabetic neuropathic arthropathy

Drug or chemical induced diabetes mellitus with Charcôt's joints

Progressive degeneration of weight-bearing joint

E09.618 Drug or chemical induced diabetes mellitus with other diabetic arthropathy

● E09.62 Drug or chemical induced diabetes mellitus with skin complications

E09.620 Drug or chemical induced diabetes mellitus with diabetic dermatitis

Drug or chemical induced diabetes mellitus with diabetic necrobiosis lipoidica

Necrotizing skin condition

E09.621 Drug or chemical induced diabetes mellitus with foot ulcer

Use additional code to identify site of ulcer (L97.4-, L97.5-)

E09.622 Drug or chemical induced diabetes mellitus with other skin ulcer

Use additional code to identify site of ulcer (L97.1-L97.9, L98.41-L98.49)

E09.628 Drug or chemical induced diabetes mellitus with other skin complications

● E09.63 Drug or chemical induced diabetes mellitus with oral complications

E09.630 Drug or chemical induced diabetes mellitus with periodontal disease

E09.638 Drug or chemical induced diabetes mellitus with other oral complications

● E09.64 Drug or chemical induced diabetes mellitus with hypoglycemia

▶ Use additional code for hypoglycemia level, if applicable (E16.A-)

E09.641 Drug or chemical induced diabetes mellitus with hypoglycemia with coma (Ex) PDX 578

E09.649 Drug or chemical induced diabetes mellitus with hypoglycemia without coma

E09.65 Drug or chemical induced diabetes mellitus with hyperglycemia

E09.69 Drug or chemical induced diabetes mellitus with other specified complication

Use additional code to identify complication

E09.8 Drug or chemical induced diabetes mellitus with unspecified complications

E09.9 Drug or chemical induced diabetes mellitus without complications

E10 Type 1 diabetes mellitus

Includes brittle diabetes (mellitus)
diabetes (mellitus) due to autoimmune process
diabetes (mellitus) due to immune mediated pancreatic islet beta-cell destruction
idiopathic diabetes (mellitus)
juvenile onset diabetes (mellitus)
ketosis-prone diabetes (mellitus)

Excludes1 diabetes mellitus due to underlying condition (E08.-)
drug or chemical induced diabetes mellitus (E09.-)
gestational diabetes (O24.4-)
hyperglycemia NOS (R73.9)
neonatal diabetes mellitus (P70.2)
postpancreatectomy diabetes mellitus (E13.-)
postprocedural diabetes mellitus (E13.-)
secondary diabetes mellitus NEC (E13.-)
type 2 diabetes mellitus (E11.-)

E10.1 Type 1 diabetes mellitus with ketoacidosis (Ex) PDX 581
Acidosis accompanied by accumulation of ketone bodies (ketosis) in body tissues and fluids

E10.10 Type 1 diabetes mellitus with ketoacidosis without coma
Coding Clinic: 2013, Q3, P20

E10.11 Type 1 diabetes mellitus with ketoacidosis with coma

E10.2 Type 1 diabetes mellitus with kidney complications

E10.21 Type 1 diabetes mellitus with diabetic nephropathy
Type 1 diabetes mellitus with intercapillary glomerulosclerosis
Type 1 diabetes mellitus with intracapillary glomerulonephrosis
Type 1 diabetes mellitus with Kimmelstiel-Wilson disease

E10.22 Type 1 diabetes mellitus with diabetic chronic kidney disease
Use additional code to identify stage of chronic kidney disease (N18.1-N18.6)

E10.29 Type 1 diabetes mellitus with other diabetic kidney complication
Type 1 diabetes mellitus with renal tubular degeneration
Coding Clinic: 2016, Q1, P13

E10.3 Type 1 diabetes mellitus with ophthalmic complications
Coding Clinic: 2016, Q4, P11

E10.31 Type 1 diabetes mellitus with unspecified diabetic retinopathy

E10.311 Type 1 diabetes mellitus with unspecified diabetic retinopathy with macular edema

E10.319 Type 1 diabetes mellitus with unspecified diabetic retinopathy without macular edema

E10.32 Type 1 diabetes mellitus with mild nonproliferative diabetic retinopathy
Type 1 diabetes mellitus with nonproliferative diabetic retinopathy NOS
One of the following 7th characters is to be assigned to codes in subcategory E10.32 to designate laterality of the disease:

1	right eye
2	left eye
3	bilateral
9	unspecified eye

E10.321 Type 1 diabetes mellitus with mild nonproliferative diabetic retinopathy with macular edema

E10.329 Type 1 diabetes mellitus with mild nonproliferative diabetic retinopathy without macular edema

E10.33 Type 1 diabetes mellitus with moderate nonproliferative diabetic retinopathy
One of the following 7th characters is to be assigned to codes in subcategory E10.33 to designate laterality of the disease:

1	right eye
2	left eye
3	bilateral
9	unspecified eye

E10.331 Type 1 diabetes mellitus with moderate nonproliferative diabetic retinopathy with macular edema

E10.339 Type 1 diabetes mellitus with moderate nonproliferative diabetic retinopathy without macular edema

E10.34 Type 1 diabetes mellitus with severe nonproliferative diabetic retinopathy
One of the following 7th characters is to be assigned to codes in subcategory E10.34 to designate laterality of the disease:

1	right eye
2	left eye
3	bilateral
9	unspecified eye

E10.341 Type 1 diabetes mellitus with severe nonproliferative diabetic retinopathy with macular edema

E10.349 Type 1 diabetes mellitus with severe nonproliferative diabetic retinopathy without macular edema

E10.35 Type 1 diabetes mellitus with proliferative diabetic retinopathy
One of the following 7th characters is to be assigned to codes in subcategory E10.35 to designate laterality of the disease:

1	right eye
2	left eye
3	bilateral
9	unspecified eye

E10.351 Type 1 diabetes mellitus with proliferative diabetic retinopathy with macular edema

E10.352 Type 1 diabetes mellitus with proliferative diabetic retinopathy with traction retinal detachment involving the macula

E10.353 Type 1 diabetes mellitus with proliferative diabetic retinopathy with traction retinal detachment not involving the macula

E10.354 Type 1 diabetes mellitus with proliferative diabetic retinopathy with combined traction retinal detachment and rhegmatogenous retinal detachment

E10.355 Type 1 diabetes mellitus with stable proliferative diabetic retinopathy

E10.359 Type 1 diabetes mellitus with proliferative diabetic retinopathy without macular edema

E10.36 Type 1 diabetes mellitus with diabetic cataract

CHAPTER 4 (E00-E89)

X● **E1Ø.37** **Type 1 diabetes mellitus with diabetic macular edema, resolved following treatment**

One of the following 7th characters is to be assigned to code E1Ø.37 to designate laterality of the disease:

1	right eye
2	left eye
3	bilateral
9	unspecified eye

E1Ø.39 **Type 1 diabetes mellitus with other diabetic ophthalmic complication**

Use additional code to identify manifestation, such as:
diabetic glaucoma (H4Ø-H42)

● **E1Ø.4** **Type 1 diabetes mellitus with neurological complications**

E1Ø.4Ø **Type 1 diabetes mellitus with diabetic neuropathy, unspecified**

E1Ø.41 **Type 1 diabetes mellitus with diabetic mononeuropathy**

E1Ø.42 **Type 1 diabetes mellitus with diabetic polyneuropathy**
Type 1 diabetes mellitus with diabetic neuralgia

E1Ø.43 **Type 1 diabetes mellitus with diabetic autonomic (poly)neuropathy**
Type 1 diabetes mellitus with diabetic gastroparesis

E1Ø.44 **Type 1 diabetes mellitus with diabetic amyotrophy**

E1Ø.49 **Type 1 diabetes mellitus with other diabetic neurological complication**

● **E1Ø.5** **Type 1 diabetes mellitus with circulatory complications**

E1Ø.51 **Type 1 diabetes mellitus with diabetic peripheral angiopathy without gangrene**

E1Ø.52 **Type 1 diabetes mellitus with diabetic peripheral angiopathy with gangrene** (Ex) PDX 582
Type 1 diabetes mellitus with diabetic gangrene
CC when PDx is its own CC

E1Ø.59 **Type 1 diabetes mellitus with other circulatory complications**

● **E1Ø.6** **Type 1 diabetes mellitus with other specified complications**

● **E1Ø.61** **Type 1 diabetes mellitus with diabetic arthropathy**

E1Ø.61Ø **Type 1 diabetes mellitus with diabetic neuropathic arthropathy**
Type 1 diabetes mellitus with Charcôt's joints

E1Ø.618 **Type 1 diabetes mellitus with other diabetic arthropathy**

● **E1Ø.62** **Type 1 diabetes mellitus with skin complications**

E1Ø.62Ø **Type 1 diabetes mellitus with diabetic dermatitis**
Type 1 diabetes mellitus with diabetic necrobiosis lipoidica

E1Ø.621 **Type 1 diabetes mellitus with foot ulcer**
Use additional code to identify site of ulcer (L97.4-, L97.5-)

E1Ø.622 **Type 1 diabetes mellitus with other skin ulcer**
Use additional code to identify site of ulcer (L97.1-L97.9, L98.41-L98.49)

E1Ø.628 **Type 1 diabetes mellitus with other skin complications**

● **E1Ø.63** **Type 1 diabetes mellitus with oral complications**

E1Ø.63Ø **Type 1 diabetes mellitus with periodontal disease**

E1Ø.638 **Type 1 diabetes mellitus with other oral complications**

● **E1Ø.64** **Type 1 diabetes mellitus with hypoglycemia**
▶Use additional code for hypoglycemia level, if applicable (E16.A-)

E1Ø.641 **Type 1 diabetes mellitus with hypoglycemia with coma** (Ex) PDX 581

E1Ø.649 **Type 1 diabetes mellitus with hypoglycemia without coma**
Coding Clinic: 2Ø16, Q1, P13

E1Ø.65 **Type 1 diabetes mellitus with hyperglycemia**
Coding Clinic: 2Ø22, Q1, P29; 2Ø13, Q3, P2Ø

E1Ø.69 **Type 1 diabetes mellitus with other specified complication**
Use additional code to identify complication
Coding Clinic: 2Ø22, Q1, P29

E1Ø.8 **Type 1 diabetes mellitus with unspecified complications**

E1Ø.9 **Type 1 diabetes mellitus without complications**

▶**E1Ø.A** **Type 1 diabetes mellitus, presymptomatic**
▶Early-stage type 1 diabetes mellitus

▶**E1Ø.AØ** **Type 1 diabetes mellitus, presymptomatic, unspecified**

▶**E1Ø.A1** **Type 1 diabetes mellitus, presymptomatic, Stage 1**
▶Multiple confirmed islet autoantibodies with normoglycemia

▶**E1Ø.A2** **Type 1 diabetes mellitus, presymptomatic, Stage 2**
▶Confirmed islet autoimmunity with dysglycemia

● **E11** **Type 2 diabetes mellitus**

Includes diabetes (mellitus) due to insulin secretory defect
diabetes NOS
insulin resistant diabetes (mellitus)

Use additional code to identify control using:
▶injectable non-insulin antidiabetic drugs (Z79.85)
insulin (Z79.4)
oral antidiabetic drugs (Z79.84)
oral hypoglycemic drugs (Z79.84)

Excludes1 diabetes mellitus due to underlying condition (EØ8.-)
drug or chemical induced diabetes mellitus (EØ9.-)
gestational diabetes (O24.4-)
neonatal diabetes mellitus (P7Ø.2)
postpancreatectomy diabetes mellitus (E13.-)
postprocedural diabetes mellitus (E13.-)
secondary diabetes mellitus NEC (E13.-)
type 1 diabetes mellitus (E1Ø.-)

Coding Clinic: 2023, Q2, P1Ø; 2Ø2Ø, Q1, P12; 2Ø16, Q4, P121, Q2, P1Ø

● **E11.Ø** **Type 2 diabetes mellitus with hyperosmolarity** (Ex) PDX 578

E11.ØØ **Type 2 diabetes mellitus with hyperosmolarity without nonketotic hyperglycemic-hyperosmolar coma (NKHHC)**
Coding Clinic: 2Ø22, Q1, P28

E11.Ø1 **Type 2 diabetes mellitus with hyperosmolarity with coma**

● **E11.1** **Type 2 diabetes mellitus with ketoacidosis** (Ex) PDX 578

E11.1Ø **Type 2 diabetes mellitus with ketoacidosis without coma**
Coding Clinic: 2Ø17, Q4, P6

E11.11 **Type 2 diabetes mellitus with ketoacidosis with coma**

CHAPTER 4 (EØØ-E89)

● **E11.2 Type 2 diabetes mellitus with kidney complications**

E11.21 Type 2 diabetes mellitus with diabetic nephropathy

Type 2 diabetes mellitus with intercapillary glomerulosclerosis

Type 2 diabetes mellitus with intracapillary glomerulonephrosis

Type 2 diabetes mellitus with Kimmelstiel-Wilson disease

Coding Clinic: 2019, Q3, P3

E11.22 Type 2 diabetes mellitus with diabetic chronic kidney disease

Use additional code to identify stage of chronic kidney disease (N18.1-N18.6)

Coding Clinic: 2022, Q3, P16; 2019, Q3, P3; 2018, Q4, P88; 2016, Q2, P36, Q1, P13

E11.29 Type 2 diabetes mellitus with other diabetic kidney complication

Type 2 diabetes mellitus with renal tubular degeneration

● **E11.3 Type 2 diabetes mellitus with ophthalmic complications**

Coding Clinic: 2016, Q4, P11

● **E11.31 Type 2 diabetes mellitus with unspecified diabetic retinopathy**

E11.311 Type 2 diabetes mellitus with unspecified diabetic retinopathy with macular edema

E11.319 Type 2 diabetes mellitus with unspecified diabetic retinopathy without macular edema

Coding Clinic: 2013, Q3, P20

● **E11.32 Type 2 diabetes mellitus with mild nonproliferative diabetic retinopathy**

Type 2 diabetes mellitus with nonproliferative diabetic retinopathy NOS

One of the following 7th characters is to be assigned to codes in subcategory E11.32 to designate laterality of the disease:

1	right eye
2	left eye
3	bilateral
9	unspecified eye

● **E11.321 Type 2 diabetes mellitus with mild nonproliferative diabetic retinopathy with macular edema**

● **E11.329 Type 2 diabetes mellitus with mild nonproliferative diabetic retinopathy without macular edema**

● **E11.33 Type 2 diabetes mellitus with moderate nonproliferative diabetic retinopathy**

One of the following 7th characters is to be assigned to codes in subcategory E11.33 to designate laterality of the disease:

1	right eye
2	left eye
3	bilateral
9	unspecified eye

● **E11.331 Type 2 diabetes mellitus with moderate nonproliferative diabetic retinopathy with macular edema**

● **E11.339 Type 2 diabetes mellitus with moderate nonproliferative diabetic retinopathy without macular edema**

● **E11.34 Type 2 diabetes mellitus with severe nonproliferative diabetic retinopathy**

One of the following 7th characters is to be assigned to codes in subcategory E11.34 to designate laterality of the disease:

1	right eye
2	left eye
3	bilateral
9	unspecified eye

● **E11.341 Type 2 diabetes mellitus with severe nonproliferative diabetic retinopathy with macular edema**

● **E11.349 Type 2 diabetes mellitus with severe nonproliferative diabetic retinopathy without macular edema**

● **E11.35 Type 2 diabetes mellitus with proliferative diabetic retinopathy**

One of the following 7th characters is to be assigned to codes in subcategory E11.35 to designate laterality of the disease:

1	right eye
2	left eye
3	bilateral
9	unspecified eye

● **E11.351 Type 2 diabetes mellitus with proliferative diabetic retinopathy with macular edema**

● **E11.352 Type 2 diabetes mellitus with proliferative diabetic retinopathy with traction retinal detachment involving the macula**

● **E11.353 Type 2 diabetes mellitus with proliferative diabetic retinopathy with traction retinal detachment not involving the macula**

● **E11.354 Type 2 diabetes mellitus with proliferative diabetic retinopathy with combined traction retinal detachment and rhegmatogenous retinal detachment**

● **E11.355 Type 2 diabetes mellitus with stable proliferative diabetic retinopathy**

● **E11.359 Type 2 diabetes mellitus with proliferative diabetic retinopathy without macular edema**

E11.36 Type 2 diabetes mellitus with diabetic cataract

Coding Clinic: 2019, Q2, P30-31; 2016, Q2, P36

X● **E11.37 Type 2 diabetes mellitus with diabetic macular edema, resolved following treatment**

One of the following 7th characters is to be assigned to code E11.37 to designate laterality of the disease:

1	right eye
2	left eye
3	bilateral
9	unspecified eye

E11.39 Type 2 diabetes mellitus with other diabetic ophthalmic complication

Use additional code to identify manifestation, such as:

diabetic glaucoma (H40-H42)

Coding Clinic: 2023, Q3, P19

CHAPTER 4 (E00-E89)

● E11.4 Type 2 diabetes mellitus with neurological complications
Coding Clinic: 2022, Q3, P16

E11.40 Type 2 diabetes mellitus with diabetic neuropathy, unspecified

E11.41 Type 2 diabetes mellitus with diabetic mononeuropathy

E11.42 Type 2 diabetes mellitus with diabetic polyneuropathy
Type 2 diabetes mellitus with diabetic neuralgia
Coding Clinic: 2020, Q1, P12; 2016, Q1, P13

E11.43 Type 2 diabetes mellitus with diabetic autonomic (poly)neuropathy
Type 2 diabetes mellitus with diabetic gastroparesis
Coding Clinic: 2023, Q2, P9; 2016, Q2, P36

E11.44 Type 2 diabetes mellitus with diabetic amyotrophy
Coding Clinic: 2022, Q3, P15; 2016, Q2, P36

E11.49 Type 2 diabetes mellitus with other diabetic neurological complication

● E11.5 Type 2 diabetes mellitus with circulatory complications

E11.51 Type 2 diabetes mellitus with diabetic peripheral angiopathy without gangrene

E11.52 Type 2 diabetes mellitus with diabetic peripheral angiopathy with gangrene (Ex) PDX 583
Type 2 diabetes mellitus with diabetic gangrene
CC when PDx is its own CC
Coding Clinic: 2017, Q4, P102

E11.59 Type 2 diabetes mellitus with other circulatory complications

● E11.6 Type 2 diabetes mellitus with other specified complications

● E11.61 Type 2 diabetes mellitus with diabetic arthropathy

E11.610 Type 2 diabetes mellitus with diabetic neuropathic arthropathy
Type 2 diabetes mellitus with Charcôt's joints
Coding Clinic: 2016, Q2, P36

E11.618 Type 2 diabetes mellitus with other diabetic arthropathy
Coding Clinic: 2018, Q2, P7; 2016, Q2, P36

● E11.62 Type 2 diabetes mellitus with skin complications

E11.620 Type 2 diabetes mellitus with diabetic dermatitis
Type 2 diabetes mellitus with diabetic necrobiosis lipoidica

E11.621 Type 2 diabetes mellitus with foot ulcer
Use additional code to identify site of ulcer (L97.4-, L97.5-)
Coding Clinic: 2020, Q1, P12; 2016, Q1, P12

E11.622 Type 2 diabetes mellitus with other skin ulcer
Use additional code to identify site of ulcer (L97.1-L97.9, L98.41-L98.49)
Coding Clinic: 2021, Q1, P8; 2017, Q4, P17

E11.628 Type 2 diabetes mellitus with other skin complications

● E11.63 Type 2 diabetes mellitus with oral complications

E11.630 Type 2 diabetes mellitus with periodontal disease

E11.638 Type 2 diabetes mellitus with other oral complications

● E11.64 Type 2 diabetes mellitus with hypoglycemia
▶ Use additional code for hypoglycemia level, if applicable (E16.A-)

E11.641 Type 2 diabetes mellitus with hypoglycemia with coma (Ex) PDX 578

E11.649 Type 2 diabetes mellitus with hypoglycemia without coma
Coding Clinic: 2016, Q3, P42; 2015, Q3, P21

E11.65 Type 2 diabetes mellitus with hyperglycemia
Coding Clinic: 2023, Q2, P10; 2022, Q1, P28; 2013, Q3, P20

E11.69 Type 2 diabetes mellitus with other specified complication
Use additional code to identify complication
Coding Clinic: 2020, Q1, P12; 2016, Q4, P142

E11.8 Type 2 diabetes mellitus with unspecified complications

E11.9 Type 2 diabetes mellitus without complications
MCE: Questionable admission when principal dx
Coding Clinic: 2023, Q3, P19; 2016, Q4, P142, Q2, P36

● E13 Other specified diabetes mellitus

Includes diabetes mellitus due to genetic defects of beta-cell function
diabetes mellitus due to genetic defects in insulin action
postpancreatectomy diabetes mellitus
postprocedural diabetes mellitus
secondary diabetes mellitus NEC

Use additional code to identify control using:
▶ injectable non-insulin antidiabetic drugs (Z79.85)
insulin (Z79.4)
oral antidiabetic drugs (Z79.84)
oral hypoglycemic drugs (Z79.84)

Excludes1 diabetes (mellitus) due to autoimmune process (E10.-)
diabetes (mellitus) due to immune mediated pancreatic islet beta-cell destruction (E10.-)
diabetes mellitus due to underlying condition (E08.-)
drug or chemical induced diabetes mellitus (E09.-)
gestational diabetes (O24.4-)
neonatal diabetes mellitus (P70.2)
type 1 diabetes mellitus (E10.-)

● E13.0 Other specified diabetes mellitus with hyperosmolarity (Ex) PDX 578

E13.00 Other specified diabetes mellitus with hyperosmolarity without nonketotic hyperglycemic-hyperosmolar coma (NKHHC)

E13.01 Other specified diabetes mellitus with hyperosmolarity with coma

● E13.1 Other specified diabetes mellitus with ketoacidosis (Ex) PDX 578

E13.10 Other specified diabetes mellitus with ketoacidosis without coma
Coding Clinic: 2016, Q2, P10; 2013, Q1, P26

E13.11 Other specified diabetes mellitus with ketoacidosis with coma

● E13.2 Other specified diabetes mellitus with kidney complications

E13.21 Other specified diabetes mellitus with diabetic nephropathy
Other specified diabetes mellitus with intercapillary glomerulosclerosis
Other specified diabetes mellitus with intracapillary glomerulonephrosis
Other specified diabetes mellitus with Kimmelstiel-Wilson disease

E13.22 Other specified diabetes mellitus with diabetic chronic kidney disease

Use additional code to identify stage of chronic kidney disease (N18.1-N18.6)

E13.29 Other specified diabetes mellitus with other diabetic kidney complication

Other specified diabetes mellitus with renal tubular degeneration

● E13.3 Other specified diabetes mellitus with ophthalmic complications

Coding Clinic: 2016, Q4, P11

● E13.31 Other specified diabetes mellitus with unspecified diabetic retinopathy

E13.311 Other specified diabetes mellitus with unspecified diabetic retinopathy with macular edema

E13.319 Other specified diabetes mellitus with unspecified diabetic retinopathy without macular edema

● E13.32 Other specified diabetes mellitus with mild nonproliferative diabetic retinopathy

Other specified diabetes mellitus with nonproliferative diabetic retinopathy NOS

One of the following 7th characters is to be assigned to codes in subcategory E13.32 to designate laterality of the disease:

1	right eye
2	left eye
3	bilateral
9	unspecified eye

● E13.321 Other specified diabetes mellitus with mild nonproliferative diabetic retinopathy with macular edema

● E13.329 Other specified diabetes mellitus with mild nonproliferative diabetic retinopathy without macular edema

● E13.33 Other specified diabetes mellitus with moderate nonproliferative diabetic retinopathy

One of the following 7th characters is to be assigned to codes in subcategory E13.33 to designate laterality of the disease:

1	right eye
2	left eye
3	bilateral
9	unspecified eye

● E13.331 Other specified diabetes mellitus with moderate nonproliferative diabetic retinopathy with macular edema

● E13.339 Other specified diabetes mellitus with moderate nonproliferative diabetic retinopathy without macular edema

● E13.34 Other specified diabetes mellitus with severe nonproliferative diabetic retinopathy

One of the following 7th characters is to be assigned to codes in subcategory E13.34 to designate laterality of the disease:

1	right eye
2	left eye
3	bilateral
9	unspecified eye

● E13.341 Other specified diabetes mellitus with severe nonproliferative diabetic retinopathy with macular edema

● E13.349 Other specified diabetes mellitus with severe nonproliferative diabetic retinopathy without macular edema

● E13.35 Other specified diabetes mellitus with proliferative diabetic retinopathy

One of the following 7th characters is to be assigned to codes in subcategory E13.35 to designate laterality of the disease:

1	right eye
2	left eye
3	bilateral
9	unspecified eye

● E13.351 Other specified diabetes mellitus with proliferative diabetic retinopathy with macular edema

● E13.352 Other specified diabetes mellitus with proliferative diabetic retinopathy with traction retinal detachment involving the macula

● E13.353 Other specified diabetes mellitus with proliferative diabetic retinopathy with traction retinal detachment not involving the macula

● E13.354 Other specified diabetes mellitus with proliferative diabetic retinopathy with combined traction retinal detachment and rhegmatogenous retinal detachment

● E13.355 Other specified diabetes mellitus with stable proliferative diabetic retinopathy

● E13.359 Other specified diabetes mellitus with proliferative diabetic retinopathy without macular edema

E13.36 Other specified diabetes mellitus with diabetic cataract

X● E13.37 Other specified diabetes mellitus with diabetic macular edema, resolved following treatment

One of the following 7th characters is to be assigned to code E13.37 to designate laterality of the disease:

1	right eye
2	left eye
3	bilateral
9	unspecified eye

E13.39 Other specified diabetes mellitus with other diabetic ophthalmic complication

Use additional code to identify manifestation, such as:

diabetic glaucoma (H40-H42)

● E13.4 Other specified diabetes mellitus with neurological complications

E13.40 Other specified diabetes mellitus with diabetic neuropathy, unspecified

E13.41 Other specified diabetes mellitus with diabetic mononeuropathy

E13.42 Other specified diabetes mellitus with diabetic polyneuropathy

Other specified diabetes mellitus with diabetic neuralgia

E13.43 Other specified diabetes mellitus with diabetic autonomic (poly)neuropathy

Other specified diabetes mellitus with diabetic gastroparesis

E13.44 Other specified diabetes mellitus with diabetic amyotrophy

E13.49 Other specified diabetes mellitus with other diabetic neurological complication

CHAPTER 4 (E00-E89)

E13.5 Other specified diabetes mellitus with circulatory complications

E13.51 **Other specified diabetes mellitus with diabetic peripheral angiopathy without gangrene**

E13.52 **Other specified diabetes mellitus with diabetic peripheral angiopathy with gangrene** PDX 584
Other specified diabetes mellitus with diabetic gangrene
CC when PDx is its own CC

E13.59 **Other specified diabetes mellitus with other circulatory complications**

E13.6 Other specified diabetes mellitus with other specified complications

E13.61 Other specified diabetes mellitus with diabetic arthropathy

E13.610 **Other specified diabetes mellitus with diabetic neuropathic arthropathy**
Other specified diabetes mellitus with Charcôt's joints

E13.618 **Other specified diabetes mellitus with other diabetic arthropathy**

E13.62 Other specified diabetes mellitus with skin complications

E13.620 **Other specified diabetes mellitus with diabetic dermatitis**
Other specified diabetes mellitus with diabetic necrobiosis lipoidica

E13.621 **Other specified diabetes mellitus with foot ulcer**
Use additional code to identify site of ulcer (L97.4-, L97.5-)

E13.622 **Other specified diabetes mellitus with other skin ulcer**
Use additional code to identify site of ulcer (L97.1-L97.9, L98.41-L98.49)

E13.628 **Other specified diabetes mellitus with other skin complications**

E13.63 Other specified diabetes mellitus with oral complications

E13.630 **Other specified diabetes mellitus with periodontal disease**

E13.638 **Other specified diabetes mellitus with other oral complications**

E13.64 Other specified diabetes mellitus with hypoglycemia
Use additional code for hypoglycemia level, if applicable (E16.A-)

E13.641 **Other specified diabetes mellitus with hypoglycemia with coma** PDX 578

E13.649 **Other specified diabetes mellitus with hypoglycemia without coma**

E13.65 **Other specified diabetes mellitus with hyperglycemia**

E13.69 **Other specified diabetes mellitus with other specified complication**
Use additional code to identify complication

E13.8 Other specified diabetes mellitus with unspecified complications

E13.9 Other specified diabetes mellitus without complications
MCE: Questionable admission when principal dx

OTHER DISORDERS OF GLUCOSE REGULATION AND PANCREATIC INTERNAL SECRETION (E15-E16)

E15 Nondiabetic hypoglycemic coma PDX 581
Includes drug-induced insulin coma in nondiabetic
hyperinsulinism with hypoglycemic coma
hypoglycemic coma NOS

E16 Other disorders of pancreatic internal secretion

E16.0 **Drug-induced hypoglycemia without coma**
Excludes1 diabetes with hypoglycemia without coma (E09.649)
Use additional ~~code for adverse effect, if applicable, to identify drug (T36-T50 with fifth or sixth character 5)~~ code for hypoglycemia level, if applicable (E16.A-)

E16.1 **Other hypoglycemia**
Functional hyperinsulinism
Functional nonhyperinsulinemic hypoglycemia
Hyperinsulinism NOS
Hyperplasia of pancreatic islet beta cells NOS
Excludes1 diabetes with hypoglycemia (E08.649, E10.649, E11.649, E13.649)
hypoglycemia in infant of diabetic mother (P70.1)
neonatal hypoglycemia (P70.4)
Use additional code for hypoglycemia level, if applicable (E16.A-)
Coding Clinic: 2024, Q2, P10

E16.2 **Hypoglycemia, unspecified**
Excludes1 diabetes with hypoglycemia (E08.649, E10.649, E11.649, E13.649)
Use additional code for hypoglycemia level, if applicable (E16.A-)
Coding Clinic: 2016, Q3, P42

E16.3 **Increased secretion of glucagon**
Hyperplasia of pancreatic endocrine cells with glucagon excess

E16.4 **Increased secretion of gastrin**
Hypergastrinemia
Hyperplasia of pancreatic endocrine cells with gastrin excess
Zollinger-Ellison syndrome

E16.8 **Other specified disorders of pancreatic internal secretion**
Increased secretion from endocrine pancreas of growth hormone-releasing hormone
Increased secretion from endocrine pancreas of pancreatic polypeptide
Increased secretion from endocrine pancreas of somatostatin
Increased secretion from endocrine pancreas of vasoactive-intestinal polypeptide

E16.9 **Disorder of pancreatic internal secretion, unspecified**
Islet-cell hyperplasia NOS
Pancreatic endocrine cell hyperplasia NOS

E16.A **Hypoglycemia level**

E16.A1 **Hypoglycemia level 1**
Decreased blood glucose level 1

E16.A2 **Hypoglycemia level 2**
Decreased blood glucose level 2

E16.A3 **Hypoglycemia level 3**
Decreased blood glucose level 3

CHAPTER 4 (E00-E89)

DISORDERS OF OTHER ENDOCRINE GLANDS (E20-E35)

Excludes1 galactorrhea (N64.3)
gynecomastia (N62)

E20 Hypoparathyroidism
Greatly reduced function of parathyroid glands; AKA parathyroid insufficiency
Excludes1 Di George's syndrome (D82.1)
postprocedural hypoparathyroidism (E89.2)
tetany NOS (R29.0)
transitory neonatal hypoparathyroidism (P71.4)

E20.0 Idiopathic hypoparathyroidism
Rare condition, unknown cause; short dwarf-like with round face

E20.1 Pseudohypoparathyroidism
Hereditary condition resembling hypoparathyroidism, but caused by inability to respond to parathyroid hormone

E20.8 Other hypoparathyroidism

E20.81 Hypoparathyroidism due to impaired parathyroid hormone secretion

E20.810 Autosomal dominant hypocalcemia
Autosomal dominant hypocalcemia type 1 (ADH1)
Autosomal dominant hypocalcemia type 2 (ADH2)
Code also, if applicable, any associated conditions, such as:
calculus of kidney (N20.0)
chronic kidney disease (N18.-)
respiratory distress (J80, R06.-)
seizure disorder (G40.-, R56.9)

E20.811 Secondary hypoparathyroidism in diseases classified elsewhere
Code first underlying condition, if known

E20.812 Autoimmune hypoparathyroidism
Code first, if applicable, underlying condition such as:
autoimmune polyglandular failure (E31.0)
Schmidt's syndrome (E31.0)

E20.818 Other specified hypoparathyroidism due to impaired parathyroid hormonesecretion
Familial isolated hypoparathyroidism

E20.819 Hypoparathyroidism due to impaired parathyroid hormone secretion,unspecified

E20.89 Other specified hypoparathyroidism
Familial hypoparathyroidism

E20.9 Hypoparathyroidism, unspecified
Parathyroid tetany

E21 Hyperparathyroidism and other disorders of parathyroid gland
Excludes1 adult osteomalacia (M83.-)
ectopic hyperparathyroidism (E34.2)
hungry bone syndrome (E83.81)
infantile and juvenile osteomalacia (E55.0)
Excludes2 familial hypocalciuric hypercalcemia (E83.52)

E21.0 Primary hyperparathyroidism
Hyperplasia of parathyroid
Osteitis fibrosa cystica generalisata [von Recklinghausen's disease of bone]

E21.1 Secondary hyperparathyroidism, not elsewhere classified
Excludes1 secondary hyperparathyroidism of renal origin (N25.81)

Item 4-4 Hyperparathyroidism is an overactive parathyroid gland that secretes excessive parathormone, causing increased levels of circulating calcium. This results in a loss of calcium in the bone (osteoporosis).

Hypoparathyroidism is an underactive parathyroid gland that results in decreased levels of circulating calcium. The primary manifestation is **tetany,** a continuous muscle spasm.

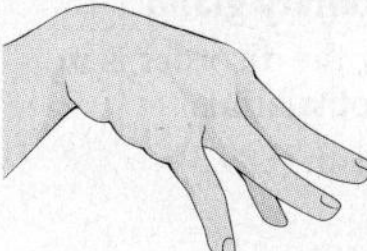

Figure 4-4 Tetany caused by hypoparathyroidism.

E21.2 Other hyperparathyroidism
Tertiary hyperparathyroidism
Excludes1 familial hypocalciuric hypercalcemia (E83.52)

E21.3 Hyperparathyroidism, unspecified

E21.4 Other specified disorders of parathyroid gland

E21.5 Disorder of parathyroid gland, unspecified

E22 Hyperfunction of pituitary gland (Ex:) PDX 585
Excludes1 Cushing's syndrome (E24.-)
Nelson's syndrome (E24.1)
overproduction of ACTH not associated with Cushing's disease (E27.0)
overproduction of pituitary ACTH (E24.0)
overproduction of thyroid-stimulating hormone (E05.8-)

E22.0 Acromegaly and pituitary gigantism
Chronic disease caused by hypersecretion of growth hormone
Overproduction of growth hormone
Excludes1 constitutional gigantism (E34.4)
constitutional tall stature (E34.4)
increased secretion from endocrine pancreas of growth hormone-releasing hormone (E16.8)

E22.1 Hyperprolactinemia
Increased levels of prolactin
Use additional code for adverse effect, if applicable, to identify drug (T36-T50 with fifth or sixth character 5)

E22.2 Syndrome of inappropriate secretion of antidiuretic hormone (Ex:) PDX 586

E22.8 Other hyperfunction of pituitary gland
Central precocious puberty

E22.9 Hyperfunction of pituitary gland, unspecified

Item 4-5 Hyperadrenalism is overactivity of the adrenal cortex, which secretes corticosteroid hormones. Excessive glucocorticoid hormone results in hyperglycemia **(Cushing's syndrome),** and excessive aldosterone results in **Conn's syndrome. Adrenogenital syndrome** is the result of excessive secretion of androgens, male hormones, which stimulates premature sexual development. **Hypoadrenalism, Addison's disease,** is a condition in which the adrenal glands atrophy.

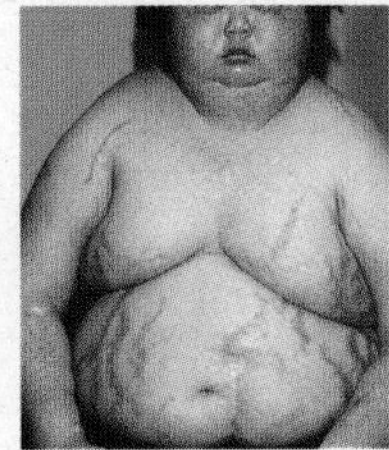

Figure 4-5 Centripetal and generalized obesity and dorsal kyphosis in a woman with Cushing's disease. (From Salvo SG: Mosby's Pathology for Massage Therapists, St. Louis, MO: Mosby/Elsevier, 2009)

CHAPTER 4 (E00-E89)

E23 Hypofunction and other disorders of the pituitary gland

Includes the listed conditions whether the disorder is in the pituitary or the hypothalamus

Excludes1 postprocedural hypopituitarism (E89.3)

E23.0 Hypopituitarism Ex: PDX 587
Fertile eunuch syndrome
Hypogonadotropic hypogonadism
Idiopathic growth hormone deficiency
Isolated deficiency of gonadotropin
Isolated deficiency of growth hormone
Isolated deficiency of pituitary hormone
Kallmann's syndrome
Lorain-Levi short stature
Necrosis of pituitary gland (postpartum)
Panhypopituitarism
Pituitary cachexia
Pituitary insufficiency NOS
Pituitary short stature
Sheehan's syndrome
Simmonds' disease
Coding Clinic: 2024, Q1, P15

E23.1 Drug-induced hypopituitarism
Use additional code for adverse effect, if applicable, to identify drug (T36-T50 with fifth or sixth character 5)

E23.2 Diabetes insipidus Ex: PDX 588
Excludes1 nephrogenic diabetes insipidus (N25.1)

E23.3 Hypothalamic dysfunction, not elsewhere classified
Excludes1 Prader-Willi syndrome (Q87.11)
Russell-Silver syndrome (Q87.19)
Coding Clinic: 2024, Q1, P15

E23.6 Other disorders of pituitary gland
Abscess of pituitary
Adiposogenital dystrophy

E23.7 Disorder of pituitary gland, unspecified

E24 Cushing's syndrome Ex: PDX 589

Excludes1 congenital adrenal hyperplasia (E25.0)

E24.0 Pituitary-dependent Cushing's disease
Overproduction of pituitary ACTH
Pituitary-dependent hypercorticalism

E24.1 Nelson's syndrome

E24.2 Drug-induced Cushing's syndrome
Use additional code for adverse effect, if applicable, to identify drug (T36-T50 with fifth or sixth character 5)

E24.3 Ectopic ACTH syndrome

E24.4 Alcohol-induced pseudo-Cushing's syndrome

E24.8 Other Cushing's syndrome

E24.9 Cushing's syndrome, unspecified

E25 Adrenogenital disorders
Disorder of production of steroid hormone in adrenal gland

Includes adrenogenital syndromes, virilizing or feminizing, whether acquired or due to adrenal hyperplasia consequent on inborn enzyme defects in hormone synthesis
female adrenal pseudohermaphroditism
female heterosexual precocious pseudopuberty
male isosexual precocious pseudopuberty
male macrogenitosomia praecox
male sexual precocity with adrenal hyperplasia
male virilization (female)

Excludes1 indeterminate sex and pseudohermaphroditism (Q56)
chromosomal abnormalities (Q90-Q99)

E25.0 Congenital adrenogenital disorders associated with enzyme deficiency
Congenital adrenal hyperplasia
21-Hydroxylase deficiency
Salt-losing congenital adrenal hyperplasia

E25.8 Other adrenogenital disorders
Idiopathic adrenogenital disorder
Use additional code for adverse effect, if applicable, to identify drug (T36-T50 with fifth or sixth character 5)

E25.9 Adrenogenital disorder, unspecified
Adrenogenital syndrome NOS

E26 Hyperaldosteronism
Abnormality of electrolyte metabolism caused by excessive secretion of aldosterone

E26.0 Primary hyperaldosteronism

E26.01 Conn's syndrome
Code also adrenal adenoma (D35.0-)

E26.02 Glucocorticoid-remediable aldosteronism
Familial aldosteronism type I

E26.09 Other primary hyperaldosteronism
Primary aldosteronism due to adrenal hyperplasia (bilateral)

E26.1 Secondary hyperaldosteronism

E26.8 Other hyperaldosteronism

E26.81 Bartter's syndrome

E26.89 Other hyperaldosteronism

E26.9 Hyperaldosteronism, unspecified
Aldosteronism NOS
Hyperaldosteronism NOS

E27 Other disorders of adrenal gland Ex: PDX 590

E27.0 Other adrenocortical overactivity
Overproduction of ACTH, not associated with Cushing's disease
Premature adrenarche
Excludes1 Cushing's syndrome (E24.-)

E27.1 Primary adrenocortical insufficiency
Addison's disease
Autoimmune adrenalitis
Excludes1 Addison only phenotype adrenoleukodystrophy (E71.528)
amyloidosis (E85.-)
tuberculous Addison's disease (A18.7)
Waterhouse-Friderichsen syndrome (A39.1)

E27.2 Addisonian crisis
Acute onset of adrenocortical insufficiency
Adrenal crisis
Adrenocortical crisis

E27.3 Drug-induced adrenocortical insufficiency
Use additional code for adverse effect, if applicable, to identify drug (T36-T50 with fifth or sixth character 5)

E27.4 Other and unspecified adrenocortical insufficiency
Excludes1 adrenoleukodystrophy [Addison-Schilder] (E71.528)
Waterhouse-Friderichsen syndrome (A39.1)

E27.40 Unspecified adrenocortical insufficiency
Adrenocortical insufficiency NOS
Hypoaldosteronism
Coding Clinic: 2024, Q1, P15

E27.49 Other adrenocortical insufficiency
Adrenal hemorrhage
Adrenal infarction
Coding Clinic: 2024, Q1, P15

E27.5 Adrenomedullary hyperfunction
Adrenomedullary hyperplasia
Catecholamine hypersecretion

E27.8 Other specified disorders of adrenal gland
Abnormality of cortisol-binding globulin

E27.9 Disorder of adrenal gland, unspecified

E28 Ovarian dysfunction
Excludes1 isolated gonadotropin deficiency (E23.0)
postprocedural ovarian failure (E89.4-)

E28.0 Estrogen excess
Use additional code for adverse effect, if applicable, to identify drug (T36-T50 with fifth or sixth character 5)

E28.1 Androgen excess
Hypersecretion of ovarian androgens
Use additional code for adverse effect, if applicable, to identify drug (T36-T50 with fifth or sixth character 5)

E28.2 Polycystic ovarian syndrome
Sclerocystic ovary syndrome
Stein-Leventhal syndrome
Coding Clinic: 2022, Q2, P16

E28.3 Primary ovarian failure
Excludes1 pure gonadal dysgenesis (Q99.1)
Turner's syndrome (Q96.-)

E28.31 Premature menopause

E28.310 Symptomatic premature menopause A
Symptoms such as flushing, sleeplessness, headache, lack of concentration, associated with premature menopause

E28.319 Asymptomatic premature menopause A
Premature menopause NOS

E28.39 Other primary ovarian failure
Decreased estrogen
Resistant ovary syndrome

E28.8 Other ovarian dysfunction
Ovarian hyperfunction NOS
Excludes1 postprocedural ovarian failure (E89.4-)

E28.9 Ovarian dysfunction, unspecified

E29 Testicular dysfunction
Excludes1 androgen insensitivity syndrome (E34.5-)
azoospermia or oligospermia NOS (N46.0-N46.1)
isolated gonadotropin deficiency (E23.0)
Klinefelter's syndrome (Q98.0-Q98.1, Q98.4)

E29.0 Testicular hyperfunction
Hypersecretion of testicular hormones

E29.1 Testicular hypofunction
Defective biosynthesis of testicular androgen NOS
5-delta-Reductase deficiency (with male pseudohermaphroditism)
Testicular hypogonadism NOS
Use additional code for adverse effect, if applicable, to identify drug (T36-T50 with fifth or sixth character 5)
Excludes1 postprocedural testicular hypofunction (E89.5)

E29.8 Other testicular dysfunction

E29.9 Testicular dysfunction, unspecified

E30 Disorders of puberty, not elsewhere classified

E30.0 Delayed puberty
Constitutional delay of puberty
Delayed sexual development

E30.1 Precocious puberty P
Sexual maturation at earlier age than normal, or before age 8 in girls and 9 in boys, usually hormonal; AKA sexual precocity or pubertas praecox
Precocious menstruation
Excludes1 Albright (-McCune) (-Sternberg) syndrome (Q78.1)
central precocious puberty (E22.8)
congenital adrenal hyperplasia (E25.0)
female heterosexual precocious pseudopuberty (E25.-)
male isosexual precocious pseudopuberty (E25.-)

E30.8 Other disorders of puberty P
Premature thelarche

E30.9 Disorder of puberty, unspecified

E31 Polyglandular dysfunction
Excludes1 ataxia telangiectasia [Louis-Bar] (G11.3)
dystrophia myotonica [Steinert] (G71.11)
pseudohypoparathyroidism (E20.1)

E31.0 Autoimmune polyglandular failure
Schmidt's syndrome

E31.1 Polyglandular hyperfunction
Excludes1 multiple endocrine adenomatosis (E31.2-)
multiple endocrine neoplasia (E31.2-)

E31.2 Multiple endocrine neoplasia [MEN] syndromes
Adenomatous hyperplasia and malignant tumors in endocrine glands
Multiple endocrine adenomatosis
Code also any associated malignancies and other conditions associated with the syndromes

E31.20 Multiple endocrine neoplasia [MEN] syndrome, unspecified
Multiple endocrine adenomatosis NOS
Multiple endocrine neoplasia [MEN] syndrome NOS

E31.21 Multiple endocrine neoplasia [MEN] type I
Wermer's syndrome

E31.22 Multiple endocrine neoplasia [MEN] type IIA
Sipple's syndrome

E31.23 Multiple endocrine neoplasia [MEN] type IIB

E31.8 Other polyglandular dysfunction

E31.9 Polyglandular dysfunction, unspecified

E32 Diseases of thymus
Excludes1 aplasia or hypoplasia of thymus with immunodeficiency (D82.1)
myasthenia gravis (G70.0)

E32.0 Persistent hyperplasia of thymus
Hypertrophy of thymus

E32.1 Abscess of thymus (Ex) PDX 591

E32.8 Other diseases of thymus
Excludes1 aplasia or hypoplasia with immunodeficiency (D82.1)
thymoma (D15.0)

E32.9 Disease of thymus, unspecified

E34 Other endocrine disorders
Excludes1 pseudohypoparathyroidism (E20.1)

E34.0 Carcinoid syndrome (Ex) PDX 592
~~Note: May be used as an additional code to identify functional activity associated with a carcinoid tumor.~~
▶Code also the underlying disorder, such as:
▶primary neuroendocrine tumors (C7A.-)
▶secondary neuroendocrine tumors (C7B.-)

▶**E34.00 Carcinoid syndrome, unspecified**
▶Carcinoid disease, unspecified

▶**E34.01 Carcinoid heart syndrome**
▶Carcinoid heart disease
▶Hedinger syndrome

▶**E34.09 Other carcinoid syndrome**
▶Carcinoid disease NEC
▶Carcinoid syndrome NEC
▶Other carcinoid disease

E34.1 Other hypersecretion of intestinal hormones

E34.2 Ectopic hormone secretion, not elsewhere classified
Excludes1 ectopic ACTH syndrome (E24.3)

CHAPTER 4 (E00-E89)

E34.3 Short stature due to endocrine disorder

Excludes1 achondroplastic short stature (Q77.4)
hypochondroplastic short stature (Q77.4)
nutritional short stature (E45)
pituitary short stature (E23.0)
progeria (E34.8)
renal short stature (N25.0)
Russell-Silver syndrome (Q87.19)
short-limbed stature with immunodeficiency (D82.2)
short stature due to endocrine disorder (E34.3-)
short stature in specific dysmorphic syndromes - code to syndrome - see Alphabetical Index
short stature NOS (R62.52)

E34.30 Short stature due to endocrine disorder, unspecified

E34.31 Constitutional short stature
Constitutional delay of growth, puberty, or maturation

● **E34.32 Genetic causes of short stature**

E34.321 Primary insulin-like growth factor-1 (IGF-1) deficiency
Acid-labile subunit gene (IGFALS) defect
Growth hormone gene 1 (GH1) defect with growth hormone neutralizing antibodies
Growth hormone insensitivity syndrome (GHIS)
Insulin-like growth factor 1 gene (IGF1) defect
Laron type short stature
Severe primary insulin-like growth factor 1 deficiency (SPIGFD)
Signal transducer and activator of transcription 5B gene (STAT5b) defect

E34.322 Insulin-like growth factor-1 (IGF-1) resistance
Genetic syndrome with resistance to insulin-like growth factor-1
Insulin-like growth factor-1 receptor (IGF-1R) defect
Post-insulin-like growth factor-1 receptor signaling defect

E34.328 Other genetic causes of short stature
Short stature due to ACAN gene variant
Short stature due to aggrecan deficiency
Short stature due to NPR-2 gene variant

E34.329 Unspecified genetic causes of short stature

● **E34.39 Other short stature due to endocrine disorder**

E34.4 Constitutional tall stature
Constitutional gigantism

● **E34.5 Androgen insensitivity syndrome**

E34.50 Androgen insensitivity syndrome, unspecified
Androgen insensitivity NOS

E34.51 Complete androgen insensitivity syndrome
Complete androgen insensitivity
de Quervain syndrome
Goldberg-Maxwell syndrome

E34.52 Partial androgen insensitivity syndrome
Partial androgen insensitivity
Reifenstein syndrome

E34.8 Other specified endocrine disorders
Pineal gland dysfunction
Progeria

Excludes2 pseudohypoparathyroidism (E20.1)

E34.9 Endocrine disorder, unspecified
Endocrine disturbance NOS
Hormone disturbance NOS

E35 *Disorders of endocrine glands in diseases classified elsewhere*

Code first underlying disease, such as:
late congenital syphilis of thymus gland [Dubois disease] (A50.9)

Use additional code, if applicable, to identify:
sequelae of tuberculosis of other organs (B90.8)

Excludes1 Echinococcus granulosus infection of thyroid gland (B67.3)
meningococcal hemorrhagic adrenalitis (A39.1)
syphilis of endocrine gland (A52.79)
tuberculosis of adrenal gland, except calcification (A18.7)
tuberculosis of endocrine gland NEC (A18.82)
tuberculosis of thyroid gland (A18.81)
Waterhouse-Friderichsen syndrome (A39.1)

INTRAOPERATIVE COMPLICATIONS OF ENDOCRINE SYSTEM (E36)

● **E36 Intraoperative complications of endocrine system**

Excludes2 postprocedural endocrine and metabolic complications and disorders, not elsewhere classified (E89.-)

● **E36.0 Intraoperative hemorrhage and hematoma of an endocrine system organ or structure complicating a procedure** Ex PDX 593

Excludes1 intraoperative hemorrhage and hematoma of an endocrine system organ or structure due to accidental puncture or laceration during a procedure (E36.1-)

E36.01 Intraoperative hemorrhage and hematoma of an endocrine system organ or structure complicating an endocrine system procedure
Coding Clinic: 2020, Q1, P19

E36.02 Intraoperative hemorrhage and hematoma of an endocrine system organ or structure complicating other procedure

● **E36.1 Accidental puncture and laceration of an endocrine system organ or structure during a procedure** Ex PDX 569

E36.11 Accidental puncture and laceration of an endocrine system organ or structure during an endocrine system procedure

E36.12 Accidental puncture and laceration of an endocrine system organ or structure during other procedure

E36.8 Other intraoperative complications of endocrine system
Use additional code, if applicable, to further specify disorder

MALNUTRITION (E40-E46)

Excludes1 intestinal malabsorption (K90.-)
sequelae of protein-calorie malnutrition (E64.0)

Excludes2 nutritional anemias (D50-D53)
starvation (T73.0)

E40 Kwashiorkor Ex PDX 594
Malnutrition produced by severe protein deficiency
Severe malnutrition with nutritional edema with dyspigmentation of skin and hair

Excludes1 marasmic kwashiorkor (E42)

Coding Clinic: 2017, Q3, P25

E41 Nutritional marasmus Ex PDX 594
Severe malnutrition with marasmus

Excludes1 marasmic kwashiorkor (E42)

Coding Clinic: 2017, Q3, P24-25

E42 Marasmic kwashiorkor Ex PDX 594
Severe protein malnutrition
Intermediate form severe protein-calorie malnutrition
Severe protein-calorie malnutrition with signs of both kwashiorkor and marasmus

Coding Clinic: 2017, Q3, P25

E43 Unspecified severe protein-calorie malnutrition (Ex) PDX 594
Starvation edema
Coding Clinic: 2023, Q4, P15; 2022, Q1, P13; 2020, Q1, P5-6; 2017, Q4, P108-109; 2017, Q3, P25

● **E44 Protein-calorie malnutrition of moderate and mild degree** (Ex) PDX 594
E44.0 Moderate protein-calorie malnutrition
E44.1 Mild protein-calorie malnutrition

E45 Retarded development following protein-calorie malnutrition (Ex) PDX 594
Nutritional short stature
Nutritional stunting
Physical retardation due to malnutrition

E46 Unspecified protein-calorie malnutrition (Ex) PDX 594
Malnutrition NOS
Protein-calorie imbalance NOS
Excludes1 nutritional deficiency NOS (E63.9)
Coding Clinic: 2017, Q3, P25

OTHER NUTRITIONAL DEFICIENCIES (E50-E64)

Excludes2 nutritional anemias (D50-D53)

● **E50 Vitamin A deficiency**
Excludes1 sequelae of vitamin A deficiency (E64.1)
E50.0 Vitamin A deficiency with conjunctival xerosis
E50.1 Vitamin A deficiency with Bitot's spot and conjunctival xerosis
Bitot's spot in the young child
E50.2 Vitamin A deficiency with corneal xerosis
E50.3 Vitamin A deficiency with corneal ulceration and xerosis
E50.4 Vitamin A deficiency with keratomalacia
Eye disorder that results in dry cornea caused by vitamin A deficiency
E50.5 Vitamin A deficiency with night blindness
E50.6 Vitamin A deficiency with xerophthalmic scars of cornea
Abnormal dryness and thickening of conjunctiva and cornea due to vitamin A deficiency
E50.7 Other ocular manifestations of vitamin A deficiency
Xerophthalmia NOS
E50.8 Other manifestations of vitamin A deficiency
Follicular keratosis
Xeroderma
E50.9 Vitamin A deficiency, unspecified
Hypovitaminosis A NOS

● **E51 Thiamine deficiency**
Excludes1 sequelae of thiamine deficiency (E64.8)
● **E51.1 Beriberi** (Ex) PDX 595
E51.11 Dry beriberi
Thiamine deficiency with nervous system manifestation most often caused by excessive alcohol consumption
Beriberi NOS
Beriberi with polyneuropathy
E51.12 Wet beriberi
Thiamine deficiency with cardiovascular manifestation most often caused by excessive alcohol consumption
Beriberi with cardiovascular manifestations
Cardiovascular beriberi
Shoshin disease
E51.2 Wernicke's encephalopathy (Ex) PDX 595
Acute disease of brain due to thiamine deficiency most often associated with excessive alcohol consumption
E51.8 Other manifestations of thiamine deficiency (Ex) PDX 595
E51.9 Thiamine deficiency, unspecified (Ex) PDX 595

E52 Niacin deficiency [pellagra]
Niacin (-tryptophan) deficiency
Nicotinamide deficiency
Pellagra (alcoholic)
Excludes1 sequelae of niacin deficiency (E64.8)

● **E53 Deficiency of other B group vitamins**
Excludes1 sequelae of vitamin B deficiency (E64.8)
E53.0 Riboflavin deficiency (Ex) PDX 595
Ariboflavinosis
Vitamin B2 deficiency
E53.1 Pyridoxine deficiency
Vitamin B6 deficiency
Excludes1 pyridoxine-responsive sideroblastic anemia (D64.3)
E53.8 Deficiency of other specified B group vitamins
Biotin deficiency
Cyanocobalamin deficiency
Folate deficiency
Folic acid deficiency
Pantothenic acid deficiency
Vitamin B12 deficiency
Excludes1 folate deficiency anemia (D52.-)
vitamin B12 deficiency anemia (D51.-)
E53.9 Vitamin B deficiency, unspecified

E54 Ascorbic acid deficiency
Deficiency of vitamin C
Scurvy
Excludes1 scorbutic anemia (D53.2)
sequelae of vitamin C deficiency (E64.2)

● **E55 Vitamin D deficiency**
Excludes1 adult osteomalacia (M83.-)
osteoporosis (M80.-)
sequelae of rickets (E64.3)
E55.0 Rickets, active (Ex) PDX 596
Infantile osteomalacia
Juvenile osteomalacia
Softening of bone
Excludes1 celiac rickets (K90.0)
Crohn's rickets (K50.-)
hereditary vitamin D-dependent rickets (E83.32)
inactive rickets (E64.3)
renal rickets (N25.0)
sequelae of rickets (E64.3)
vitamin D-resistant rickets (E83.31)
E55.9 Vitamin D deficiency, unspecified
Avitaminosis D

Item 4-6 Bitot's spots are the result of a buildup of keratin debris found on the superficial surface the conjunctiva; oval, triangular, or irregular in shape; and a sign of vitamin A deficiency and associated with night blindness. The disease may progress to **keratomalacia,** which can result in eventual prolapse of the iris and loss of the lens.

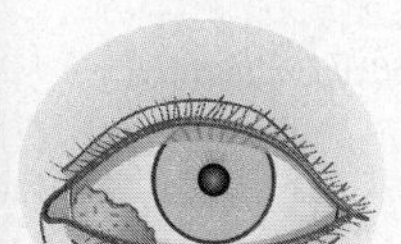

Figure 4-6 Bitot's spot on the conjunctiva.

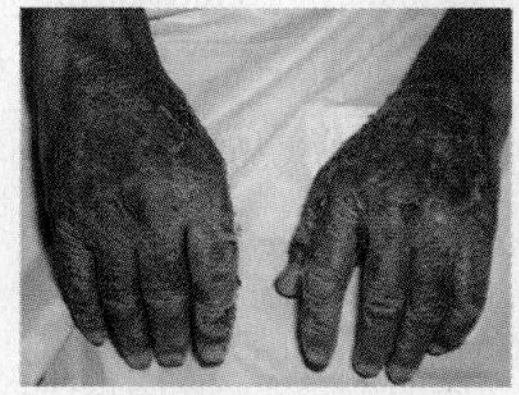

Figure 4-7 The sharply demarcated, characteristic scaling dermatitis of pellagra. (From James WD, Berger TG, Elston DM: Andrews' Diseases of the Skin: Clinical Dermatology, Philadelphia, Saunders Elsevier, 2006)

Item 4-7 Pellagra is associated with a deficiency of niacin and its precursor, **tryptophan.** Characteristics of the condition include diarrhea, dermatitis on exposed skin surfaces, dementia, and death. It is prevalent in developing countries where nutrition is inadequate. **Beriberi** is associated with thiamine deficiency.

● **E56 Other vitamin deficiencies**
Excludes1 sequelae of other vitamin deficiencies (E64.8)
E56.0 Deficiency of vitamin E
E56.1 Deficiency of vitamin K
Excludes1 deficiency of coagulation factor due to vitamin K deficiency (D68.4)
vitamin K deficiency of newborn (P53)
E56.8 Deficiency of other vitamins
E56.9 Vitamin deficiency, unspecified

E58 Dietary calcium deficiency
Excludes1 disorders of calcium metabolism (E83.5-)
sequelae of calcium deficiency (E64.8)

E59 Dietary selenium deficiency
Keshan disease
Excludes1 sequelae of selenium deficiency (E64.8)

E60 Dietary zinc deficiency

● **E61 Deficiency of other nutrient elements**
Use additional code for adverse effect, if applicable, to identify drug (T36-T50 with fifth or sixth character 5)
Excludes1 disorders of mineral metabolism (E83.-)
iodine deficiency related thyroid disorders (E00-E02)
sequelae of malnutrition and other nutritional deficiencies (E64.-)
E61.0 Copper deficiency
E61.1 Iron deficiency
Excludes1 iron deficiency anemia (D50.-)
E61.2 Magnesium deficiency
E61.3 Manganese deficiency
E61.4 Chromium deficiency
E61.5 Molybdenum deficiency
E61.6 Vanadium deficiency
E61.7 Deficiency of multiple nutrient elements
E61.8 Deficiency of other specified nutrient elements
E61.9 Deficiency of nutrient element, unspecified

● **E63 Other nutritional deficiencies**
Excludes2 dehydration (E86.0)
failure to thrive, adult (R62.7)
failure to thrive, child (R62.51)
feeding problems in newborn (P92.-)
sequelae of malnutrition and other nutritional deficiencies (E64.-)
E63.0 Essential fatty acid [EFA] deficiency
E63.1 Imbalance of constituents of food intake
E63.8 Other specified nutritional deficiencies
E63.9 Nutritional deficiency, unspecified

● **E64 Sequelae of malnutrition and other nutritional deficiencies**
Pathological condition resulting from disease, injury, or other trauma
Note: This category is to be used to indicate conditions in categories E43, E44, E46, E50-E63 as the cause of sequelae, which are themselves classified elsewhere. The "sequelae" include conditions specified as such; they also include the late effects of diseases classifiable to the above categories if the disease itself is no longer present
Code first condition resulting from (sequela) of malnutrition and other nutritional deficiencies
E64.0 Sequelae of protein-calorie malnutrition (Ex) PDX 594
Excludes2 retarded development following protein-calorie malnutrition (E45)
E64.1 Sequelae of vitamin A deficiency
E64.2 Sequelae of vitamin C deficiency
E64.3 Sequelae of rickets
E64.8 Sequelae of other nutritional deficiencies
E64.9 Sequelae of unspecified nutritional deficiency

OVERWEIGHT, OBESITY AND OTHER HYPERALIMENTATION (E65-E68)

E65 Localized adiposity
Fat pad

● **E66 Overweight and obesity**
Code first obesity complicating pregnancy, childbirth and the puerperium, if applicable (O99.21-)
Use additional code to identify body mass index (BMI), if known, for adults (Z68.1-Z68.45) or pediatrics (Z68.5-)
Excludes2 adiposogenital dystrophy E23.6)
lipomatosis NOS (E88.2)
lipomatosis dolorosa [Dercum] (E88.2)
Prader-Willi syndrome (Q87.11)
Coding Clinic: 2022, Q3, P7; 2018, Q4, P80
● **E66.0 Obesity due to excess calories**
E66.01 Morbid (severe) obesity due to excess calories
Excludes1 morbid (severe) obesity with alveolar hypoventilation (E66.2)
Coding Clinic: 2022, Q3, P6; 2022, Q2, P9; 2018, Q4, P79
E66.09 Other obesity due to excess calories
MCE: Questionable admission when principal dx
E66.1 Drug-induced obesity
MCE: Questionable admission when principal dx
Use additional code for adverse effect, if applicable, to identify drug (T36-T50 with fifth or sixth character 5)
Coding Clinic: 2022, Q3, P6
E66.2 Morbid (severe) obesity with alveolar hypoventilation (Ex) PDX 597
Uncommon condition of unknown cause leading to inadequate ventilation in lungs, even though lungs and airways are normal
Obesity hypoventilation syndrome (OHS)
Pickwickian syndrome
E66.3 Overweight
E66.8 Other obesity
MCE: Questionable admission when principal dx
▶ **E66.81 Obesity class**
▶ **E66.811 Obesity, class 1**
▶ **E66.812 Obesity, class 2**
▶ **E66.813 Obesity, class 3**
▶ **E66.89 Other obesity not elsewhere classified**
E66.9 Obesity, unspecified
Obesity NOS
MCE: Questionable admission when principal dx
Coding Clinic: 2021, Q2, P10-11

● **E67 Other hyperalimentation**
Ingestion of more than optimal amount of nutrients
Excludes1 hyperalimentation NOS (R63.2)
sequelae of hyperalimentation (E68)
E67.0 Hypervitaminosis A
E67.1 Hypercarotenemia
E67.2 Megavitamin-B6 syndrome
E67.3 Hypervitaminosis D
E67.8 Other specified hyperalimentation

E68 Sequelae of hyperalimentation
Code first condition resulting from (sequela) of hyperalimentation

METABOLIC DISORDERS (E70-E88)

Excludes1 androgen insensitivity syndrome (E34.5-)
congenital adrenal hyperplasia (E25.0)
hemolytic anemias attributable to enzyme disorders (D55.-)
Marfan syndrome (Q87.4-)
5-alpha-reductase deficiency (E29.1)

Excludes2 Ehlers-Danlos syndromes (Q79.6-)

E70 Disorders of aromatic amino-acid metabolism PDX 598

E70.0 Classical phenylketonuria
Inherited disorder that increases to harmful levels amino acid phenylalanine

E70.1 Other hyperphenylalaninemias

E70.2 Disorders of tyrosine metabolism
Excludes1 transitory tyrosinemia of newborn (P74.5)

E70.20 Disorder of tyrosine metabolism, unspecified
Tyrosine: Nonessential amino acid occurring in most proteins

E70.21 Tyrosinemia
Congenital amino acid metabolism
Hypertyrosinemia

E70.29 Other disorders of tyrosine metabolism
Alkaptonuria
Ochronosis

E70.3 Albinism
Congenital condition of reduced or absent pigment in eyes, skin, and hair

E70.30 Albinism, unspecified

E70.31 Ocular albinism

E70.310 X-linked ocular albinism

E70.311 Autosomal recessive ocular albinism

E70.318 Other ocular albinism

E70.319 Ocular albinism, unspecified

E70.32 Oculocutaneous albinism
Partial or total lack of melanin pigment in eyes
Excludes1 Chediak-Higashi syndrome (E70.330)
Hermansky-Pudlak syndrome (E70.331)

E70.320 Tyrosinase negative oculocutaneous albinism
Albinism I
Oculocutaneous albinism ty-neg

E70.321 Tyrosinase positive oculocutaneous albinism
Albinism II
Oculocutaneous albinism ty-pos

E70.328 Other oculocutaneous albinism
Cross syndrome

E70.329 Oculocutaneous albinism, unspecified

E70.33 Albinism with hematologic abnormality

E70.330 Chediak-Higashi syndrome

E70.331 Hermansky-Pudlak syndrome

E70.338 Other albinism with hematologic abnormality

E70.339 Albinism with hematologic abnormality, unspecified

E70.39 Other specified albinism
Piebaldism

E70.4 Disorders of histidine metabolism

E70.40 Disorders of histidine metabolism, unspecified

E70.41 Histidinemia

E70.49 Other disorders of histidine metabolism

E70.5 Disorders of tryptophan metabolism

E70.8 Other disorders of aromatic amino-acid metabolism

E70.81 Aromatic L-amino acid decarboxylase deficiency PDX 599
AADC deficiency

E70.89 Other disorders of aromatic amino-acid metabolism PDX 599

E70.9 Disorder of aromatic amino-acid metabolism, unspecified

E71 Disorders of branched-chain amino-acid metabolism and fatty-acid metabolism

E71.0 Maple-syrup-urine disease PDX 598
Due to defect in amino acid catabolism, causing severe ketoacidosis with smell of maple syrup in urine and on body

E71.1 Other disorders of branched-chain amino-acid metabolism PDX 598

E71.11 Branched-chain organic acidurias

E71.110 Isovaleric acidemia

E71.111 3-methylglutaconic aciduria

E71.118 Other branched-chain organic acidurias

E71.12 Disorders of propionate metabolism

E71.120 Methylmalonic acidemia

E71.121 Propionic acidemia

E71.128 Other disorders of propionate metabolism

E71.19 Other disorders of branched-chain amino-acid metabolism
Hyperleucine-isoleucinemia
Hypervalinemia

E71.2 Disorder of branched-chain amino-acid metabolism, unspecified PDX 598

E71.3 Disorders of fatty-acid metabolism
Excludes1 peroxisomal disorders (E71.5)
Refsum's disease (G60.1)
Schilder's disease (G37.0)
Excludes2 carnitine deficiency due to inborn error of metabolism (E71.42)

E71.30 Disorder of fatty-acid metabolism, unspecified

E71.31 Disorders of fatty-acid oxidation

E71.310 Long chain/very long chain acyl CoA dehydrogenase deficiency PDX 600
LCAD deficiency
VLCAD deficiency

E71.311 Medium chain acyl CoA dehydrogenase deficiency PDX 601
MCAD deficiency

E71.312 Short chain acyl CoA dehydrogenase deficiency PDX 602
SCAD deficiency

E71.313 Glutaric aciduria type II PDX 603
Glutaric aciduria type II A
Glutaric aciduria type II B
Glutaric aciduria type II C
Excludes1 glutaric aciduria (type 1) NOS (E72.3)

CHAPTER 4 (E00-E89)

E71.314 **Muscle carnitine palmitoyltransferase deficiency** (Ex) PDX 604

E71.318 **Other disorders of fatty-acid oxidation** (Ex) PDX 605

E71.32 **Disorders of ketone metabolism** (Ex) PDX 606

E71.39 **Other disorders of fatty-acid metabolism** (Ex) PDX 607

● E71.4 **Disorders of carnitine metabolism**

Excludes1 muscle carnitine palmitoyltransferase deficiency (E71.314)

E71.40 **Disorder of carnitine metabolism, unspecified**

E71.41 **Primary carnitine deficiency**

E71.42 **Carnitine deficiency due to inborn errors of metabolism**

Code also associated inborn error or metabolism

E71.43 **Iatrogenic carnitine deficiency**

Iatrogenic: Outcomes from activity of physicians

Carnitine deficiency due to hemodialysis

Carnitine deficiency due to Valproic acid therapy

● E71.44 **Other secondary carnitine deficiency**

E71.440 **Ruvalcaba-Myhre-Smith syndrome**

E71.448 **Other secondary carnitine deficiency**

● E71.5 **Peroxisomal disorders**

Class of conditions which lead to disorders of lipid metabolism

Excludes1 Schilder's disease (G37.0)

E71.50 **Peroxisomal disorder, unspecified** (Ex) PDX 608

● E71.51 **Disorders of peroxisome biogenesis**

Group 1 peroxisomal disorders

Excludes1 Refsum's disease (G60.1)

E71.510 **Zellweger syndrome** (Ex) PDX 609

E71.511 **Neonatal adrenoleukodystrophy** (Ex) PDX 610

Excludes1 X-linked adrenoleukodystrophy (E71.42-)

E71.518 **Other disorders of peroxisome biogenesis** (Ex) PDX 611

● E71.52 **X-linked adrenoleukodystrophy**

E71.520 **Childhood cerebral X-linked adrenoleukodystrophy** (Ex) PDX 612

E71.521 **Adolescent X-linked adrenoleukodystrophy** (Ex) PDX 613

E71.522 **Adrenomyeloneuropathy** (Ex) PDX 614

E71.528 **Other X-linked adrenoleukodystrophy** (Ex) PDX 615

Addison only phenotype adrenoleukodystrophy

Addison-Schilder adrenoleukodystrophy

E71.529 **X-linked adrenoleukodystrophy, unspecified type** (Ex) PDX 616

E71.53 **Other group 2 peroxisomal disorders** (Ex) PDX 617

Item 4–8 Leukodystrophy is characterized by degeneration and/or failure of the myelin formation of the central nervous system and sometimes of the peripheral nervous system. The disease is inherited and progressive.

● E71.54 **Other peroxisomal disorders**

E71.540 **Rhizomelic chondrodysplasia punctata** (Ex) PDX 618

Rare, severe, inherited disorder with limb shortening, bone and cartilage abnormalities, abnormal facial appearance, severe mental retardation, psychomotor retardation, and cataracts

Excludes1 chondrodysplasia punctata NOS (Q77.3)

E71.541 **Zellweger-like syndrome** (Ex) PDX 619

E71.542 **Other group 3 peroxisomal disorders** (Ex) PDX 620

E71.548 **Other peroxisomal disorders** (Ex) PDX 621

● E72 **Other disorders of amino-acid metabolism** (Ex) PDX 598

Excludes1 disorders of:

aromatic amino-acid metabolism (E70.-)

branched-chain amino-acid metabolism (E71.0-E71.2)

fatty-acid metabolism (E71.3)

purine and pyrimidine metabolism (E79.-)

gout (M1A.-, M10.-)

● E72.0 **Disorders of amino-acid transport**

Excludes1 disorders of tryptophan metabolism (E70.5)

E72.00 **Disorders of amino-acid transport, unspecified**

E72.01 **Cystinuria**

Hereditary aminoaciduria due to impairment of renal transport with predominant symptom of urinary cystine calculi

E72.02 **Hartnup's disease**

Inborn error of metabolism

E72.03 **Lowe's syndrome** (Ex) PDX 622

X-linked disorder with rickets, hydrophthalmia, congenital glaucoma, cataracts, mental retardation, and renal tubule dysfunction

Use additional code for associated glaucoma (H42)

E72.04 **Cystinosis**

Genetic disease with excessive depostits of amino acid cystine in cells

Fanconi (-de Toni) (-Debré) syndrome with cystinosis

Excludes1 Fanconi (-de Toni) (-Debré) syndrome without cystinosis (E72.09)

E72.09 **Other disorders of amino-acid transport**

Fanconi (-de Toni) (-Debré) syndrome, unspecified

● E72.1 **Disorders of sulfur-bearing amino-acid metabolism**

Excludes1 cystinosis (E72.04)

cystinuria (E72.01)

transcobalamin II deficiency (D51.2)

E72.10 **Disorders of sulfur-bearing amino-acid metabolism, unspecified**

E72.11 **Homocystinuria**

Cystathionine synthase deficiency

E72.12 **Methylenetetrahydrofolate reductase deficiency**

E72.19 **Other disorders of sulfur-bearing amino-acid metabolism**

Cystathioninuria

Methioninemia

Sulfite oxidase deficiency

E72.2 Disorders of urea cycle metabolism PDX 598

Excludes1 disorders of ornithine metabolism (E72.4)

E72.20 Disorder of urea cycle metabolism, unspecified

Hyperammonemia

Elevated levels of ammonia

Excludes1 hyperammonemia-hyperornithinemia-homocitrullinemia syndrome E72.4

transient hyperammonemia of newborn (P74.6)

E72.21 Argininemia

Disorder in which deficiency of enzyme arginase causes build-up of arginine and ammonia in blood

E72.22 Arginosuccinic aciduria

Gene disorder of urea cycle resulting accumulation of ammonia

E72.23 Citrullinemia

Urea cycle disorder that causes ammonia and other toxic substances to accumulate in blood

E72.29 Other disorders of urea cycle metabolism

E72.3 Disorders of lysine and hydroxylysine metabolism

Glutaric aciduria NOS

Glutaric aciduria (type I)

Hydroxylysinemia

Hyperlysinemia

Excludes1 glutaric aciduria type II (E71.313)

Refsum's disease (G60.1)

Zellweger syndrome (E71.510)

E72.4 Disorders of ornithine metabolism

Hyperammonemia-Hyperornithinemia-Homocitrullinemia syndrome

Ornithinemia (types I, II)

Ornithine transcarbamylase deficiency

Excludes1 hereditary choroidal dystrophy (H31.2-)

E72.5 Disorders of glycine metabolism PDX 598

E72.50 Disorder of glycine metabolism, unspecified

E72.51 Non-ketotic hyperglycinemia

E72.52 Trimethylaminuria

E72.53 Primary hyperoxaluria

Oxalosis

Oxaluria

E72.59 Other disorders of glycine metabolism

D-glycericacidemia

Hyperhydroxyprolinemia

Hyperprolinemia (types I, II)

Sarcosinemia

E72.8 Other specified disorders of amino-acid metabolism PDX 598

E72.81 Disorders of gamma aminobutyric acid metabolism

4-hydroxybutyric aciduria

Disorders of GABA metabolism

GABA metabolic defect

GABA transaminase deficiency

GABA-T deficiency

Gamma-hydroxybutyric aciduria

SSADHD

Succinic semialdehyde dehydrogenase deficiency

E72.89 Other specified disorders of amino-acid metabolism

Disorders of beta-amino-acid metabolism

Disorders of gamma-glutamyl cycle

E72.9 Disorder of amino-acid metabolism, unspecified PDX 598

E73 Lactose intolerance

Intolerance for lactose, due to inherited deficiency of lactase activity in intestinal mucosa

E73.0 Congenital lactase deficiency

E73.1 Secondary lactase deficiency

E73.8 Other lactose intolerance

E73.9 Lactose intolerance, unspecified

E74 Other disorders of carbohydrate metabolism

Excludes1 diabetes mellitus (E08-E13)

hypoglycemia NOS (E16.2)

increased secretion of glucagon (E16.3)

mucopolysaccharidosis (E76.0-E76.3)

E74.0 Glycogen storage disease PDX 598

E74.00 Glycogen storage disease, unspecified

E74.01 von Gierke's disease

Type I glycogen storage disease

E74.02 Pompe disease

Cardiac glycogenosis

Type II glycogen storage disease

E74.03 Cori disease

Forbes' disease

Type III glycogen storage disease

E74.04 McArdle disease

Type V glycogen storage disease

E74.05 Lysosome-associated membrane protein 2 [LAMP2] deficiency PDX 623

Danon disease

Code also, if applicable, associated manifestations such as:

dilated cardiomyopathy (I42.0)

obstructive hypertrophic cardiomyopathy (I42.1)

E74.09 Other glycogen storage disease

Andersen disease

Glycogen storage disease, types 0, IV, VI-XI

Hers disease

Liver phosphorylase deficiency

Muscle phosphofructokinase deficiency

Tauri disease

E74.1 Disorders of fructose metabolism

Excludes1 muscle phosphofructokinase deficiency (E74.09)

E74.10 Disorder of fructose metabolism, unspecified

E74.11 Essential fructosuria

Fructokinase deficiency

E74.12 Hereditary fructose intolerance

Fructosemia

E74.19 Other disorders of fructose metabolism

Fructose-1, 6-diphosphatase deficiency

E74.2 Disorders of galactose metabolism PDX 598

E74.20 Disorders of galactose metabolism, unspecified

E74.21 Galactosemia

Genetic disorders resulting from defective simple sugar (galactose) metabolism

E74.29 Other disorders of galactose metabolism

Galactokinase deficiency

E74.3 Other disorders of intestinal carbohydrate absorption

Excludes2 lactose intolerance (E73.-)

E74.31 Sucrase-isomaltase deficiency

Deficiency in metabolism in intestinal mucosa results in malabsorption of sucrose and starch

E74.39 Other disorders of intestinal carbohydrate absorption

Disorder of intestinal carbohydrate absorption NOS

Glucose-galactose malabsorption

Sucrase deficiency

CHAPTER 4 (E00-E89)

E74.4 Disorders of pyruvate metabolism and gluconeogenesis (Ex) PDX 598
Deficiency of phosphoenolpyruvate carboxykinase
Deficiency of pyruvate carboxylase
Deficiency of pyruvate dehydrogenase
Excludes1 disorders of pyruvate metabolism and gluconeogenesis with anemia (D55.-)
Leigh's syndrome (G31.82)

E74.8 Other specified disorders of carbohydrate metabolism (Ex) PDX 624

E74.81 Disorders of glucose transport, not elsewhere classified

E74.810 Glucose transporter protein type 1 deficiency
De Vivo syndrome
Glucose transport defect, blood-brain barrier
GLUT1 deficiency
GLUT1 deficiency syndrome 1, infantile onset
GLUT1 deficiency syndrome 2, childhood onset

E74.818 Other disorders of glucose transport
(Familial) renal glycosuria

E74.819 Disorders of glucose transport, unspecified

E74.82 Disorders of citrate metabolism

E74.820 SLC13A5 Citrate Transporter Disorder

E74.829 Other disorders of citrate metabolism

E74.89 Other specified disorders of carbohydrate metabolism
Essential pentosuria
Coding Clinic: 2023, Q3, P3

E74.9 Disorder of carbohydrate metabolism, unspecified

E75 Disorders of sphingolipid metabolism and other lipid storage disorders
Excludes1 mucolipidosis, types I-III (E77.0-E77.1)
Refsum's disease (G60.1)

E75.0 GM2 gangliosidosis (Ex) PDX 625
Rare metabolic disorder that causes destruction of nerve cells of brain and spinal cord

E75.00 GM2 gangliosidosis, unspecified

E75.01 Sandhoff disease

E75.02 Tay-Sachs disease

E75.09 Other GM2 gangliosidosis
Adult GM2 gangliosidosis
Juvenile GM2 gangliosidosis

E75.1 Other and unspecified gangliosidosis (Ex) PDX 625

E75.10 Unspecified gangliosidosis
Gangliosidosis NOS

E75.11 Mucolipidosis IV
Disorder with symptoms of psychomotor retardation and severe visual impairment

E75.19 Other gangliosidosis
GM1 gangliosidosis
GM3 gangliosidosis

E75.2 Other sphingolipidosis (Ex) PDX 626
Lysosomal (a particle in a cytoplasm cell that contains digestive enzymes) storage diseases with symptoms of abnormal storage of amino acids
Excludes1 adrenoleukodystrophy [Addison-Schilder] (E71.528)

E75.21 Fabry (-Anderson) disease

E75.22 Gaucher disease

E75.23 Krabbe disease

E75.24 Niemann-Pick disease
Acid sphingomyelinase deficiency (ASMD)

E75.240 Niemann-Pick disease type A
Acid sphingomyelinase deficiency type A (ASMD type A)
Infantile neurovisceral acid sphingomyelinase deficiency

E75.241 Niemann-Pick disease type B
Acid sphingomyelinase deficiency type B (ASMD type B)
Chronic visceral acid sphingomyelinase deficiency

E75.242 Niemann-Pick disease type C

E75.243 Niemann-Pick disease type D

E75.244 Niemann-Pick disease type A/B
Acid sphingomyelinase deficiency type A/B (ASMD type A/B)
Chronic neurovisceral acid sphingomyelinase deficiency

E75.248 Other Niemann-Pick disease

E75.249 Niemann-Pick disease, unspecified
Acid sphingomyelinase deficiency (ASMD) NOS

E75.25 Metachromatic leukodystrophy

E75.26 Sulfatase deficiency
Multiple sulfatase deficiency (MSD)

E75.27 Pelizaeus-Merzbacher disease

E75.28 Canavan disease

E75.29 Other sphingolipidosis
Farber's syndrome
Sulfatide lipidosis

E75.3 Sphingolipidosis, unspecified

E75.4 Neuronal ceroid lipofuscinosis (Ex) PDX 625
Batten disease
Bielschowsky-Jansky disease
Kufs disease
Spielmeyer-Vogt disease

E75.5 Other lipid storage disorders
Cerebrotendinous cholesterosis [van Bogaert-Scherer-Epstein]
Wolman's disease

E75.6 Lipid storage disorder, unspecified

E76 Disorders of glycosaminoglycan metabolism (Ex) PDX 627

E76.0 Mucopolysaccharidosis, type I
Inborn metabolic disorder of enzymes that break down carbohydrates

E76.01 Hurler's syndrome

E76.02 Hurler-Scheie syndrome

E76.03 Scheie's syndrome

E76.1 Mucopolysaccharidosis, type II
Inborn metabolic disorder of enzymes that break down carbohydrates occurs in 2-4 year old males
Hunter's syndrome

E76.2 Other mucopolysaccharidoses

E76.21 Morquio mucopolysaccharidoses

E76.210 Morquio A mucopolysaccharidoses
Classic Morquio syndrome
Morquio syndrome A
Mucopolysaccharidosis, type IVA

E76.211 Morquio B mucopolysaccharidoses
Morquio-like mucopolysaccharidoses
Morquio-like syndrome
Morquio syndrome B
Mucopolysaccharidosis, type IVB

E76.219 Morquio mucopolysaccharidoses, unspecified
Morquio syndrome
Mucopolysaccharidosis, type IV

E76.22 **Sanfilippo mucopolysaccharidoses**
Mucopolysaccharidosis, type III (A) (B) (C) (D)
Sanfilippo A syndrome
Sanfilippo B syndrome
Sanfilippo C syndrome
Sanfilippo D syndrome

E76.29 **Other mucopolysaccharidoses**
beta-Glucuronidase deficiency
Maroteaux-Lamy (mild) (severe) syndrome
Mucopolysaccharidosis, types VI, VII

E76.3 **Mucopolysaccharidosis, unspecified**

E76.8 **Other disorders of glucosaminoglycan metabolism**

E76.9 **Glucosaminoglycan metabolism disorder, unspecified**

E77 Disorders of glycoprotein metabolism

E77.0 **Defects in post-translational modification of lysosomal enzymes**
Mucolipidosis II [I-cell disease]
Mucolipidosis III [pseudo-Hurler polydystrophy]

E77.1 **Defects in glycoprotein degradation**
Aspartylglucosaminuria
Fucosidosis
Mannosidosis
Sialidosis [mucolipidosis I]

E77.8 **Other disorders of glycoprotein metabolism**

E77.9 **Disorder of glycoprotein metabolism, unspecified**

E78 Disorders of lipoprotein metabolism and other lipidemias

Excludes1 sphingolipidosis (E75.0-E75.3)

E78.0 **Pure hypercholesterolemia**
Coding Clinic: 2016, Q4, P13

E78.00 **Pure hypercholesterolemia, unspecified**
Fredrickson's hyperlipoproteinemia, type IIa
Hyperbetalipoproteinemia
Low-density-lipoprotein-type [LDL] hyperlipoproteinemia
(Pure) hypercholesterolemia NOS
Coding Clinic: 2023, Q2, P9; 2022, Q2, P6; 2016, Q4, P13

E78.01 **Familial hypercholesterolemia**
Coding Clinic: 2016, Q4, P13

E78.1 **Pure hyperglyceridemia**
Elevated fasting triglycerides
Endogenous hyperglyceridemia
Fredrickson's hyperlipoproteinemia, type IV
Hyperlipidemia, group B
Hyperprebetalipoproteinemia
Very-low-density-lipoprotein-type [VLDL] hyperlipoproteinemia

E78.2 **Mixed hyperlipidemia**
Broad- or floating-betalipoproteinemia
Combined hyperlipidemia NOS
Elevated cholesterol with elevated triglycerides NEC
Fredrickson's hyperlipoproteinemia, type IIb or III
Hyperbetalipoproteinemia with prebetalipoproteinemia
Hypercholesteremia with endogenous hyperglyceridemia
Hyperlipidemia, group C
Tubo-eruptive xanthoma
Xanthoma tuberosum

Excludes1 cerebrotendinous cholesterosis [van Bogaert-Scherer-Epstein] (E75.5)
familial combined hyperlipidemia (E78.49)

Coding Clinic: 2023, Q2, P9-10; 2022, Q2, P6-7

E78.3 **Hyperchylomicronemia**
Chylomicron retention disease
Fredrickson's hyperlipoproteinemia, type I or V
Hyperlipidemia, group D
Mixed hyperglyceridemia

E78.4 **Other hyperlipidemia**

E78.41 **Elevated Lipoprotein(a)**
Elevated Lp(a)

E78.49 **Other hyperlipidemia**
Familial combined hyperlipidemia

E78.5 **Hyperlipidemia, unspecified**
Coding Clinic: 2022, Q2, P6

E78.6 **Lipoprotein deficiency**
Abetalipoproteinemia
Depressed HDL cholesterol
High-density lipoprotein deficiency
Hypoalphalipoproteinemia
Hypobetalipoproteinemia (familial)
Lecithin cholesterol acyltransferase deficiency
Tangier disease

E78.7 **Disorders of bile acid and cholesterol metabolism**

Excludes1 Niemann-Pick disease type C (E75.242)

E78.70 **Disorder of bile acid and cholesterol metabolism, unspecified**

E78.71 **Barth syndrome** (Ex) PDX 628

E78.72 **Smith-Lemli-Opitz syndrome** (Ex) PDX 628

E78.79 **Other disorders of bile acid and cholesterol metabolism**
Coding Clinic: 2023, Q1, P27

E78.8 **Other disorders of lipoprotein metabolism**

E78.81 **Lipoid dermatoarthritis**

E78.89 **Other lipoprotein metabolism disorders**

E78.9 **Disorder of lipoprotein metabolism, unspecified**

E79 Disorders of purine and pyrimidine metabolism (Ex) PDX 573
Purines, along with pyrimidines, signal RNA and DNA production

Excludes1 Ataxia-telangiectasia (Q87.19)
Bloom's syndrome (Q82.8)
Cockayne's syndrome (Q87.19)
calculus of kidney (N20.0)
combined immunodeficiency disorders (D81.-)
Fanconi's anemia (D61.09)
gout (M1A.-, M10.-)
orotaciduric anemia (D53.0)
progeria (E34.8)
Werner's syndrome (E34.8)
xeroderma pigmentosum (Q82.1)

E79.0 **Hyperuricemia without signs of inflammatory arthritis and tophaceous disease**
Asymptomatic hyperuricemia

E79.1 **Lesch-Nyhan syndrome**
HGPRT deficiency

E79.2 **Myoadenylate deaminase deficiency**

E79.8 **Other disorders of purine and pyrimidine metabolism**

E79.81 **Aicardi-Goutières syndrome**

E79.82 **Hereditary xanthinuria**

E79.89 **Other specified disorders of purine and pyrimidine metabolism**

E79.9 **Disorder of purine and pyrimidine metabolism, unspecified**

E80 Disorders of porphyrin and bilirubin metabolism (Ex) PDX 573
Group of chemical compounds in RBCs that combine with iron to form heme

Includes defects of catalase and peroxidase

E80.0 **Hereditary erythropoietic porphyria**
Congenital erythropoietic porphyria
Erythropoietic protoporphyria

E80.1 **Porphyria cutanea tarda**

E80.2 **Other and unspecified porphyria**

E80.20 **Unspecified porphyria**
Porphyria NOS

E80.21 **Acute intermittent (hepatic) porphyria**

E80.29 **Other porphyria**
Hereditary coproporphyria

E80.3 **Defects of catalase and peroxidase** (Ex) PDX 629
Acatalasia [Takahara]

E80.4 **Gilbert syndrome**

E80.5 **Crigler-Najjar syndrome**

E80.6 Other disorders of bilirubin metabolism
Dubin-Johnson syndrome
Rotor's syndrome
Coding Clinic: 2022, Q3, P7

E80.7 Disorder of bilirubin metabolism, unspecified

E83 Disorders of mineral metabolism
Excludes1 dietary mineral deficiency (E58-E61)
parathyroid disorders (E20-E21)
vitamin D deficiency (E55.-)

E83.0 Disorders of copper metabolism
E83.00 Disorder of copper metabolism, unspecified
E83.01 Wilson's disease
Code also associated Kayser Fleischer ring (H18.04-)
E83.09 Other disorders of copper metabolism
Menkes' (kinky hair) (steely hair) disease

E83.1 Disorders of iron metabolism
Excludes1 iron deficiency anemia (D50.-)
sideroblastic anemia (D64.0-D64.3)
E83.10 Disorder of iron metabolism, unspecified
E83.11 Hemochromatosis
Excludes1 GALD (P78.84)
Gestational alloimmune liver disease (P78.84)
Neonatal hemochromatosis (P78.84)
E83.110 Hereditary hemochromatosis
Bronzed diabetes
Pigmentary cirrhosis (of liver)
Primary (hereditary) hemochromatosis
E83.111 Hemochromatosis due to repeated red blood cell transfusions
Iron overload due to repeated red blood cell transfusions
Transfusion (red blood cell) associated hemochromatosis
E83.118 Other hemochromatosis
E83.119 Hemochromatosis, unspecified
E83.19 Other disorders of iron metabolism
Use additional code, if applicable, for idiopathic pulmonary hemosiderosis (J84.03)

E83.2 Disorders of zinc metabolism
Acrodermatitis enteropathica

E83.3 Disorders of phosphorus metabolism and phosphatases
Excludes1 adult osteomalacia (M83.-)
osteoporosis (M80.-)
E83.30 Disorder of phosphorus metabolism, unspecified
E83.31 Familial hypophosphatemia
Vitamin D-resistant osteomalacia
Vitamin D-resistant rickets
Excludes1 vitamin D-deficiency rickets (E55.0)
E83.32 Hereditary vitamin D-dependent rickets (type 1) (type 2)
25-hydroxyvitamin D 1-alpha-hydroxylase deficiency
Pseudovitamin D deficiency
Vitamin D receptor defect
E83.39 Other disorders of phosphorus metabolism
Acid phosphatase deficiency
Hypophosphatasia

E83.4 Disorders of magnesium metabolism
E83.40 Disorders of magnesium metabolism, unspecified
E83.41 Hypermagnesemia
Coding Clinic: 2016, Q4, P55
E83.42 Hypomagnesemia
E83.49 Other disorders of magnesium metabolism

E83.5 Disorders of calcium metabolism
autoimmune hypoparathyroidism (E20.812)
autosomal dominant hypocalcemia (E20.810)
Excludes1 chondrocalcinosis (M11.1-M11.2)
hungry bone syndrome (E83.81)
hyperparathyroidism (E21.0-E21.3)
secondary hypoparathyroidism in diseases classified elsewhere (E20.811)
E83.50 Unspecified disorder of calcium metabolism
E83.51 Hypocalcemia
E83.52 Hypercalcemia
Familial hypocalciuric hypercalcemia
E83.59 Other disorders of calcium metabolism
Idiopathic hypercalciuria

E83.8 Other disorders of mineral metabolism
E83.81 Hungry bone syndrome
E83.89 Other disorders of mineral metabolism

E83.9 Disorder of mineral metabolism, unspecified

E84 Cystic fibrosis PDX 630
Includes mucoviscidosis
Code also exocrine pancreatic insufficiency (K86.81)
E84.0 Cystic fibrosis with pulmonary manifestations
Use additional code to identify any infectious organism present, such as:
Pseudomonas (B96.5)
Coding Clinic: 2021, Q1, P24
E84.1 Cystic fibrosis with intestinal manifestations
E84.11 Meconium ileus in cystic fibrosis N
Excludes1 meconium ileus not due to cystic fibrosis (P76.0)
E84.19 Cystic fibrosis with other intestinal manifestations
Distal intestinal obstruction syndrome
E84.8 Cystic fibrosis with other manifestations
E84.9 Cystic fibrosis, unspecified

E85 Amyloidosis PDX 631
A disorder resulting from the abnormal deposition of a particular protein (amyloid) into tissues of the body
Excludes2 Alzheimer's disease (G30.0-)
E85.0 Non-neuropathic heredofamilial amyloidosis
Hereditary amyloid nephropathy
Code also associated disorders, such as:
autoinflammatory syndromes (M04.-)
Excludes2 Transthyretin-related (ATTR) familial amyloid cardiomyopathy (E85.4)
E85.1 Neuropathic heredofamilial amyloidosis
Amyloid polyneuropathy (Portuguese)
Transthyretin-related (ATTR) familial amyloid polyneuropathy
Coding Clinic: 2012, Q4, P100
E85.2 Heredofamilial amyloidosis, unspecified

Item 4–9 Circulating fluid volume is regulated by the amount of water and sodium ingested, excreted by the kidneys into the urine, and lost through the gastrointestinal tract, lungs, and skin. To maintain blood volume within a normal range, the kidneys regulate the amount of water and sodium lost into the urine. Too much **(fluid overload)** or too little fluid volume **(volume depletion)** will affect blood pressure. Severe cases of vomiting, diarrhea, bleeding, and burns (fluid loss through exposed burn surface area) can contribute to fluid loss. Internal body environment must maintain a precise balance (homeostasis) between too much fluid and too little fluid. This complex balancing mechanism is critical to good health.

E85.3 Secondary systemic amyloidosis (Ex) PDX 631
Hemodialysis-associated amyloidosis

E85.4 Organ-limited amyloidosis (Ex) PDX 631
Localized amyloidosis
Transthyretin-related (ATTR) familial amyloid cardiomyopathy

E85.8 Other amyloidosis (Ex) PDX 631

E85.81 Light chain (AL) amyloidosis
Coding Clinic: 2024, Q2, P9

E85.82 Wild-type transthyretin-related (ATTR) amyloidosis
Senile systemic amyloidosis (SSA)

E85.89 Other amyloidosis

E85.9 Amyloidosis, unspecified

E86 Volume depletion

Excludes1 dehydration of newborn (P74.1)
postprocedural hypovolemic shock (T81.19)
traumatic hypovolemic shock (T79.4)

Excludes2 hypovolemic shock NOS (R57.1)

Use additional code(s) for any associated disorders of electrolyte and acid-base balance (E87.-)
Coding Clinic: 2019, Q2, P7

E86.0 Dehydration
Excessive loss of body water
Coding Clinic: 2019, Q2, P7-8

E86.1 Hypovolemia
Diminished volume of circulating blood
Depletion of volume of plasma

E86.9 Volume depletion, unspecified
Coding Clinic: 2019, Q2, P7-8

E87 Other disorders of fluid, electrolyte and acid-base balance (Ex) PDX 632

Excludes1 diabetes insipidus (E23.2)
electrolyte imbalance associated with hyperemesis gravidarum (O21.1)
electrolyte imbalance following ectopic or molar pregnancy (O08.5)
familial periodic paralysis (G72.3)
metabolic acidemia in newborn, unspecified (P19.9)

E87.0 Hyperosmolality and hypernatremia
Sodium [Na] excess
Sodium [Na] overload

~~**Excludes1** diabetes with hyperosmolarity (E08, E09, E11, E13 with final characters .00 or .011)~~

Excludes2 diabetes with hyperosmolarity (E08, E09, E11, E13 with final characters .00 or .01)
Coding Clinic: 2022, Q1, P29; 2018, Q2, P6

E87.1 Hypo-osmolality and hyponatremia
Sodium [Na] deficiency

Excludes1 syndrome of inappropriate secretion of antidiuretic hormone (E22.2)
Coding Clinic: 2018, Q2, P6

E87.2 Acidosis

Excludes1 diabetic acidosis - see categories E08-E10, E11, E13 with ketoacidosis

E87.20 Acidosis, unspecified
Lactic acidosis NOS
Metabolic acidosis NOS
Code also, if applicable, respiratory failure with hypercapnia (J96. with 5th character 2)

E87.21 Acute metabolic acidosis
Acute lactic acidosis

E87.22 Chronic metabolic acidosis
Chronic lactic acidosis
Code first underlying etiology, if applicable
Coding Clinic: 2022, Q4, P14

E87.29 Other acidosis
Respiratory acidosis NOS

Excludes2 acute respiratory acidosis (J96.02)
chronic respiratory acidosis (J96.12)

E87.3 Alkalosis
Alkalosis NOS
Metabolic alkalosis
Respiratory alkalosis

E87.4 Mixed disorder of acid-base balance

E87.5 Hyperkalemia
Potassium [K] excess
Potassium [K] overload

E87.6 Hypokalemia
Potassium [K] deficiency

E87.7 Fluid overload

Excludes1 edema NOS (R60.9)
fluid retention (R60.9)

E87.70 Fluid overload, unspecified
Coding Clinic: 2023, Q1, P19

E87.71 Transfusion associated circulatory overload
Fluid overload due to transfusion (blood) (blood components) TACO

E87.79 Other fluid overload

E87.8 Other disorders of electrolyte and fluid balance, not elsewhere classified
Electrolyte imbalance NOS
Hyperchloremia
Hypochloremia

E88 Other and unspecified metabolic disorders
Use additional codes for associated conditions

Excludes1 histiocytosis X (chronic) (C96.6)

E88.0 Disorders of plasma-protein metabolism, not elsewhere classified

Excludes1 monoclonal gammopathy (of undetermined significance) (D47.2)
polyclonal hypergammaglobulinemia (D89.0)
Waldenström macroglobulinemia (C88.00)

Excludes2 disorder of lipoprotein metabolism (E78.-)

E88.01 Alpha-1-antitrypsin deficiency AAT deficiency

E88.02 Plasminogen deficiency (Ex) PDX 633
Dysplasminogenemia
Hypoplasminogenemia
Type 1 plasminogen deficiency
Type 2 plasminogen deficiency
Code also, if applicable, ligneous conjunctivitis (H10.51)
Use additional code for associated findings, such as:
hydrocephalus (G91.4)
otitis media (H67.-)
respiratory disorder related to plasminogen deficiency (J99)

E88.09 Other disorders of plasma-protein metabolism, not elsewhere classified
Bisalbuminemia

E88.1 Lipodystrophy, not elsewhere classified
Defective fat metabolism resulting in absence of subcutaneous fat
Lipodystrophy NOS

Excludes1 Whipple's disease (K90.81)

E88.2 Lipomatosis, not elsewhere classified
Abnormal tumorlike accumulations of fat in tissue
Lipomatosis NOS
Lipomatosis (Check) dolorosa [Dercum]

E88.3 Tumor lysis syndrome (Ex) PDX 634
Tumor lysis syndrome (spontaneous)
Tumor lysis syndrome following antineoplastic drug chemotherapy
Use additional code for adverse effect, if applicable, to identify drug (T45.1X5)
Coding Clinic: 2019, Q2, P25

● E88.4 **Mitochondrial metabolism disorders**
Congenital disorder of metabolism
Excludes1 disorders of pyruvate metabolism (E74.4)
Kearns-Sayre syndrome (H49.81)
Leber's disease (H47.22)
Leigh's encephalopathy (G31.82)
Mitochondrial myopathy, NEC (G71.3)
Reye's syndrome (G93.7)

E88.40 **Mitochondrial metabolism disorder, unspecified** PDX 635

E88.41 **MELAS syndrome** PDX 636
Mitochondrial myopathy, encephalopathy, lactic acidosis and stroke-like episodes

E88.42 **MERRF syndrome** PDX 637
Myoclonic epilepsy associated with ragged-red fibers
Code also progressive myoclonic epilepsy (G40.3-)

E88.43 **Disorders of mitochondrial tRNA synthetases** PDX 638

E88.49 **Other mitochondrial metabolism disorders** PDX 639

● E88.8 **Other specified metabolic disorders**

● E88.81 **Metabolic syndrome and other insulin resistance**
Use additional codes for associated manifestations, such as:
obesity (E66.-)
Coding Clinic: 2022, Q3, P6-7

E88.810 **Metabolic syndrome**
Dysmetabolic syndrome

E88.811 **Insulin resistance syndrome, Type A**
Coding Clinic: 2023, Q4, P14

E88.818 **Other insulin resistance**
Insulin resistance syndrome, Type B

E88.819 **Insulin resistance, unspecified**

▶E88.82 **Obesity due to disruption of MC4R pathway**
▶Use additional code, if applicable, to identify associated manifestations, such as polyphagia (R63.2)
▶Use additional code to identify body mass index (BMI), if known (Z68.-)

E88.89 **Other specified metabolic disorders**
Launois-Bensaude adenolipomatosis
Excludes1 adult pulmonary Langerhans cell histiocytosis (J84.82)

E88.9 **Metabolic disorder, unspecified**

E88.A **Wasting disease (syndrome) due to underlying condition**
Cachexia due to underlying condition
Code first underlying condition
Excludes1 cachexia NOS (R64)
nutritional marasmus (E41)
Excludes2 failure to thrive (R62.51, R62.7)
Coding Clinic: 2023, Q4, P15

POSTPROCEDURAL ENDOCRINE AND METABOLIC COMPLICATIONS AND DISORDERS, NOT ELSEWHERE CLASSIFIED (E89)

● E89 **Postprocedural endocrine and metabolic complications and disorders, not elsewhere classified**
Excludes2 intraoperative complications of endocrine system organ or structure (E36.0-, E36.1-, E36.8)

E89.0 **Postprocedural hypothyroidism**
Postirradiation hypothyroidism
Postsurgical hypothyroidism

E89.1 **Postprocedural hypoinsulinemia** PDX 581
Postpancreatectomy hyperglycemia
Postsurgical hypoinsulinemia
▶*Code first, if applicable, diabetes mellitus (postpancreatectomy) (postprocedural) (E13.-)*
Use additional code, if applicable, to identify:
~~diabetes mellitus (postpancreatectomy) (postprocedural) (E13.)~~
acquired absence of pancreas (Z90.41-)
insulin use (Z79.4)
Excludes1 transient postprocedural hyperglycemia (R73.9)
transient postprocedural hypoglycemia (E16.2)

E89.2 **Postprocedural hypoparathyroidism**
Parathyroprival tetany
Coding Clinic: 2023, Q3, P13

E89.3 **Postprocedural hypopituitarism**
Postirradiation hypopituitarism

● E89.4 **Postprocedural ovarian failure**

E89.40 **Asymptomatic postprocedural ovarian failure**
Postprocedural ovarian failure NOS

E89.41 **Symptomatic postprocedural ovarian failure**
Symptoms such as flushing, sleeplessness, headache, lack of concentration, associated with postprocedural menopause

E89.5 **Postprocedural testicular hypofunction**

E89.6 **Postprocedural adrenocortical (-medullary) hypofunction** PDX 590

● E89.8 **Other postprocedural endocrine and metabolic complications and disorders** PDX 640
Coding Clinic: 2016, Q4, P9

● E89.81 **Postprocedural hemorrhage of an endocrine system organ or structure following a procedure**

E89.810 **Postprocedural hemorrhage of an endocrine system organ or structure following an endocrine system procedure**

E89.811 **Postprocedural hemorrhage of an endocrine system organ or structure following other procedure**

● E89.82 **Postprocedural hematoma and seroma of an endocrine system organ or structure**

E89.820 **Postprocedural hematoma of an endocrine system organ or structure following an endocrine system procedure**

E89.821 **Postprocedural hematoma of an endocrine system organ or structure following other procedure**

E89.822 **Postprocedural seroma of an endocrine system organ or structure following an endocrine system procedure**

E89.823 **Postprocedural seroma of an endocrine system organ or structure following other procedure**

E89.89 **Other postprocedural endocrine and metabolic complications and disorders**
Use additional code, if applicable, to further specify disorder

CHAPTER 5

MENTAL, BEHAVIORAL AND NEURODEVELOPMENTAL DISORDERS (FØ1-F99)

OGCR Chapter-Specific Coding Guidelines

5. **Chapter 5: Mental, Behavioral and Neurodevelopmental disorders (FØ1 – F99)**

a. **Pain disorders related to psychological factors**
Assign code F45.41, for pain that is exclusively related to psychological disorders. As indicated by the Excludes 1 note under category G89, a code from category G89 should not be assigned with code F45.41

Code F45.42, Pain disorders with related psychological factors, should be used with a code from category G89, Pain, not elsewhere classified, if there is documentation of a psychological component for a patient with acute or chronic pain.

See Section I.C.6. Pain

b. **Mental and behavioral disorders due to psychoactive substance use**

1) **In Remission**
Selection of codes for "in remission" for categories F1Ø-F19, Mental and behavioral disorders due to psychoactive substance use (categories F1Ø-F19 with -11, -.21) requires the provider's clinical judgment. The appropriate codes for "in remission" are assigned only on the basis of provider documentation (as defined in the Official Guidelines for Coding and Reporting), unless otherwise instructed by the classification.

Mild substance use disorders in early or sustained remission are classified to the appropriate codes for substance abuse in remission, and moderate or severe substance use disorders in early or sustained remission are classified to the appropriate codes for substance dependence in remission.

2) **Psychoactive Substance Use, Abuse and Dependence**
When the provider documentation refers to use, abuse and dependence of the same substance (e.g., alcohol, opioid, cannabis, etc.), only one code should be assigned to identify the pattern of use based on the following hierarchy:

- If both use and abuse are documented, assign only the code for abuse
- If both abuse and dependence are documented, assign only the code for dependence
- If use, abuse and dependence are all documented, assign only the code for dependence
- If both use and dependence are documented, assign only the code for dependence

3) **Psychoactive Substance Use, Unspecified**
As with all other unspecified diagnoses, the codes for unspecified psychoactive substance use disorders (F1Ø.9-, F11.9-, F12.9-, F13.9-, F14.9-, F15.9-, F16.9-, F19.9-, F19.9-) should only be assigned based on provider documentation and when they meet the definition of a reportable diagnosis (see Section III, Reporting Additional Diagnoses). These codes are to be used only when the psychoactive substance use is associated with a physical, mental or behavioral disorder, and such a relationship is documented by the provider.

c. **Factitious Disorder**
Factitious disorder imposed on self or Munchausen's syndrome is a disorder in which a person falsely reports or causes his or her own physical or psychological signs or symptoms. For patients with documented factitious disorder on self or Munchausen's syndrome, assign the appropriate code from subcategory F68.1-, Factitious disorder imposed on self.

Munchausen's syndrome by proxy (MSBP) is a disorder in which a caregiver (perpetrator) falsely reports or causes an illness or injury in another person (victim) under his or her care, such as a child, an elderly adult, or a person who has a disability. The condition is also referred to as "factitious disorder imposed on another" or "factitious disorder by proxy." The perpetrator, not the victim, receives this diagnosis. Assign code F68.A, Factitious disorder imposed on another, to the perpetrator's record. For the victim of a patient suffering from MSBP, assign the appropriate code from categories T74, Adult and child abuse, neglect and other maltreatment, confirmed, or T76, Adult and child abuse, neglect and other maltreatment, suspected.

See Section I.C.19.f. Adult and child abuse, neglect and other maltreatment

CHAPTER 5

MENTAL, BEHAVIORAL AND NEURODEVELOPMENTAL DISORDERS (FØ1-F99)

Includes disorders of psychological development

Excludes2 symptoms, signs and abnormal clinical laboratory findings, not elsewhere classified (RØØ-R99)

This chapter contains the following blocks:

FØ1-FØ9	Mental disorders due to known physiological conditions
F1Ø-F19	Mental and behavioral disorders due to psychoactive substance use
F2Ø-F29	Schizophrenia, schizotypal, delusional, and other non-mood psychotic disorders
F3Ø-F39	Mood [affective] disorders
F4Ø-F48	Anxiety, dissociative, stress-related, somatoform and other nonpsychotic mental disorders
F5Ø-F59	Behavioral syndromes associated with physiological disturbances and physical factors
F6Ø-F69	Disorders of adult personality and behavior
F7Ø-F79	Intellectual disabilities
F8Ø-F89	Pervasive and specific developmental disorders
F9Ø-F98	Behavioral and emotional disorders with onset usually occurring in childhood and adolescence
F99	Unspecified mental disorder

MENTAL DISORDERS DUE TO KNOWN PHYSIOLOGICAL CONDITIONS (FØ1-FØ9)

This block comprises a range of mental disorders grouped together on the basis of their having in common a demonstrable etiology in cerebral disease, brain injury, or other insult leading to cerebral dysfunction. The dysfunction may be primary, as in diseases, injuries, and insults that affect the brain directly and selectively; or secondary, as in systemic diseases and disorders that attack the brain only as one of the multiple organs or systems of the body that are involved.

● **FØ1 Vascular dementia**
Vascular dementia as a result of infarction of the brain due to vascular disease, including hypertensive cerebrovascular disease.

Includes arteriosclerotic dementia
major neurocognitive disorder due to vascular disease
multi-infarct dementia

▶ *Code first, ~~the underlying physiological condition or sequelae of cerebrovascular disease~~ if applicable, any causal condition*

● **FØ1.5 Vascular dementia, unspecified severity**

● **FØ1.5Ø Vascular dementia, unspecified severity, without behavioral disturbance, psychotic disturbance, mood disturbance, and anxiety** A
Major neurocognitive disorder due to vascular disease NOS
Vascular dementia NOS
Coding Clinic: 2021, Q2, P4

●● **FØ1.51 Vascular dementia, unspecified severity, with behavioral disturbance** A

F01.511 Vascular dementia, unspecified severity, with agitation (Ex:) PDX 5408 A
Major neurocognitive disorder due to vascular disease, unspecified severity, with aberrant motor behavior such as restlessness, rocking, pacing, or exit-seeking
Major neurocognitive disorder due to vascular disease, unspecified severity, with verbal or physical behaviors such as profanity, shouting, threatening, anger, aggression, combativeness, or violence
Vascular dementia, unspecified severity, with aberrant motor behavior such as restlessness, rocking, pacing, or exit-seeking
Vascular dementia, unspecified severity, with verbal or physical behaviors such as profanity, shouting, threatening, anger, aggression, combativeness, or violence

F01.518 Vascular dementia, unspecified severity, with other behavioral disturbance (Ex:) PDX 5419 A
Major neurocognitive disorder due to vascular disease, unspecified severity, with behavioral disturbances such as sleep disturbance, social disinhibition, or sexual disinhibition
Vascular dementia, unspecified severity, with behavioral disturbances such as sleep disturbance, social disinhibition, or sexual disinhibition

Use Additional code, if applicable, to identify wandering in vascular dementia (Z91.83)

F01.52 Vascular dementia, unspecified severity, with psychotic disturbance (Ex:) PDX 5648 A
Major neurocognitive disorder due to vascular disease, unspecified severity, with psychotic disturbance such as hallucinations, paranoia, suspiciousness, or delusional state
Vascular dementia, unspecified severity, with psychotic disturbance such as hallucinations, paranoia, suspiciousness, or delusional state

F01.53 Vascular dementia, unspecified severity, with mood disturbance (Ex:) PDX 5649 A
Major neurocognitive disorder due to vascular disease, unspecified severity, with mood disturbance such as depression, apathy, or anhedonia
Vascular dementia, unspecified severity, with mood disturbance such as depression, apathy, or anhedonia

F01.54 Vascular dementia, unspecified severity, with anxiety (Ex:) PDX 5651 A
Major neurocognitive disorder due to vascular disease, unspecified severity, with anxiety

● **F01.A Vascular dementia, mild**
Excludes1 mild neurocognitive disorder due to known physiological condition with or without behavioral disturbance (F06.7-)

F01.A0 Vascular dementia, mild, without behavioral disturbance, psychotic disturbance, mood disturbance, and anxiety A
Major neurocognitive disorder due to vascular disease, mild, NOS
Vascular dementia, mild, NOS

● **F01.A1 Vascular dementia, mild, with behavioral disturbance**

F01.A11 Vascular dementia, mild, with agitation (Ex:) PDX 4966 A
Major neurocognitive disorder due to vascular disease, mild, with aberrant motor behavior such as restlessness, rocking, pacing, or exit-seeking
Major neurocognitive disorder due to vascular disease, mild, with verbal or physical behaviors such as profanity, shouting, threatening, anger, aggression, combativeness, or violence
Vascular dementia, mild, with aberrant motor behavior such as restlessness, rocking, pacing, or exit-seeking
Vascular dementia, mild, with verbal or physical behaviors such as profanity, shouting, threatening, anger, aggression, combativeness, or violence

F01.A18 Vascular dementia, mild, with other behavioral disturbance (Ex:) PDX 5609 A
Major neurocognitive disorder due to vascular disease, mild, with behavioral disturbances such as sleep disturbance, social disinhibition, or sexual disinhibition
Vascular dementia, mild, with behavioral disturbances such as sleep disturbance, social disinhibition, or sexual disinhibition

Use Additional code, if applicable, to identify wandering in vascular dementia (Z91.83)

F01.A2 Vascular dementia, mild, with psychotic disturbance (Ex:) PDX 5428 A
Major neurocognitive disorder due to vascular disease, mild, with psychotic disturbance such as hallucinations, paranoia, suspiciousness, or delusional state
Vascular dementia, mild, with psychotic disturbance such as hallucinations, paranoia, suspiciousness, or delusional state

F01.A3 Vascular dementia, mild, with mood disturbance (Ex:) PDX 5430 A
Major neurocognitive disorder due to vascular disease, mild, with mood disturbance such as depression, apathy, or anhedonia
Vascular dementia, mild, with mood disturbance such as depression, apathy, or anhedonia

F01.A4 Vascular dementia, mild, with anxiety (Ex:) PDX 5431 A
Major neurocognitive disorder due to vascular disease, mild, with anxiety

● **F01.B Vascular dementia, moderate**

● **F01.B0 Vascular dementia, moderate, without behavioral disturbance, psychotic disturbance, mood disturbance, and anxiety** A
Major neurocognitive disorder due to vascular disease, moderate, NOS
Vascular dementia, moderate, NOS

F01.B1 Vascular dementia, moderate, with behavioral disturbance

F01.B11 Vascular dementia, moderate, with agitation (Ex) PDX 5519 A

Major neurocognitive disorder due to vascular disease, moderate, with aberrant motor behavior such as restlessness, rocking, pacing, or exit-seeking

Major neurocognitive disorder due to vascular disease, moderate, with verbal or physical behaviors such as profanity, shouting, threatening, anger, aggression, combativeness, or violence

Vascular dementia, moderate, with aberrant motor behavior such as restlessness, rocking, pacing, or exit-seeking

Vascular dementia, moderate, with verbal or physical behaviors such as profanity, shouting, threatening, anger, aggression, combativeness, or violence

F01.B18 Vascular dementia, moderate, with other behavioral disturbance (Ex) PDX 5557 A

Major neurocognitive disorder due to vascular disease, moderate, with behavioral disturbances such as sleep disturbance, social disinhibition, or sexual disinhibition

Vascular dementia, moderate, with behavioral disturbances such as sleep disturbance, social disinhibition, or sexual disinhibition

Use Additional code, if applicable, to identify wandering in vascular dementia (Z91.83)

F01.B2 Vascular dementia, moderate, with psychotic disturbance (Ex) PDX 5414 A

Major neurocognitive disorder due to vascular disease, moderate, with psychotic disturbance such as hallucinations, paranoia, suspiciousness, or delusional state

Vascular dementia, moderate, with psychotic disturbance such as hallucinations, paranoia, suspiciousness, or delusional state

F01.B3 Vascular dementia, moderate, with mood disturbance (Ex) PDX 5415 A

Major neurocognitive disorder due to vascular disease, moderate, with mood disturbance such as depression, apathy, or anhedonia

Vascular dementia, moderate, with mood disturbance such as depression, apathy, or anhedonia

F01.B4 Vascular dementia, moderate, with anxiety (Ex) PDX 5416 A

Major neurocognitive disorder due to vascular disease, moderate, with anxiety

F01.C Vascular dementia, severe

F01.C0 Vascular dementia, severe, without behavioral disturbance, psychotic disturbance, mood disturbance, and anxiety A

Major neurocognitive disorder due to vascular disease, severe, NOS

Vascular dementia, severe, NOS

F01.C1 Vascular dementia, severe, with behavioral disturbance

F01.C11 Vascular dementia, severe, with agitation (Ex) PDX 4849 A

Major neurocognitive disorder due to vascular disease, severe, with aberrant motor behavior such as restlessness, rocking, pacing, or exit-seeking

Major neurocognitive disorder due to vascular disease, severe, with verbal or physical behaviors such as profanity, shouting, threatening, anger, aggression, combativeness, or violence

Vascular dementia, severe, with aberrant motor behavior such as restlessness, rocking, pacing, or exit-seeking

Vascular dementia, severe, with verbal or physical behaviors such as profanity, shouting, threatening, anger, aggression, combativeness, or violence

F01.C18 Vascular dementia, severe, with other behavioral disturbance (Ex) PDX 4932 A

Major neurocognitive disorder due to vascular disease, severe, with behavioral disturbances such as sleep disturbance, social disinhibition, or sexual disinhibition

Vascular dementia, severe, with behavioral disturbances such as sleep disturbance, social disinhibition, or sexual disinhibition

Use Additional code, if applicable, to identify wandering in vascular dementia (Z91.83)

F01.C2 Vascular dementia, severe, with psychotic disturbance (Ex) PDX 5389 A

Major neurocognitive disorder due to vascular disease, severe, with psychotic disturbance such as hallucinations, paranoia, suspiciousness, or delusional state

Vascular dementia, severe, with psychotic disturbance such as hallucinations, paranoia, suspiciousness, or delusional state

F01.C3 Vascular dementia, severe, with mood disturbance (Ex) PDX 5390 A

Major neurocognitive disorder due to vascular disease, severe, with mood disturbance such as depression, apathy, or anhedonia

Vascular dementia, severe, with mood disturbance such as depression, apathy, or anhedonia

F01.C4 Vascular dementia, severe, with anxiety (Ex) PDX 5391 A

Major neurocognitive disorder due to vascular disease, severe, with anxiety

● **F02 Dementia in other diseases classified elsewhere**

Code first the underlying physiological condition, such as:
Alzheimer's (G30.-)
cerebral lipidosis (E75.4)
Creutzfeldt-Jakob disease (A81.0-)
~~dementia with Lewy bodies (G31.83)~~
~~dementia with Parkinsonism (G31.83)~~
epilepsy and recurrent seizures (G40.-)
frontotemporal dementia (G31.09)
hepatolenticular degeneration (E83.01)
human immunodeficiency virus [HIV] disease (B20)
Huntington's disease (G10)
hypercalcemia (E83.52)
hypothyroidism, acquired (E00-E03.-)
intoxications (T36-T65)
Jakob-Creutzfeldt disease (A81.0-)
multiple sclerosis (G35)
▶neurocognitive disorder with Lewy bodies (G31.83)
neurosyphilis (A52.17)
niacin deficiency [pellagra] (E52)
▶other frontotemporal neurocognitive disorder (G31.90)
Parkinson's disease (G20.-)
Pick's disease (G31.01)
polyarteritis nodosa (M30.0)
prion disease (A81.9)
systemic lupus erythematosus (M32.-)
traumatic brain injury (S06.-)
trypanosomiasis (B56.-, B57.-)
vitamin B deficiency (E53.8)

Includes Major neurocognitive disorder in other diseases classified elsewhere

Excludes1 mild neurocognitive disorder due to known physiological condition with or without behavioral disturbance (F06.7-)

Excludes2 dementia in alcohol and psychoactive substance disorders (F10-F19, with .17, .27, .97)
vascular dementia (F01.5-, F01.A-, F01.B-, F01.C-)

Coding Clinic: 2016, Q4, P141

● **F02.8 Dementia in other diseases classified elsewhere, unspecified severity**

F02.80 ***Dementia in other diseases classified elsewhere, unspecified severity, without behavioral disturbance, psychotic disturbance, mood disturbance, and anxiety***
Dementia in other diseases classified elsewhere NOS
Major neurocognitive disorder in other diseases classified elsewhere NOS
Coding Clinic: 2024, Q2, P9; 2017, Q1, P43; 2016, Q2, P6

● **F02.81** ***Dementia in other diseases classified elsewhere, unspecified severity, with behavioral disturbance***
Coding Clinic: 2017, Q2, P8, Q1, P43

F02.811 Dementia in other diseases classified elsewhere, unspecified severity, with agitation (Ex) PDX 5406
Dementia in other diseases classified elsewhere, unspecified severity, with aberrant motor behavior such as restlessness, rocking, pacing, or exit-seeking
Dementia in other diseases classified elsewhere, unspecified severity, with verbal or physical behaviors such as profanity, shouting, threatening, anger, aggression, combativeness, or violence
Major neurocognitive disorder in other diseases classified elsewhere, unspecified severity, with aberrant motor behavior such as restlessness, rocking, pacing, or exit-seeking
Major neurocognitive disorder in other diseases classified elsewhere, unspecified severity, with verbal or physical behaviors such as profanity, shouting, threatening, anger, aggression, combativeness, or violence

F02.818 Dementia in other diseases classified elsewhere, unspecified severity, with other behavioral disturbance (Ex) PDX 5401
Dementia in other diseases classified elsewhere with sleep disturbance, social disinhibition, or sexual disinhibition
Major neurocognitive disorder in other diseases classified elsewhere with sleep disturbance, social disinhibition, or sexual disinhibition

Use Additional code, if applicable, to identify wandering in dementia in conditions classified elsewhere (Z91.83)

F02.82 Dementia in other diseases classified elsewhere, unspecified severity, with psychotic disturbance (Ex) PDX 5042
Dementia in other diseases classified elsewhere, unspecified severity, with psychotic disturbance such as hallucinations, paranoia, suspiciousness, or delusional state
Major neurocognitive disorder in other diseases classified elsewhere, unspecified, with psychotic disturbance such as hallucinations, paranoia, suspiciousness, or delusional state

F02.83 Dementia in other diseases classified elsewhere, unspecified severity, with mood disturbance (Ex) PDX 5041
Dementia in other diseases classified elsewhere, unspecified severity, with mood disturbance such as depression, apathy, or anhedonia
Major neurocognitive disorder in other diseases classified elsewhere unspecified severity, with mood disturbance such as with depression, apathy, or anhedonia

CHAPTER 5 (F01-F99)

F02.84 Dementia in other diseases classified elsewhere, unspecified severity, with anxiety (Ex) PDX 5044
Major neurocognitive disorder in other diseases classified elsewhere unspecified severity, with anxiety

F02.A Dementia in other diseases classified elsewhere, mild
Excludes1 mild neurocognitive disorder due to known physiological condition with or without behavioral disturbance (F06.7-)

F02.A0 Dementia in other diseases classified elsewhere, mild, without behavioral disturbance, psychotic disturbance, mood disturbance, and anxiety
Dementia in other diseases classified elsewhere, mild, NOS
Major neurocognitive disorder in other diseases classified elsewhere, mild, NOS

F02.A1 Dementia in other diseases classified elsewhere, mild, with behavioral disturbance

F02.A11 Dementia in other diseases classified elsewhere, mild, with agitation (Ex) PDX 5087
Dementia in other diseases classified elsewhere, mild, with aberrant motor behavior such as restlessness, rocking, pacing, or exit-seeking
Dementia in other diseases classified elsewhere, mild, with verbal or physical behaviors such as profanity, shouting, threatening, anger, aggression, combativeness, or violence
Major neurocognitive disorder in other diseases classified elsewhere, mild, with aberrant motor behavior such as restlessness, rocking, pacing, or exit-seeking
Major neurocognitive disorder in other diseases classified elsewhere, mild, with verbal or physical behaviors such as profanity, shouting, threatening, anger, aggression, combativeness, or violence

F02.A18 Dementia in other diseases classified elsewhere, mild, with other behavioral disturbance (Ex) PDX 5062
Dementia in other diseases classified elsewhere, mild, with behavioral disturbances such as sleep disturbance, social disinhibition, or sexual disinhibition
Major neurocognitive disorder in other diseases classified elsewhere, mild, with behavioral disturbances such as sleep disturbance, social disinhibition, or sexual disinhibition
Use Additional code, if applicable, to identify wandering in dementia in conditions classified elsewhere (Z91.83)

F02.A2 Dementia in other diseases classified elsewhere, mild, with psychotic disturbance (Ex) PDX 4812
Dementia in other diseases classified elsewhere, mild, with psychotic disturbance such as hallucinations, paranoia, suspiciousness, or delusional state
Major neurocognitive disorder in other diseases classified elsewhere, mild, with psychotic disturbance such as hallucinations, paranoia, suspiciousness, or delusional state

F02.A3 Dementia in other diseases classified elsewhere, mild, with mood disturbance (Ex) PDX 4814
Dementia in other diseases classified elsewhere, mild, with mood disturbance such as depression, apathy, or anhedonia
Major neurocognitive disorder in other diseases classified elsewhere, mild, with mood disturbance such as depression, apathy, or anhedonia

F02.A4 Dementia in other diseases classified elsewhere, mild, with anxiety (Ex) PDX 4813
Major neurocognitive disorder in other diseases classified elsewhere, mild, with anxiety

F02.B Dementia in other diseases classified elsewhere, moderate

F02.B0 Dementia in other diseases classified elsewhere, moderate, without behavioral disturbance, psychotic disturbance, mood disturbance, and anxiety
Dementia in other diseases classified elsewhere, moderate, NOS
Major neurocognitive disorder in other diseases classified elsewhere, moderate, NOS

F02.B1 Dementia in other diseases classified elsewhere, moderate, with behavioral disturbance

F02.B11 Dementia in other diseases classified elsewhere, moderate, with agitation (Ex) PDX 5614
Dementia in other diseases classified elsewhere, moderate, with aberrant motor behavior such as restlessness, rocking, pacing, or exit-seeking
Dementia in other diseases classified elsewhere, moderate, with verbal or physical behaviors such as profanity, shouting, threatening, anger, aggression, combativeness, or violence
Major neurocognitive disorder in other diseases classified elsewhere, moderate, with aberrant motor behavior such as restlessness, rocking, pacing, or exit- seeking
Major neurocognitive disorder in other diseases classified elsewhere, moderate, with verbal or physical behaviors such as profanity, shouting, threatening, anger, aggression, combativeness, or violence

F02.B18 Dementia in other diseases classified elsewhere, moderate, with other behavioral disturbance (Ex) PDX 5580
Dementia in other diseases classified elsewhere, moderate, with behavioral disturbances such as sleep disturbance, social disinhibition, or sexual disinhibition
Major neurocognitive disorder in other diseases classified elsewhere, moderate, with behavioral disturbance such as sleep disturbance, social disinhibition, or sexual disinhibition
Use Additional code, if applicable, to identify wandering in dementia in conditions classified elsewhere (Z91.83)

F02.B2 Dementia in other diseases classified elsewhere, moderate, with psychotic disturbance (Ex) PDX 4793
Dementia in other diseases classified elsewhere, moderate, with psychotic disturbance such as hallucinations, paranoia, suspiciousness, or delusional state
Major neurocognitive disorder in other diseases classified elsewhere, moderate, with psychotic disturbance such as hallucinations, paranoia, suspiciousness, or delusional state

F02.B3 Dementia in other diseases classified elsewhere, moderate, with mood disturbance (Ex) PDX 4791
Dementia in other diseases classified elsewhere, moderate, with mood disturbance such as depression, apathy, or anhedonia
Major neurocognitive disorder in other diseases classified elsewhere, moderate, with mood disturbance such as depression, apathy, or anhedonia

F02.B4 Dementia in other diseases classified elsewhere, moderate, with anxiety (Ex) PDX 4796
Major neurocognitive disorder in other diseases classified elsewhere, moderate, with anxiety

F02.C Dementia in other diseases classified elsewhere, severe

F02.C0 Dementia in other diseases classified elsewhere, severe, without behavioral disturbance, psychotic disturbance, mood disturbance, and anxiety
Dementia in other diseases classified elsewhere, severe, NOS
Major neurocognitive disorder in other diseases classified elsewhere, severe, NOS

F02.C1 Dementia in other diseases classified elsewhere, severe, with behavioral disturbance

F02.C11 Dementia in other diseases classified elsewhere, severe, with agitation (Ex) PDX 5559
Dementia in other diseases classified elsewhere, severe, with aberrant motor behavior such as restlessness, rocking, pacing, or exit-seeking
Dementia in other diseases classified elsewhere, severe, with verbal or physical behaviors such as profanity, shouting, threatening, anger, aggression, combativeness, or violence
Major neurocognitive disorder in other diseases classified elsewhere, severe, with aberrant motor behavior such as restlessness, rocking, pacing, or exit-seeking
Major neurocognitive disorder in other diseases classified elsewhere, severe, with verbal or physical behaviors such as profanity, shouting, threatening, anger, aggression, combativeness, or violence
Coding Clinic: 2022, Q4, P15

F02.C18 Dementia in other diseases classified elsewhere, severe, with other behavioral disturbance (Ex) PDX 5551
Dementia in other diseases classified elsewhere, severe, with behavioral disturbances such as sleep disturbance, social disinhibition, or sexual disinhibition
Major neurocognitive disorder in other diseases classified elsewhere, severe, with behavioral disturbances such as sleep disturbance, social disinhibition, or sexual disinhibition
Use Additional code, if applicable, to identify wandering in dementia in conditions classified elsewhere (Z91.83)

F02.C2 Dementia in other diseases classified elsewhere, severe, with psychotic disturbance (Ex) PDX 4768
Dementia in other diseases classified elsewhere, severe, with psychotic disturbance such as hallucinations, paranoia, suspiciousness, or delusional state
Major neurocognitive disorder in other diseases classified elsewhere, severe, with psychotic disturbance such as hallucinations, paranoia, suspiciousness, or delusional state

F02.C3 Dementia in other diseases classified elsewhere, severe, with mood disturbance (Ex) PDX 4773
Dementia in other diseases classified elsewhere, severe, with mood disturbance such as depression, apathy, or anhedonia
Major neurocognitive disorder in other diseases classified elsewhere, severe, with mood disturbance such as depression, apathy, or anhedonia

F02.C4 Dementia in other diseases classified elsewhere, severe, with anxiety (Ex) PDX 4770
Major neurocognitive disorder in other diseases classified elsewhere, severe, with anxiety

F03 Unspecified dementia
Major neurocognitive disorder NOS
Presenile dementia NOS
Presenile psychosis NOS
Primary degenerative dementia NOS
Senile dementia NOS
Senile dementia depressed or paranoid type
Senile psychosis NOS
Excludes1 ~~senility NOS (R41.81)~~
Excludes2 dementia with delirium or acute confusional state (F05)
mild memory disturbance due to known physiological condition (F06.8)
~~senile dementia with delirium or acute confusional state (F05)~~

F03.9 Unspecified dementia, unspecified severity

F03.90 Unspecified dementia, unspecified severity, without behavioral disturbance, psychotic disturbance, mood disturbance, and anxiety A
Dementia NOS
Coding Clinic: 2024, Q2, P9; 2021, Q2, P4; 2012, Q4, P92

Item 5-1 Psychosis was a term formerly applied to any mental disorder but is now restricted to disturbances of a great magnitude in which there is a personality disintegration and loss of contact with reality.

● **F03.91 Unspecified dementia with, unspecified severity, behavioral disturbance**

F03.911 Unspecified dementia, unspecified severity, with agitation (Ex:) PDX 5384 A

Unspecified dementia, unspecified severity, with aberrant motor behavior such as restlessness, rocking, pacing, or exit-seeking

Unspecified dementia, unspecified severity, with verbal or physical behaviors such as profanity, shouting, threatening, anger, aggression, combativeness, or violence

F03.918 Unspecified dementia, unspecified severity, with other behavioral disturbance (Ex:) PDX 5381 A

Unspecified dementia, unspecified severity, with behavioral disturbances such as sleep disturbance, social disinhibition, or sexual disinhibition

Use Additional code, if applicable, to identify wandering in unspecified dementia (Z91.83)

F03.92 Unspecified dementia, unspecified severity, with psychotic disturbance (Ex:) PDX 5646 A

Unspecified dementia, unspecified severity, with psychotic disturbance such as hallucinations, paranoia, suspiciousness, or delusional state

F03.93 Unspecified dementia, unspecified severity, with mood disturbance (Ex:) PDX 5643 A

Unspecified dementia, unspecified severity, with mood disturbance such as depression, apathy, or anhedonia

F03.94 Unspecified dementia, unspecified severity, with anxiety (Ex:) PDX 5650 A

● **F03.A Unspecified dementia, mild**

Excludes1 mild neurocognitive disorder due to known physiological condition with or without behavioral disturbance (F06.7-)

F03.A0 Unspecified dementia, mild, without behavioral disturbance, psychotic disturbance, mood disturbance, and anxiety A

Dementia, mild, NOS

● **F03.A1 Unspecified dementia, mild, with behavioral disturbance**

F03.A11 Unspecified dementia, mild, with agitation (Ex:) PDX 5699 A

Unspecified dementia, mild, with aberrant motor behavior such as restlessness, rocking, pacing, or exit-seeking

Unspecified dementia, mild, with verbal or physical behaviors such as profanity, shouting, threatening, anger, aggression, combativeness, or violence

F03.A18 Unspecified dementia, mild, with other behavioral disturbance (Ex:) PDX 5694 A

Unspecified dementia, mild, with behavioral disturbances such as sleep disturbance, social disinhibition, or sexual disinhibition

Use Additional code, if applicable, to identify wandering in unspecified dementia (Z91.83)

F03.A2 Unspecified dementia, mild, with psychotic disturbance (Ex:) PDX 5505 A

Unspecified dementia, mild, with psychotic disturbance such as hallucinations, paranoia, suspiciousness, or delusional state

F03.A3 Unspecified dementia, mild, with mood disturbance (Ex:) PDX 5503 A

Unspecified dementia, mild, with mood disturbance such as depression, apathy, or anhedonia

F03.A4 Unspecified dementia, mild, with anxiety (Ex:) PDX 5506 A

● **F03.B Unspecified dementia, moderate**

F03.B0 Unspecified dementia, moderate, without behavioral disturbance, psychotic disturbance, mood disturbance, and anxiety A

Dementia, moderate, NOS

● **F03.B1 Unspecified dementia, moderate, with behavioral disturbance**

F03.B11 Unspecified dementia, moderate, with agitation (Ex:) PDX 5066 A

Unspecified dementia, moderate, with aberrant motor behavior such as restlessness, rocking, pacing, or exit-seeking

Unspecified dementia, moderate, with verbal or physical behaviors such as profanity, shouting, threatening, anger, aggression, combativeness, or violence

F03.B18 Unspecified dementia, moderate, with other behavioral disturbance (Ex:) PDX 5120 A

Unspecified dementia, moderate, with behavioral disturbances such as sleep disturbance, social disinhibition, or sexual disinhibition

Use Additional code, if applicable, to identify wandering in unspecified dementia (Z91.83)

F03.B2 Unspecified dementia, moderate, with psychotic disturbance (Ex:) PDX 5493 A

Unspecified dementia, moderate, with psychotic disturbance such as hallucinations, paranoia, suspiciousness, or delusional state

F03.B3 Unspecified dementia, moderate, with mood disturbance (Ex:) PDX 5495 A

Unspecified dementia, moderate, with mood disturbance such as depression, apathy, or anhedonia

F03.B4 Unspecified dementia, moderate, with anxiety (Ex:) PDX 5494 A

● **F03.C Unspecified dementia, severe**

F03.C0 Unspecified dementia, severe, without behavioral disturbance, psychotic disturbance, mood disturbance, and anxiety A

Dementia, severe, NOS

CHAPTER 5 (F01-F99)

● **FØ3.C1 Unspecified dementia, severe, with behavioral disturbance**

FØ3.C11 Unspecified dementia, severe, with agitation Ⓔ (Ex) PDX 5587 A

Unspecified dementia, severe, with aberrant motor behavior such as restlessness, rocking, pacing, or exit-seeking

Unspecified dementia, severe, with verbal or physical behaviors such as profanity, shouting, threatening, anger, aggression, combativeness, or violence

FØ3.C18 Unspecified dementia, severe, with other behavioral disturbance Ⓔ (Ex) PDX 5670 A

Unspecified dementia, severe, with behavioral disturbances such as sleep disturbance, social disinhibition, or sexual disinhibition

Use Additional code, if applicable, to identify wandering in unspecified dementia (Z91.83)

FØ3.C2 Unspecified dementia, severe, with psychotic disturbance Ⓔ (Ex) PDX 5471 A

Unspecified dementia, severe, with psychotic disturbance such as hallucinations, paranoia, suspiciousness, or delusional state

FØ3.C3 Unspecified dementia, severe, with mood disturbance Ⓔ (Ex) PDX 547Ø A

Unspecified dementia, severe, with mood disturbance such as depression, apathy, or anhedonia

Coding Clinic: 2Ø23, Q4, P15

FØ3.C4 Unspecified dementia, severe, with anxiety Ⓔ (Ex) PDX 5472 A

● **FØ4 Amnestic disorder due to known physiological condition**

Korsakov's psychosis or syndrome, nonalcoholic

Code first the underlying physiological condition

Excludes1 amnesia NOS (R41.3)
anterograde amnesia (R41.1)
dissociative amnesia (F44.Ø)
retrograde amnesia (R41.2)

Excludes2 alcohol-induced or unspecified Korsakov's syndrome (F1Ø.26, F1Ø.96)
Korsakov's syndrome induced by other psychoactive substances (F13.26, F13.96, F19.16, F19.26, F19.96)

● **FØ5 Delirium due to known physiological condition** Ⓔ (Ex) PDX 549

Acute or subacute brain syndrome
Acute or subacute confusional state (nonalcoholic)
Acute or subacute infective psychosis
Acute or subacute organic reaction
Acute or subacute psycho-organic syndrome
Delirium of mixed etiology
Delirium superimposed on dementia
Sundowning

Code first the underlying physiological condition, such as:
dementia (FØ3.9-)

Excludes1 delirium NOS (R41.Ø)

Excludes2 delirium tremens alcohol-induced or unspecified (F1Ø.231, F1Ø.921)

Coding Clinic: 2Ø19, Q2, P34

● **FØ6 Other mental disorders due to known physiological condition**

Includes mental disorders due to endocrine disorder
mental disorders due to exogenous hormone
mental disorders due to exogenous toxic substance
mental disorders due to primary cerebral disease
mental disorders due to somatic illness
mental disorders due to systemic disease affecting the brain

Code first the underlying physiological condition

Excludes1 unspecified dementia (FØ3.Ø-)

Excludes2 delirium due to known physiological condition (FØ5)
dementia as classified in FØ1-FØ2
other mental disorders associated with alcohol and other psychoactive substances (F1Ø-F19)

● **FØ6.Ø Psychotic disorder with hallucinations due to known physiological condition** Ⓔ (Ex) PDX 5411

Organic hallucinatory state (nonalcoholic)

Excludes2 hallucinations and perceptual disturbance induced by alcohol and other psychoactive substances (F1Ø-F19 with .151, .251, .951)
schizophrenia (F2Ø.-)

● **FØ6.1 Catatonic disorder due to known physiological condition**

Catatonia associated with another mental disorder
Catatonia NOS

Excludes1 catatonic stupor (R4Ø.1)
stupor NOS (R4Ø.1)

Excludes2 catatonic schizophrenia (F2Ø.2)
dissociative stupor (F44.2)

● **FØ6.2 Psychotic disorder with delusions due to known physiological condition** Ⓔ (Ex) PDX 5412

Paranoid and paranoid-hallucinatory organic states
Schizophrenia-like psychosis in epilepsy

Excludes2 alcohol and drug-induced psychotic disorder (F1Ø-F19 with .15Ø, .25Ø, .95Ø)
brief psychotic disorder (F23)
delusional disorder (F22)
schizophrenia (F2Ø.-)

● **FØ6.3 Mood disorder due to known physiological condition**

Excludes2 mood disorders due to alcohol and other psychoactive substances (F1Ø-F19 with .14, .24, .94)
mood disorders, not due to known physiological condition or unspecified (F3Ø-F39)

● **FØ6.3Ø Mood disorder due to known physiological condition, unspecified**

● **FØ6.31 Mood disorder due to known physiological condition with depressive features**

Depressive disorder due to known physiological condition, with depressive features

● **FØ6.32 Mood disorder due to known physiological condition with major depressive-like episode**

Depressive disorder due to known physiological condition, with major depressive-like episode

● **FØ6.33 Mood disorder due to known physiological condition with manic features**

Bipolar and related disorder due to a known physiological condition, with manic features

Bipolar and related disorder due to known physiological condition, with manic- or hypomanic-like episodes

F06.34 Mood disorder due to known physiological condition with mixed features
Bipolar and related disorder due to known physiological condition, with mixed features
Depressive disorder due to known physiological condition, with mixed features

F06.4 Anxiety disorder due to known physiological condition
Excludes2 anxiety disorders due to alcohol and other psychoactive substances (F10-F19 with .180, .280, .980)
anxiety disorders, not due to known physiological condition or unspecified (F40.-, F41.-)

F06.7 Mild neurocognitive disorder due to known physiological condition
Mild neurocognitive impairment due to a known physiological condition
Code first the underlying physiological condition, such as:
Alzheimer's disease (G30.-)
~~frontotemporal neurocognitive disorder (G31.09)~~
human immunodeficiency virus [HIV] disease (B20)
Huntington's disease (G10)
Neurocognitive disorder with Lewy bodies (G31.83)
▶other frontotemporal neurocognitive disorder (G31.09)
Parkinson's disease (G20.-)
systemic lupus erythematosus (M32.-)
traumatic brain injury (S06.-)
vitamin B deficiency (E53-)
Excludes1 age related cognitive decline (R41.81)
altered mental status (R41.82)
cerebral degeneration (G31.9)
change in mental status (R41.82)
cognitive deficits following (sequelae of) cerebral hemorrhage or infarction (I69.01- I69.11-, I69.21-I69.31-, I69.81-I69.91-)
dementia (F01.-, F02.-, F03.0-)
mild cognitive impairment due to unknown or unspecified etiology (G31.84)
neurologic neglect syndrome (R41.4)
personality change, nonpsychotic (F68.8)

F06.70 Mild neurocognitive disorder due to known physiological condition without behavioral disturbance
Mild neurocognitive disorder due to known physiological condition, NOS

F06.71 Mild neurocognitive disorder due to known physiological condition with behavioral disturbance (Ex) PDX 5210

F06.8 Other specified mental disorders due to known physiological condition
Epileptic psychosis NOS
Obsessive-compulsive and related disorder due to a known physiological condition
Organic dissociative disorder
Organic emotionally labile [asthenic] disorder

F07 Personality and behavioral disorders due to known physiological condition
Code first the underlying physiological condition

F07.0 Personality change due to known physiological condition
Frontal lobe syndrome
Limbic epilepsy personality syndrome
Lobotomy syndrome
Organic personality disorder
Organic pseudopsychopathic personality
Organic pseudoretarded personality
Postleucotomy syndrome
Excludes1 mild cognitive impairment (G31.84)
postconcussional syndrome (F07.81)
postencephalitic syndrome (F07.89)
signs and symptoms involving emotional state (R45.-)
Excludes2 specific personality disorder (F60.-)

F07.8 Other personality and behavioral disorders due to known physiological condition

F07.81 Postconcussional syndrome
Postcontusional syndrome (encephalopathy)
Post-traumatic brain syndrome, nonpsychotic
Use additional code to identify associated post-traumatic headache, if applicable (G44.3-)
Excludes1 current concussion (brain) (S06.0-)
postencephalitic syndrome (F07.89)

F07.89 Other personality and behavioral disorders due to known physiological condition
Postencephalitic syndrome
Damage to temporal brain lobes with memory loss and abnormal behavior
Right hemispheric organic affective disorder

F07.9 Unspecified personality and behavioral disorder due to known physiological condition
Organic psychosyndrome
Due to exposure to organic solvents

F09 Unspecified mental disorder due to known physiological condition
Mental disorder NOS due to known physiological condition
Organic brain syndrome NOS
Organic mental disorder NOS
Organic psychosis NOS
Symptomatic psychosis NOS
Code first the underlying physiological condition
Excludes1 mild neurocognitive disorder due to known physiological condition (F06.7-)
psychosis NOS (F29)

MENTAL AND BEHAVIORAL DISORDERS DUE TO PSYCHOACTIVE SUBSTANCE USE (F10-F19)

F10 Alcohol related disorders
Use additional code for blood alcohol level, if applicable (Y90.-)
Coding Clinic: 2019, Q3, P8

F10.1 Alcohol abuse
Excludes1 alcohol dependence (F10.2-)
alcohol use, unspecified (F10.9-)

F10.10 Alcohol abuse, uncomplicated
Alcohol use disorder, mild

F10.11 Alcohol abuse, in remission
Alcohol use disorder, mild, in early remission
Alcohol use disorder, mild, in sustained remission
Coding Clinic: 2022, Q1, P25

F10.12 Alcohol abuse with intoxication

F10.120 Alcohol abuse with intoxication, uncomplicated

F10.121 Alcohol abuse with intoxication, delirium (Ex) PDX 4806

F10.129 Alcohol abuse with intoxication, unspecified

F10.13 Alcohol abuse, with withdrawal

F10.130 Alcohol abuse with withdrawal, uncomplicated (Ex) PDX 4888

F10.131 Alcohol abuse with withdrawal delirium (Ex) PDX 4890

F10.132 Alcohol abuse with withdrawal with perceptual disturbance (Ex) PDX 4891

F10.139 Alcohol abuse with withdrawal, unspecified (Ex) PDX 4878

F10.14 Alcohol abuse with alcohol-induced mood disorder (Ex) PDX 5620
Alcohol use disorder, mild, with alcohol-induced bipolar or related disorder
Alcohol use disorder, mild, with alcohol-induced depressive disorder

F10.15 Alcohol abuse with alcohol-induced psychotic disorder

CHAPTER 5 (F01-F99)

F10.150 Alcohol abuse with alcohol-induced psychotic disorder with delusions

F10.151 Alcohol abuse with alcohol-induced psychotic disorder with hallucinations (Ex) PDX 4938

F10.159 Alcohol abuse with alcohol-induced psychotic disorder, unspecified (Ex) PDX 4928

● F10.18 Alcohol abuse with other alcohol-induced disorders

Coding Clinic: 2022, Q1, P33

F10.180 Alcohol abuse with alcohol-induced anxiety disorder (Ex) PDX 4970

Coding Clinic: 2022, Q1, P33

F10.181 Alcohol abuse with alcohol-induced sexual dysfunction (Ex) PDX 4971

F10.182 Alcohol abuse with alcohol-induced sleep disorder

F10.188 Alcohol abuse with other alcohol-induced disorder (Ex) PDX 4963

Coding Clinic: 2022, Q1, P25

F10.19 Alcohol abuse with unspecified alcohol-induced disorder (Ex) PDX 5627

● F10.2 Alcohol dependence

Excludes1 alcohol abuse (F10.1-)
alcohol use, unspecified (F10.9-)

Excludes2 toxic effect of alcohol (T51.0-)

Coding Clinic: 2019, Q3, P8

F10.20 Alcohol dependence, uncomplicated

Alcohol use disorder, moderate
Alcohol use disorder, severe

Coding Clinic: 2020, Q1, P9

F10.21 Alcohol dependence, in remission

Alcohol use disorder, moderate, in early remission
Alcohol use disorder, moderate, in sustained remission
Alcohol use disorder, severe, in early remission
Alcohol use disorder, severe, in sustained remission

● F10.22 Alcohol dependence with intoxication

Acute drunkenness (in alcoholism)

Excludes2 alcohol dependence with withdrawal (F10.23-)

F10.220 Alcohol dependence with intoxication, uncomplicated

F10.221 Alcohol dependence with intoxication delirium (Ex) PDX 5417

F10.229 Alcohol dependence with intoxication, unspecified

● F10.23 Alcohol dependence with withdrawal

Excludes2 alcohol dependence with intoxication (F10.22-)

F10.230 Alcohol dependence with withdrawal, uncomplicated (Ex) PDX 5481

F10.231 Alcohol dependence with withdrawal delirium (Ex) PDX 5482

F10.232 Alcohol dependence with withdrawal with perceptual disturbance (Ex) PDX 5477

F10.239 Alcohol dependence with withdrawal, unspecified (Ex) PDX 5475

Coding Clinic: 2015, Q2, P15

F10.24 Alcohol dependence with alcohol-induced mood disorder (Ex) PDX 5589

Alcohol use disorder, moderate, with alcohol-induced bipolar or related disorder
Alcohol use disorder, moderate, with alcohol-induced depressive disorder
Alcohol use disorder, severe, with alcohol-induced bipolar or related disorder
Alcohol use disorder, severe, with alcohol-induced depressive disorder

● F10.25 Alcohol dependence with alcohol-induced psychotic disorder

F10.250 Alcohol dependence with alcohol-induced psychotic disorder with delusions

F10.251 Alcohol dependence with alcohol-induced psychotic disorder with hallucinations (Ex) PDX 5511

F10.259 Alcohol dependence with alcohol-induced psychotic disorder, unspecified (Ex) PDX 5507

F10.26 Alcohol dependence with alcohol-induced persisting amnestic disorder

Alcohol use disorder, moderate, with alcohol-induced major neurocognitive disorder, amnestic-confabulatory type
Alcohol use disorder, severe, with alcohol-induced major neurocognitive disorder, amnestic-confabulatory type

F10.27 Alcohol dependence with alcohol-induced persisting dementia (Ex) PDX 5596

Alcohol use disorder, moderate, with alcohol-induced major neurocognitive disorder, nonamnestic-confabulatory type
Alcohol use disorder, severe, with alcohol-induced major neurocognitive disorder, nonamnestic-confabulatory type

● F10.28 Alcohol dependence with other alcohol-induced disorders

F10.280 Alcohol dependence with alcohol-induced anxiety disorder (Ex) PDX 5529

F10.281 Alcohol dependence with alcohol-induced sexual dysfunction (Ex) PDX 5532

F10.282 Alcohol dependence with alcohol-induced sleep disorder

F10.288 Alcohol dependence with other alcohol-induced disorder (Ex) PDX 5517

Alcohol use disorder, moderate, with alcohol-induced mild neurocognitive disorder
Alcohol use disorder, severe, with alcohol-induced mild neurocognitive disorder

Coding Clinic: 2020, Q1, P9

F10.29 Alcohol dependence with unspecified alcohol-induced disorder (Ex) PDX 5597

● F10.9 Alcohol use, unspecified

Excludes1 alcohol abuse (F10.1-)
alcohol dependence (F10.2-)

F10.90 Alcohol use, unspecified, uncomplicated

F10.91 Alcohol use, unspecified, in remission

● F10.92 Alcohol use, unspecified with intoxication

F10.920 Alcohol use, unspecified with intoxication, uncomplicated

F10.921 Alcohol use, unspecified with intoxication delirium (Ex) PDX 5176

F10.929 Alcohol use, unspecified with intoxication, unspecified

F10.93 Alcohol use, unspecified with withdrawal

F10.930 Alcohol use, unspecified with withdrawal, uncomplicated (Ex:) PDX 5231

F10.931 Alcohol use, unspecified with withdrawal delirium (Ex:) PDX 5233

F10.932 Alcohol use, unspecified with withdrawal with perceptual disturbance (Ex:) PDX 5234

F10.939 Alcohol use, unspecified with withdrawal, unspecified (Ex:) PDX 5224

F10.94 Alcohol use, unspecified with alcohol-induced mood disorder (Ex:) PDX 5479

Alcohol-induced bipolar or related disorder, without use disorder

Alcohol-induced depressive disorder, without use disorder

F10.95 Alcohol use, unspecified with alcohol-induced psychotic disorder

F10.950 Alcohol use, unspecified with alcohol-induced psychotic disorder with delusions

F10.951 Alcohol use, unspecified with alcohol-induced psychotic disorder with hallucinations (Ex:) PDX 5266

F10.959 Alcohol use, unspecified with alcohol-induced psychotic disorder, unspecified (Ex:) PDX 5263

Alcohol-induced psychotic disorder without use disorder

F10.96 Alcohol use, unspecified with alcohol-induced persisting amnestic disorder

Alcohol-induced major neurocognitive disorder, amnestic-confabulatory type, without use disorder

F10.97 Alcohol use, unspecified with alcohol-induced persisting dementia

Alcohol-induced major neurocognitive disorder, nonamnestic-confabulatory type, without use disorder

F10.98 Alcohol use, unspecified with other alcohol-induced disorders

F10.980 Alcohol use, unspecified with alcohol-induced anxiety disorder (Ex:) PDX 5287

Alcohol-induced anxiety disorder, without use disorder

F10.981 Alcohol use, unspecified with alcohol-induced sexual dysfunction (Ex:) PDX 5288

Alcohol-induced sexual dysfunction, without use disorder

F10.982 Alcohol use, unspecified with alcohol-induced sleep disorder

Alcohol-induced sleep disorder, without use disorder

F10.988 Alcohol use, unspecified with other alcohol-induced disorder (Ex:) PDX 5284

Alcohol-induced mild neurocognitive disorder, without use disorder

Coding Clinic: 2019, Q3, P8

F10.99 Alcohol use, unspecified with unspecified alcohol-induced disorder (Ex:) PDX 5480

F11 Opioid related disorders

F11.1 Opioid abuse

Excludes1 opioid dependence (F11.2-)
opioid use, unspecified (F11.9-)

F11.10 Opioid abuse, uncomplicated

Opioid use disorder, mild

F11.11 Opioid abuse, in remission

Opioid use disorder, mild, in early remission
Opioid use disorder, mild, in sustained remission

F11.12 Opioid abuse with intoxication

F11.120 Opioid abuse with intoxication, uncomplicated

F11.121 Opioid abuse with intoxication delirium (Ex:) PDX 5546

F11.122 Opioid abuse with intoxication with perceptual disturbance

F11.129 Opioid abuse with intoxication, unspecified

F11.13 Opioid abuse with withdrawal (Ex:) PDX 5090

F11.14 Opioid abuse with opioid-induced mood disorder

Opioid use disorder, mild, with opioid-induced depressive disorder

F11.15 Opioid abuse with opioid-induced psychotic disorder

F11.150 Opioid abuse with opioid-induced psychotic disorder with delusions (Ex:) PDX 5553

F11.151 Opioid abuse with opioid-induced psychotic disorder with hallucinations (Ex:) PDX 5555

F11.159 Opioid abuse with opioid-induced psychotic disorder, unspecified

F11.18 Opioid abuse with other opioid-induced disorder

F11.181 Opioid abuse with opioid-induced sexual dysfunction

F11.182 Opioid abuse with opioid-induced sleep disorder

F11.188 Opioid abuse with other opioid-induced disorder

Opioid-associated amnestic syndrome with opioid abuse

F11.19 Opioid abuse with unspecified opioid-induced disorder

F11.2 Opioid dependence

Excludes1 opioid abuse (F11.1-)
opioid use, unspecified (F11.9-)

Excludes2 opioid poisoning (T40.0—T40.2-)

F11.20 Opioid dependence, uncomplicated (Ex:) PDX 3215

Opioid use disorder, moderate
Opioid use disorder, severe

F11.21 Opioid dependence, in remission

Opioid use disorder, moderate, in early remission
Opioid use disorder, moderate, in sustained remission
Opioid use disorder, severe, in early remission
Opioid use disorder, severe, in sustained remission

F11.22 Opioid dependence with intoxication

Excludes1 opioid dependence with withdrawal (F11.23)

F11.220 Opioid dependence with intoxication, uncomplicated

F11.221 Opioid dependence with intoxication delirium (Ex:) PDX 4892

F11.222 Opioid dependence with intoxication with perceptual disturbance (Ex:) PDX 4880

F11.229 Opioid dependence with intoxication, unspecified

CHAPTER 5 (F01-F99)

F11.23 **Opioid dependence with withdrawal** (Ex) PDX 5067
Excludes1 opioid dependence with intoxication (F11.22-)

F11.24 **Opioid dependence with opioid-induced mood disorder**
Opioid use disorder, moderate, with opioid-induced depressive disorder

● **F11.25** **Opioid dependence with opioid-induced psychotic disorder**

F11.250 **Opioid dependence with opioid-induced psychotic disorder with delusions** (Ex) PDX 4922

F11.251 **Opioid dependence with opioid-induced psychotic disorder with hallucinations** (Ex) PDX 4916

F11.259 **Opioid dependence with opioid-induced psychotic disorder, unspecified** (Ex) PDX 4911

● **F11.28** **Opioid dependence with other opioid-induced disorder**

F11.281 **Opioid dependence with opioid-induced sexual dysfunction** (Ex) PDX 5621

F11.282 **Opioid dependence with opioid-induced sleep disorder** (Ex) PDX 5624

F11.288 **Opioid dependence with other opioid-induced disorder** (Ex) PDX 5610

F11.29 **Opioid dependence with unspecified opioid-induced disorder**

● **F11.9** **Opioid use, unspecified**
Excludes1 opioid abuse (F11.1-)
opioid dependence (F11.2-)

F11.90 **Opioid use, unspecified, uncomplicated**

F11.91 **Opioid use, unspecified, in remission**

● **F11.92** **Opioid use, unspecified with intoxication**
Excludes1 opioid use, unspecified with withdrawal (F11.93)

F11.920 **Opioid use, unspecified with intoxication, uncomplicated**

F11.921 **Opioid use, unspecified with intoxication delirium** (Ex) PDX 5967
Opioid-induced delirium

F11.922 **Opioid use, unspecified with intoxication with perceptual disturbance**

F11.929 **Opioid use, unspecified with intoxication, unspecified**

F11.93 **Opioid use, unspecified with withdrawal** (Ex) PDX 4883
Excludes1 opioid use, unspecified with intoxication (F11.92-)

F11.94 **Opioid use, unspecified with opioid-induced mood disorder**
Opioid-induced depressive disorder, without use disorder

● **F11.95** **Opioid use, unspecified with opioid-induced psychotic disorder**

F11.950 **Opioid use, unspecified with opioid-induced psychotic disorder with delusions** (Ex) PDX 6015

F11.951 **Opioid use, unspecified with opioid-induced psychotic disorder with hallucinations** (Ex) PDX 6017

F11.959 **Opioid use, unspecified with opioid-induced psychotic disorder, unspecified**

● **F11.98** **Opioid use, unspecified with other specified opioid-induced disorder**

F11.981 **Opioid use, unspecified with opioid-induced sexual dysfunction**
Opioid-induced sexual dysfunction, without use disorder

F11.982 **Opioid use, unspecified with opioid-induced sleep disorder**
Opioid-induced sleep disorder, without use disorder

F11.988 **Opioid use, unspecified with other opioid-induced disorder**
Opioid-associated amnestic syndrome with opioid abuse
Opioid-induced anxiety disorder, without use disorder

F11.99 **Opioid use, unspecified with unspecified opioid-induced disorder**

● **F12** **Cannabis related disorders**
Includes marijuana
Coding Clinic: 2020, Q1, P8

● **F12.1** **Cannabis abuse**
Excludes1 cannabis dependence (F12.2-)
cannabis use, unspecified (F12.9-)

F12.10 **Cannabis abuse, uncomplicated**
Cannabis use disorder, mild

F12.11 **Cannabis abuse, in remission**
Cannabis use disorder, mild, in early remission
Cannabis use disorder, mild, in sustained remission

● **F12.12** **Cannabis abuse with intoxication**

F12.120 **Cannabis abuse with intoxication, uncomplicated**

F12.121 **Cannabis abuse with intoxication delirium** (Ex) PDX 4967

F12.122 **Cannabis abuse with intoxication with perceptual disturbance**

F12.129 **Cannabis abuse with intoxication, unspecified**

F12.13 **Cannabis abuse with withdrawal**

● **F12.15** **Cannabis abuse with psychotic disorder**

F12.150 **Cannabis abuse with psychotic disorder with delusions** (Ex) PDX 5674

F12.151 **Cannabis abuse with psychotic disorder with hallucinations** (Ex) PDX 5678

F12.159 **Cannabis abuse with psychotic disorder, unspecified**

● **F12.18** **Cannabis abuse with other cannabis-induced disorder**

F12.180 **Cannabis abuse with cannabis-induced anxiety disorder**

F12.188 **Cannabis abuse with other cannabis-induced disorder**
Cannabis use disorder, mild, with cannabis-induced sleep disorder
Opioid-associated amnestic syndrome with opioid abuse

F12.19 **Cannabis abuse with unspecified cannabis-induced disorder**

● **F12.2** **Cannabis dependence**
Excludes1 cannabis abuse (F12.1-)
cannabis use, unspecified (F12.9-)
Excludes2 cannabis poisoning (T40.7-)

F12.20 **Cannabis dependence, uncomplicated**
Cannabis use disorder, moderate
Cannabis use disorder, severe

CHAPTER 5 (F01-F99)

F12.21 **Cannabis dependence, in remission**
Cannabis use disorder, moderate, in early remission
Cannabis use disorder, moderate, in sustained remission
Cannabis use disorder, severe, in early remission
Cannabis use disorder, severe, in sustained remission

F12.22 **Cannabis dependence with intoxication**

F12.220 **Cannabis dependence with intoxication, uncomplicated**

F12.221 **Cannabis dependence with intoxication delirium** (Ex) PDX 5524

F12.222 **Cannabis dependence with intoxication with perceptual disturbance**

F12.229 **Cannabis dependence with intoxication, unspecified**

F12.23 **Cannabis dependence with withdrawal**

F12.25 **Cannabis dependence with psychotic disorder**

F12.250 **Cannabis dependence with psychotic disorder with delusions** (Ex) PDX 5050

F12.251 **Cannabis dependence with psychotic disorder with hallucinations** (Ex) PDX 5049

F12.259 **Cannabis dependence with psychotic disorder, unspecified**

F12.28 **Cannabis dependence with other cannabis-induced disorder**

F12.280 **Cannabis dependence with cannabis-induced anxiety disorder**

F12.288 **Cannabis dependence with other cannabis-induced disorder**
Cannabis use disorder, moderate, with cannabis-induced sleep disorder
Cannabis use disorder, severe, with cannabis-induced sleep disorder

F12.29 **Cannabis dependence with unspecified cannabis-induced disorder**

F12.9 **Cannabis use, unspecified**

Excludes1 cannabis abuse (F12.1-)
cannabis dependence (F12.2-)

F12.90 **Cannabis use, unspecified, uncomplicated**
Coding Clinic: 2023, Q3, P18

F12.91 **Cannabis use, unspecified, in remission**

F12.92 **Cannabis use, unspecified with intoxication**

F12.920 **Cannabis use, unspecified with intoxication, uncomplicated**

F12.921 **Cannabis use, unspecified with intoxication delirium** (Ex) PDX 5285

F12.922 **Cannabis use, unspecified with intoxication with perceptual disturbance**

F12.929 **Cannabis use, unspecified with intoxication, unspecified**

F12.93 **Cannabis use, unspecified with withdrawal**

F12.95 **Cannabis use, unspecified with psychotic disorder**

F12.950 **Cannabis use, unspecified with psychotic disorder with delusions** (Ex) PDX 4706

F12.951 **Cannabis use, unspecified with psychotic disorder with hallucinations** (Ex) PDX 4708

F12.959 **Cannabis use, unspecified with psychotic disorder, unspecified**
Cannabis-induced psychotic disorder, without use disorder

F12.98 **Cannabis use, unspecified with other cannabis-induced disorder**

F12.980 **Cannabis use, unspecified with anxiety disorder**
Cannabis-induced anxiety disorder, without use disorder

F12.988 **Cannabis use, unspecified with other cannabis-induced disorder**
Cannabis-induced sleep disorder, without use disorder

F12.99 **Cannabis use, unspecified with unspecified cannabis-induced disorder**

F13 **Sedative, hypnotic, or anxiolytic related disorders**

F13.1 **Sedative, hypnotic or anxiolytic-related abuse**

Excludes1 sedative, hypnotic or anxiolytic-related dependence (F13.2-)
sedative, hypnotic, or anxiolytic use, unspecified (F13.9-)

F13.10 **Sedative, hypnotic or anxiolytic abuse, uncomplicated**
Sedative, hypnotic, or anxiolytic use disorder, mild

F13.11 **Sedative, hypnotic or anxiolytic abuse, in remission**
Sedative, hypnotic or anxiolytic use disorder, mild, in early remission
Sedative, hypnotic or anxiolytic use disorder, mild, in sustained remission

F13.12 **Sedative, hypnotic or anxiolytic abuse with intoxication**

F13.120 **Sedative, hypnotic or anxiolytic abuse with intoxication, uncomplicated**

F13.121 **Sedative, hypnotic or anxiolytic abuse with intoxication delirium** (Ex) PDX 5085

F13.129 **Sedative, hypnotic or anxiolytic abuse with intoxication, unspecified**

F13.13 **Sedative, hypnotic or anxiolytic abuse with withdrawal**

F13.130 **Sedative, hypnotic or anxiolytic abuse with withdrawal, uncomplicated** (Ex) PDX 5076

F13.131 **Sedative, hypnotic or anxiolytic abuse with withdrawal delirium** (Ex) PDX 5074

F13.132 **Sedative, hypnotic or anxiolytic abuse with withdrawal with perceptual disturbance** (Ex) PDX 5065

F13.139 **Sedative, hypnotic or anxiolytic abuse with withdrawal, unspecified** (Ex) PDX 5063

F13.14 **Sedative, hypnotic or anxiolytic abuse with sedative, hypnotic or anxiolytic-induced mood disorder**
Sedative, hypnotic, or anxiolytic use disorder, mild, with sedative, hypnotic, or anxiolytic-induced bipolar or related disorder
Sedative, hypnotic, or anxiolytic use disorder, mild, with sedative, hypnotic, or anxiolytic-induced depressive disorder

F13.15 **Sedative, hypnotic or anxiolytic abuse with sedative, hypnotic or anxiolytic-induced psychotic disorder**

F13.150 **Sedative, hypnotic or anxiolytic abuse with sedative, hypnotic or anxiolytic-induced psychotic disorder with delusions** (Ex) PDX 5113

F13.151 **Sedative, hypnotic or anxiolytic abuse with sedative, hypnotic or anxiolytic-induced psychotic disorder with hallucinations** (Ex) PDX 5111

CHAPTER 5 (F01-F99)

F13.159 **Sedative, hypnotic or anxiolytic abuse with sedative, hypnotic or anxiolytic-induced psychotic disorder, unspecified**

F13.18 **Sedative, hypnotic or anxiolytic abuse with other sedative, hypnotic or anxiolytic-induced disorders**

F13.180 **Sedative, hypnotic or anxiolytic abuse with sedative, hypnotic or anxiolytic-induced anxiety disorder**

F13.181 **Sedative, hypnotic or anxiolytic abuse with sedative, hypnotic or anxiolytic-induced sexual dysfunction**

F13.182 **Sedative, hypnotic or anxiolytic abuse with sedative, hypnotic or anxiolytic-induced sleep disorder**

F13.188 **Sedative, hypnotic or anxiolytic abuse with other sedative, hypnotic or anxiolytic-induced disorder**

F13.19 **Sedative, hypnotic or anxiolytic abuse with unspecified sedative, hypnotic or anxiolytic-induced disorder**

F13.2 **Sedative, hypnotic or anxiolytic-related dependence**

Excludes1 sedative, hypnotic or anxiolytic-related abuse (F13.1-)
sedative, hypnotic, or anxiolytic use, unspecified (F13.9-)

Excludes2 sedative, hypnotic, or anxiolytic poisoning (T42.-)

F13.20 **Sedative, hypnotic or anxiolytic dependence, uncomplicated** Ex: PDX 3216

F13.21 **Sedative, hypnotic or anxiolytic dependence, in remission**
Sedative, hypnotic or anxiolytic use disorder, moderate, in early remission
Sedative, hypnotic or anxiolytic use disorder, moderate, in sustained remission
Sedative, hypnotic or anxiolytic use disorder, severe, in early remission
Sedative, hypnotic or anxiolytic use disorder, severe, in sustained remission

F13.22 **Sedative, hypnotic or anxiolytic dependence with intoxication**

Excludes1 sedative, hypnotic or anxiolytic dependence with withdrawal (F13.23-)

F13.220 **Sedative, hypnotic or anxiolytic dependence with intoxication, uncomplicated**

F13.221 **Sedative, hypnotic or anxiolytic dependence with intoxication delirium** Ex: PDX 5612

F13.229 **Sedative, hypnotic or anxiolytic dependence with intoxication, unspecified**

F13.23 **Sedative, hypnotic or anxiolytic dependence with withdrawal**
Sedative, hypnotic, or anxiolytic use disorder, moderate
Sedative, hypnotic, or anxiolytic use disorder, severe

Excludes1 sedative, hypnotic or anxiolytic dependence with intoxication (F13.22-)

F13.230 **Sedative, hypnotic or anxiolytic dependence with withdrawal, uncomplicated** Ex: PDX 5595

F13.231 **Sedative, hypnotic or anxiolytic dependence with withdrawal delirium** Ex: PDX 5588

F13.232 **Sedative, hypnotic or anxiolytic dependence with withdrawal with perceptual disturbance** Ex: PDX 5585
Sedative, hypnotic, or anxiolytic withdrawal with perceptual disturbances

F13.239 **Sedative, hypnotic or anxiolytic dependence with withdrawal, unspecified** Ex: PDX 5578
Sedative, hypnotic, or anxiolytic withdrawal without perceptual disturbances

F13.24 **Sedative, hypnotic or anxiolytic dependence with sedative, hypnotic or anxiolytic-induced mood disorder**
Sedative, hypnotic, or anxiolytic use disorder, moderate, with sedative, hypnotic, or anxiolytic-induced bipolar or related disorder
Sedative, hypnotic, or anxiolytic use disorder, moderate, with sedative, hypnotic, or anxiolytic-induced depressive disorder
Sedative, hypnotic, or anxiolytic use disorder, severe, with sedative, hypnotic, or anxiolytic-induced bipolar or related disorder
Sedative, hypnotic, or anxiolytic use disorder, severe, with sedative, hypnotic, or anxiolytic-induced depressive disorder

F13.25 **Sedative, hypnotic or anxiolytic dependence with sedative, hypnotic or anxiolytic-induced psychotic disorder**

F13.250 **Sedative, hypnotic or anxiolytic dependence with sedative, hypnotic or anxiolytic-induced psychotic disorder with delusions** Ex: PDX 5653

F13.251 **Sedative, hypnotic or anxiolytic dependence with sedative, hypnotic or anxiolytic-induced psychotic disorder with hallucinations** Ex: PDX 5660

F13.259 **Sedative, hypnotic or anxiolytic dependence with sedative, hypnotic or anxiolytic-induced psychotic disorder, unspecified** Ex: PDX 5647

F13.26 **Sedative, hypnotic or anxiolytic dependence with sedative, hypnotic or anxiolytic-induced persisting amnestic disorder** Ex: PDX 5138

F13.27 **Sedative, hypnotic or anxiolytic dependence with sedative, hypnotic or anxiolytic-induced persisting dementia** Ex: PDX 5137
Sedative, hypnotic, or anxiolytic use disorder, moderate, with sedative, hypnotic, or anxiolytic-induced major neurocognitive disorder
Sedative, hypnotic, or anxiolytic use disorder, severe, with sedative, hypnotic, or anxiolytic-induced major neurocognitive disorder

F13.28 **Sedative, hypnotic or anxiolytic dependence with other sedative, hypnotic or anxiolytic-induced disorders**

F13.280 **Sedative, hypnotic or anxiolytic dependence with sedative, hypnotic or anxiolytic-induced anxiety disorder** Ex: PDX 5787

F13.281 **Sedative, hypnotic or anxiolytic dependence with sedative, hypnotic or anxiolytic-induced sexual dysfunction** Ex: PDX 5786

CHAPTER 5 (F01-F99)

F13.282 **Sedative, hypnotic or anxiolytic dependence with sedative, hypnotic or anxiolytic-induced sleep disorder** (Ex) PDX 5776

F13.288 **Sedative, hypnotic or anxiolytic dependence with other sedative, hypnotic or anxiolytic-induced disorder** (Ex) PDX 5772
Sedative, hypnotic, or anxiolytic use disorder, moderate, with sedative, hypnotic, or anxiolytic-induced mild neurocognitive disorder
Sedative, hypnotic, or anxiolytic use disorder, severe, with sedative, hypnotic, or anxiolytic-induced mild neurocognitive disorder

F13.29 **Sedative, hypnotic or anxiolytic dependence with unspecified sedative, hypnotic or anxiolytic-induced disorder**

● **F13.9** **Sedative, hypnotic or anxiolytic-related use, unspecified**
Excludes1 sedative, hypnotic or anxiolytic-related abuse (F13.1-)
sedative, hypnotic or anxiolytic-related dependence (F13.2-)

F13.90 **Sedative, hypnotic, or anxiolytic use, unspecified, uncomplicated**

F13.91 **Sedative, hypnotic or anxiolytic use, unspecified, in remission**

● **F13.92** **Sedative, hypnotic or anxiolytic use, unspecified with intoxication**
Excludes1 sedative, hypnotic or anxiolytic use, unspecified with withdrawal (F13.93-)

F13.920 **Sedative, hypnotic or anxiolytic use, unspecified with intoxication, uncomplicated**

F13.921 **Sedative, hypnotic or anxiolytic use, unspecified with intoxication delirium** (Ex) PDX 5362
Sedative, hypnotic, or anxiolytic-induced delirium

F13.929 **Sedative, hypnotic or anxiolytic use, unspecified with intoxication, unspecified**

● **F13.93** **Sedative, hypnotic or anxiolytic use, unspecified with withdrawal**
Excludes1 sedative, hypnotic or anxiolytic use, unspecified with intoxication (F13.92-)

F13.930 **Sedative, hypnotic or anxiolytic use, unspecified with withdrawal, uncomplicated** (Ex) PDX 5353

F13.931 **Sedative, hypnotic or anxiolytic use, unspecified with withdrawal delirium** (Ex) PDX 5351

F13.932 **Sedative, hypnotic or anxiolytic use, unspecified with withdrawal with perceptual disturbances** (Ex) PDX 5349

F13.939 **Sedative, hypnotic or anxiolytic use, unspecified with withdrawal, unspecified** (Ex) PDX 5347

F13.94 **Sedative, hypnotic or anxiolytic use, unspecified with sedative, hypnotic or anxiolytic-induced mood disorder**
Sedative, hypnotic, or anxiolytic-induced bipolar or related disorder, without use disorder
Sedative, hypnotic, or anxiolytic-induced depressive disorder, without use disorder

● **F13.95** **Sedative, hypnotic or anxiolytic use, unspecified with sedative, hypnotic or anxiolytic-induced psychotic disorder**

F13.950 **Sedative, hypnotic or anxiolytic use, unspecified with sedative, hypnotic or anxiolytic-induced psychotic disorder with delusions** (Ex) PDX 5379

F13.951 **Sedative, hypnotic or anxiolytic use, unspecified with sedative, hypnotic or anxiolytic-induced psychotic disorder with hallucinations** (Ex) PDX 5376

F13.959 **Sedative, hypnotic or anxiolytic use, unspecified with sedative, hypnotic or anxiolytic-induced psychotic disorder, unspecified**
Sedative, hypnotic, or anxiolytic-induced psychotic disorder, without use disorder

F13.96 **Sedative, hypnotic or anxiolytic use, unspecified with sedative, hypnotic or anxiolytic-induced persisting amnestic disorder**

F13.97 **Sedative, hypnotic or anxiolytic use, unspecified with sedative, hypnotic or anxiolytic-induced persisting dementia** (Ex) PDX 4995
Sedative, hypnotic, or anxiolytic-induced major neurocognitive disorder, without use disorder

● **F13.98** **Sedative, hypnotic or anxiolytic use, unspecified with other sedative, hypnotic or anxiolytic-induced disorders**

F13.980 **Sedative, hypnotic or anxiolytic use, unspecified with sedative, hypnotic or anxiolytic-induced anxiety disorder**
Sedative, hypnotic, or anxiolytic-induced anxiety disorder, without use disorder

F13.981 **Sedative, hypnotic or anxiolytic use, unspecified with sedative, hypnotic or anxiolytic-induced sexual dysfunction**
Sedative, hypnotic, or anxiolytic-induced sexual dysfunction disorder, without use disorder

F13.982 **Sedative, hypnotic or anxiolytic use, unspecified with sedative, hypnotic or anxiolytic-induced sleep disorder**
Sedative, hypnotic, or anxiolytic-induced sleep disorder, without use disorder

F13.988 **Sedative, hypnotic or anxiolytic use, unspecified with other sedative, hypnotic or anxiolytic-induced disorder**
Sedative, hypnotic, or anxiolytic-induced mild neurocognitive disorder

F13.99 **Sedative, hypnotic or anxiolytic use, unspecified with unspecified sedative, hypnotic or anxiolytic-induced disorder**

CHAPTER 5 (F01-F99)

F14 Cocaine related disorders
Excludes2 other stimulant-related disorders (F15.-)

F14.1 Cocaine abuse
Excludes1 cocaine dependence (F14.2-)
cocaine use, unspecified (F14.9-)

F14.10 Cocaine abuse, uncomplicated
Cocaine use disorder, mild

F14.11 Cocaine abuse, in remission
Cocaine use disorder, mild, in early remission
Cocaine use disorder, mild, in sustained remission

F14.12 Cocaine abuse with intoxication

F14.120 Cocaine abuse with intoxication, uncomplicated

F14.121 Cocaine abuse with intoxication with delirium (Ex) PDX 5701

F14.122 Cocaine abuse with intoxication with perceptual disturbance

F14.129 Cocaine abuse with intoxication, unspecified

F14.13 Cocaine abuse, unspecified with withdrawal (Ex) PDX 5834

F14.14 Cocaine abuse with cocaine-induced mood disorder
Cocaine use disorder, mild, with cocaine-induced bipolar or related disorder
Cocaine use disorder, mild, with cocaine-induced depressive disorder

F14.15 Cocaine abuse with cocaine-induced psychotic disorder

F14.150 Cocaine abuse with cocaine-induced psychotic disorder with delusions (Ex) PDX 5837

F14.151 Cocaine abuse with cocaine-induced psychotic disorder with hallucinations (Ex) PDX 5835

F14.159 Cocaine abuse with cocaine-induced psychotic disorder, unspecified

F14.18 Cocaine abuse with other cocaine-induced disorder

F14.180 Cocaine abuse with cocaine-induced anxiety disorder

F14.181 Cocaine abuse with cocaine-induced sexual dysfunction

F14.182 Cocaine abuse with cocaine-induced sleep disorder

F14.188 Cocaine abuse with other cocaine-induced disorder
Cocaine use disorder, mild, with cocaine-induced obsessive-compulsive or related disorder

F14.19 Cocaine abuse with unspecified cocaine-induced disorder

F14.2 Cocaine dependence
Excludes1 cocaine abuse (F14.1-)
cocaine use, unspecified (F14.9-)
Excludes2 cocaine poisoning (T40.5-)

F14.20 Cocaine dependence, uncomplicated (Ex) PDX 5816
Cocaine use disorder, moderate
Cocaine use disorder, severe

F14.21 Cocaine dependence, in remission
Cocaine use disorder, moderate, in early remission
Cocaine use disorder, moderate, in sustained remission
Cocaine use disorder, severe, in early remission
Cocaine use disorder, severe, in sustained remission
Coding Clinic: 2017, Q2, P27

F14.22 Cocaine dependence with intoxication
Excludes1 cocaine dependence with withdrawal (F14.23)

F14.220 Cocaine dependence with intoxication, uncomplicated

F14.221 Cocaine dependence with intoxication delirium (Ex) PDX 5068

F14.222 Cocaine dependence with intoxication with perceptual disturbance (Ex) PDX 5069

F14.229 Cocaine dependence with intoxication, unspecified (Ex) PDX 5061

F14.23 Cocaine dependence with withdrawal (Ex) PDX 5820
Excludes1 cocaine dependence with intoxication (F14.22-)

F14.24 Cocaine dependence with cocaine-induced mood disorder
Cocaine use disorder, moderate, with cocaine-induced bipolar or related disorder
Cocaine use disorder, moderate, with cocaine-induced depressive disorder
Cocaine use disorder, severe, with cocaine-induced bipolar or related disorder
Cocaine use disorder, severe, with cocaine-induced depressive disorder

F14.25 Cocaine dependence with cocaine-induced psychotic disorder

F14.250 Cocaine dependence with cocaine-induced psychotic disorder with delusions (Ex) PDX 5167

F14.251 Cocaine dependence with cocaine-induced psychotic disorder with hallucinations (Ex) PDX 5170

F14.259 Cocaine dependence with cocaine-induced psychotic disorder, unspecified (Ex) PDX 5156

F14.28 Cocaine dependence with other cocaine-induced disorder

F14.280 Cocaine dependence with cocaine-induced anxiety disorder (Ex) PDX 5188

F14.281 Cocaine dependence with cocaine-induced sexual dysfunction (Ex) PDX 5186

F14.282 Cocaine dependence with cocaine-induced sleep disorder (Ex) PDX 5187

F14.288 Cocaine dependence with other cocaine-induced disorder (Ex) PDX 5183
Cocaine use disorder, moderate, with cocaine-induced obsessive-compulsive or related disorder
Cocaine use disorder, severe, with cocaine-induced obsessive-compulsive or related disorder

F14.29 Cocaine dependence with unspecified cocaine-induced disorder

F14.9 Cocaine use, unspecified
Excludes1 cocaine abuse (F14.1-)
cocaine dependence (F14.2-)

F14.90 Cocaine use, unspecified, uncomplicated
Coding Clinic: 2018, Q2, P11

F14.91 Cocaine use, unspecified, in remission

F14.92 Cocaine use, unspecified with intoxication

F14.920 Cocaine use, unspecified with intoxication, uncomplicated

F14.921 Cocaine use, unspecified with intoxication delirium (Ex) PDX 4722

CHAPTER 5 (F01-F99)

F14.922 Cocaine use, unspecified with intoxication with perceptual disturbance

F14.929 Cocaine use, unspecified with intoxication, unspecified

F14.93 Cocaine use, unspecified with withdrawal PDX 5611

F14.94 Cocaine use, unspecified with cocaine-induced mood disorder

Cocaine-induced bipolar or related disorder, without use disorder

Cocaine-induced depressive disorder, without use disorder

F14.95 Cocaine use, unspecified with cocaine-induced psychotic disorder

F14.950 Cocaine use, unspecified with cocaine-induced psychotic disorder with delusions PDX 4823

F14.951 Cocaine use, unspecified with cocaine-induced psychotic disorder with hallucinations PDX 4821

F14.959 Cocaine use, unspecified with cocaine-induced psychotic disorder, unspecified

Cocaine-induced psychotic disorder, without use disorder

F14.98 Cocaine use, unspecified with other specified cocaine-induced disorder

F14.980 Cocaine use, unspecified with cocaine-induced anxiety disorder

Cocaine-induced anxiety disorder, without use disorder

F14.981 Cocaine use, unspecified with cocaine-induced sexual dysfunction

Cocaine-induced sexual dysfunction, without use disorder

F14.982 Cocaine use, unspecified with cocaine-induced sleep disorder

Cocaine-induced sleep disorder, without use disorder

F14.988 Cocaine use, unspecified with other cocaine-induced disorder

Cocaine-induced obsessive-compulsive or related disorder

F14.99 Cocaine use, unspecified with unspecified cocaine-induced disorder

F15 Other stimulant related disorders

Includes amphetamine-related disorders
caffeine

Excludes2 cocaine-related disorders (F14.-)

F15.1 Other stimulant abuse

Excludes1 other stimulant dependence (F15.2-)
other stimulant use, unspecified (F15.9-)

F15.10 Other stimulant abuse, uncomplicated

Amphetamine type substance use disorder, mild

Other or unspecified stimulant use disorder, mild

F15.11 Other stimulant abuse, in remission

Amphetamine type substance use disorder, mild, in early remission

Amphetamine type substance use disorder, mild, in sustained remission

Other or unspecified stimulant use disorder, mild, in early remission

Other or unspecified stimulant use disorder, mild, in sustained remission

Coding Clinic: 2021, Q3, P8

F15.12 Other stimulant abuse with intoxication

F15.120 Other stimulant abuse with intoxication, uncomplicated

F15.121 Other stimulant abuse with intoxication delirium PDX 5200

F15.122 Other stimulant abuse with intoxication with perceptual disturbance

Amphetamine or other stimulant use disorder, mild, with amphetamine or other stimulant intoxication, with perceptual disturbances

F15.129 Other stimulant abuse with intoxication, unspecified

Amphetamine or other stimulant use disorder, mild, with amphetamine or other stimulant intoxication, without perceptual disturbances

F15.13 Other stimulant abuse with withdrawal PDX 5238

F15.14 Other stimulant abuse with stimulant-induced mood disorder

Amphetamine or other stimulant use disorder, mild, with amphetamine or other stimulant-induced bipolar or related disorder

Amphetamine or other stimulant use disorder, mild, with amphetamine or other stimulant-induced depressive disorder

F15.15 Other stimulant abuse with stimulant-induced psychotic disorder

F15.150 Other stimulant abuse with stimulant-induced psychotic disorder with delusions PDX 5217

F15.151 Other stimulant abuse with stimulant-induced psychotic disorder with hallucinations PDX 5218

F15.159 Other stimulant abuse with stimulant-induced psychotic disorder, unspecified

F15.18 Other stimulant abuse with other stimulant-induced disorder

F15.180 Other stimulant abuse with stimulant-induced anxiety disorder

F15.181 Other stimulant abuse with stimulant-induced sexual dysfunction

F15.182 Other stimulant abuse with stimulant-induced sleep disorder

F15.188 Other stimulant abuse with other stimulant-induced disorder

Amphetamine or other stimulant use disorder, mild, with amphetamine or other stimulant-induced obsessive-compulsive or related disorder

F15.19 Other stimulant abuse with unspecified stimulant-induced disorder

F15.2 Other stimulant dependence

Excludes1 other stimulant abuse (F15.1-)
other stimulant use, unspecified (F15.9-)

F15.20 Other stimulant dependence, uncomplicated PDX 3218

Amphetamine type substance use disorder, moderate

Amphetamine type substance use disorder, severe

Other or unspecified stimulant use disorder, moderate

Other or unspecified stimulant use disorder, severe

F15.21 Other stimulant dependence, in remission
Amphetamine type substance use disorder, moderate, in early remission
Amphetamine type substance use disorder, moderate, in sustained remission
Amphetamine type substance use disorder, severe, in early remission
Amphetamine type substance use disorder, severe, in sustained remission
Other or unspecified stimulant use disorder, moderate, in early remission
Other or unspecified stimulant use disorder, moderate, in sustained remission
Other or unspecified stimulant use disorder, severe, in early remission
Other or unspecified stimulant use disorder, severe, in sustained remission

● F15.22 Other stimulant dependence with intoxication
Excludes1 other stimulant dependence with withdrawal (F15.23)

F15.220 Other stimulant dependence with intoxication, uncomplicated

F15.221 Other stimulant dependence with intoxication delirium (Ex) PDX 5777

F15.222 Other stimulant dependence with intoxication with perceptual disturbance (Ex) PDX 5770
Amphetamine or other stimulant use disorder, moderate, with amphetamine or other stimulant intoxication, with perceptual disturbances
Amphetamine or other stimulant use disorder, severe, with amphetamine or other stimulant intoxication, with perceptual disturbances

F15.229 Other stimulant dependence with intoxication, unspecified
Amphetamine or other stimulant use disorder, moderate, with amphetamine or other stimulant intoxication, without perceptual disturbances
Amphetamine or other stimulant use disorder, severe, with amphetamine or other stimulant intoxication, without perceptual disturbances

F15.23 Other stimulant dependence with withdrawal (Ex) PDX 5212
Amphetamine or other stimulant withdrawal
Excludes1 other stimulant dependence with intoxication (F15.22-)

F15.24 Other stimulant dependence with stimulant-induced mood disorder
Amphetamine or other stimulant use disorder, moderate, with amphetamine or other stimulant-induced bipolar or related disorder
Amphetamine or other stimulant use disorder, moderate, with amphetamine or other stimulant-induced depressive disorder
Amphetamine or other stimulant use disorder, severe, with amphetamine or other stimulant-induced bipolar or related disorder
Amphetamine or other stimulant use disorder, severe, with amphetamine or other stimulant-induced depressive disorder

● F15.25 Other stimulant dependence with stimulant-induced psychotic disorder

F15.250 Other stimulant dependence with stimulant-induced psychotic disorder with delusions (Ex) PDX 5822

F15.251 Other stimulant dependence with stimulant-induced psychotic disorder with hallucinations (Ex) PDX 5818

F15.259 Other stimulant dependence with stimulant-induced psychotic disorder, unspecified (Ex) PDX 5813

● F15.28 Other stimulant dependence with other stimulant-induced disorder

F15.280 Other stimulant dependence with stimulant-induced anxiety disorder (Ex) PDX 5990

F15.281 Other stimulant dependence with stimulant-induced sexual dysfunction (Ex) PDX 5991

F15.282 Other stimulant dependence with stimulant-induced sleep disorder (Ex) PDX 5987

F15.288 Other stimulant dependence with other stimulant-induced disorder (Ex) PDX 5976
Amphetamine or other stimulant use disorder, moderate, with amphetamine or other stimulant-induced obsessive-compulsive or related disorder
Amphetamine or other stimulant use disorder, severe, with amphetamine or other stimulant-induced obsessive-compulsive or related disorder

F15.29 Other stimulant dependence with unspecified stimulant-induced disorder

● F15.9 Other stimulant use, unspecified
Excludes1 other stimulant abuse (F15.1-)
other stimulant dependence (F15.2-)

F15.90 Other stimulant use, unspecified, uncomplicated
Coding Clinic: 2022, Q4, P46

F15.91 Other stimulant use, unspecified, in remission

● F15.92 Other stimulant use, unspecified with intoxication
Excludes1 other stimulant use, unspecified with withdrawal (F15.93)

F15.920 Other stimulant use, unspecified with intoxication, uncomplicated

F15.921 Other stimulant use, unspecified with intoxication delirium (Ex) PDX 5478
Amphetamine or other stimulant-induced delirium

F15.922 Other stimulant use, unspecified with intoxication with perceptual disturbance

F15.929 Other stimulant use, unspecified with intoxication, unspecified
Caffeine intoxication

F15.93 Other stimulant use, unspecified with withdrawal (Ex) PDX 5086
Caffeine withdrawal
Excludes1 other stimulant use, unspecified with intoxication (F15.92-)

F15.94 Other stimulant use, unspecified with stimulant-induced mood disorder
Amphetamine or other stimulant-induced bipolar or related disorder, without use disorder
Amphetamine or other stimulant-induced depressive disorder, without use disorder

● F15.95 Other stimulant use, unspecified with stimulant-induced psychotic disorder

F15.950 Other stimulant use, unspecified with stimulant-induced psychotic disorder with delusions (Ex) PDX 5496

F15.951 Other stimulant use, unspecified with stimulant-induced psychotic disorder with hallucinations (Ex) PDX 5497

F15.959 Other stimulant use, unspecified with stimulant-induced psychotic disorder, unspecified
Amphetamine or other stimulant-induced psychotic disorder, without use disorder

F15.98 Other stimulant use, unspecified with other stimulant-induced disorder

F15.980 Other stimulant use, unspecified with stimulant-induced anxiety disorder
Amphetamine or other stimulant-induced anxiety disorder, without use disorder
Caffeine-induced anxiety disorder, without use disorder

F15.981 Other stimulant use, unspecified with stimulant-induced sexual dysfunction
Amphetamine or other stimulant-induced sexual dysfunction, without use disorder

F15.982 Other stimulant use, unspecified with stimulant-induced sleep disorder
Amphetamine or other stimulant-induced sleep disorder, without use disorder
Caffeine-induced sleep disorder, without use disorder

F15.988 Other stimulant use, unspecified with other stimulant-induced disorder
Amphetamine or other stimulant-induced obsessive-compulsive or related disorder, without use disorder

F15.99 Other stimulant use, unspecified with unspecified stimulant-induced disorder

F16 Hallucinogen related disorders
Includes ecstasy
PCP
phencyclidine

F16.1 Hallucinogen abuse
Excludes1 hallucinogen dependence (F16.2-)
hallucinogen use, unspecified (F16.9-)

F16.10 Hallucinogen abuse, uncomplicated
Other hallucinogen use disorder, mild
Phencyclidine use disorder, mild
Coding Clinic: 2018, Q4, P31

F16.11 Hallucinogen abuse, in remission
Other hallucinogen use disorder, mild, in early remission
Other hallucinogen use disorder, mild, in sustained remission
Phencyclidine use disorder, mild, in early remission
Phencyclidine use disorder, mild, in sustained remission

F16.12 Hallucinogen abuse with intoxication

F16.120 Hallucinogen abuse with intoxication, uncomplicated

F16.121 Hallucinogen abuse with intoxication with delirium (Ex) PDX 5871

F16.122 Hallucinogen abuse with intoxication with perceptual disturbance

F16.129 Hallucinogen abuse with intoxication, unspecified

F16.14 Hallucinogen abuse with hallucinogen-induced mood disorder
Other hallucinogen use disorder, mild, with other hallucinogen-induced bipolar or related disorder
Other hallucinogen use disorder, mild, with other hallucinogen-induced depressive disorder
Phencyclidine use disorder, mild, with phencyclidine-induced bipolar or related disorder
Phencyclidine use disorder, mild, with phencyclidine-induced depressive disorder

F16.15 Hallucinogen abuse with hallucinogen-induced psychotic disorder

F16.150 Hallucinogen abuse with hallucinogen-induced psychotic disorder with delusions (Ex) PDX 6072

F16.151 Hallucinogen abuse with hallucinogen-induced psychotic disorder with hallucinations (Ex) PDX 6071

F16.159 Hallucinogen abuse with hallucinogen-induced psychotic disorder, unspecified

F16.18 Hallucinogen abuse with other hallucinogen-induced disorder

F16.180 Hallucinogen abuse with hallucinogen-induced anxiety disorder

F16.183 Hallucinogen abuse with hallucinogen persisting perception disorder (flashbacks)

F16.188 Hallucinogen abuse with other hallucinogen-induced disorder

F16.19 Hallucinogen abuse with unspecified hallucinogen-induced disorder

F16.2 Hallucinogen dependence
Excludes1 hallucinogen abuse (F16.1-)
hallucinogen use, unspecified (F16.9-)

F16.20 Hallucinogen dependence, uncomplicated (Ex) PDX 5939
Other hallucinogen use disorder, moderate
Other hallucinogen use disorder, severe
Phencyclidine use disorder, moderate
Phencyclidine use disorder, severe

F16.21 Hallucinogen dependence, in remission
Other hallucinogen use disorder, moderate, in early remission
Other hallucinogen use disorder, moderate, in sustained remission
Other hallucinogen use disorder, severe, in early remission
Other hallucinogen use disorder, severe, in sustained remission
Phencyclidine use disorder, moderate, in early remission
Phencyclidine use disorder, moderate, in sustained remission
Phencyclidine use disorder, severe, in early remission
Phencyclidine use disorder, severe, in sustained remission

F16.22 Hallucinogen dependence with intoxication

F16.220 Hallucinogen dependence with intoxication, uncomplicated

F16.221 Hallucinogen dependence with intoxication with delirium (Ex) PDX 5184

F16.229 Hallucinogen dependence with intoxication, unspecified

CHAPTER 5 (FØ1-F99)

F16.24 Hallucinogen dependence with hallucinogen-induced mood disorder
Other hallucinogen use disorder, moderate, with other hallucinogen-induced bipolar or related disorder
Other hallucinogen use disorder, moderate, with other hallucinogen-induced depressive disorder
Other hallucinogen use disorder, severe, with other hallucinogen-induced bipolar or related disorder
Other hallucinogen use disorder, severe, with other hallucinogen-induced depressive disorder
Phencyclidine use disorder, moderate, with phencyclidine-induced bipolar or related disorder
Phencyclidine use disorder, moderate, with phencyclidine-induced depressive disorder
Phencyclidine use disorder, severe, with phencyclidine-induced bipolar or related disorder
Phencyclidine use disorder, severe, with phencyclidine-induced depressive disorder

F16.25 Hallucinogen dependence with hallucinogen-induced psychotic disorder

F16.25Ø Hallucinogen dependence with hallucinogen-induced psychotic disorder with delusions Ex: PDX 5274

F16.251 Hallucinogen dependence with hallucinogen-induced psychotic disorder with hallucinations Ex: PDX 5273

F16.259 Hallucinogen dependence with hallucinogen-induced psychotic disorder, unspecified Ex: PDX 5272

F16.28 Hallucinogen dependence with other hallucinogen-induced disorder

F16.28Ø Hallucinogen dependence with hallucinogen-induced anxiety disorder Ex: PDX 5295

F16.283 Hallucinogen dependence with hallucinogen persisting perception disorder (flashbacks) Ex: PDX 5294

F16.288 Hallucinogen dependence with other hallucinogen-induced disorder Ex: PDX 5290

F16.29 Hallucinogen dependence with unspecified hallucinogen-induced disorder

F16.9 Hallucinogen use, unspecified
Excludes1 hallucinogen abuse (F16.1-)
hallucinogen dependence (F16.2-)

F16.9Ø Hallucinogen use, unspecified, uncomplicated

F16.91 Hallucinogen use, unspecified, in remission

F16.92 Hallucinogen use, unspecified with intoxication

F16.92Ø Hallucinogen use, unspecified with intoxication, uncomplicated

F16.921 Hallucinogen use, unspecified with intoxication with delirium Ex: PDX 4850
Other hallucinogen intoxication delirium

F16.929 Hallucinogen use, unspecified with intoxication, unspecified

F16.94 Hallucinogen use, unspecified with hallucinogen-induced mood disorder
Other hallucinogen-induced bipolar or related disorder, without use disorder
Other hallucinogen-induced depressive disorder, without use disorder
Phencyclidine-induced bipolar or related disorder, without use disorder
Phencyclidine-induced depressive disorder, without use disorder

F16.95 Hallucinogen use, unspecified with hallucinogen-induced psychotic disorder

F16.95Ø Hallucinogen use, unspecified with hallucinogen-induced psychotic disorder with delusions Ex: PDX 4994

F16.951 Hallucinogen use, unspecified with hallucinogen-induced psychotic disorder with hallucinations Ex: PDX 4993

F16.959 Hallucinogen use, unspecified with hallucinogen-induced psychotic disorder, unspecified
Other hallucinogen-induced psychotic disorder, without use disorder
Phencyclidine-induced psychotic disorder, without use disorder

F16.98 Hallucinogen use, unspecified with other specified hallucinogen-induced disorder

F16.98Ø Hallucinogen use, unspecified with hallucinogen-induced anxiety disorder
Other hallucinogen-induced anxiety disorder, without use disorder
Phencyclidine-induced anxiety disorder, without use disorder

F16.983 Hallucinogen use, unspecified with hallucinogen persisting perception disorder (flashbacks)

F16.988 Hallucinogen use, unspecified with other hallucinogen-induced disorder

F16.99 Hallucinogen use, unspecified with unspecified hallucinogen-induced disorder

F17 Nicotine dependence
Excludes1 history of tobacco dependence (Z87.891)
tobacco use NOS (Z72.Ø)
Excludes2 tobacco use (smoking) during pregnancy, childbirth and the puerperium (O99.33-)
toxic effect of nicotine (T65.2-)

F17.2 Nicotine dependence

F17.2Ø Nicotine dependence, unspecified

F17.2ØØ Nicotine dependence, unspecified, uncomplicated
Tobacco use disorder, mild
Tobacco use disorder, moderate
Tobacco use disorder, severe
Coding Clinic: 2Ø16, Q1, P37

F17.2Ø1 Nicotine dependence, unspecified, in remission
Tobacco use disorder, mild, in early remission
Tobacco use disorder, mild, in sustained remission
Tobacco use disorder, moderate, in early remission
Tobacco use disorder, moderate, in sustained remission
Tobacco use disorder, severe, in early remission
Tobacco use disorder, severe, in sustained remission

CHAPTER 5 (FØ1-F99)

F17.203 **Nicotine dependence unspecified, with withdrawal** (Ex) PDX 5901
Tobacco withdrawal

F17.208 **Nicotine dependence, unspecified, with other nicotine-induced disorders**

F17.209 **Nicotine dependence, unspecified, with unspecified nicotine-induced disorders**

● **F17.21** **Nicotine dependence, cigarettes**

● **F17.210** **Nicotine dependence, cigarettes, uncomplicated**
Coding Clinic: 2017, Q2, P28-29

● **F17.211** **Nicotine dependence, cigarettes, in remission**
Tobacco use disorder, cigarettes, mild, in early remission
Tobacco use disorder, cigarettes, mild, in sustained remission
Tobacco use disorder, cigarettes, moderate, in early remission
Tobacco use disorder, cigarettes, moderate, in sustained remission
Tobacco use disorder, cigarettes, severe, in early remission
Tobacco use disorder, cigarettes, severe, in sustained remission

F17.213 **Nicotine dependence, cigarettes, with withdrawal** (Ex) PDX 5870

F17.218 **Nicotine dependence, cigarettes, with other nicotine-induced disorders**

F17.219 **Nicotine dependence, cigarettes, with unspecified nicotine-induced disorders**

● **F17.22** **Nicotine dependence, chewing tobacco**

● **F17.220** **Nicotine dependence, chewing tobacco, uncomplicated**

● **F17.221** **Nicotine dependence, chewing tobacco, in remission**
Tobacco use disorder, chewing tobacco, mild, in early remission
Tobacco use disorder, chewing tobacco, mild, in sustained remission
Tobacco use disorder, chewing tobacco, moderate, in early remission
Tobacco use disorder, chewing tobacco, moderate, in sustained remission
Tobacco use disorder, chewing tobacco, severe, in early remission
Tobacco use disorder, chewing tobacco, severe, in sustained remission

F17.223 **Nicotine dependence, chewing tobacco, with withdrawal** (Ex) PDX 5978

F17.228 **Nicotine dependence, chewing tobacco, with other nicotine-induced disorders**

F17.229 **Nicotine dependence, chewing tobacco, with unspecified nicotine-induced disorders**

● **F17.29** **Nicotine dependence, other tobacco product**

● **F17.290** **Nicotine dependence, other tobacco product, uncomplicated**
Coding Clinic: 2017, Q2, P28-29

● **F17.291** **Nicotine dependence, other tobacco product, in remission**
Tobacco use disorder, other tobacco product, mild, in early remission
Tobacco use disorder, other tobacco product, mild, in sustained remission
Tobacco use disorder, other tobacco product, moderate, in early remission
Tobacco use disorder, other tobacco product, moderate, in sustained remission
Tobacco use disorder, other tobacco product, severe, in early remission
Tobacco use disorder, other tobacco product, severe, in sustained remission

F17.293 **Nicotine dependence, other t obacco product, with withdrawal** (Ex) PDX 5356

F17.298 **Nicotine dependence, other tobacco product, with other nicotine-induced disorders**

F17.299 **Nicotine dependence, other tobacco product, with unspecified nicotine-induced disorders**

● **F18** **Inhalant related disorders**
Includes volatile solvents

● **F18.1** **Inhalant abuse**
Excludes1 inhalant dependence (F18.2-)
inhalant use, unspecified (F18.9-)

F18.10 **Inhalant abuse, uncomplicated**
Inhalant use disorder, mild

F18.11 **Inhalant abuse, in remission**
Inhalant use disorder, mild, in early remission
Inhalant use disorder, mild, in sustained remission

● **F18.12** **Inhalant abuse with intoxication**

F18.120 **Inhalant abuse with intoxication, uncomplicated**

F18.121 **Inhalant abuse with intoxication delirium** (Ex) PDX 5333

F18.129 **Inhalant abuse with intoxication, unspecified**

F18.14 **Inhalant abuse with inhalant-induced mood disorder**
Inhalant use disorder, mild, with inhalant-induced depressive disorder

● **F18.15** **Inhalant abuse with inhalant-induced psychotic disorder**

F18.150 **Inhalant abuse with inhalant-induced psychotic disorder with delusions** (Ex) PDX 5343

F18.151 **Inhalant abuse with inhalant-induced psychotic disorder with hallucinations** (Ex) PDX 5407

F18.159 **Inhalant abuse with inhalant-induced psychotic disorder, unspecified**

F18.17 **Inhalant abuse with inhalant-induced dementia** (Ex) PDX 4664
Inhalant use disorder, mild, with inhalant-induced major neurocognitive disorder

● **F18.18** **Inhalant abuse with other inhalant-induced disorders**

F18.180 **Inhalant abuse with inhalant-induced anxiety disorder**

CHAPTER 5 (F01-F99)

F18.188 **Inhalant abuse with other inhalant-induced disorder**
Inhalant use disorder, mild, with inhalant-induced mild neurocognitive disorder

F18.19 **Inhalant abuse with unspecified inhalant-induced disorder**

● F18.2 **Inhalant dependence**
Excludes1 inhalant abuse (F18.1-)
inhalant use, unspecified (F18.9-)

F18.20 **Inhalant dependence, uncomplicated** (Ex:) PDX 3220
Inhalant use disorder, moderate
Inhalant use disorder, severe

F18.21 **Inhalant dependence, in remission**
Inhalant use disorder, moderate, in early remission
Inhalant use disorder, moderate, in sustained remission
Inhalant use disorder, severe, in early remission
Inhalant use disorder, severe, in sustained remission

● F18.22 **Inhalant dependence with intoxication**

F18.220 **Inhalant dependence with intoxication, uncomplicated**

F18.221 **Inhalant dependence with intoxication delirium** (Ex:) PDX 5292

F18.229 **Inhalant dependence with intoxication, unspecified**

F18.24 **Inhalant dependence with inhalant-induced mood disorder**
Inhalant use disorder, moderate, with inhalant-induced depressive disorder
Inhalant use disorder, severe, with inhalant-induced depressive disorder

● F18.25 **Inhalant dependence with inhalant-induced psychotic disorder**

F18.250 **Inhalant dependence with inhalant-induced psychotic disorder with delusions** (Ex:) PDX 4713

F18.251 **Inhalant dependence with inhalant-induced psychotic disorder with hallucinations** (Ex:) PDX 4712

F18.259 **Inhalant dependence with inhalant-induced psychotic disorder, unspecified** (Ex:) PDX 4709

F18.27 **Inhalant dependence with inhalant-induced dementia** (Ex:) PDX 4648
Inhalant use disorder, moderate, with inhalant-induced major neurocognitive disorder
Inhalant use disorder, severe, with inhalant-induced major neurocognitive disorder

● F18.28 **Inhalant dependence with other inhalant-induced disorders**

F18.280 **Inhalant dependence with inhalant-induced anxiety disorder** (Ex:) PDX 4733

F18.288 **Inhalant dependence with other inhalant-induced disorder** (Ex:) PDX 4724
Inhalant use disorder, moderate, with inhalant-induced mild neurocognitive disorder
Inhalant use disorder, severe, with inhalant-induced mild neurocognitive disorder

F18.29 **Inhalant dependence with unspecified inhalant-induced disorder**

● F18.9 **Inhalant use, unspecified**
Excludes1 inhalant abuse (F18.1-)
inhalant dependence (F18.2-)

F18.90 **Inhalant use, unspecified, uncomplicated**

F18.91 **Inhalant use, unspecified, in remission**

● F18.92 **Inhalant use, unspecified with intoxication**

F18.920 **Inhalant use, unspecified with intoxication, uncomplicated**

F18.921 **Inhalant use, unspecified with intoxication with delirium** (Ex:) PDX 5667

F18.929 **Inhalant use, unspecified with intoxication, unspecified**

F18.94 **Inhalant use, unspecified with inhalant-induced mood disorder**
Inhalant-induced depressive disorder

● F18.95 **Inhalant use, unspecified with inhalant-induced psychotic disorder**

F18.950 **Inhalant use, unspecified with inhalant-induced psychotic disorder with delusions** (Ex:) PDX 5738

F18.951 **Inhalant use, unspecified with inhalant-induced psychotic disorder with hallucinations** (Ex:) PDX 5740

F18.959 **Inhalant use, unspecified with inhalant-induced psychotic disorder, unspecified**

F18.97 **Inhalant use, unspecified with inhalant-induced persisting dementia** (Ex:) PDX 5836
Inhalant-induced major neurocognitive disorder

● F18.98 **Inhalant use, unspecified with other inhalant-induced disorders**

F18.980 **Inhalant use, unspecified with inhalant-induced anxiety disorder**

F18.988 **Inhalant use, unspecified with other inhalant-induced disorder**
Inhalant-induced mild neurocognitive disorder

F18.99 **Inhalant use, unspecified with unspecified inhalant-induced disorder**

● F19 **Other psychoactive substance related disorders**
Includes polysubstance drug use (indiscriminate drug use)

● F19.1 **Other psychoactive substance abuse**
Excludes1 other psychoactive substance dependence (F19.2-)
other psychoactive substance use, unspecified (F19.9-)

F19.10 **Other psychoactive substance abuse, uncomplicated**
Other (or unknown) substance use disorder, mild

F19.11 **Other psychoactive substance abuse, in remission**
Other (or unknown) substance use disorder, mild, in early remission
Other (or unknown) substance use disorder, mild, in sustained remission

● F19.12 **Other psychoactive substance abuse with intoxication**

F19.120 **Other psychoactive substance abuse with intoxication, uncomplicated**

F19.121 **Other psychoactive substance abuse with intoxication delirium** (Ex:) PDX 4756

F19.122 **Other psychoactive substance abuse with intoxication with perceptual disturbances**

F19.129 **Other psychoactive substance abuse with intoxication, unspecified**

F19.13 Other psychoactive substance abuse with withdrawal

F19.130 Other psychoactive substance abuse with withdrawal, uncomplicated PDX 4764

F19.131 Other psychoactive substance abuse with withdrawal delirium PDX 4765

F19.132 Other psychoactive substance abuse with withdrawal with perceptual disturbance PDX 4766

F19.139 Other psychoactive substance abuse with withdrawal, unspecified PDX 4774

Coding Clinic: 2023, Q3, P16

F19.14 Other psychoactive substance abuse with psychoactive substance-induced mood disorder

Other (or unknown) substance use disorder, mild, with other (or unknown) substance-induced bipolar or related disorder

Other (or unknown) substance use disorder, mild, with other (or unknown) substance-induced depressive disorder

F19.15 Other psychoactive substance abuse with psychoactive substance-induced psychotic disorder

F19.150 Other psychoactive substance abuse with psychoactive substance-induced psychotic disorder with delusions PDX 4726

F19.151 Other psychoactive substance abuse with psychoactive substance-induced psychotic disorder with hallucinations PDX 4727

F19.159 Other psychoactive substance abuse with psychoactive substance-induced psychotic disorder, unspecified

F19.16 Other psychoactive substance abuse with psychoactive substance-induced persisting amnestic disorder

F19.17 Other psychoactive substance abuse with psychoactive substance-induced persisting dementia PDX 5358

Other (or unknown) substance use disorder, mild, with other (or unknown) substance-induced major neurocognitive disorder

F19.18 Other psychoactive substance abuse with other psychoactive substance-induced disorders

F19.180 Other psychoactive substance abuse with psychoactive substance-induced anxiety disorder

F19.181 Other psychoactive substance abuse with psychoactive substance-induced sexual dysfunction

F19.182 Other psychoactive substance abuse with psychoactive substance-induced sleep disorder

F19.188 Other psychoactive substance abuse with other psychoactive substance-induced disorder

Other (or unknown) substance use disorder, mild, with other (or unknown) substance-induced mild neurocognitive disorder

Other (or unknown) substance use disorder, mild, with other (or unknown) substance-induced obsessive-compulsive or related disorder

F19.19 Other psychoactive substance abuse with unspecified psychoactive substance-induced disorder

F19.2 Other psychoactive substance dependence

Excludes1 other psychoactive substance abuse (F19.1-)
other psychoactive substance use, unspecified (F19.9-)

F19.20 Other psychoactive substance dependence, uncomplicated PDX 5355

Other (or unknown) substance use disorder, moderate

Other (or unknown) substance use disorder, severe

F19.21 Other psychoactive substance dependence, in remission

Other (or unknown) substance use disorder, moderate, in early remission

Other (or unknown) substance use disorder, moderate, in sustained remission

Other (or unknown) substance use disorder, severe, in early remission

Other (or unknown) substance use disorder, severe, in sustained remission

F19.22 Other psychoactive substance dependence with intoxication

Excludes1 other psychoactive substance dependence with withdrawal (F19.23-)

F19.220 Other psychoactive substance dependence with intoxication, uncomplicated

F19.221 Other psychoactive substance dependence with intoxication delirium PDX 5324

F19.222 Other psychoactive substance dependence with intoxication with perceptual disturbance PDX 5326

F19.229 Other psychoactive substance dependence with intoxication, unspecified

F19.23 Other psychoactive substance dependence with withdrawal

Excludes1 other psychoactive substance dependence with intoxication (F19.22-)

F19.230 Other psychoactive substance dependence with withdrawal, uncomplicated PDX 5335

F19.231 Other psychoactive substance dependence with withdrawal delirium PDX 5336

F19.232 Other psychoactive substance dependence with withdrawal with perceptual disturbance PDX 5338

F19.239 Other psychoactive substance dependence with withdrawal, unspecified PDX 5340

F19.24 Other psychoactive substance dependence with psychoactive substance-induced mood disorder

Other (or unknown) substance use disorder, moderate, with other (or unknown) substance-induced bipolar or related disorder

Other (or unknown) substance use disorder, moderate, with other (or unknown) substance-induced depressive disorder

Other (or unknown) substance use disorder, severe, with other (or unknown) substance-induced bipolar or related disorder

Other (or unknown) substance use disorder, severe, with other (or unknown) substance-induced depressive disorder

F19.25 Other psychoactive substance dependence with psychoactive substance-induced psychotic disorder

F19.250 Other psychoactive substance dependence with psychoactive substance-induced psychotic disorder with delusions (Ex) PDX 5420

F19.251 Other psychoactive substance dependence with psychoactive substance-induced psychotic disorder with hallucinations (Ex) PDX 5421

F19.259 Other psychoactive substance dependence with psychoactive substance-induced psychotic disorder, unspecified (Ex) PDX 5429

F19.26 Other psychoactive substance dependence with psychoactive substance-induced persisting amnestic disorder (Ex) PDX 5346

F19.27 Other psychoactive substance dependence with psychoactive substance-induced persisting dementia (Ex) PDX 5344

Other (or unknown) substance use disorder, moderate, with other (or unknown) substance-induced major neurocognitive disorder

Other (or unknown) substance use disorder, severe, with other (or unknown) substance-induced major neurocognitive disorder

F19.28 Other psychoactive substance dependence with other psychoactive substance-induced disorders

F19.280 Other psychoactive substance dependence with psychoactive substance-induced anxiety disorder (Ex) PDX 5403

F19.281 Other psychoactive substance dependence with psychoactive substance-induced sexual dysfunction (Ex) PDX 5404

F19.282 Other psychoactive substance dependence with psychoactive substance-induced sleep disorder (Ex) PDX 5405

F19.288 Other psychoactive substance dependence with other psychoactive substance-induced disorder (Ex) PDX 5491

Other (or unknown) substance use disorder, moderate, with other (or unknown) substance-induced mild neurocognitive disorder

Other (or unknown) substance use disorder, severe, with other (or unknown) substance-induced mild neurocognitive disorder

Other (or unknown) substance use disorder, moderate, with other (or unknown) substance-induced obsessive-compulsive or related disorder

Other (or unknown) substance use disorder, severe, with other (or unknown) substance-induced obsessive-compulsive or related disorder

F19.29 Other psychoactive substance dependence with unspecified psychoactive substance-induced disorder

F19.9 Other psychoactive substance use, unspecified

Excludes1 other psychoactive substance abuse (F19.1-)
other psychoactive substance dependence (F19.2-)

F19.90 Other psychoactive substance use, unspecified, uncomplicated

F19.91 Other psychoactive substance use, unspecified, in remission

F19.92 Other psychoactive substance use, unspecified with intoxication

Excludes1 other psychoactive substance use, unspecified with withdrawal (F19.93)

F19.920 Other psychoactive substance use, unspecified with intoxication, uncomplicated

F19.921 Other psychoactive substance use, unspecified with intoxication with delirium (Ex) PDX 5126

Other (or unknown) substance-induced delirium

F19.922 Other psychoactive substance use, unspecified with intoxication with perceptual disturbance

F19.929 Other psychoactive substance use, unspecified with intoxication, unspecified

F19.93 Other psychoactive substance use, unspecified with withdrawal

Excludes1 other psychoactive substance use, unspecified with intoxication (F19.92-)

F19.930 Other psychoactive substance use, unspecified with withdrawal, uncomplicated (Ex) PDX 5143

F19.931 Other psychoactive substance use, unspecified with withdrawal delirium (Ex) PDX 5144

F19.932 Other psychoactive substance use, unspecified with withdrawal with perceptual disturbance (Ex) PDX 5145

F19.939 Other psychoactive substance use, unspecified with withdrawal, unspecified (Ex) PDX 5152

F19.94 Other psychoactive substance use, unspecified with psychoactive substance-induced mood disorder

Other (or unknown) substance-induced bipolar or related disorder, without use disorder

Other (or unknown) substance-induced depressive disorder, without use disorder

F19.95 Other psychoactive substance use, unspecified with psychoactive substance-induced psychotic disorder

F19.950 Other psychoactive substance use, unspecified with psychoactive substance-induced psychotic disorder with delusions (Ex) PDX 5117

F19.951 Other psychoactive substance use, unspecified with psychoactive substance-induced psychotic disorder with hallucinations (Ex) PDX 5118

F19.959 Other psychoactive substance use, unspecified with psychoactive substance-induced psychotic disorder, unspecified

Other or unknown substance-induced psychotic disorder, without use disorder

F19.96 Other psychoactive substance use, unspecified with psychoactive substance-induced persisting amnestic disorder

F19.97 Other psychoactive substance use, unspecified with psychoactive substance-induced persisting dementia (Ex) PDX 5239

Other (or unknown) substance-induced major neurocognitive disorder, without use disorder

● **F19.98 Other psychoactive substance use, unspecified with other psychoactive substance-induced disorders**

F19.980 Other psychoactive substance use, unspecified with psychoactive substance-induced anxiety disorder

Other (or unknown) substance-induced anxiety disorder, without use disorder

F19.981 Other psychoactive substance use, unspecified with psychoactive substance-induced sexual dysfunction

Other (or unknown) substance-induced sexual dysfunction, without use disorder

F19.982 Other psychoactive substance use, unspecified with psychoactive substance-induced sleep disorder

Other (or unknown) substance-induced sleep disorder, without use disorder

F19.988 Other psychoactive substance use, unspecified with other psychoactive substance-induced disorder

Other (or unknown) substance-induced mild neurocognitive disorder, without use disorder

Other (or unknown) substance-induced obsessive-compulsive or related disorder, without use disorder

F19.99 Other psychoactive substance use, unspecified with unspecified psychoactive substance-induced disorder

SCHIZOPHRENIA, SCHIZOTYPAL, DELUSIONAL, AND OTHER NON-MOOD PSYCHOTIC DISORDERS (F2Ø-F29)

● **F2Ø Schizophrenia**

Personality disorders characterized by multiple mental and behavioral irregularities (may exhibit disorganized thinking, delusions, and auditory hallucinations)

Excludes1 brief psychotic disorder (F23)
cyclic schizophrenia (F25.Ø)
mood [affective] disorders with psychotic symptoms (F3Ø.2, F31.2, F31.5, F31.64, F32.3, F33.3)
schizoaffective disorder (F25.-)
schizophrenic reaction NOS (F23)

Excludes2 schizophrenic reaction in:
alcoholism (F1Ø.15-, F1Ø.25-, F1Ø.95-)
brain disease (FØ6.2)
epilepsy (FØ6.2)
psychoactive drug use (F11-F19 with .15, .25, .95)
schizotypal disorder (F21)

▶Use additional code, if applicable, to identify:
▶other specified cognitive deficit (R41.84-)

Coding Clinic: 2019, Q2, P32

F2Ø.Ø Paranoid schizophrenia (Ex) PDX 5246

Paraphrenic schizophrenia

Excludes1 involutional paranoid state (F22)
paranoia (F22)

F2Ø.1 Disorganized schizophrenia (Ex) PDX 5247

Hebephrenic schizophrenia
Hebephrenia

F2Ø.2 Catatonic schizophrenia (Ex) PDX 5248

Schizophrenic catalepsy
Schizophrenic catatonia
Schizophrenic flexibilitas cerea

Excludes1 catatonic stupor (R4Ø.1)

F2Ø.3 Undifferentiated schizophrenia

Atypical schizophrenia

Excludes1 acute schizophrenia-like psychotic disorder (F23)

Excludes2 post-schizophrenic depression (F32.89)

F2Ø.5 Residual schizophrenia (Ex) PDX 5251

Restzustand (schizophrenic)
Schizophrenic residual state

● **F2Ø.8 Other schizophrenia**

F2Ø.81 Schizophreniform disorder (Ex) PDX 4798

Schizophreniform psychosis NOS

F2Ø.89 Other schizophrenia (Ex) PDX 4782

Cenesthopathic schizophrenia
Simple schizophrenia

F2Ø.9 Schizophrenia, unspecified

Coding Clinic: 2019, Q2, P32

F21 Schizotypal disorder

Personality disorder characterized by need for social isolation, odd behavior and thinking, and often unconventional beliefs

Borderline schizophrenia
Latent schizophrenia
Latent schizophrenic reaction
Prepsychotic schizophrenia
Prodromal schizophrenia
Pseudoneurotic schizophrenia
Pseudopsychopathic schizophrenia
Schizotypal personality disorder

Excludes2 Asperger's syndrome (F84.5)
schizoid personality disorder (F6Ø.1)

F22 Delusional disorders

Delusional dysmorphophobia
Involutional paranoid state
Paranoia
Paranoia querulans
Paranoid psychosis
Paranoid state
Paraphrenia (late)
Sensitiver Beziehungswahn

Excludes1 mood [affective] disorders with psychotic symptoms (F3Ø.2, F31.2, F31.5, F31.64, F32.3, F33.3)
paranoid schizophrenia (F2Ø.Ø)

Excludes2 paranoid personality disorder (F6Ø.Ø)
paranoid psychosis, psychogenic (F23)
paranoid reaction (F23)

F23 Brief psychotic disorder (Ex) PDX 5447

Paranoid reaction
Psychogenic paranoid psychosis

Excludes2 mood [affective] disorders with psychotic symptoms (F3Ø.2, F31.2, F31.5, F31.64, F32.3, F33.3)

Coding Clinic: 2019, Q2, P32

F24 Shared psychotic disorder

Folie à deux
Induced paranoid disorder
Induced psychotic disorder

● **F25 Schizoaffective disorders**

Mental disorder exhibiting major depressive episode, manic episode, or mixed episode occurs with symptoms of schizophrenia, and mood disorder

Excludes1 mood [affective] disorders with psychotic symptoms (F3Ø.2, F31.2, F31.5, F31.64, F32.3, F33.3)
schizophrenia (F2Ø.-)

F25.Ø Schizoaffective disorder, bipolar type

Cyclic schizophrenia
Schizoaffective disorder, manic type
Schizoaffective disorder, mixed type
Schizoaffective psychosis, bipolar type

F25.1 Schizoaffective disorder, depressive type

Schizoaffective psychosis, depressive type

CHAPTER 5 (FØ1-F99)

F25.8 **Other schizoaffective disorders**

F25.9 **Schizoaffective disorder, unspecified**
Schizoaffective psychosis NOS

F28 **Other psychotic disorder not due to a substance or known physiological condition**
Chronic hallucinatory psychosis
Other specified schizophrenia spectrum and other psychotic disorder

F29 **Unspecified psychosis not due to a substance or known physiological condition**
Psychosis NOS
Unspecified schizophrenia spectrum and other psychotic disorder
Excludes1 mental disorder NOS (F99)
unspecified mental disorder due to known physiological condition (F09)

MOOD [AFFECTIVE] DISORDERS (F30-F39)

F30 **Manic episode**
Elevated, expansive, or irritable mood
Includes bipolar disorder, single manic episode
mixed affective episode
Excludes1 bipolar disorder (F31.-)
major depressive disorder, single episode (F32.-)
major depressive disorder, recurrent (F33.-)

F30.1 **Manic episode without psychotic symptoms**

F30.10 **Manic episode without psychotic symptoms, unspecified** PDX 5509

F30.11 **Manic episode without psychotic symptoms, mild** PDX 5510

F30.12 **Manic episode without psychotic symptoms, moderate** PDX 5512

F30.13 **Manic episode, severe, without psychotic symptoms** PDX 5513

F30.2 **Manic episode, severe with psychotic symptoms** PDX 5861
Manic stupor
Mania with mood-congruent psychotic symptoms
Mania with mood-incongruent psychotic symptoms

F30.3 **Manic episode in partial remission**

F30.4 **Manic episode in full remission**

F30.8 **Other manic episodes**
Abnormality of mood resembling mania but less intense
Hypomania

F30.9 **Manic episode, unspecified** PDX 5868
Mania NOS

F31 **Bipolar disorder**
Mood disorders with history of manic, mixed, or hypomanic episodes
Includes bipolar I disorder
bipolar type I disorder
manic-depressive illness
manic-depressive psychosis
manic-depressive reaction
seasonal bipolar disorder
Excludes1 bipolar disorder, single manic episode (F30.-)
major depressive disorder, single episode (F32.-)
major depressive disorder, recurrent (F33.-)
Excludes2 cyclothymia (F34.0)
Coding Clinic: 2020, Q1, P23

F31.0 **Bipolar disorder, current episode hypomanic** PDX 5965

F31.1 **Bipolar disorder, current episode manic without psychotic features**

F31.10 **Bipolar disorder, current episode manic without psychotic features, unspecified** PDX 4935

F31.11 **Bipolar disorder, current episode manic without psychotic features, mild** PDX 4941

F31.12 **Bipolar disorder, current episode manic without psychotic features, moderate** PDX 4944

F31.13 **Bipolar disorder, current episode manic without psychotic features, severe** PDX 553

F31.2 **Bipolar disorder, current episode manic severe with psychotic features** PDX 5968
Bipolar disorder, current episode manic with mood-congruent psychotic symptoms
Bipolar disorder, current episode manic with mood-incongruent psychotic symptoms
Bipolar I disorder, current or most recent episode manic with psychotic features

F31.3 **Bipolar disorder, current episode depressed, mild or moderate severity**

F31.30 **Bipolar disorder, current episode depressed, mild or moderate severity, unspecified** PDX 4886

F31.31 **Bipolar disorder, current episode depressed, mild** PDX 4881

F31.32 **Bipolar disorder, current episode depressed, moderate** PDX 4884

F31.4 **Bipolar disorder, current episode depressed, severe, without psychotic features** PDX 5969

F31.5 **Bipolar disorder, current episode depressed, severe, with psychotic features** PDX 5970
Bipolar disorder, current episode depressed with mood-incongruent psychotic symptoms
Bipolar disorder, current episode depressed with mood-congruent psychotic symptoms
Bipolar I disorder, current or most recent episode depressed, with psychotic features

F31.6 **Bipolar disorder, current episode mixed**

F31.60 **Bipolar disorder, current episode mixed, unspecified** PDX 4815

F31.61 **Bipolar disorder, current episode mixed, mild** PDX 4817

F31.62 **Bipolar disorder, current episode mixed, moderate** PDX 4804

F31.63 **Bipolar disorder, current episode mixed, severe, without psychotic features** PDX 554

F31.64 **Bipolar disorder, current episode mixed, severe, with psychotic features** PDX 4802
Bipolar disorder, current episode mixed with mood-congruent psychotic symptoms
Bipolar disorder, current episode mixed with mood-incongruent psychotic symptoms

F31.7 **Bipolar disorder, currently in remission**

F31.70 **Bipolar disorder, currently in remission, most recent episode unspecified**

F31.71 **Bipolar disorder, in partial remission, most recent episode hypomanic**

F31.72 **Bipolar disorder, in full remission, most recent episode hypomanic**

F31.73 **Bipolar disorder, in partial remission, most recent episode manic**

F31.74 **Bipolar disorder, in full remission, most recent episode manic**

F31.75 **Bipolar disorder, in partial remission, most recent episode depressed**

F31.76 **Bipolar disorder, in full remission, most recent episode depressed**

F31.77 **Bipolar disorder, in partial remission, most recent episode mixed**

F31.78 **Bipolar disorder, in full remission, most recent episode mixed**

F31.8 **Other bipolar disorders**

F31.81 **Bipolar II disorder** PDX 4781
Bipolar disorder, type 2

F31.89 **Other bipolar disorder** PDX 4763
Recurrent manic episodes NOS

F31.9 **Bipolar disorder, unspecified**
Manic depression
Coding Clinic: 2020, Q1, P23

CHAPTER 5 (F01-F99)

● **F32 Depressive episode**

Includes single episode of agitated depression
single episode of depressive reaction
single episode of major depression
single episode of psychogenic depression
single episode of reactive depression
single episode of vital depression

Excludes1 bipolar disorder (F31.-)
manic episode (F3Ø.-)
recurrent depressive disorder (F33.-)

Excludes2 adjustment disorder (F43.2)

F32.Ø Major depressive disorder, single episode, mild (Ex) PDX 5929

F32.1 Major depressive disorder, single episode, moderate (Ex) PDX 5931

F32.2 Major depressive disorder, single episode, severe without psychotic features (Ex) PDX 5933

F32.3 Major depressive disorder, single episode, severe with psychotic features (Ex) PDX 5935
Single episode of major depression with mood-congruent psychotic symptoms
Single episode of major depression with mood-incongruent psychotic symptoms
Single episode of major depression with psychotic symptoms
Single episode of psychogenic depressive psychosis
Single episode of psychotic depression
Single episode of reactive depressive psychosis

F32.4 Major depressive disorder, single episode, in partial remission

F32.5 Major depressive disorder, single episode, in full remission

● **F32.8 Other depressive episodes**

F32.81 Premenstrual dysphoric disorder
Excludes1 premenstrual tension syndrome (N94.3)
Coding Clinic: 2016, Q4, P14

F32.89 Other specified depressive episodes
Atypical depression
Post-schizophrenic depression
Single episode of 'masked' depression NOS
Coding Clinic: 2016, Q4, P14

F32.9 Major depressive disorder, single episode, unspecified
Major depression NOS
Coding Clinic: 2021, Q1, P10

F32.A Depression, unspecified
Depression NOS
Depressive disorder NOS
Coding Clinic: 2023, Q4, P15; 2021, Q4, P10

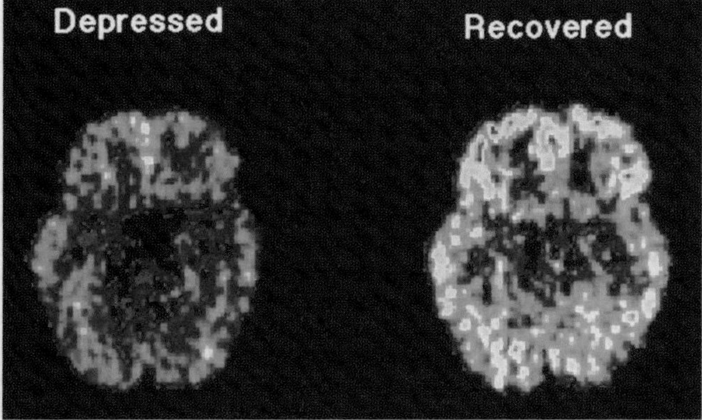

Figure 5-1 PET scan of depressed individual's brain before and after recovery. (From Fortinash KM: Psychiatric Mental Health Nursing, ed 4, St. Louis, Mosby, 2008)

● **F33 Major depressive disorder, recurrent**

Includes recurrent episodes of depressive reaction
recurrent episodes of endogenous depression
recurrent episodes of major depression
recurrent episodes of psychogenic depression
recurrent episodes of reactive depression
recurrent episodes of seasonal affective disorder
recurrent episodes of seasonal depressive disorder
recurrent episodes of vital depression

Excludes1 bipolar disorder (F31.-)
manic episode (F3Ø.-)

Coding Clinic: 2020, Q1, P23

F33.Ø Major depressive disorder, recurrent, mild (Ex) PDX 6043

F33.1 Major depressive disorder, recurrent, moderate (Ex) PDX 6046

F33.2 Major depressive disorder, recurrent severe without psychotic features (Ex) PDX 6048

F33.3 Major depressive disorder, recurrent, severe with psychotic symptoms (Ex) PDX 6050
Endogenous depression with psychotic symptoms
Major depressive disorder, recurrent, with psychotic features
Recurrent severe episodes of major depression with mood-congruent psychotic symptoms
Recurrent severe episodes of major depression with mood-incongruent psychotic symptoms
Recurrent severe episodes of major depression with psychotic symptoms
Recurrent severe episodes of psychogenic depressive psychosis
Recurrent severe episodes of psychotic depression
Recurrent severe episodes of reactive depressive psychosis

● **F33.4 Major depressive disorder, recurrent, in remission**

F33.40 Major depressive disorder, recurrent, in remission, unspecified (Ex) PDX 4964

F33.41 Major depressive disorder, recurrent, in partial remission

F33.42 Major depressive disorder, recurrent, in full remission

F33.8 Other recurrent depressive disorders (Ex) PDX 6057
Recurrent brief depressive episodes

F33.9 Major depressive disorder, recurrent, unspecified (Ex) PDX 700
Monopolar depression NOS

● **F34 Persistent mood [affective] disorders**

F34.Ø Cyclothymic disorder
Affective personality disorder
Cycloid personality
Cyclothymia
Cyclothymic personality

F34.1 Dysthymic disorder
Depressive neurosis
Depressive personality disorder
Dysthymia
Neurotic depression
Persistent anxiety depression
Persistent depressive disorder
Excludes2 anxiety depression (mild or not persistent) (F41.8)

● **F34.8 Other persistent mood [affective] disorders**

F34.81 Disruptive mood dysregulation disorder (Ex) PDX 686
Coding Clinic: 2016, Q4, P14

F34.89 Other specified persistent mood disorders (Ex) PDX 686
Coding Clinic: 2016, Q4, P14

F34.9 Persistent mood [affective] disorder, unspecified (Ex) PDX 686

F39 Unspecified mood [affective] disorder
Affective psychosis NOS

ANXIETY, DISSOCIATIVE, STRESS-RELATED, SOMATOFORM AND OTHER NONPSYCHOTIC MENTAL DISORDERS (F40-F48)

● F40 Phobic anxiety disorders
Irrational fear with avoidance of the feared subject, activity, or situation even though the individual knows that the reaction is excessive

● F40.0 Agoraphobia
Intense, irrational fear of open spaces

F40.00 Agoraphobia, unspecified

F40.01 Agoraphobia with panic disorder
Panic disorder with agoraphobia
Excludes1 panic disorder without agoraphobia (F41.0)

F40.02 Agoraphobia without panic disorder

● F40.1 Social phobias
Anthropophobia
Social anxiety disorder
Social anxiety disorder of childhood
Social neurosis

F40.10 Social phobia, unspecified

F40.11 Social phobia, generalized

● F40.2 Specific (isolated) phobias
Excludes2 dysmorphophobia (nondelusional) (F45.22)
nosophobia (F45.22)

● F40.21 Animal type phobia

F40.210 Arachnophobia
Fear of spiders

F40.218 Other animal type phobia

● F40.22 Natural environment type phobia

F40.220 Fear of thunderstorms

F40.228 Other natural environment type phobia

● F40.23 Blood, injection, injury type phobia

F40.230 Fear of blood

F40.231 Fear of injections and transfusions

F40.232 Fear of other medical care

F40.233 Fear of injury

● F40.24 Situational type phobia

F40.240 Claustrophobia
Fear of closed spaces

F40.241 Acrophobia
Fear of heights

F40.242 Fear of bridges

F40.243 Fear of flying

F40.248 Other situational type phobia

● F40.29 Other specified phobia

F40.290 Androphobia
Fear of men

F40.291 Gynephobia
Fear of women

F40.298 Other specified phobia

F40.8 Other phobic anxiety disorders
Phobic anxiety disorder of childhood

F40.9 Phobic anxiety disorder, unspecified
Phobia NOS
Phobic state NOS

● F41 Other anxiety disorders
Excludes2 anxiety in:
acute stress reaction (F43.0)
transient adjustment reaction (F43.2)
neurasthenia (F48.8)
psychophysiologic disorders (F45.-)
separation anxiety (F93.0)

F41.0 Panic disorder [episodic paroxysmal anxiety]
Panic attack
Panic state
Excludes1 panic disorder with agoraphobia (F40.01)

F41.1 Generalized anxiety disorder
Anxiety neurosis
Anxiety reaction
Anxiety state
Overanxious disorder
Excludes2 neurasthenia (F48.8)

F41.3 Other mixed anxiety disorders

F41.8 Other specified anxiety disorders
Anxiety depression (mild or not persistent)
Anxiety hysteria
Mixed anxiety and depressive disorder
Coding Clinic: 2021, Q1, P11

F41.9 Anxiety disorder, unspecified
Anxiety NOS
Coding Clinic: 2021, Q1, P11

● F42 Obsessive-compulsive disorder
Anxiety disorder with recurrent obsessions or compulsions
Excludes2 obsessive-compulsive personality (disorder) (F60.5)
obsessive-compulsive symptoms occurring in depression (F32-F33)
obsessive-compulsive symptoms occurring in schizophrenia (F20.-)

F42.2 Mixed obsessional thoughts and acts
Coding Clinic: 2016, Q4, P15

F42.3 Hoarding disorder
Coding Clinic: 2016, Q4, P14-15

F42.4 Excoriation (skin-picking) disorder
Excludes1 factitial dermatitis (L98.1)
other specified behavioral and emotional disorders with onset usually occurring in early childhood and adolescence (F98.8)
Coding Clinic: 2016, Q4, P14-15

F42.8 Other obsessive-compulsive disorder
Anancastic neurosis
Obsessive-compulsive neurosis
Coding Clinic: 2016, Q4, P15

F42.9 Obsessive-compulsive disorder, unspecified
Coding Clinic: 2016, Q4, P15

● F43 Reaction to severe stress and adjustment disorders

F43.0 Acute stress reaction
Acute crisis reaction
Acute reaction to stress
Combat and operational stress reaction
Combat fatigue
Crisis state
Psychic shock

● F43.1 Post-traumatic stress disorder (PTSD)
Traumatic neurosis

F43.10 Post-traumatic stress disorder, unspecified

F43.11 Post-traumatic stress disorder, acute

F43.12 Post-traumatic stress disorder, chronic

● F43.2 Adjustment disorders
Culture shock
Grief reaction
Hospitalism in children
Excludes2 separation anxiety disorder of childhood (F93.0)

F43.20 Adjustment disorder, unspecified

F43.21 Adjustment disorder with depressed mood

F43.22 Adjustment disorder with anxiety

F43.23 Adjustment disorder with mixed anxiety and depressed mood

F43.24 Adjustment disorder with disturbance of conduct

F43.25 Adjustment disorder with mixed disturbance of emotions and conduct

F43.29 Adjustment disorder with other symptoms

● **F43.8 Other reactions to severe stress**
Other specified trauma and stressor-related disorder

F43.81 Prolonged grief disorder
Complicated grief
Complicated grief disorder
Persistent complex bereavement disorder

F43.89 Other reactions to severe stress

F43.9 Reaction to severe stress, unspecified
Trauma and stressor-related disorder, NOS

● **F44 Dissociative and conversion disorders**
Includes conversion hysteria
conversion reaction
hysteria
hysterical psychosis
Excludes2 malingering [conscious simulation] (Z76.5)

F44.Ø Dissociative amnesia
Sudden loss of memory for personal information
Excludes1 amnesia NOS (R41.3)
anterograde amnesia (R41.1)
dissociative amnesia with dissociative fugue (F44.1)
retrograde amnesia (R41.2)
Excludes2 alcohol or other psychoactive substance-induced amnestic disorder (F1Ø, F13, F19 with .26, .96)
amnestic disorder due to known physiological condition (FØ4)
postictal amnesia in epilepsy (G4Ø.-)

F44.1 Dissociative fugue
Characterized by episode of sudden, unexpected travel with amnesia for past and partial to total confusion about identity or assumption of new identity
Dissociative amnesia with dissociative fugue
Excludes2 postictal fugue in epilepsy (G4Ø.-)

F44.2 Dissociative stupor
Profound diminution or absence of voluntary movement and responsiveness to external stimuli
Excludes1 catatonic stupor (R4Ø.1)
stupor NOS (R4Ø.1)
Excludes2 catatonic disorder due to known physiological condition (FØ6.1)
depressive stupor (F32, F33)
manic stupor (F3Ø, F31)

F44.4 Conversion disorder with motor symptom or deficit
Conversion disorder with abnormal movement
Conversion disorder with speech symptoms
Conversion disorder with swallowing symptoms
Conversion disorder with weakness/paralysis
Dissociative motor disorders
Psychogenic aphonia
Psychogenic dysphonia

F44.5 Conversion disorder with seizures or convulsions
Conversion disorder with attacks or seizures
Dissociative convulsions
Coding Clinic: 2019, Q1, P19

F44.6 Conversion disorder with sensory symptom or deficit
Conversion disorder with anesthesia or sensory loss
Conversion disorder with special sensory symptoms
Dissociative anesthesia and sensory loss
Psychogenic deafness

F44.7 Conversion disorder with mixed symptom presentation

● **F44.8 Other dissociative and conversion disorders**

F44.81 Dissociative identity disorder
Multiple personality disorder

F44.89 Other dissociative and conversion disorders
Ganser's syndrome
Psychogenic confusion
Psychogenic twilight state
Trance and possession disorders

F44.9 Dissociative and conversion disorder, unspecified
Dissociative disorder NOS

OGCR Section I.C.5.a.

Pain disorders related to psychological factors

Assign code F45.41, for pain that is exclusively related to psychological disorders. As indicated by the Excludes 1 note under category G89, a code from category G89 should not be assigned with code F45.41 Code F45.42, Pain disorders with related psychological factors, should be used with a code from category G89, Pain, not elsewhere classified, if there is documentation of a psychological component for a patient with acute or chronic pain.

See Section I.C.6. Pain

● **F45 Somatoform disorders**
Mental disorders characterized by symptoms suggesting general medical condition
Excludes2 dissociative and conversion disorders (F44.-)
factitious disorders (F68.1-, F68.A)
hair-plucking (F63.3)
lalling (F8Ø.Ø)
lisping (F8Ø.Ø)
malingering [conscious simulation] (Z76.5)
nail-biting (F98.8)
psychological or behavioral factors associated with disorders or diseases classified elsewhere (F54)
sexual dysfunction, not due to a substance or known physiological condition (F52.-)
thumb-sucking (F98.8)
tic disorders (in childhood and adolescence) (F95.-)
Tourette's syndrome (F95.2)
trichotillomania (F63.3)

F45.Ø Somatization disorder
Briquet's disorder
Multiple psychosomatic disorder

F45.1 Undifferentiated somatoform disorder
Somatic symptom disorder
Undifferentiated psychosomatic disorder

● **F45.2 Hypochondriacal disorders**
Persistent, unrealistic preoccupation with possibility of having serious disease
Excludes2 delusional dysmorphophobia (F22)
fixed delusions about bodily functions or shape (F22)

F45.2Ø Hypochondriacal disorder, unspecified

F45.21 Hypochondriasis
Hypochondriacal neurosis
Illness anxiety disorder

F45.22 Body dysmorphic disorder
▶ Bigorexia
Dysmorphophobia (nondelusional)
▶ Muscle dysmorphia
Nosophobia

F45.29 Other hypochondriacal disorders

● **F45.4 Pain disorders related to psychological factors**
Excludes1 pain NOS (R52)

F45.41 Pain disorder exclusively related to psychological factors
Somatoform pain disorder (persistent)

F45.42 Pain disorder with related psychological factors
Code also associated acute or chronic pain (G89.-)

F45.8 Other somatoform disorders
Psychogenic dysmenorrhea
Psychogenic dysphagia, including 'globus hystericus'
Psychogenic pruritus
Psychogenic torticollis
Somatoform autonomic dysfunction
Teeth grinding
Excludes1 sleep related teeth grinding (G47.63)
Coding Clinic: 2016, Q4, P118

F45.9 Somatoform disorder, unspecified
Psychosomatic disorder NOS

CHAPTER 5 (FØ1-F99)

● **F48 Other nonpsychotic mental disorders**

F48.1 Depersonalization-derealization syndrome

F48.2 Pseudobulbar affect
Involuntary emotional expression disorder
Code first underlying cause, if known, such as:
amyotrophic lateral sclerosis (G12.21)
multiple sclerosis (G35)
sequelae of cerebrovascular disease (I69.-)
sequelae of traumatic intracranial injury (S06.-)

F48.8 Other specified nonpsychotic mental disorders
Dhat syndrome
Neurasthenia
Occupational neurosis, including writer's cramp
Psychasthenia
Psychasthenic neurosis
Psychogenic syncope

F48.9 Nonpsychotic mental disorder, unspecified
Neurosis NOS

BEHAVIORAL SYNDROMES ASSOCIATED WITH PHYSIOLOGICAL DISTURBANCES AND PHYSICAL FACTORS (F50-F59)

● **F50 Eating disorders**
Excludes1 anorexia NOS (R63.0)
feeding problems of newborn (P92.-)
polyphagia (R63.2)
Excludes2 feeding difficulties (R63.3-)
feeding disorder in infancy or childhood (F98.2-)

● **F50.0 Anorexia nervosa**
Excludes1 loss of appetite (R63.0)
psychogenic loss of appetite (F50.89)

F50.00 Anorexia nervosa, unspecified (Ex) PDX 701

F50.01 Anorexia nervosa, restricting type

▶ **F50.010 Anorexia nervosa, restricting type, mild** (Ex) PDX 701
▶ Anorexia nervosa, restricting type, with a body mass index greater than or equal to 17 kg/m2

▶ **F50.011 Anorexia nervosa, restricting type, moderate** (Ex) PDX 701
▶ Anorexia nervosa, restricting type, with a body mass index of 16.0-16.99 kg/m2

▶ **F50.012 Anorexia nervosa, restricting type, severe** (Ex) PDX 701
▶ Anorexia nervosa, restricting type, with a body mass index of 15.0-15.99 kg/m2

▶ **F50.013 Anorexia nervosa, restricting type, extreme** (Ex) PDX 701
▶ Anorexia nervosa, restricting type, with a body mass index of less than 15.0 kg/m2

▶ **F50.014 Anorexia nervosa, restricting type, in remission** (Ex) PDX 701
▶ Anorexia nervosa, restricting type, in full remission
▶ Anorexia nervosa, restricting type, in partial remission

▶ **F50.019 Anorexia nervosa, restricting type, unspecified** (Ex) PDX 701

F50.02 Anorexia nervosa, binge eating/purging type
Excludes1 bulimia nervosa (F50.02-)
Coding Clinic: 2022, Q1, P13

▶ **F50.020 Anorexia nervosa, binge eating/purging type, mild** (Ex) PDX 701
▶ Anorexia nervosa, binge eating/purging type, with a body mass index greater thanor equal to 17 kg/m2

▶ **F50.021 Anorexia nervosa, binge eating/purging type, moderate** (Ex) PDX 701
▶ Anorexia nervosa, binge eating/purging type, with a body mass index of 16.0-16.99kg/m2

▶ **F50.022 Anorexia nervosa, binge eating/purging type, severe** (Ex) PDX 701
▶ Anorexia nervosa, binge eating/purging type, with a body mass index of 15.0-15.99kg/m2

▶ **F50.023 Anorexia nervosa, binge eating/purging type, extreme** (Ex) PDX 701
▶ Anorexia nervosa, binge eating/purging type, with a body mass index of less than 15.0 kg/m2

▶ **F50.024 Anorexia nervosa, binge eating/purging type, in remission** (Ex) PDX 701
▶ Anorexia nervosa, binge eating/purging type, in full remission
▶ Anorexia nervosa, binge eating/purging type, in partial remission

▶ **F50.029 Anorexia nervosa, binge eating/purging type, unspecified** (Ex) PDX 701

F50.2 Bulimia nervosa (Ex) PDX 557
Bulimia NOS
Hyperorexia nervosa
Excludes1 anorexia nervosa, binge eating/purging type (F50.02-)

▶ **F50.20 Bulimia nervosa, unspecified** (Ex) PDX 702

▶ **F50.21 Bulimia nervosa, mild** (Ex) PDX 702
▶ Bulimia nervosa with 1-3 episodes of inappropriate compensatory behavior per week

▶ **F50.22 Bulimia nervosa, moderate** (Ex) PDX 702
▶ Bulimia nervosa with 4-7 episodes of inappropriate compensatory behavior per week

▶ **F50.23 Bulimia nervosa, severe** (Ex) PDX 702
▶ Bulimia nervosa with 8-13 episodes of inappropriate compensatory behavior per week

▶ **F50.24 Bulimia nervosa, extreme** (Ex) PDX 702
▶ Bulimia nervosa with 14 or more episodes of inappropriate compensatory behavior perweek

▶ **F50.25 Bulimia nervosa, in remission** (Ex) PDX 702
▶ Bulimia nervosa, in full remission
▶ Bulimia nervosa, in partial remission

● **F50.8 Other eating disorders**
~~pica of infancy and childhood (F98.3)~~

F50.81 Binge eating disorder
Coding Clinic: 2016, Q4, P15

▶ **F50.810 Binge eating disorder, mild**
▶ Binge eating disorder with 1-3 binge eating episodes per week

▶ **F50.811 Binge eating disorder, moderate**
▶ Binge eating disorder with 4-7 binge eating episodes per week

▶ **F50.812 Binge eating disorder, severe**
▶ Binge eating disorder with 8-13 binge eating episodes per week

▶ **F50.813 Binge eating disorder, extreme**
▶ Binge eating disorder with 14 or more eating episodes per week

▶ **F50.814 Binge eating disorder, in remission**
▶ Binge eating disorder, in full remission
▶ Binge eating disorder, in partial remission

▶ **F50.819 Binge eating disorder, unspecified**

F50.82 Avoidant/restrictive food intake disorder
▶Avoidant/restrictive food intake disorder, in remission

▶**F50.83 Pica in adults** A
▶Pica in adults, in remission
▶**Excludes1** pica in infancy and childhood (F98.3)

▶**F50.84 Rumination disorder in adults** A
▶Rumination disorder in adults, in remission
▶**Excludes1** rumination disorder in infancy and childhood (F98.21)

F50.89 Other specified eating disorder
~~Pica in adults~~
Psychogenic loss of appetite
Coding Clinic: 2016, Q4, P16

F50.9 Eating disorder, unspecified
Atypical anorexia nervosa
Atypical bulimia nervosa
Feeding or eating disorder, unspecified
Other specified feeding disorder

● **F51 Sleep disorders not due to a substance or known physiological condition**
Excludes2 organic sleep disorders (G47.-)

● **F51.0 Insomnia not due to a substance or known physiological condition**
Excludes2 alcohol related insomnia (F10.182, F10.282, F10.982)
drug-related insomnia (F11.182, F11.282, F11.982, F13.182, F13.282, F13.982, F14.182, F14.282, F14.982, F15.182, F15.282, F15.982, F19.182, F19.282, F19.982)
insomnia NOS (G47.0-)
insomnia due to known physiological condition (G47.0-)
organic insomnia (G47.0-)
sleep deprivation (Z72.820)

F51.01 Primary insomnia
Idiopathic insomnia

F51.02 Adjustment insomnia

F51.03 Paradoxical insomnia

F51.04 Psychophysiologic insomnia

F51.05 Insomnia due to other mental disorder
Code also associated mental disorder

F51.09 Other insomnia not due to a substance or known physiological condition

● **F51.1 Hypersomnia not due to a substance or known physiological condition**
Hypersomnia: Excessive sleeping/sleepiness
Excludes2 alcohol related hypersomnia (F10.182, F10.282, F10.982)
drug-related hypersomnia (F11.182, F11.282, F11.982, F13.182, F13.282, F13.982, F14.182, F14.282, F14.982, F15.182, F15.282, F15.982, F19.182, F19.282, F19.982)
hypersomnia NOS (G47.10)
hypersomnia due to known physiological condition (G47.10)
idiopathic hypersomnia (G47.11, G47.12)
narcolepsy (G47.4-)

F51.11 Primary hypersomnia

F51.12 Insufficient sleep syndrome
Excludes1 sleep deprivation (Z72.820)

F51.13 Hypersomnia due to other mental disorder
Code also associated mental disorder

F51.19 Other hypersomnia not due to a substance or known physiological condition

F51.3 Sleepwalking [somnambulism]
Non-rapid eye movement sleep arousal disorders, sleepwalking type

F51.4 Sleep terrors [night terrors]
Non-rapid eye movement sleep arousal disorders, sleep terror type

F51.5 Nightmare disorder
Dream anxiety disorder

F51.8 Other sleep disorders not due to a substance or known physiological condition

F51.9 Sleep disorder not due to a substance or known physiological condition, unspecified
Emotional sleep disorder NOS

● **F52 Sexual dysfunction not due to a substance or known physiological condition**
Excludes2 Dhat syndrome (F48.8)

F52.0 Hypoactive sexual desire disorder
Total loss of feeling of sexual pleasure
Lack or loss of sexual desire
Male hypoactive sexual desire disorder
Sexual anhedonia
Excludes1 decreased libido (R68.82)

F52.1 Sexual aversion disorder
Sexual aversion and lack of sexual enjoyment

● **F52.2 Sexual arousal disorders**
Failure of genital response

F52.21 Male erectile disorder
Erectile disorder
Psychogenic impotence
Excludes1 impotence of organic origin (N52.-)
impotence NOS (N52.-)

F52.22 Female sexual arousal disorder
Female sexual interest/arousal disorder

● **F52.3 Orgasmic disorder**
Inhibited orgasm
Psychogenic anorgasmy

F52.31 Female orgasmic disorder

F52.32 Male orgasmic disorder
Delayed ejaculation

F52.4 Premature ejaculation

F52.5 Vaginismus not due to a substance or known physiological condition
Psychogenic vaginismus
Excludes2 vaginismus (due to a known physiological condition) (N94.2)

F52.6 Dyspareunia not due to a substance or known physiological condition
Dyspareunia: Difficult or painful sexual intercourse
Genito-pelvic pain penetration disorder
Psychogenic dyspareunia
Excludes2 dyspareunia (due to a known physiological condition) (N94.1-)

F52.8 Other sexual dysfunction not due to a substance or known physiological condition
Excessive sexual drive
Nymphomania
Satyriasis

● **F52.9 Unspecified sexual dysfunction not due to a substance or known physiological condition**
Sexual dysfunction NOS

● F53 **Mental and behavioral disorders associated with the puerperium, not elsewhere classified**
Acute mental illness with sudden onset following childbirth with symptoms of affective psychosis, disorientation, and confusion are prevalent
Excludes1 mood disorders with psychotic features (F3Ø.2, F31.2, F31.5, F31.64, F32.3, F33.3)
postpartum dysphoria (O9Ø.6)
psychosis in schizophrenia, schizotypal, delusional, and other psychotic disorders (F2Ø-F29)

F53.Ø **Postpartum depression** M
Postnatal depression, NOS
Postpartum depression, NOS
Coding Clinic: 2018, Q4, P8

F53.1 **Puerperal psychosis** M
Postpartum psychosis
Puerperal psychosis, NOS
Coding Clinic: 2018, Q4, P9

F54 ***Psychological and behavioral factors associated with disorders or diseases classified elsewhere***
Psychological factors affecting physical conditions
Code first the associated physical disorder, such as:
asthma (J45.-)
dermatitis (L23-L25)
gastric ulcer (K25.-)
mucous colitis (K58.-)
ulcerative colitis (K51.-)
urticaria (L5Ø.-)
Excludes2 tension-type headache (G44.2)

● F55 **Abuse of non-psychoactive substances**
Excludes2 abuse of psychoactive substances (F1Ø-F19)

F55.Ø **Abuse of antacids**

F55.1 **Abuse of herbal or folk remedies**
Coding Clinic: 2023, Q3, P16

F55.2 **Abuse of laxatives**

F55.3 **Abuse of steroids or hormones**

F55.4 **Abuse of vitamins**

F55.8 **Abuse of other non-psychoactive substances**

F59 **Unspecified behavioral syndromes associated with physiological disturbances and physical factors**
Psychogenic physiological dysfunction NOS

DISORDERS OF ADULT PERSONALITY AND BEHAVIOR (F6Ø-F69)

● F6Ø **Specific personality disorders**
Long-term patterns of thoughts and behaviors causing serious problems with relationships and work

F6Ø.Ø **Paranoid personality disorder**
Hostile, devious, and combative response to disappointments
Expansive paranoid personality (disorder)
Fanatic personality (disorder)
Querulant personality (disorder)
Paranoid personality (disorder)
Sensitive paranoid personality (disorder)
Excludes2 paranoia (F22)
paranoia querulans (F22)
paranoid psychosis (F22)
paranoid schizophrenia (F2Ø.Ø)
paranoid state (F22)

F6Ø.1 **Schizoid personality disorder**
Detachment from social relationships with minimal emotional experiences and expressions
Excludes2 Asperger's syndrome (F84.5)
delusional disorder (F22)
schizoid disorder of childhood (F84.5)
schizophrenia (F2Ø.-)
schizotypal disorder (F21)

F6Ø.2 **Antisocial personality disorder**
Continuous and chronic antisocial behavior
Amoral personality (disorder)
Asocial personality (disorder)
Dissocial personality disorder
Psychopathic personality (disorder)
Sociopathic personality (disorder)
Excludes1 conduct disorders (F91.-)
Excludes2 borderline personality disorder (F6Ø.3)

F6Ø.3 **Borderline personality disorder**
Instability of mood, self-image or sense of self, and interpersonal relationships
Aggressive personality (disorder)
Emotionally unstable personality disorder
Explosive personality (disorder)
Excludes2 antisocial personality disorder (F6Ø.2)

F6Ø.4 **Histrionic personality disorder**
Personality disorder with excessive emotional and attention-seeking behavior
Hysterical personality (disorder)
Psychoinfantile personality (disorder)

F6Ø.5 **Obsessive-compulsive personality disorder**
Anankastic personality (disorder)
Compulsive personality (disorder)
Obsessional personality (disorder)
Excludes2 obsessive-compulsive disorder (F42.-)

F6Ø.6 **Avoidant personality disorder**
Anxious personality disorder

F6Ø.7 **Dependent personality disorder**
Asthenic personality (disorder)
Inadequate personality (disorder)
Passive personality (disorder)

● F6Ø.8 **Other specific personality disorders**

F6Ø.81 **Narcissistic personality disorder**
Vanity, conceit, egotism or indifference to plight of others

F6Ø.89 **Other specific personality disorders**
Eccentric personality disorder
'Haltlose' type personality disorder
Immature personality disorder
Passive-aggressive personality disorder
Psychoneurotic personality disorder
Self-defeating personality disorder

F6Ø.9 **Personality disorder, unspecified**
Character disorder NOS
Character neurosis NOS
Pathological personality NOS

● F63 **Impulse disorders**
Excludes2 habitual excessive use of alcohol or psychoactive substances (F1Ø-F19)
impulse disorders involving sexual behavior (F65.-)

F63.Ø **Pathological gambling**
Compulsive gambling
Gambling disorder
Excludes1 gambling and betting NOS (Z72.6)
Excludes2 excessive gambling by manic patients (F3Ø, F31)
gambling in antisocial personality disorder (F6Ø.2)

F63.1 **Pyromania**
Pathological fire-setting
Excludes2 fire-setting (by) (in):
adult with antisocial personality disorder (F6Ø.2)
alcohol or psychoactive substance intoxication (F1Ø-F19)
conduct disorders (F91.-)
mental disorders due to known physiological condition (FØ1-FØ9)
schizophrenia (F2Ø.-)

F63.2 Kleptomania
Pathological stealing
Excludes1 shoplifting as the reason for observation for suspected mental disorder (Z03.8)
Excludes2 depressive disorder with stealing (F31-F33)
stealing due to underlying mental condition-code to mental condition
stealing in mental disorders due to known physiological condition (F01-F09)

F63.3 Trichotillomania
Hair plucking
Excludes2 other stereotyped movement disorder (F98.4)

● **F63.8 Other impulse disorders**
F63.81 Intermittent explosive disorder
F63.89 Other impulse disorders

F63.9 Impulse disorder, unspecified
Impulse control disorder NOS

● **F64 Gender identity disorders**

F64.0 Transsexualism
Gender identity disorder in adolescence and adulthood
Gender incongruence in adolescents and adults
Gender identity in adolescents and adults
Transgender
Excludes1 gender identity disorder of childhood (F64.2)
Coding Clinic: 2016, Q4, P16

F64.1 Dual role transvestism
Use additional code to identify sex reassignment status (Z87.890)
Excludes1 gender identity disorder in childhood (F64.2)
Excludes2 fetishistic transvestism (F65.1)
Coding Clinic: 2016, Q4, P16

F64.2 Gender identity disorder of childhood P
Gender dysphoria in children
Gender incongruence of childhood
Excludes1 gender identity disorder in adolescence and adulthood (F64.0)
Excludes2 sexual maturation disorder (F66)

F64.8 Other gender identity disorders
Other specified gender dysphoria

F64.9 Gender identity disorder, unspecified
Gender dysphoria, unspecified
Gender incongruence, unspecified
Gender-role disorder NOS

● **F65 Paraphilias**

F65.0 Fetishism
Intense sexual urges and arousing fantasies using inanimate objects
Fetishistic disorder

F65.1 Transvestic fetishism
Intense sexual urges, arousal, or orgasm associated with fantasized/actual cross-dressing
Fetishistic transvestism
Transvestic disorder

F65.2 Exhibitionism
Exhibitionistic disorder

F65.3 Voyeurism
Sexual urges or arousal involving real or fantasized observation of unsuspecting people who are naked, disrobing, or engaging in sexual activity
Voyeuristic disorder

F65.4 Pedophilia
Pedophilic disorder

● **F65.5 Sadomasochism**
F65.50 Sadomasochism, unspecified
F65.51 Sexual masochism
Sexual masochism disorder
F65.52 Sexual sadism
Sexual sadism disorder

● **F65.8 Other paraphilias**
F65.81 Frotteurism
Sexual arousal or orgasm is achieved by rubbing up against another person (or fantasies of), in crowded place with unsuspecting victim
Frotteuristic disorder
F65.89 Other paraphilias
Necrophilia
Other specified paraphilic disorder

F65.9 Paraphilia, unspecified
Paraphilic disorder, unspecified
Sexual deviation NOS

F66 Other sexual disorders
Sexual maturation disorder
Sexual relationship disorder

● **F68 Other disorders of adult personality and behavior**

● **F68.1 Factitious disorder imposed on self**
Compensation neurosis
Elaboration of physical symptoms for psychological reasons
Hospital hopper syndrome
Münchhausen's syndrome
Peregrinating patient
Excludes2 factitial dermatitis (L98.1)
person feigning illness (with obvious motivation) (Z76.5)
F68.10 Factitious disorder imposed on self, unspecified (Ex) PDX 693
F68.11 Factitious disorder imposed on self with predominantly psychological signs and symptoms
F68.12 Factitious disorder imposed on self with predominantly physical signs and symptoms (Ex) PDX 693
F68.13 Factitious disorder imposed on self with combined psychological and physical signs and symptoms

F68.8 Other specified disorders of adult personality and behavior

F68.A Factitious disorder imposed on another (Ex) PDX 693
Factitious disorder by proxy
Münchausen's by proxy

F69 Unspecified disorder of adult personality and behavior A

INTELLECTUAL DISABILITIES (F70-F79)

Code first any associated physical or developmental disorders
Excludes1 borderline intellectual functioning, IQ above 70 to 84 (R41.83)

F70 Mild intellectual disabilities
IQ level 50-55 to approximately 70
Mild mental subnormality

F71 Moderate intellectual disabilities
IQ level 35-40 to 50-55
Moderate mental subnormality

F72 Severe intellectual disabilities (Ex) PDX 703
IQ 20-25 to 35-40
Severe mental subnormality

F73 Profound intellectual disabilities (Ex) PDX 703
IQ level below 20-25
Profound mental subnormality

● F78 Other intellectual disabilities

● F78.A Other genetic related intellectual disabilities

F78.A1 SYNGAP1-related intellectual disability
Code also, if applicable, any associated:
autism spectrum disorder (F84.0)
autistic disorder (F84.0)
encephalopathy (G93.4-)
epilepsy and recurrent seizures (G40.-)
other pervasive developmental disorders (F84.8)
pervasive developmental disorder, NOS (F84.9)

F78.A9 Other genetic related intellectual disability
Code also, if applicable, any associated disorders

F79 Unspecified intellectual disabilities
Mental deficiency NOS
Mental subnormality NOS

PERVASIVE AND SPECIFIC DEVELOPMENTAL DISORDERS (F80-F89)

● F80 Specific developmental disorders of speech and language

F80.0 Phonological disorder
Communication disorder of unknown cause, characterized by failure to use age-appropriate sounds
Dyslalia
Functional speech articulation disorder
Lalling
Lisping
Phonological developmental disorder
Speech articulation developmental disorder
Speech-sound disorder
Excludes1 speech articulation impairment due to aphasia NOS (R47.01)
speech articulation impairment due to apraxia (R48.2)
Excludes2 speech articulation impairment due to hearing loss (F80.4)
speech articulation impairment due to intellectual disabilities (F70-F79)
speech articulation impairment with expressive language developmental disorder (F80.1)
speech articulation impairment with mixed receptive expressive language developmental disorder (F80.2)

F80.1 Expressive language disorder
Developmental dysphasia or aphasia, expressive type
Excludes1 mixed receptive-expressive language disorder (F80.2)
dysphasia and aphasia NOS (R47.-)
Excludes2 acquired aphasia with epilepsy [Landau-Kleffner] (G40.80-)
intellectual disabilities (F70-F79)
pervasive developmental disorders (F84.-)
selective mutism (F94.0)

F80.2 Mixed receptive-expressive language disorder
Developmental dysphasia or aphasia, receptive type
Developmental Wernicke's aphasia
Excludes1 central auditory processing disorder (H93.25)
dysphasia or aphasia NOS (R47.-)
expressive language disorder (F80.1)
expressive type dysphasia or aphasia (F80.1)
word deafness (H93.25)
Excludes2 acquired aphasia with epilepsy [Landau-Kleffner] (G40.80-)
intellectual disabilities (F70-F79)
pervasive developmental disorders (F84.-)
selective mutism (F94.0)

F80.4 Speech and language development delay due to hearing loss
Code also type of hearing loss (H90.-, H91.-)

● F80.8 Other developmental disorders of speech or language

F80.81 Childhood onset fluency disorder
Cluttering NOS
Stuttering NOS
Excludes1 adult onset fluency disorder (F98.5)
fluency disorder in conditions classified elsewhere (R47.82)
fluency disorder (stuttering) following cerebrovascular disease (I69. with final characters -23)

F80.82 Social pragmatic communication disorder
Excludes1 Asperger's syndrome (F84.5)
autistic disorder (F84.0)
Coding Clinic: 2016, Q4, P16

F80.89 Other developmental disorders of speech and language
Coding Clinic: 2017, Q1, P27

F80.9 Developmental disorder of speech and language, unspecified
Communication disorder NOS
Language disorder NOS

● F81 Specific developmental disorders of scholastic skills

F81.0 Specific reading disorder
'Backward reading'
Developmental dyslexia
Specific learning disorder, with impairment in reading
Specific reading retardation
Excludes1 alexia NOS (R48.0)
dyslexia NOS (R48.0)

F81.2 Mathematics disorder
Developmental acalculia
Developmental arithmetical disorder
Developmental Gerstmann's syndrome
Specific learning disorder, with impairment in mathematics
Excludes1 acalculia NOS (R48.8)
Excludes2 arithmetical difficulties associated with a reading disorder (F81.0)
arithmetical difficulties associated with a spelling disorder (F81.81)
arithmetical difficulties due to inadequate teaching (Z55.8)

● F81.8 Other developmental disorders of scholastic skills

F81.81 Disorder of written expression
Specific learning disorder, with impairment in written expression
Specific spelling disorder

F81.89 Other developmental disorders of scholastic skills

● F81.9 Developmental disorder of scholastic skills, unspecified
Knowledge acquisition disability NOS
Learning disability NOS
Learning disorder NOS
Coding Clinic: 2022, Q4, P41

F82 Specific developmental disorder of motor function
Clumsy child syndrome
Developmental coordination disorder
Developmental dyspraxia
Excludes1 abnormalities of gait and mobility (R26.-)
lack of coordination (R27.-)
Excludes2 lack of coordination secondary to intellectual disabilities (F70-F79)

CHAPTER 5 (F01-F99)

F84 Pervasive developmental disorders

Code also any associated medical condition and intellectual disabilities

F84.Ø Autistic disorder PDX 704

Autism spectrum disorder
Infantile autism
Infantile psychosis
Kanner's syndrome

Excludes1 Asperger's syndrome (F84.5)

Coding Clinic: 2022, Q4, P41; 2017, Q1, P27

F84.2 Rett's syndrome PDX 625

Neurodevelopmental disorder

Excludes1 Asperger's syndrome (F84.5)
Autistic disorder (F84.Ø)
other childhood disintegrative disorder (F84.3)

F84.3 Other childhood disintegrative disorder PDX 704 P

Dementia infantilis

At least two years of normal development followed by significant loss of language abilities, social skills, bowel/bladder control, motor skills

Disintegrative psychosis
Heller's syndrome

At least two years of normal development followed by significant loss of language abilities, social skills, bowel/bladder control, motor skills

Symbiotic psychosis

Abnormal relationship to mothering figure, characterized by intense separation anxiety, severe regression, giving up of useful speech, and autism

Use additional code to identify any associated neurological condition.

Excludes1 Asperger's syndrome (F84.5)
Autistic disorder (F84.Ø)
Rett's syndrome (F84.2)

F84.5 Asperger's syndrome PDX 704

Developmental disorder

Asperger's disorder
Autistic psychopathy
Schizoid disorder of childhood

F84.8 Other pervasive developmental disorders PDX 704

Overactive disorder associated with intellectual disabilities and stereotyped movements

F84.9 Pervasive developmental disorder, unspecified PDX 704

Atypical autism

F88 Other disorders of psychological development

Developmental agnosia
Global developmental delay
Other specified neurodevelopmental disorder

F89 Unspecified disorder of psychological development

Developmental disorder NOS
Neurodevelopmental disorder NOS

BEHAVIORAL AND EMOTIONAL DISORDERS WITH ONSET USUALLY OCCURRING IN CHILDHOOD AND ADOLESCENCE (F9Ø-F98)

Note: Codes within categories F9Ø-F98 may be used regardless of the age of a patient. These disorders generally have onset within the childhood or adolescent years, but may continue throughout life or not be diagnosed until adulthood.

F9Ø Attention-deficit hyperactivity disorders

Attention deficit disorder with hyperactivity=ADHD

Includes attention deficit disorder with hyperactivity
attention deficit syndrome with hyperactivity

Excludes2 anxiety disorders (F4Ø.-, F41.-)
mood [affective] disorders (F3Ø-F39)
pervasive developmental disorders (F84.-)
schizophrenia (F2Ø.-)

F9Ø.Ø Attention-deficit hyperactivity disorder, predominantly inattentive type

Attention-deficit/hyperactivity disorder, predominantly inattentive presentation

F9Ø.1 Attention-deficit hyperactivity disorder, predominantly hyperactive type

Attention-deficit/hyperactivity disorder, predominantly hyperactive impulsive presentation

F9Ø.2 Attention-deficit hyperactivity disorder, combined type

Attention-deficit/hyperactivity disorder, combined presentation

F9Ø.8 Attention-deficit hyperactivity disorder, other type

F9Ø.9 Attention-deficit hyperactivity disorder, unspecified type

Attention-deficit hyperactivity disorder of childhood or adolescence NOS
Attention-deficit hyperactivity disorder NOS

F91 Conduct disorders

Childhood/adolescence disruptive behavior disorder

Excludes1 antisocial behavior (Z72.81-)
antisocial personality disorder (F6Ø.2)

Excludes2 conduct problems associated with attention-deficit hyperactivity disorder (F9Ø.-)
mood [affective] disorders (F3Ø-F39)
pervasive developmental disorders (F84.-)
schizophrenia (F2Ø.-)

F91.Ø Conduct disorder confined to family context

F91.1 Conduct disorder, childhood-onset type

Unsocialized conduct disorder
Conduct disorder, solitary aggressive type
Unsocialized aggressive disorder

F91.2 Conduct disorder, adolescent-onset type

Socialized conduct disorder
Conduct disorder, group type

F91.3 Oppositional defiant disorder

F91.8 Other conduct disorders

Other specified conduct disorder
Other specified disruptive disorder

F91.9 Conduct disorder, unspecified

Behavioral disorder NOS
Conduct disorder NOS
Disruptive behavior disorder NOS
Disruptive disorder NOS

F93 Emotional disorders with onset specific to childhood

F93.Ø Separation anxiety disorder of childhood

Excludes2 mood [affective] disorders (F3Ø-F39)
nonpsychotic mental disorders (F4Ø-F48)
phobic anxiety disorder of childhood (F4Ø.8)
social phobia (F4Ø.1)

F93.8 Other childhood emotional disorders

Identity disorder

Excludes2 gender identity disorder of childhood (F64.2)

F93.9 Childhood emotional disorder, unspecified

F94 Disorders of social functioning with onset specific to childhood and adolescence

F94.Ø Selective mutism

Elective mutism

Excludes2 pervasive developmental disorders (F84.-)
schizophrenia (F2Ø.-)
specific developmental disorders of speech and language (F8Ø.-)
transient mutism as part of separation anxiety in young children (F93.Ø)

CHAPTER 5 (FØ1-F99)

Item 5–2 Enuresis: Bed wetting by children at night. Causes can be either psychological or medical (diabetes, urinary tract infections, or abnormalities). **Encopresis:** Overflow incontinence of bowels sometimes resulting from chronic constipation or fecal impaction. Check the documentation for additional diagnoses.

F94.1 Reactive attachment disorder of childhood
Use additional code to identify any associated failure to thrive or growth retardation
Excludes1 disinhibited attachment disorder of childhood (F94.2)
normal variation in pattern of selective attachment
Excludes2 Asperger's syndrome (F84.5)
maltreatment syndromes (T74.-)
sexual or physical abuse in childhood, resulting in psychosocial problems (Z62.81-)

F94.2 Disinhibited attachment disorder of childhood
Affectionless psychopathy
Institutional syndrome
Excludes1 reactive attachment disorder of childhood (F94.1)
Excludes2 Asperger's syndrome (F84.5)
attention-deficit hyperactivity disorders (F90.-)
hospitalism in children (F43.2-)

F94.8 Other childhood disorders of social functioning

F94.9 Childhood disorder of social functioning, unspecified

● **F95 Tic disorder**
Involuntary twitch

F95.0 Transient tic disorder
Provisional tic disorder

F95.1 Chronic motor or vocal tic disorder

F95.2 Tourette's disorder
Combined vocal and multiple motor tic disorder [de la Tourette]
Tourette's syndrome

F95.8 Other tic disorders

F95.9 Tic disorder, unspecified
Tic NOS

● **F98 Other behavioral and emotional disorders with onset usually occurring in childhood and adolescence**
Excludes2 breath-holding spells (R06.89)
gender identity disorder of childhood (F64.2)
Kleine-Levin syndrome (G47.13)
obsessive-compulsive disorder (F42.3-)
sleep disorders not due to a substance or known physiological condition (F51.-)

F98.0 Enuresis not due to a substance or known physiological condition
Enuresis: Urinary incontinence
Enuresis (primary) (secondary) of nonorganic origin
Functional enuresis
Psychogenic enuresis
Urinary incontinence of nonorganic origin
Excludes1 enuresis NOS (R32)

F98.1 Encopresis not due to a substance or known physiological condition
Encopresis: Fecal incontinence
Functional encopresis
Incontinence of feces of nonorganic origin
Psychogenic encopresis
Use additional code to identify the cause of any coexisting constipation.
Excludes1 encopresis NOS (R15.-)

● **F98.2 Other feeding disorders of infancy and childhood**
Excludes2 anorexia nervosa and other eating disorders (F50.-)
feeding difficulties (R63.3-)
feeding problems of newborn (P92.-)
pica of infancy or childhood (F98.3)

F98.21 Rumination disorder of infancy and childhood
Rumination disorder of infancy and childhood, in remission
Excludes1 rumination disorder in adults (F50.84)

F98.29 Other feeding disorders of infancy and early childhood

F98.3 Pica of infancy and childhood
Craving and eating substances such as paint, clay, or dirt to replace a nutritional deficit in the body.
Pica in infancy or childhood, in remission
Excludes1 pica in adults (F50.83)

F98.4 Stereotyped movement disorders
Stereotype/habit disorder
Excludes1 abnormal involuntary movements (R25.-)
Excludes2 compulsions in obsessive-compulsive disorder (F42.-)
hair plucking (F63.3)
movement disorders of organic origin (G20-G25)
nail-biting (F98.8)
nose-picking (F98.8)
stereotypies that are part of a broader psychiatric condition (F01-F95)
thumb-sucking (F98.8)
tic disorders (F95.-)
trichotillomania (F63.3)

F98.5 Adult onset fluency disorder
Excludes1 childhood onset fluency disorder (F80.81)
dysphasia (R47.02)
fluency disorder in conditions classified elsewhere (R47.82)
fluency disorder (stuttering) following cerebrovascular disease (I69. with final characters -23)
tic disorders (F95.-)

F98.8 Other specified behavioral and emotional disorders with onset usually occurring in childhood and adolescence
Excessive masturbation
Nail-biting
Nose-picking
Thumb-sucking

F98.9 Unspecified behavioral and emotional disorders with onset usually occurring in childhood and adolescence

UNSPECIFIED MENTAL DISORDER (F99)

F99 Mental disorder, not otherwise specified
Mental illness NOS
Excludes1 unspecified mental disorder due to known physiological condition (F09)

CHAPTER 5 (F01-F99)

CHAPTER 6

DISEASES OF THE NERVOUS SYSTEM (GØØ-G99)

OGCR Chapter-Specific Coding Guidelines

6. Chapter 6: Diseases of the Nervous System (GØØ-G99)

a. Dominant/nondominant side

Codes from category G81, Hemiplegia and hemiparesis, and subcategories, G83.1, Monoplegia of lower limb, G83.2, Monoplegia of upper limb, and G83.3, Monoplegia, unspecified, identify whether the dominant or nondominant side is affected. Should the affected side be documented, but not specified as dominant or nondominant, and the classification system does not indicate a default, code selection is as follows:

- For ambidextrous patients, the default should be dominant.
- If the left side is affected, the default is nondominant.
- If the right side is affected, the default is dominant.

b. Pain - Category G89

1) General coding information

Codes in category G89, Pain, not elsewhere classified, may be used in conjunction with codes from other categories and chapters to provide more detail about acute or chronic pain and neoplasm-related pain, unless otherwise indicated below.

If the pain is not specified as acute or chronic, post-thoracotomy, postprocedural, or neoplasm-related, do not assign codes from category G89.

A code from category G89 should not be assigned if the underlying (definitive) diagnosis is known, unless the reason for the encounter is pain control/management and not management of the underlying condition.

When an admission or encounter is for a procedure aimed at treating the underlying condition (e.g., spinal fusion, kyphoplasty), a code for the underlying condition (e.g., vertebral fracture, spinal stenosis) should be assigned as the principal diagnosis. No code from category G89 should be assigned.

(a) Category G89 Codes as Principal or First-Listed Diagnosis

Category G89 codes are acceptable as principal diagnosis or the first-listed code:

- When pain control or pain management is the reason for the admission/encounter (e.g., a patient with displaced intervertebral disc, nerve impingement and severe back pain presents for injection of steroid into the spinal canal). The underlying cause of the pain should be reported as an additional diagnosis, if known.
- When a patient is admitted for the insertion of a neurostimulator for pain control, assign the appropriate pain code as the principal or first-listed diagnosis. When an admission or encounter is for a procedure aimed at treating the underlying condition and a neurostimulator is inserted for pain control during the same admission/encounter, a code for the underlying condition should be assigned as the principal diagnosis and the appropriate pain code should be assigned as a secondary diagnosis.

(b) Use of Category G89 Codes in Conjunction with Site Specific Pain Codes

(i) Assigning Category G89 and Site-Specific Pain Codes

Codes from category G89 may be used in conjunction with codes that identify the site of pain (including codes from Chapter 18) if the category G89 code provides additional information. For example, if the code describes the site of the pain, but does not fully describe whether the pain is acute or chronic, then both codes should be assigned.

(ii) Sequencing of Category G89 Codes with Site-Specific Pain Codes

The sequencing of category G89 codes with site-specific pain codes (including Chapter 18 codes), is dependent on the circumstances of the encounter/admission as follows:

- If the encounter is for pain control or pain management, assign the code from category G89 followed by the code identifying the specific site of pain (e.g., encounter for pain management for acute neck pain from trauma is assigned code G89.11, Acute pain due to trauma, followed by code M54.2, Cervicalgia, to identify the site of pain).
- If the encounter is for any other reason except pain control or pain management, and a related definitive diagnosis has not been established (confirmed) by the provider, assign the code for the specific site of pain first, followed by the appropriate code from category G89.

2) Pain due to devices, implants and grafts

See Section I.C.19. Pain due to medical devices

3) Postoperative Pain

The provider's documentation should be used to guide the coding of postoperative pain, as well as *Section III. Reporting Additional Diagnoses* and *Section IV. Diagnostic Coding and Reporting in the Outpatient Setting.*

The default for post-thoracotomy and other postoperative pain not specified as acute or chronic is the code for the acute form.

Routine or expected postoperative pain immediately after surgery should not be coded.

(a) Postoperative pain not associated with specific postoperative complication

Postoperative pain not associated with a specific postoperative complication is assigned to the appropriate postoperative pain code in category G89.

(b) Postoperative pain associated with specific postoperative complication

Postoperative pain associated with a specific postoperative complication (such as painful wire sutures) is assigned to the appropriate code(s) found in Chapter 19, Injury, poisoning, and certain other consequences of external causes. If appropriate, use additional code(s) from category G89 to identify acute or chronic pain (G89.18 or G89.28).

4) Chronic pain

Chronic pain is classified to subcategory G89.2. There is no time frame defining when pain becomes chronic pain. The provider's documentation should be used to guide use of these codes.

5) Neoplasm Related Pain

Code G89.3 is assigned to pain documented as being related, associated or due to cancer, primary or secondary malignancy, or tumor. This code is assigned regardless of whether the pain is acute or chronic.

This code may be assigned as the principal or first-listed code when the stated reason for the admission/encounter is documented as pain control/pain management. The underlying neoplasm should be reported as an additional diagnosis.

When the reason for the admission/encounter is management of the neoplasm and the pain associated with the neoplasm is also documented, code G89.3 may be assigned as an additional diagnosis. It is not necessary to assign an additional code for the site of the pain.

See Section I.C.2 for instructions on the sequencing of neoplasms for all other stated reasons for the admission/encounter (except for pain control/pain management).

6) Chronic pain syndrome

Central pain syndrome (G89.0) and chronic pain syndrome (G89.4) are different than the term "chronic pain," and therefore codes should only be used when the provider has specifically documented this condition.

See Section I.C.5. Pain disorders related to psychological factors

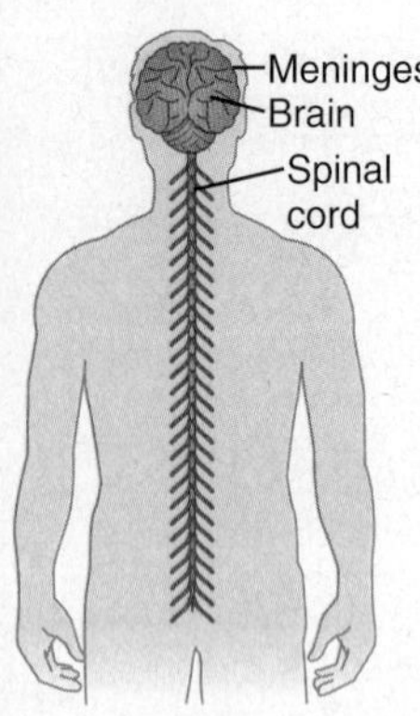

Figure 6-1 The brain and spinal cord make up the central nervous system.

Item 6–1 The two major classifications of the nervous system are the peripheral nervous system and the central nervous system (CNS). The central nervous system is composed of the brain and the spinal cord. The peripheral nervous system is composed of the parasympathetic and sympathetic systems. **Encephalitis** is the swelling of the brain. **Meningitis** is swelling of the covering of the brain, the meninges. Types and causes of brain infections are:

Type	Cause
purulent	bacterial
aseptic/abacterial	viral
chronic meningitis	mycobacterial and fungal

CHAPTER 6

DISEASES OF THE NERVOUS SYSTEM (G00-G99)

Excludes2 certain conditions originating in the perinatal period (P04-P96)
certain infectious and parasitic diseases (A00-B99)
complications of pregnancy, childbirth and the puerperium (O00-O9A)
congenital malformations, deformations, and chromosomal abnormalities (Q00-Q99)
endocrine, nutritional and metabolic diseases (E00-E88)
injury, poisoning and certain other consequences of external causes (S00-T88)
neoplasms (C00-D49)
symptoms, signs and abnormal clinical and laboratory findings, not elsewhere classified (R00-R94)

This chapter contains the following blocks:

G00-G09	Inflammatory diseases of the central nervous system
G10-G14	Systemic atrophies primarily affecting the central nervous system
G20-G26	Extrapyramidal and movement disorders
G30-G32	Other degenerative diseases of the nervous system
G35-G37	Demyelinating diseases of the central nervous system
G40-G47	Episodic and paroxysmal disorders
G50-G59	Nerve, nerve root and plexus disorders
G60-G65	Polyneuropathies and other disorders of the peripheral nervous system
G70-G73	Diseases of myoneural junction and muscle
G80-G83	Cerebral palsy and other paralytic syndromes
G89-G99	Other disorders of the nervous system

INFLAMMATORY DISEASES OF THE CENTRAL NERVOUS SYSTEM (G00-G09)

● **G00 Bacterial meningitis, not elsewhere classified**
An infection of the cerebrospinal fluid surrounding the spinal cord and brain.

Includes bacterial arachnoiditis
bacterial leptomeningitis
bacterial meningitis
bacterial pachymeningitis

Excludes1 bacterial meningoencephalitis (G04.2)
bacterial meningomyelitis (G04.2)

G00.0 Hemophilus meningitis Ex PDX 220
Meningitis due to Hemophilus influenzae

G00.1 Pneumococcal meningitis Ex PDX 220
Meningitis due to Streptococcal pneumoniae

G00.2 Streptococcal meningitis Ex PDX 220
Use additional code to further identify organism (B95.0-B95.5)

G00.3 Staphylococcal meningitis Ex PDX 220
Use additional code to further identify organism (B95.61-B95.8)

G00.8 Other bacterial meningitis Ex PDX 220
Meningitis due to Escherichia coli
Meningitis due to Friedländer bacillus
Meningitis due to Klebsiella
Use additional code to further identify organism (B96.-)

G00.9 Bacterial meningitis, unspecified Ex PDX 220
Meningitis due to gram-negative bacteria, unspecified
Purulent meningitis NOS
Pyogenic meningitis NOS
Suppurative meningitis NOS

G01 *Meningitis in bacterial diseases classified elsewhere* Ex PDX 220
Code first underlying disease

Excludes1 meningitis (in):
gonococcal (A54.81)
leptospirosis (A27.81)
listeriosis (A32.11)
Lyme disease (A69.21)
meningococcal (A39.0)
neurosyphilis (A52.13)
tuberculosis (A17.0)
meningoencephalitis and meningomyelitis in bacterial diseases classified elsewhere (G05)

G02 *Meningitis in other infectious and parasitic diseases classified elsewhere* Ex PDX 705
Code first underlying disease, such as:
African trypanosomiasis (B56.-)
poliovirus infection (A80.-)

Excludes1 candidal meningitis (B37.5)
coccidioidomycosis meningitis (B38.4)
cryptococcal meningitis (B45.1)
herpesviral [herpes simplex] meningitis (B00.3)
infectious mononucleosis complicated by meningitis (B27.- with fourth character 2)
measles complicated by meningitis (B05.1)
meningoencephalitis and meningomyelitis in other infectious and parasitic diseases classified elsewhere (G05)
mumps meningitis (B26.1)
rubella meningitis (B06.02)
varicella [chickenpox] meningitis (B01.0)
zoster meningitis (B02.1)

G03 Meningitis due to other and unspecified causes

Includes arachnoiditis NOS
leptomeningitis NOS
meningitis NOS
pachymeningitis NOS

Excludes1 meningoencephalitis (G04.-)
meningomyelitis (G04.-)

G03.0 Nonpyogenic meningitis (Ex) PDX 220
Aseptic meningitis
Nonbacterial meningitis

G03.1 Chronic meningitis (Ex) PDX 220

G03.2 Benign recurrent meningitis [Mollaret] (Ex) PDX 149

G03.8 Meningitis due to other specified causes (Ex) PDX 220

G03.9 Meningitis, unspecified (Ex) PDX 220
Arachnoiditis (spinal) NOS

G04 Encephalitis, myelitis and encephalomyelitis

Includes acute ascending myelitis
meningoencephalitis
meningomyelitis

Excludes1 encephalopathy NOS (G93.40)
other noninfectious acute disseminated encephalomyelitis (noninfectious ADEM) (G04.81)

Excludes2 acute transverse myelitis (G37.3)
alcoholic encephalopathy (G31.2)
multiple sclerosis (G35)
myalgic encephalomyelitis (G93.32)
subacute necrotizing myelitis (G37.4)
toxic encephalitis (G92.8)
toxic encephalopathy (G92.8)

G04.0 Acute disseminated encephalitis and encephalomyelitis (ADEM)

Excludes1 acute necrotizing hemorrhagic encephalopathy (G04.3-)

G04.00 Acute disseminated encephalitis and encephalomyelitis, unspecified (Ex) PDX 706

G04.01 Postinfectious acute disseminated encephalitis and encephalomyelitis (postinfectious ADEM) (Ex) PDX 707

Excludes1 post chickenpox encephalitis (B01.1)
post measles encephalitis (B05.0)
post measles myelitis (B05.1)

G04.02 Postimmunization acute disseminated encephalitis, myelitis and encephalomyelitis (Ex) PDX 708
Encephalitis, post immunization
Encephalomyelitis, post immunization
Use additional code to identify the vaccine (T50.A-, T50.B-, T50.Z-)

G04.1 Tropical spastic paraplegia (Ex) PDX 709

G04.2 Bacterial meningoencephalitis and meningomyelitis, not elsewhere classified (Ex) PDX 220

G04.3 Acute necrotizing hemorrhagic encephalopathy
Sudden and severe CNS disease with pathology of hemorrhages and necrosis of white matter

Excludes1 acute disseminated encephalitis and encephalomyelitis (G04.0-)

G04.30 Acute necrotizing hemorrhagic encephalopathy, unspecified (Ex) PDX 710

G04.31 Postinfectious acute necrotizing hemorrhagic encephalopathy (Ex) PDX 706

G04.32 Postimmunization acute necrotizing hemorrhagic encephalopathy (Ex) PDX 711
Use additional code to identify vaccine (T50.A-, T50.B-, T50.Z-)

G04.39 Other acute necrotizing hemorrhagic encephalopathy (Ex) PDX 712
Code also underlying etiology, if applicable

G04.8 Other encephalitis, myelitis and encephalomyelitis
Code also any associated seizure (G40.-, R56.9)

G04.81 Other encephalitis and encephalomyelitis (Ex) PDX 706
Noninfectious acute disseminated encephalomyelitis (noninfectious ADEM)

G04.82 Acute flaccid myelitis (Ex) PDX 713

Excludes1 transverse myelitis (G37.3)

G04.89 Other myelitis (Ex) PDX 707
Coding Clinic: 2020, Q1, P14

G04.9 Encephalitis, myelitis and encephalomyelitis, unspecified

G04.90 Encephalitis and encephalomyelitis, unspecified (Ex) PDX 714
Ventriculitis (cerebral) NOS

G04.91 Myelitis, unspecified (Ex) PDX 714

G05 Encephalitis, myelitis and encephalomyelitis in diseases classified elsewhere

Code first underlying disease, such as:
congenital toxoplasmosis encephalitis, myelitis and encephalomyelitis (P37.1)
cytomegaloviral encephalitis, myelitis and encephalomyelitis (B25.8)
encephalitis, myelitis and encephalomyelitis (in) systemic lupus erythematosus (M32.19)
eosinophilic meningoencephalitis (B83.2)
human immunodeficiency virus [HIV] disease (B20)
poliovirus (A80.-)
suppurative otitis media (H66.01-H66.4)
systemic lupus erythematosus (M32.19)
trichinellosis (B75)

Excludes1 adenoviral encephalitis, myelitis and encephalomyelitis (A85.1)
encephalitis, myelitis and encephalomyelitis (in) measles (B05.0)
enteroviral encephalitis, myelitis and encephalomyelitis (A85.0)
herpesviral [herpes simplex] encephalitis, myelitis and encephalomyelitis (B00.4)
listerial encephalitis, myelitis and encephalomyelitis (A32.12)
meningococcal encephalitis, myelitis and encephalomyelitis (A39.81)
mumps encephalitis, myelitis and encephalomyelitis (B26.2)
postchickenpox encephalitis, myelitis and encephalomyelitis (B01.1-)
rubella encephalitis, myelitis and encephalomyelitis (B06.01)
toxoplasmosis encephalitis, myelitis and encephalomyelitis (B58.2)
zoster encephalitis, myelitis and encephalomyelitis (B02.0)

G05.3 Encephalitis and encephalomyelitis in diseases classified elsewhere (Ex) PDX 707
Meningoencephalitis in diseases classified elsewhere
Code first underlying disease

G05.4 Myelitis in diseases classified elsewhere (Ex) PDX 707
Meningomyelitis in diseases classified elsewhere

G06 Intracranial and intraspinal abscess and granuloma
An accumulation of pus in either the brain or spinal cord
Use additional code (B95-B97) to identify infectious agent.

G06.0 Intracranial abscess and granuloma (Ex) PDX 715
Brain [any part] abscess (embolic)
Cerebellar abscess (embolic)
Cerebral abscess (embolic)
Intracranial epidural abscess or granuloma
Intracranial extradural abscess or granuloma
Intracranial subdural abscess or granuloma
Otogenic abscess (embolic)

Excludes1 tuberculous intracranial abscess and granuloma (A17.81)

Item 6–2 Huntington's chorea is an inherited degenerative disorder of the central nervous system and is characterized by ceaseless, jerky movements and progressive cognitive and behavioral deterioration.

G06.1 Intraspinal abscess and granuloma PDX 716
Abscess (embolic) of spinal cord [any part]
Intraspinal epidural abscess or granuloma
Intraspinal extradural abscess or granuloma
Intraspinal subdural abscess or granuloma
Excludes1 tuberculous intraspinal abscess and granuloma (A17.81)

G06.2 Extradural and subdural abscess, unspecified PDX 717

G07 Intracranial and intraspinal abscess and granuloma in diseases classified elsewhere PDX 717
Code first underlying disease, such as:
schistosomiasis granuloma of brain (B65.-)
Excludes1 abscess of brain:
amebic (A06.6)
chromomycotic (B43.1)
gonococcal (A54.82)
tuberculous (A17.81)
tuberculoma of meninges (A17.1)

G08 Intracranial and intraspinal phlebitis and thrombophlebitis PDX 717
Septic embolism of intracranial or intraspinal venous sinuses and veins
Septic endophlebitis of intracranial or intraspinal venous sinuses and veins
Septic phlebitis of intracranial or intraspinal venous sinuses and veins
Septic thrombophlebitis of intracranial or intraspinal venous sinuses and veins
Septic thrombosis of intracranial or intraspinal venous sinuses and veins
Excludes1 intracranial phlebitis and thrombophlebitis complicating:
abortion, ectopic or molar pregnancy (O00-O07, O08.7)
pregnancy, childbirth and the puerperium (O22.5, O87.3)
nonpyogenic intracranial phlebitis and thrombophlebitis (I67.6)
Excludes2 intracranial phlebitis and thrombophlebitis complicating nonpyogenic intraspinal phlebitis and thrombophlebitis (G95.1)

G09 Sequelae of inflammatory diseases of central nervous system
Note: Category G09 is to be used to indicate conditions whose primary classification is to G00-G08 as the cause of sequelae, themselves classifiable elsewhere. The 'sequelae' include conditions specified as residuals.
Code first condition resulting from (sequela) of inflammatory diseases of central nervous system

SYSTEMIC ATROPHIES PRIMARILY AFFECTING THE CENTRAL NERVOUS SYSTEM (G10-G14)

G10 Huntington's disease PDX 718
Genetic disease with degeneration of cells of the nervous system, including brain
Huntington's chorea
Huntington's dementia
Use Additional code, if applicable, to identify:
dementia with anxiety (F02.84, F02.A4, F02.B4, F02.C4)
dementia with behavioral disturbance (F02.81-, F02.A1-, F02.B1-, F02.C1-)
dementia with mood disturbance (F02.83, F02.A3, F02.B3, F02.C3)
dementia with psychotic disturbance (F02.82, F02.A2, F02.B2, F02.C2)
dementia without behavioral disturbance (F02.80, F02.A0, F02.B0, F02.C0)
mild neurocognitive disorder due to known physiological condition (F06.7-)

G11 Hereditary ataxia
Genetic neurological disorder affecting coordination
Excludes2 cerebral palsy (G80.-)
hereditary and idiopathic neuropathy (G60.-)
metabolic disorders (E70-E88)

G11.0 Congenital nonprogressive ataxia PDX 719

G11.1 Early-onset cerebellar ataxia

G11.10 Early-onset cerebellar ataxia, unspecified PDX 720

G11.11 Friedreich ataxia PDX 720
Autosomal recessive Friedreich ataxia
Friedreich ataxia with retained reflexes

G11.19 Other early-onset cerebellar ataxia PDX 720
Early-onset cerebellar ataxia with essential tremor
Early-onset cerebellar ataxia with myoclonus [Hunt's ataxia]
Early-onset cerebellar ataxia with retained tendon reflexes
X-linked recessive spinocerebellar ataxia

G11.2 Late-onset cerebellar ataxia PDX 719 A

G11.3 Cerebellar ataxia with defective DNA repair PDX 719
Ataxia telangiectasia [Louis-Bar]
Excludes2 Cockayne's syndrome (Q87.19)
other disorders of purine and pyrimidine metabolism (E79.-)
xeroderma pigmentosum (Q82.1)

G11.4 Hereditary spastic paraplegia PDX 721

G11.5 Hypomyelination - hypogonadotropic hypogonadism - hypodontia PDX 722
4H syndrome
Pol III-related leukodystrophy

G11.6 Leukodystrophy with vanishing white matter disease PDX 722

G11.8 Other hereditary ataxias PDX 719

G11.9 Hereditary ataxia, unspecified PDX 723
Hereditary cerebellar ataxia NOS
Hereditary cerebellar degeneration
Hereditary cerebellar disease
Hereditary cerebellar syndrome

G12 Spinal muscular atrophy and related syndromes

G12.0 Infantile spinal muscular atrophy, type I [Werdnig-Hoffman] PDX 724

G12.1 Other inherited spinal muscular atrophy PDX 724
Adult form spinal muscular atrophy
Childhood form, type II spinal muscular atrophy
Distal spinal muscular atrophy
Juvenile form, type III spinal muscular atrophy [Kugelberg-Welander]
Progressive bulbar palsy of childhood [Fazio-Londe]
Scapuloperoneal form spinal muscular atrophy

G12.2 Motor neuron disease
Progressive disease of motor neurons that carry impluses to muscles to move

G12.20 Motor neuron disease, unspecified PDX 724

G12.21 Amyotrophic lateral sclerosis PDX 724 A
Lou Gehrig's disease (ALS)

G12.22 Progressive bulbar palsy PDX 724

G12.23 Primary lateral sclerosis PDX 724

G12.24 Familial motor neuron disease PDX 724

G12.25 Progressive spinal muscle atrophy PDX 724

G12.29 Other motor neuron disease PDX 724

G12.8 Other spinal muscular atrophies and related syndromes PDX 724

G12.9 Spinal muscular atrophy, unspecified PDX 724

CHAPTER 6 (G00-G99)

G13 Systemic atrophies primarily affecting central nervous system in diseases classified elsewhere

G13.0 Paraneoplastic neuromyopathy and neuropathy
Carcinomatous neuromyopathy
Sensorial paraneoplastic neuropathy [Denny Brown]
Code first underlying neoplasm (C00-D49)

G13.1 Other systemic atrophy primarily affecting central nervous system in neoplastic disease
Paraneoplastic limbic encephalopathy
Code first underlying neoplasm (C00-D49)

G13.2 Systemic atrophy primarily affecting the central nervous system in myxedema
Code first underlying disease, such as:
hypothyroidism (E03.-)
myxedematous congenital iodine deficiency (E00.1)

G13.8 Systemic atrophy primarily affecting central nervous system in other diseases classified elsewhere
Code first underlying disease

G14 Postpolio syndrome
Includes Postpolio myelitic syndrome
Excludes1 sequelae of poliomyelitis (B91)

EXTRAPYRAMIDAL AND MOVEMENT DISORDERS (G20-G26)

G20 Parkinson's disease
Progressive disease of the nervous system that affects muscle coordination
Hemiparkinsonism
Idiopathic Parkinsonism or Parkinson's disease
Paralysis agitans
Parkinsonism or Parkinson's disease NOS
Primary Parkinsonism or Parkinson's disease
Use additional code, if applicable, to identify:
dementia with anxiety (F02.84, F02.A4, F02.B4, F02.C4)
dementia with behavioral disturbance (F02.81-, F02.A1-, F02.B1-, F02.C1-)
dementia with mood disturbance (F02.83, F02.A3, F02.B3, F02.C3)
dementia with psychotic disturbance (F02.82, F02.A2, F02.B2, F02.C2)
dementia without behavioral disturbance (F02.80, F02.A0, F02.B0, F02.C0)
mild neurocognitive disorder due to known physiological condition (F06.7-)
Coding Clinic: 2017, Q2, P7-8; 2016, Q2, P7

G20.A Parkinson's disease without dyskinesia

G20.A1 Parkinson's disease without dyskinesia, without mention of fluctuations
Parkinson's disease NOS
Parkinson's disease without dyskinesia, without mention of OFF episodes

G20.A2 Parkinson's disease without dyskinesia, with fluctuations
Parkinson's disease without dyskinesia, with OFF episodes
Coding Clinic: 2023, Q4, P17

G20.B Parkinson's disease with dyskinesia
Excludes1 drug induced dystonia (G24.0-)

G20.B1 Parkinson's disease with dyskinesia, without mention of fluctuations
Parkinson's disease with dyskinesia, without mention of OFF episodes
Coding Clinic: 2023, Q4, P16

G20.B2 Parkinson's disease with dyskinesia, with fluctuations
Parkinson's disease with dyskinesia, with OFF episodes
Coding Clinic: 2023, Q4, P17

G20.C Parkinsonism, unspecified
Parkinsonism, NOS
Excludes1 Parkinson's disease NOS (G20.A1)
Parkinson's disease with dyskinesia (G20.B-)
Parkinson's disease without dyskinesia (G20.A-)
secondary parkinsonism (G20.-)

G21 Secondary parkinsonism
Symptoms of Parkinson's caused by medicines, illness, or other nervous system disorder
Excludes1 ~~dementia with Parkinsonism (G31.83)~~
Huntington's disease (G10)
neurocognitive disorder with Lewy bodies (G31.83)
Shy-Drager syndrome (G90.3)
syphilitic Parkinsonism (A52.19)

G21.0 Malignant neuroleptic syndrome PDX 725
Use additional code for adverse effect, if applicable, to identify drug (T43.3X5, T43.4X5, T43.505, T43.595)
Excludes1 neuroleptic induced parkinsonism (G21.11)

G21.1 Other drug-induced secondary parkinsonism

G21.11 Neuroleptic induced parkinsonism PDX 726
Use additional code for adverse effect, if applicable, to identify drug (T43.3X5, T43.4X5, T43.505, T43.595)
Excludes1 malignant neuroleptic syndrome (G21.0)

G21.19 Other drug induced secondary parkinsonism PDX 726
Other medication-induced parkinsonism
Use additional code for adverse effect, if applicable, to identify drug (T36-T50 with fifth or sixth character 5)

G21.2 Secondary parkinsonism due to other external agents PDX 726
Code first (T51-T65) to identify external agent

G21.3 Postencephalitic parkinsonism PDX 726
G21.4 Vascular parkinsonism
G21.8 Other secondary parkinsonism PDX 726
G21.9 Secondary parkinsonism, unspecified PDX 726

G23 Other degenerative diseases of basal ganglia
Excludes2 multi-system degeneration of the autonomic nervous system (G90.3)

G23.0 Hallervorden-Spatz disease PDX 727
Pigmentary pallidal degeneration

G23.1 Progressive supranuclear ophthalmoplegia [Steele-Richardson-Olszewski] PDX 728
Progressive supranuclear palsy

G23.2 Striatonigral degeneration PDX 729

G23.3 Hypomyelination with atrophy of the basal ganglia and cerebellum PDX 730
H-ABC

G23.8 Other specified degenerative diseases of basal ganglia PDX 731
Calcification of basal ganglia

G23.9 Degenerative disease of basal ganglia, unspecified PDX 732

G24 Dystonia
Involuntary movements
Includes dyskinesia
Excludes2 athetoid cerebral palsy (G80.3)

G24.0 Drug induced dystonia
Use additional code for adverse effect, if applicable, to identify drug (T36-T50 with fifth or sixth character 5)

G24.01 Drug induced subacute dyskinesia
Drug induced blepharospasm
Drug induced orofacial dyskinesia
Neuroleptic induced tardive dyskinesia
Tardive dyskinesia

G24.02 Drug induced acute dystonia PDX 733
Acute dystonic reaction to drugs
Neuroleptic induced acute dystonia

G24.09 Other drug induced dystonia PDX 734

CHAPTER 6 (G00-G99)

G24.1 Genetic torsion dystonia
Dystonia deformans progressiva
Dystonia musculorum deformans
Familial torsion dystonia
Idiopathic familial dystonia
Idiopathic (torsion) dystonia NOS
(Schwalbe-) Ziehen-Oppenheim disease

G24.2 Idiopathic nonfamilial dystonia Ex PDX 735

G24.3 Spasmodic torticollis
Head tilts toward one side and chin is elevated and turned toward opposite side (wry neck)
Excludes1 congenital torticollis (Q68.Ø)
hysterical torticollis (F44.4)
ocular torticollis (R29.891)
psychogenic torticollis (F45.8)
torticollis NOS (M43.6)
traumatic recurrent torticollis (S13.4)

G24.4 Idiopathic orofacial dystonia
Orofacial dyskinesia
Excludes1 drug induced orofacial dyskinesia (G24.Ø1)

G24.5 Blepharospasm
Tonic spasm of orbicularis oculi muscle, producing closure of eyelids
Excludes1 drug induced blepharospasm (G24.Ø1)

G24.8 Other dystonia Ex PDX 736
Acquired torsion dystonia NOS

G24.9 Dystonia, unspecified
Dyskinesia NOS

● **G25 Other extrapyramidal and movement disorders**
Extrapyramidal: Other than pyramidal tracts
Excludes2 sleep related movement disorders (G47.6-)

G25.Ø Essential tremor
Familial tremor
Excludes1 tremor NOS (R25.1)

G25.1 Drug-induced tremor
Use additional code for adverse effect, if applicable, to identify drug (T36-T5Ø with fifth or sixth character 5)

G25.2 Other specified forms of tremor
Intention tremor

G25.3 Myoclonus
Shocklike contractions muscle(s)
Drug-induced myoclonus
Palatal myoclonus
Use additional code for adverse effect, if applicable, to identify drug (T36-T5Ø with fifth or sixth character 5)
Excludes1 facial myokymia (G51.4)
myoclonic epilepsy (G4Ø.-)

G25.4 Drug-induced chorea
Use additional code for adverse effect, if applicable, to identify drug (T36-T5Ø with fifth or sixth character 5)

G25.5 Other chorea
Continual, involuntary, jerky, movements
Chorea NOS
Excludes1 chorea NOS with heart involvement (IØ2.Ø)
Huntington's chorea (G1Ø)
rheumatic chorea (IØ2.-)
Sydenham's chorea (IØ2.-)

● **G25.6 Drug induced tics and other tics of organic origin**

G25.61 Drug induced tics
Use additional code for adverse effect, if applicable, to identify drug (T36-T5Ø with fifth or sixth character 5)

G25.69 Other tics of organic origin
Excludes1 habit spasm (F95.9)
tic NOS (F95.9)
Tourette's syndrome (F95.2)

● **G25.7 Other and unspecified drug induced movement disorders**
Use additional code for adverse effect, if applicable, to identify drug (T36-T5Ø with fifth or sixth character 5)

G25.7Ø Drug induced movement disorder, unspecified

G25.71 Drug induced akathisia
Drug induced acathisia
Neuroleptic induced acute akathisia
Tardive akathisia

G25.79 Other drug induced movement disorders

● **G25.8 Other specified extrapyramidal and movement disorders**

G25.81 Restless legs syndrome

G25.82 Stiff-man syndrome Ex PDX 737

G25.83 Benign shuddering attacks

G25.89 Other specified extrapyramidal and movement disorders

G25.9 Extrapyramidal and movement disorder, unspecified Ex PDX 737

G26 Extrapyramidal and movement disorders in diseases classified elsewhere
Code first underlying disease

OTHER DEGENERATIVE DISEASES OF THE NERVOUS SYSTEM (G3Ø-G32)

● **G3Ø Alzheimer's disease**
Progressive central neurodegenerative disorder
Includes Alzheimer's dementia senile and presenile forms
Use additional code, if applicable, to identify:
delirium, if applicable (FØ5)
dementia with anxiety (FØ2.84, FØ2.A4, FØ2.B4, FØ2.C4)
dementia with behavioral disturbance (FØ2.81-, FØ2.A1-, FØ2.B1-, FØ2.C1-)
dementia with mood disturbance (FØ2.83, FØ2.A3, FØ2.B3, FØ2.C3)
dementia with psychotic disturbance (FØ2.82, FØ2.A2, FØ2.B2, FØ2.C2)
dementia without behavioral disturbance (FØ2.8Ø, FØ2.AØ, FØ2.BØ, FØ2.CØ)
mild neurocognitive disorder due to known physiological condition (FØ6.7-)
Excludes1 senile degeneration of brain NEC (G31.1)
senile dementia NOS (FØ3.-)
senility NOS (R41.81)

G3Ø.Ø Alzheimer's disease with early onset

G3Ø.1 Alzheimer's disease with late onset A
Coding Clinic: 2022, Q4, P15

G3Ø.8 Other Alzheimer's disease

G3Ø.9 Alzheimer's disease, unspecified
Coding Clinic: 2017, Q1, P43; 2016, Q2, P6; 2012, Q4, P95

● **G31 Other degenerative diseases of nervous system, not elsewhere classified**
Use additional code, if applicable, for codes G31.Ø-G31.83, G31.85-G31.9, to identify:
dementia with behavioral disturbance (FØ2.81-, FØ2.A1-, FØ2.B1-, FØ2.C1-)
dementia with mood disturbance (FØ2.83, FØ2.A3, FØ2.B3, FØ2.C3)
dementia with psychotic disturbance (FØ2.82, FØ2.A2, FØ2.B2, FØ2.C2)
dementia without behavioral disturbance (FØ2.8Ø, FØ2.AØ, FØ2.BØ, FØ2.CØ)
mild neurocognitive disorder due to known physiological condition (FØ6.7-)
Excludes2 Reye's syndrome (G93.7)

● **G31.Ø Frontotemporal dementia**

G31.Ø1 Pick's disease
Primary progressive aphasia
Progressive isolated aphasia

G31.09 Other frontotemporal neurocognitive disorder
Frontal dementia
Use Additional code, if applicable, to identify mild neurocognitive disorders due to known physiological condition (F06.7-)

G31.1 Senile degeneration of brain, not elsewhere classified
Excludes1 Alzheimer's disease (G30.-)
senility NOS (R41.81)

G31.2 Degeneration of nervous system due to alcohol
Alcoholic cerebellar ataxia
Alcoholic cerebellar degeneration
Alcoholic cerebral degeneration
Alcoholic encephalopathy
Dysfunction of the autonomic nervous system due to alcohol
Code also associated alcoholism (F10.-)

G31.8 Other specified degenerative diseases of nervous system

G31.80 Leukodystrophy, unspecified

G31.81 Alpers' disease (Ex) PDX 625
Rare neuronal degeneration of cerebral cortex disease of young children
Grey-matter degeneration
Coding Clinic: 2017, Q2, P7

G31.82 Leigh's disease (Ex) PDX 625
Rare neurometabolic disorder that affects central nervous system
Subacute necrotizing encephalopathy

G31.83 Neurocognitive disorder with Lewy bodies
Closely allied to Parkinson's Disease
Lewy body dementia
Lewy body disease
Use Additional code, if applicable, to identify mild neurocognitive disorders due to known physiological condition (F06.7-)
Coding Clinic: 2017, Q2, P7; 2016, Q4, P141

G31.84 Mild cognitive impairment of uncertain or unknown etiology
Mild cognitive disorder NOS
Mild neurocognitive disorder of uncertain or unknown etiology
Use Additional code to identify presence of:
alcohol abuse and dependence (F10.-)
exposure to environmental tobacco smoke (Z77.22)
history of tobacco dependence (Z87.891)
hypertension (I10-I1A)
occupational exposure to environmental tobacco smoke (Z57.31)
tobacco dependence (F17.-)
tobacco use (Z72.0)

Excludes1 age related cognitive decline (R41.81)
altered mental status (R41.82)
cerebral degeneration (G31.9)
cerebrovascular diseases (I60-I69)
change in mental status (R41.82)
cognitive deficits following (sequelae of) cerebral hemorrhage or infarction (I69.01-, I69.11-, I69.21-, I69.31-, I69.81-, I69.91-)
cognitive impairment due to intracranial or head injury (S06.-)
dementia (F01.-, F02.-, F03.-)
mild neurocognitive disorder due to a known physiological condition (F06.7-)
neurologic neglect syndrome (R41.4)
personality change, nonpsychotic (F68.8)
Coding Clinic: 2021, Q3, P3

G31.85 Corticobasal degeneration

G31.86 Alexander disease

G31.89 Other specified degenerative diseases of nervous system

G31.9 Degenerative disease of nervous system, unspecified
Coding Clinic: 2021, Q3, P3

G32 Other degenerative disorders of nervous system in diseases classified elsewhere

G32.0 Subacute combined degeneration of spinal cord in diseases classified elsewhere (Ex) PDX 738
Dana-Putnam syndrome
Sclerosis of spinal cord (combined) (dorsolateral) (posterolateral)
Code first underlying disease, such as:
other dietary vitamin B12 deficiency anemia
pernicious (D51.0)
vitamin B12 deficiency anemia, unspecified (D51.8)
Excludes1 syphilitic combined degeneration of spinal cord (A52.11)

G32.8 Other specified degenerative disorders of nervous system in diseases classified elsewhere
Code first underlying disease, such as:
amyloidosis cerebral degeneration (E85.-)
cerebral degeneration (due to) hypothyroidism (E00.0-E03.9)
cerebral degeneration (due to) neoplasm (C00-D49)
cerebral degeneration (due to) vitamin B deficiency, except thiamine (E52-E53.-)
Excludes1 superior hemorrhagic polioencephalitis [Wernicke's encephalopathy] (E51.2)

G32.81 Cerebellar ataxia in diseases classified elsewhere (Ex) PDX 719
Code first underlying disease, such as:
celiac disease (with gluten ataxia) (K90.0)
cerebellar ataxia (in) neoplastic disease (paraneoplastic cerebellar degeneration) (C00-D49)
non-celiac gluten ataxia (M35.9)
Excludes1 systemic atrophy primarily affecting the central nervous system in alcoholic cerebellar ataxia (G31.2)
systemic atrophy primarily affecting the central nervous system in myxedema (G13.2)

G32.89 Other specified degenerative disorders of nervous system in diseases classified elsewhere
Degenerative encephalopathy in diseases classified elsewhere

DEMYELINATING DISEASES OF THE CENTRAL NERVOUS SYSTEM (G35-G37)

G35 Multiple sclerosis
Destruction of central nervous system; four types: relapsing remitting, secondary progressive, primary progressive, and progressive relapsing
Disseminated multiple sclerosis
Generalized multiple sclerosis
Multiple sclerosis NOS
Multiple sclerosis of brain stem
Multiple sclerosis of cord
Coding Clinic: 2021, Q1, P7

G36 Other acute disseminated demyelination
Excludes1 postinfectious encephalitis and encephalomyelitis NOS (G04.01)

G36.0 Neuromyelitis optica [Devic] (Ex) PDX 739
Inflammatory disorder in which immune system attacks optic nerves and spinal cord producing inflammation of optic nerve (optic neuritis) and spinal cord (myelitis)
Demyelination in optic neuritis
Excludes1 optic neuritis NOS (H46)

CHAPTER 6 (G00-G99)

Item 6–3 Multiple sclerosis (MS) is a nervous system disease affecting the brain and spinal cord by damaging the myelin sheath surrounding and protecting nerve cells. The damage slows down/blocks messages between the brain and body. Symptoms are visual disturbances, muscle weakness, coordination and balance issues, numbness, prickling, thinking and memory problems. The cause is unknown, though it is thought that it may be an autoimmune disease. It affects women more than men, between 20 and 40 years of age. MS can be mild, but it may cause the loss of ability to write, walk, and speak. There is no cure, but medication may slow or control symptoms.

G36.1 Acute and subacute hemorrhagic leukoencephalitis [Hurst] (Ex) PDX 740

G36.8 Other specified acute disseminated demyelination (Ex) PDX 740

G36.9 Acute disseminated demyelination, unspecified (Ex) PDX 740

● **G37 Other demyelinating diseases of central nervous system**

Destruction of central nervous system

G37.0 Diffuse sclerosis of central nervous system (Ex) PDX 741

Periaxial encephalitis

Schilder's disease

Excludes1 X linked adrenoleukodystrophy (E71.52-)

G37.1 Central demyelination of corpus callosum (Ex) PDX 740

G37.2 Central pontine myelinolysis (Ex) PDX 740

Coding Clinic: 2022, Q2, P11

G37.3 Acute transverse myelitis in demyelinating disease of central nervous system (Ex) PDX 742

Acute transverse myelitis NOS

Acute transverse myelopathy

Excludes1 acute flaccid myelitis (G04.82)
multiple sclerosis (G35)
neuromyelitis optica [Devic] (G36.0)

G37.4 Subacute necrotizing myelitis of central nervous system (Ex) PDX 714

G37.5 Concentric sclerosis [Baló] of central nervous system (Ex) PDX 743

● **G37.8 Other specified demyelinating diseases of central nervous system**

G37.81 Myelin oligodendrocyte glycoprotein antibody disease (Ex) PDX 744

MOG antibody disease

Code also associated manifestations, if known, such as:
noninfectious acute disseminated encephalomyelitis (G04.81)
neuromyelitis optica (G36.0)

G37.89 Other specified demyelinating diseases of central nervous system (Ex) PDX 744

G37.9 Demyelinating disease of central nervous system, unspecified (Ex) PDX 740

EPISODIC AND PAROXYSMAL DISORDERS (G40-G47)

● **G40 Epilepsy and recurrent seizures**

Note: The following terms are to be considered equivalent to intractable: pharmacoresistant (pharmacologically resistant), treatment resistant, refractory (medically) and poorly controlled

Excludes1 conversion disorder with seizures (F44.5)
convulsions NOS (R56.9)
post traumatic seizures (R56.1)
seizure (convulsive) NOS (R56.9)
seizure of newborn (P90)

Excludes2 hippocampal sclerosis (G93.81)
mesial temporal sclerosis (G93.81)
temporal sclerosis (G93.81)
Todd's paralysis (G83.84)

● **G40.0 Localization-related (focal) (partial) idiopathic epilepsy and epileptic syndromes with seizures of localized onset**

Benign childhood epilepsy with centrotemporal EEG spikes

Childhood epilepsy with occipital EEG paroxysms

Excludes1 adult onset localization-related epilepsy (G40.1-, G40.2-)

● **G40.00 Localization-related (focal) (partial) idiopathic epilepsy and epileptic syndromes with seizures of localized onset, not intractable**

Localization-related (focal) (partial) idiopathic epilepsy and epileptic syndromes with seizures of localized onset without intractability

G40.001 Localization-related (focal) (partial) idiopathic epilepsy and epileptic syndromes with seizures of localized onset, not intractable, with status epilepticus (Ex) PDX 745

G40.009 Localization-related (focal) (partial) idiopathic epilepsy and epileptic syndromes with seizures of localized onset, not intractable, without status epilepticus (Ex) PDX 745

Localization-related (focal) (partial) idiopathic epilepsy and epileptic syndromes with seizures of localized onset NOS

● **G40.01 Localization-related (focal) (partial) idiopathic epilepsy and epileptic syndromes with seizures of localized onset, intractable**

G40.011 Localization-related (focal) (partial) idiopathic epilepsy and epileptic syndromes with seizures of localized onset, intractable, with status epilepticus (Ex) PDX 746

G40.019 Localization-related (focal) (partial) idiopathic epilepsy and epileptic syndromes with seizures of localized onset, intractable, without status epilepticus (Ex) PDX 746

● **G40.1 Localization-related (focal) (partial) symptomatic epilepsy and epileptic syndromes with simple partial seizures**

Attacks without alteration of consciousness

Epilepsia partialis continua [Kozhevnikof]

Simple partial seizures developing into secondarily generalized seizures

● **G40.10 Localization-related (focal) (partial) symptomatic epilepsy and epileptic syndromes with simple partial seizures, not intractable**

Localization-related (focal) (partial) symptomatic epilepsy and epileptic syndromes with simple partial seizures without intractability

G40.101 Localization-related (focal) (partial) symptomatic epilepsy and epileptic syndromes with simple partial seizures, not intractable, with status epilepticus (Ex) PDX 745

G40.109 Localization-related (focal) (partial) symptomatic epilepsy and epileptic syndromes with simple partial seizures, not intractable, without status epilepticus (Ex) PDX 745

Localization-related (focal) (partial) symptomatic epilepsy and epileptic syndromes with simple partial seizures NOS

Coding Clinic: 2023, Q3, P4

CHAPTER 6 (G00-G99)

● **G40.11 Localization-related (focal) (partial) symptomatic epilepsy and epileptic syndromes with simple partial seizures, intractable**

G40.111 Localization-related (focal) (partial) symptomatic epilepsy and epileptic syndromes with simple partial seizures, intractable, with status epilepticus PDX 746

G40.119 Localization-related (focal) (partial) symptomatic epilepsy and epileptic syndromes with simple partial seizures, intractable, without status epilepticus PDX 746

● **G40.2 Localization-related (focal) (partial) symptomatic epilepsy and epileptic syndromes with complex partial seizures**

Attacks with alteration of consciousness, often with automatisms
Complex partial seizures developing into secondarily generalized seizures

● **G40.20 Localization-related (focal) (partial) symptomatic epilepsy and epileptic syndromes with complex partial seizures, not intractable**

Localization-related (focal) (partial) symptomatic epilepsy and epileptic syndromes with complex partial seizures without intractability

G40.201 Localization-related (focal) (partial) symptomatic epilepsy and epileptic syndromes with complex partial seizures, not intractable, with status epilepticus PDX 745

G40.209 Localization-related (focal) (partial) symptomatic epilepsy and epileptic syndromes with complex partial seizures, not intractable, without status epilepticus PDX 745

Localization-related (focal) (partial) symptomatic epilepsy and epileptic syndromes with complex partial seizures NOS

● **G40.21 Localization-related (focal) (partial) symptomatic epilepsy and epileptic syndromes with complex partial seizures, intractable**

G40.211 Localization-related (focal) (partial) symptomatic epilepsy and epileptic syndromes with complex partial seizures, intractable, with status epilepticus PDX 746

G40.219 Localization-related (focal) (partial) symptomatic epilepsy and epileptic syndromes with complex partial seizures, intractable, without status epilepticus PDX 746

● **G40.3 Generalized idiopathic epilepsy and epileptic syndromes**

Code also MERRF syndrome, if applicable (E88.42)

● **G40.30 Generalized idiopathic epilepsy and epileptic syndromes, not intractable**

Generalized idiopathic epilepsy and epileptic syndromes without intractability

G40.301 Generalized idiopathic epilepsy and epileptic syndromes, not intractable, with status epilepticus PDX 747

G40.309 Generalized idiopathic epilepsy and epileptic syndromes, not intractable, without status epilepticus

Generalized idiopathic epilepsy and epileptic syndromes NOS

● **G40.31 Generalized idiopathic epilepsy and epileptic syndromes, intractable**

G40.311 Generalized idiopathic epilepsy and epileptic syndromes, intractable, with status epilepticus PDX 747

G40.319 Generalized idiopathic epilepsy and epileptic syndromes, intractable, without status epilepticus PDX 747

● **G40.4 Other generalized epilepsy and epileptic syndromes**

Epilepsy with grand mal seizures on awakening
Epilepsy with myoclonic absences
Epilepsy with myoclonic-astatic seizures
Grand mal seizure NOS
Nonspecific atonic epileptic seizures
Nonspecific clonic epileptic seizures
Nonspecific myoclonic epileptic seizures
Nonspecific tonic epileptic seizures
Nonspecific tonic-clonic epileptic seizures
Symptomatic early myoclonic encephalopathy

● **G40.40 Other generalized epilepsy and epileptic syndromes, not intractable**

Other generalized epilepsy and epileptic syndromes without intractability
Other generalized epilepsy and epileptic syndromes NOS

G40.401 Other generalized epilepsy and epileptic syndromes, not intractable, with status epilepticus

G40.409 Other generalized epilepsy and epileptic syndromes, not intractable, without status epilepticus

● **G40.41 Other generalized epilepsy and epileptic syndromes, intractable**

G40.411 Other generalized epilepsy and epileptic syndromes, intractable, with status epilepticus PDX 746

G40.419 Other generalized epilepsy and epileptic syndromes, intractable, without status epilepticus PDX 746

G40.42 Cyclin-Dependent Kinase-Like 5 Deficiency Disorder

CDKL5

Use additional code, if known, to identify associated manifestations, such as:
cortical blindness (H47.61-)
global developmental delay (F88)

● **G40.5 Epileptic seizures related to external causes**

Epileptic seizures related to alcohol
Epileptic seizures related to drugs
Epileptic seizures related to hormonal changes
Epileptic seizures related to sleep deprivation
Epileptic seizures related to stress

Code also, if applicable, associated epilepsy and recurrent seizures (G40.-)

Use additional code for adverse effect, if applicable, to identify drug (T36-T50 with fifth or sixth character 5)

● **G40.50 Epileptic seizures related to external causes, not intractable**

G40.501 Epileptic seizures related to external causes, not intractable, with status epilepticus PDX 746

G40.509 Epileptic seizures related to external causes, not intractable, without status epilepticus PDX 746

Epileptic seizures related to external causes, NOS

G40.8 Other epilepsy and recurrent seizures
Epilepsies and epileptic syndromes undetermined as to whether they are focal or generalized
Landau-Kleffner syndrome

G40.80 Other epilepsy

G40.801 Other epilepsy, not intractable, with status epilepticus PDX 746
Other epilepsy without intractability with status epilepticus

G40.802 Other epilepsy, not intractable, without status epilepticus PDX 746
Other epilepsy NOS
Other epilepsy without intractability without status epilepticus

G40.803 Other epilepsy, intractable, with status epilepticus PDX 746

G40.804 Other epilepsy, intractable, without status epilepticus PDX 746

G40.81 Lennox-Gastaut syndrome

G40.811 Lennox-Gastaut syndrome, not intractable, with status epilepticus PDX 746

G40.812 Lennox-Gastaut syndrome, not intractable, without status epilepticus PDX 746

G40.813 Lennox-Gastaut syndrome, intractable, with status epilepticus PDX 746

G40.814 Lennox-Gastaut syndrome, intractable, without status epilepticus PDX 746

G40.82 Epileptic spasms
Infantile spasms
Salaam attacks
West's syndrome

G40.821 Epileptic spasms, not intractable, with status epilepticus PDX 745

G40.822 Epileptic spasms, not intractable, without status epilepticus PDX 745

G40.823 Epileptic spasms, intractable, with status epilepticus PDX 746

G40.824 Epileptic spasms, intractable, without status e pilepticus PDX 746

G40.83 Dravet syndrome
Polymorphic epilepsy in infancy (PMEI)
Severe myoclonic epilepsy in infancy (SMEI)

G40.833 Dravet syndrome, intractable, with status epilepticus PDX 748

G40.834 Dravet syndrome, intractable, without status epilepticus PDX 748
Dravet syndrome NOS

G40.84 KCNQ2-related epilepsy

G40.841 KCNQ2-related epilepsy, not intractable, with status epilepticus PDX 746

G40.842 KCNQ2-related epilepsy, not intractable, without status epilepticus PDX 746
KCNQ2-related epilepsy NOS

G40.843 KCNQ2-related epilepsy, intractable, with status epilepticus PDX 746

G40.844 KCNQ2-related epilepsy, intractable, without status epilepticus PDX 746

G40.89 Other seizures PDX 746

Excludes1 post traumatic seizures (R56.1)
recurrent seizures NOS (G40.909)
seizure NOS (R56.9)

G40.9 Epilepsy, unspecified

G40.90 Epilepsy, unspecified, not intractable
Epilepsy, unspecified, without intractability

G40.901 Epilepsy, unspecified, not intractable, with status epilepticus

G40.909 Epilepsy, unspecified, not intractable, without status epilepticus
Epilepsy NOS
Epileptic convulsions NOS
Epileptic fits NOS
Epileptic seizures NOS
Recurrent seizures NOS
Seizure disorder NOS
Coding Clinic: 2024, Q2, P9; 2021, Q2, P3

G40.91 Epilepsy, unspecified, intractable
Intractable seizure disorder NOS

G40.911 Epilepsy, unspecified, intractable, with status epilepticus PDX 746

G40.919 Epilepsy, unspecified, intractable, without status epilepticus PDX 746

G40.A Absence epileptic syndrome
Childhood absence epilepsy [pyknolepsy]
Juvenile absence epilepsy
Absence epileptic syndrome, NOS

G40.A0 Absence epileptic syndrome, not intractable

G40.A01 Absence epileptic syndrome, not intractable, with status epilepticus

G40.A09 Absence epileptic syndrome, not intractable, without status epilepticus

G40.A1 Absence epileptic syndrome, intractable

G40.A11 Absence epileptic syndrome, intractable, with status epilepticus PDX 746

G40.A19 Absence epileptic syndrome, intractable, without status epilepticus PDX 746

G40.B Juvenile myoclonic epilepsy [impulsive petit mal]

G40.B0 Juvenile myoclonic epilepsy, not intractable

G40.B01 Juvenile myoclonic epilepsy, not intractable, with status epilepticus PDX 746

G40.B09 Juvenile myoclonic epilepsy, not intractable, without status epilepticus PDX 746

G40.B1 Juvenile myoclonic epilepsy, intractable

G40.B11 Juvenile myoclonic epilepsy, intractable, with status epilepticus PDX 746

G40.B19 Juvenile myoclonic epilepsy, intractable, without status epilepticus PDX 746

G40.C Lafora progressive myoclonus epilepsy
Lafora body disease

Code also, if applicable, associated conditions such as dementia (F02.8-)

G40.C0 Lafora progressive myoclonus epilepsy, not intractable

G40.C01 Lafora progressive myoclonus epilepsy, not intractable, with status epilepticus PDX 746

G40.C09 Lafora progressive myoclonus epilepsy, not intractable, without status epilepticus PDX 746
Lafora progressive myoclonus epilepsy NOS

G40.C1 Lafora progressive myoclonus epilepsy, intractable

G40.C11 Lafora progressive myoclonus epilepsy, intractable, with status epilepticus (Ex) PDX 746

G40.C19 Lafora progressive myoclonus epilepsy, intractable, without status epilepticus (Ex) PDX 746

G43 Migraine

Note: The following terms are to be considered equivalent to intractable: pharmacoresistant (pharmacologically resistant), treatment resistant, refractory (medically) and poorly controlled

Use additional code for adverse effect, if applicable, to identify drug (T36-T50 with fifth or sixth character 5)

Excludes1 headache NOS (R51.9)
lower half migraine (G44.00)

Excludes2 headache syndromes (G44.-)

G43.0 Migraine without aura

Neurological disorder, generally recurring headaches without early symptom (aura)

Common migraine

Excludes1 chronic migraine without aura (G43.7-)

G43.00 Migraine without aura, not intractable

Neurological disorder, generally recurring headaches without early symptom (aura); resistant to cure, relief, or control

Migraine without aura without mention of refractory migraine

G43.001 Migraine without aura, not intractable, with status migrainosus

G43.009 Migraine without aura, not intractable, without status migrainosus

Migraine without aura NOS

G43.01 Migraine without aura, intractable

Intractable migraine: Not easily cured or managed; relentless pain from a migraine

Migraine without aura with refractory migraine

G43.011 Migraine without aura, intractable, with status migrainosus

G43.019 Migraine without aura, intractable, without status migrainosus

G43.1 Migraine with aura

Basilar migraine
Classical migraine
Migraine equivalents
Migraine preceded or accompanied by transient focal neurological phenomena
Migraine triggered seizures
Migraine with acute-onset aura
Migraine with aura without headache (migraine equivalents)
Migraine with prolonged aura
Migraine with typical aura
Retinal migraine

Code also any associated seizure (G40.-, R56.9)
chronic migraine with aura (G43.E-)

Excludes1 persistent migraine aura (G43.5-, G43.6-)

Item 6–4 Migraine headache is described as an intense pulsing or throbbing pain in one area of the head. It can be accompanied by extreme sensitivity to light (photophobic) and sound and is three times more common in women than in men. Symptoms include nausea and vomiting. Research indicates migraine headaches are caused by inherited abnormalities in genes that control the activities of certain cell populations in the brain.

G43.10 Migraine with aura, not intractable

Migraine with aura without mention of refractory migraine

G43.101 Migraine with aura, not intractable, with status migrainosus

G43.109 Migraine with aura, not intractable, without status migrainosus

Migraine with aura NOS

G43.11 Migraine with aura, intractable

Migraine with aura with refractory migraine

G43.111 Migraine with aura, intractable, with status migrainosus

G43.119 Migraine with aura, intractable, without status migrainosus

G43.4 Hemiplegic migraine

Inherited migraine disorder causing temporary paralysis of one side of body followed by severe headache and nausea

Familial migraine
Sporadic migraine

G43.40 Hemiplegic migraine, not intractable

Hemiplegic migraine without refractory migraine

G43.401 Hemiplegic migraine, not intractable, with status migrainosus

G43.409 Hemiplegic migraine, not intractable, without status migrainosus

Hemiplegic migraine NOS

G43.41 Hemiplegic migraine, intractable

Hemiplegic migraine with refractory migraine

G43.411 Hemiplegic migraine, intractable, with status migrainosus

G43.419 Hemiplegic migraine, intractable, without status migrainosus

G43.5 Persistent migraine aura without cerebral infarction

G43.50 Persistent migraine aura without cerebral infarction, not intractable

Persistent migraine aura without cerebral infarction, without refractory migraine

G43.501 Persistent migraine aura without cerebral infarction, not intractable, with status migrainosus

G43.509 Persistent migraine aura without cerebral infarction, not intractable, without status migrainosus

Persistent migraine aura NOS

G43.51 Persistent migraine aura without cerebral infarction, intractable

Persistent migraine aura without cerebral infarction, with refractory migraine

G43.511 Persistent migraine aura without cerebral infarction, intractable, with status migrainosus

G43.519 Persistent migraine aura without cerebral infarction, intractable, without status migrainosus

G43.6 Persistent migraine aura with cerebral infarction

Visual, motor, or psychic disturbances, paresthesias, and related neurologic abnormalities accompanying migraine

Code also the type of cerebral infarction (I63.-)

G43.60 Persistent migraine aura with cerebral infarction, not intractable

Persistent migraine aura with cerebral infarction, without refractory migraine

G43.601 Persistent migraine aura with cerebral infarction, not intractable, with status migrainosus (Ex) PDX 749

G43.609 Persistent migraine aura with cerebral infarction, not intractable, without status migrainosus (Ex) PDX 749

CHAPTER 6 (G00-G99)

G43.61 Persistent migraine aura with cerebral infarction, intractable
Persistent migraine aura with cerebral infarction, with refractory migraine
G43.611 Persistent migraine aura with cerebral infarction, intractable, with status migrainosus Ex PDX 749
G43.619 Persistent migraine aura with cerebral infarction, intractable, without status migrainosus Ex PDX 749

G43.7 Chronic migraine without aura
Transformed migraine
Excludes1 migraine without aura (G43.0-)
G43.70 Chronic migraine without aura, not intractable
Chronic migraine without aura, without refractory migraine
G43.701 Chronic migraine without aura, not intractable, with status migrainosus
G43.709 Chronic migraine without aura, not intractable, without status migrainosus
Chronic migraine without aura NOS
G43.71 Chronic migraine without aura, intractable
Chronic migraine without aura, with refractory migraine
G43.711 Chronic migraine without aura, intractable, with status migrainosus
G43.719 Chronic migraine without aura, intractable, without status migrainosus

G43.8 Other migraine
G43.80 Other migraine, not intractable
Other migraine, without refractory migraine
G43.801 Other migraine, not intractable, with status migrainosus
G43.809 Other migraine, not intractable, without status migrainosus
G43.81 Other migraine, intractable
Other migraine, with refractory migraine
G43.811 Other migraine, intractable, with status migrainosus
G43.819 Other migraine, intractable, without status migrainosus
G43.82 Menstrual migraine, not intractable
Menstrual headache, not intractable
Menstrual migraine, without refractory migraine
Menstrually related migraine, not intractable
Pre-menstrual headache, not intractable
Pre-menstrual migraine, not intractable
Pure menstrual migraine, not intractable
Code also associated premenstrual tension syndrome (N94.3)
G43.821 Menstrual migraine, not intractable, with status migrainosus ♀
G43.829 Menstrual migraine, not intractable, without status migrainosus ♀
Menstrual migraine NOS
G43.83 Menstrual migraine, intractable
Menstrual headache, intractable
Menstrual migraine, with refractory migraine
Menstrually related migraine, intractable
Pre-menstrual headache, intractable
Pre-menstrual migraine, intractable
Pure menstrual migraine, intractable
Code also associated premenstrual tension syndrome (N94.3)
G43.831 Menstrual migraine, intractable, with status migrainosus ♀
G43.839 Menstrual migraine, intractable, without status migrainosus ♀

G43.9 Migraine, unspecified
G43.90 Migraine, unspecified, not intractable
Migraine, unspecified, without refractory migraine
G43.901 Migraine, unspecified, not intractable, with status migrainosus
Status migrainosus NOS
G43.909 Migraine, unspecified, not intractable, without status migrainosus
Migraine NOS
G43.91 Migraine, unspecified, intractable
Migraine, unspecified, with refractory migraine
G43.911 Migraine, unspecified, intractable, with status migrainosus
G43.919 Migraine, unspecified, intractable, without status migrainosus

G43.A Cyclical vomiting
Excludes1 cyclical vomiting syndrome unrelated to migraine (R11.15)
G43.A0 Cyclical vomiting, in migraine, not intractable
Cyclical vomiting, without refractory migraine
G43.A1 Cyclical vomiting, in migraine, intractable
Cyclical vomiting, with refractory migraine

G43.B Ophthalmoplegic migraine
G43.B0 Ophthalmoplegic migraine, not intractable
Ophthalmoplegic migraine, without refractory migraine
G43.B1 Ophthalmoplegic migraine, intractable
Ophthalmoplegic migraine, with refractory migraine

G43.C Periodic headache syndromes in child or adult
G43.C0 Periodic headache syndromes in child or adult, not intractable
Periodic headache syndromes in child or adult, without refractory migraine
G43.C1 Periodic headache syndromes in child or adult, intractable
Periodic headache syndromes in child or adult, with refractory migraine

G43.D Abdominal migraine
G43.D0 Abdominal migraine, not intractable
Abdominal migraine, without refractory migraine
G43.D1 Abdominal migraine, intractable
Abdominal migraine, with refractory migraine

G43.E Chronic migraine with aura
Excludes1 migraine with aura (G43.1-)
G43.E0 Chronic migraine with aura, not intractable
Chronic migraine with aura, without refractory migraine
G43.E01 Chronic migraine with aura, not intractable, with status migrainosus
G43.E09 Chronic migraine with aura, not intractable, without status migrainosus
Chronic migraine with aura NOS
G43.E1 Chronic migraine with aura, intractable
Chronic migraine with aura, with refractory migraine
G43.E11 Chronic migraine with aura, intractable, with status migrainosus
G43.E19 Chronic migraine with aura, intractable, without status migrainosus

CHAPTER 6 (G00-G99)

G44 Other headache syndromes

Excludes1 headache NOS (R51.9)

Excludes2 atypical facial pain (G50.1)
headache due to lumbar puncture (G97.1)
migraines (G43.-)
trigeminal neuralgia (G50.0)

G44.0 Cluster headaches and other trigeminal autonomic cephalgias (TAC)

G44.00 Cluster headache syndrome, unspecified
Ciliary neuralgia
Cluster headache NOS
Histamine cephalgia
Lower half migraine
Migrainous neuralgia

G44.001 Cluster headache syndrome, unspecified, intractable

G44.009 Cluster headache syndrome, unspecified, not intractable
Cluster headache syndrome NOS

G44.01 Episodic cluster headache

G44.011 Episodic cluster headache, intractable

G44.019 Episodic cluster headache, not intractable
Episodic cluster headache NOS

G44.02 Chronic cluster headache

G44.021 Chronic cluster headache, intractable

G44.029 Chronic cluster headache, not intractable
Chronic cluster headache NOS

G44.03 Episodic paroxysmal hemicrania
Paroxysmal hemicrania NOS

G44.031 Episodic paroxysmal hemicrania, intractable

G44.039 Episodic paroxysmal hemicrania, not intractable
Episodic paroxysmal hemicrania NOS

G44.04 Chronic paroxysmal hemicrania
Unilateral headache

G44.041 Chronic paroxysmal hemicrania, intractable

G44.049 Chronic paroxysmal hemicrania, not intractable
Chronic paroxysmal hemicrania NOS

G44.05 Short lasting unilateral neuralgiform headache with conjunctival injection and tearing (SUNCT)

G44.051 Short lasting unilateral neuralgiform headache with conjunctival injection and tearing (SUNCT), intractable

G44.059 Short lasting unilateral neuralgiform headache with conjunctival injection and tearing (SUNCT), not intractable
Short lasting unilateral neuralgiform headache with conjunctival injection and tearing (SUNCT) NOS

G44.09 Other trigeminal autonomic cephalgias (TAC)
Cluster headaches

G44.091 Other trigeminal autonomic cephalgias (TAC), intractable

G44.099 Other trigeminal autonomic cephalgias (TAC), not intractable

G44.1 Vascular headache, not elsewhere classified

Excludes2 cluster headache (G44.0)
complicated headache syndromes (G44.5-)
drug-induced headache (G44.4-)
migraine (G43.-)
other specified headache syndromes (G44.8-)
post-traumatic headache (G44.3-)
tension-type headache (G44.2-)

G44.2 Tension-type headache

G44.20 Tension-type headache, unspecified

G44.201 Tension-type headache, unspecified, intractable

G44.209 Tension-type headache, unspecified, not intractable
Tension headache NOS

G44.21 Episodic tension-type headache

G44.211 Episodic tension-type headache, intractable

G44.219 Episodic tension-type headache, not intractable
Episodic tension-type headache NOS

G44.22 Chronic tension-type headache

G44.221 Chronic tension-type headache, intractable

G44.229 Chronic tension-type headache, not intractable
Chronic tension-type headache NOS

G44.3 Post-traumatic headache

G44.30 Post-traumatic headache, unspecified

G44.301 Post-traumatic headache, unspecified, intractable

G44.309 Post-traumatic headache, unspecified, not intractable
Post-traumatic headache NOS

G44.31 Acute post-traumatic headache

G44.311 Acute post-traumatic headache, intractable

G44.319 Acute post-traumatic headache, not intractable
Acute post-traumatic headache NOS

G44.32 Chronic post-traumatic headache

G44.321 Chronic post-traumatic headache, intractable

G44.329 Chronic post-traumatic headache, not intractable
Chronic post-traumatic headache NOS

G44.4 Drug-induced headache, not elsewhere classified
Medication overuse headache
Use additional code for adverse effect, if applicable, to identify drug (T36-T50 with fifth or sixth character 5)

G44.40 Drug-induced headache, not elsewhere classified, not intractable

G44.41 Drug-induced headache, not elsewhere classified, intractable

G44.5 Complicated headache syndromes

G44.51 Hemicrania continua
Persistent unilateral headache

G44.52 New daily persistent headache (NDPH)

G44.53 Primary thunderclap headache

G44.59 Other complicated headache syndrome

G44.8 Other specified headache syndromes

Excludes2 headache with orthostatic or positional component, not elsewhere classified (R51.0)

G44.81 Hypnic headache
Benign primary headaches

G44.82 Headache associated with sexual activity
Orgasmic headache
Preorgasmic headache

G44.83 Primary cough headache

G44.84 Primary exertional headache

G44.85 Primary stabbing headache

G44.86 Cervicogenic headache
Code also associated cervical spinal condition, if known
Coding Clinic: 2021, Q4, P12

G44.89 Other headache syndrome

G45 Transient cerebral ischemic attacks and related syndromes

Excludes1 neonatal cerebral ischemia (P91.Ø)
transient retinal artery occlusion (H34.Ø-)

Coding Clinic: 2023, Q1, P37; 2018, Q2, P9

G45.Ø Vertebro-basilar artery syndrome PDX 750

G45.1 Carotid artery syndrome (hemispheric) PDX 750

G45.2 Multiple and bilateral precerebral artery syndromes PDX 750

G45.3 Amaurosis fugax PDX 751

Transient visual loss in one eye

G45.4 Transient global amnesia

Episode of short-term memory loss, nonrecurrent, lasting few hours

Excludes1 amnesia NOS (R41.3)

G45.8 Other transient cerebral ischemic attacks and related syndromes PDX 750

G45.9 Transient cerebral ischemic attack, unspecified PDX 750

Spasm of cerebral artery
TIA
Transient cerebral ischemia NOS

G46 Vascular syndromes of brain in cerebrovascular diseases

Code first underlying cerebrovascular disease (I6Ø-I69)

G46.Ø Middle cerebral artery syndrome PDX 750

G46.1 Anterior cerebral artery syndrome PDX 750

G46.2 Posterior cerebral artery syndrome PDX 750

G46.3 Brain stem stroke syndrome

Benedikt syndrome
Claude syndrome
Foville syndrome
Millard-Gubler syndrome
Wallenberg syndrome
Weber syndrome

G46.4 Cerebellar stroke syndrome

G46.5 Pure motor lacunar syndrome

Occlusion of single deep penetrating artery

G46.6 Pure sensory lacunar syndrome

G46.7 Other lacunar syndromes

G46.8 Other vascular syndromes of brain in cerebrovascular diseases

G47 Sleep disorders

Excludes2 nightmares (F51.5)
nonorganic sleep disorders (F51.-)
sleep terrors (F51.4)
sleepwalking (F51.3)

G47.Ø Insomnia

Excludes2 alcohol related insomnia (F1Ø.182, F1Ø.282, F1Ø.982)
drug-related insomnia (F11.182, F11.282, F11.982, F13.182, F13.282, F13.982, F14.182, F14.282, F14.982, F15.182, F15.282, F15.982, F19.182, F19.282, F19.982)
idiopathic insomnia (F51.Ø1)
insomnia due to a mental disorder (F51.Ø5)
insomnia not due to a substance or known physiological condition (F51.Ø-)
nonorganic insomnia (F51.Ø-)
primary insomnia (F51.Ø1)
sleep apnea (G47.3-)

G47.ØØ Insomnia, unspecified

Insomnia NOS

G47.Ø1 Insomnia due to medical condition

Code also associated medical condition

G47.Ø9 Other insomnia

G47.1 Hypersomnia

Excludes2 alcohol-related hypersomnia (F1Ø.182, F1Ø.282, F1Ø.982)
drug-related hypersomnia (F11.182, F11.282, F11.982, F13.182, F13.282, F13.982, F14.182, F14.282, F14.982, F15.182, F15.282, F15.982, F19.182, F19.282, F19.982)
hypersomnia due to a mental disorder (F51.13)
hypersomnia not due to a substance or known physiological condition (F51.1-)
primary hypersomnia (F51.11)
sleep apnea (G47.3-)

G47.1Ø Hypersomnia, unspecified

Hypersomnia NOS

G47.11 Idiopathic hypersomnia with long sleep time

Idiopathic hypersomnia NOS

G47.12 Idiopathic hypersomnia without long sleep time

G47.13 Recurrent hypersomnia

Kleine-Levin syndrome
Menstrual related hypersomnia

G47.14 Hypersomnia due to medical condition

Code also associated medical condition

G47.19 Other hypersomnia

G47.2 Circadian rhythm sleep disorders

Disorders of the sleep wake schedule
Inversion of nyctohemeral rhythm
Inversion of sleep rhythm

G47.2Ø Circadian rhythm sleep disorder, unspecified type

Sleep wake schedule disorder NOS

G47.21 Circadian rhythm sleep disorder, delayed sleep phase type

Delayed sleep phase syndrome

G47.22 Circadian rhythm sleep disorder, advanced sleep phase type

G47.23 Circadian rhythm sleep disorder, irregular sleep wake type

Irregular sleep-wake pattern

G47.24 Circadian rhythm sleep disorder, free running type

Circadian rhythm sleep disorder, non-24-hour sleep-wake type

G47.25 Circadian rhythm sleep disorder, jet lag type

G47.26 Circadian rhythm sleep disorder, shift work type

G47.27 Circadian rhythm sleep disorder in conditions classified elsewhere

Code first underlying condition

G47.29 Other circadian rhythm sleep disorder

G47.3 Sleep apnea

Characterized by episodes in which breathing stops during sleep

Code also any associated underlying condition

Excludes1 apnea NOS (RØ6.81)
Cheyne-Stokes breathing (RØ6.3)
pickwickian syndrome (E66.2)
sleep apnea of newborn (P28.3-)

G47.3Ø Sleep apnea, unspecified

Sleep apnea NOS

G47.31 Primary central sleep apnea

Idiopathic central sleep apnea

G47.32 High altitude periodic breathing

G47.33 Obstructive sleep apnea (adult) (pediatric)

Obstructive sleep apnea hypopnea

Excludes1 obstructive sleep apnea of newborn (P28.3-)

G47.34 Idiopathic sleep related nonobstructive alveolar hypoventilation

Sleep related hypoxia

G47.35 **Congenital central alveolar hypoventilation syndrome**

G47.36 ***Sleep related hypoventilation in conditions classified elsewhere***
Sleep related hypoxemia in conditions classified elsewhere
Code first underlying condition

G47.37 ***Central sleep apnea in conditions classified elsewhere***
Code first underlying condition

G47.39 **Other sleep apnea**

G47.4 **Narcolepsy and cataplexy**
*Cataplexy is a disorder evidenced by seizures including minor slacking of the facial muscles to complete collapse and often affects people who have **narcolepsy**, a disorder in which there is great difficulty remaining awake during the daytime.*

G47.41 **Narcolepsy**

G47.411 **Narcolepsy with cataplexy**

G47.419 **Narcolepsy without cataplexy**
Narcolepsy NOS

G47.42 **Narcolepsy in conditions classified elsewhere**
Code first underlying condition

G47.421 ***Narcolepsy in conditions classified elsewhere with cataplexy***

G47.429 ***Narcolepsy in conditions classified elsewhere without cataplexy***

G47.5 **Parasomnia**
Excludes1 alcohol induced parasomnia (F10.182, F10.282, F10.982)
drug induced parasomnia (F11.182, F11.282, F11.982, F13.182, F13.282, F13.982, F14.182, F14.282, F14.982, F15.182, F15.282, F15.982, F19.182, F19.282, F19.982)
parasomnia not due to a substance or known physiological condition (F51.8)

G47.50 **Parasomnia, unspecified**
Parasomnia NOS

G47.51 **Confusional arousals**

G47.52 **REM sleep behavior disorder**

G47.53 **Recurrent isolated sleep paralysis**

G47.54 ***Parasomnia in conditions classified elsewhere***
Code first underlying condition

G47.59 **Other parasomnia**

G47.6 **Sleep related movement disorders**
Excludes2 restless legs syndrome (G25.81)

G47.61 **Periodic limb movement disorder**

G47.62 **Sleep related leg cramps**

G47.63 **Sleep related bruxism**
Excludes1 psychogenic bruxism (F45.8)
Coding Clinic: 2016, Q4, P118

G47.69 **Other sleep related movement disorders**

G47.8 **Other sleep disorders**
Other specified sleep-wake disorder

G47.9 **Sleep disorder, unspecified**
Sleep disorder NOS
Unspecified sleep-wake disorder

★**(See Plate 6 of the Anatomy Illustrations.)**

NERVE, NERVE ROOT AND PLEXUS DISORDERS (G50-G59)

Excludes1 current traumatic nerve, nerve root and plexus disorders - see Injury, nerve by body region
neuralgia NOS (M79.2)
neuritis NOS (M79.2)
peripheral neuritis in pregnancy (O26.82-)
radiculitis NOS (M54.1-)

G50 **Disorders of trigeminal nerve**
Includes disorders of 5th cranial nerve

G50.0 **Trigeminal neuralgia**
Syndrome of paroxysmal facial pain
Tic douloureux

G50.1 **Atypical facial pain**

G50.8 **Other disorders of trigeminal nerve**

G50.9 **Disorder of trigeminal nerve, unspecified**

G51 **Facial nerve disorders**
Includes disorders of 7th cranial nerve

G51.0 **Bell's palsy**
Facial palsy

G51.1 **Geniculate ganglionitis**
Rare disorder with symptoms of severe pain deep in ear, spreading to ear canal, outer ear, mastoid or eye regions
Excludes1 postherpetic geniculate ganglionitis (B02.21)

G51.2 **Melkersson's syndrome**
Melkersson-Rosenthal syndrome

G51.3 **Clonic hemifacial spasm**

G51.31 **Clonic hemifacial spasm, right**

G51.32 **Clonic hemifacial spasm, left**
Coding Clinic: 2018, Q4, P10

G51.33 **Clonic hemifacial spasm, bilateral**

G51.39 **Clonic hemifacial spasm, unspecified**

G51.4 **Facial myokymia**
Involuntary facial muscle movement

G51.8 **Other disorders of facial nerve**

G51.9 **Disorder of facial nerve, unspecified**

G52 **Disorders of other cranial nerves**
Excludes2 disorders of acoustic [8th] nerve (H93.3)
disorders of optic [2nd] nerve (H46, H47.0)
paralytic strabismus due to nerve palsy (H49.0-H49.2)

G52.0 **Disorders of olfactory nerve**
Disorders of 1st cranial nerve

G52.1 **Disorders of glossopharyngeal nerve**
Disorder of 9th cranial nerve
Glossopharyngeal neuralgia

G52.2 **Disorders of vagus nerve**
Disorders of pneumogastric [10th] nerve

G52.3 **Disorders of hypoglossal nerve**
Disorders of 12th cranial nerve

G52.7 **Disorders of multiple cranial nerves**
Polyneuritis cranialis

G52.8 **Disorders of other specified cranial nerves**

G52.9 **Cranial nerve disorder, unspecified**

G53 ***Cranial nerve disorders in diseases classified elsewhere***
Code first underlying disease, such as:
neoplasm (C00-D49)
Excludes1 multiple cranial nerve palsy in sarcoidosis (D86.82)
multiple cranial nerve palsy in syphilis (A52.15)
postherpetic geniculate ganglionitis (B02.21)
postherpetic trigeminal neuralgia (B02.22)

Item 6–5 Trigeminal neuralgia, tic douloureux, is a pain syndrome diagnosed from the patient's history alone. The condition is characterized by pain and a brief facial spasm or tic. Pain is unilateral and follows the sensory distribution of cranial nerve V, typically radiating to the maxillary (V2) or mandibular (V3) area.

Item 6–6 The most common facial nerve disorder is **Bell's Palsy,** which occurs suddenly and results in facial drooping unilaterally. This disorder is the result of a reaction to a virus that causes the facial nerve in the ear to swell, resulting in pressure in the bony canal.

● **G54 Nerve root and plexus disorders**

Raiculopathy (nerve root disorder) caused by pressure on nerve root, most common cause is herniation of intervertebral disk. Plexus disorders (plexopathies) are due to compression or injury.

Excludes1 current traumatic nerve root and plexus disorders - see nerve injury by body region
intervertebral disc disorders (M5Ø-M51)
neuralgia or neuritis NOS (M79.2)
neuritis or radiculitis brachial NOS (M54.13)
neuritis or radiculitis lumbar NOS (M54.16)
neuritis or radiculitis lumbosacral NOS (M54.17)
neuritis or radiculitis thoracic NOS (M54.14)
radiculitis NOS (M54.1Ø)
radiculopathy NOS (M54.1Ø)
spondylosis (M47.-)

G54.Ø Brachial plexus disorders
Thoracic outlet syndrome
Coding Clinic: 2023, Q2, P8

G54.1 Lumbosacral plexus disorders

G54.2 Cervical root disorders, not elsewhere classified

G54.3 Thoracic root disorders, not elsewhere classified

G54.4 Lumbosacral root disorders, not elsewhere classified

G54.5 Neuralgic amyotrophy
Parsonage-Aldren-Turner syndrome
Shoulder-girdle neuritis
Excludes1 neuralgic amyotrophy in diabetes mellitus (EØ8-E13 with .44)

G54.6 Phantom limb syndrome with pain
Sensations (cramping, itching) in a limb that no longer exists

G54.7 Phantom limb syndrome without pain
Phantom limb syndrome NOS

G54.8 Other nerve root and plexus disorders

G54.9 Nerve root and plexus disorder, unspecified

G55 Nerve root and plexus compressions in diseases classified elsewhere

Code first underlying disease, such as:
neoplasm (CØØ-D49)

Excludes1 nerve root compression (due to) (in) ankylosing spondylitis (M45.-)
nerve root compression (due to) (in)dorsopathies (M53.-, M54.-)
nerve root compression (due to) (in)intervertebral disc disorders (M5Ø.1.-, M51.1.-)
nerve root compression (due to) (in) spondylopathies (M46.-, M48.-)
nerve root compression (due to) (in) spondylosis (M47.Ø-, M47.2.-)

★**(See Plates 472 and 473 on pages 56 and 57.)**

● **G56 Mononeuropathies of upper limb**

Excludes1 current traumatic nerve disorder - see nerve injury by body region

● **G56.Ø Carpal tunnel syndrome**

G56.ØØ Carpal tunnel syndrome, unspecified upper limb

G56.Ø1 Carpal tunnel syndrome, right upper limb

G56.Ø2 Carpal tunnel syndrome, left upper limb

G56.Ø3 Carpal tunnel syndrome, bilateral upper limbs
Coding Clinic: 2016, Q4, P17

● **G56.1 Other lesions of median nerve**

G56.1Ø Other lesions of median nerve, unspecified side

G56.11 Other lesions of median nerve, right upper limb

G56.12 Other lesions of median nerve, left upper limb

G56.13 Other lesions of median nerve, bilateral upper limbs
Coding Clinic: 2016, Q4, P17

● **G56.2 Lesion of ulnar nerve**
Tardy ulnar nerve palsy

G56.2Ø Lesion of ulnar nerve, unspecified upper limb

G56.21 Lesion of ulnar nerve, right upper limb

G56.22 Lesion of ulnar nerve, left upper limb

G56.23 Lesion of ulnar nerve, bilateral upper limbs
Coding Clinic: 2016, Q4, P17

● **G56.3 Lesion of radial nerve**

G56.3Ø Lesion of radial nerve, unspecified upper limb

G56.31 Lesion of radial nerve, right upper limb

G56.32 Lesion of radial nerve, left upper limb

G56.33 Lesion of radial nerve, bilateral upper limbs
Coding Clinic: 2016, Q4, P17

● **G56.4 Causalgia of upper limb**
Intense burning pain and sensitivity to slight touch
Complex regional pain syndrome II of upper limb

Excludes1 complex regional pain syndrome I of lower limb (G9Ø.52-)
complex regional pain syndrome I of upper limb (G9Ø.51-)
complex regional pain syndrome II of lower limb (G57.7-)
reflex sympathetic dystrophy of lower limb (G9Ø.52-)
reflex sympathetic dystrophy (G9Ø.51-)

G56.4Ø Causalgia of unspecified upper limb

G56.41 Causalgia of right upper limb

G56.42 Causalgia of left upper limb

G56.43 Causalgia of bilateral upper limbs
Coding Clinic: 2016, Q4, P17

● **G56.8 Other specified mononeuropathies of upper limb**
Disease of a single nerve
Interdigital neuroma of upper limb

G56.8Ø Other specified mononeuropathies of unspecified upper limb

G56.81 Other specified mononeuropathies of right upper limb

G56.82 Other specified mononeuropathies of left upper limb

G56.83 Other specified mononeuropathies of bilateral upper limbs
Coding Clinic: 2016, Q4, P17

● **G56.9 Unspecified mononeuropathy of upper limb**
Disease of a single nerve

G56.9Ø Unspecified mononeuropathy of unspecified upper limb

G56.91 Unspecified mononeuropathy of right upper limb

G56.92 Unspecified mononeuropathy of left upper limb

G56.93 Unspecified mononeuropathy of bilateral upper limbs
Coding Clinic: 2016, Q4, P17

● **G57 Mononeuropathies of lower limb**

Excludes1 current traumatic nerve disorder - see nerve injury by body region

★(See Plates 544 and 545 on pages 58 and 59.)

● G57.0 Lesion of sciatic nerve
Excludes1 sciatica NOS (M54.3-)
Excludes2 sciatica attributed to intervertebral disc disorder (M51.1.-)
G57.00 Lesion of sciatic nerve, unspecified lower limb
G57.01 Lesion of sciatic nerve, right lower limb
G57.02 Lesion of sciatic nerve, left lower limb
G57.03 Lesion of sciatic nerve, bilateral lower limbs
Coding Clinic: 2016, Q4, P1

● G57.1 Meralgia paresthetica
Numbness or pain in outer thigh caused by injury to nerve
Lateral cutaneous nerve of thigh syndrome
G57.10 Meralgia paresthetica, unspecified lower limb
G57.11 Meralgia paresthetica, right lower limb
G57.12 Meralgia paresthetica, left lower limb
G57.13 Meralgia paresthetica, bilateral lower limbs
Coding Clinic: 2016, Q4, P1

● G57.2 Lesion of femoral nerve
G57.20 Lesion of femoral nerve, unspecified lower limb
G57.21 Lesion of femoral nerve, right lower limb
G57.22 Lesion of femoral nerve, left lower limb
G57.23 Lesion of femoral nerve, bilateral lower limbs
Coding Clinic: 2016, Q4, P1

● G57.3 Lesion of lateral popliteal nerve
Peroneal nerve palsy
G57.30 Lesion of lateral popliteal nerve, unspecified lower limb
G57.31 Lesion of lateral popliteal nerve, right lower limb
G57.32 Lesion of lateral popliteal nerve, left lower limb
G57.33 Lesion of lateral popliteal nerve, bilateral lower limbs
Coding Clinic: 2016, Q4, P1

● G57.4 Lesion of medial popliteal nerve
G57.40 Lesion of medial popliteal nerve, unspecified lower limb
G57.41 Lesion of medial popliteal nerve, right lower limb
G57.42 Lesion of medial popliteal nerve, left lower limb
G57.43 Lesion of medial popliteal nerve, bilateral lower limbs
Coding Clinic: 2016, Q4, P1

● G57.5 Tarsal tunnel syndrome
G57.50 Tarsal tunnel syndrome, unspecified lower limb
G57.51 Tarsal tunnel syndrome, right lower limb
G57.52 Tarsal tunnel syndrome, left lower limb
G57.53 Tarsal tunnel syndrome, bilateral lower limbs
Coding Clinic: 2016, Q4, P1

● G57.6 Lesion of plantar nerve
Morton's metatarsalgia
G57.60 Lesion of plantar nerve, unspecified lower limb
G57.61 Lesion of plantar nerve, right lower limb
G57.62 Lesion of plantar nerve, left lower limb
G57.63 Lesion of plantar nerve, bilateral lower limbs
Coding Clinic: 2016, Q4, P1

● G57.7 Causalgia of lower limb
Complex regional pain syndrome II of lower limb
Excludes1 complex regional pain syndrome I of lower limb (G90.52-)
complex regional pain syndrome I of upper limb (G90.51-)
complex regional pain syndrome II of upper limb (G56.4-)
reflex sympathetic dystrophy of lower limb (G90.52-)
reflex sympathetic dystrophy of upper limb (G90.51-)
G57.70 Causalgia of unspecified lower limb
G57.71 Causalgia of right lower limb
G57.72 Causalgia of left lower limb
G57.73 Causalgia of bilateral lower limbs
Coding Clinic: 2016, Q4, P1

● G57.8 Other specified mononeuropathies of lower limb
Interdigital neuroma of lower limb
G57.80 Other specified mononeuropathies of unspecified lower limb
G57.81 Other specified mononeuropathies of right lower limb
G57.82 Other specified mononeuropathies of left lower limb
G57.83 Other specified mononeuropathies of bilateral lower limbs
Coding Clinic: 2016, Q4, P17

● G57.9 Unspecified mononeuropathy of lower limb
G57.90 Unspecified mononeuropathy of unspecified lower limb
G57.91 Unspecified mononeuropathy of right lower limb
G57.92 Unspecified mononeuropathy of left lower limb
G57.93 Unspecified mononeuropathy of bilateral lower limbs
Coding Clinic: 2016, Q4, P17

● G58 Other mononeuropathies
G58.0 Intercostal neuropathy
G58.7 Mononeuritis multiplex
G58.8 Other specified mononeuropathies
G58.9 Mononeuropathy, unspecified

G59 Mononeuropathy in diseases classified elsewhere
Code first underlying disease
Excludes1 diabetic mononeuropathy (E08-E13 with .41)
syphilitic nerve paralysis (A52.19)
syphilitic neuritis (A52.15)
tuberculous mononeuropathy (A17.83)

POLYNEUROPATHIES AND OTHER DISORDERS OF THE PERIPHERAL NERVOUS SYSTEM (G60-G65)

Excludes1 neuralgia NOS (M79.2)
neuritis NOS (M79.2)
peripheral neuritis in pregnancy (O26.82-)
radiculitis NOS (M54.10)

● G60 Hereditary and idiopathic neuropathy
G60.0 Hereditary motor and sensory neuropathy
Charcot-Marie-Tooth disease
Déjerine-Sottas disease
Hereditary motor and sensory neuropathy, types I-IV
Hypertrophic neuropathy of infancy
Peroneal muscular atrophy (axonal type) (hypertrophic type)
Roussy-Lévy syndrome
G60.1 Refsum's disease (Ex) PDX 752
Genetic disorder affecting fatty acid metabolism
Infantile Refsum disease
G60.2 Neuropathy in association with hereditary ataxia
G60.3 Idiopathic progressive neuropathy
G60.8 Other hereditary and idiopathic neuropathies
Dominantly inherited sensory neuropathy
Morvan's disease
Nelaton's syndrome
Recessively inherited sensory neuropathy
G60.9 Hereditary and idiopathic neuropathy, unspecified

● G61 Inflammatory polyneuropathy
G61.0 Guillain-Barré syndrome (Ex) PDX 93
Autoimmune disease affecting peripheral nervous system
Acute (post-)infective polyneuritis
Miller Fisher Syndrome

CHAPTER 6 (G00-G99)

N Newborn Age: 0 P Pediatric Age: 0-17 M Maternity DX: 9-64 A Adult Age: 15-124
Complication\Comorbidity Major C\C (Ex) CC/MCC Exclusions Hospital-Acquired Condition Hierarchical Condition Category

G61.1 **Serum neuropathy**

Use additional code for adverse effect, if applicable, to identify serum (T5Ø.-)

● G61.8 **Other inflammatory polyneuropathies**

G61.81 **Chronic inflammatory demyelinating polyneuritis** PDX 753

G61.82 **Multifocal motor neuropathy**

MMN

G61.89 **Other inflammatory polyneuropathies**

G61.9 **Inflammatory polyneuropathy, unspecified**

● G62 **Other and unspecified polyneuropathies**

G62.Ø **Drug-induced polyneuropathy**

Use additional code for adverse effect, if applicable, to identify drug (T36-T5Ø with fifth or sixth character 5)

G62.1 **Alcoholic polyneuropathy**

Malfunction of many peripheral nerves throughout the body

Coding Clinic: 2Ø19, Q3, P8

G62.2 **Polyneuropathy due to other toxic agents**

Code first (T51-T65) to identify toxic agent

● G62.8 **Other specified polyneuropathies**

G62.81 **Critical illness polyneuropathy** PDX 754

Acute motor neuropathy

G62.82 **Radiation-induced polyneuropathy**

Use additional external cause code (W88-W9Ø, X39.Ø-) to identify cause

Coding Clinic: 2Ø16, Q4, P18

G62.89 **Other specified polyneuropathies**

Coding Clinic: 2Ø16, Q2, P11

G62.9 **Polyneuropathy, unspecified**

Neuropathy NOS

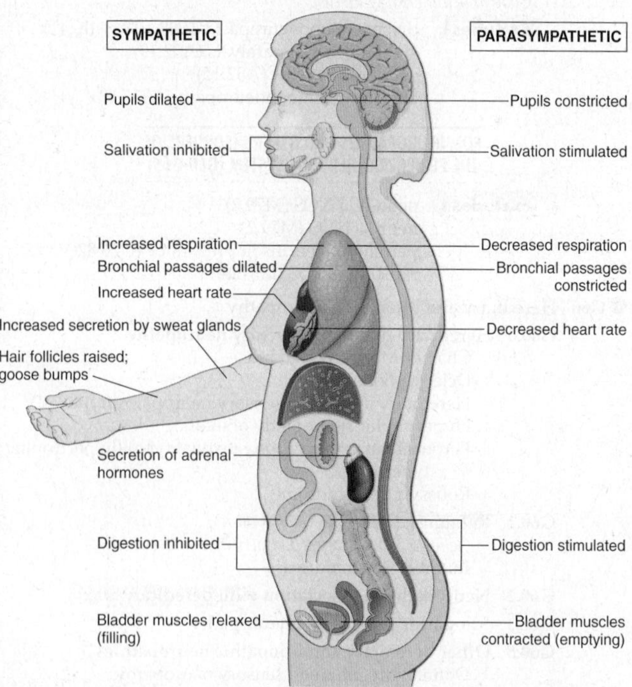

Figure 6-2 Actions of parasympathetic and sympathetic nerves. (From Chabner: The Language of Medicine, ed 9, St. Louis, Saunders, 2011)

Item 6-7 The **peripheral nervous system** consists of 31 pairs of spinal nerves, 12 pairs of cranial nerves, and the autonomic nerves, which are divided into the parasympathetic and sympathetic nerves. The cranial nerves are: olfactory (I), optic (II), oculomotor (III), trochlear (IV), trigeminal (V), abducens (VI), facial (VII), vestibulocochlear (VIII), glossopharyngeal (IX), vagus (X), accessory (XI), and hypoglossal (XII).

G63 ***Polyneuropathy in diseases classified elsewhere***

Code first underlying disease, such as:
amyloidosis (E85.-)
endocrine disease, except diabetes (EØØ-EØ7, E15-E16, E2Ø-E34)
metabolic diseases (E7Ø-E88)
neoplasm (CØØ-D49)
nutritional deficiency (E4Ø-E64)

Excludes1 polyneuropathy (in):
diabetes mellitus (EØ8-E13 with .42)
diphtheria (A36.83)
infectious mononucleosis complicated by polyneuropathy (B27.Ø-B27.9 with fifth character 1)
Lyme disease (A69.22)
mumps (B26.84)
postherpetic (BØ2.23)
rheumatoid arthritis (MØ5.5-)
scleroderma (M34.83)
systemic lupus erythematosus (M32.19)

Coding Clinic: 2Ø23, Q3, P19-2Ø; 2Ø21, Q1, P7; 2Ø12, Q4, P1ØØ

G64 **Other disorders of peripheral nervous system**

Disorder of peripheral nervous system NOS

● G65 **Sequelae of inflammatory and toxic polyneuropathies**

Code first condition resulting from (sequela) of inflammatory and toxic polyneuropathies

G65.Ø **Sequelae of Guillain-Barré syndrome**

G65.1 **Sequelae of other inflammatory polyneuropathy**

G65.2 **Sequelae of toxic polyneuropathy**

DISEASES OF MYONEURAL JUNCTION AND MUSCLE (G7Ø-G73)

● G7Ø **Myasthenia gravis and other myoneural disorders**

Excludes1 botulism (AØ5.1, A48.51-A48.52)
transient neonatal myasthenia gravis (P94.Ø)

● G7Ø.Ø **Myasthenia gravis**

Acquired and results in fatigable muscle weakness exacerbated by activity and improved with rest

G7Ø.ØØ **Myasthenia gravis without (acute) exacerbation**

Myasthenia gravis NOS

Coding Clinic: 2Ø22, Q3, P16

G7Ø.Ø1 **Myasthenia gravis with (acute) exacerbation** PDX 755

Myasthenia gravis in crisis

G7Ø.1 **Toxic myoneural disorders**

Dysfunction at junction of muscle and motor nerve (myoneural junction)

Code first (T51-T65) to identify toxic agent

G7Ø.2 **Congenital and developmental myasthenia**

● G7Ø.8 **Other specified myoneural disorders**

G7Ø.8Ø **Lambert-Eaton syndrome, unspecified** PDX 755

Lambert-Eaton syndrome NOS

G7Ø.81 ***Lambert-Eaton syndrome in disease classified elsewhere*** PDX 755

Code first underlying disease

Excludes1 Lambert-Eaton syndrome in neoplastic disease (G73.1)

G7Ø.89 **Other specified myoneural disorders**

G7Ø.9 **Myoneural disorder, unspecified**

● G71 **Primary disorders of muscles**

Excludes2 arthrogryposis multiplex congenita (Q74.3)
metabolic disorders (E7Ø-E88)
myositis (M6Ø.-)

G71.0 Muscular dystrophy

G71.00 Muscular dystrophy, unspecified

G71.01 Duchenne or Becker muscular dystrophy

Autosomal recessive, childhood type, muscular dystrophy resembling Duchenne or Becker muscular dystrophy

Benign [Becker] muscular dystrophy

Severe [Duchenne] muscular dystrophy

G71.02 Facioscapulohumeral muscular dystrophy

Scapulohumeral muscular dystrophy

Coding Clinic: 2018, Q4, P12

G71.03 Limb girdle muscular dystrophies

G71.031 Autosomal dominant limb girdle muscular dystrophy

LGMD D4 calpain-3-related

LGMD D5 collagen 6-related

Limb girdle muscular dystrophy type 1

G71.032 Autosomal recessive limb girdle muscular dystrophy due to calpain-3 dysfunction

Limb girdle muscular dystrophy type 2A

LGMD R1 calpain-3-related

Primary calpainopathy

G71.033 Limb girdle muscular dystrophy due to dysferlin dysfunction

Dysferlinopathy

LGMD R2 dysferlin-related

Limb girdle muscular dystrophy type 2B

Miyoshi Myopathy type 1

G71.034 Limb girdle muscular dystrophy due to sarcoglycan dysfunction

G71.0340 Limb girdle muscular dystrophy due to sarcoglycan dysfunction, unspecified

Sarcoglycanopathy, NOS

G71.0341 Limb girdle muscular dystrophy due to alpha sarcoglycan dysfunction

Alpha sarcoglycanopathy

Limb-girdle muscular dystrophy due to alpha-sarcoglycan deficiency

Limb girdle muscular dystrophy type 2D

G71.0342 Limb girdle muscular dystrophy due to beta sarcoglycan dysfunction

Beta sarcoglycanopathy

Limb girdle muscular dystrophy due to beta-sarcoglycan deficiency

Limb girdle muscular dystrophy type 2E

G71.0349 Limb girdle muscular dystrophy due to other sarcoglycan dysfunction

Delta sarcoglycanopathy

Delta-sarcoglycan-related LGMD R6

Gamma sarcoglycanopathy

Gamma-sarcoglycan-related LGMD R5

Limb girdle muscular dystrophy type 2C

Limb girdle muscular dystrophy type 2F

Item 6–8 Muscular dystrophies (MD) are a group of rare inherited muscle diseases. Voluntary muscles become progressively weaker. In the late stages of MD, fat and connective tissue replace muscle fibers. In some types of muscular dystrophy, heart muscles, other involuntary muscles, and other organs are affected. **Myopathies** is a general term for neuromuscular diseases in which the muscle fibers dysfunction for any one of many reasons, resulting in muscular weakness.

G71.035 Limb girdle muscular dystrophy due to anoctamin-5 dysfunction

Anoctamin-5-related LGMD R12

Anoctaminopathy

Autosomal recessive limb girdle muscular dystrophy type 2L

Miyoshi myopathy type 3

G71.038 Other limb girdle muscular dystrophy

LGMD R9 FKRP-related

LGMD R22 collagen 6-related

Limb girdle muscular dystrophy due to fukutin related protein dysfunction

Limb girdle muscular dystrophy type 2I

Other autosomal recessive limb girdle muscular dystrophy

G71.039 Limb girdle muscular dystrophy, unspecified

G71.09 Other specified muscular dystrophies

Benign scapuloperoneal muscular dystrophy with early contractures [Emery-Dreifuss]

Congenital muscular dystrophy NOS

Congenital muscular dystrophy with specific morphological abnormalities of the muscle fiber

Distal muscular dystrophy

Ocular muscular dystrophy

Oculopharyngeal muscular dystrophy

Scapuloperoneal muscular dystrophy

G71.1 Myotonic disorders

Inherited disorder that affects muscles tone

G71.11 Myotonic muscular dystrophy

Dystrophia myotonica [Steinert]

Myotonia atrophica

Myotonic dystrophy

Proximal myotonic myopathy (PROMM)

Steinert disease

G71.12 Myotonia congenita

Acetazolamide responsive myotonia congenita

Dominant myotonia congenita [Thomsen disease]

Myotonia levior

Recessive myotonia congenita [Becker disease]

G71.13 Myotonic chondrodystrophy

Chondrodystrophic myotonia

Congenital myotonic chondrodystrophy

Schwartz-Jampel disease

G71.14 Drug induced myotonia

Use additional code for adverse effect, if applicable, to identify drug (T36-T50 with fifth or sixth character 5)

G71.19 Other specified myotonic disorders

Myotonia fluctuans

Myotonia permanens

Neuromyotonia [Isaacs]

Paramyotonia congenita (of von Eulenburg)

Pseudomyotonia

Symptomatic myotonia

G71.2 Congenital myopathies

Excludes2 arthrogryposis multiplex congenita (Q74.3)

G71.20 Congenital myopathy, unspecified (Ex) PDX 756

G71.21 Nemaline myopathy (Ex) PDX 756

CHAPTER 6 (G00-G99)

G71.22 Centronuclear myopathy
- **G71.220 X-linked myotubular myopathy** PDX 756
  - Myotubular (centronuclear) myopathy
- **G71.228 Other centronuclear myopathy** PDX 756
  - Autosomal centronuclear myopathy
  - Autosomal dominant centronuclear myopathy
  - Autosomal recessive centronuclear myopathy
  - Centronuclear myopathy, NOS

G71.29 Other congenital myopathy PDX 756
- Central core disease
- Minicore disease
- Multicore disease
- Multiminicore disease

G71.3 Mitochondrial myopathy, not elsewhere classified
Myopathies associated with increased number of enlarged, often abnormal, mitochondria in muscle fibers
Excludes1 Kearns-Sayre syndrome (H49.81)
Leber's disease (H47.21)
Leigh's encephalopathy (G31.82)
mitochondrial metabolism disorders (E88.4.-)
Reye's syndrome (G93.7)

G71.8 Other primary disorders of muscles

G71.9 Primary disorder of muscle, unspecified
- Hereditary myopathy NOS

G72 Other and unspecified myopathies
Excludes1 arthrogryposis multiplex congenita (Q74.3)
dermatopolymyositis (M33.-)
ischemic infarction of muscle (M62.2-)
myositis (M60.-)
polymyositis (M33.2.-)

G72.0 Drug-induced myopathy PDX 757
Use additional code for adverse effect, if applicable, to identify drug (T36-T50 with fifth or sixth character 5)

G72.1 Alcoholic myopathy PDX 757
Use additional code to identify alcoholism (F10.-)

G72.2 Myopathy due to other toxic agents PDX 757
Code first (T51-T65) to identify toxic agent

G72.3 Periodic paralysis
- Familial periodic paralysis
- Hyperkalemic periodic paralysis (familial)
- Hypokalemic periodic paralysis (familial)
- Myotonic periodic paralysis (familial)
- Normokalemic paralysis (familial)
- Potassium sensitive periodic paralysis

Excludes1 paramyotonia congenita (of von Eulenburg) (G71.19)

G72.4 Inflammatory and immune myopathies, not elsewhere classified
- **G72.41 Inclusion body myositis [IBM]**
- **G72.49 Other inflammatory and immune myopathies, not elsewhere classified**
  - Inflammatory myopathy NOS

G72.8 Other specified myopathies
- **G72.81 Critical illness myopathy** PDX 758
  - Acute necrotizing myopathy
  - Acute quadriplegic myopathy
  - Intensive care (ICU) myopathy
  - Myopathy of critical illness
- **G72.89 Other specified myopathies**

G72.9 Myopathy, unspecified

G73 Disorders of myoneural junction and muscle in diseases classified elsewhere

G73.1 Lambert-Eaton syndrome in neoplastic disease PDX 755
Rare autoimmune disorder affecting calcium channels of nerve-muscle (neuromuscular) junction
Code first underlying neoplasm (C00-D49)
Excludes1 Lambert-Eaton syndrome not associated with neoplasm (G70.80-G70.81)

G73.3 Myasthenic syndromes in other diseases classified elsewhere PDX 755
Code first underlying disease, such as:
neoplasm (C00-D49)
thyrotoxicosis (E05.-)

G73.7 Myopathy in diseases classified elsewhere
Code first underlying disease, such as:
glycogen storage disease (E74.0-)
hyperparathyroidism (E21.0, E21.3)
hypoparathyroidism (E20.-)
lipid storage disorders (E75.-)
Excludes1 myopathy in:
rheumatoid arthritis (M05.32)
sarcoidosis (D86.87)
scleroderma (M34.82)
Sjögren syndrome (M35.03)
systemic lupus erythematosus (M32.19)

CEREBRAL PALSY AND OTHER PARALYTIC SYNDROMES (G80-G83)

G80 Cerebral palsy
Excludes1 hereditary spastic paraplegia (G11.4)

G80.0 Spastic quadriplegic cerebral palsy PDX 759
- Congenital spastic paralysis (cerebral)

G80.1 Spastic diplegic cerebral palsy PDX 760
- Spastic cerebral palsy NOS

G80.2 Spastic hemiplegic cerebral palsy PDX 761

G80.3 Athetoid cerebral palsy PDX 762
Result of damage to cerebellum or basal ganglia responsible for processing neuromuscular signals
- Double athetosis (syndrome)
- Dyskinetic cerebral palsy
- Dystonic cerebral palsy
- Vogt disease

G80.4 Ataxic cerebral palsy
Poor muscle tone and coordination

G80.8 Other cerebral palsy
- Mixed cerebral palsy syndromes

G80.9 Cerebral palsy, unspecified
- Cerebral palsy NOS

OGCR Section I.C.6.a.

Dominant/nondominant side

Codes from category G81, Hemiplegia and hemiparesis, and subcategories, G83.1, Monoplegia of lower limb, G83.2, Monoplegia of upper limb, and G83.3, Monoplegia, unspecified, identify whether the dominant and nondominant side is affected. Should the affected side be documented, but not specified as dominant or nondominant, and the classification system does not indicate a default, code selection is as follows:

- For ambidextrous patients, the default should be dominant.
- If the left side is affected, the default is nondominant.
- If the right side is affected, the default is dominant.

Item 6–9 **Hemiplegia** is complete paralysis of one side of the body—arm, leg, and trunk. **Hemiparesis** is a generalized weakness or incomplete paralysis of one side of the body. If most activities (eating, writing) are performed with the right hand, the right is the dominant side, and the left is the nondominant side. **Quadriplegia,** also called tetraplegia, is the complete paralysis of all four limbs. **Quadriparesis** is the incomplete paralysis of all four limbs. Nerve damage in C1–C4 is associated with lower limb paralysis, and C5–C7 damage is associated with upper limb paralysis. **Diplegia** is the paralysis of the upper limbs. **Monoplegia** is the complete paralysis of one limb.

G81 Hemiplegia and hemiparesis

Note: This category is to be used only when hemiplegia (complete)(incomplete) is reported without further specification, or is stated to be old or longstanding but of unspecified cause. The category is also for use in multiple coding to identify these types of hemiplegia resulting from any cause.

Excludes1 congenital cerebral palsy (G8Ø.-)
hemiplegia and hemiparesis due to sequela of cerebrovascular disease (I69.Ø5-, I69.15-, I69.25-, I69.35-, I69.85-, I69.95-)

Coding Clinic: 2Ø12, Q4, P1Ø6

G81.Ø Flaccid hemiplegia
Paralysis of half of body with loss of tone of muscles of paralyzed part and absence of tendon reflexes

G81.ØØ Flaccid hemiplegia affecting unspecified side PDX 709
G81.Ø1 Flaccid hemiplegia affecting right dominant side PDX 709
G81.Ø2 Flaccid hemiplegia affecting left dominant side PDX 709
G81.Ø3 Flaccid hemiplegia affecting right nondominant side PDX 709
G81.Ø4 Flaccid hemiplegia affecting left nondominant side PDX 709

G81.1 Spastic hemiplegia
Paralysis of half of body with spasticity of muscles of paralyzed part and increased tendon reflexes

G81.1Ø Spastic hemiplegia affecting unspecified side PDX 709
G81.11 Spastic hemiplegia affecting right dominant side PDX 709
G81.12 Spastic hemiplegia affecting left dominant side PDX 709
G81.13 Spastic hemiplegia affecting right nondominant side PDX 709
G81.14 Spastic hemiplegia affecting left nondominant side PDX 709

G81.9 Hemiplegia, unspecified

G81.9Ø Hemiplegia, unspecified affecting unspecified side PDX 709
G81.91 Hemiplegia, unspecified affecting right dominant side PDX 709
G81.92 Hemiplegia, unspecified affecting left dominant side PDX 709
G81.93 Hemiplegia, unspecified affecting right nondominant side PDX 709
G81.94 Hemiplegia, unspecified affecting left nondominant side PDX 709
Coding Clinic: 2Ø15, Q1, P26

G82 Paraplegia (paraparesis) and quadriplegia (quadriparesis)

Note: This category is to be used only when the listed conditions are reported without further specification, or are stated to be old or longstanding but of unspecified cause. The category is also for use in multiple coding to identify these conditions resulting from any cause.

Excludes1 congenital cerebral palsy (G8Ø.-)
functional quadriplegia (R53.2)
hysterical paralysis (F44.4)

G82.2 Paraplegia
Paralysis of both lower limbs NOS
Paraparesis (lower) NOS
Paraplegia (lower) NOS

G82.2Ø Paraplegia, unspecified PDX 709
Coding Clinic: 2Ø17, Q3, P3
G82.21 Paraplegia, complete PDX 709
G82.22 Paraplegia, incomplete PDX 709

G82.5 Quadriplegia
Paralysis of all limbs; AKA tetraplegia

G82.5Ø Quadriplegia, unspecified PDX 759
G82.51 Quadriplegia, C1-C4 complete PDX 759
G82.52 Quadriplegia, C1-C4 incomplete PDX 759
Coding Clinic: 2Ø24, Q2, P23
G82.53 Quadriplegia, C5-C7 complete PDX 759
G82.54 Quadriplegia, C5-C7 incomplete PDX 759

G83 Other paralytic syndromes

Note: This category is to be used only when the listed conditions are reported without further specification, or are stated to be old or longstanding but of unspecified cause. The category is also for use in multiple coding to identify these conditions resulting from any cause.

Includes paralysis (complete) (incomplete), except as in G8Ø-G82

G83.Ø Diplegia of upper limbs PDX 763
Paralysis affecting limbs on both sides; AKA bilateral paralysis
Diplegia (upper)
Paralysis of both upper limbs

G83.1 Monoplegia of lower limb
Paralysis of limb on one side
Paralysis of lower limb

Excludes1 monoplegia of lower limbs due to sequela of cerebrovascular disease (I69.Ø4-, I69.14-, I69.24-, I69.34-, I69.84-, I69.94-)

Coding Clinic: 2Ø12, Q4, P1Ø6

G83.1Ø Monoplegia of lower limb affecting unspecified side
G83.11 Monoplegia of lower limb affecting right dominant side
G83.12 Monoplegia of lower limb affecting left dominant side
G83.13 Monoplegia of lower limb affecting right nondominant side
G83.14 Monoplegia of lower limb affecting left nondominant side

G83.2 Monoplegia of upper limb
Paralysis of upper limb

Excludes1 monoplegia of upper limbs due to sequela of cerebrovascular disease (I69.Ø3-, I69.13-, I69.23-, I69.33-, I69.83-, I69.93-)

Coding Clinic: 2Ø12, Q4, P1Ø6

G83.2Ø Monoplegia of upper limb affecting unspecified side
G83.21 Monoplegia of upper limb affecting right dominant side
G83.22 Monoplegia of upper limb affecting left dominant side
G83.23 Monoplegia of upper limb affecting right nondominant side
G83.24 Monoplegia of upper limb affecting left nondominant side

G83.3 Monoplegia, unspecified
Coding Clinic: 2Ø12, Q4, P1Ø6

G83.3Ø Monoplegia, unspecified affecting unspecified side
G83.31 Monoplegia, unspecified affecting right dominant side
G83.32 Monoplegia, unspecified affecting left dominant side
G83.33 Monoplegia, unspecified affecting right nondominant side
G83.34 Monoplegia, unspecified affecting left nondominant side

G83.4 **Cauda equina syndrome** (Ex) PDX 764
Aching pain due to compression of spinal nerve roots
Neurogenic bladder due to cauda equina syndrome
Excludes1 cord bladder NOS (G95.89)
neurogenic bladder NOS (N31.9)
Coding Clinic: 2024, Q1, P18

G83.5 **Locked-in state** (Ex) PDX 765
Coding Clinic: 2022, Q2, P11

● G83.8 **Other specified paralytic syndromes**
Excludes1 paralytic syndromes due to current spinal cord injury-code to spinal cord injury (S14, S24, S34)

G83.81 **Brown-Séquard syndrome**
G83.82 **Anterior cord syndrome**
G83.83 **Posterior cord syndrome**
G83.84 **Todd's paralysis (postepileptic)**
G83.89 **Other specified paralytic syndromes**

G83.9 **Paralytic syndrome, unspecified**

OTHER DISORDERS OF THE NERVOUS SYSTEM (G89-G99)

● G89 **Pain, not elsewhere classified**
Code also related psychological factors associated with pain (F45.42)
Excludes1 generalized pain NOS (R52)
pain disorders exclusively related to psychological factors (F45.41)
pain NOS (R52)
Excludes2 atypical face pain (G50.1)
headache syndromes (G44.-)
localized pain, unspecified type - code to pain by site, such as:
abdomen pain (R10.-)
back pain (M54.9)
breast pain (N64.4)
chest pain (R07.1-R07.9)
ear pain (H92.0-)
eye pain (H57.1)
headache (R51.9)
joint pain (M25.5-)
limb pain (M79.6-)
lumbar region pain (M54.5-)
painful urination (R30.9)
pelvic and perineal pain (R10.2)
shoulder pain (M25.51-)
spine pain (M54.-)
throat pain (R07.0)
tongue pain (K14.6)
tooth pain (K08.8)
renal colic (N23)
migraines (G43.-)
myalgia (M79.1-)
pain from prosthetic devices, implants, and grafts (T82.84, T83.84, T84.84, T85.84-)
phantom limb syndrome with pain (G54.6)
vulvar vestibulitis (N94.810)
vulvodynia (N94.81-)

G89.0 **Central pain syndrome**
Neurological condition causing intractable pain resulting from damage to CNS
Déjérine-Roussy syndrome
Myelopathic pain syndrome
Thalamic pain syndrome (hyperesthetic)

● G89.1 **Acute pain, not elsewhere classified**
G89.11 **Acute pain due to trauma**
G89.12 **Acute post-thoracotomy pain**
Post-thoracotomy pain NOS
G89.18 **Other acute postprocedural pain**
Postoperative pain NOS
Postprocedural pain NOS

● G89.2 **Chronic pain, not elsewhere classified**
Excludes1 causalgia, lower limb (G57.7-)
causalgia, upper limb (G56.4-)
central pain syndrome (G89.0)
chronic pain syndrome (G89.4)
complex regional pain syndrome II, lower limb (G57.7-)
complex regional pain syndrome II, upper limb (G56.4-)
neoplasm related chronic pain (G89.3)
reflex sympathetic dystrophy (G90.5-)

G89.21 **Chronic pain due to trauma**
G89.22 **Chronic post-thoracotomy pain**
G89.28 **Other chronic postprocedural pain**
Other chronic postoperative pain
G89.29 **Other chronic pain**
Coding Clinic: 2023, Q3, P17

G89.3 **Neoplasm related pain (acute) (chronic)**
Cancer associated pain
Pain due to malignancy (primary) (secondary)
Tumor associated pain

G89.4 **Chronic pain syndrome**
Chronic pain associated with significant psychosocial dysfunction

● G90 **Disorders of autonomic nervous system**
Excludes1 dysfunction of the autonomic nervous system due to alcohol (G31.2)

● G90.0 **Idiopathic peripheral autonomic neuropathy**
G90.01 **Carotid sinus syncope**
Carotid sinus syndrome
G90.09 **Other idiopathic peripheral autonomic neuropathy**
Idiopathic peripheral autonomic neuropathy NOS

G90.1 **Familial dysautonomia [Riley-Day]**
Inherited disorder that affects nerve function

G90.2 **Horner's syndrome**
Due to damage of the sympathetic nervous system
Bernard(-Horner) syndrome
Cervical sympathetic dystrophy or paralysis

G90.3 **Multi-system degeneration of the autonomic nervous system** (Ex) PDX 766
Neurogenic orthostatic hypotension [Shy-Drager]
Excludes1 orthostatic hypotension NOS (I95.1)

G90.4 **Autonomic dysreflexia**
Syndrome resulting from lesions of spinal cord
Use additional code to identify the cause, such as:
fecal impaction (K56.41)
pressure ulcer (pressure area) (L89.-)
urinary tract infection (N39.0)

● G90.5 **Complex regional pain syndrome I (CRPS I)**
Reflex sympathetic dystrophy
Excludes1 causalgia of lower limb (G57.7-)
causalgia of upper limb (G56.4-)
complex regional pain syndrome II of lower limb (G57.7-)
complex regional pain syndrome II of upper limb (G56.4-)

G90.50 **Complex regional pain syndrome I, unspecified** (Ex) PDX 767

● G90.51 **Complex regional pain syndrome I of upper limb**
G90.511 **Complex regional pain syndrome I of right upper limb** (Ex) PDX 768
G90.512 **Complex regional pain syndrome I of left upper limb** (Ex) PDX 768
G90.513 **Complex regional pain syndrome I of upper limb, bilateral** (Ex) PDX 768
G90.519 **Complex regional pain syndrome I of unspecified upper limb** (Ex) PDX 768

CHAPTER 6 (G00-G99)

G90.52 Complex regional pain syndrome I of lower limb
- **G90.521 Complex regional pain syndrome I of right lower limb** (Ex) PDX 768
- **G90.522 Complex regional pain syndrome I of left lower limb** (Ex) PDX 768
- **G90.523 Complex regional pain syndrome I of lower limb, bilateral** (Ex) PDX 768
- **G90.529 Complex regional pain syndrome I of unspecified lower limb** (Ex) PDX 768

G90.59 Complex regional pain syndrome I of other specified site (Ex) PDX 768

G90.8 Other disorders of autonomic nervous system
Coding Clinic: 2023, Q2, P9

G90.81 Serotonin syndrome
Serotonin toxicity
Code first poisoning due to drug or toxin, such as:
- linezolid (T36.8X- with sixth character 1-4)
- monoamine oxidase inhibitors (T43.1X with sixth character 1-4)
- selective serotonin and norepinephrine reuptake inhibitors [SSNRI] (T43.21with sixth character 1-4)
- selective serotonin reuptake inhibitors [SSRI] (T43.22 with sixth character 1-4)

Use Additional code for adverse effect, if applicable, to identify drug, such as:
- linezolid (T36.8X5)
- monoamine oxidase inhibitors (T43.1X5)
- selective serotonin and norepinephrine reuptake inhibitors [SSNRI](T43.215)
- selective serotonin reuptake inhibitors [SSRI] (T43.225)

Use Additional code, if applicable, to identify:
- disseminated intravascular coagulation (D65)
- hypertensive crisis (I16.-)
- metabolic acidosis (E87.2-)
- shock, not elsewhere classified (R57.-)
- toxic encephalopathy (G92.-)
- ventricular tachycardia (I47.2-)

G90.89 Other disorders of autonomic nervous system

G90.9 Disorder of the autonomic nervous system, unspecified

G90.A Postural orthostatic tachycardia syndrome [POTS]
Chronic orthostatic intolerance
Postural tachycardia syndrome
Coding Clinic: 2022, Q4, P20

G90.B LMNB1-related autosomal dominant leukodystrophy

G91 Hydrocephalus
Dilatation of cerebral ventricles, accompanied by accumulation of cerebrospinal fluid

Includes acquired hydrocephalus

Excludes1 Arnold-Chiari syndrome with hydrocephalus (Q07.-)
congenital hydrocephalus (Q03.-)
spina bifida with hydrocephalus (Q05.-)

G91.0 Communicating hydrocephalus (Ex) PDX 769
Secondary normal pressure hydrocephalus

G91.1 Obstructive hydrocephalus (Ex) PDX 770

G91.2 (Idiopathic) normal pressure hydrocephalus (Ex) PDX 769
Normal pressure hydrocephalus NOS

G91.3 Post-traumatic hydrocephalus, unspecified (Ex) PDX 770

G91.4 Hydrocephalus in diseases classified elsewhere
Code first underlying condition, such as:
congenital syphilis (A50.4-)
neoplasm (C00-D49)
plasminogen deficiency (E88.02)

Excludes1 hydrocephalus due to congenital toxoplasmosis (P37.1)

G91.8 Other hydrocephalus (Ex) PDX 770

G91.9 Hydrocephalus, unspecified (Ex) PDX 770

G92 Toxic encephalopathy

G92.0 Immune effector cell-associated neurotoxicity syndrome
Code first underlying cause such as:
complications of immune effector cellular therapy (T80.82)

Code also, if applicable, associated signs and symptoms, such as:
cerebral edema (G93.6)
unspecified convulsions (R56.9)

G92.00 Immune effector cell-associated neurotoxicity syndrome, grade unspecified
ICANS, grade unspecified

G92.01 Immune effector cell-associated neurotoxicity syndrome, grade 1
ICANS, grade 1

G92.02 Immune effector cell-associated neurotoxicity syndrome, grade 2
ICANS, grade 2

G92.03 Immune effector cell-associated neurotoxicity syndrome, grade 3 (Ex) PDX 771
ICANS, grade 3

G92.04 Immune effector cell-associated neurotoxicity syndrome, grade 4 (Ex) PDX 771
ICANS, grade 4

G92.05 Immune effector cell-associated neurotoxicity syndrome, grade 5 (Ex) PDX 771
ICANS, grade 5

G92.8 Other toxic encephalopathy (Ex) PDX 772
Toxic encephalitis
Toxic metabolic encephalopathy

Code first poisoning due to drug or toxin, if applicable, (T36-T65 with fifth or sixth character 1-4)

Use Additional code for adverse effect, if applicable, to identify drug (T36-T50 with fifth or sixth character 5)

Coding Clinic: 2024, Q2, P15; 2022, Q1, P53

G92.9 Unspecified toxic encephalopathy (Ex) PDX 772
Code first poisoning due to drug or toxin, if applicable, (T36-T65 with fifth or sixth character 1-4)

Use Additional code for adverse effect, if applicable, to identify drug (T36-T50 with fifth or sixth character 5)

Disorder or disease of brain caused by chemicals
Coding Clinic: 2021, Q1, P13; 2017, Q1, P39-40

G93 Other disorders of brain

G93.0 Cerebral cysts
Arachnoid cyst
Porencephalic cyst, acquired

Excludes1 acquired periventricular cysts of newborn (P91.1)
congenital cerebral cysts (Q04.6)

G93.1 Anoxic brain damage, not elsewhere classified (Ex) PDX 773
Permanent brain damage by lack of oxygen perfusion through brain tissues.

Excludes1 cerebral anoxia due to anesthesia during labor and delivery (O74.3)
cerebral anoxia due to anesthesia during the puerperium (O89.2)
neonatal anoxia (P84)

G93.2 Benign intracranial hypertension
Pseudotumor

Excludes1 hypertensive encephalopathy (I67.4)
obstructive hydrocephalus (G91.1)

G93.3 Postviral and related fatigue syndromes

Excludes1 chronic fatigue NOS (R53.82)

Use Additional code, if applicable, for post COVID-19 condition, unspecified (U09.9)

Excludes1 neurasthenia (F48.8)

G93.31 Postviral fatigue syndrome

CHAPTER 6 (G00-G99)

G93.32 **Myalgic encephalomyelitis/chronic fatigue syndrome**
Chronic fatigue syndrome
ME/CFS
Myalgic encephalomyelitis

G93.39 **Other post infection and related fatigue syndromes**

● G93.4 **Other and unspecified encephalopathy**
Excludes2 alcoholic encephalopathy (G31.2)
encephalopathy in diseases classified elsewhere (G94)
hypertensive encephalopathy (I67.4)
Coding Clinic: 2024, Q2, P15; 2017, Q2, P9

G93.40 **Encephalopathy, unspecified** PDX 774

G93.41 **Metabolic encephalopathy** PDX 774
Septic encephalopathy
Coding Clinic: 2024, Q2, P15; 2017, Q2, P8; 2016, Q3, P42; 2015, Q3, P21

G93.42 **Megalencephalic leukoencephalopathy with subcortical cysts** PDX 775

G93.43 **Leukoencephalopathy with calcifications and cysts** PDX 775

G93.44 **Adult-onset leukodystrophy with axonal spheroids** PDX 775
Adult-onset leukoencephalopathy with axonal spheroids and pigmented glia

▶G93.45 **Developmental and epileptic encephalopathy** PDX 775
▶Early infantile epileptic encephalopathy
▶Code also if applicable, associated disorders such as:
▶developmental disorders of scholastic skills (F81.-)
▶developmental disorder of speech and language (F80.-)
▶epilepsy, by specific type (G40.-)
▶intellectual disabilities (F70-F79)
▶other neurodevelopmental disorder (F88)
▶pervasive developmental disorders (F84.-)

G93.49 **Other encephalopathy** PDX 775
Encephalopathy NEC
Coding Clinic: 2021, Q2, P3; 2018, Q4, P16; 2018, Q2, P22; 2017, Q2, P9

G93.5 **Compression of brain** PDX 776
Arnold-Chiari type 1 compression of brain
Compression of brain (stem)
Herniation of brain (stem)
Excludes1 traumatic compression of brain (S06.A-)

G93.6 **Cerebral edema** PDX 777
Excludes1 cerebral edema due to birth injury (P11.0)
traumatic cerebral edema (S06.1-)
Coding Clinic: 2022, Q3, P9,11

G93.7 **Reye's syndrome** PDX 778 P
Life-threatening neurological condition, usually follows viral illness
Code first (poisoning due to salicylates, if applicable (T39.0-, with sixth character 1-4)
Use additional code for adverse effect due to salicylates, if applicable (T39.0-, with sixth character 5)

● G93.8 **Other specified disorders of brain**

G93.81 **Temporal sclerosis**
Hippocampal sclerosis
Mesial temporal sclerosis

G93.82 **Brain death** PDX 575

G93.89 **Other specified disorders of brain**
Postradiation encephalopathy
Coding Clinic: 2024, Q2, P15,16; 2019, Q3, P9; 2016, Q4, P7

G93.9 **Disorder of brain, unspecified**

G94 Other disorders of brain in diseases classified elsewhere
Code first underlying disease
Excludes1 encephalopathy in congenital syphilis (A50.49)
encephalopathy in influenza (J09.X9, J10.81, J11.81)
encephalopathy in syphilis (A52.19)
hydrocephalus in diseases classified elsewhere (G91.4)
Coding Clinic: 2018, Q2, P22; 2017, Q2, P8

● G95 **Other and unspecified diseases of spinal cord**
Excludes2 myelitis (G04.-)

G95.0 **Syringomyelia and syringobulbia** PDX 779

● G95.1 **Vascular myelopathies**
Excludes2 intraspinal phlebitis and thrombophlebitis, except non-pyogenic (G08)

G95.11 **Acute infarction of spinal cord (embolic) (nonembolic)** PDX 780
Anoxia of spinal cord
Arterial thrombosis of spinal cord

G95.19 **Other vascular myelopathies** PDX 780
Edema of spinal cord
Hematomyelia
Nonpyogenic intraspinal phlebitis and thrombophlebitis
Subacute necrotic myelopathy
Coding Clinic: 2023, Q3, P21

● G95.2 **Other and unspecified cord compression**

G95.20 **Unspecified cord compression** PDX 781

G95.29 **Other cord compression** PDX 781

● G95.8 **Other specified diseases of spinal cord**
Excludes1 neurogenic bladder NOS (N31.9)
neurogenic bladder due to cauda equina syndrome (G83.4)
neuromuscular dysfunction of bladder without spinal cord lesion (N31.-)

G95.81 **Conus medullaris syndrome** PDX 780
Damage to gray matter and/or nerve roots in lower end of spinal cord

G95.89 **Other specified diseases of spinal cord** PDX 780
Cord bladder NOS
Drug-induced myelopathy
Radiation-induced myelopathy
Excludes1 myelopathy NOS (G95.9)

G95.9 **Disease of spinal cord, unspecified** PDX 781
Myelopathy NOS

● G96 **Other disorders of central nervous system**

● G96.0 **Cerebrospinal fluid leak**
Code also if applicable:
intracranial hypotension (G96.81-)
Excludes1 cerebrospinal fluid leak from spinal puncture (G97.0)
Coding Clinic: 2018, Q2, P13

G96.00 **Cerebrospinal fluid leak, unspecified** PDX 782
Code also if applicable:
head injury (S00-S09)

G96.01 **Cranial cerebrospinal fluid leak, spontaneous** PDX 782
Otorrhea due to spontaneous cerebrospinal fluid CSF leak
Rhinorrhea due to spontaneous cerebrospinal fluid CSF leak
Spontaneous cerebrospinal fluid leak from skull base

G96.02 **Spinal cerebrospinal fluid leak, spontaneous** PDX 782
Spontaneous cerebrospinal fluid leak from spine

CHAPTER 6 (G00-G99)

G96.Ø8 Other cranial cerebrospinal fluid leak (Ex) PDX 782
Postoperative cranial cerebrospinal fluid leak
Traumatic cranial cerebrospinal fluid leak
Code also if applicable:
head injury (SØØ-SØ9)

G96.Ø9 Other spinal cerebrospinal fluid leak (Ex) PDX 782
Other spinal CSF leak
Postoperative spinal cerebrospinal fluid leak
Traumatic spinal cerebrospinal fluid leak
Code also if applicable:
head injury (SØØ-SØ9)
Coding Clinic: 2022, Q3, P24

● **G96.1 Disorders of meninges, not elsewhere classified**

G96.11 Dural tear (Ex) PDX 569
Code also intracranial hypotension, if applicable (G96.81-)
Excludes1 accidental puncture or laceration of dura during a procedure (G97.41)

G96.12 Meningeal adhesions (cerebral) (spinal)

● **G96.19 Other disorders of meninges, not elsewhere classified**

G96.191 Perineural cyst
Cervical nerve root cyst
Lumbar nerve root cyst
Sacral nerve root cyst
Tarlov cyst
Thoracic nerve root cyst

G96.198 Other disorders of meninges, not elsewhere classified

● **G96.8 Other specified disorders of central nervous system**

● **G96.81 Intracranial hypotension**
Code also any associated diagnoses, such as:
Brachial amyotrophy (G54.5)
Cerebrospinal fluid leak from spine (G96.Ø2)
Cranial nerve disorders in diseases classified elsewhere (G53)
Nerve root and compressions in diseases classified elsewhere (G55)
Nonpyogenic thrombosis of intracranial venous system (I67.6)
Nontraumatic intracerebral hemorrhage (I61.-)
Nontraumatic subdural hemorrhage (I62.Ø-)
Other and unspecified cord compression (G95.2-)
Other secondary parkinsonism (G21.8)
Reversible cerebrovascular vasoconstriction syndrome (I67.841)
Spinal cord herniation (G95.89)
Stroke (I63.-)
Syringomyelia (G95.Ø)

G96.81Ø Intracranial hypotension, unspecified

G96.811 Intracranial hypotension, spontaneous

G96.819 Other intracranial hypotension

G96.89 Other specified disorders of central nervous system

G96.9 Disorder of central nervous system, unspecified

● **G97 Intraoperative and postprocedural complications and disorders of nervous system, not elsewhere classified**
Excludes2 intraoperative and postprocedural cerebrovascular infarction (I97.81-, I97.82-)
Coding Clinic: 2016, Q4, P9

G97.Ø Cerebrospinal fluid leak from spinal puncture (Ex) PDX 783
Code also any associated diagnoses or complications, such as:
intracranial hypotension following a procedure (G97.83-G97.84)

G97.1 Other reaction to spinal and lumbar puncture
Headache due to lumbar puncture
Other reaction to spinal dural puncture
Code also, if applicable, any associated headache with orthostatic component (R51.0)

G97.2 Intracranial hypotension following ventricular shunting (Ex) PDX 783
Code also any associated diagnoses or complications

● **G97.3 Intraoperative hemorrhage and hematoma of a nervous system organ or structure complicating a procedure**
Excludes1 intraoperative hemorrhage and hematoma of a nervous system organ or structure due to accidental puncture and laceration during a procedure (G97.4-)

G97.31 Intraoperative hemorrhage and hematoma of a nervous system organ or structure complicating a nervous system procedure (Ex) PDX 784

G97.32 Intraoperative hemorrhage and hematoma of a nervous system organ or structure complicating other procedure (Ex) PDX 784

● **G97.4 Accidental puncture and laceration of a nervous system organ or structure during a procedure** (Ex) PDX 569

G97.41 Accidental puncture or laceration of dura during a procedure
Incidental (inadvertent) durotomy
Code also any associated diagnoses or complications
Coding Clinic: 2024, Q1, P21

G97.48 Accidental puncture and laceration of other nervous system organ or structure during a nervous system procedure

G97.49 Accidental puncture and laceration of other nervous system organ or structure during other procedure

● **G97.5 Postprocedural hemorrhage of a nervous system organ or structure following a procedure** (Ex) PDX 785

G97.51 Postprocedural hemorrhage of a nervous system organ or structure following a nervous system procedure

G97.52 Postprocedural hemorrhage of a nervous system organ or structure following other procedure

● **G97.6 Postprocedural hematoma and seroma of a nervous system organ or structure following a procedure** (Ex) PDX 785

G97.61 Postprocedural hematoma of a nervous system organ or structure following a nervous system procedure

G97.62 Postprocedural hematoma of a nervous system organ or structure following other procedure

G97.63 Postprocedural seroma of a nervous system organ or structure following a nervous system procedure

G97.64 Postprocedural seroma of a nervous system organ or structure following other procedure

● **G97.8 Other intraoperative and postprocedural complications and disorders of nervous system**
Use additional code to further specify disorder

G97.81 Other intraoperative complications of nervous system (Ex) PDX 783

G97.82 Other postprocedural complications and disorders of nervous system (Ex) PDX 783
Coding Clinic: 2022, Q1, P35

G97.83 Intracranial hypotension following lumbar cerebrospinal fluid shunting (Ex) PDX 786
Code also any associated diagnoses or complications

G97.84 **Intracranial hypotension following other procedure** Ex PDX 786

Code also, if applicable:
accidental puncture or laceration of dura during a procedure (G97.41)
cerebrospinal fluid leak from spinal puncture (G97.0)

● G98 **Other disorders of nervous system not elsewhere classified**

Includes nervous system disorder NOS

G98.0 **Neurogenic arthritis, not elsewhere classified**
Nonsyphilitic neurogenic arthropathy NEC
Nonsyphilitic neurogenic spondylopathy NEC

Excludes1 spondylopathy (in):
syringomyelia and syringobulbia (G95.0)
tabes dorsalis (A52.11)

G98.8 **Other disorders of nervous system**
Nervous system disorder NOS

● G99 **Other disorders of nervous system in diseases classified elsewhere**

G99.0 ***Autonomic neuropathy in diseases classified elsewhere*** Ex PDX 787

Code first underlying disease, such as:
amyloidosis (E85.-)
gout (M1A.-, M10.-)
hyperthyroidism (E05.-)

Excludes1 diabetic autonomic neuropathy (E08-E13 with .43)

G99.2 ***Myelopathy in diseases classified elsewhere*** Ex PDX 768

Code first underlying disease, such as:
neoplasm (C00-D49)

Excludes1 myelopathy in:
intervertebral disease (M50.0-, M51.0-)
spondylosis (M47.0-, M47.1-)

G99.8 ***Other specified disorders of nervous system in diseases classified elsewhere***

Code first underlying disorder, such as:
amyloidosis (E85.-)
avitaminosis (E56.-)

Excludes1 nervous system involvement in:
cysticercosis (B69.0)
rubella (B06.0-)
syphilis (A52.1-)

CHAPTER 7

DISEASES OF THE EYE AND ADNEXA (HØØ-H59)

OGCR Chapter-Specific Coding Guidelines

7. Chapter 7: Diseases of the Eye and Adnexa (HØØ-H59)

a. Glaucoma

1) Assigning Glaucoma Codes

Assign as many codes from category H4Ø, Glaucoma, as needed to identify the type of glaucoma, the affected eye, and the glaucoma stage.

2) Bilateral glaucoma with same type and stage

When a patient has bilateral glaucoma and both eyes are documented as being the same type and stage, and there is a code for bilateral glaucoma, report only the code for the type of glaucoma, bilateral, with the seventh character for the stage.

When a patient has bilateral glaucoma and both eyes are documented as being the same type and stage, and the classification does not provide a code for bilateral glaucoma (i.e., subcategories H4Ø.1Ø, H4Ø.11, and H4Ø.2Ø) report only one code for the type of glaucoma with the appropriate seventh character for the stage.

3) Bilateral glaucoma stage with different types or stages

When a patient has bilateral glaucoma and each eye is documented as having a different type or stage, and the classification distinguishes laterality, assign the appropriate code for each eye rather than the code for bilateral glaucoma.

When a patient has bilateral glaucoma and each eye is documented as having a different type, and the classification does not distinguish laterality (i.e., subcategories H4Ø.1Ø, H4Ø.11 and H4Ø.2Ø), assign one code for each type of glaucoma with the appropriate seventh character for the stage.

When a patient has bilateral glaucoma and each eye is documented as having the same type, but different stage, and the classification does not distinguish laterality (i.e., subcategories H4Ø.1Ø, H4Ø.11, and H4Ø.2Ø), assign a code for the type of glaucoma for each eye with the seventh character for the specific glaucoma stage documented for each eye.

4) Patient admitted with glaucoma and stage evolves during the admission

If a patient is admitted with glaucoma and the stage progresses during the admission, assign the code for highest stage documented.

5) Indeterminate stage glaucoma

Assignment of the seventh character "4" for "indeterminate stage" should be based on the clinical documentation. The seventh character "4" is used for glaucomas whose stage cannot be clinically determined. This seventh character should not be confused with the seventh character "Ø", unspecified, which should be assigned when there is no documentation regarding the stage of the glaucoma.

b. Blindness

If "blindness" or "low vision" of both eyes is documented but the visual impairment category is not documented, assign code H54.3, Unqualified visual loss, both eyes. If "blindness" or "low vision" in one eye is documented but the visual impairment category is not documented, assign a code from H54.6-, Unqualified visual loss, one eye. If "blindness" or "visual loss" is documented without any information about whether one or both eyes are affected, assign code H54.7, Unspecified visual loss.

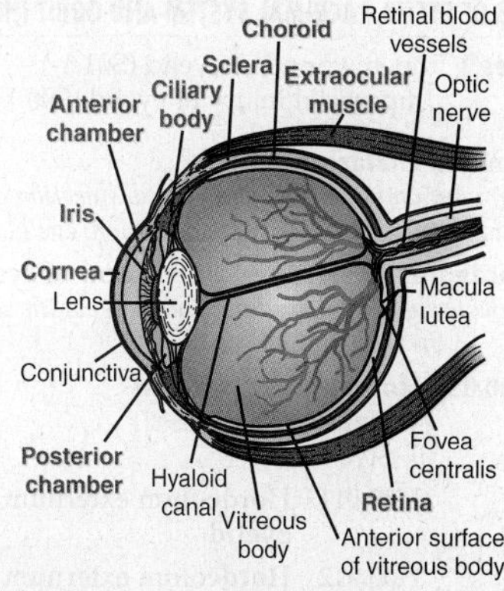

Figure 7–1 Eye and ocular adnexa. (From Buck CJ: Step-by-Step Medical Coding, ed 2016, St. Louis, Elsevier, 2016)

★**(See Plate 15 of the Anatomy Illustrations.)**

CHAPTER 7

DISEASES OF THE EYE AND ADNEXA (HØØ-H59)

Note: Use an external cause code following the code for the eye condition, if applicable, to identify the cause of the eye condition

Excludes2 certain conditions originating in the perinatal period (PØ4-P96)
certain infectious and parasitic diseases (AØØ-B99)
complications of pregnancy, childbirth and the puerperium (OØØ-O9A)
congenital malformations, deformations, and chromosomal abnormalities (QØØ-Q99)
diabetes mellitus related eye conditions (EØ9.3-, E1Ø.3-, E11.3-, E13.3-)
endocrine, nutritional and metabolic diseases (EØØ-E88)
injury (trauma) of eye and orbit (SØ5.-)
injury, poisoning and certain other consequences of external causes (SØØ-T88)
neoplasms (CØØ-D49)
symptoms, signs and abnormal clinical and laboratory findings, not elsewhere classified (RØØ-R94)
syphilis related eye disorders (A5Ø.Ø1, A5Ø.3-, A51.43, A52.71)

This chapter contains the following blocks:

HØØ-HØ5	Disorders of eyelid, lacrimal system and orbit
H1Ø-H11	Disorders of conjunctiva
H15-H22	Disorders of sclera, cornea, iris and ciliary body
H25-H28	Disorders of lens
H3Ø-H36	Disorders of choroid and retina
H4Ø-H42	Glaucoma
H43-H44	Disorders of vitreous body and globe
H46-H47	Disorders of optic nerve and visual pathways
H49-H52	Disorders of ocular muscles, binocular movement, accommodation and refraction
H53-H54	Visual disturbances and blindness
H55-H57	Other disorders of eye and adnexa
H59	Intraoperative and postprocedural complications and disorders of eye and adnexa, not elsewhere classified

DISORDERS OF EYELID, LACRIMAL SYSTEM AND ORBIT (H00-H05)

Excludes2 open wound of eyelid (S01.1-)
superficial injury of eyelid (S00.1-, S00.2-)

● **H00 Hordeolum and chalazion**
Hordeolum: inflammatory staphylococcal infection of sebaceous glands of eyelids; AKA stye. Chalazion: eyelid mass

● **H00.0 Hordeolum (externum) (internum) of eyelid**
Bacterial infection (staphylococcus) of the sebaceous gland of the eyelid (stye)

● **H00.01 Hordeolum externum**
Hordeolum NOS
Stye

H00.011 Hordeolum externum right upper eyelid
H00.012 Hordeolum externum right lower eyelid
H00.013 Hordeolum externum right eye, unspecified eyelid
H00.014 Hordeolum externum left upper eyelid
H00.015 Hordeolum externum left lower eyelid
H00.016 Hordeolum externum left eye, unspecified eyelid
H00.019 Hordeolum externum unspecified eye, unspecified eyelid

● **H00.02 Hordeolum internum**
Infection of meibomian gland

H00.021 Hordeolum internum right upper eyelid
H00.022 Hordeolum internum right lower eyelid
H00.023 Hordeolum internum right eye, unspecified eyelid
H00.024 Hordeolum internum left upper eyelid
H00.025 Hordeolum internum left lower eyelid
H00.026 Hordeolum internum left eye, unspecified eyelid
H00.029 Hordeolum internum unspecified eye, unspecified eyelid

● **H00.03 Abscess of eyelid**
Furuncle of eyelid

H00.031 Abscess of right upper eyelid
H00.032 Abscess of right lower eyelid
H00.033 Abscess of eyelid right eye, unspecified eyelid
H00.034 Abscess of left upper eyelid
H00.035 Abscess of left lower eyelid
H00.036 Abscess of eyelid left eye, unspecified eyelid
H00.039 Abscess of eyelid unspecified eye, unspecified eyelid

● **H00.1 Chalazion**
Often caused by accumulation of meibomian gland secretions resulting from a blockage of duct.
Meibomian (gland) cyst

Excludes2 infected meibomian gland (H00.02-)

H00.11 Chalazion right upper eyelid
H00.12 Chalazion right lower eyelid
H00.13 Chalazion right eye, unspecified eyelid
H00.14 Chalazion left upper eyelid
H00.15 Chalazion left lower eyelid
H00.16 Chalazion left eye, unspecified eyelid
H00.19 Chalazion unspecified eye, unspecified eyelid

● **H01 Other inflammation of eyelid**

● **H01.0 Blepharitis**
Inflammation of eyelids

Excludes1 blepharoconjunctivitis (H10.5-)

● **H01.00 Unspecified blepharitis**

H01.001 Unspecified blepharitis right upper eyelid
H01.002 Unspecified blepharitis right lower eyelid
H01.003 Unspecified blepharitis right eye, unspecified eyelid
H01.004 Unspecified blepharitis left upper eyelid
H01.005 Unspecified blepharitis left lower eyelid
H01.006 Unspecified blepharitis left eye, unspecified eyelid
H01.009 Unspecified blepharitis unspecified eye, unspecified eyelid
H01.00A Unspecified blepharitis right eye, upper and lower eyelids
H01.00B Unspecified blepharitis left eye, upper and lower eyelids

● **H01.01 Ulcerative blepharitis**

H01.011 Ulcerative blepharitis right upper eyelid
H01.012 Ulcerative blepharitis right lower eyelid
H01.013 Ulcerative blepharitis right eye, unspecified eyelid
H01.014 Ulcerative blepharitis left upper eyelid
H01.015 Ulcerative blepharitis left lower eyelid
H01.016 Ulcerative blepharitis left eye, unspecified eyelid
H01.019 Ulcerative blepharitis unspecified eye, unspecified eyelid
H01.01A Ulcerative blepharitis right eye, upper and lower eyelids
H01.01B Ulcerative blepharitis left eye, upper and lower eyelids

● **H01.02 Squamous blepharitis**

H01.021 Squamous blepharitis right upper eyelid
H01.022 Squamous blepharitis right lower eyelid
H01.023 Squamous blepharitis right eye, unspecified eyelid
H01.024 Squamous blepharitis left upper eyelid
H01.025 Squamous blepharitis left lower eyelid
H01.026 Squamous blepharitis left eye, unspecified eyelid
H01.029 Squamous blepharitis unspecified eye, unspecified eyelid
H01.02A Squamous blepharitis right eye, upper and lower eyelids
H01.02B Squamous blepharitis left eye, upper and lower eyelids

● **H01.1 Noninfectious dermatoses of eyelid**

● **H01.11 Allergic dermatitis of eyelid**
Contact dermatitis of eyelid

H01.111 Allergic dermatitis of right upper eyelid
H01.112 Allergic dermatitis of right lower eyelid
H01.113 Allergic dermatitis of right eye, unspecified eyelid

CHAPTER 7 (H00-H59)

H01.114 Allergic dermatitis of left upper eyelid

H01.115 Allergic dermatitis of left lower eyelid

H01.116 Allergic dermatitis of left eye, unspecified eyelid

H01.119 Allergic dermatitis of unspecified eye, unspecified eyelid

● H01.12 Discoid lupus erythematosus of eyelid

H01.121 Discoid lupus erythematosus of right upper eyelid

H01.122 Discoid lupus erythematosus of right lower eyelid

H01.123 Discoid lupus erythematosus of right eye, unspecified eyelid

H01.124 Discoid lupus erythematosus of left upper eyelid

H01.125 Discoid lupus erythematosus of left lower eyelid

H01.126 Discoid lupus erythematosus of left eye, unspecified eyelid

H01.129 Discoid lupus erythematosus of unspecified eye, unspecified eyelid

● H01.13 Eczematous dermatitis of eyelid

H01.131 Eczematous dermatitis of right upper eyelid

H01.132 Eczematous dermatitis of right lower eyelid

H01.133 Eczematous dermatitis of right eye, unspecified eyelid

H01.134 Eczematous dermatitis of left upper eyelid

H01.135 Eczematous dermatitis of left lower eyelid

H01.136 Eczematous dermatitis of left eye, unspecified eyelid

H01.139 Eczematous dermatitis of unspecified eye, unspecified eyelid

● H01.14 Xeroderma of eyelid

Abnormally dry

H01.141 Xeroderma of right upper eyelid

H01.142 Xeroderma of right lower eyelid

H01.143 Xeroderma of right eye, unspecified eyelid

H01.144 Xeroderma of left upper eyelid

H01.145 Xeroderma of left lower eyelid

H01.146 Xeroderma of left eye, unspecified eyelid

H01.149 Xeroderma of unspecified eye, unspecified eyelid

H01.8 Other specified inflammations of eyelid

H01.9 Unspecified inflammation of eyelid

Inflammation of eyelid NOS

● H02 Other disorders of eyelid

Turning inward (inversion) of eyelid margin and ingrowing eyelashes

Excludes1 congenital malformations of eyelid (Q10.0-Q10.3)

● H02.0 Entropion and trichiasis of eyelid

● H02.00 Unspecified entropion of eyelid

H02.001 Unspecified entropion of right upper eyelid

H02.002 Unspecified entropion of right lower eyelid

H02.003 Unspecified entropion of right eye, unspecified eyelid

H02.004 Unspecified entropion of left upper eyelid

H02.005 Unspecified entropion of left lower eyelid

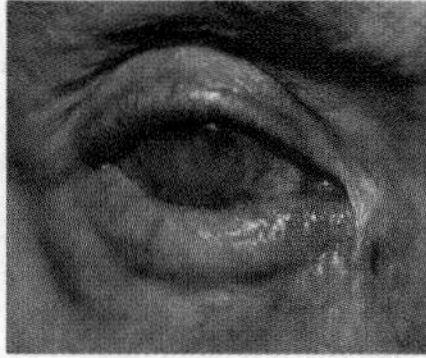

Figure 7-2 Right lower eyelid entropion. Note the inward rotation of the tarsal plate about the horizontal axis and the resultant contact between the mucocutaneous junction and ocular surface. (From Glynn M, Drake WM, Hutchison R: Hutchison's Clinical Methods: An Integrated Approach to Clinical Practice, Edinburgh, Saunders/Elsevier, 2012)

H02.006 Unspecified entropion of left eye, unspecified eyelid

H02.009 Unspecified entropion of unspecified eye, unspecified eyelid

● H02.01 Cicatricial entropion of eyelid

Scar

H02.011 Cicatricial entropion of right upper eyelid

H02.012 Cicatricial entropion of right lower eyelid

H02.013 Cicatricial entropion of right eye, unspecified eyelid

H02.014 Cicatricial entropion of left upper eyelid

H02.015 Cicatricial entropion of left lower eyelid

H02.016 Cicatricial entropion of left eye, unspecified eyelid

H02.019 Cicatricial entropion of unspecified eye, unspecified eyelid

● H02.02 Mechanical entropion of eyelid

Turning inward (inversion) of eyelid margin due to lack of support

H02.021 Mechanical entropion of right upper eyelid

H02.022 Mechanical entropion of right lower eyelid

H02.023 Mechanical entropion of right eye, unspecified eyelid

H02.024 Mechanical entropion of left upper eyelid

H02.025 Mechanical entropion of left lower eyelid

H02.026 Mechanical entropion of left eye, unspecified eyelid

H02.029 Mechanical entropion of unspecified eye, unspecified eyelid

● H02.03 Senile entropion of eyelid

Turning inward (inversion) of eyelid margin due to aging

H02.031 Senile entropion of right upper eyelid A

H02.032 Senile entropion of right lower eyelid A

H02.033 Senile entropion of right eye, unspecified eyelid A

H02.034 Senile entropion of left upper eyelid A

H02.035 Senile entropion of left lower eyelid A

H02.036 Senile entropion of left eye, unspecified eyelid A

H02.039 Senile entropion of unspecified eye, unspecified eyelid A

● H02.04 Spastic entropion of eyelid

Turning inward (inversion) of eyelid margin caused by spasm of muscle

H02.041 Spastic entropion of right upper eyelid

H02.042 Spastic entropion of right lower eyelid

H02.043 Spastic entropion of right eye, unspecified eyelid

CHAPTER 7 (H00-H59)

H02.044 Spastic entropion of left upper eyelid
H02.045 Spastic entropion of left lower eyelid
H02.046 Spastic entropion of left eye, unspecified eyelid
H02.049 Spastic entropion of unspecified eye, unspecified eyelid

● H02.05 Trichiasis without entropion
Ingrowing hairs of eyelashes
H02.051 Trichiasis without entropion right upper eyelid
H02.052 Trichiasis without entropion right lower eyelid
H02.053 Trichiasis without entropion right eye, unspecified eyelid
H02.054 Trichiasis without entropion left upper eyelid
H02.055 Trichiasis without entropion left lower eyelid
H02.056 Trichiasis without entropion left eye, unspecified eyelid
H02.059 Trichiasis without entropion unspecified eye, unspecified eyelid

● H02.1 Ectropion of eyelid
Eversion (pulling away) of eyelid

● H02.10 Unspecified ectropion of eyelid
H02.101 Unspecified ectropion of right upper eyelid
H02.102 Unspecified ectropion of right lower eyelid
H02.103 Unspecified ectropion of right eye, unspecified eyelid
H02.104 Unspecified ectropion of left upper eyelid
H02.105 Unspecified ectropion of left lower eyelid
H02.106 Unspecified ectropion of left eye, unspecified eyelid
H02.109 Unspecified ectropion of unspecified eye, unspecified eyelid

● H02.11 Cicatricial ectropion of eyelid
Pulling of eyelid down and away from eye due to scar or tightening
H02.111 Cicatricial ectropion of right upper eyelid
H02.112 Cicatricial ectropion of right lower eyelid
H02.113 Cicatricial ectropion of right eye, unspecified eyelid
H02.114 Cicatricial ectropion of left upper eyelid
H02.115 Cicatricial ectropion of left lower eyelid
H02.116 Cicatricial ectropion of left eye, unspecified eyelid
H02.119 Cicatricial ectropion of unspecified eye, unspecified eyelid

● H02.12 Mechanical ectropion of eyelid
Eversion (pulling away) of eyelid due to lack of support
H02.121 Mechanical ectropion of right upper eyelid
H02.122 Mechanical ectropion of right lower eyelid
H02.123 Mechanical ectropion of right eye, unspecified eyelid
H02.124 Mechanical ectropion of left upper eyelid
H02.125 Mechanical ectropion of left lower eyelid
H02.126 Mechanical ectropion of left eye, unspecified eyelid
H02.129 Mechanical ectropion of unspecified eye, unspecified eyelid

● H02.13 Senile ectropion of eyelid
Eversion (pulling away) of eyelid due to age
H02.131 Senile ectropion of right upper eyelid A
H02.132 Senile ectropion of right lower eyelid A
H02.133 Senile ectropion of right eye, unspecified eyelid A
H02.134 Senile ectropion of left upper eyelid A
H02.135 Senile ectropion of left lower eyelid A
H02.136 Senile ectropion of left eye, unspecified eyelid A
H02.139 Senile ectropion of unspecified eye, unspecified eyelid A

● H02.14 Spastic ectropion of eyelid
Eversion (pulling away) of eyelid due to tonic muscle spasm
H02.141 Spastic ectropion of right upper eyelid
H02.142 Spastic ectropion of right lower eyelid
H02.143 Spastic ectropion of right eye, unspecified eyelid
H02.144 Spastic ectropion of left upper eyelid
H02.145 Spastic ectropion of left lower eyelid
H02.146 Spastic ectropion of left eye, unspecified eyelid
H02.149 Spastic ectropion of unspecified eye, unspecified eyelid

● H02.15 Paralytic ectropion of eyelid
H02.151 Paralytic ectropion of right upper eyelid
H02.152 Paralytic ectropion of right lower eyelid
H02.153 Paralytic ectropion of right eye, unspecified eyelid
H02.154 Paralytic ectropion of left upper eyelid
H02.155 Paralytic ectropion of left lower eyelid
H02.156 Paralytic ectropion of left eye, unspecified eyelid
H02.159 Paralytic ectropion of unspecified eye, unspecified eyelid

● H02.2 Lagophthalmos
Condition in which eye cannot completely close

● H02.20 Unspecified lagophthalmos
H02.201 Unspecified lagophthalmos right upper eyelid
H02.202 Unspecified lagophthalmos right lower eyelid
H02.203 Unspecified lagophthalmos right eye, unspecified eyelid
H02.204 Unspecified lagophthalmos left upper eyelid
H02.205 Unspecified lagophthalmos left lower eyelid
H02.206 Unspecified lagophthalmos left eye, unspecified eyelid
H02.209 Unspecified lagophthalmos unspecified eye, unspecified eyelid
H02.20A Unspecified lagophthalmos right eye, upper and lower eyelids
H02.20B Unspecified lagophthalmos left eye, upper and lower eyelids
H02.20C Unspecified lagophthalmos, bilateral, upper and lower eyelids

CHAPTER 7 (H00-H59)

● **H02.21 Cicatricial lagophthalmos**
Upper or lower eyelid does not close due to scar or tightening
H02.211 Cicatricial lagophthalmos right upper eyelid
H02.212 Cicatricial lagophthalmos right lower eyelid
H02.213 Cicatricial lagophthalmos right eye, unspecified eyelid
H02.214 Cicatricial lagophthalmos left upper eyelid
H02.215 Cicatricial lagophthalmos left lower eyelid
H02.216 Cicatricial lagophthalmos left eye, unspecified eyelid
H02.219 Cicatricial lagophthalmos unspecified eye, unspecified eyelid
H02.21A Cicatricial lagophthalmos right eye, upper and lower eyelids
H02.21B Cicatricial lagophthalmos left eye, upper and lower eyelids
H02.21C Cicatricial lagophthalmos, bilateral, upper and lower eyelids

● **H02.22 Mechanical lagophthalmos**
Inability to close lids due to structural disorder
H02.221 Mechanical lagophthalmos right upper eyelid
H02.222 Mechanical lagophthalmos right lower eyelid
H02.223 Mechanical lagophthalmos right eye, unspecified eyelid
H02.224 Mechanical lagophthalmos left upper eyelid
H02.225 Mechanical lagophthalmos left lower eyelid
H02.226 Mechanical lagophthalmos left eye, unspecified eyelid
H02.229 Mechanical lagophthalmos unspecified eye, unspecified eyelid
H02.22A Mechanical lagophthalmos right eye, upper and lower eyelids
H02.22B Mechanical lagophthalmos left eye, upper and lower eyelids
H02.22C Mechanical lagophthalmos, bilateral, upper and lower eyelids

● **H02.23 Paralytic lagophthalmos**
Eyelids do not close due to paralysis
H02.231 Paralytic lagophthalmos right upper eyelid
H02.232 Paralytic lagophthalmos right lower eyelid
H02.233 Paralytic lagophthalmos right eye, unspecified eyelid
H02.234 Paralytic lagophthalmos left upper eyelid
H02.235 Paralytic lagophthalmos left lower eyelid
H02.236 Paralytic lagophthalmos left eye, unspecified eyelid
H02.239 Paralytic lagophthalmos unspecified eye, unspecified eyelid
H02.23A Paralytic lagophthalmos right eye, upper and lower eyelids
H02.23B Paralytic lagophthalmos left eye, upper and lower eyelids
H02.23C Paralytic lagophthalmos, bilateral, upper and lower eyelids

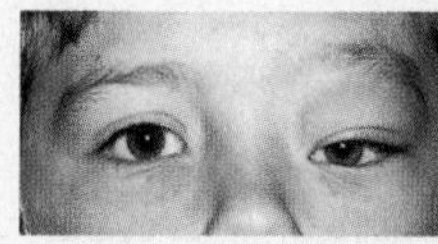

Figure 7-3 Ptosis of eyelid. (From Kanski JJ: Clinical Diagnosis in Ophthalmology, London, Elsevier Mosby, 2006)

Item 7-1 Ptosis of eyelid is drooping of the upper eyelid over the pupil when the eyes are fully opened resulting from nerve or muscle damage, which may require surgical correction.

★**(See Plate 17 of the Anatomy Illustrations.)**

● **H02.3 Blepharochalasis**
Relaxation of skin of eyelid, due to atrophy of intercellular tissue
Pseudoptosis
H02.30 Blepharochalasis unspecified eye, unspecified eyelid
H02.31 Blepharochalasis right upper eyelid
H02.32 Blepharochalasis right lower eyelid
H02.33 Blepharochalasis right eye, unspecified eyelid
H02.34 Blepharochalasis left upper eyelid
H02.35 Blepharochalasis left lower eyelid
H02.36 Blepharochalasis left eye, unspecified eyelid

● **H02.4 Ptosis of eyelid**
Falling forward, drooping, sagging of eyelid

● **H02.40 Unspecified ptosis of eyelid**
H02.401 Unspecified ptosis of right eyelid
H02.402 Unspecified ptosis of left eyelid
H02.403 Unspecified ptosis of bilateral eyelids
H02.409 Unspecified ptosis of unspecified eyelid

● **H02.41 Mechanical ptosis of eyelid**
H02.411 Mechanical ptosis of right eyelid
H02.412 Mechanical ptosis of left eyelid
H02.413 Mechanical ptosis of bilateral eyelids
H02.419 Mechanical ptosis of unspecified eyelid

● **H02.42 Myogenic ptosis of eyelid**
H02.421 Myogenic ptosis of right eyelid
H02.422 Myogenic ptosis of left eyelid
H02.423 Myogenic ptosis of bilateral eyelids
H02.429 Myogenic ptosis of unspecified eyelid

● **H02.43 Paralytic ptosis of eyelid**
Neurogenic ptosis of eyelid
H02.431 Paralytic ptosis of right eyelid
H02.432 Paralytic ptosis of left eyelid
H02.433 Paralytic ptosis of bilateral eyelids
H02.439 Paralytic ptosis unspecified eyelid

● **H02.5 Other disorders affecting eyelid function**
Excludes2 blepharospasm (G24.5)
organic tic (G25.69)
psychogenic tic (F95.-)

● **H02.51 Abnormal innervation syndrome**
H02.511 Abnormal innervation syndrome right upper eyelid
H02.512 Abnormal innervation syndrome right lower eyelid
H02.513 Abnormal innervation syndrome right eye, unspecified eyelid
H02.514 Abnormal innervation syndrome left upper eyelid
H02.515 Abnormal innervation syndrome left lower eyelid
H02.516 Abnormal innervation syndrome left eye, unspecified eyelid
H02.519 Abnormal innervation syndrome unspecified eye, unspecified eyelid

CHAPTER 7 (H00-H59)

● H02.52 Blepharophimosis
Drooping of eyelid with reduced lid size
Ankyloblepharon
H02.521 Blepharophimosis right upper eyelid
H02.522 Blepharophimosis right lower eyelid
H02.523 Blepharophimosis right eye, unspecified eyelid
H02.524 Blepharophimosis left upper eyelid
H02.525 Blepharophimosis left lower eyelid
H02.526 Blepharophimosis left eye, unspecified eyelid
H02.529 Blepharophimosis unspecified eye, unspecified lid

● H02.53 Eyelid retraction
Eyelid lag
H02.531 Eyelid retraction right upper eyelid
H02.532 Eyelid retraction right lower eyelid
H02.533 Eyelid retraction right eye, unspecified eyelid
H02.534 Eyelid retraction left upper eyelid
H02.535 Eyelid retraction left lower eyelid
H02.536 Eyelid retraction left eye, unspecified eyelid
H02.539 Eyelid retraction unspecified eye, unspecified lid

H02.59 Other disorders affecting eyelid function
Deficient blink reflex
Sensory disorders

● H02.6 Xanthelasma of eyelid
Yellow-to-orange patches or pimples clustered together on eyelid
H02.60 Xanthelasma of unspecified eye, unspecified eyelid
H02.61 Xanthelasma of right upper eyelid
H02.62 Xanthelasma of right lower eyelid
H02.63 Xanthelasma of right eye, unspecified eyelid
H02.64 Xanthelasma of left upper eyelid
H02.65 Xanthelasma of left lower eyelid
H02.66 Xanthelasma of left eye, unspecified eyelid

● H02.7 Other and unspecified degenerative disorders of eyelid and periocular area
H02.70 Unspecified degenerative disorders of eyelid and periocular area

● H02.71 Chloasma of eyelid and periocular area
Dyspigmentation of eyelid
Hyperpigmentation of eyelid
H02.711 Chloasma of right upper eyelid and periocular area
H02.712 Chloasma of right lower eyelid and periocular area
H02.713 Chloasma of right eye, unspecified eyelid and periocular area
H02.714 Chloasma of left upper eyelid and periocular area
H02.715 Chloasma of left lower eyelid and periocular area
H02.716 Chloasma of left eye, unspecified eyelid and periocular area
H02.719 Chloasma of unspecified eye, unspecified eyelid and periocular area

● H02.72 Madarosis of eyelid and periocular area
Loss of eyelashes and/or eyebrows
Hypotrichosis of eyelid
H02.721 Madarosis of right upper eyelid and periocular area
H02.722 Madarosis of right lower eyelid and periocular area
H02.723 Madarosis of right eye, unspecified eyelid and periocular area
H02.724 Madarosis of left upper eyelid and periocular area
H02.725 Madarosis of left lower eyelid and periocular area
H02.726 Madarosis of left eye, unspecified eyelid and periocular area
H02.729 Madarosis of unspecified eye, unspecified eyelid and periocular area

● H02.73 Vitiligo of eyelid and periocular area
Skin pigmentation disease characterized by white patches
Hypopigmentation of eyelid
H02.731 Vitiligo of right upper eyelid and periocular area
H02.732 Vitiligo of right lower eyelid and periocular area
H02.733 Vitiligo of right eye, unspecified eyelid and periocular area
H02.734 Vitiligo of left upper eyelid and periocular area
H02.735 Vitiligo of left lower eyelid and periocular area
H02.736 Vitiligo of left eye, unspecified eyelid and periocular area
H02.739 Vitiligo of unspecified eye, unspecified eyelid and periocular area

H02.79 Other degenerative disorders of eyelid and periocular area

● H02.8 Other specified disorders of eyelid

● H02.81 Retained foreign body in eyelid
Use additional code to identify the type of retained foreign body (Z18.-)
Excludes1 laceration of eyelid with foreign body (S01.12-)
retained intraocular foreign body (H44.6-, H44.7-)
superficial foreign body of eyelid and periocular area (S00.25-)
H02.811 Retained foreign body in right upper eyelid
H02.812 Retained foreign body in right lower eyelid
H02.813 Retained foreign body in right eye, unspecified eyelid
H02.814 Retained foreign body in left upper eyelid
H02.815 Retained foreign body in left lower eyelid
H02.816 Retained foreign body in left eye, unspecified eyelid
H02.819 Retained foreign body in unspecified eye, unspecified eyelid

● H02.82 Cysts of eyelid
Sebaceous cyst of eyelid
H02.821 Cysts of right upper eyelid
H02.822 Cysts of right lower eyelid
H02.823 Cysts of right eye, unspecified eyelid
H02.824 Cysts of left upper eyelid
H02.825 Cysts of left lower eyelid
H02.826 Cysts of left eye, unspecified eyelid
H02.829 Cysts of unspecified eye, unspecified eyelid

● H02.83 Dermatochalasis of eyelid
Skin is inelastic and hangs loosely in folds
H02.831 Dermatochalasis of right upper eyelid
H02.832 Dermatochalasis of right lower eyelid
H02.833 Dermatochalasis of right eye, unspecified eyelid
H02.834 Dermatochalasis of left upper eyelid

H02.835 Dermatochalasis of left lower eyelid
H02.836 Dermatochalasis of left eye, unspecified eyelid
H02.839 Dermatochalasis of unspecified eye, unspecified eyelid

● **H02.84 Edema of eyelid**
Hyperemia of eyelid
H02.841 Edema of right upper eyelid
H02.842 Edema of right lower eyelid
H02.843 Edema of right eye, unspecified eyelid
H02.844 Edema of left upper eyelid
H02.845 Edema of left lower eyelid
H02.846 Edema of left eye, unspecified eyelid
H02.849 Edema of unspecified eye, unspecified eyelid

● **H02.85 Elephantiasis of eyelid**
Massive secondary lymphedema with hypertrophy of skin and subcutaneous tissues (pachyderma)
H02.851 Elephantiasis of right upper eyelid
H02.852 Elephantiasis of right lower eyelid
H02.853 Elephantiasis of right eye, unspecified eyelid
H02.854 Elephantiasis of left upper eyelid
H02.855 Elephantiasis of left lower eyelid
H02.856 Elephantiasis of left eye, unspecified eyelid
H02.859 Elephantiasis of unspecified eye, unspecified eyelid

● **H02.86 Hypertrichosis of eyelid**
Excessive growth of hair
H02.861 Hypertrichosis of right upper eyelid
H02.862 Hypertrichosis of right lower eyelid
H02.863 Hypertrichosis of right eye, unspecified eyelid
H02.864 Hypertrichosis of left upper eyelid
H02.865 Hypertrichosis of left lower eyelid
H02.866 Hypertrichosis of left eye, unspecified eyelid
H02.869 Hypertrichosis of unspecified eye, unspecified eyelid

● **H02.87 Vascular anomalies of eyelid**
H02.871 Vascular anomalies of right upper eyelid
H02.872 Vascular anomalies of right lower eyelid
H02.873 Vascular anomalies of right eye, unspecified eyelid
H02.874 Vascular anomalies of left upper eyelid
H02.875 Vascular anomalies of left lower eyelid
H02.876 Vascular anomalies of left eye, unspecified eyelid
H02.879 Vascular anomalies of unspecified eye, unspecified eyelid

● **H02.88 Meibomian gland dysfunction of eyelid**
H02.881 Meibomian gland dysfunction right upper eyelid
H02.882 Meibomian gland dysfunction right lower eyelid
H02.883 Meibomian gland dysfunction of right eye, unspecified eyelid
H02.884 Meibomian gland dysfunction left upper eyelid
H02.885 Meibomian gland dysfunction left lower eyelid
H02.886 Meibomian gland dysfunction of left eye, unspecified eyelid
H02.889 Meibomian gland dysfunction of unspecified eye, unspecified eyelid
H02.88A Meibomian gland dysfunction right eye, upper and lower eyelids
H02.88B Meibomian gland dysfunction left eye, upper and lower eyelids

H02.89 Other specified disorders of eyelid
Hemorrhage of eyelid

H02.9 Unspecified disorder of eyelid
Disorder of eyelid NOS

● **H04 Disorders of lacrimal system**
Excludes1 congenital malformations of lacrimal system (Q10.4-Q10.6)

● **H04.0 Dacryoadenitis**
Inflammation of lacrimal gland

● **H04.00 Unspecified dacryoadenitis**
H04.001 Unspecified dacryoadenitis, right lacrimal gland
H04.002 Unspecified dacryoadenitis, left lacrimal gland
H04.003 Unspecified dacryoadenitis, bilateral lacrimal glands
H04.009 Unspecified dacryoadenitis, unspecified lacrimal gland

● **H04.01 Acute dacryoadenitis**
H04.011 Acute dacryoadenitis, right lacrimal gland
H04.012 Acute dacryoadenitis, left lacrimal gland
H04.013 Acute dacryoadenitis, bilateral lacrimal glands
H04.019 Acute dacryoadenitis, unspecified lacrimal gland

★**(See Plate 19 of the Anatomy Illustrations.)**

● **H04.02 Chronic dacryoadenitis**
H04.021 Chronic dacryoadenitis, right lacrimal gland
H04.022 Chronic dacryoadenitis, left lacrimal gland
H04.023 Chronic dacryoadenitis, bilateral lacrimal gland
H04.029 Chronic dacryoadenitis, unspecified lacrimal gland

● **H04.03 Chronic enlargement of lacrimal gland**
H04.031 Chronic enlargement of right lacrimal gland
H04.032 Chronic enlargement of left lacrimal gland
H04.033 Chronic enlargement of bilateral lacrimal glands
H04.039 Chronic enlargement of unspecified lacrimal gland

● **H04.1 Other disorders of lacrimal gland**

● **H04.11 Dacryops**
Watery eye or distention of lacrimal duct due to fluid
H04.111 Dacryops of right lacrimal gland
H04.112 Dacryops of left lacrimal gland
H04.113 Dacryops of bilateral lacrimal glands
H04.119 Dacryops of unspecified lacrimal gland

Iris
Lacrimal glands
Lacrimal sac
Eyelid
Sclera
Pupil
Nasolacrimal duct
Lacrimal duct

Figure 7-4 Lacrimal apparatus. (From Buck CJ: Step-by-Step Medical Coding, 2016, St. Louis, Elsevier, 2016)

CHAPTER 7 (H00-H59)

- H04.12 Dry eye syndrome
  Tear film insufficiency, NOS
  - H04.121 Dry eye syndrome of right lacrimal gland
  - H04.122 Dry eye syndrome of left lacrimal gland
  - H04.123 Dry eye syndrome of bilateral lacrimal glands
  - H04.129 Dry eye syndrome of unspecified lacrimal gland
- H04.13 Lacrimal cyst
  Lacrimal cystic degeneration
  - H04.131 Lacrimal cyst right lacrimal gland
  - H04.132 Lacrimal cyst left lacrimal gland
  - H04.133 Lacrimal cyst bilateral lacrimal glands
  - H04.139 Lacrimal cyst unspecified lacrimal gland
- H04.14 Primary lacrimal gland atrophy
  - H04.141 Primary lacrimal gland atrophy, right lacrimal gland
  - H04.142 Primary lacrimal gland atrophy, left lacrimal gland
  - H04.143 Primary lacrimal gland atrophy, bilateral lacrimal glands
  - H04.149 Primary lacrimal gland atrophy, unspecified lacrimal gland
- H04.15 Secondary lacrimal gland atrophy
  - H04.151 Secondary lacrimal gland atrophy, right lacrimal gland
  - H04.152 Secondary lacrimal gland atrophy, left lacrimal gland
  - H04.153 Secondary lacrimal gland atrophy, bilateral lacrimal glands
  - H04.159 Secondary lacrimal gland atrophy, unspecified lacrimal gland
- H04.16 Lacrimal gland dislocation
  - H04.161 Lacrimal gland dislocation, right lacrimal gland
  - H04.162 Lacrimal gland dislocation, left lacrimal gland
  - H04.163 Lacrimal gland dislocation, bilateral lacrimal glands
  - H04.169 Lacrimal gland dislocation, unspecified lacrimal gland
- H04.19 Other specified disorders of lacrimal gland

H04.2 Epiphora
Overflow of tears due to stricture of lacrimal passages; AKA lacrimation

- H04.20 Unspecified epiphora
  - H04.201 Unspecified epiphora, right side
  - H04.202 Unspecified epiphora, left side
  - H04.203 Unspecified epiphora, bilateral
  - H04.209 Unspecified epiphora, unspecified side
- H04.21 Epiphora due to excess lacrimation
  - H04.211 Epiphora due to excess lacrimation, right lacrimal gland
  - H04.212 Epiphora due to excess lacrimation, left lacrimal gland
  - H04.213 Epiphora due to excess lacrimation, bilateral lacrimal glands
  - H04.219 Epiphora due to excess lacrimation, unspecified lacrimal gland
- H04.22 Epiphora due to insufficient drainage
  - H04.221 Epiphora due to insufficient drainage, right side
  - H04.222 Epiphora due to insufficient drainage, left side
  - H04.223 Epiphora due to insufficient drainage, bilateral
  - H04.229 Epiphora due to insufficient drainage, unspecified side

H04.3 Acute and unspecified inflammation of lacrimal passages

Excludes1 neonatal dacryocystitis (P39.1)

- H04.30 Unspecified dacryocystitis
  - H04.301 Unspecified dacryocystitis of right lacrimal passage
  - H04.302 Unspecified dacryocystitis of left lacrimal passage
  - H04.303 Unspecified dacryocystitis of bilateral lacrimal passages
  - H04.309 Unspecified dacryocystitis of unspecified lacrimal passage
- H04.31 Phlegmonous dacryocystitis
  Cellulitis of lacrimal sac
  - H04.311 Phlegmonous dacryocystitis of right lacrimal passage
  - H04.312 Phlegmonous dacryocystitis of left lacrimal passage
  - H04.313 Phlegmonous dacryocystitis of bilateral lacrimal passages
  - H04.319 Phlegmonous dacryocystitis of unspecified lacrimal passage
- H04.32 Acute dacryocystitis
  Acute dacryopericystitis
  - H04.321 Acute dacryocystitis of right lacrimal passage
  - H04.322 Acute dacryocystitis of left lacrimal passage
  - H04.323 Acute dacryocystitis of bilateral lacrimal passages
  - H04.329 Acute dacryocystitis of unspecified lacrimal passage
- H04.33 Acute lacrimal canaliculitis
  - H04.331 Acute lacrimal canaliculitis of right lacrimal passage
  - H04.332 Acute lacrimal canaliculitis of left lacrimal passage
  - H04.333 Acute lacrimal canaliculitis of bilateral lacrimal passages
  - H04.339 Acute lacrimal canaliculitis of unspecified lacrimal passage

H04.4 Chronic inflammation of lacrimal passages

- H04.41 Chronic dacryocystitis
  Inflammation of lacrimal sac
  - H04.411 Chronic dacryocystitis of right lacrimal passage
  - H04.412 Chronic dacryocystitis of left lacrimal passage
  - H04.413 Chronic dacryocystitis of bilateral lacrimal passages
  - H04.419 Chronic dacryocystitis of unspecified lacrimal passage
- H04.42 Chronic lacrimal canaliculitis
  Inflammation of lacrimal ducts
  - H04.421 Chronic lacrimal canaliculitis of right lacrimal passage
  - H04.422 Chronic lacrimal canaliculitis of left lacrimal passage
  - H04.423 Chronic lacrimal canaliculitis of bilateral lacrimal passages
  - H04.429 Chronic lacrimal canaliculitis of unspecified lacrimal passage
- H04.43 Chronic lacrimal mucocele
  Accumulation of mucous secretion
  - H04.431 Chronic lacrimal mucocele of right lacrimal passage
  - H04.432 Chronic lacrimal mucocele of left lacrimal passage
  - H04.433 Chronic lacrimal mucocele of bilateral lacrimal passages
  - H04.439 Chronic lacrimal mucocele of unspecified lacrimal passage

- **H04.5 Stenosis and insufficiency of lacrimal passages**
  - **H04.51 Dacryolith**
    Concretion in lacrimal sac/duct; AKA lacrimal calculus
    - H04.511 Dacryolith of right lacrimal passage
    - H04.512 Dacryolith of left lacrimal passage
    - H04.513 Dacryolith of bilateral lacrimal passages
    - H04.519 Dacryolith of unspecified lacrimal passage
  - **H04.52 Eversion of lacrimal punctum**
    Turning out of lacrimal drainage opening
    - H04.521 Eversion of right lacrimal punctum
    - H04.522 Eversion of left lacrimal punctum
    - H04.523 Eversion of bilateral lacrimal punctum
    - H04.529 Eversion of unspecified lacrimal punctum
  - **H04.53 Neonatal obstruction of nasolacrimal duct**
    Excludes1 congenital stenosis and stricture of lacrimal duct (Q10.5)
    - H04.531 Neonatal obstruction of right nasolacrimal duct N
    - H04.532 Neonatal obstruction of left nasolacrimal duct N
    - H04.533 Neonatal obstruction of bilateral nasolacrimal duct N
    - H04.539 Neonatal obstruction of unspecified nasolacrimal duct N
  - **H04.54 Stenosis of lacrimal canaliculi**
    - H04.541 Stenosis of right lacrimal canaliculi
    - H04.542 Stenosis of left lacrimal canaliculi
    - H04.543 Stenosis of bilateral lacrimal canaliculi
    - H04.549 Stenosis of unspecified lacrimal canaliculi
  - **H04.55 Acquired stenosis of nasolacrimal duct**
    - H04.551 Acquired stenosis of right nasolacrimal duct
    - H04.552 Acquired stenosis of left nasolacrimal duct
    - H04.553 Acquired stenosis of bilateral nasolacrimal duct
    - H04.559 Acquired stenosis of unspecified nasolacrimal duct
  - **H04.56 Stenosis of lacrimal punctum**
    - H04.561 Stenosis of right lacrimal punctum
    - H04.562 Stenosis of left lacrimal punctum
    - H04.563 Stenosis of bilateral lacrimal punctum
    - H04.569 Stenosis of unspecified lacrimal punctum
  - **H04.57 Stenosis of lacrimal sac**
    - H04.571 Stenosis of right lacrimal sac
    - H04.572 Stenosis of left lacrimal sac
    - H04.573 Stenosis of bilateral lacrimal sac
    - H04.579 Stenosis of unspecified lacrimal sac
- **H04.6 Other changes of lacrimal passages**
  - **H04.61 Lacrimal fistula**
    - H04.611 Lacrimal fistula right lacrimal passage
    - H04.612 Lacrimal fistula left lacrimal passage
    - H04.613 Lacrimal fistula bilateral lacrimal passages
    - H04.619 Lacrimal fistula unspecified lacrimal passage
  - H04.69 Other changes of lacrimal passages
- **H04.8 Other disorders of lacrimal system**
  - **H04.81 Granuloma of lacrimal passages**
    Inflammatory response due to infectious or noninfectious agents
    - H04.811 Granuloma of right lacrimal passage
    - H04.812 Granuloma of left lacrimal passage
    - H04.813 Granuloma of bilateral lacrimal passages
    - H04.819 Granuloma of unspecified lacrimal passage
  - H04.89 Other disorders of lacrimal system
- H04.9 Disorder of lacrimal system, unspecified

H05 Disorders of orbit

Excludes1 congenital malformation of orbit (Q10.7)

- **H05.0 Acute inflammation of orbit**
  - H05.00 Unspecified acute inflammation of orbit
  - **H05.01 Cellulitis of orbit** (Ex) PDX 788
    Infection of soft tissue of orbit
    Abscess of orbit
    - H05.011 Cellulitis of right orbit
    - H05.012 Cellulitis of left orbit
    - H05.013 Cellulitis of bilateral orbits
    - H05.019 Cellulitis of unspecified orbit
  - **H05.02 Osteomyelitis of orbit** (Ex) PDX 789
    Infection of boney orbit of eye
    - H05.021 Osteomyelitis of right orbit
    - H05.022 Osteomyelitis of left orbit
    - H05.023 Osteomyelitis of bilateral orbits
    - H05.029 Osteomyelitis of unspecified orbit
  - **H05.03 Periostitis of orbit** (Ex) PDX 790
    Inflammation of periosteum (membrane covering bone surface)
    - H05.031 Periostitis of right orbit
    - H05.032 Periostitis of left orbit
    - H05.033 Periostitis of bilateral orbits
    - H05.039 Periostitis of unspecified orbit
  - **H05.04 Tenonitis of orbit**
    Inflammation of tenon capsule (space enclosing fascia of Tenon between eyeball and fat of orbit)
    - H05.041 Tenonitis of right orbit
    - H05.042 Tenonitis of left orbit
    - H05.043 Tenonitis of bilateral orbits
    - H05.049 Tenonitis of unspecified orbit
- **H05.1 Chronic inflammatory disorders of orbit**
  - H05.10 Unspecified chronic inflammatory disorders of orbit
  - **H05.11 Granuloma of orbit**
    Pseudotumor (inflammatory) of orbit
    - H05.111 Granuloma of right orbit
    - H05.112 Granuloma of left orbit
    - H05.113 Granuloma of bilateral orbits
    - H05.119 Granuloma of unspecified orbit
  - **H05.12 Orbital myositis**
    Inflammation of extraocular muscles of orbit
    - H05.121 Orbital myositis, right orbit
    - H05.122 Orbital myositis, left orbit
    - H05.123 Orbital myositis, bilateral
    - H05.129 Orbital myositis, unspecified orbit

CHAPTER 7 (H00-H59)

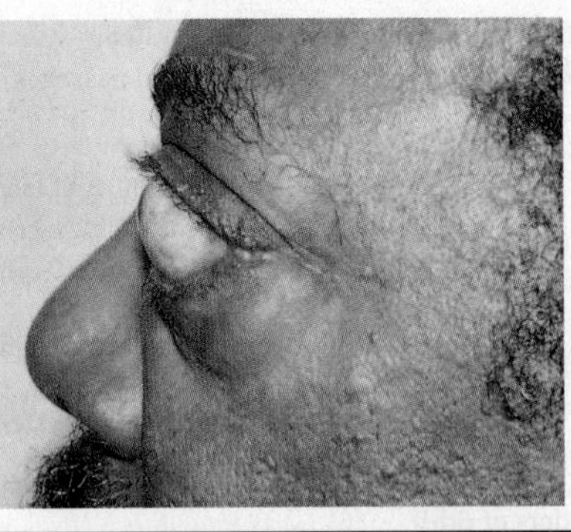

Figure 7-5 Exophthalmos. (From Black JM, Hokanson JH: Medical-Surgical Nursing: Clinical Management for Positive Outcomes, St. Louis, Saunders Elsevier, 2009)

● H05.2 Exophthalmic conditions
Bulging eyes
- H05.20 Unspecified exophthalmos
- ● H05.21 Displacement (lateral) of globe
  - H05.211 Displacement (lateral) of globe, right eye
  - H05.212 Displacement (lateral) of globe, left eye
  - H05.213 Displacement (lateral) of globe, bilateral
  - H05.219 Displacement (lateral) of globe, unspecified eye
- ● H05.22 Edema of orbit
  Orbital congestion
  - H05.221 Edema of right orbit
  - H05.222 Edema of left orbit
  - H05.223 Edema of bilateral orbit
  - H05.229 Edema of unspecified orbit
- ● H05.23 Hemorrhage of orbit
  - H05.231 Hemorrhage of right orbit
  - H05.232 Hemorrhage of left orbit
  - H05.233 Hemorrhage of bilateral orbit
  - H05.239 Hemorrhage of unspecified orbit
- ● H05.24 Constant exophthalmos
  Constant bulging eyes, often symptom of Graves disease
  - H05.241 Constant exophthalmos, right eye
  - H05.242 Constant exophthalmos, left eye
  - H05.243 Constant exophthalmos, bilateral
  - H05.249 Constant exophthalmos, unspecified eye
- ● H05.25 Intermittent exophthalmos
  Intermittent bulging eye occurring with bending forward or sharp turning of head
  - H05.251 Intermittent exophthalmos, right eye
  - H05.252 Intermittent exophthalmos, left eye
  - H05.253 Intermittent exophthalmos, bilateral
  - H05.259 Intermittent exophthalmos, unspecified eye
- ● H05.26 Pulsating exophthalmos
  Bulging eyes with pulsation and bruit, often due to aneurysm pushing eye forward
  - H05.261 Pulsating exophthalmos, right eye
  - H05.262 Pulsating exophthalmos, left eye
  - H05.263 Pulsating exophthalmos, bilateral
  - H05.269 Pulsating exophthalmos, unspecified eye

● H05.3 Deformity of orbit
Excludes1 congenital deformity of orbit (Q10.7)
hypertelorism (Q75.2)
- H05.30 Unspecified deformity of orbit
- ● H05.31 Atrophy of orbit
  - H05.311 Atrophy of right orbit
  - H05.312 Atrophy of left orbit
  - H05.313 Atrophy of bilateral orbit
  - H05.319 Atrophy of unspecified orbit
- ● H05.32 Deformity of orbit due to bone disease
  Code also associated bone disease
  - H05.321 Deformity of right orbit due to bone disease
  - H05.322 Deformity of left orbit due to bone disease
  - H05.323 Deformity of bilateral orbits due to bone disease
  - H05.329 Deformity of unspecified orbit due to bone disease
- ● H05.33 Deformity of orbit due to trauma or surgery
  - H05.331 Deformity of right orbit due to trauma or surgery
  - H05.332 Deformity of left orbit due to trauma or surgery
  - H05.333 Deformity of bilateral orbits due to trauma or surgery
  - H05.339 Deformity of unspecified orbit due to trauma or surgery
- ● H05.34 Enlargement of orbit
  - H05.341 Enlargement of right orbit
  - H05.342 Enlargement of left orbit
  - H05.343 Enlargement of bilateral orbits
  - H05.349 Enlargement of unspecified orbit
- ● H05.35 Exostosis of orbit
  - H05.351 Exostosis of right orbit
  - H05.352 Exostosis of left orbit
  - H05.353 Exostosis of bilateral orbits
  - H05.359 Exostosis of unspecified orbit

● H05.4 Enophthalmos
Recessed eyeball into orbit
- ● H05.40 Unspecified enophthalmos
  - H05.401 Unspecified enophthalmos, right eye
  - H05.402 Unspecified enophthalmos, left eye
  - H05.403 Unspecified enophthalmos, bilateral
  - H05.409 Unspecified enophthalmos, unspecified eye
- ● H05.41 Enophthalmos due to atrophy of orbital tissue
  - H05.411 Enophthalmos due to atrophy of orbital tissue, right eye
  - H05.412 Enophthalmos due to atrophy of orbital tissue, left eye
  - H05.413 Enophthalmos due to atrophy of orbital tissue, bilateral
  - H05.419 Enophthalmos due to atrophy of orbital tissue, unspecified eye
- ● H05.42 Enophthalmos due to trauma or surgery
  - H05.421 Enophthalmos due to trauma or surgery, right eye
  - H05.422 Enophthalmos due to trauma or surgery, left eye
  - H05.423 Enophthalmos due to trauma or surgery, bilateral
  - H05.429 Enophthalmos due to trauma or surgery, unspecified eye

H05.5 Retained (old) foreign body following penetrating wound of orbit
Retrobulbar foreign body
Use additional code to identify the type of retained foreign body (Z18.-)
Excludes1 current penetrating wound of orbit (S05.4-)
Excludes2 retained foreign body of eyelid (H02.81-)
retained intraocular foreign body (H44.6-, H44.7-)

H05.50 Retained (old) foreign body following penetrating wound of unspecified orbit
H05.51 Retained (old) foreign body following penetrating wound of right orbit
H05.52 Retained (old) foreign body following penetrating wound of left orbit
H05.53 Retained (old) foreign body following penetrating wound of bilateral orbits

H05.8 Other disorders of orbit

H05.81 Cyst of orbit
Encephalocele of orbit
H05.811 Cyst of right orbit
H05.812 Cyst of left orbit
H05.813 Cyst of bilateral orbits
H05.819 Cyst of unspecified orbit

H05.82 Myopathy of extraocular muscles
Weakness of muscles of eye
H05.821 Myopathy of extraocular muscles, right orbit
H05.822 Myopathy of extraocular muscles, left orbit
H05.823 Myopathy of extraocular muscles, bilateral
H05.829 Myopathy of extraocular muscles, unspecified orbit

H05.89 Other disorders of orbit

H05.9 Unspecified disorder of orbit

DISORDERS OF CONJUNCTIVA (H10-H11)

(See Plate 18 of the Anatomy Illustrations.)

H10 Conjunctivitis
Inflammation of membrane of the inside of the eyelid or on surface of eye (conjunctiva)
Excludes1 keratoconjunctivitis (H16.2-)

H10.0 Mucopurulent conjunctivitis

H10.01 Acute follicular conjunctivitis
H10.011 Acute follicular conjunctivitis, right eye
H10.012 Acute follicular conjunctivitis, left eye
H10.013 Acute follicular conjunctivitis, bilateral
H10.019 Acute follicular conjunctivitis, unspecified eye

H10.02 Other mucopurulent conjunctivitis
H10.021 Other mucopurulent conjunctivitis, right eye
H10.022 Other mucopurulent conjunctivitis, left eye
H10.023 Other mucopurulent conjunctivitis, bilateral
H10.029 Other mucopurulent conjunctivitis, unspecified eye

H10.1 Acute atopic conjunctivitis
Acute papillary conjunctivitis
H10.10 Acute atopic conjunctivitis, unspecified eye
H10.11 Acute atopic conjunctivitis, right eye
H10.12 Acute atopic conjunctivitis, left eye
H10.13 Acute atopic conjunctivitis, bilateral

H10.2 Other acute conjunctivitis

H10.21 Acute toxic conjunctivitis
Acute chemical conjunctivitis
Code first (T51-T65) to identify chemical and intent
Excludes1 burn and corrosion of eye and adnexa (T26.-)
H10.211 Acute toxic conjunctivitis, right eye
H10.212 Acute toxic conjunctivitis, left eye
H10.213 Acute toxic conjunctivitis, bilateral
H10.219 Acute toxic conjunctivitis, unspecified eye

H10.22 Pseudomembranous conjunctivitis
H10.221 Pseudomembranous conjunctivitis, right eye
H10.222 Pseudomembranous conjunctivitis, left eye
H10.223 Pseudomembranous conjunctivitis, bilateral
H10.229 Pseudomembranous conjunctivitis, unspecified eye

H10.23 Serous conjunctivitis, except viral
Excludes1 viral conjunctivitis (B30.-)
H10.231 Serous conjunctivitis, except viral, right eye
H10.232 Serous conjunctivitis, except viral, left eye
H10.233 Serous conjunctivitis, except viral, bilateral
H10.239 Serous conjunctivitis, except viral, unspecified eye

H10.3 Unspecified acute conjunctivitis
Excludes1 ophthalmia neonatorum NOS (P39.1)
H10.30 Unspecified acute conjunctivitis, unspecified eye
H10.31 Unspecified acute conjunctivitis, right eye
H10.32 Unspecified acute conjunctivitis, left eye
H10.33 Unspecified acute conjunctivitis, bilateral

H10.4 Chronic conjunctivitis

H10.40 Unspecified chronic conjunctivitis
H10.401 Unspecified chronic conjunctivitis, right eye
H10.402 Unspecified chronic conjunctivitis, left eye
H10.403 Unspecified chronic conjunctivitis, bilateral
H10.409 Unspecified chronic conjunctivitis, unspecified eye

H10.41 Chronic giant papillary conjunctivitis
Inflammation of membrane of the inside of the eyelid or on surface of eye often associated with contact lens wear
H10.411 Chronic giant papillary conjunctivitis, right eye
H10.412 Chronic giant papillary conjunctivitis, left eye
H10.413 Chronic giant papillary conjunctivitis, bilateral
H10.419 Chronic giant papillary conjunctivitis, unspecified eye

H10.42 Simple chronic conjunctivitis
H10.421 Simple chronic conjunctivitis, right eye
H10.422 Simple chronic conjunctivitis, left eye
H10.423 Simple chronic conjunctivitis, bilateral
H10.429 Simple chronic conjunctivitis, unspecified eye

CHAPTER 7 (H00-H59)

● **H10.43 Chronic follicular conjunctivitis**
Inflammation of membrane of the inside of the eyelid or on surface of eye due to topical medications or infection
H10.431 Chronic follicular conjunctivitis, right eye
H10.432 Chronic follicular conjunctivitis, left eye
H10.433 Chronic follicular conjunctivitis, bilateral
H10.439 Chronic follicular conjunctivitis, unspecified eye

H10.44 Vernal conjunctivitis
Affecting children, especially boys in which there are flattened papules with thick, gelatinous exudate on conjunctivae on inside of upper lid
Excludes1 vernal keratoconjunctivitis with limbar and corneal involvement (H16.26-)

H10.45 Other chronic allergic conjunctivitis

● **H10.5 Blepharoconjunctivitis**
Inflammation of eyelids and conjunctiva

● **H10.50 Unspecified blepharoconjunctivitis**
H10.501 Unspecified blepharoconjunctivitis, right eye
H10.502 Unspecified blepharoconjunctivitis, left eye
H10.503 Unspecified blepharoconjunctivitis, bilateral
H10.509 Unspecified blepharoconjunctivitis, unspecified eye

● **H10.51 Ligneous conjunctivitis**
Code also underlying condition if known, such as:
plasminogen deficiency (E88.02)
H10.511 Ligneous conjunctivitis, right eye
H10.512 Ligneous conjunctivitis, left eye
H10.513 Ligneous conjunctivitis, bilateral
H10.519 Ligneous conjunctivitis, unspecified eye

● **H10.52 Angular blepharoconjunctivitis**
H10.521 Angular blepharoconjunctivitis, right eye
H10.522 Angular blepharoconjunctivitis, left eye
H10.523 Angular blepharoconjunctivitis, bilateral
H10.529 Angular blepharoconjunctivitis, unspecified eye

● **H10.53 Contact blepharoconjunctivitis**
H10.531 Contact blepharoconjunctivitis, right eye
H10.532 Contact blepharoconjunctivitis, left eye
H10.533 Contact blepharoconjunctivitis, bilateral
H10.539 Contact blepharoconjunctivitis, unspecified eye

● **H10.8 Other conjunctivitis**

● **H10.81 Pingueculitis**
Inflammation of a yellow, raised thickening on the white of the eye associated with chronic dry eyes
Excludes1 pinguecula (H11.15-)
H10.811 Pingueculitis, right eye
H10.812 Pingueculitis, left eye
H10.813 Pingueculitis, bilateral
H10.819 Pingueculitis, unspecified eye

● **H10.82 Rosacea conjunctivitis**
Code first underlying rosacea dermatitis (L71.-)
H10.821 Rosacea conjunctivitis, right eye
H10.822 Rosacea conjunctivitis, left eye
H10.823 Rosacea conjunctivitis, bilateral
Coding Clinic: 2018, Q4, P15
H10.829 Rosacea conjunctivitis, unspecified eye

H10.89 Other conjunctivitis

H10.9 Unspecified conjunctivitis

● **H11 Other disorders of conjunctiva**
Excludes1 keratoconjunctivitis (H16.2-)

● **H11.0 Pterygium of eye**
Excludes1 pseudopterygium (H11.81-)

● **H11.00 Unspecified pterygium of eye**
H11.001 Unspecified pterygium of right eye
H11.002 Unspecified pterygium of left eye
H11.003 Unspecified pterygium of eye, bilateral
H11.009 Unspecified pterygium of unspecified eye

● **H11.01 Amyloid pterygium**
H11.011 Amyloid pterygium of right eye
H11.012 Amyloid pterygium of left eye
H11.013 Amyloid pterygium of eye, bilateral
H11.019 Amyloid pterygium of unspecified eye

● **H11.02 Central pterygium of eye**
H11.021 Central pterygium of right eye
H11.022 Central pterygium of left eye
H11.023 Central pterygium of eye, bilateral
H11.029 Central pterygium of unspecified eye

● **H11.03 Double pterygium of eye**
H11.031 Double pterygium of right eye
H11.032 Double pterygium of left eye
H11.033 Double pterygium of eye, bilateral
H11.039 Double pterygium of unspecified eye

● **H11.04 Peripheral pterygium of eye, stationary**
H11.041 Peripheral pterygium, stationary, right eye
H11.042 Peripheral pterygium, stationary, left eye
H11.043 Peripheral pterygium, stationary, bilateral
H11.049 Peripheral pterygium, stationary, unspecified eye

● **H11.05 Peripheral pterygium of eye, progressive**
H11.051 Peripheral pterygium, progressive, right eye
H11.052 Peripheral pterygium, progressive, left eye
H11.053 Peripheral pterygium, progressive, bilateral
H11.059 Peripheral pterygium, progressive, unspecified eye

● **H11.06 Recurrent pterygium of eye**
H11.061 Recurrent pterygium of right eye
H11.062 Recurrent pterygium of left eye
H11.063 Recurrent pterygium of eye, bilateral
H11.069 Recurrent pterygium of unspecified eye

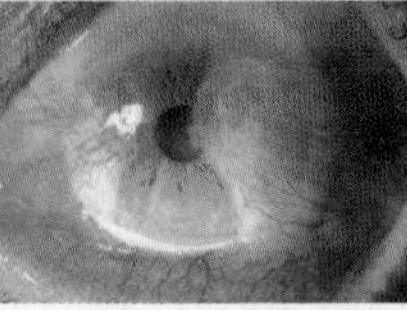

Figure 7-6 Double pterygium. Note both nasal and temporal pterygia in a 57-year-old farmer. (From Brightbill FS, McDonnell PJ: Corneal Surgery: Theory, Technique and Tissue, S.l., Mosby Elsevier, 2009)

Item 7-2 Pterygium is Greek for batlike. The condition is characterized by a membrane that extends from the limbus to the center of the cornea and resembles a wing.

● **H11.1 Conjunctival degenerations and deposits**
Excludes2 pseudopterygium (H11.81)
H11.10 Unspecified conjunctival degenerations
● **H11.11 Conjunctival deposits**
H11.111 Conjunctival deposits, right eye
H11.112 Conjunctival deposits, left eye
H11.113 Conjunctival deposits, bilateral
H11.119 Conjunctival deposits, unspecified eye
● **H11.12 Conjunctival concretions**
White to yellow nodules within or beneath conjunctiva
H11.121 Conjunctival concretions, right eye
H11.122 Conjunctival concretions, left eye
H11.123 Conjunctival concretions, bilateral
H11.129 Conjunctival concretions, unspecified eye
● **H11.13 Conjunctival pigmentations**
Conjunctival argyrosis [argyria]
H11.131 Conjunctival pigmentations, right eye
H11.132 Conjunctival pigmentations, left eye
H11.133 Conjunctival pigmentations, bilateral
H11.139 Conjunctival pigmentations, unspecified eye
● **H11.14 Conjunctival xerosis, unspecified**
Excludes1 xerosis of conjunctiva due to vitamin A deficiency (E50.0, E50.1)
H11.141 Conjunctival xerosis, unspecified, right eye
H11.142 Conjunctival xerosis, unspecified, left eye
H11.143 Conjunctival xerosis, unspecified, bilateral
H11.149 Conjunctival xerosis, unspecified, unspecified eye
● **H11.15 Pinguecula**
Yellowish spot near sclerocorneal junction, usually on nasal side; associated with aging
Excludes1 pingueculitis (H10.81-)
H11.151 Pinguecula, right eye
H11.152 Pinguecula, left eye
H11.153 Pinguecula, bilateral
H11.159 Pinguecula, unspecified eye
● **H11.2 Conjunctival scars**
● **H11.21 Conjunctival adhesions and strands (localized)**
H11.211 Conjunctival adhesions and strands (localized), right eye
H11.212 Conjunctival adhesions and strands (localized), left eye
H11.213 Conjunctival adhesions and strands (localized), bilateral
H11.219 Conjunctival adhesions and strands (localized), unspecified eye
● **H11.22 Conjunctival granuloma**
H11.221 Conjunctival granuloma, right eye
H11.222 Conjunctival granuloma, left eye
H11.223 Conjunctival granuloma, bilateral
H11.229 Conjunctival granuloma, unspecified
● **H11.23 Symblepharon**
Adhesion between tarsal conjunctiva and bulbar conjunctiva
H11.231 Symblepharon, right eye
H11.232 Symblepharon, left eye
H11.233 Symblepharon, bilateral
H11.239 Symblepharon, unspecified eye
● **H11.24 Scarring of conjunctiva**
H11.241 Scarring of conjunctiva, right eye
H11.242 Scarring of conjunctiva, left eye
H11.243 Scarring of conjunctiva, bilateral
H11.249 Scarring of conjunctiva, unspecified eye
● **H11.3 Conjunctival hemorrhage**
Subconjunctival hemorrhage
H11.30 Conjunctival hemorrhage, unspecified eye
H11.31 Conjunctival hemorrhage, right eye
H11.32 Conjunctival hemorrhage, left eye
H11.33 Conjunctival hemorrhage, bilateral
● **H11.4 Other conjunctival vascular disorders and cysts**
● **H11.41 Vascular abnormalities of conjunctiva**
Conjunctival aneurysm
H11.411 Vascular abnormalities of conjunctiva, right eye
H11.412 Vascular abnormalities of conjunctiva, left eye
H11.413 Vascular abnormalities of conjunctiva, bilateral
H11.419 Vascular abnormalities of conjunctiva, unspecified eye
● **H11.42 Conjunctival edema**
H11.421 Conjunctival edema, right eye
H11.422 Conjunctival edema, left eye
H11.423 Conjunctival edema, bilateral
H11.429 Conjunctival edema, unspecified eye
● **H11.43 Conjunctival hyperemia**
H11.431 Conjunctival hyperemia, right eye
H11.432 Conjunctival hyperemia, left eye
H11.433 Conjunctival hyperemia, bilateral
H11.439 Conjunctival hyperemia, unspecified eye
● **H11.44 Conjunctival cysts**
H11.441 Conjunctival cysts, right eye
H11.442 Conjunctival cysts, left eye
H11.443 Conjunctival cysts, bilateral
H11.449 Conjunctival cysts, unspecified eye
● **H11.8 Other specified disorders of conjunctiva**
● **H11.81 Pseudopterygium of conjunctiva**
Conjunctival scar attached to cornea
H11.811 Pseudopterygium of conjunctiva, right eye
H11.812 Pseudopterygium of conjunctiva, left eye
H11.813 Pseudopterygium of conjunctiva, bilateral
H11.819 Pseudopterygium of conjunctiva, unspecified eye
● **H11.82 Conjunctivochalasis**
Conjunctiva bulges over eyelid margin or covers lower punctum
H11.821 Conjunctivochalasis, right eye
H11.822 Conjunctivochalasis, left eye
H11.823 Conjunctivochalasis, bilateral
H11.829 Conjunctivochalasis, unspecified eye
H11.89 Other specified disorders of conjunctiva
H11.9 Unspecified disorder of conjunctiva

CHAPTER 7 (H00-H59)

DISORDERS OF SCLERA, CORNEA, IRIS AND CILIARY BODY (H15-H22)

● H15 Disorders of sclera
- ● H15.0 Scleritis
  Inflammation of the white (sclera and episclera) of the eye.
  - ● H15.00 Unspecified scleritis
    - H15.001 Unspecified scleritis, right eye
    - H15.002 Unspecified scleritis, left eye
    - H15.003 Unspecified scleritis, bilateral
    - H15.009 Unspecified scleritis, unspecified eye
  - ● H15.01 Anterior scleritis
    - H15.011 Anterior scleritis, right eye
    - H15.012 Anterior scleritis, left eye
    - H15.013 Anterior scleritis, bilateral
    - H15.019 Anterior scleritis, unspecified eye
  - ● H15.02 Brawny scleritis
    Swelling around the cornea that is gelantinous in appearance
    - H15.021 Brawny scleritis, right eye
    - H15.022 Brawny scleritis, left eye
    - H15.023 Brawny scleritis, bilateral
    - H15.029 Brawny scleritis, unspecified eye
  - ● H15.03 Posterior scleritis
    Sclerotenonitis
    - H15.031 Posterior scleritis, right eye
    - H15.032 Posterior scleritis, left eye
    - H15.033 Posterior scleritis, bilateral
    - H15.039 Posterior scleritis, unspecified eye
  - ● H15.04 Scleritis with corneal involvement
    - H15.041 Scleritis with corneal involvement, right eye
    - H15.042 Scleritis with corneal involvement, left eye
    - H15.043 Scleritis with corneal involvement, bilateral
    - H15.049 Scleritis with corneal involvement, unspecified eye
  - ● H15.05 Scleromalacia perforans
    Necrotic without inflammation; usually associated with rheumatoid arthritis
    - H15.051 Scleromalacia perforans, right eye
    - H15.052 Scleromalacia perforans, left eye
    - H15.053 Scleromalacia perforans, bilateral
    - H15.059 Scleromalacia perforans, unspecified eye
  - ● H15.09 Other scleritis
    Scleral abscess
    - H15.091 Other scleritis, right eye
    - H15.092 Other scleritis, left eye
    - H15.093 Other scleritis, bilateral
    - H15.099 Other scleritis, unspecified eye
- ● H15.1 Episcleritis
  Inflammation of the white (sclera and episclera) of the eye.
  - ● H15.10 Unspecified episcleritis
    - H15.101 Unspecified episcleritis, right eye
    - H15.102 Unspecified episcleritis, left eye
    - H15.103 Unspecified episcleritis, bilateral
    - H15.109 Unspecified episcleritis, unspecified eye
  - ● H15.11 Episcleritis periodica fugax
    Transient, recurrent inflammation of portion of episclera (connective tissue on the surface of the sclera)
    - H15.111 Episcleritis periodica fugax, right eye
    - H15.112 Episcleritis periodica fugax, left eye
    - H15.113 Episcleritis periodica fugax, bilateral
    - H15.119 Episcleritis periodica fugax, unspecified eye
  - ● H15.12 Nodular episcleritis
    Characterized by tender, localized, moveable nodule within inflamed area
    - H15.121 Nodular episcleritis, right eye
    - H15.122 Nodular episcleritis, left eye
    - H15.123 Nodular episcleritis, bilateral
    - H15.129 Nodular episcleritis, unspecified eye
- ● H15.8 Other disorders of sclera
  Excludes2 blue sclera (Q13.5)
  degenerative myopia (H44.2-)
  - ● H15.81 Equatorial staphyloma
    - H15.811 Equatorial staphyloma, right eye
    - H15.812 Equatorial staphyloma, left eye
    - H15.813 Equatorial staphyloma, bilateral
    - H15.819 Equatorial staphyloma, unspecified eye
  - ● H15.82 Localized anterior staphyloma
    - H15.821 Localized anterior staphyloma, right eye
    - H15.822 Localized anterior staphyloma, left eye
    - H15.823 Localized anterior staphyloma, bilateral
    - H15.829 Localized anterior staphyloma, unspecified eye
  - ● H15.83 Staphyloma posticum
    - H15.831 Staphyloma posticum, right eye
    - H15.832 Staphyloma posticum, left eye
    - H15.833 Staphyloma posticum, bilateral
    - H15.839 Staphyloma posticum, unspecified eye
  - ● H15.84 Scleral ectasia
    - H15.841 Scleral ectasia, right eye
    - H15.842 Scleral ectasia, left eye
    - H15.843 Scleral ectasia, bilateral
    - H15.849 Scleral ectasia, unspecified eye
  - ● H15.85 Ring staphyloma
    - H15.851 Ring staphyloma, right eye
    - H15.852 Ring staphyloma, left eye
    - H15.853 Ring staphyloma, bilateral
    - H15.859 Ring staphyloma, unspecified eye
  - H15.89 Other disorders of sclera
- H15.9 Unspecified disorder of sclera

● H16 Keratitis
- ● H16.0 Corneal ulcer
  - ● H16.00 Unspecified corneal ulcer
    - H16.001 Unspecified corneal ulcer, right eye
    - H16.002 Unspecified corneal ulcer, left eye
    - H16.003 Unspecified corneal ulcer, bilateral
    - H16.009 Unspecified corneal ulcer, unspecified eye
  - ● H16.01 Central corneal ulcer
    - H16.011 Central corneal ulcer, right eye
    - H16.012 Central corneal ulcer, left eye
    - H16.013 Central corneal ulcer, bilateral
    - H16.019 Central corneal ulcer, unspecified eye
  - ● H16.02 Ring corneal ulcer
    - H16.021 Ring corneal ulcer, right eye
    - H16.022 Ring corneal ulcer, left eye
    - H16.023 Ring corneal ulcer, bilateral
    - H16.029 Ring corneal ulcer, unspecified eye
  - ● H16.03 Corneal ulcer with hypopyon
    - H16.031 Corneal ulcer with hypopyon, right eye
    - H16.032 Corneal ulcer with hypopyon, left eye
    - H16.033 Corneal ulcer with hypopyon, bilateral
    - H16.039 Corneal ulcer with hypopyon, unspecified eye

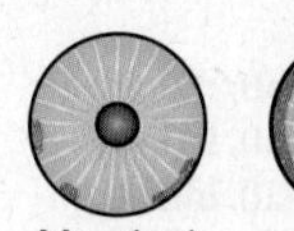

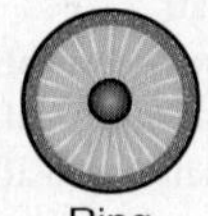

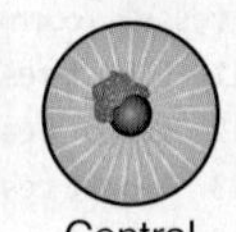

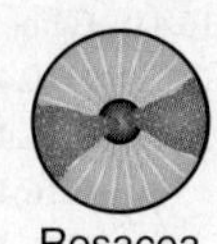

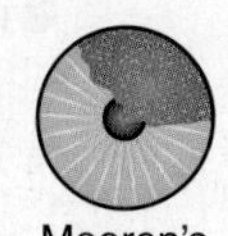

Figure 7-7 Corneal ulcers: marginal, ring, central corneal, rosacea, and Mooren's.

Item 7-3 An infected ulcer is usually called a **serpiginous** or **hypopyon** ulcer, which is a pus sac in the anterior chamber of the eye. **Marginal** ulcers are usually asymptomatic, not primary, and are often superficial and simple. More severe marginal ulcers spread to form a ring ulcer. **Ring** ulcers can extend around the entire corneal periphery. **Central corneal** ulcers develop when there is an abrasion to the epithelium and an infection develops in the eroded area. The **pyocyaneal** ulcer is the most serious corneal infection, which, if left untreated, can lead to loss of the eye.

- **H16.04 Marginal corneal ulcer**
  - **H16.041 Marginal corneal ulcer, right eye**
  - **H16.042 Marginal corneal ulcer, left eye**
  - **H16.043 Marginal corneal ulcer, bilateral**
  - **H16.049 Marginal corneal ulcer, unspecified eye**
- **H16.05 Mooren's corneal ulcer**
  - **H16.051 Mooren's corneal ulcer, right eye**
  - **H16.052 Mooren's corneal ulcer, left eye**
  - **H16.053 Mooren's corneal ulcer, bilateral**
  - **H16.059 Mooren's corneal ulcer, unspecified eye**
- **H16.06 Mycotic corneal ulcer**
  - **H16.061 Mycotic corneal ulcer, right eye**
  - **H16.062 Mycotic corneal ulcer, left eye**
  - **H16.063 Mycotic corneal ulcer, bilateral**
  - **H16.069 Mycotic corneal ulcer, unspecified eye**
- **H16.07 Perforated corneal ulcer**
  - **H16.071 Perforated corneal ulcer, right eye**
  - **H16.072 Perforated corneal ulcer, left eye**
  - **H16.073 Perforated corneal ulcer, bilateral**
  - **H16.079 Perforated corneal ulcer, unspecified eye**

H16.1 Other and unspecified superficial keratitis without conjunctivitis

- **H16.10 Unspecified superficial keratitis**
  - **H16.101 Unspecified superficial keratitis, right eye**
  - **H16.102 Unspecified superficial keratitis, left eye**
  - **H16.103 Unspecified superficial keratitis, bilateral**
  - **H16.109 Unspecified superficial keratitis, unspecified eye**
- **H16.11 Macular keratitis**
  Areolar keratitis
  Nummular keratitis
  Stellate keratitis
  Striate keratitis
  - **H16.111 Macular keratitis, right eye**
  - **H16.112 Macular keratitis, left eye**
  - **H16.113 Macular keratitis, bilateral**
  - **H16.119 Macular keratitis, unspecified eye**
- **H16.12 Filamentary keratitis**
  - **H16.121 Filamentary keratitis, right eye**
  - **H16.122 Filamentary keratitis, left eye**
  - **H16.123 Filamentary keratitis, bilateral**
  - **H16.129 Filamentary keratitis, unspecified eye**
- **H16.13 Photokeratitis**
  Snow blindness
  Welders' keratitis
  - **H16.131 Photokeratitis, right eye**
  - **H16.132 Photokeratitis, left eye**
  - **H16.133 Photokeratitis, bilateral**
  - **H16.139 Photokeratitis, unspecified eye**
- **H16.14 Punctate keratitis**
  - **H16.141 Punctate keratitis, right eye**
  - **H16.142 Punctate keratitis, left eye**
  - **H16.143 Punctate keratitis, bilateral**
  - **H16.149 Punctate keratitis, unspecified eye**

H16.2 Keratoconjunctivitis

- **H16.20 Unspecified keratoconjunctivitis**
  Superficial keratitis with conjunctivitis NOS
  - **H16.201 Unspecified keratoconjunctivitis, right eye**
  - **H16.202 Unspecified keratoconjunctivitis, left eye**
  - **H16.203 Unspecified keratoconjunctivitis, bilateral**
  - **H16.209 Unspecified keratoconjunctivitis, unspecified eye**
- **H16.21 Exposure keratoconjunctivitis**
  - **H16.211 Exposure keratoconjunctivitis, right eye**
  - **H16.212 Exposure keratoconjunctivitis, left eye**
  - **H16.213 Exposure keratoconjunctivitis, bilateral**
  - **H16.219 Exposure keratoconjunctivitis, unspecified eye**
- **H16.22 Keratoconjunctivitis sicca, not specified as Sjögren's**
  Excludes1 Sjogren's syndrome (M35.01)
  - **H16.221 Keratoconjunctivitis sicca, not specified as Sjögren's, right eye**
  - **H16.222 Keratoconjunctivitis sicca, not specified as Sjögren's, left eye**
  - **H16.223 Keratoconjunctivitis sicca, not specified as Sjögren's, bilateral**
  - **H16.229 Keratoconjunctivitis sicca, not specified as Sjögren's, unspecified eye**
- **H16.23 Neurotrophic keratoconjunctivitis**
  - **H16.231 Neurotrophic keratoconjunctivitis, right eye**
  - **H16.232 Neurotrophic keratoconjunctivitis, left eye**
  - **H16.233 Neurotrophic keratoconjunctivitis, bilateral**
  - **H16.239 Neurotrophic keratoconjunctivitis, unspecified eye**
- **H16.24 Ophthalmia nodosa**
  - **H16.241 Ophthalmia nodosa, right eye**
  - **H16.242 Ophthalmia nodosa, left eye**
  - **H16.243 Ophthalmia nodosa, bilateral**
  - **H16.249 Ophthalmia nodosa, unspecified eye**
- **H16.25 Phlyctenular keratoconjunctivitis**
  - **H16.251 Phlyctenular keratoconjunctivitis, right eye**
  - **H16.252 Phlyctenular keratoconjunctivitis, left eye**
  - **H16.253 Phlyctenular keratoconjunctivitis, bilateral**
  - **H16.259 Phlyctenular keratoconjunctivitis, unspecified eye**

H16.26 Vernal keratoconjunctivitis, with limbar and corneal involvement

Excludes1 vernal conjunctivitis without limbar and corneal involvement (H10.44)

H16.261 Vernal keratoconjunctivitis, with limbar and corneal involvement, right eye

H16.262 Vernal keratoconjunctivitis, with limbar and corneal involvement, left eye

H16.263 Vernal keratoconjunctivitis, with limbar and corneal involvement, bilateral

H16.269 Vernal keratoconjunctivitis, with limbar and corneal involvement, unspecified eye

H16.29 Other keratoconjunctivitis

H16.291 Other keratoconjunctivitis, right eye

H16.292 Other keratoconjunctivitis, left eye

H16.293 Other keratoconjunctivitis, bilateral

H16.299 Other keratoconjunctivitis, unspecified eye

H16.3 Interstitial and deep keratitis

H16.30 Unspecified interstitial keratitis

H16.301 Unspecified interstitial keratitis, right eye

H16.302 Unspecified interstitial keratitis, left eye

H16.303 Unspecified interstitial keratitis, bilateral

H16.309 Unspecified interstitial keratitis, unspecified eye

H16.31 Corneal abscess

H16.311 Corneal abscess, right eye

H16.312 Corneal abscess, left eye

H16.313 Corneal abscess, bilateral

H16.319 Corneal abscess, unspecified eye

H16.32 Diffuse interstitial keratitis

Cogan's syndrome

H16.321 Diffuse interstitial keratitis, right eye

H16.322 Diffuse interstitial keratitis, left eye

H16.323 Diffuse interstitial keratitis, bilateral

H16.329 Diffuse interstitial keratitis, unspecified eye

H16.33 Sclerosing keratitis

H16.331 Sclerosing keratitis, right eye

H16.332 Sclerosing keratitis, left eye

H16.333 Sclerosing keratitis, bilateral

H16.339 Sclerosing keratitis, unspecified eye

H16.39 Other interstitial and deep keratitis

H16.391 Other interstitial and deep keratitis, right eye

H16.392 Other interstitial and deep keratitis, left eye

H16.393 Other interstitial and deep keratitis, bilateral

H16.399 Other interstitial and deep keratitis, unspecified eye

H16.4 Corneal neovascularization

H16.40 Unspecified corneal neovascularization

H16.401 Unspecified corneal neovascularization, right eye

H16.402 Unspecified corneal neovascularization, left eye

H16.403 Unspecified corneal neovascularization, bilateral

H16.409 Unspecified corneal neovascularization, unspecified eye

H16.41 Ghost vessels (corneal)

H16.411 Ghost vessels (corneal), right eye

H16.412 Ghost vessels (corneal), left eye

H16.413 Ghost vessels (corneal), bilateral

H16.419 Ghost vessels (corneal), unspecified eye

H16.42 Pannus (corneal)

H16.421 Pannus (corneal), right eye

H16.422 Pannus (corneal), left eye

H16.423 Pannus (corneal), bilateral

H16.429 Pannus (corneal), unspecified eye

H16.43 Localized vascularization of cornea

H16.431 Localized vascularization of cornea, right eye

H16.432 Localized vascularization of cornea, left eye

H16.433 Localized vascularization of cornea, bilateral

H16.439 Localized vascularization of cornea, unspecified eye

H16.44 Deep vascularization of cornea

H16.441 Deep vascularization of cornea, right eye

H16.442 Deep vascularization of cornea, left eye

H16.443 Deep vascularization of cornea, bilateral

H16.449 Deep vascularization of cornea, unspecified eye

H16.8 Other keratitis

H16.9 Unspecified keratitis

H17 Corneal scars and opacities

H17.0 Adherent leukoma

H17.00 Adherent leukoma, unspecified eye

H17.01 Adherent leukoma, right eye

H17.02 Adherent leukoma, left eye

H17.03 Adherent leukoma, bilateral

H17.1 Central corneal opacity

H17.10 Central corneal opacity, unspecified eye

H17.11 Central corneal opacity, right eye

H17.12 Central corneal opacity, left eye

H17.13 Central corneal opacity, bilateral

H17.8 Other corneal scars and opacities

H17.81 Minor opacity of cornea

Corneal nebula

H17.811 Minor opacity of cornea, right eye

H17.812 Minor opacity of cornea, left eye

H17.813 Minor opacity of cornea, bilateral

H17.819 Minor opacity of cornea, unspecified eye

H17.82 Peripheral opacity of cornea

H17.821 Peripheral opacity of cornea, right eye

H17.822 Peripheral opacity of cornea, left eye

H17.823 Peripheral opacity of cornea, bilateral

H17.829 Peripheral opacity of cornea, unspecified eye

H17.89 Other corneal scars and opacities

H17.9 Unspecified corneal scar and opacity

H18 Other disorders of cornea

H18.0 Corneal pigmentations and deposits

H18.00 Unspecified corneal deposit

H18.001 Unspecified corneal deposit, right eye

H18.002 Unspecified corneal deposit, left eye

H18.003 Unspecified corneal deposit, bilateral

H18.009 Unspecified corneal deposit, unspecified eye

H18.01 Anterior corneal pigmentations
Staehli's line
H18.011 Anterior corneal pigmentations, right eye
H18.012 Anterior corneal pigmentations, left eye
H18.013 Anterior corneal pigmentations, bilateral
H18.019 Anterior corneal pigmentations, unspecified eye
H18.02 Argentous corneal deposits
H18.021 Argentous corneal deposits, right eye
H18.022 Argentous corneal deposits, left eye
H18.023 Argentous corneal deposits, bilateral
H18.029 Argentous corneal deposits, unspecified eye
H18.03 Corneal deposits in metabolic disorders
Code also associated metabolic disorder
H18.031 Corneal deposits in metabolic disorders, right eye
H18.032 Corneal deposits in metabolic disorders, left eye
H18.033 Corneal deposits in metabolic disorders, bilateral
H18.039 Corneal deposits in metabolic disorders, unspecified eye
H18.04 Kayser-Fleischer ring
Code also associated Wilson's disease (E83.01)
H18.041 Kayser-Fleischer ring, right eye
H18.042 Kayser-Fleischer ring, left eye
H18.043 Kayser-Fleischer ring, bilateral
H18.049 Kayser-Fleischer ring, unspecified eye
H18.05 Posterior corneal pigmentations
Krukenberg's spindle
H18.051 Posterior corneal pigmentations, right eye
H18.052 Posterior corneal pigmentations, left eye
H18.053 Posterior corneal pigmentations, bilateral
H18.059 Posterior corneal pigmentations, unspecified eye
H18.06 Stromal corneal pigmentations
Hematocornea
H18.061 Stromal corneal pigmentations, right eye
H18.062 Stromal corneal pigmentations, left eye
H18.063 Stromal corneal pigmentations, bilateral
H18.069 Stromal corneal pigmentations, unspecified eye
H18.1 Bullous keratopathy
H18.10 Bullous keratopathy, unspecified eye
H18.11 Bullous keratopathy, right eye
H18.12 Bullous keratopathy, left eye
H18.13 Bullous keratopathy, bilateral
H18.2 Other and unspecified corneal edema
H18.20 Unspecified corneal edema
H18.21 Corneal edema secondary to contact lens
Excludes2 other corneal disorders due to contact lens (H18.82-)
H18.211 Corneal edema secondary to contact lens, right eye
H18.212 Corneal edema secondary to contact lens, left eye
H18.213 Corneal edema secondary to contact lens, bilateral
H18.219 Corneal edema secondary to contact lens, unspecified eye
H18.22 Idiopathic corneal edema
H18.221 Idiopathic corneal edema, right eye
H18.222 Idiopathic corneal edema, left eye
H18.223 Idiopathic corneal edema, bilateral
H18.229 Idiopathic corneal edema, unspecified eye
H18.23 Secondary corneal edema
H18.231 Secondary corneal edema, right eye
H18.232 Secondary corneal edema, left eye
H18.233 Secondary corneal edema, bilateral
H18.239 Secondary corneal edema, unspecified eye
H18.3 Changes of corneal membranes
H18.30 Unspecified corneal membrane change
H18.31 Folds and rupture in Bowman's membrane
H18.311 Folds and rupture in Bowman's membrane, right eye
H18.312 Folds and rupture in Bowman's membrane, left eye
H18.313 Folds and rupture in Bowman's membrane, bilateral
H18.319 Folds and rupture in Bowman's membrane, unspecified eye
H18.32 Folds in Descemet's membrane
H18.321 Folds in Descemet's membrane, right eye
H18.322 Folds in Descemet's membrane, left eye
H18.323 Folds in Descemet's membrane, bilateral
H18.329 Folds in Descemet's membrane, unspecified eye
H18.33 Rupture in Descemet's membrane
H18.331 Rupture in Descemet's membrane, right eye
H18.332 Rupture in Descemet's membrane, left eye
H18.333 Rupture in Descemet's membrane, bilateral
H18.339 Rupture in Descemet's membrane, unspecified eye
H18.4 Corneal degeneration
Excludes1 Mooren's ulcer (H16.0-)
recurrent erosion of cornea (H18.83-)
H18.40 Unspecified corneal degeneration
H18.41 Arcus senilis
Senile corneal changes
H18.411 Arcus senilis, right eye
H18.412 Arcus senilis, left eye
H18.413 Arcus senilis, bilateral
H18.419 Arcus senilis, unspecified eye
H18.42 Band keratopathy
H18.421 Band keratopathy, right eye
H18.422 Band keratopathy, left eye
H18.423 Band keratopathy, bilateral
H18.429 Band keratopathy, unspecified eye
H18.43 Other calcerous corneal degeneration
H18.44 Keratomalacia
Excludes1 keratomalacia due to vitamin A deficiency (E50.4)
H18.441 Keratomalacia, right eye
H18.442 Keratomalacia, left eye
H18.443 Keratomalacia, bilateral
H18.449 Keratomalacia, unspecified eye

CHAPTER 7 (H00-H59)

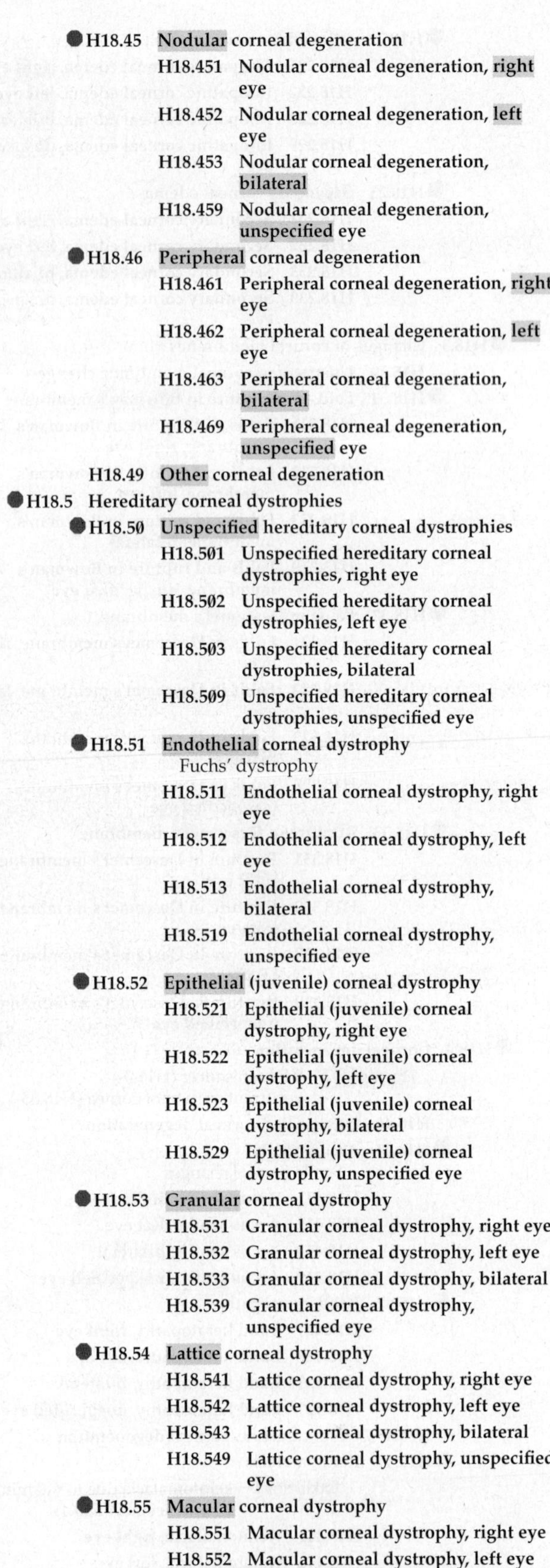

H18.45 Nodular corneal degeneration
- H18.451 Nodular corneal degeneration, right eye
- H18.452 Nodular corneal degeneration, left eye
- H18.453 Nodular corneal degeneration, bilateral
- H18.459 Nodular corneal degeneration, unspecified eye

H18.46 Peripheral corneal degeneration
- H18.461 Peripheral corneal degeneration, right eye
- H18.462 Peripheral corneal degeneration, left eye
- H18.463 Peripheral corneal degeneration, bilateral
- H18.469 Peripheral corneal degeneration, unspecified eye

H18.49 Other corneal degeneration

H18.5 Hereditary corneal dystrophies

H18.5Ø Unspecified hereditary corneal dystrophies
- H18.5Ø1 Unspecified hereditary corneal dystrophies, right eye
- H18.5Ø2 Unspecified hereditary corneal dystrophies, left eye
- H18.5Ø3 Unspecified hereditary corneal dystrophies, bilateral
- H18.5Ø9 Unspecified hereditary corneal dystrophies, unspecified eye

H18.51 Endothelial corneal dystrophy

Fuchs' dystrophy
- H18.511 Endothelial corneal dystrophy, right eye
- H18.512 Endothelial corneal dystrophy, left eye
- H18.513 Endothelial corneal dystrophy, bilateral
- H18.519 Endothelial corneal dystrophy, unspecified eye

H18.52 Epithelial (juvenile) corneal dystrophy
- H18.521 Epithelial (juvenile) corneal dystrophy, right eye
- H18.522 Epithelial (juvenile) corneal dystrophy, left eye
- H18.523 Epithelial (juvenile) corneal dystrophy, bilateral
- H18.529 Epithelial (juvenile) corneal dystrophy, unspecified eye

H18.53 Granular corneal dystrophy
- H18.531 Granular corneal dystrophy, right eye
- H18.532 Granular corneal dystrophy, left eye
- H18.533 Granular corneal dystrophy, bilateral
- H18.539 Granular corneal dystrophy, unspecified eye

H18.54 Lattice corneal dystrophy
- H18.541 Lattice corneal dystrophy, right eye
- H18.542 Lattice corneal dystrophy, left eye
- H18.543 Lattice corneal dystrophy, bilateral
- H18.549 Lattice corneal dystrophy, unspecified eye

H18.55 Macular corneal dystrophy
- H18.551 Macular corneal dystrophy, right eye
- H18.552 Macular corneal dystrophy, left eye
- H18.553 Macular corneal dystrophy, bilateral
- H18.559 Macular corneal dystrophy, unspecified eye

H18.59 Other hereditary corneal dystrophies
- H18.591 Other hereditary corneal dystrophies, right eye
- H18.592 Other hereditary corneal dystrophies, left eye
- H18.593 Other hereditary corneal dystrophies, bilateral
- H18.599 Other hereditary corneal dystrophies, unspecified eye

H18.6 Keratoconus

H18.6Ø Keratoconus, unspecified
- H18.6Ø1 Keratoconus, unspecified, right eye
- H18.6Ø2 Keratoconus, unspecified, left eye
- H18.6Ø3 Keratoconus, unspecified, bilateral
- H18.6Ø9 Keratoconus, unspecified, unspecified eye

H18.61 Keratoconus, stable
- H18.611 Keratoconus, stable, right eye
- H18.612 Keratoconus, stable, left eye
- H18.613 Keratoconus, stable, bilateral
- H18.619 Keratoconus, stable, unspecified eye

H18.62 Keratoconus, unstable

Acute hydrops
- H18.621 Keratoconus, unstable, right eye
- H18.622 Keratoconus, unstable, left eye
- H18.623 Keratoconus, unstable, bilateral
- H18.629 Keratoconus, unstable, unspecified eye

H18.7 Other and unspecified corneal deformities

Excludes1 congenital malformations of cornea (Q13.3-Q13.4)

H18.7Ø Unspecified corneal deformity

H18.71 Corneal ectasia
- H18.711 Corneal ectasia, right eye
- H18.712 Corneal ectasia, left eye
- H18.713 Corneal ectasia, bilateral
- H18.719 Corneal ectasia, unspecified eye

H18.72 Corneal staphyloma
- H18.721 Corneal staphyloma, right eye
- H18.722 Corneal staphyloma, left eye
- H18.723 Corneal staphyloma, bilateral
- H18.729 Corneal staphyloma, unspecified eye

H18.73 Descemetocele
- H18.731 Descemetocele, right eye
- H18.732 Descemetocele, left eye
- H18.733 Descemetocele, bilateral
- H18.739 Descemetocele, unspecified eye

H18.79 Other corneal deformities
- H18.791 Other corneal deformities, right eye
- H18.792 Other corneal deformities, left eye
- H18.793 Other corneal deformities, bilateral
- H18.799 Other corneal deformities, unspecified eye

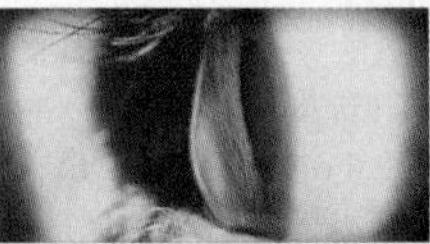

Figure 7-8 Lateral view of the displacement of the cone apex in keratoconus. (From Yanoff: Ophthalmology, ed 3, Mosby, Inc., 2008)

Item 7-4 Keratoconus results in corneal degeneration that begins in childhood, gradually changes the cornea from a round to cone shape, decreasing visual acuity. Treatment includes contact lenses. In severe cases the need for corneal transplant may be the treatment of choice; however, newer technologies may use high-frequency radio energy to shrink the edges of the cornea, pulling the central area back to a more normal shape. It can help delay or avoid the need for a corneal transplantation.

H18.8 Other specified disorders of cornea

H18.81 Anesthesia and hypoesthesia of cornea

H18.811 Anesthesia and hypoesthesia of cornea, right eye

H18.812 Anesthesia and hypoesthesia of cornea, left eye

H18.813 Anesthesia and hypoesthesia of cornea, bilateral

H18.819 Anesthesia and hypoesthesia of cornea, unspecified eye

H18.82 Corneal disorder due to contact lens

Excludes2 corneal edema due to contact lens (H18.21-)

H18.821 Corneal disorder due to contact lens, right eye

H18.822 Corneal disorder due to contact lens, left eye

H18.823 Corneal disorder due to contact lens, bilateral

H18.829 Corneal disorder due to contact lens, unspecified eye

H18.83 Recurrent erosion of cornea

H18.831 Recurrent erosion of cornea, right eye

H18.832 Recurrent erosion of cornea, left eye

H18.833 Recurrent erosion of cornea, bilateral

H18.839 Recurrent erosion of cornea, unspecified eye

H18.89 Other specified disorders of cornea

H18.891 Other specified disorders of cornea, right eye

H18.892 Other specified disorders of cornea, left eye

H18.893 Other specified disorders of cornea, bilateral

H18.899 Other specified disorders of cornea, unspecified eye

H18.9 Unspecified disorder of cornea

H20 Iridocyclitis

H20.0 Acute and subacute iridocyclitis (Ex) PDX 791

Acute anterior uveitis
Acute cyclitis
Acute iritis
Subacute anterior uveitis
Subacute cyclitis
Subacute iritis

Excludes1 iridocyclitis, iritis, uveitis (due to) (in) diabetes mellitus (E08-E13 with .39)
iridocyclitis, iritis, uveitis (due to) (in) diphtheria (A36.89)
iridocyclitis, iritis, uveitis (due to) (in) gonococcal (A54.32)
iridocyclitis, iritis, uveitis (due to) (in) herpes (simplex) (B00.51)
iridocyclitis, iritis, uveitis (due to) (in) herpes zoster (B02.32)
iridocyclitis, iritis, uveitis (due to) (in) late congenital syphilis (A50.39)
iridocyclitis, iritis, uveitis (due to) (in) late syphilis (A52.71)
iridocyclitis, iritis, uveitis (due to) (in) sarcoidosis (D86.83)
iridocyclitis, iritis, uveitis (due to) (in) syphilis (A51.43)
iridocyclitis, iritis, uveitis (due to) (in) toxoplasmosis (B58.09)
iridocyclitis, iritis, uveitis (due to) (in) tuberculosis (A18.54)

H20.00 Unspecified acute and subacute iridocyclitis

H20.01 Primary iridocyclitis

H20.011 Primary iridocyclitis, right eye

H20.012 Primary iridocyclitis, left eye

H20.013 Primary iridocyclitis, bilateral

H20.019 Primary iridocyclitis, unspecified eye

H20.02 Recurrent acute iridocyclitis

H20.021 Recurrent acute iridocyclitis, right eye

H20.022 Recurrent acute iridocyclitis, left eye

H20.023 Recurrent acute iridocyclitis, bilateral

H20.029 Recurrent acute iridocyclitis, unspecified eye

H20.03 Secondary infectious iridocyclitis

H20.031 Secondary infectious iridocyclitis, right eye

H20.032 Secondary infectious iridocyclitis, left eye

H20.033 Secondary infectious iridocyclitis, bilateral

H20.039 Secondary infectious iridocyclitis, unspecified eye

H20.04 Secondary noninfectious iridocyclitis

H20.041 Secondary noninfectious iridocyclitis, right eye

H20.042 Secondary noninfectious iridocyclitis, left eye

H20.043 Secondary noninfectious iridocyclitis, bilateral

H20.049 Secondary noninfectious iridocyclitis, unspecified eye

H20.05 Hypopyon

H20.051 Hypopyon, right eye

H20.052 Hypopyon, left eye

H20.053 Hypopyon, bilateral

H20.059 Hypopyon, unspecified eye

H20.1 Chronic iridocyclitis

Use additional code for any associated cataract (H26.21-)

Excludes2 posterior cyclitis (H30.2-)

H20.10 Chronic iridocyclitis, unspecified eye

H20.11 Chronic iridocyclitis, right eye

H20.12 Chronic iridocyclitis, left eye

H20.13 Chronic iridocyclitis, bilateral

H20.2 Lens-induced iridocyclitis

H20.20 Lens-induced iridocyclitis, unspecified eye

H20.21 Lens-induced iridocyclitis, right eye

H20.22 Lens-induced iridocyclitis, left eye

H20.23 Lens-induced iridocyclitis, bilateral

H20.8 Other iridocyclitis

Excludes2 glaucomatocyclitis crises (H40.4-)
posterior cyclitis (H30.2-)
sympathetic uveitis (H44.13-)

H20.81 Fuchs' heterochromic cyclitis

H20.811 Fuchs' heterochromic cyclitis, right eye

H20.812 Fuchs' heterochromic cyclitis, left eye

H20.813 Fuchs' heterochromic cyclitis, bilateral

H20.819 Fuchs' heterochromic cyclitis, unspecified eye

CHAPTER 7 (H00-H59)

- H20.82 **Vogt-Koyanagi syndrome**
  - H20.821 Vogt-Koyanagi syndrome, right eye
  - H20.822 Vogt-Koyanagi syndrome, left eye
  - H20.823 Vogt-Koyanagi syndrome, bilateral
  - H20.829 Vogt-Koyanagi syndrome, unspecified eye
- H20.9 **Unspecified iridocyclitis** PDX 791
  - Uveitis NOS

H21 Other disorders of iris and ciliary body

Excludes2 sympathetic uveitis (H44.1-)

- H21.0 **Hyphema**
  - **Excludes1** traumatic hyphema (S05.1-)
  - H21.00 Hyphema, unspecified eye
  - H21.01 Hyphema, right eye
  - H21.02 Hyphema, left eye
  - H21.03 Hyphema, bilateral
- H21.1 **Other vascular disorders of iris and ciliary body**
  - Neovascularization of iris or ciliary body
  - Rubeosis iridis
  - Rubeosis of iris
  - H21.1X **Other vascular disorders of iris and ciliary body**
    - H21.1X1 Other vascular disorders of iris and ciliary body, right eye
    - H21.1X2 Other vascular disorders of iris and ciliary body, left eye
    - H21.1X3 Other vascular disorders of iris and ciliary body, bilateral
    - H21.1X9 Other vascular disorders of iris and ciliary body, unspecified eye
- H21.2 **Degeneration of iris and ciliary body**
  - H21.21 **Degeneration of chamber angle**
    - H21.211 Degeneration of chamber angle, right eye
    - H21.212 Degeneration of chamber angle, left eye
    - H21.213 Degeneration of chamber angle, bilateral
    - H21.219 Degeneration of chamber angle, unspecified eye
  - H21.22 **Degeneration of ciliary body**
    - H21.221 Degeneration of ciliary body, right eye
    - H21.222 Degeneration of ciliary body, left eye
    - H21.223 Degeneration of ciliary body, bilateral
    - H21.229 Degeneration of ciliary body, unspecified eye
  - H21.23 **Degeneration of iris (pigmentary)**
    - Translucency of iris
    - H21.231 Degeneration of iris (pigmentary), right eye
    - H21.232 Degeneration of iris (pigmentary), left eye
    - H21.233 Degeneration of iris (pigmentary), bilateral
    - H21.239 Degeneration of iris (pigmentary), unspecified eye
  - H21.24 **Degeneration of pupillary margin**
    - H21.241 Degeneration of pupillary margin, right eye
    - H21.242 Degeneration of pupillary margin, left eye
    - H21.243 Degeneration of pupillary margin, bilateral
    - H21.249 Degeneration of pupillary margin, unspecified eye
  - H21.25 **Iridoschisis**
    - H21.251 Iridoschisis, right eye
    - H21.252 Iridoschisis, left eye
    - H21.253 Iridoschisis, bilateral
    - H21.259 Iridoschisis, unspecified eye
  - H21.26 **Iris atrophy (essential) (progressive)**
    - H21.261 Iris atrophy (essential) (progressive), right eye
    - H21.262 Iris atrophy (essential) (progressive), left eye
    - H21.263 Iris atrophy (essential) (progressive), bilateral
    - H21.269 Iris atrophy (essential) (progressive), unspecified eye
  - H21.27 **Miotic pupillary cyst**
    - H21.271 Miotic pupillary cyst, right eye
    - H21.272 Miotic pupillary cyst, left eye
    - H21.273 Miotic pupillary cyst, bilateral
    - H21.279 Miotic pupillary cyst, unspecified eye
  - H21.29 **Other iris atrophy**
- H21.3 **Cyst of iris, ciliary body and anterior chamber**
  - **Excludes2** miotic pupillary cyst (H21.27-)
  - H21.30 **Idiopathic cysts of iris, ciliary body or anterior chamber**
    - Cyst of iris, ciliary body or anterior chamber NOS
    - H21.301 Idiopathic cysts of iris, ciliary body or anterior chamber, right eye
    - H21.302 Idiopathic cysts of iris, ciliary body or anterior chamber, left eye
    - H21.303 Idiopathic cysts of iris, ciliary body or anterior chamber, bilateral
    - H21.309 Idiopathic cysts of iris, ciliary body or anterior chamber, unspecified eye
  - H21.31 **Exudative cysts of iris or anterior chamber**
    - H21.311 Exudative cysts of iris or anterior chamber, right eye
    - H21.312 Exudative cysts of iris or anterior chamber, left eye
    - H21.313 Exudative cysts of iris or anterior chamber, bilateral
    - H21.319 Exudative cysts of iris or anterior chamber, unspecified eye
  - H21.32 **Implantation cysts of iris, ciliary body or anterior chamber**
    - H21.321 Implantation cysts of iris, ciliary body or anterior chamber, right eye
    - H21.322 Implantation cysts of iris, ciliary body or anterior chamber, left eye
    - H21.323 Implantation cysts of iris, ciliary body or anterior chamber, bilateral
    - H21.329 Implantation cysts of iris, ciliary body or anterior chamber, unspecified eye
  - H21.33 **Parasitic cyst of iris, ciliary body or anterior chamber** PDX 792
    - H21.331 Parasitic cyst of iris, ciliary body or anterior chamber, right eye
    - H21.332 Parasitic cyst of iris, ciliary body or anterior chamber, left eye
    - H21.333 Parasitic cyst of iris, ciliary body or anterior chamber, bilateral
    - H21.339 Parasitic cyst of iris, ciliary body or anterior chamber, unspecified eye

● **H21.34 Primary cyst of pars plana**
- **H21.341 Primary cyst of pars plana, right eye**
- **H21.342 Primary cyst of pars plana, left eye**
- **H21.343 Primary cyst of pars plana, bilateral**
- **H21.349 Primary cyst of pars plana, unspecified eye**

● **H21.35 Exudative cyst of pars plana**
- **H21.351 Exudative cyst of pars plana, right eye**
- **H21.352 Exudative cyst of pars plana, left eye**
- **H21.353 Exudative cyst of pars plana, bilateral**
- **H21.359 Exudative cyst of pars plana, unspecified eye**

● **H21.4 Pupillary membranes**
Iris bombé
Pupillary occlusion
Pupillary seclusion
Excludes1 congenital pupillary membranes (Q13.8)
- **H21.40 Pupillary membranes, unspecified eye**
- **H21.41 Pupillary membranes, right eye**
- **H21.42 Pupillary membranes, left eye**
- **H21.43 Pupillary membranes, bilateral**

● **H21.5 Other and unspecified adhesions and disruptions of iris and ciliary body**
Excludes1 corectopia (Q13.2)

● **H21.50 Unspecified adhesions of iris**
Synechia (iris) NOS
- **H21.501 Unspecified adhesions of iris, right eye**
- **H21.502 Unspecified adhesions of iris, left eye**
- **H21.503 Unspecified adhesions of iris, bilateral**
- **H21.509 Unspecified adhesions of iris and ciliary body, unspecified eye**

● **H21.51 Anterior synechiae (iris)**
- **H21.511 Anterior synechiae (iris), right eye**
- **H21.512 Anterior synechiae (iris), left eye**
- **H21.513 Anterior synechiae (iris), bilateral**
- **H21.519 Anterior synechiae (iris), unspecified eye**

● **H21.52 Goniosynechiae**
- **H21.521 Goniosynechiae, right eye**
- **H21.522 Goniosynechiae, left eye**
- **H21.523 Goniosynechiae, bilateral**
- **H21.529 Goniosynechiae, unspecified eye**

● **H21.53 Iridodialysis**
- **H21.531 Iridodialysis, right eye**
- **H21.532 Iridodialysis, left eye**
- **H21.533 Iridodialysis, bilateral**
- **H21.539 Iridodialysis, unspecified eye**

● **H21.54 Posterior synechiae (iris)**
- **H21.541 Posterior synechiae (iris), right eye**
- **H21.542 Posterior synechiae (iris), left eye**
- **H21.543 Posterior synechiae (iris), bilateral**
- **H21.549 Posterior synechiae (iris), unspecified eye**

● **H21.55 Recession of chamber angle**
- **H21.551 Recession of chamber angle, right eye**
- **H21.552 Recession of chamber angle, left eye**
- **H21.553 Recession of chamber angle, bilateral**
- **H21.559 Recession of chamber angle, unspecified eye**

● **H21.56 Pupillary abnormalities**
Deformed pupil
Ectopic pupil
Rupture of sphincter, pupil
Excludes1 congenital deformity of pupil (Q13.2-)
- **H21.561 Pupillary abnormality, right eye**
- **H21.562 Pupillary abnormality, left eye**
- **H21.563 Pupillary abnormality, bilateral**
- **H21.569 Pupillary abnormality, unspecified eye**

● **H21.8 Other specified disorders of iris and ciliary body**
- **H21.81 Floppy iris syndrome**
  Intraoperative floppy iris syndrome (IFIS)
  Use additional code for adverse effect, if applicable, to identify drug (T36-T50 with fifth or sixth character 5)
- **H21.82 Plateau iris syndrome (post-iridectomy) (postprocedural)**
- **H21.89 Other specified disorders of iris and ciliary body**

H21.9 Unspecified disorder of iris and ciliary body

◗ ***H22 Disorders of iris and ciliary body in diseases classified elsewhere***
Code first underlying disease, such as:
gout (M1A.-, M10.-)
leprosy (A30.-)
parasitic disease (B89)

DISORDERS OF LENS (H25-H28)

● **H25 Age-related cataract**
Senile cataract
Excludes2 capsular glaucoma with pseudoexfoliation of lens (H40.1-)

● **H25.0 Age-related incipient cataract**

● **H25.01 Cortical age-related cataract**
- **H25.011 Cortical age-related cataract, right eye** A
- **H25.012 Cortical age-related cataract, left eye** A
- **H25.013 Cortical age-related cataract, bilateral** A
- **H25.019 Cortical age-related cataract, unspecified eye** A

● **H25.03 Anterior subcapsular polar age-related cataract**
- **H25.031 Anterior subcapsular polar age-related cataract, right eye** A
- **H25.032 Anterior subcapsular polar age-related cataract, left eye** A
- **H25.033 Anterior subcapsular polar age-related cataract, bilateral** A
- **H25.039 Anterior subcapsular polar age-related cataract, unspecified eye** A

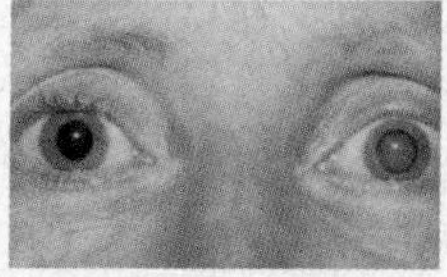

Figure 7-9 Age-related cataract. Nuclear sclerosis and cortical lens opacities are present. (From Ignatavicius DD, Workman ML: Medical-Surgical Nursing: Patient-Centered Collaborative Care, St. Louis, MO, Saunders/Elsevier, 2010)

Item 7-5 Senile cataracts are linked to the aging process. The most common area for the formation of a cataract is the cortical area of the lens. **Polar cataracts** can be either anterior or posterior. **Anterior polar cataracts** are more common and are small, white, capsular cataracts located on the anterior portion of the lens. **Total cataracts,** also called **complete** or **mature,** cause an opacity of all fibers of the lens. **Hypermature** describes a mature cataract with a swollen, milky cortex that covers the entire lens. **Immature,** also called **incipient,** cataracts have a clear cortex and are only slightly opaque. Treatment for all cataracts is the removal of the lens.

N Newborn Age: 0 **P** Pediatric Age: 0–17 **M** Maternity DX: 9–64 **A** Adult Age: 15–124
Complication\Comorbidity Major C\C CC/MCC Exclusions Hospital-Acquired Condition Hierarchical Condition Category

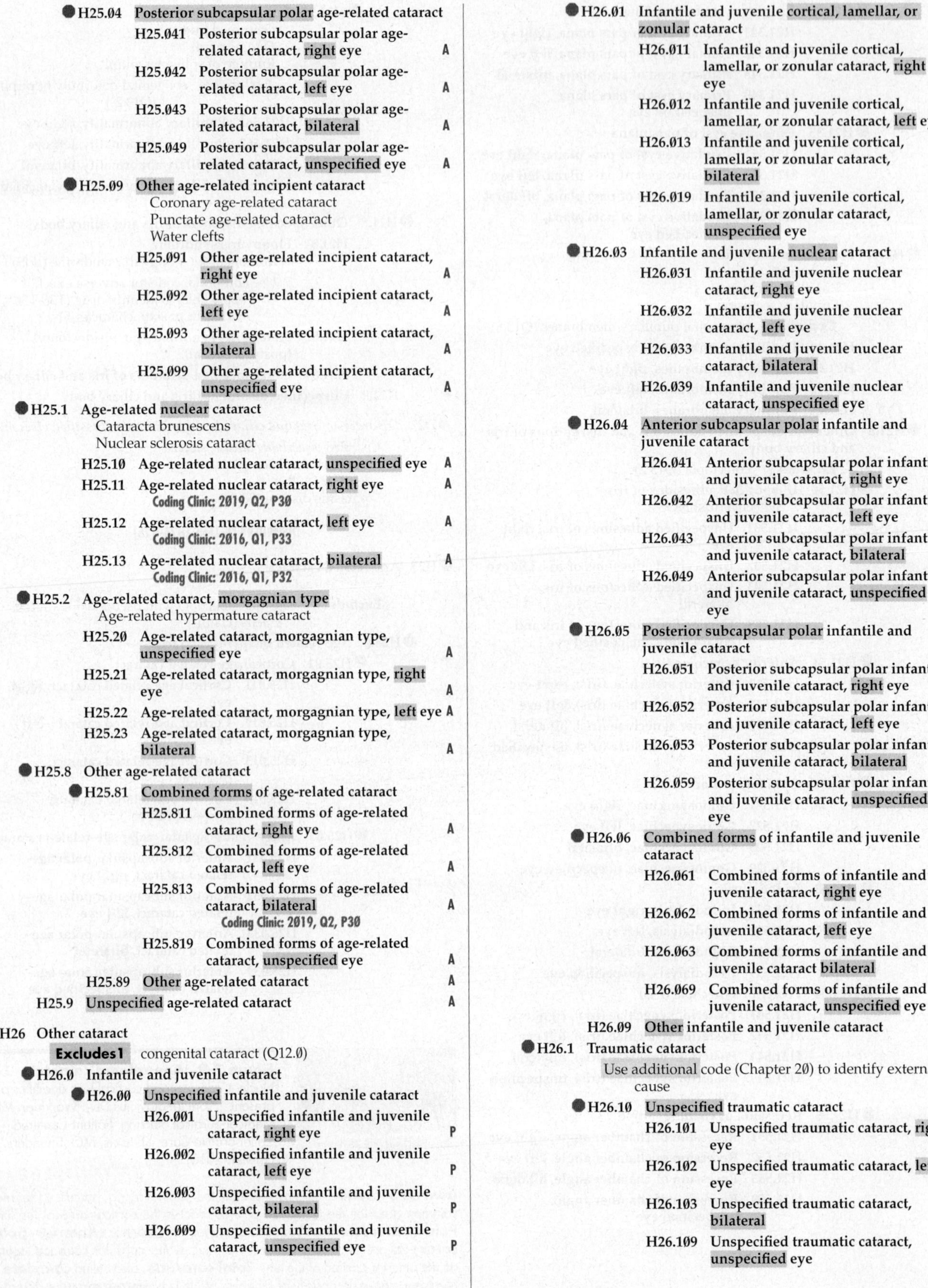

- H25.04 Posterior subcapsular polar age-related cataract
  - H25.041 Posterior subcapsular polar age-related cataract, right eye A
  - H25.042 Posterior subcapsular polar age-related cataract, left eye A
  - H25.043 Posterior subcapsular polar age-related cataract, bilateral A
  - H25.049 Posterior subcapsular polar age-related cataract, unspecified eye A
- H25.09 Other age-related incipient cataract
  Coronary age-related cataract
  Punctate age-related cataract
  Water clefts
  - H25.091 Other age-related incipient cataract, right eye A
  - H25.092 Other age-related incipient cataract, left eye A
  - H25.093 Other age-related incipient cataract, bilateral A
  - H25.099 Other age-related incipient cataract, unspecified eye A
- H25.1 Age-related nuclear cataract
  Cataracta brunescens
  Nuclear sclerosis cataract
  - H25.10 Age-related nuclear cataract, unspecified eye A
  - H25.11 Age-related nuclear cataract, right eye A
    Coding Clinic: 2019, Q2, P30
  - H25.12 Age-related nuclear cataract, left eye A
    Coding Clinic: 2016, Q1, P33
  - H25.13 Age-related nuclear cataract, bilateral A
    Coding Clinic: 2016, Q1, P32
- H25.2 Age-related cataract, morgagnian type
  Age-related hypermature cataract
  - H25.20 Age-related cataract, morgagnian type, unspecified eye A
  - H25.21 Age-related cataract, morgagnian type, right eye A
  - H25.22 Age-related cataract, morgagnian type, left eye A
  - H25.23 Age-related cataract, morgagnian type, bilateral A
- H25.8 Other age-related cataract
  - H25.81 Combined forms of age-related cataract
    - H25.811 Combined forms of age-related cataract, right eye A
    - H25.812 Combined forms of age-related cataract, left eye A
    - H25.813 Combined forms of age-related cataract, bilateral A
      Coding Clinic: 2019, Q2, P30
    - H25.819 Combined forms of age-related cataract, unspecified eye A
  - H25.89 Other age-related cataract A
- H25.9 Unspecified age-related cataract A

H26 Other cataract

Excludes1 congenital cataract (Q12.0)

- H26.0 Infantile and juvenile cataract
  - H26.00 Unspecified infantile and juvenile cataract
    - H26.001 Unspecified infantile and juvenile cataract, right eye P
    - H26.002 Unspecified infantile and juvenile cataract, left eye P
    - H26.003 Unspecified infantile and juvenile cataract, bilateral P
    - H26.009 Unspecified infantile and juvenile cataract, unspecified eye P
  - H26.01 Infantile and juvenile cortical, lamellar, or zonular cataract
    - H26.011 Infantile and juvenile cortical, lamellar, or zonular cataract, right eye P
    - H26.012 Infantile and juvenile cortical, lamellar, or zonular cataract, left eye P
    - H26.013 Infantile and juvenile cortical, lamellar, or zonular cataract, bilateral P
    - H26.019 Infantile and juvenile cortical, lamellar, or zonular cataract, unspecified eye P
  - H26.03 Infantile and juvenile nuclear cataract
    - H26.031 Infantile and juvenile nuclear cataract, right eye P
    - H26.032 Infantile and juvenile nuclear cataract, left eye P
    - H26.033 Infantile and juvenile nuclear cataract, bilateral P
    - H26.039 Infantile and juvenile nuclear cataract, unspecified eye P
  - H26.04 Anterior subcapsular polar infantile and juvenile cataract
    - H26.041 Anterior subcapsular polar infantile and juvenile cataract, right eye P
    - H26.042 Anterior subcapsular polar infantile and juvenile cataract, left eye P
    - H26.043 Anterior subcapsular polar infantile and juvenile cataract, bilateral P
    - H26.049 Anterior subcapsular polar infantile and juvenile cataract, unspecified eye P
  - H26.05 Posterior subcapsular polar infantile and juvenile cataract
    - H26.051 Posterior subcapsular polar infantile and juvenile cataract, right eye P
    - H26.052 Posterior subcapsular polar infantile and juvenile cataract, left eye P
    - H26.053 Posterior subcapsular polar infantile and juvenile cataract, bilateral P
    - H26.059 Posterior subcapsular polar infantile and juvenile cataract, unspecified eye P
  - H26.06 Combined forms of infantile and juvenile cataract
    - H26.061 Combined forms of infantile and juvenile cataract, right eye P
    - H26.062 Combined forms of infantile and juvenile cataract, left eye P
    - H26.063 Combined forms of infantile and juvenile cataract bilateral P
    - H26.069 Combined forms of infantile and juvenile cataract, unspecified eye P
  - H26.09 Other infantile and juvenile cataract P
- H26.1 Traumatic cataract
  Use additional code (Chapter 20) to identify external cause
  - H26.10 Unspecified traumatic cataract
    - H26.101 Unspecified traumatic cataract, right eye
    - H26.102 Unspecified traumatic cataract, left eye
    - H26.103 Unspecified traumatic cataract, bilateral
    - H26.109 Unspecified traumatic cataract, unspecified eye

CHAPTER 7 (H00-H59)

- H26.11 **Localized traumatic opacities**
  - H26.111 **Localized traumatic opacities, right eye**
  - H26.112 **Localized traumatic opacities, left eye**
  - H26.113 **Localized traumatic opacities, bilateral**
  - H26.119 **Localized traumatic opacities, unspecified eye**
- H26.12 **Partially resolved traumatic cataract**
  - H26.121 **Partially resolved traumatic cataract, right eye**
  - H26.122 **Partially resolved traumatic cataract, left eye**
  - H26.123 **Partially resolved traumatic cataract, bilateral**
  - H26.129 **Partially resolved traumatic cataract, unspecified eye**
- H26.13 **Total traumatic cataract**
  - H26.131 **Total traumatic cataract, right eye**
  - H26.132 **Total traumatic cataract, left eye**
  - H26.133 **Total traumatic cataract, bilateral**
  - H26.139 **Total traumatic cataract, unspecified eye**

H26.2 **Complicated cataract**
- H26.20 **Unspecified complicated cataract**
  Cataracta complicata NOS
- H26.21 **Cataract with neovascularization**
  Code also, if applicable, associated condition, such as:
  chronic iridocyclitis (H2Ø.1-)
  - H26.211 **Cataract with neovascularization, right eye**
  - H26.212 **Cataract with neovascularization, left eye**
  - H26.213 **Cataract with neovascularization, bilateral**
  - H26.219 **Cataract with neovascularization, unspecified eye**
- H26.22 **Cataract secondary to ocular disorders (degenerative) (inflammatory)**
  Code also associated ocular disorder
  - H26.221 **Cataract secondary to ocular disorders (degenerative) (inflammatory), right eye**
  - H26.222 **Cataract secondary to ocular disorders (degenerative) (inflammatory), left eye**
  - H26.223 **Cataract secondary to ocular disorders (degenerative) (inflammatory), bilateral**
  - H26.229 **Cataract secondary to ocular disorders (degenerative) (inflammatory), unspecified eye**
- H26.23 **Glaucomatous flecks (subcapsular)**
  Code first underlying glaucoma (H4Ø-H42)
  - H26.231 **Glaucomatous flecks (subcapsular), right eye**
  - H26.232 **Glaucomatous flecks (subcapsular), left eye**
  - H26.233 **Glaucomatous flecks (subcapsular), bilateral**
  - H26.239 **Glaucomatous flecks (subcapsular), unspecified eye**

H26.3 **Drug-induced cataract**
Toxic cataract
Use additional code for adverse effect, if applicable, to identify drug (T36-T5Ø with fifth or sixth character 5)
- H26.30 **Drug-induced cataract, unspecified eye**
- H26.31 **Drug-induced cataract, right eye**
- H26.32 **Drug-induced cataract, left eye**
- H26.33 **Drug-induced cataract, bilateral**

H26.4 **Secondary cataract**
Coding Clinic: 2Ø18, Q2, P14
- H26.4Ø **Unspecified secondary cataract**
- H26.41 **Soemmering's ring**
  - H26.411 **Soemmering's ring, right eye**
  - H26.412 **Soemmering's ring, left eye**
  - H26.413 **Soemmering's ring, bilateral**
  - H26.419 **Soemmering's ring, unspecified eye**
- H26.49 **Other secondary cataract**
  - H26.491 **Other secondary cataract, right eye**
  - H26.492 **Other secondary cataract, left eye**
    Coding Clinic: 2Ø18, Q2, P13
  - H26.493 **Other secondary cataract, bilateral**
  - H26.499 **Other secondary cataract, unspecified eye**

H26.8 **Other specified cataract**
H26.9 **Unspecified cataract**

H27 Other disorders of lens

Excludes1 congenital lens malformations (Q12.-)
mechanical complications of intraocular lens implant (T85.2)
pseudophakia (Z96.1)

H27.Ø **Aphakia**
Acquired absence of lens
Acquired aphakia
Aphakia due to trauma
Excludes1 cataract extraction status (Z98.4-)
congenital absence of lens (Q12.3)
congenital aphakia (Q12.3)
- H27.ØØ **Aphakia, unspecified eye**
- H27.Ø1 **Aphakia, right eye**
- H27.Ø2 **Aphakia, left eye**
- H27.Ø3 **Aphakia, bilateral**

H27.1 **Dislocation of lens**
- H27.1Ø **Unspecified dislocation of lens**
- H27.11 **Subluxation of lens**
  - H27.111 **Subluxation of lens, right eye**
  - H27.112 **Subluxation of lens, left eye**
  - H27.113 **Subluxation of lens, bilateral**
  - H27.119 **Subluxation of lens, unspecified eye**
- H27.12 **Anterior dislocation of lens**
  - H27.121 **Anterior dislocation of lens, right eye**
  - H27.122 **Anterior dislocation of lens, left eye**
  - H27.123 **Anterior dislocation of lens, bilateral**
  - H27.129 **Anterior dislocation of lens, unspecified eye**
- H27.13 **Posterior dislocation of lens**
  - H27.131 **Posterior dislocation of lens, right eye**
  - H27.132 **Posterior dislocation of lens, left eye**
  - H27.133 **Posterior dislocation of lens, bilateral**
  - H27.139 **Posterior dislocation of lens, unspecified eye**

H27.8 **Other specified disorders of lens**
H27.9 **Unspecified disorder of lens**

H28 Cataract in diseases classified elsewhere

Code first underlying disease, such as:
hypoparathyroidism (E2Ø.-)
myotonia (G71.1-)
myxedema (EØ3.-)
protein-calorie malnutrition (E4Ø-E46)

Excludes1 cataract in diabetes mellitus (EØ8.36, EØ9.36, E1Ø.36, E11.36, E13.36)

CHAPTER 7 (HØØ-H59)

DISORDERS OF CHOROID AND RETINA (H30-H36)

★ **(See Plate 16 of the Anatomy Illustrations.)**

H30 Chorioretinal inflammation

H30.0 Focal chorioretinal inflammation
Focal chorioretinitis
Focal choroiditis
Focal retinitis
Focal retinochoroiditis

H30.00 Unspecified focal chorioretinal inflammation
Focal chorioretinitis NOS
Focal choroiditis NOS
Focal retinitis NOS
Focal retinochoroiditis NOS

H30.001 Unspecified focal chorioretinal inflammation, right eye
H30.002 Unspecified focal chorioretinal inflammation, left eye
H30.003 Unspecified focal chorioretinal inflammation, bilateral
H30.009 Unspecified focal chorioretinal inflammation, unspecified eye

H30.01 Focal chorioretinal inflammation, juxtapapillary
H30.011 Focal chorioretinal inflammation, juxtapapillary, right eye
H30.012 Focal chorioretinal inflammation, juxtapapillary, left eye
H30.013 Focal chorioretinal inflammation, juxtapapillary, bilateral
H30.019 Focal chorioretinal inflammation, juxtapapillary, unspecified eye

H30.02 Focal chorioretinal inflammation of posterior pole
H30.021 Focal chorioretinal inflammation of posterior pole, right eye
H30.022 Focal chorioretinal inflammation of posterior pole, left eye
H30.023 Focal chorioretinal inflammation of posterior pole, bilateral
H30.029 Focal chorioretinal inflammation of posterior pole, unspecified eye

H30.03 Focal chorioretinal inflammation, peripheral
H30.031 Focal chorioretinal inflammation, peripheral, right eye
H30.032 Focal chorioretinal inflammation, peripheral, left eye
H30.033 Focal chorioretinal inflammation, peripheral, bilateral
H30.039 Focal chorioretinal inflammation, peripheral, unspecified eye

H30.04 Focal chorioretinal inflammation, macular or paramacular
H30.041 Focal chorioretinal inflammation, macular or paramacular, right eye
H30.042 Focal chorioretinal inflammation, macular or paramacular, left eye
H30.043 Focal chorioretinal inflammation, macular or paramacular, bilateral
H30.049 Focal chorioretinal inflammation, macular or paramacular, unspecified eye

H30.1 Disseminated chorioretinal inflammation Ex: PDX 793
Disseminated chorioretinitis
Disseminated choroiditis
Disseminated retinitis
Disseminated retinochoroiditis

Excludes2 exudative retinopathy (H35.02-)

H30.10 Unspecified disseminated chorioretinal inflammation
Disseminated chorioretinitis NOS
Disseminated choroiditis NOS
Disseminated retinitis NOS
Disseminated retinochoroiditis NOS

H30.101 Unspecified disseminated chorioretinal inflammation, right eye
H30.102 Unspecified disseminated chorioretinal inflammation, left eye
H30.103 Unspecified disseminated chorioretinal inflammation, bilateral
H30.109 Unspecified disseminated chorioretinal inflammation, unspecified eye

H30.11 Disseminated chorioretinal inflammation of posterior pole
H30.111 Disseminated chorioretinal inflammation of posterior pole, right eye
H30.112 Disseminated chorioretinal inflammation of posterior pole, left eye
H30.113 Disseminated chorioretinal inflammation of posterior pole, bilateral
H30.119 Disseminated chorioretinal inflammation of posterior pole, unspecified eye

H30.12 Disseminated chorioretinal inflammation, peripheral
H30.121 Disseminated chorioretinal inflammation, peripheral right eye
H30.122 Disseminated chorioretinal inflammation, peripheral, left eye
H30.123 Disseminated chorioretinal inflammation, peripheral, bilateral
H30.129 Disseminated chorioretinal inflammation, peripheral, unspecified eye

H30.13 Disseminated chorioretinal inflammation, generalized
H30.131 Disseminated chorioretinal inflammation, generalized, right eye
H30.132 Disseminated chorioretinal inflammation, generalized, left eye
H30.133 Disseminated chorioretinal inflammation, generalized, bilateral
H30.139 Disseminated chorioretinal inflammation, generalized, unspecified eye

H30.14 Acute posterior multifocal placoid pigment epitheliopathy
H30.141 Acute posterior multifocal placoid pigment epitheliopathy, right eye
H30.142 Acute posterior multifocal placoid pigment epitheliopathy, left eye
H30.143 Acute posterior multifocal placoid pigment epitheliopathy, bilateral
H30.149 Acute posterior multifocal placoid pigment epitheliopathy, unspecified eye

H30.2 Posterior cyclitis
Pars planitis

H30.20 Posterior cyclitis, unspecified eye
H30.21 Posterior cyclitis, right eye
H30.22 Posterior cyclitis, left eye
H30.23 Posterior cyclitis, bilateral

● **H30.8 Other chorioretinal inflammations**
- ● **H30.81 Harada's disease**
  - **H30.811 Harada's disease, right eye**
  - **H30.812 Harada's disease, left eye**
  - **H30.813 Harada's disease, bilateral**
  - **H30.819 Harada's disease, unspecified eye**
- ● **H30.89 Other chorioretinal inflammations** Ex: PDX 793
  - **H30.891 Other chorioretinal inflammations, right eye**
  - **H30.892 Other chorioretinal inflammations, left eye**
  - **H30.893 Other chorioretinal inflammations, bilateral**
  - **H30.899 Other chorioretinal inflammations, unspecified eye**

● **H30.9 Unspecified chorioretinal inflammation** Ex: PDX 793

Chorioretinitis NOS
Choroiditis NOS
Neuroretinitis NOS
Retinitis NOS
Retinochoroiditis NOS

- **H30.90 Unspecified chorioretinal inflammation, unspecified eye**
- **H30.91 Unspecified chorioretinal inflammation, right eye**
- **H30.92 Unspecified chorioretinal inflammation, left eye**
- **H30.93 Unspecified chorioretinal inflammation, bilateral**

● **H31 Other disorders of choroid**

● **H31.0 Chorioretinal scars**

Excludes2 postsurgical chorioretinal scars (H59.81-)

- ● **H31.00 Unspecified chorioretinal scars**
  - **H31.001 Unspecified chorioretinal scars, right eye**
  - **H31.002 Unspecified chorioretinal scars, left eye**
  - **H31.003 Unspecified chorioretinal scars, bilateral**
  - **H31.009 Unspecified chorioretinal scars, unspecified eye**
- ● **H31.01 Macula scars of posterior pole (postinflammatory) (post-traumatic)**

  Excludes1 postprocedural chorioretinal scar (H59.81-)
  - **H31.011 Macula scars of posterior pole (postinflammatory) (post-traumatic), right eye**
  - **H31.012 Macula scars of posterior pole (postinflammatory) (post-traumatic), left eye**
  - **H31.013 Macula scars of posterior pole (postinflammatory) (post-traumatic), bilateral**
  - **H31.019 Macula scars of posterior pole (postinflammatory) (post-traumatic), unspecified eye**
- ● **H31.02 Solar retinopathy**
  - **H31.021 Solar retinopathy, right eye**
  - **H31.022 Solar retinopathy, left eye**
  - **H31.023 Solar retinopathy, bilateral**
  - **H31.029 Solar retinopathy, unspecified eye**
- ● **H31.09 Other chorioretinal scars**
  - **H31.091 Other chorioretinal scars, right eye**
  - **H31.092 Other chorioretinal scars, left eye**
  - **H31.093 Other chorioretinal scars, bilateral**
  - **H31.099 Other chorioretinal scars, unspecified eye**

● **H31.1 Choroidal degeneration**

Excludes2 angioid streaks of macula (H35.33)

- ● **H31.10 Unspecified choroidal degeneration**

  Choroidal sclerosis NOS
  - **H31.101 Choroidal degeneration, unspecified, right eye**
  - **H31.102 Choroidal degeneration, unspecified, left eye**
  - **H31.103 Choroidal degeneration, unspecified, bilateral**
  - **H31.109 Choroidal degeneration, unspecified, unspecified eye**
- ● **H31.11 Age-related choroidal atrophy**
  - **H31.111 Age-related choroidal atrophy, right eye** A
  - **H31.112 Age-related choroidal atrophy, left eye** A
  - **H31.113 Age-related choroidal atrophy, bilateral** A
  - **H31.119 Age-related choroidal atrophy, unspecified eye** A
- ● **H31.12 Diffuse secondary atrophy of choroid**
  - **H31.121 Diffuse secondary atrophy of choroid, right eye**
  - **H31.122 Diffuse secondary atrophy of choroid, left eye**
  - **H31.123 Diffuse secondary atrophy of choroid, bilateral**
  - **H31.129 Diffuse secondary atrophy of choroid, unspecified eye**

● **H31.2 Hereditary choroidal dystrophy**

Excludes2 hyperornithinemia (E72.4)
ornithinemia (E72.4)

- **H31.20 Hereditary choroidal dystrophy, unspecified**
- **H31.21 Choroideremia**
- **H31.22 Choroidal dystrophy (central areolar) (generalized) (peripapillary)**
- **H31.23 Gyrate atrophy, choroid**
- **H31.29 Other hereditary choroidal dystrophy**

● **H31.3 Choroidal hemorrhage and rupture**
- ● **H31.30 Unspecified choroidal hemorrhage**
  - **H31.301 Unspecified choroidal hemorrhage, right eye**
  - **H31.302 Unspecified choroidal hemorrhage, left eye**
  - **H31.303 Unspecified choroidal hemorrhage, bilateral**
  - **H31.309 Unspecified choroidal hemorrhage, unspecified eye**
- ● **H31.31 Expulsive choroidal hemorrhage**
  - **H31.311 Expulsive choroidal hemorrhage, right eye**
  - **H31.312 Expulsive choroidal hemorrhage, left eye**
  - **H31.313 Expulsive choroidal hemorrhage, bilateral**
  - **H31.319 Expulsive choroidal hemorrhage, unspecified eye**

CHAPTER 7 (H00-H59)

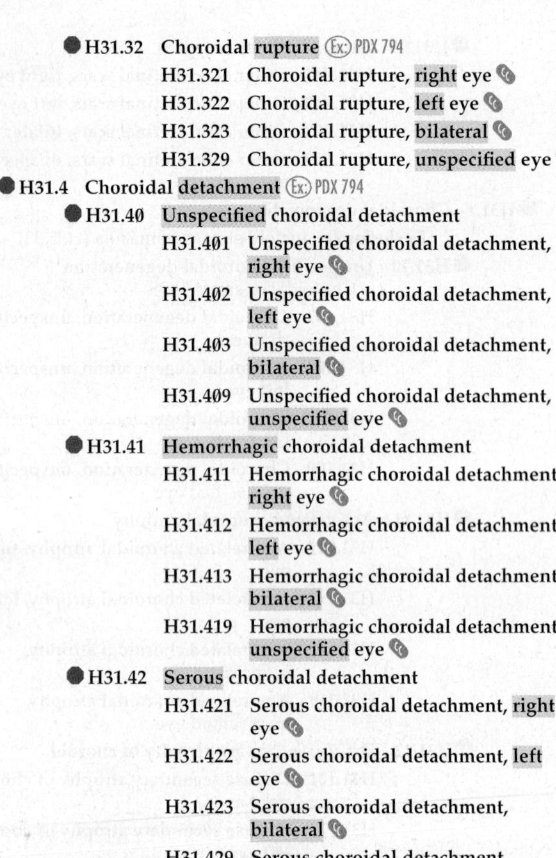

● H31.32 Choroidal rupture Ex: PDX 794
- H31.321 Choroidal rupture, right eye
- H31.322 Choroidal rupture, left eye
- H31.323 Choroidal rupture, bilateral
- H31.329 Choroidal rupture, unspecified eye

● H31.4 Choroidal detachment Ex: PDX 794

● H31.4Ø Unspecified choroidal detachment
- H31.4Ø1 Unspecified choroidal detachment, right eye
- H31.4Ø2 Unspecified choroidal detachment, left eye
- H31.4Ø3 Unspecified choroidal detachment, bilateral
- H31.4Ø9 Unspecified choroidal detachment, unspecified eye

● H31.41 Hemorrhagic choroidal detachment
- H31.411 Hemorrhagic choroidal detachment, right eye
- H31.412 Hemorrhagic choroidal detachment, left eye
- H31.413 Hemorrhagic choroidal detachment, bilateral
- H31.419 Hemorrhagic choroidal detachment, unspecified eye

● H31.42 Serous choroidal detachment
- H31.421 Serous choroidal detachment, right eye
- H31.422 Serous choroidal detachment, left eye
- H31.423 Serous choroidal detachment, bilateral
- H31.429 Serous choroidal detachment, unspecified eye

H31.8 Other specified disorders of choroid

H31.9 Unspecified disorder of choroid

H32 Chorioretinal disorders in diseases classified elsewhere

Code first underlying disease, such as:
congenital toxoplasmosis (P37.1)
histoplasmosis (B39.-)
leprosy (A3Ø.-)

Excludes1 chorioretinitis (in):
toxoplasmosis (acquired) (B58.Ø1)
tuberculosis (A18.53)

● H33 Retinal detachments and breaks

Excludes1 detachment of retinal pigment epithelium (H35.72-, H35.73-)

● H33.Ø Retinal detachment with retinal break
Rhegmatogenous retinal detachment

Excludes1 serous retinal detachment (without retinal break) (H33.2-)

● H33.ØØ Unspecified retinal detachment with retinal break
- H33.ØØ1 Unspecified retinal detachment with retinal break, right eye
- H33.ØØ2 Unspecified retinal detachment with retinal break, left eye
- H33.ØØ3 Unspecified retinal detachment with retinal break, bilateral
- H33.ØØ9 Unspecified retinal detachment with retinal break, unspecified eye

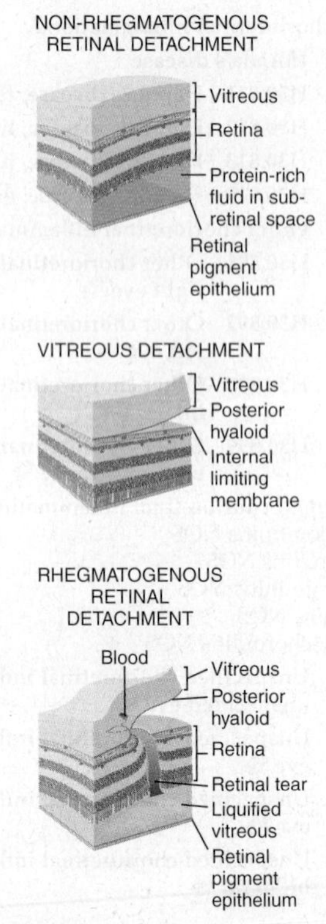

Figure 7-10 Retinal detachment. (From Kumar: Robbins and Cotran: Pathologic Basis of Disease, ed 7, Saunders, 2005)

Item 7–6 Retinal detachments and defects are conditions of the eye in which the retina separates from the underlying tissue. Initial detachment may be localized, requiring rapid treatment (medical emergency) to avoid the entire retina from detaching, which leads to vision loss and blindness.

● H33.Ø1 Retinal detachment with single break
- H33.Ø11 Retinal detachment with single break, right eye
- H33.Ø12 Retinal detachment with single break, left eye
- H33.Ø13 Retinal detachment with single break, bilateral
- H33.Ø19 Retinal detachment with single break, unspecified eye

● H33.Ø2 Retinal detachment with multiple breaks
- H33.Ø21 Retinal detachment with multiple breaks, right eye
- H33.Ø22 Retinal detachment with multiple breaks, left eye
- H33.Ø23 Retinal detachment with multiple breaks, bilateral
- H33.Ø29 Retinal detachment with multiple breaks, unspecified eye

● H33.Ø3 Retinal detachment with giant retinal tear
- H33.Ø31 Retinal detachment with giant retinal tear, right eye
- H33.Ø32 Retinal detachment with giant retinal tear, left eye
- H33.Ø33 Retinal detachment with giant retinal tear, bilateral
- H33.Ø39 Retinal detachment with giant retinal tear, unspecified eye

- H33.04 Retinal detachment with retinal dialysis
  - H33.041 Retinal detachment with retinal dialysis, right eye
  - H33.042 Retinal detachment with retinal dialysis, left eye
  - H33.043 Retinal detachment with retinal dialysis, bilateral
  - H33.049 Retinal detachment with retinal dialysis, unspecified eye
- H33.05 Total retinal detachment
  - H33.051 Total retinal detachment, right eye
  - H33.052 Total retinal detachment, left eye
  - H33.053 Total retinal detachment, bilateral
  - H33.059 Total retinal detachment, unspecified eye

H33.1 Retinoschisis and retinal cysts

Excludes1 congenital retinoschisis (Q14.1)
microcystoid degeneration of retina (H35.42-)

- H33.10 Unspecified retinoschisis
  - H33.101 Unspecified retinoschisis, right eye
  - H33.102 Unspecified retinoschisis, left eye
  - H33.103 Unspecified retinoschisis, bilateral
  - H33.109 Unspecified retinoschisis, unspecified eye
- H33.11 Cyst of ora serrata
  - H33.111 Cyst of ora serrata, right eye
  - H33.112 Cyst of ora serrata, left eye
  - H33.113 Cyst of ora serrata, bilateral
  - H33.119 Cyst of ora serrata, unspecified eye
- H33.12 Parasitic cyst of retina (Ex) PDX 792
  - H33.121 Parasitic cyst of retina, right eye
  - H33.122 Parasitic cyst of retina, left eye
  - H33.123 Parasitic cyst of retina, bilateral
  - H33.129 Parasitic cyst of retina, unspecified eye
- H33.19 Other retinoschisis and retinal cysts
  Pseudocyst of retina
  - H33.191 Other retinoschisis and retinal cysts, right eye
  - H33.192 Other retinoschisis and retinal cysts, left eye
  - H33.193 Other retinoschisis and retinal cysts, bilateral
  - H33.199 Other retinoschisis and retinal cysts, unspecified eye

H33.2 Serous retinal detachment (Ex) PDX 795

Retinal detachment NOS
Retinal detachment without retinal break

Excludes1 central serous chorioretinopathy (H35.71-)

- H33.20 Serous retinal detachment, unspecified eye
- H33.21 Serous retinal detachment, right eye
- H33.22 Serous retinal detachment, left eye
- H33.23 Serous retinal detachment, bilateral

H33.3 Retinal breaks without detachment

Excludes1 chorioretinal scars after surgery for detachment (H59.81-)
peripheral retinal degeneration without break (H35.4-)

- H33.30 Unspecified retinal break
  - H33.301 Unspecified retinal break, right eye
  - H33.302 Unspecified retinal break, left eye
  - H33.303 Unspecified retinal break, bilateral
  - H33.309 Unspecified retinal break, unspecified eye
- H33.31 Horseshoe tear of retina without detachment
  Operculum of retina without detachment
  - H33.311 Horseshoe tear of retina without detachment, right eye
  - H33.312 Horseshoe tear of retina without detachment, left eye
  - H33.313 Horseshoe tear of retina without detachment, bilateral
  - H33.319 Horseshoe tear of retina without detachment, unspecified eye
- H33.32 Round hole of retina without detachment
  - H33.321 Round hole, right eye
  - H33.322 Round hole, left eye
  - H33.323 Round hole, bilateral
  - H33.329 Round hole, unspecified eye
- H33.33 Multiple defects of retina without detachment
  - H33.331 Multiple defects of retina without detachment, right eye
  - H33.332 Multiple defects of retina without detachment, left eye
  - H33.333 Multiple defects of retina without detachment, bilateral
  - H33.339 Multiple defects of retina without detachment, unspecified eye

H33.4 Traction detachment of retina (Ex) PDX 795

Proliferative vitreo-retinopathy with retinal detachment

- H33.40 Traction detachment of retina, unspecified eye
- H33.41 Traction detachment of retina, right eye
- H33.42 Traction detachment of retina, left eye
- H33.43 Traction detachment of retina, bilateral

H33.8 Other retinal detachments (Ex) PDX 795

H34 Retinal vascular occlusions (Ex) PDX 751

Blockage in vessel of the retina

Excludes1 amaurosis fugax (G45.3)

H34.0 Transient retinal artery occlusion

- H34.00 Transient retinal artery occlusion, unspecified eye
- H34.01 Transient retinal artery occlusion, right eye
- H34.02 Transient retinal artery occlusion, left eye
- H34.03 Transient retinal artery occlusion, bilateral

H34.1 Central retinal artery occlusion

- H34.10 Central retinal artery occlusion, unspecified eye
- H34.11 Central retinal artery occlusion, right eye
- H34.12 Central retinal artery occlusion, left eye
- H34.13 Central retinal artery occlusion, bilateral

H34.2 Other retinal artery occlusions

- H34.21 Partial retinal artery occlusion
  Hollenhorst's plaque
  Retinal microembolism
  - H34.211 Partial retinal artery occlusion, right eye
  - H34.212 Partial retinal artery occlusion, left eye
  - H34.213 Partial retinal artery occlusion, bilateral
  - H34.219 Partial retinal artery occlusion, unspecified eye

- H34.23 Retinal artery branch occlusion
  - H34.231 Retinal artery branch occlusion, right eye
  - H34.232 Retinal artery branch occlusion, left eye
  - H34.233 Retinal artery branch occlusion, bilateral
  - H34.239 Retinal artery branch occlusion, unspecified eye
- H34.8 Other retinal vascular occlusions
  Coding Clinic: 2016, Q4, P19
  - H34.81 Central retinal vein occlusion
    One of the following 7th characters is to be assigned to codes in subcategory H34.81 to designate the severity of the occlusion:

0	with macular edema
1	with retinal neovascularization
2	stable Old central retinal vein occlusion

    - H34.811 Central retinal vein occlusion, right eye
    - H34.812 Central retinal vein occlusion, left eye
    - H34.813 Central retinal vein occlusion, bilateral
    - H34.819 Central retinal vein occlusion, unspecified eye
  - H34.82 Venous engorgement
    Incipient retinal vein occlusion
    Partial retinal vein occlusion
    - H34.821 Venous engorgement, right eye
    - H34.822 Venous engorgement, left eye
    - H34.823 Venous engorgement, bilateral
    - H34.829 Venous engorgement, unspecified eye
  - H34.83 Tributary (branch) retinal vein occlusion
    One of the following 7th characters is to be assigned to codes in subcategory H34.83 to designate the severity of the occlusion:

0	with macular edema
1	with retinal neovascularization
2	stable Old tributary (branch) retinal vein occlusion

    - H34.831 Tributary (branch) retinal vein occlusion, right eye
    - H34.832 Tributary (branch) retinal vein occlusion, left eye
    - H34.833 Tributary (branch) retinal vein occlusion, bilateral
    - H34.839 Tributary (branch) retinal vein occlusion, unspecified eye
- H34.9 Unspecified retinal vascular occlusion

- H35 Other retinal disorders
  Excludes2 diabetic retinal disorders (E08.311-E08.359, E09.311-E09.359, E10.311-E10.359, E11.311-E11.359, E13.311-E13.359)
  - H35.0 Background retinopathy and retinal vascular changes
    Code also any associated hypertension (I10)
    OGCR Section I. C.9.a.5.

    > Hypertensive Retinopathy
    > Subcategory H35.0, Background retinopathy and retinal vascular changes, should be used with a code from category I10–I15, Hypertensive disease to include the systemic hypertension. The sequencing is based on the reason for the encounter.

    - H35.00 Unspecified background retinopathy
    - H35.01 Changes in retinal vascular appearance
      Retinal vascular sheathing
      - H35.011 Changes in retinal vascular appearance, right eye
      - H35.012 Changes in retinal vascular appearance, left eye
      - H35.013 Changes in retinal vascular appearance, bilateral
      - H35.019 Changes in retinal vascular appearance, unspecified eye
    - H35.02 Exudative retinopathy
      Coats retinopathy
      - H35.021 Exudative retinopathy, right eye
      - H35.022 Exudative retinopathy, left eye
      - H35.023 Exudative retinopathy, bilateral
      - H35.029 Exudative retinopathy, unspecified eye
    - H35.03 Hypertensive retinopathy
      - H35.031 Hypertensive retinopathy, right eye
      - H35.032 Hypertensive retinopathy, left eye
      - H35.033 Hypertensive retinopathy, bilateral
      - H35.039 Hypertensive retinopathy, unspecified eye
    - H35.04 Retinal micro-aneurysms, unspecified
      - H35.041 Retinal micro-aneurysms, unspecified, right eye
      - H35.042 Retinal micro-aneurysms, unspecified, left eye
      - H35.043 Retinal micro-aneurysms, unspecified, bilateral
      - H35.049 Retinal micro-aneurysms, unspecified, unspecified eye
    - H35.05 Retinal neovascularization, unspecified
      - H35.051 Retinal neovascularization, unspecified, right eye
      - H35.052 Retinal neovascularization, unspecified, left eye
      - H35.053 Retinal neovascularization, unspecified, bilateral
      - H35.059 Retinal neovascularization, unspecified, unspecified eye
    - H35.06 Retinal vasculitis
      Eales disease
      Retinal perivasculitis
      - H35.061 Retinal vasculitis, right eye
      - H35.062 Retinal vasculitis, left eye
      - H35.063 Retinal vasculitis, bilateral
      - H35.069 Retinal vasculitis, unspecified eye
    - H35.07 Retinal telangiectasis
      - H35.071 Retinal telangiectasis, right eye
      - H35.072 Retinal telangiectasis, left eye
      - H35.073 Retinal telangiectasis, bilateral
      - H35.079 Retinal telangiectasis, unspecified eye
    - H35.09 Other intraretinal microvascular abnormalities
      Retinal varices
  - H35.1 Retinopathy of prematurity
    - H35.10 Retinopathy of prematurity, unspecified
      Retinopathy of prematurity NOS
      - H35.101 Retinopathy of prematurity, unspecified, right eye
      - H35.102 Retinopathy of prematurity, unspecified, left eye
      - H35.103 Retinopathy of prematurity, unspecified, bilateral
      - H35.109 Retinopathy of prematurity, unspecified, unspecified eye

CHAPTER 7 (H00-H59)

New | Revised | deleted Deleted | Excludes 1 | Excludes 2 | Includes | Use additional | Code first | Code also | Key words
OGCR Official Guidelines | Unacceptable Principal Diagnosis | X Assign placeholder X | Use Additional Character(s) | Manifestation Code | Coding Clinic

● **H35.11** Retinopathy of prematurity, stage 0
- H35.111 Retinopathy of prematurity, stage 0, right eye
- H35.112 Retinopathy of prematurity, stage 0, left eye
- H35.113 Retinopathy of prematurity, stage 0, bilateral
- H35.119 Retinopathy of prematurity, stage 0, unspecified eye

● **H35.12** Retinopathy of prematurity, stage 1
- H35.121 Retinopathy of prematurity, stage 1, right eye
- H35.122 Retinopathy of prematurity, stage 1, left eye
- H35.123 Retinopathy of prematurity, stage 1, bilateral
- H35.129 Retinopathy of prematurity, stage 1, unspecified eye

● **H35.13** Retinopathy of prematurity, stage 2
- H35.131 Retinopathy of prematurity, stage 2, right eye
- H35.132 Retinopathy of prematurity, stage 2, left eye
- H35.133 Retinopathy of prematurity, stage 2, bilateral
- H35.139 Retinopathy of prematurity, stage 2, unspecified eye

● **H35.14** Retinopathy of prematurity, stage 3
- H35.141 Retinopathy of prematurity, stage 3, right eye
- H35.142 Retinopathy of prematurity, stage 3, left eye
- H35.143 Retinopathy of prematurity, stage 3, bilateral
- H35.149 Retinopathy of prematurity, stage 3, unspecified eye

● **H35.15** Retinopathy of prematurity, stage 4
- H35.151 Retinopathy of prematurity, stage 4, right eye
- H35.152 Retinopathy of prematurity, stage 4, left eye
- H35.153 Retinopathy of prematurity, stage 4, bilateral
- H35.159 Retinopathy of prematurity, stage 4, unspecified eye

● **H35.16** Retinopathy of prematurity, stage 5
- H35.161 Retinopathy of prematurity, stage 5, right eye
- H35.162 Retinopathy of prematurity, stage 5, left eye
- H35.163 Retinopathy of prematurity, stage 5, bilateral
- H35.169 Retinopathy of prematurity, stage 5, unspecified eye

● **H35.17** Retrolental fibroplasia
- H35.171 Retrolental fibroplasia, right eye
- H35.172 Retrolental fibroplasia, left eye
- H35.173 Retrolental fibroplasia, bilateral
- H35.179 Retrolental fibroplasia, unspecified eye

● **H35.2** Other non-diabetic proliferative retinopathy

Proliferative vitreo-retinopathy

Excludes1 proliferative vitreo-retinopathy with retinal detachment (H33.4-)
Thalassemia proliferative retinopathy

Excludes2 proliferative sickle-cell retinopathy (H36.82-)

- H35.20 Other non-diabetic proliferative retinopathy, unspecified eye
- H35.21 Other non-diabetic proliferative retinopathy, right eye
- H35.22 Other non-diabetic proliferative retinopathy, left eye
- H35.23 Other non-diabetic proliferative retinopathy, bilateral

● **H35.3** Degeneration of macula and posterior pole

H35.30 Unspecified macular degeneration A
Age-related macular degeneration

● **H35.31** Nonexudative age-related macular degeneration
Atrophic age-related macular degeneration
Dry age-related macular degeneration

One of the following 7th characters is to be assigned to codes in subcategory H35.31 to designate the stage of the disease:

0	stage unspecified
1	early dry stage
2	intermediate dry stage
3	advanced atrophic without subfoveal involvement advanced dry stage
4	advanced atrophic with subfoveal involvement

● H35.311 Nonexudative age-related macular degeneration, right eye A
Coding Clinic: 2016, Q4, P20-21

● H35.312 Nonexudative age-related macular degeneration, left eye A
Coding Clinic: 2016, Q4, P20-21

● H35.313 Nonexudative age-related macular degeneration, bilateral A
Coding Clinic: 2016, Q4, P20

● H35.319 Nonexudative age-related macular degeneration, unspecified eye A
Coding Clinic: 2016, Q4, P20

● **H35.32** Exudative age-related macular degeneration
Wet age-related macular degeneration

One of the following 7th characters is to be assigned to codes in subcategory H35.32 to designate the stage of the disease:

0	stage unspecified
1	with active choroidal neovascularization
2	with inactive choroidal neovascularization with involuted or regressed neovascularization
3	with inactive scar

Coding Clinic: 2016, Q4, P20

● H35.321 Exudative age-related macular degeneration, right eye A

● H35.322 Exudative age-related macular degeneration, left eye A

● H35.323 Exudative age-related macular degeneration, bilateral A

● H35.329 Exudative age-related macular degeneration, unspecified eye A

H35.33 Angioid streaks of macula

● **H35.34** Macular cyst, hole, or pseudohole
- H35.341 Macular cyst, hole, or pseudohole, right eye
- H35.342 Macular cyst, hole, or pseudohole, left eye
- H35.343 Macular cyst, hole, or pseudohole, bilateral
- H35.349 Macular cyst, hole, or pseudohole, unspecified eye

Item 7–7 Macular degeneration is typically age-related, chronic, and is evidenced by deterioration of the macula (the part of the retina that provides for central field vision), resulting in blurred vision or a blind spot in the center of visual field while not affecting peripheral vision.

● **H35.35 Cystoid macular degeneration**
 Excludes1 cystoid macular edema following cataract surgery (H59.03-)
 H35.351 Cystoid macular degeneration, right eye
 H35.352 Cystoid macular degeneration, left eye
 H35.353 Cystoid macular degeneration, bilateral
 H35.359 Cystoid macular degeneration, unspecified eye

● **H35.36 Drusen (degenerative) of macula**
 H35.361 Drusen (degenerative) of macula, right eye
 Coding Clinic: 2016, Q4, P21
 H35.362 Drusen (degenerative) of macula, left eye
 Coding Clinic: 2016, Q4, P21
 H35.363 Drusen (degenerative) of macula, bilateral
 Coding Clinic: 2017, Q1, P51
 H35.369 Drusen (degenerative) of macula, unspecified eye

● **H35.37 Puckering of macula**
 H35.371 Puckering of macula, right eye
 H35.372 Puckering of macula, left eye
 H35.373 Puckering of macula, bilateral
 H35.379 Puckering of macula, unspecified eye

● **H35.38 Toxic maculopathy**
 Code first poisoning due to drug or toxin, if applicable (T36-T65 with fifth or sixth character 1-4)
 Use additional code for adverse effect, if applicable, to identify drug (T36-T50 with fifth or sixth character 5)
 H35.381 Toxic maculopathy, right eye
 H35.382 Toxic maculopathy, left eye
 H35.383 Toxic maculopathy, bilateral
 H35.389 Toxic maculopathy, unspecified eye

● **H35.4 Peripheral retinal degeneration**
 Excludes1 hereditary retinal degeneration (dystrophy) (H35.5-)
 peripheral retinal degeneration with retinal break (H33.3-)
 H35.40 Unspecified peripheral retinal degeneration

● **H35.41 Lattice degeneration of retina**
 Palisade degeneration of retina
 H35.411 Lattice degeneration of retina, right eye
 H35.412 Lattice degeneration of retina, left eye
 H35.413 Lattice degeneration of retina, bilateral
 H35.419 Lattice degeneration of retina, unspecified eye

● **H35.42 Microcystoid degeneration of retina**
 H35.421 Microcystoid degeneration of retina, right eye
 H35.422 Microcystoid degeneration of retina, left eye
 H35.423 Microcystoid degeneration of retina, bilateral
 H35.429 Microcystoid degeneration of retina, unspecified eye

● **H35.43 Paving stone degeneration of retina**
 H35.431 Paving stone degeneration of retina, right eye
 H35.432 Paving stone degeneration of retina, left eye
 H35.433 Paving stone degeneration of retina, bilateral
 H35.439 Paving stone degeneration of retina, unspecified eye

● **H35.44 Age-related reticular degeneration of retina**
 H35.441 Age-related reticular degeneration of retina, right eye A
 H35.442 Age-related reticular degeneration of retina, left eye A
 H35.443 Age-related reticular degeneration of retina, bilateral A
 H35.449 Age-related reticular degeneration of retina, unspecified eye A

● **H35.45 Secondary pigmentary degeneration**
 H35.451 Secondary pigmentary degeneration, right eye
 H35.452 Secondary pigmentary degeneration, left eye
 H35.453 Secondary pigmentary degeneration, bilateral
 H35.459 Secondary pigmentary degeneration, unspecified eye

● **H35.46 Secondary vitreoretinal degeneration**
 H35.461 Secondary vitreoretinal degeneration, right eye
 H35.462 Secondary vitreoretinal degeneration, left eye
 H35.463 Secondary vitreoretinal degeneration, bilateral
 H35.469 Secondary vitreoretinal degeneration, unspecified eye

● **H35.5 Hereditary retinal dystrophy**
 Excludes1 dystrophies primarily involving Bruch's membrane (H31.1-)
 H35.50 Unspecified hereditary retinal dystrophy
 H35.51 Vitreoretinal dystrophy
 H35.52 Pigmentary retinal dystrophy
 Albipunctate retinal dystrophy
 Retinitis pigmentosa
 Tapetoretinal dystrophy
 H35.53 Other dystrophies primarily involving the sensory retina
 Stargardt's disease
 H35.54 Dystrophies primarily involving the retinal pigment epithelium
 Vitelliform retinal dystrophy

● **H35.6 Retinal hemorrhage**
 H35.60 Retinal hemorrhage, unspecified eye
 H35.61 Retinal hemorrhage, right eye
 H35.62 Retinal hemorrhage, left eye
 H35.63 Retinal hemorrhage, bilateral

● **H35.7 Separation of retinal layers** Ex PDX 795
 Excludes1 retinal detachment (serous) (H33.2-)
 rhegmatogenous retinal detachment (H33.0-)
 H35.70 Unspecified separation of retinal layers

● **H35.71 Central serous chorioretinopathy**
 H35.711 Central serous chorioretinopathy, right eye
 H35.712 Central serous chorioretinopathy, left eye
 H35.713 Central serous chorioretinopathy, bilateral
 H35.719 Central serous chorioretinopathy, unspecified eye

- H35.72 Serous detachment of retinal pigment epithelium
  - H35.721 Serous detachment of retinal pigment epithelium, right eye
  - H35.722 Serous detachment of retinal pigment epithelium, left eye
  - H35.723 Serous detachment of retinal pigment epithelium, bilateral
  - H35.729 Serous detachment of retinal pigment epithelium, unspecified eye
- H35.73 Hemorrhagic detachment of retinal pigment epithelium
  - H35.731 Hemorrhagic detachment of retinal pigment epithelium, right eye
  - H35.732 Hemorrhagic detachment of retinal pigment epithelium, left eye
  - H35.733 Hemorrhagic detachment of retinal pigment epithelium, bilateral
  - H35.739 Hemorrhagic detachment of retinal pigment epithelium, unspecified eye

- H35.8 Other specified retinal disorders
  - **Excludes2** retinal hemorrhage (H35.6-)
  - H35.81 Retinal edema
    - Retinal cotton wool spots
  - H35.82 Retinal ischemia (Ex:) PDX 796
  - H35.89 Other specified retinal disorders
- H35.9 Unspecified retinal disorder

H36 Retinal disorders in diseases classified elsewhere

Code first underlying disease, such as:
lipid storage disorders (E75.-)
sickle-cell disorders (D57.-)

Excludes1 arteriosclerotic retinopathy (H35.Ø-)
diabetic retinopathy (EØ8.3-, EØ9.3-, E1Ø.3-, E11.3-, E13.3-)

- H36.8 Other retinal disorders in diseases classified elsewhere
  - H36.81 Nonproliferative sickle-cell retinopathy
    - H36.811 Nonproliferative sickle-cell retinopathy, right eye
    - H36.812 Nonproliferative sickle-cell retinopathy, left eye
    - H36.813 Nonproliferative sickle-cell retinopathy, bilateral
    - H36.819 Nonproliferative sickle-cell retinopathy, unspecified eye
  - H36.82 Proliferative sickle-cell retinopathy
    - H36.821 Proliferative sickle-cell retinopathy, right eye
    - H36.822 Proliferative sickle-cell retinopathy, left eye
    - H36.823 Proliferative sickle-cell retinopathy, bilateral
    - H36.829 Proliferative sickle-cell retinopathy, unspecified eye
  - H36.89 Other retinal disorders in diseases classified elsewhere
    - Retinal dystrophy in lipid storage disorders

GLAUCOMA (H4Ø-H42)

H4Ø Glaucoma

Intraocular pressure (IOP) that is too high results from too much aqueous humor and because of excess production or inadequate drainage, optic nerve damage and vision loss may occur.

Excludes1 absolute glaucoma (H44.51-)
congenital glaucoma (Q15.Ø)
traumatic glaucoma due to birth injury (P15.3)

- H4Ø.Ø Glaucoma suspect
  - H4Ø.ØØ Preglaucoma, unspecified
    - H4Ø.ØØ1 Preglaucoma, unspecified, right eye
    - H4Ø.ØØ2 Preglaucoma, unspecified, left eye
    - H4Ø.ØØ3 Preglaucoma, unspecified, bilateral
    - H4Ø.ØØ9 Preglaucoma, unspecified, unspecified eye
  - H4Ø.Ø1 Open angle with borderline findings, low risk
    - Open angle, low risk
    - H4Ø.Ø11 Open angle with borderline findings, low risk, right eye
    - H4Ø.Ø12 Open angle with borderline findings, low risk, left eye
    - H4Ø.Ø13 Open angle with borderline findings, low risk, bilateral
    - H4Ø.Ø19 Open angle with borderline findings, low risk, unspecified eye
  - H4Ø.Ø2 Open angle with borderline findings, high risk
    - Open angle, high risk
    - H4Ø.Ø21 Open angle with borderline findings, high risk, right eye
    - H4Ø.Ø22 Open angle with borderline findings, high risk, left eye
    - H4Ø.Ø23 Open angle with borderline findings, high risk, bilateral
    - H4Ø.Ø29 Open angle with borderline findings, high risk, unspecified eye
  - H4Ø.Ø3 Anatomical narrow angle
    - Primary angle closure suspect
    - H4Ø.Ø31 Anatomical narrow angle, right eye
    - H4Ø.Ø32 Anatomical narrow angle, left eye
    - H4Ø.Ø33 Anatomical narrow angle, bilateral
    - H4Ø.Ø39 Anatomical narrow angle, unspecified eye
  - H4Ø.Ø4 Steroid responder
    - H4Ø.Ø41 Steroid responder, right eye
    - H4Ø.Ø42 Steroid responder, left eye
    - H4Ø.Ø43 Steroid responder, bilateral
    - H4Ø.Ø49 Steroid responder, unspecified eye
  - H4Ø.Ø5 Ocular hypertension
    - H4Ø.Ø51 Ocular hypertension, right eye
    - H4Ø.Ø52 Ocular hypertension, left eye
    - H4Ø.Ø53 Ocular hypertension, bilateral
    - H4Ø.Ø59 Ocular hypertension, unspecified eye
  - H4Ø.Ø6 Primary angle closure without glaucoma damage
    - H4Ø.Ø61 Primary angle closure without glaucoma damage, right eye
    - H4Ø.Ø62 Primary angle closure without glaucoma damage, left eye
    - H4Ø.Ø63 Primary angle closure without glaucoma damage, bilateral
    - H4Ø.Ø69 Primary angle closure without glaucoma damage, unspecified eye

H40.1 Open-angle glaucoma

X **H40.10 Unspecified open-angle glaucoma**

One of the following 7th characters is to be assigned to code H40.10 to designate the stage of glaucoma

0	stage unspecified
1	mild stage
2	moderate stage
3	severe stage
4	indeterminate stage

H40.11 Primary open-angle glaucoma

Chronic simple glaucoma

One of the following 7th characters is to be assigned to each code in subcategory H40.11 to designate the stage of glaucoma

0	stage unspecified
1	mild stage
2	moderate stage
3	severe stage
4	indeterminate stage

Coding Clinic: 2016, Q4, P22

H40.111 Primary open-angle glaucoma, right eye

Coding Clinic: 2019, Q2, P31

H40.112 Primary open-angle glaucoma, left eye

H40.113 Primary open-angle glaucoma, bilateral

H40.119 Primary open-angle glaucoma, unspecified eye

H40.12 Low-tension glaucoma

One of the following 7th characters is to be assigned to each code in subcategory H40.12 to designate the stage of glaucoma

0	stage unspecified
1	mild stage
2	moderate stage
3	severe stage
4	indeterminate stage

H40.121 Low-tension glaucoma, right eye

H40.122 Low-tension glaucoma, left eye

H40.123 Low-tension glaucoma, bilateral

H40.129 Low-tension glaucoma, unspecified eye

H40.13 Pigmentary glaucoma

One of the following 7th characters is to be assigned to each code in subcategory H40.13 to designate the stage of glaucoma

0	stage unspecified
1	mild stage
2	moderate stage
3	severe stage
4	indeterminate stage

H40.131 Pigmentary glaucoma, right eye

H40.132 Pigmentary glaucoma, left eye

H40.133 Pigmentary glaucoma, bilateral

H40.139 Pigmentary glaucoma, unspecified eye

H40.14 Capsular glaucoma with pseudoexfoliation of lens

One of the following 7th characters is to be assigned to each code in subcategory H40.14 to designate the stage of glaucoma

0	stage unspecified
1	mild stage
2	moderate stage
3	severe stage
4	indeterminate stage

H40.141 Capsular glaucoma with pseudoexfoliation of lens, right eye

H40.142 Capsular glaucoma with pseudoexfoliation of lens, left eye

H40.143 Capsular glaucoma with pseudoexfoliation of lens, bilateral

H40.149 Capsular glaucoma with pseudoexfoliation of lens, unspecified eye

H40.15 Residual stage of open-angle glaucoma

H40.151 Residual stage of open-angle glaucoma, right eye

H40.152 Residual stage of open-angle glaucoma, left eye

H40.153 Residual stage of open-angle glaucoma, bilateral

H40.159 Residual stage of open-angle glaucoma, unspecified eye

H40.2 Primary angle-closure glaucoma

Excludes1 aqueous misdirection (H40.83-)
malignant glaucoma (H40.83-)

X **H40.20 Unspecified primary angle-closure glaucoma**

One of the following 7th characters is to be assigned to code H40.20 to designate the stage of glaucoma

0	stage unspecified
1	mild stage
2	moderate stage
3	severe stage
4	indeterminate stage

H40.21 Acute angle-closure glaucoma Ex: PDX 797

Acute angle-closure glaucoma attack

Acute angle-closure glaucoma crisis

H40.211 Acute angle-closure glaucoma, right eye

H40.212 Acute angle-closure glaucoma, left eye

H40.213 Acute angle-closure glaucoma, bilateral

H40.219 Acute angle-closure glaucoma, unspecified eye

H40.22 Chronic angle-closure glaucoma

Chronic primary angle closure glaucoma

One of the following 7th characters is to be assigned to each code in subcategory H40.22 to designate the stage of glaucoma

0	stage unspecified
1	mild stage
2	moderate stage
3	severe stage
4	indeterminate stage

H40.221 Chronic angle-closure glaucoma, right eye

H40.222 Chronic angle-closure glaucoma, left eye

CHAPTER 7 (H00-H59)

H40.223 **Chronic angle-closure glaucoma, bilateral**

H40.229 **Chronic angle-closure glaucoma, unspecified eye**

H40.23 **Intermittent angle-closure glaucoma**

H40.231 **Intermittent angle-closure glaucoma, right eye**

H40.232 **Intermittent angle-closure glaucoma, left eye**

H40.233 **Intermittent angle-closure glaucoma, bilateral**

H40.239 **Intermittent angle-closure glaucoma, unspecified eye**

H40.24 **Residual stage of angle-closure glaucoma**

H40.241 **Residual stage of angle-closure glaucoma, right eye**

H40.242 **Residual stage of angle-closure glaucoma, left eye**

H40.243 **Residual stage of angle-closure glaucoma, bilateral**

H40.249 **Residual stage of angle-closure glaucoma, unspecified eye**

H40.3 **Glaucoma secondary to eye trauma**

Code also underlying condition

One of the following 7th characters is to be assigned to each code in subcategory H40.3 to designate the stage of glaucoma

0	stage unspecified
1	mild stage
2	moderate stage
3	severe stage
4	indeterminate stage

X **H40.30** **Glaucoma secondary to eye trauma, unspecified eye**

X **H40.31** **Glaucoma secondary to eye trauma, right eye**

X **H40.32** **Glaucoma secondary to eye trauma, left eye**

X **H40.33** **Glaucoma secondary to eye trauma, bilateral**

H40.4 **Glaucoma secondary to eye inflammation**

Code also underlying condition

One of the following 7th characters is to be assigned to each code in subcategory H40.4 to designate the stage of glaucoma

0	stage unspecified
1	mild stage
2	moderate stage
3	severe stage
4	indeterminate stage

X **H40.40** **Glaucoma secondary to eye inflammation, unspecified eye**

X **H40.41** **Glaucoma secondary to eye inflammation, right eye**

X **H40.42** **Glaucoma secondary to eye inflammation, left eye**

X **H40.43** **Glaucoma secondary to eye inflammation, bilateral**

H40.5 **Glaucoma secondary to other eye disorders**

Code also underlying eye disorder

One of the following 7th characters is to be assigned to each code in subcategory H40.5 to designate the stage of glaucoma

0	stage unspecified
1	mild stage
2	moderate stage
3	severe stage
4	indeterminate stage

X **H40.50** **Glaucoma secondary to other eye disorders, unspecified eye**

X **H40.51** **Glaucoma secondary to other eye disorders, right eye**

X **H40.52** **Glaucoma secondary to other eye disorders, left eye**

X **H40.53** **Glaucoma secondary to other eye disorders, bilateral**

H40.6 **Glaucoma secondary to drugs**

Use additional code for adverse effect, if applicable, to identify drug (T36-T50 with fifth or sixth character 5)

One of the following 7th characters is to be assigned to each code in subcategory H40.6 to designate the stage of glaucoma

0	stage unspecified
1	mild stage
2	moderate stage
3	severe stage
4	indeterminate stage

X **H40.60** **Glaucoma secondary to drugs, unspecified eye**

X **H40.61** **Glaucoma secondary to drugs, right eye**

X **H40.62** **Glaucoma secondary to drugs, left eye**

X **H40.63** **Glaucoma secondary to drugs, bilateral**

H40.8 **Other glaucoma**

H40.81 **Glaucoma with increased episcleral venous pressure**

H40.811 **Glaucoma with increased episcleral venous pressure, right eye**

H40.812 **Glaucoma with increased episcleral venous pressure, left eye**

H40.813 **Glaucoma with increased episcleral venous pressure, bilateral**

H40.819 **Glaucoma with increased episcleral venous pressure, unspecified eye**

H40.82 **Hypersecretion glaucoma**

H40.821 **Hypersecretion glaucoma, right eye**

H40.822 **Hypersecretion glaucoma, left eye**

H40.823 **Hypersecretion glaucoma, bilateral**

H40.829 **Hypersecretion glaucoma, unspecified eye**

H40.83 **Aqueous misdirection**

Malignant glaucoma

H40.831 **Aqueous misdirection, right eye**

H40.832 **Aqueous misdirection, left eye**

H40.833 **Aqueous misdirection, bilateral**

H40.839 **Aqueous misdirection, unspecified eye**

H40.89 **Other specified glaucoma**

H40.9 **Unspecified glaucoma**

H42 ***Glaucoma in diseases classified elsewhere***

Code first underlying condition, such as:

amyloidosis (E85.-)

aniridia (Q13.1)

glaucoma (in) diabetes mellitus (E08.39, E09.39, E10.39, E11.39, E13.39)

Lowe's syndrome (E72.03)

Reiger anomaly (Q13.81)

specified metabolic disorder (E70-E88)

Excludes1 glaucoma (in) onchocerciasis (B73.02)
glaucoma (in) syphilis (A52.71)
glaucoma (in) tuberculous (A18.59)

CHAPTER 7 (H00-H59)

DISORDERS OF VITREOUS BODY AND GLOBE (H43-H44)

H43 Disorders of vitreous body

H43.Ø Vitreous prolapse

Excludes1 vitreous syndrome following cataract surgery (H59.Ø-)
traumatic vitreous prolapse (SØ5.2-)

H43.ØØ Vitreous prolapse, unspecified eye
H43.Ø1 Vitreous prolapse, right eye
H43.Ø2 Vitreous prolapse, left eye
H43.Ø3 Vitreous prolapse, bilateral

H43.1 Vitreous hemorrhage

H43.1Ø Vitreous hemorrhage, unspecified eye
H43.11 Vitreous hemorrhage, right eye
H43.12 Vitreous hemorrhage, left eye
H43.13 Vitreous hemorrhage, bilateral

H43.2 Crystalline deposits in vitreous body

H43.2Ø Crystalline deposits in vitreous body, unspecified eye
H43.21 Crystalline deposits in vitreous body, right eye
H43.22 Crystalline deposits in vitreous body, left eye
H43.23 Crystalline deposits in vitreous body, bilateral

H43.3 Other vitreous opacities

H43.31 Vitreous membranes and strands

H43.311 Vitreous membranes and strands, right eye
H43.312 Vitreous membranes and strands, left eye
H43.313 Vitreous membranes and strands, bilateral
H43.319 Vitreous membranes and strands, unspecified eye

H43.39 Other vitreous opacities

Vitreous floaters

Small clumps of cells that float in the vitreous of the eye, appearing as black specks or dots in the field of vision and common in the aging eye.

H43.391 Other vitreous opacities, right eye
H43.392 Other vitreous opacities, left eye
H43.393 Other vitreous opacities, bilateral
H43.399 Other vitreous opacities, unspecified eye

H43.8 Other disorders of vitreous body

Excludes1 proliferative vitreo-retinopathy with retinal detachment (H33.4)

Excludes2 vitreous abscess (H44.Ø2-)

H43.81 Vitreous degeneration

Vitreous detachment

H43.811 Vitreous degeneration, right eye
H43.812 Vitreous degeneration, left eye
H43.813 Vitreous degeneration, bilateral
H43.819 Vitreous degeneration, unspecified eye

H43.82 Vitreomacular adhesion

Vitreomacular traction

H43.821 Vitreomacular adhesion, right eye A
H43.822 Vitreomacular adhesion, left eye A
H43.823 Vitreomacular adhesion, bilateral A
H43.829 Vitreomacular adhesion, unspecified eye A

H43.89 Other disorders of vitreous body

H43.9 Unspecified disorder of vitreous body

H44 Disorders of globe

Includes disorders affecting multiple structures of eye

H44.Ø Purulent endophthalmitis

Use additional code to identify organism

Excludes1 bleb associated endophthalmitis (H59.4-)

H44.ØØ Unspecified purulent endophthalmitis Ex PDX 792

H44.ØØ1 Unspecified purulent endophthalmitis, right eye
H44.ØØ2 Unspecified purulent endophthalmitis, left eye
H44.ØØ3 Unspecified purulent endophthalmitis, bilateral
H44.ØØ9 Unspecified purulent endophthalmitis, unspecified eye

H44.Ø1 Panophthalmitis (acute) Ex PDX 792

H44.Ø11 Panophthalmitis (acute), right eye
H44.Ø12 Panophthalmitis (acute), left eye
H44.Ø13 Panophthalmitis (acute), bilateral
H44.Ø19 Panophthalmitis (acute), unspecified eye

H44.Ø2 Vitreous abscess (chronic) Ex PDX 798

H44.Ø21 Vitreous abscess (chronic), right eye
H44.Ø22 Vitreous abscess (chronic), left eye
H44.Ø23 Vitreous abscess (chronic), bilateral
H44.Ø29 Vitreous abscess (chronic), unspecified eye

H44.1 Other endophthalmitis

Excludes1 bleb associated endophthalmitis (H59.4-)

Excludes2 ophthalmia nodosa (H16.2-)

H44.11 Panuveitis Ex PDX 799

H44.111 Panuveitis, right eye
H44.112 Panuveitis, left eye
H44.113 Panuveitis, bilateral
H44.119 Panuveitis, unspecified eye

H44.12 Parasitic endophthalmitis, unspecified Ex DX 792

H44.121 Parasitic endophthalmitis, unspecified, right eye
H44.122 Parasitic endophthalmitis, unspecified, left eye
H44.123 Parasitic endophthalmitis, unspecified, bilateral
H44.129 Parasitic endophthalmitis, unspecified, unspecified eye

H44.13 Sympathetic uveitis Ex PDX 799

H44.131 Sympathetic uveitis, right eye
H44.132 Sympathetic uveitis, left eye
H44.133 Sympathetic uveitis, bilateral
H44.139 Sympathetic uveitis, unspecified eye

H44.19 Other endophthalmitis Ex PDX 792

H44.2 Degenerative myopia

Malignant myopia

H44.2Ø Degenerative myopia, unspecified eye
H44.21 Degenerative myopia, right eye
H44.22 Degenerative myopia, left eye
H44.23 Degenerative myopia, bilateral

CHAPTER 7 (HØØ-H59)

H44.2A Degenerative myopia with choroidal neovascularization
Use Additional code for any associated choroid disorders (H31.-)
H44.2A1 Degenerative myopia with choroidal neovascularization, right eye
H44.2A2 Degenerative myopia with choroidal neovascularization, left eye
H44.2A3 Degenerative myopia with choroidal neovascularization, bilateral
H44.2A9 Degenerative myopia with choroidal neovascularization, unspecified eye

H44.2B Degenerative myopia with macular hole
H44.2B1 Degenerative myopia with macular hole, right eye
H44.2B2 Degenerative myopia with macular hole, left eye
H44.2B3 Degenerative myopia with macular hole, bilateral
H44.2B9 Degenerative myopia with macular hole, unspecified eye

H44.2C Degenerative myopia with retinal detachment
Use Additional code to identify the retinal detachment (H33.-)
H44.2C1 Degenerative myopia with retinal detachment, right eye
H44.2C2 Degenerative myopia with retinal detachment, left eye
H44.2C3 Degenerative myopia with retinal detachment, bilateral
H44.2C9 Degenerative myopia with retinal detachment, unspecified eye

H44.2D Degenerative myopia with foveoschisis
H44.2D1 Degenerative myopia with foveoschisis, right eye
H44.2D2 Degenerative myopia with foveoschisis, left eye
H44.2D3 Degenerative myopia with foveoschisis, bilateral
H44.2D9 Degenerative myopia with foveoschisis, unspecified eye

H44.2E Degenerative myopia with other maculopathy
H44.2E1 Degenerative myopia with other maculopathy, right eye
H44.2E2 Degenerative myopia with other maculopathy, left eye
H44.2E3 Degenerative myopia with other maculopathy, bilateral
H44.2E9 Degenerative myopia with other maculopathy, unspecified eye

H44.3 Other and unspecified degenerative disorders of globe
H44.30 Unspecified degenerative disorder of globe

H44.31 Chalcosis
H44.311 Chalcosis, right eye
H44.312 Chalcosis, left eye
H44.313 Chalcosis, bilateral
H44.319 Chalcosis, unspecified eye

H44.32 Siderosis of eye
H44.321 Siderosis of eye, right eye
H44.322 Siderosis of eye, left eye
H44.323 Siderosis of eye, bilateral
H44.329 Siderosis of eye, unspecified eye

H44.39 Other degenerative disorders of globe
H44.391 Other degenerative disorders of globe, right eye
H44.392 Other degenerative disorders of globe, left eye
H44.393 Other degenerative disorders of globe, bilateral
H44.399 Other degenerative disorders of globe, unspecified eye

H44.4 Hypotony of eye
H44.40 Unspecified hypotony of eye

H44.41 Flat anterior chamber hypotony of eye
H44.411 Flat anterior chamber hypotony of right eye
H44.412 Flat anterior chamber hypotony of left eye
H44.413 Flat anterior chamber hypotony of eye, bilateral
H44.419 Flat anterior chamber hypotony of unspecified eye

H44.42 Hypotony of eye due to ocular fistula
H44.421 Hypotony of right eye due to ocular fistula
H44.422 Hypotony of left eye due to ocular fistula
H44.423 Hypotony of eye due to ocular fistula, bilateral
H44.429 Hypotony of unspecified eye due to ocular fistula

H44.43 Hypotony of eye due to other ocular disorders
H44.431 Hypotony of eye due to other ocular disorders, right eye
H44.432 Hypotony of eye due to other ocular disorders, left eye
H44.433 Hypotony of eye due to other ocular disorders, bilateral
H44.439 Hypotony of eye due to other ocular disorders, unspecified eye

H44.44 Primary hypotony of eye
H44.441 Primary hypotony of right eye
H44.442 Primary hypotony of left eye
H44.443 Primary hypotony of eye, bilateral
H44.449 Primary hypotony of unspecified eye

H44.5 Degenerated conditions of globe
H44.50 Unspecified degenerated conditions of globe

H44.51 Absolute glaucoma
H44.511 Absolute glaucoma, right eye
H44.512 Absolute glaucoma, left eye
H44.513 Absolute glaucoma, bilateral
H44.519 Absolute glaucoma, unspecified eye

H44.52 Atrophy of globe
Phthisis bulbi
H44.521 Atrophy of globe, right eye
H44.522 Atrophy of globe, left eye
H44.523 Atrophy of globe, bilateral
H44.529 Atrophy of globe, unspecified eye

H44.53 Leucocoria
H44.531 Leucocoria, right eye
H44.532 Leucocoria, left eye
H44.533 Leucocoria, bilateral
H44.539 Leucocoria, unspecified eye

H44.6 Retained (old) intraocular foreign body, magnetic

Use additional code to identify magnetic foreign body (Z18.11)

Excludes1 current intraocular foreign body (SØ5.-)

Excludes2 retained foreign body in eyelid (HØ2.81-)
retained (old) foreign body following penetrating wound of orbit (HØ5.5-)
retained (old) intraocular foreign body, nonmagnetic (H44.7-)

H44.60 Unspecified retained (old) intraocular foreign body, magnetic

- H44.601 Unspecified retained (old) intraocular foreign body, magnetic, right eye
- H44.602 Unspecified retained (old) intraocular foreign body, magnetic, left eye
- H44.603 Unspecified retained (old) intraocular foreign body, magnetic, bilateral
- H44.609 Unspecified retained (old) intraocular foreign body, magnetic, unspecified eye

H44.61 Retained (old) magnetic foreign body in anterior chamber

- H44.611 Retained (old) magnetic foreign body in anterior chamber, right eye
- H44.612 Retained (old) magnetic foreign body in anterior chamber, left eye
- H44.613 Retained (old) magnetic foreign body in anterior chamber, bilateral
- H44.619 Retained (old) magnetic foreign body in anterior chamber, unspecified eye

H44.62 Retained (old) magnetic foreign body in iris or ciliary body

- H44.621 Retained (old) magnetic foreign body in iris or ciliary body, right eye
- H44.622 Retained (old) magnetic foreign body in iris or ciliary body, left eye
- H44.623 Retained (old) magnetic foreign body in iris or ciliary body, bilateral
- H44.629 Retained (old) magnetic foreign body in iris or ciliary body, unspecified eye

H44.63 Retained (old) magnetic foreign body in lens

- H44.631 Retained (old) magnetic foreign body in lens, right eye
- H44.632 Retained (old) magnetic foreign body in lens, left eye
- H44.633 Retained (old) magnetic foreign body in lens, bilateral
- H44.639 Retained (old) magnetic foreign body in lens, unspecified eye

H44.64 Retained (old) magnetic foreign body in posterior wall of globe

- H44.641 Retained (old) magnetic foreign body in posterior wall of globe, right eye
- H44.642 Retained (old) magnetic foreign body in posterior wall of globe, left eye
- H44.643 Retained (old) magnetic foreign body in posterior wall of globe, bilateral
- H44.649 Retained (old) magnetic foreign body in posterior wall of globe, unspecified eye

H44.65 Retained (old) magnetic foreign body in vitreous body

- H44.651 Retained (old) magnetic foreign body in vitreous body, right eye
- H44.652 Retained (old) magnetic foreign body in vitreous body, left eye
- H44.653 Retained (old) magnetic foreign body in vitreous body, bilateral
- H44.659 Retained (old) magnetic foreign body in vitreous body, unspecified eye

H44.69 Retained (old) intraocular foreign body, magnetic, in other or multiple sites

- H44.691 Retained (old) intraocular foreign body, magnetic, in other or multiple sites, right eye
- H44.692 Retained (old) intraocular foreign body, magnetic, in other or multiple sites, left eye
- H44.693 Retained (old) intraocular foreign body, magnetic, in other or multiple sites, bilateral
- H44.699 Retained (old) intraocular foreign body, magnetic, in other or multiple sites, unspecified eye

H44.7 Retained (old) intraocular foreign body, nonmagnetic

Use additional code to identify nonmagnetic foreign body (Z18.Ø1-Z18.1Ø, Z18.12, Z18.2-Z18.9)

Excludes1 current intraocular foreign body (SØ5.-)

Excludes2 retained foreign body in eyelid (HØ2.81-)
retained (old) foreign body following penetrating wound of orbit (HØ5.5-)
retained (old) intraocular foreign body, magnetic (H44.6-)

H44.7Ø Unspecified retained (old) intraocular foreign body, nonmagnetic

- H44.7Ø1 Unspecified retained (old) intraocular foreign body, nonmagnetic, right eye
- H44.7Ø2 Unspecified retained (old) intraocular foreign body, nonmagnetic, left eye
- H44.7Ø3 Unspecified retained (old) intraocular foreign body, nonmagnetic, bilateral
- H44.7Ø9 Unspecified retained (old) intraocular foreign body, nonmagnetic, unspecified eye
  Retained (old) intraocular foreign body NOS

H44.71 Retained (nonmagnetic) (old) foreign body in anterior chamber

- H44.711 Retained (nonmagnetic) (old) foreign body in anterior chamber, right eye
- H44.712 Retained (nonmagnetic) (old) foreign body in anterior chamber, left eye
- H44.713 Retained (nonmagnetic) (old) foreign body in anterior chamber, bilateral
- H44.719 Retained (nonmagnetic) (old) foreign body in anterior chamber, unspecified eye

H44.72 Retained (nonmagnetic) (old) foreign body in iris or ciliary body

- H44.721 Retained (nonmagnetic) (old) foreign body in iris or ciliary body, right eye
- H44.722 Retained (nonmagnetic) (old) foreign body in iris or ciliary body, left eye
- H44.723 Retained (nonmagnetic) (old) foreign body in iris or ciliary body, bilateral
- H44.729 Retained (nonmagnetic) (old) foreign body in iris or ciliary body, unspecified eye

H44.73 Retained (nonmagnetic) (old) foreign body in lens

- H44.731 Retained (nonmagnetic) (old) foreign body in lens, right eye
- H44.732 Retained (nonmagnetic) (old) foreign body in lens, left eye
- H44.733 Retained (nonmagnetic) (old) foreign body in lens, bilateral
- H44.739 Retained (nonmagnetic) (old) foreign body in lens, unspecified eye

CHAPTER 7 (HØØ-H59)

● **H44.74 Retained (nonmagnetic) (old) foreign body in posterior wall of globe**
- **H44.741 Retained (nonmagnetic) (old) foreign body in posterior wall of globe, right eye**
- **H44.742 Retained (nonmagnetic) (old) foreign body in posterior wall of globe, left eye**
- **H44.743 Retained (nonmagnetic) (old) foreign body in posterior wall of globe, bilateral**
- **H44.749 Retained (nonmagnetic) (old) foreign body in posterior wall of globe, unspecified eye**

● **H44.75 Retained (nonmagnetic) (old) foreign body in vitreous body**
- **H44.751 Retained (nonmagnetic) (old) foreign body in vitreous body, right eye**
- **H44.752 Retained (nonmagnetic) (old) foreign body in vitreous body, left eye**
- **H44.753 Retained (nonmagnetic) (old) foreign body in vitreous body, bilateral**
- **H44.759 Retained (nonmagnetic) (old) foreign body in vitreous body, unspecified eye**

● **H44.79 Retained (old) intraocular foreign body, nonmagnetic, in other or multiple sites**
- **H44.791 Retained (old) intraocular foreign body, nonmagnetic, in other or multiple sites, right eye**
- **H44.792 Retained (old) intraocular foreign body, nonmagnetic, in other or multiple sites, left eye**
- **H44.793 Retained (old) intraocular foreign body, nonmagnetic, in other or multiple sites, bilateral**
- **H44.799 Retained (old) intraocular foreign body, nonmagnetic, in other or multiple sites, unspecified eye**

● **H44.8 Other disorders of globe**

● **H44.81 Hemophthalmos**
- **H44.811 Hemophthalmos, right eye**
- **H44.812 Hemophthalmos, left eye**
- **H44.813 Hemophthalmos, bilateral**
- **H44.819 Hemophthalmos, unspecified eye**

● **H44.82 Luxation of globe**
- **H44.821 Luxation of globe, right eye**
- **H44.822 Luxation of globe, left eye**
- **H44.823 Luxation of globe, bilateral**
- **H44.829 Luxation of globe, unspecified eye**

H44.89 Other disorders of globe

H44.9 Unspecified disorder of globe

★**(See Plate 7 of the Anatomy Illustrations.)**

DISORDERS OF OPTIC NERVE AND VISUAL PATHWAYS (H46-H47)

● **H46 Optic neuritis** (Ex) PDX 800

Excludes2 ischemic optic neuropathy (H47.01-)
neuromyelitis optica [Devic] (G36.0)

● **H46.0 Optic papillitis**
- **H46.00 Optic papillitis, unspecified eye**
- **H46.01 Optic papillitis, right eye**
- **H46.02 Optic papillitis, left eye**
- **H46.03 Optic papillitis, bilateral**

● **H46.1 Retrobulbar neuritis**
Retrobulbar neuritis NOS

Excludes1 syphilitic retrobulbar neuritis (A52.15)
- **H46.10 Retrobulbar neuritis, unspecified eye**
- **H46.11 Retrobulbar neuritis, right eye**
- **H46.12 Retrobulbar neuritis, left eye**
- **H46.13 Retrobulbar neuritis, bilateral**

H46.2 Nutritional optic neuropathy

H46.3 Toxic optic neuropathy
Code first (T51-T65) to identify cause

H46.8 Other optic neuritis

H46.9 Unspecified optic neuritis
Coding Clinic: 2023, Q3, P19

● **H47 Other disorders of optic [2nd] nerve and visual pathways**

● **H47.0 Disorders of optic nerve, not elsewhere classified**

● **H47.01 Ischemic optic neuropathy**
- **H47.011 Ischemic optic neuropathy, right eye**
- **H47.012 Ischemic optic neuropathy, left eye**
- **H47.013 Ischemic optic neuropathy, bilateral**
- **H47.019 Ischemic optic neuropathy, unspecified eye**

● **H47.02 Hemorrhage in optic nerve sheath**
- **H47.021 Hemorrhage in optic nerve sheath, right eye**
- **H47.022 Hemorrhage in optic nerve sheath, left eye**
- **H47.023 Hemorrhage in optic nerve sheath, bilateral**
- **H47.029 Hemorrhage in optic nerve sheath, unspecified eye**

● **H47.03 Optic nerve hypoplasia**
- **H47.031 Optic nerve hypoplasia, right eye**
- **H47.032 Optic nerve hypoplasia, left eye**
- **H47.033 Optic nerve hypoplasia, bilateral**
- **H47.039 Optic nerve hypoplasia, unspecified eye**

● **H47.09 Other disorders of optic nerve, not elsewhere classified**
Compression of optic nerve
- **H47.091 Other disorders of optic nerve, not elsewhere classified, right eye**
- **H47.092 Other disorders of optic nerve, not elsewhere classified, left eye**
- **H47.093 Other disorders of optic nerve, not elsewhere classified, bilateral**
- **H47.099 Other disorders of optic nerve, not elsewhere classified, unspecified eye**

● **H47.1 Papilledema**
- **H47.10 Unspecified papilledema** (Ex) PDX 801
- **H47.11 Papilledema associated with increased intracranial pressure** (Ex) PDX 801
- **H47.12 Papilledema associated with decreased ocular pressure**
- **H47.13 Papilledema associated with retinal disorder**

● **H47.14 Foster-Kennedy syndrome**
- **H47.141 Foster-Kennedy syndrome, right eye**
- **H47.142 Foster-Kennedy syndrome, left eye**
- **H47.143 Foster-Kennedy syndrome, bilateral**
- **H47.149 Foster-Kennedy syndrome, unspecified eye**

CHAPTER 7 (H00-H59)

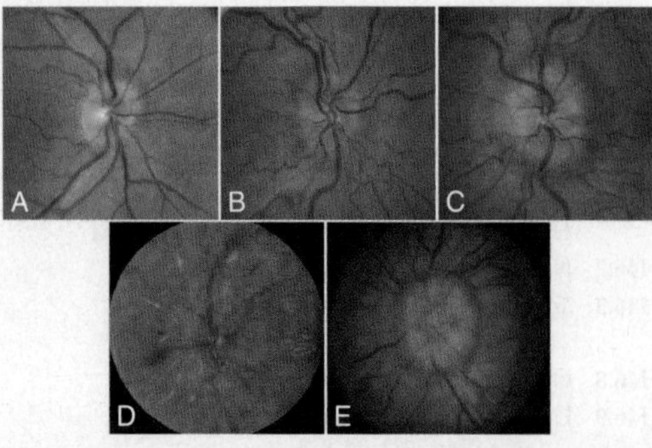

Figure 7-11 Stages of papilledema according to the Frisén grading scale. **A,** Very eary papilledema (Frisén stage 1). **B,** Early papilledema (Frisén stage 2). **C,** Moderate papilledema (Frisén stage 3). **D,** Marked papilledema (Frisén stage 4). **E,** Severe papilledema. (From Youmans JR, Winn HR: Youmans Neurological Surgery, Philadelphia, PA, Elsevier/Saunders, 2011)

Item 7-8 Papilledema is swelling of the optic disc caused by increased intracranial pressure. It is most often bilateral and occurs quickly (hours) or over weeks of time. It is a common symptom of a brain tumor. The term should not be used to describe optic disc swelling with underlying infectious, infiltrative, or inflammatory etiologies.

● H47.2 Optic atrophy
- H47.20 Unspecified optic atrophy
- ● H47.21 Primary optic atrophy
  - H47.211 Primary optic atrophy, right eye
  - H47.212 Primary optic atrophy, left eye
  - H47.213 Primary optic atrophy, bilateral
  - H47.219 Primary optic atrophy, unspecified eye
- H47.22 Hereditary optic atrophy
  - Leber's optic atrophy
- ● H47.23 Glaucomatous optic atrophy
  - H47.231 Glaucomatous optic atrophy, right eye
  - H47.232 Glaucomatous optic atrophy, left eye
  - H47.233 Glaucomatous optic atrophy, bilateral
  - H47.239 Glaucomatous optic atrophy, unspecified eye
- ● H47.29 Other optic atrophy
  - Temporal pallor of optic disc
  - H47.291 Other optic atrophy, right eye
  - H47.292 Other optic atrophy, left eye
  - H47.293 Other optic atrophy, bilateral
  - H47.299 Other optic atrophy, unspecified eye

● H47.3 Other disorders of optic disc
- ● H47.31 Coloboma of optic disc
  - H47.311 Coloboma of optic disc, right eye
  - H47.312 Coloboma of optic disc, left eye
  - H47.313 Coloboma of optic disc, bilateral
  - H47.319 Coloboma of optic disc, unspecified eye
- ● H47.32 Drusen of optic disc
  - H47.321 Drusen of optic disc, right eye
  - H47.322 Drusen of optic disc, left eye
  - H47.323 Drusen of optic disc, bilateral
  - H47.329 Drusen of optic disc, unspecified eye
- ● H47.33 Pseudopapilledema of optic disc
  - H47.331 Pseudopapilledema of optic disc, right eye
  - H47.332 Pseudopapilledema of optic disc, left eye
  - H47.333 Pseudopapilledema of optic disc, bilateral
  - H47.339 Pseudopapilledema of optic disc, unspecified eye
- ● H47.39 Other disorders of optic disc
  - H47.391 Other disorders of optic disc, right eye
  - H47.392 Other disorders of optic disc, left eye
  - H47.393 Other disorders of optic disc, bilateral
  - H47.399 Other disorders of optic disc, unspecified eye

● H47.4 Disorders of optic chiasm (Ex) DX 802
- Code also underlying condition
- H47.41 Disorders of optic chiasm in (due to) inflammatory disorders
- H47.42 Disorders of optic chiasm in (due to) neoplasm
- H47.43 Disorders of optic chiasm in (due to) vascular disorders
- H47.49 Disorders of optic chiasm in (due to) other disorders

● H47.5 Disorders of other visual pathways (Ex) PDX 802
- Disorders of optic tracts, geniculate nuclei and optic radiations
- Code also underlying condition
- ● H47.51 Disorders of visual pathways in (due to) inflammatory disorders
  - H47.511 Disorders of visual pathways in (due to) inflammatory disorders, right side
  - H47.512 Disorders of visual pathways in (due to) inflammatory disorders, left side
  - H47.519 Disorders of visual pathways in (due to) inflammatory disorders, unspecified side
- ● H47.52 Disorders of visual pathways in (due to) neoplasm
  - H47.521 Disorders of visual pathways in (due to) neoplasm, right side
  - H47.522 Disorders of visual pathways in (due to) neoplasm, left side
  - H47.529 Disorders of visual pathways in (due to) neoplasm, unspecified side
- ● H47.53 Disorders of visual pathways in (due to) vascular disorders
  - H47.531 Disorders of visual pathways in (due to) vascular disorders, right side
  - H47.532 Disorders of visual pathways in (due to) vascular disorders, left side
  - H47.539 Disorders of visual pathways in (due to) vascular disorders, unspecified side

● H47.6 Disorders of visual cortex (Ex) PDX 803
- Code also underlying condition
- **Excludes1** injury to visual cortex S04.04-
- ● H47.61 Cortical blindness
  - H47.611 Cortical blindness, right side of brain
  - H47.612 Cortical blindness, left side of brain
  - H47.619 Cortical blindness, unspecified side of brain

● H47.62 Disorders of visual cortex in (due to) inflammatory disorders
H47.621 Disorders of visual cortex in (due to) inflammatory disorders, right side of brain
H47.622 Disorders of visual cortex in (due to) inflammatory disorders, left side of brain
H47.629 Disorders of visual cortex in (due to) inflammatory disorders, unspecified side of brain
● H47.63 Disorders of visual cortex in (due to) neoplasm
H47.631 Disorders of visual cortex in (due to) neoplasm, right side of brain
H47.632 Disorders of visual cortex in (due to) neoplasm, left side of brain
H47.639 Disorders of visual cortex in (due to) neoplasm, unspecified side of brain
● H47.64 Disorders of visual cortex in (due to) vascular disorders
H47.641 Disorders of visual cortex in (due to) vascular disorders, right side of brain
H47.642 Disorders of visual cortex in (due to) vascular disorders, left side of brain
H47.649 Disorders of visual cortex in (due to) vascular disorders, unspecified side of brain
H47.9 Unspecified disorder of visual pathways

DISORDERS OF OCULAR MUSCLES, BINOCULAR MOVEMENT, ACCOMMODATION AND REFRACTION (H49-H52)

Excludes2 nystagmus and other irregular eye movements (H55)

● H49 Paralytic strabismus
Excludes2 internal ophthalmoplegia (H52.51-)
internuclear ophthalmoplegia (H51.2-)
progressive supranuclear ophthalmoplegia (G23.1)
● H49.0 Third [oculomotor] nerve palsy
H49.00 Third [oculomotor] nerve palsy, unspecified eye
H49.01 Third [oculomotor] nerve palsy, right eye
H49.02 Third [oculomotor] nerve palsy, left eye
H49.03 Third [oculomotor] nerve palsy, bilateral
● H49.1 Fourth [trochlear] nerve palsy
H49.10 Fourth [trochlear] nerve palsy, unspecified eye
H49.11 Fourth [trochlear] nerve palsy, right eye
H49.12 Fourth [trochlear] nerve palsy, left eye
H49.13 Fourth [trochlear] nerve palsy, bilateral
● H49.2 Sixth [abducent] nerve palsy
H49.20 Sixth [abducent] nerve palsy, unspecified eye
H49.21 Sixth [abducent] nerve palsy, right eye
H49.22 Sixth [abducent] nerve palsy, left eye
H49.23 Sixth [abducent] nerve palsy, bilateral
● H49.3 Total (external) ophthalmoplegia
H49.30 Total (external) ophthalmoplegia, unspecified eye
H49.31 Total (external) ophthalmoplegia, right eye
H49.32 Total (external) ophthalmoplegia, left eye
H49.33 Total (external) ophthalmoplegia, bilateral

Item 7-9 Strabismus or esotropia (crossed eyes) is a condition of the extraocular eye muscles, resulting in an inability of the eyes to focus and also affects depth perception.

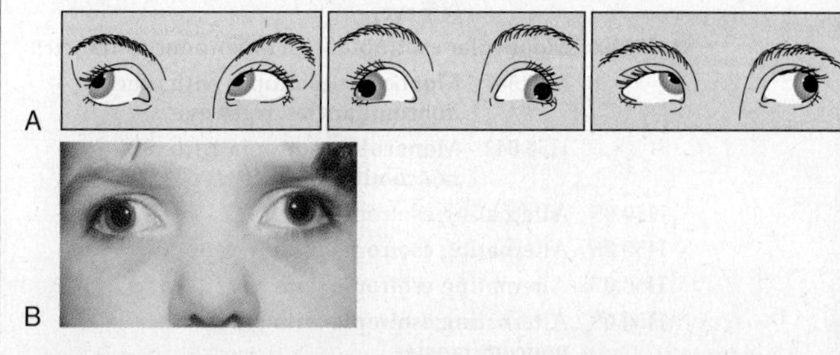

Figure 7-12 **A.** Image of strabismus. **B.** Exotropia. (**A** from Yanoff: Ophthalmology, ed 3, Mosby, Inc., 2008. **B** from Zitelli BJ, Davis HW, Pediatric Physical Diagnosis: Atlas of Pediatric Physical Diagnosis, Philadelphia, Elsevier Saunders, 2012)

● H49.4 Progressive external ophthalmoplegia
Excludes1 Kearns-Sayre syndrome (H49.81-)
H49.40 Progressive external ophthalmoplegia, unspecified eye
H49.41 Progressive external ophthalmoplegia, right eye
H49.42 Progressive external ophthalmoplegia, left eye
H49.43 Progressive external ophthalmoplegia, bilateral
● H49.8 Other paralytic strabismus
● H49.81 Kearns-Sayre syndrome
Progressive external ophthalmoplegia with pigmentary retinopathy
Code also, if applicable, other manifestations, such as:
heart block (I45.9)
H49.811 Kearns-Sayre syndrome, right eye PDX 804
H49.812 Kearns-Sayre syndrome, left eye PDX 805
H49.813 Kearns-Sayre syndrome, bilateral PDX 806
H49.819 Kearns-Sayre syndrome, unspecified eye PDX 807
● H49.88 Other paralytic strabismus
External ophthalmoplegia NOS
H49.881 Other paralytic strabismus, right eye
H49.882 Other paralytic strabismus, left eye
H49.883 Other paralytic strabismus, bilateral
H49.889 Other paralytic strabismus, unspecified eye
H49.9 Unspecified paralytic strabismus

● H50 Other strabismus
● H50.0 Esotropia
Convergent concomitant strabismus
Excludes1 intermittent esotropia (H50.31-, H50.32)
H50.00 Unspecified esotropia
● H50.01 Monocular esotropia
H50.011 Monocular esotropia, right eye
H50.012 Monocular esotropia, left eye
● H50.02 Monocular esotropia with A pattern
H50.021 Monocular esotropia with A pattern, right eye
H50.022 Monocular esotropia with A pattern, left eye

N Newborn Age: 0 P Pediatric Age: 0–17 M Maternity DX: 9–64 A Adult Age: 15–124
Complication\Comorbidity Major C\C CC/MCC Exclusions Hospital-Acquired Condition Hierarchical Condition Category

- H50.03 Monocular esotropia with V pattern
  - H50.031 Monocular esotropia with V pattern, right eye
  - H50.032 Monocular esotropia with V pattern, left eye
- H50.04 Monocular esotropia with other noncomitancies
  - H50.041 Monocular esotropia with other noncomitancies, right eye
  - H50.042 Monocular esotropia with other noncomitancies, left eye
- H50.05 Alternating esotropia
- H50.06 Alternating esotropia with A pattern
- H50.07 Alternating esotropia with V pattern
- H50.08 Alternating esotropia with other noncomitancies

H50.1 Exotropia

Misalignment in which one eye deviates outward (away from nose) while the other fixates normally

Divergent concomitant strabismus

Excludes1 intermittent exotropia (H50.33-, H50.34)

- H50.10 Unspecified exotropia
- H50.11 Monocular exotropia
  - H50.111 Monocular exotropia, right eye
  - H50.112 Monocular exotropia, left eye
- H50.12 Monocular exotropia with A pattern
  - H50.121 Monocular exotropia with A pattern, right eye
  - H50.122 Monocular exotropia with A pattern, left eye
- H50.13 Monocular exotropia with V pattern
  - H50.131 Monocular exotropia with V pattern, right eye
  - H50.132 Monocular exotropia with V pattern, left eye
- H50.14 Monocular exotropia with other noncomitancies
  - H50.141 Monocular exotropia with other noncomitancies, right eye
  - H50.142 Monocular exotropia with other noncomitancies, left eye
- H50.15 Alternating exotropia
- H50.16 Alternating exotropia with A pattern
- H50.17 Alternating exotropia with V pattern
- H50.18 Alternating exotropia with other noncomitancies

H50.2 Vertical strabismus

Hypertropia

- H50.21 Vertical strabismus, right eye
- H50.22 Vertical strabismus, left eye

H50.3 Intermittent heterotropia

Displacement of an organ or part of an organ from its normal position

- H50.30 Unspecified intermittent heterotropia
- H50.31 Intermittent monocular esotropia
  - H50.311 Intermittent monocular esotropia, right eye
  - H50.312 Intermittent monocular esotropia, left eye
- H50.32 Intermittent alternating esotropia
- H50.33 Intermittent monocular exotropia
  - H50.331 Intermittent monocular exotropia, right eye
  - H50.332 Intermittent monocular exotropia, left eye
- H50.34 Intermittent alternating exotropia

H50.4 Other and unspecified heterotropia

- H50.40 Unspecified heterotropia
- H50.41 Cyclotropia
  - H50.411 Cyclotropia, right eye
  - H50.412 Cyclotropia, left eye
- H50.42 Monofixation syndrome
- H50.43 Accommodative component in esotropia

H50.5 Heterophoria

One or both eyes wander away from the position where both eyes are looking together in the same direction

- H50.50 Unspecified heterophoria
- H50.51 Esophoria
  Eye deviates inward (toward the nose)
- H50.52 Exophoria
  Eye deviates outward (toward the ear)
- H50.53 Vertical heterophoria
- H50.54 Cyclophoria
- H50.55 Alternating heterophoria

H50.6 Mechanical strabismus

- H50.60 Mechanical strabismus, unspecified
- H50.61 Brown's sheath syndrome
  - H50.611 Brown's sheath syndrome, right eye
  - H50.612 Brown's sheath syndrome, left eye
- H50.62 Inferior oblique muscle entrapment
  - H50.621 Inferior oblique muscle entrapment, right eye
  - H50.622 Inferior oblique muscle entrapment, left eye
  - H50.629 Inferior oblique muscle entrapment, unspecified eye
- H50.63 Inferior rectus muscle entrapment
  - H50.631 Inferior rectus muscle entrapment, right eye
  - H50.632 Inferior rectus muscle entrapment, left eye
  - H50.639 Inferior rectus muscle entrapment, unspecified eye
- H50.64 Lateral rectus muscle entrapment
  - H50.641 Lateral rectus muscle entrapment, right eye
  - H50.642 Lateral rectus muscle entrapment, left eye
  - H50.649 Lateral rectus muscle entrapment, unspecified eye
- H50.65 Medial rectus muscle entrapment
  - H50.651 Medial rectus muscle entrapment, right eye
  - H50.652 Medial rectus muscle entrapment, left eye
  - H50.659 Medial rectus muscle entrapment, unspecified eye
- H50.66 Superior oblique muscle entrapment
  - H50.661 Superior oblique muscle entrapment, right eye
  - H50.662 Superior oblique muscle entrapment, left eye
  - H50.669 Superior oblique muscle entrapment, unspecified eye
- H50.67 Superior rectus muscle entrapment
  - H50.671 Superior rectus muscle entrapment, right eye
  - H50.672 Superior rectus muscle entrapment, left eye
  - H50.679 Superior rectus muscle entrapment, unspecified eye

- H50.68 Extraocular muscle entrapment, unspecified
  - H50.681 Extraocular muscle entrapment, unspecified, right eye
  - H50.682 Extraocular muscle entrapment, unspecified, left eye
  - H50.689 Extraocular muscle entrapment, unspecified, unspecified eye
- H50.69 Other mechanical strabismus
  Strabismus due to adhesions
  Traumatic limitation of duction of eye muscle

- H50.8 Other specified strabismus
  - H50.81 Duane's syndrome
    - H50.811 Duane's syndrome, right eye
    - H50.812 Duane's syndrome, left eye
  - H50.89 Other specified strabismus
- H50.9 Unspecified strabismus

H51 Other disorders of binocular movement

- H51.0 Palsy (spasm) of conjugate gaze
- H51.1 Convergence insufficiency and excess
  - H51.11 Convergence insufficiency
  - H51.12 Convergence excess
- H51.2 Internuclear ophthalmoplegia
  - H51.20 Internuclear ophthalmoplegia, unspecified eye
  - H51.21 Internuclear ophthalmoplegia, right eye
  - H51.22 Internuclear ophthalmoplegia, left eye
  - H51.23 Internuclear ophthalmoplegia, bilateral
- H51.8 Other specified disorders of binocular movement
- H51.9 Unspecified disorder of binocular movement

H52 Disorders of refraction and accommodation

- H52.0 Hypermetropia
  - H52.00 Hypermetropia, unspecified eye
  - H52.01 Hypermetropia, right eye
  - H52.02 Hypermetropia, left eye
  - H52.03 Hypermetropia, bilateral
- H52.1 Myopia
  Excludes1 degenerative myopia (H44.2-)
  - H52.10 Myopia, unspecified eye
  - H52.11 Myopia, right eye
  - H52.12 Myopia, left eye
  - H52.13 Myopia, bilateral
- H52.2 Astigmatism
  - H52.20 Unspecified astigmatism
    - H52.201 Unspecified astigmatism, right eye
    - H52.202 Unspecified astigmatism, left eye
    - H52.203 Unspecified astigmatism, bilateral
    - H52.209 Unspecified astigmatism, unspecified eye
  - H52.21 Irregular astigmatism
    - H52.211 Irregular astigmatism, right eye
    - H52.212 Irregular astigmatism, left eye
    - H52.213 Irregular astigmatism, bilateral
    - H52.219 Irregular astigmatism, unspecified eye
  - H52.22 Regular astigmatism
    - H52.221 Regular astigmatism, right eye
    - H52.222 Regular astigmatism, left eye
    - H52.223 Regular astigmatism, bilateral
    - H52.229 Regular astigmatism, unspecified eye
- H52.3 Anisometropia and aniseikonia
  - H52.31 Anisometropia
  - H52.32 Aniseikonia
- H52.4 Presbyopia
- H52.5 Disorders of accommodation
  - H52.51 Internal ophthalmoplegia (complete) (total)
    - H52.511 Internal ophthalmoplegia (complete) (total), right eye
    - H52.512 Internal ophthalmoplegia (complete) (total), left eye
    - H52.513 Internal ophthalmoplegia (complete) (total), bilateral
    - H52.519 Internal ophthalmoplegia (complete) (total), unspecified eye
  - H52.52 Paresis of accommodation
    - H52.521 Paresis of accommodation, right eye
    - H52.522 Paresis of accommodation, left eye
    - H52.523 Paresis of accommodation, bilateral
    - H52.529 Paresis of accommodation, unspecified eye
  - H52.53 Spasm of accommodation
    - H52.531 Spasm of accommodation, right eye
    - H52.532 Spasm of accommodation, left eye
    - H52.533 Spasm of accommodation, bilateral
    - H52.539 Spasm of accommodation, unspecified eye
- H52.6 Other disorders of refraction
- H52.7 Unspecified disorder of refraction

VISUAL DISTURBANCES AND BLINDNESS (H53-H54)

H53 Visual disturbances

- H53.0 Amblyopia ex anopsia
  Excludes1 amblyopia due to vitamin A deficiency (E50.5)
  - H53.00 Unspecified amblyopia
    - H53.001 Unspecified amblyopia, right eye
    - H53.002 Unspecified amblyopia, left eye
    - H53.003 Unspecified amblyopia, bilateral
    - H53.009 Unspecified amblyopia, unspecified eye
  - H53.01 Deprivation amblyopia
    - H53.011 Deprivation amblyopia, right eye
    - H53.012 Deprivation amblyopia, left eye
    - H53.013 Deprivation amblyopia, bilateral
    - H53.019 Deprivation amblyopia, unspecified eye
  - H53.02 Refractive amblyopia
    - H53.021 Refractive amblyopia, right eye
    - H53.022 Refractive amblyopia, left eye
    - H53.023 Refractive amblyopia, bilateral
    - H53.029 Refractive amblyopia, unspecified eye
  - H53.03 Strabismic amblyopia
    Excludes1 strabismus (H50.-)
    - H53.031 Strabismic amblyopia, right eye
    - H53.032 Strabismic amblyopia, left eye
    - H53.033 Strabismic amblyopia, bilateral
    - H53.039 Strabismic amblyopia, unspecified eye

Item 7–10 Disorders of refraction: **Hypermetropia,** or farsightedness, means focus at a distance is adequate but not on close objects. **Myopia** is near-sightedness or short-sightedness and means the focus on nearby objects is clear but distant objects appear blurred. **Astigmatism** is warping of the curvature of the cornea so light rays entering do not meet a single focal point, resulting in a distorted image. **Anisometropia** is unequal refractive power in which one eye may be myopic (near-sighted) and the other hyperopic (far-sighted). **Presbyopia** is the loss of focus on near objects, which occurs with age because the lens loses elasticity.

● H53.04 Amblyopia suspect
Coding Clinic: 2016, Q4, P22
H53.041 Amblyopia suspect, right eye
H53.042 Amblyopia suspect, left eye
H53.043 Amblyopia suspect, bilateral
H53.049 Amblyopia suspect, unspecified eye

● H53.1 Subjective visual disturbances (Ex) PDX 808
Excludes1 subjective visual disturbances due to vitamin A deficiency (E50.5)
visual hallucinations (R44.1)
H53.10 Unspecified subjective visual disturbances
H53.11 Day blindness
Hemeralopia
● H53.12 Transient visual loss
Scintillating scotoma
Excludes1 amaurosis fugax (G45.3-)
transient retinal artery occlusion (H34.0-)
Coding Clinic: 2022, Q1, P30
H53.121 Transient visual loss, right eye
H53.122 Transient visual loss, left eye
H53.123 Transient visual loss, bilateral
H53.129 Transient visual loss, unspecified eye
● H53.13 Sudden visual loss
H53.131 Sudden visual loss, right eye
H53.132 Sudden visual loss, left eye
H53.133 Sudden visual loss, bilateral
H53.139 Sudden visual loss, unspecified eye
● H53.14 Visual discomfort
Asthenopia
Photophobia
H53.141 Visual discomfort, right eye
H53.142 Visual discomfort, left eye
H53.143 Visual discomfort, bilateral
H53.149 Visual discomfort, unspecified
H53.15 Visual distortions of shape and size
Metamorphopsia
H53.16 Psychophysical visual disturbances
H53.19 Other subjective visual disturbances
Visual halos
Coding Clinic: 2022, Q1, P30

H53.2 Diplopia
Double vision
Coding Clinic: 2022, Q3, P10

● H53.3 Other and unspecified disorders of binocular vision
H53.30 Unspecified disorder of binocular vision
H53.31 Abnormal retinal correspondence
H53.32 Fusion with defective stereopsis
H53.33 Simultaneous visual perception without fusion
H53.34 Suppression of binocular vision

● H53.4 Visual field defects
H53.40 Unspecified visual field defects
● H53.41 Scotoma involving central area
Central scotoma
H53.411 Scotoma involving central area, right eye
H53.412 Scotoma involving central area, left eye
H53.413 Scotoma involving central area, bilateral
H53.419 Scotoma involving central area, unspecified eye
● H53.42 Scotoma of blind spot area
Enlarged blind spot
H53.421 Scotoma of blind spot area, right eye
H53.422 Scotoma of blind spot area, left eye
H53.423 Scotoma of blind spot area, bilateral
H53.429 Scotoma of blind spot area, unspecified eye
● H53.43 Sector or arcuate defects
Arcuate scotoma
Bjerrum scotoma
H53.431 Sector or arcuate defects, right eye
H53.432 Sector or arcuate defects, left eye
H53.433 Sector or arcuate defects, bilateral
H53.439 Sector or arcuate defects, unspecified eye
● H53.45 Other localized visual field defect
Peripheral visual field defect
Ring scotoma NOS
Scotoma NOS
H53.451 Other localized visual field defect, right eye
H53.452 Other localized visual field defect, left eye
H53.453 Other localized visual field defect, bilateral
H53.459 Other localized visual field defect, unspecified eye
● H53.46 Homonymous bilateral field defects
Homonymous hemianopia
Homonymous hemianopsia
Quadrant anopia
Quadrant anopsia
H53.461 Homonymous bilateral field defects, right side
H53.462 Homonymous bilateral field defects, left side
H53.469 Homonymous bilateral field defects, unspecified side
Homonymous bilateral field defects NOS
H53.47 Heteronymous bilateral field defects
Heteronymous hemianop(s)ia
● H53.48 Generalized contraction of visual field
H53.481 Generalized contraction of visual field, right eye
H53.482 Generalized contraction of visual field, left eye
H53.483 Generalized contraction of visual field, bilateral
H53.489 Generalized contraction of visual field, unspecified eye

● H53.5 Color vision deficiencies
Color blindness
Excludes2 day blindness (H53.11)
H53.50 Unspecified color vision deficiencies
Color blindness NOS
H53.51 Achromatopsia
H53.52 Acquired color vision deficiency
H53.53 Deuteranomaly
Deuteranopia
H53.54 Protanomaly
Protanopia
H53.55 Tritanomaly
Tritanopia
H53.59 Other color vision deficiencies

● H53.6 Night blindness
Excludes1 night blindness due to vitamin A deficiency (E50.5)
H53.60 Unspecified night blindness
H53.61 Abnormal dark adaptation curve

CHAPTER 7 (H00-H59)

H53.62 Acquired night blindness
H53.63 Congenital night blindness
H53.69 Other night blindness

H53.7 Vision sensitivity deficiencies
H53.71 Glare sensitivity
H53.72 Impaired contrast sensitivity

H53.8 Other visual disturbances

H53.9 Unspecified visual disturbance

H54 Blindness and low vision

Note: For definition of visual impairment categories see table below.

Code first any associated underlying cause of the blindness

Excludes1 amaurosis fugax (G45.3)

H54.0 Blindness, both eyes
Visual impairment categories 3, 4, 5 in both eyes.

H54.0X Blindness, both eyes, different category levels

H54.0X3 Blindness right eye, category 3
H54.0X33 Blindness right eye category 3, blindness left eye category 3
H54.0X34 Blindness right eye category 3, blindness left eye category 4
H54.0X35 Blindness right eye category 3, blindness left eye category 5

H54.0X4 Blindness right eye, category 4
H54.0X43 Blindness right eye category 4, blindness left eye category 3
H54.0X44 Blindness right eye category 4, blindness left eye category 4
H54.0X45 Blindness right eye category 4, blindness left eye category 5

H54.0X5 Blindness right eye, category 5
H54.0X53 Blindness right eye category 5, blindness left eye category 3
H54.0X54 Blindness right eye category 5, blindness left eye category 4
H54.0X55 Blindness right eye category 5, blindness left eye category 5

H54.1 Blindness, one eye, low vision other eye
Visual impairment categories 3, 4, 5 in one eye, with categories 1 or 2 in the other eye.

H54.10 Blindness, one eye, low vision other eye, unspecified eyes

H54.11 Blindness, right eye, low vision left eye

H54.113 Blindness right eye category 3, low vision left eye
H54.1131 Blindness right eye category 3, low vision left eye category 1
H54.1132 Blindness right eye category 3, low vision left eye category 2

H54.114 Blindness right eye category 4, low vision left eye
H54.1141 Blindness right eye category 4, low vision left eye category 1
H54.1142 Blindness right eye category 4, low vision left eye category 2

H54.115 Blindness right eye category 5, low vision left eye
H54.1151 Blindness right eye category 5, low vision left eye category 1
H54.1152 Blindness right eye category 5, low vision left eye category 2

H54.12 Blindness, left eye, low vision right eye

H54.121 Low vision right eye category 1, blindness left eye
H54.1213 Low vision right eye category 1, blindness left eye category 3
H54.1214 Low vision right eye category 1, blindness left eye category 4
H54.1215 Low vision right eye category 1, blindness left eye category 5

H54.122 Low vision right eye category 2, blindness left eye
H54.1223 Low vision right eye category 2, blindness left eye category 3
H54.1224 Low vision right eye category 2, blindness left eye category 4
H54.1225 Low vision right eye category 2, blindness left eye category 5

H54.2 Low vision, both eyes
Visual impairment categories 1 or 2 in both eyes.

H54.2X Low vision, both eyes, different category levels

H54.2X1 Low vision, right eye, category 1
H54.2X11 Low vision right eye category 1, low vision left eye category 1
H54.2X12 Low vision right eye category 1, low vision left eye category 2

H54.2X2 Low vision, right eye, category 2
H54.2X21 Low vision right eye category 2, low vision left eye category 1
H54.2X22 Low vision right eye category 2, low vision left eye category 2

H54.3 Unqualified visual loss, both eyes
Visual impairment category 9 in both eyes.

H54.4 Blindness, one eye
Visual impairment categories 3, 4, 5 in one eye [normal vision in other eye]

H54.40 Blindness, one eye, unspecified eye

H54.41 Blindness, right eye, normal vision left eye

H54.413 Blindness, right eye, category 3
H54.413A Blindness right eye category 3, normal vision left eye

H54.414 Blindness, right eye, category 4
H54.414A Blindness right eye category 4, normal vision left eye

H54.415 Blindness, right eye, category 5
H54.415A Blindness right eye category 5, normal vision left eye

CHAPTER 7 (H00-H59)

● H54.42 Blindness, left eye, normal vision right eye
● H54.42A Blindness, left eye, category 3-5
H54.42A3 Blindness left eye category 3, normal vision right eye
H54.42A4 Blindness left eye category 4, normal vision right eye
H54.42A5 Blindness left eye category 5, normal vision right eye

● H54.5 Low vision, one eye
Visual impairment categories 1 or 2 in one eye [normal vision in other eye].
H54.50 Low vision, one eye, unspecified eye
● H54.51 Low vision, right eye, normal vision left eye
● H54.511 Low vision, right eye, category 1
H54.511A Low vision right eye category 1, normal vision left eye
● H54.512 Low vision, right eye, category 2
H54.512A Low vision right eye category 2, normal vision left eye
● H54.52 Low vision, left eye, normal vision right eye
● H54.52A Low vision, left eye, category 1-2
H54.52A1 Low vision left eye category 1, normal vision right eye
H54.52A2 Low vision left eye category 2, normal vision right eye

● H54.6 Unqualified visual loss, one eye
Visual impairment category 9 in one eye [normal vision in other eye].
H54.60 Unqualified visual loss, one eye, unspecified
H54.61 Unqualified visual loss, right eye, normal vision left eye
H54.62 Unqualified visual loss, left eye, normal vision right eye

OGCR Section I.C.7.b.

Blindness

If "blindness" or "low vision" of both eyes is documented but the visual impairment category is not documented, assign code H54.3, Unqualified visual loss, both eyes. If "blindness" or "low vision" in one eye is documented but the visual impairment category is not documented, assign a code from H54.6-, Unqualified visual loss, one eye. If "blindness" or "visual loss" is documented without any information about whether one or both eyes are affected, assign code H54.7, Unspecified visual loss.

● H54.7 Unspecified visual loss
Visual impairment category 9 NOS

H54.8 Legal blindness, as defined in USA
Blindness NOS according to USA definition
Excludes1 legal blindness with specification of impairment level (H54.0-H54.7)

Note: The table below gives a classification of severity of visual impairment recommended by a WHO Study Group on the Prevention of Blindness, Geneva, 6-10 November 1972.

The term "low vision" in category H54 comprises categories 1 and 2 of the table, the term "blindness" categories 3, 4, and 5, and the term "unqualified visual loss" category 9.

If the extent of the visual field is taken into account, patients with a field no greater than 10 but greater than 5 around central fixation should be placed in category 3 and patients with a field no greater than 5 around central fixation should be placed in category 4, even if the central acuity is not impaired.

(Document 508 compliance requires all cells in the following table to be filled.)

Category of visual impairment	Visual acuity with best possible correction	
	Maximum less than:	Minimum equal to or better than:
—	6/18	6/60
3/10 (0.3)	1/10 (0.1)	—
20/70	20/200	—
—	6/60	3/60
1/10 (0.1)	1/20 (0.05)	—
20/200	20/400	—
—	3/60	1/60 (finger counting at one meter)
1/20 (0.05)	1/50 (0.02)	—
20/400	5/300 (20/1200)	—
—	1/60 (finger counting at one meter)	Light perception
1/50 (0.02)	—	—
5/300	—	—
—	No light perception	—
—	Undetermined or unspecified	—

OTHER DISORDERS OF EYE AND ADNEXA (H55-H57)

● H55 Nystagmus and other irregular eye movements
● H55.0 Nystagmus
Rapid, involuntary movements of the eyes in the horizontal or vertical direction
H55.00 Unspecified nystagmus
H55.01 Congenital nystagmus
H55.02 Latent nystagmus
H55.03 Visual deprivation nystagmus
H55.04 Dissociated nystagmus
H55.09 Other forms of nystagmus
● H55.8 Other irregular eye movements
H55.81 Deficient saccadic eye movements
H55.82 Deficient smooth pursuit eye movements
H55.89 Other irregular eye movements

● H57 Other disorders of eye and adnexa
● H57.0 Anomalies of pupillary function
H57.00 Unspecified anomaly of pupillary function
H57.01 Argyll Robertson pupil, atypical
Excludes1 syphilitic Argyll Robertson pupil (A52.19)
H57.02 Anisocoria
H57.03 Miosis
H57.04 Mydriasis
● H57.05 Tonic pupil
H57.051 Tonic pupil, right eye
H57.052 Tonic pupil, left eye
H57.053 Tonic pupil, bilateral
H57.059 Tonic pupil, unspecified eye
H57.09 Other anomalies of pupillary function
● H57.1 Ocular pain
H57.10 Ocular pain, unspecified eye
H57.11 Ocular pain, right eye
H57.12 Ocular pain, left eye
H57.13 Ocular pain, bilateral

- H57.8 Other specified disorders of eye and adnexa
  - H57.81 Brow ptosis
    - H57.811 Brow ptosis, right
    - H57.812 Brow ptosis, left
    - H57.813 Brow ptosis, bilateral
    - H57.819 Brow ptosis, unspecified
  - H57.89 Other specified disorders of eye and adnexa
  - H57.8A Foreign body sensation eye (ocular)
    - H57.8A1 Foreign body sensation, right eye
    - H57.8A2 Foreign body sensation, left eye
    - H57.8A3 Foreign body sensation, bilateral eyes
    - H57.8A9 Foreign body sensation, unspecified eye
- H57.9 Unspecified disorder of eye and adnexa

INTRAOPERATIVE AND POSTPROCEDURAL COMPLICATIONS AND DISORDERS OF EYE AND ADNEXA, NOT ELSEWHERE CLASSIFIED (H59)

- H59 Intraoperative and postprocedural complications and disorders of eye and adnexa, not elsewhere classified

  Excludes1 mechanical complication of intraocular lens (T85.2)
  mechanical complication of other ocular prosthetic devices, implants and grafts (T85.3)
  pseudophakia (Z96.1)
  secondary cataracts (H26.4-)

- H59.0 Disorders of the eye following cataract surgery (Ex) PDX 809
  - H59.01 Keratopathy (bullous aphakic) following cataract surgery
    Vitreal corneal syndrome
    Vitreous (touch) syndrome
    - H59.011 Keratopathy (bullous aphakic) following cataract surgery, right eye
    - H59.012 Keratopathy (bullous aphakic) following cataract surgery, left eye
    - H59.013 Keratopathy (bullous aphakic) following cataract surgery, bilateral
    - H59.019 Keratopathy (bullous aphakic) following cataract surgery, unspecified eye
  - H59.02 Cataract (lens) fragments in eye following cataract surgery
    - H59.021 Cataract (lens) fragments in eye following cataract surgery, right eye
    - H59.022 Cataract (lens) fragments in eye following cataract surgery, left eye
    - H59.023 Cataract (lens) fragments in eye following cataract surgery, bilateral
    - H59.029 Cataract (lens) fragments in eye following cataract surgery, unspecified eye
  - H59.03 Cystoid macular edema following cataract surgery
    - H59.031 Cystoid macular edema following cataract surgery, right eye
    - H59.032 Cystoid macular edema following cataract surgery, left eye
    - H59.033 Cystoid macular edema following cataract surgery, bilateral
    - H59.039 Cystoid macular edema following cataract surgery, unspecified eye
  - H59.09 Other disorders of the eye following cataract surgery
    - H59.091 Other disorders of the right eye following cataract surgery
    - H59.092 Other disorders of the left eye following cataract surgery
    - H59.093 Other disorders of the eye following cataract surgery, bilateral
    - H59.099 Other disorders of unspecified eye following cataract surgery
- H59.1 Intraoperative hemorrhage and hematoma of eye and adnexa complicating a procedure (Ex) PDX 810

  Excludes1 intraoperative hemorrhage and hematoma of eye and adnexa due to accidental puncture or laceration during a procedure (H59.2-)

  - H59.11 Intraoperative hemorrhage and hematoma of eye and adnexa complicating an ophthalmic procedure
    - H59.111 Intraoperative hemorrhage and hematoma of right eye and adnexa complicating an ophthalmic procedure
    - H59.112 Intraoperative hemorrhage and hematoma of left eye and adnexa complicating an ophthalmic procedure
    - H59.113 Intraoperative hemorrhage and hematoma of eye and adnexa complicating an ophthalmic procedure, bilateral
    - H59.119 Intraoperative hemorrhage and hematoma of unspecified eye and adnexa complicating an ophthalmic procedure
  - H59.12 Intraoperative hemorrhage and hematoma of eye and adnexa complicating other procedure
    - H59.121 Intraoperative hemorrhage and hematoma of right eye and adnexa complicating other procedure
    - H59.122 Intraoperative hemorrhage and hematoma of left eye and adnexa complicating other procedure
    - H59.123 Intraoperative hemorrhage and hematoma of eye and adnexa complicating other procedure, bilateral
    - H59.129 Intraoperative hemorrhage and hematoma of unspecified eye and adnexa complicating other procedure
- H59.2 Accidental puncture and laceration of eye and adnexa during a procedure (Ex) PDX 569
  - H59.21 Accidental puncture and laceration of eye and adnexa during an ophthalmic procedure
    - H59.211 Accidental puncture and laceration of right eye and adnexa during an ophthalmic procedure
    - H59.212 Accidental puncture and laceration of left eye and adnexa during an ophthalmic procedure
    - H59.213 Accidental puncture and laceration of eye and adnexa during an ophthalmic procedure, bilateral
    - H59.219 Accidental puncture and laceration of unspecified eye and adnexa during an ophthalmic procedure
  - H59.22 Accidental puncture and laceration of eye and adnexa during other procedure
    - H59.221 Accidental puncture and laceration of right eye and adnexa during other procedure
    - H59.222 Accidental puncture and laceration of left eye and adnexa during other procedure

CHAPTER 7 (H00-H59)

H59.223 Accidental puncture and laceration of eye and adnexa during other procedure, bilateral

H59.229 Accidental puncture and laceration of unspecified eye and adnexa during other procedure

● H59.3 Postprocedural hemorrhage, hematoma, and seroma of eye and adnexa following other procedure (Ex:) PDX 810

Coding Clinic: 2016, Q4, P10

● H59.31 Postprocedural hemorrhage of eye and adnexa following an ophthalmic procedure

H59.311 Postprocedural hemorrhage of right eye and adnexa following an ophthalmic procedure

H59.312 Postprocedural hemorrhage of left eye and adnexa following an ophthalmic procedure

H59.313 Postprocedural hemorrhage of eye and adnexa following an ophthalmic procedure, bilateral

H59.319 Postprocedural hemorrhage of unspecified eye and adnexa following an ophthalmic procedure

● H59.32 Postprocedural hemorrhage of eye and adnexa following other procedure

H59.321 Postprocedural hemorrhage of right eye and adnexa following other procedure

H59.322 Postprocedural hemorrhage of left eye and adnexa following other procedure

H59.323 Postprocedural hemorrhage of eye and adnexa following other procedure, bilateral

H59.329 Postprocedural hemorrhage of unspecified eye and adnexa following other procedure

● H59.33 Postprocedural hematoma of eye and adnexa following an ophthalmic procedure

H59.331 Postprocedural hematoma of right eye and adnexa following an ophthalmic procedure

H59.332 Postprocedural hematoma of left eye and adnexa following an ophthalmic procedure

H59.333 Postprocedural hematoma of eye and adnexa following an ophthalmic procedure, bilateral

H59.339 Postprocedural hematoma of unspecified eye and adnexa following an ophthalmic procedure

● H59.34 Postprocedural hematoma of eye and adnexa following other procedure

H59.341 Postprocedural hematoma of right eye and adnexa following other procedure

H59.342 Postprocedural hematoma of left eye and adnexa following other procedure

H59.343 Postprocedural hematoma of eye and adnexa following other procedure, bilateral

H59.349 Postprocedural hematoma of unspecified eye and adnexa following other procedure

● H59.35 Postprocedural seroma of eye and adnexa following an ophthalmic procedure

H59.351 Postprocedural seroma of right eye and adnexa following an ophthalmic procedure

H59.352 Postprocedural seroma of left eye and adnexa following an ophthalmic procedure

H59.353 Postprocedural seroma of eye and adnexa following an ophthalmic procedure, bilateral

H59.359 Postprocedural seroma of unspecified eye and adnexa following an ophthalmic procedure

● H59.36 Postprocedural seroma of eye and adnexa following other procedure

H59.361 Postprocedural seroma of right eye and adnexa following other procedure

H59.362 Postprocedural seroma of left eye and adnexa following other procedure

H59.363 Postprocedural seroma of eye and adnexa following other procedure, bilateral

H59.369 Postprocedural seroma of unspecified eye and adnexa following other procedure

● H59.4 Inflammation (infection) of postprocedural bleb

Postprocedural blebitis

Excludes1 filtering (vitreous) bleb after glaucoma surgery status (Z98.83)

H59.40 Inflammation (infection) of postprocedural bleb, unspecified

H59.41 Inflammation (infection) of postprocedural bleb, stage 1

H59.42 Inflammation (infection) of postprocedural bleb, stage 2

H59.43 Inflammation (infection) of postprocedural bleb, stage 3

Bleb endophthalmitis

● H59.8 Other intraoperative and postprocedural complications and disorders of eye and adnexa, not elsewhere classified (Ex:) PDX 809

● H59.81 Chorioretinal scars after surgery for detachment

H59.811 Chorioretinal scars after surgery for detachment, right eye

H59.812 Chorioretinal scars after surgery for detachment, left eye

H59.813 Chorioretinal scars after surgery for detachment, bilateral

H59.819 Chorioretinal scars after surgery for detachment, unspecified eye

H59.88 Other intraoperative complications of eye and adnexa, not elsewhere classified

H59.89 Other postprocedural complications and disorders of eye and adnexa, not elsewhere classified

CHAPTER 8

DISEASES OF THE EAR AND MASTOID PROCESS (H60-H95)

OGCR Chapter-Specific Coding Guidelines

8. Chapter 8: Diseases of the Ear and Mastoid Process (H60-H95)
Reserved for future guideline expansion

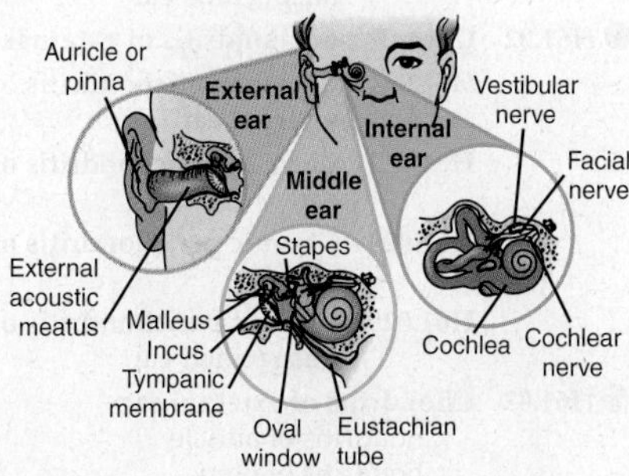

Figure 8-1 Auditory system. (From Buck CJ: Step-by-Step Medical Coding, ed 2016, St. Louis, Elsevier, 2016)

★ **(See Plate 20 of the Anatomy Illustrations.)**

CHAPTER 8

DISEASES OF THE EAR AND MASTOID PROCESS (H60-H95)

Note: Use an external cause code following the code for the ear condition, if applicable, to identify the cause of the ear condition

Excludes2 certain conditions originating in the perinatal period (P04-P96)
certain infectious and parasitic diseases (A00-B99)
complications of pregnancy, childbirth and the puerperium (O00-O9A)
congenital malformations, deformations and chromosomal abnormalities (Q00-Q99)
endocrine, nutritional and metabolic diseases (E00-E88)
injury, poisoning and certain other consequences of external causes (S00-T88)
neoplasms (C00-D49)
symptoms, signs and abnormal clinical and laboratory findings, not elsewhere classified (R00-R94)

This chapter contains the following blocks:

H60-H62	Diseases of external ear
H65-H75	Diseases of middle ear and mastoid
H80-H83	Diseases of inner ear
H90-H94	Other disorders of ear
H95	Intraoperative and postprocedural complications and disorders of ear and mastoid process, not elsewhere classified

DISEASES OF EXTERNAL EAR (H60-H62)

● **H60 Otitis externa**

● **H60.0 Abscess of external ear**
Boil of external ear
Carbuncle of auricle or external auditory canal
Furuncle of external ear

H60.00 Abscess of external ear, unspecified ear
H60.01 Abscess of right external ear
H60.02 Abscess of left external ear
H60.03 Abscess of external ear, bilateral

● **H60.1 Cellulitis of external ear**
Cellulitis of auricle
Cellulitis of external auditory canal

H60.10 Cellulitis of external ear, unspecified ear
H60.11 Cellulitis of right external ear
H60.12 Cellulitis of left external ear
H60.13 Cellulitis of external ear, bilateral

● **H60.2 Malignant otitis externa** (Ex) PDX 811

H60.20 Malignant otitis externa, unspecified ear
H60.21 Malignant otitis externa, right ear
H60.22 Malignant otitis externa, left ear
H60.23 Malignant otitis externa, bilateral

● **H60.3 Other infective otitis externa**

● **H60.31 Diffuse otitis externa**

H60.311 Diffuse otitis externa, right ear
H60.312 Diffuse otitis externa, left ear
H60.313 Diffuse otitis externa, bilateral
H60.319 Diffuse otitis externa, unspecified ear

● **H60.32 Hemorrhagic otitis externa**

H60.321 Hemorrhagic otitis externa, right ear
H60.322 Hemorrhagic otitis externa, left ear
H60.323 Hemorrhagic otitis externa, bilateral
H60.329 Hemorrhagic otitis externa, unspecified ear

● **H60.33 Swimmer's ear**

H60.331 Swimmer's ear, right ear
H60.332 Swimmer's ear, left ear
H60.333 Swimmer's ear, bilateral
H60.339 Swimmer's ear, unspecified ear

● **H60.39 Other infective otitis externa**

H60.391 Other infective otitis externa, right ear
H60.392 Other infective otitis externa, left ear
H60.393 Other infective otitis externa, bilateral
H60.399 Other infective otitis externa, unspecified ear

● **H60.4 Cholesteatoma of external ear**
Keratosis obturans of external ear (canal)

Excludes2 cholesteatoma of middle ear (H71.-)
recurrent cholesteatoma of postmastoidectomy cavity (H95.0-)

H60.40 Cholesteatoma of external ear, unspecified ear
H60.41 Cholesteatoma of right external ear
H60.42 Cholesteatoma of left external ear
H60.43 Cholesteatoma of external ear, bilateral

● **H60.5 Acute noninfective otitis externa**

● **H60.50 Unspecified acute noninfective otitis externa**
Acute otitis externa NOS

H60.501 Unspecified acute noninfective otitis externa, right ear
H60.502 Unspecified acute noninfective otitis externa, left ear
H60.503 Unspecified acute noninfective otitis externa, bilateral
H60.509 Unspecified acute noninfective otitis externa, unspecified ear

● **H60.51 Acute actinic otitis externa**

H60.511 Acute actinic otitis externa, right ear
H60.512 Acute actinic otitis externa, left ear
H60.513 Acute actinic otitis externa, bilateral
H60.519 Acute actinic otitis externa, unspecified ear

CHAPTER 8 (H60-H95)

- H60.52 Acute chemical otitis externa
  - H60.521 Acute chemical otitis externa, right ear
  - H60.522 Acute chemical otitis externa, left ear
  - H60.523 Acute chemical otitis externa, bilateral
  - H60.529 Acute chemical otitis externa, unspecified ear
- H60.53 Acute contact otitis externa
  - H60.531 Acute contact otitis externa, right ear
  - H60.532 Acute contact otitis externa, left ear
  - H60.533 Acute contact otitis externa, bilateral
  - H60.539 Acute contact otitis externa, unspecified ear
- H60.54 Acute eczematoid otitis externa
  - H60.541 Acute eczematoid otitis externa, right ear
  - H60.542 Acute eczematoid otitis externa, left ear
  - H60.543 Acute eczematoid otitis externa, bilateral
  - H60.549 Acute eczematoid otitis externa, unspecified ear
- H60.55 Acute reactive otitis externa
  - H60.551 Acute reactive otitis externa, right ear
  - H60.552 Acute reactive otitis externa, left ear
  - H60.553 Acute reactive otitis externa, bilateral
  - H60.559 Acute reactive otitis externa, unspecified ear
- H60.59 Other noninfective acute otitis externa
  - H60.591 Other noninfective acute otitis externa, right ear
  - H60.592 Other noninfective acute otitis externa, left ear
  - H60.593 Other noninfective acute otitis externa, bilateral
  - H60.599 Other noninfective acute otitis externa, unspecified ear

- H60.6 Unspecified chronic otitis externa
  - H60.60 Unspecified chronic otitis externa, unspecified ear
  - H60.61 Unspecified chronic otitis externa, right ear
  - H60.62 Unspecified chronic otitis externa, left ear
  - H60.63 Unspecified chronic otitis externa, bilateral
- H60.8 Other otitis externa
  - H60.8X Other otitis externa
    - H60.8X1 Other otitis externa, right ear
    - H60.8X2 Other otitis externa, left ear
    - H60.8X3 Other otitis externa, bilateral
    - H60.8X9 Other otitis externa, unspecified ear
- H60.9 Unspecified otitis externa
  - H60.90 Unspecified otitis externa, unspecified ear
  - H60.91 Unspecified otitis externa, right ear
  - H60.92 Unspecified otitis externa, left ear
  - H60.93 Unspecified otitis externa, bilateral

H61 Other disorders of external ear

- H61.0 Chondritis and perichondritis of external ear
  Chondrodermatitis nodularis chronica helicis
  Perichondritis of auricle
  Perichondritis of pinna
  - H61.00 Unspecified perichondritis of external ear
    - H61.001 Unspecified perichondritis of right external ear
    - H61.002 Unspecified perichondritis of left external ear
    - H61.003 Unspecified perichondritis of external ear, bilateral
    - H61.009 Unspecified perichondritis of external ear, unspecified ear
  - H61.01 Acute perichondritis of external ear
    - H61.011 Acute perichondritis of right external ear
    - H61.012 Acute perichondritis of left external ear
    - H61.013 Acute perichondritis of external ear, bilateral
    - H61.019 Acute perichondritis of external ear, unspecified ear
  - H61.02 Chronic perichondritis of external ear
    - H61.021 Chronic perichondritis of right external ear
    - H61.022 Chronic perichondritis of left external ear
    - H61.023 Chronic perichondritis of external ear, bilateral
    - H61.029 Chronic perichondritis of external ear, unspecified ear
  - H61.03 Chondritis of external ear
    Chondritis of auricle
    Chondritis of pinna
    - H61.031 Chondritis of right external ear
    - H61.032 Chondritis of left external ear
      Coding Clinic: 2015, Q1, P18
    - H61.033 Chondritis of external ear, bilateral
    - H61.039 Chondritis of external ear, unspecified ear
- H61.1 Noninfective disorders of pinna
  Excludes2 cauliflower ear (M95.1-)
  gouty tophi of ear (M1A.-)
  - H61.10 Unspecified noninfective disorders of pinna
    Disorder of pinna NOS
    - H61.101 Unspecified noninfective disorders of pinna, right ear
    - H61.102 Unspecified noninfective disorders of pinna, left ear
    - H61.103 Unspecified noninfective disorders of pinna, bilateral
    - H61.109 Unspecified noninfective disorders of pinna, unspecified ear
  - H61.11 Acquired deformity of pinna
    Acquired deformity of auricle
    Excludes2 cauliflower ear (M95.1-)
    - H61.111 Acquired deformity of pinna, right ear
    - H61.112 Acquired deformity of pinna, left ear
    - H61.113 Acquired deformity of pinna, bilateral
    - H61.119 Acquired deformity of pinna, unspecified ear
  - H61.12 Hematoma of pinna
    Hematoma of auricle
    - H61.121 Hematoma of pinna, right ear
    - H61.122 Hematoma of pinna, left ear
    - H61.123 Hematoma of pinna, bilateral
    - H61.129 Hematoma of pinna, unspecified ear
  - H61.19 Other noninfective disorders of pinna
    - H61.191 Noninfective disorders of pinna, right ear
    - H61.192 Noninfective disorders of pinna, left ear
    - H61.193 Noninfective disorders of pinna, bilateral
    - H61.199 Noninfective disorders of pinna, unspecified ear

H61.2 Impacted cerumen
Wax in ear
- H61.20 Impacted cerumen, unspecified ear
  MCE: Questionable admission when principal dx
- H61.21 Impacted cerumen, right ear
  MCE: Questionable admission when principal dx
- H61.22 Impacted cerumen, left ear
  MCE: Questionable admission when principal dx
- H61.23 Impacted cerumen, bilateral
  MCE: Questionable admission when principal dx

H61.3 Acquired stenosis of external ear canal
Collapse of external ear canal
Excludes1 postprocedural stenosis of external ear canal (H95.81-)

H61.30 Acquired stenosis of external ear canal, unspecified
- H61.301 Acquired stenosis of right external ear canal, unspecified
- H61.302 Acquired stenosis of left external ear canal, unspecified
- H61.303 Acquired stenosis of external ear canal, unspecified, bilateral
- H61.309 Acquired stenosis of external ear canal, unspecified, unspecified ear

H61.31 Acquired stenosis of external ear canal secondary to trauma
- H61.311 Acquired stenosis of right external ear canal secondary to trauma
- H61.312 Acquired stenosis of left external ear canal secondary to trauma
- H61.313 Acquired stenosis of external ear canal secondary to trauma, bilateral
- H61.319 Acquired stenosis of external ear canal secondary to trauma, unspecified ear

H61.32 Acquired stenosis of external ear canal secondary to inflammation and infection
- H61.321 Acquired stenosis of right external ear canal secondary to inflammation and infection
- H61.322 Acquired stenosis of left external ear canal secondary to inflammation and infection
- H61.323 Acquired stenosis of external ear canal secondary to inflammation and infection, bilateral
- H61.329 Acquired stenosis of external ear canal secondary to inflammation and infection, unspecified ear

H61.39 Other acquired stenosis of external ear canal
- H61.391 Other acquired stenosis of right external ear canal
- H61.392 Other acquired stenosis of left external ear canal
- H61.393 Other acquired stenosis of external ear canal, bilateral
- H61.399 Other acquired stenosis of external ear canal, unspecified ear

H61.8 Other specified disorders of external ear

H61.81 Exostosis of external canal
- H61.811 Exostosis of right external canal
- H61.812 Exostosis of left external canal
- H61.813 Exostosis of external canal, bilateral
- H61.819 Exostosis of external canal, unspecified ear

H61.89 Other specified disorders of external ear
- H61.891 Other specified disorders of right external ear
- H61.892 Other specified disorders of left external ear
- H61.893 Other specified disorders of external ear, bilateral
- H61.899 Other specified disorders of external ear, unspecified ear

H61.9 Disorder of external ear, unspecified
- H61.90 Disorder of external ear, unspecified, unspecified ear
- H61.91 Disorder of right external ear, unspecified
- H61.92 Disorder of left external ear, unspecified
- H61.93 Disorder of external ear, unspecified, bilateral

H62 Disorders of external ear in diseases classified elsewhere

H62.4 Otitis externa in other diseases classified elsewhere
Code first underlying disease, such as:
erysipelas (A46)
impetigo (L01.0-)
Excludes1 otitis externa (in):
candidiasis (B37.84)
herpes viral [herpes simplex] (B00.1)
herpes zoster (B02.8)
- *H62.40 Otitis externa in other diseases classified elsewhere, unspecified ear*
- *H62.41 Otitis externa in other diseases classified elsewhere, right ear*
- *H62.42 Otitis externa in other diseases classified elsewhere, left ear*
- *H62.43 Otitis externa in other diseases classified elsewhere, bilateral*

H62.8 Other disorders of external ear in diseases classified elsewhere
Code first underlying disease, such as:
gout (M1A.-, M10.-)

H62.8X Other disorders of external ear in diseases classified elsewhere
- *H62.8X1 Other disorders of right external ear in diseases classified elsewhere*
- *H62.8X2 Other disorders of left external ear in diseases classified elsewhere*
- *H62.8X3 Other disorders of external ear in diseases classified elsewhere, bilateral*
- *H62.8X9 Other disorders of external ear in diseases classified elsewhere, unspecified ear*

DISEASES OF MIDDLE EAR AND MASTOID (H65-H75)

★ **(See Plate 21 of the Anatomy Illustrations.)**

H65 Nonsuppurative otitis media
Bacterial or viral infection or inflammation of the middle ear; may result in fluid accumulation with pain and temporary hearing loss.
Includes nonsuppurative otitis media with myringitis
Use additional code for any associated perforated tympanic membrane (H72.-)
Use additional code to identify:
exposure to environmental tobacco smoke (Z77.22)
exposure to tobacco smoke in the perinatal period (P96.81)
history of tobacco dependence (Z87.891)
infectious agent (B95-B97)
occupational exposure to environmental tobacco smoke (Z57.31)
tobacco dependence (F17.-)
tobacco use (Z72.0)

H65.0 Acute serous otitis media
Acute and subacute secretory otitis
- H65.00 Acute serous otitis media, unspecified ear
- H65.01 Acute serous otitis media, right ear
- H65.02 Acute serous otitis media, left ear
- H65.03 Acute serous otitis media, bilateral
- H65.04 Acute serous otitis media, recurrent, right ear
- H65.05 Acute serous otitis media, recurrent, left ear
- H65.06 Acute serous otitis media, recurrent, bilateral
- H65.07 Acute serous otitis media, recurrent, unspecified ear

CHAPTER 8 (H60-H95)

H65.1 Other acute nonsuppurative otitis media

Excludes1 otitic barotrauma (T70.0)
otitis media (acute) NOS (H66.9)

H65.11 Acute and subacute allergic otitis media (mucoid) (sanguinous) (serous)

H65.111 Acute and subacute allergic otitis media (mucoid) (sanguinous) (serous), right ear

H65.112 Acute and subacute allergic otitis media (mucoid) (sanguinous) (serous), left ear

H65.113 Acute and subacute allergic otitis media (mucoid) (sanguinous) (serous), bilateral

H65.114 Acute and subacute allergic otitis media (mucoid) (sanguinous) (serous), recurrent, right ear

H65.115 Acute and subacute allergic otitis media (mucoid) (sanguinous) (serous), recurrent, left ear

H65.116 Acute and subacute allergic otitis media (mucoid) (sanguinous) (serous), recurrent, bilateral

H65.117 Acute and subacute allergic otitis media (mucoid) (sanguinous) (serous), recurrent, unspecified ear

H65.119 Acute and subacute allergic otitis media (mucoid) (sanguinous) (serous), unspecified ear

H65.19 Other acute nonsuppurative otitis media

Acute and subacute mucoid otitis media
Acute and subacute nonsuppurative otitis media NOS
Acute and subacute sanguinous otitis media
Acute and subacute seromucinous otitis media

H65.191 Other acute nonsuppurative otitis media, right ear

H65.192 Other acute nonsuppurative otitis media, left ear

H65.193 Other acute nonsuppurative otitis media, bilateral

H65.194 Other acute nonsuppurative otitis media, recurrent, right ear

H65.195 Other acute nonsuppurative otitis media, recurrent, left ear

H65.196 Other acute nonsuppurative otitis media, recurrent, bilateral

H65.197 Other acute nonsuppurative otitis media recurrent, unspecified ear

H65.199 Other acute nonsuppurative otitis media, unspecified ear

H65.2 Chronic serous otitis media

Chronic tubotympanal catarrh

H65.20 Chronic serous otitis media, unspecified ear

H65.21 Chronic serous otitis media, right ear

H65.22 Chronic serous otitis media, left ear

H65.23 Chronic serous otitis media, bilateral

H65.3 Chronic mucoid otitis media

Chronic mucinous otitis media
Chronic secretory otitis media
Chronic transudative otitis media
Glue ear

Excludes1 adhesive middle ear disease (H74.1)

H65.30 Chronic mucoid otitis media, unspecified ear

H65.31 Chronic mucoid otitis media, right ear

H65.32 Chronic mucoid otitis media, left ear

H65.33 Chronic mucoid otitis media, bilateral

H65.4 Other chronic nonsuppurative otitis media

H65.41 Chronic allergic otitis media

H65.411 Chronic allergic otitis media, right ear

H65.412 Chronic allergic otitis media, left ear

H65.413 Chronic allergic otitis media, bilateral

H65.419 Chronic allergic otitis media, unspecified ear

H65.49 Other chronic nonsuppurative otitis media

Chronic exudative otitis media
Chronic nonsuppurative otitis media NOS
Chronic otitis media with effusion (nonpurulent)
Chronic seromucinous otitis media

H65.491 Other chronic nonsuppurative otitis media, right ear

H65.492 Other chronic nonsuppurative otitis media, left ear

H65.493 Other chronic nonsuppurative otitis media, bilateral

H65.499 Other chronic nonsuppurative otitis media, unspecified ear

H65.9 Unspecified nonsuppurative otitis media

Allergic otitis media NOS
Catarrhal otitis media NOS
Exudative otitis media NOS
Mucoid otitis media NOS
Otitis media with effusion (nonpurulent) NOS
Secretory otitis media NOS
Seromucinous otitis media NOS
Serous otitis media NOS
Transudative otitis media NOS

H65.90 Unspecified nonsuppurative otitis media, unspecified ear

H65.91 Unspecified nonsuppurative otitis media, right ear

H65.92 Unspecified nonsuppurative otitis media, left ear

H65.93 Unspecified nonsuppurative otitis media, bilateral

H66 Suppurative and unspecified otitis media

Suppurative: Discharging pus

Includes suppurative and unspecified otitis media with myringitis

Use additional code to identify:
exposure to environmental tobacco smoke (Z77.22)
exposure to tobacco smoke in the perinatal period (P96.81)
history of tobacco dependence (Z87.891)
occupational exposure to environmental tobacco smoke (Z57.31)
tobacco dependence (F17.-)
tobacco use (Z72.0)

H66.0 Acute suppurative otitis media

H66.00 Acute suppurative otitis media without spontaneous rupture of ear drum

H66.001 Acute suppurative otitis media without spontaneous rupture of ear drum, right ear
Coding Clinic: 2016, Q1, P34

H66.002 Acute suppurative otitis media without spontaneous rupture of ear drum, left ear

H66.003 Acute suppurative otitis media without spontaneous rupture of ear drum, bilateral

H66.004 Acute suppurative otitis media without spontaneous rupture of ear drum, recurrent, right ear

H66.005 Acute suppurative otitis media without spontaneous rupture of ear drum, recurrent, left ear

H66.006 Acute suppurative otitis media without spontaneous rupture of ear drum, recurrent, bilateral

H66.007 Acute suppurative otitis media without spontaneous rupture of ear drum, recurrent, unspecified ear

H66.009 Acute suppurative otitis media without spontaneous rupture of ear drum, unspecified ear

H66.01 Acute suppurative otitis media with spontaneous rupture of ear drum

H66.011 Acute suppurative otitis media with spontaneous rupture of ear drum, right ear

H66.012 Acute suppurative otitis media with spontaneous rupture of ear drum, left ear

H66.013 Acute suppurative otitis media with spontaneous rupture of ear drum, bilateral

H66.014 Acute suppurative otitis media with spontaneous rupture of ear drum, recurrent, right ear

H66.015 Acute suppurative otitis media with spontaneous rupture of ear drum, recurrent, left ear

H66.016 Acute suppurative otitis media with spontaneous rupture of ear drum, recurrent, bilateral

H66.017 Acute suppurative otitis media with spontaneous rupture of ear drum, recurrent, unspecified ear

H66.019 Acute suppurative otitis media with spontaneous rupture of ear drum, unspecified ear

H66.1 Chronic tubotympanic suppurative otitis media

Benign chronic suppurative otitis media
Chronic tubotympanic disease

Use additional code for any associated perforated tympanic membrane (H72.-)

H66.10 Chronic tubotympanic suppurative otitis media, unspecified

H66.11 Chronic tubotympanic suppurative otitis media, right ear

H66.12 Chronic tubotympanic suppurative otitis media, left ear

H66.13 Chronic tubotympanic suppurative otitis media, bilateral

H66.2 Chronic atticoantral suppurative otitis media

Chronic atticoantral disease

Use additional code for any associated perforated tympanic membrane (H72.-)

H66.20 Chronic atticoantral suppurative otitis media, unspecified ear

H66.21 Chronic atticoantral suppurative otitis media, right ear

H66.22 Chronic atticoantral suppurative otitis media, left ear

H66.23 Chronic atticoantral suppurative otitis media, bilateral

H66.3 Other chronic suppurative otitis media

Chronic suppurative otitis media NOS

Use additional code for any associated perforated tympanic membrane (H72.-)

Excludes1 tuberculous otitis media (A18.6)

H66.3X Other chronic suppurative otitis media

H66.3X1 Other chronic suppurative otitis media, right ear

H66.3X2 Other chronic suppurative otitis media, left ear

H66.3X3 Other chronic suppurative otitis media, bilateral

H66.3X9 Other chronic suppurative otitis media, unspecified ear

H66.4 Suppurative otitis media, unspecified

Purulent otitis media NOS

Use additional code for any associated perforated tympanic membrane (H72.-)

H66.40 Suppurative otitis media, unspecified, unspecified ear

H66.41 Suppurative otitis media, unspecified, right ear

H66.42 Suppurative otitis media, unspecified, left ear

H66.43 Suppurative otitis media, unspecified, bilateral

H66.9 Otitis media, unspecified

Otitis media NOS
Acute otitis media NOS
Chronic otitis media NOS

Use additional code for any associated perforated tympanic membrane (H72.-)

H66.90 Otitis media, unspecified, unspecified ear

H66.91 Otitis media, unspecified, right ear

H66.92 Otitis media, unspecified, left ear

H66.93 Otitis media, unspecified, bilateral

H67 Otitis media in diseases classified elsewhere

Code first underlying disease, such as:
plasminogen deficiency (E88.02)
viral disease NEC (B00-B34)

Use additional code for any associated perforated tympanic membrane (H72.-)

Excludes1 otitis media in:
influenza (J09.X9, J10.83, J11.83)
measles (B05.3)
scarlet fever (A38.0)
tuberculosis (A18.6)

H67.1 Otitis media in diseases classified elsewhere, right ear

H67.2 Otitis media in diseases classified elsewhere, left ear

H67.3 Otitis media in diseases classified elsewhere, bilateral

H67.9 Otitis media in diseases classified elsewhere, unspecified ear

H68 Eustachian salpingitis and obstruction

H68.0 Eustachian salpingitis

H68.00 Unspecified Eustachian salpingitis

H68.001 Unspecified Eustachian salpingitis, right ear

H68.002 Unspecified Eustachian salpingitis, left ear

H68.003 Unspecified Eustachian salpingitis, bilateral

H68.009 Unspecified Eustachian salpingitis, unspecified ear

H68.01 Acute Eustachian salpingitis

H68.011 Acute Eustachian salpingitis, right ear

H68.012 Acute Eustachian salpingitis, left ear

H68.013 Acute Eustachian salpingitis, bilateral

H68.019 Acute Eustachian salpingitis, unspecified ear

H68.02 Chronic Eustachian salpingitis

H68.021 Chronic Eustachian salpingitis, right ear

H68.022 Chronic Eustachian salpingitis, left ear

H68.023 Chronic Eustachian salpingitis, bilateral

H68.029 Chronic Eustachian salpingitis, unspecified ear

CHAPTER 8 (H60-H95)

● H68.1 Obstruction of Eustachian tube
Stenosis of Eustachian tube
Stricture of Eustachian tube

● H68.10 Unspecified obstruction of Eustachian tube
H68.101 Unspecified obstruction of Eustachian tube, right ear
H68.102 Unspecified obstruction of Eustachian tube, left ear
H68.103 Unspecified obstruction of Eustachian tube, bilateral
H68.109 Unspecified obstruction of Eustachian tube, unspecified ear

● H68.11 Osseous obstruction of Eustachian tube
H68.111 Osseous obstruction of Eustachian tube, right ear
H68.112 Osseous obstruction of Eustachian tube, left ear
H68.113 Osseous obstruction of Eustachian tube, bilateral
H68.119 Osseous obstruction of Eustachian tube, unspecified ear

● H68.12 Intrinsic cartilagenous obstruction of Eustachian tube
H68.121 Intrinsic cartilagenous obstruction of Eustachian tube, right ear
H68.122 Intrinsic cartilagenous obstruction of Eustachian tube, left ear
H68.123 Intrinsic cartilagenous obstruction of Eustachian tube, bilateral
H68.129 Intrinsic cartilagenous obstruction of Eustachian tube, unspecified ear

● H68.13 Extrinsic cartilagenous obstruction of Eustachian tube
Compression of Eustachian tube
H68.131 Extrinsic cartilagenous obstruction of Eustachian tube, right ear
H68.132 Extrinsic cartilagenous obstruction of Eustachian tube, left ear
H68.133 Extrinsic cartilagenous obstruction of Eustachian tube, bilateral
H68.139 Extrinsic cartilagenous obstruction of Eustachian tube, unspecified ear

● H69 Other and unspecified disorders of Eustachian tube

● H69.0 Patulous Eustachian tube
H69.00 Patulous Eustachian tube, unspecified ear
H69.01 Patulous Eustachian tube, right ear
H69.02 Patulous Eustachian tube, left ear
H69.03 Patulous Eustachian tube, bilateral

● H69.8 Other specified disorders of Eustachian tube
H69.80 Other specified disorders of Eustachian tube, unspecified ear
H69.81 Other specified disorders of Eustachian tube, right ear
H69.82 Other specified disorders of Eustachian tube, left ear
H69.83 Other specified disorders of Eustachian tube, bilateral

● H69.9 Unspecified Eustachian tube disorder
H69.90 Unspecified Eustachian tube disorder, unspecified ear
H69.91 Unspecified Eustachian tube disorder, right ear
H69.92 Unspecified Eustachian tube disorder, left ear
H69.93 Unspecified Eustachian tube disorder, bilateral

● H70 Mastoiditis and related conditions

● H70.0 Acute mastoiditis (Ex) PDX 812
Abscess of mastoid
Empyema of mastoid

● H70.00 Acute mastoiditis without complications
H70.001 Acute mastoiditis without complications, right ear
H70.002 Acute mastoiditis without complications, left ear
H70.003 Acute mastoiditis without complications, bilateral
H70.009 Acute mastoiditis without complications, unspecified ear

● H70.01 Subperiosteal abscess of mastoid
H70.011 Subperiosteal abscess of mastoid, right ear
H70.012 Subperiosteal abscess of mastoid, left ear
H70.013 Subperiosteal abscess of mastoid, bilateral
H70.019 Subperiosteal abscess of mastoid, unspecified ear

● H70.09 Acute mastoiditis with other complications
H70.091 Acute mastoiditis with other complications, right ear
H70.092 Acute mastoiditis with other complications, left ear
H70.093 Acute mastoiditis with other complications, bilateral
H70.099 Acute mastoiditis with other complications, unspecified ear

● H70.1 Chronic mastoiditis
Caries of mastoid
Fistula of mastoid
Excludes1 tuberculous mastoiditis (A18.03)
H70.10 Chronic mastoiditis, unspecified ear
H70.11 Chronic mastoiditis, right ear
H70.12 Chronic mastoiditis, left ear
H70.13 Chronic mastoiditis, bilateral

● H70.2 Petrositis
Inflammation of petrous bone

● H70.20 Unspecified petrositis
H70.201 Unspecified petrositis, right ear
H70.202 Unspecified petrositis, left ear
H70.203 Unspecified petrositis, bilateral
H70.209 Unspecified petrositis, unspecified ear

● H70.21 Acute petrositis
H70.211 Acute petrositis, right ear
H70.212 Acute petrositis, left ear
H70.213 Acute petrositis, bilateral
H70.219 Acute petrositis, unspecified ear

● H70.22 Chronic petrositis
H70.221 Chronic petrositis, right ear
H70.222 Chronic petrositis, left ear
H70.223 Chronic petrositis, bilateral
H70.229 Chronic petrositis, unspecified ear

Item 8–1 Mastoiditis is an infection of the portion of the temporal bone of the skull that is behind the ear (mastoid process) caused by an untreated otitis media, leading to an infection of the surrounding structures which may include the brain.

● **H70.8** Other mastoiditis and related conditions

Excludes1 preauricular sinus and cyst (Q18.1)
sinus, fistula, and cyst of branchial cleft (Q18.0)

● **H70.81** Postauricular fistula
- **H70.811** Postauricular fistula, right ear
- **H70.812** Postauricular fistula, left ear
- **H70.813** Postauricular fistula, bilateral
- **H70.819** Postauricular fistula, unspecified ear

● **H70.89** Other mastoiditis and related conditions
- **H70.891** Other mastoiditis and related conditions, right ear
- **H70.892** Other mastoiditis and related conditions, left ear
- **H70.893** Other mastoiditis and related conditions, bilateral
- **H70.899** Other mastoiditis and related conditions, unspecified ear

● **H70.9** Unspecified mastoiditis
- **H70.90** Unspecified mastoiditis, unspecified ear
- **H70.91** Unspecified mastoiditis, right ear
- **H70.92** Unspecified mastoiditis, left ear
- **H70.93** Unspecified mastoiditis, bilateral

● **H71** Cholesteatoma of middle ear

Excludes2 cholesteatoma of external ear (H60.4-)
recurrent cholesteatoma of postmastoidectomy cavity (H95.0-)

● **H71.0** Cholesteatoma of attic
- **H71.00** Cholesteatoma of attic, unspecified ear
- **H71.01** Cholesteatoma of attic, right ear
- **H71.02** Cholesteatoma of attic, left ear
  Coding Clinic: 2021, Q3, P9
- **H71.03** Cholesteatoma of attic, bilateral

● **H71.1** Cholesteatoma of tympanum
- **H71.10** Cholesteatoma of tympanum, unspecified ear
- **H71.11** Cholesteatoma of tympanum, right ear
- **H71.12** Cholesteatoma of tympanum, left ear
- **H71.13** Cholesteatoma of tympanum, bilateral

● **H71.2** Cholesteatoma of mastoid
- **H71.20** Cholesteatoma of mastoid, unspecified ear
- **H71.21** Cholesteatoma of mastoid, right ear
- **H71.22** Cholesteatoma of mastoid, left ear
  Coding Clinic: 2021, Q3, P9
- **H71.23** Cholesteatoma of mastoid, bilateral

● **H71.3** Diffuse cholesteatosis
Coding Clinic: 2021, Q3, P9
- **H71.30** Diffuse cholesteatosis, unspecified ear
- **H71.31** Diffuse cholesteatosis, right ear
- **H71.32** Diffuse cholesteatosis, left ear
- **H71.33** Diffuse cholesteatosis, bilateral

● **H71.9** Unspecified cholesteatoma
- **H71.90** Unspecified cholesteatoma, unspecified ear
- **H71.91** Unspecified cholesteatoma, right ear
- **H71.92** Unspecified cholesteatoma, left ear
- **H71.93** Unspecified cholesteatoma, bilateral

★**(See Plate 22 of the Anatomy Illustrations.)**

● **H72** Perforation of tympanic membrane
Hole or rupture in ear drum

Includes persistent post-traumatic perforation of ear drum
postinflammatory perforation of ear drum

Code first any associated otitis media (H65.-, H66.1-, H66.2-, H66.3-, H66.4-, H66.9-, H67.-)

Excludes1 acute suppurative otitis media with rupture of the tympanic membrane (H66.01-)
traumatic rupture of ear drum (S09.2-)

● **H72.0** Central perforation of tympanic membrane
- **H72.00** Central perforation of tympanic membrane, unspecified ear
- **H72.01** Central perforation of tympanic membrane, right ear
- **H72.02** Central perforation of tympanic membrane, left ear
- **H72.03** Central perforation of tympanic membrane, bilateral

● **H72.1** Attic perforation of tympanic membrane
Perforation of pars flaccida
- **H72.10** Attic perforation of tympanic membrane, unspecified ear
- **H72.11** Attic perforation of tympanic membrane, right ear
- **H72.12** Attic perforation of tympanic membrane, left ear
- **H72.13** Attic perforation of tympanic membrane, bilateral

● **H72.2** Other marginal perforations of tympanic membrane

● **H72.2X** Other marginal perforations of tympanic membrane
- **H72.2X1** Other marginal perforations of tympanic membrane, right ear
- **H72.2X2** Other marginal perforations of tympanic membrane, left ear
- **H72.2X3** Other marginal perforations of tympanic membrane, bilateral
- **H72.2X9** Other marginal perforations of tympanic membrane, unspecified ear

● **H72.8** Other perforations of tympanic membrane

● **H72.81** Multiple perforations of tympanic membrane
- **H72.811** Multiple perforations of tympanic membrane, right ear
- **H72.812** Multiple perforations of tympanic membrane, left ear
- **H72.813** Multiple perforations of tympanic membrane, bilateral
- **H72.819** Multiple perforations of tympanic membrane, unspecified ear

● **H72.82** Total perforations of tympanic membrane
- **H72.821** Total perforations of tympanic membrane, right ear
- **H72.822** Total perforations of tympanic membrane, left ear
- **H72.823** Total perforations of tympanic membrane, bilateral
- **H72.829** Total perforations of tympanic membrane, unspecified ear

● **H72.9** Unspecified perforation of tympanic membrane
- **H72.90** Unspecified perforation of tympanic membrane, unspecified ear
- **H72.91** Unspecified perforation of tympanic membrane, right ear
- **H72.92** Unspecified perforation of tympanic membrane, left ear
- **H72.93** Unspecified perforation of tympanic membrane, bilateral

- H73 Other disorders of tympanic membrane
  - H73.Ø Acute myringitis
    - Excludes1 acute myringitis with otitis media (H65, H66)
    - H73.ØØ Unspecified acute myringitis
      - Acute tympanitis NOS
      - H73.ØØ1 Acute myringitis, right ear
      - H73.ØØ2 Acute myringitis, left ear
      - H73.ØØ3 Acute myringitis, bilateral
      - H73.ØØ9 Acute myringitis, unspecified ear
    - H73.Ø1 Bullous myringitis
      - H73.Ø11 Bullous myringitis, right ear
      - H73.Ø12 Bullous myringitis, left ear
      - H73.Ø13 Bullous myringitis, bilateral
      - H73.Ø19 Bullous myringitis, unspecified ear
    - H73.Ø9 Other acute myringitis
      - H73.Ø91 Other acute myringitis, right ear
      - H73.Ø92 Other acute myringitis, left ear
      - H73.Ø93 Other acute myringitis, bilateral
      - H73.Ø99 Other acute myringitis, unspecified ear
  - H73.1 Chronic myringitis
    - Chronic tympanitis
    - Excludes1 chronic myringitis with otitis media (H65, H66)
    - H73.1Ø Chronic myringitis, unspecified ear
    - H73.11 Chronic myringitis, right ear
    - H73.12 Chronic myringitis, left ear
    - H73.13 Chronic myringitis, bilateral
  - H73.2 Unspecified myringitis
    - H73.2Ø Unspecified myringitis, unspecified ear
    - H73.21 Unspecified myringitis, right ear
    - H73.22 Unspecified myringitis, left ear
    - H73.23 Unspecified myringitis, bilateral
  - H73.8 Other specified disorders of tympanic membrane
    - H73.81 Atrophic flaccid tympanic membrane
      - H73.811 Atrophic flaccid tympanic membrane, right ear
      - H73.812 Atrophic flaccid tympanic membrane, left ear
      - H73.813 Atrophic flaccid tympanic membrane, bilateral
      - H73.819 Atrophic flaccid tympanic membrane, unspecified ear
    - H73.82 Atrophic nonflaccid tympanic membrane
      - H73.821 Atrophic nonflaccid tympanic membrane, right ear
      - H73.822 Atrophic nonflaccid tympanic membrane, left ear
      - H73.823 Atrophic nonflaccid tympanic membrane, bilateral
      - H73.829 Atrophic nonflaccid tympanic membrane, unspecified ear
    - H73.89 Other specified disorders of tympanic membrane
      - H73.891 Other specified disorders of tympanic membrane, right ear
      - H73.892 Other specified disorders of tympanic membrane, left ear
      - H73.893 Other specified disorders of tympanic membrane, bilateral
      - H73.899 Other specified disorders of tympanic membrane, unspecified ear
  - H73.9 Unspecified disorder of tympanic membrane
    - H73.9Ø Unspecified disorder of tympanic membrane, unspecified ear
    - H73.91 Unspecified disorder of tympanic membrane, right ear
    - H73.92 Unspecified disorder of tympanic membrane, left ear
    - H73.93 Unspecified disorder of tympanic membrane, bilateral
- H74 Other disorders of middle ear mastoid
  - Excludes2 mastoiditis (H7Ø.-)
  - H74.Ø Tympanosclerosis
    - H74.Ø1 Tympanosclerosis, right ear
    - H74.Ø2 Tympanosclerosis, left ear
    - H74.Ø3 Tympanosclerosis, bilateral
    - H74.Ø9 Tympanosclerosis, unspecified ear
  - H74.1 Adhesive middle ear disease
    - Adhesive otitis
    - Excludes1 glue ear (H65.3-)
    - H74.11 Adhesive right middle ear disease
    - H74.12 Adhesive left middle ear disease
    - H74.13 Adhesive middle ear disease, bilateral
    - H74.19 Adhesive middle ear disease, unspecified ear
  - H74.2 Discontinuity and dislocation of ear ossicles
    - H74.2Ø Discontinuity and dislocation of ear ossicles, unspecified ear
    - H74.21 Discontinuity and dislocation of right ear ossicles
    - H74.22 Discontinuity and dislocation of left ear ossicles
    - H74.23 Discontinuity and dislocation of ear ossicles, bilateral
  - H74.3 Other acquired abnormalities of ear ossicles
    - H74.31 Ankylosis of ear ossicles
      - H74.311 Ankylosis of ear ossicles, right ear
      - H74.312 Ankylosis of ear ossicles, left ear
      - H74.313 Ankylosis of ear ossicles, bilateral
      - H74.319 Ankylosis of ear ossicles, unspecified ear
    - H74.32 Partial loss of ear ossicles
      - H74.321 Partial loss of ear ossicles, right ear
      - H74.322 Partial loss of ear ossicles, left ear
      - H74.323 Partial loss of ear ossicles, bilateral
      - H74.329 Partial loss of ear ossicles, unspecified ear
    - H74.39 Other acquired abnormalities of ear ossicles
      - H74.391 Other acquired abnormalities of right ear ossicles
      - H74.392 Other acquired abnormalities of left ear ossicles
      - H74.393 Other acquired abnormalities of ear ossicles, bilateral
      - H74.399 Other acquired abnormalities of ear ossicles, unspecified ear
  - H74.4 Polyp of middle ear
    - H74.4Ø Polyp of middle ear, unspecified ear
    - H74.41 Polyp of right middle ear
    - H74.42 Polyp of left middle ear
    - H74.43 Polyp of middle ear, bilateral

- **H74.8 Other specified disorders of middle ear and mastoid**
  - **H74.8X Other specified disorders of middle ear and mastoid**
    - H74.8X1 Other specified disorders of right middle ear and mastoid
    - H74.8X2 Other specified disorders of left middle ear and mastoid
    - H74.8X3 Other specified disorders of middle ear and mastoid, bilateral
    - H74.8X9 Other specified disorders of middle ear and mastoid, unspecified ear
- **H74.9 Unspecified disorder of middle ear and mastoid**
  - H74.90 Unspecified disorder of middle ear and mastoid, unspecified ear
  - H74.91 Unspecified disorder of right middle ear and mastoid
  - H74.92 Unspecified disorder of left middle ear and mastoid
  - H74.93 Unspecified disorder of middle ear and mastoid, bilateral

H75 Other disorders of middle ear and mastoid in diseases classified elsewhere

Code first underlying disease

- **H75.0 Mastoiditis in infectious and parasitic diseases classified elsewhere**

  Excludes1 mastoiditis (in):
  - syphilis (A52.77)
  - tuberculosis (A18.03)

  - *H75.00 Mastoiditis in infectious and parasitic diseases classified elsewhere, unspecified ear*
  - *H75.01 Mastoiditis in infectious and parasitic diseases classified elsewhere, right ear*
  - *H75.02 Mastoiditis in infectious and parasitic diseases classified elsewhere, left ear*
  - *H75.03 Mastoiditis in infectious and parasitic diseases classified elsewhere, bilateral*
- **H75.8 Other specified disorders of middle ear and mastoid in diseases classified elsewhere**
  - *H75.80 Other specified disorders of middle ear and mastoid in diseases classified elsewhere, unspecified ear*
  - *H75.81 Other specified disorders of right middle ear and mastoid in diseases classified elsewhere*
  - *H75.82 Other specified disorders of left middle ear and mastoid in diseases classified elsewhere*
  - *H75.83 Other specified disorders of middle ear and mastoid in diseases classified elsewhere, bilateral*

DISEASES OF INNER EAR (H80-H83)

★ **(See Plate 23 of the Anatomy Illustrations.)**

H80 Otosclerosis

Inherited middle ear spongelike bone growth causing hearing loss

Includes Otospongiosis

- **H80.0 Otosclerosis involving oval window, nonobliterative**
  - H80.00 Otosclerosis involving oval window, nonobliterative, unspecified ear
  - H80.01 Otosclerosis involving oval window, nonobliterative, right ear
  - H80.02 Otosclerosis involving oval window, nonobliterative, left ear
  - H80.03 Otosclerosis involving oval window, nonobliterative, bilateral
- **H80.1 Otosclerosis involving oval window, obliterative**
  - H80.10 Otosclerosis involving oval window, obliterative, unspecified ear
  - H80.11 Otosclerosis involving oval window, obliterative, right ear
  - H80.12 Otosclerosis involving oval window, obliterative, left ear
  - H80.13 Otosclerosis involving oval window, obliterative, bilateral
- **H80.2 Cochlear otosclerosis**

  Otosclerosis involving otic capsule
  Otosclerosis involving round window

  - H80.20 Cochlear otosclerosis, unspecified ear
  - H80.21 Cochlear otosclerosis, right ear
  - H80.22 Cochlear otosclerosis, left ear
  - H80.23 Cochlear otosclerosis, bilateral
- **H80.8 Other otosclerosis**
  - H80.80 Other otosclerosis, unspecified ear
  - H80.81 Other otosclerosis, right ear
  - H80.82 Other otosclerosis, left ear
  - H80.83 Other otosclerosis, bilateral
- **H80.9 Unspecified otosclerosis**
  - H80.90 Unspecified otosclerosis, unspecified ear
  - H80.91 Unspecified otosclerosis, right ear
  - H80.92 Unspecified otosclerosis, left ear
  - H80.93 Unspecified otosclerosis, bilateral

H81 Disorders of vestibular function

Excludes1 epidemic vertigo (A88.1)
vertigo NOS (R42)

- **H81.0 Ménière's disease**

  Vestibular disorder that produces recurring symptoms including severe and intermittent hearing loss including the feeling of ear pressure or pain

  Labyrinthine hydrops
  Ménière's syndrome or vertigo

  - H81.01 Ménière's disease, right ear
  - H81.02 Ménière's disease, left ear
  - H81.03 Ménière's disease, bilateral
  - H81.09 Ménière's disease, unspecified ear
- **H81.1 Benign paroxysmal vertigo**
  - H81.10 Benign paroxysmal vertigo, unspecified ear
  - H81.11 Benign paroxysmal vertigo, right ear
  - H81.12 Benign paroxysmal vertigo, left ear
  - H81.13 Benign paroxysmal vertigo, bilateral
- **H81.2 Vestibular neuronitis**
  - H81.20 Vestibular neuronitis, unspecified ear
  - H81.21 Vestibular neuronitis, right ear
  - H81.22 Vestibular neuronitis, left ear
  - H81.23 Vestibular neuronitis, bilateral
- **H81.3 Other peripheral vertigo**
  - **H81.31 Aural vertigo**
    - H81.311 Aural vertigo, right ear
    - H81.312 Aural vertigo, left ear
    - H81.313 Aural vertigo, bilateral
    - H81.319 Aural vertigo, unspecified ear
  - **H81.39 Other peripheral vertigo**

    Lermoyez' syndrome
    Otogenic vertigo
    Peripheral vertigo NOS

    - H81.391 Other peripheral vertigo, right ear
    - H81.392 Other peripheral vertigo, left ear
    - H81.393 Other peripheral vertigo, bilateral
    - H81.399 Other peripheral vertigo, unspecified ear
- H81.4 Vertigo of central origin

  Central positional nystagmus

CHAPTER 8 (H60-H95)

● H81.8 Other disorders of vestibular function
● H81.8X Other disorders of vestibular function
H81.8X1 Other disorders of vestibular function, right ear
H81.8X2 Other disorders of vestibular function, left ear
H81.8X3 Other disorders of vestibular function, bilateral
H81.8X9 Other disorders of vestibular function, unspecified ear
Coding Clinic: 2022, Q2, P12

● H81.9 Unspecified disorder of vestibular function
Vertiginous syndrome NOS
H81.90 Unspecified disorder of vestibular function, unspecified ear
H81.91 Unspecified disorder of vestibular function, right ear
H81.92 Unspecified disorder of vestibular function, left ear
H81.93 Unspecified disorder of vestibular function, bilateral

● H82 Vertiginous syndromes in diseases classified elsewhere
Code first underlying disease
Excludes1 epidemic vertigo (A88.1)
H82.1 Vertiginous syndromes in diseases classified elsewhere, right ear
H82.2 Vertiginous syndromes in diseases classified elsewhere, left ear
H82.3 Vertiginous syndromes in diseases classified elsewhere, bilateral
H82.9 Vertiginous syndromes in diseases classified elsewhere, unspecified ear

● H83 Other diseases of inner ear
● H83.0 Labyrinthitis
Balance disorder that follows URI or head injury
H83.01 Labyrinthitis, right ear
H83.02 Labyrinthitis, left ear
H83.03 Labyrinthitis, bilateral
H83.09 Labyrinthitis, unspecified ear

● H83.1 Labyrinthine fistula
H83.11 Labyrinthine fistula, right ear
H83.12 Labyrinthine fistula, left ear
H83.13 Labyrinthine fistula, bilateral
H83.19 Labyrinthine fistula, unspecified ear

● H83.2 Labyrinthine dysfunction
Labyrinthine hypersensitivity
Labyrinthine hypofunction
Labyrinthine loss of function
● H83.2X Labyrinthine dysfunction
H83.2X1 Labyrinthine dysfunction, right ear
H83.2X2 Labyrinthine dysfunction, left ear
H83.2X3 Labyrinthine dysfunction, bilateral
H83.2X9 Labyrinthine dysfunction, unspecified ear

● H83.3 Noise effects on inner ear
Acoustic trauma of inner ear
Noise-induced hearing loss of inner ear
● H83.3X Noise effects on inner ear
H83.3X1 Noise effects on right inner ear
H83.3X2 Noise effects on left inner ear
H83.3X3 Noise effects on inner ear, bilateral
H83.3X9 Noise effects on inner ear, unspecified ear

● H83.8 Other specified diseases of inner ear
● H83.8X Other specified diseases of inner ear
H83.8X1 Other specified diseases of right inner ear
H83.8X2 Other specified diseases of left inner ear
H83.8X3 Other specified diseases of inner ear, bilateral
H83.8X9 Other specified diseases of inner ear, unspecified ear

● H83.9 Unspecified disease of inner ear
H83.90 Unspecified disease of inner ear, unspecified ear
H83.91 Unspecified disease of right inner ear
H83.92 Unspecified disease of left inner ear
H83.93 Unspecified disease of inner ear, bilateral

OTHER DISORDERS OF EAR (H90-H94)

● H90 Conductive and sensorineural hearing loss
Excludes1 deaf nonspeaking NEC (H91.3)
deafness NOS (H91.9-)
hearing loss NOS (H91.9-)
noise-induced hearing loss (H83.3-)
ototoxic hearing loss (H91.0-)
sudden (idiopathic) hearing loss (H91.2-)
H90.0 Conductive hearing loss, bilateral
● H90.1 Conductive hearing loss, unilateral with unrestricted hearing on the contralateral side
H90.11 Conductive hearing loss, unilateral, right ear, with unrestricted hearing on the contralateral side
H90.12 Conductive hearing loss, unilateral, left ear, with unrestricted hearing on the contralateral side
H90.2 Conductive hearing loss, unspecified
Conductive deafness NOS
H90.3 Sensorineural hearing loss, bilateral
● H90.4 Sensorineural hearing loss, unilateral with unrestricted hearing on the contralateral side
H90.41 Sensorineural hearing loss, unilateral, right ear, with unrestricted hearing on the contralateral side
H90.42 Sensorineural hearing loss, unilateral, left ear, with unrestricted hearing on the contralateral side
H90.5 Unspecified sensorineural hearing loss
Central hearing loss NOS
Congenital deafness NOS
Neural hearing loss NOS
Perceptive hearing loss NOS
Sensorineural deafness NOS
Sensory hearing loss NOS
Excludes1 abnormal auditory perception (H93.2-)
psychogenic deafness (F44.6)
H90.6 Mixed conductive and sensorineural hearing loss, bilateral
Coding Clinic: 2015, Q2, P7
● H90.7 Mixed conductive and sensorineural hearing loss, unilateral with unrestricted hearing on the contralateral side
H90.71 Mixed conductive and sensorineural hearing loss, unilateral, right ear, with unrestricted hearing on the contralateral side
H90.72 Mixed conductive and sensorineural hearing loss, unilateral, left ear, with unrestricted hearing on the contralateral side
H90.8 Mixed conductive and sensorineural hearing loss, unspecified

● **H90.A** Conductive and sensorineural hearing loss with restricted hearing on the contralateral side
Coding Clinic: 2016, Q4, P23-24

● **H90.A1** Conductive hearing loss, unilateral, with restricted hearing on the contralateral side
- **H90.A11** Conductive hearing loss, unilateral, right ear with restricted hearing on the contralateral side
- **H90.A12** Conductive hearing loss, unilateral, left ear with restricted hearing on the contralateral side
Coding Clinic: 2016, Q4, P25

● **H90.A2** Sensorineural hearing loss, unilateral, with restricted hearing on the contralateral side
- **H90.A21** Sensorineural hearing loss, unilateral, right ear, with restricted hearing on the contralateral side
- **H90.A22** Sensorineural hearing loss, unilateral, left ear, with restricted hearing on the contralateral side

● **H90.A3** Mixed conductive and sensorineural hearing loss, unilateral with restricted hearing on the contralateral side
- **H90.A31** Mixed conductive and sensorineural hearing loss, unilateral, right ear with restricted hearing on the contralateral side
- **H90.A32** Mixed conductive and sensorineural hearing loss, unilateral, left ear with restricted hearing on the contralateral side

● **H91** Other and unspecified hearing loss
Excludes1 abnormal auditory perception (H93.2-)
hearing loss as classified in H90.-
impacted cerumen (H61.2-)
noise-induced hearing loss (H83.3-)
psychogenic deafness (F44.6)
transient ischemic deafness (H93.01-)

● **H91.0** Ototoxic hearing loss
Code first poisoning due to drug or toxin, if applicable (T36-T65 with fifth or sixth character 1-4)
Use additional code for adverse effect, if applicable, to identify drug (T36-T50 with fifth or sixth character 5)
- **H91.01** Ototoxic hearing loss, right ear
- **H91.02** Ototoxic hearing loss, left ear
- **H91.03** Ototoxic hearing loss, bilateral
- **H91.09** Ototoxic hearing loss, unspecified ear

● **H91.1** Presbycusis
Presbyacusia
- **H91.10** Presbycusis, unspecified ear
- **H91.11** Presbycusis, right ear
- **H91.12** Presbycusis, left ear
- **H91.13** Presbycusis, bilateral

● **H91.2** Sudden idiopathic hearing loss
Sudden hearing loss NOS
- **H91.20** Sudden idiopathic hearing loss, unspecified ear
- **H91.21** Sudden idiopathic hearing loss, right ear
- **H91.22** Sudden idiopathic hearing loss, left ear
- **H91.23** Sudden idiopathic hearing loss, bilateral

H91.3 Deaf nonspeaking, not elsewhere classified

● **H91.8** Other specified hearing loss

● **H91.8X** Other specified hearing loss
- **H91.8X1** Other specified hearing loss, right ear
- **H91.8X2** Other specified hearing loss, left ear
- **H91.8X3** Other specified hearing loss, bilateral
- **H91.8X9** Other specified hearing loss, unspecified ear

● **H91.9** Unspecified hearing loss
Deafness NOS
High frequency deafness
Low frequency deafness
- **H91.90** Unspecified hearing loss, unspecified ear
- **H91.91** Unspecified hearing loss, right ear
- **H91.92** Unspecified hearing loss, left ear
- **H91.93** Unspecified hearing loss, bilateral

● **H92** Otalgia and effusion of ear

● **H92.0** Otalgia
- **H92.01** Otalgia, right ear
- **H92.02** Otalgia, left ear
- **H92.03** Otalgia, bilateral
- **H92.09** Otalgia, unspecified ear

● **H92.1** Otorrhea
Excludes1 leakage of cerebrospinal fluid through ear (G96.0)
- **H92.10** Otorrhea, unspecified ear
- **H92.11** Otorrhea, right ear
- **H92.12** Otorrhea, left ear
- **H92.13** Otorrhea, bilateral

● **H92.2** Otorrhagia
Excludes1 traumatic otorrhagia - code to injury
- **H92.20** Otorrhagia, unspecified ear
- **H92.21** Otorrhagia, right ear
- **H92.22** Otorrhagia, left ear
- **H92.23** Otorrhagia, bilateral

● **H93** Other disorders of ear, not elsewhere classified

● **H93.0** Degenerative and vascular disorders of ear
Excludes1 presbycusis (H91.1)

● **H93.01** Transient ischemic deafness
- **H93.011** Transient ischemic deafness, right ear
- **H93.012** Transient ischemic deafness, left ear
- **H93.013** Transient ischemic deafness, bilateral
- **H93.019** Transient ischemic deafness, unspecified ear

● **H93.09** Unspecified degenerative and vascular disorders of ear
- **H93.091** Unspecified degenerative and vascular disorders of right ear
- **H93.092** Unspecified degenerative and vascular disorders of left ear
- **H93.093** Unspecified degenerative and vascular disorders of ear, bilateral
- **H93.099** Unspecified degenerative and vascular disorders of unspecified ear

● **H93.1** Tinnitus
Perception of sound (ringing, buzzing, humming, whistling tunes, or singing)
- **H93.11** Tinnitus, right ear
- **H93.12** Tinnitus, left ear
- **H93.13** Tinnitus, bilateral
- **H93.19** Tinnitus, unspecified ear

● **H93.A** Pulsatile tinnitus
Coding Clinic: 2016, Q4, P25
- **H93.A1** Pulsatile tinnitus, right ear
Coding Clinic: 2023, Q2, P19; 2016, Q4, P26
- **H93.A2** Pulsatile tinnitus, left ear
- **H93.A3** Pulsatile tinnitus, bilateral
- **H93.A9** Pulsatile tinnitus, unspecified ear

H93.2 Other abnormal auditory perceptions
Excludes2 auditory hallucinations (R44.Ø)

H93.21 Auditory recruitment
H93.211 Auditory recruitment, right ear
H93.212 Auditory recruitment, left ear
H93.213 Auditory recruitment, bilateral
H93.219 Auditory recruitment, unspecified ear

H93.22 Diplacusis
H93.221 Diplacusis, right ear
H93.222 Diplacusis, left ear
H93.223 Diplacusis, bilateral
H93.229 Diplacusis, unspecified ear

H93.23 Hyperacusis
H93.231 Hyperacusis, right ear
H93.232 Hyperacusis, left ear
H93.233 Hyperacusis, bilateral
H93.239 Hyperacusis, unspecified ear

H93.24 Temporary auditory threshold shift
H93.241 Temporary auditory threshold shift, right ear
H93.242 Temporary auditory threshold shift, left ear
H93.243 Temporary auditory threshold shift, bilateral
H93.249 Temporary auditory threshold shift, unspecified ear

H93.25 Central auditory processing disorder
Congenital auditory imperception
Word deafness
Excludes1 mixed receptive-expressive language disorder (F8Ø.2)

H93.29 Other abnormal auditory perceptions
H93.291 Other abnormal auditory perceptions, right ear
H93.292 Other abnormal auditory perceptions, left ear
H93.293 Other abnormal auditory perceptions, bilateral
H93.299 Other abnormal auditory perceptions, unspecified ear

H93.3 Disorders of acoustic nerve
Disorder of 8th cranial nerve
Excludes1 acoustic neuroma (D33.3)
syphilitic acoustic neuritis (A52.15)

H93.3X Disorders of acoustic nerve
H93.3X1 Disorders of right acoustic nerve
H93.3X2 Disorders of left acoustic nerve
H93.3X3 Disorders of bilateral acoustic nerves
H93.3X9 Disorders of unspecified acoustic nerve

H93.8 Other specified disorders of ear
H93.8X Other specified disorders of ear
H93.8X1 Other specified disorders of right ear
H93.8X2 Other specified disorders of left ear
H93.8X3 Other specified disorders of ear, bilateral
H93.8X9 Other specified disorders of ear, unspecified ear

H93.9 Unspecified disorder of ear
H93.90 Unspecified disorder of ear, unspecified ear
H93.91 Unspecified disorder of right ear
H93.92 Unspecified disorder of left ear
H93.93 Unspecified disorder of ear, bilateral

H94 Other disorders of ear in diseases classified elsewhere

H94.Ø Acoustic neuritis in infectious and parasitic diseases classified elsewhere
Code first underlying disease, such as:
parasitic disease (B65-B89)
Excludes1 acoustic neuritis (in):
herpes zoster (BØ2.29)
syphilis (A52.15)

H94.ØØ Acoustic neuritis in infectious and parasitic diseases classified elsewhere, unspecified ear
H94.Ø1 Acoustic neuritis in infectious and parasitic diseases classified elsewhere, right ear
H94.Ø2 Acoustic neuritis in infectious and parasitic diseases classified elsewhere, left ear
H94.Ø3 Acoustic neuritis in infectious and parasitic diseases classified elsewhere, bilateral

H94.8 Other specified disorders of ear in diseases classified elsewhere
Code first underlying disease, such as:
congenital syphilis (A5Ø.Ø)
Excludes1 aural myiasis (B87.4)
syphilitic labyrinthitis (A52.79)

H94.8Ø Other specified disorders of ear in diseases classified elsewhere, unspecified ear
H94.81 Other specified disorders of right ear in diseases classified elsewhere
H94.82 Other specified disorders of left ear in diseases classified elsewhere
H94.83 Other specified disorders of ear in diseases classified elsewhere, bilateral

INTRAOPERATIVE AND POSTPROCEDURAL COMPLICATIONS AND DISORDERS OF EAR AND MASTOID PROCESS, NOT ELSEWHERE CLASSIFIED (H95)

H95 Intraoperative and postprocedural complications and disorders of ear and mastoid process, not elsewhere classified
Coding Clinic: 2016, Q4, P1Ø

H95.Ø Recurrent cholesteatoma of postmastoidectomy cavity
H95.ØØ Recurrent cholesteatoma of postmastoidectomy cavity, unspecified ear
H95.Ø1 Recurrent cholesteatoma of postmastoidectomy cavity, right ear
H95.Ø2 Recurrent cholesteatoma of postmastoidectomy cavity, left ear
H95.Ø3 Recurrent cholesteatoma of postmastoidectomy cavity, bilateral ears

H95.1 Other disorders of ear and mastoid process following mastoidectomy

H95.11 Chronic inflammation of postmastoidectomy cavity
H95.111 Chronic inflammation of postmastoidectomy cavity, right ear
H95.112 Chronic inflammation of postmastoidectomy cavity, left ear
H95.113 Chronic inflammation of postmastoidectomy cavity, bilateral ears
H95.119 Chronic inflammation of postmastoidectomy cavity, unspecified ear

H95.12 Granulation of postmastoidectomy cavity
H95.121 Granulation of postmastoidectomy cavity, right ear
H95.122 Granulation of postmastoidectomy cavity, left ear
H95.123 Granulation of postmastoidectomy cavity, bilateral ears
H95.129 Granulation of postmastoidectomy cavity, unspecified ear

● H95.13 Mucosal cyst of postmastoidectomy cavity
- H95.131 Mucosal cyst of postmastoidectomy cavity, right ear
- H95.132 Mucosal cyst of postmastoidectomy cavity, left ear
- H95.133 Mucosal cyst of postmastoidectomy cavity, bilateral ears
- H95.139 Mucosal cyst of postmastoidectomy cavity, unspecified ear

● H95.19 Other disorders following mastoidectomy
- H95.191 Other disorders following mastoidectomy, right ear
- H95.192 Other disorders following mastoidectomy, left ear
- H95.193 Other disorders following mastoidectomy, bilateral ears
- H95.199 Other disorders following mastoidectomy, unspecified ear

● H95.2 Intraoperative hemorrhage and hematoma of ear and mastoid process complicating a procedure (Ex) PDX 813

Excludes1 intraoperative hemorrhage and hematoma of ear and mastoid process due to accidental puncture or laceration during a procedure (H95.3-)

- H95.21 Intraoperative hemorrhage and hematoma of ear and mastoid process complicating a procedure on the ear and mastoid process
- H95.22 Intraoperative hemorrhage and hematoma of ear and mastoid process complicating other procedure

● H95.3 Accidental puncture and laceration of ear and mastoid process during a procedure (Ex) PDX 569
- H95.31 Accidental puncture and laceration of the ear and mastoid process during a procedure on the ear and mastoid process
- H95.32 Accidental puncture and laceration of the ear and mastoid process during other procedure

● H95.4 Postprocedural hemorrhage of ear and mastoid process following a procedure (Ex) PDX 813
- H95.41 Postprocedural hemorrhage of ear and mastoid process following a procedure on the ear and mastoid process
- H95.42 Postprocedural hemorrhage of ear and mastoid process following other procedure

● H95.5 Postprocedural hematoma and seroma of ear and mastoid process following a procedure (Ex) PDX 813
- H95.51 Postprocedural hematoma of ear and mastoid process following a procedure on the ear and mastoid process
- H95.52 Postprocedural hematoma of ear and mastoid process following other procedure
- H95.53 Postprocedural seroma of ear and mastoid process following a procedure on the ear and mastoid process
- H95.54 Postprocedural seroma of ear and mastoid process following other procedure

● H95.8 Other intraoperative and postprocedural complications and disorders of the ear and mastoid process, not elsewhere classified (Ex) PDX 814

Excludes2 postprocedural complications and disorders following mastoidectomy (H95.Ø-, H95.1-)

● H95.81 Postprocedural stenosis of external ear canal
- H95.811 Postprocedural stenosis of right external ear canal
- H95.812 Postprocedural stenosis of left external ear canal
- H95.813 Postprocedural stenosis of external ear canal, bilateral
- H95.819 Postprocedural stenosis of unspecified external ear canal

H95.88 Other intraoperative complications and disorders of the ear and mastoid process, not elsewhere classified

Use additional code, if applicable, to further specify disorder

H95.89 Other postprocedural complications and disorders of the ear and mastoid process, not elsewhere classified

Use additional code, if applicable, to further specify disorder

CHAPTER 8 (H6Ø-H95)

CHAPTER 9

DISEASES OF THE CIRCULATORY SYSTEM (I00-I99)

OGCR Chapter-Specific Coding Guidelines

9. **Chapter 9: Diseases of the Circulatory System (I00-I99)**

a. **Hypertension**

The classification presumes a causal relationship between hypertension and heart involvement and between hypertension and kidney involvement, as the two conditions are linked by the term "with" in the Alphabetic Index. These conditions should be coded as related even in the absence of provider documentation explicitly linking them, unless the documentation clearly states the conditions are unrelated.

For hypertension and conditions not specifically linked by relational terms such as "with," "associated with" or "due to" in the classification, provider documentation must link the conditions in order to code them as related.

1) **Hypertension with Heart Disease**

Hypertension with heart conditions classified to I50.- or I51.4-I51.7, I51.89, I51.9, are assigned to, a code from category I11, Hypertensive heart disease. Use additional code(s) from category I50, Heart failure, to identify the type(s) of heart failure in those patients with heart failure.

The same heart conditions (I50.-, I51.4-I51.7, I51.89, I51.9) with hypertension, are coded separately if the provider has documented they are unrelated to the hypertension. Sequence according to the circumstances of the admission/encounter.

2) **Hypertensive Chronic Kidney Disease**

Assign codes from category I12, Hypertensive chronic kidney disease, when both hypertension and a condition classifiable to category N18, Chronic kidney disease (CKD), are present. CKD should not be coded as hypertensive if the provider indicates the CKD is not related to the hypertension.

The appropriate code from category N18 should be used as a secondary code with a code from category I12 to identify the stage of chronic kidney disease.

See Section I.C.14. Chronic kidney disease.

If a patient has hypertensive chronic kidney disease and acute renal failure, an additional code for the acute renal failure is required.

3) **Hypertensive Heart and Chronic Kidney Disease**

Assign codes from combination category I13, Hypertensive heart and chronic kidney disease, when there is hypertension with both heart and kidney involvement. If heart failure is present, assign an additional code from category I50 to identify the type of heart failure.

The appropriate code from category N18, Chronic kidney disease, should be used as a secondary code with a code from category I13 to identify the stage of chronic kidney disease.

See Section I.C.14. Chronic kidney disease.

The codes in category I13, Hypertensive heart and chronic kidney disease, are combination codes that include hypertension, heart disease and chronic kidney disease. The Includes note at I13 specifies that the conditions included at I11 and I12 are included together in I13. If a patient has hypertension, heart disease and chronic kidney disease then a code from I13 should be used, not individual codes for hypertension, heart disease and chronic kidney disease, or codes from I11 or I12.

For patients with both acute renal failure and chronic kidney disease an additional code for acute renal failure is required.

4) **Hypertensive Cerebrovascular Disease**

For hypertensive cerebrovascular disease, first assign the appropriate code from categories I60-I69, followed by the appropriate hypertension code.

5) **Hypertensive Retinopathy**

Subcategory H35.0, Background retinopathy and retinal vascular changes, should be used with a code from category I10 – I15, Hypertensive disease to include the systemic hypertension. The sequencing is based on the reason for the encounter.

6) **Hypertension, Secondary**

Secondary hypertension is due to an underlying condition. Two codes are required: one to identify the underlying etiology and one from category I15 to identify the hypertension. Sequencing of codes is determined by the reason for admission/encounter.

7) **Hypertension, Transient**

Assign code R03.0, Elevated blood pressure reading without diagnosis of hypertension, unless patient has an established diagnosis of hypertension. Assign code O13.-, Gestational [pregnancy-induced] hypertension without significant proteinuria, or O14.-, Pre-eclampsia, for transient hypertension of pregnancy.

8) **Hypertension, Controlled**

This diagnostic statement usually refers to an existing state of hypertension under control by therapy. Assign the appropriate code from categories I10-I15, Hypertensive diseases.

9) **Hypertension, Uncontrolled**

Uncontrolled hypertension may refer to untreated hypertension or hypertension not responding to current therapeutic regimen. In either case, assign the appropriate code from categories I10-I15, Hypertensive diseases.

10) **Hypertensive Crisis**

Assign a code from category I16, Hypertensive crisis, for documented hypertensive urgency, hypertensive emergency or unspecified hypertensive crisis. Code also any identified hypertensive disease (I10-I15). The sequencing is based on the reason for the encounter.

11) **Pulmonary Hypertension**

Pulmonary hypertension is classified to category I27, Other pulmonary heart diseases. For secondary pulmonary hypertension (I27.1, I27.2-), code also any associated conditions or adverse effects of drugs or toxins. The sequencing is based on the reason for the encounter, except for adverse effects of drugs.

See Section I.C.19.e ***Adverse Effects, Poisoning, Underdosing and Toxic Effects.***

b. **Atherosclerotic Coronary Artery Disease and Angina**

ICD-10-CM has combination codes for atherosclerotic heart disease with angina pectoris. The subcategories for these codes are I25.11, Atherosclerotic heart disease of native coronary artery with angina pectoris and I25.7, Atherosclerosis of coronary artery bypass graft(s) and coronary artery of transplanted heart with angina pectoris.

When using one of these combination codes it is not necessary to use an additional code for angina pectoris. A causal relationship can be assumed in a patient with both atherosclerosis and angina pectoris, unless the documentation indicates the angina is due to something other than the atherosclerosis.

If a patient with coronary artery disease is admitted due to an acute myocardial infarction (AMI), the AMI should be sequenced before the coronary artery disease.

See Section I.C.9. Acute myocardial infarction (AMI).

c. **Intraoperative and Postprocedural Cerebrovascular Accident**

Medical record documentation should clearly specify the cause-and-effect relationship between the medical intervention and the cerebrovascular accident in order to assign a code for intraoperative or postprocedural cerebrovascular accident.

Proper code assignment depends on whether it was an infarction or hemorrhage and whether it occurred intraoperatively or postoperatively. If it was a cerebral hemorrhage, code assignment depends on the type of procedure performed.

d. **Sequelae of Cerebrovascular Disease**

1) **Category I69, Sequelae of Cerebrovascular disease**

Category I69 is used to indicate conditions classifiable to categories I60-I67 as the causes of sequela (neurologic deficits), themselves classified elsewhere. These "late effects" include neurologic deficits that persist after initial onset of conditions classifiable to categories I60-I67. The neurologic deficits caused by cerebrovascular disease may be present from the onset or may arise at any time after the onset of the condition classifiable to categories I60-I67.

Codes from category I69, Sequelae of cerebrovascular disease, that specify hemiplegia, hemiparesis and monoplegia identify whether the dominant or nondominant side is affected. Should the affected side be documented, but not specified as dominant or nondominant, and the classification system does not indicate a default, code selection is as follows:

- For ambidextrous patients, the default should be dominant.
- If the left side is affected, the default is nondominant.
- If the right side is affected, the default is dominant.

2) **Codes from category I69 with codes from I60-I67**

Codes from category I69 may be assigned on a health care record with codes from I60-I67, if the patient has a current cerebrovascular disease and deficits from an old cerebrovascular disease.

3) Codes from category I69 and Personal history of transient ischemic attack (TIA) and cerebral infarction (Z86.73)

Codes from category I69 should not be assigned if the patient does not have neurologic deficits.

See Section I.C.21. 4. History (of) for use of personal history codes.

e. Acute myocardial infarction (AMI)

1) Type 1 ST elevation myocardial infarction (STEMI) and non-ST elevation myocardial infarction (NSTEMI)

The ICD-10-CM codes for acute type 1 myocardial infarction (AMI) identify the site, such as anterolateral wall or true posterior wall. Subcategories I21.0-I21.2 and code I21.3 are used for type 1 ST elevation myocardial infarction (STEMI). Code I21.4, non-ST elevation (NSTEMI) myocardial infarction, is used for type 1 non-ST elevation myocardial infarction (NSTEMI) and nontransmural MIs.

If a type 1 NSTEMI evolves to STEMI, assign the STEMI code. If a type 1 STEMI converts to NSTEMI due to thrombolytic therapy, it is still coded as STEMI.

For encounters occurring while the myocardial infarction is equal to, or less than, four weeks old, including transfers to another acute setting or a postacute setting, and the myocardial infarction meets the definition for "other diagnoses" (see Section III, Reporting Additional Diagnoses), codes from category I21 may continue to be reported. For encounters after the 4-week time frame and the patient is still receiving care related to the myocardial infarction, the appropriate aftercare code should be assigned, rather than a code from category I21. For old or healed myocardial infarctions not requiring further care, code I25.2, Old myocardial infarction, may be assigned.

2) Acute myocardial infarction, unspecified

Code I21.9, Acute myocardial infarction, unspecified, is the default for unspecified acute myocardial infarction or unspecified type. If only type 1 STEMI or transmural MI without the site is documented, assign code I21.3, ST elevation (STEMI) myocardial infarction of unspecified site.

3) AMI documented as nontransmural or subendocardial but site provided

If an AMI is documented as nontransmural or subendocardial, but the site is provided, it is still coded as a subendocardial AMI.

See Section I.C.21.3 for information on coding status post administration of tPA in a different facility within the last 24 hours.

4) Subsequent acute myocardial infarction

A code from category I22, Subsequent ST elevation (STEMI) and non-ST elevation (NSTEMI) myocardial infarction, is to be used when a patient who has suffered a type 1 or unspecified AMI has a new AMI within the 4-week time frame of the initial AMI. A code from category I22 must be used in conjunction with a code from category I21. The sequencing of the I22 and I21 codes depends on the circumstances of the encounter.

Do not assign code I22 for subsequent myocardial infarctions other than type 1 or unspecified. For subsequent type 2 AMI assign only code I21.A1. For subsequent type 4 or type 5 AMI, assign only code I21.A9.

If a subsequent myocardial infarction of one type occurs within 4 weeks of a myocardial infarction of a different type, assign the appropriate codes from category I21 to identify each type. Do not assign a code from I22. Codes from category I22 should only be assigned if both the initial and subsequent myocardial infarctions are type 1 or unspecified.

5) Other Types of Myocardial Infarction

The ICD-10-CM provides codes for different types of myocardial infarction. Type 1 myocardial infarctions are assigned to codes I21.0-I21.4 and I21.9.

Type 2 myocardial infarction, and myocardial infarction due to demand ischemia or secondary to ischemic balance, is assigned to code I21.A1, Myocardial infarction type 2 with a code for the underlying cause. Do not assign code I24.8, Other forms of acute ischemic heart disease for the demand ischemia. Sequencing of type 2 AMI or the underlying cause is dependent on the circumstances of admission. When a type 2 AMI code is described as NSTEMI or STEMI, only assign code I21.A1. Codes I21.01-I21.4 should only be assigned for type 1 AMIs.

Acute myocardial infarctions type 3, 4a, 4b, 4c, and 5 are assigned to code I21.A9, Other myocardial infarction type.

The "Code also" and "Code first" notes should be followed related to complications, and for coding of postprocedural myocardial infarctions during or following cardiac surgery.

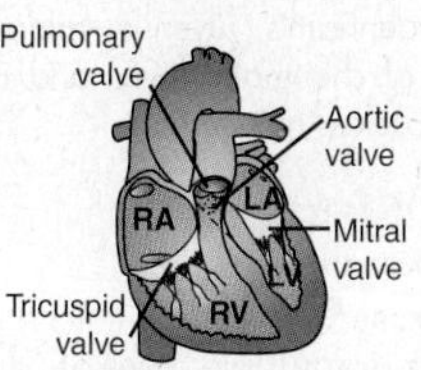

Figure 9-1 Cardiovascular valves.

Item 9-1 Rheumatic fever is the inflammation of the valve(s) of the heart, usually the mitral or aortic, which leads to valve damage. Rheumatic heart inflammations are usually **pericarditis** (sac surrounding heart), **endocarditis** (heart cavity), or **myocarditis** (heart muscle).

CHAPTER 9

DISEASES OF THE CIRCULATORY SYSTEM (I00-I99)

Excludes2 certain conditions originating in the perinatal period (P04-P96)
certain infectious and parasitic diseases (A00-B99)
complications of pregnancy, childbirth and the puerperium (O00-O9A)
congenital malformations, deformations, and chromosomal abnormalities (Q00-Q99)
endocrine, nutritional and metabolic diseases (E00-E88)
injury, poisoning and certain other consequences of external causes (S00-T88)
neoplasms (C00-D49)
symptoms, signs and abnormal clinical and laboratory findings, not elsewhere classified (R00-R94)
systemic connective tissue disorders (M30-M36)
transient cerebral ischemic attacks and related syndromes (G45.-)

This chapter contains the following blocks:

I00-I02	Acute rheumatic fever
I05-I09	Chronic rheumatic heart diseases
I10-I1A	Hypertensive diseases
I20-I25	Ischemic heart diseases
I26-I28	Pulmonary heart disease and diseases of pulmonary circulation
I30-I5A	Other forms of heart disease
I60-I69	Cerebrovascular diseases
I70-I79	Diseases of arteries, arterioles and capillaries
I80-I89	Diseases of veins, lymphatic vessels and lymph nodes, not elsewhere classified
I95-I99	Other and unspecified disorders of the circulatory system

ACUTE RHEUMATIC FEVER (I00-I02)

I00 Rheumatic fever without heart involvement

Includes arthritis, rheumatic, acute or subacute

Excludes1 rheumatic fever with heart involvement (I01.0-I01.9)

● **I01 Rheumatic fever with heart involvement**

Excludes1 chronic diseases of rheumatic origin (I05-I09) unless rheumatic fever is also present or there is evidence of reactivation or activity of the rheumatic process.

I01.0 Acute rheumatic pericarditis (Ex) PDX 201
Any condition in I00 with pericarditis
Rheumatic pericarditis (acute)

Excludes1 acute pericarditis not specified as rheumatic (I30.-)

I01.1 Acute rheumatic endocarditis (Ex) PDX 815
Any condition in I00 with endocarditis or valvulitis
Acute rheumatic valvulitis

CHAPTER 9 (I00-I99)

Item 9–2 Rheumatic chorea, also called Sydenham's, juvenile, minor, simple, or St. Vitus' dance, is a major symptom of rheumatic fever and is characterized by ceaseless, involuntary, jerky, purposeless movements.

I01.2 Acute rheumatic myocarditis (Ex:) PDX 199
Any condition in I00 with myocarditis

I01.8 Other acute rheumatic heart disease (Ex:) PDX 816
Any condition in I00 with other or multiple types of heart involvement
Acute rheumatic pancarditis

I01.9 Acute rheumatic heart disease, unspecified (Ex:) PDX 817
Any condition in I00 with unspecified type of heart involvement
Rheumatic carditis, acute
Rheumatic heart disease, active or acute

● I02 Rheumatic chorea
Includes Sydenham's chorea
Excludes1 chorea NOS (G25.5)
Huntington's chorea (G10)

I02.0 Rheumatic chorea with heart involvement (Ex:) PDX 816
Chorea NOS with heart involvement
Rheumatic chorea with heart involvement of any type classifiable under I01.-

I02.9 Rheumatic chorea without heart involvement (Ex:) PDX 817
Rheumatic chorea NOS

CHRONIC RHEUMATIC HEART DISEASES (I05-I09)

● I05 Rheumatic mitral valve diseases
Includes conditions classifiable to both I05.0 and I05.2-I05.9, whether specified as rheumatic or not
Excludes1 mitral valve disease specified as nonrheumatic (I34.-)
mitral valve disease with aortic and/or tricuspid valve involvement (I08.-)

I05.0 Rheumatic mitral stenosis
Mitral (valve) obstruction (rheumatic)

I05.1 Rheumatic mitral insufficiency
Rheumatic mitral incompetence
Rheumatic mitral regurgitation
Excludes1 mitral insufficiency not specified as rheumatic (I34.0)

I05.2 Rheumatic mitral stenosis with insufficiency
Rheumatic mitral stenosis with incompetence or regurgitation

I05.8 Other rheumatic mitral valve diseases
Rheumatic mitral (valve) failure

I05.9 Rheumatic mitral valve disease, unspecified
Rheumatic mitral (valve) disorder (chronic) NOS

● I06 Rheumatic aortic valve diseases
Excludes1 aortic valve disease not specified as rheumatic (I35.-)
aortic valve disease with mitral and/or tricuspid valve involvement (I08.-)

I06.0 Rheumatic aortic stenosis
Rheumatic aortic (valve) obstruction

I06.1 Rheumatic aortic insufficiency
Rheumatic aortic incompetence
Rheumatic aortic regurgitation

I06.2 Rheumatic aortic stenosis with insufficiency
Rheumatic aortic stenosis with incompetence or regurgitation

★ **(See Plate 33 of the Anatomy Illustrations.)**

Item 9–3 Mitral stenosis is the narrowing of the mitral valve separating the left atrium from the left ventricle. **Mitral insufficiency** is the improper closure of the mitral valve, which may lead to enlargement (hypertrophy) of the left atrium.

Item 9–4 Aortic stenosis is the narrowing of the aortic valve located between the left ventricle and the aorta. **Aortic insufficiency** is the improper closure of the aortic valve, which may lead to enlargement (hypertrophy) of the left ventricle.

I06.8 Other rheumatic aortic valve diseases

I06.9 Rheumatic aortic valve disease, unspecified
Rheumatic aortic (valve) disease NOS

● I07 Rheumatic tricuspid valve diseases
Includes rheumatic tricuspid valve diseases specified as rheumatic or unspecified
~~**Excludes1** tricuspid valve disease specified as nonrheumatic (I36.-)~~
~~tricuspid valve disease with aortic and/or mitral valve involvement (I08.-)~~
▶ **Excludes2** tricuspid valve disease specified as ▶nonrheumatic (I36.-)
▶tricuspid valve disease with aortic and/or mitral valve involvement (I08.-)

I07.0 Rheumatic tricuspid stenosis
Tricuspid (valve) stenosis (rheumatic)

I07.1 Rheumatic tricuspid insufficiency
Tricuspid (valve) insufficiency (rheumatic)

I07.2 Rheumatic tricuspid stenosis and insufficiency

I07.8 Other rheumatic tricuspid valve diseases

I07.9 Rheumatic tricuspid valve disease, unspecified
Rheumatic tricuspid valve disorder NOS

● I08 Multiple valve diseases
Includes multiple valve diseases specified as rheumatic or unspecified
Excludes1 endocarditis, valve unspecified (I38)
multiple valve disease specified a nonrheumatic (I34.-, I35.-, I36.-, I37.-, I38.-, Q22.-, Q23.-, Q24.8-)
rheumatic valve disease NOS (I09.1)

Coding Clinic: 2019, Q2, P5

I08.0 Rheumatic disorders of both mitral and aortic valves
Involvement of both mitral and aortic valves specified as rheumatic or unspecified
Coding Clinic: 2019, Q2, P5

I08.1 Rheumatic disorders of both mitral and tricuspid valves

I08.2 Rheumatic disorders of both aortic and tricuspid valves

I08.3 Combined rheumatic disorders of mitral, aortic and tricuspid valves

I08.8 Other rheumatic multiple valve diseases

I08.9 Rheumatic multiple valve disease, unspecified

● I09 Other rheumatic heart diseases

I09.0 Rheumatic myocarditis (Ex:) PDX 818
Excludes1 myocarditis not specified as rheumatic (I51.4)

I09.1 Rheumatic diseases of endocardium, valve unspecified
Rheumatic endocarditis (chronic)
Rheumatic valvulitis (chronic)
Excludes1 endocarditis, valve unspecified (I38)

I09.2 Chronic rheumatic pericarditis (Ex:) PDX 201
Adherent pericardium, rheumatic
Chronic rheumatic mediastinopericarditis
Chronic rheumatic myopericarditis
Excludes1 chronic pericarditis not specified as rheumatic (I31.-)

● I09.8 Other specified rheumatic heart diseases

I09.81 Rheumatic heart failure (Ex:) PDX 819
Use additional code to identify type of heart failure (I50.-)

I09.89 Other specified rheumatic heart diseases
Rheumatic disease of pulmonary valve

I09.9 Rheumatic heart disease, unspecified
Rheumatic carditis
Excludes1 rheumatoid carditis (M05.31)

Item 9–5 Hypertension is caused by high arterial blood pressure in the arteries. **Essential, primary,** or **idiopathic** hypertension occurs without identifiable organic cause. **Secondary** hypertension is that which has an organic cause. **Malignant** hypertension is severely elevated blood pressure. **Benign** hypertension is mildly elevated blood pressure.

HYPERTENSIVE DISEASES (I10-I16)

Use additional code to identify:
exposure to environmental tobacco smoke (Z77.22)
history of tobacco dependence (Z87.891)
occupational exposure to environmental tobacco smoke (Z57.31)
tobacco dependence (F17.-)
tobacco use (Z72.0)

Excludes1 neonatal hypertension (P29.2)
primary pulmonary hypertension (I27.0)

Excludes2 hypertensive disease complicating pregnancy, childbirth and the puerperium (O10-O11, O13-O16)

I10 Essential (primary) hypertension

Includes high blood pressure
hypertension (arterial) (benign) (essential) (malignant) (primary) (systemic)

Excludes1 hypertensive disease complicating pregnancy, childbirth and the puerperium (O10-O11, O13-O16)

Excludes2 essential (primary) hypertension involving vessels of brain (I60-I69)
essential (primary) hypertension involving vessels of eye (H35.0-)

Coding Clinic: 2023, Q4, P24-25,42

MCE: Questionable admission when principal dx

● **I11 Hypertensive heart disease**

Includes any condition in I50.- or I51.4-I51.7, I51.89, I51.9 due to hypertension

I11.0 Hypertensive heart disease with heart failure
Hypertensive heart failure
Use additional code to identify type of heart failure (I50.-)
Coding Clinic: 2017, Q1, P47

I11.9 Hypertensive heart disease without heart failure
Hypertensive heart disease NOS

OGCR Section I.C.9.a.2.

Hypertensive Chronic Kidney Disease

Assign codes from category I12, Hypertensive chronic kidney disease, when both hypertension and a condition classifiable to category N18, Chronic kidney disease (CKD), are present. **CKD sh°uld n°t be c°ded ªs hypertensive if the physiciªn hªs specificªlly d°cumented ª different cªuse.**

The appropriate code from category N18 should be used as a secondary code with a code from category I12 to identify the stage of chronic kidney disease.

See Section I.C.14. Chronic kidney disease.

If a patient has hypertensive chronic kidney disease and acute renal failure, an additional code for the acute renal failure is required.

● **I12 Hypertensive chronic kidney disease**

Includes any condition in N18 and N26 - due to hypertension
arteriosclerosis of kidney
arteriosclerotic nephritis (chronic) (interstitial)
hypertensive nephropathy
nephrosclerosis

Excludes1 hypertension due to kidney disease (I15.0, I15.1)
renovascular hypertension (I15.0)
secondary hypertension (I15.-)

Excludes2 acute kidney failure (N17.-)

Coding Clinic: 2018, Q4, P89; 2016, Q4, P123

I12.0 Hypertensive chronic kidney disease with stage 5 chronic kidney disease or end stage renal disease (Ex) PDX 820
Use additional code to identify the stage of chronic kidney disease (N18.5, N18.6)
Coding Clinic: 2016, Q3, P23

I12.9 Hypertensive chronic kidney disease with stage 1 through stage 4 chronic kidney disease, or unspecified chronic kidney disease
Hypertensive chronic kidney disease NOS
Hypertensive renal disease NOS
Use additional code to identify the stage of chronic kidney disease (N18.1-N18.4, N18.9)
Coding Clinic: 2022, Q4, P6; 2018, Q4, P88

OGCR Section I.c.9.a.3.

Hypertensive Heart and Chronic Kidney Disease

Assign codes from combination category I13, Hypertensive heart and chronic kidney disease, when **there is hypertension with both heart and kidney involvement.** If heart failure is present, assign an additional code from category I50 to identify the type of heart failure.

The appropriate code from category N18, Chronic kidney disease, should be used as a secondary code with a code from category I13 to identify the stage of chronic kidney disease.

See Section I.C.14. Chronic kidney disease.

The codes in category I13, Hypertensive heart and chronic kidney disease, are combination codes that include hypertension, heart disease and chronic kidney disease. The Includes note at I13 specifies that the conditions included at I11 and I12 are included together in I13. If a patient has hypertension, heart disease and chronic kidney disease then a code from I13 should be used, not individual codes for hypertension, heart disease and chronic kidney disease, or codes from I11 or I12.

For patients with both acute renal failure and chronic kidney disease an additional code for acute renal failure is required.

● **I13 Hypertensive heart and chronic kidney disease**

Includes any condition in I11.- with any condition in I12.-
cardiorenal disease
cardiovascular renal disease

Coding Clinic: 2022, Q4, P6

I13.0 Hypertensive heart and chronic kidney disease with heart failure and stage 1 through stage 4 chronic kidney disease, or unspecified chronic kidney disease (Ex) PDX 821
Use additional code to identify type of heart failure (I50.-)
Use additional code to identify stage of chronic kidney disease (N18.1-N18.4, N18.9)

● **I13.1 Hypertensive heart and chronic kidney disease without heart failure**

I13.10 Hypertensive heart and chronic kidney disease without heart failure, with stage 1 through stage 4 chronic kidney disease, or unspecified chronic kidney disease
Hypertensive heart disease and hypertensive chronic kidney disease NOS
Use additional code to identify the stage of chronic kidney disease (N18.1-N18.4, N18.9)

I13.11 Hypertensive heart and chronic kidney disease without heart failure, with stage 5 chronic kidney disease, or end stage renal disease (Ex) PDX 821
Use additional code to identify the stage of chronic kidney disease (N18.5, N18.6)

I13.2 Hypertensive heart and chronic kidney disease with heart failure and with stage 5 chronic kidney disease, or end stage renal disease (Ex) PDX 821
Use additional code to identify type of heart failure (I50.-)
Use additional code to identify the stage of chronic kidney disease (N18.5, N18.6)

OGCR Section I.9.a.6.

Hypertension, Secondary

Secondary hypertension is due to an underlying condition. Two codes are required: one to identify the underlying etiology and one from category I15 to identify the hypertension. Sequencing of codes is determined by the reason for admission/encounter.

● **I15 Secondary hypertension**
Code also underlying condition
Excludes1 postprocedural hypertension (I97.3)
Excludes2 secondary hypertension involving vessels of brain (I60-I69)
secondary hypertension involving vessels of eye (H35.0-)

I15.0 Renovascular hypertension

I15.1 Hypertension secondary to other renal disorders
Coding Clinic: 2016, Q3, P23

I15.2 Hypertension secondary to endocrine disorders
Coding Clinic: 2023, Q2, P16-17

I15.8 Other secondary hypertension

I15.9 Secondary hypertension, unspecified

● **I16 Hypertensive crisis**
Code also any identified hypertensive disease (I10-I15, I1A)
Coding Clinic: 2016, Q4, P26-27, 123

I16.0 Hypertensive urgency Ex: No exclusions

I16.1 Hypertensive emergency Ex: PDX 822
Coding Clinic: 2023, Q4, P25

▶ Use Additional code, if applicable, to identify specific organ dysfunction, such as:
▶acute kidney injury (N17.-)
▶acute myocardial infarction (I21.-)
▶acute pulmonary edema (left and/or right ventricular failure) (J81.0, I50.-)
▶aortic dissection (I71.0-)
▶cerebral hemorrhage (I60.-. I61.-, I62.-)
▶cerebral infarction (I63.-)
▶eclampsia (O15.-)
▶hypertensive encephalopathy (I67.4)
▶seizure (R56.9)

I16.9 Hypertensive crisis, unspecified Ex: PDX 823, I1A Other hypertension

● **I1A Other hypertension**

I1A.0 Resistant hypertension
Apparent treatment resistant hypertension
Treatment resistant hypertension
True resistant hypertension
Code first specific type of existing hypertension, if known, such as:
essential hypertension (I10)
secondary hypertension (I15.-)
Coding Clinic: 2023, Q4, P24-25

ISCHEMIC HEART DISEASES (I20-I25)

Code also the presence of hypertension (I10-I1A)

● **I20 Angina pectoris**
Chest pain/discomfort due to lack of oxygen to the heart muscle. Principal symptom of myocardial infarction.
Use additional code to identify:
exposure to environmental tobacco smoke (Z77.22)
history of tobacco dependence (Z87.891)
occupational exposure to environmental tobacco smoke (Z57.31)
tobacco dependence (F17.-)
tobacco use (Z72.0)
Excludes1 angina pectoris with atherosclerotic heart disease of native coronary arteries (I25.1-)
atherosclerosis of coronary artery bypass graft(s) and coronary artery of transplanted heart with angina pectoris (I25.7-)
postinfarction angina (I23.7)

I20.0 Unstable angina Ex: PDX 824
Accelerated angina
Crescendo angina
De novo effort angina
Intermediate coronary syndrome
Preinfarction syndrome
Worsening effort angina

I20.1 Angina pectoris with documented spasm Ex: PDX 825
Angiospastic angina
Prinzmetal angina
Spasm-induced angina
Variant angina

I20.2 Refractory angina pectoris Ex: PDX 826

● **I20.8 Other forms of angina pectoris**
Use additional code(s) for symptoms associated with angina equivalent

I20.81 Angina pectoris with coronary microvascular dysfunction
Angina pectoris with coronary microvascular disease

I20.89 Other forms of angina pectoris
Angina equivalent
Angina of effort
Coronary slow flow syndrome
Stable angina
Stenocardia

I20.9 Angina pectoris, unspecified
Angina NOS
Anginal syndrome
Cardiac angina
Ischemic chest pain

● **I21 Acute myocardial infarction**
Includes cardiac infarction
coronary (artery) embolism
coronary (artery) occlusion
coronary (artery) rupture
coronary (artery) thrombosis
infarction of heart, myocardium, or ventricle
myocardial infarction specified as acute or with a stated duration of 4 weeks (28 days) or less from onset
Use additional code, if applicable, to identify:
exposure to environmental tobacco smoke (Z77.22)
history of tobacco dependence (Z87.891)
occupational exposure to environmental tobacco smoke (Z57.31)
status post administration of tPA (rtPA) in a different facility within the last 24 hours prior to admission to current facility (Z92.82)
tobacco dependence (F17.-)
tobacco use (Z72.0)
Excludes2 old myocardial infarction (I25.2)
postmyocardial infarction syndrome (I24.1)
subsequent type 1 myocardial infarction (I22.-)
Coding Clinic: 2016, Q4, P140; 2013, Q1, P25-26; 2012, Q4, P103

● **I21.0 ST elevation (STEMI) myocardial infarction of anterior wall**
Type 1 ST elevation myocardial infarction of anterior wall
Coding Clinic: 2013, Q1, P26

I21.01 ST elevation (STEMI) myocardial infarction involving left main coronary artery Ex: PDX 827

I21.02 ST elevation (STEMI) myocardial infarction involving left anterior descending coronary artery Ex: PDX 827
ST elevation (STEMI) myocardial infarction involving diagonal coronary artery
Coding Clinic: 2013, Q1, P26

I21.09 ST elevation (STEMI) myocardial infarction involving other coronary artery of anterior wall Ex: PDX 827
Acute transmural myocardial infarction of anterior wall
Anteroapical transmural (Q wave) infarction (acute)
Anterolateral transmural (Q wave) infarction (acute)
Anteroseptal transmural (Q wave) infarction (acute)
Transmural (Q wave) infarction (acute) (of) anterior (wall) NOS
Coding Clinic: 2012, Q4, P102, 104

● **I21.1 ST elevation (STEMI) myocardial infarction of inferior wall**
Type 1 ST elevation myocardial infarction of inferior wall
Coding Clinic: 2013, Q1, P26

I21.11 ST elevation (STEMI) myocardial infarction involving right coronary artery (Ex) PDX 827
Inferoposterior transmural (Q wave) infarction (acute)

I21.19 ST elevation (STEMI) myocardial infarction involving other coronary artery of inferior wall (Ex) PDX 827
Acute transmural myocardial infarction of inferior wall
Inferolateral transmural (Q wave) infarction (acute)
Transmural (Q wave) infarction (acute) (of) diaphragmatic wall
Transmural (Q wave) infarction (acute) (of) inferior (wall) NOS

Excludes2 ST elevation (STEMI) myocardial infarction involving left circumflex coronary artery (I21.21)

Coding Clinic: 2012, Q4, P97

● **I21.2 ST elevation (STEMI) myocardial infarction of other sites**
Type 1 ST elevation myocardial infarction of other sites
Coding Clinic: 2013, Q1, P26

I21.21 ST elevation (STEMI) myocardial infarction involving left circumflex coronary artery (Ex) PDX 827
ST elevation (STEMI) myocardial infarction involving oblique marginal coronary artery

I21.29 ST elevation (STEMI) myocardial infarction involving other sites (Ex) PDX 827
Acute transmural myocardial infarction of other sites
Apical-lateral transmural (Q wave) infarction (acute)
Basal-lateral transmural (Q wave) infarction (acute)
High lateral transmural (Q wave) infarction (acute)
Lateral (wall) NOS transmural (Q wave) infarction (acute)
Posterior (true) transmural (Q wave) infarction (acute)
Posterobasal transmural (Q wave) infarction (acute)
Posterolateral transmural (Q wave) infarction (acute)
Posteroseptal transmural (Q wave) infarction (acute)
Septal transmural (Q wave) infarction (acute) NOS

OGCR Section I.c.9.e.2.

Acute myocardial infarction, unspecified

Code I21.9, Acute myocardial infarction, unspecified, is the default for unspecified acute myocardial infarction or unspecified type. If only type 1 STEMI or transmural MI without the site is documented, assign I21.3, ST elevation (STEMI) myocardial infarction of unspecified site.

I21.3 ST elevation (STEMI) myocardial infarction of unspecified site (Ex) PDX 827
Acute transmural myocardial infarction of unspecified site
Transmural (Q wave) myocardial infarction NOS
Type 1 ST elevation myocardial infarction of unspecified site
Coding Clinic: 2013, Q1, P26

I21.4 Non-ST elevation (NSTEMI) myocardial infarction (Ex) PDX 827
Acute subendocardial myocardial infarction
Non-Q wave myocardial infarction NOS
Nontransmural myocardial infarction NOS
Type 1 non-ST elevation myocardial infarction
Coding Clinic: 2024, Q1, P28; 2023, Q2, P29; 2021, Q3, P7; 2017, Q1, P44; 2015, Q2, P16; 2013, Q1, P26

I21.9 Acute myocardial infarction, unspecified (Ex) PDX 827
Myocardial infarction (acute) NOS

● **I21.A Other type of myocardial infarction**

I21.A1 Myocardial infarction type 2 (Ex) PDX 827
Myocardial infarction due to demand ischemia
Myocardial infarction secondary to ischemic imbalance

Code first, if applicable, the underlying cause, such as:
anemia (D50.0-D64.9)
chronic obstructive pulmonary disease (J44.-)
paroxysmal tachycardia (I47.0-I47.9)
shock (R57.0-R57.9)

Coding Clinic: 2017, Q4, P13-14

I21.A9 Other myocardial infarction type (Ex) PDX 827
Myocardial infarction associated with revascularization procedure
Myocardial infarction type 3
Myocardial infarction type 4a
Myocardial infarction type 4b
Myocardial infarction type 4c
Myocardial infarction type 5

Code first, if applicable, postprocedural myocardial infarction following cardiac surgery (I97.190), or postprocedural myocardial infarction during cardiac surgery (I97.790)

Code also complication, if known and applicable, such as:
(acute) stent occlusion (T82.897-)
(acute) stent stenosis (T82.857-)
(acute) stent thrombosis (T82.865-)
cardiac arrest due to underlying cardiac condition (I46.2)
complication of percutaneous coronary intervention (PCI) (I97.89)
occlusion of coronary artery bypass graft (T82.218-)

Coding Clinic: 2021, Q3, P6-7; 2019, Q2, P32-33

I21.B Myocardial infarction with coronary microvascular dysfunction (Ex) PDX 827
Myocardial infarction with coronary microvascular disease
Myocardial infarction with nonobstructive coronary arteries [MINOCA] with microvascular disease

● **I22 Subsequent ST elevation (STEMI) and non-ST elevation (NSTEMI) myocardial infarction**

Includes acute myocardial infarction occurring within four weeks (28 days) of a previous acute myocardial infarction, regardless of site
cardiac infarction
coronary (artery) embolism
coronary (artery) occlusion
coronary (artery) rupture
coronary (artery) thrombosis
infarction of heart, myocardium, or ventricle
recurrent myocardial infarction
reinfarction of myocardium
rupture of heart, myocardium, or ventricle
subsequent type 1 myocardial infarction

Excludes1 subsequent myocardial infarction, type 2 (I21.A1)
subsequent myocardial infarction of other type (type 3) (type 4) (type 5) (I21.A9)

Use additional code, if applicable, to identify:
exposure to environmental tobacco smoke (Z77.22)
history of tobacco dependence (Z87.891)
occupational exposure to environmental tobacco smoke (Z57.31)
status post administration of tPA (rtPA) in a different facility within the last 24 hours prior to admission to current facility (Z92.82)
tobacco dependence (F17.-)
tobacco use (Z72.0)

Coding Clinic: 2017, Q4, P14; 2013, Q1, P25; 2012, Q4, P103

CHAPTER 9 (I00-I99)

I22.Ø Subsequent ST elevation (STEMI) myocardial infarction of anterior wall (Ex) PDX 827
Subsequent acute transmural myocardial infarction of anterior wall
Subsequent transmural (Q wave) infarction (acute)(of) anterior (wall) NOS
Subsequent anteroapical transmural (Q wave) infarction (acute)
Subsequent anterolateral transmural (Q wave) infarction (acute)
Subsequent anteroseptal transmural (Q wave) infarction (acute)

I22.1 Subsequent ST elevation (STEMI) myocardial infarction of inferior wall (Ex) PDX 827
Subsequent acute transmural myocardial infarction of inferior wall
Subsequent transmural (Q wave) infarction (acute)(of) diaphragmatic wall
Subsequent transmural (Q wave) infarction (acute)(of) inferior (wall) NOS
Subsequent inferolateral transmural (Q wave) infarction (acute)
Subsequent inferoposterior transmural (Q wave) infarction (acute)
Coding Clinic: 2012, Q4, P97, 102, 104

I22.2 Subsequent non-ST elevation (NSTEMI) myocardial infarction (Ex) PDX 827
Subsequent acute subendocardial myocardial infarction
Subsequent non-Q wave myocardial infarction NOS
Subsequent nontransmural myocardial infarction NOS

I22.8 Subsequent ST elevation (STEMI) myocardial infarction of other sites (Ex) PDX 827
Subsequent acute transmural myocardial infarction of other sites
Subsequent apical-lateral transmural (Q wave) myocardial infarction (acute)
Subsequent basal-lateral transmural (Q wave) myocardial infarction (acute)
Subsequent high lateral transmural (Q wave) myocardial infarction (acute)
Subsequent transmural (Q wave) myocardial infarction (acute)(of) lateral (wall) NOS
Subsequent posterior (true) transmural (Q wave) myocardial infarction (acute)
Subsequent posterobasal transmural (Q wave) myocardial infarction (acute)
Subsequent posterolateral transmural (Q wave) myocardial infarction (acute)
Subsequent posteroseptal transmural (Q wave) myocardial infarction (acute)
Subsequent septal NOS transmural (Q wave) myocardial infarction (acute)

I22.9 Subsequent ST elevation (STEMI) myocardial infarction of unspecified site (Ex) PDX 827
Subsequent acute myocardial infarction of unspecified site
Subsequent myocardial infarction (acute) NOS

● **I23 Certain current complications following ST elevation (STEMI) and non-ST elevation (NSTEMI) myocardial infarction (within the 28 day period)**
Coding Clinic: 2017, Q2, P11

I23.Ø Hemopericardium as current complication following acute myocardial infarction (Ex) PDX 828 A
Excludes1 hemopericardium not specified as current complication following acute myocardial infarction (I31.2)

I23.1 Atrial septal defect as current complication following acute myocardial infarction (Ex) PDX 828 A
Excludes1 acquired atrial septal defect not specified as current complication following acute myocardial infarction (I51.Ø)

Item 9–6 Classification is based on the location of the atherosclerosis. **"Of native coronary artery"** indicates the atherosclerosis is within an original heart artery. **"Of autologous vein bypass graft"** indicates that the atherosclerosis is within a vein graft that was taken from within the patient. **"Of nonautologous biological bypass graft"** indicates the atherosclerosis is within a vessel grafted from other than the patient. **"Of artery bypass graft"** indicates the atherosclerosis is within an artery that was grafted from within the patient.

I23.2 Ventricular septal defect as current complication following acute myocardial infarction (Ex) PDX 828 A
Excludes1 acquired ventricular septal defect not specified as current complication following acute myocardial infarction (I51.Ø)

I23.3 Rupture of cardiac wall without hemopericardium as current complication following acute myocardial infarction (Ex) PDX 828 A
Coding Clinic: 2017, Q2, P11

I23.4 Rupture of chordae tendineae as current complication following acute myocardial infarction (Ex) PDX 829
Excludes1 rupture of chordae tendineae not specified as current complication following acute myocardial infarction (I51.1)

I23.5 Rupture of papillary muscle as current complication following acute myocardial infarction (Ex) PDX 830
Excludes1 rupture of papillary muscle not specified as current complication following acute myocardial infarction (I51.2)

I23.6 Thrombosis of atrium, auricular appendage, and ventricle as current complications following acute myocardial infarction (Ex) PDX 828 A
Excludes1 thrombosis of atrium, auricular appendage, and ventricle not specified as current complication following acute myocardial infarction (I51.3)

I23.7 Postinfarction angina (Ex) PDX 828 A
Coding Clinic: 2015, Q2, P16-17

I23.8 Other current complications following acute myocardial infarction (Ex) PDX 828 A

● **I24 Other acute ischemic heart diseases**
Excludes1 angina pectoris (I2Ø.-)
transient myocardial ischemia in newborn (P29.4)
Excludes2 non-ischemic myocardial injury (I5A)

I24.Ø Acute coronary thrombosis not resulting in myocardial infarction (Ex) PDX 831
Acute coronary (artery) (vein) embolism not resulting in myocardial infarction
Acute coronary (artery) (vein) occlusion not resulting in myocardial infarction
Acute coronary (artery) (vein) thromboembolism not resulting in myocardial infarction
Excludes1 atherosclerotic heart disease (I25.1-)
Coding Clinic: 2013, Q1, P24

I24.1 Dressler's syndrome (Ex) PDX 832
Postmyocardial infarction syndrome
Excludes1 postinfarction angina (I23.7)

● **I24.8 Other forms of acute ischemic heart disease**
Excludes1 myocardial infarction due to demand ischemia (I21.A1)
Coding Clinic: 2017, Q4, P13

I24.81 Acute coronary microvascular dysfunction (Ex) PDX 833
Acute (presentation of) coronary microvascular disease

I24.89 Other forms of acute ischemic heart disease (Ex) PDX 833

I24.9 Acute ischemic heart disease, unspecified (Ex:) PDX 831
Excludes1 ischemic heart disease (chronic) NOS (I25.9)

I25 Chronic ischemic heart disease
Excludes2 non-ischemic myocardial injury (I5A)
Use additional code to identify:
chronic total occlusion of coronary artery (I25.82)
exposure to environmental tobacco smoke (Z77.22)
history of tobacco dependence (Z87.891)
occupational exposure to environmental tobacco smoke (Z57.31)
tobacco dependence (F17.-)
tobacco use (Z72.Ø)

★**(See Plates 218 and 219 on pages 74 and 75.)**

I25.1 Atherosclerotic heart disease of native coronary artery
Disease in which fatty deposits form on the walls of arteries
Atherosclerotic cardiovascular disease
Coronary (artery) atheroma
Coronary (artery) atherosclerosis
Coronary (artery) disease
Coronary (artery) sclerosis
Use additional code, if applicable, to identify:
coronary atherosclerosis due to calcified coronary lesion (I25.84)
coronary atherosclerosis due to lipid rich plaque (I25.83)
Excludes2 atheroembolism (I75.-)
atherosclerosis of coronary artery bypass graft(s) and transplanted heart (I25.7-)

I25.1Ø Atherosclerotic heart disease of native coronary artery without angina pectoris A
Atherosclerotic heart disease NOS
Coding Clinic: 2Ø24, Q1, P28; 2Ø21, Q3, P6-7; 2Ø15, Q2, P17; 2Ø12, Q4, P92

OGCR See Section I.9.b.

Atherosclerotic Coronary Artery Disease and Angina

ICD-10-CM has combination codes for atherosclerotic heart disease with angina pectoris. The subcategories for these codes are I25.11, Atherosclerotic heart disease of native coronary artery with angina pectoris and I25.7, Atherosclerosis of coronary artery bypass graft(s) and coronary artery of transplanted heart with angina pectoris.

When using one of these combination codes it is not necessary to use an additional code for angina pectoris. A causal relationship can be assumed in a patient with both atherosclerosis and angina pectoris, unless the documentation indicates the angina is due to something other than the atherosclerosis.

If a patient with coronary artery disease is admitted due to an acute myocardial infarction (AMI), the AMI should be sequenced before the coronary artery disease.

See Section I.C.9. Acute myocardial infarction (AMI).

I25.11 Atherosclerotic heart disease of native coronary artery with angina pectoris

I25.11Ø Atherosclerotic heart disease of native coronary artery with unstable angina pectoris (Ex:) PDX 834 A
Excludes1 unstable angina without atherosclerotic heart disease (I2Ø.Ø)
CC when PDx is its own CC

I25.111 Atherosclerotic heart disease of native coronary artery with angina pectoris with documented spasm A
Excludes1 angina pectoris with documented spasm without atherosclerotic heart disease (I2Ø.1)

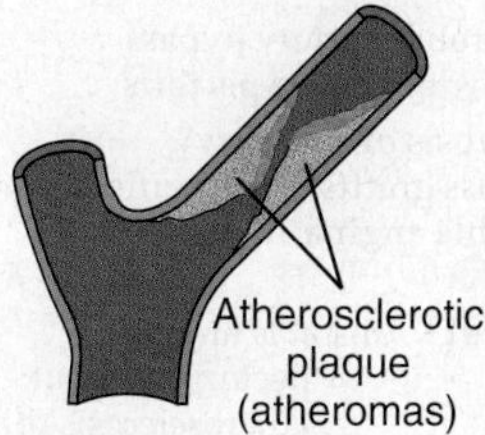

Figure 9-2 Atherosclerotic plaque.

I25.112 Atherosclerotic heart disease of native coronary artery with refractory angina pectoris (Ex:) PDX 835 A

I25.118 Atherosclerotic heart disease of native coronary artery with other forms of angina pectoris A
Excludes1 other forms of angina pectoris without atherosclerotic heart disease (I2Ø.8-)
Coding Clinic: 2Ø15, Q2, P16-17

I25.119 Atherosclerotic heart disease of native coronary artery with unspecified angina pectoris A
Atherosclerotic heart disease with angina NOS
Atherosclerotic heart disease with ischemic chest pain
Excludes1 unspecified angina pectoris without atherosclerotic heart disease (I2Ø.9)

I25.2 Old myocardial infarction
Healed myocardial infarction
Past myocardial infarction diagnosed by ECG or other investigation, but currently presenting no symptoms

I25.3 Aneurysm of heart (Ex:) PDX 836
Mural aneurysm
Ventricular aneurysm

I25.4 Coronary artery aneurysm and dissection

I25.41 Coronary artery aneurysm
Coronary arteriovenous fistula, acquired
Excludes1 congenital coronary (artery) aneurysm (Q24.5)

I25.42 Coronary artery dissection (Ex:) PDX 837

I25.5 Ischemic cardiomyopathy
Excludes2 coronary atherosclerosis (I25.1-, I25.7-)
Coding Clinic: 2Ø22, Q3, P18

I25.6 Silent myocardial ischemia

I25.7 Atherosclerosis of coronary artery bypass graft(s) and coronary artery of transplanted heart with angina pectoris
Use additional code, if applicable, to identify:
coronary atherosclerosis due to calcified coronary lesion (I25.84)
coronary atherosclerosis due to lipid rich plaque (I25.83)
Excludes1 atherosclerosis of bypass graft(s) of transplanted heart without angina pectoris (I25.812)
atherosclerosis of coronary artery bypass graft(s) without angina pectoris (I25.81Ø)
atherosclerosis of native coronary artery of transplanted heart without angina pectoris (I25.811)

● I25.70 **Atherosclerosis of coronary artery bypass graft(s), unspecified, with angina pectoris**

I25.700 **Atherosclerosis of coronary artery bypass graft(s), unspecified, with unstable angina pectoris** (Ex) PDX 838 A

Excludes1 unstable angina pectoris without atherosclerosis of coronary artery bypass graft (I20.0)

CC when PDx is its own CC

I25.701 **Atherosclerosis of coronary artery bypass graft(s), unspecified, with angina pectoris with documented spasm** A

Excludes1 angina pectoris with documented spasm without atherosclerosis of coronary artery bypass graft (I20.1)

I25.702 **Atherosclerosis of coronary artery bypass graft(s), unspecified, with refractory angina pectoris** (Ex) PDX 835 A

Coding Clinic: 2022, Q4, P22

I25.708 **Atherosclerosis of coronary artery bypass graft(s), unspecified, with other forms of angina pectoris** A

Excludes1 other forms of angina pectoris without atherosclerosis of coronary artery bypass graft (I20.8-)

I25.709 **Atherosclerosis of coronary artery bypass graft(s), unspecified, with unspecified angina pectoris** A

Excludes1 unspecified angina pectoris without atherosclerosis of coronary artery bypass graft (I20.9)

● I25.71 **Atherosclerosis of autologous vein coronary artery bypass graft(s) with angina pectoris**

I25.710 **Atherosclerosis of autologous vein coronary artery bypass graft(s) with unstable angina pectoris** (Ex) PDX 839 A

Excludes1 unstable angina without atherosclerosis of autologous vein coronary artery bypass graft(s) (I20.0)

Excludes2 embolism or thrombus of coronary artery bypass graft(s) (T82.8-)

CC when PDx is its own CC

I25.711 **Atherosclerosis of autologous vein coronary artery bypass graft(s) with angina pectoris with documented spasm** (Ex) PDX 840 A

Excludes1 angina pectoris with documented spasm without atherosclerosis of autologous vein coronary artery bypass graft(s) (I20.1)

I25.712 **Atherosclerosis of autologous vein coronary artery bypass graft(s) with refractory angina pectoris** (Ex) PDX 841 A

I25.718 **Atherosclerosis of autologous vein coronary artery bypass graft(s) with other forms of angina pectoris** (Ex) PDX 840 A

Excludes1 other forms of angina pectoris without atherosclerosis of autologous vein coronary artery bypass graft(s) (I20.8-)

I25.719 **Atherosclerosis of autologous vein coronary artery bypass graft(s) with unspecified angina pectoris** (Ex) PDX 840 A

Excludes1 unspecified angina pectoris without atherosclerosis of autologous vein coronary artery bypass graft(s) (I20.9)

● I25.72 **Atherosclerosis of autologous artery coronary artery bypass graft(s) with angina pectoris**

Atherosclerosis of internal mammary artery graft with angina pectoris

I25.720 **Atherosclerosis of autologous artery coronary artery bypass graft(s) with unstable angina pectoris** (Ex) PDX 839 A

Excludes1 unstable angina without atherosclerosis of autologous artery coronary artery bypass graft(s) (I20.0)

CC when PDx is its own CC

I25.721 **Atherosclerosis of autologous artery coronary artery bypass graft(s) with angina pectoris with documented spasm** (Ex) PDX 840 A

Excludes1 angina pectoris with documented spasm without atherosclerosis of autologous artery coronary artery bypass graft(s) (I20.1)

I25.722 **Atherosclerosis of autologous artery coronary artery bypass graft(s) with refractory angina pectoris** (Ex) PDX 841 A

CHAPTER 9 (I00-I99)

I25.728 Atherosclerosis of autologous artery coronary artery bypass graft(s) with other forms of angina pectoris (Ex) PDX 840 A

Excludes1 other forms of angina pectoris without atherosclerosis of autologous artery coronary artery bypass graft(s) (I20.8-)

I25.729 Atherosclerosis of autologous artery coronary artery bypass graft(s) with unspecified angina pectoris (Ex) PDX 840 A

Excludes1 unspecified angina pectoris without atherosclerosis of autologous artery coronary artery bypass graft(s) (I20.9)

● **I25.73 Atherosclerosis of nonautologous biological coronary artery bypass graft(s) with angina pectoris**

I25.730 Atherosclerosis of nonautologous biological coronary artery bypass graft(s) with unstable angina pectoris (Ex) PDX 839 A

Excludes1 unstable angina without atherosclerosis of nonautologous biological coronary artery bypass graft(s) (I20.0)

CC when PDx is its own CC

I25.731 Atherosclerosis of nonautologous biological coronary artery bypass graft(s) with angina pectoris with documented spasm (Ex) PDX 840 A

Excludes1 angina pectoris with documented spasm without atherosclerosis of nonautologous biological coronary artery bypass graft(s) (I20.1)

I25.732 Atherosclerosis of nonautologous biological coronary artery bypass graft(s)with refractory angina pectoris (Ex) PDX 841 A

I25.738 Atherosclerosis of nonautologous biological coronary artery bypass graft(s) with other forms of angina pectoris (Ex) PDX 840 A

Excludes1 other forms of angina pectoris without atherosclerosis of nonautologous biological coronary artery bypass graft(s) (I20.8-)

I25.739 Atherosclerosis of nonautologous biological coronary artery bypass graft(s) with unspecified angina pectoris (Ex) PDX 840 A

Excludes1 unspecified angina pectoris without atherosclerosis of nonautologous biological coronary artery bypass graft(s) (I20.9)

● **I25.75 Atherosclerosis of native coronary artery of transplanted heart with angina pectoris**

Excludes1 atherosclerosis of native coronary artery of transplanted heart without angina pectoris (I25.811)

I25.750 Atherosclerosis of native coronary artery of transplanted heart with unstable angina (Ex) PDX 842

CC when PDx is its own CC

I25.751 Atherosclerosis of native coronary artery of transplanted heart with angina pectoris with documented spasm (Ex) PDX 843

I25.752 Atherosclerosis of native coronary artery of transplanted heart with refractory angina pectoris (Ex) PDX 841 A

I25.758 Atherosclerosis of native coronary artery of transplanted heart with other forms of angina pectoris (Ex) PDX 843

I25.759 Atherosclerosis of native coronary artery of transplanted heart with unspecified angina pectoris (Ex) PDX 843

● **I25.76 Atherosclerosis of bypass graft of coronary artery of transplanted heart with angina pectoris**

Excludes1 atherosclerosis of bypass graft of coronary artery of transplanted heart without angina pectoris (I25.812)

I25.760 Atherosclerosis of bypass graft of coronary artery of transplanted heart with unstable angina (Ex) PDX 844 A

CC when PDx is its own CC

I25.761 Atherosclerosis of bypass graft of coronary artery of transplanted heart with angina pectoris with documented spasm (Ex) PDX 845 A

I25.762 Atherosclerosis of bypass graft of coronary artery of transplanted heart with refractory angina pectoris (Ex) PDX 841 A

I25.768 Atherosclerosis of bypass graft of coronary artery of transplanted heart with other forms of angina pectoris (Ex) PDX 846 A

I25.769 Atherosclerosis of bypass graft of coronary artery of transplanted heart with unspecified angina pectoris (Ex) PDX 847 A

CHAPTER 9 (I00-I99)

I25.79 Atherosclerosis of other coronary artery bypass graft(s) with angina pectoris A

I25.790 Atherosclerosis of other coronary artery bypass graft(s) with unstable angina pectoris Ex: PDX 848

Excludes1 unstable angina without atherosclerosis of other coronary artery bypass graft(s) (I20.0)

CC when PDx is its own CC

I25.791 Atherosclerosis of other coronary artery bypass graft(s) with angina pectoris with documented spasm Ex: PDX 849 A

Excludes1 angina pectoris with documented spasm without atherosclerosis of other coronary artery bypass graft(s) (I20.1)

I25.792 Atherosclerosis of other coronary artery bypass graft(s) with refractory angina pectoris Ex: PDX 841 A

I25.798 Atherosclerosis of other coronary artery bypass graft(s) with other forms of angina pectoris Ex: PDX 850 A

Excludes1 other forms of angina pectoris without atherosclerosis of other coronary artery bypass graft(s) (I20.8-)

I25.799 Atherosclerosis of other coronary artery bypass graft(s) with unspecified angina pectoris Ex: PDX 851 A

Excludes1 unspecified angina pectoris without atherosclerosis of other coronary artery bypass graft(s) (I20.9)

I25.8 Other forms of chronic ischemic heart disease

I25.81 Atherosclerosis of other coronary vessels without angina pectoris

Use additional code, if applicable, to identify:
coronary atherosclerosis due to calcified coronary lesion (I25.84)
coronary atherosclerosis due to lipid rich plaque (I25.83)

Excludes2 atherosclerotic heart disease of native coronary artery without angina pectoris (I25.10)

I25.810 Atherosclerosis of coronary artery bypass graft(s) without angina pectoris Ex: PDX 852 A

Atherosclerosis of coronary artery bypass graft NOS

Excludes1 atherosclerosis of coronary bypass graft(s) with angina pectoris (I25.70- -I25.73-, I25.79-)

Coding Clinic: 2016, Q4, P86

I25.811 Atherosclerosis of native coronary artery of transplanted heart without angina pectoris Ex: PDX 843

Atherosclerosis of native coronary artery of transplanted heart NOS

Excludes1 atherosclerosis of native coronary artery of transplanted heart with angina pectoris (I25.75-)

I25.812 Atherosclerosis of bypass graft of coronary artery of transplanted heart without angina pectoris Ex: PDX 853 A

Atherosclerosis of bypass graft of transplanted heart NOS

Excludes1 atherosclerosis of bypass graft of transplanted heart with angina pectoris (I25.76)

I25.82 Chronic total occlusion of coronary artery

Complete occlusion of coronary artery
Total occlusion of coronary artery

Code first coronary atherosclerosis (I25.1-, I25.7-, I25.81-)

Excludes1 acute coronary occlusion with myocardial infarction (I21.0-I21.B, I22.-)
acute coronary occlusion without myocardial infarction (I24.0)

I25.83 Coronary atherosclerosis due to lipid rich plaque A

Code first coronary atherosclerosis (I25.1-, I25.7-, I25.81-)

I25.84 Coronary atherosclerosis due to calcified coronary lesion

Coronary atherosclerosis due to severely calcified coronary lesion

Code first coronary atherosclerosis (I25.1-, I25.7-, I25.81-)

I25.85 Chronic coronary microvascular dysfunction

Chronic (presentation of) coronary microvascular disease
Coronary microvascular dysfunction NOS

I25.89 Other forms of chronic ischemic heart disease

I25.9 Chronic ischemic heart disease, unspecified

Ischemic heart disease (chronic) NOS

PULMONARY HEART DISEASE AND DISEASES OF PULMONARY CIRCULATION (I26-I28)

I26 Pulmonary embolism

Includes cor pulmonale without embolism (I27.81)
pulmonary (acute)(artery)(vein) infarction
pulmonary (acute)(artery)(vein) thromboembolism
pulmonary (acute)(artery)(vein) thrombosis

Excludes2 chronic pulmonary embolism (I27.82)
personal history of pulmonary embolism (Z86.711)
pulmonary embolism due to trauma (T79.0, T79.1)
pulmonary embolism due to complications of surgical and medical care (T80.0, T81.7-, T82.8-)
pulmonary embolism complicating abortion, ectopic or molar pregnancy (O00-O07, O08.2)
pulmonary embolism complicating pregnancy, childbirth and the puerperium (O88.-)
septic (non-pulmonary) arterial embolism (I76)

Coding Clinic: 2021, Q2, P10

Item 9–7 Pulmonary heart disease or **cor pulmonale** is right ventricle hypertrophy or RVH as a result of a respiratory disorder increasing back flow pressure to the right ventricle. Left untreated, cor pulmonale leads to right-heart failure and death.

CHAPTER 9 (I00-I99)

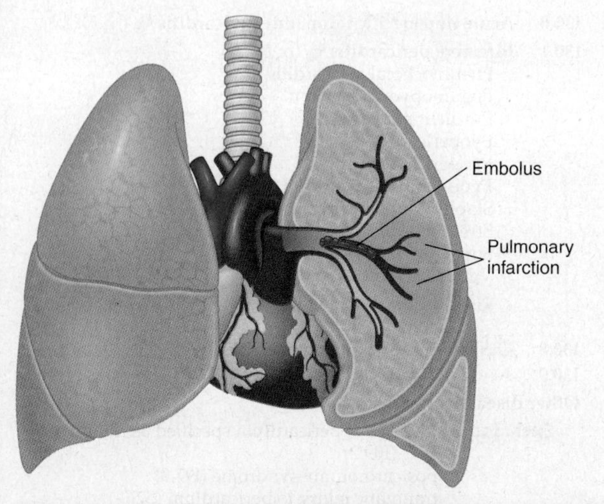

Figure 9-3 Pulmonary embolism. (From Chabner: The Language of Medicine, ed 8, St. Louis, Saunders, 2007)

I26.0 Pulmonary embolism with acute cor pulmonale (Ex) PDX 854

I26.01 Septic pulmonary embolism with acute cor pulmonale
Code first underlying infection
MCC when PDx is its own MCC

I26.02 Saddle embolus of pulmonary artery with acute cor pulmonale
MCC when PDx is its own MCC

I26.03 Cement embolism of pulmonary artery with acute cor pulmonale (Ex) PDX 854
Code first complication of other artery following a procedure (T81.718)

I26.04 Fat embolism of pulmonary artery with acute cor pulmonale (Ex) PDX 854
Code first, if applicable:
complication of other artery following a procedure (T81.718)
traumatic fat embolism (T79.1)

I26.09 Other pulmonary embolism with acute cor pulmonale
Acute cor pulmonale NOS
Other thrombotic pulmonary embolism with acute cor pulmonale
MCC when PDx is its own MCC

I26.9 Pulmonary embolism without acute cor pulmonale

I26.90 Septic pulmonary embolism without acute cor pulmonale (Ex) PDX 855
Code first underlying infection

I26.92 Saddle embolus of pulmonary artery without acute cor pulmonale (Ex) PDX 856

I26.93 Single subsegmental thrombotic pulmonary embolism without acute cor pulmonale (Ex) PDX 855
Subsegmental pulmonary embolism NOS

I26.94 Multiple subsegmental thrombotic pulmonary emboli without acute cor pulmonale (Ex) PDX 855
Coding Clinic: 2022, Q2, P13; 2021, Q2, P10

I26.95 Cement embolism of pulmonary artery without acute cor pulmonale (Ex) PDX 855
Code first complication of other artery following a procedure (T81.718)

I26.96 Fat embolism of pulmonary artery without acute cor pulmonale (Ex) PDX 855
Code first, if applicable:
complication of other artery following a procedure (T81.718)
traumatic fat embolism (T79.1)

I26.99 Other pulmonary embolism without acute cor pulmonale (Ex) PDX 855
Acute pulmonary embolism NOS
Other thrombotic pulmonary embolism with acute cor pulmonale
Pulmonary embolism NOS
Coding Clinic: 2022, Q2, P13; 2019, Q2, P22-23

I27 Other pulmonary heart diseases

I27.0 Primary pulmonary hypertension (Ex) PDX 857
Heritable pulmonary arterial hypertension
Idiopathic pulmonary arterial hypertension
Primary group 1 pulmonary hypertension
Primary pulmonary arterial hypertension
Excludes1 persistent pulmonary hypertension of newborn (P29.30)
pulmonary hypertension NOS (I27.20)
secondary pulmonary arterial hypertension (I27.21)
secondary pulmonary hypertension (I27.29)

I27.1 Kyphoscoliotic heart disease (Ex) PDX 597

I27.2 Other secondary pulmonary hypertension
Code also associated underlying condition
Excludes1 Eisenmenger's syndrome (I27.83)
Coding Clinic: 2016, Q2, P8

I27.20 Pulmonary hypertension, unspecified
Pulmonary hypertension NOS

I27.21 Secondary pulmonary arterial hypertension
(Associated) (drug-induced) (toxin-induced) pulmonary arterial hypertension NOS
(Associated) (drug-induced) (toxin-induced) (secondary) group 1 pulmonary hypertension
Code also associated conditions if applicable, or adverse effects of drugs or toxins, such as:
adverse effect of appetite depressants (T50.5X5)
congenital heart disease (Q20-Q28)
human immunodeficiency virus [HIV] disease (B20)
polymyositis (M33.2-)
portal hypertension (K76.6)
rheumatoid arthritis (M05.-)
schistosomiasis (B65.-)
Sjögren syndrome (M35.0-)
systemic sclerosis (M34.-)

I27.22 Pulmonary hypertension due to left heart disease
Group 2 pulmonary hypertension
Code also associated left heart disease, if known, such as:
multiple valve disease (I08.-)
rheumatic mitral valve diseases (I05.-)
rheumatic aortic valve diseases (I06.-)

I27.23 Pulmonary hypertension due to lung diseases and hypoxia
Group 3 pulmonary hypertension
Code also associated lung disease, if known, such as:
bronchiectasis (J47.-)
cystic fibrosis with pulmonary manifestations (E84.0)
interstitial lung disease (J84.-)
pleural effusion (J90)
sleep apnea (G47.3-)

I27.24 Chronic thromboembolic pulmonary hypertension
Group 4 pulmonary hypertension
Code also associated pulmonary embolism, if applicable (I26.-, I27.82)

I27.29 **Other secondary pulmonary hypertension**
Group 5 pulmonary hypertension
Pulmonary hypertension with unclear multifactorial mechanisms
Pulmonary hypertension due to hematologic disorders
Pulmonary hypertension due to metabolic disorders
Pulmonary hypertension due to other systemic disorders
Code also other associated disorders, if known, such as:
chronic myeloid leukemia (C92.10-C92.22)
essential thrombocythemia (D47.3)
Gaucher disease (E75.22)
hypertensive chronic kidney disease with end stage renal disease (I12.0, I13.11,I13.2)
hyperthyroidism (E05.-)
hypothyroidism (E00-E03)
polycythemia vera (D45)
sarcoidosis (D86.-)

● I27.8 **Other specified pulmonary heart diseases**

I27.81 **Cor pulmonale (chronic)**
Cor pulmonale NOS
Code also, if applicable, right heart failure (I50.81-)
Excludes1 acute cor pulmonale (I26.Ø-)

I27.82 **Chronic pulmonary embolism** Ex: PDX 856
Use additional code, if applicable, for associated long-term (current) use of anticoagulants (Z79.Ø1)
Excludes1 personal history of pulmonary embolism (Z86.711)
Coding Clinic: 2021, Q2, P1Ø

I27.83 **Eisenmenger's syndrome**
Eisenmenger's complex
(Irreversible) Eisenmenger's disease
Pulmonary hypertension with right to left shunt related to congenital heart disease
Code also underlying heart defect, if known, such as:
atrial septal defect (Q21.1-)
Eisenmenger's defect (Q21.8)
patent ductus arteriosus (Q25.0)
ventricular septal defect (Q21.0)

I27.89 **Other specified pulmonary heart diseases**

I27.9 **Pulmonary heart disease, unspecified**
Chronic cardiopulmonary disease

● I28 **Other diseases of pulmonary vessels** Ex: PDX 858

I28.Ø **Arteriovenous fistula of pulmonary vessels**
Excludes1 congenital arteriovenous fistula (Q25.72)

I28.1 **Aneurysm of pulmonary artery**
Excludes1 congenital aneurysm (Q25.79)
congenital arteriovenous aneurysm (Q25.72)

I28.8 **Other diseases of pulmonary vessels**
Pulmonary arteritis
Pulmonary endarteritis
Rupture of pulmonary vessels
Stenosis of pulmonary vessels
Stricture of pulmonary vessels

I28.9 **Disease of pulmonary vessels, unspecified**

OTHER FORMS OF HEART DISEASE (I3Ø-I5A)

● I3Ø **Acute pericarditis**
Inflammation of pericardium (sac surrounding the heart) caused by an infection
Includes acute mediastinopericarditis
acute myopericarditis
acute pericardial effusion
acute pleuropericarditis
acute pneumopericarditis
Excludes1 Dressler's syndrome (I24.1)
rheumatic pericarditis (acute) (IØ1.Ø)
viral pericarditis due to Coxsackie virus (B33.23)

I3Ø.Ø **Acute nonspecific idiopathic pericarditis** Ex: PDX 859

I3Ø.1 **Infective pericarditis** Ex: PDX 859
Pneumococcal pericarditis
Pneumopyopericardium
Purulent pericarditis
Pyopericarditis
Pyopericardium
Pyopneumopericardium
Staphylococcal pericarditis
Streptococcal pericarditis
Suppurative pericarditis
Viral pericarditis
Use additional code (B95-B97) to identify infectious agent

I3Ø.8 **Other forms of acute pericarditis** Ex: PDX 859

I3Ø.9 **Acute pericarditis, unspecified** Ex: PDX 859

● I31 **Other diseases of pericardium**
Excludes1 diseases of pericardium specified as rheumatic (IØ9.2)
postcardiotomy syndrome (I97.Ø)
traumatic injury to pericardium (S26.-)

I31.Ø **Chronic adhesive pericarditis** Ex: PDX 860
Accretio cordis
Adherent pericardium
Adhesive mediastinopericarditis

I31.1 **Chronic constrictive pericarditis** Ex: PDX 860
Concretio cordis
Pericardial calcification

I31.2 **Hemopericardium, not elsewhere classified** Ex: PDX 860
Excludes1 hemopericardium as current complication following acute myocardial infarction (I23.Ø)

● I31.3 **Pericardial effusion (noninflammatory)**
Excludes1 acute pericardial effusion (I3Ø.9)
Coding Clinic: 2Ø19, Q1, P16

I31.31 **Malignant pericardial effusion in diseases classified elsewhere** Ex: PDX 201
Code first underlying neoplasm (CØØ-D49)
Coding Clinic: 2Ø22, Q4, P24

I31.39 **Other pericardial effusion (noninflammatory)** Ex: PDX 201
Chylopericardium

● I31.4 **Cardiac tamponade** Ex: PDX 201
Code first underlying cause

I31.8 **Other specified diseases of pericardium** Ex: PDX 201
Epicardial plaques
Focal pericardial adhesions

I31.9 **Disease of pericardium, unspecified** Ex: PDX 201
Pericarditis (chronic) NOS

I32 ***Pericarditis in diseases classified elsewhere*** Ex: PDX 859
Code first underlying disease
Excludes1 pericarditis (in):
coxsackie (virus) (B33.23)
gonococcal (A54.83)
meningococcal (A39.53)
rheumatoid (arthritis) (MØ5.31)
syphilitic (A52.Ø6)
systemic lupus erythematosus (M32.12)
tuberculosis (A18.84)

● I33 **Acute and subacute endocarditis** Ex: PDX 861
Inflammation/infection of lining of heart, affecting heart valves including replacement valves and is usually caused by a bacterial infection
Excludes1 acute rheumatic endocarditis (IØ1.1)
endocarditis NOS (I38)

I33.Ø **Acute and subacute infective endocarditis**
Bacterial endocarditis (acute) (subacute)
Infective endocarditis (acute) (subacute) NOS
Endocarditis lenta (acute) (subacute)
Malignant endocarditis (acute) (subacute)
Purulent endocarditis (acute) (subacute)
Septic endocarditis (acute) (subacute)
Ulcerative endocarditis (acute) (subacute)
Vegetative endocarditis (acute) (subacute)
Use additional code (B95-B97) to identify infectious agent

CHAPTER 9 (IØØ-I99)

I33.9 Acute and subacute endocarditis, unspecified
Acute endocarditis NOS
Acute myoendocarditis NOS
Acute periendocarditis NOS
Subacute endocarditis NOS
Subacute myoendocarditis NOS
Subacute periendocarditis NOS

I34 Nonrheumatic mitral valve disorders
Code also, if applicable:
nonrheumatic mitral (valve) annulus calcification (I34.81)
Excludes1 mitral valve disease (I05.9)
mitral valve failure (I05.8)
mitral valve stenosis (I05.0)
mitral valve disorder of unspecified cause with diseases of aortic and/or tricuspid valve(s) (I08.-)
mitral valve disorder of unspecified cause with mitral stenosis or obstruction (I05.0)
mitral valve disorder specified as congenital (Q23.2, Q23.9)
mitral valve disorder specified as rheumatic (I05.-)

I34.0 Nonrheumatic mitral (valve) insufficiency
Nonrheumatic mitral (valve) incompetence NOS
Nonrheumatic mitral (valve) regurgitation NOS

I34.1 Nonrheumatic mitral (valve) prolapse
Floppy nonrheumatic mitral valve syndrome
Excludes1 Marfan's syndrome (Q87.4-)

I34.2 Nonrheumatic mitral (valve) stenosis
Code also, if applicable:
nonrheumatic mitral (valve) annulus calcification (I34.81)

I34.8 Other nonrheumatic mitral valve disorders

I34.81 Nonrheumatic mitral (valve) annulus calcification
Nonrheumatic mitral (valve) annular calcification
Mitral (valve) annulus calcification NOS
Code also, if applicable:
nonrheumatic mitral (valve) insufficiency (I34.0)
nonrheumatic mitral (valve) stenosis (I34.2)

I34.89 Other nonrheumatic mitral valve disorders

I34.9 Nonrheumatic mitral valve disorder, unspecified

I35 Nonrheumatic aortic valve disorders
~~**Excludes1** aortic valve disorder of unspecified cause but with diseases of mitral and/or tricuspid valve(s) (I08.-)~~
~~aortic valve disorder specified as congenital (Q23.0, Q23.1)~~
~~aortic valve disorder specified as rheumatic (I06.-)~~
~~hypertrophic subaortic stenosis~~
Code also, if applicable, bicuspid aortic valve (Q23.81)
Excludes2 aortic valve disorder of unspecified cause but with diseases of mitral and/or tricuspid valve(s) (I08.-)
aortic valve disorder specified as congenital (Q23.0, Q23.1)
aortic valve disorder specified as rheumatic (I06.-)
hypertrophic subaortic stenosis (I42.1)

I35.0 Nonrheumatic aortic (valve) stenosis

I35.1 Nonrheumatic aortic (valve) insufficiency
Nonrheumatic aortic (valve) incompetence NOS
Nonrheumatic aortic (valve) regurgitation NOS

I35.2 Nonrheumatic aortic (valve) stenosis with insufficiency

I35.8 Other nonrheumatic aortic valve disorders

I35.9 Nonrheumatic aortic valve disorder, unspecified

I36 Nonrheumatic tricuspid valve disorders
Excludes1 tricuspid valve disorders of unspecified cause (I07.-)
tricuspid valve disorders specified as congenital (Q22.4, Q22.8, Q22.9)
tricuspid valve disorders specified as rheumatic (I07.-)
tricuspid valve disorders with aortic and/or mitral valve involvement (I08.-)

I36.0 Nonrheumatic tricuspid (valve) stenosis

I36.1 Nonrheumatic tricuspid (valve) insufficiency
Nonrheumatic tricuspid (valve) incompetence
Nonrheumatic tricuspid (valve) regurgitation

I36.2 Nonrheumatic tricuspid (valve) stenosis with insufficiency

I36.8 Other nonrheumatic tricuspid valve disorders

I36.9 Nonrheumatic tricuspid valve disorder, unspecified

I37 Nonrheumatic pulmonary valve disorders
Excludes1 pulmonary valve disorder specified as congenital (Q22.1, Q22.2, Q22.3)
pulmonary valve disorder specified as rheumatic (I09.89)

I37.0 Nonrheumatic pulmonary valve stenosis

I37.1 Nonrheumatic pulmonary valve insufficiency
Nonrheumatic pulmonary valve incompetence
Nonrheumatic pulmonary valve regurgitation

I37.2 Nonrheumatic pulmonary valve stenosis with insufficiency

I37.8 Other nonrheumatic pulmonary valve disorders

I37.9 Nonrheumatic pulmonary valve disorder, unspecified

I38 Endocarditis, valve unspecified Ex PDX 862
Includes endocarditis (chronic) NOS
valvular incompetence NOS
valvular insufficiency NOS
valvular regurgitation NOS
valvular stenosis NOS
valvulitis (chronic) NOS
Excludes1 congenital insufficiency of cardiac valve NOS (Q24.8)
congenital stenosis of cardiac valve NOS (Q24.8)
endocardial fibroelastosis (I42.4)
endocarditis specified as rheumatic (I09.1)

I39 Endocarditis and heart valve disorders in diseases classified elsewhere Ex PDX 862
Code first underlying disease, such as:
Q fever (A78)
Excludes1 endocardial involvement in:
candidiasis (B37.6)
gonococcal infection (A54.83)
Libman-Sacks disease (M32.11)
listerosis (A32.82)
meningococcal infection (A39.51)
rheumatoid arthritis (M05.31)
syphilis (A52.03)
tuberculosis (A18.84)
typhoid fever (A01.02)

I40 Acute myocarditis Ex PDX 863
Inflammation of heart muscle due to infection (viral/bacterial)
Includes subacute myocarditis
Excludes1 acute rheumatic myocarditis (I01.2)

I40.0 Infective myocarditis
Septic myocarditis
Use additional code (B95-B97) to identify infectious agent

I40.1 Isolated myocarditis
Fiedler's myocarditis
Giant cell myocarditis
Idiopathic myocarditis

I40.8 Other acute myocarditis

I40.9 Acute myocarditis, unspecified

CHAPTER 9 (I00-I99)

I41 Myocarditis in diseases classified elsewhere PDX 863

Code first underlying disease, such as:
typhus (A75.0-A75.9)

Excludes1 myocarditis (in):
Chagas' disease (chronic) (B57.2)
acute (B57.0)
coxsackie (virus) infection (B33.22)
diphtheritic (A36.81)
gonococcal (A54.83)
influenzal (J09.X9, J10.82, J11.82)
meningococcal (A39.52)
mumps (B26.82)
rheumatoid arthritis (M05.31)
sarcoid (D86.85)
syphilis (A52.06)
toxoplasmosis (B58.81)
tuberculous (A18.84)

I42 Cardiomyopathy PDX 864

Disease of the heart muscle resulting in an abnormally enlarged, weakened, thickened, and/or stiffened muscles

Includes myocardiopathy

Code first pre-existing cardiomyopathy complicating pregnancy and puerperium (O99.4)

Excludes2 ischemic cardiomyopathy (I25.5)
peripartum cardiomyopathy (O90.3)
ventricular hypertrophy (I51.7)

I42.0 Dilated cardiomyopathy
Congestive cardiomyopathy

I42.1 Obstructive hypertrophic cardiomyopathy
Hypertrophic subaortic stenosis (idiopathic)

I42.2 Other hypertrophic cardiomyopathy
Nonobstructive hypertrophic cardiomyopathy

I42.3 Endomyocardial (eosinophilic) disease
Endomyocardial (tropical) fibrosis
Löffler's endocarditis

I42.4 Endocardial fibroelastosis
Congenital cardiomyopathy
Elastomyofibrosis

I42.5 Other restrictive cardiomyopathy
Constrictive cardiomyopathy NOS

I42.6 Alcoholic cardiomyopathy
Code also presence of alcoholism (F10.-)

I42.7 Cardiomyopathy due to drug and external agent
Code first poisoning due to drug or toxin, if applicable (T36-T65 with fifth or sixth character 1-4)
Use additional code for adverse effect, if applicable, to identify drug (T36-T50 with fifth or sixth character 5)
Coding Clinic: 2021, Q3, P8

I42.8 Other cardiomyopathies

I42.9 Cardiomyopathy, unspecified
Cardiomyopathy (primary) (secondary) NOS

I43 Cardiomyopathy in diseases classified elsewhere PDX 864

Code first underlying disease, such as:
amyloidosis (E85.-)
glycogen storage disease (E74.0-)
gout (M10.0-)
thyrotoxicosis (E05.0-E05.9-)

Excludes1 cardiomyopathy (in):
coxsackie (virus) (B33.24)
diphtheria (A36.81)
sarcoidosis (D86.85)
tuberculosis (A18.84)
Coding Clinic: 2024, Q2, P9

I44 Atrioventricular and left bundle-branch block

Conduction problem resulting in arrhythmias/dysrhythmias due to a lack of electrical impulses being transmitted normally through the heart

I44.0 Atrioventricular block, first degree

I44.1 Atrioventricular block, second degree
Atrioventricular block, type I and II
Möbitz block, type I and II
Second degree block, type I and II
Wenckebach's block

I44.2 Atrioventricular block, complete PDX 865
Complete heart block NOS
Third degree block
Coding Clinic: 2019, Q2, P4

I44.3 Other and unspecified atrioventricular block
Atrioventricular block NOS

I44.30 Unspecified atrioventricular block

I44.39 Other atrioventricular block

I44.4 Left anterior fascicular block
MCE: Questionable admission when principal dx

I44.5 Left posterior fascicular block
MCE: Questionable admission when principal dx

I44.6 Other and unspecified fascicular block

I44.60 Unspecified fascicular block
Left bundle-branch hemiblock NOS
MCE: Questionable admission when principal dx

I44.69 Other fascicular block
MCE: Questionable admission when principal dx

I44.7 Left bundle-branch block, unspecified
MCE: Questionable admission when principal dx

I45 Other conduction disorders

I45.0 Right fascicular block
MCE: Questionable admission when principal dx

I45.1 Other and unspecified right bundle-branch block

I45.10 Unspecified right bundle-branch block
Right bundle-branch block NOS
MCE: Questionable admission when principal dx

I45.19 Other right bundle-branch block
MCE: Questionable admission when principal dx

I45.2 Bifascicular block PDX 865

I45.3 Trifascicular block PDX 865

I45.4 Nonspecific intraventricular block
Bundle-branch block NOS

I45.5 Other specified heart block
Sinoatrial block
Sinoauricular block
Excludes1 heart block NOS (I45.9)

I45.6 Pre-excitation syndrome
Accelerated atrioventricular conduction
Accessory atrioventricular conduction
Anomalous atrioventricular excitation
Lown-Ganong-Levine syndrome
Pre-excitation atrioventricular conduction
Wolff-Parkinson-White syndrome

I45.8 Other specified conduction disorders

I45.81 Long QT syndrome

I45.89 Other specified conduction disorders PDX 865
Atrioventricular [AV] dissociation
Interference dissociation
Isorhythmic dissociation
Nonparoxysmal AV nodal tachycardia
Coding Clinic: 2013, Q2, P32

I45.9 Conduction disorder, unspecified
Heart block NOS
Stokes-Adams syndrome

I46 Cardiac arrest

Excludes2 cardiogenic shock (R57.0)

I46.2 Cardiac arrest due to underlying cardiac condition PDX 866
Code first underlying cardiac condition
MCC: If patient discharged alive
Coding Clinic: 2024, Q1, P27

CHAPTER 9 (I00-I99)

New · Revised · ~~deleted~~ Deleted · Excludes 1 · Excludes 2 · Includes · Use additional · Code first · Code also · Key words
OGCR Official Guidelines · Unacceptable Principal Diagnosis · X Assign placeholder X · Use Additional Character(s) · Manifestation Code · Coding Clinic

I46.8 **Cardiac arrest due to other underlying condition** (Ex) PDX 866
Code first underlying condition
MCC: If patient discharged alive

I46.9 **Cardiac arrest, cause unspecified** (Ex) PDX 866
MCC: If patient discharged alive

● **I47** **Paroxysmal tachycardia** (Ex) PDX 865
Code first tachycardia complicating:
abortion or ectopic or molar pregnancy (O00-O07, O08.8)
obstetric surgery and procedures (O75.4)
Excludes1 tachycardia NOS (R00.0)
sinoauricular tachycardia NOS (R00.0)
sinus [sinusal] tachycardia NOS (R00.0)

I47.0 **Re-entry ventricular arrhythmia**

● **I47.1** **Supraventricular tachycardia**

I47.10 **Supraventricular tachycardia, unspecified**

I47.11 **Inappropriate sinus tachycardia, so stated**
IST

I47.19 **Other supraventricular tachycardia**
Atrial (paroxysmal) tachycardia
Atrioventricular [AV] (paroxysmal) tachycardia
Atrioventricular re-entrant (nodal) tachycardia [AVNRT] [AVRT]
Junctional (paroxysmal) tachycardia
Nodal (paroxysmal) tachycardia

● **I47.2** **Ventricular tachycardia** (Ex) PDX 865

I47.20 **Ventricular tachycardia, unspecified**

I47.21 **Torsades de pointes**
Code also, if applicable, long QT syndrome (I45.81)
Use Additional code for adverse effect, if applicable, to identify drug (T36-T50 with fifth or sixth character 5)
Coding Clinic: 2022, Q4, P24

I47.29 **Other ventricular tachycardia**
Coding Clinic: 2021, Q3, P12; 2013, Q3, P23

I47.9 **Paroxysmal tachycardia, unspecified**
Bouveret (-Hoffman) syndrome

● **I48** **Atrial fibrillation and flutter** (Ex) PDX 865
Most common abnormal heart rhythm (arrhythmia) presenting as irregular, rapid beating (tachycardia) of the heart's upper chamber.

I48.0 **Paroxysmal atrial fibrillation**

● **I48.1** **Persistent atrial fibrillation**
Rapid contractions of the upper heart chamber
Excludes1 Permanent atrial fibrillation (I48.21)
Coding Clinic: 2019, Q2, P3-4

I48.11 **Longstanding persistent atrial fibrillation**

I48.19 **Other persistent atrial fibrillation**
Chronic persistent atrial fibrillation
Persistent atrial fibrillation, NOS

● **I48.2** **Chronic atrial fibrillation**
Coding Clinic: 2019, Q2, P3

I48.20 **Chronic atrial fibrillation, unspecified**
Excludes1 Chronic persistent atrial fibrillation (I48.19)

I48.21 **Permanent atrial fibrillation**

I48.3 **Typical atrial flutter**
Type I atrial flutter

I48.4 **Atypical atrial flutter**
Type II atrial flutter

● **I48.9** **Unspecified atrial fibrillation and atrial flutter**

I48.91 **Unspecified atrial fibrillation**

I48.92 **Unspecified atrial flutter**

● **I49** **Other cardiac arrhythmias** (Ex) PDX 865
Code first cardiac arrhythmia complicating:
abortion or ectopic or molar pregnancy (O00-O07, O08.8)
obstetric surgery and procedures (O75.4)
~~**Excludes1** neonatal dysrhythmia (P29.1-)~~
~~sinoatrial bradycardia (R00.1)~~
~~sinus bradycardia (R00.1)~~
~~vagal bradycardia (R00.1)~~
Excludes2 bradycardia NOS (R00.1)
▶neonatal dysrhythmia (P29.1-)
▶sinoatrial bradycardia (R00.1)
▶sinus bradycardia (R00.1)
▶vagal bradycardia (R00.1)

● **I49.0** **Ventricular fibrillation and flutter**

I49.01 **Ventricular fibrillation**
MCC: If patient discharged alive

I49.02 **Ventricular flutter**

I49.1 **Atrial premature depolarization**
Atrial premature beats

I49.2 **Junctional premature depolarization**

I49.3 **Ventricular premature depolarization**

● **I49.4** **Other and unspecified premature depolarization**

I49.40 **Unspecified premature depolarization**
Premature beats NOS

I49.49 **Other premature depolarization**
Ectopic beats
Extrasystoles
Extrasystolic arrhythmias
Premature contractions

I49.5 **Sick sinus syndrome**
Tachycardia-bradycardia syndrome
Coding Clinic: 2019, Q1, P33

I49.8 **Other specified cardiac arrhythmias**
Brugada syndrome
Coronary sinus rhythm disorder
Ectopic rhythm disorder
Nodal rhythm disorder

I49.9 **Cardiac arrhythmia, unspecified**
Arrhythmia (cardiac) NOS

● **I50** **Heart failure**
Code first heart failure complicating abortion or ectopic or molar pregnancy (O00-O07, O08.8)
heart failure due to hypertension (I11.0)
heart failure due to hypertension with chronic kidney disease (I13.-)
heart failure following surgery (I97.13-)
obstetric surgery and procedures (O75.4)
rheumatic heart failure (I09.81)
Excludes2 cardiac arrest (I46.-)
neonatal cardiac failure (P20.0)
Coding Clinic: 2017, Q1, P47; 2016, Q4, P122-123, Q1, P38; 2015, Q2, P15

I50.1 **Left ventricular failure, unspecified** (Ex) PDX 867
Cardiac asthma
Edema of lung with heart disease NOS
Edema of lung with heart failure
Left heart failure
Pulmonary edema with heart disease NOS
Pulmonary edema with heart failure
Excludes1 edema of lung without heart disease or heart failure (J81.-)
pulmonary edema without heart disease or failure (J81.-)

● **I50.2** **Systolic (congestive) heart failure**
Heart failure with reduced ejection fraction [HFrEF]
Systolic left ventricular heart failure
Code also end stage heart failure, if applicable (I50.84)
Excludes1 combined systolic (congestive) and diastolic (congestive) heart failure (I50.4-)

I50.20 **Unspecified systolic (congestive) heart failure** (Ex) PDX 868

Item 9–8 Congestive heart failure (CHF) is a condition in which the left ventricle of the heart cannot pump enough blood to the body. The blood flow from the heart slows or returns to the heart from the venous system (back flow) resulting in congestion (fluid accumulation) particularly in the abdomen. Most commonly, fluid collects in the lungs and results in shortness of breath, especially when in a reclining position.

I50.21 Acute systolic (congestive) heart failure (Ex) PDX 869
Presenting a short and relatively severe episode

I50.22 Chronic systolic (congestive) heart failure (Ex) PDX 868
Long-lasting, presenting over time

I50.23 Acute on chronic systolic (congestive) heart failure (Ex) PDX 869
Combination code. What was a chronic condition now has an acute exacerbation (to make more severe).
Coding Clinic: 2013, Q2, P33

● **I50.3 Diastolic (congestive) heart failure**
Diastolic left ventricular heart failure
Heart failure with normal ejection fraction
Heart failure with preserved ejection fraction [HFpEF]
Code also end stage heart failure, if applicable (I50.84)
Excludes1 combined systolic (congestive) and diastolic (congestive) heart failure (I50.4-)

I50.30 Unspecified diastolic (congestive) heart failure (Ex) PDX 868

I50.31 Acute diastolic (congestive) heart failure (Ex) PDX 869
Coding Clinic: 2017, Q1, P46

I50.32 Chronic diastolic (congestive) heart failure (Ex) PDX 868
Coding Clinic: 2023, Q3, P14

I50.33 Acute on chronic diastolic (congestive) heart failure (Ex) PDX 869
Coding Clinic: 2024, Q2, P10

● **I50.4 Combined systolic (congestive) and diastolic (congestive) heart failure**
Combined systolic and diastolic left ventricular heart failure
Heart failure with reduced ejection fraction and diastolic dysfunction
Code also end stage heart failure, if applicable (I50.84)

I50.40 Unspecified combined systolic (congestive) and diastolic (congestive) heart failure (Ex) PDX 868

I50.41 Acute combined systolic (congestive) and diastolic (congestive) heart failure (Ex) PDX 869

I50.42 Chronic combined systolic (congestive) and diastolic (congestive) heart failure (Ex) PDX 868

I50.43 Acute on chronic combined systolic (congestive) and diastolic (congestive) heart failure (Ex) PDX 869

● **I50.8 Other heart failure**

● **I50.81 Right heart failure**
Right ventricular failure

I50.810 Right heart failure, unspecified
Right heart failure without mention of left heart failure
Right ventricular failure NOS

I50.811 Acute right heart failure
Acute isolated right heart failure
Acute (isolated) right ventricular failure

I50.812 Chronic right heart failure
Chronic isolated right heart failure
Chronic (isolated) right ventricular failure

I50.813 Acute on chronic right heart failure
Acute on chronic isolated right heart failure
Acute on chronic (isolated) right ventricular failure
Acute decompensation of chronic (isolated) right ventricular failure
Acute exacerbation of chronic (isolated) right ventricular failure
Coding Clinic: 2023, Q3, P14

I50.814 Right heart failure due to left heart failure
Right ventricular failure secondary to left ventricular failure
Code also the type of left ventricular failure, if known (I50.2-I50.43)
Excludes1 Right heart failure with but not due to left heart failure (I50.82)

I50.82 Biventricular heart failure
Code also the type of left ventricular failure as systolic, diastolic, or combined, if known (I50.2-I50.43)

I50.83 High output heart failure

I50.84 End stage heart failure
Stage D heart failure
Code also the type of heart failure as systolic, diastolic, or combined, if known (I50.2-I50.43)
Coding Clinic: 2022, Q3, P17

I50.89 Other heart failure

I50.9 Heart failure, unspecified
Cardiac, heart or myocardial failure NOS
Congestive heart disease
Congestive heart failure NOS
Excludes2 fluid overload unrelated to congestive heart failure (E87.70)
Coding Clinic: 2017, Q1, P45-46; 2015, Q2, P15; 2012, Q4, P92

● **I51 Complications and ill-defined descriptions of heart disease**
Excludes1 any condition in I51.4-I51.9 due to hypertension (I11.-)
any condition in I51.4-I51.9 due to hypertension and chronic kidney disease (I13.-)
heart disease specified as rheumatic (I00-I09)

I51.0 Cardiac septal defect, acquired (Ex) PDX 828 A
Acquired septal atrial defect (old)
Acquired septal auricular defect (old)
Acquired septal ventricular defect (old)
Excludes1 cardiac septal defect as current complication following acute myocardial infarction (I23.1, I23.2)

I51.1 Rupture of chordae tendineae, not elsewhere classified (Ex) PDX 829
Excludes1 rupture of chordae tendineae as current complication following acute myocardial infarction (I23.4)

I51.2 Rupture of papillary muscle, not elsewhere classified (Ex) PDX 830
Excludes1 rupture of papillary muscle as current complication following acute myocardial infarction (I23.5)

I51.3 Intracardiac thrombosis, not elsewhere classified
Apical thrombosis (old)
Atrial thrombosis (old)
Auricular thrombosis (old)
Mural thrombosis (old)
Ventricular thrombosis (old)
Excludes1 intracardiac thrombosis as current complication following acute myocardial infarction (I23.6)
Coding Clinic: 2013, Q1, P24

CHAPTER 9 (I00-I99)

I51.4 Myocarditis, unspecified
Chronic (interstitial) myocarditis
Myocardial fibrosis
Myocarditis NOS
Excludes1 acute or subacute myocarditis (I4Ø.-)
Coding Clinic: 2016, Q4, P122

I51.5 Myocardial degeneration
Fatty degeneration of heart or myocardium
Myocardial disease
Senile degeneration of heart or myocardium
Coding Clinic: 2016, Q4, P122

I51.7 Cardiomegaly
Cardiac dilatation
Cardiac hypertrophy
Ventricular dilatation
Coding Clinic: 2016, Q4, P122

I51.8 Other ill-defined heart diseases
Coding Clinic: 2016, Q4, P122

I51.81 Takotsubo syndrome (Ex) PDX 870
Reversible left ventricular dysfunction following sudden emotional stress
Stress induced cardiomyopathy
Takotsubo cardiomyopathy
Transient left ventricular apical ballooning syndrome

I51.89 Other ill-defined heart diseases
Carditis (acute)(chronic)
Pancarditis (acute)(chronic)
Coding Clinic: 2019, Q2, P6

I51.9 Heart disease, unspecified
Coding Clinic: 2016, Q4, P122

I52 Other heart disorders in diseases classified elsewhere
Code first underlying disease, such as:
congenital syphilis (A5Ø.5)
mucopolysaccharidosis (E76.3)
schistosomiasis (B65.Ø-B65.9)
Excludes1 heart disease (in):
gonococcal infection (A54.83)
meningococcal infection (A39.5Ø)
rheumatoid arthritis (MØ5.31)
syphilis (A52.Ø6)

CEREBROVASCULAR DISEASES (I6Ø-I69)

Use additional code to identify presence of:
alcohol abuse and dependence (F1Ø.-)
exposure to environmental tobacco smoke (Z77.22)
history of tobacco dependence (Z87.891)
hypertension (I1Ø-I1A)
occupational exposure to environmental tobacco smoke (Z57.31)
tobacco dependence (F17.-)
tobacco use (Z72.Ø)
Excludes1 traumatic intracranial hemorrhage (SØ6.-)
Coding Clinic: 2015, Q4, P4Ø

I5A Non-ischemic myocardial injury (non-traumatic) (Ex) PDX 871
Acute (non-ischemic) myocardial injury
Chronic (non-ischemic) myocardial injury
Unspecified (non-ischemic) myocardial injury
Code first the underlying cause, if known and applicable, such as:
acute kidney failure (N17.-)
acute myocarditis (I4Ø.-)
cardiomyopathy (I42.-)
chronic kidney disease (CKD) (N18.-)
heart failure (I5Ø.-)
hypertensive urgency (I16.Ø)
nonrheumatic aortic valve disorders (I35.-)
paroxysmal tachycardia (I47.-)
pulmonary embolism (I26.-)
pulmonary hypertension (I27.Ø, I27.2-)
sepsis (A41.-)
takotsubo syndrome (I51.81)
Use additional code, if known, to indicate National Institutes of Health Stroke Scale (NIHSS) score (R29.7-)
Excludes1 acute myocardial infarction (I21.-)
injury of heart (S26.-)
Excludes2 other acute ischemic heart diseases (I24.-)
Coding Clinic: 2021, Q4, P15

I6Ø Nontraumatic subarachnoid hemorrhage
Excludes1 syphilitic ruptured cerebral aneurysm (A52.Ø5)
Excludes2 sequelae of subarachnoid hemorrhage (I69.Ø-)

I6Ø.Ø Nontraumatic subarachnoid hemorrhage from carotid siphon and bifurcation
I6Ø.ØØ Nontraumatic subarachnoid hemorrhage from unspecified carotid siphon and bifurcation (Ex) PDX 872
I6Ø.Ø1 Nontraumatic subarachnoid hemorrhage from right carotid siphon and bifurcation (Ex) PDX 872
I6Ø.Ø2 Nontraumatic subarachnoid hemorrhage from left carotid siphon and bifurcation (Ex) PDX 872

I6Ø.1 Nontraumatic subarachnoid hemorrhage from middle cerebral artery
I6Ø.1Ø Nontraumatic subarachnoid hemorrhage from unspecified middle cerebral artery (Ex) PDX 872
I6Ø.11 Nontraumatic subarachnoid hemorrhage from right middle cerebral artery (Ex) PDX 872
I6Ø.12 Nontraumatic subarachnoid hemorrhage from left middle cerebral artery (Ex) PDX 872

I6Ø.2 Nontraumatic subarachnoid hemorrhage from anterior communicating artery (Ex) PDX 872

I6Ø.3 Nontraumatic subarachnoid hemorrhage from posterior communicating artery
I6Ø.3Ø Nontraumatic subarachnoid hemorrhage from unspecified posterior communicating artery (Ex) PDX 872
I6Ø.31 Nontraumatic subarachnoid hemorrhage from right posterior communicating artery (Ex) PDX 872
I6Ø.32 Nontraumatic subarachnoid hemorrhage from left posterior communicating artery (Ex) PDX 872

I6Ø.4 Nontraumatic subarachnoid hemorrhage from basilar artery (Ex) PDX 872

I6Ø.5 Nontraumatic subarachnoid hemorrhage from vertebral artery
I6Ø.5Ø Nontraumatic subarachnoid hemorrhage from unspecified vertebral artery (Ex) PDX 872
I6Ø.51 Nontraumatic subarachnoid hemorrhage from right vertebral artery (Ex) PDX 872
I6Ø.52 Nontraumatic subarachnoid hemorrhage from left vertebral artery (Ex) PDX 872

I6Ø.6 Nontraumatic subarachnoid hemorrhage from other intracranial arteries (Ex) PDX 872

I6Ø.7 Nontraumatic subarachnoid hemorrhage from unspecified intracranial artery (Ex) PDX 872
Ruptured (congenital) berry aneurysm
Ruptured (congenital) cerebral aneurysm
Subarachnoid hemorrhage (nontraumatic) from cerebral artery NOS
Subarachnoid hemorrhage (nontraumatic) from communicating artery NOS
Excludes1 berry aneurysm, nonruptured (I67.1)

I6Ø.8 Other nontraumatic subarachnoid hemorrhage (Ex) PDX 872
Meningeal hemorrhage
Rupture of cerebral arteriovenous malformation

I6Ø.9 Nontraumatic subarachnoid hemorrhage, unspecified (Ex) PDX 872

I61 Nontraumatic intracerebral hemorrhage
Use Additional code, if known, to indicate National Institutes of Health Stroke Scale (NIHSS) score (R29.7-)
Excludes2 sequelae of intracerebral hemorrhage (I69.1-)
Coding Clinic: 2017, Q2, P1Ø

I61.Ø Nontraumatic intracerebral hemorrhage in hemisphere, subcortical (Ex) PDX 872
Deep intracerebral hemorrhage (nontraumatic)
Coding Clinic: 2016, Q4, P27

I61.1 **Nontraumatic intracerebral hemorrhage in hemisphere, cortical** (Ex:) PDX 872
Cerebral lobe hemorrhage (nontraumatic)
Superficial intracerebral hemorrhage (nontraumatic)
Coding Clinic: 2016, Q4, P28

I61.2 **Nontraumatic intracerebral hemorrhage in hemisphere, unspecified** (Ex:) PDX 872

I61.3 **Nontraumatic intracerebral hemorrhage in brain stem** (Ex:) PDX 872
Coding Clinic: 2023, Q4, P42

I61.4 **Nontraumatic intracerebral hemorrhage in cerebellum** (Ex:) PDX 872

I61.5 **Nontraumatic intracerebral hemorrhage, intraventricular** (Ex:) PDX 872

I61.6 **Nontraumatic intracerebral hemorrhage, multiple localized** (Ex:) PDX 872

I61.8 **Other nontraumatic intracerebral hemorrhage** (Ex:) PDX 872
Coding Clinic: 2024, Q2, P25

I61.9 **Nontraumatic intracerebral hemorrhage, unspecified** (Ex:) PDX 872
Coding Clinic: 2022, Q3, P9-10

● I62 **Other and unspecified nontraumatic intracranial hemorrhage** (Ex:) PDX 872
Use Additional code, if known, to indicate National Institutes of Health Stroke Scale (NIHSS) score (R29.7-)
Excludes2 sequelae of intracranial hemorrhage (I69.2)

● I62.0 **Nontraumatic subdural hemorrhage**

I62.00 **Nontraumatic subdural hemorrhage, unspecified**

I62.01 **Nontraumatic acute subdural hemorrhage**

I62.02 **Nontraumatic subacute subdural hemorrhage**

I62.03 **Nontraumatic chronic subdural hemorrhage**

I62.1 **Nontraumatic extradural hemorrhage**
Nontraumatic epidural hemorrhage
Coding Clinic: 2023, Q3, P22

I62.9 **Nontraumatic intracranial hemorrhage, unspecified**

★**(See Plate 31 of the Anatomy Illustrations.)**

● I63 **Cerebral infarction**
Excludes1 neonatal cerebral infarction (P91.82-)
Excludes2 chronic, without residual deficits (sequelae) (Z86.73)
Includes occlusion and stenosis of cerebral and precerebral arteries, resulting in cerebral infarction
Use additional code, if applicable, to identify status post administration of tPA (rtPA) in a different facility within the last 24 hours prior to admission to current facility (Z92.82)
Use additional code, if known, to indicate National Institutes of Health Stroke Scale (NIHSS) score (R29.7-)
Excludes2 sequelae of cerebral infarction (I69.3-)
Coding Clinic: 2016, Q4, P28, 61, 127

● I63.0 **Cerebral infarction due to thrombosis of precerebral arteries** (Ex:) PDX 873

I63.00 **Cerebral infarction due to thrombosis of unspecified precerebral artery**

● I63.01 **Cerebral infarction due to thrombosis of vertebral artery**

I63.011 **Cerebral infarction due to thrombosis of right vertebral artery**

I63.012 **Cerebral infarction due to thrombosis of left vertebral artery**

I63.013 **Cerebral infarction due to thrombosis of bilateral vertebral arteries**

I63.019 **Cerebral infarction due to thrombosis of unspecified vertebral artery**

I63.02 **Cerebral infarction due to thrombosis of basilar artery**

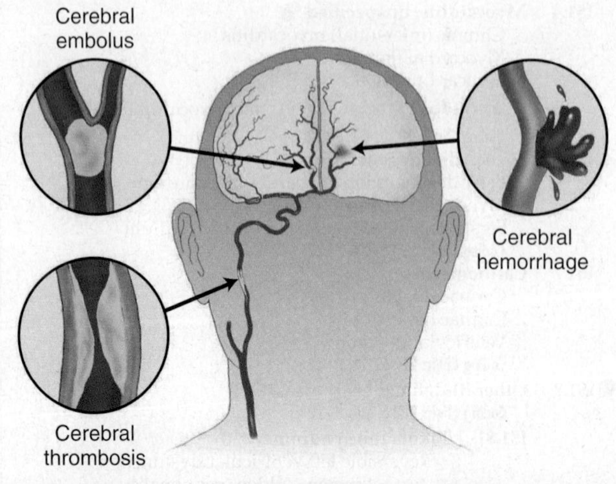

Figure 9-4 Events causing a stroke. (From Shiland: Mastering Healthcare Terminology, ed 1, St. Louis, Mosby, 2003)

● I63.03 **Cerebral infarction due to thrombosis of carotid artery**

I63.031 **Cerebral infarction due to thrombosis of right carotid artery**

I63.032 **Cerebral infarction due to thrombosis of left carotid artery**

I63.033 **Cerebral infarction due to thrombosis of bilateral carotid arteries**

I63.039 **Cerebral infarction due to thrombosis of unspecified carotid artery**

I63.09 **Cerebral infarction due to thrombosis of other precerebral artery**

● I63.1 **Cerebral infarction due to embolism of precerebral arteries** (Ex:) PDX 873

I63.10 **Cerebral infarction due to embolism of unspecified precerebral artery**

● I63.11 **Cerebral infarction due to embolism of vertebral artery**

I63.111 **Cerebral infarction due to embolism of right vertebral artery**

I63.112 **Cerebral infarction due to embolism of left vertebral artery**

I63.113 **Cerebral infarction due to embolism of bilateral vertebral arteries**

I63.119 **Cerebral infarction due to embolism of unspecified vertebral artery**

I63.12 **Cerebral infarction due to embolism of basilar artery**

● I63.13 **Cerebral infarction due to embolism of carotid artery**

I63.131 **Cerebral infarction due to embolism of right carotid artery**

I63.132 **Cerebral infarction due to embolism of left carotid artery**

I63.133 **Cerebral infarction due to embolism of bilateral carotid arteries**

I63.139 **Cerebral infarction due to embolism of unspecified carotid artery**

I63.19 **Cerebral infarction due to embolism of other precerebral artery**

- **I63.2** Cerebral infarction due to unspecified occlusion or stenosis of precerebral arteries (Ex) PDX 873
  - I63.20 Cerebral infarction due to unspecified occlusion or stenosis of unspecified precerebral arteries
  - **I63.21** Cerebral infarction due to unspecified occlusion or stenosis of vertebral arteries
    - I63.211 Cerebral infarction due to unspecified occlusion or stenosis of right vertebral artery
    - I63.212 Cerebral infarction due to unspecified occlusion or stenosis of left vertebral artery
    - I63.213 Cerebral infarction due to unspecified occlusion or stenosis of bilateral vertebral arteries
    - I63.219 Cerebral infarction due to unspecified occlusion or stenosis of unspecified vertebral artery
  - I63.22 Cerebral infarction due to unspecified occlusion or stenosis of basilar artery
  - **I63.23** Cerebral infarction due to unspecified occlusion or stenosis of carotid arteries
    - I63.231 Cerebral infarction due to unspecified occlusion or stenosis of right carotid arteries
    - I63.232 Cerebral infarction due to unspecified occlusion or stenosis of left carotid arteries
    - I63.233 Cerebral infarction due to unspecified occlusion or stenosis of bilateral carotid arteries
    - I63.239 Cerebral infarction due to unspecified occlusion or stenosis of unspecified carotid artery
  - I63.29 Cerebral infarction due to unspecified occlusion or stenosis of other precerebral arteries
- **I63.3** Cerebral infarction due to thrombosis of cerebral arteries (Ex) PDX 874
  - I63.30 Cerebral infarction due to thrombosis of unspecified cerebral artery
  - **I63.31** Cerebral infarction due to thrombosis of middle cerebral artery
    - I63.311 Cerebral infarction due to thrombosis of right middle cerebral artery
    - I63.312 Cerebral infarction due to thrombosis of left middle cerebral artery
    - I63.313 Cerebral infarction due to thrombosis of bilateral middle cerebral arteries
    - I63.319 Cerebral infarction due to thrombosis of unspecified middle cerebral artery
  - **I63.32** Cerebral infarction due to thrombosis of anterior cerebral artery
    - I63.321 Cerebral infarction due to thrombosis of right anterior cerebral artery
    - I63.322 Cerebral infarction due to thrombosis of left anterior cerebral artery
    - I63.323 Cerebral infarction due to thrombosis of bilateral anterior cerebral arteries
    - I63.329 Cerebral infarction due to thrombosis of unspecified anterior cerebral artery
  - **I63.33** Cerebral infarction due to thrombosis of posterior cerebral artery
    - I63.331 Cerebral infarction due to thrombosis of right posterior cerebral artery
    - I63.332 Cerebral infarction due to thrombosis of left posterior cerebral artery
    - I63.333 Cerebral infarction due to thrombosis of bilateral posterior cerebral arteries
    - I63.339 Cerebral infarction due to thrombosis of unspecified posterior cerebral artery
  - **I63.34** Cerebral infarction due to thrombosis of cerebellar artery
    - I63.341 Cerebral infarction due to thrombosis of right cerebellar artery
    - I63.342 Cerebral infarction due to thrombosis of left cerebellar artery
    - I63.343 Cerebral infarction due to thrombosis of bilateral cerebellar arteries
    - I63.349 Cerebral infarction due to thrombosis of unspecified cerebellar artery
  - I63.39 Cerebral infarction due to thrombosis of other cerebral artery
- **I63.4** Cerebral infarction due to embolism of cerebral arteries (Ex) PDX 874
  - I63.40 Cerebral infarction due to embolism of unspecified cerebral artery
  - **I63.41** Cerebral infarction due to embolism of middle cerebral artery
    - I63.411 Cerebral infarction due to embolism of right middle cerebral artery
    - I63.412 Cerebral infarction due to embolism of left middle cerebral artery
    - I63.413 Cerebral infarction due to embolism of bilateral middle cerebral arteries
    - I63.419 Cerebral infarction due to embolism of unspecified middle cerebral artery
  - **I63.42** Cerebral infarction due to embolism of anterior cerebral artery
    - I63.421 Cerebral infarction due to embolism of right anterior cerebral artery
    - I63.422 Cerebral infarction due to embolism of left anterior cerebral artery
    - I63.423 Cerebral infarction due to embolism of bilateral anterior cerebral arteries
    - I63.429 Cerebral infarction due to embolism of unspecified anterior cerebral artery
  - **I63.43** Cerebral infarction due to embolism of posterior cerebral artery
    - I63.431 Cerebral infarction due to embolism of right posterior cerebral artery
    - I63.432 Cerebral infarction due to embolism of left posterior cerebral artery
    - I63.433 Cerebral infarction due to embolism of bilateral posterior cerebral arteries
    - I63.439 Cerebral infarction due to embolism of unspecified posterior cerebral artery
  - **I63.44** Cerebral infarction due to embolism of cerebellar artery
    - I63.441 Cerebral infarction due to embolism of right cerebellar artery
    - I63.442 Cerebral infarction due to embolism of left cerebellar artery
    - I63.443 Cerebral infarction due to embolism of bilateral cerebellar arteries
    - I63.449 Cerebral infarction due to embolism of unspecified cerebellar artery
  - I63.49 Cerebral infarction due to embolism of other cerebral artery

● I63.5 Cerebral infarction due to unspecified occlusion or stenosis of cerebral arteries (Ex) PDX 874

I63.50 Cerebral infarction due to unspecified occlusion or stenosis of unspecified cerebral artery

● I63.51 Cerebral infarction due to unspecified occlusion or stenosis of middle cerebral artery

I63.511 Cerebral infarction due to unspecified occlusion or stenosis of right middle cerebral artery

I63.512 Cerebral infarction due to unspecified occlusion or stenosis of left middle cerebral artery

I63.513 Cerebral infarction due to unspecified occlusion or stenosis of bilateral middle cerebral arteries

I63.519 Cerebral infarction due to unspecified occlusion or stenosis of unspecified middle cerebral artery

● I63.52 Cerebral infarction due to unspecified occlusion or stenosis of anterior cerebral artery

I63.521 Cerebral infarction due to unspecified occlusion or stenosis of right anterior cerebral artery

I63.522 Cerebral infarction due to unspecified occlusion or stenosis of left anterior cerebral artery

I63.523 Cerebral infarction due to unspecified occlusion or stenosis of bilateral anterior cerebral arteries

I63.529 Cerebral infarction due to unspecified occlusion or stenosis of unspecified anterior cerebral artery

● I63.53 Cerebral infarction due to unspecified occlusion or stenosis of posterior cerebral artery

I63.531 Cerebral infarction due to unspecified occlusion or stenosis of right posterior cerebral artery

I63.532 Cerebral infarction due to unspecified occlusion or stenosis of left posterior cerebral artery

Coding Clinic: 2024, Q1, P32; 2017, Q2, P10

I63.533 Cerebral infarction due to unspecified occlusion or stenosis of bilateral posterior cerebral arteries

I63.539 Cerebral infarction due to unspecified occlusion or stenosis of unspecified posterior cerebral artery

● I63.54 Cerebral infarction due to unspecified occlusion or stenosis of cerebellar artery

I63.541 Cerebral infarction due to unspecified occlusion or stenosis of right cerebellar artery

I63.542 Cerebral infarction due to unspecified occlusion or stenosis of left cerebellar artery

I63.543 Cerebral infarction due to unspecified occlusion or stenosis of bilateral cerebellar arteries

I63.549 Cerebral infarction due to unspecified occlusion or stenosis of unspecified cerebellar artery

I63.59 Cerebral infarction due to unspecified occlusion or stenosis of other cerebral artery

I63.6 Cerebral infarction due to cerebral venous thrombosis, nonpyogenic (Ex) PDX 874

● I63.8 Other cerebral infarction (Ex) PDX 874

I63.81 Other cerebral infarction due to occlusion or stenosis of small artery

Lacunar infarction

Coding Clinic: 2018, Q4, P16

I63.89 Other cerebral infarction

Coding Clinic: 2024, Q1, P26, 32; 2022, Q1, P25; 2017, Q2, P9

I63.9 Cerebral infarction, unspecified (Ex) PDX 874

Stroke NOS

Excludes2 transient cerebral ischemic attacks and related syndromes (G45.-)

Coding Clinic: 2016, Q4, P62; 2015, Q1, P26

● I65 Occlusion and stenosis of precerebral arteries, not resulting in cerebral infarction

Includes embolism of precerebral artery
narrowing of precerebral artery
obstruction (complete) (partial) of precerebral artery
thrombosis of precerebral artery

Excludes1 insufficiency, NOS, of precerebral artery (G45.-)
insufficiency of precerebral arteries causing cerebral infarction (I63.0-I63.2)

● I65.0 Occlusion and stenosis of vertebral artery

I65.01 Occlusion and stenosis of right vertebral artery

I65.02 Occlusion and stenosis of left vertebral artery

I65.03 Occlusion and stenosis of bilateral vertebral arteries

I65.09 Occlusion and stenosis of unspecified vertebral artery

I65.1 Occlusion and stenosis of basilar artery

● I65.2 Occlusion and stenosis of carotid artery

I65.21 Occlusion and stenosis of right carotid artery

I65.22 Occlusion and stenosis of left carotid artery

I65.23 Occlusion and stenosis of bilateral carotid arteries

Coding Clinic: 2021, Q1, P4

I65.29 Occlusion and stenosis of unspecified carotid artery

I65.8 Occlusion and stenosis of other precerebral arteries

I65.9 Occlusion and stenosis of unspecified precerebral artery

Occlusion and stenosis of precerebral artery NOS

● I66 Occlusion and stenosis of cerebral arteries, not resulting in cerebral infarction

Includes embolism of cerebral artery
narrowing of cerebral artery
obstruction (complete) (partial) of cerebral artery
thrombosis of cerebral artery

Excludes1 occlusion and stenosis of cerebral artery causing cerebral infarction (I63.3-I63.5)

● I66.0 Occlusion and stenosis of middle cerebral artery

I66.01 Occlusion and stenosis of right middle cerebral artery

I66.02 Occlusion and stenosis of left middle cerebral artery

I66.03 Occlusion and stenosis of bilateral middle cerebral arteries

I66.09 Occlusion and stenosis of unspecified middle cerebral artery

● I66.1 Occlusion and stenosis of anterior cerebral artery

I66.11 Occlusion and stenosis of right anterior cerebral artery

I66.12 Occlusion and stenosis of left anterior cerebral artery

I66.13 Occlusion and stenosis of bilateral anterior cerebral arteries

I66.19 Occlusion and stenosis of unspecified anterior cerebral artery

● I66.2 Occlusion and stenosis of posterior cerebral artery

I66.21 Occlusion and stenosis of right posterior cerebral artery

I66.22 Occlusion and stenosis of left posterior cerebral artery

I66.23 Occlusion and stenosis of bilateral posterior cerebral arteries

I66.29 Occlusion and stenosis of unspecified posterior cerebral artery

I66.3 Occlusion and stenosis of cerebellar arteries
I66.8 Occlusion and stenosis of other cerebral arteries
Occlusion and stenosis of perforating arteries
I66.9 Occlusion and stenosis of unspecified cerebral artery

I67 Other cerebrovascular diseases
Excludes1 Occlusion and stenosis of cerebral artery causing cerebral infarction (I63.3-I63.5-)
Occlusion and stenosis of precerebral artery causing cerebral infarction (I63.2-)
Excludes2 sequelae of the listed conditions (I69.8)

I67.0 Dissection of cerebral arteries, nonruptured (Ex) PDX 875
Excludes1 ruptured cerebral arteries (I60.7)
Coding Clinic: 2021, Q3, P5

I67.1 Cerebral aneurysm, nonruptured
Cerebral aneurysm NOS
Cerebral arteriovenous fistula, acquired
Internal carotid artery aneurysm, intracranial portion
Internal carotid artery aneurysm, NOS
Excludes1 congenital cerebral aneurysm, nonruptured (Q28.-)
ruptured cerebral aneurysm (I60.7)

I67.2 Cerebral atherosclerosis A
Atheroma of cerebral and precerebral arteries

I67.3 Progressive vascular leukoencephalopathy (Ex) PDX 140
Binswanger's disease

I67.4 Hypertensive encephalopathy (Ex) PDX 876
Code also, if applicable, associated hypertensive conditions such as:
essential (primary) hypertension (I10)
hypertensive chronic kidney disease (I12.-)
hypertensive heart and chronic kidney disease (I13.-)
hypertensive heart disease (I11.-)
Excludes2 insufficiency, NOS, of precerebral arteries (G45.2)
Coding Clinic: 2023, Q4, P25

I67.5 Moyamoya disease (Ex) PDX 877

I67.6 Nonpyogenic thrombosis of intracranial venous system (Ex) PDX 878
Nonpyogenic thrombosis of cerebral vein
Nonpyogenic thrombosis of intracranial venous sinus
Excludes1 nonpyogenic thrombosis of intracranial venous system causing infarction (I63.6)

I67.7 Cerebral arteritis, not elsewhere classified (Ex) PDX 879
Granulomatous angiitis of the nervous system
Excludes1 allergic granulomatous angiitis (M30.1)

I67.8 Other specified cerebrovascular diseases

I67.81 Acute cerebrovascular insufficiency (Ex) PDX 880
Acute cerebrovascular insufficiency unspecified as to location or reversibility

I67.82 Cerebral ischemia (Ex) PDX 880
Chronic cerebral ischemia

I67.83 Posterior reversible encephalopathy syndrome (Ex) PDX 881
PRES

I67.84 Cerebral vasospasm and vasoconstriction (Ex) PDX 750

I67.841 Reversible cerebrovascular vasoconstriction syndrome
Call-Fleming syndrome
Code first underlying condition, if applicable, such as eclampsia (O15.00-O15.9)

I67.848 Other cerebrovascular vasospasm and vasoconstriction

I67.85 Hereditary cerebrovascular diseases (Ex) PDX 880

I67.850 Cerebral autosomal dominant arteriopathy with subcortical infarcts and leukoencephalopathy
CADASIL
Code also any associated diagnoses, such as:
epilepsy (G40.-), stroke (I63.-)
vascular dementia (F01.-)

I67.858 Other hereditary cerebrovascular disease

I67.89 Other cerebrovascular disease (Ex) PDX 879
Coding Clinic: 2023, Q2, P19

I67.9 Cerebrovascular disease, unspecified

I68 Cerebrovascular disorders in diseases classified elsewhere

I68.0 Cerebral amyloid angiopathy
Code first underlying amyloidosis (E85.-)

I68.2 Cerebral arteritis in other diseases classified elsewhere (Ex) PDX 879
Code first underlying disease
Excludes1 cerebral arteritis (in):
listerosis (A32.89)
systemic lupus erythematosus (M32.19)
syphilis (A52.04)
tuberculosis (A18.89)

I68.8 Other cerebrovascular disorders in diseases classified elsewhere
Code first underlying disease
Excludes1 syphilitic cerebral aneurysm (A52.05)

OGCR Section I.c.9.d.

Sequelae of Cerebrovascular Disease

1) Category I69, Sequelae of Cerebrovascular disease

Category I69 is used to indicate conditions classifiable to categories I60-I67 as the causes of sequela (neurologic deficits), themselves classified elsewhere. These "late effects" include neurologic deficits that persist after initial onset of conditions classifiable to categories I60-I67. The neurologic deficits caused by cerebrovascular disease may be present from the onset of may arise at any time after the onset of the condition classifiable to categories I60-I67.

Codes from category I69, Sequelae of cerebrovascular disease, that specify hemiplegia, hemiparesis and monoplegia identify whether the dominant or nondominant side is affected. Should the affected side be documented, but not specified as dominant or nondominant, and the classification system does not indicate a default, code selection is as follows:

For ambidextrous patients, the default should be dominant.

If the left side is affected, the default is nondominant.

If the right side is affected, the default is dominant.

2) Codes from category I69 with codes from I60-I67

Codes from category I69 may be assigned on a health care record with codes from I60-I67, if the patient has a current cerebrovascular disease and deficits from an old cerebrovascular disease.

I69 Sequelae of cerebrovascular disease
Note: Category I69 is to be used to indicate conditions in I60-I67 as the cause of sequelae. The 'sequelae' include conditions specified as such or as residuals which may occur at any time after the onset of the causal condition.
Excludes1 personal history of cerebral infarction without residual deficit (Z86.73)
personal history of prolonged reversible ischemic neurologic deficit (PRIND) (Z86.73)
personal history of reversible ischemic neurologcial deficit (RIND) (Z86.73)
sequelae of traumatic intracranial injury (S06.-)
Coding Clinic: 2016, Q4, P28; 2015, Q4, P40; 2012, Q4, P107

CHAPTER 9 (I00-I99)

● I69.0 Sequelae of nontraumatic subarachnoid hemorrhage

I69.00 Unspecified sequelae of nontraumatic subarachnoid hemorrhage

● I69.01 Cognitive deficits following nontraumatic subarachnoid hemorrhage

I69.010 Attention and concentration deficit following nontraumatic subarachnoid hemorrhage

I69.011 Memory deficit following nontraumatic subarachnoid hemorrhage

I69.012 Visuospatial deficit and spatial neglect following nontraumatic subarachnoid hemorrhage

I69.013 Psychomotor deficit following nontraumatic subarachnoid hemorrhage

I69.014 Frontal lobe and executive function deficit following nontraumatic subarachnoid hemorrhage

I69.015 Cognitive social or emotional deficit following nontraumatic subarachnoid hemorrhage

I69.018 Other symptoms and signs involving cognitive functions following nontraumatic subarachnoid hemorrhage

I69.019 Unspecified symptoms and signs involving cognitive functions following nontraumatic subarachnoid hemorrhage

● I69.02 Speech and language deficits following nontraumatic subarachnoid hemorrhage

I69.020 Aphasia following nontraumatic subarachnoid hemorrhage

I69.021 Dysphasia following nontraumatic subarachnoid hemorrhage

I69.022 Dysarthria following nontraumatic subarachnoid hemorrhage

I69.023 Fluency disorder following nontraumatic subarachnoid hemorrhage

Stuttering following nontraumatic subarachnoid hemorrhage

I69.028 Other speech and language deficits following nontraumatic subarachnoid hemorrhage

● I69.03 Monoplegia of upper limb following nontraumatic subarachnoid hemorrhage

I69.031 Monoplegia of upper limb following nontraumatic subarachnoid hemorrhage affecting right dominant side

I69.032 Monoplegia of upper limb following nontraumatic subarachnoid hemorrhage affecting left dominant side

I69.033 Monoplegia of upper limb following nontraumatic subarachnoid hemorrhage affecting right non-dominant side

I69.034 Monoplegia of upper limb following nontraumatic subarachnoid hemorrhage affecting left non-dominant side

I69.039 Monoplegia of upper limb following nontraumatic subarachnoid hemorrhage affecting unspecified side

● I69.04 Monoplegia of lower limb following nontraumatic subarachnoid hemorrhage

I69.041 Monoplegia of lower limb following nontraumatic subarachnoid hemorrhage affecting right dominant side

I69.042 Monoplegia of lower limb following nontraumatic subarachnoid hemorrhage affecting left dominant side

I69.043 Monoplegia of lower limb following nontraumatic subarachnoid hemorrhage affecting right non-dominant side

I69.044 Monoplegia of lower limb following nontraumatic subarachnoid hemorrhage affecting left non-dominant side

I69.049 Monoplegia of lower limb following nontraumatic subarachnoid hemorrhage affecting unspecified side

● I69.05 Hemiplegia and hemiparesis following nontraumatic subarachnoid hemorrhage

I69.051 Hemiplegia and hemiparesis following nontraumatic subarachnoid hemorrhage affecting right dominant side (Ex) PDX 882

I69.052 Hemiplegia and hemiparesis following nontraumatic subarachnoid hemorrhage affecting left dominant side (Ex) PDX 882

I69.053 Hemiplegia and hemiparesis following nontraumatic subarachnoid hemorrhage affecting right non-dominant side (Ex) PDX 883

I69.054 Hemiplegia and hemiparesis following nontraumatic subarachnoid hemorrhage affecting left non-dominant side (Ex) PDX 884

I69.059 Hemiplegia and hemiparesis following nontraumatic subarachnoid hemorrhage affecting unspecified side (Ex) PDX 884

● I69.06 Other paralytic syndrome following nontraumatic subarachnoid hemorrhage

Use additional code to identify type of paralytic syndrome, such as:
locked-in state (G83.5)
quadriplegia (G82.5-)

Excludes1 hemiplegia/hemiparesis following nontraumatic subarachnoid hemorrhage (I69.05-)
monoplegia of lower limb following nontraumatic subarachnoid hemorrhage (I69.04-)
monoplegia of upper limb following nontraumatic subarachnoid hemorrhage (I69.03-)

I69.061 Other paralytic syndrome following nontraumatic subarachnoid hemorrhage affecting right dominant side

I69.062 Other paralytic syndrome following nontraumatic subarachnoid hemorrhage affecting left dominant side

I69.063 Other paralytic syndrome following nontraumatic subarachnoid hemorrhage affecting right non-dominant side

I69.064 Other paralytic syndrome following nontraumatic subarachnoid hemorrhage affecting left nondominant side
I69.065 Other paralytic syndrome following nontraumatic subarachnoid hemorrhage, bilateral
I69.069 Other paralytic syndrome following nontraumatic subarachnoid hemorrhage affecting unspecified side

I69.09 Other sequelae of nontraumatic subarachnoid hemorrhage
I69.090 Apraxia following nontraumatic subarachnoid hemorrhage
I69.091 Dysphagia following nontraumatic subarachnoid hemorrhage
Use additional code to identify the type of dysphagia, if known (R13.11-R13.19)
I69.092 Facial weakness following nontraumatic subarachnoid hemorrhage
Facial droop following nontraumatic subarachnoid hemorrhage
I69.093 Ataxia following nontraumatic subarachnoid hemorrhage
I69.098 Other sequelae following nontraumatic subarachnoid hemorrhage
Alterations of sensation following nontraumatic subarachnoid hemorrhage
Disturbance of vision following nontraumatic subarachnoid hemorrhage
Use additional code to identify the sequelae

I69.1 Sequelae of nontraumatic intracerebral hemorrhage
I69.10 Unspecified sequelae of nontraumatic intracerebral hemorrhage

I69.11 Cognitive deficits following nontraumatic intracerebral hemorrhage
I69.110 Attention and concentration deficit following nontraumatic intracerebral hemorrhage
I69.111 Memory deficit following nontraumatic intracerebral hemorrhage
I69.112 Visuospatial deficit and spatial neglect following nontraumatic intracerebral hemorrhage
I69.113 Psychomotor deficit following nontraumatic intracerebral hemorrhage
I69.114 Frontal lobe and executive function deficit following nontraumatic intracerebral hemorrhage
I69.115 Cognitive social or emotional deficit following nontraumatic intracerebral hemorrhage
I69.118 Other symptoms and signs involving cognitive functions following nontraumatic intracerebral hemorrhage
I69.119 Unspecified symptoms and signs involving cognitive functions following nontraumatic intracerebral hemorrhage

I69.12 Speech and language deficits following nontraumatic intracerebral hemorrhage
I69.120 Aphasia following nontraumatic intracerebral hemorrhage
I69.121 Dysphasia following nontraumatic intracerebral hemorrhage
I69.122 Dysarthria following nontraumatic intracerebral hemorrhage
I69.123 Fluency disorder following nontraumatic intracerebral hemorrhage
Stuttering following nontraumatic intracerebral hemorrhage
I69.128 Other speech and language deficits following nontraumatic intracerebral hemorrhage

I69.13 Monoplegia of upper limb following nontraumatic intracerebral hemorrhage
I69.131 Monoplegia of upper limb following nontraumatic intracerebral hemorrhage affecting right dominant side
I69.132 Monoplegia of upper limb following nontraumatic intracerebral hemorrhage affecting left dominant side
I69.133 Monoplegia of upper limb following nontraumatic intracerebral hemorrhage affecting right nondominant side
I69.134 Monoplegia of upper limb following nontraumatic intracerebral hemorrhage affecting left nondominant side
I69.139 Monoplegia of upper limb following nontraumatic intracerebral hemorrhage affecting unspecified side

I69.14 Monoplegia of lower limb following nontraumatic intracerebral hemorrhage
I69.141 Monoplegia of lower limb following nontraumatic intracerebral hemorrhage affecting right dominant side
I69.142 Monoplegia of lower limb following nontraumatic intracerebral hemorrhage affecting left dominant side
I69.143 Monoplegia of lower limb following nontraumatic intracerebral hemorrhage affecting right nondominant side
I69.144 Monoplegia of lower limb following nontraumatic intracerebral hemorrhage affecting left nondominant side
I69.149 Monoplegia of lower limb following nontraumatic intracerebral hemorrhage affecting unspecified side

I69.15 Hemiplegia and hemiparesis following nontraumatic intracerebral hemorrhage
I69.151 Hemiplegia and hemiparesis following nontraumatic intracerebral hemorrhage affecting right dominant side (Ex) PDX 882
I69.152 Hemiplegia and hemiparesis following nontraumatic intracerebral hemorrhage affecting left dominant side (Ex) PDX 882
I69.153 Hemiplegia and hemiparesis following nontraumatic intracerebral hemorrhage affecting right nondominant side (Ex) PDX 883

I69.154 Hemiplegia and hemiparesis following nontraumatic intracerebral hemorrhage affecting left nondominant side (Ex) PDX 884

I69.159 Hemiplegia and hemiparesis following nontraumatic intracerebral hemorrhage affecting unspecified side (Ex) PDX 884

● I69.16 Other paralytic syndrome following nontraumatic intracerebral hemorrhage

Use additional code to identify type of paralytic syndrome, such as:
locked-in state (G83.5)
quadriplegia (G82.5-)

Excludes1 hemiplegia/hemiparesis following nontraumatic intracerebral hemorrhage (I69.15-)
monoplegia of lower limb following nontraumatic intracerebral hemorrhage (I69.14-)
monoplegia of upper limb following nontraumatic intracerebral hemorrhage (I69.13-)

I69.161 Other paralytic syndrome following nontraumatic intracerebral hemorrhage affecting right dominant side

I69.162 Other paralytic syndrome following nontraumatic intracerebral hemorrhage affecting left dominant side

I69.163 Other paralytic syndrome following nontraumatic intracerebral hemorrhage affecting right nondominant side

I69.164 Other paralytic syndrome following nontraumatic intracerebral hemorrhage affecting left nondominant side

I69.165 Other paralytic syndrome following nontraumatic intracerebral hemorrhage, bilateral

I69.169 Other paralytic syndrome following nontraumatic intracerebral hemorrhage affecting unspecified side

● I69.19 Other sequelae of nontraumatic intracerebral hemorrhage

I69.190 Apraxia following nontraumatic intracerebral hemorrhage

I69.191 Dysphagia following nontraumatic intracerebral hemorrhage

Use additional code to identify the type of dysphagia, if known (R13.11-R13.19)

I69.192 Facial weakness following nontraumatic intracerebral hemorrhage

Facial droop following nontraumatic intracerebral hemorrhage

I69.193 Ataxia following nontraumatic intracerebral hemorrhage

I69.198 Other sequelae of nontraumatic intracerebral hemorrhage

Alteration of sensations following nontraumatic intracerebral hemorrhage
Disturbance of vision following nontraumatic intracerebral hemorrhage

Use additional code to identify the sequelae

● I69.2 Sequelae of other nontraumatic intracranial hemorrhage

I69.20 Unspecified sequelae of other nontraumatic intracranial hemorrhage

● I69.21 Cognitive deficits following other nontraumatic intracranial hemorrhage

I69.210 Attention and concentration deficit following other nontraumatic intracranial hemorrhage

I69.211 Memory deficit following other nontraumatic intracranial hemorrhage

I69.212 Visuospatial deficit and spatial neglect following other nontraumatic intracranial hemorrhage

I69.213 Psychomotor deficit following other nontraumatic intracranial hemorrhage

I69.214 Frontal lobe and executive function deficit following other nontraumatic intracranial hemorrhage

I69.215 Cognitive social or emotional deficit following other nontraumatic intracranial hemorrhage

I69.218 Other symptoms and signs involving cognitive functions following other nontraumatic intracranial hemorrhage

I69.219 Unspecified symptoms and signs involving cognitive functions following other nontraumatic intracranial hemorrhage

● I69.22 Speech and language deficits following other nontraumatic intracranial hemorrhage

I69.220 Aphasia following other nontraumatic intracranial hemorrhage

I69.221 Dysphasia following other nontraumatic intracranial hemorrhage

I69.222 Dysarthria following other nontraumatic intracranial hemorrhage

I69.223 Fluency disorder following other nontraumatic intracranial hemorrhage

Stuttering following other nontraumatic intracranial hemorrhage

I69.228 Other speech and language deficits following other nontraumatic intracranial hemorrhage

● I69.23 Monoplegia of upper limb following other nontraumatic intracranial hemorrhage

I69.231 Monoplegia of upper limb following other nontraumatic intracranial hemorrhage affecting right dominant side

I69.232 Monoplegia of upper limb following other nontraumatic intracranial hemorrhage affecting left dominant side

I69.233 Monoplegia of upper limb following other nontraumatic intracranial hemorrhage affecting right nondominant side

I69.234 Monoplegia of upper limb following other nontraumatic intracranial hemorrhage affecting left nondominant side

I69.239 Monoplegia of upper limb following other nontraumatic intracranial hemorrhage affecting unspecified side

● I69.24 Monoplegia of lower limb following other nontraumatic intracranial hemorrhage

I69.241 Monoplegia of lower limb following other nontraumatic intracranial hemorrhage affecting right dominant side

I69.242 Monoplegia of lower limb following other nontraumatic intracranial hemorrhage affecting left dominant side

I69.243 Monoplegia of lower limb following other nontraumatic intracranial hemorrhage affecting right non-dominant side

I69.244 Monoplegia of lower limb following other nontraumatic intracranial hemorrhage affecting left non-dominant side

I69.249 Monoplegia of lower limb following other nontraumatic intracranial hemorrhage affecting unspecified side

● I69.25 Hemiplegia and hemiparesis following other nontraumatic intracranial hemorrhage

I69.251 Hemiplegia and hemiparesis following other nontraumatic intracranial hemorrhage affecting right dominant side (Ex) PDX 882

I69.252 Hemiplegia and hemiparesis following other nontraumatic intracranial hemorrhage affecting left dominant side (Ex) PDX 882

I69.253 Hemiplegia and hemiparesis following other nontraumatic intracranial hemorrhage affecting right non-dominant side (Ex) PDX 883

I69.254 Hemiplegia and hemiparesis following other nontraumatic intracranial hemorrhage affecting left non-dominant side (Ex) PDX 883

I69.259 Hemiplegia and hemiparesis following other nontraumatic intracranial hemorrhage affecting unspecified side (Ex) PDX 884

● I69.26 Other paralytic syndrome following other nontraumatic intracranial hemorrhage

Use additional code to identify type of paralytic syndrome, such as:
locked-in state (G83.5)
quadriplegia (G82.5-)

Excludes1 hemiplegia/hemiparesis following other nontraumatic intracranial hemorrhage (I69.25-)
monoplegia of lower limb following other nontraumatic intracranial hemorrhage (I69.24-)
monoplegia of upper limb following other nontraumatic intracranial hemorrhage (I69.23-)

I69.261 Other paralytic syndrome following other nontraumatic intracranial hemorrhage affecting right dominant side

I69.262 Other paralytic syndrome following other nontraumatic intracranial hemorrhage affecting left dominant side

I69.263 Other paralytic syndrome following other nontraumatic intracranial hemorrhage affecting right non-dominant side

I69.264 Other paralytic syndrome following other nontraumatic intracranial hemorrhage affecting left non-dominant side

I69.265 Other paralytic syndrome following other nontraumatic intracranial hemorrhage, bilateral

I69.269 Other paralytic syndrome following other nontraumatic intracranial hemorrhage affecting unspecified side

● I69.29 Other sequelae of other nontraumatic intracranial hemorrhage

I69.290 Apraxia following other nontraumatic intracranial hemorrhage

I69.291 Dysphagia following other nontraumatic intracranial hemorrhage

Use additional code to identify the type of dysphagia, if known (R13.11-R13.19)

I69.292 Facial weakness following other nontraumatic intracranial hemorrhage

Facial droop following other nontraumatic intracranial hemorrhage

I69.293 Ataxia following other nontraumatic intracranial hemorrhage

I69.298 Other sequelae of other nontraumatic intracranial hemorrhage

Alteration of sensation following other nontraumatic intracranial hemorrhage
Disturbance of vision following other nontraumatic intracranial hemorrhage

Use additional code to identify the sequelae

● I69.3 Sequelae of cerebral infarction

Sequelae of stroke NOS
Coding Clinic: 2012, Q4, P92, 95

I69.30 Unspecified sequelae of cerebral infarction

● I69.31 Cognitive deficits following cerebral infarction

I69.310 Attention and concentration deficit following cerebral infarction

I69.311 Memory deficit following cerebral infarction

I69.312 Visuospatial deficit and spatial neglect following cerebral infarction

I69.313 Psychomotor deficit following cerebral infarction

I69.314 Frontal lobe and executive function deficit following cerebral infarction

I69.315 Cognitive social or emotional deficit following cerebral infarction

I69.318 Other symptoms and signs involving cognitive functions following cerebral infarction

I69.319 Unspecified symptoms and signs involving cognitive functions following cerebral infarction

● I69.32 Speech and language deficits following cerebral infarction

I69.320 Aphasia following cerebral infarction

I69.321 Dysphasia following cerebral infarction

Coding Clinic: 2012, Q4, P91

I69.322 Dysarthria following cerebral infarction

Excludes2 transient ischemic attack (TIA) (G45.9)

I69.323 Fluency disorder following cerebral infarction

Stuttering following cerebral infarction

I69.328 Other speech and language deficits following cerebral infarction

CHAPTER 9 (I00-I99)

● I69.33 **Monoplegia of upper limb following cerebral infarction**
Coding Clinic: 2017, Q1, P47

I69.331 Monoplegia of upper limb following cerebral infarction affecting right dominant side

I69.332 Monoplegia of upper limb following cerebral infarction affecting left dominant side

I69.333 Monoplegia of upper limb following cerebral infarction affecting right non-dominant side

I69.334 Monoplegia of upper limb following cerebral infarction affecting left non-dominant side

I69.339 Monoplegia of upper limb following cerebral infarction affecting unspecified side

● I69.34 **Monoplegia of lower limb following cerebral infarction**
Coding Clinic: 2017, Q1, P47

I69.341 Monoplegia of lower limb following cerebral infarction affecting right dominant side

I69.342 Monoplegia of lower limb following cerebral infarction affecting left dominant side

I69.343 Monoplegia of lower limb following cerebral infarction affecting right non-dominant side

I69.344 Monoplegia of lower limb following cerebral infarction affecting left non-dominant side

I69.349 Monoplegia of lower limb following cerebral infarction affecting unspecified side

● I69.35 **Hemiplegia and hemiparesis following cerebral infarction**

I69.351 Hemiplegia and hemiparesis following cerebral infarction affecting right dominant side (Ex:) PDX 882

Excludes2 transient ischemic attack (TIA) (G45.9)

Coding Clinic: 2015, Q1, P25

I69.352 Hemiplegia and hemiparesis following cerebral infarction affecting left dominant side (Ex:) PDX 882

I69.353 Hemiplegia and hemiparesis following cerebral infarction affecting right non-dominant side (Ex:) PDX 883

I69.354 Hemiplegia and hemiparesis following cerebral infarction affecting left non-dominant side (Ex:) PDX 883
Coding Clinic: 2012, Q4, P91

I69.359 Hemiplegia and hemiparesis following cerebral infarction affecting unspecified side (Ex:) PDX 884

● I69.36 **Other paralytic syndrome following cerebral infarction**

Use additional code to identify type of paralytic syndrome, such as:
locked-in state (G83.5)
quadriplegia (G82.5-)

Excludes1 hemiplegia/hemiparesis following cerebral infarction (I69.35-)
monoplegia of lower limb following cerebral infarction (I69.34-)
monoplegia of upper limb following cerebral infarction (I69.33-)

I69.361 Other paralytic syndrome following cerebral infarction affecting right dominant side

I69.362 Other paralytic syndrome following cerebral infarction affecting left dominant side

I69.363 Other paralytic syndrome following cerebral infarction affecting right non-dominant side

I69.364 Other paralytic syndrome following cerebral infarction affecting left non-dominant side

I69.365 Other paralytic syndrome following cerebral infarction, bilateral

I69.369 Other paralytic syndrome following cerebral infarction affecting unspecified side

● I69.39 **Other sequelae of cerebral infarction**

I69.390 Apraxia following cerebral infarction

I69.391 Dysphagia following cerebral infarction

Use additional code to identify the type of dysphagia, if known (R13.11-R13.19)

I69.392 Facial weakness following cerebral infarction

Facial droop following cerebral infarction

Coding Clinic: 2024, Q2, P13

I69.393 Ataxia following cerebral infarction

I69.398 Other sequelae of cerebral infarction

Alteration of sensation following cerebral infarction

Disturbance of vision following cerebral infarction

Use additional code to identify the sequelae

Coding Clinic: 2024, Q2, P13

● I69.8 **Sequelae of other cerebrovascular diseases**

Excludes1 sequelae of traumatic intracranial injury (S06.-)

I69.80 Unspecified sequelae of other cerebrovascular disease

● I69.81 **Cognitive deficits following other cerebrovascular disease**

I69.810 Attention and concentration deficit following other cerebrovascular disease

I69.811 Memory deficit following other cerebrovascular disease

I69.812 Visuospatial deficit and spatial neglect following other cerebrovascular disease

I69.813 Psychomotor deficit following other cerebrovascular disease

I69.814 Frontal lobe and executive function deficit following other cerebrovascular disease

I69.815 Cognitive social or emotional deficit following other cerebrovascular disease

I69.818 Other symptoms and signs involving cognitive functions following other cerebrovascular disease

I69.819 Unspecified symptoms and signs involving cognitive functions following other cerebrovascular disease

● I69.82 **Speech and language deficits following other cerebrovascular disease**

I69.820 Aphasia following other cerebrovascular disease

CHAPTER 9 (I00-I99)

I69.821 Dysphasia following other cerebrovascular disease

I69.822 Dysarthria following other cerebrovascular disease

I69.823 Fluency disorder following other cerebrovascular disease
Stuttering following other cerebrovascular disease

I69.828 Other speech and language deficits following other cerebrovascular disease
Coding Clinic: 2019, Q3, P9

● **I69.83** Monoplegia of upper limb following other cerebrovascular disease

I69.831 Monoplegia of upper limb following other cerebrovascular disease affecting right dominant side

I69.832 Monoplegia of upper limb following other cerebrovascular disease affecting left dominant side

I69.833 Monoplegia of upper limb following other cerebrovascular disease affecting right non-dominant side

I69.834 Monoplegia of upper limb following other cerebrovascular disease affecting left non-dominant side

I69.839 Monoplegia of upper limb following other cerebrovascular disease affecting unspecified side

● **I69.84** Monoplegia of lower limb following other cerebrovascular disease

I69.841 Monoplegia of lower limb following other cerebrovascular disease affecting right dominant side

I69.842 Monoplegia of lower limb following other cerebrovascular disease affecting left dominant side

I69.843 Monoplegia of lower limb following other cerebrovascular disease affecting right non-dominant side

I69.844 Monoplegia of lower limb following other cerebrovascular disease affecting left non-dominant side

I69.849 Monoplegia of lower limb following other cerebrovascular disease affecting unspecified side

● **I69.85** Hemiplegia and hemiparesis following other cerebrovascular disease

I69.851 Hemiplegia and hemiparesis following other cerebrovascular disease affecting right dominant side (Ex) PDX 882

I69.852 Hemiplegia and hemiparesis following other cerebrovascular disease affecting left dominant side (Ex) PDX 882

I69.853 Hemiplegia and hemiparesis following other cerebrovascular disease affecting right non-dominant side (Ex) PDX 883

I69.854 Hemiplegia and hemiparesis following other cerebrovascular disease affecting left non-dominant side (Ex) PDX 883

I69.859 Hemiplegia and hemiparesis following other cerebrovascular disease affecting unspecified side (Ex) PDX 884

● **I69.86** Other paralytic syndrome following other cerebrovascular disease
Use additional code to identify type of paralytic syndrome, such as:
locked-in state (G83.5)
quadriplegia (G82.5-)

Excludes1 hemiplegia/hemiparesis following other cerebrovascular disease (I69.85-)
monoplegia of lower limb following other cerebrovascular disease (I69.84-)
monoplegia of upper limb following other cerebrovascular disease (I69.83-)

I69.861 Other paralytic syndrome following other cerebrovascular disease affecting right dominant side

I69.862 Other paralytic syndrome following other cerebrovascular disease affecting left dominant side

I69.863 Other paralytic syndrome following other cerebrovascular disease affecting right non-dominant side

I69.864 Other paralytic syndrome following other cerebrovascular disease affecting left non-dominant side

I69.865 Other paralytic syndrome following other cerebrovascular disease, bilateral

I69.869 Other paralytic syndrome following other cerebrovascular disease affecting unspecified side

● **I69.89** Other sequelae of other cerebrovascular disease

I69.890 Apraxia following other cerebrovascular disease

I69.891 Dysphagia following other cerebrovascular disease
Use additional code to identify the type of dysphagia, if known (R13.11-R13.19)

I69.892 Facial weakness following other cerebrovascular disease
Facial droop following other cerebrovascular disease

I69.893 Ataxia following other cerebrovascular disease

I69.898 Other sequelae of other cerebrovascular disease
Alteration of sensation following other cerebrovascular disease
Disturbance of vision following other cerebrovascular disease
Use additional code to identify the sequelae

● **I69.9** Sequelae of unspecified cerebrovascular diseases

Excludes1 sequelae of stroke (I69.3)
sequelae of traumatic intracranial injury (S06.-)

I69.90 Unspecified sequelae of unspecified cerebrovascular disease

● **I69.91** Cognitive deficits following unspecified cerebrovascular disease

I69.910 Attention and concentration deficit following unspecified cerebrovascular disease

I69.911 Memory deficit following unspecified cerebrovascular disease

I69.912 Visuospatial deficit and spatial neglect following unspecified cerebrovascular disease

I69.913 Psychomotor deficit following unspecified cerebrovascular disease

I69.914 Frontal lobe and executive function deficit following unspecified cerebrovascular disease

I69.915 Cognitive social or emotional deficit following unspecified cerebrovascular disease

I69.918 Other symptoms and signs involving cognitive functions following unspecified cerebrovascular disease

I69.919 Unspecified symptoms and signs involving cognitive functions following unspecified cerebrovascular disease

● I69.92 Speech and language deficits following unspecified cerebrovascular disease

I69.920 Aphasia following unspecified cerebrovascular disease

I69.921 Dysphasia following unspecified cerebrovascular disease

I69.922 Dysarthria following unspecified cerebrovascular disease

I69.923 Fluency disorder following unspecified cerebrovascular disease

Stuttering following unspecified cerebrovascular disease

I69.928 Other speech and language deficits following unspecified cerebrovascular disease

● I69.93 Monoplegia of upper limb following unspecified cerebrovascular disease

I69.931 Monoplegia of upper limb following unspecified cerebrovascular disease affecting right dominant side

I69.932 Monoplegia of upper limb following unspecified cerebrovascular disease affecting left dominant side

I69.933 Monoplegia of upper limb following unspecified cerebrovascular disease affecting right non-dominant side

I69.934 Monoplegia of upper limb following unspecified cerebrovascular disease affecting left non-dominant side

I69.939 Monoplegia of upper limb following unspecified cerebrovascular disease affecting unspecified side

● I69.94 Monoplegia of lower limb following unspecified cerebrovascular disease

I69.941 Monoplegia of lower limb following unspecified cerebrovascular disease affecting right dominant side

I69.942 Monoplegia of lower limb following unspecified cerebrovascular disease affecting left dominant side

I69.943 Monoplegia of lower limb following unspecified cerebrovascular disease affecting right non-dominant side

I69.944 Monoplegia of lower limb following unspecified cerebrovascular disease affecting left non-dominant side

I69.949 Monoplegia of lower limb following unspecified cerebrovascular disease affecting unspecified side

● I69.95 Hemiplegia and hemiparesis following unspecified cerebrovascular disease

I69.951 Hemiplegia and hemiparesis following unspecified cerebrovascular disease affecting right dominant side Ex PDX 882

I69.952 Hemiplegia and hemiparesis following unspecified cerebrovascular disease affecting left dominant side Ex PDX 882

I69.953 Hemiplegia and hemiparesis following unspecified cerebrovascular disease affecting right non-dominant side Ex PDX 883

I69.954 Hemiplegia and hemiparesis following unspecified cerebrovascular disease affecting left non-dominant side Ex PDX 884

I69.959 Hemiplegia and hemiparesis following unspecified cerebrovascular disease affecting unspecified side Ex PDX 884

● I69.96 Other paralytic syndrome following unspecified cerebrovascular disease

Use additional code to identify type of paralytic syndrome, such as:
locked-in state (G83.5)
quadriplegia (G82.5-)

Excludes1 hemiplegia/hemiparesis following unspecified cerebrovascular disease (I69.95-)
monoplegia of lower limb following unspecified cerebrovascular disease (I69.94-)
monoplegia of upper limb following unspecified cerebrovascular disease (I69.93-)

I69.961 Other paralytic syndrome following unspecified cerebrovascular disease affecting right dominant side

I69.962 Other paralytic syndrome following unspecified cerebrovascular disease affecting left dominant side

I69.963 Other paralytic syndrome following unspecified cerebrovascular disease affecting right non-dominant side

I69.964 Other paralytic syndrome following unspecified cerebrovascular disease affecting left non-dominant side

I69.965 Other paralytic syndrome following unspecified cerebrovascular disease, bilateral

I69.969 Other paralytic syndrome following unspecified cerebrovascular disease affecting unspecified side

● I69.99 Other sequelae of unspecified cerebrovascular disease

I69.990 Apraxia following unspecified cerebrovascular disease

I69.991 Dysphagia following unspecified cerebrovascular disease

Use additional code to identify the type of dysphagia, if known (R13.11-R13.19)

I69.992 Facial weakness following unspecified cerebrovascular disease

Facial droop following unspecified cerebrovascular disease

I69.993 **Ataxia following unspecified cerebrovascular disease**

I69.998 **Other sequelae following unspecified cerebrovascular disease**
Alteration in sensation following unspecified cerebrovascular disease
Disturbance of vision following unspecified cerebrovascular disease
Use additional code to identify the sequelae

DISEASES OF ARTERIES, ARTERIOLES AND CAPILLARIES (I7Ø-I79)

I7Ø Atherosclerosis
Includes arteriolosclerosis
arterial degeneration
arteriosclerosis
arteriosclerotic vascular disease
arteriovascular degeneration
atheroma
endarteritis deformans or obliterans
senile arteritis
senile endarteritis
vascular degeneration
Use additional code to identify:
exposure to environmental tobacco smoke (Z77.22)
history of tobacco dependence (Z87.891)
occupational exposure to environmental tobacco smoke (Z57.31)
tobacco dependence (F17.-)
tobacco use (Z72.Ø)
Excludes2 arteriosclerotic cardiovascular disease (I25.1-)
arteriosclerotic heart disease (I25.1-)
atheroembolism (I75.-)
cerebral atherosclerosis (I67.2)
coronary atherosclerosis (I25.1-)
mesenteric atherosclerosis (K55.1)
precerebral atherosclerosis (I67.2)
primary pulmonary atherosclerosis (I27.Ø)

I7Ø.Ø **Atherosclerosis of aorta** A

I7Ø.1 **Atherosclerosis of renal artery** A
Goldblatt's kidney
Excludes2 atherosclerosis of renal arterioles (I12.-)

★**(See Plates 500, 501, and 502 on pages 60 - 62.)**

I7Ø.2 Atherosclerosis of native arteries of the extremities
Mönckeberg's (medial) sclerosis
Use additional code, if applicable, to identify chronic total occlusion of artery of extremity (I7Ø.92)
Excludes2 atherosclerosis of bypass graft of extremities (I7Ø.3Ø-I7Ø.79)

I7Ø.2Ø Unspecified atherosclerosis of native arteries of extremities

I7Ø.2Ø1 **Unspecified atherosclerosis of native arteries of extremities, right leg** A

I7Ø.2Ø2 **Unspecified atherosclerosis of native arteries of extremities, left leg** A

I7Ø.2Ø3 **Unspecified atherosclerosis of native arteries of extremities, bilateral legs** A

I7Ø.2Ø8 **Unspecified atherosclerosis of native arteries of extremities, other extremity** A

I7Ø.2Ø9 **Unspecified atherosclerosis of native arteries of extremities, unspecified extremity** A

I7Ø.21 Atherosclerosis of native arteries of extremities with intermittent claudication

I7Ø.211 **Atherosclerosis of native arteries of extremities with intermittent claudication, right leg** A

I7Ø.212 **Atherosclerosis of native arteries of extremities with intermittent claudication, left leg** A

I7Ø.213 **Atherosclerosis of native arteries of extremities with intermittent claudication, bilateral legs** A

I7Ø.218 **Atherosclerosis of native arteries of extremities with intermittent claudication, other extremity** A

I7Ø.219 **Atherosclerosis of native arteries of extremities with intermittent claudication, unspecified extremity** A

I7Ø.22 Atherosclerosis of native arteries of extremities with rest pain
Includes any condition classifiable to I7Ø.21-
chronic limb-threatening ischemia NOS of native arteries of extremities
chronic limb-threatening ischemia of native arteries of extremities with rest pain
critical limb ischemia NOS of native arteries of extremities
critical limb ischemia of native arteries of extremities with rest pain

I7Ø.221 **Atherosclerosis of native arteries of extremities with rest pain, right leg** A

I7Ø.222 **Atherosclerosis of native arteries of extremities with rest pain, left leg** A

I7Ø.223 **Atherosclerosis of native arteries of extremities with rest pain, bilateral legs** A

I7Ø.228 **Atherosclerosis of native arteries of extremities with rest pain, other extremity** A

I7Ø.229 **Atherosclerosis of native arteries of extremities with rest pain, unspecified extremity** A

I7Ø.23 Atherosclerosis of native arteries of right leg with ulceration
Includes any condition classifiable to I7Ø.211 and I7Ø.221
chronic limb-threatening ischemia of native arteries of right leg with ulceration
critical limb ischemia of native arteries of right leg with ulceration
Use additional code to identify severity of ulcer (L97.-)

I7Ø.231 **Atherosclerosis of native arteries of right leg with ulceration of thigh** A

I7Ø.232 **Atherosclerosis of native arteries of right leg with ulceration of calf** A

I7Ø.233 **Atherosclerosis of native arteries of right leg with ulceration of ankle** A

I7Ø.234 **Atherosclerosis of native arteries of right leg with ulceration of heel and midfoot** A
Atherosclerosis of native arteries of right leg with ulceration of plantar surface of midfoot

I7Ø.235 **Atherosclerosis of native arteries of right leg with ulceration of other part of foot** A
Atherosclerosis of native arteries of right leg extremities with ulceration of toe

CHAPTER 9 (IØØ-I99)

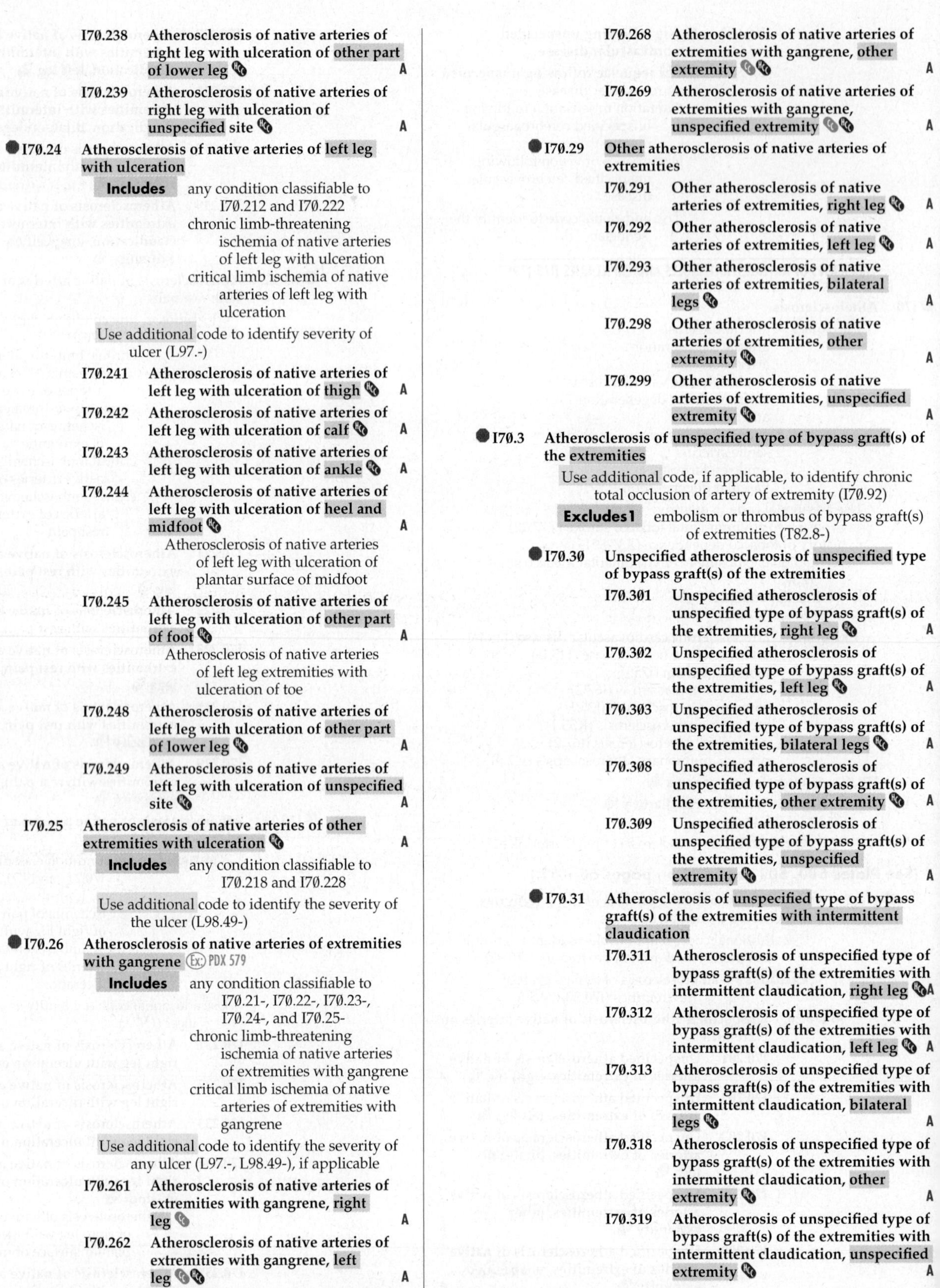

I70.238 Atherosclerosis of native arteries of right leg with ulceration of other part of lower leg A

I70.239 Atherosclerosis of native arteries of right leg with ulceration of unspecified site A

● I70.24 Atherosclerosis of native arteries of left leg with ulceration

Includes any condition classifiable to I70.212 and I70.222
chronic limb-threatening ischemia of native arteries of left leg with ulceration
critical limb ischemia of native arteries of left leg with ulceration

Use additional code to identify severity of ulcer (L97.-)

I70.241 Atherosclerosis of native arteries of left leg with ulceration of thigh A

I70.242 Atherosclerosis of native arteries of left leg with ulceration of calf A

I70.243 Atherosclerosis of native arteries of left leg with ulceration of ankle A

I70.244 Atherosclerosis of native arteries of left leg with ulceration of heel and midfoot A
Atherosclerosis of native arteries of left leg with ulceration of plantar surface of midfoot

I70.245 Atherosclerosis of native arteries of left leg with ulceration of other part of foot A
Atherosclerosis of native arteries of left leg extremities with ulceration of toe

I70.248 Atherosclerosis of native arteries of left leg with ulceration of other part of lower leg A

I70.249 Atherosclerosis of native arteries of left leg with ulceration of unspecified site A

I70.25 Atherosclerosis of native arteries of other extremities with ulceration A

Includes any condition classifiable to I70.218 and I70.228

Use additional code to identify the severity of the ulcer (L98.49-)

● I70.26 Atherosclerosis of native arteries of extremities with gangrene Ex: PDX 579

Includes any condition classifiable to I70.21-, I70.22-, I70.23-, I70.24-, and I70.25-
chronic limb-threatening ischemia of native arteries of extremities with gangrene
critical limb ischemia of native arteries of extremities with gangrene

Use additional code to identify the severity of any ulcer (L97.-, L98.49-), if applicable

I70.261 Atherosclerosis of native arteries of extremities with gangrene, right leg A

I70.262 Atherosclerosis of native arteries of extremities with gangrene, left leg A

I70.263 Atherosclerosis of native arteries of extremities with gangrene, bilateral legs A

I70.268 Atherosclerosis of native arteries of extremities with gangrene, other extremity A

I70.269 Atherosclerosis of native arteries of extremities with gangrene, unspecified extremity A

● I70.29 Other atherosclerosis of native arteries of extremities

I70.291 Other atherosclerosis of native arteries of extremities, right leg A

I70.292 Other atherosclerosis of native arteries of extremities, left leg A

I70.293 Other atherosclerosis of native arteries of extremities, bilateral legs A

I70.298 Other atherosclerosis of native arteries of extremities, other extremity A

I70.299 Other atherosclerosis of native arteries of extremities, unspecified extremity A

● I70.3 Atherosclerosis of unspecified type of bypass graft(s) of the extremities

Use additional code, if applicable, to identify chronic total occlusion of artery of extremity (I70.92)

Excludes1 embolism or thrombus of bypass graft(s) of extremities (T82.8-)

● I70.30 Unspecified atherosclerosis of unspecified type of bypass graft(s) of the extremities

I70.301 Unspecified atherosclerosis of unspecified type of bypass graft(s) of the extremities, right leg A

I70.302 Unspecified atherosclerosis of unspecified type of bypass graft(s) of the extremities, left leg A

I70.303 Unspecified atherosclerosis of unspecified type of bypass graft(s) of the extremities, bilateral legs A

I70.308 Unspecified atherosclerosis of unspecified type of bypass graft(s) of the extremities, other extremity A

I70.309 Unspecified atherosclerosis of unspecified type of bypass graft(s) of the extremities, unspecified extremity A

● I70.31 Atherosclerosis of unspecified type of bypass graft(s) of the extremities with intermittent claudication

I70.311 Atherosclerosis of unspecified type of bypass graft(s) of the extremities with intermittent claudication, right leg A

I70.312 Atherosclerosis of unspecified type of bypass graft(s) of the extremities with intermittent claudication, left leg A

I70.313 Atherosclerosis of unspecified type of bypass graft(s) of the extremities with intermittent claudication, bilateral legs A

I70.318 Atherosclerosis of unspecified type of bypass graft(s) of the extremities with intermittent claudication, other extremity A

I70.319 Atherosclerosis of unspecified type of bypass graft(s) of the extremities with intermittent claudication, unspecified extremity A

CHAPTER 9 (I00-I99)

I70.32 Atherosclerosis of unspecified type of bypass graft(s) of the extremities with rest pain

Includes any condition classifiable to I70.31-

chronic limb-threatening ischemia NOS of unspecified type of bypass graft(s) of the extremities

chronic limb-threatening ischemia of unspecified type of bypass graft(s) of the extremities with rest pain, right leg

critical limb ischemia NOS of unspecified type of bypass graft(s) of the extremities

critical limb ischemia of unspecified type of bypass graft(s) of the extremities with rest pain

I70.321 Atherosclerosis of unspecified type of bypass graft(s) of the extremities with rest pain, right leg A

I70.322 Atherosclerosis of unspecified type of bypass graft(s) of the extremities with rest pain, left leg A

I70.323 Atherosclerosis of unspecified type of bypass graft(s) of the extremities with rest pain, bilateral legs A

I70.328 Atherosclerosis of unspecified type of bypass graft(s) of the extremities with rest pain, other extremity A

I70.329 Atherosclerosis of unspecified type of bypass graft(s) of the extremities with rest pain, unspecified extremity A

I70.33 Atherosclerosis of unspecified type of bypass graft(s) of the right leg with ulceration

Includes any condition classifiable to I70.311 and I70.321

chronic limb-threatening ischemia of unspecified type of bypass graft(s) of the right leg with ulceration

critical limb ischemia of unspecified type of bypass graft(s) of the right leg with ulceration

Use additional code to identify severity of ulcer (L97.-)

I70.331 Atherosclerosis of unspecified type of bypass graft(s) of the right leg with ulceration of thigh (Ex) PDX 885 A
CC when PDx is its own CC

I70.332 Atherosclerosis of unspecified type of bypass graft(s) of the right leg with ulceration of calf (Ex) PDX 886 A
CC when PDx is its own CC

I70.333 Atherosclerosis of unspecified type of bypass graft(s) of the right leg with ulceration of ankle (Ex) PDX 887 A
CC when PDx is its own CC

I70.334 Atherosclerosis of unspecified type of bypass graft(s) of the right leg with ulceration of heel and midfoot (Ex) PDX 888 A

Atherosclerosis of unspecified type of bypass graft(s) of right leg with ulceration of plantar surface of midfoot

CC when PDx is its own CC

I70.335 Atherosclerosis of unspecified type of bypass graft(s) of the right leg with ulceration of other part of foot A

Atherosclerosis of unspecified type of bypass graft(s) of the right leg with ulceration of toe

I70.338 Atherosclerosis of unspecified type of bypass graft(s) of the right leg with ulceration of other part of lower leg (Ex) PDX 889 A
CC when PDx is its own CC

I70.339 Atherosclerosis of unspecified type of bypass graft(s) of the right leg with ulceration of unspecified site (Ex) PDX 890 A
CC when PDx is its own CC

I70.34 Atherosclerosis of unspecified type of bypass graft(s) of the left leg with ulceration

Includes any condition classifiable to I70.312 and I70.322

chronic limb-threatening ischemia of unspecified type of bypass graft(s) of the left leg with ulceration

critical limb ischemia of unspecified type of bypass graft(s) of the left leg with ulceration

Use additional code to identify severity of ulcer (L97.-)

I70.341 Atherosclerosis of unspecified type of bypass graft(s) of the left leg with ulceration of thigh (Ex) PDX 891 A
CC when PDx is its own CC

I70.342 Atherosclerosis of unspecified type of bypass graft(s) of the left leg with ulceration of calf (Ex) PDX 892 A
CC when PDx is its own CC

I70.343 Atherosclerosis of unspecified type of bypass graft(s) of the left leg with ulceration of ankle (Ex) PDX 893 A
CC when PDx is its own CC

I70.344 Atherosclerosis of unspecified type of bypass graft(s) of the left leg with ulceration of heel and midfoot (Ex) PDX 894 A

Atherosclerosis of unspecified type of bypass graft(s) of left leg with ulceration of plantar surface of midfoot

CC when PDx is its own CC

I70.345 Atherosclerosis of unspecified type of bypass graft(s) of the left leg with ulceration of other part of foot A

Atherosclerosis of unspecified type of bypass graft(s) of the left leg with ulceration of toe

I70.348 Atherosclerosis of unspecified type of bypass graft(s) of the left leg with ulceration of other part of lower leg (Ex) PDX 895 A
CC when PDx is its own CC

I70.349 Atherosclerosis of unspecified type of bypass graft(s) of the left leg with ulceration of unspecified site (Ex) PDX 896 A
CC when PDx is its own CC

I70.35 Atherosclerosis of unspecified type of bypass graft(s) of other extremity with ulceration A

Includes any condition classifiable to I70.318 and I70.328

Use additional code to identify severity of ulcer (L98.49-)

CHAPTER 9 (I00-I99)

● **I70.36 Atherosclerosis of unspecified type of bypass graft(s) of the extremities with gangrene**

Includes any condition classifiable to I70.31-, I70.32-, I70.33-, I70.34-, I70.35
chronic limb-threatening ischemia of unspecified type of bypass graft(s) of the extremities with gangrene
critical limb ischemia of unspecified type of bypass graft(s) of the extremities with gangrene

Use additional code to identify the severity of any ulcer (L97.-, L98.49-), if applicable

I70.361 Atherosclerosis of unspecified type of bypass graft(s) of the extremities with gangrene, right leg PDX 897 A
CC when PDx is its own CC

I70.362 Atherosclerosis of unspecified type of bypass graft(s) of the extremities with gangrene, left leg PDX 898 A
CC when PDx is its own CC

I70.363 Atherosclerosis of unspecified type of bypass graft(s) of the extremities with gangrene, bilateral legs PDX 899 A
CC when PDx is its own CC

I70.368 Atherosclerosis of unspecified type of bypass graft(s) of the extremities with gangrene, other extremity PDX 900 A
CC when PDx is its own CC

I70.369 Atherosclerosis of unspecified type of bypass graft(s) of the extremities with gangrene, unspecified extremity PDX 901 A
CC when PDx is its own CC

● **I70.39 Other atherosclerosis of unspecified type of bypass graft(s) of the extremities**

I70.391 Other atherosclerosis of unspecified type of bypass graft(s) of the extremities, right leg A

I70.392 Other atherosclerosis of unspecified type of bypass graft(s) of the extremities, left leg A

I70.393 Other atherosclerosis of unspecified type of bypass graft(s) of the extremities, bilateral legs A

I70.398 Other atherosclerosis of unspecified type of bypass graft(s) of the extremities, other extremity A

I70.399 Other atherosclerosis of unspecified type of bypass graft(s) of the extremities, unspecified extremity A

● **I70.4 Atherosclerosis of autologous vein bypass graft(s) of the extremities**

Use additional code, if applicable, to identify chronic total occlusion of artery of extremity (I70.92)

● **I70.40 Unspecified atherosclerosis of autologous vein bypass graft(s) of the extremities**

I70.401 Unspecified atherosclerosis of autologous vein bypass graft(s) of the extremities, right leg A

I70.402 Unspecified atherosclerosis of autologous vein bypass graft(s) of the extremities, left leg A

I70.403 Unspecified atherosclerosis of autologous vein bypass graft(s) of the extremities, bilateral legs A

I70.408 Unspecified atherosclerosis of autologous vein bypass graft(s) of the extremities, other extremity A

I70.409 Unspecified atherosclerosis of autologous vein bypass graft(s) of the extremities, unspecified extremity A

● **I70.41 Atherosclerosis of autologous vein bypass graft(s) of the extremities with intermittent claudication**

I70.411 Atherosclerosis of autologous vein bypass graft(s) of the extremities with intermittent claudication, right leg A

I70.412 Atherosclerosis of autologous vein bypass graft(s) of the extremities with intermittent claudication, left leg A

I70.413 Atherosclerosis of autologous vein bypass graft(s) of the extremities with intermittent claudication, bilateral legs A

I70.418 Atherosclerosis of autologous vein bypass graft(s) of the extremities with intermittent claudication, other extremity A

I70.419 Atherosclerosis of autologous vein bypass graft(s) of the extremities with intermittent claudication, unspecified extremity A

● **I70.42 Atherosclerosis of autologous vein bypass graft(s) of the extremities with rest pain**

Includes any condition classifiable to I70.41-
chronic limb-threatening ischemia NOS of autologous vein bypass graft(s) of the extremities
chronic limb-threatening ischemia of autologous vein bypass graft(s) of the extremities with rest pain
critical limb ischemia NOS of autologous vein bypass graft(s) of the extremities
critical limb ischemia of autologous vein bypass graft(s) of the extremities with rest pain

I70.421 Atherosclerosis of autologous vein bypass graft(s) of the extremities with rest pain, right leg A

I70.422 Atherosclerosis of autologous vein bypass graft(s) of the extremities with rest pain, left leg A

I70.423 Atherosclerosis of autologous vein bypass graft(s) of the extremities with rest pain, bilateral legs A

I70.428 Atherosclerosis of autologous vein bypass graft(s) of the extremities with rest pain, other extremity A

I70.429 Atherosclerosis of autologous vein bypass graft(s) of the extremities with rest pain, unspecified extremity A

● **I70.43 Atherosclerosis of autologous vein bypass graft(s) of the right leg with ulceration**

Includes any condition classifiable to I70.411 and I70.421
chronic limb-threatening ischemia of autologous vein bypass graft(s) of the right leg with ulceration
critical limb ischemia of autologous vein bypass graft(s) of the right leg with ulceration

Use additional code to identify severity of ulcer (L97.-)

I70.431 Atherosclerosis of autologous vein bypass graft(s) of the right leg with ulceration of thigh PDX 902 A
CC when PDx is its own CC

CHAPTER 9 (I00-I99)

I70.432 **Atherosclerosis of autologous vein bypass graft(s) of the right leg with ulceration of calf** (Ex) PDX 903 A
CC when PDx is its own CC

I70.433 **Atherosclerosis of autologous vein bypass graft(s) of the right leg with ulceration of ankle** (Ex) PDX 904 A
CC when PDx is its own CC

I70.434 **Atherosclerosis of autologous vein bypass graft(s) of the right leg with ulceration of heel and midfoot** (Ex) PDX 905 A
Atherosclerosis of autologous vein bypass graft(s) of right leg with ulceration of plantar surface of midfoot
CC when PDx is its own CC

I70.435 **Atherosclerosis of autologous vein bypass graft(s) of the right leg with ulceration of other part of foot** A
Atherosclerosis of autologous vein bypass graft(s) of right leg with ulceration of toe

I70.438 **Atherosclerosis of autologous vein bypass graft(s) of the right leg with ulceration of other part of lower leg** (Ex) PDX 906 A
CC when PDx is its own CC

I70.439 **Atherosclerosis of autologous vein bypass graft(s) of the right leg with ulceration of unspecified site** (Ex) PDX 907 A
CC when PDx is its own CC

● I70.44 **Atherosclerosis of autologous vein bypass graft(s) of the left leg with ulceration**
Includes any condition classifiable to I70.412 and I70.422
chronic limb-threatening ischemia of autologous vein bypass graft(s) of the left leg with ulceration
critical limb ischemia of autologous vein bypass graft(s) of the left leg with ulceration
Use additional code to identify severity of ulcer (L97.-)

I70.441 **Atherosclerosis of autologous vein bypass graft(s) of the left leg with ulceration of thigh** (Ex) PDX 908 A
CC when PDx is its own CC

I70.442 **Atherosclerosis of autologous vein bypass graft(s) of the left leg with ulceration of calf** (Ex) PDX 909 A
CC when PDx is its own CC

I70.443 **Atherosclerosis of autologous vein bypass graft(s) of the left leg with ulceration of ankle** (Ex) PDX 910 A
CC when PDx is its own CC

I70.444 **Atherosclerosis of autologous vein bypass graft(s) of the left leg with ulceration of heel and midfoot** (Ex) PDX 911 A
Atherosclerosis of autologous vein bypass graft(s) of left leg with ulceration of plantar surface of midfoot
CC when PDx is its own CC

I70.445 **Atherosclerosis of autologous vein bypass graft(s) of the left leg with ulceration of other part of foot** A
Atherosclerosis of autologous vein bypass graft(s) of left leg with ulceration of toe

I70.448 **Atherosclerosis of autologous vein bypass graft(s) of the left leg with ulceration of other part of lower leg** (Ex) PDX 912 A
CC when PDx is its own CC

I70.449 **Atherosclerosis of autologous vein bypass graft(s) of the left leg with ulceration of unspecified site** (Ex) PDX 913 A
CC when PDx is its own CC

I70.45 **Atherosclerosis of autologous vein bypass graft(s) of other extremity with ulceration** A
Includes any condition classifiable to I70.418, I70.428, and I70.438
Use additional code to identify severity of ulcer (L98.49-)

● I70.46 **Atherosclerosis of autologous vein bypass graft(s) of the extremities with gangrene**
Includes any condition classifiable to I70.41-, I70.42-, and I70.43-, I70.44-, I70.45
chronic limb-threatening ischemia of autologous vein bypass graft(s) of the extremities with gangrene
critical limb ischemia of autologous vein bypass graft(s) of the extremities with gangrene
Use additional code to identify the severity of any ulcer (L97.-, L98.49-), if applicable

I70.461 **Atherosclerosis of autologous vein bypass graft(s) of the extremities with gangrene, right leg** (Ex) PDX 914 A
CC when PDx is its own CC

I70.462 **Atherosclerosis of autologous vein bypass graft(s) of the extremities with gangrene, left leg** (Ex) PDX 915 A
CC when PDx is its own CC

I70.463 **Atherosclerosis of autologous vein bypass graft(s) of the extremities with gangrene, bilateral legs** (Ex) PDX 916 A
CC when PDx is its own CC

I70.468 **Atherosclerosis of autologous vein bypass graft(s) of the extremities with gangrene, other extremity** (Ex) PDX 917 A
CC when PDx is its own CC

I70.469 **Atherosclerosis of autologous vein bypass graft(s) of the extremities with gangrene, unspecified extremity** (Ex) PDX 918 A
CC when PDx is its own CC

● I70.49 **Other atherosclerosis of autologous vein bypass graft(s) of the extremities**

I70.491 **Other atherosclerosis of autologous vein bypass graft(s) of the extremities, right leg** A

I70.492 **Other atherosclerosis of autologous vein bypass graft(s) of the extremities, left leg** A

I70.493 **Other atherosclerosis of autologous vein bypass graft(s) of the extremities, bilateral legs** A

I70.498 **Other atherosclerosis of autologous vein bypass graft(s) of the extremities, other extremity** A

I70.499 **Other atherosclerosis of autologous vein bypass graft(s) of the extremities, unspecified extremity** A

CHAPTER 9 (I00-I99)

● I70.5 Atherosclerosis of nonautologous biological bypass graft(s) of the extremities
Use additional code, if applicable, to identify chronic total occlusion of artery of extremity (I70.92)

● I70.50 Unspecified atherosclerosis of nonautologous biological bypass graft(s) of the extremities

I70.501 Unspecified atherosclerosis of nonautologous biological bypass graft(s) of the extremities, right leg A

I70.502 Unspecified atherosclerosis of nonautologous biological bypass graft(s) of the extremities, left leg A

I70.503 Unspecified atherosclerosis of nonautologous biological bypass graft(s) of the extremities, bilateral legs A

I70.508 Unspecified atherosclerosis of nonautologous biological bypass graft(s) of the extremities, other extremity A

I70.509 Unspecified atherosclerosis of nonautologous biological bypass graft(s) of the extremities, unspecified extremity A

● I70.51 Atherosclerosis of nonautologous biological bypass graft(s) of the extremities intermittent claudication

I70.511 Atherosclerosis of nonautologous biological bypass graft(s) of the extremities with intermittent claudication, right leg A

I70.512 Atherosclerosis of nonautologous biological bypass graft(s) of the extremities with intermittent claudication, left leg A

I70.513 Atherosclerosis of nonautologous biological bypass graft(s) of the extremities with intermittent claudication, bilateral legs A

I70.518 Atherosclerosis of nonautologous biological bypass graft(s) of the extremities with intermittent claudication, other extremity A

I70.519 Atherosclerosis of nonautologous biological bypass graft(s) of the extremities with intermittent claudication, unspecified extremity A

● I70.52 Atherosclerosis of nonautologous biological bypass graft(s) of the extremities with rest pain

Includes any condition classifiable to I70.51-
chronic limb-threatening ischemia NOS of nonautologous biological bypass graft(s) of the extremities
chronic limb-threatening ischemia of nonautologous biological bypass graft(s) of the extremities with rest pain
critical limb ischemia NOS of nonautologous biological bypass graft(s) of the extremities
critical limb ischemia of nonautologous biological bypass graft(s) of the extremities with rest pain

I70.521 Atherosclerosis of nonautologous biological bypass graft(s) of the extremities with rest pain, right leg A

I70.522 Atherosclerosis of nonautologous biological bypass graft(s) of the extremities with rest pain, left leg A

I70.523 Atherosclerosis of nonautologous biological bypass graft(s) of the extremities with rest pain, bilateral legs A

I70.528 Atherosclerosis of nonautologous biological bypass graft(s) of the extremities with rest pain, other extremity A

I70.529 Atherosclerosis of nonautologous biological bypass graft(s) of the extremities with rest pain, unspecified extremity A

● I70.53 Atherosclerosis of nonautologous biological bypass graft(s) of the right leg with ulceration

Includes any condition classifiable to I70.511 and I70.521
chronic limb-threatening ischemia of nonautologous biological bypass graft(s) of the right leg with ulceration
critical limb ischemia of nonautologous biological bypass graft(s) of the right leg with ulceration

Use additional code to identify severity of ulcer (L97.-)

I70.531 Atherosclerosis of nonautologous biological bypass graft(s) of the right leg with ulceration of thigh (Ex) PDX 919 A
CC when PDx is its own CC

I70.532 Atherosclerosis of nonautologous biological bypass graft(s) of the right leg with ulceration of calf (Ex) PDX 920 A
CC when PDx is its own CC

I70.533 Atherosclerosis of nonautologous biological bypass graft(s) of the right leg with ulceration of ankle (Ex) PDX 921 A
CC when PDx is its own CC

I70.534 Atherosclerosis of nonautologous biological bypass graft(s) of the right leg with ulceration of heel and midfoot (Ex) PDX 922 A
Atherosclerosis of nonautologous biological bypass graft(s) of right leg with ulceration of plantar surface of midfoot
CC when PDx is its own CC

I70.535 Atherosclerosis of nonautologous biological bypass graft(s) of the right leg with ulceration of other part of foot A
Atherosclerosis of nonautologous biological bypass graft(s) of the right leg with ulceration of toe

I70.538 Atherosclerosis of nonautologous biological bypass graft(s) of the right leg with ulceration of other part of lower leg (Ex) PDX 923 A
CC when PDx is its own CC

I70.539 Atherosclerosis of nonautologous biological bypass graft(s) of the right leg with ulceration of unspecified site (Ex) PDX 924 A
CC when PDx is its own CC

● I70.54 **Atherosclerosis of nonautologous biological bypass graft(s) of the left leg with ulceration**

Includes any condition classifiable to I70.512 and I70.522

chronic limb-threatening ischemia of nonautologous biological bypass graft(s) of the left leg with ulceration

critical limb ischemia of nonautologous biological bypass graft(s) of the left leg with ulceration

Use additional code to identify severity of ulcer (L97.-)

I70.541 **Atherosclerosis of nonautologous biological bypass graft(s) of the left leg with ulceration of thigh** Ex PDX 925 A
CC when PDx is its own CC

I70.542 **Atherosclerosis of nonautologous biological bypass graft(s) of the left leg with ulceration of calf** Ex PDX 926 A
CC when PDx is its own CC

I70.543 **Atherosclerosis of nonautologous biological bypass graft(s) of the left leg with ulceration of ankle** Ex PDX 927 A
CC when PDx is its own CC

I70.544 **Atherosclerosis of nonautologous biological bypass graft(s) of the left leg with ulceration of heel and midfoot** Ex PDX 928 A
Atherosclerosis of nonautologous biological bypass graft(s) of left leg with ulceration of plantar surface of midfoot
CC when PDx is its own CC

I70.545 **Atherosclerosis of nonautologous biological bypass graft(s) of the left leg with ulceration of other part of foot** A
Atherosclerosis of nonautologous biological bypass graft(s) of the left leg with ulceration of toe

I70.548 **Atherosclerosis of nonautologous biological bypass graft(s) of the left leg with ulceration of other part of lower leg** Ex PDX 929 A
CC when PDx is its own CC

I70.549 **Atherosclerosis of nonautologous biological bypass graft(s) of the left leg with ulceration of unspecified site** Ex PDX 930 A
CC when PDx is its own CC

I70.55 **Atherosclerosis of nonautologous biological bypass graft(s) of other extremity with ulceration** A

Includes any condition classifiable to I70.518, I70.528, and I70.538

Use additional code to identify severity of ulcer (L98.49)

● I70.56 **Atherosclerosis of nonautologous biological bypass graft(s) of the extremities with gangrene**

Includes any condition classifiable to I70.51-, I70.52-, and I70.53-, I70.54-, I70.55

chronic limb-threatening ischemia of nonautologous biological bypass graft(s) of the extremities with gangrene

critical limb ischemia of nonautologous biological bypass graft(s) of the extremities with gangrene

Use additional code to identify the severity of any ulcer (L97.-, L98.49-), if applicable

I70.561 **Atherosclerosis of nonautologous biological bypass graft(s) of the extremities with gangrene, right leg** Ex PDX 931 A
CC when PDx is its own CC

I70.562 **Atherosclerosis of nonautologous biological bypass graft(s) of the extremities with gangrene, left leg** Ex PDX 932 A
CC when PDx is its own CC

I70.563 **Atherosclerosis of nonautologous biological bypass graft(s) of the extremities with gangrene, bilateral legs** Ex PDX 933 A
CC when PDx is its own CC

I70.568 **Atherosclerosis of nonautologous biological bypass graft(s) of the extremities with gangrene, other extremity** Ex PDX 934 A
CC when PDx is its own CC

I70.569 **Atherosclerosis of nonautologous biological bypass graft(s) of the extremities with gangrene, unspecified extremity** Ex PDX 935 A
CC when PDx is its own CC

● I70.59 **Other atherosclerosis of nonautologous biological bypass graft(s) of the extremities**

I70.591 **Other atherosclerosis of nonautologous biological bypass graft(s) of the extremities, right leg** A

I70.592 **Other atherosclerosis of nonautologous biological bypass graft(s) of the extremities, left leg** A

I70.593 **Other atherosclerosis of nonautologous biological bypass graft(s) of the extremities, bilateral legs** A

I70.598 **Other atherosclerosis of nonautologous biological bypass graft(s) of the extremities, other extremity** A

I70.599 **Other atherosclerosis of nonautologous biological bypass graft(s) of the extremities, unspecified extremity** A

● I70.6 **Atherosclerosis of nonbiological bypass graft(s) of the extremities**

Use additional code, if applicable, to identify chronic total occlusion of artery of extremity (I70.92)

● I70.60 **Unspecified atherosclerosis of nonbiological bypass graft(s) of the extremities**

I70.601 **Unspecified atherosclerosis of nonbiological bypass graft(s) of the extremities, right leg** A

I70.602 **Unspecified atherosclerosis of nonbiological bypass graft(s) of the extremities, left leg** A

I70.603 **Unspecified atherosclerosis of nonbiological bypass graft(s) of the extremities, bilateral legs** A

CHAPTER 9 (I00-I99)

I70.608 Unspecified atherosclerosis of nonbiological bypass graft(s) of the extremities, other extremity A

I70.609 Unspecified atherosclerosis of nonbiological bypass graft(s) of the extremities, unspecified extremity A

● I70.61 Atherosclerosis of nonbiological bypass graft(s) of the extremities with intermittent claudication

I70.611 Atherosclerosis of nonbiological bypass graft(s) of the extremities with intermittent claudication, right leg A

I70.612 Atherosclerosis of nonbiological bypass graft(s) of the extremities with intermittent claudication, left leg A

I70.613 Atherosclerosis of nonbiological bypass graft(s) of the extremities with intermittent claudication, bilateral legs A

I70.618 Atherosclerosis of nonbiological bypass graft(s) of the extremities with intermittent claudication, other extremity A

I70.619 Atherosclerosis of nonbiological bypass graft(s) of the extremities with intermittent claudication, unspecified extremity A

● I70.62 Atherosclerosis of nonbiological bypass graft(s) of the extremities with rest pain

Includes any condition classifiable to I70.61-
chronic limb-threatening ischemia NOS of nonbiological bypass graft(s) of the extremities
chronic limb-threatening ischemia of nonbiological bypass graft(s) of the extremities with rest pain
critical limb ischemia NOS of nonbiological bypass graft(s) of the extremities
critical limb ischemia of nonbiological bypass graft(s) of the extremities with rest pain

I70.621 Atherosclerosis of nonbiological bypass graft(s) of the extremities with rest pain, right leg A

I70.622 Atherosclerosis of nonbiological bypass graft(s) of the extremities with rest pain, left leg A

I70.623 Atherosclerosis of nonbiological bypass graft(s) of the extremities with rest pain, bilateral legs A

I70.628 Atherosclerosis of nonbiological bypass graft(s) of the extremities with rest pain, other extremity A

I70.629 Atherosclerosis of nonbiological bypass graft(s) of the extremities with rest pain, unspecified extremity A

● I70.63 Atherosclerosis of nonbiological bypass graft(s) of the right leg with ulceration

Includes any condition classifiable to I70.611 and I70.621
chronic limb-threatening ischemia of nonbiological bypass graft(s) of the right leg with ulceration
critical limb ischemia of nonbiological bypass graft(s) of the right leg with ulceration

Use additional code to identify severity of ulcer (L97.-)

I70.631 Atherosclerosis of nonbiological bypass graft(s) of the right leg with ulceration of thigh Ex PDX 936 A
CC when PDx is its own CC

I70.632 Atherosclerosis of nonbiological bypass graft(s) of the right leg with ulceration of calf Ex PDX 937 A
CC when PDx is its own CC

I70.633 Atherosclerosis of nonbiological bypass graft(s) of the right leg with ulceration of ankle Ex PDX 938 A
CC when PDx is its own CC

I70.634 Atherosclerosis of nonbiological bypass graft(s) of the right leg with ulceration of heel and midfoot Ex PDX 939 A
Atherosclerosis of nonbiological bypass graft(s) of right leg with ulceration of plantar surface of midfoot
CC when PDx is its own CC

I70.635 Atherosclerosis of nonbiological bypass graft(s) of the right leg with ulceration of other part of foot A
Atherosclerosis of nonbiological bypass graft(s) of the right leg with ulceration of toe

I70.638 Atherosclerosis of nonbiological bypass graft(s) of the right leg with ulceration of other part of lower leg Ex PDX 940 A
CC when PDx is its own CC

I70.639 Atherosclerosis of nonbiological bypass graft(s) of the right leg with ulceration of unspecified site Ex PDX 941 A
CC when PDx is its own CC

● I70.64 Atherosclerosis of nonbiological bypass graft(s) of the left leg with ulceration

Includes any condition classifiable to I70.612 and I70.622
chronic limb-threatening ischemia of nonbiological bypass graft(s) of the left leg with ulceration
critical limb ischemia of nonbiological bypass graft(s) of the left leg with ulceration

Use additional code to identify severity of ulcer (L97.-)

I70.641 Atherosclerosis of nonbiological bypass graft(s) of the left leg with ulceration of thigh Ex PDX 942 A
CC when PDx is its own CC

I70.642 Atherosclerosis of nonbiological bypass graft(s) of the left leg with ulceration of calf Ex PDX 943 A
CC when PDx is its own CC

I70.643 Atherosclerosis of nonbiological bypass graft(s) of the left leg with ulceration of ankle Ex PDX 944 A
CC when PDx is its own CC

I70.644 Atherosclerosis of nonbiological bypass graft(s) of the left leg with ulceration of heel and midfoot Ex PDX 945 A
Atherosclerosis of nonbiological bypass graft(s) of left leg with ulceration of plantar surface of midfoot
CC when PDx is its own CC

I70.645 Atherosclerosis of nonbiological bypass graft(s) of the left leg with ulceration of other part of foot A
Atherosclerosis of nonbiological bypass graft(s) of the left leg with ulceration of toe

I70.648 Atherosclerosis of nonbiological bypass graft(s) of the left leg with ulceration of other part of lower leg A
CC when PDx is its own CC
PDX 946

I70.649 Atherosclerosis of nonbiological bypass graft(s) of the left leg with ulceration of unspecified site PDX 947 A
CC when PDx is its own CC

I70.65 Atherosclerosis of nonbiological bypass graft(s) of other extremity with ulceration A
Includes any condition classifiable to I70.618 and I70.628
Use additional code to identify severity of ulcer (L98.49-)

● I70.66 Atherosclerosis of nonbiological bypass graft(s) of the extremities with gangrene
Includes any condition classifiable to I70.61-, I70.62-, I70.63-, I70.64-, I70.65
chronic limb-threatening ischemia of nonbiological bypass graft(s) of the extremities with gangrene
critical limb ischemia of nonbiological bypass graft(s) of the extremities with gangrene
Use additional code to identify the severity of any ulcer (L97.-, L98.49-), if applicable

I70.661 Atherosclerosis of nonbiological bypass graft(s) of the extremities with gangrene, right leg PDX 948 A
CC when PDx is its own CC

I70.662 Atherosclerosis of nonbiological bypass graft(s) of the extremities with gangrene, left leg PDX 949 A
CC when PDx is its own CC

I70.663 Atherosclerosis of nonbiological bypass graft(s) of the extremities with gangrene, bilateral legs PDX 950 A
CC when PDx is its own CC

I70.668 Atherosclerosis of nonbiological bypass graft(s) of the extremities with gangrene, other extremity PDX 951 A
CC when PDx is its own CC

I70.669 Atherosclerosis of nonbiological bypass graft(s) of the extremities with gangrene, unspecified extremity PDX 952 A
CC when PDx is its own CC

● I70.69 Other atherosclerosis of nonbiological bypass graft(s) of the extremities

I70.691 Other atherosclerosis of nonbiological bypass graft(s) of the extremities, right leg A

I70.692 Other atherosclerosis of nonbiological bypass graft(s) of the extremities, left leg A

I70.693 Other atherosclerosis of nonbiological bypass graft(s) of the extremities, bilateral legs A

I70.698 Other atherosclerosis of nonbiological bypass graft(s) of the extremities, other extremity A

I70.699 Other atherosclerosis of nonbiological bypass graft(s) of the extremities, unspecified extremity A

● I70.7 Atherosclerosis of other type of bypass graft(s) of the extremities
Use additional code, if applicable, to identify chronic total occlusion of artery of extremity (I70.92)

● I70.70 Unspecified atherosclerosis of other type of bypass graft(s) of the extremities

I70.701 Unspecified atherosclerosis of other type of bypass graft(s) of the extremities, right leg A

I70.702 Unspecified atherosclerosis of other type of bypass graft(s) of the extremities, left leg A

I70.703 Unspecified atherosclerosis of other type of bypass graft(s) of the extremities, bilateral legs A

I70.708 Unspecified atherosclerosis of other type of bypass graft(s) of the extremities, other extremity A

I70.709 Unspecified atherosclerosis of other type of bypass graft(s) of the extremities, unspecified extremity A

● I70.71 Atherosclerosis of other type of bypass graft(s) of the extremities with intermittent claudication

I70.711 Atherosclerosis of other type of bypass graft(s) of the extremities with intermittent claudication, right leg A

I70.712 Atherosclerosis of other type of bypass graft(s) of the extremities with intermittent claudication, left leg A

I70.713 Atherosclerosis of other type of bypass graft(s) of the extremities with intermittent claudication, bilateral legs A

I70.718 Atherosclerosis of other type of bypass graft(s) of the extremities with intermittent claudication, other extremity A

I70.719 Atherosclerosis of other type of bypass graft(s) of the extremities with intermittent claudication, unspecified extremity A

● I70.72 Atherosclerosis of other type of bypass graft(s) of the extremities with rest pain
Includes any condition classifiable to I70.71-
chronic limb-threatening ischemia NOS of other type of bypass graft(s) of the extremities
chronic limb-threatening ischemia of other type of bypass graft(s) of the extremities with rest pain
critical limb ischemia NOS of other type of bypass graft(s) of the extremities
critical limb ischemia of other type of bypass graft(s) of the extremities with rest pain

I70.721 Atherosclerosis of other type of bypass graft(s) of the extremities with rest pain, right leg A

I70.722 Atherosclerosis of other type of bypass graft(s) of the extremities with rest pain, left leg A

I70.723 Atherosclerosis of other type of bypass graft(s) of the extremities with rest pain, bilateral legs A

I70.728 Atherosclerosis of other type of bypass graft(s) of the extremities with rest pain, other extremity A

I70.729 Atherosclerosis of other type of bypass graft(s) of the extremities with rest pain, unspecified extremity A

● I70.73 Atherosclerosis of other type of bypass graft(s) of the right leg with ulceration

Includes any condition classifiable to I70.711 and I70.721
chronic limb-threatening ischemia of other type of bypass graft(s) of the right leg with ulceration
critical limb ischemia of other type of bypass graft(s) of the right leg with ulceration

Use additional code to identify severity of ulcer (L97.-)

I70.731 Atherosclerosis of other type of bypass graft(s) of the right leg with ulceration of thigh (Ex:) PDX 953 A
CC when PDx is its own CC

I70.732 Atherosclerosis of other type of bypass graft(s) of the right leg with ulceration of calf (Ex:) PDX 954 A
CC when PDx is its own CC

I70.733 Atherosclerosis of other type of bypass graft(s) of the right leg with ulceration of ankle (Ex:) PDX 955 A
CC when PDx is its own CC

I70.734 Atherosclerosis of other type of bypass graft(s) of the right leg with ulceration of heel and midfoot (Ex:) PDX 956 A
Atherosclerosis of other type of bypass graft(s) of right leg with ulceration of plantar surface of midfoot
CC when PDx is its own CC

I70.735 Atherosclerosis of other type of bypass graft(s) of the right leg with ulceration of other part of foot A
Atherosclerosis of other type of bypass graft(s) of right leg with ulceration of toe

I70.738 Atherosclerosis of other type of bypass graft(s) of the right leg with ulceration of other part of lower leg (Ex:) PDX 957 A
CC when PDx is its own CC

I70.739 Atherosclerosis of other type of bypass graft(s) of the right leg with ulceration of unspecified site (Ex:) PDX 958 A
CC when PDx is its own CC

● I70.74 Atherosclerosis of other type of bypass graft(s) of the left leg with ulceration

Includes any condition classifiable to I70.712 and I70.722
chronic limb-threatening ischemia of other type of bypass graft(s) of the left leg with ulceration
critical limb ischemia of other type of bypass graft(s) of the left leg with ulceration

Use additional code to identify severity of ulcer (L97.-)

I70.741 Atherosclerosis of other type of bypass graft(s) of the left leg with ulceration of thigh (Ex:) PDX 959 A
CC when PDx is its own CC

I70.742 Atherosclerosis of other type of bypass graft(s) of the left leg with ulceration of calf (Ex:) PDX 960 A
CC when PDx is its own CC

I70.743 Atherosclerosis of other type of bypass graft(s) of the left leg with ulceration of ankle (Ex:) PDX 961 A
CC when PDx is its own CC

I70.744 Atherosclerosis of other type of bypass graft(s) of the left leg with ulceration of heel and midfoot (Ex:) PDX 962 A
Atherosclerosis of other type of bypass graft(s) of left leg with ulceration of plantar surface of midfoot
CC when PDx is its own CC

I70.745 Atherosclerosis of other type of bypass graft(s) of the left leg with ulceration of other part of foot A
Atherosclerosis of other type of bypass graft(s) of left leg with ulceration of toe

I70.748 Atherosclerosis of other type of bypass graft(s) of the left leg with ulceration of other part of lower leg (Ex:) PDX 963 A
CC when PDx is its own CC

I70.749 Atherosclerosis of other type of bypass graft(s) of the left leg with ulceration of unspecified site (Ex:) PDX 964 A
CC when PDx is its own CC

I70.75 Atherosclerosis of other type of bypass graft(s) of other extremity with ulceration A

Includes any condition classifiable to I70.718 and I70.728

Use additional code to identify severity of ulcer (L98.49)

● I70.76 Atherosclerosis of other type of bypass graft(s) of the extremities with gangrene

Includes any condition classifiable to I70.71-, I70.72-, I70.73-, I70.74-, I70.75
chronic limb-threatening ischemia of other type of bypass graft(s) of the extremities with gangrene
critical limb ischemia of other type of bypass graft(s) of the extremities with gangrene

Use additional code to identify the severity of any ulcer (L97.-, L98.49-), if applicable

I70.761 Atherosclerosis of other type of bypass graft(s) of the extremities with gangrene, right leg (Ex:) PDX 965 A
CC when PDx is its own CC

I70.762 Atherosclerosis of other type of bypass graft(s) of the extremities with gangrene, left leg (Ex:) PDX 966 A
CC when PDx is its own CC

I70.763 Atherosclerosis of other type of bypass graft(s) of the extremities with gangrene, bilateral legs (Ex:) PDX 967 A
CC when PDx is its own CC

I70.768 Atherosclerosis of other type of bypass graft(s) of the extremities with gangrene, other extremity (Ex:) PDX 968 A
CC when PDx is its own CC

I70.769 **Atherosclerosis of other type of bypass graft(s) of the extremities with gangrene, unspecified extremity** (Ex) PDX 969 A
CC when PDx is its own CC

● I70.79 **Other atherosclerosis of other type of bypass graft(s) of the extremities**

I70.791 **Other atherosclerosis of other type of bypass graft(s) of the extremities, right leg** A

I70.792 **Other atherosclerosis of other type of bypass graft(s) of the extremities, left leg** A

I70.793 **Other atherosclerosis of other type of bypass graft(s) of the extremities, bilateral legs** A

I70.798 **Other atherosclerosis of other type of bypass graft(s) of the extremities, other extremity** A

I70.799 **Other atherosclerosis of other type of bypass graft(s) of the extremities, unspecified extremity** A

I70.8 **Atherosclerosis of other arteries** A

● I70.9 **Other and unspecified atherosclerosis**

I70.90 **Unspecified atherosclerosis** A

I70.91 **Generalized atherosclerosis** A

● I70.92 **Chronic total occlusion of artery of the extremities** (Ex) PDX 970 A
Complete occlusion of artery of the extremities
Total occlusion of artery of the extremities
Code first atherosclerosis of arteries of the extremities (I70.2-, I70.3-, I70.4-, I70.5-, I70.6-, I70.7-)

● I71 **Aortic aneurysm and dissection** (Ex) PDX 972
Code first, if applicable:
syphilitic aortic aneurysm (A52.01)
traumatic aortic aneurysm (S25.09, S35.09)

● I71.0 **Dissection of aorta**

I71.00 **Dissection of unspecified site of aorta** (Ex) PDX 971

● I71.01 **Dissection of thoracic aorta**

I71.010 **Dissection of ascending aorta**
Coding Clinic: 2024, Q2, P17

I71.011 **Dissection of aortic arch**
Coding Clinic: 2024, Q2, P17

I71.012 **Dissection of descending thoracic aorta**
Coding Clinic: 2024, Q2, P17

I71.019 **Dissection of thoracic aorta, unspecified**

I71.02 **Dissection of abdominal aorta** (Ex) PDX 971

I71.03 **Dissection of thoracoabdominal aorta** (Ex) PDX 971

● I71.1 **Thoracic aortic aneurysm, ruptured**

I71.10 **Thoracic aortic aneurysm, ruptured, unspecified**

I71.11 **Aneurysm of the ascending aorta, ruptured**

I71.12 **Aneurysm of the aortic arch, ruptured**

I71.13 **Aneurysm of the descending thoracic aorta, ruptured**

● I71.2 **Thoracic aortic aneurysm, without rupture**

I71.20 **Thoracic aortic aneurysm, without rupture, unspecified**

I71.21 **Aneurysm of the ascending aorta, without rupture**

I71.22 **Aneurysm of the aortic arch, without rupture**

I71.23 **Aneurysm of the descending thoracic aorta, without rupture**

● I71.3 **Abdominal aortic aneurysm, ruptured**

I71.30 **Abdominal aortic aneurysm, ruptured, unspecified**

I71.31 **Pararenal abdominal aortic aneurysm, ruptured**

I71.32 **Juxtarenal abdominal aortic aneurysm, ruptured**

I71.33 **Infrarenal abdominal aortic aneurysm, ruptured**

● I71.4 **Abdominal aortic aneurysm, without rupture**

I71.40 **Abdominal aortic aneurysm, without rupture, unspecified**

I71.41 **Pararenal abdominal aortic aneurysm, without rupture**
Coding Clinic: 2024, Q2, P16

I71.42 **Juxtarenal abdominal aortic aneurysm, without rupture**

I71.43 **Infrarenal abdominal aortic aneurysm, without rupture**

● I71.5 **Thoracoabdominal aortic aneurysm, ruptured**

I71.50 **Thoracoabdominal aortic aneurysm, ruptured, unspecified**

I71.51 **Supraceliac aneurysm of the thoracoabdominal aorta, ruptured**

I71.52 **Paravisceral aneurysm of the thoracoabdominal aorta, ruptured**

● I71.6 **Thoracoabdominal aortic aneurysm, without rupture**

I71.60 **Thoracoabdominal aortic aneurysm, without rupture, unspecified**

I71.61 **Supraceliac aneurysm of the thoracoabdominal aorta, without rupture**

I71.62 **Paravisceral aneurysm of the thoracoabdominal aorta, without rupture**

I71.8 **Aortic aneurysm of unspecified site, ruptured** (Ex) PDX 971
Rupture of aorta NOS

I71.9 **Aortic aneurysm of unspecified site, without rupture**
Aneurysm of aorta
Dilatation of aorta
Hyaline necrosis of aorta

● I72 **Other aneurysm**

Includes aneurysm (cirsoid) (false) (ruptured)

Excludes2 acquired aneurysm (I77.0)
aneurysm (of) aorta (I71.-)
aneurysm (of) arteriovenous NOS (Q27.3-)
carotid artery dissection (I77.71)
cerebral (nonruptured) aneurysm (I67.1)
coronary aneurysm (I25.4)
coronary artery dissection (I25.42)
dissection of artery NEC (I77.79)
dissection of precerebral artery, congenital (nonruptured) (Q28.1)
heart aneurysm (I25.3)
iliac artery dissection (I77.72)
precerebral artery, congential (nonruptured) (Q28.1)
pulmonary artery aneurysm (I28.1)
renal artery dissection (I77.73)
retinal aneurysm (H35.0)
ruptured cerebral aneurysm (I60.7)
varicose aneurysm (I77.0)
vertebral artery dissection (I77.74)

I72.0 **Aneurysm of carotid artery**
Aneurysm of common carotid artery
Aneurysm of external carotid artery
Aneurysm of internal carotid artery, extracranial portion

Excludes1 aneurysm of internal carotid artery, intracranial portion (I67.1)
aneurysm of internal carotid artery NOS (I67.1)

I72.1 **Aneurysm of artery of upper extremity**

I72.2 **Aneurysm of renal artery**

I72.3 **Aneurysm of iliac artery**

I72.4 **Aneurysm of artery of lower extremity**
Coding Clinic: 2019, Q2, P22

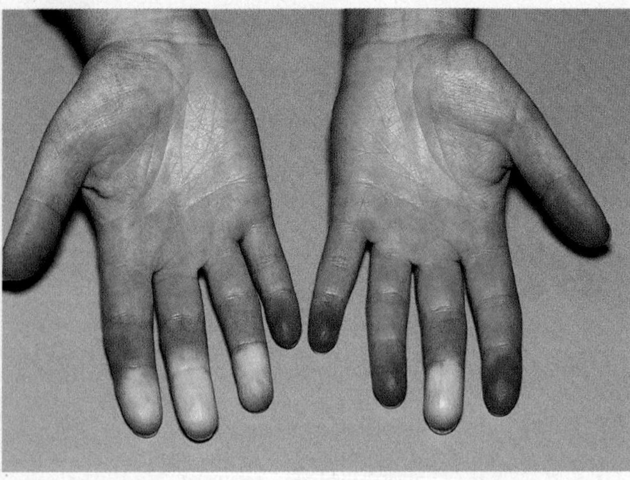

Figure 9-5 Raynaud's syndrome. (From Hallett: Comprehensive Vascular and Endovascular Surgery, ed 2, Philadelphia, Mosby Ltd., 2010)

I72.5 **Aneurysm of other precerebral arteries**
Aneurysm of basilar artery (trunk)
Excludes2 aneurysm of carotid artery (I72.Ø)
aneurysm of vertebral artery (I72.6)
dissection of carotid artery (I77.71)
dissection of other precerebral arteries (I77.75)
dissection of vertebral artery (I77.74)
Coding Clinic: 2016, Q4, P28

I72.6 **Aneurysm of vertebral artery**
Excludes2 dissection of vertebral artery (I77.74)
Coding Clinic: 2016, Q4, P28

I72.8 **Aneurysm of other specified arteries**

I72.9 **Aneurysm of unspecified site**

● I73 **Other peripheral vascular diseases**
Excludes2 chilblains (T69.1)
frostbite (T33-T34)
immersion hand or foot (T69.Ø-)
spasm of cerebral artery (G45.9)
Coding Clinic: 2018, Q4, P87-88

● I73.Ø **Raynaud's syndrome**
Diminishing oxygen supply to fingers, toes, nose, and ears when exposed to temperature changes or stress
Raynaud's disease
Raynaud's phenomenon (secondary)

I73.ØØ **Raynaud's syndrome without gangrene**

I73.Ø1 **Raynaud's syndrome with gangrene** PDX 973
CC when PDx is its own CC

I73.1 **Thromboangiitis obliterans [Buerger's disease]**
Inflammatory occlusive disease resulting in poor circulation to the legs, feet, and sometimes the hands due to progressive inflammatory narrowing and eventually obliteration of the small arteries

● I73.8 **Other specified peripheral vascular diseases**
Excludes1 diabetic (peripheral) angiopathy (EØ8-E13 with .51-.52)

I73.81 **Erythromelalgia**

I73.89 **Other specified peripheral vascular diseases**
Acrocyanosis
Erythrocyanosis
Simple acroparesthesia [Schultze's type]
Vasomotor acroparesthesia [Nothnagel's type]

Item 9-9 An **embolus** is a mass of undissolved matter present in the blood that is transported by the blood current. A **thrombus** is a blood clot that occludes or shuts off a vessel. When a thrombus is dislodged, it becomes an embolus.

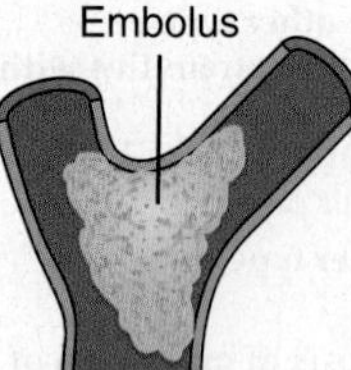

Figure 9-6 An arterial embolus.

I73.9 **Peripheral vascular disease, unspecified**
Intermittent claudication
Peripheral angiopathy NOS
Spasm of artery
Excludes1 atherosclerosis of the extremities (I7Ø.2—I7Ø.7-)
Coding Clinic: 2018, Q4, P87

● I74 **Arterial embolism and thrombosis**
Includes embolic infarction
embolic occlusion
thrombotic infarction
thrombotic occlusion
Code first embolism and thrombosis complicating abortion or ectopic or molar pregnancy (OØØ-OØ7, OØ8.2)
embolism and thrombosis complicating pregnancy, childbirth and the puerperium (O88.-)
Excludes2 atheroembolism (I75.-)
basilar embolism and thrombosis (I63.Ø-I63.2, I65.1)
carotid embolism and thrombosis (I63.Ø-I63.2, I65.2)
cerebral embolism and thrombosis (I63.3-I63.5, I66.-)
coronary embolism and thrombosis (I21-I25)
mesenteric embolism and thrombosis (K55.Ø-)
ophthalmic embolism and thrombosis (H34.-)
precerebral embolism and thrombosis NOS (I63.Ø-I63.2, I65.9)
pulmonary embolism and thrombosis (I26.-)
renal embolism and thrombosis (N28.Ø)
retinal embolism and thrombosis (H34.-)
septic embolism and thrombosis (I76)
vertebral embolism and thrombosis (I63.Ø-I63.2, I65.Ø)
Coding Clinic: 2023, Q2, P7

● I74.Ø **Embolism and thrombosis of abdominal aorta** PDX 856

I74.Ø1 **Saddle embolus of abdominal aorta**

I74.Ø9 **Other arterial embolism and thrombosis of abdominal aorta**
Aortic bifurcation syndrome
Aortoiliac obstruction
Leriche's syndrome

● I74.1 **Embolism and thrombosis of other and unspecified parts of aorta** PDX 856

I74.1Ø **Embolism and thrombosis of unspecified parts of aorta**

I74.11 **Embolism and thrombosis of thoracic aorta** PDX 974

I74.19 **Embolism and thrombosis of other parts of aorta**

I74.2 **Embolism and thrombosis of arteries of the upper extremities** PDX 975

I74.3 **Embolism and thrombosis of arteries of the lower extremities** PDX 976

I74.4 **Embolism and thrombosis of arteries of extremities, unspecified** PDX 976
Peripheral arteria l embolism NOS

I74.5 **Embolism and thrombosis of iliac artery** PDX 977
Coding Clinic: 2023, Q2, P7

I74.8 **Embolism and thrombosis of other arteries** PDX 978

I74.9 **Embolism and thrombosis of unspecified artery** PDX 978

I75 Atheroembolism
Includes atherothrombotic microembolism
cholesterol embolism

I75.0 Atheroembolism of extremities

I75.01 Atheroembolism of upper extremity PDX 979
- I75.011 Atheroembolism of right upper extremity
- I75.012 Atheroembolism of left upper extremity
- I75.013 Atheroembolism of bilateral upper extremities
- I75.019 Atheroembolism of unspecified upper extremity

I75.02 Atheroembolism of lower extremity PDX 980
- I75.021 Atheroembolism of right lower extremity
- I75.022 Atheroembolism of left lower extremity
- I75.023 Atheroembolism of bilateral lower extremities
- I75.029 Atheroembolism of unspecified lower extremity

I75.8 Atheroembolism of other sites
- I75.81 Atheroembolism of kidney PDX 981
  Use additional code for any associated acute kidney failure and chronic kidney disease (N17.-, N18.-)
- I75.89 Atheroembolism of other site PDX 982

I76 Septic arterial embolism PDX 978
Code first underlying infection, such as:
infective endocarditis (I33.0)
lung abscess (J85.-)
Use additional code to identify the site of the embolism (I74.-)
Excludes2 septic pulmonary embolism (I26.01, I26.90)

I77 Other disorders of arteries and arterioles
Excludes2 collagen (vascular) diseases (M30-M36)
hypersensitivity angiitis (M31.0)
pulmonary artery (I28.-)

I77.0 Arteriovenous fistula, acquired
Aneurysmal varix
Arteriovenous aneurysm, acquired
Excludes1 arteriovenous aneurysm NOS (Q27.3-)
presence of arteriovenous shunt (fistula) for dialysis (Z99.2)
traumatic - see injury of blood vessel by body region
Excludes2 cerebral (I67.1)
coronary (I25.4)

I77.1 Stricture of artery
Narrowing of artery
Coding Clinic: 2021, Q3, P13

I77.2 Rupture of artery PDX 983
Erosion of artery
Fistula of artery
Ulcer of artery
Excludes1 traumatic rupture of artery - see injury of blood vessel by body region

I77.3 Arterial fibromuscular dysplasia
Fibromuscular hyperplasia (of) carotid artery
Fibromuscular hyperplasia (of) renal artery

I77.4 Celiac artery compression syndrome PDX 984
Coding Clinic: 2021, Q3, P12-13

I77.5 Necrosis of artery PDX 985

I77.6 Arteritis, unspecified
Aortitis NOS
Endarteritis NOS
Excludes1 arteritis or endarteritis:
aortic arch (M31.4)
cerebral NEC (I67.7)
coronary (I25.89)
deformans (I70.-)
giant cell (M31.5, M31.6)
obliterans (I70.-)
senile (I70.-)

I77.7 Other arterial dissection
Excludes2 dissection of aorta (I71.0-)
dissection of coronary artery (I25.42)
- I77.70 Dissection of unspecified artery PDX 986
  Coding Clinic 2016, Q4, P28
- I77.71 Dissection of carotid artery PDX 987
- I77.72 Dissection of iliac artery PDX 988
- I77.73 Dissection of renal artery PDX 989
- I77.74 Dissection of vertebral artery PDX 990
  Excludes2 aneurysm of vertebral artery (I72.6)
  Coding Clinic 2024, Q1, P26
- I77.75 Dissection of other precerebral arteries PDX 991
  Dissection of basilar artery (trunk)
  Excludes2 aneurysm of carotid artery (I72.0)
  aneurysm of other precerebral arteries (I72.5)
  aneurysm of vertebral artery (I72.6)
  dissection of carotid artery (I77.71)
  dissection of vertebral artery (I77.74)
  Coding Clinic 2016, Q4, P28
- I77.76 Dissection of artery of upper extremity PDX 992
  Coding Clinic 2016, Q4, P28
- I77.77 Dissection of artery of lower extremity PDX 993
  Coding Clinic 2016, Q4, P28
- I77.79 Dissection of other specified artery PDX 994
  Coding Clinic 2016, Q4, P28

I77.8 Other specified disorders of arteries and arterioles
- I77.81 Aortic ectasia
  Ectasis aorta
  Excludes1 aortic aneurysm and dissection (I71.-)
  - I77.810 Thoracic aortic ectasia
  - I77.811 Abdominal aortic ectasia
  - I77.812 Thoracoabdominal aortic ectasia
  - I77.819 Aortic ectasia, unspecified site
- I77.82 Antineutrophilic cytoplasmic antibody [ANCA] vasculitis
  ANCA associated vasculitis
  ANCA positive vasculitis
  Excludes2 eosinophilic granulomatosis with polyangiitis (M30.1)
  granulomatosis with polyangiitis (M31.3-)
  microscopic polyangiitis (M31.7
- I77.89 Other specified disorders of arteries and arterioles
  Coding Clinic 2021, Q1, P23

I77.9 Disorder of arteries and arterioles, unspecified
Coding Clinic 2021, Q1, P4

CHAPTER 9 (I00-I99)

I78 Diseases of capillaries

I78.0 Hereditary hemorrhagic telangiectasia
Rendu-Osler-Weber disease

I78.1 Nevus, non-neoplastic
Araneus nevus
Senile nevus
Spider nevus
Stellar nevus
Excludes1 nevus NOS (D22.-)
vascular NOS (Q82.5)
Excludes2 blue nevus (D22.-)
flammeus nevus (Q82.5)
hairy nevus (D22.-)
melanocytic nevus (D22.-)
pigmented nevus (D22.-)
portwine nevus (Q82.5)
sanguineous nevus (Q82.5)
strawberry nevus (Q82.5)
verrucous nevus (Q82.5)
Coding Clinic: 2019, Q1, P21

I78.8 Other diseases of capillaries

I78.9 Disease of capillaries, unspecified

I79 Disorders of arteries, arterioles and capillaries in diseases classified elsewhere

I79.0 Aneurysm of aorta in diseases classified elsewhere
Code first underlying disease
Excludes1 syphilitic aneurysm (A52.01)

I79.1 Aortitis in diseases classified elsewhere
Code first underlying disease
Excludes1 syphilitic aortitis (A52.02)

I79.8 Other disorders of arteries, arterioles and capillaries in diseases classified elsewhere
Code first underlying disease, such as:
amyloidosis (E85.-)
Excludes1 diabetic (peripheral) angiopathy (E08-E13 with .51-.52)
syphilitic endarteritis (A52.09)
tuberculous endarteritis (A18.89)

DISEASES OF VEINS, LYMPHATIC VESSELS AND LYMPH NODES, NOT ELSEWHERE CLASSIFIED (I80-I89)

I80 Phlebitis and thrombophlebitis
Inflammation of a vein with infiltration of walls (phlebitis)
Includes endophlebitis
inflammation, vein
periphlebitis
suppurative phlebitis
Code first phlebitis and thrombophlebitis complicating abortion, ectopic or molar pregnancy (O00-O07, O08.7)
phlebitis and thrombophlebitis complicating pregnancy, childbirth and the puerperium (O22.-, O87.-)
Excludes1 venous embolism and thrombosis of lower extremities (I82.4-, I82.5-, I82.81-)

I80.0 Phlebitis and thrombophlebitis of superficial vessels of lower extremities
Phlebitis and thrombophlebitis of femoropopliteal vein

I80.00 Phlebitis and thrombophlebitis of superficial vessels of unspecified lower extremity

I80.01 Phlebitis and thrombophlebitis of superficial vessels of right lower extremity

I80.02 Phlebitis and thrombophlebitis of superficial vessels of left lower extremity

I80.03 Phlebitis and thrombophlebitis of superficial vessels of lower extremities, bilateral

I80.1 Phlebitis and thrombophlebitis of femoral vein Ex: PDX 995
Phlebitis and thrombophlebitis of common femoral vein
Phlebitis and thrombophlebitis of deep femoral vein

I80.10 Phlebitis and thrombophlebitis of unspecified femoral vein

I80.11 Phlebitis and thrombophlebitis of right femoral vein

I80.12 Phlebitis and thrombophlebitis of left femoral vein

I80.13 Phlebitis and thrombophlebitis of femoral vein, bilateral

I80.2 Phlebitis and thrombophlebitis of other and unspecified deep vessels of lower extremities

I80.20 Phlebitis and thrombophlebitis of unspecified deep vessels of lower extremities Ex: PDX 995

I80.201 Phlebitis and thrombophlebitis of unspecified deep vessels of right lower extremity

I80.202 Phlebitis and thrombophlebitis of unspecified deep vessels of left lower extremity

I80.203 Phlebitis and thrombophlebitis of unspecified deep vessels of lower extremities, bilateral

I80.209 Phlebitis and thrombophlebitis of unspecified deep vessels of unspecified lower extremity

I80.21 Phlebitis and thrombophlebitis of iliac vein Ex: PDX 995
Phlebitis and thrombophlebitis of common iliac vein
Phlebitis and thrombophlebitis of external iliac vein
Phlebitis and thrombophlebitis of internal iliac vein

I80.211 Phlebitis and thrombophlebitis of right iliac vein

I80.212 Phlebitis and thrombophlebitis of left iliac vein

I80.213 Phlebitis and thrombophlebitis of iliac vein, bilateral

I80.219 Phlebitis and thrombophlebitis of unspecified iliac vein

I80.22 Phlebitis and thrombophlebitis of popliteal vein Ex: PDX 995

I80.221 Phlebitis and thrombophlebitis of right popliteal vein

I80.222 Phlebitis and thrombophlebitis of left popliteal vein

I80.223 Phlebitis and thrombophlebitis of popliteal vein, bilateral

I80.229 Phlebitis and thrombophlebitis of unspecified popliteal vein

I80.23 Phlebitis and thrombophlebitis of tibial vein Ex: PDX 995
Phlebitis and thrombophlebitis of anterior tibial vein
Phlebitis and thrombophlebitis of posterior tibial vein

I80.231 Phlebitis and thrombophlebitis of right tibial vein

I80.232 Phlebitis and thrombophlebitis of left tibial vein

I80.233 Phlebitis and thrombophlebitis of tibial vein, bilateral

I80.239 Phlebitis and thrombophlebitis of unspecified tibial vein

I80.24 Phlebitis and thrombophlebitis of peroneal vein Ex: PDX 995

I80.241 Phlebitis and thrombophlebitis of right peroneal vein

I80.242 Phlebitis and thrombophlebitis of left peroneal vein

I80.243 Phlebitis and thrombophlebitis of peroneal vein, bilateral

I80.249 Phlebitis and thrombophlebitis of unspecified peroneal vein

I80.25 Phlebitis and thrombophlebitis of calf muscular vein
Phlebitis and thrombophlebitis of calf muscular vein, NOS
Phlebitis and thrombophlebitis of gastrocnemial vein
Phlebitis and thrombophlebitis of soleal vein

I80.251 Phlebitis and thrombophlebitis of right calf muscular vein

I80.252 Phlebitis and thrombophlebitis of left calf muscular vein

I80.253 Phlebitis and thrombophlebitis of calf muscular vein, bilateral

I80.259 Phlebitis and thrombophlebitis of unspecified calf muscular vein

I80.29 Phlebitis and thrombophlebitis of other deep vessels of lower extremities (Ex) PDX 995

I80.291 Phlebitis and thrombophlebitis of other deep vessels of right lower extremity

I80.292 Phlebitis and thrombophlebitis of other deep vessels of left lower extremity

I80.293 Phlebitis and thrombophlebitis of other deep vessels of lower extremity, bilateral

I80.299 Phlebitis and thrombophlebitis of other deep vessels of unspecified lower extremity

I80.3 Phlebitis and thrombophlebitis of lower extremities, unspecified

I80.8 Phlebitis and thrombophlebitis of other sites

I80.9 Phlebitis and thrombophlebitis of unspecified site

I81 Portal vein thrombosis (Ex) PDX 996
Portal (vein) obstruction
Excludes2 hepatic vein thrombosis (I82.0)
phlebitis of portal vein (K75.1)
Coding Clinic: 2019, Q4, P68

I82 Other venous embolism and thrombosis (Ex) PDX 999
Code first venous embolism and thrombosis complicating:
abortion, ectopic or molar pregnancy (O00-O07, O08.7)
pregnancy, childbirth and the puerperium (O22.-, O87.-)
Excludes2 venous embolism and thrombosis (of):
cerebral (I63.6, I67.6)
coronary (I21-I25)
intracranial and intraspinal, septic or NOS (G08)
intracranial, nonpyogenic (I67.6)
intraspinal, nonpyogenic (G95.1)
mesenteric (K55.0-)
portal (I81)
pulmonary (I26.-)

I82.0 Budd-Chiari syndrome (Ex) PDX 997
Hepatic vein thrombosis

I82.1 Thrombophlebitis migrans (Ex) PDX 998
"White leg" is the other term to describe a migrating thrombus.

I82.2 Embolism and thrombosis of vena cava and other thoracic veins

I82.21 Embolism and thrombosis of superior vena cava

I82.210 Acute embolism and thrombosis of superior vena cava
Embolism and thrombosis of superior vena cava NOS

I82.211 Chronic embolism and thrombosis of superior vena cava

I82.22 Embolism and thrombosis of inferior vena cava (Ex) PDX 1000

I82.220 Acute embolism and thrombosis of inferior vena cava
Embolism and thrombosis of inferior vena cava NOS

I82.221 Chronic embolism and thrombosis of inferior vena cava

I82.29 Embolism and thrombosis of other thoracic veins
Embolism and thrombosis of brachiocephalic (innominate) vein

I82.290 Acute embolism and thrombosis of other thoracic veins

I82.291 Chronic embolism and thrombosis of other thoracic veins

I82.3 Embolism and thrombosis of renal vein (Ex) PDX 1001

I82.4 Acute embolism and thrombosis of deep veins of lower extremity

I82.40 Acute embolism and thrombosis of unspecified deep veins of lower extremity
Deep vein thrombosis NOS
DVT NOS
Excludes1 acute embolism and thrombosis of unspecified deep veins of distal lower extremity (I82.4Z-)
acute embolism and thrombosis of unspecified deep veins of proximal lower extremity (I82.4Y-)

I82.401 Acute embolism and thrombosis of unspecified deep veins of right lower extremity

I82.402 Acute embolism and thrombosis of unspecified deep veins of left lower extremity

I82.403 Acute embolism and thrombosis of unspecified deep veins of lower extremity, bilateral

I82.409 Acute embolism and thrombosis of unspecified deep veins of unspecified lower extremity

I82.41 Acute embolism and thrombosis of femoral vein
Acute embolism and thrombosis of common femoral vein
Acute embolism and thrombosis of deep femoral vein

I82.411 Acute embolism and thrombosis of right femoral vein

I82.412 Acute embolism and thrombosis of left femoral vein
Coding Clinic: 2023, Q3, P12

I82.413 Acute embolism and thrombosis of femoral vein, bilateral

I82.419 Acute embolism and thrombosis of unspecified femoral vein

I82.42 Acute embolism and thrombosis of iliac vein
Acute embolism and thrombosis of common iliac vein
Acute embolism and thrombosis of external iliac vein
Acute embolism and thrombosis of internal iliac vein

I82.421 Acute embolism and thrombosis of right iliac vein

I82.422 Acute embolism and thrombosis of left iliac vein

I82.423 Acute embolism and thrombosis of iliac vein, bilateral

I82.429 Acute embolism and thrombosis of unspecified iliac vein

CHAPTER 9 (I00-I99)

● I82.43 Acute embolism and thrombosis of popliteal vein
I82.431 Acute embolism and thrombosis of right popliteal vein
I82.432 Acute embolism and thrombosis of left popliteal vein
I82.433 Acute embolism and thrombosis of popliteal vein, bilateral
I82.439 Acute embolism and thrombosis of unspecified popliteal vein

● I82.44 Acute embolism and thrombosis of tibial vein
Acute embolism and thrombosis of anterior tibial vein
Acute embolism and thrombosis of posterior tibial vein
I82.441 Acute embolism and thrombosis of right tibial vein
I82.442 Acute embolism and thrombosis of left tibial vein
I82.443 Acute embolism and thrombosis of tibial vein, bilateral
I82.449 Acute embolism and thrombosis of unspecified tibial vein

● I82.45 Acute embolism and thrombosis of peroneal vein
I82.451 Acute embolism and thrombosis of right peroneal vein
I82.452 Acute embolism and thrombosis of left peroneal vein
I82.453 Acute embolism and thrombosis of peroneal vein, bilateral
I82.459 Acute embolism and thrombosis of unspecified peroneal vein

● I82.46 Acute embolism and thrombosis of calf muscular vein
Acute embolism and thrombosis of calf muscular vein, NOS
Acute embolism and thrombosis of gastrocnemial vein
Acute embolism and thrombosis of soleal vein
I82.461 Acute embolism and thrombosis of right calf muscular vein
I82.462 Acute embolism and thrombosis of left calf muscular vein
I82.463 Acute embolism and thrombosis of calf muscular vein, bilateral
I82.469 Acute embolism and thrombosis of unspecified calf muscular vein

● I82.49 Acute embolism and thrombosis of other specified deep vein of lower extremity
I82.491 Acute embolism and thrombosis of other specified deep vein of right lower extremity
I82.492 Acute embolism and thrombosis of other specified deep vein of left lower extremity
I82.493 Acute embolism and thrombosis of other specified deep vein of lower extremity, bilateral
I82.499 Acute embolism and thrombosis of other specified deep vein of unspecified lower extremity

● I82.4Y Acute embolism and thrombosis of unspecified deep veins of proximal lower extremity
Acute embolism and thrombosis of deep vein of thigh NOS
Acute embolism and thrombosis of deep vein of upper leg NOS
I82.4Y1 Acute embolism and thrombosis of unspecified deep veins of right proximal lower extremity
I82.4Y2 Acute embolism and thrombosis of unspecified deep veins of left proximal lower extremity
I82.4Y3 Acute embolism and thrombosis of unspecified deep veins of proximal lower extremity, bilateral
I82.4Y9 Acute embolism and thrombosis of unspecified deep veins of unspecified proximal lower extremity

● I82.4Z Acute embolism and thrombosis of unspecified deep veins of distal lower extremity
Acute embolism and thrombosis of deep vein of calf NOS
Acute embolism and thrombosis of deep vein of lower leg NOS
I82.4Z1 Acute embolism and thrombosis of unspecified deep veins of right distal lower extremity
I82.4Z2 Acute embolism and thrombosis of unspecified deep veins of left distal lower extremity
I82.4Z3 Acute embolism and thrombosis of unspecified deep veins of distal lower extremity, bilateral
I82.4Z9 Acute embolism and thrombosis of unspecified deep veins of unspecified distal lower extremity

● I82.5 Chronic embolism and thrombosis of deep veins of lower extremity Ex PDX 717
Use additional code, if applicable, for associated long-term (current) use of anticoagulants (Z79.01)
Excludes1 personal history of venous embolism and thrombosis (Z86.718)

● I82.50 Chronic embolism and thrombosis of unspecified deep veins of lower extremity
Excludes1 chronic embolism and thrombosis of unspecified deep veins of distal lower extremity (I82.5Z-)
chronic embolism and thrombosis of unspecified deep veins of proximal lower extremity (I82.5Y-)
I82.501 Chronic embolism and thrombosis of unspecified deep veins of right lower extremity
I82.502 Chronic embolism and thrombosis of unspecified deep veins of left lower extremity
I82.503 Chronic embolism and thrombosis of unspecified deep veins of lower extremity, bilateral
I82.509 Chronic embolism and thrombosis of unspecified deep veins of unspecified lower extremity

● I82.51 Chronic embolism and thrombosis of femoral vein
Chronic embolism and thrombosis of common femoral vein
Chronic embolism and thrombosis of deep femoral vein
I82.511 Chronic embolism and thrombosis of right femoral vein
I82.512 Chronic embolism and thrombosis of left femoral vein
I82.513 Chronic embolism and thrombosis of femoral vein, bilateral
I82.519 Chronic embolism and thrombosis of unspecified femoral vein

Item 9–10 Varicose/Varicosities (varix = singular, varices = plural): Enlarged, engorged, tortuous, twisted vascular vessels (veins, arteries, lymphatics). As such, the condition can present in various parts of the body, although the most familiar locations are the lower extremities. A common complication of varices is thrombophlebitis. Varicosities of the anus and rectum are called hemorrhoids.

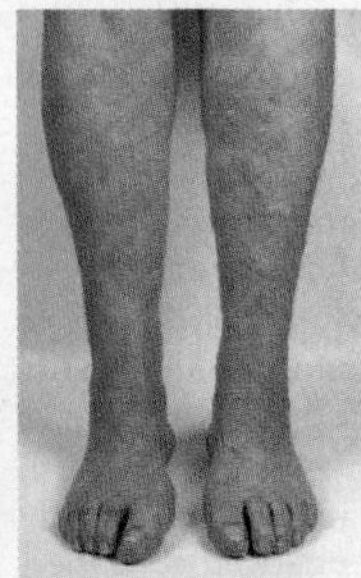

Figure 9-7 Varicose veins of the legs. (Getty Image)

● I82.52 **Chronic embolism and thrombosis of iliac vein**
Chronic embolism and thrombosis of common iliac vein
Chronic embolism and thrombosis of external iliac vein
Chronic embolism and thrombosis of internal iliac vein

I82.521 **Chronic embolism and thrombosis of right iliac vein**

I82.522 **Chronic embolism and thrombosis of left iliac vein**

I82.523 **Chronic embolism and thrombosis of iliac vein, bilateral**

I82.529 **Chronic embolism and thrombosis of unspecified iliac vein**

● I82.53 **Chronic embolism and thrombosis of popliteal vein**

I82.531 **Chronic embolism and thrombosis of right popliteal vein**

I82.532 **Chronic embolism and thrombosis of left popliteal vein**

I82.533 **Chronic embolism and thrombosis of popliteal vein, bilateral**

I82.539 **Chronic embolism and thrombosis of unspecified popliteal vein**

● I82.54 **Chronic embolism and thrombosis of tibial vein**
Chronic embolism and thrombosis of anterior tibial vein
Chronic embolism and thrombosis of posterior tibial vein

I82.541 **Chronic embolism and thrombosis of right tibial vein**

I82.542 **Chronic embolism and thrombosis of left tibial vein**

I82.543 **Chronic embolism and thrombosis of tibial vein, bilateral**

I82.549 **Chronic embolism and thrombosis of unspecified tibial vein**

● I82.55 **Chronic embolism and thrombosis of peroneal vein**

I82.551 **Chronic embolism and thrombosis of right peroneal vein**

I82.552 **Chronic embolism and thrombosis of left peroneal vein**

I82.553 **Chronic embolism and thrombosis of peroneal vein, bilateral**

I82.559 **Chronic embolism and thrombosis of unspecified peroneal vein**

● I82.56 **Chronic embolism and thrombosis of calf muscular vein**
Chronic embolism and thrombosis of calf muscular vein NOS
Chronic embolism and thrombosis of gastrocnemial vein
Chronic embolism and thrombosis of soleal vein

I82.561 **Chronic embolism and thrombosis of right calf muscular vein**

I82.562 **Chronic embolism and thrombosis of left calf muscular vein**

I82.563 **Chronic embolism and thrombosis of calf muscular vein, bilateral**

I82.569 **Chronic embolism and thrombosis of unspecified calf muscular vein**

● I82.59 **Chronic embolism and thrombosis of other specified deep vein of lower extremity**

I82.591 **Chronic embolism and thrombosis of other specified deep vein of right lower extremity**

I82.592 **Chronic embolism and thrombosis of other specified deep vein of left lower extremity**

I82.593 **Chronic embolism and thrombosis of other specified deep vein of lower extremity, bilateral**

I82.599 **Chronic embolism and thrombosis of other specified deep vein of unspecified lower extremity**

● I82.5Y **Chronic embolism and thrombosis of unspecified deep veins of proximal lower extremity**
Chronic embolism and thrombosis of deep veins of thigh NOS
Chronic embolism and thrombosis of deep veins of upper leg NOS

I82.5Y1 **Chronic embolism and thrombosis of unspecified deep veins of right proximal lower extremity**

I82.5Y2 **Chronic embolism and thrombosis of unspecified deep veins of left proximal lower extremity**

I82.5Y3 **Chronic embolism and thrombosis of unspecified deep veins of proximal lower extremity, bilateral**

I82.5Y9 **Chronic embolism and thrombosis of unspecified deep veins of unspecified proximal lower extremity**

● I82.5Z **Chronic embolism and thrombosis of unspecified deep veins of distal lower extremity**
Chronic embolism and thrombosis of deep veins of calf NOS
Chronic embolism and thrombosis of deep veins of lower leg NOS

I82.5Z1 **Chronic embolism and thrombosis of unspecified deep veins of right distal lower extremity**

I82.5Z2 **Chronic embolism and thrombosis of unspecified deep veins of left distal lower extremity**

I82.5Z3 **Chronic embolism and thrombosis of unspecified deep veins of distal lower extremity, bilateral**

I82.5Z9 **Chronic embolism and thrombosis of unspecified deep veins of unspecified distal lower extremity**

CHAPTER 9 (I00-I99)

- **I82.6 Acute embolism and thrombosis of veins of upper extremity** Ex PDX 717
  - **I82.60 Acute embolism and thrombosis of unspecified veins of upper extremity**
    - **I82.601 Acute embolism and thrombosis of unspecified veins of right upper extremity**
    - **I82.602 Acute embolism and thrombosis of unspecified veins of left upper extremity**
    - **I82.603 Acute embolism and thrombosis of unspecified veins of upper extremity, bilateral**
    - **I82.609 Acute embolism and thrombosis of unspecified veins of unspecified upper extremity**
  - **I82.61 Acute embolism and thrombosis of superficial veins of upper extremity**
    - Acute embolism and thrombosis of antecubital vein
    - Acute embolism and thrombosis of basilic vein
    - Acute embolism and thrombosis of cephalic vein
    - **I82.611 Acute embolism and thrombosis of superficial veins of right upper extremity**
    - **I82.612 Acute embolism and thrombosis of superficial veins of left upper extremity**
    - **I82.613 Acute embolism and thrombosis of superficial veins of upper extremity, bilateral**
    - **I82.619 Acute embolism and thrombosis of superficial veins of unspecified upper extremity**
  - **I82.62 Acute embolism and thrombosis of deep veins of upper extremity**
    - Acute embolism and thrombosis of brachial vein
    - Acute embolism and thrombosis of radial vein
    - Acute embolism and thrombosis of ulnar vein
    - **I82.621 Acute embolism and thrombosis of deep veins of right upper extremity**
    - **I82.622 Acute embolism and thrombosis of deep veins of left upper extremity**
    - **I82.623 Acute embolism and thrombosis of deep veins of upper extremity, bilateral**
    - **I82.629 Acute embolism and thrombosis of deep veins of unspecified upper extremity**
- **I82.7 Chronic embolism and thrombosis of veins of upper extremity** Ex PDX 717
  - Use additional code, if applicable, for associated long-term (current) use of anticoagulants (Z79.Ø1)
  - **Excludes1** personal history of venous embolism and thrombosis (Z86.718)
  - **I82.7Ø Chronic embolism and thrombosis of unspecified veins of upper extremity**
    - **I82.7Ø1 Chronic embolism and thrombosis of unspecified veins of right upper extremity**
    - **I82.7Ø2 Chronic embolism and thrombosis of unspecified veins of left upper extremity**
    - **I82.7Ø3 Chronic embolism and thrombosis of unspecified veins of upper extremity, bilateral**
    - **I82.7Ø9 Chronic embolism and thrombosis of unspecified veins of unspecified upper extremity**
  - **I82.71 Chronic embolism and thrombosis of superficial veins of upper extremity**
    - Chronic embolism and thrombosis of antecubital vein
    - Chronic embolism and thrombosis of basilic vein
    - Chronic embolism and thrombosis of cephalic vein
    - **I82.711 Chronic embolism and thrombosis of superficial veins of right upper extremity**
    - **I82.712 Chronic embolism and thrombosis of superficial veins of left upper extremity**
    - **I82.713 Chronic embolism and thrombosis of superficial veins of upper extremity, bilateral**
    - **I82.719 Chronic embolism and thrombosis of superficial veins of unspecified upper extremity**
  - **I82.72 Chronic embolism and thrombosis of deep veins of upper extremity**
    - Chronic embolism and thrombosis of brachial vein
    - Chronic embolism and thrombosis of radial vein
    - Chronic embolism and thrombosis of ulnar vein
    - **I82.721 Chronic embolism and thrombosis of deep veins of right upper extremity**
    - **I82.722 Chronic embolism and thrombosis of deep veins of left upper extremity**
    - **I82.723 Chronic embolism and thrombosis of deep veins of upper extremity, bilateral**
    - **I82.729 Chronic embolism and thrombosis of deep veins of unspecified upper extremity**
- **I82.8 Embolism and thrombosis of other specified veins**
  - Use additional code, if applicable, for associated long-term (current) use of anticoagulants (Z79.Ø1)
  - **I82.81 Embolism and thrombosis of superficial veins of lower extremities**
    - Embolism and thrombosis of saphenous vein (greater) (lesser)
    - **I82.811 Embolism and thrombosis of superficial veins of right lower extremity**
    - **I82.812 Embolism and thrombosis of superficial veins of left lower extremity**
    - **I82.813 Embolism and thrombosis of superficial veins of lower extremities, bilateral**
    - **I82.819 Embolism and thrombosis of superficial veins of unspecified lower extremity**
  - **I82.89 Embolism and thrombosis of other specified veins**
    - **I82.89Ø Acute embolism and thrombosis of other specified veins**
    - **I82.891 Chronic embolism and thrombosis of other specified veins**
- **I82.9 Embolism and thrombosis of unspecified vein**
  - **I82.9Ø Acute embolism and thrombosis of unspecified vein**
    - Embolism of vein NOS
    - Thrombosis (vein) NOS
  - **I82.91 Chronic embolism and thrombosis of unspecified vein**

CHAPTER 9 (IØØ-I99)

I82.A Embolism and thrombosis of axillary vein

I82.A1 Acute embolism and thrombosis of axillary vein

I82.A11 Acute embolism and thrombosis of right axillary vein

I82.A12 Acute embolism and thrombosis of left axillary vein

I82.A13 Acute embolism and thrombosis of axillary vein, bilateral

I82.A19 Acute embolism and thrombosis of unspecified axillary vein

I82.A2 Chronic embolism and thrombosis of axillary vein

I82.A21 Chronic embolism and thrombosis of right axillary vein

I82.A22 Chronic embolism and thrombosis of left axillary vein

I82.A23 Chronic embolism and thrombosis of axillary vein, bilateral

I82.A29 Chronic embolism and thrombosis of unspecified axillary vein

I82.B Embolism and thrombosis of subclavian vein

I82.B1 Acute embolism and thrombosis of subclavian vein

I82.B11 Acute embolism and thrombosis of right subclavian vein

I82.B12 Acute embolism and thrombosis of left subclavian vein

I82.B13 Acute embolism and thrombosis of subclavian vein, bilateral

I82.B19 Acute embolism and thrombosis of unspecified subclavian vein

I82.B2 Chronic embolism and thrombosis of subclavian vein

I82.B21 Chronic embolism and thrombosis of right subclavian vein

I82.B22 Chronic embolism and thrombosis of left subclavian vein

I82.B23 Chronic embolism and thrombosis of subclavian vein, bilateral

I82.B29 Chronic embolism and thrombosis of unspecified subclavian vein

I82.C Embolism and thrombosis of internal jugular vein

I82.C1 Acute embolism and thrombosis of internal jugular vein

I82.C11 Acute embolism and thrombosis of right internal jugular vein

I82.C12 Acute embolism and thrombosis of left internal jugular vein

I82.C13 Acute embolism and thrombosis of internal jugular vein, bilateral

I82.C19 Acute embolism and thrombosis of unspecified internal jugular vein

I82.C2 Chronic embolism and thrombosis of internal jugular vein

I82.C21 Chronic embolism and thrombosis of right internal jugular vein

I82.C22 Chronic embolism and thrombosis of left internal jugular vein

I82.C23 Chronic embolism and thrombosis of internal jugular vein, bilateral

I82.C29 Chronic embolism and thrombosis of unspecified internal jugular vein

I83 Varicose veins of lower extremities

Excludes2 varicose veins complicating pregnancy (O22.Ø-)
varicose veins complicating the puerperium (O87.4)

I83.Ø Varicose veins of lower extremities with ulcer

Use additional code to identify severity of ulcer (L97.-)

I83.ØØ Varicose veins of unspecified lower extremity with ulcer

I83.ØØ1 Varicose veins of unspecified lower extremity with ulcer of thigh A

I83.ØØ2 Varicose veins of unspecified lower extremity with ulcer of calf A

I83.ØØ3 Varicose veins of unspecified lower extremity with ulcer of ankle A

I83.ØØ4 Varicose veins of unspecified lower extremity with ulcer of heel and midfoot A

Varicose veins of unspecified lower extremity with ulcer of plantar surface of midfoot

I83.ØØ5 Varicose veins of unspecified lower extremity with ulcer other part of foot A

Varicose veins of unspecified lower extremity with ulcer of toe

I83.ØØ8 Varicose veins of unspecified lower extremity with ulcer other part of lower leg A

I83.ØØ9 Varicose veins of unspecified lower extremity with ulcer of unspecified site A

I83.Ø1 Varicose veins of right lower extremity with ulcer

I83.Ø11 Varicose veins of right lower extremity with ulcer of thigh A

I83.Ø12 Varicose veins of right lower extremity with ulcer of calf A

I83.Ø13 Varicose veins of right lower extremity with ulcer of ankle A

I83.Ø14 Varicose veins of right lower extremity with ulcer of heel and midfoot A

Varicose veins of right lower extremity with ulcer of plantar surface of midfoot

I83.Ø15 Varicose veins of right lower extremity with ulcer other part of foot A

Varicose veins of right lower extremity with ulcer of toe

I83.Ø18 Varicose veins of right lower extremity with ulcer other part of lower leg A

I83.Ø19 Varicose veins of right lower extremity with ulcer of unspecified site A

I83.Ø2 Varicose veins of left lower extremity with ulcer

I83.Ø21 Varicose veins of left lower extremity with ulcer of thigh A

I83.Ø22 Varicose veins of left lower extremity with ulcer of calf A

I83.Ø23 Varicose veins of left lower extremity with ulcer of ankle A

I83.Ø24 Varicose veins of left lower extremity with ulcer of heel and midfoot A

Varicose veins of left lower extremity with ulcer of plantar surface of midfoot

I83.Ø25 Varicose veins of left lower extremity with ulcer other part of foot A

Varicose veins of left lower extremity with ulcer of toe

I83.Ø28 Varicose veins of left lower extremity with ulcer other part of lower leg A

I83.Ø29 Varicose veins of left lower extremity with ulcer of unspecified site A

- I83.1 **Varicose veins of lower extremities with inflammation**
  - I83.1Ø **Varicose veins of unspecified lower extremity with inflammation** A
  - I83.11 **Varicose veins of right lower extremity with inflammation** A
  - I83.12 **Varicose veins of left lower extremity with inflammation** A
- I83.2 **Varicose veins of lower extremities with both ulcer and inflammation** Ex PDX 1002
  - Use additional code to identify severity of ulcer (L97.-)
  - I83.2Ø **Varicose veins of unspecified lower extremity with both ulcer and inflammation**
    - I83.2Ø1 **Varicose veins of unspecified lower extremity with both ulcer of thigh and inflammation** A
    - I83.2Ø2 **Varicose veins of unspecified lower extremity with both ulcer of calf and inflammation** A
    - I83.2Ø3 **Varicose veins of unspecified lower extremity with both ulcer of ankle and inflammation** A
    - I83.2Ø4 **Varicose veins of unspecified lower extremity with both ulcer of heel and midfoot and inflammation** A
      - Varicose veins of unspecified lower extremity with both ulcer of plantar surface of midfoot and inflammation
    - I83.2Ø5 **Varicose veins of unspecified lower extremity with both ulcer other part of foot and inflammation** A
      - Varicose veins of unspecified lower extremity with both ulcer of toe and inflammation
    - I83.2Ø8 **Varicose veins of unspecified lower extremity with both ulcer of other part of lower extremity and inflammation** A
    - I83.2Ø9 **Varicose veins of unspecified lower extremity with both ulcer of unspecified site and inflammation** A
  - I83.21 **Varicose veins of right lower extremity with both ulcer and inflammation**
    - I83.211 **Varicose veins of right lower extremity with both ulcer of thigh and inflammation** A
    - I83.212 **Varicose veins of right lower extremity with both ulcer of calf and inflammation** A
    - I83.213 **Varicose veins of right lower extremity with both ulcer of ankle and inflammation** A
    - I83.214 **Varicose veins of right lower extremity with both ulcer of heel and midfoot and inflammation** A
      - Varicose veins of right lower extremity with both ulcer of plantar surface of midfoot and inflammation
    - I83.215 **Varicose veins of right lower extremity with both ulcer other part of foot and inflammation** A
      - Varicose veins of right lower extremity with both ulcer of toe and inflammation
    - I83.218 **Varicose veins of right lower extremity with both ulcer of other part of lower extremity and inflammation** A
    - I83.219 **Varicose veins of right lower extremity with both ulcer of unspecified site and inflammation** A
  - I83.22 **Varicose veins of left lower extremity with both ulcer and inflammation**
    - I83.221 **Varicose veins of left lower extremity with both ulcer of thigh and inflammation** A
    - I83.222 **Varicose veins of left lower extremity with both ulcer of calf and inflammation** A
    - I83.223 **Varicose veins of left lower extremity with both ulcer of ankle and inflammation** A
    - I83.224 **Varicose veins of left lower extremity with both ulcer of heel and midfoot and inflammation** A
      - Varicose veins of left lower extremity with both ulcer of plantar surface of midfoot and inflammation
    - I83.225 **Varicose veins of left lower extremity with both ulcer other part of foot and inflammation** A
      - Varicose veins of left lower extremity with both ulcer of toe and inflammation
    - I83.228 **Varicose veins of left lower extremity with both ulcer of other part of lower extremity and inflammation** A
    - I83.229 **Varicose veins of left lower extremity with both ulcer of unspecified site and inflammation** A
- I83.8 **Varicose veins of lower extremities with other complications**
  - I83.81 **Varicose veins of lower extremities with pain**
    - I83.811 **Varicose veins of right lower extremity with pain** A
    - I83.812 **Varicose veins of left lower extremity with pain** A
    - I83.813 **Varicose veins of bilateral lower extremities with pain** A
    - I83.819 **Varicose veins of unspecified lower extremity with pain** A
  - I83.89 **Varicose veins of lower extremities with other complications**
    - Varicose veins of lower extremities with edema
    - Varicose veins of lower extremities with swelling
    - I83.891 **Varicose veins of right lower extremity with other complications** A
    - I83.892 **Varicose veins of left lower extremity with other complications** A
    - I83.893 **Varicose veins of bilateral lower extremities with other complications** A
    - I83.899 **Varicose veins of unspecified lower extremity with other complications** A
- I83.9 **Asymptomatic varicose veins of lower extremities**
  - Phlebectasia of lower extremities
  - Varicose veins of lower extremities
  - Varix of lower extremities
  - I83.9Ø **Asymptomatic varicose veins of unspecified lower extremity** A
    - Varicose veins NOS
  - I83.91 **Asymptomatic varicose veins of right lower extremity** A
  - I83.92 **Asymptomatic varicose veins of left lower extremity** A
  - I83.93 **Asymptomatic varicose veins of bilateral lower extremities** A

I85 Esophageal varices

Use additional code to identify:
alcohol abuse and dependence (F1Ø.-)

- I85.Ø **Esophageal varices**
  - Idiopathic esophageal varices
  - Primary esophageal varices

I85.00 Esophageal varices without bleeding (Ex) PDX 1003
Esophageal varices NOS

I85.01 Esophageal varices with bleeding (Ex) PDX 1004

● I85.1 Secondary esophageal varices
Esophageal varices secondary to alcoholic liver disease
Esophageal varices secondary to cirrhosis of liver
Esophageal varices secondary to schistosomiasis
Esophageal varices secondary to toxic liver disease
Code first underlying disease

I85.10 Secondary esophageal varices without bleeding (Ex) PDX 1005

I85.11 Secondary esophageal varices with bleeding (Ex) PDX 1006

● I86 Varicose veins of other sites
Excludes1 varicose veins of unspecified site (I83.9-)
Excludes2 retinal varices (H35.0-)

I86.0 Sublingual varices

I86.1 Scrotal varices
Varicocele

I86.2 Pelvic varices

I86.3 Vulval varices
Excludes1 vulval varices complicating childbirth and the puerperium (O87.8)
vulval varices complicating pregnancy (O22.1-)

I86.4 Gastric varices

I86.8 Varicose veins of other specified sites A
Varicose ulcer of nasal septum

● I87 Other disorders of veins

● I87.0 Postthrombotic syndrome
Chronic venous hypertension due to deep vein thrombosis
Postphlebitic syndrome
Excludes1 chronic venous hypertension without deep vein thrombosis (I87.3-)

● I87.00 Postthrombotic syndrome without complications
Asymptomatic Postthrombotic syndrome

I87.001 Postthrombotic syndrome without complications of right lower extremity

I87.002 Postthrombotic syndrome without complications of left lower extremity

I87.003 Postthrombotic syndrome without complications of bilateral lower extremity

I87.009 Postthrombotic syndrome without complications of unspecified extremity
Postthrombotic syndrome NOS

● I87.01 Postthrombotic syndrome with ulcer
Use additional code to specify site and severity of ulcer (L97.-)

I87.011 Postthrombotic syndrome with ulcer of right lower extremity (Ex) PDX 1007

I87.012 Postthrombotic syndrome with ulcer of left lower extremity (Ex) PDX 1008

I87.013 Postthrombotic syndrome with ulcer of bilateral lower extremity (Ex) PDX 1009

I87.019 Postthrombotic syndrome with ulcer of unspecified lower extremity (Ex) PDX 1010

● I87.02 Postthrombotic syndrome with inflammation

I87.021 Postthrombotic syndrome with inflammation of right lower extremity

I87.022 Postthrombotic syndrome with inflammation of left lower extremity

I87.023 Postthrombotic syndrome with inflammation of bilateral lower extremity

I87.029 Postthrombotic syndrome with inflammation of unspecified lower extremity

● I87.03 Postthrombotic syndrome with ulcer and inflammation
Use additional code to specify site and severity of ulcer (L97.-)

I87.031 Postthrombotic syndrome with ulcer and inflammation of right lower extremity (Ex) PDX 1011

I87.032 Postthrombotic syndrome with ulcer and inflammation of left lower extremity (Ex) PDX 1012

I87.033 Postthrombotic syndrome with ulcer and inflammation of bilateral lower extremity (Ex) PDX 1013

I87.039 Postthrombotic syndrome with ulcer and inflammation of unspecified lower extremity (Ex) PDX 1014

● I87.09 Postthrombotic syndrome with other complications

I87.091 Postthrombotic syndrome with other complications of right lower extremity

I87.092 Postthrombotic syndrome with other complications of left lower extremity

I87.093 Postthrombotic syndrome with other complications of bilateral lower extremity

I87.099 Postthrombotic syndrome with other complications of unspecified lower extremity

I87.1 Compression of vein (Ex) PDX 1015
Stricture of vein
Vena cava syndrome (inferior) (superior)
Excludes2 compression of pulmonary vein (I28.8)
Coding Clinic: 2023, Q2, P8

I87.2 Venous insufficiency (chronic) (peripheral)
Stasis dermatitis
Code also, if applicable, associated hypertensive conditions such as:
essential (primary) hypertension (I10)
hypertensive chronic kidney disease (I12.-)
hypertensive heart and chronic kidney disease (I13.-)
hypertensive heart disease (I11.-)
Use Additional code, if applicable, to specify site and severity of ulcer (L97.-)
Excludes1 stasis dermatitis with varicose veins of lower extremities (I83.1-, I83.2-)
Coding Clinic: 2024, Q1, P16

● I87.3 Chronic venous hypertension (idiopathic)
Stasis edema
Excludes1 chronic venous hypertension due to deep vein thrombosis (I87.0-)
varicose veins of lower extremities (I83.-)

● I87.30 Chronic venous hypertension (idiopathic) without complications
Asymptomatic chronic venous hypertension (idiopathic)

I87.301 Chronic venous hypertension (idiopathic) without complications of right lower extremity

I87.302 Chronic venous hypertension (idiopathic) without complications of left lower extremity

I87.303 Chronic venous hypertension (idiopathic) without complications of bilateral lower extremity

I87.309 Chronic venous hypertension (idiopathic) without complications of unspecified lower extremity
Chronic venous hypertension NOS

CHAPTER 9 (I00-I99)

● I87.31 Chronic venous hypertension (idiopathic) with ulcer
Use additional code to specify site and severity of ulcer (L97.-)

I87.311 **Chronic venous hypertension (idiopathic) with ulcer of right lower extremity** (Ex) PDX 1016

I87.312 **Chronic venous hypertension (idiopathic) with ulcer of left lower extremity** (Ex) PDX 1017

I87.313 **Chronic venous hypertension (idiopathic) with ulcer of bilateral lower extremity** (Ex) PDX 1018

I87.319 **Chronic venous hypertension (idiopathic) with ulcer of unspecified lower extremity** (Ex) PDX 1019

● I87.32 Chronic venous hypertension (idiopathic) with inflammation

I87.321 **Chronic venous hypertension (idiopathic) with inflammation of right lower extremity**

I87.322 **Chronic venous hypertension (idiopathic) with inflammation of left lower extremity**

I87.323 **Chronic venous hypertension (idiopathic) with inflammation of bilateral lower extremity**

I87.329 **Chronic venous hypertension (idiopathic) with inflammation of unspecified lower extremity**

● I87.33 Chronic venous hypertension (idiopathic) with ulcer and inflammation
Use additional code to specify site and severity of ulcer (L97.-)

I87.331 **Chronic venous hypertension (idiopathic) with ulcer and inflammation of right lower extremity** (Ex) PDX 1020

I87.332 **Chronic venous hypertension (idiopathic) with ulcer and inflammation of left lower extremity** (Ex) PDX 1021

I87.333 **Chronic venous hypertension (idiopathic) with ulcer and inflammation of bilateral lower extremity** (Ex) PDX 1022

I87.339 **Chronic venous hypertension (idiopathic) with ulcer and inflammation of unspecified lower extremity** (Ex) PDX 1023

● I87.39 Chronic venous hypertension (idiopathic) with other complications

I87.391 **Chronic venous hypertension (idiopathic) with other complications of right lower extremity**

I87.392 **Chronic venous hypertension (idiopathic) with other complications of left lower extremity**

I87.393 **Chronic venous hypertension (idiopathic) with other complications of bilateral lower extremity**

I87.399 **Chronic venous hypertension (idiopathic) with other complications of unspecified lower extremity**

I87.8 **Other specified disorders of veins**
Phlebosclerosis
Venofibrosis

I87.9 **Disorder of vein, unspecified**

● I88 Nonspecific lymphadenitis
Excludes1 acute lymphadenitis, except mesenteric (LØ4.-)
enlarged lymph nodes NOS (R59.-)
human immunodeficiency virus [HIV] disease resulting in generalized lymphadenopathy (B2Ø)

I88.Ø **Nonspecific mesenteric lymphadenitis**
Mesenteric lymphadenitis (acute)(chronic)

I88.1 **Chronic lymphadenitis, except mesenteric**
Adenitis
Lymphadenitis

I88.8 **Other nonspecific lymphadenitis**

I88.9 **Nonspecific lymphadenitis, unspecified**
Lymphadenitis NOS

● I89 Other noninfective disorders of lymphatic vessels and lymph nodes
Excludes1 chylocele, tunica vaginalis (nonfilarial) NOS (N5Ø.89)
enlarged lymph nodes NOS (R59.-)
filarial chylocele (B74.-)
hereditary lymphedema (Q82.Ø)

I89.Ø **Lymphedema, not elsewhere classified**
Elephantiasis (nonfilarial) NOS
Lymphangiectasis
Obliteration, lymphatic vessel
Praecox lymphedema
Secondary lymphedema
Excludes1 postmastectomy lymphedema (I97.2)
Coding Clinic: 2024, Q1, P17

I89.1 **Lymphangitis**
Chronic lymphangitis
Lymphangitis NOS
Subacute lymphangitis
Excludes1 acute lymphangitis (LØ3.-)

I89.8 **Other specified noninfective disorders of lymphatic vessels and lymph nodes**
Chylocele (nonfilarial)
Chylous ascites
Chylous cyst
Lipomelanotic reticulosis
Lymph node or vessel fistula
Lymph node or vessel infarction
Lymph node or vessel rupture

I89.9 **Noninfective disorder of lymphatic vessels and lymph nodes, unspecified**
Disease of lymphatic vessels NOS

OTHER AND UNSPECIFIED DISORDERS OF THE CIRCULATORY SYSTEM (I95-I99)

● I95 Hypotension
Subnormal arterial blood pressure
Excludes1 cardiovascular collapse (R57.9)
maternal hypotension syndrome (O26.5-)
nonspecific low blood pressure reading NOS (RØ3.1)

I95.Ø **Idiopathic hypotension**

I95.1 **Orthostatic hypotension**
Hypotension, postural
Moving from a sitting or reclining position to a standing position precipitates a sudden drop in blood pressure (hypotension).
Excludes1 neurogenic orthostatic hypotension [Shy-Drager] (G9Ø.3)
orthostatic hypotension due to drugs (I95.2)
Coding Clinic: 2023, Q2, P9

I95.2 **Hypotension due to drugs**
Orthostatic hypotension due to drugs
Use additional code for adverse effect, if applicable, to identify drug (T36-T5Ø with fifth or sixth character 5)

I95.3 **Hypotension of hemodialysis**
Intra-dialytic hypotension

I95.8 Other hypotension

I95.81 Postprocedural hypotension

I95.89 Other hypotension

Chronic hypotension

I95.9 Hypotension, unspecified

I96 Gangrene, not elsewhere classified (Ex:) PDX 579

Gangrenous cellulitis

Excludes1 gangrene in atherosclerosis of native arteries of the extremities (I70.26)
gangrene of certain specified sites - *see* Alphabetical Index
gangrene in hernia (K40.1, K40.4, K41.1, K41.4, K42.1, K43.1-, K44.1, K45.1, K46.1)
gangrene in other peripheral vascular diseases (I73.-)
gas gangrene (A48.0)
pyoderma gangrenosum (L88)

Excludes2 gangrene in diabetes mellitus (E08-E13 with .52)

Coding Clinic: 2018, Q4, P87; 2017, Q3, P6; 2013, Q2, P35

I97 Intraoperative and postprocedural complications and disorders of circulatory system, not elsewhere classified

Excludes2 postprocedural shock (T81.1-)

Coding Clinic: 2019, Q2, P22

I97.0 Postcardiotomy syndrome

I97.1 Other postprocedural cardiac functional disturbances (Ex:) PDX 1024

Excludes2 acute pulmonary insufficiency following thoracic surgery (J95.1)
intraoperative cardiac functional disturbances (I97.7-)

I97.11 Postprocedural cardiac insufficiency

I97.110 Postprocedural cardiac insufficiency following cardiac surgery

I97.111 Postprocedural cardiac insufficiency following other surgery

I97.12 Postprocedural cardiac arrest

I97.120 Postprocedural cardiac arrest following cardiac surgery

I97.121 Postprocedural cardiac arrest following other surgery

I97.13 Postprocedural heart failure

Use additional code to identify the heart failure (I50.-)

I97.130 Postprocedural heart failure following cardiac surgery

I97.131 Postprocedural heart failure following other surgery

I97.19 Other postprocedural cardiac functional disturbances

Use additional code, if applicable, to further specify disorder

I97.190 Other postprocedural cardiac functional disturbances following cardiac surgery

Use Additional code, if applicable, for type 4 or type 5 myocardial infarction, to further specify disorder

Coding Clinic: 2019, Q2, P32-33

I97.191 Other postprocedural cardiac functional disturbances following other surgery

I97.2 Postmastectomy lymphedema syndrome A

Elephantiasis due to mastectomy
Obliteration of lymphatic vessels

I97.3 Postprocedural hypertension

I97.4 Intraoperative hemorrhage and hematoma of a circulatory system organ or structure complicating a procedure (Ex:) PDX 1025

Excludes1 intraoperative hemorrhage and hematoma of a circulatory system organ or structure due to accidental puncture and laceration during a procedure (I97.5-)

Excludes2 intraoperative cerebrovascular hemorrhage complicating a procedure (G97.3-)

I97.41 Intraoperative hemorrhage and hematoma of a circulatory system organ or structure complicating a circulatory system procedure

I97.410 Intraoperative hemorrhage and hematoma of a circulatory system organ or structure complicating a cardiac catheterization

I97.411 Intraoperative hemorrhage and hematoma of a circulatory system organ or structure complicating a cardiac bypass

I97.418 Intraoperative hemorrhage and hematoma of a circulatory system organ or structure complicating other circulatory system procedure

I97.42 Intraoperative hemorrhage and hematoma of a circulatory system organ or structure complicating other procedure

Coding Clinic: 2020, Q1, P20; 2016, Q4, P100

I97.5 Accidental puncture and laceration of a circulatory system organ or structure during a procedure (Ex:) PDX 569

Excludes2 accidental puncture and laceration of brain during a procedure (G97.4-)

I97.51 Accidental puncture and laceration of a circulatory system organ or structure during a circulatory system procedure

Coding Clinic: 2019, Q2, P24

I97.52 Accidental puncture and laceration of a circulatory system organ or structure during other procedure

I97.6 Postprocedural hemorrhage, hematoma and seroma of a circulatory system organ or structure following a procedure (Ex:) PDX 1025

Excludes2 postprocedural cerebrovascular hemorrhage complicating a procedure (G97.5-)

Coding Clinic: 2016, Q4, P10

I97.61 Postprocedural hemorrhage of a circulatory system organ or structure following a circulatory system procedure

I97.610 Postprocedural hemorrhage of a circulatory system organ or structure following a cardiac catheterization

I97.611 Postprocedural hemorrhage of a circulatory system organ or structure following cardiac bypass

I97.618 Postprocedural hemorrhage of a circulatory system organ or structure following other circulatory system procedure

I97.62 Postprocedural hemorrhage, hematoma and seroma of a circulatory system organ or structure following other procedure

I97.620 Postprocedural hemorrhage of a circulatory system organ or structure following other procedure

I97.621 Postprocedural hematoma of a circulatory system organ or structure following other procedure

I97.622 Postprocedural seroma of a circulatory system organ or structure following other procedure

CHAPTER 9 (I00-I99)

- ● **I97.63** **Postprocedural hematoma of a circulatory system organ or structure following a circulatory system procedure**
  - **I97.630** **Postprocedural hematoma of a circulatory system organ or structure following a cardiac catheterization**
  - **I97.631** **Postprocedural hematoma of a circulatory system organ or structure following cardiac bypass**
  - **I97.638** **Postprocedural hematoma of a circulatory system organ or structure following other circulatory system procedure**
- ● **I97.64** **Postprocedural seroma of a circulatory system organ or structure following a circulatory system procedure**
  - **I97.640** **Postprocedural seroma of a circulatory system organ or structure following a cardiac catheterization**
  - **I97.641** **Postprocedural seroma of a circulatory system organ or structure following cardiac bypass**
  - **I97.648** **Postprocedural seroma of a circulatory system organ or structure following other circulatory system procedure**
- ● **I97.7** **Intraoperative cardiac functional disturbances** Ex PDX 1024

  Excludes2 acute pulmonary insufficiency following thoracic surgery (J95.1)
  postprocedural cardiac functional disturbances (I97.1-)
- ● **I97.71** **Intraoperative cardiac arrest**
  - **I97.710** **Intraoperative cardiac arrest during cardiac surgery**
  - **I97.711** **Intraoperative cardiac arrest during other surgery**
- ● **I97.79** **Other intraoperative cardiac functional disturbances**

  Use additional code, if applicable, to further specify disorder
  - **I97.790** **Other intraoperative cardiac functional disturbances during cardiac surgery**
  - **I97.791** **Other intraoperative cardiac functional disturbances during other surgery**
- ● **I97.8** **Other intraoperative and postprocedural complications and disorders of the circulatory system, not elsewhere classified** Ex PDX 783

  Use additional code, if applicable, to further specify disorder
- ● **I97.81** **Intraoperative cerebrovascular infarction**
  - **I97.810** **Intraoperative cerebrovascular infarction during cardiac surgery**
  - **I97.811** **Intraoperative cerebrovascular infarction during other surgery**
- ● **I97.82** **Postprocedural cerebrovascular infarction**
  - **I97.820** **Postprocedural cerebrovascular infarction following cardiac surgery**
  - **I97.821** **Postprocedural cerebrovascular infarction following other surgery**
- **I97.88** **Other intraoperative complications of the circulatory system, not elsewhere classified** Ex PDX 1024
- **I97.89** **Other postprocedural complications and disorders of the circulatory system, not elsewhere classified** Ex PDX 1024

  Coding Clinic: 2024, Q1, P26; 2019, Q2, P32-33

● **I99** **Other and unspecified disorders of circulatory system**
- **I99.8** **Other disorder of circulatory system**
- **I99.9** **Unspecified disorder of circulatory system**

CHAPTER 9 (I00-I99)

CHAPTER 10

DISEASES OF THE RESPIRATORY SYSTEM (J00-J99)

OGCR Chapter-Specific Coding Guidelines

10. Chapter 10: Diseases of the Respiratory System (J00-J99)

a. Chronic Obstructive Pulmonary Disease [COPD] and Asthma

1) Acute exacerbation of chronic obstructive bronchitis and asthma

The codes in categories J44 and J45 distinguish between uncomplicated cases and those in acute exacerbation. An acute exacerbation is a worsening or a decompensation of a chronic condition. An acute exacerbation is not equivalent to an infection superimposed on a chronic condition, though an exacerbation may be triggered by an infection.

b. Acute Respiratory Failure

1) Acute respiratory failure as principal diagnosis

A code from subcategory J96.0, Acute respiratory failure, or subcategory J96.2, Acute and chronic respiratory failure, may be assigned as a principal diagnosis when it is the condition established after study to be chiefly responsible for occasioning the admission to the hospital, and the selection is supported by the Alphabetic Index and Tabular List. However, chapter-specific coding guidelines (such as obstetrics, poisoning, HIV, newborn) that provide sequencing direction take precedence.

2) Acute respiratory failure as secondary diagnosis

Respiratory failure may be listed as a secondary diagnosis if it occurs after admission, or if it is present on admission, but does not meet the definition of principal diagnosis.

3) Sequencing of acute respiratory failure and another acute condition

When a patient is admitted with respiratory failure and another acute condition (e.g., myocardial infarction, cerebrovascular accident, aspiration pneumonia), the principal diagnosis will not be the same in every situation. This applies whether the other acute condition is a respiratory or nonrespiratory condition. Selection of the principal diagnosis will be dependent on the circumstances of admission. If both the respiratory failure and the other acute condition are equally responsible for occasioning the admission to the hospital, and there are no chapter-specific sequencing rules, the guideline regarding two or more diagnoses that equally meet the definition for principal diagnosis *(Section II, C.)* may be applied in these situations.

If the documentation is not clear as to whether acute respiratory failure and another condition are equally responsible for occasioning the admission, query the provider for clarification.

c. Influenza due to certain identified influenza viruses

Code only confirmed cases of influenza due to certain identified influenza viruses (category J09), and due to other identified influenza virus (category J10). This is an exception to the hospital inpatient guideline Section II, H. (Uncertain Diagnosis).

In this context, "confirmation" does not require documentation of positive laboratory testing specific for avian or other novel influenza A or other identified influenza virus. However, coding should be based on the provider's diagnostic statement that the patient has avian influenza, or other novel influenza A, for category J09, or has another particular identified strain of influenza, such as H1N1 or H3N2, but not identified as novel or variant, for category J10.

If the provider records "suspected" or "possible" or "probable" avian influenza, or novel influenza, or other identified influenza, then the appropriate influenza code from category J11, Influenza due to unidentified influenza virus, should be assigned. A code from category J09, Influenza due to certain identified influenza viruses, should not be assigned nor should a code from category J10, Influenza due to other identified influenza virus.

d. Ventilator associated Pneumonia

1) Documentation of Ventilator associated Pneumonia

As with all procedural or postprocedural complications, code assignment is based on the provider's documentation of the relationship between the condition and the procedure.

Code J95.851, Ventilator associated pneumonia, should be assigned only when the provider has documented ventilator associated pneumonia (VAP). An additional code to identify the organism (e.g., Pseudomonas aeruginosa, code B96.5) should also be assigned. Do not assign an additional code from categories J12-J18 to identify the type of pneumonia.

Code J95.851 should not be assigned for cases where the patient has pneumonia and is on a mechanical ventilator and the provider has not specifically stated that the pneumonia is ventilator associated pneumonia. If the documentation is unclear as to whether the patient has a pneumonia that is a complication attributable to the mechanical ventilator, query the provider.

2) Ventilator associated Pneumonia Develops after Admission

A patient may be admitted with one type of pneumonia (e.g., code J13, Pneumonia due to Streptococcus pneumonia) and subsequently develop VAP. In this instance, the principal diagnosis would be the appropriate code from categories J12-J18 for the pneumonia diagnosed at the time of admission. Code J95.851, Ventilator associated pneumonia, would be assigned as an additional diagnosis when the provider has also documented the presence of ventilator associated pneumonia.

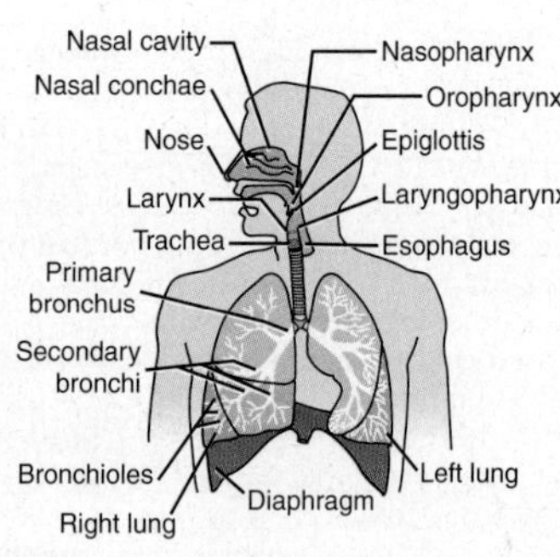

Figure 10-1 Respiratory system. (From Buck CJ: Step-by-Step Medical Coding, ed 2016, St. Louis, Elsevier, 2016)

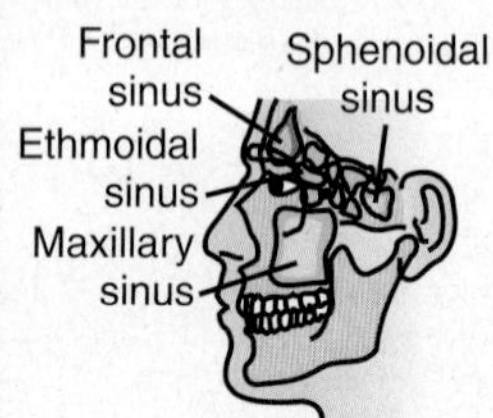

Figure 10-2 Paranasal sinuses. (From Buck CJ: Step-by-Step Medical Coding, ed 2016, St. Louis, Elsevier, 2016)

Item 10–1 Pharyngitis is painful inflammation of the pharynx (sore throat). Ninety percent of the infections are caused by a virus with the remaining being bacterial and rarely a fungus (candidiasis). Other irritants such as pollutants, chemicals, or smoke may cause similar symptoms.

CHAPTER 1Ø

DISEASES OF THE RESPIRATORY SYSTEM (JØØ-J99)

Note: When a respiratory condition is described as occurring in more than one site and is not specifically indexed, it should be classified to the lower anatomic site (e.g., tracheobronchitis to bronchitis in J4Ø).

Use additional code, where applicable, to identify:
- exposure to environmental tobacco smoke (Z77.22)
- exposure to tobacco smoke in the perinatal period (P96.81)
- history of tobacco dependence (Z87.891)
- occupational exposure to environmental tobacco smoke (Z57.31)
- tobacco dependence (F17.-)
- tobacco use (Z72.Ø)

Excludes2
- certain conditions originating in the perinatal period (PØ4-P96)
- certain infectious and parasitic diseases (AØØ-B99)
- complications of pregnancy, childbirth and the puerperium (OØØ-O99A)
- congenital malformations, deformations and chromosomal abnormalities (QØØ-Q99)
- endocrine, nutritional and metabolic diseases (EØØ-E88)
- injury, poisoning and certain other consequences of external causes (SØØ-T88)
- neoplasms (CØØ-D49)
- smoke inhalation (T59.81-)
- symptoms, signs and abnormal clinical and laboratory findings, not elsewhere classified (RØØ-R94)

This chapter contains the following blocks:

JØØ-JØ6	Acute upper respiratory infections
JØ9-J18	Influenza and pneumonia
J2Ø-J22	Other acute lower respiratory infections
J3Ø-J39	Other diseases of upper respiratory tract
J4Ø-J4A	Chronic lower respiratory diseases
J6Ø-J7Ø	Lung diseases due to external agents
J8Ø-J84	Other respiratory diseases principally affecting the interstitium
J85-J86	Suppurative and necrotic conditions of the lower respiratory tract
J9Ø-J94	Other diseases of the pleura
J95	Intraoperative and postprocedural complications and disorders of respiratory system, not elsewhere classified
J96-J99	Other diseases of the respiratory system

ACUTE UPPER RESPIRATORY INFECTIONS (JØØ-JØ6)

Use Additional code, if applicable, to identify resistance to antimicrobial drugs (Z16.-)

Excludes1 chronic obstructive pulmonary disease with acute lower respiratory infection (J44.Ø)

JØØ Acute nasopharyngitis [common cold]
- Acute rhinitis
- Coryza (acute)
- Infective nasopharyngitis NOS
- Infective rhinitis
- Nasal catarrh, acute
- Nasopharyngitis NOS

Excludes1
- acute pharyngitis (JØ2.-)
- acute sore throat NOS (JØ2.9)
- influenza virus with other respiratory manifestations (JØ9.X2, J1Ø.1, J11.1)
- pharyngitis NOS (JØ2.9)
- rhinitis NOS (J31.Ø)
- sore throat NOS (JØ2.9)

Excludes2
- allergic rhinitis (J3Ø.1-J3Ø.9)
- chronic pharyngitis (J31.2)
- chronic rhinitis (J31.Ø)
- chronic sore throat (J31.2)
- nasopharyngitis, chronic (J31.1)
- vasomotor rhinitis (J3Ø.Ø)

★**(See Plate 27 of the Anatomy Illustrations.)**

● **JØ1 Acute sinusitis**

Includes
- acute abscess of sinus
- acute empyema of sinus
- acute infection of sinus
- acute inflammation of sinus
- acute suppuration of sinus

Use additional code (B95-B97) to identify infectious agent.

Excludes1 sinusitis NOS (J32.9)

Excludes2 chronic sinusitis (J32.Ø-J32.8)

● **JØ1.Ø Acute maxillary sinusitis**
Acute antritis
- **JØ1.ØØ Acute maxillary sinusitis, unspecified**
- **JØ1.Ø1 Acute recurrent maxillary sinusitis**

● **JØ1.1 Acute frontal sinusitis**
- **JØ1.1Ø Acute frontal sinusitis, unspecified**
- **JØ1.11 Acute recurrent frontal sinusitis**

● **JØ1.2 Acute ethmoidal sinusitis**
- **JØ1.2Ø Acute ethmoidal sinusitis, unspecified**
- **JØ1.21 Acute recurrent ethmoidal sinusitis**

● **JØ1.3 Acute sphenoidal sinusitis**
- **JØ1.3Ø Acute sphenoidal sinusitis, unspecified**
- **JØ1.31 Acute recurrent sphenoidal sinusitis**

● **JØ1.4 Acute pansinusitis**
- **JØ1.4Ø Acute pansinusitis, unspecified**
- **JØ1.41 Acute recurrent pansinusitis**

● **J01.8 Other acute sinusitis**

J01.80 Other acute sinusitis
Acute sinusitis involving more than one sinus but not pansinusitis

J01.81 Other acute recurrent sinusitis
Acute recurrent sinusitis involving more than one sinus but not pansinusitis

● **J01.9 Acute sinusitis, unspecified**

J01.90 Acute sinusitis, unspecified

J01.91 Acute recurrent sinusitis, unspecified

● **J02 Acute pharyngitis**

Includes acute sore throat

Excludes1 acute laryngopharyngitis (J06.0)
peritonsillar abscess (J36)
pharyngeal abscess (J39.1)
retropharyngeal abscess (J39.0)

Excludes2 chronic pharyngitis (J31.2)

J02.0 Streptococcal pharyngitis
Septic pharyngitis
Streptococcal sore throat

Excludes2 scarlet fever (A38.-)

J02.8 Acute pharyngitis due to other specified organisms
Use additional code (B95-B97) to identify infectious agent

Excludes1 pharyngitis due to coxsackie virus (B08.5)
pharyngitis due to gonococcus (A54.5)
acute pharyngitis due to herpes [simplex] virus (B00.2)
acute pharyngitis due to infectious mononucleosis (B27.-)
enteroviral vesicular pharyngitis (B08.5)

J02.9 Acute pharyngitis, unspecified
Gangrenous pharyngitis (acute)
Infective pharyngitis (acute) NOS
Pharyngitis (acute) NOS
Sore throat (acute) NOS
Suppurative pharyngitis (acute)
Ulcerative pharyngitis (acute)

Excludes1 influenza virus with other respiratory manifestations (J09.X2, J10.1, J11.1)

● **J03 Acute tonsillitis**

Inflammation of pharyngeal tonsils caused by virus or bacteria

Excludes1 acute sore throat (J02.-)
hypertrophy of tonsils (J35.1)
peritonsillar abscess (J36)
sore throat NOS (J02.9)
streptococcal sore throat (J02.0)

Excludes2 chronic tonsillitis (J35.0)

● **J03.0 Streptococcal tonsillitis**

J03.00 Acute streptococcal tonsillitis, unspecified

J03.01 Acute recurrent streptococcal tonsillitis

● **J03.8 Acute tonsillitis due to other specified organisms**
Use additional code (B95-B97) to identify infectious agent.

Excludes1 diphtheritic tonsillitis (A36.0)
herpesviral pharyngotonsillitis (B00.2)
streptococcal tonsillitis (J03.0)
tuberculous tonsillitis (A15.8)
Vincent's tonsillitis (A69.1)

J03.80 Acute tonsillitis due to other specified organisms

J03.81 Acute recurrent tonsillitis due to other specified organisms

● **J03.9 Acute tonsillitis, unspecified**
Follicular tonsillitis (acute)
Gangrenous tonsillitis (acute)
Infective tonsillitis (acute)
Tonsillitis (acute) NOS
Ulcerative tonsillitis (acute)

Excludes1 influenza virus with other respiratory manifestations (J09.X2, J10.1, J11.1)

J03.90 Acute tonsillitis, unspecified

J03.91 Acute recurrent tonsillitis, unspecified

● **J04 Acute laryngitis and tracheitis**
Use additional code (B95-B97) to identify infectious agent.
Code also influenza, if present, such as:
influenza due to identified novel influenza A virus with other respiratory manifestations (J09.X2)
influenza due to other identified influenza virus with other respiratory manifestations (J10.1)
influenza due to unidentified influenza virus with other respiratory manifestations (J11.1)

Excludes1 acute obstructive laryngitis [croup] and epiglottitis (J05.-)

Excludes2 laryngismus (stridulus) (J38.5)

J04.0 Acute laryngitis
Edematous laryngitis (acute)
Laryngitis (acute) NOS
Subglottic laryngitis (acute)
Suppurative laryngitis (acute)
Ulcerative laryngitis (acute)

Excludes1 acute obstructive laryngitis (J05.0)

Excludes2 chronic laryngitis (J37.0)

● **J04.1 Acute tracheitis**
Acute viral tracheitis
Catarrhal tracheitis (acute)
Tracheitis (acute) NOS

Excludes2 chronic tracheitis (J42)

J04.10 Acute tracheitis without obstruction

J04.11 Acute tracheitis with obstruction (Ex) PDX 1026

J04.2 Acute laryngotracheitis
Laryngotracheitis NOS
Tracheitis (acute) with laryngitis (acute)

Excludes1 acute obstructive laryngotracheitis (J05.0)

Excludes2 chronic laryngotracheitis (J37.1)

● **J04.3 Supraglottitis, unspecified**

J04.30 Supraglottitis, unspecified, without obstruction

J04.31 Supraglottitis, unspecified, with obstruction (Ex) PDX 1027

● **J05 Acute obstructive laryngitis [croup] and epiglottitis**
Use additional code (B95-B97) to identify infectious agent.
Code also influenza, if present, such as:
influenza due to identified novel influenza A virus with other respiratory manifestations (J09.X2)
influenza due to other identified influenza virus with other respiratory manifestations (J10.1)
influenza due to unidentified influenza virus with other respiratory manifestations (J11.1)

J05.0 Acute obstructive laryngitis [croup]
Obstructive laryngitis (acute) NOS
Obstructive laryngotracheitis NOS

● **J05.1 Acute epiglottitis**

Excludes2 epiglottitis, chronic (J37.0)

J05.10 Acute epiglottitis without obstruction (Ex) PDX 1028
Epiglottitis NOS

J05.11 Acute epiglottitis with obstruction (Ex) PDX 1026

Item 10–2 Laryngitis is an inflammation of the larynx (voice box) resulting in hoarse voice or the complete loss of the voice. **Tracheitis** is an inflammation of the trachea (often following a URI) commonly caused by *staphylococcus aureus* resulting in inspiratory stridor (crowing sound on inspiration) and a crouplike cough.

● J06 Acute upper respiratory infections of multiple and unspecified sites

Excludes1 acute respiratory infection NOS (J22)
influenza virus with other respiratory manifestations (JØ9.X2, J1Ø.1, J11.1)
streptococcal pharyngitis (JØ2.Ø)

Coding Clinic: 2020, Q1, P22

JØ6.Ø Acute laryngopharyngitis

JØ6.9 Acute upper respiratory infection, unspecified
Upper respiratory disease, acute
Upper respiratory infection NOS
Use additional code (B95-B97) to identify infectious agent, if known, such as:
respiratory syncytial virus (RSV) (B97.4)

INFLUENZA AND PNEUMONIA (JØ9-J18)

Excludes2 allergic or eosinophilic pneumonia (J82)
aspiration pneumonia NOS (J69.Ø)
meconium pneumonia (P24.Ø1)
neonatal aspiration pneumonia (P24.-)
pneumonia due to solids and liquids (J69.-)
congenital pneumonia (P23.9)
lipid pneumonia (J69.1)
rheumatic pneumonia (IØØ)
ventilator associated pneumonia (J95.851)

Coding Clinic: 2020, Q1, P22

● JØ9 Influenza due to certain identified influenza viruses

Excludes1 influenza A/H1N1 (J1Ø.-)
influenza due to other influenza viruses (J1Ø.-)
influenza due to unidentified influenza virus (J11.-)
seasonal influenza due to other identified influenza virus (J1Ø.-)
seasonal influenza due to unidentified influenza virus (J11.-)

● JØ9.X Influenza due to identified novel influenza A virus
Avian influenza
Bird influenza
Influenza A/H5N1
Influenza of other animal origin, not bird or swine
Swine influenza virus (viruses that normally cause infections in pigs)

Coding Clinic: 2016, Q3, P11

JØ9.X1 Influenza due to identified novel influenza A virus with pneumonia (Ex) PDX 113
Code also , if applicable, associated:
lung abscess (J85.1)
other specified type of pneumonia

JØ9.X2 Influenza due to identified novel influenza A virus with other respiratory manifestations
Influenza due to identified novel influenza A virus NOS
Influenza due to identified novel influenza A virus with laryngitis
Influenza due to identified novel influenza A virus with pharyngitis
Influenza due to identified novel influenza A virus with upper respiratory symptoms
Use additional code, if applicable, for associated:
pleural effusion (J91.8)
sinusitis (JØ1.-)

JØ9.X3 Influenza due to identified novel influenza A virus with gastrointestinal manifestations
Influenza due to identified novel influenza A virus gastroenteritis
Excludes1 'intestinal flu' [viral gastroenteritis] (AØ8.-)

JØ9.X9 Influenza due to identified novel influenza A virus with other manifestations
Influenza due to identified novel influenza A virus with encephalopathy
Influenza due to identified novel influenza A virus with myocarditis
Influenza due to identified novel influenza A virus with otitis media
Use additional code to identify manifestation

● J1Ø Influenza due to other identified influenza virus

Includes influenza A (non-novel)
influenza B
influenza C

Excludes1 influenza due to avian influenza virus (JØ9.X-)
influenza due to swine flu (JØ9.X-)
influenza due to unidentified influenza virus (J11.-)

● J1Ø.Ø Influenza due to other identified influenza virus with pneumonia (Ex) PDX 113
Code also associated lung abscess, if applicable (J85.1)

J1Ø.ØØ Influenza due to other identified influenza virus with unspecified type of pneumonia

J1Ø.Ø1 Influenza due to other identified influenza virus with the same other identified influenza virus pneumonia

J1Ø.Ø8 Influenza due to other identified influenza virus with other specified pneumonia (Ex) PDX 1029
Code also other specified type of pneumonia
Coding Clinic: 2017, Q4, P96

J1Ø.1 Influenza due to other identified influenza virus with other respiratory manifestations
Influenza due to other identified influenza virus NOS
Influenza due to other identified influenza virus with laryngitis
Influenza due to other identified influenza virus with pharyngitis
Influenza due to other identified influenza virus with upper respiratory symptoms
Use additional code for associated pleural effusion, if applicable (J91.8)
Use additional code for associated sinusitis, if applicable (JØ1.-)
Coding Clinic: 2016, Q3, P11

J1Ø.2 Influenza due to other identified influenza virus with gastrointestinal manifestations
Influenza due to other identified influenza virus gastroenteritis
Excludes1 'intestinal flu' [viral gastroenteritis] (AØ8.-)

● J1Ø.8 Influenza due to other identified influenza virus with other manifestations

J1Ø.81 Influenza due to other identified influenza virus with encephalopathy

J1Ø.82 Influenza due to other identified influenza virus with myocarditis

J1Ø.83 Influenza due to other identified influenza virus with otitis media
Use additional code for any associated perforated tympanic membrane (H72.-)

J1Ø.89 Influenza due to other identified influenza virus with other manifestations
Use additional codes to identify the manifestations

● J11 Influenza due to unidentified influenza virus

● J11.Ø Influenza due to unidentified influenza virus with pneumonia (Ex) PDX 113
Code also associated lung abscess, if applicable (J85.1)

J11.00 Influenza due to unidentified influenza virus with unspecified type of pneumonia
Influenza with pneumonia NOS
Coding Clinic: 2016, Q3, P12

J11.08 Influenza due to unidentified influenza virus with specified pneumonia
Code also other specified type of pneumonia

J11.1 Influenza due to unidentified influenza virus with other respiratory manifestations
Influenza NOS
Influenzal laryngitis NOS
Influenzal pharyngitis NOS
Influenza with upper respiratory symptoms NOS
Use additional code for associated pleural effusion, if applicable (J91.8)
Use additional code for associated sinusitis, if applicable (J01.-)

J11.2 Influenza due to unidentified influenza virus with gastrointestinal manifestations
Influenza gastroenteritis NOS
Excludes1 'intestinal flu' [viral gastroenteritis] (A08.-)

J11.8 Influenza due to unidentified influenza virus with other manifestations

J11.81 Influenza due to unidentified influenza virus with encephalopathy
Influenzal encephalopathy NOS

J11.82 Influenza due to unidentified influenza virus with myocarditis
Influenzal myocarditis NOS

J11.83 Influenza due to unidentified influenza virus with otitis media
Influenzal otitis media NOS
Use additional code for any associated perforated tympanic membrane (H72.-)

J11.89 Influenza due to unidentified influenza virus with other manifestations
Use additional codes to identify the manifestations

J12 Viral pneumonia, not elsewhere classified (Ex) PDX 1030
Includes bronchopneumonia due to viruses other than influenza viruses
Code first associated influenza, if applicable (J09.X1, J10.0-, J11.0-)
Code also associated abscess, if applicable (J85.1)
~~**Excludes1** aspiration pneumonia due to anesthesia during labor and delivery (O74.0)~~
~~aspiration pneumonia due to anesthesia during pregnancy (O29)~~
~~aspiration pneumonia due to anesthesia during puerperium (O89.0)~~
~~aspiration pneumonia due to solids and liquids (J69.-)~~
~~aspiration pneumonia NOS (J69.0)~~
~~congenital pneumonia (P23.0)~~
~~congenital rubella pneumonitis (P35.0)~~
~~interstitial pneumonia NOS (J84.9)~~
~~lipid pneumonia (J69.1)~~
~~neonatal aspiration pneumonia (P24.-)~~
▶ **Excludes2** aspiration pneumonia due to anesthesia during labor and delivery (O74.0)
▶aspiration pneumonia due to anesthesia during pregnancy (O29)
▶aspiration pneumonia due to anesthesia during puerperium (O89.0)
▶aspiration pneumonia due to solids and liquids (J69.-)
▶aspiration pneumonia NOS (J69.0)
▶congenital pneumonia (P23.0)
▶congenital rubella pneumonitis (P35.0)
▶interstitial pneumonia NOS (J84.9)
▶lipid pneumonia (J69.1)
▶neonatal aspiration pneumonia (P24.-)
Coding Clinic: 2021, Q1, P34

Item 10-3 Pneumonia is an infection of the lungs, caused by a variety of microorganisms, including viruses, most commonly the Streptococcus pneumoniae (pneumococcus) bacteria, fungi, and parasites. Pneumonia occurs when the immune system is weakened, often by a URI or influenza.

J12.0 Adenoviral pneumonia

J12.1 Respiratory syncytial virus pneumonia
RSV pneumonia

J12.2 Parainfluenza virus pneumonia

J12.3 Human metapneumovirus pneumonia

J12.8 Other viral pneumonia

J12.81 Pneumonia due to SARS-associated coronavirus
Severe acute respiratory syndrome NOS

J12.82 Pneumonia due to coronavirus disease 2019 (Ex) No exclusions
Pneumonia due to 2019 novel coronavirus (SARS-CoV-2)
Pneumonia due to COVID-19
Code first COVID-19 (U07.1)
Coding Clinic: 2021, Q1, P33-34, 42, 47, 49

J12.89 Other viral pneumonia
Coding Clinic: 2021, Q1, P33-34

J12.9 Viral pneumonia, unspecified

J13 Pneumonia due to Streptococcus pneumoniae (Ex) PDX 113
Bronchopneumonia due to S. pneumoniae
Code first, if applicable, associated influenza, if applicable (J09.X1, J10.0-, J11.0-)
Code also, ~~associated abscess, if applicable (J85.1)~~
▶if applicable, any associated condition such as:
▶abscess (J85.1)
▶aspiration pneumonia (J69.-)
Excludes1 congenital pneumonia due to S. pneumoniae (P23.6)
lobar pneumonia, unspecified organism (J18.1)
pneumonia due to other streptococci (J15.3-J15.4)

J14 Pneumonia due to Hemophilus influenzae (Ex) PDX 113
Bronchopneumonia due to H. influenzae
Code first, if applicable, associated influenza, if applicable (J09.X1, J10.0-, J11.0-)
Code also, ~~associated abscess, if applicable (J85.1)~~
▶if applicable, any associated condition such as:
▶abscess (J85.1)
▶aspiration pneumonia (J69.-)
Excludes1 congenital pneumonia due to H. influenzae (P23.6)

J15 Bacterial pneumonia, not elsewhere classified (Ex) PDX 113
Includes bronchopneumonia due to bacteria other than S. pneumoniae and H. influenzae
Code first, if applicable, associated influenza, if applicable (J09.X1, J10.0-, J11.0-)
Code also, ~~associated abscess, if applicable (J85.1)~~
▶if applicable, any associated condition such as:
▶abscess (J85.1)
▶aspiration pneumonia (J69.-)
Excludes1 chlamydial pneumonia (J16.0)
congenital pneumonia (P23.-)
Legionnaires' disease (A48.1)
spirochetal pneumonia (A69.8)

J15.0 Pneumonia due to Klebsiella pneumoniae

J15.1 Pneumonia due to Pseudomonas

J15.2 Pneumonia due to staphylococcus

J15.20 Pneumonia due to staphylococcus, unspecified

J15.21 Pneumonia due to staphylococcus aureus

J15.211 Pneumonia due to Methicillin susceptible Staphylococcus aureus
MSSA pneumonia
Pneumonia due to Staphylococcus aureus NOS

J15.212 Pneumonia due to Methicillin resistant Staphylococcus aureus

J15.29 Pneumonia due to other staphylococcus

J15.3 Pneumonia due to streptococcus, group B

J15.4 Pneumonia due to other streptococci

Excludes1 pneumonia due to streptococcus, group B (J15.3)
pneumonia due to Streptococcus pneumoniae (J13)

J15.5 Pneumonia due to Escherichia coli

● J15.6 Pneumonia due to other Gram-negative bacteria

J15.61 Pneumonia due to Acinetobacter baumannii PDX 1032

J15.69 Pneumonia due to other Gram-negative bacteria PDX 1032
Pneumonia due to other aerobic Gram-negative bacteria
Pneumonia due to Serratia marcescens

J15.7 Pneumonia due to Mycoplasma pneumoniae

J15.8 Pneumonia due to other specified bacteria

J15.9 Unspecified bacterial pneumonia
Pneumonia due to gram-positive bacteria
Coding Clinic: 2017, Q4, P96

● J16 Pneumonia due to other infectious organisms, not elsewhere classified PDX 113

Code first, if applicable, associated influenza, if applicable (J09.X1, J10.0-, J11.0-)

Code also, ~~associated abscess, if applicable (J85.1)~~
▶if applicable, any associated condition such as:
▶abscess (J85.1)
▶aspiration pneumonia (J69.-)

Excludes1 congenital pneumonia (P23.-)
ornithosis (A70)
pneumocystosis (B59)
pneumonia NOS (J18.9)

J16.0 Chlamydial pneumonia

J16.8 Pneumonia due to other specified infectious organisms

J17 Pneumonia in diseases classified elsewhere PDX 113

Code first underlying disease, such as:
Q fever (A78)
rheumatic fever (I00)
schistosomiasis (B65.0-B65.9)

▶Code also, if applicable, any associated condition such as:
▶abscess (J85.1)
▶aspiration pneumonia (J69.-)

Excludes1 candidial pneumonia (B37.1)
chlamydial pneumonia (J16.0)
gonorrheal pneumonia (A54.84)
histoplasmosis pneumonia (B39.0-B39.2)
measles pneumonia (B05.2)
nocardiosis pneumonia (A43.0)
pneumocystosis (B59)
pneumonia due to Pneumocystis carinii (B59)
pneumonia due to Pneumocystis jiroveci (B59)
pneumonia in actinomycosis (A42.0)
pneumonia in anthrax (A22.1)
pneumonia in ascariasis (B77.81)
pneumonia in aspergillosis (B44.0-B44.1)
pneumonia in coccidioidomycosis (B38.0-B38.2)
pneumonia in cytomegalovirus disease (B25.0)
pneumonia in toxoplasmosis (B58.3)
rubella pneumonia (B06.81)
salmonella pneumonia (A02.22)
spirochetal infection NEC with pneumonia (A69.8)
tularemia pneumonia (A21.2)
typhoid fever with pneumonia (A01.03)
varicella pneumonia (B01.2)
whooping cough with pneumonia (A37 with fifth-character 1)

● J18 Pneumonia, unspecified organism PDX 113

Code first, if applicable, associated influenza, if applicable (J09.X1, J10.0-, J11.0-)

▶Code also, if applicable, any associated condition such as:
▶aspiration pneumonia (J69.-)

Excludes1 congenital pneumonia (P23.0)
drug-induced interstitial lung disorder (J70.2-J70.4)
interstitial pneumonia NOS (J84.9)
neonatal aspiration pneumonia (P24.-)
pneumonitis due to fumes and vapors (J68.0)
usual interstitial pneumonia (J84.178)

▶**Excludes2** abscess of lung with pneumonia (J85.1)
▶aspiration pneumonia due to anesthesia during labor and delivery (O74.0)
▶aspiration pneumonia due to anesthesia during pregnancy (O29)
▶aspiration pneumonia due to anesthesia during puerperium (O89.0)
▶aspiration pneumonia due to solids and liquids (J69.-)
▶aspiration pneumonia NOS (J69.0)
▶lipid pneumonia (J69.1)
▶pneumonitis due to external agents (J67-J70)

J18.0 Bronchopneumonia, unspecified organism

Excludes1 hypostatic bronchopneumonia (J18.2)
lipid pneumonia (J69.1)

Excludes2 acute bronchiolitis (J21.-)
chronic bronchiolitis (J44.89)
▶other specified chronic obstructive pulmonary disease (J44.89)

J18.1 Lobar pneumonia, unspecified organism
Coding Clinic: 2016, Q3, P15

J18.2 Hypostatic pneumonia, unspecified organism PDX 1033
Hypostatic bronchopneumonia
Passive pneumonia

J18.8 Other pneumonia, unspecified organism

J18.9 Pneumonia, unspecified organism
Coding Clinic: Q3, P15; 2019, Q2, P28; Q1, P36; 2016, Q3, P15; 2012, Q4, P94

OTHER ACUTE LOWER RESPIRATORY INFECTIONS (J20-J22)

Excludes2 chronic obstructive pulmonary disease with acute lower respiratory infection (J44.0)

● J20 Acute bronchitis

Inflammation/irritation of the bronchial tubes lasting 2-3 weeks, most commonly caused by a virus

Includes acute and subacute bronchitis (with) bronchospasm
acute and subacute bronchitis (with) tracheitis
acute and subacute bronchitis (with) tracheobronchitis, acute
acute and subacute fibrinous bronchitis
acute and subacute membranous bronchitis
acute and subacute purulent bronchitis
acute and subacute septic bronchitis

Excludes1 bronchitis NOS (J40)
tracheobronchitis NOS (J40)

Excludes2 acute bronchitis with bronchiectasis (J47.0)
acute bronchitis with chronic obstructive asthma (J44.0)
acute bronchitis with chronic obstructive pulmonary disease (J44.0)
allergic bronchitis NOS (J45.909-)
bronchitis due to chemicals, fumes and vapors (J68.0)
chronic bronchitis NOS (J42)
chronic mucopurulent bronchitis (J41.1)
chronic obstructive bronchitis (J44.-)
chronic obstructive tracheobronchitis (J44.-)
chronic simple bronchitis (J41.0)
chronic tracheobronchitis (J42)

J20.0 Acute bronchitis due to Mycoplasma pneumoniae

J20.1 Acute bronchitis due to Hemophilus influenzae

J20.2 Acute bronchitis due to streptococcus

J20.3 **Acute bronchitis due to coxsackievirus**
J20.4 **Acute bronchitis due to parainfluenza virus**
J20.5 **Acute bronchitis due to respiratory syncytial virus**
Acute bronchitis due to RSV
J20.6 **Acute bronchitis due to rhinovirus**
Coding Clinic: 2016, Q3, P10
J20.7 **Acute bronchitis due to echovirus**
J20.8 **Acute bronchitis due to other specified organisms**
Coding Clinic: 2016, Q3, P11
J20.9 **Acute bronchitis, unspecified**
Coding Clinic: 2019, Q1, P35; 2016, Q3, P16

● **J21** Acute **bronchiolitis** (Ex) PDX 1035
Bronchiolitis obliterans with organizing pneumonia (BOOP) inflammation of bronchioles and surrounding tissue in lung
Includes acute bronchiolitis with bronchospasm
Excludes2 respiratory bronchiolitis interstitial lung disease (J84.115)
J21.0 **Acute bronchiolitis due to respiratory syncytial virus** (Ex) PDX 1034
Acute bronchitis due to RSV
J21.1 **Acute bronchiolitis due to human metapneumovirus**
J21.8 **Acute bronchiolitis due to other specified organisms**
J21.9 **Acute bronchiolitis, unspecified**
Bronchiolitis (acute)
Excludes1 chronic bronchiolitis (J44.89)

J22 **Unspecified acute lower respiratory infection**
Acute (lower) respiratory (tract) infection NOS
Excludes1 upper respiratory infection (acute) (J06.9)
Coding Clinic: 2020, Q1, P22-23

OTHER DISEASES OF UPPER RESPIRATORY TRACT (J30-J39)

● **J30** **Vasomotor and allergic rhinitis**
Includes spasmodic rhinorrhea
Excludes1 allergic rhinitis with asthma (bronchial) (J45.909)
rhinitis NOS (J31.0)
J30.0 **Vasomotor rhinitis**
J30.1 **Allergic rhinitis due to pollen**
Allergy NOS due to pollen
Hay fever
Pollinosis
J30.2 **Other seasonal allergic rhinitis**
J30.5 **Allergic rhinitis due to food**
● **J30.8** **Other allergic rhinitis**
J30.81 **Allergic rhinitis due to animal (cat) (dog) hair and dander**
J30.89 **Other allergic rhinitis**
Perennial allergic rhinitis
J30.9 **Allergic rhinitis, unspecified**

● **J31** **Chronic rhinitis, nasopharyngitis and pharyngitis**
J31.0 **Chronic rhinitis**
Atrophic rhinitis (chronic)
Granulomatous rhinitis (chronic)
Hypertrophic rhinitis (chronic)
Obstructive rhinitis (chronic)
Ozena
Purulent rhinitis (chronic)
Rhinitis (chronic) NOS
Ulcerative rhinitis (chronic)
Excludes1 allergic rhinitis (J30.1-J30.9)
vasomotor rhinitis (J30.0)
J31.1 **Chronic nasopharyngitis**
Excludes2 acute nasopharyngitis (J00)
J31.2 **Chronic pharyngitis**
Chronic sore throat
Atrophic pharyngitis (chronic)
Granular pharyngitis (chronic)
Hypertrophic pharyngitis (chronic)
Excludes2 acute pharyngitis (J02.9)

● **J32** **Chronic sinusitis**
Includes sinus abscess
sinus empyema
sinus infection
sinus suppuration
Excludes2 acute sinusitis (J01.-)
J32.0 **Chronic maxillary sinusitis**
Antritis (chronic)
Maxillary sinusitis NOS
J32.1 **Chronic frontal sinusitis**
Frontal sinusitis NOS
J32.2 **Chronic ethmoidal sinusitis**
Ethmoidal sinusitis NOS
Excludes1 Woakes' ethmoiditis (J33.1)
J32.3 **Chronic sphenoidal sinusitis**
Sphenoidal sinusitis NOS
J32.4 **Chronic pansinusitis**
Pansinusitis NOS
J32.8 **Other chronic sinusitis**
Sinusitis (chronic) involving more than one sinus but not pansinusitis
J32.9 **Chronic sinusitis, unspecified**
Sinusitis (chronic) NOS

● **J33** **Nasal polyp**
Excludes1 adenomatous polyps (D14.0)
J33.0 **Polyp of nasal cavity**
Choanal polyp
Nasopharyngeal polyp
J33.1 **Polypoid sinus degeneration**
Woakes' syndrome or ethmoiditis
J33.8 **Other polyp of sinus**
Accessory polyp of sinus
Ethmoidal polyp of sinus
Maxillary polyp of sinus
Sphenoidal polyp of sinus
J33.9 **Nasal polyp, unspecified**

● **J34** **Other and unspecified disorders of nose and nasal sinuses**
Excludes2 varicose ulcer of nasal septum (I86.8)
J34.0 **Abscess, furuncle and carbuncle of nose**
Cellulitis of nose
Necrosis of nose
Ulceration of nose
J34.1 **Cyst and mucocele of nose and nasal sinus**
J34.2 **Deviated nasal septum**
Deflection or deviation of septum (nasal) (acquired)
Excludes1 congenital deviated nasal septum (Q67.4)
J34.3 **Hypertrophy of nasal turbinates**

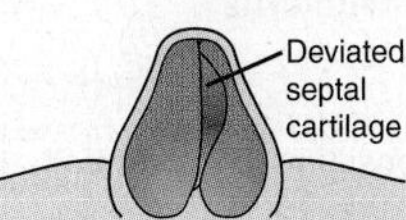

Figure 10-3 Deviated nasal septum.

Item 10-4 **Nasal polyps** are an abnormal growth of tissue (tumor) projecting from a mucous membrane and attached to the surface by a narrow elongated stalk (pedunculated). Nasal polyps usually originate in the ethmoid sinus but also may occur in the maxillary sinus. Symptoms are nasal block, sinusitis, anosmia, and secondary infections.

Item 10-5 A **deviated nasal septum** is the displacement of the septal cartilage that separates the nares. This displacement causes obstructed air flow through the nasal passages. A child can be born with this displacement (congenital), or the condition may be acquired through trauma, such as a sports injury. Symptoms include nasal block, sinusitis, and related secondary infections. Septoplasty is surgical repair of this condition.

● **J34.8 Other specified disorders of nose and nasal sinuses**

J34.81 Nasal mucositis (ulcerative)

Code also type of associated therapy, such as:
antineoplastic and immunosuppressive drugs (T45.1X-)
radiological procedure and radiotherapy (Y84.2)

Excludes2 gastrointestinal mucositis (ulcerative) (K92.81)
mucositis (ulcerative) of vagina and vulva (N76.81)
oral mucositis (ulcerative) (K12.3-)

▶● **J34.82 Nasal valve collapse**
▶Nasal valve compromise
▶Nasal valve stenosis
▶ *Code first underlying cause, such as:*
deviated nasal septum (J34.2)

▶● **J34.82Ø Internal nasal valve collapse**

▶● **J34.82ØØ Internal nasal valve collapse, unspecified**

▶● **J34.82Ø1 Internal nasal valve collapse, static**
▶Narrowing of the septum, head of the inferior turbinate and the upper lateral cartilage

▶● **J34.82Ø2 Internal nasal valve collapse, dynamic**
▶Collapse or falling of the upper, middle sidewall of the nose on inspiration

▶● **J34.821 External nasal valve collapse**

▶● **J34.821Ø External nasal valve collapse, unspecified**

▶● **J34.8211 External nasal valve collapse, static**
▶Fixed narrowing of the caudal septum, lower lateral cartilage, alar rim and nasal sill

▶● **J34.8212 External nasal valve collapse, dynamic**
▶Collapse or falling of the lower sidewall or nostril of the nose on inspiration

▶● **J34.829 Nasal valve collapse, unspecified**
▶Nasal valve collapse, NOS

J34.89 Other specified disorders of nose and nasal sinuses
Perforation of nasal septum NOS
Rhinolith

J34.9 Unspecified disorder of nose and nasal sinuses

● **J35 Chronic diseases of tonsils and adenoids**

● **J35.Ø Chronic tonsillitis and adenoiditis**

Excludes2 acute tonsillitis (JØ3.-)

J35.Ø1 Chronic tonsillitis

J35.Ø2 Chronic adenoiditis

J35.Ø3 Chronic tonsillitis and adenoiditis

J35.1 Hypertrophy of tonsils
Enlargement of tonsils

Excludes1 hypertrophy of tonsils with tonsillitis (J35.Ø-)

J35.2 Hypertrophy of adenoids
Enlargement of adenoids

Excludes1 hypertrophy of adenoids with adenoiditis (J35.Ø-)

J35.3 Hypertrophy of tonsils with hypertrophy of adenoids

Excludes1 hypertrophy of tonsils and adenoids with tonsillitis and adenoiditis (J35.Ø3)

J35.8 Other chronic diseases of tonsils and adenoids
Adenoid vegetations
Amygdalolith
Calculus, tonsil
Cicatrix of tonsil (and adenoid)
Tonsillar tag
Ulcer of tonsil

J35.9 Chronic disease of tonsils and adenoids, unspecified
Disease (chronic) of tonsils and adenoids NOS

J36 Peritonsillar abscess (Ex:) PDX 1036

Includes abscess of tonsil
peritonsillar cellulitis
quinsy

Use additional code (B95-B97) to identify infectious agent.

Excludes1 acute tonsillitis (JØ3.-)
chronic tonsillitis (J35.Ø)
retropharyngeal abscess (J39.Ø)
tonsillitis NOS (JØ3.9-)

● **J37 Chronic laryngitis and laryngotracheitis**

Use additional code to identify:
exposure to environmental tobacco smoke (Z77.22)
exposure to tobacco smoke in the perinatal period (P96.81)
history of tobacco dependence (Z87.891)
infectious agent (B95-B97)
occupational exposure to environmental tobacco smoke (Z57.31)
tobacco dependence (F17.-)
tobacco use (Z72.Ø)

J37.Ø Chronic laryngitis
Catarrhal laryngitis
Hypertrophic laryngitis
Sicca laryngitis

Excludes2 acute laryngitis (JØ4.Ø)
obstructive (acute) laryngitis (JØ5.Ø)

J37.1 Chronic laryngotracheitis
Laryngitis, chronic, with tracheitis (chronic)
Tracheitis, chronic, with laryngitis

Excludes1 chronic tracheitis (J42)

Excludes2 acute laryngotracheitis (JØ4.2)
acute tracheitis (JØ4.1)

● **J38 Diseases of vocal cords and larynx, not elsewhere classified**

Excludes1 congenital laryngeal stridor (P28.89)
obstructive laryngitis (acute) (JØ5.Ø)
postprocedural subglottic stenosis (J95.5)
stridor (RØ6.1)
ulcerative laryngitis (JØ4.Ø)

● **J38.Ø Paralysis of vocal cords and larynx**
Laryngoplegia
Paralysis of glottis

J38.ØØ Paralysis of vocal cords and larynx, unspecified

J38.Ø1 Paralysis of vocal cords and larynx, unilateral

J38.Ø2 Paralysis of vocal cords and larynx, bilateral

Figure 10-4 Coronal section of the larynx.

Item 10–6 The **larynx** extends from the tongue to the trachea and is divided into an upper and lower portion separated by folds. The framework of the larynx is cartilage composed of the single cricoid, thyroid, and epiglottic cartilages, and the paired arytenoid, cuneiform, and corniculate cartilages.

J38.1 Polyp of vocal cord and larynx
Excludes1 adenomatous polyps (D14.1)

J38.2 Nodules of vocal cords
Chorditis (fibrinous)(nodosa)(tuberosa)
Singer's nodes
Teacher's nodes

J38.3 Other diseases of vocal cords
Abscess of vocal cords
Cellulitis of vocal cords
Granuloma of vocal cords
Leukokeratosis of vocal cords
Leukoplakia of vocal cords

J38.4 Edema of larynx
Edema (of) glottis
Subglottic edema
Supraglottic edema
Excludes1 acute obstructive laryngitis [croup] (J05.0)
edematous laryngitis (J04.0)

J38.5 Laryngeal spasm
Laryngismus (stridulus)

J38.6 Stenosis of larynx

J38.7 Other diseases of larynx
Abscess of larynx
Cellulitis of larynx
Disease of larynx NOS
Necrosis of larynx
Pachyderma of larynx
Perichondritis of larynx
Ulcer of larynx

J39 Other diseases of upper respiratory tract
Excludes1 acute respiratory infection NOS (J22)
acute upper respiratory infection (J06.9)
upper respiratory inflammation due to chemicals, gases, fumes or vapors (J68.2)

J39.0 Retropharyngeal and parapharyngeal abscess (Ex) PDX 1037
Peripharyngeal abscess
Excludes1 peritonsillar abscess (J36)

J39.1 Other abscess of pharynx (Ex) PDX 1037
Cellulitis of pharynx
Nasopharyngeal abscess

J39.2 Other diseases of pharynx
Cyst of pharynx
Edema of pharynx
Excludes2 chronic pharyngitis (J31.2)
ulcerative pharyngitis (J02.9)

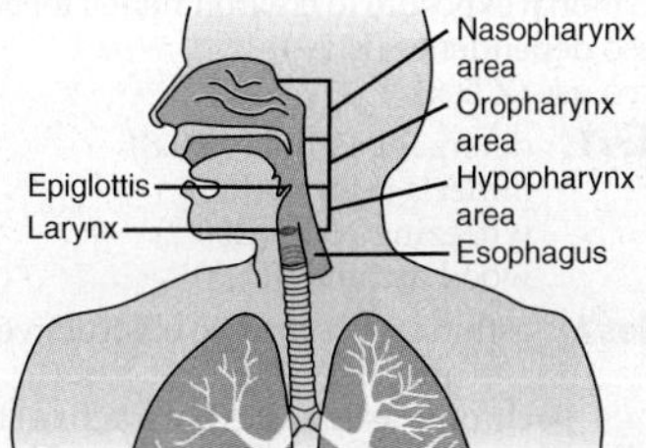

Figure 10-5 The pharynx.

Item 10–7 The **pharynx** is the passage for both food and air between the mouth and the esophagus and is divided into three areas: nasopharynx, oropharynx, and hypopharynx. The hypopharynx branches into the esophagus and the voice box.

Item 10–8 Chronic bronchitis is usually defined as being present in any patient who has persistent cough with sputum production for at least three months in at least two consecutive years. **Simple chronic bronchitis** is marked by a productive cough but no pathological airflow obstruction. **Chronic obstructive pulmonary disease (COPD)** is a group of conditions—bronchitis, emphysema, asthma, bronchiectasis, allergic alveolitis—marked by dyspnea. **Catarrhal** bronchitis is an acute form of bronchitis marked by profuse mucus and pus production (**mucopurulent** discharge). **Croupous** bronchitis, also known as pseudomembranous, fibrinous, plastic, exudative, or membranous, is marked by a violent cough and dyspnea.

J39.3 Upper respiratory tract hypersensitivity reaction, site unspecified
Excludes1 hypersensitivity reaction of upper respiratory tract, such as:
extrinsic allergic alveolitis (J67.9)
pneumoconiosis (J60-J67.9)

J39.8 Other specified diseases of upper respiratory tract
Coding Clinic: 2023, Q1, P30

J39.9 Disease of upper respiratory tract, unspecified

CHRONIC LOWER RESPIRATORY DISEASES (J40-J4A)

Excludes1 bronchitis due to chemicals, gases, fumes and vapors (J68.0)
Excludes2 cystic fibrosis (E84.-)

J40 Bronchitis, not specified as acute or chronic
Bronchitis NOS
Catarrhal bronchitis
Bronchitis with tracheitis NOS
Tracheobronchitis NOS
Use additional code to identify:
exposure to environmental tobacco smoke (Z77.22)
exposure to tobacco smoke in the perinatal period (P96.81)
history of tobacco dependence (Z87.891)
occupational exposure to environmental tobacco smoke (Z57.31)
tobacco dependence (F17.-)
tobacco use (Z72.0)
Excludes1 acute bronchitis (J20.-)
allergic bronchitis NOS (J45.909-)
asthmatic bronchitis NOS (J45.9-)
bronchitis due to chemicals, gases, fumes and vapors (J68.0)

J41 Simple and mucopurulent chronic bronchitis
Use additional code to identify:
exposure to environmental tobacco smoke (Z77.22)
exposure to tobacco smoke in the perinatal period (P96.81)
history of tobacco dependence (Z87.891)
occupational exposure to environmental tobacco smoke (Z57.31)
tobacco dependence (F17.-)
tobacco use (Z72.0)
Excludes2 chronic bronchitis NOS (J42)
chronic obstructive bronchitis (J44.-)

J41.0 Simple chronic bronchitis

J41.1 Mucopurulent chronic bronchitis

J41.8 Mixed simple and mucopurulent chronic bronchitis

J42 Unspecified chronic bronchitis
Chronic bronchitis NOS
Chronic tracheitis
Chronic tracheobronchitis
Use additional code to identify:
exposure to environmental tobacco smoke (Z77.22)
exposure to tobacco smoke in the perinatal period (P96.81)
history of tobacco dependence (Z87.891)
occupational exposure to environmental tobacco smoke (Z57.31)
tobacco dependence (F17.-)
tobacco use (Z72.0)
Excludes1 bronchiolitis obliterans and bronchiolitis obliterans syndrome (J44.81)
chronic asthmatic bronchitis (J44.-)
chronic bronchitis with airways obstruction (J44.-)
chronic emphysematous bronchitis (J44.-)
chronic obstructive pulmonary disease NOS (J44.9)
simple and mucopurulent chronic bronchitis (J41.-)

J43 Emphysema
Excludes1 compensatory emphysema (J98.3)
emphysema due to inhalation of chemicals, gases, fumes or vapors (J68.4)
interstitial emphysema (J98.2)
mediastinal emphysema (J98.2)
neonatal interstitial emphysema (P25.0)
surgical (subcutaneous) emphysema (T81.82)
Excludes2 emphysema with chronic (obstructive) bronchitis (J44.-)
emphysematous (obstructive) bronchitis (J44.-)
traumatic subcutaneous emphysema (T79.7)
Coding Clinic: 2024, Q2, P4

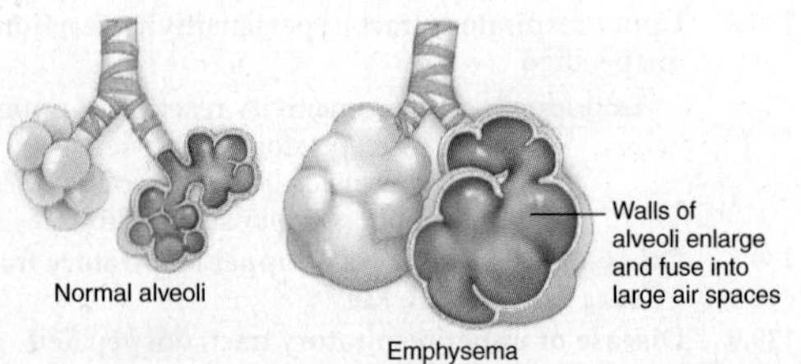

Figure 10-6 Emphysema. (From Shiland, BJ: Medical Terminology & Anatomy for ICD-10 Coding, ed 2, Mosby, 2015)

J43.Ø Unilateral pulmonary emphysema [MacLeod's syndrome]
Swyer-James syndrome
Unilateral emphysema
Unilateral hyperlucent lung
Unilateral pulmonary artery functional hypoplasia
Unilateral transparency of lung

J43.1 Panlobular emphysema
Panacinar emphysema

J43.2 Centrilobular emphysema

J43.8 Other emphysema

J43.9 Emphysema, unspecified
Bullous emphysema (lung)(pulmonary)
Emphysema (lung)(pulmonary) NOS
Emphysematous bleb
Vesicular emphysema (lung)(pulmonary)
Coding Clinic: 2Ø24, Q2, P4, 5; 2Ø19, Q1, P35-37; 2Ø17, Q4, P97-98

● J44 Other chronic obstructive pulmonary disease

Includes asthma with chronic obstructive pulmonary disease
chronic asthmatic (obstructive) bronchitis
chronic bronchitis with airway obstruction
chronic bronchitis with emphysema
chronic emphysematous bronchitis
chronic obstructive asthma
chronic obstructive bronchitis
chronic obstructive tracheobronchitis

Code also type of asthma, if applicable (J45.-)

Excludes1 chronic bronchitis NOS (J42)
chronic simple and mucopurulent bronchitis (J41.-)
chronic tracheitis (J42)
chronic tracheobronchitis (J42)

Excludes2 bronchiectasis (J47.-)
emphysema without chronic bronchitis (J43.-)

Coding Clinic: 2Ø24, Q2, P3-6; 2Ø19, Q1, P34-36; 2Ø17, Q4, P97; 2Ø17, Q1, P25; 2Ø16, Q3, P16

J44.Ø Chronic obstructive pulmonary disease with (acute) lower respiratory infection (Ex) PDX 1038
Code also to identify the infection
Coding Clinic: 2Ø24, Q2, P6; 2Ø19, Q1, P35-36; 2Ø17, Q4, P96; 2Ø17, Q2, P3Ø, Q1, P24-25; 2Ø16, Q3, P15-16

J44.1 Chronic obstructive pulmonary disease with (acute) exacerbation (Ex) PDX 1038
Decompensated COPD
Decompensated COPD with (acute) exacerbation

Excludes2 chronic obstructive pulmonary disease [COPD] with acute bronchitis (J44.Ø)
lung diseases due to external agents (J6Ø-J7Ø)

Coding Clinic: 2Ø24, Q2, P6; 2Ø19, Q1, P34-35; 2Ø17, Q4, P96; 2Ø17, Q1, P26; 2Ø16, Q3, P15-16, Q1, P36

● J44.8 Other specified chronic obstructive pulmonary disease

J44.81 Bronchiolitis obliterans and bronchiolitis obliterans syndrome
Obliterative bronchiolitis
Code first, if applicable:
complication of bone marrow transplant (T86.Ø9)
complication of stem cell transplant (T86.5)
heart-lung transplant rejection (T86.31)
lung transplant rejection (T86.81Ø)
other complications of heart-lung transplant (T86.39)
other complications of lung transplant (T86.818)

Code also, if applicable, associated conditions, such as:
chronic graft-versus-host disease (D89.811)
chronic lung allograft dysfunction (J4A.-)
chronic respiratory conditions due to chemicals, gases, fumes and vapors (J68.4)

J44.89 Other specified chronic obstructive pulmonary disease
Chronic asthmatic (obstructive) bronchitis
Chronic emphysematous bronchitis
Coding Clinic: 2Ø24, Q2, P3

J44.9 Chronic obstructive pulmonary disease, unspecified
Chronic obstructive airway disease NOS
Chronic obstructive lung disease NOS

Excludes2 lung diseases due to external agents (J6Ø-J7Ø)

Coding Clinic: 2Ø24, Q2, P3, 4, 6; 2Ø19, Q1, P36; 2Ø17, Q4, P96-97; 2Ø17, Q1, P24-25; 2Ø16, Q1, P37

● J45 Asthma (Ex) PDX 1039
Allergic (predominantly) asthma
Allergic bronchitis NOS
Allergic rhinitis with asthma
Atopic asthma
Extrinsic allergic asthma
Hay fever with asthma
Idiosyncratic asthma
Intrinsic nonallergic asthma
Nonallergic asthma

Use additional code to identify:
eosinophilic asthma (J82.83)
exposure to environmental tobacco smoke (Z77.22)
exposure to tobacco smoke in the perinatal period (P96.81)
history of tobacco dependence (Z87.891)
occupational exposure to environmental tobacco smoke (Z57.31)
tobacco dependence (F17.-)
tobacco use (Z72.Ø)

Excludes1 detergent asthma (J69.8)
miner's asthma (J6Ø)
wheezing NOS (RØ6.2)
wood asthma (J67.8)

Excludes2 asthma with chronic obstructive pulmonary disease (J44.89)
chronic asthmatic (obstructive) bronchitis (J44.89)
chronic obstructive asthma (J44.89)
other specified chronic obstructive pulmonary disease (J44.89)

Coding Clinic: 2Ø24, Q2, P3; 2Ø19, Q1, P37; 2Ø17, Q1, P25

● J45.2 Mild intermittent asthma

J45.2Ø Mild intermittent asthma, uncomplicated
Mild intermittent asthma NOS

J45.21 Mild intermittent asthma with (acute) exacerbation

J45.22 Mild intermittent asthma with status asthmaticus

Item 10-9 Asthma is a bronchial condition marked by airway obstruction, hyper-responsiveness, and inflammation. **Extrinsic** asthma, also known as allergic asthma, is characterized by the same symptoms that occur with exposure to allergens and is divided into the following types: **atopic, occupational,** and **allergic bronchopulmonary aspergillosis. Intrinsic** asthma occurs in patients who have no history of allergy or sensitivities to allergens and is divided into the following types: **nonreaginic** and **pharmacologic. Status asthmaticus** is the most severe form of asthma attack and can last for days or weeks.

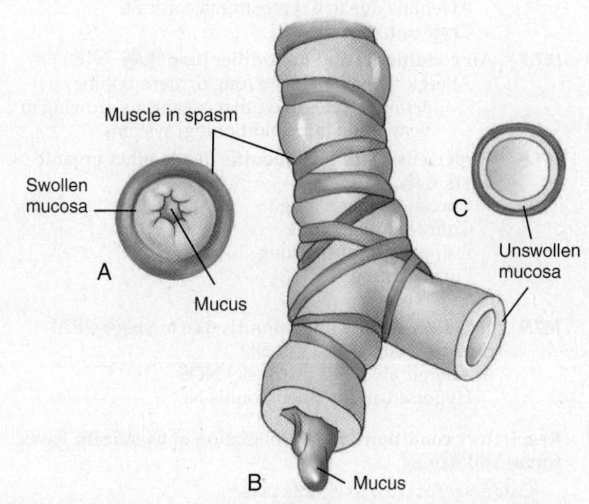

Figure 10-7 Factors causing expiratory obstruction in asthma. **A.** Cross section of a bronchiole occluded by muscle spasm, swollen mucosa, and mucus. **B.** Longitudinal section of an obstructed bronchiole. **C.** Cross section of a clear bronchiole. (From Shiland: Mastering Healthcare Terminology, ed 1, St. Louis, Mosby, 2003)

● **J45.3 Mild persistent asthma**
- **J45.30 Mild persistent asthma, uncomplicated**
  - Mild persistent asthma NOS
- **J45.31 Mild persistent asthma with (acute) exacerbation**
  - Coding Clinic: 2016, Q1, P35
- **J45.32 Mild persistent asthma with status asthmaticus**

● **J45.4 Moderate persistent asthma**
- **J45.40 Moderate persistent asthma, uncomplicated**
  - Moderate persistent asthma NOS
- **J45.41 Moderate persistent asthma with (acute) exacerbation**
  - Coding Clinic: 2017, Q1, P26
- **J45.42 Moderate persistent asthma with status asthmaticus**

● **J45.5 Severe persistent asthma**
- **J45.50 Severe persistent asthma, uncomplicated**
  - Severe persistent asthma NOS
- **J45.51 Severe persistent asthma with (acute) exacerbation**
- **J45.52 Severe persistent asthma with status asthmaticus**

● **J45.9 Other and unspecified asthma**
- ● **J45.90 Unspecified asthma**
  - Asthmatic bronchitis NOS
  - Childhood asthma NOS
  - Late onset asthma
  - **J45.901 Unspecified asthma with (acute) exacerbation**
    - Coding Clinic: 2017, Q4, P96
  - **J45.902 Unspecified asthma with status asthmaticus**
  - **J45.909 Unspecified asthma, uncomplicated**
    - Asthma NOS
    - **Excludes2** lung diseases due to external agents (J60-J70)
    - Coding Clinic: 2024, Q2, P3; 2023, Q1, P17; 2017, Q4, P96; 2017, Q1, P25
- ● **J45.99 Other asthma**
  - **J45.990 Exercise induced bronchospasm**
  - **J45.991 Cough variant asthma**
  - **J45.998 Other asthma**

● **J47 Bronchiectasis** Ex: PDX 1040

Includes bronchiolectasis

Use additional code to identify:
- exposure to environmental tobacco smoke (Z77.22)
- exposure to tobacco smoke in the perinatal period (P96.81)
- history of tobacco dependence (Z87.891)
- occupational exposure to environmental tobacco smoke (Z57.31)
- tobacco dependence (F17.-)
- tobacco use (Z72.0)

Excludes1 congenital bronchiectasis (Q33.4)
tuberculous bronchiectasis (current disease) (A15.0)

Coding Clinic: 2024, Q2, P5,6

- **J47.0 Bronchiectasis with acute lower respiratory infection**
  - Bronchiectasis with acute bronchitis
  - Code also to identify infection, if applicable
- **J47.1 Bronchiectasis with (acute) exacerbation**
  - Coding Clinic: 2021, Q1, P24
- **J47.9 Bronchiectasis, uncomplicated**
  - Bronchiectasis NOS
  - Coding Clinic: 2024, Q2, P5,6

LUNG DISEASES DUE TO EXTERNAL AGENTS (J60-J70)

Excludes2 asthma (J45.-)
malignant neoplasm of bronchus and lung (C34.-)

● **J4A Chronic lung allograft dysfunction**

Code first, if applicable:
- heart-lung transplant rejection (T86.31)
- lung transplant rejection (T86.810)
- other complications of heart-lung transplant (T86.39)
- other complications of lung transplant (T86.818)

Code also, if applicable, bronchiolitis obliterans syndrome (J44.81)

- **J4A.0 Restrictive allograft syndrome**
  - Code also, if applicable, for mixed chronic lung allograft dysfunction, bronchiolitis obliterans syndrome (J44.81)
- **J4A.8 Other chronic lung allograft dysfunction**
- **J4A.9 Chronic lung allograft dysfunction, unspecified**

J60 Coalworker's pneumoconiosis A
- Anthracosilicosis
- Anthracosis
- Black lung disease
- Coalworker's lung

Excludes1 coalworker pneumoconiosis with tuberculosis, any type in A15 (J65)

J61 Pneumoconiosis due to asbestos and other mineral fibers A
- Asbestosis

Excludes1 pleural plaque with asbestosis (J92.0)
pneumoconiosis with tuberculosis, any type in A15 (J65)

CHAPTER 10 (J00-J99)

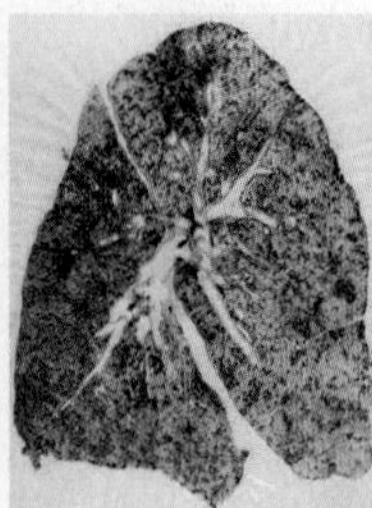

Figure 10-8 Progressive massive fibrosis superimposed on coal workers' pneumoconiosis. The large, blackened scars are located principally in the upper lobe. (From Frazier MS, Drzymkowski JW: Essentials of Human Diseases and Conditions, St. Louis, MO, Saunders, 2004)

Item 10-10 Pneumoconiosis refers to a lung condition resulting from exposure to inorganic or organic airborne particles, such as coal dust or moldy hay, as well as chemical fumes and vapors, such as insecticides. In this condition, the lungs retain the airborne particles.

● **J62 Pneumoconiosis due to dust containing silica**
Includes silicotic fibrosis (massive) of lung
Excludes1 pneumoconiosis with tuberculosis, any type in A15 (J65)
J62.0 Pneumoconiosis due to talc dust
J62.8 Pneumoconiosis due to other dust containing silica
Silicosis NOS

● **J63 Pneumoconiosis due to other inorganic dusts**
Excludes1 pneumoconiosis with tuberculosis, any type in A15 (J65)
Coding Clinic: 2019, Q3, P8
J63.0 Aluminosis (of lung)
J63.1 Bauxite fibrosis (of lung)
J63.2 Berylliosis
J63.3 Graphite fibrosis (of lung)
J63.4 Siderosis
Coding Clinic: 2019, Q3, P8
J63.5 Stannosis
J63.6 Pneumoconiosis due to other specified inorganic dusts

J64 Unspecified pneumoconiosis
Excludes1 pneumonoconiosis with tuberculosis, any type in A15 (J65)

J65 Pneumoconiosis associated with tuberculosis
Any condition in J60-J64 with tuberculosis, any type in A15
Silicotuberculosis

● **J66 Airway disease due to specific organic dust**
Excludes2 allergic alveolitis (J67.-)
asbestosis (J61)
bagassosis (J67.1)
farmer's lung (J67.0)
hypersensitivity pneumonitis due to organic dust (J67.-)
reactive airways dysfunction syndrome (J68.3)
J66.0 Byssinosis
Airway disease due to cotton dust
J66.1 Flax-dressers' disease
J66.2 Cannabinosis
J66.8 Airway disease due to other specific organic dusts

● **J67 Hypersensitivity pneumonitis due to organic dust**
Includes allergic alveolitis and pneumonitis due to inhaled organic dust and particles of fungal, actinomycetic or other origin
Excludes1 pneumonitis due to inhalation of chemicals, gases, fumes or vapors (J68.0)
J67.0 Farmer's lung
Harvester's lung
Haymaker's lung
Moldy hay disease
J67.1 Bagassosis
Bagasse disease
Bagasse pneumonitis
J67.2 Bird fancier's lung
Budgerigar fancier's disease or lung
Pigeon fancier's disease or lung
J67.3 Suberosis
Corkhandler's disease or lung
Corkworker's disease or lung
J67.4 Maltworker's lung
Alveolitis due to Aspergillus clavatus
J67.5 Mushroom-worker's lung
J67.6 Maple-bark-stripper's lung
Alveolitis due to Cryptostroma corticale
Cryptostromosis
J67.7 Air conditioner and humidifier lung Ex: PDX 1041
Allergic alveolitis due to fungal, thermophilic actinomycetes and other organisms growing in ventilation [air conditioning] systems
J67.8 Hypersensitivity pneumonitis due to other organic dusts Ex: PDX 1042
Cheese-washer's lung
Coffee-worker's lung
Fish-meal worker's lung
Furrier's lung
Sequoiosis
J67.9 Hypersensitivity pneumonitis due to unspecified organic dust Ex: PDX 1042
Allergic alveolitis (extrinsic) NOS
Hypersensitivity pneumonitis NOS

● **J68 Respiratory conditions due to inhalation of chemicals, gases, fumes and vapors**
Code first (T51-T65) to identify cause
Use additional code to identify associated respiratory conditions, such as:
acute respiratory failure (J96.0-)
J68.0 Bronchitis and pneumonitis due to chemicals, gases, fumes and vapors Ex: PDX 1042
Chemical bronchitis (acute)
Coding Clinic: 2019, Q2, P31-32
J68.1 Pulmonary edema due to chemicals, gases, fumes and vapors
Chemical pulmonary edema (acute) (chronic)
Excludes1 pulmonary edema (acute) (chronic) NOS (J81.-)
J68.2 Upper respiratory inflammation due to chemicals, gases, fumes and vapors, not elsewhere classified
J68.3 Other acute and subacute respiratory conditions due to chemicals, gases, fumes and vapors
Reactive airways dysfunction syndrome
J68.4 Chronic respiratory conditions due to chemicals, gases, fumes and vapors
Code also, if applicable, chronic conditions, such as:
emphysema (J43.-)
obliterative bronchiolitis (J44.81)
pulmonary fibrosis (J84.10)
Excludes1 chronic pulmonary edema due to chemicals, gases, fumes and vapors (J68.1)
J68.8 Other respiratory conditions due to chemicals, gases, fumes and vapors
J68.9 Unspecified respiratory condition due to chemicals, gases, fumes and vapors

CHAPTER 10 (J00-J99)

J69 Pneumonitis due to solids and liquids
Code also, if applicable, other types of pneumonias
Excludes1 neonatal aspiration syndromes (P24.-)
postprocedural pneumonitis (J95.4)

J69.0 Pneumonitis due to inhalation of food and vomit PDX 1041
Aspiration pneumonia NOS
Aspiration pneumonia (due to) food (regurgitated)
Aspiration pneumonia (due to) gastric secretions
Aspiration pneumonia (due to) milk
Aspiration pneumonia (due to) vomit
Code also any associated foreign body in respiratory tract (T17.-)
Excludes1 chemical pneumonitis due to anesthesia (J95.4)
obstetric aspiration pneumonitis (O74.0)
Coding Clinic: 2021, Q1, P34; 2019, Q2, P7, 31-32; 2017, Q1, P24

J69.1 Pneumonitis due to inhalation of oils and essences PDX 1042
Exogenous lipoid pneumonia
Lipid pneumonia NOS
Code first (T51-T65) to identify substance
Excludes1 endogenous lipoid pneumonia (J84.89)

J69.8 Pneumonitis due to inhalation of other solids and liquids PDX 1041
Pneumonitis due to aspiration of blood
Pneumonitis due to aspiration of detergent
Code first (T51-T65) to identify substance

J70 Respiratory conditions due to other external agents

J70.0 Acute pulmonary manifestations due to radiation PDX 1041
Radiation pneumonitis
Use additional code (W88-W90, X39.0-) to identify the external cause

J70.1 Chronic and other pulmonary manifestations due to radiation PDX 1041
Fibrosis of lung following radiation
Use additional code (W88-W90, X39.0-) to identify the external cause

J70.2 Acute drug-induced interstitial lung disorders
Use additional code for adverse effect, if applicable, to identify drug (T36-T50 with fifth or sixth character 5)
Excludes1 interstitial pneumonia NOS (J84.9)
lymphoid interstitial pneumonia (J84.2)
Coding Clinic: 2019, Q2, P28

J70.3 Chronic drug-induced interstitial lung disorders
Use additional code for adverse effect, if applicable, to identify drug (T36-T50 with fifth or sixth character 5)
Excludes1 interstitial pneumonia NOS (J84.9)
lymphoid interstitial pneumonia (J84.2)

J70.4 Drug-induced interstitial lung disorders, unspecified
Use additional code for adverse effect, if applicable, to identify drug (T36-T50 with fifth or sixth character 5)
Excludes1 interstitial pneumonia NOS (J84.9)
lymphoid interstitial pneumonia (J84.2)
Coding Clinic: 2019, Q2, P28

J70.5 Respiratory conditions due to smoke inhalation
Code first smoke inhalation (T59.81-)
Excludes2 smoke inhalation due to chemicals, gases, fumes and vapors (J68.9)

J70.8 Respiratory conditions due to other specified external agents
Code first (T51-T65) to identify the external agent

J70.9 Respiratory conditions due to unspecified external agent
Code first (T51-T65) to identify the external agent

OTHER RESPIRATORY DISEASES PRINCIPALLY AFFECTING THE INTERSTITIUM (J80-J84)

J80 Acute respiratory distress syndrome PDX 1043
Acute respiratory distress syndrome in adult or child
Adult hyaline membrane disease
Excludes1 respiratory distress syndrome in newborn (perinatal) (P22.0)
Coding Clinic: 2017, Q1, P26-27

J81 Pulmonary edema
Use additional code to identify:
exposure to environmental tobacco smoke (Z77.22)
history of tobacco dependence (Z87.891)
occupational exposure to environmental tobacco smoke (Z57.31)
tobacco dependence (F17.-)
tobacco use (Z72.0)
Excludes1 chemical (acute) pulmonary edema (J68.1)
hypostatic pneumonia (J18.2)
passive pneumonia (J18.2)
pulmonary edema due to external agents (J60-J70)
pulmonary edema with heart disease NOS (I50.1)
pulmonary edema with heart failure (I50.1)

J81.0 Acute pulmonary edema PDX 1044
Acute edema of lung
Coding Clinic: 2023, Q1, P25; 2017, Q1, P26

J81.1 Chronic pulmonary edema PDX 1033
Pulmonary congestion (chronic) (passive)
Pulmonary edema NOS

J82 Pulmonary eosinophilia, not elsewhere classified
Excludes2 pulmonary eosinophilia due to aspergillosis (B44.-)
pulmonary eosinophilia due to drugs (J70.2-J70.4)
pulmonary eosinophilia due to specified parasitic infection (B50-B83)
pulmonary eosinophilia due to systemic connective tissue disorders (M30-M36)
pulmonary infiltrate NOS (R91.8)

J82.8 Pulmonary eosinophilia, not elsewhere classified PDX 1045

J82.81 Chronic eosinophilic pneumonia
Eosinophilic pneumonia, NOS

J82.82 Acute eosinophilic pneumonia

J82.83 Eosinophilic asthma
Code first asthma, by type, such as:
mild intermittent asthma (J45.2-)
mild persistent asthma (J45.3-)
moderate persistent asthma (J45.4-)
severe persistent asthma (J45.5-)

J82.89 Other pulmonary eosinophilia, not elsewhere classified
Allergic pneumonia
Löffler's pneumonia
Tropical (pulmonary) eosinophilia NOS

J84 Other interstitial pulmonary diseases
Excludes1 drug-induced interstitial lung disorders (J70.2-J70.4)
interstitial emphysema (J98.2)
Excludes2 lung diseases due to external agents (J60-J70)
Coding Clinic: 2019, Q2, P28

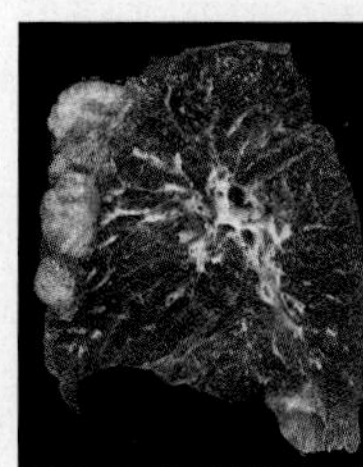

Figure 10-9 Bullous emphysema with large subpleural bullae *(upper left)*. (From Kumar: Robbins and Cotran: Pathologic Basis of Disease, ed 8, Saunders, An Imprint of Elsevier, 2009)

CHAPTER 10 (J00-J99)

J84.0 Alveolar and parieto-alveolar conditions PDX 1046

J84.01 Alveolar proteinosis

J84.02 Pulmonary alveolar microlithiasis

J84.03 Idiopathic pulmonary hemosiderosis

Essential brown induration of lung

Code first underlying disease, such as:
disorders of iron metabolism (E83.1-)

Code also, if applicable, associated condition

Excludes1 acute idiopathic pulmonary hemorrhage in infants [AIPHI] (R04.81)

J84.09 Other alveolar and parieto-alveolar conditions

J84.1 Other interstitial pulmonary diseases with fibrosis

Excludes1 pulmonary fibrosis (chronic) due to inhalation of chemicals, gases, fumes or vapors (J68.4)
pulmonary fibrosis (chronic) following radiation (J70.1)

J84.10 Pulmonary fibrosis, unspecified

Capillary fibrosis of lung
Cirrhosis of lung (chronic) NOS
Fibrosis of lung (atrophic) (chronic) (confluent) (massive) (perialveolar) (peribronchial) NOS
Induration of lung (chronic) NOS
Postinflammatory pulmonary fibrosis

Coding Clinic: 2024, Q2, P20

J84.11 Idiopathic interstitial pneumonia PDX 1046

Excludes1 lymphoid interstitial pneumonia (J84.2)
pneumocystis pneumonia (B59)

J84.111 Idiopathic interstitial pneumonia, not otherwise specified

J84.112 Idiopathic pulmonary fibrosis

Cryptogenic fibrosing alveolitis
Idiopathic fibrosing alveolitis

J84.113 Idiopathic non-specific interstitial pneumonitis

Excludes1 non-specific interstitial pneumonia NOS, or due to known underlying cause (J84.89)

J84.114 Acute interstitial pneumonitis

Hamman-Rich syndrome

Excludes1 pneumocystis pneumonia (B59)

J84.115 Respiratory bronchiolitis interstitial lung disease

J84.116 Cryptogenic organizing pneumonia

Excludes1 organizing pneumonia NOS, or due to known underlying cause (J84.89)

J84.117 Desquamative interstitial pneumonia

J84.17 Other interstitial pulmonary diseases with fibrosis in diseases classified elsewhere

J84.170 Interstitial lung disease with progressive fibrotic phenotype in diseases classified elsewhere

Progressive fibrotic interstitial lung disease

Code first underlying disease, such as:
lung diseases due to external agents (J60-J70)
rheumatoid arthritis (M05.00-M06.9)
sarcoidosis (D86.-)
systemic connective tissue disorders (M30-M36)

J84.178 Other interstitial pulmonary diseases with fibrosis in diseases classified elsewhere

Interstitial pneumonia (nonspecific) (usual) due to collagen vascular disease
Interstitial pneumonia (nonspecific) (usual) in diseases classified elsewhere
Organizing pneumonia due to collagen vascular disease
Organizing pneumonia in diseases classified elsewhere

Code first underlying disease, such as:
progressive systemic sclerosis (M34.0)
rheumatoid arthritis (M05.00-M06.9)
systemic lupus erythematosis (M32.0-M32.9)

J84.2 Lymphoid interstitial pneumonia PDX 1046

Lymphoid interstitial pneumonitis

J84.8 Other specified interstitial pulmonary diseases

Excludes1 exogenous lipoid pneumonia (J69.1)
unspecified lipoid pneumonia (J69.1)

J84.81 Lymphangioleiomyomatosis PDX 1046

Lymphangiomyomatosis

J84.82 Adult pulmonary Langerhans cell histiocytosis PDX 1046 A

Adult PLCH

J84.83 Surfactant mutations of the lung PDX 1047

J84.84 Other interstitial lung diseases of childhood PDX 1047

J84.841 Neuroendocrine cell hyperplasia of infancy

J84.842 Pulmonary interstitial glycogenosis

J84.843 Alveolar capillary dysplasia with vein misalignment

J84.848 Other interstitial lung diseases of childhood

J84.89 **Other specified interstitial pulmonary diseases**
Endogenous lipoid pneumonia
Interstitial pneumonitis
Non-specific interstitial pneumonitis NOS
Organizing pneumonia NOS
Code first, if applicable:
poisoning due to drug or toxin (T51-T65 with fifth or sixth character to indicate intent), for toxic pneumonopathy
underlying cause of pneumonopathy, if known
Use additional code, for adverse effect, to identify drug (T36-T50 with fifth or sixth character 5), if drug-induced
Excludes1 cryptogenic organizing pneumonia (J84.116)
idiopathic non-specific interstitial pneumonitis (J84.113)
lipoid pneumonia, exogenous or unspecified (J69.1)
lymphoid interstitial pneumonia (J84.2)
Coding Clinic: 2021, Q4, P106-107; 2021, Q1, P48; 2019, Q2, P28

J84.9 **Interstitial pulmonary disease, unspecified** (Ex) PDX 1046
Interstitial pneumonia NOS

SUPPURATIVE AND NECROTIC CONDITIONS OF THE LOWER RESPIRATORY TRACT (J85-J86)

J85 **Abscess of lung and mediastinum**
Use additional code (B95-B97) to identify infectious agent.
J85.0 **Gangrene and necrosis of lung** (Ex) PDX 1048
J85.1 **Abscess of lung with pneumonia** (Ex) PDX 1048
Code also the type of pneumonia
J85.2 **Abscess of lung without pneumonia** (Ex) PDX 1048
Abscess of lung NOS
J85.3 **Abscess of mediastinum** (Ex) PDX 1049

J86 **Pyothorax** (Ex) PDX 1050
▶Code also, if applicable, disruption of internal operation (surgical) wound (T81.32-)
Use additional code (B95-B97) to identify infectious agent.
Excludes1 abscess of lung (J85.-)
pyothorax due to tuberculosis (A15.6)
J86.0 **Pyothorax with fistula**
Bronchocutaneous fistula
Bronchopleural fistula
Hepatopleural fistula
Mediastinal fistula
Pleural fistula
Thoracic fistula
Any condition classifiable to J86.9 with fistula
J86.9 **Pyothorax without fistula**
Abscess of pleura
Abscess of thorax
Empyema (chest) (lung) (pleura)
Fibrinopurulent pleurisy
Purulent pleurisy
Pyopneumothorax
Septic pleurisy
Seropurulent pleurisy
Suppurative pleurisy

Item 10–11 Empyema is a condition in which pus accumulates in a body cavity. Empyema **with fistula** occurs when the pus passes from one cavity to another organ or structure.

OTHER DISEASES OF THE PLEURA (J90-J94)

J90 **Pleural effusion, not elsewhere classified** (Ex) PDX 1051
Encysted pleurisy
Pleural effusion NOS
Pleurisy with effusion (exudative) (serous)
Excludes1 chylous (pleural) effusion (J94.0)
malignant pleural effusion (J91.0))
pleurisy NOS (R09.1)
tuberculous pleural effusion (A15.6)
Coding Clinic: 2015, Q2, P16

J91 **Pleural effusion in conditions classified elsewhere**
Excludes2 pleural effusion in heart failure (I50.-)
pleural effusion in systemic lupus erythematosus (M32.13)
J91.0 ***Malignant pleural effusion*** (Ex) PDX 1051
Code first underlying neoplasm (C00-D49)
Coding Clinic: 2024, Q2, P11,12; 2022, Q3, P14-15
J91.8 ***Pleural effusion in other conditions classified elsewhere*** (Ex) PDX 1052
Code first underlying disease, such as:
filariasis (B74.0-B74.9)
influenza (J09.X2, J10.1, J11.1)
Coding Clinic: 2015, Q2, P16

J92 **Pleural plaque**
Includes pleural thickening
J92.0 **Pleural plaque with presence of asbestos**
J92.9 **Pleural plaque without asbestos**
Pleural plaque NOS

J93 **Pneumothorax and air leak**
Collapsed lung
Excludes1 congenital or perinatal pneumothorax (P25.1)
postprocedural air leak (J95.812)
postprocedural pneumothorax (J95.811)
traumatic pneumothorax (S27.0)
tuberculous (current disease) pneumothorax (A15.-)
pyopneumothorax (J86.-)
J93.0 **Spontaneous tension pneumothorax** (Ex) PDX 1053
Tension pneumothorax (most serious type) occurs when air (positive pressure) collects in the pleural space
J93.1 **Other spontaneous pneumothorax** (Ex) PDX 1053
J93.11 **Primary spontaneous pneumothorax**
J93.12 **Secondary spontaneous pneumothorax**
Code first underlying condition, such as:
catamenial pneumothorax due to endometriosis (N80.B-)
cystic fibrosis (E84.-)
eosinophilic pneumonia (J82)
lymphangioleiomyomatosis (J84.81)
malignant neoplasm of bronchus and lung (C34.-)
Marfan syndrome (Q87.4-)
pneumonia due to Pneumocystis carinii (B59)
secondary malignant neoplasm of lung (C78.0-)
spontaneous rupture of the esophagus (K22.3)
J93.8 **Other pneumothorax and air leak** (Ex) PDX 1053
J93.81 **Chronic pneumothorax**
J93.82 **Other air leak**
Persistent air leak
J93.83 **Other pneumothorax**
Acute pneumothorax
Spontaneous pneumothorax NOS
J93.9 **Pneumothorax, unspecified** (Ex) PDX 1053
Pneumothorax NOS

CHAPTER 10 (J00-J99)

J94 Other pleural conditions PDX 1051
Excludes1 pleurisy NOS (R09.1)
traumatic hemopneumothorax (S27.2)
traumatic hemothorax (S27.1)
tuberculous pleural conditions (current disease) (A15.-)

J94.0 Chylous effusion
Chyliform effusion

J94.1 Fibrothorax

J94.2 Hemothorax
Hemopneumothorax

J94.8 Other specified pleural conditions
Hydropneumothorax
Hydrothorax
Coding Clinic: 2021, Q1, P49

J94.9 Pleural condition, unspecified

INTRAOPERATIVE AND POSTPROCEDURAL COMPLICATIONS AND DISORDERS OF RESPIRATORY SYSTEM, NOT ELSEWHERE CLASSIFIED (J95)

J95 Intraoperative and postprocedural complications and disorders of respiratory system, not elsewhere classified
Excludes2 aspiration pneumonia (J69.-)
emphysema (subcutaneous) resulting from a procedure (T81.82)
hypostatic pneumonia (J18.2)
pulmonary manifestations due to radiation (J70.0- J70.1)

J95.0 Tracheostomy complications PDX 1055

J95.00 Unspecified tracheostomy complication

J95.01 Hemorrhage from tracheostomy stoma

J95.02 Infection of tracheostomy stoma
Use additional code to identify type of infection, such as:
cellulitis of neck (L03.221)
sepsis (A40, A41.-)

J95.03 Malfunction of tracheostomy stoma
Mechanical complication of tracheostomy stoma
Obstruction of tracheostomy airway
Tracheal stenosis due to tracheostomy

J95.04 Tracheo-esophageal fistula following tracheostomy

J95.09 Other tracheostomy complication

J95.1 Acute pulmonary insufficiency following thoracic surgery PDX 1056
Excludes2 functional disturbances following cardiac surgery (I97.0, I97.1-)

J95.2 Acute pulmonary insufficiency following nonthoracic surgery PDX 1057
Excludes2 functional disturbances following cardiac surgery (I97.0, I97.1-)

J95.3 Chronic pulmonary insufficiency following surgery PDX 1058
Excludes2 functional disturbances following cardiac surgery (I97.0, I97.1-)

J95.4 Chemical pneumonitis due to anesthesia PDX 1059
Mendelson's syndrome
Postprocedural aspiration pneumonia
Use additional code for adverse effect, if applicable, to identify drug (T41.- with fifth or sixth character 5)
Excludes1 aspiration pneumonitis due to anesthesia complicating labor and delivery (O74.0)
aspiration pneumonitis due to anesthesia complicating pregnancy (O29)
aspiration pneumonitis due to anesthesia complicating the puerperium (O89.01)

J95.5 Postprocedural subglottic stenosis PDX 1059

J95.6 Intraoperative hemorrhage and hematoma of a respiratory system organ or structure complicating a procedure PDX 1060
Excludes1 intraoperative hemorrhage and hematoma of a respiratory system organ or structure due to accidental puncture and laceration during procedure (J95.7-)

J95.61 Intraoperative hemorrhage and hematoma of a respiratory system organ or structure complicating a respiratory system procedure

J95.62 Intraoperative hemorrhage and hematoma of a respiratory system organ or structure complicating other procedure

J95.7 Accidental puncture and laceration of a respiratory system organ or structure during a procedure PDX 569
Excludes2 postprocedural pneumothorax (J95.811)

J95.71 Accidental puncture and laceration of a respiratory system organ or structure during a respiratory system procedure

J95.72 Accidental puncture and laceration of a respiratory system organ or structure during other procedure

J95.8 Other intraoperative and postprocedural complications and disorders of respiratory system, not elsewhere classified
Coding Clinic: 2016, Q4, P10

J95.81 Postprocedural pneumothorax and air leak

J95.811 Postprocedural pneumothorax PDX 1053
Coding Clinic: 2021, Q1, P49

J95.812 Postprocedural air leak PDX 1053

J95.82 Postprocedural respiratory failure
Excludes1 Respiratory failure in other conditions (J96.-)

J95.821 Acute postprocedural respiratory failure PDX 1056
Postprocedural respiratory failure NOS

J95.822 Acute and chronic postprocedural respiratory failure PDX 1056

J95.83 Postprocedural hemorrhage of a respiratory system organ or structure following a procedure PDX 1060

J95.830 Postprocedural hemorrhage of a respiratory system organ or structure following a respiratory system procedure

J95.831 Postprocedural hemorrhage of a respiratory system organ or structure following other procedure
Coding Clinic: 2023, Q2, P28

J95.84 Transfusion-related acute lung injury (TRALI) PDX 1059

J95.85 Complication of respirator [ventilator]

J95.850 Mechanical complication of respirator PDX 1061
Excludes1 encounter for respirator [ventilator] dependence during power failure (Z99.12)

J95.851 **Ventilator associated pneumonia** (Ex) PDX 1062
Ventilator associated pneumonitis
Use additional code to identify the organism, if known (B95.-, B96.-, B97.-)
Excludes1 ventilator lung in newborn (P27.8)
Coding Clinic: 2017, Q1, P25

J95.859 **Other complication of respirator [ventilator]** (Ex) PDX 1062
Coding Clinic: 2021, Q1, P49

● J95.86 **Postprocedural hematoma and seroma of a respiratory system organ or structure following a procedure** (Ex) PDX 1060

J95.860 **Postprocedural hematoma of a respiratory system organ or structure following a respiratory system procedure**

J95.861 **Postprocedural hematoma of a respiratory system organ or structure following other procedure**

J95.862 **Postprocedural seroma of a respiratory system organ or structure following a respiratory system procedure**

J95.863 **Postprocedural seroma of a respiratory system organ or structure following other procedure**

J95.87 **Transfusion-associated dyspnea (TAD)** (Ex) PDX 1063
Excludes1 transfusion associated circulatory overload (TACO) (E87.71)
transfusion-related acute lung injury (TRALI) (J95.84)

J95.88 **Other intraoperative complications of respiratory system, not elsewhere classified** (Ex) PDX 1059

J95.89 **Other postprocedural complications and disorders of respiratory system, not elsewhere classified** (Ex) PDX 1059
Use additional code to identify disorder, such as:
aspiration pneumonia (J69.-)
bacterial or viral pneumonia (J12-J18)
Excludes2 acute pulmonary insufficiency following thoracic surgery (J95.1)
postprocedural subglottic stenosis (J95.5)

OTHER DISEASES OF THE RESPIRATORY SYSTEM (J96-J99)

● J96 **Respiratory failure, not elsewhere classified** (Ex) PDX 1043
Excludes1 acute respiratory distress syndrome (J80)
cardiorespiratory failure (R09.2)
newborn respiratory distress syndrome (P22.0)
postprocedural respiratory failure (J95.82-)
respiratory arrest (R09.2)
respiratory arrest of newborn (P28.81)
respiratory failure of newborn (P28.5)

● J96.0 **Acute respiratory failure**

J96.00 **Acute respiratory failure, unspecified whether with hypoxia or hypercapnia**
Coding Clinic: 2016, Q3, P14

J96.01 **Acute respiratory failure with hypoxia**
Coding Clinic: 2024, Q2, P11

J96.02 **Acute respiratory failure with hypercapnia**
Acute respiratory acidosis

● J96.1 **Chronic respiratory failure**

J96.10 **Chronic respiratory failure, unspecified whether with hypoxia or hypercapnia**
Coding Clinic: 2021, Q4, P105-106; 2021, Q1, P46; 2016, Q1, P38; 2015, Q1, P21

J96.11 **Chronic respiratory failure with hypoxia**

J96.12 **Chronic respiratory failure with hypercapnia**
Chronic respiratory acidosis

● J96.2 **Acute and chronic respiratory failure**
Acute on chronic respiratory failure

J96.20 **Acute and chronic respiratory failure, unspecified whether with hypoxia or hypercapnia**

J96.21 **Acute and chronic respiratory failure with hypoxia**

J96.22 **Acute and chronic respiratory failure with hypercapnia**

● J96.9 **Respiratory failure, unspecified**

J96.90 **Respiratory failure, unspecified, unspecified whether with hypoxia or hypercapnia**
Coding Clinic: 2021, Q1, P44

J96.91 **Respiratory failure, unspecified with hypoxia**

J96.92 **Respiratory failure, unspecified with hypercapnia**

● J98 **Other respiratory disorders**
Use additional code to identify:
exposure to environmental tobacco smoke (Z77.22)
exposure to tobacco smoke in the perinatal period (P96.81)
history of tobacco dependence (Z87.891)
occupational exposure to environmental tobacco smoke (Z57.31)
tobacco dependence (F17.-)
tobacco use (Z72.0)
Excludes1 newborn apnea (P28.4-)
newborn sleep apnea (P28.3-)
Excludes2 apnea NOS (R06.81)
sleep apnea (G47.3-)

● J98.0 **Diseases of bronchus, not elsewhere classified**

J98.01 **Acute bronchospasm**
Excludes1 acute bronchiolitis with bronchospasm (J21.-)
acute bronchitis with bronchospasm (J20.-)
asthma (J45.-)
exercise induced bronchospasm (J45.990)

J98.09 **Other diseases of bronchus, not elsewhere classified**
Broncholithiasis
Calcification of bronchus
Stenosis of bronchus
Tracheobronchial collapse
Tracheobronchial dyskinesia
Ulcer of bronchus
Coding Clinic: 2022, Q3, P8

● J98.1 **Pulmonary collapse**
Excludes1 therapeutic collapse of lung status (Z98.3)

J98.11 **Atelectasis** (Ex) PDX 1064
Excludes1 newborn atelectasis
tuberculous atelectasis (current disease) (A15)

J98.19 **Other pulmonary collapse** (Ex) PDX 1064

CHAPTER 10 (J00-J99)

J98.2 Interstitial emphysema
Mediastinal emphysema
Excludes1 emphysema NOS (J43.9)
emphysema in newborn (P25.Ø)
surgical emphysema (subcutaneous) (T81.82)
traumatic subcutaneous emphysema (T79.7)

J98.3 Compensatory emphysema

J98.4 Other disorders of lung
Calcification of lung
Cystic lung disease (acquired)
Lung disease NOS
Pulmolithiasis
Excludes1 acute interstitial pneumonitis (J84.114)
pulmonary insufficiency following surgery (J95.1-J95.2)
Coding Clinic: 2Ø24, Q2, P2Ø, 21

J98.5 Diseases of mediastinum, not elsewhere classified
Excludes2 abscess of mediastinum (J85.3)
Coding Clinic: 2Ø16, Q4, P29

J98.51 Mediastinitis Ex: PDX 1065
Code first underlying condition, if applicable, such as postoperative mediastinitis (T81.-)

J98.59 Other diseases of mediastinum, not elsewhere classified Ex: PDX 1066
Fibrosis of mediastinum
Hernia of mediastinum
Retraction of mediastinum

J98.6 Disorders of diaphragm
Diaphragmatitis
Paralysis of diaphragm
Relaxation of diaphragm
Excludes1 congenital malformation of diaphragm NEC (Q79.1)
congenital diaphragmatic hernia (Q79.Ø)
Excludes2 diaphragmatic hernia (K44.-)

J98.8 Other specified respiratory disorders

J98.9 Respiratory disorder, unspecified
Respiratory disease (chronic) NOS

J99 Respiratory disorders in diseases classified elsewhere
Code first underlying disease, such as:
amyloidosis (E85.-)
ankylosing spondylitis (M45.-)
congenital syphilis (A5Ø.-)
cryoglobulinemia (D89.1)
early congenital syphilis (A5Ø.-)
plasminogen deficiency (E88.Ø2)
schistosomiasis (B65.Ø-B65.9)
Excludes1 respiratory disorders in:
amebiasis (AØ6.5)
blastomycosis (B4Ø.Ø-B4Ø.2)
candidiasis (B37.1)
coccidioidomycosis (B38.Ø-B38.2)
cystic fibrosis with pulmonary manifestations (E84.Ø)
dermatomyositis (M33.Ø1, M33.11)
histoplasmosis (B39.Ø-B39.2)
late syphilis (A52.72, A52.73)
polymyositis (M33.21)
Sjögren syndrome (M35.Ø2)
systemic lupus erythematosus (M32.13)
systemic sclerosis (M34.81)
Wegener's granulomatosis (M31.3Ø-M31.31)

CHAPTER 1Ø (JØØ-J99)

CHAPTER 11

DISEASES OF THE DIGESTIVE SYSTEM (K00-K95)

OGCR Chapter-Specific Coding Guidelines

11. Chapter 11: Diseases of the Digestive System (K00-K95)
Reserved for future guideline expansion

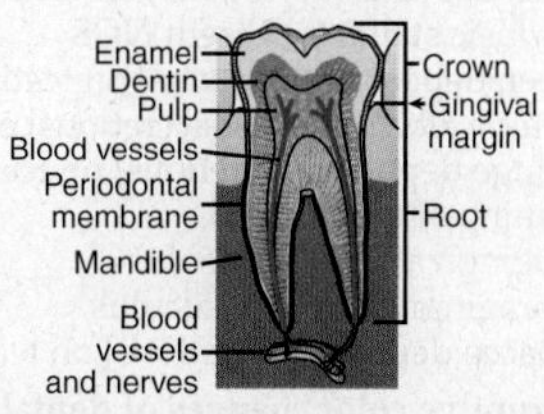

Figure 11-1 Anatomy of a tooth.

Item 11-1 **Anodontia** is the congenital absence of teeth. **Hypodontia** is partial anodontia. **Oligodontia** is the congenital absence of some teeth, whereas **supernumerary** is having more teeth than the normal number. **Mesiodens** are small extra teeth that often appear in pairs, although single small teeth are not uncommon.

CHAPTER 11

DISEASES OF THE DIGESTIVE SYSTEM (K00-K95)

Excludes2 certain conditions originating in the perinatal period (P04-P96)
certain infectious and parasitic diseases (A00-B99)
complications of pregnancy, childbirth and the puerperium (O00-O9A)
congenital malformations, deformations and chromosomal abnormalities (Q00-Q99)
endocrine, nutritional and metabolic diseases (E00-E88)
injury, poisoning and certain other consequences of external causes (S00-T88)
neoplasms (C00-D49)
symptoms, signs and abnormal clinical and laboratory findings, not elsewhere classified (R00-R94)

This chapter contains the following blocks:

K00-K14	Diseases of oral cavity and salivary glands
K20-K31	Diseases of esophagus, stomach and duodenum
K35-K38	Diseases of appendix
K40-K46	Hernia
K50-K52	Noninfective enteritis and colitis
K55-K64	Other diseases of intestines
K65-K68	Diseases of peritoneum and retroperitoneum
K70-K77	Diseases of liver
K80-K87	Disorders of gallbladder, biliary tract and pancreas
K90-K95	Other diseases of the digestive system

DISEASES OF ORAL CAVITY AND SALIVARY GLANDS (K00-K14)

K00 Disorders of tooth development and eruption
Excludes2 embedded and impacted teeth (K01.-)

K00.0 Anodontia
Hypodontia
Oligodontia
Excludes1 acquired absence of teeth (K08.1-)

K00.1 Supernumerary teeth
Distomolar
Fourth molar
Mesiodens
Paramolar
Supplementary teeth
Excludes2 supernumerary roots (K00.2)

K00.2 Abnormalities of size and form of teeth
Concrescence of teeth
Fusion of teeth
Gemination of teeth
Dens evaginatus
Dens in dente
Dens invaginatus
Enamel pearls
Macrodontia
Microdontia
Peg-shaped [conical] teeth
Supernumerary roots
Taurodontism
Tuberculum paramolare
Excludes1 abnormalities of teeth due to congenital syphilis (A50.5)
tuberculum Carabelli, which is regarded as a normal variation and should not be coded

K00.3 Mottled teeth
Dental fluorosis
Mottling of enamel
Nonfluoride enamel opacities
Excludes2 deposits [accretions] on teeth (K03.6)

K00.4 Disturbances in tooth formation
Aplasia and hypoplasia of cementum
Dilaceration of tooth
Enamel hypoplasia (neonatal) (postnatal) (prenatal)
Regional odontodysplasia
Turner's tooth
Excludes1 Hutchinson's teeth and mulberry molars in congenital syphilis (A50.5)
Excludes2 mottled teeth (K00.3)

K00.5 Hereditary disturbances in tooth structure, not elsewhere classified
Amelogenesis imperfecta
Dentinogenesis imperfecta
Odontogenesis imperfecta
Dentinal dysplasia
Shell teeth

K00.6 Disturbances in tooth eruption
Dentia praecox
Natal tooth
Neonatal tooth
Premature eruption of tooth
Premature shedding of primary [deciduous] tooth
Prenatal teeth
Retained [persistent] primary tooth
Excludes2 embedded and impacted teeth (K01.-)

K00.7 Teething syndrome

K00.8 Other disorders of tooth development
Color changes during tooth formation
Intrinsic staining of teeth NOS
Excludes2 posteruptive color changes (K03.7)

K00.9 Disorder of tooth development, unspecified
Disorder of odontogenesis NOS

K01 Embedded and impacted teeth
Excludes1 abnormal position of fully erupted teeth (M26.3-)

K01.0 Embedded teeth

K01.1 Impacted teeth

CHAPTER 11 (K00-K95)

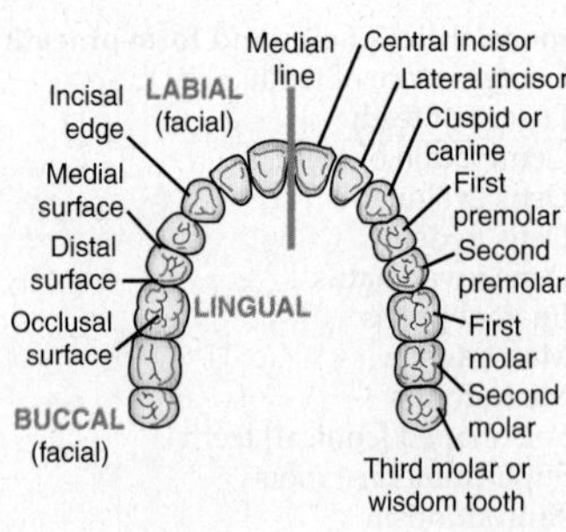

Figure 11-2 The permanent teeth within the dental arch.

Item 11-2 Each dental arch (jaw) normally contains 16 teeth. Tooth decay or **dental caries** is a disease of the enamel, dentin, and cementum of the tooth and can result in a cavity.

● **K02 Dental caries**
Includes caries of dentine
dental cavities
early childhood caries
pre-eruptive caries
recurrent caries (dentino enamel junction) (enamel) (to the pulp)
tooth decay

K02.3 Arrested dental caries
Arrested coronal and root caries

● **K02.5 Dental caries on pit and fissure surface**
Dental caries on chewing surface of tooth

K02.51 Dental caries on pit and fissure surface limited to enamel
White spot lesions [initial caries] on pit and fissure surface of tooth

K02.52 Dental caries on pit and fissure surface penetrating into dentin
Primary dental caries, cervical origin

K02.53 Dental caries on pit and fissure surface penetrating into pulp

● **K02.6 Dental caries on smooth surface**

K02.61 Dental caries on smooth surface limited to enamel
White spot lesions [initial caries] on smooth surface of tooth

K02.62 Dental caries on smooth surface penetrating into dentin

K02.63 Dental caries on smooth surface penetrating into pulp

K02.7 Dental root caries

K02.9 Dental caries, unspecified

● **K03 Other diseases of hard tissues of teeth**
Excludes2 bruxism (F45.8)
dental caries (K02.-)
teeth-grinding NOS (F45.8)

K03.0 Excessive attrition of teeth
Approximal wear of teeth
Occlusal wear of teeth

K03.1 Abrasion of teeth
Dentifrice abrasion of teeth
Habitual abrasion of teeth
Occupational abrasion of teeth
Ritual abrasion of teeth
Traditional abrasion of teeth
Wedge defect NOS

K03.2 Erosion of teeth
Erosion of teeth due to diet
Erosion of teeth due to drugs and medicaments
Erosion of teeth due to persistent vomiting
Erosion of teeth NOS
Idiopathic erosion of teeth
Occupational erosion of teeth

K03.3 Pathological resorption of teeth
Internal granuloma of pulp
Resorption of teeth (external)

K03.4 Hypercementosis
Cementation hyperplasia

K03.5 Ankylosis of teeth

K03.6 Deposits [accretions] on teeth
Betel deposits [accretions] on teeth
Black deposits [accretions] on teeth
Extrinsic staining of teeth NOS
Green deposits [accretions] on teeth
Materia alba deposits [accretions] on teeth
Orange deposits [accretions] on teeth
Staining of teeth NOS
Subgingival dental calculus
Supragingival dental calculus
Tobacco deposits [accretions] on teeth

K03.7 Posteruptive color changes of dental hard tissues
Excludes2 deposits [accretions] on teeth (K03.6)

● **K03.8 Other specified diseases of hard tissues of teeth**

K03.81 Cracked tooth
Excludes1 asymptomatic craze lines in enamel - omit code
broken or fractured tooth due to trauma (S02.5)

K03.89 Other specified diseases of hard tissues of teeth

K03.9 Disease of hard tissues of teeth, unspecified

K04 Diseases of pulp and periapical tissues
Coding Clinic: 2016, Q4, P29

● **K04.0 Pulpitis** Ex: PDX 1067
Acute pulpitis
Chronic (hyperplastic) (ulcerative) pulpitis

K04.01 Reversible pulpitis

K04.02 Irreversible pulpitis

K04.1 Necrosis of pulp
Pulpal gangrene

K04.2 Pulp degeneration
Denticles
Pulpal calcifications
Pulpal stones

K04.3 Abnormal hard tissue formation in pulp
Secondary or irregular dentine

K04.4 Acute apical periodontitis of pulpal origin Ex: PDX 1067
Acute apical periodontitis NOS
Excludes1 acute periodontitis (K05.2-)

K04.5 Chronic apical periodontitis
Apical or periapical granuloma
Apical periodontitis NOS
Excludes1 chronic periodontitis (K05.3-)

K04.6 Periapical abscess with sinus
Dental abscess with sinus
Dentoalveolar abscess with sinus

K04.7 Periapical abscess without sinus
Dental abscess without sinus
Dentoalveolar abscess without sinus

K04.8 Radicular cyst
Apical (periodontal) cyst
Periapical cyst
Residual radicular cyst
Excludes2 lateral periodontal cyst (K09.0)

● **K04.9 Other and unspecified diseases of pulp and periapical tissues**

K04.90 Unspecified diseases of pulp and periapical tissues

K04.99 Other diseases of pulp and periapical tissues

Item 11-3 **Acute gingivitis,** also known as orilitis or ulitis, is the short-term, severe inflammation of the gums (gingiva) caused by bacteria. **Chronic gingivitis** is persistent inflammation of the gums. When the gingivitis moves into the periodontium it is called periodontitis, also known as paradentitis.

● K05 Gingivitis and periodontal diseases
Use additional code to identify:
alcohol abuse and dependence (F10.-)
exposure to environmental tobacco smoke (Z77.22)
exposure to tobacco smoke in the perinatal period (P96.81)
history of tobacco dependence (Z87.891)
occupational exposure to environmental tobacco smoke (Z57.31)
tobacco dependence (F17.-)
tobacco use (Z72.0)
Coding Clinic: 2016, Q4, P29

● K05.0 Acute gingivitis
Excludes1 acute necrotizing ulcerative gingivitis (A69.1)
herpesviral [herpes simplex] gingivostomatitis (B00.2)

K05.00 Acute gingivitis, plaque induced
Acute gingivitis NOS
Plaque induced gingival disease

K05.01 Acute gingivitis, non-plaque induced

● K05.1 Chronic gingivitis
Desquamative gingivitis (chronic)
Gingivitis (chronic) NOS
Hyperplastic gingivitis (chronic)
Pregnancy associated gingivitis
Simple marginal gingivitis (chronic)
Ulcerative gingivitis (chronic)
Code first, if applicable, diseases of the digestive system complicating pregnancy (O99.61-)

K05.10 Chronic gingivitis, plaque induced
Chronic gingivitis NOS
Gingivitis NOS

K05.11 Chronic gingivitis, non-plaque induced

● K05.2 Aggressive periodontitis
Acute pericoronitis
Excludes1 acute apical periodontitis (K04.4)
periapical abscess (K04.7)
periapical abscess with sinus (K04.6)

K05.20 Aggressive periodontitis, unspecified

● K05.21 Aggressive periodontitis, localized
Periodontal abscess

K05.211 Aggressive periodontitis, localized, slight
K05.212 Aggressive periodontitis, localized, moderate
K05.213 Aggressive periodontitis, localized, severe
K05.219 Aggressive periodontitis, localized, unspecified severity

● K05.22 Aggressive periodontitis, generalized
K05.221 Aggressive periodontitis, generalized, slight
K05.222 Aggressive periodontitis, generalized, moderate
K05.223 Aggressive periodontitis, generalized, severe
K05.229 Aggressive periodontitis, generalized, unspecified severity

● K05.3 Chronic periodontitis
Chronic pericoronitis
Complex periodontitis
Periodontitis NOS
Simplex periodontitis
Excludes1 chronic apical periodontitis (K04.5)

K05.30 Chronic periodontitis, unspecified

● K05.31 Chronic periodontitis, localized
K05.311 Chronic periodontitis, localized, slight
K05.312 Chronic periodontitis, localized, moderate
K05.313 Chronic periodontitis, localized, severe
K05.319 Chronic periodontitis, localized, unspecified severity

● K05.32 Chronic periodontitis, generalized
K05.321 Chronic periodontitis, generalized, slight
K05.322 Chronic periodontitis, generalized, moderate
K05.323 Chronic periodontitis, generalized, severe
K05.329 Chronic periodontitis, generalized, unspecified severity

K05.4 Periodontosis
Juvenile periodontosis

K05.5 Other periodontal diseases
Combined periodontic-endodontic lesion
Narrow gingival width (of periodontal soft tissue)
Excludes2 leukoplakia of gingiva (K13.21)

K05.6 Periodontal disease, unspecified

● K06 Other disorders of gingiva and edentulous alveolar ridge
Excludes2 acute gingivitis (K05.0)
atrophy of edentulous alveolar ridge (K08.2)
chronic gingivitis (K05.1)
gingivitis NOS (K05.1)
Coding Clinic: 2016, Q4, P29

● K06.0 Gingival recession
Gingival recession (postinfective) (postprocedural)

● K06.01 Gingival recession, localized
K06.010 Localized gingival recession, unspecified
Localized gingival recession, NOS
K06.011 Localized gingival recession, minimal
K06.012 Localized gingival recession, moderate
K06.013 Localized gingival recession, severe

● K06.02 Gingival recession, generalized
K06.020 Generalized gingival recession, unspecified
Generalized gingival recession, NOS
K06.021 Generalized gingival recession, minimal
K06.022 Generalized gingival recession, moderate
K06.023 Generalized gingival recession, severe

K06.1 Gingival enlargement
Gingival fibromatosis

K06.2 Gingival and edentulous alveolar ridge lesions associated with trauma
Irritative hyperplasia of edentulous ridge [denture hyperplasia]
Use additional code (Chapter 20) to identify external cause or denture status (Z97.2)

K06.3 Horizontal alveolar bone loss

K06.8 Other specified disorders of gingiva and edentulous alveolar ridge
Fibrous epulis
Flabby alveolar ridge
Giant cell epulis
Peripheral giant cell granuloma of gingiva
Pyogenic granuloma of gingiva
Vertical ridge deficiency
Excludes2 gingival cyst (K09.0)

K06.9 Disorder of gingiva and edentulous alveolar ridge, unspecified

CHAPTER 11 (K00-K95)

● **K08 Other disorders of teeth and supporting structures**
Excludes2 dentofacial anomalies [including malocclusion] (M26.-)
disorders of jaw (M27.-)
Coding Clinic: 2016, Q4, P29

K08.0 Exfoliation of teeth due to systemic causes
Code also underlying systemic condition

● **K08.1 Complete loss of teeth**
Acquired loss of teeth, complete
Excludes1 congenital absence of teeth (K00.0)
exfoliation of teeth due to systemic causes (K08.0)
partial loss of teeth (K08.4-)

● **K08.10 Complete loss of teeth, unspecified cause**
K08.101 Complete loss of teeth, unspecified cause, class I
K08.102 Complete loss of teeth, unspecified cause, class II
K08.103 Complete loss of teeth, unspecified cause, class III
K08.104 Complete loss of teeth, unspecified cause, class IV
K08.109 Complete loss of teeth, unspecified cause, unspecified class
Edentulism NOS

● **K08.11 Complete loss of teeth due to trauma**
K08.111 Complete loss of teeth due to trauma, class I
K08.112 Complete loss of teeth due to trauma, class II
K08.113 Complete loss of teeth due to trauma, class III
K08.114 Complete loss of teeth due to trauma, class IV
K08.119 Complete loss of teeth due to trauma, unspecified class

● **K08.12 Complete loss of teeth due to periodontal diseases**
K08.121 Complete loss of teeth due to periodontal diseases, class I
K08.122 Complete loss of teeth due to periodontal diseases, class II
K08.123 Complete loss of teeth due to periodontal diseases, class III
K08.124 Complete loss of teeth due to periodontal diseases, class IV
K08.129 Complete loss of teeth due to periodontal diseases, unspecified class

● **K08.13 Complete loss of teeth due to caries**
K08.131 Complete loss of teeth due to caries, class I
K08.132 Complete loss of teeth due to caries, class II
K08.133 Complete loss of teeth due to caries, class III
K08.134 Complete loss of teeth due to caries, class IV
K08.139 Complete loss of teeth due to caries, unspecified class

● **K08.19 Complete loss of teeth due to other specified cause**
K08.191 Complete loss of teeth due to other specified cause, class I
K08.192 Complete loss of teeth due to other specified cause, class II
K08.193 Complete loss of teeth due to other specified cause, class III
K08.194 Complete loss of teeth due to other specified cause, class IV
K08.199 Complete loss of teeth due to other specified cause, unspecified class

● **K08.2 Atrophy of edentulous alveolar ridge**
K08.20 Unspecified atrophy of edentulous alveolar ridge
Atrophy of the mandible NOS
Atrophy of the maxilla NOS
K08.21 Minimal atrophy of the mandible
Minimal atrophy of the edentulous mandible
K08.22 Moderate atrophy of the mandible
Moderate atrophy of the edentulous mandible
K08.23 Severe atrophy of the mandible
Severe atrophy of the edentulous mandible
K08.24 Minimal atrophy of maxilla
Minimal atrophy of the edentulous maxilla
K08.25 Moderate atrophy of the maxilla
Moderate atrophy of the edentulous maxilla
K08.26 Severe atrophy of the maxilla
Severe atrophy of the edentulous maxilla

K08.3 Retained dental root

● **K08.4 Partial loss of teeth**
Acquired loss of teeth, partial
Excludes1 complete loss of teeth (K08.1-)
congenital absence of teeth (K00.0)
Excludes2 exfoliation of teeth due to systemic causes (K08.0)

● **K08.40 Partial loss of teeth, unspecified cause**
K08.401 Partial loss of teeth, unspecified cause, class I
K08.402 Partial loss of teeth, unspecified cause, class II
K08.403 Partial loss of teeth, unspecified cause, class III
K08.404 Partial loss of teeth, unspecified cause, class IV
K08.409 Partial loss of teeth, unspecified cause, unspecified class
Tooth extraction status NOS

● **K08.41 Partial loss of teeth due to trauma**
K08.411 Partial loss of teeth due to trauma, class I
K08.412 Partial loss of teeth due to trauma, class II
K08.413 Partial loss of teeth due to trauma, class III
K08.414 Partial loss of teeth due to trauma, class IV
K08.419 Partial loss of teeth due to trauma, unspecified class

● **K08.42 Partial loss of teeth due to periodontal diseases**
K08.421 Partial loss of teeth due to periodontal diseases, class I
K08.422 Partial loss of teeth due to periodontal diseases, class II
K08.423 Partial loss of teeth due to periodontal diseases, class III
K08.424 Partial loss of teeth due to periodontal diseases, class IV
K08.429 Partial loss of teeth due to periodontal diseases, unspecified class

● **K08.43 Partial loss of teeth due to caries**
K08.431 Partial loss of teeth due to caries, class I
K08.432 Partial loss of teeth due to caries, class II
K08.433 Partial loss of teeth due to caries, class III

K08.434 Partial loss of teeth due to caries, class IV

K08.439 Partial loss of teeth due to caries, unspecified class

● K08.49 Partial loss of teeth due to other specified cause

K08.491 Partial loss of teeth due to other specified cause, class I

K08.492 Partial loss of teeth due to other specified cause, class II

K08.493 Partial loss of teeth due to other specified cause, class III

K08.494 Partial loss of teeth due to other specified cause, class IV

K08.499 Partial loss of teeth due to other specified cause, unspecified class

● K08.5 Unsatisfactory restoration of tooth

Defective bridge, crown, filling
Defective dental restoration

Excludes1 dental restoration status (Z98.811)

Excludes2 endosseous dental implant failure (M27.6-)
unsatisfactory endodontic treatment (M27.5-)

K08.50 Unsatisfactory restoration of tooth, unspecified
Defective dental restoration NOS

K08.51 Open restoration margins of tooth
Dental restoration failure of marginal integrity
Open margin on tooth restoration
Poor gingival margin to tooth restoration

K08.52 Unrepairable overhanging of dental restorative materials
Overhanging of tooth restoration

● K08.53 Fractured dental restorative material

Excludes1 cracked tooth (K03.81)
traumatic fracture of tooth (S02.5)

K08.530 Fractured dental restorative material without loss of material

K08.531 Fractured dental restorative material with loss of material

K08.539 Fractured dental restorative material, unspecified

K08.54 Contour of existing restoration of tooth biologically incompatible with oral health
Dental restoration failure of periodontal anatomical integrity
Unacceptable contours of existing restoration of tooth
Unacceptable morphology of existing restoration of tooth

K08.55 Allergy to existing dental restorative material
Use additional code to identify the specific type of allergy

K08.56 Poor aesthetic of existing restoration of tooth
Dental restoration aesthetically inadequate or displeasing

K08.59 Other unsatisfactory restoration of tooth
Other defective dental restoration

● K08.8 Other specified disorders of teeth and supporting structures

K08.81 Primary occlusal trauma

K08.82 Secondary occlusal trauma

K08.89 Other specified disorders of teeth and supporting structures
Enlargement of alveolar ridge NOS
Insufficient anatomic crown height
Insufficient clinical crown length
Irregular alveolar process
Toothache NOS

K08.9 Disorder of teeth and supporting structures, unspecified

Item 11–4 **Atrophy** is wasting away of a tissue or organ, whereas **hypertrophy** is overdevelopment or enlargement of a tissue or organ. **Sialoadenitis** is salivary gland inflammation. **Parotitis** is the inflammation of the parotid gland. In the epidemic form, parotitis is also known as mumps. **Sialolithiasis** is the formation of calculus within a salivary gland. **Mucocele** is a polyp composed of mucus.

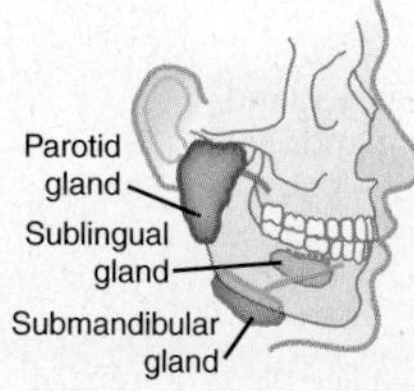

Figure 11-3 Major salivary glands.

● K09 Cysts of oral region, not elsewhere classified

Includes lesions showing histological features both of aneurysmal cyst and of another fibro-osseous lesion

Excludes2 cysts of jaw (M27.0-, M27.4-)
radicular cyst (K04.8)

K09.0 Developmental odontogenic cysts
Dentigerous cyst
Eruption cyst
Follicular cyst
Gingival cyst
Lateral periodontal cyst
Primordial cyst

Excludes2 keratocysts (D16.4, D16.5)
odontogenic keratocystic tumors (D16.4, D16.5)

K09.1 Developmental (nonodontogenic) cysts of oral region
Cyst (of) incisive canal
Cyst (of) palatine of papilla
Globulomaxillary cyst
Median palatal cyst
Nasoalveolar cyst
Nasolabial cyst
Nasopalatine duct cyst

K09.8 Other cysts of oral region, not elsewhere classified
Dermoid cyst
Epidermoid cyst
Lymphoepithelial cyst
Epstein's pearl

K09.9 Cyst of oral region, unspecified

★**(See Plate 28 of the Anatomy Illustrations.)**

● K11 Diseases of salivary glands

Use additional code to identify:
alcohol abuse and dependence (F10.-)
exposure to environmental tobacco smoke (Z77.22)
exposure to tobacco smoke in the perinatal period (P96.81)
history of tobacco dependence (Z87.891)
occupational exposure to environmental tobacco smoke (Z57.31)
tobacco dependence (F17.-)
tobacco use (Z72.0)

K11.0 Atrophy of salivary gland

K11.1 Hypertrophy of salivary gland

● K11.2 Sialoadenitis
Parotitis

Excludes1 epidemic parotitis (B26.-)
mumps (B26.-)
uveoparotid fever [Heerfordt] (D86.89)

K11.20 Sialoadenitis, unspecified

K11.21 Acute sialoadenitis

Excludes1 acute recurrent sialoadenitis (K11.22)

K11.22 Acute recurrent sialoadenitis

K11.23 Chronic sialoadenitis

K11.3 Abscess of salivary gland (Ex) PDX 1068

K11.4 Fistula of salivary gland (Ex) PDX 1068

Excludes1 congenital fistula of salivary gland (Q38.4)

K11.5 Sialolithiasis

Calculus of salivary gland or duct
Stone of salivary gland or duct

K11.6 Mucocele of salivary gland

Mucous extravasation cyst of salivary gland
Mucous retention cyst of salivary gland
Ranula

K11.7 Disturbances of salivary secretion

Hypoptyalism
Ptyalism
Xerostomia

Excludes2 dry mouth NOS (R68.2)

K11.8 Other diseases of salivary glands

Benign lymphoepithelial lesion of salivary gland
Mikulicz' disease
Necrotizing sialometaplasia
Sialectasia
Stenosis of salivary duct
Stricture of salivary duct

Excludes1 Sjögren syndrome (M35.Ø-)

K11.9 Disease of salivary gland, unspecified

Sialoadenopathy NOS

● **K12 Stomatitis and related lesions**

Use additional code to identify:
alcohol abuse and dependence (F1Ø.-)
exposure to environmental tobacco smoke (Z77.22)
exposure to tobacco smoke in the perinatal period (P96.81)
history of tobacco dependence (Z87.891)
occupational exposure to environmental tobacco smoke (Z57.31)
tobacco dependence (F17.-)
tobacco use (Z72.Ø)

Excludes1 cancrum oris (A69.Ø)
cheilitis (K13.Ø)
gangrenous stomatitis (A69.Ø)
herpesviral [herpes simplex] gingivostomatitis (BØØ.2)
noma (A69.Ø)

K12.Ø Recurrent oral aphthae

Aphthous stomatitis (major) (minor)
Bednar's aphthae
Periadenitis mucosa necrotica recurrens
Recurrent aphthous ulcer
Stomatitis herpetiformis

K12.1 Other forms of stomatitis

Stomatitis NOS
Denture stomatitis
Ulcerative stomatitis
Vesicular stomatitis

Excludes1 acute necrotizing ulcerative stomatitis (A69.1)
Vincent's stomatitis (A69.1)

K12.2 Cellulitis and abscess of mouth (Ex) PDX 1069

Cellulitis of mouth (floor)
Submandibular abscess

Excludes2 abscess of salivary gland (K11.3)
abscess of tongue (K14.Ø)
periapical abscess (KØ4.6-KØ4.7)
periodontal abscess (KØ5.21)
peritonsillar abscess (J36)

Item 11–5 Stomatitis is the inflammation of the oral mucosa. **Mucositis** is the inflammation of the mucous membranes lining the digestive tract from the mouth to the anus. It is a common side effect of chemotherapy and of radiotherapy that involves any part of the digestive tract.

● **K12.3 Oral mucositis (ulcerative)**

Mucositis (oral) (oropharyneal)

Excludes2 gastrointestinal mucositis (ulcerative) (K92.81)
mucositis (ulcerative) of vagina and vulva (N76.81)
nasal mucositis (ulcerative) (J34.81)

K12.3Ø Oral mucositis (ulcerative), unspecified

K12.31 Oral mucositis (ulcerative) due to antineoplastic therapy

Use additional code for adverse effect, if applicable, to identify antineoplastic and immunosuppressive drugs (T45.1X5)

Use additional code for other antineoplastic therapy, such as:
radiological procedure and radiotherapy (Y84.2)

K12.32 Oral mucositis (ulcerative) due to other drugs

Use additional code for adverse effect, if applicable, to identify drug (T36-T5Ø with fifth or sixth character 5)

K12.33 Oral mucositis (ulcerative) due to radiation

Use additional external cause code (W88-W9Ø, X39.Ø-) to identify cause

K12.39 Other oral mucositis (ulcerative)

Viral oral mucositis (ulcerative)

● **K13 Other diseases of lip and oral mucosa**

Includes epithelial disturbances of tongue

Use additional code to identify:
alcohol abuse and dependence (F1Ø.-)
exposure to environmental tobacco smoke (Z77.22)
exposure to tobacco smoke in the perinatal period (P96.81)
history of tobacco dependence (Z87.891)
occupational exposure to environmental tobacco smoke (Z57.31)
tobacco dependence (F17.-)
tobacco use (Z72.Ø)

Excludes2 certain disorders of gingiva and edentulous alveolar ridge (KØ5-KØ6)
cysts of oral region (KØ9.-)
diseases of tongue (K14.-)
stomatitis and related lesions (K12.-)

K13.Ø Diseases of lips

Abscess of lips
Angular cheilitis
Cellulitis of lips
Cheilitis NOS
Cheilodynia
Cheilosis
Exfoliative cheilitis
Fistula of lips
Glandular cheilitis
Hypertrophy of lips
Perlèche NEC

Excludes1 ariboflavinosis (E53.Ø)
cheilitis due to radiation-related disorders (L55-L59)
congenital fistula of lips (Q38.Ø)
congenital hypertrophy of lips (Q18.6)
Perlèche due to candidiasis (B37.83)
Perlèche due to riboflavin deficiency (E53.Ø)

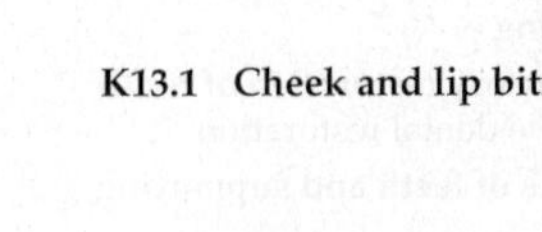

K13.1 Cheek and lip biting

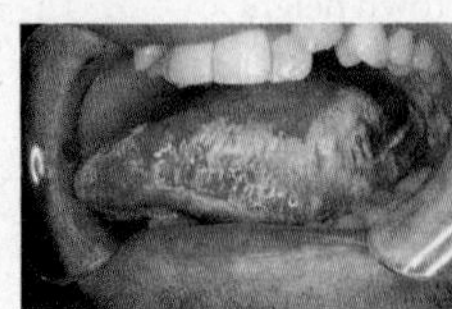

Figure 11-4 Oral leukoplakia and associated. (From Swartz MH: Textbook of Physical Diagnosis: History and Examination, Philadelphia, PA, Saunders/Elsevier, 2010)

CHAPTER 11 (KØØ-K95)

● **K13.2 Leukoplakia and other disturbances of oral epithelium, including tongue**

Excludes1 carcinoma in situ of oral epithelium (D00.0-)
hairy leukoplakia (K13.3)

K13.21 Leukoplakia of oral mucosa, including tongue

Considered precancerous and evidenced by thickened white patches of epithelium on mucous membranes

Leukokeratosis of oral mucosa
Leukoplakia of gingiva, lips, tongue

Excludes1 hairy leukoplakia (K13.3)
leukokeratosis nicotina palati (K13.24)

K13.22 Minimal keratinized residual ridge mucosa

Minimal keratinization of alveolar ridge mucosa

K13.23 Excessive keratinized residual ridge mucosa

Excessive keratinization of alveolar ridge mucosa

K13.24 Leukokeratosis nicotina palati

Smoker's palate

K13.29 Other disturbances of oral epithelium, including tongue

Erythroplakia of mouth or tongue
Focal epithelial hyperplasia of mouth or tongue
Leukoedema of mouth or tongue
Other oral epithelium disturbances

K13.3 Hairy leukoplakia

K13.4 Granuloma and granuloma-like lesions of oral mucosa

Eosinophilic granuloma
Granuloma pyogenicum
Verrucous xanthoma

K13.5 Oral submucous fibrosis

Submucous fibrosis of tongue

K13.6 Irritative hyperplasia of oral mucosa

Excludes2 irritative hyperplasia of edentulous ridge [denture hyperplasia] (K06.2)

● **K13.7 Other and unspecified lesions of oral mucosa**

K13.70 Unspecified lesions of oral mucosa

K13.79 Other lesions of oral mucosa

Focal oral mucinosis

Coding Clinic: 2022, Q2, P8

★ **(See Plate 26 of the Anatomy Illustrations.)**

● **K14 Diseases of tongue**

Use additional code to identify:
alcohol abuse and dependence (F10.-)
exposure to environmental tobacco smoke (Z77.22)
history of tobacco dependence (Z87.891)
occupational exposure to environmental tobacco smoke (Z57.31)
tobacco dependence (F17.-)
tobacco use (Z72.0)

Excludes2 erythroplakia (K13.29)
focal epithelial hyperplasia (K13.29)
leukoedema of tongue (K13.29)
leukoplakia of tongue (K13.21)
hairy leukoplakia (K13.3)
macroglossia (congenital) (Q38.2)
submucous fibrosis of tongue (K13.5)

K14.0 Glossitis

Abscess of tongue
Ulceration (traumatic) of tongue

Excludes1 atrophic glossitis (K14.4)

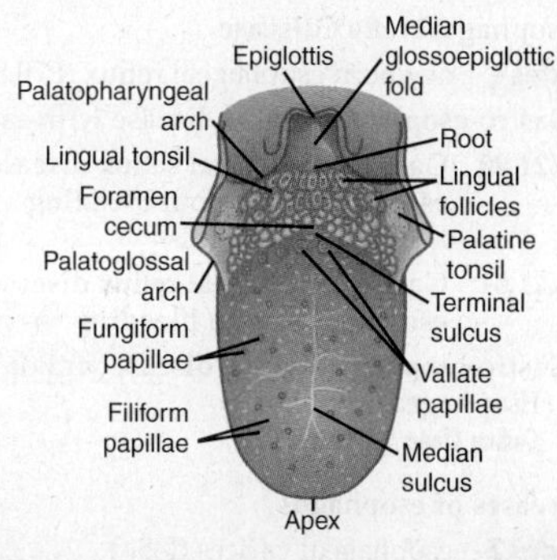

Figure 11-5 Structure of the tongue.

K14.1 Geographic tongue

Benign migratory glossitis
Glossitis areata exfoliativa

K14.2 Median rhomboid glossitis

K14.3 Hypertrophy of tongue papillae

Black hairy tongue
Coated tongue
Hypertrophy of foliate papillae
Lingua villosa nigra

K14.4 Atrophy of tongue papillae

Atrophic glossitis

K14.5 Plicated tongue

Fissured tongue
Furrowed tongue
Scrotal tongue

Excludes1 fissured tongue, congenital (Q38.3)

K14.6 Glossodynia

Glossopyrosis
Painful tongue

K14.8 Other diseases of tongue

Atrophy of tongue
Crenated tongue
Enlargement of tongue
Glossocele
Glossoptosis
Hypertrophy of tongue

K14.9 Disease of tongue, unspecified

Glossopathy NOS

DISEASES OF ESOPHAGUS, STOMACH AND DUODENUM (K20-K31)

Excludes2 hiatus hernia (K44.-)

● **K20 Esophagitis**

Use additional code to identify:
alcohol abuse and dependence (F10.-)

Excludes1 erosion of esophagus (K22.1-)
esophagitis with gastro-esophageal reflux disease (K21.0-)
reflux esophagitis (K21.0-)
ulcerative esophagitis (K22.1-)

Excludes2 eosinophilic gastritis or gastroenteritis (K52.81)

Coding Clinic: 2023, Q1, P20

K20.0 Eosinophilic esophagitis

● **K20.8 Other esophagitis**

K20.80 Other esophagitis without bleeding

Abscess of esophagus
Other esophagitis NOS

K20.81 Other esophagitis with bleeding (Ex) PDX 1070

● **K20.9 Esophagitis, unspecified**

K20.90 Esophagitis, unspecified without bleeding

Esophagitis NOS

K20.91 Esophagitis, unspecified with bleeding (Ex) PDX 1070

CHAPTER 11 (K00-K95)

●K21 **Gastro-esophageal reflux disease**
Excludes1 newborn esophageal reflux (P78.83)
●K21.0 **Gastro-esophageal reflux disease with esophagitis**
K21.00 **Gastro-esophageal reflux disease with esophagitis, without bleeding**
Reflux esophagitis
K21.01 **Gastro-esophageal reflux disease with esophagitis, with bleeding** PDX 1070
K21.9 **Gastro-esophageal reflux disease without esophagitis**
Esophageal reflux NOS
Coding Clinic: 2016, Q1, P18

●K22 **Other diseases of esophagus**
Excludes2 esophageal varices (I85.-)
K22.0 **Achalasia of cardia**
Achalasia NOS
Cardiospasm
Excludes1 congenital cardiospasm (Q39.5)
●K22.1 **Ulcer of esophagus**
Barrett's ulcer
Erosion of esophagus
Fungal ulcer of esophagus
Peptic ulcer of esophagus
Ulcer of esophagus due to ingestion of chemicals
Ulcer of esophagus due to ingestion of drugs and medicaments
Ulcerative esophagitis
Code first poisoning due to drug or toxin, if applicable (T36-T65 with fifth or sixth character 1-4)
Use additional code for adverse effect, if applicable, to identify drug (T36-T50 with fifth or sixth character 5)
Excludes1 Barrett's esophagus (K22.87-)
K22.10 **Ulcer of esophagus without bleeding** PDX 1071
Ulcer of esophagus NOS
K22.11 **Ulcer of esophagus with bleeding** PDX 1072
Excludes2 bleeding esophageal varices (I85.01, I85.11)
Coding Clinic: 2023, Q1, P20
K22.2 **Esophageal obstruction**
Compression of esophagus
Constriction of esophagus
Stenosis of esophagus
Stricture of esophagus
Excludes1 congenital stenosis or stricture of esophagus (Q39.3)
Coding Clinic: 2024, Q2, P26
K22.3 **Perforation of esophagus** PDX 1073
Rupture of esophagus
Excludes1 traumatic perforation of (thoracic) esophagus (S27.8-)
K22.4 **Dyskinesia of esophagus**
Difficulty in moving
Corkscrew esophagus
Diffuse esophageal spasm
Spasm of esophagus
Excludes1 cardiospasm (K22.0)
K22.5 **Diverticulum of esophagus, acquired**
Esophageal pouch, acquired
Excludes1 diverticulum of esophagus (congenital) (Q39.6)
K22.6 **Gastro-esophageal laceration-hemorrhage syndrome** PDX 1074
Mallory-Weiss syndrome

Item 11–6 Esophageal reflux is the return flow of the contents of the stomach to the esophagus and is referred to as GERD and/or "heartburn." **Gastroesophageal reflux** is the return flow of the contents of the stomach and duodenum to the esophagus. **Esophageal leukoplakia** are white areas on the mucous membrane of the esophagus for which no specific cause can be identified.

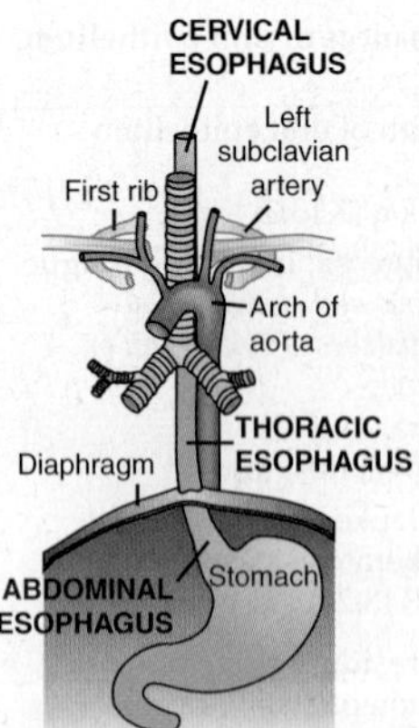

Figure 11-6 The esophagus is the muscular tube that connects the pharynx and the stomach. The 10-inch (25 cm) long esophagus is divided into three parts: **cervical, thoracic,** and **abdominal.**

Item 11–7 Achalasia is a condition in which the smooth muscle fibers of the esophagus do not relax. Most frequently, this condition occurs at the esophagogastric sphincter. **Cardiospasm,** also known as **megaesophagus,** is achalasia of the thoracic esophagus.

●K22.7 **Barrett's esophagus**
Barrett's disease
Barrett's syndrome
Excludes1 Barrett's ulcer (K22.1)
malignant neoplasm of esophagus (C15.-)
K22.70 **Barrett's esophagus without dysplasia**
Barrett's esophagus NOS
●K22.71 **Barrett's esophagus with dysplasia**
K22.710 **Barrett's esophagus with low grade dysplasia**
K22.711 **Barrett's esophagus with high grade dysplasia**
K22.719 **Barrett's esophagus with dysplasia, unspecified**
●K22.8 **Other specified diseases of esophagus**
K22.81 **Esophageal polyp**
Excludes1 benign neoplasm of esophagus (D13.0)
K22.82 **Esophagogastric junction polyp**
Excludes1 benign neoplasm of stomach (D13.1)
K22.89 **Other specified disease of esophagus**
Hemorrhage of esophagus NOS
Excludes2 esophageal varices (I85.-)
Paterson-Kelly syndrome (D50.1)
Coding Clinic: 2024, Q2, P26; 2020, Q1, P16
K22.9 **Disease of esophagus, unspecified**

K23 ***Disorders of esophagus in diseases classified elsewhere***
Code first underlying disease, such as:
congenital syphilis (A50.5)
Excludes1 late syphilis (A52.79)
megaesophagus due to Chagas' disease (B57.31)
tuberculosis (A18.83)

●K25 **Gastric ulcer** PDX 1075
Includes erosion (acute) of stomach
pylorus ulcer (peptic)
stomach ulcer (peptic)
Use additional code to identify:
alcohol abuse and dependence (F10.-)
Excludes1 acute gastritis (K29.0-)
peptic ulcer NOS (K27.-)
K25.0 **Acute gastric ulcer with hemorrhage**
Coding Clinic: 2023, Q1, P16
K25.1 **Acute gastric ulcer with perforation**
K25.2 **Acute gastric ulcer with both hemorrhage and perforation**
K25.3 **Acute gastric ulcer without hemorrhage or perforation**
K25.4 **Chronic or unspecified gastric ulcer with hemorrhage**
Coding Clinic: 2017, Q3, P27

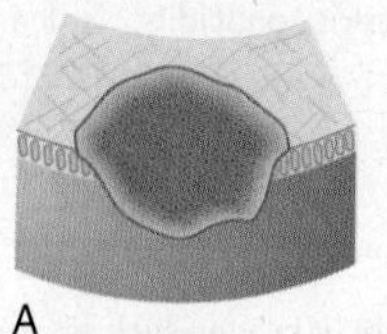

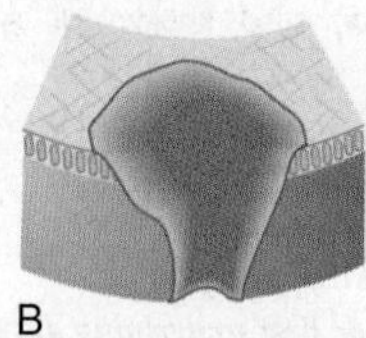

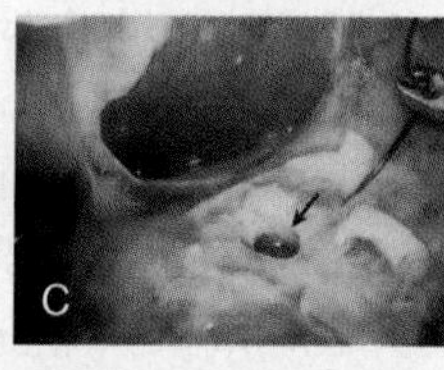

Figure 11-7 A. Ulcer. **B.** Perforated ulcer. **C.** Laparoscopic view of a perforated duodenal ulcer *(arrow)* with fibrinous exudate on the adjacent peritoneum. (**C** from Feldman: Sleisenger & Fordtran's Gastrointestinal and Liver Disease, ed 8, Saunders, An Imprint of Elsevier, 2006)

Item 11-8 Gastric ulcers are lesions of the stomach that result in the death of the tissue and a defect of the surface. **Perforated ulcers** are those in which the lesion penetrates the gastric wall, leaving a hole. **Peptic ulcers** are lesions of the stomach or the duodenum. **Peptic** refers to the gastric juice, pepsin.

K25.5 **Chronic or unspecified gastric ulcer with perforation**
K25.6 **Chronic or unspecified gastric ulcer with both hemorrhage and perforation**
K25.7 **Chronic gastric ulcer without hemorrhage or perforation**
K25.9 **Gastric ulcer, unspecified as acute or chronic, without hemorrhage or perforation**
Coding Clinic: 2021, Q1, P12

K26 Duodenal ulcer PDX 1076
Includes erosion (acute) of duodenum
duodenum ulcer (peptic)
postpyloric ulcer (peptic)
Use additional code to identify:
alcohol abuse and dependence (F1Ø.-)
Excludes1 peptic ulcer NOS (K27.-)

K26.Ø **Acute duodenal ulcer with hemorrhage**
K26.1 **Acute duodenal ulcer with perforation**
K26.2 **Acute duodenal ulcer with both hemorrhage and perforation**
K26.3 **Acute duodenal ulcer without hemorrhage or perforation** PDX 1077
K26.4 **Chronic or unspecified duodenal ulcer with hemorrhage**
Coding Clinic: 2016, Q1, P14
K26.5 **Chronic or unspecified duodenal ulcer with perforation**
K26.6 **Chronic or unspecified duodenal ulcer with both hemorrhage and perforation**
K26.7 **Chronic duodenal ulcer without hemorrhage or perforation**
Coding Clinic: 2023, Q2, P11
K26.9 **Duodenal ulcer, unspecified as acute or chronic, without hemorrhage or perforation**

K27 Peptic ulcer, site unspecified PDX 1076
Includes gastroduodenal ulcer NOS
peptic ulcer NOS
Use additional code to identify:
alcohol abuse and dependence (F1Ø.-)
Excludes1 peptic ulcer of newborn (P78.82)

K27.Ø **Acute peptic ulcer, site unspecified, with hemorrhage**
K27.1 **Acute peptic ulcer, site unspecified, with perforation**
K27.2 **Acute peptic ulcer, site unspecified, with both hemorrhage and perforation**
K27.3 **Acute peptic ulcer, site unspecified, without hemorrhage or perforation**
K27.4 **Chronic or unspecified peptic ulcer, site unspecified, with hemorrhage**
K27.5 **Chronic or unspecified peptic ulcer, site unspecified, with perforation**
K27.6 **Chronic or unspecified peptic ulcer, site unspecified, with both hemorrhage and perforation**
K27.7 **Chronic peptic ulcer, site unspecified, without hemorrhage or perforation**
K27.9 **Peptic ulcer, site unspecified, unspecified as acute or chronic, without hemorrhage or perforation**

K28 Gastrojejunal ulcer PDX 1075
Includes anastomotic ulcer (peptic) or erosion
gastrocolic ulcer (peptic) or erosion
gastrointestinal ulcer (peptic) or erosion
gastrojejunal ulcer (peptic) or erosion
jejunal ulcer (peptic) or erosion
marginal ulcer (peptic) or erosion
stomal ulcer (peptic) or erosion
Use additional code to identify:
alcohol abuse and dependence (F1Ø.-)
Excludes1 primary ulcer of small intestine (K63.3)

K28.Ø **Acute gastrojejunal ulcer with hemorrhage**
K28.1 **Acute gastrojejunal ulcer with perforation**
K28.2 **Acute gastrojejunal ulcer with both hemorrhage and perforation**
K28.3 **Acute gastrojejunal ulcer without hemorrhage or perforation**
K28.4 **Chronic or unspecified gastrojejunal ulcer with hemorrhage**
Coding Clinic: 2023, Q3, P1Ø
K28.5 **Chronic or unspecified gastrojejunal ulcer with perforation**
K28.6 **Chronic or unspecified gastrojejunal ulcer with both hemorrhage and perforation**
K28.7 **Chronic gastrojejunal ulcer without hemorrhage or perforation**
K28.9 **Gastrojejunal ulcer, unspecified as acute or chronic, without hemorrhage or perforation**

K29 Gastritis and duodenitis PDX 1078
Excludes1 eosinophilic gastritis or gastroenteritis (K52.81)
Zollinger-Ellison syndrome (E16.4)

K29.Ø Acute gastritis
Use additional code to identify:
alcohol abuse and dependence (F1Ø.-)
Excludes1 erosion (acute) of stomach (K25.-)
K29.ØØ **Acute gastritis without bleeding**
K29.Ø1 **Acute gastritis with bleeding**

K29.2 Alcoholic gastritis
Use additional code to identify:
alcohol abuse and dependence (F1Ø.-)
K29.2Ø **Alcoholic gastritis without bleeding**
K29.21 **Alcoholic gastritis with bleeding**

K29.3 Chronic superficial gastritis
K29.3Ø **Chronic superficial gastritis without bleeding**
K29.31 **Chronic superficial gastritis with bleeding**

K29.4 Chronic atrophic gastritis
Gastric atrophy
K29.4Ø **Chronic atrophic gastritis without bleeding**
K29.41 **Chronic atrophic gastritis with bleeding**

K29.5 Unspecified chronic gastritis
Chronic antral gastritis
Chronic fundal gastritis
K29.5Ø **Unspecified chronic gastritis without bleeding**
K29.51 **Unspecified chronic gastritis with bleeding**

K29.6 Other gastritis
Giant hypertrophic gastritis
Granulomatous gastritis
Ménétrier's disease
K29.6Ø **Other gastritis without bleeding**
K29.61 **Other gastritis with bleeding**

K29.7 Gastritis, unspecified
K29.7Ø **Gastritis, unspecified, without bleeding**
K29.71 **Gastritis, unspecified, with bleeding**

Item 11–9 Gastritis is a severe inflammation of the stomach. **Atrophic gastritis** is a chronic inflammation of the stomach that results in destruction of the cells of the mucosa of the stomach. Duodenitis is an inflammation of the duodenum, the first section of the small intestine.

● **K29.8 Duodenitis**
- **K29.80 Duodenitis without bleeding**
- **K29.81 Duodenitis with bleeding**

● **K29.9 Gastroduodenitis, unspecified**
- **K29.90 Gastroduodenitis, unspecified, without bleeding**
- **K29.91 Gastroduodenitis, unspecified, with bleeding**

K30 Functional dyspepsia
Indigestion
Excludes1 dyspepsia NOS (R10.13)
heartburn (R12)
nervous dyspepsia (F45.8)
neurotic dyspepsia (F45.8)
psychogenic dyspepsia (F45.8)

● **K31 Other diseases of stomach and duodenum**
Includes functional disorders of stomach
Excludes2 diabetic gastroparesis (E08.43, E09.43, E10.43, E11.43, E13.43)
diverticulum of duodenum (K57.00-K57.13)

K31.0 Acute dilatation of stomach PDX 771
Acute distention of stomach

K31.1 Adult hypertrophic pyloric stenosis PDX 772 A
Pyloric stenosis NOS
Excludes1 congenital or infantile pyloric stenosis (Q40.0)
Coding Clinic: 2023, Q3, P12

K31.2 Hourglass stricture and stenosis of stomach
Excludes1 congenital hourglass stomach (Q40.2)
hourglass contraction of stomach (K31.89)

K31.3 Pylorospasm, not elsewhere classified
Excludes1 congenital or infantile pylorospasm (Q40.0)
neurotic pylorospasm (F45.8)
psychogenic pylorospasm (F45.8)

K31.4 Gastric diverticulum
Excludes1 congenital diverticulum of stomach (Q40.2)

K31.5 Obstruction of duodenum PDX 773
Constriction of duodenum
Duodenal ileus (chronic)
Stenosis of duodenum
Narrowing
Stricture of duodenum
Narrowing
Volvulus of duodenum
Twisting/knotting
Excludes1 congenital stenosis of duodenum (Q41.0)

K31.6 Fistula of stomach and duodenum PDX 774
Gastrocolic fistula
Gastrojejunocolic fistula
Code also, if applicable, disruption of internal operation (surgical) wound (T81.32-)

K31.7 Polyp of stomach and duodenum
Excludes1 adenomatous polyp of stomach (D13.1)
Coding Clinic: 2020, Q1, P16

● **K31.8 Other specified diseases of stomach and duodenum**

● **K31.81 Angiodysplasia of stomach and duodenum**
- **K31.811 Angiodysplasia of stomach and duodenum with bleeding** PDX 770
  Coding Clinic: 2023, Q1, P16
- **K31.819 Angiodysplasia of stomach and duodenum without bleeding**
  Angiodysplasia of stomach and duodenum NOS

K31.82 Dieulafoy lesion (hemorrhagic) of stomach and duodenum PDX 775
Excludes2 Dieulafoy lesion of intestine (K63.81)

Item 11–10 Achlorhydria, also known as gastric anacidity, is the absence of gastric acid.

K31.83 Achlorhydria

K31.84 Gastroparesis
Gastroparalysis
Code first underlying disease, if known, such as:
anorexia nervosa (F50.0-)
diabetes mellitus (E08.43, E09.43, E10.43, E11.43, E13.43)
scleroderma (M34.-)

K31.89 Other diseases of stomach and duodenum
Coding Clinic: 2024, Q2, P26; 2020, Q1, P16; 2017, Q1, P28

K31.9 Disease of stomach and duodenum, unspecified

● **K31.A Gastric intestinal metaplasia**

K31.A0 Gastric intestinal metaplasia, unspecified
Gastric intestinal metaplasia indefinite for dysplasia
Gastric intestinal metaplasia NOS

● **K31.A1 Gastric intestinal metaplasia without dysplasia**
- **K31.A11 Gastric intestinal metaplasia without dysplasia, involving the antrum**
- **K31.A12 Gastric intestinal metaplasia without dysplasia, involving the body(corpus)**
- **K31.A13 Gastric intestinal metaplasia without dysplasia, involving the fundus involving the cardia**
- **K31.A14 Gastric intestinal metaplasia without dysplasia, involving the cardia**
- **K31.A15 Gastric intestinal metaplasia without dysplasia, involving multiple sites**
- **K31.A19 Gastric intestinal metaplasia without dysplasia, unspecified site**

● **K31.A2 Gastric intestinal metaplasia with dysplasia**
- **K31.A21 Gastric intestinal metaplasia with low grade dysplasia**
- **K31.A22 Gastric intestinal metaplasia with high grade dysplasia**
- **K31.A29 Gastric intestinal metaplasia with dysplasia, unspecified**

DISEASES OF APPENDIX (K35-K38)

● **K35 Acute appendicitis** PDX 1084

● **K35.2 Acute appendicitis with generalized peritonitis**

● **K35.20 Acute appendicitis with generalized peritonitis, without abscess (Acute) appendicitis with generalized peritonitis NOS**
Coding Clinic: 2018, Q4, P18

- **K35.200 Acute appendicitis with generalized peritonitis, without perforation or abscess**
  (Acute) appendicitis with generalized peritonitis without rupture or perforation of appendix NOS
- **K35.201 Acute appendicitis with generalized peritonitis, with perforation, without abscess**
  Appendicitis (acute) with generalized (diffuse) peritonitis following rupture or perforation of appendix NOS
- **K35.209 Acute appendicitis with generalized peritonitis, without abscess, unspecified as to perforation**
  (Acute) appendicitis with generalized peritonitis NOS

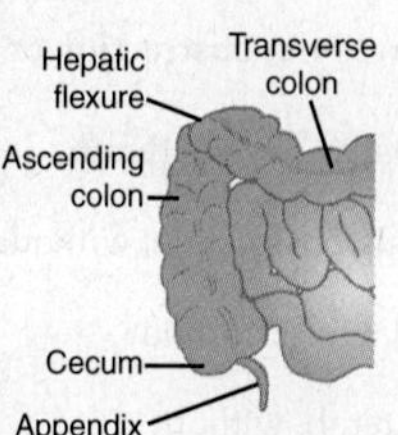

Figure 11-8 Acute appendicitis is the inflammation of the appendix, usually associated with obstruction. Most often this is a disease of adolescents and young adults.

● **K35.21 Acute appendicitis with generalized peritonitis, with abscess**

K35.210 Acute appendicitis with generalized peritonitis, without perforation, with abscess

(Acute) appendicitis with generalized peritonitis without rupture or perforation of appendix, with abscess

K35.211 Acute appendicitis with generalized peritonitis, with perforation and abscess

Appendicitis (acute) with generalized (diffuse) peritonitis following rupture or perforation of appendix, with abscess

K35.219 Acute appendicitis with generalized peritonitis, with abscess, unspecified as to perforation

(Acute) appendicitis with generalized peritonitis and abscess NOS

● **K35.3 Acute appendicitis with localized peritonitis**

K35.30 Acute appendicitis with localized peritonitis, without perforation or gangrene

Acute appendicitis with localized peritonitis NOS

K35.31 Acute appendicitis with localized peritonitis and gangrene, without perforation

K35.32 Acute appendicitis with perforation, localized peritonitis, and gangrene, without abscess

(Acute) appendicitis with perforation NOS
Perforated appendix NOS
Ruptured appendix (with localized peritonitis) NOS

Coding Clinic: 2020, Q1, P16; 2018, Q4, P18

K35.33 Acute appendicitis with perforation, localized peritonitis, and gangrene, with abscess

(Acute) appendicitis with (peritoneal) abscess NOS
Ruptured appendix with localized peritonitis and abscess

● **K35.8 Other and unspecified acute appendicitis**

K35.80 Unspecified acute appendicitis

Acute appendicitis NOS
Acute appendicitis without (localized) (generalized) peritonitis

● **K35.89 Other acute appendicitis**

K35.890 Other acute appendicitis without perforation or gangrene

K35.891 Other acute appendicitis without perforation, with gangrene

(Acute) appendicitis with gangrene NOS

K36 Other appendicitis

Chronic appendicitis
Recurrent appendicitis

K37 Unspecified appendicitis

Excludes1 unspecified appendicitis with peritonitis (K35.2-, K35.3)

● **K38 Other diseases of appendix**

K38.0 Hyperplasia of appendix

K38.1 Appendicular concretions

Fecalith of appendix
Stercolith of appendix

K38.2 Diverticulum of appendix

K38.3 Fistula of appendix

K38.8 Other specified diseases of appendix

Intussusception of appendix

K38.9 Disease of appendix, unspecified

HERNIA (K40-K46)

Note: Hernia with both gangrene and obstruction is classified to hernia with gangrene.

Includes acquired hernia
congenital [except diaphragmatic or hiatus] hernia
recurrent hernia

● **K40 Inguinal hernia** (Ex) PDX 1085

Includes bubonocele
direct inguinal hernia
double inguinal hernia
indirect inguinal hernia
inguinal hernia NOS
oblique inguinal hernia
scrotal hernia

● **K40.0 Bilateral inguinal hernia, with obstruction, without gangrene**

Inguinal hernia (bilateral) causing obstruction without gangrene
Incarcerated inguinal hernia (bilateral) without gangrene
Irreducible inguinal hernia (bilateral) without gangrene
Strangulated inguinal hernia (bilateral) without gangrene

K40.00 Bilateral inguinal hernia, with obstruction, without gangrene, not specified as recurrent

Bilateral inguinal hernia, with obstruction, without gangrene NOS

K40.01 Bilateral inguinal hernia, with obstruction, without gangrene, recurrent

Item 11-11 Hernias of the groin are the most common type, accounting for 80 percent of all hernias. There are two major types of inguinal hernias: indirect (oblique) affecting men only and direct. **Indirect inguinal hernias** result when the intestines emerge through the abdominal wall in an indirect fashion through the inguinal canal. **Direct inguinal hernias** penetrate through the abdominal wall in a direct fashion. **Femoral hernias** occur at the femoral ring where the femoral vessels enter the thigh and is most common in women. An abdominal wall hernia is also called a ventral or epigastric hernia and occurs in both sexes. Classification is based on location of the hernia and whether there is obstruction or gangrene.

Ventral, epigastric, or incisional hernia occurs on the abdominal surface caused by musculature weakness or a tear at a previous surgical site and is evidenced by a bulge that changes in size, becoming larger with exertion. An **incarcerated** hernia is one in which the intestines become trapped in the hernia. A **strangulated** hernia is one in which the blood supply to the intestines is lost. **Hiatal hernia** occurs when a loop of the stomach protrudes upward through the small opening in the diaphragm through which the esophagus passes, leaving the abdominal cavity and entering the chest. It occurs in both sexes.

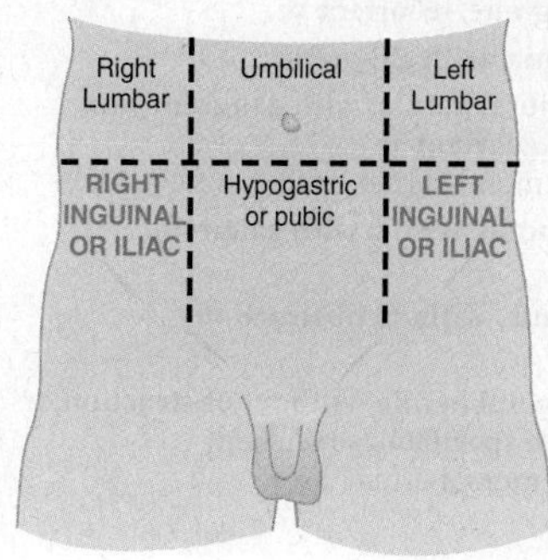

Figure 11-9 Inguinal hernias are those that are located in the inguinal or iliac areas of the abdomen.

CHAPTER 11 (K00-K95)

- K40.1 Bilateral inguinal hernia, with gangrene
  - K40.10 Bilateral inguinal hernia, with gangrene, not specified as recurrent
    - Bilateral inguinal hernia, with gangrene NOS
  - K40.11 Bilateral inguinal hernia, with gangrene, recurrent
- K40.2 Bilateral inguinal hernia, without obstruction or gangrene
  - K40.20 Bilateral inguinal hernia, without obstruction or gangrene, not specified as recurrent
    - Bilateral inguinal hernia NOS
  - K40.21 Bilateral inguinal hernia, without obstruction or gangrene, recurrent
- K40.3 Unilateral inguinal hernia, with obstruction, without gangrene
  - Inguinal hernia (unilateral) causing obstruction without gangrene
  - Incarcerated inguinal hernia (unilateral) without gangrene
  - Irreducible inguinal hernia (unilateral) without gangrene
  - Strangulated inguinal hernia (unilateral) without gangrene
  - K40.30 Unilateral inguinal hernia, with obstruction, without gangrene, not specified as recurrent
    - Inguinal hernia, with obstruction NOS
    - Unilateral inguinal hernia, with obstruction, without gangrene NOS
  - K40.31 Unilateral inguinal hernia, with obstruction, without gangrene, recurrent
- K40.4 Unilateral inguinal hernia, with gangrene
  - K40.40 Unilateral inguinal hernia, with gangrene, not specified as recurrent
    - Inguinal hernia with gangrene NOS
    - Unilateral inguinal hernia with gangrene NOS
  - K40.41 Unilateral inguinal hernia, with gangrene, recurrent
- K40.9 Unilateral inguinal hernia, without obstruction or gangrene
  - K40.90 Unilateral inguinal hernia, without obstruction or gangrene, not specified as recurrent
    - Inguinal hernia NOS
    - Unilateral inguinal hernia NOS
    - Coding Clinic: 2021, Q3, P31
  - K40.91 Unilateral inguinal hernia, without obstruction or gangrene, recurrent
    - Coding Clinic: 2021, Q3, P31

K41 Femoral hernia

- K41.0 Bilateral femoral hernia, with obstruction, without gangrene (Ex) PDX 1086
  - Femoral hernia (bilateral) causing obstruction, without gangrene
  - Incarcerated femoral hernia (bilateral), without gangrene
  - Irreducible femoral hernia (bilateral), without gangrene
  - Strangulated femoral hernia (bilateral), without gangrene
  - K41.00 Bilateral femoral hernia, with obstruction, without gangrene, not specified as recurrent
    - Bilateral femoral hernia, with obstruction, without gangrene NOS
  - K41.01 Bilateral femoral hernia, with obstruction, without gangrene, recurrent
- K41.1 Bilateral femoral hernia, with gangrene (Ex) PDX 1087
  - K41.10 Bilateral femoral hernia, with gangrene, not specified as recurrent
    - Bilateral femoral hernia, with gangrene NOS
  - K41.11 Bilateral femoral hernia, with gangrene, recurrent
- K41.2 Bilateral femoral hernia, without obstruction or gangrene
  - K41.20 Bilateral femoral hernia, without obstruction or gangrene, not specified as recurrent
    - Bilateral femoral hernia NOS
  - K41.21 Bilateral femoral hernia, without obstruction or gangrene, recurrent
- K41.3 Unilateral femoral hernia, with obstruction, without gangrene (Ex) PDX 1086
  - Femoral hernia (unilateral) causing obstruction, without gangrene
  - Incarcerated femoral hernia (unilateral), without gangrene
  - Irreducible femoral hernia (unilateral), without gangrene
  - Strangulated femoral hernia (unilateral), without gangrene
  - K41.30 Unilateral femoral hernia, with obstruction, without gangrene, not specified as recurrent
    - Femoral hernia, with obstruction NOS
    - Unilateral femoral hernia, with obstruction NOS
  - K41.31 Unilateral femoral hernia, with obstruction, without gangrene, recurrent
    - Coding Clinic: 2021, Q3, P30
- K41.4 Unilateral femoral hernia, with gangrene (Ex) PDX 1087
  - K41.40 Unilateral femoral hernia, with gangrene, not specified as recurrent
    - Femoral hernia, with gangrene NOS
    - Unilateral femoral hernia, with gangrene NOS
  - K41.41 Unilateral femoral hernia, with gangrene, recurrent
- K41.9 Unilateral femoral hernia, without obstruction or gangrene
  - K41.90 Unilateral femoral hernia, without obstruction or gangrene, not specified as recurrent
    - Femoral hernia NOS
    - Unilateral femoral hernia NOS
    - Coding Clinic: 2021, Q3, P30-31
  - K41.91 Unilateral femoral hernia, without obstruction or gangrene, recurrent

K42 Umbilical hernia

Includes paraumbilical hernia

Excludes1 omphalocele (Q79.2)

- K42.0 Umbilical hernia with obstruction, without gangrene (Ex) PDX 1088
  - Umbilical hernia causing obstruction, without gangrene
  - Incarcerated umbilical hernia, without gangrene
  - Irreducible umbilical hernia, without gangrene
  - Strangulated umbilical hernia, without gangrene
- K42.1 Umbilical hernia with gangrene (Ex) PDX 1089
  - Gangrenous umbilical hernia
- K42.9 Umbilical hernia without obstruction or gangrene
  - Umbilical hernia NOS

K43 Ventral hernia

- K43.0 Incisional hernia with obstruction, without gangrene (Ex) PDX 1088
  - Incisional hernia causing obstruction, without gangrene
  - Incarcerated incisional hernia, without gangrene
  - Irreducible incisional hernia, without gangrene
  - Strangulated incisional hernia, without gangrene
- K43.1 Incisional hernia with gangrene (Ex) PDX 1089
  - Gangrenous incisional hernia
- K43.2 Incisional hernia without obstruction or gangrene
  - Incisional hernia NOS
- K43.3 Parastomal hernia with obstruction, without gangrene (Ex) PDX 1088
  - Incarcerated parastomal hernia, without gangrene
  - Irreducible parastomal hernia, without gangrene
  - Parastomal hernia causing obstruction, without gangrene
  - Strangulated parastomal hernia, without gangrene
- K43.4 Parastomal hernia with gangrene (Ex) PDX 1089
  - Gangrenous parastomal hernia
- K43.5 Parastomal hernia without obstruction or gangrene
  - Parastomal hernia NOS

CHAPTER 11 (K00-K95)

K43.6 Other and unspecified ventral hernia with obstruction, without gangrene (Ex) PDX 1088
- Epigastric hernia causing obstruction, without gangrene
- Hypogastric hernia causing obstruction, without gangrene
- Incarcerated epigastric hernia without gangrene
- Incarcerated hypogastric hernia without gangrene
- Incarcerated midline hernia without gangrene
- Incarcerated spigelian hernia without gangrene
- Incarcerated subxiphoid hernia without gangrene
- Irreducible epigastric hernia without gangrene
- Irreducible hypogastric hernia without gangrene
- Irreducible midline hernia without gangrene
- Irreducible spigelian hernia without gangrene
- Irreducible subxiphoid hernia without gangrene
- Midline hernia causing obstruction, without gangrene
- Spigelian hernia causing obstruction, without gangrene
- Strangulated epigastric hernia without gangrene
- Strangulated hypogastric hernia without gangrene
- Strangulated midline hernia without gangrene
- Strangulated spigelian hernia without gangrene
- Strangulated subxiphoid hernia without gangrene
- Subxiphoid hernia causing obstruction, without gangrene

K43.7 Other and unspecified ventral hernia with gangrene (Ex) PDX 1089
- Any condition listed under K43.6 specified as gangrenous

K43.9 Ventral hernia without obstruction or gangrene
- Epigastric hernia
- Ventral hernia NOS

● K44 Diaphragmatic hernia (Ex) PDX 1090

Includes hiatus hernia (esophageal) (sliding)
paraesophageal hernia

Excludes1 congenital diaphragmatic hernia (Q79.Ø)
congenital hiatus hernia (Q4Ø.1)

K44.Ø Diaphragmatic hernia with obstruction, without gangrene
- Diaphragmatic hernia causing obstruction
- Incarcerated diaphragmatic hernia
- Irreducible diaphragmatic hernia
- Strangulated diaphragmatic hernia

Coding Clinic: 2Ø22, Q2, P14

K44.1 Diaphragmatic hernia with gangrene
- Gangrenous diaphragmatic hernia

K44.9 Diaphragmatic hernia without obstruction or gangrene
- Diaphragmatic hernia NOS

Coding Clinic: 2Ø17, Q1, P7

● K45 Other abdominal hernia

Includes abdominal hernia, specified site NEC
lumbar hernia
obturator hernia
pudendal hernia
retroperitoneal hernia
sciatic hernia

K45.Ø Other specified abdominal hernia with obstruction, without gangrene (Ex) PDX 1091
- Other specified abdominal hernia causing obstruction
- Other specified incarcerated abdominal hernia
- Other specified irreducible abdominal hernia
- Other specified strangulated abdominal hernia

K45.1 Other specified abdominal hernia with gangrene (Ex) PDX 1092
- Any condition listed under K45 specified as gangrenous

Coding Clinic: 2Ø24, Q2, P22, 23

K45.8 Other specified abdominal hernia without obstruction or gangrene

● K46 Unspecified abdominal hernia

Includes enterocele
epiplocele
hernia NOS
interstitial hernia
intestinal hernia
intra-abdominal hernia

Excludes1 vaginal enterocele (N81.5)

Item 11-12 Crohn's disease, also known as **regional enteritis,** is a chronic inflammatory disease of the intestines. Classification is based on location in the small (duodenum, ileum, jejunum) or large (cecum, colon, rectum, anal canal) intestine.

K46.Ø Unspecified abdominal hernia with obstruction, without gangrene (Ex) PDX 1090, 1091
- Unspecified abdominal hernia causing obstruction
- Unspecified incarcerated abdominal hernia
- Unspecified irreducible abdominal hernia
- Unspecified strangulated abdominal hernia

K46.1 Unspecified abdominal hernia with gangrene (Ex) PDX 1092
- Any condition listed under K46 specified as gangrenous

K46.9 Unspecified abdominal hernia without obstruction or gangrene
- Abdominal hernia NOS

★ **(See Plate 32 of the Anatomy Illustrations.)**

NONINFECTIVE ENTERITIS AND COLITIS (K5Ø-K52)

Includes noninfective inflammatory bowel disease

Excludes1 irritable bowel syndrome (K58.-)
megacolon (K59.3-)

● K5Ø Crohn's disease [regional enteritis] (Ex) PDX 1093

Includes granulomatous enteritis

Use additional code to identify manifestations, such as:
pyoderma gangrenosum (L88)

▶Use Additional code to identify any associated fistulas, if applicable:
- ▶anal fistula (K6Ø.3-)
- ▶anorectal fistula (K6Ø.5-)
- ▶rectal fistula (K6Ø.4-)

Excludes1 ulcerative colitis (K51.-)

● K5Ø.Ø Crohn's disease of small intestine
- Crohn's disease [regional enteritis] of duodenum
- Crohn's disease [regional enteritis] of ileum
- Crohn's disease [regional enteritis] of jejunum
- Regional ileitis
- Terminal ileitis

Excludes1 Crohn's disease of both small and large intestine (K5Ø.8-)

K5Ø.ØØ Crohn's disease of small intestine without complications

● K5Ø.Ø1 Crohn's disease of small intestine with complications

K5Ø.Ø11 Crohn's disease of small intestine with rectal bleeding

K5Ø.Ø12 Crohn's disease of small intestine with intestinal obstruction
CC when PDx is its own CC

K5Ø.Ø13 Crohn's disease of small intestine with fistula
CC when PDx is its own CC

K5Ø.Ø14 Crohn's disease of small intestine with abscess
CC when PDx is its own CC
Coding Clinic: 2Ø12, Q4, P1Ø4

K5Ø.Ø18 Crohn's disease of small intestine with other complication

K5Ø.Ø19 Crohn's disease of small intestine with unspecified complications

● K5Ø.1 Crohn's disease of large intestine
- Crohn's disease [regional enteritis] of colon
- Crohn's disease [regional enteritis] of large bowel
- Crohn's disease [regional enteritis] of rectum
- Granulomatous colitis
- Regional colitis

Excludes1 Crohn's disease of both small and large intestine (K5Ø.8)

K5Ø.1Ø Crohn's disease of large intestine without complications

CHAPTER 11 (KØØ-K95)

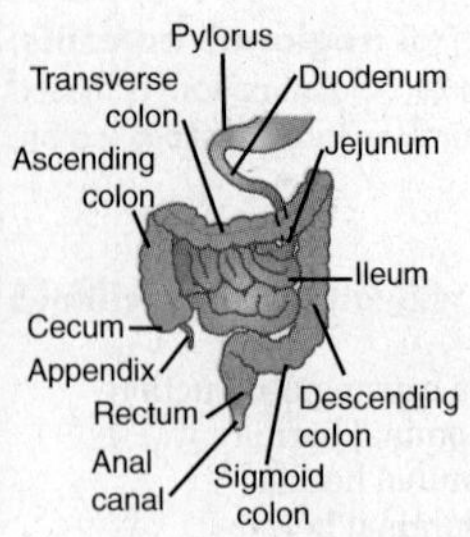

Figure 11-10 Small and large intestines.

● **K50.11** Crohn's disease of large intestine with complications

- **K50.111** Crohn's disease of large intestine with rectal bleeding
- **K50.112** Crohn's disease of large intestine with intestinal obstruction
  CC when PDx is its own CC
- **K50.113** Crohn's disease of large intestine with fistula
  CC when PDx is its own CC
- **K50.114** Crohn's disease of large intestine with abscess
  CC when PDx is its own CC
  Coding Clinic: 2012, Q4, P104
- **K50.118** Crohn's disease of large intestine with other complication
- **K50.119** Crohn's disease of large intestine with unspecified complications

● **K50.8** Crohn's disease of both small and large intestine

- **K50.80** Crohn's disease of both small and large intestine without complications

● **K50.81** Crohn's disease of both small and large intestine with complications

- **K50.811** Crohn's disease of both small and large intestine with rectal bleeding
- **K50.812** Crohn's disease of both small and large intestine with intestinal obstruction
  CC when PDx is its own CC
- **K50.813** Crohn's disease of both small and large intestine with fistula
  CC when PDx is its own CC
- **K50.814** Crohn's disease of both small and large intestine with abscess
  CC when PDx is its own CC
  Coding Clinic: 2012, Q4, P104
- **K50.818** Crohn's disease of both small and large intestine with other complication
- **K50.819** Crohn's disease of both small and large intestine with unspecified complications

● **K50.9** Crohn's disease, unspecified (Ex) PDX 1094

- **K50.90** Crohn's disease, unspecified, without complications
  Crohn's disease NOS
  Regional enteritis NOS

● **K50.91** Crohn's disease, unspecified, with complications

- **K50.911** Crohn's disease, unspecified, with rectal bleeding
- **K50.912** Crohn's disease, unspecified, with intestinal obstruction
  CC when PDx is its own CC
- **K50.913** Crohn's disease, unspecified, with fistula
  CC when PDx is its own CC
- **K50.914** Crohn's disease, unspecified, with abscess
  CC when PDx is its own CC
  Coding Clinic: 2012, Q4, P104

Item 11-13 Ulcerative colitis attacks the colonic mucosa and forms abscesses. The disease involves the intestines. Classification is based on the location:

- Enterocolitis: large and small intestine
- Ileocolitis: ileum and colon
- Proctitis: rectum
- Proctosigmoiditis: sigmoid colon and rectum

- **K50.918** Crohn's disease, unspecified, with other complication
- **K50.919** Crohn's disease, unspecified, with unspecified complications

● **K51** Ulcerative colitis (Ex) PDX 1093

Use additional code to identify manifestations, such as:
pyoderma gangrenosum (L88)

▶Use Additional code to identify any associated fistulas, if applicable:
▶anal fistula (K60.3-)
▶anorectal fistula (K60.5-)
▶rectal fistula (K60.4-)

Excludes1 Crohn's disease [regional enteritis] (K50.-)

● **K51.0** Ulcerative (chronic) pancolitis
Backwash ileitis

- **K51.00** Ulcerative (chronic) pancolitis without complications
  Ulcerative (chronic) pancolitis NOS

● **K51.01** Ulcerative (chronic) pancolitis with complications

- **K51.011** Ulcerative (chronic) pancolitis with rectal bleeding
- **K51.012** Ulcerative (chronic) pancolitis with intestinal obstruction
  CC when PDx is its own CC
- **K51.013** Ulcerative (chronic) pancolitis with fistula
  CC when PDx is its own CC
- **K51.014** Ulcerative (chronic) pancolitis with abscess
  CC when PDx is its own CC
- **K51.018** Ulcerative (chronic) pancolitis with other complication
- **K51.019** Ulcerative (chronic) pancolitis with unspecified complications

● **K51.2** Ulcerative (chronic) proctitis

- **K51.20** Ulcerative (chronic) proctitis without complications
  Ulcerative (chronic) proctitis NOS

● **K51.21** Ulcerative (chronic) proctitis with complications

- **K51.211** Ulcerative (chronic) proctitis with rectal bleeding
- **K51.212** Ulcerative (chronic) proctitis with intestinal obstruction
  CC when PDx is its own CC
- **K51.213** Ulcerative (chronic) proctitis with fistula
  CC when PDx is its own CC
- **K51.214** Ulcerative (chronic) proctitis with abscess
  CC when PDx is its own CC
- **K51.218** Ulcerative (chronic) proctitis with other complication
- **K51.219** Ulcerative (chronic) proctitis with unspecified complications

● **K51.3** Ulcerative (chronic) rectosigmoiditis

- **K51.30** Ulcerative (chronic) rectosigmoiditis without complications
  Ulcerative (chronic) rectosigmoiditis NOS

● K51.31 **Ulcerative (chronic) rectosigmoiditis with complications**
- K51.311 **Ulcerative (chronic) rectosigmoiditis with rectal bleeding**
- K51.312 **Ulcerative (chronic) rectosigmoiditis with intestinal obstruction**
  CC when PDx is its own CC
- K51.313 **Ulcerative (chronic) rectosigmoiditis with fistula**
  CC when PDx is its own CC
- K51.314 **Ulcerative (chronic) rectosigmoiditis with abscess**
  CC when PDx is its own CC
- K51.318 **Ulcerative (chronic) rectosigmoiditis with other complication**
- K51.319 **Ulcerative (chronic) rectosigmoiditis with unspecified complications**

● K51.4 **Inflammatory polyps of colon**
Excludes2 adenomatous polyp of colon (D12.6)
polyposis of colon (D12.6)
polyps of colon NOS (K63.5)
- K51.40 **Inflammatory polyps of colon without complications**
  Inflammatory polyps of colon NOS

● K51.41 **Inflammatory polyps of colon with complications**
- K51.411 **Inflammatory polyps of colon with rectal bleeding**
- K51.412 **Inflammatory polyps of colon with intestinal obstruction**
  CC when PDx is its own CC
- K51.413 **Inflammatory polyps of colon with fistula**
  CC when PDx is its own CC
- K51.414 **Inflammatory polyps of colon with abscess**
  CC when PDx is its own CC
- K51.418 **Inflammatory polyps of colon with other complication**
- K51.419 **Inflammatory polyps of colon with unspecified complications**

● K51.5 **Left sided colitis**
Left hemicolitis
- K51.50 **Left sided colitis without complications**
  Left sided colitis NOS

● K51.51 **Left sided colitis with complications**
- K51.511 **Left sided colitis with rectal bleeding**
- K51.512 **Left sided colitis with intestinal obstruction**
  CC when PDx is its own CC
- K51.513 **Left sided colitis with fistula**
  CC when PDx is its own CC
- K51.514 **Left sided colitis with abscess**
  CC when PDx is its own CC
- K51.518 **Left sided colitis with other complication**
- K51.519 **Left sided colitis with unspecified complications**

● K51.8 **Other ulcerative colitis**
- K51.80 **Other ulcerative colitis without complications**

● K51.81 **Other ulcerative colitis with complications**
- K51.811 **Other ulcerative colitis with rectal bleeding**
- K51.812 **Other ulcerative colitis with intestinal obstruction**
  CC when PDx is its own CC
- K51.813 **Other ulcerative colitis with fistula**
  CC when PDx is its own CC
- K51.814 **Other ulcerative colitis with abscess**
  CC when PDx is its own CC
- K51.818 **Other ulcerative colitis with other complication**
- K51.819 **Other ulcerative colitis with unspecified complications**

● K51.9 **Ulcerative colitis, unspecified** (Ex) PDX 1095
- K51.90 **Ulcerative colitis, unspecified, without complications**

● K51.91 **Ulcerative colitis, unspecified, with complications**
- K51.911 **Ulcerative colitis, unspecified with rectal bleeding**
- K51.912 **Ulcerative colitis, unspecified with intestinal obstruction**
  CC when PDx is its own CC
- K51.913 **Ulcerative colitis, unspecified with fistula**
  CC when PDx is its own CC
- K51.914 **Ulcerative colitis, unspecified with abscess**
  CC when PDx is its own CC
- K51.918 **Ulcerative colitis, unspecified with other complication**
- K51.919 **Ulcerative colitis, unspecified with unspecified complications**

● K52 **Other and unspecified noninfective gastroenteritis and colitis**
- K52.0 **Gastroenteritis and colitis due to radiation** (Ex) PDX 1096
- K52.1 **Toxic gastroenteritis and colitis** (Ex) PDX 1097
  Drug-induced gastroenteritis and colitis
  Code first (T51-T65) to identify toxic agent
  Use additional code for adverse effect, if applicable, to identify drug (T36-T50 with fifth or sixth character 5)
  Coding Clinic: 2019, Q1, P17

● K52.2 **Allergic and dietetic gastroenteritis and colitis**
Food hypersensitivity gastroenteritis or colitis
Use additional code to identify type of food allergy (Z91.01-, Z91.02-)
Excludes2 allergic eosinophilic colitis (K52.82)
allergic eosinophilic esophagitis (K20.0)
allergic eosinophilic gastritis (K52.81)
allergic eosinophilic gastroenteritis (K52.81)
Coding Clinic: 2016, Q4, P30-31
- K52.21 **Food protein-induced enterocolitis syndrome**
  FPIES
  Use additional code for hypovolemic shock, if present (R57.1)
- K52.22 **Food protein-induced enteropathy**
- K52.29 **Other allergic and dietetic gastroenteritis and colitis**
  Allergic proctocolitis
  Food hypersensitivity gastroenteritis or colitis
  Food-induced eosinophilic proctocolitis
  Food protein-induced proctocolitis
  Immediate gastrointestinal hypersensitivity
  Milk protein-induced proctocolitis
- K52.3 **Indeterminate colitis**
  Colonic inflammatory bowel disease unclassified (IBDU)
  Excludes1 unspecified colitis (K52.9)

● K52.8 **Other specified noninfective gastroenteritis and colitis**
- K52.81 **Eosinophilic gastritis or gastroenteritis**
  Eosinophilic enteritis
  Excludes2 eosinophilic esophagitis (K20.0)
- K52.82 **Eosinophilic colitis**
  Excludes2 allergic proctocolitis (K52.29)
  food-induced eosinophilic proctocolitis (K52.29)
  food protein-induced enterocolitis syndrome (FPIES) (K52.21)
  food protein-induced proctocolitis (K52.29)
  milk protein-induced proctocolitis (K52.29)

● K52.83 Microscopic colitis
Coding Clinic: 2016, Q4, P30-31
K52.831 Collagenous colitis
K52.832 Lymphocytic colitis
K52.838 Other microscopic colitis
K52.839 Microscopic colitis, unspecified
K52.89 Other specified noninfective gastroenteritis and colitis
Coding Clinic: 2019, Q1, P21

K52.9 Noninfective gastroenteritis and colitis, unspecified
Colitis NOS
Enteritis NOS
Gastroenteritis NOS
Ileitis NOS
Jejunitis NOS
Sigmoiditis NOS
Excludes1 diarrhea NOS (R19.7)
functional diarrhea (K59.1)
infectious gastroenteritis and colitis NOS (A09)
neonatal diarrhea (noninfective) (P78.3)
psychogenic diarrhea (F45.8)
Coding Clinic: 2021, Q3, P3-4

OTHER DISEASES OF INTESTINES (K55-K64)

● K55 Vascular disorders of intestine
Excludes1 necrotizing enterocolitis of newborn (P77.-)
Excludes2 angioectasia (angiodysplasia) duodenum (K31.81)

● K55.0 Acute vascular disorders of intestine (Ex) PDX 1098
Infarction of appendices epiploicae
Mesenteric (artery) (vein) embolism
Mesenteric (artery) (vein) infarction
Mesenteric (artery) (vein) thrombosis
Coding Clinic: 2019, Q4, P68

● K55.01 Acute (reversible) ischemia of small intestine
Coding Clinic: 2016, Q4, P32
K55.011 Focal (segmental) acute (reversible) ischemia of small intestine
K55.012 Diffuse acute (reversible) ischemia of small intestine
K55.019 Acute (reversible) ischemia of small intestine, extent unspecified

● K55.02 Acute infarction of small intestine
Gangrene of small intestine
Necrosis of small intestine
Coding Clinic: 2016, Q4, P32
K55.021 Focal (segmental) acute infarction of small intestine
K55.022 Diffuse acute infarction of small intestine
K55.029 Acute infarction of small intestine, extent unspecified

● K55.03 Acute (reversible) ischemia of large intestine
Acute fulminant ischemic colitis
Subacute ischemic colitis
Coding Clinic: 2016, Q4, P32
K55.031 Focal (segmental) acute (reversible) ischemia of large intestine
K55.032 Diffuse acute (reversible) ischemia of large intestine
K55.039 Acute (reversible) ischemia of large intestine, extent unspecified
Coding Clinic: 2019, Q4, P68

● K55.04 Acute infarction of large intestine
Gangrene of large intestine
Necrosis of large intestine
Coding Clinic: 2016, Q4, P32
K55.041 Focal (segmental) acute infarction of large intestine
K55.042 Diffuse acute infarction of large intestine
K55.049 Acute infarction of large intestine, extent unspecified

● K55.05 Acute (reversible) ischemia of intestine, part unspecified
K55.051 Focal (segmental) acute (reversible) ischemia of intestine, part unspecified
K55.052 Diffuse acute (reversible) ischemia of intestine, part unspecified
K55.059 Acute (reversible) ischemia of intestine, part and extent unspecified

● K55.06 Acute infarction of intestine, part unspecified
Acute intestinal infarction
Gangrene of intestine
Necrosis of intestine
K55.061 Focal (segmental) acute infarction of intestine, part unspecified
K55.062 Diffuse acute infarction of intestine, part unspecified
K55.069 Acute infarction of intestine, part and extent unspecified

K55.1 Chronic vascular disorders of intestine (Ex) PDX 1099
Chronic ischemic colitis
Chronic ischemic enteritis
Chronic ischemic enterocolitis
Ischemic stricture of intestine
Mesenteric atherosclerosis
Mesenteric vascular insufficiency

● K55.2 Angiodysplasia of colon
K55.20 Angiodysplasia of colon without hemorrhage
K55.21 Angiodysplasia of colon with hemorrhage (Ex) PDX 1078

● K55.3 Necrotizing enterocolitis (Ex) PDX 1098
Excludes1 necrotizing enterocolitis of newborn (P77.-)
Excludes2 necrotizing enterocolitis due to Clostridium difficile (A04.7-)
K55.30 Necrotizing enterocolitis, unspecified
Necrotizing enterocolitis, NOS
K55.31 Stage 1 necrotizing enterocolitis
Necrotizing enterocolitis without pneumatosis, without perforation
Coding Clinic: 2016, Q4, P32
K55.32 Stage 2 necrotizing enterocolitis
Necrotizing enterocolitis with pneumatosis, without perforation
Coding Clinic: 2016, Q4, P32
K55.33 Stage 3 necrotizing enterocolitis
Necrotizing enterocolitis with perforation
Necrotizing enterocolitis with pneumatosis and perforation
Coding Clinic: 2016, Q4, P32

K55.8 Other vascular disorders of intestine (Ex) PDX 1099
K55.9 Vascular disorder of intestine, unspecified (Ex) PDX 1099
Ischemic colitis
Ischemic enteritis
Ischemic enterocolitis

● K56 Paralytic ileus and intestinal obstruction without hernia (Ex) PDX 1100
Excludes1 congenital stricture or stenosis of intestine (Q41-Q42)
cystic fibrosis with meconium ileus (E84.11)
ischemic stricture of intestine (K55.1)
meconium ileus NOS (P76.0)
neonatal intestinal obstructions classifiable to P76.-
obstruction of duodenum (K31.5)
postprocedural intestinal obstruction (K91.3-)
Excludes2 stenosis of anus or rectum (K62.4)

New | Revised | ~~deleted~~ Deleted | Excludes 1 | Excludes 2 | Includes | Use additional | Code first | Code also | Key words
OGCR Official Guidelines | ● Unacceptable Principal Diagnosis | X Assign placeholder X | ● Use Additional Character(s) | Manifestation Code | Coding Clinic

K56.0 Paralytic ileus
Paralysis of bowel
Paralysis of colon
Paralysis of intestine
Excludes1 gallstone ileus (K56.3)
ileus NOS (K56.7)
obstructive ileus NOS (K56.69-)

K56.1 Intussusception
Intussusception or invagination of bowel
Intussusception or invagination of colon
Intussusception or invagination of intestine
Intussusception or invagination of rectum
Excludes2 intussusception of appendix (K38.8)
Coding Clinic: 2023, Q3, P12

K56.2 Volvulus
Strangulation of colon or intestine
Torsion of colon or intestine
Twist of colon or intestine
Excludes2 volvulus of duodenum (K31.5)
Coding Clinic: 2024, Q2, P22

K56.3 Gallstone ileus
Obstruction of intestine by gallstone

K56.4 Other impaction of intestine

K56.41 Fecal impaction
Excludes2 incomplete defecation (R15.0)
Coding Clinic: 2024, Q2, P6

K56.49 Other impaction of intestine

K56.5 Intestinal adhesions [bands] with obstruction (postinfection)
Abdominal hernia due to adhesions with obstruction
Peritoneal adhesions [bands] with intestinal obstruction (postinfection)

K56.50 Intestinal adhesions [bands], unspecified as to partial versus complete obstruction
Intestinal adhesions with obstruction NOS

K56.51 Intestinal adhesions [bands], with partial obstruction
Intestinal adhesions with incomplete obstruction

K56.52 Intestinal adhesions [bands] with complete obstruction

K56.6 Other and unspecified intestinal obstruction

K56.60 Unspecified intestinal obstruction
Coding Clinic: 2017, Q2, P12

K56.600 Partial intestinal obstruction, unspecified as to cause
Incomplete intestinal obstruction, NOS

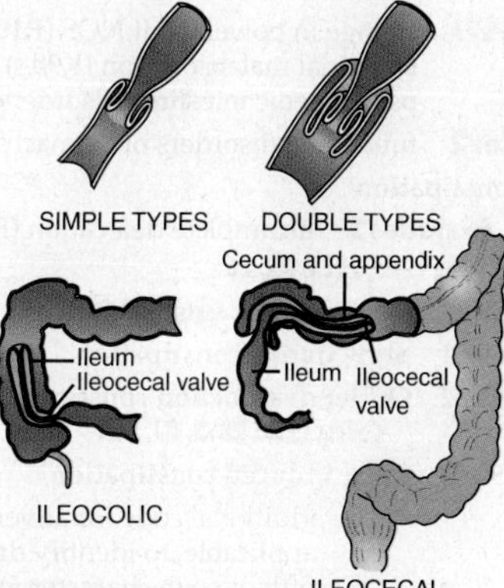

Figure 11-11 Types of intussusception.

Item 11-14 Intussusception is the prolapse (telescoping) of a part of the intestine into another adjacent part of the intestine. Intussusception may be enteric (ileoileal, jejunoileal, jejunojejunal), colic (colocolic), or intracolic (ileocecal, ileocolic).

Item 11-15 Volvulus is the twisting of a segment of the intestine, resulting in obstruction. Paralytic ileus is paralysis of the intestine. It need not be a complete paralysis, but it must prohibit the passage of food through the intestine and lead to intestinal blockage. It is a common aftermath of some types of surgery.

K56.601 Complete intestinal obstruction, unspecified as to cause

K56.609 Unspecified intestinal obstruction, unspecified as to partial versus complete obstruction
Intestinal obstruction NOS

K56.69 Other intestinal obstruction
Enterostenosis NOS
Obstructive ileus NOS
Occlusion of colon or intestine NOS
Stenosis of colon or intestine NOS
Stricture of colon or intestine NOS
Coding Clinic: 2017, Q2, P12

K56.690 Other partial intestinal obstruction
Other incomplete intestinal obstruction

K56.691 Other complete intestinal obstruction

K56.699 Other intestinal obstruction unspecified as to partial versus complete obstruction
Other intestinal obstruction, NEC
Coding Clinic: 2023, Q3, P11

K56.7 Ileus, unspecified (Ex) PDX 6752
Excludes1 obstructive ileus (K56.69-)
Excludes2 intestinal obstruction with hernia (K40-K46)
Coding Clinic: 2017, Q1, P41

K57 Diverticular disease of intestine
Code also if applicable peritonitis K65.-
Excludes1 congenital diverticulum of intestine (Q43.8)
Meckel's diverticulum (Q43.0)
Excludes2 diverticulum of appendix (K38.2)
Coding Clinic: 2022, Q1, P26

K57.0 Diverticulitis of small intestine with perforation and abscess
Excludes1 diverticulitis of both small and large intestine with perforation and abscess (K57.4-)

K57.00 Diverticulitis of small intestine with perforation and abscess without bleeding (Ex) PDX 1101
CC when PDx is its own CC

K57.01 Diverticulitis of small intestine with perforation and abscess with bleeding (Ex) PDX 1078
CC when PDx is its own CC

K57.1 Diverticular disease of small intestine without perforation or abscess
Excludes1 diverticular disease of both small and large intestine without perforation or abscess (K57.5-)

K57.10 Diverticulosis of small intestine without perforation or abscess without bleeding
Diverticular disease of small intestine NOS

K57.11 Diverticulosis of small intestine without perforation or abscess with bleeding (Ex) PDX 1078

K57.12 Diverticulitis of small intestine without perforation or abscess without bleeding (Ex) PDX 1101

K57.13 Diverticulitis of small intestine without perforation or abscess with bleeding (Ex) PDX 1078

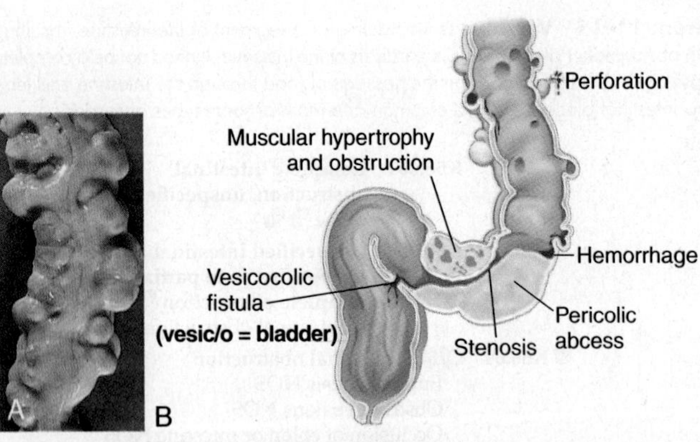

Figure 11-12 Diverticulosis. (From Shiland: Mastering Healthcare Terminology, ed 4, St. Louis, Mosby, 2012)

Item 11-16 **Diverticula** of the intestines are acquired herniations of the mucosa. Diverticulum (singular): Pocket or pouch that bulges outward through a weak spot (herniation) in the colon. Diverticula (plural). **Diverticulosis** is the condition of having diverticula. **Diverticulitis** is inflammation of these pouches or herniations. Classification is based on location (small intestine or colon) and whether it occurs with or without hemorrhage.

K57.2 Diverticulitis of large intestine with perforation and abscess
Excludes1 diverticulitis of both small and large intestine with perforation and abscess (K57.4-)
Coding Clinic: 2022, Q1, P27

K57.20 Diverticulitis of large intestine with perforation and abscess without bleeding PDX 1102
CC when PDx is its own CC
Coding Clinic: 2022, Q1, P26

K57.21 Diverticulitis of large intestine with perforation and abscess with bleeding PDX 1078
CC when PDx is its own CC

K57.3 Diverticular disease of large intestine without perforation or abscess
Excludes1 diverticular disease of both small and large intestine without perforation or abscess (K57.5-)

K57.30 Diverticulosis of large intestine without perforation or abscess without bleeding
Diverticular disease of colon NOS

K57.31 Diverticulosis of large intestine without perforation or abscess with bleeding PDX 1078

K57.32 Diverticulitis of large intestine without perforation or abscess without bleeding PDX 1102

K57.33 Diverticulitis of large intestine without perforation or abscess with bleeding PDX 1078

K57.4 Diverticulitis of both small and large intestine with perforation and abscess

K57.40 Diverticulitis of both small and large intestine with perforation and abscess without bleeding PDX 1102
CC when PDx is its own CC

K57.41 Diverticulitis of both small and large intestine with perforation and abscess with bleeding PDX 1078
CC when PDx is its own CC

K57.5 Diverticular disease of both small and large intestine without perforation or abscess

K57.50 Diverticulosis of both small and large intestine without perforation or abscess without bleeding
Diverticular disease of both small and large intestine NOS

K57.51 Diverticulosis of both small and large intestine without perforation or abscess with bleeding PDX 1078

K57.52 Diverticulitis of both small and large intestine without perforation or abscess without bleeding PDX 1102
CC when PDx is its own CC

K57.53 Diverticulitis of both small and large intestine without perforation or abscess with bleeding PDX 1078

K57.8 Diverticulitis of intestine, part unspecified, with perforation and abscess

K57.80 Diverticulitis of intestine, part unspecified, with perforation and abscess without bleeding PDX 1102
CC when PDx is its own CC

K57.81 Diverticulitis of intestine, part unspecified, with perforation and abscess with bleeding PDX 1078
CC when PDx is its own CC

K57.9 Diverticular disease of intestine, part unspecified, without perforation or abscess

K57.90 Diverticulosis of intestine, part unspecified, without perforation or abscess without bleeding
Diverticular disease of intestine NOS
Coding Clinic: 2021, Q1, P12

K57.91 Diverticulosis of intestine, part unspecified, without perforation or abscess with bleeding PDX 1078

K57.92 Diverticulitis of intestine, part unspecified, without perforation or abscess without bleeding PDX 1102

K57.93 Diverticulitis of intestine, part unspecified, without perforation or abscess with bleeding PDX 1078

K58 Irritable bowel syndrome
Includes irritable colon
spastic colon

K58.0 Irritable bowel syndrome with diarrhea

K58.1 Irritable bowel syndrome with constipation
Coding Clinic: 2016, Q4, P32

K58.2 Mixed irritable bowel syndrome
Coding Clinic: 2016, Q4, P32

K58.8 Other irritable bowel syndrome
Coding Clinic: 2016, Q4, P32

K58.9 Irritable bowel syndrome without diarrhea
Irritable bowel syndrome, unspecified

K59 Other functional intestinal disorders
Excludes1 change in bowel habit NOS (R19.4)
intestinal malabsorption (K90.-)
psychogenic intestinal disorders (F45.8)
Excludes2 functional disorders of stomach (K31.-)

K59.0 Constipation
Excludes2 incomplete defecation (R15.0)
Coding Clinic: 2024, Q2, P6

K59.00 Constipation, unspecified

K59.01 Slow transit constipation

K59.02 Outlet dysfunction constipation
Coding Clinic: 2023, Q1, P24

K59.03 Drug induced constipation
Use additional code for adverse effect, if applicable, to identify drug (T36-T50 with fifth or sixth character 5)
Coding Clinic: 2016, Q4, P33

K59.04 Chronic idiopathic constipation
Functional constipation
Coding Clinic: 2016, Q4, P33

K59.09 Other constipation
Chronic constipation

CHAPTER 11 (K00-K95)

K59.1 Functional diarrhea
Excludes1 diarrhea NOS (R19.7)
irritable bowel syndrome with diarrhea (K58.0)

K59.2 Neurogenic bowel, not elsewhere classified Ex: PDX 1103

● **K59.3 Megacolon, not elsewhere classified** Ex: PDX 1103
Dilatation of colon
Code first, if applicable (T51-T65) to identify toxic agent
Excludes1 congenital megacolon (aganglionic) (Q43.1)
megacolon (due to) (in) Chagas' disease (B57.32)
megacolon (due to) (in) Clostridium difficile (A04.7-)
megacolon (due to) (in) Hirschsprung's disease (Q43.1)
Coding Clinic: 2016, Q4, P33

K59.31 Toxic megacolon

K59.39 Other megacolon
Megacolon NOS

K59.4 Anal spasm
Proctalgia fugax

● **K59.8 Other specified functional intestinal disorders**

K59.81 Ogilvie syndrome
Acute colonic pseudo-obstruction (ACPO)

K59.89 Other specified functional intestinal disorders
Atony of colon
Pseudo-obstruction (acute) (chronic) of intestine

K59.9 Functional intestinal disorder, unspecified

● **K60 Fissure and fistula of anal and rectal regions**
Excludes1 fissure and fistula of anal and rectal regions with abscess or cellulitis (K61.-)
▶abscess or cellulitis off anal and rectal regions (K61.-)
Excludes2 anal sphincter tear (healed) (nontraumatic) (old) (K62.81)

K60.0 Acute anal fissure

K60.1 Chronic anal fissure

K60.2 Anal fissure, unspecified

K60.3 Anal fistula
▶*Code first, if applicable:*
▶Crohn's disease (K50.-)
▶ulcerative colitis (K51.-)
▶**Excludes1** congenital fistula (Q43.6)

▶ **K60.30 Anal fistula, unspecified**
▶Anal fistula NOS

▶● **K60.31 Anal fistula, simple**
▶Low intersphincteric anal fistula
▶Superficial anal fistula

▶ **K60.311 Anal fistula, simple, initial**
▶Anal fistula, simple, new

▶ **K60.312 Anal fistula, simple, persistent**
▶Anal fistula, simple, chronic

▶ **K60.313 Anal fistula, simple, recurrent**
▶Anal fistula simple, occurring following complete healing

▶ **K60.319 Anal fistula, simple, unspecified**

▶● **K60.32 Anal fistula, complex**
▶Extrasphincteric anal fistula
▶High intersphincteric anal fistula
▶Suprasphincteric anal fistula
▶Transsphincteric anal fistula
▶Code also, if applicable:
▶perianal abscess (K61.0)
▶rectovaginal fistula (N82.3)
▶stenosis of anus and rectum (K62.4)

▶ **K60.321 Anal fistula, complex, initial**
▶Anal fistula, complex, new

▶ **K60.322 Anal fistula, complex, persistent**
▶Anal fistula, complex, chronic

▶ **K60.323 Anal fistula, complex, recurrent**
▶Anal fistula complex, occurring following complete healing

▶ **K60.329 Anal fistula, complex, unspecified**

K60.4 Rectal fistula
Fistula of rectum to skin
▶*Code first, if applicable:*
▶Crohn's disease (K50.-)
▶ulcerative colitis (K51.-)
▶**Excludes1** congenital fistula (Q43.6)
rectovaginal fistula (N82.3)
vesicorectal fistula (N32.1)

▶ **K60.40 Rectal fistula, unspecified**
▶Rectal fistula NOS

▶● **K60.41 Rectal fistula, simple**
▶Low intersphincteric rectal fistula
▶Superficial rectal fistula

▶ **K60.411 Rectal fistula, simple, initial**
▶Rectal, fistula, simple, new

▶ **K60.412 Rectal fistula, simple, persistent**
▶Rectal fistula, simple, chronic

▶ **K60.413 Rectal fistula, simple, recurrent**
▶Rectal fistula simple, occurring following complete healing

▶ **K60.419 Rectal fistula, simple, unspecified**

▶● **K60.42 Rectal fistula, complex**
▶Extrasphincteric rectal fistula
▶High intersphincteric rectal fistula
▶Suprasphincteric rectal fistula
▶Transsphincteric rectal fistula
▶Code also, if applicable:
▶perianal abscess (K61.0)
▶rectovaginal fistula (N82.3)
▶stenosis of anus and rectum (K62.4)

▶ **K60.421 Rectal fistula, complex, initial**
▶Rectal fistula, complex, new

▶ **K60.422 Rectal fistula, complex, persistent**
▶Rectal fistula, complex, chronic

▶ **K60.423 Rectal fistula, complex, recurrent**
▶Rectal fistula complex occurring following complete healing

▶ **K60.429 Rectal fistula, complex, unspecified**

K60.5 Anorectal fistula
▶*Code first, if applicable:*
▶Crohn's disease (K50.-)
▶ulcerative colitis (K51.-)
▶**Excludes1** congenital fistula (Q43.6)

▶ **K60.50 Anorectal fistula, unspecified**
▶Anorectal fistula NOS

▶ **K60.51 Anorectal fistula, simple**
▶Low intersphincteric anorectal fistula
▶Superficial anorectal fistula

▶ **K60.511 Anorectal fistula, simple, initial**
▶Anorectal fistula, simple, new

▶ **K60.512 Anorectal fistula, simple, persistent**
▶Anorectal fistula, simple, chronic

▶ **K60.513 Anorectal fistula, simple, recurrent**
▶Anorectal fistula simple, occurring following complete healing

▶ **K60.519 Anorectal fistula, simple, unspecified**

▶ **K60.52 Anorectal fistula, complex**
▶Extrasphincteric anorectal fistula
▶High intersphincteric anorectal fistula
▶Suprasphincteric anorectal fistula
▶Transsphincteric anorectal fistula
▶Code also, if applicable:
▶perianal abscess (K61.0)
▶rectovaginal fistula (N82.3)
▶stenosis of anus and rectum (K62.4)

CHAPTER 11 (K00-K95)

▶ **K60.521 Anorectal fistula, complex, initial**
▶Anorectal fistula, complex, new

▶ **K60.522 Anorectal fistula, complex, persistent**
▶Anorectal fistula, complex, chronic

▶ **K60.523 Anorectal fistula, complex, recurrent**
▶Anorectal fistula complex, occurring following complete healing

▶ **K60.529 Anorectal fistula, complex, unspecified**

● **K61 Abscess of anal and rectal regions** (Ex) PDX 1104

Includes abscess of anal and rectal regions
cellulitis of anal and rectal regions

K61.0 Anal abscess
Perianal abscess
Excludes2 intrasphincteric abscess (K61.4)

K61.1 Rectal abscess
Perirectal abscess
Excludes1 ischiorectal abscess (K61.39)
Coding Clinic: 2012, Q4, P104

K61.2 Anorectal abscess

K61.3 Ischiorectal abscess

K61.31 Horseshoe abscess

K61.39 Other ischiorectal abscess
Abscess of ischiorectal fossa
Ischiorectal abscess, NOS

K61.4 Intrasphincteric abscess
Intersphincteric abscess

K61.5 Supralevator abscess

● **K62 Other diseases of anus and rectum**

Includes anal canal
Excludes2 colostomy and enterostomy malfunction (K94.0-, K91.4-)
fecal incontinence (R15.-)
hemorrhoids (K64.-)

K62.0 Anal polyp
Coding Clinic: 2018, Q1, P7

K62.1 Rectal polyp
Excludes1 adenomatous polyp (D12.8)
Coding Clinic: 2018, Q1, P7

K62.2 Anal prolapse
Prolapse of anal canal

K62.3 Rectal prolapse
Prolapse of rectal mucosa

K62.4 Stenosis of anus and rectum
Stricture of anus (sphincter)
Coding Clinic: 2019, Q2, P13

K62.5 Hemorrhage of anus and rectum (Ex) PDX 1078
Excludes1 gastrointestinal bleeding NOS (K92.2)
melena (K92.1)
neonatal rectal hemorrhage (P54.2)

K62.6 Ulcer of anus and rectum (Ex) PDX 1105
Solitary ulcer of anus and rectum
Stercoral ulcer of anus and rectum
Excludes1 fissure and fistula of anus and rectum (K60.-)
ulcerative colitis (K51.-)

K62.7 Radiation proctitis
Use additional code to identify the type of radiation (W88.-) or radiation therapy (Y84.2)
Coding Clinic: 2019, Q1, P21

Item 11–17 A **fissure** is a groove in the surface, whereas a **fistula** is an abnormal passage. An **abscess** is an accumulation of pus in a tissue cavity resulting from a bacterial or parasitic infection.

● **K62.8 Other specified diseases of anus and rectum**
Excludes2 ulcerative proctitis (K51.2)

K62.81 Anal sphincter tear (healed) (nontraumatic) (old)
Tear of anus, nontraumatic
Use additional code for any associated fecal incontinence (R15.-)
Excludes2 anal fissure (K60.-)
anal sphincter tear (healed) (old) complicating delivery (O34.7-)
traumatic tear of anal sphincter (S31.831)

K62.82 Dysplasia of anus
Anal intraepithelial neoplasia I and II (AIN I and II) (histologically confirmed)
Dysplasia of anus NOS
Mild and moderate dysplasia of anus (histologically confirmed)
Excludes1 abnormal results from anal cytologic examination without histologic confirmation (R85.61-)
anal intraepithelial neoplasia III (D01.3)
carcinoma in situ of anus (D01.3)
HGSIL of anus (R85.613)
severe dysplasia of anus (D01.3)

K62.89 Other specified diseases of anus and rectum
Proctitis NOS
Use additional code for any associated fecal incontinence (R15.-)

K62.9 Disease of anus and rectum, unspecified

● **K63 Other diseases of intestine**

K63.0 Abscess of intestine (Ex) PDX 1106
Excludes1 abscess of intestine with Crohn's disease (K50.014, K50.114, K50.814, K50.914)
abscess of intestine with diverticular disease (K57.0, K57.2, K57.4, K57.8)
abscess of intestine with ulcerative colitis (K51.014, K51.214, K51.314, K51.414, K51.514, K51.814, K51.914)
Excludes2 abscess of anal and rectal regions (K61.-)
abscess of appendix (K35.3-)

K63.1 Perforation of intestine (nontraumatic) (Ex) PDX 1107
Perforation (nontraumatic) of rectum
Excludes1 perforation (nontraumatic) of duodenum (K26.-)
perforation (nontraumatic) of intestine with diverticular disease (K57.0, K57.2, K57.4, K57.8)
Excludes2 perforation (nontraumatic) of appendix (K35.2-, K35.3)

K63.2 Fistula of intestine (Ex) PDX 1108
▶Code also, if applicable, disruption of internal operation (surgical) wound (T81.32-)
Excludes1 fistula of duodenum (K31.6)
fistula of intestine with Crohn's disease (K50.013, K50.113, K50.813, K50.913)
fistula of intestine with ulcerative colitis (K51.013, K51.213, K51.313, K51.413, K51.513, K51.813, K51.913)
Excludes2 fistula of anal and rectal regions (K60.-)
fistula of appendix (K38.3)
intestinal-genital fistula, female (N82.2-N82.4)
vesicointestinal fistula (N32.1)
Coding Clinic: 2017, Q3, P4

K63.3 Ulcer of intestine (Ex) PDX 1109
Primary ulcer of small intestine
Excludes1 duodenal ulcer (K26.-)
gastrointestinal ulcer (K28.-)
gastrojejunal ulcer (K28.-)
jejunal ulcer (K28.-)
peptic ulcer, site unspecified (K27.-)
ulcer of intestine with perforation (K63.1)
ulcer of anus or rectum (K62.6)
ulcerative colitis (K51.-)

K63.4 Enteroptosis

K63.5 Polyp of colon
Excludes2 adenomatous polyp of colon (D12.-)
inflammatory polyp of colon (K51.4-)
polyposis of colon (D12.6)
Coding Clinic: 2019, Q1, P33; 2017, Q1, P15-16; 2015, Q2, P14

● **K63.8 Other specified diseases of intestine**

K63.81 Dieulafoy lesion of intestine (Ex) PDX 1110
Excludes2 Dieulafoy lesion of stomach and duodenum (K31.82)

● **K63.82 Intestinal microbial overgrowth**

● **K63.821 Small intestinal bacterial overgrowth**

K63.8211 Small intestinal bacterial overgrowth, hydrogen-subtype

K63.8212 Small intestinal bacterial overgrowth, hydrogen sulfide-subtype

K63.8219 Small intestinal bacterial overgrowth, unspecified

K63.822 Small intestinal fungal overgrowth

K63.829 Intestinal methanogen overgrowth, unspecified

K63.89 Other specified diseases of intestine
Coding Clinic: 2013, Q2, P31

K63.9 Disease of intestine, unspecified

● **K64 Hemorrhoids and perianal venous thrombosis**
Includes piles
Excludes1 hemorrhoids complicating childbirth and the puerperium (O87.2)
hemorrhoids complicating pregnancy (O22.4)

K64.Ø First degree hemorrhoids
Grade/stage I hemorrhoids
Hemorrhoids (bleeding) without prolapse outside of anal canal

K64.1 Second degree hemorrhoids
Grade/stage II hemorrhoids
Hemorrhoids (bleeding) that prolapse with straining, but retract spontaneously

K64.2 Third degree hemorrhoids
Grade/stage III hemorrhoids
Hemorrhoids (bleeding) that prolapse with straining and require manual replacement back inside anal canal

K64.3 Fourth degree hemorrhoids
Grade/stage IV hemorrhoids
Hemorrhoids (bleeding) with prolapsed tissue that cannot be manually replaced

K64.4 Residual hemorrhoidal skin tags
External hemorrhoids, NOS
Skin tags of anus

K64.5 Perianal venous thrombosis
External hemorrhoids with thrombosis
Perianal hematoma
Thrombosed hemorrhoids NOS

K64.8 Other hemorrhoids
Internal hemorrhoids, without mention of degree
Prolapsed hemorrhoids, degree not specified

K64.9 Unspecified hemorrhoids
Hemorrhoids (bleeding) NOS
Hemorrhoids (bleeding) without mention of degree

DISEASES OF PERITONEUM AND RETROPERITONEUM (K65-K68)

● **K65 Peritonitis** (Ex) PDX 1111
Use additional code (B95-B97), to identify infectious agent, if known
Code also if applicable diverticular disease of intestine (K57.-)
Excludes1 acute appendicitis with generalized peritonitis (K35.2-)
aseptic peritonitis (T81.6)
benign paroxysmal peritonitis (E85.Ø)
chemical peritonitis (T81.6)
gonococcal peritonitis (A54.85)
neonatal peritonitis (P78.Ø-P78.1)
pelvic peritonitis, female (N73.3-N73.5)
periodic familial peritonitis (E85.Ø)
peritonitis due to talc or other foreign substance (T81.6)
peritonitis in chlamydia (A74.81)
peritonitis in diphtheria (A36.89)
peritonitis in syphilis (late) (A52.74)
peritonitis in tuberculosis (A18.31)
peritonitis with or following abortion or ectopic or molar pregnancy (OØØ-OØ7, OØ8.Ø)
peritonitis with or following appendicitis (K35.-)
puerperal peritonitis (O85)
retroperitoneal infections (K68.-)
Coding Clinic: 2022, Q1, P26

K65.Ø Generalized (acute) peritonitis
Pelvic peritonitis (acute), male
Subphrenic peritonitis (acute)
Suppurative peritonitis (acute)

K65.1 Peritoneal abscess
Abdominopelvic abscess
Abscess (of) omentum
Abscess (of) peritoneum
Mesenteric abscess
Retrocecal abscess
Subdiaphragmatic abscess
Subhepatic abscess
Subphrenic abscess
Coding Clinic: 2024, Q1, P2Ø; 2022, Q1, P26; 2019, Q1, P15

K65.2 Spontaneous bacterial peritonitis
Excludes1 bacterial peritonitis NOS (K65.9)

K65.3 Choleperitonitis
Peritonitis due to bile

K65.4 Sclerosing mesenteritis
Fat necrosis of peritoneum
(Idiopathic) sclerosing mesenteric fibrosis
Mesenteric lipodystrophy
Mesenteric panniculitis
Retractile mesenteritis

K65.8 Other peritonitis
Chronic proliferative peritonitis
Peritonitis due to urine

K65.9 Peritonitis, unspecified
Bacterial peritonitis NOS
Coding Clinic: 2013, Q2, P31

● **K66 Other disorders of peritoneum**
Excludes2 ascites (R18.-)
peritoneal effusion (chronic) (R18.8)

K66.Ø Peritoneal adhesions (postprocedural) (postinfection)
Adhesions (of) abdominal (wall)
Adhesions (of) diaphragm
Adhesions (of) intestine
Adhesions (of) male pelvis
Adhesions (of) omentum
Adhesions (of) stomach
Adhesive bands
Mesenteric adhesions
~~**Excludes1** female pelvic adhesions [bands] (N73.6)~~
~~peritoneal adhesions with intestinal obstruction (K56.5-)~~
▶ **Excludes2** female pelvic adhesions [bands] (N73.6)
▶ female pelvic postprocedural adhesions (N99.4)

Item 11-18 Peritonitis is an inflammation of the lining (peritoneum) of the abdominal cavity and surface of the intestines.

Item 11-19 Retroperitoneal infections occur between the posterior parietal peritoneum and posterior abdominal wall where the kidneys, adrenal glands, ureters, duodenum, ascending colon, descending colon, pancreas, and the large vessels and nerves are located.

K66.1 Hemoperitoneum (Ex) PDX 1112
Peritoneal hematoma
Peritoneal hemorrhage
Excludes1 traumatic hemoperitoneum (S36.8-)
Excludes2 retroperitoneal hematoma (K68.3)
retroperitoneal hemorrhage (K68.3)
Coding Clinic: 2022, Q1, P22-23

K66.8 Other specified disorders of peritoneum

K66.9 Disorder of peritoneum, unspecified

K67 ***Disorders of peritoneum in infectious diseases classified elsewhere*** (Ex) PDX 1111
Code first underlying disease, such as:
congenital syphilis (A50.0)
helminthiasis (B65.0-B83.9)
Excludes1 peritonitis in chlamydia (A74.81)
peritonitis in diphtheria (A36.89)
peritonitis in gonococcal (A54.85)
peritonitis in syphilis (late) (A52.74)
peritonitis in tuberculosis (A18.31)

● **K68 Disorders of retroperitoneum**

● **K68.1 Retroperitoneal abscess**

K68.11 Postprocedural retroperitoneal abscess (Ex) PDX 1113
Excludes2 infection following procedure (T81.44)

K68.12 Psoas muscle abscess (Ex) PDX 1114

K68.19 Other retroperitoneal abscess (Ex) PDX 1111
Coding Clinic: 2019, Q1, P15

K68.2 Retroperitoneal fibrosis (Ex) PDX 1115
Code also, if applicable, associated obstruction of ureter (N13.5)

K68.3 Retroperitoneal hematoma (Ex) PDX 1116
Retroperitoneal hemorrhage

K68.9 Other disorders of retroperitoneum (Ex) PDX 1111

DISEASES OF LIVER (K70-K77)

Excludes1 jaundice NOS (R17)
Excludes2 hemochromatosis (E83.11-)
Reye's syndrome (G93.7)
viral hepatitis (B15-B19)
Wilson's disease (E83.01)

● **K70 Alcoholic liver disease**
Use additional code to identify:
alcohol abuse and dependence (F10.-)

K70.0 Alcoholic fatty liver A

● **K70.1 Alcoholic hepatitis**

K70.10 Alcoholic hepatitis without ascites A

K70.11 Alcoholic hepatitis with ascites A

K70.2 Alcoholic fibrosis and sclerosis of liver A

● **K70.3 Alcoholic cirrhosis of liver**
Alcoholic cirrhosis NOS

K70.30 Alcoholic cirrhosis of liver without ascites A

K70.31 Alcoholic cirrhosis of liver with ascites A
Coding Clinic: 2018, Q1, P5

● **K70.4 Alcoholic hepatic failure**
Acute alcoholic hepatic failure
Alcoholic hepatic failure NOS
Chronic alcoholic hepatic failure
Subacute alcoholic hepatic failure

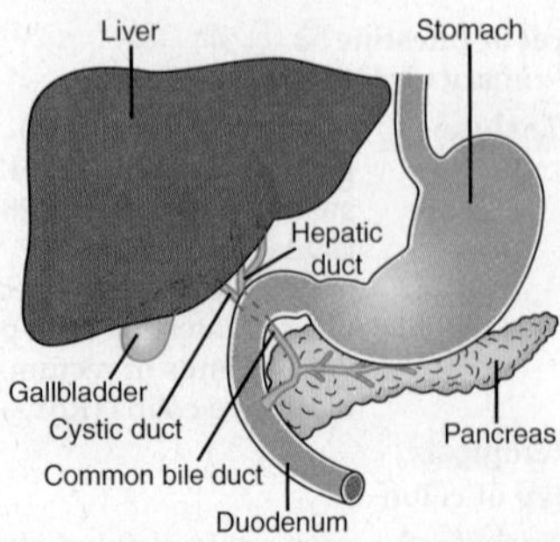

Figure 11-13 Liver and bile ducts.

Item 11-20 Cirrhosis is the progressive fibrosis of the liver resulting in loss of liver function. The main causes of cirrhosis of the liver are alcohol abuse, chronic hepatitis (inflammation of the liver), biliary disease, and excessive amounts of iron. **Alcoholic cirrhosis of the liver** is also called portal, Laënnec's, or fatty nutritional cirrhosis.

K70.40 Alcoholic hepatic failure without coma A

K70.41 Alcoholic hepatic failure with coma (Ex) PDX 1117 A
MCC when PDx is its own MCC

K70.9 Alcoholic liver disease, unspecified A

● **K71 Toxic liver disease**
Includes drug-induced idiosyncratic (unpredictable) liver disease
drug-induced toxic (predictable) liver disease
Code first poisoning due to drug or toxin, if applicable (T36-T65 with fifth or sixth character 1-4)
Use additional code for adverse effect, if applicable, to identify drug (T36-T50 with fifth or sixth character 5)
Excludes2 alcoholic liver disease (K70.-)
Budd-Chiari syndrome (I82.0)

K71.0 Toxic liver disease with cholestasis
Cholestasis with hepatocyte injury
'Pure' cholestasis

● **K71.1 Toxic liver disease with hepatic necrosis**
Hepatic failure (acute) (chronic) due to drugs

K71.10 Toxic liver disease with hepatic necrosis, without coma

K71.11 Toxic liver disease with hepatic necrosis, with coma (Ex) PDX 1118
MCC when PDx is its own MCC

K71.2 Toxic liver disease with acute hepatitis

K71.3 Toxic liver disease with chronic persistent hepatitis

K71.4 Toxic liver disease with chronic lobular hepatitis

● **K71.5 Toxic liver disease with chronic active hepatitis**
Toxic liver disease with lupoid hepatitis

K71.50 Toxic liver disease with chronic active hepatitis without ascites

K71.51 Toxic liver disease with chronic active hepatitis with ascites
Coding Clinic: 2018, Q1, P4

K71.6 Toxic liver disease with hepatitis, not elsewhere classified

K71.7 Toxic liver disease with fibrosis and cirrhosis of liver

K71.8 Toxic liver disease with other disorders of liver
Toxic liver disease with focal nodular hyperplasia
Toxic liver disease with hepatic granulomas
Toxic liver disease with peliosis hepatis
Toxic liver disease with veno-occlusive disease of liver
Coding Clinic: 2024, Q1, P25

K71.9 Toxic liver disease, unspecified

K72 Hepatic failure, not elsewhere classified

Includes fulminant hepatitis NEC, with hepatic failure
liver (cell) necrosis with hepatic failure
malignant hepatitis NEC, with hepatic failure
yellow liver atrophy or dystrophy

Excludes1 alcoholic hepatic failure (K70.4)
hepatic failure with toxic liver disease (K71.1-)
icterus of newborn (P55-P59)
postprocedural hepatic failure (K91.82)

Excludes2 hepatic failure complicating abortion or ectopic or molar pregnancy (O00-O07, O08.8)
hepatic failure complicating pregnancy, childbirth and the puerperium (O26.6-)
viral hepatitis with hepatic coma (B15-B19)

K72.0 Acute and subacute hepatic failure (Ex) PDX 1119
Acute non-viral hepatitis NOS
Coding Clinic: 2015, Q2, P17

K72.00 Acute and subacute hepatic failure without coma
Coding Clinic: 2021, Q1, P13; 2015, Q2, P17

K72.01 Acute and subacute hepatic failure with coma
MCC when PDx is its own MCC

K72.1 Chronic hepatic failure
End stage liver disease

K72.10 Chronic hepatic failure without coma
Coding Clinic: 2021, Q1, P13; 2017, Q1, P41

K72.11 Chronic hepatic failure with coma (Ex) PDX 1120
MCC when PDx is its own MCC
Coding Clinic: 2020, Q1, P15

K72.9 Hepatic failure, unspecified

K72.90 Hepatic failure, unspecified without coma
Coding Clinic: 2022, Q1, P53; 2018, Q4, P21

K72.91 Hepatic failure, unspecified with coma (Ex) PDX 1121
Hepatic coma NOS
Coding Clinic: 2016, Q2, P35

K73 Chronic hepatitis, not elsewhere classified

Excludes1 alcoholic hepatitis (chronic) (K70.1-)
drug-induced hepatitis (chronic) (K71.-)
granulomatous hepatitis (chronic) NEC (K75.3)
reactive, nonspecific hepatitis (chronic) (K75.2)
viral hepatitis (chronic) (B15-B19)

K73.0 Chronic persistent hepatitis, not elsewhere classified

K73.1 Chronic lobular hepatitis, not elsewhere classified

K73.2 Chronic active hepatitis, not elsewhere classified

K73.8 Other chronic hepatitis, not elsewhere classified

K73.9 Chronic hepatitis, unspecified

K74 Fibrosis and cirrhosis of liver

Code also, if applicable, viral hepatitis (acute) (chronic) (B15-B19)

Excludes1 alcoholic cirrhosis (of liver) (K70.3)
alcoholic fibrosis of liver (K70.2)
cardiac sclerosis of liver (K76.1)
cirrhosis (of liver) with toxic liver disease (K71.7)
congenital cirrhosis (of liver) (P78.81)
pigmentary cirrhosis (of liver) (E83.110)

K74.0 Hepatic fibrosis
Code first underlying liver disease, such as:
nonalcoholic steatohepatitis (NASH) (K75.81)

K74.00 Hepatic fibrosis, unspecified

K74.01 Hepatic fibrosis, early fibrosis
Hepatic fibrosis, stage F1 or stage F2

K74.02 Hepatic fibrosis, advanced fibrosis
Hepatic fibrosis, stage F3

Excludes1 cirrhosis of liver (K74.6-)
hepatic fibrosis, stage F4 (K74.6-)

K74.1 Hepatic sclerosis

K74.2 Hepatic fibrosis with hepatic sclerosis

K74.3 Primary biliary cirrhosis
Chronic nonsuppurative destructive cholangitis
Primary biliary cholangitis

Excludes2 primary sclerosing cholangitis (K83.01)

K74.4 Secondary biliary cirrhosis

K74.5 Biliary cirrhosis, unspecified

K74.6 Other and unspecified cirrhosis of liver

K74.60 Unspecified cirrhosis of liver
Cirrhosis (of liver) NOS
Coding Clinic: 2018, Q1, P4

K74.69 Other cirrhosis of liver
Cryptogenic cirrhosis (of liver)
Macronodular cirrhosis (of liver)
Micronodular cirrhosis (of liver)
Mixed type cirrhosis (of liver)
Portal cirrhosis (of liver)
Postnecrotic cirrhosis (of liver)

K75 Other inflammatory liver diseases

Excludes2 toxic liver disease (K71.-)

K75.0 Abscess of liver (Ex) PDX 1122
Cholangitic hepatic abscess
Hematogenic hepatic abscess
Hepatic abscess NOS
Lymphogenic hepatic abscess
Pylephlebitic hepatic abscess

Excludes1 amebic liver abscess (A06.4)
cholangitis without liver abscess (K83.09)
pylephlebitis without liver abscess (K75.1)

Excludes2 acute or subacute hepatitis NOS (B17.9)
acute or subacute non-viral hepatitis (K72.0)
chronic hepatitis NEC (K73.8)

K75.1 Phlebitis of portal vein (Ex) PDX 1122
Pylephlebitis

Excludes1 pylephlebitic liver abscess (K75.0)

K75.2 Nonspecific reactive hepatitis

Excludes1 acute or subacute hepatitis (K72.0-)
chronic hepatitis NEC (K73.-)
viral hepatitis (B15-B19)

K75.3 Granulomatous hepatitis, not elsewhere classified

Excludes1 acute or subacute hepatitis (K72.0-)
chronic hepatitis NEC (K73.-)
viral hepatitis (B15-B19)

K75.4 Autoimmune hepatitis
Lupoid hepatitis NEC

K75.8 Other specified inflammatory liver diseases

K75.81 Nonalcoholic steatohepatitis (NASH)
Use additional code, if applicable, hepatic fibrosis (K74.0-)

K75.89 Other specified inflammatory liver diseases

K75.9 Inflammatory liver disease, unspecified
Hepatitis NOS

Excludes1 acute or subacute hepatitis (K72.0-)
chronic hepatitis NEC (K73.-)
viral hepatitis (B15-B19)

Coding Clinic: 2015, Q2, P17

K76 Other diseases of liver

Excludes2 alcoholic liver disease (K70.-)
amyloid degeneration of liver (E85.-)
cystic disease of liver (congenital) (Q44.6)
hepatic vein thrombosis (I82.0)
hepatomegaly NOS (R16.0)
pigmentary cirrhosis (of liver) (E83.110)
portal vein thrombosis (I81)
toxic liver disease (K71.-)

K76.0 Fatty (change of) liver, not elsewhere classified
Nonalcoholic fatty liver disease (NAFLD)

Excludes1 nonalcoholic steatohepatitis (NASH) (K75.81)

CHAPTER 11 (K00-K95)

K76.1 Chronic passive congestion of liver
Cardiac cirrhosis
Cardiac sclerosis

K76.2 Central hemorrhagic necrosis of liver (Ex) PDX 1119
Excludes1 liver necrosis with hepatic failure (K72.-)

K76.3 Infarction of liver (Ex) PDX 1119

K76.4 Peliosis hepatis
Hepatic angiomatosis

K76.5 Hepatic veno-occlusive disease
Excludes1 Budd-Chiari syndrome (I82.0)

K76.6 Portal hypertension (Ex) PDX 1123
Use additional code for any associated complications, such as:
portal hypertensive gastropathy (K31.89)
Coding Clinic: 2020, Q1, P15

K76.7 Hepatorenal syndrome (Ex) PDX 1124
Excludes1 hepatorenal syndrome following labor and delivery (O90.41)
postprocedural hepatorenal syndrome (K91.83)

● **K76.8 Other specified diseases of liver**

● **K76.81 Hepatopulmonary syndrome**
Code first underlying liver disease, such as:
alcoholic cirrhosis of liver (K70.3-)
cirrhosis of liver without mention of alcohol (K74.6-)

K76.82 Hepatic encephalopathy
Hepatic encephalopathy, NOS
Hepatic encephalopathy without coma
Hepatocerebral intoxication
Portal-systemic encephalopathy
Code also underlying liver disease, such as:
acute and subacute hepatic failure without coma (K72.00)
alcoholic hepatic failure without coma (K70.40)
chronic hepatic failure without coma (K72.10)
hepatic failure with toxic liver disease without coma (K71.10)
hepatic failure without coma (K72.90)
icterus of newborn (P55-P59)
postprocedural hepatic failure (K91.82)
viral hepatitis without hepatic coma (B15.9, B16.1, B16.9, B17.10, B19.10, B19.20, B19.9)
Excludes1 acute and subacute hepatic failure with coma (K72.01)
alcoholic hepatic failure with coma (K70.41)
chronic hepatic failure with coma (K72.11)
hepatic failure with coma (K72.91

K76.89 Other specified diseases of liver
Cyst (simple) of liver
Focal nodular hyperplasia of liver
Hepatoptosis

K76.9 Liver disease, unspecified

K77 ***Liver disorders in diseases classified elsewhere*** (Ex) No exclusions
Code first underlying disease, such as:
amyloidosis (E85.-)
congenital syphilis (A50.0, A50.5)
congenital toxoplasmosis (P37.1)
infectious mononucleosis with liver disease (B27.0-B27.9 with fifth character 9)
schistosomiasis (B65.0-B65.9)
Excludes1 alcoholic hepatitis (K70.1-)
alcoholic liver disease (K70.-)
cytomegaloviral hepatitis (B25.1)
herpesviral [herpes simplex] hepatitis (B00.81)
mumps hepatitis (B26.81)
sarcoidosis with liver disease (D86.89)
secondary syphilis with liver disease (A51.45)
syphilis (late) with liver disease (A52.74)
toxoplasmosis (acquired) hepatitis (B58.1)
tuberculosis with liver disease (A18.83)

DISORDERS OF GALLBLADDER, BILIARY TRACT AND PANCREAS (K80–K87)

● **K80 Cholelithiasis**
Presence or formation of gallstones
Excludes1 retained cholelithiasis following cholecystectomy (K91.86)

● **K80.0 Calculus of gallbladder with acute cholecystitis**
Any condition listed in K80.2 with acute cholecystitis
Use additional code if applicable for associated gangrene of gallbladder (K82.A1), or perforation of gallbladder (K82.A2)
Check documentation for acute/chronic gallbladder/common bile duct either with or without obstruction.

K80.00 Calculus of gallbladder with acute cholecystitis without obstruction (Ex) PDX 1125
Coding Clinic: 2023, Q2, P12; 2018, Q4, P20

K80.01 Calculus of gallbladder with acute cholecystitis with obstruction (Ex) PDX 1126

● **K80.1 Calculus of gallbladder with other cholecystitis** (Ex) PDX 1126
Use additional code if applicable for associated gangrene of gallbladder (K82.A1), or perforation of gallbladder (K82.A2)

K80.10 Calculus of gallbladder with chronic cholecystitis without obstruction
Cholelithiasis with cholecystitis NOS

K80.11 Calculus of gallbladder with chronic cholecystitis with obstruction

K80.12 Calculus of gallbladder with acute and chronic cholecystitis without obstruction (Ex) PDX 1125

K80.13 Calculus of gallbladder with acute and chronic cholecystitis with obstruction

K80.18 Calculus of gallbladder with other cholecystitis without obstruction

K80.19 Calculus of gallbladder with other cholecystitis with obstruction

● **K80.2 Calculus of gallbladder without cholecystitis**
Cholecystolithiasis without cholecystitis
Cholelithiasis (without cholecystitis)
Colic (recurrent) of gallbladder (without cholecystitis)
Gallstone (impacted) of cystic duct (without cholecystitis)
Gallstone (impacted) of gallbladder (without cholecystitis)

K80.20 Calculus of gallbladder without cholecystitis without obstruction

K80.21 Calculus of gallbladder without cholecystitis with obstruction (Ex) PDX 1126

● **K80.3 Calculus of bile duct with cholangitis**
Any condition listed in K80.5 with cholangitis

K80.30 Calculus of bile duct with cholangitis, unspecified, without obstruction (Ex) PDX 1127
CC when PDx is its own CC

K80.31 Calculus of bile duct with cholangitis, unspecified, with obstruction (Ex) PDX 1128
CC when PDx is its own CC

K80.32 Calculus of bile duct with acute cholangitis without obstruction (Ex) PDX 1129
CC when PDx is its own CC

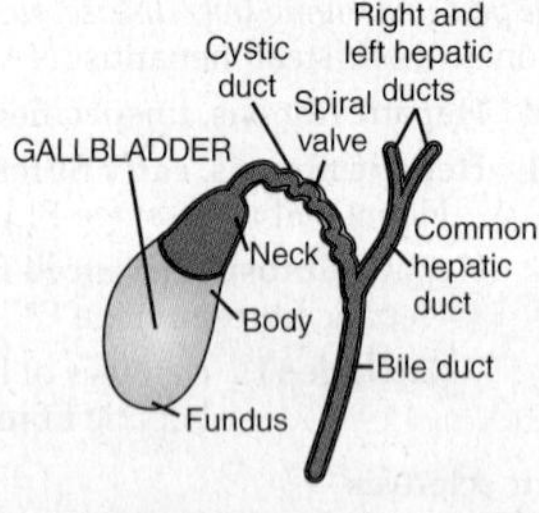

Figure 11-14 Gallbladder and bile ducts.

K80.33 **Calculus of bile duct with acute cholangitis with obstruction** (Ex:) PDX 1128
CC when PDx is its own CC

K80.34 **Calculus of bile duct with chronic cholangitis without obstruction** (Ex:) PDX 1130
CC when PDx is its own CC

K80.35 **Calculus of bile duct with chronic cholangitis with obstruction** (Ex:) PDX 1128
CC when PDx is its own CC

K80.36 **Calculus of bile duct with acute and chronic cholangitis without obstruction** (Ex:) PDX 1131
CC when PDx is its own CC

K80.37 **Calculus of bile duct with acute and chronic cholangitis with obstruction** (Ex:) PDX 1128
CC when PDx is its own CC

● **K80.4** **Calculus of bile duct with cholecystitis** (Ex:) PDX 1128
Any condition listed in K80.5 with cholecystitis (with cholangitis)
Code also, if applicable, fistula of bile duct (K83.3)
Use additional code if applicable for associated gangrene of gallbladder (K82.A1), or perforation of gallbladder (K82.A2)

K80.40 **Calculus of bile duct with cholecystitis, unspecified, without obstruction**

K80.41 **Calculus of bile duct with cholecystitis, unspecified, with obstruction**
Coding Clinic: 2019, Q1, P18

K80.42 **Calculus of bile duct with acute cholecystitis without obstruction**

K80.43 **Calculus of bile duct with acute cholecystitis with obstruction**

K80.44 **Calculus of bile duct with chronic cholecystitis without obstruction**

K80.45 **Calculus of bile duct with chronic cholecystitis with obstruction**

K80.46 **Calculus of bile duct with acute and chronic cholecystitis without obstruction**

K80.47 **Calculus of bile duct with acute and chronic cholecystitis with obstruction**

● **K80.5** **Calculus of bile duct without cholangitis or cholecystitis**
Choledocholithiasis (without cholangitis or cholecystitis)
Gallstone (impacted) of bile duct NOS (without cholangitis or cholecystitis)
Gallstone (impacted) of common duct (without cholangitis or cholecystitis)
Gallstone (impacted) of hepatic duct (without cholangitis or cholecystitis)
Hepatic cholelithiasis (without cholangitis or cholecystitis)
Hepatic colic (recurrent) (without cholangitis or cholecystitis)

K80.50 **Calculus of bile duct without cholangitis or cholecystitis without obstruction**

K80.51 **Calculus of bile duct without cholangitis or cholecystitis with obstruction** (Ex:) PDX 1128

● **K80.6** **Calculus of gallbladder and bile duct with cholecystitis**
Use additional code if applicable for associated gangrene of gallbladder (K82.A1), or perforation of gallbladder (K82.A2)

K80.60 **Calculus of gallbladder and bile duct with cholecystitis, unspecified, without obstruction** (Ex:) PDX 1128

K80.61 **Calculus of gallbladder and bile duct with cholecystitis, unspecified, with obstruction** (Ex:) PDX 1128

K80.62 **Calculus of gallbladder and bile duct with acute cholecystitis without obstruction** (Ex:) PDX 1132

K80.63 **Calculus of gallbladder and bile duct with acute cholecystitis with obstruction** (Ex:) PDX 1132

K80.64 **Calculus of gallbladder and bile duct with chronic cholecystitis without obstruction** (Ex:) PDX 1128

K80.65 **Calculus of gallbladder and bile duct with chronic cholecystitis with obstruction** (Ex:) PDX 1128

K80.66 **Calculus of gallbladder and bile duct with acute and chronic cholecystitis without obstruction** (Ex:) PDX 1133

K80.67 **Calculus of gallbladder and bile duct with acute and chronic cholecystitis with obstruction** (Ex:) PDX 1133

● **K80.7** **Calculus of gallbladder and bile duct without cholecystitis**

K80.70 **Calculus of gallbladder and bile duct without cholecystitis without obstruction**

K80.71 **Calculus of gallbladder and bile duct without cholecystitis with obstruction** (Ex:) PDX 1128

● **K80.8** **Other cholelithiasis**

K80.80 **Other cholelithiasis without obstruction**

K80.81 **Other cholelithiasis with obstruction** (Ex:) PDX 1128

● **K81** **Cholecystitis**
Chronic or acute inflammation of the gallbladder
Use additional code if applicable for associated gangrene of gallbladder (K82.A1), or perforation of gallbladder (K82.A2)
Excludes1 cholecystitis with cholelithiasis (K80.-)

K81.0 **Acute cholecystitis** (Ex:) PDX 1134
Abscess of gallbladder
Angiocholecystitis
Emphysematous (acute) cholecystitis
Empyema of gallbladder
Gangrene of gallbladder
Gangrenous cholecystitis
Suppurative cholecystitis

K81.1 **Chronic cholecystitis**

K81.2 **Acute cholecystitis with chronic cholecystitis** (Ex:) PDX 1135

K81.9 **Cholecystitis, unspecified**

● **K82** **Other diseases of gallbladder** (Ex:) PDX 1136
Excludes1 nonvisualization of gallbladder (R93.2)
postcholecystectomy syndrome (K91.5)

K82.0 **Obstruction of gallbladder**
Occlusion of cystic duct or gallbladder without cholelithiasis
Stenosis of cystic duct or gallbladder without cholelithiasis
Stricture of cystic duct or gallbladder without cholelithiasis
Excludes1 obstruction of gallbladder with cholelithiasis (K80.-)

K82.1 **Hydrops of gallbladder**
Mucocele of gallbladder

K82.2 **Perforation of gallbladder**
Rupture of cystic duct or gallbladder
Excludes1 Perforation of gallbladder in cholecystitis (K82.A2)

K82.3 **Fistula of gallbladder**
Cholecystocolic fistula
Cholecystoduodenal fistula
Coding Clinic: 2019, Q1, P18

K82.4 **Cholesterolosis of gallbladder**
Strawberry gallbladder
Excludes1 cholesterolosis of gallbladder with cholecystitis (K81.-)
cholesterolosis of gallbladder with cholelithiasis (K80.-)

K82.8 **Other specified diseases of gallbladder**
Adhesions of cystic duct or gallbladder
Atrophy of cystic duct or gallbladder
Cyst of cystic duct or gallbladder
Dyskinesia of cystic duct or gallbladder
Hypertrophy of cystic duct or gallbladder
Nonfunctioning of cystic duct or gallbladder
Ulcer of cystic duct or gallbladder

K82.9 Disease of gallbladder, unspecified

K82.A Disorders of gallbladder in diseases classified elsewhere

Code first the type of cholecystitis (K81.-), or cholelithiasis with cholecystitis (K80.00-K80.19, K80.40-K80.47, K80.60-K80.67)

K82.A1 *Gangrene of gallbladder in cholecystitis*

Coding Clinic: 2018, Q4, P20

K82.A2 Perforation of gallbladder in cholecystitis

Coding Clinic: 2018, Q4, P20

K83 Other diseases of biliary tract

Excludes1 postcholecystectomy syndrome (K91.5)

Excludes2 conditions involving the gallbladder (K81-K82)
conditions involving the cystic duct (K81-K82)

K83.0 Cholangitis

Excludes1 cholangitic liver abscess (K75.0)
cholangitis with choledocholithiasis (K80.3-, K80.4-)

Excludes2 chronic nonsuppurative destructive cholangitis (K74.3)
primary biliary cholangitis (K74.3)
primary biliary cirrhosis (K74.3)

K83.01 Primary sclerosing cholangitis (Ex:) PDX 1138

Coding Clinic: 2018, Q4, P21

K83.09 Other cholangitis (Ex:) PDX 1138

Ascending cholangitis
Cholangitis NOS
Primary cholangitis
Recurrent cholangitis
Sclerosing cholangitis
Secondary cholangitis
Stenosing cholangitis
Suppurative cholangitis

K83.1 Obstruction of bile duct (Ex:) PDX 1138

Occlusion of bile duct without cholelithiasis
Stenosis of bile duct without cholelithiasis
Stricture of bile duct without cholelithiasis

Excludes1 congenital obstruction of bile duct (Q44.3)
obstruction of bile duct with cholelithiasis (K80.-)

Coding Clinic: 2023, Q1, P27; 2016, Q1, P18

K83.2 Perforation of bile duct (Ex:) PDX 1139

Rupture of bile duct

K83.3 Fistula of bile duct (Ex:) PDX 1139

Choledochoduodenal fistula

K83.4 Spasm of sphincter of Oddi

K83.5 Biliary cyst

K83.8 Other specified diseases of biliary tract

Adhesions of biliary tract
Atrophy of biliary tract
Hypertrophy of biliary tract
Ulcer of biliary tract

K83.9 Disease of biliary tract, unspecified

K85 Acute pancreatitis (Ex:) PDX 190

Inflammatory process in which pancreatic enzymes autodigest the gland

Includes acute (recurrent) pancreatitis
subacute pancreatitis

Coding Clinic: 2016, Q4, P34

K85.0 Idiopathic acute pancreatitis

K85.00 Idiopathic acute pancreatitis without necrosis or infection

K85.01 Idiopathic acute pancreatitis with uninfected necrosis

K85.02 Idiopathic acute pancreatitis with infected necrosis

K85.1 Biliary acute pancreatitis

Gallstone pancreatitis

K85.10 Biliary acute pancreatitis without necrosis or infection

Coding Clinic: 2023, Q2, P12

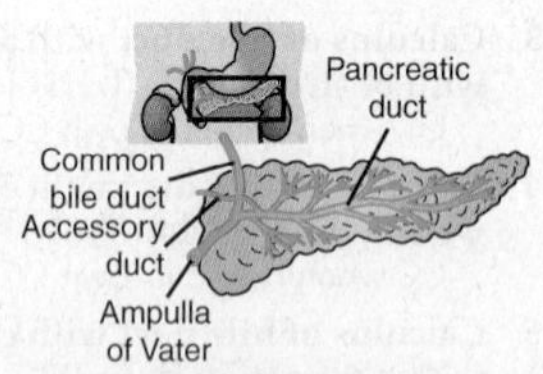

Figure 11-15 Pancreatic ductal system.

K85.11 Biliary acute pancreatitis with uninfected necrosis

K85.12 Biliary acute pancreatitis with infected necrosis

K85.2 Alcohol induced acute pancreatitis

Excludes2 alcohol induced chronic pancreatitis (K86.0)

K85.20 Alcohol induced acute pancreatitis without necrosis or infection

Coding Clinic: 2020, Q1, P9

K85.21 Alcohol induced acute pancreatitis with uninfected necrosis

K85.22 Alcohol induced acute pancreatitis with infected necrosis

K85.3 Drug induced acute pancreatitis

Use additional code for adverse effect, if applicable, to identify drug (T36-T50 with fifth or sixth character 5)

Use additional code to identify drug abuse and dependence (F11.-F17.-)

K85.30 Drug induced acute pancreatitis without necrosis or infection

K85.31 Drug induced acute pancreatitis with uninfected necrosis

K85.32 Drug induced acute pancreatitis with infected necrosis

K85.8 Other acute pancreatitis

K85.80 Other acute pancreatitis without necrosis or infection

K85.81 Other acute pancreatitis with uninfected necrosis

K85.82 Other acute pancreatitis with infected necrosis

K85.9 Acute pancreatitis, unspecified

Pancreatitis NOS

K85.90 Acute pancreatitis without necrosis or infection, unspecified

K85.91 Acute pancreatitis with uninfected necrosis, unspecified

K85.92 Acute pancreatitis with infected necrosis, unspecified

K86 Other diseases of pancreas (Ex:) PDX 1141

Excludes2 fibrocystic disease of pancreas (E84.-)
islet cell tumor (of pancreas) (D13.7)
pancreatic steatorrhea (K90.3)

K86.0 Alcohol-induced chronic pancreatitis

Use additional code to identify:
alcohol abuse and dependence (F10.-)

Code also exocrine pancreatic insufficiency (K86.81)

Excludes2 alcohol induced acute pancreatitis (K85.2-)

K86.1 Other chronic pancreatitis (Ex:) PDX 1140

Chronic pancreatitis NOS
Infectious chronic pancreatitis
Recurrent chronic pancreatitis
Relapsing chronic pancreatitis

Code also exocrine pancreatic insufficiency (K86.81)

K86.2 Cyst of pancreas

K86.3 Pseudocyst of pancreas

New Revised ~~deleted~~ Deleted Excludes 1 Excludes 2 Includes Use additional Code first Code also Key words
OGCR Official Guidelines ● Unacceptable Principal Diagnosis X Assign placeholder X ● Use Additional Character(s) Manifestation Code Coding Clinic

● **K86.8 Other specified diseases of pancreas**
Coding Clinic: 2016, Q4, P34

K86.81 Exocrine pancreatic insufficiency

K86.89 Other specified diseases of pancreas
Aseptic pancreatic necrosis, unrelated to acute pancreatitis
Atrophy of pancreas
Calculus of pancreas
Cirrhosis of pancreas
Fibrosis of pancreas
Pancreatic fat necrosis, unrelated to acute pancreatitis
Pancreatic infantilism
Pancreatic necrosis NOS, unrelated to acute pancreatitis

K86.9 Disease of pancreas, unspecified

K87 Disorders of gallbladder, biliary tract and pancreas in diseases classified elsewhere
Code first underlying disease
Excludes1 cytomegaloviral pancreatitis (B25.2)
mumps pancreatitis (B26.3)
syphilitic gallbladder (A52.74)
syphilitic pancreas (A52.74)
tuberculosis of gallbladder (A18.83)
tuberculosis of pancreas (A18.83)

OTHER DISEASES OF THE DIGESTIVE SYSTEM (K90-K95)

● **K90 Intestinal malabsorption** (Ex) PDX 1142
Excludes1 intestinal malabsorption following gastrointestinal surgery (K91.2)

K90.0 Celiac disease
Celiac disease with steatorrhea
Celiac gluten-sensitive enteropathy
Nontropical sprue
Use additional code for associated disorders including:
dermatitis herpetiformis (L13.0)
gluten ataxia (G32.81)
Code also exocrine pancreatic insufficiency (K86.81)

K90.1 Tropical sprue
Sprue NOS
Tropical steatorrhea

K90.2 Blind loop syndrome, not elsewhere classified
Blind loop syndrome NOS
Excludes1 congenital blind loop syndrome (Q43.8)
postsurgical blind loop syndrome (K91.2)

K90.3 Pancreatic steatorrhea

● **K90.4 Other malabsorption due to intolerance**
Excludes2 celiac gluten-sensitive enteropathy (K90.0)
lactose intolerance (E73.-)
Coding Clinic: 2016, Q4, P35-36

K90.41 Non-celiac gluten sensitivity
Gluten sensitivity NOS
Non-celiac gluten sensitive enteropathy

K90.49 Malabsorption due to intolerance, not elsewhere classified
Malabsorption due to intolerance to carbohydrate
Malabsorption due to intolerance to fat
Malabsorption due to intolerance to protein
Malabsorption due to intolerance to starch

● **K90.8 Other intestinal malabsorption**

K90.81 Whipple's disease (Ex) PDX 1143

● **K90.82 Short bowel syndrome**
Short gut syndrome

K90.821 Short bowel syndrome with colon in continuity (Ex) PDX 1144
Short bowel syndrome with colonic continuity
Coding Clinic: 2023, Q4, P32

K90.822 Short bowel syndrome without colon in continuity (Ex) PDX 1145
Short bowel syndrome without colonic continuity
Coding Clinic: 2023, Q4, P33

K90.829 Short bowel syndrome, unspecified (Ex) PDX 1146

K90.83 Intestinal failure (Ex) PDX 1147

K90.89 Other intestinal malabsorption (Ex) PDX 1142

K90.9 Intestinal malabsorption, unspecified (Ex) PDX 1142
Coding Clinic: 2017, Q4, P108-109

● **K91 Intraoperative and postprocedural complications and disorders of digestive system, not elsewhere classified**
Excludes2 complications of artificial opening of digestive system (K94.-)
complications of bariatric procedures (K95.-)
gastrojejunal ulcer (K28.-)
postprocedural (radiation) retroperitoneal abscess (K68.11)
radiation colitis (K52.0)
radiation gastroenteritis (K52.0)
radiation proctitis (K62.7)
Coding Clinic: 2016, Q4, P10

K91.0 Vomiting following gastrointestinal surgery

K91.1 Postgastric surgery syndromes
Dumping syndrome
Postgastrectomy syndrome
Postvagotomy syndrome

K91.2 Postsurgical malabsorption, not elsewhere classified (Ex) PDX 1148
Postsurgical blind loop syndrome
Excludes1 malabsorption osteomalacia in adults (M83.2)
malabsorption osteoporosis, postsurgical (M80.8-, M81.8)

● **K91.3 Postprocedural intestinal obstruction** (Ex) PDX 1100
Coding Clinic: 2017, Q1, P40-41

K91.30 Postprocedural intestinal obstruction, unspecified as to partial versus complete
Postprocedural intestinal obstruction NOS

K91.31 Postprocedural partial intestinal obstruction
Postprocedural incomplete intestinal obstruction

K91.32 Postprocedural complete intestinal obstruction

K91.5 Postcholecystectomy syndrome

● **K91.6 Intraoperative hemorrhage and hematoma of a digestive system organ or structure complicating a procedure** (Ex) PDX 1149
Excludes1 intraoperative hemorrhage and hematoma of a digestive system organ or structure due to accidental puncture and laceration during a procedure (K91.7-)

K91.61 Intraoperative hemorrhage and hematoma of a digestive system organ or structure complicating a digestive system procedure
Coding Clinic: 2020, Q1, P20

K91.62 Intraoperative hemorrhage and hematoma of a digestive system organ or structure complicating other procedure

● **K91.7 Accidental puncture and laceration of a digestive system organ or structure during a procedure** (Ex) PDX 569

K91.71 Accidental puncture and laceration of a digestive system organ or structure during a digestive system procedure
Coding Clinic: 2022, Q1, P51-52; 2021, Q2, P12

K91.72 Accidental puncture and laceration of a digestive system organ or structure during other procedure
Coding Clinic: 2022, Q1, P51; 2019, Q2, P24

● **K91.8 Other intraoperative and postprocedural complications and disorders of digestive system** (Ex) PDX 1150

K91.81 Other intraoperative complications of digestive system

K91.82 Postprocedural hepatic failure

K91.83 Postprocedural hepatorenal syndrome

● **K91.84 Postprocedural hemorrhage of a digestive system organ or structure following a procedure** (Ex) PDX 1149

K91.840 Postprocedural hemorrhage of a digestive system organ or structure following a digestive system procedure
Coding Clinic: 2016, Q1, P15

K91.841 Postprocedural hemorrhage of a digestive system organ or structure following other procedure

● K91.85 Complications of intestinal pouch

K91.850 Pouchitis
Inflammation of internal ileoanal pouch

K91.858 Other complications of intestinal pouch
Coding Clinic: 2019, Q2, P13

K91.86 Retained cholelithiasis following cholecystectomy

● K91.87 Postprocedural hematoma and seroma of a digestive system organ or structure following a procedure (Ex) PDX 1149

K91.870 Postprocedural hematoma of a digestive system organ or structure following a digestive system procedure
Coding Clinic: 2022, Q1, P24

K91.871 Postprocedural hematoma of a digestive system organ or structure following other procedure

K91.872 Postprocedural seroma of a digestive system organ or structure following a digestive system procedure

K91.873 Postprocedural seroma of a digestive system organ or structure following other procedure

K91.89 Other postprocedural complications and disorders of digestive system
Use additional code, if applicable, to further specify disorder
Excludes2 postprocedural retroperitoneal abscess (K68.11)
Coding Clinic: 2017, Q1, P41

● K92 Other diseases of digestive system (Ex) PDX 1078
Excludes1 neonatal gastrointestinal hemorrhage (P54.0-P54.3)

K92.0 Hematemesis

K92.1 Melena
Excludes1 occult blood in feces (R19.5)

K92.2 Gastrointestinal hemorrhage, unspecified
Gastric hemorrhage NOS
Intestinal hemorrhage NOS
Excludes1 acute hemorrhagic gastritis (K29.01)
hemorrhage of anus and rectum (K62.5)
angiodysplasia of stomach with hemorrhage (K31.811)
diverticular disease with hemorrhage (K57.-)
gastritis and duodenitis with hemorrhage (K29.-)
peptic ulcer with hemorrhage (K25-K28)
Coding Clinic: 2021, Q1, P12

● K92.8 Other specified diseases of the digestive system

K92.81 Gastrointestinal mucositis (ulcerative) (Ex) PDX 1075
Code also type of associated therapy, such as:
antineoplastic and immunosuppressive drugs (T45.1X-)
radiological procedure and radiotherapy (Y84.2)
Excludes2 mucositis (ulcerative) of vagina and vulva (N76.81)
nasal mucositis (ulcerative) (J34.81)
oral mucositis (ulcerative) (K12.3-)

K92.89 Other specified diseases of the digestive system

K92.9 Disease of digestive system, unspecified

● K94 Complications of artificial openings of the digestive system

● K94.0 Colostomy complications (Ex) PDX 1151

K94.00 Colostomy complication, unspecified

K94.01 Colostomy hemorrhage

K94.02 Colostomy infection
Use additional code to specify type of infection, such as:
cellulitis of abdominal wall (L03.311)
sepsis (A40.-, A41.-)

K94.03 Colostomy malfunction (Ex) PDX 1152
Mechanical complication of colostomy

K94.09 Other complications of colostomy

● K94.1 Enterostomy complications (Ex) PDX 1151

K94.10 Enterostomy complication, unspecified

K94.11 Enterostomy hemorrhage

K94.12 Enterostomy infection
Use additional code to specify type of infection, such as:
cellulitis of abdominal wall (L03.311)
sepsis (A40.-, A41.-)

K94.13 Enterostomy malfunction (Ex) PDX 1152
Mechanical complication of enterostomy
Coding Clinic: 2021, Q4, P18

K94.19 Other complications of enterostomy

● K94.2 Gastrostomy complications (Ex) PDX 1150

K94.20 Gastrostomy complication, unspecified

K94.21 Gastrostomy hemorrhage

K94.22 Gastrostomy infection
Use additional code to specify type of infection, such as:
cellulitis of abdominal wall (L03.311)
sepsis (A40.-, A41.-)

K94.23 Gastrostomy malfunction
Mechanical complication of gastrostomy

K94.29 Other complications of gastrostomy

● K94.3 Esophagostomy complications (Ex) PDX 1150

K94.30 Esophagostomy complications, unspecified

K94.31 Esophagostomy hemorrhage

K94.32 Esophagostomy infection
Use additional code to identify the infection

K94.33 Esophagostomy malfunction
Mechanical complication of esophagostomy

K94.39 Other complications of esophagostomy

● K95 Complications of bariatric procedures (Ex) PDX 1150

● K95.0 Complications of gastric band procedure

K95.01 Infection due to gastric band procedure
Use additional code to specify type of infection or organism, such as:
bacterial and viral infectious agents (B95.-, B96.-)
cellulitis of abdominal wall (L03.311)
sepsis (A40.-, A41.-)

K95.09 Other complications of gastric band procedure
Use additional code, if applicable, to further specify complication

● K95.8 Complications of other bariatric procedure
Excludes1 complications of gastric band surgery (K95.0-)

K95.81 Infection due to other bariatric procedure
Use additional code to specify type of infection or organism, such as:
bacterial and viral infectious agents (B95.-, B96.-)
cellulitis of abdominal wall (L03.311)
sepsis (A40.-, A41.-)

K95.89 Other complications of other bariatric procedure
Use additional code, if applicable, to further specify complication

CHAPTER 11 (K00-K95)

CHAPTER 12

DISEASES OF THE SKIN AND SUBCUTANEOUS TISSUE (L00-L99)

OGCR Chapter-Specific Coding Guidelines

12. Chapter 12: Diseases of the Skin and Subcutaneous Tissue (L00-L99)

a. Pressure ulcer stage codes

1) Pressure ulcer stages

Codes from category L89, Pressure ulcer, identify the site of the pressure ulcer as well as the stage of the ulcer.

The ICD-10-CM classifies pressure ulcer stages based on severity, which is designated by stages 1-4, unspecified stage and unstageable.

Assign as many codes from category L89 as needed to identify all the pressure ulcers the patient has, if applicable.

See Section I.B.14 for pressure ulcer stage documentation by clinicians other than patient's provider.

2) Unstageable pressure ulcers

Assignment of the code for unstageable pressure ulcer (L89.--0) should be based on the clinical documentation. These codes are used for pressure ulcers whose stage cannot be clinically determined (e.g., the ulcer is covered by eschar or has been treated with a skin or muscle graft) and pressure ulcers that are documented as deep tissue injury but not documented as due to trauma. This code should not be confused with the codes for unspecified stage (L89.--9). When there is no documentation regarding the stage of the pressure ulcer, assign the appropriate code for unspecified stage (L89.--9).

3) Documented pressure ulcer stage

Assignment of the pressure ulcer stage code should be guided by clinical documentation of the stage or documentation of the terms found in the Alphabetic Index. For clinical terms describing the stage that are not found in the Alphabetic Index, and there is no documentation of the stage, the provider should be queried.

4) Patients admitted with pressure ulcers documented as healed

No code is assigned if the documentation states that the pressure ulcer is completely healed.

5) Patients admitted with pressure ulcers documented as healing

Pressure ulcers described as healing should be assigned the appropriate pressure ulcer stage code based on the documentation in the medical record. If the documentation does not provide information about the stage of the healing pressure ulcer, assign the appropriate code for unspecified stage.

If the documentation is unclear as to whether the patient has a current (new) pressure ulcer or if the patient is being treated for a healing pressure ulcer, query the provider.

For ulcers that were present on admission but healed at the time of discharge, assign the code for the site and stage of the pressure ulcer at the time of admission.

6) Patient admitted with pressure ulcer evolving into another stage during the admission

If a patient is admitted to an inpatient hospital with a pressure ulcer at one stage and it progresses to a higher stage, two separate codes should be assigned: one code for the site and stage of the ulcer on admission and a second code for the same ulcer site and the highest stage reported during the stay.

b. Non-Pressure Chronic Ulcers

1) Patients admitted with non-pressure ulcers documented as healed

No code is assigned if the documentation states that the non-pressure ulcer is completely healed.

2) Patients admitted with non-pressure ulcers documented as healing

Non-pressure ulcers described as healing should be assigned the appropriate non-pressure ulcer code based on the documentation in the medical record. If the documentation does not provide information about the severity of the healing non-pressure ulcer, assign the appropriate code for unspecified severity.

If the documentation is unclear as to whether the patient has a current (new) non-pressure ulcer or if the patient is being treated for a healing non-pressure ulcer, query the provider.

For ulcers that were present on admission but healed at the time of discharge, assign the code for the site and severity of the non-pressure ulcer at the time of admission.

3) Patient admitted with non-pressure ulcer that progresses to another severity level during the admission

If a patient is admitted to an inpatient hospital with a non-pressure ulcer at one severity level and it progresses to a higher severity level, two separate codes should be assigned: one code for the site and severity level of the ulcer on admission and a second code for the same ulcer site and the highest severity level reported during the stay.

See Section I.B.14 for pressure ulcer stage documentation by clinicians other than patient's provider.

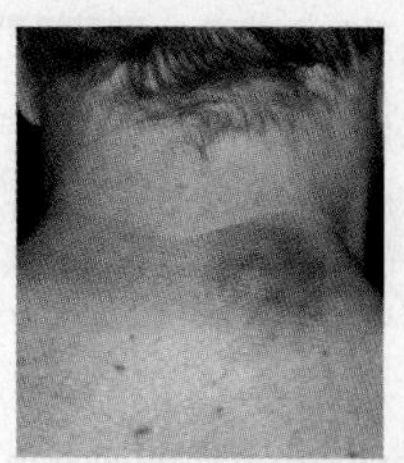

Figure 12-1 Furuncle, also known as a boil, is a staphylococcal infection. The organism enters the body through a hair follicle and so furuncles usually appear in hairy areas of the body. A cluster of furuncles is known as a carbuncle and involves infection into the deep subcutaneous fascia. These usually appear on the back and neck. (**B** from Habif TP, Binnick AN, Meyerson LB: Clinical Dermatology: A Color Guide to Diagnosis and Therapy, S.l., Mosby Elsevier, 2010)

CHAPTER 12

DISEASES OF THE SKIN AND SUBCUTANEOUS TISSUE (L00-L99)

Excludes2 certain conditions originating in the perinatal period (P04-P96)
certain infectious and parasitic diseases (A00-B99)
complications of pregnancy, childbirth and the puerperium (O00-O9A)
congenital malformations, deformations, and chromosomal abnormalities (Q00-Q99)
endocrine, nutritional and metabolic diseases (E00-E88)
lipomelanotic reticulosis (I89.8)
neoplasms (C00-D49)
symptoms, signs and abnormal clinical and laboratory findings, not elsewhere classified (R00-R94)
systemic connective tissue disorders (M30-M36)
viral warts (B07.-)

This chapter contains the following blocks:

L00-L08	Infections of the skin and subcutaneous tissue
L10-L14	Bullous disorders
L20-L30	Dermatitis and eczema
L40-L45	Papulosquamous disorders
L49-L54	Urticaria and erythema
L55-L59	Radiation-related disorders of the skin and subcutaneous tissue
L60-L75	Disorders of skin appendages
L76	Intraoperative and postprocedural complications of skin and subcutaneous tissue
L80-L99	Other disorders of the skin and subcutaneous tissue

INFECTIONS OF THE SKIN AND SUBCUTANEOUS TISSUE (L00-L08)

Use additional code (B95-B97) to identify infectious agent.

Excludes2 hordeolum (H00.0)
infective dermatitis (L30.3)
local infections of skin classified in Chapter 1
lupus panniculitis (L93.2)
panniculitis NOS (M79.3)
panniculitis of neck and back (M54.0-)
Perlèche NOS (K13.0)
Perlèche due to candidiasis (B37.0)
Perlèche due to riboflavin deficiency (E53.0)
pyogenic granuloma (L98.0)
relapsing panniculitis [Weber-Christian] (M35.6)
viral warts (B07.-)
zoster (B02.-)

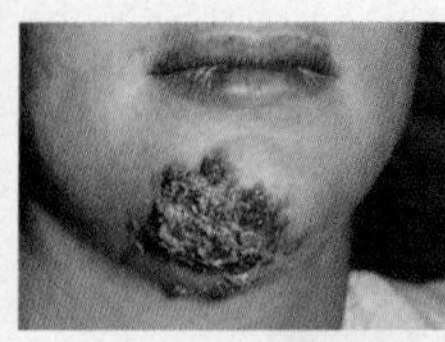

Figure 12-2 Impetigo. A thick, honey-yellow adherent crust covers the entire eroded surface. (From James WD, Elston DM, Berger TG, Andrews GC: Andrews' Diseases of the Skin: Clinical Dermatology, London, Saunders/Elsevier, 2011)

LØØ Staphylococcal scalded skin syndrome
Ritter's disease
Use additional code to identify percentage of skin exfoliation (L49.-)
Excludes1 bullous impetigo (LØ1.Ø3)
pemphigus neonatorum (LØ1.Ø3)
toxic epidermal necrolysis [Lyell] (L51.2)

●**LØ1 Impetigo**
Contagious skin infection caused by a streptococcus or staphylococcus aureus, common skin infections among children
Excludes1 impetigo herpetiformis (L4Ø.1)

●**LØ1.Ø Impetigo**
Impetigo contagiosa
Impetigo vulgaris
LØ1.ØØ Impetigo, unspecified
Impetigo NOS
LØ1.Ø1 Non-bullous impetigo
LØ1.Ø2 Bockhart's impetigo
Impetigo follicularis
Perifolliculitis NOS
Superficial pustular perifolliculitis
LØ1.Ø3 Bullous impetigo
Impetigo neonatorum
Pemphigus neonatorum
Neonate = newborn
LØ1.Ø9 Other impetigo
Ulcerative impetigo
LØ1.1 Impetiginization of other dermatoses

●**LØ2 Cutaneous abscess, furuncle and carbuncle**
Use additional code to identify organism (B95-B96)
Excludes2 abscess of anus and rectal regions (K61.-)
abscess of female genital organs (external) (N76.4)
abscess of male genital organs (external) (N48.2, N49.-)

●**LØ2.Ø Cutaneous abscess, furuncle and carbuncle of face**
Excludes2 abscess of ear, external (H6Ø.Ø)
abscess of eyelid (HØØ.Ø)
abscess of head [any part, except face] (LØ2.8)
abscess of lacrimal gland (HØ4.Ø)
abscess of lacrimal passages (HØ4.3)
abscess of mouth (K12.2)
abscess of nose (J34.Ø)
abscess of orbit (HØ5.Ø)
submandibular abscess (K12.2)
LØ2.Ø1 Cutaneous abscess of face (Ex:) PDX 1153
LØ2.Ø2 Furuncle of face
Boil of face
Folliculitis of face
LØ2.Ø3 Carbuncle of face

●**LØ2.1 Cutaneous abscess, furuncle and carbuncle of neck**
LØ2.11 Cutaneous abscess of neck (Ex:) PDX 1154
LØ2.12 Furuncle of neck
Boil of neck
Folliculitis of neck
LØ2.13 Carbuncle of neck

●**LØ2.2 Cutaneous abscess, furuncle and carbuncle of trunk**
Excludes1 non-newborn omphalitis (LØ8.82)
omphalitis of newborn (P38.-)
Excludes2 abscess of breast (N61.1)
abscess of buttocks (LØ2.3)
abscess of female external genital organs (N76.4)
abscess of male external genital organs (N48.2, N49.-)
abscess of hip (LØ2.4)

●**LØ2.21 Cutaneous abscess of trunk** (Ex:) PDX 1155
LØ2.211 Cutaneous abscess of abdominal wall
LØ2.212 Cutaneous abscess of back [any part, except buttock]
LØ2.213 Cutaneous abscess of chest wall
LØ2.214 Cutaneous abscess of groin
LØ2.215 Cutaneous abscess of perineum
LØ2.216 Cutaneous abscess of umbilicus
LØ2.219 Cutaneous abscess of trunk, unspecified

●**LØ2.22 Furuncle of trunk**
Boil of trunk
Folliculitis of trunk
LØ2.221 Furuncle of abdominal wall
LØ2.222 Furuncle of back [any part, except buttock]
LØ2.223 Furuncle of chest wall
LØ2.224 Furuncle of groin
LØ2.225 Furuncle of perineum
LØ2.226 Furuncle of umbilicus
LØ2.229 Furuncle of trunk, unspecified

●**LØ2.23 Carbuncle of trunk**
LØ2.231 Carbuncle of abdominal wall
LØ2.232 Carbuncle of back [any part, except buttock]
LØ2.233 Carbuncle of chest wall
LØ2.234 Carbuncle of groin
LØ2.235 Carbuncle of perineum
LØ2.236 Carbuncle of umbilicus
LØ2.239 Carbuncle of trunk, unspecified

●**LØ2.3 Cutaneous abscess, furuncle and carbuncle of buttock**
Excludes1 pilonidal cyst with abscess (LØ5.Ø1)
LØ2.31 Cutaneous abscess of buttock (Ex:) PDX 1156
Cutaneous abscess of gluteal region
LØ2.32 Furuncle of buttock
Boil of buttock
Folliculitis of buttock
Furuncle of gluteal region
LØ2.33 Carbuncle of buttock
Carbuncle of gluteal region

●**LØ2.4 Cutaneous abscess, furuncle and carbuncle of limb**
Excludes2 Cutaneous abscess, furuncle and carbuncle of groin (LØ2.214, LØ2.224, LØ2.234)
Cutaneous abscess, furuncle and carbuncle of hand (LØ2.5-)
Cutaneous abscess, furuncle and carbuncle of foot (LØ2.6-)

●**LØ2.41 Cutaneous abscess of limb** (Ex:) PDX 1157
LØ2.411 Cutaneous abscess of right axilla
LØ2.412 Cutaneous abscess of left axilla
LØ2.413 Cutaneous abscess of right upper limb
LØ2.414 Cutaneous abscess of left upper limb
LØ2.415 Cutaneous abscess of right lower limb (Ex:) PDX 1158

CHAPTER 12 (LØØ-L99)

L02.416 Cutaneous abscess of left lower limb (Ex) PDX 1158
L02.419 Cutaneous abscess of limb, unspecified (Ex) PDX 1158

● L02.42 Furuncle of limb
Boil of limb
Folliculitis of limb
L02.421 Furuncle of right axilla
L02.422 Furuncle of left axilla
L02.423 Furuncle of right upper limb
L02.424 Furuncle of left upper limb
L02.425 Furuncle of right lower limb
L02.426 Furuncle of left lower limb
L02.429 Furuncle of limb, unspecified

● L02.43 Carbuncle of limb
L02.431 Carbuncle of right axilla
L02.432 Carbuncle of left axilla
L02.433 Carbuncle of right upper limb
L02.434 Carbuncle of left upper limb
L02.435 Carbuncle of right lower limb
L02.436 Carbuncle of left lower limb
L02.439 Carbuncle of limb, unspecified

● L02.5 Cutaneous abscess, furuncle and carbuncle of hand

● L02.51 Cutaneous abscess of hand (Ex) PDX 1159
L02.511 Cutaneous abscess of right hand
L02.512 Cutaneous abscess of left hand
L02.519 Cutaneous abscess of unspecified hand

● L02.52 Furuncle hand
Boil of hand
Folliculitis of hand
L02.521 Furuncle right hand
L02.522 Furuncle left hand
L02.529 Furuncle unspecified hand

● L02.53 Carbuncle of hand
L02.531 Carbuncle of right hand
L02.532 Carbuncle of left hand
L02.539 Carbuncle of unspecified hand

● L02.6 Cutaneous abscess, furuncle and carbuncle of foot

● L02.61 Cutaneous abscess of foot (Ex) PDX 1160
L02.611 Cutaneous abscess of right foot
L02.612 Cutaneous abscess of left foot
L02.619 Cutaneous abscess of unspecified foot

● L02.62 Furuncle of foot
Boil of foot
Folliculitis of foot
L02.621 Furuncle of right foot
L02.622 Furuncle of left foot
L02.629 Furuncle of unspecified foot

● L02.63 Carbuncle of foot
L02.631 Carbuncle of right foot
L02.632 Carbuncle of left foot
L02.639 Carbuncle of unspecified foot

● L02.8 Cutaneous abscess, furuncle and carbuncle of other sites

● L02.81 Cutaneous abscess of other sites (Ex) PDX 1161
L02.811 Cutaneous abscess of head [any part, except face]
L02.818 Cutaneous abscess of other sites

● L02.82 Furuncle of other sites
Boil of other sites
Folliculitis of other sites
L02.821 Furuncle of head [any part, except face]
L02.828 Furuncle of other sites

Item 12-1 **Onychia** is an inflammation of the tissue surrounding the nail with pus accumulation and loss of the nail, resulting from microscopic pathogens entering through small wounds. **Paronychia** is a nail disease also known as felon or whitlow and is a bacterial or fungal infection.

● L02.83 Carbuncle of other sites
L02.831 Carbuncle of head [any part, except face]
L02.838 Carbuncle of other sites

● L02.9 Cutaneous abscess, furuncle and carbuncle, unspecified
L02.91 Cutaneous abscess, unspecified (Ex) PDX 1161
L02.92 Furuncle, unspecified
Boil NOS
Furunculosis NOS
L02.93 Carbuncle, unspecified

● L03 Cellulitis and acute lymphangitis

Excludes2 cellulitis of anal and rectal region (K61.-)
cellulitis of external auditory canal (H60.1)
cellulitis of eyelid (H00.0)
cellulitis of female external genital organs (N76.4)
cellulitis of lacrimal apparatus (H04.3)
cellulitis of male external genital organs (N48.2, N49.-)
cellulitis of mouth (K12.2)
cellulitis of nose (J34.0)
eosinophilic cellulitis [Wells] (L98.3)
febrile neutrophilic dermatosis [Sweet] (L98.2)
lymphangitis (chronic) (subacute) (I89.1)

● L03.0 Cellulitis and acute lymphangitis of finger and toe
Infection of nail
Onychia
Paronychia
Perionychia

● L03.01 Cellulitis of finger
Felon
Whitlow
Excludes1 herpetic whitlow (B00.89)
L03.011 Cellulitis of right finger
L03.012 Cellulitis of left finger
L03.019 Cellulitis of unspecified finger

● L03.02 Acute lymphangitis of finger
Hangnail with lymphangitis of finger
L03.021 Acute lymphangitis of right finger
L03.022 Acute lymphangitis of left finger
L03.029 Acute lymphangitis of unspecified finger

● L03.03 Cellulitis of toe
L03.031 Cellulitis of right toe
L03.032 Cellulitis of left toe
L03.039 Cellulitis of unspecified toe

● L03.04 Acute lymphangitis of toe
Hangnail with lymphangitis of toe
L03.041 Acute lymphangitis of right toe
L03.042 Acute lymphangitis of left toe
L03.049 Acute lymphangitis of unspecified toe

● L03.1 Cellulitis and acute lymphangitis of other parts of limb

● L03.11 Cellulitis of other parts of limb (Ex) PDX 1157
Excludes2 cellulitis of fingers (L03.01-)
cellulitis of toes (L03.03-)
groin (L03.314)
L03.111 Cellulitis of right axilla
L03.112 Cellulitis of left axilla
L03.113 Cellulitis of right upper limb

Item 12-2 **Cellulitis** is an acute spreading bacterial infection below the surface of the skin characterized by redness (erythema), warmth, swelling, pain, fever, chills, and enlarged lymph nodes ("swollen glands").

CHAPTER 12 (L00-L99)

L03.114 Cellulitis of left upper limb
Coding Clinic: 2019, Q1, P13

L03.115 Cellulitis of right lower limb (Ex) PDX 1158

L03.116 Cellulitis of left lower limb (Ex) PDX 1158

L03.119 Cellulitis of unspecified part of limb (Ex) PDX 1158

● L03.12 Acute lymphangitis of other parts of limb (Ex) PDX 1157

Excludes2 acute lymphangitis of fingers (L03.2-)
acute lymphangitis of toes (L03.04-)
acute lymphangitis of groin (L03.324)

L03.121 Acute lymphangitis of right axilla

L03.122 Acute lymphangitis of left axilla

L03.123 Acute lymphangitis of right upper limb

L03.124 Acute lymphangitis of left upper limb

L03.125 Acute lymphangitis of right lower limb (Ex) PDX 1158

L03.126 Acute lymphangitis of left lower limb (Ex) PDX 1158

L03.129 Acute lymphangitis of unspecified part of limb (Ex) PDX 1158

● L03.2 Cellulitis and acute lymphangitis of face and neck

● L03.21 Cellulitis and acute lymphangitis of face

L03.211 Cellulitis of face (Ex) PDX 1162

Excludes2 abscess of orbit (H05.01-)
cellulitis of ear (H60.1-)
cellulitis of eyelid (H00.0-)
cellulitis of head (L03.81)
cellulitis of lacrimal apparatus (H04.3)
cellulitis of lip (K13.0)
cellulitis of mouth (K12.2)
cellulitis of nose (internal) (J34.0)
cellulitis of orbit (H05.01-)
cellulitis of scalp (L03.81)

L03.212 Acute lymphangitis of face (Ex) PDX 1163

L03.213 Periorbital cellulitis (Ex) PDX 1162
Preseptal cellulitis
Coding Clinic: 2016, Q4, P36

● L03.22 Cellulitis and acute lymphangitis of neck (Ex) PDX 1154

L03.221 Cellulitis of neck

L03.222 Acute lymphangitis of neck

● L03.3 Cellulitis and acute lymphangitis of trunk

● L03.31 Cellulitis of trunk (Ex) PDX 1155

Excludes2 cellulitis of anal and rectal regions (K61.-)
cellulitis of breast NOS (N61.0)
cellulitis of female external genital organs (N76.4)
cellulitis of male external genital organs (N48.2, N49.-)
omphalitis of newborn (P38.-)
puerperal cellulitis of breast (O91.2)

L03.311 Cellulitis of abdominal wall

Excludes2 cellulitis of umbilicus (L03.316)
cellulitis of groin (L03.314)

L03.312 Cellulitis of back [any part except buttock]

L03.313 Cellulitis of chest wall

L03.314 Cellulitis of groin

L03.315 Cellulitis of perineum

L03.316 Cellulitis of umbilicus

L03.317 Cellulitis of buttock (Ex) PDX 1156

L03.319 Cellulitis of trunk, unspecified

● L03.32 Acute lymphangitis of trunk (Ex) PDX 1155

L03.321 Acute lymphangitis of abdominal wall

L03.322 Acute lymphangitis of back [any part except buttock]

L03.323 Acute lymphangitis of chest wall

L03.324 Acute lymphangitis of groin

L03.325 Acute lymphangitis of perineum

L03.326 Acute lymphangitis of umbilicus

L03.327 Acute lymphangitis of buttock (Ex) PDX 1156

L03.329 Acute lymphangitis of trunk, unspecified

● L03.8 Cellulitis and acute lymphangitis of other sites (Ex) PDX 1161

● L03.81 Cellulitis of other sites

L03.811 Cellulitis of head [any part, except face]
Cellulitis of scalp

Excludes2 cellulitis of face (L03.211)

L03.818 Cellulitis of other sites

● L03.89 Acute lymphangitis of other sites

L03.891 Acute lymphangitis of head [any part, except face]

L03.898 Acute lymphangitis of other sites

● L03.9 Cellulitis and acute lymphangitis, unspecified (Ex) PDX 1161

L03.90 Cellulitis, unspecified

L03.91 Acute lymphangitis, unspecified

Excludes1 lymphangitis NOS (I89.1)

● L04 Acute lymphadenitis

Short-term inflammation of lymph nodes which can be regionalized to involve a given area of the lymph system or systemic involving much of the body

Includes abscess (acute) of lymph nodes, except mesenteric
acute lymphadenitis, except mesenteric

Excludes1 chronic or subacute lymphadenitis, except mesenteric (I88.1)
enlarged lymph nodes (R59.-)
human immunodeficiency virus [HIV] disease resulting in generalized lymphadenopathy (B20)
lymphadenitis NOS (I88.9)
nonspecific mesenteric lymphadenitis (I88.0)

L04.0 Acute lymphadenitis of face, head and neck

New | Revised | ~~deleted~~ Deleted | Excludes 1 | Excludes 2 | Includes | Use additional | Code first | Code also | Key words
OGCR Official Guidelines | ● Unacceptable Principal Diagnosis | X Assign placeholder X | ● Use Additional Character(s) | Manifestation Code | Coding Clinic

L04.1 **Acute lymphadenitis of trunk**
L04.2 **Acute lymphadenitis of upper limb**
Acute lymphadenitis of axilla
Acute lymphadenitis of shoulder
L04.3 **Acute lymphadenitis of lower limb**
Acute lymphadenitis of hip
Excludes2 acute lymphadenitis of groin (L04.1)
L04.8 **Acute lymphadenitis of other sites**
L04.9 **Acute lymphadenitis, unspecified**

Item 12–3 Abscess is a localized collection of pus in tissues or organs and is a sign of infection, resulting in swelling and inflammation.

Item 12–4 Pilonidal cyst, also called a coccygeal cyst, is the result of a disorder called pilonidal disease. The cyst usually contains hair and pus.

● **L05** **Pilonidal cyst and sinus**
● **L05.0** **Pilonidal cyst and sinus with abscess** (Ex:) PDX 1164
L05.01 **Pilonidal cyst with abscess**
Pilonidal abscess
Pilonidal dimple with abscess
Postanal dimple with abscess
Excludes2 congenital sacral dimple (Q82.6)
parasacral dimple (Q82.6)
L05.02 **Pilonidal sinus with abscess**
Coccygeal fistula with abscess
Coccygeal sinus with abscess
Pilonidal fistula with abscess
● **L05.9** **Pilonidal cyst and sinus without abscess**
L05.91 **Pilonidal cyst without abscess**
Pilonidal dimple
Postanal dimple
Pilonidal cyst NOS
Excludes2 congenital sacral dimple (Q82.6)
parasacral dimple (Q82.6)
L05.92 **Pilonidal sinus without abscess**
Coccygeal fistula
Coccygeal sinus without abscess
Pilonidal fistula

● **L08** **Other local infections of skin and subcutaneous tissue**
L08.0 **Pyoderma**
Dermatitis gangrenosa
Purulent dermatitis
Septic dermatitis
Suppurative dermatitis
Excludes1 pyoderma gangrenosum (L88)
pyoderma vegetans (L08.81)
L08.1 **Erythrasma**
● **L08.8** **Other specified local infections of the skin and subcutaneous tissue**
L08.81 **Pyoderma vegetans**
Excludes1 pyoderma gangrenosum (L88)
pyoderma NOS (L08.0)
L08.82 **Omphalitis not of newborn**
Excludes1 omphalitis of newborn (P38.-)
L08.89 **Other specified local infections of the skin and subcutaneous tissue**
L08.9 **Local infection of the skin and subcutaneous tissue, unspecified**

BULLOUS DISORDERS (L10-L14)

Excludes1 benign familial pemphigus [Hailey-Hailey] (Q82.8)
staphylococcal scalded skin syndrome (L00)
toxic epidermal necrolysis [Lyell] (L51.2)

● **L10** **Pemphigus** (Ex:) PDX 1165
Excludes1 pemphigus neonatorum (L01.03)
L10.0 **Pemphigus vulgaris**
L10.1 **Pemphigus vegetans**
L10.2 **Pemphigus foliaceous**

Item 12–5 Dermatitis herpetiformis, also known as Duhring's disease, is a systemic disease characterized by small blisters (3 to 5 mm) and occasionally large bullae (> 5 mm).

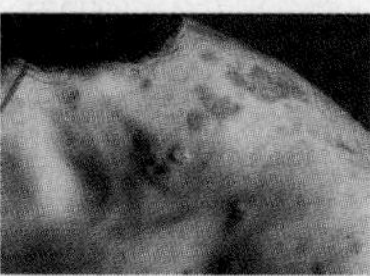

Figure 12-3 Dermatitis herpetiformis. (From Terhorst D: BASICS Dermatologie, München, Elsevier, Urban & Fischer, 2011)

L10.3 **Brazilian pemphigus [fogo selvagem]**
L10.4 **Pemphigus erythematosus**
Senear-Usher syndrome
L10.5 **Drug-induced pemphigus**
Use additional code for adverse effect, if applicable, to identify drug (T36-T50 with fifth or sixth character 5)
● **L10.8** **Other pemphigus**
L10.81 **Paraneoplastic pemphigus**
L10.89 **Other pemphigus**
L10.9 **Pemphigus, unspecified**

● **L11** **Other acantholytic disorders**
L11.0 **Acquired keratosis follicularis**
Excludes1 keratosis follicularis (congenital) [Darier-White] (Q82.8)
L11.1 **Transient acantholytic dermatosis [Grover]**
L11.8 **Other specified acantholytic disorders**
L11.9 **Acantholytic disorder, unspecified**

● **L12** **Pemphigoid** (Ex:) PDX 1165
Excludes1 herpes gestationis (O26.4-)
impetigo herpetiformis (L40.1)
L12.0 **Bullous pemphigoid**
L12.1 **Cicatricial pemphigoid**
Benign mucous membrane pemphigoid
L12.2 **Chronic bullous disease of childhood** P
Juvenile dermatitis herpetiformis
● **L12.3** **Acquired epidermolysis bullosa** (Ex:) PDX 1166
Excludes1 epidermolysis bullosa (congenital) (Q81.-)
L12.30 **Acquired epidermolysis bullosa, unspecified**
L12.31 **Epidermolysis bullosa due to drug**
Use additional code for adverse effect, if applicable, to identify drug (T36-T50 with fifth or sixth character 5)
L12.35 **Other acquired epidermolysis bullosa**
L12.8 **Other pemphigoid**
L12.9 **Pemphigoid, unspecified**

● **L13** **Other bullous disorders**
L13.0 **Dermatitis herpetiformis**
Duhring's disease
Hydroa herpetiformis
Excludes1 juvenile dermatitis herpetiformis (L12.2)
senile dermatitis herpetiformis (L12.0)
L13.1 **Subcorneal pustular dermatitis**
Sneddon-Wilkinson disease
L13.8 **Other specified bullous disorders**
L13.9 **Bullous disorder, unspecified**

L14 ***Bullous disorders in diseases classified elsewhere***
Code first underlying disease

Item 12–6 Seborrheic dermatitis is characterized by greasy, scaly, red patches and is associated with oily skin and scalp.

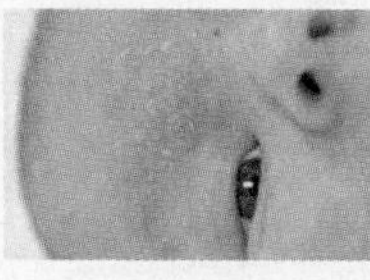

Figure 12-4 Seborrheic dermatitis. (Getty Image)

CHAPTER 12 (L00-L99)

DERMATITIS AND ECZEMA (L20-L30)

Note: In this block the terms dermatitis and eczema are used synonymously and interchangeably.

Excludes2 chronic (childhood) granulomatous disease (D71)
dermatitis gangrenosa (L08.0)
dermatitis herpetiformis (L13.0)
dry skin dermatitis (L85.3)
factitial dermatitis (L98.1)
perioral dermatitis (L71.0)
radiation-related disorders of the skin and subcutaneous tissue (L55-L59)
stasis dermatitis (I87.2)

● **L20 Atopic dermatitis**
L20.0 Besnier's prurigo
● **L20.8 Other atopic dermatitis**
Excludes2 circumscribed neurodermatitis (L28.0)
L20.81 Atopic neurodermatitis
Diffuse neurodermatitis
L20.82 Flexural eczema
L20.83 Infantile (acute) (chronic) eczema P
L20.84 Intrinsic (allergic) eczema
L20.89 Other atopic dermatitis
L20.9 Atopic dermatitis, unspecified

● **L21 Seborrheic dermatitis**
Excludes2 infective dermatitis (L30.3)
seborrheic keratosis (L82.-)
L21.0 Seborrhea capitis
Cradle cap
Coding Clinic: 2018, Q1, P6
L21.1 Seborrheic infantile dermatitis P
L21.8 Other seborrheic dermatitis
L21.9 Seborrheic dermatitis, unspecified
Seborrhea NOS

L22 Diaper dermatitis
Diaper erythema
Diaper rash
Psoriasiform diaper rash
Coding Clinic: 2021, Q4, P18

● **L23 Allergic contact dermatitis**
Excludes1 allergy NOS (T78.40)
contact dermatitis NOS (L25.9)
dermatitis NOS (L30.9)
Excludes2 dermatitis due to substances taken internally (L27.-)
dermatitis of eyelid (H01.1-)
diaper dermatitis (L22)
eczema of external ear (H60.5-)
irritant contact dermatitis (L24.-)
perioral dermatitis (L71.0)
radiation-related disorders of the skin and subcutaneous tissue (L55-L59)
L23.0 Allergic contact dermatitis due to metals
Allergic contact dermatitis due to chromium
Allergic contact dermatitis due to nickel
L23.1 Allergic contact dermatitis due to adhesives
L23.2 Allergic contact dermatitis due to cosmetics

Item 12-7 Atopic dermatitis, also known as atopic eczema, infantile eczema, disseminated neuro dermatitis, flexural eczema, and *prurigo diathesique* (Besnier), is characterized by intense itching and is often hereditary.

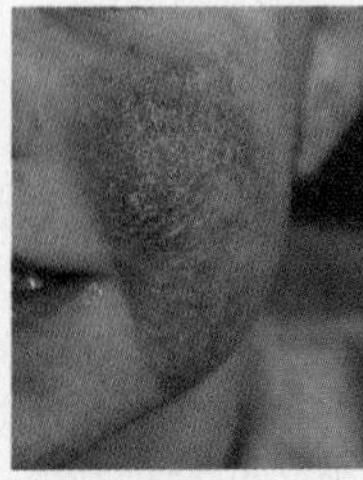

Figure 12-5 Atopic dermatitis. (From Chabner D-E: The Language of Medicine, St. Louis, MO, Saunders/Elsevier, 2007)

L23.3 Allergic contact dermatitis due to drugs in contact with skin
Use additional code for adverse effect, if applicable, to identify drug (T36-T50 with fifth or sixth character 5)
Excludes2 dermatitis due to ingested drugs and medicaments (L27.0-L27.1)
L23.4 Allergic contact dermatitis due to dyes
L23.5 Allergic contact dermatitis due to other chemical products
Allergic contact dermatitis due to cement
Allergic contact dermatitis due to insecticide
Allergic contact dermatitis due to plastic
Allergic contact dermatitis due to rubber
L23.6 Allergic contact dermatitis due to food in contact with the skin
Excludes2 dermatitis due to ingested food (L27.2)
L23.7 Allergic contact dermatitis due to plants, except food
Excludes2 allergy NOS due to pollen (J30.1)
● **L23.8 Allergic contact dermatitis due to other agents**
L23.81 Allergic contact dermatitis due to animal (cat) (dog) dander
Allergic contact dermatitis due to animal (cat) (dog) hair
L23.89 Allergic contact dermatitis due to other agents
L23.9 Allergic contact dermatitis, unspecified cause
Allergic contact eczema NOS

● **L24 Irritant contact dermatitis**
Excludes1 allergy NOS (T78.40)
contact dermatitis NOS (L25.9)
dermatitis NOS (L30.9)
Excludes2 allergic contact dermatitis (L23.-)
dermatitis due to substances taken internally (L27.-)
dermatitis of eyelid (H01.1-)
diaper dermatitis (L22)
eczema of external ear (H60.5-)
perioral dermatitis (L71.0)
radiation-related disorders of the skin and subcutaneous tissue (L55-L59)
L24.0 Irritant contact dermatitis due to detergents
L24.1 Irritant contact dermatitis due to oils and greases
L24.2 Irritant contact dermatitis due to solvents
Irritant contact dermatitis due to chlorocompound
Irritant contact dermatitis due to cyclohexane
Irritant contact dermatitis due to ester
Irritant contact dermatitis due to glycol
Irritant contact dermatitis due to hydrocarbon
Irritant contact dermatitis due to ketone
L24.3 Irritant contact dermatitis due to cosmetics
L24.4 Irritant contact dermatitis due to drugs in contact with skin
Use additional code for adverse effect, if applicable, to identify drug (T36-T50 with fifth or sixth character 5)
L24.5 Irritant contact dermatitis due to other chemical products
Irritant contact dermatitis due to cement
Irritant contact dermatitis due to insecticide
Irritant contact dermatitis due to plastic
Irritant contact dermatitis due to rubber
L24.6 Irritant contact dermatitis due to food in contact with skin
Excludes2 dermatitis due to ingested food (L27.2)
L24.7 Irritant contact dermatitis due to plants, except food
Excludes2 allergy NOS to pollen (J30.1)
● **L24.8 Irritant contact dermatitis due to other agents**
L24.81 Irritant contact dermatitis due to metals
Irritant contact dermatitis due to chromium
Irritant contact dermatitis due to nickel
L24.89 Irritant contact dermatitis due to other agents
Irritant contact dermatitis due to dyes
L24.9 Irritant contact dermatitis, unspecified cause
Irritant contact eczema NOS

CHAPTER 12 (L00-L99)

● L24.A **Irritant contact dermatitis due to friction or contact with body fluids**
Excludes1 virritant contact dermatitis related to stoma or fistula (L24.B-)
Excludes2 erythema intertrigo (L30.4)
L24.A0 **Irritant contact dermatitis due to friction or contact with body fluids, unspecified**
L24.A1 **Irritant contact dermatitis due to saliva**
L24.A2 **Irritant contact dermatitis due to fecal, urinary or dual incontinence**
Excludes1 diaper dermatitis (L22)
Coding Clinic: 2021, Q4, P18
L24.A9 **Irritant contact dermatitis due friction or contact with other specified body fluids**
Irritant contact dermatitis related to endotracheal tube
Wound fluids, exudate

● L24.B **Irritant contact dermatitis related to stoma or fistula**
Use additional code to identify any artificial opening status (Z93.-), if applicable, for contact dermatitis related to stoma secretions
L24.B0 **Irritant contact dermatitis related to unspecified stoma or fistula**
Irritant contact dermatitis related to fistula NOS
Irritant contact dermatitis related to stoma NOS
L24.B1 **Irritant contact dermatitis related to digestive stoma or fistula**
Irritant contact dermatitis related to gastrostomy
Irritant contact dermatitis related to jejunostomy
Irritant contact dermatitis related to saliva or spit fistula
L24.B2 **Irritant contact dermatitis related to respiratory stoma or fistula**
Irritant contact dermatitis related to tracheostomy
L24.B3 **Irritant contact dermatitis related to fecal or urinary stoma or fistula**
Irritant contact dermatitis related to colostomy
Irritant contact dermatitis related to enterocutaneous fistula
Irritant contact dermatitis related to ileostomy
Coding Clinic: 2021, Q4, P17,19

● L25 **Unspecified contact dermatitis**
Excludes1 allergic contact dermatitis (L23.-)
allergy NOS (T78.40)
dermatitis NOS (L30.9)
irritant contact dermatitis (L24.-)
Excludes2 dermatitis due to ingested substances (L27.-)
dermatitis of eyelid (H01.1-)
eczema of external ear (H60.5-)
perioral dermatitis (L71.0)
radiation-related disorders of the skin and subcutaneous tissue (L55-L59)
L25.0 **Unspecified contact dermatitis due to cosmetics**
L25.1 **Unspecified contact dermatitis due to drugs in contact with skin**
Use additional code for adverse effect, if applicable, to identify drug (T36-T50 with fifth or sixth character 5)
Excludes2 dermatitis due to ingested drugs and medicaments (L27.0-L27.1)
L25.2 **Unspecified contact dermatitis due to dyes**
L25.3 **Unspecified contact dermatitis due to other chemical products**
Unspecified contact dermatitis due to cement
Unspecified contact dermatitis due to insecticide
L25.4 **Unspecified contact dermatitis due to food in contact with skin**
Excludes2 dermatitis due to ingested food (L27.2)
L25.5 **Unspecified contact dermatitis due to plants, except food**
Excludes1 nettle rash (L50.9)
Excludes2 allergy NOS due to pollen (J30.1)
L25.8 **Unspecified contact dermatitis due to other agents**
L25.9 **Unspecified contact dermatitis, unspecified cause**
Contact dermatitis (occupational) NOS
Contact eczema (occupational) NOS

L26 **Exfoliative dermatitis**
Hebra's pityriasis
Excludes1 Ritter's disease (L00)

● L27 **Dermatitis due to substances taken internally**
Excludes1 allergy NOS (T78.40)
Excludes2 adverse food reaction, except dermatitis (T78.0-T78.1)
contact dermatitis (L23-L25)
drug photoallergic response (L56.1)
drug phototoxic response (L56.0)
urticaria (L50.-)
L27.0 **Generalized skin eruption due to drugs and medicaments taken internally**
Use additional code for adverse effect, if applicable, to identify drug (T36-T50 with fifth or sixth character 5)
L27.1 **Localized skin eruption due to drugs and medicaments taken internally**
Use additional code for adverse effect, if applicable, to identify drug (T36-T50 with fifth or sixth character 5)
L27.2 **Dermatitis due to ingested food**
Excludes2 dermatitis due to food in contact with skin (L23.6, L24.6, L25.4)
L27.8 **Dermatitis due to other substances taken internally**
L27.9 **Dermatitis due to unspecified substance taken internally**

● L28 **Lichen simplex chronicus and prurigo**
L28.0 **Lichen simplex chronicus**
Circumscribed neurodermatitis
Lichen NOS
L28.1 **Prurigo nodularis**
L28.2 **Other prurigo**
Prurigo NOS
Prurigo Hebra
Prurigo mitis
Urticaria papulosa

● L29 **Pruritus**
Excludes1 neurotic excoriation (L98.1)
psychogenic pruritus (F45.8)
L29.0 **Pruritus ani**
L29.1 **Pruritus scroti**
L29.2 **Pruritus vulvae**
L29.3 **Anogenital pruritus, unspecified**
L29.8 **Other pruritus**
▶L29.81 **Cholestatic pruritus**
▶Code also, if applicable, type of liver disease
▶Use Additional code for adverse effect, if applicable, to identify drug (T36-T50 with fifth or sixth character 5)
▶L29.89 **Other pruritus**
L29.9 **Pruritus, unspecified**
Itch NOS

● L30 **Other and unspecified dermatitis**
Excludes2 contact dermatitis (L23-L25)
dry skin dermatitis (L85.3)
small plaque parapsoriasis (L41.3)
stasis dermatitis (I87.2)
L30.0 **Nummular dermatitis**
L30.1 **Dyshidrosis [pompholyx]**
L30.2 **Cutaneous autosensitization**
Candidid [levurid]
Eczematid
Dermatophytid
L30.3 **Infective dermatitis**
Infectious eczematoid dermatitis
L30.4 **Erythema intertrigo**

CHAPTER 12 (L00-L99)

L30.5 Pitytiasis alba
Coding Clinic: 2018, Q1, P6
L30.8 Other specified dermatitis
L30.9 Dermatitis, unspecified
Eczema NOS

PAPULOSQUAMOUS DISORDERS (L40-L45)

● L40 Psoriasis
L40.0 Psoriasis vulgaris
Nummular psoriasis Plaque psoriasis
L40.1 Generalized pustular psoriasis
Impetigo herpetiformis Von Zumbusch's disease
L40.2 Acrodermatitis continua
L40.3 Pustulosis palmaris et plantaris
L40.4 Guttate psoriasis
● L40.5 Arthropathic psoriasis
L40.50 Arthropathic psoriasis, unspecified
L40.51 Distal interphalangeal psoriatic arthropathy
L40.52 Psoriatic arthritis mutilans
L40.53 Psoriatic spondylitis
L40.54 Psoriatic juvenile arthropathy
L40.59 Other psoriatic arthropathy
L40.8 Other psoriasis
Flexural psoriasis
L40.9 Psoriasis, unspecified

● L41 Parapsoriasis
Excludes1 poikiloderma vasculare atrophicans (L94.5)
L41.0 Pityriasis lichenoides et varioliformis acuta
Mucha-Habermann disease
L41.1 Pityriasis lichenoides chronica
L41.3 Small plaque parapsoriasis
L41.4 Large plaque parapsoriasis
L41.5 Retiform parapsoriasis
L41.8 Other parapsoriasis
L41.9 Parapsoriasis, unspecified

L42 Pityriasis rosea

● L43 Lichen planus
Excludes1 lichen planopilaris (L66.1-)
L43.0 Hypertrophic lichen planus
L43.1 Bullous lichen planus
L43.2 Lichenoid drug reaction
Use additional code for adverse effect, if applicable, to identify drug (T36-T50 with fifth or sixth character 5)
L43.3 Subacute (active) lichen planus
Lichen planus tropicus
L43.8 Other lichen planus
L43.9 Lichen planus, unspecified

● L44 Other papulosquamous disorders
L44.0 Pityriasis rubra pilaris
L44.1 Lichen nitidus
L44.2 Lichen striatus
L44.3 Lichen ruber moniliformis
L44.4 Infantile papular acrodermatitis [Gianotti-Crosti] P
L44.8 Other specified papulosquamous disorders
L44.9 Papulosquamous disorder, unspecified

L45 Papulosquamous disorders in diseases classified elsewhere
Code first underlying disease

Item 12-8 Psoriasis is a chronic, recurrent inflammatory skin disease characterized by small patches covered with thick, silvery scales. **Parapsoriasis** is a treatment-resistant erythroderma. **Pityriasis rosea** is characterized by a herald patch that is a single large lesion and that usually appears on the trunk and is followed by scattered, smaller lesions.

URTICARIA AND ERYTHEMA (L49-L54)

Excludes1 Lyme disease (A69.2-)
rosacea (L71.-)

● L49 Exfoliation due to erythematous conditions according to extent of body surface involved
Code first erythematous condition causing exfoliation, such as:
Ritter's disease (L00)
(Staphylococcal) scalded skin syndrome (L00)
Stevens-Johnson syndrome (L51.1)
Stevens-Johnson syndrome-toxic epidermal necrolysis overlap syndrome (L51.3)
Toxic epidermal necrolysis (L51.2)
● L49.0 Exfoliation due to erythematous condition involving less than 10 percent of body surface
Exfoliation due to erythematous condition NOS
● L49.1 Exfoliation due to erythematous condition involving 10-19 percent of body surface
● L49.2 Exfoliation due to erythematous condition involving 20-29 percent of body surface
● L49.3 Exfoliation due to erythematous condition involving 30-39 percent of body surface Ex: No exclusions
● L49.4 Exfoliation due to erythematous condition involving 40-49 percent of body surface Ex: No exclusions
● L49.5 Exfoliation due to erythematous condition involving 50-59 percent of body surface Ex: No exclusions
● L49.6 Exfoliation due to erythematous condition involving 60-69 percent of body surface Ex: No exclusions
● L49.7 Exfoliation due to erythematous condition involving 70-79 percent of body surface Ex: No exclusions
● L49.8 Exfoliation due to erythematous condition involving 80-89 percent of body surface Ex: No exclusions
● L49.9 Exfoliation due to erythematous condition involving 90 or more percent of body surface Ex: No exclusions

● L50 Urticaria
Excludes1 allergic contact dermatitis (L23.-)
angioneurotic edema (T78.3)
giant urticaria (T78.3)
hereditary angio-edema (D84.1)
Quincke's edema (T78.3)
serum urticaria (T80.6-)
solar urticaria (L56.3)
urticaria neonatorum (P83.8)
urticaria papulosa (L28.2)
urticaria pigmentosa (D47.01)
L50.0 Allergic urticaria
L50.1 Idiopathic urticaria
L50.2 Urticaria due to cold and heat
Excludes2 familial cold urticaria (M04.2)
L50.3 Dermatographic urticaria
L50.4 Vibratory urticaria
L50.5 Cholinergic urticaria
L50.6 Contact urticaria

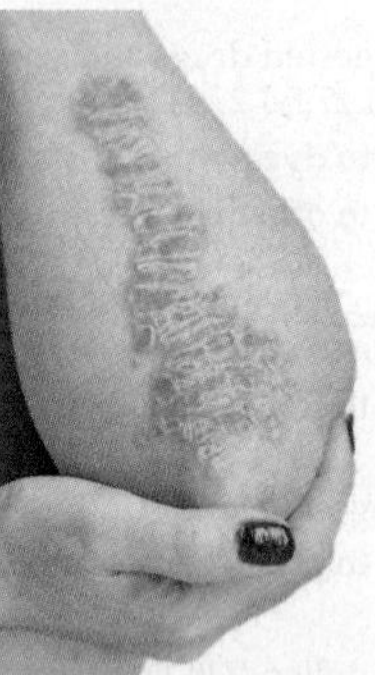

Figure 12-6 Erythematous plaques with silvery scales in a patient with psoriasis. (Getty Image)

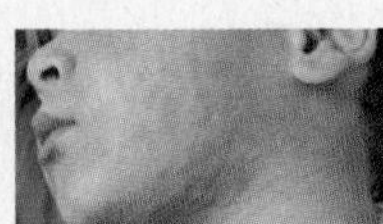

Figure 12-7 Urticaria (hives). *(Courtesy of David Effron, MD.)* (Getty Image)

Item 12-9 Urticaria is a vascular reaction in which wheals surrounded by a red halo appear and cause severe itching. The causes of urticaria or hives are extensive and varied (e.g., food, heat, cold, drugs, stress, infections).

L50.8 Other urticaria
Chronic urticaria
Recurrent periodic urticaria

L50.9 Urticaria, unspecified

● **L51 Erythema multiforme** Ex: PDX 1166
Use additional code for adverse effect, if applicable, to identify drug (T36-T50 with fifth or sixth character 5)
Use additional code to identify associated manifestations, such as:
arthropathy associated with dermatological disorders (M14.8-)
conjunctival edema (H11.42)
conjunctivitis (H10.22-)
corneal scars and opacities (H17.-)
corneal ulcer (H16.0-)
edema of eyelid (H02.84-)
inflammation of eyelid (H01.8)
keratoconjunctivitis sicca (H16.22-)
mechanical lagophthalmos (H02.22-)
stomatitis (K12.-)
symblepharon (H11.23-)
Use additional code to identify percentage of skin exfoliation (L49.-)
Excludes1 staphylococcal scalded skin syndrome (L00)
Ritter's disease (L00)

L51.0 Nonbullous erythema multiforme

L51.1 Stevens-Johnson syndrome

L51.2 Toxic epidermal necrolysis [Lyell]

L51.3 Stevens-Johnson syndrome-toxic epidermal necrolysis overlap syndrome
SJS-TEN overlap syndrome

L51.8 Other erythema multiforme

L51.9 Erythema multiforme, unspecified
Erythema iris
Erythema multiforme major NOS
Erythema multiforme minor NOS
Herpes iris

L52 Erythema nodosum
Excludes1 tuberculous erythema nodosum (A18.4)

● **L53 Other erythematous conditions** Ex: PDX 1167
Excludes1 erythema ab igne (L59.0)
erythema due to external agents in contact with skin (L23-L25)
erythema intertrigo (L30.4)

L53.0 Toxic erythema
Code first poisoning due to drug or toxin, if applicable (T36-T65 with fifth or sixth character 1-4)
Use additional code for adverse effect, if applicable, to identify drug (T36-T50 with fifth or sixth character 5)
Excludes1 neonatal erythema toxicum (P83.1)

L53.1 Erythema annulare centrifugum

L53.2 Erythema marginatum

L53.3 Other chronic figurate erythema

L53.8 Other specified erythematous conditions

L53.9 Erythematous condition, unspecified
Erythema NOS
Erythroderma NOS

L54 ***Erythema in diseases classified elsewhere***
Code first underlying disease

RADIATION-RELATED DISORDERS OF THE SKIN AND SUBCUTANEOUS TISSUE (L55-L59)

● **L55 Sunburn**

L55.0 Sunburn of first degree

L55.1 Sunburn of second degree

L55.2 Sunburn of third degree

L55.9 Sunburn, unspecified

● **L56 Other acute skin changes due to ultraviolet radiation**
Use additional code to identify the source of the ultraviolet radiation (W89, X32)

L56.0 Drug phototoxic response
Use additional code for adverse effect, if applicable, to identify drug (T36-T50 with fifth or sixth character 5)

L56.1 Drug photoallergic response
Use additional code for adverse effect, if applicable, to identify drug (T36-T50 with fifth or sixth character 5)

L56.2 Photocontact dermatitis [berloque dermatitis]

L56.3 Solar urticaria

L56.4 Polymorphous light eruption

L56.5 Disseminated superficial actinic porokeratosis (DSAP)

L56.8 Other specified acute skin changes due to ultraviolet radiation

L56.9 Acute skin change due to ultraviolet radiation, unspecified

● **L57 Skin changes due to chronic exposure to nonionizing radiation**
Use additional code to identify the source of the ultraviolet radiation (W89), or other nonionizing radiation (W90)

L57.0 Actinic keratosis
Keratosis NOS
Senile keratosis
Solar keratosis

L57.1 Actinic reticuloid

L57.2 Cutis rhomboidalis nuchae

L57.3 Poikiloderma of Civatte

L57.4 Cutis laxa senilis
Elastosis senilis

L57.5 Actinic granuloma

L57.8 Other skin changes due to chronic exposure to nonionizing radiation
Farmer's skin
Sailor's skin
Solar dermatitis

L57.9 Skin changes due to chronic exposure to nonionizing radiation, unspecified

● **L58 Radiodermatitis**
Use additional code to identify the source of the radiation (W88, W90)

L58.0 Acute radiodermatitis

L58.1 Chronic radiodermatitis

L58.9 Radiodermatitis, unspecified

● **L59 Other disorders of skin and subcutaneous tissue related to radiation**

L59.0 Erythema ab igne [dermatitis ab igne]

L59.8 Other specified disorders of the skin and subcutaneous tissue related to radiation
Coding Clinic: 2017, Q1, P34

L59.9 Disorder of the skin and subcutaneous tissue related to radiation, unspecified

DISORDERS OF SKIN APPENDAGES (L60-L75)

Excludes1 congenital malformations of integument (Q84.-)

● **L60 Nail disorders**
Excludes2 clubbing of nails (R68.3)
onychia and paronychia (L03.0-)

L60.0 Ingrowing nail

L60.1 Onycholysis

L60.2 Onychogryphosis

L6Ø.3 Nail dystrophy
L6Ø.4 Beau's lines
L6Ø.5 Yellow nail syndrome
L6Ø.8 Other nail disorders
L6Ø.9 Nail disorder, unspecified

L62 *Nail disorders in diseases classified elsewhere*
Code first underlying disease, such as:
pachydermoperiostosis (M89.4-)

● L63 **Alopecia areata**
L63.Ø Alopecia (capitis) totalis
L63.1 Alopecia universalis
L63.2 Ophiasis
L63.8 Other alopecia areata
L63.9 Alopecia areata, unspecified

● L64 **Androgenic alopecia**
Includes male-pattern baldness
L64.Ø Drug-induced androgenic alopecia
Use additional code for adverse effect, if applicable, to identify drug (T36-T5Ø with fifth or sixth character 5)
L64.8 Other androgenic alopecia
L64.9 Androgenic alopecia, unspecified

● L65 **Other nonscarring hair loss**
Use additional code for adverse effect, if applicable, to identify drug (T36-T5Ø with fifth or sixth character 5)
Excludes1 trichotillomania (F63.3)
L65.Ø Telogen effluvium
L65.1 Anagen effluvium
L65.2 Alopecia mucinosa
L65.8 Other specified nonscarring hair loss
L65.9 Nonscarring hair loss, unspecified
Alopecia NOS

● L66 **Cicatricial alopecia [scarring hair loss]**
L66.Ø Pseudopelade
L66.1 Lichen planopilaris
~~Follicular lichen planus~~
▶ L66.1Ø Lichen planopilaris, unspecified
▶ L66.11 Classic lichen planopilaris
▶ Follicular lichen planus
▶ L66.12 Frontal fibrosing alopecia
▶ FFA
▶ L66.19 Other lichen planopilaris
▶ Lassueur Graham-Little Piccardi syndrome
L66.2 Folliculitis decalvans
L66.3 Perifolliculitis capitis abscedens
L66.4 Folliculitis ulerythematosa reticulata
L66.8 Other cicatricial alopecia
Coding Clinic: 2Ø15, Q1, P19
▶ L66.81 Central centrifugal cicatricial alopecia
▶ AddCCCA
▶ L66.89 Other cicatricial alopecia
L66.9 Cicatricial alopecia, unspecified

Item 12–10 Alopecia is lack of hair and takes many forms. The most common is male pattern alopecia, also known as **androgenetic alopecia. Telogen effluvium** is early and excessive loss of hair resulting from a trauma to the hair follicle (fever, drugs, surgery, etc.).

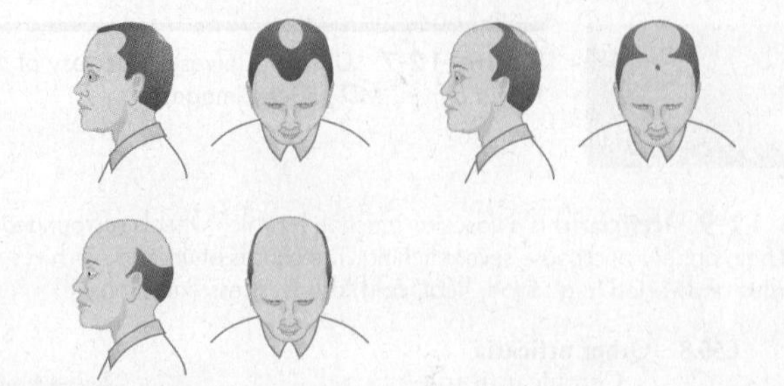

Figure 12-8 Male pattern alopecia.

● L67 **Hair color and hair shaft abnormalities**
Excludes1 monilethrix (Q84.1)
pili annulati (Q84.1)
telogen effluvium (L65.Ø)
L67.Ø Trichorrhexis nodosa
L67.1 Variations in hair color
Canities
Greyness, hair (premature)
Heterochromia of hair
Poliosis circumscripta, acquired
Poliosis NOS
L67.8 Other hair color and hair shaft abnormalities
Fragilitas crinium
L67.9 Hair color and hair shaft abnormality, unspecified

● L68 **Hypertrichosis**
Includes excess hair
Excludes1 congenital hypertrichosis (Q84.2)
persistent lanugo (Q84.2)
L68.Ø Hirsutism
Excessive growth of hair
L68.1 Acquired hypertrichosis lanuginosa
L68.2 Localized hypertrichosis
L68.3 Polytrichia
L68.8 Other hypertrichosis
L68.9 Hypertrichosis, unspecified

● L7Ø **Acne**
Excludes2 acne keloid (L73.Ø)
L7Ø.Ø Acne vulgaris
L7Ø.1 Acne conglobata
L7Ø.2 Acne varioliformis
Acne necrotica miliaris
L7Ø.3 Acne tropica
L7Ø.4 Infantile acne
L7Ø.5 Acné excoriée
Acné excoriée des jeunes filles
Picker's acne
L7Ø.8 Other acne
L7Ø.9 Acne, unspecified

● L71 **Rosacea**
Use additional code for adverse effect, if applicable, to identify drug (T36-T5Ø with fifth or sixth character 5)
L71.Ø Perioral dermatitis
L71.1 Rhinophyma
L71.8 Other rosacea
Coding Clinic: 2Ø18, Q4, P15
L71.9 Rosacea, unspecified

● L72 **Follicular cysts of skin and subcutaneous tissue**
L72.Ø Epidermal cyst
● L72.1 Pilar and trichodermal cyst
L72.11 Pilar cyst
L72.12 Trichodermal cyst
Trichilemmal (proliferating) cyst

L72.3 **Sebaceous cyst**
Excludes2 pilar cyst (L72.11)
trichilemmal (proliferating) cyst (L72.12)
L72.2 **Steatocystoma multiplex**
L72.8 **Other follicular cysts of the skin and subcutaneous tissue**
L72.9 **Follicular cyst of the skin and subcutaneous tissue, unspecified**

L73 **Other follicular disorders**
L73.0 **Acne keloid**
L73.1 **Pseudofolliculitis barbae**
L73.2 **Hidradenitis suppurativa**
L73.8 **Other specified follicular disorders**
Sycosis barbae
L73.9 **Follicular disorder, unspecified**

L74 **Eccrine sweat disorders**
Excludes2 generalized hyperhidrosis (R61)
L74.0 **Miliaria rubra**
L74.1 **Miliaria crystallina**
L74.2 **Miliaria profunda**
Miliaria tropicalis
L74.3 **Miliaria, unspecified**
L74.4 **Anhidrosis**
Hypohidrosis
L74.5 **Focal hyperhidrosis**
L74.51 **Primary focal hyperhidrosis**
L74.510 **Primary focal hyperhidrosis, axilla**
L74.511 **Primary focal hyperhidrosis, face**
L74.512 **Primary focal hyperhidrosis, palms**
L74.513 **Primary focal hyperhidrosis, soles**
L74.519 **Primary focal hyperhidrosis, unspecified**
L74.52 **Secondary focal hyperhidrosis**
Frey's syndrome
L74.8 **Other eccrine sweat disorders**
L74.9 **Eccrine sweat disorder, unspecified**
Sweat gland disorder NOS

L75 **Apocrine sweat disorders**
Excludes1 dyshidrosis (L30.1)
hidradenitis suppurativa (L73.2)
L75.0 **Bromhidrosis**
L75.1 **Chromhidrosis**
L75.2 **Apocrine miliaria**
Fox-Fordyce disease
L75.8 **Other apocrine sweat disorders**
L75.9 **Apocrine sweat disorder, unspecified**
Intraoperative and postprocedural complications of skin and subcutaneous tissue (L76)

INTRAOPERATIVE AND POSTPROCEDURAL COMPLICATIONS OF SKIN AND SUBCUTANEOUS TISSUE (L76)

L76 **Intraoperative and postprocedural complications of skin and subcutaneous tissue**
Coding Clinic: 2016, Q4, P10
L76.0 **Intraoperative hemorrhage and hematoma of skin and subcutaneous tissue complicating a procedure** (Ex) PDX 1168
Excludes1 intraoperative hemorrhage and hematoma of skin and subcutaneous tissue due to accidental puncture and laceration during a procedure (L76.1-)
L76.01 **Intraoperative hemorrhage and hematoma of skin and subcutaneous tissue complicating a dermatologic procedure**
L76.02 **Intraoperative hemorrhage and hematoma of skin and subcutaneous tissue complicating other procedure**

L76.1 **Accidental puncture and laceration of skin and subcutaneous tissue during a procedure** (Ex) PDX 569
L76.11 **Accidental puncture and laceration of skin and subcutaneous tissue during a dermatologic procedure**
L76.12 **Accidental puncture and laceration of skin and subcutaneous tissue during other procedure**
L76.2 **Postprocedural hemorrhage of skin and subcutaneous tissue following a procedure** (Ex) PDX 1168
L76.21 **Postprocedural hemorrhage of skin and subcutaneous tissue following a dermatologic procedure**
L76.22 **Postprocedural hemorrhage of skin and subcutaneous tissue following other procedure**
L76.3 **Postprocedural hematoma and seroma of skin and subcutaneous tissue following a procedure** (Ex) PDX 1168
L76.31 **Postprocedural hematoma of skin and subcutaneous tissue following a dermatologic procedure**
L76.32 **Postprocedural hematoma of skin and subcutaneous tissue following other procedure**
L76.33 **Postprocedural seroma of skin and subcutaneous tissue following a dermatologic procedure**
L76.34 **Postprocedural seroma of skin and subcutaneous tissue following other procedure**
L76.8 **Other intraoperative and postprocedural complications of skin and subcutaneous tissue**
Use additional code, if applicable, to further specify disorder
L76.81 **Other intraoperative complications of skin and subcutaneous tissue**
L76.82 **Other postprocedural complications of skin and subcutaneous tissue**
Coding Clinic: 2017, Q3, P6

OTHER DISORDERS OF THE SKIN AND SUBCUTANEOUS TISSUE (L80-L99)

L80 **Vitiligo**
Excludes2 vitiligo of eyelids (H02.73-)
vitiligo of vulva (N90.89)

L81 **Other disorders of pigmentation**
Excludes1 birthmark NOS (Q82.5)
Peutz-Jeghers syndrome (Q85.89)
Excludes2 nevus - see Alphabetical Index
L81.0 **Postinflammatory hyperpigmentation**
L81.1 **Chloasma**
L81.2 **Freckles**
L81.3 **Café au lait spots**
L81.4 **Other melanin hyperpigmentation**
Lentigo
L81.5 **Leukoderma, not elsewhere classified**
L81.6 **Other disorders of diminished melanin formation**
L81.7 **Pigmented purpuric dermatosis**
Angioma serpiginosum
L81.8 **Other specified disorders of pigmentation**
Iron pigmentation
Tattoo pigmentation
L81.9 **Disorder of pigmentation, unspecified**

L82 **Seborrheic keratosis**
Includes basal cell papilloma
dermatosis papulosa nigra
Leser-Trélat disease
Excludes2 seborrheic dermatitis (L21.-)
L82.0 **Inflamed seborrheic keratosis**
Coding Clinic: 2023, Q2, P12; 2021, Q3, P11

L82.1 Other seborrheic keratosis
Seborrheic keratosis NOS

L83 Acanthosis nigricans
Confluent and reticulated papillomatosis

L84 Corns and callosities
Callus
Clavus

L85 Other epidermal thickening
Excludes2 hypertrophic disorders of the skin (L91.-)

L85.0 Acquired ichthyosis
Excludes1 congenital ichthyosis (Q80.-)

L85.1 Acquired keratosis [keratoderma] palmaris et plantaris
Excludes1 inherited keratosis palmaris et plantaris (Q82.8)

L85.2 Keratosis punctata (palmaris et plantaris)

L85.3 Xerosis cutis
Dry skin dermatitis

L85.8 Other specified epidermal thickening
Cutaneous horn

L85.9 Epidermal thickening, unspecified

L86 *Keratoderma in diseases classified elsewhere*
Firm horny papules that have a cobblestone appearance
Code first underlying disease, such as:
Reiter's disease (M02.3-)
Excludes1 gonococcal keratoderma (A54.89)
gonococcal keratosis (A54.89)
keratoderma due to vitamin A deficiency (E50.8)
keratosis due to vitamin A deficiency (E50.8)
xeroderma due to vitamin A deficiency (E50.8)

L87 Transepidermal elimination disorders
Excludes1 granuloma annulare (perforating) (L92.0)

L87.0 Keratosis follicularis et parafollicularis in cutem penetrans
Kyrle disease
Hyperkeratosis follicularis penetrans

L87.1 Reactive perforating collagenosis

L87.2 Elastosis perforans serpiginosa

L87.8 Other transepidermal elimination disorders

L87.9 Transepidermal elimination disorder, unspecified

L88 Pyoderma gangrenosum Ex: PDX 1169
Phagedenic pyoderma
Excludes1 dermatitis gangrenosa (L08.0)

OGCR Section I.B.14.

General Coding Guidelines

Documentation for BMI, *Depth of* Non-pressure ulcers, Pressure Ulcer Stages, **Coma Scale, and** *NIH Stroke Scale*

For the Body Mass Index (BMI), depth of non-pressure chronic ulcers, pressure ulcer stage, **coma scale, and NIH stroke scale (NIHSS) codes,** code assignment may be based on medical record documentation from clinicians who are not the patient's provider (i.e., physician or other qualified healthcare practitioner legally accountable for establishing the patient's diagnosis), since this information is typically documented by other clinicians involved in the care of the patient (e.g., a dietitian often documents the BMI, a nurse often documents the pressure ulcer stages**, and an emergency medical technician often documents the coma scale**). However, the associated diagnosis (such as overweight, obesity, **acute stroke,** or pressure ulcer) must be documented by the patient's provider. If there is conflicting medical record documentation, either from the same clinician or different clinicians, the patient's attending provider should be queried for clarification.

The BMI, **coma scale, and NHSS** codes should only be reported as secondary diagnoses.

L89 Pressure ulcer Ex: PDX 1170
Includes bed sore
decubitus ulcer
plaster ulcer
pressure area
pressure sore
Code first any associated gangrene (I96)
Excludes2 decubitus (trophic) ulcer of cervix (uteri) (N86)
diabetic ulcers (E08.621, E08.622, E09.621, E09.622, E10.621, E10.622, E11.621, E11.622, E13.621, E13.622)
non-pressure chronic ulcer of skin (L97.-)
skin infections (L00-L08)
varicose ulcer (I83.0, I83.2)
Coding Clinic: 2019, Q4, P11; 2018, Q2, P22; 2016, Q4, P124

L89.0 Pressure ulcer of elbow

L89.00 Pressure ulcer of unspecified elbow

L89.000 Pressure ulcer of unspecified elbow, unstageable

L89.001 Pressure ulcer of unspecified elbow, stage 1
Healing pressure ulcer of unspecified elbow, stage 1
Pressure pre-ulcer skin changes limited to persistent focal edema, unspecified elbow

L89.002 Pressure ulcer of unspecified elbow, stage 2
Healing pressure ulcer of unspecified elbow, stage 2
Pressure ulcer with abrasion, blister, partial thickness skin loss involving epidermis and/or dermis, unspecified elbow

L89.003 Pressure ulcer of unspecified elbow, stage 3
Healing pressure ulcer of unspecified elbow, stage 3
Pressure ulcer with full thickness skin loss involving damage or necrosis of subcutaneous tissue, unspecified elbow
MCC when PDx is its own MCC

L89.004 Pressure ulcer of unspecified elbow, stage 4
Healing pressure ulcer of unspecified elbow, stage 4
Pressure ulcer with necrosis of soft tissues through to underlying muscle, tendon, or bone, unspecified elbow
MCC when PDx is its own MCC

L89.006 Pressure-induced deep tissue damage of unspecified elbow

L89.009 Pressure ulcer of unspecified elbow, unspecified stage
Healing pressure ulcer of elbow NOS
Healing pressure ulcer of unspecified elbow, unspecified stage

L89.01 Pressure ulcer of right elbow

L89.010 Pressure ulcer of right elbow, unstageable

L89.011 Pressure ulcer of right elbow, stage 1
Healing pressure ulcer of right elbow, stage 1
Pressure pre-ulcer skin changes limited to persistent focal edema, right elbow

L89.012 Pressure ulcer of right elbow, stage 2
Healing pressure ulcer of right elbow, stage 2
Pressure ulcer with abrasion, blister, partial thickness skin loss involving epidermis and/or dermis, right elbow

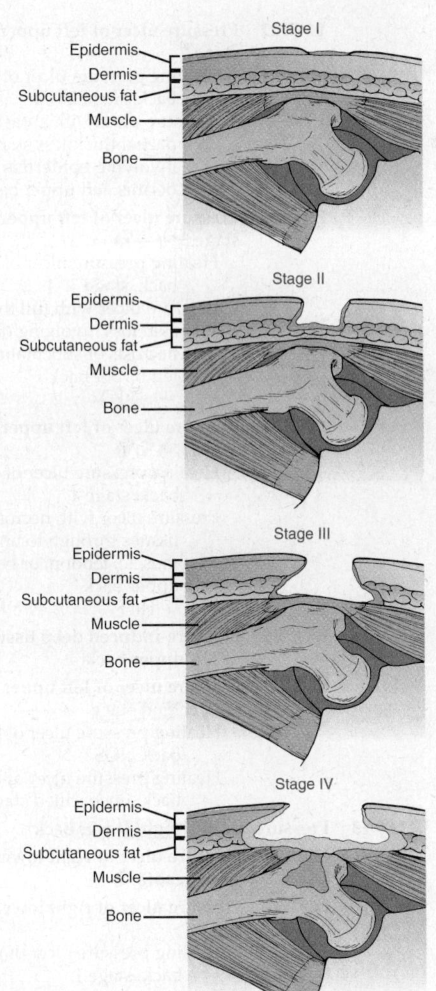

Figure 12-9 Stage I, II, III, and IV of pressure ulcers.

L89.013 Pressure ulcer of right elbow, stage 3
Healing pressure ulcer of right elbow, stage 3
Pressure ulcer with full thickness skin loss involving damage or necrosis of subcutaneous tissue, right elbow
MCC when PDx is its own MCC

L89.014 Pressure ulcer of right elbow, stage 4
Healing pressure ulcer of right elbow, stage 4
Pressure ulcer with necrosis of soft tissues through to underlying muscle, tendon, or bone, right elbow
MCC when PDx is its own MCC

L89.016 Pressure-induced deep tissue damage of right elbow

L89.019 Pressure ulcer of right elbow, unspecified stage
Healing pressure ulcer of right elbow NOS

L89.02 Pressure ulcer of left elbow

L89.020 Pressure ulcer of left elbow, unstageable

L89.021 Pressure ulcer of left elbow, stage 1
Healing pressure ulcer of left elbow, stage 1
Pressure pre-ulcer skin changes limited to persistent focal edema, left elbow

L89.022 Pressure ulcer of left elbow, stage 2
Healing pressure ulcer of left elbow, stage 2
Pressure ulcer with abrasion, blister, partial thickness skin loss involving epidermis and/or dermis, left elbow

L89.023 Pressure ulcer of left elbow, stage 3
Healing pressure ulcer of left elbow, stage 3
Pressure ulcer with full thickness skin loss involving damage or necrosis of subcutaneous tissue, left elbow
MCC when PDx is its own MCC

L89.024 Pressure ulcer of left elbow, stage 4
Healing pressure ulcer of left elbow, stage 4
Pressure ulcer with necrosis of soft tissues through to underlying muscle, tendon, or bone, left elbow
MCC when PDx is its own MCC

L89.026 Pressure-induced deep tissue damage of left elbow

L89.029 Pressure ulcer of left elbow, unspecified stage
Healing pressure ulcer of left elbow NOS

L89.1 Pressure ulcer of back

L89.10 Pressure ulcer of unspecified part of back

L89.100 Pressure ulcer of unspecified part of back, unstageable

L89.101 Pressure ulcer of unspecified part of back, stage 1
Healing pressure ulcer of unspecified part of back, stage 1
Pressure pre-ulcer skin changes limited to persistent focal edema, unspecified part of back

L89.102 Pressure ulcer of unspecified part of back, stage 2
Healing pressure ulcer of unspecified part of back, stage 2
Pressure ulcer with abrasion, blister, partial thickness skin loss involving epidermis and/or dermis, unspecified part of back

L89.103 Pressure ulcer of unspecified part of back, stage 3
Healing pressure ulcer of unspecified part of back, stage 3
Pressure ulcer with full thickness skin loss involving damage or necrosis of subcutaneous tissue, unspecified part of back
MCC when PDx is its own MCC

CHAPTER 12 (L00-L99)

L89.104 Pressure ulcer of unspecified part of back, stage 4
Healing pressure ulcer of unspecified part of back, stage 4
Pressure ulcer with necrosis of soft tissues through to underlying muscle, tendon, or bone, unspecified part of back
MCC when PDx is its own MCC

L89.106 Pressure-induced deep tissue damage of unspecified part of back

L89.109 Pressure ulcer of unspecified part of back, unspecified stage
Healing pressure ulcer of unspecified part of back NOS
Healing pressure ulcer of unspecified part of back, unspecified stage

● **L89.11 Pressure ulcer of right upper back**
Pressure ulcer of right shoulder blade

L89.110 Pressure ulcer of right upper back, unstageable

L89.111 Pressure ulcer of right upper back, stage 1
Healing pressure ulcer of right upper back, stage 1
Pressure pre-ulcer skin changes limited to persistent focal edema, right upper back

L89.112 Pressure ulcer of right upper back, stage 2
Healing pressure ulcer of right upper back, stage 2
Pressure ulcer with abrasion, blister, partial thickness skin loss involving epidermis and/or dermis, right upper back

L89.113 Pressure ulcer of right upper back, stage 3
Healing pressure ulcer of right upper back, stage 3
Pressure ulcer with full thickness skin loss involving damage or necrosis of subcutaneous tissue, right upper back
MCC when PDx is its own MCC

L89.114 Pressure ulcer of right upper back, stage 4
Healing pressure ulcer of right upper back, stage 4
Pressure ulcer with necrosis of soft tissues through to underlying muscle, tendon, or bone, right upper back
MCC when PDx is its own MCC

L89.116 Pressure-induced deep tissue damage of right upper back

L89.119 Pressure ulcer of right upper back, unspecified stage
Healing pressure ulcer of right upper back NOS
Healing pressure ulcer of right upper back, unspecified stage

● **L89.12 Pressure ulcer of left upper back**
Pressure ulcer of left shoulder blade

L89.120 Pressure ulcer of left upper back, unstageable

L89.121 Pressure ulcer of left upper back, stage 1
Healing pressure ulcer of left upper back, stage 1
Pressure pre-ulcer skin changes limited to persistent focal edema, left upper back

L89.122 Pressure ulcer of left upper back, stage 2
Healing pressure ulcer of left upper back, stage 2
Pressure ulcer with abrasion, blister, partial thickness skin loss involving epidermis and/or dermis, left upper back

L89.123 Pressure ulcer of left upper back, stage 3
Healing pressure ulcer of left upper back, stage 3
Pressure ulcer with full thickness skin loss involving damage or necrosis of subcutaneous tissue, left upper back
MCC when PDx is its own MCC

L89.124 Pressure ulcer of left upper back, stage 4
Healing pressure ulcer of left upper back, stage 4
Pressure ulcer with necrosis of soft tissues through to underlying muscle, tendon, or bone, left upper back
MCC when PDx is its own MCC

L89.126 Pressure-induced deep tissue damage of left upper back

L89.129 Pressure ulcer of left upper back, unspecified stage
Healing pressure ulcer of left upper back NOS
Healing pressure ulcer of left upper back, unspecified stage

● **L89.13 Pressure ulcer of right lower back**

L89.130 Pressure ulcer of right lower back, unstageable

L89.131 Pressure ulcer of right lower back, stage 1
Healing pressure ulcer of right lower back, stage 1
Pressure pre-ulcer skin changes limited to persistent focal edema, right lower back

L89.132 Pressure ulcer of right lower back, stage 2
Healing pressure ulcer of right lower back, stage 2
Pressure ulcer with abrasion, blister, partial thickness skin loss involving epidermis and/or dermis, right lower back

L89.133 Pressure ulcer of right lower back, stage 3
Healing pressure ulcer of right lower back, stage 3
Pressure ulcer with full thickness skin loss involving damage or necrosis of subcutaneous tissue, right lower back
MCC when PDx is its own MCC

L89.134 Pressure ulcer of right lower back, stage 4
Healing pressure ulcer of right lower back, stage 4
Pressure ulcer with necrosis of soft tissues through to underlying muscle, tendon, or bone, right lower back
MCC when PDx is its own MCC

L89.136 Pressure-induced deep tissue damage of right lower back

L89.139 Pressure ulcer of right lower back, unspecified stage
Healing pressure ulcer of right lower back NOS
Healing pressure ulcer of right lower back, unspecified stage

L89.14 Pressure ulcer of left lower back

L89.140 Pressure ulcer of left lower back, unstageable

L89.141 Pressure ulcer of left lower back, stage 1
Healing pressure ulcer of left lower back, stage 1
Pressure pre-ulcer skin changes limited to persistent focal edema, left lower back

L89.142 Pressure ulcer of left lower back, stage 2
Healing pressure ulcer of left lower back, stage 2
Pressure ulcer with abrasion, blister, partial thickness skin loss involving epidermis and/or dermis, left lower back

L89.143 Pressure ulcer of left lower back, stage 3
Healing pressure ulcer of left lower back, stage 3
Pressure ulcer with full thickness skin loss involving damage or necrosis of subcutaneous tissue, left lower back
MCC when PDx is its own MCC

L89.144 Pressure ulcer of left lower back, stage 4
Healing pressure ulcer of left lower back, stage 4
Pressure ulcer with necrosis of soft tissues through to underlying muscle, tendon, or bone, left lower back
MCC when PDx is its own MCC

L89.146 Pressure-induced deep tissue damage of left lower back

L89.149 Pressure ulcer of left lower back, unspecified stage
Healing pressure ulcer of left lower back NOS
Healing pressure ulcer of left lower back, unspecified stage

L89.15 Pressure ulcer of sacral region
Pressure ulcer of coccyx
Pressure ulcer of tailbone
Coding Clinic: 2021, Q3, P10

L89.150 Pressure ulcer of sacral region, unstageable

L89.151 Pressure ulcer of sacral region, stage 1
Healing pressure ulcer of sacral region, stage 1
Pressure pre-ulcer skin changes limited to persistent focal edema, sacral region

L89.152 Pressure ulcer of sacral region, stage 2
Healing pressure ulcer of sacral region, stage 2
Pressure ulcer with abrasion, blister, partial thickness skin loss involving epidermis and/or dermis, sacral region

L89.153 Pressure ulcer of sacral region, stage 3
Healing pressure ulcer of sacral region, stage 3
Pressure ulcer with full thickness skin loss involving damage or necrosis of subcutaneous tissue, sacral region
MCC when PDx is its own MCC
Coding Clinic: 2021, Q3, P10

L89.154 Pressure ulcer of sacral region, stage 4
Healing pressure ulcer of sacral region, stage 4
Pressure ulcer with necrosis of soft tissues through to underlying muscle, tendon, or bone, sacral region
MCC when PDx is its own MCC
Coding Clinic: 2022, Q2, P9; 2021, Q1, P24

L89.156 Pressure-induced deep tissue damage of sacral region

L89.159 Pressure ulcer of sacral region, unspecified stage
Healing pressure ulcer of sacral region NOS
Healing pressure ulcer of sacral region, unspecified stage

L89.2 Pressure ulcer of hip

L89.20 Pressure ulcer of unspecified hip

L89.200 Pressure ulcer of unspecified hip, unstageable

L89.201 Pressure ulcer of unspecified hip, stage 1
Healing pressure ulcer of unspecified hip back, stage 1
Pressure pre-ulcer skin changes limited to persistent focal edema, unspecified hip

L89.202 Pressure ulcer of unspecified hip, stage 2
Healing pressure ulcer of unspecified hip, stage 2
Pressure ulcer with abrasion, blister, partial thickness skin loss involving epidermis and/or dermis, unspecified hip

L89.203 Pressure ulcer of unspecified hip, stage 3
Healing pressure ulcer of unspecified hip, stage 3
Pressure ulcer with full thickness skin loss involving damage or necrosis of subcutaneous tissue, unspecified hip
MCC when PDx is its own MCC

L89.204 Pressure ulcer of unspecified hip, stage 4
Healing pressure ulcer of unspecified hip, stage 4
Pressure ulcer with necrosis of soft tissues through to underlying muscle, tendon, or bone, unspecified hip
MCC when PDx is its own MCC

L89.206 Pressure-induced deep tissue damage of unspecified hip

L89.209 Pressure ulcer of unspecified hip, unspecified stage
Healing pressure ulcer of unspecified hip NOS
Healing pressure ulcer of unspecified hip, unspecified stage

CHAPTER 12 (L00-L99)

- ● **L89.21 Pressure ulcer of right hip**
  - **L89.210 Pressure ulcer of right hip, unstageable**
  - **L89.211 Pressure ulcer of right hip, stage 1**
    - Healing pressure ulcer of right hip back, stage 1
    - Pressure pre-ulcer skin changes limited to persistent focal edema, right hip
  - **L89.212 Pressure ulcer of right hip, stage 2**
    - Healing pressure ulcer of right hip, stage 2
    - Pressure ulcer with abrasion, blister, partial thickness skin loss involving epidermis and/or dermis, right hip
  - **L89.213 Pressure ulcer of right hip, stage 3**
    - Healing pressure ulcer of right hip, stage 3
    - Pressure ulcer with full thickness skin loss involving damage or necrosis of subcutaneous tissue, right hip
    - MCC when PDx is its own MCC
  - **L89.214 Pressure ulcer of right hip, stage 4**
    - Healing pressure ulcer of right hip, stage 4
    - Pressure ulcer with necrosis of soft tissues through to underlying muscle, tendon, or bone, right hip
    - MCC when PDx is its own MCC
  - **L89.216 Pressure-induced deep tissue damage of right hip**
  - **L89.219 Pressure ulcer of right hip, unspecified stage**
    - Healing pressure ulcer of right hip NOS
    - Healing pressure ulcer of right hip, unspecified stage
- ● **L89.22 Pressure ulcer of left hip**
  - **L89.220 Pressure ulcer of left hip, unstageable**
  - **L89.221 Pressure ulcer of left hip, stage 1**
    - Healing pressure ulcer of left hip back, stage 1
    - Pressure pre-ulcer skin changes limited to persistent focal edema, left hip
  - **L89.222 Pressure ulcer of left hip, stage 2**
    - Healing pressure ulcer of left hip, stage 2
    - Pressure ulcer with abrasion, blister, partial thickness skin loss involving epidermis and/or dermis, left hip
  - **L89.223 Pressure ulcer of left hip, stage 3**
    - Healing pressure ulcer of left hip, stage 3
    - Pressure ulcer with full thickness skin loss involving damage or necrosis of subcutaneous tissue, left hip
    - MCC when PDx is its own MCC
  - **L89.224 Pressure ulcer of left hip, stage 4**
    - Healing pressure ulcer of left hip, stage 4
    - Pressure ulcer with necrosis of soft tissues through to underlying muscle, tendon, or bone, left hip
    - MCC when PDx is its own MCC
  - **L89.226 Pressure-induced deep tissue damage of left hip**
  - **L89.229 Pressure ulcer of left hip, unspecified stage**
    - Healing pressure ulcer of left hip NOS
    - Healing pressure ulcer of left hip, unspecified stage
- ● **L89.3 Pressure ulcer of buttock**
  - ● **L89.30 Pressure ulcer of unspecified buttock**
    - **L89.300 Pressure ulcer of unspecified buttock, unstageable**
    - **L89.301 Pressure ulcer of unspecified buttock, stage 1**
      - Healing pressure ulcer of unspecified buttock, stage 1
      - Pressure pre-ulcer skin changes limited to persistent focal edema, unspecified buttock
    - **L89.302 Pressure ulcer of unspecified buttock, stage 2**
      - Healing pressure ulcer of unspecified buttock, stage 2
      - Pressure ulcer with abrasion, blister, partial thickness skin loss involving epidermis and/or dermis, unspecified buttock
    - **L89.303 Pressure ulcer of unspecified buttock, stage 3**
      - Healing pressure ulcer of unspecified buttock, stage 3
      - Pressure ulcer with full thickness skin loss involving damage or necrosis of subcutaneous tissue, unspecified buttock
      - MCC when PDx is its own MCC
    - **L89.304 Pressure ulcer of unspecified buttock, stage 4**
      - Healing pressure ulcer of unspecified buttock, stage 4
      - Pressure ulcer with necrosis of soft tissues through to underlying muscle, tendon, or bone, unspecified buttock
      - MCC when PDx is its own MCC
    - **L89.306 Pressure-induced deep tissue damage of unspecified buttock**
    - **L89.309 Pressure ulcer of unspecified buttock, unspecified stage**
      - Healing pressure ulcer of unspecified buttock NOS
      - Healing pressure ulcer of unspecified buttock, unspecified stage
  - ● **L89.31 Pressure ulcer of right buttock**
    - **L89.310 Pressure ulcer of right buttock, unstageable**
    - **L89.311 Pressure ulcer of right buttock, stage 1**
      - Healing pressure ulcer of right buttock, stage 1
      - Pressure pre-ulcer skin changes limited to persistent focal edema, right buttock
    - **L89.312 Pressure ulcer of right buttock, stage 2**
      - Healing pressure ulcer of right buttock, stage 2
      - Pressure ulcer with abrasion, blister, partial thickness skin loss involving epidermis and/or dermis, right buttock

L89.313 Pressure ulcer of right buttock, stage 3
Healing pressure ulcer of right buttock, stage 3
Pressure ulcer with full thickness skin loss involving damage or necrosis of subcutaneous tissue, right buttock
MCC when PDx is its own MCC

L89.314 Pressure ulcer of right buttock, stage 4
Healing pressure ulcer of right buttock, stage 4
Pressure ulcer with necrosis of soft tissues through to underlying muscle, tendon, or bone, right buttock
MCC when PDx is its own MCC

L89.316 Pressure-induced deep tissue damage of right buttock

L89.319 Pressure ulcer of right buttock, unspecified stage
Healing pressure ulcer of right buttock NOS
Healing pressure ulcer of right buttock, unspecified stage

● L89.32 Pressure ulcer of left buttock

L89.320 Pressure ulcer of left buttock, unstageable

L89.321 Pressure ulcer of left buttock, stage 1
Healing pressure ulcer of left buttock, stage 1
Pressure pre-ulcer skin changes limited to persistent focal edema, left buttock

L89.322 Pressure ulcer of left buttock, stage 2
Healing pressure ulcer of left buttock, stage 2
Pressure ulcer with abrasion, blister, partial thickness skin loss involving epidermis and/or dermis, left buttock

L89.323 Pressure ulcer of left buttock, stage 3
Healing pressure ulcer of left buttock, stage 3
Pressure ulcer with full thickness skin loss involving damage or necrosis of subcutaneous tissue, left buttock
MCC when PDx is its own MCC

L89.324 Pressure ulcer of left buttock, stage 4
Healing pressure ulcer of left buttock, stage 4
Pressure ulcer with necrosis of soft tissues through to underlying muscle, tendon, or bone, left buttock
MCC when PDx is its own MCC

L89.326 Pressure-induced deep tissue damage of left buttock

L89.329 Pressure ulcer of left buttock, unspecified stage
Healing pressure ulcer of left buttock NOS
Healing pressure ulcer of left buttock, unspecified stage

● L89.4 Pressure ulcer of contiguous site of back, buttock and hip

L89.40 Pressure ulcer of contiguous site of back, buttock and hip, unspecified stage
Healing pressure ulcer of contiguous site of back, buttock and hip NOS
Healing pressure ulcer of contiguous site of back, buttock and hip, unspecified stage

L89.41 Pressure ulcer of contiguous site of back, buttock and hip, stage 1
Healing pressure ulcer of contiguous site of back, buttock and hip, stage 1
Pressure pre-ulcer skin changes limited to persistent focal edema, contiguous site of back, buttock and hip

L89.42 Pressure ulcer of contiguous site of back, buttock and hip, stage 2
Healing pressure ulcer of contiguous site of back, buttock and hip, stage 2
Pressure ulcer with abrasion, blister, partial thickness skin loss involving epidermis and/or dermis, contiguous site of back, buttock and hip

L89.43 Pressure ulcer of contiguous site of back, buttock and hip, stage 3
Healing pressure ulcer of contiguous site of back, buttock and hip, stage 3
Pressure ulcer with full thickness skin loss involving damage or necrosis of subcutaneous tissue, contiguous site of back, buttock and hip
MCC when PDx is its own MCC

L89.44 Pressure ulcer of contiguous site of back, buttock and hip, stage 4
Healing pressure ulcer of contiguous site of back, buttock and hip, stage 4
Pressure ulcer with necrosis of soft tissues through to underlying muscle, tendon, or bone, contiguous site of back, buttock and hip
MCC when PDx is its own MCC

L89.45 Pressure ulcer of contiguous site of back, buttock and hip, unstageable

L89.46 Pressure-induced deep tissue damage of contiguous site of back, buttock and hip

● L89.5 Pressure ulcer of ankle

● L89.50 Pressure ulcer of unspecified ankle

L89.500 Pressure ulcer of unspecified ankle, unstageable

L89.501 Pressure ulcer of unspecified ankle, stage 1
Healing pressure ulcer of unspecified ankle, stage 1
Pressure pre-ulcer skin changes limited to persistent focal edema, unspecified ankle

L89.502 Pressure ulcer of unspecified ankle, stage 2
Healing pressure ulcer of unspecified ankle, stage 2
Pressure ulcer with abrasion, blister, partial thickness skin loss involving epidermis and/or dermis, unspecified ankle

L89.503 Pressure ulcer of unspecified ankle, stage 3
Healing pressure ulcer of unspecified ankle, stage 3
Pressure ulcer with full thickness skin loss involving damage or necrosis of subcutaneous tissue, unspecified ankle
MCC when PDx is its own MCC

L89.504 Pressure ulcer of unspecified ankle, stage 4
Healing pressure ulcer of unspecified ankle, stage 4
Pressure ulcer with necrosis of soft tissues through to underlying muscle, tendon, or bone, unspecified ankle
MCC when PDx is its own MCC

L89.506 Pressure-induced deep tissue damage of unspecified ankle

L89.509 Pressure ulcer of unspecified ankle, unspecified stage
Healing pressure ulcer of unspecified ankle NOS
Healing pressure ulcer of unspecified ankle, unspecified stage

● **L89.51 Pressure ulcer of right ankle**

L89.510 Pressure ulcer of right ankle, unstageable

L89.511 Pressure ulcer of right ankle, stage 1
Healing pressure ulcer of right ankle, stage 1
Pressure pre-ulcer skin changes limited to persistent focal edema, right ankle

L89.512 Pressure ulcer of right ankle, stage 2
Healing pressure ulcer of right ankle, stage 2
Pressure ulcer with abrasion, blister, partial thickness skin loss involving epidermis and/or dermis, right ankle

L89.513 Pressure ulcer of right ankle, stage 3
Healing pressure ulcer of right ankle, stage 3
Pressure ulcer with full thickness skin loss involving damage or necrosis of subcutaneous tissue, right ankle
MCC when PDx is its own MCC

L89.514 Pressure ulcer of right ankle, stage 4
Healing pressure ulcer of right ankle, stage 4
Pressure ulcer with necrosis of soft tissues through to underlying muscle, tendon, or bone, right ankle
MCC when PDx is its own MCC

L89.516 Pressure-induced deep tissue damage of right ankle

L89.519 Pressure ulcer of right ankle, unspecified stage
Healing pressure ulcer of right ankle NOS
Healing pressure ulcer of right ankle, unspecified stage

● **L89.52 Pressure ulcer of left ankle**

L89.520 Pressure ulcer of left ankle, unstageable

L89.521 Pressure ulcer of left ankle, stage 1
Healing pressure ulcer of left ankle, stage 1
Pressure pre-ulcer skin changes limited to persistent focal edema, left ankle

L89.522 Pressure ulcer of left ankle, stage 2
Healing pressure ulcer of left ankle, stage 2
Pressure ulcer with abrasion, blister, partial thickness skin loss involving epidermis and/or dermis, left ankle

L89.523 Pressure ulcer of left ankle, stage 3
Healing pressure ulcer of left ankle, stage 3
Pressure ulcer with full thickness skin loss involving damage or necrosis of subcutaneous tissue, left ankle
MCC when PDx is its own MCC

L89.524 Pressure ulcer of left ankle, stage 4
Healing pressure ulcer of left ankle, stage 4
Pressure ulcer with necrosis of soft tissues through to underlying muscle, tendon, or bone, left ankle
MCC when PDx is its own MCC

L89.526 Pressure-induced deep tissue damage of left ankle

L89.529 Pressure ulcer of left ankle, unspecified stage
Healing pressure ulcer of left ankle NOS
Healing pressure ulcer of left ankle, unspecified stage

● **L89.6 Pressure ulcer of heel**

● **L89.60 Pressure ulcer of unspecified heel**

L89.600 Pressure ulcer of unspecified heel, unstageable

L89.601 Pressure ulcer of unspecified heel, stage 1
Healing pressure ulcer of unspecified heel, stage 1
Pressure pre-ulcer skin changes limited to persistent focal edema, unspecified heel

L89.602 Pressure ulcer of unspecified heel, stage 2
Healing pressure ulcer of unspecified heel, stage 2
Pressure ulcer with abrasion, blister, partial thickness skin loss involving epidermis and/or dermis, unspecified heel

L89.603 Pressure ulcer of unspecified heel, stage 3
Healing pressure ulcer of unspecified heel, stage 3
Pressure ulcer with full thickness skin loss involving damage or necrosis of subcutaneous tissue, unspecified heel
MCC when PDx is its own MCC

L89.604 Pressure ulcer of unspecified heel, stage 4
Healing pressure ulcer of unspecified heel, stage 4
Pressure ulcer with necrosis of soft tissues through to underlying muscle, tendon, or bone, unspecified heel
MCC when PDx is its own MCC

L89.606 Pressure-induced deep tissue damage of unspecified heel

L89.609 Pressure ulcer of unspecified heel, unspecified stage
Healing pressure ulcer of unspecified heel NOS
Healing pressure ulcer of unspecified heel, unspecified stage

● **L89.61 Pressure ulcer of right heel**

L89.610 Pressure ulcer of right heel, unstageable

L89.611 Pressure ulcer of right heel, stage 1
Healing pressure ulcer of right heel, stage 1
Pressure pre-ulcer skin changes limited to persistent focal edema, right heel

L89.612 Pressure ulcer of right heel, stage 2
Healing pressure ulcer of right heel, stage 2
Pressure ulcer with abrasion, blister, partial thickness skin loss involving epidermis and/or dermis, right heel

L89.613 Pressure ulcer of right heel, stage 3
Healing pressure ulcer of right heel, stage 3
Pressure ulcer with full thickness skin loss involving damage or necrosis of subcutaneous tissue, right heel
MCC when PDx is its own MCC

L89.614 Pressure ulcer of right heel, stage 4
Healing pressure ulcer of right heel, stage 4
Pressure ulcer with necrosis of soft tissues through to underlying muscle, tendon, or bone, right heel
MCC when PDx is its own MCC

L89.616 Pressure-induced deep tissue damage of right heel

L89.619 Pressure ulcer of right heel, unspecified stage
Healing pressure ulcer of right heel NOS
Healing pressure ulcer of right heel, unspecified stage

● L89.62 Pressure ulcer of left heel

L89.620 Pressure ulcer of left heel, unstageable

L89.621 Pressure ulcer of left heel, stage 1
Healing pressure ulcer of left heel, stage 1
Pressure pre-ulcer skin changes limited to persistent focal edema, left heel

L89.622 Pressure ulcer of left heel, stage 2
Healing pressure ulcer of left heel, stage 2
Pressure ulcer with abrasion, blister, partial thickness skin loss involving epidermis and/or dermis, left heel
Coding Clinic: 2016, Q4, P142

L89.623 Pressure ulcer of left heel, stage 3
Healing pressure ulcer of left heel, stage 3
Pressure ulcer with full thickness skin loss involving damage or necrosis of subcutaneous tissue, left heel
MCC when PDx is its own MCC
Coding Clinic: 2016, Q4, P142

L89.624 Pressure ulcer of left heel, stage 4
Healing pressure ulcer of left heel, stage 4
Pressure ulcer with necrosis of soft tissues through to underlying muscle, tendon, or bone, left heel
MCC when PDx is its own MCC

L89.626 Pressure-induced deep tissue damage of left heel

L89.629 Pressure ulcer of left heel, unspecified stage
Healing pressure ulcer of left heel NOS
Healing pressure ulcer of left heel, unspecified stage

● L89.8 Pressure ulcer of other site

● L89.81 Pressure ulcer of head
Pressure ulcer of face

L89.810 Pressure ulcer of head, unstageable

L89.811 Pressure ulcer of head, stage 1
Healing pressure ulcer of head, stage 1
Pressure pre-ulcer skin changes limited to persistent focal edema, head

L89.812 Pressure ulcer of head, stage 2
Healing pressure ulcer of head, stage 2
Pressure ulcer with abrasion, blister, partial thickness skin loss involving epidermis and/or dermis, head

L89.813 Pressure ulcer of head, stage 3
Healing pressure ulcer of head, stage 3
Pressure ulcer with full thickness skin loss involving damage or necrosis of subcutaneous tissue, head
MCC when PDx is its own MCC

L89.814 Pressure ulcer of head, stage 4
Healing pressure ulcer of head, stage 4
Pressure ulcer with necrosis of soft tissues through to underlying muscle, tendon, or bone, head
MCC when PDx is its own MCC

L89.816 Pressure-induced deep tissue damage of head

L89.819 Pressure ulcer of head, unspecified stage
Healing pressure ulcer of head NOS
Healing pressure ulcer of head, unspecified stage

● L89.89 Pressure ulcer of other site

L89.890 Pressure ulcer of other site, unstageable

L89.891 Pressure ulcer of other site, stage 1
Healing pressure ulcer of other site, stage 1
Pressure pre-ulcer skin changes limited to persistent focal edema, other site

L89.892 Pressure ulcer of other site, stage 2
Healing pressure ulcer of other site, stage 2
Pressure ulcer with abrasion, blister, partial thickness skin loss involving epidermis and/or dermis, other site

L89.893 Pressure ulcer of other site, stage 3
Healing pressure ulcer of other site, stage 3
Pressure ulcer with full thickness skin loss involving damage or necrosis of subcutaneous tissue, other site
MCC when PDx is its own MCC

CHAPTER 12 (L00-L99)

L89.894 **Pressure ulcer of other site, stage 4**
Healing pressure ulcer of other site, stage 4
Pressure ulcer with necrosis of soft tissues through to underlying muscle, tendon, or bone, other site
MCC when PDx is its own MCC

L89.899 **Pressure ulcer of other site, unspecified stage**
Healing pressure ulcer of other site NOS
Healing pressure ulcer of other site, unspecified stage

● **L89.9 Pressure ulcer of unspecified site**

L89.90 **Pressure ulcer of unspecified site, unspecified stage**
Healing pressure ulcer of unspecified site NOS
Healing pressure ulcer of unspecified site, unspecified stage

L89.91 **Pressure ulcer of unspecified site, stage 1**
Healing pressure ulcer of unspecified site, stage 1
Pressure pre-ulcer skin changes limited to persistent focal edema, unspecified site

L89.92 **Pressure ulcer of unspecified site, stage 2**
Healing pressure ulcer of unspecified site, stage 2
Pressure ulcer with abrasion, blister, partial thickness skin loss involving epidermis and/or dermis, unspecified site

L89.93 **Pressure ulcer of unspecified site, stage 3**
Healing pressure ulcer of unspecified site, stage 3
Pressure ulcer with full thickness skin loss involving damage or necrosis of subcutaneous tissue, unspecified site
MCC when PDx is its own MCC

L89.94 **Pressure ulcer of unspecified site, stage 4**
Healing pressure ulcer of unspecified site, stage 4
Pressure ulcer with necrosis of soft tissues through to underlying muscle, tendon, or bone, unspecified site
MCC when PDx is its own MCC

L89.95 **Pressure ulcer of unspecified site, unstageable**

L89.96 **Pressure-induced deep tissue damage of unspecified site**

● **L90 Atrophic disorders of skin**

L90.0 **Lichen sclerosus et atrophicus**
Excludes2 lichen sclerosus of external female genital organs (N90.4)
lichen sclerosus of external male genital organs (N48.0)

L90.1 **Anetoderma of Schweninger-Buzzi**

L90.2 **Anetoderma of Jadassohn-Pellizzari**

L90.3 **Atrophoderma of Pasini and Pierini**

L90.4 **Acrodermatitis chronica atrophicans**

L90.5 **Scar conditions and fibrosis of skin**
Adherent scar (skin)
Cicatrix
Disfigurement of skin due to scar
Fibrosis of skin NOS
Scar NOS
Excludes2 hypertrophic scar (L91.0)
keloid scar (L91.0)
Coding Clinic: 2016, Q2, P5; 2015, Q1, P19

Item 12–11 Scleroderma means hard skin. It is a group of diseases that causes abnormal growth of connective tissues that support the skin and organs. There are two types: localized scleroderma affecting the skin and systemic scleroderma affecting blood vessels and internal organs and the skin.

L90.6 **Striae atrophicae**

L90.8 **Other atrophic disorders of skin**

L90.9 **Atrophic disorder of skin, unspecified**

● **L91 Hypertrophic disorders of skin**

L91.0 **Keloid scar**
Hypertrophic scar
Keloid
Excludes2 acne keloid (L73.0)
scar NOS (L90.5)

L91.8 **Other hypertrophic disorders of the skin**

L91.9 **Hypertrophic disorder of the skin, unspecified**

● **L92 Granulomatous disorders of skin and subcutaneous tissue**
Excludes2 actinic granuloma (L57.5)

L92.0 **Granuloma annulare**
Perforating granuloma annulare

L92.1 **Necrobiosis lipoidica, not elsewhere classified**
Excludes1 necrobiosis lipoidica associated with diabetes mellitus (E08-E13 with .620)

L92.2 **Granuloma faciale [eosinophilic granuloma of skin]**

L92.3 **Foreign body granuloma of the skin and subcutaneous tissue**
Use additional code to identify the type of retained foreign body (Z18.-)

L92.8 **Other granulomatous disorders of the skin and subcutaneous tissue**

L92.9 **Granulomatous disorder of the skin and subcutaneous tissue, unspecified**
Excludes2 umbilical granuloma (P83.81)

● **L93 Lupus erythematosus**
Use additional code for adverse effect, if applicable, to identify drug (T36-T50 with fifth or sixth character 5)
Excludes1 lupus exedens (A18.4)
lupus vulgaris (A18.4)
scleroderma (M34.-)
systemic lupus erythematosus (M32.-)

L93.0 **Discoid lupus erythematosus**
Lupus erythematosus NOS

L93.1 **Subacute cutaneous lupus erythematosus**

L93.2 **Other local lupus erythematosus**
Lupus erythematosus profundus
Lupus panniculitis

● **L94 Other localized connective tissue disorders**
Excludes1 systemic connective tissue disorders (M30-M36)

L94.0 **Localized scleroderma [morphea]**
Circumscribed scleroderma

L94.1 **Linear scleroderma**
En coup de sabre lesion

L94.2 **Calcinosis cutis**

L94.3 **Sclerodactyly**

L94.4 **Gottron's papules**

L94.5 **Poikiloderma vasculare atrophicans**

L94.6 **Ainhum**

L94.8 **Other specified localized connective tissue disorders**

L94.9 **Localized connective tissue disorder, unspecified**

● L95 Vasculitis limited to skin, not elsewhere classified

Excludes1 angioma serpiginosum (L81.7)
Henoch(-Schönlein) purpura (D69.0)
hypersensitivity angiitis (M31.0)
lupus panniculitis (L93.2)
panniculitis NOS (M79.3)
panniculitis of neck and back (M54.0-)
polyarteritis nodosa (M30.0)
relapsing panniculitis (M35.6)
rheumatoid vasculitis (M05.2)
serum sickness (T80.6-)
urticaria (L50.-)
Wegener's granulomatosis (M31.3-)

L95.0 Livedoid vasculitis
Atrophie blanche (en plaque)

L95.1 Erythema elevatum diutinum

L95.8 Other vasculitis limited to the skin

L95.9 Vasculitis limited to the skin, unspecified

● L97 Non-pressure chronic ulcer of lower limb, not elsewhere classified (Ex) PDX 1171

Includes chronic ulcer of skin of lower limb NOS
non-healing ulcer of skin
non-infected sinus of skin
trophic ulcer NOS
tropical ulcer NOS
ulcer of skin of lower limb NOS

Code first any associated underlying condition, such as:
any associated gangrene (I96)
atherosclerosis of the lower extremities (I70.23-, I70.24-, I70.33-, I70.34-, I70.43-, I70.44-, I70.53-, I70.54-, I70.63-, I70.64-, I70.73-, I70.74-)
chronic venous hypertension (I87.31-, I87.33-)
diabetic ulcers (E08.621, E08.622, E09.621, E09.622, E10.621, E10.622, E11.621, E11.622, E13.621, E13.622)
postphlebitic syndrome (I87.01-, I87.03-)
postthrombotic syndrome (I87.01-, I87.03-)
varicose ulcer (I83.0-, I83.2-)

Excludes2 pressure ulcer (pressure area) (L89.-)
skin infections (L00-L08)
specific infections classified to A00-B99

● L97.1 Non-pressure chronic ulcer of thigh

● L97.10 Non-pressure chronic ulcer of unspecified thigh

L97.101 Non-pressure chronic ulcer of unspecified thigh limited to breakdown of skin

L97.102 Non-pressure chronic ulcer of unspecified thigh with fat layer exposed

L97.103 Non-pressure chronic ulcer of unspecified thigh with necrosis of muscle

L97.104 Non-pressure chronic ulcer of unspecified thigh with necrosis of bone

L97.105 Non-pressure chronic ulcer of unspecified thigh with muscle involvement without evidence of necrosis

L97.106 Non-pressure chronic ulcer of unspecified thigh with bone involvement without evidence of necrosis

L97.108 Non-pressure chronic ulcer of unspecified thigh with other specified severity

L97.109 Non-pressure chronic ulcer of unspecified thigh with unspecified severity

● L97.11 Non-pressure chronic ulcer of right thigh

L97.111 Non-pressure chronic ulcer of right thigh limited to breakdown of skin

L97.112 Non-pressure chronic ulcer of right thigh with fat layer exposed

L97.113 Non-pressure chronic ulcer of right thigh with necrosis of muscle

L97.114 Non-pressure chronic ulcer of right thigh with necrosis of bone

L97.115 Non-pressure chronic ulcer of right thigh with muscle involvement without evidence of necrosis

L97.116 Non-pressure chronic ulcer of right thigh with bone involvement without evidence of necrosis

L97.118 Non-pressure chronic ulcer of right thigh with other specified severity

L97.119 Non-pressure chronic ulcer of right thigh with unspecified severity

● L97.12 Non-pressure chronic ulcer of left thigh

L97.121 Non-pressure chronic ulcer of left thigh limited to breakdown of skin

L97.122 Non-pressure chronic ulcer of left thigh with fat layer exposed

L97.123 Non-pressure chronic ulcer of left thigh with necrosis of muscle

L97.124 Non-pressure chronic ulcer of left thigh with necrosis of bone

L97.125 Non-pressure chronic ulcer of left thigh with muscle involvement without evidence of necrosis

L97.126 Non-pressure chronic ulcer of left thigh with bone involvement without evidence of necrosis

L97.128 Non-pressure chronic ulcer of left thigh with other specified severity

L97.129 Non-pressure chronic ulcer of left thigh with unspecified severity

● L97.2 Non-pressure chronic ulcer of calf

● L97.20 Non-pressure chronic ulcer of unspecified calf

L97.201 Non-pressure chronic ulcer of unspecified calf limited to breakdown of skin

L97.202 Non-pressure chronic ulcer of unspecified calf with fat layer exposed

L97.203 Non-pressure chronic ulcer of unspecified calf with necrosis of muscle

L97.204 Non-pressure chronic ulcer of unspecified calf with necrosis of bone

L97.205 Non-pressure chronic ulcer of unspecified calf with muscle involvement without evidence of necrosis

L97.206 Non-pressure chronic ulcer of unspecified calf with bone involvement without evidence of necrosis

L97.208 Non-pressure chronic ulcer of unspecified calf with other specified severity

L97.209 Non-pressure chronic ulcer of unspecified calf with unspecified severity

● L97.21 Non-pressure chronic ulcer of right calf

L97.211 Non-pressure chronic ulcer of right calf limited to breakdown of skin

L97.212 Non-pressure chronic ulcer of right calf with fat layer exposed

L97.213 Non-pressure chronic ulcer of right calf with necrosis of muscle

CHAPTER 12 (L00-L99)

L97.214 Non-pressure chronic ulcer of right calf with necrosis of bone

L97.215 Non-pressure chronic ulcer of right calf with muscle involvement without evidence of necrosis

L97.216 Non-pressure chronic ulcer of right calf with bone involvement without evidence of necrosis

L97.218 Non-pressure chronic ulcer of right calf with other specified severity

L97.219 Non-pressure chronic ulcer of right calf with unspecified severity
Coding Clinic: 2024, Q1, P16

● L97.22 Non-pressure chronic ulcer of left calf

L97.221 Non-pressure chronic ulcer of left calf limited to breakdown of skin

L97.222 Non-pressure chronic ulcer of left calf with fat layer exposed

L97.223 Non-pressure chronic ulcer of left calf with necrosis of muscle

L97.224 Non-pressure chronic ulcer of left calf with necrosis of bone

L97.225 Non-pressure chronic ulcer of left calf with muscle involvement without evidence of necrosis

L97.226 Non-pressure chronic ulcer of left calf with bone involvement without evidence of necrosis

L97.228 Non-pressure chronic ulcer of left calf with other specified severity

L97.229 Non-pressure chronic ulcer of left calf with unspecified severity

● L97.3 Non-pressure chronic ulcer of ankle

● L97.30 Non-pressure chronic ulcer of unspecified ankle

L97.301 Non-pressure chronic ulcer of unspecified ankle limited to breakdown of skin

L97.302 Non-pressure chronic ulcer of unspecified ankle with fat layer exposed

L97.303 Non-pressure chronic ulcer of unspecified ankle with necrosis of muscle

L97.304 Non-pressure chronic ulcer of unspecified ankle with necrosis of bone

L97.305 Non-pressure chronic ulcer of unspecified ankle with muscle involvement without evidence of necrosis

L97.306 Non-pressure chronic ulcer of unspecified ankle with bone involvement without evidence of necrosis

L97.308 Non-pressure chronic ulcer of unspecified ankle with other specified severity

L97.309 Non-pressure chronic ulcer of unspecified ankle with unspecified severity

● L97.31 Non-pressure chronic ulcer of right ankle

L97.311 Non-pressure chronic ulcer of right ankle limited to breakdown of skin

L97.312 Non-pressure chronic ulcer of right ankle with fat layer exposed

L97.313 Non-pressure chronic ulcer of right ankle with necrosis of muscle

L97.314 Non-pressure chronic ulcer of right ankle with necrosis of bone

L97.315 Non-pressure chronic ulcer of right ankle with muscle involvement without evidence of necrosis
Coding Clinic: 2017, Q4, P17

L97.316 Non-pressure chronic ulcer of right ankle with bone involvement without evidence of necrosis

L97.318 Non-pressure chronic ulcer of right ankle with other specified severity

L97.319 Non-pressure chronic ulcer of right ankle with unspecified severity

● L97.32 Non-pressure chronic ulcer of left ankle

L97.321 Non-pressure chronic ulcer of left ankle limited to breakdown of skin

L97.322 Non-pressure chronic ulcer of left ankle with fat layer exposed
Coding Clinic: 2021, Q1, P8

L97.323 Non-pressure chronic ulcer of left ankle with necrosis of muscle

L97.324 Non-pressure chronic ulcer of left ankle with necrosis of bone

L97.325 Non-pressure chronic ulcer of left ankle with muscle involvement without evidence of necrosis

L97.326 Non-pressure chronic ulcer of left ankle with bone involvement without evidence of necrosis

L97.328 Non-pressure chronic ulcer of left ankle with other specified severity

L97.329 Non-pressure chronic ulcer of left ankle with unspecified severity

● L97.4 Non-pressure chronic ulcer of heel and midfoot
Non-pressure chronic ulcer of plantar surface of midfoot

● L97.40 Non-pressure chronic ulcer of unspecified heel and midfoot

L97.401 Non-pressure chronic ulcer of unspecified heel and midfoot limited to breakdown of skin

L97.402 Non-pressure chronic ulcer of unspecified heel and midfoot with fat layer exposed

L97.403 Non-pressure chronic ulcer of unspecified heel and midfoot with necrosis of muscle

L97.404 Non-pressure chronic ulcer of unspecified heel and midfoot with necrosis of bone

L97.405 Non-pressure chronic ulcer of unspecified heel and midfoot with muscle involvement without evidence of necrosis

L97.406 Non-pressure chronic ulcer of unspecified heel and midfoot with bone involvement without evidence of necrosis

L97.408 Non-pressure chronic ulcer of unspecified heel and midfoot with other specified severity

L97.409 Non-pressure chronic ulcer of unspecified heel and midfoot with unspecified severity

● L97.41 Non-pressure chronic ulcer of right heel and midfoot

L97.411 Non-pressure chronic ulcer of right heel and midfoot limited to breakdown of skin

L97.412 Non-pressure chronic ulcer of right heel and midfoot with fat layer exposed

L97.413 Non-pressure chronic ulcer of right heel and midfoot with necrosis of muscle

L97.414 Non-pressure chronic ulcer of right heel and midfoot with necrosis of bone

L97.415 Non-pressure chronic ulcer of right heel and midfoot with muscle involvement without evidence of necrosis

L97.416 Non-pressure chronic ulcer of right heel and midfoot with bone involvement without evidence of necrosis

L97.418 Non-pressure chronic ulcer of right heel and midfoot with other specified severity

L97.419 Non-pressure chronic ulcer of right heel and midfoot with unspecified severity

● L97.42 Non-pressure chronic ulcer of left heel and midfoot

L97.421 Non-pressure chronic ulcer of left heel and midfoot limited to breakdown of skin
Coding Clinic: 2016, Q1, P13

L97.422 Non-pressure chronic ulcer of left heel and midfoot with fat layer exposed

L97.423 Non-pressure chronic ulcer of left heel and midfoot with necrosis of muscle

L97.424 Non-pressure chronic ulcer of left heel and midfoot with necrosis of bone

L97.425 Non-pressure chronic ulcer of left heel and midfoot with muscle involvement without evidence of necrosis

L97.426 Non-pressure chronic ulcer of left heel and midfoot with bone involvement without evidence of necrosis

L97.428 Non-pressure chronic ulcer of left heel and midfoot with other specified severity

L97.429 Non-pressure chronic ulcer of left heel and midfoot with unspecified severity

● L97.5 Non-pressure chronic ulcer of other part of foot
Non-pressure chronic ulcer of toe

● L97.50 Non-pressure chronic ulcer of other part of unspecified foot

L97.501 Non-pressure chronic ulcer of other part of unspecified foot limited to breakdown of skin

L97.502 Non-pressure chronic ulcer of other part of unspecified foot with fat layer exposed

L97.503 Non-pressure chronic ulcer of other part of unspecified foot with necrosis of muscle

L97.504 Non-pressure chronic ulcer of other part of unspecified foot with necrosis of bone

L97.505 Non-pressure chronic ulcer of other part of unspecified foot with muscle involvement without evidence of necrosis

L97.506 Non-pressure chronic ulcer of other part of unspecified foot with bone involvement without evidence of necrosis

L97.508 Non-pressure chronic ulcer of other part of unspecified foot with other specified severity

L97.509 Non-pressure chronic ulcer of other part of unspecified foot with unspecified severity

● L97.51 Non-pressure chronic ulcer of other part of right foot

L97.511 Non-pressure chronic ulcer of other part of right foot limited to breakdown of skin
Coding Clinic: 2020, Q1, P12

L97.512 Non-pressure chronic ulcer of other part of right foot with fat layer exposed

L97.513 Non-pressure chronic ulcer of other part of right foot with necrosis of muscle

L97.514 Non-pressure chronic ulcer of other part of right foot with necrosis of bone

L97.515 Non-pressure chronic ulcer of other part of right foot with muscle involvement without evidence of necrosis

L97.516 Non-pressure chronic ulcer of other part of right foot with bone involvement without evidence of necrosis

L97.518 Non-pressure chronic ulcer of other part of right foot with other specified severity

L97.519 Non-pressure chronic ulcer of other part of right foot with unspecified severity

● L97.52 Non-pressure chronic ulcer of other part of left foot

L97.521 Non-pressure chronic ulcer of other part of left foot limited to breakdown of skin

L97.522 Non-pressure chronic ulcer of other part of left foot with fat layer exposed

L97.523 Non-pressure chronic ulcer of other part of left foot with necrosis of muscle

L97.524 Non-pressure chronic ulcer of other part of left foot with necrosis of bone

L97.525 Non-pressure chronic ulcer of other part of left foot with muscle involvement without evidence of necrosis

L97.526 Non-pressure chronic ulcer of other part of left foot with bone involvement without evidence of necrosis

L97.528 Non-pressure chronic ulcer of other part of left foot with other specified severity

L97.529 Non-pressure chronic ulcer of other part of left foot with unspecified severity

● L97.8 Non-pressure chronic ulcer of other part of lower leg

● L97.80 Non-pressure chronic ulcer of other part of unspecified lower leg

L97.801 Non-pressure chronic ulcer of other part of unspecified lower leg limited to breakdown of skin

L97.802 Non-pressure chronic ulcer of other part of unspecified lower leg with fat layer exposed

L97.803 Non-pressure chronic ulcer of other part of unspecified lower leg with necrosis of muscle

L97.804 Non-pressure chronic ulcer of other part of unspecified lower leg with necrosis of bone

L97.805 Non-pressure chronic ulcer of other part of unspecified lower leg with muscle involvement without evidence of necrosis

L97.806 Non-pressure chronic ulcer of other part of unspecified lower leg with bone involvement without evidence of necrosis

L97.808 Non-pressure chronic ulcer of other part of unspecified lower leg with other specified severity

L97.809 Non-pressure chronic ulcer of other part of unspecified lower leg with unspecified severity

● L97.81 Non-pressure chronic ulcer of other part of right lower leg

L97.811 Non-pressure chronic ulcer of other part of right lower leg limited to breakdown of skin

L97.812 Non-pressure chronic ulcer of other part of right lower leg with fat layer exposed

L97.813 Non-pressure chronic ulcer of other part of right lower leg with necrosis of muscle

L97.814 Non-pressure chronic ulcer of other part of right lower leg with necrosis of bone

L97.815 Non-pressure chronic ulcer of other part of right lower leg with muscle involvement without evidence of necrosis

L97.816 Non-pressure chronic ulcer of other part of right lower leg with bone involvement without evidence of necrosis

L97.818 Non-pressure chronic ulcer of other part of right lower leg with other specified severity

L97.819 Non-pressure chronic ulcer of other part of right lower leg with unspecified severity

● L97.82 Non-pressure chronic ulcer of other part of left lower leg

L97.821 Non-pressure chronic ulcer of other part of left lower leg limited to breakdown of skin

L97.822 Non-pressure chronic ulcer of other part of left lower leg with fat layer exposed

L97.823 Non-pressure chronic ulcer of other part of left lower leg with necrosis of muscle

L97.824 Non-pressure chronic ulcer of other part of left lower leg with necrosis of bone

L97.825 Non-pressure chronic ulcer of other part of left lower leg with muscle involvement without evidence of necrosis

L97.826 Non-pressure chronic ulcer of other part of left lower leg with bone involvement without evidence of necrosis

L97.828 Non-pressure chronic ulcer of other part of left lower leg with other specified severity

L97.829 Non-pressure chronic ulcer of other part of left lower leg with unspecified severity

● L97.9 Non-pressure chronic ulcer of unspecified part of lower leg

● L97.90 Non-pressure chronic ulcer of unspecified part of unspecified lower leg

L97.901 Non-pressure chronic ulcer of unspecified part of unspecified lower leg limited to breakdown of skin

L97.902 Non-pressure chronic ulcer of unspecified part of unspecified lower leg with fat layer exposed

L97.903 Non-pressure chronic ulcer of unspecified part of unspecified lower leg with necrosis of muscle

L97.904 Non-pressure chronic ulcer of unspecified part of unspecified lower leg with necrosis of bone

L97.905 Non-pressure chronic ulcer of unspecified part of unspecified lower leg with muscle involvement without evidence of necrosis

L97.906 Non-pressure chronic ulcer of unspecified part of unspecified lower leg with bone involvement without evidence of necrosis

L97.908 Non-pressure chronic ulcer of unspecified part of unspecified lower leg with other specified severity

L97.909 Non-pressure chronic ulcer of unspecified part of unspecified lower leg with unspecified severity

● L97.91 Non-pressure chronic ulcer of unspecified part of right lower leg

L97.911 Non-pressure chronic ulcer of unspecified part of right lower leg limited to breakdown of skin

L97.912 Non-pressure chronic ulcer of unspecified part of right lower leg with fat layer exposed

L97.913 Non-pressure chronic ulcer of unspecified part of right lower leg with necrosis of muscle

L97.914 Non-pressure chronic ulcer of unspecified part of right lower leg with necrosis of bone

L97.915 Non-pressure chronic ulcer of unspecified part of right lower leg with muscle involvement without evidence of necrosis

L97.916 Non-pressure chronic ulcer of unspecified part of right lower leg with bone involvement without evidence of necrosis

L97.918 Non-pressure chronic ulcer of unspecified part of right lower leg with other specified severity

L97.919 Non-pressure chronic ulcer of unspecified part of right lower leg with unspecified severity

● L97.92 Non-pressure chronic ulcer of unspecified part of left lower leg

L97.921 Non-pressure chronic ulcer of unspecified part of left lower leg limited to breakdown of skin

L97.922 Non-pressure chronic ulcer of unspecified part of left lower leg with fat layer exposed

L97.923 Non-pressure chronic ulcer of unspecified part of left lower leg with necrosis of muscle

L97.924 Non-pressure chronic ulcer of unspecified part of left lower leg with necrosis of bone

L97.925 Non-pressure chronic ulcer of unspecified part of left lower leg with muscle involvement without evidence of necrosis

L97.926 Non-pressure chronic ulcer of unspecified part of left lower leg with bone involvement without evidence of necrosis

L97.928 Non-pressure chronic ulcer of unspecified part of left lower leg with other specified severity

L97.929 Non-pressure chronic ulcer of unspecified part of left lower leg with unspecified severity

● L98 Other disorders of skin and subcutaneous tissue, not elsewhere classified

L98.0 Pyogenic granuloma

Excludes2 pyogenic granuloma of gingiva (K06.8)
pyogenic granuloma of maxillary alveolar ridge (K04.5)
pyogenic granuloma of oral mucosa (K13.4)

L98.1 Factitial dermatitis

Neurotic excoriation

Excludes1 Excoriation (skin-picking) disorder (F42.4)

Coding Clinic: 2016, Q4, P15

L98.2 Febrile neutrophilic dermatosis [Sweet]

L98.3 Eosinophilic cellulitis [Wells] Ex: PDX 1161

● L98.4 Non-pressure chronic ulcer of skin, not elsewhere classified Ex: PDX 1171

Chronic ulcer of skin NOS
Tropical ulcer NOS
Ulcer of skin NOS

Excludes2 pressure ulcer (pressure area) (L89.-)
gangrene (I96)
skin infections (L00-L08)
specific infections classified to A00-B99
ulcer of lower limb NEC (L97.-)
varicose ulcer (I83.0-I83.93)

● L98.41 Non-pressure chronic ulcer of buttock

L98.411 Non-pressure chronic ulcer of buttock limited to breakdown of skin

L98.412 Non-pressure chronic ulcer of buttock with fat layer exposed

L98.413 Non-pressure chronic ulcer of buttock with necrosis of muscle

L98.414 Non-pressure chronic ulcer of buttock with necrosis of bone

L98.415 Non-pressure chronic ulcer of buttock with muscle involvement without evidence of necrosis

L98.416 Non-pressure chronic ulcer of buttock with bone involvement without evidence of necrosis

L98.418 Non-pressure chronic ulcer of buttock with other specified severity

L98.419 Non-pressure chronic ulcer of buttock with unspecified severity

● L98.42 Non-pressure chronic ulcer of back

L98.421 Non-pressure chronic ulcer of back limited to breakdown of skin

L98.422 Non-pressure chronic ulcer of back with fat layer exposed

L98.423 Non-pressure chronic ulcer of back with necrosis of muscle

L98.424 Non-pressure chronic ulcer of back with necrosis of bone

L98.425 Non-pressure chronic ulcer of back with muscle involvement without evidence of necrosis

L98.426 Non-pressure chronic ulcer of back with bone involvement without evidence of necrosis

L98.428 Non-pressure chronic ulcer of back with other specified severity

L98.429 Non-pressure chronic ulcer of back with unspecified severity

● L98.49 Non-pressure chronic ulcer of skin of other sites Ex: PDX 698

Non-pressure chronic ulcer of skin NOS

L98.491 Non-pressure chronic ulcer of skin of other sites limited to breakdown of skin

L98.492 Non-pressure chronic ulcer of skin of other sites with fat layer exposed

L98.493 Non-pressure chronic ulcer of skin of other sites with necrosis of muscle

L98.494 Non-pressure chronic ulcer of skin of other sites with necrosis of bone

L98.495 Non-pressure chronic ulcer of skin of other sites with muscle involvement without evidence of necrosis

L98.496 Non-pressure chronic ulcer of skin of other sites with bone involvement without evidence of necrosis

L98.498 Non-pressure chronic ulcer of skin of other sites with other specified severity

L98.499 Non-pressure chronic ulcer of skin of other sites with unspecified severity

L98.5 Mucinosis of the skin

Focal mucinosis
Lichen myxedematosus
Reticular erythematous mucinosis

Excludes1 focal oral mucinosis (K13.79)
myxedema (E03.9)

L98.6 Other infiltrative disorders of the skin and subcutaneous tissue

Excludes1 hyalinosis cutis et mucosae (E78.89)

L98.7 Excessive and redundant skin and subcutaneous tissue

Loose or sagging skin following bariatric surgery weight loss
Loose or sagging skin following dietary weight loss
Loose or sagging skin, NOS

Excludes2 acquired excess or redundant skin of eyelid (H02.3-)
congenital excess or redundant skin of eyelid (Q10.3)
skin changes due to chronic exposure to nonionizing radiation (L57.-)

Coding Clinic: 2022, Q3, P11; 2016, Q4, P36

L98.8 Other specified disorders of the skin and subcutaneous tissue

Coding Clinic: 2013, Q2, P32

L98.9 Disorder of the skin and subcutaneous tissue, unspecified

L99 Other disorders of skin and subcutaneous tissue in diseases classified elsewhere

Code first underlying disease, such as:
amyloidosis (E85.-)

Excludes1 skin disorders in diabetes (E08-E13 with .62-)
skin disorders in gonorrhea (A54.89)
skin disorders in syphilis (A51.31, A52.79)

CHAPTER 12 (L00-L99)

CHAPTER 13

DISEASES OF THE MUSCULOSKELETAL SYSTEM AND CONNECTIVE TISSUE (MØØ-M99)

OGCR Chapter-Specific Coding Guidelines

13. Chapter 13: Diseases of the Musculoskeletal System and Connective Tissue (MØØ-M99)

a. Site and laterality

Most of the codes within Chapter 13 have site and laterality designations. The site represents the bone, joint or the muscle involved. For some conditions where more than one bone, joint or muscle is usually involved, such as osteoarthritis, there is a "multiple sites" code available. For categories where no multiple site code is provided and more than one bone, joint or muscle is involved, multiple codes should be used to indicate the different sites involved.

1) Bone versus joint

For certain conditions, the bone may be affected at the upper or lower end (e.g., avascular necrosis of bone, M87, Osteoporosis, M8Ø, M81). Though the portion of the bone affected may be at the joint, the site designation will be the bone, not the joint.

b. Acute traumatic versus chronic or recurrent musculoskeletal conditions

Many musculoskeletal conditions are a result of previous injury or trauma to a site, or are recurrent conditions. Bone, joint or muscle conditions that are the result of a healed injury are usually found in Chapter 13. Recurrent bone, joint or muscle conditions are also usually found in Chapter 13. Any current, acute injury should be coded to the appropriate injury code from Chapter 19. Chronic or recurrent conditions should generally be coded with a code from Chapter 13. If it is difficult to determine from the documentation in the record which code is best to describe a condition, query the provider.

c. Coding of Pathologic Fractures

7th character A is for use as long as the patient is receiving active treatment for the fracture. While the patient may be seen by a new or different provider over the course of treatment for a pathological fracture, assignment of the 7th character is based on whether the patient is undergoing active treatment and not whether the provider is seeing the patient for the first time.

7th character, D is to be used for encounters after the patient has completed active treatment for the fracture and is receiving routine care for the fracture during the healing or recovery phase. The other 7th characters, listed under each subcategory in the Tabular List, are to be used for subsequent encounters for treatment of problems associated with the healing, such as malunions, nonunions, and sequelae.

Care for complications of surgical treatment for fracture repairs during the healing or recovery phase should be coded with the appropriate complication codes.

See Section I.C.19. Coding of traumatic fractures.

d. Osteoporosis

Osteoporosis is a systemic condition, meaning that all bones of the musculoskeletal system are affected. Therefore, site is not a component of the codes under category M81, Osteoporosis without current pathological fracture. The site codes under category M8Ø, Osteoporosis with current pathological fracture, identify the site of the fracture, not the osteoporosis.

1) Osteoporosis without pathological fracture

Category M81, Osteoporosis without current pathological fracture, is for use for patients with osteoporosis who do not currently have a pathologic fracture due to the osteoporosis, even if they have had a fracture in the past. For patients with a history of osteoporosis fractures, status code Z87.31Ø, Personal history of (healed) osteoporosis fracture, should follow the code from M81.

2) Osteoporosis with current pathological fracture

Category M8Ø, Osteoporosis with current pathological fracture, is for patients who have a current pathologic fracture at the time of an encounter. The codes under M8Ø identify the site of the fracture. A code from category M8Ø, not a traumatic fracture code, should be used for any patient with known osteoporosis who suffers a fracture, even if the patient had a minor fall or trauma, if that fall or trauma would not usually break a normal, healthy bone.

CHAPTER 13

DISEASES OF THE MUSCULOSKELETAL SYSTEM AND CONNECTIVE TISSUE (MØØ-M99)

Note: Use an external cause code following the code for the musculoskeletal condition, if applicable, to identify the cause of the musculoskeletal condition

Excludes2 arthropathic psoriasis (L4Ø.5-)
certain conditions originating in the perinatal period (PØ4-P96)
certain infectious and parasitic diseases (AØØ-B99)
compartment syndrome (traumatic) (T79.A-)
complications of pregnancy, childbirth and the puerperium (OØØ-O9A)
congenital malformations, deformations, and chromosomal abnormalities (QØØ-Q99)
endocrine, nutritional and metabolic diseases (EØØ-E88)
injury, poisoning and certain other consequences of external causes (SØØ-T88)
neoplasms (CØØ-D49)
symptoms, signs and abnormal clinical and laboratory findings, not elsewhere classified (RØØ-R94)

This chapter contains the following blocks:

MØØ-MØ2	Infectious arthropathies
MØ4	Autoinflammatory syndromes
MØ5-M14	Inflammatory polyarthropathies
M15-M19	Osteoarthritis
M2Ø-M25	Other joint disorders
M26-M27	Dentofacial anomalies [including malocclusion] and other disorders of jaw
M3Ø-M36	Systemic connective tissue disorders
M4Ø-M43	Deforming dorsopathies
M45-M49	Spondylopathies
M5Ø-M54	Other dorsopathies
M6Ø-M63	Disorders of muscles
M65-M67	Disorders of synovium and tendon
M7Ø-M79	Other soft tissue disorders
M8Ø-M85	Disorders of bone density and structure
M86-M9Ø	Other osteopathies
M91-M94	Chondropathies
M95	Other disorders of the musculoskeletal system and connective tissue
M96	Intraoperative and postprocedural complications and disorders of musculoskeletal system, not elsewhere classified
M97	Periprosthetic fracture around internal prosthetic joint
M99	Biomechanical lesions, not elsewhere classified

Coding Clinic: 2Ø16, Q4, P124

ARTHROPATHIES (MØØ-M25)

Includes Disorders affecting predominantly peripheral (limb) joints

INFECTIOUS ARTHROPATHIES (MØØ-MØ2)

Note: This block comprises arthropathies due to microbiological agents.

Distinction is made between the following types of etiological relationship:

a) direct infection of joint, where organisms invade synovial tissue and microbial antigen is present in the joint;

b) indirect infection, which may be of two types: a reactive arthropathy, where microbial infection of the body is established but neither organisms nor antigens can be identified in the joint, and a postinfective arthropathy, where microbial antigen is present but recovery of an organism is inconstant and evidence of local multiplication is lacking.

MØØ Pyogenic arthritis

Excludes2 infection and inflammatory reaction due to internal joint prosthesis (T84.5-)

MØØ.Ø Staphylococcal arthritis and polyarthritis

Use additional code (B95.61-B95.8) to identify bacterial agent

MØØ.ØØ Staphylococcal arthritis, unspecified joint Ex PDX 1172

MØØ.Ø1 Staphylococcal arthritis, shoulder Ex PDX 1173

MØØ.Ø11 Staphylococcal arthritis, right shoulder

MØØ.Ø12 Staphylococcal arthritis, left shoulder

MØØ.Ø19 Staphylococcal arthritis, unspecified shoulder

MØØ.Ø2 Staphylococcal arthritis, elbow Ex PDX 1174

MØØ.Ø21 Staphylococcal arthritis, right elbow

MØØ.Ø22 Staphylococcal arthritis, left elbow

MØØ.Ø29 Staphylococcal arthritis, unspecified elbow

MØØ.Ø3 Staphylococcal arthritis, wrist Ex PDX 1175

Staphylococcal arthritis of carpal bones

MØØ.Ø31 Staphylococcal arthritis, right wrist

MØØ.Ø32 Staphylococcal arthritis, left wrist

MØØ.Ø39 Staphylococcal arthritis, unspecified wrist

MØØ.Ø4 Staphylococcal arthritis, hand Ex PDX 1176

Staphylococcal arthritis of metacarpus and phalanges

MØØ.Ø41 Staphylococcal arthritis, right hand

MØØ.Ø42 Staphylococcal arthritis, left hand

MØØ.Ø49 Staphylococcal arthritis, unspecified hand

MØØ.Ø5 Staphylococcal arthritis, hip Ex PDX 1177

MØØ.Ø51 Staphylococcal arthritis, right hip

MØØ.Ø52 Staphylococcal arthritis, left hip

MØØ.Ø59 Staphylococcal arthritis, unspecified hip

MØØ.Ø6 Staphylococcal arthritis, knee Ex PDX 1178

MØØ.Ø61 Staphylococcal arthritis, right knee

MØØ.Ø62 Staphylococcal arthritis, left knee

MØØ.Ø69 Staphylococcal arthritis, unspecified knee

MØØ.Ø7 Staphylococcal arthritis, ankle and foot Ex PDX 1179

Staphylococcal arthritis, tarsus, metatarsus and phalanges

MØØ.Ø71 Staphylococcal arthritis, right ankle and foot

MØØ.Ø72 Staphylococcal arthritis, left ankle and foot

MØØ.Ø79 Staphylococcal arthritis, unspecified ankle and foot

MØØ.Ø8 Staphylococcal arthritis, vertebrae Ex PDX 1172

MØØ.Ø9 Staphylococcal polyarthritis Ex PDX 1172

MØØ.1 Pneumococcal arthritis and polyarthritis

MØØ.1Ø Pneumococcal arthritis, unspecified joint Ex PDX 1172

MØØ.11 Pneumococcal arthritis, shoulder Ex PDX 1173

MØØ.111 Pneumococcal arthritis, right shoulder

MØØ.112 Pneumococcal arthritis, left shoulder

MØØ.119 Pneumococcal arthritis, unspecified shoulder

MØØ.12 Pneumococcal arthritis, elbow Ex PDX 1174

MØØ.121 Pneumococcal arthritis, right elbow

MØØ.122 Pneumococcal arthritis, left elbow

MØØ.129 Pneumococcal arthritis, unspecified elbow

MØØ.13 Pneumococcal arthritis, wrist Ex PDX 1175

Pneumococcal arthritis of carpal bones

MØØ.131 Pneumococcal arthritis, right wrist

MØØ.132 Pneumococcal arthritis, left wrist

MØØ.139 Pneumococcal arthritis, unspecified wrist

MØØ.14 Pneumococcal arthritis, hand Ex PDX 1176

Pneumococcal arthritis of metacarpus and phalanges

MØØ.141 Pneumococcal arthritis, right hand

MØØ.142 Pneumococcal arthritis, left hand

MØØ.149 Pneumococcal arthritis, unspecified hand

MØØ.15 Pneumococcal arthritis, hip Ex PDX 1177

MØØ.151 Pneumococcal arthritis, right hip

MØØ.152 Pneumococcal arthritis, left hip

MØØ.159 Pneumococcal arthritis, unspecified hip

MØØ.16 Pneumococcal arthritis, knee Ex PDX 1178

MØØ.161 Pneumococcal arthritis, right knee

MØØ.162 Pneumococcal arthritis, left knee

MØØ.169 Pneumococcal arthritis, unspecified knee

MØØ.17 Pneumococcal arthritis, ankle and foot Ex PDX 1179

Pneumococcal arthritis, tarsus, metatarsus and phalanges

MØØ.171 Pneumococcal arthritis, right ankle and foot

MØØ.172 Pneumococcal arthritis, left ankle and foot

MØØ.179 Pneumococcal arthritis, unspecified ankle and foot

MØØ.18 Pneumococcal arthritis, vertebrae Ex PDX 1172

MØØ.19 Pneumococcal polyarthritis Ex PDX 1172

MØØ.2 Other streptococcal arthritis and polyarthritis

Use additional code (B95.Ø-B95.2, B95.4-B95.5) to identify bacterial agent

MØØ.2Ø Other streptococcal arthritis, unspecified joint Ex PDX 1172

MØØ.21 Other streptococcal arthritis, shoulder Ex PDX 1173

MØØ.211 Other streptococcal arthritis, right shoulder

MØØ.212 Other streptococcal arthritis, left shoulder

MØØ.219 Other streptococcal arthritis, unspecified shoulder

CHAPTER 13 (MØØ-M99)

MØØ.22 Other streptococcal arthritis, elbow (Ex) PDX 1174
- **MØØ.221 Other streptococcal arthritis, right elbow**
- **MØØ.222 Other streptococcal arthritis, left elbow**
- **MØØ.229 Other streptococcal arthritis, unspecified elbow**

MØØ.23 Other streptococcal arthritis, wrist (Ex) PDX 1175
Other streptococcal arthritis of carpal bones
- **MØØ.231 Other streptococcal arthritis, right wrist**
- **MØØ.232 Other streptococcal arthritis, left wrist**
- **MØØ.239 Other streptococcal arthritis, unspecified wrist**

MØØ.24 Other streptococcal arthritis, hand (Ex) PDX 1176
Other streptococcal arthritis metacarpus and phalanges
- **MØØ.241 Other streptococcal arthritis, right hand**
- **MØØ.242 Other streptococcal arthritis, left hand**
- **MØØ.249 Other streptococcal arthritis, unspecified hand**

MØØ.25 Other streptococcal arthritis, hip (Ex) PDX 1177
- **MØØ.251 Other streptococcal arthritis, right hip**
- **MØØ.252 Other streptococcal arthritis, left hip**
- **MØØ.259 Other streptococcal arthritis, unspecified hip**

MØØ.26 Other streptococcal arthritis, knee (Ex) PDX 1178
- **MØØ.261 Other streptococcal arthritis, right knee**
- **MØØ.262 Other streptococcal arthritis, left knee**
- **MØØ.269 Other streptococcal arthritis, unspecified knee**

MØØ.27 Other streptococcal arthritis, ankle and foot (Ex) PDX 1179
Other streptococcal arthritis, tarsus, metatarsus and phalanges
- **MØØ.271 Other streptococcal arthritis, right ankle and foot**
- **MØØ.272 Other streptococcal arthritis, left ankle and foot**
- **MØØ.279 Other streptococcal arthritis, unspecified ankle and foot**

MØØ.28 Other streptococcal arthritis, vertebrae (Ex) PDX 1172

MØØ.29 Other streptococcal polyarthritis (Ex) PDX 1172

MØØ.8 Arthritis and polyarthritis due to other bacteria
Use additional code (B96) to identify bacteria

MØØ.8Ø Arthritis due to other bacteria, unspecified joint (Ex) PDX 1172

MØØ.81 Arthritis due to other bacteria, shoulder (Ex) PDX 1173
- **MØØ.811 Arthritis due to other bacteria, right shoulder**
- **MØØ.812 Arthritis due to other bacteria, left shoulder**
- **MØØ.819 Arthritis due to other bacteria, unspecified shoulder**

MØØ.82 Arthritis due to other bacteria, elbow (Ex) PDX 1174
- **MØØ.821 Arthritis due to other bacteria, right elbow**
- **MØØ.822 Arthritis due to other bacteria, left elbow**
- **MØØ.829 Arthritis due to other bacteria, unspecified elbow**

MØØ.83 Arthritis due to other bacteria, wrist (Ex) PDX 1175
Arthritis due to other bacteria, carpal bones
- **MØØ.831 Arthritis due to other bacteria, right wrist**
- **MØØ.832 Arthritis due to other bacteria, left wrist**
- **MØØ.839 Arthritis due to other bacteria, unspecified wrist**

MØØ.84 Arthritis due to other bacteria, hand (Ex) PDX 1176
Arthritis due to other bacteria, metacarpus and phalanges
- **MØØ.841 Arthritis due to other bacteria, right hand**
- **MØØ.842 Arthritis due to other bacteria, left hand**
- **MØØ.849 Arthritis due to other bacteria, unspecified hand**

MØØ.85 Arthritis due to other bacteria, hip (Ex) PDX 1177
- **MØØ.851 Arthritis due to other bacteria, right hip**
- **MØØ.852 Arthritis due to other bacteria, left hip**
- **MØØ.859 Arthritis due to other bacteria, unspecified hip**

MØØ.86 Arthritis due to other bacteria, knee (Ex) PDX 1178
- **MØØ.861 Arthritis due to other bacteria, right knee**
- **MØØ.862 Arthritis due to other bacteria, left knee**
  Coding Clinic: 2Ø19, Q3, P16
- **MØØ.869 Arthritis due to other bacteria, unspecified knee**

MØØ.87 Arthritis due to other bacteria, ankle and foot (Ex) PDX 1179
Arthritis due to other bacteria, tarsus, metatarsus, and phalanges
- **MØØ.871 Arthritis due to other bacteria, right ankle and foot**
- **MØØ.872 Arthritis due to other bacteria, left ankle and foot**
- **MØØ.879 Arthritis due to other bacteria, unspecified ankle and foot**

MØØ.88 Arthritis due to other bacteria, vertebrae (Ex) PDX 1172

MØØ.89 Polyarthritis due to other bacteria (Ex) PDX 1172

MØØ.9 Pyogenic arthritis, unspecified (Ex) PDX 1172
Infective arthritis NOS

MØ1 Direct infections of joint in infectious and parasitic diseases classified elsewhere

Code first *underlying disease, such as:*
- leprosy [Hansen's disease] (A3Ø.-)
- mycoses (B35-B49)
- O'nyong-nyong fever (A92.1)
- paratyphoid fever (AØ1.1-AØ1.4)

Excludes1
- arthropathy in Lyme disease (A69.23)
- gonococcal arthritis (A54.42)
- meningococcal arthritis (A39.83)
- mumps arthritis (B26.85)
- postinfective arthropathy (MØ2.-)
- postmeningococcal arthritis (A39.84)
- reactive arthritis (MØ2.3)
- rubella arthritis (BØ6.82)
- sarcoidosis arthritis (D86.86)
- typhoid fever arthritis (AØ1.Ø4)
- tuberculosis arthritis (A18.Ø1-A18.Ø2)

MØ1.X Direct infection of joint in infectious and parasitic diseases classified elsewhere (Ex) PDX 1180
- *MØ1.XØ Direct infection of unspecified joint in infectious and parasitic diseases classified elsewhere*

M01.X1 Direct infection of shoulder joint in infectious and parasitic diseases classified elsewhere

M01.X11 Direct infection of right shoulder in infectious and parasitic diseases classified elsewhere

M01.X12 Direct infection of left shoulder in infectious and parasitic diseases classified elsewhere

M01.X19 Direct infection of unspecified shoulder in infectious and parasitic diseases classified elsewhere

M01.X2 Direct infection of elbow in infectious and parasitic diseases classified elsewhere

M01.X21 Direct infection of right elbow in infectious and parasitic diseases classified elsewhere

M01.X22 Direct infection of left elbow in infectious and parasitic diseases classified elsewhere

M01.X29 Direct infection of unspecified elbow in infectious and parasitic diseases classified elsewhere

M01.X3 Direct infection of wrist in infectious and parasitic diseases classified elsewhere

Direct infection of carpal bones in infectious and parasitic diseases classified elsewhere

M01.X31 Direct infection of right wrist in infectious and parasitic diseases classified elsewhere

M01.X32 Direct infection of left wrist in infectious and parasitic diseases classified elsewhere

M01.X39 Direct infection of unspecified wrist in infectious and parasitic diseases classified elsewhere

M01.X4 Direct infection of hand in infectious and parasitic diseases classified elsewhere

Direct infection of metacarpus and phalanges in infectious and parasitic diseases classified elsewhere

M01.X41 Direct infection of right hand in infectious and parasitic diseases classified elsewhere

M01.X42 Direct infection of left hand in infectious and parasitic diseases classified elsewhere

M01.X49 Direct infection of unspecified hand in infectious and parasitic diseases classified elsewhere

M01.X5 Direct infection of hip in infectious and parasitic diseases classified elsewhere

M01.X51 Direct infection of right hip in infectious and parasitic diseases classified elsewhere

M01.X52 Direct infection of left hip in infectious and parasitic diseases classified elsewhere

M01.X59 Direct infection of unspecified hip in infectious and parasitic diseases classified elsewhere

M01.X6 Direct infection of knee in infectious and parasitic diseases classified elsewhere

M01.X61 Direct infection of right knee in infectious and parasitic diseases classified elsewhere

M01.X62 Direct infection of left knee in infectious and parasitic diseases classified elsewhere

M01.X69 Direct infection of unspecified knee in infectious and parasitic diseases classified elsewhere

M01.X7 Direct infection of ankle and foot in infectious and parasitic diseases classified elsewhere

Direct infection of tarsus, metatarsus and phalanges in infectious and parasitic diseases classified elsewhere

M01.X71 Direct infection of right ankle and foot in infectious and parasitic diseases classified elsewhere

M01.X72 Direct infection of left ankle and foot in infectious and parasitic diseases classified elsewhere

M01.X79 Direct infection of unspecified ankle and foot in infectious and parasitic diseases classified elsewhere

M01.X8 Direct infection of vertebrae in infectious and parasitic diseases classified elsewhere

M01.X9 Direct infection of multiple joints in infectious and parasitic diseases classified elsewhere

M02 Postinfective and reactive arthropathies (Ex) PDX 1181

Code first underlying disease, such as:
congenital syphilis [Clutton's joints] (A50.5)
enteritis due to Yersinia enterocolitica (A04.6)
infective endocarditis (I33.0)
viral hepatitis (B15-B19)

Excludes1 Behçet's disease (M35.2)
direct infections of joint in infectious and parasitic diseases classified elsewhere (M01.-)
postmeningococcal arthritis (A39.84)
mumps arthritis (B26.85)
rubella arthritis (B06.82)
syphilis arthritis (late) (A52.77)
rheumatic fever (I00)
tabetic arthropathy [Charcôt's] (A52.16)

M02.0 Arthropathy following intestinal bypass

M02.00 Arthropathy following intestinal bypass, unspecified site

M02.01 Arthropathy following intestinal bypass, shoulder

M02.011 Arthropathy following intestinal bypass, right shoulder

M02.012 Arthropathy following intestinal bypass, left shoulder

M02.019 Arthropathy following intestinal bypass, unspecified shoulder

M02.02 Arthropathy following intestinal bypass, elbow

M02.021 Arthropathy following intestinal bypass, right elbow

M02.022 Arthropathy following intestinal bypass, left elbow

M02.029 Arthropathy following intestinal bypass, unspecified elbow

M02.03 Arthropathy following intestinal bypass, wrist

Arthropathy following intestinal bypass, carpal bones

M02.031 Arthropathy following intestinal bypass, right wrist

M02.032 Arthropathy following intestinal bypass, left wrist

M02.039 Arthropathy following intestinal bypass, unspecified wrist

M02.04 Arthropathy following intestinal bypass, hand

Arthropathy following intestinal bypass, metacarpals and phalanges

M02.041 Arthropathy following intestinal bypass, right hand

M02.042 Arthropathy following intestinal bypass, left hand

M02.049 Arthropathy following intestinal bypass, unspecified hand

CHAPTER 13 (M00-M99)

MØ2.05 Arthropathy following intestinal bypass, hip
MØ2.051 Arthropathy following intestinal bypass, right hip
MØ2.052 Arthropathy following intestinal bypass, left hip
MØ2.059 Arthropathy following intestinal bypass, unspecified hip
MØ2.06 Arthropathy following intestinal bypass, knee
MØ2.061 Arthropathy following intestinal bypass, right knee
MØ2.062 Arthropathy following intestinal bypass, left knee
MØ2.069 Arthropathy following intestinal bypass, unspecified knee
MØ2.07 Arthropathy following intestinal bypass, ankle and foot
Arthropathy following intestinal bypass, tarsus, metatarsus and phalanges
MØ2.071 Arthropathy following intestinal bypass, right ankle and foot
MØ2.072 Arthropathy following intestinal bypass, left ankle and foot
MØ2.079 Arthropathy following intestinal bypass, unspecified ankle and foot
MØ2.08 Arthropathy following intestinal bypass, vertebrae
MØ2.09 Arthropathy following intestinal bypass, multiple sites
MØ2.1 Postdysenteric arthropathy
MØ2.10 Postdysenteric arthropathy, unspecified site Ex: PDX 1181
MØ2.11 Postdysenteric arthropathy, shoulder Ex: PDX 1181
MØ2.111 Postdysenteric arthropathy, right shoulder
MØ2.112 Postdysenteric arthropathy, left shoulder
MØ2.119 Postdysenteric arthropathy, unspecified shoulder
MØ2.12 Postdysenteric arthropathy, elbow Ex: PDX 1181
MØ2.121 Postdysenteric arthropathy, right elbow
MØ2.122 Postdysenteric arthropathy, left elbow
MØ2.129 Postdysenteric arthropathy, unspecified elbow
MØ2.13 Postdysenteric arthropathy, wrist Ex: PDX 1181
Postdysenteric arthropathy, carpal bones
MØ2.131 Postdysenteric arthropathy, right wrist
MØ2.132 Postdysenteric arthropathy, left wrist
MØ2.139 Postdysenteric arthropathy, unspecified wrist
MØ2.14 Postdysenteric arthropathy, hand Ex: PDX 1181
Postdysenteric arthropathy, metacarpus and phalanges
MØ2.141 Postdysenteric arthropathy, right hand
MØ2.142 Postdysenteric arthropathy, left hand
MØ2.149 Postdysenteric arthropathy, unspecified hand
MØ2.15 Postdysenteric arthropathy, hip Ex: PDX 1181
MØ2.151 Postdysenteric arthropathy, right hip
MØ2.152 Postdysenteric arthropathy, left hip
MØ2.159 Postdysenteric arthropathy, unspecified hip
MØ2.16 Postdysenteric arthropathy, knee Ex: PDX 1182
MØ2.161 Postdysenteric arthropathy, right knee
MØ2.162 Postdysenteric arthropathy, left knee
MØ2.169 Postdysenteric arthropathy, unspecified knee
MØ2.17 Postdysenteric arthropathy, ankle and foot Ex: PDX 1181
Postdysenteric arthropathy, tarsus, metatarsus and phalanges
MØ2.171 Postdysenteric arthropathy, right ankle and foot
MØ2.172 Postdysenteric arthropathy, left ankle and foot
MØ2.179 Postdysenteric arthropathy, unspecified ankle and foot
MØ2.18 Postdysenteric arthropathy, vertebrae Ex: PDX 1181
MØ2.19 Postdysenteric arthropathy, multiple sites Ex: PDX 1181
MØ2.2 Postimmunization arthropathy
MØ2.20 Postimmunization arthropathy, unspecified site
MØ2.21 Postimmunization arthropathy, shoulder
MØ2.211 Postimmunization arthropathy, right shoulder
MØ2.212 Postimmunization arthropathy, left shoulder
MØ2.219 Postimmunization arthropathy, unspecified shoulder
MØ2.22 Postimmunization arthropathy, elbow
MØ2.221 Postimmunization arthropathy, right elbow
MØ2.222 Postimmunization arthropathy, left elbow
MØ2.229 Postimmunization arthropathy, unspecified elbow
MØ2.23 Postimmunization arthropathy, wrist
Postimmunization arthropathy, carpal bones
MØ2.231 Postimmunization arthropathy, right wrist
MØ2.232 Postimmunization arthropathy, left wrist
MØ2.239 Postimmunization arthropathy, unspecified wrist
MØ2.24 Postimmunization arthropathy, hand
Postimmunization arthropathy, metacarpus and phalanges
MØ2.241 Postimmunization arthropathy, right hand
MØ2.242 Postimmunization arthropathy, left hand
MØ2.249 Postimmunization arthropathy, unspecified hand
MØ2.25 Postimmunization arthropathy, hip
MØ2.251 Postimmunization arthropathy, right hip
MØ2.252 Postimmunization arthropathy, left hip
MØ2.259 Postimmunization arthropathy, unspecified hip
MØ2.26 Postimmunization arthropathy, knee
MØ2.261 Postimmunization arthropathy, right knee
MØ2.262 Postimmunization arthropathy, left knee
MØ2.269 Postimmunization arthropathy, unspecified knee

● **M02.27 Postimmunization arthropathy, ankle and foot**
Postimmunization arthropathy, tarsus, metatarsus and phalanges
M02.271 Postimmunization arthropathy, right ankle and foot
M02.272 Postimmunization arthropathy, left ankle and foot
M02.279 Postimmunization arthropathy, unspecified ankle and foot
M02.28 Postimmunization arthropathy, vertebrae
M02.29 Postimmunization arthropathy, multiple sites

● **M02.3 Reiter's disease**
Reactive arthritis
M02.30 Reiter's disease, unspecified site (Ex:) PDX 1181
CC when PDx is its own CC

● **M02.31 Reiter's disease, shoulder**
M02.311 Reiter's disease, right shoulder (Ex:) PDX 1183
CC when PDx is its own CC
M02.312 Reiter's disease, left shoulder (Ex:) PDX 1184
CC when PDx is its own CC
M02.319 Reiter's disease, unspecified shoulder (Ex:) PDX 1181
CC when PDx is its own CC

● **M02.32 Reiter's disease, elbow**
M02.321 Reiter's disease, right elbow (Ex:) PDX 1185
CC when PDx is its own CC
M02.322 Reiter's disease, left elbow (Ex:) PDX 1186
CC when PDx is its own CC
M02.329 Reiter's disease, unspecified elbow (Ex:) PDX 1181
CC when PDx is its own CC

● **M02.33 Reiter's disease, wrist**
Reiter's disease, carpal bones
M02.331 Reiter's disease, right wrist (Ex:) PDX 1187
CC when PDx is its own CC
M02.332 Reiter's disease, left wrist (Ex:) PDX 1188
CC when PDx is its own CC
M02.339 Reiter's disease, unspecified wrist (Ex:) PDX 1181
CC when PDx is its own CC

● **M02.34 Reiter's disease, hand**
Reiter's disease, metacarpus and phalanges
M02.341 Reiter's disease, right hand (Ex:) PDX 1189
CC when PDx is its own CC
M02.342 Reiter's disease, left hand (Ex:) PDX 1190
CC when PDx is its own CC
M02.349 Reiter's disease, unspecified hand (Ex:) PDX 1181
CC when PDx is its own CC

● **M02.35 Reiter's disease, hip**
M02.351 Reiter's disease, right hip (Ex:) PDX 1190
CC when PDx is its own CC
M02.352 Reiter's disease, left hip (Ex:) PDX 1192
CC when PDx is its own CC
M02.359 Reiter's disease, unspecified hip (Ex:) PDX 1181
CC when PDx is its own CC

● **M02.36 Reiter's disease, knee**
M02.361 Reiter's disease, right knee (Ex:) PDX 1193
CC when PDx is its own CC
M02.362 Reiter's disease, left knee (Ex:) PDX 1194
CC when PDx is its own CC
M02.369 Reiter's disease, unspecified knee (Ex:) PDX 1181
CC when PDx is its own CC

● **M02.37 Reiter's disease, ankle and foot**
Reiter's disease, tarsus, metatarsus and phalanges
M02.371 Reiter's disease, right ankle and foot (Ex:) PDX 1195
CC when PDx is its own CC
M02.372 Reiter's disease, left ankle and foot (Ex:) PDX 1196
CC when PDx is its own CC
M02.379 Reiter's disease, unspecified ankle and foot (Ex:) PDX 1181
CC when PDx is its own CC
M02.38 Reiter's disease, vertebrae (Ex:) PDX 1181
CC when PDx is its own CC
M02.39 Reiter's disease, multiple sites (Ex:) PDX 1181
CC when PDx is its own CC

● **M02.8 Other reactive arthropathies** (Ex:) PDX 1181
M02.80 Other reactive arthropathies, unspecified site

● **M02.81 Other reactive arthropathies, shoulder**
M02.811 Other reactive arthropathies, right shoulder
M02.812 Other reactive arthropathies, left shoulder
M02.819 Other reactive arthropathies, unspecified shoulder

● **M02.82 Other reactive arthropathies, elbow**
M02.821 Other reactive arthropathies, right elbow
M02.822 Other reactive arthropathies, left elbow
M02.829 Other reactive arthropathies, unspecified elbow

● **M02.83 Other reactive arthropathies, wrist**
Other reactive arthropathies, carpal bones
M02.831 Other reactive arthropathies, right wrist
M02.832 Other reactive arthropathies, left wrist
M02.839 Other reactive arthropathies, unspecified wrist

● **M02.84 Other reactive arthropathies, hand**
Other reactive arthropathies, metacarpus and phalanges
M02.841 Other reactive arthropathies, right hand
M02.842 Other reactive arthropathies, left hand
M02.849 Other reactive arthropathies, unspecified hand

● **M02.85 Other reactive arthropathies, hip**
M02.851 Other reactive arthropathies, right hip
M02.852 Other reactive arthropathies, left hip
M02.859 Other reactive arthropathies, unspecified hip

MØ2.86 Other reactive arthropathies, knee
- MØ2.861 *Other reactive arthropathies, right knee*
- MØ2.862 *Other reactive arthropathies, left knee*
- MØ2.869 *Other reactive arthropathies, unspecified knee*

MØ2.87 Other reactive arthropathies, ankle and foot
Other reactive arthropathies, tarsus, metatarsus and phalanges
- MØ2.871 *Other reactive arthropathies, right ankle and foot*
- MØ2.872 *Other reactive arthropathies, left ankle and foot*
- MØ2.879 *Other reactive arthropathies, unspecified ankle and foot*

MØ2.88 *Other reactive arthropathies, vertebrae*

MØ2.89 *Other reactive arthropathies, multiple sites*

MØ2.9 *Reactive arthropathy, unspecified*

AUTOINFLAMMATORY SYNDROMES (MØ4)

MØ4 Autoinflammatory syndromes
Excludes2 Crohn's disease (K5Ø.-)
Coding Clinic: 2016, Q4, P37

MØ4.1 Periodic fever syndromes
Familial Mediterranean fever
Hyperimmunoglobin D syndrome
Mevalonate kinase deficiency
Tumor necrosis factor receptor associated periodic syndrome [TRAPS]

MØ4.2 Cryopyrin-associated periodic syndromes
Chronic infantile neurological, cutaneous and articular syndrome [CINCA]
Familial cold autoinflammatory syndrome
Familial cold urticaria
Muckle-Wells syndrome
Neonatal onset multisystemic inflammatory disorder [NOMID]

MØ4.8 Other autoinflammatory syndromes
Blau syndrome
Deficiency of interleukin 1 receptor antagonist [DIRA]
Majeed syndrome
Periodic fever, aphthous stomatitis, pharyngitis, and adenopathy syndrome [PFAPA]
Pyogenic arthritis, pyoderma gangrenosum, and acne syndrome [PAPA]

MØ4.9 Autoinflammatory syndrome, unspecified

INFLAMMATORY POLYARTHROPATHIES (MØ5-M14)

MØ5 Rheumatoid arthritis with rheumatoid factor
Excludes1 rheumatic fever (IØØ)
juvenile rheumatoid arthritis (MØ8.-)
rheumatoid arthritis of spine (M45.-)

MØ5.Ø Felty's syndrome
Rheumatoid arthritis with splenoadenomegaly and leukopenia
- MØ5.ØØ Felty's syndrome, unspecified site
- MØ5.Ø1 Felty's syndrome, shoulder
  - MØ5.Ø11 Felty's syndrome, right shoulder
  - MØ5.Ø12 Felty's syndrome, left shoulder
  - MØ5.Ø19 Felty's syndrome, unspecified shoulder
- MØ5.Ø2 Felty's syndrome, elbow
  - MØ5.Ø21 Felty's syndrome, right elbow
  - MØ5.Ø22 Felty's syndrome, left elbow
  - MØ5.Ø29 Felty's syndrome, unspecified elbow
- MØ5.Ø3 Felty's syndrome, wrist
  Felty's syndrome, carpal bones
  - MØ5.Ø31 Felty's syndrome, right wrist
  - MØ5.Ø32 Felty's syndrome, left wrist
  - MØ5.Ø39 Felty's syndrome, unspecified wrist
- MØ5.Ø4 Felty's syndrome, hand
  Felty's syndrome, metacarpus and phalanges
  - MØ5.Ø41 Felty's syndrome, right hand
  - MØ5.Ø42 Felty's syndrome, left hand
  - MØ5.Ø49 Felty's syndrome, unspecified hand
- MØ5.Ø5 Felty's syndrome, hip
  - MØ5.Ø51 Felty's syndrome, right hip
  - MØ5.Ø52 Felty's syndrome, left hip
  - MØ5.Ø59 Felty's syndrome, unspecified hip
- MØ5.Ø6 Felty's syndrome, knee
  - MØ5.Ø61 Felty's syndrome, right knee
  - MØ5.Ø62 Felty's syndrome, left knee
  - MØ5.Ø69 Felty's syndrome, unspecified knee
- MØ5.Ø7 Felty's syndrome, ankle and foot
  Felty's syndrome, tarsus, metatarsus and phalanges
  - MØ5.Ø71 Felty's syndrome, right ankle and foot
  - MØ5.Ø72 Felty's syndrome, left ankle and foot
  - MØ5.Ø79 Felty's syndrome, unspecified ankle and foot
- MØ5.Ø9 Felty's syndrome, multiple sites

MØ5.1 Rheumatoid lung disease with rheumatoid arthritis
- MØ5.1Ø Rheumatoid lung disease with rheumatoid arthritis of unspecified site
- MØ5.11 Rheumatoid lung disease with rheumatoid arthritis of shoulder
  - MØ5.111 Rheumatoid lung disease with rheumatoid arthritis of right shoulder
  - MØ5.112 Rheumatoid lung disease with rheumatoid arthritis of left shoulder
  - MØ5.119 Rheumatoid lung disease with rheumatoid arthritis of unspecified shoulder
- MØ5.12 Rheumatoid lung disease with rheumatoid arthritis of elbow
  - MØ5.121 Rheumatoid lung disease with rheumatoid arthritis of right elbow
  - MØ5.122 Rheumatoid lung disease with rheumatoid arthritis of left elbow
  - MØ5.129 Rheumatoid lung disease with rheumatoid arthritis of unspecified elbow
- MØ5.13 Rheumatoid lung disease with rheumatoid arthritis of wrist
  Rheumatoid lung disease with rheumatoid arthritis, carpal bones
  - MØ5.131 Rheumatoid lung disease with rheumatoid arthritis of right wrist
  - MØ5.132 Rheumatoid lung disease with rheumatoid arthritis of left wrist
  - MØ5.139 Rheumatoid lung disease with rheumatoid arthritis of unspecified wrist

Item 13–1 Rheumatoid arthritis (RA) is a chronic systemic inflammatory autoimmune disease of undetermined etiology involving primarily the synovial membranes and articular structures of multiple joints. It can also affect other organs, including the eyes, blood vessels, heart, and lungs. The disease is often progressive. In late stages, deformity, ankylosis, and other **inflammatory polyarthropathies** develop.

● **MØ5.14 Rheumatoid lung disease with rheumatoid arthritis of hand**
Rheumatoid lung disease with rheumatoid arthritis, metacarpus and phalanges
MØ5.141 Rheumatoid lung disease with rheumatoid arthritis of right hand
MØ5.142 Rheumatoid lung disease with rheumatoid arthritis of left hand
MØ5.149 Rheumatoid lung disease with rheumatoid arthritis of unspecified hand

● **MØ5.15 Rheumatoid lung disease with rheumatoid arthritis of hip**
MØ5.151 Rheumatoid lung disease with rheumatoid arthritis of right hip
MØ5.152 Rheumatoid lung disease with rheumatoid arthritis of left hip
MØ5.159 Rheumatoid lung disease with rheumatoid arthritis of unspecified hip

● **MØ5.16 Rheumatoid lung disease with rheumatoid arthritis of knee**
MØ5.161 Rheumatoid lung disease with rheumatoid arthritis of right knee
MØ5.162 Rheumatoid lung disease with rheumatoid arthritis of left knee
MØ5.169 Rheumatoid lung disease with rheumatoid arthritis of unspecified knee

● **MØ5.17 Rheumatoid lung disease with rheumatoid arthritis of ankle and foot**
Rheumatoid lung disease with rheumatoid arthritis, tarsus, metatarsus and phalanges
MØ5.171 Rheumatoid lung disease with rheumatoid arthritis of right ankle and foot
MØ5.172 Rheumatoid lung disease with rheumatoid arthritis of left ankle and foot
MØ5.179 Rheumatoid lung disease with rheumatoid arthritis of unspecified ankle and foot

MØ5.19 Rheumatoid lung disease with rheumatoid arthritis of multiple sites

● **MØ5.2 Rheumatoid vasculitis with rheumatoid arthritis**
MØ5.2Ø Rheumatoid vasculitis with rheumatoid arthritis of unspecified site

● **MØ5.21 Rheumatoid vasculitis with rheumatoid arthritis of shoulder**
MØ5.211 Rheumatoid vasculitis with rheumatoid arthritis of right shoulder
MØ5.212 Rheumatoid vasculitis with rheumatoid arthritis of left shoulder
MØ5.219 Rheumatoid vasculitis with rheumatoid arthritis of unspecified shoulder

● **MØ5.22 Rheumatoid vasculitis with rheumatoid arthritis of elbow**
MØ5.221 Rheumatoid vasculitis with rheumatoid arthritis of right elbow
MØ5.222 Rheumatoid vasculitis with rheumatoid arthritis of left elbow
MØ5.229 Rheumatoid vasculitis with rheumatoid arthritis of unspecified elbow

● **MØ5.23 Rheumatoid vasculitis with rheumatoid arthritis of wrist**
Rheumatoid vasculitis with rheumatoid arthritis, carpal bones
MØ5.231 Rheumatoid vasculitis with rheumatoid arthritis of right wrist
MØ5.232 Rheumatoid vasculitis with rheumatoid arthritis of left wrist
MØ5.239 Rheumatoid vasculitis with rheumatoid arthritis of unspecified wrist

● **MØ5.24 Rheumatoid vasculitis with rheumatoid arthritis of hand**
Rheumatoid vasculitis with rheumatoid arthritis, metacarpus and phalanges
MØ5.241 Rheumatoid vasculitis with rheumatoid arthritis of right hand
MØ5.242 Rheumatoid vasculitis with rheumatoid arthritis of left hand
MØ5.249 Rheumatoid vasculitis with rheumatoid arthritis of unspecified hand

● **MØ5.25 Rheumatoid vasculitis with rheumatoid arthritis of hip**
MØ5.251 Rheumatoid vasculitis with rheumatoid arthritis of right hip
MØ5.252 Rheumatoid vasculitis with rheumatoid arthritis of left hip
MØ5.259 Rheumatoid vasculitis with rheumatoid arthritis of unspecified hip

● **MØ5.26 Rheumatoid vasculitis with rheumatoid arthritis of knee**
MØ5.261 Rheumatoid vasculitis with rheumatoid arthritis of right knee
MØ5.262 Rheumatoid vasculitis with rheumatoid arthritis of left knee
MØ5.269 Rheumatoid vasculitis with rheumatoid arthritis of unspecified knee

● **MØ5.27 Rheumatoid vasculitis with rheumatoid arthritis of ankle and foot**
Rheumatoid vasculitis with rheumatoid arthritis, tarsus, metatarsus and phalanges
MØ5.271 Rheumatoid vasculitis with rheumatoid arthritis of right ankle and foot
MØ5.272 Rheumatoid vasculitis with rheumatoid arthritis of left ankle and foot
MØ5.279 Rheumatoid vasculitis with rheumatoid arthritis of unspecified ankle and foot

MØ5.29 Rheumatoid vasculitis with rheumatoid arthritis of multiple sites

● **MØ5.3 Rheumatoid heart disease with rheumatoid arthritis**
Rheumatoid carditis
Rheumatoid endocarditis
Rheumatoid myocarditis
Rheumatoid pericarditis
MØ5.3Ø Rheumatoid heart disease with rheumatoid arthritis of unspecified site

● **MØ5.31 Rheumatoid heart disease with rheumatoid arthritis of shoulder**
MØ5.311 Rheumatoid heart disease with rheumatoid arthritis of right shoulder
MØ5.312 Rheumatoid heart disease with rheumatoid arthritis of left shoulder
MØ5.319 Rheumatoid heart disease with rheumatoid arthritis of unspecified shoulder

CHAPTER 13 (MØØ-M99)

M05.32 Rheumatoid heart disease with rheumatoid arthritis of elbow

M05.321 Rheumatoid heart disease with rheumatoid arthritis of right elbow

M05.322 Rheumatoid heart disease with rheumatoid arthritis of left elbow

M05.329 Rheumatoid heart disease with rheumatoid arthritis of unspecified elbow

M05.33 Rheumatoid heart disease with rheumatoid arthritis of wrist

Rheumatoid heart disease with rheumatoid arthritis, carpal bones

M05.331 Rheumatoid heart disease with rheumatoid arthritis of right wrist

M05.332 Rheumatoid heart disease with rheumatoid arthritis of left wrist

M05.339 Rheumatoid heart disease with rheumatoid arthritis of unspecified wrist

M05.34 Rheumatoid heart disease with rheumatoid arthritis of hand

Rheumatoid heart disease with rheumatoid arthritis, metacarpus and phalanges

M05.341 Rheumatoid heart disease with rheumatoid arthritis of right hand

M05.342 Rheumatoid heart disease with rheumatoid arthritis of left hand

M05.349 Rheumatoid heart disease with rheumatoid arthritis of unspecified hand

M05.35 Rheumatoid heart disease with rheumatoid arthritis of hip

M05.351 Rheumatoid heart disease with rheumatoid arthritis of right hip

M05.352 Rheumatoid heart disease with rheumatoid arthritis of left hip

M05.359 Rheumatoid heart disease with rheumatoid arthritis of unspecified hip

M05.36 Rheumatoid heart disease with rheumatoid arthritis of knee

M05.361 Rheumatoid heart disease with rheumatoid arthritis of right knee

M05.362 Rheumatoid heart disease with rheumatoid arthritis of left knee

M05.369 Rheumatoid heart disease with rheumatoid arthritis of unspecified knee

M05.37 Rheumatoid heart disease with rheumatoid arthritis of ankle and foot

Rheumatoid heart disease with rheumatoid arthritis, tarsus, metatarsus and phalanges

M05.371 Rheumatoid heart disease with rheumatoid arthritis of right ankle and foot

M05.372 Rheumatoid heart disease with rheumatoid arthritis of left ankle and foot

M05.379 Rheumatoid heart disease with rheumatoid arthritis of unspecified ankle and foot

M05.39 Rheumatoid heart disease with rheumatoid arthritis of multiple sites

M05.4 Rheumatoid myopathy with rheumatoid arthritis

M05.40 Rheumatoid myopathy with rheumatoid arthritis of unspecified site
CC when PDx is its own CC

M05.41 Rheumatoid myopathy with rheumatoid arthritis of shoulder

M05.411 Rheumatoid myopathy with rheumatoid arthritis of right shoulder Ex PDX 1198
CC when PDx is its own CC

M05.412 Rheumatoid myopathy with rheumatoid arthritis of left shoulder Ex PDX 1199
CC when PDx is its own CC

M05.419 Rheumatoid myopathy with rheumatoid arthritis of unspecified shoulder Ex PDX 1200
CC when PDx is its own CC

M05.42 Rheumatoid myopathy with rheumatoid arthritis of elbow

M05.421 Rheumatoid myopathy with rheumatoid arthritis of right elbow Ex PDX 1201
CC when PDx is its own CC

M05.422 Rheumatoid myopathy with rheumatoid arthritis of left elbow Ex PDX 1202
CC when PDx is its own CC

M05.429 Rheumatoid myopathy with rheumatoid arthritis of unspecified elbow Ex PDX 1203
CC when PDx is its own CC

M05.43 Rheumatoid myopathy with rheumatoid arthritis of wrist

Rheumatoid myopathy with rheumatoid arthritis, carpal bones

M05.431 Rheumatoid myopathy with rheumatoid arthritis of right wrist Ex PDX 1204
CC when PDx is its own CC

M05.432 Rheumatoid myopathy with rheumatoid arthritis of left wrist Ex PDX 1205
CC when PDx is its own CC

M05.439 Rheumatoid myopathy with rheumatoid arthritis of unspecified wrist Ex PDX 1206
CC when PDx is its own CC

M05.44 Rheumatoid myopathy with rheumatoid arthritis of hand

Rheumatoid myopathy with rheumatoid arthritis, metacarpus and phalanges

M05.441 Rheumatoid myopathy with rheumatoid arthritis of right hand Ex PDX 1207
CC when PDx is its own CC

M05.442 Rheumatoid myopathy with rheumatoid arthritis of left hand Ex PDX 1208
CC when PDx is its own CC

M05.449 Rheumatoid myopathy with rheumatoid arthritis of unspecified hand Ex PDX 1209
CC when PDx is its own CC

M05.45 Rheumatoid myopathy with rheumatoid arthritis of hip

M05.451 Rheumatoid myopathy with rheumatoid arthritis of right hip Ex PDX 1210
CC when PDx is its own CC

M05.452 Rheumatoid myopathy with rheumatoid arthritis of left hip Ex PDX 1211
CC when PDx is its own CC

M05.459 Rheumatoid myopathy with rheumatoid arthritis of unspecified hip Ex PDX 1212
CC when PDx is its own CC

● M05.46 Rheumatoid myopathy with rheumatoid arthritis of knee
M05.461 Rheumatoid myopathy with rheumatoid arthritis of right knee (Ex) PDX 1213
CC when PDx is its own CC
M05.462 Rheumatoid myopathy with rheumatoid arthritis of left knee (Ex) PDX 1214
CC when PDx is its own CC
M05.469 Rheumatoid myopathy with rheumatoid arthritis of unspecified knee (Ex) PDX 1215
CC when PDx is its own CC
● M05.47 Rheumatoid myopathy with rheumatoid arthritis of ankle and foot
Rheumatoid myopathy with rheumatoid arthritis, tarsus, metatarsus and phalanges
M05.471 Rheumatoid myopathy with rheumatoid arthritis of right ankle and foot (Ex) PDX 1216
CC when PDx is its own CC
M05.472 Rheumatoid myopathy with rheumatoid arthritis of left ankle and foot (Ex) PDX 1217
CC when PDx is its own CC
M05.479 Rheumatoid myopathy with rheumatoid arthritis of unspecified ankle and foot (Ex) PDX 1218
CC when PDx is its own CC
M05.49 Rheumatoid myopathy with rheumatoid arthritis of multiple sites (Ex) PDX 1219
CC when PDx is its own CC
● M05.5 Rheumatoid polyneuropathy with rheumatoid arthritis
M05.50 Rheumatoid polyneuropathy with rheumatoid arthritis of unspecified site
● M05.51 Rheumatoid polyneuropathy with rheumatoid arthritis of shoulder
M05.511 Rheumatoid polyneuropathy with rheumatoid arthritis of right shoulder
M05.512 Rheumatoid polyneuropathy with rheumatoid arthritis of left shoulder
M05.519 Rheumatoid polyneuropathy with rheumatoid arthritis of unspecified shoulder
● M05.52 Rheumatoid polyneuropathy with rheumatoid arthritis of elbow
M05.521 Rheumatoid polyneuropathy with rheumatoid arthritis of right elbow
M05.522 Rheumatoid polyneuropathy with rheumatoid arthritis of left elbow
M05.529 Rheumatoid polyneuropathy with rheumatoid arthritis of unspecified elbow
● M05.53 Rheumatoid polyneuropathy with rheumatoid arthritis of wrist
Rheumatoid polyneuropathy with rheumatoid arthritis, carpal bones
M05.531 Rheumatoid polyneuropathy with rheumatoid arthritis of right wrist
M05.532 Rheumatoid polyneuropathy with rheumatoid arthritis of left wrist
M05.539 Rheumatoid polyneuropathy with rheumatoid arthritis of unspecified wrist
● M05.54 Rheumatoid polyneuropathy with rheumatoid arthritis of hand
Rheumatoid polyneuropathy with rheumatoid arthritis, metacarpus and phalanges
M05.541 Rheumatoid polyneuropathy with rheumatoid arthritis of right hand
M05.542 Rheumatoid polyneuropathy with rheumatoid arthritis of left hand
M05.549 Rheumatoid polyneuropathy with rheumatoid arthritis of unspecified hand
● M05.55 Rheumatoid polyneuropathy with rheumatoid arthritis of hip
M05.551 Rheumatoid polyneuropathy with rheumatoid arthritis of right hip
M05.552 Rheumatoid polyneuropathy with rheumatoid arthritis of left hip
M05.559 Rheumatoid polyneuropathy with rheumatoid arthritis of unspecified hip
● M05.56 Rheumatoid polyneuropathy with rheumatoid arthritis of knee
M05.561 Rheumatoid polyneuropathy with rheumatoid arthritis of right knee
M05.562 Rheumatoid polyneuropathy with rheumatoid arthritis of left knee
M05.569 Rheumatoid polyneuropathy with rheumatoid arthritis of unspecified knee
● M05.57 Rheumatoid polyneuropathy with rheumatoid arthritis of ankle and foot
Rheumatoid polyneuropathy with rheumatoid arthritis, tarsus, metatarsus and phalanges
M05.571 Rheumatoid polyneuropathy with rheumatoid arthritis of right ankle and foot
M05.572 Rheumatoid polyneuropathy with rheumatoid arthritis of left ankle and foot
M05.579 Rheumatoid polyneuropathy with rheumatoid arthritis of unspecified ankle and foot
M05.59 Rheumatoid polyneuropathy with rheumatoid arthritis of multiple sites
● M05.6 Rheumatoid arthritis with involvement of other organs and systems
M05.60 Rheumatoid arthritis of unspecified site with involvement of other organs and systems
● M05.61 Rheumatoid arthritis of shoulder with involvement of other organs and systems
M05.611 Rheumatoid arthritis of right shoulder with involvement of other organs and systems
M05.612 Rheumatoid arthritis of left shoulder with involvement of other organs and systems
M05.619 Rheumatoid arthritis of unspecified shoulder with involvement of other organs and systems
● M05.62 Rheumatoid arthritis of elbow with involvement of other organs and systems
M05.621 Rheumatoid arthritis of right elbow with involvement of other organs and systems
M05.622 Rheumatoid arthritis of left elbow with involvement of other organs and systems
M05.629 Rheumatoid arthritis of unspecified elbow with involvement of other organs and systems

CHAPTER 13 (M00-M99)

● M05.63 Rheumatoid arthritis of wrist with involvement of other organs and systems
Rheumatoid arthritis of carpal bones with involvement of other organs and systems
M05.631 Rheumatoid arthritis of right wrist with involvement of other organs and systems
M05.632 Rheumatoid arthritis of left wrist with involvement of other organs and systems
M05.639 Rheumatoid arthritis of unspecified wrist with involvement of other organs and systems

● M05.64 Rheumatoid arthritis of hand with involvement of other organs and systems
Rheumatoid arthritis of metacarpus and phalanges with involvement of other organs and systems
M05.641 Rheumatoid arthritis of right hand with involvement of other organs and systems
M05.642 Rheumatoid arthritis of left hand with involvement of other organs and systems
M05.649 Rheumatoid arthritis of unspecified hand with involvement of other organs and systems

● M05.65 Rheumatoid arthritis of hip with involvement of other organs and systems
M05.651 Rheumatoid arthritis of right hip with involvement of other organs and systems
M05.652 Rheumatoid arthritis of left hip with involvement of other organs and systems
M05.659 Rheumatoid arthritis of unspecified hip with involvement of other organs and systems

● M05.66 Rheumatoid arthritis of knee with involvement of other organs and systems
M05.661 Rheumatoid arthritis of right knee with involvement of other organs and systems
M05.662 Rheumatoid arthritis of left knee with involvement of other organs and systems
M05.669 Rheumatoid arthritis of unspecified knee with involvement of other organs and systems

● M05.67 Rheumatoid arthritis of ankle and foot with involvement of other organs and systems
Rheumatoid arthritis of tarsus, metatarsus and phalanges with involvement of other organs and systems
M05.671 Rheumatoid arthritis of right ankle and foot with involvement of other organs and systems
M05.672 Rheumatoid arthritis of left ankle and foot with involvement of other organs and systems
M05.679 Rheumatoid arthritis of unspecified ankle and foot with involvement of other organs and systems

M05.69 Rheumatoid arthritis of multiple sites with involvement of other organs and systems

● M05.7 Rheumatoid arthritis with rheumatoid factor without organ or systems involvement
M05.70 Rheumatoid arthritis with rheumatoid factor of unspecified site without organ or systems involvement

● M05.71 Rheumatoid arthritis with rheumatoid factor of shoulder without organ or systems involvement
M05.711 Rheumatoid arthritis with rheumatoid factor of right shoulder without organ or systems involvement
M05.712 Rheumatoid arthritis with rheumatoid factor of left shoulder without organ or systems involvement
M05.719 Rheumatoid arthritis with rheumatoid factor of unspecified shoulder without organ or systems involvement

● M05.72 Rheumatoid arthritis with rheumatoid factor of elbow without organ or systems involvement
M05.721 Rheumatoid arthritis with rheumatoid factor of right elbow without organ or systems involvement
M05.722 Rheumatoid arthritis with rheumatoid factor of left elbow without organ or systems involvement
M05.729 Rheumatoid arthritis with rheumatoid factor of unspecified elbow without organ or systems involvement

● M05.73 Rheumatoid arthritis with rheumatoid factor of wrist without organ or systems involvement
M05.731 Rheumatoid arthritis with rheumatoid factor of right wrist without organ or systems involvement
M05.732 Rheumatoid arthritis with rheumatoid factor of left wrist without organ or systems involvement
M05.739 Rheumatoid arthritis with rheumatoid factor of unspecified wrist without organ or systems involvement

● M05.74 Rheumatoid arthritis with rheumatoid factor of hand without organ or systems involvement
M05.741 Rheumatoid arthritis with rheumatoid factor of right hand without organ or systems involvement
M05.742 Rheumatoid arthritis with rheumatoid factor of left hand without organ or systems involvement
M05.749 Rheumatoid arthritis with rheumatoid factor of unspecified hand without organ or systems involvement

● M05.75 Rheumatoid arthritis with rheumatoid factor of hip without organ or systems involvement
M05.751 Rheumatoid arthritis with rheumatoid factor of right hip without organ or systems involvement
M05.752 Rheumatoid arthritis with rheumatoid factor of left hip without organ or systems involvement
M05.759 Rheumatoid arthritis with rheumatoid factor of unspecified hip without organ or systems involvement

● M05.76 Rheumatoid arthritis with rheumatoid factor of knee without organ or systems involvement
 M05.761 Rheumatoid arthritis with rheumatoid factor of right knee without organ or systems involvement
 M05.762 Rheumatoid arthritis with rheumatoid factor of left knee without organ or systems involvement
 M05.769 Rheumatoid arthritis with rheumatoid factor of unspecified knee without organ or systems involvement
● M05.77 Rheumatoid arthritis with rheumatoid factor of ankle and foot without organ or systems involvement
 M05.771 Rheumatoid arthritis with rheumatoid factor of right ankle and foot without organ or systems involvement
 M05.772 Rheumatoid arthritis with rheumatoid factor of left ankle and foot without organ or systems involvement
 M05.779 Rheumatoid arthritis with rheumatoid factor of unspecified ankle and foot without organ or systems involvement
M05.79 Rheumatoid arthritis with rheumatoid factor of multiple sites without organ or systems involvement
M05.7A Rheumatoid arthritis with rheumatoid factor of other specified site without organ or systems involvement

● M05.8 Other rheumatoid arthritis with rheumatoid factor
M05.80 Other rheumatoid arthritis with rheumatoid factor of unspecified site
● M05.81 Other rheumatoid arthritis with rheumatoid factor of shoulder
 M05.811 Other rheumatoid arthritis with rheumatoid factor of right shoulder
 M05.812 Other rheumatoid arthritis with rheumatoid factor of left shoulder
 M05.819 Other rheumatoid arthritis with rheumatoid factor of unspecified shoulder
● M05.82 Other rheumatoid arthritis with rheumatoid factor of elbow
 M05.821 Other rheumatoid arthritis with rheumatoid factor of right elbow
 M05.822 Other rheumatoid arthritis with rheumatoid factor of left elbow
 M05.829 Other rheumatoid arthritis with rheumatoid factor of unspecified elbow
● M05.83 Other rheumatoid arthritis with rheumatoid factor of wrist
 M05.831 Other rheumatoid arthritis with rheumatoid factor of right wrist
 M05.832 Other rheumatoid arthritis with rheumatoid factor of left wrist
 M05.839 Other rheumatoid arthritis with rheumatoid factor of unspecified wrist
● M05.84 Other rheumatoid arthritis with rheumatoid factor of hand
 M05.841 Other rheumatoid arthritis with rheumatoid factor of right hand
 M05.842 Other rheumatoid arthritis with rheumatoid factor of left hand
 M05.849 Other rheumatoid arthritis with rheumatoid factor of unspecified hand
● M05.85 Other rheumatoid arthritis with rheumatoid factor of hip
 M05.851 Other rheumatoid arthritis with rheumatoid factor of right hip
 M05.852 Other rheumatoid arthritis with rheumatoid factor of left hip
 M05.859 Other rheumatoid arthritis with rheumatoid factor of unspecified hip
● M05.86 Other rheumatoid arthritis with rheumatoid factor of knee
 M05.861 Other rheumatoid arthritis with rheumatoid factor of right knee
 M05.862 Other rheumatoid arthritis with rheumatoid factor of left knee
 M05.869 Other rheumatoid arthritis with rheumatoid factor of unspecified knee
● M05.87 Other rheumatoid arthritis with rheumatoid factor of ankle and foot
 M05.871 Other rheumatoid arthritis with rheumatoid factor of right ankle and foot
 M05.872 Other rheumatoid arthritis with rheumatoid factor of left ankle and foot
 M05.879 Other rheumatoid arthritis with rheumatoid factor of unspecified ankle and foot
M05.89 Other rheumatoid arthritis with rheumatoid factor of multiple sites
M05.8A Other rheumatoid arthritis with rheumatoid factor of other specified site

M05.9 Rheumatoid arthritis with rheumatoid factor, unspecified

● M06 Other rheumatoid arthritis

Coding Clinic: 2024, Q1, P17

● M06.0 Rheumatoid arthritis without rheumatoid factor
M06.00 Rheumatoid arthritis without rheumatoid factor, unspecified site
● M06.01 Rheumatoid arthritis without rheumatoid factor, shoulder
 M06.011 Rheumatoid arthritis without rheumatoid factor, right shoulder
 M06.012 Rheumatoid arthritis without rheumatoid factor, left shoulder
 M06.019 Rheumatoid arthritis without rheumatoid factor, unspecified shoulder
● M06.02 Rheumatoid arthritis without rheumatoid factor, elbow
 M06.021 Rheumatoid arthritis without rheumatoid factor, right elbow
 M06.022 Rheumatoid arthritis without rheumatoid factor, left elbow
 M06.029 Rheumatoid arthritis without rheumatoid factor, unspecified elbow

CHAPTER 13 (M00-M99)

● M06.03 Rheumatoid arthritis without rheumatoid factor, wrist
M06.031 Rheumatoid arthritis without rheumatoid factor, right wrist
M06.032 Rheumatoid arthritis without rheumatoid factor, left wrist
M06.039 Rheumatoid arthritis without rheumatoid factor, unspecified wrist

● M06.04 Rheumatoid arthritis without rheumatoid factor, hand
M06.041 Rheumatoid arthritis without rheumatoid factor, right hand
M06.042 Rheumatoid arthritis without rheumatoid factor, left hand
M06.049 Rheumatoid arthritis without rheumatoid factor, unspecified hand

● M06.05 Rheumatoid arthritis without rheumatoid factor, hip
M06.051 Rheumatoid arthritis without rheumatoid factor, right hip
M06.052 Rheumatoid arthritis without rheumatoid factor, left hip
M06.059 Rheumatoid arthritis without rheumatoid factor, unspecified hip

● M06.06 Rheumatoid arthritis without rheumatoid factor, knee
M06.061 Rheumatoid arthritis without rheumatoid factor, right knee
M06.062 Rheumatoid arthritis without rheumatoid factor, left knee
M06.069 Rheumatoid arthritis without rheumatoid factor, unspecified knee

● M06.07 Rheumatoid arthritis without rheumatoid factor, ankle and foot
M06.071 Rheumatoid arthritis without rheumatoid factor, right ankle and foot
M06.072 Rheumatoid arthritis without rheumatoid factor, left ankle and foot
M06.079 Rheumatoid arthritis without rheumatoid factor, unspecified ankle and foot

M06.08 Rheumatoid arthritis without rheumatoid factor, vertebrae
M06.09 Rheumatoid arthritis without rheumatoid factor, multiple sites
M06.0A Rheumatoid arthritis without rheumatoid factor, other specified site

M06.1 Adult-onset Still's disease A
Excludes1 Still's disease NOS (M08.2-)

● M06.2 Rheumatoid bursitis
M06.20 Rheumatoid bursitis, unspecified site

● M06.21 Rheumatoid bursitis, shoulder
M06.211 Rheumatoid bursitis, right shoulder
M06.212 Rheumatoid bursitis, left shoulder
M06.219 Rheumatoid bursitis, unspecified shoulder

● M06.22 Rheumatoid bursitis, elbow
M06.221 Rheumatoid bursitis, right elbow
M06.222 Rheumatoid bursitis, left elbow
M06.229 Rheumatoid bursitis, unspecified elbow

● M06.23 Rheumatoid bursitis, wrist
M06.231 Rheumatoid bursitis, right wrist
M06.232 Rheumatoid bursitis, left wrist
M06.239 Rheumatoid bursitis, unspecified wrist

● M06.24 Rheumatoid bursitis, hand
M06.241 Rheumatoid bursitis, right hand
M06.242 Rheumatoid bursitis, left hand
M06.249 Rheumatoid bursitis, unspecified hand

● M06.25 Rheumatoid bursitis, hip
M06.251 Rheumatoid bursitis, right hip
M06.252 Rheumatoid bursitis, left hip
M06.259 Rheumatoid bursitis, unspecified hip

● M06.26 Rheumatoid bursitis, knee
M06.261 Rheumatoid bursitis, right knee
M06.262 Rheumatoid bursitis, left knee
M06.269 Rheumatoid bursitis, unspecified knee

● M06.27 Rheumatoid bursitis, ankle and foot
M06.271 Rheumatoid bursitis, right ankle and foot
M06.272 Rheumatoid bursitis, left ankle and foot
M06.279 Rheumatoid bursitis, unspecified ankle and foot

M06.28 Rheumatoid bursitis, vertebrae
M06.29 Rheumatoid bursitis, multiple sites

● M06.3 Rheumatoid nodule
M06.30 Rheumatoid nodule, unspecified site

● M06.31 Rheumatoid nodule, shoulder
M06.311 Rheumatoid nodule, right shoulder
M06.312 Rheumatoid nodule, left shoulder
M06.319 Rheumatoid nodule, unspecified shoulder

● M06.32 Rheumatoid nodule, elbow
M06.321 Rheumatoid nodule, right elbow
M06.322 Rheumatoid nodule, left elbow
M06.329 Rheumatoid nodule, unspecified elbow

● M06.33 Rheumatoid nodule, wrist
M06.331 Rheumatoid nodule, right wrist
M06.332 Rheumatoid nodule, left wrist
M06.339 Rheumatoid nodule, unspecified wrist

● M06.34 Rheumatoid nodule, hand
M06.341 Rheumatoid nodule, right hand
M06.342 Rheumatoid nodule, left hand
M06.349 Rheumatoid nodule, unspecified hand

● M06.35 Rheumatoid nodule, hip
M06.351 Rheumatoid nodule, right hip
M06.352 Rheumatoid nodule, left hip
M06.359 Rheumatoid nodule, unspecified hip

● M06.36 Rheumatoid nodule, knee
M06.361 Rheumatoid nodule, right knee
M06.362 Rheumatoid nodule, left knee
M06.369 Rheumatoid nodule, unspecified knee

● **M06.37** Rheumatoid nodule, ankle and foot
- **M06.371** Rheumatoid nodule, right ankle and foot
- **M06.372** Rheumatoid nodule, left ankle and foot
- **M06.379** Rheumatoid nodule, unspecified ankle and foot

M06.38 Rheumatoid nodule, vertebrae

M06.39 Rheumatoid nodule, multiple sites

M06.4 Inflammatory polyarthropathy

Excludes1 polyarthritis NOS (M13.0)

Coding Clinic: 2024, Q1, P17

● **M06.8** Other specified rheumatoid arthritis

M06.80 Other specified rheumatoid arthritis, unspecified site

● **M06.81** Other specified rheumatoid arthritis, shoulder
- **M06.811** Other specified rheumatoid arthritis, right shoulder
- **M06.812** Other specified rheumatoid arthritis, left shoulder
- **M06.819** Other specified rheumatoid arthritis, unspecified shoulder

● **M06.82** Other specified rheumatoid arthritis, elbow
- **M06.821** Other specified rheumatoid arthritis, right elbow
- **M06.822** Other specified rheumatoid arthritis, left elbow
- **M06.829** Other specified rheumatoid arthritis, unspecified elbow

● **M06.83** Other specified rheumatoid arthritis, wrist
- **M06.831** Other specified rheumatoid arthritis, right wrist
- **M06.832** Other specified rheumatoid arthritis, left wrist
- **M06.839** Other specified rheumatoid arthritis, unspecified wrist

● **M06.84** Other specified rheumatoid arthritis, hand
- **M06.841** Other specified rheumatoid arthritis, right hand
- **M06.842** Other specified rheumatoid arthritis, left hand
- **M06.849** Other specified rheumatoid arthritis, unspecified hand

● **M06.85** Other specified rheumatoid arthritis, hip
- **M06.851** Other specified rheumatoid arthritis, right hip
- **M06.852** Other specified rheumatoid arthritis, left hip
- **M06.859** Other specified rheumatoid arthritis, unspecified hip

● **M06.86** Other specified rheumatoid arthritis, knee
- **M06.861** Other specified rheumatoid arthritis, right knee
- **M06.862** Other specified rheumatoid arthritis, left knee
- **M06.869** Other specified rheumatoid arthritis, unspecified knee

● **M06.87** Other specified rheumatoid arthritis, ankle and foot
- **M06.871** Other specified rheumatoid arthritis, right ankle and foot
- **M06.872** Other specified rheumatoid arthritis, left ankle and foot
- **M06.879** Other specified rheumatoid arthritis, unspecified ankle and foot

M06.88 Other specified rheumatoid arthritis, vertebrae

M06.89 Other specified rheumatoid arthritis, multiple sites

M06.8A Other specified rheumatoid arthritis, other specified site

M06.9 Rheumatoid arthritis, unspecified

Coding Clinic: 2024, Q1, P17

● **M07** Enteropathic arthropathies

Code also associated enteropathy, such as:
regional enteritis [Crohn's disease] (K50.-)
ulcerative colitis (K51.-)

Excludes1 psoriatic arthropathies (L40.5-)

● **M07.6** Enteropathic arthropathies

M07.60 Enteropathic arthropathies, unspecified site

● **M07.61** Enteropathic arthropathies, shoulder
- **M07.611** Enteropathic arthropathies, right shoulder
- **M07.612** Enteropathic arthropathies, left shoulder
- **M07.619** Enteropathic arthropathies, unspecified shoulder

● **M07.62** Enteropathic arthropathies, elbow
- **M07.621** Enteropathic arthropathies, right elbow
- **M07.622** Enteropathic arthropathies, left elbow
- **M07.629** Enteropathic arthropathies, unspecified elbow

● **M07.63** Enteropathic arthropathies, wrist
- **M07.631** Enteropathic arthropathies, right wrist
- **M07.632** Enteropathic arthropathies, left wrist
- **M07.639** Enteropathic arthropathies, unspecified wrist

● **M07.64** Enteropathic arthropathies, hand
- **M07.641** Enteropathic arthropathies, right hand
- **M07.642** Enteropathic arthropathies, left hand
- **M07.649** Enteropathic arthropathies, unspecified hand

● **M07.65** Enteropathic arthropathies, hip
- **M07.651** Enteropathic arthropathies, right hip
- **M07.652** Enteropathic arthropathies, left hip
- **M07.659** Enteropathic arthropathies, unspecified hip

● **M07.66** Enteropathic arthropathies, knee
- **M07.661** Enteropathic arthropathies, right knee
- **M07.662** Enteropathic arthropathies, left knee
- **M07.669** Enteropathic arthropathies, unspecified knee

● **M07.67** Enteropathic arthropathies, ankle and foot
- **M07.671** Enteropathic arthropathies, right ankle and foot
- **M07.672** Enteropathic arthropathies, left ankle and foot
- **M07.679** Enteropathic arthropathies, unspecified ankle and foot

M07.68 Enteropathic arthropathies, vertebrae

M07.69 Enteropathic arthropathies, multiple sites

● **M08 Juvenile arthritis**
Code also any associated underlying condition, such as:
regional enteritis [Crohn's disease] (K50.-)
ulcerative colitis (K51.-)
Excludes1 arthropathy in Whipple's disease (M14.8)
Felty's syndrome (M05.0)
juvenile dermatomyositis (M33.0-)
psoriatic juvenile arthropathy (L40.54)

● **M08.0 Unspecified juvenile rheumatoid arthritis**
Juvenile rheumatoid arthritis with or without rheumatoid factor
M08.00 Unspecified juvenile rheumatoid arthritis of unspecified site
● **M08.01 Unspecified juvenile rheumatoid arthritis, shoulder**
M08.011 Unspecified juvenile rheumatoid arthritis, right shoulder
M08.012 Unspecified juvenile rheumatoid arthritis, left shoulder
M08.019 Unspecified juvenile rheumatoid arthritis, unspecified shoulder
● **M08.02 Unspecified juvenile rheumatoid arthritis of elbow**
M08.021 Unspecified juvenile rheumatoid arthritis, right elbow
M08.022 Unspecified juvenile rheumatoid arthritis, left elbow
M08.029 Unspecified juvenile rheumatoid arthritis, unspecified elbow
● **M08.03 Unspecified juvenile rheumatoid arthritis, wrist**
M08.031 Unspecified juvenile rheumatoid arthritis, right wrist
M08.032 Unspecified juvenile rheumatoid arthritis, left wrist
M08.039 Unspecified juvenile rheumatoid arthritis, unspecified wrist
● **M08.04 Unspecified juvenile rheumatoid arthritis, hand**
M08.041 Unspecified juvenile rheumatoid arthritis, right hand
M08.042 Unspecified juvenile rheumatoid arthritis, left hand
M08.049 Unspecified juvenile rheumatoid arthritis, unspecified hand
● **M08.05 Unspecified juvenile rheumatoid arthritis, hip**
M08.051 Unspecified juvenile rheumatoid arthritis, right hip
M08.052 Unspecified juvenile rheumatoid arthritis, left hip
M08.059 Unspecified juvenile rheumatoid arthritis, unspecified hip
● **M08.06 Unspecified juvenile rheumatoid arthritis, knee**
M08.061 Unspecified juvenile rheumatoid arthritis, right knee
M08.062 Unspecified juvenile rheumatoid arthritis, left knee
M08.069 Unspecified juvenile rheumatoid arthritis, unspecified knee
● **M08.07 Unspecified juvenile rheumatoid arthritis, ankle and foot**
M08.071 Unspecified juvenile rheumatoid arthritis, right ankle and foot
M08.072 Unspecified juvenile rheumatoid arthritis, left ankle and foot
M08.079 Unspecified juvenile rheumatoid arthritis, unspecified ankle and foot
M08.08 Unspecified juvenile rheumatoid arthritis, vertebrae
M08.09 Unspecified juvenile rheumatoid arthritis, multiple sites
M08.0A Unspecified juvenile rheumatoid arthritis, other specified site

M08.1 Juvenile ankylosing spondylitis
Excludes1 ankylosing spondylitis in adults (M45.0-)

● **M08.2 Juvenile rheumatoid arthritis with systemic onset**
Still's disease NOS
Excludes1 adult-onset Still's disease (M06.1-)
M08.20 Juvenile rheumatoid arthritis with systemic onset, unspecified site
● **M08.21 Juvenile rheumatoid arthritis with systemic onset, shoulder**
M08.211 Juvenile rheumatoid arthritis with systemic onset, right shoulder
M08.212 Juvenile rheumatoid arthritis with systemic onset, left shoulder
M08.219 Juvenile rheumatoid arthritis with systemic onset, unspecified shoulder
● **M08.22 Juvenile rheumatoid arthritis with systemic onset, elbow**
M08.221 Juvenile rheumatoid arthritis with systemic onset, right elbow
M08.222 Juvenile rheumatoid arthritis with systemic onset, left elbow
M08.229 Juvenile rheumatoid arthritis with systemic onset, unspecified elbow
● **M08.23 Juvenile rheumatoid arthritis with systemic onset, wrist**
M08.231 Juvenile rheumatoid arthritis with systemic onset, right wrist
M08.232 Juvenile rheumatoid arthritis with systemic onset, left wrist
M08.239 Juvenile rheumatoid arthritis with systemic onset, unspecified wrist
● **M08.24 Juvenile rheumatoid arthritis with systemic onset, hand**
M08.241 Juvenile rheumatoid arthritis with systemic onset, right hand
M08.242 Juvenile rheumatoid arthritis with systemic onset, left hand
M08.249 Juvenile rheumatoid arthritis with systemic onset, unspecified hand
● **M08.25 Juvenile rheumatoid arthritis with systemic onset, hip**
M08.251 Juvenile rheumatoid arthritis with systemic onset, right hip
M08.252 Juvenile rheumatoid arthritis with systemic onset, left hip
M08.259 Juvenile rheumatoid arthritis with systemic onset, unspecified hip
● **M08.26 Juvenile rheumatoid arthritis with systemic onset, knee**
M08.261 Juvenile rheumatoid arthritis with systemic onset, right knee
M08.262 Juvenile rheumatoid arthritis with systemic onset, left knee
M08.269 Juvenile rheumatoid arthritis with systemic onset, unspecified knee

M08.27 Juvenile rheumatoid arthritis with systemic onset, ankle and foot

M08.271 Juvenile rheumatoid arthritis with systemic onset, right ankle and foot

M08.272 Juvenile rheumatoid arthritis with systemic onset, left ankle and foot

M08.279 Juvenile rheumatoid arthritis with systemic onset, unspecified ankle and foot

M08.28 Juvenile rheumatoid arthritis with systemic onset, vertebrae

M08.29 Juvenile rheumatoid arthritis with systemic onset, multiple sites

M08.2A Juvenile rheumatoid arthritis with systemic onset, other specified site

M08.3 Juvenile rheumatoid polyarthritis (seronegative)

M08.4 Pauciarticular juvenile rheumatoid arthritis

M08.40 Pauciarticular juvenile rheumatoid arthritis, unspecified site

M08.41 Pauciarticular juvenile rheumatoid arthritis, shoulder

M08.411 Pauciarticular juvenile rheumatoid arthritis, right shoulder

M08.412 Pauciarticular juvenile rheumatoid arthritis, left shoulder

M08.419 Pauciarticular juvenile rheumatoid arthritis, unspecified shoulder

M08.42 Pauciarticular juvenile rheumatoid arthritis, elbow

M08.421 Pauciarticular juvenile rheumatoid arthritis, right elbow

M08.422 Pauciarticular juvenile rheumatoid arthritis, left elbow

M08.429 Pauciarticular juvenile rheumatoid arthritis, unspecified elbow

M08.43 Pauciarticular juvenile rheumatoid arthritis, wrist

M08.431 Pauciarticular juvenile rheumatoid arthritis, right wrist

M08.432 Pauciarticular juvenile rheumatoid arthritis, left wrist

M08.439 Pauciarticular juvenile rheumatoid arthritis, unspecified wrist

M08.44 Pauciarticular juvenile rheumatoid arthritis, hand

M08.441 Pauciarticular juvenile rheumatoid arthritis, right hand

M08.442 Pauciarticular juvenile rheumatoid arthritis, left hand

M08.449 Pauciarticular juvenile rheumatoid arthritis, unspecified hand

M08.45 Pauciarticular juvenile rheumatoid arthritis, hip

M08.451 Pauciarticular juvenile rheumatoid arthritis, right hip

M08.452 Pauciarticular juvenile rheumatoid arthritis, left hip

M08.459 Pauciarticular juvenile rheumatoid arthritis, unspecified hip

M08.46 Pauciarticular juvenile rheumatoid arthritis, knee

M08.461 Pauciarticular juvenile rheumatoid arthritis, right knee

M08.462 Pauciarticular juvenile rheumatoid arthritis, left knee

M08.469 Pauciarticular juvenile rheumatoid arthritis, unspecified knee

M08.47 Pauciarticular juvenile rheumatoid arthritis, ankle and foot

M08.471 Pauciarticular juvenile rheumatoid arthritis, right ankle and foot

M08.472 Pauciarticular juvenile rheumatoid arthritis, left ankle and foot

M08.479 Pauciarticular juvenile rheumatoid arthritis, unspecified ankle and foot

M08.48 Pauciarticular juvenile rheumatoid arthritis, vertebrae

M08.4A Pauciarticular juvenile rheumatoid arthritis, other specified site

M08.8 Other juvenile arthritis

M08.80 Other juvenile arthritis, unspecified site

M08.81 Other juvenile arthritis, shoulder

M08.811 Other juvenile arthritis, right shoulder

M08.812 Other juvenile arthritis, left shoulder

M08.819 Other juvenile arthritis, unspecified shoulder

M08.82 Other juvenile arthritis, elbow

M08.821 Other juvenile arthritis, right elbow

M08.822 Other juvenile arthritis, left elbow

M08.829 Other juvenile arthritis, unspecified elbow

M08.83 Other juvenile arthritis, wrist

M08.831 Other juvenile arthritis, right wrist

M08.832 Other juvenile arthritis, left wrist

M08.839 Other juvenile arthritis, unspecified wrist

M08.84 Other juvenile arthritis, hand

M08.841 Other juvenile arthritis, right hand

M08.842 Other juvenile arthritis, left hand

M08.849 Other juvenile arthritis, unspecified hand

M08.85 Other juvenile arthritis, hip

M08.851 Other juvenile arthritis, right hip

M08.852 Other juvenile arthritis, left hip

M08.859 Other juvenile arthritis, unspecified hip

M08.86 Other juvenile arthritis, knee

M08.861 Other juvenile arthritis, right knee

M08.862 Other juvenile arthritis, left knee

M08.869 Other juvenile arthritis, unspecified knee

M08.87 Other juvenile arthritis, ankle and foot

M08.871 Other juvenile arthritis, right ankle and foot

M08.872 Other juvenile arthritis, left ankle and foot

M08.879 Other juvenile arthritis, unspecified ankle and foot

M08.88 Other juvenile arthritis, other specified site

Other juvenile arthritis, vertebrae

M08.89 Other juvenile arthritis, multiple sites

M08.9 Juvenile arthritis, unspecified

Excludes1 juvenile rheumatoid arthritis, unspecified (M08.0-)

M08.90 Juvenile arthritis, unspecified, unspecified site

CHAPTER 13 (M00-M99)

M08.91 Juvenile arthritis, unspecified, shoulder
M08.911 Juvenile arthritis, unspecified, right shoulder
M08.912 Juvenile arthritis, unspecified, left shoulder
M08.919 Juvenile arthritis, unspecified, unspecified shoulder
M08.92 Juvenile arthritis, unspecified, elbow
M08.921 Juvenile arthritis, unspecified, right elbow
M08.922 Juvenile arthritis, unspecified, left elbow
M08.929 Juvenile arthritis, unspecified, unspecified elbow
M08.93 Juvenile arthritis, unspecified, wrist
M08.931 Juvenile arthritis, unspecified, right wrist
M08.932 Juvenile arthritis, unspecified, left wrist
M08.939 Juvenile arthritis, unspecified, unspecified wrist
M08.94 Juvenile arthritis, unspecified, hand
M08.941 Juvenile arthritis, unspecified, right hand
M08.942 Juvenile arthritis, unspecified, left hand
M08.949 Juvenile arthritis, unspecified, unspecified hand
M08.95 Juvenile arthritis, unspecified, hip
M08.951 Juvenile arthritis, unspecified, right hip
M08.952 Juvenile arthritis, unspecified, left hip
M08.959 Juvenile arthritis, unspecified, unspecified hip
M08.96 Juvenile arthritis, unspecified, knee
M08.961 Juvenile arthritis, unspecified, right knee
M08.962 Juvenile arthritis, unspecified, left knee
M08.969 Juvenile arthritis, unspecified, unspecified knee
M08.97 Juvenile arthritis, unspecified, ankle and foot
M08.971 Juvenile arthritis, unspecified, right ankle and foot
M08.972 Juvenile arthritis, unspecified, left ankle and foot
M08.979 Juvenile arthritis, unspecified, unspecified ankle and foot
M08.98 Juvenile arthritis, unspecified, vertebrae
M08.99 Juvenile arthritis, unspecified, multiple sites
M08.9A Juvenile arthritis, unspecified, other specified site

M1A Chronic gout

Use additional code to identify:
Autonomic neuropathy in diseases classified elsewhere (G99.0)
Calculus of urinary tract in diseases classified elsewhere (N22)
Cardiomyopathy in diseases classified elsewhere (I43)
Disorders of external ear in diseases classified elsewhere (H61.1-, H62.8-)
Disorders of iris and ciliary body in diseases classified elsewhere (H22)
Glomerular disorders in diseases classified elsewhere (N08)

Excludes1 gout NOS (M10.-)
Excludes2 acute gout (M10.-)

The appropriate 7th character is to be added to each code from category M1A

0	without tophus (tophi)
1	with tophus (tophi)

M1A.0 Idiopathic chronic gout
Chronic gouty bursitis
Primary chronic gout
X M1A.00 Idiopathic chronic gout, unspecified site
M1A.01 Idiopathic chronic gout, shoulder
M1A.011 Idiopathic chronic gout, right shoulder
M1A.012 Idiopathic chronic gout, left shoulder
M1A.019 Idiopathic chronic gout, unspecified shoulder
M1A.02 Idiopathic chronic gout, elbow
M1A.021 Idiopathic chronic gout, right elbow
M1A.022 Idiopathic chronic gout, left elbow
M1A.029 Idiopathic chronic gout, unspecified elbow
M1A.03 Idiopathic chronic gout, wrist
M1A.031 Idiopathic chronic gout, right wrist
M1A.032 Idiopathic chronic gout, left wrist
M1A.039 Idiopathic chronic gout, unspecified wrist
M1A.04 Idiopathic chronic gout, hand
M1A.041 Idiopathic chronic gout, right hand
M1A.042 Idiopathic chronic gout, left hand
M1A.049 Idiopathic chronic gout, unspecified hand
M1A.05 Idiopathic chronic gout, hip
M1A.051 Idiopathic chronic gout, right hip
M1A.052 Idiopathic chronic gout, left hip
M1A.059 Idiopathic chronic gout, unspecified hip
M1A.06 Idiopathic chronic gout, knee
M1A.061 Idiopathic chronic gout, right knee
M1A.062 Idiopathic chronic gout, left knee
M1A.069 Idiopathic chronic gout, unspecified knee
M1A.07 Idiopathic chronic gout, ankle and foot
M1A.071 Idiopathic chronic gout, right ankle and foot
M1A.072 Idiopathic chronic gout, left ankle and foot
M1A.079 Idiopathic chronic gout, unspecified ankle and foot
X M1A.08 Idiopathic chronic gout, vertebrae
X M1A.09 Idiopathic chronic gout, multiple sites

M1A.1 Lead-induced chronic gout
Code first toxic effects of lead and its compounds (T56.0-)
X M1A.10 Lead-induced chronic gout, unspecified site
M1A.11 Lead-induced chronic gout, shoulder
M1A.111 Lead-induced chronic gout, right shoulder
M1A.112 Lead-induced chronic gout, left shoulder
M1A.119 Lead-induced chronic gout, unspecified shoulder
M1A.12 Lead-induced chronic gout, elbow
M1A.121 Lead-induced chronic gout, right elbow
M1A.122 Lead-induced chronic gout, left elbow
M1A.129 Lead-induced chronic gout, unspecified elbow
M1A.13 Lead-induced chronic gout, wrist
M1A.131 Lead-induced chronic gout, right wrist
M1A.132 Lead-induced chronic gout, left wrist
M1A.139 Lead-induced chronic gout, unspecified wrist
M1A.14 Lead-induced chronic gout, hand
M1A.141 Lead-induced chronic gout, right hand
M1A.142 Lead-induced chronic gout, left hand
M1A.149 Lead-induced chronic gout, unspecified hand
M1A.15 Lead-induced chronic gout, hip
M1A.151 Lead-induced chronic gout, right hip
M1A.152 Lead-induced chronic gout, left hip
M1A.159 Lead-induced chronic gout, unspecified hip
M1A.16 Lead-induced chronic gout, knee
M1A.161 Lead-induced chronic gout, right knee
M1A.162 Lead-induced chronic gout, left knee
M1A.169 Lead-induced chronic gout, unspecified knee
M1A.17 Lead-induced chronic gout, ankle and foot
M1A.171 Lead-induced chronic gout, right ankle and foot
M1A.172 Lead-induced chronic gout, left ankle and foot
M1A.179 Lead-induced chronic gout, unspecified ankle and foot
X M1A.18 Lead-induced chronic gout, vertebrae
X M1A.19 Lead-induced chronic gout, multiple sites

M1A.2 Drug-induced chronic gout
Use additional code for adverse effect, if applicable, to identify drug (T36-T50 with fifth or sixth character 5)
X M1A.20 Drug-induced chronic gout, unspecified site
M1A.21 Drug-induced chronic gout, shoulder
M1A.211 Drug-induced chronic gout, right shoulder
M1A.212 Drug-induced chronic gout, left shoulder
M1A.219 Drug-induced chronic gout, unspecified shoulder
M1A.22 Drug-induced chronic gout, elbow
M1A.221 Drug-induced chronic gout, right elbow
M1A.222 Drug-induced chronic gout, left elbow
M1A.229 Drug-induced chronic gout, unspecified elbow
M1A.23 Drug-induced chronic gout, wrist
M1A.231 Drug-induced chronic gout, right wrist
M1A.232 Drug-induced chronic gout, left wrist
M1A.239 Drug-induced chronic gout, unspecified wrist
M1A.24 Drug-induced chronic gout, hand
M1A.241 Drug-induced chronic gout, right hand
M1A.242 Drug-induced chronic gout, left hand
M1A.249 Drug-induced chronic gout, unspecified hand
M1A.25 Drug-induced chronic gout, hip
M1A.251 Drug-induced chronic gout, right hip
M1A.252 Drug-induced chronic gout, left hip
M1A.259 Drug-induced chronic gout, unspecified hip
M1A.26 Drug-induced chronic gout, knee
M1A.261 Drug-induced chronic gout, right knee
M1A.262 Drug-induced chronic gout, left knee
M1A.269 Drug-induced chronic gout, unspecified knee
M1A.27 Drug-induced chronic gout, ankle and foot
M1A.271 Drug-induced chronic gout, right ankle and foot
M1A.272 Drug-induced chronic gout, left ankle and foot
M1A.279 Drug-induced chronic gout, unspecified ankle and foot
X M1A.28 Drug-induced chronic gout, vertebrae
X M1A.29 Drug-induced chronic gout, multiple sites

M1A.3 Chronic gout due to renal impairment
Code first associated renal disease
X M1A.30 Chronic gout due to renal impairment, unspecified site
M1A.31 Chronic gout due to renal impairment, shoulder
M1A.311 Chronic gout due to renal impairment, right shoulder
M1A.312 Chronic gout due to renal impairment, left shoulder
M1A.319 Chronic gout due to renal impairment, unspecified shoulder
M1A.32 Chronic gout due to renal impairment, elbow
M1A.321 Chronic gout due to renal impairment, right elbow
M1A.322 Chronic gout due to renal impairment, left elbow
M1A.329 Chronic gout due to renal impairment, unspecified elbow
M1A.33 Chronic gout due to renal impairment, wrist
M1A.331 Chronic gout due to renal impairment, right wrist
M1A.332 Chronic gout due to renal impairment, left wrist
M1A.339 Chronic gout due to renal impairment, unspecified wrist
M1A.34 Chronic gout due to renal impairment, hand
M1A.341 Chronic gout due to renal impairment, right hand
M1A.342 Chronic gout due to renal impairment, left hand
M1A.349 Chronic gout due to renal impairment, unspecified hand

● M1A.35 Chronic gout due to renal impairment, hip
● M1A.351 Chronic gout due to renal impairment, right hip
● M1A.352 Chronic gout due to renal impairment, left hip
● M1A.359 Chronic gout due to renal impairment, unspecified hip
● M1A.36 Chronic gout due to renal impairment, knee
● M1A.361 Chronic gout due to renal impairment, right knee
● M1A.362 Chronic gout due to renal impairment, left knee
● M1A.369 Chronic gout due to renal impairment, unspecified knee
● M1A.37 Chronic gout due to renal impairment, ankle and foot
● M1A.371 Chronic gout due to renal impairment, right ankle and foot
● M1A.372 Chronic gout due to renal impairment, left ankle and foot
● M1A.379 Chronic gout due to renal impairment, unspecified ankle and foot
X● M1A.38 Chronic gout due to renal impairment, vertebrae
X● M1A.39 Chronic gout due to renal impairment, multiple sites
● M1A.4 Other secondary chronic gout
Code first associated condition
X● M1A.40 Other secondary chronic gout, unspecified site
● M1A.41 Other secondary chronic gout, shoulder
● M1A.411 Other secondary chronic gout, right shoulder
● M1A.412 Other secondary chronic gout, left shoulder
● M1A.419 Other secondary chronic gout, unspecified shoulder
● M1A.42 Other secondary chronic gout, elbow
● M1A.421 Other secondary chronic gout, right elbow
● M1A.422 Other secondary chronic gout, left elbow
● M1A.429 Other secondary chronic gout, unspecified elbow
● M1A.43 Other secondary chronic gout, wrist
● M1A.431 Other secondary chronic gout, right wrist
● M1A.432 Other secondary chronic gout, left wrist
● M1A.439 Other secondary chronic gout, unspecified wrist
● M1A.44 Other secondary chronic gout, hand
● M1A.441 Other secondary chronic gout, right hand
● M1A.442 Other secondary chronic gout, left hand
● M1A.449 Other secondary chronic gout, unspecified hand
● M1A.45 Other secondary chronic gout, hip
● M1A.451 Other secondary chronic gout, right hip
● M1A.452 Other secondary chronic gout, left hip
● M1A.459 Other secondary chronic gout, unspecified hip
● M1A.46 Other secondary chronic gout, knee
● M1A.461 Other secondary chronic gout, right knee
● M1A.462 Other secondary chronic gout, left knee
● M1A.469 Other secondary chronic gout, unspecified knee
● M1A.47 Other secondary chronic gout, ankle and foot
● M1A.471 Other secondary chronic gout, right ankle and foot
● M1A.472 Other secondary chronic gout, left ankle and foot
● M1A.479 Other secondary chronic gout, unspecified ankle and foot
X● M1A.48 Other secondary chronic gout, vertebrae
X● M1A.49 Other secondary chronic gout, multiple sites
X● M1A.9 Chronic gout, unspecified

● M10 Gout
Accumulation of uric acid that results in swollen, red, hot, painful, stiff joints
Acute gout
Gout attack
Gout flare
Podagra
Use additional code to identify:
Autonomic neuropathy in diseases classified elsewhere (G99.0)
Calculus of urinary tract in diseases classified elsewhere (N22)
Cardiomyopathy in diseases classified elsewhere (I43)
Disorders of external ear in diseases classified elsewhere (H61.1-, H62.8-)
Disorders of iris and ciliary body in diseases classified elsewhere (H22)
Glomerular disorders in diseases classified elsewhere (N08)
Excludes2 chronic gout (M1A.-)
● M10.0 Idiopathic gout
Gouty bursitis
Primary gout
M10.00 Idiopathic gout, unspecified site
● M10.01 Idiopathic gout, shoulder
M10.011 Idiopathic gout, right shoulder
M10.012 Idiopathic gout, left shoulder
M10.019 Idiopathic gout, unspecified shoulder
● M10.02 Idiopathic gout, elbow
M10.021 Idiopathic gout, right elbow
M10.022 Idiopathic gout, left elbow
M10.029 Idiopathic gout, unspecified elbow
● M10.03 Idiopathic gout, wrist
M10.031 Idiopathic gout, right wrist
M10.032 Idiopathic gout, left wrist
M10.039 Idiopathic gout, unspecified wrist
● M10.04 Idiopathic gout, hand
M10.041 Idiopathic gout, right hand
M10.042 Idiopathic gout, left hand
M10.049 Idiopathic gout, unspecified hand
● M10.05 Idiopathic gout, hip
M10.051 Idiopathic gout, right hip
M10.052 Idiopathic gout, left hip
M10.059 Idiopathic gout, unspecified hip
● M10.06 Idiopathic gout, knee
M10.061 Idiopathic gout, right knee
M10.062 Idiopathic gout, left knee
M10.069 Idiopathic gout, unspecified knee

- M10.07 Idiopathic gout, ankle and foot
  - M10.071 Idiopathic gout, right ankle and foot
  - M10.072 Idiopathic gout, left ankle and foot
  - M10.079 Idiopathic gout, unspecified ankle and foot
- M10.08 Idiopathic gout, vertebrae
- M10.09 Idiopathic gout, multiple sites

M10.1 Lead-induced gout

Code first toxic effects of lead and its compounds (T56.0-)

- M10.10 Lead-induced gout, unspecified site
- M10.11 Lead-induced gout, shoulder
  - M10.111 Lead-induced gout, right shoulder
  - M10.112 Lead-induced gout, left shoulder
  - M10.119 Lead-induced gout, unspecified shoulder
- M10.12 Lead-induced gout, elbow
  - M10.121 Lead-induced gout, right elbow
  - M10.122 Lead-induced gout, left elbow
  - M10.129 Lead-induced gout, unspecified elbow
- M10.13 Lead-induced gout, wrist
  - M10.131 Lead-induced gout, right wrist
  - M10.132 Lead-induced gout, left wrist
  - M10.139 Lead-induced gout, unspecified wrist
- M10.14 Lead-induced gout, hand
  - M10.141 Lead-induced gout, right hand
  - M10.142 Lead-induced gout, left hand
  - M10.149 Lead-induced gout, unspecified hand
- M10.15 Lead-induced gout, hip
  - M10.151 Lead-induced gout, right hip
  - M10.152 Lead-induced gout, left hip
  - M10.159 Lead-induced gout, unspecified hip
- M10.16 Lead-induced gout, knee
  - M10.161 Lead-induced gout, right knee
  - M10.162 Lead-induced gout, left knee
  - M10.169 Lead-induced gout, unspecified knee
- M10.17 Lead-induced gout, ankle and foot
  - M10.171 Lead-induced gout, right ankle and foot
  - M10.172 Lead-induced gout, left ankle and foot
  - M10.179 Lead-induced gout, unspecified ankle and foot
- M10.18 Lead-induced gout, vertebrae
- M10.19 Lead-induced gout, multiple sites

M10.2 Drug-induced gout

Use additional code for adverse effect, if applicable, to identify drug (T36-T50 with fifth or sixth character 5)

- M10.20 Drug-induced gout, unspecified site
- M10.21 Drug-induced gout, shoulder
  - M10.211 Drug-induced gout, right shoulder
  - M10.212 Drug-induced gout, left shoulder
  - M10.219 Drug-induced gout, unspecified shoulder
- M10.22 Drug-induced gout, elbow
  - M10.221 Drug-induced gout, right elbow
  - M10.222 Drug-induced gout, left elbow
  - M10.229 Drug-induced gout, unspecified elbow
- M10.23 Drug-induced gout, wrist
  - M10.231 Drug-induced gout, right wrist
  - M10.232 Drug-induced gout, left wrist
  - M10.239 Drug-induced gout, unspecified wrist
- M10.24 Drug-induced gout, hand
  - M10.241 Drug-induced gout, right hand
  - M10.242 Drug-induced gout, left hand
  - M10.249 Drug-induced gout, unspecified hand
- M10.25 Drug-induced gout, hip
  - M10.251 Drug-induced gout, right hip
  - M10.252 Drug-induced gout, left hip
  - M10.259 Drug-induced gout, unspecified hip
- M10.26 Drug-induced gout, knee
  - M10.261 Drug-induced gout, right knee
  - M10.262 Drug-induced gout, left knee
  - M10.269 Drug-induced gout, unspecified knee
- M10.27 Drug-induced gout, ankle and foot
  - M10.271 Drug-induced gout, right ankle and foot
  - M10.272 Drug-induced gout, left ankle and foot
  - M10.279 Drug-induced gout, unspecified ankle and foot
- M10.28 Drug-induced gout, vertebrae
- M10.29 Drug-induced gout, multiple sites

M10.3 Gout due to renal impairment

Code also associated renal disease

- M10.30 Gout due to renal impairment, unspecified site
- M10.31 Gout due to renal impairment, shoulder
  - M10.311 Gout due to renal impairment, right shoulder
  - M10.312 Gout due to renal impairment, left shoulder
  - M10.319 Gout due to renal impairment, unspecified shoulder
- M10.32 Gout due to renal impairment, elbow
  - M10.321 Gout due to renal impairment, right elbow
  - M10.322 Gout due to renal impairment, left elbow
  - M10.329 Gout due to renal impairment, unspecified elbow
- M10.33 Gout due to renal impairment, wrist
  - M10.331 Gout due to renal impairment, right wrist
  - M10.332 Gout due to renal impairment, left wrist
  - M10.339 Gout due to renal impairment, unspecified wrist
- M10.34 Gout due to renal impairment, hand
  - M10.341 Gout due to renal impairment, right hand
  - M10.342 Gout due to renal impairment, left hand
  - M10.349 Gout due to renal impairment, unspecified hand
- M10.35 Gout due to renal impairment, hip
  - M10.351 Gout due to renal impairment, right hip
  - M10.352 Gout due to renal impairment, left hip
  - M10.359 Gout due to renal impairment, unspecified hip
- M10.36 Gout due to renal impairment, knee
  - M10.361 Gout due to renal impairment, right knee
  - M10.362 Gout due to renal impairment, left knee
  - M10.369 Gout due to renal impairment, unspecified knee

● M10.37 Gout due to renal impairment, ankle and foot
M10.371 Gout due to renal impairment, right ankle and foot
M10.372 Gout due to renal impairment, left ankle and foot
M10.379 Gout due to renal impairment, unspecified ankle and foot
M10.38 Gout due to renal impairment, vertebrae
M10.39 Gout due to renal impairment, multiple sites

● M10.4 Other secondary gout
Code first associated condition
M10.40 Other secondary gout, unspecified site
● M10.41 Other secondary gout, shoulder
M10.411 Other secondary gout, right shoulder
M10.412 Other secondary gout, left shoulder
M10.419 Other secondary gout, unspecified shoulder
● M10.42 Other secondary gout, elbow
M10.421 Other secondary gout, right elbow
M10.422 Other secondary gout, left elbow
M10.429 Other secondary gout, unspecified elbow
● M10.43 Other secondary gout, wrist
M10.431 Other secondary gout, right wrist
M10.432 Other secondary gout, left wrist
M10.439 Other secondary gout, unspecified wrist
● M10.44 Other secondary gout, hand
M10.441 Other secondary gout, right hand
M10.442 Other secondary gout, left hand
M10.449 Other secondary gout, unspecified hand
● M10.45 Other secondary gout, hip
M10.451 Other secondary gout, right hip
M10.452 Other secondary gout, left hip
M10.459 Other secondary gout, unspecified hip
● M10.46 Other secondary gout, knee
M10.461 Other secondary gout, right knee
M10.462 Other secondary gout, left knee
M10.469 Other secondary gout, unspecified knee
● M10.47 Other secondary gout, ankle and foot
M10.471 Other secondary gout, right ankle and foot
M10.472 Other secondary gout, left ankle and foot
M10.479 Other secondary gout, unspecified ankle and foot
M10.48 Other secondary gout, vertebrae
M10.49 Other secondary gout, multiple sites

M10.9 Gout, unspecified
Gout NOS

● M11 Other crystal arthropathies

● M11.0 Hydroxyapatite deposition disease
M11.00 Hydroxyapatite deposition disease, unspecified site
● M11.01 Hydroxyapatite deposition disease, shoulder
M11.011 Hydroxyapatite deposition disease, right shoulder
M11.012 Hydroxyapatite deposition disease, left shoulder
M11.019 Hydroxyapatite deposition disease, unspecified shoulder
● M11.02 Hydroxyapatite deposition disease, elbow
M11.021 Hydroxyapatite deposition disease, right elbow
M11.022 Hydroxyapatite deposition disease, left elbow
M11.029 Hydroxyapatite deposition disease, unspecified elbow
● M11.03 Hydroxyapatite deposition disease, wrist
M11.031 Hydroxyapatite deposition disease, right wrist
M11.032 Hydroxyapatite deposition disease, left wrist
M11.039 Hydroxyapatite deposition disease, unspecified wrist
● M11.04 Hydroxyapatite deposition disease, hand
M11.041 Hydroxyapatite deposition disease, right hand
M11.042 Hydroxyapatite deposition disease, left hand
M11.049 Hydroxyapatite deposition disease, unspecified hand
● M11.05 Hydroxyapatite deposition disease, hip
M11.051 Hydroxyapatite deposition disease, right hip
M11.052 Hydroxyapatite deposition disease, left hip
M11.059 Hydroxyapatite deposition disease, unspecified hip
● M11.06 Hydroxyapatite deposition disease, knee
M11.061 Hydroxyapatite deposition disease, right knee
M11.062 Hydroxyapatite deposition disease, left knee
M11.069 Hydroxyapatite deposition disease, unspecified knee
● M11.07 Hydroxyapatite deposition disease, ankle and foot
M11.071 Hydroxyapatite deposition disease, right ankle and foot
M11.072 Hydroxyapatite deposition disease, left ankle and foot
M11.079 Hydroxyapatite deposition disease, unspecified ankle and foot
M11.08 Hydroxyapatite deposition disease, vertebrae
M11.09 Hydroxyapatite deposition disease, multiple sites

● M11.1 Familial chondrocalcinosis
M11.10 Familial chondrocalcinosis, unspecified site
● M11.11 Familial chondrocalcinosis, shoulder
M11.111 Familial chondrocalcinosis, right shoulder
M11.112 Familial chondrocalcinosis, left shoulder
M11.119 Familial chondrocalcinosis, unspecified shoulder
● M11.12 Familial chondrocalcinosis, elbow
M11.121 Familial chondrocalcinosis, right elbow
M11.122 Familial chondrocalcinosis, left elbow
M11.129 Familial chondrocalcinosis, unspecified elbow
● M11.13 Familial chondrocalcinosis, wrist
M11.131 Familial chondrocalcinosis, right wrist
M11.132 Familial chondrocalcinosis, left wrist
M11.139 Familial chondrocalcinosis, unspecified wrist

- ● M11.14 Familial chondrocalcinosis, hand
  - M11.141 Familial chondrocalcinosis, right hand
  - M11.142 Familial chondrocalcinosis, left hand
  - M11.149 Familial chondrocalcinosis, unspecified hand
- ● M11.15 Familial chondrocalcinosis, hip
  - M11.151 Familial chondrocalcinosis, right hip
  - M11.152 Familial chondrocalcinosis, left hip
  - M11.159 Familial chondrocalcinosis, unspecified hip
- ● M11.16 Familial chondrocalcinosis, knee
  - M11.161 Familial chondrocalcinosis, right knee
  - M11.162 Familial chondrocalcinosis, left knee
  - M11.169 Familial chondrocalcinosis, unspecified knee
- ● M11.17 Familial chondrocalcinosis, ankle and foot
  - M11.171 Familial chondrocalcinosis, right ankle and foot
  - M11.172 Familial chondrocalcinosis, left ankle and foot
  - M11.179 Familial chondrocalcinosis, unspecified ankle and foot
- M11.18 Familial chondrocalcinosis, vertebrae
- M11.19 Familial chondrocalcinosis, multiple sites

● M11.2 Other chondrocalcinosis
  Chondrocalcinosis NOS
- M11.20 Other chondrocalcinosis, unspecified site
- ● M11.21 Other chondrocalcinosis, shoulder
  - M11.211 Other chondrocalcinosis, right shoulder
  - M11.212 Other chondrocalcinosis, left shoulder
  - M11.219 Other chondrocalcinosis, unspecified shoulder
- ● M11.22 Other chondrocalcinosis, elbow
  - M11.221 Other chondrocalcinosis, right elbow
  - M11.222 Other chondrocalcinosis, left elbow
  - M11.229 Other chondrocalcinosis, unspecified elbow
- ● M11.23 Other chondrocalcinosis, wrist
  - M11.231 Other chondrocalcinosis, right wrist
  - M11.232 Other chondrocalcinosis, left wrist
  - M11.239 Other chondrocalcinosis, unspecified wrist
- ● M11.24 Other chondrocalcinosis, hand
  - M11.241 Other chondrocalcinosis, right hand
  - M11.242 Other chondrocalcinosis, left hand
  - M11.249 Other chondrocalcinosis, unspecified hand
- ● M11.25 Other chondrocalcinosis, hip
  - M11.251 Other chondrocalcinosis, right hip
  - M11.252 Other chondrocalcinosis, left hip
  - M11.259 Other chondrocalcinosis, unspecified hip
- ● M11.26 Other chondrocalcinosis, knee
  - M11.261 Other chondrocalcinosis, right knee
  - M11.262 Other chondrocalcinosis, left knee
  - M11.269 Other chondrocalcinosis, unspecified knee
- ● M11.27 Other chondrocalcinosis, ankle and foot
  - M11.271 Other chondrocalcinosis, right ankle and foot
  - M11.272 Other chondrocalcinosis, left ankle and foot
  - M11.279 Other chondrocalcinosis, unspecified ankle and foot
- M11.28 Other chondrocalcinosis, vertebrae
- M11.29 Other chondrocalcinosis, multiple sites

● M11.8 Other specified crystal arthropathies
- M11.80 Other specified crystal arthropathies, unspecified site
- ● M11.81 Other specified crystal arthropathies, shoulder
  - M11.811 Other specified crystal arthropathies, right shoulder
  - M11.812 Other specified crystal arthropathies, left shoulder
  - M11.819 Other specified crystal arthropathies, unspecified shoulder
- ● M11.82 Other specified crystal arthropathies, elbow
  - M11.821 Other specified crystal arthropathies, right elbow
  - M11.822 Other specified crystal arthropathies, left elbow
  - M11.829 Other specified crystal arthropathies, unspecified elbow
- ● M11.83 Other specified crystal arthropathies, wrist
  - M11.831 Other specified crystal arthropathies, right wrist
  - M11.832 Other specified crystal arthropathies, left wrist
  - M11.839 Other specified crystal arthropathies, unspecified wrist
- ● M11.84 Other specified crystal arthropathies, hand
  - M11.841 Other specified crystal arthropathies, right hand
  - M11.842 Other specified crystal arthropathies, left hand
  - M11.849 Other specified crystal arthropathies, unspecified hand
- ● M11.85 Other specified crystal arthropathies, hip
  - M11.851 Other specified crystal arthropathies, right hip
  - M11.852 Other specified crystal arthropathies, left hip
  - M11.859 Other specified crystal arthropathies, unspecified hip
- ● M11.86 Other specified crystal arthropathies, knee
  - M11.861 Other specified crystal arthropathies, right knee
  - M11.862 Other specified crystal arthropathies, left knee
  - M11.869 Other specified crystal arthropathies, unspecified knee
- ● M11.87 Other specified crystal arthropathies, ankle and foot
  - M11.871 Other specified crystal arthropathies, right ankle and foot
  - M11.872 Other specified crystal arthropathies, left ankle and foot
  - M11.879 Other specified crystal arthropathies, unspecified ankle and foot
- M11.88 Other specified crystal arthropathies, vertebrae
- M11.89 Other specified crystal arthropathies, multiple sites

M11.9 Crystal arthropathy, unspecified

● M12 Other and unspecified arthropathy
Excludes1 arthrosis (M15-M19)
cricoarytenoid arthropathy (J38.7)

● M12.0 Chronic postrheumatic arthropathy [Jaccoud]
M12.00 Chronic postrheumatic arthropathy [Jaccoud], unspecified site
● M12.01 Chronic postrheumatic arthropathy [Jaccoud], shoulder
M12.011 Chronic postrheumatic arthropathy [Jaccoud], right shoulder
M12.012 Chronic postrheumatic arthropathy [Jaccoud], left shoulder
M12.019 Chronic postrheumatic arthropathy [Jaccoud], unspecified shoulder
● M12.02 Chronic postrheumatic arthropathy [Jaccoud], elbow
M12.021 Chronic postrheumatic arthropathy [Jaccoud], right elbow
M12.022 Chronic postrheumatic arthropathy [Jaccoud], left elbow
M12.029 Chronic postrheumatic arthropathy [Jaccoud], unspecified elbow
● M12.03 Chronic postrheumatic arthropathy [Jaccoud], wrist
M12.031 Chronic postrheumatic arthropathy [Jaccoud], right wrist
M12.032 Chronic postrheumatic arthropathy [Jaccoud], left wrist
M12.039 Chronic postrheumatic arthropathy [Jaccoud], unspecified wrist
● M12.04 Chronic postrheumatic arthropathy [Jaccoud], hand
M12.041 Chronic postrheumatic arthropathy [Jaccoud], right hand
M12.042 Chronic postrheumatic arthropathy [Jaccoud], left hand
M12.049 Chronic postrheumatic arthropathy [Jaccoud], unspecified hand
● M12.05 Chronic postrheumatic arthropathy [Jaccoud], hip
M12.051 Chronic postrheumatic arthropathy [Jaccoud], right hip
M12.052 Chronic postrheumatic arthropathy [Jaccoud], left hip
M12.059 Chronic postrheumatic arthropathy [Jaccoud], unspecified hip
● M12.06 Chronic postrheumatic arthropathy [Jaccoud], knee
M12.061 Chronic postrheumatic arthropathy [Jaccoud], right knee
M12.062 Chronic postrheumatic arthropathy [Jaccoud], left knee
M12.069 Chronic postrheumatic arthropathy [Jaccoud], unspecified knee
● M12.07 Chronic postrheumatic arthropathy [Jaccoud], ankle and foot
M12.071 Chronic postrheumatic arthropathy [Jaccoud], right ankle and foot
M12.072 Chronic postrheumatic arthropathy [Jaccoud], left ankle and foot
M12.079 Chronic postrheumatic arthropathy [Jaccoud], unspecified ankle and foot
M12.08 Chronic postrheumatic arthropathy [Jaccoud], other specified site
Chronic postrheumatic arthropathy [Jaccoud], vertebrae
M12.09 Chronic postrheumatic arthropathy [Jaccoud], multiple sites

● M12.1 Kaschin-Beck disease
Osteochondroarthrosis deformans endemica
M12.10 Kaschin-Beck disease, unspecified site
● M12.11 Kaschin-Beck disease, shoulder
M12.111 Kaschin-Beck disease, right shoulder
M12.112 Kaschin-Beck disease, left shoulder
M12.119 Kaschin-Beck disease, unspecified shoulder
● M12.12 Kaschin-Beck disease, elbow
M12.121 Kaschin-Beck disease, right elbow
M12.122 Kaschin-Beck disease, left elbow
M12.129 Kaschin-Beck disease, unspecified elbow
● M12.13 Kaschin-Beck disease, wrist
M12.131 Kaschin-Beck disease, right wrist
M12.132 Kaschin-Beck disease, left wrist
M12.139 Kaschin-Beck disease, unspecified wrist
● M12.14 Kaschin-Beck disease, hand
M12.141 Kaschin-Beck disease, right hand
M12.142 Kaschin-Beck disease, left hand
M12.149 Kaschin-Beck disease, unspecified hand
● M12.15 Kaschin-Beck disease, hip
M12.151 Kaschin-Beck disease, right hip
M12.152 Kaschin-Beck disease, left hip
M12.159 Kaschin-Beck disease, unspecified hip
● M12.16 Kaschin-Beck disease, knee
M12.161 Kaschin-Beck disease, right knee
M12.162 Kaschin-Beck disease, left knee
M12.169 Kaschin-Beck disease, unspecified knee
● M12.17 Kaschin-Beck disease, ankle and foot
M12.171 Kaschin-Beck disease, right ankle and foot
M12.172 Kaschin-Beck disease, left ankle and foot
M12.179 Kaschin-Beck disease, unspecified ankle and foot
M12.18 Kaschin-Beck disease, vertebrae
M12.19 Kaschin-Beck disease, multiple sites

● M12.2 Villonodular synovitis (pigmented)
M12.20 Villonodular synovitis (pigmented), unspecified site
● M12.21 Villonodular synovitis (pigmented), shoulder
M12.211 Villonodular synovitis (pigmented), right shoulder
M12.212 Villonodular synovitis (pigmented), left shoulder
M12.219 Villonodular synovitis (pigmented), unspecified shoulder
● M12.22 Villonodular synovitis (pigmented), elbow
M12.221 Villonodular synovitis (pigmented), right elbow
M12.222 Villonodular synovitis (pigmented), left elbow
M12.229 Villonodular synovitis (pigmented), unspecified elbow
● M12.23 Villonodular synovitis (pigmented), wrist
M12.231 Villonodular synovitis (pigmented), right wrist
M12.232 Villonodular synovitis (pigmented), left wrist
M12.239 Villonodular synovitis (pigmented), unspecified wrist

● M12.24 Villonodular synovitis (pigmented), hand
M12.241 Villonodular synovitis (pigmented), right hand
M12.242 Villonodular synovitis (pigmented), left hand
M12.249 Villonodular synovitis (pigmented), unspecified hand
● M12.25 Villonodular synovitis (pigmented), hip
M12.251 Villonodular synovitis (pigmented), right hip
M12.252 Villonodular synovitis (pigmented), left hip
M12.259 Villonodular synovitis (pigmented), unspecified hip
● M12.26 Villonodular synovitis (pigmented), knee
M12.261 Villonodular synovitis (pigmented), right knee
M12.262 Villonodular synovitis (pigmented), left knee
M12.269 Villonodular synovitis (pigmented), unspecified knee
● M12.27 Villonodular synovitis (pigmented), ankle and foot
M12.271 Villonodular synovitis (pigmented), right ankle and foot
M12.272 Villonodular synovitis (pigmented), left ankle and foot
M12.279 Villonodular synovitis (pigmented), unspecified ankle and foot
M12.28 Villonodular synovitis (pigmented), other specified site
Villonodular synovitis (pigmented), vertebrae
M12.29 Villonodular synovitis (pigmented), multiple sites
● M12.3 Palindromic rheumatism
M12.30 Palindromic rheumatism, unspecified site
● M12.31 Palindromic rheumatism, shoulder
M12.311 Palindromic rheumatism, right shoulder
M12.312 Palindromic rheumatism, left shoulder
M12.319 Palindromic rheumatism, unspecified shoulder
● M12.32 Palindromic rheumatism, elbow
M12.321 Palindromic rheumatism, right elbow
M12.322 Palindromic rheumatism, left elbow
M12.329 Palindromic rheumatism, unspecified elbow
● M12.33 Palindromic rheumatism, wrist
M12.331 Palindromic rheumatism, right wrist
M12.332 Palindromic rheumatism, left wrist
M12.339 Palindromic rheumatism, unspecified wrist
● M12.34 Palindromic rheumatism, hand
M12.341 Palindromic rheumatism, right hand
M12.342 Palindromic rheumatism, left hand
M12.349 Palindromic rheumatism, unspecified hand
● M12.35 Palindromic rheumatism, hip
M12.351 Palindromic rheumatism, right hip
M12.352 Palindromic rheumatism, left hip
M12.359 Palindromic rheumatism, unspecified hip
● M12.36 Palindromic rheumatism, knee
M12.361 Palindromic rheumatism, right knee
M12.362 Palindromic rheumatism, left knee
M12.369 Palindromic rheumatism, unspecified knee
● M12.37 Palindromic rheumatism, ankle and foot
M12.371 Palindromic rheumatism, right ankle and foot
M12.372 Palindromic rheumatism, left ankle and foot
M12.379 Palindromic rheumatism, unspecified ankle and foot
M12.38 Palindromic rheumatism, other specified site
Palindromic rheumatism, vertebrae
M12.39 Palindromic rheumatism, multiple sites
● M12.4 Intermittent hydrarthrosis
M12.40 Intermittent hydrarthrosis, unspecified site
● M12.41 Intermittent hydrarthrosis, shoulder
M12.411 Intermittent hydrarthrosis, right shoulder
M12.412 Intermittent hydrarthrosis, left shoulder
M12.419 Intermittent hydrarthrosis, unspecified shoulder
● M12.42 Intermittent hydrarthrosis, elbow
M12.421 Intermittent hydrarthrosis, right elbow
M12.422 Intermittent hydrarthrosis, left elbow
M12.429 Intermittent hydrarthrosis, unspecified elbow
● M12.43 Intermittent hydrarthrosis, wrist
M12.431 Intermittent hydrarthrosis, right wrist
M12.432 Intermittent hydrarthrosis, left wrist
M12.439 Intermittent hydrarthrosis, unspecified wrist
● M12.44 Intermittent hydrarthrosis, hand
M12.441 Intermittent hydrarthrosis, right hand
M12.442 Intermittent hydrarthrosis, left hand
M12.449 Intermittent hydrarthrosis, unspecified hand
● M12.45 Intermittent hydrarthrosis, hip
M12.451 Intermittent hydrarthrosis, right hip
M12.452 Intermittent hydrarthrosis, left hip
M12.459 Intermittent hydrarthrosis, unspecified hip
● M12.46 Intermittent hydrarthrosis, knee
M12.461 Intermittent hydrarthrosis, right knee
M12.462 Intermittent hydrarthrosis, left knee
M12.469 Intermittent hydrarthrosis, unspecified knee
● M12.47 Intermittent hydrarthrosis, ankle and foot
M12.471 Intermittent hydrarthrosis, right ankle and foot
M12.472 Intermittent hydrarthrosis, left ankle and foot
M12.479 Intermittent hydrarthrosis, unspecified ankle and foot
M12.48 Intermittent hydrarthrosis, other site
M12.49 Intermittent hydrarthrosis, multiple sites
● M12.5 Traumatic arthropathy
Excludes1 current injury-see Alphabetic Index
post-traumatic osteoarthritis of first carpometacarpal joint (M18.2-M18.3)
post-traumatic osteoarthritis of hip (M16.4-M16.5)
post-traumatic osteoarthritis of knee (M17.2-M17.3)
post-traumatic osteoarthritis NOS (M19.1-)
post-traumatic osteoarthritis of other single joints (M19.1-)
M12.50 Traumatic arthropathy, unspecified site

CHAPTER 13 (MØ-M99)

●M12.51 Traumatic arthropathy, shoulder
M12.511 Traumatic arthropathy, right shoulder
M12.512 Traumatic arthropathy, left shoulder
M12.519 Traumatic arthropathy, unspecified shoulder

●M12.52 Traumatic arthropathy, elbow
M12.521 Traumatic arthropathy, right elbow
M12.522 Traumatic arthropathy, left elbow
M12.529 Traumatic arthropathy, unspecified elbow

●M12.53 Traumatic arthropathy, wrist
M12.531 Traumatic arthropathy, right wrist
M12.532 Traumatic arthropathy, left wrist
M12.539 Traumatic arthropathy, unspecified wrist

●M12.54 Traumatic arthropathy, hand
M12.541 Traumatic arthropathy, right hand
M12.542 Traumatic arthropathy, left hand
M12.549 Traumatic arthropathy, unspecified hand

●M12.55 Traumatic arthropathy, hip
M12.551 Traumatic arthropathy, right hip
M12.552 Traumatic arthropathy, left hip
Coding Clinic: 2Ø15, Q1, P17
M12.559 Traumatic arthropathy, unspecified hip

●M12.56 Traumatic arthropathy, knee
M12.561 Traumatic arthropathy, right knee
M12.562 Traumatic arthropathy, left knee
M12.569 Traumatic arthropathy, unspecified knee

●M12.57 Traumatic arthropathy, ankle and foot
M12.571 Traumatic arthropathy, right ankle and foot
M12.572 Traumatic arthropathy, left ankle and foot
M12.579 Traumatic arthropathy, unspecified ankle and foot

M12.58 Traumatic arthropathy, other specified site
Traumatic arthropathy, vertebrae

M12.59 Traumatic arthropathy, multiple sites

●M12.8 Other specific arthropathies, not elsewhere classified
Transient arthropathy

M12.8Ø Other specific arthropathies, not elsewhere classified, unspecified site

●M12.81 Other specific arthropathies, not elsewhere classified, shoulder
M12.811 Other specific arthropathies, not elsewhere classified, right shoulder
M12.812 Other specific arthropathies, not elsewhere classified, left shoulder
M12.819 Other specific arthropathies, not elsewhere classified, unspecified shoulder

●M12.82 Other specific arthropathies, not elsewhere classified, elbow
M12.821 Other specific arthropathies, not elsewhere classified, right elbow
M12.822 Other specific arthropathies, not elsewhere classified, left elbow
M12.829 Other specific arthropathies, not elsewhere classified, unspecified elbow

●M12.83 Other specific arthropathies, not elsewhere classified, wrist
M12.831 Other specific arthropathies, not elsewhere classified, right wrist
M12.832 Other specific arthropathies, not elsewhere classified, left wrist
M12.839 Other specific arthropathies, not elsewhere classified, unspecified wrist

●M12.84 Other specific arthropathies, not elsewhere classified, hand
M12.841 Other specific arthropathies, not elsewhere classified, right hand
M12.842 Other specific arthropathies, not elsewhere classified, left hand
M12.849 Other specific arthropathies, not elsewhere classified, unspecified hand

●M12.85 Other specific arthropathies, not elsewhere classified, hip
M12.851 Other specific arthropathies, not elsewhere classified, right hip
M12.852 Other specific arthropathies, not elsewhere classified, left hip
M12.859 Other specific arthropathies, not elsewhere classified, unspecified hip

●M12.86 Other specific arthropathies, not elsewhere classified, knee
M12.861 Other specific arthropathies, not elsewhere classified, right knee
M12.862 Other specific arthropathies, not elsewhere classified, left knee
M12.869 Other specific arthropathies, not elsewhere classified, unspecified knee

●M12.87 Other specific arthropathies, not elsewhere classified, ankle and foot
M12.871 Other specific arthropathies, not elsewhere classified, right ankle and foot
M12.872 Other specific arthropathies, not elsewhere classified, left ankle and foot
M12.879 Other specific arthropathies, not elsewhere classified, unspecified ankle and foot

M12.88 Other specific arthropathies, not elsewhere classified, other specified site
Other specific arthropathies, not elsewhere classified, vertebrae

M12.89 Other specific arthropathies, not elsewhere classified, multiple sites

M12.9 Arthropathy, unspecified

●M13 Other arthritis
Excludes1 arthrosis (M15-M19)
osteoarthritis (M15-M19)

M13.Ø Polyarthritis, unspecified

●M13.1 Monoarthritis, not elsewhere classified
M13.1Ø Monoarthritis, not elsewhere classified, unspecified site

●M13.11 Monoarthritis, not elsewhere classified, shoulder
M13.111 Monoarthritis, not elsewhere classified, right shoulder
M13.112 Monoarthritis, not elsewhere classified, left shoulder
M13.119 Monoarthritis, not elsewhere classified, unspecified shoulder

● M13.12 Monoarthritis, not elsewhere classified, elbow
M13.121 Monoarthritis, not elsewhere classified, right elbow
M13.122 Monoarthritis, not elsewhere classified, left elbow
M13.129 Monoarthritis, not elsewhere classified, unspecified elbow

● M13.13 Monoarthritis, not elsewhere classified, wrist
M13.131 Monoarthritis, not elsewhere classified, right wrist
M13.132 Monoarthritis, not elsewhere classified, left wrist
M13.139 Monoarthritis, not elsewhere classified, unspecified wrist

● M13.14 Monoarthritis, not elsewhere classified, hand
M13.141 Monoarthritis, not elsewhere classified, right hand
M13.142 Monoarthritis, not elsewhere classified, left hand
M13.149 Monoarthritis, not elsewhere classified, unspecified hand

● M13.15 Monoarthritis, not elsewhere classified, hip
M13.151 Monoarthritis, not elsewhere classified, right hip
M13.152 Monoarthritis, not elsewhere classified, left hip
M13.159 Monoarthritis, not elsewhere classified, unspecified hip

● M13.16 Monoarthritis, not elsewhere classified, knee
M13.161 Monoarthritis, not elsewhere classified, right knee
M13.162 Monoarthritis, not elsewhere classified, left knee
M13.169 Monoarthritis, not elsewhere classified, unspecified knee

● M13.17 Monoarthritis, not elsewhere classified, ankle and foot
M13.171 Monoarthritis, not elsewhere classified, right ankle and foot
M13.172 Monoarthritis, not elsewhere classified, left ankle and foot
M13.179 Monoarthritis, not elsewhere classified, unspecified ankle and foot

● M13.8 Other specified arthritis
Allergic arthritis
Excludes1 osteoarthritis (M15-M19)
M13.80 Other specified arthritis, unspecified site

● M13.81 Other specified arthritis, shoulder
M13.811 Other specified arthritis, right shoulder
M13.812 Other specified arthritis, left shoulder
M13.819 Other specified arthritis, unspecified shoulder

● M13.82 Other specified arthritis, elbow
M13.821 Other specified arthritis, right elbow
M13.822 Other specified arthritis, left elbow
M13.829 Other specified arthritis, unspecified elbow

● M13.83 Other specified arthritis, wrist
M13.831 Other specified arthritis, right wrist
M13.832 Other specified arthritis, left wrist
M13.839 Other specified arthritis, unspecified wrist

● M13.84 Other specified arthritis, hand
M13.841 Other specified arthritis, right hand
M13.842 Other specified arthritis, left hand
M13.849 Other specified arthritis, unspecified hand

● M13.85 Other specified arthritis, hip
M13.851 Other specified arthritis, right hip
M13.852 Other specified arthritis, left hip
M13.859 Other specified arthritis, unspecified hip

● M13.86 Other specified arthritis, knee
M13.861 Other specified arthritis, right knee
M13.862 Other specified arthritis, left knee
M13.869 Other specified arthritis, unspecified knee

● M13.87 Other specified arthritis, ankle and foot
M13.871 Other specified arthritis, right ankle and foot
M13.872 Other specified arthritis, left ankle and foot
M13.879 Other specified arthritis, unspecified ankle and foot
M13.88 Other specified arthritis, other site
M13.89 Other specified arthritis, multiple sites

● **M14 Arthropathies in other diseases classified elsewhere**
Excludes1 arthropathy in:
diabetes mellitus (EØ8-E13 with .61-)
hematological disorders (M36.2-M36.3)
hypersensitivity reactions (M36.4)
neoplastic disease (M36.1)
neurosyphillis (A52.16)
sarcoidosis (D86.86)
enteropathic arthropathies (MØ7.Ø-)
juvenile psoriatic arthropathy (L4Ø.54)
lipoid dermatoarthritis (E78.81)

● M14.6 Charcôt's joint
Neuropathic arthropathy
Excludes1 Charcôt's joint in diabetes mellitus (EØ8-E13 with .61Ø)
Charcôt's joint in tabes dorsalis (A52.16)
M14.6Ø Charcôt's joint, unspecified site

● M14.61 Charcôt's joint, shoulder
M14.611 Charcôt's joint, right shoulder
M14.612 Charcôt's joint, left shoulder
M14.619 Charcôt's joint, unspecified shoulder

● M14.62 Charcôt's joint, elbow
M14.621 Charcôt's joint, right elbow
M14.622 Charcôt's joint, left elbow
M14.629 Charcôt's joint, unspecified elbow

● M14.63 Charcôt's joint, wrist
M14.631 Charcôt's joint, right wrist
M14.632 Charcôt's joint, left wrist
M14.639 Charcôt's joint, unspecified wrist

● M14.64 Charcôt's joint, hand
M14.641 Charcôt's joint, right hand
M14.642 Charcôt's joint, left hand
M14.649 Charcôt's joint, unspecified hand

● M14.65 Charcôt's joint, hip
M14.651 Charcôt's joint, right hip
M14.652 Charcôt's joint, left hip
M14.659 Charcôt's joint, unspecified hip

● M14.66 Charcôt's joint, knee
M14.661 Charcôt's joint, right knee
M14.662 Charcôt's joint, left knee
M14.669 Charcôt's joint, unspecified knee

● M14.67 Charcôt's joint, ankle and foot
M14.671 Charcôt's joint, right ankle and foot
M14.672 Charcôt's joint, left ankle and foot
M14.679 Charcôt's joint, unspecified ankle and foot
M14.68 Charcôt's joint, vertebrae
M14.69 Charcôt's joint, multiple sites

M14.8 Arthropathies in other specified diseases classified elsewhere

Code first underlying disease, such as:
amyloidosis (E85.-)
erythema multiforme (L51.-)
erythema nodosum (L52)
hemochromatosis (E83.11-)
hyperparathyroidism (E21.-)
hypothyroidism (E00-E03)
sickle-cell disorders (D57.-)
thyrotoxicosis [hyperthyroidism] (E05.-)
Whipple's disease (K90.81)

M14.80 Arthropathies in other specified diseases classified elsewhere, unspecified site

M14.81 Arthropathies in other specified diseases classified elsewhere, shoulder

M14.811 Arthropathies in other specified diseases classified elsewhere, right shoulder

M14.812 Arthropathies in other specified diseases classified elsewhere, left shoulder

M14.819 Arthropathies in other specified diseases classified elsewhere, unspecified shoulder

M14.82 Arthropathies in other specified diseases classified elsewhere, elbow

M14.821 Arthropathies in other specified diseases classified elsewhere, right elbow

M14.822 Arthropathies in other specified diseases classified elsewhere, left elbow

M14.829 Arthropathies in other specified diseases classified elsewhere, unspecified elbow

M14.83 Arthropathies in other specified diseases classified elsewhere, wrist

M14.831 Arthropathies in other specified diseases classified elsewhere, right wrist

M14.832 Arthropathies in other specified diseases classified elsewhere, left wrist

M14.839 Arthropathies in other specified diseases classified elsewhere, unspecified wrist

M14.84 Arthropathies in other specified diseases classified elsewhere, hand

M14.841 Arthropathies in other specified diseases classified elsewhere, right hand

M14.842 Arthropathies in other specified diseases classified elsewhere, left hand

M14.849 Arthropathies in other specified diseases classified elsewhere, unspecified hand

M14.85 Arthropathies in other specified diseases classified elsewhere, hip

M14.851 Arthropathies in other specified diseases classified elsewhere, right hip

M14.852 Arthropathies in other specified diseases classified elsewhere, left hip

M14.859 Arthropathies in other specified diseases classified elsewhere, unspecified hip

M14.86 Arthropathies in other specified diseases classified elsewhere, knee

M14.861 Arthropathies in other specified diseases classified elsewhere, right knee

M14.862 Arthropathies in other specified diseases classified elsewhere, left knee

M14.869 Arthropathies in other specified diseases classified elsewhere, unspecified knee

M14.87 Arthropathies in other specified diseases classified elsewhere, ankle and foot

M14.871 Arthropathies in other specified diseases classified elsewhere, right ankle and foot

M14.872 Arthropathies in other specified diseases classified elsewhere, left ankle and foot

M14.879 Arthropathies in other specified diseases classified elsewhere, unspecified ankle and foot

M14.88 Arthropathies in other specified diseases classified elsewhere, vertebrae

M14.89 Arthropathies in other specified diseases classified elsewhere, multiple sites

OSTEOARTHRITIS (M15-M19)

Osteoarthritis is the most common degenerative joint disease and form of arthritis that breaks down the cartilage causing pain, swelling, and reduced motion in the joints.

Excludes2 osteoarthritis of spine (M47.-)

M15 Polyosteoarthritis

Includes arthritis of multiple sites

Excludes1 bilateral involvement of single joint (M16-M19)

M15.0 Primary generalized (osteo)arthritis

M15.1 Heberden's nodes (with arthropathy)
Interphalangeal distal osteoarthritis

M15.2 Bouchard's nodes (with arthropathy)
Juxtaphalangeal distal osteoarthritis

M15.3 Secondary multiple arthritis
Post-traumatic polyosteoarthritis

M15.4 Erosive (osteo)arthritis

M15.8 Other polyosteoarthritis

M15.9 Polyosteoarthritis, unspecified
Generalized osteoarthritis NOS

M16 Osteoarthritis of hip

M16.0 Bilateral primary osteoarthritis of hip
Coding Clinic: 2018, Q2, P15; 2016, Q4, P146

M16.1 Unilateral primary osteoarthritis of hip
Primary osteoarthritis of hip NOS

M16.10 Unilateral primary osteoarthritis, unspecified hip

M16.11 Unilateral primary osteoarthritis, right hip

M16.12 Unilateral primary osteoarthritis, left hip

M16.2 Bilateral osteoarthritis resulting from hip dysplasia

M16.3 Unilateral osteoarthritis resulting from hip dysplasia
Dysplastic osteoarthritis of hip NOS

M16.30 Unilateral osteoarthritis resulting from hip dysplasia, unspecified hip

M16.31 Unilateral osteoarthritis resulting from hip dysplasia, right hip

M16.32 Unilateral osteoarthritis resulting from hip dysplasia, left hip

M16.4 Bilateral post-traumatic osteoarthritis of hip

● **M16.5 Unilateral post-traumatic osteoarthritis of hip**
Post-traumatic osteoarthritis of hip NOS
M16.50 Unilateral post-traumatic osteoarthritis, unspecified hip
M16.51 Unilateral post-traumatic osteoarthritis, right hip
M16.52 Unilateral post-traumatic osteoarthritis, left hip
M16.6 Other bilateral secondary osteoarthritis of hip
M16.7 Other unilateral secondary osteoarthritis of hip
Secondary osteoarthritis of hip NOS
M16.9 Osteoarthritis of hip, unspecified

● **M17 Osteoarthritis of knee**
M17.0 Bilateral primary osteoarthritis of knee
● **M17.1 Unilateral primary osteoarthritis of knee**
Primary osteoarthritis of knee NOS
M17.10 Unilateral primary osteoarthritis, unspecified knee
Coding Clinic: 2016, Q4, P147
M17.11 Unilateral primary osteoarthritis, right knee
M17.12 Unilateral primary osteoarthritis, left knee
Coding Clinic: 2016, Q4, P146
M17.2 Bilateral post-traumatic osteoarthritis of knee
● **M17.3 Unilateral post-traumatic osteoarthritis of knee**
Post-traumatic osteoarthritis of knee NOS
M17.30 Unilateral post-traumatic osteoarthritis, unspecified knee
M17.31 Unilateral post-traumatic osteoarthritis, right knee
M17.32 Unilateral post-traumatic osteoarthritis, left knee
M17.4 Other bilateral secondary osteoarthritis of knee
M17.5 Other unilateral secondary osteoarthritis of knee
Secondary osteoarthritis of knee NOS
M17.9 Osteoarthritis of knee, unspecified
Coding Clinic: 2016, Q4, P146

● **M18 Osteoarthritis of first carpometacarpal joint**
M18.0 Bilateral primary osteoarthritis of first carpometacarpal joints
● **M18.1 Unilateral primary osteoarthritis of first carpometacarpal joint**
Primary osteoarthritis of first carpometacarpal joint NOS
M18.10 Unilateral primary osteoarthritis of first carpometacarpal joint, unspecified hand
M18.11 Unilateral primary osteoarthritis of first carpometacarpal joint, right hand
M18.12 Unilateral primary osteoarthritis of first carpometacarpal joint, left hand
M18.2 Bilateral post-traumatic osteoarthritis of first carpometacarpal joints
● **M18.3 Unilateral post-traumatic osteoarthritis of first carpometacarpal joint**
Post-traumatic osteoarthritis of first carpometacarpal joint NOS
M18.30 Unilateral post-traumatic osteoarthritis of first carpometacarpal joint, unspecified hand
M18.31 Unilateral post-traumatic osteoarthritis of first carpometacarpal joint, right hand
M18.32 Unilateral post-traumatic osteoarthritis of first carpometacarpal joint, left hand
M18.4 Other bilateral secondary osteoarthritis of first carpometacarpal joints
● **M18.5 Other unilateral secondary osteoarthritis of first carpometacarpal joint**
Secondary osteoarthritis of first carpometacarpal joint NOS
M18.50 Other unilateral secondary osteoarthritis of first carpometacarpal joint, unspecified hand
M18.51 Other unilateral secondary osteoarthritis of first carpometacarpal joint, right hand
M18.52 Other unilateral secondary osteoarthritis of first carpometacarpal joint, left hand
M18.9 Osteoarthritis of first carpometacarpal joint, unspecified

● **M19 Other and unspecified osteoarthritis**
Excludes1 polyarthritis (M15.-)
Excludes2 arthrosis of spine (M47.-)
hallux rigidus (M20.2)
osteoarthritis of spine (M47.-)
● **M19.0 Primary osteoarthritis of other joints**
● **M19.01 Primary osteoarthritis, shoulder**
M19.011 Primary osteoarthritis, right shoulder
Coding Clinic: 2016, Q4, P145
M19.012 Primary osteoarthritis, left shoulder
M19.019 Primary osteoarthritis, unspecified shoulder
● **M19.02 Primary osteoarthritis, elbow**
M19.021 Primary osteoarthritis, right elbow
M19.022 Primary osteoarthritis, left elbow
M19.029 Primary osteoarthritis, unspecified elbow
● **M19.03 Primary osteoarthritis, wrist**
M19.031 Primary osteoarthritis, right wrist
M19.032 Primary osteoarthritis, left wrist
M19.039 Primary osteoarthritis, unspecified wrist
● **M19.04 Primary osteoarthritis, hand**
Excludes2 primary osteoarthritis of first carpometacarpal joint (M18.0-, M18.1-)
M19.041 Primary osteoarthritis, right hand
M19.042 Primary osteoarthritis, left hand
M19.049 Primary osteoarthritis, unspecified hand
● **M19.07 Primary osteoarthritis ankle and foot**
M19.071 Primary osteoarthritis, right ankle and foot
M19.072 Primary osteoarthritis, left ankle and foot
M19.079 Primary osteoarthritis, unspecified ankle and foot
M19.09 Primary osteoarthritis, other specified site
● **M19.1 Post-traumatic osteoarthritis of other joints**
● **M19.11 Post-traumatic osteoarthritis, shoulder**
M19.111 Post-traumatic osteoarthritis, right shoulder
M19.112 Post-traumatic osteoarthritis, left shoulder
M19.119 Post-traumatic osteoarthritis, unspecified shoulder
● **M19.12 Post-traumatic osteoarthritis, elbow**
M19.121 Post-traumatic osteoarthritis, right elbow
M19.122 Post-traumatic osteoarthritis, left elbow
M19.129 Post-traumatic osteoarthritis, unspecified elbow

● M19.13 Post-traumatic osteoarthritis, wrist
M19.131 Post-traumatic osteoarthritis, right wrist
M19.132 Post-traumatic osteoarthritis, left wrist
M19.139 Post-traumatic osteoarthritis, unspecified wrist

● M19.14 Post-traumatic osteoarthritis, hand
Excludes2 post-traumatic osteoarthritis of first carpometacarpal joint (M18.2-, M18.3-)
M19.141 Post-traumatic osteoarthritis, right hand
M19.142 Post-traumatic osteoarthritis, left hand
M19.149 Post-traumatic osteoarthritis, unspecified hand

● M19.17 Post-traumatic osteoarthritis, ankle and foot
M19.171 Post-traumatic osteoarthritis, right ankle and foot
M19.172 Post-traumatic osteoarthritis, left ankle and foot
M19.179 Post-traumatic osteoarthritis, unspecified ankle and foot

M19.19 Post-traumatic osteoarthritis, other specified site

● M19.2 Secondary osteoarthritis of other joints

● M19.21 Secondary osteoarthritis, shoulder
M19.211 Secondary osteoarthritis, right shoulder
M19.212 Secondary osteoarthritis, left shoulder
M19.219 Secondary osteoarthritis, unspecified shoulder

● M19.22 Secondary osteoarthritis, elbow
M19.221 Secondary osteoarthritis, right elbow
M19.222 Secondary osteoarthritis, left elbow
M19.229 Secondary osteoarthritis, unspecified elbow

● M19.23 Secondary osteoarthritis, wrist
M19.231 Secondary osteoarthritis, right wrist
M19.232 Secondary osteoarthritis, left wrist
M19.239 Secondary osteoarthritis, unspecified wrist

● M19.24 Secondary osteoarthritis, hand
M19.241 Secondary osteoarthritis, right hand
M19.242 Secondary osteoarthritis, left hand
M19.249 Secondary osteoarthritis, unspecified hand

● M19.27 Secondary osteoarthritis, ankle and foot
M19.271 Secondary osteoarthritis, right ankle and foot
M19.272 Secondary osteoarthritis, left ankle and foot
M19.279 Secondary osteoarthritis, unspecified ankle and foot

M19.29 Secondary osteoarthritis, other specified site

● M19.9 Osteoarthritis, unspecified site
M19.90 Unspecified osteoarthritis, unspecified site
Arthrosis NOS
Arthritis NOS
Osteoarthritis NOS
Coding Clinic: 2016, Q4, P147
M19.91 Primary osteoarthritis, unspecified site
Primary osteoarthritis NOS
M19.92 Post-traumatic osteoarthritis, unspecified site
Post-traumatic osteoarthritis NOS
M19.93 Secondary osteoarthritis, unspecified site
Secondary osteoarthritis NOS

OTHER JOINT DISORDERS (M20-M25)

Excludes2 joints of the spine (M40-M54)

● M20 Acquired deformities of fingers and toes
Excludes1 acquired absence of fingers and toes (Z89.-)
congenital absence of fingers and toes (Q71.3-, Q72.3-)
congenital deformities and malformations of fingers and toes (Q66.-, Q68-Q70, Q74.-)

● M20.0 Deformity of finger(s)
Excludes1 clubbing of fingers (R68.3)
palmar fascial fibromatosis [Dupuytren] (M72.0)
trigger finger (M65.3)

● M20.00 Unspecified deformity of finger(s)
M20.001 Unspecified deformity of right finger(s)
M20.002 Unspecified deformity of left finger(s)
M20.009 Unspecified deformity of unspecified finger(s)

● M20.01 Mallet finger
M20.011 Mallet finger of right finger(s)
M20.012 Mallet finger of left finger(s)
M20.019 Mallet finger of unspecified finger(s)

● M20.02 Boutonnière deformity
M20.021 Boutonnière deformity of right finger(s)
M20.022 Boutonnière deformity of left finger(s)
M20.029 Boutonnière deformity of unspecified finger(s)

● M20.03 Swan-neck deformity
M20.031 Swan-neck deformity of right finger(s)
M20.032 Swan-neck deformity of left finger(s)
M20.039 Swan-neck deformity of unspecified finger(s)

● M20.09 Other deformity of finger(s)
M20.091 Other deformity of right finger(s)
M20.092 Other deformity of left finger(s)
M20.099 Other deformity of finger(s), unspecified finger(s)

● M20.1 Hallux valgus (acquired)
Excludes2 bunion (M21.6-)
Coding Clinic: 2016, Q4, P38
M20.10 Hallux valgus (acquired), unspecified foot
M20.11 Hallux valgus (acquired), right foot
M20.12 Hallux valgus (acquired), left foot

● M20.2 Hallux rigidus
M20.20 Hallux rigidus, unspecified foot
M20.21 Hallux rigidus, right foot
M20.22 Hallux rigidus, left foot

CHAPTER 13 (M00-M99)

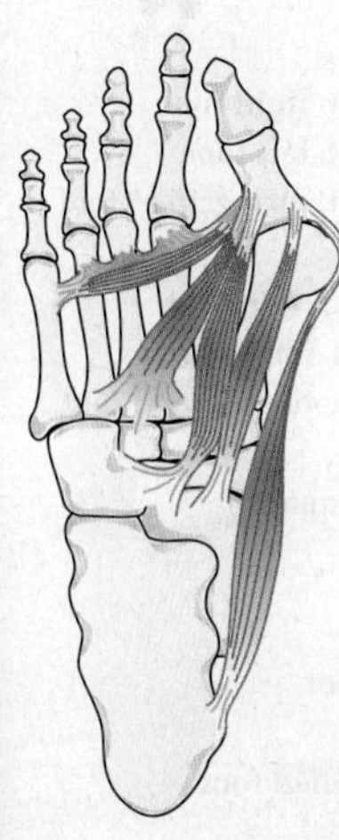

Figure 13-1 Hallux valgus.

Item 13-2 Hallux valgus is a sometimes painful structural deformity caused by an inflammation of the bursal sac at the base of the metatarsophalangeal joint (big toe). **Hallus varus** is a deviation of the great toe to the inner side of the foot or away from the next toe.

● **M20.3 Hallux varus (acquired)**
- **M20.30 Hallux varus (acquired), unspecified foot**
- **M20.31 Hallux varus (acquired), right foot**
- **M20.32 Hallux varus (acquired), left foot**

● **M20.4 Other hammer toe(s) (acquired)**
- **M20.40 Other hammer toe(s) (acquired), unspecified foot**
- **M20.41 Other hammer toe(s) (acquired), right foot**
- **M20.42 Other hammer toe(s) (acquired), left foot**

● **M20.5 Other deformities of toe(s) (acquired)**

● **M20.5X Other deformities of toe(s) (acquired)**
- **M20.5X1 Other deformities of toe(s) (acquired), right foot**
- **M20.5X2 Other deformities of toe(s) (acquired), left foot**
- **M20.5X9 Other deformities of toe(s) (acquired), unspecified foot**

● **M20.6 Acquired deformities of toe(s), unspecified**
- **M20.60 Acquired deformities of toe(s), unspecified, unspecified foot**
- **M20.61 Acquired deformities of toe(s), unspecified, right foot**
- **M20.62 Acquired deformities of toe(s), unspecified, left foot**

● **M21 Other acquired deformities of limbs**

Excludes1 acquired absence of limb (Z89.-)
congenital absence of limbs (Q71-Q73)
congenital deformities and malformations of limbs (Q65-Q66, Q68-Q74)

Excludes2 acquired deformities of fingers or toes (M20.-)
coxa plana (M91.2)

● **M21.0 Valgus deformity, not elsewhere classified**

Excludes1 metatarsus valgus (Q66.6)
talipes calcaneovalgus (Q66.4-)

- **M21.00 Valgus deformity, not elsewhere classified, unspecified site**

● **M21.02 Valgus deformity, not elsewhere classified, elbow**
Cubitus valgus
- **M21.021 Valgus deformity, not elsewhere classified, right elbow**
- **M21.022 Valgus deformity, not elsewhere classified, left elbow**
- **M21.029 Valgus deformity, not elsewhere classified, unspecified elbow**

Item 13-3 Cubitus valgus is a deformity of the elbow resulting in an increased carrying angle in which the arm extends at the side and the palm faces forward, which results in the forearm and hand extended at greater than 15 degrees.

Item 13-4 Cubitus varus is a deformity of the elbow resulting in the arm extended at the side and the palm facing forward so that the forearm and hand are held at less than 5 degrees, decreasing the carrying angle.

● **M21.05 Valgus deformity, not elsewhere classified, hip**
- **M21.051 Valgus deformity, not elsewhere classified, right hip**
- **M21.052 Valgus deformity, not elsewhere classified, left hip**
- **M21.059 Valgus deformity, not elsewhere classified, unspecified hip**

● **M21.06 Valgus deformity, not elsewhere classified, knee**
Genu valgum
Knock knee
- **M21.061 Valgus deformity, not elsewhere classified, right knee**
- **M21.062 Valgus deformity, not elsewhere classified, left knee**
- **M21.069 Valgus deformity, not elsewhere classified, unspecified knee**

● **M21.07 Valgus deformity, not elsewhere classified, ankle**
- **M21.071 Valgus deformity, not elsewhere classified, right ankle**
- **M21.072 Valgus deformity, not elsewhere classified, left ankle**
- **M21.079 Valgus deformity, not elsewhere classified, unspecified ankle**

● **M21.1 Varus deformity, not elsewhere classified**

Excludes1 metatarsus varus (Q66.22-)
tibia vara (M92.51-)

- **M21.10 Varus deformity, not elsewhere classified, unspecified site**

● **M21.12 Varus deformity, not elsewhere classified, elbow**
Cubitus varus, elbow
- **M21.121 Varus deformity, not elsewhere classified, right elbow**
- **M21.122 Varus deformity, not elsewhere classified, left elbow**
- **M21.129 Varus deformity, not elsewhere classified, unspecified elbow**

● **M21.15 Varus deformity, not elsewhere classified, hip**
- **M21.151 Varus deformity, not elsewhere classified, right hip**
- **M21.152 Varus deformity, not elsewhere classified, left hip**
- **M21.159 Varus deformity, not elsewhere classified, unspecified**

● **M21.16 Varus deformity, not elsewhere classified, knee**
Bow leg
Genu varum
- **M21.161 Varus deformity, not elsewhere classified, right knee**
- **M21.162 Varus deformity, not elsewhere classified, left knee**
- **M21.169 Varus deformity, not elsewhere classified, unspecified knee**

● **M21.17 Varus deformity, not elsewhere classified, ankle**
- **M21.171 Varus deformity, not elsewhere classified, right ankle**
- **M21.172 Varus deformity, not elsewhere classified, left ankle**
- **M21.179 Varus deformity, not elsewhere classified, unspecified ankle**

- M21.2 Flexion deformity
  - M21.2Ø Flexion deformity, unspecified site
  - M21.21 Flexion deformity, shoulder
    - M21.211 Flexion deformity, right shoulder
    - M21.212 Flexion deformity, left shoulder
    - M21.219 Flexion deformity, unspecified shoulder
  - M21.22 Flexion deformity, elbow
    - M21.221 Flexion deformity, right elbow
    - M21.222 Flexion deformity, left elbow
    - M21.229 Flexion deformity, unspecified elbow
  - M21.23 Flexion deformity, wrist
    - M21.231 Flexion deformity, right wrist
    - M21.232 Flexion deformity, left wrist
    - M21.239 Flexion deformity, unspecified wrist
  - M21.24 Flexion deformity, finger joints
    - M21.241 Flexion deformity, right finger joints
    - M21.242 Flexion deformity, left finger joints
    - M21.249 Flexion deformity, unspecified finger joints
  - M21.25 Flexion deformity, hip
    - M21.251 Flexion deformity, right hip
    - M21.252 Flexion deformity, left hip
    - M21.259 Flexion deformity, unspecified hip
  - M21.26 Flexion deformity, knee
    - M21.261 Flexion deformity, right knee
    - M21.262 Flexion deformity, left knee
    - M21.269 Flexion deformity, unspecified knee
  - M21.27 Flexion deformity, ankle and toes
    - M21.271 Flexion deformity, right ankle and toes
    - M21.272 Flexion deformity, left ankle and toes
    - M21.279 Flexion deformity, unspecified ankle and toes
- M21.3 Wrist or foot drop (acquired)
  - M21.33 Wrist drop (acquired)
    - M21.331 Wrist drop, right wrist
    - M21.332 Wrist drop, left wrist
    - M21.339 Wrist drop, unspecified wrist
  - M21.37 Foot drop (acquired)
    - M21.371 Foot drop, right foot
    - M21.372 Foot drop, left foot
    - M21.379 Foot drop, unspecified foot
- M21.4 Flat foot [pes planus] (acquired)
  - **Excludes1** congenital pes planus (Q66.5-)
  - M21.4Ø Flat foot [pes planus] (acquired), unspecified foot
  - M21.41 Flat foot [pes planus] (acquired), right foot
  - M21.42 Flat foot [pes planus] (acquired), left foot
- M21.5 Acquired clawhand, clubhand, clawfoot and clubfoot
  - **Excludes1** clubfoot, not specified as acquired (Q66.89)
  - M21.51 Acquired clawhand
    - M21.511 Acquired clawhand, right hand
    - M21.512 Acquired clawhand, left hand
    - M21.519 Acquired clawhand, unspecified hand
  - M21.52 Acquired clubhand
    - M21.521 Acquired clubhand, right hand
    - M21.522 Acquired clubhand, left hand
    - M21.529 Acquired clubhand, unspecified hand
  - M21.53 Acquired clawfoot
    - M21.531 Acquired clawfoot, right foot
    - M21.532 Acquired clawfoot, left foot
    - M21.539 Acquired clawfoot, unspecified foot
  - M21.54 Acquired clubfoot
    - M21.541 Acquired clubfoot, right foot
    - M21.542 Acquired clubfoot, left foot
    - M21.549 Acquired clubfoot, unspecified foot
- M21.6 Other acquired deformities of foot
  - **Excludes2** deformities of toe (acquired) (M2Ø.1-M2Ø.6-)
  - M21.61 Bunion
    - Coding Clinic: 2Ø16, Q4, P38
    - M21.611 Bunion of right foot
    - M21.612 Bunion of left foot
    - M21.619 Bunion of unspecified foot
  - M21.62 Bunionette
    - Coding Clinic: 2Ø16, Q4, P38
    - M21.621 Bunionette of right foot
    - M21.622 Bunionette of left foot
    - M21.629 Bunionette of unspecified foot
  - M21.6X Other acquired deformities of foot
    - M21.6X1 Other acquired deformities of right foot
      - Coding Clinic: 2Ø23, Q3, P21
    - M21.6X2 Other acquired deformities of left foot
    - M21.6X9 Other acquired deformities of unspecified foot
- M21.7 Unequal limb length (acquired)
  - **Note:** The site used should correspond to the shorter limb.
  - M21.7Ø Unequal limb length (acquired), unspecified site
  - M21.72 Unequal limb length (acquired), humerus
    - M21.721 Unequal limb length (acquired), right humerus
    - M21.722 Unequal limb length (acquired), left humerus
    - M21.729 Unequal limb length (acquired), unspecified humerus
  - M21.73 Unequal limb length (acquired), ulna and radius
    - M21.731 Unequal limb length (acquired), right ulna
    - M21.732 Unequal limb length (acquired), left ulna
    - M21.733 Unequal limb length (acquired), right radius
    - M21.734 Unequal limb length (acquired), left radius
    - M21.739 Unequal limb length (acquired), unspecified ulna and radius
  - M21.75 Unequal limb length (acquired), femur
    - M21.751 Unequal limb length (acquired), right femur
    - M21.752 Unequal limb length (acquired), left femur
    - M21.759 Unequal limb length (acquired), unspecified femur

CHAPTER 13 (MØØ-M99)

● M21.76 Unequal limb length (acquired), tibia and fibula
- M21.761 Unequal limb length (acquired), right tibia
- M21.762 Unequal limb length (acquired), left tibia
- M21.763 Unequal limb length (acquired), right fibula
- M21.764 Unequal limb length (acquired), left fibula
- M21.769 Unequal limb length (acquired), unspecified tibia and fibula

● M21.8 Other specified acquired deformities of limbs

Excludes2 coxa plana (M91.2)

- M21.80 Other specified acquired deformities of unspecified limb

● M21.82 Other specified acquired deformities of upper arm
- M21.821 Other specified acquired deformities of right upper arm
- M21.822 Other specified acquired deformities of left upper arm
- M21.829 Other specified acquired deformities of unspecified upper arm

● M21.83 Other specified acquired deformities of forearm
- M21.831 Other specified acquired deformities of right forearm
- M21.832 Other specified acquired deformities of left forearm
- M21.839 Other specified acquired deformities of unspecified forearm

● M21.85 Other specified acquired deformities of thigh
- M21.851 Other specified acquired deformities of right thigh
- M21.852 Other specified acquired deformities of left thigh
- M21.859 Other specified acquired deformities of unspecified thigh

● M21.86 Other specified acquired deformities of lower leg
- M21.861 Other specified acquired deformities of right lower leg
- M21.862 Other specified acquired deformities of left lower leg
- M21.869 Other specified acquired deformities of unspecified lower leg

● M21.9 Unspecified acquired deformity of limb and hand
- M21.90 Unspecified acquired deformity of unspecified limb

● M21.92 Unspecified acquired deformity of upper arm
- M21.921 Unspecified acquired deformity of right upper arm
- M21.922 Unspecified acquired deformity of left upper arm
- M21.929 Unspecified acquired deformity of unspecified upper arm

● M21.93 Unspecified acquired deformity of forearm
- M21.931 Unspecified acquired deformity of right forearm
- M21.932 Unspecified acquired deformity of left forearm
- M21.939 Unspecified acquired deformity of unspecified forearm

● M21.94 Unspecified acquired deformity of hand
- M21.941 Unspecified acquired deformity of hand, right hand
- M21.942 Unspecified acquired deformity of hand, left hand
- M21.949 Unspecified acquired deformity of hand, unspecified hand

● M21.95 Unspecified acquired deformity of thigh
- M21.951 Unspecified acquired deformity of right thigh
- M21.952 Unspecified acquired deformity of left thigh
- M21.959 Unspecified acquired deformity of unspecified thigh

● M21.96 Unspecified acquired deformity of lower leg
- M21.961 Unspecified acquired deformity of right lower leg
- M21.962 Unspecified acquired deformity of left lower leg
- M21.969 Unspecified acquired deformity of unspecified lower leg

● M22 Disorder of patella

Excludes2 traumatic dislocation of patella (S83.Ø-)

● M22.Ø Recurrent dislocation of patella
- M22.ØØ Recurrent dislocation of patella, unspecified knee
- M22.Ø1 Recurrent dislocation of patella, right knee
- M22.Ø2 Recurrent dislocation of patella, left knee

● M22.1 Recurrent subluxation of patella

Incomplete dislocation of patella

- M22.1Ø Recurrent subluxation of patella, unspecified knee
- M22.11 Recurrent subluxation of patella, right knee
- M22.12 Recurrent subluxation of patella, left knee

● M22.2 Patellofemoral disorders

● M22.2X Patellofemoral disorders
- M22.2X1 Patellofemoral disorders, right knee
- M22.2X2 Patellofemoral disorders, left knee
- M22.2X9 Patellofemoral disorders, unspecified knee

● M22.3 Other derangements of patella

● M22.3X Other derangements of patella
- M22.3X1 Other derangements of patella, right knee
- M22.3X2 Other derangements of patella, left knee
- M22.3X9 Other derangements of patella, unspecified knee

● M22.4 Chondromalacia patellae
- M22.4Ø Chondromalacia patellae, unspecified knee
- M22.41 Chondromalacia patellae, right knee
- M22.42 Chondromalacia patellae, left knee

● M22.8 Other disorders of patella

● M22.8X Other disorders of patella
- M22.8X1 Other disorders of patella, right knee
- M22.8X2 Other disorders of patella, left knee
- M22.8X9 Other disorders of patella, unspecified knee

● M22.9 Unspecified disorder of patella
- M22.9Ø Unspecified disorder of patella, unspecified knee
- M22.91 Unspecified disorder of patella, right knee
- M22.92 Unspecified disorder of patella, left knee

● M23 Internal derangement of knee

Excludes1 ankylosis (M24.66)
deformity of knee (M21.-)
osteochondritis dissecans (M93.2)

Excludes2 current injury - see injury of knee and lower leg (S80-S89)
recurrent dislocation or subluxation of joints (M24.4)
recurrent dislocation or subluxation of patella (M22.0-M22.1)

Coding Clinic: 2019, Q2, P26

● M23.0 Cystic meniscus

● M23.00 Cystic meniscus, unspecified meniscus
Cystic meniscus, unspecified lateral meniscus
Cystic meniscus, unspecified medial meniscus

M23.000 Cystic meniscus, unspecified lateral meniscus, right knee

M23.001 Cystic meniscus, unspecified lateral meniscus, left knee

M23.002 Cystic meniscus, unspecified lateral meniscus, unspecified knee

M23.003 Cystic meniscus, unspecified medial meniscus, right knee

M23.004 Cystic meniscus, unspecified medial meniscus, left knee

M23.005 Cystic meniscus, unspecified medial meniscus, unspecified knee

M23.006 Cystic meniscus, unspecified meniscus, right knee

M23.007 Cystic meniscus, unspecified meniscus, left knee

M23.009 Cystic meniscus, unspecified meniscus, unspecified knee

● M23.01 Cystic meniscus, anterior horn of medial meniscus

M23.011 Cystic meniscus, anterior horn of medial meniscus, right knee

M23.012 Cystic meniscus, anterior horn of medial meniscus, left knee

M23.019 Cystic meniscus, anterior horn of medial meniscus, unspecified knee

● M23.02 Cystic meniscus, posterior horn of medial meniscus

M23.021 Cystic meniscus, posterior horn of medial meniscus, right knee

M23.022 Cystic meniscus, posterior horn of medial meniscus, left knee

M23.029 Cystic meniscus, posterior horn of medial meniscus, unspecified knee

● M23.03 Cystic meniscus, other medial meniscus

M23.031 Cystic meniscus, other medial meniscus, right knee

M23.032 Cystic meniscus, other medial meniscus, left knee

M23.039 Cystic meniscus, other medial meniscus, unspecified knee

● M23.04 Cystic meniscus, anterior horn of lateral meniscus

M23.041 Cystic meniscus, anterior horn of lateral meniscus, right knee

M23.042 Cystic meniscus, anterior horn of lateral meniscus, left knee

M23.049 Cystic meniscus, anterior horn of lateral meniscus, unspecified knee

● M23.05 Cystic meniscus, posterior horn of lateral meniscus

M23.051 Cystic meniscus, posterior horn of lateral meniscus, right knee

M23.052 Cystic meniscus, posterior horn of lateral meniscus, left knee

M23.059 Cystic meniscus, posterior horn of lateral meniscus, unspecified knee

● M23.06 Cystic meniscus, other lateral meniscus

M23.061 Cystic meniscus, other lateral meniscus, right knee

M23.062 Cystic meniscus, other lateral meniscus, left knee

M23.069 Cystic meniscus, other lateral meniscus, unspecified knee

★ **(See Plate 34 of the Anatomy Illustrations.)**

● M23.2 Derangement of meniscus due to old tear or injury
Old bucket-handle tear

● M23.20 Derangement of unspecified meniscus due to old tear or injury
Derangement of unspecified lateral meniscus due to old tear or injury
Derangement of unspecified medial meniscus due to old tear or injury

M23.200 Derangement of unspecified lateral meniscus due to old tear or injury, right knee

M23.201 Derangement of unspecified lateral meniscus due to old tear or injury, left knee

M23.202 Derangement of unspecified lateral meniscus due to old tear or injury, unspecified knee

M23.203 Derangement of unspecified medial meniscus due to old tear or injury, right knee

M23.204 Derangement of unspecified medial meniscus due to old tear or injury, left knee

M23.205 Derangement of unspecified medial meniscus due to old tear or injury, unspecified knee

M23.206 Derangement of unspecified meniscus due to old tear or injury, right knee

M23.207 Derangement of unspecified meniscus due to old tear or injury, left knee

M23.209 Derangement of unspecified meniscus due to old tear or injury, unspecified knee

● M23.21 Derangement of anterior horn of medial meniscus due to old tear or injury

M23.211 Derangement of anterior horn of medial meniscus due to old tear or injury, right knee

M23.212 Derangement of anterior horn of medial meniscus due to old tear or injury, left knee

M23.219 Derangement of anterior horn of medial meniscus due to old tear or injury, unspecified knee

● M23.22 Derangement of posterior horn of medial meniscus due to old tear or injury

M23.221 Derangement of posterior horn of medial meniscus due to old tear or injury, right knee

M23.222 Derangement of posterior horn of medial meniscus due to old tear or injury, left knee

M23.229 Derangement of posterior horn of medial meniscus due to old tear or injury, unspecified knee

M23.23 Derangement of other medial meniscus due to old tear or injury
- M23.231 Derangement of other medial meniscus due to old tear or injury, right knee
- M23.232 Derangement of other medial meniscus due to old tear or injury, left knee
- M23.239 Derangement of other medial meniscus due to old tear or injury, unspecified knee

M23.24 Derangement of anterior horn of lateral meniscus due to old tear or injury
- M23.241 Derangement of anterior horn of lateral meniscus due to old tear or injury, right knee
- M23.242 Derangement of anterior horn of lateral meniscus due to old tear or injury, left knee
- M23.249 Derangement of anterior horn of lateral meniscus due to old tear or injury, unspecified knee

M23.25 Derangement of posterior horn of lateral meniscus due to old tear or injury
- M23.251 Derangement of posterior horn of lateral meniscus due to old tear or injury, right knee
- M23.252 Derangement of posterior horn of lateral meniscus due to old tear or injury, left knee
- M23.259 Derangement of posterior horn of lateral meniscus due to old tear or injury, unspecified knee

M23.26 Derangement of other lateral meniscus due to old tear or injury
- M23.261 Derangement of other lateral meniscus due to old tear or injury, right knee
- M23.262 Derangement of other lateral meniscus due to old tear or injury, left knee
- M23.269 Derangement of other lateral meniscus due to old tear or injury, unspecified knee

M23.3 Other meniscus derangements

Degenerate meniscus
Detached meniscus
Retained meniscus

M23.30 Other meniscus derangements, unspecified meniscus

Other meniscus derangements, unspecified lateral meniscus
Other meniscus derangements, unspecified medial meniscus

- M23.300 Other meniscus derangements, unspecified lateral meniscus, right knee
- M23.301 Other meniscus derangements, unspecified lateral meniscus, left knee
- M23.302 Other meniscus derangements, unspecified lateral meniscus, unspecified knee
- M23.303 Other meniscus derangements, unspecified medial meniscus, right knee
- M23.304 Other meniscus derangements, unspecified medial meniscus, left knee
- M23.305 Other meniscus derangements, unspecified medial meniscus, unspecified knee
- M23.306 Other meniscus derangements, unspecified meniscus, right knee
- M23.307 Other meniscus derangements, unspecified meniscus, left knee
- M23.309 Other meniscus derangements, unspecified meniscus, unspecified knee

M23.31 Other meniscus derangements, anterior horn of medial meniscus
- M23.311 Other meniscus derangements, anterior horn of medial meniscus, right knee
- M23.312 Other meniscus derangements, anterior horn of medial meniscus, left knee
- M23.319 Other meniscus derangements, anterior horn of medial meniscus, unspecified knee

M23.32 Other meniscus derangements, posterior horn of medial meniscus
- M23.321 Other meniscus derangements, posterior horn of medial meniscus, right knee
- M23.322 Other meniscus derangements, posterior horn of medial meniscus, left knee
- M23.329 Other meniscus derangements, posterior horn of medial meniscus, unspecified knee

M23.33 Other meniscus derangements, other medial meniscus
- M23.331 Other meniscus derangements, other medial meniscus, right knee
- M23.332 Other meniscus derangements, other medial meniscus, left knee
- M23.339 Other meniscus derangements, other medial meniscus, unspecified knee

M23.34 Other meniscus derangements, anterior horn of lateral meniscus
- M23.341 Other meniscus derangements, anterior horn of lateral meniscus, right knee
- M23.342 Other meniscus derangements, anterior horn of lateral meniscus, left knee
- M23.349 Other meniscus derangements, anterior horn of lateral meniscus, unspecified knee

M23.35 Other meniscus derangements, posterior horn of lateral meniscus
- M23.351 Other meniscus derangements, posterior horn of lateral meniscus, right knee
- M23.352 Other meniscus derangements, posterior horn of lateral meniscus, left knee
- M23.359 Other meniscus derangements, posterior horn of lateral meniscus, unspecified knee

M23.36 Other meniscus derangements, other lateral meniscus
- M23.361 Other meniscus derangements, other lateral meniscus, right knee
- M23.362 Other meniscus derangements, other lateral meniscus, left knee
- M23.369 Other meniscus derangements, other lateral meniscus, unspecified knee

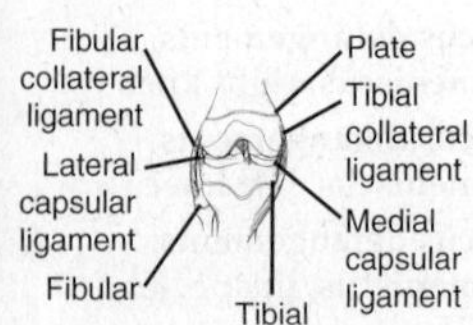

Figure 13-2 Collateral and cruciate ligament of knee. (From DeLee: DeLee and Drez's Orthopaedic Sports Medicine, ed 3, Saunders, 2009)

● **M23.4 Loose body in knee**
- M23.40 Loose body in knee, unspecified knee
- M23.41 Loose body in knee, right knee
- M23.42 Loose body in knee, left knee

● **M23.5 Chronic instability of knee**
- M23.50 Chronic instability of knee, unspecified knee
- M23.51 Chronic instability of knee, right knee
- M23.52 Chronic instability of knee, left knee

● **M23.6 Other spontaneous disruption of ligament(s) of knee**

● **M23.60 Other spontaneous disruption of unspecified ligament of knee**
- M23.601 Other spontaneous disruption of unspecified ligament of right knee
- M23.602 Other spontaneous disruption of unspecified ligament of left knee
- M23.609 Other spontaneous disruption of unspecified ligament of unspecified knee

● **M23.61 Other spontaneous disruption of anterior cruciate ligament of knee**
- M23.611 Other spontaneous disruption of anterior cruciate ligament of right knee
- M23.612 Other spontaneous disruption of anterior cruciate ligament of left knee
- M23.619 Other spontaneous disruption of anterior cruciate ligament of unspecified knee

● **M23.62 Other spontaneous disruption of posterior cruciate ligament of knee**
- M23.621 Other spontaneous disruption of posterior cruciate ligament of right knee
- M23.622 Other spontaneous disruption of posterior cruciate ligament of left knee
- M23.629 Other spontaneous disruption of posterior cruciate ligament of unspecified knee

● **M23.63 Other spontaneous disruption of medial collateral ligament of knee**
- M23.631 Other spontaneous disruption of medial collateral ligament of right knee
- M23.632 Other spontaneous disruption of medial collateral ligament of left knee
- M23.639 Other spontaneous disruption of medial collateral ligament of unspecified knee

● **M23.64 Other spontaneous disruption of lateral collateral ligament of knee**
- M23.641 Other spontaneous disruption of lateral collateral ligament of right knee
- M23.642 Other spontaneous disruption of lateral collateral ligament of left knee
- M23.649 Other spontaneous disruption of lateral collateral ligament of unspecified knee

● **M23.67 Other spontaneous disruption of capsular ligament of knee**
- M23.671 Other spontaneous disruption of capsular ligament of right knee
- M23.672 Other spontaneous disruption of capsular ligament of left knee
- M23.679 Other spontaneous disruption of capsular ligament of unspecified knee

● **M23.8 Other internal derangements of knee**

Laxity of ligament of knee
Snapping knee

● **M23.8X Other internal derangements of knee**
- M23.8X1 Other internal derangements of right knee
- M23.8X2 Other internal derangements of left knee
- M23.8X9 Other internal derangements of unspecified knee

● **M23.9 Unspecified internal derangement of knee**
- M23.90 Unspecified internal derangement of unspecified knee
- M23.91 Unspecified internal derangement of right knee
- M23.92 Unspecified internal derangement of left knee

● **M24 Other specific joint derangements**

Excludes1 current injury - see injury of joint by body region

Excludes2 ganglion (M67.4)
snapping knee (M23.8-)
temporomandibular joint disorders (M26.6-)

● **M24.0 Loose body in joint**

Excludes2 loose body in knee (M23.4)

- M24.00 Loose body in unspecified joint

● **M24.01 Loose body in shoulder**
- M24.011 Loose body in right shoulder
- M24.012 Loose body in left shoulder
- M24.019 Loose body in unspecified shoulder

● **M24.02 Loose body in elbow**
- M24.021 Loose body in right elbow
- M24.022 Loose body in left elbow
- M24.029 Loose body in unspecified elbow

● **M24.03 Loose body in wrist**
- M24.031 Loose body in right wrist
- M24.032 Loose body in left wrist
- M24.039 Loose body in unspecified wrist

● **M24.04 Loose body in finger joints**
- M24.041 Loose body in right finger joint(s)
- M24.042 Loose body in left finger joint(s)
- M24.049 Loose body in unspecified finger joint(s)

● **M24.05 Loose body in hip**
- M24.051 Loose body in right hip
- M24.052 Loose body in left hip
- M24.059 Loose body in unspecified hip

● **M24.07 Loose body in ankle and toe joints**
- M24.071 Loose body in right ankle
- M24.072 Loose body in left ankle
- M24.073 Loose body in unspecified ankle
- M24.074 Loose body in right toe joint(s)
- M24.075 Loose body in left toe joint(s)
- M24.076 Loose body in unspecified toe joints

M24.08 Loose body, other site

M24.1 Other articular cartilage disorders

Excludes2 chondrocalcinosis (M11.1-, M11.2-)
internal derangement of knee (M23.-)
metastatic calcification (E83.59)
ochronosis (E70.29)

M24.10 Other articular cartilage disorders, unspecified site

M24.11 Other articular cartilage disorders, shoulder
- **M24.111 Other articular cartilage disorders, right shoulder**
- **M24.112 Other articular cartilage disorders, left shoulder**
- **M24.119 Other articular cartilage disorders, unspecified shoulder**

M24.12 Other articular cartilage disorders, elbow
- **M24.121 Other articular cartilage disorders, right elbow**
- **M24.122 Other articular cartilage disorders, left elbow**
- **M24.129 Other articular cartilage disorders, unspecified elbow**

M24.13 Other articular cartilage disorders, wrist
- **M24.131 Other articular cartilage disorders, right wrist**
- **M24.132 Other articular cartilage disorders, left wrist**
- **M24.139 Other articular cartilage disorders, unspecified wrist**

M24.14 Other articular cartilage disorders, hand
- **M24.141 Other articular cartilage disorders, right hand**
- **M24.142 Other articular cartilage disorders, left hand**
- **M24.149 Other articular cartilage disorders, unspecified hand**

M24.15 Other articular cartilage disorders, hip
- **M24.151 Other articular cartilage disorders, right hip**
- **M24.152 Other articular cartilage disorders, left hip**
- **M24.159 Other articular cartilage disorders, unspecified hip**

M24.17 Other articular cartilage disorders, ankle and foot
- **M24.171 Other articular cartilage disorders, right ankle**
- **M24.172 Other articular cartilage disorders, left ankle**
- **M24.173 Other articular cartilage disorders, unspecified ankle**
- **M24.174 Other articular cartilage disorders, right foot**
- **M24.175 Other articular cartilage disorders, left foot**
- **M24.176 Other articular cartilage disorders, unspecified foot**

M24.19 Other articular cartilage disorders, other specified site

M24.2 Disorder of ligament

Instability secondary to old ligament injury
Ligamentous laxity NOS

Excludes1 familial ligamentous laxity (M35.7)

Excludes2 internal derangement of knee (M23.5-M23.8X9)

M24.20 Disorder of ligament, unspecified site

M24.21 Disorder of ligament, shoulder
- **M24.211 Disorder of ligament, right shoulder**
- **M24.212 Disorder of ligament, left shoulder**
- **M24.219 Disorder of ligament, unspecified shoulder**

M24.22 Disorder of ligament, elbow
- **M24.221 Disorder of ligament, right elbow**
- **M24.222 Disorder of ligament, left elbow**
- **M24.229 Disorder of ligament, unspecified elbow**

M24.23 Disorder of ligament, wrist
- **M24.231 Disorder of ligament, right wrist**
- **M24.232 Disorder of ligament, left wrist**
- **M24.239 Disorder of ligament, unspecified wrist**

M24.24 Disorder of ligament, hand
- **M24.241 Disorder of ligament, right hand**
- **M24.242 Disorder of ligament, left hand**
- **M24.249 Disorder of ligament, unspecified hand**

M24.25 Disorder of ligament, hip
- **M24.251 Disorder of ligament, right hip**
- **M24.252 Disorder of ligament, left hip**
- **M24.259 Disorder of ligament, unspecified hip**

M24.27 Disorder of ligament, ankle and foot
- **M24.271 Disorder of ligament, right ankle**
- **M24.272 Disorder of ligament, left ankle**
- **M24.273 Disorder of ligament, unspecified ankle**
- **M24.274 Disorder of ligament, right foot**
- **M24.275 Disorder of ligament, left foot**
- **M24.276 Disorder of ligament, unspecified foot**

M24.28 Disorder of ligament, vertebrae

Coding Clinic: 2023, Q2, P13-14

M24.29 Disorder of ligament, other specified site

M24.3 Pathological dislocation of joint, not elsewhere classified

Excludes1 congenital dislocation or displacement of joint - see congenital malformations and deformations of the musculoskeletal system (Q65-Q79)
current injury - see injury of joints and ligaments by body region
recurrent dislocation of joint (M24.4-)

M24.30 Pathological dislocation of unspecified joint, not elsewhere classified

M24.31 Pathological dislocation of shoulder, not elsewhere classified
- **M24.311 Pathological dislocation of right shoulder, not elsewhere classified**
- **M24.312 Pathological dislocation of left shoulder, not elsewhere classified**
- **M24.319 Pathological dislocation of unspecified shoulder, not elsewhere classified**

M24.32 Pathological dislocation of elbow, not elsewhere classified
- **M24.321 Pathological dislocation of right elbow, not elsewhere classified**
- **M24.322 Pathological dislocation of left elbow, not elsewhere classified**
- **M24.329 Pathological dislocation of unspecified elbow, not elsewhere classified**

M24.33 Pathological dislocation of wrist, not elsewhere classified
- **M24.331 Pathological dislocation of right wrist, not elsewhere classified**
- **M24.332 Pathological dislocation of left wrist, not elsewhere classified**
- **M24.339 Pathological dislocation of unspecified wrist, not elsewhere classified**

CHAPTER 13 (M00-M99)

- M24.34 Pathological dislocation of hand, not elsewhere classified
  - M24.341 Pathological dislocation of right hand, not elsewhere classified
  - M24.342 Pathological dislocation of left hand, not elsewhere classified
  - M24.349 Pathological dislocation of unspecified hand, not elsewhere classified
- M24.35 Pathological dislocation of hip, not elsewhere classified
  - M24.351 Pathological dislocation of right hip, not elsewhere classified
    Coding Clinic: 2022, Q1, P32
  - M24.352 Pathological dislocation of left hip, not elsewhere classified
    Coding Clinic: 2022, Q1, P32
  - M24.359 Pathological dislocation of unspecified hip, not elsewhere classified
- M24.36 Pathological dislocation of knee, not elsewhere classified
  - M24.361 Pathological dislocation of right knee, not elsewhere classified
  - M24.362 Pathological dislocation of left knee, not elsewhere classified
  - M24.369 Pathological dislocation of unspecified knee, not elsewhere classified
- M24.37 Pathological dislocation of ankle and foot, not elsewhere classified
  - M24.371 Pathological dislocation of right ankle, not elsewhere classified
  - M24.372 Pathological dislocation of left ankle, not elsewhere classified
  - M24.373 Pathological dislocation of unspecified ankle, not elsewhere classified
  - M24.374 Pathological dislocation of right foot, not elsewhere classified
  - M24.375 Pathological dislocation of left foot, not elsewhere classified
  - M24.376 Pathological dislocation of unspecified foot, not elsewhere classified
- M24.39 Pathological dislocation of other specified joint, not elsewhere classified

M24.4 Recurrent dislocation of joint
Recurrent subluxation of joint
Excludes2 recurrent dislocation of patella (M22.Ø-M22.1)
recurrent vertebral dislocation (M43.3-, M43.4, M43.5-)

- M24.4Ø Recurrent dislocation, unspecified joint
- M24.41 Recurrent dislocation, shoulder
  - M24.411 Recurrent dislocation, right shoulder
  - M24.412 Recurrent dislocation, left shoulder
  - M24.419 Recurrent dislocation, unspecified shoulder
- M24.42 Recurrent dislocation, elbow
  - M24.421 Recurrent dislocation, right elbow
  - M24.422 Recurrent dislocation, left elbow
  - M24.429 Recurrent dislocation, unspecified elbow
- M24.43 Recurrent dislocation, wrist
  - M24.431 Recurrent dislocation, right wrist
  - M24.432 Recurrent dislocation, left wrist
  - M24.439 Recurrent dislocation, unspecified wrist
- M24.44 Recurrent dislocation, hand and finger(s)
  - M24.441 Recurrent dislocation, right hand
  - M24.442 Recurrent dislocation, left hand
  - M24.443 Recurrent dislocation, unspecified hand
  - M24.444 Recurrent dislocation, right finger
  - M24.445 Recurrent dislocation, left finger
  - M24.446 Recurrent dislocation, unspecified finger
- M24.45 Recurrent dislocation, hip
  - M24.451 Recurrent dislocation, right hip
  - M24.452 Recurrent dislocation, left hip
  - M24.459 Recurrent dislocation, unspecified hip
- M24.46 Recurrent dislocation, knee
  - M24.461 Recurrent dislocation, right knee
  - M24.462 Recurrent dislocation, left knee
  - M24.469 Recurrent dislocation, unspecified knee
- M24.47 Recurrent dislocation, ankle, foot and toes
  - M24.471 Recurrent dislocation, right ankle
  - M24.472 Recurrent dislocation, left ankle
  - M24.473 Recurrent dislocation, unspecified ankle
  - M24.474 Recurrent dislocation, right foot
  - M24.475 Recurrent dislocation, left foot
  - M24.476 Recurrent dislocation, unspecified foot
  - M24.477 Recurrent dislocation, right toe(s)
  - M24.478 Recurrent dislocation, left toe(s)
  - M24.479 Recurrent dislocation, unspecified toe(s)
- M24.49 Recurrent dislocation, other specified joint

M24.5 Contracture of joint
Excludes1 contracture of muscle without contracture of joint (M62.4-)
contracture of tendon (sheath) without contracture of joint (M62.4-)
Dupuytren's contracture (M72.Ø)
Excludes2 acquired deformities of limbs (M2Ø-M21)

- M24.5Ø Contracture, unspecified joint
- M24.51 Contracture, shoulder
  - M24.511 Contracture, right shoulder
  - M24.512 Contracture, left shoulder
  - M24.519 Contracture, unspecified shoulder
- M24.52 Contracture, elbow
  - M24.521 Contracture, right elbow
  - M24.522 Contracture, left elbow
  - M24.529 Contracture, unspecified elbow
- M24.53 Contracture, wrist
  - M24.531 Contracture, right wrist
  - M24.532 Contracture, left wrist
  - M24.539 Contracture, unspecified wrist
- M24.54 Contracture, hand
  - M24.541 Contracture, right hand
  - M24.542 Contracture, left hand
  - M24.549 Contracture, unspecified hand
- M24.55 Contracture, hip
  - M24.551 Contracture, right hip
    Coding Clinic: 2016, Q2, P6
  - M24.552 Contracture, left hip
    Coding Clinic: 2016, Q2, P6
  - M24.559 Contracture, unspecified hip

Item 13-5 **Ankylosis** or arthrokleisis is a consolidation of a joint due to disease, injury, or surgical procedure. Spondylosis is the degeneration of the vertebral processes and formation of osteophytes and commonly occurs with age. **Spondylitis** or ankylosing spondylitis is a type of arthritis that affects the spine or backbone, causing back pain and stiffness.

● M24.56 Contracture, knee
- M24.561 Contracture, right knee
  Coding Clinic: 2016, Q2, P6
- M24.562 Contracture, left knee
  Coding Clinic: 2016, Q2, P6
- M24.569 Contracture, unspecified knee

● M24.57 Contracture, ankle and foot
- M24.571 Contracture, right ankle
- M24.572 Contracture, left ankle
- M24.573 Contracture, unspecified ankle
- M24.574 Contracture, right foot
- M24.575 Contracture, left foot
- M24.576 Contracture, unspecified foot

M24.59 Contracture, other specified joint

● M24.6 Ankylosis of joint
Excludes1 stiffness of joint without ankylosis (M25.6-)
Excludes2 spine (M43.2-)

M24.60 Ankylosis, unspecified joint

● M24.61 Ankylosis, shoulder
- M24.611 Ankylosis, right shoulder
- M24.612 Ankylosis, left shoulder
- M24.619 Ankylosis, unspecified shoulder

● M24.62 Ankylosis, elbow
- M24.621 Ankylosis, right elbow
- M24.622 Ankylosis, left elbow
- M24.629 Ankylosis, unspecified elbow

● M24.63 Ankylosis, wrist
- M24.631 Ankylosis, right wrist
- M24.632 Ankylosis, left wrist
- M24.639 Ankylosis, unspecified wrist

● M24.64 Ankylosis, hand
- M24.641 Ankylosis, right hand
- M24.642 Ankylosis, left hand
- M24.649 Ankylosis, unspecified hand

● M24.65 Ankylosis, hip
- M24.651 Ankylosis, right hip
- M24.652 Ankylosis, left hip
- M24.659 Ankylosis, unspecified hip

● M24.66 Ankylosis, knee
- M24.661 Ankylosis, right knee
- M24.662 Ankylosis, left knee
- M24.669 Ankylosis, unspecified knee

● M24.67 Ankylosis, ankle and foot
- M24.671 Ankylosis, right ankle
- M24.672 Ankylosis, left ankle
- M24.673 Ankylosis, unspecified ankle
- M24.674 Ankylosis, right foot
- M24.675 Ankylosis, left foot
- M24.676 Ankylosis, unspecified foot

M24.69 Ankylosis, other specified joint

M24.7 Protrusio acetabuli

● M24.8 Other specific joint derangements, not elsewhere classified
Excludes2 iliotibial band syndrome (M76.3)

M24.80 Other specific joint derangements of unspecified joint, not elsewhere classified

● M24.81 Other specific joint derangements of shoulder, not elsewhere classified
- M24.811 Other specific joint derangements of right shoulder, not elsewhere classified
- M24.812 Other specific joint derangements of left shoulder, not elsewhere classified
- M24.819 Other specific joint derangements of unspecified shoulder, not elsewhere classified

● M24.82 Other specific joint derangements of elbow, not elsewhere classified
- M24.821 Other specific joint derangements of right elbow, not elsewhere classified
- M24.822 Other specific joint derangements of left elbow, not elsewhere classified
- M24.829 Other specific joint derangements of unspecified elbow, not elsewhere classified

● M24.83 Other specific joint derangements of wrist, not elsewhere classified
- M24.831 Other specific joint derangements of right wrist, not elsewhere classified
- M24.832 Other specific joint derangements of left wrist, not elsewhere classified
- M24.839 Other specific joint derangements of unspecified wrist, not elsewhere classified

● M24.84 Other specific joint derangements of hand, not elsewhere classified
- M24.841 Other specific joint derangements of right hand, not elsewhere classified
- M24.842 Other specific joint derangements of left hand, not elsewhere classified
- M24.849 Other specific joint derangements of unspecified hand, not elsewhere classified

● M24.85 Other specific joint derangements of hip, not elsewhere classified
Irritable hip
- M24.851 Other specific joint derangements of right hip, not elsewhere classified
- M24.852 Other specific joint derangements of left hip, not elsewhere classified
- M24.859 Other specific joint derangements of unspecified hip, not elsewhere classified

● M24.87 Other specific joint derangements of ankle and foot, not elsewhere classified
- M24.871 Other specific joint derangements of right ankle, not elsewhere classified
- M24.872 Other specific joint derangements of left ankle, not elsewhere classified
- M24.873 Other specific joint derangements of unspecified ankle, not elsewhere classified
- M24.874 Other specific joint derangements of right foot, not elsewhere classified
- M24.875 Other specific joint derangements left foot, not elsewhere classified
- M24.876 Other specific joint derangements of unspecified foot, not elsewhere classified

M24.89 Other specific joint derangement of other specified joint, not elsewhere classified

M24.9 Joint derangement, unspecified

● M25 Other joint disorder, not elsewhere classified

Excludes2 abnormality of gait and mobility (R26.-)
acquired deformities of limb (M2Ø-M21)
calcification of bursa (M71.4-)
calcification of shoulder (joint) (M75.3)
calcification of tendon (M65.2-)
difficulty in walking (R26.2)
temporomandibular joint disorder (M26.6-)

● M25.Ø Hemarthrosis

Excludes1 current injury - see injury of joint by body region
hemophilic arthropathy (M36.2)

M25.ØØ Hemarthrosis, unspecified joint (Ex) PDX 1220
● M25.Ø1 Hemarthrosis, shoulder (Ex) PDX 1221
M25.Ø11 Hemarthrosis, right shoulder
M25.Ø12 Hemarthrosis, left shoulder
M25.Ø19 Hemarthrosis, unspecified shoulder
● M25.Ø2 Hemarthrosis, elbow (Ex) PDX 1222
M25.Ø21 Hemarthrosis, right elbow
M25.Ø22 Hemarthrosis, left elbow
M25.Ø29 Hemarthrosis, unspecified elbow
● M25.Ø3 Hemarthrosis, wrist (Ex) PDX 1223
M25.Ø31 Hemarthrosis, right wrist
M25.Ø32 Hemarthrosis, left wrist
M25.Ø39 Hemarthrosis, unspecified wrist
● M25.Ø4 Hemarthrosis, hand (Ex) PDX 1224
M25.Ø41 Hemarthrosis, right hand
M25.Ø42 Hemarthrosis, left hand
M25.Ø49 Hemarthrosis, unspecified hand
● M25.Ø5 Hemarthrosis, hip (Ex) PDX 1220
M25.Ø51 Hemarthrosis, right hip
M25.Ø52 Hemarthrosis, left hip
M25.Ø59 Hemarthrosis, unspecified hip
● M25.Ø6 Hemarthrosis, knee (Ex) PDX 1225
M25.Ø61 Hemarthrosis, right knee
M25.Ø62 Hemarthrosis, left knee
M25.Ø69 Hemarthrosis, unspecified knee
● M25.Ø7 Hemarthrosis, ankle and foot (Ex) PDX 1225
M25.Ø71 Hemarthrosis, right ankle
M25.Ø72 Hemarthrosis, left ankle
M25.Ø73 Hemarthrosis, unspecified ankle
M25.Ø74 Hemarthrosis, right foot
M25.Ø75 Hemarthrosis, left foot
M25.Ø76 Hemarthrosis, unspecified foot
M25.Ø8 Hemarthrosis, other specified site (Ex) PDX 1220
Hemarthrosis, vertebrae

● M25.1 Fistula of joint

M25.1Ø Fistula, unspecified joint
● M25.11 Fistula, shoulder
M25.111 Fistula, right shoulder
M25.112 Fistula, left shoulder
M25.119 Fistula, unspecified shoulder
● M25.12 Fistula, elbow
M25.121 Fistula, right elbow
M25.122 Fistula, left elbow
M25.129 Fistula, unspecified elbow
● M25.13 Fistula, wrist
M25.131 Fistula, right wrist
M25.132 Fistula, left wrist
M25.139 Fistula, unspecified wrist
● M25.14 Fistula, hand
M25.141 Fistula, right hand
M25.142 Fistula, left hand
M25.149 Fistula, unspecified hand
● M25.15 Fistula, hip
M25.151 Fistula, right hip
M25.152 Fistula, left hip
M25.159 Fistula, unspecified hip
● M25.16 Fistula, knee
M25.161 Fistula, right knee
M25.162 Fistula, left knee
M25.169 Fistula, unspecified knee
● M25.17 Fistula, ankle and foot
M25.171 Fistula, right ankle
M25.172 Fistula, left ankle
M25.173 Fistula, unspecified ankle
M25.174 Fistula, right foot
M25.175 Fistula, left foot
M25.176 Fistula, unspecified foot
M25.18 Fistula, other specified site
Fistula, vertebrae

● M25.2 Flail joint

M25.2Ø Flail joint, unspecified joint
● M25.21 Flail joint, shoulder
M25.211 Flail joint, right shoulder
M25.212 Flail joint, left shoulder
M25.219 Flail joint, unspecified shoulder
● M25.22 Flail joint, elbow
M25.221 Flail joint, right elbow
M25.222 Flail joint, left elbow
M25.229 Flail joint, unspecified elbow
● M25.23 Flail joint, wrist
M25.231 Flail joint, right wrist
M25.232 Flail joint, left wrist
M25.239 Flail joint, unspecified wrist
● M25.24 Flail joint, hand
M25.241 Flail joint, right hand
M25.242 Flail joint, left hand
M25.249 Flail joint, unspecified hand
● M25.25 Flail joint, hip
M25.251 Flail joint, right hip
M25.252 Flail joint, left hip
M25.259 Flail joint, unspecified hip
● M25.26 Flail joint, knee
M25.261 Flail joint, right knee
M25.262 Flail joint, left knee
M25.269 Flail joint, unspecified knee
● M25.27 Flail joint, ankle and foot
M25.271 Flail joint, right ankle and foot
M25.272 Flail joint, left ankle and foot
M25.279 Flail joint, unspecified ankle and foot
M25.28 Flail joint, other site

● M25.3 Other instability of joint

Excludes1 instability of joint secondary to old ligament injury (M24.2-)
instability of joint secondary to removal of joint prosthesis (M96.8-)

Excludes2 spinal instabilities (M53.2-)

M25.3Ø Other instability, unspecified joint
● M25.31 Other instability, shoulder
M25.311 Other instability, right shoulder
M25.312 Other instability, left shoulder
M25.319 Other instability, unspecified shoulder
● M25.32 Other instability, elbow
M25.321 Other instability, right elbow
M25.322 Other instability, left elbow
M25.329 Other instability, unspecified elbow

- ● **M25.33** Other instability, wrist
  - **M25.331** Other instability, right wrist
  - **M25.332** Other instability, left wrist
  - **M25.339** Other instability, unspecified wrist
- ● **M25.34** Other instability, hand
  - **M25.341** Other instability, right hand
  - **M25.342** Other instability, left hand
  - **M25.349** Other instability, unspecified hand
- ● **M25.35** Other instability, hip
  - **M25.351** Other instability, right hip
  - **M25.352** Other instability, left hip
  - **M25.359** Other instability, unspecified hip
- ● **M25.36** Other instability, knee
  - **M25.361** Other instability, right knee
  - **M25.362** Other instability, left knee
  - **M25.369** Other instability, unspecified knee
- ● **M25.37** Other instability, ankle and foot
  - **M25.371** Other instability, right ankle
  - **M25.372** Other instability, left ankle
  - **M25.373** Other instability, unspecified ankle
  - **M25.374** Other instability, right foot
  - **M25.375** Other instability, left foot
  - **M25.376** Other instability, unspecified foot
- **M25.39** Other instability of joint

● **M25.4** Effusion of joint

Excludes1 hydrarthrosis in yaws (A66.6)
intermittent hydrarthrosis (M12.4-)
other infective (teno)synovitis (M65.1-)

- **M25.40** Effusion, unspecified joint
- ● **M25.41** Effusion, shoulder
  - **M25.411** Effusion, right shoulder
  - **M25.412** Effusion, left shoulder
  - **M25.419** Effusion, unspecified shoulder
- ● **M25.42** Effusion, elbow
  - **M25.421** Effusion, right elbow
  - **M25.422** Effusion, left elbow
  - **M25.429** Effusion, unspecified elbow
- ● **M25.43** Effusion, wrist
  - **M25.431** Effusion, right wrist
  - **M25.432** Effusion, left wrist
  - **M25.439** Effusion, unspecified wrist
- ● **M25.44** Effusion, hand
  - **M25.441** Effusion, right hand
  - **M25.442** Effusion, left hand
  - **M25.449** Effusion, unspecified hand
- ● **M25.45** Effusion, hip
  - **M25.451** Effusion, right hip
  - **M25.452** Effusion, left hip
  - **M25.459** Effusion, unspecified hip
- ● **M25.46** Effusion, knee
  - **M25.461** Effusion, right knee
  - **M25.462** Effusion, left knee
  - **M25.469** Effusion, unspecified knee
- ● **M25.47** Effusion, ankle and foot
  - **M25.471** Effusion, right ankle
  - **M25.472** Effusion, left ankle
  - **M25.473** Effusion, unspecified ankle
  - **M25.474** Effusion, right foot
  - **M25.475** Effusion, left foot
  - **M25.476** Effusion, unspecified foot
- **M25.48** Effusion, other site

● **M25.5** Pain in joint

Excludes2 pain in hand (M79.64-)
pain in fingers (M79.64-)
pain in foot (M79.67-)
pain in limb (M79.6-)
pain in toes (M79.67-)

- **M25.50** Pain in unspecified joint
- ● **M25.51** Pain in shoulder
  - **M25.511** Pain in right shoulder
  - **M25.512** Pain in left shoulder
  - **M25.519** Pain in unspecified shoulder
- ● **M25.52** Pain in elbow
  - **M25.521** Pain in right elbow
  - **M25.522** Pain in left elbow
  - **M25.529** Pain in unspecified elbow
- ● **M25.53** Pain in wrist
  - **M25.531** Pain in right wrist
  - **M25.532** Pain in left wrist
  - **M25.539** Pain in unspecified wrist
- ● **M25.54** Pain in joints of hand
  Coding Clinic: 2016, Q4, P38
  - **M25.541** Pain in joints of right hand
  - **M25.542** Pain in joints of left hand
  - **M25.549** Pain in joints of unspecified hand
    Pain in joints of hand NOS
- ● **M25.55** Pain in hip
  - **M25.551** Pain in right hip
  - **M25.552** Pain in left hip
  - **M25.559** Pain in unspecified hip
- ● **M25.56** Pain in knee
  - **M25.561** Pain in right knee
  - **M25.562** Pain in left knee
  - **M25.569** Pain in unspecified knee
- ● **M25.57** Pain in ankle and joints of foot
  - **M25.571** Pain in right ankle and joints of right foot
  - **M25.572** Pain in left ankle and joints of left foot
  - **M25.579** Pain in unspecified ankle and joints of unspecified foot
- **M25.59** Pain in other specified joint

● **M25.6** Stiffness of joint, not elsewhere classified

Excludes1 ankylosis of joint (M24.6-)
contracture of joint (M24.5-)

- **M25.60** Stiffness of unspecified joint, not elsewhere classified
- ● **M25.61** Stiffness of shoulder, not elsewhere classified
  - **M25.611** Stiffness of right shoulder, not elsewhere classified
  - **M25.612** Stiffness of left shoulder, not elsewhere classified
  - **M25.619** Stiffness of unspecified shoulder, not elsewhere classified
- ● **M25.62** Stiffness of elbow, not elsewhere classified
  - **M25.621** Stiffness of right elbow, not elsewhere classified
  - **M25.622** Stiffness of left elbow, not elsewhere classified
  - **M25.629** Stiffness of unspecified elbow, not elsewhere classified
- ● **M25.63** Stiffness of wrist, not elsewhere classified
  - **M25.631** Stiffness of right wrist, not elsewhere classified
  - **M25.632** Stiffness of left wrist, not elsewhere classified
  - **M25.639** Stiffness of unspecified wrist, not elsewhere classified

CHAPTER 13 (M00-M99)

M25.64 Stiffness of hand, not elsewhere classified
M25.641 Stiffness of right hand, not elsewhere classified
M25.642 Stiffness of left hand, not elsewhere classified
M25.649 Stiffness of unspecified hand, not elsewhere classified
M25.65 Stiffness of hip, not elsewhere classified
M25.651 Stiffness of right hip, not elsewhere classified
M25.652 Stiffness of left hip, not elsewhere classified
M25.659 Stiffness of unspecified hip, not elsewhere classified
M25.66 Stiffness of knee, not elsewhere classified
M25.661 Stiffness of right knee, not elsewhere classified
M25.662 Stiffness of left knee, not elsewhere classified
M25.669 Stiffness of unspecified knee, not elsewhere classified
M25.67 Stiffness of ankle and foot, not elsewhere classified
M25.671 Stiffness of right ankle, not elsewhere classified
M25.672 Stiffness of left ankle, not elsewhere classified
M25.673 Stiffness of unspecified ankle, not elsewhere classified
M25.674 Stiffness of right foot, not elsewhere classified
M25.675 Stiffness of left foot, not elsewhere classified
M25.676 Stiffness of unspecified foot, not elsewhere classified
M25.69 Stiffness of other specified joint, not elsewhere classified
M25.7 Osteophyte
M25.70 Osteophyte, unspecified joint
M25.71 Osteophyte, shoulder
M25.711 Osteophyte, right shoulder
M25.712 Osteophyte, left shoulder
M25.719 Osteophyte, unspecified shoulder
M25.72 Osteophyte, elbow
M25.721 Osteophyte, right elbow
M25.722 Osteophyte, left elbow
M25.729 Osteophyte, unspecified elbow
M25.73 Osteophyte, wrist
M25.731 Osteophyte, right wrist
M25.732 Osteophyte, left wrist
M25.739 Osteophyte, unspecified wrist
M25.74 Osteophyte, hand
M25.741 Osteophyte, right hand
M25.742 Osteophyte, left hand
M25.749 Osteophyte, unspecified hand
M25.75 Osteophyte, hip
M25.751 Osteophyte, right hip
M25.752 Osteophyte, left hip
M25.759 Osteophyte, unspecified hip
M25.76 Osteophyte, knee
M25.761 Osteophyte, right knee
M25.762 Osteophyte, left knee
M25.769 Osteophyte, unspecified knee
M25.77 Osteophyte, ankle and foot
M25.771 Osteophyte, right ankle
M25.772 Osteophyte, left ankle
M25.773 Osteophyte, unspecified ankle
M25.774 Osteophyte, right foot
M25.775 Osteophyte, left foot
M25.776 Osteophyte, unspecified foot
M25.78 Osteophyte, vertebrae
M25.8 Other specified joint disorders
M25.80 Other specified joint disorders, unspecified joint
M25.81 Other specified joint disorders, shoulder
Coding Clinic: 2022, Q3, P18
M25.811 Other specified joint disorders, right shoulder
M25.812 Other specified joint disorders, left shoulder
Coding Clinic: 2022, Q3, P18
M25.819 Other specified joint disorders, unspecified shoulder
M25.82 Other specified joint disorders, elbow
M25.821 Other specified joint disorders, right elbow
M25.822 Other specified joint disorders, left elbow
M25.829 Other specified joint disorders, unspecified elbow
M25.83 Other specified joint disorders, wrist
M25.831 Other specified joint disorders, right wrist
M25.832 Other specified joint disorders, left wrist
M25.839 Other specified joint disorders, unspecified wrist
M25.84 Other specified joint disorders, hand
M25.841 Other specified joint disorders, right hand
M25.842 Other specified joint disorders, left hand
M25.849 Other specified joint disorders, unspecified hand
M25.85 Other specified joint disorders, hip
M25.851 Other specified joint disorders, right hip
M25.852 Other specified joint disorders, left hip
M25.859 Other specified joint disorders, unspecified hip
M25.86 Other specified joint disorders, knee
M25.861 Other specified joint disorders, right knee
M25.862 Other specified joint disorders, left knee
M25.869 Other specified joint disorders, unspecified knee
M25.87 Other specified joint disorders, ankle and foot
M25.871 Other specified joint disorders, right ankle and foot
M25.872 Other specified joint disorders, left ankle and foot
M25.879 Other specified joint disorders, unspecified ankle and foot
M25.9 Joint disorder, unspecified

DENTOFACIAL ANOMALIES [INCLUDING MALOCCLUSION] AND OTHER DISORDERS OF JAW (M26-M27)

Excludes1 hemifacial atrophy or hypertrophy (Q67.4)
unilateral condylar hyperplasia or hypoplasia (M27.8)

M26 Dentofacial anomalies [including malocclusion]

M26.0 Major anomalies of jaw size

Excludes1 acromegaly (E22.0)
Robin's syndrome (Q87.0)

M26.00 Unspecified anomaly of jaw size
M26.01 Maxillary hyperplasia
M26.02 Maxillary hypoplasia
M26.03 Mandibular hyperplasia
M26.04 Mandibular hypoplasia
M26.05 Macrogenia
M26.06 Microgenia
M26.07 Excessive tuberosity of jaw
Entire maxillary tuberosity
M26.09 Other specified anomalies of jaw size

M26.1 Anomalies of jaw-cranial base relationship

M26.10 Unspecified anomaly of jaw-cranial base relationship
M26.11 Maxillary asymmetry
M26.12 Other jaw asymmetry
M26.19 Other specified anomalies of jaw-cranial base relationship
Coding Clinic: 2020, Q1, P21

M26.2 Anomalies of dental arch relationship

M26.20 Unspecified anomaly of dental arch relationship

M26.21 Malocclusion, Angle's class

M26.211 Malocclusion, Angle's class I
Neutro-occlusion
M26.212 Malocclusion, Angle's class II
Disto-occlusion Division I
Disto-occlusion Division II
M26.213 Malocclusion, Angle's class III
Mesio-occlusion
M26.219 Malocclusion, Angle's class, unspecified

M26.22 Open occlusal relationship

M26.220 Open anterior occlusal relationship
Anterior open bite
M26.221 Open posterior occlusal relationship
Posterior open bite

M26.23 Excessive horizontal overlap
Excessive horizontal overjet
M26.24 Reverse articulation
Crossbite (anterior) (posterior)
M26.25 Anomalies of interarch distance
M26.29 Other anomalies of dental arch relationship
Midline deviation of dental arch
Overbite (excessive) deep
Overbite (excessive) horizontal
Overbite (excessive) vertical
Posterior lingual occlusion of mandibular teeth

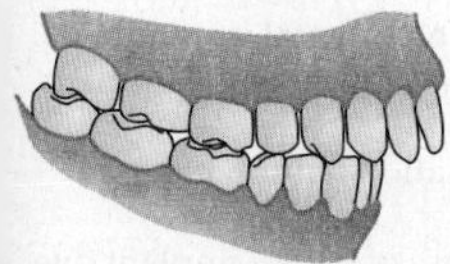

Figure 13-3 Dentofacial malocclusion.

Item 13-6 Hyperplasia is a condition of overdevelopment, whereas **hypoplasia** is a condition of underdevelopment. **Macrogenia** is overdevelopment of the chin, whereas **microgenia** is underdevelopment of the chin.

M26.3 Anomalies of tooth position of fully erupted tooth or teeth

Excludes2 embedded and impacted teeth (K01.-)

M26.30 Unspecified anomaly of tooth position of fully erupted tooth or teeth
Abnormal spacing of fully erupted tooth or teeth NOS
Displacement of fully erupted tooth or teeth NOS
Transposition of fully erupted tooth or teeth NOS
M26.31 Crowding of fully erupted teeth
M26.32 Excessive spacing of fully erupted teeth
Diastema of fully erupted tooth or teeth NOS
M26.33 Horizontal displacement of fully erupted tooth or teeth
Tipped tooth or teeth
Tipping of fully erupted tooth
M26.34 Vertical displacement of fully erupted tooth or teeth
Extruded tooth
Infraeruption of tooth or teeth
Supraeruption of tooth or teeth
M26.35 Rotation of fully erupted tooth or teeth
M26.36 Insufficient interocclusal distance of fully erupted teeth (ridge)
Lack of adequate intermaxillary vertical dimension of fully erupted teeth
M26.37 Excessive interocclusal distance of fully erupted teeth
Excessive intermaxillary vertical dimension of fully erupted teeth
Loss of occlusal vertical dimension of fully erupted teeth
M26.39 Other anomalies of tooth position of fully erupted tooth or teeth

M26.4 Malocclusion, unspecified

M26.5 Dentofacial functional abnormalities

Excludes1 bruxism (F45.8)
teeth-grinding NOS (F45.8)

M26.50 Dentofacial functional abnormalities, unspecified
M26.51 Abnormal jaw closure
M26.52 Limited mandibular range of motion
M26.53 Deviation in opening and closing of the mandible
M26.54 Insufficient anterior guidance
Insufficient anterior occlusal guidance
M26.55 Centric occlusion maximum intercuspation discrepancy
Excludes1 centric occlusion NOS (M26.59)
M26.56 Non-working side interference
Balancing side interference
M26.57 Lack of posterior occlusal support
M26.59 Other dentofacial functional abnormalities
Centric occlusion (of teeth) NOS
Malocclusion due to abnormal swallowing
Malocclusion due to mouth breathing
Malocclusion due to tongue, lip or finger habits

M26.6 Temporomandibular joint disorders

Excludes2 current temporomandibular joint dislocation (S03.0)
current temporomandibular joint sprain (S03.4)

Coding Clinic: 2016, Q4, P38-39

M26.60 Temporomandibular joint disorder, unspecified

M26.601 Right temporomandibular joint disorder, unspecified
M26.602 Left temporomandibular joint disorder, unspecified

CHAPTER 13 (M00-M99)

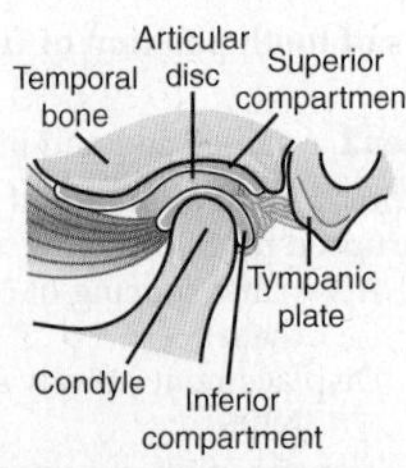

Figure 13-4 Temporomandibular joint.

Item 13–7 Dysfunction of the temporomandibular joint is termed **temporomandibular joint (TMJ) syndrome** and is characterized by pain and tenderness/spasm of the muscles of mastication, joint noise, and in the later stages, limited mandibular movement.

M26.603 Bilateral temporomandibular joint disorder, unspecified

M26.609 Unspecified temporomandibular joint disorder, unspecified side
Temporomandibular joint disorder NOS

● **M26.61 Adhesions and ankylosis of temporomandibular joint**
M26.611 Adhesions and ankylosis of right temporomandibular joint
M26.612 Adhesions and ankylosis of left temporomandibular joint
M26.613 Adhesions and ankylosis of bilateral temporomandibular joint
M26.619 Adhesions and ankylosis of temporomandibular joint, unspecified side

● **M26.62 Arthralgia of temporomandibular joint**
M26.621 Arthralgia of right temporomandibular joint
M26.622 Arthralgia of left temporomandibular joint
M26.623 Arthralgia of bilateral temporomandibular joint
M26.629 Arthralgia of temporomandibular joint, unspecified side

● **M26.63 Articular disc disorder of temporomandibular joint**
M26.631 Articular disc disorder of right temporomandibular joint
M26.632 Articular disc disorder of left temporomandibular joint
M26.633 Articular disc disorder of bilateral temporomandibular joint
M26.639 Articular disc disorder of temporomandibular joint, unspecified side

● **M26.64 Arthritis of temporomandibular joint**
M26.641 Arthritis of right temporomandibular joint
M26.642 Arthritis of left temporomandibular joint
M26.643 Arthritis of bilateral temporomandibular joint
M26.649 Arthritis of unspecified temporomandibular joint

● **M26.65 Arthropathy of temporomandibular joint**
M26.651 Arthropathy of right temporomandibular joint
M26.652 Arthropathy of left temporomandibular joint
M26.653 Arthropathy of bilateral temporomandibular joint
M26.659 Arthropathy of unspecified temporomandibular joint

M26.69 Other specified disorders of temporomandibular joint

● **M26.7 Dental alveolar anomalies**
M26.70 Unspecified alveolar anomaly
M26.71 Alveolar maxillary hyperplasia
M26.72 Alveolar mandibular hyperplasia
M26.73 Alveolar maxillary hypoplasia
M26.74 Alveolar mandibular hypoplasia
M26.79 Other specified alveolar anomalies

● **M26.8 Other dentofacial anomalies**
M26.81 Anterior soft tissue impingement
Anterior soft tissue impingement on teeth
M26.82 Posterior soft tissue impingement
Posterior soft tissue impingement on teeth
M26.89 Other dentofacial anomalies

M26.9 Dentofacial anomaly, unspecified

● **M27 Other diseases of jaws**

M27.0 Developmental disorders of jaws
Latent bone cyst of jaw
Stafne's cyst
Torus mandibularis
Torus palatinus

M27.1 Giant cell granuloma, central
Giant cell granuloma NOS
Excludes1 peripheral giant cell granuloma (K06.8)

M27.2 Inflammatory conditions of jaws
Osteitis of jaw(s)
Osteomyelitis (neonatal) jaw(s)
Osteoradionecrosis jaw(s)
Periostitis jaw(s)
Sequestrum of jaw bone
Use additional code (W88-W90, X39.0) to identify radiation, if radiation-induced
Excludes2 osteonecrosis of jaw due to drug (M87.180)

M27.3 Alveolitis of jaws
Alveolar osteitis
Dry socket

● **M27.4 Other and unspecified cysts of jaw**
Excludes1 cysts of oral region (K09.-)
latent bone cyst of jaw (M27.0)
Stafne's cyst (M27.0)
M27.40 Unspecified cyst of jaw
Cyst of jaw NOS
M27.49 Other cysts of jaw
Aneurysmal cyst of jaw
Hemorrhagic cyst of jaw
Traumatic cyst of jaw

● **M27.5 Periradicular pathology associated with previous endodontic treatment**
M27.51 Perforation of root canal space due to endodontic treatment
M27.52 Endodontic overfill
M27.53 Endodontic underfill
M27.59 Other periradicular pathology associated with previous endodontic treatment

● **M27.6 Endosseous dental implant failure**
M27.61 Osseointegration failure of dental implant
Hemorrhagic complications of dental implant placement
Iatrogenic osseointegration failure of dental implant
Osseointegration failure of dental implant due to complications of systemic disease
Osseointegration failure of dental implant due to poor bone quality
Pre-integration failure of dental implant NOS
Pre-osseointegration failure of dental implant

M27.62 Post-osseointegration biological failure of dental implant
Failure of dental implant due to lack of attached gingiva
Failure of dental implant due to occlusal trauma (caused by poor prosthetic design)
Failure of dental implant due to parafunctional habits
Failure of dental implant due to periodontal infection (peri–implantitis)
Failure of dental implant due to poor oral hygiene
Iatrogenic post-osseointegration failure of dental implant
Post-osseointegration failure of dental implant due to complications of systemic disease

M27.63 Post-osseointegration mechanical failure of dental implant
Failure of dental prosthesis causing loss of dental implant
Fracture of dental implant
Excludes2 cracked tooth (KØ3.81)
fractured dental restorative material with loss of material (KØ8.531)
fractured dental restorative material without loss of material (KØ8.53Ø)
fractured tooth (SØ2.5)

M27.69 Other endosseous dental implant failure
Dental implant failure NOS

M27.8 Other specified diseases of jaws
Cherubism
Exostosis
Fibrous dysplasia
Unilateral condylar hyperplasia
Unilateral condylar hypoplasia
Excludes1 jaw pain (R68.84)

M27.9 Disease of jaws, unspecified

SYSTEMIC CONNECTIVE TISSUE DISORDERS (M3Ø-M36)

Includes autoimmune disease NOS
collagen (vascular) disease NOS
systemic autoimmune disease
systemic collagen (vascular) disease
Excludes1 autoimmune disease, single organ or single cell-type - code to relevant condition category

● **M3Ø Polyarteritis nodosa and related conditions** (Ex) PDX 1226
Excludes1 microscopic polyarteritis (M31.7)

M3Ø.Ø Polyarteritis nodosa

M3Ø.1 Polyarteritis with lung involvement [Churg-Strauss]
Allergic granulomatous angiitis
Eosinophilic granulomatosis with polyangiitis [EGPA]
Coding Clinic: 2Ø21, Q1, P23

M3Ø.2 Juvenile polyarteritis

M3Ø.3 Mucocutaneous lymph node syndrome [Kawasaki] (Ex) PDX 1227

M3Ø.8 Other conditions related to polyarteritis nodosa
Polyangiitis overlap syndrome

● **M31 Other necrotizing vasculopathies** (Ex) PDX 1228

M31.Ø Hypersensitivity angiitis
Goodpasture's syndrome

● **M31.1 Thrombotic microangiopathy** (Ex) PDX 1229

M31.1Ø Thrombotic microangiopathy, unspecified

M31.11 Hematopoietic stem cell transplantation-associated thrombotic microangiopathy [HSCT-TMA]
Transplant-associated thrombotic microangiopathy [TA-TMA]
Code first if applicable:
complications of bone marrow transplant (T86.0-)
complications of stem cell transplant (T86.5)
Use Additional code to identify specific organ dysfunction, such as:
acute kidney failure (N17.-)
acute respiratory distress syndrome (J80)
capillary leak syndrome (I78.8)
diffuse alveolar hemorrhage (R04.89)
encephalopathy (metabolic) (septic) (G93.41)
fluid overload, unspecified (E87.70)
graft versus host disease (D89.81-)
hemolytic uremic syndrome (D59.3-)
hepatic failure (K72.-)
hepatic veno-occlusive disease (K76.5)
idiopathic interstitial pneumonia (J84.11-)
sinusoidal obstruction syndrome (K76.5)

M31.19 Other thrombotic microangiopathy
Thrombotic thrombocytopenic purpura

M31.2 Lethal midline granuloma (Ex) PDX 1226

● **M31.3 Wegener's granulomatosis** (Ex) PDX 1226
Granulomatosis with polyangiitis
Necrotizing respiratory granulomatosis
Coding Clinic: 2Ø21, Q1, P23

M31.3Ø Wegener's granulomatosis without renal involvement
Wegener's granulomatosis NOS
Coding Clinic: 2Ø21, Q2, P1Ø

M31.31 Wegener's granulomatosis with renal involvement

M31.4 Aortic arch syndrome [Takayasu] (Ex) PDX 1226

M31.5 Giant cell arteritis with polymyalgia rheumatica

M31.6 Other giant cell arteritis

M31.7 Microscopic polyangiitis (Ex) PDX 1228
Microscopic polyarteritis
Excludes1 polyarteritis nodosa (M3Ø.Ø)
Coding Clinic: 2Ø21, Q1, P23

M31.8 Other specified necrotizing vasculopathies (Ex) PDX 985
Hypocomplementemic vasculitis
Septic vasculitis

M31.9 Necrotizing vasculopathy, unspecified (Ex) PDX 985

● **M32 Systemic lupus erythematosus (SLE)**
Autoimmune inflammatory connective tissue disease of unknown cause that occurs most often in women
Excludes1 lupus erythematosus (discoid) (NOS) (L93.Ø)

M32.Ø Drug-induced systemic lupus erythematosus
Use additional code for adverse effect, if applicable, to identify drug (T36-T5Ø with fifth or sixth character 5)

● **M32.1 Systemic lupus erythematosus with organ or system involvement**

M32.1Ø Systemic lupus erythematosus, organ or system involvement unspecified

M32.11 Endocarditis in systemic lupus erythematosus (Ex) PDX 1230
Libman-Sacks disease
CC when PDx is its own CC

CHAPTER 13 (MØØ-M99)

M32.12 **Pericarditis in systemic lupus erythematosus** (Exc) PDX 1231
Lupus pericarditis
CC when PDx is its own CC

M32.13 **Lung involvement in systemic lupus erythematosus**
Pleural effusion due to systemic lupus erythematosus

M32.14 **Glomerular disease in systemic lupus erythematosus**
Lupus renal disease NOS

M32.15 **Tubulo-interstitial nephropathy in systemic lupus erythematosus**

M32.19 **Other organ or system involvement in systemic lupus erythematosus**
Use additional code(s) to identify organ or system involvement, such as encephalitis (G05.3)

M32.8 **Other forms of systemic lupus erythematosus**

M32.9 **Systemic lupus erythematosus, unspecified**
SLE NOS
Systemic lupus erythematosus NOS
Systemic lupus erythematosus without organ involvement

● **M33 Dermatopolymyositis** (Exc) PDX 1232

● **M33.0 Juvenile dermatomyositis**

M33.00 **Juvenile dermatomyositis, organ involvement unspecified**

M33.01 **Juvenile dermatomyositis with respiratory involvement**

M33.02 **Juvenile dermatomyositis with myopathy** (Exc) PDX 1233
CC when PDx is its own CC

M33.03 **Juvenile dermatomyositis without myopathy**

M33.09 **Juvenile dermatomyositis with other organ involvement**

● **M33.1 Other dermatomyositis**
Adult dermatomyositis

M33.10 **Other dermatomyositis, organ involvement unspecified**

M33.11 **Other dermatomyositis with respiratory involvement**

M33.12 **Other dermatomyositis with myopathy** (Exc) PDX 1233
CC when PDx is its own CC

M33.13 **Other dermatomyositis without myopathy**
Dermatomyositis NOS

M33.19 **Other dermatomyositis with other organ involvement**

● **M33.2 Polymyositis** (Exc) PDX 1234

M33.20 **Polymyositis, organ involvement unspecified**

M33.21 **Polymyositis with respiratory involvement**

M33.22 **Polymyositis with myopathy** (Exc) PDX 1235
CC when PDx is its own CC

M33.29 **Polymyositis with other organ involvement**

● **M33.9 Dermatopolymyositis, unspecified** (Exc) PDX 1232

M33.90 **Dermatopolymyositis, unspecified, organ involvement unspecified**

M33.91 **Dermatopolymyositis, unspecified with respiratory involvement**

M33.92 **Dermatopolymyositis, unspecified with myopathy** (Exc) PDX 1233
CC when PDx is its own CC

M33.93 **Dermatopolymyositis, unspecified without myopathy**

M33.99 **Dermatopolymyositis, unspecified with other organ involvement**

● **M34 Systemic sclerosis [scleroderma]**
Excludes1 circumscribed scleroderma (L94.0)
neonatal scleroderma (P83.88)

M34.0 **Progressive systemic sclerosis**

M34.1 **CR(E)ST syndrome**
Combination of calcinosis, Raynaud's phenomenon, esophageal dysfunction, sclerodactyly, telangiectasia

M34.2 **Systemic sclerosis induced by drug and chemical**
Code first poisoning due to drug or toxin, if applicable (T36-T65 with fifth or sixth character 1-4)
Use additional code for adverse effect, if applicable, to identify drug (T36-T50 with fifth or sixth character 5)

● **M34.8 Other forms of systemic sclerosis**

M34.81 **Systemic sclerosis with lung involvement** (Exc) PDX 1236
Code also if applicable:
other interstitial pulmonary diseases (J84.89)
secondary pulmonary arterial hypertension (I27.21)
CC when PDx is its own CC

M34.82 **Systemic sclerosis with myopathy** (Exc) PDX 1237
CC when PDx is its own CC

M34.83 **Systemic sclerosis with polyneuropathy**

M34.89 **Other systemic sclerosis**

M34.9 **Systemic sclerosis, unspecified**

● **M35 Other systemic involvement of connective tissue**
Excludes1 reactive perforating collagenosis (L87.1)

● **M35.0 Sjögren syndrome**
Sicca syndrome
Use Additional code to identify associated manifestations
Excludes1 dry mouth, unspecified (R68.2)

M35.00 **Sjögren syndrome, unspecified**

M35.01 **Sjögren syndrome with keratoconjunctivitis**

M35.02 **Sjögren syndrome with lung involvement**

M35.03 **Sjögren syndrome with myopathy** (Exc) PDX 1238
CC when PDx is its own CC

Item 13–8 Polymyalgia rheumatica is a syndrome characterized by aching and morning stiffness and is related to aging and hereditary predisposition.

M35.04 **Sjögren syndrome with tubulo-interstitial nephropathy**
Renal tubular acidosis in sicca syndrome

M35.05 **Sjögren syndrome with inflammatory arthritis**

M35.06 **Sjögren syndrome with peripheral nervous system involvement**

M35.07 **Sjögren syndrome with central nervous system involvement** (Exc) PDX 1239

M35.08 **Sjögren syndrome with gastrointestinal involvement**

M35.09 **Sjögren syndrome with other organ involvement**

M35.0A **Sjögren syndrome with glomerular disease**

M35.0B **Sjögren syndrome with vasculitis**

M35.0C **Sjögren syndrome with dental involvement**

M35.1 **Other overlap syndromes** (Exc) PDX 1240
Mixed connective tissue disease
Excludes1 polyangiitis overlap syndrome (M30.8)

M35.2 **Behçet's disease** (Exc) PDX 1181

M35.3 **Polymyalgia rheumatica**
Excludes1 polymyalgia rheumatica with giant cell arteritis (M31.5)

M35.4 **Diffuse (eosinophilic) fasciitis**

M35.5 **Multifocal fibrosclerosis** (Exc) PDX 1240

M35.6 **Relapsing panniculitis [Weber-Christian]**
Excludes1 lupus panniculitis (L93.2)
panniculitis NOS (M79.3-)

M35.7 **Hypermobility syndrome**
Familial ligamentous laxity
Excludes1 ligamentous laxity, NOS (M24.2-)
Excludes2 Ehlers-Danlos syndromes (Q79.6-)

M35.8 **Other specified systemic involvement of connective tissue** PDX 1241
Coding Clinic: 2021, Q4, P102; 2021, Q1, P36

M35.81 **Multisystem inflammatory syndrome**
MIS-A
MIS-C
Multisystem inflammatory syndrome in adults
Multisystem inflammatory syndrome in children
Pediatric inflammatory multisystem syndrome
PIMS
Code first, if applicable, COVID-19 (U07.1)
Code also any associated complications such as:
acute hepatic failure (K72.0-)
acute kidney failure (N17.-)
acute myocarditis (I40.-)
acute respiratory distress syndrome (J80)
cardiac arrhythmia (I47-I49.-)
pneumonia due to COVID-19 (J12.82)
severe sepsis (R65.2-)
viral cardiomyopathy (B33.24)
viral pericarditis (B33.23)
Use additional code, if applicable, for:
exposure to COVID-19 or SARS-C
personal history of COVID-19 (Z86.16)
post COVID-19 condition (U09.9)
Coding Clinic: 2021, Q4, P102; 2021, Q1, P36, 42

M35.89 **Other specified systemic involvement of connective tissue**

M35.9 **Systemic involvement of connective tissue, unspecified**
Autoimmune disease (systemic) NOS
Collagen (vascular) disease NOS

M36 **Systemic disorders of connective tissue in diseases classified elsewhere**
Excludes2 arthropathies in diseases classified elsewhere (M14.-)

M36.0 ***Dermato(poly)myositis in neoplastic disease*** PDX 1232
Code first underlying neoplasm (C00-D49)

M36.1 ***Arthropathy in neoplastic disease***
Code first underlying neoplasm, such as:
leukemia (C91-C95)
malignant histiocytosis (C96.A)
multiple myeloma (C90.0)

M36.2 ***Hemophilic arthropathy***
Hemarthrosis in hemophilic arthropathy
Code first underlying disease, such as:
factor VIII deficiency (D66)
with vascular defect (D68.0-)
factor IX deficiency (D67)
hemophilia (classical) (D66)
hemophilia B (D67)
hemophilia C (D68.1)

M36.3 ***Arthropathy in other blood disorders***

M36.4 ***Arthropathy in hypersensitivity reactions classified elsewhere***
Code first underlying disease, such as:
Henoch (-Schönlein) purpura (D69.0)
serum sickness (T80.6-)

M36.8 ***Systemic disorders of connective tissue in other diseases classified elsewhere***
Code first underlying disease, such as:
alkaptonuria (E70.29)
hypogammaglobulinemia (D80.-)
ochronosis (E70.29)

DORSOPATHIES (M40-M54)

DEFORMING DORSOPATHIES (M40-M43)

M40 **Kyphosis and lordosis**
Excludes1 congenital kyphosis and lordosis (Q76.4)
kyphoscoliosis (M41.-)
postprocedural kyphosis and lordosis (M96.-)
Code first underlying disease

M40.0 **Postural kyphosis**
Excludes1 osteochondrosis of spine (M42.-)
M40.00 **Postural kyphosis, site unspecified**
M40.03 **Postural kyphosis, cervicothoracic region**
M40.04 **Postural kyphosis, thoracic region**
M40.05 **Postural kyphosis, thoracolumbar region**

M40.1 **Other secondary kyphosis**
M40.10 **Other secondary kyphosis, site unspecified**
M40.12 **Other secondary kyphosis, cervical region**
M40.13 **Other secondary kyphosis, cervicothoracic region**
M40.14 **Other secondary kyphosis, thoracic region**
M40.15 **Other secondary kyphosis, thoracolumbar region**

M40.2 **Other and unspecified kyphosis**
M40.20 **Unspecified kyphosis**
M40.202 **Unspecified kyphosis, cervical region**
M40.203 **Unspecified kyphosis, cervicothoracic region**
M40.204 **Unspecified kyphosis, thoracic region**
M40.205 **Unspecified kyphosis, thoracolumbar region**
M40.209 **Unspecified kyphosis, site unspecified**
M40.29 **Other kyphosis**
M40.292 **Other kyphosis, cervical region**
M40.293 **Other kyphosis, cervicothoracic region**
M40.294 **Other kyphosis, thoracic region**
M40.295 **Other kyphosis, thoracolumbar region**
M40.299 **Other kyphosis, site unspecified**

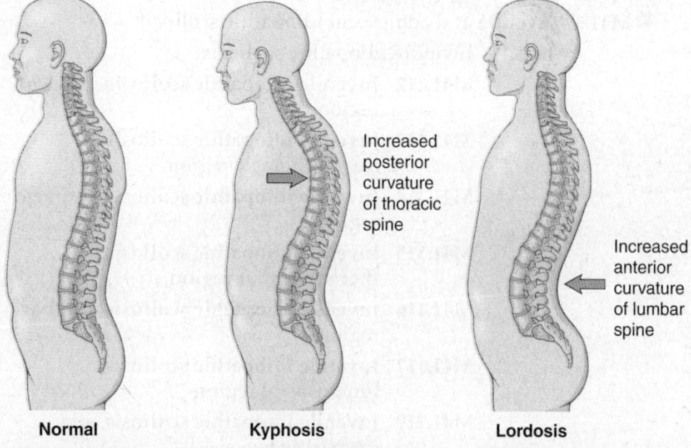

Figure 13-5 Kyphosis, Lordosis, Scoliosis. (From Chabner: The Language of Medicine, ed 8, St. Louis, Saunders, 2007)

Item 13-9 **Kyphosis** is an abnormal curvature of the spine. **Senile kyphosis** is a result of disc degeneration causing ossification (turning to bone). **Adolescent** or **juvenile** kyphosis is also known as **Scheuermann's disease,** a condition in which the discs of the lower thoracic spine herniate, causing the disc space to narrow and the spine to tilt forward. This condition is attributed to poor posture. **Lordosis or swayback** is an abnormal curvature of the spine resulting in an inward curve of the lumbar spine just above the buttocks. **Scoliosis** causes a sideways curve to the spine. The curves are S- or C-shaped, and it is most commonly acquired in late childhood and early teen years, when growth is fast.

● M40.3 Flatback syndrome
- M40.30 Flatback syndrome, site unspecified
- M40.35 Flatback syndrome, thoracolumbar region
- M40.36 Flatback syndrome, lumbar region
- M40.37 Flatback syndrome, lumbosacral region

● M40.4 Postural lordosis

Abnormal increase in the normal curvature of the lumbar spine (sway back)

Acquired lordosis
- M40.40 Postural lordosis, site unspecified
- M40.45 Postural lordosis, thoracolumbar region
- M40.46 Postural lordosis, lumbar region
- M40.47 Postural lordosis, lumbosacral region

● M40.5 Lordosis, unspecified
- M40.50 Lordosis, unspecified, site unspecified
- M40.55 Lordosis, unspecified, thoracolumbar region
- M40.56 Lordosis, unspecified, lumbar region
- M40.57 Lordosis, unspecified, lumbosacral region

● M41 Scoliosis

Includes kyphoscoliosis

Excludes1 congenital scoliosis NOS (Q67.5)
congenital scoliosis due to bony malformation (Q76.3)
postural congenital scoliosis (Q67.5)
kyphoscoliotic heart disease (I27.1)

Excludes2 postprocedural scoliosis (M96.89)
postradiation scoliosis (M96.5)

● M41.0 Infantile idiopathic scoliosis
- M41.00 Infantile idiopathic scoliosis, site unspecified
- M41.02 Infantile idiopathic scoliosis, cervical region
- M41.03 Infantile idiopathic scoliosis, cervicothoracic region
- M41.04 Infantile idiopathic scoliosis, thoracic region
- M41.05 Infantile idiopathic scoliosis, thoracolumbar region
- M41.06 Infantile idiopathic scoliosis, lumbar region
- M41.07 Infantile idiopathic scoliosis, lumbosacral region
- M41.08 Infantile idiopathic scoliosis, sacral and sacrococcygeal region

● M41.1 Juvenile and adolescent idiopathic scoliosis

● M41.11 Juvenile idiopathic scoliosis
- M41.112 Juvenile idiopathic scoliosis, cervical region
- M41.113 Juvenile idiopathic scoliosis, cervicothoracic region
- M41.114 Juvenile idiopathic scoliosis, thoracic region
- M41.115 Juvenile idiopathic scoliosis, thoracolumbar region
- M41.116 Juvenile idiopathic scoliosis, lumbar region
- M41.117 Juvenile idiopathic scoliosis, lumbosacral region
- M41.119 Juvenile idiopathic scoliosis, site unspecified

● M41.12 Adolescent idiopathic scoliosis
- M41.122 Adolescent idiopathic scoliosis, cervical region
- M41.123 Adolescent idiopathic scoliosis, cervicothoracic region
- M41.124 Adolescent idiopathic scoliosis, thoracic region
- M41.125 Adolescent idiopathic scoliosis, thoracolumbar region
  Coding Clinic: 2024, Q1, P23
- M41.126 Adolescent idiopathic scoliosis, lumbar region
- M41.127 Adolescent idiopathic scoliosis, lumbosacral region
- M41.129 Adolescent idiopathic scoliosis, site unspecified

● M41.2 Other idiopathic scoliosis
- M41.20 Other idiopathic scoliosis, site unspecified
- M41.22 Other idiopathic scoliosis, cervical region
- M41.23 Other idiopathic scoliosis, cervicothoracic region
- M41.24 Other idiopathic scoliosis, thoracic region
- M41.25 Other idiopathic scoliosis, thoracolumbar region
- M41.26 Other idiopathic scoliosis, lumbar region
- M41.27 Other idiopathic scoliosis, lumbosacral region

● M41.3 Thoracogenic scoliosis
- M41.30 Thoracogenic scoliosis, site unspecified
- M41.34 Thoracogenic scoliosis, thoracic region
- M41.35 Thoracogenic scoliosis, thoracolumbar region

● M41.4 Neuromuscular scoliosis

Scoliosis secondary to cerebral palsy, Friedreich's ataxia, poliomyelitis and other neuromuscular disorders

Code also underlying condition
- M41.40 Neuromuscular scoliosis, site unspecified
- M41.41 Neuromuscular scoliosis, occipito-atlanto-axial region
- M41.42 Neuromuscular scoliosis, cervical region
- M41.43 Neuromuscular scoliosis, cervicothoracic region
- M41.44 Neuromuscular scoliosis, thoracic region
- M41.45 Neuromuscular scoliosis, thoracolumbar region
- M41.46 Neuromuscular scoliosis, lumbar region
- M41.47 Neuromuscular scoliosis, lumbosacral region

● M41.5 Other secondary scoliosis

Coding Clinic: 2019, Q1, P19

Code first underlying disease
- ● M41.50 Other secondary scoliosis, site unspecified
- ● M41.52 Other secondary scoliosis, cervical region
- ● M41.53 Other secondary scoliosis, cervicothoracic region
- ● M41.54 Other secondary scoliosis, thoracic region
- ● M41.55 Other secondary scoliosis, thoracolumbar region
- ● M41.56 Other secondary scoliosis, lumbar region
- ● M41.57 Other secondary scoliosis, lumbosacral region

● M41.8 Other forms of scoliosis

Coding Clinic: 2022, Q1, P30
- M41.80 Other forms of scoliosis, site unspecified
- M41.82 Other forms of scoliosis, cervical region
- M41.83 Other forms of scoliosis, cervicothoracic region
- M41.84 Other forms of scoliosis, thoracic region
- M41.85 Other forms of scoliosis, thoracolumbar region
- M41.86 Other forms of scoliosis, lumbar region
- M41.87 Other forms of scoliosis, lumbosacral region

M41.9 Scoliosis, unspecified

Coding Clinic: 2022, Q1, P30

● M42 Spinal osteochondrosis

● M42.0 Juvenile osteochondrosis of spine

Calvé's disease

Scheuermann's disease

Excludes1 postural kyphosis (M40.0)
- M42.00 Juvenile osteochondrosis of spine, site unspecified
- M42.01 Juvenile osteochondrosis of spine, occipito-atlanto-axial region
- M42.02 Juvenile osteochondrosis of spine, cervical region
- M42.03 Juvenile osteochondrosis of spine, cervicothoracic region
- M42.04 Juvenile osteochondrosis of spine, thoracic region

M42.05 Juvenile osteochondrosis of spine, thoracolumbar region
M42.06 Juvenile osteochondrosis of spine, lumbar region
M42.07 Juvenile osteochondrosis of spine, lumbosacral region
M42.08 Juvenile osteochondrosis of spine, sacral and sacrococcygeal region
M42.09 Juvenile osteochondrosis of spine, multiple sites in spine

● M42.1 Adult osteochondrosis of spine
M42.10 Adult osteochondrosis of spine, site unspecified A
M42.11 Adult osteochondrosis of spine, occipitoatlanto-axial region A
M42.12 Adult osteochondrosis of spine, cervical region A
M42.13 Adult osteochondrosis of spine, cervicothoracic region A
M42.14 Adult osteochondrosis of spine, thoracic region A
M42.15 Adult osteochondrosis of spine, thoracolumbar region A
M42.16 Adult osteochondrosis of spine, lumbar region A
M42.17 Adult osteochondrosis of spine, lumbosacral region A
M42.18 Adult osteochondrosis of spine, sacral and sacrococcygeal region A
M42.19 Adult osteochondrosis of spine, multiple sites in spine A

M42.9 Spinal osteochondrosis, unspecified

● M43 Other deforming dorsopathies

Excludes1 congenital spondylolysis and spondylolisthesis (Q76.2)
hemivertebra (Q76.3-Q76.4)
Klippel-Feil syndrome (Q76.1)
lumbarization and sacralization (Q76.4)
platyspondylisis (Q76.4)
spina bifida occulta (Q76.0)
spinal curvature in osteoporosis (M80.-)
spinal curvature in Paget's disease of bone [osteitis deformans] (M88.-)

● M43.0 Spondylolysis

Excludes1 congenital spondylolysis (Q76.2)
spondylolisthesis (M43.1)

Coding Clinic: 2023, Q3, P20

M43.00 Spondylolysis, site unspecified
M43.01 Spondylolysis, occipito-atlanto-axial region
M43.02 Spondylolysis, cervical region
M43.03 Spondylolysis, cervicothoracic region
M43.04 Spondylolysis, thoracic region
M43.05 Spondylolysis, thoracolumbar region
M43.06 Spondylolysis, lumbar region
M43.07 Spondylolysis, lumbosacral region
M43.08 Spondylolysis, sacral and sacrococcygeal region
M43.09 Spondylolysis, multiple sites in spine

● M43.1 Spondylolisthesis

Excludes1 acute traumatic of lumbosacral region (S33.1)
acute traumatic of sites other than lumbosacral - code to Fracture, vertebra, by region
congenital spondylolisthesis (Q76.2)

Coding Clinic: 2023, Q3, P20

M43.10 Spondylolisthesis, site unspecified
M43.11 Spondylolisthesis, occipito-atlanto-axial region
M43.12 Spondylolisthesis, cervical region
M43.13 Spondylolisthesis, cervicothoracic region
M43.14 Spondylolisthesis, thoracic region
M43.15 Spondylolisthesis, thoracolumbar region
M43.16 Spondylolisthesis, lumbar region
Coding Clinic: 2024, Q1, P18
M43.17 Spondylolisthesis, lumbosacral region
Coding Clinic: 2023, Q3, P20
M43.18 Spondylolisthesis, sacral and sacrococcygeal region
M43.19 Spondylolisthesis, multiple sites in spine

● M43.2 Fusion of spine
Ankylosis of spinal joint

Excludes1 ankylosing spondylitis (M45.0-)
congenital fusion of spine (Q76.4)

Excludes2 arthrodesis status (Z98.1)
pseudoarthrosis after fusion or arthrodesis (M96.0)

M43.20 Fusion of spine, site unspecified
M43.21 Fusion of spine, occipito-atlanto-axial region
M43.22 Fusion of spine, cervical region
M43.23 Fusion of spine, cervicothoracic region
M43.24 Fusion of spine, thoracic region
M43.25 Fusion of spine, thoracolumbar region
M43.26 Fusion of spine, lumbar region
M43.27 Fusion of spine, lumbosacral region
M43.28 Fusion of spine, sacral and sacrococcygeal region

M43.3 Recurrent atlantoaxial dislocation with myelopathy
M43.4 Other recurrent atlantoaxial dislocation

● M43.5 Other recurrent vertebral dislocation

Excludes1 biomechanical lesions NEC (M99.-)

● M43.5X Other recurrent vertebral dislocation
M43.5X2 Other recurrent vertebral dislocation, cervical region
M43.5X3 Other recurrent vertebral dislocation, cervicothoracic region
M43.5X4 Other recurrent vertebral dislocation, thoracic region
M43.5X5 Other recurrent vertebral dislocation, thoracolumbar region
M43.5X6 Other recurrent vertebral dislocation, lumbar region
M43.5X7 Other recurrent vertebral dislocation, lumbosacral region
M43.5X8 Other recurrent vertebral dislocation, sacral and sacrococcygeal region
M43.5X9 Other recurrent vertebral dislocation, site unspecified

M43.6 Torticollis

Excludes1 congenital (sternomastoid) torticollis (Q68.0)
current injury - see Injury, of spine, by body region ocular torticollis (R29.891)
psychogenic torticollis (F45.8)
spasmodic torticollis (G24.3)
torticollis due to birth injury (P15.2)

● M43.8 Other specified deforming dorsopathies

Excludes2 kyphosis and lordosis (M40.-)
scoliosis (M41.-)

● M43.8X Other specified deforming dorsopathies
M43.8X1 Other specified deforming dorsopathies, occipito-atlanto-axial region
M43.8X2 Other specified deforming dorsopathies, cervical region
M43.8X3 Other specified deforming dorsopathies, cervicothoracic region
M43.8X4 Other specified deforming dorsopathies, thoracic region
M43.8X5 Other specified deforming dorsopathies, thoracolumbar region
M43.8X6 Other specified deforming dorsopathies, lumbar region
M43.8X7 Other specified deforming dorsopathies, lumbosacral region

Item 13–10 Spondylolisthesis is a condition caused by the slipping forward of one disc over another.

M43.8X8 Other specified deforming dorsopathies, sacral and sacrococcygeal region

M43.8X9 Other specified deforming dorsopathies, site unspecified

M43.9 Deforming dorsopathy, unspecified
Curvature of spine NOS

SPONDYLOPATHIES (M45-M49)

● M45 Ankylosing spondylitis
Rheumatoid arthritis of spine
Excludes1 arthropathy in Reiter's disease (M02.3-)
juvenile (ankylosing) spondylitis (M08.1)
Excludes2 Behçet's disease (M35.2)

M45.0 Ankylosing spondylitis of multiple sites in spine
M45.1 Ankylosing spondylitis of occipito-atlanto-axial region
M45.2 Ankylosing spondylitis of cervical region
M45.3 Ankylosing spondylitis of cervicothoracic region
M45.4 Ankylosing spondylitis of thoracic region
M45.5 Ankylosing spondylitis of thoracolumbar region
M45.6 Ankylosing spondylitis lumbar region
M45.7 Ankylosing spondylitis of lumbosacral region
M45.8 Ankylosing spondylitis sacral and sacrococcygeal region
M45.9 Ankylosing spondylitis of unspecified sites in spine

● M45.A Non-radiographic axial spondyloarthritis
M45.A0 Non-radiographic axial spondyloarthritis of unspecified sites in spine
M45.A1 Non-radiographic axial spondyloarthritis of occipito-atlanto-axial region
M45.A2 Non-radiographic axial spondyloarthritis of cervical region
M45.A3 Non-radiographic axial spondyloarthritis of cervicothoracic region
M45.A4 Non-radiographic axial spondyloarthritis of thoracic region
M45.A5 Non-radiographic axial spondyloarthritis of thoracolumbar region
M45.A6 Non-radiographic axial spondyloarthritis of lumbar region
M45.A7 Non-radiographic axial spondyloarthritis of lumbosacral region
M45.A8 Non-radiographic axial spondyloarthritis of sacral and sacrococcygeal region
M45.AB Non-radiographic axial spondyloarthritis of multiple sites in spine

● M46 Other inflammatory spondylopathies

● M46.0 Spinal enthesopathy
Disorder of ligamentous or muscular attachments of spine
M46.00 Spinal enthesopathy, site unspecified
M46.01 Spinal enthesopathy, occipito-atlanto-axial region
M46.02 Spinal enthesopathy, cervical region
M46.03 Spinal enthesopathy, cervicothoracic region
M46.04 Spinal enthesopathy, thoracic region
M46.05 Spinal enthesopathy, thoracolumbar region
M46.06 Spinal enthesopathy, lumbar region
M46.07 Spinal enthesopathy, lumbosacral region
M46.08 Spinal enthesopathy, sacral and sacrococcygeal region
M46.09 Spinal enthesopathy, multiple sites in spine

M46.1 Sacroiliitis, not elsewhere classified

● M46.2 Osteomyelitis of vertebra (Ex) PDX 1242
M46.20 Osteomyelitis of vertebra, site unspecified
M46.21 Osteomyelitis of vertebra, occipito-atlanto-axial region
M46.22 Osteomyelitis of vertebra, cervical region
M46.23 Osteomyelitis of vertebra, cervicothoracic region
M46.24 Osteomyelitis of vertebra, thoracic region
M46.25 Osteomyelitis of vertebra, thoracolumbar region
M46.26 Osteomyelitis of vertebra, lumbar region
M46.27 Osteomyelitis of vertebra, lumbosacral region
M46.28 Osteomyelitis of vertebra, sacral and sacrococcygeal region

● M46.3 Infection of intervertebral disc (pyogenic) (Ex) PDX 1243
Use additional code (B95-B97) to identify infectious agent
M46.30 Infection of intervertebral disc (pyogenic), site unspecified
M46.31 Infection of intervertebral disc (pyogenic), occipito-atlanto-axial region
M46.32 Infection of intervertebral disc (pyogenic), cervical region
M46.33 Infection of intervertebral disc (pyogenic), cervicothoracic region
M46.34 Infection of intervertebral disc (pyogenic), thoracic region
M46.35 Infection of intervertebral disc (pyogenic), thoracolumbar region
M46.36 Infection of intervertebral disc (pyogenic), lumbar region
M46.37 Infection of intervertebral disc (pyogenic), lumbosacral region
M46.38 Infection of intervertebral disc (pyogenic), sacral and sacrococcygeal region
M46.39 Infection of intervertebral disc (pyogenic), multiple sites in spine

● M46.4 Discitis, unspecified
M46.40 Discitis, unspecified, site unspecified
M46.41 Discitis, unspecified, occipito-atlanto-axial region
M46.42 Discitis, unspecified, cervical region
M46.43 Discitis, unspecified, cervicothoracic region
M46.44 Discitis, unspecified, thoracic region
M46.45 Discitis, unspecified, thoracolumbar region
M46.46 Discitis, unspecified, lumbar region
M46.47 Discitis, unspecified, lumbosacral region
M46.48 Discitis, unspecified, sacral and sacrococcygeal region
M46.49 Discitis, unspecified, multiple sites in spine

● M46.5 Other infective spondylopathies
M46.50 Other infective spondylopathies, site unspecified
M46.51 Other infective spondylopathies, occipitoatlanto-axial region
M46.52 Other infective spondylopathies, cervical region
M46.53 Other infective spondylopathies, cervicothoracic region
M46.54 Other infective spondylopathies, thoracic region
M46.55 Other infective spondylopathies, thoracolumbar region
M46.56 Other infective spondylopathies, lumbar region
M46.57 Other infective spondylopathies, lumbosacral region
M46.58 Other infective spondylopathies, sacral and sacrococcygeal region
M46.59 Other infective spondylopathies, multiple sites in spine

● M46.8 Other specified inflammatory spondylopathies
M46.80 Other specified inflammatory spondylopathies, site unspecified
M46.81 Other specified inflammatory spondylopathies, occipito-atlanto-axial region

CHAPTER 13 (M00-M99)

M46.82 Other specified inflammatory spondylopathies, cervical region
M46.83 Other specified inflammatory spondylopathies, cervicothoracic region
M46.84 Other specified inflammatory spondylopathies, thoracic region
M46.85 Other specified inflammatory spondylopathies, thoracolumbar region
M46.86 Other specified inflammatory spondylopathies, lumbar region
M46.87 Other specified inflammatory spondylopathies, lumbosacral region
M46.88 Other specified inflammatory spondylopathies, sacral and sacrococcygeal region
M46.89 Other specified inflammatory spondylopathies, multiple sites in spine

M46.9 Unspecified inflammatory spondylopathy
M46.90 Unspecified inflammatory spondylopathy, site unspecified
M46.91 Unspecified inflammatory spondylopathy, occipito-atlanto-axial region
M46.92 Unspecified inflammatory spondylopathy, cervical region
Coding Clinic: 2019, Q3, P10
M46.93 Unspecified inflammatory spondylopathy, cervicothoracic region
M46.94 Unspecified inflammatory spondylopathy, thoracic region
M46.95 Unspecified inflammatory spondylopathy, thoracolumbar region
M46.96 Unspecified inflammatory spondylopathy, lumbar region
M46.97 Unspecified inflammatory spondylopathy, lumbosacral region
M46.98 Unspecified inflammatory spondylopathy, sacral and sacrococcygeal region
M46.99 Unspecified inflammatory spondylopathy, multiple sites in spine

M47 Spondylosis

Includes arthrosis or osteoarthritis of spine
degeneration of facet joints

M47.0 Anterior spinal and vertebral artery compression syndromes (Ex) PDX 1244
Coding Clinic: 2019, Q3, P10
M47.01 Anterior spinal artery compression syndromes
M47.011 Anterior spinal artery compression syndromes, occipito-atlanto-axial region
M47.012 Anterior spinal artery compression syndromes, cervical region
Coding Clinic: 2023, Q1, P37
M47.013 Anterior spinal artery compression syndromes, cervicothoracic region
M47.014 Anterior spinal artery compression syndromes, thoracic region
M47.015 Anterior spinal artery compression syndromes, thoracolumbar region
M47.016 Anterior spinal artery compression syndromes, lumbar region
M47.019 Anterior spinal artery compression syndromes, site unspecified
M47.02 Vertebral artery compression syndromes
M47.021 Vertebral artery compression syndromes, occipito-atlanto-axial region
M47.022 Vertebral artery compression syndromes, cervical region
Coding Clinic: 2023, Q1, P37
M47.029 Vertebral artery compression syndromes, site unspecified

M47.1 Other spondylosis with myelopathy
Spondylogenic compression of spinal cord
Excludes1 vertebral subluxation (M43.3-M43.5X9)
M47.10 Other spondylosis with myelopathy, site unspecified (Ex) PDX 1245
M47.11 Other spondylosis with myelopathy, occipito-atlanto-axial region (Ex) PDX 1244
M47.12 Other spondylosis with myelopathy, cervical region (Ex) PDX 1244
Coding Clinic: 2020, Q1, P17
M47.13 Other spondylosis with myelopathy, cervicothoracic region (Ex) PDX 1244
M47.14 Other spondylosis with myelopathy, thoracic region (Ex) PDX 1246
M47.15 Other spondylosis with myelopathy, thoracolumbar region (Ex) PDX 1246
M47.16 Other spondylosis with myelopathy, lumbar region (Ex) PDX 1247

M47.2 Other spondylosis with radiculopathy
M47.20 Other spondylosis with radiculopathy, site unspecified
M47.21 Other spondylosis with radiculopathy, occipito-atlanto-axial region
M47.22 Other spondylosis with radiculopathy, cervical region
Coding Clinic: 2020, Q1, P17
M47.23 Other spondylosis with radiculopathy, cervicothoracic region
M47.24 Other spondylosis with radiculopathy, thoracic region
M47.25 Other spondylosis with radiculopathy, thoracolumbar region
M47.26 Other spondylosis with radiculopathy, lumbar region
M47.27 Other spondylosis with radiculopathy, lumbosacral region
M47.28 Other spondylosis with radiculopathy, sacral and sacrococcygeal region

M47.8 Other spondylosis
M47.81 Spondylosis without myelopathy or radiculopathy
M47.811 Spondylosis without myelopathy or radiculopathy, occipito-atlanto-axial region
M47.812 Spondylosis without myelopathy or radiculopathy, cervical region
Coding Clinic: 2019, Q3, P10-11; 2018, Q2, P15
M47.813 Spondylosis without myelopathy or radiculopathy, cervicothoracic region
M47.814 Spondylosis without myelopathy or radiculopathy, thoracic region
M47.815 Spondylosis without myelopathy or radiculopathy, thoracolumbar region
M47.816 Spondylosis without myelopathy or radiculopathy, lumbar region
M47.817 Spondylosis without myelopathy or radiculopathy, lumbosacral region
M47.818 Spondylosis without myelopathy or radiculopathy, sacral and sacrococcygeal region
M47.819 Spondylosis without myelopathy or radiculopathy, site unspecified
M47.89 Other spondylosis
M47.891 Other spondylosis, occipito-atlanto-axial region
M47.892 Other spondylosis, cervical region
M47.893 Other spondylosis, cervicothoracic region
M47.894 Other spondylosis, thoracic region

M47.895 Other spondylosis, thoracolumbar region
M47.896 Other spondylosis, lumbar region
M47.897 Other spondylosis, lumbosacral region
M47.898 Other spondylosis, sacral and sacrococcygeal region
M47.899 Other spondylosis, site unspecified
M47.9 Spondylosis, unspecified

● M48 Other spondylopathies
● M48.0 Spinal stenosis
Caudal stenosis
M48.00 Spinal stenosis, site unspecified
M48.01 Spinal stenosis, occipito-atlanto-axial region
M48.02 Spinal stenosis, cervical region
Coding Clinic: 2020, Q1, P17
M48.03 Spinal stenosis, cervicothoracic region
M48.04 Spinal stenosis, thoracic region
M48.05 Spinal stenosis, thoracolumbar region
● M48.06 Spinal stenosis, lumbar region
Coding Clinic: 2017, Q3, P24
M48.061 Spinal stenosis, lumbar region without neurogenic claudication
Spinal stenosis, lumbar region NOS
M48.062 Spinal stenosis, lumbar region with neurogenic claudication
Coding Clinic: 2017, Q4, P19
M48.07 Spinal stenosis, lumbosacral region
M48.08 Spinal stenosis, sacral and sacrococcygeal region
● M48.1 Ankylosing hyperostosis [Forestier]
Diffuse idiopathic skeletal hyperostosis [DISH]
M48.10 Ankylosing hyperostosis [Forestier], site unspecified
M48.11 Ankylosing hyperostosis [Forestier], occipito-atlanto-axial region
M48.12 Ankylosing hyperostosis [Forestier], cervical region
M48.13 Ankylosing hyperostosis [Forestier], cervicothoracic region
M48.14 Ankylosing hyperostosis [Forestier], thoracic region
M48.15 Ankylosing hyperostosis [Forestier], thoracolumbar region
M48.16 Ankylosing hyperostosis [Forestier], lumbar region
M48.17 Ankylosing hyperostosis [Forestier], lumbosacral region
M48.18 Ankylosing hyperostosis [Forestier], sacral and sacrococcygeal region
M48.19 Ankylosing hyperostosis [Forestier], multiple sites in spine
● M48.2 Kissing spine
M48.20 Kissing spine, site unspecified
M48.21 Kissing spine, occipito-atlanto-axial region
M48.22 Kissing spine, cervical region
M48.23 Kissing spine, cervicothoracic region
M48.24 Kissing spine, thoracic region
M48.25 Kissing spine, thoracolumbar region
M48.26 Kissing spine, lumbar region
M48.27 Kissing spine, lumbosacral region
● M48.3 Traumatic spondylopathy Ex PDX 1248
M48.30 Traumatic spondylopathy, site unspecified
M48.31 Traumatic spondylopathy, occipito-atlanto-axial region
M48.32 Traumatic spondylopathy, cervical region
M48.33 Traumatic spondylopathy, cervicothoracic region
M48.34 Traumatic spondylopathy, thoracic region
M48.35 Traumatic spondylopathy, thoracolumbar region
M48.36 Traumatic spondylopathy, lumbar region
M48.37 Traumatic spondylopathy, lumbosacral region
M48.38 Traumatic spondylopathy, sacral and sacrococcygeal region
● M48.4 Fatigue fracture of vertebra
Stress fracture of vertebra
Excludes1 pathological fracture NOS (M84.4-)
pathological fracture of vertebra due to neoplasm (M84.58)
pathological fracture of vertebra due to other diagnosis (M84.68)
pathological fracture of vertebra due to osteoporosis (M80.-)
traumatic fracture of vertebrae (S12.0-S12.3-, S22.0-, S32.0-)

The appropriate 7th character is to be added to each code from subcategory M48.4:

A	initial encounter for fracture
D	subsequent encounter for fracture with routine healing
G	subsequent encounter for fracture with delayed healing
S	sequela of fracture

X● M48.40 Fatigue fracture of vertebra, site unspecified
X● M48.41 Fatigue fracture of vertebra, occipitoatlanto-axial region
X● M48.42 Fatigue fracture of vertebra, cervical region
X● M48.43 Fatigue fracture of vertebra, cervicothoracic region
X● M48.44 Fatigue fracture of vertebra, thoracic region
X● M48.45 Fatigue fracture of vertebra, thoracolumbar region
X● M48.46 Fatigue fracture of vertebra, lumbar region
X● M48.47 Fatigue fracture of vertebra, lumbosacral region
X● M48.48 Fatigue fracture of vertebra, sacral and sacrococcygeal region
● M48.5 Collapsed vertebra, not elsewhere classified Ex PDX 1249
Collapsed vertebra NOS
Compression fracture of vertebra NOS
Wedging of vertebra NOS
Excludes1 current injury - see Injury of spine, by body region
fatigue fracture of vertebra (M48.4)
pathological fracture of vertebra due to neoplasm (M84.58)
pathological fracture of vertebra due to other diagnosis (M84.68)
pathological fracture of vertebra due to osteoporosis (M80.-)
pathological fracture NOS (M84.4-)
stress fracture of vertebra (M48.4-)
traumatic fracture of vertebra (S12.-, S22.-, S32.-)

The appropriate 7th character is to be added to each code from subcategory M48.5:

A	initial encounter for fracture
D	subsequent encounter for fracture with routine healing
G	subsequent encounter for fracture with delayed healing
S	sequela of fracture

X● M48.50 Collapsed vertebra, not elsewhere classified, site unspecified A, A
X● M48.51 Collapsed vertebra, not elsewhere classified, occipito-atlanto-axial region A, A
X● M48.52 Collapsed vertebra, not elsewhere classified, cervical region A, A

CHAPTER 13 (M00-M99)

X● M48.53 Collapsed vertebra, not elsewhere classified, cervicothoracic region A, A

X● M48.54 Collapsed vertebra, not elsewhere classified, thoracic region A, A

X● M48.55 Collapsed vertebra, not elsewhere classified, thoracolumbar region A, A

X● M48.56 Collapsed vertebra, not elsewhere classified, lumbar region A, A

X● M48.57 Collapsed vertebra, not elsewhere classified, lumbosacral region A, A

X● M48.58 Collapsed vertebra, not elsewhere classified, sacral and sacrococcygeal region A, A

● **M48.8 Other specified spondylopathies**

Ossification of posterior longitudinal ligament

● **M48.8X Other specified spondylopathies**

M48.8X1 Other specified spondylopathies, occipito-atlanto-axial region

M48.8X2 Other specified spondylopathies, cervical region

M48.8X3 Other specified spondylopathies, cervicothoracic region

M48.8X4 Other specified spondylopathies, thoracic region

M48.8X5 Other specified spondylopathies, thoracolumbar region

M48.8X6 Other specified spondylopathies, lumbar region

M48.8X7 Other specified spondylopathies, lumbosacral region

M48.8X8 Other specified spondylopathies, sacral and sacrococcygeal region

M48.8X9 Other specified spondylopathies, site unspecified

M48.9 Spondylopathy, unspecified

● **M49 Spondylopathies in diseases classified elsewhere**

Includes curvature of spine in diseases classified elsewhere
deformity of spine in diseases classified elsewhere
kyphosis in diseases classified elsewhere
scoliosis in diseases classified elsewhere
spondylopathy in diseases classified elsewhere

Code first underlying disease, such as:
brucellosis (A23.-)
Charcot-Marie-Tooth disease (G60.0)
enterobacterial infections (A01-A04)
osteitis fibrosa cystica (E21.0)

Excludes1 curvature of spine in tuberculosis [Pott's] (A18.01)
enteropathic arthropathies (M07.-)
gonococcal spondylitis (A54.41)
neuropathic [tabes dorsalis] spondylitis (A52.11)
neuropathic spondylopathy in syringomyelia (G95.0)
neuropathic spondylopathy in tabes dorsalis (A52.11)
nonsyphilitic neuropathic spondylopathy NEC (G98.0)
spondylitis in syphilis (acquired) (A52.77)
tuberculous spondylitis (A18.01)
typhoid fever spondylitis (A01.05)

● **M49.8 Spondylopathy in diseases classified elsewhere**

M49.80 Spondylopathy in diseases classified elsewhere, site unspecified

M49.81 Spondylopathy in diseases classified elsewhere, occipito-atlanto-axial region

M49.82 Spondylopathy in diseases classified elsewhere, cervical region

M49.83 Spondylopathy in diseases classified elsewhere, cervicothoracic region

M49.84 Spondylopathy in diseases classified elsewhere, thoracic region

M49.85 Spondylopathy in diseases classified elsewhere, thoracolumbar region

M49.86 Spondylopathy in diseases classified elsewhere, lumbar region

M49.87 Spondylopathy in diseases classified elsewhere, lumbosacral region

M49.88 Spondylopathy in diseases classified elsewhere, sacral and sacrococcygeal region

M49.89 Spondylopathy in diseases classified elsewhere, multiple sites in spine

OTHER DORSOPATHIES (M50-M54)

Excludes1 current injury - see injury of spine by body region
discitis NOS (M46.4-)

● **M50 Cervical disc disorders**

Includes cervicothoracic disc disorders with cervicalgia
cervicothoracic disc disorders

Coding Clinic: 2016, Q1, P17

● **M50.0 Cervical disc disorder with myelopathy** (Ex) PDX 1250

M50.00 Cervical disc disorder with myelopathy, unspecified cervical region

M50.01 Cervical disc disorder with myelopathy, high cervical region

C2-C3 disc disorder with myelopathy
C3-C4 disc disorder with myelopathy

Coding Clinic: 2016, Q1, P17

● **M50.02 Cervical disc disorder with myelopathy, mid-cervical region**

Coding Clinic: 2016, Q4, P39-40

M50.020 Cervical disc disorder with myelopathy, mid-cervical region, unspecified level

M50.021 Cervical disc disorder at C4-C5 level with myelopathy

C4-C5 disc disorder with myelopathy

M50.022 Cervical disc disorder at C5-C6 level with myelopathy

C5-C6 disc disorder with myelopathy

M50.023 Cervical disc disorder at C6-C7 level with myelopathy

C6-C7 disc disorder with myelopathy

M50.03 Cervical disc disorder with myelopathy, cervicothoracic region

C7-T1 disc disorder with myelopathy

● **M50.1 Cervical disc disorder with radiculopathy**

Excludes2 brachial radiculitis NOS (M54.13)

M50.10 Cervical disc disorder with radiculopathy, unspecified cervical region

M50.11 Cervical disc disorder with radiculopathy, high cervical region

C2-C3 disc disorder with radiculopathy
C3 radiculopathy due to disc disorder
C3-C4 disc disorder with radiculopathy
C4 radiculopathy due to disc disorder

● **M50.12 Cervical disc disorder with radiculopathy, mid-cervical region**

Coding Clinic: 2016, Q4, P39-40

M50.120 Mid-cervical disc disorder, unspecified level

M50.121 Cervical disc disorder at C4-C5 level with radiculopathy

C4-C5 disc disorder with radiculopathy
C5 radiculopathy due to disc disorder

M50.122 Cervical disc disorder at C5-C6 level with radiculopathy

C5-C6 disc disorder with radiculopathy
C6 radiculopathy due to disc disorder

M50.123 Cervical disc disorder at C6-C7 level with radiculopathy
C6-C7 disc disorder with radiculopathy
C7 radiculopathy due to disc disorder

M50.13 Cervical disc disorder with radiculopathy, cervicothoracic region
C7-T1 disc disorder with radiculopathy
C8 radiculopathy due to disc disorder

● M50.2 Other cervical disc displacement
Coding Clinic: 2016, Q4, P40

M50.20 Other cervical disc displacement, unspecified cervical region

M50.21 Other cervical disc displacement, high cervical region
Other C2-C3 cervical disc displacement
Other C3-C4 cervical disc displacement
Coding Clinic: 2021, Q4, P12

● M50.22 Other cervical disc displacement, mid-cervical region

M50.220 Other cervical disc displacement, mid-cervical region, unspecified level

M50.221 Other cervical disc displacement at C4-C5 level
Other C4-C5 cervical disc displacement

M50.222 Other cervical disc displacement at C5-C6 level
Other C5-C6 cervical disc displacement

M50.223 Other cervical disc displacement at C6-C7 level
Other C6-C7 cervical disc displacement

M50.23 Other cervical disc displacement, cervicothoracic region
Other C7-T1 cervical disc displacement

● M50.3 Other cervical disc degeneration
Coding Clinic: 2016, Q4, P40

M50.30 Other cervical disc degeneration, unspecified cervical region

M50.31 Other cervical disc degeneration, high cervical region
Other C2-C3 cervical disc degeneration
Other C3-C4 cervical disc degeneration

● M50.32 Other cervical disc degeneration, mid-cervical region

M50.320 Other cervical disc degeneration, mid-cervical region, unspecified level

M50.321 Other cervical disc degeneration at C4-C5 level
Other C4-C5 cervical disc degeneration

M50.322 Other cervical disc degeneration at C5-C6 level
Other C5-C6 cervical disc degeneration

M50.323 Other cervical disc degeneration at C6-C7 level
Other C6-C7 cervical disc degeneration

M50.33 Other cervical disc degeneration, cervicothoracic region
Other C7-T1 cervical disc degeneration

● M50.8 Other cervical disc disorders
Coding Clinic: 2016, Q4, P40

M50.80 Other cervical disc disorders, unspecified cervical region

M50.81 Other cervical disc disorders, high cervical region
Other C2-C3 cervical disc disorders
Other C3-C4 cervical disc disorders

● M50.82 Other cervical disc disorders, mid-cervical region

M50.820 Other cervical disc disorders, mid-cervical region, unspecified level

M50.821 Other cervical disc disorders at C4-C5 level
Other C4-C5 cervical disc disorders

M50.822 Other cervical disc disorders at C5-C6 level
Other C5-C6 cervical disc disorders

M50.823 Other cervical disc disorders at C6-C7 level
Other C6-C7 cervical disc disorders

M50.83 Other cervical disc disorders, cervicothoracic region
Other C7-T1 cervical disc disorders

● M50.9 Cervical disc disorder, unspecified
Coding Clinic: 2016, Q4, P40

M50.90 Cervical disc disorder, unspecified, unspecified cervical region

M50.91 Cervical disc disorder, unspecified, high cervical region
C2-C3 cervical disc disorder, unspecified
C3-C4 cervical disc disorder, unspecified

● M50.92 Cervical disc disorder, unspecified, mid-cervical region

M50.920 Unspecified cervical disc disorder, mid-cervical region, unspecified level

M50.921 Unspecified cervical disc disorder at C4-C5 level
Unspecified C4-C5 cervical disc disorder

M50.922 Unspecified cervical disc disorder at C5-C6 level
Unspecified C5-C6 cervical disc disorder

M50.923 Unspecified cervical disc disorder at C6-C7 level
Unspecified C6-C7 cervical disc disorder

M50.93 Cervical disc disorder, unspecified, cervicothoracic region
C7-T1 cervical disc disorder, unspecified

● M51 Thoracic, thoracolumbar, and lumbosacral intervertebral disc disorders

Excludes2 cervical and cervicothoracic disc disorders (M50.-)
sacral and sacrococcygeal disorders (M53.3)

● M51.0 Thoracic, thoracolumbar and lumbosacral intervertebral disc disorders with myelopathy

M51.04 Intervertebral disc disorders with myelopathy, thoracic region (Ex) PDX 1251

M51.05 Intervertebral disc disorders with myelopathy, thoracolumbar region (Ex) PDX 1251

M51.06 Intervertebral disc disorders with myelopathy, lumbar region (Ex) PDX 1252

● M51.1 Thoracic, thoracolumbar and lumbosacral intervertebral disc disorders with radiculopathy
Sciatica due to intervertebral disc disorder

Excludes1 lumbar radiculitis NOS (M54.16)
sciatica NOS (M54.3)

M51.14 Intervertebral disc disorders with radiculopathy, thoracic region

M51.15 Intervertebral disc disorders with radiculopathy, thoracolumbar region

M51.16 Intervertebral disc disorders with radiculopathy, lumbar region

M51.17 Intervertebral disc disorders with radiculopathy, lumbosacral region

● **M51.2 Other thoracic, thoracolumbar and lumbosacral intervertebral disc displacement**
Lumbago due to displacement of intervertebral disc
M51.24 Other intervertebral disc displacement, thoracic region
M51.25 Other intervertebral disc displacement, thoracolumbar region
M51.26 Other intervertebral disc displacement, lumbar region
M51.27 Other intervertebral disc displacement, lumbosacral region

● **M51.3 Other thoracic, thoracolumbar and lumbosacral intervertebral disc degeneration**
Coding Clinic: 2013, Q3, P22
M51.34 Other intervertebral disc degeneration, thoracic region
M51.35 Other intervertebral disc degeneration, thoracolumbar region
M51.36 Other intervertebral disc degeneration, lumbar region
Coding Clinic: 2018, Q2, P15
▶**M51.360 Other intervertebral disc degeneration, lumbar region with discogenic back pain only**
▶Other intervertebral disc degeneration, lumbar region with axial back pain only
▶**M51.361 Other intervertebral disc degeneration, lumbar region with lower extremity pain only**
▶Other intervertebral disc degeneration, lumbar region with leg pain only
▶Other intervertebral disc degeneration, lumbar region with referred sclerotomal pain only
▶**M51.362 Other intervertebral disc degeneration, lumbar region with discogenicback pain and lower extremity pain**
▶Other intervertebral disc degeneration, lumbar region with discogenic back pain and leg pain
▶Other intervertebral disc degeneration, lumbar region with axial back pain and referred sclerotomal pain
▶**M51.369 Other intervertebral disc degeneration, lumbar region without mention of lumbar back pain or lower extremity pain**
▶Other intervertebral disc degeneration, lumbar region without mention of lumbar back pain or leg pain
▶Other intervertebral disc degeneration, lumbar region, NOS
M51.37 Other intervertebral disc degeneration, lumbosacral region
Coding Clinic: 2022, Q1, P26
▶**M51.370 Other intervertebral disc degeneration, lumbosacral region with discogenic back pain only**
▶Other intervertebral disc degeneration, lumbosacral region with axial back pain only
▶**M51.371 Other intervertebral disc degeneration, lumbosacral region with lower extremity pain only**
▶Other intervertebral disc degeneration, lumbosacral region with leg pain only
▶Other intervertebral disc degeneration, lumbosacral region with referred sclerotomal pain only
▶**M51.372 Other intervertebral disc degeneration, lumbosacral region with discogenic back pain and lower extremity pain**
▶Other intervertebral disc degeneration, lumbosacral region with discogenic backpain and leg pain
▶Other intervertebral disc degeneration, lumbosacral region with axial back pain and referred sclerotomal pain
▶**M51.379 Other intervertebral disc degeneration, lumbosacral region without mention of lumbar back pain or lower extremity pain**
▶Other intervertebral disc degeneration, lumbosacral region without mention of lumbar back pain or leg pain
▶Other intervertebral disc degeneration, lumbosacral region, NOS

● **M51.4 Schmorl's nodes**
M51.44 Schmorl's nodes, thoracic region
M51.45 Schmorl's nodes, thoracolumbar region
M51.46 Schmorl's nodes, lumbar region
M51.47 Schmorl's nodes, lumbosacral region

● **M51.8 Other thoracic, thoracolumbar and lumbosacral intervertebral disc disorders**
M51.84 Other intervertebral disc disorders, thoracic region
M51.85 Other intervertebral disc disorders, thoracolumbar region
M51.86 Other intervertebral disc disorders, lumbar region
M51.87 Other intervertebral disc disorders, lumbosacral region

M51.9 Unspecified thoracic, thoracolumbar and lumbosacral intervertebral disc disorder

● **M51.A Other lumbar and lumbosacral annulus fibrosus disc defects**
M51.A0 Intervertebral annulus fibrosus defect, lumbar region, unspecified size
Code first, if applicable, lumbar disc herniation (M51.06, M51.16, M51.26)
M51.A1 Intervertebral annulus fibrosus defect, small, lumbar region
Code first, if applicable, lumbar disc herniation (M51.06, M51.16, M51.26)
M51.A2 Intervertebral annulus fibrosus defect, large, lumbar region
Code first, if applicable, lumbar disc herniation (M51.06, M51.16, M51.26)
M51.A3 Intervertebral annulus fibrosus defect, lumbosacral region, unspecified size
Code first, if applicable, lumbosacral disc herniation (M51.17, M51.27)

CHAPTER 13 (M00-M99)

M51.A4 **Intervertebral annulus fibrosus defect, small, lumbosacral region**
Code first, if applicable, lumbosacral disc herniation (M51.17, M51.27)

M51.A5 **Intervertebral annulus fibrosus defect, large, lumbosacral region**
Code first, if applicable, lumbosacral disc herniation (M51.17, M51.27)

● **M53 Other and unspecified dorsopathies, not elsewhere classified**

M53.0 Cervicocranial syndrome
Posterior cervical sympathetic syndrome

M53.1 Cervicobrachial syndrome
Excludes2 cervical disc disorder (M50.-)
thoracic outlet syndrome (G54.0)

● **M53.2 Spinal instabilities**

● **M53.2X Spinal instabilities**

M53.2X1 **Spinal instabilities, occipito-atlanto-axial region**
M53.2X2 **Spinal instabilities, cervical region**
M53.2X3 **Spinal instabilities, cervicothoracic region**
M53.2X4 **Spinal instabilities, thoracic region**
M53.2X5 **Spinal instabilities, thoracolumbar region**
M53.2X6 **Spinal instabilities, lumbar region**
M53.2X7 **Spinal instabilities, lumbosacral region**
M53.2X8 **Spinal instabilities, sacral and sacrococcygeal region**
M53.2X9 **Spinal instabilities, site unspecified**

M53.3 Sacrococcygeal disorders, not elsewhere classified
Coccygodynia

● **M53.8 Other specified dorsopathies**

M53.80 **Other specified dorsopathies, site unspecified**
M53.81 **Other specified dorsopathies, occipito-atlanto-axial region**
M53.82 **Other specified dorsopathies, cervical region**
M53.83 **Other specified dorsopathies, cervicothoracic region**
M53.84 **Other specified dorsopathies, thoracic region**
M53.85 **Other specified dorsopathies, thoracolumbar region**
M53.86 **Other specified dorsopathies, lumbar region**
M53.87 **Other specified dorsopathies, lumbosacral region**
M53.88 **Other specified dorsopathies, sacral and sacrococcygeal region**

M53.9 Dorsopathy, unspecified

● **M54 Dorsalgia**
Excludes1 psychogenic dorsalgia (F45.41)

● **M54.0 Panniculitis affecting regions of neck and back**
Excludes1 lupus panniculitis (L93.2)
panniculitis NOS (M79.3)
relapsing [Weber-Christian] panniculitis (M35.6)

M54.00 **Panniculitis affecting regions of neck and back, site unspecified**
M54.01 **Panniculitis affecting regions of neck and back, occipito-atlanto-axial region**
M54.02 **Panniculitis affecting regions of neck and back, cervical region**
M54.03 **Panniculitis affecting regions of neck and back, cervicothoracic region**
M54.04 **Panniculitis affecting regions of neck and back, thoracic region**
M54.05 **Panniculitis affecting regions of neck and back, thoracolumbar region**
M54.06 **Panniculitis affecting regions of neck and back, lumbar region**
M54.07 **Panniculitis affecting regions of neck and back, lumbosacral region**
M54.08 **Panniculitis affecting regions of neck and back, sacral and sacrococcygeal region**
M54.09 **Panniculitis affecting regions, neck and back, multiple sites in spine**

● **M54.1 Radiculopathy**
Brachial neuritis or radiculitis NOS
Lumbar neuritis or radiculitis NOS
Lumbosacral neuritis or radiculitis NOS
Thoracic neuritis or radiculitis NOS
Radiculitis NOS
Excludes1 neuralgia and neuritis NOS (M79.2)
radiculopathy with cervical disc disorder (M50.1)
radiculopathy with lumbar and other intervertebral disc disorder (M51.1-)
radiculopathy with spondylosis (M47.2-)

M54.10 **Radiculopathy, site unspecified**
M54.11 **Radiculopathy, occipito-atlanto-axial region**
M54.12 **Radiculopathy, cervical region**
M54.13 **Radiculopathy, cervicothoracic region**
M54.14 **Radiculopathy, thoracic region**
M54.15 **Radiculopathy, thoracolumbar region**
M54.16 **Radiculopathy, lumbar region**
M54.17 **Radiculopathy, lumbosacral region**
M54.18 **Radiculopathy, sacral and sacrococcygeal region**

M54.2 Cervicalgia
Excludes1 cervicalgia due to intervertebral cervical disc disorder (M50.-)

● **M54.3 Sciatica**
▶ **Excludes1** intervertebral disc degeneration, lumbar region with lower extremity pain only (M51.361)
▶intervertebral disc degeneration, lumbosacral region with lower extremity pain only (M51.371)
lesion of sciatic nerve (G57.0)
sciatica due to intervertebral disc disorder (M51.1-)
sciatica with lumbago (M54.4-)

M54.30 **Sciatica, unspecified side**
M54.31 **Sciatica, right side**
M54.32 **Sciatica, left side**

● **M54.4 Lumbago with sciatica**
▶ **Excludes1** intervertebral disc degeneration, lumbar region with discogenic back pain and lower extremity pain (M51.362)
▶intervertebral disc degeneration, lumbosacral region with discogenic back pain and lower extremity pain (M51.372)
lumbago with sciatica due to intervertebral disc disorder (M51.1-)

M54.40 **Lumbago with sciatica, unspecified side**
M54.41 **Lumbago with sciatica, right side**
M54.42 **Lumbago with sciatica, left side**
Coding Clinic: 2016, Q2, P7

● **M54.5 Low back pain**
▶ **Excludes1** intervertebral disc degeneration, lumbar region with discogenic back pain only (M51.360)
▶intervertebral disc degeneration, lumbosacral region with discogenic back pain only (M51.370)
low back strain (S39.012)
lumbago due to intervertebral disc displacement (M51.2-)
lumbago with sciatica (M54.4-)

M54.50 Low back pain, unspecified
Loin pain
Lumbago NOS
M54.51 Vertebrogenic low back pain
Low back vertebral endplate pain
Coding Clinic: 2021, Q4, P22
M54.59 Other low back pain
M54.6 Pain in thoracic spine
Excludes1 pain in thoracic spine due to intervertebral disc disorder (M51.)
● **M54.8 Other dorsalgia**
Excludes1 dorsalgia in thoracic region (M54.6)
low back pain (M54.5-)
M54.81 Occipital neuralgia
M54.89 Other dorsalgia
M54.9 Dorsalgia, unspecified
Backache NOS
Back pain NOS

SOFT TISSUE DISORDERS (M60-M79)

DISORDERS OF MUSCLES (M60-M63)

Excludes1 dermatopolymyositis (M33.-)
muscular dystrophies and myopathies (G71-G72)
myopathy in amyloidosis (E85.-)
myopathy in polyarteritis nodosa (M30.0)
myopathy in rheumatoid arthritis (M05.32)
myopathy in scleroderma (M34.-)
myopathy in Sjögren's syndrome (M35.03)
myopathy in systemic lupus erythematosus (M32.-)

● **M60 Myositis**
Excludes2 inclusion body myositis [IBM] (G72.41)
● **M60.0 Infective myositis**
Tropical pyomyositis
Use additional code (B95-B97) to identify infectious agent
● **M60.00 Infective myositis, unspecified site** Ex: PDX 1253
M60.000 Infective myositis, unspecified right arm
Infective myositis, right upper limb NOS
M60.001 Infective myositis, unspecified left arm
Infective myositis, left upper limb NOS
M60.002 Infective myositis, unspecified arm
Infective myositis, upper limb NOS
M60.003 Infective myositis, unspecified right leg
Infective myositis, right lower limb NOS
M60.004 Infective myositis, unspecified left leg
Infective myositis, left lower limb NOS
M60.005 Infective myositis, unspecified leg
Infective myositis, lower limb NOS
M60.009 Infective myositis, unspecified site Ex: PDX 1114
● **M60.01 Infective myositis, shoulder** Ex: PDX 1254
M60.011 Infective myositis, right shoulder
M60.012 Infective myositis, left shoulder
M60.019 Infective myositis, unspecified shoulder
● **M60.02 Infective myositis, upper arm** Ex: PDX 1253
M60.021 Infective myositis, right upper arm
M60.022 Infective myositis, left upper arm
M60.029 Infective myositis, unspecified upper arm
● **M60.03 Infective myositis, forearm** Ex: PDX 1253
M60.031 Infective myositis, right forearm
M60.032 Infective myositis, left forearm
M60.039 Infective myositis, unspecified forearm
● **M60.04 Infective myositis, hand and fingers** Ex: PDX 1253
M60.041 Infective myositis, right hand
M60.042 Infective myositis, left hand
M60.043 Infective myositis, unspecified hand
M60.044 Infective myositis, right finger(s)
M60.045 Infective myositis, left finger(s)
M60.046 Infective myositis, unspecified finger(s)
● **M60.05 Infective myositis, thigh** Ex: PDX 1253
M60.051 Infective myositis, right thigh
M60.052 Infective myositis, left thigh
M60.059 Infective myositis, unspecified thigh
● **M60.06 Infective myositis, lower leg** Ex: PDX 1253
M60.061 Infective myositis, right lower leg
M60.062 Infective myositis, left lower leg
M60.069 Infective myositis, unspecified lower leg
● **M60.07 Infective myositis, ankle, foot and toes** Ex: PDX 1253
M60.070 Infective myositis, right ankle
M60.071 Infective myositis, left ankle
M60.072 Infective myositis, unspecified ankle
M60.073 Infective myositis, right foot
M60.074 Infective myositis, left foot
M60.075 Infective myositis, unspecified foot
M60.076 Infective myositis, right toe(s)
M60.077 Infective myositis, left toe(s)
M60.078 Infective myositis, unspecified toe(s)
M60.08 Infective myositis, other site Ex: PDX 1253
M60.09 Infective myositis, multiple sites Ex: PDX 1253
● **M60.1 Interstitial myositis**
M60.10 Interstitial myositis of unspecified site
● **M60.11 Interstitial myositis, shoulder**
M60.111 Interstitial myositis, right shoulder
M60.112 Interstitial myositis, left shoulder
M60.119 Interstitial myositis, unspecified shoulder
● **M60.12 Interstitial myositis, upper arm**
M60.121 Interstitial myositis, right upper arm
M60.122 Interstitial myositis, left upper arm
M60.129 Interstitial myositis, unspecified upper arm
● **M60.13 Interstitial myositis, forearm**
M60.131 Interstitial myositis, right forearm
M60.132 Interstitial myositis, left forearm
M60.139 Interstitial myositis, unspecified forearm
● **M60.14 Interstitial myositis, hand**
M60.141 Interstitial myositis, right hand
M60.142 Interstitial myositis, left hand
M60.149 Interstitial myositis, unspecified hand

CHAPTER 13 (M00-M99)

- M60.15 Interstitial myositis, thigh
  - M60.151 Interstitial myositis, right thigh
  - M60.152 Interstitial myositis, left thigh
  - M60.159 Interstitial myositis, unspecified thigh
- M60.16 Interstitial myositis, lower leg
  - M60.161 Interstitial myositis, right lower leg
  - M60.162 Interstitial myositis, left lower leg
  - M60.169 Interstitial myositis, unspecified lower leg
- M60.17 Interstitial myositis, ankle and foot
  - M60.171 Interstitial myositis, right ankle and foot
  - M60.172 Interstitial myositis, left ankle and foot
  - M60.179 Interstitial myositis, unspecified ankle and foot
- M60.18 Interstitial myositis, other site
- M60.19 Interstitial myositis, multiple sites

M60.2 Foreign body granuloma of soft tissue, not elsewhere classified

Use additional code to identify the type of retained foreign body (Z18.-)

Excludes1 foreign body granuloma of skin and subcutaneous tissue (L92.3)

- M60.20 Foreign body granuloma of soft tissue, not elsewhere classified, unspecified site
- M60.21 Foreign body granuloma of soft tissue, not elsewhere classified, shoulder
  - M60.211 Foreign body granuloma of soft tissue, not elsewhere classified, right shoulder
  - M60.212 Foreign body granuloma of soft tissue, not elsewhere classified, left shoulder
  - M60.219 Foreign body granuloma of soft tissue, not elsewhere classified, unspecified shoulder
- M60.22 Foreign body granuloma of soft tissue, not elsewhere classified, upper arm
  - M60.221 Foreign body granuloma of soft tissue, not elsewhere classified, right upper arm
  - M60.222 Foreign body granuloma of soft tissue, not elsewhere classified, left upper arm
  - M60.229 Foreign body granuloma of soft tissue, not elsewhere classified, unspecified upper arm
- M60.23 Foreign body granuloma of soft tissue, not elsewhere classified, forearm
  - M60.231 Foreign body granuloma of soft tissue, not elsewhere classified, right forearm
  - M60.232 Foreign body granuloma of soft tissue, not elsewhere classified, left forearm
  - M60.239 Foreign body granuloma of soft tissue, not elsewhere classified, unspecified forearm
- M60.24 Foreign body granuloma of soft tissue, not elsewhere classified, hand
  - M60.241 Foreign body granuloma of soft tissue, not elsewhere classified, right hand
  - M60.242 Foreign body granuloma of soft tissue, not elsewhere classified, left hand
  - M60.249 Foreign body granuloma of soft tissue, not elsewhere classified, unspecified hand
- M60.25 Foreign body granuloma of soft tissue, not elsewhere classified, thigh
  - M60.251 Foreign body granuloma of soft tissue, not elsewhere classified, right thigh
  - M60.252 Foreign body granuloma of soft tissue, not elsewhere classified, left thigh
  - M60.259 Foreign body granuloma of soft tissue, not elsewhere classified, unspecified thigh
- M60.26 Foreign body granuloma of soft tissue, not elsewhere classified, lower leg
  - M60.261 Foreign body granuloma of soft tissue, not elsewhere classified, right lower leg
  - M60.262 Foreign body granuloma of soft tissue, not elsewhere classified, left lower leg
  - M60.269 Foreign body granuloma of soft tissue, not elsewhere classified, unspecified lower leg
- M60.27 Foreign body granuloma of soft tissue, not elsewhere classified, ankle and foot
  - M60.271 Foreign body granuloma of soft tissue, not elsewhere classified, right ankle and foot
  - M60.272 Foreign body granuloma of soft tissue, not elsewhere classified, left ankle and foot
  - M60.279 Foreign body granuloma of soft tissue, not elsewhere classified, unspecified ankle and foot
- M60.28 Foreign body granuloma of soft tissue, not elsewhere classified, other site

M60.8 Other myositis

- M60.80 Other myositis, unspecified site
- M60.81 Other myositis shoulder
  - M60.811 Other myositis, right shoulder
  - M60.812 Other myositis, left shoulder
  - M60.819 Other myositis, unspecified shoulder
- M60.82 Other myositis, upper arm
  - M60.821 Other myositis, right upper arm
  - M60.822 Other myositis, left upper arm
  - M60.829 Other myositis, unspecified upper arm
- M60.83 Other myositis, forearm
  - M60.831 Other myositis, right forearm
  - M60.832 Other myositis, left forearm
  - M60.839 Other myositis, unspecified forearm
- M60.84 Other myositis, hand
  - M60.841 Other myositis, right hand
  - M60.842 Other myositis, left hand
  - M60.849 Other myositis, unspecified hand
- M60.85 Other myositis, thigh
  - M60.851 Other myositis, right thigh
  - M60.852 Other myositis, left thigh
  - M60.859 Other myositis, unspecified thigh
- M60.86 Other myositis, lower leg
  - M60.861 Other myositis, right lower leg
  - M60.862 Other myositis, left lower leg
  - M60.869 Other myositis, unspecified lower leg
- M60.87 Other myositis, ankle and foot
  - M60.871 Other myositis, right ankle and foot
  - M60.872 Other myositis, left ankle and foot
  - M60.879 Other myositis, unspecified ankle and foot
- M60.88 Other myositis, other site
- M60.89 Other myositis, multiple sites

M60.9 Myositis, unspecified

● M61 Calcification and ossification of muscle
● M61.0 Myositis ossificans traumatica
M61.00 Myositis ossificans traumatica, unspecified site
● M61.01 Myositis ossificans traumatica, shoulder
M61.011 Myositis ossificans traumatica, right shoulder
M61.012 Myositis ossificans traumatica, left shoulder
M61.019 Myositis ossificans traumatica, unspecified shoulder
● M61.02 Myositis ossificans traumatica, upper arm
M61.021 Myositis ossificans traumatica, right upper arm
M61.022 Myositis ossificans traumatica, left upper arm
M61.029 Myositis ossificans traumatica, unspecified upper arm
● M61.03 Myositis ossificans traumatica, forearm
M61.031 Myositis ossificans traumatica, right forearm
M61.032 Myositis ossificans traumatica, left forearm
M61.039 Myositis ossificans traumatica, unspecified forearm
● M61.04 Myositis ossificans traumatica, hand
M61.041 Myositis ossificans traumatica, right hand
M61.042 Myositis ossificans traumatica, left hand
M61.049 Myositis ossificans traumatica, unspecified hand
● M61.05 Myositis ossificans traumatica, thigh
M61.051 Myositis ossificans traumatica, right thigh
M61.052 Myositis ossificans traumatica, left thigh
M61.059 Myositis ossificans traumatica, unspecified thigh
● M61.06 Myositis ossificans traumatica, lower leg
M61.061 Myositis ossificans traumatica, right lower leg
M61.062 Myositis ossificans traumatica, left lower leg
M61.069 Myositis ossificans traumatica, unspecified lower leg
● M61.07 Myositis ossificans traumatica, ankle and foot
M61.071 Myositis ossificans traumatica, right ankle and foot
M61.072 Myositis ossificans traumatica, left ankle and foot
M61.079 Myositis ossificans traumatica, unspecified ankle and foot
M61.08 Myositis ossificans traumatica, other site
M61.09 Myositis ossificans traumatica, multiple sites
● M61.1 Myositis ossificans progressiva
Fibrodysplasia ossificans progressiva
M61.10 Myositis ossificans progressiva, unspecified site
● M61.11 Myositis ossificans progressiva, shoulder
M61.111 Myositis ossificans progressiva, right shoulder
M61.112 Myositis ossificans progressiva, left shoulder
M61.119 Myositis ossificans progressiva, unspecified shoulder
● M61.12 Myositis ossificans progressiva, upper arm
M61.121 Myositis ossificans progressiva, right upper arm
M61.122 Myositis ossificans progressiva, left upper arm
M61.129 Myositis ossificans progressiva, unspecified arm
● M61.13 Myositis ossificans progressiva, forearm
M61.131 Myositis ossificans progressiva, right forearm
M61.132 Myositis ossificans progressiva, left forearm
M61.139 Myositis ossificans progressiva, unspecified forearm
● M61.14 Myositis ossificans progressiva, hand and finger(s)
M61.141 Myositis ossificans progressiva, right hand
M61.142 Myositis ossificans progressiva, left hand
M61.143 Myositis ossificans progressiva, unspecified hand
M61.144 Myositis ossificans progressiva, right finger(s)
M61.145 Myositis ossificans progressiva, left finger(s)
M61.146 Myositis ossificans progressiva, unspecified finger(s)
● M61.15 Myositis ossificans progressiva, thigh
M61.151 Myositis ossificans progressiva, right thigh
M61.152 Myositis ossificans progressiva, left thigh
M61.159 Myositis ossificans progressiva, unspecified thigh
● M61.16 Myositis ossificans progressiva, lower leg
M61.161 Myositis ossificans progressiva, right lower leg
M61.162 Myositis ossificans progressiva, left lower leg
M61.169 Myositis ossificans progressiva, unspecified lower leg
● M61.17 Myositis ossificans progressiva, ankle, foot and toe(s)
M61.171 Myositis ossificans progressiva, right ankle
M61.172 Myositis ossificans progressiva, left ankle
M61.173 Myositis ossificans progressiva, unspecified ankle
M61.174 Myositis ossificans progressiva, right foot
M61.175 Myositis ossificans progressiva, left foot
M61.176 Myositis ossificans progressiva, unspecified foot
M61.177 Myositis ossificans progressiva, right toe(s)
M61.178 Myositis ossificans progressiva, left toe(s)
M61.179 Myositis ossificans progressiva, unspecified toe(s)
M61.18 Myositis ossificans progressiva, other site
M61.19 Myositis ossificans progressiva, multiple sites

- ● M61.2 Paralytic calcification and ossification of muscle
  Myositis ossificans associated with quadriplegia or paraplegia
  - M61.2Ø Paralytic calcification and ossification of muscle, unspecified site
  - ● M61.21 Paralytic calcification and ossification of muscle, shoulder
    - M61.211 Paralytic calcification and ossification of muscle, right shoulder
    - M61.212 Paralytic calcification and ossification of muscle, left shoulder
    - M61.219 Paralytic calcification and ossification of muscle, unspecified shoulder
  - ● M61.22 Paralytic calcification and ossification of muscle, upper arm
    - M61.221 Paralytic calcification and ossification of muscle, right upper arm
    - M61.222 Paralytic calcification and ossification of muscle, left upper arm
    - M61.229 Paralytic calcification and ossification of muscle, unspecified upper arm
  - ● M61.23 Paralytic calcification and ossification of muscle, forearm
    - M61.231 Paralytic calcification and ossification of muscle, right forearm
    - M61.232 Paralytic calcification and ossification of muscle, left forearm
    - M61.239 Paralytic calcification and ossification of muscle, unspecified forearm
  - ● M61.24 Paralytic calcification and ossification of muscle, hand
    - M61.241 Paralytic calcification and ossification of muscle, right hand
    - M61.242 Paralytic calcification and ossification of muscle, left hand
    - M61.249 Paralytic calcification and ossification of muscle, unspecified hand
  - ● M61.25 Paralytic calcification and ossification of muscle, thigh
    - M61.251 Paralytic calcification and ossification of muscle, right thigh
    - M61.252 Paralytic calcification and ossification of muscle, left thigh
    - M61.259 Paralytic calcification and ossification of muscle, unspecified thigh
  - ● M61.26 Paralytic calcification and ossification of muscle, lower leg
    - M61.261 Paralytic calcification and ossification of muscle, right lower leg
    - M61.262 Paralytic calcification and ossification of muscle, left lower leg
    - M61.269 Paralytic calcification and ossification of muscle, unspecified lower leg
  - ● M61.27 Paralytic calcification and ossification of muscle, ankle and foot
    - M61.271 Paralytic calcification and ossification of muscle, right ankle and foot
    - M61.272 Paralytic calcification and ossification of muscle, left ankle and foot
    - M61.279 Paralytic calcification and ossification of muscle, unspecified ankle and foot
  - M61.28 Paralytic calcification and ossification of muscle, other site
  - M61.29 Paralytic calcification and ossification of muscle, multiple sites
- ● M61.3 Calcification and ossification of muscles associated with burns
  Myositis ossificans associated with burns
  - M61.3Ø Calcification and ossification of muscles associated with burns, unspecified site
  - ● M61.31 Calcification and ossification of muscles associated with burns, shoulder
    - M61.311 Calcification and ossification of muscles associated with burns, right shoulder
    - M61.312 Calcification and ossification of muscles associated with burns, left shoulder
    - M61.319 Calcification and ossification of muscles associated with burns, unspecified shoulder
  - ● M61.32 Calcification and ossification of muscles associated with burns, upper arm
    - M61.321 Calcification and ossification of muscles associated with burns, right upper arm
    - M61.322 Calcification and ossification of muscles associated with burns, left upper arm
    - M61.329 Calcification and ossification of muscles associated with burns, unspecified upper arm
  - ● M61.33 Calcification and ossification of muscles associated with burns, forearm
    - M61.331 Calcification and ossification of muscles associated with burns, right forearm
    - M61.332 Calcification and ossification of muscles associated with burns, left forearm
    - M61.339 Calcification and ossification of muscles associated with burns, unspecified forearm
  - ● M61.34 Calcification and ossification of muscles associated with burns, hand
    - M61.341 Calcification and ossification of muscles associated with burns, right hand
    - M61.342 Calcification and ossification of muscles associated with burns, left hand
    - M61.349 Calcification and ossification of muscles associated with burns, unspecified hand
  - ● M61.35 Calcification and ossification of muscles associated with burns, thigh
    - M61.351 Calcification and ossification of muscles associated with burns, right thigh
    - M61.352 Calcification and ossification of muscles associated with burns, left thigh
    - M61.359 Calcification and ossification of muscles associated with burns, unspecified thigh
  - ● M61.36 Calcification and ossification of muscles associated with burns, lower leg
    - M61.361 Calcification and ossification of muscles associated with burns, right lower leg
    - M61.362 Calcification and ossification of muscles associated with burns, left lower leg
    - M61.369 Calcification and ossification of muscles associated with burns, unspecified lower leg
  - ● M61.37 Calcification and ossification of muscles associated with burns, ankle and foot
    - M61.371 Calcification and ossification of muscles associated with burns, right ankle and foot

M61.372 Calcification and ossification of muscles associated with burns, left ankle and foot
M61.379 Calcification and ossification of muscles associated with burns, unspecified ankle and foot
M61.38 Calcification and ossification of muscles associated with burns, other site
M61.39 Calcification and ossification of muscles associated with burns, multiple sites

M61.4 Other calcification of muscle

Excludes1 calcific tendinitis NOS (M65.2-)
calcific tendinitis of shoulder (M75.3)

M61.40 Other calcification of muscle, unspecified site

M61.41 Other calcification of muscle, shoulder
M61.411 Other calcification of muscle, right shoulder
M61.412 Other calcification of muscle, left shoulder
M61.419 Other calcification of muscle, unspecified shoulder

M61.42 Other calcification of muscle, upper arm
M61.421 Other calcification of muscle, right upper arm
M61.422 Other calcification of muscle, left upper arm
M61.429 Other calcification of muscle, unspecified upper arm

M61.43 Other calcification of muscle, forearm
M61.431 Other calcification of muscle, right forearm
M61.432 Other calcification of muscle, left forearm
M61.439 Other calcification of muscle, unspecified forearm

M61.44 Other calcification of muscle, hand
M61.441 Other calcification of muscle, right hand
M61.442 Other calcification of muscle, left hand
M61.449 Other calcification of muscle, unspecified hand

M61.45 Other calcification of muscle, thigh
M61.451 Other calcification of muscle, right thigh
M61.452 Other calcification of muscle, left thigh
M61.459 Other calcification of muscle, unspecified thigh

M61.46 Other calcification of muscle, lower leg
M61.461 Other calcification of muscle, right lower leg
M61.462 Other calcification of muscle, left lower leg
M61.469 Other calcification of muscle, unspecified lower leg

M61.47 Other calcification of muscle, ankle and foot
M61.471 Other calcification of muscle, right ankle and foot
M61.472 Other calcification of muscle, left ankle and foot
M61.479 Other calcification of muscle, unspecified ankle and foot

M61.48 Other calcification of muscle, other site
M61.49 Other calcification of muscle, multiple sites

M61.5 Other ossification of muscle

M61.50 Other ossification of muscle, unspecified site

M61.51 Other ossification of muscle, shoulder
M61.511 Other ossification of muscle, right shoulder
M61.512 Other ossification of muscle, left shoulder
M61.519 Other ossification of muscle, unspecified shoulder

M61.52 Other ossification of muscle, upper arm
M61.521 Other ossification of muscle, right upper arm
M61.522 Other ossification of muscle, left upper arm
M61.529 Other ossification of muscle, unspecified upper arm

M61.53 Other ossification of muscle, forearm
M61.531 Other ossification of muscle, right forearm
M61.532 Other ossification of muscle, left forearm
M61.539 Other ossification of muscle, unspecified forearm

M61.54 Other ossification of muscle, hand
M61.541 Other ossification of muscle, right hand
M61.542 Other ossification of muscle, left hand
M61.549 Other ossification of muscle, unspecified hand

M61.55 Other ossification of muscle, thigh
M61.551 Other ossification of muscle, right thigh
M61.552 Other ossification of muscle, left thigh
M61.559 Other ossification of muscle, unspecified thigh

M61.56 Other ossification of muscle, lower leg
M61.561 Other ossification of muscle, right lower leg
M61.562 Other ossification of muscle, left lower leg
M61.569 Other ossification of muscle, unspecified lower leg

M61.57 Other ossification of muscle, ankle and foot
M61.571 Other ossification of muscle, right ankle and foot
M61.572 Other ossification of muscle, left ankle and foot
M61.579 Other ossification of muscle, unspecified ankle and foot

M61.58 Other ossification of muscle, other site
M61.59 Other ossification of muscle, multiple sites

M61.9 Calcification and ossification of muscle, unspecified

M62 Other disorders of muscle

Excludes1 alcoholic myopathy (G72.1)
cramp and spasm (R25.2)
drug-induced myopathy (G72.0)
myalgia (M79.1-)
stiff-man syndrome (G25.82)

Excludes2 nontraumatic hematoma of muscle (M79.81)

M62.0 Separation of muscle (nontraumatic)

Diastasis of muscle

Excludes1 diastasis recti complicating pregnancy, labor and delivery (O71.8)
traumatic separation of muscle - see strain of muscle by body region

M62.00 Separation of muscle (nontraumatic), unspecified site

CHAPTER 13 (M00-M99)

● M62.01 Separation of muscle (nontraumatic), shoulder
M62.011 Separation of muscle (nontraumatic), right shoulder
M62.012 Separation of muscle (nontraumatic), left shoulder
M62.019 Separation of muscle (nontraumatic), unspecified shoulder
● M62.02 Separation of muscle (nontraumatic), upper arm
M62.021 Separation of muscle (nontraumatic), right upper arm
M62.022 Separation of muscle (nontraumatic), left upper arm
M62.029 Separation of muscle (nontraumatic), unspecified upper arm
● M62.03 Separation of muscle (nontraumatic), forearm
M62.031 Separation of muscle (nontraumatic), right forearm
M62.032 Separation of muscle (nontraumatic), left forearm
M62.039 Separation of muscle (nontraumatic), unspecified forearm
● M62.04 Separation of muscle (nontraumatic), hand
M62.041 Separation of muscle (nontraumatic), right hand
M62.042 Separation of muscle (nontraumatic), left hand
M62.049 Separation of muscle (nontraumatic), unspecified hand
● M62.05 Separation of muscle (nontraumatic), thigh
M62.051 Separation of muscle (nontraumatic), right thigh
M62.052 Separation of muscle (nontraumatic), left thigh
M62.059 Separation of muscle (nontraumatic), unspecified thigh
● M62.06 Separation of muscle (nontraumatic), lower leg
M62.061 Separation of muscle (nontraumatic), right lower leg
M62.062 Separation of muscle (nontraumatic), left lower leg
M62.069 Separation of muscle (nontraumatic), unspecified lower leg
● M62.07 Separation of muscle (nontraumatic), ankle and foot
M62.071 Separation of muscle (nontraumatic), right ankle and foot
M62.072 Separation of muscle (nontraumatic), left ankle and foot
M62.079 Separation of muscle (nontraumatic), unspecified ankle and foot
M62.08 Separation of muscle (nontraumatic), other site
● M62.1 Other rupture of muscle (nontraumatic)
Excludes1 traumatic rupture of muscle - see strain of muscle by body region
Excludes2 rupture of tendon (M66.-)
M62.10 Other rupture of muscle (nontraumatic), unspecified site
● M62.11 Other rupture of muscle (nontraumatic), shoulder
M62.111 Other rupture of muscle (nontraumatic), right shoulder
M62.112 Other rupture of muscle (nontraumatic), left shoulder
M62.119 Other rupture of muscle (nontraumatic), unspecified shoulder
● M62.12 Other rupture of muscle (nontraumatic), upper arm
M62.121 Other rupture of muscle (nontraumatic), right upper arm
M62.122 Other rupture of muscle (nontraumatic), left upper arm
M62.129 Other rupture of muscle (nontraumatic), unspecified upper arm
● M62.13 Other rupture of muscle (nontraumatic), forearm
M62.131 Other rupture of muscle (nontraumatic), right forearm
M62.132 Other rupture of muscle (nontraumatic), left forearm
M62.139 Other rupture of muscle (nontraumatic), unspecified forearm
● M62.14 Other rupture of muscle (nontraumatic), hand
M62.141 Other rupture of muscle (nontraumatic), right hand
M62.142 Other rupture of muscle (nontraumatic), left hand
M62.149 Other rupture of muscle (nontraumatic), unspecified hand
● M62.15 Other rupture of muscle (nontraumatic), thigh
M62.151 Other rupture of muscle (nontraumatic), right thigh
M62.152 Other rupture of muscle (nontraumatic), left thigh
M62.159 Other rupture of muscle (nontraumatic), unspecified thigh
● M62.16 Other rupture of muscle (nontraumatic), lower leg
M62.161 Other rupture of muscle (nontraumatic), right lower leg
M62.162 Other rupture of muscle (nontraumatic), left lower leg
M62.169 Other rupture of muscle (nontraumatic), unspecified lower leg
● M62.17 Other rupture of muscle (nontraumatic), ankle and foot
M62.171 Other rupture of muscle (nontraumatic), right ankle and foot
M62.172 Other rupture of muscle (nontraumatic), left ankle and foot
M62.179 Other rupture of muscle (nontraumatic), unspecified ankle and foot
M62.18 Other rupture of muscle (nontraumatic), other site
● M62.2 Nontraumatic ischemic infarction of muscle
Excludes1 compartment syndrome (traumatic) (T79.A-)
nontraumatic compartment syndrome (M79.A-)
traumatic ischemia of muscle (T79.6)
rhabdomyolysis (M62.82)
Volkmann's ischemic contracture (T79.6)
M62.20 Nontraumatic ischemic infarction of muscle, unspecified site
● M62.21 Nontraumatic ischemic infarction of muscle, shoulder
M62.211 Nontraumatic ischemic infarction of muscle, right shoulder
M62.212 Nontraumatic ischemic infarction of muscle, left shoulder
M62.219 Nontraumatic ischemic infarction of muscle, unspecified shoulder

● M62.22 Nontraumatic ischemic infarction of muscle, upper arm
- M62.221 Nontraumatic ischemic infarction of muscle, right upper arm
- M62.222 Nontraumatic ischemic infarction of muscle, left upper arm
- M62.229 Nontraumatic ischemic infarction of muscle, unspecified upper arm

● M62.23 Nontraumatic ischemic infarction of muscle, forearm
- M62.231 Nontraumatic ischemic infarction of muscle, right forearm
- M62.232 Nontraumatic ischemic infarction of muscle, left forearm
- M62.239 Nontraumatic ischemic infarction of muscle, unspecified forearm

● M62.24 Nontraumatic ischemic infarction of muscle, hand
- M62.241 Nontraumatic ischemic infarction of muscle, right hand
- M62.242 Nontraumatic ischemic infarction of muscle, left hand
- M62.249 Nontraumatic ischemic infarction of muscle, unspecified hand

● M62.25 Nontraumatic ischemic infarction of muscle, thigh
- M62.251 Nontraumatic ischemic infarction of muscle, right thigh
- M62.252 Nontraumatic ischemic infarction of muscle, left thigh
- M62.259 Nontraumatic ischemic infarction of muscle, unspecified thigh

● M62.26 Nontraumatic ischemic infarction of muscle, lower leg
- M62.261 Nontraumatic ischemic infarction of muscle, right lower leg
- M62.262 Nontraumatic ischemic infarction of muscle, left lower leg
- M62.269 Nontraumatic ischemic infarction of muscle, unspecified lower leg

● M62.27 Nontraumatic ischemic infarction of muscle, ankle and foot
- M62.271 Nontraumatic ischemic infarction of muscle, right ankle and foot
- M62.272 Nontraumatic ischemic infarction of muscle, left ankle and foot
- M62.279 Nontraumatic ischemic infarction of muscle, unspecified ankle and foot

M62.28 Nontraumatic ischemic infarction of muscle, other site

M62.3 Immobility syndrome (paraplegic)

M62.4 Contracture of muscle

Contracture of tendon (sheath)

Excludes1 contracture of joint (M24.5-)

M62.40 Contracture of muscle, unspecified site

● M62.41 Contracture of muscle, shoulder
- M62.411 Contracture of muscle, right shoulder
- M62.412 Contracture of muscle, left shoulder
- M62.419 Contracture of muscle, unspecified shoulder

● M62.42 Contracture of muscle, upper arm
- M62.421 Contracture of muscle, right upper arm
- M62.422 Contracture of muscle, left upper arm
- M62.429 Contracture of muscle, unspecified upper arm

● M62.43 Contracture of muscle, forearm
- M62.431 Contracture of muscle, right forearm
- M62.432 Contracture of muscle, left forearm
- M62.439 Contracture of muscle, unspecified forearm

● M62.44 Contracture of muscle, hand
- M62.441 Contracture of muscle, right hand
- M62.442 Contracture of muscle, left hand
- M62.449 Contracture of muscle, unspecified hand

● M62.45 Contracture of muscle, thigh
- M62.451 Contracture of muscle, right thigh
- M62.452 Contracture of muscle, left thigh
- M62.459 Contracture of muscle, unspecified thigh

● M62.46 Contracture of muscle, lower leg
- M62.461 Contracture of muscle, right lower leg
- M62.462 Contracture of muscle, left lower leg
  Coding Clinic: 2023, Q2, P14
- M62.469 Contracture of muscle, unspecified lower leg

● M62.47 Contracture of muscle, ankle and foot
- M62.471 Contracture of muscle, right ankle and foot
- M62.472 Contracture of muscle, left ankle and foot
- M62.479 Contracture of muscle, unspecified ankle and foot

M62.48 Contracture of muscle, other site

M62.49 Contracture of muscle, multiple sites

● M62.5 Muscle wasting and atrophy, not elsewhere classified

Disuse atrophy NEC

Excludes1 neuralgic amyotrophy (G54.5)
progressive muscular atrophy (G12.21)
sarcopenia (M62.84)

Excludes2 pelvic muscle wasting (N81.84)

M62.50 Muscle wasting and atrophy, not elsewhere classified, unspecified site

● M62.51 Muscle wasting and atrophy, not elsewhere classified, shoulder
- M62.511 Muscle wasting and atrophy, not elsewhere classified, right shoulder
- M62.512 Muscle wasting and atrophy, not elsewhere classified, left shoulder
- M62.519 Muscle wasting and atrophy, not elsewhere classified, unspecified shoulder

● M62.52 Muscle wasting and atrophy, not elsewhere classified, upper arm
- M62.521 Muscle wasting and atrophy, not elsewhere classified, right upper arm
- M62.522 Muscle wasting and atrophy, not elsewhere classified, left upper arm
- M62.529 Muscle wasting and atrophy, not elsewhere classified, unspecified upper arm

● M62.53 Muscle wasting and atrophy, not elsewhere classified, forearm
- M62.531 Muscle wasting and atrophy, not elsewhere classified, right forearm
- M62.532 Muscle wasting and atrophy, not elsewhere classified, left forearm
- M62.539 Muscle wasting and atrophy, not elsewhere classified, unspecified forearm

● M62.54 Muscle wasting and atrophy, not elsewhere classified, hand
M62.541 Muscle wasting and atrophy, not elsewhere classified, right hand
M62.542 Muscle wasting and atrophy, not elsewhere classified, left hand
M62.549 Muscle wasting and atrophy, not elsewhere classified, unspecified hand

● M62.55 Muscle wasting and atrophy, not elsewhere classified, thigh
M62.551 Muscle wasting and atrophy, not elsewhere classified, right thigh
M62.552 Muscle wasting and atrophy, not elsewhere classified, left thigh
M62.559 Muscle wasting and atrophy, not elsewhere classified, unspecified thigh

● M62.56 Muscle wasting and atrophy, not elsewhere classified, lower leg
M62.561 Muscle wasting and atrophy, not elsewhere classified, right lower leg
M62.562 Muscle wasting and atrophy, not elsewhere classified, left lower leg
M62.569 Muscle wasting and atrophy, not elsewhere classified, unspecified lower leg

● M62.57 Muscle wasting and atrophy, not elsewhere classified, ankle and foot
M62.571 Muscle wasting and atrophy, not elsewhere classified, right ankle and foot
M62.572 Muscle wasting and atrophy, not elsewhere classified, left ankle and foot
M62.579 Muscle wasting and atrophy, not elsewhere classified, unspecified ankle and foot

M62.58 Muscle wasting and atrophy, not elsewhere classified, other site
M62.59 Muscle wasting and atrophy, not elsewhere classified, multiple sites

● M62.5A Muscle wasting and atrophy, not elsewhere classified, back
M62.5A0 Muscle wasting and atrophy, not elsewhere classified, back, cervical
M62.5A1 Muscle wasting and atrophy, not elsewhere classified, back, thoracic
M62.5A2 Muscle wasting and atrophy, not elsewhere classified, back, lumbosacral
M62.5A9 Muscle wasting and atrophy, not elsewhere classified, back, unspecified level

● M62.8 Other specified disorders of muscle
Excludes2 nontraumatic hematoma of muscle (M79.81)
M62.81 Muscle weakness (generalized)
Excludes1 muscle weakness in sarcopenia (M62.84)
M62.82 Rhabdomyolysis (Ex) PDX 1255
Excludes1 traumatic rhabdomyolysis (T79.6)
Coding Clinic: 2019, Q2, P12

● M62.83 Muscle spasm
M62.830 Muscle spasm of back
M62.831 Muscle spasm of calf
Charley-horse
M62.838 Other muscle spasm

M62.84 Sarcopenia
Age-related sarcopenia
Code first underlying disease, if applicable, such as:
disorders of myoneural junction and muscle disease in diseases classified elsewhere (G73.-)
other and unspecified myopathies (G72.-)
primary disorders of muscles (G71.-)
Coding Clinic: 2016, Q4, P41

▶ M62.85 Dyfunction of the multifidus muscles, lumbar region
M62.89 Other specified disorders of muscle
Muscle (sheath) hernia
M62.9 Disorder of muscle, unspecified

● M63 Disorders of muscle in diseases classified elsewhere
Code first underlying disease, such as:
leprosy (A30.-)
neoplasm (C49.-, C79.89, D21.-, D48.1-)
schistosomiasis (B65.-)
trichinellosis (B75)
Excludes1 myopathy in cysticercosis (B69.81)
myopathy in endocrine diseases (G73.7)
myopathy in metabolic diseases (G73.7)
myopathy in sarcoidosis (D86.87)
myopathy in secondary syphilis (A51.49)
myopathy in syphilis (late) (A52.78)
myopathy in toxoplasmosis (B58.82)
myopathy in tuberculosis (A18.09)

● M63.8 Disorders of muscle in diseases classified elsewhere
M63.80 Disorders of muscle in diseases classified elsewhere, unspecified site

● M63.81 Disorders of muscle in diseases classified elsewhere, shoulder
M63.811 Disorders of muscle in diseases classified elsewhere, right shoulder
M63.812 Disorders of muscle in diseases classified elsewhere, left shoulder
M63.819 Disorders of muscle in diseases classified elsewhere, unspecified shoulder

● M63.82 Disorders of muscle in diseases classified elsewhere, upper arm
M63.821 Disorders of muscle in diseases classified elsewhere, right upper arm
M63.822 Disorders of muscle in diseases classified elsewhere, left upper arm
M63.829 Disorders of muscle in diseases classified elsewhere, unspecified upper arm

● M63.83 Disorders of muscle in diseases classified elsewhere, forearm
M63.831 Disorders of muscle in diseases classified elsewhere, right forearm
M63.832 Disorders of muscle in diseases classified elsewhere, left forearm
M63.839 Disorders of muscle in diseases classified elsewhere, unspecified forearm

● M63.84 Disorders of muscle in diseases classified elsewhere, hand
M63.841 Disorders of muscle in diseases classified elsewhere, right hand
M63.842 Disorders of muscle in diseases classified elsewhere, left hand
M63.849 Disorders of muscle in diseases classified elsewhere, unspecified hand

CHAPTER 13 (M00-M99)

● **M63.85 Disorders of muscle in diseases classified elsewhere, thigh**

M63.851 Disorders of muscle in diseases classified elsewhere, right thigh

M63.852 Disorders of muscle in diseases classified elsewhere, left thigh

M63.859 Disorders of muscle in diseases classified elsewhere, unspecified thigh

● **M63.86 Disorders of muscle in diseases classified elsewhere, lower leg**

M63.861 Disorders of muscle in diseases classified elsewhere, right lower leg

M63.862 Disorders of muscle in diseases classified elsewhere, left lower leg

M63.869 Disorders of muscle in diseases classified elsewhere, unspecified lower leg

● **M63.87 Disorders of muscle in diseases classified elsewhere, ankle and foot**

M63.871 Disorders of muscle in diseases classified elsewhere, right ankle and foot

M63.872 Disorders of muscle in diseases classified elsewhere, left ankle and foot

M63.879 Disorders of muscle in diseases classified elsewhere, unspecified ankle and foot

M63.88 Disorders of muscle in diseases classified elsewhere, other site

M63.89 Disorders of muscle in diseases classified elsewhere, multiple sites

DISORDERS OF SYNOVIUM AND TENDON (M65-M67)

● **M65 Synovitis and tenosynovitis**

Excludes1 chronic crepitant synovitis of hand and wrist (M70.0-)
current injury - see injury of ligament or tendon by body region
soft tissue disorders related to use, overuse and pressure (M70.-)

● **M65.0 Abscess of tendon sheath**

Use additional code (B95-B96) to identify bacterial agent

M65.00 Abscess of tendon sheath, unspecified site

● **M65.01 Abscess of tendon sheath, shoulder**

M65.011 Abscess of tendon sheath, right shoulder

M65.012 Abscess of tendon sheath, left shoulder

M65.019 Abscess of tendon sheath, unspecified shoulder

● **M65.02 Abscess of tendon sheath, upper arm**

M65.021 Abscess of tendon sheath, right upper arm

M65.022 Abscess of tendon sheath, left upper arm

M65.029 Abscess of tendon sheath, unspecified upper arm

● **M65.03 Abscess of tendon sheath, forearm**

M65.031 Abscess of tendon sheath, right forearm

M65.032 Abscess of tendon sheath, left forearm

M65.039 Abscess of tendon sheath, unspecified forearm

● **M65.04 Abscess of tendon sheath, hand**

M65.041 Abscess of tendon sheath, right hand

M65.042 Abscess of tendon sheath, left hand

M65.049 Abscess of tendon sheath, unspecified hand

Item 13-11 Synovitis is an inflammation of a synovial membrane resulting in pain on motion and is characterized by fluctuating swelling due to effusion in a synovial sac. **Tenosynovitis** is an inflammation of a tendon sheath and occurs most commonly in the wrists, hands, and feet. Bursitis is inflammation of a bursa (fluid-filled sac) caused by repetitive use, trauma, infection, or systemic inflammatory disease. Bursae act as protectors and facilitate movement between bones and overlapping muscles (deep bursae) or between bones and tendons/skin (superficial bursae).

● **M65.05 Abscess of tendon sheath, thigh**

M65.051 Abscess of tendon sheath, right thigh

M65.052 Abscess of tendon sheath, left thigh

M65.059 Abscess of tendon sheath, unspecified thigh

● **M65.06 Abscess of tendon sheath, lower leg**

M65.061 Abscess of tendon sheath, right lower leg

M65.062 Abscess of tendon sheath, left lower leg

M65.069 Abscess of tendon sheath, unspecified lower leg

● **M65.07 Abscess of tendon sheath, ankle and foot**

M65.071 Abscess of tendon sheath, right ankle and foot

M65.072 Abscess of tendon sheath, left ankle and foot

M65.079 Abscess of tendon sheath, unspecified ankle and foot

M65.08 Abscess of tendon sheath, other site

● **M65.1 Other infective (teno)synovitis**

M65.10 Other infective (teno)synovitis, unspecified site

● **M65.11 Other infective (teno)synovitis, shoulder**

M65.111 Other infective (teno)synovitis, right shoulder

M65.112 Other infective (teno)synovitis, left shoulder

M65.119 Other infective (teno)synovitis, unspecified shoulder

● **M65.12 Other infective (teno)synovitis, elbow**

M65.121 Other infective (teno)synovitis, right elbow

M65.122 Other infective (teno)synovitis, left elbow

M65.129 Other infective (teno)synovitis, unspecified elbow

● **M65.13 Other infective (teno)synovitis, wrist**

M65.131 Other infective (teno)synovitis, right wrist

M65.132 Other infective (teno)synovitis, left wrist

M65.139 Other infective (teno)synovitis, unspecified wrist

● **M65.14 Other infective (teno)synovitis, hand**

M65.141 Other infective (teno)synovitis, right hand

M65.142 Other infective (teno)synovitis, left hand

M65.149 Other infective (teno)synovitis, unspecified hand

● **M65.15 Other infective (teno)synovitis, hip**

M65.151 Other infective (teno)synovitis, right hip

M65.152 Other infective (teno)synovitis, left hip

M65.159 Other infective (teno)synovitis, unspecified hip

M65.16 Other infective (teno)synovitis, knee
M65.161 Other infective (teno)synovitis, right knee
M65.162 Other infective (teno)synovitis, left knee
M65.169 Other infective (teno)synovitis, unspecified knee
M65.17 Other infective (teno)synovitis, ankle and foot
M65.171 Other infective (teno)synovitis, right ankle and foot
M65.172 Other infective (teno)synovitis, left ankle and foot
M65.179 Other infective (teno)synovitis, unspecified ankle and foot
M65.18 Other infective (teno)synovitis, other site
M65.19 Other infective (teno)synovitis, multiple sites
M65.2 Calcific tendinitis
Excludes1 tendinitis as classified in M75-M77
calcified tendinitis of shoulder (M75.3)
M65.20 Calcific tendinitis, unspecified site
M65.22 Calcific tendinitis, upper arm
M65.221 Calcific tendinitis, right upper arm
M65.222 Calcific tendinitis, left upper arm
M65.229 Calcific tendinitis, unspecified upper arm
M65.23 Calcific tendinitis, forearm
M65.231 Calcific tendinitis, right forearm
M65.232 Calcific tendinitis, left forearm
M65.239 Calcific tendinitis, unspecified forearm
M65.24 Calcific tendinitis, hand
M65.241 Calcific tendinitis, right hand
M65.242 Calcific tendinitis, left hand
M65.249 Calcific tendinitis, unspecified hand
M65.25 Calcific tendinitis, thigh
M65.251 Calcific tendinitis, right thigh
M65.252 Calcific tendinitis, left thigh
M65.259 Calcific tendinitis, unspecified thigh
M65.26 Calcific tendinitis, lower leg
M65.261 Calcific tendinitis, right lower leg
M65.262 Calcific tendinitis, left lower leg
M65.269 Calcific tendinitis, unspecified lower leg
M65.27 Calcific tendinitis, ankle and foot
M65.271 Calcific tendinitis, right ankle and foot
M65.272 Calcific tendinitis, left ankle and foot
M65.279 Calcific tendinitis, unspecified ankle and foot
M65.28 Calcific tendinitis, other site
M65.29 Calcific tendinitis, multiple sites
M65.3 Trigger finger
Nodular tendinous disease
M65.30 Trigger finger, unspecified finger
M65.31 Trigger thumb
M65.311 Trigger thumb, right thumb
M65.312 Trigger thumb, left thumb
M65.319 Trigger thumb, unspecified thumb
M65.32 Trigger finger, index finger
M65.321 Trigger finger, right index finger
M65.322 Trigger finger, left index finger
M65.329 Trigger finger, unspecified index finger
M65.33 Trigger finger, middle finger
M65.331 Trigger finger, right middle finger
M65.332 Trigger finger, left middle finger
M65.339 Trigger finger, unspecified middle finger
M65.34 Trigger finger, ring finger
M65.341 Trigger finger, right ring finger
M65.342 Trigger finger, left ring finger
M65.349 Trigger finger, unspecified ring finger
M65.35 Trigger finger, little finger
M65.351 Trigger finger, right little finger
M65.352 Trigger finger, left little finger
M65.359 Trigger finger, unspecified little finger
M65.4 Radial styloid tenosynovitis [de Quervain]
M65.8 Other synovitis and tenosynovitis
M65.80 Other synovitis and tenosynovitis, unspecified site
M65.81 Other synovitis and tenosynovitis, shoulder
M65.811 Other synovitis and tenosynovitis, right shoulder
M65.812 Other synovitis and tenosynovitis, left shoulder
M65.819 Other synovitis and tenosynovitis, unspecified shoulder
M65.82 Other synovitis and tenosynovitis, upper arm
M65.821 Other synovitis and tenosynovitis, right upper arm
M65.822 Other synovitis and tenosynovitis, left upper arm
M65.829 Other synovitis and tenosynovitis, unspecified upper arm
M65.83 Other synovitis and tenosynovitis, forearm
M65.831 Other synovitis and tenosynovitis, right forearm
M65.832 Other synovitis and tenosynovitis, left forearm
M65.839 Other synovitis and tenosynovitis, unspecified forearm
M65.84 Other synovitis and tenosynovitis, hand
M65.841 Other synovitis and tenosynovitis, right hand
M65.842 Other synovitis and tenosynovitis, left hand
M65.849 Other synovitis and tenosynovitis, unspecified hand
M65.85 Other synovitis and tenosynovitis, thigh
M65.851 Other synovitis and tenosynovitis, right thigh
M65.852 Other synovitis and tenosynovitis, left thigh
M65.859 Other synovitis and tenosynovitis, unspecified thigh
M65.86 Other synovitis and tenosynovitis, lower leg
M65.861 Other synovitis and tenosynovitis, right lower leg
M65.862 Other synovitis and tenosynovitis, left lower leg
M65.869 Other synovitis and tenosynovitis, unspecified lower leg
M65.87 Other synovitis and tenosynovitis, ankle and foot
M65.871 Other synovitis and tenosynovitis, right ankle and foot
M65.872 Other synovitis and tenosynovitis, left ankle and foot
M65.879 Other synovitis and tenosynovitis, unspecified ankle and foot

M65.88 Other synovitis and tenosynovitis, other site
M65.89 Other synovitis and tenosynovitis, multiple sites

M65.9 Synovitis and tenosynovitis, unspecified
M65.90 Unspecified synovitis and tenosynovitis, unspecified site
M65.91 Unspecified synovitis and tenosynovitis, shoulder
M65.911 Unspecified synovitis and tenosynovitis, right shoulder
M65.912 Unspecified synovitis and tenosynovitis, left shoulder
M65.919 Unspecified synovitis and tenosynovitis, unspecified shoulder
M65.92 Unspecified synovitis and tenosynovitis, upper arm
M65.921 Unspecified synovitis and tenosynovitis, right upper arm
M65.922 Unspecified synovitis and tenosynovitis, left upper arm
M65.929 Unspecified synovitis and tenosynovitis, unspecified upper arm
M65.93 Unspecified synovitis and tenosynovitis, forearm
M65.931 Unspecified synovitis and tenosynovitis, right forearm
M65.932 Unspecified synovitis and tenosynovitis, left forearm
M65.939 Unspecified synovitis and tenosynovitis, unspecified forearm
M65.94 Unspecified synovitis and tenosynovitis, hand
M65.941 Unspecified synovitis and tenosynovitis, right hand
M65.942 Unspecified synovitis and tenosynovitis, left hand
M65.949 Unspecified synovitis and tenosynovitis, unspecified hand
M65.95 Unspecified synovitis and tenosynovitis, thigh
M65.951 Unspecified synovitis and tenosynovitis, right thigh
M65.952 Unspecified synovitis and tenosynovitis, left thigh
M65.959 Unspecified synovitis and tenosynovitis, unspecified thigh
M65.96 Unspecified synovitis and tenosynovitis, lower leg
M65.961 Unspecified synovitis and tenosynovitis, right lower leg
M65.962 Unspecified synovitis and tenosynovitis, left lower leg
M65.969 Unspecified synovitis and tenosynovitis, unspecified lower leg
M65.97 Unspecified synovitis and tenosynovitis, ankle and foot
M65.971 Unspecified synovitis and tenosynovitis, right ankle and foot
M65.972 Unspecified synovitis and tenosynovitis, left ankle and foot
M65.979 Unspecified synovitis and tenosynovitis, unspecified ankle and foot
M65.98 Unspecified synovitis and tenosynovitis, other site
M65.99 Unspecified synovitis and tenosynovitis, multiple sites

M66 Spontaneous rupture of synovium and tendon

Includes rupture that occurs when a normal force is applied to tissues that are inferred to have less than normal strength

Excludes2 rotator cuff syndrome (M75.1-)
rupture where an abnormal force is applied to normal tissue - see injury of tendon by body region

M66.0 Rupture of popliteal cyst

M66.1 Rupture of synovium
Rupture of synovial cyst
Excludes2 rupture of popliteal cyst (M66.0)
M66.10 Rupture of synovium, unspecified joint
M66.11 Rupture of synovium, shoulder
M66.111 Rupture of synovium, right shoulder
M66.112 Rupture of synovium, left shoulder
M66.119 Rupture of synovium, unspecified shoulder
M66.12 Rupture of synovium, elbow
M66.121 Rupture of synovium, right elbow
M66.122 Rupture of synovium, left elbow
M66.129 Rupture of synovium, unspecified elbow
M66.13 Rupture of synovium, wrist
M66.131 Rupture of synovium, right wrist
M66.132 Rupture of synovium, left wrist
M66.139 Rupture of synovium, unspecified wrist
M66.14 Rupture of synovium, hand and fingers
M66.141 Rupture of synovium, right hand
M66.142 Rupture of synovium, left hand
M66.143 Rupture of synovium, unspecified hand
M66.144 Rupture of synovium, right finger(s)
M66.145 Rupture of synovium, left finger(s)
M66.146 Rupture of synovium, unspecified finger(s)
M66.15 Rupture of synovium, hip
M66.151 Rupture of synovium, right hip
M66.152 Rupture of synovium, left hip
M66.159 Rupture of synovium, unspecified hip
M66.17 Rupture of synovium, ankle, foot and toes
M66.171 Rupture of synovium, right ankle
M66.172 Rupture of synovium, left ankle
M66.173 Rupture of synovium, unspecified ankle
M66.174 Rupture of synovium, right foot
M66.175 Rupture of synovium, left foot
M66.176 Rupture of synovium, unspecified foot
M66.177 Rupture of synovium, right toe(s)
M66.178 Rupture of synovium, left toe(s)
M66.179 Rupture of synovium, unspecified toe(s)
M66.18 Rupture of synovium, other site

M66.2 Spontaneous rupture of extensor tendons
M66.20 Spontaneous rupture of extensor tendons, unspecified site
M66.21 Spontaneous rupture of extensor tendons, shoulder
M66.211 Spontaneous rupture of extensor tendons, right shoulder
M66.212 Spontaneous rupture of extensor tendons, left shoulder
M66.219 Spontaneous rupture of extensor tendons, unspecified shoulder

CHAPTER 13 (M00-M99)

● M66.22 Spontaneous rupture of extensor tendons, upper arm
M66.221 Spontaneous rupture of extensor tendons, right upper arm
M66.222 Spontaneous rupture of extensor tendons, left upper arm
M66.229 Spontaneous rupture of extensor tendons, unspecified upper arm
● M66.23 Spontaneous rupture of extensor tendons, forearm
M66.231 Spontaneous rupture of extensor tendons, right forearm
M66.232 Spontaneous rupture of extensor tendons, left forearm
M66.239 Spontaneous rupture of extensor tendons, unspecified forearm
● M66.24 Spontaneous rupture of extensor tendons, hand
M66.241 Spontaneous rupture of extensor tendons, right hand
M66.242 Spontaneous rupture of extensor tendons, left hand
M66.249 Spontaneous rupture of extensor tendons, unspecified hand
● M66.25 Spontaneous rupture of extensor tendons, thigh
M66.251 Spontaneous rupture of extensor tendons, right thigh
M66.252 Spontaneous rupture of extensor tendons, left thigh
M66.259 Spontaneous rupture of extensor tendons, unspecified thigh
● M66.26 Spontaneous rupture of extensor tendons, lower leg
M66.261 Spontaneous rupture of extensor tendons, right lower leg
M66.262 Spontaneous rupture of extensor tendons, left lower leg
M66.269 Spontaneous rupture of extensor tendons, unspecified lower leg
● M66.27 Spontaneous rupture of extensor tendons, ankle and foot
M66.271 Spontaneous rupture of extensor tendons, right ankle and foot
M66.272 Spontaneous rupture of extensor tendons, left ankle and foot
M66.279 Spontaneous rupture of extensor tendons, unspecified ankle and foot
M66.28 Spontaneous rupture of extensor tendons, other site
M66.29 Spontaneous rupture of extensor tendons, multiple sites
● M66.3 Spontaneous rupture of flexor tendons
M66.30 Spontaneous rupture of flexor tendons, unspecified site
● M66.31 Spontaneous rupture of flexor tendons, shoulder
M66.311 Spontaneous rupture of flexor tendons, right shoulder
M66.312 Spontaneous rupture of flexor tendons, left shoulder
M66.319 Spontaneous rupture of flexor tendons, unspecified shoulder
● M66.32 Spontaneous rupture of flexor tendons, upper arm
M66.321 Spontaneous rupture of flexor tendons, right upper arm
M66.322 Spontaneous rupture of flexor tendons, left upper arm
M66.329 Spontaneous rupture of flexor tendons, unspecified upper arm
● M66.33 Spontaneous rupture of flexor tendons, forearm
M66.331 Spontaneous rupture of flexor tendons, right forearm
M66.332 Spontaneous rupture of flexor tendons, left forearm
M66.339 Spontaneous rupture of flexor tendons, unspecified forearm
● M66.34 Spontaneous rupture of flexor tendons, hand
M66.341 Spontaneous rupture of flexor tendons, right hand
M66.342 Spontaneous rupture of flexor tendons, left hand
M66.349 Spontaneous rupture of flexor tendons, unspecified hand
● M66.35 Spontaneous rupture of flexor tendons, thigh
M66.351 Spontaneous rupture of flexor tendons, right thigh
M66.352 Spontaneous rupture of flexor tendons, left thigh
M66.359 Spontaneous rupture of flexor tendons, unspecified thigh
● M66.36 Spontaneous rupture of flexor tendons, lower leg
M66.361 Spontaneous rupture of flexor tendons, right lower leg
M66.362 Spontaneous rupture of flexor tendons, left lower leg
M66.369 Spontaneous rupture of flexor tendons, unspecified lower leg
● M66.37 Spontaneous rupture of flexor tendons, ankle and foot
M66.371 Spontaneous rupture of flexor tendons, right ankle and foot
M66.372 Spontaneous rupture of flexor tendons, left ankle and foot
M66.379 Spontaneous rupture of flexor tendons, unspecified ankle and foot
M66.38 Spontaneous rupture of flexor tendons, other site
M66.39 Spontaneous rupture of flexor tendons, multiple sites
● M66.8 Spontaneous rupture of other tendons
M66.80 Spontaneous rupture of other tendons, unspecified site
● M66.81 Spontaneous rupture of other tendons, shoulder
M66.811 Spontaneous rupture of other tendons, right shoulder
M66.812 Spontaneous rupture of other tendons, left shoulder
M66.819 Spontaneous rupture of other tendons, unspecified shoulder
● M66.82 Spontaneous rupture of other tendons, upper arm
M66.821 Spontaneous rupture of other tendons, right upper arm
M66.822 Spontaneous rupture of other tendons, left upper arm
M66.829 Spontaneous rupture of other tendons, unspecified upper arm
● M66.83 Spontaneous rupture of other tendons, forearm
M66.831 Spontaneous rupture of other tendons, right forearm
M66.832 Spontaneous rupture of other tendons, left forearm
M66.839 Spontaneous rupture of other tendons, unspecified forearm

CHAPTER 13 (M00-M99)

New | Revised | ~~deleted~~ Deleted | Excludes 1 | Excludes 2 | Includes | Use additional | Code first | Code also | Key words
OGCR Official Guidelines | ● Unacceptable Principal Diagnosis | X Assign placeholder X | ● Use Additional Character(s) | Manifestation Code | Coding Clinic

● M66.84 Spontaneous rupture of other tendons, hand
M66.841 Spontaneous rupture of other tendons, right hand
M66.842 Spontaneous rupture of other tendons, left hand
M66.849 Spontaneous rupture of other tendons, unspecified hand
● M66.85 Spontaneous rupture of other tendons, thigh
M66.851 Spontaneous rupture of other tendons, right thigh
M66.852 Spontaneous rupture of other tendons, left thigh
M66.859 Spontaneous rupture of other tendons, unspecified thigh
● M66.86 Spontaneous rupture of other tendons, lower leg
M66.861 Spontaneous rupture of other tendons, right lower leg
M66.862 Spontaneous rupture of other tendons, left lower leg
M66.869 Spontaneous rupture of other tendons, unspecified lower leg
● M66.87 Spontaneous rupture of other tendons, ankle and foot
M66.871 Spontaneous rupture of other tendons, right ankle and foot
M66.872 Spontaneous rupture of other tendons, left ankle and foot
M66.879 Spontaneous rupture of other tendons, unspecified ankle and foot
M66.88 Spontaneous rupture of other tendons, other sites
M66.89 Spontaneous rupture of other tendons, multiple sites
M66.9 Spontaneous rupture of unspecified tendon
Rupture at musculotendinous junction, nontraumatic

● **M67 Other disorders of synovium and tendon**

Excludes1 palmar fascial fibromatosis [Dupuytren] (M72.Ø)
tendinitis NOS (M77.9-)
xanthomatosis localized to tendons (E78.2)

● M67.Ø Short Achilles tendon (acquired)
M67.ØØ Short Achilles tendon (acquired), unspecified ankle
M67.Ø1 Short Achilles tendon (acquired), right ankle
M67.Ø2 Short Achilles tendon (acquired), left ankle
● M67.2 Synovial hypertrophy, not elsewhere classified
Excludes1 villonodular synovitis (pigmented) (M12.2-)
M67.2Ø Synovial hypertrophy, not elsewhere classified, unspecified site
● M67.21 Synovial hypertrophy, not elsewhere classified, shoulder
M67.211 Synovial hypertrophy, not elsewhere classified, right shoulder
M67.212 Synovial hypertrophy, not elsewhere classified, left shoulder
M67.219 Synovial hypertrophy, not elsewhere classified, unspecified shoulder
● M67.22 Synovial hypertrophy, not elsewhere classified, upper arm
M67.221 Synovial hypertrophy, not elsewhere classified, right upper arm
M67.222 Synovial hypertrophy, not elsewhere classified, left upper arm
M67.229 Synovial hypertrophy, not elsewhere classified, unspecified upper arm
● M67.23 Synovial hypertrophy, not elsewhere classified, forearm
M67.231 Synovial hypertrophy, not elsewhere classified, right forearm
M67.232 Synovial hypertrophy, not elsewhere classified, left forearm
M67.239 Synovial hypertrophy, not elsewhere classified, unspecified forearm
● M67.24 Synovial hypertrophy, not elsewhere classified, hand
M67.241 Synovial hypertrophy, not elsewhere classified, right hand
M67.242 Synovial hypertrophy, not elsewhere classified, left hand
M67.249 Synovial hypertrophy, not elsewhere classified, unspecified hand
● M67.25 Synovial hypertrophy, not elsewhere classified, thigh
M67.251 Synovial hypertrophy, not elsewhere classified, right thigh
M67.252 Synovial hypertrophy, not elsewhere classified, left thigh
M67.259 Synovial hypertrophy, not elsewhere classified, unspecified thigh
● M67.26 Synovial hypertrophy, not elsewhere classified, lower leg
M67.261 Synovial hypertrophy, not elsewhere classified, right lower leg
M67.262 Synovial hypertrophy, not elsewhere classified, left lower leg
M67.269 Synovial hypertrophy, not elsewhere classified, unspecified lower leg
● M67.27 Synovial hypertrophy, not elsewhere classified, ankle and foot
M67.271 Synovial hypertrophy, not elsewhere classified, right ankle and foot
M67.272 Synovial hypertrophy, not elsewhere classified, left ankle and foot
M67.279 Synovial hypertrophy, not elsewhere classified, unspecified ankle and foot
M67.28 Synovial hypertrophy, not elsewhere classified, other site
M67.29 Synovial hypertrophy, not elsewhere classified, multiple sites
● M67.3 Transient synovitis
Toxic synovitis
Excludes1 palindromic rheumatism (M12.3-)
M67.3Ø Transient synovitis, unspecified site
● M67.31 Transient synovitis, shoulder
M67.311 Transient synovitis, right shoulder
M67.312 Transient synovitis, left shoulder
M67.319 Transient synovitis, unspecified shoulder
● M67.32 Transient synovitis, elbow
M67.321 Transient synovitis, right elbow
M67.322 Transient synovitis, left elbow
M67.329 Transient synovitis, unspecified elbow
● M67.33 Transient synovitis, wrist
M67.331 Transient synovitis, right wrist
M67.332 Transient synovitis, left wrist
M67.339 Transient synovitis, unspecified wrist
● M67.34 Transient synovitis, hand
M67.341 Transient synovitis, right hand
M67.342 Transient synovitis, left hand
M67.349 Transient synovitis, unspecified hand

M67.35 Transient synovitis, hip
M67.351 Transient synovitis, right hip
M67.352 Transient synovitis, left hip
M67.359 Transient synovitis, unspecified hip
M67.36 Transient synovitis, knee
M67.361 Transient synovitis, right knee
M67.362 Transient synovitis, left knee
M67.369 Transient synovitis, unspecified knee
M67.37 Transient synovitis, ankle and foot
M67.371 Transient synovitis, right ankle and foot
M67.372 Transient synovitis, left ankle and foot
M67.379 Transient synovitis, unspecified ankle and foot
M67.38 Transient synovitis, other site
M67.39 Transient synovitis, multiple sites
M67.4 Ganglion
Ganglion of joint or tendon (sheath)
Excludes1 ganglion in yaws (A66.6)
Excludes2 cyst of bursa (M71.2-M71.3)
cyst of synovium (M71.2-M71.3)
M67.40 Ganglion, unspecified site
M67.41 Ganglion, shoulder
M67.411 Ganglion, right shoulder
M67.412 Ganglion, left shoulder
M67.419 Ganglion, unspecified shoulder
M67.42 Ganglion, elbow
M67.421 Ganglion, right elbow
M67.422 Ganglion, left elbow
M67.429 Ganglion, unspecified elbow
M67.43 Ganglion, wrist
M67.431 Ganglion, right wrist
M67.432 Ganglion, left wrist
M67.439 Ganglion, unspecified wrist
M67.44 Ganglion, hand
M67.441 Ganglion, right hand
M67.442 Ganglion, left hand
M67.449 Ganglion, unspecified hand
M67.45 Ganglion, hip
M67.451 Ganglion, right hip
M67.452 Ganglion, left hip
M67.459 Ganglion, unspecified hip
M67.46 Ganglion, knee
M67.461 Ganglion, right knee
M67.462 Ganglion, left knee
M67.469 Ganglion, unspecified knee
M67.47 Ganglion, ankle and foot
M67.471 Ganglion, right ankle and foot
M67.472 Ganglion, left ankle and foot
M67.479 Ganglion, unspecified ankle and foot
M67.48 Ganglion, other site
M67.49 Ganglion, multiple sites
M67.5 Plica syndrome
Plica knee
M67.50 Plica syndrome, unspecified knee
M67.51 Plica syndrome, right knee
M67.52 Plica syndrome, left knee
M67.8 Other specified disorders of synovium and tendon
M67.80 Other specified disorders of synovium and tendon, unspecified site
M67.81 Other specified disorders of synovium and tendon, shoulder
M67.811 Other specified disorders of synovium, right shoulder
M67.812 Other specified disorders of synovium, left shoulder
M67.813 Other specified disorders of tendon, right shoulder
M67.814 Other specified disorders of tendon, left shoulder
M67.819 Other specified disorders of synovium and tendon, unspecified shoulder
M67.82 Other specified disorders of synovium and tendon, elbow
M67.821 Other specified disorders of synovium, right elbow
M67.822 Other specified disorders of synovium, left elbow
M67.823 Other specified disorders of tendon, right elbow
M67.824 Other specified disorders of tendon, left elbow
M67.829 Other specified disorders of synovium and tendon, unspecified elbow
M67.83 Other specified disorders of synovium and tendon, wrist
M67.831 Other specified disorders of synovium, right wrist
M67.832 Other specified disorders of synovium, left wrist
M67.833 Other specified disorders of tendon, right wrist
M67.834 Other specified disorders of tendon, left wrist
M67.839 Other specified disorders of synovium and tendon, unspecified wrist
M67.84 Other specified disorders of synovium and tendon, hand
M67.841 Other specified disorders of synovium, right hand
M67.842 Other specified disorders of synovium, left hand
M67.843 Other specified disorders of tendon, right hand
M67.844 Other specified disorders of tendon, left hand
M67.849 Other specified disorders of synovium and tendon, unspecified hand
M67.85 Other specified disorders of synovium and tendon, hip
M67.851 Other specified disorders of synovium, right hip
M67.852 Other specified disorders of synovium, left hip
M67.853 Other specified disorders of tendon, right hip
M67.854 Other specified disorders of tendon, left hip
M67.859 Other specified disorders of synovium and tendon, unspecified hip
M67.86 Other specified disorders of synovium and tendon, knee
M67.861 Other specified disorders of synovium, right knee
M67.862 Other specified disorders of synovium, left knee
M67.863 Other specified disorders of tendon, right knee
M67.864 Other specified disorders of tendon, left knee
M67.869 Other specified disorders of synovium and tendon, unspecified knee

M67.87 Other specified disorders of synovium and tendon, ankle and foot
- M67.871 Other specified disorders of synovium, right ankle and foot
- M67.872 Other specified disorders of synovium, left ankle and foot
- M67.873 Other specified disorders of tendon, right ankle and foot
- M67.874 Other specified disorders of tendon, left ankle and foot
- M67.879 Other specified disorders of synovium and tendon, unspecified ankle and foot

M67.88 Other specified disorders of synovium and tendon, other site

M67.89 Other specified disorders of synovium and tendon, multiple sites

M67.9 Unspecified disorder of synovium and tendon

M67.90 Unspecified disorder of synovium and tendon, unspecified site

M67.91 Unspecified disorder of synovium and tendon, shoulder
- M67.911 Unspecified disorder of synovium and tendon, right shoulder
- M67.912 Unspecified disorder of synovium and tendon, left shoulder
- M67.919 Unspecified disorder of synovium and tendon, unspecified shoulder

M67.92 Unspecified disorder of synovium and tendon, upper arm
- M67.921 Unspecified disorder of synovium and tendon, right upper arm
- M67.922 Unspecified disorder of synovium and tendon, left upper arm
- M67.929 Unspecified disorder of synovium and tendon, unspecified upper arm

M67.93 Unspecified disorder of synovium and tendon, forearm
- M67.931 Unspecified disorder of synovium and tendon, right forearm
- M67.932 Unspecified disorder of synovium and tendon, left forearm
- M67.939 Unspecified disorder of synovium and tendon, unspecified forearm

M67.94 Unspecified disorder of synovium and tendon, hand
- M67.941 Unspecified disorder of synovium and tendon, right hand
- M67.942 Unspecified disorder of synovium and tendon, left hand
- M67.949 Unspecified disorder of synovium and tendon, unspecified hand

M67.95 Unspecified disorder of synovium and tendon, thigh
- M67.951 Unspecified disorder of synovium and tendon, right thigh
- M67.952 Unspecified disorder of synovium and tendon, left thigh
- M67.959 Unspecified disorder of synovium and tendon, unspecified thigh

M67.96 Unspecified disorder of synovium and tendon, lower leg
- M67.961 Unspecified disorder of synovium and tendon, right lower leg
- M67.962 Unspecified disorder of synovium and tendon, left lower leg
- M67.969 Unspecified disorder of synovium and tendon, unspecified lower leg

M67.97 Unspecified disorder of synovium and tendon, ankle and foot
- M67.971 Unspecified disorder of synovium and tendon, right ankle and foot
- M67.972 Unspecified disorder of synovium and tendon, left ankle and foot
- M67.979 Unspecified disorder of synovium and tendon, unspecified ankle and foot

M67.98 Unspecified disorder of synovium and tendon, other site

M67.99 Unspecified disorder of synovium and tendon, multiple sites

OTHER SOFT TISSUE DISORDERS (M70-M79)

M70 Soft tissue disorders related to use, overuse and pressure

Includes soft tissue disorders of occupational origin

Use additional external cause code to identify activity causing disorder (Y93.-)

Excludes1 bursitis NOS (M71.9-)

Excludes2 bursitis of shoulder (M75.5)
enthesopathies (M76-M77)
pressure ulcer (pressure area) (L89.-)

M70.0 Crepitant synovitis (acute) (chronic) of hand and wrist

M70.03 Crepitant synovitis (acute) (chronic), wrist
- M70.031 Crepitant synovitis (acute) (chronic), right wrist
- M70.032 Crepitant synovitis (acute) (chronic), left wrist
- M70.039 Crepitant synovitis (acute) (chronic), unspecified wrist

M70.04 Crepitant synovitis (acute) (chronic), hand
- M70.041 Crepitant synovitis (acute) (chronic), right hand
- M70.042 Crepitant synovitis (acute) (chronic), left hand
- M70.049 Crepitant synovitis (acute) (chronic), unspecified hand

M70.1 Bursitis of hand
- M70.10 Bursitis, unspecified hand
- M70.11 Bursitis, right hand
- M70.12 Bursitis, left hand

M70.2 Olecranon bursitis
- M70.20 Olecranon bursitis, unspecified elbow
- M70.21 Olecranon bursitis, right elbow
- M70.22 Olecranon bursitis, left elbow

M70.3 Other bursitis of elbow
- M70.30 Other bursitis of elbow, unspecified elbow
- M70.31 Other bursitis of elbow, right elbow
- M70.32 Other bursitis of elbow, left elbow

M70.4 Prepatellar bursitis
- M70.40 Prepatellar bursitis, unspecified knee
- M70.41 Prepatellar bursitis, right knee
- M70.42 Prepatellar bursitis, left knee

M70.5 Other bursitis of knee
- M70.50 Other bursitis of knee, unspecified knee
- M70.51 Other bursitis of knee, right knee
- M70.52 Other bursitis of knee, left knee

M70.6 Trochanteric bursitis
Trochanteric tendinitis
- M70.60 Trochanteric bursitis, unspecified hip
- M70.61 Trochanteric bursitis, right hip
- M70.62 Trochanteric bursitis, left hip

M70.7 Other bursitis of hip
Ischial bursitis
- M70.70 Other bursitis of hip, unspecified hip
- M70.71 Other bursitis of hip, right hip
- M70.72 Other bursitis of hip, left hip

CHAPTER 13 (M00-M99)

● M70.8 Other soft tissue disorders related to use, overuse and pressure
- M70.80 Other soft tissue disorders related to use, overuse and pressure of unspecified site
- ● M70.81 Other soft tissue disorders related to use, overuse and pressure of shoulder
  - M70.811 Other soft tissue disorders related to use, overuse and pressure, right shoulder
  - M70.812 Other soft tissue disorders related to use, overuse and pressure, left shoulder
  - M70.819 Other soft tissue disorders related to use, overuse and pressure, unspecified shoulder
- ● M70.82 Other soft tissue disorders related to use, overuse and pressure of upper arm
  - M70.821 Other soft tissue disorders related to use, overuse and pressure, right upper arm
  - M70.822 Other soft tissue disorders related to use, overuse and pressure, left upper arm
  - M70.829 Other soft tissue disorders related to use, overuse and pressure, unspecified upper arms
- ● M70.83 Other soft tissue disorders related to use, overuse and pressure of forearm
  - M70.831 Other soft tissue disorders related to use, overuse and pressure, right forearm
  - M70.832 Other soft tissue disorders related to use, overuse and pressure, left forearm
  - M70.839 Other soft tissue disorders related to use, overuse and pressure, unspecified forearm
- ● M70.84 Other soft tissue disorders related to use, overuse and pressure of hand
  - M70.841 Other soft tissue disorders related to use, overuse and pressure, right hand
  - M70.842 Other soft tissue disorders related to use, overuse and pressure, left hand
  - M70.849 Other soft tissue disorders related to use, overuse and pressure, unspecified hand
- ● M70.85 Other soft tissue disorders related to use, overuse and pressure of thigh
  - M70.851 Other soft tissue disorders related to use, overuse and pressure, right thigh
  - M70.852 Other soft tissue disorders related to use, overuse and pressure, left thigh
  - M70.859 Other soft tissue disorders related to use, overuse and pressure, unspecified thigh
- ● M70.86 Other soft tissue disorders related to use, overuse and pressure lower leg
  - M70.861 Other soft tissue disorders related to use, overuse and pressure, right lower leg
  - M70.862 Other soft tissue disorders related to use, overuse and pressure, left lower leg
  - M70.869 Other soft tissue disorders related to use, overuse and pressure, unspecified leg
- ● M70.87 Other soft tissue disorders related to use, overuse and pressure of ankle and foot
  - M70.871 Other soft tissue disorders related to use, overuse and pressure, right ankle and foot
  - M70.872 Other soft tissue disorders related to use, overuse and pressure, left ankle and foot
  - M70.879 Other soft tissue disorders related to use, overuse and pressure, unspecified ankle and foot
- M70.88 Other soft tissue disorders related to use, overuse and pressure other site
- M70.89 Other soft tissue disorders related to use, overuse and pressure multiple sites

● M70.9 Unspecified soft tissue disorder related to use, overuse and pressure
- M70.90 Unspecified soft tissue disorder related to use, overuse and pressure of unspecified site
- ● M70.91 Unspecified soft tissue disorder related to use, overuse and pressure of shoulder
  - M70.911 Unspecified soft tissue disorder related to use, overuse and pressure, right shoulder
  - M70.912 Unspecified soft tissue disorder related to use, overuse and pressure, left shoulder
  - M70.919 Unspecified soft tissue disorder related to use, overuse and pressure, unspecified shoulder
- ● M70.92 Unspecified soft tissue disorder related to use, overuse and pressure of upper arm
  - M70.921 Unspecified soft tissue disorder related to use, overuse and pressure, right upper arm
  - M70.922 Unspecified soft tissue disorder related to use, overuse and pressure, left upper arm
  - M70.929 Unspecified soft tissue disorder related to use, overuse and pressure, unspecified upper arm
- ● M70.93 Unspecified soft tissue disorder related to use, overuse and pressure of forearm
  - M70.931 Unspecified soft tissue disorder related to use, overuse and pressure, right forearm
  - M70.932 Unspecified soft tissue disorder related to use, overuse and pressure, left forearm
  - M70.939 Unspecified soft tissue disorder related to use, overuse and pressure, unspecified forearm
- ● M70.94 Unspecified soft tissue disorder related to use, overuse and pressure of hand
  - M70.941 Unspecified soft tissue disorder related to use, overuse and pressure, right hand
  - M70.942 Unspecified soft tissue disorder related to use, overuse and pressure, left hand
  - M70.949 Unspecified soft tissue disorder related to use, overuse and pressure, unspecified hand
- ● M70.95 Unspecified soft tissue disorder related to use, overuse and pressure of thigh
  - M70.951 Unspecified soft tissue disorder related to use, overuse and pressure, right thigh
  - M70.952 Unspecified soft tissue disorder related to use, overuse and pressure, left thigh
  - M70.959 Unspecified soft tissue disorder related to use, overuse and pressure, unspecified thigh

M70.96 Unspecified soft tissue disorder related to use, overuse and pressure lower leg
- M70.961 Unspecified soft tissue disorder related to use, overuse and pressure, right lower leg
- M70.962 Unspecified soft tissue disorder related to use, overuse and pressure, left lower leg
- M70.969 Unspecified soft tissue disorder related to use, overuse and pressure, unspecified lower leg

M70.97 Unspecified soft tissue disorder related to use, overuse and pressure of ankle and foot
- M70.971 Unspecified soft tissue disorder related to use, overuse and pressure, right ankle and foot
- M70.972 Unspecified soft tissue disorder related to use, overuse and pressure, left ankle and foot
- M70.979 Unspecified soft tissue disorder related to use, overuse and pressure, unspecified ankle and foot

M70.98 Unspecified soft tissue disorder related to use, overuse and pressure other

M70.99 Unspecified soft tissue disorder related to use, overuse and pressure multiple sites

M71 Other bursopathies

Excludes1 bunion (M20.1)
bursitis related to use, overuse or pressure (M70.-)
enthesopathies (M76-M77)

M71.0 Abscess of bursa

Use additional code (B95.-, B96.-) to identify causative organism

M71.00 Abscess of bursa, unspecified site

M71.01 Abscess of bursa, shoulder
- M71.011 Abscess of bursa, right shoulder
- M71.012 Abscess of bursa, left shoulder
- M71.019 Abscess of bursa, unspecified shoulder

M71.02 Abscess of bursa, elbow
- M71.021 Abscess of bursa, right elbow
- M71.022 Abscess of bursa, left elbow
- M71.029 Abscess of bursa, unspecified elbow

M71.03 Abscess of bursa, wrist
- M71.031 Abscess of bursa, right wrist
- M71.032 Abscess of bursa, left wrist
- M71.039 Abscess of bursa, unspecified wrist

M71.04 Abscess of bursa, hand
- M71.041 Abscess of bursa, right hand
- M71.042 Abscess of bursa, left hand
- M71.049 Abscess of bursa, unspecified hand

M71.05 Abscess of bursa, hip
- M71.051 Abscess of bursa, right hip
- M71.052 Abscess of bursa, left hip
- M71.059 Abscess of bursa, unspecified hip

M71.06 Abscess of bursa, knee
- M71.061 Abscess of bursa, right knee
- M71.062 Abscess of bursa, left knee
- M71.069 Abscess of bursa, unspecified knee

M71.07 Abscess of bursa, ankle and foot
- M71.071 Abscess of bursa, right ankle and foot
- M71.072 Abscess of bursa, left ankle and foot
- M71.079 Abscess of bursa, unspecified ankle and foot

M71.08 Abscess of bursa, other site

M71.09 Abscess of bursa, multiple sites

M71.1 Other infective bursitis

Use additional code (B95.-, B96.-) to identify causative organism

M71.10 Other infective bursitis, unspecified site

M71.11 Other infective bursitis, shoulder
- M71.111 Other infective bursitis, right shoulder
- M71.112 Other infective bursitis, left shoulder
- M71.119 Other infective bursitis, unspecified shoulder

M71.12 Other infective bursitis, elbow
- M71.121 Other infective bursitis, right elbow
- M71.122 Other infective bursitis, left elbow
- M71.129 Other infective bursitis, unspecified elbow

M71.13 Other infective bursitis, wrist
- M71.131 Other infective bursitis, right wrist
- M71.132 Other infective bursitis, left wrist
- M71.139 Other infective bursitis, unspecified wrist

M71.14 Other infective bursitis, hand
- M71.141 Other infective bursitis, right hand
- M71.142 Other infective bursitis, left hand
- M71.149 Other infective bursitis, unspecified hand

M71.15 Other infective bursitis, hip
- M71.151 Other infective bursitis, right hip
- M71.152 Other infective bursitis, left hip
- M71.159 Other infective bursitis, unspecified hip

M71.16 Other infective bursitis, knee
- M71.161 Other infective bursitis, right knee
- M71.162 Other infective bursitis, left knee
- M71.169 Other infective bursitis, unspecified knee

M71.17 Other infective bursitis, ankle and foot
- M71.171 Other infective bursitis, right ankle and foot
- M71.172 Other infective bursitis, left ankle and foot
- M71.179 Other infective bursitis, unspecified ankle and foot

M71.18 Other infective bursitis, other site

M71.19 Other infective bursitis, multiple sites

M71.2 Synovial cyst of popliteal space [Baker]

Popliteal space = popliteal cavity, popliteal fossa. Depression in the posterior aspect of the knee (behind the knee).

Excludes1 synovial cyst of popliteal space with rupture (M66.0)

M71.20 Synovial cyst of popliteal space [Baker], unspecified knee

M71.21 Synovial cyst of popliteal space [Baker], right knee

M71.22 Synovial cyst of popliteal space [Baker], left knee

M71.3 Other bursal cyst

Synovial cyst NOS

Excludes1 synovial cyst with rupture (M66.1-)

M71.30 Other bursal cyst, unspecified site

M71.31 Other bursal cyst, shoulder
- M71.311 Other bursal cyst, right shoulder
- M71.312 Other bursal cyst, left shoulder
- M71.319 Other bursal cyst, unspecified shoulder

M71.32 Other bursal cyst, elbow
- M71.321 Other bursal cyst, right elbow
- M71.322 Other bursal cyst, left elbow
- M71.329 Other bursal cyst, unspecified elbow

● M71.33 Other bursal cyst, wrist
M71.331 Other bursal cyst, right wrist
M71.332 Other bursal cyst, left wrist
M71.339 Other bursal cyst, unspecified wrist
● M71.34 Other bursal cyst, hand
M71.341 Other bursal cyst, right hand
M71.342 Other bursal cyst, left hand
M71.349 Other bursal cyst, unspecified hand
● M71.35 Other bursal cyst, hip
M71.351 Other bursal cyst, right hip
M71.352 Other bursal cyst, left hip
M71.359 Other bursal cyst, unspecified hip
● M71.37 Other bursal cyst, ankle and foot
M71.371 Other bursal cyst, right ankle and foot
M71.372 Other bursal cyst, left ankle and foot
M71.379 Other bursal cyst, unspecified ankle and foot
M71.38 Other bursal cyst, other site
M71.39 Other bursal cyst, multiple sites
● M71.4 Calcium deposit in bursa
Excludes2 calcium deposit in bursa of shoulder (M75.3)
M71.40 Calcium deposit in bursa, unspecified site
● M71.42 Calcium deposit in bursa, elbow
M71.421 Calcium deposit in bursa, right elbow
M71.422 Calcium deposit in bursa, left elbow
M71.429 Calcium deposit in bursa, unspecified elbow
● M71.43 Calcium deposit in bursa, wrist
M71.431 Calcium deposit in bursa, right wrist
M71.432 Calcium deposit in bursa, left wrist
M71.439 Calcium deposit in bursa, unspecified wrist
● M71.44 Calcium deposit in bursa, hand
M71.441 Calcium deposit in bursa, right hand
M71.442 Calcium deposit in bursa, left hand
M71.449 Calcium deposit in bursa, unspecified hand
● M71.45 Calcium deposit in bursa, hip
M71.451 Calcium deposit in bursa, right hip
M71.452 Calcium deposit in bursa, left hip
M71.459 Calcium deposit in bursa, unspecified hip
● M71.46 Calcium deposit in bursa, knee
M71.461 Calcium deposit in bursa, right knee
M71.462 Calcium deposit in bursa, left knee
M71.469 Calcium deposit in bursa, unspecified knee
● M71.47 Calcium deposit in bursa, ankle and foot
M71.471 Calcium deposit in bursa, right ankle and foot
M71.472 Calcium deposit in bursa, left ankle and foot
M71.479 Calcium deposit in bursa, unspecified ankle and foot
M71.48 Calcium deposit in bursa, other site
M71.49 Calcium deposit in bursa, multiple sites
● M71.5 Other bursitis, not elsewhere classified
Excludes1 bursitis NOS (M71.9-)
Excludes2 bursitis of shoulder (M75.5)
bursitis of tibial collateral [Pellegrini-Stieda] (M76.4-)
M71.50 Other bursitis, not elsewhere classified, unspecified site
● M71.52 Other bursitis, not elsewhere classified, elbow
M71.521 Other bursitis, not elsewhere classified, right elbow
M71.522 Other bursitis, not elsewhere classified, left elbow
M71.529 Other bursitis, not elsewhere classified, unspecified elbow
● M71.53 Other bursitis, not elsewhere classified, wrist
M71.531 Other bursitis, not elsewhere classified, right wrist
M71.532 Other bursitis, not elsewhere classified, left wrist
M71.539 Other bursitis, not elsewhere classified, unspecified wrist
● M71.54 Other bursitis, not elsewhere classified, hand
M71.541 Other bursitis, not elsewhere classified, right hand
M71.542 Other bursitis, not elsewhere classified, left hand
M71.549 Other bursitis, not elsewhere classified, unspecified hand
● M71.55 Other bursitis, not elsewhere classified, hip
M71.551 Other bursitis, not elsewhere classified, right hip
M71.552 Other bursitis, not elsewhere classified, left hip
M71.559 Other bursitis, not elsewhere classified, unspecified hip
● M71.56 Other bursitis, not elsewhere classified, knee
M71.561 Other bursitis, not elsewhere classified, right knee
M71.562 Other bursitis, not elsewhere classified, left knee
M71.569 Other bursitis, not elsewhere classified, unspecified knee
● M71.57 Other bursitis, not elsewhere classified, ankle and foot
M71.571 Other bursitis, not elsewhere classified, right ankle and foot
M71.572 Other bursitis, not elsewhere classified, left ankle and foot
M71.579 Other bursitis, not elsewhere classified, unspecified ankle and foot
M71.58 Other bursitis, not elsewhere classified, other site
● M71.8 Other specified bursopathies
M71.80 Other specified bursopathies, unspecified site
● M71.81 Other specified bursopathies, shoulder
M71.811 Other specified bursopathies, right shoulder
M71.812 Other specified bursopathies, left shoulder
M71.819 Other specified bursopathies, unspecified shoulder
● M71.82 Other specified bursopathies, elbow
M71.821 Other specified bursopathies, right elbow
M71.822 Other specified bursopathies, left elbow
M71.829 Other specified bursopathies, unspecified elbow
● M71.83 Other specified bursopathies, wrist
M71.831 Other specified bursopathies, right wrist
M71.832 Other specified bursopathies, left wrist
M71.839 Other specified bursopathies, unspecified wrist

M71.84 Other specified bursopathies, hand
- M71.841 Other specified bursopathies, right hand
- M71.842 Other specified bursopathies, left hand
- M71.849 Other specified bursopathies, unspecified hand

M71.85 Other specified bursopathies, hip
- M71.851 Other specified bursopathies, right hip
- M71.852 Other specified bursopathies, left hip
- M71.859 Other specified bursopathies, unspecified hip

M71.86 Other specified bursopathies, knee
- M71.861 Other specified bursopathies, right knee
- M71.862 Other specified bursopathies, left knee
- M71.869 Other specified bursopathies, unspecified knee

M71.87 Other specified bursopathies, ankle and foot
- M71.871 Other specified bursopathies, right ankle and foot
- M71.872 Other specified bursopathies, left ankle and foot
- M71.879 Other specified bursopathies, unspecified ankle and foot

M71.88 Other specified bursopathies, other site

M71.89 Other specified bursopathies, multiple sites

M71.9 Bursopathy, unspecified
Bursitis NOS

M72 Fibroblastic disorders

Excludes2 retroperitoneal fibromatosis (D48.3)

M72.0 Palmar fascial fibromatosis [Dupuytren] A

M72.1 Knuckle pads

M72.2 Plantar fascial fibromatosis
Plantar fasciitis

M72.4 Pseudosarcomatous fibromatosis
Nodular fasciitis

M72.6 Necrotizing fasciitis (Ex) PDX 1114
Use additional code (B95.-, B96.-) to identify causative organism

M72.8 Other fibroblastic disorders
Abscess of fascia
Fasciitis NEC
Other infective fasciitis
Use additional code to (B95.-, B96.-) identify causative organism
Excludes1 diffuse (eosinophilic) fasciitis (M35.4)
necrotizing fasciitis (M72.6)
nodular fasciitis (M72.4)
perirenal fasciitis NOS (N13.5)
perirenal fasciitis with infection (N13.6)
plantar fasciitis (M72.2)

M72.9 Fibroblastic disorder, unspecified
Fasciitis NOS
Fibromatosis NOS

M75 Shoulder lesions

Excludes2 shoulder-hand syndrome (M89.0-)

M75.0 Adhesive capsulitis of shoulder
Frozen shoulder
Periarthritis of shoulder
- M75.00 Adhesive capsulitis of unspecified shoulder
- M75.01 Adhesive capsulitis of right shoulder
- M75.02 Adhesive capsulitis of left shoulder
  Coding Clinic: 2015, Q2, P23

M75.1 Rotator cuff tear or rupture, not specified as traumatic
Rotator cuff syndrome
Supraspinatus syndrome
Supraspinatus tear or rupture, not specified as traumatic
Excludes1 tear of rotator cuff, traumatic (S46.01-)
Gradual onset due to repetitive stress to rotator cuff

M75.10 Unspecified rotator cuff tear or rupture, not specified as traumatic
- M75.100 Unspecified rotator cuff tear or rupture of unspecified shoulder, not specified as traumatic
- M75.101 Unspecified rotator cuff tear or rupture of right shoulder, not specified as traumatic
- M75.102 Unspecified rotator cuff tear or rupture of left shoulder, not specified as traumatic

M75.11 Incomplete rotator cuff tear or rupture not specified as traumatic
- M75.110 Incomplete rotator cuff tear or rupture of unspecified shoulder, not specified as traumatic
- M75.111 Incomplete rotator cuff tear or rupture of right shoulder, not specified as traumatic
- M75.112 Incomplete rotator cuff tear or rupture of left shoulder, not specified as traumatic

M75.12 Complete rotator cuff tear or rupture not specified as traumatic
- M75.120 Complete rotator cuff tear or rupture of unspecified shoulder, not specified as traumatic
- M75.121 Complete rotator cuff tear or rupture of right shoulder, not specified as traumatic
- M75.122 Complete rotator cuff tear or rupture of left shoulder, not specified as traumatic

M75.2 Bicipital tendinitis
- M75.20 Bicipital tendinitis, unspecified shoulder
- M75.21 Bicipital tendinitis, right shoulder
- M75.22 Bicipital tendinitis, left shoulder

M75.3 Calcific tendinitis of shoulder
Calcified bursa of shoulder
- M75.30 Calcific tendinitis of unspecified shoulder
- M75.31 Calcific tendinitis of right shoulder
- M75.32 Calcific tendinitis of left shoulder

M75.4 Impingement syndrome of shoulder
- M75.40 Impingement syndrome of unspecified shoulder
  Coding Clinic: 2022, Q3, P18-19
- M75.41 Impingement syndrome of right shoulder
- M75.42 Impingement syndrome of left shoulder

M75.5 Bursitis of shoulder
- M75.50 Bursitis of unspecified shoulder
- M75.51 Bursitis of right shoulder
- M75.52 Bursitis of left shoulder

M75.8 Other shoulder lesions
- M75.80 Other shoulder lesions, unspecified shoulder
- M75.81 Other shoulder lesions, right shoulder
- M75.82 Other shoulder lesions, left shoulder

M75.9 Shoulder lesion, unspecified
- M75.90 Shoulder lesion, unspecified, unspecified shoulder
- M75.91 Shoulder lesion, unspecified, right shoulder
- M75.92 Shoulder lesion, unspecified, left shoulder

CHAPTER 13 (M00-M99)

● **M76 Enthesopathies, lower limb, excluding foot**
Excludes2 bursitis due to use, overuse and pressure (M7Ø.-)
enthesopathies of ankle and foot (M77.5-)

● **M76.Ø Gluteal tendinitis**
M76.ØØ Gluteal tendinitis, unspecified hip
M76.Ø1 Gluteal tendinitis, right hip
M76.Ø2 Gluteal tendinitis, left hip

● **M76.1 Psoas tendinitis**
M76.1Ø Psoas tendinitis, unspecified hip
M76.11 Psoas tendinitis, right hip
M76.12 Psoas tendinitis, left hip

● **M76.2 Iliac crest spur**
M76.2Ø Iliac crest spur, unspecified hip
M76.21 Iliac crest spur, right hip
M76.22 Iliac crest spur, left hip

● **M76.3 Iliotibial band syndrome**
M76.3Ø Iliotibial band syndrome, unspecified leg
M76.31 Iliotibial band syndrome, right leg
M76.32 Iliotibial band syndrome, left leg

● **M76.4 Tibial collateral bursitis [Pellegrini-Stieda]**
M76.4Ø Tibial collateral bursitis [Pellegrini-Stieda], unspecified leg
M76.41 Tibial collateral bursitis [Pellegrini-Stieda], right leg
M76.42 Tibial collateral bursitis [Pellegrini-Stieda], left leg

● **M76.5 Patellar tendinitis**
M76.5Ø Patellar tendinitis, unspecified knee
M76.51 Patellar tendinitis, right knee
M76.52 Patellar tendinitis, left knee

● **M76.6 Achilles tendinitis**
Achilles bursitis
M76.6Ø Achilles tendinitis, unspecified leg
M76.61 Achilles tendinitis, right leg
M76.62 Achilles tendinitis, left leg

● **M76.7 Peroneal tendinitis**
M76.7Ø Peroneal tendinitis, unspecified leg
M76.71 Peroneal tendinitis, right leg
M76.72 Peroneal tendinitis, left leg

● **M76.8 Other specified enthesopathies of lower limb, excluding foot**

● **M76.81 Anterior tibial syndrome**
M76.811 Anterior tibial syndrome, right leg
M76.812 Anterior tibial syndrome, left leg
M76.819 Anterior tibial syndrome, unspecified leg

● **M76.82 Posterior tibial tendinitis**
M76.821 Posterior tibial tendinitis, right leg
M76.822 Posterior tibial tendinitis, left leg
M76.829 Posterior tibial tendinitis, unspecified leg

● **M76.89 Other specified enthesopathies of lower limb, excluding foot**
M76.891 Other specified enthesopathies of right lower limb, excluding foot
M76.892 Other specified enthesopathies of left lower limb, excluding foot
M76.899 Other specified enthesopathies of unspecified lower limb, excluding foot

M76.9 Unspecified enthesopathy, lower limb, excluding foot

● **M77 Other enthesopathies**
Excludes1 bursitis NOS (M71.9-)
Excludes2 bursitis due to use, overuse and pressure (M7Ø.-)
osteophyte (M25.7)
spinal enthesopathy (M46.Ø-)

● **M77.Ø Medial epicondylitis**
M77.ØØ Medial epicondylitis, unspecified elbow
M77.Ø1 Medial epicondylitis, right elbow
M77.Ø2 Medial epicondylitis, left elbow

● **M77.1 Lateral epicondylitis**
Tennis elbow
M77.1Ø Lateral epicondylitis, unspecified elbow
M77.11 Lateral epicondylitis, right elbow
M77.12 Lateral epicondylitis, left elbow

● **M77.2 Periarthritis of wrist**
M77.2Ø Periarthritis, unspecified wrist
M77.21 Periarthritis, right wrist
M77.22 Periarthritis, left wrist

● **M77.3 Calcaneal spur**
M77.3Ø Calcaneal spur, unspecified foot
M77.31 Calcaneal spur, right foot
M77.32 Calcaneal spur, left foot

● **M77.4 Metatarsalgia**
Excludes1 Morton's metatarsalgia (G57.6)
M77.4Ø Metatarsalgia, unspecified foot
M77.41 Metatarsalgia, right foot
M77.42 Metatarsalgia, left foot

● **M77.5 Other enthesopathy of foot and ankle**
M77.5Ø Other enthesopathy of unspecified foot and ankle
M77.51 Other enthesopathy of right foot and ankle
M77.52 Other enthesopathy of left foot and ankle

M77.8 Other enthesopathies, not elsewhere classified

M77.9 Enthesopathy, unspecified
Bone spur NOS
Capsulitis NOS
Periarthritis NOS
Tendinitis NOS

● **M79 Other and unspecified soft tissue disorders, not elsewhere classified**
Excludes1 psychogenic rheumatism (F45.8)
soft tissue pain, psychogenic (F45.41)

M79.Ø Rheumatism, unspecified
Excludes1 fibromyalgia (M79.7)
palindromic rheumatism (M12.3-)

● **M79.1 Myalgia**
Myofascial pain syndrome
M79.1Ø Myalgia, unspecified site
M79.11 Myalgia of mastication muscle
M79.12 Myalgia of auxiliary muscles, head and neck
M79.18 Myalgia, other site
Excludes1 fibromyalgia (M79.7)
myositis (M6Ø.-)

M79.2 Neuralgia and neuritis, unspecified
Excludes1 brachial radiculitis NOS (M54.1)
lumbosacral radiculitis NOS (M54.1)
mononeuropathies (G56-G58)
radiculitis NOS (M54.1)
sciatica (M54.3-M54.4)

M79.3 Panniculitis, unspecified
Excludes1 lupus panniculitis (L93.2)
neck and back panniculitis (M54.Ø-)
relapsing [Weber-Christian] panniculitis (M35.6)
Coding Clinic: 2Ø24, Q1, P16

M79.4 Hypertrophy of (infrapatellar) fat pad

M79.5 Residual foreign body in soft tissue

Excludes1 foreign body granuloma of skin and subcutaneous tissue (L92.3)
foreign body granuloma of soft tissue (M60.2-)

M79.6 Pain in limb, hand, foot, fingers and toes

Excludes2 pain in joint (M25.5-)

M79.60 Pain in limb, unspecified

M79.601 Pain in right arm
Pain in right upper limb NOS

M79.602 Pain in left arm
Pain in left upper limb NOS

M79.603 Pain in arm, unspecified
Pain in upper limb NOS

M79.604 Pain in right leg
Pain in right lower limb NOS

M79.605 Pain in left leg
Pain in left lower limb NOS

M79.606 Pain in leg, unspecified
Pain in lower limb NOS

M79.609 Pain in unspecified limb
Pain in limb NOS

M79.62 Pain in upper arm
Pain in axillary region

M79.621 Pain in right upper arm

M79.622 Pain in left upper arm

M79.629 Pain in unspecified upper arm

M79.63 Pain in forearm

M79.631 Pain in right forearm

M79.632 Pain in left forearm

M79.639 Pain in unspecified forearm

M79.64 Pain in hand and fingers

M79.641 Pain in right hand

M79.642 Pain in left hand

M79.643 Pain in unspecified hand

M79.644 Pain in right finger(s)

M79.645 Pain in left finger(s)

M79.646 Pain in unspecified finger(s)

M79.65 Pain in thigh

M79.651 Pain in right thigh

M79.652 Pain in left thigh

M79.659 Pain in unspecified thigh

M79.66 Pain in lower leg

M79.661 Pain in right lower leg

M79.662 Pain in left lower leg

M79.669 Pain in unspecified lower leg

M79.67 Pain in foot and toes

M79.671 Pain in right foot

M79.672 Pain in left foot

M79.673 Pain in unspecified foot

M79.674 Pain in right toe(s)

M79.675 Pain in left toe(s)

M79.676 Pain in unspecified toe(s)

M79.7 Fibromyalgia
Fibromyositis
Fibrositis
Myofibrositis

M79.A Nontraumatic compartment syndrome

Code first, if applicable, associated postprocedural complication

Excludes1 compartment syndrome NOS (T79.A-)
fibromyalgia (M79.7) nontraumatic ischemic infarction of muscle (M62.2-)
traumatic compartment syndrome (T79.A-)

M79.A1 Nontraumatic compartment syndrome of upper extremity
Nontraumatic compartment syndrome of shoulder, arm, forearm, wrist, hand, and fingers

M79.A11 Nontraumatic compartment syndrome of right upper extremity Ex PDX 1256

M79.A12 Nontraumatic compartment syndrome of left upper extremity Ex PDX 1257

M79.A19 Nontraumatic compartment syndrome of unspecified upper extremity Ex PDX 1258

M79.A2 Nontraumatic compartment syndrome of lower extremity
Nontraumatic compartment syndrome of hip, buttock, thigh, leg, foot, and toes

M79.A21 Nontraumatic compartment syndrome of right lower extremity Ex PDX 1259

M79.A22 Nontraumatic compartment syndrome of left lower extremity Ex PDX 1260

M79.A29 Nontraumatic compartment syndrome of unspecified lower extremity Ex PDX 1261

M79.A3 Nontraumatic compartment syndrome of abdomen Ex PDX 1262

M79.A9 Nontraumatic compartment syndrome of other sites Ex PDX 1263

M79.8 Other specified soft tissue disorders

M79.81 Nontraumatic hematoma of soft tissue
Nontraumatic hematoma of muscle
Nontraumatic seroma of muscle and soft tissue

M79.89 Other specified soft tissue disorders
Polyalgia

M79.9 Soft tissue disorder, unspecified

OGCR See Section I.C., Chapter 13.d.

Osteoporosis

Osteoporosis is a systemic condition, meaning that all bones of the musculoskeletal system are affected. Therefore, site is not a component of the codes under category M81, Osteoporosis without current pathological fracture. The site codes under category M80, Osteoporosis with current pathological fracture, identify the site of the fracture, not the osteoporosis.

1) Osteoporosis without pathological fracture

Category M81, Osteoporosis without current pathological fracture, is for use for patients with osteoporosis who do not currently have a pathologic fracture due to the osteoporosis, even if they have had a fracture in the past. For patients with a history of osteoporosis fractures, status code Z87.310, Personal history of (healed) osteoporosis fracture, should follow the code from M81.

2) Osteoporosis with current pathological fracture

Category M80, Osteoporosis with current pathological fracture, is for patients who have a current pathologic fracture at the time of an encounter. The codes under M80 identify the site of the fracture. A code from category M80, not a traumatic fracture code, should be used for any patient with known osteoporosis who suffers a fracture, even if the patient had a minor fall or trauma, if that fall or trauma would not usually break a normal, healthy bone.

CHAPTER 13 (M00-M99)

OSTEOPATHIES AND CHONDROPATHIES (M80-M94)

DISORDERS OF BONE DENSITY AND STRUCTURE (M80-M85)

M80 Osteoporosis with current pathological fracture (Ex) PDX 1249 [A], 1264 [K, P]

Excessive skeletal fragility (porous bone) resulting in bone fractures

Includes osteoporosis with current fragility fracture

Use additional code to identify major osseous defect, if applicable (M89.7-)

Excludes1 collapsed vertebra NOS (M48.5)
pathological fracture NOS (M84.4)
wedging of vertebra NOS (M48.5)

Excludes2 personal history of (healed) osteoporosis fracture (Z87.310)

Coding Clinic: 2018, Q2, P12

The appropriate 7th character is to be added to each code from category M80:

A	initial encounter for fracture *All encounters involving diagnosis and treatment*
D	subsequent encounter for fracture with routine healing
G	subsequent encounter for fracture with delayed healing *Encounters for attention to casting or fixation devices, medication, and follow-up visits during the healing phase*
K	subsequent encounter for fracture with nonunion *Total failure of fracture healing*
P	subsequent encounter for fracture with malunion *Fracture ends do not heal together correctly.*
S	sequela

● **M80.0 Age-related osteoporosis with current pathological fracture**
Involutional osteoporosis with current pathological fracture
Osteoporosis NOS with current pathological fracture
Postmenopausal osteoporosis with current pathological fracture
Senile osteoporosis with current pathological fracture

X● **M80.00 Age-related osteoporosis with current pathological fracture, unspecified site** A, K, P A

● **M80.01 Age-related osteoporosis with current pathological fracture, shoulder**

● **M80.011 Age-related osteoporosis with current pathological fracture, right shoulder** A, K, P A

● **M80.012 Age-related osteoporosis with current pathological fracture, left shoulder** A, K, P A

● **M80.019 Age-related osteoporosis with current pathological fracture, unspecified shoulder** A, K, P A

● **M80.02 Age-related osteoporosis with current pathological fracture, humerus**

● **M80.021 Age-related osteoporosis with current pathological fracture, right humerus** A, K, P A

● **M80.022 Age-related osteoporosis with current pathological fracture, left humerus** A, K, P A

● **M80.029 Age-related osteoporosis with current pathological fracture, unspecified humerus** A, K, P A

● **M80.03 Age-related osteoporosis with current pathological fracture, forearm**
Age-related osteoporosis with current pathological fracture of wrist

● **M80.031 Age-related osteoporosis with current pathological fracture, right forearm** A, K, P A

● **M80.032 Age-related osteoporosis with current pathological fracture, left forearm** A, K, P A

● **M80.039 Age-related osteoporosis with current pathological fracture, unspecified forearm** A, K, P A

● **M80.04 Age-related osteoporosis with current pathological fracture, hand**

● **M80.041 Age-related osteoporosis with current pathological fracture, right hand** A, K, P A

● **M80.042 Age-related osteoporosis with current pathological fracture, left hand** A, K, P A

● **M80.049 Age-related osteoporosis with current pathological fracture, unspecified hand** A, K, P A

● **M80.05 Age-related osteoporosis with current pathological fracture, femur**
Age-related osteoporosis with current pathological fracture of hip

● **M80.051 Age-related osteoporosis with current pathological fracture, right femur** A, K, P, A A

● **M80.052 Age-related osteoporosis with current pathological fracture, left femur** A, K, P, A A
Coding Clinic: 2018, Q2, P12

● **M80.059 Age-related osteoporosis with current pathological fracture, unspecified femur** A, K, P, A A

● **M80.06 Age-related osteoporosis with current pathological fracture, lower leg**

● **M80.061 Age-related osteoporosis with current pathological fracture, right lower leg** A, K, P A

● **M80.062 Age-related osteoporosis with current pathological fracture, left lower leg** A, K, P A

● **M80.069 Age-related osteoporosis with current pathological fracture, unspecified lower leg** A, K, P A

● **M80.07 Age-related osteoporosis with current pathological fracture, ankle and foot**

● **M80.071 Age-related osteoporosis with current pathological fracture, right ankle and foot** A, K, P A

● **M80.072 Age-related osteoporosis with current pathological fracture, left ankle and foot** A, K, P A

● **M80.079 Age-related osteoporosis with current pathological fracture, unspecified ankle and foot** A, K, P A

X● **M80.08 Age-related osteoporosis with current pathological fracture, vertebra(e)** A, K, P, A A

M80.0A Age-related osteoporosis with current pathological fracture, other site A, D, G, K, P, S (Ex) PDX 1265 [A], 1266 [K], 1267 [P] A

- M80.0B Age-related osteoporosis with current pathological fracture, pelvis
  - M80.0B1 Age-related osteoporosis with current pathological fracture, right pelvis A, K, P (Ex) PDX 1265 [A], 1268 [K], 1269 [P]
  - M80.0B2 Age-related osteoporosis with current pathological fracture, left pelvis A, K, P (Ex) PDX 1265 [A], 1270 [K], 1271 [P]
  - M80.0B9 Age-related osteoporosis with current pathological fracture, unspecified pelvis A, K, P (Ex) PDX 1265 [A], 1272 [K], 1273 [P]

- M80.8 Other osteoporosis with current pathological fracture (Ex) PDX 1249 [A], 1264 [K, P]

  Drug-induced osteoporosis with current pathological fracture
  Idiopathic osteoporosis with current pathological fracture
  Osteoporosis of disuse with current pathological fracture
  Postoophorectomy osteoporosis with current pathological fracture
  Postsurgical malabsorption osteoporosis with current pathological fracture
  Post-traumatic osteoporosis with current pathological fracture

  Use additional code for adverse effect, if applicable, to identify drug (T36-T50 with fifth or sixth character 5)

  - X M80.80 Other osteoporosis with current pathological fracture, unspecified site A, K, P A
  - M80.81 Other osteoporosis with pathological fracture, shoulder (Ex) PDX 888 [A], 897 [K, P]
    - M80.811 Other osteoporosis with current pathological fracture, right shoulder A, K, P
    - M80.812 Other osteoporosis with current pathological fracture, left shoulder A, K, P
    - M80.819 Other osteoporosis with current pathological fracture, unspecified shoulder A, K, P
  - M80.82 Other osteoporosis with current pathological fracture, humerus
    - M80.821 Other osteoporosis with current pathological fracture, right humerus A, K, P
    - M80.822 Other osteoporosis with current pathological fracture, left humerus A, K, P
    - M80.829 Other osteoporosis with current pathological fracture, unspecified humerus A, K, P
  - M80.83 Other osteoporosis with current pathological fracture, forearm

    Other osteoporosis with current pathological fracture of wrist
    - M80.831 Other osteoporosis with current pathological fracture, right forearm A, K, P
    - M80.832 Other osteoporosis with current pathological fracture, left forearm A, K, P
    - M80.839 Other osteoporosis with current pathological fracture, unspecified forearm A, K, P
  - M80.84 Other osteoporosis with current pathological fracture, hand
    - M80.841 Other osteoporosis with current pathological fracture, right hand A, K, P
    - M80.842 Other osteoporosis with current pathological fracture, left hand A, K, P
    - M80.849 Other osteoporosis with current pathological fracture, unspecified hand A, K, P
  - M80.85 Other osteoporosis with current pathological fracture, femur

    Other osteoporosis with current pathological fracture of hip
    - M80.851 Other osteoporosis with current pathological fracture, right femur A, K, P, A
    - M80.852 Other osteoporosis with current pathological fracture, left femur A, K, P, A
    - M80.859 Other osteoporosis with current pathological fracture, unspecified femur A, K, P, A
  - M80.86 Other osteoporosis with current pathological fracture, lower leg
    - M80.861 Other osteoporosis with current pathological fracture, right lower leg A, K, P
    - M80.862 Other osteoporosis with current pathological fracture, left lower leg A, K, P
    - M80.869 Other osteoporosis with current pathological fracture, unspecified lower leg A, K, P
  - M80.87 Other osteoporosis with current pathological fracture, ankle and foot
    - M80.871 Other osteoporosis with current pathological fracture, right ankle and foot A, K, P
    - M80.872 Other osteoporosis with current pathological fracture, left ankle and foot A, K, P
    - M80.879 Other osteoporosis with current pathological fracture, unspecified ankle and foot A, K, P
  - X M80.88 Other osteoporosis with current pathological fracture, vertebra(e) A, K, P, A
  - M80.8A Other osteoporosis with current pathological fracture, other site A, K, P (Ex) PDX 1265 [A], 1267 [K, P]
  - M80.8B Other osteoporosis with current pathological fracture, pelvis
    - M80.8B1 Other osteoporosis with current pathological fracture, right pelvis A, K, P (Ex) PDX 1265 [A], 1274 [K], 1275 [P]
    - M80.8B2 Other osteoporosis with current pathological fracture, left pelvis A, K, P (Ex) PDX 1265 [A], 1276 [K], 1277 [P]
    - M80.8B9 Other osteoporosis with current pathological fracture, unspecified pelvis A, K, P (Ex) PDX 1265 [A], 1278 [K], 1279 [P]

- M81 Osteoporosis without current pathological fracture

  Use additional code to identify:
  major osseous defect, if applicable (M89.7-)
  personal history of (healed) osteoporosis fracture, if applicable (Z87.310)

  Excludes1 osteoporosis with current pathological fracture (M80.-)
  Sudeck's atrophy (M89.0)

  - M81.0 Age-related osteoporosis without current pathological fracture A

    Involutional osteoporosis without current pathological fracture
    Osteoporosis NOS
    Postmenopausal osteoporosis without current pathological fracture
    Senile osteoporosis without current pathological fracture

CHAPTER 13 (M00-M99)

N Newborn Age: 0 P Pediatric Age: 0–17 M Maternity DX: 9–64 A Adult Age: 15–124

Complication\Comorbidity Major C\C (Ex) CC/MCC Exclusions Hospital Acquired Condition Hierarchical Condition Category

M81.6 Localized osteoporosis [Lequesne]
Excludes1 Sudeck's atrophy (M89.Ø)
M81.8 Other osteoporosis without current pathological fracture
Drug-induced osteoporosis without current pathological fracture
Idiopathic osteoporosis without current pathological fracture
Osteoporosis of disuse without current pathological fracture
Postoophorectomy osteoporosis without current pathological fracture
Postsurgical malabsorption osteoporosis without current pathological fracture
Post-traumatic osteoporosis without current pathological fracture
Use additional code for adverse effect, if applicable, to identify drug (T36-T5Ø with fifth or sixth character 5)

● **M83 Adult osteomalacia**
Excludes2 infantile and juvenile osteomalacia (E55.Ø)
renal osteodystrophy (N25.Ø)
rickets (active) (E55.Ø)
rickets (active) sequelae (E64.3)
vitamin D-resistant osteomalacia (E83.31)
vitamin D-resistant rickets (active) (E83.31)

M83.Ø Puerperal osteomalacia M
M83.1 Senile osteomalacia A
M83.2 Adult osteomalacia due to malabsorption A
Postsurgical malabsorption osteomalacia in adults
M83.3 Adult osteomalacia due to malnutrition A
M83.4 Aluminum bone disease
M83.5 Other drug-induced osteomalacia in adults A
Use additional code for adverse effect, if applicable, to identify drug (T36-T5Ø with fifth or sixth character 5)
M83.8 Other adult osteomalacia A
M83.9 Adult osteomalacia, unspecified A

● **M84 Disorder of continuity of bone**
Excludes2 traumatic fracture of bone-see fracture, by site

● **M84.3 Stress fracture** Ex PDX 1264
Fatigue fracture
March fracture
Stress fracture NOS
Stress reaction
Use additional external cause code(s) to identify the cause of the stress fracture
Excludes1 pathological fracture NOS (M84.4.-)
pathological fracture due to osteoporosis (M8Ø.-)
traumatic fracture (S12.-, S22.-, S32.-, S42.-, S52.-, S62.-, S72.-, S82.-, S92.-)
Excludes2 personal history of (healed) stress (fatigue) fracture (Z87.312)
stress fracture of vertebra (M48.4-)

The appropriate 7th character is to be added to each code from subcategory M84.3:

A	initial encounter for fracture
D	subsequent encounter for fracture with routine healing
G	subsequent encounter for fracture with delayed healing
K	subsequent encounter for fracture with nonunion
P	subsequent encounter for fracture with malunion
S	sequela

X● **M84.30 Stress fracture, unspecified site** K, P
● **M84.31 Stress fracture, shoulder**
● **M84.311 Stress fracture, right shoulder** K, P
● **M84.312 Stress fracture, left shoulder** K, P
● **M84.319 Stress fracture, unspecified shoulder** K, P
● **M84.32 Stress fracture, humerus**
● **M84.321 Stress fracture, right humerus** K, P
● **M84.322 Stress fracture, left humerus** K, P
● **M84.329 Stress fracture, unspecified humerus** K, P
● **M84.33 Stress fracture, ulna and radius**
● **M84.331 Stress fracture, right ulna** K, P
● **M84.332 Stress fracture, left ulna** K, P
● **M84.333 Stress fracture, right radius** K, P
● **M84.334 Stress fracture, left radius** K, P
● **M84.339 Stress fracture, unspecified ulna and radius** K, P
● **M84.34 Stress fracture, hand and fingers**
● **M84.341 Stress fracture, right hand** K, P
● **M84.342 Stress fracture, left hand** K, P
● **M84.343 Stress fracture, unspecified hand** K, P
● **M84.344 Stress fracture, right finger(s)** K, P
● **M84.345 Stress fracture, left finger(s)** K, P
● **M84.346 Stress fracture, unspecified finger(s)** K, P
● **M84.35 Stress fracture, pelvis and femur**
Stress fracture, hip
● **M84.350 Stress fracture, pelvis** K, P
● **M84.351 Stress fracture, right femur** K, P
● **M84.352 Stress fracture, left femur** K, P
● **M84.353 Stress fracture, unspecified femur** K, P
● **M84.359 Stress fracture, hip, unspecified** K, P
● **M84.36 Stress fracture, tibia and fibula**
● **M84.361 Stress fracture, right tibia** K, P
● **M84.362 Stress fracture, left tibia** K, P
● **M84.363 Stress fracture, right fibula** K, P
● **M84.364 Stress fracture, left fibula** K, P
● **M84.369 Stress fracture, unspecified tibia and fibula** K, P
● **M84.37 Stress fracture, ankle, foot and toes**
● **M84.371 Stress fracture, right ankle** K, P
● **M84.372 Stress fracture, left ankle** K, P
● **M84.373 Stress fracture, unspecified ankle** K, P
● **M84.374 Stress fracture, right foot** K, P
● **M84.375 Stress fracture, left foot** K, P
● **M84.376 Stress fracture, unspecified foot** K, P
● **M84.377 Stress fracture, right toe(s)** K, P
● **M84.378 Stress fracture, left toe(s)** K, P
● **M84.379 Stress fracture, unspecified toe(s)** K, P
X● **M84.38 Stress fracture, other site** K, P
Excludes2 stress fracture of vertebra (M48.4-)

● **M84.4 Pathological fracture, not elsewhere classified** Ex PDX 1249 [A], 1264 [K, P]
Chronic fracture
Pathological fracture NOS
Excludes1 collapsed vertebra NEC (M48.5)
pathological fracture in neoplastic disease (M84.5-)
pathological fracture in osteoporosis (M8Ø.-)
pathological fracture in other disease (M84.6-)
stress fracture (M84.3-)
traumatic fracture (S12.-, S22.-, S32.-, S42.-, S52.-, S62.-, S72.-, S82.-, S92.-)
Excludes2 personal history of (healed) pathological fracture (Z87.311)

The appropriate 7th character is to be added to each code from subcategory M84.4:

A	initial encounter for fracture
D	subsequent encounter for fracture with routine healing
G	subsequent encounter for fracture with delayed healing
K	subsequent encounter for fracture with nonunion
P	subsequent encounter for fracture with malunion
S	sequela

X● **M84.40** **Pathological fracture, unspecified site** A, K, P

● **M84.41** **Pathological fracture, shoulder**

● **M84.411** **Pathological fracture, right shoulder** A, K, P

● **M84.412** **Pathological fracture, left shoulder** A, K, P

● **M84.419** **Pathological fracture, unspecified shoulder** A, K, P

● **M84.42** **Pathological fracture, humerus**

● **M84.421** **Pathological fracture, right humerus** A, K, P

● **M84.422** **Pathological fracture, left humerus** A, K, P

● **M84.429** **Pathological fracture, unspecified humerus** A, K, P

● **M84.43** **Pathological fracture, ulna and radius**

● **M84.431** **Pathological fracture, right ulna** A, K, P

● **M84.432** **Pathological fracture, left ulna** A, K, P

● **M84.433** **Pathological fracture, right radius** A, K, P

● **M84.434** **Pathological fracture, left radius** A, K, P

● **M84.439** **Pathological fracture, unspecified ulna and radius** A, K, P

● **M84.44** **Pathological fracture, hand and fingers**

● **M84.441** **Pathological fracture, right hand** A, K, P

● **M84.442** **Pathological fracture, left hand** A, K, P

● **M84.443** **Pathological fracture, unspecified hand** A, K, P

● **M84.444** **Pathological fracture, right finger(s)** A, K, P

● **M84.445** **Pathological fracture, left finger(s)** A, K, P

● **M84.446** **Pathological fracture, unspecified finger(s)** A, K, P

● **M84.45** **Pathological fracture, femur and pelvis**

● **M84.451** **Pathological fracture, right femur** A, K, P, A

● **M84.452** **Pathological fracture, left femur** A, K, P, A

● **M84.453** **Pathological fracture, unspecified femur** A, K, P, A

● **M84.454** **Pathological fracture, pelvis** A, K, P, A

Coding Clinic: 2016, Q4, P43

● **M84.459** **Pathological fracture, hip, unspecified** A, K, P, A

● **M84.46** **Pathological fracture, tibia and fibula**

● **M84.461** **Pathological fracture, right tibia** A, K, P

● **M84.462** **Pathological fracture, left tibia** A, K, P

● **M84.463** **Pathological fracture, right fibula** A, K, P

● **M84.464** **Pathological fracture, left fibula** A, K, P

● **M84.469** **Pathological fracture, unspecified tibia and fibula** A, K, P

● **M84.47** **Pathological fracture, ankle, foot and toes** (Ex) PDX 888 [A], 897 [K, P]

● **M84.471** **Pathological fracture, right ankle** A, K, P

● **M84.472** **Pathological fracture, left ankle** A, K, P

● **M84.473** **Pathological fracture, unspecified ankle** A, K, P

● **M84.474** **Pathological fracture, right foot** A, K, P

● **M84.475** **Pathological fracture, left foot** A, K, P

● **M84.476** **Pathological fracture, unspecified foot** A, K, P

● **M84.477** **Pathological fracture, right toe(s)** A, K, P

● **M84.478** **Pathological fracture, left toe(s)** A, K, P

● **M84.479** **Pathological fracture, unspecified toe(s)** A, K, P

X● **M84.48** **Pathological fracture, other site** A, K, P

OGCR Section I.C. 13.C.

Coding of Pathologic Fractures

7th character A is for use as long as the patient is receiving active treatment for the fracture. While the patient may be seen by a new or different provider over the course of treatment for a pathological fracture, assignment of the 7th character is based on whether the patient is undergoing active treatment and not whether the provider is seeing the patient for the first time.

7th character, D is to be used for encounters after the patient has completed active treatment for the fracture and is receiving routine care for the fracture during the healing or recovery phase. The other 7th characters, listed under each subcategory in the Tabular List, are to be used for subsequent encounters for treatment of problems associated with the healing, such as malunions, nonunions, and sequelae.

Care for complications of surgical treatment for fracture repairs during the healing or recovery phase should be coded with the appropriate complication codes.

See Section I.C.19. Coding of traumatic fractures.

● **M84.5** **Pathological fracture in neoplastic disease**

Code also underlying neoplasm

The appropriate 7th character is to be added to each code from subcategory M84.5:

A	initial encounter for fracture
D	subsequent encounter for fracture with routine healing
G	subsequent encounter for fracture with delayed healing
K	subsequent encounter for fracture with nonunion
P	subsequent encounter for fracture with malunion
S	sequela

X● **M84.50** **Pathological fracture in neoplastic disease, unspecified site** A, K, P

CHAPTER 13 (M00-M99)

M84.51 Pathological fracture in neoplastic disease, shoulder
M84.511 Pathological fracture in neoplastic disease, right shoulder A, K, P
M84.512 Pathological fracture in neoplastic disease, left shoulder A, K, P
M84.519 Pathological fracture in neoplastic disease, unspecified shoulder A, K, P
M84.52 Pathological fracture in neoplastic disease, humerus
M84.521 Pathological fracture in neoplastic disease, right humerus A, K, P
M84.522 Pathological fracture in neoplastic disease, left humerus A, K, P
M84.529 Pathological fracture in neoplastic disease, unspecified humerus A, K, P
M84.53 Pathological fracture in neoplastic disease, ulna and radius
M84.531 Pathological fracture in neoplastic disease, right ulna A, K, P
M84.532 Pathological fracture in neoplastic disease, left ulna A, K, P
M84.533 Pathological fracture in neoplastic disease, right radius A, K, P
M84.534 Pathological fracture in neoplastic disease, left radius A, K, P
M84.539 Pathological fracture in neoplastic disease, unspecified ulna and radius A, K, P
M84.54 Pathological fracture in neoplastic disease, hand
M84.541 Pathological fracture in neoplastic disease, right hand A, K, P
M84.542 Pathological fracture in neoplastic disease, left hand A, K, P
M84.549 Pathological fracture in neoplastic disease, unspecified hand A, K, P
M84.55 Pathological fracture in neoplastic disease, pelvis and femur
M84.550 Pathological fracture in neoplastic disease, pelvis A, K, P
M84.551 Pathological fracture in neoplastic disease, right femur A, K, P, A
M84.552 Pathological fracture in neoplastic disease, left femur A, K, P, A
M84.553 Pathological fracture in neoplastic disease, unspecified femur A, K, P, A
M84.559 Pathological fracture in neoplastic disease, hip, unspecified A, K, P, A
M84.56 Pathological fracture in neoplastic disease, tibia and fibula
M84.561 Pathological fracture in neoplastic disease, right tibia A, K, P
M84.562 Pathological fracture in neoplastic disease, left tibia A, K, P
M84.563 Pathological fracture in neoplastic disease, right fibula A, K, P
M84.564 Pathological fracture in neoplastic disease, left fibula A, K, P
M84.569 Pathological fracture in neoplastic disease, unspecified tibia and fibula A, K, P
M84.57 Pathological fracture in neoplastic disease, ankle and foot
M84.571 Pathological fracture in neoplastic disease, right ankle A, K, P
M84.572 Pathological fracture in neoplastic disease, left ankle A, K, P
M84.573 Pathological fracture in neoplastic disease, unspecified ankle A, K, P
M84.574 Pathological fracture in neoplastic disease, right foot A, K, P
M84.575 Pathological fracture in neoplastic disease, left foot A, K, P
M84.576 Pathological fracture in neoplastic disease, unspecified foot A, K, P
X M84.58 Pathological fracture in neoplastic disease, other specified site A, K, P
Pathological fracture in neoplastic disease, vertebrae

M84.6 Pathological fracture in other disease
Code also underlying condition
Excludes1 pathological fracture in osteoporosis (M8Ø.-)

The appropriate 7th character is to be added to each code from subcategory M84.6:

A	initial encounter for fracture
D	subsequent encounter for fracture with routine healing
G	subsequent encounter for fracture with delayed healing
K	subsequent encounter for fracture with nonunion
P	subsequent encounter for fracture with malunion
S	sequela

X M84.6Ø Pathological fracture in other disease, unspecified site A, K, P
M84.61 Pathological fracture in other disease, shoulder
M84.611 Pathological fracture in other disease, right shoulder A, K, P
M84.612 Pathological fracture in other disease, left shoulder A, K, P
M84.619 Pathological fracture in other disease, unspecified shoulder A, K, P
M84.62 Pathological fracture in other disease, humerus
M84.621 Pathological fracture in other disease, right humerus A, K, P
M84.622 Pathological fracture in other disease, left humerus A, K, P
M84.629 Pathological fracture in other disease, unspecified humerus A, K, P
M84.63 Pathological fracture in other disease, ulna and radius
M84.631 Pathological fracture in other disease, right ulna A, K, P
M84.632 Pathological fracture in other disease, left ulna A, K, P
M84.633 Pathological fracture in other disease, right radius A, K, P
M84.634 Pathological fracture in other disease, left radius A, K, P
M84.639 Pathological fracture in other disease, unspecified ulna and radius A, K, P
M84.64 Pathological fracture in other disease, hand
M84.641 Pathological fracture in other disease, right hand A, K, P
M84.642 Pathological fracture in other disease, left hand A, K, P
M84.649 Pathological fracture in other disease, unspecified hand A, K, P
M84.65 Pathological fracture in other disease, pelvis and femur
M84.65Ø Pathological fracture in other disease, pelvis A, K, P
M84.651 Pathological fracture in other disease, right femur A, K, P, A

M84.652 Pathological fracture in other disease, left femur A, K, P, A
M84.653 Pathological fracture in other disease, unspecified femur A, K, P, A
M84.659 Pathological fracture in other disease, hip, unspecified A, K, P, A
M84.66 Pathological fracture in other disease, tibia and fibula
M84.661 Pathological fracture in other disease, right tibia A, K, P
M84.662 Pathological fracture in other disease, left tibia A, K, P
M84.663 Pathological fracture in other disease, right fibula A, K, P
M84.664 Pathological fracture in other disease, left fibula A, K, P
M84.669 Pathological fracture in other disease, unspecified tibia and fibula A, K, P
M84.67 Pathological fracture in other disease, ankle and foot
M84.671 Pathological fracture in other disease, right ankle A, K, P
M84.672 Pathological fracture in other disease, left ankle A, K, P
M84.673 Pathological fracture in other disease, unspecified ankle A, K, P
M84.674 Pathological fracture in other disease, right foot A, K, P
M84.675 Pathological fracture in other disease, left foot A, K, P
M84.676 Pathological fracture in other disease, unspecified foot A, K, P
X M84.68 Pathological fracture in other disease, other site A, K, P
M84.7 Nontraumatic fracture, not elsewhere classified
M84.75 Atypical femoral fracture

The appropriate 7th character is to be added to each code from M84.75:

A	initial encounter for fracture
D	subsequent encounter for fracture with routine healing
G	subsequent encounter for fracture with delayed healing
K	subsequent encounter for fracture with nonunion
P	subsequent encounter for fracture with malunion
S	sequela

Coding Clinic: 2016, Q4, P41

M84.750 Atypical femoral fracture, unspecified A, K, P
M84.751 Incomplete atypical femoral fracture, right leg A, K, P
M84.752 Incomplete atypical femoral fracture, left leg A, K, P
M84.753 Incomplete atypical femoral fracture, unspecified leg A, K, P
M84.754 Complete transverse atypical femoral fracture, right leg A, K, P, A
M84.755 Complete transverse atypical femoral fracture, left leg A, K, P, A
M84.756 Complete transverse atypical femoral fracture, unspecified leg A, K, P, A
M84.757 Complete oblique atypical femoral fracture, right leg A, K, P, A
M84.758 Complete oblique atypical femoral fracture, left leg A, K, P, A
M84.759 Complete oblique atypical femoral fracture, unspecified leg A, K, P, A

M84.8 Other disorders of continuity of bone
M84.80 Other disorders of continuity of bone, unspecified site
M84.81 Other disorders of continuity of bone, shoulder
M84.811 Other disorders of continuity of bone, right shoulder
M84.812 Other disorders of continuity of bone, left shoulder
M84.819 Other disorders of continuity of bone, unspecified shoulder
M84.82 Other disorders of continuity of bone, humerus
M84.821 Other disorders of continuity of bone, right humerus
M84.822 Other disorders of continuity of bone, left humerus
M84.829 Other disorders of continuity of bone, unspecified humerus
M84.83 Other disorders of continuity of bone, ulna and radius
M84.831 Other disorders of continuity of bone, right ulna
M84.832 Other disorders of continuity of bone, left ulna
M84.833 Other disorders of continuity of bone, right radius
M84.834 Other disorders of continuity of bone, left radius
M84.839 Other disorders of continuity of bone, unspecified ulna and radius
M84.84 Other disorders of continuity of bone, hand
M84.841 Other disorders of continuity of bone, right hand
M84.842 Other disorders of continuity of bone, left hand
M84.849 Other disorders of continuity of bone, unspecified hand
M84.85 Other disorders of continuity of bone, pelvic region and thigh
M84.851 Other disorders of continuity of bone, right pelvic region and thigh
M84.852 Other disorders of continuity of bone, left pelvic region and thigh
M84.859 Other disorders of continuity of bone, unspecified pelvic region and thigh
M84.86 Other disorders of continuity of bone, tibia and fibula
M84.861 Other disorders of continuity of bone, right tibia
M84.862 Other disorders of continuity of bone, left tibia
M84.863 Other disorders of continuity of bone, right fibula
M84.864 Other disorders of continuity of bone, left fibula
M84.869 Other disorders of continuity of bone, unspecified tibia and fibula
M84.87 Other disorders of continuity of bone, ankle and foot
M84.871 Other disorders of continuity of bone, right ankle and foot
M84.872 Other disorders of continuity of bone, left ankle and foot
M84.879 Other disorders of continuity of bone, unspecified ankle and foot
M84.88 Other disorders of continuity of bone, other site
M84.9 Disorder of continuity of bone, unspecified

● M85 Other disorders of bone density and structure

Excludes1 osteogenesis imperfecta (Q78.Ø)
osteopetrosis (Q78.2)
osteopoikilosis (Q78.8)
polyostotic fibrous dysplasia (Q78.1)

● M85.Ø Fibrous dysplasia (monostotic)

Excludes2 fibrous dysplasia of jaw (M27.8)

M85.ØØ Fibrous dysplasia (monostotic), unspecified site
● M85.Ø1 Fibrous dysplasia (monostotic), shoulder
M85.Ø11 Fibrous dysplasia (monostotic), right shoulder
M85.Ø12 Fibrous dysplasia (monostotic), left shoulder
M85.Ø19 Fibrous dysplasia (monostotic), unspecified shoulder
● M85.Ø2 Fibrous dysplasia (monostotic), upper arm
M85.Ø21 Fibrous dysplasia (monostotic), right upper arm
M85.Ø22 Fibrous dysplasia (monostotic), left upper arm
M85.Ø29 Fibrous dysplasia (monostotic), unspecified upper arm
● M85.Ø3 Fibrous dysplasia (monostotic), forearm
M85.Ø31 Fibrous dysplasia (monostotic), right forearm
M85.Ø32 Fibrous dysplasia (monostotic), left forearm
M85.Ø39 Fibrous dysplasia (monostotic), unspecified forearm
● M85.Ø4 Fibrous dysplasia (monostotic), hand
M85.Ø41 Fibrous dysplasia (monostotic), right hand
M85.Ø42 Fibrous dysplasia (monostotic), left hand
M85.Ø49 Fibrous dysplasia (monostotic), unspecified hand
● M85.Ø5 Fibrous dysplasia (monostotic), thigh
M85.Ø51 Fibrous dysplasia (monostotic), right thigh
M85.Ø52 Fibrous dysplasia (monostotic), left thigh
M85.Ø59 Fibrous dysplasia (monostotic), unspecified thigh
● M85.Ø6 Fibrous dysplasia (monostotic), lower leg
M85.Ø61 Fibrous dysplasia (monostotic), right lower leg
M85.Ø62 Fibrous dysplasia (monostotic), left lower leg
M85.Ø69 Fibrous dysplasia (monostotic), unspecified lower leg
● M85.Ø7 Fibrous dysplasia (monostotic), ankle and foot
M85.Ø71 Fibrous dysplasia (monostotic), right ankle and foot
M85.Ø72 Fibrous dysplasia (monostotic), left ankle and foot
M85.Ø79 Fibrous dysplasia (monostotic), unspecified ankle and foot
M85.Ø8 Fibrous dysplasia (monostotic), other site
M85.Ø9 Fibrous dysplasia (monostotic), multiple sites

● M85.1 Skeletal fluorosis

M85.1Ø Skeletal fluorosis, unspecified site
● M85.11 Skeletal fluorosis, shoulder
M85.111 Skeletal fluorosis, right shoulder
M85.112 Skeletal fluorosis, left shoulder
M85.119 Skeletal fluorosis, unspecified shoulder
● M85.12 Skeletal fluorosis, upper arm
M85.121 Skeletal fluorosis, right upper arm
M85.122 Skeletal fluorosis, left upper arm
M85.129 Skeletal fluorosis, unspecified upper arm
● M85.13 Skeletal fluorosis, forearm
M85.131 Skeletal fluorosis, right forearm
M85.132 Skeletal fluorosis, left forearm
M85.139 Skeletal fluorosis, unspecified forearm
● M85.14 Skeletal fluorosis, hand
M85.141 Skeletal fluorosis, right hand
M85.142 Skeletal fluorosis, left hand
M85.149 Skeletal fluorosis, unspecified hand
● M85.15 Skeletal fluorosis, thigh
M85.151 Skeletal fluorosis, right thigh
M85.152 Skeletal fluorosis, left thigh
M85.159 Skeletal fluorosis, unspecified thigh
● M85.16 Skeletal fluorosis, lower leg
M85.161 Skeletal fluorosis, right lower leg
M85.162 Skeletal fluorosis, left lower leg
M85.169 Skeletal fluorosis, unspecified lower leg
● M85.17 Skeletal fluorosis, ankle and foot
M85.171 Skeletal fluorosis, right ankle and foot
M85.172 Skeletal fluorosis, left ankle and foot
M85.179 Skeletal fluorosis, unspecified ankle and foot
M85.18 Skeletal fluorosis, other site
M85.19 Skeletal fluorosis, multiple sites

M85.2 Hyperostosis of skull

● M85.3 Osteitis condensans

M85.3Ø Osteitis condensans, unspecified site
● M85.31 Osteitis condensans, shoulder
M85.311 Osteitis condensans, right shoulder
M85.312 Osteitis condensans, left shoulder
M85.319 Osteitis condensans, unspecified shoulder
● M85.32 Osteitis condensans, upper arm
M85.321 Osteitis condensans, right upper arm
M85.322 Osteitis condensans, left upper arm
M85.329 Osteitis condensans, unspecified upper arm
● M85.33 Osteitis condensans, forearm
M85.331 Osteitis condensans, right forearm
M85.332 Osteitis condensans, left forearm
M85.339 Osteitis condensans, unspecified forearm
● M85.34 Osteitis condensans, hand
M85.341 Osteitis condensans, right hand
M85.342 Osteitis condensans, left hand
M85.349 Osteitis condensans, unspecified hand
● M85.35 Osteitis condensans, thigh
M85.351 Osteitis condensans, right thigh
M85.352 Osteitis condensans, left thigh
M85.359 Osteitis condensans, unspecified thigh
● M85.36 Osteitis condensans, lower leg
M85.361 Osteitis condensans, right lower leg
M85.362 Osteitis condensans, left lower leg
M85.369 Osteitis condensans, unspecified lower leg

- ● M85.37 Osteitis condensans, ankle and foot
  - M85.371 Osteitis condensans, right ankle and foot
  - M85.372 Osteitis condensans, left ankle and foot
  - M85.379 Osteitis condensans, unspecified ankle and foot
- M85.38 Osteitis condensans, other site
- M85.39 Osteitis condensans, multiple sites

● M85.4 Solitary bone cyst

Excludes2 solitary cyst of jaw (M27.4)

- M85.40 Solitary bone cyst, unspecified site
- ● M85.41 Solitary bone cyst, shoulder
  - M85.411 Solitary bone cyst, right shoulder
  - M85.412 Solitary bone cyst, left shoulder
  - M85.419 Solitary bone cyst, unspecified shoulder
- ● M85.42 Solitary bone cyst, humerus
  - M85.421 Solitary bone cyst, right humerus
  - M85.422 Solitary bone cyst, left humerus
  - M85.429 Solitary bone cyst, unspecified humerus
- ● M85.43 Solitary bone cyst, ulna and radius
  - M85.431 Solitary bone cyst, right ulna and radius
  - M85.432 Solitary bone cyst, left ulna and radius
  - M85.439 Solitary bone cyst, unspecified ulna and radius
- ● M85.44 Solitary bone cyst, hand
  - M85.441 Solitary bone cyst, right hand
  - M85.442 Solitary bone cyst, left hand
  - M85.449 Solitary bone cyst, unspecified hand
- ● M85.45 Solitary bone cyst, pelvis
  - M85.451 Solitary bone cyst, right pelvis
  - M85.452 Solitary bone cyst, left pelvis
  - M85.459 Solitary bone cyst, unspecified pelvis
- ● M85.46 Solitary bone cyst, tibia and fibula
  - M85.461 Solitary bone cyst, right tibia and fibula
  - M85.462 Solitary bone cyst, left tibia and fibula
  - M85.469 Solitary bone cyst, unspecified tibia and fibula
- ● M85.47 Solitary bone cyst, ankle and foot
  - M85.471 Solitary bone cyst, right ankle and foot
  - M85.472 Solitary bone cyst, left ankle and foot
  - M85.479 Solitary bone cyst, unspecified ankle and foot
- M85.48 Solitary bone cyst, other site

● M85.5 Aneurysmal bone cyst

Excludes2 aneurysmal cyst of jaw (M27.4)

- M85.50 Aneurysmal bone cyst, unspecified site
- ● M85.51 Aneurysmal bone cyst, shoulder
  - M85.511 Aneurysmal bone cyst, right shoulder
  - M85.512 Aneurysmal bone cyst, left shoulder
  - M85.519 Aneurysmal bone cyst, unspecified shoulder
- ● M85.52 Aneurysmal bone cyst, upper arm
  - M85.521 Aneurysmal bone cyst, right upper arm
  - M85.522 Aneurysmal bone cyst, left upper arm
  - M85.529 Aneurysmal bone cyst, unspecified upper arm
- ● M85.53 Aneurysmal bone cyst, forearm
  - M85.531 Aneurysmal bone cyst, right forearm
  - M85.532 Aneurysmal bone cyst, left forearm
  - M85.539 Aneurysmal bone cyst, unspecified forearm
- ● M85.54 Aneurysmal bone cyst, hand
  - M85.541 Aneurysmal bone cyst, right hand
  - M85.542 Aneurysmal bone cyst, left hand
  - M85.549 Aneurysmal bone cyst, unspecified hand
- ● M85.55 Aneurysmal bone cyst, thigh
  - M85.551 Aneurysmal bone cyst, right thigh
  - M85.552 Aneurysmal bone cyst, left thigh
  - M85.559 Aneurysmal bone cyst, unspecified thigh
- ● M85.56 Aneurysmal bone cyst, lower leg
  - M85.561 Aneurysmal bone cyst, right lower leg
  - M85.562 Aneurysmal bone cyst, left lower leg
  - M85.569 Aneurysmal bone cyst, unspecified lower leg
- ● M85.57 Aneurysmal bone cyst, ankle and foot
  - M85.571 Aneurysmal bone cyst, right ankle and foot
  - M85.572 Aneurysmal bone cyst, left ankle and foot
  - M85.579 Aneurysmal bone cyst, unspecified ankle and foot
- M85.58 Aneurysmal bone cyst, other site
- M85.59 Aneurysmal bone cyst, multiple sites

● M85.6 Other cyst of bone

Excludes1 cyst of jaw NEC (M27.4)
osteitis fibrosa cystica generalisata [von Recklinghausen's disease of bone] (E21.Ø)

- M85.6Ø Other cyst of bone, unspecified site
- ● M85.61 Other cyst of bone, shoulder
  - M85.611 Other cyst of bone, right shoulder
  - M85.612 Other cyst of bone, left shoulder
  - M85.619 Other cyst of bone, unspecified shoulder
- ● M85.62 Other cyst of bone, upper arm
  - M85.621 Other cyst of bone, right upper arm
  - M85.622 Other cyst of bone, left upper arm
  - M85.629 Other cyst of bone, unspecified upper arm
- ● M85.63 Other cyst of bone, forearm
  - M85.631 Other cyst of bone, right forearm
  - M85.632 Other cyst of bone, left forearm
  - M85.639 Other cyst of bone, unspecified forearm
- ● M85.64 Other cyst of bone, hand
  - M85.641 Other cyst of bone, right hand
  - M85.642 Other cyst of bone, left hand
  - M85.649 Other cyst of bone, unspecified hand
- ● M85.65 Other cyst of bone, thigh
  - M85.651 Other cyst of bone, right thigh
  - M85.652 Other cyst of bone, left thigh
  - M85.659 Other cyst of bone, unspecified thigh
- ● M85.66 Other cyst of bone, lower leg
  - M85.661 Other cyst of bone, right lower leg
  - M85.662 Other cyst of bone, left lower leg
  - M85.669 Other cyst of bone, unspecified lower leg

● M85.67 Other cyst of bone, ankle and foot
  M85.671 Other cyst of bone, right ankle and foot
  M85.672 Other cyst of bone, left ankle and foot
  M85.679 Other cyst of bone, unspecified ankle and foot
M85.68 Other cyst of bone, other site
M85.69 Other cyst of bone, multiple sites

● M85.8 Other specified disorders of bone density and structure
Hyperostosis of bones, except skull
Osteosclerosis, acquired
Excludes1 diffuse idiopathic skeletal hyperostosis [DISH] (M48.1)
osteosclerosis congenita (Q77.4)
osteosclerosis fragilitas (generalista) (Q78.2)
osteosclerosis myelofibrosis (D75.81)

M85.8Ø Other specified disorders of bone density and structure, unspecified site
● M85.81 Other specified disorders of bone density and structure, shoulder
  M85.811 Other specified disorders of bone density and structure, right shoulder
  M85.812 Other specified disorders of bone density and structure, left shoulder
  M85.819 Other specified disorders of bone density and structure, unspecified shoulder
● M85.82 Other specified disorders of bone density and structure, upper arm
  M85.821 Other specified disorders of bone density and structure, right upper arm
  M85.822 Other specified disorders of bone density and structure, left upper arm
  M85.829 Other specified disorders of bone density and structure, unspecified upper arm
● M85.83 Other specified disorders of bone density and structure, forearm
  M85.831 Other specified disorders of bone density and structure, right forearm
  M85.832 Other specified disorders of bone density and structure, left forearm
  M85.839 Other specified disorders of bone density and structure, unspecified forearm
● M85.84 Other specified disorders of bone density and structure, hand
  M85.841 Other specified disorders of bone density and structure, right hand
  M85.842 Other specified disorders of bone density and structure, left hand
  M85.849 Other specified disorders of bone density and structure, unspecified hand
● M85.85 Other specified disorders of bone density and structure, thigh
  M85.851 Other specified disorders of bone density and structure, right thigh
  M85.852 Other specified disorders of bone density and structure, left thigh
  M85.859 Other specified disorders of bone density and structure, unspecified thigh
● M85.86 Other specified disorders of bone density and structure, lower leg
  M85.861 Other specified disorders of bone density and structure, right lower leg
  M85.862 Other specified disorders of bone density and structure, left lower leg
  M85.869 Other specified disorders of bone density and structure, unspecified lower leg
● M85.87 Other specified disorders of bone density and structure, ankle and foot
  M85.871 Other specified disorders of bone density and structure, right ankle and foot
  M85.872 Other specified disorders of bone density and structure, left ankle and foot
  M85.879 Other specified disorders of bone density and structure, unspecified ankle and foot
M85.88 Other specified disorders of bone density and structure, other site
M85.89 Other specified disorders of bone density and structure, multiple sites

M85.9 Disorder of bone density and structure, unspecified
Coding Clinic: 2021, Q3, P11

OTHER OSTEOPATHIES (M86-M9Ø)

Excludes1 postprocedural osteopathies (M96.-)

● M86 Osteomyelitis
Use additional code (B95-B97) to identify infectious agent
Use additional code to identify major osseous defect, if applicable (M89.7-)
Excludes1 osteomyelitis due to:
echinococcus (B67.2)
gonococcus (A54.43)
salmonella (AØ2.24)
Excludes2 ostemyelitis of:
orbit (HØ5.Ø-)
petrous bone (H7Ø.2-)
vertebra (M46.2-)

● M86.Ø Acute hematogenous osteomyelitis
M86.ØØ Acute hematogenous osteomyelitis, unspecified site (Ex) PDX 1280
● M86.Ø1 Acute hematogenous osteomyelitis, shoulder
  M86.Ø11 Acute hematogenous osteomyelitis, right shoulder (Ex) PDX 1281
  M86.Ø12 Acute hematogenous osteomyelitis, left shoulder (Ex) PDX 1282
  M86.Ø19 Acute hematogenous osteomyelitis, unspecified shoulder (Ex) PDX 1283
● M86.Ø2 Acute hematogenous osteomyelitis, humerus
  M86.Ø21 Acute hematogenous osteomyelitis, right humerus (Ex) PDX 1284
  M86.Ø22 Acute hematogenous osteomyelitis, left humerus (Ex) PDX 1285
  M86.Ø29 Acute hematogenous osteomyelitis, unspecified humerus (Ex) PDX 1286
● M86.Ø3 Acute hematogenous osteomyelitis, radius and ulna
  M86.Ø31 Acute hematogenous osteomyelitis, right radius and ulna (Ex) PDX 1287
  M86.Ø32 Acute hematogenous osteomyelitis, left radius and ulna (Ex) PDX 1288
  M86.Ø39 Acute hematogenous osteomyelitis, unspecified radius and ulna (Ex) PDX 1289
● M86.Ø4 Acute hematogenous osteomyelitis, hand
  M86.Ø41 Acute hematogenous osteomyelitis, right hand (Ex) PDX 1290
  M86.Ø42 Acute hematogenous osteomyelitis, left hand (Ex) PDX 1291
  M86.Ø49 Acute hematogenous osteomyelitis, unspecified hand (Ex) PDX 1292

CHAPTER 13 (MØØ-M99)

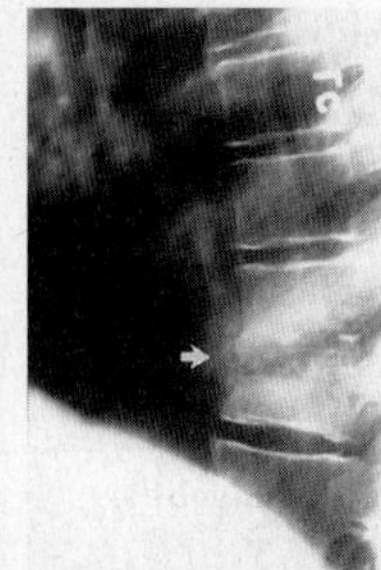

Figure 13-6 Osteomyelitis of the spine. A lateral view of the lower thoracic spine demonstrates destruction of the disk space *(arrow)* as well as destruction of the adjoining vertebral bodies. (From Mettler: Essentials of Radiology, ed 2, Saunders, An Imprint of Elsevier, 2005)

Item 13–12 Osteomyelitis is an inflammation of the bone. **Acute osteomyelitis** is a rapidly destructive, pus-producing infection capable of causing severe bone destruction. **Chronic osteomyelitis** can remain long after the initial acute episode has passed and may lead to a recurrence of the acute phase. **Brodie's abscess** is an encapsulated focal abscess that must be surgically drained. **Periostitis** is an inflammation of the periosteum, a dense membrane composed of fibrous connective tissue that closely wraps all bone, except those with articulating surfaces in joints, which are covered by synovial membranes.

● **M86.05** Acute hematogenous osteomyelitis, femur
- **M86.051** Acute hematogenous osteomyelitis, right femur Ex: PDX 1293
- **M86.052** Acute hematogenous osteomyelitis, left femur Ex: PDX 1294
- **M86.059** Acute hematogenous osteomyelitis, unspecified femur Ex: PDX 1295

● **M86.06** Acute hematogenous osteomyelitis, tibia and fibula
- **M86.061** Acute hematogenous osteomyelitis, right tibia and fibula Ex: PDX 1296
- **M86.062** Acute hematogenous osteomyelitis, left tibia and fibula Ex: PDX 1297
- **M86.069** Acute hematogenous osteomyelitis, unspecified tibia and fibula Ex: PDX 1298

● **M86.07** Acute hematogenous osteomyelitis, ankle and foot
- **M86.071** Acute hematogenous osteomyelitis, right ankle and foot Ex: PDX 1299
- **M86.072** Acute hematogenous osteomyelitis, left ankle and foot Ex: PDX 1300
- **M86.079** Acute hematogenous osteomyelitis, unspecified ankle and foot Ex: PDX 1301

M86.08 Acute hematogenous osteomyelitis, other sites Ex: PDX 1243

M86.09 Acute hematogenous osteomyelitis, multiple sites Ex: PDX 1280

● **M86.1** Other acute osteomyelitis

M86.10 Other acute osteomyelitis, unspecified site Ex: PDX 1280

● **M86.11** Other acute osteomyelitis, shoulder
- **M86.111** Other acute osteomyelitis, right shoulder Ex: PDX 1302
- **M86.112** Other acute osteomyelitis, left shoulder Ex: PDX 1303
- **M86.119** Other acute osteomyelitis, unspecified shoulder Ex: PDX 1304

● **M86.12** Other acute osteomyelitis, humerus
- **M86.121** Other acute osteomyelitis, right humerus Ex: PDX 1305
- **M86.122** Other acute osteomyelitis, left humerus Ex: PDX 1306
- **M86.129** Other acute osteomyelitis, unspecified humerus Ex: PDX 1307

● **M86.13** Other acute osteomyelitis, radius and ulna
- **M86.131** Other acute osteomyelitis, right radius and ulna Ex: PDX 1308
- **M86.132** Other acute osteomyelitis, left radius and ulna Ex: PDX 1309
- **M86.139** Other acute osteomyelitis, unspecified radius and ulna Ex: PDX 1310

● **M86.14** Other acute osteomyelitis, hand
- **M86.141** Other acute osteomyelitis, right hand Ex: PDX 1311
- **M86.142** Other acute osteomyelitis, left hand Ex: PDX 1312
- **M86.149** Other acute osteomyelitis, unspecified hand Ex: PDX 1313

● **M86.15** Other acute osteomyelitis, femur
- **M86.151** Other acute osteomyelitis, right femur Ex: PDX 1314
- **M86.152** Other acute osteomyelitis, left femur Ex: PDX 1315
- **M86.159** Other acute osteomyelitis, unspecified femur Ex: PDX 1316

● **M86.16** Other acute osteomyelitis, tibia and fibula
- **M86.161** Other acute osteomyelitis, right tibia and fibula Ex: PDX 1317
- **M86.162** Other acute osteomyelitis, left tibia and fibula Ex: PDX 1318
- **M86.169** Other acute osteomyelitis, unspecified tibia and fibula Ex: PDX 1319

● **M86.17** Other acute osteomyelitis, ankle and foot
- **M86.171** Other acute osteomyelitis, right ankle and foot Ex: PDX 1320
  Coding Clinic: 2020, Q1, P12
- **M86.172** Other acute osteomyelitis, left ankle and foot Ex: PDX 1321
- **M86.179** Other acute osteomyelitis, unspecified ankle and foot Ex: PDX 1322

M86.18 Other acute osteomyelitis, other site Ex: PDX 1243

M86.19 Other acute osteomyelitis, multiple sites Ex: PDX 1280

● **M86.2** Subacute osteomyelitis

M86.20 Subacute osteomyelitis, unspecified site Ex: PDX 1280

● **M86.21** Subacute osteomyelitis, shoulder
- **M86.211** Subacute osteomyelitis, right shoulder Ex: PDX 1323
- **M86.212** Subacute osteomyelitis, left shoulder Ex: PDX 1324
- **M86.219** Subacute osteomyelitis, unspecified shoulder Ex: PDX 1325

● **M86.22** Subacute osteomyelitis, humerus
- **M86.221** Subacute osteomyelitis, right humerus Ex: PDX 1326
- **M86.222** Subacute osteomyelitis, left humerus Ex: PDX 1327
- **M86.229** Subacute osteomyelitis, unspecified humerus Ex: PDX 1328

● **M86.23** Subacute osteomyelitis, radius and ulna
- **M86.231** Subacute osteomyelitis, right radius and ulna Ex: PDX 1329
- **M86.232** Subacute osteomyelitis, left radius and ulna Ex: PDX 1330
- **M86.239** Subacute osteomyelitis, unspecified radius and ulna Ex: PDX 1331

● M86.24 Subacute osteomyelitis, hand
M86.241 Subacute osteomyelitis, right hand (Ex:) PDX 1332
M86.242 Subacute osteomyelitis, left hand (Ex:) PDX 1333
M86.249 Subacute osteomyelitis, unspecified hand (Ex:) PDX 1334
● M86.25 Subacute osteomyelitis, femur
M86.251 Subacute osteomyelitis, right femur (Ex:) PDX 1335
M86.252 Subacute osteomyelitis, left femur (Ex:) PDX 1336
M86.259 Subacute osteomyelitis, unspecified femur (Ex:) PDX 1337
● M86.26 Subacute osteomyelitis, tibia and fibula
M86.261 Subacute osteomyelitis, right tibia and fibula (Ex:) PDX 1338
M86.262 Subacute osteomyelitis, left tibia and fibula (Ex:) PDX 1339
M86.269 Subacute osteomyelitis, unspecified tibia and fibula (Ex:) PDX 1340
● M86.27 Subacute osteomyelitis, ankle and foot
M86.271 Subacute osteomyelitis, right ankle and foot (Ex:) PDX 1341
M86.272 Subacute osteomyelitis, left ankle and foot (Ex:) PDX 1342
M86.279 Subacute osteomyelitis, unspecified ankle and foot (Ex:) PDX 1343
M86.28 Subacute osteomyelitis, other site (Ex:) PDX 1243
M86.29 Subacute osteomyelitis, multiple sites (Ex:) PDX 1280
● M86.3 Chronic multifocal osteomyelitis (Ex:) PDX 1242
M86.30 Chronic multifocal osteomyelitis, unspecified site (Ex:) PDX 1344
● M86.31 Chronic multifocal osteomyelitis, shoulder
M86.311 Chronic multifocal osteomyelitis, right shoulder
M86.312 Chronic multifocal osteomyelitis, left shoulder
M86.319 Chronic multifocal osteomyelitis, unspecified shoulder
● M86.32 Chronic multifocal osteomyelitis, humerus
M86.321 Chronic multifocal osteomyelitis, right humerus
M86.322 Chronic multifocal osteomyelitis, left humerus
M86.329 Chronic multifocal osteomyelitis, unspecified humerus
● M86.33 Chronic multifocal osteomyelitis, radius and ulna
M86.331 Chronic multifocal osteomyelitis, right radius and ulna
M86.332 Chronic multifocal osteomyelitis, left radius and ulna
M86.339 Chronic multifocal osteomyelitis, unspecified radius and ulna
● M86.34 Chronic multifocal osteomyelitis, hand
M86.341 Chronic multifocal osteomyelitis, right hand
M86.342 Chronic multifocal osteomyelitis, left hand
M86.349 Chronic multifocal osteomyelitis, unspecified hand
● M86.35 Chronic multifocal osteomyelitis, femur
M86.351 Chronic multifocal osteomyelitis, right femur
M86.352 Chronic multifocal osteomyelitis, left femur
M86.359 Chronic multifocal osteomyelitis, unspecified femur
● M86.36 Chronic multifocal osteomyelitis, tibia and fibula
M86.361 Chronic multifocal osteomyelitis, right tibia and fibula
M86.362 Chronic multifocal osteomyelitis, left tibia and fibula
M86.369 Chronic multifocal osteomyelitis, unspecified tibia and fibula
● M86.37 Chronic multifocal osteomyelitis, ankle and foot
M86.371 Chronic multifocal osteomyelitis, right ankle and foot
M86.372 Chronic multifocal osteomyelitis, left ankle and foot
M86.379 Chronic multifocal osteomyelitis, unspecified ankle and foot
M86.38 Chronic multifocal osteomyelitis, other site
M86.39 Chronic multifocal osteomyelitis, multiple sites
● M86.4 Chronic osteomyelitis with draining sinus
M86.40 Chronic osteomyelitis with draining sinus, unspecified site (Ex:) PDX 1344
● M86.41 Chronic osteomyelitis with draining sinus, shoulder
M86.411 Chronic osteomyelitis with draining sinus, right shoulder
M86.412 Chronic osteomyelitis with draining sinus, left shoulder
M86.419 Chronic osteomyelitis with draining sinus, unspecified shoulder
● M86.42 Chronic osteomyelitis with draining sinus, humerus
M86.421 Chronic osteomyelitis with draining sinus, right humerus
M86.422 Chronic osteomyelitis with draining sinus, left humerus
M86.429 Chronic osteomyelitis with draining sinus, unspecified humerus
● M86.43 Chronic osteomyelitis with draining sinus, radius and ulna
M86.431 Chronic osteomyelitis with draining sinus, right radius and ulna
M86.432 Chronic osteomyelitis with draining sinus, left radius and ulna
M86.439 Chronic osteomyelitis with draining sinus, unspecified radius and ulna
● M86.44 Chronic osteomyelitis with draining sinus, hand
M86.441 Chronic osteomyelitis with draining sinus, right hand
M86.442 Chronic osteomyelitis with draining sinus, left hand
M86.449 Chronic osteomyelitis with draining sinus, unspecified hand

CHAPTER 13 (MØØ-M99)

● **M86.45 Chronic osteomyelitis with draining sinus, femur**
- **M86.451 Chronic osteomyelitis with draining sinus, right femur**
- **M86.452 Chronic osteomyelitis with draining sinus, left femur**
- **M86.459 Chronic osteomyelitis with draining sinus, unspecified femur**

● **M86.46 Chronic osteomyelitis with draining sinus, tibia and fibula**
- **M86.461 Chronic osteomyelitis with draining sinus, right tibia and fibula**
- **M86.462 Chronic osteomyelitis with draining sinus, left tibia and fibula**
- **M86.469 Chronic osteomyelitis with draining sinus, unspecified tibia and fibula**

● **M86.47 Chronic osteomyelitis with draining sinus, ankle and foot**
- **M86.471 Chronic osteomyelitis with draining sinus, right ankle and foot**
- **M86.472 Chronic osteomyelitis with draining sinus, left ankle and foot**
- **M86.479 Chronic osteomyelitis with draining sinus, unspecified ankle and foot**

M86.48 Chronic osteomyelitis with draining sinus, other site

M86.49 Chronic osteomyelitis with draining sinus, multiple sites

● **M86.5 Other chronic hematogenous osteomyelitis**

M86.50 Other chronic hematogenous osteomyelitis, unspecified site

● **M86.51 Other chronic hematogenous osteomyelitis, shoulder**
- **M86.511 Other chronic hematogenous osteomyelitis, right shoulder**
- **M86.512 Other chronic hematogenous osteomyelitis, left shoulder**
- **M86.519 Other chronic hematogenous osteomyelitis, unspecified shoulder**

● **M86.52 Other chronic hematogenous osteomyelitis, humerus**
- **M86.521 Other chronic hematogenous osteomyelitis, right humerus**
- **M86.522 Other chronic hematogenous osteomyelitis, left humerus**
- **M86.529 Other chronic hematogenous osteomyelitis, unspecified humerus**

● **M86.53 Other chronic hematogenous osteomyelitis, radius and ulna**
- **M86.531 Other chronic hematogenous osteomyelitis, right radius and ulna**
- **M86.532 Other chronic hematogenous osteomyelitis, left radius and ulna**
- **M86.539 Other chronic hematogenous osteomyelitis, unspecified radius and ulna**

● **M86.54 Other chronic hematogenous osteomyelitis, hand**
- **M86.541 Other chronic hematogenous osteomyelitis, right hand**
- **M86.542 Other chronic hematogenous osteomyelitis, left hand**
- **M86.549 Other chronic hematogenous osteomyelitis, unspecified hand**

● **M86.55 Other chronic hematogenous osteomyelitis, femur**
- **M86.551 Other chronic hematogenous osteomyelitis, right femur**
- **M86.552 Other chronic hematogenous osteomyelitis, left femur**
- **M86.559 Other chronic hematogenous osteomyelitis, unspecified femur**

● **M86.56 Other chronic hematogenous osteomyelitis, tibia and fibula**
- **M86.561 Other chronic hematogenous osteomyelitis, right tibia and fibula**
- **M86.562 Other chronic hematogenous osteomyelitis, left tibia and fibula**
- **M86.569 Other chronic hematogenous osteomyelitis, unspecified tibia and fibula**

● **M86.57 Other chronic hematogenous osteomyelitis, ankle and foot**
- **M86.571 Other chronic hematogenous osteomyelitis, right ankle and foot**
- **M86.572 Other chronic hematogenous osteomyelitis, left ankle and foot**
- **M86.579 Other chronic hematogenous osteomyelitis, unspecified ankle and foot**

M86.58 Other chronic hematogenous osteomyelitis, other site

M86.59 Other chronic hematogenous osteomyelitis, multiple sites

● **M86.6 Other chronic osteomyelitis**

M86.60 Other chronic osteomyelitis, unspecified site Ex: PDX 1344

● **M86.61 Other chronic osteomyelitis, shoulder**
- **M86.611 Other chronic osteomyelitis, right shoulder**
- **M86.612 Other chronic osteomyelitis, left shoulder**
- **M86.619 Other chronic osteomyelitis, unspecified shoulder**

● **M86.62 Other chronic osteomyelitis, humerus**
- **M86.621 Other chronic osteomyelitis, right humerus**
- **M86.622 Other chronic osteomyelitis, left humerus**
- **M86.629 Other chronic osteomyelitis, unspecified humerus**

● **M86.63 Other chronic osteomyelitis, radius and ulna**
- **M86.631 Other chronic osteomyelitis, right radius and ulna**
- **M86.632 Other chronic osteomyelitis, left radius and ulna**
- **M86.639 Other chronic osteomyelitis, unspecified radius and ulna**

● **M86.64 Other chronic osteomyelitis, hand**
- **M86.641 Other chronic osteomyelitis, right hand**
- **M86.642 Other chronic osteomyelitis, left hand**
- **M86.649 Other chronic osteomyelitis, unspecified hand**

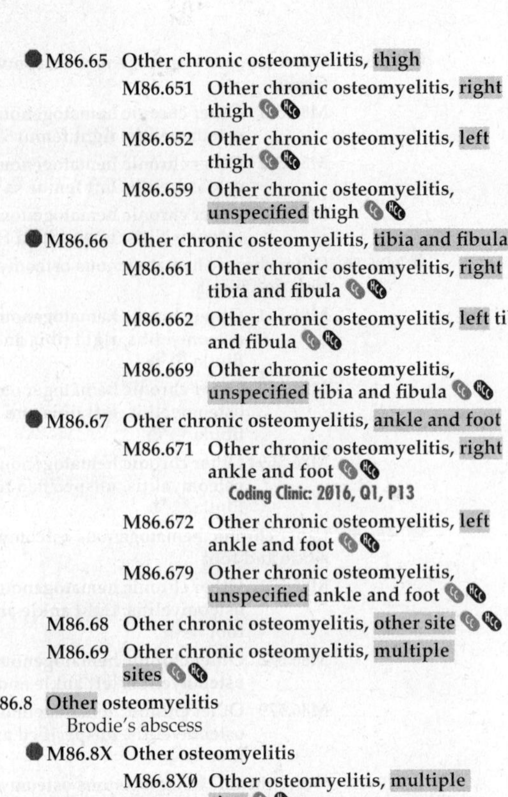

- **M86.65** Other chronic osteomyelitis, thigh
  - **M86.651** Other chronic osteomyelitis, right thigh
  - **M86.652** Other chronic osteomyelitis, left thigh
  - **M86.659** Other chronic osteomyelitis, unspecified thigh
- **M86.66** Other chronic osteomyelitis, tibia and fibula
  - **M86.661** Other chronic osteomyelitis, right tibia and fibula
  - **M86.662** Other chronic osteomyelitis, left tibia and fibula
  - **M86.669** Other chronic osteomyelitis, unspecified tibia and fibula
- **M86.67** Other chronic osteomyelitis, ankle and foot
  - **M86.671** Other chronic osteomyelitis, right ankle and foot
    Coding Clinic: 2016, Q1, P13
  - **M86.672** Other chronic osteomyelitis, left ankle and foot
  - **M86.679** Other chronic osteomyelitis, unspecified ankle and foot
- **M86.68** Other chronic osteomyelitis, other site
- **M86.69** Other chronic osteomyelitis, multiple sites

M86.8 Other osteomyelitis
Brodie's abscess

- **M86.8X** Other osteomyelitis
  - **M86.8X0** Other osteomyelitis, multiple sites
  - **M86.8X1** Other osteomyelitis, shoulder
  - **M86.8X2** Other osteomyelitis, upper arm
  - **M86.8X3** Other osteomyelitis, forearm
  - **M86.8X4** Other osteomyelitis, hand
  - **M86.8X5** Other osteomyelitis, thigh
  - **M86.8X6** Other osteomyelitis, lower leg
  - **M86.8X7** Other osteomyelitis, ankle and foot
  - **M86.8X8** Other osteomyelitis, other site
    Coding Clinic: 2022, Q1, P31
  - **M86.8X9** Other osteomyelitis, unspecified sites (Ex) PDX 1344

M86.9 Osteomyelitis, unspecified (Ex) PDX 1344
Infection of bone NOS
Periostitis without osteomyelitis

M87 Osteonecrosis (Ex) PDX 1345

Includes avascular necrosis of bone

Use additional code to identify major osseous defect, if applicable (M89.7-)

Excludes1 juvenile osteonecrosis (M91-M92)
osteochondropathies (M90-M93)

M87.0 Idiopathic aseptic necrosis of bone

- **M87.00** Idiopathic aseptic necrosis of unspecified bone
- **M87.01** Idiopathic aseptic necrosis of shoulder (Ex) PDX 1346
  Idiopathic aseptic necrosis of clavicle and scapula
  - **M87.011** Idiopathic aseptic necrosis of right shoulder
  - **M87.012** Idiopathic aseptic necrosis of left shoulder
  - **M87.019** Idiopathic aseptic necrosis of unspecified shoulder
- **M87.02** Idiopathic aseptic necrosis of humerus
  - **M87.021** Idiopathic aseptic necrosis of right humerus
  - **M87.022** Idiopathic aseptic necrosis of left humerus
  - **M87.029** Idiopathic aseptic necrosis of unspecified humerus
- **M87.03** Idiopathic aseptic necrosis of radius, ulna and carpus
  - **M87.031** Idiopathic aseptic necrosis of right radius
  - **M87.032** Idiopathic aseptic necrosis of left radius
  - **M87.033** Idiopathic aseptic necrosis of unspecified radius
  - **M87.034** Idiopathic aseptic necrosis of right ulna
  - **M87.035** Idiopathic aseptic necrosis of left ulna
  - **M87.036** Idiopathic aseptic necrosis of unspecified ulna
  - **M87.037** Idiopathic aseptic necrosis of right carpus
  - **M87.038** Idiopathic aseptic necrosis of left carpus
  - **M87.039** Idiopathic aseptic necrosis of unspecified carpus
- **M87.04** Idiopathic aseptic necrosis of hand and fingers
  Idiopathic aseptic necrosis of metacarpals and phalanges of hands
  - **M87.041** Idiopathic aseptic necrosis of right hand
  - **M87.042** Idiopathic aseptic necrosis of left hand
  - **M87.043** Idiopathic aseptic necrosis of unspecified hand
  - **M87.044** Idiopathic aseptic necrosis of right finger(s)
  - **M87.045** Idiopathic aseptic necrosis of left finger(s)
  - **M87.046** Idiopathic aseptic necrosis of unspecified finger(s)
- **M87.05** Idiopathic aseptic necrosis of pelvis and femur
  - **M87.050** Idiopathic aseptic necrosis of pelvis (Ex) PDX 907
  - **M87.051** Idiopathic aseptic necrosis of right femur (Ex) PDX 1347
  - **M87.052** Idiopathic aseptic necrosis of left femur (Ex) PDX 1347
  - **M87.059** Idiopathic aseptic necrosis of unspecified femur (Ex) PDX 1347
    Idiopathic aseptic necrosis of hip NOS

- **M87.06 Idiopathic aseptic necrosis of tibia and fibula**
  - **M87.061 Idiopathic aseptic necrosis of right tibia**
  - **M87.062 Idiopathic aseptic necrosis of left tibia**
  - **M87.063 Idiopathic aseptic necrosis of unspecified tibia**
  - **M87.064 Idiopathic aseptic necrosis of right fibula**
  - **M87.065 Idiopathic aseptic necrosis of left fibula**
  - **M87.066 Idiopathic aseptic necrosis of unspecified fibula**
- **M87.07 Idiopathic aseptic necrosis of ankle, foot and toes**
  Idiopathic aseptic necrosis of metatarsus, tarsus, and phalanges of toes
  - **M87.071 Idiopathic aseptic necrosis of right ankle**
  - **M87.072 Idiopathic aseptic necrosis of left ankle**
  - **M87.073 Idiopathic aseptic necrosis of unspecified ankle**
  - **M87.074 Idiopathic aseptic necrosis of right foot** Ex: PDX 1348
  - **M87.075 Idiopathic aseptic necrosis of left foot** Ex: PDX 1348
  - **M87.076 Idiopathic aseptic necrosis of unspecified foot** Ex: PDX 1348
  - **M87.077 Idiopathic aseptic necrosis of right toe(s)**
  - **M87.078 Idiopathic aseptic necrosis of left toe(s)**
  - **M87.079 Idiopathic aseptic necrosis of unspecified toe(s)**
- **M87.08 Idiopathic aseptic necrosis of bone, other site**
- **M87.09 Idiopathic aseptic necrosis of bone, multiple sites**

M87.1 Osteonecrosis due to drugs
Use additional code for adverse effect, if applicable, to identify drug (T36-T50 with fifth or sixth character 5)

- **M87.10 Osteonecrosis due to drugs, unspecified bone**
- **M87.11 Osteonecrosis due to drugs, shoulder**
  - **M87.111 Osteonecrosis due to drugs, right shoulder**
  - **M87.112 Osteonecrosis due to drugs, left shoulder**
  - **M87.119 Osteonecrosis due to drugs, unspecified shoulder**
- **M87.12 Osteonecrosis due to drugs, humerus** Ex: PDX 1346
  - **M87.121 Osteonecrosis due to drugs, right humerus**
  - **M87.122 Osteonecrosis due to drugs, left humerus**
  - **M87.129 Osteonecrosis due to drugs, unspecified humerus**
- **M87.13 Osteonecrosis due to drugs of radius, ulna and carpus**
  - **M87.131 Osteonecrosis due to drugs of right radius**
  - **M87.132 Osteonecrosis due to drugs of left radius**
  - **M87.133 Osteonecrosis due to drugs of unspecified radius**
  - **M87.134 Osteonecrosis due to drugs of right ulna**
  - **M87.135 Osteonecrosis due to drugs of left ulna**
  - **M87.136 Osteonecrosis due to drugs of unspecified ulna**
  - **M87.137 Osteonecrosis due to drugs of right carpus**
  - **M87.138 Osteonecrosis due to drugs of left carpus**
  - **M87.139 Osteonecrosis due to drugs of unspecified carpus**
- **M87.14 Osteonecrosis due to drugs, hand and fingers**
  - **M87.141 Osteonecrosis due to drugs, right hand**
  - **M87.142 Osteonecrosis due to drugs, left hand**
  - **M87.143 Osteonecrosis due to drugs, unspecified hand**
  - **M87.144 Osteonecrosis due to drugs, right finger(s)**
  - **M87.145 Osteonecrosis due to drugs, left finger(s)**
  - **M87.146 Osteonecrosis due to drugs, unspecified finger(s)**
- **M87.15 Osteonecrosis due to drugs, pelvis and femur** Ex: PDX 1347
  - **M87.150 Osteonecrosis due to drugs, pelvis**
  - **M87.151 Osteonecrosis due to drugs, right femur**
  - **M87.152 Osteonecrosis due to drugs, left femur**
  - **M87.159 Osteonecrosis due to drugs, unspecified femur**
- **M87.16 Osteonecrosis due to drugs, tibia and fibula**
  - **M87.161 Osteonecrosis due to drugs, right tibia**
  - **M87.162 Osteonecrosis due to drugs, left tibia**
  - **M87.163 Osteonecrosis due to drugs, unspecified tibia**
  - **M87.164 Osteonecrosis due to drugs, right fibula**
  - **M87.165 Osteonecrosis due to drugs, left fibula**
  - **M87.166 Osteonecrosis due to drugs, unspecified fibula**
- **M87.17 Osteonecrosis due to drugs, ankle, foot and toes**
  - **M87.171 Osteonecrosis due to drugs, right ankle**
  - **M87.172 Osteonecrosis due to drugs, left ankle**
  - **M87.173 Osteonecrosis due to drugs, unspecified ankle**
  - **M87.174 Osteonecrosis due to drugs, right foot** Ex: PDX 1348
  - **M87.175 Osteonecrosis due to drugs, left foot** Ex: PDX 1348
  - **M87.176 Osteonecrosis due to drugs, unspecified foot** Ex: PDX 1348
  - **M87.177 Osteonecrosis due to drugs, right toe(s)**
  - **M87.178 Osteonecrosis due to drugs, left toe(s)**
  - **M87.179 Osteonecrosis due to drugs, unspecified toe(s)**

● M87.18 Osteonecrosis due to drugs, other site
  M87.180 Osteonecrosis due to drugs, jaw
  M87.188 Osteonecrosis due to drugs, other site
M87.19 Osteonecrosis due to drugs, multiple sites

● M87.2 Osteonecrosis due to previous trauma
  M87.20 Osteonecrosis due to previous trauma, unspecified bone
  ● M87.21 Osteonecrosis due to previous trauma, shoulder
    M87.211 Osteonecrosis due to previous trauma, right shoulder
    M87.212 Osteonecrosis due to previous trauma, left shoulder
    M87.219 Osteonecrosis due to previous trauma, unspecified shoulder
  ● M87.22 Osteonecrosis due to previous trauma, humerus (Ex) PDX 1346
    M87.221 Osteonecrosis due to previous trauma, right humerus
    M87.222 Osteonecrosis due to previous trauma, left humerus
    M87.229 Osteonecrosis due to previous trauma, unspecified humerus
  ● M87.23 Osteonecrosis due to previous trauma of radius, ulna and carpus
    M87.231 Osteonecrosis due to previous trauma of right radius
    M87.232 Osteonecrosis due to previous trauma of left radius
    M87.233 Osteonecrosis due to previous trauma of unspecified radius
    M87.234 Osteonecrosis due to previous trauma of right ulna
    M87.235 Osteonecrosis due to previous trauma of left ulna
    M87.236 Osteonecrosis due to previous trauma of unspecified ulna
    M87.237 Osteonecrosis due to previous trauma of right carpus
    M87.238 Osteonecrosis due to previous trauma of left carpus
    M87.239 Osteonecrosis due to previous trauma of unspecified carpus
  ● M87.24 Osteonecrosis due to previous trauma, hand and fingers
    M87.241 Osteonecrosis due to previous trauma, right hand
    M87.242 Osteonecrosis due to previous trauma, left hand
    M87.243 Osteonecrosis due to previous trauma, unspecified hand
    M87.244 Osteonecrosis due to previous trauma, right finger(s)
    M87.245 Osteonecrosis due to previous trauma, left finger(s)
    M87.246 Osteonecrosis due to previous trauma, unspecified finger(s)
  ● M87.25 Osteonecrosis due to previous trauma, pelvis and femur (Ex) PDX 1347
    M87.250 Osteonecrosis due to previous trauma, pelvis
    M87.251 Osteonecrosis due to previous trauma, right femur
    M87.252 Osteonecrosis due to previous trauma, left femur
    M87.256 Osteonecrosis due to previous trauma, unspecified femur
  ● M87.26 Osteonecrosis due to previous trauma, tibia and fibula
    M87.261 Osteonecrosis due to previous trauma, right tibia
    M87.262 Osteonecrosis due to previous trauma, left tibia
    M87.263 Osteonecrosis due to previous trauma, unspecified tibia
    M87.264 Osteonecrosis due to previous trauma, right fibula
    M87.265 Osteonecrosis due to previous trauma, left fibula
    M87.266 Osteonecrosis due to previous trauma, unspecified fibula
  ● M87.27 Osteonecrosis due to previous trauma, ankle, foot and toes
    M87.271 Osteonecrosis due to previous trauma, right ankle
    M87.272 Osteonecrosis due to previous trauma, left ankle
    M87.273 Osteonecrosis due to previous trauma, unspecified ankle
    M87.274 Osteonecrosis due to previous trauma, right foot (Ex) PDX 1348
    M87.275 Osteonecrosis due to previous trauma, left foot (Ex) PDX 1348
    M87.276 Osteonecrosis due to previous trauma, unspecified foot (Ex) PDX 1348
    M87.277 Osteonecrosis due to previous trauma, right toe(s)
    M87.278 Osteonecrosis due to previous trauma, left toe(s)
    M87.279 Osteonecrosis due to previous trauma, unspecified toe(s)
  M87.28 Osteonecrosis due to previous trauma, other site
  M87.29 Osteonecrosis due to previous trauma, multiple sites

● M87.3 Other secondary osteonecrosis
  M87.30 Other secondary osteonecrosis, unspecified bone
  ● M87.31 Other secondary osteonecrosis, shoulder
    M87.311 Other secondary osteonecrosis, right shoulder
    M87.312 Other secondary osteonecrosis, left shoulder
    M87.319 Other secondary osteonecrosis, unspecified shoulder
  ● M87.32 Other secondary osteonecrosis, humerus (Ex) PDX 1346
    M87.321 Other secondary osteonecrosis, right humerus
    M87.322 Other secondary osteonecrosis, left humerus
    M87.329 Other secondary osteonecrosis, unspecified humerus
  ● M87.33 Other secondary osteonecrosis of radius, ulna and carpus
    M87.331 Other secondary osteonecrosis of right radius
    M87.332 Other secondary osteonecrosis of left radius
    M87.333 Other secondary osteonecrosis of unspecified radius
    M87.334 Other secondary osteonecrosis of right ulna
    M87.335 Other secondary osteonecrosis of left ulna

CHAPTER 13 (M00-M99)

M87.336 Other secondary osteonecrosis of unspecified ulna
M87.337 Other secondary osteonecrosis of right carpus
M87.338 Other secondary osteonecrosis of left carpus
M87.339 Other secondary osteonecrosis of unspecified carpus

● M87.34 Other secondary osteonecrosis, hand and fingers
M87.341 Other secondary osteonecrosis, right hand
M87.342 Other secondary osteonecrosis, left hand
M87.343 Other secondary osteonecrosis, unspecified hand
M87.344 Other secondary osteonecrosis, right finger(s)
M87.345 Other secondary osteonecrosis, left finger(s)
M87.346 Other secondary osteonecrosis, unspecified finger(s)

● M87.35 Other secondary osteonecrosis, pelvis and femur (Ex) PDX 1347
M87.350 Other secondary osteonecrosis, pelvis
M87.351 Other secondary osteonecrosis, right femur
M87.352 Other secondary osteonecrosis, left femur
M87.353 Other secondary osteonecrosis, unspecified femur

● M87.36 Other secondary osteonecrosis, tibia and fibula
M87.361 Other secondary osteonecrosis, right tibia
M87.362 Other secondary osteonecrosis, left tibia
M87.363 Other secondary osteonecrosis, unspecified tibia
M87.364 Other secondary osteonecrosis, right fibula
M87.365 Other secondary osteonecrosis, left fibula
M87.366 Other secondary osteonecrosis, unspecified fibula

● M87.37 Other secondary osteonecrosis, ankle and foot
M87.371 Other secondary osteonecrosis, right ankle
M87.372 Other secondary osteonecrosis, left ankle
M87.373 Other secondary osteonecrosis, unspecified ankle
M87.374 Other secondary osteonecrosis, right foot (Ex) PDX 1348
M87.375 Other secondary osteonecrosis, left foot (Ex) PDX 1348
M87.376 Other secondary osteonecrosis, unspecified foot (Ex) PDX 1348
M87.377 Other secondary osteonecrosis, right toe(s)
M87.378 Other secondary osteonecrosis, left toe(s)
M87.379 Other secondary osteonecrosis, unspecified toe(s)

M87.38 Other secondary osteonecrosis, other site
M87.39 Other secondary osteonecrosis, multiple sites

● M87.8 Other osteonecrosis
M87.80 Other osteonecrosis, unspecified bone

● M87.81 Other osteonecrosis, shoulder
M87.811 Other osteonecrosis, right shoulder
M87.812 Other osteonecrosis, left shoulder
M87.819 Other osteonecrosis, unspecified shoulder

● M87.82 Other osteonecrosis, humerus (Ex) PDX 1346
M87.821 Other osteonecrosis, right humerus
M87.822 Other osteonecrosis, left humerus
M87.829 Other osteonecrosis, unspecified humerus

● M87.83 Other osteonecrosis of radius, ulna and carpus
M87.831 Other osteonecrosis of right radius
M87.832 Other osteonecrosis of left radius
M87.833 Other osteonecrosis of unspecified radius
M87.834 Other osteonecrosis of right ulna
M87.835 Other osteonecrosis of left ulna
M87.836 Other osteonecrosis of unspecified ulna
M87.837 Other osteonecrosis of right carpus
M87.838 Other osteonecrosis of left carpus
M87.839 Other osteonecrosis of unspecified carpus

● M87.84 Other osteonecrosis, hand and fingers
M87.841 Other osteonecrosis, right hand
M87.842 Other osteonecrosis, left hand
M87.843 Other osteonecrosis, unspecified hand
M87.844 Other osteonecrosis, right finger(s)
M87.845 Other osteonecrosis, left finger(s)
M87.849 Other osteonecrosis, unspecified finger(s)

● M87.85 Other osteonecrosis, pelvis and femur (Ex) PDX 1347
M87.850 Other osteonecrosis, pelvis
M87.851 Other osteonecrosis, right femur
M87.852 Other osteonecrosis, left femur
M87.859 Other osteonecrosis, unspecified femur

● M87.86 Other osteonecrosis, tibia and fibula
M87.861 Other osteonecrosis, right tibia
M87.862 Other osteonecrosis, left tibia
M87.863 Other osteonecrosis, unspecified tibia
M87.864 Other osteonecrosis, right fibula
M87.865 Other osteonecrosis, left fibula
M87.869 Other osteonecrosis, unspecified fibula

● M87.87 Other osteonecrosis, ankle, foot and toes
M87.871 Other osteonecrosis, right ankle
M87.872 Other osteonecrosis, left ankle
M87.873 Other osteonecrosis, unspecified ankle

CHAPTER 13 (M00-M99)

M87.874 Other osteonecrosis, right foot PDX 1348
M87.875 Other osteonecrosis, left foot PDX 1348
M87.876 Other osteonecrosis, unspecified foot PDX 1348
M87.877 Other osteonecrosis, right toe(s)
M87.878 Other osteonecrosis, left toe(s)
M87.879 Other osteonecrosis, unspecified toe(s)
M87.88 Other osteonecrosis, other site
M87.89 Other osteonecrosis, multiple sites
M87.9 Osteonecrosis, unspecified
Necrosis of bone NOS

M88 Osteitis deformans [Paget's disease of bone]

Chronic disorder that results in enlarged and deformed bones. The excessive breakdown and formation of bone tissue causes bones to weaken and results in bone pain, arthritis, deformities, and fractures.

Excludes1 osteitis deformans in neoplastic disease (M90.6)

M88.0 Osteitis deformans of skull
M88.1 Osteitis deformans of vertebrae
M88.8 Osteitis deformans of other bones
M88.81 Osteitis deformans of shoulder
M88.811 Osteitis deformans of right shoulder
M88.812 Osteitis deformans of left shoulder
M88.819 Osteitis deformans of unspecified shoulder
M88.82 Osteitis deformans of upper arm
M88.821 Osteitis deformans of right upper arm
M88.822 Osteitis deformans of left upper arm
M88.829 Osteitis deformans of unspecified upper arm
M88.83 Osteitis deformans of forearm
M88.831 Osteitis deformans of right forearm
M88.832 Osteitis deformans of left forearm
M88.839 Osteitis deformans of unspecified forearm
M88.84 Osteitis deformans of hand
M88.841 Osteitis deformans of right hand
M88.842 Osteitis deformans of left hand
M88.849 Osteitis deformans of unspecified hand
M88.85 Osteitis deformans of thigh
M88.851 Osteitis deformans of right thigh
M88.852 Osteitis deformans of left thigh
M88.859 Osteitis deformans of unspecified thigh
M88.86 Osteitis deformans of lower leg
M88.861 Osteitis deformans of right lower leg
M88.862 Osteitis deformans of left lower leg
M88.869 Osteitis deformans of unspecified lower leg
M88.87 Osteitis deformans of ankle and foot
M88.871 Osteitis deformans of right ankle and foot
M88.872 Osteitis deformans of left ankle and foot
M88.879 Osteitis deformans of unspecified ankle and foot
M88.88 Osteitis deformans of other bones

Excludes2 osteitis deformans of skull (M88.0)
osteitis deformans of vertebrae (M88.1)

M88.89 Osteitis deformans of multiple sites
M88.9 Osteitis deformans of unspecified bone

M89 Other disorders of bone

M89.0 Algoneurodystrophy
Shoulder-hand syndrome
Sudeck's atrophy

Excludes1 causalgia, lower limb (G57.7-)
causalgia, upper limb (G56.4-)
complex regional pain syndrome II, lower limb (G57.7-)
complex regional pain syndrome II, upper limb (G56.4-)
reflex sympathetic dystrophy (G90.5-)

M89.00 Algoneurodystrophy, unspecified site
M89.01 Algoneurodystrophy, shoulder
M89.011 Algoneurodystrophy, right shoulder
M89.012 Algoneurodystrophy, left shoulder
M89.019 Algoneurodystrophy, unspecified shoulder
M89.02 Algoneurodystrophy, upper arm
M89.021 Algoneurodystrophy, right upper arm
M89.022 Algoneurodystrophy, left upper arm
M89.029 Algoneurodystrophy, unspecified upper arm
M89.03 Algoneurodystrophy, forearm
M89.031 Algoneurodystrophy, right forearm
M89.032 Algoneurodystrophy, left forearm
M89.039 Algoneurodystrophy, unspecified forearm
M89.04 Algoneurodystrophy, hand
M89.041 Algoneurodystrophy, right hand
M89.042 Algoneurodystrophy, left hand
M89.049 Algoneurodystrophy, unspecified hand
M89.05 Algoneurodystrophy, thigh
M89.051 Algoneurodystrophy, right thigh
M89.052 Algoneurodystrophy, left thigh
M89.059 Algoneurodystrophy, unspecified thigh
M89.06 Algoneurodystrophy, lower leg
M89.061 Algoneurodystrophy, right lower leg
M89.062 Algoneurodystrophy, left lower leg
M89.069 Algoneurodystrophy, unspecified lower leg
M89.07 Algoneurodystrophy, ankle and foot
M89.071 Algoneurodystrophy, right ankle and foot
M89.072 Algoneurodystrophy, left ankle and foot
M89.079 Algoneurodystrophy, unspecified ankle and foot
M89.08 Algoneurodystrophy, other site
M89.09 Algoneurodystrophy, multiple sites
M89.1 Physeal arrest
Arrest of growth plate
Epiphyseal arrest
Growth plate arrest

CHAPTER 13 (M00-M99)

- ● M89.12 Physeal arrest, humerus
  - M89.121 Complete physeal arrest, right proximal humerus
  - M89.122 Complete physeal arrest, left proximal humerus
  - M89.123 Partial physeal arrest, right proximal humerus
  - M89.124 Partial physeal arrest, left proximal humerus
  - M89.125 Complete physeal arrest, right distal humerus
  - M89.126 Complete physeal arrest, left distal humerus
  - M89.127 Partial physeal arrest, right distal humerus
  - M89.128 Partial physeal arrest, left distal humerus
  - M89.129 Physeal arrest, humerus, unspecified
- ● M89.13 Physeal arrest, forearm
  - M89.131 Complete physeal arrest, right distal radius
  - M89.132 Complete physeal arrest, left distal radius
  - M89.133 Partial physeal arrest, right distal radius
  - M89.134 Partial physeal arrest, left distal radius
  - M89.138 Other physeal arrest of forearm
  - M89.139 Physeal arrest, forearm, unspecified
- ● M89.15 Physeal arrest, femur
  - M89.151 Complete physeal arrest, right proximal femur
  - M89.152 Complete physeal arrest, left proximal femur
  - M89.153 Partial physeal arrest, right proximal femur
  - M89.154 Partial physeal arrest, left proximal femur
  - M89.155 Complete physeal arrest, right distal femur
  - M89.156 Complete physeal arrest, left distal femur
  - M89.157 Partial physeal arrest, right distal femur
  - M89.158 Partial physeal arrest, left distal femur
  - M89.159 Physeal arrest, femur, unspecified
- ● M89.16 Physeal arrest, lower leg
  - M89.160 Complete physeal arrest, right proximal tibia
  - M89.161 Complete physeal arrest, left proximal tibia
  - M89.162 Partial physeal arrest, right proximal tibia
  - M89.163 Partial physeal arrest, left proximal tibia
  - M89.164 Complete physeal arrest, right distal tibia
  - M89.165 Complete physeal arrest, left distal tibia
  - M89.166 Partial physeal arrest, right distal tibia
  - M89.167 Partial physeal arrest, left distal tibia
  - M89.168 Other physeal arrest of lower leg
  - M89.169 Physeal arrest, lower leg, unspecified
- M89.18 Physeal arrest, other site

● M89.2 Other disorders of bone development and growth

- M89.20 Other disorders of bone development and growth, unspecified site
- ● M89.21 Other disorders of bone development and growth, shoulder
  - M89.211 Other disorders of bone development and growth, right shoulder
  - M89.212 Other disorders of bone development and growth, left shoulder
  - M89.219 Other disorders of bone development and growth, unspecified shoulder
- ● M89.22 Other disorders of bone development and growth, humerus
  - M89.221 Other disorders of bone development and growth, right humerus
  - M89.222 Other disorders of bone development and growth, left humerus
  - M89.229 Other disorders of bone development and growth, unspecified humerus
- ● M89.23 Other disorders of bone development and growth, ulna and radius
  - M89.231 Other disorders of bone development and growth, right ulna
  - M89.232 Other disorders of bone development and growth, left ulna
  - M89.233 Other disorders of bone development and growth, right radius
  - M89.234 Other disorders of bone development and growth, left radius
  - M89.239 Other disorders of bone development and growth, unspecified ulna and radius
- ● M89.24 Other disorders of bone development and growth, hand
  - M89.241 Other disorders of bone development and growth, right hand
  - M89.242 Other disorders of bone development and growth, left hand
  - M89.249 Other disorders of bone development and growth, unspecified hand
- ● M89.25 Other disorders of bone development and growth, femur
  - M89.251 Other disorders of bone development and growth, right femur
  - M89.252 Other disorders of bone development and growth, left femur
  - M89.259 Other disorders of bone development and growth, unspecified femur
- ● M89.26 Other disorders of bone development and growth, tibia and fibula
  - M89.261 Other disorders of bone development and growth, right tibia
  - M89.262 Other disorders of bone development and growth, left tibia
  - M89.263 Other disorders of bone development and growth, right fibula
  - M89.264 Other disorders of bone development and growth, left fibula
  - M89.269 Other disorders of bone development and growth, unspecified lower leg
- ● M89.27 Other disorders of bone development and growth, ankle and foot
  - M89.271 Other disorders of bone development and growth, right ankle and foot
  - M89.272 Other disorders of bone development and growth, left ankle and foot
  - M89.279 Other disorders of bone development and growth, unspecified ankle and foot
- M89.28 Other disorders of bone development and growth, other site
- M89.29 Other disorders of bone development and growth, multiple sites

● M89.3 Hypertrophy of bone
M89.30 Hypertrophy of bone, unspecified site
● M89.31 Hypertrophy of bone, shoulder
M89.311 Hypertrophy of bone, right shoulder
M89.312 Hypertrophy of bone, left shoulder
M89.319 Hypertrophy of bone, unspecified shoulder
● M89.32 Hypertrophy of bone, humerus
M89.321 Hypertrophy of bone, right humerus
M89.322 Hypertrophy of bone, left humerus
M89.329 Hypertrophy of bone, unspecified humerus
● M89.33 Hypertrophy of bone, ulna and radius
M89.331 Hypertrophy of bone, right ulna
M89.332 Hypertrophy of bone, left ulna
M89.333 Hypertrophy of bone, right radius
M89.334 Hypertrophy of bone, left radius
M89.339 Hypertrophy of bone, unspecified ulna and radius
● M89.34 Hypertrophy of bone, hand
M89.341 Hypertrophy of bone, right hand
M89.342 Hypertrophy of bone, left hand
M89.349 Hypertrophy of bone, unspecified hand
● M89.35 Hypertrophy of bone, femur
M89.351 Hypertrophy of bone, right femur
M89.352 Hypertrophy of bone, left femur
M89.359 Hypertrophy of bone, unspecified femur
● M89.36 Hypertrophy of bone, tibia and fibula
M89.361 Hypertrophy of bone, right tibia
M89.362 Hypertrophy of bone, left tibia
M89.363 Hypertrophy of bone, right fibula
M89.364 Hypertrophy of bone, left fibula
M89.369 Hypertrophy of bone, unspecified tibia and fibula
● M89.37 Hypertrophy of bone, ankle and foot
M89.371 Hypertrophy of bone, right ankle and foot
M89.372 Hypertrophy of bone, left ankle and foot
M89.379 Hypertrophy of bone, unspecified ankle and foot
M89.38 Hypertrophy of bone, other site
M89.39 Hypertrophy of bone, multiple sites
● M89.4 Other hypertrophic osteoarthropathy
Marie-Bamberger disease
Pachydermoperiostosis
M89.40 Other hypertrophic osteoarthropathy, unspecified site
● M89.41 Other hypertrophic osteoarthropathy, shoulder
M89.411 Other hypertrophic osteoarthropathy, right shoulder
M89.412 Other hypertrophic osteoarthropathy, left shoulder
M89.419 Other hypertrophic osteoarthropathy, unspecified shoulder
● M89.42 Other hypertrophic osteoarthropathy, upper arm
M89.421 Other hypertrophic osteoarthropathy, right upper arm
M89.422 Other hypertrophic osteoarthropathy, left upper arm
M89.429 Other hypertrophic osteoarthropathy, unspecified upper arm
● M89.43 Other hypertrophic osteoarthropathy, forearm
M89.431 Other hypertrophic osteoarthropathy, right forearm
M89.432 Other hypertrophic osteoarthropathy, left forearm
M89.439 Other hypertrophic osteoarthropathy, unspecified forearm
● M89.44 Other hypertrophic osteoarthropathy, hand
M89.441 Other hypertrophic osteoarthropathy, right hand
M89.442 Other hypertrophic osteoarthropathy, left hand
M89.449 Other hypertrophic osteoarthropathy, unspecified hand
● M89.45 Other hypertrophic osteoarthropathy, thigh
M89.451 Other hypertrophic osteoarthropathy, right thigh
M89.452 Other hypertrophic osteoarthropathy, left thigh
M89.459 Other hypertrophic osteoarthropathy, unspecified thigh
● M89.46 Other hypertrophic osteoarthropathy, lower leg
M89.461 Other hypertrophic osteoarthropathy, right lower leg
M89.462 Other hypertrophic osteoarthropathy, left lower leg
M89.469 Other hypertrophic osteoarthropathy, unspecified lower leg
● M89.47 Other hypertrophic osteoarthropathy, ankle and foot
M89.471 Other hypertrophic osteoarthropathy, right ankle and foot
M89.472 Other hypertrophic osteoarthropathy, left ankle and foot
M89.479 Other hypertrophic osteoarthropathy, unspecified ankle and foot
M89.48 Other hypertrophic osteoarthropathy, other site
M89.49 Other hypertrophic osteoarthropathy, multiple sites
● M89.5 Osteolysis
Use additional code to identify major osseous defect, if applicable (M89.7-)
Excludes2 periprosthetic osteolysis of internal prosthetic joint (T84.05-)
M89.50 Osteolysis, unspecified site
● M89.51 Osteolysis, shoulder
M89.511 Osteolysis, right shoulder
M89.512 Osteolysis, left shoulder
M89.519 Osteolysis, unspecified shoulder
● M89.52 Osteolysis, upper arm
M89.521 Osteolysis, right upper arm
M89.522 Osteolysis, left upper arm
M89.529 Osteolysis, unspecified upper arm
● M89.53 Osteolysis, forearm
M89.531 Osteolysis, right forearm
M89.532 Osteolysis, left forearm
M89.539 Osteolysis, unspecified forearm
● M89.54 Osteolysis, hand
M89.541 Osteolysis, right hand
M89.542 Osteolysis, left hand
M89.549 Osteolysis, unspecified hand
● M89.55 Osteolysis, thigh
M89.551 Osteolysis, right thigh
M89.552 Osteolysis, left thigh
M89.559 Osteolysis, unspecified thigh

● M89.56 Osteolysis, lower leg
M89.561 Osteolysis, right lower leg
M89.562 Osteolysis, left lower leg
M89.569 Osteolysis, unspecified lower leg
● M89.57 Osteolysis, ankle and foot
M89.571 Osteolysis, right ankle and foot
M89.572 Osteolysis, left ankle and foot
M89.579 Osteolysis, unspecified ankle and foot
M89.58 Osteolysis, other site
M89.59 Osteolysis, multiple sites
● M89.6 Osteopathy after poliomyelitis
Use additional code (B91) to identify previous poliomyelitis
Excludes1 postpolio syndrome (G14)
M89.60 Osteopathy after poliomyelitis, unspecified site
● M89.61 Osteopathy after poliomyelitis, shoulder
M89.611 Osteopathy after poliomyelitis, right shoulder
M89.612 Osteopathy after poliomyelitis, left shoulder
M89.619 Osteopathy after poliomyelitis, unspecified shoulder
● M89.62 Osteopathy after poliomyelitis, upper arm
M89.621 Osteopathy after poliomyelitis, right upper arm
M89.622 Osteopathy after poliomyelitis, left upper arm
M89.629 Osteopathy after poliomyelitis, unspecified upper arm
● M89.63 Osteopathy after poliomyelitis, forearm
M89.631 Osteopathy after poliomyelitis, right forearm
M89.632 Osteopathy after poliomyelitis, left forearm
M89.639 Osteopathy after poliomyelitis, unspecified forearm
● M89.64 Osteopathy after poliomyelitis, hand
M89.641 Osteopathy after poliomyelitis, right hand
M89.642 Osteopathy after poliomyelitis, left hand
M89.649 Osteopathy after poliomyelitis, unspecified hand
● M89.65 Osteopathy after poliomyelitis, thigh
M89.651 Osteopathy after poliomyelitis, right thigh
M89.652 Osteopathy after poliomyelitis, left thigh
M89.659 Osteopathy after poliomyelitis, unspecified thigh
● M89.66 Osteopathy after poliomyelitis, lower leg
M89.661 Osteopathy after poliomyelitis, right lower leg
M89.662 Osteopathy after poliomyelitis, left lower leg
M89.669 Osteopathy after poliomyelitis, unspecified lower leg
● M89.67 Osteopathy after poliomyelitis, ankle and foot
M89.671 Osteopathy after poliomyelitis, right ankle and foot
M89.672 Osteopathy after poliomyelitis, left ankle and foot
M89.679 Osteopathy after poliomyelitis, unspecified ankle and foot
M89.68 Osteopathy after poliomyelitis, other site
M89.69 Osteopathy after poliomyelitis, multiple sites
● M89.7 Major osseous defect
Code first underlying disease, if known, such as:
aseptic necrosis of bone (M87.-)
malignant neoplasm of bone (C4Ø.-)
osteolysis (M89.5-)
osteomyelitis (M86.-)
osteonecrosis (M87.-)
osteoporosis (M8Ø.-, M81.-)
periprosthetic osteolysis (T84.Ø5-)
M89.7Ø Major osseous defect, unspecified site
● M89.71 Major osseous defect, shoulder region
Major osseous defect clavicle or scapula
M89.711 Major osseous defect, right shoulder region
M89.712 Major osseous defect, left shoulder region
M89.719 Major osseous defect, unspecified shoulder region
● M89.72 Major osseous defect, humerus
M89.721 Major osseous defect, right humerus
M89.722 Major osseous defect, left humerus
M89.729 Major osseous defect, unspecified humerus
● M89.73 Major osseous defect, forearm
Major osseous defect of radius and ulna
M89.731 Major osseous defect, right forearm
M89.732 Major osseous defect, left forearm
M89.739 Major osseous defect, unspecified forearm
● M89.74 Major osseous defect, hand
Major osseous defect of carpus, fingers, metacarpus
M89.741 Major osseous defect, right hand
M89.742 Major osseous defect, left hand
M89.749 Major osseous defect, unspecified hand
● M89.75 Major osseous defect, pelvic region and thigh
Major osseous defect of femur and pelvis
M89.751 Major osseous defect, right pelvic region and thigh
M89.752 Major osseous defect, left pelvic region and thigh
M89.759 Major osseous defect, unspecified pelvic region and thigh
● M89.76 Major osseous defect, lower leg
Major osseous defect of fibula and tibia
M89.761 Major osseous defect, right lower leg
M89.762 Major osseous defect, left lower leg
M89.769 Major osseous defect, unspecified lower leg
● M89.77 Major osseous defect, ankle and foot
Major osseous defect of metatarsus, tarsus, toes
M89.771 Major osseous defect, right ankle and foot
M89.772 Major osseous defect, left ankle and foot
M89.779 Major osseous defect, unspecified ankle and foot
M89.78 Major osseous defect, other site
M89.79 Major osseous defect, multiple sites
● M89.8 Other specified disorders of bone
Infantile cortical hyperostoses
Post-traumatic subperiosteal ossification
Coding Clinic: 2Ø22, Q2, P1Ø
● M89.8X Other specified disorders of bone

CHAPTER 13 (MØØ-M99)

M89.8XØ Other specified disorders of bone, multiple sites

M89.8X1 Other specified disorders of bone, shoulder

M89.8X2 Other specified disorders of bone, upper arm

M89.8X3 Other specified disorders of bone, forearm
Coding Clinic: 2Ø19, Q3, P1Ø

M89.8X4 Other specified disorders of bone, hand

M89.8X5 Other specified disorders of bone, thigh

M89.8X6 Other specified disorders of bone, lower leg

M89.8X7 Other specified disorders of bone, ankle and foot

M89.8X8 Other specified disorders of bone, other site
Coding Clinic: 2Ø23, Q2, P19

M89.8X9 Other specified disorders of bone, unspecified site

M89.9 Disorder of bone, unspecified

M9Ø Osteopathies in diseases classified elsewhere

Excludes1 osteochondritis, osteomyelitis, and osteopathy (in):
- cryptococcosis (B45.3)
- diabetes mellitus (EØ8-E13 with .69-)
- gonococcal (A54.43)
- neurogenic syphilis (A52.11)
- renal osteodystrophy (N25.Ø)
- salmonellosis (AØ2.24)
- secondary syphilis (A51.46)
- syphilis (late) (A52.77)

M9Ø.5 Osteonecrosis in diseases classified elsewhere

Code first underlying disease, such as:
- caisson disease (T7Ø.3)
- hemoglobinopathy (D5Ø-D64)

M9Ø.5Ø Osteonecrosis in diseases classified elsewhere, unspecified site Ex PDX 1345
CC when PDx is its own CC

M9Ø.51 Osteonecrosis in diseases classified elsewhere, shoulder Ex PDX 1346

M9Ø.511 Osteonecrosis in diseases classified elsewhere, right shoulder
CC when PDx is its own CC

M9Ø.512 Osteonecrosis in diseases classified elsewhere, left shoulder
CC when PDx is its own CC

M9Ø.519 Osteonecrosis in diseases classified elsewhere, unspecified shoulder
CC when PDx is its own CC

M9Ø.52 Osteonecrosis in diseases classified elsewhere, upper arm Ex PDX 1345

M9Ø.521 Osteonecrosis in diseases classified elsewhere, right upper arm
CC when PDx is its own CC

M9Ø.522 Osteonecrosis in diseases classified elsewhere, left upper arm
CC when PDx is its own CC

M9Ø.529 Osteonecrosis in diseases classified elsewhere, unspecified upper arm
CC when PDx is its own CC

M9Ø.53 Osteonecrosis in diseases classified elsewhere, forearm Ex PDX 1345

M9Ø.531 Osteonecrosis in diseases classified elsewhere, right forearm
CC when PDx is its own CC

M9Ø.532 Osteonecrosis in diseases classified elsewhere, left forearm
CC when PDx is its own CC

M9Ø.539 Osteonecrosis in diseases classified elsewhere, unspecified forearm
CC when PDx is its own CC

M9Ø.54 Osteonecrosis in diseases classified elsewhere, hand Ex PDX 1345

M9Ø.541 Osteonecrosis in diseases classified elsewhere, right hand
CC when PDx is its own CC

M9Ø.542 Osteonecrosis in diseases classified elsewhere, left hand
CC when PDx is its own CC

M9Ø.549 Osteonecrosis in diseases classified elsewhere, unspecified hand
CC when PDx is its own CC

M9Ø.55 Osteonecrosis in diseases classified elsewhere, thigh Ex PDX 1347

M9Ø.551 Osteonecrosis in diseases classified elsewhere, right thigh
CC when PDx is its own CC

M9Ø.552 Osteonecrosis in diseases classified elsewhere, left thigh
CC when PDx is its own CC

M9Ø.559 Osteonecrosis in diseases classified elsewhere, unspecified thigh
CC when PDx is its own CC

M9Ø.56 Osteonecrosis in diseases classified elsewhere, lower leg Ex PDX 1345

M9Ø.561 Osteonecrosis in diseases classified elsewhere, right lower leg
CC when PDx is its own CC

M9Ø.562 Osteonecrosis in diseases classified elsewhere, left lower leg
CC when PDx is its own CC

M9Ø.569 Osteonecrosis in diseases classified elsewhere, unspecified lower leg
CC when PDx is its own CC

M9Ø.57 Osteonecrosis in diseases classified elsewhere, ankle and foot Ex PDX 1345

M9Ø.571 Osteonecrosis in diseases classified elsewhere, right ankle and foot
CC when PDx is its own CC

M9Ø.572 Osteonecrosis in diseases classified elsewhere, left ankle and foot
CC when PDx is its own CC

M9Ø.579 Osteonecrosis in diseases classified elsewhere, unspecified ankle and foot
CC when PDx is its own CC

M9Ø.58 Osteonecrosis in diseases classified elsewhere, other site Ex PDX 1345
CC when PDx is its own CC

M9Ø.59 Osteonecrosis in diseases classified elsewhere, multiple sites Ex PDX 1345
CC when PDx is its own CC

M9Ø.6 Osteitis deformans in neoplastic diseases

Osteitis deformans in malignant neoplasm of bone

Code first the neoplasm (C4Ø.-, C41.-)

Excludes1 osteitis deformans [Paget's disease of bone] (M88.-)

M9Ø.6Ø Osteitis deformans in neoplastic diseases, unspecified site

M90.61 Osteitis deformans in neoplastic diseases, shoulder
M90.611 Osteitis deformans in neoplastic diseases, right shoulder
M90.612 Osteitis deformans in neoplastic diseases, left shoulder
M90.619 Osteitis deformans in neoplastic diseases, unspecified shoulder

M90.62 Osteitis deformans in neoplastic diseases, upper arm
M90.621 Osteitis deformans in neoplastic diseases, right upper arm
M90.622 Osteitis deformans in neoplastic diseases, left upper arm
M90.629 Osteitis deformans in neoplastic diseases, unspecified upper arm

M90.63 Osteitis deformans in neoplastic diseases, forearm
M90.631 Osteitis deformans in neoplastic diseases, right forearm
M90.632 Osteitis deformans in neoplastic diseases, left forearm
M90.639 Osteitis deformans in neoplastic diseases, unspecified forearm

M90.64 Osteitis deformans in neoplastic diseases, hand
M90.641 Osteitis deformans in neoplastic diseases, right hand
M90.642 Osteitis deformans in neoplastic diseases, left hand
M90.649 Osteitis deformans in neoplastic diseases, unspecified hand

M90.65 Osteitis deformans in neoplastic diseases, thigh
M90.651 Osteitis deformans in neoplastic diseases, right thigh
M90.652 Osteitis deformans in neoplastic diseases, left thigh
M90.659 Osteitis deformans in neoplastic diseases, unspecified thigh

M90.66 Osteitis deformans in neoplastic diseases, lower leg
M90.661 Osteitis deformans in neoplastic diseases, right lower leg
M90.662 Osteitis deformans in neoplastic diseases, left lower leg
M90.669 Osteitis deformans in neoplastic diseases, unspecified lower leg

M90.67 Osteitis deformans in neoplastic diseases, ankle and foot
M90.671 Osteitis deformans in neoplastic diseases, right ankle and foot
M90.672 Osteitis deformans in neoplastic diseases, left ankle and foot
M90.679 Osteitis deformans in neoplastic diseases, unspecified ankle and foot

M90.68 Osteitis deformans in neoplastic diseases, other site

M90.69 Osteitis deformans in neoplastic diseases, multiple sites

M90.8 Osteopathy in diseases classified elsewhere

Code first underlying disease, such as:
rickets (E55.0)
vitamin-D-resistant rickets (E83.31)

M90.80 Osteopathy in diseases classified elsewhere, unspecified site

M90.81 Osteopathy in diseases classified elsewhere, shoulder
M90.811 Osteopathy in diseases classified elsewhere, right shoulder
M90.812 Osteopathy in diseases classified elsewhere, left shoulder
M90.819 Osteopathy in diseases classified elsewhere, unspecified shoulder

M90.82 Osteopathy in diseases classified elsewhere, upper arm
M90.821 Osteopathy in diseases classified elsewhere, right upper arm
M90.822 Osteopathy in diseases classified elsewhere, left upper arm
M90.829 Osteopathy in diseases classified elsewhere, unspecified upper arm

M90.83 Osteopathy in diseases classified elsewhere, forearm
M90.831 Osteopathy in diseases classified elsewhere, right forearm
M90.832 Osteopathy in diseases classified elsewhere, left forearm
M90.839 Osteopathy in diseases classified elsewhere, unspecified forearm

M90.84 Osteopathy in diseases classified elsewhere, hand
M90.841 Osteopathy in diseases classified elsewhere, right hand
M90.842 Osteopathy in diseases classified elsewhere, left hand
M90.849 Osteopathy in diseases classified elsewhere, unspecified hand

M90.85 Osteopathy in diseases classified elsewhere, thigh
M90.851 Osteopathy in diseases classified elsewhere, right thigh
M90.852 Osteopathy in diseases classified elsewhere, left thigh
M90.859 Osteopathy in diseases classified elsewhere, unspecified thigh

M90.86 Osteopathy in diseases classified elsewhere, lower leg
M90.861 Osteopathy in diseases classified elsewhere, right lower leg
M90.862 Osteopathy in diseases classified elsewhere, left lower leg
M90.869 Osteopathy in diseases classified elsewhere, unspecified lower leg

M90.87 Osteopathy in diseases classified elsewhere, ankle and foot
M90.871 Osteopathy in diseases classified elsewhere, right ankle and foot
M90.872 Osteopathy in diseases classified elsewhere, left ankle and foot
M90.879 Osteopathy in diseases classified elsewhere, unspecified ankle and foot

M90.88 Osteopathy in diseases classified elsewhere, other site

M90.89 Osteopathy in diseases classified elsewhere, multiple sites

CHONDROPATHIES (M91-M94)

Excludes1 postprocedural chondropathies (M96.-)

M91 Juvenile osteochondrosis of hip and pelvis

Excludes1 slipped upper femoral epiphysis (nontraumatic) (M93.Ø-)

M91.Ø Juvenile osteochondrosis of pelvis
Osteochondrosis (juvenile) of acetabulum
Osteochondrosis (juvenile) of iliac crest [Buchanan]
Osteochondrosis (juvenile) of ischiopubic synchondrosis [van Neck]
Osteochondrosis (juvenile) of symphysis pubis [Pierson]

M91.1 Juvenile osteochondrosis of head of femur [Legg-Calvé-Perthes]
- **M91.1Ø** Juvenile osteochondrosis of head of femur [Legg-Calvé-Perthes], unspecified leg
- **M91.11** Juvenile osteochondrosis of head of femur [Legg-Calvé-Perthes], right leg
- **M91.12** Juvenile osteochondrosis of head of femur [Legg-Calvé-Perthes], left leg

M91.2 Coxa plana
Hip deformity due to previous juvenile osteochondrosis
- **M91.2Ø** Coxa plana, unspecified hip
- **M91.21** Coxa plana, right hip
- **M91.22** Coxa plana, left hip

M91.3 Pseudocoxalgia
- **M91.3Ø** Pseudocoxalgia, unspecified hip
- **M91.31** Pseudocoxalgia, right hip
- **M91.32** Pseudocoxalgia, left hip

M91.4 Coxa magna
- **M91.4Ø** Coxa magna, unspecified hip
- **M91.41** Coxa magna, right hip
- **M91.42** Coxa magna, left hip

M91.8 Other juvenile osteochondrosis of hip and pelvis
Juvenile osteochondrosis after reduction of congenital dislocation of hip
- **M91.8Ø** Other juvenile osteochondrosis of hip and pelvis, unspecified leg
- **M91.81** Other juvenile osteochondrosis of hip and pelvis, right leg
- **M91.82** Other juvenile osteochondrosis of hip and pelvis, left leg

M91.9 Juvenile osteochondrosis of hip and pelvis, unspecified
- **M91.9Ø** Juvenile osteochondrosis of hip and pelvis, unspecified, unspecified leg
- **M91.91** Juvenile osteochondrosis of hip and pelvis, unspecified, right leg
- **M91.92** Juvenile osteochondrosis of hip and pelvis, unspecified, left leg

M92 Other juvenile osteochondrosis

M92.Ø Juvenile osteochondrosis of humerus
Osteochondrosis (juvenile) of capitulum of humerus [Panner]
Osteochondrosis (juvenile) of head of humerus [Haas]
- **M92.ØØ** Juvenile osteochondrosis of humerus, unspecified arm
- **M92.Ø1** Juvenile osteochondrosis of humerus, right arm
- **M92.Ø2** Juvenile osteochondrosis of humerus, left arm

M92.1 Juvenile osteochondrosis of radius and ulna
Osteochondrosis (juvenile) of lower ulna [Burns]
Osteochondrosis (juvenile) of radial head [Brailsford]
- **M92.1Ø** Juvenile osteochondrosis of radius and ulna, unspecified arm
- **M92.11** Juvenile osteochondrosis of radius and ulna, right arm
- **M92.12** Juvenile osteochondrosis of radius and ulna, left arm

M92.2 Juvenile osteochondrosis, hand

M92.2Ø Unspecified juvenile osteochondrosis, hand
- **M92.2Ø1** Unspecified juvenile osteochondrosis, right hand
- **M92.2Ø2** Unspecified juvenile osteochondrosis, left hand
- **M92.2Ø9** Unspecified juvenile osteochondrosis, unspecified hand

M92.21 Osteochondrosis (juvenile) of carpal lunate [Kienböck]
- **M92.211** Osteochondrosis (juvenile) of carpal lunate [Kienböck], right hand
- **M92.212** Osteochondrosis (juvenile) of carpal lunate [Kienböck], left hand
- **M92.219** Osteochondrosis (juvenile) of carpal lunate [Kienböck], unspecified hand

M92.22 Osteochondrosis (juvenile) of metacarpal heads [Mauclaire]
- **M92.221** Osteochondrosis (juvenile) of metacarpal heads [Mauclaire], right hand
- **M92.222** Osteochondrosis (juvenile) of metacarpal heads [Mauclaire], left hand
- **M92.229** Osteochondrosis (juvenile) of metacarpal heads [Mauclaire], unspecified hand

M92.29 Other juvenile osteochondrosis, hand
- **M92.291** Other juvenile osteochondrosis, right hand
- **M92.292** Other juvenile osteochondrosis, left hand
- **M92.299** Other juvenile osteochondrosis, unspecified hand

M92.3 Other juvenile osteochondrosis, upper limb
- **M92.3Ø** Other juvenile osteochondrosis, unspecified upper limb
- **M92.31** Other juvenile osteochondrosis, right upper limb
- **M92.32** Other juvenile osteochondrosis, left upper limb

M92.4 Juvenile osteochondrosis of patella
Osteochondrosis (juvenile) of primary patellar center [Köhler]
Osteochondrosis (juvenile) of secondary patellar center [Sinding Larsen]
- **M92.4Ø** Juvenile osteochondrosis of patella, unspecified knee
- **M92.41** Juvenile osteochondrosis of patella, right knee
- **M92.42** Juvenile osteochondrosis of patella, left knee

M92.5 Juvenile osteochondrosis of tibia and fibula

M92.5Ø Unspecified juvenile osteochondrosis of tibia and fibula
- **M92.5Ø1** Unspecified juvenile osteochondrosis, right leg
- **M92.5Ø2** Unspecified juvenile osteochondrosis, left leg
- **M92.5Ø3** Unspecified juvenile osteochondrosis, bilateral leg
- **M92.5Ø9** Unspecified juvenile osteochondrosis, unspecified leg

M92.51 Juvenile osteochondrosis of proximal tibia
Blount disease
Tibia vara
- **M92.511** Juvenile osteochondrosis of proximal tibia, right leg
- **M92.512** Juvenile osteochondrosis of proximal tibia, left leg

M92.513 Juvenile osteochondrosis of proximal tibia, bilateral

M92.519 Juvenile osteochondrosis of proximal tibia, unspecified leg

● M92.52 Juvenile osteochondrosis of tibia tubercle
Osgood-Schlatter disease

M92.521 Juvenile osteochondrosis of tibia tubercle, right leg

M92.522 Juvenile osteochondrosis of tibia tubercle, left leg

M92.523 Juvenile osteochondrosis of tibia tubercle, bilateral

M92.529 Juvenile osteochondrosis of tibia tubercle, unspecified leg

M92.59 Other juvenile osteochondrosis of tibia and fibula

M92.591 Other juvenile osteochondrosis of tibia and fibula, right leg

M92.592 Other juvenile osteochondrosis of tibia and fibula, left leg

M92.593 Other juvenile osteochondrosis of tibia and fibula, bilateral

M92.599 Other juvenile osteochondrosis of tibia and fibula, unspecified leg

● M92.6 Juvenile osteochondrosis of tarsus
Osteochondrosis (juvenile) of calcaneum [Sever]
Osteochondrosis (juvenile) of os tibiale externum [Haglund]
Osteochondrosis (juvenile) of talus [Diaz]
Osteochondrosis (juvenile) of tarsal navicular [Köhler]

M92.60 Juvenile osteochondrosis of tarsus, unspecified ankle

M92.61 Juvenile osteochondrosis of tarsus, right ankle

M92.62 Juvenile osteochondrosis of tarsus, left ankle

● M92.7 Juvenile osteochondrosis of metatarsus
Osteochondrosis (juvenile) of fifth metatarsus [Iselin]
Osteochondrosis (juvenile) of second metatarsus [Freiberg]

M92.70 Juvenile osteochondrosis of metatarsus, unspecified foot

M92.71 Juvenile osteochondrosis of metatarsus, right foot

M92.72 Juvenile osteochondrosis of metatarsus, left foot

M92.8 Other specified juvenile osteochondrosis
~~Calcaneal apophysitis~~

M92.9 Juvenile osteochondrosis, unspecified
Juvenile apophysitis NOS
Juvenile epiphysitis NOS
Juvenile osteochondritis NOS
Juvenile osteochondrosis NOS

● M93 Other osteochondropathies
Excludes2 osteochondrosis of spine (M42.-)

● M93.0 Slipped upper femoral epiphysis (nontraumatic)
Slipped capital femoral epiphysis (SCFE)
Slipped upper femoral epiphysis (SUFE)
Use additional code for associated chondrolysis (M94.3)

● M93.00 Unspecified slipped upper femoral epiphysis (nontraumatic)

M93.001 Unspecified slipped upper femoral epiphysis (nontraumatic), right hip

M93.002 Unspecified slipped upper femoral epiphysis (nontraumatic), left hip

M93.003 Unspecified slipped upper femoral epiphysis (nontraumatic), unspecified hip

M93.004 Unspecified slipped upper femoral epiphysis (nontraumatic), bilateral hips

● M93.01 Acute slipped upper femoral epiphysis, stable (nontraumatic)

M93.011 Acute slipped upper femoral epiphysis, stable (nontraumatic), right hip

M93.012 Acute slipped upper femoral epiphysis, stable (nontraumatic), left hip

M93.013 Acute slipped upper femoral epiphysis, stable (nontraumatic), unspecified hip

M93.014 Acute slipped upper femoral epiphysis, stable (nontraumatic), bilateral hips

● M93.02 Chronic slipped upper femoral epiphysis, stable (nontraumatic)

M93.021 Chronic slipped upper femoral epiphysis, stable (nontraumatic), right hip

M93.022 Chronic slipped upper femoral epiphysis, stable (nontraumatic), left hip

M93.023 Chronic slipped upper femoral epiphysis, stable (nontraumatic), unspecified hip

M93.024 Chronic slipped upper femoral epiphysis, stable (nontraumatic), bilateral hips

● M93.03 Acute on chronic slipped upper femoral epiphysis, stable (nontraumatic)

M93.031 Acute on chronic slipped upper femoral epiphysis, stable (nontraumatic), right hip

M93.032 Acute on chronic slipped upper femoral epiphysis, stable (nontraumatic), left hip

M93.033 Acute on chronic slipped upper femoral epiphysis, stable (nontraumatic), unspecified hip

M93.034 Acute on chronic slipped upper femoral epiphysis, stable (nontraumatic), bilateral hips

● M93.04 Acute slipped upper femoral epiphysis, unstable (nontraumatic)

M93.041 Acute slipped upper femoral epiphysis, unstable (nontraumatic), right hip

M93.042 Acute slipped upper femoral epiphysis, unstable (nontraumatic), left hip

M93.043 Acute slipped upper femoral epiphysis, unstable (nontraumatic), unspecified hip

M93.044 Acute slipped upper femoral epiphysis, unstable (nontraumatic), bilateral hips

● M93.05 Acute on chronic slipped upper femoral epiphysis, unstable (nontraumatic)

M93.051 Acute on chronic slipped upper femoral epiphysis, unstable (nontraumatic), right hip

M93.052 Acute on chronic slipped upper femoral epiphysis, unstable (nontraumatic), left hip

M93.053 Acute on chronic slipped upper femoral epiphysis, unstable (nontraumatic), unspecified hip

M93.054 Acute on chronic slipped upper femoral epiphysis, unstable (nontraumatic), bilateral hips

CHAPTER 13 (M00-M99)

●M93.Ø6 Acute slipped upper femoral epiphysis, unspecified stability (nontraumatic)
M93.Ø61 Acute slipped upper femoral epiphysis, unspecified stability (nontraumatic), right hip
M93.Ø62 Acute slipped upper femoral epiphysis, unspecified stability (nontraumatic), left hip
M93.Ø63 Acute slipped upper femoral epiphysis, unspecified stability (nontraumatic), unspecified hip
M93.Ø64 Acute slipped upper femoral epiphysis, unspecified stability (nontraumatic), bilateral hips
●M93.Ø7 Acute on chronic slipped upper femoral epiphysis, unspecified stability (nontraumatic)
M93.Ø71 Acute on chronic slipped upper femoral epiphysis, unspecified stability (nontraumatic), right hip
M93.Ø72 Acute on chronic slipped upper femoral epiphysis, unspecified stability (nontraumatic), left hip
M93.Ø73 Acute on chronic slipped upper femoral epiphysis, unspecified stability (nontraumatic), unspecified hip
M93.Ø74 Acute on chronic slipped upper femoral epiphysis, unspecified stability (nontraumatic), bilateral hips
M93.1 Kienböck's disease of adults A
Adult osteochondrosis of carpal lunates
●M93.2 Osteochondritis dissecans
M93.2Ø Osteochondritis dissecans of unspecified site
●M93.21 Osteochondritis dissecans of shoulder
M93.211 Osteochondritis dissecans, right shoulder
M93.212 Osteochondritis dissecans, left shoulder
M93.219 Osteochondritis dissecans, unspecified shoulder
●M93.22 Osteochondritis dissecans of elbow
M93.221 Osteochondritis dissecans, right elbow
M93.222 Osteochondritis dissecans, left elbow
M93.229 Osteochondritis dissecans, unspecified elbow
●M93.23 Osteochondritis dissecans of wrist
M93.231 Osteochondritis dissecans, right wrist
M93.232 Osteochondritis dissecans, left wrist
M93.239 Osteochondritis dissecans, unspecified wrist
●M93.24 Osteochondritis dissecans of joints of hand
M93.241 Osteochondritis dissecans, joints of right hand
M93.242 Osteochondritis dissecans, joints of left hand
M93.249 Osteochondritis dissecans, joints of unspecified hand
●M93.25 Osteochondritis dissecans of hip
M93.251 Osteochondritis dissecans, right hip
M93.252 Osteochondritis dissecans, left hip
M93.259 Osteochondritis dissecans, unspecified hip
●M93.26 Osteochondritis dissecans knee
M93.261 Osteochondritis dissecans, right knee
M93.262 Osteochondritis dissecans, left knee
M93.269 Osteochondritis dissecans, unspecified knee
●M93.27 Osteochondritis dissecans of ankle and joints of foot
M93.271 Osteochondritis dissecans, right ankle and joints of right foot
M93.272 Osteochondritis dissecans, left ankle and joints of left foot
M93.279 Osteochondritis dissecans, unspecified ankle and joints of foot
M93.28 Osteochondritis dissecans other site
M93.29 Osteochondritis dissecans multiple sites
●M93.8 Other specified osteochondropathies
M93.8Ø Other specified osteochondropathies of unspecified site
●M93.81 Other specified osteochondropathies of shoulder
M93.811 Other specified osteochondropathies, right shoulder
M93.812 Other specified osteochondropathies, left shoulder
M93.819 Other specified osteochondropathies, unspecified shoulder
●M93.82 Other specified osteochondropathies of upper arm
M93.821 Other specified osteochondropathies, right upper arm
M93.822 Other specified osteochondropathies, left upper arm
M93.829 Other specified osteochondropathies, unspecified upper arm
●M93.83 Other specified osteochondropathies of forearm
M93.831 Other specified osteochondropathies, right forearm
M93.832 Other specified osteochondropathies, left forearm
M93.839 Other specified osteochondropathies, unspecified forearm
●M93.84 Other specified osteochondropathies of hand
M93.841 Other specified osteochondropathies, right hand
M93.842 Other specified osteochondropathies, left hand
M93.849 Other specified osteochondropathies, unspecified hand
●M93.85 Other specified osteochondropathies of thigh
M93.851 Other specified osteochondropathies, right thigh
M93.852 Other specified osteochondropathies, left thigh
M93.859 Other specified osteochondropathies, unspecified thigh
●M93.86 Other specified osteochondropathies lower leg
M93.861 Other specified osteochondropathies, right lower leg
M93.862 Other specified osteochondropathies, left lower leg
M93.869 Other specified osteochondropathies, unspecified lower leg
●M93.87 Other specified osteochondropathies of ankle and foot
M93.871 Other specified osteochondropathies, right ankle and foot
M93.872 Other specified osteochondropathies, left ankle and foot
M93.879 Other specified osteochondropathies, unspecified ankle and foot
M93.88 Other specified osteochondropathies other
M93.89 Other specified osteochondropathies multiple sites

M93.9 Osteochondropathy, unspecified
Apophysitis NOS
Epiphysitis NOS
Osteochondritis NOS
Osteochondrosis NOS
M93.90 Osteochondropathy, unspecified of unspecified site
● M93.91 Osteochondropathy, unspecified of shoulder
M93.911 Osteochondropathy, unspecified, right shoulder
M93.912 Osteochondropathy, unspecified, left shoulder
M93.919 Osteochondropathy, unspecified, unspecified shoulder
● M93.92 Osteochondropathy, unspecified of upper arm
M93.921 Osteochondropathy, unspecified, right upper arm
M93.922 Osteochondropathy, unspecified, left upper arm
M93.929 Osteochondropathy, unspecified, unspecified upper arm
● M93.93 Osteochondropathy, unspecified of forearm
M93.931 Osteochondropathy, unspecified, right forearm
M93.932 Osteochondropathy, unspecified, left forearm
M93.939 Osteochondropathy, unspecified, unspecified forearm
● M93.94 Osteochondropathy, unspecified of hand
M93.941 Osteochondropathy, unspecified, right hand
M93.942 Osteochondropathy, unspecified, left hand
M93.949 Osteochondropathy, unspecified, unspecified hand
● M93.95 Osteochondropathy, unspecified of thigh
M93.951 Osteochondropathy, unspecified, right thigh
M93.952 Osteochondropathy, unspecified, left thigh
M93.959 Osteochondropathy, unspecified, unspecified thigh
● M93.96 Osteochondropathy, unspecified lower leg
M93.961 Osteochondropathy, unspecified, right lower leg
M93.962 Osteochondropathy, unspecified, left lower leg
M93.969 Osteochondropathy, unspecified, unspecified lower leg
● M93.97 Osteochondropathy, unspecified of ankle and foot
M93.971 Osteochondropathy, unspecified, right ankle and foot
M93.972 Osteochondropathy, unspecified, left ankle and foot
M93.979 Osteochondropathy, unspecified, unspecified ankle and foot
M93.98 Osteochondropathy, unspecified other
M93.99 Osteochondropathy, unspecified multiple sites

● M94 Other disorders of cartilage
M94.0 Chondrocostal junction syndrome [Tietze]
Costochondritis
M94.1 Relapsing polychondritis
● M94.2 Chondromalacia
Excludes1 chondromalacia patellae (M22.4)
M94.20 Chondromalacia, unspecified site
● M94.21 Chondromalacia, shoulder
M94.211 Chondromalacia, right shoulder
M94.212 Chondromalacia, left shoulder
M94.219 Chondromalacia, unspecified shoulder
● M94.22 Chondromalacia, elbow
M94.221 Chondromalacia, right elbow
M94.222 Chondromalacia, left elbow
M94.229 Chondromalacia, unspecified elbow
● M94.23 Chondromalacia, wrist
M94.231 Chondromalacia, right wrist
M94.232 Chondromalacia, left wrist
M94.239 Chondromalacia, unspecified wrist
● M94.24 Chondromalacia, joints of hand
M94.241 Chondromalacia, joints of right hand
M94.242 Chondromalacia, joints of left hand
M94.249 Chondromalacia, joints of unspecified hand
● M94.25 Chondromalacia, hip
M94.251 Chondromalacia, right hip
M94.252 Chondromalacia, left hip
M94.259 Chondromalacia, unspecified hip
● M94.26 Chondromalacia, knee
M94.261 Chondromalacia, right knee
M94.262 Chondromalacia, left knee
M94.269 Chondromalacia, unspecified knee
● M94.27 Chondromalacia, ankle and joints of foot
M94.271 Chondromalacia, right ankle and joints of right foot
M94.272 Chondromalacia, left ankle and joints of left foot
M94.279 Chondromalacia, unspecified ankle and joints of foot
M94.28 Chondromalacia, other site
M94.29 Chondromalacia, multiple sites
● M94.3 Chondrolysis
Code first any associated slipped upper femoral epiphysis (nontraumatic) (M93.0-)
● M94.35 Chondrolysis, hip
M94.351 Chondrolysis, right hip
M94.352 Chondrolysis, left hip
M94.359 Chondrolysis, unspecified hip
● M94.8 Other specified disorders of cartilage
● M94.8X Other specified disorders of cartilage
M94.8X0 Other specified disorders of cartilage, multiple sites
M94.8X1 Other specified disorders of cartilage, shoulder
M94.8X2 Other specified disorders of cartilage, upper arm
M94.8X3 Other specified disorders of cartilage, forearm
M94.8X4 Other specified disorders of cartilage, hand
M94.8X5 Other specified disorders of cartilage, thigh
M94.8X6 Other specified disorders of cartilage, lower leg
M94.8X7 Other specified disorders of cartilage, ankle and foot
M94.8X8 Other specified disorders of cartilage, other site
M94.8X9 Other specified disorders of cartilage, unspecified sites
M94.9 Disorder of cartilage, unspecified

CHAPTER 13 (M00-M99)

OTHER DISORDERS OF THE MUSCULOSKELETAL SYSTEM AND CONNECTIVE TISSUE (M95)

● **M95 Other acquired deformities of musculoskeletal system and connective tissue**

Excludes2 acquired absence of limbs and organs (Z89-Z90)
acquired deformities of limbs (M20-M21)
congenital malformations and deformations of the musculoskeletal system (Q65-Q79)
deforming dorsopathies (M40-M43)
dentofacial anomalies [including malocclusion] (M26.-)
postprocedural musculoskeletal disorders (M96.-)

M95.0 Acquired deformity of nose
Excludes2 deviated nasal septum (J34.2)

● **M95.1 Cauliflower ear**
Excludes2 other acquired deformities of ear (H61.1)

M95.10 Cauliflower ear, unspecified ear
M95.11 Cauliflower ear, right ear
M95.12 Cauliflower ear, left ear

M95.2 Other acquired deformity of head
Coding Clinic: 2023, Q1, P31

M95.3 Acquired deformity of neck

M95.4 Acquired deformity of chest and rib
Coding Clinic: 2022, Q2, P14

M95.5 Acquired deformity of pelvis
Excludes1 maternal care for known or suspected disproportion (O33.-)

M95.8 Other specified acquired deformities of musculoskeletal system

M95.9 Acquired deformity of musculoskeletal system, unspecified

INTRAOPERATIVE AND POSTPROCEDURAL COMPLICATIONS AND DISORDERS OF MUSCULOSKELETAL SYSTEM, NOT ELSEWHERE CLASSIFIED (M96)

● **M96 Intraoperative and postprocedural complications and disorders of musculoskeletal system, not elsewhere classified**

Excludes2 arthropathy following intestinal bypass (M02.0-)
complications of internal orthopedic prosthetic devices, implants and grafts (T84.-)
disorders associated with osteoporosis (M80)
periprosthetic fracture around internal prosthetic joint (M97.-)
presence of functional implants and other devices (Z96-Z97)

M96.0 Pseudarthrosis after fusion or arthrodesis (Ex) PDX 1349

M96.1 Postlaminectomy syndrome, not elsewhere classified
Coding Clinic: 2024, Q1, P18

M96.2 Postradiation kyphosis
M96.3 Postlaminectomy kyphosis
M96.4 Postsurgical lordosis
M96.5 Postradiation scoliosis

● **M96.6 Fracture of bone following insertion of orthopedic implant, joint prosthesis, or bone plate** (Ex) PDX 1350
Intraoperative fracture of bone during insertion of orthopedic implant, joint prosthesis, or bone plate
Excludes2 complication of internal orthopedic devices, implants or grafts (T84.-)

● **M96.62 Fracture of humerus following insertion of orthopedic implant, joint prosthesis, or bone plate**

M96.621 Fracture of humerus following insertion of orthopedic implant, joint prosthesis, or bone plate, right arm
M96.622 Fracture of humerus following insertion of orthopedic implant, joint prosthesis, or bone plate, left arm
M96.629 Fracture of humerus following insertion of orthopedic implant, joint prosthesis, or bone plate, unspecified arm

● **M96.63 Fracture of radius or ulna following insertion of orthopedic implant, joint prosthesis, or bone plate**

M96.631 Fracture of radius or ulna following insertion of orthopedic implant, joint prosthesis, or bone plate, right arm
M96.632 Fracture of radius or ulna following insertion of orthopedic implant, joint prosthesis, or bone plate, left arm
M96.639 Fracture of radius or ulna following insertion of orthopedic implant, joint prosthesis, or bone plate, unspecified arm

M96.65 Fracture of pelvis following insertion of orthopedic implant, joint prosthesis, or bone plate

● **M96.66 Fracture of femur following insertion of orthopedic implant, joint prosthesis, or bone plate**

M96.661 Fracture of femur following insertion of orthopedic implant, joint prosthesis, or bone plate, right leg
M96.662 Fracture of femur following insertion of orthopedic implant, joint prosthesis, or bone plate, left leg
M96.669 Fracture of femur following insertion of orthopedic implant, joint prosthesis, or bone plate, unspecified leg

● **M96.67 Fracture of tibia or fibula following insertion of orthopedic implant, joint prosthesis, or bone plate**

M96.671 Fracture of tibia or fibula following insertion of orthopedic implant, joint prosthesis, or bone plate, right leg
M96.672 Fracture of tibia or fibula following insertion of orthopedic implant, joint prosthesis, or bone plate, left leg
M96.679 Fracture of tibia or fibula following insertion of orthopedic implant, joint prosthesis, or bone plate, unspecified leg

M96.69 Fracture of other bone following insertion of orthopedic implant, joint prosthesis, or bone plate

● **M96.8 Other intraoperative and postprocedural complications and disorders of musculoskeletal system, not elsewhere classified**
Coding Clinic: 2016, Q4, P10

● **M96.81 Intraoperative hemorrhage and hematoma of a musculoskeletal structure complicating a procedure** (Ex) PDX 1351
Excludes1 intraoperative hemorrhage and hematoma of a musculoskeletal structure due to accidental puncture and laceration during a procedure (M96.82-)

M96.810 Intraoperative hemorrhage and hematoma of a musculoskeletal structure complicating a musculoskeletal system procedure
M96.811 Intraoperative hemorrhage and hematoma of a musculoskeletal structure complicating other procedure

● **M96.82 Accidental puncture and laceration of a musculoskeletal structure during a procedure** (Ex) PDX 569

M96.820 Accidental puncture and laceration of a musculoskeletal structure during a musculoskeletal system procedure

M96.821 Accidental puncture and laceration of a musculoskeletal structure during other procedure

● **M96.83 Postprocedural hemorrhage of a musculoskeletal structure following a procedure** (Ex) PDX 1351

M96.830 Postprocedural hemorrhage of a musculoskeletal structure following a musculoskeletal system procedure

M96.831 Postprocedural hemorrhage of a musculoskeletal structure following other procedure

● **M96.84 Postprocedural hematoma and seroma of a musculoskeletal structure following a procedure** (Ex) PDX 1351

M96.840 Postprocedural hematoma of a musculoskeletal structure following a musculoskeletal system procedure

M96.841 Postprocedural hematoma of a musculoskeletal structure following other procedure
Coding Clinic: 2016, Q4, P10

M96.842 Postprocedural seroma of a musculoskeletal structure following a musculoskeletal system procedure

M96.843 Postprocedural seroma of a musculoskeletal structure following other procedure
Coding Clinic: 2023, Q2, P13

M96.89 Other intraoperative and postprocedural complications and disorders of the musculoskeletal system (Ex) PDX 814
Instability of joint secondary to removal of joint prosthesis
Use additional code, if applicable, to further specify disorder
Coding Clinic: 2 2024, Q1, P18, 23; 023, Q2, P14; 2022, Q2, P14; 2021, Q1, P5

● **M96.A Fracture of ribs, sternum and thorax associated with compression of the chest and cardiopulmonary resuscitation** (Ex) PDX 1352

M96.A1 Fracture of sternum associated with chest compression and cardiopulmonary resuscitation
Fracture of xiphoid process associated with chest compression and cardiopulmonary resuscitation

M96.A2 Fracture of one rib associated with chest compression and cardiopulmonary resuscitation

M96.A3 Multiple fractures of ribs associated with chest compression and cardiopulmonary resuscitation
Coding Clinic: 2022, Q4, P32-33

M96.A4 Flail chest associated with chest compression and cardiopulmonary resuscitation

M96.A9 Other fracture associated with chest compression and cardiopulmonary resuscitation

PERIPROSTHETIC FRACTURE AROUND INTERNAL PROSTHETIC JOINT (M97)

● **M97 Periprosthetic fracture around internal prosthetic joint** (Ex) PDX 1350

Code first if known, the specific type and cause of fracture, such as traumatic or pathological

Excludes2 fracture of bone following insertion of orthopedic implant, joint prosthesis or bone plate (M96.6-)
breakage (fracture) of prosthetic joint (T84.01-)

Coding Clinic: 2016, Q4, P42

The appropriate 7th character is to be added to each code from category M97:

A	initial encounter
D	subsequent encounter
S	sequela

● **M97.0 Periprosthetic fracture around internal prosthetic hip joint**

X● **M97.01 Periprosthetic fracture around internal prosthetic right hip joint** A
Coding Clinic: 2016, Q4, P43

X● **M97.02 Periprosthetic fracture around internal prosthetic left hip joint** A

● **M97.1 Periprosthetic fracture around internal prosthetic knee joint**

X● **M97.11 Periprosthetic fracture around internal prosthetic right knee joint** A

X● **M97.12 Periprosthetic fracture around internal prosthetic left knee joint** A

● **M97.2 Periprosthetic fracture around internal prosthetic ankle joint**

X● **M97.21 Periprosthetic fracture around internal prosthetic right ankle joint** A

X● **M97.22 Periprosthetic fracture around internal prosthetic left ankle joint** A

● **M97.3 Periprosthetic fracture around internal prosthetic shoulder joint**

X● **M97.31 Periprosthetic fracture around internal prosthetic right shoulder joint** A

X● **M97.32 Periprosthetic fracture around internal prosthetic left shoulder joint** A

● **M97.4 Periprosthetic fracture around internal prosthetic elbow joint**

X● **M97.41 Periprosthetic fracture around internal prosthetic right elbow joint** A

X● **M97.42 Periprosthetic fracture around internal prosthetic left elbow joint** A

X● **M97.8 Periprosthetic fracture around other internal prosthetic joint** A
Periprosthetic fracture around internal prosthetic finger joint
Periprosthetic fracture around internal prosthetic spinal joint
Periprosthetic fracture around internal prosthetic toe joint
Periprosthetic fracture around internal prosthetic wrist joint
Use additional code to identify the joint (Z96.6-)

X● **M97.9 Periprosthetic fracture around unspecified internal prosthetic joint** A

CHAPTER 13 (M00-M99)

BIOMECHANICAL LESIONS, NOT ELSEWHERE CLASSIFIED (M99)

● M99 Biomechanical lesions, not elsewhere classified

Note: This category should not be used if the condition can be classified elsewhere.

● M99.0 Segmental and somatic dysfunction

M99.00 Segmental and somatic dysfunction of head region

M99.01 Segmental and somatic dysfunction of cervical region

M99.02 Segmental and somatic dysfunction of thoracic region

M99.03 Segmental and somatic dysfunction of lumbar region

M99.04 Segmental and somatic dysfunction of sacral region

M99.05 Segmental and somatic dysfunction of pelvic region

M99.06 Segmental and somatic dysfunction of lower extremity

M99.07 Segmental and somatic dysfunction of upper extremity

M99.08 Segmental and somatic dysfunction of rib cage

M99.09 Segmental and somatic dysfunction of abdomen and other regions

● M99.1 Subluxation complex (vertebral)

M99.10 Subluxation complex (vertebral) of head region (Ex:) PDX 913

M99.11 Subluxation complex (vertebral) of cervical region (Ex:) PDX 913

M99.12 Subluxation complex (vertebral) of thoracic region

M99.13 Subluxation complex (vertebral) of lumbar region

M99.14 Subluxation complex (vertebral) of sacral region

M99.15 Subluxation complex (vertebral) of pelvic region

M99.16 Subluxation complex (vertebral) of lower extremity

M99.17 Subluxation complex (vertebral) of upper extremity

M99.18 Subluxation complex (vertebral) of rib cage (Ex:) PDX 914

M99.19 Subluxation complex (vertebral) of abdomen and other regions

● M99.2 Subluxation stenosis of neural canal

M99.20 Subluxation stenosis of neural canal of head region

M99.21 Subluxation stenosis of neural canal of cervical region

M99.22 Subluxation stenosis of neural canal of thoracic region

M99.23 Subluxation stenosis of neural canal of lumbar region

M99.24 Subluxation stenosis of neural canal of sacral region

M99.25 Subluxation stenosis of neural canal of pelvic region

M99.26 Subluxation stenosis of neural canal of lower extremity

M99.27 Subluxation stenosis of neural canal of upper extremity

M99.28 Subluxation stenosis of neural canal of rib cage

M99.29 Subluxation stenosis of neural canal of abdomen and other regions

● M99.3 Osseous stenosis of neural canal

M99.30 Osseous stenosis of neural canal of head region

M99.31 Osseous stenosis of neural canal of cervical region

M99.32 Osseous stenosis of neural canal of thoracic region

M99.33 Osseous stenosis of neural canal of lumbar region

M99.34 Osseous stenosis of neural canal of sacral region

M99.35 Osseous stenosis of neural canal of pelvic region

M99.36 Osseous stenosis of neural canal of lower extremity

M99.37 Osseous stenosis of neural canal of upper extremity

M99.38 Osseous stenosis of neural canal of rib cage

M99.39 Osseous stenosis of neural canal of abdomen and other regions

● M99.4 Connective tissue stenosis of neural canal

M99.40 Connective tissue stenosis of neural canal of head region

M99.41 Connective tissue stenosis of neural canal of cervical region

M99.42 Connective tissue stenosis of neural canal of thoracic region

M99.43 Connective tissue stenosis of neural canal of lumbar region

M99.44 Connective tissue stenosis of neural canal of sacral region

M99.45 Connective tissue stenosis of neural canal of pelvic region

M99.46 Connective tissue stenosis of neural canal of lower extremity

M99.47 Connective tissue stenosis of neural canal of upper extremity

M99.48 Connective tissue stenosis of neural canal of rib cage

M99.49 Connective tissue stenosis of neural canal of abdomen and other regions

● M99.5 Intervertebral disc stenosis of neural canal

M99.50 Intervertebral disc stenosis of neural canal of head region

M99.51 Intervertebral disc stenosis of neural canal of cervical region

M99.52 Intervertebral disc stenosis of neural canal of thoracic region

M99.53 Intervertebral disc stenosis of neural canal of lumbar region

M99.54 Intervertebral disc stenosis of neural canal of sacral region

M99.55 Intervertebral disc stenosis of neural canal of pelvic region

M99.56 Intervertebral disc stenosis of neural canal of lower extremity

M99.57 Intervertebral disc stenosis of neural canal of upper extremity

M99.58 Intervertebral disc stenosis of neural canal of rib cage

M99.59 Intervertebral disc stenosis of neural canal of abdomen and other regions

● M99.6 Osseous and subluxation stenosis of intervertebral foramina

M99.60 Osseous and subluxation stenosis of intervertebral foramina of head region

M99.61 Osseous and subluxation stenosis of intervertebral foramina of cervical region

M99.62 Osseous and subluxation stenosis of intervertebral foramina of thoracic region
M99.63 Osseous and subluxation stenosis of intervertebral foramina of lumbar region
M99.64 Osseous and subluxation stenosis of intervertebral foramina of sacral region
M99.65 Osseous and subluxation stenosis of intervertebral foramina of pelvic region
M99.66 Osseous and subluxation stenosis of intervertebral foramina of lower extremity
M99.67 Osseous and subluxation stenosis of intervertebral foramina of upper extremity
M99.68 Osseous and subluxation stenosis of intervertebral foramina of rib cage
M99.69 Osseous and subluxation stenosis of intervertebral foramina of abdomen and other regions

● M99.7 Connective tissue and disc stenosis of intervertebral foramina

M99.70 Connective tissue and disc stenosis of intervertebral foramina of head region
M99.71 Connective tissue and disc stenosis of intervertebral foramina of cervical region
M99.72 Connective tissue and disc stenosis of intervertebral foramina of thoracic region
M99.73 Connective tissue and disc stenosis of intervertebral foramina of lumbar region
M99.74 Connective tissue and disc stenosis of intervertebral foramina of sacral region
M99.75 Connective tissue and disc stenosis of intervertebral foramina of pelvic region
M99.76 Connective tissue and disc stenosis of intervertebral foramina of lower extremity
M99.77 Connective tissue and disc stenosis of intervertebral foramina of upper extremity
M99.78 Connective tissue and disc stenosis of intervertebral foramina of rib cage
M99.79 Connective tissue and disc stenosis of intervertebral foramina of abdomen and other regions

● M99.8 Other biomechanical lesions

M99.80 Other biomechanical lesions of head region
M99.81 Other biomechanical lesions of cervical region
M99.82 Other biomechanical lesions of thoracic region
M99.83 Other biomechanical lesions of lumbar region
M99.84 Other biomechanical lesions of sacral region
M99.85 Other biomechanical lesions of pelvic region
M99.86 Other biomechanical lesions of lower extremity
M99.87 Other biomechanical lesions of upper extremity
M99.88 Other biomechanical lesions of rib cage
M99.89 Other biomechanical lesions of abdomen and other regions

M99.9 Biomechanical lesion, unspecified

CHAPTER 13 (MØØ-M99)

CHAPTER 14

DISEASES OF THE GENITOURINARY SYSTEM (N00-N99)

OGCR Chapter-Specific Coding Guidelines

14. Chapter 14: Diseases of Genitourinary System (N00-N99)

a. Chronic kidney disease

1) Stages of chronic kidney disease (CKD)

The ICD-10-CM classifies CKD based on severity. The severity of CKD is designated by stages 1-5. Stage 2, code N18.2, equates to mild CKD; stage 3, code N18.3, equates to moderate CKD; and stage 4, code N18.4, equates to severe CKD. Code N18.6, End stage renal disease (ESRD), is assigned when the provider has documented end-stage-renal disease (ESRD).

If both a stage of CKD and ESRD are documented, assign code N18.6 only.

2) Chronic kidney disease and kidney transplant status

Patients who have undergone kidney transplant may still have some form of chronic kidney disease CKD because the kidney transplant may not fully restore kidney function. Therefore, the presence of CKD alone does not constitute a transplant complication. Assign the appropriate N18 code for the patient's stage of CKD and code Z94.0, Kidney transplant status. If a transplant complication such as failure or rejection or other transplant complication is documented, see Section I.C.19.g for information on coding complications of a kidney transplant. If the documentation is unclear as to whether the patient has a complication of the transplant, query the provider.

3) Chronic kidney disease with other conditions

Patients with CKD may also suffer from other serious conditions, most commonly diabetes mellitus and hypertension. The sequencing of the CKD code in relationship to codes for other contributing conditions is based on the conventions in the Tabular List.

See I.C.9. Hypertensive chronic kidney disease.

See I.C.19. Chronic kidney disease and kidney transplant complications.

Item 14–1 Nephritis (inflammation) or **nephropathy** (disease) **with lesion of proliferative glomerulonephritis** results from a streptococcal infection.

Nephritis (inflammation) or **nephropathy** (disease) **with lesion of membranous glomerulonephritis** is characterized by deposits along the epithelial side of the basement membrane.

Nephritis (inflammation) or **nephropathy** (disease) **with lesion of membranoproliferative glomerulonephritis** is characterized by alterations in the basement membranes of the kidney and the glomerular cells.

Nephritis (inflammation) or **nephropathy** (disease) **with lesion of rapidly progressive glomerulonephritis** is characterized by rapid and progressive decline in renal function.

Nephritis (inflammation) or **nephropathy** (disease) **with lesion of renal cortical necrosis** is characterized by death of the cortical tissues.

Nephritis (inflammation) or **nephropathy** (disease) **with lesion of renal medullary necrosis** is characterized by death of the tissues that collect urine.

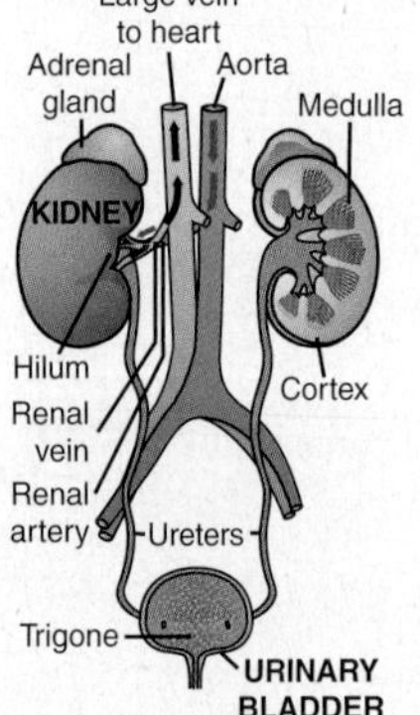

Figure 14-1 Kidneys within the urinary system.

Item 14–2 Glomerulonephritis is nephritis accompanied by inflammation of the glomeruli of the kidney, resulting in the degeneration of the glomeruli and the nephrons.

Acute glomerulonephritis primarily affects children and young adults and is usually a result of a streptococcal infection.

Proliferative glomerulonephritis is the acute form of the disease resulting from a streptococcal infection.

Rapidly progressive glomerulonephritis, also known as **crescentic** or **malignant glomerulonephritis**, is the acute form of the disease, which leads quickly to rapid and progressive decline in renal function.

CHAPTER 14

DISEASES OF THE GENITOURINARY SYSTEM (N00-N99)

Excludes2 certain conditions originating in the perinatal period (P04-P96)
certain infectious and parasitic diseases (A00-B99)
complications of pregnancy, childbirth and the puerperium (O00-O9A)
congenital malformations, deformations and chromosomal abnormalities (Q00-Q99)
endocrine, nutritional and metabolic diseases (E00-E88)
injury, poisoning and certain other consequences of external causes (S00-T88)
neoplasms (C00-D49)
symptoms, signs and abnormal clinical and laboratory findings, not elsewhere classified (R00-R94)

This chapter contains the following blocks:

N00-N08	Glomerular diseases
N10-N16	Renal tubulo-interstitial diseases
N17-N19	Acute kidney failure and chronic kidney disease
N20-N23	Urolithiasis
N25-N29	Other disorders of kidney and ureter
N30-N39	Other diseases of the urinary system
N40-N53	Diseases of male genital organs
N60-N65	Disorders of breast
N70-N77	Inflammatory diseases of female pelvic organs
N80-N98	Noninflammatory disorders of female genital tract
N99	Intraoperative and postprocedural complications and disorders of genitourinary system, not elsewhere classified

GLOMERULAR DISEASES (N00-N08)

Code also any associated kidney failure (N17-N19)

Excludes1 hypertensive chronic kidney disease (I12.-)

● **N00 Acute nephritic syndrome** (Ex) PDX 1355

Includes acute glomerular disease
acute glomerulonephritis
acute nephritis

Excludes1 acute tubulo-interstitial nephritis (N10)
nephritic syndrome NOS (N05.-)

N00.0 Acute nephritic syndrome with minor glomerular abnormality
Acute nephritic syndrome with minimal change lesion

N00.1 Acute nephritic syndrome with focal and segmental glomerular lesions
Acute nephritic syndrome with focal and segmental hyalinosis
Acute nephritic syndrome with focal and segmental sclerosis
Acute nephritic syndrome with focal glomerulonephritis

N00.2 Acute nephritic syndrome with diffuse membranous glomerulonephritis

N00.3 Acute nephritic syndrome with diffuse mesangial proliferative glomerulonephritis

N00.4 Acute nephritic syndrome with diffuse endocapillary proliferative glomerulonephritis

N00.5 Acute nephritic syndrome with diffuse mesangiocapillary glomerulonephritis
Acute nephritic syndrome with membranoproliferative glomerulonephritis, types 1 and 3, or NOS
Excludes1 Acute nephritic syndrome with C3 glomerulonephritis (N00.A)
Acute nephritic syndrome with C3 glomerulopathy (N00.A)

N00.6 Acute nephritic syndrome with dense deposit disease
Acute nephritic syndrome with C3 glomerulopathy with dense deposit disease
Acute nephritic syndrome with membranoproliferative glomerulonephritis, type 2

N00.7 Acute nephritic syndrome with diffuse crescentic glomerulonephritis
Acute nephritic syndrome with extracapillary glomerulonephritis

N00.8 Acute nephritic syndrome with other morphologic changes
Acute nephritic syndrome with proliferative glomerulonephritis NOS

N00.9 Acute nephritic syndrome with unspecified morphologic changes

N00.A Acute nephritic syndrome with C3 glomerulonephritis (Ex) PDX 1357
Acute nephritic syndrome with C3 glomerulopathy, NOS
Excludes1 Acute nephritic syndrome (with C3 glomerulopathy) with dense deposit disease(N00.6)

N01 Rapidly progressive nephritic syndrome (Ex) PDX 1355
Includes rapidly progressive glomerular disease
rapidly progressive glomerulonephritis
rapidly progressive nephritis
Excludes1 nephritic syndrome NOS (N05.-)

N01.0 Rapidly progressive nephritic syndrome with minor glomerular abnormality
Rapidly progressive nephritic syndrome with minimal change lesion

N01.1 Rapidly progressive nephritic syndrome with focal and segmental glomerular lesions
Rapidly progressive nephritic syndrome with focal and segmental hyalinosis
Rapidly progressive nephritic syndrome with focal and segmental sclerosis
Rapidly progressive nephritic syndrome with focal glomerulonephritis

N01.2 Rapidly progressive nephritic syndrome with diffuse membranous glomerulonephritis

N01.3 Rapidly progressive nephritic syndrome with diffuse mesangial proliferative glomerulonephritis

N01.4 Rapidly progressive nephritic syndrome with diffuse endocapillary proliferative glomerulonephritis

N01.5 Rapidly progressive nephritic syndrome with diffuse mesangiocapillary glomerulonephritis
Rapidly progressive nephritic syndrome with membranoproliferative glomerulonephritis, types 1 and 3, or NOS
Excludes1 Rapidly progressive nephritic syndrome with C3 glomerulonephritis (N01.A)
Rapidly progressive nephritic syndrome with C3 glomerulopathy (N01.A)

N01.6 Rapidly progressive nephritic syndrome with dense deposit disease
Rapidly progressive nephritic syndrome with C3 glomerulopathy with dense deposit disease
Rapidly progressive nephritic syndrome with membranoproliferative glomerulonephritis, type 2

N01.7 Rapidly progressive nephritic syndrome with diffuse crescentic glomerulonephritis
Rapidly progressive nephritic syndrome with extracapillary glomerulonephritis

N01.8 Rapidly progressive nephritic syndrome with other morphologic changes
Rapidly progressive nephritic syndrome with proliferative glomerulonephritis NOS

N01.9 Rapidly progressive nephritic syndrome with unspecified morphologic changes

N01.A Rapidly progressive nephritic syndrome with C3 glomerulonephritis (Ex) PDX 1357
Rapidly progressive nephritic syndrome with C3 glomerulopathy, NOS
Excludes1 Rapidly progressive nephritic syndrome (with C3 glomerulopathy) with dense deposit disease (N01.6)

N02 Recurrent and persistent hematuria (Ex) PDX 1358
Excludes1 acute cystitis with hematuria (N30.01)
hematuria NOS (R31.9)
hematuria not associated with specified morphologic lesions (R31.-)

N02.0 Recurrent and persistent hematuria with minor glomerular abnormality
Recurrent and persistent hematuria with minimal change lesion

N02.1 Recurrent and persistent hematuria with focal and segmental glomerular lesions
Recurrent and persistent hematuria with focal and segmental hyalinosis
Recurrent and persistent hematuria with focal and segmental sclerosis
Recurrent and persistent hematuria with focal glomerulonephritis

N02.2 Recurrent and persistent hematuria with diffuse membranous glomerulonephritis

N02.3 Recurrent and persistent hematuria with diffuse mesangial proliferative glomerulonephritis

N02.4 Recurrent and persistent hematuria with diffuse endocapillary proliferative glomerulonephritis

N02.5 Recurrent and persistent hematuria with diffuse mesangiocapillary glomerulonephritis
Recurrent and persistent hematuria with membranoproliferative glomerulonephritis, types 1 and 3, or NOS
Excludes1 Recurrent and persistent hematuria with C3 glomerulonephritis (N02.A)
Recurrent and persistent hematuria with C3 glomerulopathy (N02.A)

N02.6 Recurrent and persistent hematuria with dense deposit disease
Recurrent and persistent hematuria with C3 glomerulopathy with dense deposit disease
Recurrent and persistent hematuria with membranoproliferative glomerulonephritis, type 2

N02.7 Recurrent and persistent hematuria with diffuse crescentic glomerulonephritis
Recurrent and persistent hematuria with extracapillary glomerulonephritis

N02.8 Recurrent and persistent hematuria with other morphologic changes (Ex) PDX 1355
Recurrent and persistent hematuria with proliferative glomerulonephritis NOS

N02.9 Recurrent and persistent hematuria with unspecified morphologic changes (Ex) PDX 1355
Coding Clinic: 2017, Q2, P5

Item 14–3 Chronic glomerulonephritis (GN) persists over a period of years, with remissions and exacerbation.

Chronic GN with lesion of proliferative glomerulonephritis results from a streptococcal infection.

Chronic GN with lesion of membranous glomerulonephritis, also known as membranous nephropathy, is characterized by deposits along the epithelial side of the basement membrane.

Chronic GN with lesion of membrano-proliferative glomerulonephritis (MPGN) is a group of disorders characterized by alterations in the basement membranes of the kidney and the glomerular cells.

Chronic GN with lesion of rapidly progressive glomerulonephritis is characterized by necrosis, endothelial proliferation, and mesangial proliferation. The condition is marked by rapid and progressive decline in renal function.

N02.A Recurrent and persistent hematuria with C3 glomerulonephritis (Ex) PDX 1359
Recurrent and persistent hematuria with C3 glomerulopathy
Excludes1 Recurrent and persistent hematuria (with C3 glomerulopathy) with dense deposit disease (N02.6)

● **N02.B Recurrent and persistent immunoglobulin A nephropathy**

N02.B1 Recurrent and persistent immunoglobulin A nephropathy with glomerular lesion (Ex) PDX 1360

N02.B2 Recurrent and persistent immunoglobulin A nephropathy with focal and segmentalglomerular lesion (Ex) PDX 1361
Recurrent and persistent immunoglobulin A nephropathy with focal and segmentalhyalinosis or sclerosis

N02.B3 Recurrent and persistent immunoglobulin A nephropathy with diffuse membranoproliferative glomerulonephritis (Ex) PDX 1362

N02.B4 Recurrent and persistent immunoglobulin A nephropathy with diffuse membranous glomerulonephritis (Ex) PDX 1363

N02.B5 Recurrent and persistent immunoglobulin A nephropathy with diffuse mesangialproliferative glomerulonephritis (Ex) PDX 1364

N02.B6 Recurrent and persistent immunoglobulin A nephropathy with diffuse mesangiocapillary glomerulonephritis (Ex) PDX 1365

N02.B9 Other recurrent and persistent immunoglobulin A nephropathy (Ex) PDX 1366

● **N03 Chronic nephritic syndrome** (Ex) PDX 160

Includes chronic glomerular disease
chronic glomerulonephritis
chronic nephritis

Excludes1 chronic tubulo-interstitial nephritis (N11.-)
diffuse sclerosing glomerulonephritis (N05.8-)
nephritic syndrome NOS (N05.-)

N03.0 Chronic nephritic syndrome with minor glomerular abnormality
Chronic nephritic syndrome with minimal change lesion

N03.1 Chronic nephritic syndrome with focal and segmental glomerular lesions
Chronic nephritic syndrome with focal and segmental hyalinosis
Chronic nephritic syndrome with focal and segmental sclerosis
Chronic nephritic syndrome with focal glomerulonephritis

N03.2 Chronic nephritic syndrome with diffuse membranous glomerulonephritis

N03.3 Chronic nephritic syndrome with diffuse mesangial proliferative glomerulonephritis

N03.4 Chronic nephritic syndrome with diffuse endocapillary proliferative glomerulonephritis

N03.5 Chronic nephritic syndrome with diffuse mesangiocapillary glomerulonephritis
Chronic nephritic syndrome with membranoproliferative glomerulonephritis, types 1 and 3, or NOS
Excludes1 Chronic nephritic syndrome with C3 glomerulonephritis (N03.A)
Chronic nephritic syndrome with C3 glomerulopathy (N03.A)

N03.6 Chronic nephritic syndrome with dense deposit disease
Chronic nephritic syndrome with C3 glomerulopathy with dense deposit disease
Chronic nephritic syndrome with membranoproliferative glomerulonephritis, type 2

N03.7 Chronic nephritic syndrome with diffuse crescentic glomerulonephritis
Chronic nephritic syndrome with extracapillary glomerulonephritis

N03.8 Chronic nephritic syndrome with other morphologic changes
Chronic nephritic syndrome with proliferative glomerulonephritis NOS

N03.9 Chronic nephritic syndrome with unspecified morphologic changes

N03.A Chronic nephritic syndrome with C3 glomerulonephritis (Ex) PDX 1359
Chronic nephritic syndrome with C3 glomerulopathy
Excludes1 Chronic nephritic syndrome (with C3 glomerulopathy) with dense deposit disease(N03.6)

● **N04 Nephrotic syndrome**

Includes congenital nephrotic syndrome
lipoid nephrosis

N04.0 Nephrotic syndrome with minor glomerular abnormality (Ex) PDX 1358
Nephrotic syndrome with minimal change lesion

N04.1 Nephrotic syndrome with focal and segmental glomerular lesions (Ex) PDX 1358
Nephrotic syndrome with focal and segmental hyalinosis
Nephrotic syndrome with focal and segmental sclerosis
Nephrotic syndrome with focal glomerulonephritis

● **N04.2 Nephrotic syndrome with diffuse membranous glomerulonephritis** (Ex) PDX 1367

N04.20 Nephrotic syndrome with diffuse membranous glomerulonephritis, unspecified
Membranous nephropathy NOS with nephrotic syndrome

N04.21 Primary membranous nephropathy with nephrotic syndrome
Idiopathic membranous nephropathy with nephrotic syndrome

N04.22 Secondary membranous nephropathy with nephrotic syndrome
Code first, if applicable, other disease or disorder or poisoning causing membranous nephropathy
Use Additional code, if applicable, for adverse effect of drug causing membranous nephropathy

N04.29 Other nephrotic syndrome with diffuse membranous glomerulonephritis

N04.3 Nephrotic syndrome with diffuse mesangial proliferative glomerulonephritis (Ex) PDX 1358

N04.4 Nephrotic syndrome with diffuse endocapillary proliferative glomerulonephritis (Ex) PDX 1358

N04.5 Nephrotic syndrome with diffuse mesangiocapillary glomerulonephritis (Ex) PDX 1358
Nephrotic syndrome with membranoproliferative glomerulonephritis, types 1 and 3, or NOS
Excludes1 Nephrotic syndrome with C3 glomerulonephritis (N04.A)
Nephrotic syndrome with C3 glomerulopathy (N04.A)

CHAPTER 14 (N00-N99)

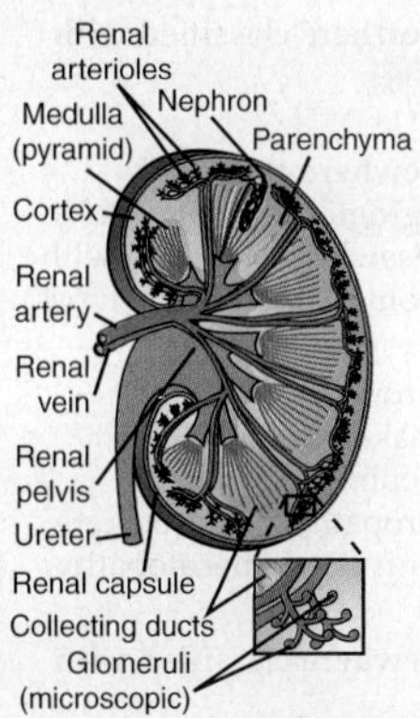

Figure 14-2 Kidney cross section.

Item 14–4 Nephrotic syndrome (NS) is marked by massive proteinuria (protein in the urine) and water retention. Patients with NS are particularly vulnerable to staphylococcal and pneumococcal infections. NS with lesion of proliferative glomerulonephritis results from a streptococcal infection. NS with lesion of membranous glomerulonephritis results in thickening of the capillary walls. NS with lesion of minimal change glomerulonephritis is usually a benign disorder that occurs mostly in children and requires electron microscopy (biopsy) to verify changes in the glomeruli.

N04.6 Nephrotic syndrome with dense deposit disease (Ex) PDX 1358
- Nephrotic syndrome with C3 glomerulopathy with dense deposit disease
- Nephrotic syndrome with membranoproliferative glomerulonephritis, type 2

N04.7 Nephrotic syndrome with diffuse crescentic glomerulonephritis (Ex) PDX 1355
- Nephrotic syndrome with extracapillary glomerulonephritis

N04.8 Nephrotic syndrome with other morphologic changes (Ex) PDX 1355
- Nephrotic syndrome with proliferative glomerulonephritis NOS

N04.9 Nephrotic syndrome with unspecified morphologic changes (Ex) PDX 1355

N04.A Nephrotic syndrome with C3 glomerulonephritis (Ex) PDX 1359
- Nephrotic syndrome with C3 glomerulopathy

Excludes1 Nephrotic syndrome (with C3 glomerulopathy) with dense deposit disease (N04.6)

● N05 Unspecified nephritic syndrome (Ex) PDX 160

Includes glomerular disease NOS
glomerulonephritis NOS
nephritis NOS
nephropathy NOS and renal disease NOS with morphological lesion specified in .0-.8

Excludes1 nephropathy NOS with no stated morphological lesion (N28.9)
renal disease NOS with no stated morphological lesion (N28.9)
tubulo-interstitial nephritis NOS (N12)

N05.0 Unspecified nephritic syndrome with minor glomerular abnormality
- Unspecified nephritic syndrome with minimal change lesion

N05.1 Unspecified nephritic syndrome with focal and segmental glomerular lesions
- Unspecified nephritic syndrome with focal and segmental hyalinosis
- Unspecified nephritic syndrome with focal and segmental sclerosis
- Unspecified nephritic syndrome with focal glomerulonephritis

N05.2 Unspecified nephritic syndrome with diffuse membranous glomerulonephritis

N05.3 Unspecified nephritic syndrome with diffuse mesangial proliferative glomerulonephritis

N05.4 Unspecified nephritic syndrome with diffuse endocapillary proliferative glomerulonephritis

N05.5 Unspecified nephritic syndrome with diffuse mesangiocapillary glomerulonephritis
- Unspecified nephritic syndrome with membranoproliferative glomerulonephritis, types 1 and 3, or NOS

Excludes1 Unspecified nephritic syndrome with C3 glomerulonephritis (N05.A)
Unspecified nephritic syndrome with C3 glomerulopathy (N05.A)

N05.6 Unspecified nephritic syndrome with dense deposit disease
- Unspecified nephritic syndrome with C3 glomerulopathy with dense deposit disease
- Unspecified nephritic syndrome with membranoproliferative glomerulonephritis, type 2

N05.7 Unspecified nephritic syndrome with diffuse crescentic glomerulonephritis
- Unspecified nephritic syndrome with extracapillary glomerulonephritis

N05.8 Unspecified nephritic syndrome with other morphologic changes
- Unspecified nephritic syndrome with proliferative glomerulonephritis NOS

N05.9 Unspecified nephritic syndrome with unspecified morphologic changes

N05.A Unspecified nephritic syndrome with C3 glomerulonephritis (Ex) PDX 1359
- Unspecified nephritic syndrome with C3 glomerulopathy

Excludes1 Unspecified nephritic syndrome (with C3 glomerulopathy) with dense deposit disease(N05.6)

● N06 Isolated proteinuria with specified morphological lesion (Ex) PDX 1368

Excludes1 proteinuria not associated with specific morphologic lesions (R80.0)

N06.0 Isolated proteinuria with minor glomerular abnormality
- Isolated proteinuria with minimal change lesion

N06.1 Isolated proteinuria with focal and segmental glomerular lesions
- Isolated proteinuria with focal and segmental hyalinosis
- Isolated proteinuria with focal and segmental sclerosis
- Isolated proteinuria with focal glomerulonephritis

N06.2 Isolated proteinuria with diffuse membranous glomerulonephritis

● N06.20 Isolated proteinuria with diffuse membranous glomerulonephritis, unspecified
- Membranous nephropathy, NOS

Excludes1 membranous nephropathy NOS with nephrotic syndrome (N04.20)

N06.21 Primary membranous nephropathy with isolated proteinuria
- Idiopathic membranous nephropathy (with isolated proteinuria)
- Primary membranous nephropathy, NOS

Excludes1 primary membranous nephropathy with nephrotic syndrome (N04.21)

CHAPTER 14 (N00-N99)

N06.22 **Secondary membranous nephropathy with isolated proteinuria**
Secondary membranous nephropathy, NOS
Code first, if applicable, other disease or disorder or poisoning causing membranous nephropathy
Use Additional code, if applicable, for adverse effect of drug causing membranous nephropathy
Excludes1 secondary membranous nephropathy with nephrotic syndrome (N04.22)

N06.29 **Other isolated proteinuria with diffuse membranous glomerulonephritis**

N06.3 **Isolated proteinuria with diffuse mesangial proliferative glomerulonephritis** Ex: PDX 160

N06.4 **Isolated proteinuria with diffuse endocapillary proliferative glomerulonephritis** Ex: PDX 160

N06.5 **Isolated proteinuria with diffuse mesangiocapillary glomerulonephritis** Ex: PDX 160
Isolated proteinuria with membranoproliferative glomerulonephritis, types 1 and 3, or NOS
Excludes1 Isolated proteinuria with C3 glomerulonephritis (N06.A)
Isolated proteinuria with C3 glomerulopathy (N06.A)

N06.6 **Isolated proteinuria with dense deposit disease**
Isolated proteinuria with C3 glomerulopathy with dense deposit disease
Isolated proteinuria with membranoproliferative glomerulonephritis, type 2

N06.7 **Isolated proteinuria with diffuse crescentic glomerulonephritis**
Isolated proteinuria with extracapillary glomerulonephritis

N06.8 **Isolated proteinuria with other morphologic lesion**
Isolated proteinuria with proliferative glomerulonephritis NOS

N06.9 **Isolated proteinuria with unspecified morphologic lesion**

N06.A **Isolated proteinuria with C3 glomerulonephritis** Ex: PDX 1359
Isolated proteinuria with C3 glomerulopathy
Excludes1 Isolated proteinuria (with C3 glomerulopathy) with dense deposit disease (N06.6)

● N07 **Hereditary nephropathy, not elsewhere classified** Ex: PDX 160
Excludes2 Alport's syndrome (Q87.81-)
hereditary amyloid nephropathy (E85.-)
nail patella syndrome (Q87.2)
non-neuropathic heredofamilial amyloidosis (E85.-)

N07.0 **Hereditary nephropathy, not elsewhere classified with minor glomerular abnormality**
Hereditary nephropathy, not elsewhere classified with minimal change lesion

N07.1 **Hereditary nephropathy, not elsewhere classified with focal and segmental glomerular lesions**
Hereditary nephropathy, not elsewhere classified with focal and segmental hyalinosis
Hereditary nephropathy, not elsewhere classified with focal and segmental sclerosis
Hereditary nephropathy, not elsewhere classified with focal glomerulonephritis

N07.2 **Hereditary nephropathy, not elsewhere classified with diffuse membranous glomerulonephritis**

N07.3 **Hereditary nephropathy, not elsewhere classified with diffuse mesangial proliferative glomerulonephritis**

N07.4 **Hereditary nephropathy, not elsewhere classified with diffuse endocapillary proliferative glomerulonephritis**

N07.5 **Hereditary nephropathy, not elsewhere classified with diffuse mesangiocapillary glomerulonephritis**
Hereditary nephropathy, not elsewhere classified with membranoproliferative glomerulonephritis, types 1 and 3, or NOS
Excludes1 Hereditary nephropathy, not elsewhere classified with C3 glomerulonephritis (N07.A)
Hereditary nephropathy, not elsewhere classified with C3 glomerulopathy (N07.A)

N07.6 **Hereditary nephropathy, not elsewhere classified with dense deposit disease**
Hereditary nephropathy, not elsewhere classified with C3 glomerulopathy with dense deposit disease
Hereditary nephropathy, not elsewhere classified with membranoproliferative glomerulonephritis, type 2

N07.7 **Hereditary nephropathy, not elsewhere classified with diffuse crescentic glomerulonephritis**
Hereditary nephropathy, not elsewhere classified with extracapillary glomerulonephritis

N07.8 **Hereditary nephropathy, not elsewhere classified with other morphologic lesions**
Hereditary nephropathy, not elsewhere classified with proliferative glomerulonephritis NOS

N07.9 **Hereditary nephropathy, not elsewhere classified with unspecified morphologic lesions**

N07.A **Hereditary nephropathy, not elsewhere classified with C3 glomerulonephritis** Ex: PDX 1359
Hereditary nephropathy, not elsewhere classified with C3 glomerulopathy
Excludes1 Hereditary nephropathy, not elsewhere classified (with C3 glomerulopathy) with dense deposit disease (N07.6)

N08 ***Glomerular disorders in diseases classified elsewhere***
Glomerulonephritis
Nephritis
Nephropathy
Code first underlying disease, such as:
amyloidosis (E85.-)
congenital syphilis (A50.5)
cryoglobulinemia (D89.1)
disseminated intravascular coagulation (D65)
gout (M1A.-, M10.-)
microscopic polyangiitis (M31.7)
multiple myeloma (C90.0-)
sepsis (A40.0-A41.9)
sickle-cell disease (D57.0-D57.8)
Excludes1 glomerulonephritis, nephritis and nephropathy (in):
antiglomerular basement membrane disease (M31.0)
diabetes (E08-E13 with .21)
gonococcal (A54.21)
Goodpasture's syndrome (M31.0)
hemolytic-uremic syndrome (D59.3)
lupus (M32.14)
mumps (B26.83)
syphilis (A52.75)
systemic lupus erythematosus (M32.14)
Wegener's granulomatosis (M31.31)
pyelonephritis in diseases classified elsewhere (N16)
renal tubulo-interstitial disorders classified elsewhere (N16)

RENAL TUBULO-INTERSTITIAL DISEASES (N10-N16)

Includes pyelonephritis

Excludes1 pyeloureteritis cystica (N28.85)

N10 Acute pyelonephritis (Ex) PDX 1369
Acute infectious interstitial nephritis
Acute pyelitis
Acute tubulo-interstitial nephritis
Hemoglobin nephrosis
Myoglobin nephrosis
Use additional code (B95-B97), to identify infectious agent
Coding Clinic: 2019, Q3, P13-14

● **N11 Chronic tubulo-interstitial nephritis**

Includes chronic infectious interstitial nephritis
chronic pyelitis
chronic pyelonephritis

Use additional code (B95-B97), to identify infectious agent

N11.0 Nonobstructive reflux-associated chronic pyelonephritis
Pyelonephritis (chronic) associated with (vesicoureteral) reflux
Excludes1 vesicoureteral reflux NOS (N13.70)

N11.1 Chronic obstructive pyelonephritis (Ex) PDX 1370
Pyelonephritis (chronic) associated with anomaly of pelviureteric junction
Pyelonephritis (chronic) associated with anomaly of pyeloureteric junction
Pyelonephritis (chronic) associated with crossing of vessel
Pyelonephritis (chronic) associated with kinking of ureter
Pyelonephritis (chronic) associated with obstruction of ureter
Pyelonephritis (chronic) associated with stricture of pelviureteric junction
Pyelonephritis (chronic) associated with stricture of ureter
Excludes1 calculous pyelonephritis (N20.9)
obstructive uropathy (N13.-)
CC when PDx is its own CC

N11.8 Other chronic tubulo-interstitial nephritis (Ex) PDX 1371
Nonobstructive chronic pyelonephritis NOS

N11.9 Chronic tubulo-interstitial nephritis, unspecified (Ex) PDX 1372
Chronic interstitial nephritis NOS
Chronic pyelitis NOS
Chronic pyelonephritis NOS

N12 Tubulo-interstitial nephritis, not specified as acute or chronic (Ex) PDX 1372
Interstitial nephritis NOS
Pyelitis NOS
Pyelonephritis NOS
Excludes1 calculous pyelonephritis (N20.9)

● **N13 Obstructive and reflux uropathy** (Ex) PDX 1373

Excludes2 calculus of kidney and ureter without hydronephrosis (N20.-)
congenital obstructive defects of renal pelvis and ureter (Q62.0-Q62.3)
hydronephrosis with ureteropelvic junction obstruction (Q62.11)
obstructive pyelonephritis (N11.1)

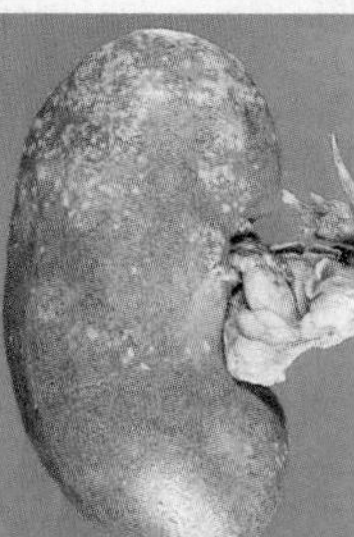

Figure 14-3 Acute pyelonephritis. Cortical surface exhibits grayish white areas of inflammation and abscess formation. (From Frazier MS, Drzymkowski JW: Essentials of Human Diseases and Conditions, St. Louis, Saunders/Elsevier, 2009)

Item 14-5 Pyelonephritis is an infection of the kidneys and ureters and may be chronic or acute in one or both kidneys.

N13.0 Hydronephrosis with ureteropelvic junction obstruction
Hydronephrosis due to acquired occlusion of ureteropelvic junction
Excludes2 Hydronephrosis with ureteropelvic junction obstruction due to calculus (N13.2)
CC when PDx is its own CC
Coding Clinic: 2016, Q4, P43

N13.1 Hydronephrosis with ureteral stricture, not elsewhere classified
Excludes1 hydronephrosis with ureteral stricture with infection (N13.6)
CC when PDx is its own CC

N13.2 Hydronephrosis with renal and ureteral calculous obstruction
Excludes1 hydronephrosis with renal and ureteral calculous obstruction with infection (N13.6)
CC when PDx is its own CC

● **N13.3 Other and unspecified hydronephrosis**
Excludes1 hydronephrosis with infection (N13.6)
N13.30 Unspecified hydronephrosis
N13.39 Other hydronephrosis

N13.4 Hydroureter (Ex) PDX 1374
Excludes1 congenital hydroureter (Q62.3-)
hydroureter with infection (N13.6)
vesicoureteral-reflux with hydroureter (N13.73-)

N13.5 Crossing vessel and stricture of ureter without hydronephrosis
Kinking and stricture of ureter without hydronephrosis
Excludes1 crossing vessel and stricture of ureter without hydronephrosis with infection (N13.6)
Coding Clinic: 2016, Q4, P43

N13.6 Pyonephrosis
Conditions in N13.0-N13.5 with infection
Obstructive uropathy with infection
Use additional code (B95-B97), to identify infectious agent
Coding Clinic: 2018, Q2, P21

● **N13.7 Vesicoureteral-reflux**
Excludes1 reflux-associated pyelonephritis (N11.0)
N13.70 Vesicoureteral-reflux, unspecified
Occurs when urine flows from bladder back into ureters
Vesicoureteral-reflux NOS
N13.71 Vesicoureteral-reflux without reflux nephropathy

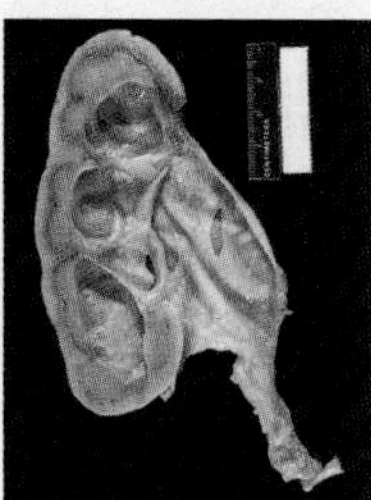

Figure 14-4 Hydronephrosis of the kidney, with marked dilatation of pelvis and calyces and thinning of renal parenchyma. (From Kumar: Robbins and Cotran: Pathologic Basis of Disease, ed 8, Saunders, An Imprint of Elsevier, 2009)

CHAPTER 14 (N00-N99)

N13.72 Vesicoureteral-reflux with reflux nephropathy without hydroureter
- **N13.721 Vesicoureteral-reflux with reflux nephropathy without hydroureter, unilateral**
- **N13.722 Vesicoureteral-reflux with reflux nephropathy without hydroureter, bilateral**
- **N13.729 Vesicoureteral-reflux with reflux nephropathy without hydroureter, unspecified**

N13.73 Vesicoureteral-reflux with reflux nephropathy with hydroureter
- **N13.731 Vesicoureteral-reflux with reflux nephropathy with hydroureter, unilateral**
- **N13.732 Vesicoureteral-reflux with reflux nephropathy with hydroureter, bilateral**
- **N13.739 Vesicoureteral-reflux with reflux nephropathy with hydroureter, unspecified**

N13.8 Other obstructive and reflux uropathy (Ex) PDX 1374
Urinary tract obstruction due to specified cause
Code first, if applicable, any causal condition first, such as:
enlarged prostate (N40.1)

N13.9 Obstructive and reflux uropathy, unspecified
Urinary tract obstruction NOS

N14 Drug- and heavy-metal-induced tubulo-interstitial and tubular conditions
Code first poisoning due to drug or toxin, if applicable (T36-T65 with fifth or sixth character 1-4)
Use additional code for adverse effect, if applicable, to identify drug (T36-T50 with fifth or sixth character 5)

N14.0 Analgesic nephropathy

N14.1 Nephropathy induced by other drugs, medicaments and biological substances
Coding Clinic: 2021, Q3, P9-10
- **N14.11 Contrast-induced nephropathy**
  Contrast medium, radiography nephropathy
  Excludes2 acute kidney failure (N17.-)
  Coding Clinic: 2022, Q4, P33
- **N14.19 Nephropathy induced by other drugs, medicaments and biological substances**

N14.2 Nephropathy induced by unspecified drug, medicament or biological substance

N14.3 Nephropathy induced by heavy metals

N14.4 Toxic nephropathy, not elsewhere classified

N15 Other renal tubulo-interstitial diseases

N15.0 Balkan nephropathy
Balkan endemic nephropathy

N15.1 Renal and perinephric abscess (Ex) PDX 1375

N15.8 Other specified renal tubulo-interstitial diseases

N15.9 Renal tubulo-interstitial disease, unspecified
Infection of kidney NOS
Excludes1 urinary tract infection NOS (N39.0)

N16 Renal tubulo-interstitial disorders in diseases classified elsewhere
Pyelonephritis
Tubulo-interstitial nephritis
Code first underlying disease, such as:
brucellosis (A23.0-A23.9)
cryoglobulinemia (D89.1)
glycogen storage disease (E74.0-)
leukemia (C91-C95)
lymphoma (C81.0-C85.9, C96.0-C96.9)
multiple myeloma (C90.0-)
sepsis (A40.0-A41.9)
Wilson's disease (E83.01)

Excludes1 diphtheritic pyelonephritis and tubulo-interstitial nephritis (A36.84)
pyelonephritis and tubulo-interstitial nephritis in candidiasis (B37.49)
pyelonephritis and tubulo-interstitial nephritis in cystinosis (E72.04)
pyelonephritis and tubulo-interstitial nephritis in salmonella infection (A02.25)
pyelonephritis and tubulo-interstitial nephritis in sarcoidosis (D86.84)
pyelonephritis and tubulo-interstitial nephritis in Sjögren syndrome (M35.04)
pyelonephritis and tubulo-interstitial nephritis in systemic lupus erythematosus (M32.15)
pyelonephritis and tubulo-interstitial nephritis in toxoplasmosis (B58.83)
renal tubular degeneration in diabetes (E08-E13 with .29)
syphilitic pyelonephritis and tubulo-interstitial nephritis (A52.75)

ACUTE KIDNEY FAILURE AND CHRONIC KIDNEY DISEASE (N17-N19)

Excludes2 congenital renal failure (P96.0)
drug- and heavy-metal-induced tubulo-interstitial and tubular conditions (N14.-)
extrarenal uremia (R39.2)
hemolytic-uremic syndrome (D59.3-)
hepatorenal syndrome (K76.7)
postpartum hepatorenal syndrome (O90.41)
posttraumatic renal failure (T79.5)
prerenal uremia (R39.2)
renal failure complicating abortion or ectopic or molar pregnancy (O00-O07, O08.4)
renal failure following labor and delivery (O90.41)
renal failure postprocedural (N99.0)

N17 Acute kidney failure (Ex) PDX 1376
Code also associated underlying condition
Excludes1 posttraumatic renal failure (T79.5)

N17.0 Acute kidney failure with tubular necrosis
Acute tubular necrosis
Renal tubular necrosis
Tubular necrosis NOS
Coding Clinic: 2022, Q4, P33 ; 2021, Q3, P10

N17.1 Acute kidney failure with acute cortical necrosis
Acute cortical necrosis
Cortical necrosis NOS
Renal cortical necrosis

N17.2 Acute kidney failure with medullary necrosis
Medullary [papillary] necrosis NOS
Acute medullary [papillary] necrosis
Renal medullary [papillary] necrosis

N17.8 Other acute kidney failure (Ex) PDX 1377

N17.9 Acute kidney failure, unspecified
Acute kidney injury (nontraumatic)
Excludes2 traumatic kidney injury (S37.0-)
Coding Clinic: 2023, Q3, P5; 2019, Q2, P7,25

Item 14-6 Decreased blood flow is the usual cause of **acute renal failure** that offers a good prognosis for recovery.
Chronic renal failure is usually the result of long-standing kidney disease and is a very serious condition that generally results in death.

● **N18 Chronic kidney disease (CKD)** PDX 1378
Code first any associated:
diabetic chronic kidney disease (E08.22, E09.22, E10.22, E11.22, E13.22)
hypertensive chronic kidney disease (I12.-, I13.-)
Use additional code to identify kidney transplant status, if applicable, (Z94.0)
Coding Clinic: 2018, Q4, P89; 2016, Q4, P123
N18.1 Chronic kidney disease, stage 1
N18.2 Chronic kidney disease, stage 2 (mild)
● **N18.3 Chronic kidney disease, stage 3 (moderate)**
Coding Clinic: 2022, Q4, P6
N18.30 Chronic kidney disease, stage 3 unspecified
N18.31 Chronic kidney disease, stage 3a
N18.32 Chronic kidney disease, stage 3b
N18.4 Chronic kidney disease, stage 4 (severe)
Coding Clinic: 2023, Q1, P18; 2022, Q4, P14; 2013, Q1, P24
N18.5 Chronic kidney disease, stage 5
Excludes1 chronic kidney disease, stage 5 requiring chronic dialysis (N18.6)
N18.6 End stage renal disease PDX 1379
Chronic kidney disease requiring chronic dialysis
Use additional code to identify dialysis status (Z99.2)
Coding Clinic: 2022, Q3, P16; 2016, Q3, P23, Q1, P13
N18.9 Chronic kidney disease, unspecified
Chronic renal disease
Chronic renal failure NOS
Chronic renal insufficiency
Chronic uremia NOS
Diffuse sclerosing glomerulonephritis NOS
Coding Clinic: 2018, Q4, P88

N19 Unspecified kidney failure
Uremia NOS
Excludes1 acute kidney failure (N17.-)
chronic kidney disease (N18.-)
chronic uremia (N18.9)
extrarenal uremia (R39.2)
prerenal uremia (R39.2)
renal insufficiency (acute) (N28.9)
uremia of newborn (P96.0)

UROLITHIASIS (N20-N23)

● **N20 Calculus of kidney and ureter** PDX 1380
Calculous pyelonephritis
Excludes1 nephrocalcinosis (E83.59)
that with hydronephrosis (N13.2)
Coding Clinic: 2019, Q3, P14
N20.0 Calculus of kidney
Nephrolithiasis NOS
Renal calculus
Renal stone
Staghorn calculus
Stone in kidney
Coding Clinic: 2019, Q3, P13; 2017, Q1, P5
N20.1 Calculus of ureter
Calculus of the ureteropelvic junction
Ureteric stone
Coding Clinic: 2016, Q3, P24

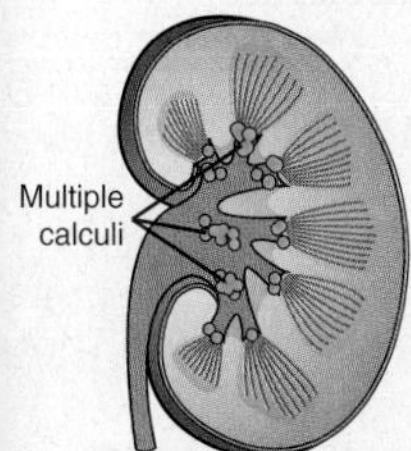

Figure 14-5 Multiple urinary calculi.

N20.2 Calculus of kidney with calculus of ureter
N20.9 Urinary calculus, unspecified

● **N21 Calculus of lower urinary tract**
Includes calculus of lower urinary tract with cystitis and urethritis
N21.0 Calculus in bladder
Calculus in diverticulum of bladder
Urinary bladder stone
Excludes2 staghorn calculus (N20.0)
Coding Clinic: 2015, Q2, P9
N21.1 Calculus in urethra
Excludes2 calculus of prostate (N42.0)
N21.8 Other lower urinary tract calculus
N21.9 Calculus of lower urinary tract, unspecified
Excludes1 calculus of urinary tract NOS (N20.9)

N22 ***Calculus of urinary tract in diseases classified elsewhere***
Code first underlying disease, such as:
gout (M1A.-, M10.-)
schistosomiasis (B65.0-B65.9)

N23 Unspecified renal colic

OTHER DISORDERS OF KIDNEY AND URETER (N25-N29)

Excludes2 disorders of kidney and ureter with urolithiasis (N20-N23)

● **N25 Disorders resulting from impaired renal tubular function**
N25.0 Renal osteodystrophy
Azotemic osteodystrophy
Phosphate-losing tubular disorders
Renal rickets
Renal short stature
Excludes2 metabolic disorders classifiable to E70-E88
N25.1 Nephrogenic diabetes insipidus PDX 1381
Excludes1 diabetes insipidus NOS (E23.2)
● **N25.8 Other disorders resulting from impaired renal tubular function**
N25.81 Secondary hyperparathyroidism of renal origin PDX 1382
Excludes1 secondary hyperparathyroidism, non-renal (E21.1)
Excludes2 metabolic disorders classifiable to E70-E88
N25.89 Other disorders resulting from impaired renal tubular function
Hypokalemic nephropathy
Lightwood-Albright syndrome
Renal tubular acidosis NOS
N25.9 Disorder resulting from impaired renal tubular function, unspecified

● **N26 Unspecified contracted kidney**
Excludes1 contracted kidney due to hypertension (I12.-)
diffuse sclerosing glomerulonephritis (N05.8.-)
hypertensive nephrosclerosis (arteriolar) (arteriosclerotic) (I12.-)
small kidney of unknown cause (N27.-)
N26.1 Atrophy of kidney (terminal)
N26.2 Page kidney
N26.9 Renal sclerosis, unspecified

● **N27 Small kidney of unknown cause**
Includes oligonephronia
N27.0 Small kidney, unilateral
N27.1 Small kidney, bilateral
N27.9 Small kidney, unspecified

CHAPTER 14 (N00-N99)

N28 Other disorders of kidney and ureter, not elsewhere classified

N28.Ø Ischemia and infarction of kidney PDX 1383
Renal artery embolism
Renal artery obstruction
Renal artery occlusion
Renal artery thrombosis
Renal infarct
Excludes1 atherosclerosis of renal artery (extrarenal part) (I7Ø.1)
congenital stenosis of renal artery (Q27.1)
Goldblatt's kidney (I7Ø.1)

N28.1 Cyst of kidney, acquired
Cyst (multiple) (solitary) of kidney, (acquired)
Excludes1 cystic kidney disease (congenital) (Q61.-)

N28.8 Other specified disorders of kidney and ureter PDX 1373
Excludes1 hydroureter (N13.4)
ureteric stricture with hydronephrosis (N13.1)
ureteric stricture without hydronephrosis (N13.5)

N28.81 Hypertrophy of kidney
N28.82 Megaloureter
N28.83 Nephroptosis
N28.84 Pyelitis cystica
N28.85 Pyeloureteritis cystica
N28.86 Ureteritis cystica
N28.89 Other specified disorders of kidney and ureter
Coding Clinic: 2023, Q3, P5

N28.9 Disorder of kidney and ureter, unspecified
Nephropathy NOS
Renal disease (acute) NOS
Renal insufficiency (acute)
Excludes1 chronic renal insufficiency (N18.9)
unspecified nephritic syndrome (NØ5.-)
Coding Clinic: 2Ø16, Q1, P13

N29 Other disorders of kidney and ureter in diseases classified elsewhere
Code first underlying disease, such as:
amyloidosis (E85.-)
nephrocalcinosis (E83.59)
schistosomiasis (B65.Ø-B65.9)
Excludes1 disorders of kidney and ureter in:
cystinosis (E72.Ø)
gonorrhea (A54.21)
syphilis (A52.75)
tuberculosis (A18.11)

OTHER DISEASES OF THE URINARY SYSTEM (N3Ø-N39)

Excludes2 urinary infection (complicating):
abortion or ectopic or molar pregnancy (OØØ-OØ7, OØ8.8)
pregnancy, childbirth and the puerperium (O23.-, O75.3, O86.2-)

N3Ø Cystitis PDX 1384
Infection of bladder and irritation in lower urinary tract
Use additional code to identify infectious agent (B95-B97)
Excludes1 prostatocystitis (N41.3)

N3Ø.Ø Acute cystitis
Excludes1 irradiation cystitis (N3Ø.4-)
trigonitis (N3Ø.3-)
N3Ø.ØØ Acute cystitis without hematuria
N3Ø.Ø1 Acute cystitis with hematuria

N3Ø.1 Interstitial cystitis (chronic)
Ongoing infection of kidney glomeruli and tubules
N3Ø.1Ø Interstitial cystitis (chronic) without hematuria
N3Ø.11 Interstitial cystitis (chronic) with hematuria

N3Ø.2 Other chronic cystitis
N3Ø.2Ø Other chronic cystitis without hematuria
N3Ø.21 Other chronic cystitis with hematuria

N3Ø.3 Trigonitis
Inflammation of triangular area of bladder (where the ureters and urethra come together)
Urethrotrigonitis
N3Ø.3Ø Trigonitis without hematuria
N3Ø.31 Trigonitis with hematuria

N3Ø.4 Irradiation cystitis
N3Ø.4Ø Irradiation cystitis without hematuria
N3Ø.41 Irradiation cystitis with hematuria

N3Ø.8 Other cystitis
Abscess of bladder
N3Ø.8Ø Other cystitis without hematuria
N3Ø.81 Other cystitis with hematuria

N3Ø.9 Cystitis, unspecified
N3Ø.9Ø Cystitis, unspecified without hematuria
N3Ø.91 Cystitis, unspecified with hematuria

N31 Neuromuscular dysfunction of bladder, not elsewhere classified
Use additional code to identify any associated urinary incontinence (N39.3-N39.4-)
Excludes1 cord bladder NOS (G95.89)
neurogenic bladder due to cauda equina syndrome (G83.4)
neuromuscular dysfunction due to spinal cord lesion (G95.89)

N31.Ø Uninhibited neuropathic bladder, not elsewhere classified
N31.1 Reflex neuropathic bladder, not elsewhere classified
N31.2 Flaccid neuropathic bladder, not elsewhere classified
Atonic (motor) (sensory) neuropathic bladder
Diminished tone of bladder muscle
Autonomous neuropathic bladder
Nonreflex neuropathic bladder
N31.8 Other neuromuscular dysfunction of bladder
N31.9 Neuromuscular dysfunction of bladder, unspecified
Neurogenic bladder dysfunction NOS

N32 Other disorders of bladder PDX 1385
Excludes2 calculus of bladder (N21.Ø)
cystocele (N81.1-)
hernia or prolapse of bladder, female (N81.1-)

N32.Ø Bladder-neck obstruction
Bladder-neck stenosis (acquired)
Excludes1 congenital bladder-neck obstruction (Q64.3-)

N32.1 Vesicointestinal fistula
Vesicorectal fistula

N32.2 Vesical fistula, not elsewhere classified
Excludes1 fistula between bladder and female genital tract (N82.Ø-N82.1)

N32.3 Diverticulum of bladder
Formation of sac from a herniation of wall of bladder
Excludes1 congenital diverticulum of bladder (Q64.6)
diverticulitis of bladder (N3Ø.8-)

N32.8 Other specified disorders of bladder
N32.81 Overactive bladder
Detrusor muscle hyperactivity
Excludes1 frequent urination due to specified bladder condition- code to condition
N32.89 Other specified disorders of bladder
Bladder hemorrhage
Bladder hypertrophy
Calcified bladder
Contracted bladder

N32.9 Bladder disorder, unspecified

N33 Bladder disorders in diseases classified elsewhere

Code first underlying disease, such as:
schistosomiasis (B65.Ø-B65.9)

Excludes1 bladder disorder in syphilis (A52.76)
bladder disorder in tuberculosis (A18.12)
candidal cystitis (B37.41)
chlamydial cystitis(A56.Ø1)
cystitis in gonorrhea (A54.Ø1)
cystitis in neurogenic bladder (N31.-)
diphtheritic cystitis (A36.85)
syphilitic cystitis (A52.76)
trichomonal cystitis (A59.Ø3)

N34 Urethritis and urethral syndrome

Use additional code (B95-B97), to identify infectious agent

Excludes2 Reiter's disease (MØ2.3-)
urethritis in diseases with a predominantly sexual mode of transmission (A5Ø-A64)
urethrotrigonitis (N3Ø.3-)

N34.Ø Urethral abscess (Ex:) PDX 1386
Abscess (of) Cowper's gland
Abscess (of) Littré's gland
Abscess (of) urethral (gland)
Periurethral abscess

Excludes1 urethral caruncle (N36.2)

N34.1 Nonspecific urethritis
Nongonococcal urethritis
Nonvenereal urethritis

N34.2 Other urethritis
Inflammation of urethra
Meatitis, urethral
Postmenopausal urethritis
Ulcer of urethra (meatus)
Urethritis NOS

N34.3 Urethral syndrome, unspecified

N35 Urethral stricture

Narrowing of lumen of urethra caused by scarring due to infection or injury

Excludes1 congenital urethral stricture (Q64.3-)
postprocedural urethral stricture (N99.1-)

N35.Ø Post-traumatic urethral stricture
Urethral stricture due to injury

Excludes1 postprocedural urethral stricture (N99.1-)

N35.Ø1 Post-traumatic urethral stricture, male

N35.Ø1Ø Post-traumatic urethral stricture, male, meatal

N35.Ø11 Post-traumatic bulbous urethral stricture

N35.Ø12 Post-traumatic membranous urethral stricture

N35.Ø13 Post-traumatic anterior urethral stricture

N35.Ø14 Post-traumatic urethral stricture, male, unspecified

N35.Ø16 Post-traumatic urethral stricture, male, overlapping sites (Ex:) PDX 934

N35.Ø2 Post-traumatic urethral stricture, female

N35.Ø21 Urethral stricture due to childbirth

N35.Ø28 Other post-traumatic urethral stricture, female

N35.1 Postinfective urethral stricture, not elsewhere classified

Excludes1 urethral stricture associated with schistosomiasis (B65.-, N29)
gonococcal urethral stricture (A54.Ø1)
syphilitic urethral stricture (A52.76)

N35.11 Postinfective urethral stricture, not elsewhere classified, male

N35.111 Postinfective urethral stricture, not elsewhere classified, male, meatal

N35.112 Postinfective bulbous urethral stricture, not elsewhere classified, male

N35.113 Postinfective membranous urethral stricture, not elsewhere classified, male

N35.114 Postinfective anterior urethral stricture, not elsewhere classified, male

N35.116 Postinfective urethral stricture, not elsewhere classified, male, overlapping sites

N35.119 Postinfective urethral stricture, not elsewhere classified, male, unspecified

N35.12 Postinfective urethral stricture, not elsewhere classified, female

N35.8 Other urethral stricture

Excludes1 postprocedural urethral stricture (N99.1-)

N35.81 Other urethral stricture, male

N35.811 Other urethral stricture, male, meatal

N35.812 Other bulbous urethral stricture, male

N35.813 Other membranous urethral stricture, male

N35.814 Other anterior urethral stricture, male

N35.816 Other urethral stricture, male, overlapping sites

N35.819 Other urethral stricture, male, unspecified site

N35.82 Other urethral stricture, female

N35.9 Urethral stricture, unspecified

N35.91 Urethral stricture, unspecified, male

N35.911 Unspecified urethral stricture, male, meatal

N35.912 Unspecified bulbous urethral stricture, male

N35.913 Unspecified membranous urethral stricture, male

N35.914 Unspecified anterior urethral stricture, male

N35.916 Unspecified urethral stricture, male, overlapping sites

N35.919 Unspecified urethral stricture, male, unspecified site
Pinhole meatus NOS
Urethral stricture NOS

N35.92 Unspecified urethral stricture, female

N36 Other disorders of urethra

N36.Ø Urethral fistula (Ex:) PDX 1387
Urethroperineal fistula
Urethrorectal fistula
Urinary fistula NOS

Excludes1 urethroscrotal fistula (N5Ø.89)
urethrovaginal fistula (N82.1)
urethrovesicovaginal fistula (N82.1)

N36.1 Urethral diverticulum

N36.2 Urethral caruncle

N36.4 Urethral functional and muscular disorders

Use additional code to identify associated urinary stress incontinence (N39.3)

N36.41 Hypermobility of urethra

N36.42 Intrinsic sphincter deficiency (ISD)

N36.43 Combined hypermobility of urethra and intrinsic sphincter deficiency

N36.44 Muscular disorders of urethra
Bladder sphincter dyssynergy

N36.5 Urethral false passage

N36.8 Other specified disorders of urethra

Excludes1 congenital urethrocele (Q64.7)
female urethrocele (N81.Ø)

Coding Clinic: 2Ø22, Q2, P7

N36.9 Urethral disorder, unspecified

N37 *Urethral disorders in diseases classified elsewhere*
Code first underlying disease
Excludes1 urethritis (in):
candidal infection (B37.41)
chlamydial (A56.01)
gonorrhea (A54.01)
syphilis (A52.76)
trichomonal infection (A59.03)
tuberculosis (A18.13)

N39 Other disorders of urinary system
Excludes2 hematuria NOS (R31.-)
recurrent or persistent hematuria (N02.-)
recurrent or persistent hematuria with specified morphological lesion (N02.-)
proteinuria NOS (R80.-)

N39.0 Urinary tract infection, site not specified (Ex:) PDX 1388
Use additional code (B95-B97), to identify infectious agent
Excludes1 candidiasis of urinary tract (B37.4-)
neonatal urinary tract infection (P39.3)
pyonephrosis (N13.6)
pyuria (R82.81)
urinary tract infection of specified site, such as:
cystitis (N30.-)
urethritis (N34.-)
Coding Clinic: 2018, Q2, P22; Q1, P16; 2012, Q4, P94

N39.3 Stress incontinence (female) (male)
Code also any associated overactive bladder (N32.81)
Excludes1 mixed incontinence (N39.46)
Coding Clinic: 2021, Q4, P18

N39.4 Other specified urinary incontinence
Code also any associated overactive bladder (N32.81)
Excludes1 enuresis NOS (R32)
functional urinary incontinence (R39.81)
urinary incontinence associated with cognitive impairment (R39.81)
urinary incontinence NOS (R32)
urinary incontinence of nonorganic origin (F98.0)

N39.41 Urge incontinence
Excludes1 mixed incontinence (N39.46)

N39.42 Incontinence without sensory awareness
Insensible (urinary) incontinence

N39.43 Post-void dribbling

N39.44 Nocturnal enuresis
Excludes2 nocturnal polyuria (R35.81)

N39.45 Continuous leakage

N39.46 Mixed incontinence
Urge and stress incontinence

N39.49 Other specified urinary incontinence

N39.490 Overflow incontinence

N39.491 Coital incontinence
Coding Clinic: 2016, Q4, P44

N39.492 Postural (urinary) incontinence
Coding Clinic: 2016, Q4, P44

N39.498 Other specified urinary incontinence
Reflex incontinence
Total incontinence

N39.8 Other specified disorders of urinary system

N39.9 Disorder of urinary system, unspecified

DISEASES OF MALE GENITAL ORGANS (N40-N53)

★(See Plate 5 of the Anatomy Illustrations.)

N40 Benign prostatic hyperplasia
Includes adenofibromatous hypertrophy of prostate
benign hypertrophy of the prostate
Enlargement of prostate gland usually occurring with age and causing obstructed urine flow
benign prostatic hypertrophy
BPH
enlarged prostate
nodular prostate
polyp of prostate
Excludes1 benign neoplasms of prostate (adenoma, benign) (fibroadenoma) (fibroma) (myoma) (D29.1)
malignant neoplasm of prostate (C61)

N40.0 Benign prostatic hyperplasia without lower urinary tract symptoms A
Enlarged prostate without LUTS
Enlarged prostate NOS

N40.1 Benign prostatic hyperplasia with lower urinary tract symptoms A
Enlarged prostate with LUTS
Use additional code for associated symptoms, when specified:
incomplete bladder emptying (R39.14)
nocturia (R35.1)
straining on urination (R39.16)
urinary frequency (R35.0)
urinary hesitancy (R39.11)
urinary incontinence (N39.4-)
urinary obstruction (N13.8)
urinary retention (R33.8)
urinary urgency (R39.15)
weak urinary stream (R39.12)
Coding Clinic: 2018, Q4, P55

N40.2 Nodular prostate without lower urinary tract symptoms A
Nodular prostate without LUTS

N40.3 Nodular prostate with lower urinary tract symptoms A
Use additional code for associated symptoms, when specified:
incomplete bladder emptying (R39.14)
nocturia (R35.1)
straining on urination (R39.16)
urinary frequency (R35.0)
urinary hesitancy (R39.11)
urinary incontinence (N39.4-)
urinary obstruction (N13.8)
urinary retention (R33.8)
urinary urgency (R39.15)
weak urinary stream (R39.12)

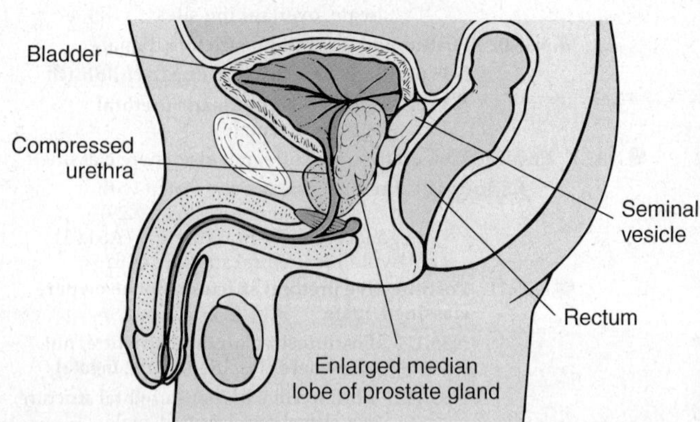

Figure 14-6 Benign prostatic hyperplasia. (From Shiland: Mastering Healthcare Terminology, ed 3, St. Louis, Mosby, 2010)

CHAPTER 14 (N00-N99)

Item 14–7 Hydrocele is a sac of fluid accumulating in the testes membrane.

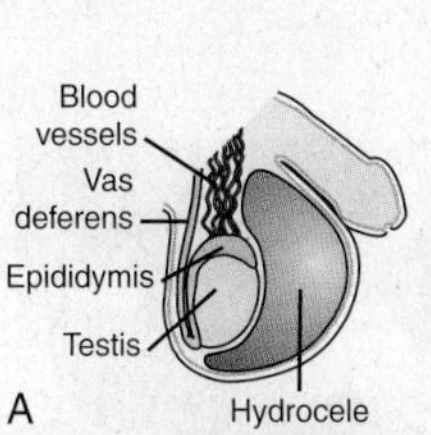

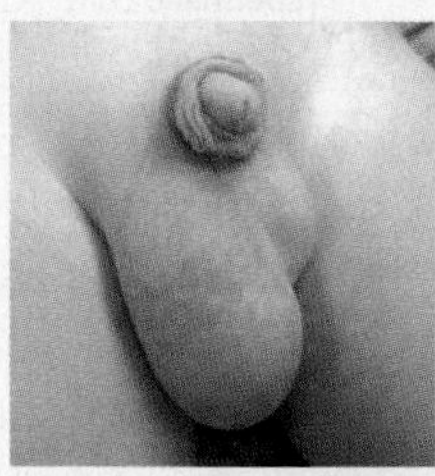

Figure 14-7 A. Hydrocele. **B.** Newborn with large right hydrocele. (**B** from Nelson WE, Kliegman R: Nelson Textbook of Pediatrics, Philadelphia, Saunders Elsevier, 2011)

● **N41 Inflammatory diseases of prostate**
Use additional code (B95-B97), to identify infectious agent
- **N41.0 Acute prostatitis** CC (Ex) PDX 1389 A
  Coding Clinic: 2024, Q1, P16
- **N41.1 Chronic prostatitis** A
- **N41.2 Abscess of prostate** CC (Ex) PDX 1389 A
- **N41.3 Prostatocystitis** A
  Coding Clinic: 2024, Q1, P16
- **N41.4 Granulomatous prostatitis** A
- **N41.8 Other inflammatory diseases of prostate** A
- **N41.9 Inflammatory disease of prostate, unspecified** A
  Prostatitis NOS

● **N42 Other and unspecified disorders of prostate**
- **N42.0 Calculus of prostate** A
  Prostatic stone
- **N42.1 Congestion and hemorrhage of prostate** A
  Excludes1 enlarged prostate (N40.-)
  hematuria (R31.-)
  hyperplasia of prostate (N40.-)
  inflammatory diseases of prostate (N41.-)
- ● **N42.3 Dysplasia of prostate**
  Coding Clinic: 2016, Q4, P44
  - **N42.30 Unspecified dysplasia of prostate**
  - **N42.31 Prostatic intraepithelial neoplasia**
    PIN
    Prostatic intraepithelial neoplasia I (PIN I)
    Prostatic intraepithelial neoplasia II (PIN II)
    Excludes1 prostatic intraepithelial neoplasia III (PIN III) (D07.5)
  - **N42.32 Atypical small acinar proliferation of prostate**
  - **N42.39 Other dysplasia of prostate**
- ● **N42.8 Other specified disorders of prostate**
  - **N42.81 Prostatodynia syndrome** A
    Painful prostate syndrome
  - **N42.82 Prostatosis syndrome** A
  - **N42.83 Cyst of prostate** A
  - **N42.89 Other specified disorders of prostate** A
- **N42.9 Disorder of prostate, unspecified** A

● **N43 Hydrocele and spermatocele**
Includes hydrocele of spermatic cord, testis or tunica vaginalis
Excludes1 congenital hydrocele (P83.5)
- **N43.0 Encysted hydrocele**
- **N43.1 Infected hydrocele** CC (Ex) PDX 1390
  Use additional code (B95-B97), to identify infectious agent
- **N43.2 Other hydrocele**
- **N43.3 Hydrocele, unspecified**
- ● **N43.4 Spermatocele of epididymis**
  Spermatic cyst
  - **N43.40 Spermatocele of epididymis, unspecified**
  - **N43.41 Spermatocele of epididymis, single**
  - **N43.42 Spermatocele of epididymis, multiple**

● **N44 Noninflammatory disorders of testis**
- ● **N44.0 Torsion of testis** (Ex) PDX 1391
  - **N44.00 Torsion of testis, unspecified** CC
  - **N44.01 Extravaginal torsion of spermatic cord** CC
  - **N44.02 Intravaginal torsion of spermatic cord** CC
    Torsion of spermatic cord NOS
  - **N44.03 Torsion of appendix testis** CC
  - **N44.04 Torsion of appendix epididymis** CC
- **N44.1 Cyst of tunica albuginea testis**
- **N44.2 Benign cyst of testis**
- **N44.8 Other noninflammatory disorders of the testis**

● **N45 Orchitis and epididymitis**
*Orchitis is inflammation of one or both of the testes as a result of mumps or other infection, trauma, or metastasis. **Epididymitis** is inflammation of the tubular structure that connects the testicle with the vas deferens.*
Use additional code (B95-B97), to identify infectious agent
- **N45.1 Epididymitis**
- **N45.2 Orchitis**
- **N45.3 Epididymo-orchitis**
- **N45.4 Abscess of epididymis or testis** CC (Ex) PDX 1392

● **N46 Male infertility**
Excludes1 vasectomy status (Z98.52)
- ● **N46.0 Azoospermia**
  Absolute male infertility
  Male infertility due to germinal (cell) aplasia
  Male infertility due to spermatogenic arrest (complete)
  - **N46.01 Organic azoospermia** A
    Azoospermia NOS
  - ● **N46.02 Azoospermia due to extratesticular causes**
    Code also associated cause
    - **N46.021 Azoospermia due to drug therapy** A
    - **N46.022 Azoospermia due to infection** A
    - **N46.023 Azoospermia due to obstruction of efferent ducts** A
    - **N46.024 Azoospermia due to radiation** A
    - **N46.025 Azoospermia due to systemic disease** A
    - **N46.029 Azoospermia due to other extratesticular causes** A
- ● **N46.1 Oligospermia**
  Male infertility due to germinal cell desquamation
  Male infertility due to hypospermatogenesis
  Male infertility due to incomplete spermatogenic arrest
  - **N46.11 Organic oligospermia** A
    Oligospermia NOS
  - ● **N46.12 Oligospermia due to extratesticular causes**
    Code also associated cause
    - **N46.121 Oligospermia due to drug therapy** A
    - **N46.122 Oligospermia due to infection** A
    - **N46.123 Oligospermia due to obstruction of efferent ducts** A
    - **N46.124 Oligospermia due to radiation** A
    - **N46.125 Oligospermia due to systemic disease** A
    - **N46.129 Oligospermia due to other extratesticular causes** A
- **N46.8 Other male infertility** A
- **N46.9 Male infertility, unspecified** A

Item 14–8 Male infertility is the inability of the female sex partner to conceive after one year of unprotected intercourse.

Azoospermia is no sperm ejaculated and **oligospermia** is few sperm ejaculated—both resulting in infertility. Extratesticular causes such as injury, infections, radiation, and chemotherapy may also cause male infertility.

● N47 **Disorders of prepuce**
N47.0 **Adherent prepuce, newborn** N
N47.1 **Phimosis**
N47.2 **Paraphimosis**
N47.3 **Deficient foreskin**
N47.4 **Benign cyst of prepuce**
N47.5 **Adhesions of prepuce and glans penis**
N47.6 **Balanoposthitis**
Use additional code (B95-B97), to identify infectious agent
Excludes1 balanitis (N48.1)
N47.7 **Other inflammatory diseases of prepuce**
Use additional code (B95-B97), to identify infectious agent
N47.8 **Other disorders of prepuce**

● N48 **Other disorders of penis**
N48.0 **Leukoplakia of penis**
Balanitis xerotica obliterans
Kraurosis of penis
Lichen sclerosus of external male genital organs
Excludes1 carcinoma in situ of penis (D07.4)
N48.1 **Balanitis**
Use additional code (B95-B97), to identify infectious agent
Excludes1 amebic balanitis (A06.8)
balanitis xerotica obliterans (N48.0)
candidal balanitis (B37.42)
gonococcal balanitis (A54.23)
herpesviral [herpes simplex] balanitis (A60.01)
● N48.2 **Other inflammatory disorders of penis**
Use additional code (B95-B97), to identify infectious agent
Excludes1 balanitis (N48.1)
balanitis xerotica obliterans (N48.0)
balanoposthitis (N47.6)
N48.21 **Abscess of corpus cavernosum and penis**
N48.22 **Cellulitis of corpus cavernosum and penis**
N48.29 **Other inflammatory disorders of penis**
● N48.3 **Priapism** Ex PDX 1393
Painful erection
Code first underlying cause
N48.30 **Priapism, unspecified**
N48.31 **Priapism due to trauma**
N48.32 *Priapism due to disease classified elsewhere*
N48.33 **Priapism, drug-induced**
N48.39 **Other priapism**
N48.5 **Ulcer of penis**
N48.6 **Induration penis plastica**
Peyronie's disease
Plastic induration of penis
● N48.8 **Other specified disorders of penis**
N48.81 **Thrombosis of superficial vein of penis**
N48.82 **Acquired torsion of penis**
Acquired torsion of penis NOS
Excludes1 congenital torsion of penis (Q55.63)
N48.83 **Acquired buried penis**
Excludes1 congenital hidden penis (Q55.64)
N48.89 **Other specified disorders of penis**
N48.9 **Disorder of penis, unspecified**

Item 14–9 Seminal vesiculitis is an inflammation of the seminal vesicle. **Spermatocele** is a benign cystic accumulation of sperm arising from the head of the epididymis. **Torsion of the testis** is a medical emergency occurring most commonly in boys 7 to 12 years of age and results from a congenital abnormality of the covering of the testis allowing the testis to twist within its sac and cutting off the blood supply to the testis.

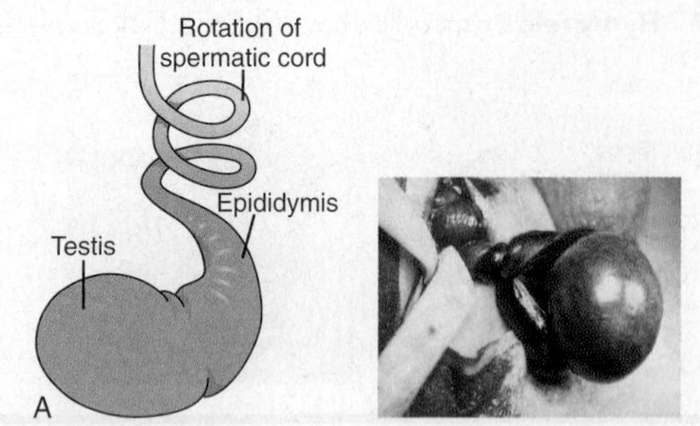

Figure 14-8 A. Torsion of testis. **B.** Torsion of the testis. (**B** from Kliegman R, Nelson WE: Nelson Textbook of Pediatrics, Philadelphia, Saunders, 2007)

● N49 **Inflammatory disorders of male genital organs, not elsewhere classified**
Use additional code (B95-B97), to identify infectious agent
Excludes1 inflammation of penis (N48.1, N48.2-)
orchitis and epididymitis (N45.-)
N49.0 **Inflammatory disorders of seminal vesicle**
Vesiculitis NOS
N49.1 **Inflammatory disorders of spermatic cord, tunica vaginalis and vas deferens**
Vasitis
N49.2 **Inflammatory disorders of scrotum**
N49.3 **Fournier gangrene**
N49.8 **Inflammatory disorders of other specified male genital organs**
Inflammation of multiple sites in male genital organs
N49.9 **Inflammatory disorder of unspecified male genital organ**
Abscess of unspecified male genital organ
Boil of unspecified male genital organ
Carbuncle of unspecified male genital organ
Cellulitis of unspecified male genital organ

● N50 **Other and unspecified disorders of male genital organs**
Excludes2 torsion of testis (N44.0-)
N50.0 **Atrophy of testis**
N50.1 **Vascular disorders of male genital organs**
Hematocele, NOS, of male genital organs
Hemorrhage of male genital organs
Thrombosis of male genital organs
N50.3 **Cyst of epididymis**
● N50.8 **Other specified disorders of male genital organs**
Coding Clinic: 2016, Q4, P45
● N50.81 **Testicular pain**
N50.811 **Right testicular pain**
N50.812 **Left testicular pain**
N50.819 **Testicular pain, unspecified**
N50.82 **Scrotal pain**
N50.89 **Other specified disorders of the male genital organs**
Atrophy of scrotum, seminal vesicle, spermatic cord, tunica vaginalis and vas deferens
Chylocele, tunica vaginalis (nonfilarial) NOS
Edema of scrotum, seminal vesicle, spermatic cord, tunica vaginalis and vas deferens
Hypertrophy of scrotum, seminal vesicle, spermatic cord, tunica vaginalis and vas deferens
Stricture of spermatic cord, tunica vaginalis, and vas deferens
Ulcer of scrotum, seminal vesicle, spermatic cord, testis, tunica vaginalis and vas deferens
Urethroscrotal fistula
N50.9 **Disorder of male genital organs, unspecified**

N51 Disorders of male genital organs in diseases classified elsewhere
Code first underlying disease, such as:
filariasis (B74.0-B74.9)
Excludes1 amebic balanitis (A06.8)
candidal balanitis (B37.42)
gonococcal balanitis (A54.23)
gonococcal prostatitis (A54.22)
herpesviral [herpes simplex] balanitis (A60.01)
trichomonal prostatitis (A59.02)
tuberculous prostatitis (A18.14)

N52 Male erectile dysfunction
Excludes1 psychogenic impotence (F52.21)
N52.0 Vasculogenic erectile dysfunction
N52.01 Erectile dysfunction due to arterial insufficiency A
N52.02 Corporo-venous occlusive erectile dysfunction A
N52.03 Combined arterial insufficiency and corporo-venous occlusive erectile dysfunction A
N52.1 Erectile dysfunction due to diseases classified elsewhere A
Code first underlying disease
N52.2 Drug-induced erectile dysfunction A
N52.3 Postprocedural erectile dysfunction
N52.31 Erectile dysfunction following radical prostatectomy A
N52.32 Erectile dysfunction following radical cystectomy A
N52.33 Erectile dysfunction following urethral surgery A
N52.34 Erectile dysfunction following simple prostatectomy A
N52.35 Erectile dysfunction following radiation therapy A
Coding Clinic: 2016, Q4, P45
N52.36 Erectile dysfunction following interstitial seed therapy A
Coding Clinic: 2016, Q4, P45
N52.37 Erectile dysfunction following prostate ablative therapy A
Erectile dysfunction following cryotherapy
Erectile dysfunction following other prostate ablative therapies
Erectile dysfunction following ultrasound ablative therapies
Coding Clinic: 2016, Q4, P45
N52.39 Other and unspecified postprocedural erectile dysfunction A
N52.8 Other male erectile dysfunction A
N52.9 Male erectile dysfunction, unspecified A
Impotence NOS

N53 Other male sexual dysfunction
Excludes1 psychogenic sexual dysfunction (F52.-)
N53.1 Ejaculatory dysfunction
Excludes1 premature ejaculation (F52.4)
N53.11 Retarded ejaculation
N53.12 Painful ejaculation
N53.13 Anejaculatory orgasm
N53.14 Retrograde ejaculation
N53.19 Other ejaculatory dysfunction
Ejaculatory dysfunction NOS
N53.8 Other male sexual dysfunction
N53.9 Unspecified male sexual dysfunction

DISORDERS OF BREAST (N60-N65)

Excludes1 disorders of breast associated with childbirth (O91-O92)

N60 Benign mammary dysplasia
Benign lumpiness of breast
Includes fibrocystic mastopathy
N60.0 Solitary cyst of breast
Cyst of breast
N60.01 Solitary cyst of right breast
N60.02 Solitary cyst of left breast
N60.09 Solitary cyst of unspecified breast
N60.1 Diffuse cystic mastopathy
Cystic breast
Fibrocystic disease of breast
Excludes1 diffuse cystic mastopathy with epithelial proliferation (N60.3-)
N60.11 Diffuse cystic mastopathy of right breast A
N60.12 Diffuse cystic mastopathy of left breast A
N60.19 Diffuse cystic mastopathy of unspecified breast A
N60.2 Fibroadenosis of breast
Adenofibrosis of breast
Excludes2 fibroadenoma of breast (D24.-)
N60.21 Fibroadenosis of right breast
N60.22 Fibroadenosis of left breast
N60.29 Fibroadenosis of unspecified breast
N60.3 Fibrosclerosis of breast
Cystic mastopathy with epithelial proliferation
N60.31 Fibrosclerosis of right breast
N60.32 Fibrosclerosis of left breast
N60.39 Fibrosclerosis of unspecified breast
N60.4 Mammary duct ectasia
N60.41 Mammary duct ectasia of right breast
N60.42 Mammary duct ectasia of left breast
N60.49 Mammary duct ectasia of unspecified breast
N60.8 Other benign mammary dysplasias
N60.81 Other benign mammary dysplasias of right breast
N60.82 Other benign mammary dysplasias of left breast
N60.89 Other benign mammary dysplasias of unspecified breast
N60.9 Unspecified benign mammary dysplasia
N60.91 Unspecified benign mammary dysplasia of right breast
N60.92 Unspecified benign mammary dysplasia of left breast
N60.99 Unspecified benign mammary dysplasia of unspecified breast

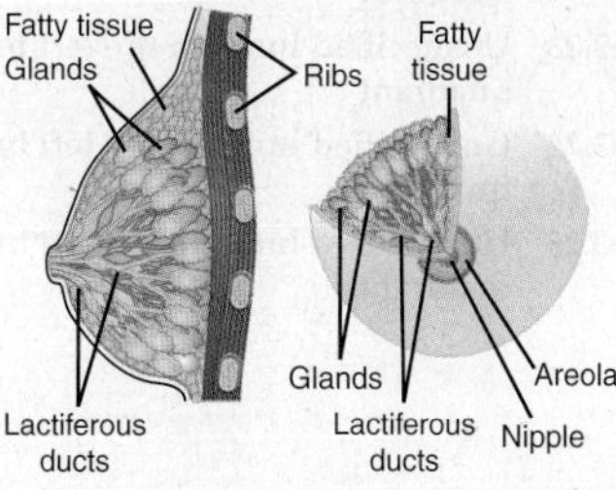

Figure 14-9 Breast.

CHAPTER 14 (N00-N99)

N61 Inflammatory disorders of breast

Excludes1 inflammatory carcinoma of breast (C50.9)
inflammatory disorder of breast associated with childbirth (O91.-)
neonatal infective mastitis (P39.0)
thrombophlebitis of breast [Mondor's disease] (I80.8)

N61.0 Mastitis without abscess
Infective mastitis (acute) (nonpuerperal) (subacute)
Mastitis (acute) (nonpuerperal) (subacute) NOS
Cellulitis (acute) (nonpuerperal) (subacute) of breast NOS
Cellulitis (acute) (nonpuerperal) (subacute) of nipple NOS

N61.1 Abscess of the breast and nipple
Abscess (acute) (chronic) (nonpuerperal) of areola
Abscess (acute) (chronic) (nonpuerperal) of breast
Carbuncle of breast
Mastitis with abscess

N61.2 Granulomatous mastitis
N61.20 Granulomatous mastitis, unspecified breast
N61.21 Granulomatous mastitis, right breast
N61.22 Granulomatous mastitis, left breast
N61.23 Granulomatous mastitis, bilateral breast

N62 Hypertrophy of breast
Gynecomastia
Hypertrophy of breast NOS
Massive pubertal hypertrophy of breast

Excludes1 breast engorgement of newborn (P83.4)
disproportion of reconstructed breast (N65.1)

N63 Unspecified lump in breast
Nodule(s) NOS in breast

N63.0 Unspecified lump in unspecified breast

N63.1 Unspecified lump in the right breast
N63.10 Unspecified lump in the right breast, unspecified quadrant
Coding Clinic: 2022, Q3, P8
N63.11 Unspecified lump in the right breast, upper outer quadrant
Coding Clinic: 2017, Q4, P19
N63.12 Unspecified lump in the right breast, upper inner quadrant
N63.13 Unspecified lump in the right breast, lower outer quadrant
N63.14 Unspecified lump in the right breast, lower inner quadrant
N63.15 Unspecified lump in the right breast, overlapping quadrants

N63.2 Unspecified lump in the left breast
N63.20 Unspecified lump in the left breast, unspecified quadrant
N63.21 Unspecified lump in the left breast, upper outer quadrant
N63.22 Unspecified lump in the left breast, upper inner quadrant
N63.23 Unspecified lump in the left breast, lower outer quadrant
N63.24 Unspecified lump in the left breast, lower inner quadrant
N63.25 Unspecified lump in the left breast, overlapping quadrants

N63.3 Unspecified lump in axillary tail
N63.31 Unspecified lump in axillary tail of the right breast
N63.32 Unspecified lump in axillary tail of the left breast

N63.4 Unspecified lump in breast, subareolar
N63.41 Unspecified lump in right breast, subareolar
N63.42 Unspecified lump in left breast, subareolar

N64 Other disorders of breast

Excludes2 mechanical complication of breast prosthesis and implant (T85.4-)

N64.0 Fissure and fistula of nipple

N64.1 Fat necrosis of breast
Fat necrosis (segmental) of breast
Code first breast necrosis due to breast graft (T85.898)

N64.2 Atrophy of breast

N64.3 Galactorrhea not associated with childbirth
Excessive or spontaneous flow of milk

N64.4 Mastodynia

N64.5 Other signs and symptoms in breast

Excludes2 abnormal findings on diagnostic imaging of breast (R92.-)

N64.51 Induration of breast
N64.52 Nipple discharge

Excludes1 abnormal findings in nipple discharge (R89.-)

N64.53 Retraction of nipple
N64.59 Other signs and symptoms in breast

N64.8 Other specified disorders of breast
N64.81 Ptosis of breast A

Excludes1 ptosis of native breast in relation to reconstructed breast (N65.1)

N64.82 Hypoplasia of breast A
Micromastia

Excludes1 congenital absence of breast (Q83.0)
hypoplasia of native breast in relation to reconstructed breast (N65.1)

N64.89 Other specified disorders of breast
Galactocele
Subinvolution of breast (postlactational)
Coding Clinic: 2019, Q1, P32; 2018, Q1, P4

N64.9 Disorder of breast, unspecified
Coding Clinic: 2018, Q1, P4

N65 Deformity and disproportion of reconstructed breast

N65.0 Deformity of reconstructed breast A
Contour irregularity in reconstructed breast
Excess tissue in reconstructed breast
Misshapen reconstructed breast

N65.1 Disproportion of reconstructed breast A
Breast asymmetry between native breast and reconstructed breast
Disproportion between native breast and reconstructed breast

CHAPTER 14 (N00-N99)

INFLAMMATORY DISEASES OF FEMALE PELVIC ORGANS (N70-N77)

Excludes1 inflammatory diseases of female pelvic organs complicating:
abortion or ectopic or molar pregnancy (O00-O07, O08.0)
pregnancy, childbirth and the puerperium (O23.-, O75.3, O85, O86.-)

★ **(See Plate 35 of the Anatomy Illustrations.)**

● **N70 Salpingitis and oophoritis** (Ex:) PDX 1394
Oophoritis = inflammation of ovary
Salpingitis = inflammation of falloplan tube
Includes abscess (of) fallopian tube
abscess (of) ovary
pyosalpinx
salpingo-oophoritis
tubo-ovarian abscess
tubo-ovarian inflammatory disease
Use additional code (B95-B97), to identify infectious agent
Excludes1 gonococcal infection (A54.24)
tuberculous infection (A18.17)

● **N70.0 Acute salpingitis and oophoritis**
N70.01 Acute salpingitis
N70.02 Acute oophoritis
N70.03 Acute salpingitis and oophoritis

● **N70.1 Chronic salpingitis and oophoritis**
Hydrosalpinx
N70.11 Chronic salpingitis
N70.12 Chronic oophoritis
N70.13 Chronic salpingitis and oophoritis

● **N70.9 Salpingitis and oophoritis, unspecified**
N70.91 Salpingitis, unspecified
N70.92 Oophoritis, unspecified
N70.93 Salpingitis and oophoritis, unspecified

● **N71 Inflammatory disease of uterus, except cervix**
Includes endo (myo) metritis
metritis
myometritis
pyometra
uterine abscess
Use additional code (B95-B97), to identify infectious agent
Excludes1 hyperplastic endometritis (N85.0-)
infection of uterus following delivery (O85, O86.-)

N71.0 Acute inflammatory disease of uterus (Ex:) PDX 1395
N71.1 Chronic inflammatory disease of uterus
N71.9 Inflammatory disease of uterus, unspecified

N72 Inflammatory disease of cervix uteri
Includes cervicitis (with or without erosion or ectropion)
endocervicitis (with or without erosion or ectropion)
exocervicitis (with or without erosion or ectropion)
Use additional code (B95-B97), to identify infectious agent
Excludes1 erosion and ectropion of cervix without cervicitis (N86)

● **N73 Other female pelvic inflammatory diseases** (Ex:) PDX 1394
Use additional code (B95-B97), to identify infectious agent

N73.0 Acute parametritis and pelvic cellulitis
Abscess of broad ligament
Abscess of parametrium
Pelvic cellulitis, female

N73.1 Chronic parametritis and pelvic cellulitis
Any condition in N73.0 specified as chronic
Excludes1 tuberculous parametritis and pelvic cellutitis (A18.17)

N73.2 Unspecified parametritis and pelvic cellulitis
Any condition in N73.0 unspecified whether acute or chronic

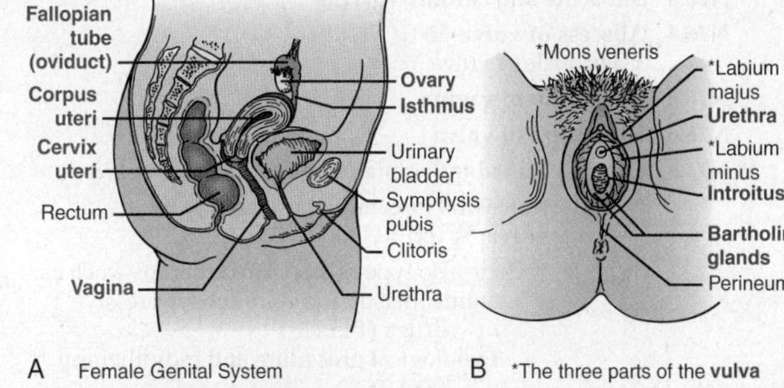

Figure 14-10 A. Female genital system. **B.** External female genital system. (From Buck CJ: Step-by-Step Medical Coding, ed 2016, St. Louis, Elsevier, 2016)

Item 14-10 Salpingitis is an infection of one or both fallopian tubes. **Oophoritis** is an infection of one or both ovaries.

N73.3 Female acute pelvic peritonitis
N73.4 Female chronic pelvic peritonitis
Excludes1 tuberculous pelvic (female) peritonitis (A18.17)
N73.5 Female pelvic peritonitis, unspecified
N73.6 Female pelvic peritoneal adhesions (postinfective)
Excludes2 postprocedural pelvic peritoneal adhesions (N99.4)
N73.8 Other specified female pelvic inflammatory diseases
N73.9 Female pelvic inflammatory disease, unspecified
Female pelvic infection or inflammation NOS

◗ ***N74 Female pelvic inflammatory disorders in diseases classified elsewhere***
Code first underlying disease
Excludes1 chlamydial cervicitis (A56.02)
chlamydial pelvic inflammatory disease (A56.11)
gonococcal cervicitis (A54.03)
gonococcal pelvic inflammatory disease (A54.24)
herpesviral [herpes simplex] cervicitis (A60.03)
herpesviral [herpes simplex] pelvic inflammatory disease (A60.09)
syphilitic cervicitis (A52.76)
syphilitic pelvic inflammatory disease (A52.76)
trichomonal cervicitis (A59.09)
tuberculous cervicitis (A18.16)
tuberculous pelvic inflammatory disease (A18.17)

● **N75 Diseases of Bartholin's gland**
N75.0 Cyst of Bartholin's gland
Cysts filled with liquid or semisolid material
N75.1 Abscess of Bartholin's gland (Ex:) PDX 1396
Localized collection of pus
N75.8 Other diseases of Bartholin's gland
Bartholinitis
N75.9 Disease of Bartholin's gland, unspecified

● **N76 Other inflammation of vagina and vulva**
Use additional code (B95-B97), to identify infectious agent
Excludes2 senile (atrophic) vaginitis (N95.2)
vulvar vestibulitis (N94.810)

N76.0 Acute vaginitis
Acute vulvovaginitis
Vaginitis NOS
Vulvovaginitis NOS

N76.1 Subacute and chronic vaginitis
Chronic vulvovaginitis
Subacute vulvovaginitis

N76.2 Acute vulvitis
Vulvitis NOS

CHAPTER 14 (N00-N99)

N76.3 **Subacute and chronic vulvitis**

N76.4 **Abscess of vulva** (Ex:) PDX 1396
Furuncle of vulva

N76.5 **Ulceration of vagina**

N76.6 **Ulceration of vulva**

N76.8 **Other specified inflammation of vagina and vulva**

N76.81 **Mucositis (ulcerative) of vagina and vulva** (Ex:) PDX 1397
Code also type of associated therapy, such as:
antineoplastic and immunosuppressive drugs (T45.1X-)
radiological procedure and radiotherapy (Y84.2)
Excludes2 gastrointestinal mucositis (ulcerative) (K92.81)
nasal mucositis (ulcerative) (J34.81)
oral mucositis (ulcerative) (K12.3-)

N76.82 **Fournier disease of vagina and vulva**
Fournier gangrene of vagina and vulva
Code also, if applicable, diabetes mellitus (E08-E13 with .9)
Excludes1 gangrene in diabetes mellitus (E08-E13 with .52)

N76.89 **Other specified inflammation of vagina and vulva**

N77 **Vulvovaginal ulceration and inflammation in diseases classified elsewhere**

N77.0 ***Ulceration of vulva in diseases classified elsewhere***
Code first underlying disease, such as:
Behçet's disease (M35.2)
Excludes1 ulceration of vulva in gonococcal infection (A54.02)
ulceration of vulva in herpesviral [herpes simplex] infection (A60.04)
ulceration of vulva in syphilis (A51.0)
ulceration of vulva in tuberculosis (A18.18)

N77.1 ***Vaginitis, vulvitis and vulvovaginitis in diseases classified elsewhere***
Code first underlying disease, such as:
pinworm (B80)
Excludes1 candidial vulvovaginitis (B37.3-)
chlamydial vulvovaginitis (A56.02)
gonococcal vulvovaginitis (A54.02)
herpesviral [herpes simplex] vulvovaginitis (A60.04)
trichomonal vulvovaginitis (A59.01)
tuberculous vulvovaginitis (A18.18)
vulvovaginitis in early syphilis (A51.0)
vulvovaginitis in late syphilis (A52.76)

NONINFLAMMATORY DISORDERS OF FEMALE GENITAL TRACT (N80-N98)

N80 **Endometriosis**

N80.0 **Endometriosis of uterus**
Endometriosis of the cervix
Excludes1 stromal endometriosis (D39.0)

N80.00 **Endometriosis of the uterus, unspecified**

N80.01 **Superficial endometriosis of the uterus**

N80.02 **Deep endometriosis of the uterus**
Deep retrocervical endometriosis

N80.03 **Adenomyosis of the uterus**
Adenomyosis NOS

N80.1 **Endometriosis of ovary**

N80.10 **Endometriosis of ovary, unspecified depth**

N80.101 **Endometriosis of right ovary, unspecified depth**

N80.102 **Endometriosis of left ovary, unspecified depth**

N80.103 **Endometriosis of bilateral ovaries, unspecified depth**

N80.109 **Endometriosis of ovary, unspecified side, unspecified depth**
Endometriosis of ovary NOS

N80.11 **Superficial endometriosis of the ovary**

N80.111 **Superficial endometriosis of right ovary**
Coding Clinic: 2022, Q4, P36

N80.112 **Superficial endometriosis of left ovary**

N80.113 **Superficial endometriosis of bilateral ovaries**

N80.119 **Superficial endometriosis of ovary, unspecified ovary**

N80.12 **Deep endometriosis of ovary**
Deep ovarian endometriosis
Endometrioma

N80.121 **Deep endometriosis of right ovary**

N80.122 **Deep endometriosis of left ovary**

N80.123 **Deep endometriosis of bilateral ovaries**

N80.129 **Deep endometriosis of ovary, unspecified ovary**

N80.2 **Endometriosis of fallopian tube**

N80.20 **Endometriosis of fallopian tube, unspecified depth**

N80.201 **Endometriosis of right fallopian tube, unspecified depth**

N80.202 **Endometriosis of left fallopian tube, unspecified depth**

N80.203 **Endometriosis of bilateral fallopian tubes, unspecified depth**

N80.209 **Endometriosis of unspecified fallopian tube, unspecified depth**
Endometriosis fallopian tube NOS

N80.21 **Superficial endometriosis of fallopian tube**

N80.211 **Superficial endometriosis of right fallopian tube**

N80.212 **Superficial endometriosis of left fallopian tube**

N80.213 **Superficial endometriosis of bilateral fallopian tubes**

N80.219 **Superficial endometriosis of unspecified fallopian tube**

N80.22 **Deep endometriosis of the fallopian tube**
Deep endometriosis involving muscular wall of fallopian tube

N80.221 **Deep endometriosis of right fallopian tube**

N80.222 **Deep endometriosis of left fallopian tube**

N80.223 **Deep endometriosis of bilateral fallopian tubes**

N80.229 **Deep endometriosis of unspecified fallopian tube**

N80.3 **Endometriosis of pelvic peritoneum**

N80.30 **Endometriosis of pelvic peritoneum, unspecified**
Endometriosis of the retroperitoneum NOS

N80.31 **Endometriosis of the anterior cul-de-sac**

N80.311 **Superficial endometriosis of the anterior cul-de-sac**

N80.312 **Deep endometriosis of the anterior cul-de-sac**

N80.319 **Endometriosis of the anterior cul-de-sac, unspecified depth**
Endometriosis of the anterior cul-de-sac NOS

- **N80.32 Endometriosis of the posterior cul-de-sac**
  - **N80.321 Superficial endometriosis of the posterior cul-de-sac**
  - **N80.322 Deep endometriosis of the posterior cul-de-sac**
  - **N80.329 Endometriosis of the posterior cul-de-sac, unspecified depth**
    Endometriosis of the posterior cul-de-sac NOS
- **N80.33 Superficial endometriosis of the pelvic sidewall**
  - **N80.331 Superficial endometriosis of the right pelvic sidewall**
  - **N80.332 Superficial endometriosis of the left pelvic sidewall**
  - **N80.333 Superficial endometriosis of bilateral pelvic sidewall**
  - **N80.339 Superficial endometriosis of pelvic sidewall, unspecified side**
- **N80.34 Deep endometriosis of the pelvic sidewall**
  - **N80.341 Deep endometriosis of the right pelvic sidewall**
  - **N80.342 Deep endometriosis of the left pelvic sidewall**
  - **N80.343 Deep endometriosis of the bilateral pelvic sidewall**
  - **N80.349 Deep endometriosis of the pelvic sidewall, unspecified side**
    Coding Clinic: 2022, Q4, P36
- **N80.35 Endometriosis of the pelvic sidewall, unspecified depth**
  - **N80.351 Endometriosis of the right pelvic sidewall, unspecified depth**
  - **N80.352 Endometriosis of the left pelvic sidewall, unspecified depth**
  - **N80.353 Endometriosis of bilateral pelvic sidewall, unspecified depth**
  - **N80.359 Endometriosis of pelvic sidewall, unspecified side, unspecified depth**
    Endometriosis of the pelvic sidewall NOS
- **N80.36 Superficial endometriosis of the pelvic brim**
  - **N80.361 Superficial endometriosis of the right pelvic brim**
  - **N80.362 Superficial endometriosis of the left pelvic brim**
  - **N80.363 Superficial endometriosis of bilateral pelvic brim**
  - **N80.369 Superficial endometriosis of the pelvic brim, unspecified side**
- **N80.37 Deep endometriosis of the pelvic brim**
  - **N80.371 Deep endometriosis of the right pelvic brim**
  - **N80.372 Deep endometriosis of the left pelvic brim**
  - **N80.373 Deep endometriosis of bilateral pelvic brim**
  - **N80.379 Deep endometriosis of the pelvic brim, unspecified side**
- **N80.38 Endometriosis of the pelvic brim, unspecified depth**
  - **N80.381 Endometriosis of the right pelvic brim, unspecified depth**
  - **N80.382 Endometriosis of the left pelvic brim, unspecified depth**
  - **N80.383 Endometriosis of bilateral pelvic brim, unspecified depth**
  - **N80.389 Endometriosis of the pelvic brim, unspecified side, unspecified depth**
    Endometriosis of the pelvic brim NOS
- **N80.39 Endometriosis of other pelvic peritoneum**
  - **N80.391 Superficial endometriosis of the pelvic peritoneum, other specified sites**
  - **N80.392 Deep endometriosis of the pelvic peritoneum, other specified sites**
  - **N80.399 Endometriosis of the pelvic peritoneum, other specified sites, unspecified depth**
- **N80.3A Superficial endometriosis of the uterosacral ligament(s)**
  - **N80.3A1 Superficial endometriosis of the right uterosacral ligament**
  - **N80.3A2 Superficial endometriosis of the left uterosacral ligament**
  - **N80.3A3 Superficial endometriosis of the bilateral uterosacral ligament(s)**
  - **N80.3A9 Superficial endometriosis of the uterosacral ligament(s), unspecified side**
- **N80.3B Deep endometriosis of the uterosacral ligament(s)**
  - **N80.3B1 Deep endometriosis of the right uterosacral ligament**
  - **N80.3B2 Deep endometriosis of the left uterosacral ligament**
  - **N80.3B3 Deep endometriosis of bilateral uterosacral ligament(s)**
  - **N80.3B9 Deep endometriosis of the uterosacral ligament(s), unspecified side**
- **N80.3C Endometriosis of the uterosacral ligament(s), unspecified depth**
  - **N80.3C1 Endometriosis of the right uterosacral ligament, unspecified depth**
  - **N80.3C2 Endometriosis of the left uterosacral ligament, unspecified depth**
  - **N80.3C3 Endometriosis of bilateral uterosacral ligament(s), unspecified depth**
  - **N80.3C9 Endometriosis of the uterosacral ligament(s), unspecified side, unspecified depth**
    Endometriosis of the uterosacral ligament(s) NOS
- **N80.4 Endometriosis of rectovaginal septum and vagina**
  - **N80.40 Endometriosis of rectovaginal septum, unspecified involvement of vagina**
    Endometriosis of the rectovaginal septum, NOS
  - **N80.41 Endometriosis of rectovaginal septum without involvement of vagina**
  - **N80.42 Endometriosis of rectovaginal septum with involvement of vagina**
- **N80.5 Endometriosis of intestine**
  - **N80.50 Endometriosis of intestine, unspecified**
  - **N80.51 Endometriosis of the rectum**
    - **N80.511 Superficial endometriosis of the rectum**
    - **N80.512 Deep endometriosis of the rectum**
      Deep endometriosis of the rectum, multifocal
    - **N80.519 Endometriosis of the rectum, unspecified depth**
      Endometriosis of the rectum NOS
  - **N80.52 Endometriosis of the sigmoid colon**
    - **N80.521 Superficial endometriosis of the sigmoid colon**
    - **N80.522 Deep endometriosis of the sigmoid colon**
    - **N80.529 Endometriosis of the sigmoid colon, unspecified depth**
      Endometriosis of the sigmoid colon NOS

CHAPTER 14 (N00-N99)

● N80.53 Endometriosis of the cecum
- N80.531 Superficial endometriosis of the cecum
- N80.532 Deep endometriosis of the cecum
- N80.539 Endometriosis of the cecum, unspecified depth
  - Endometriosis of the cecum NOS

● N80.54 Endometriosis of the appendix
- N80.541 Superficial endometriosis of the appendix
- N80.542 Deep endometriosis of the appendix
- N80.549 Endometriosis of the appendix, unspecified depth
  - Endometriosis of the appendix NOS

● N80.55 Endometriosis of other parts of the colon
  - Endometriosis of descending colon
  - Endometriosis of transverse colon
- N80.551 Superficial endometriosis of other parts of the colon
- N80.552 Deep endometriosis of other parts of the colon
- N80.559 Endometriosis of other parts of the colon, unspecified depth
  - Endometriosis of colon NOS

N80.6 Endometriosis in cutaneous scar

N80.8 Other endometriosis
  - Endometriosis of other sites

N80.9 Endometriosis, unspecified

● N80.A Endometriosis of bladder and ureters
- N80.A0 Endometriosis of bladder, unspecified depth
  - Endometriosis of bladder NOS
- N80.A1 Superficial endometriosis of bladder
- N80.A2 Deep endometriosis of bladder
- ● N80.A4 Superficial endometriosis of ureter
  - Extrinsic endometriosis of ureter
  - Code also, if applicable, obstructive and reflux uropathy (N13.-)
  - N80.A41 Superficial endometriosis of right ureter
  - N80.A42 Superficial endometriosis of left ureter
  - N80.A43 Superficial endometriosis of bilateral ureters
  - N80.A49 Superficial endometriosis of unspecified ureter
- ● N80.A5 Deep endometriosis of ureter
  - Intrinsic endometriosis of ureter
  - Code also, if applicable, obstructive and reflux uropathy (N13.-)
  - N80.A51 Deep endometriosis of right ureter
  - N80.A52 Deep endometriosis of left ureter
  - N80.A53 Deep endometriosis of bilateral ureters
  - N80.A59 Deep endometriosis of unspecified ureter
- ● N80.A6 Endometriosis of ureter, unspecified depth
  - Code also, if applicable, obstructive and reflux uropathy (N13.-)
  - N80.A61 Endometriosis of right ureter, unspecified depth
  - N80.A62 Endometriosis of left ureter, unspecified depth
  - N80.A63 Endometriosis of bilateral ureters, unspecified depth
  - N80.A69 Endometriosis of unspecified ureter, unspecified depth

● N80.B Endometriosis of cardiothoracic space
  - Endometriosis of thorax
  - Code also, if applicable:
    - catamenial hemothorax (J94.2)
    - catamenial pneumothorax (J93.12)
- N80.B1 Endometriosis of pleura
- N80.B2 Endometriosis of lung
- ● N80.B3 Endometriosis of diaphragm
  - N80.B31 Superficial endometriosis of diaphragm
  - N80.B32 Deep endometriosis of diaphragm
  - N80.B39 Endometriosis of diaphragm, unspecified depth
    - Endometriosis of the diaphragm NOS
- N80.B4 Endometriosis of the pericardial space
- N80.B5 Endometriosis of the mediastinal space
- N80.B6 Endometriosis of cardiothoracic space

N80.C Endometriosis of the abdomen
- N80.C0 Endometriosis of the abdomen, unspecified
  - Endometriosis of the abdomen NOS
- ● N80.C1 Endometriosis of the anterior abdominal wall
  - N80.C10 Endometriosis of the anterior abdominal wall, subcutaneous tissue
  - N80.C11 Endometriosis of the anterior abdominal wall, fascia and muscular layers
  - N80.C19 Endometriosis of the anterior abdominal wall, unspecified depth
    - Endometriosis of the anterior abdominal wall NOS
- N80.C2 Endometriosis of the umbilicus
- N80.C3 Endometriosis of the inguinal canal
- N80.C4 Endometriosis of extra-pelvic abdominal peritoneum
- N80.C9 Endometriosis of other site of abdomen

● N80.D Endometriosis of the pelvic nerves
  - Endometriosis of the nerves of the retroperitoneum
- N80.D0 Endometriosis of the pelvic nerves, unspecified
  - Endometriosis of nerve of the retroperitoneum, NOS
- N80.D1 Endometriosis of the sacral splanchnic nerves
  - Endometriosis of the pelvic splanchnic nerves
- N80.D2 Endometriosis of the sacral nerve roots
- N80.D3 Endometriosis of the obturator nerve
- N80.D4 Endometriosis of the sciatic nerve
- N80.D5 Endometriosis of the pudendal nerve
- N80.D6 Endometriosis of the femoral nerve
- N80.D9 Endometriosis of other pelvic nerve
  - Endometriosis of the other nerves of the retroperitoneum

● N81 Female genital prolapse

Excludes1 genital prolapse complicating pregnancy, labor or delivery (O34.5-)
prolapse and hernia of ovary and fallopian tube (N83.4-)
prolapse of vaginal vault after hysterectomy (N99.3)

N81.0 Urethrocele

Excludes1 urethrocele with cystocele (N81.1-)
urethrocele with prolapse of uterus (N81.2-N81.4)

Item 14–11 Endometriosis is a condition for which no clear cause has been identified. Endometrial tissue is expelled from the uterus into the abdominal cavity and can implant onto a variety of organs. Classification is based on the site of implant of the endometrial tissue.

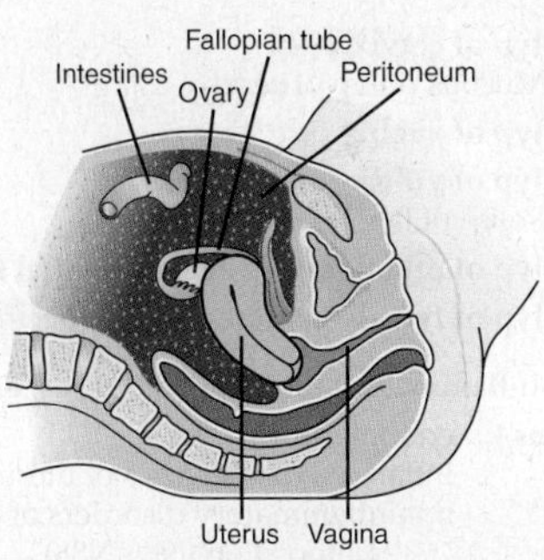

Figure 14-11 Sites of potential endometrial implants.

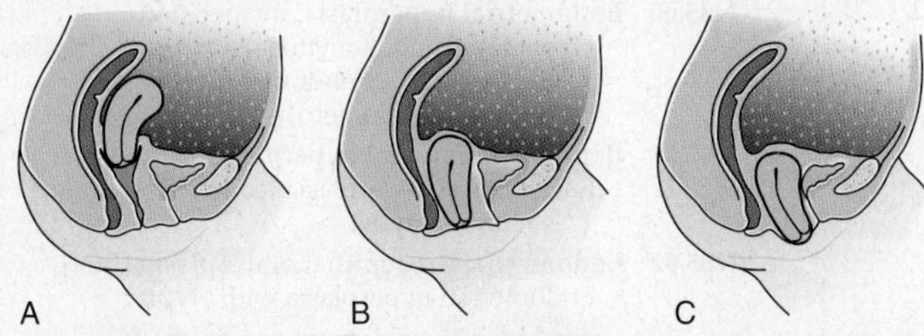

Figure 14-12 Three stages of uterine prolapse. **A.** Uterus is prolapsed. **B.** Vagina and uterus are prolapsed (incomplete uterovaginal prolapse). **C.** Vagina and uterus are completely prolapsed and are exposed through the external genitalia (complete uterovaginal prolapse).

● **N81.1 Cystocele**
Cystocele with urethrocele
Cystourethrocele
Excludes1 cystocele with prolapse of uterus (N81.2-N81.4)

N81.10 Cystocele, unspecified
Prolapse of (anterior) vaginal wall NOS

N81.11 Cystocele, midline

N81.12 Cystocele, lateral
Paravaginal cystocele

N81.2 Incomplete uterovaginal prolapse
First degree uterine prolapse
Prolapse of cervix NOS
Second degree uterine prolapse
Excludes1 cervical stump prolapse (N81.85)

N81.3 Complete uterovaginal prolapse
Procidentia (uteri) NOS
Third degree uterine prolapse

N81.4 Uterovaginal prolapse, unspecified
Prolapse of uterus NOS

N81.5 Vaginal enterocele
Excludes1 enterocele with prolapse of uterus (N81.2-N81.4)

N81.6 Rectocele
Prolapse of posterior vaginal wall
Use additional code for any associated fecal incontinence, if applicable (R15.-)
Excludes1 rectocele with prolapse of uterus (N81.2-N81.4)
Excludes2 perineocele (N81.81)
rectal prolapse (K62.3)

● **N81.8 Other female genital prolapse**

N81.81 Perineocele

N81.82 Incompetence or weakening of pubocervical tissue

N81.83 Incompetence or weakening of rectovaginal tissue

N81.84 Pelvic muscle wasting
Disuse atrophy of pelvic muscles and anal sphincter

N81.85 Cervical stump prolapse

N81.89 Other female genital prolapse
Deficient perineum
Old laceration of muscles of pelvic floor

N81.9 Female genital prolapse, unspecified

● **N82 Fistulae involving female genital tract** (Ex) PDX 1398
Excludes1 vesicointestinal fistulae (N32.1)

N82.0 Vesicovaginal fistula

N82.1 Other female urinary-genital tract fistulae
Cervicovesical fistula
Ureterovaginal fistula
Urethrovaginal fistula
Uteroureteric fistula
Uterovesical fistula
Coding Clinic: 2017, Q3, P4

N82.2 Fistula of vagina to small intestine

N82.3 Fistula of vagina to large intestine
Rectovaginal fistula

N82.4 Other female intestinal-genital tract fistulae
Intestinouterine fistula

N82.5 Female genital tract-skin fistulae
Uterus to abdominal wall fistula
Vaginoperineal fistula

N82.8 Other female genital tract fistulae

N82.9 Female genital tract fistula, unspecified

● **N83 Noninflammatory disorders of ovary, fallopian tube and broad ligament**
Excludes2 hydrosalpinx (N70.1-)

● **N83.0 Follicular cyst of ovary**
Cyst of graafian follicle
Hemorrhagic follicular cyst (of ovary)
Coding Clinic: 2016, Q4, P46

N83.00 Follicular cyst of ovary, unspecified side

N83.01 Follicular cyst of right ovary

N83.02 Follicular cyst of left ovary

● **N83.1 Corpus luteum cyst**
Hemorrhagic corpus luteum cyst
Coding Clinic: 2016, Q4, P46

N83.10 Corpus luteum cyst of ovary, unspecified side

N83.11 Corpus luteum cyst of right ovary

N83.12 Corpus luteum cyst of left ovary
Coding Clinic: 2022, Q1, P23

● **N83.2 Other and unspecified ovarian cysts**
Excludes1 developmental ovarian cyst (Q50.1)
neoplastic ovarian cyst (D27.-)
polycystic ovarian syndrome (E28.2)
Stein-Leventhal syndrome (E28.2)
Coding Clinic: 2016, Q4, P46

● **N83.20 Unspecified ovarian cysts**
Coding Clinic: 2022, Q1, P23

N83.201 Unspecified ovarian cyst, right side

N83.202 Unspecified ovarian cyst, left side
Coding Clinic: 2022, Q1, P23

N83.209 Unspecified ovarian cyst, unspecified side
Ovarian cyst, NOS

● **N83.29 Other ovarian cysts**
Retention cyst of ovary
Simple cyst of ovary

N83.291 Other ovarian cyst, right side

N83.292 Other ovarian cyst, left side

N83.299 Other ovarian cyst, unspecified side

● **N83.3 Acquired atrophy of ovary and fallopian tube**
Coding Clinic: 2016, Q4, P46

● **N83.31 Acquired atrophy of ovary**

N83.311 Acquired atrophy of right ovary

N83.312 Acquired atrophy of left ovary

N83.319 Acquired atrophy of ovary, unspecified side
Acquired atrophy of ovary, NOS

● N83.32 Acquired atrophy of fallopian tube
N83.321 Acquired atrophy of right fallopian tube
N83.322 Acquired atrophy of left fallopian tube
N83.329 Acquired atrophy of fallopian tube, unspecified side
Acquired atrophy of fallopian tube, NOS
● N83.33 Acquired atrophy of ovary and fallopian tube
N83.331 Acquired atrophy of right ovary and fallopian tube
N83.332 Acquired atrophy of left ovary and fallopian tube
N83.339 Acquired atrophy of ovary and fallopian tube, unspecified side
Acquired atrophy of ovary and fallopian tube, NOS
● N83.4 Prolapse and hernia of ovary and fallopian tube
Coding Clinic: 2016, Q4, P46
N83.40 Prolapse and hernia of ovary and fallopian tube, unspecified side
Prolapse and hernia of ovary and fallopian tube, NOS
N83.41 Prolapse and hernia of right ovary and fallopian tube
N83.42 Prolapse and hernia of left ovary and fallopian tube
● N83.5 Torsion of ovary, ovarian pedicle and fallopian tube (Ex) PDX 1399
Torsion of accessory tube
Coding Clinic: 2016, Q4, P46
● N83.51 Torsion of ovary and ovarian pedicle
N83.511 Torsion of right ovary and ovarian pedicle
N83.512 Torsion of left ovary and ovarian pedicle
N83.519 Torsion of ovary and ovarian pedicle, unspecified side
Torsion of ovary and ovarian pedicle, NOS
● N83.52 Torsion of fallopian tube
Torsion of hydatid of Morgagni
N83.521 Torsion of right fallopian tube
N83.522 Torsion of left fallopian tube
N83.529 Torsion of fallopian tube, unspecified side
Torsion of fallopian tube, NOS
N83.53 Torsion of ovary, ovarian pedicle and fallopian tube
N83.6 Hematosalpinx
Excludes1 hematosalpinx (with) (in):
hematocolpos (N89.7)
hematometra (N85.7)
tubal pregnancy (O00.1-)
N83.7 Hematoma of broad ligament
N83.8 Other noninflammatory disorders of ovary, fallopian tube and broad ligament
Broad ligament laceration syndrome [Allen-Masters]
N83.9 Noninflammatory disorder of ovary, fallopian tube and broad ligament, unspecified

● N84 Polyp of female genital tract
Excludes1 adenomatous polyp (D28.-)
placental polyp (O90.89)
N84.0 Polyp of corpus uteri
Polyp of endometrium
Polyp of uterus NOS
Excludes1 polypoid endometrial hyperplasia (N85.0-)
N84.1 Polyp of cervix uteri
Mucous polyp of cervix
N84.2 Polyp of vagina
N84.3 Polyp of vulva
Polyp of labia
N84.8 Polyp of other parts of female genital tract
N84.9 Polyp of female genital tract, unspecified

● N85 Other noninflammatory disorders of uterus, except cervix
Excludes1 endometriosis (N80.-)
inflammatory diseases of uterus (N71.-)
noninflammatory disorders of cervix, except malposition (N86-N88)
polyp of corpus uteri (N84.0)
uterine prolapse (N81.-)
● N85.0 Endometrial hyperplasia
N85.00 Endometrial hyperplasia, unspecified
Hyperplasia (adenomatous) (cystic) (glandular) of endometrium
Hyperplastic endometritis
N85.01 Benign endometrial hyperplasia
Endometrial hyperplasia (complex) (simple) without atypia
N85.02 Endometrial intraepithelial neoplasia [EIN]
Endometrial hyperplasia with atypia
Excludes1 malignant neoplasm of endometrium (with endometrial intraepithelial neoplasia [EIN]) (C54.1)
N85.2 Hypertrophy of uterus
Bulky or enlarged uterus
Excludes1 puerperal hypertrophy of uterus (O90.89)
N85.3 Subinvolution of uterus
Excludes1 puerperal subinvolution of uterus (O90.89)
N85.4 Malposition of uterus
Anteversion of uterus
Retroflexion of uterus
Retroversion of uterus
Excludes1 malposition of uterus complicating pregnancy, labor or delivery (O34.5-, O65.5)
N85.5 Inversion of uterus
Excludes1 current obstetric trauma (O71.2)
postpartum inversion of uterus (O71.2)
N85.6 Intrauterine synechiae
N85.7 Hematometra
Hematosalpinx with hematometra
Excludes1 hematometra with hematocolpos (N89.7)
N85.8 Other specified noninflammatory disorders of uterus
Atrophy of uterus, acquired
Fibrosis of uterus NOS
N85.9 Noninflammatory disorder of uterus, unspecified
Disorder of uterus NOS
N85.A Isthmocele
Isthmocele (non-pregnant state)
Code also any associated conditions such as:
abnormal uterine and vaginal bleeding, unspecified (N93.9)
female infertility of uterine origin (N97.2)
pelvic and perineal pain (R10.2)
Excludes1 maternal care for cesarean scar defect (isthmocele) (O34.22)
Coding Clinic: 2022, Q4, P37

N86 Erosion and ectropion of cervix uteri
Decubitus (trophic) ulcer of cervix
Eversion of cervix
Excludes1 erosion and ectropion of cervix with cervicitis (N72)

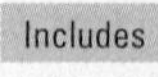
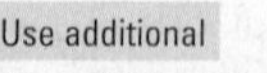
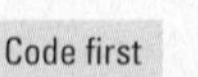
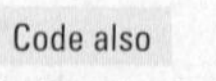

N87 Dysplasia of cervix uteri

Excludes1 abnormal results from cervical cytologic examination without histologic confirmation (R87.61-)
carcinoma in situ of cervix uteri (D06.-)
cervical intraepithelial neoplasia III [CIN III] (D06.-)
HGSIL of cervix (R87.613)
severe dysplasia of cervix uteri (D06.-)

N87.0 Mild cervical dysplasia
Cervical intraepithelial neoplasia I [CIN I]

N87.1 Moderate cervical dysplasia
Cervical intraepithelial neoplasia II [CIN II]

N87.9 Dysplasia of cervix uteri, unspecified
Anaplasia of cervix
Cervical atypism
Cervical dysplasia NOS

N88 Other noninflammatory disorders of cervix uteri

Excludes2 inflammatory disease of cervix (N72)
polyp of cervix (N84.1)

N88.0 Leukoplakia of cervix uteri

N88.1 Old laceration of cervix uteri
Adhesions of cervix

Excludes1 current obstetric trauma (O71.3)

N88.2 Stricture and stenosis of cervix uteri

Excludes1 stricture and stenosis of cervix uteri complicating labor (O65.5)

N88.3 Incompetence of cervix uteri
Investigation and management of (suspected) cervical incompetence in a nonpregnant woman

Excludes1 cervical incompetence complicating pregnancy (O34.3-)

N88.4 Hypertrophic elongation of cervix uteri

N88.8 Other specified noninflammatory disorders of cervix uteri

Excludes1 current obstetric trauma (O71.3)

N88.9 Noninflammatory disorder of cervix uteri, unspecified

N89 Other noninflammatory disorders of vagina

Excludes1 abnormal results from vaginal cytologic examination without histologic confirmation (R87.62-)
carcinoma in situ of vagina (D07.2)
HGSIL of vagina (R87.623)
inflammation of vagina (N76.-)
senile (atrophic) vaginitis (N95.2)
severe dysplasia of vagina (D07.2)
trichomonal leukorrhea (A59.00)
vaginal intraepithelial neoplasia [VAIN], grade III (D07.2)

N89.0 Mild vaginal dysplasia
Vaginal intraepithelial neoplasia [VAIN], grade I

N89.1 Moderate vaginal dysplasia
Vaginal intraepithelial neoplasia [VAIN], grade II

N89.3 Dysplasia of vagina, unspecified

N89.4 Leukoplakia of vagina

N89.5 Stricture and atresia of vagina
Vaginal adhesions
Vaginal stenosis

Excludes1 congenital atresia or stricture (Q52.4)
postprocedural adhesions of vagina (N99.2)

N89.6 Tight hymenal ring
Rigid hymen
Tight introitus

Excludes1 imperforate hymen (Q52.3)

N89.7 Hematocolpos
Hematocolpos with hematometra or hematosalpinx
Coding Clinic: 2016, Q4, P59

N89.8 Other specified noninflammatory disorders of vagina
Leukorrhea NOS
Old vaginal laceration
Pessary ulcer of vagina

Excludes1 current obstetric trauma (O70.-, O71.4, O71.7-O71.8)
old laceration involving muscles of pelvic floor (N81.8)

N89.9 Noninflammatory disorder of vagina, unspecified

N90 Other noninflammatory disorders of vulva and perineum

Excludes1 anogenital (venereal) warts (A63.0)
carcinoma in situ of vulva (D07.1)
condyloma acuminatum (A63.0)
current obstetric trauma (O70.-, O71.7-O71.8)
inflammation of vulva (N76.-)
severe dysplasia of vulva (D07.1)
vulvar intraepithelial neoplasm III [VIN III] (D07.1)

N90.0 Mild vulvar dysplasia
Vulvar intraepithelial neoplasia [VIN], grade I

N90.1 Moderate vulvar dysplasia
Vulvar intraepithelial neoplasia [VIN], grade II

N90.3 Dysplasia of vulva, unspecified

N90.4 Leukoplakia of vulva
Dystrophy of vulva
Kraurosis of vulva
Lichen sclerosus of external female genital organs

N90.5 Atrophy of vulva
Stenosis of vulva

N90.6 Hypertrophy of vulva
Coding Clinic: 2016, Q4, P46

N90.60 Unspecified hypertrophy of vulva
Unspecified hypertrophy of labia

N90.61 Childhood asymmetric labium majus enlargement
CALME

N90.69 Other specified hypertrophy of vulva
Other specified hypertrophy of labia

N90.7 Vulvar cyst

N90.8 Other specified noninflammatory disorders of vulva and perineum

N90.81 Female genital mutilation status
Female genital cutting status

N90.810 Female genital mutilation status, unspecified
Female genital cutting status, unspecified
Female genital mutilation status NOS

N90.811 Female genital mutilation Type I status
Clitorectomy status
Female genital cutting Type I status

N90.812 Female genital mutilation Type II status
Clitorectomy with excision of labia minora status
Female genital cutting Type II status

N90.813 Female genital mutilation Type III status
Female genital cutting Type III status
Infibulation status

N90.818 Other female genital mutilation status
Female genital cutting Type IV status
Female genital mutilation Type IV status
Other female genital cutting status

N90.89 Other specified noninflammatory disorders of vulva and perineum
Adhesions of vulva
Hypertrophy of clitoris

N90.9 Noninflammatory disorder of vulva and perineum, unspecified

● **N91 Absent, scanty and rare menstruation**
Excludes1 ovarian dysfunction (E28.-)
N91.0 Primary amenorrhea
N91.1 Secondary amenorrhea
N91.2 Amenorrhea, unspecified
N91.3 Primary oligomenorrhea
N91.4 Secondary oligomenorrhea
N91.5 Oligomenorrhea, unspecified
Hypomenorrhea NOS

● **N92 Excessive, frequent and irregular menstruation**
Excludes1 postmenopausal bleeding (N95.0)
precocious puberty (menstruation) (E30.1)
N92.0 Excessive and frequent menstruation with regular cycle
Heavy periods NOS
Polymenorrhea
Menorrhagia NOS
N92.1 Excessive and frequent menstruation with irregular cycle
Irregular intermenstrual bleeding
Irregular, shortened intervals between menstrual bleeding
Menometrorrhagia
Metrorrhagia
N92.2 Excessive menstruation at puberty P
Excessive bleeding associated with onset of menstrual periods
Pubertal menorrhagia
Puberty bleeding
N92.3 Ovulation bleeding
Regular intermenstrual bleeding
N92.4 Excessive bleeding in the premenopausal period
Climacteric menorrhagia or metrorrhagia
Menopausal menorrhagia or metrorrhagia
Perimenopausal bleeding
Perimenopausal menorrhagia or metrorrhagia
Preclimacteric menorrhagia or metrorrhagia
Premenopausal menorrhagia or metrorrhagia
N92.5 Other specified irregular menstruation
N92.6 Irregular menstruation, unspecified
Irregular bleeding NOS
Irregular periods NOS
Excludes1 irregular menstruation with:
lengthened intervals or scanty bleeding (N91.3-N91.5)
shortened intervals or excessive bleeding (N92.1)

● **N93 Other abnormal uterine and vaginal bleeding**
Excludes1 neonatal vaginal hemorrhage (P54.6)
precocious puberty (menstruation) (E30.1)
pseudomenses (P54.6)
N93.0 Postcoital and contact bleeding
N93.1 Pre-pubertal vaginal bleeding
Coding Clinic: 2016, Q4, P47
N93.8 Other specified abnormal uterine and vaginal bleeding
Dysfunctional or functional uterine or vaginal bleeding NOS
N93.9 Abnormal uterine and vaginal bleeding, unspecified

● **N94 Pain and other conditions associated with female genital organs and menstrual cycle**
N94.0 Mittelschmerz
Ovulation pain
● **N94.1 Dyspareunia**
Painful intercourse/coitus
Excludes1 psychogenic dyspareunia (F52.6)
Coding Clinic: 2016, Q4, P47
N94.10 Unspecified dyspareunia
N94.11 Superficial (introital) dyspareunia
N94.12 Deep dyspareunia
N94.19 Other specified dyspareunia
N94.2 Vaginismus
Vagina tightness
Excludes1 psychogenic vaginismus (F52.5)
N94.3 Premenstrual tension syndrome
AKA: PMS
Code also associated menstrual migraine (G43.82-, G43.83-)
Excludes1 Premenstrual dysphoric disorder (F32.81)
Coding Clinic: 2016, Q4, P14
N94.4 Primary dysmenorrhea
Lifelong painful menstruation
N94.5 Secondary dysmenorrhea
Later onset of painful menstruation
N94.6 Dysmenorrhea, unspecified
Excludes1 psychogenic dysmenorrhea (F45.8)
● **N94.8 Other specified conditions associated with female genital organs and menstrual cycle**
● **N94.81 Vulvodynia**
N94.810 Vulvar vestibulitis
N94.818 Other vulvodynia
N94.819 Vulvodynia, unspecified
Vulvodynia NOS
N94.89 Other specified conditions associated with female genital organs and menstrual cycle
N94.9 Unspecified condition associated with female genital organs and menstrual cycle

● **N95 Menopausal and other perimenopausal disorders**
Menopausal and other perimenopausal disorders due to naturally occurring (age-related) menopause and perimenopause
Excludes1 excessive bleeding in the premenopausal period (N92.4)
menopausal and perimenopausal disorders due to artificial or premature menopause (E89.4-, E28.31-)
premature menopause (E28.31-)
Excludes2 postmenopausal osteoporosis (M81.0-)
postmenopausal osteoporosis with current pathological fracture (M80.0-)
postmenopausal urethritis (N34.2)
N95.0 Postmenopausal bleeding
N95.1 Menopausal and female climacteric states
Symptoms such as flushing, sleeplessness, headache, lack of concentration, associated with natural (age-related) menopause
Use additional code for associated symptoms
Excludes1 asymptomatic menopausal state (Z78.0)
symptoms associated with artificial menopause (E89.41)
symptoms associated with premature menopause (E28.310)
N95.2 Postmenopausal atrophic vaginitis
Senile (atrophic) vaginitis
N95.8 Other specified menopausal and perimenopausal disorders
N95.9 Unspecified menopausal and perimenopausal disorder

N96 Recurrent pregnancy loss
Investigation or care in a nonpregnant woman with history of recurrent pregnancy loss
Excludes1 recurrent pregnancy loss with current pregnancy (O26.2-)

● **N97 Female infertility**
Includes inability to achieve a pregnancy
sterility, female NOS
Excludes2 female infertility associated with:
hypopituitarism (E23.0)
Stein-Leventhal syndrome (E28.2)
incompetence of cervix uteri (N88.3)
Coding Clinic: 2022, Q2, P16

N97.0 **Female infertility associated with anovulation**
Coding Clinic: 2022, Q2, P16

N97.1 **Female infertility of tubal origin**
Female infertility associated with congenital anomaly of tube
Female infertility due to tubal block
Female infertility due to tubal occlusion
Female infertility due to tubal stenosis

N97.2 **Female infertility of uterine origin**
Female infertility associated with congenital anomaly of uterus
Female infertility due to nonimplantation of ovum

N97.8 **Female infertility of other origin**

N97.9 **Female infertility, unspecified**

● **N98** **Complications associated with artificial fertilization** (Ex:) PDX 814

N98.0 **Infection associated with artificial insemination** (Ex:) PDX 1400

N98.1 **Hyperstimulation of ovaries**
Hyperstimulation of ovaries NOS
Hyperstimulation of ovaries associated with induced ovulation

N98.2 **Complications of attempted introduction of fertilized ovum following in vitro fertilization**

N98.3 **Complications of attempted introduction of embryo in embryo transfer**

N98.8 **Other complications associated with artificial fertilization**

N98.9 **Complication associated with artificial fertilization, unspecified**

INTRAOPERATIVE AND POSTPROCEDURAL COMPLICATIONS AND DISORDERS OF GENITOURINARY SYSTEM, NOT ELSEWHERE CLASSIFIED (N99)

● **N99** **Intraoperative and postprocedural complications and disorders of genitourinary system, not elsewhere classified**
Excludes2 irradiation cystitis (N30.4-)
postoophorectomy osteoporosis with current pathological fracture (M80.8-)
postoophorectomy osteoporosis without current pathological fracture (M81.8)

N99.0 **Postprocedural (acute) (chronic) kidney failure**
Use additional code to type of kidney disease

● **N99.1** **Postprocedural urethral stricture**
Postcatheterization urethral stricture

● **N99.11** **Postprocedural urethral stricture, male**

N99.110 **Postprocedural urethral stricture, male, meatal**

N99.111 **Postprocedural bulbous urethral stricture, male**

N99.112 **Postprocedural membranous urethral stricture, male**

N99.113 **Postprocedural anterior bulbous urethral stricture, male**
Coding Clinic: 2016, Q4, P48

N99.114 **Postprocedural urethral stricture, male, unspecified**

N99.115 **Postprocedural fossa navicularis urethral stricture**
Coding Clinic: 2016, Q4, P47

N99.116 **Postprocedural urethral stricture, male, overlapping sites**

N99.12 **Postprocedural urethral stricture, female**

N99.2 **Postprocedural adhesions of vagina**

N99.3 **Prolapse of vaginal vault after hysterectomy**

N99.4 **Postprocedural pelvic peritoneal adhesions**
Excludes2 pelvic peritoneal adhesions NOS (N73.6)
postinfective pelvic peritoneal adhesions (N73.6)

● **N99.5** **Complications of stoma of urinary tract**
Excludes2 mechanical complication of urinary catheter (T83.0-)

● **N99.51** **Complication of cystostomy**

N99.510 **Cystostomy hemorrhage** (Ex:) PDX 1401

N99.511 **Cystostomy infection** (Ex:) PDX 1402

N99.512 **Cystostomy malfunction** (Ex:) PDX 1403

N99.518 **Other cystostomy complication** (Ex:) PDX 1401

● **N99.52** **Complication of incontinent external stoma of urinary tract**

N99.520 **Hemorrhage of incontinent external stoma of urinary tract**

N99.521 **Infection of incontinent external stoma of urinary tract**
Coding Clinic: 2016, Q4, P48

N99.522 **Malfunction of incontinent external stoma of urinary tract**

N99.523 **Herniation of incontinent stoma of urinary tract**
Coding Clinic: 2016, Q4, P48

N99.524 **Stenosis of incontinent stoma of urinary tract**
Coding Clinic: 2016, Q4, P48

N99.528 **Other complication of incontinent external stoma of urinary tract**

● **N99.53** **Complication of continent stoma of urinary tract**

N99.530 **Hemorrhage of continent stoma of urinary tract**

N99.531 **Infection of continent stoma of urinary tract**

N99.532 **Malfunction of continent stoma of urinary tract**

N99.533 **Herniation of continent stoma of urinary tract**
Coding Clinic: 2016, Q4, P48

N99.534 **Stenosis of continent stoma of urinary tract**
Coding Clinic: 2016, Q4, P48

N99.538 **Other complication of continent stoma of urinary tract**

● **N99.6** **Intraoperative hemorrhage and hematoma of a genitourinary system organ or structure complicating a procedure** (Ex:) PDX 1404
Excludes1 intraoperative hemorrhage and hematoma of a genitourinary system organ or structure due to accidental puncture or laceration during a procedure (N99.7-)

N99.61 **Intraoperative hemorrhage and hematoma of a genitourinary system organ or structure complicating a genitourinary system procedure**

N99.62 **Intraoperative hemorrhage and hematoma of a genitourinary system organ or structure complicating other procedure**

● **N99.7** **Accidental puncture and laceration of a genitourinary system organ or structure during a procedure** (Ex:) PDX 569

N99.71 **Accidental puncture and laceration of a genitourinary system organ or structure during a genitourinary system procedure**

N99.72 **Accidental puncture and laceration of a genitourinary system organ or structure during other procedure**

● N99.8 Other intraoperative and postprocedural complications and disorders of genitourinary system (Ex) PDX 1404
Coding Clinic: 2016, Q4, P10

N99.81 Other intraoperative complications of genitourinary system

● N99.82 Postprocedural hemorrhage of a genitourinary system organ or structure following a procedure

N99.820 Postprocedural hemorrhage of a genitourinary system organ or structure following a genitourinary system procedure

N99.821 Postprocedural hemorrhage of a genitourinary system organ or structure following other procedure

N99.83 Residual ovary syndrome

● N99.84 Postprocedural hematoma and seroma of a genitourinary system organ or structure following a procedure

N99.840 Postprocedural hematoma of a genitourinary system organ or structure following a genitourinary system procedure

N99.841 Postprocedural hematoma of a genitourinary system organ or structure following other procedure

N99.842 Postprocedural seroma of a genitourinary system organ or structure following a genitourinary system procedure

N99.843 Postprocedural seroma of a genitourinary system organ or structure following other procedure

N99.85 Post endometrial ablation syndrome
Coding Clinic: 2019, Q4, P12

N99.89 Other postprocedural complications and disorders of genitourinary system

CHAPTER 14 (N00-N99)

CHAPTER 15

PREGNANCY, CHILDBIRTH, AND THE PUERPERIUM (O00-O9A)

OGCR Chapter-Specific Coding Guidelines

15. **Chapter 15: Pregnancy, Childbirth, and the Puerperium (O00-O9A)**

a. **General Rules for Obstetric Cases**

1) **Codes from Chapter 15 and sequencing priority**

Obstetric cases require codes from Chapter 15, codes in the range O00-O9A, Pregnancy, Childbirth, and the Puerperium. Chapter 15 codes have sequencing priority over codes from other chapters. Additional codes from other chapters may be used in conjunction with Chapter 15 codes to further specify conditions. Should the provider document that the pregnancy is incidental to the encounter, then code Z33.1, Pregnant state, incidental, should be used in place of any Chapter 15 codes. It is the provider's responsibility to state that the condition being treated is not affecting the pregnancy.

2) **Chapter 15 codes used only on the maternal record**

Chapter 15 codes are to be used only on the maternal record, never on the record of the newborn.

3) **Final character for trimester**

The majority of codes in Chapter 15 have a final character indicating the trimester of pregnancy. The timeframes for the trimesters are indicated at the beginning of the chapter. If trimester is not a component of a code it is because the condition always occurs in a specific trimester, or the concept of trimester of pregnancy is not applicable. Certain codes have characters for only certain trimesters because the condition does not occur in all trimesters, but it may occur in more than just one.

Assignment of the final character for trimester should be based on the provider's documentation of the trimester (or number of weeks) for the current admission/encounter. This applies to the assignment of trimester for pre-existing conditions as well as those that develop during or are due to the pregnancy. The provider's documentation of the number of weeks may be used to assign the appropriate code identifying the trimester.

Whenever delivery occurs during the current admission, and there is an "in childbirth" option for the obstetric complication being coded, the "in childbirth" code should be assigned.

4) **Selection of trimester for inpatient admissions that encompass more than one trimester**

In instances when a patient is admitted to a hospital for complications of pregnancy during one trimester and remains in the hospital into a subsequent trimester, the trimester character for the antepartum complication code should be assigned on the basis of the trimester when the complication developed, not the trimester of the discharge. If the condition developed prior to the current admission/encounter or represents a pre-existing condition, the trimester character for the trimester at the time of the admission/encounter should be assigned.

5) **Unspecified trimester**

Each category that includes codes for trimester has a code for "unspecified trimester." The "unspecified trimester" code should rarely be used, such as when the documentation in the record is insufficient to determine the trimester and it is not possible to obtain clarification.

6) **7th character for Fetus Identification**

Where applicable, a 7th character is to be assigned for certain categories (O31, O32, O33.3 - O33.6, O35, O36, O40, O41, O60.1, O60.2, O64, and O69) to identify the fetus for which the complication code applies.

Assign 7th character "0":

- For single gestations
- When the documentation in the record is insufficient to determine the fetus affected and it is not possible to obtain clarification.
- When it is not possible to clinically determine which fetus is affected.

b. **Selection of OB Principal or First-listed Diagnosis**

1) **Routine outpatient prenatal visits**

For routine outpatient prenatal visits when no complications are present, a code from category Z34, Encounter for supervision of normal pregnancy, should be used as the first-listed diagnosis. These codes should not be used in conjunction with Chapter 15 codes.

2) **Supervision of High-Risk Pregnancy**

Codes from category O09, Supervision of high-risk pregnancy, are intended for use only during the prenatal period. For complications during the labor or delivery episode as a result of a high-risk pregnancy, assign the applicable complication codes from Chapter 15. If there are no complications during the labor or delivery episode, assign code O80, Encounter for full-term uncomplicated delivery.

For routine prenatal outpatient visits for patients with high-risk pregnancies, a code from category O09, Supervision of high-risk pregnancy, should be used as the first-listed diagnosis. Secondary Chapter 15 codes may be used in conjunction with these codes if appropriate.

3) **Episodes when no delivery occurs**

In episodes when no delivery occurs, the principal diagnosis should correspond to the principal complication of the pregnancy which necessitated the encounter. Should more than one complication exist, all of which are treated or monitored, any of the complications codes may be sequenced first.

4) **When a delivery occurs**

When an obstetric patient is admitted and delivers during that admission, the condition that prompted the admission should be sequenced as the principal diagnosis. If multiple conditions prompted the admission, sequence the one most related to the delivery as the principal diagnosis. A code for any complication of the delivery should be assigned as an additional diagnosis. In cases of cesarean delivery, if the patient was admitted with a condition that resulted in the performance of a cesarean procedure, that condition should be selected as the principal diagnosis. If the reason for the admission was unrelated to the condition resulting in the cesarean delivery, the condition related to the reason for the admission should be selected as the principal diagnosis.

5) **Outcome of delivery**

A code from category Z37, Outcome of delivery, should be included on every maternal record when a delivery has occurred. These codes are not to be used on subsequent records or on the newborn record.

c. **Pre-existing conditions versus conditions due to the pregnancy**

Certain categories in Chapter 15 distinguish between conditions of the mother that existed prior to pregnancy (pre-existing) and those that are a direct result of pregnancy. When assigning codes from Chapter 15, it is important to assess if a condition was pre-existing prior to pregnancy or developed during or due to the pregnancy in order to assign the correct code.

Categories that do not distinguish between pre-existing and pregnancy-related conditions may be used for either. It is acceptable to use codes specifically for the puerperium with codes complicating pregnancy and childbirth if a condition arises postpartum during the delivery encounter.

d. **Pre-existing hypertension in pregnancy**

Category O10, Pre-existing hypertension complicating pregnancy, childbirth and the puerperium, includes codes for hypertensive heart and hypertensive chronic kidney disease. When assigning one of the O10 codes that includes hypertensive heart disease or hypertensive chronic kidney disease, it is necessary to add a secondary code from the appropriate hypertension category to specify the type of heart failure or chronic kidney disease.

See Section I.C.9. Hypertension.

e. **Fetal Conditions Affecting the Management of the Mother**

1) **Codes from categories O35 and O36**

Codes from categories O35, Maternal care for known or suspected fetal abnormality and damage, and O36, Maternal care for other fetal problems, are assigned only when the fetal condition is actually responsible for modifying the management of the mother, i.e., by requiring diagnostic studies, additional observation, special care, or termination of pregnancy. The fact that the fetal condition exists does not justify assigning a code from this series to the mother's record.

2) **In utero surgery**

In cases when surgery is performed on the fetus, a diagnosis code from category O35, Maternal care for known or suspected fetal abnormality and damage, should be assigned identifying the fetal condition. Assign the appropriate procedure code for the procedure performed.

No code from Chapter 16, the perinatal codes, should be used on the mother's record to identify fetal conditions. Surgery performed in utero on a fetus is still to be coded as an obstetric encounter.

f. **HIV Infection in Pregnancy, Childbirth, and the Puerperium**

During pregnancy, childbirth or the puerperium, a patient admitted because of an HIV-related illness should receive a principal diagnosis from subcategory O98.7-, Human immunodeficiency [HIV] disease complicating pregnancy, childbirth and the puerperium, followed by the code(s) for the HIV-related illness(es).

Patients with asymptomatic HIV infection status admitted during pregnancy, childbirth, or the puerperium should receive codes of O98.7- and Z21, Asymptomatic human immunodeficiency virus [HIV] infection status.

g. **Diabetes mellitus in pregnancy**

Diabetes mellitus is a significant complicating factor in pregnancy. Pregnant women who are diabetic should be assigned a code from category O24, Diabetes mellitus in pregnancy, childbirth, and the puerperium, first, followed by the appropriate diabetes code(s) (E08-E13) from Chapter 4.

h. Long-term use of insulin and oral hypoglycemics
See Section I.C.4.a.3 for information on the long-term use of insulin and oral hypoglycemic.

i. Gestational (pregnancy induced) diabetes
Gestational (pregnancy induced) diabetes can occur during the second and third trimester of pregnancy in women who were not diabetic prior to pregnancy. Gestational diabetes can cause complications in the pregnancy similar to those of pre-existing diabetes mellitus. It also puts the woman at greater risk of developing diabetes after the pregnancy. Codes for gestational diabetes are in subcategory O24.4, Gestational diabetes mellitus. No other code from category O24, Diabetes mellitus in pregnancy, childbirth, and the puerperium, should be used with a code from O24.4.

The codes under subcategory O24.4 include diet controlled, insulin controlled, and controlled by oral hypoglycemic drugs. If a patient with gestational diabetes is treated with both diet and insulin, only the code for insulin-controlled is required. If a patient with gestational diabetes is treated with both diet and oral hypoglycemic medications, only the code for "controlled by oral hypoglycemic drugs" is required. Code Z79.4, Long-term (current) use of insulin or code Z79.84, Long-term (current) use of oral hypoglycemic drugs, should not be assigned with codes from subcategory O24.4.

An abnormal glucose tolerance in pregnancy is assigned a code from subcategory O99.81, Abnormal glucose complicating pregnancy, childbirth, and the puerperium.

j. Sepsis and septic shock complicating abortion, pregnancy, childbirth and the puerperium
When assigning a Chapter 15 code for sepsis complicating abortion, pregnancy, childbirth, and the puerperium, a code for the specific type of infection should be assigned as an additional diagnosis. If severe sepsis is present, a code from subcategory R65.2, Severe sepsis, and code(s) for associated organ dysfunction(s) should also be assigned as additional diagnoses.

k. Puerperal sepsis
Code O85, Puerperal sepsis, should be assigned with a secondary code to identify the causal organism (e.g., for a bacterial infection, assign a code from category B95-B96, Bacterial infections in conditions classified elsewhere). A code from category A40, Streptococcal sepsis, or A41, Other sepsis, should not be used for puerperal sepsis. If applicable, use additional codes to identify severe sepsis (R65.2-) and any associated acute organ dysfunction.

l. Alcohol, tobacco and drug use during pregnancy, childbirth and the puerperium

1) Alcohol use during pregnancy, childbirth and the puerperium
Codes under subcategory O99.31, Alcohol use complicating pregnancy, childbirth, and the puerperium, should be assigned for any pregnancy case when a mother uses alcohol during the pregnancy or postpartum. A secondary code from category F10, Alcohol-related disorders, should also be assigned to identify manifestations of the alcohol use.

2) Tobacco use during pregnancy, childbirth, and the puerperium
Codes under subcategory O99.33, Smoking (tobacco) complicating pregnancy, childbirth, and the puerperium, should be assigned for any pregnancy case when a mother uses any type of tobacco product during the pregnancy or postpartum. A secondary code from category F17, Nicotine dependence, should also be assigned to identify the type of nicotine dependence.

3) Drug use during pregnancy, childbirth and the puerperium
Codes under subcategory O99.32, Drug use complicating pregnancy, childbirth, and the puerperium, should be assigned for any pregnancy case when a mother uses drugs during the pregnancy or postpartum. This can involve illegal drugs, or inappropriate use or abuse of prescription drugs. Secondary code(s) from categories F11-F16 and F18F19 should also be assigned to identify manifestations of the drug use.

m. Poisoning, toxic effects, adverse effects and underdosing in a pregnant patient
A code from subcategory O9A.2, Injury, poisoning and certain other consequences of external causes complicating pregnancy, childbirth, and the puerperium, should be sequenced first, followed by the appropriate injury, poisoning, toxic effect, adverse effect or underdosing code, and then the additional code(s) that specifies the condition caused by the poisoning, toxic effect, adverse effect or underdosing.

See Section I.C.19. Adverse effects, poisoning, underdosing and toxic effects.

n. Normal Delivery, Code O80

1) Encounter for full-term uncomplicated delivery
Code O80 should be assigned when a woman is admitted for a full-term normal delivery and delivers a single, healthy infant without any complications antepartum, during the delivery, or postpartum during the delivery episode. Code O80 is always a principal diagnosis. It is not to be used if any other code from Chapter 15 is needed to describe a current complication of the antenatal, delivery, or perinatal period. Additional codes from other chapters may be used with code O80 if they are not related to or are in any way complicating the pregnancy.

2) Uncomplicated delivery with resolved antepartum complication
Code O80 may be used if the patient had a complication at some point during the pregnancy, but the complication is not present at the time of the admission for delivery.

3) Outcome of delivery for O80
Z37.0, Single live birth, is the only outcome of delivery code appropriate for use with O80.

o. The Peripartum and Postpartum Periods

1) Peripartum and Postpartum periods
The postpartum period begins immediately after delivery and continues for six weeks following delivery. The peripartum period is defined as the last month of pregnancy to five months postpartum.

2) Peripartum and postpartum complication
A postpartum complication is any complication occurring within the six-week period.

3) Pregnancy-related complications after 6 week period
Chapter 15 codes may also be used to describe pregnancy-related complications after the peripartum or postpartum period if the provider documents that a condition is pregnancy related.

4) Admission for routine postpartum care following delivery outside hospital
When the mother delivers outside the hospital prior to admission and is admitted for routine postpartum care and no complications are noted, code Z39.0, Encounter for care and examination of mother immediately after delivery, should be assigned as the principal diagnosis.

5) Pregnancy associated cardiomyopathy
Pregnancy associated cardiomyopathy, code O90.3, is unique in that it may be diagnosed in the third trimester of pregnancy but may continue to progress months after delivery. For this reason, it is referred to as peripartum cardiomyopathy. Code O90.3 is only for use when the cardiomyopathy develops as a result of pregnancy in a woman who did not have pre-existing heart disease.

p. Code O94, Sequelae of complication of pregnancy, childbirth, and the puerperium

1) Code O94
Code O94, Sequelae of complication of pregnancy, childbirth, and the puerperium, is for use in those cases when an initial complication of a pregnancy develops a sequelae requiring care or treatment at a future date.

2) After the initial postpartum period
This code may be used at any time after the initial postpartum period.

3) Sequencing of Code O94
This code, like all sequela codes, is to be sequenced following the code describing the sequelae of the complication.

q. Termination of Pregnancy and Spontaneous abortions

1) Abortion with Liveborn Fetus
When an attempted termination of pregnancy results in a liveborn fetus assign code Z33.2, Encounter for elective termination of pregnancy and a code from category Z37, Outcome of Delivery.

2) Retained Products of Conception following an abortion
Subsequent encounters for retained products of conception following a spontaneous abortion or elective termination of pregnancy, without complications are assigned O03.4, Incomplete spontaneous, abortion without complication, or codes O07.4, Failed attempted termination of pregnancy without complication. This advice is appropriate even when the patient was discharged previously with a discharge diagnosis of complete abortion. If the patient has a specific complication associated with the spontaneous abortion or elective termination of pregnancy in addition to retained products of conception, assign the appropriate complication in category O03 or O07 instead of code O03.4 or O07.4

3) Complications leading to abortion
Codes from Chapter 15 may be used as additional codes to identify any documented complications of the pregnancy in conjunction with codes in categories in O04, O07 and O08.

r. Abuse in a pregnant patient
For suspected or confirmed cases of abuse of a pregnant patient, a code(s) from subcategories O9A.3, Physical abuse complicating pregnancy, childbirth, and the puerperium, O9A.4, Sexual abuse complicating pregnancy, childbirth, and the puerperium, and O9A.5, Psychological abuse complicating pregnancy, childbirth, and the puerperium, should be sequenced first, followed by the appropriate codes (if applicable) to identify any associated current injury due to physical abuse, sexual abuse, and the perpetrator of abuse.

See Section I.C.19. Adult and child abuse, neglect and other maltreatment.

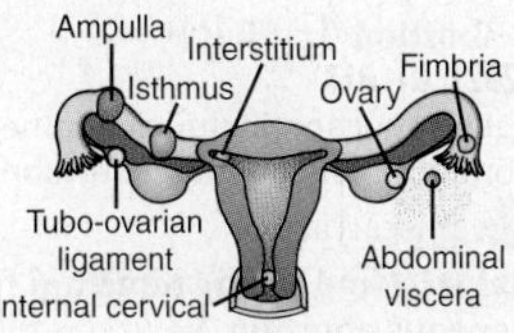

Figure 15-1 Implantation sites of ectopic pregnancy.

Item 15–1 **Ectopic** pregnancy most often occurs in the fallopian tube. Pregnancy outside the uterus may end in a lifethreatening rupture.

★**(See Plate 4 of the Anatomy Illustrations.)**

CHAPTER 15

PREGNANCY, CHILDBIRTH, AND THE PUERPERIUM (O00-O9A)

Note: CODES FROM THIS CHAPTER ARE FOR USE ONLY ON MATERNAL RECORDS, NEVER ON NEWBORN RECORDS

Codes from this chapter are for use for conditions related to or aggravated by the pregnancy, childbirth, or by the puerperium (maternal causes or obstetric causes)

Trimesters are counted from the first day of the last menstrual period. They are defined as follows:

1st trimester - less than 14 weeks 0 days

2nd trimester - 14 weeks 0 days to less than 28 weeks 0 days

3rd trimester - 28 weeks 0 days until delivery

Use additional code , if applicable, from category Z3A, Weeks of gestation, to identify the specific week of the pregnancy, if known.

Excludes1 supervision of normal pregnancy (Z34.-)

Excludes2 mental and behavioral disorders associated with the puerperium (F53.-)
obstetrical tetanus (A34)
postpartum necrosis of pituitary gland (E23.0)
puerperal osteomalacia (M83.0)

This chapter contains the following blocks:

O00-O08	Pregnancy with abortive outcome
O09	Supervision of high risk pregnancy
O10-O16	Edema, proteinuria and hypertensive disorders in pregnancy, childbirth and the puerperium
O20-O29	Other maternal disorders predominantly related to pregnancy
O30-O48	Maternal care related to the fetus and amniotic cavity and possible delivery problems
O60-O77	Complications of labor and delivery
O80, O82	Encounter for delivery
O85-O92	Complications predominantly related to the puerperium
O94-O9A	Other obstetric conditions, not elsewhere classified

PREGNANCY WITH ABORTIVE OUTCOME (O00-O08)

Excludes1 continuing pregnancy in multiple gestation after abortion of one fetus or more (O31.1-, O31.3-)

Coding Clinic: 2016, Q4, P130

● **O00 Ectopic pregnancy** (Ex) PDX 1405

Includes ruptured ectopic pregnancy

Use additional code from category O08 to identify any associated complication

● **O00.0 Abdominal pregnancy**

Excludes1 maternal care for viable fetus in abdominal pregnancy (O36.7-)

Coding Clinic: 2016, Q4, P49

O00.00 Abdominal pregnancy **without intrauterine pregnancy** M
Abdominal pregnancy NOS

O00.01 Abdominal pregnancy **with intrauterine pregnancy** M

● **O00.1 Tubal pregnancy**
Fallopian pregnancy
Rupture of (fallopian) tube due to pregnancy
Tubal abortion
Coding Clinic: 2016, Q4, P49

● **O00.10** Tubal pregnancy **without intrauterine pregnancy**
Tubal pregnancy NOS

O00.101 **Right** tubal pregnancy without intrauterine pregnancy M

O00.102 **Left** tubal pregnancy without intrauterine pregnancy M

O00.109 **Unspecified** tubal pregnancy without intrauterine pregnancy M

● **O00.11** Tubal pregnancy **with intrauterine pregnancy**

O00.111 **Right** tubal pregnancy with intrauterine pregnancy M

O00.112 **Left** tubal pregnancy with intrauterine pregnancy M

O00.119 **Unspecified** tubal pregnancy with intrauterine pregnancy M

● **O00.2 Ovarian pregnancy**
Coding Clinic: 2016, Q4, P49

● **O00.20** Ovarian pregnancy **without intrauterine pregnancy**
Ovarian pregnancy NOS

O00.201 **Right** ovarian pregnancy without intrauterine pregnancy M

O00.202 **Left** ovarian pregnancy without intrauterine pregnancy M

O00.209 **Unspecified** ovarian pregnancy without intrauterine pregnancy M

● **O00.21** Ovarian pregnancy **with intrauterine pregnancy**

O00.211 **Right** ovarian pregnancy with intrauterine pregnancy M

O00.212 **Left** ovarian pregnancy with intrauterine pregnancy M

O00.219 **Unspecified** ovarian pregnancy with intrauterine pregnancy M

● **O00.8 Other ectopic pregnancy**
Cervical pregnancy
Cornual pregnancy
Intraligamentous pregnancy
Mural pregnancy
Coding Clinic: 2016, Q4, P49

O00.80 Other ectopic pregnancy **without intrauterine pregnancy** M
Other ectopic pregnancy NOS

O00.81 Other ectopic pregnancy **with intrauterine pregnancy** M

● O00.9 Ectopic pregnancy, unspecified
Coding Clinic: 2016, Q4, P49

O00.90 Unspecified ectopic pregnancy without intrauterine pregnancy M
Ectopic pregnancy NOS

O00.91 Unspecified ectopic pregnancy with intrauterine pregnancy M

● O01 Hydatidiform mole
Use additional code from category O08 to identify any associated complication
Excludes1 chorioadenoma (destruens) (D39.2)
malignant hydatidiform mole (D39.2)

O01.0 Classical hydatidiform mole M
Complete hydatidiform mole

O01.1 Incomplete and partial hydatidiform mole M

O01.9 Hydatidiform mole, unspecified M
Trophoblastic disease NOS
Vesicular mole NOS

● O02 Other abnormal products of conception
Use additional code from category O08 to identify any associated complication
Excludes1 papyraceous fetus (O31.0-)

O02.0 Blighted ovum and nonhydatidiform mole M
Carneous mole
Fleshy mole
Intrauterine mole NOS
Molar pregnancy NEC
Pathological ovum

O02.1 Missed abortion M
Early fetal death, before completion of 20 weeks of gestation, with retention of dead fetus
Excludes1 failed induced abortion (O07.-)
fetal death (intrauterine) (late) (O36.4)
missed abortion with blighted ovum (O02.0)
missed abortion with hydatidiform mole (O01.-)
missed abortion with nonhydatidiform (O02.0)
missed abortion with other abnormal products of conception (O02.8-)
missed delivery (O36.4)
stillbirth (P95)
Coding Clinic: 2022, Q2, P3-4; 2019, Q3, P12

● O02.8 Other specified abnormal products of conception
Excludes1 abnormal products of conception with blighted ovum (O02.0)
abnormal products of conception with hydatidiform mole (O01.-)
abnormal products of conception with nonhydatidiform mole (O02.0)

O02.81 Inappropriate change in quantitative human chorionic gonadotropin (hCG) in early pregnancy M
Biochemical pregnancy
Chemical pregnancy
Inappropriate level of quantitative human chorionic gonadotropin (hCG) for gestational age in early pregnancy

O02.89 Other abnormal products of conception M

O02.9 Abnormal product of conception, unspecified M

Item 15–2 A **hydatidiform** mole is an overproduction of placental tissue. The tumor secretes a hormone, chorionic gonadotropic hormone (CGH), that indicates a positive pregnancy test. There is no viable fetus. More than 80% of hydatidiform moles are noncancerous.

● O03 Spontaneous abortion Ex: PDX 1406
Coding Clinic: 2023, Q1, P17
Note: Incomplete abortion includes retained products of conception following spontaneous abortion.
Includes miscarriage

O03.0 Genital tract and pelvic infection following incomplete spontaneous abortion M
Endometritis following incomplete spontaneous abortion
Oophoritis following incomplete spontaneous abortion
Parametritis following incomplete spontaneous abortion
Pelvic peritonitis following incomplete spontaneous abortion
Salpingitis following incomplete spontaneous abortion
Salpingo-oophoritis following incomplete spontaneous abortion
Excludes1 sepsis following incomplete spontaneous abortion (O03.37)
urinary tract infection following incomplete spontaneous abortion (O03.38)

O03.1 Delayed or excessive hemorrhage following incomplete spontaneous abortion M
Afibrinogenemia following incomplete spontaneous abortion
Defibrination syndrome following incomplete spontaneous abortion
Hemolysis following incomplete spontaneous abortion
Intravascular coagulation following incomplete spontaneous abortion

O03.2 Embolism following incomplete spontaneous abortion M
Air embolism following incomplete spontaneous abortion
Amniotic fluid embolism following incomplete spontaneous abortion
Blood-clot embolism following incomplete spontaneous abortion
Embolism NOS following incomplete spontaneous abortion
Fat embolism following incomplete spontaneous abortion
Pulmonary embolism following incomplete spontaneous abortion
Pyemic embolism following incomplete spontaneous abortion
Septic or septicopyemic embolism following incomplete spontaneous abortion
Soap embolism following incomplete spontaneous abortion

● O03.3 Other and unspecified complications following incomplete spontaneous abortion

O03.30 Unspecified complication following incomplete spontaneous abortion M

O03.31 Shock following incomplete spontaneous abortion M
Circulatory collapse following incomplete spontaneous abortion
Shock (postprocedural) following incomplete spontaneous abortion
Excludes1 shock due to infection following incomplete spontaneous abortion (O03.37)

O03.32 Renal failure following incomplete spontaneous abortion M
Kidney failure (acute) following incomplete spontaneous abortion
Oliguria following incomplete spontaneous abortion
Renal shutdown following incomplete spontaneous abortion
Renal tubular necrosis following incomplete spontaneous abortion
Uremia following incomplete spontaneous abortion

O03.33 Metabolic disorder following incomplete spontaneous abortion M

O03.34 Damage to pelvic organs following incomplete spontaneous abortion M

Laceration, perforation, tear or chemical damage of bladder following incomplete spontaneous abortion

Laceration, perforation, tear or chemical damage of bowel following incomplete spontaneous abortion

Laceration, perforation, tear or chemical damage of broad ligament following incomplete spontaneous abortion

Laceration, perforation, tear or chemical damage of cervix following incomplete spontaneous abortion

Laceration, perforation, tear or chemical damage of periurethral tissue following incomplete spontaneous abortion

Laceration, perforation, tear or chemical damage of uterus following incomplete spontaneous abortion

Laceration, perforation, tear or chemical damage of vagina following incomplete spontaneous abortion

O03.35 Other venous complications following incomplete spontaneous abortion M

O03.36 Cardiac arrest following incomplete spontaneous abortion M

O03.37 Sepsis following incomplete spontaneous abortion M

Use additional code to identify infectious agent (B95-B97)

Use additional code to identify severe sepsis, if applicable (R65.2-)

Excludes1 septic or septicopyemic embolism following incomplete spontaneous abortion (O03.2)

O03.38 Urinary tract infection following incomplete spontaneous abortion M

Cystitis following incomplete spontaneous abortion

O03.39 Incomplete spontaneous abortion with other complications M

O03.4 Incomplete spontaneous abortion without complication M

Coding Clinic: 2023, Q1, P17

O03.5 Genital tract and pelvic infection following complete or unspecified spontaneous abortion M

Endometritis following complete or unspecified spontaneous abortion

Oophoritis following complete or unspecified spontaneous abortion

Parametritis following complete or unspecified spontaneous abortion

Pelvic peritonitis following complete or unspecified spontaneous abortion

Salpingitis following complete or unspecified spontaneous abortion

Salpingo-oophoritis following complete or unspecified spontaneous abortion

Excludes1 sepsis following complete or unspecified spontaneous abortion (O03.87)
urinary tract infection following complete or unspecified spontaneous abortion (O03.88)

O03.6 Delayed or excessive hemorrhage following complete or unspecified spontaneous abortion M

Afibrinogenemia following complete or unspecified spontaneous abortion

Defibrination syndrome following complete or unspecified spontaneous abortion

Hemolysis following complete or unspecified spontaneous abortion

Intravascular coagulation following complete or unspecified spontaneous abortion

Coding Clinic: 2022, Q1, P19

O03.7 Embolism following complete or unspecified spontaneous abortion M

Air embolism following complete or unspecified spontaneous abortion

Amniotic fluid embolism following complete or unspecified spontaneous abortion

Blood-clot embolism following complete or unspecified spontaneous abortion

Embolism NOS following complete or unspecified spontaneous abortion

Fat embolism following complete or unspecified spontaneous abortion

Pulmonary embolism following complete or unspecified spontaneous abortion

Pyemic embolism following complete or unspecified spontaneous abortion

Septic or septicopyemic embolism following complete or unspecified spontaneous abortion

Soap embolism following complete or unspecified spontaneous abortion

● **O03.8 Other and unspecified complications following complete or unspecified spontaneous abortion**

O03.80 Unspecified complication following complete or unspecified spontaneous abortion M

O03.81 Shock following complete or unspecified spontaneous abortion M

Circulatory collapse following complete or unspecified spontaneous abortion

Shock (postprocedural) following complete or unspecified spontaneous abortion

Excludes1 shock due to infection following complete or unspecified spontaneous abortion (O03.87)

O03.82 Renal failure following complete or unspecified spontaneous abortion M

Kidney failure (acute) following complete or unspecified spontaneous abortion

Oliguria following complete or unspecified spontaneous abortion

Renal shutdown following complete or unspecified spontaneous abortion

Renal tubular necrosis following complete or unspecified spontaneous abortion

Uremia following complete or unspecified spontaneous abortion

O03.83 Metabolic disorder following complete or unspecified spontaneous abortion M

O03.84 Damage to pelvic organs following complete or unspecified spontaneous abortion M

Laceration, perforation, tear or chemical damage of bladder following complete or unspecified spontaneous abortion

Laceration, perforation, tear or chemical damage of bowel following complete or unspecified spontaneous abortion

Laceration, perforation, tear or chemical damage of broad ligament following complete or unspecified spontaneous abortion

Laceration, perforation, tear or chemical damage of cervix following complete or unspecified spontaneous abortion

Laceration, perforation, tear or chemical damage of periurethral tissue following complete or unspecified spontaneous abortion

Laceration, perforation, tear or chemical damage of uterus following complete or unspecified spontaneous abortion

Laceration, perforation, tear or chemical damage of vagina following complete or unspecified spontaneous abortion

O03.85 Other venous complications following complete or unspecified spontaneous abortion M

O03.86 **Cardiac arrest following complete or unspecified spontaneous abortion** M

O03.87 **Sepsis following complete or unspecified spontaneous abortion** M

Use additional code to identify infectious agent (B95-B97)

Use additional code to identify severe sepsis, if applicable (R65.2-)

Excludes1 septic or septicopyemic embolism following complete or unspecified spontaneous abortion (O03.7)

O03.88 **Urinary tract infection following complete or unspecified spontaneous abortion** M

Cystitis following complete or unspecified spontaneous abortion

O03.89 **Complete or unspecified spontaneous abortion with other complications** M

O03.9 **Complete or unspecified spontaneous abortion without complication** M

Miscarriage NOS

Spontaneous abortion NOS

● O04 **Complications following (induced) termination of pregnancy** Ex: PDX 1406

Includes complications following (induced) termination of pregnancy

Excludes2 encounter for elective termination of pregnancy, uncomplicated (Z33.2)

failed attempted termination of pregnancy (O07.-)

Coding Clinic: 2023, Q2, P15-16; 2023, Q1, P17

O04.5 **Genital tract and pelvic infection following (induced) termination of pregnancy** M

Endometritis following (induced) termination of pregnancy

Oophoritis following (induced) termination of pregnancy

Parametritis following (induced) termination of pregnancy

Pelvic peritonitis following (induced) termination of pregnancy

Salpingitis following (induced) termination of pregnancy

Salpingo-oophoritis following (induced) termination of pregnancy

Excludes1 sepsis following (induced) termination of pregnancy (O04.87)

urinary tract infection following (induced) termination of pregnancy (O04.88)

O04.6 **Delayed or excessive hemorrhage following (induced) termination of pregnancy** M

Afibrinogenemia following (induced) termination of pregnancy

Defibrination syndrome following (induced) termination of pregnancy

Hemolysis following (induced) termination of pregnancy

Intravascular coagulation following (induced) termination of pregnancy

Coding Clinic: 2023, Q2, P15-16; 2019, Q3, P12

O04.7 **Embolism following (induced) termination of pregnancy** M

Air embolism following (induced) termination of pregnancy

Amniotic fluid embolism following (induced) termination of pregnancy

Blood-clot embolism following (induced) termination of pregnancy

Embolism NOS following (induced) termination of pregnancy

Fat embolism following (induced) termination of pregnancy

Pulmonary embolism following (induced) termination of pregnancy

Pyemic embolism following (induced) termination of pregnancy

Septic or septicopyemic embolism following (induced) termination of pregnancy

Soap embolism following (induced) termination of pregnancy

● O04.8 **(Induced) termination of pregnancy with other and unspecified complications**

O04.80 **(Induced) termination of pregnancy with unspecified complications** M

O04.81 **Shock following (induced) termination of pregnancy** M

Circulatory collapse following (induced) termination of pregnancy

Shock (postprocedural) following (induced) termination of pregnancy

Excludes1 shock due to infection following (induced) termination of pregnancy (O04.87)

O04.82 **Renal failure following (induced) termination of pregnancy** M

Kidney failure (acute) following (induced) termination of pregnancy

Oliguria following (induced) termination of pregnancy

Renal shutdown following (induced) termination of pregnancy

Renal tubular necrosis following (induced) termination of pregnancy

Uremia following (induced) termination of pregnancy

O04.83 **Metabolic disorder following (induced) termination of pregnancy** M

O04.84 **Damage to pelvic organs following (induced) termination of pregnancy** M

Laceration, perforation, tear or chemical damage of bladder following (induced) termination of pregnancy

Laceration, perforation, tear or chemical damage of bowel following (induced) termination of pregnancy

Laceration, perforation, tear or chemical damage of broad ligament following (induced) termination of pregnancy

Laceration, perforation, tear or chemical damage of cervix following (induced) termination of pregnancy

Laceration, perforation, tear or chemical damage of periurethral tissue following (induced) termination of pregnancy

Laceration, perforation, tear or chemical damage of uterus following (induced) termination of pregnancy

Laceration, perforation, tear or chemical damage of vagina following (induced) termination of pregnancy

O04.85 **Other venous complications following (induced) termination of pregnancy** M

O04.86 **Cardiac arrest following (induced) termination of pregnancy** M

O04.87 Sepsis following (induced) termination of pregnancy M
Use additional code to identify infectious agent (B95-B97)
Use additional code to identify severe sepsis, if applicable (R65.2-)
Excludes1 septic or septicopyemic embolism following (induced) termination of pregnancy (O04.7)

O04.88 Urinary tract infection following (induced) termination of pregnancy M
Cystitis following (induced) termination of pregnancy

O04.89 (Induced) termination of pregnancy with other complications M

● O07 Failed attempted termination of pregnancy
Includes failure of attempted induction of termination of pregnancy
incomplete elective abortion
Excludes1 incomplete spontaneous abortion (O03.0-)
Coding Clinic: 2023, Q1, P17

O07.0 Genital tract and pelvic infection following failed attempted termination of pregnancy (Ex) PDX 1407 M
Endometritis following failed attempted termination of pregnancy
Oophoritis following failed attempted termination of pregnancy
Parametritis following failed attempted termination of pregnancy
Pelvic peritonitis following failed attempted termination of pregnancy
Salpingitis following failed attempted termination of pregnancy
Salpingo-oophoritis following failed attempted termination of pregnancy
Excludes1 sepsis following failed attempted termination of pregnancy (O07.37)
urinary tract infection following failed attempted termination of pregnancy (O07.38)

O07.1 Delayed or excessive hemorrhage following failed attempted termination of pregnancy (Ex) PDX 1408 M
Afibrinogenemia following failed attempted termination of pregnancy
Defibrination syndrome following failed attempted termination of pregnancy
Hemolysis following failed attempted termination of pregnancy
Intravascular coagulation following failed attempted termination of pregnancy

O07.2 Embolism following failed attempted termination of pregnancy (Ex) PDX 1409 M
Air embolism following failed attempted termination of pregnancy
Amniotic fluid embolism following failed attempted termination of pregnancy
Blood-clot embolism following failed attempted termination of pregnancy
Embolism NOS following failed attempted termination of pregnancy
Fat embolism following failed attempted termination of pregnancy
Pulmonary embolism following failed attempted termination of pregnancy
Pyemic embolism following failed attempted termination of pregnancy
Septic or septicopyemic embolism following failed attempted termination of pregnancy
Soap embolism following failed attempted termination of pregnancy

● O07.3 Failed attempted termination of pregnancy with other and unspecified complications

O07.30 Failed attempted termination of pregnancy with unspecified complications (Ex) PDX 1406 M

O07.31 Shock following failed attempted termination of pregnancy (Ex) PDX 1410 M
Circulatory collapse following failed attempted termination of pregnancy
Shock (postprocedural) following failed attempted termination of pregnancy
Excludes1 shock due to infection following failed attempted termination of pregnancy (O07.37)

O07.32 Renal failure following failed attempted termination of pregnancy (Ex) PDX 1411 M
Kidney failure (acute) following failed attempted termination of pregnancy
Oliguria following failed attempted termination of pregnancy
Renal shutdown following failed attempted termination of pregnancy
Renal tubular necrosis following failed attempted termination of pregnancy
Uremia following failed attempted termination of pregnancy

O07.33 Metabolic disorder following failed attempted termination of pregnancy (Ex) PDX 1406 M

O07.34 Damage to pelvic organs following failed attempted termination of pregnancy (Ex) PDX 1412 M
Laceration, perforation, tear or chemical damage of bladder following failed attempted termination of pregnancy
Laceration, perforation, tear or chemical damage of bowel following failed attempted termination of pregnancy
Laceration, perforation, tear or chemical damage of broad ligament following failed attempted termination of pregnancy
Laceration, perforation, tear or chemical damage of cervix following failed attempted termination of pregnancy
Laceration, perforation, tear or chemical damage of periurethral tissue following failed attempted termination of pregnancy
Laceration, perforation, tear or chemical damage of uterus following failed attempted termination of pregnancy
Laceration, perforation, tear or chemical damage of vagina following failed attempted termination of pregnancy

O07.35 Other venous complications following failed attempted termination of pregnancy (Ex) PDX 1406 M

O07.36 Cardiac arrest following failed attempted termination of pregnancy (Ex) PDX 1406 M

O07.37 Sepsis following failed attempted termination of pregnancy (Ex) PDX 1407 M
Use additional code (B95-B97), to identify infectious agent
Use additional code (R65.2-) to identify severe sepsis, if applicable
Excludes1 septic or septicopyemic embolism following failed attempted termination of pregnancy (O07.2)

O07.38 Urinary tract infection following failed attempted termination of pregnancy (Ex) PDX 1406 M
Cystitis following failed attempted termination of pregnancy

O07.39 Failed attempted termination of pregnancy with other complications (Ex) PDX 1406 M

O07.4 Failed attempted termination of pregnancy without complication M

CHAPTER 15 (O00-O9A)

O08 Complications following ectopic and molar pregnancy (Ex) PDX 1414
This category is for use with categories O00-O02 to identify any associated complications.
Coding Clinic: 2023, Q1, P17

O08.0 Genital tract and pelvic infection following ectopic and molar pregnancy (Ex) PDX 86 M
Endometritis following ectopic and molar pregnancy
Oophoritis following ectopic and molar pregnancy
Parametritis following ectopic and molar pregnancy
Pelvic peritonitis following ectopic and molar pregnancy
Salpingitis following ectopic and molar pregnancy
Salpingo-oophoritis following ectopic and molar pregnancy
Excludes1 sepsis following ectopic and molar pregnancy (O08.82)
urinary tract infection (O08.83)

O08.1 Delayed or excessive hemorrhage following ectopic and molar pregnancy (Ex) PDX 1413 M
Afibrinogenemia following ectopic and molar pregnancy
Defibrination syndrome following ectopic and molar pregnancy
Hemolysis following ectopic and molar pregnancy
Intravascular coagulation following ectopic and molar pregnancy
Excludes1 delayed or excessive hemorrhage due to incomplete abortion (O03.1)

O08.2 Embolism following ectopic and molar pregnancy M
Air embolism following ectopic and molar pregnancy
Amniotic fluid embolism following ectopic and molar pregnancy
Blood-clot embolism following ectopic and molar pregnancy
Embolism NOS following ectopic and molar pregnancy
Fat embolism following ectopic and molar pregnancy
Pulmonary embolism following ectopic and molar pregnancy
Pyemic embolism following ectopic and molar pregnancy
Septic or septicopyemic embolism following ectopic and molar pregnancy
Soap embolism following ectopic and molar pregnancy

O08.3 Shock following ectopic and molar pregnancy M
Circulatory collapse following ectopic and molar pregnancy
Shock (postprocedural) following ectopic and molar pregnancy
Excludes1 shock due to infection following ectopic and molar pregnancy (O08.82)

O08.4 Renal failure following ectopic and molar pregnancy M
Kidney failure (acute) following ectopic and molar pregnancy
Oliguria following ectopic and molar pregnancy
Renal shutdown following ectopic and molar pregnancy
Renal tubular necrosis following ectopic and molar pregnancy
Uremia following ectopic and molar pregnancy

O08.5 Metabolic disorders following an ectopic and molar pregnancy M

O08.6 Damage to pelvic organs and tissues following an ectopic and molar pregnancy M
Laceration, perforation, tear or chemical damage of bladder following an ectopic and molar pregnancy
Laceration, perforation, tear or chemical damage of bowel following an ectopic and molar pregnancy
Laceration, perforation, tear or chemical damage of broad ligament following an ectopic and molar pregnancy
Laceration, perforation, tear or chemical damage of cervix following an ectopic and molar pregnancy
Laceration, perforation, tear or chemical damage of periurethral tissue following an ectopic and molar pregnancy
Laceration, perforation, tear or chemical damage of uterus following an ectopic and molar pregnancy
Laceration, perforation, tear or chemical damage of vagina following an ectopic and molar pregnancy

O08.7 Other venous complications following an ectopic and molar pregnancy M

O08.8 Other complications following an ectopic and molar pregnancy

O08.81 Cardiac arrest following an ectopic and molar pregnancy M

O08.82 Sepsis following ectopic and molar pregnancy (Ex) PDX 86 M
Use additional code (B95-B97), to identify infectious agent
Use additional code (R65.2-) to identify severe sepsis, if applicable
Excludes1 septic or septicopyemic embolism following ectopic and molar pregnancy (O08.2)

O08.83 Urinary tract infection following an ectopic and molar pregnancy M
Cystitis following an ectopic and molar pregnancy

O08.89 Other complications following an ectopic and molar pregnancy M

O08.9 Unspecified complication following an ectopic and molar pregnancy M

SUPERVISION OF HIGH RISK PREGNANCY (O09)

O09 Supervision of high risk pregnancy
Coding Clinic: 2016, Q4, P125, 150

O09.0 Supervision of pregnancy with history of infertility

O09.00 Supervision of pregnancy with history of infertility, unspecified trimester M

O09.01 Supervision of pregnancy with history of infertility, first trimester M

O09.02 Supervision of pregnancy with history of infertility, second trimester M

O09.03 Supervision of pregnancy with history of infertility, third trimester M

O09.1 Supervision of pregnancy with history of ectopic pregnancy
Coding Clinic: 2016, Q4, P49-50

O09.10 Supervision of pregnancy with history of ectopic pregnancy, unspecified trimester M

O09.11 Supervision of pregnancy with history of ectopic pregnancy, first trimester M

O09.12 Supervision of pregnancy with history of ectopic pregnancy, second trimester M

O09.13 Supervision of pregnancy with history of ectopic pregnancy, third trimester M

O09.A Supervision of pregnancy with history of molar pregnancy
Coding Clinic: 2016, Q4, P50

O09.A0 Supervision of pregnancy with history of molar pregnancy, unspecified trimester M

O09.A1 Supervision of pregnancy with history of molar pregnancy, first trimester M

O09.A2 Supervision of pregnancy with history of molar pregnancy, second trimester M

O09.A3 Supervision of pregnancy with history of molar pregnancy, third trimester M

O09.2 Supervision of pregnancy with other poor reproductive or obstetric history

Excludes2 pregnancy care for patient with history of recurrent pregnancy loss (O26.2-)

O09.21 Supervision of pregnancy with history of pre-term labor

O09.211 Supervision of pregnancy with history of pre-term labor, first trimester M

O09.212 Supervision of pregnancy with history of pre-term labor, second trimester M

O09.213 Supervision of pregnancy with history of pre-term labor, third trimester M

O09.219 Supervision of pregnancy with history of pre-term labor, unspecified trimester M

O09.29 Supervision of pregnancy with other poor reproductive or obstetric history

Supervision of pregnancy with history of neonatal death

Supervision of pregnancy with history of stillbirth

O09.291 Supervision of pregnancy with other poor reproductive or obstetric history, first trimester M

O09.292 Supervision of pregnancy with other poor reproductive or obstetric history, second trimester M

O09.293 Supervision of pregnancy with other poor reproductive or obstetric history, third trimester M

O09.299 Supervision of pregnancy with other poor reproductive or obstetric history, unspecified trimester M

O09.3 Supervision of pregnancy with insufficient antenatal care

Supervision of concealed pregnancy

Supervision of hidden pregnancy

O09.30 Supervision of pregnancy with insufficient antenatal care, unspecified trimester M

O09.31 Supervision of pregnancy with insufficient antenatal care, first trimester M

O09.32 Supervision of pregnancy with insufficient antenatal care, second trimester M

O09.33 Supervision of pregnancy with insufficient antenatal care, third trimester M

O09.4 Supervision of pregnancy with grand multiparity

O09.40 Supervision of pregnancy with grand multiparity, unspecified trimester M

O09.41 Supervision of pregnancy with grand multiparity, first trimester M

O09.42 Supervision of pregnancy with grand multiparity, second trimester M

O09.43 Supervision of pregnancy with grand multiparity, third trimester M

O09.5 Supervision of elderly primigravida and multigravida

Pregnancy for a female 35 years and older at expected date of delivery

O09.51 Supervision of elderly primigravida

O09.511 Supervision of elderly primigravida, first trimester M

O09.512 Supervision of elderly primigravida, second trimester M

O09.513 Supervision of elderly primigravida, third trimester M

O09.519 Supervision of elderly primigravida, unspecified trimester M

O09.52 Supervision of elderly multigravida

O09.521 Supervision of elderly multigravida, first trimester M

O09.522 Supervision of elderly multigravida, second trimester M

O09.523 Supervision of elderly multigravida, third trimester M

Coding Clinic: 2016, Q4, P150

O09.529 Supervision of elderly multigravida, unspecified trimester M

O09.6 Supervision of young primigravida and multigravida

Supervision of pregnancy for a female less than 16 years old at expected date of delivery

O09.61 Supervision of young primigravida

O09.611 Supervision of young primigravida, first trimester M

O09.612 Supervision of young primigravida, second trimester M

O09.613 Supervision of young primigravida, third trimester M

O09.619 Supervision of young primigravida, unspecified trimester M

O09.62 Supervision of young multigravida

O09.621 Supervision of young multigravida, first trimester M

O09.622 Supervision of young multigravida, second trimester M

O09.623 Supervision of young multigravida, third trimester M

O09.629 Supervision of young multigravida, unspecified trimester M

O09.7 Supervision of high risk pregnancy due to social problems

O09.70 Supervision of high risk pregnancy due to social problems, unspecified trimester M

O09.71 Supervision of high risk pregnancy due to social problems, first trimester M

O09.72 Supervision of high risk pregnancy due to social problems, second trimester M

O09.73 Supervision of high risk pregnancy due to social problems, third trimester M

O09.8 Supervision of other high risk pregnancies

O09.81 Supervision of pregnancy resulting from assisted reproductive technology

Supervision of pregnancy resulting from in-vitro fertilization

Excludes2 gestational carrier status (Z33.3)

O09.811 Supervision of pregnancy resulting from assisted reproductive technology, first trimester M

O09.812 Supervision of pregnancy resulting from assisted reproductive technology, second trimester M

O09.813 Supervision of pregnancy resulting from assisted reproductive technology, third trimester M

O09.819 Supervision of pregnancy resulting from assisted reproductive technology, unspecified trimester M

O09.82 Supervision of pregnancy with history of in utero procedure during previous pregnancy

O09.821 Supervision of pregnancy with history of in utero procedure during previous pregnancy, first trimester M

O09.822 Supervision of pregnancy with history of in utero procedure during previous pregnancy, second trimester M

CHAPTER 15 (O00-O9A)

● O09.823 Supervision of pregnancy with history of in utero procedure during previous pregnancy, third trimester M

● O09.829 Supervision of pregnancy with history of in utero procedure during previous pregnancy, unspecified trimester M

Excludes1 supervision of pregnancy affected by in utero procedure during current pregnancy (O35.7)

● O09.89 Supervision of other high risk pregnancies

● O09.891 Supervision of other high risk pregnancies, first trimester M

● O09.892 Supervision of other high risk pregnancies, second trimester M

● O09.893 Supervision of other high risk pregnancies, third trimester M

● O09.899 Supervision of other high risk pregnancies, unspecified trimester M

● O09.9 Supervision of high risk pregnancy, unspecified

● O09.90 Supervision of high risk pregnancy, unspecified, unspecified trimester M

● O09.91 Supervision of high risk pregnancy, unspecified, first trimester M

● O09.92 Supervision of high risk pregnancy, unspecified, second trimester M

● O09.93 Supervision of high risk pregnancy, unspecified, third trimester M

EDEMA, PROTEINURIA AND HYPERTENSIVE DISORDERS IN PREGNANCY, CHILDBIRTH AND THE PUERPERIUM (O10-O16)

● O10 Pre-existing hypertension complicating pregnancy, childbirth and the puerperium Ex: PDX 1415

Includes pre-existing hypertension with pre-existing proteinuria complicating pregnancy, childbirth and the puerperium

Excludes2 pre-existing hypertension with superimposed pre-eclampsia complicating pregnancy, childbirth and the puerperium (O11.-)

Coding Clinic: 2016, Q4, P50

● O10.0 Pre-existing essential hypertension complicating pregnancy, childbirth and the puerperium

Any condition in I10 specified as a reason for obstetric care during pregnancy, childbirth or the puerperium

● O10.01 Pre-existing essential hypertension complicating pregnancy

O10.011 Pre-existing essential hypertension complicating pregnancy, first trimester M

O10.012 Pre-existing essential hypertension complicating pregnancy, second trimester M

O10.013 Pre-existing essential hypertension complicating pregnancy, third trimester M

O10.019 Pre-existing essential hypertension complicating pregnancy, unspecified trimester M

O10.02 Pre-existing essential hypertension complicating childbirth M

O10.03 Pre-existing essential hypertension complicating the puerperium M

● O10.1 Pre-existing hypertensive heart disease complicating pregnancy, childbirth and the puerperium

Any condition in I11 specified as a reason for obstetric care during pregnancy, childbirth or the puerperium

Use additional code from I11 to identify the type of hypertensive heart disease

● O10.11 Pre-existing hypertensive heart disease complicating pregnancy

O10.111 Pre-existing hypertensive heart disease complicating pregnancy, first trimester M

O10.112 Pre-existing hypertensive heart disease complicating pregnancy, second trimester M

O10.113 Pre-existing hypertensive heart disease complicating pregnancy, third trimester M

O10.119 Pre-existing hypertensive heart disease complicating pregnancy, unspecified trimester M

O10.12 Pre-existing hypertensive heart disease complicating childbirth M

O10.13 Pre-existing hypertensive heart disease complicating the puerperium M

● O10.2 Pre-existing hypertensive chronic kidney disease complicating pregnancy, childbirth and the puerperium

Any condition in I12 specified as a reason for obstetric care during pregnancy, childbirth or the puerperium

Use additional code from I12 to identify the type of hypertensive chronic kidney disease

● O10.21 Pre-existing hypertensive chronic kidney disease complicating pregnancy

O10.211 Pre-existing hypertensive chronic kidney disease complicating pregnancy, first trimester M

O10.212 Pre-existing hypertensive chronic kidney disease complicating pregnancy, second trimester M

O10.213 Pre-existing hypertensive chronic kidney disease complicating pregnancy, third trimester M

O10.219 Pre-existing hypertensive chronic kidney disease complicating pregnancy, unspecified trimester M

O10.22 Pre-existing hypertensive chronic kidney disease complicating childbirth M

O10.23 Pre-existing hypertensive chronic kidney disease complicating the puerperium M

● O10.3 Pre-existing hypertensive heart and chronic kidney disease complicating pregnancy, childbirth and the puerperium

Any condition in I13 specified as a reason for obstetric care during pregnancy, childbirth or the puerperium

Use additional code from I13 to identify the type of hypertensive heart and chronic kidney disease

● O10.31 Pre-existing hypertensive heart and chronic kidney disease complicating pregnancy

O10.311 Pre-existing hypertensive heart and chronic kidney disease complicating pregnancy, first trimester M

O10.312 Pre-existing hypertensive heart and chronic kidney disease complicating pregnancy, second trimester M

O10.313 Pre-existing hypertensive heart and chronic kidney disease complicating pregnancy, third trimester M

O10.319 Pre-existing hypertensive heart and chronic kidney disease complicating pregnancy, unspecified trimester M

CHAPTER 15 (O00-O9A)

O10.32 Pre-existing hypertensive heart and chronic kidney disease complicating childbirth M

O10.33 Pre-existing hypertensive heart and chronic kidney disease complicating the puerperium M

● O10.4 Pre-existing secondary hypertension complicating pregnancy, childbirth and the puerperium

Any condition in I15 specified as a reason for obstetric care during pregnancy, childbirth or the puerperium

Use additional code from I15 to identify the type of secondary hypertension

● O10.41 Pre-existing secondary hypertension complicating pregnancy

O10.411 Pre-existing secondary hypertension complicating pregnancy, first trimester M

O10.412 Pre-existing secondary hypertension complicating pregnancy, second trimester M

O10.413 Pre-existing secondary hypertension complicating pregnancy, third trimester M

O10.419 Pre-existing secondary hypertension complicating pregnancy, unspecified trimester M

O10.42 Pre-existing secondary hypertension complicating childbirth M

O10.43 Pre-existing secondary hypertension complicating the puerperium M

● O10.9 Unspecified pre-existing hypertension complicating pregnancy, childbirth and the puerperium

● O10.91 Unspecified pre-existing hypertension complicating pregnancy

O10.911 Unspecified pre-existing hypertension complicating pregnancy, first trimester M

O10.912 Unspecified pre-existing hypertension complicating pregnancy, second trimester M

O10.913 Unspecified pre-existing hypertension complicating pregnancy, third trimester M

O10.919 Unspecified pre-existing hypertension complicating pregnancy, unspecified trimester M

O10.92 Unspecified pre-existing hypertension complicating childbirth M

O10.93 Unspecified pre-existing hypertension complicating the puerperium M

● O11 Pre-existing hypertension with pre-eclampsia (Ex:) PDX 1415

Includes conditions in O10 complicated by pre-eclampsia
pre-eclampsia superimposed pre-existing hypertension

Use additional code from O10 to identify the type of hypertension

Coding Clinic: 2016, Q4, P50

O11.1 Pre-existing hypertension with pre-eclampsia, first trimester M

O11.2 Pre-existing hypertension with pre-eclampsia, second trimester M

O11.3 Pre-existing hypertension with pre-eclampsia, third trimester M

O11.4 Pre-existing hypertension with pre-eclampsia, complicating childbirth M

O11.5 Pre-existing hypertension with pre-eclampsia, complicating the puerperium M

O11.9 Pre-existing hypertension with pre-eclampsia, unspecified trimester M

● O12 Gestational [pregnancy-induced] edema and proteinuria without hypertension (Ex:) PDX 1416

Coding Clinic: 2016, Q4, P50

● O12.0 Gestational edema

O12.00 Gestational edema, unspecified trimester M

O12.01 Gestational edema, first trimester M

O12.02 Gestational edema, second trimester M

O12.03 Gestational edema, third trimester M

O12.04 Gestational edema, complicating childbirth M

O12.05 Gestational edema, complicating the puerperium M

● O12.1 Gestational proteinuria

O12.10 Gestational proteinuria, unspecified trimester M

O12.11 Gestational proteinuria, first trimester M

O12.12 Gestational proteinuria, second trimester M

O12.13 Gestational proteinuria, third trimester M

O12.14 Gestational proteinuria, complicating childbirth M

O12.15 Gestational proteinuria, complicating the puerperium M

● O12.2 Gestational edema with proteinuria

O12.20 Gestational edema with proteinuria, unspecified trimester M

O12.21 Gestational edema with proteinuria, first trimester M
CC when PDx is its own CC

O12.22 Gestational edema with proteinuria, second trimester M
CC when PDx is its own CC

O12.23 Gestational edema with proteinuria, third trimester M
CC when PDx is its own CC

O12.24 Gestational edema with proteinuria, complicating childbirth M

O12.25 Gestational edema with proteinuria, complicating the puerperium M

● O13 Gestational [pregnancy-induced] hypertension without significant proteinuria

Includes gestational hypertension NOS
transient hypertension of pregnancy

Coding Clinic: 2016, Q4, P50

O13.1 Gestational [pregnancy-induced] hypertension without significant proteinuria, first trimester M

O13.2 Gestational [pregnancy-induced] hypertension without significant proteinuria, second trimester M

O13.3 Gestational [pregnancy-induced] hypertension without significant proteinuria, third trimester M

O13.4 Gestational [pregnancy-induced] hypertension without significant proteinuria, complicating childbirth M

O13.5 Gestational [pregnancy-induced] hypertension without significant proteinuria, complicating the puerperium M

O13.9 Gestational [pregnancy-induced] hypertension without significant proteinuria, unspecified trimester M

● O14 Pre-eclampsia (Ex:) PDX 1415

Excludes1 pre-existing hypertension with pre-eclampsia (O11)

Coding Clinic: 2016, Q4, P50

● O14.0 Mild to moderate pre-eclampsia

O14.00 Mild to moderate pre-eclampsia, unspecified trimester M

O14.02 Mild to moderate pre-eclampsia, second trimester M

O14.03 Mild to moderate pre-eclampsia, third trimester M

O14.04 Mild to moderate pre-eclampsia, complicating childbirth M
Coding Clinic: 2019, Q2, P8

O14.05 Mild to moderate pre-eclampsia, complicating the puerperium M

● O14.1 Severe pre-eclampsia
Excludes1 HELLP syndrome (O14.2-)
H=hemolysis, EL=elevated liver enzymes, LP=low platelet count
Coding Clinic: 2019, Q3, P12
- O14.10 Severe pre-eclampsia, unspecified trimester M
- O14.12 Severe pre-eclampsia, second trimester M
- O14.13 Severe pre-eclampsia, third trimester M
- O14.14 Severe pre-eclampsia complicating childbirth M
- O14.15 Severe pre-eclampsia, complicating the puerperium M

● O14.2 HELLP syndrome
Severe pre-eclampsia with hemolysis, elevated liver enzymes and low platelet count (HELLP)
- O14.20 HELLP syndrome (HELLP), unspecified trimester M
- O14.22 HELLP syndrome (HELLP), second trimester M
- O14.23 HELLP syndrome (HELLP), third trimester M
- O14.24 HELLP syndrome, complicating childbirth M
- O14.25 HELLP syndrome, complicating the puerperium M

● O14.9 Unspecified pre-eclampsia
- O14.90 Unspecified pre-eclampsia, unspecified trimester M
- O14.92 Unspecified pre-eclampsia, second trimester M
- O14.93 Unspecified pre-eclampsia, third trimester M
- O14.94 Unspecified pre-eclampsia, complicating childbirth M
- O14.95 Unspecified pre-eclampsia, complicating the puerperium M

● O15 Eclampsia (Ex) PDX 1415
Includes convulsions following conditions in O10-O14 and O16

● O15.0 Eclampsia complicating pregnancy
Coding Clinic: 2016, Q4, P50
- O15.00 Eclampsia complicating pregnancy, unspecified trimester M
- O15.02 Eclampsia complicating pregnancy, second trimester M
- O15.03 Eclampsia complicating pregnancy, third trimester M

O15.1 Eclampsia complicating labor M
O15.2 Eclampsia complicating the puerperium M
O15.9 Eclampsia, unspecified as to time period M
Eclampsia NOS

● O16 Unspecified maternal hypertension (Ex) PDX 1415
Coding Clinic: 2016, Q4, P50
- O16.1 Unspecified maternal hypertension, first trimester M
- O16.2 Unspecified maternal hypertension, second trimester M
- O16.3 Unspecified maternal hypertension, third trimester M
- O16.4 Unspecified maternal hypertension, complicating childbirth M
- O16.5 Unspecified maternal hypertension, complicating the puerperium M
- O16.9 Unspecified maternal hypertension, unspecified trimester M

OTHER MATERNAL DISORDERS PREDOMINANTLY RELATED TO PREGNANCY (O20-O29)

Excludes2 maternal care related to the fetus and amniotic cavity and possible delivery problems (O30-O48)
maternal diseases classifiable elsewhere but complicating pregnancy, labor and delivery, and the puerperium (O98-O99)

● O20 Hemorrhage in early pregnancy (Ex) PDX 1417
Includes hemorrhage before completion of 20 weeks gestation
Excludes1 pregnancy with abortive outcome (O00-O08)

O20.0 Threatened abortion M
Hemorrhage specified as due to threatened abortion
O20.8 Other hemorrhage in early pregnancy M
Coding Clinic: 2023, Q3, P18
O20.9 Hemorrhage in early pregnancy, unspecified M

● O21 Excessive vomiting in pregnancy
O21.0 Mild hyperemesis gravidarum M
Hyperemesis gravidarum, mild or unspecified, starting before the end of the 20th week of gestation
O21.1 Hyperemesis gravidarum with metabolic disturbance M
Hyperemesis gravidarum, starting before the end of the 20th week of gestation, with metabolic disturbance such as carbohydrate depletion
Hyperemesis gravidarum, starting before the end of the 20th week of gestation, with metabolic disturbance such as dehydration
Hyperemesis gravidarum, starting before the end of the 20th week of gestation, with metabolic disturbance such as electrolyte imbalance
O21.2 Late vomiting of pregnancy M
Excessive vomiting starting after 20 completed weeks of gestation
O21.8 Other vomiting complicating pregnancy M
Vomiting due to diseases classified elsewhere, complicating pregnancy
Use additional code, to identify cause
O21.9 Vomiting of pregnancy, unspecified M

● O22 Venous complications and hemorrhoids in pregnancy (Ex) PDX 1418
Excludes1 venous complications of:
abortion NOS (O03.9)
ectopic or molar pregnancy (O08.7)
failed attempted abortion (O07.35)
induced abortion (O04.85)
spontaneous abortion (O03.89)
Excludes2 obstetric pulmonary embolism (O88.-)
venous complications and hemorrhoids of childbirth and the puerperium (O87.-)

● O22.0 Varicose veins of lower extremity in pregnancy
Varicose veins NOS in pregnancy
- O22.00 Varicose veins of lower extremity in pregnancy, unspecified trimester M
- O22.01 Varicose veins of lower extremity in pregnancy, first trimester M
- O22.02 Varicose veins of lower extremity in pregnancy, second trimester M
- O22.03 Varicose veins of lower extremity in pregnancy, third trimester M

● O22.1 Genital varices in pregnancy
Perineal varices in pregnancy
Vaginal varices in pregnancy
Vulval varices in pregnancy
- O22.10 Genital varices in pregnancy, unspecified trimester M
- O22.11 Genital varices in pregnancy, first trimester M

CHAPTER 15 (O00-O9A)

O22.12 Genital varices in pregnancy, second trimester M
O22.13 Genital varices in pregnancy, third trimester M

O22.2 Superficial thrombophlebitis in pregnancy
Phlebitis in pregnancy NOS
Thrombophlebitis of legs in pregnancy
Thrombosis in pregnancy NOS
Use additional code to identify the superficial thrombophlebitis (I80.0-)
O22.20 Superficial thrombophlebitis in pregnancy, unspecified trimester M
O22.21 Superficial thrombophlebitis in pregnancy, first trimester M
O22.22 Superficial thrombophlebitis in pregnancy, second trimester M
O22.23 Superficial thrombophlebitis in pregnancy, third trimester M

O22.3 Deep phlebothrombosis in pregnancy
Deep vein thrombosis, antepartum
Use additional code to identify the deep vein thrombosis (I82.4-, I82.5-, I82.62-, I82.72-)
Use additional code, if applicable, for associated long-term (current) use of anticoagulants (Z79.01)
O22.30 Deep phlebothrombosis in pregnancy, unspecified trimester M
O22.31 Deep phlebothrombosis in pregnancy, first trimester M
O22.32 Deep phlebothrombosis in pregnancy, second trimester M
O22.33 Deep phlebothrombosis in pregnancy, third trimester M

O22.4 Hemorrhoids in pregnancy
O22.40 Hemorrhoids in pregnancy, unspecified trimester M
O22.41 Hemorrhoids in pregnancy, first trimester M
O22.42 Hemorrhoids in pregnancy, second trimester M
O22.43 Hemorrhoids in pregnancy, third trimester M

O22.5 Cerebral venous thrombosis in pregnancy
Cerebrovenous sinus thrombosis in pregnancy
O22.50 Cerebral venous thrombosis in pregnancy, unspecified trimester M
O22.51 Cerebral venous thrombosis in pregnancy, first trimester M
O22.52 Cerebral venous thrombosis in pregnancy, second trimester M
O22.53 Cerebral venous thrombosis in pregnancy, third trimester M

O22.8 Other venous complications in pregnancy
O22.8X Other venous complications in pregnancy
O22.8X1 Other venous complications in pregnancy, first trimester M
O22.8X2 Other venous complications in pregnancy, second trimester M
O22.8X3 Other venous complications in pregnancy, third trimester M
O22.8X9 Other venous complications in pregnancy, unspecified trimester M

O22.9 Venous complication in pregnancy, unspecified
Gestational phlebitis NOS
Gestational phlebopathy NOS
Gestational thrombosis NOS
O22.90 Venous complication in pregnancy, unspecified, unspecified trimester M
O22.91 Venous complication in pregnancy, unspecified, first trimester M
O22.92 Venous complication in pregnancy, unspecified, second trimester M
O22.93 Venous complication in pregnancy, unspecified, third trimester M

O23 Infections of genitourinary tract in pregnancy
Use additional code to identify organism (B95.-, B96.-)
Excludes2 gonococcal infections complicating pregnancy, childbirth and the puerperium (O98.2)
infections with a predominantly sexual mode of transmission NOS complicating pregnancy, childbirth and the puerperium (O98.3)
syphilis complicating pregnancy, childbirth and the puerperium (O98.1)
tuberculosis of genitourinary system complicating pregnancy, childbirth and the puerperium (O98.0)
venereal disease NOS complicating pregnancy, childbirth and the puerperium (O98.3)

O23.0 Infections of kidney in pregnancy Ex: PDX 1419
Pyelonephritis in pregnancy
O23.00 Infections of kidney in pregnancy, unspecified trimester M
O23.01 Infections of kidney in pregnancy, first trimester M
O23.02 Infections of kidney in pregnancy, second trimester M
O23.03 Infections of kidney in pregnancy, third trimester M

O23.1 Infections of bladder in pregnancy
O23.10 Infections of bladder in pregnancy, unspecified trimester M
O23.11 Infections of bladder in pregnancy, first trimester M
O23.12 Infections of bladder in pregnancy, second trimester M
O23.13 Infections of bladder in pregnancy, third trimester M

O23.2 Infections of urethra in pregnancy
O23.20 Infections of urethra in pregnancy, unspecified trimester M
O23.21 Infections of urethra in pregnancy, first trimester M
O23.22 Infections of urethra in pregnancy, second trimester M
O23.23 Infections of urethra in pregnancy, third trimester M

O23.3 Infections of other parts of urinary tract in pregnancy
O23.30 Infections of other parts of urinary tract in pregnancy, unspecified trimester M
O23.31 Infections of other parts of urinary tract in pregnancy, first trimester M
O23.32 Infections of other parts of urinary tract in pregnancy, second trimester M
O23.33 Infections of other parts of urinary tract in pregnancy, third trimester M

O23.4 Unspecified infection of urinary tract in pregnancy
O23.40 Unspecified infection of urinary tract in pregnancy, unspecified trimester M
O23.41 Unspecified infection of urinary tract in pregnancy, first trimester M
O23.42 Unspecified infection of urinary tract in pregnancy, second trimester M
O23.43 Unspecified infection of urinary tract in pregnancy, third trimester M

O23.5 Infections of the genital tract in pregnancy
O23.51 Infection of cervix in pregnancy
O23.511 Infections of cervix in pregnancy, first trimester M
O23.512 Infections of cervix in pregnancy, second trimester M
O23.513 Infections of cervix in pregnancy, third trimester M
O23.519 Infections of cervix in pregnancy, unspecified trimester M

CHAPTER 15 (O00-O9A)

● O23.52 Salpingo-oophoritis in pregnancy
Oophoritis = inflammation of ovary
Salpingitis = inflammation of fallopian tube
Oophoritis in pregnancy
Salpingitis in pregnancy
O23.521 Salpingo-oophoritis in pregnancy, first trimester M
O23.522 Salpingo-oophoritis in pregnancy, second trimester M
O23.523 Salpingo-oophoritis in pregnancy, third trimester M
O23.529 Salpingo-oophoritis in pregnancy, unspecified trimester M
● O23.59 Infection of other part of genital tract in pregnancy
Coding Clinic: 2022, Q1, P20
O23.591 Infection of other part of genital tract in pregnancy, first trimester M
O23.592 Infection of other part of genital tract in pregnancy, second trimester M
O23.593 Infection of other part of genital tract in pregnancy, third trimester M
Coding Clinic: 2022, Q1, P20
O23.599 Infection of other part of genital tract in pregnancy, unspecified trimester M
● O23.9 Unspecified genitourinary tract infection in pregnancy
Genitourinary tract infection in pregnancy NOS
O23.90 Unspecified genitourinary tract infection in pregnancy, unspecified trimester M
O23.91 Unspecified genitourinary tract infection in pregnancy, first trimester M
O23.92 Unspecified genitourinary tract infection in pregnancy, second trimester M
O23.93 Unspecified genitourinary tract infection in pregnancy, third trimester M

OGCR Section I.C.15.g.

Diabetes mellitus in pregnancy
Diabetes mellitus is a significant complicating factor in pregnancy. Pregnant women who are diabetic should be assigned a code from category O24, Diabetes mellitus in pregnancy, childbirth, and the puerperium, first, followed by the appropriate diabetes code(s) (E08-E13) from Chapter 4.

● O24 Diabetes mellitus in pregnancy, childbirth, and the puerperium (Ex) PDX 1420
● O24.0 Pre-existing type 1 diabetes mellitus, in pregnancy, childbirth and the puerperium
Juvenile onset diabetes mellitus, in pregnancy, childbirth and the puerperium
Ketosis-prone diabetes mellitus in pregnancy, childbirth and the puerperium
Use additional code from category E10 to further identify any manifestations
● O24.01 Pre-existing type 1 diabetes mellitus, in pregnancy
O24.011 Pre-existing type 1 diabetes mellitus, in pregnancy, first trimester M
O24.012 Pre-existing type 1 diabetes mellitus, in pregnancy, second trimester M
O24.013 Pre-existing type 1 diabetes mellitus, in pregnancy, third trimester M
O24.019 Pre-existing type 1 diabetes mellitus, in pregnancy, unspecified trimester M
O24.02 Pre-existing type 1 diabetes mellitus, in childbirth M
O24.03 Pre-existing type 1 diabetes mellitus, in the puerperium M

● O24.1 Pre-existing type 2 diabetes mellitus, in pregnancy, childbirth and the puerperium
Insulin-resistant diabetes mellitus in pregnancy, childbirth and the puerperium
Use additional code (for):
from category E11 to further identify any manifestations
long-term (current) use of insulin (Z79.4)
▶ Use additional injectable non-insulin antidiabetic drugs (Z79.85)
● O24.11 Pre-existing type 2 diabetes mellitus, in pregnancy
O24.111 Pre-existing type 2 diabetes mellitus, in pregnancy, first trimester M
O24.112 Pre-existing type 2 diabetes mellitus, in pregnancy, second trimester M
O24.113 Pre-existing type 2 diabetes mellitus, in pregnancy, third trimester M
O24.119 Pre-existing type 2 diabetes mellitus, in pregnancy, unspecified trimester M
O24.12 Pre-existing type 2 diabetes mellitus, in childbirth M
O24.13 Pre-existing type 2 diabetes mellitus, in the puerperium M
● O24.3 Unspecified pre-existing diabetes mellitus in pregnancy, childbirth and the puerperium
Use additional code (for):
from category E11 to further identify any manifestation
long-term (current) use of insulin (Z79.4)
▶ Use additional injectable non-insulin antidiabetic drugs (Z79.85)
● O24.31 Unspecified pre-existing diabetes mellitus in pregnancy
O24.311 Unspecified pre-existing diabetes mellitus in pregnancy, first trimester M
O24.312 Unspecified pre-existing diabetes mellitus in pregnancy, second trimester M
O24.313 Unspecified pre-existing diabetes mellitus in pregnancy, third trimester M
O24.319 Unspecified pre-existing diabetes mellitus in pregnancy, unspecified trimester M
O24.32 Unspecified pre-existing diabetes mellitus in childbirth M
O24.33 Unspecified pre-existing diabetes mellitus in the puerperium M
● O24.4 Gestational diabetes mellitus
Diabetes mellitus arising in pregnancy
Gestational diabetes mellitus NOS
Coding Clinic: 2016, Q4, P50, 126
● O24.41 Gestational diabetes mellitus in pregnancy
O24.410 Gestational diabetes mellitus in pregnancy, diet controlled M
O24.414 Gestational diabetes mellitus in pregnancy, insulin controlled M
O24.415 Gestational diabetes mellitus in pregnancy, controlled by oral hypoglycemic drugs M
Gestational diabetes mellitus in pregnancy, controlled by oral antidiabetic drugs
Coding Clinic: 2016, Q4, P50
O24.419 Gestational diabetes mellitus in pregnancy, unspecified control M
Coding Clinic: 2015, Q4, P34

● O24.42 Gestational diabetes mellitus in childbirth
- O24.420 Gestational diabetes mellitus in childbirth, diet controlled M
- O24.424 Gestational diabetes mellitus in childbirth, insulin controlled M
- O24.425 Gestational diabetes mellitus in childbirth, controlled by oral hypoglycemic drugs M
  - Gestational diabetes mellitus in childbirth, controlled by oral antidiabetic drugs
  - **Coding Clinic: 2016, Q4, P50**
- O24.429 Gestational diabetes mellitus in childbirth, unspecified control M

OGCR Section I.C.15.i.

Gestational (pregnancy induced) diabetes

Gestational (pregnancy induced) diabetes can occur during the second and third trimester of pregnancy in women who were not diabetic prior to pregnancy. Gestational diabetes can cause complications in the pregnancy similar to those of pre-existing diabetes mellitus. It also puts the woman at greater risk of developing diabetes after the pregnancy. Codes for gestational diabetes are in subcategory O24.4, Gestational diabetes mellitus. No other code from category O24, Diabetes mellitus in pregnancy, childbirth, and the puerperium, should be used with a code from O24.4

The codes under subcategory O24.4 include diet controlled, insulin controlled, **and controlled by oral hypoglycemic drugs.** If a patient with gestational diabetes is treated with both diet and insulin, only the code for insulin-controlled is required. **If a patient with gestational diabetes is treated with both diet and oral hypoglycemic medications, only the code for "controlled by oral hypoglycemic drugs" is required.** Code Z79.4, Long-term (current) use of insulin **or code Z79.84, Long-term (current) use of oral hypoglycemic drugs,** should not be assigned with codes from subcategory O24.4.

An abnormal glucose tolerance in pregnancy is assigned a code from subcategory O99.81, Abnormal glucose complicating pregnancy, childbirth, and the puerperium.

● O24.43 Gestational diabetes mellitus in the puerperium
- O24.430 Gestational diabetes mellitus in the puerperium, diet controlled M
- O24.434 Gestational diabetes mellitus in the puerperium, insulin controlled M
- O24.435 Gestational diabetes mellitus in puerperium, controlled by oral hypoglycemic drugs M
  - Gestational diabetes mellitus in puerperium, controlled by oral antidiabetic drugs
  - **Coding Clinic: 2016, Q4, P50**
- O24.439 Gestational diabetes mellitus in the puerperium, unspecified control M

● O24.8 Other pre-existing diabetes mellitus in pregnancy, childbirth, and the puerperium

Use additional code (for):
- from categories E08, E09 and E13 to further identify any manifestation
- long-term (current) use of insulin (Z79.4)

▶ Use additional injectable non-insulin antidiabetic drugs (Z79.85)

● O24.81 Other pre-existing diabetes mellitus in pregnancy
- O24.811 Other pre-existing diabetes mellitus in pregnancy, first trimester M
- O24.812 Other pre-existing diabetes mellitus in pregnancy, second trimester M
- O24.813 Other pre-existing diabetes mellitus in pregnancy, third trimester M
- O24.819 Other pre-existing diabetes mellitus in pregnancy, unspecified trimester M

O24.82 Other pre-existing diabetes mellitus in childbirth M

O24.83 Other pre-existing diabetes mellitus in the puerperium M

● O24.9 Unspecified diabetes mellitus in pregnancy, childbirth and the puerperium

Use additional code (for):
- ▶ from categories E08, E09 and E13 to further identify any manifestation
- ▶ injectable non-insulin antidiabetic drugs (Z79.85)
- ▶ long-term (current) use of insulin (Z79.4)

Unknown whether patient was diabetic before pregnancy occurred

● O24.91 Unspecified diabetes mellitus in pregnancy
- O24.911 Unspecified diabetes mellitus in pregnancy, first trimester M
- O24.912 Unspecified diabetes mellitus in pregnancy, second trimester M
- O24.913 Unspecified diabetes mellitus in pregnancy, third trimester M
- O24.919 Unspecified diabetes mellitus in pregnancy, unspecified trimester M

O24.92 Unspecified diabetes mellitus in childbirth M

O24.93 Unspecified diabetes mellitus in the puerperium M

● O25 Malnutrition in pregnancy, childbirth and the puerperium

● O25.1 Malnutrition in pregnancy
- O25.10 Malnutrition in pregnancy, unspecified trimester M
- O25.11 Malnutrition in pregnancy, first trimester M
- O25.12 Malnutrition in pregnancy, second trimester M
- O25.13 Malnutrition in pregnancy, third trimester M

O25.2 Malnutrition in childbirth M

O25.3 Malnutrition in the puerperium M

● O26 Maternal care for other conditions predominantly related to pregnancy

● O26.0 Excessive weight gain in pregnancy

Excludes2 gestational edema (O12.0, O12.2)
- O26.00 Excessive weight gain in pregnancy, unspecified trimester M
- O26.01 Excessive weight gain in pregnancy, first trimester M
- O26.02 Excessive weight gain in pregnancy, second trimester M
- O26.03 Excessive weight gain in pregnancy, third trimester M

● O26.1 Low weight gain in pregnancy
- O26.10 Low weight gain in pregnancy, unspecified trimester M
- O26.11 Low weight gain in pregnancy, first trimester M
- O26.12 Low weight gain in pregnancy, second trimester M
- O26.13 Low weight gain in pregnancy, third trimester M

● O26.2 Pregnancy care for patient with recurrent pregnancy loss
- O26.20 Pregnancy care for patient with recurrent pregnancy loss, unspecified trimester M
- O26.21 Pregnancy care for patient with recurrent pregnancy loss, first trimester M
- O26.22 Pregnancy care for patient with recurrent pregnancy loss, second trimester M
- O26.23 Pregnancy care for patient with recurrent pregnancy loss, third trimester M

● O26.3 Retained intrauterine contraceptive device in pregnancy
- O26.30 Retained intrauterine contraceptive device in pregnancy, unspecified trimester M
- O26.31 Retained intrauterine contraceptive device in pregnancy, first trimester M
- O26.32 Retained intrauterine contraceptive device in pregnancy, second trimester M
- O26.33 Retained intrauterine contraceptive device in pregnancy, third trimester M

● O26.4 Herpes gestationis
- O26.40 Herpes gestationis, unspecified trimester M
- O26.41 Herpes gestationis, first trimester M
- O26.42 Herpes gestationis, second trimester M
- O26.43 Herpes gestationis, third trimester M

● O26.5 Maternal hypotension syndrome
Supine hypotensive syndrome
- O26.50 Maternal hypotension syndrome, unspecified trimester M
- O26.51 Maternal hypotension syndrome, first trimester M
- O26.52 Maternal hypotension syndrome, second trimester M
- O26.53 Maternal hypotension syndrome, third trimester M

● O26.6 Liver and biliary tract disorders in pregnancy, childbirth and the puerperium
Use additional code to identify the specific disorder
Excludes2 hepatorenal syndrome following labor and delivery (O90.41)

● O26.61 Liver and biliary tract disorders in pregnancy (Ex) PDX 1421
- O26.611 Liver and biliary tract disorders in pregnancy, first trimester M
- O26.612 Liver and biliary tract disorders in pregnancy, second trimester M
- O26.613 Liver and biliary tract disorders in pregnancy, third trimester M
- O26.619 Liver and biliary tract disorders in pregnancy, unspecified trimester M

O26.62 Liver and biliary tract disorders in childbirth (Ex) PDX 1421 M
Coding Clinic: 2023, Q1, P26-27

O26.63 Liver and biliary tract disorders in the puerperium M

● O26.64 Intrahepatic cholestasis of pregnancy
- O26.641 Intrahepatic cholestasis of pregnancy, first trimester (Ex) PDX 1422 M
- O26.642 Intrahepatic cholestasis of pregnancy, second trimester (Ex) PDX 1423 M
- O26.643 Intrahepatic cholestasis of pregnancy, third trimester (Ex) PDX 1424 M
- O26.649 Intrahepatic cholestasis of pregnancy, unspecified trimester M

● O26.7 Subluxation of symphysis (pubis) in pregnancy, childbirth and the puerperium
Excludes1 traumatic separation of symphysis (pubis) during childbirth (O71.6)

● O26.71 Subluxation of symphysis (pubis) in pregnancy
- O26.711 Subluxation of symphysis (pubis) in pregnancy, first trimester M
- O26.712 Subluxation of symphysis (pubis) in pregnancy, second trimester M
- O26.713 Subluxation of symphysis (pubis) in pregnancy, third trimester M
- O26.719 Subluxation of symphysis (pubis) in pregnancy, unspecified trimester M

O26.72 Subluxation of symphysis (pubis) in childbirth M

O26.73 Subluxation of symphysis (pubis) in the puerperium M

● O26.8 Other specified pregnancy related conditions

● O26.81 Pregnancy related exhaustion and fatigue
- O26.811 Pregnancy related exhaustion and fatigue, first trimester M
- O26.812 Pregnancy related exhaustion and fatigue, second trimester M
- O26.813 Pregnancy related exhaustion and fatigue, third trimester M
- O26.819 Pregnancy related exhaustion and fatigue, unspecified trimester M

● O26.82 Pregnancy related peripheral neuritis
- O26.821 Pregnancy related peripheral neuritis, first trimester M
- O26.822 Pregnancy related peripheral neuritis, second trimester M
- O26.823 Pregnancy related peripheral neuritis, third trimester M
- O26.829 Pregnancy related peripheral neuritis, unspecified trimester M

● O26.83 Pregnancy related renal disease (Ex) PDX 1416
Use additional code to identify the specific disorder
- O26.831 Pregnancy related renal disease, first trimester M
- O26.832 Pregnancy related renal disease, second trimester M
- O26.833 Pregnancy related renal disease, third trimester M
- O26.839 Pregnancy related renal disease, unspecified trimester M

● O26.84 Uterine size-date discrepancy complicating pregnancy
Excludes1 encounter for suspected problem with fetal growth ruled out (Z03.74)
- O26.841 Uterine size-date discrepancy, first trimester M
- O26.842 Uterine size-date discrepancy, second trimester M
- O26.843 Uterine size-date discrepancy, third trimester M
- O26.849 Uterine size-date discrepancy, unspecified trimester M

● O26.85 Spotting complicating pregnancy
- O26.851 Spotting complicating pregnancy, first trimester M
- O26.852 Spotting complicating pregnancy, second trimester M
- O26.853 Spotting complicating pregnancy, third trimester M
- O26.859 Spotting complicating pregnancy, unspecified trimester M

O26.86 Pruritic urticarial papules and plaques of pregnancy (PUPPP) M
Polymorphic eruption of pregnancy

● O26.87 Cervical shortening (Ex) PDX 1425
Excludes1 encounter for suspected cervical shortening ruled out (Z03.75)
- O26.872 Cervical shortening, second trimester M
- O26.873 Cervical shortening, third trimester M
- O26.879 Cervical shortening, unspecified trimester M

● O26.89 Other specified pregnancy related conditions
Use Additional code, if applicable, to identify specific condition such as insulin resistance(E88.81-)
- O26.891 Other specified pregnancy related conditions, first trimester M
- O26.892 Other specified pregnancy related conditions, second trimester M

O26.893 Other specified pregnancy related conditions, third trimester **M**
Coding Clinic: 2015, Q3, P40

O26.899 Other specified pregnancy related conditions, unspecified trimester **M**

● O26.9 Pregnancy related conditions, unspecified

O26.90 Pregnancy related conditions, unspecified, unspecified trimester **M**

O26.91 Pregnancy related conditions, unspecified, first trimester **M**

O26.92 Pregnancy related conditions, unspecified, second trimester **M**

O26.93 Pregnancy related conditions, unspecified, third trimester **M**

● O28 Abnormal findings on antenatal screening of mother

Excludes1 diagnostic findings classified elsewhere - see Alphabetical Index

O28.0 Abnormal hematological finding on antenatal screening of mother **M**

O28.1 Abnormal biochemical finding on antenatal screening of mother **M**

O28.2 Abnormal cytological finding on antenatal screening of mother **M**

O28.3 Abnormal ultrasonic finding on antenatal screening of mother **M**
Coding Clinic: 2016, Q4, P5

O28.4 Abnormal radiological finding on antenatal screening of mother **M**

O28.5 Abnormal chromosomal and genetic finding on antenatal screening of mother **M**

O28.8 Other abnormal findings on antenatal screening of mother **M**

O28.9 Unspecified abnormal findings on antenatal screening of mother **M**

● O29 Complications of anesthesia during pregnancy

Includes maternal complications arising from the administration of a general, regional or local anesthetic, analgesic or other sedation during pregnancy

Use additional code, if necessary, to identify the complication

Excludes2 complications of anesthesia during labor and delivery (O74.-)
complications of anesthesia during the puerperium (O89.-)

● O29.0 Pulmonary complications of anesthesia during pregnancy

● O29.01 Aspiration pneumonitis due to anesthesia during pregnancy
Inhalation of stomach contents or secretions NOS due to anesthesia during pregnancy
Mendelson's syndrome due to anesthesia during pregnancy

O29.011 Aspiration pneumonitis due to anesthesia during pregnancy, first trimester **M**

O29.012 Aspiration pneumonitis due to anesthesia during pregnancy, second trimester **M**

O29.013 Aspiration pneumonitis due to anesthesia during pregnancy, third trimester **M**

O29.019 Aspiration pneumonitis due to anesthesia during pregnancy, unspecified trimester **M**

● O29.02 Pressure collapse of lung due to anesthesia during pregnancy

O29.021 Pressure collapse of lung due to anesthesia during pregnancy, first trimester **M**

O29.022 Pressure collapse of lung due to anesthesia during pregnancy, second trimester **M**

O29.023 Pressure collapse of lung due to anesthesia during pregnancy, third trimester **M**

O29.029 Pressure collapse of lung due to anesthesia during pregnancy, unspecified trimester **M**

● O29.09 Other pulmonary complications of anesthesia during pregnancy

O29.091 Other pulmonary complications of anesthesia during pregnancy, first trimester **M**

O29.092 Other pulmonary complications of anesthesia during pregnancy, second trimester **M**

O29.093 Other pulmonary complications of anesthesia during pregnancy, third trimester **M**

O29.099 Other pulmonary complications of anesthesia during pregnancy, unspecified trimester **M**

● O29.1 Cardiac complications of anesthesia during pregnancy

● O29.11 Cardiac arrest due to anesthesia during pregnancy

O29.111 Cardiac arrest due to anesthesia during pregnancy, first trimester **M**

O29.112 Cardiac arrest due to anesthesia during pregnancy, second trimester **M**

O29.113 Cardiac arrest due to anesthesia during pregnancy, third trimester **M**

O29.119 Cardiac arrest due to anesthesia during pregnancy, unspecified trimester **M**

● O29.12 Cardiac failure due to anesthesia during pregnancy

O29.121 Cardiac failure due to anesthesia during pregnancy, first trimester **M**

O29.122 Cardiac failure due to anesthesia during pregnancy, second trimester **M**

O29.123 Cardiac failure due to anesthesia during pregnancy, third trimester **M**

O29.129 Cardiac failure due to anesthesia during pregnancy, unspecified trimester **M**

● O29.19 Other cardiac complications of anesthesia during pregnancy

O29.191 Other cardiac complications of anesthesia during pregnancy, first trimester **M**

O29.192 Other cardiac complications of anesthesia during pregnancy, second trimester **M**

O29.193 Other cardiac complications of anesthesia during pregnancy, third trimester **M**

O29.199 Other cardiac complications of anesthesia during pregnancy, unspecified trimester **M**

● O29.2 Central nervous system complications of anesthesia during pregnancy

● O29.21 Cerebral anoxia due to anesthesia during pregnancy

O29.211 Cerebral anoxia due to anesthesia during pregnancy, first trimester **M**

O29.212 Cerebral anoxia due to anesthesia during pregnancy, second trimester **M**

O29.213 Cerebral anoxia due to anesthesia during pregnancy, third trimester **M**

O29.219 Cerebral anoxia due to anesthesia during pregnancy, unspecified trimester **M**

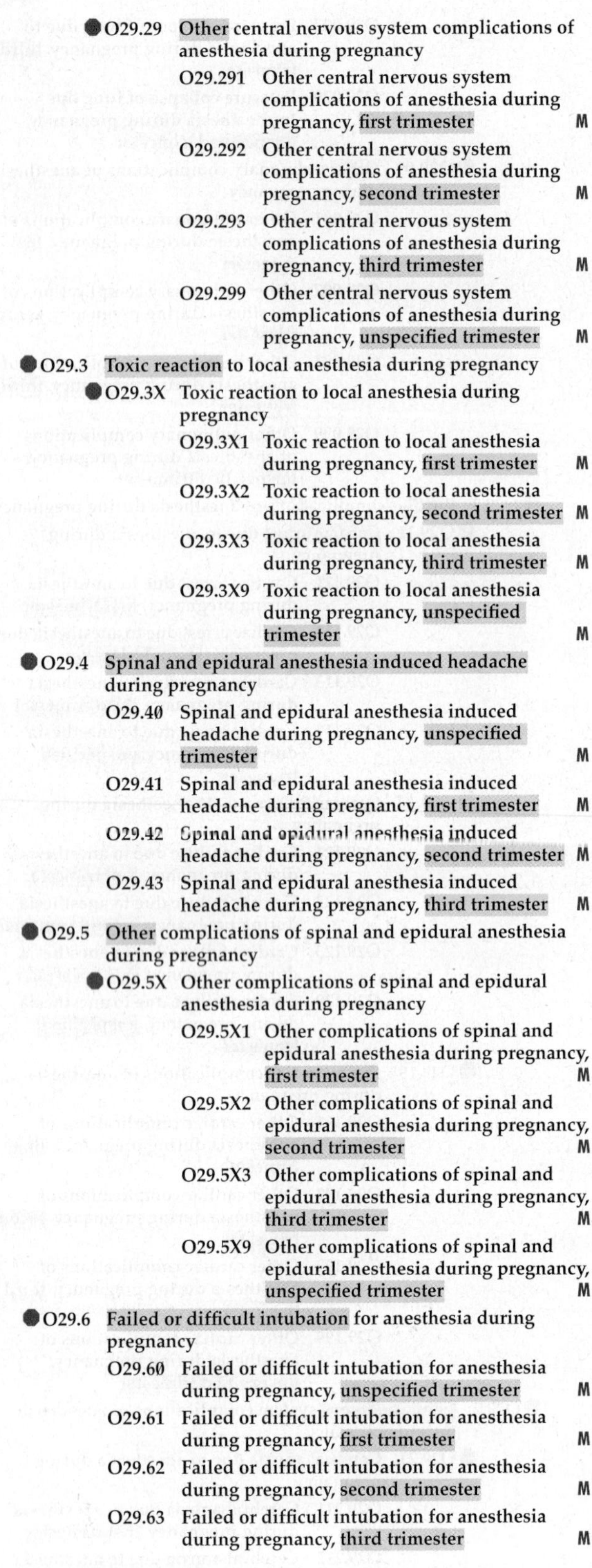

● O29.29 Other central nervous system complications of anesthesia during pregnancy

O29.291 Other central nervous system complications of anesthesia during pregnancy, first trimester M

O29.292 Other central nervous system complications of anesthesia during pregnancy, second trimester M

O29.293 Other central nervous system complications of anesthesia during pregnancy, third trimester M

O29.299 Other central nervous system complications of anesthesia during pregnancy, unspecified trimester M

● O29.3 Toxic reaction to local anesthesia during pregnancy

● O29.3X Toxic reaction to local anesthesia during pregnancy

O29.3X1 Toxic reaction to local anesthesia during pregnancy, first trimester M

O29.3X2 Toxic reaction to local anesthesia during pregnancy, second trimester M

O29.3X3 Toxic reaction to local anesthesia during pregnancy, third trimester M

O29.3X9 Toxic reaction to local anesthesia during pregnancy, unspecified trimester M

● O29.4 Spinal and epidural anesthesia induced headache during pregnancy

O29.4Ø Spinal and epidural anesthesia induced headache during pregnancy, unspecified trimester M

O29.41 Spinal and epidural anesthesia induced headache during pregnancy, first trimester M

O29.42 Spinal and epidural anesthesia induced headache during pregnancy, second trimester M

O29.43 Spinal and epidural anesthesia induced headache during pregnancy, third trimester M

● O29.5 Other complications of spinal and epidural anesthesia during pregnancy

● O29.5X Other complications of spinal and epidural anesthesia during pregnancy

O29.5X1 Other complications of spinal and epidural anesthesia during pregnancy, first trimester M

O29.5X2 Other complications of spinal and epidural anesthesia during pregnancy, second trimester M

O29.5X3 Other complications of spinal and epidural anesthesia during pregnancy, third trimester M

O29.5X9 Other complications of spinal and epidural anesthesia during pregnancy, unspecified trimester M

● O29.6 Failed or difficult intubation for anesthesia during pregnancy

O29.6Ø Failed or difficult intubation for anesthesia during pregnancy, unspecified trimester M

O29.61 Failed or difficult intubation for anesthesia during pregnancy, first trimester M

O29.62 Failed or difficult intubation for anesthesia during pregnancy, second trimester M

O29.63 Failed or difficult intubation for anesthesia during pregnancy, third trimester M

● O29.8 Other complications of anesthesia during pregnancy

● O29.8X Other complications of anesthesia during pregnancy

O29.8X1 Other complications of anesthesia during pregnancy, first trimester M

O29.8X2 Other complications of anesthesia during pregnancy, second trimester M

O29.8X3 Other complications of anesthesia during pregnancy, third trimester M

O29.8X9 Other complications of anesthesia during pregnancy, unspecified trimester M

● O29.9 Unspecified complication of anesthesia during pregnancy

O29.9Ø Unspecified complication of anesthesia during pregnancy, unspecified trimester M

O29.91 Unspecified complication of anesthesia during pregnancy, first trimester M

O29.92 Unspecified complication of anesthesia during pregnancy, second trimester M

O29.93 Unspecified complication of anesthesia during pregnancy, third trimester M

MATERNAL CARE RELATED TO THE FETUS AND AMNIOTIC CAVITY AND POSSIBLE DELIVERY PROBLEMS (O3Ø-O48)

● O3Ø Multiple gestation

Code also any complications specific to multiple gestation

Coding Clinic: 2Ø16, Q4, P51

● O3Ø.Ø Twin pregnancy

● O3Ø.ØØ Twin pregnancy, unspecified number of placenta and unspecified number of amniotic sacs

O3Ø.ØØ1 Twin pregnancy, unspecified number of placenta and unspecified number of amniotic sacs, first trimester M

O3Ø.ØØ2 Twin pregnancy, unspecified number of placenta and unspecified number of amniotic sacs, second trimester M

O3Ø.ØØ3 Twin pregnancy, unspecified number of placenta and unspecified number of amniotic sacs, third trimester M

O3Ø.ØØ9 Twin pregnancy, unspecified number of placenta and unspecified number of amniotic sacs, unspecified trimester M

● O3Ø.Ø1 Twin pregnancy, monochorionic/monoamniotic

Twin pregnancy, one placenta, one amniotic sac

Excludes1 conjoined twins (O3Ø.Ø2-)

O3Ø.Ø11 Twin pregnancy, monochorionic/monoamniotic, first trimester M

O3Ø.Ø12 Twin pregnancy, monochorionic/monoamniotic, second trimester M

O3Ø.Ø13 Twin pregnancy, monochorionic/monoamniotic, third trimester M

O3Ø.Ø19 Twin pregnancy, monochorionic/monoamniotic, unspecified trimester M

● O3Ø.Ø2 Conjoined twin pregnancy

O3Ø.Ø21 Conjoined twin pregnancy, first trimester M

O3Ø.Ø22 Conjoined twin pregnancy, second trimester M

O3Ø.Ø23 Conjoined twin pregnancy, third trimester M

O3Ø.Ø29 Conjoined twin pregnancy, unspecified trimester M

● **O30.03** Twin pregnancy, monochorionic/diamniotic
Twin pregnancy, one placenta, two amniotic sacs
- **O30.031** Twin pregnancy, monochorionic/diamniotic, first trimester M
- **O30.032** Twin pregnancy, monochorionic/diamniotic, second trimester M
- **O30.033** Twin pregnancy, monochorionic/diamniotic, third trimester M
- **O30.039** Twin pregnancy, monochorionic/diamniotic, unspecified trimester M

● **O30.04** Twin pregnancy, dichorionic/diamniotic
Twin pregnancy, two placentae, two amniotic sacs
- **O30.041** Twin pregnancy, dichorionic/diamniotic, first trimester M
- **O30.042** Twin pregnancy, dichorionic/diamniotic, second trimester M
- **O30.043** Twin pregnancy, dichorionic/diamniotic, third trimester M
- **O30.049** Twin pregnancy, dichorionic/diamniotic, unspecified trimester M

● **O30.09** Twin pregnancy, unable to determine number of placenta and number of amniotic sacs
- **O30.091** Twin pregnancy, unable to determine number of placenta and number of amniotic sacs, first trimester M
- **O30.092** Twin pregnancy, unable to determine number of placenta and number of amniotic sacs, second trimester M
- **O30.093** Twin pregnancy, unable to determine number of placenta and number of amniotic sacs, third trimester M
- **O30.099** Twin pregnancy, unable to determine number of placenta and number of amniotic sacs, unspecified trimester M

● **O30.1 Triplet pregnancy** (Ex) PDX 1426

● **O30.10** Triplet pregnancy, unspecified number of placenta and unspecified number of amniotic sacs
- **O30.101** Triplet pregnancy, unspecified number of placenta and unspecified number of amniotic sacs, first trimester M
- **O30.102** Triplet pregnancy, unspecified number of placenta and unspecified number of amniotic sacs, second trimester M
- **O30.103** Triplet pregnancy, unspecified number of placenta and unspecified number of amniotic sacs, third trimester M
  Coding Clinic: 2016, Q2, P8
- **O30.109** Triplet pregnancy, unspecified number of placenta and unspecified number of amniotic sacs, unspecified trimester M

● **O30.11** Triplet pregnancy with two or more monochorionic fetuses
- **O30.111** Triplet pregnancy with two or more monochorionic fetuses, first trimester M
- **O30.112** Triplet pregnancy with two or more monochorionic fetuses, second trimester M
- **O30.113** Triplet pregnancy with two or more monochorionic fetuses, third trimester M
- **O30.119** Triplet pregnancy with two or more monochorionic fetuses, unspecified trimester M

● **O30.12** Triplet pregnancy with two or more monoamniotic fetuses
- **O30.121** Triplet pregnancy with two or more monoamniotic fetuses, first trimester M
- **O30.122** Triplet pregnancy with two or more monoamniotic fetuses, second trimester M
- **O30.123** Triplet pregnancy with two or more monoamniotic fetuses, third trimester M
- **O30.129** Triplet pregnancy with two or more monoamniotic fetuses, unspecified trimester M

● **O30.13** Triplet pregnancy, trichorionic/triamniotic
- **O30.131** Triplet pregnancy, trichorionic/triamniotic, first trimester M
- **O30.132** Triplet pregnancy, trichorionic/triamniotic, second trimester M
- **O30.133** Triplet pregnancy, trichorionic/triamniotic, third trimester M
- **O30.139** Triplet pregnancy, trichorionic/triamniotic, unspecified trimester M

● **O30.19** Triplet pregnancy, unable to determine number of placenta and number of amniotic sacs
- **O30.191** Triplet pregnancy, unable to determine number of placenta and number of amniotic sacs, first trimester M
- **O30.192** Triplet pregnancy, unable to determine number of placenta and number of amniotic sacs, second trimester M
- **O30.193** Triplet pregnancy, unable to determine number of placenta and number of amniotic sacs, third trimester M
- **O30.199** Triplet pregnancy, unable to determine number of placenta and number of amniotic sacs, unspecified trimester M

● **O30.2 Quadruplet pregnancy** (Ex) PDX 1426

● **O30.20** Quadruplet pregnancy, unspecified number of placenta and unspecified number of amniotic sacs
- **O30.201** Quadruplet pregnancy, unspecified number of placenta and unspecified number of amniotic sacs, first trimester M
- **O30.202** Quadruplet pregnancy, unspecified number of placenta and unspecified number of amniotic sacs, second trimester M
- **O30.203** Quadruplet pregnancy, unspecified number of placenta and unspecified number of amniotic sacs, third trimester M
- **O30.209** Quadruplet pregnancy, unspecified number of placenta and unspecified number of amniotic sacs, unspecified trimester M

● **O30.21** Quadruplet pregnancy with two or more monochorionic fetuses
- **O30.211** Quadruplet pregnancy with two or more monochorionic fetuses, first trimester M
- **O30.212** Quadruplet pregnancy with two or more monochorionic fetuses, second trimester M

O30.213 Quadruplet pregnancy with two or more monochorionic fetuses, third trimester M

O30.219 Quadruplet pregnancy with two or more monochorionic fetuses, unspecified trimester M

● O30.22 Quadruplet pregnancy with two or more monoamniotic fetuses

O30.221 Quadruplet pregnancy with two or more monoamniotic fetuses, first trimester M

O30.222 Quadruplet pregnancy with two or more monoamniotic fetuses, second trimester M

O30.223 Quadruplet pregnancy with two or more monoamniotic fetuses, third trimester M

O30.229 Quadruplet pregnancy with two or more monoamniotic fetuses, unspecified trimester M

● O30.23 Quadruplet pregnancy, quadrachorionic/quadra-amniotic

O30.231 Quadruplet pregnancy, quadrachorionic/quadra-amniotic, first trimester M

O30.232 Quadruplet pregnancy, quadrachorionic/quadra-amniotic, second trimester M

O30.233 Quadruplet pregnancy, quadrachorionic/quadra-amniotic, third trimester M

O30.239 Quadruplet pregnancy, quadrachorionic/quadra-amniotic, unspecifiedtrimester M

● O30.29 Quadruplet pregnancy, unable to determine number of placenta and number of amniotic sacs

O30.291 Quadruplet pregnancy, unable to determine number of placenta and number of amniotic sacs, first trimester M

O30.292 Quadruplet pregnancy, unable to determine number of placenta and number of amniotic sacs, second trimester M

O30.293 Quadruplet pregnancy, unable to determine number of placenta and number of amniotic sacs, third trimester M

O30.299 Quadruplet pregnancy, unable to determine number of placenta and number of amniotic sacs, unspecified trimester M

● O30.8 Other specified multiple gestation (Ex:) PDX 1426

Multiple gestation pregnancy greater then quadruplets

● O30.80 Other specified multiple gestation, unspecified number of placenta and unspecified number of amniotic sacs

O30.801 Other specified multiple gestation, unspecified number of placenta and unspecified number of amniotic sacs, first trimester M

O30.802 Other specified multiple gestation, unspecified number of placenta and unspecified number of amniotic sacs, second trimester M

O30.803 Other specified multiple gestation, unspecified number of placenta and unspecified number of amniotic sacs, third trimester M

O30.809 Other specified multiple gestation, unspecified number of placenta and unspecified number of amniotic sacs, unspecified trimester M

● O30.81 Other specified multiple gestation with two or more monochorionic fetuses

O30.811 Other specified multiple gestation with two or more monochorionic fetuses, first trimester M

O30.812 Other specified multiple gestation with two or more monochorionic fetuses, second trimester M

O30.813 Other specified multiple gestation with two or more monochorionic fetuses, third trimester M

O30.819 Other specified multiple gestation with two or more monochorionic fetuses, unspecified trimester M

● O30.82 Other specified multiple gestation with two or more monoamniotic fetuses

O30.821 Other specified multiple gestation with two or more monoamniotic fetuses, first trimester M

O30.822 Other specified multiple gestation with two or more monoamniotic fetuses, second trimester M

O30.823 Other specified multiple gestation with two or more monoamniotic fetuses, third trimester M

O30.829 Other specified multiple gestation with two or more monoamniotic fetuses, unspecified trimester M

● O30.83 Other specified multiple gestation, number of chorions and amnions are both equalto the number of fetuses

Pentachorionic, penta-amniotic pregnancy (quintuplets)

Hexachorionic, hexa-amniotic pregnancy (sextuplets)

Heptachorionic, hepta-amniotic pregnancy (septuplets)

O30.831 Other specified multiple gestation, number of chorions and amnions are both equal to the number of fetuses, first trimester M

O30.832 Other specified multiple gestation, number of chorions and amnions are both equal to the number of fetuses, second trimester M

O30.833 Other specified multiple gestation, number of chorions and amnions are both equal to the number of fetuses, third trimester M

O30.839 Other specified multiple gestation, number of chorions and amnions are both equal to the number of fetuses, unspecified trimester M

● O30.89 Other specified multiple gestation, unable to determine number of placenta and number of amniotic sacs

O30.891 Other specified multiple gestation, unable to determine number of placenta and number of amniotic sacs, first trimester M

O30.892 Other specified multiple gestation, unable to determine number of placenta and number of amniotic sacs, second trimester M

O30.893 Other specified multiple gestation, unable to determine number of placenta and number of amniotic sacs, third trimester M

O30.899 Other specified multiple gestation, unable to determine number of placenta and number of amniotic sacs, unspecified trimester M

CHAPTER 15 (O00-O9A)

● O30.9 Multiple gestation, unspecified
Multiple pregnancy NOS
O30.90 Multiple gestation, unspecified, unspecified trimester M
O30.91 Multiple gestation, unspecified, first trimester M
O30.92 Multiple gestation, unspecified, second trimester M
O30.93 Multiple gestation, unspecified, third trimester M

● O31 Complications specific to multiple gestation
Excludes2 delayed delivery of second twin, triplet, etc. (O63.2)
malpresentation of one fetus or more (O32.9)
placental transfusion syndromes (O43.0-)

Coding Clinic: 2012, Q4, P107

One of the following 7th characters is to be assigned to each code under category O31. 7th character 0 is for single gestations and multiple gestations where the fetus is unspecified. 7th characters 1 through 9 are for cases of multiple gestations to identify the fetus for which the code applies. The appropriate code from category O30, Multiple gestation, must also be assigned when assigning a code from category O31 that has a 7th character of 1 through 9.

0	not applicable or unspecified
1	fetus 1
2	fetus 2
3	fetus 3
4	fetus 4
5	fetus 5
9	other fetus

● O31.0 Papyraceous fetus
Fetus compressus
X● O31.00 Papyraceous fetus, unspecified trimester M
X● O31.01 Papyraceous fetus, first trimester M
X● O31.02 Papyraceous fetus, second trimester M
X● O31.03 Papyraceous fetus, third trimester M

● O31.1 Continuing pregnancy after spontaneous abortion of one fetus or more
X● O31.10 Continuing pregnancy after spontaneous abortion of one fetus or more, unspecified trimester M
X● O31.11 Continuing pregnancy after spontaneous abortion of one fetus or more, first trimester M
X● O31.12 Continuing pregnancy after spontaneous abortion of one fetus or more, second trimester M
X● O31.13 Continuing pregnancy after spontaneous abortion of one fetus or more, third trimester M

● O31.2 Continuing pregnancy after intrauterine death of one fetus or more
X● O31.20 Continuing pregnancy after intrauterine death of one fetus or more, unspecified trimester M
X● O31.21 Continuing pregnancy after intrauterine death of one fetus or more, first trimester M
X● O31.22 Continuing pregnancy after intrauterine death of one fetus or more, second trimester M
X● O31.23 Continuing pregnancy after intrauterine death of one fetus or more, third trimester M

● O31.3 Continuing pregnancy after elective fetal reduction of one fetus or more
Continuing pregnancy after selective termination of one fetus or more
X● O31.30 Continuing pregnancy after elective fetal reduction of one fetus or more, unspecified trimester M
X● O31.31 Continuing pregnancy after elective fetal reduction of one fetus or more, first trimester M
X● O31.32 Continuing pregnancy after elective fetal reduction of one fetus or more, second trimester M
X● O31.33 Continuing pregnancy after elective fetal reduction of one fetus or more, third trimester M

● O31.8 Other complications specific to multiple gestation (Ex) PDX 1426
● O31.8X Other complications specific to multiple gestation
● O31.8X1 Other complications specific to multiple gestation, first trimester M
● O31.8X2 Other complications specific to multiple gestation, second trimester M
● O31.8X3 Other complications specific to multiple gestation, third trimester M
● O31.8X9 Other complications specific to multiple gestation, unspecified trimester M

● O32 Maternal care for malpresentation of fetus
Includes the listed conditions as a reason for observation, hospitalization or other obstetric care of the mother, or for cesarean delivery before onset of labor
Excludes1 malpresentation of fetus with obstructed labor (O64.-)

Coding Clinic: 2012, Q4, P107

One of the following 7th characters is to be assigned to each code under category O32. 7th character 0 is for single gestations and multiple gestations where the fetus is unspecified. 7th characters 1 through 9 are for cases of multiple gestations to identify the fetus for which the code applies. The appropriate code from category O30, Multiple gestation, must also be assigned when assigning a code from category O32 that has a 7th character of 1 through 9.

0	not applicable or unspecified
1	fetus 1
2	fetus 2
3	fetus 3
4	fetus 4
5	fetus 5
9	other fetus

X● O32.0 Maternal care for unstable lie M
X● O32.1 Maternal care for breech presentation M
Maternal care for buttocks presentation
Maternal care for complete breech
Maternal care for frank breech
Excludes1 footling presentation (O32.8)
incomplete breech (O32.8)
X● O32.2 Maternal care for transverse and oblique lie M
Maternal care for oblique presentation
Maternal care for transverse presentation
X● O32.3 Maternal care for face, brow and chin presentation M
X● O32.4 Maternal care for high head at term M
Maternal care for failure of head to enter pelvic brim
X● O32.6 Maternal care for compound presentation M
X● O32.8 Maternal care for other malpresentation of fetus M
Maternal care for footling presentation
Maternal care for incomplete breech
X● O32.9 Maternal care for malpresentation of fetus, unspecified M

CHAPTER 15 (O00-O9A)

●O33 **Maternal care for disproportion**

Includes the listed conditions as a reason for observation, hospitalization or other obstetric care of the mother, or for cesarean delivery before onset of labor

Excludes1 disproportion with obstructed labor (O65-O66)

O33.0 **Maternal care for disproportion due to deformity of maternal pelvic bones** (Ex) PDX 1427 M

Maternal care for disproportion due to pelvic deformity causing disproportion NOS

O33.1 **Maternal care for disproportion due to generally contracted pelvis** M

Maternal care for disproportion due to contracted pelvis NOS causing disproportion

O33.2 **Maternal care for disproportion due to inlet contraction of pelvis** M

Maternal care for disproportion due to inlet contraction (pelvis) causing disproportion

X●O33.3 **Maternal care for disproportion due to outlet contraction of pelvis** M

Maternal care for disproportion due to mid-cavity contraction (pelvis)

Maternal care for disproportion due to outlet contraction (pelvis)

One of the following 7th characters is to be assigned to code O33.3. 7th character Ø is for single gestations and multiple gestations where the fetus is unspecified. 7th characters 1 through 9 are for cases of multiple gestations to identify the fetus for which the code applies. The appropriate code from category O3Ø, Multiple gestation, must also be assigned when assigning code O33.3 with a 7th character of 1 through 9.

Ø not applicable or unspecified
1 fetus 1
2 fetus 2
3 fetus 3
4 fetus 4
5 fetus 5
9 other fetus

X●O33.4 **Maternal care for disproportion of mixed maternal and fetal origin** M

One of the following 7th characters is to be assigned to code O33.4. 7th character Ø is for single gestations and multiple gestations where the fetus is unspecified. 7th characters 1 through 9 are for cases of multiple gestations to identify the fetus for which the code applies. The appropriate code from category O3Ø, Multiple gestation, must also be assigned when assigning code O33.4 with a 7th character of 1 through 9.

Ø not applicable or unspecified
1 fetus 1
2 fetus 2
3 fetus 3
4 fetus 4
5 fetus 5
9 other fetus

X●O33.5 **Maternal care for disproportion due to unusually large fetus** M

Maternal care for disproportion due to disproportion of fetal origin with normally formed fetus

Maternal care for disproportion due to fetal disproportion NOS

One of the following 7th characters is to be assigned to code O33.5. 7th character Ø is for single gestations and multiple gestations where the fetus is unspecified. 7th characters 1 through 9 are for cases of multiple gestations to identify the fetus for which the code applies. The appropriate code from category O3Ø, Multiple gestation, must also be assigned when assigning code O33.5 with a 7th character of 1 through 9.

Ø not applicable or unspecified
1 fetus 1
2 fetus 2
3 fetus 3
4 fetus 4
5 fetus 5
9 other fetus

X●O33.6 **Maternal care for disproportion due to hydrocephalic fetus** M

One of the following 7th characters is to be assigned to code O33.6. 7th character Ø is for single gestations and multiple gestations where the fetus is unspecified. 7th characters 1 through 9 are for cases of multiple gestations to identify the fetus for which the code applies. The appropriate code from category O3Ø, Multiple gestation, must also be assigned when assigning code O33.6 with a 7th character of 1 through 9.

Ø not applicable or unspecified
1 fetus 1
2 fetus 2
3 fetus 3
4 fetus 4
5 fetus 5
9 other fetus

X●O33.7 **Maternal care for disproportion due to other fetal deformities** M

Maternal care for disproportion due to fetal ascites

Maternal care for disproportion due to fetal hydrops

Maternal care for disproportion due to fetal meningomyelocele

Maternal care for disproportion due to fetal sacral teratoma

Maternal care for disproportion due to fetal tumor

Excludes1 obstructed labor due to other fetal deformities (O66.3)

Coding Clinic: 2016, Q4, P51

One of the following 7th characters is to be assigned to code O33.7. 7th character Ø is for single gestations and multiple gestations where the fetus is unspecified. 7th characters 1 through 9 are for cases of multiple gestations to identify the fetus for which the code applies. The appropriate code from category O3Ø, Multiple gestation, must also be assigned when assigning code O33.7 with a 7th character of 1 through 9.

Ø not applicable or unspecified
1 fetus 1
2 fetus 2
3 fetus 3
4 fetus 4
5 fetus 5
9 other fetus

O33.8 **Maternal care for disproportion of other origin** M

O33.9 **Maternal care for disproportion, unspecified** M
Maternal care for disproportion due to cephalopelvic disproportion NOS
Maternal care for disproportion due to fetopelvic disproportion NOS

● O34 **Maternal care for abnormality of pelvic organs**
Includes the listed conditions as a reason for hospitalization or other obstetric care of the mother, or for cesarean delivery before onset of labor
Code first any associated obstructed labor (O65.5)
Use additional code for specific condition

● O34.0 **Maternal care for congenital malformation of uterus**
Maternal care for double uterus
Maternal care for uterus bicornis

O34.00 **Maternal care for unspecified congenital malformation of uterus, unspecified trimester** M

O34.01 **Maternal care for unspecified congenital malformation of uterus, first trimester** M

O34.02 **Maternal care for unspecified congenital malformation of uterus, second trimester** M

O34.03 **Maternal care for unspecified congenital malformation of uterus, third trimester** M

● O34.1 **Maternal care for benign tumor of corpus uteri**
Excludes2 maternal care for benign tumor of cervix (O34.4-)
maternal care for malignant neoplasm of uterus (O9A.1-)

O34.10 **Maternal care for benign tumor of corpus uteri, unspecified trimester** M

O34.11 **Maternal care for benign tumor of corpus uteri, first trimester** M

O34.12 **Maternal care for benign tumor of corpus uteri, second trimester** M

O34.13 **Maternal care for benign tumor of corpus uteri, third trimester** M

● O34.2 **Maternal care due to uterine scar from previous surgery**
Coding Clinic: 2016, Q4, P76

● O34.21 **Maternal care for scar from previous cesarean delivery**
Coding Clinic: 2016, Q4, P51

O34.211 **Maternal care for low transverse scar from previous cesarean delivery** M

O34.212 **Maternal care for vertical scar from previous cesarean delivery** M
Maternal care for classical scar from previous cesarean delivery

O34.218 **Maternal care for other type scar from previous cesarean delivery** M
Mid-transverse T incision

O34.219 **Maternal care for unspecified type scar from previous cesarean delivery** M

O34.22 **Maternal care for cesarean scar defect (isthmocele)** M

O34.29 **Maternal care due to uterine scar from other previous surgery** M
Maternal care due to uterine scar from other transmural uterine incision

● O34.3 **Maternal care for cervical incompetence** (Ex) PDX 1425
Maternal care for cerclage with or without cervical incompetence
Maternal care for Shirodkar suture with or without cervical incompetence

O34.30 **Maternal care for cervical incompetence, unspecified trimester** M

O34.31 **Maternal care for cervical incompetence, first trimester** M

O34.32 **Maternal care for cervical incompetence, second trimester** M

O34.33 **Maternal care for cervical incompetence, third trimester** M

● O34.4 **Maternal care for other abnormalities of cervix**

O34.40 **Maternal care for other abnormalities of cervix, unspecified trimester** M

O34.41 **Maternal care for other abnormalities of cervix, first trimester** M

O34.42 **Maternal care for other abnormalities of cervix, second trimester** M

O34.43 **Maternal care for other abnormalities of cervix, third trimester** M

● O34.5 **Maternal care for other abnormalities of gravid uterus**

● O34.51 **Maternal care for incarceration of gravid uterus**

O34.511 **Maternal care for incarceration of gravid uterus, first trimester** M

O34.512 **Maternal care for incarceration of gravid uterus, second trimester** M

O34.513 **Maternal care for incarceration of gravid uterus, third trimester** M

O34.519 **Maternal care for incarceration of gravid uterus, unspecified trimester** M

● O34.52 **Maternal care for prolapse of gravid uterus**

O34.521 **Maternal care for prolapse of gravid uterus, first trimester** M

O34.522 **Maternal care for prolapse of gravid uterus, second trimester** M

O34.523 **Maternal care for prolapse of gravid uterus, third trimester** M

O34.529 **Maternal care for prolapse of gravid uterus, unspecified trimester** M

● O34.53 **Maternal care for retroversion of gravid uterus**

O34.531 **Maternal care for retroversion of gravid uterus, first trimester** M

O34.532 **Maternal care for retroversion of gravid uterus, second trimester** M

O34.533 **Maternal care for retroversion of gravid uterus, third trimester** M

O34.539 **Maternal care for retroversion of gravid uterus, unspecified trimester** M

● O34.59 **Maternal care for other abnormalities of gravid uterus**

O34.591 **Maternal care for other abnormalities of gravid uterus, first trimester** M

O34.592 **Maternal care for other abnormalities of gravid uterus, second trimester** M

O34.593 **Maternal care for other abnormalities of gravid uterus, third trimester** M

O34.599 **Maternal care for other abnormalities of gravid uterus, unspecified trimester** M

● O34.6 **Maternal care for abnormality of vagina**
Excludes2 maternal care for vaginal varices in pregnancy (O22.1-)

O34.60 **Maternal care for abnormality of vagina, unspecified trimester** M

O34.61 **Maternal care for abnormality of vagina, first trimester** M

O34.62 **Maternal care for abnormality of vagina, second trimester** M

O34.63 **Maternal care for abnormality of vagina, third trimester** M

CHAPTER 15 (O00-O9A)

●O34.7 Maternal care for abnormality of vulva and perineum

Excludes2 maternal care for perineal and vulval varices in pregnancy (O22.1-)

O34.70 **Maternal care for abnormality of vulva and perineum, unspecified trimester** M

O34.71 **Maternal care for abnormality of vulva and perineum, first trimester** M

O34.72 **Maternal care for abnormality of vulva and perineum, second trimester** M

O34.73 **Maternal care for abnormality of vulva and perineum, third trimester** M

●O34.8 Maternal care for other abnormalities of pelvic organs

O34.80 **Maternal care for other abnormalities of pelvic organs, unspecified trimester** M

O34.81 **Maternal care for other abnormalities of pelvic organs, first trimester** M

O34.82 **Maternal care for other abnormalities of pelvic organs, second trimester** M

O34.83 **Maternal care for other abnormalities of pelvic organs, third trimester** M

●O34.9 Maternal care for abnormality of pelvic organ, unspecified

O34.90 **Maternal care for abnormality of pelvic organ, unspecified, unspecified trimester** M

O34.91 **Maternal care for abnormality of pelvic organ, unspecified, first trimester** M

O34.92 **Maternal care for abnormality of pelvic organ, unspecified, second trimester** M

O34.93 **Maternal care for abnormality of pelvic organ, unspecified, third trimester** M

●O35 **Maternal care for known or suspected fetal abnormality and damage**

Includes the listed conditions in the fetus as a reason for hospitalization or other obstetric care to the mother, or for termination of pregnancy

Code also any associated maternal condition

Excludes1 encounter for suspected maternal and fetal conditions ruled out (Z03.7-)

One of the following 7th characters is to be assigned to each code under category O35. 7th character 0 is for single gestations and multiple gestations where the fetus is unspecified. 7th characters 1 through 9 are for cases of multiple gestations to identify the fetus for which the code applies. The appropriate code from category O30, Multiple gestation, must also be assigned when assigning a code from category O35 that has a 7th character of 1 through 9.

0	not applicable or unspecified
1	fetus 1
2	fetus 2
3	fetus 3
4	fetus 4
5	fetus 5
9	other fetus

X●O35.0 Maternal care for (suspected) central nervous system malformation in fetus M

Excludes2 chromosomal abnormality in fetus (O35.1-)

X●O35.00 **Maternal care for (suspected) central nervous system malformation or damage in fetus, unspecified** M

X●O35.01 **Maternal care for (suspected) central nervous system malformation or damage in fetus, agenesis of the corpus callosum** M

X●O35.02 **Maternal care for (suspected) central nervous system malformation or damage in fetus, anencephaly** M

X●O35.03 **Maternal care for (suspected) central nervous system malformation or damage in fetus, choroid plexus cysts** M

X●O35.04 **Maternal care for (suspected) central nervous system malformation or damage in fetus, encephalocele** M

X●O35.05 **Maternal care for (suspected) central nervous system malformation or damage in fetus, holoprosencephaly** M

X●O35.06 **Maternal care for (suspected) central nervous system malformation or damage in fetus, hydrocephaly** M

Maternal care for fetal hydrocephalus

X●O35.07 **Maternal care for (suspected) central nervous system malformation or damage in fetus, microcephaly** M

X●O35.08 **Maternal care for (suspected) central nervous system malformation or damage in fetus, spina bifida** M

X●O35.09 **Maternal care for (suspected) other central nervous system malformation or damage in Fetus** M

X●O35.1 Maternal care for (suspected) chromosomal abnormality in fetus M

X●O35.10 **Maternal care for (suspected) chromosomal abnormality in fetus, unspecified** M

X●O35.11 **Maternal care for (suspected) chromosomal abnormality in fetus, Trisomy 13** M

X●O35.12 **Maternal care for (suspected) chromosomal abnormality in fetus, Trisomy 18** M

X●O35.13 **Maternal care for (suspected) chromosomal abnormality in fetus, Trisomy 21** M

X●O35.14 **Maternal care for (suspected) chromosomal abnormality in fetus, Turner Syndrome** M

X●O35.15 **Maternal care for (suspected) chromosomal abnormality in fetus, sex chromosome Abnormality** M

X●O35.19 **Maternal care for (suspected) chromosomal abnormality in fetus, other chromosomal abnormality** M

X●O35.2 Maternal care for (suspected) hereditary disease in fetus M

Excludes2 chromosomal abnormality in fetus (O35.1-)

X●O35.3 Maternal care for (suspected) damage to fetus from viral disease in mother M

Maternal care for damage to fetus from maternal cytomegalovirus infection

Maternal care for damage to fetus from maternal rubella

Coding Clinic: 2016, Q4, P6

X●O35.4 Maternal care for (suspected) damage to fetus from alcohol M

X●O35.5 Maternal care for (suspected) damage to fetus by drugs M

Maternal care for damage to fetus from drug addiction

X●O35.6 Maternal care for (suspected) damage to fetus by radiation M

X●O35.7 Maternal care for (suspected) damage to fetus by other medical procedures M

Maternal care for damage to fetus by amniocentesis

Maternal care for damage to fetus by biopsy procedures

Maternal care for damage to fetus by hematological investigation

Maternal care for damage to fetus by intrauterine contraceptive device

Maternal care for damage to fetus by intrauterine surgery

X●O35.8 Maternal care for other (suspected) fetal abnormality and damage M

Maternal care for damage to fetus from maternal listeriosis

Maternal care for damage to fetus from maternal toxoplasmosis

X●O35.9 Maternal care for (suspected) fetal abnormality and damage, unspecified M

X●O35.A Maternal care for other (suspected) fetal abnormality and damage, fetal facial anomalies M

X●O35.B Maternal care for other (suspected) fetal abnormality and damage, fetal cardiac anomalies M

X● O35.C Maternal care for other (suspected) fetal abnormality and damage, fetal pulmonary anomalies M

X● O35.D Maternal care for other (suspected) fetal abnormality and damage, fetal gastrointestinal anomalies M

X● O35.E Maternal care for other (suspected) fetal abnormality and damage, fetal genitourinary anomalies M

X● O35.F Maternal care for other (suspected) fetal abnormality and damage, fetal musculoskeletal anomalies of trunk M

Excludes2 maternal care for other (suspected) fetal abnormality and damage, fetal lower extremities anomalies (O35.H)
maternal care for other (suspected) fetal abnormality and damage, fetal upper extremities anomalies (O35.G)

X● O35.G Maternal care for other (suspected) fetal abnormality and damage, fetal upper extremities anomalies M

X● O35.H Maternal care for other (suspected) fetal abnormality and damage, fetal lower extremities Anomalies M

OGCR Section I.C.15.e.l.

Fetal Conditions Affecting the Management of the Mother

1) Code from categories O35 and O36

Codes from categories O35, Maternal care for known or suspected fetal abnormality and damage, and O36, Maternal care for other fetal problems, are assigned only when the fetal condition is actually responsible for modifying the management of the mother, i.e., by requiring diagnostic studies, additional observation, special care, or termination of pregnancy. The fact that the fetal condition exists does not justify assigning a code from this series to the mother's record.

2) In utero surgery

In cases when surgery is performed on the fetus, a diagnosis code from category O35, Maternal care for known or suspected fetal abnormality and damage, should be assigned identifying the fetal condition. Assign the appropriate procedure code for the procedure performed.

No code from Chapter 16, the perinatal codes, should be used on the mother's record to identify fetal conditions. Surgery performed in utero on a fetus is still to be coded as an obstetric encounter.

● O36 Maternal care for other fetal problems

Includes the listed conditions in the fetus as a reason for hospitalization or other obstetric care of the mother, or for termination of pregnancy

Excludes1 encounter for suspected maternal and fetal conditions ruled out (Z03.7-)
placental transfusion syndromes (O43.0-)

Excludes2 labor and delivery complicated by fetal stress (O77.-)

One of the following 7th characters is to be assigned to each code under category O36. 7th character 0 is for single gestations and multiple gestations where the fetus is unspecified. 7th characters 1 through 9 are for cases of multiple gestations to identify the fetus for which the code applies. The appropriate code from category O30, Multiple gestation, must also be assigned when assigning a code from category O36 that has a 7th character of 1 through 9.

0	not applicable or unspecified
1	fetus 1
2	fetus 2
3	fetus 3
4	fetus 4
5	fetus 5
9	other fetus

Coding Clinic: 2015, Q3, P40

● O36.0 Maternal care for rhesus isoimmunization (Ex) PDX 1428
Maternal care for Rh incompatibility (with hydrops fetalis)

● O36.01 Maternal care for anti-D [Rh] antibodies

● O36.011 Maternal care for anti-D [Rh] antibodies, first trimester M

● O36.012 Maternal care for anti-D [Rh] antibodies, second trimester M

● O36.013 Maternal care for anti-D [Rh] antibodies, third trimester M

● O36.019 Maternal care for anti-D [Rh] antibodies, unspecified trimester M

● O36.09 Maternal care for other rhesus isoimmunization

● O36.091 Maternal care for other rhesus isoimmunization, first trimester M

● O36.092 Maternal care for other rhesus isoimmunization, second trimester M

● O36.093 Maternal care for other rhesus isoimmunization, third trimester M
Coding Clinic: 2015, Q3, P40

● O36.099 Maternal care for other rhesus isoimmunization, unspecified trimester M

● O36.1 Maternal care for other isoimmunization
Maternal care for ABO isoimmunization

● O36.11 Maternal care for Anti-A sensitization
Maternal care for isoimmunization NOS (with hydrops fetalis)

● O36.111 Maternal care for Anti-A sensitization, first trimester M

● O36.112 Maternal care for Anti-A sensitization, second trimester M

● O36.113 Maternal care for Anti-A sensitization, third trimester M

● O36.119 Maternal care for Anti-A sensitization, unspecified trimester M

● O36.19 Maternal care for other isoimmunization
Maternal care for Anti-B sensitization

● O36.191 Maternal care for other isoimmunization, first trimester M

● O36.192 Maternal care for other isoimmunization, second trimester M

● O36.193 Maternal care for other isoimmunization, third trimester M

● O36.199 Maternal care for other isoimmunization, unspecified trimester M

● O36.2 Maternal care for hydrops fetalis
Maternal care for hydrops fetalis NOS
Maternal care for hydrops fetalis not associated with isoimmunization

Excludes1 hydrops fetalis associated with ABO isoimmunization (O36.1-)
hydrops fetalis associated with rhesus isoimmunization (O36.0-)

● O36.20 Maternal care for hydrops fetalis, unspecified trimester M

● O36.21 Maternal care for hydrops fetalis, first trimester M

● O36.22 Maternal care for hydrops fetalis, second trimester M

● O36.23 Maternal care for hydrops fetalis, third trimester M

● O36.4 Maternal care for intrauterine death (Ex) PDX 1429 M
Maternal care for intrauterine fetal death NOS
Maternal care for intrauterine fetal death after completion of 20 weeks of gestation
Maternal care for late fetal death
Maternal care for missed delivery

Excludes1 missed abortion (O02.1)
stillbirth (P95)

Coding Clinic: 2022, Q2, P3-4

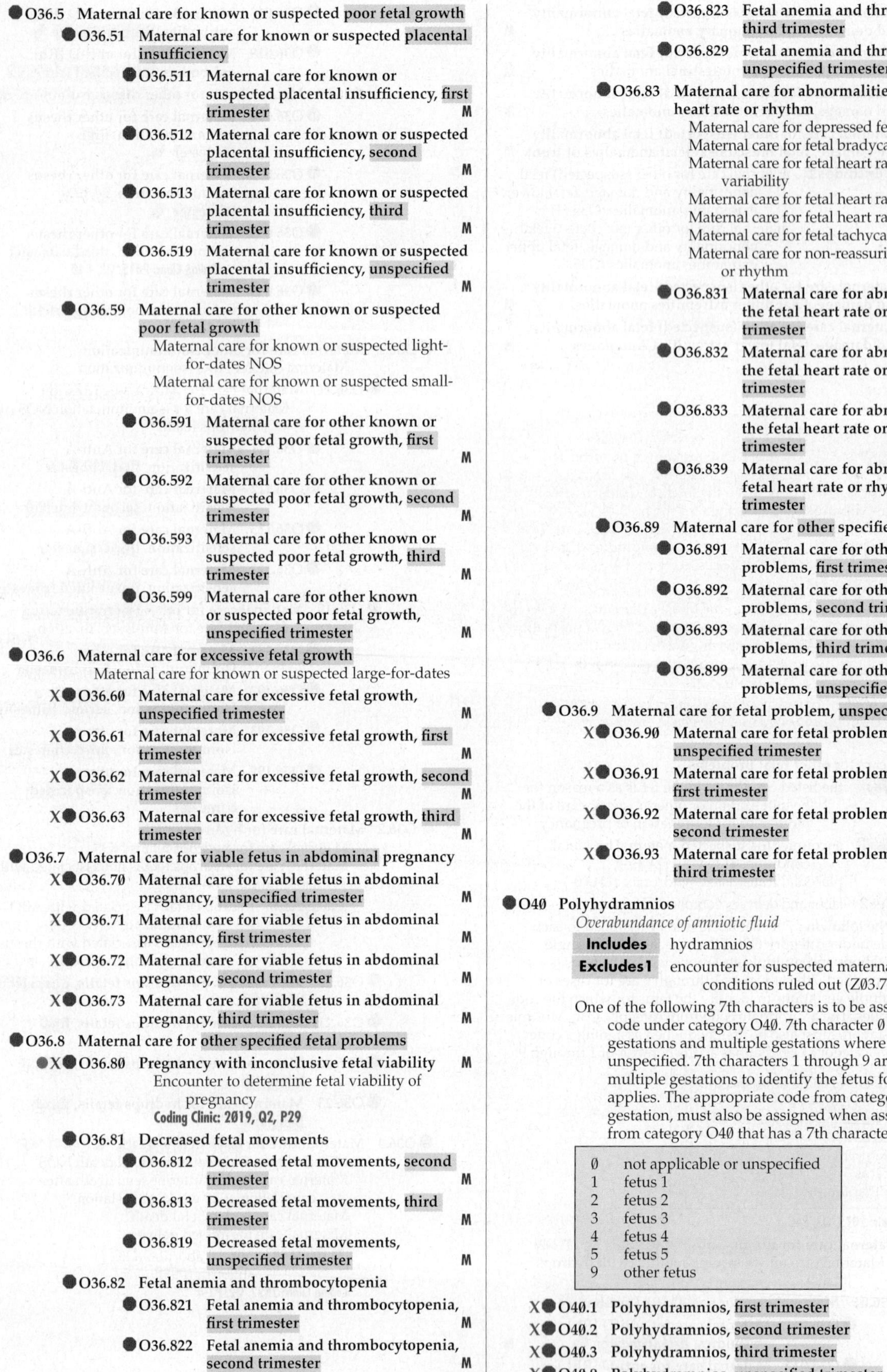

- O36.5 Maternal care for known or suspected poor fetal growth
  - O36.51 Maternal care for known or suspected placental insufficiency
    - O36.511 Maternal care for known or suspected placental insufficiency, first trimester M
    - O36.512 Maternal care for known or suspected placental insufficiency, second trimester M
    - O36.513 Maternal care for known or suspected placental insufficiency, third trimester M
    - O36.519 Maternal care for known or suspected placental insufficiency, unspecified trimester M
  - O36.59 Maternal care for other known or suspected poor fetal growth
    - Maternal care for known or suspected light-for-dates NOS
    - Maternal care for known or suspected small-for-dates NOS
    - O36.591 Maternal care for other known or suspected poor fetal growth, first trimester M
    - O36.592 Maternal care for other known or suspected poor fetal growth, second trimester M
    - O36.593 Maternal care for other known or suspected poor fetal growth, third trimester M
    - O36.599 Maternal care for other known or suspected poor fetal growth, unspecified trimester M
- O36.6 Maternal care for excessive fetal growth
  - Maternal care for known or suspected large-for-dates
  - X O36.60 Maternal care for excessive fetal growth, unspecified trimester M
  - X O36.61 Maternal care for excessive fetal growth, first trimester M
  - X O36.62 Maternal care for excessive fetal growth, second trimester M
  - X O36.63 Maternal care for excessive fetal growth, third trimester M
- O36.7 Maternal care for viable fetus in abdominal pregnancy
  - X O36.70 Maternal care for viable fetus in abdominal pregnancy, unspecified trimester M
  - X O36.71 Maternal care for viable fetus in abdominal pregnancy, first trimester M
  - X O36.72 Maternal care for viable fetus in abdominal pregnancy, second trimester M
  - X O36.73 Maternal care for viable fetus in abdominal pregnancy, third trimester M
- O36.8 Maternal care for other specified fetal problems
  - X O36.80 Pregnancy with inconclusive fetal viability M
    - Encounter to determine fetal viability of pregnancy
    - Coding Clinic: 2019, Q2, P29
  - O36.81 Decreased fetal movements
    - O36.812 Decreased fetal movements, second trimester M
    - O36.813 Decreased fetal movements, third trimester M
    - O36.819 Decreased fetal movements, unspecified trimester M
  - O36.82 Fetal anemia and thrombocytopenia
    - O36.821 Fetal anemia and thrombocytopenia, first trimester M
    - O36.822 Fetal anemia and thrombocytopenia, second trimester M
    - O36.823 Fetal anemia and thrombocytopenia, third trimester M
    - O36.829 Fetal anemia and thrombocytopenia, unspecified trimester M
  - O36.83 Maternal care for abnormalities of the fetal heart rate or rhythm
    - Maternal care for depressed fetal heart rate tones
    - Maternal care for fetal bradycardia
    - Maternal care for fetal heart rate abnormal variability
    - Maternal care for fetal heart rate decelerations
    - Maternal care for fetal heart rate irregularity
    - Maternal care for fetal tachycardia
    - Maternal care for non-reassuring fetal heart rate or rhythm
    - O36.831 Maternal care for abnormalities of the fetal heart rate or rhythm, first trimester M
    - O36.832 Maternal care for abnormalities of the fetal heart rate or rhythm, second trimester M
    - O36.833 Maternal care for abnormalities of the fetal heart rate or rhythm, third trimester M
    - O36.839 Maternal care for abnormalities of the fetal heart rate or rhythm, unspecified trimester M
  - O36.89 Maternal care for other specified fetal problems
    - O36.891 Maternal care for other specified fetal problems, first trimester M
    - O36.892 Maternal care for other specified fetal problems, second trimester M
    - O36.893 Maternal care for other specified fetal problems, third trimester M
    - O36.899 Maternal care for other specified fetal problems, unspecified trimester M
- O36.9 Maternal care for fetal problem, unspecified
  - X O36.90 Maternal care for fetal problem, unspecified, unspecified trimester M
  - X O36.91 Maternal care for fetal problem, unspecified, first trimester M
  - X O36.92 Maternal care for fetal problem, unspecified, second trimester M
  - X O36.93 Maternal care for fetal problem, unspecified, third trimester M

O40 Polyhydramnios

Overabundance of amniotic fluid

Includes hydramnios

Excludes1 encounter for suspected maternal and fetal conditions ruled out (Z03.7-)

One of the following 7th characters is to be assigned to each code under category O40. 7th character 0 is for single gestations and multiple gestations where the fetus is unspecified. 7th characters 1 through 9 are for cases of multiple gestations to identify the fetus for which the code applies. The appropriate code from category O30, Multiple gestation, must also be assigned when assigning a code from category O40 that has a 7th character of 1 through 9.

0	not applicable or unspecified
1	fetus 1
2	fetus 2
3	fetus 3
4	fetus 4
5	fetus 5
9	other fetus

- X O40.1 Polyhydramnios, first trimester M
- X O40.2 Polyhydramnios, second trimester M
- X O40.3 Polyhydramnios, third trimester M
- X O40.9 Polyhydramnios, unspecified trimester M

CHAPTER 15 (O00-O9A)

O41 Other disorders of amniotic fluid and membranes

Excludes1 encounter for suspected maternal and fetal conditions ruled out (Z03.7-)

One of the following 7th characters is to be assigned to each code under category O41. 7th character 0 is for single gestations and multiple gestations where the fetus is unspecified. 7th characters 1 through 9 are for cases of multiple gestations to identify the fetus for which the code applies. The appropriate code from category O30, Multiple gestation, must also be assigned when assigning a code from category O41 that has a 7th character of 1 through 9.

0	not applicable or unspecified
1	fetus 1
2	fetus 2
3	fetus 3
4	fetus 4
5	fetus 5
9	other fetus

O41.0 Oligohydramnios (Ex) PDX 1430
Scant volume of amniotic fluid
Oligohydramnios without rupture of membranes

X **O41.00** Oligohydramnios, unspecified trimester M
X **O41.01** Oligohydramnios, first trimester M
X **O41.02** Oligohydramnios, second trimester M
X **O41.03** Oligohydramnios, third trimester M

O41.1 Infection of amniotic sac and membranes (Ex) PDX 1431

O41.10 Infection of amniotic sac and membranes, unspecified
O41.101 Infection of amniotic sac and membranes, unspecified, first trimester M
O41.102 Infection of amniotic sac and membranes, unspecified, second trimester M
O41.103 Infection of amniotic sac and membranes, unspecified, third trimester M
O41.109 Infection of amniotic sac and membranes, unspecified, unspecified trimester M

O41.12 Chorioamnionitis
Coding Clinic: 2019, Q2, P34-35
O41.121 Chorioamnionitis, first trimester M
O41.122 Chorioamnionitis, second trimester M
O41.123 Chorioamnionitis, third trimester M
O41.129 Chorioamnionitis, unspecified trimester M

O41.14 Placentitis
O41.141 Placentitis, first trimester M
O41.142 Placentitis, second trimester M
O41.143 Placentitis, third trimester M
O41.149 Placentitis, unspecified trimester M

O41.8 Other specified disorders of amniotic fluid and membranes

O41.8X Other specified disorders of amniotic fluid and membranes
O41.8X1 Other specified disorders of amniotic fluid and membranes, first trimester M
O41.8X2 Other specified disorders of amniotic fluid and membranes, second trimester M
O41.8X3 Other specified disorders of amniotic fluid and membranes, third trimester M
Coding Clinic: 2024, Q1, P14
O41.8X9 Other specified disorders of amniotic fluid and membranes, unspecified trimester M

O41.9 Disorder of amniotic fluid and membranes, unspecified

X **O41.90** Disorder of amniotic fluid and membranes, unspecified, unspecified trimester M
X **O41.91** Disorder of amniotic fluid and membranes, unspecified, first trimester M
X **O41.92** Disorder of amniotic fluid and membranes, unspecified, second trimester M
X **O41.93** Disorder of amniotic fluid and membranes, unspecified, third trimester M

O42 Premature rupture of membranes
Coding Clinic: 2023, Q3, P17

O42.0 Premature rupture of membranes, onset of labor within 24 hours of rupture

O42.00 Premature rupture of membranes, onset of labor within 24 hours of rupture, unspecified weeks of gestation M

O42.01 Preterm premature rupture of membranes, onset of labor within 24 hours of rupture
Premature rupture of membranes before 37 completed weeks of gestation
O42.011 Preterm premature rupture of membranes, onset of labor within 24 hours of rupture, first trimester M
O42.012 Preterm premature rupture of membranes, onset of labor within 24 hours of rupture, second trimester M
O42.013 Preterm premature rupture of membranes, onset of labor within 24 hours of rupture, third trimester M
O42.019 Preterm premature rupture of membranes, onset of labor within 24 hours of rupture, unspecified trimester M

O42.02 Full-term premature rupture of membranes, onset of labor within 24 hours of rupture M
Premature rupture of membranes at or after 37 completed weeks of gestation, onset of labor within 24 hours of rupture

O42.1 Premature rupture of membranes, onset of labor more than 24 hours following rupture

O42.10 Premature rupture of membranes, onset of labor more than 24 hours following rupture, unspecified weeks of gestation M

O42.11 Preterm premature rupture of membranes, onset of labor more than 24 hours following rupture
Premature rupture of membranes before 37 completed weeks of gestation
O42.111 Preterm premature rupture of membranes, onset of labor more than 24 hours following rupture, first trimester M
O42.112 Preterm premature rupture of membranes, onset of labor more than 24 hours following rupture, second trimester M
O42.113 Preterm premature rupture of membranes, onset of labor more than 24 hours following rupture, third trimester M
O42.119 Preterm premature rupture of membranes, onset of labor more than 24 hours following rupture, unspecified trimester M

O42.12 Full-term premature rupture of membranes, onset of labor more than 24 hours following rupture M
Premature rupture of membranes at or after 37 completed weeks of gestation, onset of labor more than 24 hours following rupture

O42.9 Premature rupture of membranes, unspecified as to length of time between rupture and onset of labor

O42.90 Premature rupture of membranes, unspecified as to length of time between rupture and onset of labor, unspecified weeks of gestation M

O42.91 Preterm premature rupture of membranes, unspecified as to length of time between rupture and onset of labor

Premature rupture of membranes before 37 completed weeks of gestation

O42.911 Preterm premature rupture of membranes, unspecified as to length of time between rupture and onset of labor, first trimester M

O42.912 Preterm premature rupture of membranes, unspecified as to length of time between rupture and onset of labor, second trimester M

O42.913 Preterm premature rupture of membranes, unspecified as to length of time between rupture and onset of labor, third trimester M

O42.919 Preterm premature rupture of membranes, unspecified as to length of time between rupture and onset of labor, unspecified trimester M

O42.92 Full-term premature rupture of membranes, unspecified as to length of time between rupture and onset of labor M

Premature rupture of membranes at or after 37 completed weeks of gestation, unspecified as to length of time between rupture and onset of labor

O43 Placental disorders

Excludes2 maternal care for poor fetal growth due to placental insufficiency (O36.5-)
placenta previa (O44.-)
placental polyp (O90.89)
placentitis (O41.14-)
premature separation of placenta [abruptio placentae] (O45.-)

O43.0 Placental transfusion syndromes

O43.01 Fetomaternal placental transfusion syndrome

Maternofetal placental transfusion syndrome

O43.011 Fetomaternal placental transfusion syndrome, first trimester M

O43.012 Fetomaternal placental transfusion syndrome, second trimester M

O43.013 Fetomaternal placental transfusion syndrome, third trimester M

O43.019 Fetomaternal placental transfusion syndrome, unspecified trimester M

O43.02 Fetus-to-fetus placental transfusion syndrome

O43.021 Fetus-to-fetus placental transfusion syndrome, first trimester M

O43.022 Fetus-to-fetus placental transfusion syndrome, second trimester M

O43.023 Fetus-to-fetus placental transfusion syndrome, third trimester M

O43.029 Fetus-to-fetus placental transfusion syndrome, unspecified trimester M

O43.1 Malformation of placenta

O43.10 Malformation of placenta, unspecified

Abnormal placenta NOS

O43.101 Malformation of placenta, unspecified, first trimester M

O43.102 Malformation of placenta, unspecified, second trimester M

O43.103 Malformation of placenta, unspecified, third trimester M

O43.109 Malformation of placenta, unspecified, unspecified trimester M

O43.11 Circumvallate placenta

O43.111 Circumvallate placenta, first trimester M

O43.112 Circumvallate placenta, second trimester M

O43.113 Circumvallate placenta, third trimester M

O43.119 Circumvallate placenta, unspecified trimester M

O43.12 Velamentous insertion of umbilical cord

O43.121 Velamentous insertion of umbilical cord, first trimester M

O43.122 Velamentous insertion of umbilical cord, second trimester M

O43.123 Velamentous insertion of umbilical cord, third trimester M

O43.129 Velamentous insertion of umbilical cord, unspecified trimester M

O43.19 Other malformation of placenta

O43.191 Other malformation of placenta, first trimester M

O43.192 Other malformation of placenta, second trimester M

O43.193 Other malformation of placenta, third trimester M

O43.199 Other malformation of placenta, unspecified trimester M

O43.2 Morbidly adherent placenta

Code also associated third stage postpartum hemorrhage, if applicable (O72.0)

Excludes1 retained placenta (O73.-)

O43.21 Placenta accreta

O43.211 Placenta accreta, first trimester M

O43.212 Placenta accreta, second trimester M

O43.213 Placenta accreta, third trimester M

O43.219 Placenta accreta, unspecified trimester M

O43.22 Placenta increta

O43.221 Placenta increta, first trimester M

O43.222 Placenta increta, second trimester M

Coding Clinic: 2022, Q1, P21

O43.223 Placenta increta, third trimester M

O43.229 Placenta increta, unspecified trimester M

O43.23 Placenta percreta

O43.231 Placenta percreta, first trimester M

O43.232 Placenta percreta, second trimester M

O43.233 Placenta percreta, third trimester M

O43.239 Placenta percreta, unspecified trimester M

O43.8 Other placental disorders

O43.81 Placental infarction

O43.811 Placental infarction, first trimester M

O43.812 Placental infarction, second trimester M

O43.813 Placental infarction, third trimester M

O43.819 Placental infarction, unspecified trimester M

O43.89 Other placental disorders

Placental dysfunction

O43.891 Other placental disorders, first trimester M

O43.892 Other placental disorders, second trimester M

O43.893 Other placental disorders, third trimester M

O43.899 Other placental disorders, unspecified trimester M

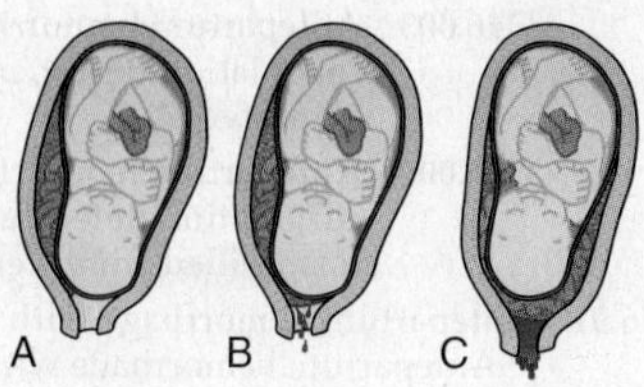

Figure 15-2 **A.** Marginal placento previa. **B.** Partial placenta previa. **C.** Total placento previa.

Item 15-3 **Placenta previa** is a condition in which the opening of the cervix is obstructed by the displaced placenta. The three types, marginal, partial, and total, are varying degrees of placenta displacement. Placenta abruption is the premature breaking away of the placenta from the site of the uterine implant before the delivery of the fetus.

● **O43.9** **Unspecified placental disorder**
- **O43.90** **Unspecified placental disorder, unspecified trimester** M
- **O43.91** **Unspecified placental disorder, first trimester** M
- **O43.92** **Unspecified placental disorder, second trimester** M
- **O43.93** **Unspecified placental disorder, third trimester** M

● **O44** **Placenta previa** (Ex) PDX 1417
Coding Clinic: 2016, Q4, P52

● **O44.0** **Complete placenta previa NOS or without hemorrhage**
Placenta previa NOS
- **O44.00** **Complete placenta previa NOS or without hemorrhage, unspecified trimester** M
- **O44.01** **Complete placenta previa NOS or without hemorrhage, first trimester** M
- **O44.02** **Complete placenta previa NOS or without hemorrhage, second trimester** M
- **O44.03** **Complete placenta previa NOS or without hemorrhage, third trimester** M

● **O44.1** **Complete placenta previa with hemorrhage**
Excludes1 labor and delivery complicated by hemorrhage from vasa previa (O69.4)
- **O44.10** **Complete placenta previa with hemorrhage, unspecified trimester** M
- **O44.11** **Complete placenta previa with hemorrhage, first trimester** M
- **O44.12** **Complete placenta previa with hemorrhage, second trimester** M
- **O44.13** **Complete placenta previa with hemorrhage, third trimester** M

● **O44.2** **Partial placenta previa without hemorrhage**
Marginal placenta previa, NOS or without hemorrhage
- **O44.20** **Partial placenta previa NOS or without hemorrhage, unspecified trimester** M
- **O44.21** **Partial placenta previa NOS or without hemorrhage, first trimester** M
- **O44.22** **Partial placenta previa NOS or without hemorrhage, second trimester** M
- **O44.23** **Partial placenta previa NOS or without hemorrhage, third trimester** M

● **O44.3** **Partial placenta previa with hemorrhage**
Marginal placenta previa with hemorrhage
- **O44.30** **Partial placenta previa with hemorrhage, unspecified trimester** M
- **O44.31** **Partial placenta previa with hemorrhage, first trimester** M
- **O44.32** **Partial placenta previa with hemorrhage, second trimester** M
- **O44.33** **Partial placenta previa with hemorrhage, third trimester** M

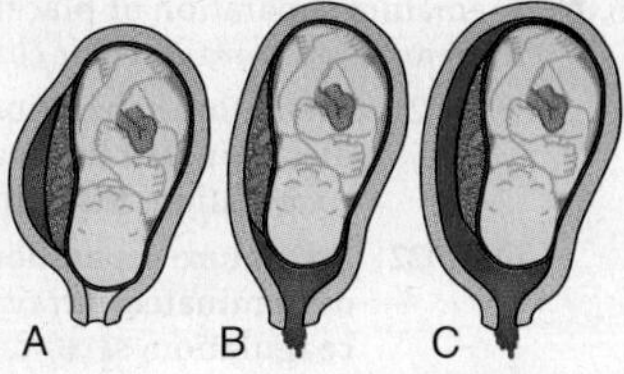

Figure 15-3 Abruptio placentae is classified according to the grade of separation of the placenta from the uterine wall. **A.** Mild separation in which hemorrhage is internal. **B.** Moderate separation in which there is external hemorrhage. **C.** Severe separation in which there is external hemorrhage and extreme separation.

● **O44.4** **Low lying placenta NOS or without hemorrhage**
Low implantation of placenta NOS or without hemorrhage
- **O44.40** **Low lying placenta NOS or without hemorrhage, unspecified trimester** M
- **O44.41** **Low lying placenta NOS or without hemorrhage, first trimester** M
- **O44.42** **Low lying placenta NOS or without hemorrhage, second trimester** M
- **O44.43** **Low lying placenta NOS or without hemorrhage, third trimester** M

● **O44.5** **Low lying placenta with hemorrhage**
Low implantation of placenta with hemorrhage
- **O44.50** **Low lying placenta with hemorrhage, unspecified trimester** M
- **O44.51** **Low lying placenta with hemorrhage, first trimester** M
- **O44.52** **Low lying placenta with hemorrhage, second trimester** M
- **O44.53** **Low lying placenta with hemorrhage, third trimester** M

● **O45** **Premature separation of placenta [abruptio placentae]**

● **O45.0** **Premature separation of placenta with coagulation defect** (Ex) PDX 1432

● **O45.00** **Premature separation of placenta with coagulation defect, unspecified**
- **O45.001** **Premature separation of placenta with coagulation defect, unspecified, first trimester** M
- **O45.002** **Premature separation of placenta with coagulation defect, unspecified, second trimester** M
- **O45.003** **Premature separation of placenta with coagulation defect, unspecified, third trimester** M
- **O45.009** **Premature separation of placenta with coagulation defect, unspecified, unspecified trimester** M

● **O45.01** **Premature separation of placenta with afibrinogenemia**
Premature separation of placenta with hypofibrinogenemia
- **O45.011** **Premature separation of placenta with afibrinogenemia, first trimester** M
- **O45.012** **Premature separation of placenta with afibrinogenemia, second trimester** M
- **O45.013** **Premature separation of placenta with afibrinogenemia, third trimester** M
- **O45.019** **Premature separation of placenta with afibrinogenemia, unspecified trimester** M

CHAPTER 15 (O00-O9A)

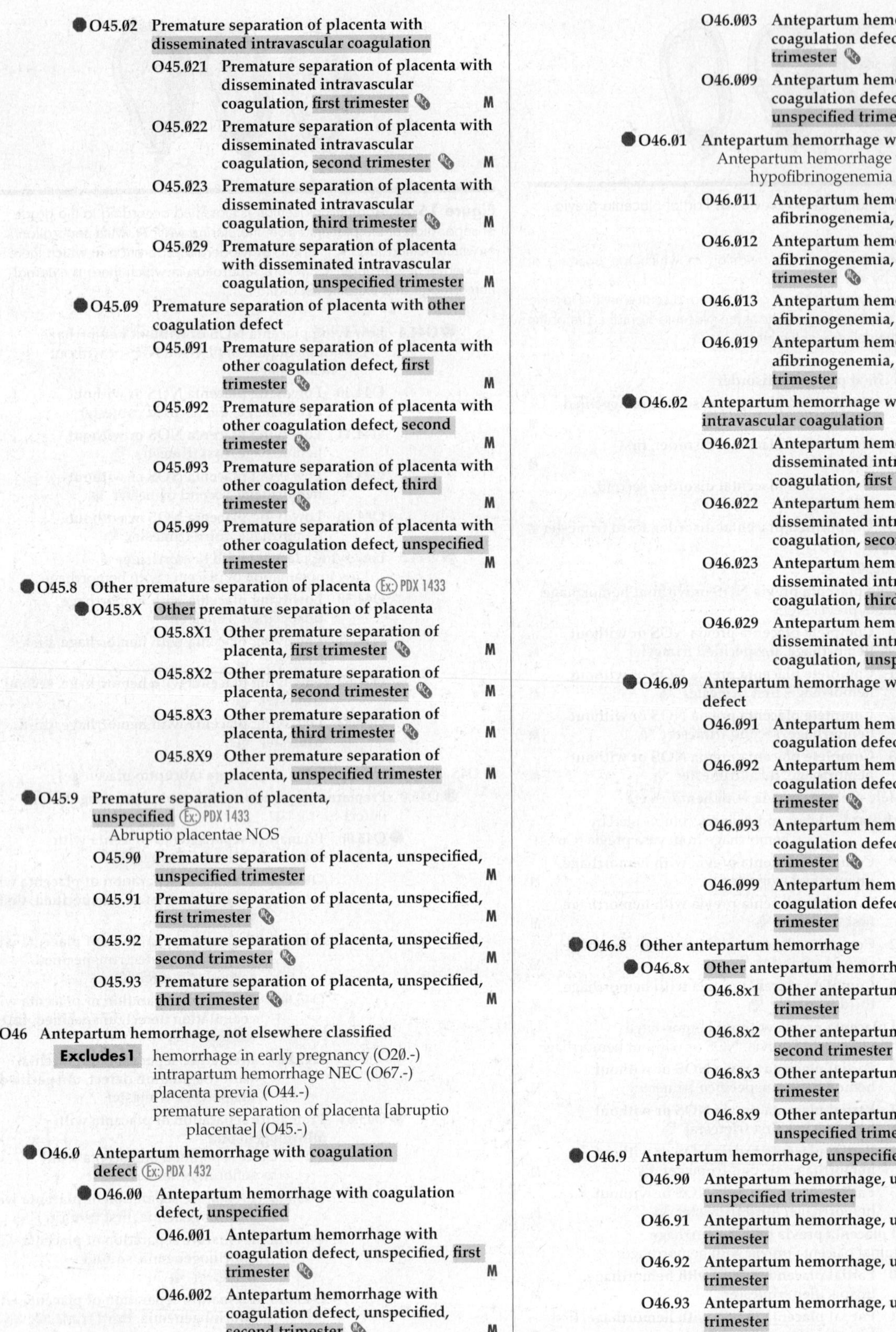

● O45.02 Premature separation of placenta with disseminated intravascular coagulation
- O45.021 Premature separation of placenta with disseminated intravascular coagulation, first trimester M
- O45.022 Premature separation of placenta with disseminated intravascular coagulation, second trimester M
- O45.023 Premature separation of placenta with disseminated intravascular coagulation, third trimester M
- O45.029 Premature separation of placenta with disseminated intravascular coagulation, unspecified trimester M

● O45.09 Premature separation of placenta with other coagulation defect
- O45.091 Premature separation of placenta with other coagulation defect, first trimester M
- O45.092 Premature separation of placenta with other coagulation defect, second trimester M
- O45.093 Premature separation of placenta with other coagulation defect, third trimester M
- O45.099 Premature separation of placenta with other coagulation defect, unspecified trimester M

● O45.8 Other premature separation of placenta Ex: PDX 1433

● O45.8X Other premature separation of placenta
- O45.8X1 Other premature separation of placenta, first trimester M
- O45.8X2 Other premature separation of placenta, second trimester M
- O45.8X3 Other premature separation of placenta, third trimester M
- O45.8X9 Other premature separation of placenta, unspecified trimester M

● O45.9 Premature separation of placenta, unspecified Ex: PDX 1433
Abruptio placentae NOS
- O45.90 Premature separation of placenta, unspecified, unspecified trimester M
- O45.91 Premature separation of placenta, unspecified, first trimester M
- O45.92 Premature separation of placenta, unspecified, second trimester M
- O45.93 Premature separation of placenta, unspecified, third trimester M

● O46 Antepartum hemorrhage, not elsewhere classified

Excludes1 hemorrhage in early pregnancy (O20.-)
intrapartum hemorrhage NEC (O67.-)
placenta previa (O44.-)
premature separation of placenta [abruptio placentae] (O45.-)

● O46.0 Antepartum hemorrhage with coagulation defect Ex: PDX 1432

● O46.00 Antepartum hemorrhage with coagulation defect, unspecified
- O46.001 Antepartum hemorrhage with coagulation defect, unspecified, first trimester M
- O46.002 Antepartum hemorrhage with coagulation defect, unspecified, second trimester M
- O46.003 Antepartum hemorrhage with coagulation defect, unspecified, third trimester M
- O46.009 Antepartum hemorrhage with coagulation defect, unspecified, unspecified trimester M

● O46.01 Antepartum hemorrhage with afibrinogenemia
Antepartum hemorrhage with hypofibrinogenemia
- O46.011 Antepartum hemorrhage with afibrinogenemia, first trimester M
- O46.012 Antepartum hemorrhage with afibrinogenemia, second trimester M
- O46.013 Antepartum hemorrhage with afibrinogenemia, third trimester M
- O46.019 Antepartum hemorrhage with afibrinogenemia, unspecified trimester M

● O46.02 Antepartum hemorrhage with disseminated intravascular coagulation
- O46.021 Antepartum hemorrhage with disseminated intravascular coagulation, first trimester M
- O46.022 Antepartum hemorrhage with disseminated intravascular coagulation, second trimester M
- O46.023 Antepartum hemorrhage with disseminated intravascular coagulation, third trimester M
- O46.029 Antepartum hemorrhage with disseminated intravascular coagulation, unspecified trimester M

● O46.09 Antepartum hemorrhage with other coagulation defect
- O46.091 Antepartum hemorrhage with other coagulation defect, first trimester M
- O46.092 Antepartum hemorrhage with other coagulation defect, second trimester M
- O46.093 Antepartum hemorrhage with other coagulation defect, third trimester M
- O46.099 Antepartum hemorrhage with other coagulation defect, unspecified trimester M

● O46.8 Other antepartum hemorrhage

● O46.8x Other antepartum hemorrhage
- O46.8x1 Other antepartum hemorrhage, first trimester M
- O46.8x2 Other antepartum hemorrhage, second trimester M
- O46.8x3 Other antepartum hemorrhage, third trimester M
- O46.8x9 Other antepartum hemorrhage, unspecified trimester M

● O46.9 Antepartum hemorrhage, unspecified
- O46.90 Antepartum hemorrhage, unspecified, unspecified trimester M
- O46.91 Antepartum hemorrhage, unspecified, first trimester M
- O46.92 Antepartum hemorrhage, unspecified, second trimester M
- O46.93 Antepartum hemorrhage, unspecified, third trimester M

CHAPTER 15 (O00-O9A)

O47 False labor (Ex) PDX 1434
Includes Braxton Hicks contractions
threatened labor
Excludes1 preterm labor (O60.-)

O47.0 False labor before 37 completed weeks of gestation
O47.00 False labor before 37 completed weeks of gestation, unspecified trimester M
O47.02 False labor before 37 completed weeks of gestation, second trimester M
O47.03 False labor before 37 completed weeks of gestation, third trimester M

O47.1 False labor at or after 37 completed weeks of gestation M
Coding Clinic: 2021, Q1, P10

O47.9 False labor, unspecified M

O48 Late pregnancy
O48.0 Post-term pregnancy M
Pregnancy over 40 completed weeks to 42 completed weeks gestation
Coding Clinic: 2022, Q2 P3-4

O48.1 Prolonged pregnancy M
Pregnancy which has advanced beyond 42 completed weeks gestation
Coding Clinic: 2022, Q2 P3-4

COMPLICATIONS OF LABOR AND DELIVERY (O60-O77)

O60 Preterm labor (Ex) PDX 1434
Includes onset (spontaneous) of labor before 37 completed weeks of gestation
Excludes1 false labor (O47.0-)
threatened labor NOS (O47.0-)

O60.0 Preterm labor without delivery
O60.00 Preterm labor without delivery, unspecified trimester M
O60.02 Preterm labor without delivery, second trimester M
O60.03 Preterm labor without delivery, third trimester M

O60.1 Preterm labor with preterm delivery
One of the following 7th characters is to be assigned to each code under subcategory O60.1. 7th character 0 is for single gestations and multiple gestations where the fetus is unspecified. 7th characters 1 through 9 are for cases of multiple gestations to identify the fetus for which the code applies. The appropriate code from category O30, Multiple gestation, must also be assigned when assigning a code from subcategory O60.1 that has a 7th character of 1 through 9.

0	not applicable or unspecified
1	fetus 1
2	fetus 2
3	fetus 3
4	fetus 4
5	fetus 5
9	other fetus

Coding Clinic: 2016, Q2, P11

X **O60.10 Preterm labor with preterm delivery, unspecified trimester** M
Preterm labor with delivery NOS
X **O60.12 Preterm labor second trimester with preterm delivery second trimester** M
X **O60.13 Preterm labor second trimester with preterm delivery third trimester** M
X **O60.14 Preterm labor third trimester with preterm delivery third trimester** M
Coding Clinic: 2016, Q2, P10

O60.2 Term delivery with preterm labor
One of the following 7th characters is to be assigned to each code under subcategory O60.2. 7th character 0 is for single gestations and multiple gestations where the fetus is unspecified. 7th characters 1 through 9 are for cases of multiple gestations to identify the fetus for which the code applies. The appropriate code from category O30, Multiple gestation, must also be assigned when assigning a code from subcategory O60.2 that has a 7th character of 1 through 9.

0	not applicable or unspecified
1	fetus 1
2	fetus 2
3	fetus 3
4	fetus 4
5	fetus 5
9	other fetus

X **O60.20 Term delivery with preterm labor, unspecified trimester** M
X **O60.22 Term delivery with preterm labor, second trimester** M
X **O60.23 Term delivery with preterm labor, third trimester** M

O61 Failed induction of labor
O61.0 Failed medical induction of labor M
Failed induction (of labor) by oxytocin
Failed induction (of labor) by prostaglandins
O61.1 Failed instrumental induction of labor M
Failed mechanical induction (of labor)
Failed surgical induction (of labor)
O61.8 Other failed induction of labor M
O61.9 Failed induction of labor, unspecified M

O62 Abnormalities of forces of labor
O62.0 Primary inadequate contractions M
Failure of cervical dilatation
Primary hypotonic uterine dysfunction
Uterine inertia during latent phase of labor
Coding Clinic: 2024, Q1, P13
O62.1 Secondary uterine inertia M
Arrested active phase of labor
Secondary hypotonic uterine dysfunction
O62.2 Other uterine inertia M
Atony of uterus without hemorrhage
Atony of uterus NOS
Desultory labor
Hypotonic uterine dysfunction NOS
Irregular labor
Poor contractions
Slow slope active phase of labor
Uterine inertia NOS
Excludes1 atony of uterus with hemorrhage (postpartum) (O72.1)
postpartum atony of uterus without hemorrhage (O75.89)
O62.3 Precipitate labor M
O62.4 Hypertonic, incoordinate, and prolonged uterine contractions M
Cervical spasm
Contraction ring dystocia
Dyscoordinate labor
Hour-glass contraction of uterus
Hypertonic uterine dysfunction
Incoordinate uterine action
Tetanic contractions
Uterine dystocia NOS
Uterine spasm
Excludes1 dystocia (fetal) (maternal) NOS (O66.9)
O62.8 Other abnormalities of forces of labor M
O62.9 Abnormality of forces of labor, unspecified M

CHAPTER 15 (O00-O9A)

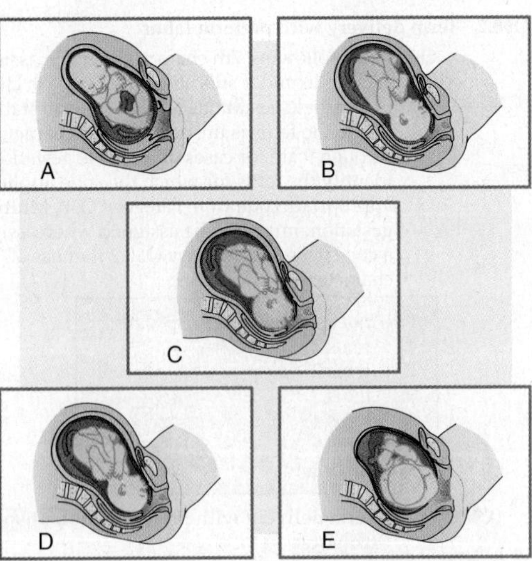

Figure 15-4 Five types of malposition and malpresentation of the fetus: **A.** Breech. **B.** Vertex. **C.** Face. **D.** Brow. **E.** Shoulder.

● **O63 Long labor**

O63.0 Prolonged first stage (of labor) M

O63.1 Prolonged second stage (of labor) M

O63.2 Delayed delivery of second twin, triplet, etc. M

O63.9 Long labor, unspecified (Ex) PDX 1435 M
Prolonged labor NOS

● **O64 Obstructed labor due to malposition and malpresentation of fetus**

One of the following 7th characters is to be assigned to each code under category O64. 7th character 0 is for single gestations and multiple gestations where the fetus is unspecified. 7th characters 1 through 9 are for cases of multiple gestations to identify the fetus for which the code applies. The appropriate code from category O30, Multiple gestation, must also be assigned when assigning a code from category O64 that has a 7th character of 1 through 9.

0	not applicable or unspecified
1	fetus 1
2	fetus 2
3	fetus 3
4	fetus 4
5	fetus 5
9	other fetus

X● **O64.0 Obstructed labor due to incomplete rotation of fetal head** M
Deep transverse arrest
Obstructed labor due to persistent occipitoiliac (position)
Obstructed labor due to persistent occipitoposterior (position)
Obstructed labor due to persistent occipitosacral (position)
Obstructed labor due to persistent occipitotransverse (position)

X● **O64.1 Obstructed labor due to breech presentation** M
Obstructed labor due to buttocks presentation
Obstructed labor due to complete breech presentation
Obstructed labor due to frank breech presentation

X● **O64.2 Obstructed labor due to face presentation** M
Obstructed labor due to chin presentation

X● **O64.3 Obstructed labor due to brow presentation** M

X● **O64.4 Obstructed labor due to shoulder presentation** M
Prolapsed arm
Excludes1 impacted shoulders (O66.0)
shoulder dystocia (O66.0)

X● **O64.5 Obstructed labor due to compound presentation** M

X● **O64.8 Obstructed labor due to other malposition and malpresentation** M
Obstructed labor due to footling presentation
Obstructed labor due to incomplete breech presentation

X● **O64.9 Obstructed labor due to malposition and malpresentation, unspecified** M

● **O65 Obstructed labor due to maternal pelvic abnormality**

O65.0 Obstructed labor due to deformed pelvis M

O65.1 Obstructed labor due to generally contracted pelvis M

O65.2 Obstructed labor due to pelvic inlet contraction M

O65.3 Obstructed labor due to pelvic outlet and mid-cavity contraction M

O65.4 Obstructed labor due to fetopelvic disproportion, unspecified M
Excludes1 dystocia due to abnormality of fetus (O66.2-O66.3)

O65.5 Obstructed labor due to abnormality of maternal pelvic organs M
Obstructed labor due to conditions listed in O34.-
Use additional code to identify abnormality of pelvic organs O34.-

O65.8 Obstructed labor due to other maternal pelvic abnormalities M

O65.9 Obstructed labor due to maternal pelvic abnormality, unspecified M

● **O66 Other obstructed labor**

O66.0 Obstructed labor due to shoulder dystocia M
Impacted shoulders

O66.1 Obstructed labor due to locked twins M

O66.2 Obstructed labor due to unusually large fetus M

O66.3 Obstructed labor due to other abnormalities of fetus M
Dystocia due to fetal ascites
Dystocia due to fetal hydrops
Dystocia due to fetal meningomyelocele
Dystocia due to fetal sacral teratoma
Dystocia due to fetal tumor
Dystocia due to hydrocephalic fetus
Use additional code to identify cause of obstruction

● **O66.4 Failed trial of labor**

O66.40 Failed trial of labor, unspecified M

O66.41 Failed attempted vaginal birth after previous cesarean delivery M
Code first rupture of uterus, if applicable (O71.0-, O71.1)

O66.5 Attempted application of vacuum extractor and forceps M
Attempted application of vacuum or forceps, with subsequent delivery by forceps or cesarean delivery

O66.6 Obstructed labor due to other multiple fetuses M

O66.8 Other specified obstructed labor M
Use additional code to identify cause of obstruction

O66.9 Obstructed labor, unspecified M
Dystocia NOS
Fetal dystocia NOS
Maternal dystocia NOS

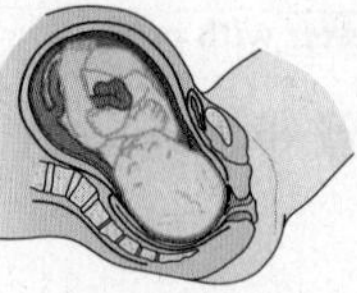

Figure 15-5 Hydrocephalic fetus causing disproportion.

CHAPTER 15 (O00-O9A)

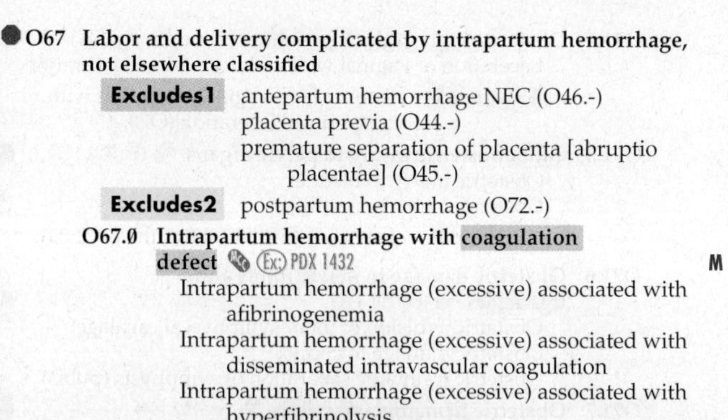

● **O67 Labor and delivery complicated by intrapartum hemorrhage, not elsewhere classified**

Excludes1 antepartum hemorrhage NEC (O46.-)
placenta previa (O44.-)
premature separation of placenta [abruptio placentae] (O45.-)

Excludes2 postpartum hemorrhage (O72.-)

O67.Ø Intrapartum hemorrhage with coagulation defect (Ex) PDX 1432 **M**
Intrapartum hemorrhage (excessive) associated with afibrinogenemia
Intrapartum hemorrhage (excessive) associated with disseminated intravascular coagulation
Intrapartum hemorrhage (excessive) associated with hyperfibrinolysis
Intrapartum hemorrhage (excessive) associated with hypofibrinogenemia

O67.8 Other intrapartum hemorrhage **M**
Excessive intrapartum hemorrhage

O67.9 Intrapartum hemorrhage, unspecified **M**

O68 Labor and delivery complicated by abnormality of fetal acid-base balance (Ex) PDX 1436 **M**
Fetal acidemia complicating labor and delivery
Fetal acidosis complicating labor and delivery
Fetal alkalosis complicating labor and delivery
Fetal metabolic acidemia complicating labor and delivery

Excludes1 fetal stress NOS (O77.9)
labor and delivery complicated by electrocardiographic evidence of fetal stress (O77.8)
labor and delivery complicated by ultrasonic evidence of fetal stress (O77.8)

Excludes2 abnormality in fetal heart rate or rhythm (O76)
labor and delivery complicated by meconium in amniotic fluid (O77.Ø)

● **O69 Labor and delivery complicated by umbilical cord complications**

One of the following 7th characters is to be assigned to each code under category O69. 7th character Ø is for single gestations and multiple gestations where the fetus is unspecified. 7th characters 1 through 9 are for cases of multiple gestations to identify the fetus for which the code applies. The appropriate code from category O3Ø, Multiple gestation, must also be assigned when assigning a code from category O69 that has a 7th character of 1 through 9.

Ø	not applicable or unspecified
1	fetus 1
2	fetus 2
3	fetus 3
4	fetus 4
5	fetus 5
9	other fetus

X● **O69.Ø Labor and delivery complicated by prolapse of cord** **M**

X● **O69.1 Labor and delivery complicated by cord around neck, with compression** **M**

Excludes1 labor and delivery complicated by cord around neck, without compression (O69.81)

X● **O69.2 Labor and delivery complicated by other cord entanglement, with compression** **M**
Labor and delivery complicated by compression of cord NOS
Labor and delivery complicated by entanglement of cords of twins in monoamniotic sac
Labor and delivery complicated by knot in cord

Excludes1 labor and delivery complicated by other cord entanglement, without compression (O69.82)

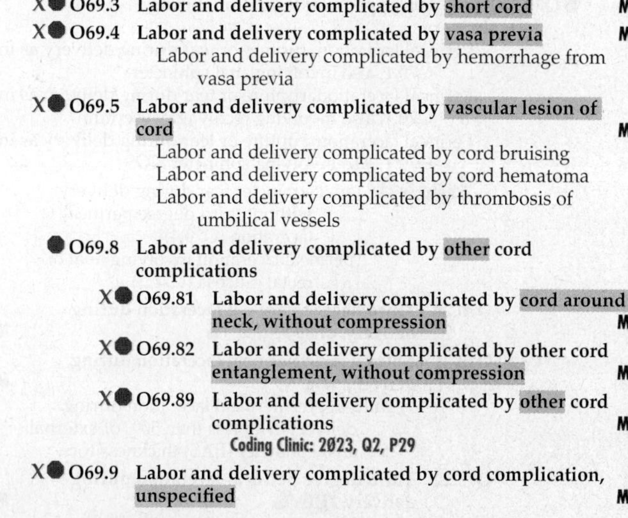

X● **O69.3 Labor and delivery complicated by short cord** **M**

X● **O69.4 Labor and delivery complicated by vasa previa** **M**
Labor and delivery complicated by hemorrhage from vasa previa

X● **O69.5 Labor and delivery complicated by vascular lesion of cord** **M**
Labor and delivery complicated by cord bruising
Labor and delivery complicated by cord hematoma
Labor and delivery complicated by thrombosis of umbilical vessels

● **O69.8 Labor and delivery complicated by other cord complications**

X● **O69.81 Labor and delivery complicated by cord around neck, without compression** **M**

X● **O69.82 Labor and delivery complicated by other cord entanglement, without compression** **M**

X● **O69.89 Labor and delivery complicated by other cord complications** **M**
Coding Clinic: 2Ø23, Q2, P29

X● **O69.9 Labor and delivery complicated by cord complication, unspecified** **M**

● **O7Ø Perineal laceration during delivery**

Includes episiotomy extended by laceration

Excludes1 obstetric high vaginal laceration alone (O71.4)

O7Ø.Ø First degree perineal laceration during delivery **M**
Perineal laceration, rupture or tear involving fourchette during delivery
Perineal laceration, rupture or tear involving labia during delivery
Perineal laceration, rupture or tear involving skin during delivery
Perineal laceration, rupture or tear involving vagina during delivery
Perineal laceration, rupture or tear involving vulva during delivery
Slight perineal laceration, rupture or tear during delivery

O7Ø.1 Second degree perineal laceration during delivery **M**
Perineal laceration, rupture or tear during delivery as in O7Ø.Ø, also involving pelvic floor
Perineal laceration, rupture or tear during delivery as in O7Ø.Ø, also involving perineal muscles
Perineal laceration, rupture or tear during delivery as in O7Ø.Ø, also involving vaginal muscles

Excludes1 perineal laceration involving anal sphincter (O7Ø.2)

Coding Clinic: 2Ø16, Q4, P53; Q2, P34

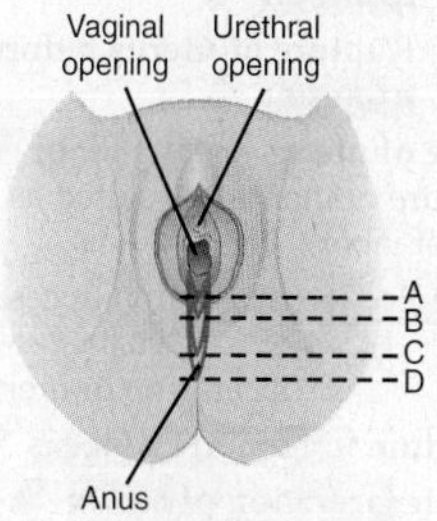

Figure 15-6 Perineal lacerations: **A.** First-degree is laceration of superficial tissues. **B.** Second-degree is limited to the pelvic floor and may involve the perineal or vaginal muscles. **C.** Third-degree involves the anal sphincter. **D.** Fourth-degree involves anal or rectal mucosa.

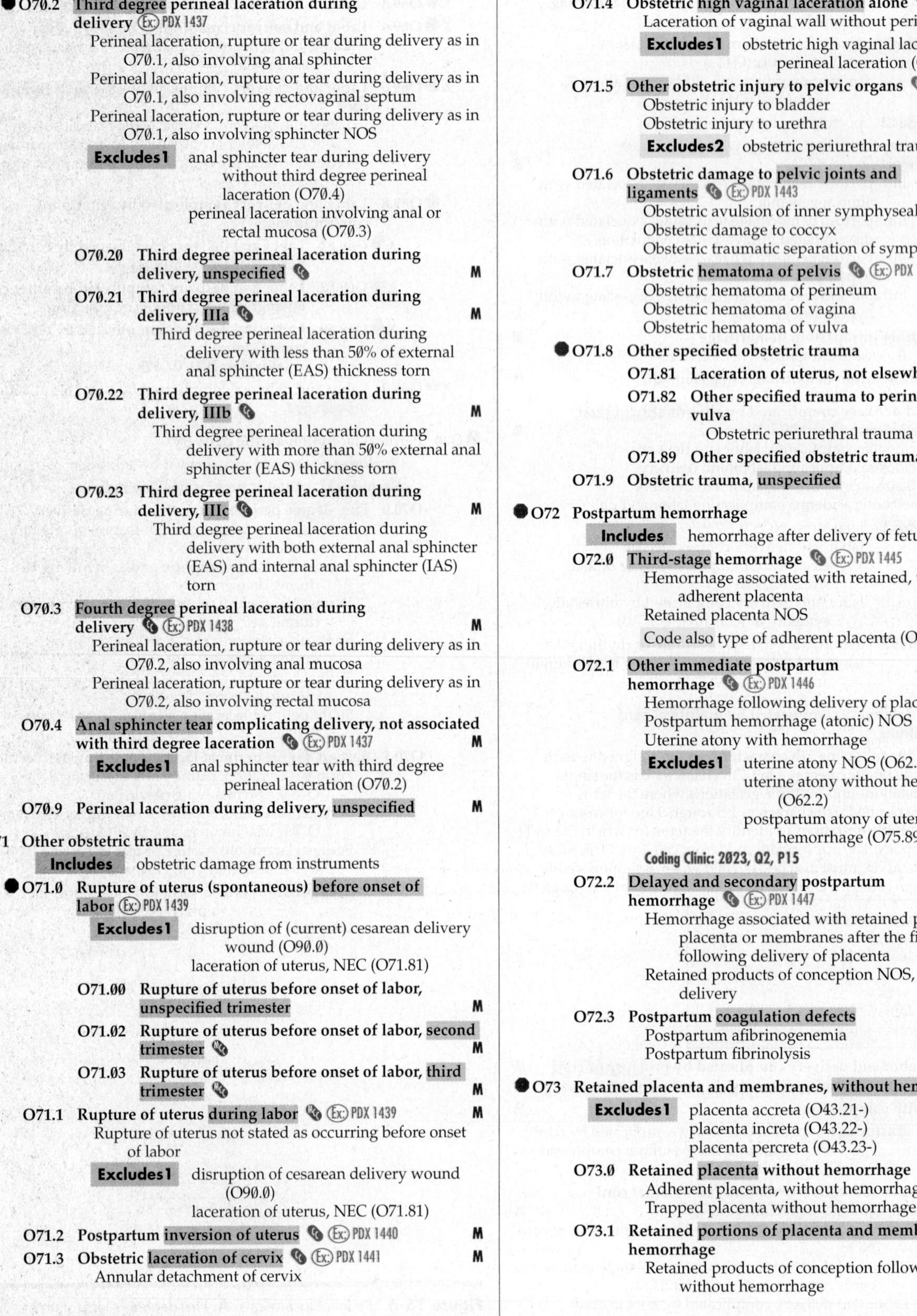

● O70.2 **Third degree perineal laceration during delivery** Ex PDX 1437
Perineal laceration, rupture or tear during delivery as in O70.1, also involving anal sphincter
Perineal laceration, rupture or tear during delivery as in O70.1, also involving rectovaginal septum
Perineal laceration, rupture or tear during delivery as in O70.1, also involving sphincter NOS
Excludes1 anal sphincter tear during delivery without third degree perineal laceration (O70.4)
perineal laceration involving anal or rectal mucosa (O70.3)

O70.20 **Third degree perineal laceration during delivery, unspecified** M

O70.21 **Third degree perineal laceration during delivery, IIIa** M
Third degree perineal laceration during delivery with less than 50% of external anal sphincter (EAS) thickness torn

O70.22 **Third degree perineal laceration during delivery, IIIb** M
Third degree perineal laceration during delivery with more than 50% external anal sphincter (EAS) thickness torn

O70.23 **Third degree perineal laceration during delivery, IIIc** M
Third degree perineal laceration during delivery with both external anal sphincter (EAS) and internal anal sphincter (IAS) torn

O70.3 **Fourth degree perineal laceration during delivery** Ex PDX 1438 M
Perineal laceration, rupture or tear during delivery as in O70.2, also involving anal mucosa
Perineal laceration, rupture or tear during delivery as in O70.2, also involving rectal mucosa

O70.4 **Anal sphincter tear complicating delivery, not associated with third degree laceration** Ex PDX 1437 M
Excludes1 anal sphincter tear with third degree perineal laceration (O70.2)

O70.9 **Perineal laceration during delivery, unspecified** M

● O71 **Other obstetric trauma**
Includes obstetric damage from instruments

● O71.0 **Rupture of uterus (spontaneous) before onset of labor** Ex PDX 1439
Excludes1 disruption of (current) cesarean delivery wound (O90.0)
laceration of uterus, NEC (O71.81)

O71.00 **Rupture of uterus before onset of labor, unspecified trimester** M

O71.02 **Rupture of uterus before onset of labor, second trimester** M

O71.03 **Rupture of uterus before onset of labor, third trimester** M

O71.1 **Rupture of uterus during labor** Ex PDX 1439 M
Rupture of uterus not stated as occurring before onset of labor
Excludes1 disruption of cesarean delivery wound (O90.0)
laceration of uterus, NEC (O71.81)

O71.2 **Postpartum inversion of uterus** Ex PDX 1440 M

O71.3 **Obstetric laceration of cervix** Ex PDX 1441 M
Annular detachment of cervix

O71.4 **Obstetric high vaginal laceration alone** Ex PDX 1442 M
Laceration of vaginal wall without perineal laceration
Excludes1 obstetric high vaginal laceration with perineal laceration (O70.-)

O71.5 **Other obstetric injury to pelvic organs** Ex PDX 1439 M
Obstetric injury to bladder
Obstetric injury to urethra
Excludes2 obstetric periurethral trauma (O71.82)

O71.6 **Obstetric damage to pelvic joints and ligaments** Ex PDX 1443 M
Obstetric avulsion of inner symphyseal cartilage
Obstetric damage to coccyx
Obstetric traumatic separation of symphysis (pubis)

O71.7 **Obstetric hematoma of pelvis** Ex PDX 1444 M
Obstetric hematoma of perineum
Obstetric hematoma of vagina
Obstetric hematoma of vulva

● O71.8 **Other specified obstetric trauma**

O71.81 **Laceration of uterus, not elsewhere classified** M

O71.82 **Other specified trauma to perineum and vulva** M
Obstetric periurethral trauma

O71.89 **Other specified obstetric trauma** M

O71.9 **Obstetric trauma, unspecified** M

● O72 **Postpartum hemorrhage**
Includes hemorrhage after delivery of fetus or infant

O72.0 **Third-stage hemorrhage** Ex PDX 1445 M
Hemorrhage associated with retained, trapped or adherent placenta
Retained placenta NOS
Code also type of adherent placenta (O43.2-)

O72.1 **Other immediate postpartum hemorrhage** Ex PDX 1446 M
Hemorrhage following delivery of placenta
Postpartum hemorrhage (atonic) NOS
Uterine atony with hemorrhage
Excludes1 uterine atony NOS (O62.2)
uterine atony without hemorrhage (O62.2)
postpartum atony of uterus without hemorrhage (O75.89)
Coding Clinic: 2023, Q2, P15

O72.2 **Delayed and secondary postpartum hemorrhage** Ex PDX 1447 M
Hemorrhage associated with retained portions of placenta or membranes after the first 24 hours following delivery of placenta
Retained products of conception NOS, following delivery

O72.3 **Postpartum coagulation defects** M
Postpartum afibrinogenemia
Postpartum fibrinolysis

● O73 **Retained placenta and membranes, without hemorrhage**
Excludes1 placenta accreta (O43.21-)
placenta increta (O43.22-)
placenta percreta (O43.23-)

O73.0 **Retained placenta without hemorrhage** M
Adherent placenta, without hemorrhage
Trapped placenta without hemorrhage

O73.1 **Retained portions of placenta and membranes, without hemorrhage** M
Retained products of conception following delivery, without hemorrhage

● **O74 Complications of anesthesia during labor and delivery**

Includes maternal complications arising from the administration of a general, regional or local anesthetic, analgesic or other sedation during labor and delivery

Use additional code, if applicable, to identify specific complication

O74.0 Aspiration pneumonitis due to anesthesia during labor and delivery M
Inhalation of stomach contents or secretions NOS due to anesthesia during labor and delivery
Mendelson's syndrome due to anesthesia during labor and delivery

O74.1 Other pulmonary complications of anesthesia during labor and delivery M

O74.2 Cardiac complications of anesthesia during labor and delivery M

O74.3 Central nervous system complications of anesthesia during labor and delivery M

O74.4 Toxic reaction to local anesthesia during labor and delivery M

O74.5 Spinal and epidural anesthesia-induced headache during labor and delivery M

O74.6 Other complications of spinal and epidural anesthesia during labor and delivery M

O74.7 Failed or difficult intubation for anesthesia during labor and delivery M

O74.8 Other complications of anesthesia during labor and delivery M

O74.9 Complication of anesthesia during labor and delivery, unspecified M

● **O75 Other complications of labor and delivery, not elsewhere classified**

Excludes2 puerperal (postpartum) infection (O86.-)
puerperal (postpartum) sepsis (O85)

O75.Ø Maternal distress during labor and delivery M

O75.1 Shock during or following labor and delivery (Ex) PDX 1448 M
Obstetric shock following labor and delivery

O75.2 Pyrexia during labor, not elsewhere classified (Ex) PDX 1448 M

O75.3 Other infection during labor (Ex) PDX 1450 M
Sepsis during labor
Use additional code (B95-B97), to identify infectious agent

O75.4 Other complications of obstetric surgery and procedures M
Cardiac arrest following obstetric surgery or procedures
Cardiac failure following obstetric surgery or procedures
Cerebral anoxia following obstetric surgery or procedures
Pulmonary edema following obstetric surgery or procedures
Use additional code to identify specific complication

Excludes2 complications of anesthesia during labor and delivery (O74.-)
disruption of obstetrical (surgical) wound (O9Ø.Ø-O9Ø.1)
hematoma of obstetrical (surgical) wound (O9Ø.2)
infection of obstetrical (surgical) wound (O86.Ø-)

O75.5 Delayed delivery after artificial rupture of membranes M

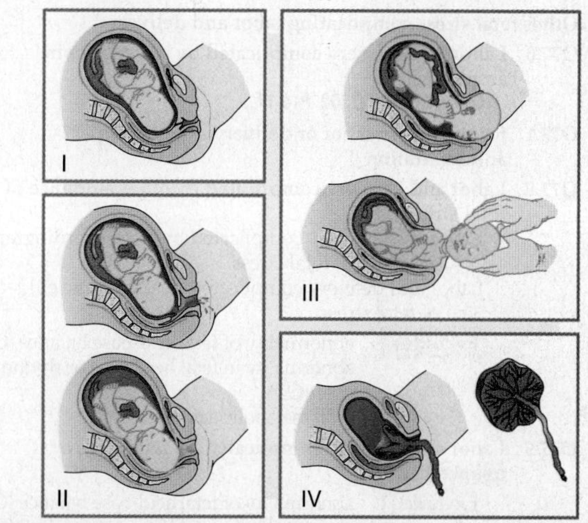

Figure 15-7 The four stages of normal delivery: **I.** Lightening, which occurs 2 to 4 weeks before birth, at which time the fetus turns with head toward the vagina. **II.** Regular contractions begin, the amniotic sac ruptures, and dilation is complete. **III.** Delivery of the head and rotation. **IV.** Expulsion of placenta.

● **O75.8 Other specified complications of labor and delivery**

O75.81 Maternal exhaustion complicating labor and delivery M

O75.82 Onset (spontaneous) of labor after 37 completed weeks of gestation but before 39 completed weeks gestation, with delivery by (planned) cesarean section M
Delivery by (planned) cesarean section occurring after 37 completed weeks of gestation but before 39 completed weeks gestation due to (spontaneous) onset of labor
Code first to specify reason for planned cesarean section such as:
cephalopelvic disproportion (normally formed fetus) (O33.9)
previous cesarean delivery (O34.21-)
Coding Clinic: 2022, Q2, P3-4

O75.89 Other specified complications of labor and delivery M

O75.9 Complication of labor and delivery, unspecified M

O76 Abnormality in fetal heart rate and rhythm complicating labor and delivery M
Depressed fetal heart rate tones complicating labor and delivery
Fetal bradycardia complicating labor and delivery
Fetal heart rate decelerations complicating labor and delivery
Fetal heart rate irregularity complicating labor and delivery
Fetal heart rate abnormal variability complicating labor and delivery
Fetal tachycardia complicating labor and delivery
Non-reassuring fetal heart rate or rhythm complicating labor and delivery

Excludes1 fetal stress NOS (O77.9)
labor and delivery complicated by electrocardiographic evidence of fetal stress (O77.8)
labor and delivery complicated by ultrasonic evidence of fetal stress (O77.8)

Excludes2 fetal metabolic acidemia (O68)
other fetal stress (O77.Ø-O77.1)

CHAPTER 15 (OØØ-O9A)

● O77 **Other fetal stress complicating labor and delivery**

O77.Ø **Labor and delivery complicated by meconium in amniotic fluid** M
Coding Clinic: 2022, Q2, P16-17

O77.1 **Fetal stress in labor or delivery due to drug administration** M

O77.8 **Labor and delivery complicated by other evidence of fetal stress** M
Labor and delivery complicated by electrocardiographic evidence of fetal stress
Labor and delivery complicated by ultrasonic evidence of fetal stress
Excludes1 abnormality of fetal acid-base balance (O68)
abnormality in fetal heart rate or rhythm (O76)
fetal metabolic acidemia (O68)

O77.9 **Labor and delivery complicated by fetal stress, unspecified** M
Excludes1 abnormality of fetal acid-base balance (O68)
abnormality in fetal heart rate or rhythm (O76)
fetal metabolic acidemia (O68)

OGCR Section I.C., Chapter 15.n.

Normal Delivery, Code O8Ø

1) Encounter for full-term uncomplicated delivery

Code O8Ø should be assigned when a woman is admitted for a full-term normal delivery and delivers a single, healthy infant without any complications antepartum, during the delivery, or postpartum during the delivery episode. Code O8Ø is always a principal diagnosis. It is not to be used if any other code from Chapter 15 is needed to describe a current complication of the antenatal, delivery, or perinatal period. Additional codes from other chapters may be used with code O8Ø if they are not related to or are in any way complicating the pregnancy.

2) Uncomplicated delivery with resolved antepartum complication

Code O8Ø may be used if the patient had a complication at some point during the pregnancy, but the complication is not present at the time of the admission for delivery.

3) Outcome of delivery for O8Ø

Z37.Ø, Single live brith, is the only outcome of delivery code appropriate for use with O8Ø.

ENCOUNTER FOR DELIVERY (O8Ø-O82)

O8Ø **Encounter for full-term uncomplicated delivery** M
Delivery requiring minimal or no assistance, with or without episiotomy, without fetal manipulation [e.g., rotation version] or instrumentation [forceps] of a spontaneous, cephalic, vaginal, full-term, single, live-born infant. This code is for use as a single diagnosis code and is not to be used with any other code from Chapter 15.
Use additional code to indicate outcome of delivery (Z37.Ø)
Coding Clinic: 2016, Q4, P124, 150

O82 **Encounter for cesarean delivery without indication** M
Use additional code to indicate outcome of delivery (Z37.Ø)

COMPLICATIONS PREDOMINANTLY RELATED TO THE PUERPERIUM (O85-O92)

Excludes2 mental and behavioral disorders associated with the puerperium (F53.-)
obstetrical tetanus (A34)
puerperal osteomalacia (M83.Ø)

O85 **Puerperal sepsis** (Ex) PDX 1451 M
Postpartum sepsis
Puerperal peritonitis
Puerperal pyemia
Use additional code (B95-B97), to identify infectious agent
Use additional code (R65.2-) to identify severe sepsis, if applicable
Excludes1 fever of unknown origin following delivery (O86.4)
~~genital tract infection following delivery (O86.1-)~~
obstetric pyemic and septic embolism (O88.3-)
puerperal septic thrombophlebitis (O86.81)
~~urinary tract infection following delivery (O86.2-)~~
▶ **Excludes2** genital tract infection following delivery (O86.1-)
▶sepsis during labor (O75.3)
▶urinary tract infection following delivery (O86.2-)
Coding Clinic: 2022, Q2, P5; 2018, Q4, P23

● O86 **Other puerperal infections**
Use additional code (B95-B97), to identify infectious agent
Excludes2 infection during labor (O75.3)
obstetrical tetanus (A34)

● O86.Ø **Infection of obstetric surgical wound**
Infected cesarean delivery wound following delivery
Infected perineal repair following delivery
Excludes1 complications of procedures, not elsewhere classified (T81.44)
postprocedural fever NOS (R5Ø.82)
postprocedural retroperitoneal abscess (K68.11)

O86.ØØ **Infection of obstetric surgical wound, unspecified** M

O86.Ø1 **Infection of obstetric surgical wound, superficial incisional site** M
Subcutaneous abscess following an obstetrical procedure
Stitch abscess following an obstetrical procedure

O86.Ø2 **Infection of obstetric surgical wound, deep incisional site** M
Intramuscular abscess following an obstetrical procedure
Sub-fascial abscess following an obstetrical procedure
Coding Clinic: 2018, Q4, P23

O86.Ø3 **Infection of obstetric surgical wound, organ and space site** M
Intraabdominal abscess following an obstetrical procedure
Subphrenic abscess following an obstetrical procedure

O86.Ø4 **Sepsis following an obstetrical procedure** (Ex) PDX 1451 M
Use additional code to identify the sepsis

O86.Ø9 **Infection of obstetric surgical wound, other surgical site** M

● O86.1 **Other infection of genital tract following delivery** (Ex) PDX 1419

O86.11 **Cervicitis following delivery** M

O86.12 **Endometritis following delivery** (Ex) PDX 1451 M

O86.13 **Vaginitis following delivery** M

O86.19 **Other infection of genital tract following delivery** M

CHAPTER 15 (OØØ-O9A)

▶ New ➡ Revised ~~deleted~~ Deleted Excludes 1 Excludes 2 Includes Use additional Code first Code also Key words
OGCR Official Guidelines ● Unacceptable Principal Diagnosis X Assign placeholder X ● Use Additional Character(s) Manifestation Code Coding Clinic

● O86.2 Urinary tract infection following delivery (Ex) PDX 1419
O86.20 Urinary tract infection following delivery, unspecified M
Puerperal urinary tract infection NOS
Coding Clinic: 2022, Q2, P5
O86.21 Infection of kidney following delivery M
O86.22 Infection of bladder following delivery M
Infection of urethra following delivery
O86.29 Other urinary tract infection following delivery M
O86.4 Pyrexia of unknown origin following delivery (Ex) PDX 1452 M
Puerperal infection NOS following delivery
Puerperal pyrexia NOS following delivery
Excludes2 pyrexia during labor (O75.2)
● O86.8 Other specified puerperal infections (Ex) PDX 1451
O86.81 Puerperal septic thrombophlebitis M
O86.89 Other specified puerperal infections M

● **O87 Venous complications and hemorrhoids in the puerperium** (Ex) PDX 1418
Includes venous complications in labor, delivery and the puerperium
Excludes2 obstetric embolism (O88.-)
puerperal septic thrombophlebitis (O86.81)
venous complications in pregnancy (O22.-)
O87.0 Superficial thrombophlebitis in the puerperium M
Puerperal phlebitis NOS
Puerperal thrombosis NOS
Use additional code, if applicable, to identify the superficial vein thrombosis, such as thrombosis of superficial vessels of lower extremities (I80.0-)
O87.1 Deep phlebothrombosis in the puerperium M
Deep vein thrombosis, postpartum
Pelvic thrombophlebitis, postpartum
Use additional code to identify the deep vein thrombosis (I82.4-, I82.5-, I82.62-, I82.72-)
Use additional code, if applicable, for associated long-term (current) use of anticoagulants (Z79.01)
O87.2 Hemorrhoids in the puerperium M
O87.3 Cerebral venous thrombosis in the puerperium M
Cerebrovenous sinus thrombosis in the puerperium
O87.4 Varicose veins of lower extremity in the puerperium M
O87.8 Other venous complications in the puerperium M
Genital varices in the puerperium
O87.9 Venous complication in the puerperium, unspecified M
Puerperal phlebopathy NOS

O88 Obstetric embolism (Ex) PDX 1453
Excludes1 embolism complicating abortion NOS (O03.2)
embolism complicating ectopic or molar pregnancy (O08.2)
embolism complicating failed attempted abortion (O07.2)
embolism complicating induced abortion (O04.7)
embolism complicating spontaneous abortion (O03.2, O03.7)
● O88.0 Obstetric air embolism
● O88.01 Obstetric air embolism in pregnancy
O88.011 Air embolism in pregnancy, first trimester M
O88.012 Air embolism in pregnancy, second trimester M
O88.013 Air embolism in pregnancy, third trimester M
O88.019 Air embolism in pregnancy, unspecified trimester M
O88.02 Air embolism in childbirth M
O88.03 Air embolism in the puerperium M
● O88.1 Amniotic fluid embolism
Anaphylactoid syndrome in pregnancy
● O88.11 Amniotic fluid embolism in pregnancy
O88.111 Amniotic fluid embolism in pregnancy, first trimester M
O88.112 Amniotic fluid embolism in pregnancy, second trimester M
O88.113 Amniotic fluid embolism in pregnancy, third trimester M
O88.119 Amniotic fluid embolism in pregnancy, unspecified trimester M
O88.12 Amniotic fluid embolism in childbirth M
O88.13 Amniotic fluid embolism in the puerperium M
● O88.2 Obstetric thromboembolism
● O88.21 Thromboembolism in pregnancy
Obstetric (pulmonary) embolism NOS
O88.211 Thromboembolism in pregnancy, first trimester M
O88.212 Thromboembolism in pregnancy, second trimester M
O88.213 Thromboembolism in pregnancy, third trimester M
O88.219 Thromboembolism in pregnancy, unspecified trimester M
O88.22 Thromboembolism in childbirth M
O88.23 Thromboembolism in the puerperium M
Puerperal (pulmonary) embolism NOS
● O88.3 Obstetric pyemic and septic embolism
● O88.31 Pyemic and septic embolism in pregnancy
O88.311 Pyemic and septic embolism in pregnancy, first trimester M
O88.312 Pyemic and septic embolism in pregnancy, second trimester M
O88.313 Pyemic and septic embolism in pregnancy, third trimester M
O88.319 Pyemic and septic embolism in pregnancy, unspecified trimester M
O88.32 Pyemic and septic embolism in childbirth M
O88.33 Pyemic and septic embolism in the puerperium M
● O88.8 Other obstetric embolism
Obstetric fat embolism
● O88.81 Other embolism in pregnancy
O88.811 Other embolism in pregnancy, first trimester M
O88.812 Other embolism in pregnancy, second trimester M
O88.813 Other embolism in pregnancy, third trimester M
O88.819 Other embolism in pregnancy, unspecified trimester M
O88.82 Other embolism in childbirth M
O88.83 Other embolism in the puerperium M

● **O89 Complications of anesthesia during the puerperium**
Includes maternal complications arising from the administration of a general, regional or local anesthetic, analgesic or other sedation during the puerperium
Use additional code, if applicable, to identify specific complication
● O89.0 Pulmonary complications of anesthesia during the puerperium
O89.01 Aspiration pneumonitis due to anesthesia during the puerperium M
Inhalation of stomach contents or secretions NOS due to anesthesia during the puerperium
Mendelson's syndrome due to anesthesia during the puerperium
O89.09 Other pulmonary complications of anesthesia during the puerperium M

O89.1 Cardiac complications of anesthesia during the puerperium M
O89.2 Central nervous system complications of anesthesia during the puerperium M
O89.3 Toxic reaction to local anesthesia during the puerperium M
O89.4 Spinal and epidural anesthesia-induced headache during the puerperium M
O89.5 Other complications of spinal and epidural anesthesia during the puerperium M
O89.6 Failed or difficult intubation for anesthesia during the puerperium M
O89.8 Other complications of anesthesia during the puerperium M
O89.9 Complication of anesthesia during the puerperium, unspecified M

● O9Ø Complications of the puerperium, not elsewhere classified

O9Ø.Ø Disruption of cesarean delivery wound M
Dehiscence of cesarean delivery wound
Excludes1 rupture of uterus (spontaneous) before onset of labor (O71.Ø-)
rupture of uterus during labor (O71.1)

O9Ø.1 Disruption of perineal obstetric wound M
Disruption of wound of episiotomy
Disruption of wound of perineal laceration
Secondary perineal tear

O9Ø.2 Hematoma of obstetric wound M

O9Ø.3 Peripartum cardiomyopathy (Ex) PDX 1454 M
Conditions in I42.- arising during pregnancy and the puerperium
Excludes1 pre-existing heart disease complicating pregnancy and the puerperium (O99.4-)
Coding Clinic: 2022, Q3, P16-18

● O9Ø.4 Postpartum acute kidney failure (Ex) PDX 1455 M
Excludes1 non-anuria and oliguria (R34)

O9Ø.41 Hepatorenal syndrome following labor and delivery M
O9Ø.49 Other postpartum acute kidney failure M
Postpartum acute kidney failure
Puerperal anuria
Puerperal oliguria

O9Ø.5 Postpartum thyroiditis M

O9Ø.6 Postpartum mood disturbance M
Postpartum blues
Postpartum sadness
Postpartum dysphoria
Excludes1 postpartum depression (F53.Ø)
puerperal psychosis (F53.1)

● O9Ø.8 Other complications of the puerperium, not elsewhere classified

O9Ø.81 Anemia of the puerperium M
Postpartum anemia NOS
Excludes1 pre-existing anemia complicating the puerperium (O99.Ø3)

O9Ø.89 Other complications of the puerperium, not elsewhere classified M
Placental polyp

O9Ø.9 Complication of the puerperium, unspecified M

● O91 Infections of breast associated with pregnancy, the puerperium and lactation
Use additional code to identify infection

● O91.Ø Infection of nipple associated with pregnancy, the puerperium and lactation

● O91.Ø1 Infection of nipple associated with pregnancy
Gestational abscess of nipple
O91.Ø11 Infection of nipple associated with pregnancy, first trimester M
O91.Ø12 Infection of nipple associated with pregnancy, second trimester M
O91.Ø13 Infection of nipple associated with pregnancy, third trimester M
O91.Ø19 Infection of nipple associated with pregnancy, unspecified trimester M

O91.Ø2 Infection of nipple associated with the puerperium M
Puerperal abscess of nipple

O91.Ø3 Infection of nipple associated with lactation M
Abscess of nipple associated with lactation

● O91.1 Abscess of breast associated with pregnancy, the puerperium and lactation

● O91.11 Abscess of breast associated with pregnancy
Gestational mammary abscess
Gestational purulent mastitis
Gestational subareolar abscess
O91.111 Abscess of breast associated with pregnancy, first trimester M
O91.112 Abscess of breast associated with pregnancy, second trimester M
O91.113 Abscess of breast associated with pregnancy, third trimester M
O91.119 Abscess of breast associated with pregnancy, unspecified trimester M

O91.12 Abscess of breast associated with the puerperium M
Puerperal mammary abscess
Puerperal purulent mastitis
Puerperal subareolar abscess

O91.13 Abscess of breast associated with lactation M
Mammary abscess associated with lactation
Purulent mastitis associated with lactation
Subareolar abscess associated with lactation

● O91.2 Nonpurulent mastitis associated with pregnancy, the puerperium and lactation

● O91.21 Nonpurulent mastitis associated with pregnancy
Gestational interstitial mastitis
Gestational lymphangitis of breast
Gestational mastitis NOS
Gestational parenchymatous mastitis
O91.211 Nonpurulent mastitis associated with pregnancy, first trimester M
O91.212 Nonpurulent mastitis associated with pregnancy, second trimester M
O91.213 Nonpurulent mastitis associated with pregnancy, third trimester M
O91.219 Nonpurulent mastitis associated with pregnancy, unspecified trimester M

O91.22 Nonpurulent mastitis associated with the puerperium M
Puerperal interstitial mastitis
Puerperal lymphangitis of breast
Puerperal mastitis NOS
Puerperal parenchymatous mastitis

O91.23 Nonpurulent mastitis associated with lactation M
Interstitial mastitis associated with lactation
Lymphangitis of breast associated with lactation
Mastitis NOS associated with lactation
Parenchymatous mastitis associated with lactation

● O92 Other disorders of breast and disorders of lactation associated with pregnancy and the puerperium

● O92.Ø Retracted nipple associated with pregnancy, the puerperium, and lactation

● O92.Ø1 Retracted nipple associated with pregnancy
O92.Ø11 Retracted nipple associated with pregnancy, first trimester M
O92.Ø12 Retracted nipple associated with pregnancy, second trimester M

O92.013 Retracted nipple associated with pregnancy, third trimester M

O92.019 Retracted nipple associated with pregnancy, unspecified trimester M

O92.02 Retracted nipple associated with the puerperium M

O92.03 Retracted nipple associated with lactation M

● O92.1 Cracked nipple associated with pregnancy, the puerperium, and lactation
Fissure of nipple, gestational or puerperal

● O92.11 Cracked nipple associated with pregnancy

O92.111 Cracked nipple associated with pregnancy, first trimester M

O92.112 Cracked nipple associated with pregnancy, second trimester M

O92.113 Cracked nipple associated with pregnancy, third trimester M

O92.119 Cracked nipple associated with pregnancy, unspecified trimester M

O92.12 Cracked nipple associated with the puerperium M

O92.13 Cracked nipple associated with lactation M

● O92.2 Other and unspecified disorders of breast associated with pregnancy and the puerperium

O92.20 Unspecified disorder of breast associated with pregnancy and the puerperium M

O92.29 Other disorders of breast associated with pregnancy and the puerperium M

O92.3 Agalactia M
Primary agalactia
Excludes1 elective agalactia (O92.5)
secondary agalactia (O92.5)
therapeutic agalactia (O92.5)

O92.4 Hypogalactia M

O92.5 Suppressed lactation M
Elective agalactia
Therapeutic agalactia
Secondary agalactia
Excludes1 primary agalactia (O92.3)

O92.6 Galactorrhea M

● O92.7 Other and unspecified disorders of lactation

O92.70 Unspecified disorders of lactation M

O92.79 Other disorders of lactation M
Puerperal galactocele

OTHER OBSTETRIC CONDITIONS, NOT ELSEWHERE CLASSIFIED (O94-O9A)

● O94 Sequelae of complication of pregnancy, childbirth, and the puerperium M

Note: This category is to be used to indicate conditions in O00-O77.-, O85-O94 and O98-O9A.- as the cause of late effects. The "sequelae" include conditions specified as such, or as late effects, which may occur at any time after the puerperium.

Code first condition resulting from (sequela) of complication of pregnancy, childbirth, and the puerperium

Coding Clinic: 2022, Q3, P17-18

O98 Maternal infectious and parasitic diseases classifiable elsewhere but complicating pregnancy, childbirth and the puerperium

Includes the listed conditions when complicating the pregnant state, when aggravated by the pregnancy, or as a reason for obstetric care

Use additional code (Chapter 1), to identify specific infectious or parasitic disease

Excludes2 herpes gestationis (O26.4-)
infectious carrier state (O99.82-, O99.83-)
obstetrical tetanus (A34)
puerperal infection (O86.-)
puerperal sepsis (O85)
when the reason for maternal care is that the disease is known or suspected to have affected the fetus (O35-O36)

● O98.0 Tuberculosis complicating pregnancy, childbirth and the puerperium (Ex) PDX 1456
Conditions in A15-A19

● O98.01 Tuberculosis complicating pregnancy

O98.011 Tuberculosis complicating pregnancy, first trimester M

O98.012 Tuberculosis complicating pregnancy, second trimester M

O98.013 Tuberculosis complicating pregnancy, third trimester M

O98.019 Tuberculosis complicating pregnancy, unspecified trimester M

O98.02 Tuberculosis complicating childbirth M

O98.03 Tuberculosis complicating the puerperium M

● O98.1 Syphilis complicating pregnancy, childbirth and the puerperium (Ex) PDX 1457
Conditions in A50-A53

● O98.11 Syphilis complicating pregnancy

O98.111 Syphilis complicating pregnancy, first trimester M

O98.112 Syphilis complicating pregnancy, second trimester M

O98.113 Syphilis complicating pregnancy, third trimester M

O98.119 Syphilis complicating pregnancy, unspecified trimester M

O98.12 Syphilis complicating childbirth M

O98.13 Syphilis complicating the puerperium M

● O98.2 Gonorrhea complicating pregnancy, childbirth and the puerperium (Ex) PDX 1457
Conditions in A54.-

● O98.21 Gonorrhea complicating pregnancy

O98.211 Gonorrhea complicating pregnancy, first trimester M

O98.212 Gonorrhea complicating pregnancy, second trimester M

O98.213 Gonorrhea complicating pregnancy, third trimester M

O98.219 Gonorrhea complicating pregnancy, unspecified trimester M

O98.22 Gonorrhea complicating childbirth M

O98.23 Gonorrhea complicating the puerperium M

● O98.3 Other infections with a predominantly sexual mode of transmission complicating pregnancy, childbirth and the puerperium (Ex) PDX 1457
Conditions in A55-A64

● O98.31 Other infections with a predominantly sexual mode of transmission complicating pregnancy

O98.311 Other infections with a predominantly sexual mode of transmission complicating pregnancy, first trimester M

O98.312 Other infections with a predominantly sexual mode of transmission complicating pregnancy, second trimester M

O98.313 Other infections with a predominantly sexual mode of transmission complicating pregnancy, third trimester M

O98.319 Other infections with a predominantly sexual mode of transmission complicating pregnancy, unspecified trimester M

O98.32 Other infections with a predominantly sexual mode of transmission complicating childbirth M
Coding Clinic: 2020, Q1, P20

O98.33 Other infections with a predominantly sexual mode of transmission complicating the puerperium M

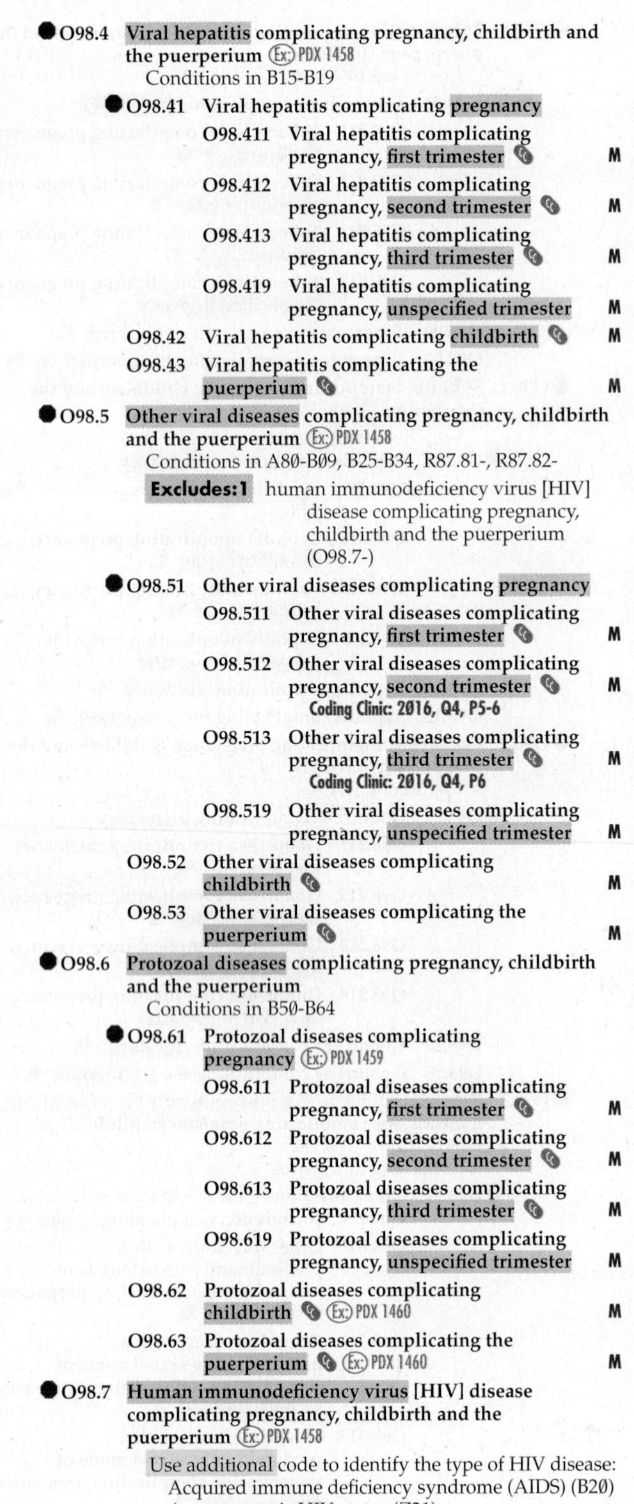

● O98.4 Viral hepatitis complicating pregnancy, childbirth and the puerperium Ex PDX 1458
Conditions in B15-B19

● O98.41 Viral hepatitis complicating pregnancy
O98.411 Viral hepatitis complicating pregnancy, first trimester M
O98.412 Viral hepatitis complicating pregnancy, second trimester M
O98.413 Viral hepatitis complicating pregnancy, third trimester M
O98.419 Viral hepatitis complicating pregnancy, unspecified trimester M

O98.42 Viral hepatitis complicating childbirth M
O98.43 Viral hepatitis complicating the puerperium M

● O98.5 Other viral diseases complicating pregnancy, childbirth and the puerperium Ex PDX 1458
Conditions in A80-B09, B25-B34, R87.81-, R87.82-
Excludes:1 human immunodeficiency virus [HIV] disease complicating pregnancy, childbirth and the puerperium (O98.7-)

● O98.51 Other viral diseases complicating pregnancy
O98.511 Other viral diseases complicating pregnancy, first trimester M
O98.512 Other viral diseases complicating pregnancy, second trimester M
Coding Clinic: 2016, Q4, P5-6
O98.513 Other viral diseases complicating pregnancy, third trimester M
Coding Clinic: 2016, Q4, P6
O98.519 Other viral diseases complicating pregnancy, unspecified trimester M

O98.52 Other viral diseases complicating childbirth M
O98.53 Other viral diseases complicating the puerperium M

● O98.6 Protozoal diseases complicating pregnancy, childbirth and the puerperium
Conditions in B50-B64

● O98.61 Protozoal diseases complicating pregnancy Ex PDX 1459
O98.611 Protozoal diseases complicating pregnancy, first trimester M
O98.612 Protozoal diseases complicating pregnancy, second trimester M
O98.613 Protozoal diseases complicating pregnancy, third trimester M
O98.619 Protozoal diseases complicating pregnancy, unspecified trimester M

O98.62 Protozoal diseases complicating childbirth Ex PDX 1460 M
O98.63 Protozoal diseases complicating the puerperium Ex PDX 1460 M

● O98.7 Human immunodeficiency virus [HIV] disease complicating pregnancy, childbirth and the puerperium Ex PDX 1458
Use additional code to identify the type of HIV disease:
Acquired immune deficiency syndrome (AIDS) (B20)
Asymptomatic HIV status (Z21)
HIV positive NOS (Z21)
Symptomatic HIV disease (B20)

OGCR Section I.C.15.f.

HIV Infection in Pregnancy, Childbirth and the Puerperium

During pregnancy, childbirth or the puerperium, a patient admitted because of an HIV-related illness should receive a principal diagnosis from subcategory O98.7-. Human immunodeficiency [HIV] disease complicating pregnancy, childbirth and the puerperium, followed by the code(s) for the HIV-related illness(es).

Patients with asymptomatic HIV infection status admitted during pregnancy, childbirth, or the puerperium should receive codes of O98.7- and Z21, Asymptomatic human immunodeficiency virus [HIV] infection status.

● O98.71 Human immunodeficiency virus [HIV] disease complicating pregnancy
O98.711 Human immunodeficiency virus [HIV] disease complicating pregnancy, first trimester M
O98.712 Human immunodeficiency virus [HIV] disease complicating pregnancy, second trimester M
O98.713 Human immunodeficiency virus [HIV] disease complicating pregnancy, third trimester M
O98.719 Human immunodeficiency virus [HIV] disease complicating pregnancy, unspecified trimester M

O98.72 Human immunodeficiency virus [HIV] disease complicating childbirth M
O98.73 Human immunodeficiency virus [HIV] disease complicating the puerperium M

● O98.8 Other maternal infectious and parasitic diseases complicating pregnancy, childbirth and the puerperium Ex PDX 1458

● O98.81 Other maternal infectious and parasitic diseases complicating pregnancy
O98.811 Other maternal infectious and parasitic diseases complicating pregnancy, first trimester M
O98.812 Other maternal infectious and parasitic diseases complicating pregnancy, second trimester M
O98.813 Other maternal infectious and parasitic diseases complicating pregnancy, third trimester M
O98.819 Other maternal infectious and parasitic diseases complicating pregnancy, unspecified trimester M

O98.82 Other maternal infectious and parasitic diseases complicating childbirth M
Coding Clinic: 2020, Q1, P10
O98.83 Other maternal infectious and parasitic diseases complicating the puerperium M
Coding Clinic: 2022, Q2, P5

● O98.9 Unspecified maternal infectious and parasitic disease complicating pregnancy, childbirth and the puerperium Ex PDX 1458

● O98.91 Unspecified maternal infectious and parasitic disease complicating pregnancy
O98.911 Unspecified maternal infectious and parasitic disease complicating pregnancy, first trimester M
O98.912 Unspecified maternal infectious and parasitic disease complicating pregnancy, second trimester M
O98.913 Unspecified maternal infectious and parasitic disease complicating pregnancy, third trimester M

O98.919 Unspecified maternal infectious and parasitic disease complicating pregnancy, unspecified trimester M

O98.92 Unspecified maternal infectious and parasitic disease complicating childbirth M

O98.93 Unspecified maternal infectious and parasitic disease complicating the puerperium M

O99 Other maternal diseases classifiable elsewhere but complicating pregnancy, childbirth and the puerperium

Includes: conditions which complicate the pregnant state, are aggravated by the pregnancy or are a main reason for obstetric care

Use additional code to identify specific condition

Excludes2 when the reason for maternal care is that the condition is known or suspected to have affected the fetus (O35-O36)

Coding Clinic: 2018, Q4, P8-9

O99.0 Anemia complicating pregnancy, childbirth and the puerperium

Conditions in D50-D64

Excludes1 anemia arising in the puerperium (O90.81)
postpartum anemia NOS (O90.81)

O99.01 Anemia complicating pregnancy

O99.011 Anemia complicating pregnancy, first trimester M

O99.012 Anemia complicating pregnancy, second trimester M

O99.013 Anemia complicating pregnancy, third trimester M

O99.019 Anemia complicating pregnancy, unspecified trimester M

O99.02 Anemia complicating childbirth M

O99.03 Anemia complicating the puerperium M

Excludes1 postpartum anemia not pre-existing prior to delivery (O90.81)

O99.1 Other diseases of the blood and blood-forming organs and certain disorders involving the immune mechanism complicating pregnancy, childbirth and the puerperium

Conditions in D65-D89

Excludes1 hemorrhage with coagulation defects (O45.-, O46.0-, O67.0, O72.3)

O99.11 Other diseases of the blood and blood-forming organs and certain disorders involving the immune mechanism complicating pregnancy

O99.111 Other diseases of the blood and blood-forming organs and certain disorders involving the immune mechanism complicating pregnancy, first trimester (Ex) PDX 1461 M

O99.112 Other diseases of the blood and blood-forming organs and certain disorders involving the immune mechanism complicating pregnancy, second trimester (Ex) PDX 1462 M

O99.113 Other diseases of the blood and blood-forming organs and certain disorders involving the immune mechanism complicating pregnancy, third trimester (Ex) PDX 1463 M

O99.119 Other diseases of the blood and blood-forming organs and certain disorders involving the immune mechanism complicating pregnancy, unspecified trimester (Ex) PDX 1464 M

O99.12 Other diseases of the blood and blood-forming organs and certain disorders involving the immune mechanism complicating childbirth (Ex) PDX 1465 M

O99.13 Other diseases of the blood and blood-forming organs and certain disorders involving the immune mechanism complicating the puerperium (Ex) PDX 1466 M

O99.2 Endocrine, nutritional and metabolic diseases complicating pregnancy, childbirth and the puerperium

Conditions in E00-E89

Excludes2 diabetes mellitus (O24.-)
malnutrition (O25.-)
postpartum thyroiditis (O90.5)

O99.21 Obesity complicating pregnancy, childbirth, and the puerperium

Use additional code to identify the type of obesity (E66.-)

O99.210 Obesity complicating pregnancy, unspecified trimester M

O99.211 Obesity complicating pregnancy, first trimester M

O99.212 Obesity complicating pregnancy, second trimester M

O99.213 Obesity complicating pregnancy, third trimester M

O99.214 Obesity complicating childbirth M
Coding Clinic: 2021, Q2, P10-11; 2018, Q4, P80

O99.215 Obesity complicating the puerperium M

O99.28 Other endocrine, nutritional and metabolic diseases complicating pregnancy, childbirth and the puerperium

O99.280 Endocrine, nutritional and metabolic diseases complicating pregnancy, unspecified trimester M

O99.281 Endocrine, nutritional and metabolic diseases complicating pregnancy, first trimester M

O99.282 Endocrine, nutritional and metabolic diseases complicating pregnancy, second trimester M

O99.283 Endocrine, nutritional and metabolic diseases complicating pregnancy, third trimester M

O99.284 Endocrine, nutritional and metabolic diseases complicating childbirth M

O99.285 Endocrine, nutritional and metabolic diseases complicating the puerperium M
Coding Clinic: 2021, Q1, P9

O99.3 Mental disorders and diseases of the nervous system complicating pregnancy, childbirth and the puerperium

O99.31 Alcohol use complicating pregnancy, childbirth, and the puerperium

Use additional code(s) from F10 to identify manifestations of the alcohol use

O99.310 Alcohol use complicating pregnancy, unspecified trimester M

O99.311 Alcohol use complicating pregnancy, first trimester M

O99.312 Alcohol use complicating pregnancy, second trimester M

O99.313 Alcohol use complicating pregnancy, third trimester M

O99.314 Alcohol use complicating childbirth M

O99.315 Alcohol use complicating the puerperium M

CHAPTER 15 (O00-O9A)

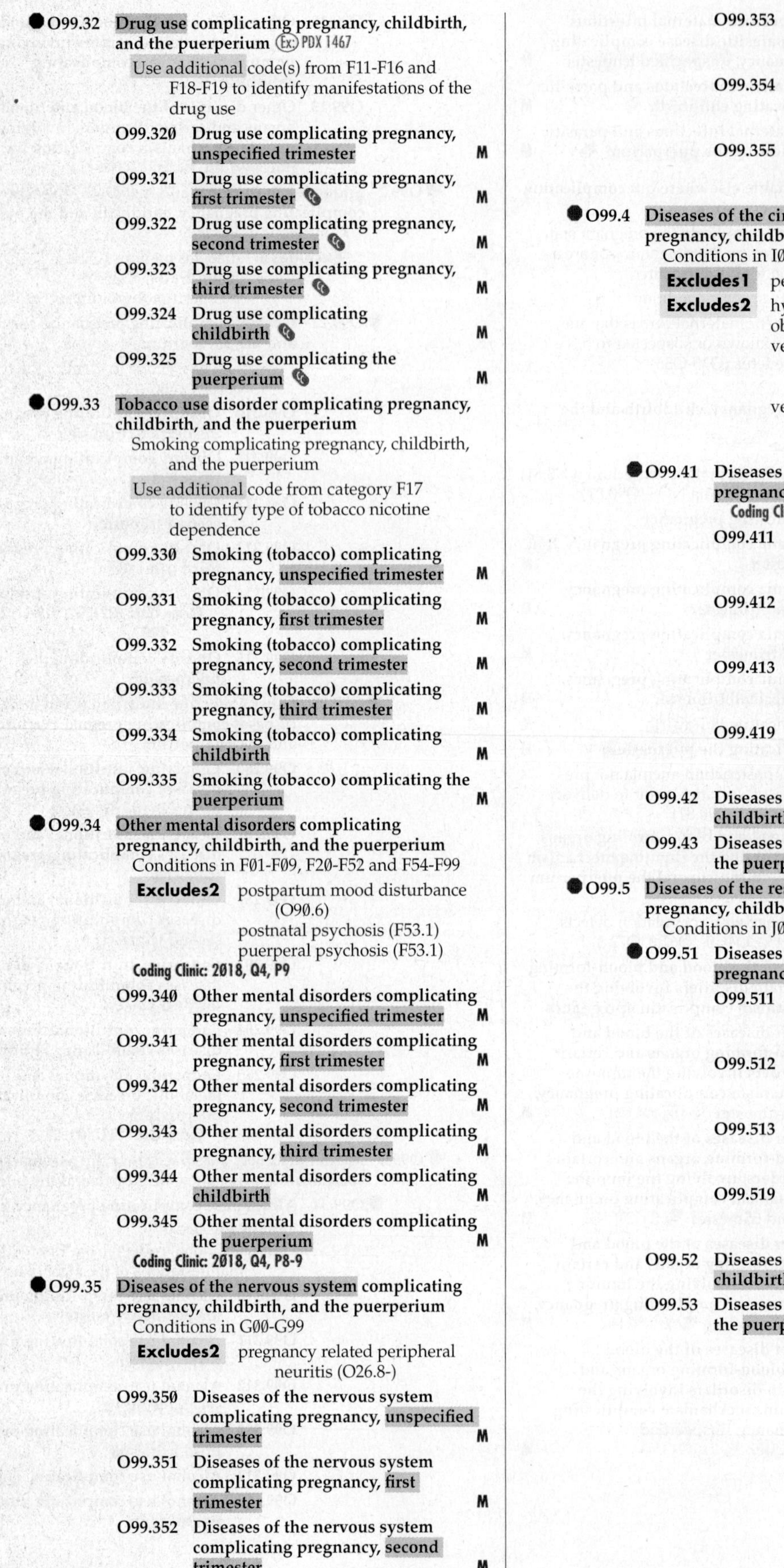

● O99.32 **Drug use complicating pregnancy, childbirth, and the puerperium** Ex: PDX 1467

Use additional code(s) from F11-F16 and F18-F19 to identify manifestations of the drug use

O99.320 **Drug use complicating pregnancy, unspecified trimester** M

O99.321 **Drug use complicating pregnancy, first trimester** M

O99.322 **Drug use complicating pregnancy, second trimester** M

O99.323 **Drug use complicating pregnancy, third trimester** M

O99.324 **Drug use complicating childbirth** M

O99.325 **Drug use complicating the puerperium** M

● O99.33 **Tobacco use disorder complicating pregnancy, childbirth, and the puerperium**

Smoking complicating pregnancy, childbirth, and the puerperium

Use additional code from category F17 to identify type of tobacco nicotine dependence

O99.330 **Smoking (tobacco) complicating pregnancy, unspecified trimester** M

O99.331 **Smoking (tobacco) complicating pregnancy, first trimester** M

O99.332 **Smoking (tobacco) complicating pregnancy, second trimester** M

O99.333 **Smoking (tobacco) complicating pregnancy, third trimester** M

O99.334 **Smoking (tobacco) complicating childbirth** M

O99.335 **Smoking (tobacco) complicating the puerperium** M

● O99.34 **Other mental disorders complicating pregnancy, childbirth, and the puerperium**

Conditions in F01-F09, F20-F52 and F54-F99

Excludes2 postpartum mood disturbance (O90.6)
postnatal psychosis (F53.1)
puerperal psychosis (F53.1)

Coding Clinic: 2018, Q4, P9

O99.340 **Other mental disorders complicating pregnancy, unspecified trimester** M

O99.341 **Other mental disorders complicating pregnancy, first trimester** M

O99.342 **Other mental disorders complicating pregnancy, second trimester** M

O99.343 **Other mental disorders complicating pregnancy, third trimester** M

O99.344 **Other mental disorders complicating childbirth** M

O99.345 **Other mental disorders complicating the puerperium** M

Coding Clinic: 2018, Q4, P8-9

● O99.35 **Diseases of the nervous system complicating pregnancy, childbirth, and the puerperium**

Conditions in G00-G99

Excludes2 pregnancy related peripheral neuritis (O26.8-)

O99.350 **Diseases of the nervous system complicating pregnancy, unspecified trimester** M

O99.351 **Diseases of the nervous system complicating pregnancy, first trimester** M

O99.352 **Diseases of the nervous system complicating pregnancy, second trimester** M

O99.353 **Diseases of the nervous system complicating pregnancy, third trimester** M

O99.354 **Diseases of the nervous system complicating childbirth** Ex: PDX 1468 M

O99.355 **Diseases of the nervous system complicating the puerperium** Ex: PDX 1469 M

● O99.4 **Diseases of the circulatory system complicating pregnancy, childbirth and the puerperium** Ex: PDX 1454

Conditions in I00-I99

Excludes1 peripartum cardiomyopathy (O90.3)

Excludes2 hypertensive disorders (O10-O16)
obstetric embolism (O88.-)
venous complications and cerebrovenous sinus thrombosis in labor, childbirth and the puerperium (O87.-)
venous complications and cerebrovenous sinus thrombosis in pregnancy (O22.-)

● O99.41 **Diseases of the circulatory system complicating pregnancy**

Coding Clinic: 2016, Q2, P8

O99.411 **Diseases of the circulatory system complicating pregnancy, first trimester** M

O99.412 **Diseases of the circulatory system complicating pregnancy, second trimester** M

O99.413 **Diseases of the circulatory system complicating pregnancy, third trimester** M

O99.419 **Diseases of the circulatory system complicating pregnancy, unspecified trimester** M

O99.42 **Diseases of the circulatory system complicating childbirth** M

O99.43 **Diseases of the circulatory system complicating the puerperium** M

● O99.5 **Diseases of the respiratory system complicating pregnancy, childbirth and the puerperium**

Conditions in J00-J99

● O99.51 **Diseases of the respiratory system complicating pregnancy**

O99.511 **Diseases of the respiratory system complicating pregnancy, first trimester** M

O99.512 **Diseases of the respiratory system complicating pregnancy, second trimester** M

O99.513 **Diseases of the respiratory system complicating pregnancy, third trimester** M

O99.519 **Diseases of the respiratory system complicating pregnancy, unspecified trimester** M

O99.52 **Diseases of the respiratory system complicating childbirth** M

O99.53 **Diseases of the respiratory system complicating the puerperium** M

● O99.6 **Diseases of the digestive system complicating pregnancy, childbirth and the puerperium**
Conditions in KØØ-K93
Excludes2 hemorrhoids in pregnancy (O22.4-)
liver and biliary tract disorders in pregnancy, childbirth and the puerperium (O26.6-)

● O99.61 **Diseases of the digestive system complicating pregnancy**

O99.611 **Diseases of the digestive system complicating pregnancy, first trimester** M

O99.612 **Diseases of the digestive system complicating pregnancy, second trimester** M

O99.613 **Diseases of the digestive system complicating pregnancy, third trimester** M

O99.619 **Diseases of the digestive system complicating pregnancy, unspecified trimester** M

O99.62 **Diseases of the digestive system complicating childbirth** M

O99.63 **Diseases of the digestive system complicating the puerperium** M

● O99.7 **Diseases of the skin and subcutaneous tissue complicating pregnancy, childbirth and the puerperium**
Conditions in LØØ-L99
Excludes2 herpes gestationis (O26.4)
pruritic urticarial papules and plaques of pregnancy (PUPPP) (O26.86)

● O99.71 **Diseases of the skin and subcutaneous tissue complicating pregnancy**

O99.711 **Diseases of the skin and subcutaneous tissue complicating pregnancy, first trimester** M

O99.712 **Diseases of the skin and subcutaneous tissue complicating pregnancy, second trimester** M

O99.713 **Diseases of the skin and subcutaneous tissue complicating pregnancy, third trimester** M

O99.719 **Diseases of the skin and subcutaneous tissue complicating pregnancy, unspecified trimester** M

O99.72 **Diseases of the skin and subcutaneous tissue complicating childbirth** M

O99.73 **Diseases of the skin and subcutaneous tissue complicating the puerperium** M

● O99.8 **Other specified diseases and conditions complicating pregnancy, childbirth and the puerperium**
Conditions in DØØ-D48, HØØ-H95, MØØ-N99, and QØØ-Q99
Use additional code to identify condition
Excludes2 genitourinary infections in pregnancy (O23.-)
infection of genitourinary tract following delivery (O86.1-O86.4)
malignant neoplasm complicating pregnancy, childbirth and the puerperium (O9A.1-)
maternal care for known or suspected abnormality of maternal pelvic organs (O34.-)
postpartum acute kidney failure (O9Ø.49)
traumatic injuries in pregnancy (O9A.2-)

● O99.81 **Abnormal glucose complicating pregnancy, childbirth and the puerperium**
Excludes1 gestational diabetes (O24.4-)

O99.81Ø **Abnormal glucose complicating pregnancy** M

O99.814 **Abnormal glucose complicating childbirth** M

O99.815 **Abnormal glucose complicating the puerperium** M

● O99.82 **Streptococcus B carrier state complicating pregnancy, childbirth and the puerperium**
Excludes1 Carrier of streptococcus group B (GBS) in a nonpregnant woman (Z22.33Ø)

● O99.82Ø **Streptococcus B carrier state complicating pregnancy** M

O99.824 **Streptococcus B carrier state complicating childbirth** M
Coding Clinic: 2019, Q2, P9

● O99.825 **Streptococcus B carrier state complicating the puerperium** M

● O99.83 **Other infection carrier state complicating pregnancy, childbirth and the puerperium** (Ex) PDX 1458
Use additional code to identify the carrier state (Z22.-)

O99.83Ø **Other infection carrier state complicating pregnancy** M

O99.834 **Other infection carrier state complicating childbirth** M

O99.835 **Other infection carrier state complicating the puerperium** M

● O99.84 **Bariatric surgery status complicating pregnancy, childbirth and the puerperium**
Gastric banding status complicating pregnancy, childbirth and the puerperium
Gastric bypass status for obesity complicating pregnancy, childbirth and the puerperium
Obesity surgery status complicating pregnancy, childbirth and the puerperium

O99.84Ø **Bariatric surgery status complicating pregnancy, unspecified trimester** M

O99.841 **Bariatric surgery status complicating pregnancy, first trimester** M

O99.842 **Bariatric surgery status complicating pregnancy, second trimester** M

O99.843 **Bariatric surgery status complicating pregnancy, third trimester** M

O99.844 **Bariatric surgery status complicating childbirth** M

O99.845 **Bariatric surgery status complicating the puerperium** M

● O99.89 **Other specified diseases and conditions complicating pregnancy, childbirth and the puerperium** M

O99.891 **Other specified diseases and conditions complicating pregnancy** M

O99.892 **Other specified diseases and conditions complicating childbirth** M
Coding Clinic: 2023, Q3, P17

O99.893 **Other specified diseases and conditions complicating puerperium** M

CHAPTER 15 (OØØ-O9A)

OGCR Section I.C.2.l.3.

Malignant neoplasm in a pregnant patient

When a pregnant woman has a malignant neoplasm, a code from subcategory O9A.1-, Malignant neoplasm complicating pregnancy, childbirth, and the puerperium, should be sequenced first, followed by the appropriate code from Chapter 2 to indicate the type of neoplasm.

● **O9A Maternal malignant neoplasms, traumatic injuries and abuse classifiable elsewhere but complicating pregnancy, childbirth and the puerperium**

● **O9A.1 Malignant neoplasm complicating pregnancy, childbirth and the puerperium**

Conditions in CØØ-C96

Use additional code to identify neoplasm

Excludes2 maternal care for benign tumor of corpus uteri (O34.1-)
maternal care for benign tumor of cervix (O34.4-)

● **O9A.11 Malignant neoplasm complicating pregnancy**

O9A.111 Malignant neoplasm complicating pregnancy, first trimester M

O9A.112 Malignant neoplasm complicating pregnancy, second trimester M

O9A.113 Malignant neoplasm complicating pregnancy, third trimester M

O9A.119 Malignant neoplasm complicating pregnancy, unspecified trimester M

O9A.12 Malignant neoplasm complicating childbirth M

O9A.13 Malignant neoplasm complicating the puerperium M

Coding Clinic: 2015, Q3, P19

● **O9A.2 Injury, poisoning and certain other consequences of external causes complicating pregnancy, childbirth and the puerperium**

Conditions in SØØ-T88, except T74 and T76

Use additional code(s) to identify the injury or poisoning

Excludes2 physical, sexual and psychological abuse complicating pregnancy, childbirth and the puerperium (O9A.3-, O9A.4-, O9A.5-)

● **O9A.21 Injury, poisoning and certain other consequences of external causes complicating pregnancy**

O9A.211 Injury, poisoning and certain other consequences of external causes complicating pregnancy, first trimester M

O9A.212 Injury, poisoning and certain other consequences of external causes complicating pregnancy, second trimester M

O9A.213 Injury, poisoning and certain other consequences of external causes complicating pregnancy, third trimester M

O9A.219 Injury, poisoning and certain other consequences of external causes complicating pregnancy, unspecified trimester M

O9A.22 Injury, poisoning and certain other consequences of external causes complicating childbirth M

O9A.23 Injury, poisoning and certain other consequences of external causes complicating the puerperium M

● **O9A.3 Physical abuse complicating pregnancy, childbirth and the puerperium**

Conditions in T74.11 or T76.11

Use additional code (if applicable):
to identify any associated current injury due to physical abuse
to identify the perpetrator of abuse (YØ7.-)

Excludes2 sexual abuse complicating pregnancy, childbirth and the puerperium (O9A.4)

● **O9A.31 Physical abuse complicating pregnancy**

O9A.311 Physical abuse complicating pregnancy, first trimester M

O9A.312 Physical abuse complicating pregnancy, second trimester M

O9A.313 Physical abuse complicating pregnancy, third trimester M

O9A.319 Physical abuse complicating pregnancy, unspecified trimester M

O9A.32 Physical abuse complicating childbirth M

O9A.33 Physical abuse complicating the puerperium M

● **O9A.4 Sexual abuse complicating pregnancy, childbirth and the puerperium**

Conditions in T74.21 or T76.21

Use additional code (if applicable):
to identify any associated current injury due to sexual abuse
to identify the perpetrator of abuse (YØ7.-)

● **O9A.41 Sexual abuse complicating pregnancy**

O9A.411 Sexual abuse complicating pregnancy, first trimester M

O9A.412 Sexual abuse complicating pregnancy, second trimester M

O9A.413 Sexual abuse complicating pregnancy, third trimester M

O9A.419 Sexual abuse complicating pregnancy, unspecified trimester M

O9A.42 Sexual abuse complicating childbirth M

O9A.43 Sexual abuse complicating the puerperium M

● **O9A.5 Psychological abuse complicating pregnancy, childbirth and the puerperium**

Conditions in T74.31 or T76.31

Use additional code to identify the perpetrator of abuse (YØ7.-)

● **O9A.51 Psychological abuse complicating pregnancy**

O9A.511 Psychological abuse complicating pregnancy, first trimester M

O9A.512 Psychological abuse complicating pregnancy, second trimester M

O9A.513 Psychological abuse complicating pregnancy, third trimester M

O9A.519 Psychological abuse complicating pregnancy, unspecified trimester M

O9A.52 Psychological abuse complicating childbirth M

O9A.53 Psychological abuse complicating the puerperium M

CHAPTER 16

CERTAIN CONDITIONS ORIGINATING IN THE PERINATAL PERIOD (P00-P96)

OGCR Chapter-Specific Coding Guidelines

16. Chapter 16: Certain Conditions Originating in the Perinatal Period (P00-P96)

For coding and reporting purposes the perinatal period is defined as before birth through the 28th day following birth. The following guidelines are provided for reporting purposes

a. General Perinatal Rules

1) Use of Chapter 16 Codes

Codes in this chapter are never for use on the maternal record. Codes from Chapter 15, the obstetric chapter, are never permitted on the newborn record. Chapter 16 codes may be used throughout the life of the patient if the condition is still present.

2) Principal Diagnosis for Birth Record

When coding the birth episode in a newborn record, assign a code from category Z38, Liveborn infants according to place of birth and type of delivery, as the principal diagnosis. A code from category Z38 is assigned only once, to a newborn at the time of birth. If a newborn is transferred to another institution, a code from category Z38 should not be used at the receiving hospital.

A code from category Z38 is used only on the newborn record, not on the mother's record.

3) Use of Codes from other Chapters with Codes from Chapter 16

Codes from other chapters may be used with codes from chapter 16 if the codes from the other chapters provide more specific detail. Codes for signs and symptoms may be assigned when a definitive diagnosis has not been established. If the reason for the encounter is a perinatal condition, the code from Chapter 16 should be sequenced first.

4) Use of Chapter 16 Codes after the Perinatal Period

Should a condition originate in the perinatal period, and continue throughout the life of the patient, the perinatal code should continue to be used regardless of the patient's age.

5) Birth process or community acquired conditions

If a newborn has a condition that may be either due to the birth process or community acquired and the documentation does not indicate which it is, the default is due to the birth process and the code from Chapter 16 should be used. If the condition is community-acquired, a code from Chapter 16 should not be assigned.

6) Code all clinically significant conditions

All clinically significant conditions noted on routine newborn examination should be coded. A condition is clinically significant if it requires:

- clinical evaluation; or
- therapeutic treatment; or
- diagnostic procedures; or
- extended length of hospital stay; or
- increased nursing care and/or monitoring; or
- has implications for future health care needs

Note: The perinatal guidelines listed above are the same as the general coding guidelines for "additional diagnoses", except for the final point regarding implications for future health care needs. Codes should be assigned for conditions that have been specified by the provider as having implications for future health care needs.

b. Observation and Evaluation of Newborns for Suspected Conditions Not Found

1) Use of Z05 codes

Assign a code from category Z05, Observation and evaluation of newborns and infants for suspected conditions ruled out, to identify those instances when a healthy newborn is evaluated for a suspected condition that is determined after study not to be present. Do not use a code from category Z05 when the patient has identified signs or symptoms of a suspected problem; in such cases code the sign or symptom.

2) Z05 on Other than the Birth Record

A code from category Z05 may also be assigned as a principal or first-listed code for readmissions or encounters when the code from category Z38 code no longer applies. Codes from category Z05 are for use only for healthy newborns and infants for which no condition after study is found to be present.

3) Z05 on a birth record

A code from category Z05 is to be used as a secondary code after the code from category Z38, Liveborn infants according to place of birth and type of delivery.

c. Coding Additional Perinatal Diagnoses

1) Assigning codes for conditions that require treatment

Assign codes for conditions that require treatment or further investigation, prolong the length of stay, or require resource utilization.

2) Codes for conditions specified as having implications for future health care needs

Assign codes for conditions that have been specified by the provider as having implications for future health care needs.

Note: This guideline should not be used for adult patients.

d. Prematurity and Fetal Growth Retardation

Providers utilize different criteria in determining prematurity. A code for prematurity should not be assigned unless it is documented. Assignment of codes in categories P05, Disorders of newborn related to slow fetal growth and fetal malnutrition, and P07, Disorders of newborn related to short gestation and low birth weight, not elsewhere classified, should be based on the recorded birth weight and estimated gestational age.

When both birth weight and gestational age are available, two codes from category P07 should be assigned, with the code for birth weight sequenced before the code for gestational age.

e. Low birth weight and immaturity status

Codes from category P07, Disorders of newborn related to short gestation and low birth weight, not elsewhere classified, are for use for a child or adult who was premature or had a low birth weight as a newborn and this is affecting the patient's current health status.

See Section I.C.21. Factors influencing health status and contact with health services, Status.

f. Bacterial Sepsis of Newborn

Category P36, Bacterial sepsis of newborn, includes congenital sepsis. If a perinate is documented as having sepsis without documentation of congenital or community acquired, the default is congenital and a code from category P36 should be assigned. If the P36 code includes the causal organism, an additional code from category B95, Streptococcus, Staphylococcus, and Enterococcus as the cause of diseases classified elsewhere, or B96, Other bacterial agents as the cause of diseases classified elsewhere, should not be assigned. If the P36 code does not include the causal organism, assign an additional code from category B96. If applicable, use additional codes to identify severe sepsis (R65.2-) and any associated acute organ dysfunction.

g. Stillbirth

Code P95, Stillbirth, is only for use in institutions that maintain separate records for stillbirths. No other code should be used with P95. Code P95 should not be used on the mother's record.

CHAPTER 16

CERTAIN CONDITIONS ORIGINATING IN THE PERINATAL PERIOD (P00-P96)

Note: Codes from this chapter are for use on newborn records only, never on maternal records.

Includes conditions that have their origin in the fetal or perinatal period (before birth through the first 28 days after birth) even if morbidity occurs later

Excludes2 congenital malformations, deformations and chromosomal abnormalities (Q00-Q99)
endocrine, nutritional and metabolic diseases (E00-E88)
injury, poisoning and certain other consequences of external causes (S00-T88)
neoplasms (C00-D49)
tetanus neonatorum (A33)

This chapter contains the following blocks:

P00-P04	Newborn affected by maternal factors and by complications of pregnancy, labor, and delivery
P05-P08	Disorders of newborns related to length of gestation and fetal growth
P09	Abnormal findings on neonatal screening
P10-P15	Birth trauma
P19-P29	Respiratory and cardiovascular disorders specific to the perinatal period
P35-P39	Infections specific to the perinatal period
P50-P61	Hemorrhagic and hematological disorders of newborn
P70-P74	Transitory endocrine and metabolic disorders specific to newborn
P76-P78	Digestive system disorders of newborn
P80-P83	Conditions involving the integument and temperature regulation of newborn
P84	Other problems with newborn
P90-P96	Other disorders originating in the perinatal period

NEWBORN AFFECTED BY MATERNAL FACTORS AND BY COMPLICATIONS OF PREGNANCY, LABOR, AND DELIVERY (P00–P04)

Note: These codes are for use when the listed maternal conditions are specified as the cause of confirmed morbidity or potential morbidity which have their origin in the perinatal period (before birth through the first 28 days after birth).

● **P00 Newborn affected by maternal conditions that may be unrelated to present pregnancy**
Code first any current condition in newborn
Excludes2 encounter for observation of newborn for suspected diseases and conditions ruled out (Z05.-)
newborn affected by maternal complications of pregnancy (P01.-)
newborn affected by maternal endocrine and metabolic disorders (P70–P74)
newborn affected by noxious substances transmitted via placenta or breast milk (P04.-)
Coding Clinic: 2016, Q4, P54

P00.0 Newborn affected by maternal hypertensive disorders
Newborn affected by maternal conditions classifiable to O10-O11, O13-O16

P00.1 Newborn affected by maternal renal and urinary tract diseases
Newborn affected by maternal conditions classifiable to N00-N39

P00.2 Newborn affected by maternal infectious and parasitic diseases
Newborn affected by maternal infectious disease classifiable to A00-B99, J09 and J10
Excludes1 maternal genital tract or other localized infections (P00.8)
Excludes2 infections specific to the perinatal period (P35-P39)
newborn affected by (positive) maternal group B streptococcus (GBS) colonization (P00.82)
Coding Clinic: 2019, Q2, P10; 2015, Q3, P21

P00.3 Newborn affected by other maternal circulatory and respiratory diseases
Newborn affected by maternal conditions classifiable to I00-I99, J00-J99, Q20-Q34 and not included in P00.0, P00.2

P00.4 Newborn affected by maternal nutritional disorders
Newborn affected by maternal disorders classifiable to E40-E64
Maternal malnutrition NOS

P00.5 Newborn affected by maternal injury
Newborn affected by maternal conditions classifiable to O9A.2-

P00.6 Newborn affected by surgical procedure on mother
Newborn affected by amniocentesis
Excludes1 Cesarean delivery for present delivery (P03.4)
damage to placenta from amniocentesis, cesarean delivery or surgical induction (P02.1)
previous surgery to uterus or pelvic organs (P03.89)
Excludes2 newborn affected by complication of (fetal) intrauterine procedure (P96.5)

P00.7 Newborn affected by other medical procedures on mother, not elsewhere classified
Newborn affected by radiation to mother
Excludes1 damage to placenta from amniocentesis, cesarean delivery or surgical induction (P02.1)
newborn affected by other complications of labor and delivery (P03.-)

● **P00.8 Newborn affected by other maternal conditions**

P00.81 Newborn affected by periodontal disease in mother

P00.82 Newborn affected by (positive) maternal group B streptococcus (GBS) colonization
Contact with positive maternal group B streptococcus
Coding Clinic: 2021, Q4, P23

P00.89 Newborn affected by other maternal conditions
Newborn affected by conditions classifiable to T80-T88
Newborn affected by maternal genital tract or other localized infections
Newborn affected by maternal systemic lupus erythematosus
Use additional code to identify infectious agent, if known
Excludes2 newborn affected by positive maternal group B streptococcus (GBS) colonization (P00.82)
Coding Clinic: 2019, Q2, P9

P00.9 Newborn affected by unspecified maternal condition

● **P01 Newborn affected by maternal complications of pregnancy**
Code first any current condition in newborn
Excludes2 encounter for observation of newborn for suspected diseases and conditions ruled out (Z05.-)
Coding Clinic: 2016, Q4, P54

P01.0 Newborn affected by incompetent cervix

P01.1 Newborn affected by premature rupture of membranes

P01.2 Newborn affected by oligohydramnios
Excludes1 oligohydramnios due to premature rupture of membranes (P01.1)

P01.3 Newborn affected by polyhydramnios
Excess of amniotic fluid, usually > 2000 mL
Newborn affected by hydramnios

P01.4 Newborn affected by ectopic pregnancy
Newborn affected by abdominal pregnancy

P01.5 Newborn affected by multiple pregnancy
Newborn affected by triplet (pregnancy)
Newborn affected by twin (pregnancy)

P01.6 Newborn affected by maternal death

P01.7 Newborn affected by malpresentation before labor
Newborn affected by breech presentation before labor
Newborn affected by external version before labor
Newborn affected by face presentation before labor
Newborn affected by transverse lie before labor
Newborn affected by unstable lie before labor

P01.8 Newborn affected by other maternal complications of pregnancy

P01.9 Newborn affected by maternal complication of pregnancy, unspecified

● P02 Newborn affected by complications of placenta, cord and membranes
Code first any current condition in newborn
Excludes2 encounter for observation of newborn for suspected diseases and conditions ruled out (Z05.-)
Coding Clinic: 2016, Q4, P54

P02.0 Newborn affected by placenta previa

P02.1 Newborn affected by other forms of placental separation and hemorrhage
Newborn affected by abruptio placenta
Newborn affected by accidental hemorrhage
Newborn affected by antepartum hemorrhage
Newborn affected by damage to placenta from amniocentesis, cesarean delivery or surgical induction
Newborn affected by maternal blood loss
Newborn affected by premature separation of placenta

● P02.2 Newborn affected by other and unspecified morphological and functional abnormalities of placenta

P02.20 Newborn affected by unspecified morphological and functional abnormalities of placenta

P02.29 Newborn affected by other morphological and functional abnormalities of placenta
Newborn affected by placental dysfunction
Newborn affected by placental infarction
Newborn affected by placental insufficiency

P02.3 Newborn affected by placental transfusion syndromes
Newborn affected by placental and cord abnormalities resulting in twin-to-twin or other transplacental transfusion

P02.4 Newborn affected by prolapsed cord

P02.5 Newborn affected by other compression of umbilical cord
Newborn affected by umbilical cord (tightly) around neck
Newborn affected by entanglement of umbilical cord
Newborn affected by knot in umbilical cord
Coding Clinic: 2022, Q1, P22

● P02.6 Newborn affected by other and unspecified conditions of umbilical cord

P02.60 Newborn affected by unspecified conditions of umbilical cord

P02.69 Newborn affected by other conditions of umbilical cord
Newborn affected by short umbilical cord
Newborn affected by vasa previa
Excludes1 newborn affected by single umbilical artery (Q27.0)

● P02.7 Newborn affected by chorioamnionitis
Inflammation of chorion and amnion

P02.70 Newborn affected by fetal inflammatory response syndrome
Newborn affected by FIRS

P02.78 Newborn affected by other conditions from chorioamnionitis
Newborn affected by amnionitis
Newborn affected by membranitis
Newborn affected by placentitis

P02.8 Newborn affected by other abnormalities of membranes

P02.9 Newborn affected by abnormality of membranes, unspecified

● P03 Newborn affected by other complications of labor and delivery
Code first any current condition in newborn
Excludes2 encounter for observation of newborn for suspected diseases and conditions ruled out (Z05.-)
Coding Clinic: 2016, Q4, P54

P03.0 Newborn affected by breech delivery and extraction

P03.1 Newborn affected by other malpresentation, malposition and disproportion during labor and delivery
Newborn affected by contracted pelvis
Newborn affected by conditions classifiable to O64-O66
Newborn affected by persistent occipitoposterior
Newborn affected by transverse lie

P03.2 Newborn affected by forceps delivery

P03.3 Newborn affected by delivery by vacuum extractor [ventouse]

P03.4 Newborn affected by Cesarean delivery

P03.5 Newborn affected by precipitate delivery
Newborn affected by rapid second stage

P03.6 Newborn affected by abnormal uterine contractions
Newborn affected by conditions classifiable to O62.-, except O62.3
Newborn affected by hypertonic labor
Newborn affected by uterine inertia

● P03.8 Newborn affected by other specified complications of labor and delivery

● P03.81 Newborn affected by abnormality in fetal (intrauterine) heart rate or rhythm
Excludes1 neonatal cardiac dysrhythmia (P29.1-)

P03.810 Newborn affected by abnormality in fetal (intrauterine) heart rate or rhythm before the onset of labor

P03.811 Newborn affected by abnormality in fetal (intrauterine) heart rate or rhythm during labor

P03.819 Newborn affected by abnormality in fetal (intrauterine) heart rate or rhythm, unspecified as to time of onset

P03.82 Meconium passage during delivery
Excludes1 meconium aspiration (P24.00, P24.01)
meconium staining (P96.83)

P03.89 Newborn affected by other specified complications of labor and delivery
Newborn affected by abnormality of maternal soft tissues
Newborn affected by conditions classifiable to O60-O75 and by procedures used in labor and delivery not included in P02.- and P03.0-P03.6
Newborn affected by induction of labor

P03.9 Newborn affected by complication of labor and delivery, unspecified

CHAPTER 16 (P00-P96)

● **P04 Newborn affected by noxious substances transmitted via placenta or breast milk**

Code first any current condition in newborn, if applicable

Includes nonteratogenic effects of substances transmitted via placenta

Excludes2 congenital malformations (Q00-Q99)
encounter for observation of newborn for suspected diseases and conditions ruled out (Z05.-)
neonatal jaundice from excessive hemolysis due to drugs or toxins transmitted from mother (P58.4)
newborn in contact with and (suspected) exposures hazardous to health not transmitted via placenta or breast milk (Z77.-)

Coding Clinic: 2016, Q4, P54

P04.0 Newborn affected by maternal anesthesia and analgesia in pregnancy, labor and delivery
Newborn affected by reactions and intoxications from maternal opiates and tranquilizers administered for procedures during pregnancy or labor and delivery

Excludes2 newborn affected by other maternal medication (P04.1-)

● **P04.1 Newborn affected by other maternal medication**

Code first, if applicable, withdrawal symptoms from maternal use of drugs of addiction (P96.1)
withdrawal symptoms from therapeutic use of drugs in newborn (P96.2)

Excludes1 dysmorphism due to warfarin (Q86.2)
fetal hydantoin syndrome (Q86.1)

Excludes2 maternal anesthesia and analgesia in pregnancy, labor and delivery (P04.0)
maternal use of drugs of addiction (P04.4-)

P04.11 Newborn affected by maternal antineoplastic chemotherapy
P04.12 Newborn affected by maternal cytotoxic drugs
P04.13 Newborn affected by maternal use of anticonvulsants
P04.14 Newborn affected by maternal use of opiates
P04.15 Newborn affected by maternal use of antidepressants
P04.16 Newborn affected by maternal use of amphetamines
P04.17 Newborn affected by maternal use of sedative-hypnotics
P04.1A Newborn affected by maternal use of anxiolytics
P04.18 Newborn affected by other maternal medication
P04.19 Newborn affected by maternal use of unspecified medication

Coding Clinic: 2016, Q4, P55

P04.2 Newborn affected by maternal use of tobacco
Newborn affected by exposure in utero to tobacco smoke

Excludes2 newborn exposure to environmental tobacco smoke (P96.81)

P04.3 Newborn affected by maternal use of alcohol

Excludes1 fetal alcohol syndrome (Q86.0)

● **P04.4 Newborn affected by maternal use of drugs of addiction**

P04.40 Newborn affected by maternal use of unspecified drugs of addiction
P04.41 Newborn affected by maternal use of cocaine
P04.42 Newborn affected by maternal use of hallucinogens

Excludes2 newborn affected by other maternal medication (P04.1-)

P04.49 Newborn affected by maternal use of other drugs of addiction

Excludes2 newborn affected by maternal anesthesia and analgesia (P04.0)
withdrawal symptoms from maternal use of drugs of addiction (P96.1)

P04.5 Newborn affected by maternal use of nutritional chemical substances

P04.6 Newborn affected by maternal exposure to environmental chemical substances

● **P04.8 Newborn affected by other maternal noxious substances**

P04.81 Newborn affected by maternal use of cannabis
P04.89 Newborn affected by other maternal noxious substances

P04.9 Newborn affected by maternal noxious substance, unspecified

OGCR Section I.C.16.d.

Prematurity and Fetal Growth Retardation

Providers utilize different criteria in determining prematurity. A code for prematurity should not be assigned unless it is documented. Assignment of codes in categories P05, Disorders of newborn related to slow fetal growth and fetal malnutrition, and P07, Disorders of newborn related to short gestation and low birth weight, not elsewhere classified, should be based on the recorded birth weight and estimated gestational age.

When both birth weight and gestational age are available, two codes from category P07 should be assigned, with the code for birth weight sequenced before the code for gestational age.

DISORDERS OF NEWBORN RELATED TO LENGTH OF GESTATION AND FETAL GROWTH (P05-P08)

● **P05 Disorders of newborn related to slow fetal growth and fetal malnutrition**

Coding Clinic: 2016, Q4, P56

● **P05.0 Newborn light for gestational age**
Newborn light-for-dates
Weight below but length above 10th percentile for gestational age

P05.00 Newborn light for gestational age, unspecified weight
P05.01 Newborn light for gestational age, less than 500 grams
P05.02 Newborn light for gestational age, 500-749 grams
P05.03 Newborn light for gestational age, 750-999 grams
P05.04 Newborn light for gestational age, 1000-1249 grams
P05.05 Newborn light for gestational age, 1250-1499 grams
P05.06 Newborn light for gestational age, 1500-1749 grams
P05.07 Newborn light for gestational age, 1750-1999 grams
P05.08 Newborn light for gestational age, 2000-2499 grams
P05.09 Newborn light for gestational age, 2500 grams and over
Newborn light for gestational age, other

Coding Clinic: 2016, Q4, P55

● **P05.1 Newborn small for gestational age**
Newborn small-and-light-for-dates
Newborn small-for-dates
Weight and length below 10th percentile for gestational age

P05.10 Newborn small for gestational age, unspecified weight

P05.11 Newborn small for gestational age, less than 500 grams

P05.12 Newborn small for gestational age, 500-749 grams

P05.13 Newborn small for gestational age, 750-999 grams

P05.14 Newborn small for gestational age, 1000-1249 grams

P05.15 Newborn small for gestational age, 1250-1499 grams

P05.16 Newborn small for gestational age, 1500-1749 grams

P05.17 Newborn small for gestational age, 1750-1999 grams

P05.18 Newborn small for gestational age, 2000-2499 grams

P05.19 Newborn small for gestational age, other
Newborn small for gestational age, 2500 grams and over
Coding Clinic: 2016, Q4, P55

P05.2 Newborn affected by fetal (intrauterine) malnutrition not light or small for gestational age
Infant, not light or small for gestational age, showing signs of fetal malnutrition, such as dry, peeling skin and loss of subcutaneous tissue
Excludes1 newborn affected by fetal malnutrition with light for gestational age (P05.0-)
newborn affected by fetal malnutrition with small for gestational age (P05.1-)

P05.9 Newborn affected by slow intrauterine growth, unspecified
Newborn affected by fetal growth retardation NOS

● **P07 Disorders of newborn related to short gestation and low birth weight, not elsewhere classified**
Note: When both birth weight and gestational age of the newborn are available, both should be coded with birth weight sequenced before gestational age.
Includes the listed conditions, without further specification, as the cause of morbidity or additional care, in newborn

● **P07.0 Extremely low birth weight newborn**
Newborn birth weight 999 g. or less
Excludes1 low birth weight due to slow fetal growth and fetal malnutrition (P05.-)

P07.00 Extremely low birth weight newborn, unspecified weight

P07.01 Extremely low birth weight newborn, less than 500 grams

P07.02 Extremely low birth weight newborn, 500-749 grams

P07.03 Extremely low birth weight newborn, 750-999 grams

● **P07.1 Other low birth weight newborn**
Newborn birth weight 1000-2499 g.
Excludes1 low birth weight due to slow fetal growth and fetal malnutrition (P05.-)

P07.10 Other low birth weight newborn, unspecified weight

P07.14 Other low birth weight newborn, 1000-1249 grams

P07.15 Other low birth weight newborn, 1250-1499 grams

P07.16 Other low birth weight newborn, 1500-1749 grams

P07.17 Other low birth weight newborn, 1750-1999 grams

P07.18 Other low birth weight newborn, 2000-2499 grams

● **P07.2 Extreme immaturity of newborn**
Less than 28 completed weeks (less than 196 completed days) of gestation

P07.20 Extreme immaturity of newborn, unspecified weeks of gestation
Gestational age less than 28 completed weeks NOS

P07.21 Extreme immaturity of newborn, gestational age less than 23 completed weeks
Extreme immaturity of newborn, gestational age less than 23 weeks, 0 days

P07.22 Extreme immaturity of newborn, gestational age 23 completed weeks
Extreme immaturity of newborn, gestational age 23 weeks, 0 days through 23 weeks, 6 days

P07.23 Extreme immaturity of newborn, gestational age 24 completed weeks
Extreme immaturity of newborn, gestational age 24 weeks, 0 days through 24 weeks, 6 days

P07.24 Extreme immaturity of newborn, gestational age 25 completed weeks
Extreme immaturity of newborn, gestational age 25 weeks, 0 days through 25 weeks, 6 days

P07.25 Extreme immaturity of newborn, gestational age 26 completed weeks
Extreme immaturity of newborn, gestational age 26 weeks, 0 days through 26 weeks, 6 days

P07.26 Extreme immaturity of newborn, gestational age 27 completed weeks
Extreme immaturity of newborn, gestational age 27 weeks, 0 days through 27 weeks, 6 days

● **P07.3 Preterm [premature] newborn [other]**
28 completed weeks or more but less than 37 completed weeks (196 completed days but less than 259 completed days) of gestation
Prematurity NOS

P07.30 Preterm newborn, unspecified weeks of gestation

P07.31 Preterm newborn, gestational age 28 completed weeks
Preterm newborn, gestational age 28 weeks, 0 days through 28 weeks, 6 days

P07.32 Preterm newborn, gestational age 29 completed weeks
Preterm newborn, gestational age 29 weeks, 0 days through 29 weeks, 6 days

P07.33 Preterm newborn, gestational age 30 completed weeks
Preterm newborn, gestational age 30 weeks, 0 days through 30 weeks, 6 days

P07.34 Preterm newborn, gestational age 31 completed weeks
Preterm newborn, gestational age 31 weeks, 0 days through 31 weeks, 6 days

P07.35 Preterm newborn, gestational age 32 completed weeks
Preterm newborn, gestational age 32 weeks, 0 days through 32 weeks, 6 days

P07.36 Preterm newborn, gestational age 33 completed weeks
Preterm newborn, gestational age 33 weeks, 0 days through 33 weeks, 6 days

P07.37 **Preterm newborn, gestational age 34 completed weeks**
Preterm newborn, gestational age 34 weeks, 0 days through 34 weeks, 6 days
Coding Clinic: 2017, Q2, P7

P07.38 **Preterm newborn, gestational age 35 completed weeks**
Preterm newborn, gestational age 35 weeks, 0 days through 35 weeks, 6 days

P07.39 **Preterm newborn, gestational age 36 completed weeks**
Preterm newborn, gestational age 36 weeks, 0 days through 36 weeks, 6 days
Coding Clinic: 2017, Q3, P26

● P08 **Disorders of newborn related to long gestation and high birth weight**
Note: When both birth weight and gestational age of the newborn are available, priority of assignment should be given to birth weight.
Includes the listed conditions, without further specification, as causes of morbidity or additional care, in newborn

P08.0 **Exceptionally large newborn baby**
Usually implies a birth weight of 4500 g. or more
Excludes1 syndrome of infant of diabetic mother (P70.1)
syndrome of infant of mother with gestational diabetes (P70.0)

P08.1 **Other heavy for gestational age newborn**
Other newborn heavy- or large-for-dates regardless of period of gestation
Usually implies a birth weight of 4000 g. to 4499 g.
Excludes1 newborn with a birth weight of 4500 or more (P08.0)
syndrome of infant of diabetic mother (P70.1)
syndrome of infant of mother with gestational diabetes (P70.0)

● P08.2 **Late newborn, not heavy for gestational age**

P08.21 **Post-term newborn**
Newborn with gestation period over 40 completed weeks to 42 completed weeks

P08.22 **Prolonged gestation of newborn**
Newborn with gestation period over 42 completed weeks (294 days or more), not heavy- or large-for-dates
Postmaturity NOS

ABNORMAL FINDINGS ON NEONATAL SCREENING (P09)

● P09 **Abnormal findings on neonatal screening**
Includes: Abnormal findings on state mandated newborn screens
Failed newborn screening
Excludes2 nonspecific serologic evidence of human immunodeficiency virus [HIV] (R75)

P09.1 **Abnormal findings on neonatal screening for inborn errors of metabolism**

P09.2 **Abnormal findings on neonatal screening for congenital endocrine disease**
Abnormal findings on neonatal screening for congenital adrenal hyperplasia
Abnormal findings on neonatal screening for hypothyroidism screen

P09.3 **Abnormal findings on neonatal screening for congenital hematologic disorders**
Abnormal findings for hemoglobinopathy screening
Abnormal findings on red cell membrane defects screen
Abnormal findings on sickle cell screen

P09.4 **Abnormal findings on neonatal screening for cystic fibrosis**

P09.5 **Abnormal findings on neonatal screening for critical congenital heart disease**
Neonatal congenital heart disease screening failure

P09.6 **Abnormal findings on neonatal screening for neonatal hearing loss**
Excludes2 encounter for hearing examination following failed hearing screening (Z01.110)

P09.8 **Other abnormal findings on neonatal screening**

P09.9 **Abnormal findings on neonatal screening, unspecified**

BIRTH TRAUMA (P10-P15)

● P10 **Intracranial laceration and hemorrhage due to birth injury** Ex PDX 1470
Excludes1 intracranial hemorrhage of newborn NOS (P52.9)
intracranial hemorrhage of newborn due to anoxia or hypoxia (P52.-)
nontraumatic intracranial hemorrhage of newborn (P52.-)

P10.0 **Subdural hemorrhage due to birth injury**
Subdural hematoma (localized) due to birth injury
Excludes1 subdural hemorrhage accompanying tentorial tear (P10.4)

P10.1 **Cerebral hemorrhage due to birth injury**

P10.2 **Intraventricular hemorrhage due to birth injury** Ex PDX 1471

P10.3 **Subarachnoid hemorrhage due to birth injury** Ex PDX 1472

P10.4 **Tentorial tear due to birth injury**
Pertaining to tentorium of cerebellum (extension of dura mater that separates cerebellum from inferior portion of occipital lobes)

P10.8 **Other intracranial lacerations and hemorrhages due to birth injury**

P10.9 **Unspecified intracranial laceration and hemorrhage due to birth injury**

● P11 **Other birth injuries to central nervous system**

P11.0 **Cerebral edema due to birth injury** Ex PDX 1470

P11.1 **Other specified brain damage due to birth injury**

P11.2 **Unspecified brain damage due to birth injury** Ex PDX 1470

P11.3 **Birth injury to facial nerve**
Facial palsy due to birth injury

P11.4 **Birth injury to other cranial nerves**

P11.5 **Birth injury to spine and spinal cord**
Fracture of spine due to birth injury

P11.9 **Birth injury to central nervous system, unspecified** Ex PDX 1470

● P12 **Birth injury to scalp**

P12.0 **Cephalhematoma due to birth injury**

P12.1 **Chignon (from vacuum extraction) due to birth injury**

P12.2 **Epicranial subaponeurotic hemorrhage due to birth injury** Ex PDX 1473
Subgaleal hemorrhage

P12.3 **Bruising of scalp due to birth injury**

P12.4 **Injury of scalp of newborn due to monitoring equipment**
Sampling incision of scalp of newborn
Scalp clip (electrode) injury of newborn

● P12.8 **Other birth injuries to scalp**

P12.81 **Caput succedaneum**

P12.89 **Other birth injuries to scalp**

P12.9 **Birth injury to scalp, unspecified**

● P13 **Birth injury to skeleton**
Excludes2 birth injury to spine (P11.5)

P13.0 **Fracture of skull due to birth injury**

P13.1 **Other birth injuries to skull**
Excludes1 cephalhematoma (P12.0)

P13.2 **Birth injury to femur**

P13.3 **Birth injury to other long bones**

Item 16-1 The **peripheral nervous system** consists of 31 pairs of spinal nerves, 12 pairs of cranial nerves, and the autonomic nerves, which are divided into the parasympathetic and sympathetic nerves. The cranial nerves are: olfactory (I), optic (II), oculomotor (III), trochlear (IV), trigeminal (V), abducens (VI), facial (VII), vestibulocochlear (VIII), glossopharyngeal (IX), vagus (X), accessory (XI), and hypoglossal (XII).

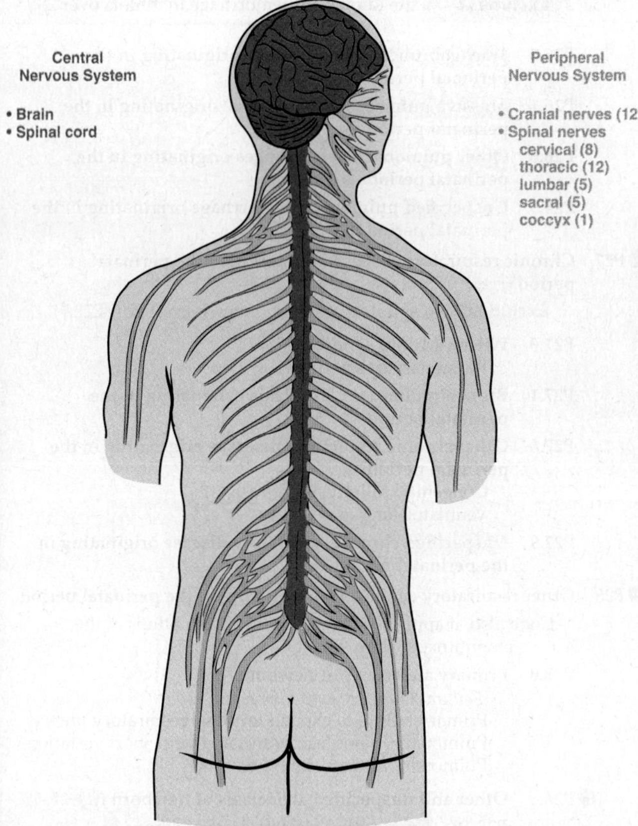

Figure 16-1 The central nervous system consists of the brain and spinal cord. The peripheral nervous system consists of nerves that lie outside the skull and spinal cord. (From Stoy: Mosby's EMT-Basic Textbook, ed 2, St. Louis, Mosby, 2007)

P13.4 **Fracture of clavicle due to birth injury**
P13.8 **Birth injuries to other parts of skeleton**
P13.9 **Birth injury to skeleton, unspecified**

● **P14** **Birth injury to peripheral nervous system**
P14.0 **Erb's paralysis due to birth injury**
P14.1 **Klumpke's paralysis due to birth injury**
P14.2 **Phrenic nerve paralysis due to birth injury**
P14.3 **Other brachial plexus birth injuries**
P14.8 **Birth injuries to other parts of peripheral nervous system**
P14.9 **Birth injury to peripheral nervous system, unspecified**

● **P15** **Other birth injuries**
P15.0 **Birth injury to liver**
Rupture of liver due to birth injury
P15.1 **Birth injury to spleen**
Rupture of spleen due to birth injury
P15.2 **Sternomastoid injury due to birth injury**
P15.3 **Birth injury to eye**
Subconjunctival hemorrhage due to birth injury
Traumatic glaucoma due to birth injury
P15.4 **Birth injury to face**
Facial congestion due to birth injury
P15.5 **Birth injury to external genitalia**
P15.6 **Subcutaneous fat necrosis due to birth injury**
P15.8 **Other specified birth injuries**
P15.9 **Birth injury, unspecified**

RESPIRATORY AND CARDIOVASCULAR DISORDERS SPECIFIC TO THE PERINATAL PERIOD (P19-P29)

● **P19** **Metabolic acidemia in newborn**
Includes metabolic acidemia in newborn
P19.0 **Metabolic acidemia in newborn first noted before onset of labor**
P19.1 **Metabolic acidemia in newborn first noted during labor**
P19.2 **Metabolic acidemia noted at birth**
P19.9 **Metabolic acidemia in newborn, unspecified**

● **P22** **Respiratory distress of newborn**
Coding Clinic: 2019, Q2, P29
P22.0 **Respiratory distress syndrome of newborn** (Ex) PDX 1047
Cardiorespiratory distress syndrome of newborn
Hyaline membrane disease
Idiopathic respiratory distress syndrome [IRDS or RDS] of newborn
Pulmonary hypoperfusion syndrome
Respiratory distress syndrome, type I
Excludes2 respiratory arrest of newborn (P28.81)
respiratory failure of newborn NOS (P28.5)
Coding Clinic: 2019, Q2, P29
P22.1 **Transient tachypnea of newborn**
Idiopathic tachypnea of newborn
Respiratory distress syndrome, type II
Wet lung syndrome
P22.8 **Other respiratory distress of newborn**
Excludes1 respiratory arrest of newborn (P28.81)
respiratory failure of newborn NOS (P28.5)
P22.9 **Respiratory distress of newborn, unspecified**
Excludes1 respiratory arrest of newborn (P28.81)
respiratory failure of newborn NOS (P28.5)

● **P23** **Congenital pneumonia** (Ex) PDX 1474
Includes infective pneumonia acquired in utero or during birth
Excludes1 neonatal pneumonia resulting from aspiration (P24.-)
P23.0 **Congenital pneumonia due to viral agent**
Use additional code (B97) to identify organism
Excludes1 congenital rubella pneumonitis (P35.0)
P23.1 **Congenital pneumonia due to Chlamydia**
P23.2 **Congenital pneumonia due to staphylococcus**
P23.3 **Congenital pneumonia due to streptococcus, group B**
P23.4 **Congenital pneumonia due to Escherichia coli**
P23.5 **Congenital pneumonia due to Pseudomonas**
P23.6 **Congenital pneumonia due to other bacterial agents**
Congenital pneumonia due to Hemophilus influenzae
Congenital pneumonia due to Klebsiella pneumoniae
Congenital pneumonia due to Mycoplasma
Congenital pneumonia due to Streptococcus, except group B
Use additional code (B95-B96) to identify organism
P23.8 **Congenital pneumonia due to other organisms**
P23.9 **Congenital pneumonia, unspecified**

● **P24** **Neonatal aspiration**
Includes aspiration in utero and during delivery
● **P24.0** **Meconium aspiration**
Excludes1 meconium passage (without aspiration) during delivery (P03.82)
meconium staining (P96.83)
P24.00 **Meconium aspiration without respiratory symptoms**
Meconium aspiration NOS

CHAPTER 16 (P00-P96)

P24.01 **Meconium aspiration with respiratory symptoms** (Ex) PDX 1474
Meconium aspiration pneumonia
Meconium aspiration pneumonitis
Meconium aspiration syndrome NOS
Use additional code to identify any secondary pulmonary hypertension, if applicable (I27.2-)

● P24.1 **Neonatal aspiration of (clear) amniotic fluid and mucus**
Neonatal aspiration of liquor (amnii)

P24.10 **Neonatal aspiration of (clear) amniotic fluid and mucus without respiratory symptoms**
Neonatal aspiration of amniotic fluid and mucus NOS

P24.11 **Neonatal aspiration of (clear) amniotic fluid and mucus with respiratory symptoms** (Ex) PDX 1474
Neonatal aspiration of amniotic fluid and mucus with pneumonia
Neonatal aspiration of amniotic fluid and mucus with pneumonitis
Use additional code to identify any secondary pulmonary hypertension, if applicable (I27.2-)

● P24.2 **Neonatal aspiration of blood**

P24.20 **Neonatal aspiration of blood without respiratory symptoms**
Neonatal aspiration of blood NOS

P24.21 **Neonatal aspiration of blood with respiratory symptoms** (Ex) PDX 1474
Neonatal aspiration of blood with pneumonia
Neonatal aspiration of blood with pneumonitis
Use additional code to identify any secondary pulmonary hypertension, if applicable (I27.2-)

● P24.3 **Neonatal aspiration of milk and regurgitated food**
Neonatal aspiration of stomach contents

P24.30 **Neonatal aspiration of milk and regurgitated food without respiratory symptoms**
Neonatal aspiration of milk and regurgitated food NOS

P24.31 **Neonatal aspiration of milk and regurgitated food with respiratory symptoms** (Ex) PDX 1474
Neonatal aspiration of milk and regurgitated food with pneumonia
Neonatal aspiration of milk and regurgitated food with pneumonitis
Use additional code to identify any secondary pulmonary hypertension, if applicable (I27.2-)

● P24.8 **Other neonatal aspiration**

P24.80 **Other neonatal aspiration without respiratory symptoms**
Neonatal aspiration NEC

P24.81 **Other neonatal aspiration with respiratory symptoms** (Ex) PDX 1474
Neonatal aspiration pneumonia NEC
Neonatal aspiration with pneumonitis NEC
Neonatal aspiration with pneumonia NOS
Neonatal aspiration with pneumonitis NOS
Use additional code to identify any secondary pulmonary hypertension, if applicable (I27.2-)

P24.9 **Neonatal aspiration, unspecified**

● P25 **Interstitial emphysema and related conditions originating in the perinatal period** (Ex) PDX 1047

P25.0 **Interstitial emphysema originating in the perinatal period**

P25.1 **Pneumothorax originating in the perinatal period**

P25.2 **Pneumomediastinum originating in the perinatal period**

P25.3 **Pneumopericardium originating in the perinatal period**

P25.8 **Other conditions related to interstitial emphysema originating in the perinatal period**

● P26 **Pulmonary hemorrhage originating in the perinatal period** (Ex) PDX 1047
Excludes1 acute idiopathic hemorrhage in infants over 28 days old (R04.81)

P26.0 **Tracheobronchial hemorrhage originating in the perinatal period**

P26.1 **Massive pulmonary hemorrhage originating in the perinatal period**

P26.8 **Other pulmonary hemorrhages originating in the perinatal period**

P26.9 **Unspecified pulmonary hemorrhage originating in the perinatal period**

● P27 **Chronic respiratory disease originating in the perinatal period** (Ex) PDX 1047
Excludes2 respiratory distress of newborn (P22.0-P22.9)

P27.0 **Wilson-Mikity syndrome**
Pulmonary dysmaturity

P27.1 **Bronchopulmonary dysplasia originating in the perinatal period**

P27.8 **Other chronic respiratory diseases originating in the perinatal period**
Congenital pulmonary fibrosis
Ventilator lung in newborn

P27.9 **Unspecified chronic respiratory disease originating in the perinatal period**

● P28 **Other respiratory conditions originating in the perinatal period**
Code also, if applicable, congenital malformations of the respiratory system (Q30-Q34)

P28.0 **Primary atelectasis of newborn** (Ex) PDX 1047
Failure of lungs to expand properly at birth
Primary failure to expand terminal respiratory units
Pulmonary hypoplasia associated with short gestation
Pulmonary immaturity NOS

● P28.1 **Other and unspecified atelectasis of newborn** (Ex) PDX 1047

P28.10 **Unspecified atelectasis of newborn**
Atelectasis of newborn NOS

P28.11 **Resorption atelectasis without respiratory distress syndrome**
Excludes1 resorption atelectasis with respiratory distress syndrome (P22.0)

P28.19 **Other atelectasis of newborn**
Partial atelectasis of newborn
Secondary atelectasis of newborn

P28.2 **Cyanotic attacks of newborn** (Ex) PDX 1475
Excludes1 apnea of newborn (P28.3- - P28.4-)

● P28.3 **Primary sleep apnea of newborn** (Ex) PDX 1476
Sleep apnea of newborn NOS
Excludes2 other apnea of newborn (P28.4-)

P28.30 **Primary sleep apnea of newborn, unspecified**
Transient oxygen desaturation spells of newborn during sleep

P28.31 **Primary central sleep apnea of newborn**

P28.32 **Primary obstructive sleep apnea of newborn**

P28.33 **Primary mixed sleep apnea of newborn**

P28.39 **Other primary sleep apnea of newborn**

● **P28.4 Other apnea of newborn** PDX 1476
Excludes2 primary sleep apnea of newborn (P28.3-)
P28.40 Unspecified apnea of newborn
Apnea of newborn, NOS
Transient oxygen desaturation spells of newborn
P28.41 Central neonatal apnea of newborn
P28.42 Obstructive apnea of newborn
P28.43 Mixed neonatal apnea of newborn
P28.49 Other apnea of newborn
Apnea of prematurity
P28.5 Respiratory failure of newborn PDX 1047
Excludes2 respiratory arrest of newborn (P28.81)
respiratory distress of newborn (P22.Ø)
Coding Clinic: 2019, Q2, P29
● **P28.8 Other specified respiratory conditions of newborn**
P28.81 Respiratory arrest of newborn PDX 1477
Coding Clinic: 2017, Q2, P6
P28.89 Other specified respiratory conditions of newborn
Congenital laryngeal stridor
Sniffles in newborn
Snuffles in newborn
Excludes1 early congenital syphilitic rhinitis (A5Ø.Ø5)
P28.9 Respiratory condition of newborn, unspecified
Respiratory depression in newborn
Code also associated underlying condition
● **P29 Cardiovascular disorders originating in the perinatal period**
Excludes2 congenital malformations of the circulatory system (Q2Ø-Q28)
P29.Ø Neonatal cardiac failure
● **P29.1 Neonatal cardiac dysrhythmia**
P29.11 Neonatal tachycardia
P29.12 Neonatal bradycardia
P29.2 Neonatal hypertension
● **P29.3 Persistent fetal circulation**
P29.3Ø Pulmonary hypertension of newborn PDX 1478
Persistent pulmonary hypertension of newborn
P29.38 Other persistent fetal circulation PDX 1479
Delayed closure of ductus arteriosus
P29.4 Transient myocardial ischemia in newborn
● **P29.8 Other cardiovascular disorders originating in the perinatal period**
P29.81 Cardiac arrest of newborn PDX 1480
P29.89 Other cardiovascular disorders originating in the perinatal period
P29.9 Cardiovascular disorder originating in the perinatal period, unspecified

INFECTIONS SPECIFIC TO THE PERINATAL PERIOD (P35-P39)

Infections acquired in utero, during birth via the umbilicus, or during the first 28 days after birth
Excludes2 asymptomatic human immunodeficiency virus [HIV] infection status (Z21)
congenital gonococcal infection (A54.-)
congenital pneumonia (P23.-)
congenital syphilis (A5Ø.-)
human immunodeficiency virus [HIV] disease (B2Ø)
infant botulism (A48.51)
infectious diseases not specific to the perinatal period (AØØ-B99, JØ9, J1Ø.-)
intestinal infectious disease (AØØ-AØ9)
laboratory evidence of human immunodeficiency virus [HIV] (R75)
tetanus neonatorum (A33)

● **P35 Congenital viral diseases** PDX 1482
Includes infections acquired in utero or during birth
P35.Ø Congenital rubella syndrome PDX 1481
Congenital rubella pneumonitis
P35.1 Congenital cytomegalovirus infection PDX 1481
Viruses transmitted by multiple routes that cause mild/subclinical infection
P35.2 Congenital herpesviral [herpes simplex] infection
P35.3 Congenital viral hepatitis
P35.4 Congenital Zika virus disease
Use additional code to identify manifestations of congenital Zika virus disease
Coding Clinic: 2018, Q4, P26
P35.8 Other congenital viral diseases
Congenital varicella [chickenpox]
Coding Clinic: 2016, Q4, P7
P35.9 Congenital viral disease, unspecified
● **P36 Bacterial sepsis of newborn** PDX 1483
Includes congenital sepsis
Use additional code(s), if applicable, to identify severe sepsis (R65.2-) and associated acute organ dysfunction(s)
P36.Ø Sepsis of newborn due to streptococcus, group B
● **P36.1 Sepsis of newborn due to other and unspecified streptococci**
P36.1Ø Sepsis of newborn due to unspecified streptococci
P36.19 Sepsis of newborn due to other streptococci
P36.2 Sepsis of newborn due to Staphylococcus aureus
● **P36.3 Sepsis of newborn due to other and unspecified staphylococci**
P36.3Ø Sepsis of newborn due to unspecified staphylococci
P36.39 Sepsis of newborn due to other staphylococci
P36.4 Sepsis of newborn due to Escherichia coli
P36.5 Sepsis of newborn due to anaerobes
P36.8 Other bacterial sepsis of newborn
Use additional code from category B96 to identify organism
P36.9 Bacterial sepsis of newborn, unspecified
● **P37 Other congenital infectious and parasitic diseases** PDX 1484
Excludes2 congenital syphilis (A5Ø.-)
infectious neonatal diarrhea (AØØ-AØ9)
necrotizing enterocolitis in newborn (P77.-)
noninfectious neonatal diarrhea (P78.3)
ophthalmia neonatorum due to gonococcus (A54.31)
tetanus neonatorum (A33)
P37.Ø Congenital tuberculosis PDX 1482
P37.1 Congenital toxoplasmosis
Parasitic infection, often causing mild flu-like illness
Hydrocephalus due to congenital toxoplasmosis
P37.2 Neonatal (disseminated) listeriosis
Acquired transplacentally or during/after parturition in which symptoms are those of sepsis
P37.3 Congenital falciparum malaria
P37.4 Other congenital malaria
P37.5 Neonatal candidiasis
P37.8 Other specified congenital infectious and parasitic diseases
P37.9 Congenital infectious or parasitic disease, unspecified
● **P38 Omphalitis of newborn**
Inflammation of umbilicus
Excludes1 omphalitis not of newborn (LØ8.82)
tetanus omphalitis (A33)
umbilical hemorrhage of newborn (P51.-)
P38.1 Omphalitis with mild hemorrhage PDX 1485
P38.9 Omphalitis without hemorrhage PDX 1486
Omphalitis of newborn NOS

● P39 **Other infections specific to the perinatal period**
Use additional code to identify organism or specific infection

P39.Ø **Neonatal infective mastitis**
Excludes1 breast engorgement of newborn (P83.4)
noninfective mastitis of newborn (P83.4)

P39.1 **Neonatal conjunctivitis and dacryocystitis**
Neonatal chlamydial conjunctivitis
Ophthalmia neonatorum NOS
Neonate = newborn
Excludes1 gonococcal conjunctivitis (A54.31)

P39.2 **Intra-amniotic infection affecting newborn, not elsewhere classified**

P39.3 **Neonatal urinary tract infection**

P39.4 **Neonatal skin infection**
Neonatal pyoderma
Excludes1 pemphigus neonatorum (LØØ)
staphylococcal scalded skin syndrome (LØØ)

P39.8 **Other specified infections specific to the perinatal period**

P39.9 **Infection specific to the perinatal period, unspecified**

HEMORRHAGIC AND HEMATOLOGICAL DISORDERS OF NEWBORN (P5Ø-P61)

Excludes1 congenital stenosis and stricture of bile ducts (Q44.3)
Crigler-Najjar syndrome (E8Ø.5)
Dubin-Johnson syndrome (E8Ø.6)
Gilbert syndrome (E8Ø.4)
hereditary hemolytic anemias (D55-D58)

● P5Ø **Newborn affected by intrauterine (fetal) blood loss**
Excludes1 congenital anemia from intrauterine (fetal) blood loss (P61.3)

P5Ø.Ø **Newborn affected by intrauterine (fetal) blood loss from vasa previa**

P5Ø.1 **Newborn affected by intrauterine (fetal) blood loss from ruptured cord**

P5Ø.2 **Newborn affected by intrauterine (fetal) blood loss from placenta**

P5Ø.3 **Newborn affected by hemorrhage into co-twin**

P5Ø.4 **Newborn affected by hemorrhage into maternal circulation**

P5Ø.5 **Newborn affected by intrauterine (fetal) blood loss from cut end of co-twin's cord**

P5Ø.8 **Newborn affected by other intrauterine (fetal) blood loss**

P5Ø.9 **Newborn affected by intrauterine (fetal) blood loss, unspecified**
Newborn affected by fetal hemorrhage NOS

● P51 **Umbilical hemorrhage of newborn**
Excludes1 omphalitis with mild hemorrhage (P38.1)
umbilical hemorrhage from cut end of co-twins cord (P5Ø.5)

P51.Ø **Massive umbilical hemorrhage of newborn**

P51.8 **Other umbilical hemorrhages of newborn**
Slipped umbilical ligature NOS

P51.9 **Umbilical hemorrhage of newborn, unspecified**

● P52 **Intracranial nontraumatic hemorrhage of newborn**
Includes intracranial hemorrhage due to anoxia or hypoxia
Excludes1 intracranial hemorrhage due to birth injury (P1Ø.-)
intracranial hemorrhage due to other injury (SØ6.-)

P52.Ø **Intraventricular (nontraumatic) hemorrhage, grade 1, of newborn** (Ex) PDX 1471
Subependymal hemorrhage (without intraventricular extension)
Bleeding into germinal matrix

P52.1 **Intraventricular (nontraumatic) hemorrhage, grade 2, of newborn** (Ex) PDX 1471
Subependymal hemorrhage with intraventricular extension
Bleeding into ventricle

● P52.2 **Intraventricular (nontraumatic) hemorrhage, grade 3 and grade 4, of newborn** (Ex) PDX 1471

P52.21 **Intraventricular (nontraumatic) hemorrhage, grade 3, of newborn**
Subependymal hemorrhage with intraventricular extension with enlargement of ventricle

P52.22 **Intraventricular (nontraumatic) hemorrhage, grade 4, of newborn**
Bleeding into cerebral cortex
Subependymal hemorrhage with intracerebral extension

P52.3 **Unspecified intraventricular (nontraumatic) hemorrhage of newborn** (Ex) PDX 1471

P52.4 **Intracerebral (nontraumatic) hemorrhage of newborn** (Ex) PDX 1470

P52.5 **Subarachnoid (nontraumatic) hemorrhage of newborn** (Ex) PDX 1472

P52.6 **Cerebellar (nontraumatic) and posterior fossa hemorrhage of newborn** (Ex) PDX 1471

P52.8 **Other intracranial (nontraumatic) hemorrhages of newborn** (Ex) PDX 1470

P52.9 **Intracranial (nontraumatic) hemorrhage of newborn, unspecified** (Ex) PDX 1470

P53 **Hemorrhagic disease of newborn** (Ex) PDX 1490
Vitamin K deficiency of newborn

● P54 **Other neonatal hemorrhages** (Ex) PDX 1491
Excludes1 newborn affected by (intrauterine) blood loss (P5Ø.-)
pulmonary hemorrhage originating in the perinatal period (P26.-)

P54.Ø **Neonatal hematemesis**
Vomiting of blood
Excludes1 neonatal hematemesis due to swallowed maternal blood (P78.2)

P54.1 **Neonatal melena**
Dark-colored feces stained with blood pigments
Excludes1 neonatal melena due to swallowed maternal blood (P78.2)

P54.2 **Neonatal rectal hemorrhage**

P54.3 **Other neonatal gastrointestinal hemorrhage**

P54.4 **Neonatal adrenal hemorrhage**

P54.5 **Neonatal cutaneous hemorrhage**
Neonatal bruising
Neonatal ecchymoses
Neonatal petechiae
Neonatal superficial hematomata
Excludes2 bruising of scalp due to birth injury (P12.3)
cephalhematoma due to birth injury (P12.Ø)

P54.6 **Neonatal vaginal hemorrhage**
Neonatal pseudomenses

P54.8 **Other specified neonatal hemorrhages**

P54.9 **Neonatal hemorrhage, unspecified**

● P55 **Hemolytic disease of newborn**
AKA erythroblastosis fetalis and is due to Rh isoimmunization, result of Rh blood factor incompatibilities between mother (Rh negative) and fetus (Rh positive)

P55.Ø **Rh isoimmunization of newborn**

P55.1 **ABO isoimmunization of newborn**
Coding Clinic: 2Ø15, Q3, P2Ø

P55.8 **Other hemolytic diseases of newborn**

P55.9 **Hemolytic disease of newborn, unspecified**

● P56 **Hydrops fetalis due to hemolytic disease** (Ex) PDX 1492
Caused by maternal sensitization to fetal blood group antigen
Excludes1 hydrops fetalis NOS (P83.2)

P56.Ø **Hydrops fetalis due to isoimmunization**

● **P56.9 Hydrops fetalis due to other and unspecified hemolytic disease**

P56.90 Hydrops fetalis due to unspecified hemolytic disease

P56.99 Hydrops fetalis due to other hemolytic disease

● **P57 Kernicterus** (Ex) PDX 1493

High levels of bilirubin in blood, with severe neural symptoms

P57.0 Kernicterus due to isoimmunization (Ex) PDX 1492

P57.8 Other specified kernicterus

Excludes1 Crigler-Najjar syndrome (E80.5)

P57.9 Kernicterus, unspecified

● **P58 Neonatal jaundice due to other excessive hemolysis**

Excludes1 jaundice due to isoimmunization (P55-P57)

P58.0 Neonatal jaundice due to bruising

P58.1 Neonatal jaundice due to bleeding

P58.2 Neonatal jaundice due to infection

P58.3 Neonatal jaundice due to polycythemia

● **P58.4 Neonatal jaundice due to drugs or toxins transmitted from mother or given to newborn**

Code first poisoning due to drug or toxin, if applicable (T36-T65 with fifth or sixth character 1-4)

Use additional code for adverse effect, if applicable, to identify drug (T36-T50 with fifth or sixth character 5)

● **P58.41 Neonatal jaundice due to drugs or toxins transmitted from mother**

● **P58.42 Neonatal jaundice due to drugs or toxins given to newborn**

P58.5 Neonatal jaundice due to swallowed maternal blood

P58.8 Neonatal jaundice due to other specified excessive hemolysis

P58.9 Neonatal jaundice due to excessive hemolysis, unspecified

● **P59 Neonatal jaundice from other and unspecified causes**

Excludes1 jaundice due to inborn errors of metabolism (E70-E88)
kernicterus (P57.-)

P59.0 Neonatal jaundice associated with preterm delivery

Hyperbilirubinemia of prematurity

Jaundice due to delayed conjugation associated with preterm delivery

P59.1 Inspissated bile syndrome (Ex) PDX 1493

● **P59.2 Neonatal jaundice from other and unspecified hepatocellular damage** (Ex) PDX 1493

Excludes1 congenital viral hepatitis (P35.3)

P59.20 Neonatal jaundice from unspecified hepatocellular damage

P59.29 Neonatal jaundice from other hepatocellular damage (Ex) PDX 1493

Neonatal giant cell hepatitis

Neonatal (idiopathic) hepatitis

P59.3 Neonatal jaundice from breast milk inhibitor

P59.8 Neonatal jaundice from other specified causes

P59.9 Neonatal jaundice, unspecified

Neonatal physiological jaundice (intense)(prolonged) NOS

Coding Clinic: 2015, Q3, P20

P60 Disseminated intravascular coagulation of newborn (Ex) PDX 1490

Defibrination syndrome of newborn

● **P61 Other perinatal hematological disorders**

Excludes1 transient hypogammaglobulinemia of infancy (D80.7)

P61.0 Transient neonatal thrombocytopenia

Lack of sufficient numbers of circulating thrombocytes (platelets) (Ex) PDX 1490

Neonatal thrombocytopenia due to exchange transfusion

Neonatal thrombocytopenia due to idiopathic maternal thrombocytopenia

Neonatal thrombocytopenia due to isoimmunization

P61.1 Polycythemia neonatorum

Neonate = newborn

P61.2 Anemia of prematurity (Ex) PDX 1494

P61.3 Congenital anemia from fetal blood loss (Ex) PDX 1494

P61.4 Other congenital anemias, not elsewhere classified (Ex) PDX 1495

Congenital anemia NOS

P61.5 Transient neonatal neutropenia (Ex) PDX 1496

Low levels of granulocytic neutrophilic white blood cells

Excludes1 congenital neutropenia (nontransient) (D70.0)

P61.6 Other transient neonatal disorders of coagulation (Ex) PDX 1497

P61.8 Other specified perinatal hematological disorders

P61.9 Perinatal hematological disorder, unspecified

TRANSITORY ENDOCRINE AND METABOLIC DISORDERS SPECIFIC TO NEWBORN (P70-P74)

Includes transitory endocrine and metabolic disturbances caused by the infant's response to maternal endocrine and metabolic factors, or its adjustment to extrauterine environment

● **P70 Transitory disorders of carbohydrate metabolism specific to newborn**

P70.0 Syndrome of infant of mother with gestational diabetes

Newborn (with hypoglycemia) affected by maternal gestational diabetes

Excludes1 newborn (with hypoglycemia) affected by maternal (pre-existing) diabetes mellitus (P70.1)
syndrome of infant of a diabetic mother (P70.1)

P70.1 Syndrome of infant of a diabetic mother

Newborn (with hypoglycemia) affected by maternal (pre-existing) diabetes mellitus

Excludes1 newborn (with hypoglycemia) affected by maternal gestational diabetes (P70.0)
syndrome of infant of mother with gestational diabetes (P70.0)

P70.2 Neonatal diabetes mellitus (Ex) PDX 1498

P70.3 Iatrogenic neonatal hypoglycemia

P70.4 Other neonatal hypoglycemia

Transitory neonatal hypoglycemia

P70.8 Other transitory disorders of carbohydrate metabolism of newborn (Ex) PDX 1499

P70.9 Transitory disorder of carbohydrate metabolism of newborn, unspecified

● **P71 Transitory neonatal disorders of calcium and magnesium metabolism** (Ex) PDX 1498

P71.0 Cow's milk hypocalcemia in newborn

P71.1 Other neonatal hypocalcemia

Excludes1 neonatal hypoparathyroidism (P71.4)

P71.2 Neonatal hypomagnesemia

P71.3 Neonatal tetany without calcium or magnesium deficiency

Neonatal tetany NOS

P71.4 Transitory neonatal hypoparathyroidism

P71.8 Other transitory neonatal disorders of calcium and magnesium metabolism
Coding Clinic: 2016, Q4, P55

P71.9 Transitory neonatal disorder of calcium and magnesium metabolism, unspecified

● P72 Other transitory neonatal endocrine disorders
Excludes1 congenital hypothyroidism with or without goiter (E03.0-E03.1)
dyshormogenetic goiter (E07.1)
Pendred's syndrome (E07.1)

P72.0 Neonatal goiter, not elsewhere classified (Ex) PDX 1500
Transitory congenital goiter with normal functioning

P72.1 Transitory neonatal hyperthyroidism (Ex) PDX 1498
Neonatal thyrotoxicosis

P72.2 Other transitory neonatal disorders of thyroid function, not elsewhere classified (Ex) PDX 1501
Transitory neonatal hypothyroidism

P72.8 Other specified transitory neonatal endocrine disorders (Ex) PDX 1502

P72.9 Transitory neonatal endocrine disorder, unspecified

● P74 Other transitory neonatal electrolyte and metabolic disturbances

P74.0 Late metabolic acidosis of newborn (Ex) PDX 1498
Excludes1 (fetal) metabolic acidosis of newborn (P19)

P74.1 Dehydration of newborn

● P74.2 Disturbances of sodium balance of newborn
Coding Clinic: 2018, Q2, P6

P74.21 Hypernatremia of newborn

P74.22 Hyponatremia of newborn

● P74.3 Disturbances of potassium balance of newborn

P74.31 Hyperkalemia of newborn

P74.32 Hypokalemia of newborn

● P74.4 Other transitory electrolyte disturbances of newborn

P74.41 Alkalosis of newborn (Ex) PDX 1503
Hyperbicarbonatemia

● P74.42 Disturbances of chlorine balance of newborn

P74.421 Hyperchloremia of newborn
Hyperchloremic metabolic acidosis
Excludes2 late metabolic acidosis of the newborn (P74.0)

P74.422 Hypochloremia of newborn

P74.49 Other transitory electrolyte disturbance of newborn

P74.5 Transitory tyrosinemia of newborn (Ex) PDX 1504

P74.6 Transitory hyperammonemia of newborn (Ex) PDX 1505

P74.8 Other transitory metabolic disturbances of newborn (Ex) PDX 1506
Amino-acid metabolic disorders described as transitory

P74.9 Transitory metabolic disturbance of newborn, unspecified

DIGESTIVE SYSTEM DISORDERS OF NEWBORN (P76-P78)

● P76 Other intestinal obstruction of newborn

P76.0 Meconium plug syndrome
Fetal stool obstruction in large intestine, present at birth; may be symptom of organic disease.
Meconium ileus NOS
Excludes1 meconium ileus in cystic fibrosis (E84.11)

P76.1 Transitory ileus of newborn (Ex) PDX 1507
Temporary obstruction of ileus (small intestine)
Excludes1 Hirschsprung's disease (Q43.1)

P76.2 Intestinal obstruction due to inspissated milk
Being thickened, dried, or made less fluid

P76.8 Other specified intestinal obstruction of newborn
Excludes1 intestinal obstruction classifiable to K56.-

P76.9 Intestinal obstruction of newborn, unspecified

● P77 Necrotizing enterocolitis of newborn (Ex) PDX 1508

P77.1 Stage 1 necrotizing enterocolitis in newborn
Necrotizing enterocolitis without pneumatosis, without perforation

P77.2 Stage 2 necrotizing enterocolitis in newborn
Necrotizing enterocolitis with pneumatosis, without perforation

P77.3 Stage 3 necrotizing enterocolitis in newborn
Necrotizing enterocolitis with perforation
Necrotizing enterocolitis with pneumatosis and perforation

P77.9 Necrotizing enterocolitis in newborn, unspecified
Necrotizing enterocolitis in newborn, NOS

● P78 Other perinatal digestive system disorders
Excludes1 cystic fibrosis (E84.0-E84.9)
neonatal gastrointestinal hemorrhages (P54.0-P54.3)

P78.0 Perinatal intestinal perforation (Ex) PDX 1508
Meconium peritonitis

P78.1 Other neonatal peritonitis
Neonatal peritonitis NOS

P78.2 Neonatal hematemesis and melena due to swallowed maternal blood

P78.3 Noninfective neonatal diarrhea
Neonatal diarrhea NOS

● P78.8 Other specified perinatal digestive system disorders

P78.81 Congenital cirrhosis (of liver)

P78.82 Peptic ulcer of newborn

P78.83 Newborn esophageal reflux
Neonatal esophageal reflux

P78.84 Gestational alloimmune liver disease
GALD
Neonatal hemochromatosis
Excludes1 hemochromatosis (E83.11-)

P78.89 Other specified perinatal digestive system disorders

P78.9 Perinatal digestive system disorder, unspecified

CONDITIONS INVOLVING THE INTEGUMENT AND TEMPERATURE REGULATION OF NEWBORN (P80-P83)

● P80 Hypothermia of newborn

P80.0 Cold injury syndrome
Severe and usually chronic hypothermia associated with a pink flushed appearance, edema and neurological and biochemical abnormalities.
Excludes1 mild hypothermia of newborn (P80.8)

P80.8 Other hypothermia of newborn
Mild hypothermia of newborn

P80.9 Hypothermia of newborn, unspecified

● P81 Other disturbances of temperature regulation of newborn

P81.0 Environmental hyperthermia of newborn

P81.8 Other specified disturbances of temperature regulation of newborn

P81.9 Disturbance of temperature regulation of newborn, unspecified
Fever of newborn NOS

● P83 Other conditions of integument specific to newborn
Excludes1 congenital malformations of skin and integument (Q80-Q84)
hydrops fetalis due to hemolytic disease (P56.-)
neonatal skin infection (P39.4)
staphylococcal scalded skin syndrome (L00)
Excludes2 cradle cap (L21.0)
diaper [napkin] dermatitis (L22)

P83.0 Sclerema neonatorum (Ex) PDX 1509
Neonate = newborn

P83.1 Neonatal erythema toxicum
Benign, generalized, transient pustules that become firm vesicles

P83.2 Hydrops fetalis not due to hemolytic disease (Ex) PDX 1510
Severe, life-threatening problem of severe edema (swelling) as a result of too much fluid leaving blood and entering tissue
Hydrops fetalis NOS

● P83.3 Other and unspecified edema specific to newborn (Ex) PDX 1511
P83.30 Unspecified edema specific to newborn
P83.39 Other edema specific to newborn

P83.4 Breast engorgement of newborn
Noninfective mastitis of newborn

P83.5 Congenital hydrocele

P83.6 Umbilical polyp of newborn

● P83.8 Other specified conditions of integument specific to newborn
P83.81 Umbilical granuloma
Excludes2 Granulomatous disorder of the skin and subcutaneous tissue, unspecified (L92.9)
P83.88 Other specified conditions of integument specific to newborn
Bronze baby syndrome
Neonatal scleroderma
Urticaria neonatorum

P83.9 Condition of the integument specific to newborn, unspecified

OTHER PROBLEMS WITH NEWBORN (P84)

P84 Other problems with newborn
Acidemia of newborn
Acidosis of newborn
Anoxia of newborn NOS
Asphyxia of newborn NOS
Hypercapnia of newborn
Hypoxemia of newborn
Hypoxia of newborn NOS
Mixed metabolic and respiratory acidosis of newborn
Excludes1 intracranial hemorrhage due to anoxia or hypoxia (P52.-)
hypoxic ischemic encephalopathy [HIE] (P91.6-)
late metabolic acidosis of newborn (P74.0)

OTHER DISORDERS ORIGINATING IN THE PERINATAL PERIOD (P90-P96)

P90 Convulsions of newborn (Ex) PDX 1512
Excludes1 benign myoclonic epilepsy in infancy (G40.3-)
benign neonatal convulsions (familial) (G40.3-)

● P91 Other disturbances of cerebral status of newborn

P91.0 Neonatal cerebral ischemia (Ex) PDX 1513
Excludes1 Neonatal cerebral infarction (P91.82-)

P91.1 Acquired periventricular cysts of newborn (Ex) PDX 1513

P91.2 Neonatal cerebral leukomalacia (Ex) PDX 1472
Degeneration of white matter adjacent to cerebral ventricles following cerebral hypoxia or brain ischemia in neonates
Periventricular leukomalacia

P91.3 Neonatal cerebral irritability (Ex) PDX 1513

P91.4 Neonatal cerebral depression (Ex) PDX 1513

P91.5 Neonatal coma (Ex) PDX 1513

● P91.6 Hypoxic ischemic encephalopathy [HIE] (Ex) PDX 1514
Excludes1 Neonatal cerebral depression (P91.4)
Neonatal cerebral irritability (P91.3)
Neonatal coma (P91.5)

P91.60 Hypoxic ischemic encephalopathy [HIE], unspecified
P91.61 Mild hypoxic ischemic encephalopathy [HIE]
P91.62 Moderate hypoxic ischemic encephalopathy [HIE]
P91.63 Severe hypoxic ischemic encephalopathy [HIE]

● P91.8 Other specified disturbances of cerebral status of newborn

● P91.81 Neonatal encephalopathy
P91.811 Neonatal encephalopathy in diseases classified elsewhere
Code first underlying condition, if known, such as:
congenital cirrhosis (of liver) (P78.81)
intracranial nontraumatic hemorrhage of newborn (P52.-)
kernicterus (P57.-)
P91.819 Neonatal encephalopathy, unspecified

● P91.82 Neonatal cerebral infarction (Ex) PDX 1515
Neonatal stroke
Perinatal arterial ischemic stroke
Perinatal cerebral infarction
Excludes1 cerebral infarction (I63.-)
Excludes2 intracranial hemorrhage of newborn (P52.-)
P91.821 Neonatal cerebral infarction, right side of brain
P91.822 Neonatal cerebral infarction, left side of brain
P91.823 Neonatal cerebral infarction, bilateral
P91.829 Neonatal cerebral infarction, unspecified side

P91.88 Other specified disturbances of cerebral status of newborn

P91.9 Disturbance of cerebral status of newborn, unspecified

● P92 Feeding problems of newborn
Excludes2 feeding problems in child over 28 days old (R63.3-)
Coding Clinic: 2017, Q1, P28; 2016, Q3, P19

● P92.0 Vomiting of newborn
Excludes1 vomiting of child over 28 days old (R11.-)
P92.01 Bilious vomiting of newborn (Ex) PDX 1516
Excludes1 bilious vomiting in child over 28 days old (R11.14)
P92.09 Other vomiting of newborn
Excludes1 regurgitation of food in newborn (P92.1)

P92.1 Regurgitation and rumination of newborn

P92.2 Slow feeding of newborn

P92.3 Underfeeding of newborn

P92.4 Overfeeding of newborn

P92.5 Neonatal difficulty in feeding at breast
Coding Clinic: 2017, Q1, P28; 2016, Q3, P19

P92.6 Failure to thrive in newborn
Excludes1 failure to thrive in child over 28 days old (R62.51)

P92.8 Other feeding problems of newborn

P92.9 Feeding problem of newborn, unspecified

● **P93 Reactions and intoxications due to drugs administered to newborn** Ex PDX 1517

Includes reactions and intoxications due to drugs administered to fetus affecting newborn

Excludes1 jaundice due to drugs or toxins transmitted from mother or given to newborn (P58.4-)
reactions and intoxications from maternal opiates, tranquilizers and other medication (P04.0-P04.1, P04.4-)
withdrawal symptoms from maternal use of drugs of addiction (P96.1)
withdrawal symptoms from therapeutic use of drugs in newborn (P96.2)

P93.0 Grey baby syndrome
Grey syndrome from chloramphenicol administration in newborn

P93.8 Other reactions and intoxications due to drugs administered to newborn
Use additional code for adverse effect, if applicable, to identify drug (T36-T50 with fifth or sixth character 5)

● **P94 Disorders of muscle tone of newborn**

P94.0 Transient neonatal myasthenia gravis Ex PDX 1498
Excludes1 myasthenia gravis (G70.0)

P94.1 Congenital hypertonia

P94.2 Congenital hypotonia
Floppy baby syndrome, unspecified

P94.8 Other disorders of muscle tone of newborn

P94.9 Disorder of muscle tone of newborn, unspecified

OGCR Section I.C.16.g.

Stillbirth

Code P95, Stillbirth, is only for use for institutions that maintain separate records for stillbirths. No other code should be used with P95. Code P95 should not be used on the mother's record.

P95 Stillbirth
Deadborn fetus NOS
Fetal death of unspecified cause
Stillbirth NOS

Excludes1 maternal care for intrauterine death (O36.4)
missed abortion (O02.1)
outcome of delivery, stillbirth (Z37.1, Z37.3, Z37.4, Z37.7)

● **P96 Other conditions originating in the perinatal period**

P96.0 Congenital renal failure
Uremia of newborn

P96.1 Neonatal withdrawal symptoms from maternal use of drugs of addiction Ex PDX 1517
Drug withdrawal syndrome in infant of dependent mother
Neonatal abstinence syndrome

Excludes1 reactions and intoxications from maternal opiates and tranquilizers administered during labor and delivery (P04.0)

P96.2 Withdrawal symptoms from therapeutic use of drugs in newborn Ex PDX 1517

P96.3 Wide cranial sutures of newborn
Neonatal craniotabes

P96.5 Complication to newborn due to (fetal) intrauterine procedure
Excludes2 newborn affected by amniocentesis (P00.6)

● **P96.8 Other specified conditions originating in the perinatal period**

P96.81 Exposure to (parental) (environmental) tobacco smoke in the perinatal period
Excludes2 newborn affected by in utero exposure to tobacco (P04.2)
exposure to environmental tobacco smoke after the perinatal period (Z77.22)

P96.82 Delayed separation of umbilical cord

P96.83 Meconium staining
Excludes1 meconium aspiration (P24.00, P24.01)
meconium passage during delivery (P03.82)

P96.89 Other specified conditions originating in the perinatal period
Use additional code to specify condition

P96.9 Condition originating in the perinatal period, unspecified
Congenital debility NOS

CHAPTER 16 (P00-P96)

CHAPTER 17

CONGENITAL MALFORMATIONS, DEFORMATIONS, AND CHROMOSOMAL ABNORMALITIES (Q00-Q99)

OGCR Chapter-Specific Coding Guidelines

17. **Chapter 17: Congenital malformations, deformations, and chromosomal abnormalities (Q00-Q99)**
Assign an appropriate code(s) from categories Q00-Q99, Congenital malformations, deformations, and chromosomal abnormalities when a malformation/deformation or chromosomal abnormality is documented. A malformation/deformation/ or chromosomal abnormality may be the principal/first-listed diagnosis on a record or a secondary diagnosis.
When a malformation/deformation/or chromosomal abnormality does not have a unique code assignment, assign additional code(s) for any manifestations that may be present.
When the code assignment specifically identifies the malformation/deformation/or chromosomal abnormality, manifestations that are an inherent component of the anomaly should not be coded separately. Additional codes should be assigned for manifestations that are not an inherent component.
Codes from Chapter 17 may be used throughout the life of the patient. If a congenital malformation or deformity has been corrected, a personal history code should be used to identify the history of the malformation or deformity. Although present at birth, malformation/deformation/or chromosomal abnormality may not be identified until later in life. Whenever the condition is diagnosed by the physician, it is appropriate to assign a code from codes Q00-Q99.
For the birth admission, the appropriate code from category Z38, Liveborn infants, according to place of birth and type of delivery, should be sequenced as the principal diagnosis, followed by any congenital anomaly codes, Q00-Q99.

CHAPTER 17

CONGENITAL MALFORMATIONS, DEFORMATIONS, AND CHROMOSOMAL ABNORMALITIES (Q00-Q99)

Note: Codes from this chapter are not for use on maternal records

Excludes2 inborn errors of metabolism (E70-E88)

This chapter contains the following blocks:

Q00-Q07	Congenital malformations of the nervous system
Q10-Q18	Congenital malformations of eye, ear, face and neck
Q20-Q28	Congenital malformations of the circulatory system
Q30-Q34	Congenital malformations of the respiratory system
Q35-Q37	Cleft lip and cleft palate
Q38-Q45	Other congenital malformations of the digestive system
Q50-Q56	Congenital malformations of genital organs
Q60-Q64	Congenital malformations of the urinary system
Q65-Q79	Congenital malformations and deformations of the musculoskeletal system
Q80-Q89	Other congenital malformations
Q90-Q99	Chromosomal abnormalities, not elsewhere classified

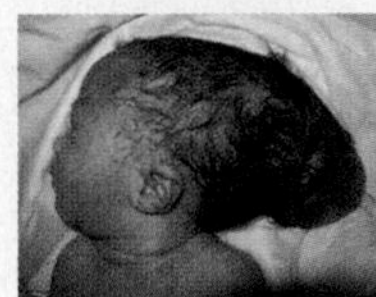

Figure 17-1 An infant with a large occipital encephalocele. The large skin-covered encephalocele is visible. (From Swaiman KF, Ashwal S, Ferriero DM: Pediatric Neurology: Principles and Practice, Philadelphia, Saunders, 2012)

CONGENITAL MALFORMATIONS OF THE NERVOUS SYSTEM (Q00–Q07)

● Q00 Anencephaly and similar malformations (Ex) PDX 1518

Q00.0 Anencephaly
Absence of skull with cerebral hemispheres missing or reduced to small masses attached to base of cranium
Acephaly
Acrania
Amyelencephaly
Hemianencephaly
Hemicephaly

Q00.1 Craniorachischisis
Developmental anomaly consisting of fissure of cranium and vertebral column

Q00.2 Iniencephaly
Developmental anomaly characterized by enlargement of foramen magnum and absence of laminae and spinous processes of cervical, dorsal

● Q01 Encephalocele (Ex) PDX 1519
Sac-like protrusions of brain and membranes visible through an opening in skull

Includes Arnold-Chiari syndrome, type III
encephalocystocele
encephalomyelocele
hydroencephalocele
hydromeningocele, cranial
meningocele, cerebral
meningoencephalocele

Excludes1 Meckel-Gruber syndrome (Q61.9)

Q01.0 Frontal encephalocele
Q01.1 Nasofrontal encephalocele
Q01.2 Occipital encephalocele
Q01.8 Encephalocele of other sites
Q01.9 Encephalocele, unspecified

Q02 Microcephaly
Head size measures significantly below normal based on standardized charts

Includes hydromicrocephaly
micrencephalon

Code first, if applicable, congenital Zika virus disease

Excludes1 Meckel-Gruber syndrome (Q61.9)

Coding Clinic: 2018, Q4, P26; 2016, Q4, P7

● Q03 Congenital hydrocephalus
Accumulation of cerebrospinal fluid in ventricles resulting in swelling and enlargement

Includes hydrocephalus in newborn

Excludes1 Arnold-Chiari syndrome, type II (Q07.0-)
acquired hydrocephalus (G91.-)
hydrocephalus due to congenital toxoplasmosis (P37.1)
hydrocephalus with spina bifida (Q05.0-Q05.4)

Q03.0 Malformations of aqueduct of Sylvius
Anomaly of aqueduct of Sylvius
Obstruction of aqueduct of Sylvius, congenital
Stenosis of aqueduct of Sylvius

Q03.1 Atresia of foramina of Magendie and Luschka
Dandy-Walker syndrome

Q03.8 Other congenital hydrocephalus

Q03.9 Congenital hydrocephalus, unspecified

CHAPTER 17 (Q00-Q99)

Q04 Other congenital malformations of brain (Ex) PDX 1519
Excludes1 cyclopia (Q87.0)
macrocephaly (Q75.3)

Q04.0 Congenital malformations of corpus callosum
Agenesis of corpus callosum

Q04.1 Arhinencephaly
Congenital absence of olfactory bulbs, tract, or nerves

Q04.2 Holoprosencephaly
Failure of cleavage of forebrain (prosencephalon) resulting in incomplete or absent cortical separation and deficits in midline facial development

Q04.3 Other reduction deformities of brain
Absence of part of brain
Agenesis of part of brain
Cerebral cortex are not fully formed, brain surface is smooth
Agyria
Aplasia of part of brain
Hydranencephaly
Hypoplasia of part of brain
Lissencephaly
Congenital malformation or absence of convolutions of cerebral cortex
Microgyria
Malformation of brain characterized by excessive number of small convolutions (gyri) on surface
Pachygyria
Reduction in number of sulci of cerebrum
Excludes1 congenital malformations of corpus callosum (Q04.0)

Q04.4 Septo-optic dysplasia of brain (Ex) PDX 1520

Q04.5 Megalencephaly (Ex) PDX 1520
Abnormally large brain

Q04.6 Congenital cerebral cysts (Ex) PDX 1520
Porencephaly Schizencephaly
Excludes1 acquired porencephalic cyst (G93.0)

Q04.8 Other specified congenital malformations of brain (Ex) PDX 1520
Arnold-Chiari syndrome, type IV
Macrogyria

Q04.9 Congenital malformation of brain, unspecified
Congenital anomaly NOS of brain
Congenital deformity NOS of brain
Congenital disease or lesion NOS of brain
Multiple anomalies NOS of brain, congenital

Q05 Spina bifida (Ex) PDX 1521
Developmental anomaly characterized by defective closure of vertebral arch, through which spinal cord and meninges may protrude
Includes hydromeningocele (spinal)
meningocele (spinal)
meningomyelocele
myelocele
myelomeningocele
rachischisis
spina bifida (aperta)(cystica)
syringomyelocele
Use additional code for any associated paraplegia (paraparesis) (G82.2-)
Excludes1 Arnold-Chiari syndrome, type II (Q07.0-)
spina bifida occulta (Q76.0)

Q05.0 Cervical spina bifida with hydrocephalus

Q05.1 Thoracic spina bifida with hydrocephalus
Dorsal spina bifida with hydrocephalus
Thoracolumbar spina bifida with hydrocephalus

Q05.2 Lumbar spina bifida with hydrocephalus
Lumbosacral spina bifida with hydrocephalus

Q05.3 Sacral spina bifida with hydrocephalus

Q05.4 Unspecified spina bifida with hydrocephalus

Q05.5 Cervical spina bifida without hydrocephalus

Q05.6 Thoracic spina bifida without hydrocephalus
Dorsal spina bifida NOS
Thoracolumbar spina bifida NOS

Q05.7 Lumbar spina bifida without hydrocephalus
Lumbosacral spina bifida NOS

Q05.8 Sacral spina bifida without hydrocephalus

Q05.9 Spina bifida, unspecified

Q06 Other congenital malformations of spinal cord

Q06.0 Amyelia
Congenital absence of spinal cord

Q06.1 Hypoplasia and dysplasia of spinal cord
Underdevelopment of spinal cord
Atelomyelia
Congenitally incomplete development of spinal cord
Myelatelia
Myelodysplasia of spinal cord
Defective development of spinal cord, especially lower segments

Q06.2 Diastematomyelia
Congenital anomaly, associated with spina bifida, in which spinal cord is split into halves and surrounded by dural sac

Q06.3 Other congenital cauda equina malformations

Q06.4 Hydromyelia
Dilation of central canal of spinal cord with increased fluid accumulation
Hydrorachis

Q06.8 Other specified congenital malformations of spinal cord

Q06.9 Congenital malformation of spinal cord, unspecified
Congenital anomaly NOS of spinal cord
Congenital deformity NOS of spinal cord
Congenital disease or lesion NOS of spinal cord

Q07 Other congenital malformations of nervous system
Excludes2 congenital central alveolar hypoventilation syndrome (G47.35)
familial dysautonomia [Riley-Day] (G90.1)
neurofibromatosis (nonmalignant) (Q85.0-)

Q07.0 Arnold-Chiari syndrome
Herniation of cerebellar tonsils and vermis through foramen magnum into spinal canal
Arnold-Chiari syndrome, type II
Excludes1 Arnold-Chiari syndrome, type III (Q01.-)
Arnold-Chiari syndrome, type IV (Q04.8)

Q07.00 Arnold-Chiari syndrome without spina bifida or hydrocephalus

Q07.01 Arnold-Chiari syndrome with spina bifida

Q07.02 Arnold-Chiari syndrome with hydrocephalus (Ex) PDX 1521

Q07.03 Arnold-Chiari syndrome with spina bifida and hydrocephalus (Ex) PDX 1521

Q07.8 Other specified congenital malformations of nervous system
Agenesis of nerve
Displacement of brachial plexus
Jaw-winking syndrome
Marcus Gunn's syndrome

Q07.9 Congenital malformation of nervous system, unspecified
Congenital anomaly NOS of nervous system
Congenital deformity NOS of nervous system
Congenital disease or lesion NOS of nervous system

CONGENITAL MALFORMATIONS OF EYE, EAR, FACE AND NECK (Q10-Q18)

Excludes2 cleft lip and cleft palate (Q35-Q37)
congenital malformation of cervical spine (Q05.0, Q05.5, Q67.5, Q76.0-Q76.4)
congenital malformation of larynx (Q31.-)
congenital malformation of lip NEC (Q38.0)
congenital malformation of nose (Q30.-)
congenital malformation of parathyroid gland (Q89.2)
congenital malformation of thyroid gland (Q89.2)

● **Q10 Congenital malformations of eyelid, lacrimal apparatus and orbit**
Excludes1 cryptophthalmos NOS (Q11.2)
cryptophthalmos syndrome (Q87.0)

Q10.0 Congenital ptosis
Prolapse or drooping of upper eyelid from paralysis of third nerve or from sympathetic innervations

Q10.1 Congenital ectropion
Outward turning of eyelid

Q10.2 Congenital entropion
Inward turning of eyelid

Q10.3 Other congenital malformations of eyelid
Ablepharon
Blepharophimosis, congenital
Coloboma of eyelid
Congenital absence or agenesis of cilia
Congenital absence or agenesis of eyelid
Congenital accessory eyelid
Congenital accessory eye muscle
Congenital malformation of eyelid NOS

Q10.4 Absence and agenesis of lacrimal apparatus
Congenital absence of punctum lacrimale

Q10.5 Congenital stenosis and stricture of lacrimal duct

Q10.6 Other congenital malformations of lacrimal apparatus
Congenital malformation of lacrimal apparatus NOS

Q10.7 Congenital malformation of orbit

● **Q11 Anophthalmos, microphthalmos and macrophthalmos**
Absence of eye and optic pit

Q11.0 Cystic eyeball

Q11.1 Other anophthalmos
Anophthalmos NOS
Agenesis of eye
Absence of eye
Aplasia of eye

Q11.2 Microphthalmos
Partial absence of eye and optic pit
Cryptophthalmos NOS
Dysplasia of eye
Hypoplasia of eye
Rudimentary eye
Excludes1 cryptophthalmos syndrome (Q87.0)

Q11.3 Macrophthalmos
Congenital enlargement of eyes
Excludes1 macrophthalmos in congenital glaucoma (Q15.0)

● **Q12 Congenital lens malformations**

Q12.0 Congenital cataract

Q12.1 Congenital displaced lens

Q12.2 Coloboma of lens

Q12.3 Congenital aphakia

Q12.4 Spherophakia
Smaller, more spherical optic lens than normal

Q12.8 Other congenital lens malformations
Microphakia

Q12.9 Congenital lens malformation, unspecified

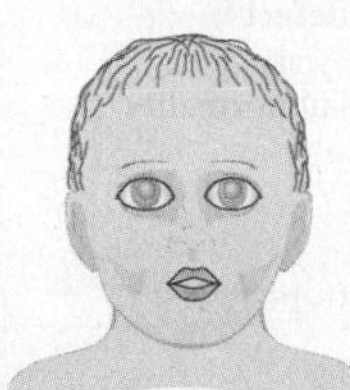

Figure 17-2 Bilateral congenital **hydrophthalmia,** in which the eyes are very large in comparison to the other facial features due to glaucoma.

● **Q13 Congenital malformations of anterior segment of eye**

Q13.0 Coloboma of iris
Coloboma NOS

Q13.1 Absence of iris
Aniridia
Use additional code for associated glaucoma (H42)

Q13.2 Other congenital malformations of iris
Anisocoria, congenital
Atresia of pupil
Congenital malformation of iris NOS
Corectopia

Q13.3 Congenital corneal opacity

Q13.4 Other congenital corneal malformations
Congenital malformation of cornea NOS
Microcornea
Peter's anomaly

Q13.5 Blue sclera
Condition of unusual blueness of sclera; not harmful

● **Q13.8 Other congenital malformations of anterior segment of eye**

Q13.81 Rieger anomaly
▶Axenfeld-Rieger syndrome
▶Code also any other associated congenital malformations such as cardiac defects
Use additional code for associated glaucoma (H42)

Q13.89 Other congenital malformations of anterior segment of eye

Q13.9 Congenital malformation of anterior segment of eye, unspecified

● **Q14 Congenital malformations of posterior segment of eye**
Excludes2 optic nerve hypoplasia (H47.03-)

Q14.0 Congenital malformation of vitreous humor
Congenital vitreous opacity

Q14.1 Congenital malformation of retina
Congenital retinal aneurysm

Q14.2 Congenital malformation of optic disc
Coloboma of optic disc

Q14.3 Congenital malformation of choroid

Q14.8 Other congenital malformations of posterior segment of eye
Coloboma of the fundus

Q14.9 Congenital malformation of posterior segment of eye, unspecified

● **Q15 Other congenital malformations of eye**
Excludes1 congenital nystagmus (H55.01)
ocular albinism (E70.31-)
optic nerve hypoplasia (H47.03-)
retinitis pigmentosa (H35.52)

Q15.0 Congenital glaucoma
Axenfeld's anomaly
Buphthalmos
Congenital syndrome characterized by enlargement of the eye with symptoms of glaucoma.
Glaucoma of childhood
Glaucoma of newborn
Hydrophthalmos
Keratoglobus, congenital, with glaucoma
Macrocornea with glaucoma
Macrophthalmos in congenital glaucoma
Megalocornea with glaucoma

Q15.8 Other specified congenital malformations of eye

Q15.9 Congenital malformation of eye, unspecified
Congenital anomaly of eye
Congenital deformity of eye

● **Q16 Congenital malformations of ear causing impairment of hearing**
Excludes1 congenital deafness (H90.-)

Q16.0 Congenital absence of (ear) auricle

Q16.1 Congenital absence, atresia and stricture of auditory canal (external)
Congenital atresia or stricture of osseous meatus

Q16.2 Absence of eustachian tube

Q16.3 Congenital malformation of ear ossicles
Congenital fusion of ear ossicles

Q16.4 Other congenital malformations of middle ear
Congenital malformation of middle ear NOS

Q16.5 Congenital malformation of inner ear
Congenital anomaly of membranous labyrinth
Congenital anomaly of organ of Corti

Q16.9 Congenital malformation of ear causing impairment of hearing, unspecified
Congenital absence of ear NOS

● **Q17 Other congenital malformations of ear**
Excludes1 congenital malformations of ear with impairment of hearing (Q16.Ø-Q16.9)
preauricular sinus (Q18.1)

Q17.Ø Accessory auricle
Accessory tragus
Polyotia
Preauricular appendage or tag
Supernumerary ear
Supernumerary lobule

Q17.1 Macrotia
Enlarged ears

Q17.2 Microtia
An abnormally small or underdeveloped external ear

Q17.3 Other misshapen ear
Pointed ear

Q17.4 Misplaced ear
Low-set ears
Excludes1 cervical auricle (Q18.2)

Q17.5 Prominent ear
Bat ear

Q17.8 Other specified congenital malformations of ear
Congenital absence of lobe of ear

Q17.9 Congenital malformation of ear, unspecified
Congenital anomaly of ear NOS

● **Q18 Other congenital malformations of face and neck**
Excludes1 cleft lip and cleft palate (Q35-Q37)
conditions classified to Q67.Ø-Q67.4
congenital malformations of skull and face bones (Q75.-)
cyclopia (Q87.Ø)
dentofacial anomalies [including malocclusion] (M26.-)
malformation syndromes affecting facial appearance (Q87.Ø)
persistent thyroglossal duct (Q89.2)

Q18.Ø Sinus, fistula and cyst of branchial cleft
Branchial vestige
Brachial remnants (cysts, fistula, skin tags) that are developmental anomalies

Q18.1 Preauricular sinus and cyst
Fistula of auricle, congenital
Cervicoaural fistula
Abnormal passage in neck originating from first branchial cleft

Q18.2 Other branchial cleft malformations
Branchial cleft malformation NOS
Cervical auricle
Otocephaly

Q18.3 Webbing of neck
Pterygium colli
Thick fold of skin on side of neck

Q18.4 Macrostomia
Results from failure of union of maxillary and mandibular processes, results in abnormally large mouth

Q18.5 Microstomia

Q18.6 Macrocheilia
Excessive size of lips
Hypertrophy of lip, congenital

Q18.7 Microcheilia
Abnormal smallness of lips

Q18.8 Other specified congenital malformations of face and neck
Medial cyst of face and neck
Medial fistula of face and neck
Medial sinus of face and neck

Q18.9 Congenital malformation of face and neck, unspecified
Congenital anomaly NOS of face and neck

CONGENITAL MALFORMATIONS OF THE CIRCULATORY SYSTEM (Q2Ø-Q28)

● **Q2Ø Congenital malformations of cardiac chambers and connections** Ex PDX 1522
Excludes1 dextrocardia with situs inversus (Q89.3)
mirror-image atrial arrangement with situs inversus (Q89.3)

Q2Ø.Ø Common arterial trunk
Persistent truncus arteriosus
Excludes1 aortic septal defect (Q21.4)

Q2Ø.1 Double outlet right ventricle
Taussig-Bing syndrome

Q2Ø.2 Double outlet left ventricle

Q2Ø.3 Discordant ventriculoarterial connection
Dextrotransposition of aorta
Transposition of great vessels (complete)

Q2Ø.4 Double inlet ventricle
Common ventricle
Cor triloculare biatriatum
Single ventricle

Q2Ø.5 Discordant atrioventricular connection
Corrected transposition
Levotransposition
Ventricular inversion

Q2Ø.6 Isomerism of atrial appendages
Isomerism of atrial appendages with asplenia or polysplenia

Q2Ø.8 Other congenital malformations of cardiac chambers and connections
Cor binoculare

Q2Ø.9 Congenital malformation of cardiac chambers and connections, unspecified

● **Q21 Congenital malformations of cardiac septa**
Excludes1 acquired cardiac septal defect (I51.Ø)

Q21.Ø Ventricular septal defect Ex PDX 1523
Roger's disease

Q21.1 Atrial septal defect Ex PDX 1524
Excludes 2 ostium primum atrial septal defect (type I) (Q21.2Ø)

Q21.1Ø Atrial septal defect, unspecified

Q21.11 Secundum atrial septal defect
Fenestrated atrial septum
Patent or persistent ostium secundum defect (type II)

Q21.12 Patent foramen ovale
Persistent foramen ovale

Q21.13 Coronary sinus atrial septal defect
Coronary sinus defect
Unroofed coronary sinus

Q21.14 Superior sinus venosus atrial septal defect
Superior vena cava type atrial septal defect

Q21.15 Inferior sinus venosus atrial septal defect
Inferior vena cava type atrial septal defect

Q21.16 Sinus venosus atrial septal defect, unspecified
Sinus venosus defect, NOS

Q21.19 Other specified atrial septal defect
Common atrium
Other specified atrial septal abnormality

Q21.2 Atrioventricular septal defect Ex PDX 1525
Atrioventricular canal defect
Endocardial cushion defect
Ostium primum atrial septal defect (type I)

Q21.2Ø Atrioventricular septal defect, unspecified as to partial or complete
Atrioventricular canal, NOS
Endocardial cushion defect NOS
Ostium primum atrial septal defect (type I) NOS

Q21.21 Partial atrioventricular septal defect
Incomplete atrioventricular canal
Incomplete atrioventricular septal defect
Incomplete endocardial cushion defect
Ostium primum atrial septal defect (type I) with separate atrioventricular valves
Partial atrioventricular canal
Partial endocardial cushion defect

Q21.22 Transitional atrioventricular septal defect
Intermediate atrioventricular canal
Intermediate atrioventricular septal defect
Intermediate endocardial cushion defect
Ostium primum atrial septal defect (type I) with separate atrioventricular valves and a small or restrictive inlet VSD
Transitional atrioventricular canal
Transitional endocardial cushion defect

Q21.23 Complete atrioventricular septal defect
Common atrioventricular canal
Common atrioventricular septal defect
Common endocardial cushion defect
Ostium primum atrial septal defect (type I) with common atrioventricular valve and a moderate or larger inlet VSD

Q21.3 Tetralogy of Fallot Ex: PDX 1522
Ventricular septal defect with pulmonary stenosis or atresia, dextroposition of aorta and hypertrophy of right ventricle.

Q21.4 Aortopulmonary septal defect
Aortic septal defect
Aortopulmonary window

Q21.8 Other congenital malformations of cardiac septa
Eisenmenger's defect
Pentalogy of Fallot
Code also, if applicable:
Eisenmenger's complex (I27.83)
Eisenmenger's syndrome (I27.83)

Q21.9 Congenital malformation of cardiac septum, unspecified
Septal (heart) defect NOS

Q22 Congenital malformations of pulmonary and tricuspid valves

Q22.Ø Pulmonary valve atresia Ex: PDX 1526

Q22.1 Congenital pulmonary valve stenosis Ex: PDX 1526

Q22.2 Congenital pulmonary valve insufficiency Ex: PDX 1527
Congenital pulmonary valve regurgitation

Q22.3 Other congenital malformations of pulmonary valve Ex: PDX 1527
Congenital malformation of pulmonary valve NOS
Supernumerary cusps of pulmonary valve

Q22.4 Congenital tricuspid stenosis Ex: PDX 1528
Congenital tricuspid atresia

Q22.5 Ebstein's anomaly Ex: PDX 1528
Malformation of tricuspid valve

Q22.6 Hypoplastic right heart syndrome Ex: PDX 1528

Q22.8 Other congenital malformations of tricuspid valve Ex: PDX 1528

Q22.9 Congenital malformation of tricuspid valve, unspecified Ex: PDX 1528

Q23 Congenital malformations of aortic and mitral valves

Q23.Ø Congenital stenosis of aortic valve Ex: PDX 1529
Congenital aortic atresia
Congenital aortic stenosis NOS
Excludes1 congenital stenosis of aortic valve in hypoplastic left heart syndrome (Q23.4)
congenital subaortic stenosis (Q24.4)
supravalvular aortic stenosis (congenital) (Q25.3)

Q23.1 Congenital insufficiency of aortic valve Ex: PDX 1529
~~Bicuspid aortic valve~~
Congenital aortic insufficiency

Q23.2 Congenital mitral stenosis Ex: PDX 1529
Congenital mitral atresia

Q23.3 Congenital mitral insufficiency Ex: PDX 1529

Q23.4 Hypoplastic left heart syndrome Ex: PDX 1528

Q23.8 Other congenital malformations of aortic and mitral valves

▶**Q23.81 Bicuspid aortic valve**
▶Congenital bicuspid aortic valve
▶Unicuspid (congenital) aortic valve (at birth)
▶Code also, if applicable, acquired aortic valve disorders, such as:
▶aortic (valve) insufficiency (nonrheumatic) (I35.1)
▶aortic (valve) stenosis (nonrheumatic) (I35.0)
▶aortic (valve) stenosis with insufficiency (nonrheumatic) (I35.2)

▶**Q23.82 Congenital mitral valve cleft leaflet**
▶Cleft mitral valve leaflet at birth

▶**Q23.88 Other congenital malformations of aortic and mitral valves**

Q23.9 Congenital malformation of aortic and mitral valves, unspecified

Q24 Other congenital malformations of heart
Excludes1 endocardial fibroelastosis (I42.4)

Q24.Ø Dextrocardia Ex: PDX 1530
Heart is located in right hemithorax
Excludes1 dextrocardia with situs inversus (Q89.3)
isomerism of atrial appendages (with asplenia or polysplenia) (Q2Ø.6)
mirror-image atrial arrangement with situs inversus (Q89.3)

Q24.1 Levocardia Ex: PDX 1530
Normal position of heart but related structures on wrong side

Q24.2 Cor triatriatum Ex: PDX 1531
Congenital heart defect; left atrium is subdivided

Q24.3 Pulmonary infundibular stenosis Ex: PDX 1531
Subvalvular pulmonic stenosis

Q24.4 Congenital subaortic stenosis Ex: PDX 1531

Q24.5 Malformation of coronary vessels Ex: PDX 1532
Congenital coronary (artery) aneurysm

Q24.6 Congenital heart block Ex: PDX 1533

Q24.8 Other specified congenital malformations of heart
Congenital diverticulum of left ventricle
Congenital malformation of myocardium
Congenital malformation of pericardium
Malposition of heart
Uhl's disease

Q24.9 Congenital malformation of heart, unspecified
Congenital anomaly of heart
Congenital disease of heart

Q25 Congenital malformations of great arteries

Q25.Ø Patent ductus arteriosus Ex: PDX 1534
Fetal blood vessel connecting left pulmonary artery directly to descending aorta
Patent ductus Botallo
Persistent ductus arteriosus

Q25.1 Coarctation of aorta Ex: PDX 1535
Coarctation of aorta (preductal) (postductal)
Stenosis of aorta
Coding Clinic: 2Ø16, Q4, P56-57

Q25.2 Atresia of aorta Ex: PDX 1536
Coding Clinic: 2Ø16, Q4, P56

Q25.21 Interruption of aortic arch
Atresia of aortic arch

Q25.29 Other atresia of aorta
Atresia of aorta

Q25.3 Supravalvular aortic stenosis Ex: PDX 1536
Excludes1 congenital aortic stenosis NOS (Q23.Ø)
congenital stenosis of aortic valve (Q23.Ø)

CHAPTER 17 (QØØ-Q99)

● Q25.4 **Other congenital malformations of aorta** (Ex) PDX 1537
  Excludes1 hypoplasia of aorta in hypoplastic left heart syndrome (Q23.4)
  Coding Clinic: 2016, Q4, P57
  Q25.40 **Congenital malformation of aorta unspecified**
  Q25.41 **Absence and aplasia of aorta**
  Q25.42 **Hypoplasia of aorta**
  Q25.43 **Congenital aneurysm of aorta**
    Congenital aneurysm of aortic root
    Congenital aneurysm of aortic sinus
  Q25.44 **Congenital dilation of aorta**
  Q25.45 **Double aortic arch**
    Vascular ring of aorta
  Q25.46 **Tortuous aortic arch**
    Persistent convolutions of aortic arch
  Q25.47 **Right aortic arch**
    Persistent right aortic arch
  Q25.48 **Anomalous origin of subclavian artery**
  Q25.49 **Other congenital malformations of aorta**
    Aortic arch
    Bovine arch
Q25.5 **Atresia of pulmonary artery** (Ex) PDX 1538
Q25.6 **Stenosis of pulmonary artery** (Ex) PDX 1538
  Supravalvular pulmonary stenosis
● Q25.7 **Other congenital malformations of pulmonary artery** (Ex) PDX 1538
  Q25.71 **Coarctation of pulmonary artery**
  Q25.72 **Congenital pulmonary arteriovenous malformation**
    Congenital pulmonary arteriovenous aneurysm
  Q25.79 **Other congenital malformations of pulmonary artery**
    Aberrant pulmonary artery
    Agenesis of pulmonary artery
    Congenital aneurysm of pulmonary artery
    Congenital anomaly of pulmonary artery
    Hypoplasia of pulmonary artery
Q25.8 **Other congenital malformations of other great arteries** (Ex) PDX 1537
Q25.9 **Congenital malformation of great arteries, unspecified** (Ex) PDX 1537

● **Q26 Congenital malformations of great veins**
Q26.Ø **Congenital stenosis of vena cava** (Ex) PDX 1539
  Congenital stenosis of vena cava (inferior)(superior)
Q26.1 **Persistent left superior vena cava** (Ex) PDX 1539
Q26.2 **Total anomalous pulmonary venous connection** (Ex) PDX 1540
  Total anomalous pulmonary venous return [TAPVR], subdiaphragmatic
  Total anomalous pulmonary venous return [TAPVR], supradiaphragmatic
Q26.3 **Partial anomalous pulmonary venous connection** (Ex) PDX 1541
  Partial anomalous pulmonary venous return
Q26.4 **Anomalous pulmonary venous connection, unspecified** (Ex) PDX 1541
Q26.5 **Anomalous portal venous connection**
Q26.6 **Portal vein-hepatic artery fistula**
Q26.8 **Other congenital malformations of great veins** (Ex) PDX 1539
  Absence of vena cava (inferior) (superior)
  Azygos continuation of inferior vena cava
  Persistent left posterior cardinal vein
  Scimitar syndrome
Q26.9 **Congenital malformation of great vein, unspecified** (Ex) PDX 1542
  Congenital anomaly of vena cava (inferior) (superior) NOS

● **Q27 Other congenital malformations of peripheral vascular system**
  Excludes2 anomalies of cerebral and precerebral vessels (Q28.Ø-Q28.3)
  anomalies of coronary vessels (Q24.5)
  anomalies of pulmonary artery (Q25.5-Q25.7)
  congenital retinal aneurysm (Q14.1)
  hemangioma and lymphangioma (D18.-)
Q27.Ø **Congenital absence and hypoplasia of umbilical artery**
  Single umbilical artery
Q27.1 **Congenital renal artery stenosis**
Q27.2 **Other congenital malformations of renal artery**
  Congenital malformation of renal artery NOS
  Multiple renal arteries
● Q27.3 **Arteriovenous malformation (peripheral)**
  Arteriovenous aneurysm
  Excludes1 acquired arteriovenous aneurysm (I77.Ø)
  Excludes2 arteriovenous malformation of cerebral vessels (Q28.2)
  arteriovenous malformation of precerebral vessels (Q28.Ø)
  Q27.3Ø **Arteriovenous malformation, site unspecified** (Ex) PDX 1543
  Q27.31 **Arteriovenous malformation of vessel of upper limb**
  Q27.32 **Arteriovenous malformation of vessel of lower limb**
  Q27.33 **Arteriovenous malformation of digestive system vessel**
  Q27.34 **Arteriovenous malformation of renal vessel**
  Q27.39 **Arteriovenous malformation, other site**
Q27.4 **Congenital phlebectasia** (Ex) PDX 1543
Q27.8 **Other specified congenital malformations of peripheral vascular system**
  Absence of peripheral vascular system
  Atresia of peripheral vascular system
  Congenital aneurysm (peripheral)
  Congenital stricture, artery
  Congenital varix
  Excludes1 arteriovenous malformation (Q27.3-)
Q27.9 **Congenital malformation of peripheral vascular system, unspecified**
  Anomaly of artery or vein NOS

● **Q28 Other congenital malformations of circulatory system**
  Excludes1 congenital aneurysm NOS (Q27.8)
  congenital coronary aneurysm (Q24.5)
  ruptured cerebral arteriovenous malformation (I6Ø.8)
  ruptured malformation of precerebral vessels (I72.Ø)
  Excludes2 congenital peripheral aneurysm (Q27.8)
  congenital pulmonary aneurysm (Q25.79)
  congenital retinal aneurysm (Q14.1)
Q28.Ø **Arteriovenous malformation of precerebral vessels** (Ex) PDX 1543
  Congenital arteriovenous precerebral aneurysm (nonruptured)
Q28.1 **Other malformations of precerebral vessels** (Ex) PDX 1543
  Congenital malformation of precerebral vessels NOS
  Congenital precerebral aneurysm (nonruptured)
Q28.2 **Arteriovenous malformation of cerebral vessels** (Ex) PDX 1544
  Arteriovenous malformation of brain NOS
  Congenital arteriovenous cerebral aneurysm (nonruptured)
Q28.3 **Other malformations of cerebral vessels** (Ex) PDX 1544
  Congenital cerebral aneurysm (nonruptured)
  Congenital malformation of cerebral vessels NOS
  Developmental venous anomaly

Q28.8 **Other specified congenital malformations of circulatory system** (Ex) PDX 1543
Congenital aneurysm, specified site NEC
Spinal vessel anomaly

Q28.9 **Congenital malformation of circulatory system, unspecified** (Ex) PDX 1545

CONGENITAL MALFORMATIONS OF THE RESPIRATORY SYSTEM (Q30-Q34)

● **Q30 Congenital malformations of nose**
Excludes1 congenital deviation of nasal septum (Q67.4)

Q30.0 **Choanal atresia**
Atresia of nares (anterior) (posterior)
Congenital stenosis of nares (anterior) (posterior)

Q30.1 **Agenesis and underdevelopment of nose**
Congenital absent of nose

Q30.2 **Fissured, notched and cleft nose**

Q30.3 **Congenital perforated nasal septum**

Q30.8 **Other congenital malformations of nose**
Accessory nose
Congenital anomaly of nasal sinus wall
Coding Clinic: 2022, Q2, P17

Q30.9 **Congenital malformation of nose, unspecified**

● **Q31 Congenital malformations of larynx** (Ex) PDX 1546
Excludes1 congenital laryngeal stridor NOS (P28.89)

Q31.0 **Web of larynx**
Glottic web of larynx
Subglottic web of larynx
Web of larynx NOS

Q31.1 **Congenital subglottic stenosis**

Q31.2 **Laryngeal hypoplasia**

Q31.3 **Laryngocele**

Q31.5 **Congenital laryngomalacia**

Q31.8 **Other congenital malformations of larynx**
Absence of larynx
Agenesis of larynx
Atresia of larynx
Congenital cleft thyroid cartilage
Congenital fissure of epiglottis
Congenital stenosis of larynx NEC
Posterior cleft of cricoid cartilage

Q31.9 **Congenital malformation of larynx, unspecified**

● **Q32 Congenital malformations of trachea and bronchus** (Ex) PDX 1546
Excludes1 congenital bronchiectasis (Q33.4)

Q32.0 **Congenital tracheomalacia**

Q32.1 **Other congenital malformations of trachea**
Atresia of trachea
Congenital anomaly of tracheal cartilage
Congenital dilatation of trachea
Congenital malformation of trachea
Congenital stenosis of trachea
Congenital tracheocele

Q32.2 **Congenital bronchomalacia**

Q32.3 **Congenital stenosis of bronchus**

Q32.4 **Other congenital malformations of bronchus**
Absence of bronchus
Agenesis of bronchus
Atresia of bronchus
Congenital diverticulum of bronchus
Congenital malformation of bronchus NOS

● **Q33 Congenital malformations of lung** (Ex) PDX 1547

Q33.0 **Congenital cystic lung**
Congenital cystic lung disease
Congenital honeycomb lung
Congenital polycystic lung disease
Excludes1 cystic fibrosis (E84.0)
cystic lung disease, acquired or unspecified (J98.4)

Q33.1 **Accessory lobe of lung**
Azygos lobe (fissured), lung

Q33.2 **Sequestration of lung**

Q33.3 **Agenesis of lung**
Congenital absence of lung (lobe)

Q33.4 **Congenital bronchiectasis** (Ex) PDX 1548

Q33.5 **Ectopic tissue in lung**

Q33.6 **Congenital hypoplasia and dysplasia of lung**
Excludes1 pulmonary hypoplasia associated with short gestation (P28.0)

Q33.8 **Other congenital malformations of lung**

Q33.9 **Congenital malformation of lung, unspecified**

● **Q34 Other congenital malformations of respiratory system**
Excludes2 congenital central alveolar hypoventilation syndrome (G47.35)

Q34.0 **Anomaly of pleura**

Q34.1 **Congenital cyst of mediastinum**

Q34.8 **Other specified congenital malformations of respiratory system**
Atresia of nasopharynx

Q34.9 **Congenital malformation of respiratory system, unspecified**
Congenital absence of respiratory system
Congenital anomaly of respiratory system NOS

CLEFT LIP AND CLEFT PALATE (Q35-Q37)

Use additional code to identify associated malformation of the nose (Q30.2)

Excludes2 Robin's syndrome (Q87.0)

● **Q35 Cleft palate**
Includes fissure of palate
palatoschisis
Excludes1 cleft palate with cleft lip (Q37.-)

Q35.1 **Cleft hard palate**

Q35.3 **Cleft soft palate**

Q35.5 **Cleft hard palate with cleft soft palate**

Q35.7 **Cleft uvula**

Q35.9 **Cleft palate, unspecified**
Cleft palate NOS

● **Q36 Cleft lip**
Includes cheiloschisis
congenital fissure of lip
harelip
labium leporinum
Excludes1 cleft lip with cleft palate (Q37.-)

Q36.0 **Cleft lip, bilateral**

Q36.1 **Cleft lip, median**

Q36.9 **Cleft lip, unilateral**
Cleft lip NOS

● **Q37 Cleft palate with cleft lip**
Includes cheilopalatoschisis

Q37.0 **Cleft hard palate with bilateral cleft lip**

Q37.1 **Cleft hard palate with unilateral cleft lip**
Cleft hard palate with cleft lip NOS

Q37.2 **Cleft soft palate with bilateral cleft lip**

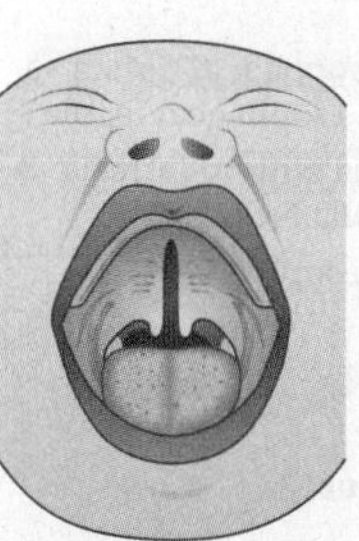

Figure 17-3 Cleft palate.

CHAPTER 17 (Q00-Q99)

Q37.3 **Cleft soft palate with unilateral cleft lip**
Cleft soft palate with cleft lip NOS
Q37.4 **Cleft hard and soft palate with bilateral cleft lip**
Q37.5 **Cleft hard and soft palate with unilateral cleft lip**
Cleft hard and soft palate with cleft lip NOS
Q37.8 **Unspecified cleft palate with bilateral cleft lip**
Q37.9 **Unspecified cleft palate with unilateral cleft lip**
Cleft palate with cleft lip NOS

OTHER CONGENITAL MALFORMATIONS OF THE DIGESTIVE SYSTEM (Q38-Q45)

● Q38 **Other congenital malformations of tongue, mouth and pharynx**
Excludes1 dentofacial anomalies (M26.-)
macrostomia (Q18.4)
microstomia (Q18.5)

Q38.0 **Congenital malformations of lips, not elsewhere classified**
Congenital fistula of lip
Congenital malformation of lip NOS
Van der Woude's syndrome
Excludes1 cleft lip (Q36.-)
cleft lip with cleft palate (Q37.-)
macrocheilia (Q18.6)
microcheilia (Q18.7)

Q38.1 **Ankyloglossia**
Restricted movement of tongue resulting in speech difficulty
Tongue tie

Q38.2 **Macroglossia**
Excessive size of tongue
Congenital hypertrophy of tongue

Q38.3 **Other congenital malformations of tongue**
Aglossia
Bifid tongue
Congenital adhesion of tongue
Congenital fissure of tongue
Congenital malformation of tongue NOS
Double tongue
Hypoglossia
Hypoplasia of tongue
Microglossia

Q38.4 **Congenital malformations of salivary glands and ducts**
Atresia of salivary glands and ducts
Congenital absence of salivary glands and ducts
Congenital accessory salivary glands and ducts
Congenital fistula of salivary gland

Q38.5 **Congenital malformations of palate, not elsewhere classified**
Congenital absence of uvula
Congenital malformation of palate NOS
Congenital high arched palate
Excludes1 cleft palate (Q35.-)
cleft palate with cleft lip (Q37.-)

Q38.6 **Other congenital malformations of mouth**
Congenital malformation of mouth NOS

Q38.7 **Congenital pharyngeal pouch**
Congenital diverticulum of pharynx
Excludes1 pharyngeal pouch syndrome (D82.1)

Q38.8 **Other congenital malformations of pharynx**
Congenital malformation of pharynx NOS
Imperforate pharynx

● Q39 **Congenital malformations of esophagus** (Ex:) PDX 1549, 1550

Q39.0 **Atresia of esophagus without fistula**
Atresia of esophagus NOS

Q39.1 **Atresia of esophagus with tracheo-esophageal fistula**
Atresia of esophagus with broncho-esophageal fistula

Q39.2 **Congenital tracheo-esophageal fistula without atresia**
Congenital tracheo-esophageal fistula NOS

Q39.3 **Congenital stenosis and stricture of esophagus**

Q39.4 **Esophageal web**

Q39.5 **Congenital dilatation of esophagus**
Congenital cardiospasm

Q39.6 **Congenital diverticulum of esophagus**
Congenital esophageal pouch

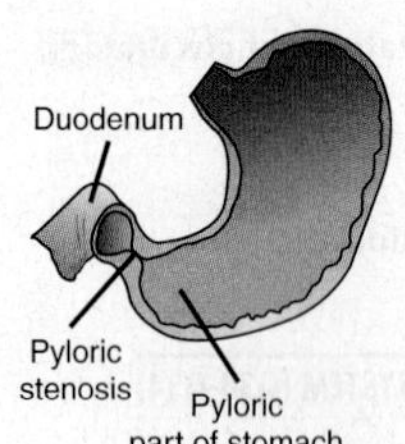

Figure 17-4 Pyloric stenosis.

Q39.8 **Other congenital malformations of esophagus**
Congenital absence of esophagus
Congenital displacement of esophagus
Congenital duplication of esophagus

Q39.9 **Congenital malformation of esophagus, unspecified**

● Q40 **Other congenital malformations of upper alimentary tract**

Q40.0 **Congenital hypertrophic pyloric stenosis**
Congenital or infantile constriction
Congenital or infantile hypertrophy
Congenital or infantile spasm
Congenital or infantile stenosis
Congenital or infantile stricture

Q40.1 **Congenital hiatus hernia**
Congenital displacement of cardia through esophageal hiatus
Excludes1 congenital diaphragmatic hernia (Q79.0)

Q40.2 **Other specified congenital malformations of stomach**
Congenital displacement of stomach
Congenital diverticulum of stomach
Congenital hourglass stomach
Congenital duplication of stomach
Megalogastria
Microgastria

Q40.3 **Congenital malformation of stomach, unspecified**

Q40.8 **Other specified congenital malformations of upper alimentary tract**

Q40.9 **Congenital malformation of upper alimentary tract, unspecified**
Congenital anomaly of upper alimentary tract
Congenital deformity of upper alimentary tract

● Q41 **Congenital absence, atresia and stenosis of small intestine** (Ex:) PDX 1551
Includes congenital obstruction, occlusion or stricture of small intestine or intestine NOS
Excludes1 cystic fibrosis with intestinal manifestation (E84.11)
meconium ileus NOS (without cystic fibrosis) (P76.0)

Q41.0 **Congenital absence, atresia and stenosis of duodenum**

Q41.1 **Congenital absence, atresia and stenosis of jejunum**
Apple peel syndrome
Imperforate jejunum

Q41.2 **Congenital absence, atresia and stenosis of ileum**

Q41.8 **Congenital absence, atresia and stenosis of other specified parts of small intestine**

Q41.9 **Congenital absence, atresia and stenosis of small intestine, part unspecified**
Congenital absence, atresia and stenosis of intestine NOS

● Q42 **Congenital absence, atresia and stenosis of large intestine** (Ex:) PDX 1552
Includes congenital obstruction, occlusion and stricture of large intestine

Q42.0 **Congenital absence, atresia and stenosis of rectum with fistula**

Q42.1 **Congenital absence, atresia and stenosis of rectum without fistula**
Imperforate rectum

Q42.2 **Congenital absence, atresia and stenosis of anus with fistula**

Q42.3 Congenital absence, atresia and stenosis of anus without fistula
Imperforate anus

Q42.8 Congenital absence, atresia and stenosis of other parts of large intestine

Q42.9 Congenital absence, atresia and stenosis of large intestine, part unspecified

● **Q43 Other congenital malformations of intestine** (Ex) PDX 1555

Q43.0 Meckel's diverticulum (displaced) (hypertrophic)
Congenital abnormality in which a pouch remains on the lower end of the small intestine
Persistent omphalomesenteric duct
Persistent vitelline duct

Q43.1 Hirschsprung's disease (Ex) PDX 1553
Developmental disorder of enteric nervous system characterized by absence of ganglion cells in distal colon resulting in functional obstruction
Aganglionosis
Congenital (aganglionic) megacolon

Q43.2 Other congenital functional disorders of colon (Ex) PDX 1553
Congenital dilatation of colon

Q43.3 Congenital malformations of intestinal fixation (Ex) PDX 1554
Congenital omental, anomalous adhesions [bands]
Congenital peritoneal adhesions [bands]
Incomplete rotation of cecum and colon
Insufficient rotation of cecum and colon
Jackson's membrane
Malrotation of colon
Rotation failure of cecum and colon
Universal mesentery

Q43.4 Duplication of intestine

Q43.5 Ectopic anus
Anal opening in abnormal location

Q43.6 Congenital fistula of rectum and anus
Excludes1 congenital fistula of anus with absence, atresia and stenosis (Q42.2)
congenital fistula of rectum with absence, atresia and stenosis (Q42.0)
congenital rectovaginal fistula (Q52.2)
congenital urethrorectal fistula (Q64.73)
pilonidal fistula or sinus (L05.-)

Q43.7 Persistent cloaca
Malformation in which rectum, vagina, and urinary tract form one channel; AKA congenital cloaca
Cloaca NOS

Q43.8 Other specified congenital malformations of intestine
Congenital blind loop syndrome
Congenital diverticulitis, colon
Congenital diverticulum, intestine
Dolichocolon
Megaloappendix
Megaloduodenum
Microcolon
Transposition of appendix
Transposition of colon
Transposition of intestine

Q43.9 Congenital malformation of intestine, unspecified

● **Q44 Congenital malformations of gallbladder, bile ducts and liver**

Q44.0 Agenesis, aplasia and hypoplasia of gallbladder (Ex) PDX 1556
Congenital absence of gallbladder

Q44.1 Other congenital malformations of gallbladder (Ex) PDX 1556
Congenital malformation of gallbladder NOS
Intrahepatic gallbladder

Q44.2 Atresia of bile ducts (Ex) PDX 1557

Q44.3 Congenital stenosis and stricture of bile ducts (Ex) PDX 1557

Q44.4 Choledochal cyst (Ex) PDX 1556

Q44.5 Other congenital malformations of bile ducts (Ex) PDX 1556
Accessory hepatic duct
Biliary duct duplication
Congenital malformation of bile duct NOS
Cystic duct duplication

Q44.6 Cystic disease of liver (Ex) PDX 1558
Fibrocystic disease of liver

● **Q44.7 Other congenital malformations of liver** (Ex) PDX 1556
Code also associated underlying condition

Q44.70 Other congenital malformation of liver, unspecified
Congenital malformation of liver, NOS

Q44.71 Alagille syndrome
Alagille-Watson syndrome

Q44.79 Other congenital malformations of liver
Accessory liver
Congenital absence of liver
Congenital hepatomegaly

● **Q45 Other congenital malformations of digestive system** (Ex) PDX 1559
Excludes2 congenital diaphragmatic hernia (Q79.0)
congenital hiatus hernia (Q40.1)

Q45.0 Agenesis, aplasia and hypoplasia of pancreas
Congenital absence of pancreas

Q45.1 Annular pancreas

Q45.2 Congenital pancreatic cyst

Q45.3 Other congenital malformations of pancreas and pancreatic duct
Accessory pancreas
Congenital malformation of pancreas or pancreatic duct NOS
Excludes1 congenital diabetes mellitus (E10.-)
cystic fibrosis (E84.0-E84.9)
fibrocystic disease of pancreas (E84.-)
neonatal diabetes mellitus (P70.2)

Q45.8 Other specified congenital malformations of digestive system
Absence (complete) (partial) of alimentary tract NOS
Duplication of digestive system
Malposition, congenital of digestive system

Q45.9 Congenital malformation of digestive system, unspecified
Congenital anomaly of digestive system
Congenital deformity of digestive system

CONGENITAL MALFORMATIONS OF GENITAL ORGANS (Q50-Q56)

Excludes1 androgen insensitivity syndrome (E34.5-)
syndromes associated with anomalies in the number and form of chromosomes (Q90-Q99)

● **Q50 Congenital malformations of ovaries, fallopian tubes and broad ligaments**

● **Q50.0 Congenital absence of ovary**
Excludes1 Turner's syndrome (Q96.-)

Q50.01 Congenital absence of ovary, unilateral

Q50.02 Congenital absence of ovary, bilateral

Q50.1 Developmental ovarian cyst

Q50.2 Congenital torsion of ovary

● **Q50.3 Other congenital malformations of ovary**

Q50.31 Accessory ovary

Q50.32 Ovarian streak
Inadequate ovaries with absent follicular and hormonal function
46, XX with streak gonads

Q50.39 Other congenital malformation of ovary
Congenital malformation of ovary NOS

Q50.4 Embryonic cyst of fallopian tube
Fimbrial cyst

Q50.5 **Embryonic cyst of broad ligament**
Epoophoron cyst
Parovarian cyst

Q50.6 **Other congenital malformations of fallopian tube and broad ligament**
Absence of fallopian tube and broad ligament
Accessory fallopian tube and broad ligament
Atresia of fallopian tube and broad ligament
Congenital malformation of fallopian tube or broad ligament NOS

● Q51 Congenital malformations of uterus and cervix

Q51.0 **Agenesis and aplasia of uterus**
Congenital absence of uterus

● Q51.1 **Doubling of uterus with doubling of cervix and vagina**

Q51.10 **Doubling of uterus with doubling of cervix and vagina without obstruction**
Doubling of uterus with doubling of cervix and vagina NOS

Q51.11 **Doubling of uterus with doubling of cervix and vagina with obstruction**

● Q51.2 **Other doubling of uterus**
Doubling of uterus NOS
Septate uterus

Q51.21 **Complete doubling of uterus**
Complete septate uterus

Q51.22 **Partial doubling of uterus**
Partial septate uterus

Q51.28 **Other and unspecified doubling of uterus**
Septate uterus NOS

Q51.3 **Bicornate uterus**
Bicornate uterus, complete or partial
Birth defect in which uterus has two separate "horns" that form top of uterus

Q51.4 **Unicornate uterus**
Unicornate uterus with or without a separate uterine horn
Uterus with only one functioning horn
Uterus with half being undeveloped

Q51.5 **Agenesis and aplasia of cervix**
Congenital absence of cervix

Q51.6 **Embryonic cyst of cervix**

Q51.7 **Congenital fistulae between uterus and digestive and urinary tracts**

● Q51.8 **Other congenital malformations of uterus and cervix**

● Q51.81 **Other congenital malformations of uterus**

Q51.810 **Arcuate uterus**
Arcuatus uterus

Q51.811 **Hypoplasia of uterus**

Q51.818 **Other congenital malformations of uterus**
Müllerian anomaly of uterus NEC

● Q51.82 **Other congenital malformations of cervix**

Q51.820 **Cervical duplication**

Q51.821 **Hypoplasia of cervix**

Q51.828 **Other congenital malformations of cervix**

Q51.9 **Congenital malformation of uterus and cervix, unspecified**

● Q52 Other congenital malformations of female genitalia

Q52.0 **Congenital absence of vagina**
Vaginal agenesis, total or partial

● Q52.1 **Doubling of vagina**
Excludes1 doubling of vagina with doubling of uterus and cervix (Q51.1-)

Q52.10 **Doubling of vagina, unspecified**
Septate vagina NOS

Q52.11 **Transverse vaginal septum**

● Q52.12 **Longitudinal vaginal septum**
Coding Clinic: 2016, Q4, P58

Q52.120 **Longitudinal vaginal septum, nonobstructing**

Q52.121 **Longitudinal vaginal septum, obstructing, right side**

Q52.122 **Longitudinal vaginal septum, obstructing, left side**

Q52.123 **Longitudinal vaginal septum, microperforate, right side**

Q52.124 **Longitudinal vaginal septum, microperforate, left side**
Coding Clinic: 2016, Q4, P59

Q52.129 **Other and unspecified longitudinal vaginal septum**

Q52.2 **Congenital rectovaginal fistula**
Excludes1 cloaca (Q43.7)

Q52.3 **Imperforate hymen**
Membrane (hymen) completely closes vaginal orifice

Q52.4 **Other congenital malformations of vagina**
Canal of Nuck cyst, congenital
Congenital malformation of vagina NOS
Embryonic vaginal cyst
Gartner's duct cyst
Coding Clinic: 2022, Q2, P16

Q52.5 **Fusion of labia**

Q52.6 **Congenital malformation of clitoris**

● Q52.7 **Other and unspecified congenital malformations of vulva**

Q52.70 **Unspecified congenital malformations of vulva**
Congenital malformation of vulva NOS

Q52.71 **Congenital absence of vulva**

Q52.79 **Other congenital malformations of vulva**
Congenital cyst of vulva

Q52.8 **Other specified congenital malformations of female genitalia**

Q52.9 **Congenital malformation of female genitalia, unspecified**

● Q53 Undescended and ectopic testicle

● Q53.0 **Ectopic testis**

Q53.00 **Ectopic testis, unspecified**

Q53.01 **Ectopic testis, unilateral**

Q53.02 **Ectopic testes, bilateral**

● Q53.1 **Undescended testicle, unilateral**

Q53.10 **Unspecified undescended testicle, unilateral**

● Q53.11 **Abdominal testis, unilateral**

Q53.111 **Unilateral intraabdominal testis**

Q53.112 **Unilateral inguinal testis**

Q53.12 **Ectopic perineal testis, unilateral**

Q53.13 **Unilateral high scrotal testis**

● Q53.2 **Undescended testicle, bilateral**

Item 17–1 Testes form in the abdomen of the male and only descend into the scrotum during normal embryonic development. "Ectopic" testes are out of their normal place or "retained" (left behind) in the abdomen. Crypto (hidden) orchism (testicle) is a major risk factor for testicular cancer.

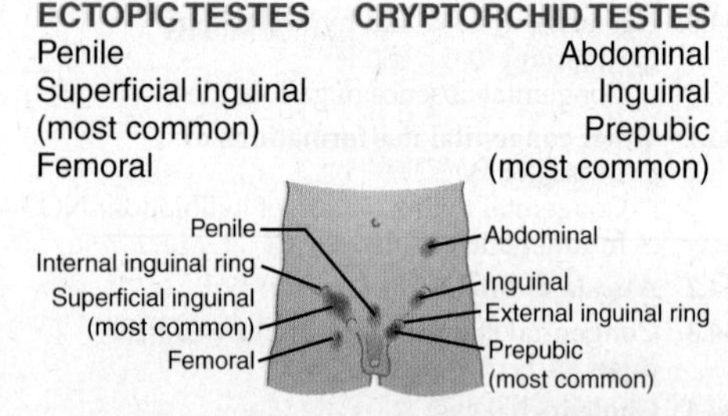

Figure 17-5 Undescended testes and the positions of the testes in various types of cryptorchidism or abnormal paths of descent.

Q53.2Ø **Undescended testicle, unspecified, bilateral**

● Q53.21 **Abdominal testis, bilateral**

Q53.211 **Bilateral intraabdominal testes**

Q53.212 **Bilateral inguinal testes**

Q53.22 **Ectopic perineal testis, bilateral**

Q53.23 **Bilateral high scrotal testes**

Q53.9 **Undescended testicle, unspecified**
Cryptorchism NOS

● Q54 **Hypospadias**
Birth defect of male; urethra opens in abnormal location on shaft
Excludes1 epispadias (Q64.Ø)

Q54.Ø **Hypospadias, balanic**
Hypospadias, coronal
Hypospadias, glandular

Q54.1 **Hypospadias, penile**

Q54.2 **Hypospadias, penoscrotal**

Q54.3 **Hypospadias, perineal**

Q54.4 **Congenital chordee**
Chordee without hypospadias

Q54.8 **Other hypospadias**
Hypospadias with intersex state

Q54.9 **Hypospadias, unspecified**

● Q55 **Other congenital malformations of male genital organs**
Excludes1 congenital hydrocele (P83.5)
hypospadias (Q54.-)

Q55.Ø **Absence and aplasia of testis**
Monorchism

Q55.1 **Hypoplasia of testis and scrotum**
Fusion of testes

● Q55.2 **Other and unspecified congenital malformations of testis and scrotum**

Q55.2Ø **Unspecified congenital malformations of testis and scrotum**
Congenital malformation of testis or scrotum NOS

Q55.21 **Polyorchism**
Developmental anomaly characterized by presence of more than two testes

Q55.22 **Retractile testis**

Q55.23 **Scrotal transposition**

Q55.29 **Other congenital malformations of testis and scrotum**

Q55.3 **Atresia of vas deferens**
Code first any associated cystic fibrosis (E84.-)

Q55.4 **Other congenital malformations of vas deferens, epididymis, seminal vesicles and prostate**
Absence or aplasia of prostate
Absence or aplasia of spermatic cord
Congenital malformation of vas deferens, epididymis, seminal vesicles or prostate NOS

Q55.5 **Congenital absence and aplasia of penis**

● Q55.6 **Other congenital malformations of penis**

Q55.61 **Curvature of penis (lateral)**

Q55.62 **Hypoplasia of penis**
Underdevelopment penis
Micropenis

Q55.63 **Congenital torsion of penis**
Excludes1 acquired torsion of penis (N48.82)

Q55.64 **Hidden penis**
Buried penis
Concealed penis
Excludes1 acquired buried penis (N48.83)

Q55.69 **Other congenital malformation of penis**
Congenital malformation of penis NOS

Q55.7 **Congenital vasocutaneous fistula**
Abnormal opening between vas deferens and skin

Q55.8 **Other specified congenital malformations of male genital organs**

Q55.9 **Congenital malformation of male genital organ, unspecified**
Congenital anomaly of male genital organ
Congenital deformity of male genital organ

● Q56 **Indeterminate sex and pseudohermaphroditism**
Internal reproductive organs are opposite external physical characteristics.
Excludes1 46,XX true hermaphrodite (Q99.1)
androgen insensitivity syndrome (E34.5-)
chimera 46,XX/46,XY true hermaphrodite (Q99.Ø)
female pseudohermaphroditism with adrenocortical disorder (E25.-)
pseudohermaphroditism with specified chromosomal anomaly (Q96-Q99)
pure gonadal dysgenesis (Q99.1)

Q56.Ø **Hermaphroditism, not elsewhere classified**
Ovotestis

Q56.1 **Male pseudohermaphroditism, not elsewhere classified**
46, XY with streak gonads
Male pseudohermaphroditism NOS

Q56.2 **Female pseudohermaphroditism, not elsewhere classified**
Female pseudohermaphroditism NOS

Q56.3 **Pseudohermaphroditism, unspecified**

Q56.4 **Indeterminate sex, unspecified**
Ambiguous genitalia

CONGENITAL MALFORMATIONS OF THE URINARY SYSTEM (Q6Ø-Q64)

● Q6Ø **Renal agenesis and other reduction defects of kidney** (Ex) PDX 1560
Includes congenital absence of kidney
congenital atrophy of kidney
infantile atrophy of kidney

Q6Ø.Ø **Renal agenesis, unilateral**

Q6Ø.1 **Renal agenesis, bilateral**

Q6Ø.2 **Renal agenesis, unspecified**

Q6Ø.3 **Renal hypoplasia, unilateral**

Q6Ø.4 **Renal hypoplasia, bilateral**

Q6Ø.5 **Renal hypoplasia, unspecified**

Q6Ø.6 **Potter's syndrome**

● Q61 **Cystic kidney disease**
Cysts that develop in failing kidney due to end-stage renal disease
Excludes1 acquired cyst of kidney (N28.1)
Potter's syndrome (Q6Ø.6)

● Q61.Ø **Congenital renal cyst**

Q61.ØØ **Congenital renal cyst, unspecified** (Ex) PDX 1561
Cyst of kidney NOS (congenital)

Q61.Ø1 **Congenital single renal cyst** (Ex) PDX 1562

Q61.Ø2 **Congenital multiple renal cysts** (Ex) PDX 1563

● Q61.1 **Polycystic kidney, infantile type** (Ex) PDX 1564
Polycystic kidney, autosomal recessive

Q61.11 **Cystic dilatation of collecting ducts**

Q61.19 **Other polycystic kidney, infantile type**

Q61.2 **Polycystic kidney, adult type** (Ex) PDX 1564
Polycystic kidney, autosomal dominant

Q61.3 **Polycystic kidney, unspecified** (Ex) PDX 1564
Coding Clinic: 2016, Q3, P23

Q61.4 **Renal dysplasia** (Ex) PDX 1565
Multicystic dysplastic kidney
Multicystic kidney (development)
Multicystic kidney disease
Multicystic renal dysplasia
Excludes1 polycystic kidney disease (Q61.11-Q61.3)

Q61.5 **Medullary cystic kidney** (Ex) PDX 1563
Nephronophthisis
Sponge kidney NOS

Q61.8 Other cystic kidney diseases Ex: PDX 1563
Fibrocystic kidney
Fibrocystic renal degeneration or disease

Q61.9 Cystic kidney disease, unspecified Ex: PDX 1561
Meckel-Gruber syndrome

● Q62 Congenital obstructive defects of renal pelvis and congenital malformations of ureter

Q62.0 Congenital hydronephrosis Ex: PDX 1566

● Q62.1 Congenital occlusion of ureter Ex: PDX 1566
Atresia and stenosis of ureter

Q62.10 Congenital occlusion of ureter, unspecified

Q62.11 Congenital occlusion of ureteropelvic junction

Q62.12 Congenital occlusion of ureterovesical orifice

Q62.2 Congenital megaureter Ex: PDX 1566
Congenital dilatation of ureter

● Q62.3 Other obstructive defects of renal pelvis and ureter

Q62.31 Congenital ureterocele, orthotopic Ex: PDX 1567

Q62.32 Cecoureterocele Ex: PDX 1568
Ectopic ureterocele

Q62.39 Other obstructive defects of renal pelvis and ureter Ex: PDX 1566
Ureteropelvic junction obstruction NOS

Q62.4 Agenesis of ureter
Congenital absence ureter

Q62.5 Duplication of ureter
Accessory ureter
Double ureter

● Q62.6 Malposition of ureter

Q62.60 Malposition of ureter, unspecified

Q62.61 Deviation of ureter

Q62.62 Displacement of ureter

Q62.63 Anomalous implantation of ureter
Ectopia of ureter
Ectopic ureter

Q62.69 Other malposition of ureter

Q62.7 Congenital vesico-uretero-renal reflux

Q62.8 Other congenital malformations of ureter
Anomaly of ureter NOS

● Q63 Other congenital malformations of kidney

Excludes1 congenital nephrotic syndrome (N04.-)

Q63.0 Accessory kidney

Q63.1 Lobulated, fused and horseshoe kidney

Q63.2 Ectopic kidney
Congenital displaced kidney
Malrotation of kidney

Q63.3 Hyperplastic and giant kidney
Compensatory hypertrophy of kidney

Q63.8 Other specified congenital malformations of kidney
Congenital renal calculi

Q63.9 Congenital malformation of kidney, unspecified

● Q64 Other congenital malformations of urinary system

Q64.0 Epispadias
Urethral opening somewhere on dorsum of penis

Excludes1 hypospadias (Q54.-)

● Q64.1 Exstrophy of urinary bladder Ex: PDX 1569
Bladder is exposed, inside out, and protrudes through abdominal wall

Q64.10 Exstrophy of urinary bladder, unspecified
Ectopia vesicae

Q64.11 Supravesical fissure of urinary bladder

Q64.12 Cloacal exstrophy of urinary bladder

Q64.19 Other exstrophy of urinary bladder
Extroversion of bladder

Q64.2 Congenital posterior urethral valves Ex: PDX 1570

● Q64.3 Other atresia and stenosis of urethra and bladder neck Ex: PDX 1570

Q64.31 Congenital bladder neck obstruction
Congenital obstruction of vesicourethral orifice

Q64.32 Congenital stricture of urethra

Q64.33 Congenital stricture of urinary meatus

Q64.39 Other atresia and stenosis of urethra and bladder neck
Atresia and stenosis of urethra and bladder neck NOS

Q64.4 Malformation of urachus
Cyst of urachus
Patent urachus
Prolapse of urachus

Q64.5 Congenital absence of bladder and urethra

Q64.6 Congenital diverticulum of bladder

● Q64.7 Other and unspecified congenital malformations of bladder and urethra

Excludes1 congenital prolapse of bladder (mucosa) (Q79.4)

Q64.70 Unspecified congenital malformation of bladder and urethra
Malformation of bladder or urethra NOS

Q64.71 Congenital prolapse of urethra

Q64.72 Congenital prolapse of urinary meatus

Q64.73 Congenital urethrorectal fistula

Q64.74 Double urethra

Q64.75 Double urinary meatus

Q64.79 Other congenital malformations of bladder and urethra

Q64.8 Other specified congenital malformations of urinary system

Q64.9 Congenital malformation of urinary system, unspecified
Congenital anomaly NOS of urinary system
Congenital deformity NOS of urinary system

CONGENITAL MALFORMATIONS AND DEFORMATIONS OF THE MUSCULOSKELETAL SYSTEM (Q65-Q79)

● Q65 Congenital deformities of hip

Excludes1 clicking hip (R29.4)

● Q65.0 Congenital dislocation of hip, unilateral

Q65.00 Congenital dislocation of unspecified hip, unilateral

Q65.01 Congenital dislocation of right hip, unilateral

Q65.02 Congenital dislocation of left hip, unilateral

Q65.1 Congenital dislocation of hip, bilateral

Q65.2 Congenital dislocation of hip, unspecified

● Q65.3 Congenital partial dislocation of hip, unilateral

Q65.30 Congenital partial dislocation of unspecified hip, unilateral

Q65.31 Congenital partial dislocation of right hip, unilateral

Q65.32 Congenital partial dislocation of left hip, unilateral

Q65.4 Congenital partial dislocation of hip, bilateral

Q65.5 Congenital partial dislocation of hip, unspecified

Q65.6 Congenital unstable hip
Congenital dislocatable hip

● Q65.8 Other congenital deformities of hip

Q65.81 Congenital coxa valga

Q65.82 Congenital coxa vara

Q65.89 Other specified congenital deformities of hip
Anteversion of femoral neck
Congenital acetabular dysplasia

Q65.9 Congenital deformity of hip, unspecified

Item 17-2 **Equinus foot** is a term referring to the hoof of a horse. The deformity is usually congenital or spastic. **Talipes equinovarus** is referred to as clubfoot. The foot tends to be smaller than normal, with the heel pointing downward and the forefoot turning inward. The heel cord (Achilles tendon) is tight, causing the heel to be drawn up toward the leg.

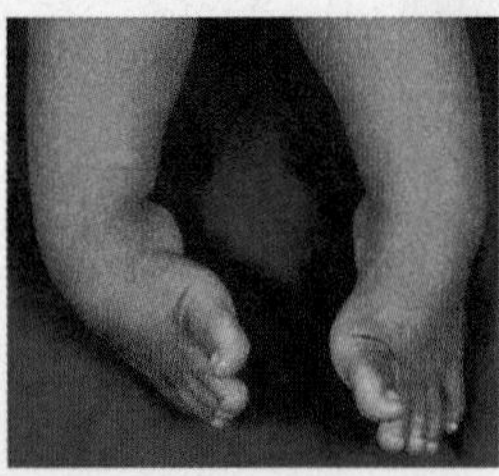

Figure 17-6 Supination and cavus deformity of forefoot. (From Kliegman R, Nelson WE: Nelson Textbook of Pediatrics, Philadelphia, Saunders, 2007)

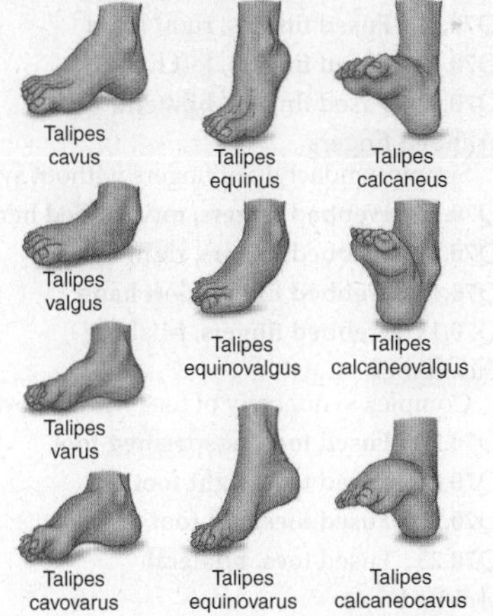

Figure 17-7 Talipes. (From Dorland: Dorland's Illustrated Medical Dictionary, ed 31, Saunders, 2007, p 1893)

Q66 Congenital deformities of feet
Excludes1 reduction defects of feet (Q72.-)
valgus deformities (acquired) (M21.0-)
varus deformities (acquired) (M21.1-)

Q66.0 Congenital talipes equinovarus
Heel is turned inward from midline and foot is plantar flexed; AKA clubfoot
Q66.00 Congenital talipes equinovarus, unspecified foot
Q66.01 Congenital talipes equinovarus, right foot
Q66.02 Congenital talipes equinovarus, left foot

Q66.1 Congenital talipes calcaneovarus
Deformity of foot in which heel is turned toward midline of body and anterior of foot is elevated
Q66.10 Congenital talipes calcaneovarus, unspecified foot
Q66.11 Congenital talipes calcaneovarus, right foot
Q66.12 Congenital talipes calcaneovarus, left foot

Q66.2 Congenital metatarsus (primus) varus
Angulation of first metatarsal bone toward midline of body
Coding Clinic: 2016, Q4, P59
Q66.21 Congenital metatarsus primus varus
Q66.211 Congenital metatarsus primus varus, right foot
Q66.212 Congenital metatarsus primus varus, left foot
Q66.219 Congenital metatarsus primus varus, unspecified foot
Q66.22 Congenital metatarsus adductus
Congenital metatarsus varus
Q66.221 Congenital metatarsus adductus, right foot
Q66.222 Congenital metatarsus adductus, left foot
Q66.229 Congenital metatarsus adductus, unspecified foot

Q66.3 Other congenital varus deformities of feet
Hallux varus, congenital
Q66.30 Other congenital varus deformities of feet, unspecified foot
Q66.31 Other congenital varus deformities of feet, right foot
Q66.32 Other congenital varus deformities of feet, left foot

Q66.4 Congenital talipes calcaneovalgus
Q66.40 Congenital talipes calcaneovalgus, unspecified foot
Q66.41 Congenital talipes calcaneovalgus, right foot
Q66.42 Congenital talipes calcaneovalgus, left foot

Q66.5 Congenital pes planus
Congenital flat foot
Congenital rigid flat foot
Congenital spastic (everted) flat foot
Excludes1 pes planus, acquired (M21.4)
Q66.50 Congenital pes planus, unspecified foot
Q66.51 Congenital pes planus, right foot
Q66.52 Congenital pes planus, left foot

Q66.6 Other congenital valgus deformities of feet
Inward angulation
Congenital metatarsus valgus

Q66.7 Congenital pes cavus
Q66.70 Congenital pes cavus, unspecified foot
Q66.71 Congenital pes cavus, right foot
Q66.72 Congenital pes cavus, left foot

Q66.8 Other congenital deformities of feet
Q66.80 Congenital vertical talus deformity, unspecified foot
Q66.81 Congenital vertical talus deformity, right foot
Q66.82 Congenital vertical talus deformity, left foot
Q66.89 Other specified congenital deformities of feet
Congenital asymmetric talipes
Congenital clubfoot NOS
Congenital talipes NOS
Congenital tarsal coalition
Hammer toe, congenital

Q66.9 Congenital deformity of feet, unspecified
Q66.90 Congenital deformity of feet, unspecified, unspecified foot
Q66.91 Congenital deformity of feet, unspecified, right foot
Q66.92 Congenital deformity of feet, unspecified, left foot

Q67 Congenital musculoskeletal deformities of head, face, spine and chest
Excludes1 congenital malformation syndromes classified to Q87.-
Potter's syndrome (Q60.6)

Q67.0 Congenital facial asymmetry
Q67.1 Congenital compression facies
Q67.2 Dolichocephaly
Long head dimension
Excludes1 sagittal craniosynostosis (Q75.01)
Q67.3 Plagiocephaly
Asymmetric shape of head resulting from irregular closure of cranial sutures
Excludes1 coronal craniosynostosis (Q75.02-)
lambdoid craniosynostosis (Q75.04-)

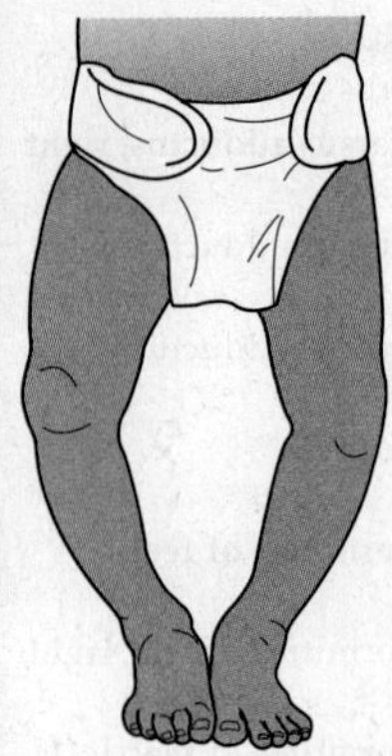

Figure 17-8 Mild to moderate inbowing of the lower leg. (From Lissauer T, Clayden G: Illustrated Textbook of Paediatrics, Edinburgh, Mosby, 2011)

Q67.4 Other congenital deformities of skull, face and jaw
Congenital depressions in skull
Congenital hemifacial atrophy or hypertrophy
Deviation of nasal septum, congenital
Squashed or bent nose, congenital
Excludes1 dentofacial anomalies [including malocclusion] (M26.-)
syphilitic saddle nose (A50.5)

Q67.5 Congenital deformity of spine PDX 1571
Congenital postural scoliosis
Congenital scoliosis NOS
Excludes1 infantile idiopathic scoliosis (M41.0)
scoliosis due to congenital bony malformation (Q76.3)

Q67.6 Pectus excavatum
Congenital funnel chest
Funnel-shaped chest depression

Q67.7 Pectus carinatum
Congenital pigeon chest

Q67.8 Other congenital deformities of chest PDX 1572
Congenital deformity of chest wall NOS

● **Q68 Other congenital musculoskeletal deformities**
Excludes1 reduction defects of limb(s) (Q71-Q73)
Excludes2 congenital myotonic chondrodystrophy (G71.13)

Q68.0 Congenital deformity of sternocleidomastoid muscle
Congenital contracture of sternocleidomastoid (muscle)
Congenital (sternomastoid) torticollis
Sternomastoid tumor (congenital)

Q68.1 Congenital deformity of finger(s) and hand PDX 1572
Congenital clubfinger
Spade-like hand (congenital)

Q68.2 Congenital deformity of knee
Congenital dislocation of knee
Congenital genu recurvatum
Hyperextension of knee resulting from hypermobility

Q68.3 Congenital bowing of femur
Excludes1 anteversion of femur (neck) (Q65.89)

Q68.4 Congenital bowing of tibia and fibula

Q68.5 Congenital bowing of long bones of leg, unspecified

Q68.6 Discoid meniscus

Q68.8 Other specified congenital musculoskeletal deformities
Congenital deformity of clavicle
Congenital deformity of elbow
Congenital deformity of forearm
Congenital deformity of scapula
Congenital deformity of wrist
Congenital dislocation of elbow
Congenital dislocation of shoulder
Congenital dislocation of wrist

● **Q69 Polydactyly**
AKA hyperdactyly, consists of supernumerary fingers or toes

Q69.0 Accessory finger(s)

Q69.1 Accessory thumb(s)

Q69.2 Accessory toe(s)
Accessory hallux

Q69.9 Polydactyly, unspecified
Supernumerary digit(s) NOS

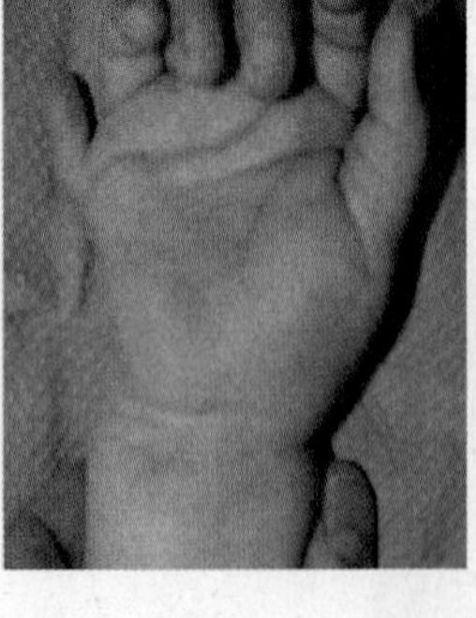

Figure 17-9 Thumb and index finger. (From Chung K: Hand and Upper Extremity Reconstruction, 1e, Saunders, 2008)

● **Q70 Syndactyly**
Webbing between distal phalanges of adjacent digits

● **Q70.0 Fused fingers**
Complex syndactyly of fingers with synostosis
Q70.00 Fused fingers, unspecified hand
Q70.01 Fused fingers, right hand
Q70.02 Fused fingers, left hand
Q70.03 Fused fingers, bilateral

● **Q70.1 Webbed fingers**
Simple syndactyly of fingers without synostosis
Q70.10 Webbed fingers, unspecified hand
Q70.11 Webbed fingers, right hand
Q70.12 Webbed fingers, left hand
Q70.13 Webbed fingers, bilateral

● **Q70.2 Fused toes**
Complex syndactyly of toes with synostosis
Q70.20 Fused toes, unspecified foot
Q70.21 Fused toes, right foot
Q70.22 Fused toes, left foot
Q70.23 Fused toes, bilateral

● **Q70.3 Webbed toes**
Simple syndactyly of toes without synostosis
Q70.30 Webbed toes, unspecified foot
Q70.31 Webbed toes, right foot
Q70.32 Webbed toes, left foot
Q70.33 Webbed toes, bilateral

Q70.4 Polysyndactyly, unspecified
Excludes1 specified syndactyly of hand and feet - code to specified conditions (Q70.0- -Q70.3-)
Extra and webbed digits

Q70.9 Syndactyly, unspecified
Symphalangy NOS

● **Q71 Reduction defects of upper limb**

● **Q71.0 Congenital complete absence of upper limb**
Q71.00 Congenital complete absence of unspecified upper limb
Q71.01 Congenital complete absence of right upper limb
Q71.02 Congenital complete absence of left upper limb
Q71.03 Congenital complete absence of upper limb, bilateral

● **Q71.1 Congenital absence of upper arm and forearm with hand present**
Q71.10 Congenital absence of unspecified upper arm and forearm with hand present
Q71.11 Congenital absence of right upper arm and forearm with hand present
Q71.12 Congenital absence of left upper arm and forearm with hand present
Q71.13 Congenital absence of upper arm and forearm with hand present, bilateral

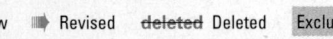

Q71.2 Congenital absence of both forearm and hand
- Q71.20 Congenital absence of both forearm and hand, unspecified upper limb
- Q71.21 Congenital absence of both forearm and hand, right upper limb
- Q71.22 Congenital absence of both forearm and hand, left upper limb
- Q71.23 Congenital absence of both forearm and hand, bilateral

Q71.3 Congenital absence of hand and finger
- Q71.30 Congenital absence of unspecified hand and finger
- Q71.31 Congenital absence of right hand and finger
- Q71.32 Congenital absence of left hand and finger
- Q71.33 Congenital absence of hand and finger, bilateral

Q71.4 Longitudinal reduction defect of radius
Clubhand (congenital)
Radial clubhand
- Q71.40 Longitudinal reduction defect of unspecified radius
- Q71.41 Longitudinal reduction defect of right radius
- Q71.42 Longitudinal reduction defect of left radius
- Q71.43 Longitudinal reduction defect of radius, bilateral

Q71.5 Longitudinal reduction defect of ulna
- Q71.50 Longitudinal reduction defect of unspecified ulna
- Q71.51 Longitudinal reduction defect of right ulna
- Q71.52 Longitudinal reduction defect of left ulna
- Q71.53 Longitudinal reduction defect of ulna, bilateral

Q71.6 Lobster-claw hand
- Q71.60 Lobster-claw hand, unspecified hand
- Q71.61 Lobster-claw right hand
- Q71.62 Lobster-claw left hand
- Q71.63 Lobster-claw hand, bilateral

Q71.8 Other reduction defects of upper limb
- Q71.81 Congenital shortening of upper limb
  - Q71.811 Congenital shortening of right upper limb
  - Q71.812 Congenital shortening of left upper limb
  - Q71.813 Congenital shortening of upper limb, bilateral
  - Q71.819 Congenital shortening of unspecified upper limb
- Q71.89 Other reduction defects of upper limb
  - Q71.891 Other reduction defects of right upper limb
  - Q71.892 Other reduction defects of left upper limb
  - Q71.893 Other reduction defects of upper limb, bilateral
  - Q71.899 Other reduction defects of unspecified upper limb

Q71.9 Unspecified reduction defect of upper limb
- Q71.90 Unspecified reduction defect of unspecified upper limb
- Q71.91 Unspecified reduction defect of right upper limb
- Q71.92 Unspecified reduction defect of left upper limb
- Q71.93 Unspecified reduction defect of upper limb, bilateral

Q72 Reduction defects of lower limb

Q72.Ø Congenital complete absence of lower limb
- Q72.ØØ Congenital complete absence of unspecified lower limb
- Q72.Ø1 Congenital complete absence of right lower limb
- Q72.Ø2 Congenital complete absence of left lower limb
- Q72.Ø3 Congenital complete absence of lower limb, bilateral

Q72.1 Congenital absence of thigh and lower leg with foot present
- Q72.1Ø Congenital absence of unspecified thigh and lower leg with foot present
- Q72.11 Congenital absence of right thigh and lower leg with foot present
- Q72.12 Congenital absence of left thigh and lower leg with foot present
- Q72.13 Congenital absence of thigh and lower leg with foot present, bilateral

Q72.2 Congenital absence of both lower leg and foot
- Q72.2Ø Congenital absence of both lower leg and foot, unspecified lower limb
- Q72.21 Congenital absence of both lower leg and foot, right lower limb
- Q72.22 Congenital absence of both left lower leg and foot, left lower limb
- Q72.23 Congenital absence of both lower leg and foot, bilateral

Q72.3 Congenital absence of foot and toe(s)
- Q72.3Ø Congenital absence of unspecified foot and toe(s)
- Q72.31 Congenital absence of right foot and toe(s)
- Q72.32 Congenital absence of left foot and toe(s)
- Q72.33 Congenital absence of foot and toe(s), bilateral

Q72.4 Longitudinal reduction defect of femur
Proximal femoral focal deficiency
- Q72.4Ø Longitudinal reduction defect of unspecified femur
- Q72.41 Longitudinal reduction defect of right femur
- Q72.42 Longitudinal reduction defect of left femur
- Q72.43 Longitudinal reduction defect of femur, bilateral

Q72.5 Longitudinal reduction defect of tibia
- Q72.5Ø Longitudinal reduction defect of unspecified tibia
- Q72.51 Longitudinal reduction defect of right tibia
- Q72.52 Longitudinal reduction defect of left tibia
- Q72.53 Longitudinal reduction defect of tibia, bilateral

Q72.6 Longitudinal reduction defect of fibula
- Q72.6Ø Longitudinal reduction defect of unspecified fibula
- Q72.61 Longitudinal reduction defect of right fibula
- Q72.62 Longitudinal reduction defect of left fibula
- Q72.63 Longitudinal reduction defect of fibula, bilateral

Q72.7 Split foot
- Q72.7Ø Split foot, unspecified lower limb
- Q72.71 Split foot, right lower limb
- Q72.72 Split foot, left lower limb
- Q72.73 Split foot, bilateral

Q72.8 Other reduction defects of lower limb
- Q72.81 Congenital shortening of lower limb
  - Q72.811 Congenital shortening of right lower limb
  - Q72.812 Congenital shortening of left lower limb
  - Q72.813 Congenital shortening of lower limb, bilateral
  - Q72.819 Congenital shortening of unspecified lower limb

CHAPTER 17 (QØØ-Q99)

● Q72.89 Other reduction defects of lower limb
Q72.891 Other reduction defects of right lower limb
Q72.892 Other reduction defects of left lower limb
Q72.893 Other reduction defects of lower limb, bilateral
Q72.899 Other reduction defects of unspecified lower limb

● Q72.9 Unspecified reduction defect of lower limb
Q72.90 Unspecified reduction defect of unspecified lower limb
Q72.91 Unspecified reduction defect of right lower limb
Q72.92 Unspecified reduction defect of left lower limb
Q72.93 Unspecified reduction defect of lower limb, bilateral

● Q73 Reduction defects of unspecified limb
Q73.0 Congenital absence of unspecified limb(s)
Amelia NOS
Q73.1 Phocomelia, unspecified limb(s)
Phocomelia NOS
Absence/shortening of long bones primarily as a result of thalidomide
Q73.8 Other reduction defects of unspecified limb(s)
Longitudinal reduction deformity of unspecified limb(s)
Ectromelia of limb NOS
Gross hypoplasia or aplasia of one or more long bones of limb(s)
Hemimelia of limb NOS
Absence of one-half of long bone
Reduction defect of limb NOS

● Q74 Other congenital malformations of limb(s)
Excludes1 polydactyly (Q69.-)
reduction defect of limb (Q71-Q73)
syndactyly (Q70.-)
Q74.0 Other congenital malformations of upper limb(s), including shoulder girdle
Accessory carpal bones
Cleidocranial dysostosis
Congenital pseudarthrosis of clavicle
Macrodactylia (fingers)
Madelung's deformity
Radioulnar synostosis
Sprengel's deformity
Triphalangeal thumb
Q74.1 Congenital malformation of knee
Congenital absence of patella
Congenital dislocation of patella
Congenital genu valgum
Congenital genu varum
Rudimentary patella
Excludes1 congenital dislocation of knee (Q68.2)
congenital genu recurvatum (Q68.2)
nail patella syndrome (Q87.2)
Q74.2 Other congenital malformations of lower limb(s), including pelvic girdle
Congenital fusion of sacroiliac joint
Congenital malformation of ankle joint
Congenital malformation of sacroiliac joint
Excludes1 anteversion of femur (neck) (Q65.89)
Q74.3 Arthrogryposis multiplex congenita Ex: PDX 1572
Q74.8 Other specified congenital malformations of limb(s)
Q74.9 Unspecified congenital malformation of limb(s)
Congenital anomaly of limb(s) NOS

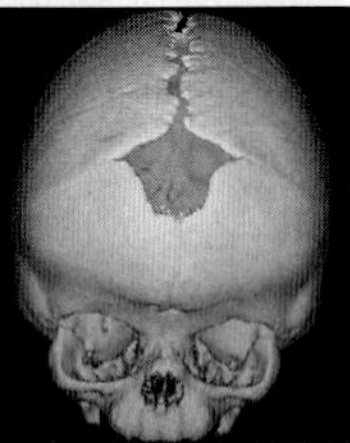

Figure 17-10 Generalized craniosynostosis without symptoms or signs of increased intracranial pressure. (From Goetz C: Textbook of Clinical Neurology, St. Louis, MO, Elsevier, 2007)

Item 17-3 Anencephalus is a congenital deformity of the cranial vault. **Craniosynostosis,** also known as craniostenosis and stenocephaly, signifies any form of congenital deformity of the skull that results from the premature closing of the sutures of the skull. **Iniencephaly** is a deformity in which the head and neck are flexed backward to a great extent and the head is very large in comparison to the shortened body.

● Q75 Other congenital malformations of skull and face bones
Excludes1 congenital malformation of face NOS (Q18.-)
congenital malformation syndromes classified to Q87.-
dentofacial anomalies [including malocclusion] (M26.-)
musculoskeletal deformities of head and face (Q67.0-Q67.4)
skull defects associated with congenital anomalies of brain such as:
anencephaly (Q00.0)
encephalocele (Q01.-)
hydrocephalus (Q03.-)
microcephaly (Q02)

● Q75.0 Craniosynostosis
Premature closure of sutures of skull
● Q75.00 Craniosynostosis unspecified
Craniosynostosis NOS
Q75.001 Craniosynostosis unspecified, unilateral
Q75.002 Craniosynostosis unspecified, bilateral
Q75.009 Craniosynostosis unspecified
Imperfect fusion of skull
● Q75.01 Sagittal craniosynostosis
Non-deformational dolichocephaly
Non-deformational scaphocephaly
Excludes1 plagiocephaly (Q67.3)
● Q75.02 Coronal craniosynostosis
Non-deformational anterior plagiocephaly
Excludes1 dolichocephaly (Q67.2)
Q75.021 Coronal craniosynostosis unilateral
Non-deformational anterior plagiocephaly
Q75.022 Coronal craniosynostosis bilateral
Non-deformational brachycephaly
Q75.029 Coronal craniosynostosis unspecified
● Q75.03 Metopic craniosynostosis
Trigonocephaly
● Q75.04 Lambdoid craniosynostosis
Non-deformational posterior plagiocephaly
Excludes1 dolichocephaly (Q67.2)
Q75.041 Lambdoid craniosynostosis, unilateral
Q75.042 Lambdoid craniosynostosis, bilateral
Q75.049 Lambdoid craniosynostosis, unspecified

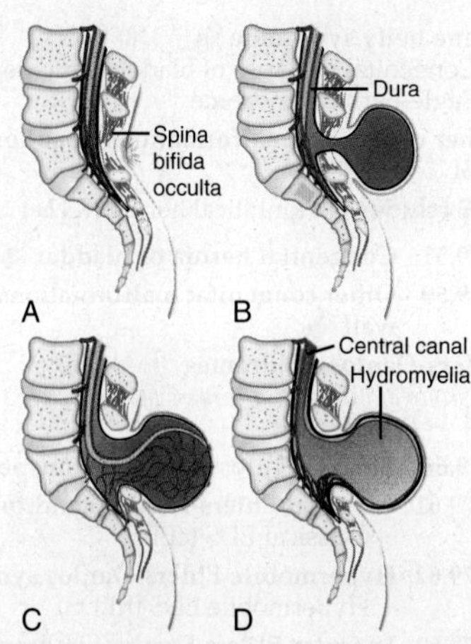

Figure 17-11 **A.** Spina bifida occulta. **B.** Meningocele. **C.** Myelomeningocele. **D.** Myelocystocele (syringomyelocele) or hydromyelia.

Item 17-4 **Spina bifida** is a midline spinal defect in which one or more vertebrae fail to fuse, leaving an opening in the vertebral canal. When the defect is not visible, it is called spina bifida occulta, and when it is visible, it is called spina bifida cystica.

● **Q75.05 Multi-suture craniosynostosis**
- **Q75.051 Cloverleaf skull**
  Kleeblattschaedel skull
- **Q75.052 Pansynostosis**
- **Q75.058 Other multi-suture craniosynostosis**
  Excludes1 coronal craniosynostosis, bilateral (Q75.022)
  lambdoid craniosynostosis, bilateral (Q75.042)

Q75.08 Other single-suture craniosynostosis

Q75.1 Craniofacial dysostosis
Congential deformity of head
Crouzon's disease

Q75.2 Hypertelorism

Q75.3 Macrocephaly
Unusually large size of head; AKA megalocephaly

Q75.4 Mandibulofacial dysostosis
Franceschetti syndrome
Treacher Collins syndrome

Q75.5 Oculomandibular dysostosis
Ossification of occular and mandibular bones

Q75.8 Other specified congenital malformations of skull and face bones
Absence of skull bone, congenital
Congenital deformity of forehead
Platybasia

Q75.9 Congenital malformation of skull and face bones, unspecified
Congenital anomaly of face bones NOS
Congenital anomaly of skull NOS

● **Q76 Congenital malformations of spine and bony thorax**
Excludes1 congenital musculoskeletal deformities of spine and chest (Q67.5-Q67.8)

Q76.0 Spina bifida occulta
Excludes1 meningocele (spinal) (Q05.-)
spina bifida (aperta) (cystica) (Q05.-)

Q76.1 Klippel-Feil syndrome
Cervical fusion syndrome

Q76.2 Congenital spondylolisthesis
Congenital spondylolysis
Excludes1 spondylolisthesis (acquired) (M43.1-)
spondylolysis (acquired) (M43.0-)

Q76.3 Congenital scoliosis due to congenital bony malformation (Ex) PDX 1571
Hemivertebra fusion or failure of segmentation with scoliosis
Coding Clinic: 2022, Q4, P41

● **Q76.4 Other congenital malformations of spine, not associated with scoliosis**

● **Q76.41 Congenital kyphosis**
Abnormal increase in convexity curvature of thoracic spinal column; AKA humpback
- **Q76.411 Congenital kyphosis, occipito-atlanto-axial region**
- **Q76.412 Congenital kyphosis, cervical region**
- **Q76.413 Congenital kyphosis, cervicothoracic region**
- **Q76.414 Congenital kyphosis, thoracic region**
- **Q76.415 Congenital kyphosis, thoracolumbar region**
- **Q76.419 Congenital kyphosis, unspecified region**

● **Q76.42 Congenital lordosis** (Ex) PDX 1571
An abnormal increase in curvature of lumbar spine (sway back)
- **Q76.425 Congenital lordosis, thoracolumbar region**
- **Q76.426 Congenital lordosis, lumbar region**
- **Q76.427 Congenital lordosis, lumbosacral region**
- **Q76.428 Congenital lordosis, sacral and sacrococcygeal region**
- **Q76.429 Congenital lordosis, unspecified region**

Q76.49 Other congenital malformations of spine, not associated with scoliosis
Congenital absence of vertebra NOS
Congenital fusion of spine NOS
Congenital malformation of lumbosacral (joint) (region) NOS
Congenital malformation of spine NOS
Hemivertebra NOS
Malformation of spine NOS
Platyspondylisis NOS
Supernumerary vertebra NOS

Q76.5 Cervical rib
Supernumerary rib in cervical region

Q76.6 Other congenital malformations of ribs (Ex) PDX 1573
Accessory rib
Congenital absence of rib
Congenital fusion of ribs
Congenital malformation of ribs NOS
Excludes1 short rib syndrome (Q77.2)

Q76.7 Congenital malformation of sternum (Ex) PDX 1573
Congenital absence of sternum
Sternum bifidum

Q76.8 Other congenital malformations of bony thorax (Ex) PDX 1573

Q76.9 Congenital malformation of bony thorax, unspecified (Ex) PDX 1573

● **Q77 Osteochondrodysplasia with defects of growth of tubular bones and spine**
Excludes1 mucopolysaccharidosis (E76.0-E76.3)
Excludes2 congenital myotonic chondrodystrophy (G71.13)

Q77.0 Achondrogenesis
Hypochondrogenesis

Q77.1 Thanatophoric short stature

Q77.2 Short rib syndrome (Ex) PDX 1573
Asphyxiating thoracic dysplasia [Jeune]

CHAPTER 17 (Q00-Q99)

Q77.3 **Chondrodysplasia punctata**
Benign cartilaginous neoplasms
Excludes1 rhizomelic chondrodysplasia punctata (E71.43)

Q77.4 **Achondroplasia**
Disturbance of epiphyseal chondroblastic growth and maturation, results in dwarfism
Hypochondroplasia
Osteosclerosis congenita

Q77.5 **Diastrophic dysplasia**

Q77.6 **Chondroectodermal dysplasia**
Defective development of skin, hair, teeth, with polydactyly and defect of cardiac septum
Ellis-van Creveld syndrome

Q77.7 **Spondyloepiphyseal dysplasia**

Q77.8 **Other osteochondrodysplasia with defects of growth of tubular bones and spine**

Q77.9 **Osteochondrodysplasia with defects of growth of tubular bones and spine, unspecified**

● Q78 **Other osteochondrodysplasias**
Disorder of development of bone and cartilage; common cause of dwarfism
Excludes2 congenital myotonic chondrodystrophy (G71.13)

Q78.0 **Osteogenesis imperfecta** (Ex) PDX 1574
Fragilitas ossium
Osteopsathyrosis

Q78.1 **Polyostotic fibrous dysplasia**
Albright(-McCune)(-Sternberg) syndrome

Q78.2 **Osteopetrosis** (Ex) PDX 1574
Abnormally dense bone; AKA marble bones disease, ivory bones
Albers-Schönberg syndrome
Osteosclerosis NOS

Q78.3 **Progressive diaphyseal dysplasia**
Camurati-Engelmann syndrome

Q78.4 **Enchondromatosis**
Thinning of overlying cortex of bone and distorted length
Maffucci's syndrome
Ollier's disease

Q78.5 **Metaphyseal dysplasia**
Disturbance in enchondral bone growth, causing ends of shafts to remain larger than normal in circumference
Pyle's syndrome

Q78.6 **Multiple congenital exostoses**
Diaphyseal aclasis

Q78.8 **Other specified osteochondrodysplasias**
Osteopoikilosis

Q78.9 **Osteochondrodysplasia, unspecified**
Chondrodystrophy NOS
AKA skeletal dysplasia (dwarfism) caused by genetic mutations affecting hyaline cartilage capping long bones and vertebrae
Osteodystrophy NOS

● Q79 **Congenital malformations of musculoskeletal system, not elsewhere classified**
Excludes2 congenital (sternomastoid) torticollis (Q68.0)

Q79.0 **Congenital diaphragmatic hernia** (Ex) PDX 1575
Excludes1 congenital hiatus hernia (Q40.1)

Q79.1 **Other congenital malformations of diaphragm** (Ex) PDX 1575
Absence of diaphragm
Congenital malformation of diaphragm NOS
Eventration of diaphragm

Q79.2 **Exomphalos** (Ex) PDX 1576
Abdominal hernia in which part of intestine protrudes at umbilicus; AKA exomphalos and exumbilication
Omphalocele
Excludes1 umbilical hernia (K42.-)

Q79.3 **Gastroschisis** (Ex) PDX 1576
Congenital fissure of anterior abdominal wall often with protrusion of small/large intestine

Q79.4 **Prune belly syndrome** (Ex) PDX 1576
Congenital prolapse of bladder mucosa
Eagle-Barrett syndrome

● Q79.5 **Other congenital malformations of abdominal wall** (Ex) PDX 1576
Excludes1 umbilical hernia (K42.-)

Q79.51 **Congenital hernia of bladder**

Q79.59 **Other congenital malformations of abdominal wall**

● Q79.6 **Ehlers-Danlos syndromes** (Ex) PDX 1577
Group of inherited disorders of connective tissue; AKA cutis hyperelastica

Q79.60 **Ehlers-Danlos syndrome, unspecified**

Q79.61 **Classical Ehlers-Danlos syndrome**
Classical EDS (cEDS)

Q79.62 **Hypermobile Ehlers-Danlos syndrome**
Hypermobile EDS (hEDS)

Q79.63 **Vascular Ehlers-Danlos syndrome**
Vascular EDS (vEDS)

Q79.69 **Other Ehlers-Danlos syndromes**

Q79.8 **Other congenital malformations of musculoskeletal system**
Absence of muscle
Absence of tendon
Accessory muscle
Amyotrophia congenita
Congenital constricting bands
Congenital shortening of tendon
Poland syndrome

Q79.9 **Congenital malformation of musculoskeletal system, unspecified**
Congenital anomaly of musculoskeletal system NOS
Congenital deformity of musculoskeletal system NOS

OTHER CONGENITAL MALFORMATIONS (Q80-Q89)

● Q80 **Congenital ichthyosis**
Characterized by increased keratinization, resulting in noninflammatory scaling of skin
Excludes1 Refsum's disease (G60.1)

Q80.0 **Ichthyosis vulgaris**

Q80.1 **X-linked ichthyosis**

Q80.2 **Lamellar ichthyosis**
Collodion baby

Q80.3 **Congenital bullous ichthyosiform erythroderma**

Q80.4 **Harlequin fetus**

Q80.8 **Other congenital ichthyosis**

Q80.9 **Congenital ichthyosis, unspecified**

● Q81 **Epidermolysis bullosa**
Loosening of epidermis

Q81.0 **Epidermolysis bullosa simplex**
Excludes1 Cockayne's syndrome (Q87.19)

Q81.1 **Epidermolysis bullosa letalis**
Herlitz' syndrome

Q81.2 **Epidermolysis bullosa dystrophica**

Q81.8 **Other epidermolysis bullosa**

Q81.9 **Epidermolysis bullosa, unspecified**

● Q82 **Other congenital malformations of skin**
Excludes1 acrodermatitis enteropathica (E83.2)
congenital erythropoietic porphyria (E80.0)
pilonidal cyst or sinus (L05.-)
Sturge-Weber (-Dimitri) syndrome (Q85.89)

Q82.0 **Hereditary lymphedema**
Characterized by swelling of subcutaneous tissue caused by obstruction of lymphatic vessels and resulting edema of lymph fluid

Q82.1 **Xeroderma pigmentosum**
Extreme sensitivity to ultraviolet rays that most commonly affects the eyes and skin, but may also involve the nervous system

Q82.2 Congenital cutaneous mastocytosis
Characterized by infiltrates of mast cells in tissues/organs
Congenital diffuse cutaneous mastocytosis
Congenital maculopapular cutaneous mastocytosis
Congenital urticaria pigmentosa
Excludes1 cutaneous mastocytosis NOS (D47.Ø1)
diffuse cutaneous mastocytosis (with onset after newborn period) (D47.Ø1)
malignant mastocytosis (C96.2-)
systemic mastocytosis (D47.Ø2)
urticaria pigmentosa (non-congenital) (with onset after newborn period) (D47.Ø1)

Q82.3 Incontinentia pigmenti
Characterized by hypopigmented cutaneous in adults and early childhood

Q82.4 Ectodermal dysplasia (anhidrotic)
Absence/deficiency of tissues/structures, including teeth, hair, nails, and certain glands
Excludes1 Ellis-van Creveld syndrome (Q77.6)

Q82.5 Congenital non-neoplastic nevus
Birthmark NOS
Flammeus Nevus
Portwine Nevus
Sanguineous Nevus
Strawberry Nevus
Vascular Nevus NOS
Verrucous Nevus
Excludes2 Café au lait spots (L81.3)
lentigo (L81.4)
nevus NOS (D22.-)
araneus nevus (I78.1)
melanocytic nevus (D22.-)
pigmented nevus (D22.-)
spider nevus (I78.1)
stellar nevus (I78.1)

Q82.6 Congenital sacral dimple
Parasacral dimple
Excludes2 pilonidal cyst with abscess (LØ5.Ø1)
pilonidal cyst without abscess (LØ5.91)
Coding Clinic: 2Ø16, Q4, P6Ø

Q82.8 Other specified congenital malformations of skin
Abnormal palmar creases
Accessory skin tags
Benign familial pemphigus [Hailey-Hailey]
Congenital poikiloderma
Cutis laxa (hyperelastica)
Dermatoglyphic anomalies
Inherited keratosis palmaris et plantaris
Keratosis follicularis [Darier-White]
Excludes1 Ehlers-Danlos syndromes (Q79.6-)
Coding Clinic: 2Ø16, Q1, P17

Q82.9 Congenital malformation of skin, unspecified

● **Q83 Congenital malformations of breast**
Excludes2 absence of pectoral muscle (Q79.8)
hypoplasia of breast (N64.82)
micromastia (N64.82)

Q83.Ø Congenital absence of breast with absent nipple

Q83.1 Accessory breast
Supernumerary breast

Q83.2 Absent nipple

Q83.3 Accessory nipple
Supernumerary nipple

Q83.8 Other congenital malformations of breast

Q83.9 Congenital malformation of breast, unspecified

● **Q84 Other congenital malformations of integument**

Q84.Ø Congenital alopecia
Congenital atrichosis

Q84.1 Congenital morphological disturbances of hair, not elsewhere classified
Beaded hair
Monilethrix
Pili annulati
Excludes1 Menkes' kinky hair syndrome (E83.Ø9)

Q84.2 Other congenital malformations of hair
Congenital hypertrichosis
Congenital malformation of hair NOS
Persistent lanugo

Q84.3 Anonychia
Absence of nail
Excludes1 nail patella syndrome (Q87.2)

Q84.4 Congenital leukonychia
Opaque, whitish discoloration of nails; AKA leukopathia unguium

Q84.5 Enlarged and hypertrophic nails
Congenital onychauxis
Pachyonychia

Q84.6 Other congenital malformations of nails
Congenital clubnail
Congenital koilonychia
Congenital malformation of nail NOS

Q84.8 Other specified congenital malformations of integument
Aplasia cutis congenita

Q84.9 Congenital malformation of integument, unspecified
Congenital anomaly of integument NOS
Congenital deformity of integument NOS

● **Q85 Phakomatoses, not elsewhere classified**
Excludes1 ataxia telangiectasia [Louis-Bar] (G11.3)
familial dysautonomia [Riley-Day] (G9Ø.1)

● **Q85.Ø Neurofibromatosis (nonmalignant)**
Developmental changes in nervous system and other structures, with formation of neurofibromas

Q85.ØØ Neurofibromatosis, unspecified

Q85.Ø1 Neurofibromatosis, type 1
Von Recklinghausen disease

Q85.Ø2 Neurofibromatosis, type 2
Acoustic neurofibromatosis

Q85.Ø3 Schwannomatosis

Q85.Ø9 Other neurofibromatosis

Q85.1 Tuberous sclerosis (Ex:) PDX 1578
Bourneville's disease
Epiloia

● **Q85.8 Other phakomatoses, not elsewhere classified** (Ex:) PDX 1579
Excludes1 Meckel-Gruber syndrome (Q61.9)
Coding Clinic: 2Ø21, Q3, P12

Q85.81 PTEN hamartoma tumor syndrome
PHTS
PTEN related Cowden syndrome
Code also, if applicable, genetic susceptibility to malignant neoplasm (Z15.0-)
Coding Clinic: 2Ø22, Q4, P41

Q85.82 Other Cowden syndrome

Q85.83 Von Hippel-Lindau syndrome
Code also manifestations
Coding Clinic: 2Ø23, Q2, P16

Q85.89 Other phakomatoses, not elsewhere classified
Peutz-Jeghers syndrome
Sturge-Weber(-Dimitri) syndrome

Q85.9 Phakomatosis, unspecified (Ex:) PDX 1579
Hamartosis NOS

CHAPTER 17 (QØØ-Q99)

● Q86 **Congenital malformation syndromes due to known exogenous causes, not elsewhere classified**
 Excludes2 iodine-deficiency-related hypothyroidism (E00-E02)
 nonteratogenic effects of substances transmitted via placenta or breast milk (P04.-)
 Q86.0 **Fetal alcohol syndrome (dysmorphic)**
 Q86.1 **Fetal hydantoin syndrome**
 Meadow's syndrome
 Q86.2 **Dysmorphism due to warfarin**
 Q86.8 **Other congenital malformation syndromes due to known exogenous causes**

● Q87 **Other specified congenital malformation syndromes affecting multiple systems**
 Use additional code(s) to identify all associated manifestations
 Q87.0 **Congenital malformation syndromes predominantly affecting facial appearance**
 Acrocephalopolysyndactyly
 Acrocephalosyndactyly [Apert]
 Cryptophthalmos syndrome
 Cyclopia
 Goldenhar syndrome
 Moebius syndrome
 Oro-facial-digital syndrome
 Robin syndrome
 Whistling face
 ● Q87.1 **Congenital malformation syndromes predominantly associated with short stature** (Ex) PDX 1580
 Q87.11 **Prader-Willi syndrome**
 Q87.19 **Other congenital malformation syndromes predominantly associated with short stature**
 Aarskog syndrome
 Cockayne syndrome
 De Lange syndrome
 Dubowitz syndrome
 Noonan syndrome
 Robinow-Silverman-Smith syndrome
 Russell-Silver syndrome
 Seckel syndrome
 Excludes1 Ellis-van Creveld syndrome (Q77.6)
 Smith-Lemli-Opitz syndrome (E78.72)
 Q87.2 **Congenital malformation syndromes predominantly involving limbs** (Ex) PDX 1581
 Holt-Oram syndrome
 Klippel-Trenaunay-Weber syndrome
 Nail patella syndrome
 Rubinstein-Taybi syndrome
 Sirenomelia syndrome
 Thrombocytopenia with absent radius [TAR] syndrome
 VATER syndrome
 Q87.3 **Congenital malformation syndromes involving early overgrowth** (Ex) PDX 1581
 Beckwith-Wiedemann syndrome
 Sotos' syndrome
 Weaver syndrome
 ● Q87.4 **Marfan's syndrome** (Ex) PDX 1582
 Q87.40 **Marfan's syndrome, unspecified**
 ● Q87.41 **Marfan syndrome with cardiovascular manifestations**
 Q87.410 **Marfan syndrome with aortic dilation**
 Q87.418 **Marfan syndrome with other cardiovascular manifestations**
 Q87.42 **Marfan syndrome with ocular manifestations**
 Q87.43 **Marfan syndrome with skeletal manifestation**
 Q87.5 **Other congenital malformation syndromes with other skeletal changes** (Ex) PDX 1583
 ● Q87.8 **Other specified congenital malformation syndromes, not elsewhere classified** (Ex) PDX 1581
 Excludes1 Zellweger syndrome (E71.510)
 Q87.81 **Alport syndrome**
 Progressive sensorineural hearing loss, progressive pyelonephritis or glomerulonephritis, and ocular defects
 Use additional code to identify stage of chronic kidney disease (N18.1-N18.6)
 Q87.82 **Arterial tortuosity syndrome**
 Coding Clinic: 2016, Q4, P60-61
 Q87.83 **Bardet-Biedl syndrome**
 Q87.84 **Laurence-Moon syndrome**
 Q87.85 **MED13L syndrome**
 Asadollahi-Rauch syndrome
 Mediator complex subunit 13L syndrome
 Code also, if applicable, any associated manifestations such as:
 autism spectrum disorder (F84.0-)
 congenital malformations of cardiac septa (Q21.-)
 epilepsy and recurrent seizures (G40.-)
 intellectual disability (F70-F79)
 ▶ Q87.86 **Kleefstra syndrome**
 Q87.89 **Other specified congenital malformation syndromes, not elsewhere classified**

● Q89 **Other congenital malformations, not elsewhere classified**
 ● Q89.0 **Congenital absence and malformations of spleen** (Ex) PDX 1584
 Excludes1 isomerism of atrial appendages (with asplenia or polysplenia) (Q20.6)
 Q89.01 **Asplenia (congenital)**
 Q89.09 **Congenital malformations of spleen**
 Congenital splenomegaly
 Q89.1 **Congenital malformations of adrenal gland**
 Excludes1 adrenogenital disorders (E25.-)
 congenital adrenal hyperplasia (E25.0)
 Q89.2 **Congenital malformations of other endocrine glands**
 Congenital malformation of parathyroid or thyroid gland
 Persistent thyroglossal duct
 Thyroglossal cyst
 Excludes1 congenital goiter (E03.0)
 congenital hypothyroidism (E03.1)
 Q89.3 **Situs inversus** (Ex) PDX 1585
 Lateral transposition of viscera of thorax and abdomen
 Dextrocardia with situs inversus
 Mirror-image atrial arrangement with situs inversus
 Situs inversus or transversus abdominalis
 Situs inversus or transversus thoracis
 Transposition of abdominal viscera
 Transposition of thoracic viscera
 Excludes1 dextrocardia NOS (Q24.0)
 Q89.4 **Conjoined twins** (Ex) PDX 1586
 Craniopagus
 Dicephaly
 Pygopagus
 Thoracopagus
 Q89.7 **Multiple congenital malformations, not elsewhere classified** (Ex) PDX 1585
 Multiple congenital anomalies NOS
 Multiple congenital deformities NOS
 Excludes1 congenital malformation syndromes affecting multiple systems (Q87.-)
 Q89.8 **Other specified congenital malformations** (Ex) PDX 1581
 Use additional code(s) to identify all associated manifestations
 Coding Clinic: 2021, Q3, P12
 Q89.9 **Congenital malformation, unspecified**
 Congenital anomaly NOS
 Congenital deformity NOS

CHAPTER 17 (Q00-Q99)

CHROMOSOMAL ABNORMALITIES, NOT ELSEWHERE CLASSIFIED (Q90-Q99)

Excludes2 mitochondrial metabolic disorders (E88.4-)

Q90 Down syndrome
Code also associated physical condition(s), such as atrioventricular septal defect (Q21.2-)
Use additional code(s) to identify any associated and degree of intellectual disabilities (F70-F79)

Q90.0 Trisomy 21, nonmosaicism (meiotic nondisjunction)
Trisomy 21, nondisjunction, accounts for 95% of Downs syndrome cases

Q90.1 Trisomy 21, mosaicism (mitotic nondisjunction)

Q90.2 Trisomy 21, translocation

Q90.9 Down syndrome, unspecified
Trisomy 21 NOS

Q91 Trisomy 18 and Trisomy 13 Ex PDX 1587

Q91.0 Trisomy 18, nonmosaicism (meiotic nondisjunction)

Q91.1 Trisomy 18, mosaicism (mitotic nondisjunction)

Q91.2 Trisomy 18, translocation

Q91.3 Trisomy 18, unspecified

Q91.4 Trisomy 13, nonmosaicism (meiotic nondisjunction)

Q91.5 Trisomy 13, mosaicism (mitotic nondisjunction)

Q91.6 Trisomy 13, translocation

Q91.7 Trisomy 13, unspecified

Q92 Other trisomies and partial trisomies of the autosomes, not elsewhere classified
Includes unbalanced translocations and insertions
Excludes1 trisomies of chromosomes 13, 18, 21 (Q90-Q91)

Q92.0 Whole chromosome trisomy, nonmosaicism (meiotic nondisjunction)

Q92.1 Whole chromosome trisomy, mosaicism (mitotic nondisjunction)

Q92.2 Partial trisomy
Less than whole arm duplicated
Whole arm or more duplicated
Excludes1 partial trisomy due to unbalanced translocation (Q92.5)

Q92.5 Duplications with other complex rearrangements
Partial trisomy due to unbalanced translocations
Code also any associated deletions due to unbalanced translocations, inversions and insertions (Q93.7)

Q92.6 Marker chromosomes
Trisomies due to dicentrics
Trisomies due to extra rings
Trisomies due to isochromosomes
Individual with marker heterochromatin

Q92.61 Marker chromosomes in normal individual

Q92.62 Marker chromosomes in abnormal individual

Q92.7 Triploidy and polyploidy

Q92.8 Other specified trisomies and partial trisomies of autosomes
Duplications identified by fluorescence in situ hybridization (FISH)
Duplications identified by in situ hybridization (ISH)
Duplications seen only at prometaphase

Q92.9 Trisomy and partial trisomy of autosomes, unspecified

Q93 Monosomies and deletions from the autosomes, not elsewhere classified

Q93.0 Whole chromosome monosomy, nonmosaicism (meiotic nondisjunction)

Q93.1 Whole chromosome monosomy, mosaicism (mitotic nondisjunction)

Q93.2 Chromosome replaced with ring, dicentric or isochromosome

Q93.3 Deletion of short arm of chromosome 4 Ex PDX 1588
Wolff-Hirschorn syndrome

Q93.4 Deletion of short arm of chromosome 5 Ex PDX 1587
Cri-du-chat syndrome

Q93.5 Other deletions of part of a chromosome Ex PDX 1587

Q93.51 Angelman syndrome

Q93.52 Phelan-McDermid syndrome
22q13.3 deletion syndrome
Use additional code(s) to identify any associated conditions, such as:
autism spectrum disorder (F84.0)
degree of intellectual disabilities (F70-F79)
epilepsy and recurrent seizures (G40.-)
lymphedema (I89.0)

Q93.59 Other deletions of part of a chromosome

Q93.7 Deletions with other complex rearrangements Ex PDX 1589
Deletions due to unbalanced translocations, inversions and insertions
Code also any associated duplications due to unbalanced translocations, inversions and insertions (Q92.5)

Q93.8 Other deletions from the autosomes Ex PDX 1587

Q93.81 Velo-cardio-facial syndrome
Deletion 22q11.2
Coding Clinic: 2019, Q3, P14

Q93.82 Williams syndrome

Q93.88 Other microdeletions Miller-Dieker syndrome
Smith-Magenis syndrome

Q93.89 Other deletions from the autosomes Ex PDX 1590
Deletions identified by fluorescence in situ hybridization (FISH)
Deletions identified by in situ hybridization (ISH)
Deletions seen only at prometaphase

Q93.9 Deletion from autosomes, unspecified Ex PDX 1591

Q95 Balanced rearrangements and structural markers, not elsewhere classified
Includes Robertsonian and balanced reciprocal translocations and insertions

Q95.0 Balanced translocation and insertion in normal individual

Q95.1 Chromosome inversion in normal individual

Q95.2 Balanced autosomal rearrangement in abnormal individual

Q95.3 Balanced sex/autosomal rearrangement in abnormal individual

Q95.5 Individual with autosomal fragile site

Q95.8 Other balanced rearrangements and structural markers

Q95.9 Balanced rearrangement and structural marker, unspecified

Q96 Turner's syndrome
Caused by missing or incomplete X chromosome affecting growth and sexual development
Excludes1 Noonan syndrome (Q87.19)

Q96.0 Karyotype 45, X

Q96.1 Karyotype 46, X iso (Xq)
Karyotype 46, isochromosome Xq

Q96.2 Karyotype 46, X with abnormal sex chromosome, except iso (Xq)
Karyotype 46, X with abnormal sex chromosome, except isochromosome Xq

Q96.3 Mosaicism, 45, X/46, XX or XY

Q96.4 Mosaicism, 45, X/other cell line(s) with abnormal sex chromosome

Q96.8 Other variants of Turner's syndrome

Q96.9 Turner's syndrome, unspecified

CHAPTER 17 (Q00-Q99)

● Q97 **Other sex chromosome abnormalities, female phenotype, not elsewhere classified**

Excludes1 Turner's syndrome (Q96.-)

Q97.0 **Karyotype 47, XXX**

Q97.1 **Female with more than three X chromosomes**

Q97.2 **Mosaicism, lines with various numbers of X chromosomes**

Q97.3 **Female with 46, XY karyotype**

Q97.8 **Other specified sex chromosome abnormalities, female phenotype**

Q97.9 **Sex chromosome abnormality, female phenotype, unspecified**

● Q98 **Other sex chromosome abnormalities, male phenotype, not elsewhere classified**

Q98.0 **Klinefelter syndrome karyotype 47, XXY**

Q98.1 **Klinefelter syndrome, male with more than two X chromosomes**

Q98.3 **Other male with 46, XX karyotype**

Q98.4 **Klinefelter syndrome, unspecified**

Q98.5 **Karyotype 47, XYY**

Q98.6 **Male with structurally abnormal sex chromosome**

Q98.7 **Male with sex chromosome mosaicism**

Q98.8 **Other specified sex chromosome abnormalities, male phenotype**

Q98.9 **Sex chromosome abnormality, male phenotype, unspecified**

● Q99 **Other chromosome abnormalities, not elsewhere classified**

Q99.0 **Chimera 46, XX/46, XY**

Chimera 46, XX/46, XY true hermaphrodite

Q99.1 **46, XX true hermaphrodite**

46, XX with streak gonads

46, XY with streak gonads

Pure gonadal dysgenesis

Q99.2 **Fragile X chromosome**

Fragile X syndrome

Q99.8 **Other specified chromosome abnormalities**

Q99.9 **Chromosomal abnormality, unspecified**

CHAPTER 18

SYMPTOMS, SIGNS, AND ABNORMAL CLINICAL AND LABORATORY FINDINGS, NOT ELSEWHERE CLASSIFIED (RØØ-R99)

OGCR Chapter-Specific Coding Guidelines

18. **Chapter 18: Symptoms, signs, and abnormal clinical and laboratory findings, not elsewhere classified (RØØ-R99)**
Chapter 18 includes symptoms, signs, abnormal results of clinical or other investigative procedures, and ill-defined conditions regarding which no diagnosis classifiable elsewhere is recorded. Signs and symptoms that point to a specific diagnosis have been assigned to a category in other chapters of the classification.

a. Use of symptom codes
Codes that describe symptoms and signs are acceptable for reporting purposes when a related definitive diagnosis has not been established (confirmed) by the provider.

b. Use of a symptom code with a definitive diagnosis code
Codes for signs and symptoms may be reported in addition to a related definitive diagnosis when the sign or symptom is not routinely associated with that diagnosis, such as the various signs and symptoms associated with complex syndromes. The definitive diagnosis code should be sequenced before the symptom code.

Signs or symptoms that are associated routinely with a disease process should not be assigned as additional codes, unless otherwise instructed by the classification.

c. Combination codes that include symptoms
ICD-10-CM contains a number of combination codes that identify both the definitive diagnosis and common symptoms of that diagnosis. When using one of these combination codes, an additional code should not be assigned for the symptom.

d. Repeated falls
Code R29.6, Repeated falls, is for use for encounters when a patient has recently fallen and the reason for the fall is being investigated.

Code Z91.81, History of falling, is for use when a patient has fallen in the past and is at risk for future falls. When appropriate, both codes R29.6 and Z91.81 may be assigned together.

e. Coma scale
The coma scale codes (R4Ø.2-) can be used in conjunction with traumatic brain injury codes, acute cerebrovascular disease or sequelae of cerebrovascular disease codes. These codes are primarily for use by trauma registries, but they may be used in any setting where this information is collected. The coma scale may also be used to assess the status of the central nervous system for other non-trauma conditions, such as monitoring patients in the intensive care unit regardless of medical condition. The coma scale codes should be sequenced after the diagnosis code(s).

These codes, one from each subcategory, are needed to complete the scale. The 7th character indicates when the scale was recorded. The 7th character should match for all three codes.

At a minimum, report the initial score documented on presentation at your facility. This may be a score from the emergency medicine technician (EMT) or in the emergency department. If desired, a facility may choose to capture multiple coma scale scores.

Assign code R4Ø.24, Glasgow coma scale, total score, when only the total score is documented in the medical record and not the individual score(s).

Do not report codes for individual or total Glasgow coma scale scores for a patient with a medically induced coma or a sedated patient.

See Section I.B.14 for coma scale documentation by clinicians other than patient's provider.

f. Functional quadriplegia
GUIDELINE HAS BEEN DELETED EFFECTIVE OCTOBER 1, 2Ø17

g. SIRS due to Non-Infectious Process
The systemic inflammatory response syndrome (SIRS) can develop as a result of certain non-infectious disease processes, such as trauma, malignant neoplasm, or pancreatitis. When SIRS is documented with a noninfectious condition, and no subsequent infection is documented, the code for the underlying condition, such as an injury, should be assigned, followed by code R65.1Ø, Systemic inflammatory response syndrome (SIRS) of non-infectious origin without acute organ dysfunction, or code R65.11, Systemic inflammatory response syndrome (SIRS) of non-infectious origin with acute organ dysfunction. If an associated acute organ dysfunction is documented, the appropriate code(s) for the specific type of organ dysfunction(s) should be assigned in addition to code R65.11. If acute organ dysfunction is documented, but it cannot be determined if the acute organ dysfunction is associated with SIRS or due to another condition (e.g., directly due to the trauma), the provider should be queried.

h. Death NOS
Code R99, Ill-defined and unknown cause of mortality, is only for use in the very limited circumstance when a patient who has already died is brought into an emergency department or other healthcare facility and is pronounced dead upon arrival. It does not represent the discharge disposition of death.

i. NIHSS Stroke Scale
The NIH stroke scale (NIHSS) codes (R29.7- -) can be used in conjunction with acute stroke codes (I63) to identify the patient's neurological status and the severity of the stroke. The stroke scale codes should be sequenced after the acute stroke diagnosis code(s).

At a minimum, report the initial score documented. If desired, a facility may choose to capture multiple stroke scale scores.

See Section I.B.14 for NIHSS stroke scale documentation by clinicians other than patient's provider.

OGCR Section I.B.4.

Signs and symptoms

Codes that describe symptoms and signs, as opposed to diagnoses, are acceptable for reporting purposes when a related definitive diagnosis has not been established (confirmed) by the provider. Chapter 18 of ICD-10-CM, Symptoms, Signs, and Abnormal Clinical and Laboratory Findings, Not Elsewhere Classified (codes RØØ.Ø-R99) contains many, but not all codes for symptoms.

CHAPTER 18

SYMPTOMS, SIGNS, AND ABNORMAL CLINICAL AND LABORATORY FINDINGS, NOT ELSEWHERE CLASSIFIED (RØØ-R99)

Note: This chapter includes symptoms, signs, abnormal results of clinical or other investigative procedures, and ill-defined conditions regarding which no diagnosis classifiable elsewhere is recorded.

Signs and symptoms that point rather definitely to a given diagnosis have been assigned to a category in other chapters of the classification. In general, categories in this chapter include the less well-defined conditions and symptoms that, without the necessary study of the case to establish a final diagnosis, point perhaps equally to two or more diseases or to two or more systems of the body. Practically all categories in the chapter could be designated "not otherwise specified", "unknown etiology" or "transient". The Alphabetical Index should be consulted to determine which symptoms and signs are to be allocated here and which to other chapters. The residual subcategories, numbered .8, are generally provided for other relevant symptoms that cannot be allocated elsewhere in the classification.

The conditions and signs or symptoms included in categories RØØ-R94 consist of:

(a) cases for which no more specific diagnosis can be made even after all the facts bearing on the case have been investigated;

(b) signs or symptoms existing at the time of initial encounter that proved to be transient and whose causes could not be determined;

(c) provisional diagnosis in a patient who failed to return for further investigation or care;

(d) cases referred elsewhere for investigation or treatment before the diagnosis was made;

(e) cases in which a more precise diagnosis was not available for any other reason;

(f) certain symptoms, for which supplementary information is provided, that represent important problems in medical care in their own right.

Excludes2 abnormal findings on antenatal screening of mother (O28.-)
certain conditions originating in the perinatal period (PØ4-P96)
signs and symptoms classified in the body system chapters
signs and symptoms of breast (N63, N64.5)

This chapter contains the following blocks:

RØØ-RØ9	Symptoms and signs involving the circulatory and respiratory systems
R1Ø-R19	Symptoms and signs involving the digestive system and abdomen
R2Ø-R23	Symptoms and signs involving the skin and subcutaneous tissue
R25-R29	Symptoms and signs involving the nervous and musculoskeletal systems
R3Ø-R39	Symptoms and signs involving the genitourinary system
R4Ø-R46	Symptoms and signs involving cognition, perception, emotional state and behavior
R47-R49	Symptoms and signs involving speech and voice
R5Ø-R69	General symptoms and signs
R7Ø-R79	Abnormal findings on examination of blood, without diagnosis
R8Ø-R82	Abnormal findings on examination of urine, without diagnosis
R83-R89	Abnormal findings on examination of other body fluids, substances and tissues, without diagnosis
R9Ø-R94	Abnormal findings on diagnostic imaging and in function studies, without diagnosis
R97	Abnormal tumor markers
R99	Ill-defined and unknown cause of mortality

SYMPTOMS AND SIGNS INVOLVING THE CIRCULATORY AND RESPIRATORY SYSTEMS (RØØ-RØ9)

● **RØØ Abnormalities of heart beat**

Excludes1 abnormalities originating in the perinatal period (P29.1-)
inappropriate sinus tachycardia, so stated (I47.11)

Excludes2 specified arrhythmias (I47-I49)

RØØ.Ø Tachycardia, unspecified
Rapid heart rate >1ØØ beats
Rapid heart beat
Sinoauricular tachycardia NOS
Sinus [sinusal] tachycardia NOS

Excludes1 neonatal tachycardia (P29.11)
paroxysmal tachycardia (I47.-)

Coding Clinic: 2022, Q4, P47

RØØ.1 Bradycardia, unspecified
Slow heart rate, <6Ø
Sinoatrial bradycardia
Sinus bradycardia
Slow heart beat
Vagal bradycardia

Use additional code for adverse effect, if applicable, to identify drug (T36-T5Ø with fifth or sixth character 5)

Excludes1 neonatal bradycardia (P29.12)

RØØ.2 Palpitations
Awareness of heart beat

RØØ.8 Other abnormalities of heart beat

RØØ.9 Unspecified abnormalities of heart beat

● **R01 Cardiac murmurs and other cardiac sounds**

Excludes1 cardiac murmurs and sounds originating in the perinatal period (P29.8)

R01.0 Benign and innocent cardiac murmurs
Functional cardiac murmur

R01.1 Cardiac murmur, unspecified
Cardiac bruit NOS
Heart murmur NOS
Systolic murmur NOS

R01.2 Other cardiac sounds
Cardiac dullness, increased or decreased
Precordial friction

OGCR Section I.C.9.a.7.

Hypertension, Transient

Assign code R03.0, Elevated blood pressure reading without diagnosis of hypertension, unless patient has an established diagnosis of hypertension. Assign code O13.-, Gestational [pregnancy-induced] hypertension with significant proteinuria, or O14.-, Pre-eclampsia, for transient hypertension of pregnancy.

● **R03 Abnormal blood-pressure reading, without diagnosis**

R03.0 Elevated blood-pressure reading, without diagnosis of hypertension
Note: This category is to be used to record an episode of elevated blood pressure in a patient in whom no formal diagnosis of hypertension has been made, or as an isolated incidental finding.
MCE: Questionable admission when principal dx

R03.1 Nonspecific low blood-pressure reading
Excludes1 hypotension (I95.-)
maternal hypotension syndrome (O26.5-)
neurogenic orthostatic hypotension (G90.3)

● **R04 Hemorrhage from respiratory passages** (Ex) PDX 1592

R04.0 Epistaxis
Hemorrhage from nose
Nosebleed
Coding Clinic: 2023, Q2, P28; 2018, Q4, P38

R04.1 Hemorrhage from throat
Excludes2 hemoptysis (R04.2)

R04.2 Hemoptysis
Blood-stained sputum
Cough with hemorrhage

● **R04.8 Hemorrhage from other sites in respiratory passages**

R04.81 Acute idiopathic pulmonary hemorrhage in infants **P**
AIPHI
Acute idiopathic hemorrhage in infants over 28 days old
Excludes1 perinatal pulmonary hemorrhage (P26.-)
von Willebrand's disease (D68.0-)

R04.89 Hemorrhage from other sites in respiratory passages
Pulmonary hemorrhage NOS

R04.9 Hemorrhage from respiratory passages, unspecified

● **R05 Cough**

Excludes1 paroxysmal cough due to Bordetella pertussis (A37.0-)
smoker's cough (J41.0)
Excludes2 cough with hemorrhage (R04.2))

R05.1 Acute cough

R05.2 Subacute cough

R05.3 Chronic cough
Persistent cough
Refractory cough
Unexplained cough

● **R05.4 Cough syncope**
Code first syncope and collapse (R55)

R05.8 Other specified cough

R05.9 Cough, unspecified

● **R06 Abnormalities of breathing**

Excludes1 acute respiratory distress syndrome (J80)
respiratory arrest (R09.2)
respiratory arrest of newborn (P28.81)
respiratory distress syndrome of newborn (P22.-)
respiratory failure (J96.-)
respiratory failure of newborn (P28.5)

● **R06.0 Dyspnea**
Excludes1 tachypnea NOS (R06.82)
transient tachypnea of newborn (P22.1)

R06.00 Dyspnea, unspecified
Coding Clinic: 2017, Q1, P26-27

R06.01 Orthopnea

R06.02 Shortness of breath

R06.03 Acute respiratory distress

R06.09 Other forms of dyspnea

R06.1 Stridor
Harsh, high-pitched breath sound
Excludes1 congenital laryngeal stridor (P28.89)
laryngismus (stridulus) (J38.5)

R06.2 Wheezing
Excludes1 Asthma (J45.-)
Coding Clinic: 2016, Q2, P34

R06.3 Periodic breathing (Ex) PDX 1593
Cheyne-Stokes breathing
An abnormal pattern of breathing with gradually increasing and decreasing tidal volume with some periods of apnea

R06.4 Hyperventilation
Excludes1 psychogenic hyperventilation (F45.8)

R06.5 Mouth breathing
Excludes2 dry mouth NOS (R68.2)

R06.6 Hiccough
Excludes1 psychogenic hiccough (F45.8)

R06.7 Sneezing

● **R06.8 Other abnormalities of breathing**

R06.81 Apnea, not elsewhere classified
Apnea NOS
Excludes1 apnea (of) newborn (P28.4-)
sleep apnea (G47.3-)
sleep apnea of newborn (primary) (P28.3-)

R06.82 Tachypnea, not elsewhere classified
Tachypnea NOS
Excludes1 transitory tachypnea of newborn (P22.1)

R06.83 Snoring

R06.89 Other abnormalities of breathing
Breath-holding (spells)
Sighing

R06.9 Unspecified abnormalities of breathing

● **R07 Pain in throat and chest**

Excludes1 epidemic myalgia (B33.0)
Excludes2 jaw pain R68.84
pain in breast (N64.4)

R07.0 Pain in throat
Excludes1 chronic sore throat (J31.2)
sore throat (acute) NOS (J02.9)
Excludes2 dysphagia (R13.1-)
pain in neck (M54.2)

R07.1 Chest pain on breathing
Painful respiration

R07.2 Precordial pain

CHAPTER 18 (R00-R99)

N Newborn Age: 0 P Pediatric Age: 0–17 M Maternity DX: 9–64 A Adult Age: 15–124
Complication\Comorbidity Major C\C (Ex) CC/MCC Exclusions Hospital-Acquired Condition Hierarchical Condition Category

● R07.8 **Other chest pain**

R07.81 **Pleurodynia**
Pleurodynia NOS
Excludes1 epidemic pleurodynia (B33.0)

R07.82 **Intercostal pain**

R07.89 **Other chest pain**
Anterior chest-wall pain NOS
Coding Clinic: 2021, Q1, P42

R07.9 **Chest pain, unspecified**

● R09 **Other symptoms and signs involving the circulatory and respiratory system**
Excludes1 acute respiratory distress syndrome (J80)
respiratory arrest of newborn (P28.81)
respiratory distress syndrome of newborn (P22.0)
respiratory failure (J96.-)
respiratory failure of newborn (P28.5)

● R09.0 **Asphyxia and hypoxemia**
Excludes1 asphyxia due to carbon monoxide (T58.-)
asphyxia due to foreign body in respiratory tract (T17.-)
birth (intrauterine) asphyxia (P84)
hyperventilation (R06.4)
traumatic asphyxia (T71.-)
Excludes2 hypercapnia (R06.89)

R09.01 **Asphyxia** (Ex) PDX 1594

R09.02 **Hypoxemia**
Coding Clinic: 2019, Q3, P15

R09.1 **Pleurisy**
Occurs when double membrane (pleura) lining chest cavity and lung surface becomes inflamed, causing sharp pain on inspiration/expiration
Excludes1 pleurisy with effusion (J90)

R09.2 **Respiratory arrest** (Ex) PDX 1594
Cardiorespiratory failure
Excludes1 cardiac arrest (I46.-)
respiratory arrest of newborn (P28.81)
respiratory distress of newborn (P22.0)
respiratory failure (J96.-)
respiratory failure of newborn (P28.5)
respiratory insufficiency (R06.89)
respiratory insufficiency of newborn (P28.5)
MCC: Only if patient discharged alive

R09.3 **Abnormal sputum**
Abnormal amount of sputum
Abnormal color of sputum
Abnormal odor of sputum
Excessive sputum
Excludes1 blood-stained sputum (R04.2)

● R09.8 **Other specified symptoms and signs involving the circulatory and respiratory systems**

R09.81 **Nasal congestion**

R09.82 **Postnasal drip**

R09.89 **Other specified symptoms and signs involving the circulatory and respiratory systems**
Bruit (arterial)
Abnormal chest percussion
Friction sounds in chest
Chest tympany
Choking sensation
Rales
Wet rattling, clicking, crackling sounds on auscultation
Weak pulse
Excludes2 foreign body in throat (T17.2-)
wheezing (R06.2)
Coding Clinic: 2021, Q1, P42

● R09.A **Foreign body sensation of the circulatory and respiratory system**

R09.A0 **Foreign body sensation, unspecified**

R09.A1 **Foreign body sensation, nose**

R09.A2 **Foreign body sensation, throat**
Foreign body sensation globus

R09.A9 **Foreign body sensation, other site**

SYMPTOMS AND SIGNS INVOLVING THE DIGESTIVE SYSTEM AND ABDOMEN (R10-R19)

Excludes2 congenital or infantile pylorospasm (Q40.0)
gastrointestinal hemorrhage (K92.0-K92.2)
intestinal obstruction (K56.-)
newborn gastrointestinal hemorrhage (P54.0-P54.3)
newborn intestinal obstruction (P76.-)
pylorospasm (K31.3)
signs and symptoms involving the urinary system (R30-R39)
symptoms referable to female genital organs (N94.-)
symptoms referable to male genital organs (N48-N50)

● R10 **Abdominal and pelvic pain**
Excludes1 renal colic (N23)
Excludes2 dorsalgia (M54.-)
flatulence and related conditions (R14.-)

R10.0 **Acute abdomen**
Severe abdominal pain (generalized) (with abdominal rigidity)
Excludes1 abdominal rigidity NOS (R19.3)
generalized abdominal pain NOS (R10.84)
localized abdominal pain (R10.1-R10.3-)

● R10.1 **Pain localized to upper abdomen**

R10.10 **Upper abdominal pain, unspecified**

R10.11 **Right upper quadrant pain**

R10.12 **Left upper quadrant pain**

R10.13 **Epigastric pain**
Dyspepsia
Excludes1 functional dyspepsia (K30)

R10.2 **Pelvic and perineal pain**
Excludes1 vulvodynia (N94.81)

● R10.3 **Pain localized to other parts of lower abdomen**

R10.30 **Lower abdominal pain, unspecified**

R10.31 **Right lower quadrant pain**

R10.32 **Left lower quadrant pain**

R10.33 **Periumbilical pain**

● R10.8 **Other abdominal pain**

● R10.81 **Abdominal tenderness**
Abdominal tenderness NOS

R10.811 **Right upper quadrant abdominal tenderness**

R10.812 **Left upper quadrant abdominal tenderness**

R10.813 **Right lower quadrant abdominal tenderness**

R10.814 **Left lower quadrant abdominal tenderness**

R10.815 **Periumbilic abdominal tenderness**

R10.816 **Epigastric abdominal tenderness**

R10.817 **Generalized abdominal tenderness**

R10.819 **Abdominal tenderness, unspecified site**

● R10.82 **Rebound abdominal tenderness**

R10.821 **Right upper quadrant rebound abdominal tenderness**

R10.822 **Left upper quadrant rebound abdominal tenderness**

R10.823 **Right lower quadrant rebound abdominal tenderness**

R10.824 **Left lower quadrant rebound abdominal tenderness**

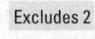

R10.825 **Periumbilic rebound abdominal tenderness**
R10.826 **Epigastric rebound abdominal tenderness**
R10.827 **Generalized rebound abdominal tenderness**
R10.829 **Rebound abdominal tenderness, unspecified site**

R10.83 **Colic** P
Colic NOS
Infantile colic
Excludes1 colic in adult and child over 12 months old (R10.84)

R10.84 **Generalized abdominal pain**
Excludes1 generalized abdominal pain associated with acute abdomen (R10.0)

R10.9 **Unspecified abdominal pain**

● R11 **Nausea and vomiting**
Excludes1 cyclical vomiting associated with migraine (G43.A-)
excessive vomiting in pregnancy (O21.-)
hematemesis (K92.0)
neonatal hematemesis (P54.0)
newborn vomiting (P92.0-)
psychogenic vomiting (F50.89)
vomiting associated with bulimia nervosa (F50.2-)
vomiting following gastrointestinal surgery (K91.0)
Coding Clinic: 2017, Q1, P27

● R11.0 **Nausea**
Nausea NOS
Nausea without vomiting

● R11.1 **Vomiting**
R11.10 **Vomiting, unspecified**
Vomiting NOS
R11.11 **Vomiting without nausea**
R11.12 **Projectile vomiting**
R11.13 **Vomiting of fecal matter**
R11.14 **Bilious vomiting**
Bilious emesis
R11.15 **Cyclical vomiting syndrome unrelated to migraine**
Cyclic vomiting syndrome NOS
Persistent vomiting
Excludes1 cyclical vomiting in migraine (G43.A-)
Excludes2 bulimia nervosa (F50.20)
diabetes mellitus due to underlying condition (E08.-)

R11.2 **Nausea with vomiting, unspecified**
Persistent nausea with vomiting NOS
Coding Clinic: 2020, Q1, P8

R12 **Heartburn**
Excludes1 dyspepsia NOS (R10.13)
functional dyspepsia (K30)

● R13 **Aphagia and dysphagia**
R13.0 **Aphagia**
Inability to swallow
Excludes1 psychogenic aphagia (F50.9)

● R13.1 **Dysphagia**
Difficulty swallowing
Code first, if applicable, dysphagia following cerebrovascular disease (I69. with final characters -91)
Excludes1 psychogenic dysphagia (F45.8)
R13.10 **Dysphagia, unspecified**
Difficulty in swallowing NOS
R13.11 **Dysphagia, oral phase**
R13.12 **Dysphagia, oropharyngeal phase**
R13.13 **Dysphagia, pharyngeal phase**
R13.14 **Dysphagia, pharyngoesophageal phase**
R13.19 **Other dysphagia**
Cervical dysphagia
Neurogenic dysphagia

● R14 **Flatulence and related conditions**
Excludes1 psychogenic aerophagy (F45.8)
R14.0 **Abdominal distension (gaseous)**
Bloating
Tympanites (abdominal) (intestinal)
R14.1 **Gas pain**
R14.2 **Eructation**
Belching air from stomach through mouth
R14.3 **Flatulence**

● R15 **Fecal incontinence**
Includes encopresis NOS
Excludes1 fecal incontinence of nonorganic origin (F98.1)
R15.0 **Incomplete defecation**
Excludes1 constipation (K59.0-)
fecal impaction (K56.41)
R15.1 **Fecal smearing**
Fecal soiling
R15.2 **Fecal urgency**
R15.9 **Full incontinence of feces**
Fecal incontinence NOS

● R16 **Hepatomegaly and splenomegaly, not elsewhere classified**
Enlargement of liver or spleen
R16.0 **Hepatomegaly, not elsewhere classified**
Hepatomegaly NOS
R16.1 **Splenomegaly, not elsewhere classified**
Splenomegaly NOS
R16.2 **Hepatomegaly with splenomegaly, not elsewhere classified**
Hepatosplenomegaly NOS

R17 **Unspecified jaundice** (Ex) PDX 1595
Excludes1 neonatal jaundice (P55, P57-P59)

● R18 **Ascites** (Ex) PDX 1596
Includes fluid in peritoneal cavity
Excludes1 ascites in alcoholic cirrhosis (K70.31)
ascites in alcoholic hepatitis (K70.11)
ascites in toxic liver disease with chronic active hepatitis (K71.51)

● R18.0 **Malignant ascites**
Code first malignancy, such as:
malignant neoplasm of ovary (C56.-)
secondary malignant neoplasm of retroperitoneum and peritoneum (C78.6)
R18.8 **Other ascites**
Ascites NOS
Peritoneal effusion (chronic)
Coding Clinic: 2018, Q1, P4

● R19 **Other symptoms and signs involving the digestive system and abdomen**
Excludes1 acute abdomen (R10.0)

● R19.0 **Intra-abdominal and pelvic swelling, mass and lump**
Excludes1 abdominal distension (gaseous) (R14.-)
ascites (R18.-)
R19.00 **Intra-abdominal and pelvic swelling, mass and lump, unspecified site**
R19.01 **Right upper quadrant abdominal swelling, mass and lump**
R19.02 **Left upper quadrant abdominal swelling, mass and lump**
R19.03 **Right lower quadrant abdominal swelling, mass and lump**
R19.04 **Left lower quadrant abdominal swelling, mass and lump**

CHAPTER 18 (R00-R99)

R19.05 **Periumbilic swelling, mass or lump**
Diffuse or generalized umbilical swelling or mass

R19.06 **Epigastric swelling, mass or lump**

R19.07 **Generalized intra-abdominal and pelvic swelling, mass and lump**
Diffuse or generalized intra-abdominal swelling or mass NOS
Diffuse or generalized pelvic swelling or mass NOS

R19.09 **Other intra-abdominal and pelvic swelling, mass and lump**

● R19.1 **Abnormal bowel sounds**

R19.11 **Absent bowel sounds**

R19.12 **Hyperactive bowel sounds**

R19.15 **Other abnormal bowel sounds**
Abnormal bowel sounds NOS

R19.2 **Visible peristalsis**
Hyperperistalsis

● R19.3 **Abdominal rigidity**
Excludes1 abdominal rigidity with severe abdominal pain (R10.0)

R19.30 **Abdominal rigidity, unspecified site**

R19.31 **Right upper quadrant abdominal rigidity**

R19.32 **Left upper quadrant abdominal rigidity**

R19.33 **Right lower quadrant abdominal rigidity**

R19.34 **Left lower quadrant abdominal rigidity**

R19.35 **Periumbilic abdominal rigidity**

R19.36 **Epigastric abdominal rigidity**

R19.37 **Generalized abdominal rigidity**

R19.4 **Change in bowel habit**
Excludes1 constipation (K59.0-)
functional diarrhea (K59.1)

R19.5 **Other fecal abnormalities**
Abnormal stool color
Bulky stools
Mucus in stools
Occult blood in feces
Occult blood in stools
Excludes1 melena (K92.1)
neonatal melena (P54.1)
Coding Clinic: 2021, Q1, P10; 2019, Q1, P32

R19.6 **Halitosis**

R19.7 **Diarrhea, unspecified**
Diarrhea NOS
Excludes1 functional diarrhea (K59.1)
neonatal diarrhea (P78.3)
psychogenic diarrhea (F45.8)
Coding Clinic: 2021, Q3, P4

R19.8 **Other specified symptoms and signs involving the digestive system and abdomen**

SYMPTOMS AND SIGNS INVOLVING THE SKIN AND SUBCUTANEOUS TISSUE (R20-R23)

Excludes2 symptoms relating to breast (N64.4-N64.5)

● R20 **Disturbances of skin sensation**
Excludes1 dissociative anesthesia and sensory loss (F44.6)
psychogenic disturbances (F45.8)

R20.0 **Anesthesia of skin**
Loss of sensation

R20.1 **Hypoesthesia of skin**
Unpleasant abnormal sensation

R20.2 **Paresthesia of skin**
Abnormal touch sensation, including burning, prickling, often in absence of external stimulus
Formication   Tingling skin
Pins and needles
Excludes1 acroparesthesia (I73.8)

R20.3 **Hyperesthesia**

R20.8 **Other disturbances of skin sensation**

R20.9 **Unspecified disturbances of skin sensation**

R21 **Rash and other nonspecific skin eruption**
Includes rash NOS
Excludes1 specified type of rash- code to condition
vesicular eruption (R23.8)

● R22 **Localized swelling, mass and lump of skin and subcutaneous tissue**
Includes subcutaneous nodules (localized) (superficial)
Excludes1 abnormal findings on diagnostic imaging (R90-R93)
edema (R60.-)
enlarged lymph nodes (R59.-)
localized adiposity (E65)
swelling of joint (M25.4-)

R22.0 **Localized swelling, mass and lump, head**

R22.1 **Localized swelling, mass and lump, neck**

R22.2 **Localized swelling, mass and lump, trunk**
Excludes1 intra-abdominal or pelvic mass and lump (R19.0-)
intra-abdominal or pelvic swelling (R19.0-)
Excludes2 breast mass and lump (N63)
Coding Clinic: 2022, Q3, P8

● R22.3 **Localized swelling, mass and lump, upper limb**

R22.30 **Localized swelling, mass and lump, unspecified upper limb**

R22.31 **Localized swelling, mass and lump, right upper limb**

R22.32 **Localized swelling, mass and lump, left upper limb**

R22.33 **Localized swelling, mass and lump, upper limb, bilateral**

● R22.4 **Localized swelling, mass and lump, lower limb**

R22.40 **Localized swelling, mass and lump, unspecified lower limb**

R22.41 **Localized swelling, mass and lump, right lower limb**

R22.42 **Localized swelling, mass and lump, left lower limb**

R22.43 **Localized swelling, mass and lump, lower limb, bilateral**

R22.9 **Localized swelling, mass and lump, unspecified**

● R23 **Other skin changes**

R23.0 **Cyanosis**
Excludes1 acrocyanosis (I73.8)
cyanotic attacks of newborn (P28.2)

R23.1 **Pallor**
Clammy skin

R23.2 **Flushing**
Excessive blushing
Code first, if applicable, menopausal and female climacteric states (N95.1)

R23.3 **Spontaneous ecchymoses**
Small hemorrhagic spot of skin; AKA black and blue spot
Petechiae
Excludes1 ecchymoses of newborn (P54.5)
purpura (D69.-)

R23.4 **Changes in skin texture**
Desquamation of skin   Scaling of skin
Induration of skin
Excludes1 epidermal thickening NOS (L85.9)

R23.8 **Other skin changes**

R23.9 **Unspecified skin changes**

▶ New ➡ Revised ~~deleted~~ Deleted | Excludes 1 | Excludes 2 | Includes | Use additional | Code first | Code also | Key words
OGCR Official Guidelines ● Unacceptable Principal Diagnosis X Assign placeholder X ● Use Additional Character(s) ◗ Manifestation Code Coding Clinic

SYMPTOMS AND SIGNS INVOLVING THE NERVOUS AND MUSCULOSKELETAL SYSTEMS (R25-R29)

● **R25 Abnormal involuntary movements**
Excludes1 specific movement disorders (G20-G26)
stereotyped movement disorders (F98.4)
tic disorders (F95.-)

R25.Ø Abnormal head movements
R25.1 Tremor, unspecified
Excludes1 chorea NOS (G25.5)
essential tremor (G25.Ø)
hysterical tremor (F44.4)
intention tremor (G25.2)

R25.2 Cramp and spasm
Excludes2 carpopedal spasm (R29.Ø)
charley-horse (M62.831)
infantile spasms (G4Ø.4-)
muscle spasm of back (M62.83Ø)
muscle spasm of calf (M62.831)

R25.3 Fasciculation
Twitching NOS

R25.8 Other abnormal involuntary movements
R25.9 Unspecified abnormal involuntary movements

● **R26 Abnormalities of gait and mobility**
Excludes1 ataxia NOS (R27.Ø)
hereditary ataxia (G11.-)
locomotor (syphilitic) ataxia (A52.11)
immobility syndrome (paraplegic) (M62.3)

R26.Ø Ataxic gait
Staggering gait
Coding Clinic: 2Ø22, Q2, P12

R26.1 Paralytic gait
Spastic gait

R26.2 Difficulty in walking, not elsewhere classified
Excludes1 falling (R29.6)
unsteadiness on feet (R26.81)
Coding Clinic: 2Ø16, Q2, P7

● **R26.8 Other abnormalities of gait and mobility**
R26.81 Unsteadiness on feet
R26.89 Other abnormalities of gait and mobility

R26.9 Unspecified abnormalities of gait and mobility

● **R27 Other lack of coordination**
Excludes1 ataxic gait (R26.Ø)
hereditary ataxia (G11.-)
vertigo NOS (R42)

R27.Ø Ataxia, unspecified
Excludes1 ataxia following cerebrovascular disease (I69. with final characters -93)
Coding Clinic: 2Ø22, Q3, P1Ø

R27.8 Other lack of coordination
R27.9 Unspecified lack of coordination

● **R29 Other symptoms and signs involving the nervous and musculoskeletal systems**

R29.Ø Tetany (Ex) PDX 6194
Hyperexcitability of nerves and muscles characterized by spasm, twitching, and cramps
Carpopedal spasm
Excludes1 hysterical tetany (F44.5)
neonatal tetany (P71.3)
parathyroid tetany (E2Ø.9)
post-thyroidectomy tetany (E89.2)

R29.1 Meningismus (Ex) PDX 1598

R29.2 Abnormal reflex
Excludes2 abnormal pupillary reflex (H57.Ø)
hyperactive gag reflex (J39.2)
vasovagal reaction or syncope (R55)

R29.3 Abnormal posture

R29.4 Clicking hip
Excludes1 congenital deformities of hip (Q65.-)

R29.5 Transient paralysis (Ex) PDX 1599
Code first any associated spinal cord injury (S14.Ø, S14.1-, S24.Ø, S24.1-, S34.Ø-, S34.1-)
Excludes1 transient ischemic attack (G45.9)

R29.6 Repeated falls
Falling
Tendency to fall
Excludes2 at risk for falling (Z91.81)
history of falling (Z91.81)

OGCR Section I.C.18.d.

Repeated falls

Code R29.6, Repeated falls, is for use for encounters when a patient has recently fallen and the reason for the fall is being investigated.

Code Z91.81, History of falling, is for use when a patient has fallen in the past and is at risk for future falls.When appropriate, both codes R29.6 and Z91.81 may be assigned together.

Coding Clinic: 2Ø16, Q2, P7

● **R29.7 National Institutes of Health Stroke Scale (NIHSS) score**
Code first the type of cerebral infarction (I63.-)
Coding Clinic: 2Ø16, Q4, P61, 127

● **R29.7Ø NIHSS score Ø-9**
● **R29.7ØØ NIHSS score Ø**
● **R29.7Ø1 NIHSS score 1**
● **R29.7Ø2 NIHSS score 2**
● **R29.7Ø3 NIHSS score 3**
● **R29.7Ø4 NIHSS score 4**
● **R29.7Ø5 NIHSS score 5**
● **R29.7Ø6 NIHSS score 6**
● **R29.7Ø7 NIHSS score 7**
● **R29.7Ø8 NIHSS score 8**
● **R29.7Ø9 NIHSS score 9**

● **R29.71 NIHSS score 1Ø-19**
● **R29.71Ø NIHSS score 1Ø**
● **R29.711 NIHSS score 11**
● **R29.712 NIHSS score 12**
● **R29.713 NIHSS score 13**
● **R29.714 NIHSS score 14**
● **R29.715 NIHSS score 15**
● **R29.716 NIHSS score 16**
● **R29.717 NIHSS score 17**
● **R29.718 NIHSS score 18**
● **R29.719 NIHSS score 19**

● **R29.72 NIHSS score 2Ø-29**
● **R29.72Ø NIHSS score 2Ø**
● **R29.721 NIHSS score 21**
● **R29.722 NIHSS score 22**
● **R29.723 NIHSS score 23**
● **R29.724 NIHSS score 24**
● **R29.725 NIHSS score 25**
● **R29.726 NIHSS score 26**
● **R29.727 NIHSS score 27**
● **R29.728 NIHSS score 28**
● **R29.729 NIHSS score 29**

OGCR Section I.C.18.i.

NIHSS Stroke Scale

The NIH stroke scale (NIHSS) codes (R29.7- -) can be used in conjunction with acute stroke codes (I63) to identify the patient's neurological status and the severity of the stroke. The stroke scale codes should be sequenced after the acute stroke diagnosis code(s).

At a minimum, report the initial score documented. If desired, a facility may choose to capture multiple stroke scale scores.

CHAPTER 18 (RØØ-R99)

● R29.73 NIHSS score 30-39
- ● R29.730 NIHSS score 30
  Coding Clinic: 2016, Q4, P62
- ● R29.731 NIHSS score 31
- ● R29.732 NIHSS score 32
- ● R29.733 NIHSS score 33
- ● R29.734 NIHSS score 34
- ● R29.735 NIHSS score 35
- ● R29.736 NIHSS score 36
- ● R29.737 NIHSS score 37
- ● R29.738 NIHSS score 38
- ● R29.739 NIHSS score 39

● R29.74 NIHSS score 40-42
- ● R29.740 NIHSS score 40
- ● R29.741 NIHSS score 41
- ● R29.742 NIHSS score 42

● R29.8 Other symptoms and signs involving the nervous and musculoskeletal systems

● R29.81 Other symptoms and signs involving the nervous system

R29.810 Facial weakness
Facial droop
Excludes1 Bell's palsy (G51.0)
facial weakness following cerebrovascular disease (I69. with final characters -92)
Coding Clinic: 2022, Q3, P9

R29.818 Other symptoms and signs involving the nervous system

● R29.89 Other symptoms and signs involving the musculoskeletal system
Excludes2 pain in limb (M79.6-)

R29.890 Loss of height
Excludes1 osteoporosis (M80-M81)

R29.891 Ocular torticollis
Excludes1 congenital (sternomastoid) torticollis Q68.0
psychogenic torticollis (F45.8)
spasmodic torticollis (G24.3)
torticollis due to birth injury (P15.8)
torticollis NOS M43.6

R29.898 Other symptoms and signs involving the musculoskeletal system

● R29.9 Unspecified symptoms and signs involving the nervous and musculoskeletal systems

R29.90 Unspecified symptoms and signs involving the nervous system

R29.91 Unspecified symptoms and signs involving the musculoskeletal system

SYMPTOMS AND SIGNS INVOLVING THE GENITOURINARY SYSTEM (R30-R39)

● R30 Pain associated with micturition
Excludes1 psychogenic pain associated with micturition (F45.8)

R30.0 Dysuria
Painful urination
Strangury

R30.1 Vesical tenesmus
Straining to urinate, with sensation of a full bladder even when empty

R30.9 Painful micturition, unspecified
Painful urination NOS

● R31 Hematuria
Excludes1 hematuria included with underlying conditions, such as:
acute cystitis with hematuria (N30.01)
recurrent and persistent hematuria in glomerular diseases (N02.-)

R31.0 Gross hematuria
Coding Clinic: 2017, Q1, P17

R31.1 Benign essential microscopic hematuria

● R31.2 Other microscopic hematuria
Coding Clinic: 2016, Q4, P62

R31.21 Asymptomatic microscopic hematuria
AMH

R31.29 Other microscopic hematuria

R31.9 Hematuria, unspecified
Coding Clinic: 2017, Q1, P6

R32 Unspecified urinary incontinence
Enuresis NOS
Excludes1 functional urinary incontinence (R39.81)
nonorganic enuresis (F98.0)
stress incontinence and other specified urinary incontinence (N39.3-N39.4-)
urinary incontinence associated with cognitive impairment (R39.81)
Coding Clinic: 2021, Q4, P18

● R33 Retention of urine
Excludes1 psychogenic retention of urine (F45.8)

R33.0 Drug induced retention of urine
Use additional code for adverse effect, if applicable, to identify drug (T36-T50 with fifth or sixth character 5)

R33.8 Other retention of urine
Code first, if applicable, any causal condition, such as:
enlarged prostate (N40.1)
Coding Clinic: 2018, Q4, P55

R33.9 Retention of urine, unspecified

R34 Anuria and oliguria
Excludes1 anuria and oliguria complicating abortion or ectopic or molar pregnancy (O00-O07, O08.4)
anuria and oliguria complicating pregnancy (O26.83-)
anuria and oliguria complicating the puerperium (O90.49)

● R35 Polyuria
Passage of excessive volume of urine
Code first, if applicable, any causal condition, such as:
enlarged prostate (N40.1)
Excludes1 psychogenic polyuria (F45.8)

R35.0 Frequency of micturition
Discharge or passage of urine; AKA uresis

R35.1 Nocturia
Urinary frequency at night

● R35.8 Other polyuria

R35.81 Nocturnal polyuria
Excludes2 nocturnal enuresis (N39.44)

R35.89 Other polyuria
Polyuria NOS

● R36 Urethral discharge

R36.0 Urethral discharge without blood

R36.1 Hematospermia
Presence of blood in semen

R36.9 Urethral discharge, unspecified
Penile discharge NOS
Urethrorrhea

R37 Sexual dysfunction, unspecified

CHAPTER 18 (R00-R99)

● **R39 Other and unspecified symptoms and signs involving the genitourinary system**

R39.0 Extravasation of urine (Ex) PDX 1600
Leakage, discharge

● **R39.1 Other difficulties with micturition**
Code first, if applicable, any causal condition, such as:
enlarged prostate (N40.1)

R39.11 Hesitancy of micturition

R39.12 Poor urinary stream
Weak urinary steam

R39.13 Splitting of urinary stream

R39.14 Feeling of incomplete bladder emptying

R39.15 Urgency of urination
Excludes1 urge incontinence (N39.41, N39.46)

R39.16 Straining to void

● **R39.19 Other difficulties with micturition**
Coding Clinic: 2016, Q4, P63

R39.191 Need to immediately re-void

R39.192 Position dependent micturition

R39.198 Other difficulties with micturition

R39.2 Extrarenal uremia
Prerenal uremia
Excludes1 uremia NOS (N19)

● **R39.8 Other symptoms and signs involving the genitourinary system**

R39.81 Functional urinary incontinence
Urinary incontinence due to cognitive impairment, or severe physical disability or immobility
Excludes1 stress incontinence and other specified urinary incontinence (N39.3-N39.4-)
urinary incontinence NOS (R32)

R39.82 Chronic bladder pain
Coding Clinic: 2016, Q4, P64

R39.83 Unilateral non-palpable testicle

R39.84 Bilateral non-palpable testicles

R39.89 Other symptoms and signs involving the genitourinary system
Coding Clinic: 2016, Q4, P64

R39.9 Unspecified symptoms and signs involving the genitourinary system

SYMPTOMS AND SIGNS INVOLVING COGNITION, PERCEPTION, EMOTIONAL STATE AND BEHAVIOR (R40-R46)

Excludes2 symptoms and signs constituting part of a pattern of mental disorder (F01-F99)
Coding Clinic: 2015, Q4, P40

● **R40 Somnolence, stupor and coma** (Ex) PDX 575
Excludes1 neonatal coma (P91.5)
somnolence, stupor and coma in diabetes (E08-E13)
somnolence, stupor and coma in hepatic failure (K72.-)
somnolence, stupor and coma in hypoglycemia (nondiabetic) (E15)

R40.0 Somnolence
Drowsiness
Excludes1 coma (R40.2-)

R40.1 Stupor
Lowered level of consciousness
Catatonic stupor
Semicoma
Excludes1 catatonic schizophrenia (F20.2)
coma (R40.2-)
depressive stupor (F31-F33)
dissociative stupor (F44.2)
manic stupor (F30.2)

OGCR Section I.C.18.e.

Coma scale

The coma scale codes (R40.2-) can be used in conjunction with traumatic brain injury codes, acute cerebrovascular disease or sequelae of cerebrovascular disease codes. These codes are primarily for use by trauma registries, but they may be used in any setting where this information is collected. The coma scale may also be used to assess the status of the central nervous system for other non-trauma conditions, such as monitoring patients in the intensive care unit regardless of medical condition. The coma scale codes should be sequenced after the diagnosis code(s).

These codes, one from each subcategory, are needed to complete the scale. The 7th character indicates when the scale was recorded. The 7th character should match for all three codes.

At a minimum, report the initial score documented on presentation at your facility. This may be a score from the emergency medicine technician (EMT) or in the emergency department. If desired, a facility may choose to capture multiple coma scale scores.

Assign code R40.24, Glasgow coma scale, total score, when only the total score is documented in the medical record and not the individual score(s).

● **R40.2 Coma**
Code first any associated:
fracture of skull (S02.-)
intracranial injury (S06.-)

Note: One code from each subcategory R40.21-R40-23 is required to complete the coma scale
Coding Clinic: 2021, Q4, P112; 2016, Q4, P127

● **R40.20 Unspecified coma**
Coma NOS
Unconsciousness NOS
Coding Clinic: 2021, Q4, P112

● **R40.21 Coma scale, eyes open**
The following appropriate 7th character is to be added to subcategory R40.21-:

0 unspecified time
1 in the field [EMT or ambulance]
2 at arrival to emergency department
3 at hospital admission
4 24 hours or more after hospital admission

Coding Clinic: 2021, Q4, P112; 2017, Q4, P25; 2015, Q2, P18

●● **R40.211 Coma scale, eyes open, never**
Coma scale eye opening score of 1

●● **R40.212 Coma scale, eyes open, to pain**
Coma scale eye opening score of 2

●● **R40.213 Coma scale, eyes open, to sound**
Coma scale eye opening score of 3

●● **R40.214 Coma scale, eyes open, spontaneous**
Coma scale eye opening score of 4

● **R40.22 Coma scale, best verbal response**
The following appropriate 7th character is to be added to subcategory R40.22-:

0 unspecified time
1 in the field [EMT or ambulance]
2 at arrival to emergency department
3 at hospital admission
4 24 hours or more after hospital admission

Coding Clinic: 2021, Q4, P112; 2017, Q4, P25; 2015, Q2, P18

●● **R40.221 Coma scale, best verbal response, none**
Coma scale verbal score of 1

●● **R40.222 Coma scale, best verbal response, incomprehensible words**
Coma scale verbal score of 2
Incomprehensible sounds (2-5 years of age)
Moans/grunts to pain; restless (< 2 years old)

R40.223 Coma scale, best verbal response, **inappropriate words**
Coma scale verbal score of 3
Inappropriate crying or screaming (< 2 years of age)
Screaming (2-5 years of age)

R40.224 Coma scale, best verbal response, **confused conversation**
Coma scale verbal score of 4
Inappropriate words (2-5 years of age)
Irritable cries (< 2 years of age)

R40.225 Coma scale, best verbal response, **oriented**
Coma scale verbal score of 5
Cooing or babbling or crying appropriately (< 2 years of age)
Uses appropriate words (2- 5 years of age)

R40.23 Coma scale, best motor response
The following appropriate 7th character is to be added to subcategory R40.23-:

0	unspecified time
1	in the field [EMT or ambulance]
2	at arrival to emergency department
3	at hospital admission
4	24 hours or more after hospital admission

Coding Clinic: 2017, Q4, P25; 2015, Q2, P18

R40.231 Coma scale, best motor response, **none**
Coma scale motor score of 1

Glasgow Coma Scale

Eye Opening Response	
• Spontaneous--open with blinking at baseline	4 points
• To verbal stimuli, command, speech	3 points
• To pain only (not applied to face)	2 points
• No response	1 point
Verbal Response	
• Oriented	5 points
• Confused conversation, but able to answer questions	4 points
• Inappropriate words	3 points
• Incomprehensible speech	2 points
• No response	1 point
Motor Response	
• Obeys commands for movement	6 points
• Purposeful movement to painful stimulus	5 points
• Withdraws in response to pain	4 points
• Flexion in response to pain (decorticate posturing)	3 points
• Extension response in response to pain (decerebrate posturing)	2 points
• No response	1 point
Categorization: Coma: No eye opening, no ability to follow commands, no word verbalizations (3-8)	
Head Injury Classification: Severe Head Injury--GCS score of 8 or less; Moderate Head Injury--GCS score of 9 to 12; Mild head injury--GCS score of 13 to 15	
(Adapted from: Advanced Trauma Life Support: Course for Physicians, American College of Surgeons, 1993). http://www.bt.cdc.gov/masscasulatires/gscale.asp	

Figure 18-1

R40.232 Coma scale, best motor response, **extension**
Abnormal extensor posturing to pain or noxious stimuli (< 2 years of age)
Coma scale motor score of 2
Extensor posturing to pain or noxious stimuli (2-5 years of age)

R40.233 Coma scale, best motor response, **abnormal flexion**
Coma scale motor score of 3
Abnormal flexure posturing to pain or noxious stimuli (2-5 years of age)
Flexion/decorticate posturing (< 2 years of age)

R40.234 Coma scale, best motor response, **flexion withdrawal**
Coma scale motor score of 4
Withdraws from pain or noxious stimuli (2-5 years of age)

R40.235 Coma scale, best motor response, **localizes pain**
Coma scale motor score of 5
Localizes pain (2-5 years of age)
Withdraws to touch (< 2 years of age)

R40.236 Coma scale, best motor response, **obeys commands**
Coma scale motor score of 6
Normal or spontaneous movement (< 2 years of age)
Obeys commands (2-5 years of age)

R40.24 Glasgow coma scale, total score
Note: Assign a code from subcategory R40.24, when only the total coma score is documented
The following appropriate 7th character is to be added to subcategory R40.24-:

0	unspecified time
1	in the field [EMT or ambulance]
2	at arrival to emergency department
3	at hospital admission
4	24 hours or more after hospital admission

Coding Clinic: 2016, Q4, P64; 2015, Q2, P18

R40.241 Glasgow coma scale score **13-15**
R40.242 Glasgow coma scale score **9-12**
R40.243 Glasgow coma scale score **3-8**
R40.244 **Other** coma, without documented Glasgow coma scale score, or with partial score reported

R40.2A Nontraumatic coma due to underlying condition
Secondary coma
Code first underlying condition
Coding Clinic: 2023, Q4, P42

R40.3 Persistent vegetative state
R40.4 Transient alteration of awareness

R41 Other symptoms and signs involving cognitive functions and awareness
Excludes1 dissociative [conversion] disorders (F44.-)
mild cognitive impairment, of uncertain or unknown etiology (G31.84)

R41.0 Disorientation, **unspecified**
Confusion NOS
Delirium NOS
Excludes1 delirium due to known physiological condition (F05)
Coding Clinic: 2022, Q2, P11; 2019, Q2, P34; 2016, Q4, P71

R41.1 **Anterograde** amnesia
R41.2 **Retrograde** amnesia

R41.3 Other amnesia
Amnesia NOS
Memory loss NOS
Excludes1 amnestic disorder due to known physiologic condition (F04)
amnestic syndrome due to psychoactive substance use (F10-F19 with 5th character .6)
mild memory disturbance due to known physiological condition (F06.8)
transient global amnesia (G45.4)

R41.4 Neurologic neglect syndrome (Ex) PDX 1601
Asomatognosia
Hemi-akinesia
Hemi-inattention
Hemispatial neglect
Left-sided neglect
Sensory neglect
Visuospatial neglect
Excludes1 visuospatial deficit (R41.842)

● **R41.8 Other symptoms and signs involving cognitive functions and awareness**

R41.81 Age-related cognitive decline A
Senility NOS

R41.82 Altered mental status, unspecified
Change in mental status NOS
Excludes1 altered level of consciousness (R40.-)
altered mental status due to known condition - code to condition
delirium NOS (R41.0)
Coding Clinic: 2012, Q4, P98

● **R41.83 Borderline intellectual functioning**
IQ level 71 to 84
Excludes1 intellectual disabilities (F70-F79)

● **R41.84 Other specified cognitive deficit**
▶ *Code first the underlying condition, if known, such as:*
▶ schizophrenia (F20.-)
Excludes1 cognitive deficits as sequelae of cerebrovascular disease (I69.01-, I69.11-, I69.21-, I69.31-, I69.81-, I69.91-)

R41.840 Attention and concentration deficit
Excludes1 attention-deficit hyperactivity disorders (F90.-)

R41.841 Cognitive communication deficit
R41.842 Visuospatial deficit
R41.843 Psychomotor deficit
R41.844 Frontal lobe and executive function deficit

▶ **R41.85 Anosognosia**

R41.89 Other symptoms and signs involving cognitive functions and awareness
~~Anosognosia~~

R41.9 Unspecified symptoms and signs involving cognitive functions and awareness
Unspecified neurocognitive disorder

R42 Dizziness and giddiness
Light-headedness
Vertigo NOS
Excludes1 vertiginous syndromes (H81.-)
vertigo from infrasound (T75.23)
Coding Clinic: 2015, Q4, P40

● **R43 Disturbances of smell and taste**

R43.0 Anosmia
Absence of sense of smell; AKA anosphresia and olfactory anesthesia

R43.1 Parosmia

R43.2 Parageusia
Perversion of sense of taste or bad taste in mouth; AKA dysgeusia

R43.8 Other disturbances of smell and taste
Mixed disturbance of smell and taste

R43.9 Unspecified disturbances of smell and taste

● **R44 Other symptoms and signs involving general sensations and perceptions**
Excludes1 alcoholic hallucinations (F10.151, F10.251, F10.951)
hallucinations in drug psychosis (F11-F19 with fifth to sixth characters 51)
hallucinations in mood disorders with psychotic symptoms (F30.2, F31.5, F32.3, F33.3)
hallucinations in schizophrenia, schizotypal and delusional disorders (F20-F29)
Excludes2 disturbances of skin sensation (R20.-)

R44.0 Auditory hallucinations (Ex) PDX 1602
R44.1 Visual hallucinations
R44.2 Other hallucinations (Ex) PDX 1602
R44.3 Hallucinations, unspecified (Ex) PDX 1602
Coding Clinic: 2022, Q2, P11
R44.8 Other symptoms and signs involving general sensations and perceptions
R44.9 Unspecified symptoms and signs involving general sensations and perceptions

● **R45 Symptoms and signs involving emotional state**

R45.0 Nervousness
Nervous tension
R45.1 Restlessness and agitation
R45.2 Unhappiness
R45.3 Demoralization and apathy
Excludes1 anhedonia (R45.84)
R45.4 Irritability and anger
R45.5 Hostility
R45.6 Violent behavior
R45.7 State of emotional shock and stress, unspecified

● **R45.8 Other symptoms involving emotional state**

R45.81 Low self-esteem
R45.82 Worries
R45.83 Excessive crying of child, adolescent or adult
Excludes1 excessive crying of infant (baby) R68.11
R45.84 Anhedonia
Total loss of feeling of pleasure in pleasurable acts

● **R45.85 Homicidal and suicidal ideations**
Excludes1 suicide attempt (T14.91)
● **R45.850 Homicidal ideations**
R45.851 Suicidal ideations (Ex) PDX 642
Coding Clinic: 2022, Q1, P29

R45.86 Emotional lability
R45.87 Impulsiveness
R45.88 Nonsuicidal self-harm
Nonsuicidal self-injury
Nonsuicidal self-mutilation
Self-inflicted injury without suicidal intent
Code also injury, if known
Coding Clinic: 2021, Q4, P27

R45.89 Other symptoms and signs involving emotional state
Flat affect
Loneliness

R46 Symptoms and signs involving appearance and behavior

Excludes1 appearance and behavior in schizophrenia, schizotypal and delusional disorders (F20-F29)
mental and behavioral disorders (F01-F99)

R46.0 Very low level of personal hygiene

R46.1 Bizarre personal appearance

R46.2 Strange and inexplicable behavior

R46.3 Overactivity

R46.4 Slowness and poor responsiveness

Excludes1 stupor (R40.1)

R46.5 Suspiciousness and marked evasiveness

R46.6 Undue concern and preoccupation with stressful events

R46.7 Verbosity and circumstantial detail obscuring reason for contact

R46.8 Other symptoms and signs involving appearance and behavior

R46.81 Obsessive-compulsive behavior

Excludes1 obsessive-compulsive disorder (F42.-)

R46.89 Other symptoms and signs involving appearance and behavior

SYMPTOMS AND SIGNS INVOLVING SPEECH AND VOICE (R47-R49)

R47 Speech disturbances, not elsewhere classified

Excludes1 autism (F84.0)
cluttering (F80.81)
specific developmental disorders of speech and language (F80.-)
stuttering (F80.81)

R47.0 Dysphasia and aphasia

R47.01 Aphasia (Ex: PDX 1603

Excludes1 aphasia following cerebrovascular disease (I69. with final characters -20)
progressive isolated aphasia (G31.01)

Coding Clinic: 2022, Q3, P9

R47.02 Dysphasia

Impairment in comprehension of speech, caused by left-sided brain damage

Excludes1 dysphasia following cerebrovascular disease (I69. with final characters -21)

R47.1 Dysarthria and anarthria

Motor speech disorder

Excludes1 dysarthria following cerebrovascular disease (I69. with final characters -22)

Coding Clinic: 2022, Q3, P9

R47.8 Other speech disturbances

Excludes1 dysarthria following cerebrovascular disease (I69. with final characters -28)

R47.81 Slurred speech

R47.82 Fluency disorder in conditions classified elsewhere

Stuttering in conditions classified elsewhere

Code first underlying disease or condition, such as:
Parkinson's disease (G20.-)

Excludes1 adult onset fluency disorder (F98.5)
childhood onset fluency disorder (F80.81)
fluency disorder (stuttering) following cerebrovascular disease (I69. with final characters -23)

R47.89 Other speech disturbances

R47.9 Unspecified speech disturbances

R48 Dyslexia and other symbolic dysfunctions, not elsewhere classified

Excludes1 specific developmental disorders of scholastic skills (F81.-)

R48.0 Dyslexia and alexia

R48.1 Agnosia

Loss of ability to recognize objects, persons, sounds, shapes, or smells

Astereognosia (astereognosis)
Autotopagnosia

Excludes1 visual object agnosia (R48.3)

R48.2 Apraxia

Loss of ability to execute or carry out learned purposeful movements

Excludes1 apraxia following cerebrovascular disease (I69. with final characters -90)

R48.3 Visual agnosia

Prosopagnosia
Simultanagnosia (asimultagnosia)

R48.8 Other symbolic dysfunctions

Acalculia

Difficulty performing simple mathematical tasks resulting from neurological injury

Agraphia

Coding Clinic: 2017, Q1, P27

R48.9 Unspecified symbolic dysfunctions

R49 Voice and resonance disorders

Excludes1 psychogenic voice and resonance disorders (F44.4)

R49.0 Dysphonia

Hoarseness

R49.1 Aphonia

Loss of voice

R49.2 Hypernasality and hyponasality

R49.21 Hypernasality

R49.22 Hyponasality

R49.8 Other voice and resonance disorders

R49.9 Unspecified voice and resonance disorder

Change in voice NOS
Resonance disorder NOS

GENERAL SYMPTOMS AND SIGNS (R50-R69)

R50 Fever of other and unknown origin

Excludes1 chills without fever (R68.83)
febrile convulsions (R56.0-)
fever of unknown origin during labor (O75.2)
fever of unknown origin in newborn (P81.9)
hypothermia due to illness (R68.0)
malignant hyperthermia due to anesthesia (T88.3)
puerperal pyrexia NOS (O86.4)

R50.2 Drug induced fever

Use additional code for adverse effect, if applicable, to identify drug (T36-T50 with fifth or sixth character 5)

Excludes1 postvaccination (postimmunization) fever (R50.83)

R50.8 Other specified fever

R50.81 Fever presenting with conditions classified elsewhere

Code first underlying condition when associated fever is present, such as with:
leukemia (C91-C95)
neutropenia (D70.-)
sickle-cell disease (D57.-)

Coding Clinic: 2023, Q4, P7; 2019, Q2, P25

R50.82 Postprocedural fever

Excludes1 postprocedural infection (T81.44)
posttransfusion fever (R50.84)
postvaccination (postimmunization) fever (R50.83)

R50.83 Postvaccination fever
Postimmunization fever

R50.84 Febrile nonhemolytic transfusion reaction
FNHTR
Posttransfusion fever

R50.9 Fever, unspecified
Fever NOS
Fever of unknown origin [FUO]
Fever with chills
Fever with rigors
Hyperpyrexia NOS
Persistent fever
Pyrexia NOS

● R51 Headache
Excludes2 atypical face pain (G50.1)
migraine and other headache syndromes (G43-G44)
trigeminal neuralgia (G50.0)

R51.0 Headache with orthostatic component, not elsewhere classified
Headache with positional component, not elsewhere classified

R51.9 Headache, unspecified
Facial pain NOS

R52 Pain, unspecified
Acute pain NOS
Generalized pain NOS
Excludes1 acute and chronic pain, not elsewhere classified (G89.-)
localized pain, unspecified type - code to pain by site, such as:
abdomen pain (R10.-)
back pain (M54.9)
breast pain (N64.4)
chest pain (R07.1-R07.9)
ear pain (H92.0-)
eye pain (H57.1)
headache (R51.9)
joint pain (M25.5-)
limb pain (M79.6-)
lumbar region pain (M54.5-)
pelvic and perineal pain (R10.2)
shoulder pain (M25.51-)
spine pain (M54.-)
throat pain (R07.0)
tongue pain (K14.6)
tooth pain (K08.8)
renal colic (N23)
pain disorders exclusively related to psychological factors (F45.41)

● R53 Malaise and fatigue

R53.0 Neoplastic (malignant) related fatigue
Code first associated neoplasm

R53.1 Weakness
Asthenia NOS
Excludes1 age-related weakness (R54)
muscle weakness (generalized) (M62.81)
sarcopenia (M62.84)
senile asthenia (R54)
Coding Clinic: 2021, Q4, P103; 2017, Q1, P7

R53.2 Functional quadriplegia (Ex) PDX 759
Complete immobility due to severe physical disability or frailty
Excludes1 frailty NOS (R54)
hysterical paralysis (F44.4)
immobility syndrome (M62.3)
neurologic quadriplegia (G82.5-)
quadriplegia (G82.50)
Coding Clinic: 2022, Q4, P15; 2016, Q2, P6

● R53.8 Other malaise and fatigue
Excludes1 combat exhaustion and fatigue (F43.0)
congenital debility (P96.9)
exhaustion and fatigue due to excessive exertion (T73.3)
exhaustion and fatigue due to exposure (T73.2)
exhaustion and fatigue due to heat (T67.-)
exhaustion and fatigue due to pregnancy (O26.8-)
exhaustion and fatigue due to recurrent depressive episode (F33)
exhaustion and fatigue due to senile debility (R54)

R53.81 Other malaise
Chronic debility
Debility NOS
General physical deterioration
Malaise NOS
Nervous debility
Excludes1 age-related physical debility (R54)
Coding Clinic: 2021, Q1, P43

R53.82 Chronic fatigue, unspecified
Excludes1 chronic fatigue syndrome (G93.32)
myalgic encephalomyelitis (G93.32)
other post infection and related fatigue syndromes (G93.39)
postviral fatigue syndrome (G93.31)

R53.83 Other fatigue
Fatigue NOS
Lack of energy
Lethargy
Tiredness
Excludes2 exhaustion and fatigue due to depressive episode (F32.-)
Coding Clinic: 2017, Q1, P7

R54 Age-related physical debility A
Frailty
Old age
Senescence
Senile asthenia
Senile debility
Excludes1 age-related cognitive decline (R41.81)
sarcopenia (M62.84)
senile psychosis (F03.-)
senility NOS (R41.81)

R55 Syncope and collapse
Blackout
Fainting
Vasovagal attack
Excludes1 cardiogenic shock (R57.0)
carotid sinus syncope (G90.01)
heat syncope (T67.1)
neurocirculatory asthenia (F45.8)
neurogenic orthostatic hypotension (G90.3)
orthostatic hypotension (I95.1)
postprocedural shock (T81.1-)
psychogenic syncope (F48.8)
shock NOS (R57.9)
shock complicating or following abortion or ectopic or molar pregnancy (O00-O07, O08.3)
shock complicating or following labor and delivery (O75.1)
Stokes-Adams attack (I45.9)
unconsciousness NOS (R40.2-)

CHAPTER 18 (R00-R99)

R56 Convulsions, not elsewhere classified
Excludes1 dissociative convulsions and seizures (F44.5)
epileptic convulsions and seizures (G40.-)
newborn convulsions and seizures (P90)

R56.0 Febrile convulsions PDX 1604

R56.00 Simple febrile convulsions
Febrile convulsion NOS
Febrile seizure NOS

R56.01 Complex febrile convulsions
Atypical febrile seizure
Complex febrile seizure
Complicated febrile seizure
Excludes1 status epilepticus (G40.901)

R56.1 Post traumatic seizures PDX 749
Excludes1 post traumatic epilepsy (G40.-)

R56.9 Unspecified convulsions
Convulsion disorder
Fit NOS
Recurrent convulsions
Seizure(s) (convulsive) NOS
Coding Clinic: 2022, Q4, P46; 2021, Q1, P3; 2019, Q4, P18

R57 Shock, not elsewhere classified PDX 1605
Excludes1 anaphylactic shock NOS (T78.2)
anaphylactic reaction or shock due to adverse food reaction (T78.0-)
anaphylactic shock due to adverse effect of correct drug or medicament properly administered (T88.6)
anaphylactic shock due to serum (T80.5-)
electric shock (T75.4)
obstetric shock (O75.1)
postprocedural shock (T81.1-)
psychic shock (F43.0)
shock complicating or following ectopic or molar pregnancy (O00-O07, O08.3)
shock due to anesthesia (T88.2)
shock due to lightning (T75.01)
traumatic shock (T79.4)
toxic shock syndrome (A48.3)

R57.0 Cardiogenic shock
Excludes2 septic shock (R65.21)
MCC: Only if patient discharged alive

R57.1 Hypovolemic shock
Decreased blood volume (loss)
MCC: Only if patient discharged alive
Coding Clinic: 2019, Q2, P7-8

R57.8 Other shock
MCC: Only if patient discharged alive

R57.9 Shock, unspecified
Failure of peripheral circulation NOS
Resulting in significant blood pressure drop

R58 Hemorrhage, not elsewhere classified
Hemorrhage NOS
Excludes1 hemorrhage included with underlying conditions, such as:
acute duodenal ulcer with hemorrhage (K26.0)
acute gastritis with bleeding (K29.01)
ulcerative enterocolitis with rectal bleeding (K51.01)

R59 Enlarged lymph nodes
Includes swollen glands
Excludes1 lymphadenitis NOS (I88.9)
acute lymphadenitis (L04.-)
chronic lymphadenitis (I88.1)
mesenteric (acute) (chronic) lymphadenitis (I88.0)

R59.0 Localized enlarged lymph nodes

R59.1 Generalized enlarged lymph nodes
Lymphadenopathy NOS

R59.9 Enlarged lymph nodes, unspecified

R60 Edema, not elsewhere classified
Excludes1 angioneurotic edema (T78.3)
ascites (R18.-)
cerebral edema (G93.6)
cerebral edema due to birth injury (P11.0)
edema of larynx (J38.4)
edema of nasopharynx (J39.2)
edema of pharynx (J39.2)
gestational edema (O12.0-)
hereditary edema (Q82.0)
hydrops fetalis NOS (P83.2)
hydrothorax (J94.8)
hydrops fetalis NOS (P83.2)
newborn edema (P83.3)
pulmonary edema (J81.-)

R60.0 Localized edema

R60.1 Generalized edema
Excludes2 nutritional edema (E40-E46)

R60.9 Edema, unspecified
Fluid retention NOS

R61 Generalized hyperhidrosis
Excessive sweating
Night sweats
Secondary hyperhidrosis
Code first, if applicable, menopausal and female climacteric states (N95.1)
Excludes1 focal (primary) (secondary) hyperhidrosis (L74.5-)
Frey's syndrome (L74.52)
localized (primary) (secondary) hyperhidrosis (L74.5-)

R62 Lack of expected normal physiological development in childhood and adults
Excludes1 delayed puberty (E30.0)
gonadal dysgenesis (Q99.1)
hypopituitarism (E23.0)

R62.0 Delayed milestone in childhood P
Delayed attainment of expected physiological developmental stage
Late talker
Late walker

R62.5 Other and unspecified lack of expected normal physiological development in childhood
Excludes1 HIV disease resulting in failure to thrive (B20)
physical retardation due to malnutrition (E45)

R62.50 Unspecified lack of expected normal physiological development in childhood
Infantilism NOS

R62.51 Failure to thrive (child) P
Failure to gain weight
Excludes1 failure to thrive in child under 28 days old (P92.6)
Coding Clinic: 2018, Q4, P82

R62.52 Short stature (child)
Lack of growth
Physical retardation
Short stature NOS
Excludes1 short stature due to endocrine disorder (E34.3-)

R62.59 Other lack of expected normal physiological development in childhood

R62.7 Adult failure to thrive A

R63 Symptoms and signs concerning food and fluid intake

Excludes1 bulimia NOS (F5Ø.2-)

R63.Ø Anorexia
Loss of appetite
Excludes1 anorexia nervosa (F5Ø.Ø-)
loss of appetite of nonorganic origin (F5Ø.89)

R63.1 Polydipsia
Excessive thirst

R63.2 Polyphagia
Excessive eating
Hyperalimentation NOS

R63.3 Feeding difficulties
Excludes2 eating disorders (F5Ø.-)
feeding problems of newborn (P92.-)
infant feeding disorder of nonorganic origin (F98.2-)

R63.3Ø Feeding difficulties, unspecified P

R63.31 Pediatric feeding disorder, acute
Pediatric feeding dysfunction, acute
Code also, if applicable, associated conditions such as:
aspiration pneumonia (J69.Ø)
dysphagia (R13.1-)
gastro-esophageal reflux disease (K21.-)
malnutrition (E4Ø-E46)

R63.32 Pediatric feeding disorder, chronic P
Pediatric feeding dysfunction, chronic
Code also, if applicable, associated conditions such as:
aspiration pneumonia (J69.Ø)
dysphagia (R13.1-)
gastro-esophageal reflux disease (K21.-)
malnutrition (E4Ø-E46)

R63.39 Other feeding difficulties
Feeding problem (elderly) (infant) NOS
Picky eater
Coding Clinic: 2Ø17, Q1, P27; 2Ø16, Q3, P19

R63.4 Abnormal weight loss

R63.5 Abnormal weight gain
Excludes1 excessive weight gain in pregnancy (O26.Ø-)
obesity (E66.-)

R63.6 Underweight
Use additional code to identify body mass index (BMI), if known (Z68.-)
Excludes1 abnormal weight loss (R63.4)
anorexia nervosa (F5Ø.Ø-)
malnutrition (E4Ø-E46)

R63.8 Other symptoms and signs concerning food and fluid intake

R64 Cachexia (Ex) PDX 1606
Excludes1 abnormal weight loss (R63.4)
cachexia due to underlying condition (E88.A)
nutritional marasmus (E41)
Coding Clinic: 2Ø17, Q3, P25

R65 Symptoms and signs specifically associated with systemic inflammation and infection

R65.1 Systemic inflammatory response syndrome (SIRS) of non-infectious origin
Code first underlying condition, such as:
heatstroke (T67.Ø-)
injury and trauma (SØØ-T88)
Excludes1 sepsis - code to infection
severe sepsis (R65.2)
Coding Clinic: 2Ø19, Q2, P38

R65.1Ø Systemic inflammatory response syndrome (SIRS) of non-infectious origin without acute organ dysfunction (Ex) PDX 72
Systemic inflammatory response syndrome (SIRS) NOS
Coding Clinic: 2Ø19, Q2, P25, 38

R65.11 Systemic inflammatory response syndrome (SIRS) of non-infectious origin with acute organ dysfunction (Ex) PDX 72
Use additional code to identify specific acute organ dysfunction, such as:
acute kidney failure (N17.-)
acute respiratory failure (J96.Ø-)
critical illness myopathy (G72.81)
critical illness polyneuropathy (G62.81)
disseminated intravascular coagulopathy [DIC] (D65)
encephalopathy (metabolic) (septic) (G93.41)
hepatic failure (K72.Ø-)

OGCR Section I.C.18.g.

SIRS due to Non-Infectious Process

The systemic inflammatory response syndrome (SIRS) can develop as a result of certain non-infectious disease processes, such as trauma, malignant neoplasm, or pancreatitis. When SIRS is documented with a noninfectious condition, and no subsequent infection is documented, the code for the underlying condition, such as an injury, should be assigned, followed by code R65.1Ø, Systemic inflammatory response syndrome (SIRS) of non-infectious origin without acute organ dysfunction, or code R65.11, Systemic inflammatory response syndrome (SIRS) of non-infectious origin with acute organ dysfunction. If an associated acute organ dysfunction is documented, the appropriate code(s) for the specific type of organ dysfunction(s) should be assigned in addition to code R65.11. If acute organ dysfunction is documented, but it cannot be determined if the acute organ dysfunction is associated with SIRS or due to another condition (e.g., directly due to the trauma), the provider should be queried.

R65.2 Severe sepsis
Infection with associated acute organ dysfunction
Sepsis with acute organ dysfunction
Sepsis with multiple organ dysfunction
Systemic inflammatory response syndrome due to infectious process with acute organ dysfunction
Code first underlying infection, such as:
infection following a procedure (T81.44)
infections following infusion, transfusion and therapeutic injection (T8Ø.2-)
puerperal sepsis (O85)
sepsis following complete or unspecified spontaneous abortion (OØ3.87)
sepsis following ectopic and molar pregnancy (OØ8.82)
sepsis following incomplete spontaneous abortion (OØ3.37)
sepsis following (induced) termination of pregnancy (OØ4.87)
sepsis NOS (A41.9)
Use additional code to identify specific acute organ dysfunction, such as:
acute kidney failure (N17.-)
acute respiratory failure (J96.Ø-)
critical illness myopathy (G72.81)
critical illness polyneuropathy (G62.81)
disseminated intravascular coagulopathy [DIC] (D65)
encephalopathy (metabolic) (septic) (G93.41)
hepatic failure (K72.Ø-)
Coding Clinic: 2Ø17, Q4, P99; 2Ø16, Q3, P8

R65.2Ø Severe sepsis without septic shock (Ex) PDX 72
Severe sepsis NOS
Coding Clinic: 2Ø19, Q1, P14; 2Ø18, Q4, P9Ø; 2Ø16, Q3, P14

R65.21 Severe sepsis with septic shock (Ex) PDX 1605
MCC when PDx is its own MCC

● **R68 Other general symptoms and signs**

R68.Ø Hypothermia, not associated with low environmental temperature

Excludes1 hypothermia NOS (accidental) (T68)
hypothermia due to anesthesia (T88.51)
hypothermia due to low environmental temperature (T68)
newborn hypothermia (P8Ø.-)

● **R68.1 Nonspecific symptoms peculiar to infancy**

Excludes1 colic, infantile (R1Ø.83)
neonatal cerebral irritability (P91.3)
teething syndrome (KØØ.7)

R68.11 Excessive crying of infant (baby) P

Excludes1 excessive crying of child, adolescent, or adult (R45.83)

R68.12 Fussy infant (baby) P
Irritable infant

R68.13 Apparent life threatening event in infant (ALTE) P
Apparent life threatening event in newborn
Brief resolved unexplained event (BRUE)

Code first confirmed diagnosis, if known

Use additional code(s) for associated signs and symptoms if no confirmed diagnosis established, or if signs and symptoms are not associated routinely with confirmed diagnosis, or provide additional information for cause of ALTE

R68.19 Other nonspecific symptoms peculiar to infancy P

R68.2 Dry mouth, unspecified

Excludes1 dry mouth due to dehydration (E86.Ø)
dry mouth due to Sjögren syndrome (M35.Ø-)
~~salivary gland hyposecretion (K11.7)~~

▶ **Excludes2** salivary gland hyposecretion (K11.7)

R68.3 Clubbing of fingers
Clubbing of nails

Excludes1 congenital clubfinger (Q68.1)

● **R68.8 Other general symptoms and signs**

R68.81 Early satiety

R68.82 Decreased libido A
Decreased sexual desire

R68.83 Chills (without fever)
Chills NOS

Excludes1 chills with fever (R5Ø.9)

R68.84 Jaw pain
Mandibular pain
Maxilla pain

Excludes1 temporomandibular joint arthralgia (M26.62-)

R68.89 Other general symptoms and signs

R69 Illness, unspecified
Unknown and unspecified cases of morbidity

ABNORMAL FINDINGS ON EXAMINATION OF BLOOD, WITHOUT DIAGNOSIS (R7Ø-R79)

Excludes2 abnormal findings on antenatal screening of mother (O28.-)
abnormalities of lipids (E78.-)
abnormalities of platelets and thrombocytes (D69.-)
abnormalities of white blood cells classified elsewhere (D7Ø-D72)
coagulation hemorrhagic disorders (D65-D68)
diagnostic abnormal findings classified elsewhere —*see* Alphabetical Index
hemorrhagic and hematological disorders of newborn (P5Ø-P61)

● **R7Ø Elevated erythrocyte sedimentation rate and abnormality of plasma viscosity**

R7Ø.Ø Elevated erythrocyte sedimentation rate

R7Ø.1 Abnormal plasma viscosity

● **R71 Abnormality of red blood cells**

Excludes1 anemias (D5Ø-D64)
anemia of premature infant (P61.2)
benign (familial) polycythemia (D75.Ø)
congenital anemias (P61.2-P61.4)
newborn anemia due to isoimmunization (P55.-)
polycythemia neonatorum (P61.1)
polycythemia NOS (D75.1)
polycythemia vera (D45)
secondary polycythemia (D75.1)

R71.Ø Precipitous drop in hematocrit (Ex:) PDX 1607
Drop (precipitous) in hemoglobin
Drop in hematocrit
Blood volume that has decreased red blood cells

R71.8 Other abnormality of red blood cells
Abnormal red-cell morphology NOS
Abnormal red-cell volume NOS
Anisocytosis
Red blood cells of unequal size
Poikilocytosis
Red blood cells of abnormal shape

● **R73 Elevated blood glucose level**

Excludes1 diabetes mellitus (EØ8-E13)
diabetes mellitus in pregnancy, childbirth and the puerperium (O24.-)
neonatal disorders (P7Ø.Ø-P7Ø.2)
postsurgical hypoinsulinemia (E89.1)

● **R73.Ø Abnormal glucose**

Excludes1 abnormal glucose in pregnancy (O99.81-)
diabetes mellitus (EØ8-E13)
dysmetabolic syndrome X (E88.81-)
gestational diabetes (O24.4-)
glycosuria (R81)
hypoglycemia (E16.2)
▶type 1 diabetes mellitus, presymptomatic (E1Ø.A-)

R73.Ø1 Impaired fasting glucose
Elevated fasting glucose

R73.Ø2 Impaired glucose tolerance (oral)
Elevated glucose tolerance

R73.Ø3 Prediabetes
Latent diabetes
Coding Clinic: 2Ø16, Q4, P65

R73.Ø9 Other abnormal glucose
Abnormal glucose NOS
Abnormal non-fasting glucose tolerance
Coding Clinic: 2Ø16, Q4, P65

R73.9 Hyperglycemia, unspecified

● **R74 Abnormal serum enzyme levels**

● **R74.Ø Nonspecific elevation of levels of transaminase and lactic acid dehydrogenase [LDH]**

R74.Ø1 Elevation of levels of liver transaminase levels
Elevation of levels of alanine transaminase (ALT)
Elevation of levels of aspartate transaminase (AST)

R74.Ø2 Elevation of levels of lactic acid dehydrogenase [LDH]

R74.8 Abnormal levels of other serum enzymes
Abnormal level of acid phosphatase
Abnormal level of alkaline phosphatase
Abnormal level of amylase
Abnormal level of lipase [triacylglycerol lipase]
Coding Clinic: 2Ø19, Q2, P6

R74.9 Abnormal serum enzyme level, unspecified

R75 Inconclusive laboratory evidence of human immunodeficiency virus [HIV]
Nonconclusive HIV-test finding in infants

Excludes1 asymptomatic human immunodeficiency virus [HIV] infection status (Z21)
human immunodeficiency virus [HIV] disease (B2Ø)

OGCR Section I.C.1.e and f.

Patients with inconclusive HIV serology

e. Patients with inconclusive HIV serology, but no definitive diagnosis or manifestations of the illness, may be assigned code R75, Inconclusive laboratory evidence of human immunodeficiency virus [HIV].

f. Previously diagnosed HIV-related illness

Patients with any known prior diagnosis of an HIV-related illness should be coded to B2Ø. Once a patient has developed an HIV-related illness, the patient should always be assigned code B2Ø on every subsequent admission/encounter. Patients previously diagnosed with any HIV illness (B2Ø) should never be assigned to R75 or Z21, Asymptomatic human immunodeficiency virus [HIV] infection status.

● **R76 Other abnormal immunological findings in serum**

R76.Ø Raised antibody titer

Excludes1 isoimmunization in pregnancy (O36.Ø-O36.1)
isoimmunization affecting newborn (P55.-)

Coding Clinic: 2021, Q1, P7

● **R76.1 Nonspecific reaction to test for tuberculosis**

R76.11 Nonspecific reaction to tuberculin skin test without active tuberculosis

Abnormal result of Mantoux test
PPD positive
Tuberculin (skin test) positive
Tuberculin (skin test) reactor

Excludes1 nonspecific reaction to cell mediated immunity measurement of gamma interferon antigen response without active tuberculosis (R76.12)

R76.12 Nonspecific reaction to cell mediated immunity measurement of gamma interferon antigen response without active tuberculosis

Nonspecific reaction to QuantiFERON-TB test (QFT) without active tuberculosis

Excludes1 nonspecific reaction to tuberculin skin test without active tuberculosis (R76.11)
positive tuberculin skin test (R76.11)

R76.8 Other specified abnormal immunological findings in serum

Raised level of immunoglobulins NOS

Coding Clinic: 2021, Q1, P7

R76.9 Abnormal immunological finding in serum, unspecified

● **R77 Other abnormalities of plasma proteins**

Excludes1 disorders of plasma-protein metabolism (E88.Ø-)

R77.Ø Abnormality of albumin

R77.1 Abnormality of globulin

Hyperglobulinemia NOS

R77.2 Abnormality of alphafetoprotein

R77.8 Other specified abnormalities of plasma proteins

Coding Clinic: 2019, Q2, P6

R77.9 Abnormality of plasma protein, unspecified

Coding Clinic: 2019, Q2, P6

● **R78 Findings of drugs and other substances, not normally found in blood**

Use additional code to identify any retained foreign body, if applicable (Z18.-)

Excludes2 mental or behavioral disorders due to psychoactive substance use (F1Ø-F19)

R78.Ø Finding of alcohol in blood

Use additional external cause code (Y9Ø.-), for detail regarding alcohol level.

R78.1 Finding of opiate drug in blood

R78.2 Finding of cocaine in blood

R78.3 Finding of hallucinogen in blood

R78.4 Finding of other drugs of addictive potential in blood

R78.5 Finding of other psychotropic drug in blood

R78.6 Finding of steroid agent in blood

● **R78.7 Finding of abnormal level of heavy metals in blood**

R78.71 Abnormal lead level in blood

Excludes1 lead poisoning (T56.Ø-)

R78.79 Finding of abnormal level of heavy metals in blood

● **R78.8 Finding of other specified substances, not normally found in blood**

R78.81 Bacteremia (Ex) PDX 1608

Blood poisoning/bacteremia

Excludes1 sepsis-code to specified infection

R78.89 Finding of other specified substances, not normally found in blood

Finding of abnormal level of lithium in blood

R78.9 Finding of unspecified substance, not normally found in blood

● **R79 Other abnormal findings of blood chemistry**

Use additional code to identify any retained foreign body, if applicable (Z18.-)

Excludes1 asymptomatic hyperuricemia (E79.Ø)
hyperglycemia NOS (R73.9)
hypoglycemia NOS (E16.2)
neonatal hypoglycemia (P7Ø.3-P7Ø.4)
specific findings indicating disorder of amino-acid metabolism (E7Ø-E72)
specific findings indicating disorder of carbohydrate metabolism (E73-E74)
specific findings indicating disorder of lipid metabolism (E75.-)

R79.Ø Abnormal level of blood mineral

Abnormal blood level of cobalt
Abnormal blood level of copper
Abnormal blood level of iron
Abnormal blood level of magnesium
Abnormal blood level of mineral NEC
Abnormal blood level of zinc

Excludes1 abnormal level of lithium (R78.89)
disorders of mineral metabolism (E83.-)
neonatal hypomagnesemia (P71.2)
nutritional mineral deficiency (E58-E61)

R79.1 Abnormal coagulation profile

Abnormal or prolonged bleeding time
Abnormal or prolonged coagulation time
Abnormal or prolonged partial thromboplastin time [PTT]
Abnormal or prolonged prothrombin time [PT]
Low von Willebrand factor

Excludes1 coagulation defects (D68.-)

Excludes2 abnormality of fluid, electrolyte or acid-base balance (E86-E87)

● **R79.8 Other specified abnormal findings of blood chemistry**

R79.81 Abnormal blood-gas level

R79.82 Elevated C-reactive protein (CRP)

R79.83 Abnormal findings of blood amino-acid level

Homocysteinemia

Excludes1 disorders of amino-acid metabolism (E7Ø-E72)

Coding Clinic: 2021, Q4, P28

R79.89 Other specified abnormal findings of blood chemistry

Coding Clinic: 2019, Q2, P6

R79.9 Abnormal finding of blood chemistry, unspecified

ABNORMAL FINDINGS ON EXAMINATION OF URINE, WITHOUT DIAGNOSIS (R8Ø-R82)

Excludes1 abnormal findings on antenatal screening of mother (O28.-)
diagnostic abnormal findings classified elsewhere - see Alphabetical Index
specific findings indicating disorder of amino-acid metabolism (E7Ø-E72)
specific findings indicating disorder of carbohydrate metabolism (E73-E74)

● R80 Proteinuria
Excludes1 gestational proteinuria (O12.1-)
R80.0 Isolated proteinuria
Idiopathic proteinuria
Excludes1 isolated proteinuria with specific morphological lesion (N06.-)
R80.1 Persistent proteinuria, unspecified
R80.2 Orthostatic proteinuria, unspecified
Postural proteinuria
R80.3 Bence Jones proteinuria
R80.8 Other proteinuria
R80.9 Proteinuria, unspecified
Albuminuria NOS

R81 Glycosuria
Excludes1 renal glycosuria (E74.818)

● R82 Other and unspecified abnormal findings in urine
Includes chromoabnormalities in urine
Use additional code to identify any retained foreign body, if applicable (Z18.-)
Excludes2 hematuria (R31.-)
R82.0 Chyluria (Ex) PDX 1609
White milky urine
Excludes1 filarial chyluria (B74.-)
R82.1 Myoglobinuria (Ex) PDX 1610
Presence of myoglobin (iron containing protein) in urine
R82.2 Biliuria
Presence of bile pigments/salts in urine
R82.3 Hemoglobinuria
Presence of hemoglobin in urine
Excludes1 hemoglobinuria due to hemolysis from external causes NEC (D59.6)
hemoglobinuria due to paroxysmal nocturnal [Marchiafava-Micheli] (D59.5)
R82.4 Acetonuria
Ketonuria
R82.5 Elevated urine levels of drugs, medicaments and biological substances
Elevated urine levels of catecholamines
Elevated urine levels of indoleacetic acid
Elevated urine levels of 17-ketosteroids
Elevated urine levels of steroids
R82.6 Abnormal urine levels of substances chiefly nonmedicinal as to source
Abnormal urine level of heavy metals
● R82.7 Abnormal findings on microbiological examination of urine
Excludes1 colonization status (Z22.-)
Coding Clinic: 2016, Q4, P65
R82.71 Bacteriuria
R82.79 Other abnormal findings on microbiological examination of urine
Positive culture findings of urine
● R82.8 Abnormal findings on cytological and histological examination of urine
R82.81 Pyuria
Sterile pyuria
Coding Clinic: 2019, Q4, P16
R82.89 Other abnormal findings on cytological and histological examination of urine
● R82.9 Other and unspecified abnormal findings in urine
R82.90 Unspecified abnormal findings in urine
R82.91 Other chromoabnormalities of urine
Chromoconversion (dipstick)
Idiopathic dipstick converts positive for blood with no cellular forms in sediment
Excludes1 hemoglobinuria (R82.3)
myoglobinuria (R82.1)
● R82.99 Other abnormal findings in urine (Ex) PDX 1609
R82.991 Hypocitraturia
R82.992 Hyperoxaluria
Excludes1 Primary hyperoxaluria (E72.53)
R82.993 Hyperuricosuria
R82.994 Hypercalciuria
Idiopathic hypercalciuria
R82.998 Other abnormal findings in urine
Cells and casts in urine
Crystalluria
Melanuria

ABNORMAL FINDINGS ON EXAMINATION OF OTHER BODY FLUIDS, SUBSTANCES AND TISSUES, WITHOUT DIAGNOSIS (R83-R89)

Excludes1 abnormal findings on antenatal screening of mother (O28.-)
diagnostic abnormal findings classified elsewhere - see Alphabetical Index
Excludes2 abnormal findings on examination of blood, without diagnosis (R70-R79)
abnormal findings on examination of urine, without diagnosis (R80-R82)
abnormal tumor markers (R97.-)

● R83 Abnormal findings in cerebrospinal fluid
R83.0 Abnormal level of enzymes in cerebrospinal fluid
R83.1 Abnormal level of hormones in cerebrospinal fluid
R83.2 Abnormal level of other drugs, medicaments and biological substances in cerebrospinal fluid
R83.3 Abnormal level of substances chiefly nonmedicinal as to source in cerebrospinal fluid
R83.4 Abnormal immunological findings in cerebrospinal fluid
R83.5 Abnormal microbiological findings in cerebrospinal fluid
Positive culture findings in cerebrospinal fluid
Excludes1 colonization status (Z22.-)
R83.6 Abnormal cytological findings in cerebrospinal fluid
R83.8 Other abnormal findings in cerebrospinal fluid
Abnormal chromosomal findings in cerebrospinal fluid
R83.9 Unspecified abnormal finding in cerebrospinal fluid

● R84 Abnormal findings in specimens from respiratory organs and thorax
Includes abnormal findings in bronchial washings
abnormal findings in nasal secretions
abnormal findings in pleural fluid
abnormal findings in sputum
abnormal findings in throat scrapings
Excludes1 blood-stained sputum (R04.2)
R84.0 Abnormal level of enzymes in specimens from respiratory organs and thorax
R84.1 Abnormal level of hormones in specimens from respiratory organs and thorax
R84.2 Abnormal level of other drugs, medicaments and biological substances in specimens from respiratory organs and thorax
R84.3 Abnormal level of substances chiefly nonmedicinal as to source in specimens from respiratory organs and thorax
R84.4 Abnormal immunological findings in specimens from respiratory organs and thorax
R84.5 Abnormal microbiological findings in specimens from respiratory organs and thorax
Positive culture findings in specimens from respiratory organs and thorax
Excludes1 colonization status (Z22.-)
R84.6 Abnormal cytological findings in specimens from respiratory organs and thorax

R84.7 **Abnormal histological findings in specimens from respiratory organs and thorax**

R84.8 **Other abnormal findings in specimens from respiratory organs and thorax**
Abnormal chromosomal findings in specimens from respiratory organs and thorax

R84.9 **Unspecified abnormal finding in specimens from respiratory organs and thorax**

R85 **Abnormal findings in specimens from digestive organs and abdominal cavity**

Includes abnormal findings in peritoneal fluid
abnormal findings in saliva

Excludes1 cloudy peritoneal dialysis effluent (R88.Ø)
fecal abnormalities (R19.5)

R85.Ø **Abnormal level of enzymes in specimens from digestive organs and abdominal cavity**

R85.1 **Abnormal level of hormones in specimens from digestive organs and abdominal cavity**

R85.2 **Abnormal level of other drugs, medicaments and biological substances in specimens from digestive organs and abdominal cavity**

R85.3 **Abnormal level of substances chiefly nonmedicinal as to source in specimens from digestive organs and abdominal cavity**

R85.4 **Abnormal immunological findings in specimens from digestive organs and abdominal cavity**

R85.5 **Abnormal microbiological findings in specimens from digestive organs and abdominal cavity**
Positive culture findings in specimens from digestive organs and abdominal cavity

Excludes1 colonization status (Z22.-)

R85.6 **Abnormal cytological findings in specimens from digestive organs and abdominal cavity**

R85.61 **Abnormal cytologic smear of anus**

Excludes1 abnormal cytological findings in specimens from other digestive organs and abdominal cavity (R85.69)
carcinoma in situ of anus (histologically confirmed) (DØ1.3)
anal intraepithelial neoplasia I [AIN I] (K62.82)
anal intraepithelial neoplasia II [AIN II] (K62.82)
anal intraepithelial neoplasia III [AIN III] (DØ1.3)
dysplasia (mild) (moderate) of anus (histologically confirmed) (K62.82)
severe dysplasia of anus (histologically confirmed) (DØ1.3)

Excludes2 anal high risk human papillomavirus (HPV) DNA test positive (R85.81)
anal low risk human papillomavirus (HPV) DNA test positive (R85.82)

R85.61Ø **Atypical squamous cells of undetermined significance on cytologic smear of anus (ASC-US)**

R85.611 **Atypical squamous cells cannot exclude high grade squamous intraepithelial lesion on cytologic smear of anus (ASC-H)**

R85.612 **Low grade squamous intraepithelial lesion on cytologic smear of anus (LGSIL)**

R85.613 **High grade squamous intraepithelial lesion on cytologic smear of anus (HGSIL)**

R85.614 **Cytologic evidence of malignancy on smear of anus**

R85.615 **Unsatisfactory cytologic smear of anus**
Inadequate sample of cytologic smear of anus

R85.616 **Satisfactory anal smear but lacking transformation zone**

R85.618 **Other abnormal cytological findings on specimens from anus**

R85.619 **Unspecified abnormal cytological findings in specimens from anus**
Abnormal anal cytology NOS
Atypical glandular cells of anus NOS

R85.69 **Abnormal cytological findings in specimens from other digestive organs and abdominal cavity**

R85.7 **Abnormal histological findings in specimens from digestive organs and abdominal cavity**

R85.8 **Other abnormal findings in specimens from digestive organs and abdominal cavity**

R85.81 **Anal high risk human papillomavirus (HPV) DNA test positive**

Excludes1 anogenital warts due to human papillomavirus (HPV) (A63.Ø)
condyloma acuminatum (A63.Ø)

R85.82 **Anal low risk human papillomavirus (HPV) DNA test positive**
Use additional code for associated human papillomavirus (B97.7)

R85.89 **Other abnormal findings in specimens from digestive organs and abdominal cavity**
Abnormal chromosomal findings in specimens from digestive organs and abdominal cavity

R85.9 **Unspecified abnormal finding in specimens from digestive organs and abdominal cavity**

R86 **Abnormal findings in specimens from male genital organs**

Includes abnormal findings in prostatic secretions
abnormal findings in semen, seminal fluid
abnormal spermatozoa

Excludes1 azoospermia (N46.Ø-)
oligospermia (N46.1-)

R86.Ø **Abnormal level of enzymes in specimens from male genital organs**

R86.1 **Abnormal level of hormones in specimens from male genital organs**

R86.2 **Abnormal level of other drugs, medicaments and biological substances in specimens from male genital organs**

R86.3 **Abnormal level of substances chiefly nonmedicinal as to source in specimens from male genital organs**

R86.4 **Abnormal immunological findings in specimens from male genital organs**

R86.5 **Abnormal microbiological findings in specimens from male genital organs**
Positive culture findings in specimens from male genital organs

Excludes1 colonization status (Z22.-)

R86.6 **Abnormal cytological findings in specimens from male genital organs**

R86.7 **Abnormal histological findings in specimens from male genital organs**

R86.8 **Other abnormal findings in specimens from male genital organs**
Abnormal chromosomal findings in specimens from male genital organs

R86.9 **Unspecified abnormal finding in specimens from male genital organs**

● **R87 Abnormal findings in specimens from female genital organs**

Includes abnormal findings in secretion and smears from cervix uteri
abnormal findings in secretion and smears from vagina
abnormal findings in secretion and smears from vulva

R87.0 Abnormal level of enzymes in specimens from female genital organs

R87.1 Abnormal level of hormones in specimens from female genital organs

R87.2 Abnormal level of other drugs, medicaments and biological substances in specimens from female genital organs

R87.3 Abnormal level of substances chiefly nonmedicinal as to source in specimens from female genital organs

R87.4 Abnormal immunological findings in specimens from female genital organs

R87.5 Abnormal microbiological findings in specimens from female genital organs

Positive culture findings in specimens from female genital organs

Excludes1 colonization status (Z22.-)

● **R87.6 Abnormal cytological findings in specimens from female genital organs**

● **R87.61 Abnormal cytological findings in specimens from cervix uteri**

Excludes1 abnormal cytological findings in specimens from other female genital organs (R87.69)
abnormal cytological findings in specimens from vagina (R87.62-)
carcinoma in situ of cervix uteri (histologically confirmed) (D06.-)
cervical intraepithelial neoplasia I [CIN I] (N87.0)
cervical intraepithelial neoplasia II [CIN II] (N87.1)
cervical intraepithelial neoplasia III [CIN III] (D06.-)
dysplasia (mild) (moderate) of cervix uteri (histologically confirmed) (N87.-)
severe dysplasia of cervix uteri (histologically confirmed) (D06.-)

Excludes2 cervical high risk human papillomavirus (HPV) DNA test positive (R87.810)
cervical low risk human papillomavirus (HPV) DNA test positive (R87.820)

R87.610 Atypical squamous cells of undetermined significance on cytologic smear of cervix (ASC-US)

R87.611 Atypical squamous cells cannot exclude high grade squamous intraepithelial lesion on cytologic smear of cervix (ASC-H)

R87.612 Low grade squamous intraepithelial lesion on cytologic smear of cervix (LGSIL)

R87.613 High grade squamous intraepithelial lesion on cytologic smear of cervix (HGSIL)

R87.614 Cytologic evidence of malignancy on smear of cervix

R87.615 Unsatisfactory cytologic smear of cervix

Inadequate sample of cytologic smear of cervix

R87.616 Satisfactory cervical smear but lacking transformation zone

R87.618 Other abnormal cytological findings on specimens from cervix uteri

R87.619 Unspecified abnormal cytological findings in specimens from cervix uteri

Abnormal cervical cytology NOS
Abnormal Papanicolaou smear of cervix NOS
Abnormal thin preparation smear of cervix NOS
Atypical endocervical cells of cervix NOS
Atypical endometrial cells of cervix NOS
Atypical glandular cells of cervix NOS

● **R87.62 Abnormal cytological findings in specimens from vagina**

Use additional code to identify acquired absence of uterus and cervix, if applicable (Z90.71-)

Excludes1 abnormal cytological findings in specimens from cervix uteri (R87.61-)
abnormal cytological findings in specimens from other female genital organs (R87.69)
carcinoma in situ of vagina (histologically confirmed) (D07.2)
vaginal intraepithelial neoplasia I [VAIN I] (N89.0)
vaginal intraepithelial neoplasia II [VAIN II] (N89.1)
vaginal intraepithelial neoplasia III [VAIN III] (D07.2)
dysplasia (mild) (moderate) of vagina (histologically confirmed) (N89.-)
severe dysplasia of vagina (histologically confirmed) (D07.2)

Excludes2 vaginal high risk human papillomavirus (HPV) DNA test positive (R87.811)
vaginal low risk human papillomavirus (HPV) DNA test positive (R87.821)

R87.620 Atypical squamous cells of undetermined significance on cytologic smear of vagina (ASC-US)

R87.621 Atypical squamous cells cannot exclude high grade squamous intraepithelial lesion on cytologic smear of vagina (ASC-H)

R87.622 Low grade squamous intraepithelial lesion on cytologic smear of vagina (LGSIL)

R87.623 High grade squamous intraepithelial lesion on cytologic smear of vagina (HGSIL)

R87.624 Cytologic evidence of malignancy on smear of vagina

R87.625 Unsatisfactory cytologic smear of vagina

Inadequate sample of cytologic smear of vagina

R87.628 Other abnormal cytological findings on specimens from vagina

R87.629 **Unspecified abnormal cytological findings in specimens from vagina**
Abnormal Papanicolaou smear of vagina NOS
Abnormal thin preparation smear of vagina NOS
Abnormal vaginal cytology NOS
Atypical endocervical cells of vagina NOS
Atypical endometrial cells of vagina NOS
Atypical glandular cells of vagina NOS

R87.69 **Abnormal cytological findings in specimens from other female genital organs**
Abnormal cytological findings in specimens from female genital organs NOS
Excludes1 dysplasia of vulva (histologically confirmed) (N90.0-N90.3)

R87.7 **Abnormal histological findings in specimens from female genital organs**
Excludes1 carcinoma in situ (histologically confirmed) of female genital organs (D06-D07.3)
cervical intraepithelial neoplasia I [CIN I] (N87.0)
cervical intraepithelial neoplasia II [CIN II] (N87.1)
cervical intraepithelial neoplasia III [CIN III] (D06.-)
dysplasia (mild) (moderate) of cervix uteri (histologically confirmed) (N87.-)
dysplasia (mild) (moderate) of vagina (histologically confirmed) (N89.-)
vaginal intraepithelial neoplasia I [VAIN I] (N89.0)
vaginal intraepithelial neoplasia II [VAIN II] (N89.1)
vaginal intraepithelial neoplasia III [VAIN III] (D07.2)
severe dysplasia of cervix uteri (histologically confirmed) (D06.-)
severe dysplasia of vagina (histologically confirmed) (D07.2)

● R87.8 **Other abnormal findings in specimens from female genital organs**

● R87.81 **High risk human papillomavirus (HPV) DNA test positive from female genital organs**
Excludes1 anogenital warts due to human papillomavirus (HPV) (A63.0)
condyloma acuminatum (A63.0)

R87.810 **Cervical high risk human papillomavirus (HPV) DNA test positive**

R87.811 **Vaginal high risk human papillomavirus (HPV) DNA test positive**

● R87.82 **Low risk human papillomavirus (HPV) DNA test positive from female genital organs**
Use additional code for associated human papillomavirus (B97.7)

R87.820 **Cervical low risk human papillomavirus (HPV) DNA test positive**

R87.821 **Vaginal low risk human papillomavirus (HPV) DNA test positive**

R87.89 **Other abnormal findings in specimens from female genital organs**
Abnormal chromosomal findings in specimens from female genital organs

R87.9 **Unspecified abnormal finding in specimens from female genital organs**

● R88 **Abnormal findings in other body fluids and substances**

R88.0 **Cloudy (hemodialysis) (peritoneal) dialysis effluent**

R88.8 **Abnormal findings in other body fluids and substances**

● R89 **Abnormal findings in specimens from other organs, systems and tissues**
Includes abnormal findings in nipple discharge
abnormal findings in synovial fluid
abnormal findings in wound secretions

R89.0 **Abnormal level of enzymes in specimens from other organs, systems and tissues**

R89.1 **Abnormal level of hormones in specimens from other organs, systems and tissues**

R89.2 **Abnormal level of other drugs, medicaments and biological substances in specimens from other organs, systems and tissues**

R89.3 **Abnormal level of substances chiefly nonmedicinal as to source in specimens from other organs, systems and tissues**

R89.4 **Abnormal immunological findings in specimens from other organs, systems and tissues**

R89.5 **Abnormal microbiological findings in specimens from other organs, systems and tissues**
Positive culture findings in specimens from other organs, systems and tissues
Excludes1 colonization status (Z22.-)

R89.6 **Abnormal cytological findings in specimens from other organs, systems and tissues**

R89.7 **Abnormal histological findings in specimens from other organs, systems and tissues**

R89.8 **Other abnormal findings in specimens from other organs, systems and tissues**
Abnormal chromosomal findings in specimens from other organs, systems and tissues

R89.9 **Unspecified abnormal finding in specimens from other organs, systems and tissues**

ABNORMAL FINDINGS ON DIAGNOSTIC IMAGING AND IN FUNCTION STUDIES, WITHOUT DIAGNOSIS (R90-R94)

Includes nonspecific abnormal findings on diagnostic imaging by computerized axial tomography [CAT scan]
nonspecific abnormal findings on diagnostic imaging by magnetic resonance imaging [MRI][NMR]
nonspecific abnormal findings on diagnostic imaging by positron emission tomography [PET scan]
nonspecific abnormal findings on diagnostic imaging by thermography
nonspecific abnormal findings on diagnostic imaging by ultrasound [echogram]
nonspecific abnormal findings on diagnostic imaging by X-ray examination

Excludes1 abnormal findings on antenatal screening of mother (O28.-)
diagnostic abnormal findings classified elsewhere - see Alphabetical Index

● R90 **Abnormal findings on diagnostic imaging of central nervous system**

R90.0 **Intracranial space-occupying lesion found on diagnostic imaging of central nervous system**

● R90.8 **Other abnormal findings on diagnostic imaging of central nervous system**

R90.81 **Abnormal echoencephalogram**

R90.82 **White matter disease, unspecified**

R90.89 **Other abnormal findings on diagnostic imaging of central nervous system**
Other cerebrovascular abnormality found on diagnostic imaging of central nervous system

● R91 **Abnormal findings on diagnostic imaging of lung**

R91.1 **Solitary pulmonary nodule**
Coin lesion lung
Solitary pulmonary nodule, subsegmental branch of the bronchial tree

R91.8 **Other nonspecific abnormal finding of lung field**
Lung mass NOS found on diagnostic imaging of lung
Pulmonary infiltrate NOS
Shadow, lung

● R92 **Abnormal and inconclusive findings on diagnostic imaging of breast**

R92.Ø **Mammographic microcalcification found on diagnostic imaging of breast**
Excludes2 mammographic calcification (calculus) found on diagnostic imaging of breast (R92.1)

R92.1 **Mammographic calcification found on diagnostic imaging of breast**
Mammographic calculus found on diagnostic imaging of breast

R92.2 **Inconclusive mammogram**
Inconclusive mammogram NEC
Inconclusive mammography NEC
Coding Clinic: 2Ø15, Q1, P24

● R92.3 **Mammographic density found on imaging of breast**
Code also, if applicable, inconclusive mammogram (R92.2)

R92.3Ø **Dense breasts, unspecified**
Dense breasts NOS
Low density

● R92.31 **Mammographic fatty tissue density of breast**
Breast Imaging Reporting and Data System (BI-RADS): A
Breast Imaging Reporting and Data System (BI-RADS): 1

R92.311 **Mammographic fatty tissue density, right breast**

R92.312 **Mammographic fatty tissue density, left breast**

R92.313 **Mammographic fatty tissue density, bilateral breasts**

● R92.32 **Mammographic fibroglandular density of breast**
Breast Imaging Reporting and Data System (BI-RADS): B
Breast Imaging Reporting and Data System (BI-RADS): 2

R92.321 **Mammographic fibroglandular density, right breast**

R92.322 **Mammographic fibroglandular density, left breast**

R92.323 **Mammographic fibroglandular density, bilateral breasts**

● R92.33 **Mammographic heterogeneous density of breast**
Breast Imaging Reporting and Data System (BI-RADS): C
Breast Imaging Reporting and Data System (BI-RADS): 3

R92.331 **Mammographic heterogeneous density, right breast**

R92.332 **Mammographic heterogeneous density, left breast**

R92.333 **Mammographic heterogeneous density, bilateral breasts**
Coding Clinic: 2Ø23, Q4, P44

● R92.34 **Mammographic extreme density of breast**
Breast Imaging Reporting and Data System (BI-RADS): D
Breast Imaging Reporting and Data System (BI-RADS): 4

R92.341 **Mammographic extreme density, right breast**

R92.342 **Mammographic extreme density, left breast**

R92.343 **Mammographic extreme density, bilateral breasts**

R92.8 **Other abnormal and inconclusive findings on diagnostic imaging of breast**

● R93 **Abnormal findings on diagnostic imaging of other body structures**

R93.Ø **Abnormal findings on diagnostic imaging of skull and head, not elsewhere classified**
Excludes1 intracranial space-occupying lesion found on diagnostic imaging (R9Ø.Ø)

R93.1 **Abnormal findings on diagnostic imaging of heart and coronary circulation**
Abnormal echocardiogram NOS
Abnormal heart shadow

R93.2 **Abnormal findings on diagnostic imaging of liver and biliary tract**
Nonvisualization of gallbladder

R93.3 **Abnormal findings on diagnostic imaging of other parts of digestive tract**

● R93.4 **Abnormal findings on diagnostic imaging of urinary organs**
Excludes2 hypertrophy of kidney (N28.81)
Coding Clinic: 2Ø16, Q4, P66

R93.41 **Abnormal radiologic findings on diagnostic imaging of renal pelvis, ureter, or bladder**
Filling defect of bladder found on diagnostic imaging
Filling defect of renal pelvis found on diagnostic imaging
Filling defect of ureter found on diagnostic imaging

● R93.42 **Abnormal radiologic findings on diagnostic imaging of kidney**

R93.421 **Abnormal radiologic findings on diagnostic imaging of right kidney**

R93.422 **Abnormal radiologic findings on diagnostic imaging of left kidney**

R93.429 **Abnormal radiologic findings on diagnostic imaging of unspecified kidney**

R93.49 **Abnormal radiologic findings on diagnostic imaging of other urinary organs**

R93.5 **Abnormal findings on diagnostic imaging of other abdominal regions, including retroperitoneum**

R93.6 **Abnormal findings on diagnostic imaging of limbs**
Excludes2 abnormal finding in skin and subcutaneous tissue (R93.8-)
Coding Clinic: 2Ø2Ø, Q1, P14

R93.7 **Abnormal findings on diagnostic imaging of other parts of musculoskeletal system**
Excludes2 abnormal findings on diagnostic imaging of skull (R93.Ø)

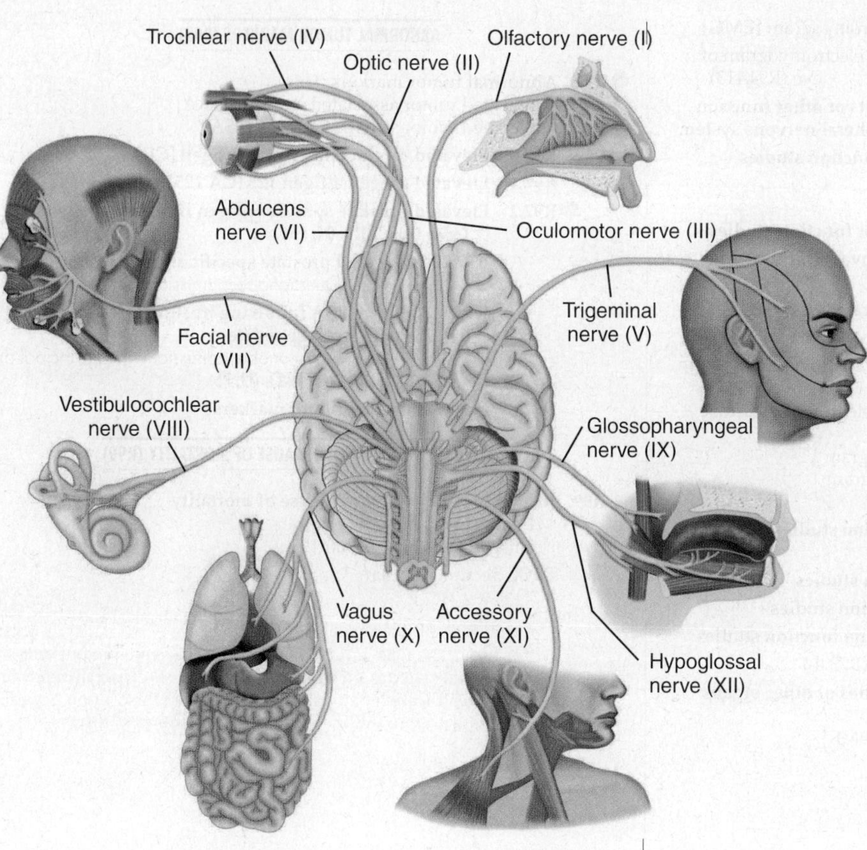

Figure 18-2 Cranial nerves. (From Patton and Thibodeau: Anatomy and physiology, ed 7, St. Louis, Mosby, 2009)

Item 18-1 The **peripheral nervous system** consists of 31 pairs of spinal nerves, 12 pairs of cranial nerves, and the autonomic nerves, which are divided into the parasympathetic and sympathetic nerves. The cranial nerves are: olfactory (I), optic (II), oculomotor (III), trochlear (IV), trigeminal (V), abducens (VI), facial (VII), vestibulocochlear (VIII), glossopharyngeal (IX), vagus (X), accessory (XI), and hypoglossal (XII).

● **R93.8 Abnormal findings on diagnostic imaging of other specified body structures**

● **R93.81 Abnormal radiologic findings on diagnostic imaging of testis**

R93.811 Abnormal radiologic findings on diagnostic imaging of right testicle

R93.812 Abnormal radiologic findings on diagnostic imaging of left testicle

R93.813 Abnormal radiologic findings on diagnostic imaging of testicles, bilateral

R93.819 Abnormal radiologic findings on diagnostic imaging of unspecified testicle

R93.89 Abnormal findings on diagnostic imaging of other specified body structures

Abnormal finding by radioisotope localization of placenta

Abnormal radiological finding in skin and subcutaneous tissue

Mediastinal shift

R93.9 Diagnostic imaging inconclusive due to excess body fat of patient

● **R94 Abnormal results of function studies**

Includes abnormal results of radionuclide [radioisotope] uptake studies

abnormal results of scintigraphy

● **R94.0 Abnormal results of function studies of central nervous system**

R94.01 Abnormal electroencephalogram [EEG]

R94.02 Abnormal brain scan

R94.09 Abnormal results of other function studies of central nervous system

● **R94.1 Abnormal results of function studies of peripheral nervous system and special senses**

● **R94.11 Abnormal results of function studies of eye**

R94.110 Abnormal electro-oculogram [EOG]

R94.111 Abnormal electroretinogram [ERG]

Abnormal retinal function study

R94.112 Abnormal visually evoked potential [VEP]

R94.113 Abnormal oculomotor study

R94.118 Abnormal results of other function studies of eye

● **R94.12 Abnormal results of function studies of ear and other special senses**

R94.120 Abnormal auditory function study

Coding Clinic: 2016, Q3, P17

R94.121 Abnormal vestibular function study

R94.128 Abnormal results of other function studies of ear and other special senses

● **R94.13 Abnormal results of function studies of peripheral nervous system**

R94.130 Abnormal response to nerve stimulation, unspecified

R94.131 **Abnormal electromyogram [EMG]**
Excludes1 electromyogram of eye (R94.113)

R94.138 **Abnormal results of other function studies of peripheral nervous system**

R94.2 **Abnormal results of pulmonary function studies**
Reduced ventilatory capacity
Reduced vital capacity

● R94.3 **Abnormal results of cardiovascular function studies**

R94.30 **Abnormal result of cardiovascular function study, unspecified**

R94.31 **Abnormal electrocardiogram [ECG] [EKG]**
Excludes1 long QT syndrome (I45.81)

R94.39 **Abnormal result of other cardiovascular function study**
Abnormal electrophysiological intracardiac studies
Abnormal phonocardiogram
Abnormal vectorcardiogram
Coding Clinic: 2023, Q1, P25

R94.4 **Abnormal results of kidney function studies**
Abnormal renal function test

R94.5 **Abnormal results of liver function studies**

R94.6 **Abnormal results of thyroid function studies**

R94.7 **Abnormal results of other endocrine function studies**
Excludes2 abnormal glucose (R73.0-)

R94.8 **Abnormal results of function studies of other organs and systems**
Abnormal basal metabolic rate [BMR]
Abnormal bladder function test
Abnormal splenic function test

ABNORMAL TUMOR MARKERS (R97)

● R97 **Abnormal tumor markers**
Elevated tumor associated antigens [TAA]
Elevated tumor specific antigens [TSA]

R97.0 **Elevated carcinoembryonic antigen [CEA]**

R97.1 **Elevated cancer antigen 125 [CA 125]**

● R97.2 **Elevated prostate specific antigen [PSA]**
Coding Clinic: 2016, Q4, P66

R97.20 **Elevated prostate specific antigen [PSA]** A
MCE: Questionable admission when principal dx

R97.21 **Rising PSA following treatment for malignant neoplasm of prostate** A
MCE: Questionable admission when principal dx
Coding Clinic: 2023, Q2, P5

R97.8 **Other abnormal tumor markers**

ILL-DEFINED AND UNKNOWN CAUSE OF MORTALITY (R99)

R99 **Ill-defined and unknown cause of mortality**
Death (unexplained) NOS
Unspecified cause of mortality

OGCR **Section I.C.18.h.**

Death NOS

Code R99, Ill-defined and unknown cause of mortality, is only for use in the very limited circumstance when a patient who has already died is brought into the emergency department or other healthcare facility and is pronounced dead upon arrival. It does not represent the discharge disposition of death.

CHAPTER 19

INJURY, POISONING AND CERTAIN OTHER CONSEQUENCES OF EXTERNAL CAUSES (S00-T88)

OGCR Chapter-Specific Coding Guidelines

19. Chapter 19: Injury, poisoning, and certain other consequences of external causes (S00-T88)

a. Application of 7th Characters in Chapter 19

Most categories in Chapter 19 have a 7th character requirement for each applicable code. Most categories in this chapter have three 7th character values (with the exception of fractures): A, initial encounter, D, subsequent encounter and S, sequela. Categories for traumatic fractures have additional 7th character values. While the patient may be seen by a new or different provider over the course of treatment for an injury, assignment of the 7th character is based on whether the patient is undergoing active treatment and not whether the provider is seeing the patient for the first time.

For complication codes, active treatment refers to treatment for the condition described by the code, even though it may be related to an earlier precipitating problem. For example, code T84.50XA, Infection and inflammatory reaction due to unspecified internal joint prosthesis, initial encounter, is used when active treatment is provided for the infection, even though the condition relates to the prosthetic device, implant or graft that was placed at a previous encounter.

7th character "A", initial encounter is used for each encounter where the patient is receiving active treatment for the condition.

7th character "D" subsequent encounter is used for encounters after the patient has completed active treatment of the condition and is receiving routine care for the condition during the healing or recovery phase.

The aftercare Z codes should not be used for aftercare for conditions such as injuries or poisonings, where 7th characters are provided to identify subsequent care. For example, for aftercare of an injury, assign the acute injury code with the 7th character "D" (subsequent encounter).

7th character "S", sequela, is for use for complications or conditions that arise as a direct result of a condition, such as scar formation after a burn. The scars are sequelae of the burn. When using 7th character "S", it is necessary to use both the injury code that precipitated the sequela and the code for the sequela itself. The "S" is added only to the injury code, not the sequela code. The 7th character "S" identifies the injury responsible for the sequela. The specific type of sequela (e.g. scar) is sequenced first, followed by the injury code.

See Section I.B.10. Sequelae, (Late Effects).

b. Coding of Injuries

When coding injuries, assign separate codes for each injury unless a combination code is provided, in which case the combination code is assigned. Codes from category T07, Unspecified multiple injuries should not be assigned in the inpatient setting unless information for a more specific code is not available. Traumatic injury codes (S00-T14.9) are not to be used for normal, healing surgical wounds or to identify complications of surgical wounds.

The code for the most serious injury, as determined by the provider and the focus of treatment, is sequenced first.

1) Superficial injuries

Superficial injuries such as abrasions or contusions are not coded when associated with more severe injuries of the same site.

2) Primary injury with damage to nerves/blood vessels

When a primary injury results in minor damage to peripheral nerves or blood vessels, the primary injury is sequenced first with additional code(s) for injuries to nerves and spinal cord (such as category S04), and/or injury to blood vessels (such as category S15). When the primary injury is to the blood vessels or nerves, that injury should be sequenced first.

c. Coding of Traumatic Fractures

The principles of multiple coding of injuries should be followed in coding fractures. Fractures of specified sites are coded individually by site in accordance with both the provisions within categories S02, S12, S22, S32, S42, S49, S52, S59, S62, S72, S79, S82, S89, S92 and the level of detail furnished by medical record content.

A fracture not indicated as open or closed should be coded to closed. A fracture not indicated whether displaced or not displaced should be coded to displaced.

More specific guidelines are as follows:

1) Initial vs. Subsequent Encounter for Fractures

Traumatic fractures are coded using the appropriate 7th character for initial encounter (A, B, C) for each encounter where the patient is receiving active treatment for the fracture. The appropriate 7th character for initial encounter should also be assigned for a patient who delayed seeking treatment for the fracture or nonunion.

Fractures are coded using the appropriate 7th character for subsequent care for encounters after the patient has completed active treatment of the fracture and is receiving routine care for the fracture during the healing or recovery phase.

Care for complications of surgical treatment for fracture repairs during the healing or recovery phase should be coded with the appropriate complication codes.

Care of complications of fractures, such as malunion and nonunion, should be reported with the appropriate 7th character for subsequent care with nonunion (K, M, N,) or subsequent care with malunion (P, Q, R).

Malunion/nonunion: The appropriate 7th character for initial encounter should also be assigned for a patient who delayed seeking treatment for the fracture or nonunion.

The open fracture designations in the assignment of the 7th character for fractures of the forearm, femur and lower leg, including ankle are based on the Gustilo open fracture classification. When the Gustilo classification type is not specified for an open fracture, the 7th character for open fracture type I or II should be assigned (B, E, H, M, Q).

A code from category M80, not a traumatic fracture code, should be used for any patient with known osteoporosis who suffers a fracture, even if the patient had a minor fall or trauma, if that fall or trauma would not usually break a normal, healthy bone.

See Section I.C.13. Osteoporosis.

The aftercare Z codes should not be used for aftercare for traumatic fractures. For aftercare of a traumatic fracture, assign the acute fracture code with the appropriate 7th character.

2) Multiple fractures sequencing

Multiple fractures are sequenced in accordance with the severity of the fracture.

d. Coding of Burns and Corrosions

The ICD-10-CM makes a distinction between burns and corrosions. The burn codes are for thermal burns, except sunburns, that come from a heat source, such as a fire or hot appliance. The burn codes are also for burns resulting from electricity and radiation. Corrosions are burns due to chemicals. The guidelines are the same for burns and corrosions.

Current burns (T20-T25) are classified by depth, extent and by agent (X code). Burns are classified by depth as first degree (erythema), second degree (blistering), and third degree (full-thickness involvement). Burns of the eye and internal organs (T26-T28) are classified by site, but not by degree.

1) Sequencing of burn and related condition codes

Sequence first the code that reflects the highest degree of burn when more than one burn is present.

a. When the reason for the admission or encounter is for treatment of external multiple burns, sequence first the code that reflects the burn of the highest degree.

b. When a patient has both internal and external burns, the circumstances of admission govern the selection of the principal diagnosis or first-listed diagnosis.

c. When a patient is admitted for burn injuries and other related conditions such as smoke inhalation and/or respiratory failure, the circumstances of admission govern the selection of the principal or first-listed diagnosis.

2) Burns of the same *anatomic* site
Classify burns of the same anatomic site and on the same side but of different degrees to the subcategory identifying the highest degree recorded in the diagnosis (e.g., for second- and third-degree burns of right thigh, assign only code T24.311-).

3) Non-healing burns
Non-healing burns are coded as acute burns.

Necrosis of burned skin should be coded as a non-healed burn.

4) Infected Burn
For any documented infected burn site, use an additional code for the infection.

5) Assign separate codes for each burn site
When coding burns, assign separate codes for each burn site. Category T3Ø, Burn and corrosion, body region unspecified is extremely vague and should rarely be used.

Codes for burns of "multiple sites" should only be assigned when the medical record documentation does not specify the individual sites.

6) Burns and Corrosions Classified According to Extent of Body Surface Involved
Assign codes from category T31, Burns classified according to extent of body surface involved, or T32, Corrosions classified according to extent of body surface involved, when the site of the burn is not specified or when there is a need for additional data. It is advisable to use category T31 as additional coding when needed to provide data for evaluating burn mortality, such as that needed by burn units. It is also advisable to use category T31 as an additional code for reporting purposes when there is mention of a third-degree burn involving 2Ø percent or more of the body surface.

Categories T31 and T32 are based on the classic "rule of nines" in estimating body surface involved: head and neck are assigned nine percent, each arm nine percent, each leg 18 percent, the anterior trunk 18 percent, posterior trunk 18 percent, and genitalia one percent. Providers may change these percentage assignments where necessary to accommodate infants and children who have proportionately larger heads than adults, and patients who have large buttocks, thighs, or abdomen that involve burns.

7) Encounters for treatment of sequela of burns
Encounters for the treatment of the late effects of burns or corrosions (i.e., scars or joint contractures) should be coded with a burn or corrosion code with the 7th character "S" for sequela.

8) Sequelae with a late effect code and current burn
When appropriate, both a code for a current burn or corrosion with 7th character "A" or "D" and a burn or corrosion code with 7th character "S" may be assigned on the same record (when both a current burn and sequelae of an old burn exist). Burns and corrosions do not heal at the same rate and a current healing wound may still exist with sequela of a healed burn or corrosion.

See Section I.B.1Ø. Sequela, (Late Effects).

9) Use of an external cause code with burns and corrosions
An external cause code should be used with burns and corrosions to identify the source and intent of the burn, as well as the place where it occurred.

e. Adverse Effects, Poisoning , Underdosing and Toxic Effects
Codes in categories T36-T65 are combination codes that include the substance that was taken as well as the intent. No additional external cause code is required for poisonings, toxic effects, adverse effects and underdosing codes.

1) Do not code directly from the Table of Drugs
Do not code directly from the Table of Drugs and Chemicals. Always refer back to the Tabular List.

2) Use as many codes as necessary to describe
Use as many codes as necessary to describe completely all drugs, medicinal or biological substances.

3) If the same code would describe the causative agent
If the same code would describe the causative agent for more than one adverse reaction, poisoning, toxic effect or underdosing, assign the code only once.

4) If two or more drugs, medicinal or biological substances
If two or more drugs, medicinal or biological substances are reported, code each individually unless a combination code is listed in the Table of Drugs and Chemicals.

5) The occurrence of drug toxicity is classified in ICD-10-CM as follows:

(a) Adverse Effect
When coding an adverse effect of a drug that has been correctly prescribed and properly administered, assign the appropriate code for the nature of the adverse effect followed by the appropriate code for the adverse effect of the drug (T36-T5Ø). The code for the drug should have a 5th or 6th character "5" (for example T36.ØX5-) Examples of the nature of an adverse effect are tachycardia, delirium, gastrointestinal hemorrhaging, vomiting, hypokalemia, hepatitis, renal failure, or respiratory failure.

(b) Poisoning
When coding a poisoning or reaction to the improper use of a medication (e.g., overdose, wrong substance given or taken in error, wrong route of administration), first assign the appropriate code from categories T36-T5Ø. The poisoning codes have an associated intent as their 5th or 6th character (accidental, intentional self-harm, assault and undetermined). If the intent of the poisoning is unknown or unspecified, code the intent as accidental intent. The undetermined intent is only for use if the documentation in the record specifies that the intent cannot be determined. Use additional code(s) for all manifestations of poisonings.

If there is also a diagnosis of abuse or dependence of the substance, the abuse or dependence is assigned as an additional code.

Examples of poisoning include:

(i) Error was made in drug prescription
Errors made in drug prescription or in the administration of the drug by provider, nurse, patient, or other person.

(ii) Overdose of a drug intentionally taken If an overdose of a drug was intentionally taken or administered and resulted in drug toxicity, it would be coded as a poisoning.

(iii) Nonprescribed drug taken with correctly prescribed and properly administered drug.
If a nonprescribed drug or medicinal agent was taken in combination with a correctly prescribed and properly administered drug, any drug toxicity or other reaction resulting from the interaction of the two drugs would be classified as a poisoning.

(iv) Interaction of drug(s) and alcohol.
When a reaction results from the interaction of a drug(s) and alcohol, this would be classified as poisoning.

See Section I.C.4. if poisoning is the result of insulin pump malfunctions.

(c) Underdosing
Underdosing refers to taking less of a medication than is prescribed by a provider or a manufacturer's instruction. Discontinuing the use of a prescribed medication on the patient's own initiative (not directed by the patient's provider) is also classified as an underdosing. For underdosing, assign the code from categories T36-T5Ø (fifth or sixth character "6").

Codes for underdosing should never be assigned as principal or first-listed codes. If a patient has a relapse or exacerbation of the medical condition for which the drug is prescribed because of the reduction in dose, then the medical condition itself should be coded.

Noncompliance (Z91.12-, Z91.13- and Z91.14-) or complication of care (Y63.6-Y63.9) codes are to be used with an underdosing code to indicate intent, if known.

(d) Toxic Effects

When a harmful substance is ingested or comes in contact with a person, this is classified as a toxic effect. The toxic effect codes are in categories T51-T65.

Toxic effect codes have an associated intent: accidental, intentional self-harm, assault and undetermined.

f. Adult and child abuse, neglect and other maltreatment

Sequence first the appropriate code from categories T74 (Adult and child abuse, neglect and other maltreatment, confirmed) or T76 (Adult and child abuse, neglect and other maltreatment, suspected) for abuse, neglect and other maltreatment, followed by any accompanying mental health or injury code(s).

If the documentation in the medical record states abuse or neglect it is coded as confirmed (T74.-). It is coded as suspected if it is documented as suspected (T76.-).

For cases of confirmed abuse or neglect an external cause code from the assault section (X92-Y09) should be added to identify the cause of any physical injuries. A perpetrator code (Y07) should be added when the perpetrator of the abuse is known. For suspected cases of abuse or neglect, do not report external cause or perpetrator code.

If a suspected case of abuse, neglect or mistreatment is ruled out during an encounter code Z04.71, Encounter for examination and observation following alleged physical adult abuse, ruled out, or code Z04.72, Encounter for examination and observation following alleged child physical abuse, ruled out, should be used, not a code from T76.

If a suspected case of alleged rape or sexual abuse is ruled out during an encounter code Z04.41, Encounter for examination and observation following alleged adult rape or code Z04.42, Encounter for examination and observation following alleged child rape, should be used, not a code from T76.

If a suspected case of forced sexual exploitation or forced labor exploitation is ruled out during an encounter, code Z04.81, Encounter for examination and observation of victim following forced sexual exploitation, or code Z04.82, Encounter for examination and observation of victim following forced labor exploitation, should be used, not a code from T76.

See Section I.C.15. Abuse in a pregnant patient.

g. Complications of care

1) General guidelines for complications of care

(a) Documentation of complications of care

See Section I.B.16. for information on documentation of complications of care.

2) Pain due to medical devices

Pain associated with devices, implants or grafts left in a surgical site (for example painful hip prosthesis) is assigned to the appropriate code(s) found in Chapter 19, Injury, poisoning, and certain other consequences of external causes. Specific codes for pain due to medical devices are found in the T code section of the ICD-10-CM. Use additional code(s) from category G89 to identify acute or chronic pain due to presence of the device, implant or graft (G89.18 or G89.28).

3) Transplant complications

(a) Transplant complications other than kidney

Codes under category T86, Complications of transplanted organs and tissues, are for use for both complications and rejection of transplanted organs. A transplant complication code is only assigned if the complication affects the function of the transplanted organ. Two codes are required to fully describe a transplant complication: the appropriate code from category T86 and a secondary code that identifies the complication.

Pre-existing conditions or conditions that develop after the transplant are not coded as complications unless they affect the function of the transplanted organs.

See I.C.21. for transplant organ removal status.

See I.C.2. for malignant neoplasm associated with transplanted organ.

(b) Kidney transplant complications

Patients who have undergone kidney transplant may still have some form of chronic kidney disease (CKD) because the kidney transplant may not fully restore kidney function. Code T86.1- should be assigned for documented complications of a kidney transplant, such as transplant failure or rejection or other transplant complication. Code T86.1- should not be assigned for post kidney transplant patients who have chronic kidney (CKD) unless a transplant complication such as transplant failure or rejection is documented. If the documentation is unclear as to whether the patient has a complication of the transplant, query the provider.

Conditions that affect the function of the transplanted kidney, other than CKD, should be assigned a code from subcategory T86.1, Complications of transplanted organ, Kidney, and a secondary code that identifies the complication.

For patients with CKD following a kidney transplant, but who do not have a complication such as failure or rejection, *see Section I.C.14. Chronic kidney disease and kidney transplant status.*

4) Complication codes that include the external cause

As with certain other T codes, some of the complications of care codes have the external cause included in the code. The code includes the nature of the complication as well as the type of procedure that caused the complication. No external cause code indicating the type of procedure is necessary for these codes.

5) Complications of care codes within the body system chapters

Intraoperative and postprocedural complication codes are found within the body system chapters with codes specific to the organs and structures of that body system. These codes should be sequenced first, followed by a code(s) for the specific complication, if applicable.

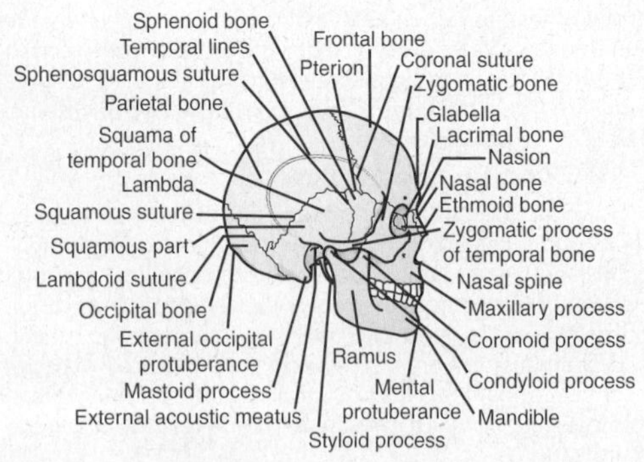

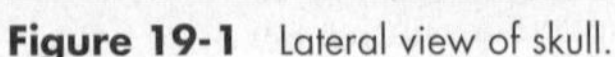

Figure 19-1 Lateral view of skull.

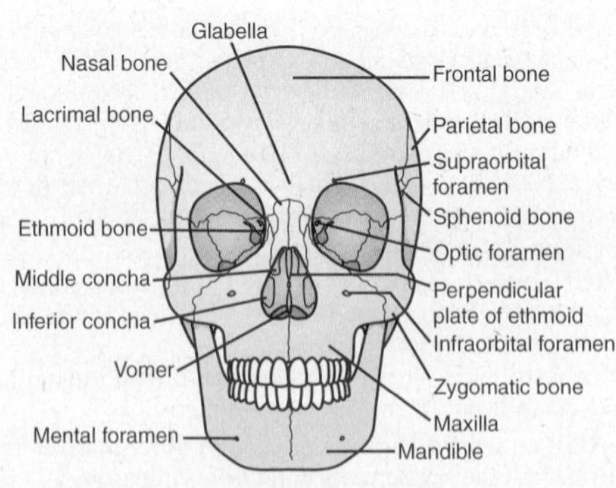

Figure 19-2 Frontal view of skull.

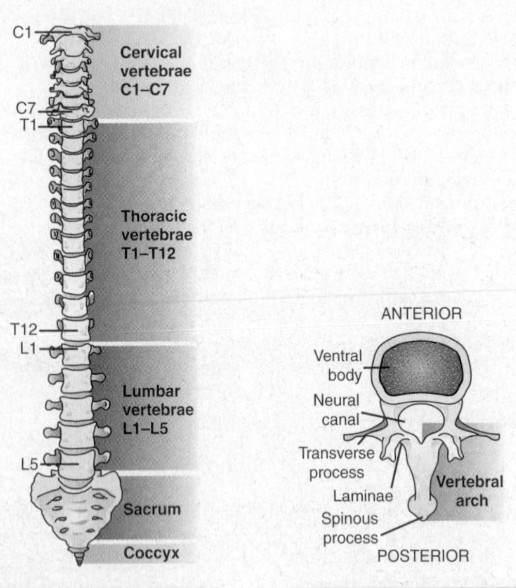

Figure 19-3 Anterior view of vertebral column.

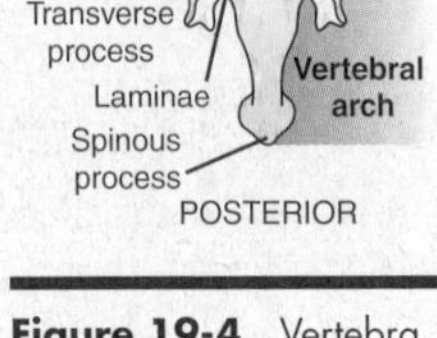

Figure 19-4 Vertebra viewed from above.

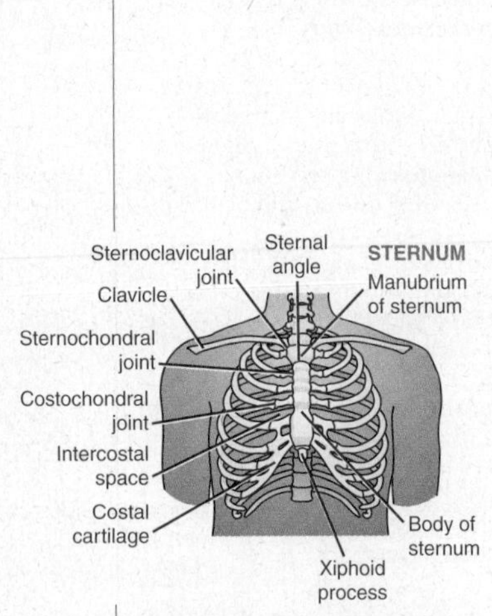

Figure 19-5 Anterior view of rib cage.

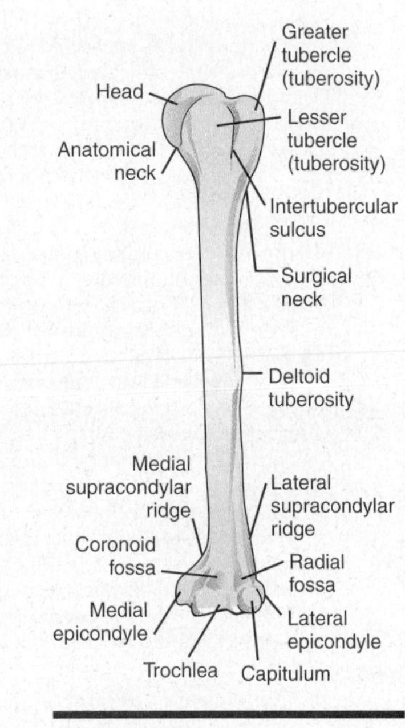

Figure 19-6 Anterior aspect of left humerus.

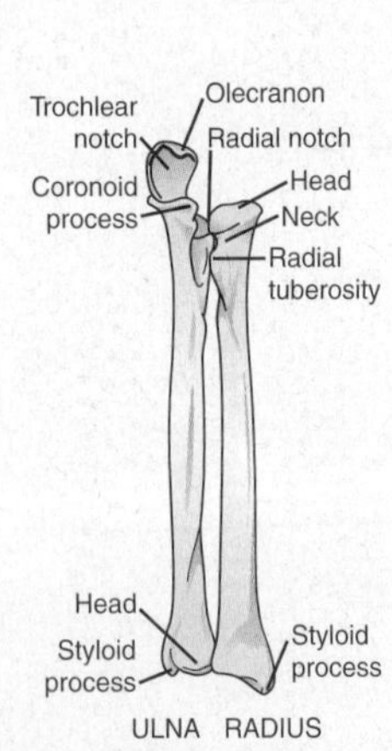

Figure 19-7 Anterior aspect of left radius and ulna.

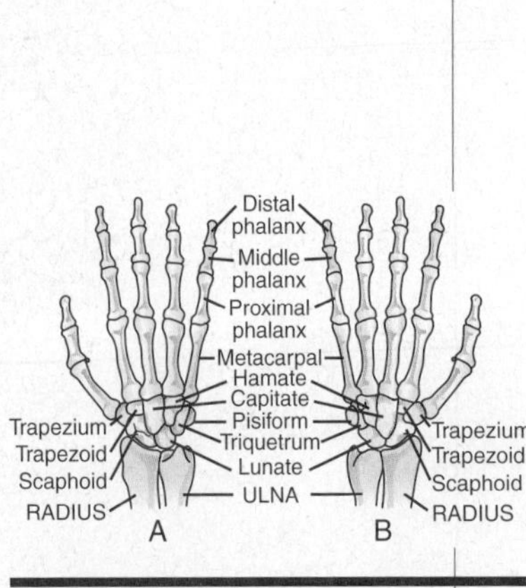

Figure 19-8 Right hand and wrist: **A.** Dorsal surface. **B.** Palmar surface.

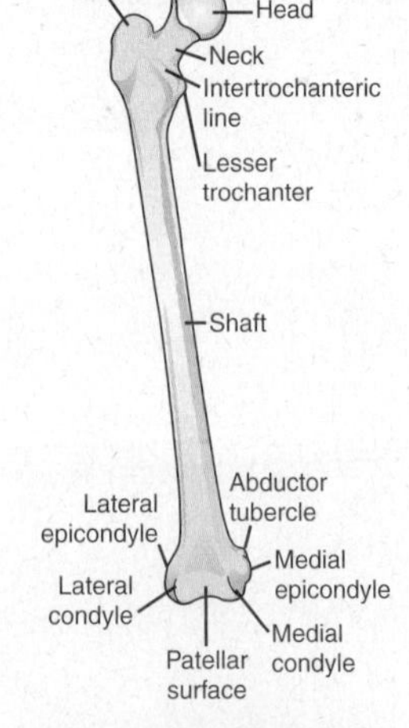

Figure 19-9 Anterior aspect of right femur.

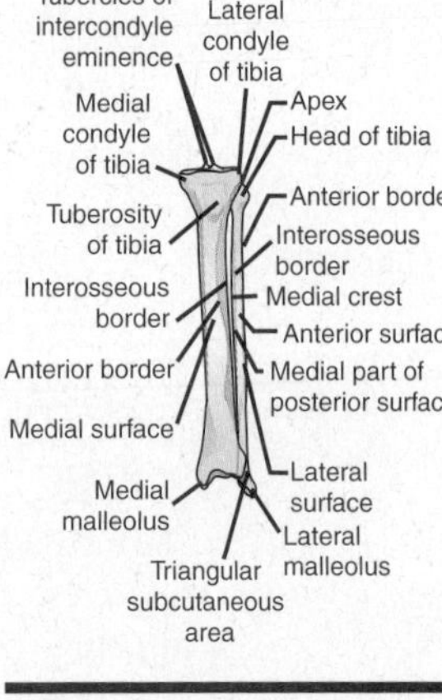

Figure 19-10 Anterior aspect of left tibia and fibula.

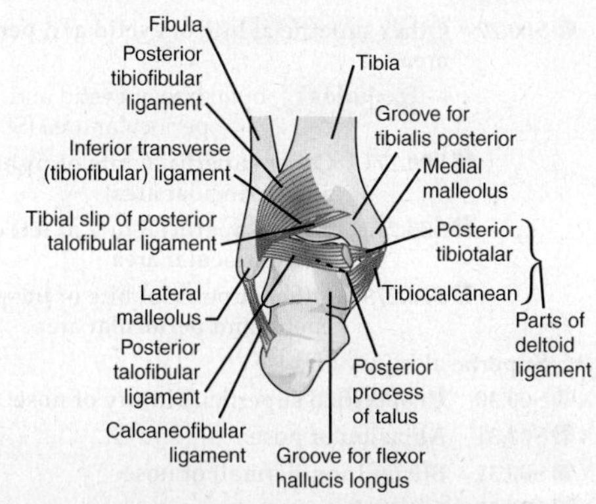

Figure 19-11 Posterior aspect of the left ankle joint.

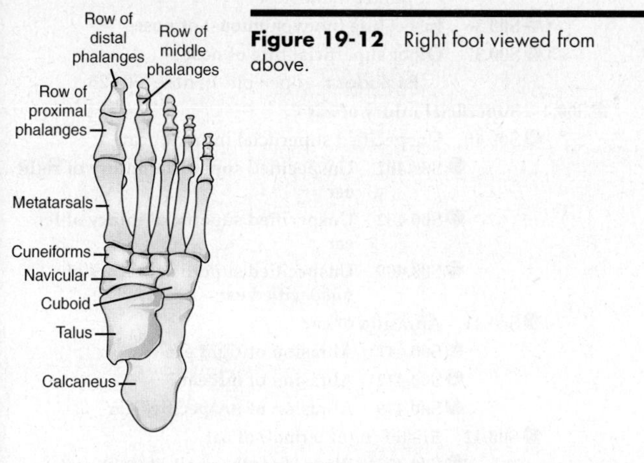

Figure 19-12 Right foot viewed from above.

CHAPTER 19

INJURY, POISONING AND CERTAIN OTHER CONSEQUENCES OF EXTERNAL CAUSES (S00-T88)

Note: Use secondary code(s) from Chapter 20, External causes of morbidity, to indicate cause of injury. Codes within the T section that include the external cause do not require an additional external cause code.

Use additional code to identify any retained foreign body, if applicable (Z18.-)

Excludes1 birth trauma (P10-P15)
obstetric trauma (O70-O71)

Note: The chapter uses the S-section for coding different types of injuries related to single body regions and the T-section to cover injuries to unspecified body regions as well as poisoning and certain other consequences of external causes.

This chapter contains the following blocks:

S00-S09	Injuries to the head
S10-S19	Injuries to the neck
S20-S29	Injuries to the thorax
S30-S39	Injuries to the abdomen, lower back, lumbar spine, pelvis and external genitals
S40-S49	Injuries to the shoulder and upper arm
S50-S59	Injuries to the elbow and forearm
S60-S69	Injuries to the wrist, hand, and fingers
S70-S79	Injuries to the hip and thigh
S80-S89	Injuries to the knee and lower leg
S90-S99	Injuries to the ankle and foot
T07	Injuries involving multiple body regions
T14	Injury of unspecified body region
T15-T19	Effects of foreign body entering through natural orifice
T20-T25	Burns and corrosions of external body surface, specified by site
T26-T28	Burns and corrosions confined to eye and internal organs
T30-T32	Burns and corrosions of multiple and unspecified body regions
T33-T34	Frostbite
T36-T50	Poisoning by, adverse effect of and underdosing of drugs, medicaments and biological substances
T51-T65	Toxic effects of substances chiefly nonmedicinal as to source
T66-T78	Other and unspecified effects of external causes
T79	Certain early complications of trauma
T80-T88	Complications of surgical and medical care, not elsewhere classified

INJURIES TO THE HEAD (S00-S09)

Includes injuries of ear
injuries of eye
injuries of face [any part]
injuries of gum
injuries of jaw
injuries of oral cavity
injuries of palate
injuries of periocular area
injuries of scalp
injuries of temporomandibular joint area
injuries of tongue
injuries of tooth

Code also for any associated infection

Excludes2 burns and corrosions (T20-T32)
effects of foreign body in ear (T16)
effects of foreign body in larynx (T17.3)
effects of foreign body in mouth NOS (T18.0)
effects of foreign body in nose (T17.0-T17.1)
effects of foreign body in pharynx (T17.2)
effects of foreign body on external eye (T15.-)
frostbite (T33-T34)
insect bite or sting, venomous (T63.4)

● **S00 Superficial injury of head**

Excludes1 diffuse cerebral contusion (S06.2-)
focal cerebral contusion (S06.3-)
injury of eye and orbit (S05.-)
open wound of head (S01.-)

The appropriate 7th character is to be added to each code from category S00

A	initial encounter *All encounters involving diagnosis and treatment*
D	subsequent encounter *Encounters during the healing phase*
S	sequela

● **S00.0 Superficial injury of scalp**

X● **S00.00 Unspecified superficial injury of scalp**

X● **S00.01 Abrasion of scalp**

X● **S00.02 Blister (nonthermal) of scalp**

X● **S00.03 Contusion of scalp**
Bruise of scalp
Hematoma of scalp

X● **S00.04 External constriction of part of scalp**

X● **S00.05 Superficial foreign body of scalp**
Splinter in the scalp

X● **S00.06 Insect bite (nonvenomous) of scalp**

X● **S00.07 Other superficial bite of scalp**
Excludes1 open bite of scalp (S01.05)

S00.1 Contusion of eyelid and periocular area
Black eye
Excludes2 contusion of eyeball and orbital tissues (S05.1-)
X S00.10 Contusion of unspecified eyelid and periocular area
X S00.11 Contusion of right eyelid and periocular area
X S00.12 Contusion of left eyelid and periocular area
S00.2 Other and unspecified superficial injuries of eyelid and periocular area
Excludes2 superficial injury of conjunctiva and cornea (S05.0-)
S00.20 Unspecified superficial injury of eyelid and periocular area
S00.201 Unspecified superficial injury of right eyelid and periocular area
S00.202 Unspecified superficial injury of left eyelid and periocular area
S00.209 Unspecified superficial injury of unspecified eyelid and periocular area
S00.21 Abrasion of eyelid and periocular area
S00.211 Abrasion of right eyelid and periocular area
S00.212 Abrasion of left eyelid and periocular area
S00.219 Abrasion of unspecified eyelid and periocular area
S00.22 Blister (nonthermal) of eyelid and periocular area
S00.221 Blister (nonthermal) of right eyelid and periocular area
S00.222 Blister (nonthermal) of left eyelid and periocular area
S00.229 Blister (nonthermal) of unspecified eyelid and periocular area
S00.24 External constriction of eyelid and periocular area
S00.241 External constriction of right eyelid and periocular area
S00.242 External constriction of left eyelid and periocular area
S00.249 External constriction of unspecified eyelid and periocular area
S00.25 Superficial foreign body of eyelid and periocular area
Splinter of eyelid and periocular area
Excludes2 retained foreign body in eyelid (H02.81-)
S00.251 Superficial foreign body of right eyelid and periocular area
S00.252 Superficial foreign body of left eyelid and periocular area
S00.259 Superficial foreign body of unspecified eyelid and periocular area
S00.26 Insect bite (nonvenomous) of eyelid and periocular area
S00.261 Insect bite (nonvenomous) of right eyelid and periocular area
S00.262 Insect bite (nonvenomous) of left eyelid and periocular area
S00.269 Insect bite (nonvenomous) of unspecified eyelid and periocular area
S00.27 Other superficial bite of eyelid and periocular area
Excludes1 open bite of eyelid and periocular area (S01.15)
S00.271 Other superficial bite of right eyelid and periocular area
S00.272 Other superficial bite of left eyelid and periocular area
S00.279 Other superficial bite of unspecified eyelid and periocular area
S00.3 Superficial injury of nose
X S00.30 Unspecified superficial injury of nose
X S00.31 Abrasion of nose
X S00.32 Blister (nonthermal) of nose
X S00.33 Contusion of nose
Bruise of nose
Hematoma of nose
X S00.34 External constriction of nose
X S00.35 Superficial foreign body of nose
Splinter in the nose
X S00.36 Insect bite (nonvenomous) of nose
X S00.37 Other superficial bite of nose
Excludes1 open bite of nose (S01.25)
S00.4 Superficial injury of ear
S00.40 Unspecified superficial injury of ear
S00.401 Unspecified superficial injury of right ear
S00.402 Unspecified superficial injury of left ear
S00.409 Unspecified superficial injury of unspecified ear
S00.41 Abrasion of ear
S00.411 Abrasion of right ear
S00.412 Abrasion of left ear
S00.419 Abrasion of unspecified ear
S00.42 Blister (nonthermal) of ear
S00.421 Blister (nonthermal) of right ear
S00.422 Blister (nonthermal) of left ear
S00.429 Blister (nonthermal) of unspecified ear
S00.43 Contusion of ear
Bruise of ear
Hematoma of ear
S00.431 Contusion of right ear
S00.432 Contusion of left ear
S00.439 Contusion of unspecified ear
S00.44 External constriction of ear
S00.441 External constriction of right ear
S00.442 External constriction of left ear
S00.449 External constriction of unspecified ear
S00.45 Superficial foreign body of ear
Splinter in the ear
S00.451 Superficial foreign body of right ear
S00.452 Superficial foreign body of left ear
S00.459 Superficial foreign body of unspecified ear
S00.46 Insect bite (nonvenomous) of ear
S00.461 Insect bite (nonvenomous) of right ear
S00.462 Insect bite (nonvenomous) of left ear
S00.469 Insect bite (nonvenomous) of unspecified ear

● S00.47 Other superficial bite of ear
Excludes1 open bite of ear (S01.35)
● S00.471 Other superficial bite of right ear
● S00.472 Other superficial bite of left ear
● S00.479 Other superficial bite of unspecified ear
● S00.5 Superficial injury of lip and oral cavity
● S00.50 Unspecified superficial injury of lip and oral cavity
● S00.501 Unspecified superficial injury of lip
● S00.502 Unspecified superficial injury of oral cavity
● S00.51 Abrasion of lip and oral cavity
● S00.511 Abrasion of lip
● S00.512 Abrasion of oral cavity
● S00.52 Blister (nonthermal) of lip and oral cavity
● S00.521 Blister (nonthermal) of lip
● S00.522 Blister (nonthermal) of oral cavity
● S00.53 Contusion of lip and oral cavity
● S00.531 Contusion of lip
Bruise of lip
Hematoma of lip
● S00.532 Contusion of oral cavity
Bruise of oral cavity
Hematoma of oral cavity
● S00.54 External constriction of lip and oral cavity
● S00.541 External constriction of lip
● S00.542 External constriction of oral cavity
● S00.55 Superficial foreign body of lip and oral cavity
● S00.551 Superficial foreign body of lip
Splinter of lip and oral cavity
● S00.552 Superficial foreign body of oral cavity
Splinter of lip and oral cavity
● S00.56 Insect bite (nonvenomous) of lip and oral cavity
● S00.561 Insect bite (nonvenomous) of lip
● S00.562 Insect bite (nonvenomous) of oral cavity
● S00.57 Other superficial bite of lip and oral cavity
● S00.571 Other superficial bite of lip
Excludes1 open bite of lip (S01.551)
● S00.572 Other superficial bite of oral cavity
Excludes1 open bite of oral cavity (S01.552)
● S00.8 Superficial injury of other parts of head
Superficial injuries of face [any part]
X● S00.80 Unspecified superficial injury of other part of head
X● S00.81 Abrasion of other part of head
X● S00.82 Blister (nonthermal) of other part of head
X● S00.83 Contusion of other part of head
Bruise of other part of head
Hematoma of other part of head
X● S00.84 External constriction of other part of head
X● S00.85 Superficial foreign body of other part of head
Splinter in other part of head
X● S00.86 Insect bite (nonvenomous) of other part of head
X● S00.87 Other superficial bite of other part of head
Excludes1 open bite of other part of head (S01.85)
● S00.9 Superficial injury of unspecified part of head
X● S00.90 Unspecified superficial injury of unspecified part of head
X● S00.91 Abrasion of unspecified part of head
X● S00.92 Blister (nonthermal) of unspecified part of head
X● S00.93 Contusion of unspecified part of head
Bruise of head
Hematoma of head
X● S00.94 External constriction of unspecified part of head
X● S00.95 Superficial foreign body of unspecified part of head
Splinter of head
X● S00.96 Insect bite (nonvenomous) of unspecified part of head
X● S00.97 Other superficial bite of unspecified part of head
Excludes1 open bite of head (S01.95)

● S01 Open wound of head
Code also any associated:
injury of cranial nerve (S04.-)
injury of muscle and tendon of head (S09.1-)
intracranial injury (S06.-)
wound infection
Excludes1 open skull fracture (S02.- with 7th character B)
Excludes2 injury of eye and orbit (S05.-)
traumatic amputation of part of head (S08.-)
The appropriate 7th character is to be added to each code from category S01

A	initial encounter
D	subsequent encounter
S	sequela

● S01.0 Open wound of scalp
Excludes1 avulsion of scalp (S08.0-)
X● S01.00 Unspecified open wound of scalp
X● S01.01 Laceration without foreign body of scalp
X● S01.02 Laceration with foreign body of scalp
Coding Clinic: 2015, Q1, P5-7
X● S01.03 Puncture wound without foreign body of scalp
X● S01.04 Puncture wound with foreign body of scalp
X● S01.05 Open bite of scalp
Bite of scalp NOS
Excludes1 superficial bite of scalp (S00.06, S00.07-)
● S01.1 Open wound of eyelid and periocular area
Open wound of eyelid and periocular area with or without involvement of lacrimal passages
● S01.10 Unspecified open wound of eyelid and periocular area (Ex) PDX 1611
● S01.101 Unspecified open wound of right eyelid and periocular area A
● S01.102 Unspecified open wound of left eyelid and periocular area A
● S01.109 Unspecified open wound of unspecified eyelid and periocular area A
● S01.11 Laceration without foreign body of eyelid and periocular area
● S01.111 Laceration without foreign body of right eyelid and periocular area
● S01.112 Laceration without foreign body of left eyelid and periocular area
● S01.119 Laceration without foreign body of unspecified eyelid and periocular area
● S01.12 Laceration with foreign body of eyelid and periocular area
● S01.121 Laceration with foreign body of right eyelid and periocular area
● S01.122 Laceration with foreign body of left eyelid and periocular area
● S01.129 Laceration with foreign body of unspecified eyelid and periocular area

CHAPTER 19 (S00-T88)

● S01.13 Puncture wound without foreign body of eyelid and periocular area
● S01.131 Puncture wound without foreign body of right eyelid and periocular area
● S01.132 Puncture wound without foreign body of left eyelid and periocular area
● S01.139 Puncture wound without foreign body of unspecified eyelid and periocular area
● S01.14 Puncture wound with foreign body of eyelid and periocular area
● S01.141 Puncture wound with foreign body of right eyelid and periocular area
● S01.142 Puncture wound with foreign body of left eyelid and periocular area
● S01.149 Puncture wound with foreign body of unspecified eyelid and periocular area
● S01.15 Open bite of eyelid and periocular area
Bite of eyelid and periocular area NOS
Excludes1 superficial bite of eyelid and periocular area (S00.26, S00.27)
● S01.151 Open bite of right eyelid and periocular area
● S01.152 Open bite of left eyelid and periocular area
● S01.159 Open bite of unspecified eyelid and periocular area
● S01.2 Open wound of nose
X● S01.20 Unspecified open wound of nose
X● S01.21 Laceration without foreign body of nose
Coding Clinic: 2015, Q1, P5-6
X● S01.22 Laceration with foreign body of nose
X● S01.23 Puncture wound without foreign body of nose
X● S01.24 Puncture wound with foreign body of nose
X● S01.25 Open bite of nose
Bite of nose NOS
Excludes1 superficial bite of nose (S00.36, S00.37)
● S01.3 Open wound of ear
● S01.30 Unspecified open wound of ear
● S01.301 Unspecified open wound of right ear
● S01.302 Unspecified open wound of left ear
● S01.309 Unspecified open wound of unspecified ear
● S01.31 Laceration without foreign body of ear
● S01.311 Laceration without foreign body of right ear
● S01.312 Laceration without foreign body of left ear
● S01.319 Laceration without foreign body of unspecified ear
● S01.32 Laceration with foreign body of ear
● S01.321 Laceration with foreign body of right ear
● S01.322 Laceration with foreign body of left ear
● S01.329 Laceration with foreign body of unspecified ear
● S01.33 Puncture wound without foreign body of ear
● S01.331 Puncture wound without foreign body of right ear
● S01.332 Puncture wound without foreign body of left ear
● S01.339 Puncture wound without foreign body of unspecified ear
● S01.34 Puncture wound with foreign body of ear
● S01.341 Puncture wound with foreign body of right ear
● S01.342 Puncture wound with foreign body of left ear
● S01.349 Puncture wound with foreign body of unspecified ear
● S01.35 Open bite of ear
Bite of ear NOS
Excludes1 superficial bite of ear (S00.46, S00.47)
● S01.351 Open bite of right ear
● S01.352 Open bite of left ear
● S01.359 Open bite of unspecified ear
● S01.4 Open wound of cheek and temporomandibular area
● S01.40 Unspecified open wound of cheek and temporomandibular area
● S01.401 Unspecified open wound of right cheek and temporomandibular area
● S01.402 Unspecified open wound of left cheek and temporomandibular area
● S01.409 Unspecified open wound of unspecified cheek and temporomandibular area
● S01.41 Laceration without foreign body of cheek and temporomandibular area
● S01.411 Laceration without foreign body of right cheek and temporomandibular area
Coding Clinic: 2015, Q1, P5-7
● S01.412 Laceration without foreign body of left cheek and temporomandibular area
● S01.419 Laceration without foreign body of unspecified cheek and temporomandibular area
● S01.42 Laceration with foreign body of cheek and temporomandibular area
● S01.421 Laceration with foreign body of right cheek and temporomandibular area
● S01.422 Laceration with foreign body of left cheek and temporomandibular area
● S01.429 Laceration with foreign body of unspecified cheek and temporomandibular area
● S01.43 Puncture wound without foreign body of cheek and temporomandibular area
● S01.431 Puncture wound without foreign body of right cheek and temporomandibular area
● S01.432 Puncture wound without foreign body of left cheek and temporomandibular area
● S01.439 Puncture wound without foreign body of unspecified cheek and temporomandibular area
● S01.44 Puncture wound with foreign body of cheek and temporomandibular area
● S01.441 Puncture wound with foreign body of right cheek and temporomandibular area
● S01.442 Puncture wound with foreign body of left cheek and temporomandibular area
● S01.449 Puncture wound with foreign body of unspecified cheek and temporomandibular area

- **S01.45** Open bite of cheek and temporomandibular area
  Bite of cheek and temporomandibular area NOS
  Excludes2 superficial bite of cheek and temporomandibular area (S00.86, S00.87)
  - **S01.451** Open bite of right cheek and temporomandibular area
  - **S01.452** Open bite of left cheek and temporomandibular area
  - **S01.459** Open bite of unspecified cheek and temporomandibular area
- **S01.5** Open wound of lip and oral cavity
  Excludes2 tooth dislocation (S03.2)
  tooth fracture (S02.5)
  - **S01.50** Unspecified open wound of lip and oral cavity
    - **S01.501** Unspecified open wound of lip
    - **S01.502** Unspecified open wound of oral cavity
  - **S01.51** Laceration of lip and oral cavity without foreign body
    - **S01.511** Laceration without foreign body of lip
    - **S01.512** Laceration without foreign body of oral cavity
  - **S01.52** Laceration of lip and oral cavity with foreign body
    - **S01.521** Laceration with foreign body of lip
    - **S01.522** Laceration with foreign body of oral cavity
  - **S01.53** Puncture wound of lip and oral cavity without foreign body
    - **S01.531** Puncture wound without foreign body of lip
    - **S01.532** Puncture wound without foreign body of oral cavity
  - **S01.54** Puncture wound of lip and oral cavity with foreign body
    - **S01.541** Puncture wound with foreign body of lip
    - **S01.542** Puncture wound with foreign body of oral cavity
  - **S01.55** Open bite of lip and oral cavity
    - **S01.551** Open bite of lip
      Bite of lip NOS
      Excludes1 superficial bite of lip (S00.571)
    - **S01.552** Open bite of oral cavity
      Bite of oral cavity NOS
      Excludes1 superficial bite of oral cavity (S00.572)
- **S01.8** Open wound of other parts of head
  - X **S01.80** Unspecified open wound of other part of head
  - X **S01.81** Laceration without foreign body of other part of head
  - X **S01.82** Laceration with foreign body of other part of head
  - X **S01.83** Puncture wound without foreign body of other part of head
  - X **S01.84** Puncture wound with foreign body of other part of head
  - X **S01.85** Open bite of other part of head
    Bite of other part of head NOS
    Excludes1 superficial bite of other part of head (S00.87)
- **S01.9** Open wound of unspecified part of head
  - X **S01.90** Unspecified open wound of unspecified part of head
  - X **S01.91** Laceration without foreign body of unspecified part of head
  - X **S01.92** Laceration with foreign body of unspecified part of head
  - X **S01.93** Puncture wound without foreign body of unspecified part of head
  - X **S01.94** Puncture wound with foreign body of unspecified part of head
  - X **S01.95** Open bite of unspecified part of head
    Bite of head NOS
    Excludes1 superficial bite of head NOS (S00.97)

S02 Fracture of skull and facial bones

Note: A fracture not indicated as open or closed should be coded to closed
The appropriate 7th character is to be added to each code from category S02

A	initial encounter for closed fracture
B	initial encounter for open fracture
D	subsequent encounter for fracture with routine healing
G	subsequent encounter for fracture with delayed healing
K	subsequent encounter for fracture with nonunion
S	sequela

Code also any associated intracranial injury (S06.-)

- X **S02.0** Fracture of vault of skull A, K, B, A, B, A, B, S (Ex) PDX 1264 [K], 1612 [A, B]
  Fracture of frontal bone
  Fracture of parietal bone
- **S02.1** Fracture of base of skull (Ex) PDX 1264 [K], 1612 [A, B]
  Excludes2 lateral orbital wall (S02.84-)
  medial orbital wall (S02.83-)
  orbital floor (S02.3-)
  Coding Clinic: 2016, Q4, P66
  - **S02.10** Unspecified fracture of base of skull
    - **S02.101** Fracture of base of skull, right side A, K, B, A, B, A, B, S
    - **S02.102** Fracture of base of skull, left side A, K, B, A, B, A, B, S
    - **S02.109** Fracture of base of skull, unspecified side A, K, B, A, B, A, B, S
  - **S02.11** Fracture of occiput
    - **S02.110** Type I occipital condyle fracture, unspecified side A, K, B, A, B, A, B, S
    - **S02.111** Type II occipital condyle fracture, unspecified side A, K, B, A, B, A, B, S
    - **S02.112** Type III occipital condyle fracture, unspecified side A, K, B, A, B, A, B, S
    - **S02.113** Unspecified occipital condyle fracture A, K, B, A, B, A, B, S
    - **S02.118** Other fracture of occiput, unspecified side A, K, B, A, B, A, B, S
    - **S02.119** Unspecified fracture of occiput A, K, B, A, B, A, B, S
    - **S02.11A** Type I occipital condyle fracture, right side A, K, B, A, B, A, B, S

CHAPTER 19 (S00-T88)

- SØ2.11B **Type I occipital condyle fracture, left side** A, K, B, A, B, A, B, S
- SØ2.11C **Type II occipital condyle fracture, right side** A, K, B, A, B, A, B, S
- SØ2.11D **Type II occipital condyle fracture, left side** A, K, B, A, B, A, B, S
- SØ2.11E **Type III occipital condyle fracture, right side** A, K, B, A, B, A, B, S
- SØ2.11F **Type III occipital condyle fracture, left side** A, K, B, A, B, A, B, S
- SØ2.11G **Other fracture of occiput, right side** A, K, B, A, B, A, B, S
- SØ2.11H **Other fracture of occiput, left side** A, K, B, A, B, A, B, S

SØ2.12 **Fracture of orbital roof**

- SØ2.121 **Fracture of orbital roof, right side** A, K, B, A, B
- SØ2.122 **Fracture of orbital roof, left side** A, K, B, A, B
- SØ2.129 **Fracture of orbital roof, unspecified side** A, K, B, A, B

X SØ2.19 **Other fracture of base of skull** A, K, B, A, B, A, B, S
Fracture of anterior fossa of base of skull
Fracture of ethmoid sinus
Fracture of frontal sinus
Fracture of middle fossa of base of skull
Fracture of posterior fossa of base of skull
Fracture of sphenoid
Fracture of temporal bone
Coding Clinic: 2024, Q2, P15

X SØ2.2 **Fracture of nasal bones** B, K, B (Ex) PDX 1264 [K], 1613 [B]

SØ2.3 **Fracture of orbital floor** (Ex) PDX 1264 [K], 1614 [A, B]
Fracture of inferior orbital wall
Excludes1 orbit NOS (SØ2.85)
Excludes2 lateral orbital wall (SØ2.84-)
medial orbital wall (SØ2.83-)
orbital roof (SØ2.1-)
Coding Clinic: 2016, Q4, P66

- X SØ2.30 **Fracture of orbital floor, unspecified side** A, B, K, A, B, A, B, S
- X SØ2.31 **Fracture of orbital floor, right side** A, B, K, A, B, A, B, S
- X SØ2.32 **Fracture of orbital floor, left side** A, B, K, A, B, A, B, S

SØ2.4 **Fracture of malar, maxillary and zygoma bones**
Fracture of superior maxilla
Fracture of upper jaw (bone)
Fracture of zygomatic process of temporal bone
Coding Clinic: 2016, Q4, P66

SØ2.40 **Fracture of malar, maxillary and zygoma bones, unspecified** (Ex) PDX 1264 [K], 1615 [A, B]

- SØ2.400 **Malar fracture unspecified side** A, B, K, A, B, A, B, S
- SØ2.401 **Maxillary fracture, unspecified side** A, B, K, A, B, A, B, S
- SØ2.402 **Zygomatic fracture, unspecified side** A, B, K, A, B, A, B, S
- SØ2.40A **Malar fracture, right side** A, B, K, A, B, A, B, S
- SØ2.40B **Malar fracture, left side** A, B, K, A, B, A, B, S
- SØ2.40C **Maxillary fracture, right side** A, B, K, A, B, A, B, S
- SØ2.40D **Maxillary fracture, left side** A, B, K, A, B, A, B, S
- SØ2.40E **Zygomatic fracture, right side** A, B, K, A, B, A, B, S
- SØ2.40F **Zygomatic fracture, left side** A, B, K, A, B, A, B, S

SØ2.41 **LeFort fracture** (Ex) PDX 1264 [K], 1615 [A, B]

- SØ2.411 **LeFort I fracture** A, B, K, A, B, A, B, S
- SØ2.412 **LeFort II fracture** A, B, K, A, B, A, B, S
- SØ2.413 **LeFort III fracture** A, B, K, A, B, A, B, S

X SØ2.42 **Fracture of alveolus of maxilla** A, B, K, A, B, A, B, S (Ex) PDX 1264 [K], 1614 [A, B]

X SØ2.5 **Fracture of tooth (traumatic) Broken tooth** K (Ex) PDX 1264
Excludes1 cracked tooth (nontraumatic) (KØ3.81)

SØ2.6 **Fracture of mandible** (Ex) PDX 1264 [K], 1615 [A, B]
Fracture of lower jaw (bone)
Coding Clinic: 2016, Q4, P66

SØ2.60 **Fracture of mandible of unspecified site**

- SØ2.600 **Fracture of unspecified part of body of mandible, unspecified side** A, B, K, A, B, A, B, S
- SØ2.601 **Fracture of unspecified part of body of right mandible** A, B, K, A, B, A, B, S
- SØ2.602 **Fracture of unspecified part of body of left mandible** A, B, K, A, B, A, B, S
- SØ2.609 **Fracture of mandible, unspecified** A, B, K, A, B, A, B, S

SØ2.61 **Fracture of condylar process of mandible**

- SØ2.610 **Fracture of condylar process of mandible, unspecified side** A, B, K, A, B, A, B, S
- SØ2.611 **Fracture of condylar process of right mandible** A, B, K, A, B, A, B, S
  Coding Clinic: 2021, Q1, P6
- SØ2.612 **Fracture of condylar process of left mandible** A, B, K, A, B, A, B, S

SØ2.62 **Fracture of subcondylar process of mandible**

- SØ2.620 **Fracture of subcondylar process of mandible, unspecified side** A, B, K, A, B, A, B, S
- SØ2.621 **Fracture of subcondylar process of right mandible** A, B, K, A, B, A, B, S
- SØ2.622 **Fracture of subcondylar process of left mandible** A, B, K, A, B, A, B, S

SØ2.63 **Fracture of coronoid process of mandible**

- SØ2.630 **Fracture of coronoid process of mandible, unspecified side** A, B, K, A, B, A, B, S
- SØ2.631 **Fracture of coronoid process of right mandible** A, B, K, A, B, A, B, S
- SØ2.632 **Fracture of coronoid process of left mandible** A, B, K, A, B, A, B, S

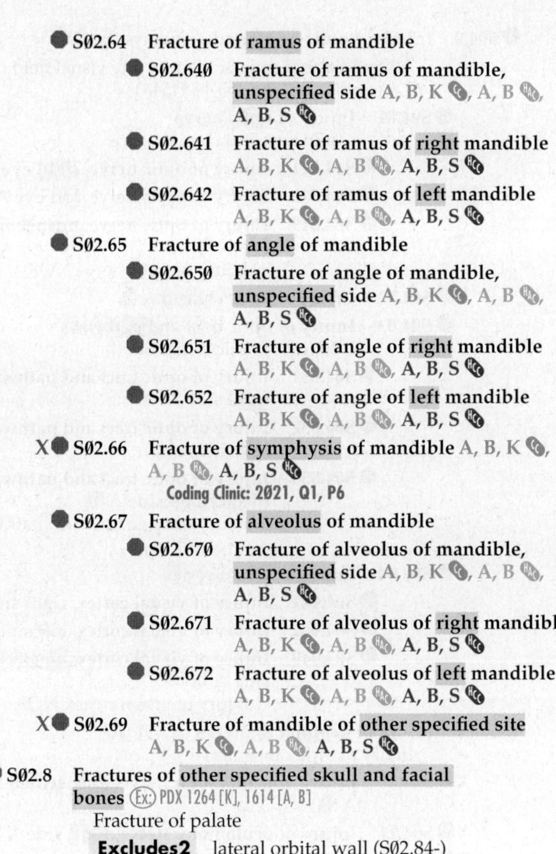

● **SØ2.64 Fracture of ramus of mandible**
● **SØ2.640 Fracture of ramus of mandible, unspecified side** A, B, K, A, B, A, B, S
● **SØ2.641 Fracture of ramus of right mandible** A, B, K, A, B, A, B, S
● **SØ2.642 Fracture of ramus of left mandible** A, B, K, A, B, A, B, S
● **SØ2.65 Fracture of angle of mandible**
● **SØ2.650 Fracture of angle of mandible, unspecified side** A, B, K, A, B, A, B, S
● **SØ2.651 Fracture of angle of right mandible** A, B, K, A, B, A, B, S
● **SØ2.652 Fracture of angle of left mandible** A, B, K, A, B, A, B, S
X● **SØ2.66 Fracture of symphysis of mandible** A, B, K, A, B, A, B, S
Coding Clinic: 2Ø21, Q1, P6
● **SØ2.67 Fracture of alveolus of mandible**
● **SØ2.670 Fracture of alveolus of mandible, unspecified side** A, B, K, A, B, A, B, S
● **SØ2.671 Fracture of alveolus of right mandible** A, B, K, A, B, A, B, S
● **SØ2.672 Fracture of alveolus of left mandible** A, B, K, A, B, A, B, S
X● **SØ2.69 Fracture of mandible of other specified site** A, B, K, A, B, A, B, S
● **SØ2.8 Fractures of other specified skull and facial bones** (Ex:) PDX 1264 [K], 1614 [A, B]
Fracture of palate
Excludes2 lateral orbital wall (SØ2.84-)
medial orbital wall (SØ2.83-)
Coding Clinic: 2Ø16, Q4, P66

X● **SØ2.8Ø Fracture of other specified skull and facial bones, unspecified side** A, B, K, A, B, A, B, S
X● **SØ2.81 Fracture of other specified skull and facial bones, right side** A, B, K, A, B, A, B, S
X● **SØ2.82 Fracture of other specified skull and facial bones, left side** A, B, K, A, B, A, B, S
● **SØ2.83 Fracture of medial orbital wall**
Excludes2 orbital floor (SØ2.3-)
orbital roof (SØ2.12-)
SØ2.831 Fracture of medial orbital wall, right side A, B, K, A, B
SØ2.832 Fracture of medial orbital wall, left side A, B, K, A, B
SØ2.839 Fracture of medial orbital wall, unspecified side A, B, K, A, B
● **SØ2.84 Fracture of lateral orbital wall**
Excludes2 orbital floor (SØ2.3-)
orbital roof (SØ2.12-)
SØ2.841 Fracture of lateral orbital wall, right side A, B, K, A, B
SØ2.842 Fracture of lateral orbital wall, left side A, B, K, A, B
SØ2.849 Fracture of lateral orbital wall, unspecified side A, B, K, A, B
SØ2.85 Fracture of orbit, unspecified A, B, K, A, B
Fracture of orbit NOS
Fracture of orbit wall NOS
Excludes1 lateral orbital wall (SØ2.84-)
medial orbital wall (SØ2.83-)
orbital floor (SØ2.3-)
orbital roof (SØ2.12-)

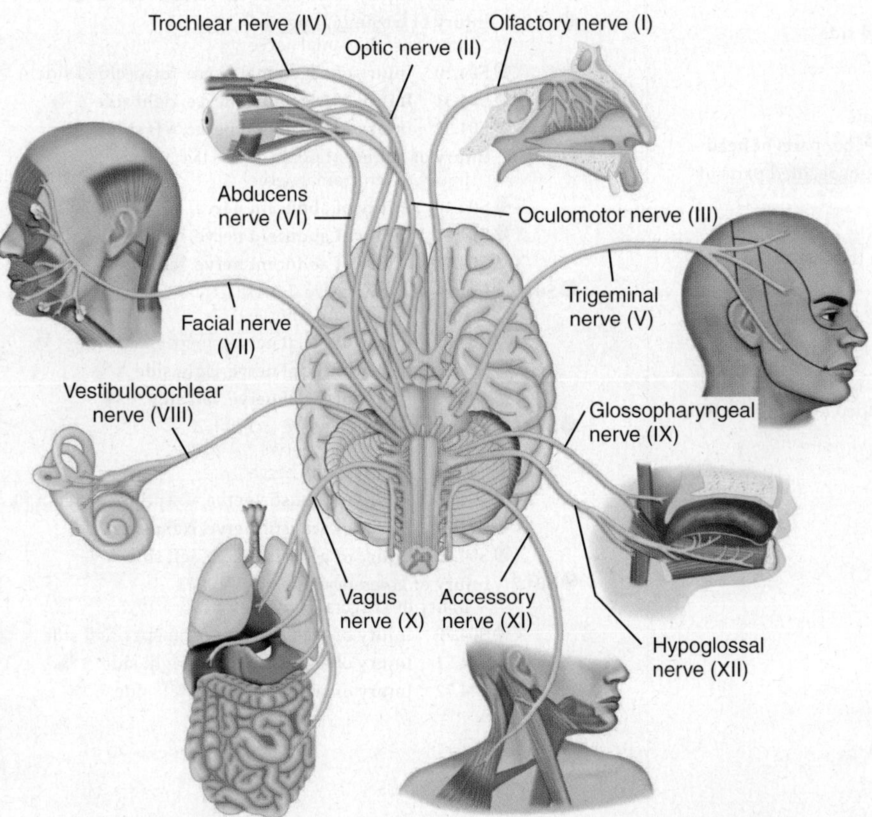

Figure 19-13 Cranial nerves. (From Patton and Thibodeau: Anatomy and physiology, ed 7, St. Louis, Mosby, 2009)

● S02.9 Fracture of unspecified skull and facial bones Ex: PDX 1264 [K], 1612, 1614 [A, B]

X● S02.91 Unspecified fracture of skull A, K, B, A, B, A, B, S

X● S02.92 Unspecified fracture of facial bones A, B, K, A, B, A, B, S

● S03 Dislocation and sprain of joints and ligaments of head

Includes avulsion of joint (capsule) or ligament of head
laceration of cartilage, joint (capsule) or ligament of head
sprain of cartilage, joint (capsule) or ligament of head
traumatic hemarthrosis of joint or ligament of head
traumatic rupture of joint or ligament of head
traumatic subluxation of joint or ligament of head
traumatic tear of joint or ligament of head

Code also any associated open wound

Excludes2 Strain of muscle or tendon of head (S09.1)

The appropriate 7th character is to be added to each code from category S03

A	initial encounter
D	subsequent encounter
S	sequela

● S03.0 Dislocation of jaw
Dislocation of jaw (cartilage) (meniscus)
Dislocation of mandible
Dislocation of temporomandibular (joint)
Coding Clinic: 2016, Q4, P67

X● S03.00 Dislocation of jaw, unspecified side

X● S03.01 Dislocation of jaw, right side

X● S03.02 Dislocation of jaw, left side

X● S03.03 Dislocation of jaw, bilateral side

X● S03.1 Dislocation of septal cartilage of nose

X● S03.2 Dislocation of tooth

● S03.4 Sprain of jaw
Sprain of temporomandibular (joint) (ligament)
Coding Clinic: 2016, Q4, P67

X● S03.40 Sprain of jaw, unspecified side

X● S03.41 Sprain of jaw, right side

X● S03.42 Sprain of jaw, left side

X● S03.43 Sprain of jaw, bilateral side

X● S03.8 Sprain of joints and ligaments of other parts of head

X● S03.9 Sprain of joints and ligaments of unspecified parts of head

● S04 Injury of cranial nerve

The selection of side should be based on the side of the body being affected

Code first any associated intracranial injury (S06.-)

Code also any associated:
open wound of head (S01.-)
skull fracture (S02.-)

The appropriate 7th character is to be added to each code from category S04

A	initial encounter
D	subsequent encounter
S	sequela

● S04.0 Injury of optic nerve and pathways Ex: PDX 1616
Use additional code to identify any visual field defect or blindness (H53.4-, H54.-)

● S04.01 Injury of optic nerve
Injury of 2nd cranial nerve

● S04.011 Injury of optic nerve, right eye A

● S04.012 Injury of optic nerve, left eye A

● S04.019 Injury of optic nerve, unspecified eye A
Injury of optic nerve NOS

X● S04.02 Injury of optic chiasm A

● S04.03 Injury of optic tract and pathways
Injury of optic radiation

● S04.031 Injury of optic tract and pathways, right side A

● S04.032 Injury of optic tract and pathways, left side A

● S04.039 Injury of optic tract and pathways, unspecified side A
Injury of optic tract and pathways NOS

● S04.04 Injury of visual cortex

● S04.041 Injury of visual cortex, right side A

● S04.042 Injury of visual cortex, left side A

● S04.049 Injury of visual cortex, unspecified side A
Injury of visual cortex NOS

● S04.1 Injury of oculomotor nerve Ex: PDX 1617
Injury of 3rd cranial nerve

X● S04.10 Injury of oculomotor nerve, unspecified side A

X● S04.11 Injury of oculomotor nerve, right side A

X● S04.12 Injury of oculomotor nerve, left side A

● S04.2 Injury of trochlear nerve Ex: PDX 1618
Injury of 4th cranial nerve

X● S04.20 Injury of trochlear nerve, unspecified side A

X● S04.21 Injury of trochlear nerve, right side A

X● S04.22 Injury of trochlear nerve, left side A

● S04.3 Injury of trigeminal nerve Ex: PDX 1619
Injury of 5th cranial nerve

X● S04.30 Injury of trigeminal nerve, unspecified side A

X● S04.31 Injury of trigeminal nerve, right side A

X● S04.32 Injury of trigeminal nerve, left side A

● S04.4 Injury of abducent nerve Ex: PDX 1620
Injury of 6th cranial nerve

X● S04.40 Injury of abducent nerve, unspecified side A

X● S04.41 Injury of abducent nerve, right side A

X● S04.42 Injury of abducent nerve, left side A

● S04.5 Injury of facial nerve Ex: PDX 1621
Injury of 7th cranial nerve

X● S04.50 Injury of facial nerve, unspecified side A

X● S04.51 Injury of facial nerve, right side A

X● S04.52 Injury of facial nerve, left side A

● S04.6 Injury of acoustic nerve Ex: PDX 1622
Injury of auditory nerve
Injury of 8th cranial nerve

X● S04.60 Injury of acoustic nerve, unspecified side A

X● S04.61 Injury of acoustic nerve, right side A

X● S04.62 Injury of acoustic nerve, left side A

● S04.7 Injury of accessory nerve Ex: PDX 1623
Injury of 11th cranial nerve

X● S04.70 Injury of accessory nerve, unspecified side A

X● S04.71 Injury of accessory nerve, right side A

X● S04.72 Injury of accessory nerve, left side A

● **S04.8 Injury of other cranial nerves** (Ex:) PDX 1624
● **S04.81 Injury of olfactory [1st] nerve**
● **S04.811 Injury of olfactory [1st] nerve, right side** A
● **S04.812 Injury of olfactory [1st] nerve, left side** A
● **S04.819 Injury of olfactory [1st] nerve, unspecified side** A
● **S04.89 Injury of other cranial nerves**
Injury of vagus [10th] nerve
● **S04.891 Injury of other cranial nerves, right side** A
● **S04.892 Injury of other cranial nerves, left side** A
● **S04.899 Injury of other cranial nerves, unspecified side** A
X● **S04.9 Injury of unspecified cranial nerve** A (Ex:) PDX 1624

● **S05 Injury of eye and orbit**
Includes open wound of eye and orbit
Excludes2 2nd cranial [optic] nerve injury (S04.0-)
3rd cranial [oculomotor] nerve injury (S04.1-)
open wound of eyelid and periocular area (S01.1-)
orbital bone fracture (S02.1-, S02.3-, S02.8-)
superficial injury of eyelid (S00.1-S00.2)

The appropriate 7th character is to be added to each code from category S05

A initial encounter
D subsequent encounter
S sequela

● **S05.0 Injury of conjunctiva and corneal abrasion without foreign body**
Excludes1 foreign body in conjunctival sac (T15.1)
foreign body in cornea (T15.0)
X● **S05.00 Injury of conjunctiva and corneal abrasion without foreign body, unspecified eye**
X● **S05.01 Injury of conjunctiva and corneal abrasion without foreign body, right eye**
X● **S05.02 Injury of conjunctiva and corneal abrasion without foreign body, left eye**
● **S05.1 Contusion of eyeball and orbital tissues**
Traumatic hyphema
Excludes2 black eye NOS (S00.1)
contusion of eyelid and periocular area (S00.1)
X● **S05.10 Contusion of eyeball and orbital tissues, unspecified eye**
X● **S05.11 Contusion of eyeball and orbital tissues, right eye**
X● **S05.12 Contusion of eyeball and orbital tissues, left eye**
● **S05.2 Ocular laceration and rupture with prolapse or loss of intraocular tissue** (Ex:) PDX 1611
X● **S05.20 Ocular laceration and rupture with prolapse or loss of intraocular tissue, unspecified eye** A
X● **S05.21 Ocular laceration and rupture with prolapse or loss of intraocular tissue, right eye** A
X● **S05.22 Ocular laceration and rupture with prolapse or loss of intraocular tissue, left eye** A
● **S05.3 Ocular laceration without prolapse or loss of intraocular tissue** (Ex:) PDX 1611
Laceration of eye NOS
X● **S05.30 Ocular laceration without prolapse or loss of intraocular tissue, unspecified eye** A
X● **S05.31 Ocular laceration without prolapse or loss of intraocular tissue, right eye** A
X● **S05.32 Ocular laceration without prolapse or loss of intraocular tissue, left eye** A
● **S05.4 Penetrating wound of orbit with or without foreign body** (Ex:) PDX 1611
Excludes2 retained (old) foreign body following penetrating wound in orbit (H05.5-)
X● **S05.40 Penetrating wound of orbit with or without foreign body, unspecified eye** A
X● **S05.41 Penetrating wound of orbit with or without foreign body, right eye** A
X● **S05.42 Penetrating wound of orbit with or without foreign body, left eye** A
● **S05.5 Penetrating wound with foreign body of eyeball** (Ex:) PDX 1625
Excludes2 retained (old) intraocular foreign body (H44.6-, H44.7)
X● **S05.50 Penetrating wound with foreign body of unspecified eyeball** A
X● **S05.51 Penetrating wound with foreign body of right eyeball** A
X● **S05.52 Penetrating wound with foreign body of left eyeball** A
● **S05.6 Penetrating wound without foreign body of eyeball**
Ocular penetration NOS
X● **S05.60 Penetrating wound without foreign body of unspecified eyeball**
X● **S05.61 Penetrating wound without foreign body of right eyeball**
X● **S05.62 Penetrating wound without foreign body of left eyeball**
● **S05.7 Avulsion of eye** (Ex:) PDX 1611
Traumatic enucleation
X● **S05.70 Avulsion of unspecified eye** A
X● **S05.71 Avulsion of right eye** A
X● **S05.72 Avulsion of left eye** A
● **S05.8 Other injuries of eye and orbit** (Ex:) PDX 1611
Lacrimal duct injury
● **S05.8X Other injuries of eye and orbit**
● **S05.8X1 Other injuries of right eye and orbit** A
● **S05.8X2 Other injuries of left eye and orbit** A
● **S05.8X9 Other injuries of unspecified eye and orbit** A
● **S05.9 Unspecified injury of eye and orbit** (Ex:) PDX 1611
Injury of eye NOS
X● **S05.90 Unspecified injury of unspecified eye and orbit**
X● **S05.91 Unspecified injury of right eye and orbit** A
X● **S05.92 Unspecified injury of left eye and orbit** A

● **S06 Intracranial injury**
Includes traumatic brain injury
Code also any associated:
open wound of head (S01.-)
skull fracture (S02.-)
Excludes1 head injury NOS (S09.90)

The appropriate 7th character is to be added to each code from category S06

A initial encounter
D subsequent encounter
S sequela

Note: 7th characters D and S do not apply to codes in category S06 with 6th character 7 - death due to brain injury prior to regaining consciousness, or 8 - death due to other cause prior to regaining consciousness.

Coding Clinic: 2015, Q4, P40

CHAPTER 19 (S00-T88)

S06.0 Concussion
Commotio cerebri
Excludes1 concussion with other intracranial injuries classified in subcategories S06.1- to S06.6- , and S06.81- to S06.82-, code to specified intracranial injury
Coding Clinic: 2016, Q4, P67

S06.0X Concussion

S06.0X0 Concussion without loss of consciousness S
S06.0X1 Concussion with loss of consciousness of 30 minutes or less A, A, S (Ex:) PDX 1612
Concussion with brief loss of consciousness
S06.0X9 Concussion with loss of consciousness of unspecified duration A, A, S (Ex:) PDX 1612
Coding Clinic: 2016, Q4, P68
S06.0XA Concussion with loss of consciousness status unknown A, A, (Ex:) PDX 1626
Concussion NOS

S06.1 Traumatic cerebral edema
Diffuse traumatic cerebral edema
Focal traumatic cerebral edema
Coding Clinic: 2016, Q4, P67

S06.1X Traumatic cerebral edema

S06.1X0 Traumatic cerebral edema without loss of consciousness A, A, S (Ex:) PDX 1627
MCC when PDx is its own MCC
Coding Clinic: 2015, Q1, P12
S06.1X1 Traumatic cerebral edema with loss of consciousness of 30 minutes or less A, A, A, S (Ex:) PDX 1628
Traumatic cerebral edema with brief loss of consciousness
MCC when PDx is its own MCC
S06.1X2 Traumatic cerebral edema with loss of consciousness of 31 minutes to 59 minutes A, A, A, S (Ex:) PDX 1628
MCC when PDx is its own MCC
S06.1X3 Traumatic cerebral edema with loss of consciousness of 1 hour to 5 hours 59 minutes A, A, A, S (Ex:) PDX 1628
MCC when PDx is its own MCC
S06.1X4 Traumatic cerebral edema with loss of consciousness of 6 hours to 24 hours A, A, A, S (Ex:) PDX 1628
MCC when PDx is its own MCC
S06.1X5 Traumatic cerebral edema with loss of consciousness greater than 24 hours with return to pre-existing conscious level A, A, A, S (Ex:) PDX 1628
MCC when PDx is its own MCC
S06.1X6 Traumatic cerebral edema with loss of consciousness greater than 24 hours without return to pre-existing conscious level with patient surviving A, A, A, S (Ex:) PDX 1612
MCC when PDx is its own MCC
S06.1X7 Traumatic cerebral edema with loss of consciousness of any duration with death due to brain injury prior to regaining consciousness A, A (Ex:) PDX 1612
MCC when PDx is its own MCC
S06.1X8 Traumatic cerebral edema with loss of consciousness of any duration with death due to other cause prior to regaining consciousness A, A (Ex:) PDX 1612
MCC when PDx is its own MCC
S06.1X9 Traumatic cerebral edema with loss of consciousness of unspecified duration A, A, A, S (Ex:) PDX 1628
MCC when PDx is its own MCC
S06.1XA Traumatic cerebral edema with loss of consciousness status unknown A, A (Ex:) PDX 1629
Traumatic cerebral edema NOS

S06.2 Diffuse traumatic brain injury
Diffuse axonal brain injury
Excludes1 traumatic diffuse cerebral edema (S06.1X-)
Use Additional code, if applicable, for traumatic brain compression or herniation (S06.A-)

S06.2X Diffuse traumatic brain injury

S06.2X0 Diffuse traumatic brain injury without loss of consciousness A, S
S06.2X1 Diffuse traumatic brain injury with loss of consciousness of 30 minutes or less A, A, A, S (Ex:) PDX 1612
Diffuse traumatic brain injury with brief loss of consciousness
S06.2X2 Diffuse traumatic brain injury with loss of consciousness of 31 minutes to 59 minutes A, A, A, S (Ex:) PDX 1612
S06.2X3 Diffuse traumatic brain injury with loss of consciousness of 1 hour to 5 hours 59 minutes A, A, A, S (Ex:) PDX 1612
S06.2X4 Diffuse traumatic brain injury with loss of consciousness of 6 hours to 24 hours A, A, A, S (Ex:) PDX 1612
S06.2X5 Diffuse traumatic brain injury with loss of consciousness greater than 24 hours with return to pre-existing conscious levels A, A, A, S (Ex:) PDX 1612
S06.2X6 Diffuse traumatic brain injury with loss of consciousness greater than 24 hours without return to pre-existing conscious level with patient surviving A, A, A, S (Ex:) PDX 1612
S06.2X7 Diffuse traumatic brain injury with loss of consciousness of any duration with death due to brain injury prior to regaining consciousness A, A (Ex:) PDX 1612
S06.2X8 Diffuse traumatic brain injury with loss of consciousness of any duration with death due to other cause prior to regaining consciousness A, A (Ex:) PDX 1612
S06.2X9 Diffuse traumatic brain injury with loss of consciousness of unspecified duration A, A, A, S (Ex:) PDX 1612
Diffuse traumatic brain injury NOS
S06.2XA Diffuse traumatic brain injury with loss of consciousness status unknown A, A, (Ex:) PDX 1626
Diffuse traumatic brain injury NOS

CHAPTER 19 (S00-T88)

S06.3 Focal traumatic brain injury

Excludes2 any condition classifiable to S06.4-S06.6
focal cerebral edema (S06.1)

Use Additional code, if applicable, for traumatic brain compression or herniation (S06.A-)

S06.30 Unspecified focal traumatic brain injury

S06.300 Unspecified focal traumatic brain injury without loss of consciousness A, S

S06.301 Unspecified focal traumatic brain injury with loss of consciousness of 30 minutes or less A, A, A, S (Ex:) PDX 1612

Unspecified focal traumatic brain injury with brief loss of consciousness

S06.302 Unspecified focal traumatic brain injury with loss of consciousness of 31 minutes to 59 minutes A, A, A, S (Ex:) PDX 1612

S06.303 Unspecified focal traumatic brain injury with loss of consciousness of 1 hour to 5 hours 59 minutes A, A, A, S (Ex:) PDX 1612

S06.304 Unspecified focal traumatic brain injury with loss of consciousness of 6 hours to 24 hours A, A, A, S (Ex:) PDX 1612

S06.305 Unspecified focal traumatic brain injury with loss of consciousness greater than 24 hours with return to pre-existing conscious level A, A, A, S (Ex:) PDX 1612

S06.306 Unspecified focal traumatic brain injury with loss of consciousness greater than 24 hours without return to pre-existing conscious level with patient surviving A, A, A, S (Ex:) PDX 1612

S06.307 Unspecified focal traumatic brain injury with loss of consciousness of any duration with death due to brain injury prior to regaining consciousness A, A (Ex:) PDX 1612

S06.308 Unspecified focal traumatic brain injury with loss of consciousness of any duration with death due to other cause prior to regaining consciousness A, A (Ex:) PDX 1612

S06.309 Unspecified focal traumatic brain injury with loss of consciousness of unspecified duration A, A, A, S (Ex:) PDX 1612

S06.30A Unspecified focal traumatic brain injury with loss of consciousness status unknown A, A, (Ex:) PDX 1626

Unspecified focal traumatic brain injury NOS

S06.31 Contusion and laceration of right cerebrum

S06.310 Contusion and laceration of right cerebrum without loss of consciousness A, A, A, S (Ex:) PDX 1612

S06.311 Contusion and laceration of right cerebrum with loss of consciousness of 30 minutes or less A, A, A, S (Ex:) PDX 1612

Contusion and laceration of right cerebrum with brief loss of consciousness

S06.312 Contusion and laceration of right cerebrum with loss of consciousness of 31 minutes to 59 minutes A, A, A, S (Ex:) PDX 1612

S06.313 Contusion and laceration of right cerebrum with loss of consciousness of 1 hour to 5 hours 59 minutes A, A, A, S (Ex:) PDX 1612

S06.314 Contusion and laceration of right cerebrum with loss of consciousness of 6 hours to 24 hours A, A, A, S (Ex:) PDX 1612

S06.315 Contusion and laceration of right cerebrum with loss of consciousness greater than 24 hours with return to pre-existing conscious level A, A, A, S (Ex:) PDX 1612

S06.316 Contusion and laceration of right cerebrum with loss of consciousness greater than 24 hours without return to pre-existing conscious level with patient surviving A, A, A, S (Ex:) PDX 1612

S06.317 Contusion and laceration of right cerebrum with loss of consciousness of any duration with death due to brain injury prior to regaining consciousness A, A (Ex:) PDX 1612

S06.318 Contusion and laceration of right cerebrum with loss of consciousness of any duration with death due to other cause prior to regaining consciousness A, A (Ex:) PDX 1612

S06.319 Contusion and laceration of right cerebrum with loss of consciousness of unspecified duration A, A, A, S (Ex:) PDX 1612

S06.31A Contusion and laceration of right cerebrum with loss of consciousness status unknown A, A, (Ex:) PDX 1626

Contusion and laceration of right cerebrum NOS

S06.32 Contusion and laceration of left cerebrum

S06.320 Contusion and laceration of left cerebrum without loss of consciousness A, A, A, S (Ex:) PDX 1612

S06.321 Contusion and laceration of left cerebrum with loss of consciousness of 30 minutes or less A, A, A, S (Ex:) PDX 1612

Contusion and laceration of left cerebrum with brief loss of consciousness

S06.322 Contusion and laceration of left cerebrum with loss of consciousness of 31 minutes to 59 minutes A, A, A, S (Ex:) PDX 1612

S06.323 Contusion and laceration of left cerebrum with loss of consciousness of 1 hour to 5 hours 59 minutes A, A, A, S (Ex:) PDX 1612

S06.324 Contusion and laceration of left cerebrum with loss of consciousness of 6 hours to 24 hours A, A, A, S (Ex:) PDX 1612

S06.325 Contusion and laceration of left cerebrum with loss of consciousness greater than 24 hours with return to pre-existing conscious level A, A, A, S (Ex:) PDX 1612

S06.326 Contusion and laceration of left cerebrum with loss of consciousness greater than 24 hours without return to pre-existing conscious level with patient surviving A, A, A, S (Ex:) PDX 1612

S06.327 Contusion and laceration of left cerebrum with loss of consciousness of any duration with death due to brain injury prior to regaining consciousness A, A (Ex:) PDX 1612

S06.328 Contusion and laceration of left cerebrum with loss of consciousness of any duration with death due to other cause prior to regaining consciousness A, A (Ex:) PDX 1612

S06.329 Contusion and laceration of left cerebrum with loss of consciousness of unspecified duration A, A, A, S (Ex:) PDX 1612

S06.32A Contusion and laceration of left cerebrum with loss of consciousness status unknown A, A (Ex:) PDX 1626

Contusion and laceration of left cerebrum NOS

S06.33 Contusion and laceration of cerebrum, unspecified

S06.330 Contusion and laceration of cerebrum, unspecified, without loss of consciousness A, A, A, S (Ex:) PDX 1612

S06.331 Contusion and laceration of cerebrum, unspecified, with loss of consciousness of 30 minutes or less A, A, A, S (Ex:) PDX 1612

Contusion and laceration of cerebrum, unspecified, with brief loss of consciousness

S06.332 Contusion and laceration of cerebrum, unspecified, with loss of consciousness of 31 minutes to 59 minutes A, A, A, S (Ex:) PDX 1612

S06.333 Contusion and laceration of cerebrum, unspecified, with loss of consciousness of 1 hour to 5 hours 59 minutes A, A, A, S (Ex:) PDX 1612

S06.334 Contusion and laceration of cerebrum, unspecified, with loss of consciousness of 6 hours to 24 hours A, A, A, S (Ex:) PDX 1612

S06.335 Contusion and laceration of cerebrum, unspecified, with loss of consciousness greater than 24 hours with return to pre-existing conscious level A, A, A, S (Ex:) PDX 1612

S06.336 Contusion and laceration of cerebrum, unspecified, with loss of consciousness greater than 24 hours without return to pre-existing conscious level with patient surviving A, A, A, S (Ex:) PDX 1612

S06.337 Contusion and laceration of cerebrum, unspecified, with loss of consciousness of any duration with death due to brain injury prior to regaining consciousness A, A (Ex:) PDX 1612

S06.338 Contusion and laceration of cerebrum, unspecified, with loss of consciousness of any duration with death due to other cause prior to regaining consciousness A, A (Ex:) PDX 1612

S06.339 Contusion and laceration of cerebrum, unspecified, with loss of consciousness of unspecified duration A, A, A, S (Ex:) PDX 1612

S06.33A Contusion and laceration of cerebrum, unspecified, with loss of consciousness status unknown A, A (Ex:) PDX 1626

Contusion and laceration of cerebrum NOS

S06.34 Traumatic hemorrhage of right cerebrum

Traumatic intracerebral hemorrhage and hematoma of right cerebrum

S06.340 Traumatic hemorrhage of right cerebrum without loss of consciousness A, A, A, S (Ex:) PDX 1612

Coding Clinic: 2015, Q1, P12

S06.341 Traumatic hemorrhage of right cerebrum with loss of consciousness of 30 minutes or less A, A, A, S (Ex:) PDX 1612

Traumatic hemorrhage of right cerebrum with brief loss of consciousness

S06.342 Traumatic hemorrhage of right cerebrum with loss of consciousness of 31 minutes to 59 minutes A, A, A, S (Ex:) PDX 1612

S06.343 Traumatic hemorrhage of right cerebrum with loss of consciousness of 1 hours to 5 hours 59 minutes A, A, A, S (Ex:) PDX 1612

S06.344 Traumatic hemorrhage of right cerebrum with loss of consciousness of 6 hours to 24 hours A, A, A, S (Ex:) PDX 1612

S06.345 Traumatic hemorrhage of right cerebrum with loss of consciousness greater than 24 hours with return to pre-existing conscious level A, A, A, S (Ex:) PDX 1612

S06.346 Traumatic hemorrhage of right cerebrum with loss of consciousness greater than 24 hours without return to pre-existing conscious level with patient surviving A, A, A, S (Ex:) PDX 1612

S06.347 Traumatic hemorrhage of right cerebrum with loss of consciousness of any duration with death due to brain injury prior to regaining consciousness A, A (Ex:) PDX 1612

S06.348 Traumatic hemorrhage of right cerebrum with loss of consciousness of any duration with death due to other cause prior to regaining consciousness A, A (Ex:) PDX 1612

S06.349 Traumatic hemorrhage of right cerebrum with loss of consciousness of unspecified duration A, A, A, S (Ex:) PDX 1612

S06.34A Traumatic hemorrhage of right cerebrum with loss of consciousness status unknown A, A (Ex:) PDX 1626

Traumatic hemorrhage of right cerebrum NOS

- S06.35 Traumatic hemorrhage of left cerebrum
  Traumatic intracerebral hemorrhage and hematoma of left cerebrum
  - S06.350 Traumatic hemorrhage of left cerebrum without loss of consciousness A, A, A, S (Ex) PDX 1612
  - S06.351 Traumatic hemorrhage of left cerebrum with loss of consciousness of 30 minutes or less A, A, A, S (Ex) PDX 1612
    Traumatic hemorrhage of left cerebrum with brief loss of consciousness
  - S06.352 Traumatic hemorrhage of left cerebrum with loss of consciousness of 31 minutes to 59 minutes A, A, A, S (Ex) PDX 1612
  - S06.353 Traumatic hemorrhage of left cerebrum with loss of consciousness of 1 hours to 5 hours 59 minutes A, A, A, S (Ex) PDX 1612
  - S06.354 Traumatic hemorrhage of left cerebrum with loss of consciousness of 6 hours to 24 hours A, A, A, S (Ex) PDX 1612
  - S06.355 Traumatic hemorrhage of left cerebrum with loss of consciousness greater than 24 hours with return to pre-existing conscious level A, A, A, S (Ex) PDX 1612
  - S06.356 Traumatic hemorrhage of left cerebrum with loss of consciousness greater than 24 hours without return to pre-existing conscious level with patient surviving A, A, A, S (Ex) PDX 1612
  - S06.357 Traumatic hemorrhage of left cerebrum with loss of consciousness of any duration with death due to brain injury prior to regaining consciousness A, A (Ex) PDX 1612
  - S06.358 Traumatic hemorrhage of left cerebrum with loss of consciousness of any duration with death due to other cause prior to regaining consciousness A, A (Ex) PDX 1612
  - S06.359 Traumatic hemorrhage of left cerebrum with loss of consciousness of unspecified duration A, A, A, S (Ex) PDX 1612
  - S06.35A Traumatic hemorrhage of left cerebrum with loss of consciousness status unknown A, A (Ex) PDX 1626
    Traumatic hemorrhage of left cerebrum NOS
- S06.36 Traumatic hemorrhage of cerebrum, unspecified
  Traumatic intracerebral hemorrhage and hematoma, unspecified
  - S06.360 Traumatic hemorrhage of cerebrum, unspecified, without loss of consciousness A, A, A, S (Ex) PDX 1612
  - S06.361 Traumatic hemorrhage of cerebrum, unspecified, with loss of consciousness of 30 minutes or less A, A, A, S (Ex) PDX 1612
    Traumatic hemorrhage of cerebrum, unspecified, with brief loss of consciousness
  - S06.362 Traumatic hemorrhage of cerebrum, unspecified, with loss of consciousness of 31 minutes to 59 minutes A, A, A, S (Ex) PDX 1612
  - S06.363 Traumatic hemorrhage of cerebrum, unspecified, with loss of consciousness of 1 hours to 5 hours 59 minutes A, A, A, S (Ex) PDX 1612
  - S06.364 Traumatic hemorrhage of cerebrum, unspecified, with loss of consciousness of 6 hours to 24 hours A, A, A, S (Ex) PDX 1612
  - S06.365 Traumatic hemorrhage of cerebrum, unspecified, with loss of consciousness greater than 24 hours with return to pre-existing conscious level A, A, A, S (Ex) PDX 1612
  - S06.366 Traumatic hemorrhage of cerebrum, unspecified, with loss of consciousness greater than 24 hours without return to pre-existing conscious level with patient surviving A, A, A, S (Ex) PDX 1612
  - S06.367 Traumatic hemorrhage of cerebrum, unspecified, with loss of consciousness of any duration with death due to brain injury prior to regaining consciousness A, A (Ex) PDX 1612
  - S06.368 Traumatic hemorrhage of cerebrum, unspecified, with loss of consciousness of any duration with death due to other cause prior to regaining consciousness A, A (Ex) PDX 1612
  - S06.369 Traumatic hemorrhage of cerebrum, unspecified, with loss of consciousness of unspecified duration A, A, A, S (Ex) PDX 1612
  - S06.36A Traumatic hemorrhage of cerebrum, unspecified, with loss of consciousness status unknownA, A (Ex) PDX 1626
    Traumatic hemorrhage of cerebrum NOS
- S06.37 Contusion, laceration, and hemorrhage of cerebellum
  - S06.370 Contusion, laceration, and hemorrhage of cerebellum without loss of consciousness A, A, A, S (Ex) PDX 1630
  - S06.371 Contusion, laceration, and hemorrhage of cerebellum with loss of consciousness of 30 minutes or less A, A, A, S (Ex) PDX 1612
    Contusion, laceration, and hemorrhage of cerebellum with brief loss of consciousness
  - S06.372 Contusion, laceration, and hemorrhage of cerebellum with loss of consciousness of 31 minutes to 59 minutes A, A, A, S (Ex) PDX 1612
  - S06.373 Contusion, laceration, and hemorrhage of cerebellum with loss of consciousness of 1 hour to 5 hours 59 minutes A, A, A, S (Ex) PDX 1612
  - S06.374 Contusion, laceration, and hemorrhage of cerebellum with loss of consciousness of 6 hours to 24 hours A, A, A, S (Ex) PDX 1612
  - S06.375 Contusion, laceration, and hemorrhage of cerebellum with loss of consciousness greater than 24 hours with return to pre-existing conscious level A, A, A, S (Ex) PDX 1612

CHAPTER 19 (S00-T88)

● S06.376 Contusion, laceration, and hemorrhage of cerebellum with loss of consciousness greater than 24 hours without return to pre-existing conscious level with patient surviving A, A, A, S (Ex) PDX 1612

● S06.377 Contusion, laceration, and hemorrhage of cerebellum with loss of consciousness of any duration with death due to brain injury prior to regaining consciousness A, A (Ex) PDX 1612

● S06.378 Contusion, laceration, and hemorrhage of cerebellum with loss of consciousness of any duration with death due to other cause prior to regaining consciousness A, A (Ex) PDX 1612

● S06.379 Contusion, laceration, and hemorrhage of cerebellum with loss of consciousness of unspecified duration A, A, A, S (Ex) PDX 1612

● S06.37A Contusion, laceration, and hemorrhage of cerebellum with loss of consciousness status unknown A, A (Ex) PDX 1626
Contusion, laceration, and hemorrhage of cerebellum NOS

● S06.38 Contusion, laceration, and hemorrhage of brainstem

● S06.380 Contusion, laceration, and hemorrhage of brainstem without loss of consciousness A, A, A, S (Ex) PDX 1631

● S06.381 Contusion, laceration, and hemorrhage of brainstem with loss of consciousness of 30 minutes or less A, A, A, S (Ex) PDX 1612
Contusion, laceration, and hemorrhage of brainstem with brief loss of consciousness

● S06.382 Contusion, laceration, and hemorrhage of brainstem with loss of consciousness of 31 minutes to 59 minutes A, A, A, S (Ex) PDX 1612

● S06.383 Contusion, laceration, and hemorrhage of brainstem with loss of consciousness of 1 hour to 5 hours 59 minutes A, A, A, S (Ex) PDX 1612

● S06.384 Contusion, laceration, and hemorrhage of brainstem with loss of consciousness of 6 hours to 24 hours A, A, A, S (Ex) PDX 1612

● S06.385 Contusion, laceration, and hemorrhage of brainstem with loss of consciousness greater than 24 hours with return to pre-existing conscious level A, A, A, S (Ex) PDX 1612

● S06.386 Contusion, laceration, and hemorrhage of brainstem with loss of consciousness greater than 24 hours without return to pre-existing conscious level with patient surviving A, A, A, S (Ex) PDX 1612

● S06.387 Contusion, laceration, and hemorrhage of brainstem with loss of consciousness of any duration with death due to brain injury prior to regaining consciousness A, A (Ex) PDX 1612

● S06.388 Contusion, laceration, and hemorrhage of brainstem with loss of consciousness of any duration with death due to other cause prior to regaining consciousness A, A (Ex) PDX 1612

● S06.389 Contusion, laceration, and hemorrhage of brainstem with loss of consciousness of unspecified duration A, A, A, S (Ex) PDX 1612

● S06.38A Contusion, laceration, and hemorrhage of brainstem with loss of consciousness status unknown A, A (Ex) PDX 1626
Contusion, laceration, and hemorrhage of brainstem NOS

● S06.4 Epidural hemorrhage
Situated outside dura mater
Extradural hemorrhage NOS
Intracranial hemorrhage due to trauma
Extradural hemorrhage (traumatic)

● S06.4X Epidural hemorrhage

● S06.4X0 Epidural hemorrhage without loss of consciousness A, A, A, S (Ex) PDX 1612

● S06.4X1 Epidural hemorrhage with loss of consciousness of 30 minutes or less A, A, A, S (Ex) PDX 1612
Epidural hemorrhage with brief loss of consciousness

● S06.4X2 Epidural hemorrhage with loss of consciousness of 31 minutes to 59 minutes A, A, A, S (Ex) PDX 1612

● S06.4X3 Epidural hemorrhage with loss of consciousness of 1 hour to 5 hours 59 minutes A, A, A, S (Ex) PDX 1612

● S06.4X4 Epidural hemorrhage with loss of consciousness of 6 hours to 24 hours A, A, A, S (Ex) PDX 1612

● S06.4X5 Epidural hemorrhage with loss of consciousness greater than 24 hours with return to pre-existing conscious level A, A, A, S (Ex) PDX 1612

● S06.4X6 Epidural hemorrhage with loss of consciousness greater than 24 hours without return to pre-existing conscious level with patient surviving A, A, A, S (Ex) PDX 1612

● S06.4X7 Epidural hemorrhage with loss of consciousness of any duration with death due to brain injury prior to regaining consciousness A, A (Ex) PDX 1612

● S06.4X8 Epidural hemorrhage with loss of consciousness of any duration with death due to other causes prior to regaining consciousness A, A (Ex) PDX 1612

● S06.4X9 Epidural hemorrhage with loss of consciousness of unspecified duration A, A, A, S (Ex) PDX 1612

● S06.4XA Epidural hemorrhage with loss of consciousness status unknown A, A (Ex) PDX 1632
Epidural hemorrhage NOS

● **S06.5 Traumatic subdural hemorrhage**
Use Additional code, if applicable, for traumatic brain compression or herniation (S06.A-)
Coding Clinic: 2024, Q2, P15

● **S06.5X Traumatic subdural hemorrhage**

● **S06.5X0 Traumatic subdural hemorrhage without loss of consciousness** A, A, A, S Ex: PDX 1612
Coding Clinic: 2021, Q1, P4; 2018, Q2, P13; 2015, Q3, P37

● **S06.5X1 Traumatic subdural hemorrhage with loss of consciousness of 30 minutes or less** A, A, A, S Ex: PDX 1612
Traumatic subdural hemorrhage with brief loss of consciousness

● **S06.5X2 Traumatic subdural hemorrhage with loss of consciousness of 31 minutes to 59 minutes** A, A, A, S Ex: PDX 1612

● **S06.5X3 Traumatic subdural hemorrhage with loss of consciousness of 1 hour to 5 hours 59 minutes** A, A, A, S Ex: PDX 1612

● **S06.5X4 Traumatic subdural hemorrhage with loss of consciousness of 6 hours to 24 hours** A, A, A, S Ex: PDX 1612

● **S06.5X5 Traumatic subdural hemorrhage with loss of consciousness greater than 24 hours with return to pre-existing conscious level** A, A, A, S Ex: PDX 1612

● **S06.5X6 Traumatic subdural hemorrhage with loss of consciousness greater than 24 hours without return to pre-existing conscious level with patient surviving** A, A, A, S Ex: PDX 1612
Coding Clinic: 2021, Q2, P5

● **S06.5X7 Traumatic subdural hemorrhage with loss of consciousness of any duration with death due to brain injury before regaining consciousness** A, A Ex: PDX 1612

● **S06.5X8 Traumatic subdural hemorrhage with loss of consciousness of any duration with death due to other cause before regaining consciousness** A, A Ex: PDX 1612

● **S06.5X9 Traumatic subdural hemorrhage with loss of consciousness of unspecified duration** A, A, A, S Ex: PDX 1612

● **S06.5XA Traumatic subdural hemorrhage with loss of consciousness status unknown** A, A Ex: PDX 1626
Traumatic subdural hemorrhage NOS
Coding Clinic: 2022, Q4, P45

● **S06.6 Traumatic subarachnoid hemorrhage**
Between arachnoid and pia mater
Use Additional code, if applicable, for traumatic brain compression or herniation (S06.A-)
Coding Clinic: 2016, Q4, P67

● **S06.6X Traumatic subarachnoid hemorrhage**

● **S06.6X0 Traumatic subarachnoid hemorrhage without loss of consciousness** A, A, A, S Ex: PDX 1612
Coding Clinic: 2015, Q3, P37

● **S06.6X1 Traumatic subarachnoid hemorrhage with loss of consciousness of 30 minutes or less** A, A, A, S Ex: PDX 1612
Traumatic subarachnoid hemorrhage with brief loss of consciousness

● **S06.6X2 Traumatic subarachnoid hemorrhage with loss of consciousness of 31 minutes to 59 minutes** A, A, A, S Ex: PDX 1612

● **S06.6X3 Traumatic subarachnoid hemorrhage with loss of consciousness of 1 hour to 5 hours 59 minutes** A, A, A, S Ex: PDX 1612

● **S06.6X4 Traumatic subarachnoid hemorrhage with loss of consciousness of 6 hours to 24 hours** A, A, A, S Ex: PDX 1612

● **S06.6X5 Traumatic subarachnoid hemorrhage with loss of consciousness greater than 24 hours with return to pre-existing conscious level** A, A, A, S Ex: PDX 1612

● **S06.6X6 Traumatic subarachnoid hemorrhage with loss of consciousness greater than 24 hours without return to pre-existing conscious level with patient surviving** A, A, A, S Ex: PDX 1612
Coding Clinic: 2021, Q2, P5

● **S06.6X7 Traumatic subarachnoid hemorrhage with loss of consciousness of any duration with death due to brain injury prior to regaining consciousness** A, A Ex: PDX 1612

● **S06.6X8 Traumatic subarachnoid hemorrhage with loss of consciousness of any duration with death due to other cause prior to regaining consciousness** A, A Ex: PDX 1612

● **S06.6X9 Traumatic subarachnoid hemorrhage with loss of consciousness of unspecified duration** A, A, A, S Ex: PDX 1612

● **S06.6XA Traumatic subarachnoid hemorrhage with loss of consciousness status unknown** A, A Ex: PDX 1626
Traumatic subarachnoid hemorrhage NOS
Coding Clinic: 2022, Q4, P45

● **S06.8 Other specified intracranial injuries**

● **S06.81 Injury of right internal carotid artery, intracranial portion, not elsewhere classified**
Coding Clinic: 2016, Q4, P67

● **S06.810 Injury of right internal carotid artery, intracranial portion, not elsewhere classified without loss of consciousness** A, S

● **S06.811 Injury of right internal carotid artery, intracranial portion, not elsewhere classified with loss of consciousness of 30 minutes or less** A, A, A, S Ex: PDX 1612
Injury of right internal carotid artery, intracranial portion, not elsewhere classified with brief loss of consciousness

● **S06.812 Injury of right internal carotid artery, intracranial portion, not elsewhere classified with loss of consciousness of 31 minutes to 59 minutes** A, A, A, S Ex: PDX 1612

● **S06.813 Injury of right internal carotid artery, intracranial portion, not elsewhere classified with loss of consciousness of 1 hour to 5 hours 59 minutes** A, A, A, S Ex: PDX 1612

- S06.814 Injury of right internal carotid artery, intracranial portion, not elsewhere classified with loss of consciousness of 6 hours to 24 hours A, A, A, S Ex PDX 1612
- S06.815 Injury of right internal carotid artery, intracranial portion, not elsewhere classified with loss of consciousness greater than 24 hours with return to pre-existing conscious level A, A, A, S Ex PDX 1612
- S06.816 Injury of right internal carotid artery, intracranial portion, not elsewhere classified with loss of consciousness greater than 24 hours without return to pre-existing conscious level with patient surviving A, A, A, S Ex PDX 1612
- S06.817 Injury of right internal carotid artery, intracranial portion, not elsewhere classified with loss of consciousness of any duration with death due to brain injury prior to regaining consciousness A, A Ex PDX 1612
- S06.818 Injury of right internal carotid artery, intracranial portion, not elsewhere classified with loss of consciousness of any duration with death due to other cause prior to regaining consciousness A, A Ex PDX 1612
- S06.819 Injury of right internal carotid artery, intracranial portion, not elsewhere classified with loss of consciousness of unspecified duration A, A, A, S Ex PDX 1612
- S06.81A Injury of right internal carotid artery, intracranial portion, not elsewhere classified with loss of consciousness status unknown A, A Ex PDX 1626
  Injury of right internal carotid artery, intracranial portion, not elsewhere classified NOS

S06.82 Injury of left internal carotid artery, intracranial portion, not elsewhere classified
Coding Clinic: 2016, Q4, P67

- S06.820 Injury of left internal carotid artery, intracranial portion, not elsewhere classified without loss of consciousness A, S
- S06.821 Injury of left internal carotid artery, intracranial portion, not elsewhere classified with loss of consciousness of 30 minutes or less A, A, A, S Ex PDX 1612
  Injury of left internal carotid artery, intracranial portion, not elsewhere classified with brief loss of consciousness
- S06.822 Injury of left internal carotid artery, intracranial portion, not elsewhere classified with loss of consciousness of 31 minutes to 59 minutes A, A, A, S Ex PDX 1612
- S06.823 Injury of left internal carotid artery, intracranial portion, not elsewhere classified with loss of consciousness of 1 hour to 5 hours 59 minutes A, A, A, S Ex PDX 1612
- S06.824 Injury of left internal carotid artery, intracranial portion, not elsewhere classified with loss of consciousness of 6 hours to 24 hours A, A, A, S Ex PDX 1612
- S06.825 Injury of left internal carotid artery, intracranial portion, not elsewhere classified with loss of consciousness greater than 24 hours with return to pre-existing conscious level A, A Ex PDX 1612
- S06.826 Injury of left internal carotid artery, intracranial portion, not elsewhere classified with loss of consciousness greater than 24 hours without return to pre-existing conscious level with patient surviving A, A, A, S Ex PDX 1612
- S06.827 Injury of left internal carotid artery, intracranial portion, not elsewhere classified with loss of consciousness of any duration with death due to brain injury prior to regaining consciousness A, A Ex PDX 1612
- S06.828 Injury of left internal carotid artery, intracranial portion, not elsewhere classified with loss of consciousness of any duration with death due to other cause prior to regaining consciousness A, A Ex PDX 1612
- S06.829 Injury of left internal carotid artery, intracranial portion, not elsewhere classified with loss of consciousness of unspecified duration A, A, A, S Ex PDX 1612
- S06.82A Injury of left internal carotid artery, intracranial portion, not elsewhere classified with loss of consciousness status unknown A, A Ex PDX 1626
  Injury of left internal carotid artery, intracranial portion, not elsewhere classified NOS

S06.89 Other specified intracranial injury
Excludes1 concussion (S06.0X-)

- S06.890 Other specified intracranial injury without loss of consciousness A, S
  Coding Clinic: 2024, Q2, P16
- S06.891 Other specified intracranial injury with loss of consciousness of 30 minutes or less A, A, A, S Ex PDX 1612
  Other specified intracranial injury with brief loss of consciousness
- S06.892 Other specified intracranial injury with loss of consciousness of 31 minutes to 59 minutes A, A, A, S Ex PDX 1612
- S06.893 Other specified intracranial injury with loss of consciousness of 1 hour to 5 hours 59 minutes A, A, A, S Ex PDX 1612
- S06.894 Other specified intracranial injury with loss of consciousness of 6 hours to 24 hours A, A, A, S Ex PDX 1612
- S06.895 Other specified intracranial injury with loss of consciousness greater than 24 hours with return to pre-existing conscious level A, A, A, S Ex PDX 1612
- S06.896 Other specified intracranial injury with loss of consciousness greater than 24 hours without return to pre-existing conscious level with patient surviving A, A, A, S Ex PDX 1612
- S06.897 Other specified intracranial injury with loss of consciousness of any duration with death due to brain injury prior to regaining consciousness A, A Ex PDX 1612

S06.898 Other specified intracranial injury with loss of consciousness of any duration with death due to other cause prior to regaining consciousness A, A Ex PDX 1612

S06.899 Other specified intracranial injury with loss of consciousness of unspecified duration A, A, A, S Ex PDX 1612

S06.89A Other specified intracranial injury with loss of consciousness status unknown A, A Ex PDX 1626

S06.8A Primary blast injury of brain, not elsewhere classified Ex PDX 1626

Code also, if applicable, focal traumatic brain injury (S06.3-)

Excludes2 traumatic cerebral edema (S06.1)

S06.8A0 Primary blast injury of brain, not elsewhere classified without loss of consciousness A, A

S06.8A1 Primary blast injury of brain, not elsewhere classified with loss of consciousness of 30 minutes or less A, A

Primary blast injury of brain, not elsewhere classified with brief loss of consciousness

S06.8A2 Primary blast injury of brain, not elsewhere classified with loss of consciousness of 31 minutes to 59 minutes A, A

S06.8A3 Primary blast injury of brain, not elsewhere classified with loss of consciousness of 1 hour to 5 hours 59 minutes A, A

S06.8A4 Primary blast injury of brain, not elsewhere classified with loss of consciousness of 6 hours to 24 hours A, A

S06.8A5 Primary blast injury of brain, not elsewhere classified with loss of consciousness greater than 24 hours with return to pre-existing conscious level A, A

S06.8A6 Primary blast injury of brain, not elsewhere classified with loss of consciousness greater than 24 hours without return to pre-existing conscious level with patient surviving A, A

S06.8A7 Primary blast injury of brain, not elsewhere classified with loss of consciousness of any duration with death due to brain injury prior to regaining consciousness A, A

S06.8A8 Primary blast injury of brain, not elsewhere classified with loss of consciousness of any duration with death due to other cause prior to regaining consciousness A, A

S06.8AA Primary blast injury of brain, not elsewhere classified with loss of consciousness status unknown A, A

Primary blast injury of brain NOS

S06.8A9 Primary blast injury of brain, not elsewhere classified with loss of consciousness of unspecified duration A, A

S06.9 Unspecified intracranial injury

Brain injury NOS

Head injury NOS with loss of consciousness

Traumatic brain injury NOS

Excludes1 conditions classifiable to S06.0- to S06.8- code to specified intracranial injury

head injury NOS (S09.90)

S06.9X Unspecified intracranial injury

S06.9X0 Unspecified intracranial injury without loss of consciousness A, S

S06.9X1 Unspecified intracranial injury with loss of consciousness of 30 minutes or less A, A, A, S Ex PDX 1612

Unspecified intracranial injury with brief loss of consciousness

S06.9X2 Unspecified intracranial injury with loss of consciousness of 31 minutes to 59 minutes A, A, A, S Ex PDX 1612

S06.9X3 Unspecified intracranial injury with loss of consciousness of 1 hour to 5 hours 59 minutes A, A, A, S Ex PDX 1612

S06.9X4 Unspecified intracranial injury with loss of consciousness of 6 hours to 24 hours A, A, A, S Ex PDX 1612

S06.9X5 Unspecified intracranial injury with loss of consciousness greater than 24 hours with return to pre-existing conscious level A, A, A, S Ex PDX 1612

S06.9X6 Unspecified intracranial injury with loss of consciousness greater than 24 hours without return to pre-existing conscious level with patient surviving A, A, A, S Ex PDX 1612

S06.9X7 Unspecified intracranial injury with loss of consciousness of any duration with death due to brain injury prior to regaining consciousness A, A Ex PDX 1612

S06.9X8 Unspecified intracranial injury with loss of consciousness of any duration with death due to other cause prior to regaining consciousness A, A Ex PDX 1612

S06.9X9 Unspecified intracranial injury with loss of consciousness of unspecified duration A, A, A, S Ex PDX 1612

S06.9XA Unspecified intracranial injury with loss of consciousness status unknown A, A Ex PDX 1626

S06.A Traumatic brain compression and herniation A Ex PDX 1627

Traumatic cerebral compression

Code first the underlying traumatic brain injury, such as:

- diffuse traumatic brain injury (S06.2-)
- focal traumatic brain injury (S06.3-)
- traumatic subdural hemorrhage (S06.5-)
- traumatic subarachnoid hemorrhage (S06.6-)

S06.A0 Traumatic brain compression without herniation A

Traumatic brain compression NOS

Traumatic cerebral compression NOS

S06.A1 Traumatic brain compression with herniation

Traumatic brain herniation

Traumatic brainstem compression with herniation

Traumatic cerebellar compression with herniation

Traumatic cerebral compression with herniation

CHAPTER 19 (S00-T88)

● **S07 Crushing injury of head** (Ex) PDX 1633

Use additional code for all associated injuries, such as:
intracranial injuries (S06.-)
skull fractures (S02.-)

The appropriate 7th character is to be added to each code from category S07

A	initial encounter
D	subsequent encounter
S	sequela

X● **S07.0** Crushing injury of face A, A
X● **S07.1** Crushing injury of skull A, A
X● **S07.8** Crushing injury of other parts of head A, A
X● **S07.9** Crushing injury of head, part unspecified A, A

● **S08 Avulsion and traumatic amputation of part of head**

An amputation not identified as partial or complete should be coded to complete

The appropriate 7th character is to be added to each code from category S08

A	initial encounter
D	subsequent encounter
S	sequela

X● **S08.0** Avulsion of scalp
● **S08.1** Traumatic amputation of ear
● **S08.11** Complete traumatic amputation of ear
● **S08.111** Complete traumatic amputation of right ear
● **S08.112** Complete traumatic amputation of left ear
● **S08.119** Complete traumatic amputation of unspecified ear
● **S08.12** Partial traumatic amputation of ear
● **S08.121** Partial traumatic amputation of right ear
● **S08.122** Partial traumatic amputation of left ear
● **S08.129** Partial traumatic amputation of unspecified ear
● **S08.8** Traumatic amputation of other parts of head
● **S08.81** Traumatic amputation of nose
● **S08.811** Complete traumatic amputation of nose
● **S08.812** Partial traumatic amputation of nose
X● **S08.89** Traumatic amputation of other parts of head

● **S09 Other and unspecified injuries of head**

The appropriate 7th character is to be added to each code from category S09

A	initial encounter
D	subsequent encounter
S	sequela

X● **S09.0** Injury of blood vessels of head, not elsewhere classified A (Ex) PDX 1634

Excludes1 injury of cerebral blood vessels (S06.-)
injury of precerebral blood vessels (S15.-)

● **S09.1** Injury of muscle and tendon of head

Code also any associated open wound (S01.-)

Excludes2 sprain to joints and ligament of head (S03.9)

X● **S09.10** Unspecified injury of muscle and tendon of head
Injury of muscle and tendon of head NOS
X● **S09.11** Strain of muscle and tendon of head
X● **S09.12** Laceration of muscle and tendon of head
X● **S09.19** Other specified injury of muscle and tendon of head

● **S09.2** Traumatic rupture of ear drum (Ex) PDX 1635

Excludes1 traumatic rupture of ear drum due to blast injury (S09.31-)

X● **S09.20** Traumatic rupture of unspecified ear drum A
X● **S09.21** Traumatic rupture of right ear drum A
X● **S09.22** Traumatic rupture of left ear drum A

● **S09.3** Other specified and unspecified injury of middle and inner ear (Ex) PDX 1635

Excludes1 injury to ear NOS (S09.91-)

Excludes2 injury to external ear (S00.4-, S01.3-, S08.1-)

● **S09.30** Unspecified injury of middle and inner ear
● **S09.301** Unspecified injury of right middle and inner ear A
● **S09.302** Unspecified injury of left middle and inner ear A
● **S09.309** Unspecified injury of unspecified middle and inner ear A
● **S09.31** Primary blast injury of ear
Blast injury of ear NOS
● **S09.311** Primary blast injury of right ear A
● **S09.312** Primary blast injury of left ear A
● **S09.313** Primary blast injury of ear, bilateral A
● **S09.319** Primary blast injury of unspecified ear A
● **S09.39** Other specified injury of middle and inner ear
Secondary blast injury to ear
● **S09.391** Other specified injury of right middle and inner ear A
● **S09.392** Other specified injury of left middle and inner ear A
● **S09.399** Other specified injury of unspecified middle and inner ear A

X● **S09.8** Other specified injuries of head
● **S09.9** Unspecified injury of face and head
X● **S09.90** Unspecified injury of head
Head injury NOS

Excludes1 brain injury NOS (S06.9-)
head injury NOS with loss of consciousness (S06.9-)
intracranial injury NOS (S06.9-)

X● **S09.91** Unspecified injury of ear
Injury of ear NOS
X● **S09.92** Unspecified injury of nose
Injury of nose NOS
X● **S09.93** Unspecified injury of face
Injury of face NOS

INJURIES TO THE NECK (S10-S19)

Includes injuries of nape
injuries of supraclavicular region
injuries of throat

Excludes2 burns and corrosions (T20-T32)
effects of foreign body in esophagus (T18.1)
effects of foreign body in larynx (T17.3)
effects of foreign body in pharynx (T17.2)
effects of foreign body in trachea (T17.4)
frostbite (T33-T34)
insect bite or sting, venomous (T63.4)

● **S10 Superficial injury of neck**

The appropriate 7th character is to be added to each code from category S10

A	initial encounter
D	subsequent encounter
S	sequela

X● S10.Ø Contusion of throat
Contusion of cervical esophagus
Contusion of larynx
Contusion of pharynx
Contusion of trachea

● S10.1 Other and unspecified superficial injuries of throat
X● S10.10 Unspecified superficial injuries of throat
X● S10.11 Abrasion of throat
X● S10.12 Blister (nonthermal) of throat
X● S10.14 External constriction of part of throat
X● S10.15 Superficial foreign body of throat
Splinter in the throat
X● S10.16 Insect bite (nonvenomous) of throat
X● S10.17 Other superficial bite of throat
Excludes1 open bite of throat (S11.85)

● S10.8 Superficial injury of other specified parts of neck
X● S10.80 Unspecified superficial injury of other specified part of neck
X● S10.81 Abrasion of other specified part of neck
X● S10.82 Blister (nonthermal) of other specified part of neck
X● S10.83 Contusion of other specified part of neck
X● S10.84 External constriction of other specified part of neck
X● S10.85 Superficial foreign body of other specified part of neck
Splinter in other part of neck
X● S10.86 Insect bite of other specified part of neck
X● S10.87 Other superficial bite of other specified part of neck
Excludes1 open bite of other specified parts of neck (S11.85)

● S10.9 Superficial injury of unspecified part of neck
X● S10.90 Unspecified superficial injury of unspecified part of neck
X● S10.91 Abrasion of unspecified part of neck
X● S10.92 Blister (nonthermal) of unspecified part of neck
X● S10.93 Contusion of unspecified part of neck
X● S10.94 External constriction of unspecified part of neck
X● S10.95 Superficial foreign body of unspecified part of neck
X● S10.96 Insect bite of unspecified part of neck
X● S10.97 Other superficial bite of unspecified part of neck

● S11 Open wound of neck
Code also any associated:
spinal cord injury (S14.Ø, S14.1-)
wound infection
Excludes2 open fracture of vertebra (S12.- with 7th character B)
The appropriate 7th character is to be added to each code from category S11

A	initial encounter
D	subsequent encounter
S	sequela

● S11.Ø Open wound of larynx and trachea (Ex:) PDX 1636
● S11.Ø1 Open wound of larynx
Excludes2 open wound of vocal cord (S11.Ø3)
● S11.Ø11 Laceration without foreign body of larynx A
● S11.Ø12 Laceration with foreign body of larynx A
● S11.Ø13 Puncture wound without foreign body of larynx A
● S11.Ø14 Puncture wound with foreign body of larynx A
● S11.Ø15 Open bite of larynx A
Bite of larynx NOS
● S11.Ø19 Unspecified open wound of larynx A
● S11.Ø2 Open wound of trachea
Open wound of cervical trachea
Open wound of trachea NOS
Excludes2 open wound of thoracic trachea (S27.5-)
● S11.Ø21 Laceration without foreign body of trachea A
● S11.Ø22 Laceration with foreign body of trachea A
● S11.Ø23 Puncture wound without foreign body of trachea A
● S11.Ø24 Puncture wound with foreign body of trachea A
● S11.Ø25 Open bite of trachea A
Bite of trachea NOS
● S11.Ø29 Unspecified open wound of trachea A
● S11.Ø3 Open wound of vocal cord
● S11.Ø31 Laceration without foreign body of vocal cord A
● S11.Ø32 Laceration with foreign body of vocal cord A
● S11.Ø33 Puncture wound without foreign body of vocal cord A
● S11.Ø34 Puncture wound with foreign body of vocal cord A
● S11.Ø35 Open bite of vocal cord A
Bite of vocal cord NOS
● S11.Ø39 Unspecified open wound of vocal cord A

● S11.1 Open wound of thyroid gland
X● S11.10 Unspecified open wound of thyroid gland A (Ex:) PDX 1637
X● S11.11 Laceration without foreign body of thyroid gland A (Ex:) PDX 1637
X● S11.12 Laceration with foreign body of thyroid gland A (Ex:) PDX 1638
X● S11.13 Puncture wound without foreign body of thyroid gland A (Ex:) PDX 1637
X● S11.14 Puncture wound with foreign body of thyroid gland A (Ex:) PDX 1638
X● S11.15 Open bite of thyroid gland A (Ex:) PDX 1637
Bite of thyroid gland NOS

● S11.2 Open wound of pharynx and cervical esophagus
Excludes1 open wound of esophagus NOS (S27.8-)
X● S11.20 Unspecified open wound of pharynx and cervical esophagus A (Ex:) PDX 1639
X● S11.21 Laceration without foreign body of pharynx and cervical esophagus A (Ex:) PDX 1639
X● S11.22 Laceration with foreign body of pharynx and cervical esophagus A (Ex:) PDX 1640
X● S11.23 Puncture wound without foreign body of pharynx and cervical esophagus A (Ex:) PDX 1639
X● S11.24 Puncture wound with foreign body of pharynx and cervical esophagus A (Ex:) PDX 1640
X● S11.25 Open bite of pharynx and cervical esophagus A (Ex:) PDX 1639
Bite of pharynx and cervical esophagus NOS

● S11.8 Open wound of other specified parts of neck
X● S11.80 Unspecified open specified wound of other part of neck
X● S11.81 Laceration without foreign body of other specified part of neck
X● S11.82 Laceration with foreign body of other specified part of neck
X● S11.83 Puncture wound without foreign body of other specified part of neck

X S11.84 **Puncture wound with foreign body** of other specified part of neck

X S11.85 **Open bite** of other specified part of neck
Bite of other part of neck NOS
Excludes1 superficial bite of other specified part of neck (S10.87)

X S11.89 **Other** open wound of other part of neck

S11.9 Open wound of **unspecified** part of neck

X S11.90 **Unspecified** open wound of unspecified part of neck

X S11.91 **Laceration without foreign body** of unspecified part of neck

X S11.92 **Laceration with foreign body** of unspecified part of neck

X S11.93 **Puncture wound without foreign body** of unspecified part of neck

X S11.94 **Puncture wound with foreign body** of unspecified part of neck

X S11.95 **Open bite** of unspecified part of neck
Bite of neck NOS
Excludes1 superficial bite of neck (S10.97)

S12 Fracture of cervical vertebra and other parts of neck

Note: A fracture not indicated as displaced or nondisplaced should be coded to displaced

A fracture not indicated as open or closed should be coded to closed

Includes fracture of cervical neural arch
fracture of cervical spine
fracture of cervical spinous process
fracture of cervical transverse process
fracture of cervical vertebral arch
fracture of neck

Code first any associated cervical spinal cord injury (S14.0, S14.1-)

The appropriate 7th character is to be added to all codes from subcategories S12.0-S12.6

A	initial encounter for closed fracture
B	initial encounter for open fracture
D	subsequent encounter for fracture with routine healing
G	subsequent encounter for fracture with delayed healing
K	subsequent encounter for fracture with nonunion
S	sequela

S12.0 Fracture of first **cervical vertebra** (Ex) PDX 1264 [K], 1641 [A, B]
Atlas

S12.00 **Unspecified** fracture of **first** cervical vertebra

S12.000 Unspecified **displaced** fracture of first cervical vertebra A, K, B, A, B, A, B

S12.001 Unspecified **nondisplaced** fracture of first cervical vertebra A, K, B, A, B, A, B

X S12.01 **Stable burst** fracture of first cervical vertebra A, K, B, A, B, A, B

X S12.02 **Unstable burst** fracture of first cervical vertebra A, K, B, A, B, A, B

S12.03 **Posterior arch** fracture of first cervical vertebra

S12.030 **Displaced** posterior arch fracture of first cervical vertebra A, K, B, A, B, A, B

S12.031 **Nondisplaced** posterior arch fracture of first cervical vertebra A, K, B, A, B, A, B

S12.04 **Lateral mass** fracture of first cervical vertebra

S12.040 **Displaced** lateral mass fracture of first cervical vertebra A, K, B, A, B, A, B

S12.041 **Nondisplaced** lateral mass fracture of first cervical vertebra A, K, B, A, B, A, B

S12.09 **Other** fracture of first cervical vertebra

S12.090 Other **displaced** fracture of first cervical vertebra A, K, B, A, B, A, B

S12.091 Other **nondisplaced** fracture of first cervical vertebra A, K, B, A, B, A, B

S12.1 Fracture of **second** cervical vertebra (Ex) PDX 1264 [K], 1641 [A, B]
Axis

S12.10 **Unspecified** fracture of second cervical vertebra

S12.100 Unspecified **displaced** fracture of second cervical vertebra A, K, B, A, B, A, B
Coding Clinic: 2024, Q2, P23

S12.101 Unspecified **nondisplaced** fracture of second cervical vertebra A, K, B, A, B, A, B

S12.11 **Type II dens** fracture

S12.110 **Anterior** displaced Type II dens fracture A, K, B, A, B, A, B

S12.111 **Posterior** displaced Type II dens fracture A, K, B, A, B, A, B

S12.112 **Nondisplaced** Type II dens fracture A, K, B, A, B, A, B

S12.12 **Other dens** fracture

S12.120 Other **displaced** dens fracture A, K, B, A, B, A, B

S12.121 Other **nondisplaced** dens fracture A, K, B, A, B, A, B

S12.13 **Unspecified traumatic spondylolisthesis** of second cervical vertebra

S12.130 Unspecified traumatic **displaced** spondylolisthesis of second cervical vertebra A, K, B, A, B, A, B

S12.131 Unspecified traumatic **nondisplaced** spondylolisthesis of second cervical vertebra A, K, B, A, B, A, B

X S12.14 **Type III traumatic spondylolisthesis** of second cervical vertebra A, K, B, A, B, A, B

S12.15 **Other traumatic spondylolisthesis** of second cervical vertebra

S12.150 Other traumatic **displaced** spondylolisthesis of second cervical vertebra A, K, B, A, B, A, B

S12.151 Other traumatic **nondisplaced** spondylolisthesis of second cervical vertebra A, K, B, A, B, A, B

S12.19 **Other** fracture of second cervical vertebra

S12.190 Other **displaced** fracture of second cervical vertebra A, K, B, A, B, A, B

S12.191 Other **nondisplaced** fracture of second cervical vertebra A, K, B, A, B, A, B

S12.2 Fracture of **third** cervical vertebra (Ex) PDX 1264 [K], 1641 [A, B]

S12.20 **Unspecified** fracture of third cervical vertebra

S12.200 Unspecified **displaced** fracture of third cervical vertebra A, K, B, A, B, A, B

S12.201 Unspecified **nondisplaced** fracture of third cervical vertebra A, K, B, A, B, A, B

S12.23 **Unspecified** traumatic **spondylolisthesis** of **third** cervical vertebra

S12.230 Unspecified traumatic **displaced** spondylolisthesis of third cervical vertebra A, K, B, A, B, A, B

S12.231 Unspecified traumatic **nondisplaced** spondylolisthesis of third cervical vertebra A, K, B, A, B, A, B

X S12.24 Type III traumatic spondylolisthesis of third cervical vertebra A, K, B, A, B, A, B

S12.25 Other traumatic spondylolisthesis of third cervical vertebra

S12.250 Other traumatic displaced spondylolisthesis of third cervical vertebra A, K, B, A, B, A, B

S12.251 Other traumatic nondisplaced spondylolisthesis of third cervical vertebra A, K, B, A, B, A, B

S12.29 Other fracture of third cervical vertebra

S12.290 Other displaced fracture of third cervical vertebra A, K, B, A, B, A, B

S12.291 Other nondisplaced fracture of third cervical vertebra A, K, B, A, B, A, B

S12.3 Fracture of fourth cervical vertebra (Ex:) PDX 1264 [K], 1641 [A, B]

S12.30 Unspecified fracture of fourth cervical vertebra

S12.300 Unspecified displaced fracture of fourth cervical vertebra A, K, B, A, B, A, B

S12.301 Unspecified nondisplaced fracture of fourth cervical vertebra A, K, B, A, B, A, B

S12.33 Unspecified traumatic spondylolisthesis of fourth cervical vertebra

S12.330 Unspecified traumatic displaced spondylolisthesis of fourth cervical vertebra A, K, B, A, B, A, B

S12.331 Unspecified traumatic nondisplaced spondylolisthesis of fourth cervical vertebra A, K, B, A, B, A, B

X S12.34 Type III traumatic spondylolisthesis of fourth cervical vertebra A, K, B, A, B, A, B

S12.35 Other traumatic spondylolisthesis of fourth cervical vertebra

S12.350 Other traumatic displaced spondylolisthesis of fourth cervical vertebra A, K, B, A, B, A, B

S12.351 Other traumatic nondisplaced spondylolisthesis of fourth cervical vertebra A, K, B, A, B, A, B

S12.39 Other fracture of fourth cervical vertebra

S12.390 Other displaced fracture of fourth cervical vertebra A, K, B, A, B, A, B

S12.391 Other nondisplaced fracture of fourth cervical vertebra A, K, B, A, B, A, B

S12.4 Fracture of fifth cervical vertebra (Ex:) PDX 1264 [K], 1641 [A, B]

S12.40 Unspecified fracture of fifth cervical vertebra

S12.400 Unspecified displaced fracture of fifth cervical vertebra A, K, B, A, B, A, B

S12.401 Unspecified nondisplaced fracture of fifth cervical vertebra A, K, B, A, B, A, B

S12.43 Unspecified traumatic spondylolisthesis of fifth cervical vertebra

S12.430 Unspecified traumatic displaced spondylolisthesis of fifth cervical vertebra A, K, B, A, B, A, B

S12.431 Unspecified traumatic nondisplaced spondylolisthesis of fifth cervical vertebra A, K, B, A, B, A, B

X S12.44 Type III traumatic spondylolisthesis of fifth cervical vertebra A, K, B, A, B, A, B

S12.45 Other traumatic spondylolisthesis of fifth cervical vertebra

S12.450 Other traumatic displaced spondylolisthesis of fifth cervical vertebra A, K, B, A, B, A, B

S12.451 Other traumatic nondisplaced spondylolisthesis of fifth cervical vertebra A, K, B, A, B, A, B

S12.49 Other fracture of fifth cervical vertebra

S12.490 Other displaced fracture of fifth cervical vertebra A, K, B, A, B, A, B

S12.491 Other nondisplaced fracture of fifth cervical vertebra A, K, B, A, B, A, B

S12.5 Fracture of sixth cervical vertebra (Ex:) PDX 1264 [K], 1641 [A, B]

S12.50 Unspecified fracture of sixth cervical vertebra

S12.500 Unspecified displaced fracture of sixth cervical vertebra A, K, B, A, B, A, B

S12.501 Unspecified nondisplaced fracture of sixth cervical vertebra A, K, B, A, B, A, B

S12.53 Unspecified traumatic spondylolisthesis of sixth cervical vertebra

S12.530 Unspecified traumatic displaced spondylolisthesis of sixth cervical vertebra A, K, B, A, B, A, B

S12.531 Unspecified traumatic nondisplaced spondylolisthesis of sixth cervical vertebra A, K, B, A, B, A, B

X S12.54 Type III traumatic spondylolisthesis of sixth cervical vertebra A, K, B, A, B, A, B

S12.55 Other traumatic spondylolisthesis of sixth cervical vertebra

S12.550 Other traumatic displaced spondylolisthesis of sixth cervical vertebra A, K, B, A, B, A, B

S12.551 Other traumatic nondisplaced spondylolisthesis of sixth cervical vertebra A, K, B, A, B, A, B

S12.59 Other fracture of sixth cervical vertebra

S12.590 Other displaced fracture of sixth cervical vertebra A, K, B, A, B, A, B

S12.591 Other nondisplaced fracture of sixth cervical vertebra A, K, B, A, B, A, B

S12.6 Fracture of seventh cervical vertebra (Ex:) PDX 1264 [K], 1641 [A, B]

S12.60 Unspecified fracture of seventh cervical vertebra

S12.600 Unspecified displaced fracture of seventh cervical vertebra A, K, B, A, B, A, B

S12.601 Unspecified nondisplaced fracture of seventh cervical vertebra A, K, B, A, B, A, B

S12.63 Unspecified traumatic spondylolisthesis of seventh cervical vertebra

S12.630 Unspecified traumatic displaced spondylolisthesis of seventh cervical vertebra A, K, B, A, B, A, B

S12.631 Unspecified traumatic nondisplaced spondylolisthesis of seventh cervical vertebra A, K, B, A, B, A, B

X S12.64 Type III traumatic spondylolisthesis of seventh cervical vertebra A, K, B, A, B, A, B

S12.65 Other traumatic spondylolisthesis of seventh cervical vertebra

● S12.650 Other traumatic displaced spondylolisthesis of seventh cervical vertebra A, K, B, A, B, A, B

● S12.651 Other traumatic nondisplaced spondylolisthesis of seventh cervical vertebra A, K, B, A, B, A, B

● S12.69 Other fracture of seventh cervical vertebra

● S12.690 Other displaced fracture of seventh cervical vertebra A, K, B, A, B, A, B

● S12.691 Other nondisplaced fracture of seventh cervical vertebra A, K, B, A, B, A, B

X● S12.8 Fracture of other parts of neck A, A, A (Ex) PDX 1642

Hyoid bone
Larynx
Thyroid cartilage
Trachea

The appropriate 7th character is to be added to code S12.8

A	initial encounter
D	subsequent encounter
S	sequela

X● S12.9 Fracture of neck, unspecified A, A, A (Ex) PDX 1641

Fracture of neck NOS
Fracture of cervical spine NOS
Fracture of cervical vertebra NOS

The appropriate 7th character is to be added to code S12.9

A	initial encounter
D	subsequent encounter
S	sequela

● S13 Dislocation and sprain of joints and ligaments at neck level (Ex) PDX 1353

Includes avulsion of joint or ligament at neck level
laceration of cartilage, joint or ligament at neck level
sprain of cartilage, joint or ligament at neck level
traumatic hemarthrosis of joint or ligament at neck level
traumatic rupture of joint or ligament at neck level
traumatic subluxation of joint or ligament at neck level
traumatic tear of joint or ligament at neck level

Code also any associated open wound

Excludes2 strain of muscle or tendon at neck level (S16.1)

The appropriate 7th character is to be added to each code from category S13

A	initial encounter
D	subsequent encounter
S	sequela

X● S13.0 Traumatic rupture of cervical intervertebral disc A, A

Excludes1 rupture or displacement (nontraumatic) of cervical intervertebral disc NOS (M50.-)

● S13.1 Subluxation and dislocation of cervical vertebrae

Code also any associated:
open wound of neck (S11.-)
spinal cord injury (S14.1-)

Excludes2 fracture of cervical vertebrae (S12.0-S12.3-)

● S13.10 Subluxation and dislocation of unspecified cervical vertebrae

● S13.100 Subluxation of unspecified cervical vertebrae A, A

● S13.101 Dislocation of unspecified cervical vertebrae A, A

● S13.11 Subluxation and dislocation of C0/C1 cervical vertebrae

Subluxation and dislocation of atlantooccipital joint
Subluxation and dislocation of atloidooccipital joint
Subluxation and dislocation of occipitoatloid joint

● S13.110 Subluxation of C0/C1 cervical vertebrae A, A

● S13.111 Dislocation of C0/C1 cervical vertebrae A, A

● S13.12 Subluxation and dislocation of C1/C2 cervical vertebrae

Subluxation and dislocation of atlantoaxial joint

● S13.120 Subluxation of C1/C2 cervical vertebrae A, A

● S13.121 Dislocation of C1/C2 cervical vertebrae A, A

● S13.13 Subluxation and dislocation of C2/C3 cervical vertebrae

● S13.130 Subluxation of C2/C3 cervical vertebrae A, A

● S13.131 Dislocation of C2/C3 cervical vertebrae A, A

● S13.14 Subluxation and dislocation of C3/C4 cervical vertebrae

● S13.140 Subluxation of C3/C4 cervical vertebrae A, A

● S13.141 Dislocation of C3/C4 cervical vertebrae A, A

● S13.15 Subluxation and dislocation of C4/C5 cervical vertebrae

● S13.150 Subluxation of C4/C5 cervical vertebrae A, A

● S13.151 Dislocation of C4/C5 cervical vertebrae A, A

● S13.16 Subluxation and dislocation of C5/C6 cervical vertebrae

● S13.160 Subluxation of C5/C6 cervical vertebrae A, A

● S13.161 Dislocation of C5/C6 cervical vertebrae A, A

● S13.17 Subluxation and dislocation of C6/C7 cervical vertebrae

● S13.170 Subluxation of C6/C7 cervical vertebrae A, A

● S13.171 Dislocation of C6/C7 cervical vertebrae A, A

● S13.18 Subluxation and dislocation of C7/T1 cervical vertebrae

● S13.180 Subluxation of C7/T1 cervical vertebrae A, A

● S13.181 Dislocation of C7/T1 cervical vertebrae A, A

● S13.2 Dislocation of other and unspecified parts of neck

X● S13.20 Dislocation of unspecified parts of neck A, A

X● S13.29 Dislocation of other parts of neck A, A

X● S13.4 Sprain of ligaments of cervical spine

Sprain of anterior longitudinal (ligament), cervical
Sprain of atlanto-axial (joints)
Sprain of atlanto-occipital (joints)
Whiplash injury of cervical spine

X● S13.5 Sprain of thyroid region

Sprain of cricoarytenoid (joint) (ligament)
Sprain of cricothyroid (joint) (ligament)
Sprain of thyroid cartilage

X● S13.8 Sprain of joints and ligaments of other parts of neck

X● S13.9 Sprain of joints and ligaments of unspecified parts of neck

● **S14 Injury of nerves and spinal cord at neck level** (Ex) PDX 1643

Note: Code to highest level of cervical cord injury

Code also any associated:
fracture of cervical vertebra (S12.0--S12.6.-)
open wound of neck (S11.-)
transient paralysis (R29.5)

The appropriate 7th character is to be added to each code from category S14

A	initial encounter
D	subsequent encounter
S	sequela

X● **S14.0 Concussion and edema of cervical spinal cord** A, A, D, S
Coding Clinic: 2024, Q2, P24

● **S14.1 Other and unspecified injuries of cervical spinal cord**

● **S14.10 Unspecified injury of cervical spinal cord**

● **S14.101 Unspecified injury at C1 level of cervical spinal cord** A, A, A, D, S

● **S14.102 Unspecified injury at C2 level of cervical spinal cord** A, A, A, D, S

● **S14.103 Unspecified injury at C3 level of cervical spinal cord** A, A, A, D, S

● **S14.104 Unspecified injury at C4 level of cervical spinal cord** A, A, A, D, S

● **S14.105 Unspecified injury at C5 level of cervical spinal cord** A, A, A, D, S

● **S14.106 Unspecified injury at C6 level of cervical spinal cord** A, A, A, D, S

● **S14.107 Unspecified injury at C7 level of cervical spinal cord** A, A, A, D, S

● **S14.108 Unspecified injury at C8 level of cervical spinal cord** A, A, D, S

● **S14.109 Unspecified injury at unspecified level of cervical spinal cord** A, D, S
Injury of cervical spinal cord NOS

● **S14.11 Complete lesion of cervical spinal cord**

● **S14.111 Complete lesion at C1 level of cervical spinal cord** A, A, A, D, S

● **S14.112 Complete lesion at C2 level of cervical spinal cord** A, A, A, D, S

● **S14.113 Complete lesion at C3 level of cervical spinal cord** A, A, A, D, S

● **S14.114 Complete lesion at C4 level of cervical spinal cord** A, A, A, D, S

● **S14.115 Complete lesion at C5 level of cervical spinal cord** A, A, A, D, S

● **S14.116 Complete lesion at C6 level of cervical spinal cord** A, A, A, D, S

● **S14.117 Complete lesion at C7 level of cervical spinal cord** A, A, A, D, S

● **S14.118 Complete lesion at C8 level of cervical spinal cord** A, A, D, S

● **S14.119 Complete lesion at unspecified level of cervical spinal cord** A, D, S

● **S14.12 Central cord syndrome of cervical spinal cord**

● **S14.121 Central cord syndrome at C1 level of cervical spinal cord** A, A, A, D, S

● **S14.122 Central cord syndrome at C2 level of cervical spinal cord** A, A, A, D, S

● **S14.123 Central cord syndrome at C3 level of cervical spinal cord** A, A, A, D, S
Coding Clinic: 2024, Q2, P23

● **S14.124 Central cord syndrome at C4 level of cervical spinal cord** A, A, A, D, S

● **S14.125 Central cord syndrome at C5 level of cervical spinal cord** A, A, A, D, S

● **S14.126 Central cord syndrome at C6 level of cervical spinal cord** A, A, A, D, S

● **S14.127 Central cord syndrome at C7 level of cervical spinal cord** A, A, A, D, S

● **S14.128 Central cord syndrome at C8 level of cervical spinal cord** A, A, D, S

● **S14.129 Central cord syndrome at unspecified level of cervical spinal cord** A, D, S

● **S14.13 Anterior cord syndrome of cervical spinal cord**

● **S14.131 Anterior cord syndrome at C1 level of cervical spinal cord** A, A, A, D, S

● **S14.132 Anterior cord syndrome at C2 level of cervical spinal cord** A, A, A, D, S

● **S14.133 Anterior cord syndrome at C3 level of cervical spinal cord** A, A, A, D, S

● **S14.134 Anterior cord syndrome at C4 level of cervical spinal cord** A, A, A, D, S

● **S14.135 Anterior cord syndrome at C5 level of cervical spinal cord** A, A, A, D, S

● **S14.136 Anterior cord syndrome at C6 level of cervical spinal cord** A, A, A, D, S

● **S14.137 Anterior cord syndrome at C7 level of cervical spinal cord** A, A, A, D, S

● **S14.138 Anterior cord syndrome at C8 level of cervical spinal cord** A, A, D, S

● **S14.139 Anterior cord syndrome at unspecified level of cervical spinal cord**, A, D, S

● **S14.14 Brown-Séquard syndrome of cervical spinal cord**

● **S14.141 Brown-Séquard syndrome at C1 level of cervical spinal cord** A, A, D, S

● **S14.142 Brown-Séquard syndrome at C2 level of cervical spinal cord** A, A, D, S

● **S14.143 Brown-Séquard syndrome at C3 level of cervical spinal cord** A, A, D, S

● **S14.144 Brown-Séquard syndrome at C4 level of cervical spinal cord** A, A, D, S

● **S14.145 Brown-Séquard syndrome at C5 level of cervical spinal cord** A, A, D, S

● **S14.146 Brown-Séquard syndrome at C6 level of cervical spinal cord** A, A, D, S

● **S14.147 Brown-Séquard syndrome at C7 level of cervical spinal cord** A, A, D, S

● **S14.148 Brown-Séquard syndrome at C8 level of cervical spinal cord** A, A, D, S

● **S14.149 Brown-Séquard syndrome at unspecified level of cervical spinal cord** A, D, S

CHAPTER 19 (S00-T88)

- S14.15 Other incomplete lesions of cervical spinal cord
  - Incomplete lesion of cervical spinal cord NOS
  - Posterior cord syndrome of cervical spinal cord
  - S14.151 Other incomplete lesion at C1 level of cervical spinal cord A, A, A, D, S
  - S14.152 Other incomplete lesion at C2 level of cervical spinal cord A, A, A, D, S
  - S14.153 Other incomplete lesion at C3 level of cervical spinal cord A, A, A, D, S
  - S14.154 Other incomplete lesion at C4 level of cervical spinal cord A, A, A, D, S
  - S14.155 Other incomplete lesion at C5 level of cervical spinal cord A, A, A, D, S
  - S14.156 Other incomplete lesion at C6 level of cervical spinal cord A, A, A, D, S
  - S14.157 Other incomplete lesion at C7 level of cervical spinal cord A, A, A, D, S
  - S14.158 Other incomplete lesion at C8 level of cervical spinal cord A, A, D, S
  - S14.159 Other incomplete lesion at unspecified level of cervical spinal cord A, D, S
- X S14.2 Injury of nerve root of cervical spine
- X S14.3 Injury of brachial plexus
- X S14.4 Injury of peripheral nerves of neck
- X S14.5 Injury of cervical sympathetic nerves
- X S14.8 Injury of other specified nerves of neck
- X S14.9 Injury of unspecified nerves of neck

S15 Injury of blood vessels at neck level

Code also any associated open wound (S11.-)

The appropriate 7th character is to be added to each code from category S15

A	initial encounter
D	subsequent encounter
S	sequela

- S15.0 Injury of carotid artery of neck
  - Injury of carotid artery (common) (external) (internal, extracranial portion)
  - Injury of carotid artery NOS
  - **Excludes1** injury of internal carotid artery, intracranial portion (S06.8)
  - S15.00 Unspecified injury of carotid artery
    - S15.001 Unspecified injury of right carotid artery A (Ex:) PDX 1644
    - S15.002 Unspecified injury of left carotid artery A (Ex:) PDX 1645
    - S15.009 Unspecified injury of unspecified carotid artery A (Ex:) PDX 1646
  - S15.01 Minor laceration of carotid artery
    - Incomplete transection of carotid artery
    - Laceration of carotid artery NOS
    - Superficial laceration of carotid artery
    - S15.011 Minor laceration of right carotid artery A (Ex:) PDX 1647
    - S15.012 Minor laceration of left carotid artery A (Ex:) PDX 1648
    - S15.019 Minor laceration of unspecified carotid artery A (Ex:) PDX 1649
  - S15.02 Major laceration of carotid artery
    - Complete transection of carotid artery
    - Traumatic rupture of carotid artery
    - S15.021 Major laceration of right carotid artery A (Ex:) PDX 1650
    - S15.022 Major laceration of left carotid artery A (Ex:) PDX 1651
    - S15.029 Major laceration of unspecified carotid artery A (Ex:) PDX 1646
  - S15.09 Other specified injury of carotid artery
    - S15.091 Other specified injury of right carotid artery A (Ex:) PDX 1652
    - S15.092 Other specified injury of left carotid artery A (Ex:) PDX 1653
    - S15.099 Other specified injury of unspecified carotid artery A (Ex:) PDX 1646
- S15.1 Injury of vertebral artery (Ex:) PDX 1634
  - S15.10 Unspecified injury of vertebral artery
    - S15.101 Unspecified injury of right vertebral artery A
    - S15.102 Unspecified injury of left vertebral artery A
    - S15.109 Unspecified injury of unspecified vertebral artery A
  - S15.11 Minor laceration of vertebral artery
    - Incomplete transection of vertebral artery
    - Laceration of vertebral artery NOS
    - Superficial laceration of vertebral artery
    - S15.111 Minor laceration of right vertebral artery A
    - S15.112 Minor laceration of left vertebral artery A
    - S15.119 Minor laceration of unspecified vertebral artery A
  - S15.12 Major laceration of vertebral artery
    - Complete transection of vertebral artery
    - Traumatic rupture of vertebral artery
    - S15.121 Major laceration of right vertebral artery A
    - S15.122 Major laceration of left vertebral artery A
    - S15.129 Major laceration of unspecified vertebral artery A
  - S15.19 Other specified injury of vertebral artery
    - S15.191 Other specified injury of right vertebral artery A
    - S15.192 Other specified injury of left vertebral artery A
    - S15.199 Other specified injury of unspecified vertebral artery A
- S15.2 Injury of external jugular vein
  - S15.20 Unspecified injury of external jugular vein
    - S15.201 Unspecified injury of right external jugular vein A (Ex:) PDX 1654
    - S15.202 Unspecified injury of left external jugular vein A (Ex:) PDX 1655
    - S15.209 Unspecified injury of unspecified external jugular vein A (Ex:) PDX 1656
  - S15.21 Minor laceration of external jugular vein
    - Incomplete transection of external jugular vein
    - Laceration of external jugular vein NOS
    - Superficial laceration of external jugular vein
    - S15.211 Minor laceration of right external jugular vein A (Ex:) PDX 1657
    - S15.212 Minor laceration of left external jugular vein A (Ex:) PDX 1658
    - S15.219 Minor laceration of unspecified external jugular vein A (Ex:) PDX 1659

● **S15.22 Major laceration of external jugular vein**
Complete transection of external jugular vein
Traumatic rupture of external jugular vein
● **S15.221 Major laceration of right external jugular vein** A (Ex) PDX 1660
● **S15.222 Major laceration of left external jugular vein** A (Ex) PDX 1661
● **S15.229 Major laceration of unspecified external jugular vein** A (Ex) PDX 1662
● **S15.29 Other specified injury of external jugular vein**
● **S15.291 Other specified injury of right external jugular vein** A (Ex) PDX 1663
● **S15.292 Other specified injury of left external jugular vein** A (Ex) PDX 1664
● **S15.299 Other specified injury of unspecified external jugular vein** A (Ex) PDX 1665
● **S15.3 Injury of internal jugular vein**
● **S15.30 Unspecified injury of internal jugular vein**
● **S15.301 Unspecified injury of right internal jugular vein** A (Ex) PDX 1666
● **S15.302 Unspecified injury of left internal jugular vein** A (Ex) PDX 1667
● **S15.309 Unspecified injury of unspecified internal jugular vein** A (Ex) PDX 1668
● **S15.31 Minor laceration of internal jugular vein**
Incomplete transection of internal jugular vein
Laceration of internal jugular vein NOS
Superficial laceration of internal jugular vein
● **S15.311 Minor laceration of right internal jugular vein** A (Ex) PDX 1669
● **S15.312 Minor laceration of left internal jugular vein** A (Ex) PDX 1670
● **S15.319 Minor laceration of unspecified internal jugular vein** A (Ex) PDX 1671
● **S15.32 Major laceration of internal jugular vein**
Complete transection of internal jugular vein
Traumatic rupture of internal jugular vein
● **S15.321 Major laceration of right internal jugular vein** A (Ex) PDX 1672
● **S15.322 Major laceration of left internal jugular vein** A (Ex) PDX 1673
● **S15.329 Major laceration of unspecified internal jugular vein** A (Ex) PDX 1674
● **S15.39 Other specified injury of internal jugular vein**
● **S15.391 Other specified injury of right internal jugular vein** A (Ex) PDX 1675
● **S15.392 Other specified injury of left internal jugular vein** A (Ex) PDX 1676
● **S15.399 Other specified injury of unspecified internal jugular vein** A (Ex) PDX 1677
X● **S15.8 Injury of other specified blood vessels at neck level** A (Ex) PDX 1634
X● **S15.9 Injury of unspecified blood vessel at neck level** A (Ex) PDX 1634

● **S16 Injury of muscle, fascia and tendon at neck level**
Code also any associated open wound (S11.-)
Excludes2 sprain of joint or ligament at neck level (S13.9)
The appropriate 7th character is to be added to each code from category S16

A	initial encounter
D	subsequent encounter
S	sequela

X● **S16.1 Strain of muscle, fascia and tendon at neck level**
X● **S16.2 Laceration of muscle, fascia and tendon at neck level**
X● **S16.8 Other specified injury of muscle, fascia and tendon at neck level**
X● **S16.9 Unspecified injury of muscle, fascia and tendon at neck level**

● **S17 Crushing injury of neck** (Ex) PDX 1633
Use additional code for all associated injuries, such as:
injury of blood vessels (S15.-)
open wound of neck (S11.-)
spinal cord injury (S14.0, S14.1-)
vertebral fracture (S12.0--S12.3-)
The appropriate 7th character is to be added to each code from category S17

A	initial encounter
D	subsequent encounter
S	sequela

X● **S17.0 Crushing injury of larynx and trachea** A, A
X● **S17.8 Crushing injury of other specified parts of neck** A, A
X● **S17.9 Crushing injury of neck, part unspecified** A, A

● **S19 Other and unspecified injuries of neck**
The appropriate 7th character is to be added to each code from category S19

A	initial encounter
D	subsequent encounter
S	sequela

● **S19.8 Other specified injuries of neck**
X● **S19.80 Other specified injuries of unspecified part of neck**
X● **S19.81 Other specified injuries of larynx**
X● **S19.82 Other specified injuries of cervical trachea**
Excludes2 other specified injury of thoracic trachea (S27.5-)
X● **S19.83 Other specified injuries of vocal cord**
X● **S19.84 Other specified injuries of thyroid gland**
X● **S19.85 Other specified injuries of pharynx and cervical esophagus**
Coding Clinic: 2022, Q1, P27
X● **S19.89 Other specified injuries of other specified part of neck**
X● **S19.9 Unspecified injury of neck**

INJURIES TO THE THORAX (S20-S29)

Includes injuries of breast
injuries of chest (wall)
injuries of interscapular area

Excludes2 burns and corrosions (T20-T32)
effects of foreign body in bronchus (T17.5)
effects of foreign body in esophagus (T18.1)
effects of foreign body in lung (T17.8)
effects of foreign body in trachea (T17.4)
frostbite (T33-T34)
injuries of axilla
injuries of clavicle
injuries of scapular region
injuries of shoulder
insect bite or sting, venomous (T63.4)

● **S20 Superficial injury of thorax**
The appropriate 7th character is to be added to each code from category S20

A	initial encounter
D	subsequent encounter
S	sequela

● **S20.0 Contusion of breast**
X● **S20.00 Contusion of breast, unspecified breast**
X● **S20.01 Contusion of right breast**
X● **S20.02 Contusion of left breast**

CHAPTER 19 (S00-T88)

S20.1 Other and unspecified superficial injuries of breast
- S20.10 Unspecified superficial injuries of breast
  - S20.101 Unspecified superficial injuries of breast, right breast
  - S20.102 Unspecified superficial injuries of breast, left breast
  - S20.109 Unspecified superficial injuries of breast, unspecified breast
- S20.11 Abrasion of breast
  - S20.111 Abrasion of breast, right breast
  - S20.112 Abrasion of breast, left breast
  - S20.119 Abrasion of breast, unspecified breast
- S20.12 Blister (nonthermal) of breast
  - S20.121 Blister (nonthermal) of breast, right breast
  - S20.122 Blister (nonthermal) of breast, left breast
  - S20.129 Blister (nonthermal) of breast, unspecified breast
- S20.14 External constriction of part of breast
  - S20.141 External constriction of part of breast, right breast
  - S20.142 External constriction of part of breast, left breast
  - S20.149 External constriction of part of breast, unspecified breast
- S20.15 Superficial foreign body of breast
  Splinter in the breast
  - S20.151 Superficial foreign body of breast, right breast
  - S20.152 Superficial foreign body of breast, left breast
  - S20.159 Superficial foreign body of breast, unspecified breast
- S20.16 Insect bite (nonvenomous) of breast
  - S20.161 Insect bite (nonvenomous) of breast, right breast
  - S20.162 Insect bite (nonvenomous) of breast, left breast
  - S20.169 Insect bite (nonvenomous) of breast, unspecified breast
- S20.17 Other superficial bite of breast
  Excludes1 open bite of breast (S21.05-)
  - S20.171 Other superficial bite of breast, right breast
  - S20.172 Other superficial bite of breast, left breast
  - S20.179 Other superficial bite of breast, unspecified breast

S20.2 Contusion of thorax
- X S20.20 Contusion of thorax, unspecified
- S20.21 Contusion of front wall of thorax
  - S20.211 Contusion of right front wall of thorax
  - S20.212 Contusion of left front wall of thorax
  - S20.213 Contusion of bilateral front wall of thorax
  - S20.214 Contusion of middle front wall of thorax
  - S20.219 Contusion of unspecified front wall of thorax
- S20.22 Contusion of back wall of thorax
  - S20.221 Contusion of right back wall of thorax
  - S20.222 Contusion of left back wall of thorax
  - S20.223 Contusion of bilateral back wall of thorax
  - S20.224 Contusion of middle back wall of thorax
  - S20.229 Contusion of unspecified back wall of thorax

S20.3 Other and unspecified superficial injuries of front wall of thorax
- S20.30 Unspecified superficial injuries of front wall of thorax
  - S20.301 Unspecified superficial injuries of right front wall of thorax
  - S20.302 Unspecified superficial injuries of left front wall of thorax
  - S20.303 Unspecified superficial injuries of bilateral front wall of thorax
  - S20.304 Unspecified superficial injuries of middle front wall of thorax
  - S20.309 Unspecified superficial injuries of unspecified front wall of thorax
- S20.31 Abrasion of front wall of thorax
  - S20.311 Abrasion of right front wall of thorax
  - S20.312 Abrasion of left front wall of thorax
  - S20.313 Abrasion of bilateral front wall of thorax
  - S20.314 Abrasion of middle front wall of thorax
  - S20.319 Abrasion of unspecified front wall of thorax
- S20.32 Blister (nonthermal) of front wall of thorax
  - S20.321 Blister (nonthermal) of right front wall of thorax
  - S20.322 Blister (nonthermal) of left front wall of thorax
  - S20.323 Blister (nonthermal) of bilateral front wall of thorax
  - S20.324 Blister (nonthermal) of middle front wall of thorax
  - S20.329 Blister (nonthermal) of unspecified front wall of thorax
- S20.34 External constriction of front wall of thorax
  - S20.341 External constriction of right front wall of thorax
  - S20.342 External constriction of left front wall of thorax
  - S20.343 External constriction of bilateral front wall of thorax
  - S20.344 External constriction of middle front wall of thorax
  - S20.349 External constriction of unspecified front wall of thorax
- S20.35 Superficial foreign body of front wall of thorax
  Splinter in front wall of thorax
  - S20.351 Superficial foreign body of right front wall of thorax
  - S20.352 Superficial foreign body of left front wall of thorax
  - S20.353 Superficial foreign body of bilateral front wall of thorax
  - S20.354 Superficial foreign body of middle front wall of thorax
  - S20.359 Superficial foreign body of unspecified front wall of thorax
- S20.36 Insect bite (nonvenomous) of front wall of thorax
  - S20.361 Insect bite (nonvenomous) of right front wall of thorax
  - S20.362 Insect bite (nonvenomous) of left front wall of thorax
  - S20.363 Insect bite (nonvenomous) of bilateral front wall of thorax
  - S20.364 Insect bite (nonvenomous) of middle front wall of thorax
  - S20.369 Insect bite (nonvenomous) of unspecified front wall of thorax

- S20.37 Other superficial bite of front wall of thorax
  Excludes1 open bite of front wall of thorax (S21.14)
  - S20.371 Other superficial bite of right front wall of thorax
  - S20.372 Other superficial bite of left front wall of thorax
  - S20.373 Other superficial bite of bilateral front wall of thorax
  - S20.374 Other superficial bite of middle front wall of thorax
  - S20.379 Other superficial bite of unspecified front wall of thorax

- S20.4 Other and unspecified superficial injuries of back wall of thorax
  - S20.40 Unspecified superficial injuries of back wall of thorax
    - S20.401 Unspecified superficial injuries of right back wall of thorax
    - S20.402 Unspecified superficial injuries of left back wall of thorax
    - S20.409 Unspecified superficial injuries of unspecified back wall of thorax
  - S20.41 Abrasion of back wall of thorax
    - S20.411 Abrasion of right back wall of thorax
    - S20.412 Abrasion of left back wall of thorax
    - S20.419 Abrasion of unspecified back wall of thorax
  - S20.42 Blister (nonthermal) of back wall of thorax
    - S20.421 Blister (nonthermal) of right back wall of thorax
    - S20.422 Blister (nonthermal) of left back wall of thorax
    - S20.429 Blister (nonthermal) of unspecified back wall of thorax
  - S20.44 External constriction of back wall of thorax
    - S20.441 External constriction of right back wall of thorax
    - S20.442 External constriction of left back wall of thorax
    - S20.449 External constriction of unspecified back wall of thorax
  - S20.45 Superficial foreign body of back wall of thorax
    Splinter of back wall of thorax
    - S20.451 Superficial foreign body of right back wall of thorax
    - S20.452 Superficial foreign body of left back wall of thorax
    - S20.459 Superficial foreign body of unspecified back wall of thorax
  - S20.46 Insect bite (nonvenomous) of back wall of thorax
    - S20.461 Insect bite (nonvenomous) of right back wall of thorax
    - S20.462 Insect bite (nonvenomous) of left back wall of thorax
    - S20.469 Insect bite (nonvenomous) of unspecified back wall of thorax
  - S20.47 Other superficial bite of back wall of thorax
    Excludes1 open bite of back wall of thorax (S21.24)
    - S20.471 Other superficial bite of right back wall of thorax
    - S20.472 Other superficial bite of left back wall of thorax
    - S20.479 Other superficial bite of unspecified back wall of thorax

- S20.9 Superficial injury of unspecified parts of thorax
  Excludes1 contusion of thorax NOS (S20.20)
  - X S20.90 Unspecified superficial injury of unspecified parts of thorax
    Superficial injury of thoracic wall NOS
  - X S20.91 Abrasion of unspecified parts of thorax
  - X S20.92 Blister (nonthermal) of unspecified parts of thorax
  - X S20.94 External constriction of unspecified parts of thorax
  - X S20.95 Superficial foreign body of unspecified parts of thorax
    Splinter in thorax NOS
  - X S20.96 Insect bite (nonvenomous) of unspecified parts of thorax
  - X S20.97 Other superficial bite of unspecified parts of thorax
    Excludes1 open bite of thorax NOS (S21.95)

- S21 Open wound of thorax
  Code also any associated injury such as:
  injury of heart (S26.-)
  injury of intrathoracic organs (S27.-)
  rib fracture (S22.3-, S22.4-)
  spinal cord injury (S24.0-, S24.1-)
  traumatic hemothorax (S27.1)
  traumatic hemopneumothorax (S27.3)
  traumatic pneumothorax (S27.0)
  wound infection
  Excludes1 traumatic amputation (partial) of thorax (S28.1)
  The appropriate 7th character is to be added to each code from category S21

A	initial encounter
D	subsequent encounter
S	sequela

- S21.0 Open wound of breast
  - S21.00 Unspecified open wound of breast
    - S21.001 Unspecified open wound of right breast
    - S21.002 Unspecified open wound of left breast
    - S21.009 Unspecified open wound of unspecified breast
  - S21.01 Laceration without foreign body of breast
    - S21.011 Laceration without foreign body of right breast
    - S21.012 Laceration without foreign body of left breast
    - S21.019 Laceration without foreign body of unspecified breast
  - S21.02 Laceration with foreign body of breast
    - S21.021 Laceration with foreign body of right breast
    - S21.022 Laceration with foreign body of left breast
    - S21.029 Laceration with foreign body of unspecified breast
  - S21.03 Puncture wound without foreign body of breast
    - S21.031 Puncture wound without foreign body of right breast
    - S21.032 Puncture wound without foreign body of left breast
    - S21.039 Puncture wound without foreign body of unspecified breast

Item 19–1 Pneumothorax is a collection of gas (positive air pressure) in the pleural space, resulting in the lung collapsing. A **tension pneumothorax** is life-threatening and is a result of air in the pleural space causing a displacement in the mediastinal structures and cardiopulmonary function compromise. A **traumatic pneumothorax** results from blunt or penetrating injury that disrupts the parietal/visceral pleura. **Hemothorax** is blood or bloody fluid in the pleural cavity as a result of traumatic blood vessel rupture or inflammation of the lungs from pneumonia.

- S21.04 Puncture wound with foreign body of breast
  - S21.041 Puncture wound with foreign body of right breast
  - S21.042 Puncture wound with foreign body of left breast
  - S21.049 Puncture wound with foreign body of unspecified breast
- S21.05 Open bite of breast
  Bite of breast NOS
  Excludes1 superficial bite of breast (S20.17)
  - S21.051 Open bite of right breast
  - S21.052 Open bite of left breast
  - S21.059 Open bite of unspecified breast

S21.1 Open wound of front wall of thorax without penetration into thoracic cavity (Ex:) PDX 1678
Open wound of chest without penetration into thoracic cavity

- S21.10 Unspecified open wound of front wall of thorax without penetration into thoracic cavity
  - S21.101 Unspecified open wound of right front wall of thorax without penetration into thoracic cavity A
  - S21.102 Unspecified open wound of left front wall of thorax without penetration into thoracic cavity A
  - S21.109 Unspecified open wound of unspecified front wall of thorax without penetration into thoracic cavity A
- S21.11 Laceration without foreign body of front wall of thorax without penetration into thoracic cavity
  - S21.111 Laceration without foreign body of right front wall of thorax without penetration into thoracic cavity A
  - S21.112 Laceration without foreign body of left front wall of thorax without penetration into thoracic cavity A
  - S21.119 Laceration without foreign body of unspecified front wall of thorax without penetration into thoracic cavity A
- S21.12 Laceration with foreign body of front wall of thorax without penetration into thoracic cavity
  - S21.121 Laceration with foreign body of right front wall of thorax without penetration into thoracic cavity A
  - S21.122 Laceration with foreign body of left front wall of thorax without penetration into thoracic cavity A
  - S21.129 Laceration with foreign body of unspecified front wall of thorax without penetration into thoracic cavity A
- S21.13 Puncture wound without foreign body of front wall of thorax without penetration into thoracic cavity
  - S21.131 Puncture wound without foreign body of right front wall of thorax without penetration into thoracic cavity A
  - S21.132 Puncture wound without foreign body of left front wall of thorax without penetration into thoracic cavity A
  - S21.139 Puncture wound without foreign body of unspecified front wall of thorax without penetration into thoracic cavity A
- S21.14 Puncture wound with foreign body of front wall of thorax without penetration into thoracic cavity
  - S21.141 Puncture wound with foreign body of right front wall of thorax without penetration into thoracic cavity A
  - S21.142 Puncture wound with foreign body of left front wall of thorax without penetration into thoracic cavity A
  - S21.149 Puncture wound with foreign body of unspecified front wall of thorax without penetration into thoracic cavity A
- S21.15 Open bite of front wall of thorax without penetration into thoracic cavity
  Bite of front wall of thorax NOS
  Excludes1 superficial bite of front wall of thorax (S20.37)
  - S21.151 Open bite of right front wall of thorax without penetration into thoracic cavity A
  - S21.152 Open bite of left front wall of thorax without penetration into thoracic cavity A
  - S21.159 Open bite of unspecified front wall of thorax without penetration into thoracic cavity A

S21.2 Open wound of back wall of thorax without penetration into thoracic cavity

- S21.20 Unspecified open wound of back wall of thorax without penetration into thoracic cavity
  - S21.201 Unspecified open wound of right back wall of thorax without penetration into thoracic cavity
  - S21.202 Unspecified open wound of left back wall of thorax without penetration into thoracic cavity
  - S21.209 Unspecified open wound of unspecified back wall of thorax without penetration into thoracic cavity
- S21.21 Laceration without foreign body of back wall of thorax without penetration into thoracic cavity
  - S21.211 Laceration without foreign body of right back wall of thorax without penetration into thoracic cavity
  - S21.212 Laceration without foreign body of left back wall of thorax without penetration into thoracic cavity
  - S21.219 Laceration without foreign body of unspecified back wall of thorax without penetration into thoracic cavity
- S21.22 Laceration with foreign body of back wall of thorax without penetration into thoracic cavity
  - S21.221 Laceration with foreign body of right back wall of thorax without penetration into thoracic cavity
  - S21.222 Laceration with foreign body of left back wall of thorax without penetration into thoracic cavity
  - S21.229 Laceration with foreign body of unspecified back wall of thorax without penetration into thoracic cavity

CHAPTER 19 (S00-T88)

- **S21.23** Puncture wound without foreign body of back wall of thorax without penetration into thoracic cavity
  - **S21.231** Puncture wound without foreign body of right back wall of thorax without penetration into thoracic cavity
  - **S21.232** Puncture wound without foreign body of left back wall of thorax without penetration into thoracic cavity
  - **S21.239** Puncture wound without foreign body of unspecified back wall of thorax without penetration into thoracic cavity
- **S21.24** Puncture wound with foreign body of back wall of thorax without penetration into thoracic cavity
  - **S21.241** Puncture wound with foreign body of right back wall of thorax without penetration into thoracic cavity
  - **S21.242** Puncture wound with foreign body of left back wall of thorax without penetration into thoracic cavity
  - **S21.249** Puncture wound with foreign body of unspecified back wall of thorax without penetration into thoracic cavity
- **S21.25** Open bite of back wall of thorax without penetration into thoracic cavity
  Bite of back wall of thorax NOS
  Excludes1 superficial bite of back wall of thorax (S2Ø.47)
  - **S21.251** Open bite of right back wall of thorax without penetration into thoracic cavity
  - **S21.252** Open bite of left back wall of thorax without penetration into thoracic cavity
  - **S21.259** Open bite of unspecified back wall of thorax without penetration into thoracic cavity

S21.3 Open wound of front wall of thorax with penetration into thoracic cavity
Open wound of chest with penetration into thoracic cavity

- **S21.3Ø** Unspecified open wound of front wall of thorax with penetration into thoracic cavity
  - **S21.3Ø1** Unspecified open wound of right front wall of thorax with penetration into thoracic cavity A (Ex) PDX 1679
  - **S21.3Ø2** Unspecified open wound of left front wall of thorax with penetration into thoracic cavity A (Ex) PDX 1679
  - **S21.3Ø9** Unspecified open wound of unspecified front wall of thorax with penetration into thoracic cavity A (Ex) PDX 1680
- **S21.31** Laceration without foreign body of front wall of thorax with penetration into thoracic cavity (Ex) PDX 1679
  - **S21.311** Laceration without foreign body of right front wall of thorax with penetration into thoracic cavity A
  - **S21.312** Laceration without foreign body of left front wall of thorax with penetration into thoracic cavity A
  - **S21.319** Laceration without foreign body of unspecified front wall of thorax with penetration into thoracic cavity A
- **S21.32** Laceration with foreign body of front wall of thorax with penetration into thoracic cavity (Ex) PDX 1679
  - **S21.321** Laceration with foreign body of right front wall of thorax with penetration into thoracic cavity A
  - **S21.322** Laceration with foreign body of left front wall of thorax with penetration into thoracic cavity A
  - **S21.329** Laceration with foreign body of unspecified front wall of thorax with penetration into thoracic cavity A
- **S21.33** Puncture wound without foreign body of front wall of thorax with penetration into thoracic cavity (Ex) PDX 1679
  - **S21.331** Puncture wound without foreign body of right front wall of thorax with penetration into thoracic cavity A
  - **S21.332** Puncture wound without foreign body of left front wall of thorax with penetration into thoracic cavity A
  - **S21.339** Puncture wound without foreign body of unspecified front wall of thorax with penetration into thoracic cavity A
- **S21.34** Puncture wound with foreign body of front wall of thorax with penetration into thoracic cavity (Ex) PDX 1679
  - **S21.341** Puncture wound with foreign body of right front wall of thorax with penetration into thoracic cavity A
  - **S21.342** Puncture wound with foreign body of left front wall of thorax with penetration into thoracic cavity A
  - **S21.349** Puncture wound with foreign body of unspecified front wall of thorax with penetration into thoracic cavity A
- **S21.35** Open bite of front wall of thorax with penetration into thoracic cavity (Ex) PDX 1679
  Excludes1 superficial bite of front wall of thorax (S2Ø.37)
  - **S21.351** Open bite of right front wall of thorax with penetration into thoracic cavity A
  - **S21.352** Open bite of left front wall of thorax with penetration into thoracic cavity A
  - **S21.359** Open bite of unspecified front wall of thorax with penetration into thoracic cavity A

S21.4 Open wound of back wall of thorax with penetration into thoracic cavity (Ex) PDX 1679

- **S21.4Ø** Unspecified open wound of back wall of thorax with penetration into thoracic cavity
  - **S21.4Ø1** Unspecified open wound of right back wall of thorax with penetration into thoracic cavity A
  - **S21.4Ø2** Unspecified open wound of left back wall of thorax with penetration into thoracic cavity A
  - **S21.4Ø9** Unspecified open wound of unspecified back wall of thorax with penetration into thoracic cavity A
- **S21.41** Laceration without foreign body of back wall of thorax with penetration into thoracic cavity
  - **S21.411** Laceration without foreign body of right back wall of thorax with penetration into thoracic cavity A
  - **S21.412** Laceration without foreign body of left back wall of thorax with penetration into thoracic cavity A
  - **S21.419** Laceration without foreign body of unspecified back wall of thorax with penetration into thoracic cavity A

CHAPTER 19 (SØØ-T88)

CHAPTER 19 (SØØ-T88)

● S21.42 Laceration with foreign body of back wall of thorax with penetration into thoracic cavity

● S21.421 Laceration with foreign body of right back wall of thorax with penetration into thoracic cavity A

● S21.422 Laceration with foreign body of left back wall of thorax with penetration into thoracic cavity A

● S21.429 Laceration with foreign body of unspecified back wall of thorax with penetration into thoracic cavity A

● S21.43 Puncture wound without foreign body of back wall of thorax with penetration into thoracic cavity

● S21.431 Puncture wound without foreign body of right back wall of thorax with penetration into thoracic cavity A

● S21.432 Puncture wound without foreign body of left back wall of thorax with penetration into thoracic cavity A

● S21.439 Puncture wound without foreign body of unspecified back wall of thorax with penetration into thoracic cavity A

● S21.44 Puncture wound with foreign body of back wall of thorax with penetration into thoracic cavity

● S21.441 Puncture wound with foreign body of right back wall of thorax with penetration into thoracic cavity A

● S21.442 Puncture wound with foreign body of left back wall of thorax with penetration into thoracic cavity A

● S21.449 Puncture wound with foreign body of unspecified back wall of thorax with penetration into thoracic cavity A

● S21.45 Open bite of back wall of thorax with penetration into thoracic cavity

Bite of back wall of thorax NOS

Excludes1 superficial bite of back wall of thorax (S2Ø.47)

● S21.451 Open bite of right back wall of thorax with penetration into thoracic cavity A

● S21.452 Open bite of left back wall of thorax with penetration into thoracic cavity A

● S21.459 Open bite of unspecified back wall of thorax with penetration into thoracic cavity A

● S21.9 Open wound of unspecified part of thorax (Ex) PDX 1678

Open wound of thoracic wall NOS

X● S21.9Ø Unspecified open wound of unspecified part of thorax A

X● S21.91 Laceration without foreign body of unspecified part of thorax A

X● S21.92 Laceration with foreign body of unspecified part of thorax A

X● S21.93 Puncture wound without foreign body of unspecified part of thorax A

X● S21.94 Puncture wound with foreign body of unspecified part of thorax A

X● S21.95 Open bite of unspecified part of thorax A

Excludes1 superficial bite of thorax (S2Ø.97)

● S22 Fracture of rib(s), sternum and thoracic spine

Note: A fracture not indicated as displaced or nondisplaced should be coded to displaced

A fracture not indicated as open or closed should be coded to closed

Includes fracture of thoracic neural arch
fracture of thoracic spinous process
fracture of thoracic transverse process
fracture of thoracic vertebra
fracture of thoracic vertebral arch

Code also, if applicable, any associated condition such as:
- injury of intrathoracic organ (S27.-)
- spinal cord injury (S24.Ø-, S24.1-)
- ▶traumatic hemopneumothorax (S27.2)
- ▶traumatic hemothorax (S27.1-)
- ▶traumatic pneumothorax (S27.Ø)

Excludes1 transection of thorax (S28.1)

Excludes2 fracture of clavicle (S42.Ø-)
fracture of scapula (S42.1-)

The appropriate 7th character is to be added to each code from category S22

A	initial encounter for closed fracture
B	initial encounter for open fracture
D	subsequent encounter for fracture with routine healing
G	subsequent encounter for fracture with delayed healing
K	subsequent encounter for fracture with nonunion
S	sequela

● S22.Ø Fracture of thoracic vertebra (Ex) PDX 1264 [K], 1681 [A, B]

● S22.ØØ Fracture of unspecified thoracic vertebra

● S22.ØØØ Wedge compression fracture of unspecified thoracic vertebra A, K, B, A, B, A, B

● S22.ØØ1 Stable burst fracture of unspecified thoracic vertebra A, K, B, A, B, A, B

● S22.ØØ2 Unstable burst fracture of unspecified thoracic vertebra A, K, B, A, B, A, B

● S22.ØØ8 Other fracture of unspecified thoracic vertebra A, K, B, A, B, A, B

● S22.ØØ9 Unspecified fracture of unspecified thoracic vertebra A, K, B, A, B, A, B

● S22.Ø1 Fracture of first thoracic vertebra

● S22.Ø1Ø Wedge compression fracture of first thoracic vertebra A, K, B, A, B, A, B

● S22.Ø11 Stable burst fracture of first thoracic vertebra A, K, B, A, B, A, B

● S22.Ø12 Unstable burst fracture of first thoracic vertebra A, K, B, A, B, A, B

● S22.Ø18 Other fracture of first thoracic vertebra A, K, B, A, B, A, B

● S22.Ø19 Unspecified fracture of first thoracic vertebra A, K, B, A, B, A, B

● S22.Ø2 Fracture of second thoracic vertebra

● S22.Ø2Ø Wedge compression fracture of second thoracic vertebra A, K, B, A, B, A, B

● S22.Ø21 Stable burst fracture of second thoracic vertebra A, K, B, A, B, A, B

● S22.022 Unstable burst fracture of second thoracic vertebra A, K, B, A, B, A, B

● S22.028 Other fracture of second thoracic vertebra A, K, B, A, B, A, B

● S22.029 Unspecified fracture of second thoracic vertebra A, K, B, A, B, A, B

● S22.03 Fracture of third thoracic vertebra

● S22.030 Wedge compression fracture of third thoracic vertebra A, K, B, A, B, A, B

● S22.031 Stable burst fracture of third thoracic vertebra A, K, B, A, B, A, B

● S22.032 Unstable burst fracture of third thoracic vertebra A, K, B, A, B, A, B

● S22.038 Other fracture of third thoracic vertebra A, K, B, A, B, A, B

● S22.039 Unspecified fracture of third thoracic vertebra A, K, B, A, B, A, B

● S22.04 Fracture of fourth thoracic vertebra

● S22.040 Wedge compression fracture of fourth thoracic vertebra A, K, B, A, B, A, B

● S22.041 Stable burst fracture of fourth thoracic vertebra A, K, B, A, B, A, B

● S22.042 Unstable burst fracture of fourth thoracic vertebra A, K, B, A, B, A, B

● S22.048 Other fracture of fourth thoracic vertebra A, K, B, A, B, A, B

● S22.049 Unspecified fracture of fourth thoracic vertebra A, K, B, A, B, A, B

● S22.05 Fracture of T5-T6 vertebra

● S22.050 Wedge compression fracture of T5-T6 vertebra A, K, B, A, B, A, B

● S22.051 Stable burst fracture of T5-T6 vertebra A, K, B, A, B, A, B

● S22.052 Unstable burst fracture of T5-T6 vertebra A, K, B, A, B, A, B

● S22.058 Other fracture of T5-T6 vertebra A, K, B, A, B, A, B

● S22.059 Unspecified fracture of T5-T6 vertebra A, K, B, A, B, A, B

● S22.06 Fracture of T7-T8 vertebra

● S22.060 Wedge compression fracture of T7-T8 vertebra A, K, B, A, B, A, B

● S22.061 Stable burst fracture of T7-T8 vertebra A, K, B, A, B, A, B

● S22.062 Unstable burst fracture of T7-T8 vertebra A, K, B, A, B, A, B

● S22.068 Other fracture of T7-T8 thoracic vertebra A, K, B, A, B, A, B

● S22.069 Unspecified fracture of T7-T8 vertebra A, K, B, A, B, A, B

● S22.07 Fracture of T9-T10 vertebra

● S22.070 Wedge compression fracture of T9-T10 vertebra A, K, B, A, B, A, B

● S22.071 Stable burst fracture of T9-T10 vertebra A, K, B, A, B, A, B

● S22.072 Unstable burst fracture of T9-T10 vertebra A, K, B, A, B, A, B

● S22.078 Other fracture of T9-T10 vertebra A, K, B, A, B, A, B

● S22.079 Unspecified fracture of T9-T10 vertebra A, K, B, A, B, A, B

● S22.08 Fracture of T11-T12 vertebra

● S22.080 Wedge compression fracture of T11-T12 vertebra A, K, B, A, B, A, B

● S22.081 Stable burst fracture of T11-T12 vertebra A, K, B, A, B, A, B

● S22.082 Unstable burst fracture of T11-T12 vertebra A, K, B, A, B, A, B

● S22.088 Other fracture of T11-T12 vertebra A, K, B, A, B, A, B

● S22.089 Unspecified fracture of T11-T12 vertebra A, K, B, A, B, A, B

● S22.2 Fracture of sternum (Ex:) PDX 1264 [K], 1682 [A, B]

X● S22.20 Unspecified fracture of sternum A, K, B, A, B

X● S22.21 Fracture of manubrium A, K, B, A, B

X● S22.22 Fracture of body of sternum A, K, B, A, B

X● S22.23 Sternal manubrial dissociation A, K, B, A, B

X● S22.24 Fracture of xiphoid process A, K, B, A, B

● S22.3 Fracture of one rib (Ex:) PDX 1264 [K], 1683 [A], 1684 [B]

X● S22.31 Fracture of one rib, right side A, K, B, A, B

X● S22.32 Fracture of one rib, left side A, K, B, A, B

X● S22.39 Fracture of one rib, unspecified side A, K, B, A, B

● S22.4 Multiple fractures of ribs

Fractures of two or more ribs

Excludes1 flail chest (S22.5-)

X● S22.41 Multiple fractures of ribs, right side A, K, B, A, B (Ex:) PDX 1264 [K], 1684 [A, B]

X● S22.42 Multiple fractures of ribs, left side A, K, B, A, B (Ex:) PDX 1264 [K], 1684 [A, B]

X● S22.43 Multiple fractures of ribs, bilateral A, K, B, A, B (Ex:) PDX 1264 [K], 1684 [A, B]

X● S22.49 Multiple fractures of ribs, unspecified side A, K, B, A, B (Ex:) PDX 1264 [K], 1684 [A], 1685 [B]

X● S22.5 Flail chest K, A, B, A, B (Ex:) PDX 1264 [K], 1683 [A, B]

Unstable chest due to sternum and/or rib fracture

X● S22.9 Fracture of bony thorax, part unspecified A, K, B, A, B (Ex:) PDX 1264 [K], 1686 [A, B]

● S23 **Dislocation and sprain of joints and ligaments of thorax**

Includes avulsion of joint or ligament of thorax
laceration of cartilage, joint or ligament of thorax
sprain of cartilage, joint or ligament of thorax
traumatic hemarthrosis of joint or ligament of thorax
traumatic rupture of joint or ligament of thorax
traumatic subluxation of joint or ligament of thorax
traumatic tear of joint or ligament of thorax

Code also any associated: open wound

Excludes2 dislocation, sprain of sternoclavicular joint (S43.2, S43.6)
strain of muscle or tendon of thorax (S29.01-)

The appropriate 7th character is to be added to each code from category S23

A	initial encounter
D	subsequent encounter
S	sequela

X● S23.0 **Traumatic rupture of thoracic intervertebral disc**

Excludes1 rupture or displacement (nontraumatic) of thoracic intervertebral disc NOS (M51.- with fifth character 4)

● S23.1 **Subluxation and dislocation of thoracic vertebra**

Code also any associated
open wound of thorax (S21.-)
spinal cord injury (S24.0-, S24.1-)

Excludes2 fracture of thoracic vertebrae (S22.0-)

● S23.10 **Subluxation and dislocation of unspecified thoracic vertebra**

● S23.100 **Subluxation of unspecified thoracic vertebra**

● S23.101 **Dislocation of unspecified thoracic vertebra**

● S23.11 **Subluxation and dislocation of T1/T2 thoracic vertebra**

● S23.110 **Subluxation of T1/T2 thoracic vertebra**

● S23.111 **Dislocation of T1/T2 thoracic vertebra**

● S23.12 **Subluxation and dislocation of T2/T3-T3/T4 thoracic vertebra**

● S23.120 **Subluxation of T2/T3 thoracic vertebra**

● S23.121 **Dislocation of T2/T3 thoracic vertebra**

● S23.122 **Subluxation of T3/T4 thoracic vertebra**

● S23.123 **Dislocation of T3/T4 thoracic vertebra**

● S23.13 **Subluxation and dislocation of T4/T5-T5/T6 thoracic vertebra**

● S23.130 **Subluxation of T4/T5 thoracic vertebra**

● S23.131 **Dislocation of T4/T5 thoracic vertebra**

● S23.132 **Subluxation of T5/T6 thoracic vertebra**

● S23.133 **Dislocation of T5/T6 thoracic vertebra**

● S23.14 **Subluxation and dislocation of T6/T7-T7/T8 thoracic vertebra**

● S23.140 **Subluxation of T6/T7 thoracic vertebra**

● S23.141 **Dislocation of T6/T7 thoracic vertebra**

● S23.142 **Subluxation of T7/T8 thoracic vertebra**

● S23.143 **Dislocation of T7/T8 thoracic vertebra**

● S23.15 **Subluxation and dislocation of T8/T9-T9/T10 thoracic vertebra**

● S23.150 **Subluxation of T8/T9 thoracic vertebra**

● S23.151 **Dislocation of T8/T9 thoracic vertebra**

● S23.152 **Subluxation of T9/T10 thoracic vertebra**

● S23.153 **Dislocation of T9/T10 thoracic vertebra**

● S23.16 **Subluxation and dislocation of T10/T11-T11/T12 thoracic vertebra**

● S23.160 **Subluxation of T10/T11 thoracic vertebra**

● S23.161 **Dislocation of T10/T11 thoracic vertebra**

● S23.162 **Subluxation of T11/T12 thoracic vertebra**

● S23.163 **Dislocation of T11/T12 thoracic vertebra**

● S23.17 **Subluxation and dislocation of T12/L1 thoracic vertebra**

● S23.170 **Subluxation of T12/L1 thoracic vertebra**

● S23.171 **Dislocation of T12/L1 thoracic vertebra**

● S23.2 **Dislocation of other and unspecified parts of thorax**

X● S23.20 **Dislocation of unspecified part of thorax**

X● S23.29 **Dislocation of other parts of thorax**

X● S23.3 **Sprain of ligaments of thoracic spine**

● S23.4 **Sprain of ribs and sternum**

X● S23.41 **Sprain of ribs**

● S23.42 **Sprain of sternum**

● S23.420 **Sprain of sternoclavicular (joint) (ligament)**

● S23.421 **Sprain of chondrosternal joint**

● S23.428 **Other sprain of sternum**

● S23.429 **Unspecified sprain of sternum**

X● S23.8 **Sprain of other specified parts of thorax**

X● S23.9 **Sprain of unspecified parts of thorax**

● S24 **Injury of nerves and spinal cord at thorax level** Ex: PDX 1687

Note: Code to highest level of thoracic spinal cord injury.
Injuries to the spinal cord (S24.0 and S24.1) refer to the cord level and not bone level injury, and can affect nerve roots at and below the level given.

Code also any associated:
fracture of thoracic vertebra (S22.0-)
open wound of thorax (S21.-)
transient paralysis (R29.5)

Excludes2 injury of brachial plexus (S14.3)

The appropriate 7th character is to be added to each code from category S24

A	initial encounter
D	subsequent encounter
S	sequela

X● S24.0 **Concussion and edema of thoracic spinal cord A, A, D, S**

● S24.1 **Other and unspecified injuries of thoracic spinal cord**

● S24.10 **Unspecified injury of thoracic spinal cord**

● S24.101 **Unspecified injury at T1 level of thoracic spinal cord A, A, A, D, S**

● S24.102 **Unspecified injury at T2-T6 level of thoracic spinal cord A, A, A, D, S**

- **S24.103 Unspecified injury at T7-T10 level of thoracic spinal cord** A, A, A, D, S
- **S24.104 Unspecified injury at T11-T12 level of thoracic spinal cord** A, A, A, D, S
- **S24.109 Unspecified injury at unspecified level of thoracic spinal cord** A, D, S
  Injury of thoracic spinal cord NOS

S24.11 Complete lesion of thoracic spinal cord

- **S24.111 Complete lesion at T1 level of thoracic spinal cord** A, A, A, D, S
- **S24.112 Complete lesion at T2-T6 level of thoracic spinal cord** A, A, A, D, S
- **S24.113 Complete lesion at T7-T10 level of thoracic spinal cord** A, A, A, D, S
- **S24.114 Complete lesion at T11-T12 level of thoracic spinal cord** A, A, A, D, S
- **S24.119 Complete lesion at unspecified level of thoracic spinal cord** A, D, S

S24.13 Anterior cord syndrome of thoracic spinal cord

- **S24.131 Anterior cord syndrome at T1 level of thoracic spinal cord** A, A, A, D, S
- **S24.132 Anterior cord syndrome at T2-T6 level of thoracic spinal cord** A, A, A, D, S
- **S24.133 Anterior cord syndrome at T7-T10 level of thoracic spinal cord** A, A, A, D, S
- **S24.134 Anterior cord syndrome at T11-T12 level of thoracic spinal cord** A, A, A, D, S
- **S24.139 Anterior cord syndrome at unspecified level of thoracic spinal cord** A, D, S

S24.14 Brown-Séquard syndrome of thoracic spinal cord

- **S24.141 Brown-Séquard syndrome at T1 level of thoracic spinal cord** A, A, D, S
- **S24.142 Brown-Séquard syndrome at T2-T6 level of thoracic spinal cord** A, A, D, S
- **S24.143 Brown-Séquard syndrome at T7-T10 level of thoracic spinal cord** A, A, D, S
- **S24.144 Brown-Séquard syndrome at T11-T12 level of thoracic spinal cord** A, A, D, S
- **S24.149 Brown-Séquard syndrome at unspecified level of thoracic spinal cord** A, D, S

S24.15 Other incomplete lesions of thoracic spinal cord
Incomplete lesion of thoracic spinal cord NOS
Posterior cord syndrome of thoracic spinal cord

- **S24.151 Other incomplete lesion at T1 level of thoracic spinal cord** A, A, A, D, S
- **S24.152 Other incomplete lesion at T2-T6 level of thoracic spinal cord** A, A, A, D, S
- **S24.153 Other incomplete lesion at T7-T10 level of thoracic spinal cord** A, A, A, D, S
- **S24.154 Other incomplete lesion at T11-T12 level of thoracic spinal cord** A, A, A, D, S
- **S24.159 Other incomplete lesion at unspecified level of thoracic spinal cord** A, D, S

X **S24.2 Injury of nerve root of thoracic spine**

X **S24.3 Injury of peripheral nerves of thorax**

X **S24.4 Injury of thoracic sympathetic nervous system**
Injury of cardiac plexus
Injury of esophageal plexus
Injury of pulmonary plexus
Injury of stellate ganglion
Injury of thoracic sympathetic ganglion

X **S24.8 Injury of other specified nerves of thorax**

X **S24.9 Injury of unspecified nerve of thorax**

S25 Injury of blood vessels of thorax

The appropriate 7th character is to be added to each code from category S25

A	initial encounter
D	subsequent encounter
S	sequela

Code also any associated open wound (S21.-)

S25.0 Injury of thoracic aorta Ex: PDX 1688
Injury of aorta NOS

- X **S25.00 Unspecified injury of thoracic aorta** A
- X **S25.01 Minor laceration of thoracic aorta** A
  Incomplete transection of thoracic aorta
  Laceration of thoracic aorta NOS
  Superficial laceration of thoracic aorta
- X **S25.02 Major laceration of thoracic aorta** A
  Complete transection of thoracic aorta
  Traumatic rupture of thoracic aorta
- X **S25.09 Other specified injury of thoracic aorta** A

S25.1 Injury of innominate or subclavian artery Ex: PDX 1689

S25.10 Unspecified injury of innominate or subclavian artery

- **S25.101 Unspecified injury of right innominate or subclavian artery** A
- **S25.102 Unspecified injury of left innominate or subclavian artery** A
- **S25.109 Unspecified injury of unspecified innominate or subclavian artery** A

S25.11 Minor laceration of innominate or subclavian artery
Incomplete transection of innominate or subclavian artery
Laceration of innominate or subclavian artery NOS
Superficial laceration of innominate or subclavian artery

- **S25.111 Minor laceration of right innominate or subclavian artery** A
- **S25.112 Minor laceration of left innominate or subclavian artery** A
- **S25.119 Minor laceration of unspecified innominate or subclavian artery** A

S25.12 Major laceration of innominate or subclavian artery
Complete transection of innominate or subclavian artery
Traumatic rupture of innominate or subclavian artery

- **S25.121 Major laceration of right innominate or subclavian artery** A
- **S25.122 Major laceration of left innominate or subclavian artery** A
- **S25.129 Major laceration of unspecified innominate or subclavian artery** A

CHAPTER 19 (S00-T88)

S25.19 Other specified injury of innominate or subclavian artery
S25.191 Other specified injury of right innominate or subclavian artery A
S25.192 Other specified injury of left innominate or subclavian artery A
S25.199 Other specified injury of unspecified innominate or subclavian artery A

S25.2 Injury of superior vena cava Ex: PDX 1690
Injury of vena cava NOS
X S25.20 Unspecified injury of superior vena cava A
X S25.21 Minor laceration of superior vena cava A
Incomplete transection of superior vena cava
Laceration of superior vena cava NOS
Superficial laceration of superior vena cava
X S25.22 Major laceration of superior vena cava A
Complete transection of superior vena cava
Traumatic rupture of superior vena cava
X S25.29 Other specified injury of superior vena cava A

S25.3 Injury of innominate or subclavian vein Ex: PDX 1691
S25.30 Unspecified injury of innominate or subclavian vein
S25.301 Unspecified injury of right innominate or subclavian vein A
S25.302 Unspecified injury of left innominate or subclavian vein A
S25.309 Unspecified injury of unspecified innominate or subclavian vein A
S25.31 Minor laceration of innominate or subclavian vein
Incomplete transection of innominate or subclavian vein
Laceration of innominate or subclavian vein NOS
Superficial laceration of innominate or subclavian vein
S25.311 Minor laceration of right innominate or subclavian vein A
S25.312 Minor laceration of left innominate or subclavian vein A
S25.319 Minor laceration of unspecified innominate or subclavian vein A
S25.32 Major laceration of innominate or subclavian vein
Complete transection of innominate or subclavian vein
Traumatic rupture of innominate or subclavian vein
S25.321 Major laceration of right innominate or subclavian vein A
S25.322 Major laceration of left innominate or subclavian vein A
S25.329 Major laceration of unspecified innominate or subclavian vein A
S25.39 Other specified injury of innominate or subclavian vein
S25.391 Other specified injury of right innominate or subclavian vein A
S25.392 Other specified injury of left innominate or subclavian vein A
S25.399 Other specified injury of unspecified innominate or subclavian vein A

S25.4 Injury of pulmonary blood vessels Ex: PDX 1692
S25.40 Unspecified injury of pulmonary blood vessels
S25.401 Unspecified injury of right pulmonary blood vessels A
S25.402 Unspecified injury of left pulmonary blood vessels A
S25.409 Unspecified injury of unspecified pulmonary blood vessels A
S25.41 Minor laceration of pulmonary blood vessels
Incomplete transection of pulmonary blood vessels
Laceration of pulmonary blood vessels NOS
Superficial laceration of pulmonary blood vessels
S25.411 Minor laceration of right pulmonary blood vessels A
S25.412 Minor laceration of left pulmonary blood vessels A
S25.419 Minor laceration of unspecified pulmonary blood vessels A
S25.42 Major laceration of pulmonary blood vessels
Complete transection of pulmonary blood vessels
Traumatic rupture of pulmonary blood vessels
S25.421 Major laceration of right pulmonary blood vessels A
S25.422 Major laceration of left pulmonary blood vessels A
S25.429 Major laceration of unspecified pulmonary blood vessels A
S25.49 Other specified injury of pulmonary blood vessels
S25.491 Other specified injury of right pulmonary blood vessels A
S25.492 Other specified injury of left pulmonary blood vessels A
S25.499 Other specified injury of unspecified pulmonary blood vessels A

S25.5 Injury of intercostal blood vessels Ex: PDX 1693
S25.50 Unspecified injury of intercostal blood vessels
S25.501 Unspecified injury of intercostal blood vessels, right side A
S25.502 Unspecified injury of intercostal blood vessels, left side A
S25.509 Unspecified injury of intercostal blood vessels, unspecified side A
S25.51 Laceration of intercostal blood vessels
S25.511 Laceration of intercostal blood vessels, right side A
S25.512 Laceration of intercostal blood vessels, left side A
S25.519 Laceration of intercostal blood vessels, unspecified side A
S25.59 Other specified injury of intercostal blood vessels
S25.591 Other specified injury of intercostal blood vessels, right side A
S25.592 Other specified injury of intercostal blood vessels, left side A
S25.599 Other specified injury of intercostal blood vessels, unspecified side A

S25.8 Injury of other blood vessels of thorax (Ex) PDX 1694
Injury of azygos vein
Injury of mammary artery or vein

S25.80 Unspecified injury of other blood vessels of thorax

S25.801 Unspecified injury of other blood vessels of thorax, right side A

S25.802 Unspecified injury of other blood vessels of thorax, left side A

S25.809 Unspecified injury of other blood vessels of thorax, unspecified side A

S25.81 Laceration of other blood vessels of thorax

S25.811 Laceration of other blood vessels of thorax, right side A

S25.812 Laceration of other blood vessels of thorax, left side A

S25.819 Laceration of other blood vessels of thorax, unspecified side A

S25.89 Other specified injury of other blood vessels of thorax

S25.891 Other specified injury of other blood vessels of thorax, right side A

S25.892 Other specified injury of other blood vessels of thorax, left side A

S25.899 Other specified injury of other blood vessels of thorax, unspecified side A

S25.9 Injury of unspecified blood vessel of thorax (Ex) PDX 1694

X **S25.90** Unspecified injury of unspecified blood vessel of thorax A

X **S25.91** Laceration of unspecified blood vessel of thorax A

X **S25.99** Other specified injury of unspecified blood vessel of thorax A

S26 Injury of heart

The appropriate 7th character is to be added to each code from category S26

A	initial encounter
D	subsequent encounter
S	sequela

Code also any associated:
open wound of thorax (S21.-)
traumatic hemopneumothorax (S27.2)
traumatic hemothorax (S27.1)
traumatic pneumothorax (S27.0)

S26.0 Injury of heart with hemopericardium
Hemopericardium: effusion of blood within pericardium

X **S26.00** Unspecified injury of heart with hemopericardium A (Ex) PDX 1695

X **S26.01** Contusion of heart with hemopericardium A (Ex) PDX 1696

S26.02 Laceration of heart with hemopericardium (Ex) PDX 1696

S26.020 Mild laceration of heart with hemopericardium A
Laceration of heart without penetration of heart chamber

S26.021 Moderate laceration of heart with hemopericardium A
Laceration of heart with penetration of heart chamber

S26.022 Major laceration of heart with hemopericardium A
Laceration of heart with penetration of multiple heart chambers

X **S26.09** Other injury of heart with hemopericardium A (Ex) PDX 1695

Item 19-2 Pneumothorax is a collection of gas (positive air pressure) in the pleural space resulting in the lung collapsing. A **tension pneumothorax** is life-threatening and is a result of air in the pleural space causing a displacement in the mediastinal structures and cardiopulmonary function compromise. A **traumatic pneumothorax** results from blunt or penetrating injury that disrupts the parietal/visceral pleura. **Hemothorax** is blood or bloody fluid in the pleural cavity as a result of traumatic blood vessel rupture or inflammation of the lungs from pneumonia.

S26.1 Injury of heart without hemopericardium
Hemopericardium: effusion of blood within pericardium

X **S26.10** Unspecified injury of heart without hemopericardium A (Ex) PDX 1695

X **S26.11** Contusion of heart without hemopericardium A (Ex) PDX 1696

X **S26.12** Laceration of heart without hemopericardium A (Ex) PDX 1696

X **S26.19** Other injury of heart without hemopericardium A (Ex) PDX 1695

S26.9 Injury of heart, unspecified with or without hemopericardium
Hemopericardium: effusion of blood within pericardium

X **S26.90** Unspecified injury of heart, unspecified with or without hemopericardium A (Ex) PDX 1695

X **S26.91** Contusion of heart, unspecified with or without hemopericardium A (Ex) PDX 1696

X **S26.92** Laceration of heart, unspecified with or without hemopericardium A (Ex) PDX 1696
Laceration of heart NOS

X **S26.99** Other injury of heart, unspecified with or without hemopericardium A (Ex) PDX 1695

S27 Injury of other and unspecified intrathoracic organs

Code also any associated open wound of thorax (S21.-)

Excludes2 injury of cervical esophagus (S10-S19)
injury of trachea (cervical) (S10-S19)

The appropriate 7th character is to be added to each code from category S27

A	initial encounter
D	subsequent encounter
S	sequela

X **S27.0** Traumatic pneumothorax A (Ex) PDX 1697

Excludes1 spontaneous pneumothorax (J93.-)

X **S27.1** Traumatic hemothorax A (Ex) PDX 1697

X **S27.2** Traumatic hemopneumothorax A (Ex) PDX 1697

S27.3 Other and unspecified injuries of lung

S27.30 Unspecified injury of lung (Ex) PDX 1698

S27.301 Unspecified injury of lung, unilateral A

S27.302 Unspecified injury of lung, bilateral A

S27.309 Unspecified injury of lung, unspecified A

S27.31 Primary blast injury of lung (Ex) PDX 1698
Blast injury of lung NOS

S27.311 Primary blast injury of lung, unilateral A

S27.312 Primary blast injury of lung, bilateral A

S27.319 Primary blast injury of lung, unspecified A

S27.32 Contusion of lung (Ex) PDX 1698

S27.321 Contusion of lung, unilateral A

S27.322 Contusion of lung, bilateral A

S27.329 Contusion of lung, unspecified A

CHAPTER 19 (S00-T88)

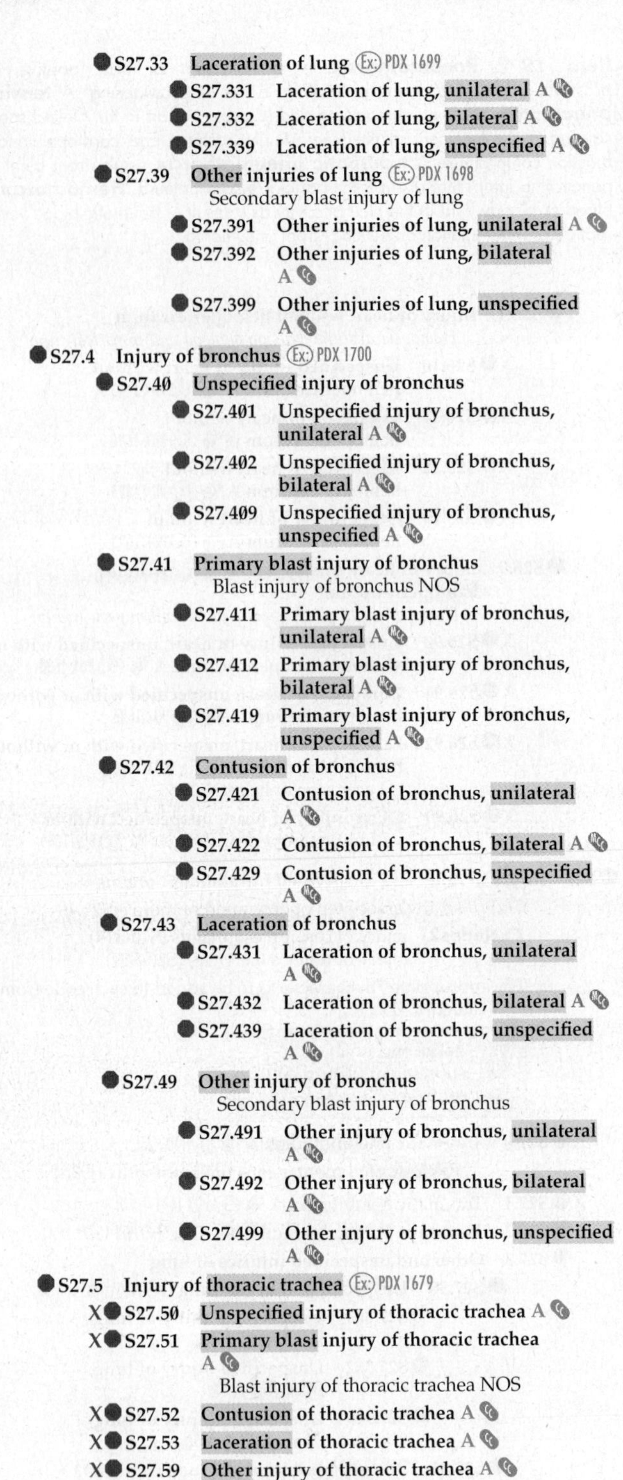

- ● S27.33 **Laceration** of lung Ex: PDX 1699
  - ● S27.331 Laceration of lung, **unilateral** A
  - ● S27.332 Laceration of lung, **bilateral** A
  - ● S27.339 Laceration of lung, **unspecified** A
- ● S27.39 **Other** injuries of lung Ex: PDX 1698
  Secondary blast injury of lung
  - ● S27.391 Other injuries of lung, **unilateral** A
  - ● S27.392 Other injuries of lung, **bilateral** A
  - ● S27.399 Other injuries of lung, **unspecified** A

● S27.4 Injury of **bronchus** Ex: PDX 1700

- ● S27.40 **Unspecified** injury of bronchus
  - ● S27.401 Unspecified injury of bronchus, **unilateral** A
  - ● S27.402 Unspecified injury of bronchus, **bilateral** A
  - ● S27.409 Unspecified injury of bronchus, **unspecified** A
- ● S27.41 **Primary blast** injury of bronchus
  Blast injury of bronchus NOS
  - ● S27.411 Primary blast injury of bronchus, **unilateral** A
  - ● S27.412 Primary blast injury of bronchus, **bilateral** A
  - ● S27.419 Primary blast injury of bronchus, **unspecified** A
- ● S27.42 **Contusion** of bronchus
  - ● S27.421 Contusion of bronchus, **unilateral** A
  - ● S27.422 Contusion of bronchus, **bilateral** A
  - ● S27.429 Contusion of bronchus, **unspecified** A
- ● S27.43 **Laceration** of bronchus
  - ● S27.431 Laceration of bronchus, **unilateral** A
  - ● S27.432 Laceration of bronchus, **bilateral** A
  - ● S27.439 Laceration of bronchus, **unspecified** A
- ● S27.49 **Other** injury of bronchus
  Secondary blast injury of bronchus
  - ● S27.491 Other injury of bronchus, **unilateral** A
  - ● S27.492 Other injury of bronchus, **bilateral** A
  - ● S27.499 Other injury of bronchus, **unspecified** A

● S27.5 Injury of **thoracic trachea** Ex: PDX 1679

- X● S27.50 **Unspecified** injury of thoracic trachea A
- X● S27.51 **Primary blast** injury of thoracic trachea A
  Blast injury of thoracic trachea NOS
- X● S27.52 **Contusion** of thoracic trachea A
- X● S27.53 **Laceration** of thoracic trachea A
- X● S27.59 **Other** injury of thoracic trachea A
  Secondary blast injury of thoracic trachea

● S27.6 Injury of **pleura** Ex: PDX 1679

- X● S27.60 **Unspecified** injury of pleura A
- X● S27.63 **Laceration** of pleura A
- X● S27.69 **Other** injury of pleura A

● S27.8 Injury of other specified intrathoracic organs

- ● S27.80 Injury of **diaphragm** Ex: PDX 1701
  - ● S27.802 **Contusion** of diaphragm A
  - ● S27.803 **Laceration** of diaphragm A
  - ● S27.808 **Other** injury of diaphragm A
  - ● S27.809 **Unspecified** injury of diaphragm A
- ● S27.81 Injury of **esophagus** (thoracic part) Ex: PDX 1702
  - ● S27.812 **Contusion** of esophagus (thoracic part) A
  - ● S27.813 **Laceration** of esophagus (thoracic part) A
  - ● S27.818 **Other** injury of esophagus (thoracic part) A
  - ● S27.819 **Unspecified** injury of esophagus (thoracic part) A
- ● S27.89 Injury of **other** specified intrathoracic organs Ex: PDX 1679
  Injury of lymphatic thoracic duct
  Injury of thymus gland
  - ● S27.892 **Contusion** of other specified intrathoracic organs A
  - ● S27.893 **Laceration** of other specified intrathoracic organs A
  - ● S27.898 **Other** injury of other specified intrathoracic organs A
  - ● S27.899 **Unspecified** injury of other specified intrathoracic organs A

X● S27.9 Injury of **unspecified** intrathoracic organ A Ex: PDX 1703

● S28 Crushing injury of thorax, and traumatic amputation of part of thorax

The appropriate 7th character is to be added to each code from category S28

A	initial encounter
D	subsequent encounter
S	sequela

X● S28.0 **Crushed chest**
Use additional code for all associated injuries
Excludes1 flail chest (S22.5)

X● S28.1 Traumatic amputation (partial) of **part of thorax, except breast** A Ex: PDX 1678

● S28.2 Traumatic amputation of **breast**

- ● S28.21 **Complete** traumatic amputation of breast
  Traumatic amputation of breast NOS
  - ● S28.211 Complete traumatic amputation of **right** breast
  - ● S28.212 Complete traumatic amputation of **left** breast
  - ● S28.219 Complete traumatic amputation of **unspecified** breast
- ● S28.22 **Partial** traumatic amputation of breast
  - ● S28.221 Partial traumatic amputation of **right** breast
  - ● S28.222 Partial traumatic amputation of **left** breast
  - ● S28.229 Partial traumatic amputation of **unspecified** breast

● S29 Other and unspecified injuries of thorax
Code also any associated open wound (S21.-)
The appropriate 7th character is to be added to each code from category S29
A initial encounter
D subsequent encounter
S sequela

● S29.0 Injury of muscle and tendon at thorax level
● S29.00 Unspecified injury of muscle and tendon of thorax
● S29.001 Unspecified injury of muscle and tendon of front wall of thorax
● S29.002 Unspecified injury of muscle and tendon of back wall of thorax
● S29.009 Unspecified injury of muscle and tendon of unspecified wall of thorax
● S29.01 Strain of muscle and tendon of thorax
● S29.011 Strain of muscle and tendon of front wall of thorax
● S29.012 Strain of muscle and tendon of back wall of thorax
● S29.019 Strain of muscle and tendon of unspecified wall of thorax
● S29.02 Laceration of muscle and tendon of thorax (Ex:) PDX 1678
● S29.021 Laceration of muscle and tendon of front wall of thorax A
● S29.022 Laceration of muscle and tendon of back wall of thorax
● S29.029 Laceration of muscle and tendon of unspecified wall of thorax A
● S29.09 Other injury of muscle and tendon of thorax
● S29.091 Other injury of muscle and tendon of front wall of thorax
● S29.092 Other injury of muscle and tendon of back wall of thorax
● S29.099 Other injury of muscle and tendon of unspecified wall of thorax
X● S29.8 Other specified injuries of thorax
X● S29.9 Unspecified injury of thorax

INJURIES TO THE ABDOMEN, LOWER BACK, LUMBAR SPINE PELVIS AND EXTERNAL GENITALS (S30-S39)

Includes injuries to the abdominal wall
injuries to the anus
injuries to the buttock
injuries to the external genitalia
injuries to the flank
injuries to the groin

Excludes2 burns and corrosions (T20-T32)
effects of foreign body in anus and rectum (T18.5)
effects of foreign body in genitourinary tract (T19.-)
effects of foreign body in stomach, small intestine and colon (T18.2-T18.4)
frostbite (T33-T34)
insect bite or sting, venomous (T63.4)

● S30 Superficial injury of abdomen, lower back, pelvis and external genitals
Excludes2 superficial injury of hip (S70.-)
The appropriate 7th character is to be added to each code from category S30
A initial encounter
D subsequent encounter
S sequela

X● S30.0 Contusion of lower back and pelvis
Contusion of buttock
X● S30.1 Contusion of abdominal wall
Contusion of flank
Contusion of groin
● S30.2 Contusion of external genital organs
● S30.20 Contusion of unspecified external genital organ
● S30.201 Contusion of unspecified external genital organ, male
● S30.202 Contusion of unspecified external genital organ, female
X● S30.21 Contusion of penis
X● S30.22 Contusion of scrotum and testes
X● S30.23 Contusion of vagina and vulva
X● S30.3 Contusion of anus
● S30.8 Other superficial injuries of abdomen, lower back, pelvis and external genitals
● S30.81 Abrasion of abdomen, lower back, pelvis and external genitals
● S30.810 Abrasion of lower back and pelvis
● S30.811 Abrasion of abdominal wall
● S30.812 Abrasion of penis
● S30.813 Abrasion of scrotum and testes
● S30.814 Abrasion of vagina and vulva
● S30.815 Abrasion of unspecified external genital organs, male
● S30.816 Abrasion of unspecified external genital organs, female
● S30.817 Abrasion of anus
● S30.82 Blister (nonthermal) of abdomen, lower back, pelvis and external genitals
● S30.820 Blister (nonthermal) of lower back and pelvis
● S30.821 Blister (nonthermal) of abdominal wall
● S30.822 Blister (nonthermal) of penis
● S30.823 Blister (nonthermal) of scrotum and testes
● S30.824 Blister (nonthermal) of vagina and vulva
● S30.825 Blister (nonthermal) of unspecified external genital organs, male
● S30.826 Blister (nonthermal) of unspecified external genital organs, female
● S30.827 Blister (nonthermal) of anus
● S30.84 External constriction of abdomen, lower back, pelvis and external genitals
● S30.840 External constriction of lower back and pelvis
● S30.841 External constriction of abdominal wall
● S30.842 External constriction of penis
Hair tourniquet syndrome of penis
Use additional cause code to identify the constricting item (W49.0-)

CHAPTER 19 (S00-T88)

- S30.843 External constriction of scrotum and testes
- S30.844 External constriction of vagina and vulva
- S30.845 External constriction of unspecified external genital organs, male
- S30.846 External constriction of unspecified external genital organs, female

S30.85 Superficial foreign body of abdomen, lower back, pelvis and external genitals
Splinter in the abdomen, lower back, pelvis and external genitals

- S30.850 Superficial foreign body of lower back and pelvis
- S30.851 Superficial foreign body of abdominal wall
- S30.852 Superficial foreign body of penis
- S30.853 Superficial foreign body of scrotum and testes
- S30.854 Superficial foreign body of vagina and vulva
- S30.855 Superficial foreign body of unspecified external genital organs, male
- S30.856 Superficial foreign body of unspecified external genital organs, female
- S30.857 Superficial foreign body of anus

S30.86 Insect bite (nonvenomous) of abdomen, lower back, pelvis and external genitals

- S30.860 Insect bite (nonvenomous) of lower back and pelvis
- S30.861 Insect bite (nonvenomous) of abdominal wall
- S30.862 Insect bite (nonvenomous) of penis
- S30.863 Insect bite (nonvenomous) of scrotum and testes
- S30.864 Insect bite (nonvenomous) of vagina and vulva
- S30.865 Insect bite (nonvenomous) of unspecified external genital organs, male
- S30.866 Insect bite (nonvenomous) of unspecified external genital organs, female
- S30.867 Insect bite (nonvenomous) of anus

S30.87 Other superficial bite of abdomen, lower back, pelvis and external genitals

Excludes1 open bite of abdomen, lower back, pelvis and external genitals (S31.05, S31.15, S31.25, S31.35, S31.45, S31.55)

- S30.870 Other superficial bite of lower back and pelvis
- S30.871 Other superficial bite of abdominal wall
- S30.872 Other superficial bite of penis
- S30.873 Other superficial bite of scrotum and testes
- S30.874 Other superficial bite of vagina and vulva
- S30.875 Other superficial bite of unspecified external genital organs, male
- S30.876 Other superficial bite of unspecified external genital organs, female
- S30.877 Other superficial bite of anus

S30.9 Unspecified superficial injury of abdomen, lower back, pelvis and external genitals

- X S30.91 Unspecified superficial injury of lower back and pelvis
- X S30.92 Unspecified superficial injury of abdominal wall
- X S30.93 Unspecified superficial injury of penis
- X S30.94 Unspecified superficial injury of scrotum and testes
- X S30.95 Unspecified superficial injury of vagina and vulva
- X S30.96 Unspecified superficial injury of unspecified external genital organs, male
- X S30.97 Unspecified superficial injury of unspecified external genital organs, female
- X S30.98 Unspecified superficial injury of anus

S31 Open wound of abdomen, lower back, pelvis and external genitals

Code also any associated:
spinal cord injury (S24.0, S24.1-, S34.0-, S34.1-)
wound infection

Excludes1 traumatic amputation of part of abdomen, lower back and pelvis (S38.2-, S38.3)

Excludes2 open wound of hip (S71.00-S71.02)
open fracture of pelvis (S32.1--S32.9 with 7th character B)

The appropriate 7th character is to be added to each code from category S31

A initial encounter
D subsequent encounter
S sequela

S31.0 Open wound of lower back and pelvis Ex: PDX 1704

S31.00 Unspecified open wound of lower back and pelvis

- S31.000 Unspecified open wound of lower back and pelvis without penetration into retroperitoneum
  Unspecified open wound of lower back and pelvis NOS
- S31.001 Unspecified open wound of lower back and pelvis with penetration into retroperitoneum A

S31.01 Laceration without foreign body of lower back and pelvis

- S31.010 Laceration without foreign body of lower back and pelvis without penetration into retroperitoneum
  Laceration without foreign body of lower back and pelvis NOS
- S31.011 Laceration without foreign body of lower back and pelvis with penetration into retroperitoneum A

S31.02 Laceration with foreign body of lower back and pelvis

- S31.020 Laceration with foreign body of lower back and pelvis without penetration into retroperitoneum
  Laceration with foreign body of lower back and pelvis NOS
- S31.021 Laceration with foreign body of lower back and pelvis with penetration into retroperitoneum A

CHAPTER 19 (S00-T88)

● **S31.03 Puncture wound without foreign body of lower back and pelvis**

● **S31.030 Puncture wound without foreign body of lower back and pelvis without penetration into retroperitoneum**
Puncture wound without foreign body of lower back and pelvis NOS

● **S31.031 Puncture wound without foreign body of lower back and pelvis with penetration into retroperitoneum** A

● **S31.04 Puncture wound with foreign body of lower back and pelvis**

● **S31.040 Puncture wound with foreign body of lower back and pelvis without penetration into retroperitoneum**
Puncture wound with foreign body of lower back and pelvis NOS

● **S31.041 Puncture wound with foreign body of lower back and pelvis with penetration into retroperitoneum** A

● **S31.05 Open bite of lower back and pelvis**
Bite of lower back and pelvis NOS
Excludes1 superficial bite of lower back and pelvis (S30.860, S30.870)

● **S31.050 Open bite of lower back and pelvis without penetration into retroperitoneum**
Open bite of lower back and pelvis NOS

● **S31.051 Open bite of lower back and pelvis with penetration into retroperitoneum** A

● **S31.1 Open wound of abdominal wall without penetration into peritoneal cavity**
Open wound of abdominal wall NOS
Excludes2 open wound of abdominal wall with penetration into peritoneal cavity (S31.6-)

● **S31.10 Unspecified open wound of abdominal wall without penetration into peritoneal cavity**

● **S31.100 Unspecified open wound of abdominal wall, right upper quadrant without penetration into peritoneal cavity**

● **S31.101 Unspecified open wound of abdominal wall, left upper quadrant without penetration into peritoneal cavity**

CHAPTER 19 (S00-T88)

S31.1Ø2 Unspecified open wound of abdominal wall, epigastric region without penetration into peritoneal cavity

S31.1Ø3 Unspecified open wound of abdominal wall, right lower quadrant without penetration into peritoneal cavity

S31.1Ø4 Unspecified open wound of abdominal wall, left lower quadrant without penetration into peritoneal cavity

S31.1Ø5 Unspecified open wound of abdominal wall, periumbilic region without penetration into peritoneal cavity

S31.1Ø9 Unspecified open wound of abdominal wall, unspecified quadrant without penetration into peritoneal cavity

Unspecified open wound of abdominal wall NOS

S31.11 Laceration without foreign body of abdominal wall without penetration into peritoneal cavity

S31.11Ø Laceration without foreign body of abdominal wall, right upper quadrant without penetration into peritoneal cavity

S31.111 Laceration without foreign body of abdominal wall, left upper quadrant without penetration into peritoneal cavity

S31.112 Laceration without foreign body of abdominal wall, epigastric region without penetration into peritoneal cavity

S31.113 Laceration without foreign body of abdominal wall, right lower quadrant without penetration into peritoneal cavity

S31.114 Laceration without foreign body of abdominal wall, left lower quadrant without penetration into peritoneal cavity

S31.115 Laceration without foreign body of abdominal wall, periumbilic region without penetration into peritoneal cavity

S31.119 Laceration without foreign body of abdominal wall, unspecified quadrant without penetration into peritoneal cavity

S31.12 Laceration with foreign body of abdominal wall without penetration into peritoneal cavity

S31.12Ø Laceration of abdominal wall with foreign body, right upper quadrant without penetration into peritoneal cavity

S31.121 Laceration of abdominal wall with foreign body, left upper quadrant without penetration into peritoneal cavity

S31.122 Laceration of abdominal wall with foreign body, epigastric region without penetration into peritoneal cavity

S31.123 Laceration of abdominal wall with foreign body, right lower quadrant without penetration into peritoneal cavity

S31.124 Laceration of abdominal wall with foreign body, left lower quadrant without penetration into peritoneal cavity

S31.125 Laceration of abdominal wall with foreign body, periumbilic region without penetration into peritoneal cavity

S31.129 Laceration of abdominal wall with foreign body, unspecified quadrant without penetration into peritoneal cavity

S31.13 Puncture wound of abdominal wall without foreign body without penetration into peritoneal cavity

S31.13Ø Puncture wound of abdominal wall without foreign body, right upper quadrant without penetration into peritoneal cavity

S31.131 Puncture wound of abdominal wall without foreign body, left upper quadrant without penetration into peritoneal cavity

S31.132 Puncture wound of abdominal wall without foreign body, epigastric region without penetration into peritoneal cavity

S31.133- Puncture wound of abdominal wall without foreign body, right lower quadrant without penetration into peritoneal cavity

S31.134 Puncture wound of abdominal wall without foreign body, left lower quadrant without penetration into peritoneal cavity

S31.135 Puncture wound of abdominal wall without foreign body, periumbilic region without penetration into peritoneal cavity

S31.139 Puncture wound of abdominal wall without foreign body, unspecified quadrant without penetration into peritoneal cavity

S31.14 Puncture wound of abdominal wall with foreign body without penetration into peritoneal cavity

S31.14Ø Puncture wound of abdominal wall with foreign body, right upper quadrant without penetration into peritoneal cavity

S31.141 Puncture wound of abdominal wall with foreign body, left upper quadrant without penetration into peritoneal cavity

S31.142 Puncture wound of abdominal wall with foreign body, epigastric region without penetration into peritoneal cavity

S31.143 Puncture wound of abdominal wall with foreign body, right lower quadrant without penetration into peritoneal cavity

S31.144 Puncture wound of abdominal wall with foreign body, left lower quadrant without penetration into peritoneal cavity

S31.145 Puncture wound of abdominal wall with foreign body, periumbilic region without penetration into peritoneal cavity

S31.149 Puncture wound of abdominal wall with foreign body, unspecified quadrant without penetration into peritoneal cavity

● S31.15 **Open bite of abdominal wall without penetration into peritoneal cavity**
Bite of abdominal wall NOS
Excludes1 superficial bite of abdominal wall (S30.871)

● S31.150 **Open bite of abdominal wall, right upper quadrant without penetration into peritoneal cavity**

● S31.151 **Open bite of abdominal wall, left upper quadrant without penetration into peritoneal cavity**

● S31.152 **Open bite of abdominal wall, epigastric region without penetration into peritoneal cavity**

● S31.153 **Open bite of abdominal wall, right lower quadrant without penetration into peritoneal cavity**

● S31.154 **Open bite of abdominal wall, left lower quadrant without penetration into peritoneal cavity**

● S31.155 **Open bite of abdominal wall, periumbilic region without penetration into peritoneal cavity**

● S31.159 **Open bite of abdominal wall, unspecified quadrant without penetration into peritoneal cavity**

● S31.2 Open wound of penis

X● S31.20 **Unspecified open wound of penis**

X● S31.21 **Laceration without foreign body of penis**

X● S31.22 **Laceration with foreign body of penis**

X● S31.23 **Puncture wound without foreign body of penis**

X● S31.24 **Puncture wound with foreign body of penis**

X● S31.25 **Open bite of penis**
Bite of penis NOS
Excludes1 superficial bite of penis (S30.862, S30.872)

● S31.3 Open wound of scrotum and testes

X● S31.30 **Unspecified open wound of scrotum and testes**

X● S31.31 **Laceration without foreign body of scrotum and testes**

X● S31.32 **Laceration with foreign body of scrotum and testes**

X● S31.33 **Puncture wound without foreign body of scrotum and testes**

X● S31.34 **Puncture wound with foreign body of scrotum and testes**

X● S31.35 **Open bite of scrotum and testes**
Bite of scrotum and testes NOS
Excludes1 superficial bite of scrotum and testes (S30.863, S30.873)

● S31.4 Open wound of vagina and vulva
Excludes1 injury to vagina and vulva during delivery (O70.-, O71.4)

X● S31.40 **Unspecified open wound of vagina and vulva**

X● S31.41 **Laceration without foreign body of vagina and vulva**

X● S31.42 **Laceration with foreign body of vagina and vulva**

X● S31.43 **Puncture wound without foreign body of vagina and vulva**

X● S31.44 **Puncture wound with foreign body of vagina and vulva**

X● S31.45 **Open bite of vagina and vulva**
Bite of vagina and vulva NOS
Excludes1 superficial bite of vagina and vulva (S30.864, S30.874)

● S31.5 Open wound of unspecified external genital organs
Excludes1 traumatic amputation of external genital organs (S38.21, S38.22)

● S31.50 **Unspecified open wound of unspecified external genital organs**

● S31.501 **Unspecified open wound of unspecified external genital organs, male**

● S31.502 **Unspecified open wound of unspecified external genital organs, female**

● S31.51 **Laceration without foreign body of unspecified external genital organs**

● S31.511 **Laceration without foreign body of unspecified external genital organs, male**

● S31.512 **Laceration without foreign body of unspecified external genital organs, female**

● S31.52 **Laceration with foreign body of unspecified external genital organs**

● S31.521 **Laceration with foreign body of unspecified external genital organs, male**

● S31.522 **Laceration with foreign body of unspecified external genital organs, female**

● S31.53 **Puncture wound without foreign body of unspecified external genital organs**

● S31.531 **Puncture wound without foreign body of unspecified external genital organs, male**

● S31.532 **Puncture wound without foreign body of unspecified external genital organs, female**

● S31.54 **Puncture wound with foreign body of unspecified external genital organs**

● S31.541 **Puncture wound with foreign body of unspecified external genital organs, male**

● S31.542 **Puncture wound with foreign body of unspecified external genital organs, female**

● S31.55 **Open bite of unspecified external genital organs**
Bite of unspecified external genital organs NOS
Excludes1 superficial bite of unspecified external genital organs (S30.865, S30.866, S30.875, S30.876)

● S31.551 **Open bite of unspecified external genital organs, male**

● S31.552 **Open bite of unspecified external genital organs, female**

● S31.6 Open wound of abdominal wall with penetration into peritoneal cavity (Ex) PDX 1704
Coding Clinic: 2023, Q3, P9

● S31.60 **Unspecified open wound of abdominal wall with penetration into peritoneal cavity**

● S31.600 **Unspecified open wound of abdominal wall, right upper quadrant with penetration into peritoneal cavity** A

● S31.601 **Unspecified open wound of abdominal wall, left upper quadrant with penetration into peritoneal cavity** A

● S31.602 **Unspecified open wound of abdominal wall, epigastric region with penetration into peritoneal cavity** A

● S31.603 Unspecified open wound of abdominal wall, right lower quadrant with penetration into peritoneal cavity A

● S31.604 Unspecified open wound of abdominal wall, left lower quadrant with penetration into peritoneal cavity A

● S31.605 Unspecified open wound of abdominal wall, periumbilic region with penetration into peritoneal cavity A

● S31.609 Unspecified open wound of abdominal wall, unspecified quadrant with penetration into peritoneal cavity A

● S31.61 Laceration without foreign body of abdominal wall with penetration into peritoneal cavity

● S31.610 Laceration without foreign body of abdominal wall, right upper quadrant with penetration into peritoneal cavity A

● S31.611 Laceration without foreign body of abdominal wall, left upper quadrant with penetration into peritoneal cavity A

● S31.612 Laceration without foreign body of abdominal wall, epigastric region with penetration into peritoneal cavity A

● S31.613 Laceration without foreign body of abdominal wall, right lower quadrant with penetration into peritoneal cavity A,
Coding Clinic: 2015, Q4, P37

● S31.614 Laceration without foreign body of abdominal wall, left lower quadrant with penetration into peritoneal cavity A

● S31.615 Laceration without foreign body of abdominal wall, periumbilic region with penetration into peritoneal cavity A

● S31.619 Laceration without foreign body of abdominal wall, unspecified quadrant with penetration into peritoneal cavity A

● S31.62 Laceration with foreign body of abdominal wall with penetration into peritoneal cavity

● S31.620 Laceration with foreign body of abdominal wall, right upper quadrant with penetration into peritoneal cavity A

● S31.621 Laceration with foreign body of abdominal wall, left upper quadrant with penetration into peritoneal cavity A

● S31.622 Laceration with foreign body of abdominal wall, epigastric region with penetration into peritoneal cavity A

● S31.623 Laceration with foreign body of abdominal wall, right lower quadrant with penetration into peritoneal cavity A

● S31.624 Laceration with foreign body of abdominal wall, left lower quadrant with penetration into peritoneal cavity A

● S31.625 Laceration with foreign body of abdominal wall, periumbilic region with penetration into peritoneal cavity A

● S31.629 Laceration with foreign body of abdominal wall, unspecified quadrant with penetration into peritoneal cavity A

● S31.63 Puncture wound without foreign body of abdominal wall with penetration into peritoneal cavity

● S31.630 Puncture wound without foreign body of abdominal wall, right upper quadrant with penetration into peritoneal cavity A

● S31.631 Puncture wound without foreign body of abdominal wall, left upper quadrant with penetration into peritoneal cavity A

● S31.632 Puncture wound without foreign body of abdominal wall, epigastric region with penetration into peritoneal cavity A

● S31.633 Puncture wound without foreign body of abdominal wall, right lower quadrant with penetration into peritoneal cavity A

● S31.634 Puncture wound without foreign body of abdominal wall, left lower quadrant with penetration into peritoneal cavity A

● S31.635 Puncture wound without foreign body of abdominal wall, periumbilic region with penetration into peritoneal cavity A

● S31.639 Puncture wound without foreign body of abdominal wall, unspecified quadrant with penetration into peritoneal cavity A

● S31.64 Puncture wound with foreign body of abdominal wall with penetration into peritoneal cavity

● S31.640 Puncture wound with foreign body of abdominal wall, right upper quadrant with penetration into peritoneal cavity A

● S31.641 Puncture wound with foreign body of abdominal wall, left upper quadrant with penetration into peritoneal cavity A

● S31.642 Puncture wound with foreign body of abdominal wall, epigastric region with penetration into peritoneal cavity A

● S31.643 Puncture wound with foreign body of abdominal wall, right lower quadrant with penetration into peritoneal cavity A

● S31.644 Puncture wound with foreign body of abdominal wall, left lower quadrant with penetration into peritoneal cavity A

● S31.645 Puncture wound with foreign body of abdominal wall, periumbilic region with penetration into peritoneal cavity A

● S31.649 Puncture wound with foreign body of abdominal wall, unspecified quadrant with penetration into peritoneal cavity A

S31.65 Open bite of abdominal wall with penetration into peritoneal cavity

Excludes1 superficial bite of abdominal wall (S3Ø.861, S3Ø.871)

S31.65Ø Open bite of abdominal wall, right upper quadrant with penetration into peritoneal cavity A

S31.651 Open bite of abdominal wall, left upper quadrant with penetration into peritoneal cavity A

S31.652 Open bite of abdominal wall, epigastric region with penetration into peritoneal cavity A

S31.653 Open bite of abdominal wall, right lower quadrant with penetration into peritoneal cavity A

S31.654 Open bite of abdominal wall, left lower quadrant with penetration into peritoneal cavity A

S31.655 Open bite of abdominal wall, periumbilic region with penetration into peritoneal cavity A

S31.659 Open bite of abdominal wall, unspecified quadrant with penetration into peritoneal cavity A

S31.8 Open wound of other parts of abdomen, lower back and pelvis

S31.8Ø Open wound of unspecified buttock

S31.8Ø1 Laceration without foreign body of unspecified buttock

S31.8Ø2 Laceration with foreign body of unspecified buttock

S31.8Ø3 Puncture wound without foreign body of unspecified buttock

S31.8Ø4 Puncture wound with foreign body of unspecified buttock

S31.8Ø5 Open bite of unspecified buttock

Bite of buttock NOS

Excludes1 superficial bite of buttock (S3Ø.87Ø)

S31.8Ø9 Unspecified open wound of unspecified buttock

S31.81 Open wound of right buttock

S31.811 Laceration without foreign body of right buttock

S31.812 Laceration with foreign body of right buttock

S31.813 Puncture wound without foreign body of right buttock

S31.814 Puncture wound with foreign body of right buttock

S31.815 Open bite of right buttock

Bite of right buttock NOS

Excludes1 superficial bite of buttock (S3Ø.87Ø)

S31.819 Unspecified open wound of right buttock

S31.82 Open wound of left buttock

S31.821 Laceration without foreign body of left buttock

S31.822 Laceration with foreign body of left buttock

S31.823 Puncture wound without foreign body of left buttock

S31.824 Puncture wound with foreign body of left buttock

S31.825 Open bite of left buttock

Bite of left buttock NOS

Excludes1 superficial bite of buttock (S3Ø.87Ø)

S31.829 Unspecified open wound of left buttock

S31.83 Open wound of anus

S31.831 Laceration without foreign body of anus

S31.832 Laceration with foreign body of anus

S31.833 Puncture wound without foreign body of anus

S31.834 Puncture wound with foreign body of anus

S31.835 Open bite of anus

Bite of anus NOS

Excludes1 superficial bite of anus (S3Ø.877)

S31.839 Unspecified open wound of anus

S32 Fracture of lumbar spine and pelvis

Note: A fracture not indicated as displaced or nondisplaced should be coded to displaced

A fracture not indicated as opened or closed should be coded to closed

Includes fracture of lumbosacral neural arch
fracture of lumbosacral spinous process
fracture of lumbosacral transverse process
fracture of lumbosacral vertebra
fracture of lumbosacral vertebral arch

Code first any associated spinal cord and spinal nerve injury (S34.-)

Excludes1 transection of abdomen (S38.3)

Excludes2 fracture of hip NOS (S72.Ø-)

The appropriate 7th character is to be added to each code from category S32

A	initial encounter for closed fracture
B	initial encounter for open fracture
D	subsequent encounter for fracture with routine healing
G	subsequent encounter for fracture with delayed healing
K	subsequent encounter for fracture with nonunion
S	sequela

S32.Ø Fracture of lumbar vertebra (Ex:) PDX 1264 [K], 1705 [A, B]

Fracture of lumbar spine NOS

S32.ØØ Fracture of unspecified lumbar vertebra

S32.ØØØ Wedge compression fracture of unspecified lumbar vertebra A, K, B, A, B, A, B

S32.ØØ1 Stable burst fracture of unspecified lumbar vertebra A, K, B, A, B, A, B

S32.ØØ2 Unstable burst fracture of unspecified lumbar vertebra A, K, B, A, B, A, B

S32.ØØ8 Other fracture of unspecified lumbar vertebra A, K, B, A, B, A, B

S32.ØØ9 Unspecified fracture of unspecified lumbar vertebra A, K, B, A, B, A, B

S32.Ø1 Fracture of first lumbar vertebra

S32.Ø1Ø Wedge compression fracture of first lumbar vertebra A, K, B, A, B, A, B

S32.Ø11 Stable burst fracture of first lumbar vertebra A, K, B, A, B, A, B

S32.Ø12 Unstable burst fracture of first lumbar vertebra A, K, B, A, B, A, B

S32.Ø18 Other fracture of first lumbar vertebra A, K, B, A, B, A, B

S32.Ø19 Unspecified fracture of first lumbar vertebra A, K, B, A, B, A, B

● S32.02 Fracture of second lumbar vertebra
● S32.020 Wedge compression fracture of second lumbar vertebra A, K, B, A, B, A, B
● S32.021 Stable burst fracture of second lumbar vertebra A, K, B, A, B, A, B
● S32.022 Unstable burst fracture of second lumbar vertebra A, K, B, A, B, A, B
● S32.028 Other fracture of second lumbar vertebra A, K, B, A, B, A, B
● S32.029 Unspecified fracture of second lumbar vertebra A, K, B, A, B, A, B
● S32.03 Fracture of third lumbar vertebra
● S32.030 Wedge compression fracture of third lumbar vertebra A, K, B, A, B, A, B
● S32.031 Stable burst fracture of third lumbar vertebra A, K, B, A, B, A, B
● S32.032 Unstable burst fracture of third lumbar vertebra A, K, B, A, B, A, B
● S32.038 Other fracture of third lumbar vertebra A, K, B, A, B, A, B
● S32.039 Unspecified fracture of third lumbar vertebra A, K, B, A, B, A, B
● S32.04 Fracture of fourth lumbar vertebra
● S32.040 Wedge compression fracture of fourth lumbar vertebra A, K, B, A, B, A, B
● S32.041 Stable burst fracture of fourth lumbar vertebra A, K, B, A, B, A, B
● S32.042 Unstable burst fracture of fourth lumbar vertebra A, K, B, A, B, A, B
● S32.048 Other fracture of fourth lumbar vertebra A, K, B, A, B, A, B
● S32.049 Unspecified fracture of fourth lumbar vertebra A, K, B, A, B, A, B
● S32.05 Fracture of fifth lumbar vertebra
● S32.050 Wedge compression fracture of fifth lumbar vertebra A, K, B, A, B, A, B
● S32.051 Stable burst fracture of fifth lumbar vertebra A, K, B, A, B, A, B
● S32.052 Unstable burst fracture of fifth lumbar vertebra A, K, B, A, B, A, B
● S32.058 Other fracture of fifth lumbar vertebra A, K, B, A, B, A, B
● S32.059 Unspecified fracture of fifth lumbar vertebra A, K, B, A, B, A, B
● S32.1 Fracture of sacrum Ex PDX 1264 [K], 1706 [A, B]
For vertical fractures, code to most medial fracture extension
Use two codes if both a vertical and transverse fracture are present
Code also any associated fracture of pelvic ring (S32.8-)
X● S32.10 Unspecified fracture of sacrum A, K, B, A, B, A, B
● S32.11 Zone I fracture of sacrum
Vertical sacral ala fracture of sacrum
● S32.110 Nondisplaced Zone I fracture of sacrum A, K, B, A, B, A, B
● S32.111 Minimally displaced Zone I fracture of sacrum A, K, B, A, B, A, B
● S32.112 Severely displaced Zone I fracture of sacrum A, K, B, A, B, A, B
● S32.119 Unspecified Zone I fracture of sacrum A, K, B, A, B, A, B
● S32.12 Zone II fracture of sacrum
Vertical foraminal region fracture of sacrum
● S32.120 Nondisplaced Zone II fracture of sacrum A, K, B, A, B, A, B
● S32.121 Minimally displaced Zone II fracture of sacrum A, K, B, A, B, A, B
● S32.122 Severely displaced Zone II fracture of sacrum A, K, B, A, B, A, B
● S32.129 Unspecified Zone II fracture of sacrum A, K, B, A, B, A, B
● S32.13 Zone III fracture of sacrum
Vertical fracture into spinal canal region of sacrum
● S32.130 Nondisplaced Zone III fracture of sacrum A, K, B, A, B, A, B
● S32.131 Minimally displaced Zone III fracture of sacrum A, K, B, A, B, A, B
● S32.132 Severely displaced Zone III fracture of sacrum A, K, B, A, B, A, B
● S32.139 Unspecified Zone III fracture of sacrum A, K, B, A, B, A, B
X● S32.14 Type 1 fracture of sacrum A, K, B, A, B, A, B
Transverse flexion fracture of sacrum without displacement
X● S32.15 Type 2 fracture of sacrum A, K, B, A, B, A, B
Transverse flexion fracture of sacrum with posterior displacement
X● S32.16 Type 3 fracture of sacrum A, K, B, A, B, A, B
Transverse extension fracture of sacrum with anterior displacement
X● S32.17 Type 4 fracture of sacrum A, K, B, A, B, A, B
Transverse segmental comminution of upper sacrum
X● S32.19 Other fracture of sacrum A, K, B, A, B, A, B
X● S32.2 Fracture of coccyx A, K, B, A, B, A, B Ex PDX 1264 [K], 1706 [A, B]
● S32.3 Fracture of ilium Ex PDX 1264 [K], 1686 [A], 1707 [B]
Excludes1 fracture of ilium with associated disruption of pelvic ring (S32.8-)
● S32.30 Unspecified fracture of ilium
● S32.301 Unspecified fracture of right ilium A, K, B, A, B, A, B
● S32.302 Unspecified fracture of left ilium A, K, B, A, B, A, B
● S32.309 Unspecified fracture of unspecified ilium A, K, B, A, B, A, B
● S32.31 Avulsion fracture of ilium
● S32.311 Displaced avulsion fracture of right ilium A, K, B, A, B, A, B
● S32.312 Displaced avulsion fracture of left ilium A, K, B, A, B, A, B
● S32.313 Displaced avulsion fracture of unspecified ilium A, K, B, A, B, A, B
● S32.314 Nondisplaced avulsion fracture of right ilium A, K, B, A, B, A, B

- S32.315 Nondisplaced avulsion fracture of left ilium A, K, B, A, B, A, B
- S32.316 Nondisplaced avulsion fracture of unspecified ilium A, K, B, A, B, A, B
- S32.39 Other fracture of ilium
  - S32.391 Other fracture of right ilium A, K, B, A, B, A, B
  - S32.392 Other fracture of left ilium A, K, B, A, B, A, B
  - S32.399 Other fracture of unspecified ilium A, K, B, A, B, A, B

S32.4 Fracture of acetabulum (Ex) PDX 1264 [K], 1708 [A], 1709 [B]

Code also any associated fracture of pelvic ring (S32.8-)

- S32.40 Unspecified fracture of acetabulum
  - S32.401 Unspecified fracture of right acetabulum K, A, B, A, B, A, B
  - S32.402 Unspecified fracture of left acetabulum K, A, B, A, B, A, B
  - S32.409 Unspecified fracture of unspecified acetabulum K, A, B, A, B, A, B
- S32.41 Fracture of anterior wall of acetabulum
  - S32.411 Displaced fracture of anterior wall of right acetabulum K, A, B, A, B, A, B
  - S32.412 Displaced fracture of anterior wall of left acetabulum K, A, B, A, B, A, B
  - S32.413 Displaced fracture of anterior wall of unspecified acetabulum K, A, B, A, B, A, B
  - S32.414 Nondisplaced fracture of anterior wall of right acetabulum K, A, B, A, B, A, B
  - S32.415 Nondisplaced fracture of anterior wall of left acetabulum K, A, B, A, B, A, B
  - S32.416 Nondisplaced fracture of anterior wall of unspecified acetabulum K, A, B, A, B, A, B
- S32.42 Fracture of posterior wall of acetabulum
  - S32.421 Displaced fracture of posterior wall of right acetabulum K, A, B, A, B, A, B
  - S32.422 Displaced fracture of posterior wall of left acetabulum K, A, B, A, B, A, B
  - S32.423 Displaced fracture of posterior wall of unspecified acetabulum K, A, B, A, B, A, B
  - S32.424 Nondisplaced fracture of posterior wall of right acetabulum K, A, B, A, B, A, B
  - S32.425 Nondisplaced fracture of posterior wall of left acetabulum K, A, B, A, B, A, B
  - S32.426 Nondisplaced fracture of posterior wall of unspecified acetabulum K, A, B, A, B, A, B
- S32.43 Fracture of anterior column [iliopubic] of acetabulum
  - S32.431 Displaced fracture of anterior column [iliopubic] of right acetabulum K, A, B, A, B, A, B
  - S32.432 Displaced fracture of anterior column [iliopubic] of left acetabulum K, A, B, A, B, A, B
  - S32.433 Displaced fracture of anterior column [iliopubic] of unspecified acetabulum K, A, B, A, B, A, B
  - S32.434 Nondisplaced fracture of anterior column [iliopubic] of right acetabulum K, A, B, A, B, A, B
  - S32.435 Nondisplaced fracture of anterior column [iliopubic] of left acetabulum K, A, B, A, B, A, B
  - S32.436 Nondisplaced fracture of anterior column [iliopubic] of unspecified acetabulum K, A, B, A, B, A, B
- S32.44 Fracture of posterior column [ilioischial] of acetabulum
  - S32.441 Displaced fracture of posterior column [ilioischial] of right acetabulum K, A, B, A, B, A, B
  - S32.442 Displaced fracture of posterior column [ilioischial] of left acetabulum K, A, B, A, B, A, B
  - S32.443 Displaced fracture of posterior column [ilioischial] of unspecified acetabulum K, A, B, A, B, A, B
  - S32.444 Nondisplaced fracture of posterior column [ilioischial] of right acetabulum K, A, B, A, B, A, B
  - S32.445 Nondisplaced fracture of posterior column [ilioischial] of left acetabulum K, A, B, A, B, A, B
  - S32.446 Nondisplaced fracture of posterior column [ilioischial] of unspecified acetabulum K, A, B, A, B, A, B
- S32.45 Transverse fracture of acetabulum
  - S32.451 Displaced transverse fracture of right acetabulum K, A, B, A, B, A, B
  - S32.452 Displaced transverse fracture of left acetabulum K, A, B, A, B, A, B
  - S32.453 Displaced transverse fracture of unspecified acetabulum K, A, B, A, B, A, B
  - S32.454 Nondisplaced transverse fracture of right acetabulum K, A, B, A, B, A, B
  - S32.455 Nondisplaced transverse fracture of left acetabulum K, A, B, A, B, A, B
  - S32.456 Nondisplaced transverse fracture of unspecified acetabulum K, A, B, A, B, A, B
- S32.46 Associated transverse-posterior fracture of acetabulum
  - S32.461 Displaced associated transverse-posterior fracture of right acetabulum K, A, B, A, B, A, B
  - S32.462 Displaced associated transverse-posterior fracture of left acetabulum K, A, B, A, B, A, B
  - S32.463 Displaced associated transverse-posterior fracture of unspecified acetabulum K, A, B, A, B, A, B
  - S32.464 Nondisplaced associated transverse-posterior fracture of right acetabulum K, A, B, A, B, A, B

CHAPTER 19 (SØØ-T88)

S32.465 Nondisplaced associated transverse-posterior fracture of left acetabulum K, A, B, A, B, A, B

S32.466 Nondisplaced associated transverse-posterior fracture of unspecified acetabulum K, A, B, A, B, A, B

S32.47 Fracture of medial wall of acetabulum

S32.471 Displaced fracture of medial wall of right acetabulum K, A, B, A, B, A, B

S32.472 Displaced fracture of medial wall of left acetabulum K, A, B, A, B, A, B

S32.473 Displaced fracture of medial wall of unspecified acetabulum K, A, B, A, B, A, B

S32.474 Nondisplaced fracture of medial wall of right acetabulum K, A, B, A, B, A, B

S32.475 Nondisplaced fracture of medial wall of left acetabulum K, A, B, A, B, A, B

S32.476 Nondisplaced fracture of medial wall of unspecified acetabulum K, A, B, A, B, A, B

S32.48 Dome fracture of acetabulum

S32.481 Displaced dome fracture of right acetabulum K, A, B, A, B, A, B

S32.482 Displaced dome fracture of left acetabulum K, A, B, A, B, A, B

S32.483 Displaced dome fracture of unspecified acetabulum K, A, B, A, B, A, B

S32.484 Nondisplaced dome fracture of right acetabulum K, A, B, A, B, A, B

S32.485 Nondisplaced dome fracture of left acetabulum K, A, B, A, B, A, B

S32.486 Nondisplaced dome fracture of unspecified acetabulum K, A, B, A, B, A, B

S32.49 Other fracture of acetabulum

S32.491 Other fracture of right acetabulum K, A, B, A, B, A, B

S32.492 Other fracture of left acetabulum K, A, B, A, B, A, B

S32.499 Other fracture of unspecified acetabulum K, A, B, A, B, A, B

S32.5 Fracture of pubis (Ex) PDX 1264 [K], 1710 [A, B]

Excludes1 fracture of pubis with associated disruption of pelvic ring (S32.8-)

S32.50 Unspecified fracture of pubis

S32.501 Unspecified fracture of right pubis A, K, B, A, B, A, B

S32.502 Unspecified fracture of left pubis A, K, B, A, B, A, B

S32.509 Unspecified fracture of unspecified pubis A, K, B, A, B, A, B

S32.51 Fracture of superior rim of pubis

S32.511 Fracture of superior rim of right pubis A, K, B, A, B, A, B

S32.512 Fracture of superior rim of left pubis A, K, B, A, B, A, B

S32.519 Fracture of superior rim of unspecified pubis A, K, B, A, B, A, B

S32.59 Other specified fracture of pubis

S32.591 Other specified fracture of right pubis A, K, B, A, B, A, B

S32.592 Other specified fracture of left pubis A, K, B, A, B, A, B

S32.599 Other specified fracture of unspecified pubis A, K, B, A, B, A, B

S32.6 Fracture of ischium (Ex) PDX 1264 [K], 1711 [A], 1712 [B]

Excludes1 fracture of ischium with associated disruption of pelvic ring (S32.8-)

S32.60 Unspecified fracture of ischium

S32.601 Unspecified fracture of right ischium A, K, B, A, B, A, B

S32.602 Unspecified fracture of left ischium A, K, B, A, B, A, B

S32.609 Unspecified fracture of unspecified ischium A, K, B, A, B, A, B

S32.61 Avulsion fracture of ischium

S32.611 Displaced avulsion fracture of right ischium A, K, B, A, B, A, B

S32.612 Displaced avulsion fracture of left ischium A, K, B, A, B, A, B

S32.613 Displaced avulsion fracture of unspecified ischium A, K, B, A, B, A, B

S32.614 Nondisplaced avulsion fracture of right ischium A, K, B, A, B, A, B

S32.615 Nondisplaced avulsion fracture of left ischium A, K, B, A, B, A, B

S32.616 Nondisplaced avulsion fracture of unspecified ischium A, K, B, A, B, A, B

S32.69 Other specified fracture of ischium

S32.691 Other specified fracture of right ischium A, K, B, A, B, A, B

S32.692 Other specified fracture of left ischium A, K, B, A, B, A, B

S32.699 Other specified fracture of unspecified ischium A, K, B, A, B, A, B

S32.8 Fracture of other parts of pelvis

Code also any associated:
fracture of acetabulum (S32.4-)
sacral fracture (S32.1-)

S32.81 Multiple fractures of pelvis with disruption of pelvic ring (Ex) PDX 1264 [K], 1713 [A, B]

Multiple pelvic fractures with disruption of pelvic circle

S32.810 Multiple fractures of pelvis with stable disruption of pelvic ring A, K, B, A, B, A, B

S32.811 Multiple fractures of pelvis with unstable disruption of pelvic ring A, K, B, A, B, A, B

X S32.82 Multiple fractures of pelvis without disruption of pelvic ring A, K, B, A, B, A, B (Ex) PDX 1264 [K], 1714 [A], 1715 [B]

Multiple pelvic fractures without disruption of pelvic circle

X S32.89 Fracture of other parts of pelvis A, K, B, A, B, A, B (Ex) PDX 1264 [K], 1716 [A, B]

X S32.9 Fracture of unspecified parts of lumbosacral spine and pelvis A, K, B, A, B, A, B (Ex) PDX 1264 [K], 1713 [A, B]

Fracture of lumbosacral spine NOS
Fracture of pelvis NOS
Coding Clinic: 2012, Q4, P93

● S33 Dislocation and sprain of joints and ligaments of lumbar spine and pelvis

Includes avulsion of joint or ligament of lumbar spine and pelvis
laceration of cartilage, joint or ligament of lumbar spine and pelvis
sprain of cartilage, joint or ligament of lumbar spine and pelvis
traumatic hemarthrosis of joint or ligament of lumbar spine and pelvis
traumatic rupture of joint or ligament of lumbar spine and pelvis
traumatic subluxation of joint or ligament of lumbar spine and pelvis
traumatic tear of joint or ligament of lumbar spine and pelvis

Code also any associated open wound

Excludes1 nontraumatic rupture or displacement of lumbar intervertebral disc NOS (M51.-)
obstetric damage to pelvic joints and ligaments (O71.6)

Excludes2 dislocation and sprain of joints and ligaments of hip (S73.-)
strain of muscle of lower back and pelvis (S39.01-)

The appropriate 7th character is to be added to each code from category S33

A	initial encounter
D	subsequent encounter
S	sequela

X● **S33.0 Traumatic rupture of lumbar intervertebral disc**

Excludes1 rupture or displacement (nontraumatic) of lumbar intervertebral disc NOS (M51.- with fifth character 6)

● **S33.1 Subluxation and dislocation of lumbar vertebra**

Code also any associated:
open wound of abdomen, lower back and pelvis (S31)
spinal cord injury (S24.0, S24.1-, S34.0-, S34.1-)

Excludes2 fracture of lumbar vertebrae (S32.0-)

● **S33.10 Subluxation and dislocation of unspecified lumbar vertebra**

● **S33.100 Subluxation of unspecified lumbar vertebra**

● **S33.101 Dislocation of unspecified lumbar vertebra**

● **S33.11 Subluxation and dislocation of L1/L2 lumbar vertebra**

● **S33.110 Subluxation of L1/L2 lumbar vertebra**

● **S33.111 Dislocation of L1/L2 lumbar vertebra**

● **S33.12 Subluxation and dislocation of L2/L3 lumbar vertebra**

● **S33.120 Subluxation of L2/L3 lumbar vertebra**

● **S33.121 Dislocation of L2/L3 lumbar vertebra**

● **S33.13 Subluxation and dislocation of L3/L4 lumbar vertebra**

● **S33.130 Subluxation of L3/L4 lumbar vertebra**

● **S33.131 Dislocation of L3/L4 lumbar vertebra**

● **S33.14 Subluxation and dislocation of L4/L5 lumbar vertebra**

● **S33.140 Subluxation of L4/L5 lumbar vertebra**

● **S33.141 Dislocation of L4/L5 lumbar vertebra**

X● **S33.2 Dislocation of sacroiliac and sacrococcygeal joint**

● **S33.3 Dislocation of other and unspecified parts of lumbar spine and pelvis**

X● **S33.30 Dislocation of unspecified parts of lumbar spine and pelvis**

X● **S33.39 Dislocation of other parts of lumbar spine and pelvis**

X● **S33.4 Traumatic rupture of symphysis pubis**

X● **S33.5 Sprain of ligaments of lumbar spine**

X● **S33.6 Sprain of sacroiliac joint**

X● **S33.8 Sprain of other parts of lumbar spine and pelvis**

X● **S33.9 Sprain of unspecified parts of lumbar spine and pelvis**

● S34 Injury of lumbar and sacral spinal cord and nerves at abdomen, lower back and pelvis level

Note: Code to highest level of lumbar cord injury
Injuries to the spinal cord (S34.0 and S34.1) refer to the cord level and not bone level injury, and can affect nerve roots at and below the level given.

The appropriate 7th character is to be added to each code from category S34

A	initial encounter
D	subsequent encounter
S	sequela

Code also any associated:
fracture of vertebra (S22.0-, S32.0-)
open wound of abdomen, lower back and pelvis (S31.-)
transient paralysis (R29.5)

● **S34.0 Concussion and edema of lumbar and sacral spinal cord**

X● **S34.01 Concussion and edema of lumbar spinal cord** A, A, D, S (Ex) PDX 1717

X● **S34.02 Concussion and edema of sacral spinal cord** A, A, D, S (Ex) PDX 1718
Concussion and edema of conus medullaris

● **S34.1 Other and unspecified injury of lumbar and sacral spinal cord**

● **S34.10 Unspecified injury to lumbar spinal cord** (Ex) PDX 1717

● **S34.101 Unspecified injury to L_1 level of lumbar spinal cord** A, A, A, D, S
Unspecified injury to lumbar spinal cord level 1

● **S34.102 Unspecified injury to L_2 level of lumbar spinal cord** A, A, A, D, S
Unspecified injury to lumbar spinal cord level 2

● **S34.103 Unspecified injury to L_3 level of lumbar spinal cord** A, A, A, D, S
Unspecified injury to lumbar spinal cord level 3

● **S34.104 Unspecified injury to L_4 level of lumbar spinal cord** A, A, A, D, S
Unspecified injury to lumbar spinal cord level 4

● **S34.105 Unspecified injury to L_5 level of lumbar spinal cord** A, A, A, D, S
Unspecified injury to lumbar spinal cord level 5

● **S34.109 Unspecified injury to unspecified level of lumbar spinal cord** A, A, A, D, S

● **S34.11 Complete lesion of lumbar spinal cord** (Ex) PDX 1717

● **S34.111 Complete lesion of L_1 level of lumbar spinal cord** A, A, A, D, S
Complete lesion of lumbar spinal cord level 1

● **S34.112 Complete lesion of L_2 level of lumbar spinal cord** A, A, A, D, S
Complete lesion of lumbar spinal cord level 2

● **S34.113 Complete lesion of L_3 level of lumbar spinal cord** A, A, A, D, S
Complete lesion of lumbar spinal cord level 3

● S34.114 **Complete lesion of L_4 level of lumbar spinal cord** A, A, A, D, S
Complete lesion of lumbar spinal cord level 4

● S34.115 **Complete lesion of L_5 level of lumbar spinal cord** A, A, A, D, S
Complete lesion of lumbar spinal cord level 5

● S34.119 **Complete lesion of unspecified level of lumbar spinal cord** A, A, A, D, S

● S34.12 **Incomplete lesion of lumbar spinal cord** (Ex:) PDX 1717

● S34.121 **Incomplete lesion of L_1 level of lumbar spinal cord** A, A, A, D, S
Incomplete lesion of lumbar spinal cord level 1

● S34.122 **Incomplete lesion of L_2 level of lumbar spinal cord** A, A, A, D, S
Incomplete lesion of lumbar spinal cord level 2

● S34.123 **Incomplete lesion of L_3 level of lumbar spinal cord** A, A, A, D, S
Incomplete lesion of lumbar spinal cord level 3

● S34.124 **Incomplete lesion of L_4 level of lumbar spinal cord** A, A, A, D, S
Incomplete lesion of lumbar spinal cord level 4

● S34.125 **Incomplete lesion of L_5 level of lumbar spinal cord** A, A, A, D, S
Incomplete lesion of lumbar spinal cord level 5

● S34.129 **Incomplete lesion of unspecified level of lumbar spinal cord** A, A, A, D, S

● S34.13 **Other and unspecified injury to sacral spinal cord** (Ex:) PDX 1718
Other injury to conus medullaris

● S34.131 **Complete lesion of sacral spinal cord** A, A, A, D, S
Complete lesion of conus medullaris

● S34.132 **Incomplete lesion of sacral spinal cord** A, A, A, D, S
Incomplete lesion of conus medullaris

● S34.139 **Unspecified injury to sacral spinal cord** A, A, A, D, S
Unspecified injury of conus medullaris

● S34.2 **Injury of nerve root of lumbar and sacral spine**

X● S34.21 **Injury of nerve root of lumbar spine**

X● S34.22 **Injury of nerve root of sacral spine**

X● S34.3 **Injury of cauda equina** A, A, A, D, S (Ex:) PDX 1718

X● S34.4 **Injury of lumbosacral plexus**

X● S34.5 **Injury of lumbar, sacral and pelvic sympathetic nerves**
Injury of celiac ganglion or plexus
Injury of hypogastric plexus
Injury of mesenteric plexus (inferior) (superior)
Injury of splanchnic nerve

X● S34.6 **Injury of peripheral nerve(s) at abdomen, lower back and pelvis level**

X● S34.8 **Injury of other nerves at abdomen, lower back and pelvis level**

X● S34.9 **Injury of unspecified nerves at abdomen, lower back and pelvis level**

● S35 **Injury of blood vessels at abdomen, lower back and pelvis level**

The appropriate 7th character is to be added to each code from category S35

A	initial encounter
D	subsequent encounter
S	sequela

Code also any associated open wound (S31.-)

● S35.Ø **Injury of abdominal aorta** (Ex:) PDX 1719

Excludes1 injury of aorta NOS (S25.Ø)

X● S35.ØØ **Unspecified injury of abdominal aorta** A

X● S35.Ø1 **Minor laceration of abdominal aorta** A
Incomplete transection of abdominal aorta
Laceration of abdominal aorta NOS
Superficial laceration of abdominal aorta

X● S35.Ø2 **Major laceration of abdominal aorta** A
Complete transection of abdominal aorta
Traumatic rupture of abdominal aorta

X● S35.Ø9 **Other injury of abdominal aorta** A

● S35.1 **Injury of inferior vena cava** (Ex:) PDX 1720
Injury of hepatic vein

Excludes1 injury of vena cava NOS (S25.2)

X● S35.1Ø **Unspecified injury of inferior vena cava** A

X● S35.11 **Minor laceration of inferior vena cava** A
Incomplete transection of inferior vena cava
Laceration of inferior vena cava NOS
Superficial laceration of inferior vena cava

X● S35.12 **Major laceration of inferior vena cava** A
Complete transection of inferior vena cava
Traumatic rupture of inferior vena cava

X● S35.19 **Other injury of inferior vena cava** A

● S35.2 **Injury of celiac or mesenteric artery and branches**

● S35.21 **Injury of celiac artery** (Ex:) PDX 1721

● S35.211 **Minor laceration of celiac artery** A
Incomplete transection of celiac artery
Laceration of celiac artery NOS
Superficial laceration of celiac artery

● S35.212 **Major laceration of celiac artery** A
Complete transection of celiac artery
Traumatic rupture of celiac artery

● S35.218 **Other injury of celiac artery** A

● S35.219 **Unspecified injury of celiac artery** A

● S35.22 **Injury of superior mesenteric artery** (Ex:) PDX 1722

● S35.221 **Minor laceration of superior mesenteric artery** A
Incomplete transection of superior mesenteric artery
Laceration of superior mesenteric artery NOS
Superficial laceration of superior mesenteric artery

● S35.222 **Major laceration of superior mesenteric artery** A
Complete transection of superior mesenteric artery
Traumatic rupture of superior mesenteric artery

● S35.228 **Other injury of superior mesenteric artery** A

● S35.229 **Unspecified injury of superior mesenteric artery** A

- **S35.23** Injury of inferior mesenteric artery (Ex) PDX 1723
  - **S35.231** **Minor laceration of inferior mesenteric artery** A
    - Incomplete transection of inferior mesenteric artery
    - Laceration of inferior mesenteric artery NOS
    - Superficial laceration of inferior mesenteric artery
  - **S35.232** **Major laceration of inferior mesenteric artery** A
    - Complete transection of inferior mesenteric artery
    - Traumatic rupture of inferior mesenteric artery
  - **S35.238** **Other injury of inferior mesenteric artery** A
  - **S35.239** **Unspecified injury of inferior mesenteric artery** A
- **S35.29** Injury of branches of celiac and mesenteric artery
  - Injury of gastric artery
  - Injury of gastroduodenal artery
  - Injury of hepatic artery
  - Injury of splenic artery
  - **S35.291** **Minor laceration of branches of celiac and mesenteric artery** A (Ex) PDX 1724
    - Incomplete transection of branches of celiac and mesenteric artery
    - Laceration of branches of celiac and mesenteric artery NOS
    - Superficial laceration of branches of celiac and mesenteric artery
  - **S35.292** **Major laceration of branches of celiac and mesenteric artery** A (Ex) PDX 1725
    - Complete transection of branches of celiac and mesenteric artery
    - Traumatic rupture of branches of celiac and mesenteric artery
  - **S35.298** **Other injury of branches of celiac and mesenteric artery** A (Ex) PDX 1725
  - **S35.299** **Unspecified injury of branches of celiac and mesenteric artery** A (Ex) PDX 1726
- **S35.3** Injury of portal or splenic vein and branches
  - **S35.31** Injury of portal vein (Ex) PDX 1727
    - **S35.311** **Laceration of portal vein** A
    - **S35.318** **Other specified injury of portal vein** A
    - **S35.319** **Unspecified injury of portal vein** A
  - **S35.32** Injury of splenic vein (Ex) PDX 1728
    - **S35.321** **Laceration of splenic vein** A
    - **S35.328** **Other specified injury of splenic vein** A
    - **S35.329** **Unspecified injury of splenic vein** A
  - **S35.33** Injury of superior mesenteric vein (Ex) PDX 1729
    - **S35.331** **Laceration of superior mesenteric vein** A
    - **S35.338** **Other specified injury of superior mesenteric vein** A
    - **S35.339** **Unspecified injury of superior mesenteric vein** A
  - **S35.34** Injury of inferior mesenteric vein (Ex) PDX 1730
    - **S35.341** **Laceration of inferior mesenteric vein** A
    - **S35.348** **Other specified injury of inferior mesenteric vein** A
    - **S35.349** **Unspecified injury of inferior mesenteric vein** A
- **S35.4** Injury of renal blood vessels
  - **S35.40** Unspecified injury of renal blood vessel
    - **S35.401** **Unspecified injury of right renal artery** A (Ex) PDX 1731
    - **S35.402** **Unspecified injury of left renal artery** A (Ex) PDX 1731
    - **S35.403** **Unspecified injury of unspecified renal artery** A (Ex) PDX 1731
    - **S35.404** **Unspecified injury of right renal vein** A (Ex) PDX 1732
    - **S35.405** **Unspecified injury of left renal vein** A (Ex) PDX 1732
    - **S35.406** **Unspecified injury of unspecified renal vein** A (Ex) PDX 1732
  - **S35.41** Laceration of renal blood vessel
    - **S35.411** **Laceration of right renal artery** A (Ex) PDX 1731
    - **S35.412** **Laceration of left renal artery** A (Ex) PDX 1731
    - **S35.413** **Laceration of unspecified renal artery** A (Ex) PDX 1731
    - **S35.414** **Laceration of right renal vein** A (Ex) PDX 1732
    - **S35.415** **Laceration of left renal vein** A (Ex) PDX 1732
    - **S35.416** **Laceration of unspecified renal vein** A (Ex) PDX 1732
  - **S35.49** Other specified injury of renal blood vessel (Ex) PDX 1731, 1732
    - **S35.491** **Other specified injury of right renal artery** A (Ex) PDX 1731
    - **S35.492** **Other specified injury of left renal artery** A (Ex) PDX 1731
    - **S35.493** **Other specified injury of unspecified renal artery** A (Ex) PDX 1731
    - **S35.494** **Other specified injury of right renal vein** A (Ex) PDX 1732
    - **S35.495** **Other specified injury of left renal vein** A (Ex) PDX 1732
    - **S35.496** **Other specified injury of unspecified renal vein** A (Ex) PDX 1732
- **S35.5** Injury of iliac blood vessels
  - X **S35.50** **Injury of unspecified iliac blood vessel(s)** A (Ex) PDX 1733
  - **S35.51** Injury of iliac artery or vein
    - Injury of hypogastric artery or vein
    - **S35.511** **Injury of right iliac artery** A (Ex) PDX 1734
    - **S35.512** **Injury of left iliac artery** A (Ex) PDX 1734
    - **S35.513** **Injury of unspecified iliac artery** A (Ex) PDX 1734
    - **S35.514** **Injury of right iliac vein** A (Ex) PDX 1735
    - **S35.515** **Injury of left iliac vein** A (Ex) PDX 1735
    - **S35.516** **Injury of unspecified iliac vein** A (Ex) PDX 1735
  - **S35.53** Injury of uterine artery or vein
    - **S35.531** **Injury of right uterine artery** A (Ex) PDX 1736
    - **S35.532** **Injury of left uterine artery** A (Ex) PDX 1736
    - **S35.533** **Injury of unspecified uterine artery** A (Ex) PDX 1736
    - **S35.534** **Injury of right uterine vein** A (Ex) PDX 1737
    - **S35.535** **Injury of left uterine vein** A (Ex) PDX 1737
    - **S35.536** **Injury of unspecified uterine vein** A (Ex) PDX 1737
  - X **S35.59** **Injury of other iliac blood vessels** A (Ex) PDX 1733

CHAPTER 19 (SØØ-T88)

● S35.8 Injury of other blood vessels at abdomen, lower back and pelvis level (Ex) PDX 1738
Injury of ovarian artery or vein

● S35.8X Injury of other blood vessels at abdomen, lower back and pelvis level

● S35.8X1 Laceration of other blood vessels at abdomen, lower back and pelvis level A

● S35.8X8 Other specified injury of other blood vessels at abdomen, lower back and pelvis level A

● S35.8X9 Unspecified injury of other blood vessels at abdomen, lower back and pelvis level A

● S35.9 Injury of unspecified blood vessel at abdomen, lower back and pelvis level (Ex) PDX 1739

X● S35.90 Unspecified injury of unspecified blood vessel at abdomen, lower back and pelvis level A

X● S35.91 Laceration of unspecified blood vessel at abdomen, lower back and pelvis level A

X● S35.99 Other specified injury of unspecified blood vessel at abdomen, lower back and pelvis level A

● S36 Injury of intra-abdominal organs
The appropriate 7th character is to be added to each code from category S36

A	initial encounter
D	subsequent encounter
S	sequela

Code also any associated open wound (S31.-)

● S36.0 Injury of spleen (Ex) PDX 1740

X● S36.00 Unspecified injury of spleen A

● S36.02 Contusion of spleen

● S36.020 Minor contusion of spleen A
Contusion of spleen less than 2 cm

● S36.021 Major contusion of spleen A
Contusion of spleen greater than 2 cm

● S36.029 Unspecified contusion of spleen A
Coding Clinic: 2015, Q2, P36, Q1, P11

● S36.03 Laceration of spleen

● S36.030 Superficial (capsular) laceration of spleen A
Laceration of spleen less than 1 cm
Minor laceration of spleen

● S36.031 Moderate laceration of spleen A
Laceration of spleen 1 to 3 cm
Coding Clinic: 2022, Q1, P23; 2015, Q2, P36, Q1, P11

● S36.032 Major laceration of spleen A
Avulsion of spleen
Laceration of spleen greater than 3 cm
Massive laceration of spleen
Multiple moderate lacerations of spleen
Stellate laceration of spleen

● S36.039 Unspecified laceration of spleen A

X● S36.09 Other injury of spleen A

● S36.1 Injury of liver and gallbladder and bile duct

● S36.11 Injury of liver (Ex) PDX 1741
Coding Clinic: 2024, Q1, P25

● S36.112 Contusion of liver A

● S36.113 Laceration of liver, unspecified degree A

● S36.114 Minor laceration of liver A
Laceration involving capsule only, or, without significant involvement of hepatic parenchyma [i.e., less than 1 cm deep]

● S36.115 Moderate laceration of liver A
Laceration involving parenchyma but without major disruption of parenchyma [i.e., less than 10 cm long and less than 3 cm deep]

● S36.116 Major laceration of liver A
Laceration with significant disruption of hepatic parenchyma [i.e., greater than 10 cm long and 3 cm deep]
Multiple moderate lacerations, with or without hematoma
Stellate laceration of liver

● S36.118 Other injury of liver A

● S36.119 Unspecified injury of liver A
Coding Clinic: 2015, Q2, P17

● S36.12 Injury of gallbladder (Ex) PDX 1742

● S36.122 Contusion of gallbladder A

● S36.123 Laceration of gallbladder A

● S36.128 Other injury of gallbladder A

● S36.129 Unspecified injury of gallbladder A

X● S36.13 Injury of bile duct A (Ex) PDX 1742

● S36.2 Injury of pancreas (Ex) PDX 1743

● S36.20 Unspecified injury of pancreas

● S36.200 Unspecified injury of head of pancreas A

● S36.201 Unspecified injury of body of pancreas A

● S36.202 Unspecified injury of tail of pancreas A

● S36.209 Unspecified injury of unspecified part of pancreas A

● S36.22 Contusion of pancreas

● S36.220 Contusion of head of pancreas A

● S36.221 Contusion of body of pancreas A

● S36.222 Contusion of tail of pancreas A

● S36.229 Contusion of unspecified part of pancreas A

● S36.23 Laceration of pancreas, unspecified degree

● S36.230 Laceration of head of pancreas, unspecified degree A

● S36.231 Laceration of body of pancreas, unspecified degree A

● S36.232 Laceration of tail of pancreas, unspecified degree A

● S36.239 Laceration of unspecified part of pancreas, unspecified degree A

● S36.24 Minor laceration of pancreas

● S36.240 Minor laceration of head of pancreas A

● S36.241 Minor laceration of body of pancreas A

● S36.242 Minor laceration of tail of pancreas A

● S36.249 Minor laceration of unspecified part of pancreas A

● S36.25 Moderate laceration of pancreas

● S36.250 Moderate laceration of head of pancreas A

● S36.251 Moderate laceration of body of pancreas A

● S36.252 Moderate laceration of tail of pancreas A

● S36.259 Moderate laceration of unspecified part of pancreas A

CHAPTER 19 (S00-T88)

S36.26 Major laceration of pancreas
S36.260 Major laceration of head of pancreas A
S36.261 Major laceration of body of pancreas A
S36.262 Major laceration of tail of pancreas A
S36.269 Major laceration of unspecified part of pancreas A
S36.29 Other injury of pancreas
S36.290 Other injury of head of pancreas A
S36.291 Other injury of body of pancreas A
S36.292 Other injury of tail of pancreas A
S36.299 Other injury of unspecified part of pancreas A
S36.3 Injury of stomach (Ex) PDX 1744
X S36.30 Unspecified injury of stomach A
X S36.32 Contusion of stomach A
X S36.33 Laceration of stomach A
X S36.39 Other injury of stomach A
S36.4 Injury of small intestine (Ex) PDX 1745
S36.40 Unspecified injury of small intestine
S36.400 Unspecified injury of duodenum A
S36.408 Unspecified injury of other part of small intestine A
S36.409 Unspecified injury of unspecified part of small intestine A
S36.41 Primary blast injury of small intestine
Blast injury of small intestine NOS
S36.410 Primary blast injury of duodenum A
S36.418 Primary blast injury of other part of small intestine A
S36.419 Primary blast injury of unspecified part of small intestine A
S36.42 Contusion of small intestine
S36.420 Contusion of duodenum A
S36.428 Contusion of other part of small intestine A
S36.429 Contusion of unspecified part of small intestine A
S36.43 Laceration of small intestine
S36.430 Laceration of duodenum A
S36.438 Laceration of other part of small intestine A
S36.439 Laceration of unspecified part of small intestine A
S36.49 Other injury of small intestine
S36.490 Other injury of duodenum A
S36.498 Other injury of other part of small intestine A
Coding Clinic: 2023, Q3, P8-9
S36.499 Other injury of unspecified part of small intestine A
S36.5 Injury of colon (Ex) PDX 1746
Excludes2 injury of rectum (S36.6-)
S36.50 Unspecified injury of colon
S36.500 Unspecified injury of ascending [right] colon A
S36.501 Unspecified injury of transverse colon A
S36.502 Unspecified injury of descending [left] colon A
S36.503 Unspecified injury of sigmoid colon A
S36.508 Unspecified injury of other part of colon A
S36.509 Unspecified injury of unspecified part of colon A
S36.51 Primary blast injury of colon
Blast injury of colon NOS
S36.510 Primary blast injury of ascending [right] colon A
S36.511 Primary blast injury of transverse colon A
S36.512 Primary blast injury of descending [left] colon A
S36.513 Primary blast injury of sigmoid colon A
S36.518 Primary blast injury of other part of colon A
S36.519 Primary blast injury of unspecified part of colon A
S36.52 Contusion of colon
S36.520 Contusion of ascending [right] colon A
S36.521 Contusion of transverse colon A
S36.522 Contusion of descending [left] colon A
S36.523 Contusion of sigmoid colon A
S36.528 Contusion of other part of colon A
S36.529 Contusion of unspecified part of colon A
S36.53 Laceration of colon
S36.530 Laceration of ascending [right] colon A
S36.531 Laceration of transverse colon A
S36.532 Laceration of descending [left] colon A
S36.533 Laceration of sigmoid colon A
S36.538 Laceration of other part of colon A
S36.539 Laceration of unspecified part of colon A
S36.59 Other injury of colon
Secondary blast injury of colon
S36.590 Other injury of ascending [right] colon A
Coding Clinic: 2023, Q3, P8-9
S36.591 Other injury of transverse colon A
S36.592 Other injury of descending [left] colon A
S36.593 Other injury of sigmoid colon A
S36.598 Other injury of other part of colon A
S36.599 Other injury of unspecified part of colon A
S36.6 Injury of rectum (Ex) PDX 1746
X S36.60 Unspecified injury of rectum A
X S36.61 Primary blast injury of rectum A
Blast injury of rectum NOS
X S36.62 Contusion of rectum A
X S36.63 Laceration of rectum A
X S36.69 Other injury of rectum A
Secondary blast injury of rectum
S36.8 Injury of other intra-abdominal organs (Ex) PDX 1705
X S36.81 Injury of peritoneum A
S36.89 Injury of other intra-abdominal organs
Injury of retroperitoneum
S36.892 Contusion of other intra-abdominal organs A
S36.893 Laceration of other intra-abdominal organs A

CHAPTER 19 (S00-T88)

● S36.898 Other injury of other intra-abdominal organs A
S36.899 Unspecified injury of other intra-abdominal organs A

● S36.9 Injury of unspecified intra-abdominal organ (Ex) PDX 1705
X● S36.90 Unspecified injury of unspecified intra-abdominal organ A
X● S36.92 Contusion of unspecified intra-abdominal organ A
X● S36.93 Laceration of unspecified intra-abdominal organ A
X● S36.99 Other injury of unspecified intra-abdominal organ A

● S37 Injury of urinary and pelvic organs

Code also any associated open wound (S31.-)

Excludes1 obstetric trauma to pelvic organs (O71.-)

Excludes2 injury of peritoneum (S36.81)
injury of retroperitoneum (S36.89-)

The appropriate 7th character is to be added to each code from category S37

A	initial encounter
D	subsequent encounter
S	sequela

● S37.0 Injury of kidney (Ex) PDX 1747

Excludes2 acute kidney injury (nontraumatic) (N17.9)

● S37.00 Unspecified injury of kidney
● S37.001 Unspecified injury of right kidney A
● S37.002 Unspecified injury of left kidney A
● S37.009 Unspecified injury of unspecified kidney A

● S37.01 Minor contusion of kidney
Contusion of kidney less than 2 cm
Contusion of kidney NOS
● S37.011 Minor contusion of right kidney A
● S37.012 Minor contusion of left kidney A
● S37.019 Minor contusion of unspecified kidney A

● S37.02 Major contusion of kidney
Contusion of kidney greater than 2 cm
● S37.021 Major contusion of right kidney A
● S37.022 Major contusion of left kidney A
● S37.029 Major contusion of unspecified kidney A

● S37.03 Laceration of kidney, unspecified degree
● S37.031 Laceration of right kidney, unspecified degree A
● S37.032 Laceration of left kidney, unspecified degree A
● S37.039 Laceration of unspecified kidney, unspecified degree A

● S37.04 Minor laceration of kidney
Laceration of kidney less than 1 cm
● S37.041 Minor laceration of right kidney A
● S37.042 Minor laceration of left kidney A
● S37.049 Minor laceration of unspecified kidney A

● S37.05 Moderate laceration of kidney
Laceration of kidney 1 to 3 cm
● S37.051 Moderate laceration of right kidney A
● S37.052 Moderate laceration of left kidney A
● S37.059 Moderate laceration of unspecified kidney A

● S37.06 Major laceration of kidney
Avulsion of kidney
Laceration of kidney greater than 3 cm
Massive laceration of kidney
Multiple moderate lacerations of kidney
Stellate laceration of kidney
● S37.061 Major laceration of right kidney A
● S37.062 Major laceration of left kidney A
● S37.069 Major laceration of unspecified kidney A

● S37.09 Other injury of kidney
● S37.091 Other injury of right kidney A
● S37.092 Other injury of left kidney A
● S37.099 Other injury of unspecified kidney A

● S37.1 Injury of ureter (Ex) PDX 1748
X● S37.10 Unspecified injury of ureter A
X● S37.12 Contusion of ureter A
X● S37.13 Laceration of ureter A
X● S37.19 Other injury of ureter A

● S37.2 Injury of bladder (Ex) PDX 1749
X● S37.20 Unspecified injury of bladder A
X● S37.22 Contusion of bladder A
X● S37.23 Laceration of bladder A
X● S37.29 Other injury of bladder A

● S37.3 Injury of urethra (Ex) PDX 1749
X● S37.30 Unspecified injury of urethra A
X● S37.32 Contusion of urethra A
X● S37.33 Laceration of urethra A
X● S37.39 Other injury of urethra A

● S37.4 Injury of ovary
● S37.40 Unspecified injury of ovary
● S37.401 Unspecified injury of ovary, unilateral
● S37.402 Unspecified injury of ovary, bilateral
● S37.409 Unspecified injury of ovary, unspecified

● S37.42 Contusion of ovary
● S37.421 Contusion of ovary, unilateral
● S37.422 Contusion of ovary, bilateral
● S37.429 Contusion of ovary, unspecified

● S37.43 Laceration of ovary
● S37.431 Laceration of ovary, unilateral
● S37.432 Laceration of ovary, bilateral
● S37.439 Laceration of ovary, unspecified

● S37.49 Other injury of ovary
● S37.491 Other injury of ovary, unilateral
● S37.492 Other injury of ovary, bilateral
● S37.499 Other injury of ovary, unspecified

● S37.5 Injury of fallopian tube
● S37.50 Unspecified injury of fallopian tube
● S37.501 Unspecified injury of fallopian tube, unilateral
● S37.502 Unspecified injury of fallopian tube, bilateral
● S37.509 Unspecified injury of fallopian tube, unspecified

● S37.51 Primary blast injury of fallopian tube
Blast injury of fallopian tube NOS
● S37.511 Primary blast injury of fallopian tube, unilateral
● S37.512 Primary blast injury of fallopian tube, bilateral
● S37.519 Primary blast injury of fallopian tube, unspecified

CHAPTER 19 (SØ-T88)

S37.52 Contusion of fallopian tube
- S37.521 Contusion of fallopian tube, unilateral
- S37.522 Contusion of fallopian tube, bilateral
- S37.529 Contusion of fallopian tube, unspecified

S37.53 Laceration of fallopian tube
- S37.531 Laceration of fallopian tube, unilateral
- S37.532 Laceration of fallopian tube, bilateral
- S37.539 Laceration of fallopian tube, unspecified

S37.59 Other injury of fallopian tube
Secondary blast injury of fallopian tube
- S37.591 Other injury of fallopian tube, unilateral
- S37.592 Other injury of fallopian tube, bilateral
- S37.599 Other injury of fallopian tube, unspecified

S37.6 Injury of uterus (Ex) PDX 1750
Excludes1 injury to gravid uterus (O9A.2-)
injury to uterus during delivery (O71.-)
- X S37.60 Unspecified injury of uterus A
- X S37.62 Contusion of uterus A
- X S37.63 Laceration of uterus A
- X S37.69 Other injury of uterus A

S37.8 Injury of other urinary and pelvic organs

S37.81 Injury of adrenal gland (Ex) PDX 1751
- S37.812 Contusion of adrenal gland A
- S37.813 Laceration of adrenal gland A
- S37.818 Other injury of adrenal gland A
- S37.819 Unspecified injury of adrenal gland A

S37.82 Injury of prostate
- S37.822 Contusion of prostate
- S37.823 Laceration of prostate
- S37.828 Other injury of prostate
- S37.829 Unspecified injury of prostate

S37.89 Injury of other urinary and pelvic organ (Ex) PDX 1752
- S37.892 Contusion of other urinary and pelvic organ A
- S37.893 Laceration of other urinary and pelvic organ A
- S37.898 Other injury of other urinary and pelvic organ A
- S37.899 Unspecified injury of other urinary and pelvic organ A

S37.9 Injury of unspecified urinary and pelvic organ (Ex) PDX 1752
- X S37.90 Unspecified injury of unspecified urinary and pelvic organ A
- X S37.92 Contusion of unspecified urinary and pelvic organ A
- X S37.93 Laceration of unspecified urinary and pelvic organ A
- X S37.99 Other injury of unspecified urinary and pelvic organ A

S38 Crushing injury and traumatic amputation of abdomen, lower back, pelvis and external genitals

An amputation not identified as partial or complete should be coded to complete

The appropriate 7th character is to be added to each code from category S38

A	initial encounter
D	subsequent encounter
S	sequela

S38.0 Crushing injury of external genital organs
Use additional code for any associated injuries

S38.00 Crushing injury of unspecified external genital organs
- S38.001 Crushing injury of unspecified external genital organs, male
- S38.002 Crushing injury of unspecified external genital organs, female

- X S38.01 Crushing injury of penis
- X S38.02 Crushing injury of scrotum and testis
- X S38.03 Crushing injury of vulva

X S38.1 Crushing injury of abdomen, lower back, and pelvis
Use additional code for all associated injuries, such as:
fracture of thoracic or lumbar spine and pelvis (S22.0-, S32.-)
injury to intra-abdominal organs (S36.-)
injury to urinary and pelvic organs (S37.-)
open wound of abdominal wall (S31.-)
spinal cord injury (S34.0, S34.1-)
Excludes2 crushing injury of external genital organs (S38.0-)

S38.2 Traumatic amputation of external genital organs

S38.21 Traumatic amputation of female external genital organs
Traumatic amputation of clitoris
Traumatic amputation of labium (majus) (minus)
Traumatic amputation of vulva
- S38.211 Complete traumatic amputation of female external genital organs
- S38.212 Partial traumatic amputation of female external genital organs

S38.22 Traumatic amputation of penis
- S38.221 Complete traumatic amputation of penis
- S38.222 Partial traumatic amputation of penis

S38.23 Traumatic amputation of scrotum and testis
- S38.231 Complete traumatic amputation of scrotum and testis
- S38.232 Partial traumatic amputation of scrotum and testis

X S38.3 Transection (partial) of abdomen

S39 Other and unspecified injuries of abdomen, lower back, pelvis and external genitals

Code also any associated open wound (S31.-)
Excludes2 sprain of joints and ligaments of lumbar spine and pelvis (S33.-)

The appropriate 7th character is to be added to each code from category S39

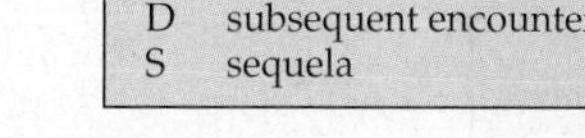

A	initial encounter
D	subsequent encounter
S	sequela

CHAPTER 19 (S00-T88)

● S39.0 Injury of muscle, fascia and tendon of abdomen, lower back and pelvis
● S39.00 Unspecified injury of muscle, fascia and tendon of abdomen, lower back and pelvis
● S39.001 Unspecified injury of muscle, fascia and tendon of abdomen
● S39.002 Unspecified injury of muscle, fascia and tendon of lower back
● S39.003 Unspecified injury of muscle, fascia and tendon of pelvis
● S39.01 Strain of muscle, fascia and tendon of abdomen, lower back and pelvis
● S39.011 Strain of muscle, fascia and tendon of abdomen
● S39.012 Strain of muscle, fascia and tendon of lower back
Coding Clinic: 2016, Q4, P74
● S39.013 Strain of muscle, fascia and tendon of pelvis
● S39.02 Laceration of muscle, fascia and tendon of abdomen, lower back and pelvis
● S39.021 Laceration of muscle, fascia and tendon of abdomen
● S39.022 Laceration of muscle, fascia and tendon of lower back
● S39.023 Laceration of muscle, fascia and tendon of pelvis
● S39.09 Other injury of muscle, fascia and tendon of abdomen, lower back and pelvis
● S39.091 Other injury of muscle, fascia and tendon of abdomen
● S39.092 Other injury of muscle, fascia and tendon of lower back
● S39.093 Other injury of muscle, fascia and tendon of pelvis
● S39.8 Other specified injuries of abdomen, lower back, pelvis and external genitals
X● S39.81 Other specified injuries of abdomen
X● S39.82 Other specified injuries of lower back
X● S39.83 Other specified injuries of pelvis
● S39.84 Other specified injuries of external genitals
● S39.840 Fracture of corpus cavernosum penis
● S39.848 Other specified injuries of external genitals
● S39.9 Unspecified injury of abdomen, lower back, pelvis and external genitals
X● S39.91 Unspecified injury of abdomen
X● S39.92 Unspecified injury of lower back
X● S39.93 Unspecified injury of pelvis
X● S39.94 Unspecified injury of external genitals

INJURIES TO THE SHOULDER AND UPPER ARM (S40-S49)

Includes injuries of axilla injuries of scapular region

Excludes2 burns and corrosions (T20-T32)
frostbite (T33-T34)
injuries of elbow (S50-S59)
insect bite or sting, venomous (T63.4)

● S40 Superficial injury of shoulder and upper arm

The appropriate 7th character is to be added to each code from category S40

A	initial encounter
D	subsequent encounter
S	sequela

● S40.0 Contusion of shoulder and upper arm
● S40.01 Contusion of shoulder
● S40.011 Contusion of right shoulder
● S40.012 Contusion of left shoulder
● S40.019 Contusion of unspecified shoulder
● S40.02 Contusion of upper arm
● S40.021 Contusion of right upper arm
● S40.022 Contusion of left upper arm
● S40.029 Contusion of unspecified upper arm
● S40.2 Other superficial injuries of shoulder
● S40.21 Abrasion of shoulder
● S40.211 Abrasion of right shoulder
● S40.212 Abrasion of left shoulder
● S40.219 Abrasion of unspecified shoulder
● S40.22 Blister (nonthermal) of shoulder
● S40.221 Blister (nonthermal) of right shoulder
● S40.222 Blister (nonthermal) of left shoulder
● S40.229 Blister (nonthermal) of unspecified shoulder
● S40.24 External constriction of shoulder
● S40.241 External constriction of right shoulder
● S40.242 External constriction of left shoulder
● S40.249 External constriction of unspecified shoulder
● S40.25 Superficial foreign body of shoulder
Splinter in the shoulder
● S40.251 Superficial foreign body of right shoulder
● S40.252 Superficial foreign body of left shoulder
● S40.259 Superficial foreign body of unspecified shoulder
● S40.26 Insect bite (nonvenomous) of shoulder
● S40.261 Insect bite (nonvenomous) of right shoulder
● S40.262 Insect bite (nonvenomous) of left shoulder
● S40.269 Insect bite (nonvenomous) of unspecified shoulder
● S40.27 Other superficial bite of shoulder
Excludes1 open bite of shoulder (S41.05)
● S40.271 Other superficial bite of right shoulder
● S40.272 Other superficial bite of left shoulder
● S40.279 Other superficial bite of unspecified shoulder
● S40.8 Other superficial injuries of upper arm
● S40.81 Abrasion of upper arm
● S40.811 Abrasion of right upper arm
● S40.812 Abrasion of left upper arm
● S40.819 Abrasion of unspecified upper arm
● S40.82 Blister (nonthermal) of upper arm
● S40.821 Blister (nonthermal) of right upper arm
● S40.822 Blister (nonthermal) of left upper arm
● S40.829 Blister (nonthermal) of unspecified upper arm
● S40.84 External constriction of upper arm
● S40.841 External constriction of right upper arm
● S40.842 External constriction of left upper arm
● S40.849 External constriction of unspecified upper arm

S40.85 Superficial foreign body of upper arm
Splinter in the upper arm
S40.851 Superficial foreign body of right upper arm
S40.852 Superficial foreign body of left upper arm
S40.859 Superficial foreign body of unspecified upper arm
S40.86 Insect bite (nonvenomous) of upper arm
S40.861 Insect bite (nonvenomous) of right upper arm
S40.862 Insect bite (nonvenomous) of left upper arm
S40.869 Insect bite (nonvenomous) of unspecified upper arm
S40.87 Other superficial bite of upper arm
Excludes1 open bite of upper arm (S41.14)
Excludes2 other superficial bite of shoulder (S40.27-)
S40.871 Other superficial bite of right upper arm
S40.872 Other superficial bite of left upper arm
S40.879 Other superficial bite of unspecified upper arm
S40.9 Unspecified superficial injury of shoulder and upper arm
S40.91 Unspecified superficial injury of shoulder
S40.911 Unspecified superficial injury of right shoulder
S40.912 Unspecified superficial injury of left shoulder
S40.919 Unspecified superficial injury of unspecified shoulder
S40.92 Unspecified superficial injury of upper arm
S40.921 Unspecified superficial injury of right upper arm
S40.922 Unspecified superficial injury of left upper arm
S40.929 Unspecified superficial injury of unspecified upper arm

S41 Open wound of shoulder and upper arm
Code also any associated wound infection
Excludes1 traumatic amputation of shoulder and upper arm (S48.-)
Excludes2 open fracture of shoulder and upper arm (S42.- with 7th character B or C)
The appropriate 7th character is to be added to each code from category S41

A	initial encounter
D	subsequent encounter
S	sequela

S41.0 Open wound of shoulder
S41.00 Unspecified open wound of shoulder
S41.001 Unspecified open wound of right shoulder
S41.002 Unspecified open wound of left shoulder
S41.009 Unspecified open wound of unspecified shoulder
S41.01 Laceration without foreign body of shoulder
S41.011 Laceration without foreign body of right shoulder
S41.012 Laceration without foreign body of left shoulder
S41.019 Laceration without foreign body of unspecified shoulder
S41.02 Laceration with foreign body of shoulder
S41.021 Laceration with foreign body of right shoulder
S41.022 Laceration with foreign body of left shoulder
S41.029 Laceration with foreign body of unspecified shoulder
S41.03 Puncture wound without foreign body of shoulder
S41.031 Puncture wound without foreign body of right shoulder
S41.032 Puncture wound without foreign body of left shoulder
S41.039 Puncture wound without foreign body of unspecified shoulder
S41.04 Puncture wound with foreign body of shoulder
S41.041 Puncture wound with foreign body of right shoulder
S41.042 Puncture wound with foreign body of left shoulder
S41.049 Puncture wound with foreign body of unspecified shoulder
S41.05 Open bite of shoulder
Bite of shoulder NOS
Excludes1 superficial bite of shoulder (S40.27)
S41.051 Open bite of right shoulder
S41.052 Open bite of left shoulder
S41.059 Open bite of unspecified shoulder
S41.1 Open wound of upper arm
S41.10 Unspecified open wound of upper arm
S41.101 Unspecified open wound of right upper arm
S41.102 Unspecified open wound of left upper arm
S41.109 Unspecified open wound of unspecified upper arm
S41.11 Laceration without foreign body of upper arm
S41.111 Laceration without foreign body of right upper arm
S41.112 Laceration without foreign body of left upper arm
S41.119 Laceration without foreign body of unspecified upper arm
S41.12 Laceration with foreign body of upper arm
S41.121 Laceration with foreign body of right upper arm
S41.122 Laceration with foreign body of left upper arm
S41.129 Laceration with foreign body of unspecified upper arm
S41.13 Puncture wound without foreign body of upper arm
S41.131 Puncture wound without foreign body of right upper arm
S41.132 Puncture wound without foreign body of left upper arm
S41.139 Puncture wound without foreign body of unspecified upper arm
S41.14 Puncture wound with foreign body of upper arm
S41.141 Puncture wound with foreign body of right upper arm
S41.142 Puncture wound with foreign body of left upper arm
S41.149 Puncture wound with foreign body of unspecified upper arm

S41.15 **Open bite of upper arm**
Bite of upper arm NOS
Excludes1 superficial bite of upper arm (S40.87)
S41.151 Open bite of right upper arm
S41.152 Open bite of left upper arm
S41.159 Open bite of unspecified upper arm

S42 **Fracture of shoulder and upper arm**
Note: A fracture not indicated as displaced or nondisplaced should be coded to displaced
A fracture not indicated as open or closed should be coded to closed
Excludes1 periprosthetic fracture around internal prosthetic shoulder joint (M97.3)
traumatic amputation of shoulder and upper arm (S48.-)
The appropriate 7th character is to be added to all codes from category S42

A	initial encounter for closed fracture
B	initial encounter for open fracture
D	subsequent encounter for fracture with routine healing
G	subsequent encounter for fracture with delayed healing
K	subsequent encounter for fracture with nonunion
P	subsequent encounter for fracture with malunion
S	sequela

S42.0 **Fracture of clavicle** Ex PDX 1264 [K, P], 1754 [B]
S42.00 Fracture of unspecified part of clavicle
S42.001 Fracture of unspecified part of right clavicle B, K, P, B
S42.002 Fracture of unspecified part of left clavicle B, K, P, B
S42.009 Fracture of unspecified part of unspecified clavicle B, K, P, B
Coding Clinic: 2012, Q4, P3
S42.01 Fracture of sternal end of clavicle
S42.011 Anterior displaced fracture of sternal end of right clavicle B, K, P, B
S42.012 Anterior displaced fracture of sternal end of left clavicle B, K, P, B
S42.013 Anterior displaced fracture of sternal end of unspecified clavicle B, K, P, B
Displaced fracture of sternal end of clavicle NOS
S42.014 Posterior displaced fracture of sternal end of right clavicle B, K, P, B
S42.015 Posterior displaced fracture of sternal end of left clavicle B, K, P, B
S42.016 Posterior displaced fracture of sternal end of unspecified clavicle B, K, P, B
S42.017 Nondisplaced fracture of sternal end of right clavicle B, K, P, B
S42.018 Nondisplaced fracture of sternal end of left clavicle B, K, P, B
S42.019 Nondisplaced fracture of sternal end of unspecified clavicle B, K, P, B
S42.02 Fracture of shaft of clavicle
S42.021 Displaced fracture of shaft of right clavicle B, K, P, B
S42.022 Displaced fracture of shaft of left clavicle B, K, P, B
S42.023 Displaced fracture of shaft of unspecified clavicle B, K, P, B
S42.024 Nondisplaced fracture of shaft of right clavicle B, K, P, B
S42.025 Nondisplaced fracture of shaft of left clavicle B, K, P, B
S42.026 Nondisplaced fracture of shaft of unspecified clavicle B, K, P, B
S42.03 Fracture of lateral end of clavicle
Fracture of acromial end of clavicle
S42.031 Displaced fracture of lateral end of right clavicle B, K, P, B
S42.032 Displaced fracture of lateral end of left clavicle B, K, P, B
S42.033 Displaced fracture of lateral end of unspecified clavicle B, K, P, B
S42.034 Nondisplaced fracture of lateral end of right clavicle B, K, P, B
S42.035 Nondisplaced fracture of lateral end of left clavicle B, K, P, B
S42.036 Nondisplaced fracture of lateral end of unspecified clavicle B, K, P, B

S42.1 **Fracture of scapula** Ex PDX 1264 [K, P], 1754 [B]
S42.10 Fracture of unspecified part of scapula
S42.101 Fracture of unspecified part of scapula, right shoulder B, K, P, B
S42.102 Fracture of unspecified part of scapula, left shoulder B, K, P, B
S42.109 Fracture of unspecified part of scapula, unspecified shoulder B, K, P, B
S42.11 Fracture of body of scapula
S42.111 Displaced fracture of body of scapula, right shoulder B, K, P, B
S42.112 Displaced fracture of body of scapula, left shoulder B, K, P, B
S42.113 Displaced fracture of body of scapula, unspecified shoulder B, K, P, B
S42.114 Nondisplaced fracture of body of scapula, right shoulder B, K, P, B
S42.115 Nondisplaced fracture of body of scapula, left shoulder B, K, P, B
S42.116 Nondisplaced fracture of body of scapula, unspecified shoulder B, K, P, B
S42.12 Fracture of acromial process
S42.121 Displaced fracture of acromial process, right shoulder B, K, P, B
S42.122 Displaced fracture of acromial process, left shoulder B, K, P, B
S42.123 Displaced fracture of acromial process, unspecified shoulder B, K, P, B
S42.124 Nondisplaced fracture of acromial process, right shoulder B, K, P, B
S42.125 Nondisplaced fracture of acromial process, left shoulder B, K, P, B
S42.126 Nondisplaced fracture, of acromial process, unspecified shoulder B, K, P, B
S42.13 Fracture of coracoid process
S42.131 Displaced fracture of coracoid process, right shoulder B, K, P, B
S42.132 Displaced fracture of coracoid process, left shoulder B, K, P, B
S42.133 Displaced fracture of coracoid process, unspecified shoulder B, K, P, B
S42.134 Nondisplaced fracture of coracoid process, right shoulder B, K, P, B

S42.135 Nondisplaced fracture of coracoid process, left shoulder B, K, P, B

S42.136 Nondisplaced fracture of coracoid process, unspecified shoulder B, K, P, B

S42.14 Fracture of glenoid cavity of scapula

S42.141 Displaced fracture of glenoid cavity of scapula, right shoulder B, K, P, B

S42.142 Displaced fracture of glenoid cavity of scapula, left shoulder B, K, P, B

S42.143 Displaced fracture of glenoid cavity of scapula, unspecified shoulder B, K, P, B

S42.144 Nondisplaced fracture of glenoid cavity of scapula, right shoulder B, K, P, B

S42.145 Nondisplaced fracture of glenoid cavity of scapula, left shoulder B, K, P, B

S42.146 Nondisplaced fracture of glenoid cavity of scapula, unspecified shoulder B, K, P, B

S42.15 Fracture of neck of scapula

S42.151 Displaced fracture of neck of scapula, right shoulder B, K, P, B

S42.152 Displaced fracture of neck of scapula, left shoulder B, K, P, B

S42.153 Displaced fracture of neck of scapula, unspecified shoulder B, K, P, B

S42.154 Nondisplaced fracture of neck of scapula, right shoulder B, K, P, B

S42.155 Nondisplaced fracture of neck of scapula, left shoulder B, K, P, B

S42.156 Nondisplaced fracture of neck of scapula, unspecified shoulder B, K, P, B

S42.19 Fracture of other part of scapula

S42.191 Fracture of other part of scapula, right shoulder B, K, P, B

S42.192 Fracture of other part of scapula, left shoulder B, K, P, B

S42.199 Fracture of other part of scapula, unspecified shoulder B, K, P, B

S42.2 Fracture of upper end of humerus

Fracture of proximal end of humerus

Excludes2 fracture of shaft of humerus (S42.3-)
physeal fracture of upper end of humerus (S49.0-)

S42.20 Unspecified fracture of upper end of humerus

S42.201 Unspecified fracture of upper end of right humerus A, K, P, B, A, B (Ex) PDX 1264 [K, P], 1755 [A], 1756 [B]

S42.202 Unspecified fracture of upper end of left humerus A, K, P, B, A, B (Ex) PDX 1264 [K, P], 1756 [B], 1757 [A]

S42.209 Unspecified fracture of upper end of unspecified humerus A, K, P, B, A, B (Ex) PDX 1264 [K, P], 1756 [B], 1758 [A]

S42.21 Unspecified fracture of surgical neck of humerus

Fracture of neck of humerus NOS

S42.211 Unspecified displaced fracture of surgical neck of right humerus A, K, P, B, A, B (Ex) PDX 1264 [K, P], 1755 [A], 1756 [B]

S42.212 Unspecified displaced fracture of surgical neck of left humerus A, K, P, B, A, B (Ex) PDX 1264 [K, P], 1756 [B], 1757 [A]

S42.213 Unspecified displaced fracture of surgical neck of unspecified humerus A, K, P, B, A, B (Ex) PDX 1264 [K, P], 1756 [B], 1758 [A]

S42.214 Unspecified nondisplaced fracture of surgical neck of right humerus A, K, P, B, A, B (Ex) PDX 1264 [K, P], 1755 [A], 1756 [B]

S42.215 Unspecified nondisplaced fracture of surgical neck of left humerus A, K, P, B, A, B (Ex) PDX 1264 [K, P], 1756 [B], 1757 [A]

S42.216 Unspecified nondisplaced fracture of surgical neck of unspecified humerus A, K, P, B, A, B (Ex) PDX 1264 [K, P], 1756 [B], 1758 [A]

S42.22 2-part fracture of surgical neck of humerus

S42.221 2-part displaced fracture of surgical neck of right humerus A, K, P, B, A, B (Ex) PDX 1264 [K, P], 1755 [A], 1756 [B]

S42.222 2-part displaced fracture of surgical neck of left humerus A, K, P, B, A, B (Ex) PDX 1264 [K, P], 1756 [B], 1757 [A]

S42.223 2-part displaced fracture of surgical neck of unspecified humerus A, K, P, B, A, B (Ex) PDX 1264 [K, P], 1756 [B], 1758 [A]

S42.224 2-part nondisplaced fracture of surgical neck of right humerus A, K, P, B, A, B (Ex) PDX 1264 [K, P], 1755 [A], 1756 [B]

S42.225 2-part nondisplaced fracture of surgical neck of left humerus A, K, P, B, A, B (Ex) PDX 1264 [K, P], 1756 [B], 1757 [A]

S42.226 2-part nondisplaced fracture of surgical neck of unspecified humerus A, K, P, B, A, B (Ex) PDX 1264 [K, P], 1756 [B], 1758 [A]

S42.23 3-part fracture of surgical neck of humerus

S42.231 3-part fracture of surgical neck of right humerus A, K, P, B, A, B (Ex) PDX 1264 [K, P], 1755 [A], 1756 [B]

S42.232 3-part fracture of surgical neck of left humerus A, K, P, B, A, B (Ex) PDX 1264 [K, P], 1756 [B], 1757 [A]

S42.239 3-part fracture of surgical neck of unspecified humerus A, K, P, B, A, B (Ex) PDX 1264 [K, P], 1756 [B], 1758 [A]

S42.24 4-part fracture of surgical neck of humerus

S42.241 4-part fracture of surgical neck of right humerus A, K, P, B, A, B (Ex) PDX 1264 [K, P], 1755 [A], 1756 [B]

S42.242 4-part fracture of surgical neck of left humerus A, K, P, B, A, B (Ex) PDX 1264 [K, P], 1756 [B], 1757 [A]

S42.249 4-part fracture of surgical neck of unspecified humerus A, K, P, B, A, B (Ex) PDX 1264 [K, P], 1756 [B], 1758 [A]

S42.25 Fracture of greater tuberosity of humerus

S42.251 Displaced fracture of greater tuberosity of right humerus A, K, P, B, A, B (Ex) PDX 1264 [K, P], 1755 [A], 1756 [B]

S42.252 Displaced fracture of greater tuberosity of left humerus A, K, P, B, A, B (Ex) PDX 1264 [K, P], 1756 [B], 1757 [A]

S42.253 Displaced fracture of greater tuberosity of unspecified humerus A, K, P, B, A, B (Ex) PDX 1264 [K, P], 1756 [B], 1758 [A]

S42.254 Nondisplaced fracture of greater tuberosity of right humerus A, K, P, B, A, B (Ex) PDX 1264 [K, P], 1755 [A], 1756 [B]

S42.255 **Nondisplaced fracture of greater tuberosity of left humerus** A, K, P, B, A, B (Ex) PDX 1264 [K, P], 1756 [B], 1757 [A]

S42.256 **Nondisplaced fracture of greater tuberosity of unspecified humerus** A, K, P, B, A, B (Ex) PDX 1264 [K, P], 1756 [B], 1758 [A]

S42.26 **Fracture of lesser tuberosity of humerus**

S42.261 **Displaced fracture of lesser tuberosity of right humerus** A, K, P, B, A, B (Ex) PDX 1264 [K, P], 1755 [A], 1756 [B]

S42.262 **Displaced fracture of lesser tuberosity of left humerus** A, K, P, B, A, B (Ex) PDX 1264 [K, P], 1756 [B], 1757 [A]

S42.263 **Displaced fracture of lesser tuberosity of unspecified humerus** A, K, P, B, A, B (Ex) PDX 1264 [K, P], 1756 [B], 1758 [A]

S42.264 **Nondisplaced fracture of lesser tuberosity of right humerus** A, K, P, B, A, B (Ex) PDX 1264 [K, P], 1755 [A], 1756 [B]

S42.265 **Nondisplaced fracture of lesser tuberosity of left humerus** A, K, P, B, A, B (Ex) PDX 1264 [K, P], 1756 [B], 1757 [A]

S42.266 **Nondisplaced fracture of lesser tuberosity of unspecified humerus** A, K, P, B, A, B (Ex) PDX 1264 [K, P], 1756 [B], 1758 [A]

S42.27 **Torus fracture of upper end of humerus**

The appropriate 7th character is to be added to all codes in subcategory S42.27

A	initial encounter for closed fracture
D	subsequent encounter for fracture with routine healing
G	subsequent encounter for fracture with delayed healing
K	subsequent encounter for fracture with nonunion
P	subsequent encounter for fracture with malunion
S	sequela

S42.271 **Torus fracture of upper end of right humerus** A, K, P, A (Ex) PDX 1264 [K, P], 1755 [A], 1756 [B]

S42.272 **Torus fracture of upper end of left humerus** A, K, P, A (Ex) PDX 1264 [K, P], 1756 [B], 1757 [A]

S42.279 **Torus fracture of upper end of unspecified humerus** A, K, P, A (Ex) PDX 1264 [K, P], 1756 [B], 1758 [A]

S42.29 **Other fracture of upper end of humerus**

Fracture of anatomical neck of humerus
Fracture of articular head of humerus

S42.291 **Other displaced fracture of upper end of right humerus** A, K, P, B, A, B (Ex) PDX 1264 [K, P], 1755 [A], 1756 [B]

S42.292 **Other displaced fracture of upper end of left humerus** A, K, P, B, A, B (Ex) PDX 1264 [K, P], 1756 [B], 1757 [A]

Coding Clinic: 2024, Q2, P24

S42.293 **Other displaced fracture of upper end of unspecified humerus** A, K, P, B, A, B (Ex) PDX 1264 [K, P], 1756 [B], 1758 [A]

S42.294 **Other nondisplaced fracture of upper end of right humerus** A, K, P, B, A, B (Ex) PDX 1264 [K, P], 1755 [A], 1756 [B]

S42.295 **Other nondisplaced fracture of upper end of left humerus** A, K, P, B, A, B (Ex) PDX 1264 [K, P], 1756 [B], 1757 [A]

Coding Clinic: 2019, Q1, P19

S42.296 **Other nondisplaced fracture of upper end of unspecified humerus** A, K, P, B, A, B (Ex) PDX 1264 [K, P], 1756 [B], 1758 [A]

S42.3 **Fracture of shaft of humerus**

Fracture of humerus NOS
Fracture of upper arm NOS

Excludes2 physeal fractures of upper end of humerus (S49.0-)
physeal fractures of lower end of humerus (S49.1-)

S42.30 **Unspecified fracture of shaft of humerus**

S42.301 **Unspecified fracture of shaft of humerus, right arm** A, K, P, B, A, B (Ex) PDX 1264 [K, P], 1755 [A], 1756 [B]

S42.302 **Unspecified fracture of shaft of humerus, left arm** A, K, P, B, A, B (Ex) PDX 1264 [K, P], 1756 [B], 1757 [A]

S42.309 **Unspecified fracture of shaft of humerus, unspecified arm** A, K, P, B, A, B (Ex) PDX 1264 [K, P], 1756 [B], 1758 [A]

S42.31 **Greenstick fracture of shaft of humerus**

The appropriate 7th character is to be added to all codes in subcategory S42.3

A	initial encounter for closed fracture
D	subsequent encounter for fracture with routine healing
G	subsequent encounter for fracture with delayed healing
K	subsequent encounter for fracture with nonunion
P	subsequent encounter for fracture with malunion
S	sequela

S42.311 **Greenstick fracture of shaft of humerus, right arm** A, K, P, A (Ex) PDX 1264 [K, P], 1759 [A]

S42.312 **Greenstick fracture of shaft of humerus, left arm** A, K, P, A (Ex) PDX 1264 [K, P], 1760 [A]

S42.319 **Greenstick fracture of shaft of humerus, unspecified arm** A, K, P, A (Ex) PDX 1264 [K, P], 1761 [A]

S42.32 **Transverse fracture of shaft of humerus**

S42.321 **Displaced transverse fracture of shaft of humerus, right arm** A, K, P, B, A, B (Ex) PDX 1264 [K, P], 1756 [B], 1759 [A]

S42.322 **Displaced transverse fracture of shaft of humerus, left arm** A, K, P, B, A, B (Ex) PDX 1264 [K, P], 1756 [B], 1760 [A]

S42.323 **Displaced transverse fracture of shaft of humerus, unspecified arm** A, K, P, B, A, B (Ex) PDX 1264 [K, P], 1756 [B], 1761 [A]

S42.324 **Nondisplaced transverse fracture of shaft of humerus, right arm** A, K, P, B, A, B (Ex) PDX 1264 [K, P], 1756 [B], 1759 [A]

S42.325 **Nondisplaced transverse fracture of shaft of humerus, left arm** A, K, P, B, A, B (Ex) PDX 1264 [K, P], 1756 [B], 1760 [A]

S42.326 **Nondisplaced transverse fracture of shaft of humerus, unspecified arm** A, K, P, B, A, B (Ex) PDX 1264 [K, P], 1756 [B], 1761 [A]

- **S42.33 Oblique fracture of shaft of humerus**
  - **S42.331** Displaced oblique fracture of shaft of humerus, right arm A, K, P, B, A, B (Ex) PDX 1264 [K, P], 1756 [B], 1759 [A]
  - **S42.332** Displaced oblique fracture of shaft of humerus, left arm A, K, P, B, A, B (Ex) PDX 1264 [K, P], 1756 [B], 1760 [A]
  - **S42.333** Displaced oblique fracture of shaft of humerus, unspecified arm A, K, P, B, A, B (Ex) PDX 1264 [K, P], 1756 [B], 1761 [A]
  - **S42.334** Nondisplaced oblique fracture of shaft of humerus, right arm A, K, P, B, A, B (Ex) PDX 1264 [K, P], 1756 [B], 1759 [A]
  - **S42.335** Nondisplaced oblique fracture of shaft of humerus, left arm A, K, P, B, A, B (Ex) PDX 1264 [K, P], 1756 [B], 1760 [A]
  - **S42.336** Nondisplaced oblique fracture of shaft of humerus, unspecified arm A, K, P, B, A, B (Ex) PDX 1264 [K, P], 1756 [B], 1761 [A]
- **S42.34 Spiral fracture of shaft of humerus**
  - **S42.341** Displaced spiral fracture of shaft of humerus, right arm A, K, P, B, A, B (Ex) PDX 1264 [K, P], 1756 [B], 1759 [A]
  - **S42.342** Displaced spiral fracture of shaft of humerus, left arm A, K, P, B, A, B (Ex) PDX 1264 [K, P], 1756 [B], 1760 [A]
  - **S42.343** Displaced spiral fracture of shaft of humerus, unspecified arm A, K, P, B, A, B (Ex) PDX 1264 [K, P], 1756 [B], 1761 [A]
  - **S42.344** Nondisplaced spiral fracture of shaft of humerus, right arm A, K, P, B, A, B (Ex) PDX 1264 [K, P], 1756 [B], 1759 [A]
  - **S42.345** Nondisplaced spiral fracture of shaft of humerus, left arm A, K, P, B, A, B (Ex) PDX 1264 [K, P], 1756 [B], 1760 [A]
  - **S42.346** Nondisplaced spiral fracture of shaft of humerus, unspecified arm A, K, P, B, A, B (Ex) PDX 1264 [K, P], 1756 [B], 1761 [A]
- **S42.35 Comminuted fracture of shaft of humerus**
  - **S42.351** Displaced comminuted fracture of shaft of humerus, right arm A, K, P, B, A, B (Ex) PDX 1264 [K, P], 1756 [B], 1759 [A]
  - **S42.352** Displaced comminuted fracture of shaft of humerus, left arm A, K, P, B, A, B (Ex) PDX 1264 [K, P], 1756 [B], 1760 [A]
  - **S42.353** Displaced comminuted fracture of shaft of humerus, unspecified arm A, K, P, B, A, B (Ex) PDX 1264 [K, P], 1756 [B], 1761 [A]
  - **S42.354** Nondisplaced comminuted fracture of shaft of humerus, right arm A, K, P, B, A, B (Ex) PDX 1264 [K, P], 1756 [B], 1759 [A]
  - **S42.355** Nondisplaced comminuted fracture of shaft of humerus, left arm A, K, P, B, A, B (Ex) PDX 1264 [K, P], 1756 [B], 1760 [A]
  - **S42.356** Nondisplaced comminuted fracture of shaft of humerus, unspecified arm A, K, P, B, A, B (Ex) PDX 1264 [K, P], 1756 [B], 1761 [A]
- **S42.36 Segmental fracture of shaft of humerus**
  - **S42.361** Displaced segmental fracture of shaft of humerus, right arm A, K, P, B, A, B (Ex) PDX 1264 [K, P], 1756 [B], 1759 [A]
  - **S42.362** Displaced segmental fracture of shaft of humerus, left arm A, K, P, B, A, B (Ex) PDX 1264 [K, P], 1756 [B], 1760 [A]
  - **S42.363** Displaced segmental fracture of shaft of humerus, unspecified arm A, K, P, B, A, B (Ex) PDX 1264 [K, P], 1756 [B], 1761 [A]
  - **S42.364** Nondisplaced segmental fracture of shaft of humerus, right arm A, K, P, B, A, B (Ex) PDX 1264 [K, P], 1756 [B], 1759 [A]
  - **S42.365** Nondisplaced segmental fracture of shaft of humerus, left arm A, K, P, B, A, B (Ex) PDX 1264 [K, P], 1756 [B], 1760 [A]
  - **S42.366** Nondisplaced segmental fracture of shaft of humerus, unspecified arm A, K, P, B, A, B (Ex) PDX 1264 [K, P], 1756 [B], 1761 [A]
- **S42.39 Other fracture of shaft of humerus**
  - **S42.391** Other fracture of shaft of right humerus A, K, P, B, A, B (Ex) PDX 1264 [K, P], 1756 [B], 1759 [A]
  - **S42.392** Other fracture of shaft of left humerus A, K, P, B, A, B (Ex) PDX 1264 [K, P], 1756 [B], 1760 [A]
  - **S42.399** Other fracture of shaft of unspecified humerus A, K, P, B, A, B (Ex) PDX 1264 [K, P], 1756 [B], 1761 [A]

S42.4 Fracture of lower end of humerus
Fracture of distal end of humerus

Excludes2 fracture of shaft of humerus (S42.3-)
physeal fracture of lower end of humerus (S49.1-)

- **S42.40 Unspecified fracture of lower end of humerus**
  Fracture of elbow NOS
  - **S42.401** Unspecified fracture of lower end of right humerus A, K, P, B, A, B (Ex) PDX 1264 [K], 1264 [P], 1755 [A], 1756 [B]
  - **S42.402** Unspecified fracture of lower end of left humerus A, K, P, B, A, B (Ex) PDX 1264 [K], 1264 [P], 1756 [B], 1757 [A]
  - **S42.409** Unspecified fracture of lower end of unspecified humerus A, K, P, B, A, B (Ex) PDX 1264 [K], 1264 [P], 1756 [B], 1758 [A]
- **S42.41 Simple supracondylar fracture without intercondylar fracture of humerus**
  - **S42.411** Displaced simple supracondylar fracture without intercondylar fracture of right humerus A, K, P, B, A, B (Ex) PDX 1264 [K], 1264 [P], 1755 [A], 1756 [B]
  - **S42.412** Displaced simple supracondylar fracture without intercondylar fracture of left humerus A, K, P, B, A, B (Ex) PDX 1264 [K], 1264 [P], 1756 [B], 1757 [A]
  - **S42.413** Displaced simple supracondylar fracture without intercondylar fracture of unspecified humerus A, K, P, B, A, B (Ex) PDX 1264 [K], 1264 [P], 1756 [B], 1758 [A]
  - **S42.414** Nondisplaced simple supracondylar fracture without intercondylar fracture of right humerus A, K, P, B, A, B (Ex) PDX 1264 [K], 1264 [P], 1755 [A], 1756 [B]
  - **S42.415** Nondisplaced simple supracondylar fracture without intercondylar fracture of left humerus A, K, P, B, A, B (Ex) PDX 1264 [K], 1264 [P], 1756 [B], 1757 [A]

CHAPTER 19 (S00-T88)

- S42.416 Nondisplaced simple supracondylar fracture without intercondylar fracture of unspecified humerus A, K, P, B, A, B (Ex) PDX 1264 [K], 1264 [P], 1756 [B], 1758 [A]
- S42.42 Comminuted supracondylar fracture without intercondylar fracture of humerus
  - S42.421 Displaced comminuted supracondylar fracture without intercondylar fracture of right humerus A, K, P, B, A, B (Ex) PDX 1264 [K], 1264 [P], 1755 [A], 1756 [B]
  - S42.422 Displaced comminuted supracondylar fracture without intercondylar fracture of left humerus A, K, P, B, A, B (Ex) PDX 1264 [K], 1264 [P], 1756 [B], 1757 [A]
  - S42.423 Displaced comminuted supracondylar fracture without intercondylar fracture of unspecified humerus A, K, P, B, A, B (Ex) PDX 1264 [K, P], 1756 [B], 1248 [A]
  - S42.424 Nondisplaced comminuted supracondylar fracture without intercondylar fracture of right humerus A, K, P, B, A, B (Ex) PDX 1264 [K, P], 1755 [A], 1756 [B]
  - S42.425 Nondisplaced comminuted supracondylar fracture without intercondylar fracture of left humerus A, K, P, B, A, B (Ex) PDX 1264 [K, P], 1756 [B], 1757 [A]
  - S42.426 Nondisplaced comminuted supracondylar fracture without intercondylar fracture of unspecified humerus A, K, P, B, A, B (Ex) PDX 1264 [K, P], 1756 [B], 1758 [A]
- S42.43 Fracture (avulsion) of lateral epicondyle of humerus
  - S42.431 Displaced fracture (avulsion) of lateral epicondyle of right humerus A, K, P, B, A, B (Ex) PDX 1264 [K, P], 1755 [A], 1756 [B]
  - S42.432 Displaced fracture (avulsion) of lateral epicondyle of left humerus A, K, P, B, A, B (Ex) PDX 1264 [K, P], 1756 [B], 1757 [A]
  - S42.433 Displaced fracture (avulsion) of lateral epicondyle of unspecified humerus A, K, P, B, A, B (Ex) PDX 1264 [K, P], 1756 [B], 1758 [A]
  - S42.434 Nondisplaced fracture (avulsion) of lateral epicondyle of right humerus A, K, P, B, A, B (Ex) PDX 1264 [K, P], 1755 [A], 1756 [B]
  - S42.435 Nondisplaced fracture (avulsion) of lateral epicondyle of left humerus A, K, P, B, A, B (Ex) PDX 1264 [K, P], 1756 [B], 1757 [A]
  - S42.436 Nondisplaced fracture (avulsion) of lateral epicondyle of unspecified humerus A, K, P, B, A, B (Ex) PDX 1264 [K, P], 1756 [B], 1758 [A]
- S42.44 Fracture (avulsion) of medial epicondyle of humerus
  - S42.441 Displaced fracture (avulsion) of medial epicondyle of right humerus A, K, P, B, A, B (Ex) PDX 1264 [K, P], 1755 [A], 1756 [B]
  - S42.442 Displaced fracture (avulsion) of medial epicondyle of left humerus A, K, P, B, A, B (Ex) PDX 1264 [K, P], 1756 [B], 1757 [A]
  - S42.443 Displaced fracture (avulsion) of medial epicondyle of unspecified humerus A, K, P, B, A, B (Ex) PDX 1264 [K, P], 1756 [B], 1758 [A]
  - S42.444 Nondisplaced fracture (avulsion) of medial epicondyle of right humerus A, K, P, B, A, B (Ex) PDX 1264 [K, P], 1755 [A], 1756 [B]
  - S42.445 Nondisplaced fracture (avulsion) of medial epicondyle of left humerus A, K, P, B, A, B (Ex) PDX 1264 [K, P], 1756 [B], 1757 [A]
  - S42.446 Nondisplaced fracture (avulsion) of medial epicondyle of unspecified humerus A, K, P, B, A, B (Ex) PDX 1264 [K, P], 1756 [B], 1758 [A]
  - S42.447 Incarcerated fracture (avulsion) of medial epicondyle of right humerus A, K, P, B, A, B (Ex) PDX 1264 [K, P], 1755 [A], 1756 [B]
  - S42.448 Incarcerated fracture (avulsion) of medial epicondyle of left humerus A, K, P, B, A, B (Ex) PDX 1264 [K, P], 1756 [B], 1757 [A]
  - S42.449 Incarcerated fracture (avulsion) of medial epicondyle of unspecified humerus A, K, P, B, A, B (Ex) PDX 1264 [K, P], 1756 [B], 1758 [A]
- S42.45 Fracture of lateral condyle of humerus
  Fracture of capitellum of humerus
  - S42.451 Displaced fracture of lateral condyle of right humerus A, K, P, B, A, B (Ex) PDX 1264 [K, P], 1755 [A], 1756 [B]
  - S42.452 Displaced fracture of lateral condyle of left humerus A, K, P, B, A, B (Ex) PDX 1264 [K, P], 1756 [B], 1757 [A]
  - S42.453 Displaced fracture of lateral condyle of unspecified humerus A, K, P, B, A, B (Ex) PDX 1264 [K, P], 1756 [B], 1758 [A]
  - S42.454 Nondisplaced fracture of lateral condyle of right humerus A, K, P, B, A, B (Ex) PDX 1264 [K, P], 1755 [A], 1756 [B]
  - S42.455 Nondisplaced fracture of lateral condyle of left humerus A, K, P, B, A, B (Ex) PDX 1264 [K, P], 1756 [B], 1757 [A]
  - S42.456 Nondisplaced fracture of lateral condyle of unspecified humerus A, K, P, B, A, B (Ex) PDX 1264 [K, P], 1756 [B], 1758 [A]
- S42.46 Fracture of medial condyle of humerus
  Trochlea fracture of humerus
  - S42.461 Displaced fracture of medial condyle of right humerus A, K, P, B, A, B (Ex) PDX 1264 [K, P], 1755 [A], 1756 [B]
  - S42.462 Displaced fracture of medial condyle of left humerus A, K, P, B, A, B (Ex) PDX 1264 [K, P], 1756 [B], 1757 [A]
  - S42.463 Displaced fracture of medial condyle of unspecified humerus A, K, P, B, A, B (Ex) PDX 1264 [K, P], 1756 [B], 1758 [A]
  - S42.464 Nondisplaced fracture of medial condyle of right humerus A, K, P, B, A, B (Ex) PDX 1264 [K, P], 1755 [A], 1756 [B]
  - S42.465 Nondisplaced fracture of medial condyle of left humerus A, K, P, B, A, B (Ex) PDX 1264 [K, P], 1756 [B], 1757 [A]

● S42.466 **Nondisplaced fracture of medial condyle of unspecified humerus** A, K, P, B, A, B (Ex) PDX 1264 [K, P], 1756 [B], 1758 [A]

● **S42.47 Transcondylar fracture of humerus**

● S42.471 **Displaced transcondylar fracture of right humerus** A, K, P, B, A, B (Ex) PDX 1264 [K, P], 1755 [A], 1756 [B]

● S42.472 **Displaced transcondylar fracture of left humerus** A, K, P, B, A, B (Ex) PDX 1264 [K, P], 1756 [B], 1757 [A]

● S42.473 **Displaced transcondylar fracture of unspecified humerus** A, K, P, B, A, B (Ex) PDX 1264 [K, P], 1756 [B], 1758 [A]

● S42.474 **Nondisplaced transcondylar fracture of right humerus** A, K, P, B, A, B (Ex) PDX 1264 [K, P], 1755 [A], 1756 [B]

● S42.475 **Nondisplaced transcondylar fracture of left humerus** A, K, P, B, A, B (Ex) PDX 1264 [K, P], 1756 [B], 1757 [A]

● S42.476 **Nondisplaced transcondylar fracture of unspecified humerus** A, K, P, B, A, B (Ex) PDX 1264 [K, P], 1756 [B], 1758 [A]

● **S42.48 Torus fracture of lower end of humerus**

The appropriate 7th character is to be added to all codes in subcategory S42.48

A	initial encounter for closed fracture
D	subsequent encounter for fracture with routine healing
G	subsequent encounter for fracture with delayed healing
K	subsequent encounter for fracture with nonunion
P	subsequent encounter for fracture with malunion
S	sequela

● S42.481 **Torus fracture of lower end of right humerus** A, K, P, A (Ex) PDX 1264 [K, P], 1755 [A]

● S42.482 **Torus fracture of lower end of left humerus** A, K, P, A (Ex) PDX 1264 [K, P], 1756 [B], 1757 [A]

● S42.489 **Torus fracture of lower end of unspecified humerus** A, K, P, A (Ex) PDX 1264 [K, P], 1756 [B], 1758 [A]

● **S42.49 Other fracture of lower end of humerus**

● S42.491 **Other displaced fracture of lower end of right humerus** A, K, P, B, A, B (Ex) PDX 1264 [K, P], 1756 [B], 1757 [A]

● S42.492 **Other displaced fracture of lower end of left humerus** A, K, P, B, A, B (Ex) PDX 1264 [K, P], 1756 [B], 1758 [A]

● S42.493 **Other displaced fracture of lower end of unspecified humerus** A, K, P, B, A, B (Ex) PDX 1264 [K, P], 1755 [A], 1756 [B]

● S42.494 **Other nondisplaced fracture of lower end of right humerus** A, K, P, B, A, B (Ex) PDX 1264 [K, P], 1756 [B], 1757 [A]

● S42.495 **Other nondisplaced fracture of lower end of left humerus** A, K, P, B, A, B (Ex) PDX 1264 [K, P], 1756 [B], 1758 [A]

● S42.496 **Other nondisplaced fracture of lower end of unspecified humerus** A, K, P, B, A, B (Ex) PDX 1264 [K, P], 1755 [A], 1756 [B]

● **S42.9 Fracture of shoulder girdle, part unspecified** (Ex) PDX 1264 [K, P], 1756 [B], 1758 [A]

Fracture of shoulder NOS

X● S42.90 **Fracture of unspecified shoulder girdle, part unspecified** A, K, P, B, A, B

X● S42.91 **Fracture of right shoulder girdle, part unspecified** A, K, P, B, A, B

X● S42.92 **Fracture of left shoulder girdle, part unspecified** A, K, P, B, A, B

● **S43 Dislocation and sprain of joints and ligaments of shoulder girdle**

Includes avulsion of joint or ligament of shoulder girdle
laceration of cartilage, joint or ligament of shoulder girdle
sprain of cartilage, joint or ligament of shoulder girdle
traumatic hemarthrosis of joint or ligament of shoulder girdle
traumatic rupture of joint or ligament of shoulder girdle
traumatic subluxation of joint or ligament of shoulder girdle
traumatic tear of joint or ligament of shoulder girdle

Code also any associated open wound

Excludes2 strain of muscle, fascia and tendon of shoulder and upper arm (S46.-)

The appropriate 7th character is to be added to each code from category S43

A	initial encounter
D	subsequent encounter
S	sequela

● **S43.0 Subluxation and dislocation of shoulder joint**

Dislocation of glenohumeral joint
Subluxation of glenohumeral joint

● S43.00 **Unspecified subluxation and dislocation of shoulder joint**

Dislocation of humerus NOS
Subluxation of humerus NOS

● S43.001 **Unspecified subluxation of right shoulder joint**

● S43.002 **Unspecified subluxation of left shoulder joint**

● S43.003 **Unspecified subluxation of unspecified shoulder joint**

● S43.004 **Unspecified dislocation of right shoulder joint**

● S43.005 **Unspecified dislocation of left shoulder joint**

● S43.006 **Unspecified dislocation of unspecified shoulder joint**

● S43.01 **Anterior subluxation and dislocation of humerus**

● S43.011 **Anterior subluxation of right humerus**

● S43.012 **Anterior subluxation of left humerus**

● S43.013 **Anterior subluxation of unspecified humerus**

● S43.014 **Anterior dislocation of right humerus**

● S43.015 **Anterior dislocation of left humerus**

● S43.016 **Anterior dislocation of unspecified humerus**

● S43.02 **Posterior subluxation and dislocation of humerus**

● S43.021 **Posterior subluxation of right humerus**

● S43.022 **Posterior subluxation of left humerus**

● S43.023 **Posterior subluxation of unspecified humerus**

● S43.024 **Posterior dislocation of right humerus**

● S43.025 **Posterior dislocation of left humerus**

● S43.026 **Posterior dislocation of unspecified humerus**

- S43.03 Inferior subluxation and dislocation of humerus
  - S43.031 Inferior subluxation of right humerus
  - S43.032 Inferior subluxation of left humerus
  - S43.033 Inferior subluxation of unspecified humerus
  - S43.034 Inferior dislocation of right humerus
  - S43.035 Inferior dislocation of left humerus
  - S43.036 Inferior dislocation of unspecified humerus
- S43.08 Other subluxation and dislocation of shoulder joint
  - S43.081 Other subluxation of right shoulder joint
  - S43.082 Other subluxation of left shoulder joint
  - S43.083 Other subluxation of unspecified shoulder joint
  - S43.084 Other dislocation of right shoulder joint
  - S43.085 Other dislocation of left shoulder joint
  - S43.086 Other dislocation of unspecified shoulder joint

S43.1 Subluxation and dislocation of acromioclavicular joint

- S43.10 Unspecified dislocation of acromioclavicular joint
  - S43.101 Unspecified dislocation of right acromioclavicular joint
  - S43.102 Unspecified dislocation of left acromioclavicular joint
  - S43.109 Unspecified dislocation of unspecified acromioclavicular joint
- S43.11 Subluxation of acromioclavicular joint
  - S43.111 Subluxation of right acromioclavicular joint
  - S43.112 Subluxation of left acromioclavicular joint
  - S43.119 Subluxation of unspecified acromioclavicular joint
- S43.12 Dislocation of acromioclavicular joint, 100%-200% displacement
  - S43.121 Dislocation of right acromioclavicular joint, 100%-200% displacement
  - S43.122 Dislocation of left acromioclavicular joint, 100%-200% displacement
  - S43.129 Dislocation of unspecified acromioclavicular joint, 100%-200% displacement
- S43.13 Dislocation of acromioclavicular joint, greater than 200% displacement
  - S43.131 Dislocation of right acromioclavicular joint, greater than 200% displacement
  - S43.132 Dislocation of left acromioclavicular joint, greater than 200% displacement
  - S43.139 Dislocation of unspecified acromioclavicular joint, greater than 200% displacement
- S43.14 Inferior dislocation of acromioclavicular joint
  - S43.141 Inferior dislocation of right acromioclavicular joint
  - S43.142 Inferior dislocation of left acromioclavicular joint
  - S43.149 Inferior dislocation of unspecified acromioclavicular joint
- S43.15 Posterior dislocation of acromioclavicular joint
  - S43.151 Posterior dislocation of right acromioclavicular joint
  - S43.152 Posterior dislocation of left acromioclavicular joint
  - S43.159 Posterior dislocation of unspecified acromioclavicular joint

S43.2 Subluxation and dislocation of sternoclavicular joint

- S43.20 Unspecified subluxation and dislocation of sternoclavicular joint
  - S43.201 Unspecified subluxation of right sternoclavicular joint A, A Ex PDX 1762
  - S43.202 Unspecified subluxation of left sternoclavicular joint A, A Ex PDX 1763
  - S43.203 Unspecified subluxation of unspecified sternoclavicular joint A, A Ex PDX 1354
  - S43.204 Unspecified dislocation of right sternoclavicular joint A, A Ex PDX 1762
  - S43.205 Unspecified dislocation of left sternoclavicular joint A, A Ex PDX 1763
  - S43.206 Unspecified dislocation of unspecified sternoclavicular joint A, A Ex PDX 1354
- S43.21 Anterior subluxation and dislocation of sternoclavicular joint
  - S43.211 Anterior subluxation of right sternoclavicular joint A, A Ex PDX 1762
  - S43.212 Anterior subluxation of left sternoclavicular joint A, A Ex PDX 1763
  - S43.213 Anterior subluxation of unspecified sternoclavicular joint A, A Ex PDX 1354
  - S43.214 Anterior dislocation of right sternoclavicular joint A, A Ex PDX 1762
  - S43.215 Anterior dislocation of left sternoclavicular joint A, A Ex PDX 1763
  - S43.216 Anterior dislocation of unspecified sternoclavicular joint A, A Ex PDX 1354
- S43.22 Posterior subluxation and dislocation of sternoclavicular joint
  - S43.221 Posterior subluxation of right sternoclavicular joint A, A Ex PDX 1762
  - S43.222 Posterior subluxation of left sternoclavicular joint A, A Ex PDX 1763
  - S43.223 Posterior subluxation of unspecified sternoclavicular joint A, A Ex PDX 1354
  - S43.224 Posterior dislocation of right sternoclavicular joint A, A Ex PDX 1762
  - S43.225 Posterior dislocation of left sternoclavicular joint A, A Ex PDX 1763
  - S43.226 Posterior dislocation of unspecified sternoclavicular joint A, A Ex PDX 1354

S43.3 Subluxation and dislocation of other and unspecified parts of shoulder girdle

- S43.30 Subluxation and dislocation of unspecified parts of shoulder girdle
  Dislocation of shoulder girdle NOS
  Subluxation of shoulder girdle NOS
  - S43.301 Subluxation of unspecified parts of right shoulder girdle
  - S43.302 Subluxation of unspecified parts of left shoulder girdle
  - S43.303 Subluxation of unspecified parts of unspecified shoulder girdle
  - S43.304 Dislocation of unspecified parts of right shoulder girdle

S43.305 **Dislocation of unspecified parts of left shoulder girdle**
S43.306 **Dislocation of unspecified parts of unspecified shoulder girdle**
S43.31 **Subluxation and dislocation of scapula**
S43.311 **Subluxation of right scapula**
S43.312 **Subluxation of left scapula**
S43.313 **Subluxation of unspecified scapula**
S43.314 **Dislocation of right scapula**
S43.315 **Dislocation of left scapula**
S43.316 **Dislocation of unspecified scapula**
S43.39 **Subluxation and dislocation of other parts of shoulder girdle**
S43.391 **Subluxation of other parts of right shoulder girdle**
S43.392 **Subluxation of other parts of left shoulder girdle**
S43.393 **Subluxation of other parts of unspecified shoulder girdle**
S43.394 **Dislocation of other parts of right shoulder girdle**
S43.395 **Dislocation of other parts of left shoulder girdle**
S43.396 **Dislocation of other parts of unspecified shoulder girdle**
S43.4 **Sprain of shoulder joint**
S43.40 **Unspecified sprain of shoulder joint**
S43.401 **Unspecified sprain of right shoulder joint**
S43.402 **Unspecified sprain of left shoulder joint**
S43.409 **Unspecified sprain of unspecified shoulder joint**
S43.41 **Sprain of coracohumeral (ligament)**
S43.411 **Sprain of right coracohumeral (ligament)**
S43.412 **Sprain of left coracohumeral (ligament)**
S43.419 **Sprain of unspecified coracohumeral (ligament)**
S43.42 **Sprain of rotator cuff capsule**
Encounters during the healing phase
Excludes1 rotator cuff syndrome (complete) (incomplete), not specified as traumatic (M75.1-)
Excludes2 injury of tendon of rotator cuff (S46.0-)
S43.421 **Sprain of right rotator cuff capsule**
S43.422 **Sprain of left rotator cuff capsule**
S43.429 **Sprain of unspecified rotator cuff capsule**
S43.43 **Superior glenoid labrum lesion**
SLAP lesion
Coding Clinic: 2019, Q2, P27
S43.431 **Superior glenoid labrum lesion of right shoulder**
S43.432 **Superior glenoid labrum lesion of left shoulder**
Coding Clinic: 2024, Q2, P24
S43.439 **Superior glenoid labrum lesion of unspecified shoulder**
S43.49 **Other sprain of shoulder joint**
S43.491 **Other sprain of right shoulder joint**
S43.492 **Other sprain of left shoulder joint**
S43.499 **Other sprain of unspecified shoulder joint**
S43.5 **Sprain of acromioclavicular joint**
Sprain of acromioclavicular ligament
X S43.50 **Sprain of unspecified acromioclavicular joint**
X S43.51 **Sprain of right acromioclavicular joint**
X S43.52 **Sprain of left acromioclavicular joint**
S43.6 **Sprain of sternoclavicular joint**
X S43.60 **Sprain of unspecified sternoclavicular joint**
X S43.61 **Sprain of right sternoclavicular joint**
X S43.62 **Sprain of left sternoclavicular joint**
S43.8 **Sprain of other specified parts of shoulder girdle**
X S43.80 **Sprain of other specified parts of unspecified shoulder girdle**
X S43.81 **Sprain of other specified parts of right shoulder girdle**
X S43.82 **Sprain of other specified parts of left shoulder girdle**
S43.9 **Sprain of unspecified parts of shoulder girdle**
X S43.90 **Sprain of unspecified parts of unspecified shoulder girdle**
Sprain of shoulder girdle NOS
X S43.91 **Sprain of unspecified parts of right shoulder girdle**
X S43.92 **Sprain of unspecified parts of left shoulder girdle**

S44 **Injury of nerves at shoulder and upper arm level**
Code also any associated open wound (S41.-)
Excludes2 injury of brachial plexus (S14.3-)
The appropriate 7th character is to be added to each code from category S44

A	initial encounter
D	subsequent encounter
S	sequela

S44.0 **Injury of ulnar nerve at upper arm level**
Excludes1 ulnar nerve NOS (S54.0)
X S44.00 **Injury of ulnar nerve at upper arm level, unspecified arm**
X S44.01 **Injury of ulnar nerve at upper arm level, right arm**
X S44.02 **Injury of ulnar nerve at upper arm level, left arm**
S44.1 **Injury of median nerve at upper arm level**
Excludes1 median nerve NOS (S54.1)
X S44.10 **Injury of median nerve at upper arm level, unspecified arm**
X S44.11 **Injury of median nerve at upper arm level, right arm**
X S44.12 **Injury of median nerve at upper arm level, left arm**
S44.2 **Injury of radial nerve at upper arm level**
Excludes1 radial nerve NOS (S54.2)
X S44.20 **Injury of radial nerve at upper arm level, unspecified arm**
X S44.21 **Injury of radial nerve at upper arm level, right arm**
X S44.22 **Injury of radial nerve at upper arm level, left arm**
S44.3 **Injury of axillary nerve**
X S44.30 **Injury of axillary nerve, unspecified arm**
X S44.31 **Injury of axillary nerve, right arm**
X S44.32 **Injury of axillary nerve, left arm**
S44.4 **Injury of musculocutaneous nerve**
X S44.40 **Injury of musculocutaneous nerve, unspecified arm**
X S44.41 **Injury of musculocutaneous nerve, right arm**
X S44.42 **Injury of musculocutaneous nerve, left arm**
S44.5 **Injury of cutaneous sensory nerve at shoulder and upper arm level**
X S44.50 **Injury of cutaneous sensory nerve at shoulder and upper arm level, unspecified arm**
X S44.51 **Injury of cutaneous sensory nerve at shoulder and upper arm level, right arm**
X S44.52 **Injury of cutaneous sensory nerve at shoulder and upper arm level, left arm**

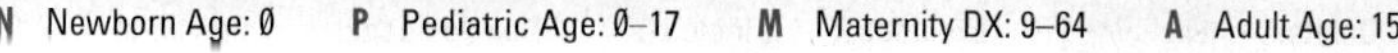
N Newborn Age: 0 P Pediatric Age: 0–17 M Maternity DX: 9–64 A Adult Age: 15–124

S44.8 Injury of other nerves at shoulder and upper arm level
- S44.8X Injury of other nerves at shoulder and upper arm level
  - S44.8X1 Injury of other nerves at shoulder and upper arm level, right arm
  - S44.8X2 Injury of other nerves at shoulder and upper arm level, left arm
  - S44.8X9 Injury of other nerves at shoulder and upper arm level, unspecified arm

S44.9 Injury of unspecified nerve at shoulder and upper arm level
- X S44.90 Injury of unspecified nerve at shoulder and upper arm level, unspecified arm
- X S44.91 Injury of unspecified nerve at shoulder and upper arm level, right arm
- X S44.92 Injury of unspecified nerve at shoulder and upper arm level, left arm

S45 Injury of blood vessels at shoulder and upper arm level

Code also any associated open wound (S41.-)

Excludes2 injury of subclavian artery (S25.1)
injury of subclavian vein (S25.3)

The appropriate 7th character is to be added to each code from category S45

A	initial encounter
D	subsequent encounter
S	sequela

S45.0 Injury of axillary artery
- S45.00 Unspecified injury of axillary artery
  - S45.001 Unspecified injury of axillary artery, right side A (Ex) PDX 1764
  - S45.002 Unspecified injury of axillary artery, left side A (Ex) PDX 1765
  - S45.009 Unspecified injury of axillary artery, unspecified side A (Ex) PDX 1766
- S45.01 Laceration of axillary artery
  - S45.011 Laceration of axillary artery, right side A (Ex) PDX 1764
  - S45.012 Laceration of axillary artery, left side A (Ex) PDX 1765
  - S45.019 Laceration of axillary artery, unspecified side A (Ex) PDX 1766
- S45.09 Other specified injury of axillary artery
  - S45.091 Other specified injury of axillary artery, right side A (Ex) PDX 1764
  - S45.092 Other specified injury of axillary artery, left side A (Ex) PDX 1765
  - S45.099 Other specified injury of axillary artery, unspecified side A (Ex) PDX 1766

S45.1 Injury of brachial artery
- S45.10 Unspecified injury of brachial artery
  - S45.101 Unspecified injury of brachial artery, right side A (Ex) PDX 1767
  - S45.102 Unspecified injury of brachial artery, left side A (Ex) PDX 1768
  - S45.109 Unspecified injury of brachial artery, unspecified side A (Ex) PDX 1769
- S45.11 Laceration of brachial artery
  - S45.111 Laceration of brachial artery, right side A (Ex) PDX 1767
  - S45.112 Laceration of brachial artery, left side A (Ex) PDX 1768
  - S45.119 Laceration of brachial artery, unspecified side A (Ex) PDX 1769
- S45.19 Other specified injury of brachial artery
  - S45.191 Other specified injury of brachial artery, right side A (Ex) PDX 1767
  - S45.192 Other specified injury of brachial artery, left side A (Ex) PDX 1768
  - S45.199 Other specified injury of brachial artery, unspecified side A (Ex) PDX 1769

S45.2 Injury of axillary or brachial vein
- S45.20 Unspecified injury of axillary or brachial vein
  - S45.201 Unspecified injury of axillary or brachial vein, right side A (Ex) PDX 1767
  - S45.202 Unspecified injury of axillary or brachial vein, left side A (Ex) PDX 1768
  - S45.209 Unspecified injury of axillary or brachial vein, unspecified side A (Ex) PDX 1769
- S45.21 Laceration of axillary or brachial vein
  - S45.211 Laceration of axillary or brachial vein, right side A (Ex) PDX 1767
  - S45.212 Laceration of axillary or brachial vein, left side A (Ex) PDX 1768
  - S45.219 Laceration of axillary or brachial vein, unspecified side A (Ex) PDX 1769
- S45.29 Other specified injury of axillary or brachial vein
  - S45.291 Other specified injury of axillary or brachial vein, right side A (Ex) PDX 1767
  - S45.292 Other specified injury of axillary or brachial vein, left side A (Ex) PDX 1768
  - S45.299 Other specified injury of axillary or brachial vein, unspecified side A (Ex) PDX 1769

S45.3 Injury of superficial vein at shoulder and upper arm level
- S45.30 Unspecified injury of superficial vein at shoulder and upper arm level
  - S45.301 Unspecified injury of superficial vein at shoulder and upper arm level, right arm A (Ex) PDX 1770
  - S45.302 Unspecified injury of superficial vein at shoulder and upper arm level, left arm A (Ex) PDX 1771
  - S45.309 Unspecified injury of superficial vein at shoulder and upper arm level, unspecified arm A (Ex) PDX 1772
- S45.31 Laceration of superficial vein at shoulder and upper arm level
  - S45.311 Laceration of superficial vein at shoulder and upper arm level, right arm A (Ex) PDX 1770
  - S45.312 Laceration of superficial vein at shoulder and upper arm level, left arm A (Ex) PDX 1771
  - S45.319 Laceration of superficial vein at shoulder and upper arm level, unspecified arm A (Ex) PDX 1772
- S45.39 Other specified injury of superficial vein at shoulder and upper arm level
  - S45.391 Other specified injury of superficial vein at shoulder and upper arm level, right arm A (Ex) PDX 1770
  - S45.392 Other specified injury of superficial vein at shoulder and upper arm level, left arm A (Ex) PDX 1771
  - S45.399 Other specified injury of superficial vein at shoulder and upper arm level, unspecified arm A (Ex) PDX 1772

CHAPTER 19 (S00-T88)

- **S45.8** Injury of other specified blood vessels at shoulder and upper arm level
  - **S45.80** Unspecified injury of other specified blood vessels at shoulder and upper arm level
    - **S45.801** Unspecified injury of other specified blood vessels at shoulder and upper arm level, right arm A (Ex) PDX 1770
    - **S45.802** Unspecified injury of other specified blood vessels at shoulder and upper arm level, left arm A (Ex) PDX 1771
    - **S45.809** Unspecified injury of other specified blood vessels at shoulder and upper arm level, unspecified arm A (Ex) PDX 1772
  - **S45.81** Laceration of other specified blood vessels at shoulder and upper arm level
    - **S45.811** Laceration of other specified blood vessels at shoulder and upper arm level, right arm A (Ex) PDX 1770
    - **S45.812** Laceration of other specified blood vessels at shoulder and upper arm level, left arm A (Ex) PDX 1771
    - **S45.819** Laceration of other specified blood vessels at shoulder and upper arm level, unspecified arm A (Ex) PDX 1772
  - **S45.89** Other specified injury of other specified blood vessels at shoulder and upper arm level
    - **S45.891** Other specified injury of other specified blood vessels at shoulder and upper arm level, right arm A (Ex) PDX 1770
    - **S45.892** Other specified injury of other specified blood vessels at shoulder and upper arm level, left arm A (Ex) PDX 1771
    - **S45.899** Other specified injury of other specified blood vessels at shoulder and upper arm level, unspecified arm A (Ex) PDX 1772
- **S45.9** Injury of unspecified blood vessel at shoulder and upper arm level
  - **S45.90** Unspecified injury of unspecified blood vessel at shoulder and upper arm level
    - **S45.901** Unspecified injury of unspecified blood vessel at shoulder and upper arm level, right arm A (Ex) PDX 1770
    - **S45.902** Unspecified injury of unspecified blood vessel at shoulder and upper arm level, left arm A (Ex) PDX 1771
    - **S45.909** Unspecified injury of unspecified blood vessel at shoulder and upper arm level, unspecified arm A (Ex) PDX 1772
  - **S45.91** Laceration of unspecified blood vessel at shoulder and upper arm level
    - **S45.911** Laceration of unspecified blood vessel at shoulder and upper arm level, right arm A (Ex) PDX 1770
    - **S45.912** Laceration of unspecified blood vessel at shoulder and upper arm level, left arm A (Ex) PDX 1771
    - **S45.919** Laceration of unspecified blood vessel at shoulder and upper arm level, unspecified arm A (Ex) PDX 1772
  - **S45.99** Other specified injury of unspecified blood vessel at shoulder and upper arm level
    - **S45.991** Other specified injury of unspecified blood vessel at shoulder and upper arm level, right arm A (Ex) PDX 1770
    - **S45.992** Other specified injury of unspecified blood vessel at shoulder and upper arm level, left arm A (Ex) PDX 1771
    - **S45.999** Other specified injury of unspecified blood vessel at shoulder and upper arm level, unspecified arm A (Ex) PDX 1772

S46 Injury of muscle, fascia and tendon at shoulder and upper arm level

Code also any associated open wound (S41.-)

Excludes2 injury of muscle, fascia and tendon at elbow (S56.-)
sprain of joints and ligaments of shoulder girdle (S43.9)

The appropriate 7th character is to be added to each code from category S46

A	initial encounter
D	subsequent encounter
S	sequela

- **S46.0** Injury of muscle(s) and tendon(s) of the rotator cuff of shoulder
  - **S46.00** Unspecified injury of muscle(s) and tendon(s) of the rotator cuff of shoulder
    - **S46.001** Unspecified injury of muscle(s) and tendon(s) of the rotator cuff of right shoulder
    - **S46.002** Unspecified injury of muscle(s) and tendon(s) of the rotator cuff of left shoulder
    - **S46.009** Unspecified injury of muscle(s) and tendon(s) of the rotator cuff of unspecified shoulder
  - **S46.01** Strain of muscle(s) and tendon(s) of the rotator cuff of shoulder
    Acute onset due to trauma to rotator cuff muscle/tendon
    - **S46.011** Strain of muscle(s) and tendon(s) of the rotator cuff of right shoulder
    - **S46.012** Strain of muscle(s) and tendon(s) of the rotator cuff of left shoulder
    - **S46.019** Strain of muscle(s) and tendon(s) of the rotator cuff of unspecified shoulder
  - **S46.02** Laceration of muscle(s) and tendon(s) of the rotator cuff of shoulder
    - **S46.021** Laceration of muscle(s) and tendon(s) of the rotator cuff of right shoulder A (Ex) PDX 1773
    - **S46.022** Laceration of muscle(s) and tendon(s) of the rotator cuff of left shoulder A (Ex) PDX 1774
    - **S46.029** Laceration of muscle(s) and tendon(s) of the rotator cuff of unspecified shoulder A (Ex) PDX 1775
  - **S46.09** Other injury of muscle(s) and tendon(s) of the rotator cuff of shoulder
    - **S46.091** Other injury of muscle(s) and tendon(s) of the rotator cuff of right shoulder
    - **S46.092** Other injury of muscle(s) and tendon(s) of the rotator cuff of left shoulder
    - **S46.099** Other injury of muscle(s) and tendon(s) of the rotator cuff of unspecified shoulder

CHAPTER 19 (S00-T88)

- S46.1 Injury of muscle, fascia and tendon of long head of biceps
  - S46.10 Unspecified injury of muscle, fascia and tendon of long head of biceps
    - S46.101 Unspecified injury of muscle, fascia and tendon of long head of biceps, right arm
    - S46.102 Unspecified injury of muscle, fascia and tendon of long head of biceps, left arm
    - S46.109 Unspecified injury of muscle, fascia and tendon of long head of biceps, unspecified arm
  - S46.11 Strain of muscle, fascia and tendon of long head of biceps
    Coding Clinic: 2019, Q2, P27
    - S46.111 Strain of muscle, fascia and tendon of long head of biceps, right arm
    - S46.112 Strain of muscle, fascia and tendon of long head of biceps, left arm
    - S46.119 Strain of muscle, fascia and tendon of long head of biceps, unspecified arm
  - S46.12 Laceration of muscle, fascia and tendon of long head of biceps
    - S46.121 Laceration of muscle, fascia and tendon of long head of biceps, right arm A (Ex) PDX 1773
    - S46.122 Laceration of muscle, fascia and tendon of long head of biceps, left arm A (Ex) PDX 1774
    - S46.129 Laceration of muscle, fascia and tendon of long head of biceps, unspecified arm A (Ex) PDX 1775
  - S46.19 Other injury of muscle, fascia and tendon of long head of biceps
    - S46.191 Other injury of muscle, fascia and tendon of long head of biceps, right arm
    - S46.192 Other injury of muscle, fascia and tendon of long head of biceps, left arm
    - S46.199 Other injury of muscle, fascia and tendon of long head of biceps, unspecified arm
- S46.2 Injury of muscle, fascia and tendon of other parts of biceps
  - S46.20 Unspecified injury of muscle, fascia and tendon of other parts of biceps
    - S46.201 Unspecified injury of muscle, fascia and tendon of other parts of biceps, right arm
    - S46.202 Unspecified injury of muscle, fascia and tendon of other parts of biceps, left arm
    - S46.209 Unspecified injury of muscle, fascia and tendon of other parts of biceps, unspecified arm
  - S46.21 Strain of muscle, fascia and tendon of other parts of biceps
    - S46.211 Strain of muscle, fascia and tendon of other parts of biceps, right arm
    - S46.212 Strain of muscle, fascia and tendon of other parts of biceps, left arm
    - S46.219 Strain of muscle, fascia and tendon of other parts of biceps, unspecified arm
  - S46.22 Laceration of muscle, fascia and tendon of other parts of biceps
    - S46.221 Laceration of muscle, fascia and tendon of other parts of biceps, right arm A (Ex) PDX 1773
    - S46.222 Laceration of muscle, fascia and tendon of other parts of biceps, left arm A (Ex) PDX 1774
    - S46.229 Laceration of muscle, fascia and tendon of other parts of biceps, unspecified arm A (Ex) PDX 1775
  - S46.29 Other injury of muscle, fascia and tendon of other parts of biceps
    - S46.291 Other injury of muscle, fascia and tendon of other parts of biceps, right arm
    - S46.292 Other injury of muscle, fascia and tendon of other parts of biceps, left arm
    - S46.299 Other injury of muscle, fascia and tendon of other parts of biceps, unspecified arm
- S46.3 Injury of muscle, fascia and tendon of triceps
  - S46.30 Unspecified injury of muscle, fascia and tendon of triceps
    - S46.301 Unspecified injury of muscle, fascia and tendon of triceps, right arm
    - S46.302 Unspecified injury of muscle, fascia and tendon of triceps, left arm
    - S46.309 Unspecified injury of muscle, fascia and tendon of triceps, unspecified arm
  - S46.31 Strain of muscle, fascia and tendon of triceps
    - S46.311 Strain of muscle, fascia and tendon of triceps, right arm
    - S46.312 Strain of muscle, fascia and tendon of triceps, left arm
    - S46.319 Strain of muscle, fascia and tendon of triceps, unspecified arm
  - S46.32 Laceration of muscle, fascia and tendon of triceps
    - S46.321 Laceration of muscle, fascia and tendon of triceps, right arm A (Ex) PDX 1773
    - S46.322 Laceration of muscle, fascia and tendon of triceps, left arm A (Ex) PDX 1774
    - S46.329 Laceration of muscle, fascia and tendon of triceps, unspecified arm A (Ex) PDX 1775
  - S46.39 Other injury of muscle, fascia and tendon of triceps
    - S46.391 Other injury of muscle, fascia and tendon of triceps, right arm
    - S46.392 Other injury of muscle, fascia and tendon of triceps, left arm
    - S46.399 Other injury of muscle, fascia and tendon of triceps, unspecified arm
- S46.8 Injury of other muscles, fascia and tendons at shoulder and upper arm level
  - S46.80 Unspecified injury of other muscles, fascia and tendons at shoulder and upper arm level
    - S46.801 Unspecified injury of other muscles, fascia and tendons at shoulder and upper arm level, right arm
    - S46.802 Unspecified injury of other muscles, fascia and tendons at shoulder and upper arm level, left arm
    - S46.809 Unspecified injury of other muscles, fascia and tendons at shoulder and upper arm level, unspecified arm

● S46.81 Strain of other muscles, fascia and tendons at shoulder and upper arm level
● S46.811 Strain of other muscles, fascia and tendons at shoulder and upper arm level, right arm
● S46.812 Strain of other muscles, fascia and tendons at shoulder and upper arm level, left arm
● S46.819 Strain of other muscles, fascia and tendons at shoulder and upper arm level, unspecified arm
● S46.82 Laceration of other muscles, fascia and tendons at shoulder and upper arm level
● S46.821 Laceration of other muscles, fascia and tendons at shoulder and upper arm level, right arm A (Ex) PDX 1773
● S46.822 Laceration of other muscles, fascia and tendons at shoulder and upper arm level, left arm A (Ex) PDX 1774
● S46.829 Laceration of other muscles, fascia and tendons at shoulder and upper arm level, unspecified arm A (Ex) PDX 1775
● S46.89 Other injury of other muscles, fascia and tendons at shoulder and upper arm level
● S46.891 Other injury of other muscles, fascia and tendons at shoulder and upper arm level, right arm
● S46.892 Other injury of other muscles, fascia and tendons at shoulder and upper arm level, left arm
● S46.899 Other injury of other muscles, fascia and tendons at shoulder and upper arm level, unspecified arm
● S46.9 Injury of unspecified muscle, fascia and tendon at shoulder and upper arm level
● S46.90 Unspecified injury of unspecified muscle, fascia and tendon at shoulder and upper arm level
● S46.901 Unspecified injury of unspecified muscle, fascia and tendon at shoulder and upper arm level, right arm
● S46.902 Unspecified injury of unspecified muscle, fascia and tendon at shoulder and upper arm level, left arm
● S46.909 Unspecified injury of unspecified muscle, fascia and tendon at shoulder and upper arm level, unspecified arm
● S46.91 Strain of unspecified muscle, fascia and tendon at shoulder and upper arm level
● S46.911 Strain of unspecified muscle, fascia and tendon at shoulder and upper arm level, right arm
● S46.912 Strain of unspecified muscle, fascia and tendon at shoulder and upper arm level, left arm
● S46.919 Strain of unspecified muscle, fascia and tendon at shoulder and upper arm level, unspecified arm
● S46.92 Laceration of unspecified muscle, fascia and tendon at shoulder and upper arm level
● S46.921 Laceration of unspecified muscle, fascia and tendon at shoulder and upper arm level, right arm A (Ex) PDX 1773
● S46.922 Laceration of unspecified muscle, fascia and tendon at shoulder and upper arm level, left arm A (Ex) PDX 1774
● S46.929 Laceration of unspecified muscle, fascia and tendon at shoulder and upper arm level, unspecified arm A (Ex) PDX 1775
● S46.99 Other injury of unspecified muscle, fascia and tendon at shoulder and upper arm level
● S46.991 Other injury of unspecified muscle, fascia and tendon at shoulder and upper arm level, right arm
● S46.992 Other injury of unspecified muscle, fascia and tendon at shoulder and upper arm level, left arm
● S46.999 Other injury of unspecified muscle, fascia and tendon at shoulder and upper arm level, unspecified arm

● S47 Crushing injury of shoulder and upper arm

Use additional code for all associated injuries

Excludes2 crushing injury of elbow (S57.Ø-)

The appropriate 7th character is to be added to each code from category S47

A	initial encounter
D	subsequent encounter
S	sequela

X● S47.1 Crushing injury of right shoulder and upper arm
X● S47.2 Crushing injury of left shoulder and upper arm
X● S47.9 Crushing injury of shoulder and upper arm, unspecified arm

● S48 Traumatic amputation of shoulder and upper arm

An amputation not identified as partial or complete should be coded to complete

Excludes1 traumatic amputation at elbow level (S58.Ø)

The appropriate 7th character is to be added to each code from category S48

A	initial encounter
D	subsequent encounter
S	sequela

● S48.Ø Traumatic amputation at shoulder joint
● S48.Ø1 Complete traumatic amputation at shoulder joint
● S48.Ø11 Complete traumatic amputation at right shoulder joint A, A, S (Ex) PDX 1776
● S48.Ø12 Complete traumatic amputation at left shoulder joint A, A, S (Ex) PDX 1777
● S48.Ø19 Complete traumatic amputation at unspecified shoulder joint A, A, S (Ex) PDX 1778
● S48.Ø2 Partial traumatic amputation at shoulder joint
● S48.Ø21 Partial traumatic amputation at right shoulder joint A, A, S (Ex) PDX 1776
● S48.Ø22 Partial traumatic amputation at left shoulder joint A, A, S (Ex) PDX 1777
● S48.Ø29 Partial traumatic amputation at unspecified shoulder joint A, A, S (Ex) PDX 1778
● S48.1 Traumatic amputation at level between shoulder and elbow
● S48.11 Complete traumatic amputation at level between shoulder and elbow
● S48.111 Complete traumatic amputation at level between right shoulder and elbow A, A, S (Ex) PDX 1776
● S48.112 Complete traumatic amputation at level between left shoulder and elbow A, A, S (Ex) PDX 1777
● S48.119 Complete traumatic amputation at level between unspecified shoulder and elbow A, A, S (Ex) PDX 1778

CHAPTER 19 (SØØ-T88)

S48.12 Partial traumatic amputation at level between shoulder and elbow

S48.121 Partial traumatic amputation at level between right shoulder and elbow A, A, S PDX 1776

S48.122 Partial traumatic amputation at level between left shoulder and elbow A, A, S PDX 1777

S48.129 Partial traumatic amputation at level between unspecified shoulder and elbow A, A, S PDX 1778

S48.9 Traumatic amputation of shoulder and upper arm, level unspecified

S48.91 Complete traumatic amputation of shoulder and upper arm, level unspecified

S48.911 Complete traumatic amputation of right shoulder and upper arm, level unspecified A, A, S PDX 1776

S48.912 Complete traumatic amputation of left shoulder and upper arm, level unspecified A, A, S PDX 1777

S48.919 Complete traumatic amputation of unspecified shoulder and upper arm, level unspecified A, A, S PDX 1778

S48.92 Partial traumatic amputation of shoulder and upper arm, level unspecified

S48.921 Partial traumatic amputation of right shoulder and upper arm, level unspecified A, A, S PDX 1776

S48.922 Partial traumatic amputation of left shoulder and upper arm, level unspecified A, A, S PDX 1777

S48.929 Partial traumatic amputation of unspecified shoulder and upper arm, level unspecified A, A, S PDX 1778

S49 Other and unspecified injuries of shoulder and upper arm

The appropriate 7th character is to be added to each code from subcategories S49.0 and S49.1

A	initial encounter for closed fracture
D	subsequent encounter for fracture with routine healing
G	subsequent encounter for fracture with delayed healing
K	subsequent encounter for fracture with nonunion
P	subsequent encounter for fracture with malunion
S	sequela

S49.0 Physeal fracture of upper end of humerus

S49.00 Unspecified physeal fracture of upper end of humerus

S49.001 Unspecified physeal fracture of upper end of humerus, right arm A, K, P, A PDX 1264 [K, P], 1755 [A]

S49.002 Unspecified physeal fracture of upper end of humerus, left arm A, K, P, A PDX 1264 [K, P], 1757 [A]

S49.009 Unspecified physeal fracture of upper end of humerus, unspecified arm A, K, P, A PDX 1264 [K, P], 1758 [A]

S49.01 Salter-Harris Type I physeal fracture of upper end of humerus

S49.011 Salter-Harris Type I physeal fracture of upper end of humerus, right arm A, K, P, A PDX 1264 [K, P], 1755 [A]

S49.012 Salter-Harris Type I physeal fracture of upper end of humerus, left arm A, K, P, A PDX 1264 [K, P], 1757 [A]

S49.019 Salter-Harris Type I physeal fracture of upper end of humerus, unspecified arm A, K, P, A PDX 1264 [K, P], 1758 [A]

Item 19–3 SALTER-HARRIS TYPE 1: epiphysis is completely separated from end of bone, or metaphysic growth plate remains attached to epiphysis

SALTER-HARRIS TYPE 2: epiphysis and growth plate are partially separated from metaphysis, which is cracked—most common type

SALTER-HARRIS TYPE 3: fracture occurring through epiphysis and separates part of epiphysis and growth plate from metaphysis fracture, usually at distal end of tibia

SALTER-HARRIS TYPE 4: fracture runs through epiphysis, across growth plate, into metaphysic, surgery is required to restore joint surface to normal and align growth plate

S49.02 Salter-Harris Type II physeal fracture of upper end of humerus

S49.021 Salter-Harris Type II physeal fracture of upper end of humerus, right arm A, K, P, A PDX 1264 [K, P], 1755 [A]

S49.022 Salter-Harris Type II physeal fracture of upper end of humerus, left arm A, K, P, A PDX 1264 [K, P], 1757 [A]

S49.029 Salter-Harris Type II physeal fracture of upper end of humerus, unspecified arm A, K, P, A PDX 1264 [K, P], 1758 [A]

S49.03 Salter-Harris Type III physeal fracture of upper end of humerus

S49.031 Salter-Harris Type III physeal fracture of upper end of humerus, right arm A, K, P, A PDX 1264 [K, P], 1755 [A]

S49.032 Salter-Harris Type III physeal fracture of upper end of humerus, left arm A, K, P, A PDX 1264 [K, P], 1757 [A]

S49.039 Salter-Harris Type III physeal fracture of upper end of humerus, unspecified arm A, K, P, A PDX 1264 [K, P], 1758 [A]

S49.04 Salter-Harris Type IV physeal fracture of upper end of humerus

S49.041 Salter-Harris Type IV physeal fracture of upper end of humerus, right arm A, K, P, A PDX 1264 [K, P], 1755 [A]

S49.042 Salter-Harris Type IV physeal fracture of upper end of humerus, left arm A, K, P, A PDX 1264 [K, P], 1757 [A]

S49.049 Salter-Harris Type IV physeal fracture of upper end of humerus, unspecified arm A, K, P, A PDX 1264 [K, P], 1758 [A]

S49.09 Other physeal fracture of upper end of humerus

S49.091 Other physeal fracture of upper end of humerus, right arm A, K, P, A PDX 1264 [K, P], 1755 [A]

S49.092 Other physeal fracture of upper end of humerus, left arm A, K, P, A PDX 1264 [K, P], 1757 [A]

S49.099 Other physeal fracture of upper end of humerus, unspecified arm A, K, P, A PDX 1264 [K, P], 1758 [A]

S49.1 Physeal fracture of lower end of humerus

S49.10 Unspecified physeal fracture of lower end of humerus

S49.101 Unspecified physeal fracture of lower end of humerus, right arm A, K, P, A PDX 1264 [K, P], 1755 [A]

S49.102 Unspecified physeal fracture of lower end of humerus, left arm A, K, P, A PDX 1264 [K, P], 1757 [A]

S49.109 Unspecified physeal fracture of lower end of humerus, unspecified arm A, K, P, A PDX 1264 [K, P], 1758 [A]

- S49.11 Salter-Harris Type I physeal fracture of lower end of humerus
  - S49.111 Salter-Harris Type I physeal fracture of lower end of humerus, right arm A, K, P, A (Ex) PDX 1264 [K, P], 1757 [A]
  - S49.112 Salter-Harris Type I physeal fracture of lower end of humerus, left arm A, K, P, A (Ex) PDX 1264 [K, P], 1755 [A]
  - S49.119 Salter-Harris Type I physeal fracture of lower end of humerus, unspecified arm A, K, P, A (Ex) PDX 1264 [K, P], 1758 [A]
- S49.12 Salter-Harris Type II physeal fracture of lower end of humerus
  - S49.121 Salter-Harris Type II physeal fracture of lower end of humerus, right arm A, K, P, A (Ex) PDX 1264 [K, P], 1757 [A]
  - S49.122 Salter-Harris Type II physeal fracture of lower end of humerus, left arm A, K, P, A (Ex) PDX 1264 [K, P], 1755 [A]
  - S49.129 Salter-Harris Type II physeal fracture of lower end of humerus, unspecified arm A, K, P, A (Ex) PDX 1264 [K, P], 1758 [A]
- S49.13 Salter-Harris Type III physeal fracture of lower end of humerus
  - S49.131 Salter-Harris Type III physeal fracture of lower end of humerus, right arm A, K, P, A (Ex) PDX 1264 [K, P], 1757 [A]
  - S49.132 Salter-Harris Type III physeal fracture of lower end of humerus, left arm A, K, P, A (Ex) PDX 1264 [K, P], 1755 [A]
  - S49.139 Salter-Harris Type III physeal fracture of lower end of humerus, unspecified arm A, K, P, A (Ex) PDX 1264 [K, P], 1758 [A]
- S49.14 Salter-Harris Type IV physeal fracture of lower end of humerus
  - S49.141 Salter-Harris Type IV physeal fracture of lower end of humerus, right arm A, K, P (Ex) PDX 1264 [K, P], 1757 [A]
  - S49.142 Salter-Harris Type IV physeal fracture of lower end of humerus, left arm A, K, P, A (Ex) PDX 1264 [K, P], 1755 [A]
  - S49.149 Salter-Harris Type IV physeal fracture of lower end of humerus, unspecified arm A, K, P, A (Ex) PDX 1264 [K, P], 1758 [A]
- S49.19 Other physeal fracture of lower end of humerus
  - S49.191 Other physeal fracture of lower end of humerus, right arm A, K, P, A (Ex) PDX 1264 [K, P], 1757 [A]
  - S49.192 Other physeal fracture of lower end of humerus, left arm A, K, P, A (Ex) PDX 1264 [K, P], 1755 [A]
  - S49.199 Other physeal fracture of lower end of humerus, unspecified arm A, K, P, A (Ex) PDX 1264 [K, P], 1758 [A]

S49.8 Other specified injuries of shoulder and upper arm

The appropriate 7th character is to be added to each code in subcategory S49.8

A	initial encounter
D	subsequent encounter
S	sequela

- X S49.80 Other specified injuries of shoulder and upper arm, unspecified arm
- X S49.81 Other specified injuries of right shoulder and upper arm
- X S49.82 Other specified injuries of left shoulder and upper arm

S49.9 Unspecified injury of shoulder and upper arm

The appropriate 7th character is to be added to each code in subcategory S49.9

A	initial encounter
D	subsequent encounter
S	sequela

- X S49.90 Unspecified injury of shoulder and upper arm, unspecified arm
- X S49.91 Unspecified injury of right shoulder and upper arm
- X S49.92 Unspecified injury of left shoulder and upper arm

INJURIES TO THE ELBOW AND FOREARM (S50-S59)

Excludes2 burns and corrosions (T20-T32)
frostbite (T33-T34)
injuries of wrist and hand (S60-S69)
insect bite or sting, venomous (T63.4)

S50 Superficial injury of elbow and forearm

Excludes2 superficial injury of wrist and hand (S60.-)

The appropriate 7th character is to be added to each code from category S50

A	initial encounter
D	subsequent encounter
S	sequela

- S50.0 Contusion of elbow
  - X S50.00 Contusion of unspecified elbow
  - X S50.01 Contusion of right elbow
  - X S50.02 Contusion of left elbow
- S50.1 Contusion of forearm
  - X S50.10 Contusion of unspecified forearm
  - X S50.11 Contusion of right forearm
  - X S50.12 Contusion of left forearm
- S50.3 Other superficial injuries of elbow
  - S50.31 Abrasion of elbow
    - S50.311 Abrasion of right elbow
    - S50.312 Abrasion of left elbow
    - S50.319 Abrasion of unspecified elbow
  - S50.32 Blister (nonthermal) of elbow
    - S50.321 Blister (nonthermal) of right elbow
    - S50.322 Blister (nonthermal) of left elbow
    - S50.329 Blister (nonthermal) of unspecified elbow
  - S50.34 External constriction of elbow
    - S50.341 External constriction of right elbow
    - S50.342 External constriction of left elbow
    - S50.349 External constriction of unspecified elbow
  - S50.35 Superficial foreign body of elbow
    Splinter in the elbow
    - S50.351 Superficial foreign body of right elbow
    - S50.352 Superficial foreign body of left elbow
    - S50.359 Superficial foreign body of unspecified elbow
  - S50.36 Insect bite (nonvenomous) of elbow
    - S50.361 Insect bite (nonvenomous) of right elbow
    - S50.362 Insect bite (nonvenomous) of left elbow
    - S50.369 Insect bite (nonvenomous) of unspecified elbow

CHAPTER 19 (S00-T88)

S50.37 Other superficial bite of elbow
Excludes1 open bite of elbow (S51.04)
S50.371 Other superficial bite of right elbow
S50.372 Other superficial bite of left elbow
S50.379 Other superficial bite of unspecified elbow

S50.8 Other superficial injuries of forearm
S50.81 Abrasion of forearm
S50.811 Abrasion of right forearm
S50.812 Abrasion of left forearm
S50.819 Abrasion of unspecified forearm
S50.82 Blister (nonthermal) of forearm
S50.821 Blister (nonthermal) of right forearm
S50.822 Blister (nonthermal) of left forearm
S50.829 Blister (nonthermal) of unspecified forearm
S50.84 External constriction of forearm
S50.841 External constriction of right forearm
S50.842 External constriction of left forearm
S50.849 External constriction of unspecified forearm
S50.85 Superficial foreign body of forearm
Splinter in the forearm
S50.851 Superficial foreign body of right forearm
S50.852 Superficial foreign body of left forearm
S50.859 Superficial foreign body of unspecified forearm
S50.86 Insect bite (nonvenomous) of forearm
S50.861 Insect bite (nonvenomous) of right forearm
S50.862 Insect bite (nonvenomous) of left forearm
S50.869 Insect bite (nonvenomous) of unspecified forearm
S50.87 Other superficial bite of forearm
Excludes1 open bite of forearm (S51.84)
S50.871 Other superficial bite of right forearm
S50.872 Other superficial bite of left forearm
S50.879 Other superficial bite of unspecified forearm

S50.9 Unspecified superficial injury of elbow and forearm
S50.90 Unspecified superficial injury of elbow
S50.901 Unspecified superficial injury of right elbow
S50.902 Unspecified superficial injury of left elbow
S50.909 Unspecified superficial injury of unspecified elbow
S50.91 Unspecified superficial injury of forearm
S50.911 Unspecified superficial injury of right forearm
S50.912 Unspecified superficial injury of left forearm
S50.919 Unspecified superficial injury of unspecified forearm

S51 Open wound of elbow and forearm
Code also any associated wound infection
Excludes1 open fracture of elbow and forearm (S52.- with open fracture 7th character)
traumatic amputation of elbow and forearm (S58.-)
Excludes2 open wound of wrist and hand (S61.-)
The appropriate 7th character is to be added to each code from category S51

A	initial encounter
D	subsequent encounter
S	sequela

S51.0 Open wound of elbow
S51.00 Unspecified open wound of elbow
S51.001 Unspecified open wound of right elbow
Coding Clinic: 2012, Q4, P108
S51.002 Unspecified open wound of left elbow
S51.009 Unspecified open wound of unspecified elbow
Open wound of elbow NOS
S51.01 Laceration without foreign body of elbow
S51.011 Laceration without foreign body of right elbow
S51.012 Laceration without foreign body of left elbow
S51.019 Laceration without foreign body of unspecified elbow
S51.02 Laceration with foreign body of elbow
S51.021 Laceration with foreign body of right elbow
S51.022 Laceration with foreign body of left elbow
S51.029 Laceration with foreign body of unspecified elbow
S51.03 Puncture wound without foreign body of elbow
S51.031 Puncture wound without foreign body of right elbow
S51.032 Puncture wound without foreign body of left elbow
S51.039 Puncture wound without foreign body of unspecified elbow
S51.04 Puncture wound with foreign body of elbow
S51.041 Puncture wound with foreign body of right elbow
S51.042 Puncture wound with foreign body of left elbow
S51.049 Puncture wound with foreign body of unspecified elbow
S51.05 Open bite of elbow
Bite of elbow NOS
Excludes1 superficial bite of elbow (S50.36, S50.37)
S51.051 Open bite, right elbow
S51.052 Open bite, left elbow
S51.059 Open bite, unspecified elbow

S51.8 Open wound of forearm
Excludes2 open wound of elbow (S51.0-)
S51.80 Unspecified open wound of forearm
S51.801 Unspecified open wound of right forearm
S51.802 Unspecified open wound of left forearm
S51.809 Unspecified open wound of unspecified forearm
Open wound of forearm NOS
S51.81 Laceration without foreign body of forearm
S51.811 Laceration without foreign body of right forearm
S51.812 Laceration without foreign body of left forearm
S51.819 Laceration without foreign body of unspecified forearm
S51.82 Laceration with foreign body of forearm
S51.821 Laceration with foreign body of right forearm
S51.822 Laceration with foreign body of left forearm
S51.829 Laceration with foreign body of unspecified forearm

● **S51.83 Puncture wound without foreign body of forearm**

● **S51.831 Puncture wound without foreign body of right forearm**

● **S51.832 Puncture wound without foreign body of left forearm**

● **S51.839 Puncture wound without foreign body of unspecified forearm**

● **S51.84 Puncture wound with foreign body of forearm**

● **S51.841 Puncture wound with foreign body of right forearm**

● **S51.842 Puncture wound with foreign body of left forearm**

● **S51.849 Puncture wound with foreign body of unspecified forearm**

● **S51.85 Open bite of forearm**

Bite of forearm NOS

Excludes1 superficial bite of forearm (S50.86, S50.87)

● **S51.851 Open bite of right forearm**

● **S51.852 Open bite of left forearm**

● **S51.859 Open bite of unspecified forearm**

● **S52 Fracture of forearm**

Note: A fracture not identified as displaced or nondisplaced should be coded to displaced

A fracture not designated as open or closed should be coded to closed

The open fracture designations are based on the Gustilo open fracture classification

Excludes1 traumatic amputation of forearm (S58.-)

Excludes2 fracture at wrist and hand level (S62.-)

periprosthetic fracture around internal prosthetic elbow joint (M97.4)

The appropriate 7th character is to be added to all codes from category S52

A	initial encounter for closed fracture
B	initial encounter for open fracture type I or II initial encounter for open fracture NOS
C	initial encounter for open fracture type IIIA, IIIB, or IIIC
D	subsequent encounter for closed fracture with routine healing
E	subsequent encounter for open fracture type I or II with routine healing
F	subsequent encounter for open fracture type IIIA, IIIB, or IIIC with routine healing
G	subsequent encounter for closed fracture with delayed healing
H	subsequent encounter for open fracture type I or II with delayed healing
J	subsequent encounter for open fracture type IIIA, IIIB, or IIIC with delayed healing
K	subsequent encounter for closed fracture with nonunion
M	subsequent encounter for open fracture type I or II with nonunion
N	subsequent encounter for open fracture type IIIA, IIIB, or IIIC with nonunion
P	subsequent encounter for closed fracture with malunion
Q	subsequent encounter for open fracture type I or II with malunion
R	subsequent encounter for open fracture type IIIA, IIIB, or IIIC with malunion
S	sequela

Coding Clinic: 2016, Q1, P33

● **S52.0 Fracture of upper end of ulna**

Fracture of proximal end of ulna

Excludes2 fracture of elbow NOS (S42.40-)
fractures of shaft of ulna (S52.2-)

● **S52.00 Unspecified fracture of upper end of ulna** Ex PDX 1264 [K, M, N, P, Q, R], 1779 [B, C]

● **S52.001 Unspecified fracture of upper end of right ulna** K, M, N, P, Q, R, B, C, B, C

● **S52.002 Unspecified fracture of upper end of left ulna** K, M, N, P, Q, R, B, C, B, C

● **S52.009 Unspecified fracture of upper end of unspecified ulna** K, M, N, P, Q, R, B, C, B, C

● **S52.01 Torus fracture of upper end of ulna**

The appropriate 7th character is to be added to all codes in subcategory S52.01

A	initial encounter for closed fracture
D	subsequent encounter for fracture with routine healing
G	subsequent encounter for fracture with delayed healing
K	subsequent encounter for fracture with nonunion
P	subsequent encounter for fracture with malunion
S	sequela

● **S52.011 Torus fracture of upper end of right ulna** A, K, P, A Ex PDX 1264 [K, P], 1780 [A]

● **S52.012 Torus fracture of upper end of left ulna** A, K, P, A Ex PDX 1264 [K, P], 1781 [A]

● **S52.019 Torus fracture of upper end of unspecified ulna** A, K, P, A Ex PDX 1264 [K, P], 1782 [A]

● **S52.02 Fracture of olecranon process without intraarticular extension of ulna** Ex PDX 1264 [K, M, N, P, Q, R], 1783 [B, C]

● **S52.021 Displaced fracture of olecranon process without intraarticular extension of right ulna** K, M, N, P, Q, R, B, C, B, C

● **S52.022 Displaced fracture of olecranon process without intraarticular extension of left ulna** K, M, N, P, Q, R, B, C, B, C

● **S52.023 Displaced fracture of olecranon process without intraarticular extension of unspecified ulna** K, M, N, P, Q, R, B, C, B, C

● **S52.024 Nondisplaced fracture of olecranon process without intraarticular extension of right ulna** K, M, N, P, Q, R, B, C, B, C

● **S52.025 Nondisplaced fracture of olecranon process without intraarticular extension of left ulna** K, M, N, P, Q, R, B, C, B, C

● **S52.026 Nondisplaced fracture of olecranon process without intraarticular extension of unspecified ulna** K, M, N, P, Q, R, B, C, B, C

● **S52.03 Fracture of olecranon process with intraarticular extension of ulna** Ex PDX 1264 [K, M, N, P, Q, R], 1783 [B, C]

● **S52.031 Displaced fracture of olecranon process with intraarticular extension of right ulna** K, M, N, P, Q, R, B, C, B, C

CHAPTER 19 (S00-T88)

S52.032 **Displaced** fracture of olecranon process with intraarticular extension of **left** ulna K, M, N, P, Q, R, B, C, B, C

S52.033 **Displaced** fracture of olecranon process with intraarticular extension of **unspecified** ulna K, M, N, P, Q, R, B, C, B, C

S52.034 **Nondisplaced** fracture of olecranon process with intraarticular extension of **right** ulna K, M, N, P, Q, R, B, C, B, C

S52.035 **Nondisplaced** fracture of olecranon process with intraarticular extension of **left** ulna K, M, N, P, Q, R, B, C, B, C

S52.036 **Nondisplaced** fracture of olecranon process with intraarticular extension of **unspecified** ulna K, M, N, P, Q, R, B, C, B, C

S52.04 Fracture of **coronoid process** of ulna Ex PDX 1264 [K, M, N, P, Q, R], 1779 [B, C]

S52.041 **Displaced** fracture of coronoid process of **right** ulna K, M, N, P, Q, R, B, C, B, C

S52.042 **Displaced** fracture of coronoid process of **left** ulna K, M, N, P, Q, R, B, C, B, C

S52.043 **Displaced** fracture of coronoid process of **unspecified** ulna K, M, N, P, Q, R, B, C, B, C

S52.044 **Nondisplaced** fracture of coronoid process of **right** ulna K, M, N, P, Q, R, B, C, B, C

S52.045 **Nondisplaced** fracture of coronoid process of **left** ulna K, M, N, P, Q, R, B, C, B, C

S52.046 **Nondisplaced** fracture of coronoid process of **unspecified** ulna K, M, N, P, Q, R, B, C, B, C

S52.09 **Other** fracture of upper end of ulna Ex PDX 1264 [K, M, N, P, Q, R], 1779 [B, C]

S52.091 Other fracture of upper end of **right** ulna K, M, N, P, Q, R, B, C, B, C

S52.092 Other fracture of upper end of **left** ulna K, M, N, P, Q, R, B, C, B, C

S52.099 Other fracture of upper end of **unspecified** ulna K, M, N, P, Q, R, B, C, B, C

S52.1 Fracture of **upper end of radius**

Fracture of proximal end of radius

Excludes2 physeal fractures of upper end of radius (S59.2-)
fracture of shaft of radius (S52.3-)

S52.10 **Unspecified** fracture of upper end of radius Ex PDX 1264 [K, M, N, P, Q, R], 1779 [B, C]

S52.101 Unspecified fracture of upper end of **right** radius K, M, N, P, Q, R, B, C, B, C

S52.102 Unspecified fracture of upper end of **left** radius K, M, N, P, Q, R, B, C, B, C

S52.109 Unspecified fracture of upper end of **unspecified** radius K, M, N, P, Q, R, B, C, B, C

S52.11 **Torus** fracture of upper end of radius

The appropriate 7th character is to be added to all codes in subcategory S52.11

A	initial encounter for closed fracture
D	subsequent encounter for fracture with routine healing
G	subsequent encounter for fracture with delayed healing
K	subsequent encounter for fracture with nonunion
P	subsequent encounter for fracture with malunion
S	sequela

S52.111 Torus fracture of upper end of **right** radius A, K, P, A Ex PDX 1264 [K, P], 1780 [A]

S52.112 Torus fracture of upper end of **left** radius A, K, P, A Ex PDX 1264 [K, P], 1781 [A]

S52.119 Torus fracture of upper end of **unspecified** radius A, K, P, A Ex PDX 1264 [K, P], 1782 [A]

S52.12 Fracture of **head** of radius Ex PDX 1264 [K, M, N, P, Q, R], 1269 [B, C]

S52.121 **Displaced** fracture of head of **right** radius K, M, N, P, Q, R, B, C, B, C

S52.122 **Displaced** fracture of head of **left** radius K, M, N, P, Q, R, B, C, B, C

S52.123 **Displaced** fracture of head of **unspecified** radius K, M, N, P, Q, R, B, C, B, C

S52.124 **Nondisplaced** fracture of head of **right** radius K, M, N, P, Q, R, B, C, B, C

S52.125 **Nondisplaced** fracture of head of **left** radius K, M, N, P, Q, R, B, C, B, C

S52.126 **Nondisplaced** fracture of head of **unspecified** radius K, M, N, P, Q, R, B, C, B, C

S52.13 Fracture of **neck** of radius Ex PDX 1264 [K, M, N, P, Q, R], 1779 [B, C]

S52.131 **Displaced** fracture of neck of **right** radius K, M, N, P, Q, R, B, C, B, C

S52.132 **Displaced** fracture of neck of **left** radius K, M, N, P, Q, R, B, C, B, C

S52.133 **Displaced** fracture of neck of **unspecified** radius K, M, N, P, Q, R, B, C, B, C

S52.134 **Nondisplaced** fracture of neck of **right** radius K, M, N, P, Q, R, B, C, B, C

S52.135 **Nondisplaced** fracture of neck of **left** radius K, M, N, P, Q, R, B, C, B, C

S52.136 **Nondisplaced** fracture of neck of **unspecified** radius K, M, N, P, Q, R, B, C, B, C

S52.18 **Other** fracture of upper end of radius Ex PDX 1264 [K, M, N, P, Q, R], 1779 [B, C]

S52.181 Other fracture of upper end of **right** radius K, M, N, P, Q, R, B, C, B, C

S52.182 Other fracture of upper end of **left** radius K, M, N, P, Q, R, B, C, B, C

S52.189 Other fracture of upper end of unspecified radius K, M, N, P, Q, R, B, C, B, C

S52.2 Fracture of shaft of ulna

S52.20 Unspecified fracture of shaft of ulna
Fracture of ulna NOS

S52.201 Unspecified fracture of shaft of right ulna A, K, M, N, P, Q, R, B, C, A, B, C (Ex:) PDX 1264 [K, M, N, P, Q, R], 1779 [B, C], 1780 [A]

S52.202 Unspecified fracture of shaft of left ulna A, K, M, N, P, Q, R, B, C, A, B, C (Ex:) PDX 1264 [K, M, N, P, Q, R], 1779 [B, C], 1781 [A]

S52.209 Unspecified fracture of shaft of unspecified ulna A, K, M, N, P, Q, R, B, C, A, B, C (Ex:) PDX 1264 [K, M, N, P, Q, R], 1779 [B, C], 1782 [A]

S52.21 Greenstick fracture of shaft of ulna

The appropriate 7th character is to be added to all codes in subcategory S52.21

A	initial encounter for closed fracture
D	subsequent encounter for fracture with routine healing
G	subsequent encounter for fracture with delayed healing
K	subsequent encounter for fracture with nonunion
P	subsequent encounter for fracture with malunion
S	sequela

S52.211 Greenstick fracture of shaft of right ulna A, K, P, A (Ex:) PDX 1774 [K, P], 1780 [A]

S52.212 Greenstick fracture of shaft of left ulna A, K, P, A (Ex:) PDX 1774 [K, P], 1781 [A]

S52.219 Greenstick fracture of shaft of unspecified ulna A, K, P, A (Ex:) PDX 1774 [K, P], 1782 [A]

S52.22 Transverse fracture of shaft of ulna

S52.221 Displaced transverse fracture of shaft of right ulna A, K, M, N, P, Q, R, B, C, A, B, C (Ex:) PDX 1264 [K, M, N, P, Q, R], 1779 [B, C], 1780 [A]

S52.222 Displaced transverse fracture of shaft of left ulna A, K, M, N, P, Q, R, B, C, A, B, C (Ex:) PDX 1264 [K, M, N, P, Q, R], 1779 [B, C], 1781 [A]

S52.223 Displaced transverse fracture of shaft of unspecified ulna A, K, M, N, P, Q, R, B, C, A, B, C (Ex:) PDX 1264 [K, M, N, P, Q, R], 1779 [B, C], 1782 [A]

S52.224 Nondisplaced transverse fracture of shaft of right ulna A, K, M, N, P, Q, R, B, C, A, B, C (Ex:) PDX 1264 [K, M, N, P, Q, R], 1779 [B, C], 1780 [A]

S52.225 Nondisplaced transverse fracture of shaft of left ulna A, K, M, N, P, Q, R, B, C, A, B, C (Ex:) PDX 1264 [K, M, N, P, Q, R], 1779 [B, C], 1781 [A]

S52.226 Nondisplaced transverse fracture of shaft of unspecified ulna A, K, M, N, P, Q, R, B, C, A, B, C (Ex:) PDX 1264 [K, M, N, P, Q, R], 1779 [B, C], 1782 [A]

S52.23 Oblique fracture of shaft of ulna

S52.231 Displaced oblique fracture of shaft of right ulna A, K, M, N, P, Q, R, B, C, A, B, C (Ex:) PDX 1264 [K, M, N, P, Q, R], 1779 [B, C], 1780 [A]

S52.232 Displaced oblique fracture of shaft of left ulna A, K, M, N, P, Q, R, B, C, A, B, C (Ex:) PDX 1264 [K, M, N, P, Q, R], 1779 [B, C], 1781 [A]

S52.233 Displaced oblique fracture of shaft of unspecified ulna A, K, M, N, P, Q, R, B, C, A, B, C (Ex:) PDX 1264 [K, M, N, P, Q, R], 1779 [B, C], 1782 [A]

S52.234 Nondisplaced oblique fracture of shaft of right ulna A, K, M, N, P, Q, R, B, C, A, B, C (Ex:) PDX 1264 [K, M, N, P, Q, R], 1779 [B, C], 1780 [A]

S52.235 Nondisplaced oblique fracture of shaft of left ulna A, K, M, N, P, Q, R, B, C, A, B, C (Ex:) PDX 1264 [K, M, N, P, Q, R], 1779 [B, C], 1781 [A]

S52.236 Nondisplaced oblique fracture of shaft of unspecified ulna A, K, M, N, P, Q, R, B, C, A, B, C (Ex:) PDX 1264 [K, M, N, P, Q, R], 1779 [B, C], 1782 [A]

S52.24 Spiral fracture of shaft of ulna

S52.241 Displaced spiral fracture of shaft of ulna, right arm A, K, M, N, P, Q, R, B, C, A, B, C (Ex:) PDX 1264 [K, M, N, P, Q, R], 1779 [B, C], 1780 [A]

S52.242 Displaced spiral fracture of shaft of ulna, left arm A, K, M, N, P, Q, R, B, C, A, B, C (Ex:) PDX 1264 [K, M, N, P, Q, R], 1779 [B, C], 1781 [A]

S52.243 Displaced spiral fracture of shaft of ulna, unspecified arm A, K, M, N, P, Q, R, B, C, A, B, C (Ex:) PDX 1264 [K, M, N, P, Q, R], 1779 [B, C], 1782 [A]

S52.244 Nondisplaced spiral fracture of shaft of ulna, right arm A, K, M, N, P, Q, R, B, C, A, B, C (Ex:) PDX 1264 [K, M, N, P, Q, R], 1779 [B, C], 1780 [A]

S52.245 Nondisplaced spiral fracture of shaft of ulna, left arm A, K, M, N, P, Q, R, B, C, A, B, C (Ex:) PDX 1264 [K, M, N, P, Q, R], 1779 [B, C], 1781 [A]

S52.246 Nondisplaced spiral fracture of shaft of ulna, unspecified arm A, K, M, N, P, Q, R, B, C, A, B, C (Ex:) PDX 1264 [K, M, N, P, Q, R], 1779 [B, C], 1782 [A]

S52.25 Comminuted fracture of shaft of ulna

S52.251 Displaced comminuted fracture of shaft of ulna, right arm A, K, M, N, P, Q, R, B, C, A, B, C (Ex:) PDX 1264 [K, M, N, P, Q, R], 1779 [B, C], 1780 [A]

S52.252 Displaced comminuted fracture of shaft of ulna, left arm A, K, M, N, P, Q, R, B, C, A, B, C (Ex:) PDX 1264 [K, M, N, P, Q, R], 1779 [B, C], 1781 [A]

S52.253 Displaced comminuted fracture of shaft of ulna, unspecified arm A, K, M, N, P, Q, R, B, C, A, B, C (Ex:) PDX 1264 [K, M, N, P, Q, R], 1779 [B, C], 1782 [A]

CHAPTER 19 (SØØ-T88)

S52.254 **Nondisplaced** comminuted fracture of shaft of ulna, **right** arm
A, K, M, N, P, Q, R, B, C, A, B, C (Ex) PDX 1264 [K, M, N, P, Q, R], 1779 [B, C], 1780 [A]

S52.255 **Nondisplaced** comminuted fracture of shaft of ulna, **left** arm
A, K, M, N, P, Q, R, B, C, A, B, C (Ex) PDX 1264 [K, M, N, P, Q, R], 1779 [B, C], 1781 [A]

S52.256 **Nondisplaced** comminuted fracture of shaft of ulna, **unspecified** arm
A, K, M, N, P, Q, R, B, C, A, B, C (Ex) PDX 1264 [K, M, N, P, Q, R], 1779 [B, C], 1782 [A]

S52.26 **Segmental** fracture of shaft of ulna

S52.261 **Displaced** segmental fracture of shaft of ulna, **right** arm
A, K, M, N, P, Q, R, B, C, A, B, C (Ex) PDX 1264 [K, M, N, P, Q, R], 1779 [B, C], 1780 [A]

S52.262 **Displaced** segmental fracture of shaft of ulna, **left** arm A, K, M, N, P, Q, R, B, C, A, B, C (Ex) PDX 1264 [K, M, N, P, Q, R], 1779 [B, C], 1781 [A]

S52.263 **Displaced** segmental fracture of shaft of ulna, **unspecified** arm
A, K, M, N, P, Q, R, B, C, A, B, C (Ex) PDX 1264 [K, M, N, P, Q, R], 1779 [B, C], 1782 [A]

S52.264 **Nondisplaced** segmental fracture of shaft of ulna, **right** arm
A, K, M, N, P, Q, R, B, C, A, B, C (Ex) PDX 1264 [K, M, N, P, Q, R], 1779 [B, C], 1780 [A]

S52.265 **Nondisplaced** segmental fracture of shaft of ulna, **left** arm
A, K, M, N, P, Q, R, B, C, A, B, C (Ex) PDX 1264 [K, M, N, P, Q, R], 1779 [B, C], 1781 [A]

S52.266 **Nondisplaced** segmental fracture of shaft of ulna, **unspecified** arm
A, K, M, N, P, Q, R, B, C, A, B, C (Ex) PDX 1264 [K, M, N, P, Q, R], 1779 [B, C], 1782 [A]

S52.27 **Monteggia's** fracture of ulna
Fracture of upper shaft of ulna with dislocation of radial head (Ex) PDX 1264 [K, M, N, P, Q, R], 1779 [B, C]

S52.271 Monteggia's fracture of **right** ulna
K, M, N, P, Q, R, B, C, B, C

S52.272 Monteggia's fracture of **left** ulna
K, M, N, P, Q, R, B, C, B, C

S52.279 Monteggia's fracture of **unspecified** ulna K, M, N, P, Q, R, B, C, B, C

S52.28 **Bent bone** of ulna

S52.281 Bent bone of **right** ulna
A, K, M, N, P, Q, R, B, C, A, B, C (Ex) PDX 1264 [K, M, N, P, Q, R], 1779 [B, C], 1780 [A]

S52.282 Bent bone of **left** ulna
A, K, M, N, P, Q, R, B, C, A, B, C (Ex) PDX 1264 [K, M, N, P, Q, R], 1779 [B, C], 1781 [A]

S52.283 Bent bone of **unspecified** ulna
A, K, M, N, P, Q, R, B, C, A, B, C (Ex) PDX 1264 [K, M, N, P, Q, R], 1779 [B, C], 1782 [A]

S52.29 **Other** fracture of shaft of ulna

S52.291 Other fracture of shaft of **right** ulna
A, K, M, N, P, Q, R, B, C, A, B, C (Ex) PDX 1264 [K, M, N, P, Q, R], 1779 [B, C], 1780 [A]

S52.292 Other fracture of shaft of **left** ulna
A, K, M, N, P, Q, R, B, C, A, B, C (Ex) PDX 1264 [K, M, N, P, Q, R], 1779 [B, C], 1781 [A]

S52.299 Other fracture of shaft of **unspecified** ulna A, K, M, N, P, Q, R, B, C, A, B, C (Ex) PDX 1264 [K, M, N, P, Q, R], 1779 [B, C], 1782 [A]

S52.3 Fracture of **shaft of radius**

S52.30 **Unspecified** fracture of shaft of radius

S52.301 Unspecified fracture of shaft of **right** radius A, K, M, N, P, Q, R, B, C, A, B, C (Ex) PDX 1264 [K, M, N, P, Q, R], 1779 [B, C], 1780 [A]

S52.302 Unspecified fracture of shaft of **left** radius A, K, M, N, P, Q, R, B, C, A, B, C (Ex) PDX 1264 [K, M, N, P, Q, R], 1779 [B, C], 1781 [A]

S52.309 Unspecified fracture of shaft of **unspecified** radius
A, K, M, N, P, Q, R, B, C, A, B, C (Ex) PDX 1264 [K, M, N, P, Q, R], 1779 [B, C], 1782 [A]

S52.31 **Greenstick** fracture of shaft of radius
The appropriate 7th character is to be added to all codes in subcategory S52.31

A	initial encounter for closed fracture
D	subsequent encounter for fracture with routine healing
G	subsequent encounter for fracture with delayed healing
K	subsequent encounter for fracture with nonunion
P	subsequent encounter for fracture with malunion
S	sequela

S52.311 Greenstick fracture of shaft of radius, **right** arm A, K, P, A (Ex) PDX 1264 [K, P], 1780 [A]

S52.312 Greenstick fracture of shaft of radius, **left** arm A, K, P, A (Ex) PDX 1264 [K, P], 1781 [A]

S52.319 Greenstick fracture of shaft of radius, **unspecified** arm A, K, P, A (Ex) PDX 1264 [K, P], 1782 [A]

S52.32 **Transverse** fracture of shaft of radius

S52.321 **Displaced** transverse fracture of shaft of **right** radius A, K, M, N, P, Q, R, B, C, A, B, C (Ex) PDX 1264 [K, M, N, P, Q, R], 1779 [B, C], 1780 [A]

S52.322 **Displaced** transverse fracture of shaft of **left** radius A, K, M, N, P, Q, R, B, C, A, B, C (Ex) PDX 1264 [K, M, N, P, Q, R], 1779 [B, C], 1781 [A]

S52.323 **Displaced** transverse fracture of shaft of **unspecified** radius
A, K, M, N, P, Q, R, B, C, A, B, C (Ex) PDX 1264 [K, M, N, P, Q, R], 1779 [B, C], 1782 [A]

S52.324 **Nondisplaced** transverse fracture of shaft of **right** radius
A, K, M, N, P, Q, R, B, C, A, B, C (Ex) PDX 1264 [K, M, N, P, Q, R], 1779 [B, C], 1780 [A]

S52.325 **Nondisplaced** transverse fracture of shaft of **left** radius
A, K, M, N, P, Q, R, B, C, A, B, C (Ex) PDX 1264 [K, M, N, P, Q, R], 1779 [B, C], 1781 [A]

S52.326 **Nondisplaced** transverse fracture of shaft of **unspecified** radius
A, K, M, N, P, Q, R, B, C, A, B, C (Ex) PDX 1264 [K, M, N, P, Q, R], 1779 [B, C], 1782 [A]

S52.33 Oblique fracture of shaft of radius

S52.331 Displaced oblique fracture of shaft of right radius A, K, M, N, P, Q, R, B, C, A, B, C PDX 1264 [K, M, N, P, Q, R], 1779 [B, C], 1780 [A]

S52.332 Displaced oblique fracture of shaft of left radius A, K, M, N, P, Q, R, B, C, A, B, C PDX 1264 [K, M, N, P, Q, R], 1779 [B, C], 1781 [A]

S52.333 Displaced oblique fracture of shaft of unspecified radius A, K, M, N, P, Q, R, B, C, A, B, C PDX 1264 [K, M, N, P, Q, R], 1779 [B, C], 1782 [A]

S52.334 Nondisplaced oblique fracture of shaft of right radius A, K, M, N, P, Q, R, B, C, A, B, C PDX 1264 [K, M, N, P, Q, R], 1779 [B, C], 1780 [A]

S52.335 Nondisplaced oblique fracture of shaft of left radius A, K, M, N, P, Q, R, B, C, A, B, C PDX 1264 [K, M, N, P, Q, R], 1779 [B, C], 1781 [A]

S52.336 Nondisplaced oblique fracture of shaft of unspecified radius A, K, M, N, P, Q, R, B, C, A, B, C PDX 1264 [K, M, N, P, Q, R], 1779 [B, C], 1782 [A]

S52.34 Spiral fracture of shaft of radius

S52.341 Displaced spiral fracture of shaft of radius, right arm A, K, M, N, P, Q, R, B, C, A, B, C PDX 1264 [K, M, N, P, Q, R], 1779 [B, C], 1780 [A]

S52.342 Displaced spiral fracture of shaft of radius, left arm A, K, M, N, P, Q, R, B, C, A, B, C PDX 1264 [K, M, N, P, Q, R], 1779 [B, C], 1781 [A]

S52.343 Displaced spiral fracture of shaft of radius, unspecified arm A, K, M, N, P, Q, R, B, C, A, B, C PDX 1264 [K, M, N, P, Q, R], 1779 [B, C], 1782 [A]

S52.344 Nondisplaced spiral fracture of shaft of radius, right arm A, K, M, N, P, Q, R, B, C, A, B, C PDX 1264 [K, M, N, P, Q, R], 1779 [B, C], 1780 [A]

S52.345 Nondisplaced spiral fracture of shaft of radius, left arm A, K, M, N, P, Q, R, B, C, A, B, C PDX 1264 [K, M, N, P, Q, R], 1779 [B, C], 1781 [A]

S52.346 Nondisplaced spiral fracture of shaft of radius, unspecified arm A, K, M, N, P, Q, R, B, C, A, B, C PDX 1264 [K, M, N, P, Q, R], 1779 [B, C], 1782 [A]

S52.35 Comminuted fracture of shaft of radius

S52.351 Displaced comminuted fracture of shaft of radius, right arm A, K, M, N, P, Q, R, B, C, A, B, C PDX 1264 [K, M, N, P, Q, R], 1779 [B, C], 1780 [A]

S52.352 Displaced comminuted fracture of shaft of radius, left arm A, K, M, N, P, Q, R, B, C, A, B, C PDX 1264 [K, M, N, P, Q, R], 1779 [B, C], 1781 [A]

S52.353 Displaced comminuted fracture of shaft of radius, unspecified arm A, K, M, N, P, Q, R, B, C, A, B, C PDX 1264 [K, M, N, P, Q, R], 1779 [B, C], 1782 [A]

S52.354 Nondisplaced comminuted fracture of shaft of radius, right arm A, K, M, N, P, Q, R, B, C, A, B, C PDX 1264 [K, M, N, P, Q, R], 1779 [B, C], 1780 [A]

S52.355 Nondisplaced comminuted fracture of shaft of radius, left arm A, K, M, N, P, Q, R, B, C, A, B, C PDX 1264 [K, M, N, P, Q, R], 1779 [B, C], 1781 [A]

S52.356 Nondisplaced comminuted fracture of shaft of radius, unspecified arm A, K, M, N, P, Q, R, B, C, A, B, C PDX 1264 [K, M, N, P, Q, R], 1779 [B, C], 1782 [A]

S52.36 Segmental fracture of shaft of radius

S52.361 Displaced segmental fracture of shaft of radius, right arm A, K, M, N, P, Q, R, B, C, A, B, C PDX 1264 [K, M, N, P, Q, R], 1779 [B, C], 1780 [A]

S52.362 Displaced segmental fracture of shaft of radius, left arm A, K, M, N, P, Q, R, B, C, A, B, C PDX 1264 [K, M, N, P, Q, R], 1779 [B, C], 1781 [A]

S52.363 Displaced segmental fracture of shaft of radius, unspecified arm A, K, M, N, P, Q, R, B, C, A, B, C PDX 1264 [K, M, N, P, Q, R], 1779 [B, C], 1782 [A]

S52.364 Nondisplaced segmental fracture of shaft of radius, right arm A, K, M, N, P, Q, R, B, C, A, B, C PDX 1264 [K, M, N, P, Q, R], 1779 [B, C], 1780 [A]

S52.365 Nondisplaced segmental fracture of shaft of radius, left arm A, K, M, N, P, Q, R, B, C, A, B, C PDX 1264 [K, M, N, P, Q, R], 1779 [B, C], 1781 [A]

S52.366 Nondisplaced segmental fracture of shaft of radius, unspecified arm A, K, M, N, P, Q, R, B, C, A, B, C PDX 1264 [K, M, N, P, Q, R], 1779 [B, C], 1782 [A]

S52.37 Galeazzi's fracture

Fracture of lower shaft of radius with radioulnar joint dislocation

S52.371 Galeazzi's fracture of right radius A, K, M, N, P, Q, R, B, C, A, B, C PDX 1264 [K, M, N, P, Q, R], 1779 [B, C], 1780 [A]

S52.372 Galeazzi's fracture of left radius A, K, M, N, P, Q, R, B, C, A, B, C PDX 1264 [K, M, N, P, Q, R], 1779 [B, C], 1781 [A]

S52.379 Galeazzi's fracture of unspecified radius A, K, M, N, P, Q, R, B, C, A, B, C PDX 1264 [K, M, N, P, Q, R], 1779 [B, C], 1782 [A]

S52.38 Bent bone of radius

S52.381 Bent bone of right radius A, K, M, N, P, Q, R, B, C, A, B, C PDX 1264 [K, M, N, P, Q, R], 1779 [B, C], 1780 [A]

S52.382 Bent bone of left radius A, K, M, N, P, Q, R, B, C, A, B, C PDX 1264 [K, M, N, P, Q, R], 1779 [B, C], 1781 [A]

S52.389 Bent bone of unspecified radius A, K, M, N, P, Q, R, B, C, A, B, C PDX 1264 [K, M, N, P, Q, R], 1779 [B, C], 1782 [A]

CHAPTER 19 (S00-T88)

● S52.39 Other fracture of shaft of radius

● S52.391 Other fracture of shaft of radius, right arm A, K, M, N, P, Q, R, B, C, A, B, C (Ex) PDX 1264 [K, M, N, P, Q, R], 1779 [B, C], 1780 [A]

● S52.392 Other fracture of shaft of radius, left arm A, K, M, N, P, Q, R, B, C, A, B, C (Ex) PDX 1264 [K, M, N, P, Q, R], 1779 [B, C], 1781 [A]

● S52.399 Other fracture of shaft of radius, unspecified arm A, K, M, N, P, Q, R, B, C, A, B, C (Ex) PDX 1264 [K, M, N, P, Q, R], 1779 [B, C], 1782 [A]

● S52.5 Fracture of lower end of radius

Fracture of distal end of radius

Excludes2 physeal fractures of lower end of radius (S59.2-)

● S52.50 Unspecified fracture of the lower end of radius

● S52.501 Unspecified fracture of the lower end of right radius A, K, M, N, P, Q, R, B, C, A, B, C (Ex) PDX 1264 [K, M, N, P, Q, R], 1779 [B, C], 1780 [A]

● S52.502 Unspecified fracture of the lower end of left radius A, K, M, N, P, Q, R, B, C, A, B, C (Ex) PDX 1264 [K, M, N, P, Q, R], 1779 [B, C], 1781 [A]

● S52.509 Unspecified fracture of the lower end of unspecified radius A, K, M, N, P, Q, R, B, C, A, B, C (Ex) PDX 1264 [K, M, N, P, Q, R], 1779 [B, C], 1782 [A]

● S52.51 Fracture of radial styloid process

● S52.511 Displaced fracture of right radial styloid process A, K, M, N, P, Q, R, B, C, A, B, C (Ex) PDX 1264 [K, M, N, P, Q, R], 1779 [B, C], 1780 [A]

● S52.512 Displaced fracture of left radial styloid process A, K, M, N, P, Q, R, B, C, A, B, C (Ex) PDX 1264 [K, M, N, P, Q, R], 1779 [B, C], 1781 [A]

● S52.513 Displaced fracture of unspecified radial styloid process A, K, M, N, P, Q, R, B, C, A, B, C (Ex) PDX 1264 [K, M, N, P, Q, R], 1779 [B, C], 1782 [A]

● S52.514 Nondisplaced fracture of right radial styloid process A, K, M, N, P, Q, R, B, C, A, B, C (Ex) PDX 1264 [K, M, N, P, Q, R], 1779 [B, C], 1780 [A]

● S52.515 Nondisplaced fracture of left radial styloid process A, K, M, N, P, Q, R, B, C, A, B, C (Ex) PDX 1264 [K, M, N, P, Q, R], 1779 [B, C], 1781 [A]

● S52.516 Nondisplaced fracture of unspecified radial styloid process A, K, M, N, P, Q, R, B, C, A, B, C (Ex) PDX 1264 [K, M, N, P, Q, R], 1779 [B, C], 1782 [A]

● S52.52 Torus fracture of lower end of radius

The appropriate 7th character is to be added to all codes in subcategory S52.52

A	initial encounter for closed fracture
D	subsequent encounter for fracture with routine healing
G	subsequent encounter for fracture with delayed healing
K	subsequent encounter for fracture with nonunion
P	subsequent encounter for fracture with malunion
S	sequela

● S52.521 Torus fracture of lower end of right radius A, K, P, A (Ex) PDX 1264 [K, P], 1780 [A]

● S52.522 Torus fracture of lower end of left radius A, K, P, A (Ex) PDX 1264 [K, P], 1781 [A]

● S52.529 Torus fracture of lower end of unspecified radius A, K, P, A (Ex) PDX 1264 [K, P], 1782 [A]

● S52.53 Colles' fracture

● S52.531 Colles' fracture of right radius A, K, M, N, P, Q, R, B, C, A, B, C (Ex) PDX 1264 [K, M, N, P, Q, R], 1779 [B, C], 1780 [A]

● S52.532 Colles' fracture of left radius A, K, M, N, P, Q, R, B, C, A, B, C (Ex) PDX 1264 [K, M, N, P, Q, R], 1779 [B, C], 1781 [A]

Coding Clinic: 2016, Q2, P5

● S52.539 Colles' fracture of unspecified radius A, K, M, N, P, Q, R, B, C, A, B, C (Ex) PDX 1264 [K, M, N, P, Q, R], 1779 [B, C], 1782 [A]

● S52.54 Smith's fracture

● S52.541 Smith's fracture of right radius A, K, M, N, P, Q, R, B, C, A, B, C (Ex) PDX 1264 [K, M, N, P, Q, R], 1779 [B, C], 1780 [A]

● S52.542 Smith's fracture of left radius A, K, M, N, P, Q, R, B, C, A, B, C (Ex) PDX 1264 [K, M, N, P, Q, R], 1779 [B, C], 1781 [A]

● S52.549 Smith's fracture of unspecified radius A, K, M, N, P, Q, R, B, C, A, B, C (Ex) PDX 1264 [K, M, N, P, Q, R], 1779 [B, C], 1782 [A]

● S52.55 Other extraarticular fracture of lower end of radius

● S52.551 Other extraarticular fracture of lower end of right radius A, K, M, N, P, Q, R, B, C, A, B, C (Ex) PDX 1264 [K, M, N, P, Q, R], 1779 [B, C], 1780 [A]

● S52.552 Other extraarticular fracture of lower end of left radius A, K, M, N, P, Q, R, B, C, A, B, C (Ex) PDX 1264 [K, M, N, P, Q, R], 1779 [B, C], 1781 [A]

● S52.559 Other extraarticular fracture of lower end of unspecified radius A, K, M, N, P, Q, R, B, C, A, B, C (Ex) PDX 1264 [K, M, N, P, Q, R], 1779 [B, C], 1782 [A]

● S52.56 Barton's fracture

● S52.561 Barton's fracture of right radius A, K, M, N, P, Q, R, B, C, A, B, C (Ex) PDX 1264 [K, M, N, P, Q, R], 1779 [B, C], 1780 [A]

● S52.562 Barton's fracture of left radius A, K, M, N, P, Q, R, B, C, A, B, C (Ex) PDX 1264 [K, M, N, P, Q, R], 1779 [B, C], 1781 [A]

● S52.569 Barton's fracture of unspecified radius A, K, M, N, P, Q, R, B, C, A, B, C (Ex) PDX 1264 [K, M, N, P, Q, R], 1779 [B, C], 1782 [A]

● S52.57 Other intraarticular fracture of lower end of radius

● S52.571 Other intraarticular fracture of lower end of right radius A, K, M, N, P, Q, R, B, C, A, B, C (Ex) PDX 1264 [K, M, N, P, Q, R], 1779 [B, C], 1780 [A]

- S52.572 **Other intraarticular fracture of lower end of left radius** A, K, M, N, P, Q, R, B, C, A, B, C (Ex) PDX 1264 [K, M, N, P, Q, R], 1779 [B, C], 1781 [A]
- S52.579 **Other intraarticular fracture of lower end of unspecified radius** A, K, M, N, P, Q, R, B, C, A, B, C (Ex) PDX 1264 [K, M, N, P, Q, R], 1779 [B, C], 1782 [A]
- S52.59 **Other fractures of lower end of radius**
  - S52.591 **Other fractures of lower end of right radius** A, K, M, N, P, Q, R, B, C, A, B, C (Ex) PDX 1264 [K, M, N, P, Q, R], 1779 [B, C], 1780 [A]
    Coding Clinic: 2019, Q3, P10
  - S52.592 **Other fractures of lower end of left radius** A, K, M, N, P, Q, R, B, C, A, B, C (Ex) PDX 1264 [K, M, N, P, Q, R], 1779 [B, C], 1781 [A]
  - S52.599 **Other fractures of lower end of unspecified radius** A, K, M, N, P, Q, R, B, C, A, B, C (Ex) PDX 1264 [K, M, N, P, Q, R], 1779 [B, C], 1782 [A]

S52.6 Fracture of lower end of ulna

- S52.60 **Unspecified fracture of lower end of ulna**
  - S52.601 **Unspecified fracture of lower end of right ulna** A, K, M, N, P, Q, R, B, C, A, B, C (Ex) PDX 1264 [K, M, N, P, Q, R], 1779 [B, C], 1780 [A]
  - S52.602 **Unspecified fracture of lower end of left ulna** A, K, M, N, P, Q, R, B, C, A, B, C (Ex) PDX 1264 [K, M, N, P, Q, R], 1779 [B, C], 1781 [A]
  - S52.609 **Unspecified fracture of lower end of unspecified ulna** A, K, M, N, P, Q, R, B, C, A, B, C (Ex) PDX 1264 [K, M, N, P, Q, R], 1779 [B, C], 1782 [A]
- S52.61 **Fracture of ulna styloid process**
  - S52.611 **Displaced fracture of right ulna styloid process** A, K, M, N, P, Q, R, B, C, A, B, C (Ex) PDX 1264 [K, M, N, P, Q, R], 1779 [B, C], 1780 [A]
  - S52.612 **Displaced fracture of left ulna styloid process** A, K, M, N, P, Q, R, B, C, A, B, C (Ex) PDX 1264 [K, M, N, P, Q, R], 1779 [B, C], 1781 [A]
  - S52.613 **Displaced fracture of unspecified ulna styloid process** A, K, M, N, P, Q, R, B, C, A, B, C (Ex) PDX 1264 [K, M, N, P, Q, R], 1779 [B, C], 1782 [A]
  - S52.614 **Nondisplaced fracture of right ulna styloid process** A, K, M, N, P, Q, R, B, C, A, B, C (Ex) PDX 1264 [K, M, N, P, Q, R], 1779 [B, C], 1780 [A]
  - S52.615 **Nondisplaced fracture of left ulna styloid process** A, K, M, N, P, Q, R, B, C, A, B, C (Ex) PDX 1264 [K, M, N, P, Q, R], 1779 [B, C], 1781 [A]
  - S52.616 **Nondisplaced fracture of unspecified ulna styloid process** A, K, M, N, P, Q, R, B, C, A, B, C (Ex) PDX 1264 [K, M, N, P, Q, R], 1779 [B, C], 1782 [A]
- S52.62 **Torus fracture of lower end of ulna**
  The appropriate 7th character is to be added to all codes in subcategory S52.62

A	initial encounter for closed fracture
D	subsequent encounter for fracture with routine healing
G	subsequent encounter for fracture with delayed healing
K	subsequent encounter for fracture with nonunion
P	subsequent encounter for fracture with malunion
S	sequela

  - S52.621 **Torus fracture of lower end of right ulna** A, K, P, A (Ex) PDX 1264 [K, P], 1780 [A]
  - S52.622 **Torus fracture of lower end of left ulna** A, K, P, A (Ex) PDX 1264 [K, P], 1781 [A]
  - S52.629 **Torus fracture of lower end of unspecified ulna** A, K, P, A (Ex) PDX 1264 [K, P], 1782 [A]
- S52.69 **Other fracture of lower end of ulna**
  - S52.691 **Other fracture of lower end of right ulna** A, K, M, N, P, Q, R, B, C, A, B, C (Ex) PDX 1264 [K, M, N, P, Q, R], 1779 [B, C], 1780 [A]
    Coding Clinic: 2019, Q3, P10
  - S52.692 **Other fracture of lower end of left ulna** A, K, M, N, P, Q, R, B, C, A, B, C (Ex) PDX 1264 [K, M, N, P, Q, R], 1779 [B, C], 1781 [A]
  - S52.699 **Other fracture of lower end of unspecified ulna** A, K, M, N, P, Q, R, B, C, A, B, C (Ex) PDX 1264 [K, M, N, P, Q, R], 1779 [B, C], 1782 [A]

S52.9 Unspecified fracture of forearm (Ex) PDX 1264 [K, M, N, P, Q, R], 1779 [B, C], 1782 [A]

- X S52.90 **Unspecified fracture of unspecified forearm** A, K, M, N, P, Q, R, B, C, A, B, C
- X S52.91 **Unspecified fracture of right forearm** A, K, M, N, P, Q, R, B, C, A, B, C
- X S52.92 **Unspecified fracture of left forearm** A, K, M, N, P, Q, R, B, C, A, B, C

S53 Dislocation and sprain of joints and ligaments of elbow

Includes avulsion of joint or ligament of elbow
laceration of cartilage, joint or ligament of elbow
sprain of cartilage, joint or ligament of elbow
traumatic hemarthrosis of joint or ligament of elbow
traumatic rupture of joint or ligament of elbow
traumatic subluxation of joint or ligament of elbow
traumatic tear of joint or ligament of elbow

Code also any associated open wound

Excludes2 strain of muscle, fascia and tendon at forearm level (S56.-)

The appropriate 7th character is to be added to each code from category S53

A	initial encounter
D	subsequent encounter
S	sequela

S53.0 Subluxation and dislocation of radial head
Dislocation of radiohumeral joint
Subluxation of radiohumeral joint
Excludes1 Monteggia's fracture-dislocation (S52.27-)

- S53.00 **Unspecified subluxation and dislocation of radial head**
  - S53.001 **Unspecified subluxation of right radial head**
  - S53.002 **Unspecified subluxation of left radial head**

N Newborn Age: 0 **P** Pediatric Age: 0–17 **M** Maternity DX: 9–64 **A** Adult Age: 15–124

Complication\Comorbidity · Major C\C · CC/MCC Exclusions · Hospital-Acquired Condition · Hierarchical Condition Category

S53.003 Unspecified subluxation of unspecified radial head
S53.004 Unspecified dislocation of right radial head
S53.005 Unspecified dislocation of left radial head
S53.006 Unspecified dislocation of unspecified radial head
S53.01 Anterior subluxation and dislocation of radial head
Anteriomedial subluxation and dislocation of radial head
S53.011 Anterior subluxation of right radial head
S53.012 Anterior subluxation of left radial head
S53.013 Anterior subluxation of unspecified radial head
S53.014 Anterior dislocation of right radial head
S53.015 Anterior dislocation of left radial head
S53.016 Anterior dislocation of unspecified radial head
S53.02 Posterior subluxation and dislocation of radial head
Posteriolateral subluxation and dislocation of radial head
S53.021 Posterior subluxation of right radial head
S53.022 Posterior subluxation of left radial head
S53.023 Posterior subluxation of unspecified radial head
S53.024 Posterior dislocation of right radial head
S53.025 Posterior dislocation of left radial head
S53.026 Posterior dislocation of unspecified radial head
S53.03 Nursemaid's elbow
S53.031 Nursemaid's elbow, right elbow
Coding Clinic: 2015, Q1, P7-8
S53.032 Nursemaid's elbow, left elbow
S53.033 Nursemaid's elbow, unspecified elbow
S53.09 Other subluxation and dislocation of radial head
S53.091 Other subluxation of right radial head
S53.092 Other subluxation of left radial head
S53.093 Other subluxation of unspecified radial head
S53.094 Other dislocation of right radial head
S53.095 Other dislocation of left radial head
S53.096 Other dislocation of unspecified radial head
S53.1 Subluxation and dislocation of ulnohumeral joint
Subluxation and dislocation of elbow NOS
Excludes1 dislocation of radial head alone (S53.0-)
S53.10 Unspecified subluxation and dislocation of ulnohumeral joint
S53.101 Unspecified subluxation of right ulnohumeral joint
S53.102 Unspecified subluxation of left ulnohumeral joint
S53.103 Unspecified subluxation of unspecified ulnohumeral joint
S53.104 Unspecified dislocation of right ulnohumeral joint
S53.105 Unspecified dislocation of left ulnohumeral joint
S53.106 Unspecified dislocation of unspecified ulnohumeral joint
S53.11 Anterior subluxation and dislocation of ulnohumeral joint
S53.111 Anterior subluxation of right ulnohumeral joint
S53.112 Anterior subluxation of left ulnohumeral joint
S53.113 Anterior subluxation of unspecified ulnohumeral joint
S53.114 Anterior dislocation of right ulnohumeral joint
Coding Clinic: 2012, Q4, P108
S53.115 Anterior dislocation of left ulnohumeral joint
S53.116 Anterior dislocation of unspecified ulnohumeral joint
S53.12 Posterior subluxation and dislocation of ulnohumeral joint
S53.121 Posterior subluxation of right ulnohumeral joint
S53.122 Posterior subluxation of left ulnohumeral joint
S53.123 Posterior subluxation of unspecified ulnohumeral joint
S53.124 Posterior dislocation of right ulnohumeral joint
S53.125 Posterior dislocation of left ulnohumeral joint
S53.126 Posterior dislocation of unspecified ulnohumeral joint
S53.13 Medial subluxation and dislocation of ulnohumeral joint
S53.131 Medial subluxation of right ulnohumeral joint
S53.132 Medial subluxation of left ulnohumeral joint
S53.133 Medial subluxation of unspecified ulnohumeral joint
S53.134 Medial dislocation of right ulnohumeral joint
S53.135 Medial dislocation of left ulnohumeral joint
S53.136 Medial dislocation of unspecified ulnohumeral joint
S53.14 Lateral subluxation and dislocation of ulnohumeral joint
S53.141 Lateral subluxation of right ulnohumeral joint
S53.142 Lateral subluxation of left ulnohumeral joint
S53.143 Lateral subluxation of unspecified ulnohumeral joint
S53.144 Lateral dislocation of right ulnohumeral joint
S53.145 Lateral dislocation of left ulnohumeral joint
S53.146 Lateral dislocation of unspecified ulnohumeral joint
S53.19 Other subluxation and dislocation of ulnohumeral joint
S53.191 Other subluxation of right ulnohumeral joint
S53.192 Other subluxation of left ulnohumeral joint
S53.193 Other subluxation of unspecified ulnohumeral joint
S53.194 Other dislocation of right ulnohumeral joint

- S53.195 Other dislocation of left ulnohumeral joint
- S53.196 Other dislocation of unspecified ulnohumeral joint

S53.2 Traumatic rupture of radial collateral ligament

Excludes1 sprain of radial collateral ligament NOS (S53.43-)

- X S53.2Ø Traumatic rupture of unspecified radial collateral ligament
- X S53.21 Traumatic rupture of right radial collateral ligament
- X S53.22 Traumatic rupture of left radial collateral ligament

S53.3 Traumatic rupture of ulnar collateral ligament

Excludes1 sprain of ulnar collateral ligament (S53.44-)

- X S53.3Ø Traumatic rupture of unspecified ulnar collateral ligament
- X S53.31 Traumatic rupture of right ulnar collateral ligament
- X S53.32 Traumatic rupture of left ulnar collateral ligament

S53.4 Sprain of elbow

Excludes2 traumatic rupture of radial collateral ligament (S53.2-)
traumatic rupture of ulnar collateral ligament (S53.3-)

S53.4Ø Unspecified sprain of elbow
- S53.4Ø1 Unspecified sprain of right elbow
- S53.4Ø2 Unspecified sprain of left elbow
- S53.4Ø9 Unspecified sprain of unspecified elbow
  Sprain of elbow NOS

S53.41 Radiohumeral (joint) sprain
- S53.411 Radiohumeral (joint) sprain of right elbow
- S53.412 Radiohumeral (joint) sprain of left elbow
- S53.419 Radiohumeral (joint) sprain of unspecified elbow

S53.42 Ulnohumeral (joint) sprain
- S53.421 Ulnohumeral (joint) sprain of right elbow
- S53.422 Ulnohumeral (joint) sprain of left elbow
- S53.429 Ulnohumeral (joint) sprain of unspecified elbow

S53.43 Radial collateral ligament sprain
- S53.431 Radial collateral ligament sprain of right elbow
- S53.432 Radial collateral ligament sprain of left elbow
- S53.439 Radial collateral ligament sprain of unspecified elbow

S53.44 Ulnar collateral ligament sprain
- S53.441 Ulnar collateral ligament sprain of right elbow
- S53.442 Ulnar collateral ligament sprain of left elbow
- S53.449 Ulnar collateral ligament sprain of unspecified elbow

S53.49 Other sprain of elbow
- S53.491 Other sprain of right elbow
- S53.492 Other sprain of left elbow
- S53.499 Other sprain of unspecified elbow

S54 Injury of nerves at forearm level

Code also any associated open wound (S51.-)

Excludes2 injury of nerves at wrist and hand level (S64.-)

The appropriate 7th character is to be added to each code from category S54

A	initial encounter
D	subsequent encounter
S	sequela

S54.Ø Injury of ulnar nerve at forearm level
Injury of ulnar nerve NOS
- X S54.ØØ Injury of ulnar nerve at forearm level, unspecified arm
- X S54.Ø1 Injury of ulnar nerve at forearm level, right arm
- X S54.Ø2 Injury of ulnar nerve at forearm level, left arm

S54.1 Injury of median nerve at forearm level
Injury of median nerve NOS
- X S54.1Ø Injury of median nerve at forearm level, unspecified arm
- X S54.11 Injury of median nerve at forearm level, right arm
- X S54.12 Injury of median nerve at forearm level, left arm

S54.2 Injury of radial nerve at forearm level
Injury of radial nerve NOS
- X S54.2Ø Injury of radial nerve at forearm level, unspecified arm
- X S54.21 Injury of radial nerve at forearm level, right arm
- X S54.22 Injury of radial nerve at forearm level, left arm

S54.3 Injury of cutaneous sensory nerve at forearm level
- X S54.3Ø Injury of cutaneous sensory nerve at forearm level, unspecified arm
- X S54.31 Injury of cutaneous sensory nerve at forearm level, right arm
- X S54.32 Injury of cutaneous sensory nerve at forearm level, left arm

S54.8 Injury of other nerves at forearm level
- S54.8X Injury of other nerves at forearm level
  - S54.8X1 Injury of other nerves at forearm level, right arm
  - S54.8X2 Injury of other nerves at forearm level, left arm
  - S54.8X9 Injury of other nerves at forearm level, unspecified arm

S54.9 Injury of unspecified nerve at forearm level
- X S54.9Ø Injury of unspecified nerve at forearm level, unspecified arm
- X S54.91 Injury of unspecified nerve at forearm level, right arm
- X S54.92 Injury of unspecified nerve at forearm level, left arm

S55 Injury of blood vessels at forearm level

Code also any associated open wound (S51.-)

Excludes2 injury of blood vessels at wrist and hand level (S65.-)
injury of brachial vessels (S45.1-S45.2)

The appropriate 7th character is to be added to each code from category S55

A	initial encounter
D	subsequent encounter
S	sequela

S55.Ø Injury of ulnar artery at forearm level
- S55.ØØ Unspecified injury of ulnar artery at forearm level
  - S55.ØØ1 Unspecified injury of ulnar artery at forearm level, right arm
    A Ex PDX 1784

CHAPTER 19 (SØØ-T88)

- S55.002 Unspecified injury of ulnar artery at forearm level, left arm A Ex PDX 1785
- S55.009 Unspecified injury of ulnar artery at forearm level, unspecified arm A Ex PDX 1786

S55.01 Laceration of ulnar artery at forearm level
- S55.011 Laceration of ulnar artery at forearm level, right arm A Ex PDX 1784
- S55.012 Laceration of ulnar artery at forearm level, left arm A Ex PDX 1785
- S55.019 Laceration of ulnar artery at forearm level, unspecified arm A Ex PDX 1786

S55.09 Other specified injury of ulnar artery at forearm level
- S55.091 Other specified injury of ulnar artery at forearm level, right arm A Ex PDX 1784
- S55.092 Other specified injury of ulnar artery at forearm level, left arm A Ex PDX 1785
- S55.099 Other specified injury of ulnar artery at forearm level, unspecified arm A Ex PDX 1786

S55.1 Injury of radial artery at forearm level

S55.10 Unspecified injury of radial artery at forearm level
- S55.101 Unspecified injury of radial artery at forearm level, right arm A Ex PDX 1787
- S55.102 Unspecified injury of radial artery at forearm level, left arm A Ex PDX 1788
- S55.109 Unspecified injury of radial artery at forearm level, unspecified arm A Ex PDX 1789

S55.11 Laceration of radial artery at forearm level
- S55.111 Laceration of radial artery at forearm level, right arm A Ex PDX 1787
- S55.112 Laceration of radial artery at forearm level, left arm A Ex PDX 1788
- S55.119 Laceration of radial artery at forearm level, unspecified arm A Ex PDX 1789

S55.19 Other specified injury of radial artery at forearm level
- S55.191 Other specified injury of radial artery at forearm level, right arm A Ex PDX 1787
- S55.192 Other specified injury of radial artery at forearm level, left arm A Ex PDX 1788
- S55.199 Other specified injury of radial artery at forearm level, unspecified arm A Ex PDX 1789

S55.2 Injury of vein at forearm level

S55.20 Unspecified injury of vein at forearm level
- S55.201 Unspecified injury of vein at forearm level, right arm A Ex PDX 1770
- S55.202 Unspecified injury of vein at forearm level, left arm A Ex PDX 1771
- S55.209 Unspecified injury of vein at forearm level, unspecified arm A Ex PDX 1772

S55.21 Laceration of vein at forearm level
- S55.211 Laceration of vein at forearm level, right arm A Ex PDX 1770
- S55.212 Laceration of vein at forearm level, left arm A Ex PDX 1771
- S55.219 Laceration of vein at forearm level, unspecified arm A Ex PDX 1772

S55.29 Other specified injury of vein at forearm level
- S55.291 Other specified injury of vein at forearm level, right arm A Ex PDX 1770
- S55.292 Other specified injury of vein at forearm level, left arm A Ex PDX 1771
- S55.299 Other specified injury of vein at forearm level, unspecified arm A Ex PDX 1772

S55.8 Injury of other blood vessels at forearm level

S55.80 Unspecified injury of other blood vessels at forearm level
- S55.801 Unspecified injury of other blood vessels at forearm level, right arm A Ex PDX 1770
- S55.802 Unspecified injury of other blood vessels at forearm level, left arm A Ex PDX 1771
- S55.809 Unspecified injury of other blood vessels at forearm level, unspecified arm A Ex PDX 1772

S55.81 Laceration of other blood vessels at forearm level
- S55.811 Laceration of other blood vessels at forearm level, right arm A Ex PDX 1770
- S55.812 Laceration of other blood vessels at forearm level, left arm A Ex PDX 1771
- S55.819 Laceration of other blood vessels at forearm level, unspecified arm A Ex PDX 1772

S55.89 Other specified injury of other blood vessels at forearm level
- S55.891 Other specified injury of other blood vessels at forearm level, right arm A Ex PDX 1770
- S55.892 Other specified injury of other blood vessels at forearm level, left arm A Ex PDX 1771
- S55.899 Other specified injury of other blood vessels at forearm level, unspecified arm A Ex PDX 1772

S55.9 Injury of unspecified blood vessel at forearm level

S55.90 Unspecified injury of unspecified blood vessel at forearm level
- S55.901 Unspecified injury of unspecified blood vessel at forearm level, right arm A Ex PDX 1770
- S55.902 Unspecified injury of unspecified blood vessel at forearm level, left arm A Ex PDX 1771
- S55.909 Unspecified injury of unspecified blood vessel at forearm level, unspecified arm A Ex PDX 1772

S55.91 Laceration of unspecified blood vessel at forearm level
- S55.911 Laceration of unspecified blood v essel at forearm level, right arm A Ex PDX 1770
- S55.912 Laceration of unspecified blood vessel at forearm level, left arm A Ex PDX 1771
- S55.919 Laceration of unspecified blood vessel at forearm level, unspecified arm A Ex PDX 1772

S55.99 Other specified injury of unspecified blood vessel at forearm level
- S55.991 Other specified injury of unspecified blood vessel at forearm level, right arm A Ex PDX 1770
- S55.992 Other specified injury of unspecified blood vessel at forearm level, left arm A Ex PDX 1771

CHAPTER 19 (S00-T88)

- **S55.999** Other specified injury of unspecified blood vessel at forearm level, unspecified arm A PDX 1772

S56 Injury of muscle, fascia and tendon at forearm level

Code also any associated open wound (S51.-)

Excludes2 injury of muscle, fascia and tendon at or below wrist (S66.-)
sprain of joints and ligaments of elbow (S53.4-)

The appropriate 7th character is to be added to each code from category S56

A	initial encounter
D	subsequent encounter
S	sequela

- **S56.0** Injury of flexor muscle, fascia and tendon of thumb at forearm level
  - **S56.00** Unspecified injury of flexor muscle, fascia and tendon of thumb at forearm level
    - **S56.001** Unspecified injury of flexor muscle, fascia and tendon of right thumb at forearm level
    - **S56.002** Unspecified injury of flexor muscle, fascia and tendon of left thumb at forearm level
    - **S56.009** Unspecified injury of flexor muscle, fascia and tendon of unspecified thumb at forearm level
  - **S56.01** Strain of flexor muscle, fascia and tendon of thumb at forearm level
    - **S56.011** Strain of flexor muscle, fascia and tendon of right thumb at forearm level
    - **S56.012** Strain of flexor muscle, fascia and tendon of left thumb at forearm level
    - **S56.019** Strain of flexor muscle, fascia and tendon of unspecified thumb at forearm level
  - **S56.02** Laceration of flexor muscle, fascia and tendon of thumb at forearm level
    - **S56.021** Laceration of flexor muscle, fascia and tendon of right thumb at forearm level A PDX 1790
    - **S56.022** Laceration of flexor muscle, fascia and tendon of left thumb at forearm level A PDX 1791
    - **S56.029** Laceration of flexor muscle, fascia and tendon of unspecified thumb at forearm level A PDX 1792
  - **S56.09** Other injury of flexor muscle, fascia and tendon of thumb at forearm level
    - **S56.091** Other injury of flexor muscle, fascia and tendon of right thumb at forearm level
    - **S56.092** Other injury of flexor muscle, fascia and tendon of left thumb at forearm level
    - **S56.099** Other injury of flexor muscle, fascia and tendon of unspecified thumb at forearm level
- **S56.1** Injury of flexor muscle, fascia and tendon of other and unspecified finger at forearm level
  - **S56.10** Unspecified injury of flexor muscle, fascia and tendon of other and unspecified finger at forearm level
    - **S56.101** Unspecified injury of flexor muscle, fascia and tendon of right index finger at forearm level
    - **S56.102** Unspecified injury of flexor muscle, fascia and tendon of left index finger at forearm level
    - **S56.103** Unspecified injury of flexor muscle, fascia and tendon of right middle finger at forearm level
    - **S56.104** Unspecified injury of flexor muscle, fascia and tendon of left middle finger at forearm level
    - **S56.105** Unspecified injury of flexor muscle, fascia and tendon of right ring finger at forearm level
    - **S56.106** Unspecified injury of flexor muscle, fascia and tendon of left ring finger at forearm level
    - **S56.107** Unspecified injury of flexor muscle, fascia and tendon of right little finger at forearm level
    - **S56.108** Unspecified injury of flexor muscle, fascia and tendon of left little finger at forearm level
    - **S56.109** Unspecified injury of flexor muscle, fascia and tendon of unspecified finger at forearm level
  - **S56.11** Strain of flexor muscle, fascia and tendon of other and unspecified finger at forearm level
    - **S56.111** Strain of flexor muscle, fascia and tendon of right index finger at forearm level
    - **S56.112** Strain of flexor muscle, fascia and tendon of left index finger at forearm level
    - **S56.113** Strain of flexor muscle, fascia and tendon of right middle finger at forearm level
    - **S56.114** Strain of flexor muscle, fascia and tendon of left middle finger at forearm level
    - **S56.115** Strain of flexor muscle, fascia and tendon of right ring finger at forearm level
    - **S56.116** Strain of flexor muscle, fascia and tendon of left ring finger at forearm level
    - **S56.117** Strain of flexor muscle, fascia and tendon of right little finger at forearm level
    - **S56.118** Strain of flexor muscle, fascia and tendon of left little finger at forearm level
    - **S56.119** Strain of flexor muscle, fascia and tendon of finger of unspecified finger at forearm level
  - **S56.12** Laceration of flexor muscle, fascia and tendon of other and unspecified finger at forearm level
    - **S56.121** Laceration of flexor muscle, fascia and tendon of right index finger at forearm level A PDX 1790
    - **S56.122** Laceration of flexor muscle, fascia and tendon of left index finger at forearm level A PDX 1791
    - **S56.123** Laceration of flexor muscle, fascia and tendon of right middle finger at forearm level A PDX 1790
    - **S56.124** Laceration of flexor muscle, fascia and tendon of left middle finger at forearm level A PDX 1791
    - **S56.125** Laceration of flexor muscle, fascia and tendon of right ring finger at forearm level A PDX 1790
    - **S56.126** Laceration of flexor muscle, fascia and tendon of left ring finger at forearm level A PDX 1791
    - **S56.127** Laceration of flexor muscle, fascia and tendon of right little finger at forearm level A PDX 1790

S56.128 Laceration of flexor muscle, fascia and tendon of left little finger at forearm level A (Ex) PDX 1791

S56.129 Laceration of flexor muscle, fascia and tendon of unspecified finger at forearm level A (Ex) PDX 1792

S56.19 Other injury of flexor muscle, fascia and tendon of other and unspecified finger at forearm level

S56.191 Other injury of flexor muscle, fascia and tendon of right index finger at forearm level

S56.192 Other injury of flexor muscle, fascia and tendon of left index finger at forearm level

S56.193 Other injury of flexor muscle, fascia and tendon of right middle finger at forearm level

S56.194 Other injury of flexor muscle, fascia and tendon of left middle finger at forearm level

S56.195 Other injury of flexor muscle, fascia and tendon of right ring finger at forearm level

S56.196 Other injury of flexor muscle, fascia and tendon of left ring finger at forearm level

S56.197 Other injury of flexor muscle, fascia and tendon of right little finger at forearm level

S56.198 Other injury of flexor muscle, fascia and tendon of left little finger at forearm level

S56.199 Other injury of flexor muscle, fascia and tendon of unspecified finger at forearm level

S56.2 Injury of other flexor muscle, fascia and tendon at forearm level

S56.20 Unspecified injury of other flexor muscle, fascia and tendon at forearm level

S56.201 Unspecified injury of other flexor muscle, fascia and tendon at forearm level, right arm

S56.202 Unspecified injury of other flexor muscle, fascia and tendon at forearm level, left arm

S56.209 Unspecified injury of other flexor muscle, fascia and tendon at forearm level, unspecified arm

S56.21 Strain of other flexor muscle, fascia and tendon at forearm level

S56.211 Strain of other flexor muscle, fascia and tendon at forearm level, right arm

S56.212 Strain of other flexor muscle, fascia and tendon at forearm level, left arm

S56.219 Strain of other flexor muscle, fascia and tendon at forearm level, unspecified arm

S56.22 Laceration of other flexor muscle, fascia and tendon at forearm level

S56.221 Laceration of other flexor muscle, fascia and tendon at forearm level, right arm A (Ex) PDX 1790

S56.222 Laceration of other flexor muscle, fascia and tendon at forearm level, left arm A (Ex) PDX 1791

S56.229 Laceration of other flexor muscle, fascia and tendon at forearm level, unspecified arm A (Ex) PDX 1792

S56.29 Other injury of other flexor muscle, fascia and tendon at forearm level

S56.291 Other injury of other flexor muscle, fascia and tendon at forearm level, right arm

S56.292 Other injury of other flexor muscle, fascia and tendon at forearm level, left arm

S56.299 Other injury of other flexor muscle, fascia and tendon at forearm level, unspecified arm

S56.3 Injury of extensor or abductor muscles, fascia and tendons of thumb at forearm level

S56.30 Unspecified injury of extensor or abductor muscles, fascia and tendons of thumb at forearm level

S56.301 Unspecified injury of extensor or abductor muscles, fascia and tendons of right thumb at forearm level

S56.302 Unspecified injury of extensor or abductor muscles, fascia and tendons of left thumb at forearm level

S56.309 Unspecified injury of extensor or abductor muscles, fascia and tendons of unspecified thumb at forearm level

S56.31 Strain of extensor or abductor muscles, fascia and tendons of thumb at forearm level

S56.311 Strain of extensor or abductor muscles, fascia and tendons of right thumb at forearm level

S56.312 Strain of extensor or abductor muscles, fascia and tendons of left thumb at forearm level

S56.319 Strain of extensor or abductor muscles, fascia and tendons of unspecified thumb at forearm level

S56.32 Laceration of extensor or abductor muscles, fascia and tendons of thumb at forearm level

S56.321 Laceration of extensor or abductor muscles, fascia and tendons of right thumb at forearm level A (Ex) PDX 1790

S56.322 Laceration of extensor or abductor muscles, fascia and tendons of left thumb at forearm level A (Ex) PDX 1791

S56.329 Laceration of extensor or abductor muscles, fascia and tendons of unspecified thumb at forearm level A (Ex) PDX 1792

S56.39 Other injury of extensor or abductor muscles, fascia and tendons of thumb at forearm level

S56.391 Other injury of extensor or abductor muscles, fascia and tendons of right thumb at forearm level

S56.392 Other injury of extensor or abductor muscles, fascia and tendons of left thumb at forearm level

S56.399 Other injury of extensor or abductor muscles, fascia and tendons of unspecified thumb at forearm level

S56.4 Injury of extensor muscle, fascia and tendon of other and unspecified finger at forearm level

S56.40 Unspecified injury of extensor muscle, fascia and tendon of other and unspecified finger at forearm level

S56.401 Unspecified injury of extensor muscle, fascia and tendon of right index finger at forearm level

S56.402 Unspecified injury of extensor muscle, fascia and tendon of left index finger at forearm level

S56.403 Unspecified injury of extensor muscle, fascia and tendon of right middle finger at forearm level

S56.404 Unspecified injury of extensor muscle, fascia and tendon of left middle finger at forearm level

S56.405 Unspecified injury of extensor muscle, fascia and tendon of right ring finger at forearm level

S56.406 Unspecified injury of extensor muscle, fascia and tendon of left ring finger at forearm level

S56.407 Unspecified injury of extensor muscle, fascia and tendon of right little finger at forearm level

S56.408 Unspecified injury of extensor muscle, fascia and tendon of left little finger at forearm level

S56.409 Unspecified injury of extensor muscle, fascia and tendon of unspecified finger at forearm level

S56.41 Strain of extensor muscle, fascia and tendon of other and unspecified finger at forearm level

S56.411 Strain of extensor muscle, fascia and tendon of right index finger at forearm level

S56.412 Strain of extensor muscle, fascia and tendon of left index finger at forearm level

S56.413 Strain of extensor muscle, fascia and tendon of right middle finger at forearm level

S56.414 Strain of extensor muscle, fascia and tendon of left middle finger at forearm level

S56.415 Strain of extensor muscle, fascia and tendon of right ring finger at forearm level

S56.416 Strain of extensor muscle, fascia and tendon of left ring finger at forearm level

S56.417 Strain of extensor muscle, fascia and tendon of right little finger at forearm level

S56.418 Strain of extensor muscle, fascia and tendon of left little finger at forearm level

S56.419 Strain of extensor muscle, fascia and tendon of finger, unspecified finger at forearm level

S56.42 Laceration of extensor muscle, fascia and tendon of other and unspecified finger at forearm level

S56.421 Laceration of extensor muscle, fascia and tendon of right index finger at forearm level A (Ex) PDX 1790

S56.422 Laceration of extensor muscle, fascia and tendon of left index finger at forearm level A (Ex) PDX 1791

S56.423 Laceration of extensor muscle, fascia and tendon of right middle finger at forearm level A (Ex) PDX 1790

S56.424 Laceration of extensor muscle, fascia and tendon of left middle finger at forearm level A (Ex) PDX 1791

S56.425 Laceration of extensor muscle, fascia and tendon of right ring finger at forearm level A (Ex) PDX 1790

S56.426 Laceration of extensor muscle, fascia and tendon of left ring finger at forearm level A (Ex) PDX 1791

S56.427 Laceration of extensor muscle, fascia and tendon of right little finger at forearm level A (Ex) PDX 1790

S56.428 Laceration of extensor muscle, fascia and tendon of left little finger at forearm level A (Ex) PDX 1791

S56.429 Laceration of extensor muscle, fascia and tendon of unspecified finger at forearm level A (Ex) PDX 1792

S56.49 Other injury of extensor muscle, fascia and tendon of other and unspecified finger at forearm level

S56.491 Other injury of extensor muscle, fascia and tendon of right index finger at forearm level

S56.492 Other injury of extensor muscle, fascia and tendon of left index finger at forearm level

S56.493 Other injury of extensor muscle, fascia and tendon of right middle finger at forearm level

S56.494 Other injury of extensor muscle, fascia and tendon of left middle finger at forearm level

S56.495 Other injury of extensor muscle, fascia and tendon of right ring finger at forearm level

S56.496 Other injury of extensor muscle, fascia and tendon of left ring finger at forearm level

S56.497 Other injury of extensor muscle, fascia and tendon of right little finger at forearm level

S56.498 Other injury of extensor muscle, fascia and tendon of left little finger at forearm level

S56.499 Other injury of extensor muscle, fascia and tendon of unspecified finger at forearm level

S56.5 Injury of other extensor muscle, fascia and tendon at forearm level

S56.50 Unspecified injury of other extensor muscle, fascia and tendon at forearm level

S56.501 Unspecified injury of other extensor muscle, fascia and tendon at forearm level, right arm

S56.502 Unspecified injury of other extensor muscle, fascia and tendon at forearm level, left arm

S56.509 Unspecified injury of other extensor muscle, fascia and tendon at forearm level, unspecified arm

S56.51 Strain of other extensor muscle, fascia and tendon at forearm level

S56.511 Strain of other extensor muscle, fascia and tendon at forearm level, right arm

S56.512 Strain of other extensor muscle, fascia and tendon at forearm level, left arm

S56.519 Strain of other extensor muscle, fascia and tendon at forearm level, unspecified arm

S56.52 Laceration of other extensor muscle, fascia and tendon at forearm level

S56.521 Laceration of other extensor muscle, fascia and tendon at forearm level, right arm A (Ex) PDX 1790

S56.522 Laceration of other extensor muscle, fascia and tendon at forearm level, left arm A (Ex) PDX 1791

S56.529 Laceration of other extensor muscle, fascia and tendon at forearm level, unspecified arm A (Ex) PDX 1792

S56.59 Other injury of other extensor muscle, fascia and tendon at forearm level

S56.591 Other injury of other extensor muscle, fascia and tendon at forearm level, right arm

S56.592 Other injury of other extensor muscle, fascia and tendon at forearm level, left arm

S56.599 Other injury of other extensor muscle, fascia and tendon at forearm level, unspecified arm

CHAPTER 19 (S00-T88)

● S56.8 Injury of other muscles, fascia and tendons at forearm level

● S56.80 Unspecified injury of other muscles, fascia and tendons at forearm level

● S56.801 Unspecified injury of other muscles, fascia and tendons at forearm level, right arm

● S56.802 Unspecified injury of other muscles, fascia and tendons at forearm level, left arm

● S56.809 Unspecified injury of other muscles, fascia and tendons at forearm level, unspecified arm

● S56.81 Strain of other muscles, fascia and tendons at forearm level

● S56.811 Strain of other muscles, fascia and tendons at forearm level, right arm

● S56.812 Strain of other muscles, fascia and tendons at forearm level, left arm

● S56.819 Strain of other muscles, fascia and tendons at forearm level, unspecified arm

● S56.82 Laceration of other muscles, fascia and tendons at forearm level

● S56.821 Laceration of other muscles, fascia and tendons at forearm level, right arm A (Ex) PDX 1790

● S56.822 Laceration of other muscles, fascia and tendons at forearm level, left arm A (Ex) PDX 1791

● S56.829 Laceration of other muscles, fascia and tendons at forearm level, unspecified arm A (Ex) PDX 1792

● S56.89 Other injury of other muscles, fascia and tendons at forearm level

● S56.891 Other injury of other muscles, fascia and tendons at forearm level, right arm

● S56.892 Other injury of other muscles, fascia and tendons at forearm level, left arm

● S56.899 Other injury of other muscles, fascia and tendons at forearm level, unspecified arm

● S56.9 Injury of unspecified muscles, fascia and tendons at forearm level

● S56.90 Unspecified injury of unspecified muscles, fascia and tendons at forearm level

● S56.901 Unspecified injury of unspecified muscles, fascia and tendons at forearm level, right arm

● S56.902 Unspecified injury of unspecified muscles, fascia and tendons at forearm level, left arm

● S56.909 Unspecified injury of unspecified muscles, fascia and tendons at forearm level, unspecified arm

● S56.91 Strain of unspecified muscles, fascia and tendons at forearm level

● S56.911 Strain of unspecified muscles, fascia and tendons at forearm level, right arm

● S56.912 Strain of unspecified muscles, fascia and tendons at forearm level, left arm

● S56.919 Strain of unspecified muscles, fascia and tendons at forearm level, unspecified arm

● S56.92 Laceration of unspecified muscles, fascia and tendons at forearm level

● S56.921 Laceration of unspecified muscles, fascia and tendons at forearm level, right arm A (Ex) PDX 1790

● S56.922 Laceration of unspecified muscles, fascia and tendons at forearm level, left arm A (Ex) PDX 1791

● S56.929 Laceration of unspecified muscles, fascia and tendons at forearm level, unspecified arm A (Ex) PDX 1792

● S56.99 Other injury of unspecified muscles, fascia and tendons at forearm level

● S56.991 Other injury of unspecified muscles, fascia and tendons at forearm level, right arm

● S56.992 Other injury of unspecified muscles, fascia and tendons at forearm level, left arm

● S56.999 Other injury of unspecified muscles, fascia and tendons at forearm level, unspecified arm

● S57 Crushing injury of elbow and forearm

Use additional code(s) for all associated injuries

Excludes2 crushing injury of wrist and hand (S67.-)

The appropriate 7th character is to be added to each code from category S57

A initial encounter
D subsequent encounter
S sequela

● S57.0 Crushing injury of elbow

X● S57.00 Crushing injury of unspecified elbow

X● S57.01 Crushing injury of right elbow

X● S57.02 Crushing injury of left elbow

● S57.8 Crushing injury of forearm

X● S57.80 Crushing injury of unspecified forearm

X● S57.81 Crushing injury of right forearm

X● S57.82 Crushing injury of left forearm

● S58 Traumatic amputation of elbow and forearm

An amputation not identified as partial or complete should be coded to complete

Excludes1 traumatic amputation of wrist and hand (S68.-)

The appropriate 7th character is to be added to each code from category S58

A initial encounter
D subsequent encounter
S sequela

● S58.0 Traumatic amputation at elbow level

● S58.01 Complete traumatic amputation at elbow level

● S58.011 Complete traumatic amputation at elbow level, right arm A, A, S (Ex) PDX 1776

● S58.012 Complete traumatic amputation at elbow level, left arm A, A, S (Ex) PDX 1777

● S58.019 Complete traumatic amputation at elbow level, unspecified arm A, A, S (Ex) PDX 1778

● S58.02 Partial traumatic amputation at elbow level

● S58.021 Partial traumatic amputation at elbow level, right arm A, A, S (Ex) PDX 1776

● S58.022 Partial traumatic amputation at elbow level, left arm A, A, S (Ex) PDX 1777

● S58.029 Partial traumatic amputation at elbow level, unspecified arm A, A, S (Ex) PDX 1778

● S58.1 Traumatic amputation at level between elbow and wrist

● S58.11 Complete traumatic amputation at level between elbow and wrist

● S58.111 Complete traumatic amputation at level between elbow and wrist, right arm A, A, S (Ex) PDX 1776

● S58.112 Complete traumatic amputation at level between elbow and wrist, left arm A, A, S (Ex) PDX 1777

● S58.119 Complete traumatic amputation at level between elbow and wrist, unspecified arm A, A, S (Ex) PDX 1778

- S58.12 Partial traumatic amputation at level between elbow and wrist
  - S58.121 Partial traumatic amputation at level between elbow and wrist, right arm A, A, S (Ex) PDX 1776
  - S58.122 Partial traumatic amputation at level between elbow and wrist, left arm A, A, S (Ex) PDX 1777
  - S58.129 Partial traumatic amputation at level between elbow and wrist, unspecified arm A, A, S (Ex) PDX 1778
- S58.9 Traumatic amputation of forearm, level unspecified

  Excludes1 traumatic amputation of wrist (S68.-)
  - S58.91 Complete traumatic amputation of forearm, level unspecified
    - S58.911 Complete traumatic amputation of right forearm, level unspecified A, A, S (Ex) PDX 1776
    - S58.912 Complete traumatic amputation of left forearm, level unspecified A, A, S (Ex) PDX 1777
    - S58.919 Complete traumatic amputation of unspecified forearm, level unspecified A, A, S (Ex) PDX 1778
  - S58.92 Partial traumatic amputation of forearm, level unspecified
    - S58.921 Partial traumatic amputation of right forearm, level unspecified A, A, S (Ex) PDX 1776
    - S58.922 Partial traumatic amputation of left forearm, level unspecified A, A, S (Ex) PDX 1777
    - S58.929 Partial traumatic amputation of unspecified forearm, level unspecified A, A, S (Ex) PDX 1778

S59 Other and unspecified injuries of elbow and forearm

Excludes2 other and unspecified injuries of wrist and hand (S69.-)

The appropriate 7th character is to be added to each code from subcategories S59.Ø, S59.1, and S59.2

A	initial encounter for closed fracture
D	subsequent encounter for fracture with routine healing
G	subsequent encounter for fracture with delayed healing
K	subsequent encounter for fracture with nonunion
P	subsequent encounter for fracture with malunion
S	sequela

- S59.Ø Physeal fracture of lower end of ulna
  - S59.ØØ Unspecified physeal fracture of lower end of ulna
    - S59.ØØ1 Unspecified physeal fracture of lower end of ulna, right arm A, K, P, A (Ex) PDX 1264 [K, P], 1780 [A]
    - S59.ØØ2 Unspecified physeal fracture of lower end of ulna, left arm A, K, P, A (Ex) PDX 1264 [K, P], 1781 [A]
    - S59.ØØ9 Unspecified physeal fracture of lower end of ulna, unspecified arm A, K, P, A (Ex) PDX 1264 [K, P], 1782 [A]

Item 19–4 SALTER-HARRIS TYPE 1: epiphysis is completely separated from end of bone, or metaphysic growth plate remains attached to epiphysis

SALTER-HARRIS TYPE 2: epiphysis and growth plate are partially separated from metaphysis, which is cracked—most common type

SALTER-HARRIS TYPE 3: fracture occurring through epiphysis and separates part of epiphysis and growth plate from metaphysis fracture, usually at distal end of tibia

SALTER-HARRIS TYPE 4: fracture runs through epiphysis, across growth plate, into metaphysic, surgery is required to restore joint surface to normal and align growth plate

  - S59.Ø1 Salter-Harris Type I physeal fracture of lower end of ulna
    - S59.Ø11 Salter-Harris Type I physeal fracture of lower end of ulna, right arm A, K, P, A (Ex) PDX 1264 [K, P], 1780 [A]
    - S59.Ø12 Salter-Harris Type I physeal fracture of lower end of ulna, left arm A, K, P, A (Ex) PDX 1264 [K, P], 1781 [A]
    - S59.Ø19 Salter-Harris Type I physeal fracture of lower end of ulna, unspecified arm A, K, P, A (Ex) PDX 1264 [K, P], 1782 [A]
  - S59.Ø2 Salter-Harris Type II physeal fracture of lower end of ulna
    - S59.Ø21 Salter-Harris Type II physeal fracture of lower end of ulna, right arm A, K, P, A (Ex) PDX 1264 [K, P], 1780 [A]
    - S59.Ø22 Salter-Harris Type II physeal fracture of lower end of ulna, left arm A, K, P, A (Ex) PDX 1264 [K, P], 1781 [A]
    - S59.Ø29 Salter-Harris Type II physeal fracture of lower end of ulna, unspecified arm A, K, P, A (Ex) PDX 1264 [K, P], 1782 [A]
  - S59.Ø3 Salter-Harris Type III physeal fracture of lower end of ulna
    - S59.Ø31 Salter-Harris Type III physeal fracture of lower end of ulna, right arm A, K, P, A (Ex) PDX 1264 [K, P], 1780 [A]
    - S59.Ø32 Salter-Harris Type III physeal fracture of lower end of ulna, left arm A, K, P, A (Ex) PDX 1264 [K, P], 1781 [A]
    - S59.Ø39 Salter-Harris Type III physeal fracture of lower end of ulna, unspecified arm A, K, P, A (Ex) PDX 1264 [K, P], 1782 [A]
  - S59.Ø4 Salter-Harris Type IV physeal fracture of lower end of ulna
    - S59.Ø41 Salter-Harris Type IV physeal fracture of lower end of ulna, right arm A, K, P, A (Ex) PDX 1264 [K, P], 1780 [A]
    - S59.Ø42 Salter-Harris Type IV physeal fracture of lower end of ulna, left arm A, K, P, A (Ex) PDX 1264 [K, P], 1781 [A]
    - S59.Ø49 Salter-Harris Type IV physeal fracture of lower end of ulna, unspecified arm A, K, P, A (Ex) PDX 1264 [K, P], 1782 [A]
  - S59.Ø9 Other physeal fracture of lower end of ulna
    - S59.Ø91 Other physeal fracture of lower end of ulna, right arm A, K, P, A (Ex) PDX 1264 [K, P], 1780 [A]
    - S59.Ø92 Other physeal fracture of lower end of ulna, left arm A, K, P, A (Ex) PDX 1264 [K, P], 1781 [A]
    - S59.Ø99 Other physeal fracture of lower end of ulna, unspecified arm A, K, P, A (Ex) PDX 1264 [K, P], 1782 [A]
- S59.1 Physeal fracture of upper end of radius (Ex) PDX 1264
  - S59.1Ø Unspecified physeal fracture of upper end of radius
    - S59.1Ø1 Unspecified physeal fracture of upper end of radius, right arm K, P
    - S59.1Ø2 Unspecified physeal fracture of upper end of radius, left arm K, P
    - S59.1Ø9 Unspecified physeal fracture of upper end of radius, unspecified arm K, P
  - S59.11 Salter-Harris Type I physeal fracture of upper end of radius
    - S59.111 Salter-Harris Type I physeal fracture of upper end of radius, right arm K, P
    - S59.112 Salter-Harris Type I physeal fracture of upper end of radius, left arm K, P
    - S59.119 Salter-Harris Type I physeal fracture of upper end of radius, unspecified arm K, P

CHAPTER 19 (SØØ-T88)

- S59.12 Salter-Harris Type II physeal fracture of upper end of radius
  - S59.121 Salter-Harris Type II physeal fracture of upper end of radius, right arm K, P
  - S59.122 Salter-Harris Type II physeal fracture of upper end of radius, left arm K, P
  - S59.129 Salter-Harris Type II physeal fracture of upper end of radius, unspecified arm K, P
- S59.13 Salter-Harris Type III physeal fracture of upper end of radius
  - S59.131 Salter-Harris Type III physeal fracture of upper end of radius, right arm K, P
  - S59.132 Salter-Harris Type III physeal fracture of upper end of radius, left arm K, P
  - S59.139 Salter-Harris Type III physeal fracture of upper end of radius, unspecified arm K, P
- S59.14 Salter-Harris Type IV physeal fracture of upper end of radius
  - S59.141 Salter-Harris Type IV physeal fracture of upper end of radius, right arm K, P
  - S59.142 Salter-Harris Type IV physeal fracture of upper end of radius, left arm K, P
  - S59.149 Salter-Harris Type IV physeal fracture of upper end of radius, unspecified arm K, P
- S59.19 Other physeal fracture of upper end of radius
  - S59.191 Other physeal fracture of upper end of radius, right arm K, P
  - S59.192 Other physeal fracture of upper end of radius, left arm K, P
  - S59.199 Other physeal fracture of upper end of radius, unspecified arm K, P

- S59.2 Physeal fracture of lower end of radius
  - S59.20 Unspecified physeal fracture of lower end of radius
    - S59.201 Unspecified physeal fracture of lower end of radius, right arm A, K, P, A (Ex:) PDX 1264 [K, P], 1780 [A]
    - S59.202 Unspecified physeal fracture of lower end of radius, left arm A, K, P, A (Ex:) PDX 1264 [K, P], 1781 [A]
    - S59.209 Unspecified physeal fracture of lower end of radius, unspecified arm A, K, P, A (Ex:) PDX 1264 [K, P], 1782 [A]
  - S59.21 Salter-Harris Type I physeal fracture of lower end of radius
    - S59.211 Salter-Harris Type I physeal fracture of lower end of radius, right arm A, K, P, A (Ex:) PDX 1264 [K, P], 1780 [A]
    - S59.212 Salter-Harris Type I physeal fracture of lower end of radius, left arm A, K, P, A (Ex:) PDX 1264 [K, P], 1781 [A]
    - S59.219 Salter-Harris Type I physeal fracture of lower end of radius, unspecified arm A, K, P, A (Ex:) PDX 1264 [K, P], 1782 [A]
  - S59.22 Salter-Harris Type II physeal fracture of lower end of radius
    - S59.221 Salter-Harris Type II physeal fracture of lower end of radius, right arm A, K, P, A (Ex:) PDX 1264 [K, P], 1780 [A]
    - S59.222 Salter-Harris Type II physeal fracture of lower end of radius, left arm A, K, P, A (Ex:) PDX 1264 [K, P], 1781 [A]
    - S59.229 Salter-Harris Type II physeal fracture of lower end of radius, unspecified arm A, K, P, A (Ex:) PDX 1264 [K, P], 1782 [A]
  - S59.23 Salter-Harris Type III physeal fracture of lower end of radius
    - S59.231 Salter-Harris Type III physeal fracture of lower end of radius, right arm A, K, P, A (Ex:) PDX 1264 [K, P], 1780 [A]
    - S59.232 Salter-Harris Type III physeal fracture of lower end of radius, left arm A, K, P, A (Ex:) PDX 1264 [K, P], 1781 [A]
    - S59.239 Salter-Harris Type III physeal fracture of lower end of radius, unspecified arm A, K, P, A (Ex:) PDX 1264 [K, P], 1782 [A]
  - S59.24 Salter-Harris Type IV physeal fracture of lower end of radius
    - S59.241 Salter-Harris Type IV physeal fracture of lower end of radius, right arm A, K, P, A (Ex:) PDX 1264 [K, P], 1780 [A]
    - S59.242 Salter-Harris Type IV physeal fracture of lower end of radius, left arm A, K, P, A (Ex:) PDX 1264 [K, P], 1781 [A]
    - S59.249 Salter-Harris Type IV physeal fracture of lower end of radius, unspecified arm A, K, P, A (Ex:) PDX 1264 [K, P], 1782 [A]
  - S59.29 Other physeal fracture of lower end of radius
    - S59.291 Other physeal fracture of lower end of radius, right arm A, K, P, A (Ex:) PDX 1264 [K, P], 1780 [A]
    - S59.292 Other physeal fracture of lower end of radius, left arm A, K, P, A (Ex:) PDX 1264 [K, P], 1781 [A]
    - S59.299 Other physeal fracture of lower end of radius, unspecified arm A, K, P, A (Ex:) PDX 1264 [K, P], 1782 [A]

- S59.8 Other specified injuries of elbow and forearm

The appropriate 7th character is to be added to each code in subcategory S59.8

A	initial encounter
D	subsequent encounter
S	sequela

  - S59.80 Other specified injuries of elbow
    - S59.801 Other specified injuries of right elbow
    - S59.802 Other specified injuries of left elbow
    - S59.809 Other specified injuries of unspecified elbow
  - S59.81 Other specified injuries of forearm
    - S59.811 Other specified injuries right forearm
    - S59.812 Other specified injuries left forearm
    - S59.819 Other specified injuries unspecified forearm

- S59.9 Unspecified injury of elbow and forearm

The appropriate 7th character is to be added to each code in subcategory S59.9

A	initial encounter
D	subsequent encounter
S	sequela

  - S59.90 Unspecified injury of elbow
    - S59.901 Unspecified injury of right elbow
    - S59.902 Unspecified injury of left elbow
    - S59.909 Unspecified injury of unspecified elbow
  - S59.91 Unspecified injury of forearm
    - S59.911 Unspecified injury of right forearm
    - S59.912 Unspecified injury of left forearm
    - S59.919 Unspecified injury of unspecified forearm

INJURIES TO THE WRIST, HAND AND FINGERS (S60-S69)

Excludes2 burns and corrosions (T20-T32)
frostbite (T33-T34)
insect bite or sting, venomous (T63.4)

S60 Superficial injury of wrist, hand and fingers
The appropriate 7th character is to be added to each code from category S60

A initial encounter
D subsequent encounter
S sequela

S60.0 Contusion of finger without damage to nail
Excludes1 contusion involving nail (matrix) (S60.1)
X **S60.00 Contusion of unspecified finger without damage to nail**
Contusion of finger(s) NOS
S60.01 Contusion of thumb without damage to nail
S60.011 Contusion of right thumb without damage to nail
S60.012 Contusion of left thumb without damage to nail
S60.019 Contusion of unspecified thumb without damage to nail
S60.02 Contusion of index finger without damage to nail
S60.021 Contusion of right index finger without damage to nail
S60.022 Contusion of left index finger without damage to nail
S60.029 Contusion of unspecified index finger without damage to nail
S60.03 Contusion of middle finger without damage to nail
S60.031 Contusion of right middle finger without damage to nail
S60.032 Contusion of left middle finger without damage to nail
S60.039 Contusion of unspecified middle finger without damage to nail
S60.04 Contusion of ring finger without damage to nail
S60.041 Contusion of right ring finger without damage to nail
S60.042 Contusion of left ring finger without damage to nail
S60.049 Contusion of unspecified ring finger without damage to nail
S60.05 Contusion of little finger without damage to nail
S60.051 Contusion of right little finger without damage to nail
S60.052 Contusion of left little finger without damage to nail
S60.059 Contusion of unspecified little finger without damage to nail
S60.1 Contusion of finger with damage to nail
X **S60.10 Contusion of unspecified finger with damage to nail**
S60.11 Contusion of thumb with damage to nail
S60.111 Contusion of right thumb with damage to nail
S60.112 Contusion of left thumb with damage to nail
S60.119 Contusion of unspecified thumb with damage to nail
S60.12 Contusion of index finger with damage to nail
S60.121 Contusion of right index finger with damage to nail
S60.122 Contusion of left index finger with damage to nail
S60.129 Contusion of unspecified index finger with damage to nail
S60.13 Contusion of middle finger with damage to nail
S60.131 Contusion of right middle finger with damage to nail
S60.132 Contusion of left middle finger with damage to nail
S60.139 Contusion of unspecified middle finger with damage to nail
S60.14 Contusion of ring finger with damage to nail
S60.141 Contusion of right ring finger with damage to nail
S60.142 Contusion of left ring finger with damage to nail
S60.149 Contusion of unspecified ring finger with damage to nail
S60.15 Contusion of little finger with damage to nail
S60.151 Contusion of right little finger with damage to nail
S60.152 Contusion of left little finger with damage to nail
S60.159 Contusion of unspecified little finger with damage to nail
S60.2 Contusion of wrist and hand
Excludes2 contusion of fingers (S60.0-, S60.1-)
S60.21 Contusion of wrist
S60.211 Contusion of right wrist
S60.212 Contusion of left wrist
S60.219 Contusion of unspecified wrist
S60.22 Contusion of hand
S60.221 Contusion of right hand
S60.222 Contusion of left hand
S60.229 Contusion of unspecified hand
S60.3 Other superficial injuries of thumb
S60.31 Abrasion of thumb
S60.311 Abrasion of right thumb
S60.312 Abrasion of left thumb
S60.319 Abrasion of unspecified thumb
S60.32 Blister (nonthermal) of thumb
S60.321 Blister (nonthermal) of right thumb
S60.322 Blister (nonthermal) of left thumb
S60.329 Blister (nonthermal) of unspecified thumb
S60.34 External constriction of thumb
Hair tourniquet syndrome of thumb
Use additional cause code to identify the constricting item (W49.0-)
S60.341 External constriction of right thumb
S60.342 External constriction of left thumb
S60.349 External constriction of unspecified thumb
S60.35 Superficial foreign body of thumb
Splinter in the thumb
S60.351 Superficial foreign body of right thumb
S60.352 Superficial foreign body of left thumb
S60.359 Superficial foreign body of unspecified thumb

CHAPTER 19 (S00-T88)

- S60.36 Insect bite (nonvenomous) of thumb
  - S60.361 Insect bite (nonvenomous) of right thumb
  - S60.362 Insect bite (nonvenomous) of left thumb
  - S60.369 Insect bite (nonvenomous) of unspecified thumb
- S60.37 Other superficial bite of thumb
  - **Excludes1** open bite of thumb (S61.05-, S61.15-)
  - S60.371 Other superficial bite of right thumb
  - S60.372 Other superficial bite of left thumb
  - S60.379 Other superficial bite of unspecified thumb
- S60.39 Other superficial injuries of thumb
  - S60.391 Other superficial injuries of right thumb
  - S60.392 Other superficial injuries of left thumb
  - S60.399 Other superficial injuries of unspecified thumb

S60.4 Other superficial injuries of other fingers

- S60.41 Abrasion of fingers
  - S60.410 Abrasion of right index finger
  - S60.411 Abrasion of left index finger
  - S60.412 Abrasion of right middle finger
  - S60.413 Abrasion of left middle finger
  - S60.414 Abrasion of right ring finger
  - S60.415 Abrasion of left ring finger
  - S60.416 Abrasion of right little finger
  - S60.417 Abrasion of left little finger
  - S60.418 Abrasion of other finger
    - Abrasion of specified finger with unspecified laterality
  - S60.419 Abrasion of unspecified finger
- S60.42 Blister (nonthermal) of fingers
  - S60.420 Blister (nonthermal) of right index finger
  - S60.421 Blister (nonthermal) of left index finger
  - S60.422 Blister (nonthermal) of right middle finger
  - S60.423 Blister (nonthermal) of left middle finger
  - S60.424 Blister (nonthermal) of right ring finger
  - S60.425 Blister (nonthermal) of left ring finger
  - S60.426 Blister (nonthermal) of right little finger
  - S60.427 Blister (nonthermal) of left little finger
  - S60.428 Blister (nonthermal) of other finger
    - Blister (nonthermal) of specified finger with unspecified laterality
  - S60.429 Blister (nonthermal) of unspecified finger
- S60.44 External constriction of fingers
  - Hair tourniquet syndrome of finger
  - Use additional cause code to identify the constricting item (W49.0-)
  - S60.440 External constriction of right index finger
  - S60.441 External constriction of left index finger
  - S60.442 External constriction of right middle finger
  - S60.443 External constriction of left middle finger
  - S60.444 External constriction of right ring finger
  - S60.445 External constriction of left ring finger
  - S60.446 External constriction of right little finger
  - S60.447 External constriction of left little finger
  - S60.448 External constriction of other finger
    - External constriction of specified finger with unspecified laterality
  - S60.449 External constriction of unspecified finger
- S60.45 Superficial foreign body of fingers
  - Splinter in the finger(s)
  - S60.450 Superficial foreign body of right index finger
  - S60.451 Superficial foreign body of left index finger
  - S60.452 Superficial foreign body of right middle finger
  - S60.453 Superficial foreign body of left middle finger
  - S60.454 Superficial foreign body of right ring finger
  - S60.455 Superficial foreign body of left ring finger
  - S60.456 Superficial foreign body of right little finger
  - S60.457 Superficial foreign body of left little finger
  - S60.458 Superficial foreign body of other finger
    - Superficial foreign body of specified finger with unspecified laterality
  - S60.459 Superficial foreign body of unspecified finger
- S60.46 Insect bite (nonvenomous) of fingers
  - S60.460 Insect bite (nonvenomous) of right index finger
  - S60.461 Insect bite (nonvenomous) of left index finger
  - S60.462 Insect bite (nonvenomous) of right middle finger
  - S60.463 Insect bite (nonvenomous) of left middle finger
  - S60.464 Insect bite (nonvenomous) of right ring finger
  - S60.465 Insect bite (nonvenomous) of left ring finger
  - S60.466 Insect bite (nonvenomous) of right little finger
  - S60.467 Insect bite (nonvenomous) of left little finger
  - S60.468 Insect bite (nonvenomous) of other finger
    - Insect bite (nonvenomous) of specified finger with unspecified laterality
  - S60.469 Insect bite (nonvenomous) of unspecified finger
- S60.47 Other superficial bite of fingers
  - **Excludes1** open bite of fingers (S61.25-, S61.35-)
  - S60.470 Other superficial bite of right index finger
  - S60.471 Other superficial bite of left index finger
  - S60.472 Other superficial bite of right middle finger

- **S60.473 Other superficial bite of left middle finger**
- **S60.474 Other superficial bite of right ring finger**
- **S60.475 Other superficial bite of left ring finger**
- **S60.476 Other superficial bite of right little finger**
- **S60.477 Other superficial bite of left little finger**
- **S60.478 Other superficial bite of other finger**
  Other superficial bite of specified finger with unspecified laterality
- **S60.479 Other superficial bite of unspecified finger**

S60.5 Other superficial injuries of hand
Excludes2 superficial injuries of fingers (S60.3-, S60.4-)

S60.51 Abrasion of hand
- **S60.511 Abrasion of right hand**
- **S60.512 Abrasion of left hand**
- **S60.519 Abrasion of unspecified hand**

S60.52 Blister (nonthermal) of hand
- **S60.521 Blister (nonthermal) of right hand**
- **S60.522 Blister (nonthermal) of left hand**
- **S60.529 Blister (nonthermal) of unspecified hand**

S60.54 External constriction of hand
- **S60.541 External constriction of right hand**
- **S60.542 External constriction of left hand**
- **S60.549 External constriction of unspecified hand**

S60.55 Superficial foreign body of hand
Splinter in the hand
- **S60.551 Superficial foreign body of right hand**
- **S60.552 Superficial foreign body of left hand**
- **S60.559 Superficial foreign body of unspecified hand**

S60.56 Insect bite (nonvenomous) of hand
- **S60.561 Insect bite (nonvenomous) of right hand**
- **S60.562 Insect bite (nonvenomous) of left hand**
- **S60.569 Insect bite (nonvenomous) of unspecified hand**

S60.57 Other superficial bite of hand
Excludes1 open bite of hand (S61.45-)
- **S60.571 Other superficial bite of hand of right hand**
- **S60.572 Other superficial bite of hand of left hand**
- **S60.579 Other superficial bite of hand of unspecified hand**

S60.8 Other superficial injuries of wrist

S60.81 Abrasion of wrist
- **S60.811 Abrasion of right wrist**
- **S60.812 Abrasion of left wrist**
- **S60.819 Abrasion of unspecified wrist**

S60.82 Blister (nonthermal) of wrist
- **S60.821 Blister (nonthermal) of right wrist**
- **S60.822 Blister (nonthermal) of left wrist**
- **S60.829 Blister (nonthermal) of unspecified wrist**

S60.84 External constriction of wrist
- **S60.841 External constriction of right wrist**
- **S60.842 External constriction of left wrist**
- **S60.849 External constriction of unspecified wrist**

S60.85 Superficial foreign body of wrist
Splinter in the wrist
- **S60.851 Superficial foreign body of right wrist**
- **S60.852 Superficial foreign body of left wrist**
- **S60.859 Superficial foreign body of unspecified wrist**

S60.86 Insect bite (nonvenomous) of wrist
- **S60.861 Insect bite (nonvenomous) of right wrist**
- **S60.862 Insect bite (nonvenomous) of left wrist**
- **S60.869 Insect bite (nonvenomous) of unspecified wrist**

S60.87 Other superficial bite of wrist
Excludes1 open bite of wrist (S61.55)
- **S60.871 Other superficial bite of right wrist**
- **S60.872 Other superficial bite of left wrist**
- **S60.879 Other superficial bite of unspecified wrist**

S60.9 Unspecified superficial injury of wrist, hand and fingers

S60.91 Unspecified superficial injury of wrist
- **S60.911 Unspecified superficial injury of right wrist**
- **S60.912 Unspecified superficial injury of left wrist**
- **S60.919 Unspecified superficial injury of unspecified wrist**

S60.92 Unspecified superficial injury of hand
- **S60.921 Unspecified superficial injury of right hand**
- **S60.922 Unspecified superficial injury of left hand**
- **S60.929 Unspecified superficial injury of unspecified hand**

S60.93 Unspecified superficial injury of thumb
- **S60.931 Unspecified superficial injury of right thumb**
- **S60.932 Unspecified superficial injury of left thumb**
- **S60.939 Unspecified superficial injury of unspecified thumb**

S60.94 Unspecified superficial injury of other fingers
- **S60.940 Unspecified superficial injury of right index finger**
- **S60.941 Unspecified superficial injury of left index finger**
- **S60.942 Unspecified superficial injury of right middle finger**
- **S60.943 Unspecified superficial injury of left middle finger**
- **S60.944 Unspecified superficial injury of right ring finger**
- **S60.945 Unspecified superficial injury of left ring finger**
- **S60.946 Unspecified superficial injury of right little finger**
- **S60.947 Unspecified superficial injury of left little finger**
- **S60.948 Unspecified superficial injury of other finger**
  Unspecified superficial injury of specified finger with unspecified laterality
- **S60.949 Unspecified superficial injury of unspecified finger**

S61 Open wound of wrist, hand and fingers
Code also any associated wound infection
Excludes1 open fracture of wrist, hand and finger (S62.- with 7th character B)
traumatic amputation of wrist and hand (S68.-)
The appropriate 7th character is to be added to each code from category S61

A	initial encounter
D	subsequent encounter
S	sequela

S61.0 Open wound of thumb without damage to nail
Excludes1 open wound of thumb with damage to nail (S61.1-)

S61.00 Unspecified open wound of thumb without damage to nail
S61.001 Unspecified open wound of right thumb without damage to nail
S61.002 Unspecified open wound of left thumb without damage to nail
S61.009 Unspecified open wound of unspecified thumb without damage to nail

S61.01 Laceration without foreign body of thumb without damage to nail
S61.011 Laceration without foreign body of right thumb without damage to nail
S61.012 Laceration without foreign body of left thumb without damage to nail
S61.019 Laceration without foreign body of unspecified thumb without damage to nail

S61.02 Laceration with foreign body of thumb without damage to nail
S61.021 Laceration with foreign body of right thumb without damage to nail
S61.022 Laceration with foreign body of left thumb without damage to nail
S61.029 Laceration with foreign body of unspecified thumb without damage to nail

S61.03 Puncture wound without foreign body of thumb without damage to nail
S61.031 Puncture wound without foreign body of right thumb without damage to nail
S61.032 Puncture wound without foreign body of left thumb without damage to nail
S61.039 Puncture wound without foreign body of unspecified thumb without damage to nail

S61.04 Puncture wound with foreign body of thumb without damage to nail
S61.041 Puncture wound with foreign body of right thumb without damage to nail
S61.042 Puncture wound with foreign body of left thumb without damage to nail
S61.049 Puncture wound with foreign body of unspecified thumb without damage to nail

S61.05 Open bite of thumb without damage to nail
Bite of thumb NOS
Excludes1 superficial bite of thumb (S60.36-, S60.37-)
S61.051 Open bite of right thumb without damage to nail
S61.052 Open bite of left thumb without damage to nail
S61.059 Open bite of unspecified thumb without damage to nail

S61.1 Open wound of thumb with damage to nail

S61.10 Unspecified open wound of thumb with damage to nail
S61.101 Unspecified open wound of right thumb with damage to nail
S61.102 Unspecified open wound of left thumb with damage to nail
S61.109 Unspecified open wound of unspecified thumb with damage to nail

S61.11 Laceration without foreign body of thumb with damage to nail
S61.111 Laceration without foreign body of right thumb with damage to nail
S61.112 Laceration without foreign body of left thumb with damage to nail
S61.119 Laceration without foreign body of unspecified thumb with damage to nail

S61.12 Laceration with foreign body of thumb with damage to nail
S61.121 Laceration with foreign body of right thumb with damage to nail
S61.122 Laceration with foreign body of left thumb with damage to nail
S61.129 Laceration with foreign body of unspecified thumb with damage to nail

S61.13 Puncture wound without foreign body of thumb with damage to nail
S61.131 Puncture wound without foreign body of right thumb with damage to nail
S61.132 Puncture wound without foreign body of left thumb with damage to nail
S61.139 Puncture wound without foreign body of unspecified thumb with damage to nail

S61.14 Puncture wound with foreign body of thumb with damage to nail
S61.141 Puncture wound with foreign body of right thumb with damage to nail
S61.142 Puncture wound with foreign body of left thumb with damage to nail
S61.149 Puncture wound with foreign body of unspecified thumb with damage to nail

S61.15 Open bite of thumb with damage to nail
Bite of thumb with damage to nail NOS
Excludes1 superficial bite of thumb (S60.36-, S60.37-)
S61.151 Open bite of right thumb with damage to nail
S61.152 Open bite of left thumb with damage to nail
S61.159 Open bite of unspecified thumb with damage to nail

S61.2 Open wound of other finger without damage to nail
Excludes1 open wound of finger involving nail (matrix) (S61.3-)
Excludes2 open wound of thumb without damage to nail (S61.0-)

S61.20 Unspecified open wound of other finger without damage to nail
S61.200 Unspecified open wound of right index finger without damage to nail
S61.201 Unspecified open wound of left index finger without damage to nail
S61.202 Unspecified open wound of right middle finger without damage to nail

- S61.203 **Unspecified open wound of left middle finger without damage to nail**
- S61.204 **Unspecified open wound of right ring finger without damage to nail**
- S61.205 **Unspecified open wound of left ring finger without damage to nail**
- S61.206 **Unspecified open wound of right little finger without damage to nail**
- S61.207 **Unspecified open wound of left little finger without damage to nail**
- S61.208 **Unspecified open wound of other finger without damage to nail**
  Unspecified open wound of specified finger with unspecified laterality without damage to nail
- S61.209 **Unspecified open wound of unspecified finger without damage to nail**

S61.21 **Laceration without foreign body of finger without damage to nail**

- S61.210 **Laceration without foreign body of right index finger without damage to nail**
- S61.211 **Laceration without foreign body of left index finger without damage to nail**
- S61.212 **Laceration without foreign body of right middle finger without damage to nail**
- S61.213 **Laceration without foreign body of left middle finger without damage to nail**
- S61.214 **Laceration without foreign body of right ring finger without damage to nail**
- S61.215 **Laceration without foreign body of left ring finger without damage to nail**
- S61.216 **Laceration without foreign body of right little finger without damage to nail**
- S61.217 **Laceration without foreign body of left little finger without damage to nail**
- S61.218 **Laceration without foreign body of other finger without damage to nail**
  Laceration without foreign body of specified finger with unspecified laterality without damage to nail
- S61.219 **Laceration without foreign body of unspecified finger without damage to nail**

S61.22 **Laceration with foreign body of finger without damage to nail**

- S61.220 **Laceration with foreign body of right index finger without damage to nail**
- S61.221 **Laceration with foreign body of left index finger without damage to nail**
- S61.222 **Laceration with foreign body of right middle finger without damage to nail**
- S61.223 **Laceration with foreign body of left middle finger without damage to nail**
- S61.224 **Laceration with foreign body of right ring finger without damage to nail**
- S61.225 **Laceration with foreign body of left ring finger without damage to nail**
- S61.226 **Laceration with foreign body of right little finger without damage to nail**
- S61.227 **Laceration with foreign body of left little finger without damage to nail**
- S61.228 **Laceration with foreign body of other finger without damage to nail**
  Laceration with foreign body of specified finger with unspecified laterality without damage to nail
- S61.229 **Laceration with foreign body of unspecified finger without damage to nail**

S61.23 **Puncture wound without foreign body of finger without damage to nail**

- S61.230 **Puncture wound without foreign body of right index finger without damage to nail**
- S61.231 **Puncture wound without foreign body of left index finger without damage to nail**
- S61.232 **Puncture wound without foreign body of right middle finger without damage to nail**
- S61.233 **Puncture wound without foreign body of left middle finger without damage to nail**
- S61.234 **Puncture wound without foreign body of right ring finger without damage to nail**
- S61.235 **Puncture wound without foreign body of left ring finger without damage to nail**
- S61.236 **Puncture wound without foreign body of right little finger without damage to nail**
- S61.237 **Puncture wound without foreign body of left little finger without damage to nail**
- S61.238 **Puncture wound without foreign body of other finger without damage to nail**
  Puncture wound without foreign body of specified finger with unspecified laterality without damage to nail
- S61.239 **Puncture wound without foreign body of unspecified finger without damage to nail**

S61.24 **Puncture wound with foreign body of finger without damage to nail**

- S61.240 **Puncture wound with foreign body of right index finger without damage to nail**
- S61.241 **Puncture wound with foreign body of left index finger without damage to nail**
- S61.242 **Puncture wound with foreign body of right middle finger without damage to nail**
- S61.243 **Puncture wound with foreign body of left middle finger without damage to nail**
- S61.244 **Puncture wound with foreign body of right ring finger without damage to nail**
- S61.245 **Puncture wound with foreign body of left ring finger without damage to nail**
- S61.246 **Puncture wound with foreign body of right little finger without damage to nail**
- S61.247 **Puncture wound with foreign body of left little finger without damage to nail**

CHAPTER 19 (S00-T88)

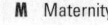

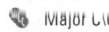

- ● S61.248 Puncture wound with foreign body of other finger without damage to nail
  - Puncture wound with foreign body of specified finger with unspecified laterality without damage to nail
- ● S61.249 Puncture wound with foreign body of unspecified finger without damage to nail

● S61.25 Open bite of finger without damage to nail
- Bite of finger without damage to nail NOS
- **Excludes1** superficial bite of finger (S60.46-, S60.47-)

- ● S61.250 Open bite of right index finger without damage to nail
- ● S61.251 Open bite of left index finger without damage to nail
- ● S61.252 Open bite of right middle finger without damage to nail
- ● S61.253 Open bite of left middle finger without damage to nail
- ● S61.254 Open bite of right ring finger without damage to nail
- ● S61.255 Open bite of left ring finger without damage to nail
- ● S61.256 Open bite of right little finger without damage to nail
- ● S61.257 Open bite of left little finger without damage to nail
- ● S61.258 Open bite of other finger without damage to nail
  - Open bite of specified finger with unspecified laterality without damage to nail
- ● S61.259 Open bite of unspecified finger without damage to nail

● S61.3 Open wound of other finger with damage to nail

● S61.30 Unspecified open wound of finger with damage to nail
- ● S61.300 Unspecified open wound of right index finger with damage to nail
- ● S61.301 Unspecified open wound of left index finger with damage to nail
- ● S61.302 Unspecified open wound of right middle finger with damage to nail
- ● S61.303 Unspecified open wound of left middle finger with damage to nail
- ● S61.304 Unspecified open wound of right ring finger with damage to nail
- ● S61.305 Unspecified open wound of left ring finger with damage to nail
- ● S61.306 Unspecified open wound of right little finger with damage to nail
- ● S61.307 Unspecified open wound of left little finger with damage to nail
- ● S61.308 Unspecified open wound of other finger with damage to nail
  - Unspecified open wound of specified finger with unspecified laterality with damage to nail
- ● S61.309 Unspecified open wound of unspecified finger with damage to nail

● S61.31 Laceration without foreign body of finger with damage to nail
- ● S61.310 Laceration without foreign body of right index finger with damage to nail
- ● S61.311 Laceration without foreign body of left index finger with damage to nail
- ● S61.312 Laceration without foreign body of right middle finger with damage to nail
- ● S61.313 Laceration without foreign body of left middle finger with damage to nail
- ● S61.314 Laceration without foreign body of right ring finger with damage to nail
- ● S61.315 Laceration without foreign body of left ring finger with damage to nail
- ● S61.316 Laceration without foreign body of right little finger with damage to nail
- ● S61.317 Laceration without foreign body of left little finger with damage to nail
- ● S61.318 Laceration without foreign body of other finger with damage to nail
  - Laceration without foreign body of specified finger with unspecified laterality with damage to nail
- ● S61.319 Laceration without foreign body of unspecified finger with damage to nail

● S61.32 Laceration with foreign body of finger with damage to nail
- ● S61.320 Laceration with foreign body of right index finger with damage to nail
- ● S61.321 Laceration with foreign body of left index finger with damage to nail
- ● S61.322 Laceration with foreign body of right middle finger with damage to nail
- ● S61.323 Laceration with foreign body of left middle finger with damage to nail
- ● S61.324 Laceration with foreign body of right ring finger with damage to nail
- ● S61.325 Laceration with foreign body of left ring finger with damage to nail
- ● S61.326 Laceration with foreign body of right little finger with damage to nail
- ● S61.327 Laceration with foreign body of left little finger with damage to nail
- ● S61.328 Laceration with foreign body of other finger with damage to nail
  - Laceration with foreign body of specified finger with unspecified laterality with damage to nail
- ● S61.329 Laceration with foreign body of unspecified finger with damage to nail

● S61.33 Puncture wound without foreign body of finger with damage to nail
- ● S61.330 Puncture wound without foreign body of right index finger with damage to nail
- ● S61.331 Puncture wound without foreign body of left index finger with damage to nail
- ● S61.332 Puncture wound without foreign body of right middle finger with damage to nail
- ● S61.333 Puncture wound without foreign body of left middle finger with damage to nail
- ● S61.334 Puncture wound without foreign body of right ring finger with damage to nail
- ● S61.335 Puncture wound without foreign body of left ring finger with damage to nail
- ● S61.336 Puncture wound without foreign body of right little finger with damage to nail

S61.337 Puncture wound without foreign body of left little finger with damage to nail
S61.338 Puncture wound without foreign body of other finger with damage to nail
Puncture wound without foreign body of specified finger with unspecified laterality with damage to nail
S61.339 Puncture wound without foreign body of unspecified finger with damage to nail
S61.34 Puncture wound with foreign body of finger with damage to nail
S61.340 Puncture wound with foreign body of right index finger with damage to nail
S61.341 Puncture wound with foreign body of left index finger with damage to nail
S61.342 Puncture wound with foreign body of right middle finger with damage to nail
S61.343 Puncture wound with foreign body of left middle finger with damage to nail
S61.344 Puncture wound with foreign body of right ring finger with damage to nail
S61.345 Puncture wound with foreign body of left ring finger with damage to nail
S61.346 Puncture wound with foreign body of right little finger with damage to nail
S61.347 Puncture wound with foreign body of left little finger with damage to nail
S61.348 Puncture wound with foreign body of other finger with damage to nail
Puncture wound with foreign body of specified finger with unspecified laterality with damage to nail
S61.349 Puncture wound with foreign body of unspecified finger with damage to nail
S61.35 Open bite of finger with damage to nail
Bite of finger with damage to nail NOS
Excludes1 superficial bite of finger (S6Ø.46-, S6Ø.47-)
S61.350 Open bite of right index finger with damage to nail
S61.351 Open bite of left index finger with damage to nail
S61.352 Open bite of right middle finger with damage to nail
S61.353 Open bite of left middle finger with damage to nail
S61.354 Open bite of right ring finger with damage to nail
S61.355 Open bite of left ring finger with damage to nail
S61.356 Open bite of right little finger with damage to nail
S61.357 Open bite of left little finger with damage to nail
S61.358 Open bite of other finger with damage to nail
Open bite of specified finger with unspecified laterality with damage to nail
S61.359 Open bite of unspecified finger with damage to nail

S61.4 Open wound of hand
S61.4Ø Unspecified open wound of hand
S61.4Ø1 Unspecified open wound of right hand
S61.4Ø2 Unspecified open wound of left hand
S61.4Ø9 Unspecified open wound of unspecified hand
S61.41 Laceration without foreign body of hand
S61.411 Laceration without foreign body of right hand
S61.412 Laceration without foreign body of left hand
S61.419 Laceration without foreign body of unspecified hand
S61.42 Laceration with foreign body of hand
S61.421 Laceration with foreign body of right hand
S61.422 Laceration with foreign body of left hand
S61.429 Laceration with foreign body of unspecified hand
S61.43 Puncture wound without foreign body of hand
S61.431 Puncture wound without foreign body of right hand
S61.432 Puncture wound without foreign body of left hand
S61.439 Puncture wound without foreign body of unspecified hand
S61.44 Puncture wound with foreign body of hand
S61.441 Puncture wound with foreign body of right hand
S61.442 Puncture wound with foreign body of left hand
S61.449 Puncture wound with foreign body of unspecified hand
S61.45 Open bite of hand
Bite of hand NOS
Excludes1 superficial bite of hand (S6Ø.56-, S6Ø.57-)
S61.451 Open bite of right hand
S61.452 Open bite of left hand
S61.459 Open bite of unspecified hand
S61.5 Open wound of wrist
S61.5Ø Unspecified open wound of wrist
S61.5Ø1 Unspecified open wound of right wrist
S61.5Ø2 Unspecified open wound of left wrist
S61.5Ø9 Unspecified open wound of unspecified wrist
S61.51 Laceration without foreign body of wrist
S61.511 Laceration without foreign body of right wrist
S61.512 Laceration without foreign body of left wrist
S61.519 Laceration without foreign body of unspecified wrist
S61.52 Laceration with foreign body of wrist
S61.521 Laceration with foreign body of right wrist
S61.522 Laceration with foreign body of left wrist
S61.529 Laceration with foreign body of unspecified wrist

CHAPTER 19 (SØØ-T88)

S61.53 Puncture wound without foreign body of wrist
S61.531 Puncture wound without foreign body of right wrist
S61.532 Puncture wound without foreign body of left wrist
S61.539 Puncture wound without foreign body of unspecified wrist
S61.54 Puncture wound with foreign body of wrist
S61.541 Puncture wound with foreign body of right wrist
S61.542 Puncture wound with foreign body of left wrist
S61.549 Puncture wound with foreign body of unspecified wrist
S61.55 Open bite of wrist
Bite of wrist NOS
Excludes1 superficial bite of wrist (S60.86-, S60.87-)
S61.551 Open bite of right wrist
S61.552 Open bite of left wrist
S61.559 Open bite of unspecified wrist

S62 Fracture at wrist and hand level
Note: A fracture not indicated as displaced or nondisplaced should be coded to displaced
A fracture not indicated as open or closed should be coded to closed
Excludes1 traumatic amputation of wrist and hand (S68.-)
Excludes2 fracture of distal parts of ulna and radius (S52.-)
The appropriate 7th character is to be added to each code from category S62

A	initial encounter for closed fracture
B	initial encounter for open fracture
D	subsequent encounter for fracture with routine healing
G	subsequent encounter for fracture with delayed healing
K	subsequent encounter for fracture with nonunion
P	subsequent encounter for fracture with malunion
S	sequela

S62.0 Fracture of navicular [scaphoid] bone of wrist (Ex:) PDX 1264 [K, P], 1793 [B]
S62.00 Unspecified fracture of navicular [scaphoid] bone of wrist
S62.001 Unspecified fracture of navicular [scaphoid] bone of right wrist B, K, P, B
S62.002 Unspecified fracture of navicular [scaphoid] bone of left wrist B, K, P, B
Coding Clinic: 2012, Q4, P106
S62.009 Unspecified fracture of navicular [scaphoid] bone of unspecified wrist B, K, P, B
S62.01 Fracture of distal pole of navicular [scaphoid] bone of wrist
Fracture of volar tuberosity of navicular [scaphoid] bone of wrist
S62.011 Displaced fracture of distal pole of navicular [scaphoid] bone of right wrist B, K, P, B
S62.012 Displaced fracture of distal pole of navicular [scaphoid] bone of left wrist B, K, P, B
S62.013 Displaced fracture of distal pole of navicular [scaphoid] bone of unspecified wrist B, K, P, B
S62.014 Nondisplaced fracture of distal pole of navicular [scaphoid] bone of right wrist B, K, P, B
S62.015 Nondisplaced fracture of distal pole of navicular [scaphoid] bone of left wrist B, K, P, B
S62.016 Nondisplaced fracture of distal pole of navicular [scaphoid] bone of unspecified wrist B, K, P, B
S62.02 Fracture of middle third of navicular [scaphoid] bone of wrist
S62.021 Displaced fracture of middle third of navicular [scaphoid] bone of right wrist B, K, P, B
S62.022 Displaced fracture of middle third of navicular [scaphoid] bone of left wrist B, K, P, B
S62.023 Displaced fracture of middle third of navicular [scaphoid] bone of unspecified wrist B, K, P, B
S62.024 Nondisplaced fracture of middle third of navicular [scaphoid] bone of right wrist B, K, P, B
S62.025 Nondisplaced fracture of middle third of navicular [scaphoid] bone of left wrist B, K, P, B
S62.026 Nondisplaced fracture of middle third of navicular [scaphoid] bone of unspecified wrist B, K, P, B
S62.03 Fracture of proximal third of navicular [scaphoid] bone of wrist
S62.031 Displaced fracture of proximal third of navicular [scaphoid] bone of right wrist B, K, P, B
S62.032 Displaced fracture of proximal third of navicular [scaphoid] bone of left wrist B, K, P, B
S62.033 Displaced fracture of proximal third of navicular [scaphoid] bone of unspecified wrist B, K, P, B
S62.034 Nondisplaced fracture of proximal third of navicular [scaphoid] bone of right wrist B, K, P, B
S62.035 Nondisplaced fracture of proximal third of navicular [scaphoid] bone of left wrist B, K, P, B
S62.036 Nondisplaced fracture of proximal third of navicular [scaphoid] bone of unspecified wrist B, K, P, B
S62.1 Fracture of other and unspecified carpal bone(s) (Ex:) PDX 1264 [K, P], 1793 [B]
Excludes2 fracture of scaphoid of wrist (S62.0-)
S62.10 Fracture of unspecified carpal bone
Fracture of wrist NOS
S62.101 Fracture of unspecified carpal bone, right wrist B, K, P, B
S62.102 Fracture of unspecified carpal bone, left wrist B, K, P, B
Coding Clinic: 2012, Q4, P95
S62.109 Fracture of unspecified carpal bone, unspecified wrist B, K, P, B
S62.11 Fracture of triquetrum [cuneiform] bone of wrist
S62.111 Displaced fracture of triquetrum [cuneiform] bone, right wrist B, K, P, B
S62.112 Displaced fracture of triquetrum [cuneiform] bone, left wrist B, K, P, B
S62.113 Displaced fracture of triquetrum [cuneiform] bone, unspecified wrist B, K, P, B
S62.114 Nondisplaced fracture of triquetrum [cuneiform] bone, right wrist B, K, P, B

S62.115 Nondisplaced fracture of triquetrum [cuneiform] bone, left wrist B, K, P, B

S62.116 Nondisplaced fracture of triquetrum [cuneiform] bone, unspecified wrist B, K, P, B

S62.12 Fracture of lunate [semilunar]

S62.121 Displaced fracture of lunate [semilunar], right wrist B, K, P, B

S62.122 Displaced fracture of lunate [semilunar], left wrist B, K, P, B

S62.123 Displaced fracture of lunate [semilunar], unspecified wrist B, K, P, B

S62.124 Nondisplaced fracture of lunate [semilunar], right wrist B, K, P, B

S62.125 Nondisplaced fracture of lunate [semilunar], left wrist B, K, P, B

S62.126 Nondisplaced fracture of lunate [semilunar], unspecified wrist B, K, P, B

S62.13 Fracture of capitate [os magnum] bone

S62.131 Displaced fracture of capitate [os magnum] bone, right wrist B, K, P, B

S62.132 Displaced fracture of capitate [os magnum] bone, left wrist B, K, P, B

S62.133 Displaced fracture of capitate [os magnum] bone, unspecified wrist B, K, P, B

S62.134 Nondisplaced fracture of capitate [os magnum] bone, right wrist B, K, P, B

S62.135 Nondisplaced fracture of capitate [os magnum] bone, left wrist B, K, P, B

S62.136 Nondisplaced fracture of capitate [os magnum] bone, unspecified wrist B, K, P, B

S62.14 Fracture of body of hamate [unciform] bone

Fracture of hamate [unciform] bone NOS

S62.141 Displaced fracture of body of hamate [unciform] bone, right wrist B, K, P, B

S62.142 Displaced fracture of body of hamate [unciform] bone, left wrist B, K, P, B

S62.143 Displaced fracture of body of hamate [unciform] bone, unspecified wrist B, K, P, B

S62.144 Nondisplaced fracture of body of hamate [unciform] bone, right wrist B, K, P, B

S62.145 Nondisplaced fracture of body of hamate [unciform] bone, left wrist B, K, P, B

S62.146 Nondisplaced fracture of body of hamate [unciform] bone, unspecified wrist B, K, P, B

S62.15 Fracture of hook process of hamate [unciform] bone

Fracture of unciform process of hamate [unciform] bone

S62.151 Displaced fracture of hook process of hamate [unciform] bone, right wrist B, K, P, B

S62.152 Displaced fracture of hook process of hamate [unciform] bone, left wrist B, K, P, B

S62.153 Displaced fracture of hook process of hamate [unciform] bone, unspecified wrist B, K, P, B

S62.154 Nondisplaced fracture of hook process of hamate [unciform] bone, right wrist B, K, P, B

S62.155 Nondisplaced fracture of hook process of hamate [unciform] bone, left wrist B, K, P, B

S62.156 Nondisplaced fracture of hook process of hamate [unciform] bone, unspecified wrist B, K, P, B

S62.16 Fracture of pisiform

S62.161 Displaced fracture of pisiform, right wrist B, K, P, B

S62.162 Displaced fracture of pisiform, left wrist B, K, P, B

S62.163 Displaced fracture of pisiform, unspecified wrist B, K, P, B

S62.164 Nondisplaced fracture of pisiform, right wrist B, K, P, B

S62.165 Nondisplaced fracture of pisiform, left wrist B, K, P, B

S62.166 Nondisplaced fracture of pisiform, unspecified wrist B, K, P, B

S62.17 Fracture of trapezium [larger multangular]

S62.171 Displaced fracture of trapezium [larger multangular], right wrist B, K, P, B

S62.172 Displaced fracture of trapezium [larger multangular], left wrist B, K, P, B

S62.173 Displaced fracture of trapezium [larger multangular], unspecified wrist B, K, P, B

S62.174 Nondisplaced fracture of trapezium [larger multangular], right wrist B, K, P, B

S62.175 Nondisplaced fracture of trapezium [larger multangular], left wrist B, K, P, B

S62.176 Nondisplaced fracture of trapezium [larger multangular], unspecified wrist B, K, P, B

S62.18 Fracture of trapezoid [smaller multangular]

S62.181 Displaced fracture of trapezoid [smaller multangular], right wrist B, K, P, B

S62.182 Displaced fracture of trapezoid [smaller multangular], left wrist B, K, P, B

S62.183 Displaced fracture of trapezoid [smaller multangular], unspecified wrist B, K, P, B

S62.184 Nondisplaced fracture of trapezoid [smaller multangular], right wrist B, K, P, B

S62.185 Nondisplaced fracture of trapezoid [smaller multangular], left wrist B, K, P, B

S62.186 Nondisplaced fracture of trapezoid [smaller multangular], unspecified wrist B, K, P, B

CHAPTER 19 (SØØ-T88)

S62.2 Fracture of first metacarpal bone PDX 1264 [K, P], 1794 [B]
S62.20 Unspecified fracture of first metacarpal bone
S62.201 Unspecified fracture of first metacarpal bone, right hand B, K, P, B
S62.202 Unspecified fracture of first metacarpal bone, left hand B, K, P, B
S62.209 Unspecified fracture of first metacarpal bone, unspecified hand B, K, P, B
S62.21 Bennett's fracture
S62.211 Bennett's fracture, right hand B, K, P, B
S62.212 Bennett's fracture, left hand B, K, P, B
S62.213 Bennett's fracture, unspecified hand B, K, P, B
S62.22 Rolando's fracture
S62.221 Displaced Rolando's fracture, right hand B, K, P, B
S62.222 Displaced Rolando's fracture, left hand B, K, P, B
S62.223 Displaced Rolando's fracture, unspecified hand B, K, P, B
S62.224 Nondisplaced Rolando's fracture, right hand B, K, P, B
S62.225 Nondisplaced Rolando's fracture, left hand B, K, P, B
S62.226 Nondisplaced Rolando's fracture, unspecified hand B, K, P, B
S62.23 Other fracture of base of first metacarpal bone
S62.231 Other displaced fracture of base of first metacarpal bone, right hand B, K, P, B
S62.232 Other displaced fracture of base of first metacarpal bone, left hand B, K, P, B
S62.233 Other displaced fracture of base of first metacarpal bone, unspecified hand B, K, P, B
S62.234 Other nondisplaced fracture of base of first metacarpal bone, right hand B, K, P, B
S62.235 Other nondisplaced fracture of base of first metacarpal bone, left hand B, K, P, B
S62.236 Other nondisplaced fracture of base of first metacarpal bone, unspecified hand B, K, P, B
S62.24 Fracture of shaft of first metacarpal bone
S62.241 Displaced fracture of shaft of first metacarpal bone, right hand B, K, P, B
S62.242 Displaced fracture of shaft of first metacarpal bone, left hand B, K, P, B
S62.243 Displaced fracture of shaft of first metacarpal bone, unspecified hand B, K, P, B
S62.244 Nondisplaced fracture of shaft of first metacarpal bone, right hand B, K, P, B
S62.245 Nondisplaced fracture of shaft of first metacarpal bone, left hand B, K, P, B
S62.246 Nondisplaced fracture of shaft of first metacarpal bone, unspecified hand B, K, P, B
S62.25 Fracture of neck of first metacarpal bone
S62.251 Displaced fracture of neck of first metacarpal bone, right hand B, K, P, B
S62.252 Displaced fracture of neck of first metacarpal bone, left hand B, K, P, B
S62.253 Displaced fracture of neck of first metacarpal bone, unspecified hand B, K, P, B
S62.254 Nondisplaced fracture of neck of first metacarpal bone, right hand B, K, P, B
S62.255 Nondisplaced fracture of neck of first metacarpal bone, left hand B, K, P, B
S62.256 Nondisplaced fracture of neck of first metacarpal bone, unspecified hand B, K, P, B
S62.29 Other fracture of first metacarpal bone
S62.291 Other fracture of first metacarpal bone, right hand B, K, P, B
S62.292 Other fracture of first metacarpal bone, left hand B, K, P, B
S62.299 Other fracture of first metacarpal bone, unspecified hand B, K, P, B
S62.3 Fracture of other and unspecified metacarpal bone PDX 1264 [K, P], 1794 [B]
Excludes2 fracture of first metacarpal bone (S62.2-)
S62.30 Unspecified fracture of other metacarpal bone
S62.300 Unspecified fracture of second metacarpal bone, right hand B, K, P, B
S62.301 Unspecified fracture of second metacarpal bone, left hand B, K, P, B
S62.302 Unspecified fracture of third metacarpal bone, right hand B, K, P, B
S62.303 Unspecified fracture of third metacarpal bone, left hand B, K, P, B
S62.304 Unspecified fracture of fourth metacarpal bone, right hand B, K, P, B
S62.305 Unspecified fracture of fourth metacarpal bone, left hand B, K, P, B
S62.306 Unspecified fracture of fifth metacarpal bone, right hand B, K, P, B
S62.307 Unspecified fracture of fifth metacarpal bone, left hand B, K, P, B
S62.308 Unspecified fracture of other metacarpal bone B, K, P, B
Unspecified fracture of specified metacarpal bone with unspecified laterality
S62.309 Unspecified fracture of unspecified metacarpal bone B, K, P, B
S62.31 Displaced fracture of base of other metacarpal bone
S62.310 Displaced fracture of base of second metacarpal bone, right hand B, K, P, B
S62.311 Displaced fracture of base of second metacarpal bone, left hand B, K, P, B

CHAPTER 19 (SØØ-T88)

S62.312 Displaced fracture of base of third metacarpal bone, right hand B, K, P, B

S62.313 Displaced fracture of base of third metacarpal bone, left hand B, K, P, B

S62.314 Displaced fracture of base of fourth metacarpal bone, right hand B, K, P, B

S62.315 Displaced fracture of base of fourth metacarpal bone, left hand B, K, P, B

S62.316 Displaced fracture of base of fifth metacarpal bone, right hand B, K, P, B

S62.317 Displaced fracture of base of fifth metacarpal bone, left hand B, K, P, B

S62.318 Displaced fracture of base of other metacarpal bone B, K, P, B
Displaced fracture of base of specified metacarpal bone with unspecified laterality

S62.319 Displaced fracture of base of unspecified metacarpal bone B, K, P, B

S62.32 Displaced fracture of shaft of other metacarpal bone

S62.320 Displaced fracture of shaft of second metacarpal bone, right hand B, K, P, B

S62.321 Displaced fracture of shaft of second metacarpal bone, left hand B, K, P, B

S62.322 Displaced fracture of shaft of third metacarpal bone, right hand B, K, P, B

S62.323 Displaced fracture of shaft of third metacarpal bone, left hand B, K, P, B

S62.324 Displaced fracture of shaft of fourth metacarpal bone, right hand B, K, P, B

S62.325 Displaced fracture of shaft of fourth metacarpal bone, left hand B, K, P, B

S62.326 Displaced fracture of shaft of fifth metacarpal bone, right hand B, K, P, B

S62.327 Displaced fracture of shaft of fifth metacarpal bone, left hand B, K, P, B

S62.328 Displaced fracture of shaft of other metacarpal bone B, K, P, B
Displaced fracture of shaft of specified metacarpal bone with unspecified laterality

S62.329 Displaced fracture of shaft of unspecified metacarpal bone B, K, P, B

S62.33 Displaced fracture of neck of other metacarpal bone

S62.330 Displaced fracture of neck of second metacarpal bone, right hand B, K, P, B

S62.331 Displaced fracture of neck of second metacarpal bone, left hand B, K, P, B

S62.332 Displaced fracture of neck of third metacarpal bone, right hand B, K, P, B

S62.333 Displaced fracture of neck of third metacarpal bone, left hand B, K, P, B

S62.334 Displaced fracture of neck of fourth metacarpal bone, right hand B, K, P, B

S62.335 Displaced fracture of neck of fourth metacarpal bone, left hand B, K, P, B

S62.336 Displaced fracture of neck of fifth metacarpal bone, right hand B, K, P, B

S62.337 Displaced fracture of neck of fifth metacarpal bone, left hand B, K, P, B

S62.338 Displaced fracture of neck of other metacarpal bone B, K, P, B
Displaced fracture of neck of specified metacarpal bone with unspecified laterality

S62.339 Displaced fracture of neck of unspecified metacarpal bone B, K, P, B

S62.34 Nondisplaced fracture of base of other metacarpal bone

S62.340 Nondisplaced fracture of base of second metacarpal bone, right hand B, K, P, B

S62.341 Nondisplaced fracture of base of second metacarpal bone, left hand B, K, P, B

S62.342 Nondisplaced fracture of base of third metacarpal bone, right hand B, K, P, B

S62.343 Nondisplaced fracture of base of third metacarpal bone, left hand B, K, P, B

S62.344 Nondisplaced fracture of base of fourth metacarpal bone, right hand B, K, P, B

S62.345 Nondisplaced fracture of base of fourth metacarpal bone, left hand B, K, P, B

S62.346 Nondisplaced fracture of base of fifth metacarpal bone, right hand B, K, P, B

S62.347 Nondisplaced fracture of base of fifth metacarpal bone, left hand B, K, P, B

S62.348 Nondisplaced fracture of base of other metacarpal bone B, K, P, B
Nondisplaced fracture of base of specified metacarpal bone with unspecified laterality

S62.349 Nondisplaced fracture of base of unspecified metacarpal bone B, K, P, B

S62.35 Nondisplaced fracture of shaft of other metacarpal bone

S62.350 Nondisplaced fracture of shaft of second metacarpal bone, right hand B, K, P, B

S62.351 Nondisplaced fracture of shaft of second metacarpal bone, left hand B, K, P, B

S62.352 Nondisplaced fracture of shaft of third metacarpal bone, right hand B, K, P, B

S62.353 Nondisplaced fracture of shaft of third metacarpal bone, left hand B, K, P, B

S62.354 Nondisplaced fracture of shaft of fourth metacarpal bone, right hand B, K, P, B

S62.355 Nondisplaced fracture of shaft of fourth metacarpal bone, left hand B, K, P, B

S62.356 Nondisplaced fracture of shaft of fifth metacarpal bone, right hand B, K, P, B

S62.357 Nondisplaced fracture of shaft of fifth metacarpal bone, left hand B, K, P, B

S62.358 Nondisplaced fracture of shaft of other metacarpal bone B, K, P, B
Nondisplaced fracture of shaft of specified metacarpal bone with unspecified laterality

S62.359 Nondisplaced fracture of shaft of unspecified metacarpal bone B, K, P, B

S62.36 Nondisplaced fracture of neck of other metacarpal bone

S62.360 Nondisplaced fracture of neck of second metacarpal bone, right hand B, K, P, B

S62.361 Nondisplaced fracture of neck of second metacarpal bone, left hand B, K, P, B

S62.362 Nondisplaced fracture of neck of third metacarpal bone, right hand B, K, P, B

S62.363 Nondisplaced fracture of neck of third metacarpal bone, left hand B, K, P, B

S62.364 Nondisplaced fracture of neck of fourth metacarpal bone, right hand B, K, P, B

S62.365 Nondisplaced fracture of neck of fourth metacarpal bone, left hand B, K, P, B

S62.366 Nondisplaced fracture of neck of fifth metacarpal bone, right hand B, K, P, B

S62.367 Nondisplaced fracture of neck of fifth metacarpal bone, left hand B, K, P, B

S62.368 Nondisplaced fracture of neck of other metacarpal bone B, K, P, B
Nondisplaced fracture of neck of specified metacarpal bone with unspecified laterality

S62.369 Nondisplaced fracture of neck of unspecified metacarpal bone B, K, P, B

S62.39 Other fracture of other metacarpal bone

S62.390 Other fracture of second metacarpal bone, right hand B, K, P, B

S62.391 Other fracture of second metacarpal bone, left hand B, K, P, B

S62.392 Other fracture of third metacarpal bone, right hand B, K, P, B

S62.393 Other fracture of third metacarpal bone, left hand B, K, P, B

S62.394 Other fracture of fourth metacarpal bone, right hand B, K, P, B

S62.395 Other fracture of fourth metacarpal bone, left hand B, K, P, B

S62.396 Other fracture of fifth metacarpal bone, right hand B, K, P, B

S62.397 Other fracture of fifth metacarpal bone, left hand B, K, P, B

S62.398 Other fracture of other metacarpal bone B, K, P, B
Other fracture of specified metacarpal bone with unspecified laterality

S62.399 Other fracture of unspecified metacarpal bone B, K, P, B

S62.5 Fracture of thumb Ex: PDX 1264 [K, P], 1795 [B]

S62.50 Fracture of unspecified phalanx of thumb

S62.501 Fracture of unspecified phalanx of right thumb B, K, P, B

S62.502 Fracture of unspecified phalanx of left thumb B, K, P, B

S62.509 Fracture of unspecified phalanx of unspecified thumb B, K, P, B

S62.51 Fracture of proximal phalanx of thumb

S62.511 Displaced fracture of proximal phalanx of right thumb B, K, P, B

S62.512 Displaced fracture of proximal phalanx of left thumb B, K, P, B

S62.513 Displaced fracture of proximal phalanx of unspecified thumb B, K, P, B

S62.514 Nondisplaced fracture of proximal phalanx of right thumb B, K, P, B

S62.515 Nondisplaced fracture of proximal phalanx of left thumb B, K, P, B

S62.516 Nondisplaced fracture of proximal phalanx of unspecified thumb B, K, P, B

S62.52 Fracture of distal phalanx of thumb

S62.521 Displaced fracture of distal phalanx of right thumb B, K, P, B

S62.522 Displaced fracture of distal phalanx of left thumb B, K, P, B

S62.523 Displaced fracture of distal phalanx of unspecified thumb B, K, P, B

S62.524 Nondisplaced fracture of distal phalanx of right thumb B, K, P, B

S62.525 Nondisplaced fracture of distal phalanx of left thumb B, K, P, B

S62.526 Nondisplaced fracture of distal phalanx of unspecified thumb B, K, P, B

S62.6 Fracture of other and unspecified finger(s) Ex: PDX 1264 [K, P], 1795 [B]

Excludes2 fracture of thumb (S62.5-)

S62.60 Fracture of unspecified phalanx of finger

S62.600 Fracture of unspecified phalanx of right index finger B, K, P, B

S62.601 Fracture of unspecified phalanx of left index finger B, K, P, B

S62.602 Fracture of unspecified phalanx of right middle finger B, K, P, B

S62.603 Fracture of unspecified phalanx of left middle finger B, K, P, B

S62.604 Fracture of unspecified phalanx of right ring finger B, K, P, B

S62.605 Fracture of unspecified phalanx of left ring finger B, K, P, B

S62.606 Fracture of unspecified phalanx of right little finger B, K, P, B

S62.607 Fracture of unspecified phalanx of left little finger B, K, P, B

- S62.608 Fracture of unspecified phalanx of other finger B, K, P, B
  Fracture of unspecified phalanx of specified finger with unspecified laterality
- S62.609 Fracture of unspecified phalanx of unspecified finger B, K, P, B

- S62.61 Displaced fracture of proximal phalanx of finger
  - S62.610 Displaced fracture of proximal phalanx of right index finger B, K, P, B
  - S62.611 Displaced fracture of proximal phalanx of left index finger B, K, P, B
  - S62.612 Displaced fracture of proximal phalanx of right middle finger B, K, P, B
  - S62.613 Displaced fracture of proximal phalanx of left middle finger B, K, P, B
  - S62.614 Displaced fracture of proximal phalanx of right ring finger B, K, P, B
  - S62.615 Displaced fracture of proximal phalanx of left ring finger B, K, P, B
  - S62.616 Displaced fracture of proximal phalanx of right little finger B, K, P, B
  - S62.617 Displaced fracture of proximal phalanx of left little finger B, K, P, B
  - S62.618 Displaced fracture of proximal phalanx of other finger B, K, P, B
    Displaced fracture of proximal phalanx of specified finger with unspecified laterality
  - S62.619 Displaced fracture of proximal phalanx of unspecified finger B, K, P, B
- S62.62 Displaced fracture of middle phalanx of finger
  - S62.620 Displaced fracture of middle phalanx of right index finger B, K, P, B
  - S62.621 Displaced fracture of middle phalanx of left index finger B, K, P, B
  - S62.622 Displaced fracture of middle phalanx of right middle finger B, K, P, B
  - S62.623 Displaced fracture of middle phalanx of left middle finger B, K, P, B
  - S62.624 Displaced fracture of middle phalanx of right ring finger B, K, P, B
  - S62.625 Displaced fracture of middle phalanx of left ring finger B, K, P, B
  - S62.626 Displaced fracture of middle phalanx of right little finger B, K, P, B
  - S62.627 Displaced fracture of middle phalanx of left little finger B, K, P, B
  - S62.628 Displaced fracture of middle phalanx of other finger B, K, P, B
    Displaced fracture of middle phalanx of specified finger with unspecified laterality
  - S62.629 Displaced fracture of middle phalanx of unspecified finger B, K, P, B
- S62.63 Displaced fracture of distal phalanx of finger
  - S62.630 Displaced fracture of distal phalanx of right index finger B, K, P, B
  - S62.631 Displaced fracture of distal phalanx of left index finger B, K, P, B
  - S62.632 Displaced fracture of distal phalanx of right middle finger B, K, P, B
  - S62.633 Displaced fracture of distal phalanx of left middle finger B, K, P, B
  - S62.634 Displaced fracture of distal phalanx of right ring finger B, K, P, B
  - S62.635 Displaced fracture of distal phalanx of left ring finger B, K, P, B
  - S62.636 Displaced fracture of distal phalanx of right little finger B, K, P, B
  - S62.637 Displaced fracture of distal phalanx of left little finger B, K, P, B
  - S62.638 Displaced fracture of distal phalanx of other finger B, K, P, B
    Displaced fracture of distal phalanx of specified finger with unspecified laterality
  - S62.639 Displaced fracture of distal phalanx of unspecified finger B, K, P, B
- S62.64 Nondisplaced fracture of proximal phalanx of finger
  - S62.640 Nondisplaced fracture of proximal phalanx of right index finger B, K, P, B
  - S62.641 Nondisplaced fracture of proximal phalanx of left index finger B, K, P, B
  - S62.642 Nondisplaced fracture of proximal phalanx of right middle finger B, K, P, B
  - S62.643 Nondisplaced fracture of proximal phalanx of left middle finger B, K, P, B
  - S62.644 Nondisplaced fracture of proximal phalanx of right ring finger B, K, P, B
  - S62.645 Nondisplaced fracture of proximal phalanx of left ring finger B, K, P, B
  - S62.646 Nondisplaced fracture of proximal phalanx of right little finger B, K, P, B
  - S62.647 Nondisplaced fracture of proximal phalanx of left little finger B, K, P, B
  - S62.648 Nondisplaced fracture of proximal phalanx of other finger B, K, P, B
    Nondisplaced fracture of proximal phalanx of specified finger with unspecified laterality
  - S62.649 Nondisplaced fracture of proximal phalanx of unspecified finger B, K, P, B
- S62.65 Nondisplaced fracture of middle phalanx of finger
  - S62.650 Nondisplaced fracture of middle phalanx of right index finger B, K, P, B
  - S62.651 Nondisplaced fracture of middle phalanx of left index finger B, K, P, B
  - S62.652 Nondisplaced fracture of middle phalanx of right middle finger B, K, P, B
  - S62.653 Nondisplaced fracture of middle phalanx of left middle finger B, K, P, B
  - S62.654 Nondisplaced fracture of middle phalanx of right ring finger B, K, P, B
  - S62.655 Nondisplaced fracture of middle phalanx of left ring finger B, K, P, B

CHAPTER 19 (S00-T88)

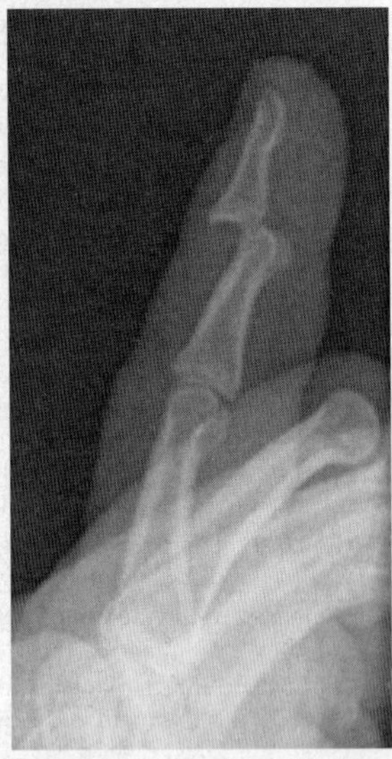

Figure 19-14 Dorsal dislocation of the distal phalanx of the index finger. (From Hardy M, Snaith B: Musculoskeletal Trauma: A Guide to Assessment and Diagnosis, 1e, Elsevier, 2011)

● **S62.656** **Nondisplaced fracture of middle phalanx of right little finger** B, K, P, B

● **S62.657** **Nondisplaced fracture of middle phalanx of left little finger** B, K, P, B

● **S62.658** **Nondisplaced fracture of middle phalanx of other finger** B, K, P, B
Nondisplaced fracture of middle phalanx of specified finger with unspecified laterality

● **S62.659** **Nondisplaced fracture of middle phalanx of unspecified finger** B, K, P, B

● **S62.66** **Nondisplaced fracture of distal phalanx of finger**

● **S62.660** **Nondisplaced fracture of distal phalanx of right index finger** B, K, P, B

● **S62.661** **Nondisplaced fracture of distal phalanx of left index finger** B, K, P, B

● **S62.662** **Nondisplaced fracture of distal phalanx of right middle finger** B, K, P, B

● **S62.663** **Nondisplaced fracture of distal phalanx of left middle finger** B, K, P, B

● **S62.664** **Nondisplaced fracture of distal phalanx of right ring finger** B, K, P, B

● **S62.665** **Nondisplaced fracture of distal phalanx of left ring finger** B, K, P, B

● **S62.666** **Nondisplaced fracture of distal phalanx of right little finger** B, K, P, B

● **S62.667** **Nondisplaced fracture of distal phalanx of left little finger** B, K, P, B

● **S62.668** **Nondisplaced fracture of distal phalanx of other finger** B, K, P, B
Nondisplaced fracture of distal phalanx of specified finger with unspecified laterality

● **S62.669** **Nondisplaced fracture of distal phalanx of unspecified finger** B, K, P, B

● **S62.9** **Unspecified fracture of wrist and hand**

X● **S62.90** **Unspecified fracture of unspecified wrist and hand** B, K, P, B (Ex) PDX 1264 [K, P], 1796 [B]

X● **S62.91** **Unspecified fracture of right wrist and hand** B, K, P, B (Ex) PDX 1264 [K, P], 1797 [B]

X● **S62.92** **Unspecified fracture of left wrist and hand** B, K, P, B (Ex) DX 1264 [K, P], 1797 [B]

● **S63** **Dislocation and sprain of joints and ligaments at wrist and hand level**

Includes avulsion of joint or ligament at wrist and hand level
laceration of cartilage, joint or ligament at wrist and hand level
sprain of cartilage, joint or ligament at wrist and hand level
traumatic hemarthrosis of joint or ligament at wrist and hand level
traumatic rupture of joint or ligament at wrist and hand level
traumatic subluxation of joint or ligament at wrist and hand level
traumatic tear of joint or ligament at wrist and hand level

Code also any associated open wound

Excludes2 strain of muscle, fascia and tendon of wrist and hand (S66.-)

The appropriate 7th character is to be added to each code from category S63

A	initial encounter
D	subsequent encounter
S	sequela

● **S63.0** **Subluxation and dislocation of wrist and hand joints**

● **S63.00** **Unspecified subluxation and dislocation of wrist and hand**
Dislocation of carpal bone NOS
Dislocation of distal end of radius NOS
Subluxation of carpal bone NOS
Subluxation of distal end of radius NOS

● **S63.001** **Unspecified subluxation of right wrist and hand**

● **S63.002** **Unspecified subluxation of left wrist and hand**

● **S63.003** **Unspecified subluxation of unspecified wrist and hand**

● **S63.004** **Unspecified dislocation of right wrist and hand**

● **S63.005** **Unspecified dislocation of left wrist and hand**

● **S63.006** **Unspecified dislocation of unspecified wrist and hand**

● **S63.01** **Subluxation and dislocation of distal radioulnar joint**

● **S63.011** **Subluxation of distal radioulnar joint of right wrist**

● **S63.012** **Subluxation of distal radioulnar joint of left wrist**

● **S63.013** **Subluxation of distal radioulnar joint of unspecified wrist**

● **S63.014** **Dislocation of distal radioulnar joint of right wrist**

● **S63.015** **Dislocation of distal radioulnar joint of left wrist**

● **S63.016** **Dislocation of distal radioulnar joint of unspecified wrist**

● **S63.02** **Subluxation and dislocation of radiocarpal joint**

● **S63.021** **Subluxation of radiocarpal joint of right wrist**

● **S63.022** **Subluxation of radiocarpal joint of left wrist**

S63.023 Subluxation of radiocarpal joint of unspecified wrist
S63.024 Dislocation of radiocarpal joint of right wrist
S63.025 Dislocation of radiocarpal joint of left wrist
S63.026 Dislocation of radiocarpal joint of unspecified wrist

S63.03 Subluxation and dislocation of midcarpal joint
S63.031 Subluxation of midcarpal joint of right wrist
S63.032 Subluxation of midcarpal joint of left wrist
S63.033 Subluxation of midcarpal joint of unspecified wrist
S63.034 Dislocation of midcarpal joint of right wrist
S63.035 Dislocation of midcarpal joint of left wrist
S63.036 Dislocation of midcarpal joint of unspecified wrist

S63.04 Subluxation and dislocation of carpometacarpal joint of thumb
Excludes2 interphalangeal subluxation and dislocation of thumb (S63.1-)
S63.041 Subluxation of carpometacarpal joint of right thumb
S63.042 Subluxation of carpometacarpal joint of left thumb
S63.043 Subluxation of carpometacarpal joint of unspecified thumb
S63.044 Dislocation of carpometacarpal joint of right thumb
S63.045 Dislocation of carpometacarpal joint of left thumb
S63.046 Dislocation of carpometacarpal joint of unspecified thumb

S63.05 Subluxation and dislocation of other carpometacarpal joint
Excludes2 subluxation and dislocation of carpometacarpal joint of thumb (S63.04-)
S63.051 Subluxation of other carpometacarpal joint of right hand
S63.052 Subluxation of other carpometacarpal joint of left hand
S63.053 Subluxation of other carpometacarpal joint of unspecified hand
S63.054 Dislocation of other carpometacarpal joint of right hand
S63.055 Dislocation of other carpometacarpal joint of left hand
S63.056 Dislocation of other carpometacarpal joint of unspecified hand

S63.06 Subluxation and dislocation of metacarpal (bone), proximal end
S63.061 Subluxation of metacarpal (bone), proximal end of right hand
S63.062 Subluxation of metacarpal (bone), proximal end of left hand
S63.063 Subluxation of metacarpal (bone), proximal end of unspecified hand
S63.064 Dislocation of metacarpal (bone), proximal end of right hand
S63.065 Dislocation of metacarpal (bone), proximal end of left hand
S63.066 Dislocation of metacarpal (bone), proximal end of unspecified hand

S63.07 Subluxation and dislocation of distal end of ulna
S63.071 Subluxation of distal end of right ulna
S63.072 Subluxation of distal end of left ulna
S63.073 Subluxation of distal end of unspecified ulna
S63.074 Dislocation of distal end of right ulna
S63.075 Dislocation of distal end of left ulna
S63.076 Dislocation of distal end of unspecified ulna

S63.09 Other subluxation and dislocation of wrist and hand
S63.091 Other subluxation of right wrist and hand
S63.092 Other subluxation of left wrist and hand
S63.093 Other subluxation of unspecified wrist and hand
S63.094 Other dislocation of right wrist and hand
S63.095 Other dislocation of left wrist and hand
S63.096 Other dislocation of unspecified wrist and hand

S63.1 Subluxation and dislocation of thumb

S63.10 Unspecified subluxation and dislocation of thumb
S63.101 Unspecified subluxation of right thumb
S63.102 Unspecified subluxation of left thumb
S63.103 Unspecified subluxation of unspecified thumb
S63.104 Unspecified dislocation of right thumb
S63.105 Unspecified dislocation of left thumb
S63.106 Unspecified dislocation of unspecified thumb

S63.11 Subluxation and dislocation of metacarpophalangeal joint of thumb
S63.111 Subluxation of metacarpophalangeal joint of right thumb
S63.112 Subluxation of metacarpophalangeal joint of left thumb
S63.113 Subluxation of metacarpophalangeal joint of unspecified thumb
S63.114 Dislocation of metacarpophalangeal joint of right thumb
S63.115 Dislocation of metacarpophalangeal joint of left thumb
S63.116 Dislocation of metacarpophalangeal joint of unspecified thumb

S63.12 Subluxation and dislocation of interphalangeal joint of thumb
S63.121 Subluxation of interphalangeal joint of right thumb
S63.122 Subluxation of interphalangeal joint of left thumb
S63.123 Subluxation of interphalangeal joint of unspecified thumb
S63.124 Dislocation of interphalangeal joint of right thumb
S63.125 Dislocation of interphalangeal joint of left thumb
S63.126 Dislocation of interphalangeal joint of unspecified thumb

CHAPTER 19 (SØØ-T88)

S63.2 Subluxation and dislocation of other finger(s)
Excludes2 subluxation and dislocation of thumb (S63.1-)
S63.20 Unspecified subluxation of other finger
S63.200 Unspecified subluxation of right index finger
S63.201 Unspecified subluxation of left index finger
S63.202 Unspecified subluxation of right middle finger
S63.203 Unspecified subluxation of left middle finger
S63.204 Unspecified subluxation of right ring finger
S63.205 Unspecified subluxation of left ring finger
S63.206 Unspecified subluxation of right little finger
S63.207 Unspecified subluxation of left little finger
S63.208 Unspecified subluxation of other finger
Unspecified subluxation of specified finger with unspecified laterality
S63.209 Unspecified subluxation of unspecified finger
S63.21 Subluxation of metacarpophalangeal joint of finger
S63.210 Subluxation of metacarpophalangeal joint of right index finger
S63.211 Subluxation of metacarpophalangeal joint of left index finger
S63.212 Subluxation of metacarpophalangeal joint of right middle finger
S63.213 Subluxation of metacarpophalangeal joint of left middle finger
S63.214 Subluxation of metacarpophalangeal joint of right ring finger
S63.215 Subluxation of metacarpophalangeal joint of left ring finger
S63.216 Subluxation of metacarpophalangeal joint of right little finger
S63.217 Subluxation of metacarpophalangeal joint of left little finger
S63.218 Subluxation of metacarpophalangeal joint of other finger
Subluxation of metacarpophalangeal joint of specified finger with unspecified laterality
S63.219 Subluxation of metacarpophalangeal joint of unspecified finger
S63.22 Subluxation of unspecified interphalangeal joint of finger
S63.220 Subluxation of unspecified interphalangeal joint of right index finger
S63.221 Subluxation of unspecified interphalangeal joint of left index finger
S63.222 Subluxation of unspecified interphalangeal joint of right middle finger
S63.223 Subluxation of unspecified interphalangeal joint of left middle finger
S63.224 Subluxation of unspecified interphalangeal joint of right ring finger
S63.225 Subluxation of unspecified interphalangeal joint of left ring finger
S63.226 Subluxation of unspecified interphalangeal joint of right little finger
S63.227 Subluxation of unspecified interphalangeal joint of left little finger
S63.228 Subluxation of unspecified interphalangeal joint of other finger
Subluxation of unspecified interphalangeal joint of specified finger with unspecified laterality
S63.229 Subluxation of unspecified interphalangeal joint of unspecified finger
S63.23 Subluxation of proximal interphalangeal joint of finger
S63.230 Subluxation of proximal interphalangeal joint of right index finger
S63.231 Subluxation of proximal interphalangeal joint of left index finger
S63.232 Subluxation of proximal interphalangeal joint of right middle finger
S63.233 Subluxation of proximal interphalangeal joint of left middle finger
S63.234 Subluxation of proximal interphalangeal joint of right ring finger
S63.235 Subluxation of proximal interphalangeal joint of left ring finger
S63.236 Subluxation of proximal interphalangeal joint of right little finger
S63.237 Subluxation of proximal interphalangeal joint of left little finger
S63.238 Subluxation of proximal interphalangeal joint of other finger
Subluxation of proximal interphalangeal joint of specified finger with unspecified laterality
S63.239 Subluxation of proximal interphalangeal joint of unspecified finger
S63.24 Subluxation of distal interphalangeal joint of finger
S63.240 Subluxation of distal interphalangeal joint of right index finger
S63.241 Subluxation of distal interphalangeal joint of left index finger
S63.242 Subluxation of distal interphalangeal joint of right middle finger
S63.243 Subluxation of distal interphalangeal joint of left middle finger
S63.244 Subluxation of distal interphalangeal joint of right ring finger
S63.245 Subluxation of distal interphalangeal joint of left ring finger
S63.246 Subluxation of distal interphalangeal joint of right little finger
S63.247 Subluxation of distal interphalangeal joint of left little finger

- **S63.248 Subluxation of distal interphalangeal joint of other finger**
  Subluxation of distal interphalangeal joint of specified finger with unspecified laterality
- **S63.249 Subluxation of distal interphalangeal joint of unspecified finger**

S63.25 Unspecified dislocation of other finger

- **S63.250 Unspecified dislocation of right index finger**
- **S63.251 Unspecified dislocation of left index finger**
- **S63.252 Unspecified dislocation of right middle finger**
- **S63.253 Unspecified dislocation of left middle finger**
- **S63.254 Unspecified dislocation of right ring finger**
- **S63.255 Unspecified dislocation of left ring finger**
- **S63.256 Unspecified dislocation of right little finger**
- **S63.257 Unspecified dislocation of left little finger**
- **S63.258 Unspecified dislocation of other finger**
  Unspecified dislocation of specified finger with unspecified laterality
- **S63.259 Unspecified dislocation of unspecified finger**
  Unspecified dislocation of unspecified finger with unspecified laterality

S63.26 Dislocation of metacarpophalangeal joint of finger

- **S63.260 Dislocation of metacarpophalangeal joint of right index finger**
- **S63.261 Dislocation of metacarpophalangeal joint of left index finger**
- **S63.262 Dislocation of metacarpophalangeal joint of right middle finger**
- **S63.263 Dislocation of metacarpophalangeal joint of left middle finger**
- **S63.264 Dislocation of metacarpophalangeal joint of right ring finger**
- **S63.265 Dislocation of metacarpophalangeal joint of left ring finger**
- **S63.266 Dislocation of metacarpophalangeal joint of right little finger**
- **S63.267 Dislocation of metacarpophalangeal joint of left little finger**
- **S63.268 Dislocation of metacarpophalangeal joint of other finger**
  Dislocation of metacarpophalangeal joint of specified finger with unspecified laterality
- **S63.269 Dislocation of metacarpophalangeal joint of unspecified finger**

S63.27 Dislocation of unspecified interphalangeal joint of finger

- **S63.270 Dislocation of unspecified interphalangeal joint of right index finger**
- **S63.271 Dislocation of unspecified interphalangeal joint of left index finger**
- **S63.272 Dislocation of unspecified interphalangeal joint of right middle finger**
- **S63.273 Dislocation of unspecified interphalangeal joint of left middle finger**
- **S63.274 Dislocation of unspecified interphalangeal joint of right ring finger**
- **S63.275 Dislocation of unspecified interphalangeal joint of left ring finger**
- **S63.276 Dislocation of unspecified interphalangeal joint of right little finger**
- **S63.277 Dislocation of unspecified interphalangeal joint of left little finger**
- **S63.278 Dislocation of unspecified interphalangeal joint of other finger**
  Dislocation of unspecified interphalangeal joint of specified finger with unspecified laterality
- **S63.279 Dislocation of unspecified interphalangeal joint of unspecified finger**
  Dislocation of unspecified interphalangeal joint of unspecified finger without specified laterality

S63.28 Dislocation of proximal interphalangeal joint of finger

- **S63.280 Dislocation of proximal interphalangeal joint of right index finger**
- **S63.281 Dislocation of proximal interphalangeal joint of left index finger**
- **S63.282 Dislocation of proximal interphalangeal joint of right middle finger**
- **S63.283 Dislocation of proximal interphalangeal joint of left middle finger**
- **S63.284 Dislocation of proximal interphalangeal joint of right ring finger**
- **S63.285 Dislocation of proximal interphalangeal joint of left ring finger**
- **S63.286 Dislocation of proximal interphalangeal joint of right little finger**
- **S63.287 Dislocation of proximal interphalangeal joint of left little finger**
- **S63.288 Dislocation of proximal interphalangeal joint of other finger**
  Dislocation of proximal interphalangeal joint of specified finger with unspecified laterality
- **S63.289 Dislocation of proximal interphalangeal joint of unspecified finger**

S63.29 Dislocation of distal interphalangeal joint of finger

- **S63.290 Dislocation of distal interphalangeal joint of right index finger**
- **S63.291 Dislocation of distal interphalangeal joint of left index finger**
- **S63.292 Dislocation of distal interphalangeal joint of right middle finger**
- **S63.293 Dislocation of distal interphalangeal joint of left middle finger**

S63.294 Dislocation of distal interphalangeal joint of right ring finger

S63.295 Dislocation of distal interphalangeal joint of left ring finger

S63.296 Dislocation of distal interphalangeal joint of right little finger

S63.297 Dislocation of distal interphalangeal joint of left little finger

S63.298 Dislocation of distal interphalangeal joint of other finger
Dislocation of distal interphalangeal joint of specified finger with unspecified laterality

S63.299 Dislocation of distal interphalangeal joint of unspecified finger

S63.3 Traumatic rupture of ligament of wrist

S63.30 Traumatic rupture of unspecified ligament of wrist

S63.301 Traumatic rupture of unspecified ligament of right wrist

S63.302 Traumatic rupture of unspecified ligament of left wrist

S63.309 Traumatic rupture of unspecified ligament of unspecified wrist

S63.31 Traumatic rupture of collateral ligament of wrist

S63.311 Traumatic rupture of collateral ligament of right wrist

S63.312 Traumatic rupture of collateral ligament of left wrist

S63.319 Traumatic rupture of collateral ligament of unspecified wrist

S63.32 Traumatic rupture of radiocarpal ligament

S63.321 Traumatic rupture of right radiocarpal ligament

S63.322 Traumatic rupture of left radiocarpal ligament

S63.329 Traumatic rupture of unspecified radiocarpal ligament

S63.33 Traumatic rupture of ulnocarpal (palmar) ligament

S63.331 Traumatic rupture of right ulnocarpal (palmar) ligament

S63.332 Traumatic rupture of left ulnocarpal (palmar) ligament

S63.339 Traumatic rupture of unspecified ulnocarpal (palmar) ligament

S63.39 Traumatic rupture of other ligament of wrist

S63.391 Traumatic rupture of other ligament of right wrist

S63.392 Traumatic rupture of other ligament of left wrist

S63.399 Traumatic rupture of other ligament of unspecified wrist

S63.4 Traumatic rupture of ligament of finger at metacarpophalangeal and interphalangeal joint(s)

S63.40 Traumatic rupture of unspecified ligament of finger at metacarpophalangeal and interphalangeal joint

S63.400 Traumatic rupture of unspecified ligament of right index finger at metacarpophalangeal and interphalangeal joint

S63.401 Traumatic rupture of unspecified ligament of left index finger at metacarpophalangeal and interphalangeal joint

S63.402 Traumatic rupture of unspecified ligament of right middle finger at metacarpophalangeal and interphalangeal joint

S63.403 Traumatic rupture of unspecified ligament of left middle finger at metacarpophalangeal and interphalangeal joint

S63.404 Traumatic rupture of unspecified ligament of right ring finger at metacarpophalangeal and interphalangeal joint

S63.405 Traumatic rupture of unspecified ligament of left ring finger at metacarpophalangeal and interphalangeal joint

S63.406 Traumatic rupture of unspecified ligament of right little finger at metacarpophalangeal and interphalangeal joint

S63.407 Traumatic rupture of unspecified ligament of left little finger at metacarpophalangeal and interphalangeal joint

S63.408 Traumatic rupture of unspecified ligament of other finger at metacarpophalangeal and interphalangeal joint
Traumatic rupture of unspecified ligament of specified finger with unspecified laterality at metacarpophalangeal and interphalangeal joint

S63.409 Traumatic rupture of unspecified ligament of unspecified finger at metacarpophalangeal and interphalangeal joint

S63.41 Traumatic rupture of collateral ligament of finger at metacarpophalangeal and interphalangeal joint

S63.410 Traumatic rupture of collateral ligament of right index finger at metacarpophalangeal and interphalangeal joint

S63.411 Traumatic rupture of collateral ligament of left index finger at metacarpophalangeal and interphalangeal joint

S63.412 Traumatic rupture of collateral ligament of right middle finger at metacarpophalangeal and interphalangeal joint

S63.413 Traumatic rupture of collateral ligament of left middle finger at metacarpophalangeal and interphalangeal joint

S63.414 Traumatic rupture of collateral ligament of right ring finger at metacarpophalangeal and interphalangeal joint

S63.415 Traumatic rupture of collateral ligament of left ring finger at metacarpophalangeal and interphalangeal joint

S63.416 Traumatic rupture of collateral ligament of right little finger at metacarpophalangeal and interphalangeal joint

S63.417 Traumatic rupture of collateral ligament of left little finger at metacarpophalangeal and interphalangeal joint

- **S63.418 Traumatic rupture of collateral ligament of other finger at metacarpophalangeal and interphalangeal joint**
  Traumatic rupture of collateral ligament of specified finger with unspecified laterality at metacarpophalangeal and interphalangeal joint
- **S63.419 Traumatic rupture of collateral ligament of unspecified finger at metacarpophalangeal and interphalangeal joint**

S63.42 Traumatic rupture of palmar ligament of finger at metacarpophalangeal and interphalangeal joint

- **S63.420 Traumatic rupture of palmar ligament of right index finger at metacarpophalangeal and interphalangeal joint**
- **S63.421 Traumatic rupture of palmar ligament of left index finger at metacarpophalangeal and interphalangeal joint**
- **S63.422 Traumatic rupture of palmar ligament of right middle finger at metacarpophalangeal and interphalangeal joint**
- **S63.423 Traumatic rupture of palmar ligament of left middle finger at metacarpophalangeal and interphalangeal joint**
- **S63.424 Traumatic rupture of palmar ligament of right ring finger at metacarpophalangeal and interphalangeal joint**
- **S63.425 Traumatic rupture of palmar ligament of left ring finger at metacarpophalangeal and interphalangeal joint**
- **S63.426 Traumatic rupture of palmar ligament of right little finger at metacarpophalangeal and interphalangeal joint**
- **S63.427 Traumatic rupture of palmar ligament of left little finger at metacarpophalangeal and interphalangeal joint**
- **S63.428 Traumatic rupture of palmar ligament of other finger at metacarpophalangeal and interphalangeal joint**
  Traumatic rupture of palmar ligament of specified finger with unspecified laterality at metacarpophalangeal and interphalangeal joint
- **S63.429 Traumatic rupture of palmar ligament of unspecified finger at metacarpophalangeal and interphalangeal joint**

S63.43 Traumatic rupture of volar plate of finger at metacarpophalangeal and interphalangeal joint

- **S63.430 Traumatic rupture of volar plate of right index finger at metacarpophalangeal and interphalangeal joint**
- **S63.431 Traumatic rupture of volar plate of left index finger at metacarpophalangeal and interphalangeal joint**
- **S63.432 Traumatic rupture of volar plate of right middle finger at metacarpophalangeal and interphalangeal joint**
- **S63.433 Traumatic rupture of volar plate of left middle finger at metacarpophalangeal and interphalangeal joint**
- **S63.434 Traumatic rupture of volar plate of right ring finger at metacarpophalangeal and interphalangeal joint**
- **S63.435 Traumatic rupture of volar plate of left ring finger at metacarpophalangeal and interphalangeal joint**
- **S63.436 Traumatic rupture of volar plate of right little finger at metacarpophalangeal and interphalangeal joint**
- **S63.437 Traumatic rupture of volar plate of left little finger at metacarpophalangeal and interphalangeal joint**
- **S63.438 Traumatic rupture of volar plate of other finger at metacarpophalangeal and interphalangeal joint**
  Traumatic rupture of volar plate of specified finger with unspecified laterality at metacarpophalangeal and interphalangeal joint
- **S63.439 Traumatic rupture of volar plate of unspecified finger at metacarpophalangeal and interphalangeal joint**

S63.49 Traumatic rupture of other ligament of finger at metacarpophalangeal and interphalangeal joint

- **S63.490 Traumatic rupture of other ligament of right index finger at metacarpophalangeal and interphalangeal joint**
- **S63.491 Traumatic rupture of other ligament of left index finger at metacarpophalangeal and interphalangeal joint**
- **S63.492 Traumatic rupture of other ligament of right middle finger at metacarpophalangeal and interphalangeal joint**
- **S63.493 Traumatic rupture of other ligament of left middle finger at metacarpophalangeal and interphalangeal joint**
- **S63.494 Traumatic rupture of other ligament of right ring finger at metacarpophalangeal and interphalangeal joint**
- **S63.495 Traumatic rupture of other ligament of left ring finger at metacarpophalangeal and interphalangeal joint**
- **S63.496 Traumatic rupture of other ligament of right little finger at metacarpophalangeal and interphalangeal joint**
- **S63.497 Traumatic rupture of other ligament of left little finger at metacarpophalangeal and interphalangeal joint**

S63.498 Traumatic rupture of other ligament of other finger at metacarpophalangeal and interphalangeal joint
Traumatic rupture of ligament of specified finger with unspecified laterality at metacarpophalangeal and interphalangeal joint
S63.499 Traumatic rupture of other ligament of unspecified finger at metacarpophalangeal and interphalangeal joint

S63.5 Other and unspecified sprain of wrist
S63.50 Unspecified sprain of wrist
S63.501 Unspecified sprain of right wrist
S63.502 Unspecified sprain of left wrist
S63.509 Unspecified sprain of unspecified wrist
S63.51 Sprain of carpal (joint)
S63.511 Sprain of carpal joint of right wrist
S63.512 Sprain of carpal joint of left wrist
S63.519 Sprain of carpal joint of unspecified wrist
S63.52 Sprain of radiocarpal joint
Excludes1 traumatic rupture of radiocarpal ligament (S63.32-)
S63.521 Sprain of radiocarpal joint of right wrist
S63.522 Sprain of radiocarpal joint of left wrist
S63.529 Sprain of radiocarpal joint of unspecified wrist
S63.59 Other specified sprain of wrist
S63.591 Other specified sprain of right wrist
S63.592 Other specified sprain of left wrist
S63.599 Other specified sprain of unspecified wrist

S63.6 Other and unspecified sprain of finger(s)
Excludes1 traumatic rupture of ligament of finger at metacarpophalangeal and interphalangeal joint(s) (S63.4-)
S63.60 Unspecified sprain of thumb
S63.601 Unspecified sprain of right thumb
S63.602 Unspecified sprain of left thumb
S63.609 Unspecified sprain of unspecified thumb
S63.61 Unspecified sprain of other and unspecified finger(s)
S63.610 Unspecified sprain of right index finger
S63.611 Unspecified sprain of left index finger
S63.612 Unspecified sprain of right middle finger
S63.613 Unspecified sprain of left middle finger
S63.614 Unspecified sprain of right ring finger
S63.615 Unspecified sprain of left ring finger
S63.616 Unspecified sprain of right little finger
S63.617 Unspecified sprain of left little finger
S63.618 Unspecified sprain of other finger
Unspecified sprain of specified finger with unspecified laterality
S63.619 Unspecified sprain of unspecified finger
S63.62 Sprain of interphalangeal joint of thumb
S63.621 Sprain of interphalangeal joint of right thumb
S63.622 Sprain of interphalangeal joint of left thumb
S63.629 Sprain of interphalangeal joint of unspecified thumb
S63.63 Sprain of interphalangeal joint of other and unspecified finger(s)
S63.630 Sprain of interphalangeal joint of right index finger
S63.631 Sprain of interphalangeal joint of left index finger
S63.632 Sprain of interphalangeal joint of right middle finger
S63.633 Sprain of interphalangeal joint of left middle finger
S63.634 Sprain of interphalangeal joint of right ring finger
S63.635 Sprain of interphalangeal joint of left ring finger
S63.636 Sprain of interphalangeal joint of right little finger
S63.637 Sprain of interphalangeal joint of left little finger
S63.638 Sprain of interphalangeal joint of other finger
S63.639 Sprain of interphalangeal joint of unspecified finger
S63.64 Sprain of metacarpophalangeal joint of thumb
S63.641 Sprain of metacarpophalangeal joint of right thumb
S63.642 Sprain of metacarpophalangeal joint of left thumb
S63.649 Sprain of metacarpophalangeal joint of unspecified thumb
S63.65 Sprain of metacarpophalangeal joint of other and unspecified finger(s)
S63.650 Sprain of metacarpophalangeal joint of right index finger
S63.651 Sprain of metacarpophalangeal joint of left index finger
S63.652 Sprain of metacarpophalangeal joint of right middle finger
S63.653 Sprain of metacarpophalangeal joint of left middle finger
S63.654 Sprain of metacarpophalangeal joint of right ring finger
S63.655 Sprain of metacarpophalangeal joint of left ring finger
S63.656 Sprain of metacarpophalangeal joint of right little finger
S63.657 Sprain of metacarpophalangeal joint of left little finger
S63.658 Sprain of metacarpophalangeal joint of other finger
Sprain of metacarpophalangeal joint of specified finger with unspecified laterality
S63.659 Sprain of metacarpophalangeal joint of unspecified finger
S63.68 Other sprain of thumb
S63.681 Other sprain of right thumb
S63.682 Other sprain of left thumb
S63.689 Other sprain of unspecified thumb
S63.69 Other sprain of other and unspecified finger(s)
S63.690 Other sprain of right index finger
S63.691 Other sprain of left index finger
S63.692 Other sprain of right middle finger

CHAPTER 19 (SØØ-T88)

● S63.693 Other sprain of left middle finger
● S63.694 Other sprain of right ring finger
● S63.695 Other sprain of left ring finger
● S63.696 Other sprain of right little finger
● S63.697 Other sprain of left little finger
● S63.698 Other sprain of other finger
Other sprain of specified finger with unspecified laterality
● S63.699 Other sprain of unspecified finger
● **S63.8 Sprain of other part of wrist and hand**
● S63.8X Sprain of other part of wrist and hand
● S63.8X1 Sprain of other part of right wrist and hand
● S63.8X2 Sprain of other part of left wrist and hand
● S63.8X9 Sprain of other part of unspecified wrist and hand
● **S63.9 Sprain of unspecified part of wrist and hand**
X● S63.90 Sprain of unspecified part of unspecified wrist and hand
X● S63.91 Sprain of unspecified part of right wrist and hand
X● S63.92 Sprain of unspecified part of left wrist and hand

● S64 Injury of nerves at wrist and hand level

The appropriate 7th character is to be added to each code from category S64

A	initial encounter
D	subsequent encounter
S	sequela

Code also any associated open wound (S61.-)

● **S64.0 Injury of ulnar nerve at wrist and hand level**
X● S64.00 Injury of ulnar nerve at wrist and hand level of unspecified arm
X● S64.01 Injury of ulnar nerve at wrist and hand level of right arm
X● S64.02 Injury of ulnar nerve at wrist and hand level of left arm
● **S64.1 Injury of median nerve at wrist and hand level**
X● S64.10 Injury of median nerve at wrist and hand level of unspecified arm
X● S64.11 Injury of median nerve at wrist and hand level of right arm
X● S64.12 Injury of median nerve at wrist and hand level of left arm
● **S64.2 Injury of radial nerve at wrist and hand level**
X● S64.20 Injury of radial nerve at wrist and hand level of unspecified arm
X● S64.21 Injury of radial nerve at wrist and hand level of right arm
X● S64.22 Injury of radial nerve at wrist and hand level of left arm
● **S64.3 Injury of digital nerve of thumb**
X● S64.30 Injury of digital nerve of unspecified thumb
X● S64.31 Injury of digital nerve of right thumb
X● S64.32 Injury of digital nerve of left thumb
● **S64.4 Injury of digital nerve of other and unspecified finger**
X● S64.40 Injury of digital nerve of unspecified finger
● S64.49 Injury of digital nerve of other finger
● S64.490 Injury of digital nerve of right index finger
● S64.491 Injury of digital nerve of left index finger
● S64.492 Injury of digital nerve of right middle finger
● S64.493 Injury of digital nerve of left middle finger
● S64.494 Injury of digital nerve of right ring finger
● S64.495 Injury of digital nerve of left ring finger
● S64.496 Injury of digital nerve of right little finger
● S64.497 Injury of digital nerve of left little finger
● S64.498 Injury of digital nerve of other finger
Injury of digital nerve of specified finger with unspecified laterality
● **S64.8 Injury of other nerves at wrist and hand level**
● S64.8X Injury of other nerves at wrist and hand level
● S64.8X1 Injury of other nerves at wrist and hand level of right arm
● S64.8X2 Injury of other nerves at wrist and hand level of left arm
● S64.8X9 Injury of other nerves at wrist and hand level of unspecified arm
● **S64.9 Injury of unspecified nerve at wrist and hand level**
X● S64.90 Injury of unspecified nerve at wrist and hand level of unspecified arm
X● S64.91 Injury of unspecified nerve at wrist and hand level of right arm
X● S64.92 Injury of unspecified nerve at wrist and hand level of left arm

● S65 Injury of blood vessels at wrist and hand level

The appropriate 7th character is to be added to each code from category S65

A	initial encounter
D	subsequent encounter
S	sequela

Code also any associated open wound (S61.-)

● **S65.0 Injury of ulnar artery at wrist and hand level**
● S65.00 Unspecified injury of ulnar artery at wrist and hand level
● S65.001 Unspecified injury of ulnar artery at wrist and hand level of right arm
A (Ex) PDX 1784
● S65.002 Unspecified injury of ulnar artery at wrist and hand level of left arm
A (Ex) PDX 1785
● S65.009 Unspecified injury of ulnar artery at wrist and hand level of unspecified arm A (Ex) PDX 1786
● S65.01 Laceration of ulnar artery at wrist and hand level
● S65.011 Laceration of ulnar artery at wrist and hand level of right arm
A (Ex) PDX 1784
● S65.012 Laceration of ulnar artery at wrist and hand level of left arm A (Ex) PDX 1785
● S65.019 Laceration of ulnar artery at wrist and hand level of unspecified arm
A (Ex) PDX 1786
● S65.09 Other specified injury of ulnar artery at wrist and hand level
● S65.091 Other specified injury of ulnar artery at wrist and hand level of right arm
A (Ex) PDX 1784
● S65.092 Other specified injury of ulnar artery at wrist and hand level of left arm
A (Ex) PDX 1785
● S65.099 Other specified injury of ulnar artery at wrist and hand level of unspecified arm A (Ex) PDX 1786

CHAPTER 19 (S00-T88)

S65.1 Injury of radial artery at wrist and hand level

S65.10 Unspecified injury of radial artery at wrist and hand level

S65.101 Unspecified injury of radial artery at wrist and hand level of right arm A PDX 1787

S65.102 Unspecified injury of radial artery at wrist and hand level of left arm A PDX 1788

S65.109 Unspecified injury of radial artery at wrist and hand level of unspecified arm A PDX 1789

S65.11 Laceration of radial artery at wrist and hand level

S65.111 Laceration of radial artery at wrist and hand level of right arm A PDX 1787

S65.112 Laceration of radial artery at wrist and hand level of left arm A PDX 1788

S65.119 Laceration of radial artery at wrist and hand level of unspecified arm A PDX 1789

S65.19 Other specified injury of radial artery at wrist and hand level

S65.191 Other specified injury of radial artery at wrist and hand level of right arm A PDX 1787

S65.192 Other specified injury of radial artery at wrist and hand level of left arm A PDX 1788

S65.199 Other specified injury of radial artery at wrist and hand level of unspecified arm A PDX 1789

S65.2 Injury of superficial palmar arch

S65.20 Unspecified injury of superficial palmar arch

S65.201 Unspecified injury of superficial palmar arch of right hand A PDX 1798

S65.202 Unspecified injury of superficial palmar arch of left hand A PDX 1799

S65.209 Unspecified injury of superficial palmar arch of unspecified hand A PDX 1800

S65.21 Laceration of superficial palmar arch

S65.211 Laceration of superficial palmar arch of right hand A PDX 1798

S65.212 Laceration of superficial palmar arch of left hand A PDX 1799

S65.219 Laceration of superficial palmar arch of unspecified hand A PDX 1800

S65.29 Other specified injury of superficial palmar arch

S65.291 Other specified injury of superficial palmar arch of right hand A PDX 1798

S65.292 Other specified injury of superficial palmar arch of left hand A PDX 1799

S65.299 Other specified injury of superficial palmar arch of unspecified hand A PDX 1800

S65.3 Injury of deep palmar arch

S65.30 Unspecified injury of deep palmar arch

S65.301 Unspecified injury of deep palmar arch of right hand A PDX 1798

S65.302 Unspecified injury of deep palmar arch of left hand A PDX 1799

S65.309 Unspecified injury of deep palmar arch of unspecified hand A PDX 1800

S65.31 Laceration of deep palmar arch

S65.311 Laceration of deep palmar arch of right hand A PDX 1798

S65.312 Laceration of deep palmar arch of left hand A PDX 1799

S65.319 Laceration of deep palmar arch of unspecified hand A PDX 1800

S65.39 Other specified injury of deep palmar arch

S65.391 Other specified injury of deep palmar arch of right hand A PDX 1798

S65.392 Other specified injury of deep palmar arch of left hand A PDX 1799

S65.399 Other specified injury of deep palmar arch of unspecified hand A PDX 1800

S65.4 Injury of blood vessel of thumb

S65.40 Unspecified injury of blood vessel of thumb

S65.401 Unspecified injury of blood vessel of right thumb A PDX 1801

S65.402 Unspecified injury of blood vessel of left thumb A PDX 1802

S65.409 Unspecified injury of blood vessel of unspecified thumb A PDX 1803

S65.41 Laceration of blood vessel of thumb

S65.411 Laceration of blood vessel of right thumb A PDX 1801

S65.412 Laceration of blood vessel of left thumb A PDX 1802

S65.419 Laceration of blood vessel of unspecified thumb A PDX 1803

S65.49 Other specified injury of blood vessel of thumb

S65.491 Other specified injury of blood vessel of right thumb A PDX 1801

S65.492 Other specified injury of blood vessel of left thumb A PDX 1802

S65.499 Other specified injury of blood vessel of unspecified thumb A PDX 1803

S65.5 Injury of blood vessel of other and unspecified finger

S65.50 Unspecified injury of blood vessel of other and unspecified finger

S65.500 Unspecified injury of blood vessel of right index finger A PDX 1801

S65.501 Unspecified injury of blood vessel of left index finger A PDX 1802

S65.502 Unspecified injury of blood vessel of right middle finger A PDX 1801

S65.503 Unspecified injury of blood vessel of left middle finger A PDX 1802

S65.504 Unspecified injury of blood vessel of right ring finger A PDX 1801

S65.505 Unspecified injury of blood vessel of left ring finger A PDX 1802

S65.506 Unspecified injury of blood vessel of right little finger A PDX 1801

S65.507 Unspecified injury of blood vessel of left little finger A PDX 1802

S65.508 Unspecified injury of blood vessel of other finger A PDX 1803
Unspecified injury of blood vessel of specified finger with unspecified laterality

S65.509 Unspecified injury of blood vessel of unspecified finger A PDX 1803

S65.51 Laceration of blood vessel of other and unspecified finger

S65.510 Laceration of blood vessel of right index finger A PDX 1801

S65.511 Laceration of blood vessel of left index finger A PDX 1802

S65.512 Laceration of blood vessel of right middle finger A PDX 1801

S65.513 Laceration of blood vessel of left middle finger A PDX 1802

S65.514 Laceration of blood vessel of right ring finger A PDX 1801

S65.515 Laceration of blood vessel of left ring finger A PDX 1802

S65.516 Laceration of blood vessel of right little finger A PDX 1801

S65.517 Laceration of blood vessel of left little finger A PDX 1802

S65.518 Laceration of blood vessel of other finger A PDX 1803

Laceration of blood vessel of specified finger with unspecified laterality

S65.519 Laceration of blood vessel of unspecified finger A PDX 1803

S65.59 Other specified injury of blood vessel of other and unspecified finger

S65.590 Other specified injury of blood vessel of right index finger A PDX 1801

S65.591 Other specified injury of blood vessel of left index finger A PDX 1802

S65.592 Other specified injury of blood vessel of right middle finger A PDX 1801

S65.593 Other specified injury of blood vessel of left middle finger A PDX 1802

S65.594 Other specified injury of blood vessel of right ring finger A PDX 1801

S65.595 Other specified injury of blood vessel of left ring finger A PDX 1802

S65.596 Other specified injury of blood vessel of right little finger A PDX 1801

S65.597 Other specified injury of blood vessel of left little finger A PDX 1802

S65.598 Other specified injury of blood vessel of other finger A PDX 1803

Other specified injury of blood vessel of specified finger with unspecified laterality

S65.599 Other specified injury of blood vessel of unspecified finger A PDX 1803

S65.8 Injury of other blood vessels at wrist and hand level

S65.80 Unspecified injury of other blood vessels at wrist and hand level

S65.801 Unspecified injury of other blood vessels at wrist and hand level of right arm A PDX 1770

S65.802 Unspecified injury of other blood vessels at wrist and hand level of left arm A PDX 1771

S65.809 Unspecified injury of other blood vessels at wrist and hand level of unspecified arm A PDX 1772

S65.81 Laceration of other blood vessels at wrist and hand level

S65.811 Laceration of other blood vessels at wrist and hand level of right arm A PDX 1770

S65.812 Laceration of other blood vessels at wrist and hand level of left arm A PDX 1771

S65.819 Laceration of other blood vessels at wrist and hand level of unspecified arm A PDX 1772

S65.89 Other specified injury of other blood vessels at wrist and hand level

S65.891 Other specified injury of other blood vessels at wrist and hand level of right arm A PDX 1770

S65.892 Other specified injury of other blood vessels at wrist and hand level of left arm A PDX 1771

S65.899 Other specified injury of other blood vessels at wrist and hand level of unspecified arm A PDX 1772

S65.9 Injury of unspecified blood vessel at wrist and hand level

S65.90 Unspecified injury of unspecified blood vessel at wrist and hand level

S65.901 Unspecified injury of unspecified blood vessel at wrist and hand level of right arm A PDX 1770

S65.902 Unspecified injury of unspecified blood vessel at wrist and hand level of left arm A PDX 1771

S65.909 Unspecified injury of unspecified blood vessel at wrist and hand level of unspecified arm A PDX 1772

S65.91 Laceration of unspecified blood vessel at wrist and hand level

S65.911 Laceration of unspecified blood vessel at wrist and hand level of right arm A PDX 1770

S65.912 Laceration of unspecified blood vessel at wrist and hand level of left arm A PDX 1771

S65.919 Laceration of unspecified blood vessel at wrist and hand level of unspecified arm A PDX 1772

S65.99 Other specified injury of unspecified blood vessel at wrist and hand level

S65.991 Other specified injury of unspecified blood vessel at wrist and hand of right arm A PDX 1770

S65.992 Other specified injury of unspecified blood vessel at wrist and hand of left arm A PDX 1771

S65.999 Other specified injury of unspecified blood vessel at wrist and hand of unspecified arm A PDX 1772

S66 Injury of muscle, fascia and tendon at wrist and hand level

Code also any associated open wound (S61.-)

Excludes2 sprain of joints and ligaments of wrist and hand (S63.-)

The appropriate 7th character is to be added to each code from category S66

A initial encounter
D subsequent encounter
S sequela

S66.0 Injury of long flexor muscle, fascia and tendon of thumb at wrist and hand level

S66.00 Unspecified injury of long flexor muscle, fascia and tendon of thumb at wrist and hand level

S66.001 Unspecified injury of long flexor muscle, fascia and tendon of right thumb at wrist and hand level

S66.002 Unspecified injury of long flexor muscle, fascia and tendon of left thumb at wrist and hand level

S66.009 Unspecified injury of long flexor muscle, fascia and tendon of unspecified thumb at wrist and hand level

CHAPTER 19 (S00-T88)

● S66.Ø1 Strain of long flexor muscle, fascia and tendon of thumb at wrist and hand level
● S66.Ø11 Strain of long flexor muscle, fascia and tendon of right thumb at wrist and hand level
● S66.Ø12 Strain of long flexor muscle, fascia and tendon of left thumb at wrist and hand level
● S66.Ø19 Strain of long flexor muscle, fascia and tendon of unspecified thumb at wrist and hand level
● S66.Ø2 Laceration of long flexor muscle, fascia and tendon of thumb at wrist and hand level
● S66.Ø21 Laceration of long flexor muscle, fascia and tendon of right thumb at wrist and hand level A (Ex) PDX 1804
● S66.Ø22 Laceration of long flexor muscle, fascia and tendon of left thumb at wrist and hand level A (Ex) PDX 1805
● S66.Ø29 Laceration of long flexor muscle, fascia and tendon of unspecified thumb at wrist and hand level A (Ex) PDX 1806
● S66.Ø9 Other specified injury of long flexor muscle, fascia and tendon of thumb at wrist and hand level
● S66.Ø91 Other specified injury of long flexor muscle, fascia and tendon of right thumb at wrist and hand level
● S66.Ø92 Other specified injury of long flexor muscle, fascia and tendon of left thumb at wrist and hand level
● S66.Ø99 Other specified injury of long flexor muscle, fascia and tendon of unspecified thumb at wrist and hand level
● S66.1 Injury of flexor muscle, fascia and tendon of other and unspecified finger at wrist and hand level
Excludes2 injury of long flexor muscle, fascia and tendon of thumb at wrist and hand level (S66.Ø-)
● S66.1Ø Unspecified injury of flexor muscle, fascia and tendon of other and unspecified finger at wrist and hand level
● S66.1ØØ Unspecified injury of flexor muscle, fascia and tendon of right index finger at wrist and hand level
● S66.1Ø1 Unspecified injury of flexor muscle, fascia and tendon of left index finger at wrist and hand level
● S66.1Ø2 Unspecified injury of flexor muscle, fascia and tendon of right middle finger at wrist and hand level
● S66.1Ø3 Unspecified injury of flexor muscle, fascia and tendon of left middle finger at wrist and hand level
● S66.1Ø4 Unspecified injury of flexor muscle, fascia and tendon of right ring finger at wrist and hand level
● S66.1Ø5 Unspecified injury of flexor muscle, fascia and tendon of left ring finger at wrist and hand level
● S66.1Ø6 Unspecified injury of flexor muscle, fascia and tendon of right little finger at wrist and hand level
● S66.1Ø7 Unspecified injury of flexor muscle, fascia and tendon of left little finger at wrist and hand level
● S66.1Ø8 Unspecified injury of flexor muscle, fascia and tendon of other finger at wrist and hand level
Unspecified injury of flexor muscle, fascia and tendon of specified finger with unspecified laterality at wrist and hand level
● S66.1Ø9 Unspecified injury of flexor muscle, fascia and tendon of unspecified finger at wrist and hand level
● S66.11 Strain of flexor muscle, fascia and tendon of other and unspecified finger at wrist and hand level
● S66.11Ø Strain of flexor muscle, fascia and tendon of right index finger at wrist and hand level
● S66.111 Strain of flexor muscle, fascia and tendon of left index finger at wrist and hand level
● S66.112 Strain of flexor muscle, fascia and tendon of right middle finger at wrist and hand level
● S66.113 Strain of flexor muscle, fascia and tendon of left middle finger at wrist and hand level
● S66.114 Strain of flexor muscle, fascia and tendon of right ring finger at wrist and hand level
● S66.115 Strain of flexor muscle, fascia and tendon of left ring finger at wrist and hand level
● S66.116 Strain of flexor muscle, fascia and tendon of right little finger at wrist and hand level
● S66.117 Strain of flexor muscle, fascia and tendon of left little finger at wrist and hand level
● S66.118 Strain of flexor muscle, fascia and tendon of other finger at wrist and hand level
Strain of flexor muscle, fascia and tendon of specified finger with unspecified laterality at wrist and hand level
● S66.119 Strain of flexor muscle, fascia and tendon of unspecified finger at wrist and hand level
● S66.12 Laceration of flexor muscle, fascia and tendon of other and unspecified finger at wrist and hand level
● S66.12Ø Laceration of flexor muscle, fascia and tendon of right index finger at wrist and hand level A (Ex) PDX 1804
● S66.121 Laceration of flexor muscle, fascia and tendon of left index finger at wrist and hand level A (Ex) PDX 1805
● S66.122 Laceration of flexor muscle, fascia and tendon of right middle finger at wrist and hand level A (Ex) PDX 1804
● S66.123 Laceration of flexor muscle, fascia and tendon of left middle finger at wrist and hand level A (Ex) PDX 1805
● S66.124 Laceration of flexor muscle, fascia and tendon of right ring finger at wrist and hand level A (Ex) PDX 1804
● S66.125 Laceration of flexor muscle, fascia and tendon of left ring finger at wrist and hand level A (Ex) PDX 1805
● S66.126 Laceration of flexor muscle, fascia and tendon of right little finger at wrist and hand level A (Ex) PDX 1804
● S66.127 Laceration of flexor muscle, fascia and tendon of left little finger at wrist and hand level A (Ex) PDX 1805

S66.128 Laceration of flexor muscle, fascia and tendon of other finger at wrist and hand level A (Ex) PDX 1806
Laceration of flexor muscle, fascia and tendon of specified finger with unspecified laterality at wrist and hand level

S66.129 Laceration of flexor muscle, fascia and tendon of unspecified finger at wrist and hand level A (Ex) PDX 1806

S66.19 Other injury of flexor muscle, fascia and tendon of other and unspecified finger at wrist and hand level

S66.190 Other injury of flexor muscle, fascia and tendon of right index finger at wrist and hand level

S66.191 Other injury of flexor muscle, fascia and tendon of left index finger at wrist and hand level

S66.192 Other injury of flexor muscle, fascia and tendon of right middle finger at wrist and hand level

S66.193 Other injury of flexor muscle, fascia and tendon of left middle finger at wrist and hand level

S66.194 Other injury of flexor muscle, fascia and tendon of right ring finger at wrist and hand level

S66.195 Other injury of flexor muscle, fascia and tendon of left ring finger at wrist and hand level

S66.196 Other injury of flexor muscle, fascia and tendon of right little finger at wrist and hand level

S66.197 Other injury of flexor muscle, fascia and tendon of left little finger at wrist and hand level

S66.198 Other injury of flexor muscle, fascia and tendon of other finger at wrist and hand level
Other injury of flexor muscle, fascia and tendon of specified finger with unspecified laterality at wrist and hand level

S66.199 Other injury of flexor muscle, fascia and tendon of unspecified finger at wrist and hand level

S66.2 Injury of extensor muscle, fascia and tendon of thumb at wrist and hand level

S66.20 Unspecified injury of extensor muscle, fascia and tendon of thumb at wrist and hand level

S66.201 Unspecified injury of extensor muscle, fascia and tendon of right thumb at wrist and hand level

S66.202 Unspecified injury of extensor muscle, fascia and tendon of left thumb at wrist and hand level

S66.209 Unspecified injury of extensor muscle, fascia and tendon of unspecified thumb at wrist and hand level

S66.21 Strain of extensor muscle, fascia and tendon of thumb at wrist and hand level

S66.211 Strain of extensor muscle, fascia and tendon of right thumb at wrist and hand level

S66.212 Strain of extensor muscle, fascia and tendon of left thumb at wrist and hand level

S66.219 Strain of extensor muscle, fascia and tendon of unspecified thumb at wrist and hand level

S66.22 Laceration of extensor muscle, fascia and tendon of thumb at wrist and hand level

S66.221 Laceration of extensor muscle, fascia and tendon of right thumb at wrist and hand level A (Ex) PDX 1804

S66.222 Laceration of extensor muscle, fascia and tendon of left thumb at wrist and hand level A (Ex) PDX 1805

S66.229 Laceration of extensor muscle, fascia and tendon of unspecified thumb at wrist and hand level A (Ex) PDX 1806

S66.29 Other specified injury of extensor muscle, fascia and tendon of thumb at wrist and hand level

S66.291 Other specified injury of extensor muscle, fascia and tendon of right thumb at wrist and hand level

S66.292 Other specified injury of extensor muscle, fascia and tendon of left thumb at wrist and hand level

S66.299 Other specified injury of extensor muscle, fascia and tendon of unspecified thumb at wrist and hand level

S66.3 Injury of extensor muscle, fascia and tendon of other and unspecified finger at wrist and hand level
Excludes2 injury of extensor muscle, fascia and tendon of thumb at wrist and hand level (S66.2-)

S66.30 Unspecified injury of extensor muscle, fascia and tendon of other and unspecified finger at wrist and hand level

S66.300 Unspecified injury of extensor muscle, fascia and tendon of right index finger at wrist and hand level

S66.301 Unspecified injury of extensor muscle, fascia and tendon of left index finger at wrist and hand level

S66.302 Unspecified injury of extensor muscle, fascia and tendon of right middle finger at wrist and hand level

S66.303 Unspecified injury of extensor muscle, fascia and tendon of left middle finger at wrist and hand level

S66.304 Unspecified injury of extensor muscle, fascia and tendon of right ring finger at wrist and hand level

S66.305 Unspecified injury of extensor muscle, fascia and tendon of left ring finger at wrist and hand level

S66.306 Unspecified injury of extensor muscle, fascia and tendon of right little finger at wrist and hand level

S66.307 Unspecified injury of extensor muscle, fascia and tendon of left little finger at wrist and hand level

S66.308 Unspecified injury of extensor muscle, fascia and tendon of other finger at wrist and hand level
Unspecified injury of extensor muscle, fascia and tendon of specified finger with unspecified laterality at wrist and hand level

S66.309 Unspecified injury of extensor muscle, fascia and tendon of unspecified finger at wrist and hand level

CHAPTER 19 (SØØ-T88)

- S66.31 Strain of extensor muscle, fascia and tendon of other and unspecified finger at wrist and hand level
  - S66.310 Strain of extensor muscle, fascia and tendon of right index finger at wrist and hand level
  - S66.311 Strain of extensor muscle, fascia and tendon of left index finger at wrist and hand level
  - S66.312 Strain of extensor muscle, fascia and tendon of right middle finger at wrist and hand level
  - S66.313 Strain of extensor muscle, fascia and tendon of left middle finger at wrist and hand level
  - S66.314 Strain of extensor muscle, fascia and tendon of right ring finger at wrist and hand level
  - S66.315 Strain of extensor muscle, fascia and tendon of left ring finger at wrist and hand level
  - S66.316 Strain of extensor muscle, fascia and tendon of right little finger at wrist and hand level
  - S66.317 Strain of extensor muscle, fascia and tendon of left little finger at wrist and hand level
  - S66.318 Strain of extensor muscle, fascia and tendon of other finger at wrist and hand level
    Strain of extensor muscle, fascia and tendon of specified finger with unspecified laterality at wrist and hand level
  - S66.319 Strain of extensor muscle, fascia and tendon of unspecified finger at wrist and hand level
- S66.32 Laceration of extensor muscle, fascia and tendon of other and unspecified finger at wrist and hand level
  - S66.320 Laceration of extensor muscle, fascia and tendon of right index finger at wrist and hand level A Ex: PDX 1804
  - S66.321 Laceration of extensor muscle, fascia and tendon of left index finger at wrist and hand level A Ex: PDX 1805
  - S66.322 Laceration of extensor muscle, fascia and tendon of right middle finger at wrist and hand level A Ex: PDX 1804
  - S66.323 Laceration of extensor muscle, fascia and tendon of left middle finger at wrist and hand level A Ex: PDX 1805
  - S66.324 Laceration of extensor muscle, fascia and tendon of right ring finger at wrist and hand level A Ex: PDX 1804
  - S66.325 Laceration of extensor muscle, fascia and tendon of left ring finger at wrist and hand level A Ex: PDX 1805
  - S66.326 Laceration of extensor muscle, fascia and tendon of right little finger at wrist and hand level A Ex: PDX 1804
  - S66.327 Laceration of extensor muscle, fascia and tendon of left little finger at wrist and hand level A Ex: PDX 1805
  - S66.328 Laceration of extensor muscle, fascia and tendon of other finger at wrist and hand level A Ex: PDX 1806
    Laceration of extensor muscle, fascia and tendon of specified finger with unspecified laterality at wrist and hand level
  - S66.329 Laceration of extensor muscle, fascia and tendon of unspecified finger at wrist and hand level A Ex: PDX 1806
- S66.39 Other injury of extensor muscle, fascia and tendon of other and unspecified finger at wrist and hand level
  - S66.390 Other injury of extensor muscle, fascia and tendon of right index finger at wrist and hand level
  - S66.391 Other injury of extensor muscle, fascia and tendon of left index finger at wrist and hand level
  - S66.392 Other injury of extensor muscle, fascia and tendon of right middle finger at wrist and hand level
  - S66.393 Other injury of extensor muscle, fascia and tendon of left middle finger at wrist and hand level
  - S66.394 Other injury of extensor muscle, fascia and tendon of right ring finger at wrist and hand level
  - S66.395 Other injury of extensor muscle, fascia and tendon of left ring finger at wrist and hand level
  - S66.396 Other injury of extensor muscle, fascia and tendon of right little finger at wrist and hand level
  - S66.397 Other injury of extensor muscle, fascia and tendon of left little finger at wrist and hand level
  - S66.398 Other injury of extensor muscle, fascia and tendon of other finger at wrist and hand level
    Other injury of extensor muscle, fascia and tendon of specified finger with unspecified laterality at wrist and hand level
  - S66.399 Other injury of extensor muscle, fascia and tendon of unspecified finger at wrist and hand level

S66.4 Injury of intrinsic muscle, fascia and tendon of thumb at wrist and hand level

- S66.40 Unspecified injury of intrinsic muscle, fascia and tendon of thumb at wrist and hand level
  - S66.401 Unspecified injury of intrinsic muscle, fascia and tendon of right thumb at wrist and hand level
  - S66.402 Unspecified injury of intrinsic muscle, fascia and tendon of left thumb at wrist and hand level
  - S66.409 Unspecified injury of intrinsic muscle, fascia and tendon of unspecified thumb at wrist and hand level
- S66.41 Strain of intrinsic muscle, fascia and tendon of thumb at wrist and hand level
  - S66.411 Strain of intrinsic muscle, fascia and tendon of right thumb at wrist and hand level
  - S66.412 Strain of intrinsic muscle, fascia and tendon of left thumb at wrist and hand level
  - S66.419 Strain of intrinsic muscle, fascia and tendon of unspecified thumb at wrist and hand level
- S66.42 Laceration of intrinsic muscle, fascia and tendon of thumb at wrist and hand level
  - S66.421 Laceration of intrinsic muscle, fascia and tendon of right thumb at wrist and hand level A Ex: PDX 1804
  - S66.422 Laceration of intrinsic muscle, fascia and tendon of left thumb at wrist and hand level A Ex: PDX 1805
  - S66.429 Laceration of intrinsic muscle, fascia and tendon of unspecified thumb at wrist and hand level A Ex: PDX 1806

● S66.49 **Other specified injury of intrinsic muscle, fascia and tendon of thumb at wrist and hand level**

● S66.491 **Other specified injury of intrinsic muscle, fascia and tendon of right thumb at wrist and hand level**

● S66.492 **Other specified injury of intrinsic muscle, fascia and tendon of left thumb at wrist and hand level**

● S66.499 **Other specified injury of intrinsic muscle, fascia and tendon of unspecified thumb at wrist and hand level**

● S66.5 **Injury of intrinsic muscle, fascia and tendon of other and unspecified finger at wrist and hand level**

Excludes2 injury of intrinsic muscle, fascia and tendon of thumb at wrist and hand level (S66.4-)

● S66.5Ø **Unspecified injury of intrinsic muscle, fascia and tendon of other and unspecified finger at wrist and hand level**

● S66.5ØØ **Unspecified injury of intrinsic muscle, fascia and tendon of right index finger at wrist and hand level**

● S66.5Ø1 **Unspecified injury of intrinsic muscle, fascia and tendon of left index finger at wrist and hand level**

● S66.5Ø2 **Unspecified injury of intrinsic muscle, fascia and tendon of right middle finger at wrist and hand level**

● S66.5Ø3 **Unspecified injury of intrinsic muscle, fascia and tendon of left middle finger at wrist and hand level**

● S66.5Ø4 **Unspecified injury of intrinsic muscle, fascia and tendon of right ring finger at wrist and hand level**

● S66.5Ø5 **Unspecified injury of intrinsic muscle, fascia and tendon of left ring finger at wrist and hand level**

● S66.5Ø6 **Unspecified injury of intrinsic muscle, fascia and tendon of right little finger at wrist and hand level**

● S66.5Ø7 **Unspecified injury of intrinsic muscle, fascia and tendon of left little finger at wrist and hand level**

● S66.5Ø8 **Unspecified injury of intrinsic muscle, fascia and tendon of other finger at wrist and hand level**

Unspecified injury of intrinsic muscle, fascia and tendon of specified finger with unspecified laterality at wrist and hand level

● S66.5Ø9 **Unspecified injury of intrinsic muscle, fascia and tendon of unspecified finger at wrist and hand level**

● S66.51 **Strain of intrinsic muscle, fascia and tendon of other and unspecified finger at wrist and hand level**

● S66.51Ø **Strain of intrinsic muscle, fascia and tendon of right index finger at wrist and hand level**

● S66.511 **Strain of intrinsic muscle, fascia and tendon of left index finger at wrist and hand level**

● S66.512 **Strain of intrinsic muscle, fascia and tendon of right middle finger at wrist and hand level**

● S66.513 **Strain of intrinsic muscle, fascia and tendon of left middle finger at wrist and hand level**

● S66.514 **Strain of intrinsic muscle, fascia and tendon of right ring finger at wrist and hand level**

● S66.515 **Strain of intrinsic muscle, fascia and tendon of left ring finger at wrist and hand level**

● S66.516 **Strain of intrinsic muscle, fascia and tendon of right little finger at wrist and hand level**

● S66.517 **Strain of intrinsic muscle, fascia and tendon of left little finger at wrist and hand level**

● S66.518 **Strain of intrinsic muscle, fascia and tendon of other finger at wrist and hand level**

Strain of intrinsic muscle, fascia and tendon of specified finger with unspecified laterality at wrist and hand level

● S66.519 **Strain of intrinsic muscle, fascia and tendon of unspecified finger at wrist and hand level**

● S66.52 **Laceration of intrinsic muscle, fascia and tendon of other and unspecified finger at wrist and hand level**

● S66.52Ø **Laceration of intrinsic muscle, fascia and tendon of right index finger at wrist and hand level** A (Ex) PDX 1804

● S66.521 **Laceration of intrinsic muscle, fascia and tendon of left index finger at wrist and hand level** A (Ex) PDX 1805

● S66.522 **Laceration of intrinsic muscle, fascia and tendon of right middle finger at wrist and hand level** A (Ex) PDX 1804

● S66.523 **Laceration of intrinsic muscle, fascia and tendon of left middle finger at wrist and hand level** A (Ex) PDX 1805

● S66.524 **Laceration of intrinsic muscle, fascia and tendon of right ring finger at wrist and hand level** A (Ex) PDX 1804

● S66.525 **Laceration of intrinsic muscle, fascia and tendon of left ring finger at wrist and hand level** A (Ex) PDX 1805

● S66.526 **Laceration of intrinsic muscle, fascia and tendon of right little finger at wrist and hand level** A (Ex) PDX 1804

● S66.527 **Laceration of intrinsic muscle, fascia and tendon of left little finger at wrist and hand level** A (Ex) PDX 1805

● S66.528 **Laceration of intrinsic muscle, fascia and tendon of other finger at wrist and hand level** A (Ex) PDX 1806

Laceration of intrinsic muscle, fascia and tendon of specified finger with unspecified laterality at wrist and hand level

● S66.529 **Laceration of intrinsic muscle, fascia and tendon of unspecified finger at wrist and hand level** A (Ex) PDX 1806

● S66.59 **Other injury of intrinsic muscle, fascia and tendon of other and unspecified finger at wrist and hand level**

● S66.59Ø **Other injury of intrinsic muscle, fascia and tendon of right index finger at wrist and hand level**

● S66.591 **Other injury of intrinsic muscle, fascia and tendon of left index finger at wrist and hand level**

● S66.592 **Other injury of intrinsic muscle, fascia and tendon of right middle finger at wrist and hand level**

● S66.593 **Other injury of intrinsic muscle, fascia and tendon of left middle finger at wrist and hand level**

● S66.594 **Other injury of intrinsic muscle, fascia and tendon of right ring finger at wrist and hand level**

CHAPTER 19 (SØØ-T88)

- S66.595 Other injury of intrinsic muscle, fascia and tendon of **left ring** finger at wrist and hand level
- S66.596 Other injury of intrinsic muscle, fascia and tendon of **right little** finger at wrist and hand level
- S66.597 Other injury of intrinsic muscle, fascia and tendon of **left little** finger at wrist and hand level
- S66.598 Other injury of intrinsic muscle, fascia and tendon of **other** finger at wrist and hand level
  Other injury of intrinsic muscle, fascia and tendon of specified finger with unspecified laterality at wrist and hand level
- S66.599 Other injury of intrinsic muscle, fascia and tendon of **unspecified** finger at wrist and hand level

S66.8 Injury of **other specified** muscles, fascia and tendons at wrist and hand level

- S66.80 **Unspecified** injury of other specified muscles, fascia and tendons at wrist and hand level
  - S66.801 Unspecified injury of other specified muscles, fascia and tendons at wrist and hand level, **right** hand
  - S66.802 Unspecified injury of other specified muscles, fascia and tendons at wrist and hand level, **left** hand
  - S66.809 Unspecified injury of other specified muscles, fascia and tendons at wrist and hand level, **unspecified** hand
- S66.81 **Strain** of other specified muscles, fascia and tendons at wrist and hand level
  - S66.811 Strain of other specified muscles, fascia and tendons at wrist and hand level, **right** hand
  - S66.812 Strain of other specified muscles, fascia and tendons at wrist and hand level, **left** hand
  - S66.819 Strain of other specified muscles, fascia and tendons at wrist and hand level, **unspecified** hand
- S66.82 **Laceration** of other specified muscles, fascia and tendons at wrist and hand level
  - S66.821 Laceration of other specified muscles, fascia and tendons at wrist and hand level, **right** hand A (Ex) PDX 1804
  - S66.822 Laceration of other specified muscles, fascia and tendons at wrist and hand level, **left** hand A (Ex) PDX 1805
  - S66.829 Laceration of other specified muscles, fascia and tendons at wrist and hand level, **unspecified** hand A (Ex) PDX 1806
- S66.89 **Other** injury of other specified muscles, fascia and tendons at wrist and hand level
  - S66.891 Other injury of other specified muscles, fascia and tendons at wrist and hand level, **right** hand
  - S66.892 Other injury of other specified muscles, fascia and tendons at wrist and hand level, **left** hand
  - S66.899 Other injury of other specified muscles, fascia and tendons at wrist and hand level, **unspecified** hand

S66.9 Injury of **unspecified** muscle, fascia and tendon at wrist and hand level

- S66.90 **Unspecified** injury of unspecified muscle, fascia and tendon at wrist and hand level
  - S66.901 Unspecified injury of unspecified muscle, fascia and tendon at wrist and hand level, **right** hand
  - S66.902 Unspecified injury of unspecified muscle, fascia and tendon at wrist and hand level, **left** hand
  - S66.909 Unspecified injury of unspecified muscle, fascia and tendon at wrist and hand level, **unspecified** hand
- S66.91 **Strain** of unspecified muscle, fascia and tendon at wrist and hand level
  - S66.911 Strain of unspecified muscle, fascia and tendon at wrist and hand level, **right** hand
  - S66.912 Strain of unspecified muscle, fascia and tendon at wrist and hand level, **left** hand
  - S66.919 Strain of unspecified muscle, fascia and tendon at wrist and hand level, **unspecified** hand
- S66.92 **Laceration** of unspecified muscle, fascia and tendon at wrist and hand level
  - S66.921 Laceration of unspecified muscle, fascia and tendon at wrist and hand level, **right** hand A (Ex) PDX 1804
  - S66.922 Laceration of unspecified muscle, fascia and tendon at wrist and hand level, **left** hand A (Ex) PDX 1805
  - S66.929 Laceration of unspecified muscle, fascia and tendon at wrist and hand level, **unspecified** hand A (Ex) PDX 1806
- S66.99 **Other** injury of unspecified muscle, fascia and tendon at wrist and hand level
  - S66.991 Other injury of unspecified muscle, fascia and tendon at wrist and hand level, **right** hand
  - S66.992 Other injury of unspecified muscle, fascia and tendon at wrist and hand level, **left** hand
  - S66.999 Other injury of unspecified muscle, fascia and tendon at wrist and hand level, **unspecified** hand

S67 **Crushing injury** of wrist, hand and fingers

Use additional code for all associated injuries, such as:
fracture of wrist and hand (S62.-)
open wound of wrist and hand (S61.-)

The appropriate 7th character is to be added to each code from category S67

A	initial encounter
D	subsequent encounter
S	sequela

- S67.0 Crushing injury of **thumb**
  - X S67.00 Crushing injury of **unspecified** thumb
  - X S67.01 Crushing injury of **right** thumb
  - X S67.02 Crushing injury of **left** thumb
- S67.1 Crushing injury of other and unspecified **finger**(s)
  Excludes2 crushing injury of thumb (S67.0-)
  - X S67.10 Crushing injury of **unspecified** finger(s)
  - S67.19 Crushing injury of other finger(s)
    - S67.190 Crushing injury of **right index** finger
    - S67.191 Crushing injury of **left index** finger
    - S67.192 Crushing injury of **right middle** finger
    - S67.193 Crushing injury of **left middle** finger

CHAPTER 19 (S00-T88)

S67.194 Crushing injury of right ring finger
S67.195 Crushing injury of left ring finger
S67.196 Crushing injury of right little finger
S67.197 Crushing injury of left little finger
S67.198 Crushing injury of other finger
Crushing injury of specified finger with unspecified laterality

S67.2 Crushing injury of hand
Excludes2 crushing injury of fingers (S67.1-)
crushing injury of thumb (S67.Ø-)
X S67.2Ø Crushing injury of unspecified hand
X S67.21 Crushing injury of right hand
X S67.22 Crushing injury of left hand

S67.3 Crushing injury of wrist
X S67.3Ø Crushing injury of unspecified wrist
X S67.31 Crushing injury of right wrist
X S67.32 Crushing injury of left wrist

S67.4 Crushing injury of wrist and hand
Excludes1 crushing injury of hand alone (S67.2-)
crushing injury of wrist alone (S67.3-)
Excludes2 crushing injury of fingers (S67.1-)
crushing injury of thumb (S67.Ø-)
X S67.4Ø Crushing injury of unspecified wrist and hand
X S67.41 Crushing injury of right wrist and hand
X S67.42 Crushing injury of left wrist and hand

S67.9 Crushing injury of unspecified part(s) of wrist, hand and fingers
X S67.9Ø Crushing injury of unspecified part(s) of unspecified wrist, hand and fingers
X S67.91 Crushing injury of unspecified part(s) of right wrist, hand and fingers
X S67.92 Crushing injury of unspecified part(s) of left wrist, hand and fingers

S68 Traumatic amputation of wrist, hand and fingers

An amputation not identified as partial or complete should be coded to complete

The appropriate 7th character is to be added to each code from category S68

A initial encounter
D subsequent encounter
S sequela

S68.Ø Traumatic metacarpophalangeal amputation of thumb
Traumatic amputation of thumb NOS

S68.Ø1 Complete traumatic metacarpophalangeal amputation of thumb
S68.Ø11 Complete traumatic metacarpophalangeal amputation of right thumb S
S68.Ø12 Complete traumatic metacarpophalangeal amputation of left thumb S
S68.Ø19 Complete traumatic metacarpophalangeal amputation of unspecified thumb S

S68.Ø2 Partial traumatic metacarpophalangeal amputation of thumb
S68.Ø21 Partial traumatic metacarpophalangeal amputation of right thumb S
S68.Ø22 Partial traumatic metacarpophalangeal amputation of left thumb S
S68.Ø29 Partial traumatic metacarpophalangeal amputation of unspecified thumb S

S68.1 Traumatic metacarpophalangeal amputation of other and unspecified finger
Traumatic amputation of finger NOS
Excludes2 traumatic metacarpophalangeal amputation of thumb (S68.Ø-)

S68.11 Complete traumatic metacarpophalangeal amputation of other and unspecified finger
S68.11Ø Complete traumatic metacarpophalangeal amputation of right index finger S
S68.111 Complete traumatic metacarpophalangeal amputation of left index finger S
S68.112 Complete traumatic metacarpophalangeal amputation of right middle finger S
S68.113 Complete traumatic metacarpophalangeal amputation of left middle finger S
S68.114 Complete traumatic metacarpophalangeal amputation of right ring finger S
S68.115 Complete traumatic metacarpophalangeal amputation of left ring finger S
S68.116 Complete traumatic metacarpophalangeal amputation of right little finger S
S68.117 Complete traumatic metacarpophalangeal amputation of left little finger S
S68.118 Complete traumatic metacarpophalangeal amputation of other finger S
Complete traumatic metacarpophalangeal amputation of specified finger with unspecified laterality
S68.119 Complete traumatic metacarpophalangeal amputation of unspecified finger S

S68.12 Partial traumatic metacarpophalangeal amputation of other and unspecified finger
S68.12Ø Partial traumatic metacarpophalangeal amputation of right index finger S
S68.121 Partial traumatic metacarpophalangeal amputation of left index finger S
S68.122 Partial traumatic metacarpophalangeal amputation of right middle finger S
S68.123 Partial traumatic metacarpophalangeal amputation of left middle finger S
S68.124 Partial traumatic metacarpophalangeal amputation of right ring finger S
S68.125 Partial traumatic metacarpophalangeal amputation of left ring finger S
S68.126 Partial traumatic metacarpophalangeal amputation of right little finger S
S68.127 Partial traumatic metacarpophalangeal amputation of left little finger S

CHAPTER 19 (SØØ-T88)

S68.128 Partial traumatic metacarpophalangeal amputation of **other** finger S
Partial traumatic metacarpophalangeal amputation of specified finger with unspecified laterality

S68.129 Partial traumatic metacarpophalangeal amputation of **unspecified** finger S

S68.4 Traumatic amputation of **hand** at wrist level
Traumatic amputation of hand NOS
Traumatic amputation of wrist

S68.41 **Complete** traumatic amputation of hand at wrist level

S68.411 Complete traumatic amputation of **right** hand at wrist level A, A, S (Ex) PDX 1776

S68.412 Complete traumatic amputation of **left** hand at wrist level A, A, S (Ex) PDX 1777

S68.419 Complete traumatic amputation of **unspecified** hand at wrist level A, A, S (Ex) PDX 1778

S68.42 **Partial** traumatic amputation of hand at wrist level

S68.421 Partial traumatic amputation of **right** hand at wrist level A, A, S (Ex) PDX 1776

S68.422 Partial traumatic amputation of **left** hand at wrist level A, A, S (Ex) PDX 1777

S68.429 Partial traumatic amputation of **unspecified** hand at wrist level A, A, S (Ex) PDX 1778

S68.5 Traumatic **transphalangeal** amputation of **thumb**
Traumatic interphalangeal joint amputation of thumb

S68.51 **Complete** traumatic transphalangeal amputation of thumb

S68.511 Complete traumatic transphalangeal amputation of **right** thumb S

S68.512 Complete traumatic transphalangeal amputation of **left** thumb S

S68.519 Complete traumatic transphalangeal amputation of **unspecified** thumb S

S68.52 **Partial** traumatic transphalangeal amputation of thumb

S68.521 Partial traumatic transphalangeal amputation of **right** thumb S

S68.522 Partial traumatic transphalangeal amputation of **left** thumb S

S68.529 Partial traumatic transphalangeal amputation of **unspecified** thumb S

S68.6 Traumatic **transphalangeal** amputation of other and unspecified **finger**

S68.61 **Complete** traumatic transphalangeal amputation of other and unspecified finger(s)

S68.610 Complete traumatic transphalangeal amputation of **right index** finger S

S68.611 Complete traumatic transphalangeal amputation of **left index** finger S

S68.612 Complete traumatic transphalangeal amputation of **right middle** finger S

S68.613 Complete traumatic transphalangeal amputation of **left middle** finger S

S68.614 Complete traumatic transphalangeal amputation of **right ring** finger S

S68.615 Complete traumatic transphalangeal amputation of **left ring** finger S

S68.616 Complete traumatic transphalangeal amputation of **right little** finger S

S68.617 Complete traumatic transphalangeal amputation of **left little** finger S

S68.618 Complete traumatic transphalangeal amputation of **other** finger S
Complete traumatic transphalangeal amputation of specified finger with unspecified laterality

S68.619 Complete traumatic transphalangeal amputation of **unspecified** finger S

S68.62 **Partial** traumatic transphalangeal amputation of other and unspecified finger

S68.620 Partial traumatic transphalangeal amputation of **right index** finger S

S68.621 Partial traumatic transphalangeal amputation of **left index** finger S

S68.622 Partial traumatic transphalangeal amputation of **right middle** finger S

S68.623 Partial traumatic transphalangeal amputation of **left middle** finger S

S68.624 Partial traumatic transphalangeal amputation of **right ring** finger S

S68.625 Partial traumatic transphalangeal amputation of **left ring** finger S

S68.626 Partial traumatic transphalangeal amputation of **right little** finger S

S68.627 Partial traumatic transphalangeal amputation of **left little** finger S

S68.628 Partial traumatic transphalangeal amputation of **other** finger S
Partial traumatic transphalangeal amputation of specified finger with unspecified laterality

S68.629 Partial traumatic transphalangeal amputation of **unspecified** finger S

S68.7 Traumatic **transmetacarpal** amputation of **hand**

S68.71 **Complete** traumatic transmetacarpal amputation of hand

S68.711 Complete traumatic transmetacarpal amputation of **right** hand A, A, S (Ex) PDX 1776

S68.712 Complete traumatic transmetacarpal amputation of **left** hand A, A, S (Ex) PDX 1777

S68.719 Complete traumatic transmetacarpal amputation of **unspecified** hand A, A, S (Ex) PDX 1778

S68.72 **Partial** traumatic transmetacarpal amputation of hand

S68.721 Partial traumatic transmetacarpal amputation of **right** hand A, A, S (Ex) PDX 1776

S68.722 Partial traumatic transmetacarpal amputation of **left** hand A, A, S (Ex) PDX 1777

S68.729 Partial traumatic transmetacarpal amputation of **unspecified** hand A, A, S (Ex) PDX 1778

S69 Other and unspecified injuries of wrist, hand and finger(s)
The appropriate 7th character is to be added to each code from category S69

A	initial encounter
D	subsequent encounter
S	sequela

S69.8 **Other** specified injuries of wrist, hand and finger(s)

X S69.80 Other specified injuries of **unspecified** wrist, hand and finger(s)

X S69.81 Other specified injuries of **right** wrist, hand and finger(s)

X S69.82 Other specified injuries of **left** wrist, hand and finger(s)

CHAPTER 19 (SØØ-T88)

● **S69.9 Unspecified injury of wrist, hand and finger(s)**
- X● **S69.90 Unspecified injury of unspecified wrist, hand and finger(s)**
- X● **S69.91 Unspecified injury of right wrist, hand and finger(s)**
- X● **S69.92 Unspecified injury of left wrist, hand and finger(s)**

INJURIES TO THE HIP AND THIGH (S7Ø-S79)

Excludes2 burns and corrosions (T2Ø-T32)
frostbite (T33-T34)
snake bite (T63.Ø-)
venomous insect bite or sting (T63.4-)

● **S7Ø Superficial injury of hip and thigh**

The appropriate 7th character is to be added to each code from category S7Ø

A	initial encounter
D	subsequent encounter
S	sequela

● **S7Ø.Ø Contusion of hip**
- X● **S7Ø.ØØ Contusion of unspecified hip**
- X● **S7Ø.Ø1 Contusion of right hip**
- X● **S7Ø.Ø2 Contusion of left hip**

● **S7Ø.1 Contusion of thigh**
- X● **S7Ø.1Ø Contusion of unspecified thigh**
- X● **S7Ø.11 Contusion of right thigh**
- X● **S7Ø.12 Contusion of left thigh**

● **S7Ø.2 Other superficial injuries of hip**
- ● **S7Ø.21 Abrasion of hip**
  - ● **S7Ø.211 Abrasion, right hip**
  - ● **S7Ø.212 Abrasion, left hip**
  - ● **S7Ø.219 Abrasion, unspecified hip**
- ● **S7Ø.22 Blister (nonthermal) of hip**
  - ● **S7Ø.221 Blister (nonthermal), right hip**
  - ● **S7Ø.222 Blister (nonthermal), left hip**
  - ● **S7Ø.229 Blister (nonthermal), unspecified hip**
- ● **S7Ø.24 External constriction of hip**
  - ● **S7Ø.241 External constriction, right hip**
  - ● **S7Ø.242 External constriction, left hip**
  - ● **S7Ø.249 External constriction, unspecified hip**
- ● **S7Ø.25 Superficial foreign body of hip**
  Splinter in the hip
  - ● **S7Ø.251 Superficial foreign body, right hip**
  - ● **S7Ø.252 Superficial foreign body, left hip**
  - ● **S7Ø.259 Superficial foreign body, unspecified hip**
- ● **S7Ø.26 Insect bite (nonvenomous) of hip**
  - ● **S7Ø.261 Insect bite (nonvenomous), right hip**
  - ● **S7Ø.262 Insect bite (nonvenomous), left hip**
  - ● **S7Ø.269 Insect bite (nonvenomous), unspecified hip**
- ● **S7Ø.27 Other superficial bite of hip**
  Excludes1 open bite of hip (S71.Ø5-)
  - ● **S7Ø.271 Other superficial bite of hip, right hip**
  - ● **S7Ø.272 Other superficial bite of hip, left hip**
  - ● **S7Ø.279 Other superficial bite of hip, unspecified hip**

● **S7Ø.3 Other superficial injuries of thigh**
- ● **S7Ø.31 Abrasion of thigh**
  - ● **S7Ø.311 Abrasion, right thigh**
  - ● **S7Ø.312 Abrasion, left thigh**
  - ● **S7Ø.319 Abrasion, unspecified thigh**
- ● **S7Ø.32 Blister (nonthermal) of thigh**
  - ● **S7Ø.321 Blister (nonthermal), right thigh**
  - ● **S7Ø.322 Blister (nonthermal), left thigh**
  - ● **S7Ø.329 Blister (nonthermal), unspecified thigh**
- ● **S7Ø.34 External constriction of thigh**
  - ● **S7Ø.341 External constriction, right thigh**
  - ● **S7Ø.342 External constriction, left thigh**
  - ● **S7Ø.349 External constriction, unspecified thigh**
- ● **S7Ø.35 Superficial foreign body of thigh**
  Splinter in the thigh
  - ● **S7Ø.351 Superficial foreign body, right thigh**
  - ● **S7Ø.352 Superficial foreign body, left thigh**
  - ● **S7Ø.359 Superficial foreign body, unspecified thigh**
- ● **S7Ø.36 Insect bite (nonvenomous) of thigh**
  - ● **S7Ø.361 Insect bite (nonvenomous), right thigh**
  - ● **S7Ø.362 Insect bite (nonvenomous), left thigh**
  - ● **S7Ø.369 Insect bite (nonvenomous), unspecified thigh**
- ● **S7Ø.37 Other superficial bite of thigh**
  Excludes1 open bite of thigh (S71.15)
  - ● **S7Ø.371 Other superficial bite of right thigh**
  - ● **S7Ø.372 Other superficial bite of left thigh**
  - ● **S7Ø.379 Other superficial bite of unspecified thigh**

● **S7Ø.9 Unspecified superficial injury of hip and thigh**
- ● **S7Ø.91 Unspecified superficial injury of hip**
  - ● **S7Ø.911 Unspecified superficial injury of right hip**
  - ● **S7Ø.912 Unspecified superficial injury of left hip**
  - ● **S7Ø.919 Unspecified superficial injury of unspecified hip**
- ● **S7Ø.92 Unspecified superficial injury of thigh**
  - ● **S7Ø.921 Unspecified superficial injury of right thigh**
  - ● **S7Ø.922 Unspecified superficial injury of left thigh**
  - ● **S7Ø.929 Unspecified superficial injury of unspecified thigh**

● **S71 Open wound of hip and thigh**

Code also any associated wound infection

Excludes1 open fracture of hip and thigh (S72.-)
traumatic amputation of hip and thigh (S78.-)

Excludes2 bite of venomous animal (T63.-)
open wound of ankle, foot and toes (S91.-)
open wound of knee and lower leg (S81.-)

The appropriate 7th character is to be added to each code from category S71

A	initial encounter
D	subsequent encounter
S	sequela

● **S71.Ø Open wound of hip**
- ● **S71.ØØ Unspecified open wound of hip**
  - ● **S71.ØØ1 Unspecified open wound, right hip**
  - ● **S71.ØØ2 Unspecified open wound, left hip**
  - ● **S71.ØØ9 Unspecified open wound, unspecified hip**
- ● **S71.Ø1 Laceration without foreign body of hip**
  - ● **S71.Ø11 Laceration without foreign body, right hip**
  - ● **S71.Ø12 Laceration without foreign body, left hip**
  - ● **S71.Ø19 Laceration without foreign body, unspecified hip**

CHAPTER 19 (SØØ-T88)

- S71.02 Laceration with foreign body of hip
  - S71.021 Laceration with foreign body, right hip
  - S71.022 Laceration with foreign body, left hip
  - S71.029 Laceration with foreign body, unspecified hip
- S71.03 Puncture wound without foreign body of hip
  - S71.031 Puncture wound without foreign body, right hip
  - S71.032 Puncture wound without foreign body, left hip
  - S71.039 Puncture wound without foreign body, unspecified hip
- S71.04 Puncture wound with foreign body of hip
  - S71.041 Puncture wound with foreign body, right hip
  - S71.042 Puncture wound with foreign body, left hip
  - S71.049 Puncture wound with foreign body, unspecified hip
- S71.05 Open bite of hip
  Bite of hip NOS
  Excludes1 superficial bite of hip (S7Ø.26, S7Ø.27)
  - S71.051 Open bite, right hip
  - S71.052 Open bite, left hip
  - S71.059 Open bite, unspecified hip

S71.1 Open wound of thigh

- S71.10 Unspecified open wound of thigh
  - S71.101 Unspecified open wound, right thigh
  - S71.102 Unspecified open wound, left thigh
  - S71.109 Unspecified open wound, unspecified thigh
- S71.11 Laceration without foreign body of thigh
  - S71.111 Laceration without foreign body, right thigh
  - S71.112 Laceration without foreign body, left thigh
  - S71.119 Laceration without foreign body, unspecified thigh
- S71.12 Laceration with foreign body of thigh
  - S71.121 Laceration with foreign body, right thigh
  - S71.122 Laceration with foreign body, left thigh
  - S71.129 Laceration with foreign body, unspecified thigh
- S71.13 Puncture wound without foreign body of thigh
  - S71.131 Puncture wound without foreign body, right thigh
  - S71.132 Puncture wound without foreign body, left thigh
    Coding Clinic: 2023, Q3, P12
  - S71.139 Puncture wound without foreign body, unspecified thigh
- S71.14 Puncture wound with foreign body of thigh
  - S71.141 Puncture wound with foreign body, right thigh
  - S71.142 Puncture wound with foreign body, left thigh
  - S71.149 Puncture wound with foreign body, unspecified thigh
- S71.15 Open bite of thigh
  Bite of thigh NOS
  Excludes1 superficial bite of thigh (S7Ø.37-)
  - S71.151 Open bite, right thigh
  - S71.152 Open bite, left thigh
  - S71.159 Open bite, unspecified thigh

S72 Fracture of femur

Note: A fracture not indicated as displaced or nondisplaced should be coded to displaced
A fracture not indicated as open or closed should be coded to closed
The open fracture designations are based on the Gustilo open fracture classification

Excludes1 traumatic amputation of hip and thigh (S78.-)

Excludes2 fracture of lower leg and ankle (S82.-)
fracture of foot (S92.-)
periprosthetic fracture of prosthetic implant of hip (M97.Ø-)

The appropriate 7th character is to be added to all codes from category S72

A	initial encounter for closed fracture
B	initial encounter for open fracture type I or II initial encounter for open fracture NOS
C	initial encounter for open fracture type IIIA, IIIB, or IIIC
D	subsequent encounter for closed fracture with routine healing
E	subsequent encounter for open fracture type I or II with routine healing
F	subsequent encounter for open fracture type IIIA, IIIB, or IIIC with routine healing
G	subsequent encounter for closed fracture with delayed healing
H	subsequent encounter for open fracture type I or II with delayed healing
J	subsequent encounter for open fracture type IIIA, IIIB, or IIIC with delayed healing
K	subsequent encounter for closed fracture with nonunion
M	subsequent encounter for open fracture type I or II with nonunion
N	subsequent encounter for open fracture type IIIA, IIIB, or IIIC with nonunion
P	subsequent encounter for closed fracture with malunion
Q	subsequent encounter for open fracture type I or II with malunion
R	subsequent encounter for open fracture type IIIA, IIIB, or IIIC with malunion
S	sequela

S72.Ø Fracture of head and neck of femur
Excludes2 physeal fracture of lower end of femur (S79.1-)
physeal fracture of upper end of femur (S79.Ø-)

- S72.ØØ Fracture of unspecified part of neck of femur
  Fracture of hip NOS
  Fracture of neck of femur NOS
  - S72.ØØ1 Fracture of unspecified part of neck of right femur K, M, N, P, Q, R, A, B, C, A, B, C, A, B, C (Ex) PDX 1264 [K, M, N, P, Q, R], 1807 [A], 1808 [B, C]
  - S72.ØØ2 Fracture of unspecified part of neck of left femur K, M, N, P, Q, R, A, B, C, A, B, C, A, B, C (Ex) PDX 1264 [K, M, N, P, Q, R], 1808 [B, C], 1809 [A]
    Coding Clinic: 2015, Q4, P37, Q1, P17
  - S72.ØØ9 Fracture of unspecified part of neck of unspecified femur K, M, N, P, Q, R, A, B, C, A, B, C, A, B, C (Ex) PDX 1264 [K, M, N, P, Q, R], 1808 [A, B, C]

S72.01 Unspecified intracapsular fracture of femur
Subcapital fracture of femur

S72.011 Unspecified intracapsular fracture of right femur K, M, N, P, Q, R, A, B, C, A, B, C, A, B, C (Ex) PDX 1264 [K, M, N, P, Q, R], 1807 [A], 1808 [B, C]

S72.012 Unspecified intracapsular fracture of left femur K, M, N, P, Q, R, A, B, C, A, B, C, A, B, C (Ex) PDX 1264 [K, M, N, P, Q, R], 1808 [B, C], 1809 [A]

S72.019 Unspecified intracapsular fracture of unspecified femur K, M, N, P, Q, R, A, B, C, A, B, C, A, B, C (Ex) PDX 1264 [K, M, N, P, Q, R], 1808 [A, B, C]

S72.02 Fracture of epiphysis (separation) (upper) of femur
Transepiphyseal fracture of femur
Fracture and separation across growth plate

Excludes1 capital femoral epiphyseal fracture (pediatric) of femur (S79.01-)
Salter-Harris Type I physeal fracture of upper end of femur (S79.01-)

S72.021 Displaced fracture of epiphysis (separation) (upper) of right femur K, M, N, P, Q, R, A, B, C, A, B, C, A, B, C (Ex) PDX 1264 [K, M, N, P, Q, R], 1807 [A], 1808 [B, C]

S72.022 Displaced fracture of epiphysis (separation) (upper) of left femur K, M, N, P, Q, R, A, B, C, A, B, C, A, B, C (Ex) PDX 1264 [K, M, N, P, Q, R], 1808 [B, C], 1809 [A]

S72.023 Displaced fracture of epiphysis (separation) (upper) of unspecified femur K, M, N, P, Q, R, A, B, C, A, B, C, A, B, C (Ex) PDX 1264 [K, M, N, P, Q, R], 1808 [A, B, C]

S72.024 Nondisplaced fracture of epiphysis (separation) (upper) of right femur K, M, N, P, Q, R, A, B, C, A, B, C, A, B, C (Ex) PDX 1264 [K, M, N, P, Q, R], 1807 [A], 1808 [B, C]

S72.025 Nondisplaced fracture of epiphysis (separation) (upper) of left femur K, M, N, P, Q, R, A, B, C, A, B, C, A, B, C
(Ex) For S72.025[A]: PDX 1809
For S72.025[B,C]: PDX 1808
For S72.025[K,M,N,P,Q,R]: PDX 1264

S72.026 Nondisplaced fracture of epiphysis (separation) (upper) of unspecified femur K, M, N, P, Q, R, A, B, C, A, B, C, A, B, C (Ex) PDX 1264 [K, M, N, P, Q, R], 1808 [A, B, C]

S72.03 Midcervical fracture of femur
Transcervical fracture of femur NOS

S72.031 Displaced midcervical fracture of right femur K, M, N, P, Q, R, A, B, C, A, B, C, A, B, C (Ex:) PDX 1264 [K, M, N, P, Q, R], 1807 [A], 1808 [B, C]

S72.032 Displaced midcervical fracture of left femur K, M, N, P, Q, R, A, B, C, A, B, C, A, B, C (Ex:) PDX 1264 [K, M, N, P, Q, R], 1808 [B, C], 1809 [A]

S72.033 Displaced midcervical fracture of unspecified femur K, M, N, P, Q, R, A, B, C, A, B, C, A, B, C (Ex:) PDX 1264 [K, M, N, P, Q, R], 1808 [A, B, C]

S72.034 Nondisplaced midcervical fracture of right femur K, M, N, P, Q, R, A, B, C, A, B, C, A, B, C (Ex:) PDX 1264 [K, M, N, P, Q, R], 1807 [A], 1808 [B, C]

S72.035 Nondisplaced midcervical fracture of left femur K, M, N, P, Q, R, A, B, C, A, B, C, A, B, C (Ex:) PDX 1264 [K, M, N, P, Q, R], 1808 [B, C], 1809 [A]

S72.036 Nondisplaced midcervical fracture of unspecified femur K, M, N, P, Q, R, A, B, C, A, B, C, A, B, C (Ex:) PDX 1264 [K, M, N, P, Q, R], 1808 [A, B, C]

S72.04 Fracture of base of neck of femur
Cervicotrochanteric fracture of femur

S72.041 Displaced fracture of base of neck of right femur K, M, N, P, Q, R, A, B, C, A, B, C, A, B, C (Ex:) PDX 1264 [K, M, N, P, Q, R], 1807 [A], 1808 [B, C]

S72.042 Displaced fracture of base of neck of left femur K, M, N, P, Q, R, A, B, C, A, B, C, A, B, C (Ex:) PDX 1264 [K, M, N, P, Q, R], 1808 [B, C], 1809 [A]

S72.043 Displaced fracture of base of neck of unspecified femur K, M, N, P, Q, R, A, B, C, A, B, C, A, B, C (Ex:) PDX 1264 [K, M, N, P, Q, R], 1808 [A, B, C]

S72.044 Nondisplaced fracture of base of neck of right femur K, M, N, P, Q, R, A, B, C, A, B, C, A, B, C (Ex:) PDX 1264 [K, M, N, P, Q, R], 1807 [A], 1808 [B, C]

S72.045 Nondisplaced fracture of base of neck of left femur K, M, N, P, Q, R, A, B, C, A, B, C, A, B, C (Ex:) PDX 1264 [K, M, N, P, Q, R], 1808 [B, C], 1809 [A]

S72.046 Nondisplaced fracture of base of neck of unspecified femur K, M, N, P, Q, R, A, B, C, A, B, C, A, B, C (Ex:) PDX 1264 [K, M, N, P, Q, R], 1808 [A, B, C]

S72.05 Unspecified fracture of head of femur
Fracture of head of femur NOS

S72.051 Unspecified fracture of head of right femur K, M, N, P, Q, R, A, B, C, A, B, C, A, B, C (Ex:) PDX 1807, 1264 [K, M, N, P, Q, R], 1808 [A, B, C]

S72.052 Unspecified fracture of head of left femur K, M, N, P, Q, R, A, B, C, A, B, C, A, B, C (Ex:) PDX 1809, 1264 [K, M, N, P, Q, R], 1808 [A, B, C]

S72.059 Unspecified fracture of head of unspecified femur K, M, N, P, Q, R, A, B, C, A, B, C, A, B, C (Ex:) PDX 1264 [K, M, N, P, Q, R], 1808 [A, B, C]

S72.06 Articular fracture of head of femur

S72.061 Displaced articular fracture of head of right femur K, M, N, P, Q, R, A, B, C, A, B, C, A, B, C (Ex:) PDX 1264 [K, M, N, P, Q, R], 1807 [A], 1808 [B, C]

S72.062 Displaced articular fracture of head of left femur K, M, N, P, Q, R, A, B, C, A, B, C, A, B, C (Ex:) PDX 1264 [K, M, N, P, Q, R], 1808 [B, C], 1809 [A]

S72.063 Displaced articular fracture of head of unspecified femur K, M, N, P, Q, R, A, B, C, A, B, C, A, B, C (Ex:) PDX 1264 [K, M, N, P, Q, R], 1808 [A, B, C]

S72.064 Nondisplaced articular fracture of head of right femur K, M, N, P, Q, R, A, B, C, A, B, C, A, B, C (Ex:) PDX 1264 [K, M, N, P, Q, R], 1807 [A], 1808 [B, C]

S72.065 Nondisplaced articular fracture of head of left femur K, M, N, P, Q, R, A, B, C, A, B, C, A, B, C (Ex:) PDX 1264 [K, M, N, P, Q, R], 1808 [B, C], 1809 [A]

S72.066 Nondisplaced articular fracture of head of unspecified femur K, M, N, P, Q, R, A, B, C, A, B, C, A, B, C (Ex:) PDX 1264 [K, M, N, P, Q, R], 1808 [A, B, C]

S72.09 Other fracture of head and neck of femur

S72.091 Other fracture of head and neck of right femur K, M, N, P, Q, R, A, B, C, A, B, C, A, B, C (Ex:) PDX 1264 [K, M, N, P, Q, R], 1807 [A], 1808 [B, C]

S72.092 Other fracture of head and neck of left femur K, M, N, P, Q, R, A, B, C, A, B, C, A, B, C (Ex:) PDX 1264 [K, M, N, P, Q, R], 1808 [B, C], 1809 [A]

S72.099 Other fracture of head and neck of unspecified femur K, M, N, P, Q, R, A, B, C, A, B, C, A, B, C (Ex:) PDX 1264 [K, M, N, P, Q, R], 1808 [A, B, C]

S72.1 Pertrochanteric fracture
Fracture extending close to, but not into, joint

S72.10 Unspecified trochanteric fracture of femur
Fracture of trochanter NOS

S72.101 Unspecified trochanteric fracture of right femur K, M, N, P, Q, R, A, B, C, A, B, C, A, B, C (Ex:) PDX 1264 [K, M, N, P, Q, R], 1807 [A], 1808 [B, C]

S72.102 Unspecified trochanteric fracture of left femur K, M, N, P, Q, R, A, B, C, A, B, C, A, B, C (Ex:) PDX 1264 [K, M, N, P, Q, R], 1808 [B, C], 1809 [A]

S72.109 Unspecified trochanteric fracture of unspecified femur K, M, N, P, Q, R, A, B, C, A, B, C, A, B, C (Ex:) PDX 1264 [K, M, N, P, Q, R], 1808 [A, B, C]

S72.11 Fracture of greater trochanter of femur

S72.111 Displaced fracture of greater trochanter of right femur K, M, N, P, Q, R, A, B, C, A, B, C, A, B, C (Ex:) PDX 1264 [K, M, N, P, Q, R], 1807 [A], 1808 [B, C]

S72.112 Displaced fracture of greater trochanter of left femur K, M, N, P, Q, R, A, B, C, A, B, C, A, B, C (Ex:) PDX 1264 [K, M, N, P, Q, R], 1808 [B, C], 1809 [A]

S72.113 Displaced fracture of greater trochanter of unspecified femur K, M, N, P, Q, R, A, B, C, A, B, C, A, B, C (Ex:) PDX 1264 [K, M, N, P, Q, R], 1808 [A, B, C]

S72.114 Nondisplaced fracture of greater trochanter of right femur K, M, N, P, Q, R, A, B, C, A, B, C, A, B, C (Ex:) PDX 1264 [K, M, N, P, Q, R], 1807 [A], 1808 [B, C]

● **S72.115** **Nondisplaced fracture of greater trochanter of left femur** K, M, N, P, Q, R, A, B, C, A, B, C, A, B, C (Ex) PDX 1264 [K, M, N, P, Q, R], 1808 [B, C], 1809 [A]

● **S72.116** **Nondisplaced fracture of greater trochanter of unspecified femur** K, M, N, P, Q, R, A, B, C, A, B, C, A, B, C (Ex) PDX 1264 [K, M, N, P, Q, R], 1808 [A, B, C]

● **S72.12** Fracture of lesser trochanter of femur

● **S72.121** **Displaced fracture of lesser trochanter of right femur** K, M, N, P, Q, R, A, B, C, A, B, C, A, B, C (Ex) PDX 1264 [K, M, N, P, Q, R], 1807 [A], 1808 [B, C]

● **S72.122** **Displaced fracture of lesser trochanter of left femur** K, M, N, P, Q, R, A, B, C, A, B, C, A, B, C (Ex) PDX 1264 [K, M, N, P, Q, R], 1808 [B, C], 1809 [A]

● **S72.123** **Displaced fracture of lesser trochanter of unspecified femur** K, M, N, P, Q, R, A, B, C, A, B, C, A, B, C (Ex) PDX 1264 [K, M, N, P, Q, R], 1808 [A, B, C]

● **S72.124** **Nondisplaced fracture of lesser trochanter of right femur** K, M, N, P, Q, R, A, B, C, A, B, C, A, B, C (Ex) PDX 1264 [K, M, N, P, Q, R], 1807 [A], 1808 [B, C]

● **S72.125** **Nondisplaced fracture of lesser trochanter of left femur** K, M, N, P, Q, R, A, B, C, A, B, C, A, B, C (Ex) PDX 1264 [K, M, N, P, Q, R], 1808 [B, C], 1809 [A]

● **S72.126** **Nondisplaced fracture of lesser trochanter of unspecified femur** K, M, N, P, Q, R, A, B, C, A, B, C, A, B, C (Ex) PDX 1264 [K, M, N, P, Q, R], 1808 [A, B, C]

● **S72.13** Apophyseal fracture of femur

Pertaining to articulations between articular facets of adjacent vertebrae

Excludes1 chronic (nontraumatic) slipped upper femoral epiphysis (M93.Ø-)

● **S72.131** **Displaced apophyseal fracture of right femur** K, M, N, P, Q, R, A, B, C, A, B, C, A, B, C (Ex) PDX 1264 [K, M, N, P, Q, R], 1807 [A], 1808 [B, C]

● **S72.132** **Displaced apophyseal fracture of left femur** K, M, N, P, Q, R, A, B, C, A, B, C, A, B, C (Ex) PDX 1264 [K, M, N, P, Q, R], 1808 [B, C], 1809 [A]

● **S72.133** **Displaced apophyseal fracture of unspecified femur** K, M, N, P, Q, R, A, B, C, A, B, C, A, B, C (Ex) PDX 1264 [K, M, N, P, Q, R], 1808 [A, B, C]

● **S72.134** **Nondisplaced apophyseal fracture of right femur** K, M, N, P, Q, R, A, B, C, A, B, C, A, B, C (Ex) PDX 1264 [K, M, N, P, Q, R], 1807 [A], 1808 [B, C]

● **S72.135** **Nondisplaced apophyseal fracture of left femur** K, M, N, P, Q, R, A, B, C, A, B, C, A, B, C (Ex) PDX 1264 [K, M, N, P, Q, R], 1808 [B, C], 1809 [A]

● **S72.136** **Nondisplaced apophyseal fracture of unspecified femur** K, M, N, P, Q, R, A, B, C, A, B, C, A, B, C (Ex) PDX 1264 [K, M, N, P, Q, R], 1808 [A, B, C]

● **S72.14** Intertrochanteric fracture of femur

● **S72.141** **Displaced intertrochanteric fracture of right femur** K, M, N, P, Q, R, A, B, C, A, B, C, A, B, C (Ex) PDX 1264 [K, M, N, P, Q, R], 1807 [A], 1808 [B, C]

Coding Clinic: 2Ø16, Q3, P17

● **S72.142** **Displaced intertrochanteric fracture of left femur** K, M, N, P, Q, R, A, B, C, A, B, C, A, B, C (Ex) PDX 1264 [K, M, N, P, Q, R], 1808 [B, C], 1809 [A]

● **S72.143** **Displaced intertrochanteric fracture of unspecified femur** K, M, N, P, Q, R, A, B, C, A, B, C, A, B, C (Ex) PDX 1264 [K, M, N, P, Q, R], 1808 [A, B, C]

● **S72.144** **Nondisplaced intertrochanteric fracture of right femur** K, M, N, P, Q, R, A, B, C, A, B, C, A, B, C (Ex) PDX 1264 [K, M, N, P, Q, R], 1807 [A], 1808 [B, C]

● **S72.145** **Nondisplaced intertrochanteric fracture of left femur** K, M, N, P, Q, R, A, B, C, A, B, C, A, B, C (Ex) PDX 1264 [K, M, N, P, Q, R], 1808 [B, C], 1809 [A]

● **S72.146** **Nondisplaced intertrochanteric fracture of unspecified femur** K, M, N, P, Q, R, A, B, C, A, B, C, A, B, C (Ex) PDX 1264 [K, M, N, P, Q, R], 1808 [A, B, C]

● **S72.2** Subtrochanteric fracture of femur (Ex) PDX 1264 [K, M, N, P, Q, R], 1808 [A, B, C]

Subtrochanteric: inferior to trochanter

X● **S72.21** **Displaced subtrochanteric fracture of right femur** K, M, N, P, Q, R, A, B, C, A, B, C, A, B, C

X● **S72.22** **Displaced subtrochanteric fracture of left femur** K, M, N, P, Q, R, A, B, C, A, B, C, A, B, C

X● **S72.23** **Displaced subtrochanteric fracture of unspecified femur** K, M, N, P, Q, R, A, B, C, A, B, C, A, B, C

X● **S72.24** **Nondisplaced subtrochanteric fracture of right femur** K, M, N, P, Q, R, A, B, C, A, B, C, A, B, C

X● **S72.25** **Nondisplaced subtrochanteric fracture of left femur** K, M, N, P, Q, R, A, B, C, A, B, C, A, B, C

X● **S72.26** **Nondisplaced subtrochanteric fracture of unspecified femur** K, M, N, P, Q, R, A, B, C, A, B, C, A, B, C

● **S72.3** Fracture of shaft of femur

● **S72.30** **Unspecified fracture of shaft of femur**

● **S72.301** **Unspecified fracture of shaft of right femur** K, M, N, P, Q, R, A, B, C, A, B, C, A, B, C (Ex) PDX 1264 [K, M, N, P, Q, R], 1807 [A, 1808 [B, C]

Coding Clinic: 2Ø18, Q2, P12

● **S72.302** **Unspecified fracture of shaft of left femur** K, M, N, P, Q, R, A, B, C, A, B, C, A, B, C (Ex) PDX 1264 [K, M, N, P, Q, R], 1808 [B, C], 1809 [A]

● **S72.309** **Unspecified fracture of shaft of unspecified femur** K, M, N, P, Q, R, A, B, C, A, B, C, A, B, C (Ex) PDX 1264 [K, M, N, P, Q, R], 1808 [A, B, C]

● **S72.32** **Transverse fracture of shaft of femur**

● **S72.321** **Displaced transverse fracture of shaft of right femur** K, M, N, P, Q, R, A, B, C, A, B, C, A, B, C (Ex) PDX 1264 [K, M, N, P, Q, R], 1807 [A], 1808 [B, C]

● **S72.322** **Displaced transverse fracture of shaft of left femur** K, M, N, P, Q, R, A, B, C, A, B, C, A, B, C (Ex) PDX 1264 [K, M, N, P, Q, R], 1808 [B, C], 1809 [A]

CHAPTER 19 (SØØ-T88)

S72.323 Displaced transverse fracture of shaft of unspecified femur K, M, N, P, Q, R, A, B, C, A, B, C, A, B, C (Ex:) PDX 1264 [K, M, N, P, Q, R], 1808 [A, B, C]

S72.324 Nondisplaced transverse fracture of shaft of right femur K, M, N, P, Q, R, A, B, C, A, B, C, A, B, C (Ex:) PDX 1264 [K, M, N, P, Q, R], 1807 [A], 1808 [B, C]

S72.325 Nondisplaced transverse fracture of shaft of left femur K, M, N, P, Q, R, A, B, C, A, B, C, A, B, C (Ex:) PDX 1264 [K, M, N, P, Q, R], 1808 [B, C], 1809 [A]

S72.326 Nondisplaced transverse fracture of shaft of unspecified femur K, M, N, P, Q, R, A, B, C, A, B, C, A, B, C (Ex:) PDX 1264 [K, M, N, P, Q, R], 1808 [A, B, C]

S72.33 Oblique fracture of shaft of femur

S72.331 Displaced oblique fracture of shaft of right femur K, M, N, P, Q, R, A, B, C, A, B, C, A, B, C (Ex:) PDX 1264 [K, M, N, P, Q, R], 1807 [A], 1808 [B, C]

S72.332 Displaced oblique fracture of shaft of left femur K, M, N, P, Q, R, A, B, C, A, B, C, A, B, C (Ex:) PDX 1264 [K, M, N, P, Q, R], 1808 [B, C], 1809 [A]

S72.333 Displaced oblique fracture of shaft of unspecified femur K, M, N, P, Q, R, A, B, C, A, B, C, A, B, C (Ex:) PDX 1264 [K, M, N, P, Q, R], 1808 [A, B, C]

S72.334 Nondisplaced oblique fracture of shaft of right femur K, M, N, P, Q, R, A, B, C, A, B, C, A, B, C (Ex:) PDX 1264 [K, M, N, P, Q, R], 1807 [A], 1808 [B, C]

S72.335 Nondisplaced oblique fracture of shaft of left femur K, M, N, P, Q, R, A, B, C, A, B, C, A, B, C (Ex:) PDX 1264 [K, M, N, P, Q, R], 1808 [B, C], 1809 [A]

S72.336 Nondisplaced oblique fracture of shaft of unspecified femur K, M, N, P, Q, R, A, B, C, A, B, C, A, B, C (Ex:) PDX 1264 [K, M, N, P, Q, R], 1808 [A, B, C]

S72.34 Spiral fracture of shaft of femur

S72.341 Displaced spiral fracture of shaft of right femur K, M, N, P, Q, R, A, B, C, A, B, C, A, B, C (Ex:) PDX 1264 [K, M, N, P, Q, R], 1807 [A], 1808 [B, C]

S72.342 Displaced spiral fracture of shaft of left femur K, M, N, P, Q, R, A, B, C, A, B, C, A, B, C (Ex:) PDX 1264 [K, M, N, P, Q, R], 1808 [B, C], 1809 [A]

S72.343 Displaced spiral fracture of shaft of unspecified femur K, M, N, P, Q, R, A, B, C, A, B, C, A, B, C (Ex:) PDX 1264 [K, M, N, P, Q, R], 1808 [A, B, C]

S72.344 Nondisplaced spiral fracture of shaft of right femur K, M, N, P, Q, R, A, B, C, A, B, C, A, B, C (Ex:) PDX 1264 [K, M, N, P, Q, R], 1807 [A], 1808 [B, C]

S72.345 Nondisplaced spiral fracture of shaft of left femur K, M, N, P, Q, R, A, B, C, A, B, C, A, B, C (Ex:) PDX 1264 [K, M, N, P, Q, R], 1808 [B, C], 1809 [A]

S72.346 Nondisplaced spiral fracture of shaft of unspecified femur K, M, N, P, Q, R, A, B, C, A, B, C, A, B, C (Ex:) PDX 1264 [K, M, N, P, Q, R], 1808 [A, B, C]

S72.35 Comminuted fracture of shaft of femur

S72.351 Displaced comminuted fracture of shaft of right femur K, M, N, P, Q, R, A, B, C, A, B, C, A, B, C (Ex:) PDX 1264 [K, M, N, P, Q, R], 1807 [A], 1808 [B, C]

S72.352 Displaced comminuted fracture of shaft of left femur K, M, N, P, Q, R, A, B, C, A, B, C, A, B, C (Ex:) PDX 1264 [K, M, N, P, Q, R], 1808 [B, C], 1809 [A]

S72.353 Displaced comminuted fracture of shaft of unspecified femur K, M, N, P, Q, R, A, B, C, A, B, C, A, B, C (Ex:) PDX 1264 [K, M, N, P, Q, R], 1808 [A, B, C]

S72.354 Nondisplaced comminuted fracture of shaft of right femur K, M, N, P, Q, R, A, B, C, A, B, C, A, B, C (Ex:) PDX 1264 [K, M, N, P, Q, R], 1807 [A], 1808 [B, C]

S72.355 Nondisplaced comminuted fracture of shaft of left femur K, M, N, P, Q, R, A, B, C, A, B, C, A, B, C (Ex:) PDX 1264 [K, M, N, P, Q, R], 1808 [B, C], 1809 [A]

S72.356 Nondisplaced comminuted fracture of shaft of unspecified femur K, M, N, P, Q, R, A, B, C, A, B, C, A, B, C (Ex:) PDX 1264 [K, M, N, P, Q, R], 1808 [A, B, C]

S72.36 Segmental fracture of shaft of femur

S72.361 Displaced segmental fracture of shaft of right femur K, M, N, P, Q, R, A, B, C, A, B, C, A, B, C (Ex:) PDX 1264 [K, M, N, P, Q, R], 1807 [A], 1808 [B, C]

S72.362 Displaced segmental fracture of shaft of left femur K, M, N, P, Q, R, A, B, C, A, B, C, A, B, C (Ex:) PDX 1264 [K, M, N, P, Q, R], 1808 [B, C], 1809 [A]

S72.363 Displaced segmental fracture of shaft of unspecified femur K, M, N, P, Q, R, A, B, C, A, B, C, A, B, C (Ex:) PDX 1264 [K, M, N, P, Q, R], 1808 [A, B, C]

S72.364 Nondisplaced segmental fracture of shaft of right femur K, M, N, P, Q, R, A, B, C, A, B, C, A, B, C (Ex:) PDX 1264 [K, M, N, P, Q, R], 1807 [A], 1808 [B, C]

S72.365 Nondisplaced segmental fracture of shaft of left femur K, M, N, P, Q, R, A, B, C, A, B, C, A, B, C (Ex:) PDX 1264 [K, M, N, P, Q, R], 1808 [B, C], 1809 [A]

S72.366 Nondisplaced segmental fracture of shaft of unspecified femur K, M, N, P, Q, R, A, B, C, A, B, C, A, B, C (Ex:) PDX 1264 [K, M, N, P, Q, R], 1808 [A, B, C]

S72.39 Other fracture of shaft of femur

S72.391 Other fracture of shaft of right femur K, M, N, P, Q, R, A, B, C, A, B, C, A, B, C (Ex:) PDX 1264 [K, M, N, P, Q, R], 1807 [A], 1808 [B, C]

S72.392 Other fracture of shaft of left femur K, M, N, P, Q, R, A, B, C, A, B, C, A, B, C (Ex:) PDX 1264 [K, M, N, P, Q, R], 1808 [B, C], 1809 [A]

S72.399 Other fracture of shaft of unspecified femur K, M, N, P, Q, R, A, B, C, A, B, C, A, B, C (Ex:) PDX 1264 [K, M, N, P, Q, R], 1808 [A, B, C]

S72.4 Fracture of lower end of femur
Fracture of distal end of femur

Excludes2 fracture of shaft of femur (S72.3-)
physeal fracture of lower end of femur (S79.1-)

S72.40 Unspecified fracture of lower end of femur

S72.401 Unspecified fracture of lower end of right femur A, K, M, N, P, Q, R, B, C, A, B, C, A, B, C Ex: PDX 1264 [K, M, N, P, Q, R], 1810 [A], 1811 [B, C]
Coding Clinic: 2016, Q4, P43

S72.402 Unspecified fracture of lower end of left femur A, K, M, N, P, Q, R, B, C, A, B, C, A, B, C Ex: PDX 1264 [K, M, N, P, Q, R], 1811 [B, C], 1812 [A]

S72.409 Unspecified fracture of lower end of unspecified femur A, K, M, N, P, Q, R, B, C, A, B, C, A, B, C Ex: PDX 1264 [K, M, N, P, Q, R], 1811 [A, B, C]

S72.41 Unspecified condyle fracture of lower end of femur
Condyle fracture of femur NOS

S72.411 Displaced unspecified condyle fracture of lower end of right femur A, K, M, N, P, Q, R, B, C, A, B, C, A, B, C Ex: PDX 1264 [K, M, N, P, Q, R], 1810 [A], 1811 [B, C]

S72.412 Displaced unspecified condyle fracture of lower end of left femur A, K, M, N, P, Q, R, B, C, A, B, C, A, B, C Ex: PDX 1264 [K, M, N, P, Q, R], 1811 [B, C], 1812 [A]

S72.413 Displaced unspecified condyle fracture of lower end of unspecified femur A, K, M, N, P, Q, R, B, C, A, B, C, A, B, C Ex: PDX 1264 [K, M, N, P, Q, R], 1811 [A, B, C]

S72.414 Nondisplaced unspecified condyle fracture of lower end of right femur A, K, M, N, P, Q, R, B, C, A, B, C, A, B, C Ex: PDX 1264 [K, M, N, P, Q, R], 1810 [A], 1811 [B, C]

S72.415 Nondisplaced unspecified condyle fracture of lower end of left femur A, K, M, N, P, Q, R, B, C, A, B, C, A, B, C Ex: PDX 1264 [K, M, N, P, Q, R], 1811 [B, C], 1812 [A]

S72.416 Nondisplaced unspecified condyle fracture of lower end of unspecified femur A, K, M, N, P, Q, R, B, C, A, B, C, A, B, C Ex: PDX 1264 [K, M, N, P, Q, R], 1811 [A, B, C]

S72.42 Fracture of lateral condyle of femur

S72.421 Displaced fracture of lateral condyle of right femur A, K, M, N, P, Q, R, B, C, A, B, C, A, B, C Ex: PDX 1264 [K, M, N, P, Q, R], 1810 [A], 1811 [B, C]

S72.422 Displaced fracture of lateral condyle of left femur A, K, M, N, P, Q, R, B, C, A, B, C, A, B, C Ex: PDX 1264 [K, M, N, P, Q, R], 1811 [B, C], 1812 [A]

S72.423 Displaced fracture of lateral condyle of unspecified femur A, K, M, N, P, Q, R, B, C, A, B, C, A, B, C Ex: PDX 1264 [K, M, N, P, Q, R], 1811 [A, B, C]

S72.424 Nondisplaced fracture of lateral condyle of right femur A, K, M, N, P, Q, R, B, C, A, B, C, A, B, C Ex: PDX 1264 [K, M, N, P, Q, R], 1810 [A], 1811 [B, C]

S72.425 Nondisplaced fracture of lateral condyle of left femur A, K, M, N, P, Q, R, B, C, A, B, C, A, B, C Ex: PDX 1264 [K, M, N, P, Q, R], 1811 [B, C], 1812 [A]

S72.426 Nondisplaced fracture of lateral condyle of unspecified femur A, K, M, N, P, Q, R, B, C, A, B, C, A, B, C Ex: PDX 1264 [K, M, N, P, Q, R], 1811 [A, B, C]

S72.43 Fracture of medial condyle of femur

S72.431 Displaced fracture of medial condyle of right femur A, K, M, N, P, Q, R, B, C, A, B, C, A, B, C Ex: PDX 1264 [K, M, N, P, Q, R], 1810 [A], 1811 [B, C]

S72.432 Displaced fracture of medial condyle of left femur A, K, M, N, P, Q, R, B, C, A, B, C, A, B, C Ex: PDX 1264 [K, M, N, P, Q, R], 1811 [B, C], 1812 [A]

S72.433 Displaced fracture of medial condyle of unspecified femur A, K, M, N, P, Q, R, B, C, A, B, C, A, B, C Ex: PDX 1264 [K, M, N, P, Q, R], 1811 [A, B, C]

S72.434 Nondisplaced fracture of medial condyle of right femur A, K, M, N, P, Q, R, B, C, A, B, C, A, B, C Ex: PDX 1264 [K, M, N, P, Q, R], 1810 [A], 1811 [B, C]

S72.435 Nondisplaced fracture of medial condyle of left femur A, K, M, N, P, Q, R, B, C, A, B, C, A, B, C Ex: PDX 1264 [K, M, N, P, Q, R], 1811 [B, C], 1812 [A]

S72.436 Nondisplaced fracture of medial condyle of unspecified femur A, K, M, N, P, Q, R, B, C, A, B, C, A, B, C Ex: PDX 1264 [K, M, N, P, Q, R], 1811 [A, B, C]

S72.44 Fracture of lower epiphysis (separation) of femur

Excludes1 Salter-Harris Type I physeal fracture of lower end of femur (S79.11-)

S72.441 Displaced fracture of lower epiphysis (separation) of right femur A, K, M, N, P, Q, R, B, C, A, B, C, A, B, C Ex: PDX 1264 [K, M, N, P, Q, R], 1810 [A], 1811 [B, C]

S72.442 Displaced fracture of lower epiphysis (separation) of left femur A, K, M, N, P, Q, R, B, C, A, B, C, A, B, C Ex: PDX 1264 [K, M, N, P, Q, R], 1811 [B, C], 1812 [A]

S72.443 Displaced fracture of lower epiphysis (separation) of unspecified femur A, K, M, N, P, Q, R, B, C, A, B, C, A, B, C Ex: PDX 1264 [K, M, N, P, Q, R], 1811 [A, B, C]

S72.444 Nondisplaced fracture of lower epiphysis (separation) of right femur A, K, M, N, P, Q, R, B, C, A, B, C, A, B, C Ex: PDX 1264 [K, M, N, P, Q, R], 1810 [A], 1811 [B, C]

S72.445 Nondisplaced fracture of lower epiphysis (separation) of left femur A, K, M, N, P, Q, R, B, C, A, B, C, A, B, C Ex: PDX 1264 [K, M, N, P, Q, R], 1811 [B, C], 1812 [A]

● S72.446 **Nondisplaced** fracture of lower epiphysis (separation) of **unspecified** femur A, K, M, N, P, Q, R, B, C, A, B, C, A, B, C (Ex) PDX 1264 [K, M, N, P, Q, R], 1811 [A, B, C]

● S72.45 **Supracondylar fracture without intracondylar extension of lower end of femur**

Supracondylar fracture of lower end of femur NOS

Excludes1 supracondylar fracture with intracondylar extension of lower end of femur (S72.46-)

● S72.451 **Displaced** supracondylar fracture without intracondylar extension of lower end of **right** femur A, K, M, N, P, Q, R, B, C, A, B, C, A, B, C (Ex) PDX 1264 [K, M, N, P, Q, R], 1810 [A], 1811 [B, C]

● S72.452 **Displaced** supracondylar fracture without intracondylar extension of lower end of **left** femur A, K, M, N, P, Q, R, B, C, A, B, C, A, B, C (Ex) PDX 1264 [K, M, N, P, Q, R], 1811 [B, C], 1812 [A]

● S72.453 **Displaced** supracondylar fracture without intracondylar extension of lower end of **unspecified** femur A, K, M, N, P, Q, R, B, C, A, B, C, A, B, C (Ex) PDX 1264 [K, M, N, P, Q, R], 1811 [A, B, C]

● S72.454 **Nondisplaced** supracondylar fracture without intracondylar extension of lower end of **right** femur A, K, M, N, P, Q, R, B, C, A, B, C, A, B, C (Ex) PDX 1264 [K, M, N, P, Q, R], 1810 [A], 1811 [B, C]

● S72.455 **Nondisplaced** supracondylar fracture without intracondylar extension of lower end of **left** femur A, K, M, N, P, Q, R, B, C, A, B, C, A, B, C (Ex) PDX 1264 [K, M, N, P, Q, R], 1811 [B, C], 1812 [A]

● S72.456 **Nondisplaced** supracondylar fracture without intracondylar extension of lower end of **unspecified** femur A, K, M, N, P, Q, R, B, C, A, B, C, A, B, C (Ex) PDX 1264 [K, M, N, P, Q, R], 1811 [A, B, C]

● S72.46 **Supracondylar fracture with intracondylar extension of lower end of femur**

Excludes1 supracondylar fracture without intracondylar extension of lower end of femur (S72.45-)

● S72.461 **Displaced** supracondylar fracture with intracondylar extension of lower end of **right** femur A, K, M, N, P, Q, R, B, C, A, B, C, A, B, C (Ex) PDX 1264 [K, M, N, P, Q, R], 1810 [A], 1811 [B, C]

● S72.462 **Displaced** supracondylar fracture with intracondylar extension of lower end of **left** femur A, K, M, N, P, Q, R, B, C, A, B, C, A, B, C (Ex) PDX 1264 [K, M, N, P, Q, R], 1811 [B, C], 1812 [A]

● S72.463 **Displaced** supracondylar fracture with intracondylar extension of lower end of **unspecified** femur A, K, M, N, P, Q, R, B, C, A, B, C, A, B, C (Ex) PDX 1264 [K, M, N, P, Q, R], 1811 [A, B, C]

● S72.464 **Nondisplaced** supracondylar fracture with intracondylar extension of lower end of **right** femur A, K, M, N, P, Q, R, B, C, A, B, C, A, B, C (Ex) PDX 1264 [K, M, N, P, Q, R], 1810 [A], 1811 [B, C]

● S72.465 **Nondisplaced** supracondylar fracture with intracondylar extension of lower end of **left** femur A, K, M, N, P, Q, R, B, C, A, B, C, A, B, C (Ex) PDX 1264 [K, M, N, P, Q, R], 1811 [B, C], 1812 [A]

● S72.466 **Nondisplaced** supracondylar fracture with intracondylar extension of lower end of **unspecified** femur A, K, M, N, P, Q, R, B, C, A, B, C, A, B, C (Ex) PDX 1264 [K, M, N, P, Q, R], 1811 [A, B, C]

● S72.47 **Torus fracture of lower end of femur**

The appropriate 7th character is to be added to all codes in subcategory S72.47

A	initial encounter for closed fracture
D	subsequent encounter for fracture with routine healing
G	subsequent encounter for fracture with delayed healing
K	subsequent encounter for fracture with nonunion
P	subsequent encounter for fracture with malunion
S	sequela

● S72.471 Torus fracture of lower end of **right** femur A, K, P, A, A (Ex) PDX 1264 [K, P], 1810 [A]

● S72.472 Torus fracture of lower end of **left** femur A, K, P, A, A (Ex) PDX 1264 [K, P], 1812 [A]

● S72.479 Torus fracture of lower end of **unspecified** femur A, K, P, A, A (Ex) PDX 1264 [K, P], 1811 [A]

● S72.49 **Other** fracture of lower end of femur

● S72.491 Other fracture of lower end of **right** femur A, K, M, N, P, Q, R, B, C, A, B, C, A, B, C (Ex) PDX 1810, 1813, 1264

● S72.492 Other fracture of lower end of **left** femur A, K, M, N, P, Q, R, B, C, A, B, C, A, B, C (Ex) PDX 1812, 1813, 1264

● S72.499 Other fracture of lower end of **unspecified** femur A, K, M, N, P, Q, R, B, C, A, B, C, A, B, C (Ex) PDX 1812, 1813, 1264

● S72.8 Other fracture of femur (Ex) PDX 1264 [K, M, N, P, Q, R], 1808 [A, B, C]

● S72.8X **Other** fracture of femur

● S72.8X1 Other fracture of **right** femur K, M, N, P, Q, R, A, B, C, A, B, C, A, B, C

● S72.8X2 Other fracture of **left** femur K, M, N, P, Q, R, A, B, C, A, B, C, A, B, C

● S72.8X9 Other fracture of **unspecified** femur K, M, N, P, Q, R, A, B, C, A, B, C, A, B, C

● S72.9 **Unspecified** fracture of femur (Ex) PDX 1264 [K, M, N, P, Q, R], 1808 [A, B, C]

Fracture of thigh NOS

Fracture of upper leg NOS

Excludes1 fracture of hip NOS (S72.ØØ-, S72.Ø1-)

X ● S72.9Ø Unspecified fracture of **unspecified** femur K, M, N, P, Q, R, A, B, C, A, B, C, A, B, C

Coding Clinic: 2Ø12, Q4, P94

X ● S72.91 Unspecified fracture of **right** femur K, M, N, P, Q, R, A, B, C, A, B, C, A, B, C

X ● S72.92 Unspecified fracture of **left** femur K, M, N, P, Q, R, A, B, C, A, B, C, A, B, C

S73 Dislocation and sprain of joint and ligaments of hip

Includes avulsion of joint or ligament of hip
laceration of cartilage, joint or ligament of hip
sprain of cartilage, joint or ligament of hip
traumatic hemarthrosis of joint or ligament of hip
traumatic rupture of joint or ligament of hip
traumatic subluxation of joint or ligament of hip
traumatic tear of joint or ligament of hip

Code also any associated open wound

Excludes2 strain of muscle, fascia and tendon of hip and thigh (S76.-)

The appropriate 7th character is to be added to each code from category S73

A	initial encounter
D	subsequent encounter
S	sequela

S73.0 Subluxation and dislocation of hip
Out of position
Excludes2 dislocation and subluxation of hip prosthesis (T84.020, T84.021)

S73.00 Unspecified subluxation and dislocation of hip
Dislocation of hip NOS
Subluxation of hip NOS

S73.001 Unspecified subluxation of right hip A, A, A (Ex) PDX 1814
S73.002 Unspecified subluxation of left hip A, A, A (Ex) PDX 1815
S73.003 Unspecified subluxation of unspecified hip A, A, A (Ex) PDX 1306
S73.004 Unspecified dislocation of right hip A, A, A (Ex) PDX 1814
S73.005 Unspecified dislocation of left hip A, A, A (Ex) PDX 1815
S73.006 Unspecified dislocation of unspecified hip A, A, A (Ex) PDX 1816

S73.01 Posterior subluxation and dislocation of hip
S73.011 Posterior subluxation of right hip A, A, A (Ex) PDX 1817
S73.012 Posterior subluxation of left hip A, A, A (Ex) PDX 1818
S73.013 Posterior subluxation of unspecified hip A, A, A (Ex) PDX 1819
S73.014 Posterior dislocation of right hip A, A, A (Ex) PDX 1817
S73.015 Posterior dislocation of left hip A, A, A (Ex) PDX 1818
S73.016 Posterior dislocation of unspecified hip A, A, A (Ex) PDX 1819

S73.02 Obturator subluxation and dislocation of hip
S73.021 Obturator subluxation of right hip A, A, A (Ex) PDX 1820
S73.022 Obturator subluxation of left hip A, A, A (Ex) PDX 1821
S73.023 Obturator subluxation of unspecified hip A, A, A (Ex) PDX 1822
S73.024 Obturator dislocation of right hip A, A, A (Ex) PDX 1820
S73.025 Obturator dislocation of left hip A, A, A (Ex) PDX 1821
S73.026 Obturator dislocation of unspecified hip A, A, A (Ex) PDX 1822

S73.03 Other anterior subluxation and dislocation of hip
S73.031 Other anterior subluxation of right hip A, A, A (Ex) PDX 1823
S73.032 Other anterior subluxation of left hip A, A, A (Ex) PDX 1824
S73.033 Other anterior subluxation of unspecified hip A, A, A (Ex) PDX 1825
S73.034 Other anterior dislocation of right hip A, A, A (Ex) PDX 1823
S73.035 Other anterior dislocation of left hip A, A, A (Ex) PDX 1824
S73.036 Other anterior dislocation of unspecified hip A, A, A (Ex) PDX 1825

S73.04 Central subluxation and dislocation of hip
S73.041 Central subluxation of right hip A, A, A (Ex) PDX 1814
S73.042 Central subluxation of left hip A, A, A (Ex) PDX 1815
S73.043 Central subluxation of unspecified hip A, A, A (Ex) PDX 1816
S73.044 Central dislocation of right hip A, A, A (Ex) PDX 1814
S73.045 Central dislocation of left hip A, A, A (Ex) PDX 1815
S73.046 Central dislocation of unspecified hip A, A, A (Ex) PDX 1816

S73.1 Sprain of hip
S73.10 Unspecified sprain of hip
S73.101 Unspecified sprain of right hip
S73.102 Unspecified sprain of left hip
S73.109 Unspecified sprain of unspecified hip

S73.11 Iliofemoral ligament sprain of hip
S73.111 Iliofemoral ligament sprain of right hip
S73.112 Iliofemoral ligament sprain of left hip
S73.119 Iliofemoral ligament sprain of unspecified hip

S73.12 Ischiocapsular (ligament) sprain of hip
S73.121 Ischiocapsular ligament sprain of right hip
S73.122 Ischiocapsular ligament sprain of left hip
S73.129 Ischiocapsular ligament sprain of unspecified hip

S73.19 Other sprain of hip
S73.191 Other sprain of right hip
S73.192 Other sprain of left hip
S73.199 Other sprain of unspecified hip

S74 Injury of nerves at hip and thigh level

Code also any associated open wound (S71.-)

Excludes2 injury of nerves at ankle and foot level (S94.-)
injury of nerves at lower leg level (S84.-)

The appropriate 7th character is to be added to each code from category S74

A	initial encounter
D	subsequent encounter
S	sequela

S74.0 Injury of sciatic nerve at hip and thigh level
X **S74.00** Injury of sciatic nerve at hip and thigh level, unspecified leg
X **S74.01** Injury of sciatic nerve at hip and thigh level, right leg
X **S74.02** Injury of sciatic nerve at hip and thigh level, left leg

S74.1 Injury of femoral nerve at hip and thigh level
X **S74.10** Injury of femoral nerve at hip and thigh level, unspecified leg
X **S74.11** Injury of femoral nerve at hip and thigh level, right leg
X **S74.12** Injury of femoral nerve at hip and thigh level, left leg

CHAPTER 19 (S00-T88)

● S74.2 Injury of cutaneous sensory nerve at hip and thigh level

X● S74.2Ø Injury of cutaneous sensory nerve at hip and thigh level, unspecified leg

X● S74.21 Injury of cutaneous sensory nerve at hip and high level, right leg

X● S74.22 Injury of cutaneous sensory nerve at hip and thigh level, left leg

● S74.8 Injury of other nerves at hip and thigh level

● S74.8X Injury of other nerves at hip and thigh level

● S74.8X1 Injury of other nerves at hip and thigh level, right leg

● S74.8X2 Injury of other nerves at hip and thigh level, left leg

● S74.8X9 Injury of other nerves at hip and thigh level, unspecified leg

● S74.9 Injury of unspecified nerve at hip and thigh level

X● S74.9Ø Injury of unspecified nerve at hip and thigh level, unspecified leg

X● S74.91 Injury of unspecified nerve at hip and thigh level, right leg

X● S74.92 Injury of unspecified nerve at hip and thigh level, left leg

● S75 Injury of blood vessels at hip and thigh level

Code also any associated open wound (S71.-)

Excludes2 injury of blood vessels at lower leg level (S85.-)
injury of popliteal artery (S85.Ø)

The appropriate 7th character is to be added to each code from category S75

A	initial encounter
D	subsequent encounter
S	sequela

● S75.Ø Injury of femoral artery

● S75.ØØ Unspecified injury of femoral artery

● S75.ØØ1 Unspecified injury of femoral artery, right leg A (Ex:) PDX 1826

● S75.ØØ2 Unspecified injury of femoral artery, left leg A (Ex:) PDX 1827

● S75.ØØ9 Unspecified injury of femoral artery, unspecified leg A (Ex:) PDX 1828

● S75.Ø1 Minor laceration of femoral artery

Incomplete transection of femoral artery
Laceration of femoral artery NOS
Superficial laceration of femoral artery

● S75.Ø11 Minor laceration of femoral artery, right leg A (Ex:) PDX 1826

● S75.Ø12 Minor laceration of femoral artery, left leg A (Ex:) PDX 1827

● S75.Ø19 Minor laceration of femoral artery, unspecified leg A (Ex:) PDX 1828

● S75.Ø2 Major laceration of femoral artery

Complete transection of femoral artery
Traumatic rupture of femoral artery

● S75.Ø21 Major laceration of femoral artery, right leg A (Ex:) PDX 1826

● S75.Ø22 Major laceration of femoral artery, left leg A (Ex:) PDX 1827
Coding Clinic: 2Ø23, Q3, P12

● S75.Ø29 Major laceration of femoral artery, unspecified leg A (Ex:) PDX 1828

● S75.Ø9 Other specified injury of femoral artery

● S75.Ø91 Other specified injury of femoral artery, right leg A (Ex:) PDX 1826

● S75.Ø92 Other specified injury of femoral artery, left leg A (Ex:) PDX 1827

● S75.Ø99 Other specified injury of femoral artery, unspecified leg A (Ex:) PDX 1828

● S75.1 Injury of femoral vein at hip and thigh level

● S75.1Ø Unspecified injury of femoral vein at hip and thigh level

● S75.1Ø1 Unspecified injury of femoral vein at hip and thigh level, right leg A (Ex:) PDX 1829

● S75.1Ø2 Unspecified injury of femoral vein at hip and thigh level, left leg A (Ex:) PDX 1830

● S75.1Ø9 Unspecified injury of femoral vein at hip and thigh level, unspecified leg A (Ex:) PDX 1831

● S75.11 Minor laceration of femoral vein at hip and thigh level

Incomplete transection of femoral vein at hip and thigh level
Laceration of femoral vein at hip and thigh level NOS
Superficial laceration of femoral vein at hip and thigh level

● S75.111 Minor laceration of femoral vein at hip and thigh level, right leg A (Ex:) PDX 1829

● S75.112 Minor laceration of femoral vein at hip and thigh level, left leg A (Ex:) PDX 1830

● S75.119 Minor laceration of femoral vein at hip and thigh level, unspecified leg A (Ex:) PDX 1831

● S75.12 Major laceration of femoral vein at hip and thigh level

Complete transection of femoral vein at hip and thigh level
Traumatic rupture of femoral vein at hip and thigh level

● S75.121 Major laceration of femoral vein at hip and thigh level, right leg A (Ex:) PDX 1829

● S75.122 Major laceration of femoral vein at hip and thigh level, left leg A (Ex:) PDX 1830
Coding Clinic: 2Ø23, Q3, P12

● S75.129 Major laceration of femoral vein at hip and thigh level, unspecified leg A (Ex:) PDX 1831

● S75.19 Other specified injury of femoral vein at hip and thigh level

● S75.191 Other specified injury of femoral vein at hip and thigh level, right leg A (Ex:) PDX 1829

● S75.192 Other specified injury of femoral vein at hip and thigh level, left leg A (Ex:) PDX 1830

● S75.199 Other specified injury of femoral vein at hip and thigh level, unspecified leg A (Ex:) PDX 1831

● S75.2 Injury of greater saphenous vein at hip and thigh level

Excludes1 greater saphenous vein NOS (S85.3)

● S75.2Ø Unspecified injury of greater saphenous vein at hip and thigh level

● S75.2Ø1 Unspecified injury of greater saphenous vein at hip and thigh level, right leg A (Ex:) PDX 1822

● S75.2Ø2 Unspecified injury of greater saphenous vein at hip and thigh level, left leg A (Ex:) PDX 1823

● S75.2Ø9 Unspecified injury of greater saphenous vein at hip and thigh level, unspecified leg A (Ex:) PDX 1834

● S75.21 **Minor laceration of greater saphenous vein at hip and thigh level**
Incomplete transection of greater saphenous vein at hip and thigh level
Laceration of greater saphenous vein at hip and thigh level NOS
Superficial laceration of greater saphenous vein at hip and thigh level

● S75.211 **Minor laceration of greater saphenous vein at hip and thigh level, right leg** A (Ex:) PDX 1832

● S75.212 **Minor laceration of greater saphenous vein at hip and thigh level, left leg** A (Ex:) PDX 1833

● S75.219 **Minor laceration of greater saphenous vein at hip and thigh level, unspecified leg** A (Ex:) PDX 1834

● S75.22 **Major laceration of greater saphenous vein at hip and thigh level**
Complete transection of greater saphenous vein at hip and thigh level
Traumatic rupture of greater saphenous vein at hip and thigh level

● S75.221 **Major laceration of greater saphenous vein at hip and thigh level, right leg** A (Ex:) PDX 1832

● S75.222 **Major laceration of greater saphenous vein at hip and thigh level, left leg** A (Ex:) PDX 1833

● S75.229 **Major laceration of greater saphenous vein at hip and thigh level, unspecified leg** A (Ex:) PDX 1834

● S75.29 **Other specified injury of greater saphenous vein at hip and thigh level**

● S75.291 **Other specified injury of greater saphenous vein at hip and thigh level, right leg** A (Ex:) PDX 1832

● S75.292 **Other specified injury of greater saphenous vein at hip and thigh level, left leg** A (Ex:) PDX 1833

● S75.299 **Other specified injury of greater saphenous vein at hip and thigh level, unspecified leg** A (Ex:) PDX 1834

● S75.8 **Injury of other blood vessels at hip and thigh level**

● S75.80 **Unspecified injury of other blood vessels at hip and thigh level**

● S75.801 **Unspecified injury of other blood vessels at hip and thigh level, right leg** A (Ex:) PDX 1835

● S75.802 **Unspecified injury of other blood vessels at hip and thigh level, left leg** A (Ex:) PDX 1836

● S75.809 **Unspecified injury of other blood vessels at hip and thigh level, unspecified leg** A (Ex:) PDX 1837

● S75.81 **Laceration of other blood vessels at hip and thigh level**

● S75.811 **Laceration of other blood vessels at hip and thigh level, right leg** A (Ex:) PDX 1835

● S75.812 **Laceration of other blood vessels at hip and thigh level, left leg** A (Ex:) PDX 1836

● S75.819 **Laceration of other blood vessels at hip and thigh level, unspecified leg** A (Ex:) PDX 1837

● S75.89 **Other specified injury of other blood vessels at hip and thigh level**

● S75.891 **Other specified injury of other blood vessels at hip and thigh level, right leg** A (Ex:) PDX 1835

● S75.892 **Other specified injury of other blood vessels at hip and thigh level, left leg** A (Ex:) PDX 1836

● S75.899 **Other specified injury of other blood vessels at hip and thigh level, unspecified leg** A (Ex:) PDX 1837

● S75.9 **Injury of unspecified blood vessel at hip and thigh level**

● S75.90 **Unspecified injury of unspecified blood vessel at hip and thigh level**

● S75.901 **Unspecified injury of unspecified blood vessel at hip and thigh level, right leg** A (Ex:) PDX 1835

● S75.902 **Unspecified injury of unspecified blood vessel at hip and thigh level, left leg** A (Ex:) PDX 1836

● S75.909 **Unspecified injury of unspecified blood vessel at hip and thigh level, unspecified leg** A (Ex:) PDX 1837

● S75.91 **Laceration of unspecified blood vessel at hip and thigh level**

● S75.911 **Laceration of unspecified blood vessel at hip and thigh level, right leg** A (Ex:) PDX 1835

● S75.912 **Laceration of unspecified blood vessel at hip and thigh level, left leg** A (Ex:) PDX 1836

● S75.919 **Laceration of unspecified blood vessel at hip and thigh level, unspecified leg** A (Ex:) PDX 1837

● S75.99 **Other specified injury of unspecified blood vessel at hip and thigh level**

● S75.991 **Other specified injury of unspecified blood vessel at hip and thigh level, right leg** A (Ex:) PDX 1835

● S75.992 **Other specified injury of unspecified blood vessel at hip and thigh level, left leg** A (Ex:) PDX 1836

● S75.999 **Other specified injury of unspecified blood vessel at hip and thigh level, unspecified leg** A (Ex:) PDX 1837

● S76 **Injury of muscle, fascia and tendon at hip and thigh level**
Code also any associated open wound (S71.-)
Excludes2 injury of muscle, fascia and tendon at lower leg level (S86)
sprain of joint and ligament of hip (S73.1)
The appropriate 7th character is to be added to each code from category S76

A	initial encounter
D	subsequent encounter
S	sequela

● S76.0 **Injury of muscle, fascia and tendon of hip**

● S76.00 **Unspecified injury of muscle, fascia and tendon of hip**

● S76.001 **Unspecified injury of muscle, fascia and tendon of right hip**

● S76.002 **Unspecified injury of muscle, fascia and tendon of left hip**

● S76.009 **Unspecified injury of muscle, fascia and tendon of unspecified hip**

● S76.01 **Strain of muscle, fascia and tendon of hip**

● S76.011 **Strain of muscle, fascia and tendon of right hip**

● S76.012 **Strain of muscle, fascia and tendon of left hip**

● S76.019 **Strain of muscle, fascia and tendon of unspecified hip**

● S76.02 **Laceration of muscle, fascia and tendon of hip**

● S76.021 **Laceration of muscle, fascia and tendon of right hip** A (Ex:) PDX 1838

CHAPTER 19 (S00-T88)

S76.022 Laceration of muscle, fascia and tendon of left hip A (Ex:) PDX 1839

S76.029 Laceration of muscle, fascia and tendon of unspecified hip A (Ex:) PDX 1840

S76.09 Other specified injury of muscle, fascia and tendon of hip

S76.091 Other specified injury of muscle, fascia and tendon of right hip

S76.092 Other specified injury of muscle, fascia and tendon of left hip

S76.099 Other specified injury of muscle, fascia and tendon of unspecified hip

S76.1 Injury of quadriceps muscle, fascia and tendon
Injury of patellar ligament (tendon)

S76.10 Unspecified injury of quadriceps muscle, fascia and tendon

S76.101 Unspecified injury of right quadriceps muscle, fascia and tendon

S76.102 Unspecified injury of left quadriceps muscle, fascia and tendon

S76.109 Unspecified injury of unspecified quadriceps muscle, fascia and tendon

S76.11 Strain of quadriceps muscle, fascia and tendon

S76.111 Strain of right quadriceps muscle, fascia and tendon

S76.112 Strain of left quadriceps muscle, fascia and tendon

S76.119 Strain of unspecified quadriceps muscle, fascia and tendon

S76.12 Laceration of quadriceps muscle, fascia and tendon

S76.121 Laceration of right quadriceps muscle, fascia and tendon A (Ex:) PDX 1838

S76.122 Laceration of left quadriceps muscle, fascia and tendon A (Ex:) PDX 1839

S76.129 Laceration of unspecified quadriceps muscle, fascia and tendon A (Ex:) PDX 1840

S76.19 Other specified injury of quadriceps muscle, fascia and tendon

S76.191 Other specified injury of right quadriceps muscle, fascia and tendon

S76.192 Other specified injury of left quadriceps muscle, fascia and tendon

S76.199 Other specified injury of unspecified quadriceps muscle, fascia and tendon

S76.2 Injury of adductor muscle, fascia and tendon of thigh

S76.20 Unspecified injury of adductor muscle, fascia and tendon of thigh

S76.201 Unspecified injury of adductor muscle, fascia and tendon of right thigh

S76.202 Unspecified injury of adductor muscle, fascia and tendon of left thigh

S76.209 Unspecified injury of adductor muscle, fascia and tendon of unspecified thigh

S76.21 Strain of adductor muscle, fascia and tendon of thigh

S76.211 Strain of adductor muscle, fascia and tendon of right thigh

S76.212 Strain of adductor muscle, fascia and tendon of left thigh

S76.219 Strain of adductor muscle, fascia and tendon of unspecified thigh

S76.22 Laceration of adductor muscle, fascia and tendon of thigh

S76.221 Laceration of adductor muscle, fascia and tendon of right thigh A (Ex:) PDX 1838

S76.222 Laceration of adductor muscle, fascia and tendon of left thigh A (Ex:) PDX 1839

S76.229 Laceration of adductor muscle, fascia and tendon of unspecified thigh A (Ex:) PDX 1840

S76.29 Other injury of adductor muscle, fascia and tendon of thigh

S76.291 Other injury of adductor muscle, fascia and tendon of right thigh

S76.292 Other injury of adductor muscle, fascia and tendon of left thigh

S76.299 Other injury of adductor muscle, fascia and tendon of unspecified thigh

S76.3 Injury of muscle, fascia and tendon of the posterior muscle group at thigh level

S76.30 Unspecified injury of muscle, fascia and tendon of the posterior muscle group at thigh level

S76.301 Unspecified injury of muscle, fascia and tendon of the posterior muscle group at thigh level, right thigh

S76.302 Unspecified injury of muscle, fascia and tendon of the posterior muscle group at thigh level, left thigh

S76.309 Unspecified injury of muscle, fascia and tendon of the posterior muscle group at thigh level, unspecified thigh

S76.31 Strain of muscle, fascia and tendon of the posterior muscle group at thigh level

S76.311 Strain of muscle, fascia and tendon of the posterior muscle group at thigh level, right thigh

S76.312 Strain of muscle, fascia and tendon of the posterior muscle group at thigh level, left thigh

S76.319 Strain of muscle, fascia and tendon of the posterior muscle group at thigh level, unspecified thigh

S76.32 Laceration of muscle, fascia and tendon of the posterior muscle group at thigh level

S76.321 Laceration of muscle, fascia and tendon of the posterior muscle group at thigh level, right thigh A (Ex:) PDX 1838

S76.322 Laceration of muscle, fascia and tendon of the posterior muscle group at thigh level, left thigh A (Ex:) PDX 1839

S76.329 Laceration of muscle, fascia and tendon of the posterior muscle group at thigh level, unspecified thigh A (Ex:) PDX 1840

S76.39 Other specified injury of muscle, fascia and tendon of the posterior muscle group at thigh level

S76.391 Other specified injury of muscle, fascia and tendon of the posterior muscle group at thigh level, right thigh

S76.392 Other specified injury of muscle, fascia and tendon of the posterior muscle group at thigh level, left thigh

S76.399 Other specified injury of muscle, fascia and tendon of the posterior muscle group at thigh level, unspecified thigh

- **S76.8** Injury of other specified muscles, fascia and tendons at thigh level
  - **S76.80** Unspecified injury of other specified muscles, fascia and tendons at thigh level
    - **S76.801** Unspecified injury of other specified muscles, fascia and tendons at thigh level, right thigh
    - **S76.802** Unspecified injury of other specified muscles, fascia and tendons at thigh level, left thigh
    - **S76.809** Unspecified injury of other specified muscles, fascia and tendons at thigh level, unspecified thigh
  - **S76.81** Strain of other specified specified muscles, fascia and tendons at thigh level
    - **S76.811** Strain of other specified muscles, fascia and tendons at thigh level, right thigh
    - **S76.812** Strain of other specified muscles, fascia and tendons at thigh level, left thigh
    - **S76.819** Strain of other specified muscles, fascia and tendons at thigh level, unspecified thigh
  - **S76.82** Laceration of other specified muscles, fascia and tendons at thigh level
    - **S76.821** Laceration of other specified muscles, fascia and tendons at thigh level, right thigh A (Ex) PDX 1838
    - **S76.822** Laceration of other specified muscles, fascia and tendons at thigh level, left thigh A (Ex) PDX 1839
    - **S76.829** Laceration of other specified muscles, fascia and tendons at thigh level, unspecified thigh A (Ex) PDX 1840
  - **S76.89** Other injury of other specified muscles, fascia and tendons at thigh level
    - **S76.891** Other injury of other specified muscles, fascia and tendons at thigh level, right thigh
    - **S76.892** Other injury of other specified muscles, fascia and tendons at thigh level, left thigh
    - **S76.899** Other injury of other specified muscles, fascia and tendons at thigh level, unspecified thigh
- **S76.9** Injury of unspecified muscles, fascia and tendons at thigh level
  - **S76.90** Unspecified injury of unspecified muscles, fascia and tendons at thigh level
    - **S76.901** Unspecified injury of unspecified muscles, fascia and tendons at thigh level, right thigh
    - **S76.902** Unspecified injury of unspecified muscles, fascia and tendons at thigh level, left thigh
    - **S76.909** Unspecified injury of unspecified muscles, fascia and tendons at thigh level, unspecified thigh
  - **S76.91** Strain of unspecified muscles, fascia and tendons at thigh level
    - **S76.911** Strain of unspecified muscles, fascia and tendons at thigh level, right thigh
    - **S76.912** Strain of unspecified muscles, fascia and tendons at thigh level, left thigh
    - **S76.919** Strain of unspecified muscles fascia and tendons at thigh level, unspecified thigh
  - **S76.92** Laceration of unspecified muscles, fascia and tendons at thigh level
    - **S76.921** Laceration of unspecified muscles, fascia and tendons at thigh level, right thigh A (Ex) PDX 1838
    - **S76.922** Laceration of unspecified muscles, fascia and tendons at thigh level, left thigh A (Ex) PDX 1839
    - **S76.929** Laceration of unspecified muscles, fascia and tendons at thigh level, unspecified thigh A (Ex) PDX 1840
  - **S76.99** Other specified injury of unspecified muscles, fascia and tendons at thigh level
    - **S76.991** Other specified injury of unspecified muscles, fascia and tendons at thigh level, right thigh
    - **S76.992** Other specified injury of unspecified muscles, fascia and tendons at thigh level, left thigh
    - **S76.999** Other specified injury of unspecified muscles, fascia and tendons at thigh level, unspecified thigh

S77 Crushing injury of hip and thigh

Use additional code(s) for all associated injuries

Excludes2 crushing injury of ankle and foot (S97.-)
crushing injury of lower leg (S87.-)

The appropriate 7th character is to be added to each code from category S77

A	initial encounter
D	subsequent encounter
S	sequela

- **S77.0** Crushing injury of hip (Ex) PDX 1841
  - X **S77.00** Crushing injury of unspecified hip A, A
  - X **S77.01** Crushing injury of right hip A, A
  - X **S77.02** Crushing injury of left hip A, A
- **S77.1** Crushing injury of thigh (Ex) PDX 1842
  - X **S77.10** Crushing injury of unspecified thigh A, A
  - X **S77.11** Crushing injury of right thigh A, A
  - X **S77.12** Crushing injury of left thigh A, A
- **S77.2** Crushing injury of hip with thigh
  - X **S77.20** Crushing injury of unspecified hip with thigh
  - X **S77.21** Crushing injury of right hip with thigh
  - X **S77.22** Crushing injury of left hip with thigh

S78 Traumatic amputation of hip and thigh

An amputation not identified as partial or complete should be coded to complete

Excludes1 traumatic amputation of knee (S88.0-)

The appropriate 7th character is to be added to each code from category S78

A	initial encounter
D	subsequent encounter
S	sequela

- **S78.0** Traumatic amputation at hip joint
  - **S78.01** Complete traumatic amputation at hip joint
    - **S78.011** Complete traumatic amputation at right hip joint A, A, D, S (Ex) PDX 1843
    - **S78.012** Complete traumatic amputation at left hip joint A, A, D, S (Ex) PDX 1844
    - **S78.019** Complete traumatic amputation at unspecified hip joint A, A, D, S (Ex) PDX 1845

S78.02 Partial traumatic amputation at hip joint
- **S78.021** Partial traumatic amputation at right hip joint A, A, D, S (Ex) PDX 1843
- **S78.022** Partial traumatic amputation at left hip joint A, A, D, S (Ex) PDX 1844
- **S78.029** Partial traumatic amputation at unspecified hip joint A, A, D, S (Ex) PDX 1845

S78.1 Traumatic amputation at level between hip and knee
Excludes1 traumatic amputation of knee (S88.0-)

S78.11 Complete traumatic amputation at level between hip and knee
- **S78.111** Complete traumatic amputation at level between right hip and knee A, A, D, S (Ex) PDX 1843
- **S78.112** Complete traumatic amputation at level between left hip and knee A, A, D, S (Ex) PDX 1844
- **S78.119** Complete traumatic amputation at level between unspecified hip and knee A, A, D, S (Ex) PDX 1845

S78.12 Partial traumatic amputation at level between hip and knee
- **S78.121** Partial traumatic amputation at level between right hip and knee A, A, D, S (Ex) PDX 1843
- **S78.122** Partial traumatic amputation at level between left hip and knee A, A, D, S (Ex) PDX 1844
- **S78.129** Partial traumatic amputation at level between unspecified hip and knee A, A, D, S (Ex) PDX 1845

S78.9 Traumatic amputation of hip and thigh, level unspecified

S78.91 Complete traumatic amputation of hip and thigh, level unspecified
- **S78.911** Complete traumatic amputation of right hip and thigh, level unspecified A, A, D, S (Ex) PDX 1843
- **S78.912** Complete traumatic amputation of left hip and thigh, level unspecified A, A, D, S (Ex) PDX 1844
- **S78.919** Complete traumatic amputation of unspecified hip and thigh, level unspecified A, A, D, S (Ex) PDX 1845

S78.92 Partial traumatic amputation of hip and thigh, level unspecified
- **S78.921** Partial traumatic amputation of right hip and thigh, level unspecified A, A, D, S (Ex) PDX 1843
- **S78.922** Partial traumatic amputation of left hip and thigh, level unspecified A, A, D, S (Ex) PDX 1844
- **S78.929** Partial traumatic amputation of unspecified hip and thigh, level unspecified A, A, D, S (Ex) PDX 1845

S79 Other and unspecified injuries of hip and thigh

Note: A fracture not indicated as open or closed should be coded to closed

The appropriate 7th character is to be added to each code from subcategories S79.0 and S79.1

A	initial encounter for closed fracture
D	subsequent encounter for fracture with routine healing
G	subsequent encounter for fracture with delayed healing
K	subsequent encounter for fracture with nonunion
P	subsequent encounter for fracture with malunion
S	sequela

Item 19-5 SALTER-HARRIS TYPE 1: epiphysis is completely separated from end of bone, or metaphysic growth plate remains attached to epiphysis
SALTER-HARRIS TYPE 2: epiphysis and growth plate are partially separated from metaphysis, which is cracked—most common type
SALTER-HARRIS TYPE 3: fracture occurring through epiphysis and separates part of epiphysis and growth plate from metaphysis fracture, usually at distal end of tibia
SALTER-HARRIS TYPE 4: fracture runs through epiphysis, across growth plate, into metaphysic; surgery is required to restore joint surface to normal and align growth plate

S79.0 Physeal fracture of upper end of femur
Excludes1 apophyseal fracture of upper end of femur (S72.13-)
nontraumatic slipped upper femoral epiphysis (M93.0-)

S79.00 Unspecified physeal fracture of upper end of femur
- **S79.001** Unspecified physeal fracture of upper end of right femur K, P, A, A, A (Ex) PDX 1264 [K, P], 1807 [A]
- **S79.002** Unspecified physeal fracture of upper end of left femur K, P, A, A, A (Ex) PDX 1264 [K, P], 1809 [A]
- **S79.009** Unspecified physeal fracture of upper end of unspecified femur K, P, A, A, A (Ex) PDX 1264 [K, P], 1808 [A]

S79.01 Salter-Harris Type I physeal fracture of upper end of femur
Acute on chronic slipped capital femoral epiphysis (traumatic)
Acute slipped capital femoral epiphysis (traumatic)
Capital femoral epiphyseal fracture
Excludes1 chronic slipped upper femoral epiphysis (nontraumatic) (M93.02-)
- **S79.011** Salter-Harris Type I physeal fracture of upper end of right femur K, P, A, A, A (Ex) PDX 1264 [K, P], 1807 [A]
- **S79.012** Salter-Harris Type I physeal fracture of upper end of left femur K, P, A, A, A (Ex) PDX 1264 [K, P], 1809 [A]
- **S79.019** Salter-Harris Type I physeal fracture of upper end of unspecified femur K, P, A, A, A (Ex) PDX 1264 [K, P], 1808 [A]

S79.09 Other physeal fracture of upper end of femur
- **S79.091** Other physeal fracture of upper end of right femur K, P, A, A, A (Ex) PDX 1264 [K, P], 1807 [A]
- **S79.092** Other physeal fracture of upper end of left femur K, P, A, A, A (Ex) PDX 1264 [K, P], 1809 [A]
- **S79.099** Other physeal fracture of upper end of unspecified femur K, P, A, A, A (Ex) PDX 1264 [K, P], 1808 [A]

S79.1 Physeal fracture of lower end of femur

S79.10 Unspecified physeal fracture of lower end of femur
- **S79.101** Unspecified physeal fracture of lower end of right femur A, K, P, A, A (Ex) PDX 1264 [K, P], 1810 [A]
- **S79.102** Unspecified physeal fracture of lower end of left femur A, K, P, A, A (Ex) PDX 1264 [K, P], 1812 [A]
- **S79.109** Unspecified physeal fracture of lower end of unspecified femur A, K, P, A, A (Ex) PDX 1264 [K, P], 1811 [A]

- **S79.11** Salter-Harris Type I physeal fracture of lower end of femur
  - **S79.111** Salter-Harris Type I physeal fracture of lower end of right femur A, K, P, A, A (Ex:) PDX 1264 [K, P], 1810 [A]
  - **S79.112** Salter-Harris Type I physeal fracture of lower end of left femur A, K, P, A, A (Ex:) PDX 1264 [K, P], 1812 [A]
  - **S79.119** Salter-Harris Type I physeal fracture of lower end of unspecified femur A, K, P, A, A (Ex:) PDX 1264 [K, P], 1811 [A]
- **S79.12** Salter-Harris Type II physeal fracture of lower end of femur
  - **S79.121** Salter-Harris Type II physeal fracture of lower end of right femur A, K, P, A, A (Ex:) PDX 1264 [K, P], 1810 [A]
  - **S79.122** Salter-Harris Type II physeal fracture of lower end of left femur A, K, P, A, A (Ex:) PDX 1264 [K, P], 1812 [A]
  - **S79.129** Salter-Harris Type II physeal fracture of lower end of unspecified femur A, K, P, A, A (Ex:) PDX 1264 [K, P], 1811 [A]
- **S79.13** Salter-Harris Type III physeal fracture of lower end of femur
  - **S79.131** Salter-Harris Type III physeal fracture of lower end of right femur A, K, P, A, A (Ex:) PDX 1264 [K, P], 1810 [A]
  - **S79.132** Salter-Harris Type III physeal fracture of lower end of left femur A, K, P, A, A (Ex:) PDX 1264 [K, P], 1812 [A]
  - **S79.139** Salter-Harris Type III physeal fracture of lower end of unspecified femur A, K, P, A, A (Ex:) PDX 1264 [K, P], 1811 [A]
- **S79.14** Salter-Harris Type IV physeal fracture of lower end of femur
  - **S79.141** Salter-Harris Type IV physeal fracture of lower end of right femur A, K, P, A, A (Ex:) PDX 1264 [K, P], 1810 [A]
  - **S79.142** Salter-Harris Type IV physeal fracture of lower end of left femur A, K, P, A, A (Ex:) PDX 1264 [K, P], 1812 [A]
  - **S79.149** Salter-Harris Type IV physeal fracture of lower end of unspecified femur A, K, P, A, A (Ex:) PDX 1264 [K, P], 1811 [A]
- **S79.19** Other physeal fracture of lower end of femur
  - **S79.191** Other physeal fracture of lower end of right femur A, K, P, A, A (Ex:) PDX 1264 [K, P], 1810 [A]
  - **S79.192** Other physeal fracture of lower end of left femur A, K, P, A, A (Ex:) PDX 1264 [K, P], 1812 [A]
  - **S79.199** Other physeal fracture of lower end of unspecified femur A, K, P, A, A (Ex:) PDX 1264 [K, P], 1811 [A]

S79.8 Other specified injuries of hip and thigh

The appropriate 7th character is to be added to each code in subcategory S79.8

A	initial encounter
D	subsequent encounter
S	sequela

- **S79.81** Other specified injuries of hip
  - **S79.811** Other specified injuries of right hip
  - **S79.812** Other specified injuries of left hip
  - **S79.819** Other specified injuries of unspecified hip
- **S79.82** Other specified injuries of thigh
  - **S79.821** Other specified injuries of right thigh
  - **S79.822** Other specified injuries of left thigh
  - **S79.829** Other specified injuries of unspecified thigh

S79.9 Unspecified injury of hip and thigh

The appropriate 7th character is to be added to each code in subcategory S79.9

A	initial encounter
D	subsequent encounter
S	sequela

- **S79.91** Unspecified injury of hip
  - **S79.911** Unspecified injury of right hip
  - **S79.912** Unspecified injury of left hip
  - **S79.919** Unspecified injury of unspecified hip
- **S79.92** Unspecified injury of thigh
  - **S79.921** Unspecified injury of right thigh
  - **S79.922** Unspecified injury of left thigh
  - **S79.929** Unspecified injury of unspecified thigh

INJURIES TO THE KNEE AND LOWER LEG (S80-S89)

Excludes2 burns and corrosions (T20-T32)
frostbite (T33-T34)
injuries of ankle and foot, except fracture of ankle and malleolus (S90-S99)
insect bite or sting, venomous (T63.4)

S80 Superficial injury of knee and lower leg

Excludes2 superficial injury of ankle and foot (S90.-)

The appropriate 7th character is to be added to each code from category S80

A	initial encounter
D	subsequent encounter
S	sequela

- **S80.0** Contusion of knee
  - X **S80.00** Contusion of unspecified knee
  - X **S80.01** Contusion of right knee
  - X **S80.02** Contusion of left knee
- **S80.1** Contusion of lower leg
  - X **S80.10** Contusion of unspecified lower leg
  - X **S80.11** Contusion of right lower leg
  - X **S80.12** Contusion of left lower leg
- **S80.2** Other superficial injuries of knee
  - **S80.21** Abrasion of knee
    - **S80.211** Abrasion, right knee
    - **S80.212** Abrasion, left knee
    - **S80.219** Abrasion, unspecified knee
  - **S80.22** Blister (nonthermal) of knee
    - **S80.221** Blister (nonthermal), right knee
    - **S80.222** Blister (nonthermal), left knee
    - **S80.229** Blister (nonthermal), unspecified knee
  - **S80.24** External constriction of knee
    - **S80.241** External constriction, right knee
    - **S80.242** External constriction, left knee
    - **S80.249** External constriction, unspecified knee
  - **S80.25** Superficial foreign body of knee
    Splinter in the knee
    - **S80.251** Superficial foreign body, right knee
    - **S80.252** Superficial foreign body, left knee
    - **S80.259** Superficial foreign body, unspecified knee
  - **S80.26** Insect bite (nonvenomous) of knee
    - **S80.261** Insect bite (nonvenomous), right knee
    - **S80.262** Insect bite (nonvenomous), left knee
    - **S80.269** Insect bite (nonvenomous), unspecified knee

CHAPTER 19 (S00-T88)

● S80.27 Other superficial bite of knee
Excludes1 open bite of knee (S81.05-)
● S80.271 Other superficial bite of right knee
● S80.272 Other superficial bite of left knee
● S80.279 Other superficial bite of unspecified knee

● S80.8 Other superficial injuries of lower leg
● S80.81 Abrasion of lower leg
● S80.811 Abrasion, right lower leg
● S80.812 Abrasion, left lower leg
● S80.819 Abrasion, unspecified lower leg
● S80.82 Blister (nonthermal) of lower leg
● S80.821 Blister (nonthermal), right lower leg
● S80.822 Blister (nonthermal), left lower leg
● S80.829 Blister (nonthermal), unspecified lower leg
● S80.84 External constriction of lower leg
● S80.841 External constriction, right lower leg
● S80.842 External constriction, left lower leg
● S80.849 External constriction, unspecified lower leg
● S80.85 Superficial foreign body of lower leg
Splinter in the lower leg
● S80.851 Superficial foreign body, right lower leg
● S80.852 Superficial foreign body, left lower leg
● S80.859 Superficial foreign body, unspecified lower leg
● S80.86 Insect bite (nonvenomous) of lower leg
● S80.861 Insect bite (nonvenomous), right lower leg
● S80.862 Insect bite (nonvenomous), left lower leg
● S80.869 Insect bite (nonvenomous), unspecified lower leg
● S80.87 Other superficial bite of lower leg
Excludes1 open bite of lower leg (S81.85-)
● S80.871 Other superficial bite, right lower leg
● S80.872 Other superficial bite, left lower leg
● S80.879 Other superficial bite, unspecified lower leg

● S80.9 Unspecified superficial injury of knee and lower leg
● S80.91 Unspecified superficial injury of knee
● S80.911 Unspecified superficial injury of right knee
● S80.912 Unspecified superficial injury of left knee
● S80.919 Unspecified superficial injury of unspecified knee
● S80.92 Unspecified superficial injury of lower leg
● S80.921 Unspecified superficial injury of right lower leg
● S80.922 Unspecified superficial injury of left lower leg
● S80.929 Unspecified superficial injury of unspecified lower leg

● S81 Open wound of knee and lower leg
Code also any associated wound infection
Excludes1 open fracture of knee and lower leg (S82.-)
traumatic amputation of lower leg (S88.-)
Excludes2 open wound of ankle and foot (S91.-)

The appropriate 7th character is to be added to each code from category S81

A	initial encounter
D	subsequent encounter
S	sequela

● S81.0 Open wound of knee
● S81.00 Unspecified open wound of knee
● S81.001 Unspecified open wound, right knee
● S81.002 Unspecified open wound, left knee
● S81.009 Unspecified open wound, unspecified knee
● S81.01 Laceration without foreign body of knee
● S81.011 Laceration without foreign body, right knee
● S81.012 Laceration without foreign body, left knee
● S81.019 Laceration without foreign body, unspecified knee
● S81.02 Laceration with foreign body of knee
● S81.021 Laceration with foreign body, right knee
● S81.022 Laceration with foreign body, left knee
● S81.029 Laceration with foreign body, unspecified knee
● S81.03 Puncture wound without foreign body of knee
● S81.031 Puncture wound without foreign body, right knee
● S81.032 Puncture wound without foreign body, left knee
● S81.039 Puncture wound without foreign body, unspecified knee
● S81.04 Puncture wound with foreign body of knee
● S81.041 Puncture wound with foreign body, right knee
● S81.042 Puncture wound with foreign body, left knee
● S81.049 Puncture wound with foreign body, unspecified knee
● S81.05 Open bite of knee
Bite of knee NOS
Excludes1 superficial bite of knee (S80.27-)
● S81.051 Open bite, right knee
● S81.052 Open bite, left knee
● S81.059 Open bite, unspecified knee

● S81.8 Open wound of lower leg
● S81.80 Unspecified open wound of lower leg
● S81.801 Unspecified open wound, right lower leg
● S81.802 Unspecified open wound, left lower leg
● S81.809 Unspecified open wound, unspecified lower leg
● S81.81 Laceration without foreign body of lower leg
● S81.811 Laceration without foreign body, right lower leg
● S81.812 Laceration without foreign body, left lower leg
● S81.819 Laceration without foreign body, unspecified lower leg
● S81.82 Laceration with foreign body of lower leg
● S81.821 Laceration with foreign body, right lower leg
● S81.822 Laceration with foreign body, left lower leg
● S81.829 Laceration with foreign body, unspecified lower leg

● S81.83 Puncture wound without foreign body of lower leg
- ● S81.831 Puncture wound without foreign body, right lower leg
- ● S81.832 Puncture wound without foreign body, left lower leg
- ● S81.839 Puncture wound without foreign body, unspecified lower leg

● S81.84 Puncture wound with foreign body of lower leg
- ● S81.841 Puncture wound with foreign body, right lower leg
  Coding Clinic: 2016, Q3, P46
- ● S81.842 Puncture wound with foreign body, left lower leg
- ● S81.849 Puncture wound with foreign body, unspecified lower leg

● S81.85 Open bite of lower leg
Bite of lower leg NOS
Excludes1 superficial bite of lower leg (S80.86-, S80.87-)
- ● S81.851 Open bite, right lower leg
- ● S81.852 Open bite, left lower leg
- ● S81.859 Open bite, unspecified lower leg

● **S82 Fracture of lower leg, including ankle**

Note: A fracture not indicated as displaced or nondisplaced should be coded to displaced

A fracture not indicated as open or closed should be coded to closed

The open fracture designations are based on the Gustilo open fracture classification

Includes fracture of malleolus
Excludes1 traumatic amputation of lower leg (S88.-)
Excludes2 fracture of foot, except ankle (S92.-)
periprosthetic fracture around internal prosthetic ankle joint (M97.2)
periprosthetic fracture around internal of prosthetic implant of knee joint (M97.1-)

The appropriate 7th character is to be added to all codes from category S82

A	initial encounter for closed fracture
B	initial encounter for open fracture type I or II initial encounter for open fracture NOS
C	initial encounter for open fracture type IIIA, IIIB, or IIIC
D	subsequent encounter for closed fracture with routine healing
E	subsequent encounter for open fracture type I or II with routine healing
F	subsequent encounter for open fracture type IIIA, IIIB, or IIIC with routine healing
G	subsequent encounter for closed fracture with delayed healing
H	subsequent encounter for open fracture type I or II with delayed healing
J	subsequent encounter for open fracture type IIIA, IIIB, or IIIC with delayed healing
K	subsequent encounter for closed fracture with nonunion
M	subsequent encounter for open fracture type I or II with nonunion
N	subsequent encounter for open fracture type IIIA, IIIB, or IIIC with nonunion
P	subsequent encounter for closed fracture with malunion
Q	subsequent encounter for open fracture type I or II with malunion
R	subsequent encounter for open fracture type IIIA, IIIB, or IIIC with malunion
S	sequela

● S82.0 Fracture of patella
Knee cap

● S82.00 Unspecified fracture of patella
- ● S82.001 Unspecified fracture of right patella A, B, C,K,M, N, P, Q, R, A, B, C (Ex) PDX 1264 [K, M, N, P, Q, R], 1846 [A], 1847 [B, C]
- ● S82.002 Unspecified fracture of left patella A, B, C,K,M, N, P, Q, R, A, B, C (Ex) PDX 1264 [K, M, N, P, Q, R], 1847 [B, C], 1848 [A]
- ● S82.009 Unspecified fracture of unspecified patella A, B, C,K,M, N, P, Q, R, A, B, C (Ex) PDX 1264 [K, M, N, P, Q, R], 1847 [B, C], 1849 [A]

● S82.01 Osteochondral fracture of patella
- ● S82.011 Displaced osteochondral fracture of right patella A, B, C,K,M, N, P, Q, R, A, B, C (Ex) PDX 1264 [K, M, N, P, Q, R], 1846 [A], 1847 [B, C]
- ● S82.012 Displaced osteochondral fracture of left patella A, B, C,K,M, N, P, Q, R, A, B, C (Ex) PDX 1264 [K, M, N, P, Q, R], 1847 [B, C], 1848 [A]
- ● S82.013 Displaced osteochondral fracture of unspecified patella A, B, C,K,M, N, P, Q, R, A, B, C (Ex) PDX 1264 [K, M, N, P, Q, R], 1847 [B, C], 1849 [A]
- ● S82.014 Nondisplaced osteochondral fracture of right patella A, B, C,K,M, N, P, Q, R, A, B, C (Ex) PDX 1264 [K, M, N, P, Q, R], 1846 [A], 1847 [B, C]
- ● S82.015 Nondisplaced osteochondral fracture of left patella A, B, C,K,M, N, P, Q, R, A, B, C (Ex) PDX 1264 [K, M, N, P, Q, R], 1847 [B, C], 1848 [A]
- ● S82.016 Nondisplaced osteochondral fracture of unspecified patella A, B, C,K,M, N, P, Q, R, A, B, C (Ex) PDX 1264 [K, M, N, P, Q, R], 1847 [B, C], 1849 [A]

● S82.02 Longitudinal fracture of patella
- ● S82.021 Displaced longitudinal fracture of right patella A, B, C,K,M, N, P, Q, R, A, B, C (Ex) PDX 1264 [K, M, N, P, Q, R], 1846 [A], 1847 [B, C]
- ● S82.022 Displaced longitudinal fracture of left patella A, B, C,K,M, N, P, Q, R, A, B, C (Ex) PDX 1264 [K, M, N, P, Q, R], 1847 [B, C], 1848 [A]
- ● S82.023 Displaced longitudinal fracture of unspecified patella A, B, C,K,M, N, P, Q, R, A, B, C (Ex) PDX 1264 [K, M, N, P, Q, R], 1847 [B, C], 1849 [A]
- ● S82.024 Nondisplaced longitudinal fracture of right patella A, B, C,K,M, N, P, Q, R, A, B, C (Ex) PDX 1264 [K, M, N, P, Q, R], 1846 [A], 1847 [B, C]
- ● S82.025 Nondisplaced longitudinal fracture of left patella A, B, C,K,M, N, P, Q, R, A, B, C (Ex) PDX 1264 [K, M, N, P, Q, R], 1847 [B, C], 1848 [A]
- ● S82.026 Nondisplaced longitudinal fracture of unspecified patella A, B, C,K,M, N, P, Q, R, A, B, C (Ex) PDX 1264 [K, M, N, P, Q, R], 1847 [B, C], 1849 [A]

● S82.03 Transverse fracture of patella
- ● S82.031 Displaced transverse fracture of right patella A, B, C,K,M, N, P, Q, R, A, B, C (Ex) PDX 1264 [K, M, N, P, Q, R], 1846 [A], 1847 [B, C]
- ● S82.032 Displaced transverse fracture of left patella A, B, C,K,M, N, P, Q, R, A, B, C (Ex) PDX 1264 [K, M, N, P, Q, R], 1847 [B, C], 1848 [A]

CHAPTER 19 (S00-T88)

S82.033 **Displaced transverse fracture of unspecified patella** A, B, C,K,M, N, P, Q, R, A, B, C (Ex) PDX 1264 [K, M, N, P, Q, R], 1847 [B, C], 1849 [A]

S82.034 **Nondisplaced transverse fracture of right patella** A, B, C,K,M, N, P, Q, R, A, B, C (Ex) PDX 1264 [K, M, N, P, Q, R], 1846 [A], 1847 [B, C]

S82.035 **Nondisplaced transverse fracture of left patella** A, B, C,K,M, N, P, Q, R, A, B, C (Ex) PDX 1264 [K, M, N, P, Q, R], 1847 [B, C], 1848 [A]

S82.036 **Nondisplaced transverse fracture of unspecified patella** A, B, C,K,M, N, P, Q, R, A, B, C (Ex) PDX 1264 [K, M, N, P, Q, R], 1847 [B, C], 1849 [A]

S82.04 Comminuted fracture of patella

S82.041 **Displaced comminuted fracture of right patella** A, B, C,K,M, N, P, Q, R, A, B, C (Ex) PDX 1264 [K, M, N, P, Q, R], 1846 [A], 1847 [B, C]

S82.042 **Displaced comminuted fracture of left patella** A, B, C,K,M, N, P, Q, R, A, B, C (Ex) PDX 1264 [K, M, N, P, Q, R], 1847 [B, C], 1848 [A]

S82.043 **Displaced comminuted fracture of unspecified patella** A, B, C,K,M, N, P, Q, R, A, B, C (Ex) PDX 1264 [K, M, N, P, Q, R], 1847 [B, C], 1849 [A]

S82.044 **Nondisplaced comminuted fracture of right patella** A, B, C,K,M, N, P, Q, R, A, B, C (Ex) PDX 1264 [K, M, N, P, Q, R], 1846 [A], 1847 [B, C]

S82.045 **Nondisplaced comminuted fracture of left patella** A, B, C,K,M, N, P, Q, R, A, B, C (Ex) PDX 1264 [K, M, N, P, Q, R], 1847 [B, C], 1848 [A]

S82.046 **Nondisplaced comminuted fracture of unspecified patella** A, B, C,K,M, N, P, Q, R, A, B, C (Ex) PDX 1264 [K, M, N, P, Q, R], 1847 [B, C], 1849 [A]

S82.09 Other fracture of patella

S82.091 **Other fracture of right patella** A, B, C,K,M, N, P, Q, R, A, B, C (Ex) PDX 1264 [K, M, N, P, Q, R], 1846 [A], 1847 [B, C]

S82.092 **Other fracture of left patella** A, B, C,K,M, N, P, Q, R, A, B, C (Ex) PDX 1264 [K, M, N, P, Q, R], 1847 [B, C], 1848 [A]

S82.099 **Other fracture of unspecified patella** A, B, C,K,M, N, P, Q, R, A, B, C (Ex) PDX 1264 [K, M, N, P, Q, R], 1847 [B, C], 1849 [A]

S82.1 Fracture of upper end of tibia

Fracture of proximal end of tibia

Excludes2 fracture of shaft of tibia (S82.2-)
physeal fracture of upper end of tibia (S89.Ø-)

S82.1Ø Unspecified fracture of upper end of tibia

S82.1Ø1 **Unspecified fracture of upper end of right tibia** A, K, M, N, P, Q, R, B, C, A, B, C (Ex) PDX 1264 [K, M, N, P, Q, R], 1850 [A], 1851 [B, C]

S82.1Ø2 **Unspecified fracture of upper end of left tibia** A, K, M, N, P, Q, R, B, C, A, B, C (Ex) PDX 1264 [K, M, N, P, Q, R], 1851 [B, C], 1852 [A]

S82.1Ø9 **Unspecified fracture of upper end of unspecified tibia** A, K, M, N, P, Q, R, B, C, A, B, C (Ex) PDX 1264 [K, M, N, P, Q, R], 1851 [A, B, C]

S82.11 Fracture of tibial spine

S82.111 **Displaced fracture of right tibial spine** A, K, M, N, P, Q, R, B, C, A, B, C (Ex) PDX 1264 [K, M, N, P, Q, R], 1850 [A], 1851 [B, C]

S82.112 **Displaced fracture of left tibial spine** A, K, M, N, P, Q, R, B, C, A, B, C (Ex) PDX 1264 [K, M, N, P, Q, R], 1851 [B, C], 1852 [A]

S82.113 **Displaced fracture of unspecified tibial spine** A, K, M, N, P, Q, R, B, C, A, B, C (Ex) PDX 1264 [K, M, N, P, Q, R], 1851 [A, B, C]

S82.114 **Nondisplaced fracture of right tibial spine** A, K, M, N, P, Q, R, B, C, A, B, C (Ex) PDX 1264 [K, M, N, P, Q, R], 1850 [A], 1851 [B, C]

S82.115 **Nondisplaced fracture of left tibial spine** A, K, M, N, P, Q, R, B, C, A, B, C (Ex) PDX 1264 [K, M, N, P, Q, R], 1851 [B, C], 1852 [A]

S82.116 **Nondisplaced fracture of unspecified tibial spine** A, K, M, N, P, Q, R, B, C, A, B, C (Ex) PDX 1264 [K, M, N, P, Q, R], 1851 [A, B, C]

S82.12 Fracture of lateral condyle of tibia

S82.121 **Displaced fracture of lateral condyle of right tibia** A, K, M, N, P, Q, R, B, C, A, B, C (Ex) PDX 1264 [K, M, N, P, Q, R], 1850 [A], 1851 [B, C]

S82.122 **Displaced fracture of lateral condyle of left tibia** A, K, M, N, P, Q, R, B, C, A, B, C (Ex) PDX 1264 [K, M, N, P, Q, R], 1851 [B, C], 1852 [A]

S82.123 **Displaced fracture of lateral condyle of unspecified tibia** A, K, M, N, P, Q, R, B, C, A, B, C (Ex) PDX 1264 [K, M, N, P, Q, R], 1851 [A, B, C]

S82.124 **Nondisplaced fracture of lateral condyle of right tibia** A, K, M, N, P, Q, R, B, C, A, B, C (Ex) PDX 1264 [K, M, N, P, Q, R], 1850 [A], 1851 [B, C]

S82.125 **Nondisplaced fracture of lateral condyle of left tibia** A, K, M, N, P, Q, R, B, C, A, B, C (Ex) PDX 1264 [K, M, N, P, Q, R], 1851 [B, C], 1852 [A]

S82.126 **Nondisplaced fracture of lateral condyle of unspecified tibia** A, K, M, N, P, Q, R, B, C, A, B, C (Ex) PDX 1264 [K, M, N, P, Q, R], 1851 [A, B, C]

S82.13 Fracture of medial condyle of tibia

S82.131 **Displaced fracture of medial condyle of right tibia** A, K, M, N, P, Q, R, B, C, A, B, C (Ex) PDX 1264 [K, M, N, P, Q, R], 1850 [A], 1851 [B, C]

S82.132 **Displaced fracture of medial condyle of left tibia** A, K, M, N, P, Q, R, B, C, A, B, C (Ex) PDX 1264 [K, M, N, P, Q, R], 1851 [B, C], 1852 [A]

S82.133 **Displaced fracture of medial condyle of unspecified tibia** A, K, M, N, P, Q, R, B, C, A, B, C (Ex) PDX 1264 [K, M, N, P, Q, R], 1851 [A, B, C]

S82.134 **Nondisplaced fracture of medial condyle of right tibia** A, K, M, N, P, Q, R, B, C, A, B, C (Ex) PDX 1264 [K, M, N, P, Q, R], 1850 [A], 1851 [B, C]

S82.135 **Nondisplaced fracture of medial condyle of left tibia** A, K, M, N, P, Q, R, B, C, A, B, C (Ex) PDX 1264 [K, M, N, P, Q, R], 1851 [B, C], 1852 [A]

S82.136 **Nondisplaced fracture of medial condyle of unspecified tibia** A, K, M, N, P, Q, R, B, C, A, B, C (Ex) PDX 1264 [K, M, N, P, Q, R], 1851 [A, B, C]

S82.14 Bicondylar fracture of tibia
Fracture of tibial plateau NOS

S82.141 Displaced bicondylar fracture of right tibia A, K, M, N, P, Q, R, B, C, A, B, C (Ex:) PDX 1264 [K, M, N, P, Q, R], 1850 [A], 1851 [B, C]

S82.142 Displaced bicondylar fracture of left tibia A, K, M, N, P, Q, R, B, C, A, B, C (Ex:) PDX 1264 [K, M, N, P, Q, R], 1851 [B, C], 1852 [A]

S82.143 Displaced bicondylar fracture of unspecified tibia A, K, M, N, P, Q, R, B, C, A, B, C (Ex:) PDX 1264 [K, M, N, P, Q, R], 1851 [A, B, C]

S82.144 Nondisplaced bicondylar fracture of right tibia A, K, M, N, P, Q, R, B, C, A, B, C (Ex:) PDX 1264 [K, M, N, P, Q, R], 1850 [A], 1851 [B, C]

S82.145 Nondisplaced bicondylar fracture of left tibia A, K, M, N, P, Q, R, B, C, A, B, C (Ex:) PDX 1264 [K, M, N, P, Q, R], 1851 [B, C], 1852 [A]

S82.146 Nondisplaced bicondylar fracture of unspecified tibia A, K, M, N, P, Q, R, B, C, A, B, C (Ex:) PDX 1264 [K, M, N, P, Q, R], 1851 [A, B, C]

S82.15 Fracture of tibial tuberosity

S82.151 Displaced fracture of right tibial tuberosity A, K, M, N, P, Q, R, B, C, A, B, C (Ex:) PDX 1264 [K, M, N, P, Q, R], 1850 [A], 1851 [B, C]

S82.152 Displaced fracture of left tibial tuberosity A, K, M, N, P, Q, R, B, C, A, B, C (Ex:) PDX 1264 [K, M, N, P, Q, R], 1851 [B, C], 1852 [A]

S82.153 Displaced fracture of unspecified tibial tuberosity A, K, M, N, P, Q, R, B, C, A, B, C (Ex:) PDX 1264 [K, M, N, P, Q, R], 1851 [A, B, C]

S82.154 Nondisplaced fracture of right tibial tuberosity A, K, M, N, P, Q, R, B, C, A, B, C (Ex:) PDX 1264 [K, M, N, P, Q, R], 1850 [A], 1851 [B, C]

S82.155 Nondisplaced fracture of left tibial tuberosity A, K, M, N, P, Q, R, B, C, A, B, C (Ex:) PDX 1264 [K, M, N, P, Q, R], 1851 [B, C], 1852 [A]

S82.156 Nondisplaced fracture of unspecified tibial tuberosity A, K, M, N, P, Q, R, B, C, A, B, C (Ex:) PDX 1264 [K, M, N, P, Q, R], 1851 [A, B, C]

S82.16 Torus fracture of upper end of tibia

The appropriate 7th character is to be added to all codes in subcategory S82.16

A	initial encounter for closed fracture
D	subsequent encounter for fracture with routine healing
G	subsequent encounter for fracture with delayed healing
K	subsequent encounter for fracture with nonunion
P	subsequent encounter for fracture with malunion
S	sequela

S82.161 Torus fracture of upper end of right tibia A, K, P, A (Ex:) PDX 1853, 1264

S82.162 Torus fracture of upper end of left tibia A, K, P, A (Ex:) PDX 1854, 1264

S82.169 Torus fracture of upper end of unspecified tibia A, K, P, A (Ex:) PDX 1855, 1264

S82.19 Other fracture of upper end of tibia

S82.191 Other fracture of upper end of right tibia A, K, M, N, P, Q, R, B, C, A, B, C (Ex:) PDX 1264 [K, M, N, P, Q, R], 1850 [A], 1851 [B, C]

S82.192 Other fracture of upper end of left tibia A, K, M, N, P, Q, R, B, C, A, B, C (Ex:) PDX 1264 [K, M, N, P, Q, R], 1851 [B, C], 1852 [A]

S82.199 Other fracture of upper end of unspecified tibia A, K, M, N, P, Q, R, B, C, A, B, C (Ex:) PDX 1264 [K, M, N, P, Q, R], 1851 [A, B, C]

S82.2 Fracture of shaft of tibia

S82.20 Unspecified fracture of shaft of tibia
Fracture of tibia NOS

S82.201 Unspecified fracture of shaft of right tibia A, K, M, N, P, Q, R, B, C, A, B, C (Ex:) PDX 1856, 1851, 1264

S82.202 Unspecified fracture of shaft of left tibia A, K, M, N, P, Q, R, B, C, A, B, C (Ex:) PDX 1264 [K, M, N, P, Q, R], 1851 [B, C], 1852 [A]

S82.209 Unspecified fracture of shaft of unspecified tibia A, K, M, N, P, Q, R, B, C, A, B, C (Ex:) PDX 1264 [K, M, N, P, Q, R], 1851 [A, B, C]

S82.22 Transverse fracture of shaft of tibia

S82.221 Displaced transverse fracture of shaft of right tibia A, K, M, N, P, Q, R, B, C, A, B, C (Ex:) PDX 1264 [K, M, N, P, Q, R], 1850 [A], 1851 [B, C]

S82.222 Displaced transverse fracture of shaft of left tibia A, K, M, N, P, Q, R, B, C, A, B, C (Ex:) PDX 1264 [K, M, N, P, Q, R], 1851 [B, C], 1852 [A]

S82.223 Displaced transverse fracture of shaft of unspecified tibia A, K, M, N, P, Q, R, B, C, A, B, C (Ex:) PDX 1264 [K, M, N, P, Q, R], 1851 [A, B, C]

S82.224 Nondisplaced transverse fracture of shaft of right tibia A, K, M, N, P, Q, R, B, C, A, B, C (Ex:) PDX 1264 [K, M, N, P, Q, R], 1850 [A], 1851 [B, C]

S82.225 Nondisplaced transverse fracture of shaft of left tibia A, K, M, N, P, Q, R, B, C, A, B, C (Ex:) PDX 1264 [K, M, N, P, Q, R], 1851 [B, C], 1852 [A]

S82.226 Nondisplaced transverse fracture of shaft of unspecified tibia A, K, M, N, P, Q, R, B, C, A, B, C (Ex:) PDX 1264 [K, M, N, P, Q, R], 1851 [A, B, C]

S82.23 Oblique fracture of shaft of tibia

S82.231 Displaced oblique fracture of shaft of right tibia A, K, M, N, P, Q, R, B, C, A, B, C (Ex:) PDX 1264 [K, M, N, P, Q, R], 1850 [A], 1851 [B, C]

S82.232 Displaced oblique fracture of shaft of left tibia A, K, M, N, P, Q, R, B, C, A, B, C (Ex:) PDX 1264 [K, M, N, P, Q, R], 1851 [B, C], 1852 [A]

S82.233 Displaced oblique fracture of shaft of unspecified tibia A, K, M, N, P, Q, R, B, C, A, B, C (Ex:) PDX 1264 [K, M, N, P, Q, R], 1851 [A, B, C]

S82.234 Nondisplaced oblique fracture of shaft of right tibia A, K, M, N, P, Q, R, B, C, A, B, C (Ex:) PDX 1264 [K, M, N, P, Q, R], 1850 [A], 1851 [B, C]
Coding Clinic: 2015, Q1, P9-10

CHAPTER 19 (S00-T88)

● S82.235 Nondisplaced oblique fracture of shaft of left tibia A, K, M, N, P, Q, R, B, C, A, B, C (Ex:) PDX 1264 [K, M, N, P, Q, R], 1851 [B, C], 1852 [A]

● S82.236 Nondisplaced oblique fracture of shaft of unspecified tibia A, K, M, N, P, Q, R, B, C, A, B, C (Ex:) PDX 1264 [K, M, N, P, Q, R], 1851 [A, B, C]

● S82.24 Spiral fracture of shaft of tibia
Toddler fracture

● S82.241 Displaced spiral fracture of shaft of right tibia A, K, M, N, P, Q, R, B, C, A, B, C (Ex:) PDX 1264 [K, M, N, P, Q, R], 1850 [A], 1851 [B, C]

● S82.242 Displaced spiral fracture of shaft of left tibia A, K, M, N, P, Q, R, B, C, A, B, C (Ex:) PDX 1264 [K, M, N, P, Q, R], 1851 [B, C], 1852 [A]

● S82.243 Displaced spiral fracture of shaft of unspecified tibia A, K, M, N, P, Q, R, B, C, A, B, C (Ex:) PDX 1264 [K, M, N, P, Q, R], 1851 [A, B, C]

● S82.244 Nondisplaced spiral fracture of shaft of right tibia A, K, M, N, P, Q, R, B, C, A, B, C (Ex:) PDX 1264 [K, M, N, P, Q, R], 1850 [A], 1851 [B, C]

● S82.245 Nondisplaced spiral fracture of shaft of left tibia A, K, M, N, P, Q, R, B, C, A, B, C (Ex:) PDX 1264 [K, M, N, P, Q, R], 1851 [B, C], 1852 [A]

● S82.246 Nondisplaced spiral fracture of shaft of unspecified tibia A, K, M, N, P, Q, R, B, C, A, B, C (Ex:) PDX 1264 [K, M, N, P, Q, R], 1851 [A, B, C]

● S82.25 Comminuted fracture of shaft of tibia

● S82.251 Displaced comminuted fracture of shaft of right tibia A, K, M, N, P, Q, R, B, C, A, B, C (Ex:) PDX 1264 [K, M, N, P, Q, R], 1850 [A], 1851 [B, C]
Coding Clinic: 2015, Q2, P6

● S82.252 Displaced comminuted fracture of shaft of left tibia A, K, M, N, P, Q, R, B, C, A, B, C (Ex:) PDX 1264 [K, M, N, P, Q, R], 1851 [B, C], 1852 [A]

● S82.253 Displaced comminuted fracture of shaft of unspecified tibia A, K, M, N, P, Q, R, B, C, A, B, C (Ex:) PDX 1264 [K, M, N, P, Q, R], 1851 [A, B, C]

● S82.254 Nondisplaced comminuted fracture of shaft of right tibia A, K, M, N, P, Q, R, B, C, A, B, C (Ex:) PDX 1264 [K, M, N, P, Q, R], 1850 [A], 1851 [B, C]

● S82.255 Nondisplaced comminuted fracture of shaft of left tibia A, K, M, N, P, Q, R, B, C, A, B, C (Ex:) PDX 1264 [K, M, N, P, Q, R], 1851 [B, C], 1852 [A]

● S82.256 Nondisplaced comminuted fracture of shaft of unspecified tibia A, K, M, N, P, Q, R, B, C, A, B, C (Ex:) PDX 1264 [K, M, N, P, Q, R], 1851 [A, B, C]

● S82.26 Segmental fracture of shaft of tibia

● S82.261 Displaced segmental fracture of shaft of right tibia A, K, M, N, P, Q, R, B, C, A, B, C (Ex:) PDX 1264 [K, M, N, P, Q, R], 1850 [A], 1851 [B, C]

● S82.262 Displaced segmental fracture of shaft of left tibia A, K, M, N, P, Q, R, B, C, A, B, C (Ex:) PDX 1264 [K, M, N, P, Q, R], 1851 [B, C], 1852 [A]

● S82.263 Displaced segmental fracture of shaft of unspecified tibia A, K, M, N, P, Q, R, B, C, A, B, C (Ex:) PDX 1264 [K, M, N, P, Q, R], 1851 [A, B, C]

● S82.264 Nondisplaced segmental fracture of shaft of right tibia A, K, M, N, P, Q, R, B, C, A, B, C (Ex:) PDX 1264 [K, M, N, P, Q, R], 1850 [A], 1851 [B, C]

● S82.265 Nondisplaced segmental fracture of shaft of left tibia A, K, M, N, P, Q, R, B, C, A, B, C (Ex:) PDX 1264 [K, M, N, P, Q, R], 1851 [B, C], 1852 [A]

● S82.266 Nondisplaced segmental fracture of shaft of unspecified tibia A, K, M, N, P, Q, R, B, C, A, B, C (Ex:) PDX 1264 [K, M, N, P, Q, R], 1851 [A, B, C]

● S82.29 Other fracture of shaft of tibia

● S82.291 Other fracture of shaft of right tibia A, K, M, N, P, Q, R, B, C, A, B, C (Ex:) PDX 1264 [K, M, N, P, Q, R], 1850 [A], 1851 [B, C]

● S82.292 Other fracture of shaft of left tibia A, K, M, N, P, Q, R, B, C, A, B, C (Ex:) PDX 1264 [K, M, N, P, Q, R], 1851 [B, C], 1852 [A]

● S82.299 Other fracture of shaft of unspecified tibia A, K, M, N, P, Q, R, B, C, A, B, C (Ex:) PDX 1264 [K, M, N, P, Q, R], 1851 [A, B, C]

● S82.3 Fracture of lower end of tibia

Excludes1 bimalleolar fracture of lower leg (S82.84-)
fracture of medial malleolus alone (S82.5-)
Maisonneuve's fracture (S82.86-)
pilon fracture of distal tibia (S82.87-)
trimalleolar fractures of lower leg (S82.85-)

● S82.30 Unspecified fracture of lower end of tibia (Ex:) PDX 1264 [K, M, N, P, Q, R], 1857 [B, C]

● S82.301 Unspecified fracture of lower end of right tibia B, C, K, M, N, P, Q, R, B, C

● S82.302 Unspecified fracture of lower end of left tibia B, C, K, M, N, P, Q, R, B, C

● S82.309 Unspecified fracture of lower end of unspecified tibia B, C, K, M, N, P, Q, R, B, C

● S82.31 Torus fracture of lower end of tibia

The appropriate 7th character is to be added to all codes in subcategory S82.31

A	initial encounter for closed fracture
D	subsequent encounter for fracture with routine healing
G	subsequent encounter for fracture with delayed healing
K	subsequent encounter for fracture with nonunion
P	subsequent encounter for fracture with malunion
S	sequela

● S82.311 Torus fracture of lower end of right tibia A, K, P, A (Ex:) PDX 1264 [K, P], 1853 [A]

● S82.312 Torus fracture of lower end of left tibia A, K, P, A (Ex:) PDX 1264 [K, P], 1854 [A]

● S82.319 Torus fracture of lower end of unspecified tibia A, K, P, A (Ex:) PDX 1264 [K, P], 1855 [A]

● S82.39 Other fracture of lower end of tibia (Ex) PDX 1264 [K, M, N, P, Q, R], 1857 [B, C]
  ● S82.391 Other fracture of lower end of right tibia B, C, K, M, N, P, Q, R, B, C
  ● S82.392 Other fracture of lower end of left tibia B, C, K, M, N, P, Q, R, B, C
  Coding Clinic: 2015, Q1, P25
  ● S82.399 Other fracture of lower end of unspecified tibia B, C, K, M, N, P, Q, R, B, C

● S82.4 Fracture of shaft of fibula (Ex) PDX 1264 [K, M, N, P, Q, R], 1851 [B, C]
Excludes2 fracture of lateral malleolus alone (S82.6-)

● S82.40 Unspecified fracture of shaft of fibula
  ● S82.401 Unspecified fracture of shaft of right fibula K, M, N, P, Q, R, B, C, B, C
  ● S82.402 Unspecified fracture of shaft of left fibula K, M, N, P, Q, R, B, C, B, C
  ● S82.409 Unspecified fracture of shaft of unspecified fibula K, M, N, P, Q, R, B, C, B, C

● S82.42 Transverse fracture of shaft of fibula
  ● S82.421 Displaced transverse fracture of shaft of right fibula K, M, N, P, Q, R, B, C, B, C
  ● S82.422 Displaced transverse fracture of shaft of left fibula K, M, N, P, Q, R, B, C, B, C
  ● S82.423 Displaced transverse fracture of shaft of unspecified fibula K, M, N, P, Q, R, B, C, B, C
  ● S82.424 Nondisplaced transverse fracture of shaft of right fibula K, M, N, P, Q, R, B, C, B, C
  ● S82.425 Nondisplaced transverse fracture of shaft of left fibula K, M, N, P, Q, R, B, C, B, C
  ● S82.426 Nondisplaced transverse fracture of shaft of unspecified fibula K, M, N, P, Q, R, B, C, B, C

● S82.43 Oblique fracture of shaft of fibula
  ● S82.431 Displaced oblique fracture of shaft of right fibula K, M, N, P, Q, R, B, C, B, C
  ● S82.432 Displaced oblique fracture of shaft of left fibula K, M, N, P, Q, R, B, C, B, C
  ● S82.433 Displaced oblique fracture of shaft of unspecified fibula K, M, N, P, Q, R, B, C, B, C
  ● S82.434 Nondisplaced oblique fracture of shaft of right fibula K, M, N, P, Q, R, B, C, B, C
  ● S82.435 Nondisplaced oblique fracture of shaft of left fibula K, M, N, P, Q, R, B, C, B, C
  ● S82.436 Nondisplaced oblique fracture of shaft of unspecified fibula K, M, N, P, Q, R, B, C, B, C

● S82.44 Spiral fracture of shaft of fibula
  ● S82.441 Displaced spiral fracture of shaft of right fibula K, M, N, P, Q, R, B, C, B, C
  ● S82.442 Displaced spiral fracture of shaft of left fibula K, M, N, P, Q, R, B, C, B, C
  ● S82.443 Displaced spiral fracture of shaft of unspecified fibula K, M, N, P, Q, R, B, C, B, C
  ● S82.444 Nondisplaced spiral fracture of shaft of right fibula K, M, N, P, Q, R, B, C, B, C
  ● S82.445 Nondisplaced spiral fracture of shaft of left fibula K, M, N, P, Q, R, B, C, B, C
  ● S82.446 Nondisplaced spiral fracture of shaft of unspecified fibula K, M, N, P, Q, R, B, C, B, C

● S82.45 Comminuted fracture of shaft of fibula
  ● S82.451 Displaced comminuted fracture of shaft of right fibula K, M, N, P, Q, R, B, C, B, C
  ● S82.452 Displaced comminuted fracture of shaft of left fibula K, M, N, P, Q, R, B, C, B, C
  ● S82.453 Displaced comminuted fracture of shaft of unspecified fibula K, M, N, P, Q, R, B, C, B, C
  ● S82.454 Nondisplaced comminuted fracture of shaft of right fibula K, M, N, P, Q, R, B, C, B, C
  ● S82.455 Nondisplaced comminuted fracture of shaft of left fibula K, M, N, P, Q, R, B, C, B, C
  ● S82.456 Nondisplaced comminuted fracture of shaft of unspecified fibula K, M, N, P, Q, R, B, C, B, C

● S82.46 Segmental fracture of shaft of fibula
  ● S82.461 Displaced segmental fracture of shaft of right fibula K, M, N, P, Q, R, B, C, B, C
  ● S82.462 Displaced segmental fracture of shaft of left fibula K, M, N, P, Q, R, B, C, B, C
  ● S82.463 Displaced segmental fracture of shaft of unspecified fibula K, M, N, P, Q, R, B, C, B, C
  ● S82.464 Nondisplaced segmental fracture of shaft of right fibula K, M, N, P, Q, R, B, C, B, C
  ● S82.465 Nondisplaced segmental fracture of shaft of left fibula K, M, N, P, Q, R, B, C, B, C
  ● S82.466 Nondisplaced segmental fracture of shaft of unspecified fibula K, M, N, P, Q, R, B, C, B, C

● S82.49 Other fracture of shaft of fibula
  ● S82.491 Other fracture of shaft of right fibula K, M, N, P, Q, R, B, C, B, C
  ● S82.492 Other fracture of shaft of left fibula K, M, N, P, Q, R, B, C, B, C
  ● S82.499 Other fracture of shaft of unspecified fibula K, M, N, P, Q, R, B, C, B, C

● S82.5 Fracture of medial malleolus (Ex) PDX 1264 [K, M, N, P, Q, R], 1857 [B, C]
Excludes1 pilon fracture of distal tibia (S82.87-)
Salter-Harris type III of lower end of tibia (S89.13-)
Salter-Harris type IV of lower end of tibia (S89.14-)

  X● S82.51 Displaced fracture of medial malleolus of right tibia B, C, K, M, N, P, Q, R, B, C
  X● S82.52 Displaced fracture of medial malleolus of left tibia B, C, K, M, N, P, Q, R, B, C
  X● S82.53 Displaced fracture of medial malleolus of unspecified tibia B, C, K, M, N, P, Q, R, B, C
  X● S82.54 Nondisplaced fracture of medial malleolus of right tibia B, C, K, M, N, P, Q, R, B, C

CHAPTER 19 (S00-T88)

X● S82.55 Nondisplaced fracture of medial malleolus of left tibia B, C, K, M, N, P, Q, R, B, C

X● S82.56 Nondisplaced fracture of medial malleolus of unspecified tibia B, C, K, M, N, P, Q, R, B, C

● S82.6 Fracture of lateral malleolus (Ex) PDX 1264 [K, M, N, P, Q, R], 1857 [B, C]

Excludes1 pilon fracture of distal tibia (S82.87-)

X● S82.61 Displaced fracture of lateral malleolus of right fibula B, C, K, M, N, P, Q, R, B, C

X● S82.62 Displaced fracture of lateral malleolus of left fibula B, C, K, M, N, P, Q, R, B, C

X● S82.63 Displaced fracture of lateral malleolus of unspecified fibula B, C, K, M, N, P, Q, R, B, C

X● S82.64 Nondisplaced fracture of lateral malleolus of right fibula B, C, K, M, N, P, Q, R, B, C

X● S82.65 Nondisplaced fracture of lateral malleolus of left fibula B, C, K, M, N, P, Q, R, B, C

X● S82.66 Nondisplaced fracture of lateral malleolus of unspecified fibula B, C, K, M, N, P, Q, R, B, C

● S82.8 Other fractures of lower leg

● S82.81 Torus fracture of upper end of fibula (Ex) PDX 1264

The appropriate 7th character is to be added to all codes in subcategory S82.81

A	initial encounter for closed fracture
D	subsequent encounter for fracture with routine healing
G	subsequent encounter for fracture with delayed healing
K	subsequent encounter for fracture with nonunion
P	subsequent encounter for fracture with malunion
S	sequela

● S82.811 Torus fracture of upper end of right fibula K, P

● S82.812 Torus fracture of upper end of left fibula K, P

● S82.819 Torus fracture of upper end of unspecified fibula K, P

● S82.82 Torus fracture of lower end of fibula (Ex) PDX 1264

The appropriate 7th character is to be added to all codes in subcategory S82.82

A	initial encounter for closed fracture
D	subsequent encounter for fracture with routine healing
G	subsequent encounter for fracture with delayed healing
K	subsequent encounter for fracture with nonunion
P	subsequent encounter for fracture with malunion
S	sequela

● S82.821 Torus fracture of lower end of right fibula K, P

● S82.822 Torus fracture of lower end of left fibula K, P

● S82.829 Torus fracture of lower end of unspecified fibula K, P

● S82.83 Other fracture of upper and lower end of fibula (Ex) PDX 1264 [K, M, N, P, Q, R], 1857 [B, C]

● S82.831 Other fracture of upper and lower end of right fibula K, M, N, P, Q, R, B, C, B, C

● S82.832 Other fracture of upper and lower end of left fibula K, M, N, P, Q, R, B, C, B, C

Coding Clinic: 2015, Q1, P9-10

● S82.839 Other fracture of upper and lower end of unspecified fibula K, M, N, P, Q, R, B, C, B, C

● S82.84 Bimalleolar fracture of lower leg (Ex) PDX 1264 [K, M, N, P, Q, R], 1857 [B, C]

● S82.841 Displaced bimalleolar fracture of right lower leg B, C, K, M, N, P, Q, R, B, C

● S82.842 Displaced bimalleolar fracture of left lower leg B, C, K, M, N, P, Q, R, B, C

● S82.843 Displaced bimalleolar fracture of unspecified lower leg B, C, K, M, N, P, Q, R, B, C

● S82.844 Nondisplaced bimalleolar fracture of right lower leg B, C, K, M, N, P, Q, R, B, C

● S82.845 Nondisplaced bimalleolar fracture of left lower leg B, C, K, M, N, P, Q, R, B, C

● S82.846 Nondisplaced bimalleolar fracture of unspecified lower leg B, C, K, M, N, P, Q, R, B, C

● S82.85 Trimalleolar fracture of lower leg (Ex) PDX 1264 [K, M, N, P, Q, R], 1857 [B, C]

● S82.851 Displaced trimalleolar fracture of right lower leg B, C, K, M, N, P, Q, R, B, C

● S82.852 Displaced trimalleolar fracture of left lower leg B, C, K, M, N, P, Q, R, B, C

● S82.853 Displaced trimalleolar fracture of unspecified lower leg B, C, K, M, N, P, Q, R, B, C

● S82.854 Nondisplaced trimalleolar fracture of right lower leg B, C, K, M, N, P, Q, R, B, C

● S82.855 Nondisplaced trimalleolar fracture of left lower leg B, C, K, M, N, P, Q, R, B, C

● S82.856 Nondisplaced trimalleolar fracture of unspecified lower leg B, C, K, M, N, P, Q, R, B, C

● S82.86 Maisonneuve's fracture (Ex) PDX 1264 [K, M, N, P, Q, R], 1851 [B, C]

● S82.861 Displaced Maisonneuve's fracture of right leg K, M, N, P, Q, R, B, C, B, C

● S82.862 Displaced Maisonneuve's fracture of left leg K, M, N, P, Q, R, B, C, B, C

● S82.863 Displaced Maisonneuve's fracture of unspecified leg K, M, N, P, Q, R, B, C, B, C

● S82.864 Nondisplaced Maisonneuve's fracture of right leg K, M, N, P, Q, R, B, C, B, C

● S82.865 Nondisplaced Maisonneuve's fracture of left leg K, M, N, P, Q, R, B, C, B, C

● S82.866 Nondisplaced Maisonneuve's fracture of unspecified leg K, M, N, P, Q, R, B, C, B, C

● S82.87 Pilon fracture of tibia (Ex) PDX 1264 [K, M, N, P, Q, R], 1857 [B, C]

● S82.871 Displaced pilon fracture of right tibia B, C, K, M, N, P, Q, R, B, C

● S82.872 Displaced pilon fracture of left tibia B, C, K, M, N, P, Q, R, B, C

● S82.873 Displaced pilon fracture of unspecified tibia B, C, K, M, N, P, Q, R, B, C

CHAPTER 19 (S00-T88)

S82.874 Nondisplaced pilon fracture of right tibia B, C, K, M, N, P, Q, R, B, C
S82.875 Nondisplaced pilon fracture of left tibia B, C, K, M, N, P, Q, R, B, C
S82.876 Nondisplaced pilon fracture of unspecified tibia B, C, K, M, N, P, Q, R, B, C
S82.89 Other fractures of lower leg (Ex) PDX 1264 [K, M, N, P, Q, R], 1857 [B, C]
Fracture of ankle NOS
S82.891 Other fracture of right lower leg B, C, K, M, N, P, Q, R, B, C
S82.892 Other fracture of left lower leg B, C, K, M, N, P, Q, R, B, C
S82.899 Other fracture of unspecified lower leg B, C, K, M, N, P, Q, R, B, C
S82.9 Unspecified fracture of lower leg (Ex) PDX 1264 [K, M, N, P, Q, R], 1858 [B, C]
X S82.90 Unspecified fracture of unspecified lower leg A, K, M, N, P, Q, R, B, C
X S82.91 Unspecified fracture of right lower leg A, K, M, N, P, Q, R, B, C
X S82.92 Unspecified fracture of left lower leg A, K, M, N, P, Q, R, B, C

S83 Dislocation and sprain of joints and ligaments of knee

Includes avulsion of joint or ligament of knee
laceration of cartilage, joint or ligament of knee
sprain of cartilage, joint or ligament of knee
traumatic hemarthrosis of joint or ligament of knee
traumatic rupture of joint or ligament of knee
traumatic subluxation of joint or ligament of knee
traumatic tear of joint or ligament of knee

Code also any associated open wound

Excludes2 derangement of patella (M22.0-M22.3)
injury of patellar ligament (tendon) (S76.1-)
internal derangement of knee (M23.-)
old dislocation of knee (M24.36)
pathological dislocation of knee (M24.36)
recurrent dislocation of knee (M22.0)
strain of muscle, fascia and tendon of lower leg (S86.-)

Coding Clinic: 2019, Q2, P26

The appropriate 7th character is to be added to each code from category S83

A	initial encounter
D	subsequent encounter
S	sequela

S83.0 Subluxation and dislocation of patella
S83.00 Unspecified subluxation and dislocation of patella
S83.001 Unspecified subluxation of right patella
S83.002 Unspecified subluxation of left patella
S83.003 Unspecified subluxation of unspecified patella
S83.004 Unspecified dislocation of right patella
S83.005 Unspecified dislocation of left patella
S83.006 Unspecified dislocation of unspecified patella
S83.01 Lateral subluxation and dislocation of patella
S83.011 Lateral subluxation of right patella
S83.012 Lateral subluxation of left patella
S83.013 Lateral subluxation of unspecified patella
S83.014 Lateral dislocation of right patella
S83.015 Lateral dislocation of left patella
S83.016 Lateral dislocation of unspecified patella
S83.09 Other subluxation and dislocation of patella
S83.091 Other subluxation of right patella
S83.092 Other subluxation of left patella
S83.093 Other subluxation of unspecified patella
S83.094 Other dislocation of right patella
S83.095 Other dislocation of left patella
S83.096 Other dislocation of unspecified patella
S83.1 Subluxation and dislocation of knee
Excludes2 instability of knee prosthesis (T84.022, T84.023)
S83.10 Unspecified subluxation and dislocation of knee
S83.101 Unspecified subluxation of right knee
S83.102 Unspecified subluxation of left knee
S83.103 Unspecified subluxation of unspecified knee
S83.104 Unspecified dislocation of right knee
S83.105 Unspecified dislocation of left knee
S83.106 Unspecified dislocation of unspecified knee
S83.11 Anterior subluxation and dislocation of proximal end of tibia
Posterior subluxation and dislocation of distal end of femur
S83.111 Anterior subluxation of proximal end of tibia, right knee
S83.112 Anterior subluxation of proximal end of tibia, left knee
S83.113 Anterior subluxation of proximal end of tibia, unspecified knee
S83.114 Anterior dislocation of proximal end of tibia, right knee
S83.115 Anterior dislocation of proximal end of tibia, left knee
S83.116 Anterior dislocation of proximal end of tibia, unspecified knee
S83.12 Posterior subluxation and dislocation of proximal end of tibia
Anterior dislocation of distal end of femur
S83.121 Posterior subluxation of proximal end of tibia, right knee
S83.122 Posterior subluxation of proximal end of tibia, left knee
S83.123 Posterior subluxation of proximal end of tibia, unspecified knee
S83.124 Posterior dislocation of proximal end of tibia, right knee
S83.125 Posterior dislocation of proximal end of tibia, left knee
S83.126 Posterior dislocation of proximal end of tibia, unspecified knee
S83.13 Medial subluxation and dislocation of proximal end of tibia
S83.131 Medial subluxation of proximal end of tibia, right knee
S83.132 Medial subluxation of proximal end of tibia, left knee
S83.133 Medial subluxation of proximal end of tibia, unspecified knee
S83.134 Medial dislocation of proximal end of tibia, right knee
S83.135 Medial dislocation of proximal end of tibia, left knee
S83.136 Medial dislocation of proximal end of tibia, unspecified knee

CHAPTER 19 (S00-T88)

- ● S83.14 Lateral subluxation and dislocation of proximal end of tibia
  - ● S83.141 Lateral subluxation of proximal end of tibia, right knee
  - ● S83.142 Lateral subluxation of proximal end of tibia, left knee
  - ● S83.143 Lateral subluxation of proximal end of tibia, unspecified knee
  - ● S83.144 Lateral dislocation of proximal end of tibia, right knee
  - ● S83.145 Lateral dislocation of proximal end of tibia, left knee
  - ● S83.146 Lateral dislocation of proximal end of tibia, unspecified knee
- ● S83.19 Other subluxation and dislocation of knee
  - ● S83.191 Other subluxation of right knee
  - ● S83.192 Other subluxation of left knee
  - ● S83.193 Other subluxation of unspecified knee
  - ● S83.194 Other dislocation of right knee
  - ● S83.195 Other dislocation of left knee
  - ● S83.196 Other dislocation of unspecified knee

● S83.2 Tear of meniscus, current injury

Excludes1 old bucket-handle tear (M23.2)

- ● S83.20 Tear of unspecified meniscus, current injury
  Tear of meniscus of knee NOS
  - ● S83.200 Bucket-handle tear of unspecified meniscus, current injury, right knee
  - ● S83.201 Bucket-handle tear of unspecified meniscus, current injury, left knee
  - ● S83.202 Bucket-handle tear of unspecified meniscus, current injury, unspecified knee
  - ● S83.203 Other tear of unspecified meniscus, current injury, right knee
  - ● S83.204 Other tear of unspecified meniscus, current injury, left knee
  - ● S83.205 Other tear of unspecified meniscus, current injury, unspecified knee
  - ● S83.206 Unspecified tear of unspecified meniscus, current injury, right knee
  - ● S83.207 Unspecified tear of unspecified meniscus, current injury, left knee
  - ● S83.209 Unspecified tear of unspecified meniscus, current injury, unspecified knee
- ● S83.21 Bucket-handle tear of medial meniscus, current injury
  - ● S83.211 Bucket-handle tear of medial meniscus, current injury, right knee
  - ● S83.212 Bucket-handle tear of medial meniscus, current injury, left knee
  - ● S83.219 Bucket-handle tear of medial meniscus, current injury, unspecified knee
- ● S83.22 Peripheral tear of medial meniscus, current injury
  - ● S83.221 Peripheral tear of medial meniscus, current injury, right knee
  - ● S83.222 Peripheral tear of medial meniscus, current injury, left knee
  - ● S83.229 Peripheral tear of medial meniscus, current injury, unspecified knee
- ● S83.23 Complex tear of medial meniscus, current injury
  - ● S83.231 Complex tear of medial meniscus, current injury, right knee
  - ● S83.232 Complex tear of medial meniscus, current injury, left knee
    Coding Clinic: 2019, Q2, P26
  - ● S83.239 Complex tear of medial meniscus, current injury, unspecified knee
- ● S83.24 Other tear of medial meniscus, current injury
  - ● S83.241 Other tear of medial meniscus, current injury, right knee
  - ● S83.242 Other tear of medial meniscus, current injury, left knee
  - ● S83.249 Other tear of medial meniscus, current injury, unspecified knee
- ● S83.25 Bucket-handle tear of lateral meniscus, current injury
  - ● S83.251 Bucket-handle tear of lateral meniscus, current injury, right knee
  - ● S83.252 Bucket-handle tear of lateral meniscus, current injury, left knee
  - ● S83.259 Bucket-handle tear of lateral meniscus, current injury, unspecified knee
- ● S83.26 Peripheral tear of lateral meniscus, current injury
  - ● S83.261 Peripheral tear of lateral meniscus, current injury, right knee
  - ● S83.262 Peripheral tear of lateral meniscus, current injury, left knee
  - ● S83.269 Peripheral tear of lateral meniscus, current injury, unspecified knee
- ● S83.27 Complex tear of lateral meniscus, current injury
  - ● S83.271 Complex tear of lateral meniscus, current injury, right knee
  - ● S83.272 Complex tear of lateral meniscus, current injury, left knee
  - ● S83.279 Complex tear of lateral meniscus, current injury, unspecified knee
- ● S83.28 Other tear of lateral meniscus, current injury
  - ● S83.281 Other tear of lateral meniscus, current injury, right knee
  - ● S83.282 Other tear of lateral meniscus, current injury, left knee
  - ● S83.289 Other tear of lateral meniscus, current injury, unspecified knee

● S83.3 Tear of articular cartilage of knee, current

- X● S83.30 Tear of articular cartilage of unspecified knee, current
- X● S83.31 Tear of articular cartilage of right knee, current
- X● S83.32 Tear of articular cartilage of left knee, current

● S83.4 Sprain of collateral ligament of knee

- ● S83.40 Sprain of unspecified collateral ligament of knee
  - ● S83.401 Sprain of unspecified collateral ligament of right knee
  - ● S83.402 Sprain of unspecified collateral ligament of left knee
  - ● S83.409 Sprain of unspecified collateral ligament of unspecified knee
- ● S83.41 Sprain of medial collateral ligament of knee
  Sprain of tibial collateral ligament
  - ● S83.411 Sprain of medial collateral ligament of right knee
  - ● S83.412 Sprain of medial collateral ligament of left knee
  - ● S83.419 Sprain of medial collateral ligament of unspecified knee
- ● S83.42 Sprain of lateral collateral ligament of knee
  Sprain of fibular collateral ligament
  - ● S83.421 Sprain of lateral collateral ligament of right knee
  - ● S83.422 Sprain of lateral collateral ligament of left knee
  - ● S83.429 Sprain of lateral collateral ligament of unspecified knee

S83.5 Sprain of cruciate ligament of knee
S83.50 Sprain of unspecified cruciate ligament of knee
S83.501 Sprain of unspecified cruciate ligament of right knee
S83.502 Sprain of unspecified cruciate ligament of left knee
S83.509 Sprain of unspecified cruciate ligament of unspecified knee
S83.51 Sprain of anterior cruciate ligament of knee
S83.511 Sprain of anterior cruciate ligament of right knee
Coding Clinic: 2016, Q2, P4
S83.512 Sprain of anterior cruciate ligament of left knee
S83.519 Sprain of anterior cruciate ligament of unspecified knee
S83.52 Sprain of posterior cruciate ligament of knee
S83.521 Sprain of posterior cruciate ligament of right knee
S83.522 Sprain of posterior cruciate ligament of left knee
S83.529 Sprain of posterior cruciate ligament of unspecified knee
S83.6 Sprain of the superior tibiofibular joint and ligament
X S83.60 Sprain of the superior tibiofibular joint and ligament, unspecified knee
X S83.61 Sprain of the superior tibiofibular joint and ligament, right knee
X S83.62 Sprain of the superior tibiofibular joint and ligament, left knee
S83.8 Sprain of other specified parts of knee
S83.8X Sprain of other specified parts of knee
S83.8X1 Sprain of other specified parts of right knee
S83.8X2 Sprain of other specified parts of left knee
S83.8X9 Sprain of other specified parts of unspecified knee
S83.9 Sprain of unspecified site of knee
X S83.90 Sprain of unspecified site of unspecified knee
X S83.91 Sprain of unspecified site of right knee
X S83.92 Sprain of unspecified site of left knee

S84 Injury of nerves at lower leg level
Code also any associated open wound (S81.-)
Excludes2 injury of nerves at ankle and foot level (S94.-)
The appropriate 7th character is to be added to each code from category S84

A initial encounter
D subsequent encounter
S sequela

S84.0 Injury of tibial nerve at lower leg level
X S84.00 Injury of tibial nerve at lower leg level, unspecified leg
X S84.01 Injury of tibial nerve at lower leg level, right leg
X S84.02 Injury of tibial nerve at lower leg level, left leg
S84.1 Injury of peroneal nerve at lower leg level
X S84.10 Injury of peroneal nerve at lower leg level, unspecified leg
X S84.11 Injury of peroneal nerve at lower leg level, right leg
X S84.12 Injury of peroneal nerve at lower leg level, left leg
S84.2 Injury of cutaneous sensory nerve at lower leg level
X S84.20 Injury of cutaneous sensory nerve at lower leg level, unspecified leg
X S84.21 Injury of cutaneous sensory nerve at lower leg level, right leg
X S84.22 Injury of cutaneous sensory nerve at lower leg level, left leg
S84.8 Injury of other nerves at lower leg level
S84.80 Injury of other nerves at lower leg level
S84.801 Injury of other nerves at lower leg level, right leg
S84.802 Injury of other nerves at lower leg level, left leg
S84.809 Injury of other nerves at lower leg level, unspecified leg
S84.9 Injury of unspecified nerve at lower leg level
X S84.90 Injury of unspecified nerve at lower leg level, unspecified leg
X S84.91 Injury of unspecified nerve at lower leg level, right leg
X S84.92 Injury of unspecified nerve at lower leg level, left leg

S85 Injury of blood vessels at lower leg level
Code also any associated open wound (S81.-)
Excludes2 injury of blood vessels at ankle and foot level (S95.-)
The appropriate 7th character is to be added to each code from category S85

A initial encounter
D subsequent encounter
S sequela

S85.0 Injury of popliteal artery
S85.00 Unspecified injury of popliteal artery
S85.001 Unspecified injury of popliteal artery, right leg A Ex PDX 1859
S85.002 Unspecified injury of popliteal artery, left leg A Ex PDX 1860
S85.009 Unspecified injury of popliteal artery, unspecified leg A Ex PDX 1861
S85.01 Laceration of popliteal artery
S85.011 Laceration of popliteal artery, right leg A Ex PDX 1859
S85.012 Laceration of popliteal artery, left leg A Ex PDX 1860
S85.019 Laceration of popliteal artery, unspecified leg A Ex PDX 1861
S85.09 Other specified injury of popliteal artery
S85.091 Other specified injury of popliteal artery, right leg A Ex PDX 1859
S85.092 Other specified injury of popliteal artery, left leg A Ex PDX 1860
S85.099 Other specified injury of popliteal artery, unspecified leg A Ex PDX 1861
S85.1 Injury of tibial artery
S85.10 Unspecified injury of unspecified tibial artery
Injury of tibial artery NOS
S85.101 Unspecified injury of unspecified tibial artery, right leg A Ex PDX 1862
S85.102 Unspecified injury of unspecified tibial artery, left leg A Ex PDX 1863
S85.109 Unspecified injury of unspecified tibial artery, unspecified leg A Ex PDX 1864
S85.11 Laceration of unspecified tibial artery
S85.111 Laceration of unspecified tibial artery, right leg A Ex PDX 1862
S85.112 Laceration of unspecified tibial artery, left leg A Ex PDX 1863
S85.119 Laceration of unspecified tibial artery, unspecified leg A Ex PDX 1864

CHAPTER 19 (S00-T88)

● S85.12 Other specified injury of unspecified tibial artery
● S85.121 Other specified injury of unspecified tibial artery, right leg A Ex: PDX 1862
● S85.122 Other specified injury of unspecified tibial artery, left leg A Ex: PDX 1863
● S85.129 Other specified injury of unspecified tibial artery, unspecified leg A Ex: PDX 1864
● S85.13 Unspecified injury of anterior tibial artery
● S85.131 Unspecified injury of anterior tibial artery, right leg A Ex: PDX 1865
● S85.132 Unspecified injury of anterior tibial artery, left leg A Ex: PDX 1866
● S85.139 Unspecified injury of anterior tibial artery, unspecified leg A Ex: PDX 1867
● S85.14 Laceration of anterior tibial artery
● S85.141 Laceration of anterior tibial artery, right leg A Ex: PDX 1865
● S85.142 Laceration of anterior tibial artery, left leg A Ex: PDX 1866
● S85.149 Laceration of anterior tibial artery, unspecified leg A Ex: PDX 1867
● S85.15 Other specified injury of anterior tibial artery
● S85.151 Other specified injury of anterior tibial artery, right leg A Ex: PDX 1865
● S85.152 Other specified injury of anterior tibial artery, left leg A Ex: PDX 1866
● S85.159 Other specified injury of anterior tibial artery, unspecified leg A Ex: PDX 1867
● S85.16 Unspecified injury of posterior tibial artery
● S85.161 Unspecified injury of posterior tibial artery, right leg A Ex: PDX 1868
● S85.162 Unspecified injury of posterior tibial artery, left leg A Ex: PDX 1869
● S85.169 Unspecified injury of posterior tibial artery, unspecified leg A Ex: PDX 1860
● S85.17 Laceration of posterior tibial artery
● S85.171 Laceration of posterior tibial artery, right leg A Ex: PDX 1868
● S85.172 Laceration of posterior tibial artery, left leg A Ex: PDX 1869
● S85.179 Laceration of posterior tibial artery, unspecified leg A Ex: PDX 1870
● S85.18 Other specified injury of posterior tibial artery
● S85.181 Other specified injury of posterior tibial artery, right leg A Ex: PDX 1868
● S85.182 Other specified injury of posterior tibial artery, left leg A Ex: PDX 1869
● S85.189 Other specified injury of posterior tibial artery, unspecified leg A Ex: PDX 1870
● S85.2 Injury of peroneal artery
● S85.20 Unspecified injury of peroneal artery
● S85.201 Unspecified injury of peroneal artery, right leg A Ex: PDX 1835
● S85.202 Unspecified injury of peroneal artery, left leg A Ex: PDX 1836
● S85.209 Unspecified injury of peroneal artery, unspecified leg A Ex: PDX 1837
● S85.21 Laceration of peroneal artery
● S85.211 Laceration of peroneal artery, right leg A Ex: PDX 1835
● S85.212 Laceration of peroneal artery, left leg A Ex: PDX 1836
● S85.219 Laceration of peroneal artery, unspecified leg A Ex: PDX 1837
● S85.29 Other specified injury of peroneal artery
● S85.291 Other specified injury of peroneal artery, right leg A Ex: PDX 1835
● S85.292 Other specified injury of peroneal artery, left leg A Ex: PDX 1836
● S85.299 Other specified injury of peroneal artery, unspecified leg A Ex: PDX 1837
● S85.3 Injury of greater saphenous vein at lower leg level
Injury of greater saphenous vein NOS
Injury of saphenous vein NOS
● S85.30 Unspecified injury of greater saphenous vein at lower leg level
● S85.301 Unspecified injury of greater saphenous vein at lower leg level, right leg A Ex: PDX 1832
● S85.302 Unspecified injury of greater saphenous vein at lower leg level, left leg A Ex: PDX 1833
● S85.309 Unspecified injury of greater saphenous vein at lower leg level, unspecified leg A Ex: PDX 1834
● S85.31 Laceration of greater saphenous vein at lower leg level
● S85.311 Laceration of greater saphenous vein at lower leg level, right leg A Ex: PDX 1832
● S85.312 Laceration of greater saphenous vein at lower leg level, left leg A Ex: PDX 1833
● S85.319 Laceration of greater saphenous vein at lower leg level, unspecified leg A Ex: PDX 1834
● S85.39 Other specified injury of greater saphenous vein at lower leg level
● S85.391 Other specified injury of greater saphenous vein at lower leg level, right leg A Ex: PDX 1832
● S85.392 Other specified injury of greater saphenous vein at lower leg level, left leg A Ex: PDX 1833
● S85.399 Other specified injury of greater saphenous vein at lower leg level, unspecified leg A Ex: PDX 1834
● S85.4 Injury of lesser saphenous vein at lower leg level
● S85.40 Unspecified injury of lesser saphenous vein at lower leg level
● S85.401 Unspecified injury of lesser saphenous vein at lower leg level, right leg A Ex: PDX 1832
● S85.402 Unspecified injury of lesser saphenous vein at lower leg level, left leg A Ex: PDX 1833
● S85.409 Unspecified injury of lesser saphenous vein at lower leg level, unspecified leg A Ex: PDX 1834
● S85.41 Laceration of lesser saphenous vein at lower leg level
● S85.411 Laceration of lesser saphenous vein at lower leg level, right leg A Ex: PDX 1832
● S85.412 Laceration of lesser saphenous vein at lower leg level, left leg A Ex: PDX 1833
● S85.419 Laceration of lesser saphenous vein at lower leg level, unspecified leg A Ex: PDX 1834
● S85.49 Other specified injury of lesser saphenous vein at lower leg level
● S85.491 Other specified injury of lesser saphenous vein at lower leg level, right leg A Ex: PDX 1832

S85.492 Other specified injury of lesser saphenous vein at lower leg level, left leg A (Ex) PDX 1833

S85.499 Other specified injury of lesser saphenous vein at lower leg level, unspecified leg A (Ex) PDX 1834

S85.5 Injury of popliteal vein

S85.50 Unspecified injury of popliteal vein

S85.501 Unspecified injury of popliteal vein, right leg A (Ex) PDX 1871

S85.502 Unspecified injury of popliteal vein, left leg A (Ex) PDX 1872

S85.509 Unspecified injury of popliteal vein, unspecified leg A (Ex) PDX 1873

S85.51 Laceration of popliteal vein

S85.511 Laceration of popliteal vein, right leg A (Ex) PDX 1871

S85.512 Laceration of popliteal vein, left leg A (Ex) PDX 1872

S85.519 Laceration of popliteal vein, unspecified leg A (Ex) PDX 1873

S85.59 Other specified injury of popliteal vein

S85.591 Other specified injury of popliteal vein, right leg A (Ex) PDX 1871

S85.592 Other specified injury of popliteal vein, left leg A (Ex) PDX 1872

S85.599 Other specified injury of popliteal vein, unspecified leg A (Ex) PDX 1873

S85.8 Injury of other blood vessels at lower leg level

S85.80 Unspecified injury of other blood vessels at lower leg level

S85.801 Unspecified injury of other blood vessels at lower leg level, right leg A (Ex) PDX 1835

S85.802 Unspecified injury of other blood vessels at lower leg level, left leg A (Ex) PDX 1836

S85.809 Unspecified injury of other blood vessels at lower leg level, unspecified leg A (Ex) PDX 1837

S85.81 Laceration of other blood vessels at lower leg level

S85.811 Laceration of other blood vessels at lower leg level, right leg A (Ex) PDX 1835

S85.812 Laceration of other blood vessels at lower leg level, left leg A (Ex) PDX 1836

S85.819 Laceration of other blood vessels at lower leg level, unspecified leg A (Ex) PDX 1837

S85.89 Other specified injury of other blood vessels at lower leg level

S85.891 Other specified injury of other blood vessels at lower leg level, right leg A (Ex) PDX 1835

S85.892 Other specified injury of other blood vessels at lower leg level, left leg A (Ex) PDX 1836

S85.899 Other specified injury of other blood vessels at lower leg level, unspecified leg A (Ex) PDX 1837

S85.9 Injury of unspecified blood vessel at lower leg level

S85.90 Unspecified injury of unspecified blood vessel at lower leg level

S85.901 Unspecified injury of unspecified blood vessel at lower leg level, right leg A (Ex) PDX 1835

S85.902 Unspecified injury of unspecified blood vessel at lower leg level, left leg A (Ex) PDX 1836

S85.909 Unspecified injury of unspecified blood vessel at lower leg level, unspecified leg A (Ex) PDX 1837

S85.91 Laceration of unspecified blood vessel at lower leg level

S85.911 Laceration of unspecified blood vessel at lower leg level, right leg A (Ex) PDX 1835

S85.912 Laceration of unspecified blood vessel at lower leg level, left leg A (Ex) PDX 1836

S85.919 Laceration of unspecified blood vessel at lower leg level, unspecified leg A (Ex) PDX 1837

S85.99 Other specified injury of unspecified blood vessel at lower leg level

S85.991 Other specified injury of unspecified blood vessel at lower leg level, right leg A (Ex) PDX 1835

S85.992 Other specified injury of unspecified blood vessel at lower leg level, left leg A (Ex) PDX 1836

S85.999 Other specified injury of unspecified blood vessel at lower leg level, unspecified leg A (Ex) PDX 1837

S86 Injury of muscle, fascia and tendon at lower leg level

Code also any associated open wound (S81.-)

Excludes2 injury of muscle, fascia and tendon at ankle (S96.-)
injury of patellar ligament (tendon) (S76.1-)
sprain of joints and ligaments of knee (S83.-)

The appropriate 7th character is to be added to each code from category S86

A	initial encounter
D	subsequent encounter
S	sequela

S86.0 Injury of Achilles tendon

S86.00 Unspecified injury of Achilles tendon

S86.001 Unspecified injury of right Achilles tendon

S86.002 Unspecified injury of left Achilles tendon

S86.009 Unspecified injury of unspecified Achilles tendon

S86.01 Strain of Achilles tendon

S86.011 Strain of right Achilles tendon

S86.012 Strain of left Achilles tendon

S86.019 Strain of unspecified Achilles tendon

S86.02 Laceration of Achilles tendon

S86.021 Laceration of right Achilles tendon A (Ex) PDX 1874

S86.022 Laceration of left Achilles tendon A (Ex) PDX 1875

S86.029 Laceration of unspecified Achilles tendon A (Ex) PDX 1876

S86.09 Other specified injury of Achilles tendon

S86.091 Other specified injury of right Achilles tendon

S86.092 Other specified injury of left Achilles tendon

S86.099 Other specified injury of unspecified Achilles tendon

S86.1 Injury of other muscle(s) and tendon(s) of posterior muscle group at lower leg level

S86.10 Unspecified injury of other muscle(s) and tendon(s) of posterior muscle group at lower leg level

S86.101 Unspecified injury of other muscle(s) and tendon(s) of posterior muscle group at lower leg level, right leg

CHAPTER 19 (S00-T88)

- S86.102 Unspecified injury of other muscle(s) and tendon(s) of posterior muscle group at lower leg level, left leg
- S86.109 Unspecified injury of other muscle(s) and tendon(s) of posterior muscle group at lower leg level, unspecified leg
- S86.11 Strain of other muscle(s) and tendon(s) of posterior muscle group at lower leg level
  - S86.111 Strain of other muscle(s) and tendon(s) of posterior muscle group at lower leg level, right leg
  - S86.112 Strain of other muscle(s) and tendon(s) of posterior muscle group at lower leg level, left leg
  - S86.119 Strain of other muscle(s) and tendon(s) of posterior muscle group at lower leg level, unspecified leg
- S86.12 Laceration of other muscle(s) and tendon(s) of posterior muscle group at lower leg level
  - S86.121 Laceration of other muscle(s) and tendon(s) of posterior muscle group at lower leg level, right leg A (Ex:) PDX 1874
  - S86.122 Laceration of other muscle(s) and tendon(s) of posterior muscle group at lower leg level, left leg A (Ex:) PDX 1875
  - S86.129 Laceration of other muscle(s) and tendon(s) of posterior muscle group at lower leg level, unspecified leg A (Ex:) PDX 1876
- S86.19 Other injury of other muscle(s) and tendon(s) of posterior muscle group at lower leg level
  - S86.191 Other injury of other muscle(s) and tendon(s) of posterior muscle group at lower leg level, right leg
  - S86.192 Other injury of other muscle(s) and tendon(s) of posterior muscle group at lower leg level, left leg
  - S86.199 Other injury of other muscle(s) and tendon(s) of posterior muscle group at lower leg level, unspecified leg

S86.2 Injury of muscle(s) and tendon(s) of anterior muscle group at lower leg level

- S86.20 Unspecified injury of muscle(s) and tendon(s) of anterior muscle group at lower leg level
  - S86.201 Unspecified injury of muscle(s) and tendon(s) of anterior muscle group at lower leg level, right leg
  - S86.202 Unspecified injury of muscle(s) and tendon(s) of anterior muscle group at lower leg level, left leg
  - S86.209 Unspecified injury of muscle(s) and tendon(s) of anterior muscle group at lower leg level, unspecified leg
- S86.21 Strain of muscle(s) and tendon(s) of anterior muscle group at lower leg level
  - S86.211 Strain of muscle(s) and tendon(s) of anterior muscle group at lower leg level, right leg
  - S86.212 Strain of muscle(s) and tendon(s) of anterior muscle group at lower leg level, left leg
  - S86.219 Strain of muscle(s) and tendon(s) of anterior muscle group at lower leg level, unspecified leg
- S86.22 Laceration of muscle(s) and tendon(s) of anterior muscle group at lower leg level
  - S86.221 Laceration of muscle(s) and tendon(s) of anterior muscle group at lower leg level, right leg A (Ex:) PDX 1874
  - S86.222 Laceration of muscle(s) and tendon(s) of anterior muscle group at lower leg level, left leg A (Ex:) PDX 1875
  - S86.229 Laceration of muscle(s) and tendon(s) of anterior muscle group at lower leg level, unspecified leg A (Ex:) PDX 1876
- S86.29 Other injury of muscle(s) and tendon(s) of anterior muscle group at lower leg level
  - S86.291 Other injury of muscle(s) and tendon(s) of anterior muscle group at lower leg level, right leg
  - S86.292 Other injury of muscle(s) and tendon(s) of anterior muscle group at lower leg level, left leg
  - S86.299 Other injury of muscle(s) and tendon(s) of anterior muscle group at lower leg level, unspecified leg

S86.3 Injury of muscle(s) and tendon(s) of peroneal muscle group at lower leg level

- S86.30 Unspecified injury of muscle(s) and tendon(s) of peroneal muscle group at lower leg level
  - S86.301 Unspecified injury of muscle(s) and tendon(s) of peroneal muscle group at lower leg level, right leg
  - S86.302 Unspecified injury of muscle(s) and tendon(s) of peroneal muscle group at lower leg level, left leg
  - S86.309 Unspecified injury of muscle(s) and tendon(s) of peroneal muscle group at lower leg level, unspecified leg
- S86.31 Strain of muscle(s) and tendon(s) of peroneal muscle group at lower leg level
  - S86.311 Strain of muscle(s) and tendon(s) of peroneal muscle group at lower leg level, right leg
  - S86.312 Strain of muscle(s) and tendon(s) of peroneal muscle group at lower leg level, left leg
  - S86.319 Strain of muscle(s) and tendon(s) of peroneal muscle group at lower leg level, unspecified leg
- S86.32 Laceration of muscle(s) and tendon(s) of peroneal muscle group at lower leg level
  - S86.321 Laceration of muscle(s) and tendon(s) of peroneal muscle group at lower leg level, right leg A (Ex:) PDX 1874
  - S86.322 Laceration of muscle(s) and tendon(s) of peroneal muscle group at lower leg level, left leg A (Ex:) PDX 1875
  - S86.329 Laceration of muscle(s) and tendon(s) of peroneal muscle group at lower leg level, unspecified leg A (Ex:) PDX 1876
- S86.39 Other injury of muscle(s) and tendon(s) of peroneal muscle group at lower leg level
  - S86.391 Other injury of muscle(s) and tendon(s) of peroneal muscle group at lower leg level, right leg
  - S86.392 Other injury of muscle(s) and tendon(s) of peroneal muscle group at lower leg level, left leg
  - S86.399 Other injury of muscle(s) and tendon(s) of peroneal muscle group at lower leg level, unspecified leg

S86.8 Injury of other muscles and tendons at lower leg level

- S86.80 Unspecified injury of other muscles and tendons at lower leg level
  - S86.801 Unspecified injury of other muscle(s) and tendon(s) at lower leg level, right leg
  - S86.802 Unspecified injury of other muscle(s) and tendon(s) at lower leg level, left leg

S86.809 Unspecified injury of other muscle(s) and tendon(s) at lower leg level, unspecified leg

S86.81 Strain of other muscles and tendons at lower leg level

S86.811 Strain of other muscle(s) and tendon(s) at lower leg level, right leg

S86.812 Strain of other muscle(s) and tendon(s) at lower leg level, left leg

S86.819 Strain of other muscle(s) and tendon(s) at lower leg level, unspecified leg

S86.82 Laceration of other muscles and tendons at lower leg level

S86.821 Laceration of other muscle(s) and tendon(s) at lower leg level, right leg A (Ex) PDX 1874

S86.822 Laceration of other muscle(s) and tendon(s) at lower leg level, left leg A (Ex) PDX 1875

S86.829 Laceration of other muscle(s) and tendon(s) at lower leg level, unspecified leg A (Ex) PDX 1876

S86.89 Other injury of other muscles and tendons at lower leg level

S86.891 Other injury of other muscle(s) and tendon(s) at lower leg level, right leg

S86.892 Other injury of other muscle(s) and tendon(s) at lower leg level, left leg

S86.899 Other injury of other muscle(s) and tendon(s) at lower leg level, unspecified leg

S86.9 Injury of unspecified muscle and tendon at lower leg level

S86.90 Unspecified injury of unspecified muscle and tendon at lower leg level

S86.901 Unspecified injury of unspecified muscle(s) and tendon(s) at lower leg level, right leg

S86.902 Unspecified injury of unspecified muscle(s) and tendon(s) at lower leg level, left leg

S86.909 Unspecified injury of unspecified muscle(s) and tendon(s) at lower leg level, unspecified leg

S86.91 Strain of unspecified muscle and tendon at lower leg level

S86.911 Strain of unspecified muscle(s) and tendon(s) at lower leg level, right leg

S86.912 Strain of unspecified muscle(s) and tendon(s) at lower leg level, left leg

S86.919 Strain of unspecified muscle(s) and tendon(s) at lower leg level, unspecified leg

S86.92 Laceration of unspecified muscle and tendon at lower leg level

S86.921 Laceration of unspecified muscle(s) and tendon(s) at lower leg level, right leg A (Ex) PDX 1874

S86.922 Laceration of unspecified muscle(s) and tendon(s) at lower leg level, left leg A (Ex) PDX 1875

S86.929 Laceration of unspecified muscle(s) and tendon(s) at lower leg level, unspecified leg A (Ex) PDX 1876

S86.99 Other injury of unspecified muscle and tendon at lower leg level

S86.991 Other injury of unspecified muscle(s) and tendon(s) at lower leg level, right leg

S86.992 Other injury of unspecified muscle(s) and tendon(s) at lower leg level, left leg

S86.999 Other injury of unspecified muscle(s) and tendon(s) at lower leg level, unspecified leg

S87 Crushing injury of lower leg

Use additional code(s) for all associated injuries

Excludes2 crushing injury of ankle and foot (S97.-)

The appropriate 7th character is to be added to each code from category S87

A	initial encounter
D	subsequent encounter
S	sequela

S87.0 Crushing injury of knee

X S87.00 Crushing injury of unspecified knee

X S87.01 Crushing injury of right knee

X S87.02 Crushing injury of left knee

S87.8 Crushing injury of lower leg

X S87.80 Crushing injury of unspecified lower leg

X S87.81 Crushing injury of right lower leg

X S87.82 Crushing injury of left lower leg

S88 Traumatic amputation of lower leg

An amputation not identified as partial or complete should be coded to complete

Excludes1 traumatic amputation of ankle and foot (S98.-)

The appropriate 7th character is to be added to each code from category S88

A	initial encounter
D	subsequent encounter
S	sequela

S88.0 Traumatic amputation at knee level

S88.01 Complete traumatic amputation at knee level

S88.011 Complete traumatic amputation at knee level, right lower leg A, A, D, S (Ex) PDX 1843
Coding Clinic: 2023, Q1, P28-29

S88.012 Complete traumatic amputation at knee level, left lower leg A, A, D, S (Ex) PDX 1844
Coding Clinic: 2023, Q1, P28-29

S88.019 Complete traumatic amputation at knee level, unspecified lower leg A, A, D, S (Ex) PDX 1845

S88.02 Partial traumatic amputation at knee level

S88.021 Partial traumatic amputation at knee level, right lower leg A, A, D, S (Ex) PDX 1843

S88.022 Partial traumatic amputation at knee level, left lower leg A, A, D, S (Ex) PDX 1844

S88.029 Partial traumatic amputation at knee level, unspecified lower leg A, A, D, S (Ex) PDX 1845

S88.1 Traumatic amputation at level between knee and ankle

S88.11 Complete traumatic amputation at level between knee and ankle

S88.111 Complete traumatic amputation at level between knee and ankle, right lower leg A, A, D, S (Ex) PDX 1843

S88.112 Complete traumatic amputation at level between knee and ankle, left lower leg A, A, D, S (Ex) PDX 1844

S88.119 Complete traumatic amputation at level between knee and ankle, unspecified lower leg A, A, D, S (Ex) PDX 1845

CHAPTER 19 (S00-T88)

- S88.12 Partial traumatic amputation at level between knee and ankle
  - S88.121 Partial traumatic amputation at level between knee and ankle, right lower leg A, A, D, S (Ex:) PDX 1843
  - S88.122 Partial traumatic amputation at level between knee and ankle, left lower leg A, A, D, S (Ex:) PDX 1844
  - S88.129 Partial traumatic amputation at level between knee and ankle, unspecified lower leg A, A, D, S (Ex:) PDX 1845
- S88.9 Traumatic amputation of lower leg, level unspecified
  - S88.91 Complete traumatic amputation of lower leg, level unspecified
    - S88.911 Complete traumatic amputation of right lower leg, level unspecified A, A, D, S (Ex:) PDX 1843
    - S88.912 Complete traumatic amputation of left lower leg, level unspecified A, A, D, S (Ex:) PDX 1844
    - S88.919 Complete traumatic amputation of unspecified lower leg, level unspecified A, A, D, S (Ex:) PDX 1845
  - S88.92 Partial traumatic amputation of lower leg, level unspecified
    - S88.921 Partial traumatic amputation of right lower leg, level unspecified A, A, D, S (Ex:) PDX 1843
    - S88.922 Partial traumatic amputation of left lower leg, level unspecified A, A, D, S (Ex:) PDX 1844
    - S88.929 Partial traumatic amputation of unspecified lower leg, level unspecified A, A, D, S (Ex:) PDX 1845

S89 Other and unspecified injuries of lower leg

Note: A fracture not indicated as open or closed should be coded to closed

Excludes2 other and unspecified injuries of ankle and foot (S99.-)

The appropriate 7th character is to be added to each code from subcategories S89.0, S89.1, S89.2, and S89.3

A	initial encounter for closed fracture
D	subsequent encounter for fracture with routine healing
G	subsequent encounter for fracture with delayed healing
K	subsequent encounter for fracture with nonunion
P	subsequent encounter for fracture with malunion
S	sequela

- S89.0 Physeal fracture of upper end of tibia
  - S89.00 Unspecified physeal fracture of upper end of tibia
    - S89.001 Unspecified physeal fracture of upper end of right tibia A, K, P, A (Ex:) PDX 1264 [K, P], 1850 [A]
    - S89.002 Unspecified physeal fracture of upper end of left tibia A, K, P, A (Ex:) PDX 1264 [K, P], 1852 [A]
    - S89.009 Unspecified physeal fracture of upper end of unspecified tibia A, K, P, A (Ex:) PDX 1264 [K, P], 1851 [A]
  - S89.01 Salter-Harris Type I physeal fracture of upper end of tibia
    - S89.011 Salter-Harris Type I physeal fracture of upper end of right tibia A, K, P, A (Ex:) PDX 1264 [K, P], 1850 [A]
    - S89.012 Salter-Harris Type I physeal fracture of upper end of left tibia A, K, P, A (Ex:) PDX 1264 [K, P], 1852 [A]
    - S89.019 Salter-Harris Type I physeal fracture of upper end of unspecified tibia A, K, P, A (Ex:) PDX 1264 [K, P], 1851 [A]
  - S89.02 Salter-Harris Type II physeal fracture of upper end of tibia
    - S89.021 Salter-Harris Type II physeal fracture of upper end of right tibia A, K, P, A (Ex:) PDX 1264 [K, P], 1850 [A]
    - S89.022 Salter-Harris Type II physeal fracture of upper end of left tibia A, K, P, A (Ex:) PDX 1264 [K, P], 1852 [A]
    - S89.029 Salter-Harris Type II physeal fracture of upper end of unspecified tibia A, K, P, A (Ex:) PDX 1264 [K, P], 1851 [A]
  - S89.03 Salter-Harris Type III physeal fracture of upper end of tibia
    - S89.031 Salter-Harris Type III physeal fracture of upper end of right tibia A, K, P, A (Ex:) PDX 1264 [K, P], 1850 [A]
    - S89.032 Salter-Harris Type III physeal fracture of upper end of left tibia A, K, P, A (Ex:) PDX 1264 [K, P], 1852 [A]
    - S89.039 Salter-Harris Type III physeal fracture of upper end of unspecified tibia A, K, P, A (Ex:) PDX 1264 [K, P], 1851 [A]
  - S89.04 Salter-Harris Type IV physeal fracture of upper end of tibia
    - S89.041 Salter-Harris Type IV physeal fracture of upper end of right tibia A, K, P, A (Ex:) PDX 1264 [K, P], 1850 [A]
    - S89.042 Salter-Harris Type IV physeal fracture of upper end of left tibia A, K, P, A (Ex:) PDX 1264 [K, P], 1852 [A]
    - S89.049 Salter-Harris Type IV physeal fracture of upper end of unspecified tibia A, K, P, A (Ex:) PDX 1264 [K, P], 1851 [A]
  - S89.09 Other physeal fracture of upper end of tibia
    - S89.091 Other physeal fracture of upper end of right tibia A, K, P, A (Ex:) PDX 1264 [K, P], 1850 [A]
    - S89.092 Other physeal fracture of upper end of left tibia A, K, P, A (Ex:) PDX 1264 [K, P], 1852 [A]
    - S89.099 Other physeal fracture of upper end of unspecified tibia A, K, P, A (Ex:) PDX 1264 [K, P], 1851 [A]
- S89.1 Physeal fracture of lower end of tibia (Ex:) PDX 1264
  - S89.10 Unspecified physeal fracture of lower end of tibia
    - S89.101 Unspecified physeal fracture of lower end of right tibia K, P
    - S89.102 Unspecified physeal fracture of lower end of left tibia K, P
    - S89.109 Unspecified physeal fracture of lower end of unspecified tibia K, P
  - S89.11 Salter-Harris Type I physeal fracture of lower end of tibia
    - S89.111 Salter-Harris Type I physeal fracture of lower end of right tibia K, P
    - S89.112 Salter-Harris Type I physeal fracture of lower end of left tibia K, P
    - S89.119 Salter-Harris Type I physeal fracture of lower end of unspecified tibia K, P
  - S89.12 Salter-Harris Type II physeal fracture of lower end of tibia
    - S89.121 Salter-Harris Type II physeal fracture of lower end of right tibia K, P
    - S89.122 Salter-Harris Type II physeal fracture of lower end of left tibia K, P
    - S89.129 Salter-Harris Type II physeal fracture of lower end of unspecified tibia K, P

CHAPTER 19 (SØØ-T88)

- S89.13 **Salter-Harris Type III physeal fracture of lower end of tibia**
  - **Excludes1** fracture of medial malleolus (adult) (S82.5-)
  - S89.131 Salter-Harris Type III physeal fracture of lower end of right tibia K, P
  - S89.132 Salter-Harris Type III physeal fracture of lower end of left tibia K, P
  - S89.139 Salter-Harris Type III physeal fracture of lower end of unspecified tibia K, P
- S89.14 **Salter-Harris Type IV physeal fracture of lower end of tibia**
  - **Excludes1** fracture of medial malleolus (adult) (S82.5-)
  - S89.141 Salter-Harris Type IV physeal fracture of lower end of right tibia K, P
  - S89.142 Salter-Harris Type IV physeal fracture of lower end of left tibia K, P
  - S89.149 Salter-Harris Type IV physeal fracture of lower end of unspecified tibia K, P
- S89.19 **Other physeal fracture of lower end of tibia**
  - S89.191 Other physeal fracture of lower end of right tibia K, P
  - S89.192 Other physeal fracture of lower end of left tibia K, P
  - S89.199 Other physeal fracture of lower end of unspecified tibia K, P

S89.2 Physeal fracture of upper end of fibula (Ex) PDX 1264

- S89.20 **Unspecified physeal fracture of upper end of fibula**
  - S89.201 Unspecified physeal fracture of upper end of right fibula K, P
  - S89.202 Unspecified physeal fracture of upper end of left fibula K, P
  - S89.209 Unspecified physeal fracture of upper end of unspecified fibula K, P
- S89.21 **Salter-Harris Type I physeal fracture of upper end of fibula**
  - S89.211 Salter-Harris Type I physeal fracture of upper end of right fibula K, P
  - S89.212 Salter-Harris Type I physeal fracture of upper end of left fibula K, P
  - S89.219 Salter-Harris Type I physeal fracture of upper end of unspecified fibula K, P
- S89.22 **Salter-Harris Type II physeal fracture of upper end of fibula**
  - S89.221 Salter-Harris Type II physeal fracture of upper end of right fibula K, P
  - S89.222 Salter-Harris Type II physeal fracture of upper end of left fibula K, P
  - S89.229 Salter-Harris Type II physeal fracture of upper end of unspecified fibula K, P
- S89.29 **Other physeal fracture of upper end of fibula**
  - S89.291 Other physeal fracture of upper end of right fibula K, P
  - S89.292 Other physeal fracture of upper end of left fibula K, P
  - S89.299 Other physeal fracture of upper end of unspecified fibula K, P

S89.3 Physeal fracture of lower end of fibula (Ex) PDX 1264

- S89.30 **Unspecified physeal fracture of lower end of fibula**
  - S89.301 Unspecified physeal fracture of lower end of right fibula K, P
  - S89.302 Unspecified physeal fracture of lower end of left fibula K, P
  - S89.309 Unspecified physeal fracture of lower end of unspecified fibula K, P
- S89.31 **Salter-Harris Type I physeal fracture of lower end of fibula**
  - S89.311 Salter-Harris Type I physeal fracture of lower end of right fibula K, P
  - S89.312 Salter-Harris Type I physeal fracture of lower end of left fibula K, P
  - S89.319 Salter-Harris Type I physeal fracture of lower end of unspecified fibula K, P
- S89.32 **Salter-Harris Type II physeal fracture of lower end of fibula**
  - S89.321 Salter-Harris Type II physeal fracture of lower end of right fibula K, P
  - S89.322 Salter-Harris Type II physeal fracture of lower end of left fibula K, P
  - S89.329 Salter-Harris Type II physeal fracture of lower end of unspecified fibula K, P
- S89.39 **Other physeal fracture of lower end of fibula**
  - S89.391 Other physeal fracture of lower end of right fibula K, P
  - S89.392 Other physeal fracture of lower end of left fibula K, P
  - S89.399 Other physeal fracture of lower end of unspecified fibula K, P

S89.8 Other specified injuries of lower leg

The appropriate 7th character is to be added to each code in subcategory S89.8

- A initial encounter
- D subsequent encounter
- S sequela

- X S89.80 Other specified injuries of unspecified lower leg
- X S89.81 Other specified injuries of right lower leg
- X S89.82 Other specified injuries of left lower leg

S89.9 Unspecified injury of lower leg

The appropriate 7th character is to be added to each code in subcategory S89.9

- A initial encounter
- D subsequent encounter
- S sequela

- X S89.90 Unspecified injury of unspecified lower leg
- X S89.91 Unspecified injury of right lower leg
- X S89.92 Unspecified injury of left lower leg

INJURIES TO THE ANKLE AND FOOT (S90-S99)

Excludes2 burns and corrosions (T20-T32)
fracture of ankle and malleolus (S82.-)
frostbite (T33-T34)
insect bite or sting, venomous (T63.4)

S90 Superficial injury of ankle, foot and toes

The appropriate 7th character is to be added to each code from category S90

- A initial encounter
- D subsequent encounter
- S sequela

S90.0 Contusion of ankle

- X S90.00 Contusion of unspecified ankle
- X S90.01 Contusion of right ankle
- X S90.02 Contusion of left ankle

- S90.1 Contusion of toe without damage to nail
  - S90.11 Contusion of great toe without damage to nail
    - S90.111 Contusion of right great toe without damage to nail
    - S90.112 Contusion of left great toe without damage to nail
    - S90.119 Contusion of unspecified great toe without damage to nail
  - S90.12 Contusion of lesser toe without damage to nail
    - S90.121 Contusion of right lesser toe(s) without damage to nail
    - S90.122 Contusion of left lesser toe(s) without damage to nail
    - S90.129 Contusion of unspecified lesser toe(s) without damage to nail
      Contusion of toe NOS
- S90.2 Contusion of toe with damage to nail
  - S90.21 Contusion of great toe with damage to nail
    - S90.211 Contusion of right great toe with damage to nail
    - S90.212 Contusion of left great toe with damage to nail
    - S90.219 Contusion of unspecified great toe with damage to nail
  - S90.22 Contusion of lesser toe with damage to nail
    - S90.221 Contusion of right lesser toe(s) with damage to nail
    - S90.222 Contusion of left lesser toe(s) with damage to nail
    - S90.229 Contusion of unspecified lesser toe(s) with damage to nail
- S90.3 Contusion of foot
  Excludes2 contusion of toes (S90.1-, S90.2-)
  - X S90.30 Contusion of unspecified foot
    Contusion of foot NOS
  - X S90.31 Contusion of right foot
  - X S90.32 Contusion of left foot
- S90.4 Other superficial injuries of toe
  - S90.41 Abrasion of toe
    - S90.411 Abrasion, right great toe
    - S90.412 Abrasion, left great toe
    - S90.413 Abrasion, unspecified great toe
    - S90.414 Abrasion, right lesser toe(s)
    - S90.415 Abrasion, left lesser toe(s)
    - S90.416 Abrasion, unspecified lesser toe(s)
  - S90.42 Blister (nonthermal) of toe
    - S90.421 Blister (nonthermal), right great toe
    - S90.422 Blister (nonthermal), left great toe
    - S90.423 Blister (nonthermal), unspecified great toe
    - S90.424 Blister (nonthermal), right lesser toe(s)
    - S90.425 Blister (nonthermal), left lesser toe(s)
    - S90.426 Blister (nonthermal), unspecified lesser toe(s)
  - S90.44 External constriction of toe
    Hair tourniquet syndrome of toe
    - S90.441 External constriction, right great toe
    - S90.442 External constriction, left great toe
    - S90.443 External constriction, unspecified great toe
    - S90.444 External constriction, right lesser toe(s)
    - S90.445 External constriction, left lesser toe(s)
    - S90.446 External constriction, unspecified lesser toe(s)
  - S90.45 Superficial foreign body of toe
    Splinter in the toe
    - S90.451 Superficial foreign body, right great toe
    - S90.452 Superficial foreign body, left great toe
    - S90.453 Superficial foreign body, unspecified great toe
    - S90.454 Superficial foreign body, right lesser toe(s)
    - S90.455 Superficial foreign body, left lesser toe(s)
    - S90.456 Superficial foreign body, unspecified lesser toe(s)
  - S90.46 Insect bite (nonvenomous) of toe
    - S90.461 Insect bite (nonvenomous), right great toe
    - S90.462 Insect bite (nonvenomous), left great toe
    - S90.463 Insect bite (nonvenomous), unspecified great toe
    - S90.464 Insect bite (nonvenomous), right lesser toe(s)
    - S90.465 Insect bite (nonvenomous), left lesser toe(s)
    - S90.466 Insect bite (nonvenomous), unspecified lesser toe(s)
  - S90.47 Other superficial bite of toe
    Excludes1 open bite of toe (S91.15-, S91.25-)
    - S90.471 Other superficial bite of right great toe
    - S90.472 Other superficial bite of left great toe
    - S90.473 Other superficial bite of unspecified great toe
    - S90.474 Other superficial bite of right lesser toe(s)
    - S90.475 Other superficial bite of left lesser toe(s)
    - S90.476 Other superficial bite of unspecified lesser toe(s)
- S90.5 Other superficial injuries of ankle
  - S90.51 Abrasion of ankle
    - S90.511 Abrasion, right ankle
    - S90.512 Abrasion, left ankle
    - S90.519 Abrasion, unspecified ankle
  - S90.52 Blister (nonthermal) of ankle
    - S90.521 Blister (nonthermal), right ankle
    - S90.522 Blister (nonthermal), left ankle
    - S90.529 Blister (nonthermal), unspecified ankle
  - S90.54 External constriction of ankle
    - S90.541 External constriction, right ankle
    - S90.542 External constriction, left ankle
    - S90.549 External constriction, unspecified ankle
  - S90.55 Superficial foreign body of ankle
    Splinter in the ankle
    - S90.551 Superficial foreign body, right ankle
    - S90.552 Superficial foreign body, left ankle
    - S90.559 Superficial foreign body, unspecified ankle
  - S90.56 Insect bite (nonvenomous) of ankle
    - S90.561 Insect bite (nonvenomous), right ankle
    - S90.562 Insect bite (nonvenomous), left ankle
    - S90.569 Insect bite (nonvenomous), unspecified ankle

- **S90.57 Other superficial bite of ankle**
  - **Excludes1** open bite of ankle (S91.05-)
  - **S90.571 Other superficial bite of ankle, right ankle**
  - **S90.572 Other superficial bite of ankle, left ankle**
  - **S90.579 Other superficial bite of ankle, unspecified ankle**
- **S90.8 Other superficial injuries of foot**
  - **S90.81 Abrasion of foot**
    - **S90.811 Abrasion, right foot**
    - **S90.812 Abrasion, left foot**
    - **S90.819 Abrasion, unspecified foot**
  - **S90.82 Blister (nonthermal) of foot**
    - **S90.821 Blister (nonthermal), right foot**
    - **S90.822 Blister (nonthermal), left foot**
    - **S90.829 Blister (nonthermal), unspecified foot**
  - **S90.84 External constriction of foot**
    - **S90.841 External constriction, right foot**
    - **S90.842 External constriction, left foot**
    - **S90.849 External constriction, unspecified foot**
  - **S90.85 Superficial foreign body of foot**
    - Splinter in the foot
    - **S90.851 Superficial foreign body, right foot**
    - **S90.852 Superficial foreign body, left foot**
    - **S90.859 Superficial foreign body, unspecified foot**
  - **S90.86 Insect bite (nonvenomous) of foot**
    - **S90.861 Insect bite (nonvenomous), right foot**
    - **S90.862 Insect bite (nonvenomous), left foot**
    - **S90.869 Insect bite (nonvenomous), unspecified foot**
  - **S90.87 Other superficial bite of foot**
    - **Excludes1** open bite of foot (S91.35-)
    - **S90.871 Other superficial bite of right foot**
    - **S90.872 Other superficial bite of left foot**
    - **S90.879 Other superficial bite of unspecified foot**
- **S90.9 Unspecified superficial injury of ankle, foot and toe**
  - **S90.91 Unspecified superficial injury of ankle**
    - **S90.911 Unspecified superficial injury of right ankle**
    - **S90.912 Unspecified superficial injury of left ankle**
    - **S90.919 Unspecified superficial injury of unspecified ankle**
  - **S90.92 Unspecified superficial injury of foot**
    - **S90.921 Unspecified superficial injury of right foot**
    - **S90.922 Unspecified superficial injury of left foot**
    - **S90.929 Unspecified superficial injury of unspecified foot**
  - **S90.93 Unspecified superficial injury of toes**
    - **S90.931 Unspecified superficial injury of right great toe**
    - **S90.932 Unspecified superficial injury of left great toe**
    - **S90.933 Unspecified superficial injury of unspecified great toe**
    - **S90.934 Unspecified superficial injury of right lesser toe(s)**
    - **S90.935 Unspecified superficial injury of left lesser toe(s)**
    - **S90.936 Unspecified superficial injury of unspecified lesser toe(s)**

S91 Open wound of ankle, foot and toes

Code also any associated wound infection

Excludes1 open fracture of ankle, foot and toes (S92.-with 7th character B)
traumatic amputation of ankle and foot (S98.-)

The appropriate 7th character is to be added to each code from category S91

A	initial encounter
D	subsequent encounter
S	sequela

- **S91.0 Open wound of ankle**
  - **S91.00 Unspecified open wound of ankle**
    - **S91.001 Unspecified open wound, right ankle**
    - **S91.002 Unspecified open wound, left ankle**
    - **S91.009 Unspecified open wound, unspecified ankle**
  - **S91.01 Laceration without foreign body of ankle**
    - **S91.011 Laceration without foreign body, right ankle**
    - **S91.012 Laceration without foreign body, left ankle**
      - **Coding Clinic: 2021, Q1, P8**
    - **S91.019 Laceration without foreign body, unspecified ankle**
  - **S91.02 Laceration with foreign body of ankle**
    - **S91.021 Laceration with foreign body, right ankle**
    - **S91.022 Laceration with foreign body, left ankle**
    - **S91.029 Laceration with foreign body, unspecified ankle**
  - **S91.03 Puncture wound without foreign body of ankle**
    - **S91.031 Puncture wound without foreign body, right ankle**
    - **S91.032 Puncture wound without foreign body, left ankle**
    - **S91.039 Puncture wound without foreign body, unspecified ankle**
  - **S91.04 Puncture wound with foreign body of ankle**
    - **S91.041 Puncture wound with foreign body, right ankle**
    - **S91.042 Puncture wound with foreign body, left ankle**
    - **S91.049 Puncture wound with foreign body, unspecified ankle**
  - **S91.05 Open bite of ankle**
    - **Excludes1** superficial bite of ankle (S90.56-, S90.57-)
    - **S91.051 Open bite, right ankle**
    - **S91.052 Open bite, left ankle**
    - **S91.059 Open bite, unspecified ankle**
- **S91.1 Open wound of toe without damage to nail**
  - **S91.10 Unspecified open wound of toe without damage to nail**
    - **S91.101 Unspecified open wound of right great toe without damage to nail**
    - **S91.102 Unspecified open wound of left great toe without damage to nail**
    - **S91.103 Unspecified open wound of unspecified great toe without damage to nail**
    - **S91.104 Unspecified open wound of right lesser toe(s) without damage to nail**
    - **S91.105 Unspecified open wound of left lesser toe(s) without damage to nail**

CHAPTER 19 (S00-T88)

- S91.106 Unspecified open wound of unspecified lesser toe(s) without damage to nail
- S91.109 Unspecified open wound of unspecified toe(s) without damage to nail

S91.11 Laceration without foreign body of toe without damage to nail

- S91.111 Laceration without foreign body of right great toe without damage to nail
- S91.112 Laceration without foreign body of left great toe without damage to nail
- S91.113 Laceration without foreign body of unspecified great toe without damage to nail
- S91.114 Laceration without foreign body of right lesser toe(s) without damage to nail
- S91.115 Laceration without foreign body of left lesser toe(s) without damage to nail
- S91.116 Laceration without foreign body of unspecified lesser toe(s) without damage to nail
- S91.119 Laceration without foreign body of unspecified toe without damage to nail

S91.12 Laceration with foreign body of toe without damage to nail

- S91.121 Laceration with foreign body of right great toe without damage to nail
- S91.122 Laceration with foreign body of left great toe without damage to nail
- S91.123 Laceration with foreign body of unspecified great toe without damage to nail
- S91.124 Laceration with foreign body of right lesser toe(s) without damage to nail
- S91.125 Laceration with foreign body of left lesser toe(s) without damage to nail
- S91.126 Laceration with foreign body of unspecified lesser toe(s) without damage to nail
- S91.129 Laceration with foreign body of unspecified toe(s) without damage to nail

S91.13 Puncture wound without foreign body of toe without damage to nail

- S91.131 Puncture wound without foreign body of right great toe without damage to nail
- S91.132 Puncture wound without foreign body of left great toe without damage to nail
- S91.133 Puncture wound without foreign body of unspecified great toe without damage to nail
- S91.134 Puncture wound without foreign body of right lesser toe(s) without damage to nail
- S91.135 Puncture wound without foreign body of left lesser toe(s) without damage to nail
- S91.136 Puncture wound without foreign body of unspecified lesser toe(s) without damage to nail
- S91.139 Puncture wound without foreign body of unspecified toe(s) without damage to nail

S91.14 Puncture wound with foreign body of toe without damage to nail

- S91.141 Puncture wound with foreign body of right great toe without damage to nail
- S91.142 Puncture wound with foreign body of left great toe without damage to nail
- S91.143 Puncture wound with foreign body of unspecified great toe without damage to nail
- S91.144 Puncture wound with foreign body of right lesser toe(s) without damage to nail
- S91.145 Puncture wound with foreign body of left lesser toe(s) without damage to nail
- S91.146 Puncture wound with foreign body of unspecified lesser toe(s) without damage to nail
- S91.149 Puncture wound with foreign body of unspecified toe(s) without damage to nail

S91.15 Open bite of toe without damage to nail

Bite of toe NOS

Excludes1 superficial bite of toe (S90.46-, S90.47-)

- S91.151 Open bite of right great toe without damage to nail
- S91.152 Open bite of left great toe without damage to nail
- S91.153 Open bite of unspecified great toe without damage to nail
- S91.154 Open bite of right lesser toe(s) without damage to nail
- S91.155 Open bite of left lesser toe(s) without damage to nail
- S91.156 Open bite of unspecified lesser toe(s) without damage to nail
- S91.159 Open bite of unspecified toe(s) without damage to nail

S91.2 Open wound of toe with damage to nail

S91.20 Unspecified open wound of toe with damage to nail

- S91.201 Unspecified open wound of right great toe with damage to nail
- S91.202 Unspecified open wound of left great toe with damage to nail
- S91.203 Unspecified open wound of unspecified great toe with damage to nail
- S91.204 Unspecified open wound of right lesser toe(s) with damage to nail
- S91.205 Unspecified open wound of left lesser toe(s) with damage to nail
- S91.206 Unspecified open wound of unspecified lesser toe(s) with damage to nail
- S91.209 Unspecified open wound of unspecified toe(s) with damage to nail

S91.21 Laceration without foreign body of toe with damage to nail

- S91.211 Laceration without foreign body of right great toe with damage to nail
- S91.212 Laceration without foreign body of left great toe with damage to nail
- S91.213 Laceration without foreign body of unspecified great toe with damage to nail
- S91.214 Laceration without foreign body of right lesser toe(s) with damage to nail
- S91.215 Laceration without foreign body of left lesser toe(s) with damage to nail
- S91.216 Laceration without foreign body of unspecified lesser toe(s) with damage to nail
- S91.219 Laceration without foreign body of unspecified toe(s) with damage to nail

CHAPTER 19 (S00-T88)

● S91.22 Laceration with foreign body of toe with damage to nail
- ● S91.221 Laceration with foreign body of right great toe with damage to nail
- ● S91.222 Laceration with foreign body of left great toe with damage to nail
- ● S91.223 Laceration with foreign body of unspecified great toe with damage to nail
- ● S91.224 Laceration with foreign body of right lesser toe(s) with damage to nail
- ● S91.225 Laceration with foreign body of left lesser toe(s) with damage to nail
- ● S91.226 Laceration with foreign body of unspecified lesser toe(s) with damage to nail
- ● S91.229 Laceration with foreign body of unspecified toe(s) with damage to nail

● S91.23 Puncture wound without foreign body of toe with damage to nail
- ● S91.231 Puncture wound without foreign body of right great toe with damage to nail
- ● S91.232 Puncture wound without foreign body of left great toe with damage to nail
- ● S91.233 Puncture wound without foreign body of unspecified great toe with damage to nail
- ● S91.234 Puncture wound without foreign body of right lesser toe(s) with damage to nail
- ● S91.235 Puncture wound without foreign body of left lesser toe(s) with damage to nail
- ● S91.236 Puncture wound without foreign body of unspecified lesser toe(s) with damage to nail
- ● S91.239 Puncture wound without foreign body of unspecified toe(s) with damage to nail

● S91.24 Puncture wound with foreign body of toe with damage to nail
- ● S91.241 Puncture wound with foreign body of right great toe with damage to nail
- ● S91.242 Puncture wound with foreign body of left great toe with damage to nail
- ● S91.243 Puncture wound with foreign body of unspecified great toe with damage to nail
- ● S91.244 Puncture wound with foreign body of right lesser toe(s) with damage to nail
- ● S91.245 Puncture wound with foreign body of left lesser toe(s) with damage to nail
- ● S91.246 Puncture wound with foreign body of unspecified lesser toe(s) with damage to nail
- ● S91.249 Puncture wound with foreign body of unspecified toe(s) with damage to nail

● S91.25 Open bite of toe with damage to nail

Bite of toe with damage to nail NOS

Excludes1 superficial bite of toe (S90.46-, S90.47-)

- ● S91.251 Open bite of right great toe with damage to nail
- ● S91.252 Open bite of left great toe with damage to nail
- ● S91.253 Open bite of unspecified great toe with damage to nail
- ● S91.254 Open bite of right lesser toe(s) with damage to nail
- ● S91.255 Open bite of left lesser toe(s) with damage to nail
- ● S91.256 Open bite of unspecified lesser toe(s) with damage to nail
- ● S91.259 Open bite of unspecified toe(s) with damage to nail

● S91.3 Open wound of foot

● S91.30 Unspecified open wound of foot
- ● S91.301 Unspecified open wound, right foot
- ● S91.302 Unspecified open wound, left foot
- ● S91.309 Unspecified open wound, unspecified foot

● S91.31 Laceration without foreign body of foot
- ● S91.311 Laceration without foreign body, right foot
- ● S91.312 Laceration without foreign body, left foot
- ● S91.319 Laceration without foreign body, unspecified foot

● S91.32 Laceration with foreign body of foot
- ● S91.321 Laceration with foreign body, right foot
- ● S91.322 Laceration with foreign body, left foot
- ● S91.329 Laceration with foreign body, unspecified foot

● S91.33 Puncture wound without foreign body of foot
- ● S91.331 Puncture wound without foreign body, right foot
- ● S91.332 Puncture wound without foreign body, left foot
- ● S91.339 Puncture wound without foreign body, unspecified foot

● S91.34 Puncture wound with foreign body of foot
- ● S91.341 Puncture wound with foreign body, right foot
- ● S91.342 Puncture wound with foreign body, left foot
- ● S91.349 Puncture wound with foreign body, unspecified foot

● S91.35 Open bite of foot

Excludes1 superficial bite of foot (S90.86-, S90.87-)

- ● S91.351 Open bite, right foot
- ● S91.352 Open bite, left foot
- ● S91.359 Open bite, unspecified foot

● S92 Fracture of foot and toe, except ankle

Note: A fracture not indicated as displaced or nondisplaced should be coded to displaced

A fracture not indicated as open or closed should be coded to closed

Excludes2 fracture of ankle (S82.-)
fracture of malleolus (S82.-)
traumatic amputation of ankle and foot (S98.-)

The appropriate 7th character is to be added to each code from category S92

A	initial encounter for closed fracture
B	initial encounter for open fracture
D	subsequent encounter for fracture with routine healing
G	subsequent encounter for fracture with delayed healing
K	subsequent encounter for fracture with nonunion
P	subsequent encounter for fracture with malunion
S	sequela

- S92.0 Fracture of calcaneus (Ex:) PDX 1264 [K, P], 1877 [B]
  Heel bone Os calcis
  Excludes2 Physeal fracture of calcaneus (S99.0-)
  - S92.00 Unspecified fracture of calcaneus
    - S92.001 Unspecified fracture of right calcaneus B, K, P, B
    - S92.002 Unspecified fracture of left calcaneus B, K, P, B
    - S92.009 Unspecified fracture of unspecified calcaneus B, K, P, B
  - S92.01 Fracture of body of calcaneus
    - S92.011 Displaced fracture of body of right calcaneus B, K, P, B
    - S92.012 Displaced fracture of body of left calcaneus B, K, P, B
    - S92.013 Displaced fracture of body of unspecified calcaneus B, K, P, B
    - S92.014 Nondisplaced fracture of body of right calcaneus B, K, P, B
    - S92.015 Nondisplaced fracture of body of left calcaneus B, K, P, B
    - S92.016 Nondisplaced fracture of body of unspecified calcaneus B, K, P, B
  - S92.02 Fracture of anterior process of calcaneus
    - S92.021 Displaced fracture of anterior process of right calcaneus B, K, P, B
    - S92.022 Displaced fracture of anterior process of left calcaneus B, K, P, B
    - S92.023 Displaced fracture of anterior process of unspecified calcaneus B, K, P, B
    - S92.024 Nondisplaced fracture of anterior process of right calcaneus B, K, P, B
    - S92.025 Nondisplaced fracture of anterior process of left calcaneus B, K, P, B
    - S92.026 Nondisplaced fracture of anterior process of unspecified calcaneus B, K, P, B
  - S92.03 Avulsion fracture of tuberosity of calcaneus
    - S92.031 Displaced avulsion fracture of tuberosity of right calcaneus B, K, P, B
    - S92.032 Displaced avulsion fracture of tuberosity of left calcaneus B, K, P, B
    - S92.033 Displaced avulsion fracture of tuberosity of unspecified calcaneus B, K, P, B
    - S92.034 Nondisplaced avulsion fracture of tuberosity of right calcaneus B, K, P, B
    - S92.035 Nondisplaced avulsion fracture of tuberosity of left calcaneus B, K, P, B
    - S92.036 Nondisplaced avulsion fracture of tuberosity of unspecified calcaneus B, K, P, B
  - S92.04 Other fracture of tuberosity of calcaneus
    - S92.041 Displaced other fracture of tuberosity of right calcaneus B, K, P, B
    - S92.042 Displaced other fracture of tuberosity of left calcaneus B, K, P, B
    - S92.043 Displaced other fracture of tuberosity of unspecified calcaneus B, K, P, B
    - S92.044 Nondisplaced other fracture of tuberosity of right calcaneus B, K, P, B
    - S92.045 Nondisplaced other fracture of tuberosity of left calcaneus B, K, P, B
    - S92.046 Nondisplaced other fracture of tuberosity of unspecified calcaneus B, K, P, B
  - S92.05 Other extraarticular fracture of calcaneus
    - S92.051 Displaced other extraarticular fracture of right calcaneus B, K, P, B
    - S92.052 Displaced other extraarticular fracture of left calcaneus B, K, P, B
    - S92.053 Displaced other extraarticular fracture of unspecified calcaneus B, K, P, B
    - S92.054 Nondisplaced other extraarticular fracture of right calcaneus B, K, P, B
    - S92.055 Nondisplaced other extraarticular fracture of left calcaneus B, K, P, B
    - S92.056 Nondisplaced other extraarticular fracture of unspecified calcaneus B, K, P, B
  - S92.06 Intraarticular fracture of calcaneus
    - S92.061 Displaced intraarticular fracture of right calcaneus B, K, P, B
    - S92.062 Displaced intraarticular fracture of left calcaneus B, K, P, B
    - S92.063 Displaced intraarticular fracture of unspecified calcaneus B, K, P, B
    - S92.064 Nondisplaced intraarticular fracture of right calcaneus B, K, P, B
    - S92.065 Nondisplaced intraarticular fracture of left calcaneus B, K, P, B
    - S92.066 Nondisplaced intraarticular fracture of unspecified calcaneus B, K, P, B
- S92.1 Fracture of talus (Ex:) PDX 1264 [K, P], 1878 [B]
  Astragalus
  - S92.10 Unspecified fracture of talus
    - S92.101 Unspecified fracture of right talus B, K, P, B
    - S92.102 Unspecified fracture of left talus B, K, P, B
    - S92.109 Unspecified fracture of unspecified talus B, K, P, B
  - S92.11 Fracture of neck of talus
    - S92.111 Displaced fracture of neck of right talus B, K, P, B
    - S92.112 Displaced fracture of neck of left talus B, K, P, B
    - S92.113 Displaced fracture of neck of unspecified talus B, K, P, B
    - S92.114 Nondisplaced fracture of neck of right talus B, K, P, B
    - S92.115 Nondisplaced fracture of neck of left talus B, K, P, B
    - S92.116 Nondisplaced fracture of neck of unspecified talus B, K, P, B
  - S92.12 Fracture of body of talus
    - S92.121 Displaced fracture of body of right talus B, K, P, B
    - S92.122 Displaced fracture of body of left talus B, K, P, B
    - S92.123 Displaced fracture of body of unspecified talus B, K, P, B
    - S92.124 Nondisplaced fracture of body of right talus B, K, P, B
    - S92.125 Nondisplaced fracture of body of left talus B, K, P, B
    - S92.126 Nondisplaced fracture of body of unspecified talus B, K, P, B

- S92.13 Fracture of posterior process of talus
  - S92.131 Displaced fracture of posterior process of right talus B, K, P, B
  - S92.132 Displaced fracture of posterior process of left talus B, K, P, B
  - S92.133 Displaced fracture of posterior process of unspecified talus B, K, P, B
  - S92.134 Nondisplaced fracture of posterior process of right talus B, K, P, B
  - S92.135 Nondisplaced fracture of posterior process of left talus B, K, P, B
  - S92.136 Nondisplaced fracture of posterior process of unspecified talus B, K, P, B
- S92.14 Dome fracture of talus
  - **Excludes1** osteochondritis dissecans (M93.2)
  - S92.141 Displaced dome fracture of right talus B, K, P, B
  - S92.142 Displaced dome fracture of left talus B, K, P, B
  - S92.143 Displaced dome fracture of unspecified talus B, K, P, B
  - S92.144 Nondisplaced dome fracture of right talus B, K, P, B
  - S92.145 Nondisplaced dome fracture of left talus B, K, P, B
  - S92.146 Nondisplaced dome fracture of unspecified talus B, K, P, B
- S92.15 Avulsion fracture (chip fracture) of talus
  - S92.151 Displaced avulsion fracture (chip fracture) of right talus B, K, P, B
  - S92.152 Displaced avulsion fracture (chip fracture) of left talus B, K, P, B
  - S92.153 Displaced avulsion fracture (chip fracture) of unspecified talus B, K, P, B
  - S92.154 Nondisplaced avulsion fracture (chip fracture) of right talus B, K, P, B
  - S92.155 Nondisplaced avulsion fracture (chip fracture) of left talus B, K, P, B
  - S92.156 Nondisplaced avulsion fracture (chip fracture) of unspecified talus B, K, P, B
- S92.19 Other fracture of talus
  - S92.191 Other fracture of right talus B, K, P, B
  - S92.192 Other fracture of left talus B, K, P, B
  - S92.199 Other fracture of unspecified talus B, K, P, B

S92.2 Fracture of other and unspecified tarsal bone(s)

- S92.20 Fracture of unspecified tarsal bone(s) (Ex) PDX 1264 [K, P], 1879 [B]
  - S92.201 Fracture of unspecified tarsal bone(s) of right foot B, K, P, B
  - S92.202 Fracture of unspecified tarsal bone(s) of left foot B, K, P, B
  - S92.209 Fracture of unspecified tarsal bone(s) of unspecified foot B, K, P, B
- S92.21 Fracture of cuboid bone (Ex) PDX 1264 [K, P], 1878 [B]
  - S92.211 Displaced fracture of cuboid bone of right foot B, K, P, B
  - S92.212 Displaced fracture of cuboid bone of left foot B, K, P, B
  - S92.213 Displaced fracture of cuboid bone of unspecified foot B, K, P, B
  - S92.214 Nondisplaced fracture of cuboid bone of right foot B, K, P, B
  - S92.215 Nondisplaced fracture of cuboid bone of left foot B, K, P, B
  - S92.216 Nondisplaced fracture of cuboid bone of unspecified foot B, K, P, B
- S92.22 Fracture of lateral cuneiform (Ex) PDX 1264 [K, P], 1878 [B]
  - S92.221 Displaced fracture of lateral cuneiform of right foot B, K, P, B
  - S92.222 Displaced fracture of lateral cuneiform of left foot B, K, P, B
  - S92.223 Displaced fracture of lateral cuneiform of unspecified foot B, K, P, B
  - S92.224 Nondisplaced fracture of lateral cuneiform of right foot B, K, P, B
  - S92.225 Nondisplaced fracture of lateral cuneiform of left foot B, K, P, B
  - S92.226 Nondisplaced fracture of lateral cuneiform of unspecified foot B, K, P, B
- S92.23 Fracture of intermediate cuneiform (Ex) PDX 897 [K, P], 1368 [B]
  - S92.231 Displaced fracture of intermediate cuneiform of right foot B, K, P, B
  - S92.232 Displaced fracture of intermediate cuneiform of left foot B, K, P, B
  - S92.233 Displaced fracture of intermediate cuneiform of unspecified foot B, K, P, B
  - S92.234 Nondisplaced fracture of intermediate cuneiform of right foot B, K, P, B
  - S92.235 Nondisplaced fracture of intermediate cuneiform of left foot B, K, P, B
  - S92.236 Nondisplaced fracture of intermediate cuneiform of unspecified foot B, K, P, B
- S92.24 Fracture of medial cuneiform (Ex) PDX 1264 [K, P], 1878 [B]
  - S92.241 Displaced fracture of medial cuneiform of right foot B, K, P, B
  - S92.242 Displaced fracture of medial cuneiform of left foot B, K, P, B
  - S92.243 Displaced fracture of medial cuneiform of unspecified foot B, K, P, B
  - S92.244 Nondisplaced fracture of medial cuneiform of right foot B, K, P, B
  - S92.245 Nondisplaced fracture of medial cuneiform of left foot B, K, P, B
  - S92.246 Nondisplaced fracture of medial cuneiform of unspecified foot B, K, P, B
- S92.25 Fracture of navicular [scaphoid] of foot (Ex) 1264 [K, P], 1878 [B]
  - S92.251 Displaced fracture of navicular [scaphoid] of right foot B, K, P, B
  - S92.252 Displaced fracture of navicular [scaphoid] of left foot B, K, P, B
  - S92.253 Displaced fracture of navicular [scaphoid] of unspecified foot B, K, P, B
  - S92.254 Nondisplaced fracture of navicular [scaphoid] of right foot B, K, P, B
  - S92.255 Nondisplaced fracture of navicular [scaphoid] of left foot B, K, P, B

S92.256 Nondisplaced fracture of navicular [scaphoid] of unspecified foot B, K, P, B

S92.3 Fracture of metatarsal bone(s) (Ex) PDX 1264 [K, P], 1878 [B]

Excludes2 Physeal fracture of metatarsal (S99.1-)

S92.30 Fracture of unspecified metatarsal bone(s)

S92.301 Fracture of unspecified metatarsal bone(s), right foot B, K, P, B

S92.302 Fracture of unspecified metatarsal bone(s), left foot B, K, P, B

S92.309 Fracture of unspecified metatarsal bone(s), unspecified foot B, K, P, B

S92.31 Fracture of first metatarsal bone

S92.311 Displaced fracture of first metatarsal bone, right foot B, K, P, B

S92.312 Displaced fracture of first metatarsal bone, left foot B, K, P, B

S92.313 Displaced fracture of first metatarsal bone, unspecified foot B, K, P, B

S92.314 Nondisplaced fracture of first metatarsal bone, right foot B, K, P, B

S92.315 Nondisplaced fracture of first metatarsal bone, left foot B, K, P, B

S92.316 Nondisplaced fracture of first metatarsal bone, unspecified foot B, K, P, B

S92.32 Fracture of second metatarsal bone

S92.321 Displaced fracture of second metatarsal bone, right foot B, K, P, B

S92.322 Displaced fracture of second metatarsal bone, left foot B, K, P, B

S92.323 Displaced fracture of second metatarsal bone, unspecified foot B, K, P, B

S92.324 Nondisplaced fracture of second metatarsal bone, right foot B, K, P, B

S92.325 Nondisplaced fracture of second metatarsal bone, left foot B, K, P, B

S92.326 Nondisplaced fracture of second metatarsal bone, unspecified foot B, K, P, B

S92.33 Fracture of third metatarsal bone

Coding Clinic: 2018, Q1, P3

S92.331 Displaced fracture of third metatarsal bone, right foot B, K, P, B

S92.332 Displaced fracture of third metatarsal bone, left foot B, K, P, B

S92.333 Displaced fracture of third metatarsal bone, unspecified foot B, K, P, B

S92.334 Nondisplaced fracture of third metatarsal bone, right foot B, K, P, B

S92.335 Nondisplaced fracture of third metatarsal bone, left foot B, K, P, B

S92.336 Nondisplaced fracture of third metatarsal bone, unspecified foot B, K, P, B

S92.34 Fracture of fourth metatarsal bone

S92.341 Displaced fracture of fourth metatarsal bone, right foot B, K, P, B

S92.342 Displaced fracture of fourth metatarsal bone, left foot B, K, P, B

S92.343 Displaced fracture of fourth metatarsal bone, unspecified foot B, K, P, B

S92.344 Nondisplaced fracture of fourth metatarsal bone, right foot B, K, P, B

S92.345 Nondisplaced fracture of fourth metatarsal bone, left foot B, K, P, B

S92.346 Nondisplaced fracture of fourth metatarsal bone, unspecified foot B, K, P, B

S92.35 Fracture of fifth metatarsal bone

S92.351 Displaced fracture of fifth metatarsal bone, right foot B, K, P, B

S92.352 Displaced fracture of fifth metatarsal bone, left foot B, K, P, B

S92.353 Displaced fracture of fifth metatarsal bone, unspecified foot B, K, P, B

S92.354 Nondisplaced fracture of fifth metatarsal bone, right foot B, K, P, B

S92.355 Nondisplaced fracture of fifth metatarsal bone, left foot B, K, P, B

S92.356 Nondisplaced fracture of fifth metatarsal bone, unspecified foot B, K, P, B

S92.4 Fracture of great toe (Ex) PDX 1264

Excludes2 Physeal fracture of phalanx of toe (S99.2-)

S92.40 Unspecified fracture of great toe

S92.401 Displaced unspecified fracture of right great toe K, P

S92.402 Displaced unspecified fracture of left great toe K, P

S92.403 Displaced unspecified fracture of unspecified great toe K, P

S92.404 Nondisplaced unspecified fracture of right great toe K, P

S92.405 Nondisplaced unspecified fracture of left great toe K, P

S92.406 Nondisplaced unspecified fracture of unspecified great toe K, P

S92.41 Fracture of proximal phalanx of great toe

S92.411 Displaced fracture of proximal phalanx of right great toe K, P

S92.412 Displaced fracture of proximal phalanx of left great toe K, P

S92.413 Displaced fracture of proximal phalanx of unspecified great toe K, P

S92.414 Nondisplaced fracture of proximal phalanx of right great toe K, P

S92.415 Nondisplaced fracture of proximal phalanx of left great toe K, P

S92.416 Nondisplaced fracture of proximal phalanx of unspecified great toe K, P

S92.42 Fracture of distal phalanx of great toe

S92.421 Displaced fracture of distal phalanx of right great toe K, P

S92.422 Displaced fracture of distal phalanx of left great toe K, P

S92.423 Displaced fracture of distal phalanx of unspecified great toe K, P

S92.424 Nondisplaced fracture of distal phalanx of right great toe K, P

CHAPTER 19 (SØØ-T88)

- S92.425 Nondisplaced fracture of distal phalanx of left great toe K, P
- S92.426 Nondisplaced fracture of distal phalanx of unspecified great toe K, P
- S92.49 Other fracture of great toe
  - S92.491 Other fracture of right great toe K, P
  - S92.492 Other fracture of left great toe K, P
  - S92.499 Other fracture of unspecified great toe K, P

S92.5 Fracture of lesser toe(s) (Ex) PDX 1264

Excludes2 Physeal fracture of phalanx of toe (S99.2-)

- S92.50 Unspecified fracture of lesser toe(s)
  - S92.501 Displaced unspecified fracture of right lesser toe(s) K, P
  - S92.502 Displaced unspecified fracture of left lesser toe(s) K, P
  - S92.503 Displaced unspecified fracture of unspecified lesser toe(s) K, P
  - S92.504 Nondisplaced unspecified fracture of right lesser toe(s) K, P
  - S92.505 Nondisplaced unspecified fracture of left lesser toe(s) K, P
  - S92.506 Nondisplaced unspecified fracture of unspecified lesser toe(s) K, P
- S92.51 Fracture of proximal phalanx of lesser toe(s)
  - S92.511 Displaced fracture of proximal phalanx of right lesser toe(s) K, P
  - S92.512 Displaced fracture of proximal phalanx of left lesser toe(s) K, P
  - S92.513 Displaced fracture of proximal phalanx of unspecified lesser toe(s) K, P
  - S92.514 Nondisplaced fracture of proximal phalanx of right lesser toe(s) K, P
  - S92.515 Nondisplaced fracture of proximal phalanx of left lesser toe(s) K, P
  - S92.516 Nondisplaced fracture of proximal phalanx of unspecified lesser toe(s) K, P
- S92.52 Fracture of middle phalanx of lesser toe(s)
  - S92.521 Displaced fracture of middle phalanx of right lesser toe(s) K, P
  - S92.522 Displaced fracture of middle phalanx of left lesser toe(s) K, P
  - S92.523 Displaced fracture of middle phalanx of unspecified lesser toe(s) K, P
  - S92.524 Nondisplaced fracture of middle phalanx of right lesser toe(s) K, P
  - S92.525 Nondisplaced fracture of middle phalanx of left lesser toe(s) K, P
  - S92.526 Nondisplaced fracture of middle phalanx of unspecified lesser toe(s) K, P
- S92.53 Fracture of distal phalanx of lesser toe(s)
  - S92.531 Displaced fracture of distal phalanx of right lesser toe(s) K, P
  - S92.532 Displaced fracture of distal phalanx of left lesser toe(s) K, P
  - S92.533 Displaced fracture of distal phalanx of unspecified lesser toe(s) K, P
  - S92.534 Nondisplaced fracture of distal phalanx of right lesser toe(s) K, P
  - S92.535 Nondisplaced fracture of distal phalanx of left lesser toe(s) K, P
  - S92.536 Nondisplaced fracture of distal phalanx of unspecified lesser toe(s) K, P
- S92.59 Other fracture of lesser toe(s)
  - S92.591 Other fracture of right lesser toe(s) K, P
  - S92.592 Other fracture of left lesser toe(s) K, P
  - S92.599 Other fracture of unspecified lesser toe(s) K, P

S92.8 Other fracture of foot, except ankle (Ex) PDX 1264 [K, P], 1879 [B]

- S92.81 Other fracture of foot
  Sesamoid fracture of foot
  Coding Clinic: 2016, Q4, P68
  - S92.811 Other fracture of right foot B, K, P, B
  - S92.812 Other fracture of left foot B, K, P, B
  - S92.819 Other fracture of unspecified foot B, K, P, B

S92.9 Unspecified fracture of foot and toe

- S92.90 Unspecified fracture of foot (Ex) PDX 1264 [K, P], 1879 [B]
  - S92.901 Unspecified fracture of right foot B, K, P, B
  - S92.902 Unspecified fracture of left foot B, K, P, B
  - S92.909 Unspecified fracture of unspecified foot B, K, P, B
- S92.91 Unspecified fracture of toe (Ex) PDX 1264
  - S92.911 Unspecified fracture of right toe(s) K, P
  - S92.912 Unspecified fracture of left toe(s) K, P
  - S92.919 Unspecified fracture of unspecified toe(s) K, P

S93 Dislocation and sprain of joints and ligaments at ankle, foot and toe level

Includes
- avulsion of joint or ligament of ankle, foot and toe
- laceration of cartilage, joint or ligament of ankle, foot and toe
- sprain of cartilage, joint or ligament of ankle, foot and toe
- traumatic hemarthrosis of joint or ligament of ankle, foot and toe
- traumatic rupture of joint or ligament of ankle, foot and toe
- traumatic subluxation of joint or ligament of ankle, foot and toe
- traumatic tear of joint or ligament of ankle, foot and toe

Code also any associated open wound

Excludes2 strain of muscle and tendon of ankle and foot (S96.-)

The appropriate 7th character is to be added to each code from category S93

A	initial encounter
D	subsequent encounter
S	sequela

S93.0 Subluxation and dislocation of ankle joint
Subluxation and dislocation of astragalus
Subluxation and dislocation of fibula, lower end
Subluxation and dislocation of talus
Subluxation and dislocation of tibia, lower end

- X S93.01 Subluxation of right ankle joint
- X S93.02 Subluxation of left ankle joint
- X S93.03 Subluxation of unspecified ankle joint
- X S93.04 Dislocation of right ankle joint
- X S93.05 Dislocation of left ankle joint
- X S93.06 Dislocation of unspecified ankle joint

S93.1 Subluxation and dislocation of toe

- S93.10 Unspecified subluxation and dislocation of toe
  Dislocation of toe NOS
  Subluxation of toe NOS

- S93.101 Unspecified subluxation of right toe(s)
- S93.102 Unspecified subluxation of left toe(s)
- S93.103 Unspecified subluxation of unspecified toe(s)
- S93.104 Unspecified dislocation of right toe(s)
- S93.105 Unspecified dislocation of left toe(s)
- S93.106 Unspecified dislocation of unspecified toe(s)

S93.11 Dislocation of interphalangeal joint
- S93.111 Dislocation of interphalangeal joint of right great toe
- S93.112 Dislocation of interphalangeal joint of left great toe
- S93.113 Dislocation of interphalangeal joint of unspecified great toe
- S93.114 Dislocation of interphalangeal joint of right lesser toe(s)
- S93.115 Dislocation of interphalangeal joint of left lesser toe(s)
- S93.116 Dislocation of interphalangeal joint of unspecified lesser toe(s)
- S93.119 Dislocation of interphalangeal joint of unspecified toe(s)

S93.12 Dislocation of metatarsophalangeal joint
- S93.121 Dislocation of metatarsophalangeal joint of right great toe
- S93.122 Dislocation of metatarsophalangeal joint of left great toe
- S93.123 Dislocation of metatarsophalangeal joint of unspecified great toe
- S93.124 Dislocation of metatarsophalangeal joint of right lesser toe(s)
- S93.125 Dislocation of metatarsophalangeal joint of left lesser toe(s)
- S93.126 Dislocation of metatarsophalangeal joint of unspecified lesser toe(s)
- S93.129 Dislocation of metatarsophalangeal joint of unspecified toe(s)

S93.13 Subluxation of interphalangeal joint
- S93.131 Subluxation of interphalangeal joint of right great toe
- S93.132 Subluxation of interphalangeal joint of left great toe
- S93.133 Subluxation of interphalangeal joint of unspecified great toe
- S93.134 Subluxation of interphalangeal joint of right lesser toe(s)
- S93.135 Subluxation of interphalangeal joint of left lesser toe(s)
- S93.136 Subluxation of interphalangeal joint of unspecified lesser toe(s)
- S93.139 Subluxation of interphalangeal joint of unspecified toe(s)

S93.14 Subluxation of metatarsophalangeal joint
- S93.141 Subluxation of metatarsophalangeal joint of right great toe
- S93.142 Subluxation of metatarsophalangeal joint of left great toe
- S93.143 Subluxation of metatarsophalangeal joint of unspecified great toe
- S93.144 Subluxation of metatarsophalangeal joint of right lesser toe(s)
- S93.145 Subluxation of metatarsophalangeal joint of left lesser toe(s)
- S93.146 Subluxation of metatarsophalangeal joint of unspecified lesser toe(s)
- S93.149 Subluxation of metatarsophalangeal joint of unspecified toe(s)

S93.3 Subluxation and dislocation of foot
Excludes2 dislocation of toe (S93.1-)

S93.30 Unspecified subluxation and dislocation of foot
Dislocation of foot NOS
Subluxation of foot NOS
- S93.301 Unspecified subluxation of right foot
- S93.302 Unspecified subluxation of left foot
- S93.303 Unspecified subluxation of unspecified foot
- S93.304 Unspecified dislocation of right foot
- S93.305 Unspecified dislocation of left foot
- S93.306 Unspecified dislocation of unspecified foot

S93.31 Subluxation and dislocation of tarsal joint
- S93.311 Subluxation of tarsal joint of right foot
- S93.312 Subluxation of tarsal joint of left foot
- S93.313 Subluxation of tarsal joint of unspecified foot
- S93.314 Dislocation of tarsal joint of right foot
- S93.315 Dislocation of tarsal joint of left foot
- S93.316 Dislocation of tarsal joint of unspecified foot

S93.32 Subluxation and dislocation of tarsometatarsal joint
- S93.321 Subluxation of tarsometatarsal joint of right foot
- S93.322 Subluxation of tarsometatarsal joint of left foot
- S93.323 Subluxation of tarsometatarsal joint of unspecified foot
- S93.324 Dislocation of tarsometatarsal joint of right foot
- S93.325 Dislocation of tarsometatarsal joint of left foot
- S93.326 Dislocation of tarsometatarsal joint of unspecified foot

S93.33 Other subluxation and dislocation of foot
- S93.331 Other subluxation of right foot
- S93.332 Other subluxation of left foot
- S93.333 Other subluxation of unspecified foot
- S93.334 Other dislocation of right foot
- S93.335 Other dislocation of left foot
- S93.336 Other dislocation of unspecified foot

S93.4 Sprain of ankle
Injury to ligaments when one or more is stretched/torn
Excludes2 injury of Achilles tendon (S86.0-)

S93.40 Sprain of unspecified ligament of ankle
Sprain of ankle NOS
Sprained ankle NOS
- S93.401 Sprain of unspecified ligament of right ankle
- S93.402 Sprain of unspecified ligament of left ankle
- S93.409 Sprain of unspecified ligament of unspecified ankle

S93.41 Sprain of calcaneofibular ligament
- S93.411 Sprain of calcaneofibular ligament of right ankle
- S93.412 Sprain of calcaneofibular ligament of left ankle
- S93.419 Sprain of calcaneofibular ligament of unspecified ankle

S93.42 Sprain of deltoid ligament
- S93.421 Sprain of deltoid ligament of right ankle
- S93.422 Sprain of deltoid ligament of left ankle
- S93.429 Sprain of deltoid ligament of unspecified ankle

S93.43 Sprain of tibiofibular ligament
S93.431 Sprain of tibiofibular ligament of right ankle
S93.432 Sprain of tibiofibular ligament of left ankle
S93.439 Sprain of tibiofibular ligament of unspecified ankle
S93.49 Sprain of other ligament of ankle
Sprain of internal collateral ligament
Sprain of talofibular ligament
S93.491 Sprain of other ligament of right ankle
S93.492 Sprain of other ligament of left ankle
S93.499 Sprain of other ligament of unspecified ankle
S93.5 Sprain of toe
S93.50 Unspecified sprain of toe
S93.501 Unspecified sprain of right great toe
S93.502 Unspecified sprain of left great toe
S93.503 Unspecified sprain of unspecified great toe
S93.504 Unspecified sprain of right lesser toe(s)
S93.505 Unspecified sprain of left lesser toe(s)
S93.506 Unspecified sprain of unspecified lesser toe(s)
S93.509 Unspecified sprain of unspecified toe(s)
S93.51 Sprain of interphalangeal joint of toe
S93.511 Sprain of interphalangeal joint of right great toe
S93.512 Sprain of interphalangeal joint of left great toe
S93.513 Sprain of interphalangeal joint of unspecified great toe
S93.514 Sprain of interphalangeal joint of right lesser toe(s)
S93.515 Sprain of interphalangeal joint of left lesser toe(s)
S93.516 Sprain of interphalangeal joint of unspecified lesser toe(s)
S93.519 Sprain of interphalangeal joint of unspecified toe(s)
S93.52 Sprain of metatarsophalangeal joint of toe
S93.521 Sprain of metatarsophalangeal joint of right great toe
S93.522 Sprain of metatarsophalangeal joint of left great toe
S93.523 Sprain of metatarsophalangeal joint of unspecified great toe
S93.524 Sprain of metatarsophalangeal joint of right lesser toe(s)
S93.525 Sprain of metatarsophalangeal joint of left lesser toe(s)
S93.526 Sprain of metatarsophalangeal joint of unspecified lesser toe(s)
S93.529 Sprain of metatarsophalangeal joint of unspecified toe(s)
S93.6 Sprain of foot
Excludes2 sprain of metatarsophalangeal joint of toe (S93.52-)
sprain of toe (S93.5-)
S93.60 Unspecified sprain of foot
S93.601 Unspecified sprain of right foot
S93.602 Unspecified sprain of left foot
S93.609 Unspecified sprain of unspecified foot
S93.61 Sprain of tarsal ligament of foot
S93.611 Sprain of tarsal ligament of right foot
S93.612 Sprain of tarsal ligament of left foot
S93.619 Sprain of tarsal ligament of unspecified foot
S93.62 Sprain of tarsometatarsal ligament of foot
S93.621 Sprain of tarsometatarsal ligament of right foot
S93.622 Sprain of tarsometatarsal ligament of left foot
S93.629 Sprain of tarsometatarsal ligament of unspecified foot
S93.69 Other sprain of foot
S93.691 Other sprain of right foot
S93.692 Other sprain of left foot
S93.699 Other sprain of unspecified foot

S94 Injury of nerves at ankle and foot level

The appropriate 7th character is to be added to each code from category S94

A	initial encounter
D	subsequent encounter
S	sequela

Code also any associated open wound (S91.-)

S94.0 Injury of lateral plantar nerve
X S94.00 Injury of lateral plantar nerve, unspecified leg
X S94.01 Injury of lateral plantar nerve, right leg
X S94.02 Injury of lateral plantar nerve, left leg
S94.1 Injury of medial plantar nerve
X S94.10 Injury of medial plantar nerve, unspecified leg
X S94.11 Injury of medial plantar nerve, right leg
X S94.12 Injury of medial plantar nerve, left leg
S94.2 Injury of deep peroneal nerve at ankle and foot level
Injury of terminal, lateral branch of deep peroneal nerve
X S94.20 Injury of deep peroneal nerve at ankle and foot level, unspecified leg
X S94.21 Injury of deep peroneal nerve at ankle and foot level, right leg
X S94.22 Injury of deep peroneal nerve at ankle and foot level, left leg
S94.3 Injury of cutaneous sensory nerve at ankle and foot level
X S94.30 Injury of cutaneous sensory nerve at ankle and foot level, unspecified leg
X S94.31 Injury of cutaneous sensory nerve at ankle and foot level, right leg
X S94.32 Injury of cutaneous sensory nerve at ankle and foot level, left leg
S94.8 Injury of other nerves at ankle and foot level
S94.8X Injury of other nerves at ankle and foot level
S94.8X1 Injury of other nerves at ankle and foot level, right leg
S94.8X2 Injury of other nerves at ankle and foot level, left leg
S94.8X9 Injury of other nerves at ankle and foot level, unspecified leg
S94.9 Injury of unspecified nerve at ankle and foot level
X S94.90 Injury of unspecified nerve at ankle and foot level, unspecified leg
X S94.91 Injury of unspecified nerve at ankle and foot level, right leg
X S94.92 Injury of unspecified nerve at ankle and foot level, left leg

S95 Injury of blood vessels at ankle and foot level

Code also any associated open wound (S91.-)

Excludes2 injury of posterior tibial artery and vein (S85.1-, S85.8-)

The appropriate 7th character is to be added to each code from category S95

A	initial encounter
D	subsequent encounter
S	sequela

S95.0 Injury of dorsal artery of foot
S95.00 Unspecified injury of dorsal artery of foot
S95.001 Unspecified injury of dorsal artery of right foot A (Ex) PDX 1835

S95.002 Unspecified injury of dorsal artery of left foot A Ex: PDX 1836
S95.009 Unspecified injury of dorsal artery of unspecified foot A Ex: PDX 1837
S95.01 Laceration of dorsal artery of foot
S95.011 Laceration of dorsal artery of right foot A Ex: PDX 1835
S95.012 Laceration of dorsal artery of left foot A Ex: PDX 1836
S95.019 Laceration of dorsal artery of unspecified foot A Ex: PDX 1837
S95.09 Other specified injury of dorsal artery of foot
S95.091 Other specified injury of dorsal artery of right foot A Ex: PDX 1835
S95.092 Other specified injury of dorsal artery of left foot A Ex: PDX 1836
S95.099 Other specified injury of dorsal artery of unspecified foot A Ex: PDX 1837
S95.1 Injury of plantar artery of foot
S95.10 Unspecified injury of plantar artery of foot
S95.101 Unspecified injury of plantar artery of right foot A Ex: PDX 1880
S95.102 Unspecified injury of plantar artery of left foot A Ex: PDX 1881
S95.109 Unspecified injury of plantar artery of unspecified foot A Ex: PDX 1832
S95.11 Laceration of plantar artery of foot
S95.111 Laceration of plantar artery of right foot A Ex: PDX 1880
S95.112 Laceration of plantar artery of left foot A Ex: PDX 1881
S95.119 Laceration of plantar artery of unspecified foot A Ex: PDX 1882
S95.19 Other specified injury of plantar artery of foot
S95.191 Other specified injury of plantar artery of right foot A Ex: PDX 1880
S95.192 Other specified injury of plantar artery of left foot A Ex: PDX 1881
S95.199 Other specified injury of plantar artery of unspecified foot A Ex: PDX 1882
S95.2 Injury of dorsal vein of foot
S95.20 Unspecified injury of dorsal vein of foot
S95.201 Unspecified injury of dorsal vein of right foot A Ex: PDX 1835
S95.202 Unspecified injury of dorsal vein of left foot A Ex: PDX 1836
S95.209 Unspecified injury of dorsal vein of unspecified foot A Ex: PDX 1837
S95.21 Laceration of dorsal vein of foot
S95.211 Laceration of dorsal vein of right foot A Ex: PDX 1835
S95.212 Laceration of dorsal vein of left foot A Ex: PDX 1836
S95.219 Laceration of dorsal vein of unspecified foot A Ex: PDX 1837
S95.29 Other specified injury of dorsal vein of foot
S95.291 Other specified injury of dorsal vein of right foot A Ex: PDX 1835
S95.292 Other specified injury of dorsal vein of left foot A Ex: PDX 1836
S95.299 Other specified injury of dorsal vein of unspecified foot A Ex: PDX 1837
S95.8 Injury of other blood vessels at ankle and foot level
S95.80 Unspecified injury of other blood vessels at ankle and foot level
S95.801 Unspecified injury of other blood vessels at ankle and foot level, right leg A Ex: PDX 1835
S95.802 Unspecified injury of other blood vessels at ankle and foot level, left leg A Ex: PDX 1836
S95.809 Unspecified injury of other blood vessels at ankle and foot level, unspecified leg A Ex: PDX 1837
S95.81 Laceration of other blood vessels at ankle and foot level
S95.811 Laceration of other blood vessels at ankle and foot level, right leg A Ex: PDX 1835
S95.812 Laceration of other blood vessels at ankle and foot level, left leg A Ex: PDX 1836
S95.819 Laceration of other blood vessels at ankle and foot level, unspecified leg A Ex: PDX 1837
S95.89 Other specified injury of other blood vessels at ankle and foot level
S95.891 Other specified injury of other blood vessels at ankle and foot level, right leg A Ex: PDX 1835
S95.892 Other specified injury of other blood vessels at ankle and foot level, left leg A Ex: PDX 1836
S95.899 Other specified injury of other blood vessels at ankle and foot level, unspecified leg A Ex: PDX 1837
S95.9 Injury of unspecified blood vessel at ankle and foot level
S95.90 Unspecified injury of unspecified blood vessel at ankle and foot level
S95.901 Unspecified injury of unspecified blood vessel at ankle and foot level, right leg A Ex: PDX 1835
S95.902 Unspecified injury of unspecified blood vessel at ankle and foot level, left leg A Ex: PDX 1836
S95.909 Unspecified injury of unspecified blood vessel at ankle and foot level, unspecified leg A Ex: PDX 1837
S95.91 Laceration of unspecified blood vessel at ankle and foot level
S95.911 Laceration of unspecified blood vessel at ankle and foot level, right leg A Ex: PDX 1835
S95.912 Laceration of unspecified blood vessel at ankle and foot level, left leg A Ex: PDX 1836
S95.919 Laceration of unspecified blood vessel at ankle and foot level, unspecified leg A Ex: PDX 1837
S95.99 Other specified injury of unspecified blood vessel at ankle and foot level
S95.991 Other specified injury of unspecified blood vessel at ankle and foot level, right leg A Ex: PDX 1835
S95.992 Other specified injury of unspecified blood vessel at ankle and foot level, left leg A Ex: PDX 1836
S95.999 Other specified injury of unspecified blood vessel at ankle and foot level, unspecified leg A Ex: PDX 1837

S96 Injury of muscle and tendon at ankle and foot level
Code also any associated open wound (S91.-)
Excludes2 injury of Achilles tendon (S86.0-)
sprain of joints and ligaments of ankle and foot (S93.-)
The appropriate 7th character is to be added to each code from category S96

A initial encounter
D subsequent encounter
S sequela

S96.0 Injury of muscle and tendon of long flexor muscle of toe at ankle and foot level

S96.00 Unspecified injury of muscle and tendon of long flexor muscle of toe at ankle and foot level

S96.001 Unspecified injury of muscle and tendon of long flexor muscle of toe at ankle and foot level, right foot

S96.002 Unspecified injury of muscle and tendon of long flexor muscle of toe at ankle and foot level, left foot

S96.009 Unspecified injury of muscle and tendon of long flexor muscle of toe at ankle and foot level, unspecified foot

S96.01 Strain of muscle and tendon of long flexor muscle of toe at ankle and foot level

S96.011 Strain of muscle and tendon of long flexor muscle of toe at ankle and foot level, right foot

S96.012 Strain of muscle and tendon of long flexor muscle of toe at ankle and foot level, left foot

S96.019 Strain of muscle and tendon of long flexor muscle of toe at ankle and foot level, unspecified foot

S96.02 Laceration of muscle and tendon of long flexor muscle of toe at ankle and foot level

S96.021 Laceration of muscle and tendon of long flexor muscle of toe at ankle and foot level, right foot A (Ex) PDX 1874

S96.022 Laceration of muscle and tendon of long flexor muscle of toe at ankle and foot level, left foot A (Ex) PDX 1875

S96.029 Laceration of muscle and tendon of long flexor muscle of toe at ankle and foot level, unspecified foot A (Ex) PDX 1876

S96.09 Other injury of muscle and tendon of long flexor muscle of toe at ankle and foot level

S96.091 Other injury of muscle and tendon of long flexor muscle of toe at ankle and foot level, right foot

S96.092 Other injury of muscle and tendon of long flexor muscle of toe at ankle and foot level, left foot

S96.099 Other injury of muscle and tendon of long flexor muscle of toe at ankle and foot level, unspecified foot

S96.1 Injury of muscle and tendon of long extensor muscle of toe at ankle and foot level

S96.10 Unspecified injury of muscle and tendon of long extensor muscle of toe at ankle and foot level

S96.101 Unspecified injury of muscle and tendon of long extensor muscle of toe at ankle and foot level, right foot

S96.102 Unspecified injury of muscle and tendon of long extensor muscle of toe at ankle and foot level, left foot

S96.109 Unspecified injury of muscle and tendon of long extensor muscle of toe at ankle and foot level, unspecified foot

S96.11 Strain of muscle and tendon of long extensor muscle of toe at ankle and foot level

S96.111 Strain of muscle and tendon of long extensor muscle of toe at ankle and foot level, right foot

S96.112 Strain of muscle and tendon of long extensor muscle of toe at ankle and foot level, left foot

S96.119 Strain of muscle and tendon of long extensor muscle of toe at ankle and foot level, unspecified foot

S96.12 Laceration of muscle and tendon of long extensor muscle of toe at ankle and foot level

S96.121 Laceration of muscle and tendon of long extensor muscle of toe at ankle and foot level, right foot A (Ex) PDX 1874

S96.122 Laceration of muscle and tendon of long extensor muscle of toe at ankle and foot level, left foot A (Ex) PDX 1875

S96.129 Laceration of muscle and tendon of long extensor muscle of toe at ankle and foot level, unspecified foot A (Ex) PDX 1876

S96.19 Other specified injury of muscle and tendon of long extensor muscle of toe at ankle and foot level

S96.191 Other specified injury of muscle and tendon of long extensor muscle of toe at ankle and foot level, right foot

S96.192 Other specified injury of muscle and tendon of long extensor muscle of toe at ankle and foot level, left foot

S96.199 Other specified injury of muscle and tendon of long extensor muscle of toe at ankle and foot level, unspecified foot

S96.2 Injury of intrinsic muscle and tendon at ankle and foot level

S96.20 Unspecified injury of intrinsic muscle and tendon at ankle and foot level

S96.201 Unspecified injury of intrinsic muscle and tendon at ankle and foot level, right foot

S96.202 Unspecified injury of intrinsic muscle and tendon at ankle and foot level, left foot

S96.209 Unspecified injury of intrinsic muscle and tendon at ankle and foot level, unspecified foot

S96.21 Strain of intrinsic muscle and tendon at ankle and foot level

S96.211 Strain of intrinsic muscle and tendon at ankle and foot level, right foot

S96.212 Strain of intrinsic muscle and tendon at ankle and foot level, left foot

S96.219 Strain of intrinsic muscle and tendon at ankle and foot level, unspecified foot

S96.22 Laceration of intrinsic muscle and tendon at ankle and foot level

S96.221 Laceration of intrinsic muscle and tendon at ankle and foot level, right foot A (Ex) PDX 1874

S96.222 Laceration of intrinsic muscle and tendon at left ankle and foot level, left foot A (Ex) PDX 1875

S96.229 Laceration of intrinsic muscle and tendon at ankle and foot level, unspecified foot A (Ex) PDX 1876

S96.29 Other specified injury of intrinsic muscle and tendon at ankle and foot level

S96.291 Other specified injury of intrinsic muscle and tendon at ankle and foot level, right foot

S96.292 Other specified injury of intrinsic muscle and tendon at ankle and foot level, left foot

S96.299 Other specified injury of intrinsic muscle and tendon at ankle and foot level, unspecified foot

- S96.8 Injury of other specified muscles and tendons at ankle and foot level
  - S96.80 Unspecified injury of other specified muscles and tendons at ankle and foot level
    - S96.801 Unspecified injury of other specified muscles and tendons at ankle and foot level, right foot
    - S96.802 Unspecified injury of other specified muscles and tendons at ankle and foot level, left foot
    - S96.809 Unspecified injury of other specified muscles and tendons at ankle and foot level, unspecified foot
  - S96.81 Strain of other specified muscles and tendons at ankle and foot level
    - S96.811 Strain of other specified muscles and tendons at ankle and foot level, right foot
    - S96.812 Strain of other specified muscles and tendons at ankle and foot level, left foot
    - S96.819 Strain of other specified muscles and tendons at ankle and foot level, unspecified foot
  - S96.82 Laceration of other specified muscles and tendons at ankle and foot level
    - S96.821 Laceration of other specified muscles and tendons at ankle and foot level, right foot A (Ex:) PDX 1874
    - S96.822 Laceration of other specified muscles and tendons at ankle and foot level, left foot A (Ex:) PDX 1875
    - S96.829 Laceration of other specified muscles and tendons at ankle and foot level, unspecified foot A (Ex:) PDX 1876
  - S96.89 Other specified injury of other specified muscles and tendons at ankle and foot level
    - S96.891 Other specified injury of other specified muscles and tendons at ankle and foot level, right foot
    - S96.892 Other specified injury of other specified muscles and tendons at ankle and foot level, left foot
    - S96.899 Other specified injury of other specified muscles and tendons at ankle and foot level, unspecified foot
- S96.9 Injury of unspecified muscle and tendon at ankle and foot level
  - S96.90 Unspecified injury of unspecified muscle and tendon at ankle and foot level
    - S96.901 Unspecified injury of unspecified muscle and tendon at ankle and foot level, right foot
    - S96.902 Unspecified injury of unspecified muscle and tendon at ankle and foot level, left foot
    - S96.909 Unspecified injury of unspecified muscle and tendon at ankle and foot level, unspecified foot
  - S96.91 Strain of unspecified muscle and tendon at ankle and foot level
    - S96.911 Strain of unspecified muscle and tendon at ankle and foot level, right foot
    - S96.912 Strain of unspecified muscle and tendon at ankle and foot level, left foot
    - S96.919 Strain of unspecified muscle and tendon at ankle and foot level, unspecified foot
  - S96.92 Laceration of unspecified muscle and tendon at ankle and foot level
    - S96.921 Laceration of unspecified muscle and tendon at ankle and foot level, right foot A (Ex:) PDX 1874
    - S96.922 Laceration of unspecified muscle and tendon at ankle and foot level, left foot A (Ex:) PDX 1875
    - S96.929 Laceration of unspecified muscle and tendon at ankle and foot level, unspecified foot A (Ex:) PDX 1876
  - S96.99 Other specified injury of unspecified muscle and tendon at ankle and foot level
    - S96.991 Other specified injury of unspecified muscle and tendon at ankle and foot level, right foot
    - S96.992 Other specified injury of unspecified muscle and tendon at ankle and foot level, left foot
    - S96.999 Other specified injury of unspecified muscle and tendon at ankle and foot level, unspecified foot

S97 Crushing injury of ankle and foot

Use additional code(s) for all associated injuries

The appropriate 7th character is to be added to each code from category S97

A	initial encounter
D	subsequent encounter
S	sequela

- S97.0 Crushing injury of ankle
  - X S97.00 Crushing injury of unspecified ankle
  - X S97.01 Crushing injury of right ankle
  - X S97.02 Crushing injury of left ankle
- S97.1 Crushing injury of toe
  - S97.10 Crushing injury of unspecified toe(s)
    - S97.101 Crushing injury of unspecified right toe(s)
    - S97.102 Crushing injury of unspecified left toe(s)
    - S97.109 Crushing injury of unspecified toe(s)
      Crushing injury of toe NOS
  - S97.11 Crushing injury of great toe
    - S97.111 Crushing injury of right great toe
    - S97.112 Crushing injury of left great toe
    - S97.119 Crushing injury of unspecified great toe
  - S97.12 Crushing injury of lesser toe(s)
    - S97.121 Crushing injury of right lesser toe(s)
    - S97.122 Crushing injury of left lesser toe(s)
    - S97.129 Crushing injury of lesser toe(s), unspecified toe(s)
- S97.8 Crushing injury of foot
  - X S97.80 Crushing injury of foot, unspecified side
    Crushing injury of foot NOS
  - X S97.81 Crushing injury of right foot
  - X S97.82 Crushing injury of left foot

S98 Traumatic amputation of ankle and foot

An amputation not identified as partial or complete should be coded to complete

The appropriate 7th character is to be added to each code from category S98

A	initial encounter
D	subsequent encounter
S	sequela

CHAPTER 19 (SØØ-T88)

- **S98.0** Traumatic amputation of **foot at ankle level**
  - **S98.01** **Complete** traumatic amputation of foot at ankle level
    - **S98.011** Complete traumatic amputation of **right** foot at ankle level A, A, D, S (Ex) PDX 1843
    - **S98.012** Complete traumatic amputation of **left** foot at ankle level A, A, D, S (Ex) PDX 1844
    - **S98.019** Complete traumatic amputation of **unspecified** foot at ankle level A, A, D, S (Ex) PDX 1845
  - **S98.02** **Partial** traumatic amputation of foot at ankle level
    - **S98.021** Partial traumatic amputation of **right** foot at ankle level A, A, D, S (Ex) PDX 1843
    - **S98.022** Partial traumatic amputation of **left** foot at ankle level A, A, D, S (Ex) PDX 1844
    - **S98.029** Partial traumatic amputation of **unspecified** foot at ankle level A, A, D, S (Ex) PDX 1845
- **S98.1** Traumatic amputation of **one toe**
  - **S98.11** **Complete** traumatic amputation of **great toe**
    - **S98.111** Complete traumatic amputation of **right** great toe A, D, S
    - **S98.112** Complete traumatic amputation of **left** great toe A, D, S
    - **S98.119** Complete traumatic amputation of **unspecified** great toe A, D, S
  - **S98.12** **Partial** traumatic amputation of **great toe**
    - **S98.121** Partial traumatic amputation of **right** great toe A, D, S
    - **S98.122** Partial traumatic amputation of **left** great toe A, D, S
    - **S98.129** Partial traumatic amputation of **unspecified** great toe A, D, S
  - **S98.13** **Complete** traumatic amputation of one **lesser toe**

    Traumatic amputation of toe NOS
    - **S98.131** Complete traumatic amputation of one **right** lesser toe A, D, S
    - **S98.132** Complete traumatic amputation of one **left** lesser toe A, D, S
    - **S98.139** Complete traumatic amputation of one **unspecified** lesser toe A, D, S
  - **S98.14** **Partial** traumatic amputation of one **lesser toe**
    - **S98.141** Partial traumatic amputation of one **right** lesser toe A, D, S
    - **S98.142** Partial traumatic amputation of one **left** lesser toe A, D, S
    - **S98.149** Partial traumatic amputation of one **unspecified** lesser toe A, D, S
- **S98.2** Traumatic amputation of **two or more lesser toes**
  - **S98.21** **Complete** traumatic amputation of two or more **lesser toes**
    - **S98.211** Complete traumatic amputation of two or more **right** lesser toes A, D, S
    - **S98.212** Complete traumatic amputation of two or more **left** lesser toes A, D, S
    - **S98.219** Complete traumatic amputation of two or more **unspecified** lesser toes A, D, S
  - **S98.22** **Partial** traumatic amputation of two or more **lesser toes**
    - **S98.221** Partial traumatic amputation of two or more **right** lesser toes A, D, S
    - **S98.222** Partial traumatic amputation of two or more **left** lesser toes A, D, S
    - **S98.229** Partial traumatic amputation of two or more **unspecified** lesser toes A, D, S
- **S98.3** Traumatic amputation of **midfoot**
  - **S98.31** **Complete** traumatic amputation of midfoot
    - **S98.311** Complete traumatic amputation of **right** midfoot A, A, D, S (Ex) PDX 1843
    - **S98.312** Complete traumatic amputation of **left** midfoot A, A, D, S (Ex) PDX 1844
    - **S98.319** Complete traumatic amputation of **unspecified** midfoot A, A, D, S (Ex) PDX 1845
  - **S98.32** **Partial** traumatic amputation of midfoot
    - **S98.321** Partial traumatic amputation of **right** midfoot A, A, D, S (Ex) PDX 1843
    - **S98.322** Partial traumatic amputation of **left** midfoot A, A, D, S (Ex) PDX 1844
    - **S98.329** Partial traumatic amputation of **unspecified** midfoot A, A, D, S (Ex) PDX 1845
- **S98.9** Traumatic amputation of foot, **level unspecified**
  - **S98.91** **Complete** traumatic amputation of foot, level unspecified
    - **S98.911** Complete traumatic amputation of **right** foot, level unspecified A, A, D, S (Ex) PDX 1843
    - **S98.912** Complete traumatic amputation of **left** foot, level unspecified A, A, D, S (Ex) PDX 1844
    - **S98.919** Complete traumatic amputation of **unspecified** foot, level unspecified A, A, D, S (Ex) PDX 1845
  - **S98.92** **Partial** traumatic amputation of foot, level unspecified
    - **S98.921** Partial traumatic amputation of **right** foot, level unspecified A, A, D, S (Ex) PDX 1843
    - **S98.922** Partial traumatic amputation of **left** foot, level unspecified A, A, D, S (Ex) PDX 1844
    - **S98.929** Partial traumatic amputation of **unspecified** foot, level unspecified A, A, D, S (Ex) PDX 1845

S99 Other and unspecified injuries of ankle and foot

Coding Clinic: 2016, Q4, P68

- **S99.0** **Physeal** fracture of **calcaneus**

  The appropriate 7th character is to be added to each code from subcategories S99.0

A	initial encounter for closed fracture
B	initial encounter for open fracture
D	subsequent encounter for fracture with routine healing
G	subsequent encounter for fracture with delayed healing
K	subsequent encounter for fracture with nonunion
P	subsequent encounter for fracture with malunion
S	sequela

  - **S99.00** **Unspecified** physeal fracture of calcaneus
    - **S99.001** Unspecified physeal fracture of **right** calcaneus
    - **S99.002** Unspecified physeal fracture of **left** calcaneus
    - **S99.009** Unspecified physeal fracture of **unspecified** calcaneus

S99.01 Salter-Harris Type I physeal fracture of calcaneus
Coding Clinic: 2016, Q4, P69
S99.011 Salter-Harris Type I physeal fracture of right calcaneus
S99.012 Salter-Harris Type I physeal fracture of left calcaneus
S99.019 Salter-Harris Type I physeal fracture of unspecified calcaneus
S99.02 Salter-Harris Type II physeal fracture of calcaneus
Coding Clinic: 2016, Q4, P69
S99.021 Salter-Harris Type II physeal fracture of right calcaneus
S99.022 Salter-Harris Type II physeal fracture of left calcaneus
S99.029 Salter-Harris Type II physeal fracture of unspecified calcaneus
S99.03 Salter-Harris Type III physeal fracture of calcaneus
Coding Clinic: 2016, Q4, P69
S99.031 Salter-Harris Type III physeal fracture of right calcaneus
S99.032 Salter-Harris Type III physeal fracture of left calcaneus
S99.039 Salter-Harris Type III physeal fracture of unspecified calcaneus
S99.04 Salter-Harris Type IV physeal fracture of calcaneus
Coding Clinic: 2016, Q4, P69
S99.041 Salter-Harris Type IV physeal fracture of right calcaneus
S99.042 Salter-Harris Type IV physeal fracture of left calcaneus
S99.049 Salter-Harris Type IV physeal fracture of unspecified calcaneus
S99.09 Other physeal fracture of calcaneus
Coding Clinic: 2016, Q4, P69
S99.091 Other physeal fracture of right calcaneus
S99.092 Other physeal fracture of left calcaneus
S99.099 Other physeal fracture of unspecified calcaneus

S99.1 Physeal fracture of metatarsal
The appropriate 7th character is to be added to each code from subcategories S99.1

A	initial encounter for closed fracture
B	initial encounter for open fracture
D	subsequent encounter for fracture with routine healing
G	subsequent encounter for fracture with delayed healing
K	subsequent encounter for fracture with nonunion
P	subsequent encounter for fracture with malunion
S	sequela

S99.10 Unspecified physeal fracture of metatarsal
S99.101 Unspecified physeal fracture of right metatarsal
S99.102 Unspecified physeal fracture of left metatarsal
S99.109 Unspecified physeal fracture of unspecified metatarsal
S99.11 Salter-Harris Type I physeal fracture of metatarsal
Coding Clinic: 2016, Q4, P69
S99.111 Salter-Harris Type I physeal fracture of right metatarsal
S99.112 Salter-Harris Type I physeal fracture of left metatarsal
Coding Clinic: 2018, Q1, P3
S99.119 Salter-Harris Type I physeal fracture of unspecified metatarsal
S99.12 Salter-Harris Type II physeal fracture of metatarsal
Coding Clinic: 2016, Q4, P69
S99.121 Salter-Harris Type II physeal fracture of right metatarsal
S99.122 Salter-Harris Type II physeal fracture of left metatarsal
S99.129 Salter-Harris Type II physeal fracture of unspecified metatarsal
S99.13 Salter-Harris Type III physeal fracture of metatarsal
Coding Clinic: 2016, Q4, P69
S99.131 Salter-Harris Type III physeal fracture of right metatarsal
S99.132 Salter-Harris Type III physeal fracture of left metatarsal
S99.139 Salter-Harris Type III physeal fracture of unspecified metatarsal
S99.14 Salter-Harris Type IV physeal fracture of metatarsal
Coding Clinic: 2016, Q4, P69
S99.141 Salter-Harris Type IV physeal fracture of right metatarsal
S99.142 Salter-Harris Type IV physeal fracture of left metatarsal
S99.149 Salter-Harris Type IV physeal fracture of unspecified metatarsal
S99.19 Other physeal fracture of metatarsal
Coding Clinic: 2016, Q4, P69
S99.191 Other physeal fracture of right metatarsal
S99.192 Other physeal fracture of left metatarsal
S99.199 Other physeal fracture of unspecified metatarsal

S99.2 Physeal fracture of phalanx of toe
The appropriate 7th character is to be added to each code from subcategories S99.2

A	initial encounter for closed fracture
B	initial encounter for open fracture
D	subsequent encounter for fracture with routine healing
G	subsequent encounter for fracture with delayed healing
K	subsequent encounter for fracture with nonunion
P	subsequent encounter for fracture with malunion
S	sequela

S99.20 Unspecified physeal fracture of phalanx of toe
S99.201 Unspecified physeal fracture of phalanx of right toe
S99.202 Unspecified physeal fracture of phalanx of right toe
S99.209 Unspecified physeal fracture of phalanx of unspecified toe

CHAPTER 19 (S00-T88)

New | Revised | deleted Deleted | Excludes 1 | Excludes 2 | Includes | Use additional | Code first | Code also | Key words
OGCR Official Guidelines | Unacceptable Principal Diagnosis | X Assign placeholder X | Use Additional Character(s) | Manifestation Code | Coding Clinic

● S99.21 Salter-Harris Type I physeal fracture of phalanx of toe
Coding Clinic: 2016, Q4, P69
● S99.211 Salter-Harris Type I physeal fracture of phalanx of right toe
● S99.212 Salter-Harris Type I physeal fracture of phalanx of left toe
● S99.219 Salter-Harris Type I physeal fracture of phalanx of unspecified toe

● S99.22 Salter-Harris Type II physeal fracture of phalanx of toe
Coding Clinic: 2016, Q4, P69
● S99.221 Salter-Harris Type II physeal fracture of phalanx of right toe
● S99.222 Salter-Harris Type II physeal fracture of phalanx of left toe
● S99.229 Salter-Harris Type II physeal fracture of phalanx of unspecified toe

● S99.23 Salter-Harris Type III physeal fracture of phalanx of toe
Coding Clinic: 2016, Q4, P69
● S99.231 Salter-Harris Type III physeal fracture of phalanx of right toe
● S99.232 Salter-Harris Type III physeal fracture of phalanx of left toe
● S99.239 Salter-Harris Type III physeal fracture of phalanx of unspecified toe

● S99.24 Salter-Harris Type IV physeal fracture of phalanx of toe
Coding Clinic: 2016, Q4, P69
● S99.241 Salter-Harris Type IV physeal fracture of phalanx of right toe
● S99.242 Salter-Harris Type IV physeal fracture of phalanx of left toe
● S99.249 Salter-Harris Type IV physeal fracture of phalanx of unspecified toe

● S99.29 Other physeal fracture of phalanx of toe
Coding Clinic: 2016, Q4, P69
● S99.291 Other physeal fracture of phalanx of right toe
● S99.292 Other physeal fracture of phalanx of left toe
● S99.299 Other physeal fracture of phalanx of unspecified toe

● S99.8 Other specified injuries of ankle and foot
The appropriate 7th character is to be added to each code from subcategory S99.8

A initial encounter
D subsequent encounter
S sequela

● S99.81 Other specified injuries of ankle
● S99.811 Other specified injuries of right ankle
● S99.812 Other specified injuries of left ankle
● S99.819 Other specified injuries of unspecified ankle

● S99.82 Other specified injuries of foot
● S99.821 Other specified injuries of right foot
● S99.822 Other specified injuries of left foot
● S99.829 Other specified injuries of unspecified foot

● S99.9 Unspecified injury of ankle and foot
The appropriate 7th character is to be added to each code from subcategory S99.9

A initial encounter
D subsequent encounter
S sequela

● S99.91 Unspecified injury of ankle
● S99.911 Unspecified injury of right ankle
● S99.912 Unspecified injury of left ankle
● S99.919 Unspecified injury of unspecified ankle

● S99.92 Unspecified injury of foot
● S99.921 Unspecified injury of right foot
● S99.922 Unspecified injury of left foot
● S99.929 Unspecified injury of unspecified foot

INJURY, POISONING AND CERTAIN OTHER CONSEQUENCES OF EXTERNAL CAUSES (T07-T88)

INJURIES INVOLVING MULTIPLE BODY REGIONS (T07)

Excludes1 burns and corrosions (T20-T32)
frostbite (T33-T34)
insect bite or sting, venomous (T63.4)
sunburn (L55.-)

X● T07 Unspecified multiple injuries
The appropriate 7th character is to be added to code T07

A initial encounter
D subsequent encounter
S sequela

Excludes1 injury NOS (T14.90)

INJURY OF UNSPECIFIED BODY REGION (T14)

● T14 Injury of unspecified body region
The appropriate 7th character is to be added to each code from category T14

A initial encounter
D subsequent encounter
S sequela

Excludes1 multiple unspecified injuries (T07)

X● T14.8 Other injury of unspecified body region
Abrasion NOS
Contusion NOS
Crush injury NOS
Fracture NOS
Skin injury NOS
Vascular injury NOS
Wound NOS

● T14.9 Unspecified injury
X● T14.90 Injury, unspecified
Injury NOS
X● T14.91 Suicide attempt A, D, S
Attempted suicide NOS

CHAPTER 19 (S00-T88)

EFFECTS OF FOREIGN BODY ENTERING THROUGH NATURAL ORIFICE (T15-T19)

Use additional code, if known, for foreign body entering into or through a natural orifice (W44.-)

Excludes2 foreign body accidentally left in operation wound (T81.5-)
foreign body in penetrating wound - see open wound by body region
residual foreign body in soft tissue (M79.5)
splinter, without open wound - see superficial injury by body region

●**T15 Foreign body on external eye**

Excludes2 foreign body in penetrating wound of orbit and eye ball (S05.4-, S05.5-)
open wound of eyelid and periocular area (S01.1-)
retained foreign body in eyelid (H02.8-)
retained (old) foreign body in penetrating wound of orbit and eye ball (H05.5-, H44.6-, H44.7-)
superficial foreign body of eyelid and periocular area (S00.25-)

The appropriate 7th character is to be added to each code from category T15

A	initial encounter
D	subsequent encounter
S	sequela

●**T15.0 Foreign body in cornea**
X●**T15.00 Foreign body in cornea, unspecified eye**
X●**T15.01 Foreign body in cornea, right eye**
X●**T15.02 Foreign body in cornea, left eye**

●**T15.1 Foreign body in conjunctival sac**
X●**T15.10 Foreign body in conjunctival sac, unspecified eye**
X●**T15.11 Foreign body in conjunctival sac, right eye**
X●**T15.12 Foreign body in conjunctival sac, left eye**

●**T15.8 Foreign body in other and multiple parts of external eye**
Foreign body in lacrimal punctum
X●**T15.80 Foreign body in other and multiple parts of external eye, unspecified eye**
X●**T15.81 Foreign body in other and multiple parts of external eye, right eye**
X●**T15.82 Foreign body in other and multiple parts of external eye, left eye**

●**T15.9 Foreign body on external eye, part unspecified**
X●**T15.90 Foreign body on external eye, part unspecified, unspecified eye**
X●**T15.91 Foreign body on external eye, part unspecified, right eye**
X●**T15.92 Foreign body on external eye, part unspecified, left eye**

●**T16 Foreign body in ear**

Includes foreign body in auditory canal

The appropriate 7th character is to be added to each code from category T16

A	initial encounter
D	subsequent encounter
S	sequela

X●**T16.1 Foreign body in right ear**
X●**T16.2 Foreign body in left ear**
X●**T16.9 Foreign body in ear, unspecified ear**

●**T17 Foreign body in respiratory tract**

The appropriate 7th character is to be added to each code from category T17

A	initial encounter
D	subsequent encounter
S	sequela

X●**T17.0 Foreign body in nasal sinus**
X●**T17.1 Foreign body in nostril**
Foreign body in nose NOS

●**T17.2 Foreign body in pharynx**
Foreign body in nasopharynx
Foreign body in throat NOS
●**T17.20 Unspecified foreign body in pharynx**
●**T17.200 Unspecified foreign body in pharynx causing asphyxiation**
●**T17.208 Unspecified foreign body in pharynx causing other injury**
●**T17.21 Gastric contents in pharynx**
Aspiration of gastric contents into pharynx
Vomitus in pharynx
●**T17.210 Gastric contents in pharynx causing asphyxiation**
●**T17.218 Gastric contents in pharynx causing other injury**
●**T17.22 Food in pharynx**
Bones in pharynx
Seeds in pharynx
●**T17.220 Food in pharynx causing asphyxiation**
●**T17.228 Food in pharynx causing other injury**
●**T17.29 Other foreign object in pharynx**
●**T17.290 Other foreign object in pharynx causing asphyxiation**
●**T17.298 Other foreign object in pharynx causing other injury**

●**T17.3 Foreign body in larynx**
●**T17.30 Unspecified foreign body in larynx**
●**T17.300 Unspecified foreign body in larynx causing asphyxiation**
●**T17.308 Unspecified foreign body in larynx causing other injury**
●**T17.31 Gastric contents in larynx**
Aspiration of gastric contents into larynx
Vomitus in larynx
●**T17.310 Gastric contents in larynx causing asphyxiation**
●**T17.318 Gastric contents in larynx causing other injury**
●**T17.32 Food in larynx**
Bones in larynx
Seeds in larynx
●**T17.320 Food in larynx causing asphyxiation**
●**T17.328 Food in larynx causing other injury**
●**T17.39 Other foreign object in larynx**
●**T17.390 Other foreign object in larynx causing asphyxiation**
●**T17.398 Other foreign object in larynx causing other injury**

●**T17.4 Foreign body in trachea** (Ex) PDX 1883
●**T17.40 Unspecified foreign body in trachea**
●**T17.400 Unspecified foreign body in trachea causing asphyxiation** A
●**T17.408 Unspecified foreign body in trachea causing other injury** A

● T17.41 Gastric contents in trachea
Aspiration of gastric contents into trachea
Vomitus in trachea
● T17.410 Gastric contents in trachea causing asphyxiation A
● T17.418 Gastric contents in trachea causing other injury A
● T17.42 Food in trachea
Bones in trachea
Seeds in trachea
● T17.420 Food in trachea causing asphyxiation A
● T17.428 Food in trachea causing other injury A
● T17.49 Other foreign object in trachea
● T17.490 Other foreign object in trachea causing asphyxiation A
● T17.498 Other foreign object in trachea causing other injury A
● T17.5 Foreign body in bronchus (Ex:) PDX 1884
● T17.50 Unspecified foreign body in bronchus
● T17.500 Unspecified foreign body in bronchus causing asphyxiation A
● T17.508 Unspecified foreign body in bronchus causing other injury A
● T17.51 Gastric contents in bronchus
Aspiration of gastric contents into bronchus
Vomitus in bronchus
● T17.510 Gastric contents in bronchus causing asphyxiation A
● T17.518 Gastric contents in bronchus causing other injury A
● T17.52 Food in bronchus
Bones in bronchus
Seeds in bronchus
● T17.520 Food in bronchus causing asphyxiation A
● T17.528 Food in bronchus causing other injury A
● T17.59 Other foreign object in bronchus
● T17.590 Other foreign object in bronchus causing asphyxiation A
● T17.598 Other foreign object in bronchus causing other injury A
● T17.8 Foreign body in other parts of respiratory tract (Ex:) PDX 1884
Foreign body in bronchioles
Foreign body in lung
● T17.80 Unspecified foreign body in other parts of respiratory tract
● T17.800 Unspecified foreign body in other parts of respiratory tract causing asphyxiation A
● T17.808 Unspecified foreign body in other parts of respiratory tract causing other injury A
● T17.81 Gastric contents in other parts of respiratory tract
Aspiration of gastric contents into other parts of respiratory tract
Vomitus in other parts of respiratory tract
● T17.810 Gastric contents in other parts of respiratory tract causing asphyxiation A
● T17.818 Gastric contents in other parts of respiratory tract causing other injury A
● T17.82 Food in other parts of respiratory tract
Bones in other parts of respiratory tract
Seeds in other parts of respiratory tract
● T17.820 Food in other parts of respiratory tract causing asphyxiation A
● T17.828 Food in other parts of respiratory tract causing other injury A
● T17.89 Other foreign object in other parts of respiratory tract
● T17.890 Other foreign object in other parts of respiratory tract causing asphyxiation A
● T17.898 Other foreign object in other parts of respiratory tract causing other injury A
● T17.9 Foreign body in respiratory tract, part unspecified
● T17.90 Unspecified foreign body in respiratory tract, part unspecified
● T17.900 Unspecified foreign body in respiratory tract, part unspecified causing asphyxiation
● T17.908 Unspecified foreign body in respiratory tract, part unspecified causing other injury
● T17.91 Gastric contents in respiratory tract, part unspecified
Aspiration of gastric contents into respiratory tract, part unspecified
Vomitus in trachea respiratory tract, part unspecified
● T17.910 Gastric contents in respiratory tract, part unspecified causing asphyxiation
● T17.918 Gastric contents in respiratory tract, part unspecified causing other injury
● T17.92 Food in respiratory tract, part unspecified
Bones in respiratory tract, part unspecified
Seeds in respiratory tract, part unspecified
● T17.920 Food in respiratory tract, part unspecified causing asphyxiation
● T17.928 Food in respiratory tract, part unspecified causing other injury
● T17.99 Other foreign object in respiratory tract, part unspecified
● T17.990 Other foreign object in respiratory tract, part unspecified in causing asphyxiation
Coding Clinic: 2019, Q3, P15
● T17.998 Other foreign object in respiratory tract, part unspecified causing other injury

● T18 Foreign body in alimentary tract
Excludes2 foreign body in pharynx (T17.2-)
The appropriate 7th character is to be added to each code from category T18

A	initial encounter
D	subsequent encounter
S	sequela

X● T18.0 Foreign body in mouth
X● T18.1 Foreign body in esophagus
Excludes2 foreign body in respiratory tract (T17.-)
● T18.10 Unspecified foreign body in esophagus
● T18.100 Unspecified foreign body in esophagus causing compression of trachea
Unspecified foreign body in esophagus causing obstruction of respiration
● T18.108 Unspecified foreign body in esophagus causing other injury

CHAPTER 19 (S00-T88)

- ● T18.11 **Gastric contents in esophagus**
  Vomitus in esophagus
  - ● T18.110 **Gastric contents in esophagus causing compression of trachea**
    Gastric contents in esophagus causing obstruction of respiration
  - ● T18.118 **Gastric contents in esophagus causing other injury**
- ● T18.12 **Food in esophagus**
  Bones in esophagus
  Seeds in esophagus
  - ● T18.120 **Food in esophagus causing compression of trachea**
    Food in esophagus causing obstruction of respiration
  - ● T18.128 **Food in esophagus causing other injury**
- ● T18.19 **Other foreign object in esophagus**
  - ● T18.190 **Other foreign object in esophagus causing compression of trachea**
    Other foreign body in esophagus causing obstruction of respiration
    Coding Clinic: 2015, Q1, P24
  - ● T18.198 **Other foreign object in esophagus causing other injury**
    Coding Clinic: 2015, Q1, P24
- X● T18.2 **Foreign body in stomach**
- X● T18.3 **Foreign body in small intestine**
- X● T18.4 **Foreign body in colon**
- X● T18.5 **Foreign body in anus and rectum**
  Foreign body in rectosigmoid (junction)
- X● T18.8 **Foreign body in other parts of alimentary tract**
- X● T18.9 **Foreign body of alimentary tract, part unspecified**
  Foreign body in digestive system NOS
  Swallowed foreign body NOS

● T19 **Foreign body in genitourinary tract**

Excludes2 complications due to implanted mesh (T83.7-)
mechanical complications of contraceptive device (intrauterine) (vaginal) (T83.3-)
presence of contraceptive device (intrauterine) (vaginal) (Z97.5)

The appropriate 7th character is to be added to each code from category T19

A	initial encounter
D	subsequent encounter
S	sequela

- X● T19.0 **Foreign body in urethra**
- X● T19.1 **Foreign body in bladder**
- X● T19.2 **Foreign body in vulva and vagina**
- X● T19.3 **Foreign body in uterus**
- X● T19.4 **Foreign body in penis**
- X● T19.8 **Foreign body in other parts of genitourinary tract**
- X● T19.9 **Foreign body in genitourinary tract, part unspecified**

BURNS AND CORROSIONS (T20-T32)

Includes burns (thermal) from electrical heating appliances
burns (thermal) from electricity
burns (thermal) from flame
burns (thermal) from friction
burns (thermal) from hot air and hot gases
burns (thermal) from hot objects
burns (thermal) from lightning
burns (thermal) from radiation chemical
burn [corrosion] (external) (internal) scalds

Excludes2 erythema [dermatitis] ab igne (L59.0)
radiation-related disorders of the skin and subcutaneous tissue (L55-L59)
sunburn (L55.-)

OGCR Section I.C.19.d.

Burns and Corrosions

The ICD-10-CM makes a distinction between burn and corrosions. The burn codes are for thermal burns, except sunburns, that come from a heat source, such as a fire or hot appliance. The burn codes are also for burns resulting from electricity and radiation. Corrosions are burns due to chemicals. The guidelines for burns and corrosions are the same.

Current burns (T20-T25) are classified by depth, extent and by agent (X code). Burns are classified by depth as first degree (erythema), second degree (blistering), and third degree (full-thickness involvement). Burns of the eye and internal organs (T26-T28) are classified by site, but not by degree.

1) Sequencing of burn and related condition codes

Sequence first the code that reflects the highest degree of burn when more than one burn is present.

a. When the reason for the admission or encounter is for treatment of external multiple burns, sequence first the code that reflects the burn of the highest degree.

b. When a patient has both internal and external burns, the circumstances of admission govern the selection of the principal diagnosis or first-listed diagnosis.

c. When a patient is admitted for burn injuries and other related conditions such as smoke inhalation and/or respiratory failure, the circumstances of admission govern the selection of the principal or first-listed diagnosis.

2) Burns of the same local site

Classify burns of the same local site (three-character category level, T20-T28) but of different degrees to the subcategory identifying the highest degree recorded in the diagnosis.

BURNS AND CORROSIONS OF EXTERNAL BODY SURFACE, SPECIFIED BY SITE (T20-T25)

Includes burns and corrosions of first degree [erythema]
burns and corrosions of second degree [blisters] [epidermal loss]
burns and corrosions of third degree [deep necrosis of underlying tissue] [full-thickness skin loss]

Use additional code from category T31 or T32 to identify extent of body surface involved

● T20 **Burn and corrosion of head, face, and neck**

Excludes2 burn and corrosion of ear drum (T28.41, T28.91)
burn and corrosion of eye and adnexa (T26.-)
burn and corrosion of mouth and pharynx (T28.0)

The appropriate 7th character is to be added to each code from category T20

A	initial encounter
D	subsequent encounter
S	sequela

- ● T20.0 **Burn of unspecified degree of head, face, and neck**
  Use additional external cause code to identify the source, place and intent of the burn (X00-X19, X75-X77, X96-X98, Y92)
  - X● T20.00 **Burn of unspecified degree of head, face, and neck, unspecified site**
  - ● T20.01 **Burn of unspecified degree of ear [any part, except ear drum]**
    Excludes2 burn of ear drum (T28.41-)
    - ● T20.011 **Burn of unspecified degree of right ear [any part, except ear drum]**
    - ● T20.012 **Burn of unspecified degree of left ear [any part, except ear drum]**
    - ● T20.019 **Burn of unspecified degree of unspecified ear [any part, except ear drum]**

▶ New ➡ Revised ~~deleted~~ Deleted Excludes 1 Excludes 2 Includes Use additional Code first Code also Key words
OGCR Official Guidelines ● Unacceptable Principal Diagnosis X Assign placeholder X ● Use Additional Character(s) ◗ Manifestation Code Coding Clinic

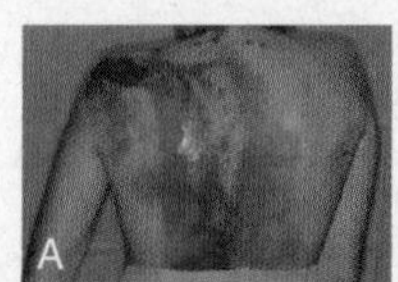

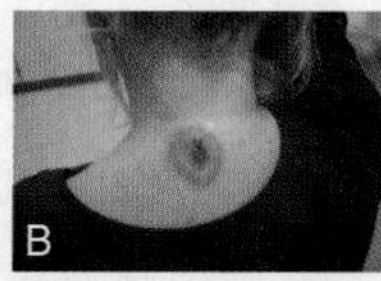

Figure 19-15 **A.** Second-degree burn. **B.** Third-degree burn. (A. From Black J, Hawks J: Medical-Surgical Nursing: Clinical Management for Positive Outcomes, 8e, Saunders, 2008. B. From Marx J, Hockberger R, Walls R: Rosen's Emergency Medicine - Concepts and Clinical Practice, 7e, Mosby, 2009)

X● **T20.02** **Burn of unspecified degree of lip(s)**
X● **T20.03** **Burn of unspecified degree of chin**
X● **T20.04** **Burn of unspecified degree of nose (septum)**
X● **T20.05** **Burn of unspecified degree of scalp [any part]**
X● **T20.06** **Burn of unspecified degree of forehead and cheek**
X● **T20.07** **Burn of unspecified degree of neck**
X● **T20.09** **Burn of unspecified degree of multiple sites of head, face, and neck**

● **T20.1** **Burn of first degree of head, face, and neck**
Use additional external cause code to identify the source, place and intent of the burn (X00-X19, X75-X77, X96-X98, Y92)

X● **T20.10** **Burn of first degree of head, face, and neck, unspecified site**
● **T20.11** **Burn of first degree of ear [any part, except ear drum]**
Excludes2 burn of ear drum (T28.41-)
● **T20.111** **Burn of first degree of right ear [any part, except ear drum]**
● **T20.112** **Burn of first degree of left ear [any part, except ear drum]**
● **T20.119** **Burn of first degree of unspecified ear [any part, except ear drum]**
X● **T20.12** **Burn of first degree of lip(s)**
X● **T20.13** **Burn of first degree of chin**
X● **T20.14** **Burn of first degree of nose (septum)**
X● **T20.15** **Burn of first degree of scalp [any part]**
X● **T20.16** **Burn of first degree of forehead and cheek**
X● **T20.17** **Burn of first degree of neck**
X● **T20.19** **Burn of first degree of multiple sites of head, face, and neck**

● **T20.2** **Burn of second degree of head, face, and neck**
Use additional external cause code to identify the source, place and intent of the burn (X00-X19, X75-X77, X96-X98, Y92)

X● **T20.20** **Burn of second degree of head, face, and neck, unspecified site**
● **T20.21** **Burn of second degree of ear [any part, except ear drum]**
Excludes2 burn of ear drum (T28.41-)
● **T20.211** **Burn of second degree of right ear [any part, except ear drum]**
● **T20.212** **Burn of second degree of left ear [any part, except ear drum]**
● **T20.219** **Burn of second degree of unspecified ear [any part, except ear drum]**
X● **T20.22** **Burn of second degree of lip(s)**
X● **T20.23** **Burn of second degree of chin**
X● **T20.24** **Burn of second degree of nose (septum)**
X● **T20.25** **Burn of second degree of scalp [any part]**
Coding Clinic: 2015, Q1, P19
X● **T20.26** **Burn of second degree of forehead and cheek**
X● **T20.27** **Burn of second degree of neck**
X● **T20.29** **Burn of second degree of multiple sites of head, face, and neck**

● **T20.3** **Burn of third degree of head, face, and neck**
Use additional external cause code to identify the source, place and intent of the burn (X00-X19, X75-X77, X96-X98, Y92)

X● **T20.30** **Burn of third degree of head, face, and neck, unspecified site** A, A (Ex) See PDX 1885
● **T20.31** **Burn of third degree of ear [any part, except ear drum]** (Ex) PDX 1886
Excludes2 burn of ear drum (T28.41-)
● **T20.311** **Burn of third degree of right ear [any part, except ear drum]** A, A
● **T20.312** **Burn of third degree of left ear [any part, except ear drum]** A, A
Coding Clinic: 2015, Q1, P18
● **T20.319** **Burn of third degree of unspecified ear [any part, except ear drum]** A, A
X● **T20.32** **Burn of third degree of lip(s)** A, A (Ex) PDX 1887
X● **T20.33** **Burn of third degree of chin** A, A (Ex) PDX 1888
X● **T20.34** **Burn of third degree of nose (septum)** A, A (Ex) PDX 1889
X● **T20.35** **Burn of third degree of scalp [any part]** A, A (Ex) PDX 1890
X● **T20.36** **Burn of third degree of forehead and cheek** A, A (Ex) PDX 1891
X● **T20.37** **Burn of third degree of neck** A, A (Ex) PDX 1892
X● **T20.39** **Burn of third degree of multiple sites of head, face, and neck** A, A (Ex) PDX 1893

● **T20.4** **Corrosion of unspecified degree of head, face, and neck**
Code first (T51-T65) to identify chemical and intent
Use additional external cause code to identify place (Y92)

X● **T20.40** **Corrosion of unspecified degree of head, face, and neck, unspecified site**
● **T20.41** **Corrosion of unspecified degree of ear [any part, except ear drum]**
Excludes2 corrosion of ear drum (T28.91-)
● **T20.411** **Corrosion of unspecified degree of right ear [any part, except ear drum]**
● **T20.412** **Corrosion of unspecified degree of left ear [any part, except ear drum]**
● **T20.419** **Corrosion of unspecified degree of unspecified ear [any part, except ear drum]**
X● **T20.42** **Corrosion of unspecified degree of lip(s)**
X● **T20.43** **Corrosion of unspecified degree of chin**
X● **T20.44** **Corrosion of unspecified degree of nose (septum)**
X● **T20.45** **Corrosion of unspecified degree of scalp [any part]**
X● **T20.46** **Corrosion of unspecified degree of forehead and cheek**
X● **T20.47** **Corrosion of unspecified degree of neck**
X● **T20.49** **Corrosion of unspecified degree of multiple sites of head, face, and neck**

● **T20.5** Corrosion of **first degree** of head, face, and neck
Code first (T51-T65) *to identify chemical and intent*
Use additional external cause code to identify place (Y92)

X● **T20.50** Corrosion of first degree of head, face, and neck, **unspecified** site

● **T20.51** Corrosion of first degree of **ear** [any part, except ear drum]
Excludes2 corrosion of ear drum (T28.91-)

● **T20.511** Corrosion of first degree of **right** ear [any part, except ear drum]

● **T20.512** Corrosion of first degree of **left** ear [any part, except ear drum]

● **T20.519** Corrosion of first degree of **unspecified** ear [any part, except ear drum]

X● **T20.52** Corrosion of first degree of **lip(s)**

X● **T20.53** Corrosion of first degree of **chin**

X● **T20.54** Corrosion of first degree of **nose** (septum)

X● **T20.55** Corrosion of first degree of **scalp** [any part]

X● **T20.56** Corrosion of first degree of **forehead and cheek**

X● **T20.57** Corrosion of first degree of **neck**

X● **T20.59** Corrosion of first degree of **multiple sites** of head, face, and neck

● **T20.6** Corrosion of **second degree** of head, face, and neck
Code first (T51-T65) *to identify chemical and intent*
Use additional external cause code to identify place (Y92)

X● **T20.60** Corrosion of second degree of head, face, and neck, **unspecified** site

● **T20.61** Corrosion of second degree of **ear** [any part, except ear drum]
Excludes2 corrosion of ear drum (T28.91-)

● **T20.611** Corrosion of second degree of **right** ear [any part, except ear drum]

● **T20.612** Corrosion of second degree of **left** ear [any part, except ear drum]

● **T20.619** Corrosion of second degree of **unspecified** ear [any part, except ear drum]

X● **T20.62** Corrosion of second degree of **lip(s)**

X● **T20.63** Corrosion of second degree of **chin**

X● **T20.64** Corrosion of second degree of **nose** (septum)

X● **T20.65** Corrosion of second degree of **scalp** [any part]

X● **T20.66** Corrosion of second degree of **forehead and cheek**

X● **T20.67** Corrosion of second degree of **neck**

X● **T20.69** Corrosion of second degree of **multiple sites** of head, face, and neck

● **T20.7** Corrosion of **third degree** of head, face, and neck
Code first (T51-T65) *to identify chemical and intent*
Use additional external cause code to identify place (Y92)

X● **T20.70** Corrosion of third degree of head, face, and neck, **unspecified** site A, A Ex PDX 1885

● **T20.71** Corrosion of third degree of **ear** [any part, except ear drum] Ex PDX 1886
Excludes2 corrosion of ear drum (T28.91-)

● **T20.711** Corrosion of third degree of **right** ear [any part, except ear drum] A, A

● **T20.712** Corrosion of third degree of **left** ear [any part, except ear drum] A, A

● **T20.719** Corrosion of third degree of **unspecified** ear [any part, except ear drum] A, A

X● **T20.72** Corrosion of third degree of **lip(s)** A, A Ex PDX 1887

X● **T20.73** Corrosion of third degree of **chin** A, A Ex PDX 1888

X● **T20.74** Corrosion of third degree of **nose** (septum) A, A Ex PDX 1889

X● **T20.75** Corrosion of third degree of **scalp** [any part] A, A Ex PDX 1890

X● **T20.76** Corrosion of third degree of **forehead and cheek** A, A Ex PDX 1891

X● **T20.77** Corrosion of third degree of **neck** A, A Ex PDX 1892

X● **T20.79** Corrosion of third degree of **multiple sites** of head, face, and neck A, A Ex PDX 1893

● **T21** **Burn and corrosion of trunk**
Includes burns and corrosion of hip region
Excludes2 burns and corrosion of axilla (T22.- with fifth character 4)
burns and corrosion of scapular region (T22.- with fifth character 6)
burns and corrosion of shoulder (T22.- with fifth character 5)

The appropriate 7th character is to be added to each code from category T21

A initial encounter
D subsequent encounter
S sequela

● **T21.0** Burn of **unspecified degree** of trunk
Use additional external cause code to identify the source, place and intent of the burn (X00-X19, X75-X77, X96-X98, Y92)

X● **T21.00** Burn of unspecified degree of trunk, **unspecified** site

X● **T21.01** Burn of unspecified degree of **chest wall**
Burn of unspecified degree of breast

X● **T21.02** Burn of unspecified degree of **abdominal wall**
Burn of unspecified degree of flank
Burn of unspecified degree of groin

X● **T21.03** Burn of unspecified degree of **upper back**
Burn of unspecified degree of interscapular region

X● **T21.04** Burn of unspecified degree of **lower back**

X● **T21.05** Burn of unspecified degree of **buttock**
Burn of unspecified degree of anus

X● **T21.06** Burn of unspecified degree of **male genital region**
Burn of unspecified degree of penis
Burn of unspecified degree of scrotum
Burn of unspecified degree of testis

X● **T21.07** Burn of unspecified degree of **female genital region**
Burn of unspecified degree of labium (majus) (minus)
Burn of unspecified degree of perineum
Burn of unspecified degree of vulva
Excludes2 burn of vagina (T28.3)

X● **T21.09** Burn of unspecified degree of **other site** of trunk

● **T21.1** Burn of **first degree** of trunk
Use additional external cause code to identify the source, place and intent of the burn (X00-X19, X75-X77, X96-X98, Y92)

X● **T21.10** Burn of first degree of trunk, **unspecified** site

X● **T21.11** Burn of first degree of **chest wall**
Burn of first degree of breast

X● **T21.12** Burn of first degree of **abdominal wall**
Burn of first degree of flank
Burn of first degree of groin

X● **T21.13** Burn of first degree of **upper back**
Burn of first degree of interscapular region

X● T21.14 **Burn of first degree of lower back**

X● T21.15 **Burn of first degree of buttock**
Burn of first degree of anus

X● T21.16 **Burn of first degree of male genital region**
Burn of first degree of penis
Burn of first degree of scrotum
Burn of first degree of testis

X● T21.17 **Burn of first degree of female genital region**
Burn of first degree of labium (majus) (minus)
Burn of first degree of perineum
Burn of first degree of vulva
Excludes2 burn of vagina (T28.3)

X● T21.19 **Burn of first degree of other site of trunk**

● T21.2 **Burn of second degree of trunk**
Use additional external cause code to identify the source, place and intent of the burn (X00-X19, X75-X77, X96-X98, Y92)

X● T21.20 **Burn of second degree of trunk, unspecified site**

X● T21.21 **Burn of second degree of chest wall**
Burn of second degree of breast

X● T21.22 **Burn of second degree of abdominal wall**
Burn of second degree of flank
Burn of second degree of groin

X● T21.23 **Burn of second degree of upper back**
Burn of second degree of interscapular region

X● T21.24 **Burn of second degree of lower back**

X● T21.25 **Burn of second degree of buttock**
Burn of second degree of anus

X● T21.26 **Burn of second degree of male genital region**
Burn of second degree of penis
Burn of second degree of scrotum
Burn of second degree of testis

X● T21.27 **Burn of second degree of female genital region**
Burn of second degree of labium (majus) (minus)
Burn of second degree of perineum
Burn of second degree of vulva
Excludes2 burn of vagina (T28.3)

X● T21.29 **Burn of second degree of other site of trunk**

● T21.3 **Burn of third degree of trunk**
Use additional external cause code to identify the source, place and intent of the burn (X00-X19, X75-X77, X96-X98, Y92)

X● T21.30 **Burn of third degree of trunk, unspecified site**
A, A (Ex) PDX 1894

X● T21.31 **Burn of third degree of chest wall** A, A
Burn of third degree of breast (Ex) PDX 1895
Coding Clinic: 2016, Q2, P6

X● T21.32 **Burn of third degree of abdominal wall** A, A (Ex) PDX 1896
Burn of third degree of flank
Burn of third degree of groin

X● T21.33 **Burn of third degree of upper back**
A, A (Ex) PDX 1897
Burn of third degree of interscapular region

X● T21.34 **Burn of third degree of lower back** A, A (Ex) PDX 1897

X● T21.35 **Burn of third degree of buttock** A, A (Ex) PDX 1897
Burn of third degree of anus

X● T21.36 **Burn of third degree of male genital region**
A, A (Ex) PDX 1898
Burn of third degree of penis
Burn of third degree of scrotum
Burn of third degree of testis

X● T21.37 **Burn of third degree of female genital region**
A, A (Ex) PDX 1898
Burn of third degree of labium (majus) (minus)
Burn of third degree of perineum
Burn of third degree of vulva
Excludes2 burn of vagina (T28.3)

X● T21.39 **Burn of third degree of other site of trunk** A, A (Ex) PDX 1894

● T21.4 **Corrosion of unspecified degree of trunk**
Code first *(T51-T65) to identify chemical and intent*
Use additional external cause code to identify place (Y92)

X● T21.40 **Corrosion of unspecified degree of trunk, unspecified site**

X● T21.41 **Corrosion of unspecified degree of chest wall**
Corrosion of unspecified degree of breast

X● T21.42 **Corrosion of unspecified degree of abdominal wall**
Corrosion of unspecified degree of flank
Corrosion of unspecified degree of groin

X● T21.43 **Corrosion of unspecified degree of upper back**
Corrosion of unspecified degree of interscapular region

X● T21.44 **Corrosion of unspecified degree of lower back**

X● T21.45 **Corrosion of unspecified degree of buttock**
Corrosion of unspecified degree of anus

X● T21.46 **Corrosion of unspecified degree of male genital region**
Corrosion of unspecified degree of penis
Corrosion of unspecified degree of scrotum
Corrosion of unspecified degree of testis

X● T21.47 **Corrosion of unspecified degree of female genital region**
Corrosion of unspecified degree of labium (majus) (minus)
Corrosion of unspecified degree of perineum
Corrosion of unspecified degree of vulva
Excludes2 corrosion of vagina (T28.8)

X● T21.49 **Corrosion of unspecified degree of other site of trunk**

● T21.5 **Corrosion of first degree of trunk**
Code first *(T51-T65) to identify chemical and intent*
Use additional external cause code to identify place (Y92)

X● T21.50 **Corrosion of first degree of trunk, unspecified site**

X● T21.51 **Corrosion of first degree of chest wall**
Corrosion of first degree of breast

X● T21.52 **Corrosion of first degree of abdominal wall**
Corrosion of first degree of flank
Corrosion of first degree of groin

X● T21.53 **Corrosion of first degree of upper back**
Corrosion of first degree of interscapular region

X● T21.54 **Corrosion of first degree of lower back**

X● T21.55 **Corrosion of first degree of buttock**
Corrosion of first degree of anus

X● T21.56 **Corrosion of first degree of male genital region**
Corrosion of first degree of penis
Corrosion of first degree of scrotum
Corrosion of first degree of testis

X● T21.57 **Corrosion of first degree of female genital region**
Corrosion of first degree of labium (majus) (minus)
Corrosion of first degree of perineum
Corrosion of first degree of vulva
Excludes2 corrosion of vagina (T28.8)

X● T21.59 **Corrosion of first degree of other site of trunk**

● T21.6 Corrosion of second degree of trunk
Code first (T51-T65) to identify chemical and intent
Use additional external cause code to identify place (Y92)

X● T21.60 **Corrosion of second degree of trunk, unspecified site**

X● T21.61 **Corrosion of second degree of chest wall**
Corrosion of second degree of breast

X● T21.62 **Corrosion of second degree of abdominal wall**
Corrosion of second degree of flank
Corrosion of second degree of groin

X● T21.63 **Corrosion of second degree of upper back**
Corrosion of second degree of interscapular region

X● T21.64 **Corrosion of second degree of lower back**

X● T21.65 **Corrosion of second degree of buttock**
Corrosion of second degree of anus

X● T21.66 **Corrosion of second degree of male genital region**
Corrosion of second degree of penis
Corrosion of second degree of scrotum
Corrosion of second degree of testis

X● T21.67 **Corrosion of second degree of female genital region**
Corrosion of second degree of labium (majus) (minus)
Corrosion of second degree of perineum
Corrosion of second degree of vulva
Excludes2 corrosion of vagina (T28.8)

X● T21.69 **Corrosion of second degree of other site of trunk**

● T21.7 Corrosion of third degree of trunk
Code first (T51-T65) to identify chemical and intent
Use additional external cause code to identify place (Y92)

X● T21.70 **Corrosion of third degree of trunk, unspecified site** A, A (Ex:) PDX 1894

X● T21.71 **Corrosion of third degree of chest wall** A, A (Ex:) PDX 1895
Corrosion of third degree of breast

X● T21.72 **Corrosion of third degree of abdominal wall** A, A (Ex:) PDX 1896
Corrosion of third degree of flank
Corrosion of third degree of groin

X● T21.73 **Corrosion of third degree of upper back** A, A (Ex:) PDX 1897
Corrosion of third degree of interscapular region

X● T21.74 **Corrosion of third degree of lower back** A, A (Ex:) PDX 1897

X● T21.75 **Corrosion of third degree of buttock** A, A (Ex:) PDX 1897
Corrosion of third degree of anus

X● T21.76 **Corrosion of third degree of male genital region** A, A (Ex:) PDX 1898
Corrosion of third degree of penis
Corrosion of third degree of scrotum
Corrosion of third degree of testis

X● T21.77 **Corrosion of third degree of female genital region** A, A (Ex:) PDX 1898
Corrosion of third degree of labium (majus) (minus)
Corrosion of third degree of perineum
Corrosion of third degree of vulva
Excludes2 corrosion of vagina (T28.8)

X● T21.79 **Corrosion of third degree of other site of trunk** A, A (Ex:) PDX 1894

● T22 **Burn and corrosion of shoulder and upper limb, except wrist and hand**
Excludes2 burn and corrosion of interscapular region (T21.-)
burn and corrosion of wrist and hand (T23.-)

The appropriate 7th character is to be added to each code from category T22

A	initial encounter
D	subsequent encounter
S	sequela

● T22.Ø Burn of unspecified degree of shoulder and upper limb, except wrist and hand
Use additional external cause code to identify the source, place and intent of the burn (XØØ-X19, X75-X77, X96-X98, Y92)

X● T22.ØØ **Burn of unspecified degree of shoulder and upper limb, except wrist and hand, unspecified site**

● T22.Ø1 **Burn of unspecified degree of forearm**
● T22.Ø11 **Burn of unspecified degree of right forearm**
● T22.Ø12 **Burn of unspecified degree of left forearm**
● T22.Ø19 **Burn of unspecified degree of unspecified forearm**

● T22.Ø2 **Burn of unspecified degree of elbow**
● T22.Ø21 **Burn of unspecified degree of right elbow**
● T22.Ø22 **Burn of unspecified degree of left elbow**
● T22.Ø29 **Burn of unspecified degree of unspecified elbow**

● T22.Ø3 **Burn of unspecified degree of upper arm**
● T22.Ø31 **Burn of unspecified degree of right upper arm**
● T22.Ø32 **Burn of unspecified degree of left upper arm**
● T22.Ø39 **Burn of unspecified degree of unspecified upper arm**

● T22.Ø4 **Burn of unspecified degree of axilla**
● T22.Ø41 **Burn of unspecified degree of right axilla**
● T22.Ø42 **Burn of unspecified degree of left axilla**
● T22.Ø49 **Burn of unspecified degree of unspecified axilla**

● T22.Ø5 **Burn of unspecified degree of shoulder**
● T22.Ø51 **Burn of unspecified degree of right shoulder**
● T22.Ø52 **Burn of unspecified degree of left shoulder**
● T22.Ø59 **Burn of unspecified degree of unspecified shoulder**

● T22.Ø6 **Burn of unspecified degree of scapular region**
● T22.Ø61 **Burn of unspecified degree of right scapular region**
● T22.Ø62 **Burn of unspecified degree of left scapular region**
● T22.Ø69 **Burn of unspecified degree of unspecified scapular region**

T22.09 Burn of unspecified degree of multiple sites of shoulder and upper limb, except wrist and hand
T22.091 Burn of unspecified degree of multiple sites of right shoulder and upper limb, except wrist and hand
T22.092 Burn of unspecified degree of multiple sites of left shoulder and upper limb, except wrist and hand
T22.099 Burn of unspecified degree of multiple sites of unspecified shoulder and upper limb, except wrist and hand

T22.1 Burn of first degree of shoulder and upper limb, except wrist and hand
Use additional external cause code to identify the source, place and intent of the burn (X00-X19, X75-X77, X96-X98, Y92)
X T22.10 Burn of first degree of shoulder and upper limb, except wrist and hand, unspecified site
T22.11 Burn of first degree of forearm
T22.111 Burn of first degree of right forearm
T22.112 Burn of first degree of left forearm
T22.119 Burn of first degree of unspecified forearm
T22.12 Burn of first degree of elbow
T22.121 Burn of first degree of right elbow
T22.122 Burn of first degree of left elbow
T22.129 Burn of first degree of unspecified elbow
T22.13 Burn of first degree of upper arm
T22.131 Burn of first degree of right upper arm
T22.132 Burn of first degree of left upper arm
T22.139 Burn of first degree of unspecified upper arm
T22.14 Burn of first degree of axilla
T22.141 Burn of first degree of right axilla
T22.142 Burn of first degree of left axilla
T22.149 Burn of first degree of unspecified axilla
T22.15 Burn of first degree of shoulder
T22.151 Burn of first degree of right shoulder
T22.152 Burn of first degree of left shoulder
T22.159 Burn of first degree of unspecified shoulder
T22.16 Burn of first degree of scapular region
T22.161 Burn of first degree of right scapular region
T22.162 Burn of first degree of left scapular region
T22.169 Burn of first degree of unspecified scapular region
T22.19 Burn of first degree of multiple sites of shoulder and upper limb, except wrist and hand
T22.191 Burn of first degree of multiple sites of right shoulder and upper limb, except wrist and hand
T22.192 Burn of first degree of multiple sites of left shoulder and upper limb, except wrist and hand
T22.199 Burn of first degree of multiple sites of unspecified shoulder and upper limb, except wrist and hand

T22.2 Burn of second degree of shoulder and upper limb, except wrist and hand
Use additional external cause code to identify the source, place and intent of the burn (X00-X19, X75-X77, X96-X98, Y92)
X T22.20 Burn of second degree of shoulder and upper limb, except wrist and hand, unspecified site
T22.21 Burn of second degree of forearm
T22.211 Burn of second degree of right forearm
T22.212 Burn of second degree of left forearm
T22.219 Burn of second degree of unspecified forearm
T22.22 Burn of second degree of elbow
T22.221 Burn of second degree of right elbow
T22.222 Burn of second degree of left elbow
T22.229 Burn of second degree of unspecified elbow
T22.23 Burn of second degree of upper arm
T22.231 Burn of second degree of right upper arm
T22.232 Burn of second degree of left upper arm
T22.239 Burn of second degree of unspecified upper arm
T22.24 Burn of second degree of axilla
T22.241 Burn of second degree of right axilla
T22.242 Burn of second degree of left axilla
T22.249 Burn of second degree of unspecified axilla
T22.25 Burn of second degree of shoulder
T22.251 Burn of second degree of right shoulder
T22.252 Burn of second degree of left shoulder
T22.259 Burn of second degree of unspecified shoulder
T22.26 Burn of second degree of scapular region
T22.261 Burn of second degree of right scapular region
T22.262 Burn of second degree of left scapular region
T22.269 Burn of second degree of unspecified scapular region
T22.29 Burn of second degree of multiple sites of shoulder and upper limb, except wrist and hand
T22.291 Burn of second degree of multiple sites of right shoulder and upper limb, except wrist and hand
T22.292 Burn of second degree of multiple sites of left shoulder and upper limb, except wrist and hand
T22.299 Burn of second degree of multiple sites of unspecified shoulder and upper limb, except wrist and hand

● T22.3 Burn of third degree of shoulder and upper limb, except wrist and hand
Use additional external cause code to identify the source, place and intent of the burn (X00-X19, X75-X77, X96-X98, Y92)

X ● T22.30 Burn of third degree of shoulder and upper limb, except wrist and hand, unspecified site A, A (Ex:) PDX 1899

● T22.31 Burn of third degree of forearm (Ex:) PDX 1900
● T22.311 Burn of third degree of right forearm A, A
● T22.312 Burn of third degree of left forearm A, A
● T22.319 Burn of third degree of unspecified forearm A, A

● T22.32 Burn of third degree of elbow (Ex:) PDX 1901
● T22.321 Burn of third degree of right elbow A, A
● T22.322 Burn of third degree of left elbow A, A
● T22.329 Burn of third degree of unspecified elbow A, A

● T22.33 Burn of third degree of upper arm (Ex:) PDX 1902
● T22.331 Burn of third degree of right upper arm A, A
● T22.332 Burn of third degree of left upper arm A, A
● T22.339 Burn of third degree of unspecified upper arm A, A

● T22.34 Burn of third degree of axilla (Ex:) PDX 1903
● T22.341 Burn of third degree of right axilla A, A
● T22.342 Burn of third degree of left axilla A, A
● T22.349 Burn of third degree of unspecified axilla A, A

● T22.35 Burn of third degree of shoulder (Ex:) PDX 1904
● T22.351 Burn of third degree of right shoulder A, A
● T22.352 Burn of third degree of left shoulder A, A
● T22.359 Burn of third degree of unspecified shoulder A, A

● T22.36 Burn of third degree of scapular region (Ex:) PDX 1905
● T22.361 Burn of third degree of right scapular region A, A
● T22.362 Burn of third degree of left scapular region A, A
● T22.369 Burn of third degree of unspecified scapular region A, A

● T22.39 Burn of third degree of multiple sites of shoulder and upper limb, except wrist and hand (Ex:) PDX 1899
● T22.391 Burn of third degree of multiple sites of right shoulder and upper limb, except wrist and hand A, A
● T22.392 Burn of third degree of multiple sites of left shoulder and upper limb, except wrist and hand A, A
● T22.399 Burn of third degree of multiple sites of unspecified shoulder and upper limb, except wrist and hand A, A

● T22.4 Corrosion of unspecified degree of shoulder and upper limb, except wrist and hand
Code first (T51-T65) to identify chemical and intent
Use additional external cause code to identify place (Y92)

X ● T22.40 Corrosion of unspecified degree of shoulder and upper limb, except wrist and hand, unspecified site

● T22.41 Corrosion of unspecified degree of forearm
● T22.411 Corrosion of unspecified degree of right forearm
● T22.412 Corrosion of unspecified degree of left forearm
● T22.419 Corrosion of unspecified degree of unspecified forearm

● T22.42 Corrosion of unspecified degree of elbow
● T22.421 Corrosion of unspecified degree of right elbow
● T22.422 Corrosion of unspecified degree of left elbow
● T22.429 Corrosion of unspecified degree of unspecified elbow

● T22.43 Corrosion of unspecified degree of upper arm
● T22.431 Corrosion of unspecified degree of right upper arm
● T22.432 Corrosion of unspecified degree of left upper arm
● T22.439 Corrosion of unspecified degree of unspecified upper arm

● T22.44 Corrosion of unspecified degree of axilla
● T22.441 Corrosion of unspecified degree of right axilla
● T22.442 Corrosion of unspecified degree of left axilla
● T22.449 Corrosion of unspecified degree of unspecified axilla

● T22.45 Corrosion of unspecified degree of shoulder
● T22.451 Corrosion of unspecified degree of right shoulder
● T22.452 Corrosion of unspecified degree of left shoulder
● T22.459 Corrosion of unspecified degree of unspecified shoulder

● T22.46 Corrosion of unspecified degree of scapular region
● T22.461 Corrosion of unspecified degree of right scapular region
● T22.462 Corrosion of unspecified degree of left scapular region
● T22.469 Corrosion of unspecified degree of unspecified scapular region

● T22.49 Corrosion of unspecified degree of multiple sites of shoulder and upper limb, except wrist and hand
● T22.491 Corrosion of unspecified degree of multiple sites of right shoulder and upper limb, except wrist and hand
● T22.492 Corrosion of unspecified degree of multiple sites of left shoulder and upper limb, except wrist and hand
● T22.499 Corrosion of unspecified degree of multiple sites of unspecified shoulder and upper limb, except wrist and hand

T22.5 Corrosion of first degree of shoulder and upper limb, except wrist and hand

Code first (T51-T65) to identify chemical and intent

Use additional external cause code to identify place (Y92)

X **T22.50** Corrosion of first degree of shoulder and upper limb, except wrist and hand unspecified site

T22.51 Corrosion of first degree of forearm

T22.511 Corrosion of first degree of right forearm

T22.512 Corrosion of first degree of left forearm

T22.519 Corrosion of first degree of unspecified forearm

T22.52 Corrosion of first degree of elbow

T22.521 Corrosion of first degree of right elbow

T22.522 Corrosion of first degree of left elbow

T22.529 Corrosion of first degree of unspecified elbow

T22.53 Corrosion of first degree of upper arm

T22.531 Corrosion of first degree of right upper arm

T22.532 Corrosion of first degree of left upper arm

T22.539 Corrosion of first degree of unspecified upper arm

T22.54 Corrosion of first degree of axilla

T22.541 Corrosion of first degree of right axilla

T22.542 Corrosion of first degree of left axilla

T22.549 Corrosion of first degree of unspecified axilla

T22.55 Corrosion of first degree of shoulder

T22.551 Corrosion of first degree of right shoulder

T22.552 Corrosion of first degree of left shoulder

T22.559 Corrosion of first degree of unspecified shoulder

T22.56 Corrosion of first degree of scapular region

T22.561 Corrosion of first degree of right scapular region

T22.562 Corrosion of first degree of left scapular region

T22.569 Corrosion of first degree of unspecified scapular region

T22.59 Corrosion of first degree of multiple sites of shoulder and upper limb, except wrist and hand

T22.591 Corrosion of first degree of multiple sites of right shoulder and upper limb, except wrist and hand

T22.592 Corrosion of first degree of multiple sites of left shoulder and upper limb, except wrist and hand

T22.599 Corrosion of first degree of multiple sites of unspecified shoulder and upper limb, except wrist and hand

T22.6 Corrosion of second degree of shoulder and upper limb, except wrist and hand

Code first (T51-T65) to identify chemical and intent

Use additional external cause code to identify place (Y92)

X **T22.60** Corrosion of second degree of shoulder and upper limb, except wrist and hand, unspecified site

T22.61 Corrosion of second degree of forearm

T22.611 Corrosion of second degree of right forearm

T22.612 Corrosion of second degree of left forearm

T22.619 Corrosion of second degree of unspecified forearm

T22.62 Corrosion of second degree of elbow

T22.621 Corrosion of second degree of right elbow

T22.622 Corrosion of second degree of left elbow

T22.629 Corrosion of second degree of unspecified elbow

T22.63 Corrosion of second degree of upper arm

T22.631 Corrosion of second degree of right upper arm

T22.632 Corrosion of second degree of left upper arm

T22.639 Corrosion of second degree of unspecified upper arm

T22.64 Corrosion of second degree of axilla

T22.641 Corrosion of second degree of right axilla

T22.642 Corrosion of second degree of left axilla

T22.649 Corrosion of second degree of unspecified axilla

T22.65 Corrosion of second degree of shoulder

T22.651 Corrosion of second degree of right shoulder

T22.652 Corrosion of second degree of left shoulder

T22.659 Corrosion of second degree of unspecified shoulder

T22.66 Corrosion of second degree of scapular region

T22.661 Corrosion of second degree of right scapular region

T22.662 Corrosion of second degree of left scapular region

T22.669 Corrosion of second degree of unspecified scapular region

T22.69 Corrosion of second degree of multiple sites of shoulder and upper limb, except wrist and hand

T22.691 Corrosion of second degree of multiple sites of right shoulder and upper limb, except wrist and hand

T22.692 Corrosion of second degree of multiple sites of left shoulder and upper limb, except wrist and hand

T22.699 Corrosion of second degree of multiple sites of unspecified shoulder and upper limb, except wrist and hand

T22.7 Corrosion of third degree of shoulder and upper limb, except wrist and hand

Code first (T51-T65) to identify chemical and intent

Use additional external cause code to identify place (Y92)

X **T22.70** Corrosion of third degree of shoulder and upper limb, except wrist and hand, unspecified site A, A (Ex) PDX 1899

T22.71 Corrosion of third degree of forearm (Ex) PDX 1900

T22.711 Corrosion of third degree of right forearm A, A

T22.712 Corrosion of third degree of left forearm A, A

T22.719 Corrosion of third degree of unspecified forearm A, A

CHAPTER 19 (SØ-T88)

- T22.72 Corrosion of third degree of elbow Ex: PDX 1901
  - T22.721 Corrosion of third degree of right elbow A, A
  - T22.722 Corrosion of third degree of left elbow A, A
  - T22.729 Corrosion of third degree of unspecified elbow A, A
- T22.73 Corrosion of third degree of upper arm Ex: PDX 1902
  - T22.731 Corrosion of third degree of right upper arm A, A
  - T22.732 Corrosion of third degree of left upper arm A, A
  - T22.739 Corrosion of third degree of unspecified upper arm A, A
- T22.74 Corrosion of third degree of axilla Ex: PDX 1903
  - T22.741 Corrosion of third degree of right axilla A, A
  - T22.742 Corrosion of third degree of left axilla A, A
  - T22.749 Corrosion of third degree of unspecified axilla A, A
- T22.75 Corrosion of third degree of shoulder Ex: PDX 1904
  - T22.751 Corrosion of third degree of right shoulder A, A
  - T22.752 Corrosion of third degree of left shoulder A, A
  - T22.759 Corrosion of third degree of unspecified shoulder A, A
- T22.76 Corrosion of third degree of scapular region Ex: PDX 1905
  - T22.761 Corrosion of third degree of right scapular region A, A
  - T22.762 Corrosion of third degree of left scapular region A, A
  - T22.769 Corrosion of third degree of unspecified scapular region A, A
- T22.79 Corrosion of third degree of multiple sites of shoulder and upper limb, except wrist and hand Ex: PDX 1899
  - T22.791 Corrosion of third degree of multiple sites of right shoulder and upper limb, except wrist and hand A, A
  - T22.792 Corrosion of third degree of multiple sites of left shoulder and upper limb, except wrist and hand A, A
  - T22.799 Corrosion of third degree of multiple sites of unspecified shoulder and upper limb, except wrist and hand A, A

T23 Burn and corrosion of wrist and hand

The appropriate 7th character is to be added to each code from category T23

A	initial encounter
D	subsequent encounter
S	sequela

- T23.0 Burn of unspecified degree of wrist and hand

  Use additional external cause code to identify the source, place and intent of the burn (X00-X19, X75-X77, X96-X98, Y92)

  - T23.00 Burn of unspecified degree of hand, unspecified site
    - T23.001 Burn of unspecified degree of right hand, unspecified site
    - T23.002 Burn of unspecified degree of left hand, unspecified site
    - T23.009 Burn of unspecified degree of unspecified hand, unspecified site
  - T23.01 Burn of unspecified degree of thumb (nail)
    - T23.011 Burn of unspecified degree of right thumb (nail)
    - T23.012 Burn of unspecified degree of left thumb (nail)
    - T23.019 Burn of unspecified degree of unspecified thumb (nail)
  - T23.02 Burn of unspecified degree of single finger (nail) except thumb
    - T23.021 Burn of unspecified degree of single right finger (nail) except thumb
    - T23.022 Burn of unspecified degree of single left finger (nail) except thumb
    - T23.029 Burn of unspecified degree of unspecified single finger (nail) except thumb
  - T23.03 Burn of unspecified degree of multiple fingers (nail), not including thumb
    - T23.031 Burn of unspecified degree of multiple right fingers (nail), not including thumb
    - T23.032 Burn of unspecified degree of multiple left fingers (nail), not including thumb
    - T23.039 Burn of unspecified degree of unspecified multiple fingers (nail), not including thumb
  - T23.04 Burn of unspecified degree of multiple fingers (nail), including thumb
    - T23.041 Burn of unspecified degree of multiple right fingers (nail), including thumb
    - T23.042 Burn of unspecified degree of multiple left fingers (nail), including thumb
    - T23.049 Burn of unspecified degree of unspecified multiple fingers (nail), including thumb
  - T23.05 Burn of unspecified degree of palm
    - T23.051 Burn of unspecified degree of right palm
    - T23.052 Burn of unspecified degree of left palm
    - T23.059 Burn of unspecified degree of unspecified palm
  - T23.06 Burn of unspecified degree of back of hand
    - T23.061 Burn of unspecified degree of back of right hand
    - T23.062 Burn of unspecified degree of back of left hand
    - T23.069 Burn of unspecified degree of back of unspecified hand
  - T23.07 Burn of unspecified degree of wrist
    - T23.071 Burn of unspecified degree of right wrist
    - T23.072 Burn of unspecified degree of left wrist
    - T23.079 Burn of unspecified degree of unspecified wrist
  - T23.09 Burn of unspecified degree of multiple sites of wrist and hand
    - T23.091 Burn of unspecified degree of multiple sites of right wrist and hand
    - T23.092 Burn of unspecified degree of multiple sites of left wrist and hand
    - T23.099 Burn of unspecified degree of multiple sites of unspecified wrist and hand

- T23.1 Burn of first degree of wrist and hand
  Use additional external cause code to identify the source, place and intent of the burn (X00-X19, X75-X77, X96-X98, Y92)
  - T23.10 Burn of first degree of hand, unspecified site
    - T23.101 Burn of first degree of right hand, unspecified site
    - T23.102 Burn of first degree of left hand, unspecified site
    - T23.109 Burn of first degree of unspecified hand, unspecified site
  - T23.11 Burn of first degree of thumb (nail)
    - T23.111 Burn of first degree of right thumb (nail)
    - T23.112 Burn of first degree of left thumb (nail)
    - T23.119 Burn of first degree of unspecified thumb (nail)
  - T23.12 Burn of first degree of single finger (nail) except thumb
    - T23.121 Burn of first degree of single right finger (nail) except thumb
    - T23.122 Burn of first degree of single left finger (nail) except thumb
    - T23.129 Burn of first degree of unspecified single finger (nail) except thumb
  - T23.13 Burn of first degree of multiple fingers (nail), not including thumb
    - T23.131 Burn of first degree of multiple right fingers (nail), not including thumb
    - T23.132 Burn of first degree of multiple left fingers (nail), not including thumb
    - T23.139 Burn of first degree of unspecified multiple fingers (nail), not including thumb
  - T23.14 Burn of first degree of multiple fingers (nail), including thumb
    - T23.141 Burn of first degree of multiple right fingers (nail), including thumb
    - T23.142 Burn of first degree of multiple left fingers (nail), including thumb
    - T23.149 Burn of first degree of unspecified multiple fingers (nail), including thumb
  - T23.15 Burn of first degree of palm
    - T23.151 Burn of first degree of right palm
    - T23.152 Burn of first degree of left palm
    - T23.159 Burn of first degree of unspecified palm
  - T23.16 Burn of first degree of back of hand
    - T23.161 Burn of first degree of back of right hand
    - T23.162 Burn of first degree of back of left hand
    - T23.169 Burn of first degree of back of unspecified hand
  - T23.17 Burn of first degree of wrist
    - T23.171 Burn of first degree of right wrist
    - T23.172 Burn of first degree of left wrist
    - T23.179 Burn of first degree of unspecified wrist
  - T23.19 Burn of first degree of multiple sites of wrist and hand
    - T23.191 Burn of first degree of multiple sites of right wrist and hand
    - T23.192 Burn of first degree of multiple sites of left wrist and hand
    - T23.199 Burn of first degree of multiple sites of unspecified wrist and hand

- T23.2 Burn of second degree of wrist and hand
  Use additional external cause code to identify the source, place and intent of the burn (X00-X19, X75-X77, X96-X98, Y92)
  - T23.20 Burn of second degree of hand, unspecified site
    - T23.201 Burn of second degree of right hand, unspecified site
    - T23.202 Burn of second degree of left hand, unspecified site
    - T23.209 Burn of second degree of unspecified hand, unspecified site
  - T23.21 Burn of second degree of thumb (nail)
    - T23.211 Burn of second degree of right thumb (nail)
    - T23.212 Burn of second degree of left thumb (nail)
    - T23.219 Burn of second degree of unspecified thumb (nail)
  - T23.22 Burn of second degree of single finger (nail) except thumb
    - T23.221 Burn of second degree of single right finger (nail) except thumb
    - T23.222 Burn of second degree of single left finger (nail) except thumb
    - T23.229 Burn of second degree of unspecified single finger (nail) except thumb
  - T23.23 Burn of second degree of multiple fingers (nail), not including thumb
    - T23.231 Burn of second degree of multiple right fingers (nail), not including thumb
    - T23.232 Burn of second degree of multiple left fingers (nail), not including thumb
    - T23.239 Burn of second degree of unspecified multiple fingers (nail), not including thumb
  - T23.24 Burn of second degree of multiple fingers (nail), including thumb
    - T23.241 Burn of second degree of multiple right fingers (nail), including thumb
    - T23.242 Burn of second degree of multiple left fingers (nail), including thumb
    - T23.249 Burn of second degree of unspecified multiple fingers (nail), including thumb
  - T23.25 Burn of second degree of palm
    - T23.251 Burn of second degree of right palm
    - T23.252 Burn of second degree of left palm
    - T23.259 Burn of second degree of unspecified palm
  - T23.26 Burn of second degree of back of hand
    - T23.261 Burn of second degree of back of right hand
    - T23.262 Burn of second degree of back of left hand
    - T23.269 Burn of second degree of back of unspecified hand
  - T23.27 Burn of second degree of wrist
    - T23.271 Burn of second degree of right wrist
    - T23.272 Burn of second degree of left wrist
    - T23.279 Burn of second degree of unspecified wrist
  - T23.29 Burn of second degree of multiple sites of wrist and hand
    - T23.291 Burn of second degree of multiple sites of right wrist and hand
    - T23.292 Burn of second degree of multiple sites of left wrist and hand
    - T23.299 Burn of second degree of multiple sites of unspecified wrist and hand

● T23.3 Burn of third degree of wrist and hand
Use additional external cause code to identify the source, place and intent of the burn (XØØ-X19, X75-X77, X96-X98, Y92)

● T23.30 Burn of third degree of hand, unspecified site (Ex) PDX 1906
● T23.301 Burn of third degree of right hand, unspecified site A, A
Coding Clinic: 2015, Q1, P19
● T23.302 Burn of third degree of left hand, unspecified site A, A
Coding Clinic: 2016, Q2, P5
● T23.309 Burn of third degree of unspecified hand, unspecified site A, A

● T23.31 Burn of third degree of thumb (nail) (Ex) PDX 1907
● T23.311 Burn of third degree of right thumb (nail) A, A
● T23.312 Burn of third degree of left thumb (nail) A, A
● T23.319 Burn of third degree of unspecified thumb (nail) A, A

● T23.32 Burn of third degree of single finger (nail) except thumb (Ex) PDX 1908
● T23.321 Burn of third degree of single right finger (nail) except thumb A, A
● T23.322 Burn of third degree of single left finger (nail) except thumb A, A
● T23.329 Burn of third degree of unspecified single finger (nail) except thumb A, A

● T23.33 Burn of third degree of multiple fingers (nail), not including thumb (Ex) PDX 1909
● T23.331 Burn of third degree of multiple right fingers (nail), not including thumb A, A
● T23.332 Burn of third degree of multiple left fingers (nail), not including thumb A, A
● T23.339 Burn of third degree of unspecified multiple fingers (nail), not including thumb A, A

● T23.34 Burn of third degree of multiple fingers (nail), including thumb (Ex) PDX 1910
● T23.341 Burn of third degree of multiple right fingers (nail), including thumb A, A
● T23.342 Burn of third degree of multiple left fingers (nail), including thumb A, A
● T23.349 Burn of third degree of unspecified multiple fingers (nail), including thumb A, A

● T23.35 Burn of third degree of palm (Ex) PDX 1911
● T23.351 Burn of third degree of right palm A, A
● T23.352 Burn of third degree of left palm A, A
● T23.359 Burn of third degree of unspecified palm A, A

● T23.36 Burn of third degree of back of hand (Ex) PDX 1912
● T23.361 Burn of third degree of back of right hand A, A
● T23.362 Burn of third degree of back of left hand A, A
● T23.369 Burn of third degree of back of unspecified hand A, A

● T23.37 Burn of third degree of wrist (Ex) PDX 1913
● T23.371 Burn of third degree of right wrist A, A
● T23.372 Burn of third degree of left wrist A, A
● T23.379 Burn of third degree of unspecified wrist A, A

● T23.39 Burn of third degree of multiple sites of wrist and hand (Ex) PDX 1906
● T23.391 Burn of third degree of multiple sites of right wrist and hand A, A
● T23.392 Burn of third degree of multiple sites of left wrist and hand A, A
● T23.399 Burn of third degree of multiple sites of unspecified wrist and hand A, A

● T23.4 Corrosion of unspecified degree of wrist and hand
Code first (T51-T65) *to identify chemical and intent*
Use additional external cause code to identify place (Y92)

● T23.40 Corrosion of unspecified degree of hand, unspecified site
● T23.401 Corrosion of unspecified degree of right hand, unspecified site
● T23.402 Corrosion of unspecified degree of left hand, unspecified site
● T23.409 Corrosion of unspecified degree of unspecified hand, unspecified site

● T23.41 Corrosion of unspecified degree of thumb (nail)
● T23.411 Corrosion of unspecified degree of right thumb (nail)
● T23.412 Corrosion of unspecified degree of left thumb (nail)
● T23.419 Corrosion of unspecified degree of unspecified thumb (nail)

● T23.42 Corrosion of unspecified degree of single finger (nail) except thumb
● T23.421 Corrosion of unspecified degree of single right finger (nail) except thumb
● T23.422 Corrosion of unspecified degree of single left finger (nail) except thumb
● T23.429 Corrosion of unspecified degree of unspecified single finger (nail) except thumb

● T23.43 Corrosion of unspecified degree of multiple fingers (nail), not including thumb
● T23.431 Corrosion of unspecified degree of multiple right fingers (nail), not including thumb
● T23.432 Corrosion of unspecified degree of multiple left fingers (nail), not including thumb
● T23.439 Corrosion of unspecified degree of unspecified multiple fingers (nail), not including thumb

● T23.44 Corrosion of unspecified degree of multiple fingers (nail), including thumb
● T23.441 Corrosion of unspecified degree of multiple right fingers (nail), including thumb
● T23.442 Corrosion of unspecified degree of multiple left fingers (nail), including thumb
● T23.449 Corrosion of unspecified degree of unspecified multiple fingers (nail), including thumb

- T23.45 Corrosion of unspecified degree of palm
  - T23.451 Corrosion of unspecified degree of right palm
  - T23.452 Corrosion of unspecified degree of left palm
  - T23.459 Corrosion of unspecified degree of unspecified palm
- T23.46 Corrosion of unspecified degree of back of hand
  - T23.461 Corrosion of unspecified degree of back of right hand
  - T23.462 Corrosion of unspecified degree of back of left hand
  - T23.469 Corrosion of unspecified degree of back of unspecified hand
- T23.47 Corrosion of unspecified degree of wrist
  - T23.471 Corrosion of unspecified degree of right wrist
  - T23.472 Corrosion of unspecified degree of left wrist
  - T23.479 Corrosion of unspecified degree of unspecified wrist
- T23.49 Corrosion of unspecified degree of multiple sites of wrist and hand
  - T23.491 Corrosion of unspecified degree of multiple sites of right wrist and hand
  - T23.492 Corrosion of unspecified degree of multiple sites of left wrist and hand
  - T23.499 Corrosion of unspecified degree of multiple sites of unspecified wrist and hand

- T23.5 Corrosion of first degree of wrist and hand

  Code first (T51-T65) to identify chemical and intent

  Use additional external cause code to identify place (Y92)

- T23.50 Corrosion of first degree of hand, unspecified site
  - T23.501 Corrosion of first degree of right hand, unspecified site
  - T23.502 Corrosion of first degree of left hand, unspecified site
  - T23.509 Corrosion of first degree of unspecified hand, unspecified site
- T23.51 Corrosion of first degree of thumb (nail)
  - T23.511 Corrosion of first degree of right thumb (nail)
  - T23.512 Corrosion of first degree of left thumb (nail)
  - T23.519 Corrosion of first degree of unspecified thumb (nail)
- T23.52 Corrosion of first degree of single finger (nail) except thumb
  - T23.521 Corrosion of first degree of single right finger (nail) except thumb
  - T23.522 Corrosion of first degree of single left finger (nail) except thumb
  - T23.529 Corrosion of first degree of unspecified single finger (nail) except thumb
- T23.53 Corrosion of first degree of multiple fingers (nail), not including thumb
  - T23.531 Corrosion of first degree of multiple right fingers (nail), not including thumb
  - T23.532 Corrosion of first degree of multiple left fingers (nail), not including thumb
  - T23.539 Corrosion of first degree of unspecified multiple fingers (nail), not including thumb
- T23.54 Corrosion of first degree of multiple fingers (nail), including thumb
  - T23.541 Corrosion of first degree of multiple right fingers (nail), including thumb
  - T23.542 Corrosion of first degree of multiple left fingers (nail), including thumb
  - T23.549 Corrosion of first degree of unspecified multiple fingers (nail), including thumb
- T23.55 Corrosion of first degree of palm
  - T23.551 Corrosion of first degree of right palm
  - T23.552 Corrosion of first degree of left palm
  - T23.559 Corrosion of first degree of unspecified palm
- T23.56 Corrosion of first degree of back of hand
  - T23.561 Corrosion of first degree of back of right hand
  - T23.562 Corrosion of first degree of back of left hand
  - T23.569 Corrosion of first degree of back of unspecified hand
- T23.57 Corrosion of first degree of wrist
  - T23.571 Corrosion of first degree of right wrist
  - T23.572 Corrosion of first degree of left wrist
  - T23.579 Corrosion of first degree of unspecified wrist
- T23.59 Corrosion of first degree of multiple sites of wrist and hand
  - T23.591 Corrosion of first degree of multiple sites of right wrist and hand
  - T23.592 Corrosion of first degree of multiple sites of left wrist and hand
  - T23.599 Corrosion of first degree of multiple sites of unspecified wrist and hand

- T23.6 Corrosion of second degree of wrist and hand

  Code first (T51-T65) to identify chemical and intent

  Use additional external cause code to identify place (Y92)

- T23.60 Corrosion of second degree of hand, unspecified site
  - T23.601 Corrosion of second degree of right hand, unspecified site
  - T23.602 Corrosion of second degree of left hand, unspecified site
  - T23.609 Corrosion of second degree of unspecified hand, unspecified site
- T23.61 Corrosion of second degree of thumb (nail)
  - T23.611 Corrosion of second degree of right thumb (nail)
  - T23.612 Corrosion of second degree of left thumb (nail)
  - T23.619 Corrosion of second degree of unspecified thumb (nail)
- T23.62 Corrosion of second degree of single finger (nail) except thumb
  - T23.621 Corrosion of second degree of single right finger (nail) except thumb
  - T23.622 Corrosion of second degree of single left finger (nail) except thumb
  - T23.629 Corrosion of second degree of unspecified single finger (nail) except thumb

- ● T23.63 Corrosion of second degree of multiple fingers (nail), not including thumb
  - ● T23.631 Corrosion of second degree of multiple right fingers (nail), not including thumb
  - ● T23.632 Corrosion of second degree of multiple left fingers (nail), not including thumb
  - ● T23.639 Corrosion of second degree of unspecified multiple fingers (nail), not including thumb
- ● T23.64 Corrosion of second degree of multiple fingers (nail), including thumb
  - ● T23.641 Corrosion of second degree of multiple right fingers (nail), including thumb
  - ● T23.642 Corrosion of second degree of multiple left fingers (nail), including thumb
  - ● T23.649 Corrosion of second degree of unspecified multiple fingers (nail), including thumb
- ● T23.65 Corrosion of second degree of palm
  - ● T23.651 Corrosion of second degree of right palm
  - ● T23.652 Corrosion of second degree of left palm
  - ● T23.659 Corrosion of second degree of unspecified palm
- ● T23.66 Corrosion of second degree of back of hand
  - ● T23.661 Corrosion of second degree back of right hand
  - ● T23.662 Corrosion of second degree back of left hand
  - ● T23.669 Corrosion of second degree back of unspecified hand
- ● T23.67 Corrosion of second degree of wrist
  - ● T23.671 Corrosion of second degree of right wrist
  - ● T23.672 Corrosion of second degree of left wrist
  - ● T23.679 Corrosion of second degree of unspecified wrist
- ● T23.69 Corrosion of second degree of multiple sites of wrist and hand
  - ● T23.691 Corrosion of second degree of multiple sites of right wrist and hand
  - ● T23.692 Corrosion of second degree of multiple sites of left wrist and hand
  - ● T23.699 Corrosion of second degree of multiple sites of unspecified wrist and hand

● T23.7 Corrosion of third degree of wrist and hand

Code first (T51-T65) to identify chemical and intent

Use additional external cause code to identify place (Y92)

- ● T23.70 Corrosion of third degree of hand, unspecified site Ex: PDX 1906
  - ● T23.701 Corrosion of third degree of right hand, unspecified site A, A
  - ● T23.702 Corrosion of third degree of left hand, unspecified site A, A
  - ● T23.709 Corrosion of third degree of unspecified hand, unspecified site A, A
- ● T23.71 Corrosion of third degree of thumb (nail) Ex: PDX 1907
  - ● T23.711 Corrosion of third degree of right thumb (nail) A, A
  - ● T23.712 Corrosion of third degree of left thumb (nail) A, A
  - ● T23.719 Corrosion of third degree of unspecified thumb (nail) A, A
- ● T23.72 Corrosion of third degree of single finger (nail) except thumb Ex: PDX 1908
  - ● T23.721 Corrosion of third degree of single right finger (nail) except thumb A, A
  - ● T23.722 Corrosion of third degree of single left finger (nail) except thumb A, A
  - ● T23.729 Corrosion of third degree of unspecified single finger (nail) except thumb A, A
- ● T23.73 Corrosion of third degree of multiple fingers (nail), not including thumb Ex: PDX 1909
  - ● T23.731 Corrosion of third degree of multiple right fingers (nail), not including thumb A, A
  - ● T23.732 Corrosion of third degree of multiple left fingers (nail), not including thumb A, A
  - ● T23.739 Corrosion of third degree of unspecified multiple fingers (nail), not including thumb A, A
- ● T23.74 Corrosion of third degree of multiple fingers (nail), including thumb Ex: PDX 1910
  - ● T23.741 Corrosion of third degree of multiple right fingers (nail), including thumb A, A
  - ● T23.742 Corrosion of third degree of multiple left fingers (nail), including thumb A, A
  - ● T23.749 Corrosion of third degree of unspecified multiple fingers (nail), including thumb A, A
- ● T23.75 Corrosion of third degree of palm Ex: PDX 1911
  - ● T23.751 Corrosion of third degree of right palm A, A
  - ● T23.752 Corrosion of third degree of left palm A, A
  - ● T23.759 Corrosion of third degree of unspecified palm A, A
- ● T23.76 Corrosion of third degree of back of hand Ex: PDX 1912
  - ● T23.761 Corrosion of third degree of back of right hand A, A
  - ● T23.762 Corrosion of third degree of back of left hand A, A
  - ● T23.769 Corrosion of third degree of back of unspecified hand A, A
- ● T23.77 Corrosion of third degree of wrist Ex: PDX 1913
  - ● T23.771 Corrosion of third degree of right wrist A, A
  - ● T23.772 Corrosion of third degree of left wrist A, A
  - ● T23.779 Corrosion of third degree of unspecified wrist A, A

T23.79 Corrosion of third degree of multiple sites of wrist and hand Ex PDX 1906

T23.791 Corrosion of third degree of multiple sites of right wrist and hand A, A

T23.792 Corrosion of third degree of multiple sites of left wrist and hand A, A

T23.799 Corrosion of third degree of multiple sites of unspecified wrist and hand A, A

T24 Burn and corrosion of lower limb, except ankle and foot

Excludes2 burn and corrosion of ankle and foot (T25.-)
burn and corrosion of hip region (T21.-)

The appropriate 7th character is to be added to each code from category T24

A	initial encounter
D	subsequent encounter
S	sequela

T24.0 Burn of unspecified degree of lower limb, except ankle and foot

Use additional external cause code to identify the source, place and intent of the burn (X00-X19, X75-X77, X96-X98, Y92)

T24.00 Burn of unspecified degree of unspecified site of lower limb, except ankle and foot

T24.001 Burn of unspecified degree of unspecified site of right lower limb, except ankle and foot

T24.002 Burn of unspecified degree of unspecified site of left lower limb, except ankle and foot

T24.009 Burn of unspecified degree of unspecified site of unspecified lower limb, except ankle and foot

T24.01 Burn of unspecified degree of thigh

T24.011 Burn of unspecified degree of right thigh

T24.012 Burn of unspecified degree of left thigh

T24.019 Burn of unspecified degree of unspecified thigh

T24.02 Burn of unspecified degree of knee

T24.021 Burn of unspecified degree of right knee

T24.022 Burn of unspecified degree of left knee

T24.029 Burn of unspecified degree of unspecified knee

T24.03 Burn of unspecified degree of lower leg

T24.031 Burn of unspecified degree of right lower leg

T24.032 Burn of unspecified degree of left lower leg

T24.039 Burn of unspecified degree of unspecified lower leg

T24.09 Burn of unspecified degree of multiple sites of lower limb, except ankle and foot

T24.091 Burn of unspecified degree of multiple sites of right lower limb, except ankle and foot

T24.092 Burn of unspecified degree of multiple sites of left lower limb, except ankle and foot

T24.099 Burn of unspecified degree of multiple sites of unspecified lower limb, except ankle and foot

T24.1 Burn of first degree of lower limb, except ankle and foot

Use additional external cause code to identify the source, place and intent of the burn (X00-X19, X75-X77, X96-X98, Y92)

T24.10 Burn of first degree of unspecified site of lower limb, except ankle and foot

T24.101 Burn of first degree of unspecified site of right lower limb, except ankle and foot

T24.102 Burn of first degree of unspecified site of left lower limb, except ankle and foot

T24.109 Burn of first degree of unspecified site of unspecified lower limb, except ankle and foot

T24.11 Burn of first degree of thigh

T24.111 Burn of first degree of right thigh

T24.112 Burn of first degree of left thigh

T24.119 Burn of first degree of unspecified thigh

T24.12 Burn of first degree of knee

T24.121 Burn of first degree of right knee

T24.122 Burn of first degree of left knee

T24.129 Burn of first degree of unspecified knee

T24.13 Burn of first degree of lower leg

T24.131 Burn of first degree of right lower leg

T24.132 Burn of first degree of left lower leg

T24.139 Burn of first degree of unspecified lower leg

T24.19 Burn of first degree of multiple sites of lower limb, except ankle and foot

T24.191 Burn of first degree of multiple sites of right lower limb, except ankle and foot

T24.192 Burn of first degree of multiple sites of left lower limb, except ankle and foot

T24.199 Burn of first degree of multiple sites of unspecified lower limb, except ankle and foot

T24.2 Burn of second degree of lower limb, except ankle and foot

Use additional external cause code to identify the source, place and intent of the burn (X00-X19, X75-X77, X96-X98, Y92)

T24.20 Burn of second degree of unspecified site of lower limb, except ankle and foot

T24.201 Burn of second degree of unspecified site of right lower limb, except ankle and foot

T24.202 Burn of second degree of unspecified site of left lower limb, except ankle and foot

T24.209 Burn of second degree of unspecified site of unspecified lower limb, except ankle and foot

T24.21 Burn of second degree of thigh

T24.211 Burn of second degree of right thigh

T24.212 Burn of second degree of left thigh

T24.219 Burn of second degree of unspecified thigh

T24.22 Burn of second degree of knee

T24.221 Burn of second degree of right knee

T24.222 Burn of second degree of left knee

T24.229 Burn of second degree of unspecified knee

CHAPTER 19 (S00-T88)

- T24.23 Burn of second degree of lower leg
  - T24.231 Burn of second degree of right lower leg
  - T24.232 Burn of second degree of left lower leg
  - T24.239 Burn of second degree of unspecified lower leg
- T24.29 Burn of second degree of multiple sites of lower limb, except ankle and foot
  - T24.291 Burn of second degree of multiple sites of right lower limb, except ankle and foot
  - T24.292 Burn of second degree of multiple sites of left lower limb, except ankle and foot
  - T24.299 Burn of second degree of multiple sites of unspecified lower limb, except ankle and foot
- T24.3 Burn of third degree of lower limb, except ankle and foot

  Use additional external cause code to identify the source, place and intent of the burn (X00-X19, X75-X77, X96-X98, Y92)
  - T24.30 Burn of third degree of unspecified site of lower limb, except ankle and foot Ex: PDX 1914
    - T24.301 Burn of third degree of unspecified site of right lower limb, except ankle and foot A, A
    - T24.302 Burn of third degree of unspecified site of left lower limb, except ankle and foot A, A
    - T24.309 Burn of third degree of unspecified site of unspecified lower limb, except ankle and foot A, A
  - T24.31 Burn of third degree of thigh Ex: PDX 1915
    - T24.311 Burn of third degree of right thigh A, A
    - T24.312 Burn of third degree of left thigh A, A
    - T24.319 Burn of third degree of unspecified thigh A, A
  - T24.32 Burn of third degree of knee Ex: PDX 1916
    - T24.321 Burn of third degree of right knee A, A
    - T24.322 Burn of third degree of left knee A, A
    - T24.329 Burn of third degree of unspecified knee A, A
  - T24.33 Burn of third degree of lower leg Ex: PDX 1917
    - T24.331 Burn of third degree of right lower leg A, A
    - T24.332 Burn of third degree of left lower leg A, A
    - T24.339 Burn of third degree of unspecified lower leg A, A
  - T24.39 Burn of third degree of multiple sites of lower limb, except ankle and foot Ex: PDX 1914
    - T24.391 Burn of third degree of multiple sites of right lower limb, except ankle and foot A, A

      Coding Clinic: 2016, Q2, P5
    - T24.392 Burn of third degree of multiple sites of left lower limb, except ankle and foot A, A
    - T24.399 Burn of third degree of multiple sites of unspecified lower limb, except ankle and foot A, A
- T24.4 Corrosion of unspecified degree of lower limb, except ankle and foot

  Code first (T51-T65) to identify chemical and intent

  Use additional external cause code to identify place (Y92)
  - T24.40 Corrosion of unspecified degree of unspecified site of lower limb, except ankle and foot
    - T24.401 Corrosion of unspecified degree of unspecified site of right lower limb, except ankle and foot
    - T24.402 Corrosion of unspecified degree of unspecified site of left lower limb, except ankle and foot
    - T24.409 Corrosion of unspecified degree of unspecified site of unspecified lower limb, except ankle and foot
  - T24.41 Corrosion of unspecified degree of thigh
    - T24.411 Corrosion of unspecified degree of right thigh
    - T24.412 Corrosion of unspecified degree of left thigh
    - T24.419 Corrosion of unspecified degree of unspecified thigh
  - T24.42 Corrosion of unspecified degree of knee
    - T24.421 Corrosion of unspecified degree of right knee
    - T24.422 Corrosion of unspecified degree of left knee
    - T24.429 Corrosion of unspecified degree of unspecified knee
  - T24.43 Corrosion of unspecified degree of lower leg
    - T24.431 Corrosion of unspecified degree of right lower leg
    - T24.432 Corrosion of unspecified degree of left lower leg
    - T24.439 Corrosion of unspecified degree of unspecified lower leg
  - T24.49 Corrosion of unspecified degree of multiple sites of lower limb, except ankle and foot
    - T24.491 Corrosion of unspecified degree of multiple sites of right lower limb, except ankle and foot
    - T24.492 Corrosion of unspecified degree of multiple sites of left lower limb, except ankle and foot
    - T24.499 Corrosion of unspecified degree of multiple sites of unspecified lower limb, except ankle and foot
- T24.5 Corrosion of first degree of lower limb, except ankle and foot

  Code first (T51-T65) to identify chemical and intent

  Use additional external cause code to identify place (Y92)
  - T24.50 Corrosion of first degree of unspecified site of lower limb, except ankle and foot
    - T24.501 Corrosion of first degree of unspecified site of right lower limb, except ankle and foot
    - T24.502 Corrosion of first degree of unspecified site of left lower limb, except ankle and foot
    - T24.509 Corrosion of first degree of unspecified site of unspecified lower limb, except ankle and foot
  - T24.51 Corrosion of first degree of thigh
    - T24.511 Corrosion of first degree of right thigh
    - T24.512 Corrosion of first degree of left thigh
    - T24.519 Corrosion of first degree of unspecified thigh

CHAPTER 19 (S00-T88)

- T24.52 Corrosion of first degree of knee
  - T24.521 Corrosion of first degree of right knee
  - T24.522 Corrosion of first degree of left knee
  - T24.529 Corrosion of first degree of unspecified knee
- T24.53 Corrosion of first degree of lower leg
  - T24.531 Corrosion of first degree of right lower leg
  - T24.532 Corrosion of first degree of left lower leg
  - T24.539 Corrosion of first degree of unspecified lower leg
- T24.59 Corrosion of first degree of multiple sites of lower limb, except ankle and foot
  - T24.591 Corrosion of first degree of multiple sites of right lower limb, except ankle and foot
  - T24.592 Corrosion of first degree of multiple sites of left lower limb, except ankle and foot
  - T24.599 Corrosion of first degree of multiple sites of unspecified lower limb, except ankle and foot

T24.6 Corrosion of second degree of lower limb, except ankle and foot

Code first (*T51-T65*) *to identify chemical and intent*

Use additional external cause code to identify place (Y92)

- T24.6Ø Corrosion of second degree of unspecified site of lower limb, except ankle and foot
  - T24.6Ø1 Corrosion of second degree of unspecified site of right lower limb, except ankle and foot
  - T24.6Ø2 Corrosion of second degree of unspecified site of left lower limb, except ankle and foot
  - T24.6Ø9 Corrosion of second degree of unspecified site of unspecified lower limb, except ankle and foot
- T24.61 Corrosion of second degree of thigh
  - T24.611 Corrosion of second degree of right thigh
  - T24.612 Corrosion of second degree of left thigh
  - T24.619 Corrosion of second degree of unspecified thigh
- T24.62 Corrosion of second degree of knee
  - T24.621 Corrosion of second degree of right knee
  - T24.622 Corrosion of second degree of left knee
  - T24.629 Corrosion of second degree of unspecified knee
- T24.63 Corrosion of second degree of lower leg
  - T24.631 Corrosion of second degree of right lower leg
  - T24.632 Corrosion of second degree of left lower leg
  - T24.639 Corrosion of second degree of unspecified lower leg
- T24.69 Corrosion of second degree of multiple sites of lower limb, except ankle and foot
  - T24.691 Corrosion of second degree of multiple sites of right lower limb, except ankle and foot
  - T24.692 Corrosion of second degree of multiple sites of left lower limb, except ankle and foot
  - T24.699 Corrosion of second degree of multiple sites of unspecified lower limb, except ankle and foot

T24.7 Corrosion of third degree of lower limb, except ankle and foot

Code first (*T51-T65*) *to identify chemical and intent*

Use additional external cause code to identify place (Y92)

- T24.7Ø Corrosion of third degree of unspecified site of lower limb, except ankle and foot Ex PDX 1914
  - T24.7Ø1 Corrosion of third degree of unspecified site of right lower limb, except ankle and foot A CC, A HCC
  - T24.7Ø2 Corrosion of third degree of unspecified site of left lower limb, except ankle and foot A CC, A HCC
  - T24.7Ø9 Corrosion of third degree of unspecified site of unspecified lower limb, except ankle and foot A CC, A HCC
- T24.71 Corrosion of third degree of thigh Ex PDX 1915
  - T24.711 Corrosion of third degree of right thigh A CC, A HCC
  - T24.712 Corrosion of third degree of left thigh A CC, A HCC
  - T24.719 Corrosion of third degree of unspecified thigh A CC, A HCC
- T24.72 Corrosion of third degree of knee Ex PDX 1916
  - T24.721 Corrosion of third degree of right knee A CC, A HCC
  - T24.722 Corrosion of third degree of left knee A CC, A HCC
  - T24.729 Corrosion of third degree of unspecified knee A CC, A HCC
- T24.73 Corrosion of third degree of lower leg Ex PDX 1917
  - T24.731 Corrosion of third degree of right lower leg A CC, A HCC
  - T24.732 Corrosion of third degree of left lower leg A CC, A HCC
  - T24.739 Corrosion of third degree of unspecified lower leg A CC, A HCC
- T24.79 Corrosion of third degree of multiple sites of lower limb, except ankle and foot Ex PDX 1914
  - T24.791 Corrosion of third degree of multiple sites of right lower limb, except ankle and foot A CC, A HCC
  - T24.792 Corrosion of third degree of multiple sites of left lower limb, except ankle and foot A CC, A HCC
  - T24.799 Corrosion of third degree of multiple sites of unspecified lower limb, except ankle and foot A CC, A HCC

T25 Burn and corrosion of ankle and foot

The appropriate 7th character is to be added to each code from category T25

A	initial encounter
D	subsequent encounter
S	sequela

T25.Ø Burn of unspecified degree of ankle and foot

Use additional external cause code to identify the source, place and intent of the burn (XØØ-X19, X75-X77, X96-X98, Y92)

- T25.Ø1 Burn of unspecified degree of ankle
  - T25.Ø11 Burn of unspecified degree of right ankle
  - T25.Ø12 Burn of unspecified degree of left ankle
  - T25.Ø19 Burn of unspecified degree of unspecified ankle

CHAPTER 19 (SØØ-T88)

- T25.02 Burn of unspecified degree of foot
  - Excludes2 burn of unspecified degree of toe(s) (nail) (T25.03-)
  - T25.021 Burn of unspecified degree of right foot
  - T25.022 Burn of unspecified degree of left foot
  - T25.029 Burn of unspecified degree of unspecified foot
- T25.03 Burn of unspecified degree of toe(s) (nail)
  - T25.031 Burn of unspecified degree of right toe(s) (nail)
  - T25.032 Burn of unspecified degree of left toe(s) (nail)
  - T25.039 Burn of unspecified degree of unspecified toe(s) (nail)
- T25.09 Burn of unspecified degree of multiple sites of ankle and foot
  - T25.091 Burn of unspecified degree of multiple sites of right ankle and foot
  - T25.092 Burn of unspecified degree of multiple sites of left ankle and foot
  - T25.099 Burn of unspecified degree of multiple sites of unspecified ankle and foot

T25.1 Burn of first degree of ankle and foot

Use additional external cause code to identify the source, place and intent of the burn (X00-X19, X75-X77, X96-X98, Y92)

- T25.11 Burn of first degree of ankle
  - T25.111 Burn of first degree of right ankle
  - T25.112 Burn of first degree of left ankle
  - T25.119 Burn of first degree of unspecified ankle
- T25.12 Burn of first degree of foot
  - Excludes2 burn of first degree of toe(s) (nail) (T25.13-)
  - T25.121 Burn of first degree of right foot
  - T25.122 Burn of first degree of left foot
  - T25.129 Burn of first degree of unspecified foot
- T25.13 Burn of first degree of toe(s) (nail)
  - T25.131 Burn of first degree of right toe(s) (nail)
  - T25.132 Burn of first degree of left toe(s) (nail)
  - T25.139 Burn of first degree of unspecified toe(s) (nail)
- T25.19 Burn of first degree of multiple sites of ankle and foot
  - T25.191 Burn of first degree of multiple sites of right ankle and foot
  - T25.192 Burn of first degree of multiple sites of left ankle and foot
  - T25.199 Burn of first degree of multiple sites of unspecified ankle and foot

T25.2 Burn of second degree of ankle and foot

Use additional external cause code to identify the source, place and intent of the burn (X00-X19, X75-X77, X96-X98, Y92)

- T25.21 Burn of second degree of ankle
  - T25.211 Burn of second degree of right ankle
  - T25.212 Burn of second degree of left ankle
  - T25.219 Burn of second degree of unspecified ankle
- T25.22 Burn of second degree of foot
  - Excludes2 burn of second degree of toe(s) (nail) (T25.23-)
  - T25.221 Burn of second degree of right foot
  - T25.222 Burn of second degree of left foot
  - T25.229 Burn of second degree of unspecified foot
- T25.23 Burn of second degree of toe(s) (nail)
  - T25.231 Burn of second degree of right toe(s) (nail)
  - T25.232 Burn of second degree of left toe(s) (nail)
  - T25.239 Burn of second degree of unspecified toe(s) (nail)
- T25.29 Burn of second degree of multiple sites of ankle and foot
  - T25.291 Burn of second degree of multiple sites of right ankle and foot
  - T25.292 Burn of second degree of multiple sites of left ankle and foot
  - T25.299 Burn of second degree of multiple sites of unspecified ankle and foot

T25.3 Burn of third degree of ankle and foot

Use additional external cause code to identify the source, place and intent of the burn (X00-X19, X75-X77, X96-X98, Y92)

- T25.31 Burn of third degree of ankle Ex PDX 1918
  - T25.311 Burn of third degree of right ankle A, A
  - T25.312 Burn of third degree of left ankle A, A
  - T25.319 Burn of third degree of unspecified ankle A, A
- T25.32 Burn of third degree of foot Ex PDX 1919
  - Excludes2 burn of third degree of toe(s) (nail) (T25.33-)
  - T25.321 Burn of third degree of right foot A, A
  - T25.322 Burn of third degree of left foot A, A
  - T25.329 Burn of third degree of unspecified foot A, A
- T25.33 Burn of third degree of toe(s) (nail) Ex PDX 1920
  - T25.331 Burn of third degree of right toe(s) (nail) A, A
  - T25.332 Burn of third degree of left toe(s) (nail) A, A
  - T25.339 Burn of third degree of unspecified toe(s) (nail) A, A
- T25.39 Burn of third degree of multiple sites of ankle and foot Ex PDX 1914
  - T25.391 Burn of third degree of multiple sites of right ankle and foot A, A
  - T25.392 Burn of third degree of multiple sites of left ankle and foot A, A
  - T25.399 Burn of third degree of multiple sites of unspecified ankle and foot A, A

T25.4 Corrosion of unspecified degree of ankle and foot

Code first (T51-T65) to identify chemical and intent

Use additional external cause code to identify place (Y92)

- T25.41 Corrosion of unspecified degree of ankle
  - T25.411 Corrosion of unspecified degree of right ankle
  - T25.412 Corrosion of unspecified degree of left ankle
  - T25.419 Corrosion of unspecified degree of unspecified ankle

● T25.42 Corrosion of unspecified degree of foot
Excludes2 corrosion of unspecified degree of toe(s) (nail) (T25.43-)
● T25.421 Corrosion of unspecified degree of right foot
● T25.422 Corrosion of unspecified degree of left foot
● T25.429 Corrosion of unspecified degree of unspecified foot
● T25.43 Corrosion of unspecified degree of toe(s) (nail)
● T25.431 Corrosion of unspecified degree of right toe(s) (nail)
● T25.432 Corrosion of unspecified degree of left toe(s) (nail)
● T25.439 Corrosion of unspecified degree of unspecified toe(s) (nail)
● T25.49 Corrosion of unspecified degree of multiple sites of ankle and foot
● T25.491 Corrosion of unspecified degree of multiple sites of right ankle and foot
● T25.492 Corrosion of unspecified degree of multiple sites of left ankle and foot
● T25.499 Corrosion of unspecified degree of multiple sites of unspecified ankle and foot

● T25.5 Corrosion of first degree of ankle and foot
Code first (T51-T65) to identify chemical and intent
Use additional external cause code to identify place (Y92)
● T25.51 Corrosion of first degree of ankle
● T25.511 Corrosion of first degree of right ankle
● T25.512 Corrosion of first degree of left ankle
● T25.519 Corrosion of first degree of unspecified ankle
● T25.52 Corrosion of first degree of foot
Excludes2 corrosion of first degree of toe(s) (nail) (T25.53-)
● T25.521 Corrosion of first degree of right foot
● T25.522 Corrosion of first degree of left foot
● T25.529 Corrosion of first degree of unspecified foot
● T25.53 Corrosion of first degree of toe(s) (nail)
● T25.531 Corrosion of first degree of right toe(s) (nail)
● T25.532 Corrosion of first degree of left toe(s) (nail)
● T25.539 Corrosion of first degree of unspecified toe(s) (nail)
● T25.59 Corrosion of first degree of multiple sites of ankle and foot
● T25.591 Corrosion of first degree of multiple sites of right ankle and foot
● T25.592 Corrosion of first degree of multiple sites of left ankle and foot
● T25.599 Corrosion of first degree of multiple sites of unspecified ankle and foot

● T25.6 Corrosion of second degree of ankle and foot
Code first (T51-T65) to identify chemical and intent
Use additional external cause code to identify place (Y92)
● T25.61 Corrosion of second degree of ankle
● T25.611 Corrosion of second degree of right ankle
● T25.612 Corrosion of second degree of left ankle
● T25.619 Corrosion of second degree of unspecified ankle
● T25.62 Corrosion of second degree of foot
Excludes2 corrosion of second degree of toe(s) (nail) (T25.63-)
● T25.621 Corrosion of second degree of right foot
● T25.622 Corrosion of second degree of left foot
● T25.629 Corrosion of second degree of unspecified foot
● T25.63 Corrosion of second degree of toe(s) (nail)
● T25.631 Corrosion of second degree of right toe(s) (nail)
● T25.632 Corrosion of second degree of left toe(s) (nail)
● T25.639 Corrosion of second degree of unspecified toe(s) (nail)
● T25.69 Corrosion of second degree of multiple sites of ankle and foot
● T25.691 Corrosion of second degree of right ankle and foot
● T25.692 Corrosion of second degree of left ankle and foot
● T25.699 Corrosion of second degree of unspecified ankle and foot

● T25.7 Corrosion of third degree of ankle and foot
Code first (T51-T65) to identify chemical and intent
Use additional external cause code to identify place (Y92)
● T25.71 Corrosion of third degree of ankle Ex PDX 1918
● T25.711 Corrosion of third degree of right ankle A, A
● T25.712 Corrosion of third degree of left ankle A, A
● T25.719 Corrosion of third degree of unspecified ankle A, A
● T25.72 Corrosion of third degree of foot Ex PDX 1919
Excludes2 corrosion of third degree of toe(s) (nail) (T25.73-)
● T25.721 Corrosion of third degree of right foot A, A
● T25.722 Corrosion of third degree of left foot A, A
● T25.729 Corrosion of third degree of unspecified foot A, A
● T25.73 Corrosion of third degree of toe(s) (nail) Ex PDX 1920
● T25.731 Corrosion of third degree of right toe(s) (nail) A, A
● T25.732 Corrosion of third degree of left toe(s) (nail) A, A
● T25.739 Corrosion of third degree of unspecified toe(s) (nail) A, A
● T25.79 Corrosion of third degree of multiple sites of ankle and foot Ex PDX 1914
● T25.791 Corrosion of third degree of multiple sites of right ankle and foot A, A
● T25.792 Corrosion of third degree of multiple sites of left ankle and foot A, A
● T25.799 Corrosion of third degree of multiple sites of unspecified ankle and foot A, A

CHAPTER 19 (S00-T88)

BURNS AND CORROSIONS CONFINED TO EYE AND INTERNAL ORGANS (T26-T28)

T26 Burn and corrosion confined to eye and adnexa

The appropriate 7th character is to be added to each code from category T26

A initial encounter
D subsequent encounter
S sequela

T26.0 Burn of eyelid and periocular area

Use additional external cause code to identify the source, place and intent of the burn (X00-X19, X75-X77, X96-X98, Y92)

X T26.00 Burn of unspecified eyelid and periocular area
X T26.01 Burn of right eyelid and periocular area
X T26.02 Burn of left eyelid and periocular area

T26.1 Burn of cornea and conjunctival sac

Use additional external cause code to identify the source, place and intent of the burn (X00-X19, X75-X77, X96-X98, Y92)

X T26.10 Burn of cornea and conjunctival sac, unspecified eye
X T26.11 Burn of cornea and conjunctival sac, right eye
X T26.12 Burn of cornea and conjunctival sac, left eye

T26.2 Burn with resulting rupture and destruction of eyeball

Use additional external cause code to identify the source, place and intent of the burn (X00-X19, X75-X77, X96-X98, Y92)

X T26.20 Burn with resulting rupture and destruction of unspecified eyeball A, A (Ex) PDX 1921
X T26.21 Burn with resulting rupture and destruction of right eyeball A, A (Ex) PDX 1922
X T26.22 Burn with resulting rupture and destruction of left eyeball A, A (Ex) PDX 1923

T26.3 Burns of other specified parts of eye and adnexa

Use additional external cause code to identify the source, place and intent of the burn (X00-X19, X75-X77, X96-X98, Y92)

X T26.30 Burns of other specified parts of unspecified eye and adnexa
X T26.31 Burns of other specified parts of right eye and adnexa
X T26.32 Burns of other specified parts of left eye and adnexa

T26.4 Burn of eye and adnexa, part unspecified

Use additional external cause code to identify the source, place and intent of the burn (X00-X19, X75-X77, X96-X98, Y92)

X T26.40 Burn of unspecified eye and adnexa, part unspecified
X T26.41 Burn of right eye and adnexa, part unspecified
X T26.42 Burn of left eye and adnexa, part unspecified

T26.5 Corrosion of eyelid and periocular area

Code first (T51-T65) to identify chemical and intent

Use additional external cause code to identify place (Y92)

X T26.50 Corrosion of unspecified eyelid and periocular area
X T26.51 Corrosion of right eyelid and periocular area
X T26.52 Corrosion of left eyelid and periocular area

T26.6 Corrosion of cornea and conjunctival sac

Code first (T51-T65) to identify chemical and intent

Use additional external cause code to identify place (Y92)

X T26.60 Corrosion of cornea and conjunctival sac, unspecified eye
X T26.61 Corrosion of cornea and conjunctival sac, right eye
X T26.62 Corrosion of cornea and conjunctival sac, left eye

T26.7 Corrosion with resulting rupture and destruction of eyeball

Code first (T51-T65) to identify chemical and intent

Use additional external cause code to identify place (Y92)

X T26.70 Corrosion with resulting rupture and destruction of unspecified eyeball A, A (Ex) PDX 1924
X T26.71 Corrosion with resulting rupture and destruction of right eyeball A, A (Ex) PDX 1925
X T26.72 Corrosion with resulting rupture and destruction of left eyeball A, A (Ex) PDX 1926

T26.8 Corrosions of other specified parts of eye and adnexa

Code first (T51-T65) to identify chemical and intent

Use additional external cause code to identify place (Y92)

X T26.80 Corrosions of other specified parts of unspecified eye and adnexa
X T26.81 Corrosions of other specified parts of right eye and adnexa
X T26.82 Corrosions of other specified parts of left eye and adnexa

T26.9 Corrosion of eye and adnexa, part unspecified

Code first (T51-T65) to identify chemical and intent

Use additional external cause code to identify place (Y92)

X T26.90 Corrosion of unspecified eye and adnexa, part unspecified
X T26.91 Corrosion of right eye and adnexa, part unspecified
X T26.92 Corrosion of left eye and adnexa, part unspecified

T27 Burn and corrosion of respiratory tract (Ex) PDX 1927

Use additional external cause code to identify the source and intent of the burn (X00-X19, X75-X77, X96-X98)

Use additional external cause code to identify place (Y92)

The appropriate 7th character is to be added to each code from category T27

A initial encounter
D subsequent encounter
S sequela

X T27.0 Burn of larynx and trachea A, A
X T27.1 Burn involving larynx and trachea with lung A, A
X T27.2 Burn of other parts of respiratory tract A, A
Burn of thoracic cavity
X T27.3 Burn of respiratory tract, part unspecified A, A
X T27.4 Corrosion of larynx and trachea A, A
Code first (T51-T65) to identify chemical and intent
X T27.5 Corrosion involving larynx and trachea with lung A, A
Code first (T51-T65) to identify chemical and intent
X T27.6 Corrosion of other parts of respiratory tract A, A
Code first (T51-T65) to identify chemical and intent
X T27.7 Corrosion of respiratory tract, part unspecified A, A
Code first (T51-T65) to identify chemical and intent

T28 Burn and corrosion of other internal organs

Use additional external cause code to identify the source and intent of the burn (X00-X19, X75-X77, X96-X98)

Use additional external cause code to identify place (Y92)

The appropriate 7th character is to be added to each code from category T28

A initial encounter
D subsequent encounter
S sequela

X T28.0 Burn of mouth and pharynx
X T28.1 Burn of esophagus A, A (Ex) PDX 1928

X● T28.2 Burn of other parts of alimentary tract A, A (Ex) PDX 1929
X● T28.3 Burn of internal genitourinary organs
X● T28.4 Burns of other and unspecified internal organs
X● T28.40 Burn of unspecified internal organ
● T28.41 Burn of ear drum
● T28.411 Burn of right ear drum
● T28.412 Burn of left ear drum
● T28.419 Burn of unspecified ear drum
X● T28.49 Burn of other internal organ
X● T28.5 Corrosion of mouth and pharynx
Code first (T51-T65) to identify chemical and intent
X● T28.6 Corrosion of esophagus A, A (Ex) PDX 1928
Code first (T51-T65) to identify chemical and intent
X● T28.7 Corrosion of other parts of alimentary tract A, A (Ex) PDX 1929
Code first (T51-T65) to identify chemical and intent
X● T28.8 Corrosion of internal genitourinary organs
Code first (T51-T65) to identify chemical and intent
● T28.9 Corrosions of other and unspecified internal organs
Code first (T51-T65) to identify chemical and intent
X● T28.90 Corrosions of unspecified internal organs
● T28.91 Corrosions of ear drum
● T28.911 Corrosions of right ear drum
● T28.912 Corrosions of left ear drum
● T28.919 Corrosions of unspecified ear drum
X● T28.99 Corrosions of other internal organs

OGCR Section I.C.19.d.5.

Assign separate code for each burn site

When coding burns, assign separate codes for each burn site. Category T30, Burn and corrosion, body region unspecified is extremely vague and should rarely be used.

BURNS AND CORROSIONS OF MULTIPLE AND UNSPECIFIED BODY REGIONS (T30-T32)

● T30 Burn and corrosion, body region unspecified
T30.0 Burn of unspecified body region, unspecified degree
This code is not for inpatient use. Code to specified site and degree of burns
Burn NOS
Multiple burns NOS
T30.4 Corrosion of unspecified body region, unspecified degree
This code is not for inpatient use. Code to specified site and degree of corrosion
Corrosion NOS
Multiple corrosion NOS

● T31 Burns classified according to extent of body surface involved (Ex) PDX 1930
Note: This category is to be used as the primary code only when the site of the burn is unspecified. It should be used as a supplementary code with categories T20-T25 when the site is specified.
T31.0 Burns involving less than 10% of body surface
● T31.1 Burns involving 10-19% of body surface
T31.10 Burns involving 10-19% of body surface with 0% to 9% third degree burns
Burns involving 10-19% of body surface NOS
T31.11 Burns involving 10-19% of body surface with 10-19% third degree burns
● T31.2 Burns involving 20-29% of body surface
T31.20 Burns involving 20-29% of body surface with 0% to 9% third degree burns
Burns involving 20-29% of body surface NOS
T31.21 Burns involving 20-29% of body surface with 10-19% third degree burns
T31.22 Burns involving 20-29% of body surface with 20-29% third degree burns

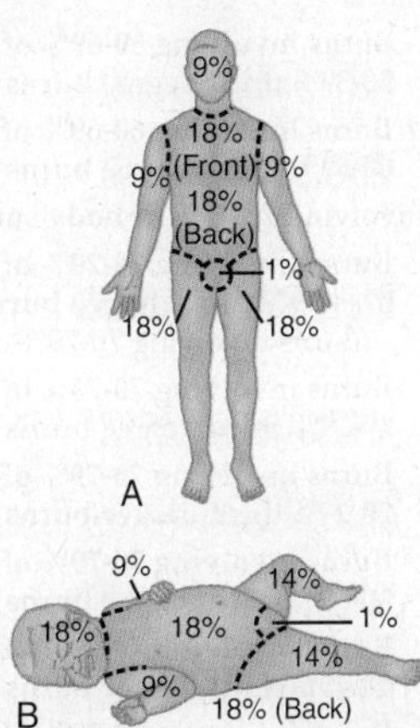

Figure 19-16 Rule of nines: percentages of total body area. (From Marx: Rosen's Emergency Medicine: Concepts and Clinical Practice, ed 6, Mosby, 2006)

● T31.3 Burns involving 30-39% of body surface
T31.30 Burns involving 30-39% of body surface with 0% to 9% third degree burns
Burns involving 30-39% of body surface NOS
T31.31 Burns involving 30-39% of body surface with 10-19% third degree burns
T31.32 Burns involving 30-39% of body surface with 20-29% third degree burns
T31.33 Burns involving 30-39% of body surface with 30-39% third degree burns
● T31.4 Burns involving 40-49% of body surface
T31.40 Burns involving 40-49% of body surface with 0% to 9% third degree burns
Burns involving 40-49% of body surface NOS
T31.41 Burns involving 40-49% of body surface with 10-19% third degree burns
T31.42 Burns involving 40-49% of body surface with 20-29% third degree burns
T31.43 Burns involving 40-49% of body surface with 30-39% third degree burns
T31.44 Burns involving 40-49% of body surface with 40-49% third degree burns
● T31.5 Burns involving 50-59% of body surface
T31.50 Burns involving 50-59% of body surface with 0% to 9% third degree burns
Burns involving 50-59% of body surface NOS
T31.51 Burns involving 50-59% of body surface with 10-19% third degree burns
T31.52 Burns involving 50-59% of body surface with 20-29% third degree burns
T31.53 Burns involving 50-59% of body surface with 30-39% third degree burns
T31.54 Burns involving 50-59% of body surface with 40-49% third degree burns
T31.55 Burns involving 50-59% of body surface with 50-59% third degree burns
● T31.6 Burns involving 60-69% of body surface
T31.60 Burns involving 60-69% of body surface with 0% to 9% third degree burns
Burns involving 60-69% of body surface NOS
T31.61 Burns involving 60-69% of body surface with 10-19% third degree burns
T31.62 Burns involving 60-69% of body surface with 20-29% third degree burns
T31.63 Burns involving 60-69% of body surface with 30-39% third degree burns
T31.64 Burns involving 60-69% of body surface with 40-49% third degree burns

CHAPTER 19 (S00-T88)

T31.65 Burns involving 60-69% of body surface with 50-59% third degree burns

T31.66 Burns involving 60-69% of body surface with 60-69% third degree burns

● T31.7 Burns involving 70-79% of body surface

T31.70 Burns involving 70-79% of body surface with 0% to 9% third degree burns
Burns involving 70-79% of body surface NOS

T31.71 Burns involving 70-79% of body surface with 10-19% third degree burns

T31.72 Burns involving 70-79% of body surface with 20-29% third degree burns

T31.73 Burns involving 70-79% of body surface with 30-39% third degree burns

T31.74 Burns involving 70-79% of body surface with 40-49% third degree burns

T31.75 Burns involving 70-79% of body surface with 50-59% third degree burns

T31.76 Burns involving 70-79% of body surface with 60-69% third degree burns

T31.77 Burns involving 70-79% of body surface with 70-79% third degree burns

● T31.8 Burns involving 80-89% of body surface

T31.80 Burns involving 80-89% of body surface with 0% to 9% third degree burns
Burns involving 80-89% of body surface NOS

T31.81 Burns involving 80-89% of body surface with 10-19% third degree burns

T31.82 Burns involving 80-89% of body surface with 20-29% third degree burns

T31.83 Burns involving 80-89% of body surface with 30-39% third degree burns

T31.84 Burns involving 80-89% of body surface with 40-49% third degree burns

T31.85 Burns involving 80-89% of body surface with 50-59% third degree burns

T31.86 Burns involving 80-89% of body surface with 60-69% third degree burns

T31.87 Burns involving 80-89% of body surface with 70-79% third degree burns

T31.88 Burns involving 80-89% of body surface with 80-89% third degree burns

● T31.9 Burns involving 90% or more of body surface

T31.90 Burns involving 90% or more of body surface with 0% to 9% third degree burns
Burns involving 90% or more of body surface NOS

T31.91 Burns involving 90% or more of body surface with 10-19% third degree burns

T31.92 Burns involving 90% or more of body surface with 20-29% third degree burns

T31.93 Burns involving 90% or more of body surface with 30-39% third degree burns

T31.94 Burns involving 90% or more of body surface with 40-49% third degree burns

T31.95 Burns involving 90% or more of body surface with 50-59% third degree burns

T31.96 Burns involving 90% or more of body surface with 60-69% third degree burns

T31.97 Burns involving 90% or more of body surface with 70-79% third degree burns

T31.98 Burns involving 90% or more of body surface with 80-89% third degree burns

T31.99 Burns involving 90% or more of body surface with 90% or more third degree burns

● T32 Corrosions classified according to extent of body surface involved Ex: PDX 1930

Note: This category is to be used as the primary code only when the site of the corrosion is unspecified. It may be used as a supplementary code with categories T20-T25 when the site is specified.

T32.0 Corrosions involving less than 10% of body surface

● T32.1 Corrosions involving 10-19% of body surface

T32.10 Corrosions involving 10-19% of body surface with 0% to 9% third degree corrosion
Corrosions involving 10-19% of body surface NOS

T32.11 Corrosions involving 10-19% of body surface with 10-19% third degree corrosion

● T32.2 Corrosions involving 20-29% of body surface

T32.20 Corrosions involving 20-29% of body surface with 0% to 9% third degree corrosion

T32.21 Corrosions involving 20-29% of body surface with 10-19% third degree corrosion

T32.22 Corrosions involving 20-29% of body surface with 20-29% third degree corrosion

● T32.3 Corrosions involving 30-39% of body surface

T32.30 Corrosions involving 30-39% of body surface with 0% to 9% third degree corrosion

T32.31 Corrosions involving 30-39% of body surface with 10-19% third degree corrosion

T32.32 Corrosions involving 30-39% of body surface with 20-29% third degree corrosion

T32.33 Corrosions involving 30-39% of body surface with 30-39% third degree corrosion

● T32.4 Corrosions involving 40-49% of body surface

T32.40 Corrosions involving 40-49% of body surface with 0% to 9% third degree corrosion

T32.41 Corrosions involving 40-49% of body surface with 10-19% third degree corrosion

T32.42 Corrosions involving 40-49% of body surface with 20-29% third degree corrosion

T32.43 Corrosions involving 40-49% of body surface with 30-39% third degree corrosion

T32.44 Corrosions involving 40-49% of body surface with 40-49% third degree corrosion

● T32.5 Corrosions involving 50-59% of body surface

T32.50 Corrosions involving 50-59% of body surface with 0% to 9% third degree corrosion

T32.51 Corrosions involving 50-59% of body surface with 10-19% third degree corrosion

T32.52 Corrosions involving 50-59% of body surface with 20-29% third degree corrosion

T32.53 Corrosions involving 50-59% of body surface with 30-39% third degree corrosion

T32.54 Corrosions involving 50-59% of body surface with 40-49% third degree corrosion

T32.55 Corrosions involving 50-59% of body surface with 50-59% third degree corrosion

● T32.6 Corrosions involving 60-69% of body surface

T32.60 Corrosions involving 60-69% of body surface with 0% to 9% third degree corrosion

T32.61 Corrosions involving 60-69% of body surface with 10-19% third degree corrosion

T32.62 Corrosions involving 60-69% of body surface with 20-29% third degree corrosion

T32.63 Corrosions involving 60-69% of body surface with 30-39% third degree corrosion

T32.64 Corrosions involving 60-69% of body surface with 40-49% third degree corrosion

T32.65 Corrosions involving 60-69% of body surface with 50-59% third degree corrosion

T32.66 Corrosions involving 60-69% of body surface with 60-69% third degree corrosion

T32.7 Corrosions involving **70-79%** of body surface
- T32.70 Corrosions involving 70-79% of body surface with **0% to 9% third degree** corrosion
- T32.71 Corrosions involving 70-79% of body surface with **10-19% third degree** corrosion
- T32.72 Corrosions involving 70-79% of body surface with **20-29% third degree** corrosion
- T32.73 Corrosions involving 70-79% of body surface with **30-39% third degree** corrosion
- T32.74 Corrosions involving 70-79% of body surface with **40-49% third degree** corrosion
- T32.75 Corrosions involving 70-79% of body surface with **50-59% third degree** corrosion
- T32.76 Corrosions involving 70-79% of body surface with **60-69% third degree** corrosion
- T32.77 Corrosions involving 70-79% of body surface with **70-79% third degree** corrosion

T32.8 Corrosions involving **80-89%** of body surface
- T32.80 Corrosions involving 80-89% of body surface with **0% to 9% third degree** corrosion
- T32.81 Corrosions involving 80-89% of body surface with **10-19% third degree** corrosion
- T32.82 Corrosions involving 80-89% of body surface with **20-29% third degree** corrosion
- T32.83 Corrosions involving 80-89% of body surface with **30-39% third degree** corrosion
- T32.84 Corrosions involving 80-89% of body surface with **40-49% third degree** corrosion
- T32.85 Corrosions involving 80-89% of body surface with **50-59% third degree** corrosion
- T32.86 Corrosions involving 80-89% of body surface with **60-69% third degree** corrosion
- T32.87 Corrosions involving 80-89% of body surface with **70-79% third degree** corrosion
- T32.88 Corrosions involving 80-89% of body surface with **80-89% third degree** corrosion

T32.9 Corrosions involving **90% or more** of body surface
- T32.90 Corrosions involving 90% or more of body surface with **0% to 9% third degree** corrosion
- T32.91 Corrosions involving 90% or more of body surface with **10-19% third degree** corrosion
- T32.92 Corrosions involving 90% or more of body surface with **20-29% third degree** corrosion
- T32.93 Corrosions involving 90% or more of body surface with **30-39% third degree** corrosion
- T32.94 Corrosions involving 90% or more of body surface with **40-49% third degree** corrosion
- T32.95 Corrosions involving 90% or more of body surface with **50-59% third degree** corrosion
- T32.96 Corrosions involving 90% or more of body surface with **60-69% third degree** corrosion
- T32.97 Corrosions involving 90% or more of body surface with **70-79% third degree** corrosion
- T32.98 Corrosions involving 90% or more of body surface with **80-89% third degree** corrosion
- T32.99 Corrosions involving 90% or more of body surface with **90% or more** third degree corrosion

FROSTBITE (T33-T34)

Excludes2 hypothermia and other effects of reduced temperature (T68, T69.-)

T33 Superficial frostbite

Includes frostbite with partial thickness skin loss

The appropriate 7th character is to be added to each code from category T33

- A initial encounter
- D subsequent encounter
- S sequela

T33.0 Superficial frostbite of **head** (Ex) PDX 1931
- T33.01 Superficial frostbite of **ear**
  - T33.011 Superficial frostbite of **right** ear A, A
  - T33.012 Superficial frostbite of **left** ear A, A
  - T33.019 Superficial frostbite of **unspecified** ear A, A
- X T33.02 Superficial frostbite of **nose** A, A
- X T33.09 Superficial frostbite of **other part** of head A, A

X **T33.1** Superficial frostbite of **neck** A, A (Ex) PDX 1931

X **T33.2** Superficial frostbite of **thorax** A, A (Ex) PDX 1932

X **T33.3** Superficial frostbite of **abdominal wall, lower back and pelvis** A, A (Ex) PDX 1932

T33.4 Superficial frostbite of **arm** (Ex) PDX 1932

Excludes2 superficial frostbite of wrist and hand (T33.5-)
- X T33.40 Superficial frostbite of **unspecified** arm A, A
- X T33.41 Superficial frostbite of **right** arm A, A
- X T33.42 Superficial frostbite of **left** arm A, A

T33.5 Superficial frostbite of wrist, hand, and fingers (Ex) PDX 1933
- T33.51 Superficial frostbite of **wrist**
  - T33.511 Superficial frostbite of **right** wrist A, A
  - T33.512 Superficial frostbite of **left** wrist A, A
  - T33.519 Superficial frostbite of **unspecified** wrist A, A
- T33.52 Superficial frostbite of **hand**

  Excludes2 superficial frostbite of fingers (T33.53-)
  - T33.521 Superficial frostbite of **right** hand A, A
  - T33.522 Superficial frostbite of **left** hand A, A
  - T33.529 Superficial frostbite of **unspecified** hand A, A
- T33.53 Superficial frostbite of **finger(s)**
  - T33.531 Superficial frostbite of **right** finger(s) A, A
  - T33.532 Superficial frostbite of **left** finger(s) A, A
  - T33.539 Superficial frostbite of **unspecified** finger(s) A, A

T33.6 Superficial frostbite of **hip and thigh** (Ex) PDX 1932
- X T33.60 Superficial frostbite of **unspecified** hip and thigh A, A
- X T33.61 Superficial frostbite of **right** hip and thigh A, A
- X T33.62 Superficial frostbite of **left** hip and thigh A, A

CHAPTER 19 (S00-T88)

● T33.7 Superficial frostbite of knee and lower leg (Ex) PDX 1932
Excludes2 superficial frostbite of ankle and foot (T33.8-)
X● T33.70 Superficial frostbite of unspecified knee and lower leg A, A
X● T33.71 Superficial frostbite of right knee and lower leg A, A
X● T33.72 Superficial frostbite of left knee and lower leg A, A
● T33.8 Superficial frostbite of ankle, foot, and toe(s) (Ex) PDX 1934
● T33.81 Superficial frostbite of ankle
● T33.811 Superficial frostbite of right ankle A, A
● T33.812 Superficial frostbite of left ankle A, A
● T33.819 Superficial frostbite of unspecified ankle A, A
● T33.82 Superficial frostbite of foot
● T33.821 Superficial frostbite of right foot A, A
● T33.822 Superficial frostbite of left foot A, A
● T33.829 Superficial frostbite of unspecified foot A, A
● T33.83 Superficial frostbite of toe(s)
● T33.831 Superficial frostbite of right toe(s) A, A
● T33.832 Superficial frostbite of left toe(s) A, A
● T33.839 Superficial frostbite of unspecified toe(s) A, A
● T33.9 Superficial frostbite of other and unspecified sites (Ex) PDX 1932
X● T33.90 Superficial frostbite of unspecified sites A, A
Superficial frostbite NOS
X● T33.99 Superficial frostbite of other sites A, A
Superficial frostbite of leg NOS
Superficial frostbite of trunk NOS

● T34 Frostbite with tissue necrosis
The appropriate 7th character is to be added to each code from category T34

A	initial encounter
D	subsequent encounter
S	sequela

● T34.0 Frostbite with tissue necrosis of head (Ex) PDX 1931
● T34.01 Frostbite with tissue necrosis of ear
● T34.011 Frostbite with tissue necrosis of right ear A, A
● T34.012 Frostbite with tissue necrosis of left ear A, A
● T34.019 Frostbite with tissue necrosis of unspecified ear A, A
X● T34.02 Frostbite with tissue necrosis of nose A, A
X● T34.09 Frostbite with tissue necrosis of other part of head A, A
X● T34.1 Frostbite with tissue necrosis of neck A, A (Ex) PDX 1931
X● T34.2 Frostbite with tissue necrosis of thorax A, A (Ex) PDX 1932
X● T34.3 Frostbite with tissue necrosis of abdominal wall, lower back and pelvis A, A (Ex) PDX 1932
● T34.4 Frostbite with tissue necrosis of arm (Ex) PDX 1932
Excludes2 frostbite with tissue necrosis of wrist and hand (T34.5-)
X● T34.40 Frostbite with tissue necrosis of unspecified arm A, A
X● T34.41 Frostbite with tissue necrosis of right arm A, A
X● T34.42 Frostbite with tissue necrosis of left arm A, A
● T34.5 Frostbite with tissue necrosis of wrist, hand, and finger(s) (Ex) PDX 1933
● T34.51 Frostbite with tissue necrosis of wrist
● T34.511 Frostbite with tissue necrosis of right wrist A, A
● T34.512 Frostbite with tissue necrosis of left wrist A, A
● T34.519 Frostbite with tissue necrosis of unspecified wrist A, A
● T34.52 Frostbite with tissue necrosis of hand
Excludes2 frostbite with tissue necrosis of finger(s) (T34.53-)
● T34.521 Frostbite with tissue necrosis of right hand A, A
● T34.522 Frostbite with tissue necrosis of left hand A, A
● T34.529 Frostbite with tissue necrosis of unspecified hand A, A
● T34.53 Frostbite with tissue necrosis of finger(s)
● T34.531 Frostbite with tissue necrosis of right finger(s) A, A
● T34.532 Frostbite with tissue necrosis of left finger(s) A, A
● T34.539 Frostbite with tissue necrosis of unspecified finger(s) A, A
● T34.6 Frostbite with tissue necrosis of hip and thigh (Ex) PDX 1932
X● T34.60 Frostbite with tissue necrosis of unspecified hip and thigh A, A
X● T34.61 Frostbite with tissue necrosis of right hip and thigh A, A
X● T34.62 Frostbite with tissue necrosis of left hip and thigh A, A
● T34.7 Frostbite with tissue necrosis of knee and lower leg (Ex) PDX 1932
Excludes2 frostbite with tissue necrosis of ankle and foot (T34.8-)
X● T34.70 Frostbite with tissue necrosis of unspecified knee and lower leg A, A
X● T34.71 Frostbite with tissue necrosis of right knee and lower leg A, A
X● T34.72 Frostbite with tissue necrosis of left knee and lower leg A, A
● T34.8 Frostbite with tissue necrosis of ankle, foot, and toe(s) (Ex) PDX 1934
● T34.81 Frostbite with tissue necrosis of ankle
● T34.811 Frostbite with tissue necrosis of right ankle A, A
● T34.812 Frostbite with tissue necrosis of left ankle A, A
● T34.819 Frostbite with tissue necrosis of unspecified ankle A, A
● T34.82 Frostbite with tissue necrosis of foot
● T34.821 Frostbite with tissue necrosis of right foot A, A
● T34.822 Frostbite with tissue necrosis of left foot A, A
● T34.829 Frostbite with tissue necrosis of unspecified foot A, A

CHAPTER 19 (SØ-T88)

- T34.83 **Frostbite with tissue necrosis of toe(s)**
  - T34.831 **Frostbite with tissue necrosis of right toe(s)** A, A
  - T34.832 **Frostbite with tissue necrosis of left toe(s)** A, A
  - T34.839 **Frostbite with tissue necrosis of unspecified toe(s)** A, A
- T34.9 **Frostbite with tissue necrosis of other and unspecified sites** PDX 1932
  - X T34.90 **Frostbite with tissue necrosis of unspecified sites** A, A
    Frostbite with tissue necrosis NOS
  - X T34.99 **Frostbite with tissue necrosis of other sites** A, A
    Frostbite with tissue necrosis of leg NOS
    Frostbite with tissue necrosis of trunk NOS

OGCR See Section I.C.19.e.

Adverse Effects, Poisoning, Underdosing and Toxic Effects
Codes in categories T36-T65 are combination codes that include the substance that was taken as well as the intent. No additional external cause code is required for poisonings, toxic effects, adverse effects and underdosing codes.

POISONING BY, ADVERSE EFFECTS OF AND UNDERDOSING OF DRUGS MEDICAMENTS AND BIOLOGICAL SUBSTANCES (T36-T5Ø)

Includes adverse effect of correct substance properly administered
poisoning by overdose of substance
poisoning by wrong substance given or taken in error
underdosing by (inadvertently) (deliberately) taking less substance than prescribed or instructed

Code first, for adverse effects, the nature of the adverse effect, such as:
adverse effect NOS (T88.7)
aspirin gastritis (K29.-)
blood disorders (D56-D76)
contact dermatitis (L23-L25)
dermatitis due to substances taken internally (L27.-)
nephropathy (N14.Ø-N14.2)

Note: The drug giving rise to the adverse effect should be identified by use of codes from categories T36-T5Ø with fifth or sixth character 5.

Use additional code(s) to specify:
manifestations of poisoning
underdosing or failure in dosage during medical and surgical care (Y63.6, Y63.8-Y63.9)
underdosing of medication regimen (Z91.12-, Z91.13-)

Excludes1 toxic reaction to local anesthesia in pregnancy (O29.3-)

Excludes2 abuse and dependence of psychoactive substances (F1Ø-F19)
abuse of non-dependence-producing substances (F55.-)
drug reaction and poisoning affecting newborn (PØØ-P96)
immunodeficiency due to drugs (D84.821)
pathological drug intoxication (inebriation) (F1Ø-F19)

T36 Poisoning by, adverse effect of and underdosing of systemic antibiotics

Excludes1 antineoplastic antibiotics (T45.1-)
locally applied antibiotic NEC (T49.Ø)
topically used antibiotic for ear, nose and throat (T49.6)
topically used antibiotic for eye (T49.5)

The appropriate 7th character is to be added to each code from category T36

A	initial encounter
D	subsequent encounter
S	sequela

- T36.Ø **Poisoning by, adverse effect of and underdosing of penicillins**
  - T36.ØX **Poisoning by, adverse effect of and underdosing of penicillins**
    - T36.ØX1 **Poisoning by penicillins, accidental (unintentional)**
      Poisoning by penicillins NOS
    - T36.ØX2 **Poisoning by penicillins, intentional self-harm** A, S
    - T36.ØX3 **Poisoning by penicillins, assault**
    - T36.ØX4 **Poisoning by penicillins, undetermined**
    - T36.ØX5 **Adverse effect of penicillins**
    - T36.ØX6 **Underdosing of penicillins**
- T36.1 **Poisoning by, adverse effect of and underdosing of cephalosporins and other betalactam antibiotics**
  - T36.1X **Poisoning by, adverse effect of and underdosing of cephalosporins and other beta-lactam antibiotics**
    - T36.1X1 **Poisoning by cephalosporins and other beta-lactam antibiotics, accidental (unintentional)**
      Poisoning by cephalosporins and other beta-lactam antibiotics NOS
    - T36.1X2 **Poisoning by cephalosporins and other beta-lactam antibiotics, intentional self-harm** A, S
    - T36.1X3 **Poisoning by cephalosporins and other beta-lactam antibiotics, assault**
    - T36.1X4 **Poisoning by cephalosporins and other beta-lactam antibiotics, undetermined**
    - T36.1X5 **Adverse effect of cephalosporins and other beta-lactam antibiotics**
    - T36.1X6 **Underdosing of cephalosporins and other beta-lactam antibiotics**
- T36.2 **Poisoning by, adverse effect of and underdosing of chloramphenicol group**
  - T36.2X **Poisoning by, adverse effect of and underdosing of chloramphenicol group**
    - T36.2X1 **Poisoning by chloramphenicol group, accidental (unintentional)**
      Poisoning by chloramphenicol group NOS
    - T36.2X2 **Poisoning by chloramphenicol group, intentional self-harm** A, S
    - T36.2X3 **Poisoning by chloramphenicol group, assault**
    - T36.2X4 **Poisoning by chloramphenicol group, undetermined**
    - T36.2X5 **Adverse effect of chloramphenicol group**
    - T36.2X6 **Underdosing of chloramphenicol group**
- T36.3 **Poisoning by, adverse effect of and underdosing of macrolides**
  - T36.3X **Poisoning by, adverse effect of and underdosing of macrolides**
    - T36.3X1 **Poisoning by macrolides, accidental (unintentional)**
      Poisoning by macrolides NOS
    - T36.3X2 **Poisoning by macrolides, intentional self-harm** A, S
    - T36.3X3 **Poisoning by macrolides, assault**
    - T36.3X4 **Poisoning by macrolides, undetermined**
    - T36.3X5 **Adverse effect of macrolides**
    - T36.3X6 **Underdosing of macrolides**

T36.4 Poisoning by, adverse effect of and underdosing of tetracyclines

T36.4X Poisoning by, adverse effect of and underdosing of tetracyclines

T36.4X1 Poisoning by tetracyclines, accidental (unintentional)
Poisoning by tetracyclines NOS

T36.4X2 Poisoning by tetracyclines, intentional self-harm A, S

T36.4X3 Poisoning by tetracyclines, assault

T36.4X4 Poisoning by tetracyclines, undetermined

T36.4X5 Adverse effect of tetracyclines

T36.4X6 Underdosing of tetracyclines

T36.5 Poisoning by, adverse effect of and underdosing of aminoglycosides
Poisoning by, adverse effect of and underdosing of streptomycin

T36.5X Poisoning by, adverse effect of and underdosing of aminoglycosides

T36.5X1 Poisoning by aminoglycosides, accidental (unintentional)
Poisoning by aminoglycosides NOS

T36.5X2 Poisoning by aminoglycosides, intentional self-harm A, S

T36.5X3 Poisoning by aminoglycosides, assault

T36.5X4 Poisoning by aminoglycosides, undetermined

T36.5X5 Adverse effect of aminoglycosides

T36.5X6 Underdosing of aminoglycosides

T36.6 Poisoning by, adverse effect of and underdosing of rifampicins

T36.6X Poisoning by, adverse effect of and underdosing of rifampicins

T36.6X1 Poisoning by rifampicins, accidental (unintentional)
Poisoning by rifampicins NOS

T36.6X2 Poisoning by rifampicins, intentional self-harm A, S

T36.6X3 Poisoning by rifampicins, assault

T36.6X4 Poisoning by rifampicins, undetermined

T36.6X5 Adverse effect of rifampicins

T36.6X6 Underdosing of rifampicins

T36.7 Poisoning by, adverse effect of and underdosing of antifungal antibiotics, systemically used

T36.7X Poisoning by, adverse effect of and underdosing of antifungal antibiotics, systemically used

T36.7X1 Poisoning by antifungal antibiotics, systemically used, accidental (unintentional)
Poisoning by antifungal antibiotics, systemically used NOS

T36.7X2 Poisoning by antifungal antibiotics, systemically used, intentional self-harm A, S

T36.7X3 Poisoning by antifungal antibiotics, systemically used, assault

T36.7X4 Poisoning by antifungal antibiotics, systemically used, undetermined

T36.7X5 Adverse effect of antifungal antibiotics, systemically used

T36.7X6 Underdosing of antifungal antibiotics, systemically used

T36.8 Poisoning by, adverse effect of and underdosing of other systemic antibiotics

T36.8X Poisoning by, adverse effect of and underdosing of other systemic antibiotics

T36.8X1 Poisoning by other systemic antibiotics, accidental (unintentional)
Poisoning by other systemic antibiotics NOS

T36.8X2 Poisoning by other systemic antibiotics, intentional self-harm A, S

T36.8X3 Poisoning by other systemic antibiotics, assault

T36.8X4 Poisoning by other systemic antibiotics, undetermined

T36.8X5 Adverse effect of other systemic antibiotics
Coding Clinic: 2017, Q1, P39

T36.8X6 Underdosing of other systemic antibiotics

T36.9 Poisoning by, adverse effect of and underdosing of unspecified systemic antibiotic

X T36.91 Poisoning by unspecified systemic antibiotic, accidental (unintentional)
Poisoning by systemic antibiotic NOS

X T36.92 Poisoning by unspecified systemic antibiotic, intentional self-harm A, S

X T36.93 Poisoning by unspecified systemic antibiotic, assault

X T36.94 Poisoning by unspecified systemic antibiotic, undetermined

X T36.95 Adverse effect of unspecified systemic antibiotic

X T36.96 Underdosing of unspecified systemic antibiotic

T37 Poisoning by, adverse effect of and underdosing of other systemic anti-infectives and antiparasitics

Excludes1 anti-infectives topically used for ear, nose and throat (T49.6-)
anti-infectives topically used for eye (T49.5-)
locally applied anti-infectives NEC (T49.0-)

The appropriate 7th character is to be added to each code from category T37

A	initial encounter
D	subsequent encounter
S	sequela

T37.0 Poisoning by, adverse effect of and underdosing of sulfonamides

T37.0X Poisoning by, adverse effect of and underdosing of sulfonamides

T37.0X1 Poisoning by sulfonamides, accidental (unintentional)
Poisoning by sulfonamides NOS

T37.0X2 Poisoning by sulfonamides, intentional self-harm A, S

T37.0X3 Poisoning by sulfonamides, assault

T37.0X4 Poisoning by sulfonamides, undetermined

T37.0X5 Adverse effect of sulfonamides

T37.0X6 Underdosing of sulfonamides

T37.1 Poisoning by, adverse effect of and underdosing of antimycobacterial drugs

Excludes1 rifampicins (T36.6-) streptomycin (T36.5-)

T37.1X Poisoning by, adverse effect of and underdosing of antimycobacterial drugs

T37.1X1 Poisoning by antimycobacterial drugs, accidental (unintentional)
Poisoning by antimycobacterial drugs NOS

T37.1X2 Poisoning by antimycobacterial drugs, intentional self-harm A, S

T37.1X3 Poisoning by antimycobacterial drugs, assault

T37.1X4 Poisoning by antimycobacterial drugs, undetermined

T37.1X5 Adverse effect of antimycobacterial drugs

T37.1X6 Underdosing of antimycobacterial drugs

T37.2 Poisoning by, adverse effect of and underdosing of antimalarials and drugs acting on other blood protozoa

Excludes1 hydroxyquinoline derivatives (T37.8-)

T37.2X Poisoning by, adverse effect of and underdosing of antimalarials and drugs acting on other blood protozoa

T37.2X1 Poisoning by antimalarials and drugs acting on other blood protozoa, accidental (unintentional)
Poisoning by antimalarials and drugs acting on other blood protozoa NOS

T37.2X2 Poisoning by antimalarials and drugs acting on other blood protozoa, intentional self-harm A, S

T37.2X3 Poisoning by antimalarials and drugs acting on other blood protozoa, assault

T37.2X4 Poisoning by antimalarials and drugs acting on other blood protozoa, undetermined

T37.2X5 Adverse effect of antimalarials and drugs acting on other blood protozoa

T37.2X6 Underdosing of antimalarials and drugs acting on other blood protozoa

T37.3 Poisoning by, adverse effect of and underdosing of other antiprotozoal drugs

T37.3X Poisoning by, adverse effect of and underdosing of other antiprotozoal drugs

T37.3X1 Poisoning by other antiprotozoal drugs, accidental (unintentional)
Poisoning by other antiprotozoal drugs NOS

T37.3X2 Poisoning by other antiprotozoal drugs, intentional self-harm A, S

T37.3X3 Poisoning by other antiprotozoal drugs, assault

T37.3X4 Poisoning by other antiprotozoal drugs, undetermined

T37.3X5 Adverse effect of other antiprotozoal drugs

T37.3X6 Underdosing of other antiprotozoal drugs

T37.4 Poisoning by, adverse effect of and underdosing of anthelminthics

T37.4X Poisoning by, adverse effect of and underdosing of anthelminthics

T37.4X1 Poisoning by anthelminthics, accidental (unintentional)
Poisoning by anthelminthics NOS

T37.4X2 Poisoning by anthelminthics, intentional self-harm A, S

T37.4X3 Poisoning by anthelminthics, assault

T37.4X4 Poisoning by anthelminthics, undetermined

T37.4X5 Adverse effect of anthelminthics

T37.4X6 Underdosing of anthelminthics

T37.5 Poisoning by, adverse effect of and underdosing of antiviral drugs

Excludes1 amantadine (T42.8-)
cytarabine (T45.1-)

T37.5X Poisoning by, adverse effect of and underdosing of antiviral drugs

T37.5X1 Poisoning by antiviral drugs, accidental (unintentional)
Poisoning by antiviral drugs NOS

T37.5X2 Poisoning by antiviral drugs, intentional self-harm A, S

T37.5X3 Poisoning by antiviral drugs, assault

T37.5X4 Poisoning by antiviral drugs, undetermined

T37.5X5 Adverse effect of antiviral drugs

T37.5X6 Underdosing of antiviral drugs

T37.8 Poisoning by, adverse effect of and underdosing of other specified systemic anti-infectives and antiparasitics
Poisoning by, adverse effect of and underdosing of hydroxyquinoline derivatives

Excludes1 antimalarial drugs (T37.2-)

T37.8X Poisoning by, adverse effect of and underdosing of other specified systemic anti-infectives and antiparasitics

T37.8X1 Poisoning by other specified systemic anti-infectives and antiparasitics, accidental (unintentional)
Poisoning by other specified systemic anti-infectives and antiparasitics NOS

T37.8X2 Poisoning by other specified systemic anti-infectives and antiparasitics, intentional self-harm A, S

T37.8X3 Poisoning by other specified systemic anti-infectives and antiparasitics, assault

T37.8X4 Poisoning by other specified systemic anti-infectives and antiparasitics, undetermined

T37.8X5 Adverse effect of other specified systemic anti-infectives and antiparasitics

T37.8X6 Underdosing of other specified systemic anti-infectives and antiparasitics

T37.9 Poisoning by, adverse effect of and underdosing of unspecified systemic anti-infective and antiparasitics

X T37.91 Poisoning by unspecified systemic anti-infective and antiparasitics, accidental (unintentional)
Poisoning by, adverse effect of and underdosing of systemic anti-infective and antiparasitics NOS

X T37.92 Poisoning by unspecified systemic anti-infective and antiparasitics, intentional self-harm A, S

X T37.93 Poisoning by unspecified systemic anti-infective and antiparasitics, assault

X T37.94 Poisoning by unspecified systemic anti-infective and antiparasitics, undetermined

X T37.95 Adverse effect of unspecified systemic anti-infective and antiparasitic

X T37.96 Underdosing of unspecified systemic anti-infectives and antiparasitics

CHAPTER 19 (SØ-T88)

T38 Poisoning by, adverse effect of and underdosing of hormones and their synthetic substitutes and antagonists, not elsewhere classified

Excludes1 mineralocorticoids and their antagonists (T5Ø.Ø-)
oxytocic hormones (T48.Ø-)
parathyroid hormones and derivatives (T5Ø.9-)

The appropriate 7th character is to be added to each code from category T38

A initial encounter
D subsequent encounter
S sequela

T38.Ø Poisoning by, adverse effect of and underdosing of glucocorticoids and synthetic analogues

Excludes1 glucocorticoids, topically used (T49.-)

T38.ØX Poisoning by, adverse effect of and underdosing of glucocorticoids and synthetic analogues

T38.ØX1 Poisoning by glucocorticoids and synthetic analogues, accidental (unintentional)
Poisoning by glucocorticoids and synthetic analogues NOS

T38.ØX2 Poisoning by glucocorticoids and synthetic analogues, intentional self-harm A, S

T38.ØX3 Poisoning by glucocorticoids and synthetic analogues, assault

T38.ØX4 Poisoning by glucocorticoids and synthetic analogues, undetermined

T38.ØX5 Adverse effect of glucocorticoids and synthetic analogues

T38.ØX6 Underdosing of glucocorticoids and synthetic analogues

T38.1 Poisoning by, adverse effect of and underdosing of thyroid hormones and substitutes

T38.1X Poisoning by, adverse effect of and underdosing of thyroid hormones and substitutes

T38.1X1 Poisoning by thyroid hormones and substitutes, accidental (unintentional)
Poisoning by thyroid hormones and substitutes NOS

T38.1X2 Poisoning by thyroid hormones and substitutes, intentional self-harm A, S

T38.1X3 Poisoning by thyroid hormones and substitutes, assault

T38.1X4 Poisoning by thyroid hormones and substitutes, undetermined

T38.1X5 Adverse effect of thyroid hormones and substitutes

T38.1X6 Underdosing of thyroid hormones and substitutes

T38.2 Poisoning by, adverse effect of and underdosing of antithyroid drugs

T38.2X Poisoning by, adverse effect of and underdosing of antithyroid drugs

T38.2X1 Poisoning by antithyroid drugs, accidental (unintentional)
Poisoning by antithyroid drugs NOS

T38.2X2 Poisoning by antithyroid drugs, intentional self-harm A, S

T38.2X3 Poisoning by antithyroid drugs, assault

T38.2X4 Poisoning by antithyroid drugs, undetermined

T38.2X5 Adverse effect of antithyroid drugs

T38.2X6 Underdosing of antithyroid drugs

T38.3 Poisoning by, adverse effect of and underdosing of insulin and oral hypoglycemic [antidiabetic] drugs

T38.3X Poisoning by, adverse effect of and underdosing of insulin and oral hypoglycemic [antidiabetic] drugs

T38.3X1 Poisoning by insulin and oral hypoglycemic [antidiabetic] drugs, accidental (unintentional)
Poisoning by insulin and oral hypoglycemic [antidiabetic] drugs NOS

T38.3X2 Poisoning by insulin and oral hypoglycemic [antidiabetic] drugs, intentional self-harm

T38.3X3 Poisoning by insulin and oral hypoglycemic [antidiabetic] drugs, assault A, S

T38.3X4 Poisoning by insulin and oral hypoglycemic [antidiabetic] drugs, undetermined

T38.3X5 Adverse effect of insulin and oral hypoglycemic [antidiabetic] drugs

T38.3X6 Underdosing of insulin and oral hypoglycemic [antidiabetic] drugs

T38.4 Poisoning by, adverse effect of and underdosing of oral contraceptives
Poisoning by, adverse effect of and underdosing of multiple- and single-ingredient oral contraceptive preparations

T38.4X Poisoning by, adverse effect of and underdosing of oral contraceptives

T38.4X1 Poisoning by oral contraceptives, accidental (unintentional)
Poisoning by oral contraceptives NOS

T38.4X2 Poisoning by oral contraceptives, intentional self-harm A, S

T38.4X3 Poisoning by oral contraceptives, assault

T38.4X4 Poisoning by oral contraceptives, undetermined

T38.4X5 Adverse effect of oral contraceptives

T38.4X6 Underdosing of oral contraceptives

T38.5 Poisoning by, adverse effect of and underdosing of other estrogens and progestogens
Poisoning by, adverse effect of and underdosing of estrogens and progestogens mixtures and substitutes

T38.5X Poisoning by, adverse effect of and underdosing of other estrogens and progestogens

T38.5X1 Poisoning by other estrogens and progestogens, accidental (unintentional)
Poisoning by other estrogens and progestogens NOS

T38.5X2 Poisoning by other estrogens and progestogens, intentional self-harm A, S

T38.5X3 Poisoning by other estrogens and progestogens, assault

T38.5X4 Poisoning by other estrogens and progestogens, undetermined

T38.5X5 Adverse effect of other estrogens and progestogens

T38.5X6 Underdosing of other estrogens and progestogens

CHAPTER 19 (SØØ-T88)

T38.6 Poisoning by, adverse effect of and underdosing of antigonadotrophins, antiestrogens, antiandrogens, not elsewhere classified
Poisoning by, adverse effect of and underdosing of tamoxifen

T38.6X Poisoning by, adverse effect of and underdosing of antigonadotrophins, antiestrogens, antiandrogens, not elsewhere classified

T38.6X1 Poisoning by antigonadotrophins, antiestrogens, antiandrogens, not elsewhere classified, accidental (unintentional)
Poisoning by antigonadotrophins, antiestrogens, antiandrogens, not elsewhere classified NOS

T38.6X2 Poisoning by antigonadotrophins, antiestrogens, antiandrogens, not elsewhere classified, intentional self-harm A, S

T38.6X3 Poisoning by antigonadotrophins, antiestrogens, antiandrogens, not elsewhere classified, assault

T38.6X4 Poisoning by antigonadotrophins, antiestrogens, antiandrogens, not elsewhere classified, undetermined

T38.6X5 Adverse effect of antigonadotrophins, antiestrogens, antiandrogens, not elsewhere classified

T38.6X6 Underdosing of antigonadotrophins, antiestrogens, antiandrogens, not elsewhere classified

T38.7 Poisoning by, adverse effect of and underdosing of androgens and anabolic congeners

T38.7X Poisoning by, adverse effect of and underdosing of androgens and anabolic congeners

T38.7X1 Poisoning by androgens and anabolic congeners, accidental (unintentional)
Poisoning by androgens and anabolic congeners NOS

T38.7X2 Poisoning by androgens and anabolic congeners, intentional self-harm A, S

T38.7X3 Poisoning by androgens and anabolic congeners, assault

T38.7X4 Poisoning by androgens and anabolic congeners, undetermined

T38.7X5 Adverse effect of androgens and anabolic congeners

T38.7X6 Underdosing of androgens and anabolic congeners

T38.8 Poisoning by, adverse effect of and underdosing of other and unspecified hormones and synthetic substitutes

T38.80 Poisoning by, adverse effect of and underdosing of unspecified hormones and synthetic substitutes

T38.801 Poisoning by unspecified hormones and synthetic substitutes, accidental (unintentional)
Poisoning by unspecified hormones and synthetic substitutes NOS

T38.802 Poisoning by unspecified hormones and synthetic substitutes, intentional self-harm A, S

T38.803 Poisoning by unspecified hormones and synthetic substitutes, assault

T38.804 Poisoning by unspecified hormones and synthetic substitutes, undetermined

T38.805 Adverse effect of unspecified hormones and synthetic substitutes

T38.806 Underdosing of unspecified hormones and synthetic substitutes

T38.81 Poisoning by, adverse effect of and underdosing of anterior pituitary [adenohypophyseal] hormones

T38.811 Poisoning by anterior pituitary [adenohypophyseal] hormones, accidental (unintentional)
Poisoning by anterior pituitary [adenohypophyseal] hormones NOS

T38.812 Poisoning by anterior pituitary [adenohypophyseal] hormones, intentional self-harm A, S

T38.813 Poisoning by anterior pituitary [adenohypophyseal] hormones, assault

T38.814 Poisoning by anterior pituitary [adenohypophyseal] hormones, undetermined

T38.815 Adverse effect of anterior pituitary [adenohypophyseal] hormones

T38.816 Underdosing of anterior pituitary [adenohypophyseal] hormones

T38.89 Poisoning by, adverse effect of and underdosing of other hormones and synthetic substitutes

T38.891 Poisoning by other hormones and synthetic substitutes, accidental (unintentional)
Poisoning by other hormones and synthetic substitutes NOS

T38.892 Poisoning by other hormones and synthetic substitutes, intentional self-harm A, S

T38.893 Poisoning by other hormones and synthetic substitutes, assault

T38.894 Poisoning by other hormones and synthetic substitutes, undetermined

T38.895 Adverse effect of other hormones and synthetic substitutes

T38.896 Underdosing of other hormones and synthetic substitutes

T38.9 Poisoning by, adverse effect of and underdosing of other and unspecified hormone antagonists

T38.90 Poisoning by, adverse effect of and underdosing of unspecified hormone antagonists

T38.901 Poisoning by unspecified hormone antagonists, accidental (unintentional)
Poisoning by unspecified hormone antagonists NOS

T38.902 Poisoning by unspecified hormone antagonists, intentional self-harm A, S

T38.903 Poisoning by unspecified hormone antagonists, assault

T38.904 Poisoning by unspecified hormone antagonists, undetermined

T38.905 Adverse effect of unspecified hormone antagonists

T38.906 Underdosing of unspecified hormone antagonists

CHAPTER 19 (S00-T88)

T38.99 Poisoning by, adverse effect of and underdosing of other hormone antagonists

T38.991 Poisoning by other hormone antagonists, accidental (unintentional)
Poisoning by other hormone antagonists NOS

T38.992 Poisoning by other hormone antagonists, intentional self-harm A, S

T38.993 Poisoning by other hormone antagonists, assault

T38.994 Poisoning by other hormone antagonists, undetermined

T38.995 Adverse effect of other hormone antagonists

T38.996 Underdosing of other hormone antagonists

T39 Poisoning by, adverse effect of and underdosing of nonopioid analgesics, antipyretics and antirheumatics

The appropriate 7th character is to be added to each code from category T39

A	initial encounter
D	subsequent encounter
S	sequela

T39.0 Poisoning by, adverse effect of and underdosing of salicylates

T39.01 Poisoning by, adverse effect of and underdosing of aspirin
Poisoning by, adverse effect of and underdosing of acetylsalicylic acid

T39.011 Poisoning by aspirin, accidental (unintentional)

T39.012 Poisoning by aspirin, intentional self-harm A, S

T39.013 Poisoning by aspirin, assault

T39.014 Poisoning by aspirin, undetermined

T39.015 Adverse effect of aspirin
Coding Clinic: 2016, Q1, P15

T39.016 Underdosing of aspirin

T39.09 Poisoning by, adverse effect of and underdosing of other salicylates

T39.091 Poisoning by salicylates, accidental (unintentional)
Poisoning by salicylates NOS

T39.092 Poisoning by salicylates, intentional self-harm A, S

T39.093 Poisoning by salicylates, assault

T39.094 Poisoning by salicylates, undetermined

T39.095 Adverse effect of salicylates

T39.096 Underdosing of salicylates

T39.1 Poisoning by, adverse effect of and underdosing of 4-Aminophenol derivatives

T39.1X Poisoning by, adverse effect of and underdosing of 4-Aminophenol derivatives

T39.1X1 Poisoning by 4-Aminophenol derivatives, accidental (unintentional)
Poisoning by 4-Aminophenol derivatives NOS

T39.1X2 Poisoning by 4-Aminophenol derivatives, intentional self-harm A, S

T39.1X3 Poisoning by 4-Aminophenol derivatives, assault

T39.1X4 Poisoning by 4-Aminophenol derivatives, undetermined

T39.1X5 Adverse effect of 4-Aminophenol derivatives

T39.1X6 Underdosing of 4-Aminophenol derivatives

T39.2 Poisoning by, adverse effect of and underdosing of pyrazolone derivatives

T39.2X Poisoning by, adverse effect of and underdosing of pyrazolone derivatives

T39.2X1 Poisoning by pyrazolone derivatives, accidental (unintentional)
Poisoning by pyrazolone derivatives NOS

T39.2X2 Poisoning by pyrazolone derivatives, intentional self-harm A, S

T39.2X3 Poisoning by pyrazolone derivatives, assault

T39.2X4 Poisoning by pyrazolone derivatives, undetermined

T39.2X5 Adverse effect of pyrazolone derivatives

T39.2X6 Underdosing of pyrazolone derivatives

T39.3 Poisoning by, adverse effect of and underdosing of other nonsteroidal anti-inflammatory drugs [NSAID]

T39.31 Poisoning by, adverse effect of and underdosing of propionic acid derivatives
Poisoning by, adverse effect of and underdosing of fenoprofen
Poisoning by, adverse effect of and underdosing of flurbiprofen
Poisoning by, adverse effect of and underdosing of ibuprofen
Poisoning by, adverse effect of and underdosing of ketoprofen
Poisoning by, adverse effect of and underdosing of naproxen
Poisoning by, adverse effect of and underdosing of oxaprozin

T39.311 Poisoning by propionic acid derivatives, accidental (unintentional)

T39.312 Poisoning by propionic acid derivatives, intentional self-harm A, S

T39.313 Poisoning by propionic acid derivatives, assault

T39.314 Poisoning by propionic acid derivatives, undetermined

T39.315 Adverse effect of propionic acid derivatives

T39.316 Underdosing of propionic acid derivatives

T39.39 Poisoning by, adverse effect of and underdosing of other nonsteroidal anti-inflammatory drugs [NSAID]

T39.391 Poisoning by other nonsteroidal anti-inflammatory drugs [NSAID], accidental (unintentional)
Poisoning by other nonsteroidal anti-inflammatory drugs NOS

T39.392 Poisoning by other nonsteroidal anti-inflammatory drugs [NSAID], intentional self-harm A, S

T39.393 Poisoning by other nonsteroidal anti-inflammatory drugs [NSAID], assault

T39.394 Poisoning by other nonsteroidal anti-inflammatory drugs [NSAID], undetermined

T39.395 Adverse effect of other nonsteroidal anti-inflammatory drugs [NSAID]

T39.396 Underdosing of other nonsteroidal anti-inflammatory drugs [NSAID]

T39.4 Poisoning by, adverse effect of and underdosing of antirheumatics, not elsewhere classified

Excludes1 poisoning by, adverse effect of and underdosing of glucocorticoids (T38.0-)
poisoning by, adverse effect of and underdosing of salicylates (T39.0-)

T39.4X Poisoning by, adverse effect of and underdosing of antirheumatics, not elsewhere classified

T39.4X1 Poisoning by antirheumatics, not elsewhere classified, accidental (unintentional)
Poisoning by antirheumatics, not elsewhere classified NOS

T39.4X2 Poisoning by antirheumatics, not elsewhere classified, intentional self-harm A, S

T39.4X3 Poisoning by antirheumatics, not elsewhere classified, assault

T39.4X4 Poisoning by antirheumatics, not elsewhere classified, undetermined

T39.4X5 Adverse effect of antirheumatics, not elsewhere classified

T39.4X6 Underdosing of antirheumatics, not elsewhere classified

T39.8 Poisoning by, adverse effect of and underdosing of other nonopioid analgesics and antipyretics, not elsewhere classified

T39.8X Poisoning by, adverse effect of and underdosing of other nonopioid analgesics and antipyretics, not elsewhere classified

T39.8X1 Poisoning by other nonopioid analgesics and antipyretics, not elsewhere classified, accidental (unintentional)
Poisoning by other nonopioid analgesics and antipyretics, not elsewhere classified NOS

T39.8X2 Poisoning by other nonopioid analgesics and antipyretics, not elsewhere classified, intentional self-harm A, S

T39.8X3 Poisoning by other nonopioid analgesics and antipyretics, not elsewhere classified, assault

T39.8X4 Poisoning by other nonopioid analgesics and antipyretics, not elsewhere classified, undetermined

T39.8X5 Adverse effect of other nonopioid analgesics and antipyretics, not elsewhere classified

T39.8X6 Underdosing of other nonopioid analgesics and antipyretics, not elsewhere classified

T39.9 Poisoning by, adverse effect of and underdosing of unspecified nonopioid analgesic, antipyretic and antirheumatic

X T39.91 Poisoning by unspecified nonopioid analgesic, antipyretic and antirheumatic, accidental (unintentional)
Poisoning by nonopioid analgesic, antipyretic and antirheumatic NOS

X T39.92 Poisoning by unspecified nonopioid analgesic, antipyretic and antirheumatic, intentional self-harm A, S

X T39.93 Poisoning by unspecified nonopioid analgesic, antipyretic and antirheumatic, assault

X T39.94 Poisoning by unspecified nonopioid analgesic, antipyretic and antirheumatic, undetermined

X T39.95 Adverse effect of unspecified nonopioid analgesic, antipyretic and antirheumatic

X T39.96 Underdosing of unspecified nonopioid analgesic, antipyretic and antirheumatic

T40 Poisoning by, adverse effect of and underdosing of narcotics and psychodysleptics [hallucinogens]

Excludes2 drug dependence and related mental and behavioral disorders due to psychoactive substance use (F10.-F19.-)

The appropriate 7th character is to be added to each code from category T40

A	initial encounter
D	subsequent encounter
S	sequela

T40.0 Poisoning by, adverse effect of and underdosing of opium

T40.0X Poisoning by, adverse effect of and underdosing of opium

T40.0X1 Poisoning by opium, accidental (unintentional)
Poisoning by opium NOS

T40.0X2 Poisoning by opium, intentional self-harm A, S

T40.0X3 Poisoning by opium, assault

T40.0X4 Poisoning by opium, undetermined

T40.0X5 Adverse effect of opium

T40.0X6 Underdosing of opium

T40.1 Poisoning by and adverse effect of heroin

T40.1X Poisoning by and adverse effect of heroin

T40.1X1 Poisoning by heroin, accidental (unintentional)
Poisoning by heroin NOS

T40.1X2 Poisoning by heroin, intentional self-harm A, S

T40.1X3 Poisoning by heroin, assault

T40.1X4 Poisoning by heroin, undetermined

T40.2 Poisoning by, adverse effect of and underdosing of other opioids

T40.2X Poisoning by, adverse effect of and underdosing of other opioids

T40.2X1 Poisoning by other opioids, accidental (unintentional)
Poisoning by other opioids NOS

T40.2X2 Poisoning by other opioids, intentional self-harm A, S

T40.2X3 Poisoning by other opioids, assault

T40.2X4 Poisoning by other opioids, undetermined

T40.2X5 Adverse effect of other opioids

T40.2X6 Underdosing of other opioids

T40.3 Poisoning by, adverse effect of and underdosing of methadone

T40.3X Poisoning by, adverse effect of and underdosing of methadone

T40.3X1 Poisoning by methadone, accidental (unintentional)
Poisoning by methadone NOS

T40.3X2 Poisoning by methadone, intentional self-harm A, S

T40.3X3 Poisoning by methadone, assault

T40.3X4 Poisoning by methadone, undetermined

T40.3X5 Adverse effect of methadone

T40.3X6 Underdosing of methadone

T40.4 Poisoning by, adverse effect of and underdosing of other synthetic narcotics

T40.41 Poisoning by, adverse effect of and underdosing of fentanyl or fentanyl analogs

T40.411 Poisoning by fentanyl or fentanyl analogs, accidental (unintentional)

T40.412 Poisoning by fentanyl or fentanyl analogs, intentional self-harm

T40.413 Poisoning by fentanyl or fentanyl analogs, assault

T40.414 Poisoning by fentanyl or fentanyl analogs, undetermined

T40.415 Adverse effect of fentanyl or fentanyl analogs

T40.416 Underdosing of fentanyl or fentanyl analogs

T40.42 Poisoning by, adverse effect of and underdosing of tramadol

T40.421 Poisoning by tramadol, accidental (unintentional)

T40.422 Poisoning by tramadol, intentional self-harm

T40.423 Poisoning by tramadol, assault

T40.424 Poisoning by tramadol, undetermined

T40.425 Adverse effect of tramadol

T40.426 Underdosing of tramadol

T40.49 Poisoning by, adverse effect of and underdosing of other synthetic narcotics

T40.491 Poisoning by other synthetic narcotics, accidental (unintentional)

T40.492 Poisoning by other synthetic narcotics, intentional self-harm

T40.493 Poisoning by other synthetic narcotics, assault

T40.494 Poisoning by other synthetic narcotics, undetermined

T40.495 Adverse effect of other synthetic narcotics

T40.496 Underdosing of other synthetic narcotics

T40.5 Poisoning by, adverse effect of and underdosing of cocaine

T40.5X Poisoning by, adverse effect of and underdosing of cocaine

T40.5X1 Poisoning by cocaine, accidental (unintentional)
Poisoning by cocaine NOS
Coding Clinic: 2016, Q2, P9

T40.5X2 Poisoning by cocaine, intentional self-harm A, S

T40.5X3 Poisoning by cocaine, assault

T40.5X4 Poisoning by cocaine, undetermined

T40.5X5 Adverse effect of cocaine

T40.5X6 Underdosing of cocaine

T40.6 Poisoning by, adverse effect of and underdosing of other and unspecified narcotics

T40.60 Poisoning by, adverse effect of and underdosing of unspecified narcotics

T40.601 Poisoning by unspecified narcotics, accidental (unintentional)
Poisoning by narcotics NOS

T40.602 Poisoning by unspecified narcotics, intentional self-harm A, S

T40.603 Poisoning by unspecified narcotics, assault

T40.604 Poisoning by unspecified narcotics, undetermined

T40.605 Adverse effect of unspecified narcotics

T40.606 Underdosing of unspecified narcotics

T40.69 Poisoning by, adverse effect of and underdosing of other narcotics

T40.691 Poisoning by other narcotics, accidental (unintentional)
Poisoning by other narcotics NOS

T40.692 Poisoning by other narcotics, intentional self-harm A, S

T40.693 Poisoning by other narcotics, assault

T40.694 Poisoning by other narcotics, undetermined

T40.695 Adverse effect of other narcotics

T40.696 Underdosing of other narcotics

T40.7 Poisoning by, adverse effect of and underdosing of cannabis (derivatives)

T40.71 Poisoning by, adverse effect of and underdosing of cannabis (derivatives)

T40.711 Poisoning by cannabis, accidental (unintentional)

T40.712 Poisoning by cannabis, intentional self-harm

T40.713 Poisoning by cannabis, assault

T40.714 Poisoning by cannabis, undetermined

T40.715 Adverse effect of cannabis

T40.716 Underdosing of cannabis

T40.72 Poisoning by, adverse effect of and underdosing of synthetic cannabinoids

T40.721 Poisoning by synthetic cannabinoids, accidental (unintentional)

T40.722 Poisoning by synthetic cannabinoids, intentional self-harm

T40.723 Poisoning by synthetic cannabinoids, assault

T40.724 Poisoning by synthetic cannabinoids, undetermined

T40.725 Adverse effect of synthetic cannabinoids

T40.726 Underdosing of synthetic cannabinoids

T40.8 Poisoning by and adverse effect of lysergide [LSD]

T40.8X Poisoning by and adverse effect of lysergide [LSD]

T40.8X1 Poisoning by lysergide [LSD], accidental (unintentional)
Poisoning by lysergide [LSD] NOS

T40.8X2 Poisoning by lysergide [LSD], intentional self-harm A, S

T40.8X3 Poisoning by lysergide [LSD], assault

T40.8X4 Poisoning by lysergide [LSD], undetermined

T40.9 Poisoning by, adverse effect of and underdosing of other and unspecified psychodysleptics [hallucinogens]

T40.90 Poisoning by, adverse effect of and underdosing of unspecified psychodysleptics [hallucinogens]

T40.901 Poisoning by unspecified psychodysleptics [hallucinogens], accidental (unintentional)

T40.902 Poisoning by unspecified psychodysleptics [hallucinogens], intentional self-harm A, S

T40.903 Poisoning by unspecified psychodysleptics [hallucinogens], assault

T40.904 Poisoning by unspecified psychodysleptics [hallucinogens], undetermined

T40.905 Adverse effect of unspecified psychodysleptics [hallucinogens]
T40.906 Underdosing of unspecified psychodysleptics [hallucinogens]

T40.99 Poisoning by, adverse effect of and underdosing of other psychodysleptics [hallucinogens]
T40.991 Poisoning by other psychodysleptics [hallucinogens], accidental (unintentional)
Poisoning by other psychodysleptics [hallucinogens] NOS
T40.992 Poisoning by other psychodysleptics [hallucinogens], intentional self-harm A, S
T40.993 Poisoning by other psychodysleptics [hallucinogens], assault
T40.994 Poisoning by other psychodysleptics [hallucinogens], undetermined
T40.995 Adverse effect of other psychodysleptics [hallucinogens]
T40.996 Underdosing of other psychodysleptics [hallucinogens]

T41 Poisoning by, adverse effect of and underdosing of anesthetics and therapeutic gases

Excludes1 benzodiazepines (T42.4-)
cocaine (T40.5-)
complications of anesthesia during pregnancy (O29.-)
complications of anesthesia during labor and delivery (O74.-)
complications of anesthesia during the puerperium (O89.-) opioids (T40.0-T40.2-)

The appropriate 7th character is to be added to each code from category T41

A	initial encounter
D	subsequent encounter
S	sequela

T41.0 Poisoning by, adverse effect of and underdosing of inhaled anesthetics
Excludes1 oxygen (T41.5-)

T41.0X Poisoning by, adverse effect of and underdosing of inhaled anesthetics
T41.0X1 Poisoning by inhaled anesthetics, accidental (unintentional)
Poisoning by inhaled anesthetics NOS
T41.0X2 Poisoning by inhaled anesthetics, intentional self-harm A, S
T41.0X3 Poisoning by inhaled anesthetics, assault
T41.0X4 Poisoning by inhaled anesthetics, undetermined
T41.0X5 Adverse effect of inhaled anesthetics
T41.0X6 Underdosing of inhaled anesthetics

T41.1 Poisoning by, adverse effect of and underdosing of intravenous anesthetics
Poisoning by, adverse effect of and underdosing of thiobarbiturates

T41.1X Poisoning by, adverse effect of and underdosing of intravenous anesthetics
T41.1X1 Poisoning by intravenous anesthetics, accidental (unintentional)
Poisoning by intravenous anesthetics NOS
T41.1X2 Poisoning by intravenous anesthetics, intentional self-harm A, S
T41.1X3 Poisoning by intravenous anesthetics, assault
T41.1X4 Poisoning by intravenous anesthetics, undetermined
T41.1X5 Adverse effect of intravenous anesthetics
T41.1X6 Underdosing of intravenous anesthetics

T41.2 Poisoning by, adverse effect of and underdosing of other and unspecified general anesthetics

T41.20 Poisoning by, adverse effect of and underdosing of unspecified general anesthetics
T41.201 Poisoning by unspecified general anesthetics, accidental (unintentional)
Poisoning by general anesthetics NOS
T41.202 Poisoning by unspecified general anesthetics, intentional self-harm A, S
T41.203 Poisoning by unspecified general anesthetics, assault
T41.204 Poisoning by unspecified general anesthetics, undetermined
T41.205 Adverse effect of unspecified general anesthetics
Coding Clinic: 2016, Q4, P73
T41.206 Underdosing of unspecified general anesthetics

T41.29 Poisoning by, adverse effect of and underdosing of other general anesthetics
T41.291 Poisoning by other general anesthetics, accidental (unintentional)
Poisoning by other general anesthetics NOS
T41.292 Poisoning by other general anesthetics, intentional self-harm A, S
T41.293 Poisoning by other general anesthetics, assault
T41.294 Poisoning by other general anesthetics, undetermined
T41.295 Adverse effect of other general anesthetics
T41.296 Underdosing of other general anesthetics

T41.3 Poisoning by, adverse effect of and underdosing of local anesthetics
Cocaine (topical)
Excludes2 poisoning by cocaine used as a central nervous system stimulant (T40.5X1-T40.5X4)

T41.3X Poisoning by, adverse effect of and underdosing of local anesthetics
T41.3X1 Poisoning by local anesthetics, accidental (unintentional)
Poisoning by local anesthetics NOS
T41.3X2 Poisoning by local anesthetics, intentional self-harm A, S
T41.3X3 Poisoning by local anesthetics, assault
T41.3X4 Poisoning by local anesthetics, undetermined
T41.3X5 Adverse effect of local anesthetics
T41.3X6 Underdosing of local anesthetics

T41.4 Poisoning by, adverse effect of and underdosing of unspecified anesthetic
X T41.41 Poisoning by unspecified anesthetic, accidental (unintentional)
Poisoning by anesthetic NOS
X T41.42 Poisoning by unspecified anesthetic, intentional self-harm A, S
X T41.43 Poisoning by unspecified anesthetic, assault
X T41.44 Poisoning by unspecified anesthetic, undetermined
X T41.45 Adverse effect of unspecified anesthetic
X T41.46 Underdosing of unspecified anesthetics

CHAPTER 19 (S00-T88)

● T41.5 **Poisoning by, adverse effect of and underdosing of therapeutic gases**

● T41.5X **Poisoning by, adverse effect of and underdosing of therapeutic gases**

● T41.5X1 **Poisoning by therapeutic gases, accidental (unintentional)**
Poisoning by therapeutic gases NOS

● T41.5X2 **Poisoning by therapeutic gases, intentional self-harm A, S**

● T41.5X3 **Poisoning by therapeutic gases, assault**

● T41.5X4 **Poisoning by therapeutic gases, undetermined**

●● T41.5X5 **Adverse effect of therapeutic gases**

●● T41.5X6 **Underdosing of therapeutic gases**

● T42 **Poisoning by, adverse effect of and underdosing of antiepileptic, sedative-hypnotic and antiparkinsonism drugs**

Excludes2 drug dependence and related mental and behavioral disorders due to psychoactive substance use (F1Ø.--F19.-)

The appropriate 7th character is to be added to each code from category T42

A	initial encounter
D	subsequent encounter
S	sequela

● T42.Ø **Poisoning by, adverse effect of and underdosing of hydantoin derivatives**

● T42.ØX **Poisoning by, adverse effect of and underdosing of hydantoin derivatives**

● T42.ØX1 **Poisoning by hydantoin derivatives, accidental (unintentional)**
Poisoning by hydantoin derivatives NOS

● T42.ØX2 **Poisoning by hydantoin derivatives, intentional self-harm A, S**

● T42.ØX3 **Poisoning by hydantoin derivatives, assault**

● T42.ØX4 **Poisoning by hydantoin derivatives, undetermined**

●● T42.ØX5 **Adverse effect of hydantoin derivatives**

●● T42.ØX6 **Underdosing of hydantoin derivatives**

● T42.1 **Poisoning by, adverse effect of and underdosing of iminostilbenes**
Poisoning by, adverse effect of and underdosing of carbamazepine

● T42.1X **Poisoning by, adverse effect of and underdosing of iminostilbenes**

● T42.1X1 **Poisoning by iminostilbenes, accidental (unintentional)**
Poisoning by iminostilbenes NOS

● T42.1X2 **Poisoning by iminostilbenes, intentional self-harm A, S**

● T42.1X3 **Poisoning by iminostilbenes, assault**

● T42.1X4 **Poisoning by iminostilbenes, undetermined**

●● T42.1X5 **Adverse effect of iminostilbenes**

●● T42.1X6 **Underdosing of iminostilbenes**

● T42.2 **Poisoning by, adverse effect of and underdosing of succinimides and oxazolidinediones**

● T42.2X **Poisoning by, adverse effect of and underdosing of succinimides and oxazolidinediones**

● T42.2X1 **Poisoning by succinimides and oxazolidinediones, accidental (unintentional)**
Poisoning by succinimides and oxazolidinediones NOS

● T42.2X2 **Poisoning by succinimides and oxazolidinediones, intentional self-harm A, S**

● T42.2X3 **Poisoning by succinimides and oxazolidinediones, assault**

● T42.2X4 **Poisoning by succinimides and oxazolidinediones, undetermined**

●● T42.2X5 **Adverse effect of succinimides and oxazolidinediones**

●● T42.2X6 **Underdosing of succinimides and oxazolidinediones**

● T42.3 **Poisoning by, adverse effect of and underdosing of barbiturates**

Excludes1 poisoning by, adverse effect of and underdosing of thiobarbiturates (T41.1-)

● T42.3X **Poisoning by, adverse effect of and underdosing of barbiturates**

● T42.3X1 **Poisoning by barbiturates, accidental (unintentional)**
Poisoning by barbiturates NOS

● T42.3X2 **Poisoning by barbiturates, intentional self-harm A, S**

● T42.3X3 **Poisoning by barbiturates, assault**

● T42.3X4 **Poisoning by barbiturates, undetermined**

●● T42.3X5 **Adverse effect of barbiturates**

●● T42.3X6 **Underdosing of barbiturates**

● T42.4 **Poisoning by, adverse effect of and underdosing of benzodiazepines**

● T42.4X **Poisoning by, adverse effect of and underdosing of benzodiazepines**

● T42.4X1 **Poisoning by benzodiazepines, accidental (unintentional)**
Poisoning by benzodiazepines NOS

● T42.4X2 **Poisoning by benzodiazepines, intentional self-harm A, S**

● T42.4X3 **Poisoning by benzodiazepines, assault**

● T42.4X4 **Poisoning by benzodiazepines, undetermined**

●● T42.4X5 **Adverse effect of benzodiazepines**

●● T42.4X6 **Underdosing of benzodiazepines**

● T42.5 **Poisoning by, adverse effect of and underdosing of mixed antiepileptics**

● T42.5X **Poisoning by, adverse effect of and underdosing of antiepileptics**

● T42.5X1 **Poisoning by mixed antiepileptics, accidental (unintentional)**
Poisoning by mixed antiepileptics NOS

● T42.5X2 **Poisoning by mixed antiepileptics, intentional self-harm A, S**

● T42.5X3 **Poisoning by mixed antiepileptics, assault**

● T42.5X4 **Poisoning by mixed antiepileptics, undetermined**

●● T42.5X5 **Adverse effect of mixed antiepileptics**

●● T42.5X6 **Underdosing of mixed antiepileptics**

● T42.6 **Poisoning by, adverse effect of and underdosing of other antiepileptic and sedative-hypnotic drugs**
Poisoning by, adverse effect of and underdosing of methaqualone
Poisoning by, adverse effect of and underdosing of valproic acid

Excludes1 poisoning by, adverse effect of and underdosing of carbamazepine (T42.1-)

T42.6X Poisoning by, adverse effect of and underdosing of other antiepileptic and sedative-hypnotic drugs

T42.6X1 Poisoning by other antiepileptic and sedative-hypnotic drugs, accidental (unintentional)
Poisoning by other antiepileptic and sedative-hypnotic drugs NOS

T42.6X2 Poisoning by other antiepileptic and sedative-hypnotic drugs, intentional self-harm A, S

T42.6X3 Poisoning by other antiepileptic and sedative-hypnotic drugs, assault

T42.6X4 Poisoning by other antiepileptic and sedative-hypnotic drugs, undetermined

T42.6X5 Adverse effect of other antiepileptic and sedative-hypnotic drugs

T42.6X6 Underdosing of other antiepileptic and sedative-hypnotic drugs

T42.7 Poisoning by, adverse effect of and underdosing of unspecified antiepileptic and sedative-hypnotic drugs

X T42.71 Poisoning by unspecified antiepileptic and sedative-hypnotic drugs, accidental (unintentional)
Poisoning by antiepileptic and sedative-hypnotic drugs NOS

X T42.72 Poisoning by unspecified antiepileptic and sedative-hypnotic drugs, intentional self-harm A, S

X T42.73 Poisoning by unspecified antiepileptic and sedative-hypnotic drugs, assault

X T42.74 Poisoning by unspecified antiepileptic and sedative-hypnotic drugs, undetermined

X T42.75 Adverse effect of unspecified antiepileptic and sedative-hypnotic drugs

X T42.76 Underdosing of unspecified antiepileptic and sedative-hypnotic drugs

T42.8 Poisoning by, adverse effect of and underdosing of antiparkinsonism drugs and other central muscle-tone depressants
Poisoning by, adverse effect of and underdosing of amantadine

T42.8X Poisoning by, adverse effect of and underdosing of antiparkinsonism drugs and other central muscle-tone depressants

T42.8X1 Poisoning by antiparkinsonism drugs and other central muscle-tone depressants, accidental (unintentional)
Poisoning by antiparkinsonism drugs and other central muscle-tone depressants NOS

T42.8X2 Poisoning by antiparkinsonism drugs and other central muscle-tone depressants, intentional self-harm A, S

T42.8X3 Poisoning by antiparkinsonism drugs and other central muscle-tone depressants, assault

T42.8X4 Poisoning by antiparkinsonism drugs and other central muscle-tone depressants, undetermined

T42.8X5 Adverse effect of antiparkinsonism drugs and other central muscle-tone depressants

T42.8X6 Underdosing of antiparkinsonism drugs and other central muscle-tone depressants

T43 Poisoning by, adverse effect of and underdosing of psychotropic drugs, not elsewhere classified

Excludes1 appetite depressants (T50.5-)
barbiturates (T42.3-)
benzodiazepines (T42.4-)
methaqualone (T42.6-)
psychodysleptics [hallucinogens] (T40.7-T40.9-)

Excludes2 drug dependence and related mental and behavioral disorders due to psychoactive substance use (F10.--F19.-)

The appropriate 7th character is to be added to each code from category T43

A	initial encounter
D	subsequent encounter
S	sequela

T43.0 Poisoning by, adverse effect of and underdosing of tricyclic and tetracyclic antidepressants

T43.01 Poisoning by, adverse effect of and underdosing of tricyclic antidepressants

T43.011 Poisoning by tricyclic antidepressants, accidental (unintentional)
Poisoning by tricyclic antidepressants NOS

T43.012 Poisoning by tricyclic antidepressants, intentional self-harm A, S

T43.013 Poisoning by tricyclic antidepressants, assault

T43.014 Poisoning by tricyclic antidepressants, undetermined

T43.015 Adverse effect of tricyclic antidepressants

T43.016 Underdosing of tricyclic antidepressants

T43.02 Poisoning by, adverse effect of and underdosing of tetracyclic antidepressants

T43.021 Poisoning by tetracyclic antidepressants, accidental (unintentional)
Poisoning by tetracyclic antidepressants NOS

T43.022 Poisoning by tetracyclic antidepressants, intentional self-harm A, S

T43.023 Poisoning by tetracyclic antidepressants, assault

T43.024 Poisoning by tetracyclic antidepressants, undetermined

T43.025 Adverse effect of tetracyclic antidepressants

T43.026 Underdosing of tetracyclic antidepressants

T43.1 Poisoning by, adverse effect of and underdosing of monoamine-oxidase-inhibitor antidepressants

T43.1X Poisoning by, adverse effect of and underdosing of monoamine-oxidase-inhibitor antidepressants

T43.1X1 Poisoning by monoamine-oxidase-inhibitor antidepressants, accidental (unintentional)
Poisoning by monoamine-oxidase-inhibitor antidepressants NOS

T43.1X2 Poisoning by monoamine-oxidase-inhibitor antidepressants, intentional self-harm A, S

T43.1X3 Poisoning by monoamine-oxidase-inhibitor antidepressants, assault

T43.1X4 Poisoning by monoamine-oxidase-inhibitor antidepressants, undetermined

T43.1X5 **Adverse effect** of monoamine-oxidase-inhibitor antidepressants

T43.1X6 **Underdosing** of monoamine-oxidase-inhibitor antidepressants

T43.2 Poisoning by, adverse effect of and underdosing of other and unspecified antidepressants

T43.20 Poisoning by, adverse effect of and underdosing of **unspecified antidepressants**

T43.201 Poisoning by unspecified antidepressants, **accidental** (unintentional)
Poisoning by antidepressants NOS

T43.202 Poisoning by unspecified antidepressants, **intentional** self-harm A, S

T43.203 Poisoning by unspecified antidepressants, **assault**

T43.204 Poisoning by unspecified antidepressants, **undetermined**

T43.205 **Adverse effect** of unspecified antidepressants
Antidepressant discontinuation syndrome

T43.206 **Underdosing** of unspecified antidepressants

T43.21 Poisoning by, adverse effect of and underdosing of **selective serotonin and norepinephrine reuptake inhibitors**
Poisoning by, adverse effect of and underdosing of SSNRI antidepressants

T43.211 Poisoning by selective serotonin and norepinephrine reuptake inhibitors, **accidental** (unintentional)

T43.212 Poisoning by selective serotonin and norepinephrine reuptake inhibitors, **intentional** self-harm A, S

T43.213 Poisoning by selective serotonin and norepinephrine reuptake inhibitors, **assault**

T43.214 Poisoning by selective serotonin and norepinephrine reuptake inhibitors, **undetermined**

T43.215 **Adverse effect** of selective serotonin and norepinephrine reuptake inhibitors

T43.216 **Underdosing** of selective serotonin and norepinephrine reuptake inhibitors

T43.22 Poisoning by, adverse effect of and underdosing of **selective serotonin reuptake inhibitors**
Poisoning by, adverse effect of and underdosing of SSRI antidepressants

T43.221 Poisoning by selective serotonin reuptake inhibitors, **accidental** (unintentional)

T43.222 Poisoning by selective serotonin reuptake inhibitors, **intentional** self-harm A, S

T43.223 Poisoning by selective serotonin reuptake inhibitors, **assault**

T43.224 Poisoning by selective serotonin reuptake inhibitors, undetermined

T43.225 **Adverse effect** of selective serotonin reuptake inhibitors
Coding Clinic: 2022, Q2, P11

T43.226 **Underdosing** of selective serotonin reuptake inhibitors

T43.29 Poisoning by, adverse effect of and underdosing of **other antidepressants**

T43.291 Poisoning by other antidepressants, **accidental** (unintentional)
Poisoning by other antidepressants NOS

T43.292 Poisoning by other antidepressants, **intentional** self-harm A, S

T43.293 Poisoning by other antidepressants, **assault**

T43.294 Poisoning by other antidepressants, **undetermined**

T43.295 **Adverse effect** of other antidepressants

T43.296 **Underdosing** of other antidepressants

T43.3 Poisoning by, adverse effect of and underdosing of phenothiazine antipsychotics and neuroleptics

T43.3X Poisoning by, adverse effect of and underdosing of **phenothiazine antipsychotics and neuroleptics**

T43.3X1 Poisoning by phenothiazine antipsychotics and neuroleptics, **accidental** (unintentional)
Poisoning by phenothiazine antipsychotics and neuroleptics NOS

T43.3X2 Poisoning by phenothiazine antipsychotics and neuroleptics, **intentional** self-harm A, S

T43.3X3 Poisoning by phenothiazine antipsychotics and neuroleptics, **assault**

T43.3X4 Poisoning by phenothiazine antipsychotics and neuroleptics, **undetermined**

T43.3X5 **Adverse effect** of phenothiazine antipsychotics and neuroleptics

T43.3X6 **Underdosing** of phenothiazine antipsychotics and neuroleptics

T43.4 Poisoning by, adverse effect of and underdosing of butyrophenone and thiothixene neuroleptics

T43.4X Poisoning by, adverse effect of and underdosing of **butyrophenone and thiothixene neuroleptics**

T43.4X1 Poisoning by butyrophenone and thiothixene neuroleptics, **accidental** (unintentional)
Poisoning by butyrophenone and thiothixene neuroleptics NOS

T43.4X2 Poisoning by butyrophenone and thiothixene neuroleptics, **intentional** self-harm A, S

T43.4X3 Poisoning by butyrophenone and thiothixene neuroleptics, **assault**

T43.4X4 Poisoning by butyrophenone and thiothixene neuroleptics, **undetermined**

T43.4X5 **Adverse effect** of butyrophenone and thiothixene neuroleptics

T43.4X6 **Underdosing** of butyrophenone and thiothixene neuroleptics

T43.5 Poisoning by, adverse effect of and underdosing of other and unspecified antipsychotics and neuroleptics
Excludes1 poisoning by, adverse effect of and underdosing of rauwolfia (T46.5-)

T43.50 Poisoning by, adverse effect of and underdosing of unspecified antipsychotics and neuroleptics

T43.501 Poisoning by unspecified antipsychotics and neuroleptics, accidental (unintentional)
Poisoning by antipsychotics and neuroleptics NOS

T43.502 Poisoning by unspecified antipsychotics and neuroleptics, intentional self-harm A, S

T43.503 Poisoning by unspecified antipsychotics and neuroleptics, assault

T43.504 Poisoning by unspecified antipsychotics and neuroleptics, undetermined

T43.505 Adverse effect of unspecified antipsychotics and neuroleptics
Coding Clinic: 2022, Q4, P24

T43.506 Underdosing of unspecified antipsychotics and neuroleptics

T43.59 Poisoning by, adverse effect of and underdosing of other antipsychotics and neuroleptics

T43.591 Poisoning by other antipsychotics and neuroleptics, accidental (unintentional)
Poisoning by other antipsychotics and neuroleptics NOS

T43.592 Poisoning by other antipsychotics and neuroleptics, intentional self-harm A, S
Coding Clinic: 2017, Q1, P40

T43.593 Poisoning by other antipsychotics and neuroleptics, assault

T43.594 Poisoning by other antipsychotics and neuroleptics, undetermined

T43.595 Adverse effect of other antipsychotics and neuroleptics
Coding Clinic: 2022, Q2, P11

T43.596 Underdosing of other antipsychotics and neuroleptics

T43.6 Poisoning by, adverse effect of and underdosing of psychostimulants
Excludes1 poisoning by, adverse effect of and underdosing of cocaine (T40.5-)

T43.60 Poisoning by, adverse effect of and underdosing of unspecified psychostimulant

T43.601 Poisoning by unspecified psychostimulants, accidental (unintentional)
Poisoning by psychostimulants NOS

T43.602 Poisoning by unspecified psychostimulants, intentional self-harm A, S

T43.603 Poisoning by unspecified psychostimulants, assault

T43.604 Poisoning by unspecified psychostimulants, undetermined

T43.605 Adverse effect of unspecified psychostimulants

T43.606 Underdosing of unspecified psychostimulants

T43.61 Poisoning by, adverse effect of and underdosing of caffeine

T43.611 Poisoning by caffeine, accidental (unintentional)
Poisoning by caffeine NOS

T43.612 Poisoning by caffeine, intentional self-harm A, S

T43.613 Poisoning by caffeine, assault

T43.614 Poisoning by caffeine, undetermined

T43.615 Adverse effect of caffeine

T43.616 Underdosing of caffeine

T43.62 Poisoning by, adverse effect of and underdosing of amphetamines

T43.621 Poisoning by amphetamines, accidental (unintentional)
Poisoning by amphetamines NOS
Coding Clinic: 2021, Q3, P8

T43.622 Poisoning by amphetamines, intentional self-harm A, S

T43.623 Poisoning by amphetamines, assault

T43.624 Poisoning by amphetamines, undetermined

T43.625 Adverse effect of amphetamines

T43.626 Underdosing of amphetamines

T43.63 Poisoning by, adverse effect of and underdosing of methylphenidate

T43.631 Poisoning by methylphenidate, accidental (unintentional)
Poisoning by methylphenidate NOS

T43.632 Poisoning by methylphenidate, intentional self-harm A, S

T43.633 Poisoning by methylphenidate, assault

T43.634 Poisoning by methylphenidate, undetermined

T43.635 Adverse effect of methylphenidate

T43.636 Underdosing of methylphenidate

T43.64 Poisoning by ecstasy
Poisoning by MDMA
Poisoning by 3,4-methylenedioxymethamphetamine

T43.641 Poisoning by ecstasy, accidental (unintentional)
Poisoning by ecstasy NOS
Coding Clinic: 2018, Q4, P31

T43.642 Poisoning by ecstasy, intentional self-harm A, S

T43.643 Poisoning by ecstasy, assault

T43.644 Poisoning by ecstasy, undetermined

T43.65 Poisoning by, adverse effect of and underdosing of methamphetamines

T43.651 Poisoning by methamphetamines accidental (unintentional)
Poisoning by methamphetamines NOS
Coding Clinic: 2022, Q4, P46

T43.652 Poisoning by methamphetamines intentional self-harm

T43.653 Poisoning by methamphetamines, assault

T43.654 Poisoning by methamphetamines, undetermined

T43.655 Adverse effect of methamphetamines
Coding Clinic: 2022, Q4, P47

T43.656 Underdosing of methamphetamines

CHAPTER 19 (S00-T88)

T43.69 Poisoning by, adverse effect of and underdosing of other psychostimulants

T43.691 Poisoning by other psychostimulants, accidental (unintentional)
Poisoning by other psychostimulants NOS

T43.692 Poisoning by other psychostimulants, intentional self-harm A, S

T43.693 Poisoning by other psychostimulants, assault

T43.694 Poisoning by other psychostimulants, undetermined

T43.695 Adverse effect of other psychostimulants

T43.696 Underdosing of other psychostimulants

T43.8 Poisoning by, adverse effect of and underdosing of other psychotropic drugs

T43.8X Poisoning by, adverse effect of and underdosing of other psychotropic drugs

T43.8X1 Poisoning by other psychotropic drugs, accidental (unintentional)
Poisoning by other psychotropic drugs NOS

T43.8X2 Poisoning by other psychotropic drugs, intentional self-harm A, S

T43.8X3 Poisoning by other psychotropic drugs, assault

T43.8X4 Poisoning by other psychotropic drugs, undetermined

T43.8X5 Adverse effect of other psychotropic drugs

T43.8X6 Underdosing of other psychotropic drugs

T43.9 Poisoning by, adverse effect of and underdosing of unspecified psychotropic drug

X T43.91 Poisoning by unspecified psychotropic drug, accidental (unintentional)
Poisoning by psychotropic drug NOS

X T43.92 Poisoning by unspecified psychotropic drug, intentional self-harm A, S

X T43.93 Poisoning by unspecified psychotropic drug, assault

X T43.94 Poisoning by unspecified psychotropic drug, undetermined

X T43.95 Adverse effect of unspecified psychotropic drug

X T43.96 Underdosing of unspecified psychotropic drug

T44 Poisoning by, adverse effect of and underdosing of drugs primarily affecting the autonomic nervous system

The appropriate 7th character is to be added to each code from category T44

A	initial encounter
D	subsequent encounter
S	sequela

T44.Ø Poisoning by, adverse effect of and underdosing of anticholinesterase agents

T44.ØX Poisoning by, adverse effect of and underdosing of anticholinesterase agents

T44.ØX1 Poisoning by anticholinesterase agents, accidental (unintentional)
Poisoning by anticholinesterase agents NOS

T44.ØX2 Poisoning by anticholinesterase agents, intentional self-harm A, S

T44.ØX3 Poisoning by anticholinesterase agents, assault

T44.ØX4 Poisoning by anticholinesterase agents, undetermined

T44.ØX5 Adverse effect of anticholinesterase agents

T44.ØX6 Underdosing of anticholinesterase agents

T44.1 Poisoning by, adverse effect of and underdosing of other parasympathomimetics [cholinergics]

T44.1X Poisoning by, adverse effect of and underdosing of other parasympathomimetics [cholinergics]

T44.1X1 Poisoning by other parasympathomimetics [cholinergics], accidental (unintentional)
Poisoning by other parasympathomimetics [cholinergics] NOS

T44.1X2 Poisoning by other parasympathomimetics [cholinergics], intentional self-harm A, S

T44.1X3 Poisoning by other parasympathomimetics [cholinergics], assault

T44.1X4 Poisoning by other parasympathomimetics [cholinergics], undetermined

T44.1X5 Adverse effect of other parasympathomimetics [cholinergics]

T44.1X6 Underdosing of other parasympathomimetics [cholinergics]

T44.2 Poisoning by, adverse effect of and underdosing of ganglionic blocking drugs

T44.2X Poisoning by, adverse effect of and underdosing of ganglionic blocking drugs

T44.2X1 Poisoning by ganglionic blocking drugs, accidental (unintentional)
Poisoning by ganglionic blocking drugs NOS

T44.2X2 Poisoning by ganglionic blocking drugs, intentional self-harm A, S

T44.2X3 Poisoning by ganglionic blocking drugs, assault

T44.2X4 Poisoning by ganglionic blocking drugs, undetermined

T44.2X5 Adverse effect of ganglionic blocking drugs

T44.2X6 Underdosing of ganglionic blocking drugs

T44.3 Poisoning by, adverse effect of and underdosing of other parasympatholytics [anticholinergics and antimuscarinics] and spasmolytics
Poisoning by, adverse effect of and underdosing of papaverine

T44.3X Poisoning by, adverse effect of and underdosing of other parasympatholytics [anticholinergics and antimuscarinics] and spasmolytics

T44.3X1 Poisoning by other parasympatholytics [anticholinergics and antimuscarinics] and spasmolytics, accidental (unintentional)
Poisoning by other parasympatholytics [anticholinergics and antimuscarinics] and spasmolytics NOS

T44.3X2 Poisoning by other parasympatholytics [anticholinergics and antimuscarinics] and spasmolytics, intentional self-harm A, S

T44.3X3 Poisoning by other parasympatholytics [anticholinergics and antimuscarinics] and spasmolytics, assault

T44.3X4 Poisoning by other parasympatholytics [anticholinergics and antimuscarinics] and spasmolytics, undetermined

T44.3X5 Adverse effect of other parasympatholytics [anticholinergics and antimuscarinics] and spasmolytics

T44.3X6 Underdosing of other parasympatholytics [anticholinergics and antimuscarinics] and spasmolytics

T44.4 Poisoning by, adverse effect of and underdosing of predominantly alpha-adrenoreceptor agonists

Poisoning by, adverse effect of and underdosing of metaraminol

T44.4X Poisoning by, adverse effect of and underdosing of predominantly alpha-adrenoreceptor agonists

T44.4X1 Poisoning by predominantly alpha-adrenoreceptor agonists, accidental (unintentional)

Poisoning by predominantly alpha-adrenoreceptor agonists NOS

T44.4X2 Poisoning by predominantly alpha-adrenoreceptor agonists, intentional self-harm A, S

T44.4X3 Poisoning by predominantly alpha-adrenoreceptor agonists, assault

T44.4X4 Poisoning by predominantly alpha-adrenoreceptor agonists, undetermined

T44.4X5 Adverse effect of predominantly alpha-adrenoreceptor agonists

T44.4X6 Underdosing of predominantly alpha-adrenoreceptor agonists

T44.5 Poisoning by, adverse effect of and underdosing of predominantly beta-adrenoreceptor agonists

Excludes1 poisoning by, adverse effect of and underdosing of beta-adrenoreceptor agonists used in asthma therapy (T48.6-)

T44.5X Poisoning by, adverse effect of and underdosing of predominantly beta-adrenoreceptor agonists

T44.5X1 Poisoning by predominantly beta-adrenoreceptor agonists, accidental (unintentional)

Poisoning by predominantly beta-adrenoreceptor agonists NOS

T44.5X2 Poisoning by predominantly beta-adrenoreceptor agonists, intentional self-harm A, S

T44.5X3 Poisoning by predominantly beta-adrenoreceptor agonists, assault

T44.5X4 Poisoning by predominantly beta-adrenoreceptor agonists, undetermined

T44.5X5 Adverse effect of predominantly beta-adrenoreceptor agonists

T44.5X6 Underdosing of predominantly beta-adrenoreceptor agonists

T44.6 Poisoning by, adverse effect of and underdosing of alpha-adrenoreceptor antagonists

Excludes1 poisoning by, adverse effect of and underdosing of ergot alkaloids (T48.Ø)

T44.6X Poisoning by, adverse effect of and underdosing of alpha-adrenoreceptor antagonists

T44.6X1 Poisoning by alpha-adrenoreceptor antagonists, accidental (unintentional)

Poisoning by alpha-adrenoreceptor antagonists NOS

T44.6X2 Poisoning by alpha-adrenoreceptor antagonists, intentional self-harm A, S

T44.6X3 Poisoning by alpha-adrenoreceptor antagonists, assault

T44.6X4 Poisoning by alpha-adrenoreceptor antagonists, undetermined

T44.6X5 Adverse effect of alpha-adrenoreceptor antagonists

T44.6X6 Underdosing of alpha-adrenoreceptor antagonists

T44.7 Poisoning by, adverse effect of and underdosing of beta-adrenoreceptor antagonists

T44.7X Poisoning by, adverse effect of and underdosing of beta-adrenoreceptor antagonists

T44.7X1 Poisoning by beta-adrenoreceptor antagonists, accidental (unintentional)

Poisoning by beta-adrenoreceptor antagonists NOS

T44.7X2 Poisoning by beta-adrenoreceptor antagonists, intentional self-harm A, S

T44.7X3 Poisoning by beta-adrenoreceptor antagonists, assault

T44.7X4 Poisoning by beta-adrenoreceptor antagonists, undetermined

T44.7X5 Adverse effect of beta-adrenoreceptor antagonists

T44.7X6 Underdosing of beta-adrenoreceptor antagonists

T44.8 Poisoning by, adverse effect of and underdosing of centrally-acting and adrenergic-neuron-blocking agents

Excludes2 poisoning by, adverse effect of and underdosing of clonidine (T46.5)
poisoning by, adverse effect of and underdosing of guanethidine (T46.5)

T44.8X Poisoning by, adverse effect of and underdosing of centrally-acting and adrenergic-neuron-blocking agents

T44.8X1 Poisoning by centrally-acting and adrenergic-neuron-blocking agents, accidental (unintentional)

Poisoning by centrally-acting and adrenergic-neuron-blocking agents NOS

T44.8X2 Poisoning by centrally-acting and adrenergic-neuron-blocking agents, intentional self-harm A, S

T44.8X3 Poisoning by centrally-acting and adrenergic-neuron-blocking agents, assault

T44.8X4 Poisoning by centrally-acting and adrenergic-neuron-blocking agents, undetermined

T44.8X5 Adverse effect of centrally-acting and adrenergic-neuron-blocking agents

T44.8X6 Underdosing of centrally-acting and adrenergic-neuron-blocking agents

CHAPTER 19 (SØØ-T88)

T44.9 Poisoning by, adverse effect of and underdosing of other and unspecified drugs primarily affecting the autonomic nervous system

Poisoning by, adverse effect of and underdosing of drug stimulating both alpha and beta-adrenoreceptors

T44.90 Poisoning by, adverse effect of and underdosing of unspecified drugs primarily affecting the autonomic nervous system

T44.901 Poisoning by unspecified drugs primarily affecting the autonomic nervous system, accidental (unintentional)

Poisoning by unspecified drugs primarily affecting the autonomic nervous system NOS

T44.902 Poisoning by unspecified drugs primarily affecting the autonomic nervous system, intentional self-harm A, S

T44.903 Poisoning by unspecified drugs primarily affecting the autonomic nervous system, assault

T44.904 Poisoning by unspecified drugs primarily affecting the autonomic nervous system, undetermined

T44.905 Adverse effect of unspecified drugs primarily affecting the autonomic nervous system

T44.906 Underdosing of unspecified drugs primarily affecting the autonomic nervous system

T44.99 Poisoning by, adverse effect of and underdosing of other drugs primarily affecting the autonomic nervous system

T44.991 Poisoning by other drug primarily affecting the autonomic nervous system, accidental (unintentional)

Poisoning by other drugs primarily affecting the autonomic nervous system NOS

T44.992 Poisoning by other drug primarily affecting the autonomic nervous system, intentional self-harm A, S

T44.993 Poisoning by other drug primarily affecting the autonomic nervous system, assault

T44.994 Poisoning by other drug primarily affecting the autonomic nervous system, undetermined

T44.995 Adverse effect of other drug primarily affecting the autonomic nervous system

T44.996 Underdosing of other drug primarily affecting the autonomic nervous system

T45 Poisoning by, adverse effect of and underdosing of primarily systemic and hematological agents, not elsewhere classified

The appropriate 7th character is to be added to each code from category T45

A	initial encounter
D	subsequent encounter
S	sequela

T45.Ø Poisoning by, adverse effect of and underdosing of antiallergic and antiemetic drugs

Excludes1 poisoning by, adverse effect of and underdosing of phenothiazine-based neuroleptics (T43.3)

T45.ØX Poisoning by, adverse effect of and underdosing of antiallergic and antiemetic drugs

T45.ØX1 Poisoning by antiallergic and antiemetic drugs, accidental (unintentional)

Poisoning by antiallergic and antiemetic drugs NOS

T45.ØX2 Poisoning by antiallergic and antiemetic drugs, intentional self-harm A, S

T45.ØX3 Poisoning by antiallergic and antiemetic drugs, assault

T45.ØX4 Poisoning by antiallergic and antiemetic drugs, undetermined

T45.ØX5 Adverse effect of antiallergic and antiemetic drugs

T45.ØX6 Underdosing of antiallergic and antiemetic drugs

T45.1 Poisoning by, adverse effect of and underdosing of antineoplastic and immunosuppressive drugs

▶ **Excludes1** poisoning by, adverse effect of and underdosing of immune checkpoint inhibitors andimmunostimulant drugs (T45.A)

Coding Clinic: 2Ø23, Q2, P1Ø

T45.1X Poisoning by, adverse effect of and underdosing of antineoplastic and immunosuppressive drugs

T45.1X1 Poisoning by antineoplastic and immunosuppressive drugs, accidental (unintentional)

Poisoning by antineoplastic and immunosuppressive drugs NOS

T45.1X2 Poisoning by antineoplastic and immunosuppressive drugs, intentional self-harm A, S

T45.1X3 Poisoning by antineoplastic and immunosuppressive drugs, assault

T45.1X4 Poisoning by antineoplastic and immunosuppressive drugs, undetermined

T45.1X5 Adverse effect of antineoplastic and immunosuppressive drugs

Coding Clinic: 2Ø24, Q1, P25; 2Ø21, Q3, P4; 2Ø19, Q2, P25, 28; Q1, P17, 21

T45.1X6 Underdosing of antineoplastic and immunosuppressive drugs

T45.2 Poisoning by, adverse effect of and underdosing of vitamins

Excludes2 poisoning by, adverse effect of and underdosing of nicotinic acid (derivatives) (T46.7)
poisoning by, adverse effect of and underdosing of iron (T45.4)
poisoning by, adverse effect of and underdosing of vitamin K (T45.7)

T45.2X Poisoning by, adverse effect of and underdosing of vitamins

T45.2X1 Poisoning by vitamins, accidental (unintentional)
Poisoning by vitamins NOS

T45.2X2 Poisoning by vitamins, intentional self-harm A, S

T45.2X3 Poisoning by vitamins, assault

T45.2X4 Poisoning by vitamins, undetermined

T45.2X5 Adverse effect of vitamins

T45.2X6 Underdosing of vitamins
Excludes1 vitamin deficiencies (E50-E56)

T45.3 Poisoning by, adverse effect of and underdosing of enzymes

T45.3X Poisoning by, adverse effect of and underdosing of enzymes

T45.3X1 Poisoning by enzymes, accidental (unintentional)
Poisoning by enzymes NOS

T45.3X2 Poisoning by enzymes, intentional self-harm A, S

T45.3X3 Poisoning by enzymes, assault

T45.3X4 Poisoning by enzymes, undetermined

T45.3X5 Adverse effect of enzymes

T45.3X6 Underdosing of enzymes

T45.4 Poisoning by, adverse effect of and underdosing of iron and its compounds

T45.4X Poisoning by, adverse effect of and underdosing of iron and its compounds

T45.4X1 Poisoning by iron and its compounds, accidental (unintentional)
Poisoning by iron and its compounds NOS

T45.4X2 Poisoning by iron and its compounds, intentional self-harm A, S

T45.4X3 Poisoning by iron and its compounds, assault

T45.4X4 Poisoning by iron and its compounds, undetermined

T45.4X5 Adverse effect of iron and its compounds

T45.4X6 Underdosing of iron and its compounds
Excludes1 iron deficiency (E61.1)

T45.5 Poisoning by, adverse effect of and underdosing of anticoagulants and antithrombotic drugs

T45.51 Poisoning by, adverse effect of and underdosing of anticoagulants

T45.511 Poisoning by anticoagulants, accidental (unintentional)
Poisoning by anticoagulants NOS

T45.512 Poisoning by anticoagulants, intentional self-harm A, S

T45.513 Poisoning by anticoagulants, assault

T45.514 Poisoning by anticoagulants, undetermined

T45.515 Adverse effect of anticoagulants
Coding Clinic: 2021, Q1, P5; 2016, Q1, P14; 2013, Q2, P35

T45.516 Underdosing of anticoagulants

T45.52 Poisoning by, adverse effect of and underdosing of antithrombotic drugs
Poisoning by, adverse effect of and underdosing of antiplatelet drugs
Excludes2 poisoning by, adverse effect of and underdosing of aspirin (T39.01-)
poisoning by, adverse effect of and underdosing of acetylsalicylic acid (T39.01-)

T45.521 Poisoning by antithrombotic drugs, accidental (unintentional)
Poisoning by antithrombotic drug NOS

T45.522 Poisoning by antithrombotic drugs, intentional self-harm A, S

T45.523 Poisoning by antithrombotic drugs, assault

T45.524 Poisoning by antithrombotic drugs, undetermined

T45.525 Adverse effect of antithrombotic drugs
Coding Clinic: 2016, Q1, P15

T45.526 Underdosing of antithrombotic drugs

T45.6 Poisoning by, adverse effect of and underdosing of fibrinolysis-affecting drugs

T45.60 Poisoning by, adverse effect of and underdosing of unspecified fibrinolysis-affecting drugs

T45.601 Poisoning by unspecified fibrinolysis-affecting drugs, accidental (unintentional)
Poisoning by fibrinolysis-affecting drug NOS

T45.602 Poisoning by unspecified fibrinolysis-affecting drugs, intentional self-harm A, S

T45.603 Poisoning by unspecified fibrinolysis-affecting drugs, assault

T45.604 Poisoning by unspecified fibrinolysis-affecting drugs, undetermined

T45.605 Adverse effect of unspecified fibrinolysis-affecting drugs

T45.606 Underdosing of unspecified fibrinolysis-affecting drugs

T45.61 Poisoning by, adverse effect of and underdosing of thrombolytic drugs

T45.611 Poisoning by thrombolytic drug, accidental (unintentional)
Poisoning by thrombolytic drug NOS

T45.612 Poisoning by thrombolytic drug, intentional self-harm A, S

T45.613 Poisoning by thrombolytic drug, assault

T45.614 Poisoning by thrombolytic drug, undetermined

T45.615 Adverse effect of thrombolytic drugs
Coding Clinic: 2017, Q2, P10

T45.616 Underdosing of thrombolytic drugs

T45.62 Poisoning by, adverse effect of and underdosing of hemostatic drugs

T45.621 Poisoning by hemostatic drug, accidental (unintentional)
Poisoning by hemostatic drug NOS

T45.622 Poisoning by hemostatic drug, intentional self-harm A, S

T45.623 Poisoning by hemostatic drug, assault

T45.624 Poisoning by hemostatic drug, undetermined

T45.625 Adverse effect of hemostatic drug

T45.626 Underdosing of hemostatic drugs

T45.69 Poisoning by, adverse effect of and underdosing of other fibrinolysis-affecting drugs

T45.691 Poisoning by other fibrinolysis-affecting drugs, accidental (unintentional)

Poisoning by other fibrinolysis-affecting drug NOS

T45.692 Poisoning by other fibrinolysis-affecting drugs, intentional self-harm A, S

T45.693 Poisoning by other fibrinolysis-affecting drugs, assault

T45.694 Poisoning by other fibrinolysis-affecting drugs, undetermined

T45.695 Adverse effect of other fibrinolysis-affecting drugs

T45.696 Underdosing of other fibrinolysis-affecting drugs

T45.7 Poisoning by, adverse effect of and underdosing of anticoagulant antagonists, vitamin K and other coagulants

T45.7X Poisoning by, adverse effect of and underdosing of anticoagulant antagonists, vitamin K and other coagulants

T45.7X1 Poisoning by anticoagulant antagonists, vitamin K and other coagulants, accidental (unintentional)

Poisoning by anticoagulant antagonists, vitamin K and other coagulants NOS

T45.7X2 Poisoning by anticoagulant antagonists, vitamin K and other coagulants, intentional self-harm A, S

T45.7X3 Poisoning by anticoagulant antagonists, vitamin K and other coagulants, assault

T45.7X4 Poisoning by anticoagulant antagonists, vitamin K and other coagulants, undetermined

T45.7X5 Adverse effect of anticoagulant antagonists, vitamin K and other coagulants

T45.7X6 Underdosing of anticoagulant antagonist, vitamin K and other coagulants

Excludes1 vitamin K deficiency (E56.1)

T45.8 Poisoning by, adverse effect of and underdosing of other primarily systemic and hematological agents

Poisoning by, adverse effect of and underdosing of liver preparations and other antianemic agents

Poisoning by, adverse effect of and underdosing of natural blood and blood products

Poisoning by, adverse effect of and underdosing of plasma substitute

Excludes2 poisoning by, adverse effect of and underdosing of immunoglobulin (T50.Z1)

poisoning by, adverse effect of and underdosing of iron (T45.4)

transfusion reactions (T80.-)

T45.8X Poisoning by, adverse effect of and underdosing of other primarily systemic and hematological agents

T45.8X1 Poisoning by other primarily systemic and hematological agents, accidental (unintentional)

Poisoning by other primarily systemic and hematological agents NOS

T45.8X2 Poisoning by other primarily systemic and hematological agents, intentional self-harm A, S

T45.8X3 Poisoning by other primarily systemic and hematological agents, assault

T45.8X4 Poisoning by other primarily systemic and hematological agents, undetermined

T45.8X5 Adverse effect of other primarily systemic and hematological agents

Coding Clinic: 2016, Q4, P42

T45.8X6 Underdosing of other primarily systemic and hematological agents

T45.9 Poisoning by, adverse effect of and underdosing of unspecified primarily systemic and hematological agent

X **T45.91 Poisoning by unspecified primarily systemic and hematological agent, accidental (unintentional)**

Poisoning by primarily systemic and hematological agent NOS

X **T45.92 Poisoning by unspecified primarily systemic and hematological agent, intentional self-harm A, S**

X **T45.93 Poisoning by unspecified primarily systemic and hematological agent, assault**

X **T45.94 Poisoning by unspecified primarily systemic and hematological agent, undetermined**

X **T45.95 Adverse effect of unspecified primarily systemic and hematological agent**

X **T45.96 Underdosing of unspecified primarily systemic and hematological agent**

T45.A Poisoning by, adverse effect of and underdosing of immune checkpoint inhibitors andimmunostimulant drugs

Excludes1 poisoning by, adverse effect of and underdosing of antineoplastic andimmunosuppressive drug (T45.1)

T45.AX Poisoning by, adverse effect of and underdosing of immune checkpoint inhibitorsand immunostimulant drugs

T45.AX1 Poisoning by immune checkpoint inhibitors and immunostimulant drugs,accidental (unintentional)

Poisoning by immune checkpoint inhibitors and immunosuppressive drugs NOS

T45.AX2 Poisoning by immune checkpoint inhibitors and immunostimulant drugs, intentional self-harm

T45.AX3 Poisoning by immune checkpoint inhibitors and immunostimulant drugs, assault

T45.AX4 Poisoning by immune checkpoint inhibitors and immunostimulant drugs, undetermined

T45.AX5 Adverse effect of immune checkpoint inhibitors and immunostimulant drugs

T45.AX6 Underdosing of immune checkpoint inhibitors and immunostimulant drugs

T46 Poisoning by, adverse effect of and underdosing of agents primarily affecting the cardiovascular system

Excludes1 poisoning by, adverse effect of and underdosing of metaraminol (T44.4)

The appropriate 7th character is to be added to each code from category T46

A	initial encounter
D	subsequent encounter
S	sequela

CHAPTER 19 (S00-T88)

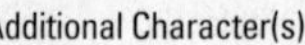

T46.Ø Poisoning by, adverse effect of and underdosing of cardiac-stimulant glycosides and drugs of similar action

T46.ØX Poisoning by, adverse effect of and underdosing of cardiac-stimulant glycosides and drugs of similar action

T46.ØX1 Poisoning by cardiac-stimulant glycosides and drugs of similar action, accidental (unintentional)
Poisoning by cardiac-stimulant glycosides and drugs of similar action NOS

T46.ØX2 Poisoning by cardiac-stimulant glycosides and drugs of similar action, intentional self-harm A, S

T46.ØX3 Poisoning by cardiac-stimulant glycosides and drugs of similar action, assault

T46.ØX4 Poisoning by cardiac-stimulant glycosides and drugs of similar action, undetermined

T46.ØX5 Adverse effect of cardiac-stimulant glycosides and drugs of similar action

T46.ØX6 Underdosing of cardiac-stimulant glycosides and drugs of similar action

T46.1 Poisoning by, adverse effect of and underdosing of calcium-channel blockers

T46.1X Poisoning by, adverse effect of and underdosing of calcium-channel blockers

T46.1X1 Poisoning by calcium-channel blockers, accidental (unintentional)
Poisoning by calcium-channel blockers NOS

T46.1X2 Poisoning by calcium-channel blockers, intentional self-harm A, S

T46.1X3 Poisoning by calcium-channel blockers, assault

T46.1X4 Poisoning by calcium-channel blockers, undetermined

T46.1X5 Adverse effect of calcium-channel blockers

T46.1X6 Underdosing of calcium-channel blockers

T46.2 Poisoning by, adverse effect of and underdosing of other antidysrhythmic drugs, not elsewhere classified

Excludes1 poisoning by, adverse effect of and underdosing of beta-adrenoreceptor antagonists (T44.7-)

T46.2X Poisoning by, adverse effect of and underdosing of other antidysrhythmic drugs

T46.2X1 Poisoning by other antidysrhythmic drugs, accidental (unintentional)
Poisoning by other antidysrhythmic drugs NOS

T46.2X2 Poisoning by other antidysrhythmic drugs, intentional self-harm A, S

T46.2X3 Poisoning by other antidysrhythmic drugs, assault

T46.2X4 Poisoning by other antidysrhythmic drugs, undetermined

T46.2X5 Adverse effect of other antidysrhythmic drugs

T46.2X6 Underdosing of other antidysrhythmic drugs

T46.3 Poisoning by, adverse effect of and underdosing of coronary vasodilators
Poisoning by, adverse effect of and underdosing of dipyridamole

Excludes1 poisoning by, adverse effect of and underdosing of calcium-channel blockers (T46.1)

T46.3X Poisoning by, adverse effect of and underdosing of coronary vasodilators

T46.3X1 Poisoning by coronary vasodilators, accidental (unintentional)
Poisoning by coronary vasodilators NOS

T46.3X2 Poisoning by coronary vasodilators, intentional self-harm A, S

T46.3X3 Poisoning by coronary vasodilators, assault

T46.3X4 Poisoning by coronary vasodilators, undetermined

T46.3X5 Adverse effect of coronary vasodilators

T46.3X6 Underdosing of coronary vasodilators

T46.4 Poisoning by, adverse effect of and underdosing of angiotensin-converting-enzyme inhibitors

T46.4X Poisoning by, adverse effect of and underdosing of angiotensin-converting-enzyme inhibitors

T46.4X1 Poisoning by angiotensin-converting-enzyme inhibitors, accidental (unintentional)
Poisoning by angiotensin-converting-enzyme inhibitors NOS

T46.4X2 Poisoning by angiotensin-converting-enzyme inhibitors, intentional self-harm A, S

T46.4X3 Poisoning by angiotensin-converting-enzyme inhibitors, assault

T46.4X4 Poisoning by angiotensin-converting-enzyme inhibitors, undetermined

T46.4X5 Adverse effect of angiotensin-converting-enzyme inhibitors

T46.4X6 Underdosing of angiotensin-converting-enzyme inhibitors

T46.5 Poisoning by, adverse effect of and underdosing of other antihypertensive drugs

Excludes2 poisoning by, adverse effect of and underdosing of beta-adrenoreceptor antagonists (T44.7)
poisoning by, adverse effect of and underdosing of calcium-channel blockers (T46.1)
poisoning by, adverse effect of and underdosing of diuretics (T5Ø.Ø-T5Ø.2)

T46.5X Poisoning by, adverse effect of and underdosing of other antihypertensive drugs

T46.5X1 Poisoning by other antihypertensive drugs, accidental (unintentional)
Poisoning by other antihypertensive drugs NOS

T46.5X2 Poisoning by other antihypertensive drugs, intentional self-harm A, S

T46.5X3 Poisoning by other antihypertensive drugs, assault

T46.5X4 Poisoning by other antihypertensive drugs, undetermined

T46.5X5 Adverse effect of other antihypertensive drugs

T46.5X6 Underdosing of other antihypertensive drugs
Coding Clinic: 2022, Q1, P36

T46.6 Poisoning by, adverse effect of and underdosing of antihyperlipidemic and antiarteriosclerotic drugs

T46.6X Poisoning by, adverse effect of and underdosing of antihyperlipidemic and antiarteriosclerotic drugs

CHAPTER 19 (SØØ-T88)

T46.6X1 Poisoning by antihyperlipidemic and antiarteriosclerotic drugs, accidental (unintentional)
Poisoning by antihyperlipidemic and antiarteriosclerotic drugs NOS

T46.6X2 Poisoning by antihyperlipidemic and antiarteriosclerotic drugs, intentional self-harm A, S

T46.6X3 Poisoning by antihyperlipidemic and antiarteriosclerotic drugs, assault

T46.6X4 Poisoning by antihyperlipidemic and antiarteriosclerotic drugs, undetermined

T46.6X5 Adverse effect of antihyperlipidemic and antiarteriosclerotic drugs

T46.6X6 Underdosing of antihyperlipidemic and antiarteriosclerotic drugs

T46.7 Poisoning by, adverse effect of and underdosing of peripheral vasodilators
Poisoning by, adverse effect of and underdosing of nicotinic acid (derivatives)
Excludes1 poisoning by, adverse effect of and underdosing of papaverine (T44.3)

T46.7X Poisoning by, adverse effect of and underdosing of peripheral vasodilators

T46.7X1 Poisoning by peripheral vasodilators, accidental (unintentional)
Poisoning by peripheral vasodilators NOS

T46.7X2 Poisoning by peripheral vasodilators, intentional self-harm A, S

T46.7X3 Poisoning by peripheral vasodilators, assault

T46.7X4 Poisoning by peripheral vasodilators, undetermined

T46.7X5 Adverse effect of peripheral vasodilators

T46.7X6 Underdosing of peripheral vasodilators

T46.8 Poisoning by, adverse effect of and underdosing of antivaricose drugs, including sclerosing agents

T46.8X Poisoning by, adverse effect of and underdosing of antivaricose drugs, including sclerosing agents

T46.8X1 Poisoning by antivaricose drugs, including sclerosing agents, accidental (unintentional)
Poisoning by antivaricose drugs, including sclerosing agents NOS

T46.8X2 Poisoning by antivaricose drugs, including sclerosing agents, intentional self-harm A, S

T46.8X3 Poisoning by antivaricose drugs, including sclerosing agents, assault

T46.8X4 Poisoning by antivaricose drugs, including sclerosing agents, undetermined

T46.8X5 Adverse effect of antivaricose drugs, including sclerosing agents

T46.8X6 Underdosing of antivaricose drugs, including sclerosing agents

T46.9 Poisoning by, adverse effect of and underdosing of other and unspecified agents primarily affecting the cardiovascular system

T46.90 Poisoning by, adverse effect of and underdosing of unspecified agents primarily affecting the cardiovascular system

T46.901 Poisoning by unspecified agents primarily affecting the cardiovascular system, accidental (unintentional)

T46.902 Poisoning by unspecified agents primarily affecting the cardiovascular system, intentional self-harm A, S

T46.903 Poisoning by unspecified agents primarily affecting the cardiovascular system, assault

T46.904 Poisoning by unspecified agents primarily affecting the cardiovascular system, undetermined

T46.905 Adverse effect of unspecified agents primarily affecting the cardiovascular system

T46.906 Underdosing of unspecified agents primarily affecting the cardiovascular system

T46.99 Poisoning by, adverse effect of and underdosing of other agents primarily affecting the cardiovascular system

T46.991 Poisoning by other agents primarily affecting the cardiovascular system, accidental (unintentional)

T46.992 Poisoning by other agents primarily affecting the cardiovascular system, intentional self-harm A, S

T46.993 Poisoning by other agents primarily affecting the cardiovascular system, assault

T46.994 Poisoning by other agents primarily affecting the cardiovascular system, undetermined

T46.995 Adverse effect of other agents primarily affecting the cardiovascular system

T46.996 Underdosing of other agents primarily affecting the cardiovascular system

T47 Poisoning by, adverse effect of and underdosing of agents primarily affecting the gastrointestinal system

The appropriate 7th character is to be added to each code from category T47

A initial encounter
D subsequent encounter
S sequela

T47.0 Poisoning by, adverse effect of and underdosing of histamine H2-receptor blockers

T47.0X Poisoning by, adverse effect of and underdosing of histamine H2-receptor blockers

T47.0X1 Poisoning by histamine H2-receptor blockers, accidental (unintentional)
Poisoning by histamine H2-receptor blockers NOS

T47.0X2 Poisoning by histamine H2-receptor blockers, intentional self-harm A, S

T47.0X3 Poisoning by histamine H2-receptor blockers, assault

T47.0X4 Poisoning by histamine H2-receptor blockers, undetermined

T47.0X5 Adverse effect of histamine H2-receptor blockers

T47.0X6 Underdosing of histamine H2-receptor blockers

T47.1 Poisoning by, adverse effect of and underdosing of other antacids and anti-gastric-secretion drugs

T47.1X Poisoning by, adverse effect of and underdosing of other antacids and anti-gastric-secretion drugs

- T47.1X1 Poisoning by other antacids and anti-gastric-secretion drugs, accidental (unintentional)
  - Poisoning by other antacids and anti-gastric-secretion drugs NOS
- T47.1X2 Poisoning by other antacids and anti-gastric-secretion drugs, intentional self-harm A, S
- T47.1X3 Poisoning by other antacids and anti-gastric-secretion drugs, assault
- T47.1X4 Poisoning by other antacids and anti-gastric-secretion drugs, undetermined
- T47.1X5 Adverse effect of other antacids and anti-gastric-secretion drugs
- T47.1X6 Underdosing of other antacids and anti-gastric-secretion drugs

T47.2 Poisoning by, adverse effect of and underdosing of stimulant laxatives

- T47.2X Poisoning by, adverse effect of and underdosing of stimulant laxatives
  - T47.2X1 Poisoning by stimulant laxatives, accidental (unintentional)
    - Poisoning by stimulant laxatives NOS
  - T47.2X2 Poisoning by stimulant laxatives, intentional self-harm A, S
  - T47.2X3 Poisoning by stimulant laxatives, assault
  - T47.2X4 Poisoning by stimulant laxatives, undetermined
  - T47.2X5 Adverse effect of stimulant laxatives
  - T47.2X6 Underdosing of stimulant laxatives

T47.3 Poisoning by, adverse effect of and underdosing of saline and osmotic laxatives

- T47.3X Poisoning by and adverse effect of saline and osmotic laxatives
  - T47.3X1 Poisoning by saline and osmotic laxatives, accidental (unintentional)
    - Poisoning by saline and osmotic laxatives NOS
  - T47.3X2 Poisoning by saline and osmotic laxatives, intentional self-harm
  - T47.3X3 Poisoning by saline and osmotic laxatives, assault A, S
  - T47.3X4 Poisoning by saline and osmotic laxatives, undetermined
  - T47.3X5 Adverse effect of saline and osmotic laxatives
  - T47.3X6 Underdosing of saline and osmotic laxatives

T47.4 Poisoning by, adverse effect of and underdosing of other laxatives

- T47.4X Poisoning by, adverse effect of and underdosing of other laxatives
  - T47.4X1 Poisoning by other laxatives, accidental (unintentional)
    - Poisoning by other laxatives NOS
  - T47.4X2 Poisoning by other laxatives, intentional self-harm A, S
  - T47.4X3 Poisoning by other laxatives, assault
  - T47.4X4 Poisoning by other laxatives, undetermined
  - T47.4X5 Adverse effect of other laxatives
  - T47.4X6 Underdosing of other laxatives

T47.5 Poisoning by, adverse effect of and underdosing of digestants

- T47.5X Poisoning by, adverse effect of and underdosing of digestants
  - T47.5X1 Poisoning by digestants, accidental (unintentional)
    - Poisoning by digestants NOS
  - T47.5X2 Poisoning by digestants, intentional self-harm A, S
  - T47.5X3 Poisoning by digestants, assault
  - T47.5X4 Poisoning by digestants, undetermined
  - T47.5X5 Adverse effect of digestants
  - T47.5X6 Underdosing of digestants

T47.6 Poisoning by, adverse effect of and underdosing of antidiarrheal drugs

Excludes2 poisoning by, adverse effect of and underdosing of systemic antibiotics and other anti-infectives (T36-T37)

- T47.6X Poisoning by, adverse effect of and underdosing of antidiarrheal drugs
  - T47.6X1 Poisoning by antidiarrheal drugs, accidental (unintentional)
    - Poisoning by antidiarrheal drugs NOS
  - T47.6X2 Poisoning by antidiarrheal drugs, intentional self-harm A, S
  - T47.6X3 Poisoning by antidiarrheal drugs, assault
  - T47.6X4 Poisoning by antidiarrheal drugs, undetermined
  - T47.6X5 Adverse effect of antidiarrheal drugs
  - T47.6X6 Underdosing of antidiarrheal drugs

T47.7 Poisoning by, adverse effect of and underdosing of emetics

- T47.7X Poisoning by, adverse effect of and underdosing of emetics
  - T47.7X1 Poisoning by emetics, accidental (unintentional)
    - Poisoning by emetics NOS
  - T47.7X2 Poisoning by emetics, intentional self-harm A, S
  - T47.7X3 Poisoning by emetics, assault
  - T47.7X4 Poisoning by emetics, undetermined
  - T47.7X5 Adverse effect of emetics
  - T47.7X6 Underdosing of emetics

T47.8 Poisoning by, adverse effect of and underdosing of other agents primarily affecting gastrointestinal system

- T47.8X Poisoning by, adverse effect of and underdosing of other agents primarily affecting gastrointestinal system
  - T47.8X1 Poisoning by other agents primarily affecting gastrointestinal system, accidental (unintentional)
    - Poisoning by other agents primarily affecting gastrointestinal system NOS
  - T47.8X2 Poisoning by other agents primarily affecting gastrointestinal system, intentional self-harm A, S
  - T47.8X3 Poisoning by other agents primarily affecting gastrointestinal system, assault
  - T47.8X4 Poisoning by other agents primarily affecting gastrointestinal system, undetermined
  - T47.8X5 Adverse effect of other agents primarily affecting gastrointestinal system
  - T47.8X6 Underdosing of other agents primarily affecting gastrointestinal system

T47.9 Poisoning by, adverse effect of and underdosing of unspecified agents primarily affecting the gastrointestinal system

X T47.91 Poisoning by unspecified agents primarily affecting the gastrointestinal system, accidental (unintentional)
Poisoning by agents primarily affecting the gastrointestinal system NOS

X T47.92 Poisoning by unspecified agents primarily affecting the gastrointestinal system, intentional self-harm A, S

X T47.93 Poisoning by unspecified agents primarily affecting the gastrointestinal system, assault

X T47.94 Poisoning by unspecified agents primarily affecting the gastrointestinal system, undetermined

X T47.95 Adverse effect of unspecified agents primarily affecting the gastrointestinal system

X T47.96 Underdosing of unspecified agents primarily affecting the gastrointestinal system

T48 Poisoning by, adverse effect of and underdosing of agents primarily acting on smooth and skeletal muscles and the respiratory system

The appropriate 7th character is to be added to each code from category T48

A initial encounter
D subsequent encounter
S sequela

T48.Ø Poisoning by, adverse effect of and underdosing of oxytocic drugs

Excludes1 poisoning by, adverse effect of and underdosing of estrogens, progestogens and antagonists (T38.4-T38.6)

T48.ØX Poisoning by, adverse effect of and underdosing of oxytocic drugs

T48.ØX1 Poisoning by oxytocic drugs, accidental (unintentional)
Poisoning by oxytocic drugs NOS

T48.ØX2 Poisoning by oxytocic drugs, intentional self-harm A, S

T48.ØX3 Poisoning by oxytocic drugs, assault

T48.ØX4 Poisoning by oxytocic drugs, undetermined

T48.ØX5 Adverse effect of oxytocic drugs

T48.ØX6 Underdosing of oxytocic drugs

T48.1 Poisoning by, adverse effect of and underdosing of skeletal muscle relaxants [neuromuscular blocking agents]

T48.1X Poisoning by, adverse effect of and underdosing of skeletal muscle relaxants [neuromuscular blocking agents]

T48.1X1 Poisoning by skeletal muscle relaxants [neuromuscular blocking agents], accidental (unintentional)
Poisoning by skeletal muscle relaxants [neuromuscular blocking agents] NOS

T48.1X2 Poisoning by skeletal muscle relaxants [neuromuscular blocking agents], intentional self-harm A, S

T48.1X3 Poisoning by skeletal muscle relaxants [neuromuscular blocking agents], assault

T48.1X4 Poisoning by skeletal muscle relaxants [neuromuscular blocking agents], undetermined

T48.1X5 Adverse effect of skeletal muscle relaxants [neuromuscular blocking agents]

T48.1X6 Underdosing of skeletal muscle relaxants [neuromuscular blocking agents]

T48.2 Poisoning by, adverse effect of and underdosing of other and unspecified drugs acting on muscles

T48.2Ø Poisoning by, adverse effect of and underdosing of unspecified drugs acting on muscles

T48.2Ø1 Poisoning by unspecified drugs acting on muscles, accidental (unintentional)
Poisoning by unspecified drugs acting on muscles NOS

T48.2Ø2 Poisoning by unspecified drugs acting on muscles, intentional self-harm A, S

T48.2Ø3 Poisoning by unspecified drugs acting on muscles, assault

T48.2Ø4 Poisoning by unspecified drugs acting on muscles, undetermined

T48.2Ø5 Adverse effect of unspecified drugs acting on muscles

T48.2Ø6 Underdosing of unspecified drugs acting on muscles

T48.29 Poisoning by, adverse effect of and underdosing of other drugs acting on muscles

T48.291 Poisoning by other drugs acting on muscles, accidental (unintentional)
Poisoning by other drugs acting on muscles NOS

T48.292 Poisoning by other drugs acting on muscles, intentional self-harm A, S

T48.293 Poisoning by other drugs acting on muscles, assault

T48.294 Poisoning by other drugs acting on muscles, undetermined

T48.295 Adverse effect of other drugs acting on muscles

T48.296 Underdosing of other drugs acting on muscles

T48.3 Poisoning by, adverse effect of and underdosing of antitussives

T48.3X Poisoning by, adverse effect of and underdosing of antitussives

T48.3X1 Poisoning by antitussives, accidental (unintentional)
Poisoning by antitussives NOS

T48.3X2 Poisoning by antitussives, intentional self-harm A, S

T48.3X3 Poisoning by antitussives, assault

T48.3X4 Poisoning by antitussives, undetermined

T48.3X5 Adverse effect of antitussives

T48.3X6 Underdosing of antitussives

T48.4 Poisoning by, adverse effect of and underdosing of expectorants

T48.4X Poisoning by, adverse effect of and underdosing of expectorants

T48.4X1 Poisoning by expectorants, accidental (unintentional)
Poisoning by expectorants NOS

T48.4X2 Poisoning by expectorants, intentional self-harm A, S

T48.4X3 Poisoning by expectorants, assault

T48.4X4 Poisoning by expectorants, undetermined

T48.4X5 Adverse effect of expectorants

T48.4X6 Underdosing of expectorants

T48.5 Poisoning by, adverse effect of and underdosing of other anti-common-cold drugs
Poisoning by, adverse effect of and underdosing of decongestants
Excludes2 poisoning by, adverse effect of and underdosing of antipyretics, NEC (T39.9-)
poisoning by, adverse effect of and underdosing of non-steroidal antiinflammatory drugs (T39.3-)
poisoning by, adverse effect of and underdosing of salicylates (T39.Ø-)

T48.5X Poisoning by, adverse effect of and underdosing of other anti-common-cold drugs

T48.5X1 Poisoning by other anti-common-cold drugs, accidental (unintentional)
Poisoning by other anti-common-cold drugs NOS

T48.5X2 Poisoning by other anti-common-cold drugs, intentional self-harm A, S

T48.5X3 Poisoning by other anti-common-cold drugs, assault

T48.5X4 Poisoning by other anti-common-cold drugs, undetermined

T48.5X5 Adverse effect of other anti-common-cold drugs

T48.5X6 Underdosing of other anti-common-cold drugs

T48.6 Poisoning by, adverse effect of and underdosing of antiasthmatics, not elsewhere classified
Poisoning by, adverse effect of and underdosing of beta-adrenoreceptor agonists used in asthma therapy
Excludes1 poisoning by, adverse effect of and underdosing of beta-adrenoreceptor agonists not used in asthma therapy (T44.5)
poisoning by, adverse effect of and underdosing of anterior pituitary [adenohypophyseal] hormones (T38.8)

T48.6X Poisoning by, adverse effect of and underdosing of antiasthmatics

T48.6X1 Poisoning by antiasthmatics, accidental (unintentional)
Poisoning by antiasthmatics NOS

T48.6X2 Poisoning by antiasthmatics, intentional self-harm A, S

T48.6X3 Poisoning by antiasthmatics, assault

T48.6X4 Poisoning by antiasthmatics, undetermined

T48.6X5 Adverse effect of antiasthmatics

T48.6X6 Underdosing of antiasthmatics

T48.9 Poisoning by, adverse effect of and underdosing of other and unspecified agents primarily acting on the respiratory system

T48.90 Poisoning by, adverse effect of and underdosing of unspecified agents primarily acting on the respiratory system

T48.901 Poisoning by unspecified agents primarily acting on the respiratory system, accidental (unintentional)

T48.902 Poisoning by unspecified agents primarily acting on the respiratory system, intentional self-harm A, S

T48.903 Poisoning by unspecified agents primarily acting on the respiratory system, assault

T48.904 Poisoning by unspecified agents primarily acting on the respiratory system, undetermined

T48.905 Adverse effect of unspecified agents primarily acting on the respiratory system

T48.906 Underdosing of unspecified agents primarily acting on the respiratory system

T48.99 Poisoning by, adverse effect of and underdosing of other agents primarily acting on the respiratory system

T48.991 Poisoning by other agents primarily acting on the respiratory system, accidental (unintentional)

T48.992 Poisoning by other agents primarily acting on the respiratory system, intentional self-harm A, S

T48.993 Poisoning by other agents primarily acting on the respiratory system, assault

T48.994 Poisoning by other agents primarily acting on the respiratory system, undetermined

T48.995 Adverse effect of other agents primarily acting on the respiratory system

T48.996 Underdosing of other agents primarily acting on the respiratory system

T49 Poisoning by, adverse effect of and underdosing of topical agents primarily affecting skin and mucous membrane and by ophthalmological, otorhinorlaryngological and dental drugs
Includes poisoning by, adverse effect of and underdosing of glucocorticoids, topically used

The appropriate 7th character is to be added to each code from category T49

A initial encounter
D subsequent encounter
S sequela

T49.Ø Poisoning by, adverse effect of and underdosing of local antifungal, anti-infective and anti-inflammatory drugs

T49.ØX Poisoning by, adverse effect of and underdosing of local antifungal, anti-infective and anti-inflammatory drugs

T49.ØX1 Poisoning by local antifungal, anti-infective and anti-inflammatory drugs, accidental (unintentional)
Poisoning by local antifungal, anti-infective and anti-inflammatory drugs NOS

T49.ØX2 Poisoning by local antifungal, anti-infective and anti-inflammatory drugs, intentional self-harm A, S

T49.ØX3 Poisoning by local antifungal, anti-infective and anti-inflammatory drugs, assault

T49.ØX4 Poisoning by local antifungal, anti-infective and anti-inflammatory drugs, undetermined

T49.ØX5 Adverse effect of local antifungal, anti-infective and anti-inflammatory drugs

T49.ØX6 Underdosing of local antifungal, anti-infective and anti-inflammatory drugs

T49.1 Poisoning by, adverse effect of and underdosing of antipruritics

T49.1X Poisoning by, adverse effect of and underdosing of antipruritics

T49.1X1 Poisoning by antipruritics, accidental (unintentional)
Poisoning by antipruritics NOS

T49.1X2 Poisoning by antipruritics, intentional self-harm A, S

T49.1X3 Poisoning by antipruritics, assault

T49.1X4 Poisoning by antipruritics, undetermined

T49.1X5 Adverse effect of antipruritics

T49.1X6 Underdosing of antipruritics

T49.2 Poisoning by, adverse effect of and underdosing of local astringents and local detergents

T49.2X Poisoning by, adverse effect of and underdosing of local astringents and local detergents

T49.2X1 Poisoning by local astringents and local detergents, accidental (unintentional)

Poisoning by local astringents and local detergents NOS

T49.2X2 Poisoning by local astringents and local detergents, intentional self-harm A, S

T49.2X3 Poisoning by local astringents and local detergents, assault

T49.2X4 Poisoning by local astringents and local detergents, undetermined

T49.2X5 Adverse effect of local astringents and local detergents

T49.2X6 Underdosing of local astringents and local detergents

T49.3 Poisoning by, adverse effect of and underdosing of emollients, demulcents and protectants

T49.3X Poisoning by, adverse effect of and underdosing of emollients, demulcents and protectants

T49.3X1 Poisoning by emollients, demulcents and protectants, accidental (unintentional)

Poisoning by emollients, demulcents and protectants NOS

T49.3X2 Poisoning by emollients, demulcents and protectants, intentional self-harm A, S

T49.3X3 Poisoning by emollients, demulcents and protectants, assault

T49.3X4 Poisoning by emollients, demulcents and protectants, undetermined

T49.3X5 Adverse effect of emollients, demulcents and protectants

T49.3X6 Underdosing of emollients, demulcents and protectants

T49.4 Poisoning by, adverse effect of and underdosing of keratolytics, keratoplastics, and other hair treatment drugs and preparations

T49.4X Poisoning by, adverse effect of and underdosing of keratolytics, keratoplastics, and other hair treatment drugs and preparations

T49.4X1 Poisoning by keratolytics, keratoplastics, and other hair treatment drugs and preparations, accidental (unintentional)

Poisoning by keratolytics, keratoplastics, and other hair treatment drugs and preparations NOS

T49.4X2 Poisoning by keratolytics, keratoplastics, and other hair treatment drugs and preparations, intentional self-harm A, S

T49.4X3 Poisoning by keratolytics, keratoplastics, and other hair treatment drugs and preparations, assault

T49.4X4 Poisoning by keratolytics, keratoplastics, and other hair treatment drugs and preparations, undetermined

T49.4X5 Adverse effect of keratolytics, keratoplastics, and other hair treatment drugs and preparations

T49.4X6 Underdosing of keratolytics, keratoplastics, and other hair treatment drugs and preparations

T49.5 Poisoning by, adverse effect of and underdosing of ophthalmological drugs and preparations

T49.5X Poisoning by, adverse effect of and underdosing of ophthalmological drugs and preparations

T49.5X1 Poisoning by ophthalmological drugs and preparations, accidental (unintentional)

Poisoning by ophthalmological drugs and preparations NOS

T49.5X2 Poisoning by ophthalmological drugs and preparations, intentional self-harm A, S

T49.5X3 Poisoning by ophthalmological drugs and preparations, assault

T49.5X4 Poisoning by ophthalmological drugs and preparations, undetermined

T49.5X5 Adverse effect of ophthalmological drugs and preparations

T49.5X6 Underdosing of ophthalmological drugs and preparations

T49.6 Poisoning by, adverse effect of and underdosing of otorhinolaryngological drugs and preparations

T49.6X Poisoning by, adverse effect of and underdosing of otorhinolaryngological drugs and preparations

T49.6X1 Poisoning by otorhinolaryngological drugs and preparations, accidental (unintentional)

Poisoning by otorhinolaryngological drugs and preparations NOS

T49.6X2 Poisoning by otorhinolaryngological drugs and preparations, intentional self-harm A, S

T49.6X3 Poisoning by otorhinolaryngological drugs and preparations, assault

T49.6X4 Poisoning by otorhinolaryngological drugs and preparations, undetermined

T49.6X5 Adverse effect of otorhinolaryngological drugs and preparations

T49.6X6 Underdosing of otorhinolaryngological drugs and preparations

T49.7 Poisoning by, adverse effect of and underdosing of dental drugs, topically applied

T49.7X Poisoning by, adverse effect of and underdosing of dental drugs, topically applied

T49.7X1 Poisoning by dental drugs, topically applied, accidental (unintentional)

Poisoning by dental drugs, topically applied NOS

T49.7X2 Poisoning by dental drugs, topically applied, intentional self-harm A, S

T49.7X3 Poisoning by dental drugs, topically applied, assault

T49.7X4 Poisoning by dental drugs, topically applied, undetermined

T49.7X5 Adverse effect of dental drugs, topically applied

T49.7X6 Underdosing of dental drugs, topically applied

T49.8 Poisoning by, adverse effect of and underdosing of other topical agents

Poisoning by, adverse effect of and underdosing of spermicides

T49.8X Poisoning by, adverse effect of and underdosing of other topical agents

T49.8X1 Poisoning by other topical agents, accidental (unintentional)

Poisoning by other topical agents NOS

T49.8X2 Poisoning by other topical agents, intentional self-harm A, S

T49.8X3 Poisoning by other topical agents, assault

T49.8X4 Poisoning by other topical agents, undetermined

T49.8X5 Adverse effect of other topical agents

T49.8X6 Underdosing of other topical agents

T49.9 Poisoning by, adverse effect of and underdosing of unspecified topical agent

X T49.91 Poisoning by unspecified topical agent, accidental (unintentional)

X T49.92 Poisoning by unspecified topical agent, intentional self-harm A, S

X T49.93 Poisoning by unspecified topical agent, assault

X T49.94 Poisoning by unspecified topical agent, undetermined

X T49.95 Adverse effect of unspecified topical agent

X T49.96 Underdosing of unspecified topical agent

T50 Poisoning by, adverse effect of and underdosing of diuretics and other and unspecified drugs, medicaments and biological substances

The appropriate 7th character is to be added to each code from category T50

A initial encounter
D subsequent encounter
S sequela

T50.0 Poisoning by, adverse effect of and underdosing of mineralocorticoids and their antagonists

T50.0X Poisoning by, adverse effect of and underdosing of mineralocorticoids and their antagonists

T50.0X1 Poisoning by mineralocorticoids and their antagonists, accidental (unintentional)
Poisoning by mineralocorticoids and their antagonists NOS

T50.0X2 Poisoning by mineralocorticoids and their antagonists, intentional self-harm A, S

T50.0X3 Poisoning by mineralocorticoids and their antagonists, assault

T50.0X4 Poisoning by mineralocorticoids and their antagonists, undetermined

T50.0X5 Adverse effect of mineralocorticoids and their antagonists

T50.0X6 Underdosing of mineralocorticoids and their antagonists

T50.1 Poisoning by, adverse effect of and underdosing of loop [high-ceiling] diuretics

T50.1X Poisoning by, adverse effect of and underdosing of loop [high-ceiling] diuretics

T50.1X1 Poisoning by loop [high-ceiling] diuretics, accidental (unintentional)
Poisoning by loop [high-ceiling] diuretics NOS

T50.1X2 Poisoning by loop [high-ceiling] diuretics, intentional self-harm A, S

T50.1X3 Poisoning by loop [high-ceiling] diuretics, assault

T50.1X4 Poisoning by loop [high-ceiling] diuretics, undetermined

T50.1X5 Adverse effect of loop [high-ceiling] diuretics

T50.1X6 Underdosing of loop [high-ceiling] diuretics

T50.2 Poisoning by, adverse effect of and underdosing of carbonic-anhydrase inhibitors, benzothiadiazides and other diuretics
Poisoning by, adverse effect of and underdosing of acetazolamide

T50.2X Poisoning by, adverse effect of and underdosing of carbonic-anhydrase inhibitors, benzothiadiazides and other diuretics

T50.2X1 Poisoning by carbonic-anhydrase inhibitors, benzothiadiazides and other diuretics, accidental (unintentional)
Poisoning by carbonic-anhydrase inhibitors, benzothiadiazides and other diuretics NOS

T50.2X2 Poisoning by carbonic-anhydrase inhibitors, benzothiadiazides and other diuretics, intentional self-harm A, S

T50.2X3 Poisoning by carbonic-anhydrase inhibitors, benzothiadiazides and other diuretics, assault

T50.2X4 Poisoning by carbonic-anhydrase inhibitors, benzothiadiazides and other diuretics, undetermined

T50.2X5 Adverse effect of carbonic-anhydrase inhibitors, benzothiadiazides and other diuretics

T50.2X6 Underdosing of carbonic-anhydrase inhibitors, benzothiadiazides and other diuretics

T50.3 Poisoning by, adverse effect of and underdosing of electrolytic, caloric and water-balance agents
Poisoning by, adverse effect of and underdosing of oral rehydration salts

T50.3X Poisoning by, adverse effect of and underdosing of electrolytic, caloric and water-balance agents

T50.3X1 Poisoning by electrolytic, caloric and water-balance agents, accidental (unintentional)
Poisoning by electrolytic, caloric and water-balance agents NOS

T50.3X2 Poisoning by electrolytic, caloric and water-balance agents, intentional self-harm A, S

T50.3X3 Poisoning by electrolytic, caloric and water-balance agents, assault

T50.3X4 Poisoning by electrolytic, caloric and water-balance agents, undetermined

T50.3X5 Adverse effect of electrolytic, caloric and water-balance agents
Coding Clinic: 2022, Q2, P11

T50.3X6 Underdosing of electrolytic, caloric and water-balance agents

T50.4 Poisoning by, adverse effect of and underdosing of drugs affecting uric acid metabolism

T50.4X Poisoning by, adverse effect of and underdosing of drugs affecting uric acid metabolism

T50.4X1 Poisoning by drugs affecting uric acid metabolism, accidental (unintentional)
Poisoning by drugs affecting uric acid metabolism NOS

T50.4X2 Poisoning by drugs affecting uric acid metabolism, intentional self-harm A, S

T50.4X3 Poisoning by drugs affecting uric acid metabolism, assault

T50.4X4 Poisoning by drugs affecting uric acid metabolism, undetermined

T50.4X5 Adverse effect of drugs affecting uric acid metabolism

T50.4X6 Underdosing of drugs affecting uric acid metabolism

CHAPTER 19 (S00-T88)

T50.5 Poisoning by, adverse effect of and underdosing of appetite depressants

T50.5X Poisoning by, adverse effect of and underdosing of appetite depressants

T50.5X1 Poisoning by appetite depressants, accidental (unintentional)
Poisoning by appetite depressants NOS

T50.5X2 Poisoning by appetite depressants, intentional self-harm A, S

T50.5X3 Poisoning by appetite depressants, assault

T50.5X4 Poisoning by appetite depressants, undetermined

T50.5X5 Adverse effect of appetite depressants

T50.5X6 Underdosing of appetite depressants

T50.6 Poisoning by, adverse effect of and underdosing of antidotes and chelating agents
Poisoning by, adverse effect of and underdosing of alcohol deterrents

T50.6X Poisoning by, adverse effect of and underdosing of antidotes and chelating agents

T50.6X1 Poisoning by antidotes and chelating agents, accidental (unintentional)
Poisoning by antidotes and chelating agents NOS

T50.6X2 Poisoning by antidotes and chelating agents, intentional self-harm A, S

T50.6X3 Poisoning by antidotes and chelating agents, assault

T50.6X4 Poisoning by antidotes and chelating agents, undetermined

T50.6X5 Adverse effect of antidotes and chelating agents

T50.6X6 Underdosing of antidotes and chelating agents

T50.7 Poisoning by, adverse effect of and underdosing of analeptics and opioid receptor antagonists

T50.7X Poisoning by, adverse effect of and underdosing of analeptics and opioid receptor antagonists

T50.7X1 Poisoning by analeptics and opioid receptor antagonists, accidental (unintentional)
Poisoning by analeptics and opioid receptor antagonists NOS

T50.7X2 Poisoning by analeptics and opioid receptor antagonists, intentional self-harm A, S

T50.7X3 Poisoning by analeptics and opioid receptor antagonists, assault

T50.7X4 Poisoning by analeptics and opioid receptor antagonists, undetermined

T50.7X5 Adverse effect of analeptics and opioid receptor antagonists

T50.7X6 Underdosing of analeptics and opioid receptor antagonists

T50.8 Poisoning by, adverse effect of and underdosing of diagnostic agents

T50.8X Poisoning by, adverse effect of and underdosing of diagnostic agents

T50.8X1 Poisoning by diagnostic agents, accidental (unintentional)
Poisoning by diagnostic agents NOS

T50.8X2 Poisoning by diagnostic agents, intentional self-harm A, S

T50.8X3 Poisoning by diagnostic agents, assault

T50.8X4 Poisoning by diagnostic agents, undetermined

T50.8X5 Adverse effect of diagnostic agents
Coding Clinic: 2023, Q3, P4-5; 2022, Q4, P33; 2021, Q3, P9-10

T50.8X6 Underdosing of diagnostic agents

T50.A Poisoning by, adverse effect of and underdosing of bacterial vaccines

T50.A1 Poisoning by, adverse effect of and underdosing of pertussis vaccine, including combinations with a pertussis component

T50.A11 Poisoning by pertussis vaccine, including combinations with a pertussis component, accidental (unintentional)

T50.A12 Poisoning by pertussis vaccine, including combinations with a pertussis component, intentional self-harm A, S

T50.A13 Poisoning by pertussis vaccine, including combinations with a pertussis component, assault

T50.A14 Poisoning by pertussis vaccine, including combinations with a pertussis component, undetermined

T50.A15 Adverse effect of pertussis vaccine, including combinations with a pertussis component

T50.A16 Underdosing of pertussis vaccine, including combinations with a pertussis component

T50.A2 Poisoning by, adverse effect of and underdosing of mixed bacterial vaccines without a pertussis component

T50.A21 Poisoning by mixed bacterial vaccines without a pertussis component, accidental (unintentional)

T50.A22 Poisoning by mixed bacterial vaccines without a pertussis component, intentional self-harm A, S

T50.A23 Poisoning by mixed bacterial vaccines without a pertussis component, assault

T50.A24 Poisoning by mixed bacterial vaccines without a pertussis component, undetermined

T50.A25 Adverse effect of mixed bacterial vaccines without a pertussis component

T50.A26 Underdosing of mixed bacterial vaccines without a pertussis component

T50.A9 Poisoning by, adverse effect of and underdosing of other bacterial vaccines

T50.A91 Poisoning by other bacterial vaccines, accidental (unintentional)

T50.A92 Poisoning by other bacterial vaccines, intentional self-harm A, S

T50.A93 Poisoning by other bacterial vaccines, assault

T50.A94 Poisoning by other bacterial vaccines, undetermined

T50.A95 Adverse effect of other bacterial vaccines

T50.A96 Underdosing of other bacterial vaccines

T50.B Poisoning by, adverse effect of and underdosing of viral vaccines

T50.B1 Poisoning by, adverse effect of and underdosing of smallpox vaccines

T50.B11 Poisoning by smallpox vaccines, accidental (unintentional)

T50.B12 Poisoning by smallpox vaccines, intentional self-harm A, S

- T50.B13 **Poisoning by smallpox vaccines, assault**
- T50.B14 **Poisoning by smallpox vaccines, undetermined**
- T50.B15 **Adverse effect of smallpox vaccines**
- T50.B16 **Underdosing of smallpox vaccines**

T50.B9 **Poisoning by, adverse effect of and underdosing of other viral vaccines**
- T50.B91 **Poisoning by other viral vaccines, accidental (unintentional)**
- T50.B92 **Poisoning by other viral vaccines, intentional self-harm A, S**
- T50.B93 **Poisoning by other viral vaccines, assault**
- T50.B94 **Poisoning by other viral vaccines, undetermined**
- T50.B95 **Adverse effect of other viral vaccines**
  Coding Clinic: 2021, Q1, P43-44
- T50.B96 **Underdosing of other viral vaccines**

T50.Z **Poisoning by, adverse effect of and underdosing of other vaccines and biological substances**

T50.Z1 **Poisoning by, adverse effect of and underdosing of immunoglobulin**
- T50.Z11 **Poisoning by immunoglobulin, accidental (unintentional)**
- T50.Z12 **Poisoning by immunoglobulin, intentional self-harm A, S**
- T50.Z13 **Poisoning by immunoglobulin, assault**
- T50.Z14 **Poisoning by immunoglobulin, undetermined**
- T50.Z15 **Adverse effect of immunoglobulin**
- T50.Z16 **Underdosing of immunoglobulin**

T50.Z9 **Poisoning by, adverse effect of and underdosing of other vaccines and biological substances**
- T50.Z91 **Poisoning by other vaccines and biological substances, accidental (unintentional)**
- T50.Z92 **Poisoning by other vaccines and biological substances, intentional self-harm A, S**
- T50.Z93 **Poisoning by other vaccines and biological substances, assault**
- T50.Z94 **Poisoning by other vaccines and biological substances, undetermined**
- T50.Z95 **Adverse effect of other vaccines and biological substances**
  Coding Clinic: 2020, Q1, P19
- T50.Z96 **Underdosing of other vaccines and biological substances**

T50.9 **Poisoning by, adverse effect of and underdosing of other and unspecified drugs, medicaments and biological substances**

T50.90 **Poisoning by, adverse effect of and underdosing of unspecified drugs, medicaments and biological substances**
- T50.901 **Poisoning by unspecified drugs, medicaments and biological substances, accidental (unintentional)**
  Coding Clinic: 2015, Q1, P21
- T50.902 **Poisoning by unspecified drugs, medicaments and biological substances, intentional self-harm A, S**
- T50.903 **Poisoning by unspecified drugs, medicaments and biological substances, assault**
- T50.904 **Poisoning by unspecified drugs, medicaments and biological substances, undetermined**
- T50.905 **Adverse effect of unspecified drugs, medicaments and biological substances**
- T50.906 **Underdosing of unspecified drugs, medicaments and biological substances**

T50.91 **Poisoning by, adverse effect of and underdosing of multiple unspecified drugs, medicaments and biological substances**
Multiple drug ingestion NOS
Code also any specific drugs, medicaments and biological substances
- T50.911 **Poisoning by multiple unspecified drugs, medicaments and biological substances, accidental (unintentional)**
- T50.912 **Poisoning by multiple unspecified drugs, medicaments and biological substances, intentional self-harm**
- T50.913 **Poisoning by multiple unspecified drugs, medicaments and biological substances, assault**
- T50.914 **Poisoning by multiple unspecified drugs, medicaments and biological substances, undetermined**
- T50.915 **Adverse effect of multiple unspecified drugs, medicaments and biological substances**
- T50.916 **Underdosing of multiple unspecified drugs, medicaments and biological substances**

T50.99 **Poisoning by, adverse effect of and underdosing of other drugs, medicaments and biological substances**
- T50.991 **Poisoning by other drugs, medicaments and biological substances, accidental (unintentional)**
- T50.992 **Poisoning by other drugs, medicaments and biological substances, intentional self-harm A, S**
- T50.993 **Poisoning by other drugs, medicaments and biological substances, assault**
- T50.994 **Poisoning by other drugs, medicaments and biological substances, undetermined**
- T50.995 **Adverse effect of other drugs, medicaments and biological substances**
  Coding Clinic: 2023, Q3, P4-5
- T50.996 **Underdosing of other drugs, medicaments and biological substances**

TOXIC EFFECTS OF SUBSTANCES CHIEFLY NONMEDICINAL AS TO SOURCE (T51-T65)

Note: When no intent is indicated code to accidental. Undetermined intent is only for use when there is specific documentation in the record that the intent of the toxic effect cannot be determined.

Use additional code(s): for all associated manifestations of toxic effect, such as:
respiratory conditions due to external agents (J60-J70)
personal history of foreign body fully removed (Z87.821)
to identify any retained foreign body, if applicable (Z18.-)

Excludes1 contact with and (suspected) exposure to toxic substances (Z77.-)

T51 **Toxic effect of alcohol**

The appropriate 7th character is to be added to each code from category T51

A	initial encounter
D	subsequent encounter
S	sequela

CHAPTER 19 (S00-T88)

T51.Ø Toxic effect of ethanol
Toxic effect of ethyl alcohol
Excludes2 acute alcohol intoxication or 'hangover' effects (F1Ø.129, F1Ø.229, F1Ø.929)
drunkenness (F1Ø.129, F1Ø.229, F1Ø.929)
pathological alcohol intoxication (F1Ø.129, F1Ø.229, F1Ø.929)

T51.ØX Toxic effect of ethanol

T51.ØX1 Toxic effect of ethanol, accidental (unintentional)
Toxic effect of ethanol NOS

T51.ØX2 Toxic effect of ethanol, intentional self-harm A, S

T51.ØX3 Toxic effect of ethanol, assault

T51.ØX4 Toxic effect of ethanol, undetermined

T51.1 Toxic effect of methanol
Toxic effect of methyl alcohol

T51.1X Toxic effect of methanol

T51.1X1 Toxic effect of methanol, accidental (unintentional)
Toxic effect of methanol NOS

T51.1X2 Toxic effect of methanol, intentional self-harm A, S

T51.1X3 Toxic effect of methanol, assault

T51.1X4 Toxic effect of methanol, undetermined

T51.2 Toxic effect of 2-Propanol
Toxic effect of isopropyl alcohol

T51.2X Toxic effect of 2-Propanol

T51.2X1 Toxic effect of 2-Propanol, accidental (unintentional)
Toxic effect of 2-Propanol NOS

T51.2X2 Toxic effect of 2-Propanol, intentional self-harm A, S

T51.2X3 Toxic effect of 2-Propanol, assault

T51.2X4 Toxic effect of 2-Propanol, undetermined

T51.3 Toxic effect of fusel oil
Toxic effect of amyl alcohol
Toxic effect of butyl [1-butanol] alcohol
Toxic effect of propyl [1-propanol] alcohol

T51.3X Toxic effect of fusel oil

T51.3X1 Toxic effect of fusel oil, accidental (unintentional)
Toxic effect of fusel oil NOS

T51.3X2 Toxic effect of fusel oil, intentional self-harm A, S

T51.3X3 Toxic effect of fusel oil, assault

T51.3X4 Toxic effect of fusel oil, undetermined

T51.8 Toxic effect of other alcohols

T51.8X Toxic effect of other alcohols

T51.8X1 Toxic effect of other alcohols, accidental (unintentional)
Toxic effect of other alcohols NOS

T51.8X2 Toxic effect of other alcohols, intentional self-harm A, S

T51.8X3 Toxic effect of other alcohols, assault

T51.8X4 Toxic effect of other alcohols, undetermined

T51.9 Toxic effect of unspecified alcohol

X **T51.91 Toxic effect of unspecified alcohol, accidental (unintentional)**

X **T51.92 Toxic effect of unspecified alcohol, intentional self-harm A, S**

X **T51.93 Toxic effect of unspecified alcohol, assault**

X **T51.94 Toxic effect of unspecified alcohol, undetermined**

T52 Toxic effect of organic solvents
Excludes1 halogen derivatives of aliphatic and aromatic hydrocarbons (T53.-)

The appropriate 7th character is to be added to each code from category T52

A	initial encounter
D	subsequent encounter
S	sequela

T52.Ø Toxic effects of petroleum products
Toxic effects of gasoline [petrol]
Toxic effects of kerosene [paraffin oil]
Toxic effects of paraffin wax
Toxic effects of ether petroleum
Toxic effects of naphtha petroleum
Toxic effects of spirit petroleum

T52.ØX Toxic effects of petroleum products

T52.ØX1 Toxic effect of petroleum products, accidental (unintentional)
Toxic effects of petroleum products NOS

T52.ØX2 Toxic effect of petroleum products, intentional self-harm A, S

T52.ØX3 Toxic effect of petroleum products, assault

T52.ØX4 Toxic effect of petroleum products, undetermined

T52.1 Toxic effects of benzene
Excludes1 homologues of benzene (T52.2)
nitroderivatives and aminoderivatives of benzene and its homologues (T65.3)

T52.1X Toxic effects of benzene

T52.1X1 Toxic effect of benzene, accidental (unintentional)
Toxic effects of benzene NOS

T52.1X2 Toxic effect of benzene, intentional self-harm A, S

T52.1X3 Toxic effect of benzene, assault

T52.1X4 Toxic effect of benzene, undetermined

T52.2 Toxic effects of homologues of benzene
Toxic effects of toluene [methylbenzene]
Toxic effects of xylene [dimethylbenzene]

T52.2X Toxic effects of homologues of benzene

T52.2X1 Toxic effect of homologues of benzene, accidental (unintentional)
Toxic effects of homologues of benzene NOS

T52.2X2 Toxic effect of homologues of benzene, intentional self-harm A, S

T52.2X3 Toxic effect of homologues of benzene, assault

T52.2X4 Toxic effect of homologues of benzene, undetermined

T52.3 Toxic effects of glycols

T52.3X Toxic effects of glycols

T52.3X1 Toxic effect of glycols, accidental (unintentional)
Toxic effects of glycols NOS

T52.3X2 Toxic effect of glycols, intentional self-harm A, S

T52.3X3 Toxic effect of glycols, assault

T52.3X4 Toxic effect of glycols, undetermined

T52.4 Toxic effects of ketones

T52.4X Toxic effects of ketones

T52.4X1 Toxic effect of ketones, accidental (unintentional)
Toxic effects of ketones NOS

T52.4X2 Toxic effect of ketones, intentional self-harm A, S

T52.4X3 Toxic effect of ketones, assault

T52.4X4 Toxic effect of ketones, undetermined

T52.8 Toxic effects of other organic solvents

T52.8X Toxic effects of other organic solvents

T52.8X1 Toxic effect of other organic solvents, accidental (unintentional)
Toxic effects of other organic solvents NOS

T52.8X2 Toxic effect of other organic solvents, intentional self-harm A, S

T52.8X3 Toxic effect of other organic solvents, assault

T52.8X4 Toxic effect of other organic solvents, undetermined

T52.9 Toxic effects of unspecified organic solvent

X **T52.91 Toxic effect of unspecified organic solvent, accidental (unintentional)**

X **T52.92 Toxic effect of unspecified organic solvent, intentional self-harm A, S**

X **T52.93 Toxic effect of unspecified organic solvent, assault**

X **T52.94 Toxic effect of unspecified organic solvent, undetermined**

T53 Toxic effect of halogen derivatives of aliphatic and aromatic hydrocarbons

The appropriate 7th character is to be added to each code from category T53

A	initial encounter
D	subsequent encounter
S	sequela

T53.0 Toxic effects of carbon tetrachloride
Toxic effects of tetrachloromethane

T53.0X Toxic effects of carbon tetrachloride

T53.0X1 Toxic effect of carbon tetrachloride, accidental (unintentional)
Toxic effects of carbon tetrachloride NOS

T53.0X2 Toxic effect of carbon tetrachloride, intentional self-harm A, S

T53.0X3 Toxic effect of carbon tetrachloride, assault

T53.0X4 Toxic effect of carbon tetrachloride, undetermined

T53.1 Toxic effects of chloroform
Toxic effects of trichloromethane

T53.1X Toxic effects of chloroform

T53.1X1 Toxic effect of chloroform, accidental (unintentional)
Toxic effects of chloroform NOS

T53.1X2 Toxic effect of chloroform, intentional self-harm A, S

T53.1X3 Toxic effect of chloroform, assault

T53.1X4 Toxic effect of chloroform, undetermined

T53.2 Toxic effects of trichloroethylene
Toxic effects of trichloroethene

T53.2X Toxic effects of trichloroethylene

T53.2X1 Toxic effect of trichloroethylene, accidental (unintentional)
Toxic effects of trichloroethylene NOS

T53.2X2 Toxic effect of trichloroethylene, intentional self-harm A, S

T53.2X3 Toxic effect of trichloroethylene, assault

T53.2X4 Toxic effect of trichloroethylene, undetermined

T53.3 Toxic effects of tetrachloroethylene
Toxic effects of perchloroethylene
Toxic effect of tetrachloroethene

T53.3X Toxic effects of tetrachloroethylene

T53.3X1 Toxic effect of tetrachloroethylene, accidental (unintentional)
Toxic effects of tetrachloroethylene NOS

T53.3X2 Toxic effect of tetrachloroethylene, intentional self-harm A, S

T53.3X3 Toxic effect of tetrachloroethylene, assault

T53.3X4 Toxic effect of tetrachloroethylene, undetermined

T53.4 Toxic effects of dichloromethane
Toxic effects of methylene chloride

T53.4X Toxic effects of dichloromethane

T53.4X1 Toxic effect of dichloromethane, accidental (unintentional)
Toxic effects of dichloromethane NOS

T53.4X2 Toxic effect of dichloromethane, intentional self-harm A, S

T53.4X3 Toxic effect of dichloromethane, assault

T53.4X4 Toxic effect of dichloromethane, undetermined

T53.5 Toxic effects of chlorofluorocarbons

T53.5X Toxic effects of chlorofluorocarbons

T53.5X1 Toxic effect of chlorofluorocarbons, accidental (unintentional)
Toxic effects of chlorofluorocarbons NOS

T53.5X2 Toxic effect of chlorofluorocarbons, intentional self-harm A, S

T53.5X3 Toxic effect of chlorofluorocarbons, assault

T53.5X4 Toxic effect of chlorofluorocarbons, undetermined

T53.6 Toxic effects of other halogen derivatives of aliphatic hydrocarbons

T53.6X Toxic effects of other halogen derivatives of aliphatic hydrocarbons

T53.6X1 Toxic effect of other halogen derivatives of aliphatic hydrocarbons, accidental (unintentional)
Toxic effects of other halogen derivatives of aliphatic hydrocarbons NOS

T53.6X2 Toxic effect of other halogen derivatives of aliphatic hydrocarbons, intentional self-harm A, S

T53.6X3 Toxic effect of other halogen derivatives of aliphatic hydrocarbons, assault

T53.6X4 Toxic effect of other halogen derivatives of aliphatic hydrocarbons, undetermined

T53.7 Toxic effects of other halogen derivatives of aromatic hydrocarbons

T53.7X Toxic effects of other halogen derivatives of aromatic hydrocarbons

T53.7X1 Toxic effect of other halogen derivatives of aromatic hydrocarbons, accidental (unintentional)
Toxic effects of other halogen derivatives of aromatic hydrocarbons NOS

T53.7X2 Toxic effect of other halogen derivatives of aromatic hydrocarbons, intentional self-harm A, S

T53.7X3 Toxic effect of other halogen derivatives of aromatic hydrocarbons, assault

T53.7X4 Toxic effect of other halogen derivatives of aromatic hydrocarbons, undetermined

T53.9 Toxic effects of unspecified halogen derivatives of aliphatic and aromatic hydrocarbons

X T53.91 Toxic effect of unspecified halogen derivatives of aliphatic and aromatic hydrocarbons, accidental (unintentional)

X T53.92 Toxic effect of unspecified halogen derivatives of aliphatic and aromatic hydrocarbons, intentional self-harm A, S

X T53.93 Toxic effect of unspecified halogen derivatives of aliphatic and aromatic hydrocarbons, assault

X T53.94 Toxic effect of unspecified halogen derivatives of aliphatic and aromatic hydrocarbons, undetermined

T54 Toxic effect of corrosive substances

The appropriate 7th character is to be added to each code from category T54

A	initial encounter
D	subsequent encounter
S	sequela

T54.Ø Toxic effects of phenol and phenol homologues

T54.ØX Toxic effects of phenol and phenol homologues

T54.ØX1 Toxic effect of phenol and phenol homologues, accidental (unintentional)
Toxic effects of phenol and phenol homologues NOS

T54.ØX2 Toxic effect of phenol and phenol homologues, intentional self-harm A, S

T54.ØX3 Toxic effect of phenol and phenol homologues, assault

T54.ØX4 Toxic effect of phenol and phenol homologues, undetermined

T54.1 Toxic effects of other corrosive organic compounds

T54.1X Toxic effects of other corrosive organic compounds

T54.1X1 Toxic effect of other corrosive organic compounds, accidental (unintentional)
Toxic effects of other corrosive organic compounds NOS

T54.1X2 Toxic effect of other corrosive organic compounds, intentional self-harm A, S

T54.1X3 Toxic effect of other corrosive organic compounds, assault

T54.1X4 Toxic effect of other corrosive organic compounds, undetermined

T54.2 Toxic effects of corrosive acids and acid-like substances
Toxic effects of hydrochloric acid
Toxic effects of sulfuric acid

T54.2X Toxic effects of corrosive acids and acid-like substances

T54.2X1 Toxic effect of corrosive acids and acid-like substances, accidental (unintentional)
Toxic effects of corrosive acids and acid-like substances NOS

T54.2X2 Toxic effect of corrosive acids and acid-like substances, intentional self-harm A, S

T54.2X3 Toxic effect of corrosive acids and acid-like substances, assault

T54.2X4 Toxic effect of corrosive acids and acid-like substances, undetermined

T54.3 Toxic effects of corrosive alkalis and alkali-like substances
Toxic effects of potassium hydroxide
Toxic effects of sodium hydroxide

T54.3X Toxic effects of corrosive alkalis and alkali-like substances

T54.3X1 Toxic effect of corrosive alkalis and alkali-like substances, accidental (unintentional)
Toxic effects of corrosive alkalis and alkali-like substances NOS

T54.3X2 Toxic effect of corrosive alkalis and alkali-like substances, intentional self-harm A, S

T54.3X3 Toxic effect of corrosive alkalis and alkali-like substances, assault

T54.3X4 Toxic effect of corrosive alkalis and alkali-like substances, undetermined

T54.9 Toxic effects of unspecified corrosive substance

X T54.91 Toxic effect of unspecified corrosive substance, accidental (unintentional)

X T54.92 Toxic effect of unspecified corrosive substance, intentional self-harm A, S

X T54.93 Toxic effect of unspecified corrosive substance, assault

X T54.94 Toxic effect of unspecified corrosive substance, undetermined

T55 Toxic effect of soaps and detergents

The appropriate 7th character is to be added to each code from category T55

A	initial encounter
D	subsequent encounter
S	sequela

T55.Ø Toxic effect of soaps

T55.ØX Toxic effect of soaps

T55.ØX1 Toxic effect of soaps, accidental (unintentional)
Toxic effect of soaps NOS

T55.ØX2 Toxic effect of soaps, intentional self-harm A, S

T55.ØX3 Toxic effect of soaps, assault

T55.ØX4 Toxic effect of soaps, undetermined

T55.1 Toxic effect of detergents

T55.1X Toxic effect of detergents

T55.1X1 Toxic effect of detergents, accidental (unintentional)
Toxic effect of detergents NOS

T55.1X2 Toxic effect of detergents, intentional self-harm A, S

T55.1X3 Toxic effect of detergents, assault

T55.1X4 Toxic effect of detergents, undetermined

T56 Toxic effect of metals

Includes toxic effects of fumes and vapors of metals
toxic effects of metals from all sources, except medicinal substances

Use additional code to identify any retained metal foreign body, if applicable (Z18.Ø-, T18.1-)

Excludes1 arsenic and its compounds (T57.Ø)
manganese and its compounds (T57.2)

The appropriate 7th character is to be added to each code from category T56

A	initial encounter
D	subsequent encounter
S	sequela

T56.Ø Toxic effects of lead and its compounds

T56.ØX Toxic effects of lead and its compounds

T56.ØX1 Toxic effect of lead and its compounds, accidental (unintentional)
Toxic effects of lead and its compounds NOS

CHAPTER 19 (SØØ-T88)

T56.0X2 Toxic effect of lead and its compounds, intentional self-harm A, S
T56.0X3 Toxic effect of lead and its compounds, assault
T56.0X4 Toxic effect of lead and its compounds, undetermined

T56.1 Toxic effects of mercury and its compounds
T56.1X Toxic effects of mercury and its compounds
T56.1X1 Toxic effect of mercury and its compounds, accidental (unintentional)
Toxic effects of mercury and its compounds NOS
T56.1X2 Toxic effect of mercury and its compounds, intentional self-harm A, S
T56.1X3 Toxic effect of mercury and its compounds, assault
T56.1X4 Toxic effect of mercury and its compounds, undetermined

T56.2 Toxic effects of chromium and its compounds
T56.2X Toxic effects of chromium and its compounds
T56.2X1 Toxic effect of chromium and its compounds, accidental (unintentional)
Toxic effects of chromium and its compounds NOS
T56.2X2 Toxic effect of chromium and its compounds, intentional self-harm A, S
T56.2X3 Toxic effect of chromium and its compounds, assault
T56.2X4 Toxic effect of chromium and its compounds, undetermined

T56.3 Toxic effects of cadmium and its compounds
T56.3X Toxic effects of cadmium and its compounds
T56.3X1 Toxic effect of cadmium and its compounds, accidental (unintentional)
Toxic effects of cadmium and its compounds NOS
T56.3X2 Toxic effect of cadmium and its compounds, intentional self-harm A, S
T56.3X3 Toxic effect of cadmium and its compounds, assault
T56.3X4 Toxic effect of cadmium and its compounds, undetermined

T56.4 Toxic effects of copper and its compounds
T56.4X Toxic effects of copper and its compounds
T56.4X1 Toxic effect of copper and its compounds, accidental (unintentional)
Toxic effects of copper and its compounds NOS
T56.4X2 Toxic effect of copper and its compounds, intentional self-harm A, S
T56.4X3 Toxic effect of copper and its compounds, assault
T56.4X4 Toxic effect of copper and its compounds, undetermined

T56.5 Toxic effects of zinc and its compounds
T56.5X Toxic effects of zinc and its compounds
T56.5X1 Toxic effect of zinc and its compounds, accidental (unintentional)
Toxic effects of zinc and its compounds NOS
T56.5X2 Toxic effect of zinc and its compounds, intentional self-harm A, S
T56.5X3 Toxic effect of zinc and its compounds, assault
T56.5X4 Toxic effect of zinc and its compounds, undetermined

T56.6 Toxic effects of tin and its compounds
T56.6X Toxic effects of tin and its compounds
T56.6X1 Toxic effect of tin and its compounds, accidental (unintentional)
Toxic effects of tin and its compounds NOS
T56.6X2 Toxic effect of tin and its compounds, intentional self-harm A, S
T56.6X3 Toxic effect of tin and its compounds, assault
T56.6X4 Toxic effect of tin and its compounds, undetermined

T56.7 Toxic effects of beryllium and its compounds
T56.7X Toxic effects of beryllium and its compounds
T56.7X1 Toxic effect of beryllium and its compounds, accidental (unintentional)
Toxic effects of beryllium and its compounds NOS
T56.7X2 Toxic effect of beryllium and its compounds, intentional self-harm A, S
T56.7X3 Toxic effect of beryllium and its compounds, assault
T56.7X4 Toxic effect of beryllium and its compounds, undetermined

T56.8 Toxic effects of other metals
T56.81 Toxic effect of thallium
T56.811 Toxic effect of thallium, accidental (unintentional)
Toxic effect of thallium NOS
T56.812 Toxic effect of thallium, intentional self-harm A, S
T56.813 Toxic effect of thallium, assault
T56.814 Toxic effect of thallium, undetermined
T56.82 Toxic effect of gadolinium
Excludes1 adverse effect of diagnostic agents (T50.8X5-)
T56.821 Toxic effect of gadolinium, accidental (unintentional)
Toxic effect of gadolinium NOS
T56.822 Toxic effect of gadolinium, intentional self-harm
T56.823 Toxic effect of gadolinium, assault
T56.824 Toxic effect of gadolinium, undetermined
T56.89 Toxic effects of other metals
T56.891 Toxic effect of other metals, accidental (unintentional)
Toxic effects of other metals NOS
T56.892 Toxic effect of other metals, intentional self-harm A, S
T56.893 Toxic effect of other metals, assault
T56.894 Toxic effect of other metals, undetermined

T56.9 Toxic effects of unspecified metal
X T56.91 Toxic effect of unspecified metal, accidental (unintentional)
X T56.92 Toxic effect of unspecified metal, intentional self-harm A, S
X T56.93 Toxic effect of unspecified metal, assault
X T56.94 Toxic effect of unspecified metal, undetermined

CHAPTER 19 (S00-T88)

T57 Toxic effect of other inorganic substances

The appropriate 7th character is to be added to each code from category T57

A initial encounter
D subsequent encounter
S sequela

T57.Ø Toxic effect of arsenic and its compounds

T57.ØX Toxic effect of arsenic and its compounds

T57.ØX1 Toxic effect of arsenic and its compounds, accidental (unintentional)

Toxic effect of arsenic and its compounds NOS

T57.ØX2 Toxic effect of arsenic and its compounds, intentional self-harm A, S

T57.ØX3 Toxic effect of arsenic and its compounds, assault

T57.ØX4 Toxic effect of arsenic and its compounds, undetermined

T57.1 Toxic effect of phosphorus and its compounds

Excludes1 organophosphate insecticides (T6Ø.Ø)

T57.1X Toxic effect of phosphorus and its compounds

T57.1X1 Toxic effect of phosphorus and its compounds, accidental (unintentional)

Toxic effect of phosphorus and its compounds NOS

T57.1X2 Toxic effect of phosphorus and its compounds, intentional self-harm A, S

T57.1X3 Toxic effect of phosphorus and its compounds, assault

T57.1X4 Toxic effect of phosphorus and its compounds, undetermined

T57.2 Toxic effect of manganese and its compounds

T57.2X Toxic effect of manganese and its compounds

T57.2X1 Toxic effect of manganese and its compounds, accidental (unintentional)

Toxic effect of manganese and its compounds NOS

T57.2X2 Toxic effect of manganese and its compounds, intentional self-harm A, S

T57.2X3 Toxic effect of manganese and its compounds, assault

T57.2X4 Toxic effect of manganese and its compounds, undetermined

T57.3 Toxic effect of hydrogen cyanide

T57.3X Toxic effect of hydrogen cyanide

T57.3X1 Toxic effect of hydrogen cyanide, accidental (unintentional)

Toxic effect of hydrogen cyanide NOS

T57.3X2 Toxic effect of hydrogen cyanide, intentional self-harm A, S

T57.3X3 Toxic effect of hydrogen cyanide, assault

T57.3X4 Toxic effect of hydrogen cyanide, undetermined

T57.8 Toxic effect of other specified inorganic substances

T57.8X Toxic effect of other specified inorganic substances

T57.8X1 Toxic effect of other specified inorganic substances, accidental (unintentional)

Toxic effect of other specified inorganic substances NOS

T57.8X2 Toxic effect of other specified inorganic substances, intentional self-harm A, S

T57.8X3 Toxic effect of other specified inorganic substances, assault

T57.8X4 Toxic effect of other specified inorganic substances, undetermined

T57.9 Toxic effect of unspecified inorganic substance

X T57.91 Toxic effect of unspecified inorganic substance, accidental (unintentional)

X T57.92 Toxic effect of unspecified inorganic substance, intentional self-harm A, S

X T57.93 Toxic effect of unspecified inorganic substance, assault

X T57.94 Toxic effect of unspecified inorganic substance, undetermined

T58 Toxic effect of carbon monoxide

Includes asphyxiation from carbon monoxide
toxic effect of carbon monoxide from all sources

The appropriate 7th character is to be added to each code from category T58

A initial encounter
D subsequent encounter
S sequela

T58.Ø Toxic effect of carbon monoxide from motor vehicle exhaust

Toxic effect of exhaust gas from gas engine
Toxic effect of exhaust gas from motor pump

X T58.Ø1 Toxic effect of carbon monoxide from motor vehicle exhaust, accidental (unintentional)

X T58.Ø2 Toxic effect of carbon monoxide from motor vehicle exhaust, intentional self-harm A, S

X T58.Ø3 Toxic effect of carbon monoxide from motor vehicle exhaust, assault

X T58.Ø4 Toxic effect of carbon monoxide from motor vehicle exhaust, undetermined

T58.1 Toxic effect of carbon monoxide from utility gas

Toxic effect of acetylene
Toxic effect of gas NOS used for lighting, heating, cooking
Toxic effect of water gas

X T58.11 Toxic effect of carbon monoxide from utility gas, accidental (unintentional)

X T58.12 Toxic effect of carbon monoxide from utility gas, intentional self-harm A, S

X T58.13 Toxic effect of carbon monoxide from utility gas, assault

X T58.14 Toxic effect of carbon monoxide from utility gas, undetermined

T58.2 Toxic effect of carbon monoxide from incomplete combustion of other domestic fuels

Toxic effect of carbon monoxide from incomplete combustion of coal, coke, kerosene, wood

T58.2X Toxic effect of carbon monoxide from incomplete combustion of other domestic fuels

T58.2X1 Toxic effect of carbon monoxide from incomplete combustion of other domestic fuels, accidental (unintentional)

T58.2X2 Toxic effect of carbon monoxide from incomplete combustion of other domestic fuels, intentional self-harm A, S

T58.2X3 **Toxic effect of carbon monoxide from incomplete combustion of other domestic fuels, assault**

T58.2X4 **Toxic effect of carbon monoxide from incomplete combustion of other domestic fuels, undetermined**

T58.8 **Toxic effect of carbon monoxide from other source**
Toxic effect of carbon monoxide from blast furnace gas
Toxic effect of carbon monoxide from fuels in industrial use
Toxic effect of carbon monoxide from kiln vapor

T58.8X **Toxic effect of carbon monoxide from other source**

T58.8X1 **Toxic effect of carbon monoxide from other source, accidental (unintentional)**

T58.8X2 **Toxic effect of carbon monoxide from other source, intentional self-harm A, S**

T58.8X3 **Toxic effect of carbon monoxide from other source, assault**

T58.8X4 **Toxic effect of carbon monoxide from other source, undetermined**

T58.9 **Toxic effect of carbon monoxide from unspecified source**

X T58.91 **Toxic effect of carbon monoxide from unspecified source, accidental (unintentional)**

X T58.92 **Toxic effect of carbon monoxide from unspecified source, intentional self-harm A, S**

X T58.93 **Toxic effect of carbon monoxide from unspecified source, assault**

X T58.94 **Toxic effect of carbon monoxide from unspecified source, undetermined**

T59 **Toxic effect of other gases, fumes and vapors**

Includes aerosol propellants
Excludes1 chlorofluorocarbons (T53.5)

The appropriate 7th character is to be added to each code from category T59

A	initial encounter
D	subsequent encounter
S	sequela

T59.0 **Toxic effect of nitrogen oxides**

T59.0X **Toxic effect of nitrogen oxides**

T59.0X1 **Toxic effect of nitrogen oxides, accidental (unintentional)**
Toxic effect of nitrogen oxides NOS

T59.0X2 **Toxic effect of nitrogen oxides, intentional self-harm A, S**

T59.0X3 **Toxic effect of nitrogen oxides, assault**

T59.0X4 **Toxic effect of nitrogen oxides, undetermined**

T59.1 **Toxic effect of sulfur dioxide**

T59.1X **Toxic effect of sulfur dioxide**

T59.1X1 **Toxic effect of sulfur dioxide, accidental (unintentional)**
Toxic effect of sulfur dioxide NOS

T59.1X2 **Toxic effect of sulfur dioxide, intentional self-harm A, S**

T59.1X3 **Toxic effect of sulfur dioxide, assault**

T59.1X4 **Toxic effect of sulfur dioxide, undetermined**

T59.2 **Toxic effect of formaldehyde**

T59.2X **Toxic effect of formaldehyde**

T59.2X1 **Toxic effect of formaldehyde, accidental (unintentional)**
Toxic effect of formaldehyde NOS

T59.2X2 **Toxic effect of formaldehyde, intentional self-harm A, S**

T59.2X3 **Toxic effect of formaldehyde, assault**

T59.2X4 **Toxic effect of formaldehyde, undetermined**

T59.3 **Toxic effect of lacrimogenic gas**
Toxic effect of tear gas

T59.3X **Toxic effect of lacrimogenic gas**

T59.3X1 **Toxic effect of lacrimogenic gas, accidental (unintentional)**
Toxic effect of lacrimogenic gas NOS

T59.3X2 **Toxic effect of lacrimogenic gas, intentional self-harm A, S**

T59.3X3 **Toxic effect of lacrimogenic gas, assault**

T59.3X4 **Toxic effect of lacrimogenic gas, undetermined**

T59.4 **Toxic effect of chlorine gas**

T59.4X **Toxic effect of chlorine gas**

T59.4X1 **Toxic effect of chlorine gas, accidental (unintentional)**
Toxic effect of chlorine gas NOS

T59.4X2 **Toxic effect of chlorine gas, intentional self-harm A, S**

T59.4X3 **Toxic effect of chlorine gas, assault**

T59.4X4 **Toxic effect of chlorine gas, undetermined**

T59.5 **Toxic effect of fluorine gas and hydrogen fluoride**

T59.5X **Toxic effect of fluorine gas and hydrogen fluoride**

T59.5X1 **Toxic effect of fluorine gas and hydrogen fluoride, accidental (unintentional)**
Toxic effect of fluorine gas and hydrogen fluoride NOS

T59.5X2 **Toxic effect of fluorine gas and hydrogen fluoride, intentional self-harm A, S**

T59.5X3 **Toxic effect of fluorine gas and hydrogen fluoride, assault**

T59.5X4 **Toxic effect of fluorine gas and hydrogen fluoride, undetermined**

T59.6 **Toxic effect of hydrogen sulfide**

T59.6X **Toxic effect of hydrogen sulfide**

T59.6X1 **Toxic effect of hydrogen sulfide, accidental (unintentional)**
Toxic effect of hydrogen sulfide NOS

T59.6X2 **Toxic effect of hydrogen sulfide, intentional self-harm A, S**

T59.6X3 **Toxic effect of hydrogen sulfide, assault**

T59.6X4 **Toxic effect of hydrogen sulfide, undetermined**

T59.7 **Toxic effect of carbon dioxide**

T59.7X **Toxic effect of carbon dioxide**

T59.7X1 **Toxic effect of carbon dioxide, accidental (unintentional)**
Toxic effect of carbon dioxide NOS

T59.7X2 **Toxic effect of carbon dioxide, intentional self-harm A, S**

T59.7X3 **Toxic effect of carbon dioxide, assault**

T59.7X4 **Toxic effect of carbon dioxide, undetermined**

T59.8 **Toxic effect of other specified gases, fumes and vapors**

T59.81 **Toxic effect of smoke**
Smoke inhalation
Excludes2 toxic effect of cigarette (tobacco) smoke (T65.22-)

T59.811 **Toxic effect of smoke, accidental (unintentional)**
Toxic effect of smoke NOS

T59.812 **Toxic effect of smoke, intentional self-harm A, S**

T59.813 Toxic effect of smoke, assault

T59.814 Toxic effect of smoke, undetermined

T59.89 Toxic effect of other specified gases, fumes and vapors

T59.891 Toxic effect of other specified gases, fumes and vapors, accidental (unintentional)

T59.892 Toxic effect of other specified gases, fumes and vapors, intentional self-harm A, S

T59.893 Toxic effect of other specified gases, fumes and vapors, assault

T59.894 Toxic effect of other specified gases, fumes and vapors, undetermined

T59.9 Toxic effect of unspecified gases, fumes and vapors

X T59.91 Toxic effect of unspecified gases, fumes and vapors, accidental (unintentional)

X T59.92 Toxic effect of unspecified gases, fumes and vapors, intentional self-harm A, S

X T59.93 Toxic effect of unspecified gases, fumes and vapors, assault

X T59.94 Toxic effect of unspecified gases, fumes and vapors, undetermined

T6Ø Toxic effect of pesticides

Includes toxic effect of wood preservatives

The appropriate 7th character is to be added to each code from category T6Ø

A initial encounter
D subsequent encounter
S sequela

T6Ø.Ø Toxic effect of organophosphate and carbamate insecticides

T6Ø.ØX Toxic effect of organophosphate and carbamate insecticides

T6Ø.ØX1 Toxic effect of organophosphate and carbamate insecticides, accidental (unintentional)
Toxic effect of organophosphate and carbamate insecticides NOS

T6Ø.ØX2 Toxic effect of organophosphate and carbamate insecticides, intentional self-harm A, S

T6Ø.ØX3 Toxic effect of organophosphate and carbamate insecticides, assault

T6Ø.ØX4 Toxic effect of organophosphate and carbamate insecticides, undetermined

T6Ø.1 Toxic effect of halogenated insecticides

Excludes1 chlorinated hydrocarbon (T53.-)

T6Ø.1X Toxic effect of halogenated insecticides

T6Ø.1X1 Toxic effect of halogenated insecticides, accidental (unintentional)
Toxic effect of halogenated insecticides NOS

T6Ø.1X2 Toxic effect of halogenated insecticides, intentional self-harm A, S

T6Ø.1X3 Toxic effect of halogenated insecticides, assault

T6Ø.1X4 Toxic effect of halogenated insecticides, undetermined

T6Ø.2 Toxic effect of other insecticides

T6Ø.2X Toxic effect of other insecticides

T6Ø.2X1 Toxic effect of other insecticides, accidental (unintentional)
Toxic effect of other insecticides NOS

T6Ø.2X2 Toxic effect of other insecticides, intentional self-harm A, S

T6Ø.2X3 Toxic effect of other insecticides, assault

T6Ø.2X4 Toxic effect of other insecticides, undetermined

T6Ø.3 Toxic effect of herbicides and fungicides

T6Ø.3X Toxic effect of herbicides and fungicides

T6Ø.3X1 Toxic effect of herbicides and fungicides, accidental (unintentional)
Toxic effect of herbicides and fungicides NOS

T6Ø.3X2 Toxic effect of herbicides and fungicides, intentional self-harm A, S

T6Ø.3X3 Toxic effect of herbicides and fungicides, assault

T6Ø.3X4 Toxic effect of herbicides and fungicides, undetermined

T6Ø.4 Toxic effect of rodenticides

Excludes1 strychnine and its salts (T65.1)
thallium (T56.81-)

T6Ø.4X Toxic effect of rodenticides

T6Ø.4X1 Toxic effect of rodenticides, accidental (unintentional)
Toxic effect of rodenticides NOS

T6Ø.4X2 Toxic effect of rodenticides, intentional self-harm A, S

T6Ø.4X3 Toxic effect of rodenticides, assault

T6Ø.4X4 Toxic effect of rodenticides, undetermined

T6Ø.8 Toxic effect of other pesticides

T6Ø.8X Toxic effect of other pesticides

T6Ø.8X1 Toxic effect of other pesticides, accidental (unintentional)
Toxic effect of other pesticides NOS

T6Ø.8X2 Toxic effect of other pesticides, intentional self-harm A, S

T6Ø.8X3 Toxic effect of other pesticides, assault

T6Ø.8X4 Toxic effect of other pesticides, undetermined

T6Ø.9 Toxic effect of unspecified pesticide

X T6Ø.91 Toxic effect of unspecified pesticide, accidental (unintentional)

X T6Ø.92 Toxic effect of unspecified pesticide, intentional self-harm A, S

X T6Ø.93 Toxic effect of unspecified pesticide, assault

X T6Ø.94 Toxic effect of unspecified pesticide, undetermined

T61 Toxic effect of noxious substances eaten as seafood

Excludes1 allergic reaction to food, such as:
anaphylactic reaction or shock due to adverse food reaction (T78.Ø-)
bacterial foodborne intoxications (AØ5.-)
dermatitis (L23.6, L25.4, L27.2)
food protein-induced enterocolitis syndrome (K52.21)
food protein-induced enteropathy (K52.22)
gastroenteritis (noninfective) (K52.29)
toxic effect of aflatoxin and other mycotoxins (T64)
toxic effect of cyanides (T65.Ø-)
toxic effect of harmful algae bloom (T65.82-)
toxic effect of hydrogen cyanide (T57.3-)
toxic effect of mercury (T56.1-)
toxic effect of red tide (T65.82-)

The appropriate 7th character is to be added to each code from category T61

A initial encounter
D subsequent encounter
S sequela

● T61.Ø Ciguatera fish poisoning
X● T61.Ø1 Ciguatera fish poisoning, accidental (unintentional)
X● T61.Ø2 Ciguatera fish poisoning, intentional self-harm A, S
X● T61.Ø3 Ciguatera fish poisoning, assault
X● T61.Ø4 Ciguatera fish poisoning, undetermined
● T61.1 Scombroid fish poisoning
Histamine-like syndrome
X● T61.11 Scombroid fish poisoning, accidental (unintentional)
X● T61.12 Scombroid fish poisoning, intentional self-harm A, S
X● T61.13 Scombroid fish poisoning, assault
X● T61.14 Scombroid fish poisoning, undetermined
● T61.7 Other fish and shellfish poisoning
● T61.77 Other fish poisoning
● T61.771 Other fish poisoning, accidental (unintentional)
● T61.772 Other fish poisoning, intentional self-harm A, S
● T61.773 Other fish poisoning, assault
● T61.774 Other fish poisoning, undetermined
● T61.78 Other shellfish poisoning
● T61.781 Other shellfish poisoning, accidental (unintentional)
● T61.782 Other shellfish poisoning, intentional self-harm A, S
● T61.783 Other shellfish poisoning, assault
● T61.784 Other shellfish poisoning, undetermined
● T61.8 Toxic effect of other seafood
● T61.8X Toxic effect of other seafood
● T61.8X1 Toxic effect of other seafood, accidental (unintentional)
● T61.8X2 Toxic effect of other seafood, intentional self-harm A, S
● T61.8X3 Toxic effect of other seafood, assault
● T61.8X4 Toxic effect of other seafood, undetermined
● T61.9 Toxic effect of unspecified seafood
X● T61.91 Toxic effect of unspecified seafood, accidental (unintentional)
X● T61.92 Toxic effect of unspecified seafood, intentional self-harm A, S
X● T61.93 Toxic effect of unspecified seafood, assault
X● T61.94 Toxic effect of unspecified seafood, undetermined

● T62 Toxic effect of other noxious substances eaten as food

Excludes1 allergic reaction to food, such as:
anaphylactic shock (reaction) due to adverse food reaction (T78.Ø-)
dermatitis (L23.6, L25.4, L27.2)
food protein-induced enterocolitis syndrome (K52.21)
food protein-induced enteropathy (K52.22)
gastroenteritis (noninfective) (K52.29)
bacterial food borne intoxications (AØ5.-)
toxic effect of aflatoxin and other mycotoxins (T64)
toxic effect of cyanides (T65.Ø-)
toxic effect of hydrogen cyanide (T57.3-)
toxic effect of mercury (T56.1-)

The appropriate 7th character is to be added to each code from category T62

A	initial encounter
D	subsequent encounter
S	sequela

● T62.Ø Toxic effect of ingested mushrooms
● T62.ØX Toxic effect of ingested mushrooms
● T62.ØX1 Toxic effect of ingested mushrooms, accidental (unintentional)
Toxic effect of ingested mushrooms NOS
● T62.ØX2 Toxic effect of ingested mushrooms, intentional self-harm A, S
● T62.ØX3 Toxic effect of ingested mushrooms, assault
● T62.ØX4 Toxic effect of ingested mushrooms, undetermined
● T62.1 Toxic effect of ingested berries
● T62.1X Toxic effect of ingested berries
● T62.1X1 Toxic effect of ingested berries, accidental (unintentional)
Toxic effect of ingested berries NOS
● T62.1X2 Toxic effect of ingested berries, intentional self-harm A, S
● T62.1X3 Toxic effect of ingested berries, assault
● T62.1X4 Toxic effect of ingested berries, undetermined
● T62.2 Toxic effect of other ingested (parts of) plant(s)
● T62.2X Toxic effect of other ingested (parts of) plant(s)
● T62.2X1 Toxic effect of other ingested (parts of) plant(s), accidental (unintentional)
Toxic effect of other ingested (parts of) plant(s) NOS
● T62.2X2 Toxic effect of other ingested (parts of) plant(s), intentional self-harm A, S
● T62.2X3 Toxic effect of other ingested (parts of) plant(s), assault
● T62.2X4 Toxic effect of other ingested (parts of) plant(s), undetermined
● T62.8 Toxic effect of other specified noxious substances eaten as food
● T62.8X Toxic effect of other specified noxious substances eaten as food
● T62.8X1 Toxic effect of other specified noxious substances eaten as food, accidental (unintentional)
Toxic effect of other specified noxious substances eaten as food NOS
● T62.8X2 Toxic effect of other specified noxious substances eaten as food, intentional self-harm A, S
● T62.8X3 Toxic effect of other specified noxious substances eaten as food, assault
● T62.8X4 Toxic effect of other specified noxious substances eaten as food, undetermined
● T62.9 Toxic effect of unspecified noxious substance eaten as food
X● T62.91 Toxic effect of unspecified noxious substance eaten as food, accidental (unintentional)
Toxic effect of unspecified noxious substance eaten as food NOS
X● T62.92 Toxic effect of unspecified noxious substance eaten as food, intentional self-harm A, S
X● T62.93 Toxic effect of unspecified noxious substance eaten as food, assault
X● T62.94 Toxic effect of unspecified noxious substance eaten as food, undetermined

T63 Toxic effect of contact with venomous animals and plants

Includes bite or touch of venomous animal
pricked or stuck by thorn or leaf

Excludes2 ingestion of toxic animal or plant (T61.-, T62.-)

The appropriate 7th character is to be added to each code from category T63

A initial encounter
D subsequent encounter
S sequela

T63.0 Toxic effect of snake venom

T63.00 Toxic effect of unspecified snake venom

T63.001 Toxic effect of unspecified snake venom, accidental (unintentional)
Toxic effect of unspecified snake venom NOS

T63.002 Toxic effect of unspecified snake venom, intentional self-harm A, S

T63.003 Toxic effect of unspecified snake venom, assault

T63.004 Toxic effect of unspecified snake venom, undetermined

T63.01 Toxic effect of rattlesnake venom

T63.011 Toxic effect of rattlesnake venom, accidental (unintentional)
Toxic effect of rattlesnake venom NOS

T63.012 Toxic effect of rattlesnake venom, intentional self-harm A, S

T63.013 Toxic effect of rattlesnake venom, assault

T63.014 Toxic effect of rattlesnake venom, undetermined

T63.02 Toxic effect of coral snake venom

T63.021 Toxic effect of coral snake venom, accidental (unintentional)
Toxic effect of coral snake venom NOS

T63.022 Toxic effect of coral snake venom, intentional self-harm A, S

T63.023 Toxic effect of coral snake venom, assault

T63.024 Toxic effect of coral snake venom, undetermined

T63.03 Toxic effect of taipan venom

T63.031 Toxic effect of taipan venom, accidental (unintentional)
Toxic effect of taipan venom NOS

T63.032 Toxic effect of taipan venom, intentional self-harm A, S

T63.033 Toxic effect of taipan venom, assault

T63.034 Toxic effect of taipan venom, undetermined

T63.04 Toxic effect of cobra venom

T63.041 Toxic effect of cobra venom, accidental (unintentional)
Toxic effect of cobra venom NOS

T63.042 Toxic effect of cobra venom, intentional self-harm A, S

T63.043 Toxic effect of cobra venom, assault

T63.044 Toxic effect of cobra venom, undetermined

T63.06 Toxic effect of venom of other North and South American snake

T63.061 Toxic effect of venom of other North and South American snake, accidental (unintentional)
Toxic effect of venom of other North and South American snake NOS

T63.062 Toxic effect of venom of other North and South American snake, intentional self-harm A, S

T63.063 Toxic effect of venom of other North and South American snake, assault

T63.064 Toxic effect of venom of other North and South American snake, undetermined

T63.07 Toxic effect of venom of other Australian snake

T63.071 Toxic effect of venom of other Australian snake, accidental (unintentional)
Toxic effect of venom of other Australian snake NOS

T63.072 Toxic effect of venom of other Australian snake, intentional self-harm A, S

T63.073 Toxic effect of venom of other Australian snake, assault

T63.074 Toxic effect of venom of other Australian snake, undetermined

T63.08 Toxic effect of venom of other African and Asian snake

T63.081 Toxic effect of venom of other African and Asian snake, accidental (unintentional)
Toxic effect of venom of other African and Asian snake NOS

T63.082 Toxic effect of venom of other African and Asian snake, intentional self-harm A, S

T63.083 Toxic effect of venom of other African and Asian snake, assault

T63.084 Toxic effect of venom of other African and Asian snake, undetermined

T63.09 Toxic effect of venom of other snake

T63.091 Toxic effect of venom of other snake, accidental (unintentional)
Toxic effect of venom of other snake NOS

T63.092 Toxic effect of venom of other snake, intentional self-harm A, S

T63.093 Toxic effect of venom of other snake, assault

T63.094 Toxic effect of venom of other snake, undetermined

T63.1 Toxic effect of venom of other reptiles

T63.11 Toxic effect of venom of gila monster

T63.111 Toxic effect of venom of gila monster, accidental (unintentional)
Toxic effect of venom of gila monster NOS

T63.112 Toxic effect of venom of gila monster, intentional self-harm A, S

T63.113 Toxic effect of venom of gila monster, assault

T63.114 Toxic effect of venom of gila monster, undetermined

T63.12 Toxic effect of venom of other venomous lizard

T63.121 Toxic effect of venom of other venomous lizard, accidental (unintentional)
Toxic effect of venom of other venomous lizard NOS

T63.122 Toxic effect of venom of other venomous lizard, intentional self-harm A, S

T63.123 Toxic effect of venom of other venomous lizard, assault

T63.124 Toxic effect of venom of other venomous lizard, undetermined

T63.19 Toxic effect of venom of other reptiles
T63.191 Toxic effect of venom of other reptiles, accidental (unintentional)
Toxic effect of venom of other reptiles NOS
T63.192 Toxic effect of venom of other reptiles, intentional self-harm A, S
T63.193 Toxic effect of venom of other reptiles, assault
T63.194 Toxic effect of venom of other reptiles, undetermined
T63.2 Toxic effect of venom of scorpion
T63.2X Toxic effect of venom of scorpion
T63.2X1 Toxic effect of venom of scorpion, accidental (unintentional)
Toxic effect of venom of scorpion NOS
T63.2X2 Toxic effect of venom of scorpion, intentional self-harm A, S
T63.2X3 Toxic effect of venom of scorpion, assault
T63.2X4 Toxic effect of venom of scorpion, undetermined
T63.3 Toxic effect of venom of spider
T63.30 Toxic effect of unspecified spider venom
T63.301 Toxic effect of unspecified spider venom, accidental (unintentional)
T63.302 Toxic effect of unspecified spider venom, intentional self-harm A, S
T63.303 Toxic effect of unspecified spider venom, assault
T63.304 Toxic effect of unspecified spider venom, undetermined
T63.31 Toxic effect of venom of black widow spider
T63.311 Toxic effect of venom of black widow spider, accidental (unintentional)
T63.312 Toxic effect of venom of black widow spider, intentional self-harm A, S
T63.313 Toxic effect of venom of black widow spider, assault
T63.314 Toxic effect of venom of black widow spider, undetermined
T63.32 Toxic effect of venom of tarantula
T63.321 Toxic effect of venom of tarantula, accidental (unintentional)
T63.322 Toxic effect of venom of tarantula, intentional self-harm A, S
T63.323 Toxic effect of venom of tarantula, assault
T63.324 Toxic effect of venom of tarantula, undetermined
T63.33 Toxic effect of venom of brown recluse spider
T63.331 Toxic effect of venom of brown recluse spider, accidental (unintentional)
T63.332 Toxic effect of venom of brown recluse spider, intentional self-harm A, S
T63.333 Toxic effect of venom of brown recluse spider, assault
T63.334 Toxic effect of venom of brown recluse spider, undetermined
T63.39 Toxic effect of venom of other spider
T63.391 Toxic effect of venom of other spider, accidental (unintentional)
T63.392 Toxic effect of venom of other spider, intentional self-harm A, S
T63.393 Toxic effect of venom of other spider, assault
T63.394 Toxic effect of venom of other spider, undetermined
T63.4 Toxic effect of venom of other arthropods
Use additional code, if applicable, for anaphylactic shock (T78.2)
T63.41 Toxic effect of venom of centipedes and venomous millipedes
T63.411 Toxic effect of venom of centipedes and venomous millipedes, accidental (unintentional)
T63.412 Toxic effect of venom of centipedes and venomous millipedes, intentional self-harm A, S
T63.413 Toxic effect of venom of centipedes and venomous millipedes, assault
T63.414 Toxic effect of venom of centipedes and venomous millipedes, undetermined
T63.42 Toxic effect of venom of ants
T63.421 Toxic effect of venom of ants, accidental (unintentional)
T63.422 Toxic effect of venom of ants, intentional self-harm A, S
T63.423 Toxic effect of venom of ants, assault
T63.424 Toxic effect of venom of ants, undetermined
T63.43 Toxic effect of venom of caterpillars
T63.431 Toxic effect of venom of caterpillars, accidental (unintentional)
T63.432 Toxic effect of venom of caterpillars, intentional self-harm A, S
T63.433 Toxic effect of venom of caterpillars, assault
T63.434 Toxic effect of venom of caterpillars, undetermined
T63.44 Toxic effect of venom of bees
T63.441 Toxic effect of venom of bees, accidental (unintentional)
T63.442 Toxic effect of venom of bees, intentional self-harm A, S
T63.443 Toxic effect of venom of bees, assault
T63.444 Toxic effect of venom of bees, undetermined
T63.45 Toxic effect of venom of hornets
T63.451 Toxic effect of venom of hornets, accidental (unintentional)
T63.452 Toxic effect of venom of hornets, intentional self-harm A, S
T63.453 Toxic effect of venom of hornets, assault
T63.454 Toxic effect of venom of hornets, undetermined
T63.46 Toxic effect of venom of wasps
Toxic effect of yellow jacket
T63.461 Toxic effect of venom of wasps, accidental (unintentional)
T63.462 Toxic effect of venom of wasps, intentional self-harm A, S
T63.463 Toxic effect of venom of wasps, assault
T63.464 Toxic effect of venom of wasps, undetermined
T63.48 Toxic effect of venom of other arthropod
T63.481 Toxic effect of venom of other arthropod, accidental (unintentional)
T63.482 Toxic effect of venom of other arthropod, intentional self-harm A, S

CHAPTER 19 (S00-T88)

- T63.483 Toxic effect of venom of other arthropod, assault
- T63.484 Toxic effect of venom of other arthropod, undetermined

T63.5 Toxic effect of contact with venomous fish
  Excludes2 poisoning by ingestion of fish (T61.-)

T63.51 Toxic effect of contact with stingray
- T63.511 Toxic effect of contact with stingray, accidental (unintentional)
- T63.512 Toxic effect of contact with stingray, intentional self-harm A, S
- T63.513 Toxic effect of contact with stingray, assault
- T63.514 Toxic effect of contact with stingray, undetermined

T63.59 Toxic effect of contact with other venomous fish
- T63.591 Toxic effect of contact with other venomous fish, accidental (unintentional)
- T63.592 Toxic effect of contact with other venomous fish, intentional self-harm A, S
- T63.593 Toxic effect of contact with other venomous fish, assault
- T63.594 Toxic effect of contact with other venomous fish, undetermined

T63.6 Toxic effect of contact with other venomous marine animals
  Excludes1 sea-snake venom (T63.Ø9)
  Excludes2 poisoning by ingestion of shellfish (T61.78-)

T63.61 Toxic effect of contact with Portuguese Man-o-war
  Toxic effect of contact with bluebottle
- T63.611 Toxic effect of contact with Portuguese Man-o-war, accidental (unintentional)
- T63.612 Toxic effect of contact with Portuguese Man-o-war, intentional self-harm A, S
- T63.613 Toxic effect of contact with Portuguese Man-o-war, assault
- T63.614 Toxic effect of contact with Portuguese Man-o-war, undetermined

T63.62 Toxic effect of contact with other jellyfish
- T63.621 Toxic effect of contact with other jellyfish, accidental (unintentional)
- T63.622 Toxic effect of contact with other jellyfish, intentional self-harm A, S
- T63.623 Toxic effect of contact with other jellyfish, assault
- T63.624 Toxic effect of contact with other jellyfish, undetermined

T63.63 Toxic effect of contact with sea anemone
- T63.631 Toxic effect of contact with sea anemone, accidental (unintentional)
- T63.632 Toxic effect of contact with sea anemone, intentional self-harm A, S
- T63.633 Toxic effect of contact with sea anemone, assault
- T63.634 Toxic effect of contact with sea anemone, undetermined

T63.69 Toxic effect of contact with other venomous marine animals
- T63.691 Toxic effect of contact with other venomous marine animals, accidental (unintentional)
- T63.692 Toxic effect of contact with other venomous marine animals, intentional self-harm A, S
- T63.693 Toxic effect of contact with other venomous marine animals, assault
- T63.694 Toxic effect of contact with other venomous marine animals, undetermined

T63.7 Toxic effect of contact with venomous plant

T63.71 Toxic effect of contact with venomous marine plant
- T63.711 Toxic effect of contact with venomous marine plant, accidental (unintentional)
- T63.712 Toxic effect of contact with venomous marine plant, intentional self-harm A, S
- T63.713 Toxic effect of contact with venomous marine plant, assault
- T63.714 Toxic effect of contact with venomous marine plant, undetermined

T63.79 Toxic effect of contact with other venomous plant
- T63.791 Toxic effect of contact with other venomous plant, accidental (unintentional)
- T63.792 Toxic effect of contact with other venomous plant, intentional self-harm A, S
- T63.793 Toxic effect of contact with other venomous plant, assault
- T63.794 Toxic effect of contact with other venomous plant, undetermined

T63.8 Toxic effect of contact with other venomous animals

T63.81 Toxic effect of contact with venomous frog
  Excludes1 contact with nonvenomous frog (W62.Ø)
- T63.811 Toxic effect of contact with venomous frog, accidental (unintentional)
- T63.812 Toxic effect of contact with venomous frog, intentional self-harm A, S
- T63.813 Toxic effect of contact with venomous frog, assault
- T63.814 Toxic effect of contact with venomous frog, undetermined

T63.82 Toxic effect of contact with venomous toad
  Excludes1 contact with nonvenomous toad (W62.1)
- T63.821 Toxic effect of contact with venomous toad, accidental (unintentional)
- T63.822 Toxic effect of contact with venomous toad, intentional self-harm A, S
- T63.823 Toxic effect of contact with venomous toad, assault
- T63.824 Toxic effect of contact with venomous toad, undetermined

T63.83 Toxic effect of contact with other venomous amphibian
  Excludes1 contact with nonvenomous amphibian (W62.9)
- T63.831 Toxic effect of contact with other venomous amphibian, accidental (unintentional)
- T63.832 Toxic effect of contact with other venomous amphibian, intentional self-harm A, S
- T63.833 Toxic effect of contact with other venomous amphibian, assault
- T63.834 Toxic effect of contact with other venomous amphibian, undetermined

T63.89 Toxic effect of contact with other venomous animals
- T63.891 Toxic effect of contact with other venomous animals, accidental (unintentional)
- T63.892 Toxic effect of contact with other venomous animals, intentional self-harm A, S
- T63.893 Toxic effect of contact with other venomous animals, assault
- T63.894 Toxic effect of contact with other venomous animals, undetermined

T63.9 Toxic effect of contact with unspecified venomous animal
- X T63.91 Toxic effect of contact with unspecified venomous animal, accidental (unintentional)
- X T63.92 Toxic effect of contact with unspecified venomous animal, intentional self-harm A, S
- X T63.93 Toxic effect of contact with unspecified venomous animal, assault
- X T63.94 Toxic effect of contact with unspecified venomous animal, undetermined

T64 Toxic effect of aflatoxin and other mycotoxin food contaminants

The appropriate 7th character is to be added to each code from category T64

A	initial encounter
D	subsequent encounter
S	sequela

T64.Ø Toxic effect of aflatoxin
- X T64.Ø1 Toxic effect of aflatoxin, accidental (unintentional)
- X T64.Ø2 Toxic effect of aflatoxin, intentional self-harm A, S
- X T64.Ø3 Toxic effect of aflatoxin, assault
- X T64.Ø4 Toxic effect of aflatoxin, undetermined

T64.8 Toxic effect of other mycotoxin food contaminants
- X T64.81 Toxic effect of other mycotoxin food contaminants, accidental (unintentional)
- X T64.82 Toxic effect of other mycotoxin food contaminants, intentional self-harm A, S
- X T64.83 Toxic effect of other mycotoxin food contaminants, assault
- X T64.84 Toxic effect of other mycotoxin food contaminants, undetermined

T65 Toxic effect of other and unspecified substances

The appropriate 7th character is to be added to each code from category T65

A	initial encounter
D	subsequent encounter
S	sequela

T65.Ø Toxic effect of cyanides

Excludes1 hydrogen cyanide (T57.3-)

T65.ØX Toxic effect of cyanides
- T65.ØX1 Toxic effect of cyanides, accidental (unintentional)
  - Toxic effect of cyanides NOS
- T65.ØX2 Toxic effect of cyanides, intentional self-harm A, S
- T65.ØX3 Toxic effect of cyanides, assault
- T65.ØX4 Toxic effect of cyanides, undetermined

T65.1 Toxic effect of strychnine and its salts

T65.1X Toxic effect of strychnine and its salts
- T65.1X1 Toxic effect of strychnine and its salts, accidental (unintentional)
  - Toxic effect of strychnine and its salts NOS
- T65.1X2 Toxic effect of strychnine and its salts, intentional self-harm A, S
- T65.1X3 Toxic effect of strychnine and its salts, assault
- T65.1X4 Toxic effect of strychnine and its salts, undetermined

T65.2 Toxic effect of tobacco and nicotine

Excludes2 nicotine dependence (F17.-)

T65.21 Toxic effect of chewing tobacco
- T65.211 Toxic effect of chewing tobacco, accidental (unintentional)
  - Toxic effect of chewing tobacco NOS
- T65.212 Toxic effect of chewing tobacco, intentional self-harm A, S
- T65.213 Toxic effect of chewing tobacco, assault
- T65.214 Toxic effect of chewing tobacco, undetermined

T65.22 Toxic effect of tobacco cigarettes

Toxic effect of tobacco smoke

Use additional code for exposure to second hand tobacco smoke (Z57.31, Z77.22)
- T65.221 Toxic effect of tobacco cigarettes, accidental (unintentional)
  - Toxic effect of tobacco cigarettes NOS
- T65.222 Toxic effect of tobacco cigarettes, intentional self-harm A, S
- T65.223 Toxic effect of tobacco cigarettes, assault
- T65.224 Toxic effect of tobacco cigarettes, undetermined

T65.29 Toxic effect of other tobacco and nicotine
- T65.291 Toxic effect of other tobacco and nicotine, accidental (unintentional)
  - Toxic effect of other tobacco and nicotine NOS
- T65.292 Toxic effect of other tobacco and nicotine, intentional self-harm A, S
- T65.293 Toxic effect of other tobacco and nicotine, assault
- T65.294 Toxic effect of other tobacco and nicotine, undetermined

T65.3 Toxic effect of nitroderivatives and aminoderivatives of benzene and its homologues

Toxic effect of aniline [benzenamine]

Toxic effect of nitrobenzene

Toxic effect of trinitrotoluene

T65.3X Toxic effect of nitroderivatives and aminoderivatives of benzene and its homologues
- T65.3X1 Toxic effect of nitroderivatives and aminoderivatives of benzene and its homologues, accidental (unintentional)
  - Toxic effect of nitroderivatives and aminoderivatives of benzene and its homologues NOS
- T65.3X2 Toxic effect of nitroderivatives and aminoderivatives of benzene and its homologues, intentional self-harm A, S

CHAPTER 19 (SØØ-T88)

T65.3X3 Toxic effect of nitroderivatives and aminoderivatives of benzene and its homologues, assault

T65.3X4 Toxic effect of nitroderivatives and aminoderivatives of benzene and its homologues, undetermined

T65.4 Toxic effect of carbon disulfide

T65.4X Toxic effect of carbon disulfide

T65.4X1 Toxic effect of carbon disulfide, accidental (unintentional)
Toxic effect of carbon disulfide NOS

T65.4X2 Toxic effect of carbon disulfide, intentional self-harm A, S

T65.4X3 Toxic effect of carbon disulfide, assault

T65.4X4 Toxic effect of carbon disulfide, undetermined

T65.5 Toxic effect of nitroglycerin and other nitric acids and esters
Toxic effect of 1,2,3-Propanetriol trinitrate

T65.5X Toxic effect of nitroglycerin and other nitric acids and esters

T65.5X1 Toxic effect of nitroglycerin and other nitric acids and esters, accidental (unintentional)
Toxic effect of nitroglycerin and other nitric acids and esters NOS

T65.5X2 Toxic effect of nitroglycerin and other nitric acids and esters, intentional self-harm A, S

T65.5X3 Toxic effect of nitroglycerin and other nitric acids and esters, assault

T65.5X4 Toxic effect of nitroglycerin and other nitric acids and esters, undetermined

T65.6 Toxic effect of paints and dyes, not elsewhere classified

T65.6X Toxic effect of paints and dyes, not elsewhere classified

T65.6X1 Toxic effect of paints and dyes, not elsewhere classified, accidental (unintentional)
Toxic effect of paints and dyes NOS

T65.6X2 Toxic effect of paints and dyes, not elsewhere classified, intentional self-harm A, S

T65.6X3 Toxic effect of paints and dyes, not elsewhere classified, assault

T65.6X4 Toxic effect of paints and dyes, not elsewhere classified, undetermined

T65.8 Toxic effect of other specified substances

T65.81 Toxic effect of latex

T65.811 Toxic effect of latex, accidental (unintentional)
Toxic effect of latex NOS

T65.812 Toxic effect of latex, intentional self-harm A, S

T65.813 Toxic effect of latex, assault

T65.814 Toxic effect of latex, undetermined

T65.82 Toxic effect of harmful algae and algae toxins
Toxic effect of (harmful) algae bloom NOS
Toxic effect of blue-green algae bloom
Toxic effect of brown tide
Toxic effect of cyanobacteria bloom
Toxic effect of Florida red tide
Toxic effect of pfiesteria piscicida
Toxic effect of red tide

T65.821 Toxic effect of harmful algae and algae toxins, accidental (unintentional)
Toxic effect of harmful algae and algae toxins NOS

T65.822 Toxic effect of harmful algae and algae toxins, intentional self-harm A, S

T65.823 Toxic effect of harmful algae and algae toxins, assault

T65.824 Toxic effect of harmful algae and algae toxins, undetermined

T65.83 Toxic effect of fiberglass

T65.831 Toxic effect of fiberglass, accidental (unintentional)
Toxic effect of fiberglass NOS

T65.832 Toxic effect of fiberglass, intentional self-harm A, S

T65.833 Toxic effect of fiberglass, assault

T65.834 Toxic effect of fiberglass, undetermined

T65.89 Toxic effect of other specified substances

T65.891 Toxic effect of other specified substances, accidental (unintentional)
Toxic effect of other specified substances NOS
Coding Clinic: 2018, Q1, P5

T65.892 Toxic effect of other specified substances, intentional self-harm A, S

T65.893 Toxic effect of other specified substances, assault

T65.894 Toxic effect of other specified substances, undetermined

T65.9 Toxic effect of unspecified substance

X T65.91 Toxic effect of unspecified substance, accidental (unintentional)
Poisoning NOS

X T65.92 Toxic effect of unspecified substance, intentional self-harm A, S

X T65.93 Toxic effect of unspecified substance, assault

X T65.94 Toxic effect of unspecified substance, undetermined

OTHER AND UNSPECIFIED EFFECTS OF EXTERNAL CAUSES (T66-T78)

T66 Radiation sickness, unspecified

Excludes1 specified adverse effects of radiation, such as:
burns (T20-T31)
leukemia (C91-C95)
radiation gastroenteritis and colitis (K52.0)
radiation pneumonitis (J70.0)
radiation related disorders of the skin and subcutaneous tissue (L55-L59)
sunburn (L55.-)

The appropriate 7th character is to be added to code T66

A initial encounter
D subsequent encounter
S sequela

T67 Effects of heat and light

Excludes1 erythema [dermatitis] ab igne (L59.0)
malignant hyperpyrexia due to anesthesia (T88.3)
radiation-related disorders of the skin and subcutaneous tissue (L55-L59)

Excludes2 burns (T20-T31)
sunburn (L55.-)
sweat disorder due to heat (L74-L75)

The appropriate 7th character is to be added to each code from category T67

A initial encounter
D subsequent encounter
S sequela

X **T67.0 Heatstroke and sunstroke** A (Ex) PDX 1935

Use additional code(s) to identify any associated complications of heatstroke, such as:
coma and stupor (R40.-)
rhabdomyolysis (M62.82)
systemic inflammatory response syndrome (R65.1-)

Coding Clinic: 2019, Q4, P18

X **T67.01 Heatstroke and sunstroke** A
Heat apoplexy
Heat pyrexia
Siriasis
Thermoplegia

X **T67.02 Exertional heatstroke** A
Coding Clinic: 2019, Q4, P18

X **T67.09 Other heatstroke and sunstroke** A

X **T67.1 Heat syncope**
Heat collapse

X **T67.2 Heat cramp**

X **T67.3 Heat exhaustion, anhydrotic**
Heat prostration due to water depletion
Excludes1 heat exhaustion due to salt depletion (T67.4)

X **T67.4 Heat exhaustion due to salt depletion**
Heat prostration due to salt (and water) depletion

X **T67.5 Heat exhaustion, unspecified**
Heat prostration NOS

X **T67.6 Heat fatigue, transient**

X **T67.7 Heat edema**

X **T67.8 Other effects of heat and light**

X **T67.9 Effect of heat and light, unspecified**

X **T68 Hypothermia**
Accidental hypothermia
Hypothermia NOS

Use additional code to identify source of exposure:
Exposure to excessive cold of man-made origin (W93)
Exposure to excessive cold of natural origin (X31)

Excludes1 hypothermia following anesthesia (T88.51)
hypothermia not associated with low environmental temperature (R68.0)
hypothermia of newborn (P80.-)

Excludes2 frostbite (T33-T34)

The appropriate 7th character is to be added to code T68

A initial encounter
D subsequent encounter
S sequela

T69 Other effects of reduced temperature

Use additional code to identify source of exposure:
Exposure to excessive cold of man-made origin (W93)
Exposure to excessive cold of natural origin (X31)

Excludes2 frostbite (T33-T34)

The appropriate 7th character is to be added to each code from category T69

A initial encounter
D subsequent encounter
S sequela

T69.0 Immersion hand and foot

T69.01 Immersion hand

T69.011 Immersion hand, right hand

T69.012 Immersion hand, left hand

T69.019 Immersion hand, unspecified hand

T69.02 Immersion foot (Ex) PDX 1936
Trench foot

T69.021 Immersion foot, right foot A, A

T69.022 Immersion foot, left foot A, A

T69.029 Immersion foot, unspecified foot A, A

X **T69.1 Chilblains**

X **T69.8 Other specified effects of reduced temperature**

X **T69.9 Effect of reduced temperature, unspecified**

T70 Effects of air pressure and water pressure

The appropriate 7th character is to be added to each code from category T70

A initial encounter
D subsequent encounter
S sequela

X **T70.0 Otitic barotrauma**
Aero-otitis media
Effects of change in ambient atmospheric pressure or water pressure on ears

X **T70.1 Sinus barotrauma**
Aerosinusitis
Effects of change in ambient atmospheric pressure on sinuses

T70.2 Other and unspecified effects of high altitude

Excludes2 polycythemia due to high altitude (D75.1)

X **T70.20 Unspecified effects of high altitude**

X **T70.29 Other effects of high altitude**
Alpine sickness
Anoxia due to high altitude
Barotrauma NOS
Hypobaropathy
Mountain sickness

X **T70.3 Caisson disease [decompression sickness]** A, A (Ex) PDX 1937
Compressed-air disease
Diver's palsy or paralysis

X● **T70.4 Effects of high-pressure fluids**
Hydraulic jet injection (industrial)
Pneumatic jet injection (industrial)
Traumatic jet injection (industrial)

X● **T70.8 Other effects of air pressure and water pressure**

X● **T70.9 Effect of air pressure and water pressure, unspecified**

● **T71 Asphyxiation** Ex PDX 1938
Mechanical suffocation
Traumatic suffocation

Excludes1 acute respiratory distress (syndrome) (J80)
anoxia due to high altitude (T70.2)
asphyxia NOS (R09.01)
asphyxia from carbon monoxide (T58.-)
asphyxia from inhalation of food or foreign body (T17.-)
asphyxia from other gases, fumes and vapors (T59.-)
respiratory distress (syndrome) in newborn (P22.-)

The appropriate 7th character is to be added to each code from category T71

A	initial encounter
D	subsequent encounter
S	sequela

● **T71.1 Asphyxiation due to mechanical threat to breathing**
Suffocation due to mechanical threat to breathing

● **T71.11 Asphyxiation due to smothering under pillow**

● **T71.111 Asphyxiation due to smothering under pillow, accidental** A, A
Asphyxiation due to smothering under pillow NOS

● **T71.112 Asphyxiation due to smothering under pillow, intentional self-harm** A, A, A, S

● **T71.113 Asphyxiation due to smothering under pillow, assault** A, A

● **T71.114 Asphyxiation due to smothering under pillow, undetermined** A, A

● **T71.12 Asphyxiation due to plastic bag**

● **T71.121 Asphyxiation due to plastic bag, accidental** A, A
Asphyxiation due to plastic bag NOS

● **T71.122 Asphyxiation due to plastic bag, intentional self-harm** A, A, A, S

● **T71.123 Asphyxiation due to plastic bag, assault** A, A

● **T71.124 Asphyxiation due to plastic bag, undetermined** A, A

● **T71.13 Asphyxiation due to being trapped in bed linens**

● **T71.131 Asphyxiation due to being trapped in bed linens, accidental** A, A
Asphyxiation due to being trapped in bed linens NOS

● **T71.132 Asphyxiation due to being trapped in bed linens, intentional self-harm** A, A, A, S

● **T71.133 Asphyxiation due to being trapped in bed linens, assault** A, A

● **T71.134 Asphyxiation due to being trapped in bed linens, undetermined** A, A

● **T71.14 Asphyxiation due to smothering under another person's body (in bed)**

● **T71.141 Asphyxiation due to smothering under another person's body (in bed), accidental** A, A
Asphyxiation due to smothering under another person's body (in bed) NOS

● **T71.143 Asphyxiation due to smothering under another person's body (in bed), assault** A, A

● **T71.144 Asphyxiation due to smothering under another person's body (in bed), undetermined** A, A

● **T71.15 Asphyxiation due to smothering in furniture**

● **T71.151 Asphyxiation due to smothering in furniture, accidental** A, A
Asphyxiation due to smothering in furniture NOS

● **T71.152 Asphyxiation due to smothering in furniture, intentional self-harm** A, A, A, S

● **T71.153 Asphyxiation due to smothering in furniture, assault** A, A

● **T71.154 Asphyxiation due to smothering in furniture, undetermined** A, A

● **T71.16 Asphyxiation due to hanging**
Hanging by window shade cord
Use additional code for any associated injuries, such as:
crushing injury of neck (S17.-)
fracture of cervical vertebrae (S12.0-S12.2-)
open wound of neck (S11.-)

● **T71.161 Asphyxiation due to hanging, accidental** A, A
Asphyxiation due to hanging NOS
Hanging NOS

● **T71.162 Asphyxiation due to hanging, intentional self-harm** A, A, A, S

● **T71.163 Asphyxiation due to hanging, assault** A, A

● **T71.164 Asphyxiation due to hanging, undetermined** A, A

● **T71.19 Asphyxiation due to mechanical**
Threat to breathing due to other causes

● **T71.191 Asphyxiation due to mechanical threat to breathing due to other causes, accidental** A, A
Asphyxiation due to other causes NOS
Coding Clinic: 2016, Q4, P76

● **T71.192 Asphyxiation due to mechanical threat to breathing due to other causes, intentional self-harm** A, A, A, S

● **T71.193 Asphyxiation due to mechanical threat to breathing due to other causes, assault** A, A

● **T71.194 Asphyxiation due to mechanical threat to breathing due to other causes, undetermined** A, A

● **T71.2 Asphyxiation due to systemic oxygen deficiency due to low oxygen content in ambient air**
Suffocation due to systemic oxygen deficiency due to low oxygen content in ambient air

X● **T71.20 Asphyxiation due to systemic oxygen deficiency due to low oxygen content in ambient air due to unspecified cause** A, A

X● **T71.21 Asphyxiation due to cave-in or falling earth** A, A
Use additional code for any associated cataclysm (X34-X38)

● **T71.22 Asphyxiation due to being trapped in a car trunk**

● **T71.221 Asphyxiation due to being trapped in a car trunk, accidental** A

● **T71.222 Asphyxiation due to being trapped in a car trunk, intentional self-harm** A, A, S

● T71.223 Asphyxiation due to being trapped in a car trunk, assault A
● T71.224 Asphyxiation due to being trapped in a car trunk, undetermined A
● T71.23 Asphyxiation due to being trapped in a (discarded) refrigerator
● T71.231 Asphyxiation due to being trapped in a (discarded) refrigerator, accidental A
● T71.232 Asphyxiation due to being trapped in a (discarded) refrigerator, intentional self-harm A, A, S
● T71.233 Asphyxiation due to being trapped in a (discarded) refrigerator, assault A
● T71.234 Asphyxiation due to being trapped in a (discarded) refrigerator, undetermined A
X● T71.29 Asphyxiation due to being trapped in other low oxygen environment A, A
X● T71.9 Asphyxiation due to unspecified cause A, A
Suffocation (by strangulation) due to unspecified cause
Suffocation NOS
Systemic oxygen deficiency due to low oxygen content in ambient air due to unspecified cause
Systemic oxygen deficiency due to mechanical threat to breathing due to unspecified cause
Traumatic asphyxia NOS

● T73 Effects of other deprivation
The appropriate 7th character is to be added to each code from category T73
A initial encounter
D subsequent encounter
S sequela

X● T73.0 Starvation
Deprivation of food
X● T73.1 Deprivation of water
X● T73.2 Exhaustion due to exposure
X● T73.3 Exhaustion due to excessive exertion
Exhaustion due to overexertion
X● T73.8 Other effects of deprivation
X● T73.9 Effect of deprivation, unspecified

● T74 Adult and child abuse, neglect and other maltreatment, confirmed
Use additional code, if applicable, to identify any associated current injury
Use additional external cause code to identify perpetrator, if known (Y07.-)
Excludes1 abuse and maltreatment in pregnancy (O9A.3-, O9A.4-, O9A.5-)
adult and child maltreatment, suspected (T76.-)
The appropriate 7th character is to be added to each code from category T74
A initial encounter
D subsequent encounter
S sequela

● T74.0 Neglect or abandonment, confirmed (Ex) PDX 1939
X● T74.01 Adult neglect or abandonment, confirmed A — A
X● T74.02 Child neglect or abandonment, confirmed A — P
● T74.1 Physical abuse, confirmed (Ex) PDX 1939
Excludes2 sexual abuse (T74.2-)
X● T74.11 Adult physical abuse, confirmed A — A
X● T74.12 Child physical abuse, confirmed A — P
Excludes2 shaken infant syndrome (T74.4)
● T74.2 Sexual abuse, confirmed (Ex) PDX 1939
Rape, confirmed
Sexual assault, confirmed
X● T74.21 Adult sexual abuse, confirmed A — A
X● T74.22 Child sexual abuse, confirmed A — P
● T74.3 Psychological abuse, confirmed (Ex) PDX 1939
Bullying and intimidation, confirmed
Intimidation through social media, confirmed
Target of threatened harm, confirmed
Target of threatened physical violence, confirmed
Target of threatened sexual abuse, confirmed
X● T74.31 Adult psychological abuse, confirmed — A
X● T74.32 Child psychological abuse, confirmed A — P
X● T74.4 Shaken infant syndrome A (Ex) PDX 1939 — P
● T74.5 Forced sexual exploitation, confirmed (Ex) PDX 1940
X● T74.51 Adult forced sexual exploitation, confirmed — P
X● T74.52 Child sexual exploitation, confirmed — P
● T74.6 Forced labor exploitation, confirmed (Ex) PDX 1940
X● T74.61 Adult forced labor exploitation, confirmed — P
X● T74.62 Child forced labor exploitation, confirmed — P
● T74.9 Unspecified maltreatment, confirmed (Ex) PDX 1939
X● T74.91 Unspecified adult maltreatment, confirmed A — A
X● T74.92 Unspecified child maltreatment, confirmed A — P
● T74.A Financial abuse, confirmed
T74.A1 Adult financial abuse, confirmed
T74.A2 Child financial abuse, confirmed

● T75 Other and unspecified effects of other external causes
Excludes1 adverse effects NEC (T78.-)
Excludes2 burns (electric) (T20-T31)
The appropriate 7th character is to be added to each code from category T75
A initial encounter
D subsequent encounter
S sequela

● T75.0 Effects of lightning
Struck by lightning
X● T75.00 Unspecified effects of lightning
Struck by lightning NOS
X● T75.01 Shock due to being struck by lightning
X● T75.09 Other effects of lightning
Use additional code for other effects of lightning
X● T75.1 Unspecified effects of drowning and nonfatal submersion A, A (Ex) PDX 1941
Immersion
Excludes1 specified effects of drowning code to effects
Coding Clinic: 2023, Q1, P26
● T75.2 Effects of vibration
X● T75.20 Unspecified effects of vibration
X● T75.21 Pneumatic hammer syndrome
X● T75.22 Traumatic vasospastic syndrome
X● T75.23 Vertigo from infrasound
Excludes1 vertigo NOS (R42)
X● T75.29 Other effects of vibration
X● T75.3 Motion sickness
Airsickness
Seasickness
Travel sickness
Use additional external cause code to identify vehicle or type of motion (Y92.81-)
X● T75.4 Electrocution
Shock from electric current
Shock from electroshock gun (taser)

● T75.8 Other specified effects of external causes
- X● T75.81 Effects of abnormal gravitation [G] forces
- X● T75.82 Effects of weightlessness
- X● T75.89 Other specified effects of external causes

● T76 Adult and child abuse, neglect and other maltreatment, suspected (Ex) PDX 1423

Use additional code, if applicable, to identify any associated current injury

Excludes1 adult and child maltreatment, confirmed (T74.-)
suspected abuse and maltreatment in pregnancy (O9A.3-, O9A.4-, O9A.5-)
suspected adult physical abuse, ruled out (Z04.71)
suspected adult sexual abuse, ruled out (Z04.41)
suspected child physical abuse, ruled out (Z04.72)
suspected child sexual abuse, ruled out (Z04.42)

The appropriate 7th character is to be added to each code from category T76

A	initial encounter
D	subsequent encounter
S	sequela

Coding Clinic: 2016, Q4, P129

● T76.0 Neglect or abandonment, suspected (Ex) PDX 1939
- X● T76.01 Adult neglect or abandonment, suspected A — A
- X● T76.02 Child neglect or abandonment, suspected A — P

● T76.1 Physical abuse, suspected (Ex) PDX 1939
- X● T76.11 Adult physical abuse, suspected A — A
- X● T76.12 Child physical abuse, suspected A — P
  Coding Clinic: 2019, Q2, P12

● T76.2 Sexual abuse, suspected (Ex) PDX 1939
Rape, suspected
Excludes1 alleged abuse, ruled out (Z04.7)
- X● T76.21 Adult sexual abuse, suspected A — A
- X● T76.22 Child sexual abuse, suspected A — P

● T76.3 Psychological abuse, suspected (Ex) PDX 1939
Bullying and intimidation, suspected
Intimidation through social media, suspected
Target of threatened harm, suspected
Target of threatened physical violence, suspected
Target of threatened sexual abuse, suspected
- X● T76.31 Adult psychological abuse, suspected — A
- X● T76.32 Child psychological abuse, suspected A — P

● T76.5 Forced sexual exploitation, suspected (Ex) PDX 1940
- X● T76.51 Adult forced sexual exploitation, suspected — P
- X● T76.52 Child sexual exploitation, suspected — P

● T76.6 Forced labor exploitation, suspected (Ex) PDX 1940
- X● T76.61 Adult forced labor exploitation, suspected — P
- X● T76.62 Child forced labor exploitation, suspected — P

● T76.9 Unspecified maltreatment, suspected (Ex) PDX 1939
- X● T76.91 Unspecified adult maltreatment, suspected A — A
- X● T76.92 Unspecified child maltreatment, suspected A — P

● T76.A Financial abuse, suspected
- X● T76.A1 Adult financial abuse, suspected
- X● T76.A2 Child financial abuse, suspected

● T78 Adverse effects, not elsewhere classified

Excludes2 complications of surgical and medical care NEC (T80-T88)

The appropriate 7th character is to be added to each code from category T78

A	initial encounter
D	subsequent encounter
S	sequela

● T78.0 Anaphylactic reaction due to food (Ex) PDX 1942
Anaphylactic reaction due to adverse food reaction
Anaphylactic shock or reaction due to nonpoisonous foods
Anaphylactoid reaction due to food
- X● T78.00 Anaphylactic reaction due to unspecified food A
- X● T78.01 Anaphylactic reaction due to peanuts A
- X● T78.02 Anaphylactic reaction due to shellfish (crustaceans) A
- X● T78.03 Anaphylactic reaction due to other fish A
- X● T78.04 Anaphylactic reaction due to fruits and vegetables A
- X● T78.05 Anaphylactic reaction due to tree nuts and seeds A
  Excludes2 anaphylactic reaction due to peanuts (T78.01)
- X● T78.06 Anaphylactic reaction due to food additives A
- X● T78.07 Anaphylactic reaction due to milk and dairy products A
- X● T78.08 Anaphylactic reaction due to eggs A
- X● T78.09 Anaphylactic reaction due to other food products A

X● T78.1 Other adverse food reactions, not elsewhere classified
Use additional code to identify the type of reaction, if applicable

Excludes1 anaphylactic reaction or shock due to adverse food reaction (T78.0-)
anaphylactic reaction due to food (T78.0-)
bacterial food borne intoxications (A05.-)

Excludes2 allergic and dietetic gastroenteritis and colitis (K52.29)
allergic rhinitis due to food (J30.5)
dermatitis due to food in contact with skin (L23.6, L24.6, L25.4)
dermatitis due to ingested food (L27.2)
food protein-induced enterocolitis syndrome (K52.21)
food protein-induced enteropathy (K52.22)

X● T78.2 Anaphylactic shock, unspecified A (Ex) PDX 1943
Occurs when allergic response triggers large quantities of histamines, prostaglandins, leukotrienes resulting in systemic vasodilation
Allergic shock
Anaphylactic reaction
Anaphylaxis

Excludes1 anaphylactic reaction or shock due to adverse effect of correct medicinal substance properly administered (T88.6)
anaphylactic reaction or shock due to adverse food reaction (T78.0-)
anaphylactic reaction or shock due to serum (T80.5-)

X● T78.3 Angioneurotic edema
Allergic angioedema
Giant urticaria
Vascular disorder resulting from abnormalities of autonomic nervous system fibers supplying blood vessels
Quincke's edema

Excludes1 serum urticaria (T80.6-)
urticaria (L50.-)

● **T78.4 Other and unspecified allergy**
Excludes1 specified types of allergic reaction such as:
allergic diarrhea (K52.29)
allergic gastroenteritis and colitis (K52.29)
dermatitis (L23-L25, L27.-)
food protein-induced enterocolitis syndrome (K52.21)
food protein-induced enteropathy (K52.22)
hay fever (J30.1)

X● **T78.40 Allergy, unspecified**
Allergic reaction NOS
Hypersensitivity NOS

X● **T78.41 Arthus phenomenon**
Arthus reaction

X● **T78.49 Other allergy**
Coding Clinic: 2021, Q1, P42

X● **T78.8 Other adverse effects, not elsewhere classified**

CERTAIN EARLY COMPLICATIONS OF TRAUMA (T79)

● **T79 Certain early complications of trauma, not elsewhere classified**
Excludes2 acute respiratory distress syndrome (J80)
complications occurring during or following medical procedures (T80-T88)
complications of surgical and medical care NEC (T80-T88)
newborn respiratory distress syndrome (P22.0)

The appropriate 7th character is to be added to each code from category T79

A initial encounter
D subsequent encounter
S sequela

X● **T79.0 Air embolism (traumatic)** A, A (Ex) PDX 1944
Excludes1 air embolism complicating abortion or ectopic or molar pregnancy (O00-O07, O08.2)
air embolism complicating pregnancy, childbirth and the puerperium (O88.0)
air embolism following infusion, transfusion, and therapeutic injection (T80.0)
air embolism following procedure NEC (T81.7-)
Coding Clinic: 2024, Q2, P16

X● **T79.1 Fat embolism (traumatic)** A, A (Ex) PDX 1945
Excludes1 fat embolism complicating:
abortion or ectopic or molar pregnancy (O00-O07, O08.2)
pregnancy, childbirth and the puerperium (O88.8)

X● **T79.2 Traumatic secondary and recurrent hemorrhage and seroma** A, A (Ex) PDX 1946

X● **T79.4 Traumatic shock** A, A (Ex) PDX 1947
Shock (immediate) (delayed) following injury
Excludes1 anaphylactic shock due to adverse food reaction (T78.0-)
anaphylactic shock due to correct medicinal substance properly administered (T88.6)
anaphylactic shock due to serum (T80.5-)
anaphylactic shock NOS (T78.2)
electric shock (T75.4)
nontraumatic shock NEC (R57.-)
obstetric shock (O75.1)
postprocedural shock (T81.1-)
septic shock (R65.21)
shock complicating abortion or ectopic or molar pregnancy (O00-O07, O08.3)
shock due to anesthesia (T88.2)
shock due to lightning (T75.01)
shock NOS (R57.9)

X● **T79.5 Traumatic anuria** A, A (Ex) PDX 1948
Crush syndrome
Renal failure following crushing

X● **T79.6 Traumatic ischemia of muscle** A
Traumatic rhabdomyolysis
Volkmann's ischemic contracture
Excludes2 anterior tibial syndrome (M76.8)
compartment syndrome (traumatic) (T79.A-)
nontraumatic ischemia of muscle (M62.2-)

X● **T79.7 Traumatic subcutaneous emphysema** A, A (Ex) PDX 1949
Excludes2 emphysema NOS (J43)
emphysema (subcutaneous) resulting from a procedure (T81.82)

X● **T79.8 Other early complications of trauma** A
Coding Clinic: 2024, Q2, P16

X● **T79.9 Unspecified early complication of trauma** A

● **T79.A Traumatic compartment syndrome**
Excludes1 fibromyalgia (M79.7)
nontraumatic compartment syndrome (M79.A-)
Excludes2 traumatic ischemic infarction of muscle (T79.6)

X● **T79.A0 Compartment syndrome, unspecified** A (Ex) PDX 1950
Compartment syndrome NOS

● **T79.A1 Traumatic compartment syndrome of upper extremity**
Traumatic compartment syndrome of shoulder, arm, forearm, wrist, hand, and fingers

● **T79.A11 Traumatic compartment syndrome of right upper extremity** A, A (Ex) PDX 1951

● **T79.A12 Traumatic compartment syndrome of left upper extremity** A, A (Ex) PDX 1952

● **T79.A19 Traumatic compartment syndrome of unspecified upper extremity** A, A (Ex) PDX 1953

● **T79.A2 Traumatic compartment syndrome of lower extremity**
Traumatic compartment syndrome of hip, buttock, thigh, leg, foot, and toes

● **T79.A21 Traumatic compartment syndrome of right lower extremity** A, A (Ex) PDX 1954

● **T79.A22 Traumatic compartment syndrome of left lower extremity** A, A (Ex) PDX 1955

● **T79.A29 Traumatic compartment syndrome of unspecified lower extremity** A (Ex) PDX 1956

X● **T79.A3 Traumatic compartment syndrome of abdomen** A, A (Ex) PDX 1957

X● **T79.A9 Traumatic compartment syndrome of other sites** A, A (Ex) PDX 1958

CHAPTER 19 (S00-T88)

COMPLICATIONS OF SURGICAL AND MEDICAL CARE NOT ELSEWHERE CLASSIFIED (T80-T88)

Use additional code for adverse effect, if applicable, to identify drug (T36-T50 with fifth or sixth character 5)

Use additional code(s) to identify the specified condition resulting from the complication.

Use additional code to identify devices involved and details of circumstances (Y62-Y82)

Excludes2 any encounters with medical care for postprocedural conditions in which no complications are present, such as:
- artificial opening status (Z93.-)
- closure of external stoma (Z43.-)
- fitting and adjustment of external prosthetic device (Z44.-)

burns and corrosions from local applications and irradiation (T20-T32)
complications of surgical procedures during pregnancy, childbirth and the puerperium (O00-O9A)
mechanical complication of respirator [ventilator] (J95.850)
poisoning and toxic effects of drugs and chemicals (T36-T65 with fifth or sixth character 1-4 or 6)
postprocedural fever (R50.82)
specified complications classified elsewhere, such as:
- cerebrospinal fluid leak from spinal puncture (G97.0)
- colostomy malfunction (K94.0-)
- disorders of fluid and electrolyte imbalance (E86-E87)
- functional disturbances following cardiac surgery (I97.0-I97.1)
- intraoperative and postprocedural complications of specified body systems (D78.-, E36.-, E89.-, G97.3-, G97.4, H59.3-, H59.-, H95.2-, H95.3, I97.4-, I97.5, J95.6-, J95.7, K91.6-, L76.-, M96.-, N99.-)
- ostomy complications (J95.0-, K94.-, N99.5-)
- postgastric surgery syndromes (K91.1)
- postlaminectomy syndrome NEC (M96.1)
- postmastectomy lymphedema syndrome (I97.2)
- postsurgical blind-loop syndrome (K91.2)
- ventilator associated pneumonia (J95.851)

● T80 Complications following infusion, transfusion and therapeutic injection

Includes complications following perfusion

Excludes2 bone marrow transplant rejection (T86.01)
febrile nonhemolytic transfusion reaction (R50.84)
fluid overload due to transfusion (E87.71)
posttransfusion purpura (D69.51)
transfusion associated circulatory overload (TACO) (E87.71)
transfusion (red blood cell) associated hemochromatosis (E83.111)
transfusion related acute lung injury (TRALI) (J95.84)

The appropriate 7th character is to be added to each code from category T80

A	initial encounter
D	subsequent encounter
S	sequela

X● T80.0 Air embolism following infusion, transfusion and therapeutic injection A, A (Ex) PDX 1959

X● T80.1 Vascular complications following infusion, transfusion and therapeutic injection A (Ex) PDX 1960

Use additional code to identify the vascular complication

Excludes2 extravasation of vesicant agent (T80.81-)
infiltration of vesicant agent (T80.81-)
vascular complications specified as due to prosthetic devices, implants and grafts (T82.8- T83.8-, T84.8-, T85.8-)
postprocedural vascular complications (T81.7-)

● T80.2 Infections following infusion, transfusion and therapeutic injection

Use additional code to identify the specific infection, such as:
sepsis (A41.9)

Use additional code (R65.2-) to identify severe sepsis, if applicable

Excludes2 infections specified as due to prosthetic devices, implants and grafts (T82.6-T82.7, T83.5-T83.6, T84.5-T84.7, T85.7)
postprocedural infections (T81.44)

Coding Clinic: 2018, Q4, P89

● T80.21 Infection due to central venous catheter (Ex) PDX 1400

Infection due to pulmonary artery catheter (Swan-Ganz catheter)

Coding Clinic: 2019, Q1, P13-14; 2018, Q4, P89

● T80.211 Bloodstream infection due to central venous catheter A, A
- Catheter-related bloodstream infection (CRBSI) NOS
- Central line-associated bloodstream infection (CLABSI)
- Bloodstream infection due to Hickman catheter
- Bloodstream infection due to peripherally inserted central catheter (PICC)
- Bloodstream infection due to portacath (port-a-cath)
- Bloodstream infection due to pulmonary artery catheter
- Bloodstream infection due to triple lumen catheter
- Bloodstream infection due to umbilical venous catheter

Coding Clinic: 2018, Q4, P89

● T80.212 Local infection due to central venous catheter A, A
- Exit or insertion site infection
- Local infection due to Hickman catheter
- Local infection due to peripherally inserted central catheter (PICC)
- Local infection due to portacath (port-a-cath)
- Local infection due to pulmonary artery catheter
- Local infection due to triple lumen catheter
- Local infection due to umbilical venous catheter
- Port or reservoir infection
- Tunnel infection

● T80.218 Other infection due to central venous catheter A, A
- Other central line-associated infection
- Other infection due to Hickman catheter
- Other infection due to peripherally inserted central catheter (PICC)
- Other infection due to portacath (port-a-cath)
- Other infection due to pulmonary artery catheter
- Other infection due to triple lumen catheter
- Other infection due to umbilical venous catheter

● **T80.219 Unspecified infection due to central venous catheter** A, A
Central line-associated infection NOS
Unspecified infection due to Hickman catheter
Unspecified infection due to peripherally inserted central catheter (PICC)
Unspecified infection due to portacath (port-a-cath)
Unspecified infection due to pulmonary artery catheter
Unspecified infection due to triple lumen catheter
Unspecified infection due to umbilical venous catheter

X● **T80.22 Acute infection following transfusion, infusion, or injection of blood and blood products** A (Ex) PDX 1961

X● **T80.29 Infection following other infusion, transfusion and therapeutic injection** A (Ex) PDX 1961

● **T80.3 ABO incompatibility reaction due to transfusion of blood or blood products** (Ex) PDX 1962
Excludes1 minor blood group antigens reactions (Duffy) (E) (K) (Kell) (Kidd) (Lewis) (M) (N) (P) (S) (T80.A-)

X● **T80.30 ABO incompatibility reaction due to transfusion of blood or blood products, unspecified** A, A
ABO incompatibility blood transfusion NOS
Reaction to ABO incompatibility from transfusion NOS

● **T80.31 ABO incompatibility with hemolytic transfusion reaction**

● **T80.310 ABO incompatibility with acute hemolytic transfusion reaction** A, A
ABO incompatibility with hemolytic transfusion reaction less than 24 hours after transfusion
Acute hemolytic transfusion reaction (AHTR) due to ABO incompatibility

● **T80.311 ABO incompatibility with delayed hemolytic transfusion reaction** A, A
ABO incompatibility with hemolytic transfusion reaction 24 hours or more after transfusion
Delayed hemolytic transfusion reaction (DHTR) due to ABO incompatibility

● **T80.319 ABO incompatibility with hemolytic transfusion reaction, unspecified** A, A
ABO incompatibility with hemolytic transfusion reaction at unspecified time after transfusion
Hemolytic transfusion reaction (HTR) due to ABO incompatibility NOS

X● **T80.39 Other ABO incompatibility reaction due to transfusion of blood or blood products** A, A
Delayed serologic transfusion reaction (DSTR) from ABO incompatibility
Other ABO incompatible blood transfusion
Other reaction to ABO incompatible blood transfusion

● **T80.4 Rh incompatibility reaction due to transfusion of blood or blood products**
Reaction due to incompatibility of Rh antigens (C) (c) (D) (E) (e)

X● **T80.40 Rh incompatibility reaction due to transfusion of blood or blood products, unspecified** A (Ex) PDX 1962
Reaction due to Rh factor in transfusion NOS
Rh incompatible blood transfusion NOS

● **T80.41 Rh incompatibility with hemolytic transfusion reaction** (Ex) PDX 1962

● **T80.410 Rh incompatibility with acute hemolytic transfusion reaction** A
Acute hemolytic transfusion reaction (AHTR) due to Rh incompatibility
Rh incompatibility with hemolytic transfusion reaction less than 24 hours after transfusion

● **T80.411 Rh incompatibility with delayed hemolytic transfusion reaction** A
Delayed hemolytic transfusion reaction (DHTR) due to Rh incompatibility
Rh incompatibility with hemolytic transfusion reaction 24 hours or more after transfusion

● **T80.419 Rh incompatibility with hemolytic transfusion reaction, unspecified** A
Rh incompatibility with hemolytic transfusion reaction at unspecified time after transfusion
Hemolytic transfusion reaction (HTR) due to Rh incompatibility NOS

X● **T80.49 Other Rh incompatibility reaction due to transfusion of blood or blood products** A (Ex) PDX 1963
Delayed serologic transfusion reaction (DSTR) from Rh incompatibility
Other reaction to Rh incompatible blood transfusion

● **T80.5 Anaphylactic reaction due to serum** (Ex) PDX 1964
Allergic reaction due to serum
Anaphylactic shock due to serum
Anaphylactoid reaction due to serum
Anaphylaxis due to serum
Excludes1 ABO incompatibility reaction due to transfusion of blood or blood products (T80.3-)
allergic reaction or shock NOS (T78.2)
anaphylactic reaction or shock NOS (T78.2)
anaphylactic reaction or shock due to adverse effect of correct medicinal substance properly administered (T88.6)
other serum reaction (T80.6-)

X● **T80.51 Anaphylactic reaction due to administration of blood and blood products** A

X● **T80.52 Anaphylactic reaction due to vaccination** A
Coding Clinic: 2021, Q1, P43

X● **T80.59 Anaphylactic reaction due to other serum** A

● **T80.6 Other serum reactions**
Intoxication by serum
Protein sickness
Serum rash
Serum sickness
Serum urticaria
Excludes2 serum hepatitis (B16-B19)

X● **T80.61 Other serum reaction due to administration of blood and blood products** A (Ex) PDX 1964

X● **T80.62 Other serum reaction due to vaccination** A (Ex) PDX 1964
Coding Clinic: 2021, Q1, P42

X● **T80.69 Other serum reaction due to other serum** A (Ex) PDX 1965
Code also, if applicable, arthropathy in hypersensitivity reactions classified elsewhere (M36.4)

● T80.8 **Other complications following infusion, transfusion and therapeutic injection**

● T80.81 **Extravasation of vesicant agent** Ex: PDX 1966
Infiltration of vesicant agent

● T80.810 **Extravasation of vesicant antineoplastic chemotherapy** A
Infiltration of vesicant antineoplastic chemotherapy

● T80.818 **Extravasation of other vesicant agent** A
Infiltration of other vesicant agent

T80.82 **Complication of immune effector cellular therapy**
Complication of chimeric antigen receptor (CAR-T) cell therapy
Complication of IEC therapy

▶ **Excludes2** adverse effect of immune checkpoint inhibitors and immunostimulant drugs (T45.AX5)
complication of bone marrow transplant (T86.0)
complication of stem cell transplant (T86.5)

Use additional code to identify the specific complication, such as:
cytokine release syndrome (D89.83-)
immune effector cell-associated neurotoxicity syndrome (G92.0-)

X● T80.89 **Other complications following infusion, transfusion and therapeutic injection**
Delayed serologic transfusion reaction (DSTR), unspecified incompatibility
Use additional code to identify graft-versus-host reaction, if applicable, (D89.81-)

● T80.9 **Unspecified complication following infusion, transfusion and therapeutic injection**

X● T80.90 **Unspecified complication following infusion and therapeutic injection**

● T80.91 **Hemolytic transfusion reaction, unspecified incompatibility** Ex: PDX 1962

Excludes1 ABO incompatibility with hemolytic transfusion reaction (T80.31-)
Non-ABO incompatibility with hemolytic transfusion reaction (T80.A1-)
Rh incompatibility with hemolytic transfusion reaction (T80.41-)

● T80.910 **Acute hemolytic transfusion reaction, unspecified incompatibility** A

● T80.911 **Delayed hemolytic transfusion reaction, unspecified incompatibility** A

● T80.919 **Hemolytic transfusion reaction, unspecified incompatibility, unspecified as acute or delayed** A
Hemolytic transfusion reaction NOS

X● T80.92 **Unspecified transfusion reaction**
Transfusion reaction NOS

● T80.A **Non-ABO incompatibility reaction due to transfusion of blood or blood products**
Reaction due to incompatibility of minor antigens (Duffy) (Kell) (Kidd) (Lewis) (M) (N) (P) (S)

X● T80.A0 **Non-ABO incompatibility reaction due to transfusion of blood or blood products, unspecified** A Ex: PDX 1967
Non-ABO antigen incompatibility reaction from transfusion NOS

● T80.A1 **Non-ABO incompatibility with hemolytic transfusion reaction**

● T80.A10 **Non-ABO incompatibility with acute hemolytic transfusion reaction** A Ex: PDX 1968
Acute hemolytic transfusion reaction (AHTR) due to non-ABO incompatibility
Non-ABO incompatibility with hemolytic transfusion reaction less than 24 hours after transfusion

● T80.A11 **Non-ABO incompatibility with delayed hemolytic transfusion reaction** A Ex: PDX 1969
Delayed hemolytic transfusion reaction (DHTR) due to non-ABO incompatibility
Non-ABO incompatibility with hemolytic transfusion reaction 24 or more hours after transfusion

● T80.A19 **Non-ABO incompatibility with hemolytic transfusion reaction, unspecified** A Ex: PDX 1970
Hemolytic transfusion reaction (HTR) due to non-ABO incompatibility NOS
Non-ABO incompatibility with hemolytic transfusion reaction at unspecified time after transfusion

X● T80.A9 **Other non-ABO incompatibility reaction due to transfusion of blood or blood products** A Ex: PDX 1962
Delayed serologic transfusion reaction (DSTR) from non-ABO incompatibility
Other reaction to non-ABO incompatible blood transfusion

● T81 **Complications of procedures, not elsewhere classified**
Use additional code for adverse effect, if applicable, to identify drug (T36-T50 with fifth or sixth character 5)

Excludes2 complications following immunization (T88.0-T88.1)
complications following infusion, transfusion and therapeutic injection (T80.-)
complications of transplanted organs and tissue (T86.-)
poisoning and toxic effects of drugs and chemicals (T36-T65 with fifth or sixth character 1-4)
specified complications classified elsewhere, such as:
complication of prosthetic devices, implants and grafts (T82-T85)
dermatitis due to drugs and medicaments (L23.3, L24.4, L25.1, L27.0-L27.1)
endosseous dental implant failure (M27.6-)
floppy iris syndrome (IFIS) (intraoperative) H21.81
intraoperative and postprocedural complications of specific body system (D78.-, E36.-, E89.-, G97.3-, G97.4, H59.3-, H59.-, H95.2-, H95.3, I97.4-, I97.5, J95, K91.-, L76.-, M96.-, N99.-)
ostomy complications (J95.0-, K94.-, N99.5-)
plateau iris syndrome (post-iridectomy) (postprocedural) H21.82

Coding Clinic: 2019, Q2, P21-22; 2016, Q4, P29

The appropriate 7th character is to be added to each code from category T81

A	initial encounter
D	subsequent encounter
S	sequela

CHAPTER 19 (S00-T88)

● T81.1 **Postprocedural shock** (Ex) PDX 1971
Shock during or resulting from a procedure, not elsewhere classified

Excludes1 anaphylactic shock NOS (T78.2)
anaphylactic shock due to correct substance properly administered (T88.6)
anaphylactic shock due to serum (T80.5-)
electric shock (T75.4)
obstetric shock (O75.1)
septic shock (R65.21)
shock due to anesthesia (T88.2)
shock following abortion or ectopic or molar pregnancy (O00-O07, O08.3)
traumatic shock (T79.4)

X● T81.10 **Postprocedural shock unspecified** A
Collapse NOS during or resulting from a procedure, not elsewhere classified
Postprocedural failure of peripheral circulation
Postprocedural shock NOS

X● T81.11 **Postprocedural cardiogenic shock** A, A

●X● T81.12 **Postprocedural septic shock** A, A
Postprocedural endotoxic shock resulting from a procedure, not elsewhere classified
Postprocedural gram-negative shock resulting from a procedure, not elsewhere classified
Code first underlying infection
Use additional code, to identify any associated acute organ dysfunction, if applicable

X● T81.19 **Other postprocedural shock** A
Postprocedural hypovolemic shock
Coding Clinic: 2021, Q1, P14

● T81.3 **Disruption of wound, not elsewhere classified** (Ex) PDX 1972
Disruption of any suture materials or other closure methods

Excludes1 breakdown (mechanical) of permanent sutures (T85.612)
displacement of permanent sutures (T85.622)
disruption of cesarean delivery wound (O90.0)
disruption of perineal obstetric wound (O90.1)
mechanical complication of permanent sutures NEC (T85.692)

X● T81.30 **Disruption of wound, unspecified** A
Disruption of wound NOS

X● T81.31 **Disruption of external operation (surgical) wound, not elsewhere classified** A

Excludes1 dehiscence of amputation stump (T87.81)

Dehiscence of operation wound NOS
Disruption of operation wound NOS
Disruption or dehiscence of closure of cornea
Disruption or dehiscence of closure of mucosa
Disruption or dehiscence of closure of skin and subcutaneous tissue
Full-thickness skin disruption or dehiscence
Superficial disruption or dehiscence of operation wound
Coding Clinic: 2015, Q1, P20

X● T81.32 **Disruption of internal operation (surgical) wound, not elsewhere classified** A
~~Deep disruption or dehiscence of operation wound NOS~~
~~Disruption or dehiscence of closure of internal organ or other internal tissue~~
~~Disruption or dehiscence of closure of muscle or muscle flap~~
~~Disruption or dehiscence of closure of ribs or rib cage~~
~~Disruption or dehiscence of closure of skull or craniotomy~~
~~Disruption or dehiscence of closure of sternum or sternotomy~~
~~Disruption or dehiscence of closure of tendon or ligament~~
~~Disruption or dehiscence of closure of superficial or muscular fascia~~
Coding Clinic: 2017, Q3, P4

▶● T81.320 **Disruption or dehiscence of gastrointestinal tract anastomosis, repair, or closure** A

▶● T81.321 **Disruption or dehiscence of closure of internal operation (surgical) wound ofabdominal wall muscle or fascia** A

▶● T81.328 **Disruption or dehiscence of closure of other specified internal operation(surgical) wound** A
▶Disruption or dehiscence of closure of muscle or muscle flap (other than abdominal wall muscle)
▶Disruption or dehiscence of closure of ribs or rib cage
▶Disruption or dehiscence of closure of skull or craniotomy
▶Disruption or dehiscence of closure of sternum or sternotomy
▶Disruption or dehiscence of closure of tendon or ligament
▶Disruption or dehiscence of closure of superficial or muscular fascia (other than abdominal wall fascia)

▶● T81.329 **Deep disruption or dehiscence of operation wound, unspecified** A
▶Deep disruption or dehiscence of operation wound NOS

X● T81.33 **Disruption of traumatic injury wound repair** A
Disruption or dehiscence of closure of traumatic laceration (external) (internal)

● T81.4 **Infection following a procedure** A (Ex) PDX 1113
▶ Code also, if applicable, disruption of internal operation (surgical) wound (T81.32-)
Use additional code to identify infection
Use additional code (R65.2-) to identify severe sepsis, if applicable

Excludes2 bleb associated endophthalmitis (H59.4-)
infection due to infusion, transfusion and therapeutic injection (T80.2-)
infection due to prosthetic devices, implants and grafts (T82.6-T82.7, T83.5-T83.6, T84.5-T84.7, T85.7)
obstetric surgical wound infection (O86.0-)
postprocedural fever NOS (R50.82)
postprocedural retroperitoneal abscess (K68.11)

X● T81.40 **Infection following a procedure, unspecified** A, A
Coding Clinic: 2024, Q1, P19

X● T81.41 **Infection following a procedure, superficial incisional surgical site** A, A
Subcutaneous abscess following a procedure
Stitch abscess following a procedure
Coding Clinic: 2024, Q1, P19; 2018, Q4, P34

X● T81.42 **Infection following a procedure, deep incisional surgical site** A, A
Intra-muscular abscess following a procedure
Coding Clinic: 2024, Q1, P19

X● T81.43 **Infection following a procedure, organ and space surgical site** A, A
Intra-abdominal abscess following a procedure
Subphrenic abscess following a procedure
Coding Clinic: 2024, Q1, P19,20

X● T81.44 **Sepsis following a procedure** A, A, A
Use additional code to identify the sepsis
Coding Clinic: 2024, Q1, P19

X● T81.49 **Infection following a procedure, other surgical site** A, A
Coding Clinic: 2024, Q1, P19; 2015, Q4, P37

CHAPTER 19 (S00-T88)

● **T81.5 Complications of foreign body accidentally left in body following procedure**

● **T81.50 Unspecified complication of foreign body accidentally left in body following procedure**

● **T81.500 Unspecified complication of foreign body accidentally left in body following surgical operation** A, A (Ex) PDX 1973

● **T81.501 Unspecified complication of foreign body accidentally left in body following infusion or transfusion** A, A (Ex) PDX 1974

● **T81.502 Unspecified complication of foreign body accidentally left in body following kidney dialysis** A, A, A, D, S (Ex) PDX 1973

● **T81.503 Unspecified complication of foreign body accidentally left in body following injection or immunization** A, A (Ex) PDX 1973

● **T81.504 Unspecified complication of foreign body accidentally left in body following endoscopic examination** A, A (Ex) PDX 1973

● **T81.505 Unspecified complication of foreign body accidentally left in body following heart catheterization** A, A (Ex) PDX 1973

● **T81.506 Unspecified complication of foreign body accidentally left in body following aspiration, puncture or other catheterization** A, A (Ex) PDX 1973

● **T81.507 Unspecified complication of foreign body accidentally left in body following removal of catheter or packing** A, A (Ex) PDX 1973

● **T81.508 Unspecified complication of foreign body accidentally left in body following other procedure** A, A (Ex) PDX 1973

● **T81.509 Unspecified complication of foreign body accidentally left in body following unspecified procedure** A, A (Ex) PDX 1973

● **T81.51 Adhesions due to foreign body accidentally left in body following procedure**

● **T81.510 Adhesions due to foreign body accidentally left in body following surgical operation** A, A (Ex) PDX 1973

● **T81.511 Adhesions due to foreign body accidentally left in body following infusion or transfusion** A, A (Ex) PDX 1974

● **T81.512 Adhesions due to foreign body accidentally left in body following kidney dialysis** A, A, A, D, S (Ex) PDX 1973

● **T81.513 Adhesions due to foreign body accidentally left in body following injection or immunization** A, A (Ex) PDX 1973

● **T81.514 Adhesions due to foreign body accidentally left in body following endoscopic examination** A, A (Ex) PDX 1973

● **T81.515 Adhesions due to foreign body accidentally left in body following heart catheterization** A, A (Ex) PDX 1973

● **T81.516 Adhesions due to foreign body accidentally left in body following aspiration, puncture or other catheterization** A, A (Ex) PDX 1973

● **T81.517 Adhesions due to foreign body accidentally left in body following removal of catheter or packing** A, A (Ex) PDX 1973

● **T81.518 Adhesions due to foreign body accidentally left in body following other procedure** A, A (Ex) PDX 1973

● **T81.519 Adhesions due to foreign body accidentally left in body following unspecified procedure** A, A (Ex) PDX 1973

● **T81.52 Obstruction due to foreign body accidentally left in body following procedure**

● **T81.520 Obstruction due to foreign body accidentally left in body following surgical operation** A, A (Ex) PDX 1973

● **T81.521 Obstruction due to foreign body accidentally left in body following infusion or transfusion** A, A (Ex) PDX 1974

● **T81.522 Obstruction due to foreign body accidentally left in body following kidney dialysis** A, A, A, D, S (Ex) PDX 1973

● **T81.523 Obstruction due to foreign body accidentally left in body following injection or immunization** A, A (Ex) PDX 1973

● **T81.524 Obstruction due to foreign body accidentally left in body following endoscopic examination** A, A (Ex) PDX 1973

● **T81.525 Obstruction due to foreign body accidentally left in body following heart catheterization** A, A (Ex) PDX 1973

● **T81.526 Obstruction due to foreign body accidentally left in body following aspiration, puncture or other catheterization** A, A (Ex) PDX 1973

● **T81.527 Obstruction due to foreign body accidentally left in body following removal of catheter or packing** A, A (Ex) PDX 1973

● **T81.528 Obstruction due to foreign body accidentally left in body following other procedure** A, A (Ex) PDX 1973

● **T81.529 Obstruction due to foreign body accidentally left in body following unspecified procedure** A, A (Ex) PDX 1973

● **T81.53 Perforation due to foreign body accidentally left in body following procedure**

● **T81.530 Perforation due to foreign body accidentally left in body following surgical operation** A, A (Ex) PDX 1973

● **T81.531 Perforation due to foreign body accidentally left in body following infusion or transfusion** A, A (Ex) PDX 1974

● **T81.532 Perforation due to foreign body accidentally left in body following kidney dialysis** A, A, A, D, S (Ex) PDX 1973

● **T81.533 Perforation due to foreign body accidentally left in body following injection or immunization** A, A (Ex) PDX 1973

● **T81.534 Perforation due to foreign body accidentally left in body following endoscopic examination** A, A (Ex) PDX 1973

T81.535 Perforation due to foreign body accidentally left in body following heart catheterization A, A (Ex) PDX 1973

T81.536 Perforation due to foreign body accidentally left in body following aspiration, puncture or other catheterization A, A (Ex) PDX 1973

T81.537 Perforation due to foreign body accidentally left in body following removal of catheter or packing A, A (Ex) PDX 1973

T81.538 Perforation due to foreign body accidentally left in body following other procedure A, A (Ex) PDX 1973

T81.539 Perforation due to foreign body accidentally left in body following unspecified procedure A, A (Ex) PDX 1973

T81.59 Other complications of foreign body accidentally left in body following procedure

Excludes2 obstruction or perforation due to prosthetic devices and implants intentionally left in body (T82.Ø-T82.5, T83.Ø-T83.4, T83.7, T84.Ø-T84.4, T85.Ø-T85.6)

T81.59Ø Other complications of foreign body accidentally left in body following surgical operation A, A (Ex) PDX 1973

T81.591 Other complications of foreign body accidentally left in body following infusion or transfusion A, A (Ex) PDX 1974

T81.592 Other complications of foreign body accidentally left in body following kidney dialysis A, A, A, D, S (Ex) PDX 1973

T81.593 Other complications of foreign body accidentally left in body following injection or immunization A, A (Ex) PDX 1973

T81.594 Other complications of foreign body accidentally left in body following endoscopic examination A, A (Ex) PDX 1973

T81.595 Other complications of foreign body accidentally left in body following heart catheterization A, A (Ex) PDX 1973

T81.596 Other complications of foreign body accidentally left in body following aspiration, puncture or other catheterization A, A (Ex) PDX 1973

T81.597 Other complications of foreign body accidentally left in body following removal of catheter or packing A, A (Ex) PDX 1973

T81.598 Other complications of foreign body accidentally left in body following other procedure A, A (Ex) PDX 1973

T81.599 Other complications of foreign body accidentally left in body following unspecified procedure A, A (Ex) PDX 1973

T81.6 Acute reaction to foreign substance accidentally left during a procedure (Ex) PDX 1975

Excludes2 complications of foreign body accidentally left in body cavity or operation wound following procedure (T81.5-)

X **T81.6Ø Unspecified acute reaction to foreign substance accidentally left during a procedure** A, A

X **T81.61 Aseptic peritonitis due to foreign substance accidentally left during a procedure** A, A
Chemical peritonitis

X **T81.69 Other acute reaction to foreign substance accidentally left during a procedure** A, A

T81.7 Vascular complications following a procedure, not elsewhere classified
Air embolism following procedure NEC
Phlebitis or thrombophlebitis resulting from a procedure

Excludes1 embolism complicating abortion or ectopic or molar pregnancy (OØØ-OØ7, OØ8.2)
embolism complicating pregnancy, childbirth and the puerperium (O88.-)
traumatic embolism (T79.Ø)

Excludes2 embolism due to prosthetic devices, implants and grafts (T82.8, T83.81, T84.8-, T85.1-)
embolism following infusion, transfusion and therapeutic injection (T8Ø.Ø)

Coding Clinic: 2Ø19, Q2, P23

T81.71 Complication of artery following a procedure, not elsewhere classified
Coding Clinic: 2Ø19, Q2, P22

T81.71Ø Complication of mesenteric artery following a procedure, not elsewhere classified A (Ex) PDX 1976

T81.711 Complication of renal artery following a procedure, not elsewhere classified A (Ex) PDX 1976

T81.718 Complication of other artery following a procedure, not elsewhere classified A (Ex) PDX 1977
Coding Clinic: 2Ø19, Q2, P22-23

T81.719 Complication of unspecified artery following a procedure, not elsewhere classified A (Ex) PDX 1977

X **T81.72 Complication of vein following a procedure, not elsewhere classified** A (Ex) PDX 1977
Coding Clinic: 2Ø19, Q2, P22

T81.8 Other complications of procedures, not elsewhere classified

Excludes2 hypothermia following anesthesia (T88.51)
malignant hyperpyrexia due to anesthesia (T88.3)

X **T81.81 Complication of inhalation therapy**

X **T81.82 Emphysema (subcutaneous) resulting from a procedure**

X **T81.83 Persistent postprocedural fistula** A (Ex) PDX 1978
▶ Code also, if applicable, disruption of internal operation (surgical) wound (T81.32-)
Use additional code, if known, for site of fistula such as:
anal fistula (K6Ø.3-)
anorectal fistula (K6Ø.5-)
bladder fistula (N32.2)
other female intestinal-genital tract fistulae (N82.4)
Coding Clinic: 2Ø23, Q1, P3Ø; 2Ø17, Q3, P3-5

X **T81.89 Other complications of procedures, not elsewhere classified**
Use additional code to specify complication, such as:
postprocedural delirium (FØ5)

X **T81.9 Unspecified complication of procedure**

T82 Complications of cardiac and vascular prosthetic devices, implants and grafts

Excludes2 failure and rejection of transplanted organs and tissue (T86.-)

The appropriate 7th character is to be added to each code from category T82

A	initial encounter
D	subsequent encounter
S	sequela

T82.0 Mechanical complication of heart valve prosthesis PDX 1979
Mechanical complication of artificial heart valve
Excludes1 mechanical complication of biological heart valve graft (T82.22-)

X **T82.01 Breakdown (mechanical) of heart valve prosthesis** A

X **T82.02 Displacement of heart valve prosthesis** A
Malposition of heart valve prosthesis

X **T82.03 Leakage of heart valve prosthesis** A

X **T82.09 Other mechanical complication of heart valve prosthesis** A
Obstruction (mechanical) of heart valve prosthesis
Perforation of heart valve prosthesis
Protrusion of heart valve prosthesis

T82.1 Mechanical complication of cardiac electronic device

T82.11 Breakdown (mechanical) of cardiac electronic device

T82.110 Breakdown (mechanical) of cardiac electrode A PDX 1980

T82.111 Breakdown (mechanical) of cardiac pulse generator (battery) A PDX 1980

T82.118 Breakdown (mechanical) of other cardiac electronic device A PDX 1981

T82.119 Breakdown (mechanical) of unspecified cardiac electronic device A PDX 1982

T82.12 Displacement of cardiac electronic device
Malposition of cardiac electronic device

T82.120 Displacement of cardiac electrode A PDX 1980

T82.121 Displacement of cardiac pulse generator (battery) A PDX 1980

T82.128 Displacement of other cardiac electronic device A PDX 1981

T82.129 Displacement of unspecified cardiac electronic device A PDX 1983

T82.19 Other mechanical complication of cardiac electronic device
Leakage of cardiac electronic device
Obstruction of cardiac electronic device
Perforation of cardiac electronic device
Protrusion of cardiac electronic device

T82.190 Other mechanical complication of cardiac electrode A PDX 1980

T82.191 Other mechanical complication of cardiac pulse generator (battery) A PDX 1980

T82.198 Other mechanical complication of other cardiac electronic device A PDX 1981

T82.199 Other mechanical complication of unspecified cardiac device A PDX 1984

T82.2 Mechanical complication of coronary artery bypass graft and biological heart valve graft
Excludes1 mechanical complication of artificial heart valve prosthesis (T82.0-)

T82.21 Mechanical complication of coronary artery bypass graft PDX 1985

T82.211 Breakdown (mechanical) of coronary artery bypass graft A

T82.212 Displacement of coronary artery bypass graft A
Malposition of coronary artery bypass graft

T82.213 Leakage of coronary artery bypass graft A

T82.218 Other mechanical complication of coronary artery bypass graft A
Obstruction, mechanical of coronary artery bypass graft
Perforation of coronary artery bypass graft
Protrusion of coronary artery bypass graft

T82.22 Mechanical complication of biological heart valve graft PDX 1981

T82.221 Breakdown (mechanical) of biological heart valve graft A

T82.222 Displacement of biological heart valve graft A
Malposition of biological heart valve graft

T82.223 Leakage of biological heart valve graft A

T82.228 Other mechanical complication of biological heart valve graft A
Obstruction of biological heart valve graft
Perforation of biological heart valve graft
Protrusion of biological heart valve graft

T82.3 Mechanical complication of other vascular grafts PDX 1986

T82.31 Breakdown (mechanical) of other vascular grafts

T82.310 Breakdown (mechanical) of aortic (bifurcation) graft (replacement) A, A

T82.311 Breakdown (mechanical) of carotid arterial graft (bypass) A, A

T82.312 Breakdown (mechanical) of femoral arterial graft (bypass) A, A

T82.318 Breakdown (mechanical) of other vascular grafts A, A

T82.319 Breakdown (mechanical) of unspecified vascular grafts A, A

T82.32 Displacement of other vascular grafts
Malposition of other vascular grafts

T82.320 Displacement of aortic (bifurcation) graft (replacement) A, A

T82.321 Displacement of carotid arterial graft (bypass) A, A

T82.322 Displacement of femoral arterial graft (bypass) A, A

T82.328 Displacement of other vascular grafts A, A

T82.329 Displacement of unspecified vascular grafts A, A

T82.33 Leakage of other vascular grafts

T82.330 Leakage of aortic (bifurcation) graft (replacement) A, A

T82.331 Leakage of carotid arterial graft (bypass) A, A

CHAPTER 19 (S00-T88)

● T82.332 Leakage of femoral arterial graft (bypass) A, A

● T82.338 Leakage of other vascular grafts A, A

● T82.339 Leakage of unspecified vascular graft A, A

● T82.39 Other mechanical complication of other vascular grafts
Obstruction (mechanical) of other vascular grafts
Perforation of other vascular grafts
Protrusion of other vascular grafts

● T82.390 Other mechanical complication of aortic (bifurcation) graft (replacement) A, A

● T82.391 Other mechanical complication of carotid arterial graft (bypass) A, A

● T82.392 Other mechanical complication of femoral arterial graft (bypass) A, A

● T82.398 Other mechanical complication of other vascular grafts A, A

● T82.399 Other mechanical complication of unspecified vascular grafts A, A

● T82.4 Mechanical complication of vascular dialysis catheter (Ex) PDX 1986
Mechanical complication of hemodialysis catheter
Excludes1 mechanical complication of intraperitoneal dialysis catheter (T85.62)

X● T82.41 Breakdown (mechanical) of vascular dialysis catheter A, A, D, S

X● T82.42 Displacement of vascular dialysis catheter A, A, D, S
Malposition of vascular dialysis catheter

X● T82.43 Leakage of vascular dialysis catheter A, A, D, S

X● T82.49 Other complication of vascular dialysis catheter A, A, D, S
Obstruction (mechanical) of vascular dialysis catheter
Perforation of vascular dialysis catheter
Protrusion of vascular dialysis catheter

● T82.5 Mechanical complication of other cardiac and vascular devices and implants
Excludes2 mechanical complication of epidural and subdural infusion catheter (T85.61)

● T82.51 Breakdown (mechanical) of other cardiac and vascular devices and implants

● T82.510 Breakdown (mechanical) of surgically created arteriovenous fistula A, A (Ex) PDX 1986

● T82.511 Breakdown (mechanical) of surgically created arteriovenous shunt A, A (Ex) PDX 1986

● T82.512 Breakdown (mechanical) of artificial heart A (Ex) PDX 1981

● T82.513 Breakdown (mechanical) of balloon (counterpulsation) device A, A (Ex) PDX 1986

● T82.514 Breakdown (mechanical) of infusion catheter A, A (Ex) PDX 1986

● T82.515 Breakdown (mechanical) of umbrella device A, A (Ex) PDX 1986

● T82.518 Breakdown (mechanical) of other cardiac and vascular devices and implants A, A (Ex) PDX 1986

● T82.519 Breakdown (mechanical) of unspecified cardiac and vascular devices and implants A (Ex) PDX 1987

● T82.52 Displacement of other cardiac and vascular devices and implants
Malposition of other cardiac and vascular devices and implants

● T82.520 Displacement of surgically created arteriovenous fistula A, A (Ex) PDX 1986

● T82.521 Displacement of surgically created arteriovenous shunt A, A (Ex) PDX 1986

● T82.522 Displacement of artificial heart A (Ex) PDX 1981

● T82.523 Displacement of balloon (counterpulsation) device A, A (Ex) PDX 1986

● T82.524 Displacement of infusion catheter A, A (Ex) PDX 1986
Coding Clinic: 2019, Q3, P15

● T82.525 Displacement of umbrella device A, A (Ex) PDX 1986

● T82.528 Displacement of other cardiac and vascular devices and implants A, A (Ex) PDX 1986

● T82.529 Displacement of unspecified cardiac and vascular devices and implants A (Ex) PDX 1986

● T82.53 Leakage of other cardiac and vascular devices and implants

● T82.530 Leakage of surgically created arteriovenous fistula A, A (Ex) PDX 1986

● T82.531 Leakage of surgically created arteriovenous shunt A, A (Ex) PDX 1986

● T82.532 Leakage of artificial heart A (Ex) PDX 1981

● T82.533 Leakage of balloon (counterpulsation) device A, A (Ex) PDX 1986

● T82.534 Leakage of infusion catheter A, A (Ex) PDX 1986

● T82.535 Leakage of umbrella device A, A (Ex) PDX 1986

● T82.538 Leakage of other cardiac and vascular devices and implants A, A (Ex) PDX 1986

● T82.539 Leakage of unspecified cardiac and vascular devices and implants A (Ex) PDX 1987

● T82.59 Other mechanical complication of other cardiac and vascular devices and implants
Obstruction (mechanical) of other cardiac and vascular devices and implants
Perforation of other cardiac and vascular devices and implants
Protrusion of other cardiac and vascular devices and implants

● T82.590 Other mechanical complication of surgically created arteriovenous fistula A, A (Ex) PDX 1986

● T82.591 Other mechanical complication of surgically created arteriovenous shunt A, A (Ex) PDX 1986

● T82.592 Other mechanical complication of artificial heart A (Ex) PDX 1981

● T82.593 Other mechanical complication of balloon (counterpulsation) device A, A (Ex) PDX 1986

● T82.594 Other mechanical complication of infusion catheter A, A (Ex) PDX 1981

● T82.595 Other mechanical complication of umbrella device A, A (Ex) PDX 1986

CHAPTER 19 (S00-T88)

T82.598 Other mechanical complication of other cardiac and vascular devices and implants A, A PDX 1981

T82.599 Other mechanical complication of unspecified cardiac and vascular devices and implants A PDX 1987

X T82.6 Infection and inflammatory reaction due to cardiac valve prosthesis A, A, A PDX 1988

Use additional code to identify infection

X T82.7 Infection and inflammatory reaction due to other cardiac and vascular devices, implants and grafts A, A, A PDX 1988

Use additional code to identify infection

Coding Clinic: 2019, Q1, P13-14; 2018, Q4, P89

T82.8 Other specified complications of cardiac and vascular prosthetic devices, implants and grafts

T82.81 Embolism due to cardiac and vascular prosthetic devices, implants and grafts

Coding Clinic: 2016, Q4, P70

T82.817 Embolism due to cardiac prosthetic devices, implants and grafts A PDX 1989

Coding Clinic: 2016, Q4, P70; 2015, Q1, P20

T82.818 Embolism due to vascular prosthetic devices, implants and grafts A, A PDX 1988

T82.82 Fibrosis due to cardiac and vascular prosthetic devices, implants and grafts

Coding Clinic: 2016, Q4, P70

T82.827 Fibrosis due to cardiac prosthetic devices, implants and grafts A PDX 1989

T82.828 Fibrosis due to vascular prosthetic devices, implants and grafts A, A PDX 1988

T82.83 Hemorrhage due to cardiac and vascular prosthetic devices, implants and grafts

Coding Clinic: 2016, Q4, P70

T82.837 Hemorrhage due to cardiac prosthetic devices, implants and grafts A PDX 1989

T82.838 Hemorrhage due to vascular prosthetic devices, implants and grafts A, A PDX 1988

T82.84 Pain due to cardiac and vascular prosthetic devices, implants and grafts

Coding Clinic: 2016, Q4, P70

T82.847 Pain due to cardiac prosthetic devices, implants and grafts A PDX 1989

T82.848 Pain due to vascular prosthetic devices, implants and grafts A, A PDX 1988

T82.85 Stenosis due to cardiac and vascular prosthetic devices, implants and grafts

T82.855 Stenosis of coronary artery stent A PDX 1989

In-stent stenosis (restenosis) of coronary artery stent

Restenosis of coronary artery stent

Coding Clinic: 2021, Q3, P6-7; 2016, Q4, P70

T82.856 Stenosis of peripheral vascular stent A, A PDX 1988

In-stent stenosis (restenosis) of peripheral vascular stent

Restenosis of peripheral vascular stent

Coding Clinic: 2016, Q4, P70

T82.857 Stenosis of other cardiac prosthetic devices, implants and grafts A PDX 1989

Coding Clinic: 2016, Q4, P70

T82.858 Stenosis of other vascular prosthetic devices, implants and grafts A, A PDX 1988

Coding Clinic: 2016, Q4, P70

T82.86 Thrombosis of cardiac and vascular prosthetic devices, implants and grafts

T82.867 Thrombosis due to cardiac prosthetic devices, implants and grafts A PDX 1989

T82.868 Thrombosis due to vascular prosthetic devices, implants and grafts A, A PDX 1988

Coding Clinic: 2023, Q2, P7

T82.89 Other specified complication of cardiac and vascular prosthetic devices, implants and grafts

T82.897 Other specified complication of cardiac prosthetic devices, implants and grafts A PDX 1989

Coding Clinic: 2019, Q2, P32-33

T82.898 Other specified complication of vascular prosthetic devices, implants and grafts A, A PDX 1988

X T82.9 Unspecified complication of cardiac and vascular prosthetic device, implant and graft A PDX 1989

T83 Complications of genitourinary prosthetic devices, implants and grafts

Excludes2 failure and rejection of transplanted organs and tissue (T86.-)

The appropriate 7th character is to be added to each code from category T83

A	initial encounter
D	subsequent encounter
S	sequela

Coding Clinic: 2016, Q4, P70-71

T83.0 Mechanical complication of urinary catheter PDX 1990

Excludes2 complications of stoma of urinary tract (N99.5-)

Coding Clinic: 2016, Q4, P70

T83.01 Breakdown (mechanical) of urinary catheter

T83.010 Breakdown (mechanical) of cystostomy catheter A, A

T83.011 Breakdown (mechanical) of indwelling urethral catheter A

T83.012 Breakdown (mechanical) of nephrostomy catheter A

T83.018 Breakdown (mechanical) of other urinary catheter A

Breakdown (mechanical) of Hopkins catheter

Breakdown (mechanical) of ileostomy catheter

Breakdown (mechanical) urostomy catheter

T83.02 Displacement of urinary catheter

Malposition of urinary catheter

T83.020 Displacement of cystostomy catheter A, A

T83.021 Displacement of indwelling urethral catheter A

T83.022 Displacement of nephrostomy catheter A

T83.028 Displacement of other urinary catheter A

Displacement of Hopkins catheter

Displacement of ileostomy catheter

Displacement of urostomy catheter

T83.03 Leakage of urinary catheter

T83.030 Leakage of cystostomy catheter A, A

Coding Clinic: 2021, Q4, P19

T83.031 Leakage of indwelling urethral catheter A

T83.032 Leakage of nephrostomy catheter A

● **T83.038 Leakage of other urinary catheter** A
Leakage of Hopkins catheter
Leakage of ileostomy catheter
Leakage of urostomy catheter

● **T83.09 Other mechanical complication of urinary catheter**
Obstruction (mechanical) of urinary catheter
Perforation of urinary catheter
Protrusion of urinary catheter

● **T83.090 Other mechanical complication of cystostomy catheter** A, A

● **T83.091 Other mechanical complication of indwelling urethral catheter** A

● **T83.092 Other mechanical complication of nephrostomy catheter** A

● **T83.098 Other mechanical complication of other urinary catheter** A
Other mechanical complication of Hopkins catheter
Other mechanical complication of ileostomy catheter
Other mechanical complication of urostomy catheter

● **T83.1 Mechanical complication of other urinary devices and implants** Ex PDX 1990
Coding Clinic: 2016, Q4, P70

● **T83.11 Breakdown (mechanical) of other urinary devices and implants**

● **T83.110 Breakdown (mechanical) of urinary electronic stimulator device** A, A
Excludes2 Breakdown (mechanical) of electrode (lead) for sacral nerve neurostimulator (T85.111)
Breakdown (mechanical) of implanted electronic sacral neurostimulator, pulse generator or receiver (T85.113)

● **T83.111 Breakdown (mechanical) of implanted urinary sphincter** A, A

● **T83.112 Breakdown (mechanical) of indwelling ureteral stent** A, A

● **T83.113 Breakdown (mechanical) of other urinary stents** A, A
Breakdown (mechanical) of ileal conduit stent
Breakdown (mechanical) of nephroureteral stent

● **T83.118 Breakdown (mechanical) of other urinary devices and implants** A, A

● **T83.12 Displacement of other urinary devices and implants**
Malposition of other urinary devices and implants

● **T83.120 Displacement of urinary electronic stimulator device** A, A
Excludes2 Displacement of electrode (lead) for sacral nerve neurostimulator (T85.121)
Displacement of implanted electronic sacral neurostimulator, pulse generator or receiver (T85.123)

● **T83.121 Displacement of implanted urinary sphincter** A, A

● **T83.122 Displacement of indwelling ureteral stent** A, A

● **T83.123 Displacement of other urinary stents** A, A
Displacement of ileal conduit stent
Displacement of nephroureteral stent

● **T83.128 Displacement of other urinary devices and implants** A, A

● **T83.19 Other mechanical complication of other urinary devices and implants**
Leakage of other urinary devices and implants
Obstruction (mechanical) of other urinary devices and implants
Perforation of other urinary devices and implants
Protrusion of other urinary devices and implants

● **T83.190 Other mechanical complication of urinary electronic stimulator device** A, A
Excludes2 Other mechanical complication of electrode (lead) for sacral nerve neurostimulator (T85.191)
Other mechanical complication of implanted electronic sacral neurostimulator, pulse generator or receiver (T85.193)

● **T83.191 Other mechanical complication of implanted urinary sphincter** A, A

● **T83.192 Other mechanical complication of indwelling ureteral stent** A, A

● **T83.193 Other mechanical complication of other urinary stent** A, A
Other mechanical complication of ileal conduit stent
Other mechanical complication of nephroureteral stent

● **T83.198 Other mechanical complication of other urinary devices and implants** A, A

● **T83.2 Mechanical complication of graft of urinary organ** Ex PDX 1990
Coding Clinic: 2016, Q4, P70

X● **T83.21 Breakdown (mechanical) of graft of urinary organ** A, A

X● **T83.22 Displacement of graft of urinary organ** A, A
Malposition of graft of urinary organ

X● **T83.23 Leakage of graft of urinary organ** A, A

X● **T83.24 Erosion of graft of urinary organ** A, A
Coding Clinic: 2016, Q4, P70

X● **T83.25 Exposure of graft of urinary organ** A, A
Coding Clinic: 2016, Q4, P70

X● **T83.29 Other mechanical complication of graft of urinary organ** A, A
Obstruction (mechanical) of graft of urinary organ
Perforation of graft of urinary organ
Protrusion of graft of urinary organ

CHAPTER 19 (S00-T88)

● T83.3 Mechanical complication of intrauterine contraceptive device (Ex) PDX 1990

X● T83.31 Breakdown (mechanical) of intrauterine contraceptive device

X● T83.32 Displacement of intrauterine contraceptive device
Malposition of intrauterine contraceptive device
Missing string of intrauterine contraceptive device

X● T83.39 Other mechanical complication of intrauterine contraceptive device
Leakage of intrauterine contraceptive device
Obstruction (mechanical) of intrauterine contraceptive device
Perforation of intrauterine contraceptive device
Protrusion of intrauterine contraceptive device

● T83.4 Mechanical complication of other prosthetic devices, implants and grafts of genital tract (Ex) PDX 1990
Coding Clinic: 2016, Q4, P71

● T83.41 Breakdown (mechanical) of other prosthetic devices, implants and grafts of genital tract

● T83.410 Breakdown (mechanical) of implanted penile prosthesis
A, A
Breakdown (mechanical) of penile prosthesis cylinder
Breakdown (mechanical) of penile prosthesis pump
Breakdown (mechanical) of penile prosthesis reservoir

● T83.411 Breakdown (mechanical) of implanted testicular prosthesis
A, A

● T83.418 Breakdown (mechanical) of other prosthetic devices, implants and grafts of genital tract A, A

● T83.42 Displacement of other prosthetic devices, implants and grafts of genital tract
Malposition of other prosthetic devices, implants and grafts of genital tract

● T83.420 Displacement of implanted penile prosthesis A, A
Displacement of penile prosthesis cylinder
Displacement of penile prosthesis pump
Displacement of penile prosthesis reservoir

● T83.421 Displacement of implanted testicular prosthesis A, A

● T83.428 Displacement of other prosthetic devices, implants and grafts of genital tract A, A
Coding Clinic: 2018, Q1, P6

● T83.49 Other mechanical complication of other prosthetic devices, implants and grafts of genital tract
Leakage of other prosthetic devices, implants and grafts of genital tract
Obstruction, mechanical of other prosthetic devices, implants and grafts of genital tract
Perforation of other prosthetic devices, implants and grafts of genital tract
Protrusion of other prosthetic devices, implants and grafts of genital tract

● T83.490 Other mechanical complication of implanted penile prosthesis
A, A
Other mechanical complication of penile prosthesis cylinder
Other mechanical complication of penile prosthesis pump
Other mechanical complication of penile prosthesis reservoir

● T83.491 Other mechanical complication of implanted testicular prosthesis
A, A

● T83.498 Other mechanical complication of other prosthetic devices, implants and grafts of genital tract A, A

● T83.5 Infection and inflammatory reaction due to prosthetic device, implant and graft in urinary system
Use additional code to identify infection
Coding Clinic: 2016, Q4, P71

● T83.51 Infection and inflammatory reaction due to urinary catheter
Excludes2 complications of stoma of urinary tract (N99.5-)

● T83.510 Infection and inflammatory reaction due to cystostomy catheter
A, A (Ex) PDX 1991

● T83.511 Infection and inflammatory reaction due to indwelling urethral catheter A, A (Ex) PDX 1992
Coding Clinic: 2022, Q2, P7

● T83.512 Infection and inflammatory reaction due to nephrostomy catheter A, A (Ex) PDX 1991

● T83.518 Infection and inflammatory reaction due to other urinary catheter A, A (Ex) PDX 1991
Infection and inflammatory reaction due to Hopkins catheter
Infection and inflammatory reaction due to ileostomy catheter
Infection and inflammatory reaction due to urostomy catheter

● T83.59 Infection and inflammatory reaction due to prosthetic device, implant and graft in urinary system (Ex) PDX 1991

● T83.590 Infection and inflammatory reaction due to implanted urinary neurostimulation device A, A
Excludes2 Infection and inflammatory reaction due to electrode lead of sacral nerve neurostimulator (T85.732)
Infection and inflammatory reaction due to pulse generator or receiver of sacral nerve neurostimulator (T85.734)

● T83.591 Infection and inflammatory reaction due to implanted urinary sphincter
A, A

● T83.592 Infection and inflammatory reaction due to indwelling ureteral stent
A, A

● T83.593 Infection and inflammatory reaction due to other urinary stents A, A
Infection and inflammatory reaction due to ileal conduit stents
Infection and inflammatory reaction due to nephroureteral stent

T83.598 Infection and inflammatory reaction due to other prosthetic device, implant and graft in urinary system A, A

T83.6 Infection and inflammatory reaction due to prosthetic device, implant and graft in genital tract (Ex:) PDX 1991
Use additional code to identify infection
Coding Clinic: 2016, Q4, P71

T83.61 Infection and inflammatory reaction due to implanted penile prosthesis A, A
Infection and inflammatory reaction due to penile prosthesis cylinder
Infection and inflammatory reaction due to penile prosthesis pump
Infection and inflammatory reaction due to penile prosthesis reservoir

T83.62 Infection and inflammatory reaction due to implanted testicular prosthesis A, A

T83.69 Infection and inflammatory reaction due to other prosthetic device, implant and graft in genital tract A, A

T83.7 Complications due to implanted mesh and other prosthetic materials
Coding Clinic: 2016, Q4, P71

T83.71 Erosion of implanted mesh and other prosthetic materials to surrounding organ or tissue (Ex:) PDX 1990
Coding Clinic: 2016, Q4, P71

T83.711 Erosion of implanted vaginal mesh to surrounding organ or tissue A
Erosion of implanted vaginal mesh into pelvic floor muscles
Coding Clinic: 2016, Q4, P71

T83.712 Erosion of implanted urethral mesh to surrounding organ or tissue A, A
Erosion of implanted female urethral sling
Erosion of implanted male urethral sling
Erosion of implanted urethral mesh into pelvic floor muscles

T83.713 Erosion of implanted urethral bulking agent to surrounding organ or tissue A, A

T83.714 Erosion of implanted ureteral bulking agent to surrounding organ or tissue A, A

T83.718 Erosion of other implanted mesh to organ or tissue A, A
Coding Clinic: 2016, Q4, P71

T83.719 Erosion of other prosthetic materials to surrounding organ or tissue A, A
Coding Clinic: 2016, Q4, P71

T83.72 Exposure of implanted mesh and other prosthetic materials into surrounding organ or tissue (Ex:) PDX 1990
Extrusion of implanted mesh
Coding Clinic: 2016, Q4, P71

T83.721 Exposure of implanted vaginal mesh into vagina A
Exposure of implanted vaginal mesh through vaginal wall

T83.722 Exposure of implanted urethral mesh into urethra A, A
Exposure of implanted female urethral sling
Exposure of implanted male urethral sling
Exposure of implanted urethral mesh through urethral wall

T83.723 Exposure of implanted urethral bulking agent into urethra A, A

T83.724 Exposure of implanted ureteral bulking agent into ureter A, A

T83.728 Exposure of other implanted mesh into organ or tissue A, A
Coding Clinic: 2016, Q4, P71

T83.729 Exposure of other prosthetic materials into organ or tissue A, A
Coding Clinic: 2016, Q4, P71

X T83.79 Other specified complications due to other genitourinary prosthetic materials A, A (Ex:) PDX 1991

T83.8 Other specified complications of genitourinary prosthetic devices, implants and grafts (Ex:) PDX 1991

X T83.81 Embolism due to genitourinary prosthetic devices, implants and grafts A, A

X T83.82 Fibrosis due to genitourinary prosthetic devices, implants and grafts A, A

X T83.83 Hemorrhage due to genitourinary prosthetic devices, implants and grafts A, A

X T83.84 Pain due to genitourinary prosthetic devices, implants and grafts A, A

X T83.85 Stenosis due to genitourinary prosthetic devices, implants and grafts A, A

X T83.86 Thrombosis due to genitourinary prosthetic devices, implants and grafts A, A

X T83.89 Other specified complication of genitourinary prosthetic devices, implants and grafts A, A
Coding Clinic: 2022, Q3, P13

X T83.9 Unspecified complication of genitourinary prosthetic device, implant and graft A, A (Ex:) PDX 1991

T84 Complications of internal orthopedic prosthetic devices, implants and grafts
Excludes2 failure and rejection of transplanted organs and tissues (T86.-)
fracture of bone following insertion of orthopedic implant, joint prosthesis or bone plate (M96.6)

The appropriate 7th character is to be added to each code from category T84

A	initial encounter
D	subsequent encounter
S	sequela

T84.0 Mechanical complication of internal joint prosthesis (Ex:) PDX 1350

T84.01 Broken internal joint prosthesis
Breakage (fracture) of prosthetic joint
Broken prosthetic joint implant
Excludes1 periprosthetic joint implant fracture (M97.-)
Coding Clinic: 2016, Q4, P42

T84.010 Broken internal right hip prosthesis A, A

T84.011 Broken internal left hip prosthesis A, A

T84.012 Broken internal right knee prosthesis A, A

T84.013 Broken internal left knee prosthesis A, A

T84.018 Broken internal joint prosthesis, other site A, A
Use additional code to identify the joint (Z96.6-)

T84.019 Broken internal joint prosthesis, unspecified site A, A

T84.02 Dislocation of internal joint prosthesis
Instability of internal joint prosthesis
Subluxation of internal joint prosthesis

T84.020 Dislocation of internal right hip prosthesis A, A

T84.021 Dislocation of internal left hip prosthesis A, A
Coding Clinic: 2019, Q2, P27

T84.022 Instability of internal right knee prosthesis A, A

T84.023 Instability of internal left knee prosthesis A, A

T84.028 Dislocation of other internal joint prosthesis A, A

Use additional code to identify the joint (Z96.6-)

T84.029 Dislocation of unspecified internal joint prosthesis A, A

T84.03 Mechanical loosening of internal prosthetic joint

Aseptic loosening of prosthetic joint

T84.030 Mechanical loosening of internal right hip prosthetic joint A, A

T84.031 Mechanical loosening of internal left hip prosthetic joint A, A

T84.032 Mechanical loosening of internal right knee prosthetic joint A, A

T84.033 Mechanical loosening of internal left knee prosthetic joint A, A

T84.038 Mechanical loosening of other internal prosthetic joint A, A

Use additional code to identify the joint (Z96.6-)

T84.039 Mechanical loosening of unspecified internal prosthetic joint A, A

T84.05 Periprosthetic osteolysis of internal prosthetic joint

Use additional code to identify major osseous defect, if applicable (M89.7-)

T84.050 Periprosthetic osteolysis of internal prosthetic right hip joint A, A

T84.051 Periprosthetic osteolysis of internal prosthetic left hip joint A, A

T84.052 Periprosthetic osteolysis of internal prosthetic right knee joint A, A

T84.053 Periprosthetic osteolysis of internal prosthetic left knee joint A, A

T84.058 Periprosthetic osteolysis of other internal prosthetic joint A, A

Use additional code to identify the joint (Z96.6-)

T84.059 Periprosthetic osteolysis of unspecified internal prosthetic joint A, A

T84.06 Wear of articular bearing surface of internal prosthetic joint

T84.060 Wear of articular bearing surface of internal prosthetic right hip joint A, A

T84.061 Wear of articular bearing surface of internal prosthetic left hip joint A, A

T84.062 Wear of articular bearing surface of internal prosthetic right knee joint A, A

T84.063 Wear of articular bearing surface of internal prosthetic left knee joint A, A

T84.068 Wear of articular bearing surface of other internal prosthetic joint A, A

Use additional code to identify the joint (Z96.6-)

T84.069 Wear of articular bearing surface of unspecified internal prosthetic joint A, A

T84.09 Other mechanical complication of internal joint prosthesis

Prosthetic joint implant failure NOS

T84.090 Other mechanical complication of internal right hip prosthesis A, A

Coding Clinic: 2019, Q1, P20

T84.091 Other mechanical complication of internal left hip prosthesis A, A

T84.092 Other mechanical complication of internal right knee prosthesis A, A

T84.093 Other mechanical complication of internal left knee prosthesis A, A

T84.098 Other mechanical complication of other internal joint prosthesis A, A

Use additional code to identify the joint (Z96.6-)

T84.099 Other mechanical complication of unspecified internal joint prosthesis A, A

T84.1 Mechanical complication of internal fixation device of bones of limb (Ex) PDX 1350

Excludes2 mechanical complication of internal fixation device of bones of feet (T84.2-)
mechanical complication of internal fixation device of bones of fingers (T84.2-)
mechanical complication of internal fixation device of bones of hands (T84.2-)
mechanical complication of internal fixation device of bones of toes (T84.2-)

T84.11 Breakdown (mechanical) of internal fixation device of bones of limb

T84.110 Breakdown (mechanical) of internal fixation device of right humerus A, A

T84.111 Breakdown (mechanical) of internal fixation device of left humerus A, A

T84.112 Breakdown (mechanical) of internal fixation device of bone of right forearm A, A

T84.113 Breakdown (mechanical) of internal fixation device of bone of left forearm A, A

T84.114 Breakdown (mechanical) of internal fixation device of right femur A, A

T84.115 Breakdown (mechanical) of internal fixation device of left femur A, A

T84.116 Breakdown (mechanical) of internal fixation device of bone of right lower leg A, A

T84.117 Breakdown (mechanical) of internal fixation device of bone of left lower leg A, A

T84.119 Breakdown (mechanical) of internal fixation device of unspecified bone of limb A, A

T84.12 Displacement of internal fixation device of bones of limb

Malposition of internal fixation device of bones of limb

T84.120 Displacement of internal fixation device of right humerus A, A

T84.121 Displacement of internal fixation device of left humerus A, A

T84.122 Displacement of internal fixation device of bone of right forearm A, A

T84.123 Displacement of internal fixation device of bone of left forearm A, A

T84.124 Displacement of internal fixation device of right femur A, A

CHAPTER 19 (S00-T88)

- T84.125 **Displacement of internal fixation device of left femur** A, A
- T84.126 **Displacement of internal fixation device of bone of right lower leg** A, A
- T84.127 **Displacement of internal fixation device of bone of left lower leg** A, A
- T84.129 **Displacement of internal fixation device of unspecified bone of limb** A, A

T84.19 **Other mechanical complication of internal fixation device of bones of limb**
Obstruction (mechanical) of internal fixation device of bones of limb
Perforation of internal fixation device of bones of limb
Protrusion of internal fixation device of bones of limb

- T84.190 **Other mechanical complication of internal fixation device of right humerus** A, A
- T84.191 **Other mechanical complication of internal fixation device of left humerus** A, A
- T84.192 **Other mechanical complication of internal fixation device of bone of right forearm** A, A
- T84.193 **Other mechanical complication of internal fixation device of bone of left forearm** A, A
- T84.194 **Other mechanical complication of internal fixation device of right femur** A, A
- T84.195 **Other mechanical complication of internal fixation device of left femur** A, A
- T84.196 **Other mechanical complication of internal fixation device of bone of right lower leg** A, A
- T84.197 **Other mechanical complication of internal fixation device of bone of left lower leg** A, A
- T84.199 **Other mechanical complication of internal fixation device of unspecified bone of limb** A, A

T84.2 **Mechanical complication of internal fixation device of other bones** (Ex) PDX 1350

T84.21 **Breakdown (mechanical) of internal fixation device of other bones**

- T84.210 **Breakdown (mechanical) of internal fixation device of bones of hand and fingers** A, A
- T84.213 **Breakdown (mechanical) of internal fixation device of bones of foot and toes** A, A
- T84.216 **Breakdown (mechanical) of internal fixation device of vertebrae** A, A
- T84.218 **Breakdown (mechanical) of internal fixation device of other bones** A, A

T84.22 **Displacement of internal fixation device of other bones**
Malposition of internal fixation device of other bones

- T84.220 **Displacement of internal fixation device of bones of hand and fingers** A, A
- T84.223 **Displacement of internal fixation device of bones of foot and toes** A, A
- T84.226 **Displacement of internal fixation device of vertebrae** A, A
- T84.228 **Displacement of internal fixation device of other bones** A, A

T84.29 **Other mechanical complication of internal fixation device of other bones**
Obstruction (mechanical) of internal fixation device of other bones
Perforation of internal fixation device of other bones
Protrusion of internal fixation device of other bones

- T84.290 **Other mechanical complication of internal fixation device of bones of hand and fingers** A, A
- T84.293 **Other mechanical complication of internal fixation device of bones of foot and toes** A, A
- T84.296 **Other mechanical complication of internal fixation device of vertebrae** A, A
  Coding Clinic: 2024, Q2, P12
- T84.298 **Other mechanical complication of internal fixation device of other bones** A, A

T84.3 **Mechanical complication of other bone devices, implants and grafts** (Ex) PDX 1350
Excludes2 other complications of bone graft (T86.83-)

T84.31 **Breakdown (mechanical) of other bone devices, implants and grafts**

- T84.310 **Breakdown (mechanical) of electronic bone stimulator** A, A
- T84.318 **Breakdown (mechanical) of other bone devices, implants and grafts** A, A

T84.32 **Displacement of other bone devices, implants and grafts**
Malposition of other bone devices, implants and grafts

- T84.320 **Displacement of electronic bone stimulator** A, A
- T84.328 **Displacement of other bone devices, implants and grafts** A, A

T84.39 **Other mechanical complication of other bone devices, implants and grafts**
Obstruction (mechanical) of other bone devices, implants and grafts
Perforation of other bone devices, implants and grafts
Protrusion of other bone devices, implants and grafts

- T84.390 **Other mechanical complication of electronic bone stimulator** A, A
- T84.398 **Other mechanical complication of other bone devices, implants and grafts** A, A

T84.4 **Mechanical complication of other internal orthopedic devices, implants and grafts** (Ex) PDX 1350

T84.41 **Breakdown (mechanical) of other internal orthopedic devices, implants and grafts**

- T84.410 **Breakdown (mechanical) of muscle and tendon graft** A, A
- T84.418 **Breakdown (mechanical) of other internal orthopedic devices, implants and grafts** A, A

T84.42 **Displacement of other internal orthopedic devices, implants and grafts**
Malposition of other internal orthopedic devices, implants and grafts

- T84.420 **Displacement of muscle and tendon graft** A, A
- T84.428 **Displacement of other internal orthopedic devices, implants and grafts** A, A

T84.49 Other mechanical complication of other internal orthopedic devices, implants and grafts
Mechanical complication of other internal orthopedic devices, implants and grafts NOS
Obstruction (mechanical) of other internal orthopedic devices, implants and grafts
Perforation of other internal orthopedic devices, implants and grafts
Protrusion of other internal orthopedic devices, implants and grafts

T84.490 Other mechanical complication of muscle and tendon graft A, A

T84.498 Other mechanical complication of other internal orthopedic devices, implants and grafts A, A

T84.5 Infection and inflammatory reaction due to internal joint prosthesis (Ex) PDX 1993
Use additional code to identify infection
Coding Clinic: 2015, Q1, P16

X T84.50 Infection and inflammatory reaction due to unspecified internal joint prosthesis A, A
Coding Clinic: 2015, Q1, P3

X T84.51 Infection and inflammatory reaction due to internal right hip prosthesis A, A
Coding Clinic: 2015, Q4, P36

X T84.52 Infection and inflammatory reaction due to internal left hip prosthesis A, A
Coding Clinic: 2015, Q1, P16-17

X T84.53 Infection and inflammatory reaction due to internal right knee prosthesis A, A

X T84.54 Infection and inflammatory reaction due to internal left knee prosthesis A, A
Coding Clinic: 2019, Q3, P16

X T84.59 Infection and inflammatory reaction due to other internal joint prosthesis A, A

T84.6 Infection and inflammatory reaction due to internal fixation device (Ex) PDX 1993
Use additional code to identify infection

X T84.60 Infection and inflammatory reaction due to internal fixation device of unspecified site A, A, A

T84.61 Infection and inflammatory reaction due to internal fixation device of arm

T84.610 Infection and inflammatory reaction due to internal fixation device of right humerus A, A, A

T84.611 Infection and inflammatory reaction due to internal fixation device of left humerus A, A, A

T84.612 Infection and inflammatory reaction due to internal fixation device of right radius A, A, A

T84.613 Infection and inflammatory reaction due to internal fixation device of left radius A, A, A

T84.614 Infection and inflammatory reaction due to internal fixation device of right ulna A, A, A

T84.615 Infection and inflammatory reaction due to internal fixation device of left ulna A, A, A

T84.619 Infection and inflammatory reaction due to internal fixation device of unspecified bone of arm A, A, A

T84.62 Infection and inflammatory reaction due to internal fixation device of leg

T84.620 Infection and inflammatory reaction due to internal fixation device of right femur A, A

T84.621 Infection and inflammatory reaction due to internal fixation device of left femur A, A

T84.622 Infection and inflammatory reaction due to internal fixation device of right tibia A, A

T84.623 Infection and inflammatory reaction due to internal fixation device of left tibia A, A

T84.624 Infection and inflammatory reaction due to internal fixation device of right fibula A, A

T84.625 Infection and inflammatory reaction due to internal fixation device of left fibula A, A

T84.629 Infection and inflammatory reaction due to internal fixation device of unspecified bone of leg A, A

X T84.63 Infection and inflammatory reaction due to internal fixation device of spine A, A, A

X T84.69 Infection and inflammatory reaction due to internal fixation device of other site A, A, A

T84.7 Infection and inflammatory reaction due to other internal orthopedic prosthetic devices, implants and grafts A, A, A (Ex) PDX 1993
Use additional code to identify infection

T84.8 Other specified complications of internal orthopedic prosthetic devices, implants and grafts (Ex) PDX 1993

X T84.81 Embolism due to internal orthopedic prosthetic devices, implants and grafts A, A

X T84.82 Fibrosis due to internal orthopedic prosthetic devices, implants and grafts A, A

X T84.83 Hemorrhage due to internal orthopedic prosthetic devices, implants and grafts A, A

X T84.84 Pain due to internal orthopedic prosthetic devices, implants and grafts A, A
Coding Clinic: 2024, Q2, P13

X T84.85 Stenosis due to internal orthopedic prosthetic devices, implants and grafts A, A

X T84.86 Thrombosis due to internal orthopedic prosthetic devices, implants and grafts A, A

X T84.89 Other specified complication of internal orthopedic prosthetic devices, implants and grafts A, A

X T84.9 Unspecified complication of internal orthopedic prosthetic device, implant and graft A, A (Ex) PDX 1993

T85 Complications of other internal prosthetic devices, implants and grafts
Excludes2 failure and rejection of transplanted organs and tissue (T86.-)
The appropriate 7th character is to be added to each code from category T85

A	initial encounter
D	subsequent encounter
S	sequela

Coding Clinic: 2016, Q4, P71

T85.0 Mechanical complication of ventricular intracranial (communicating) shunt (Ex) PDX 1994

X T85.01 Breakdown (mechanical) of ventricular intracranial (communicating) shunt A, A

X T85.02 Displacement of ventricular intracranial (communicating) shunt A, A
Malposition of ventricular intracranial (communicating) shunt

X T85.03 Leakage of ventricular intracranial (communicating) shunt A, A

CHAPTER 19 (S00-T88)

X● T85.09 **Other mechanical complication of ventricular intracranial (communicating) shunt** A, A
Obstruction (mechanical) of ventricular intracranial (communicating) shunt
Perforation of ventricular intracranial (communicating) shunt
Protrusion of ventricular intracranial (communicating) shunt

● T85.1 **Mechanical complication of implanted electronic stimulator of nervous system** (Ex) PDX 1994
Coding Clinic: 2016, Q4, P71

● T85.11 **Breakdown (mechanical) of implanted electronic stimulator of nervous system**

● T85.110 **Breakdown (mechanical) of implanted electronic neurostimulator of brain electrode (lead)** A, A

● T85.111 **Breakdown (mechanical) of implanted electronic neurostimulator of peripheral nerve electrode (lead)** A, A
Breakdown of electrode (lead) for cranial nerve neurostimulators
Breakdown of electrode (lead) for gastric neurostimulator
Breakdown of electrode (lead) for sacral nerve neurostimulator
Breakdown of electrode (lead) for vagal nerve neurostimulators

● T85.112 **Breakdown (mechanical) of implanted electronic neurostimulator of spinal cord electrode (lead)** A, A

● T85.113 **Breakdown (mechanical) of implanted electronic neurostimulator, generator** A, A
Breakdown (mechanical) of implanted electronic neurostimulator generator, brain, peripheral, gastric, spinal
Breakdown (mechanical) of implanted electronic sacral neurostimulator, pulse generator or receiver

● T85.118 **Breakdown (mechanical) of other implanted electronic stimulator of nervous system** A, A

● T85.12 **Displacement of implanted electronic stimulator of nervous system**
Malposition of implanted electronic stimulator of nervous system

● T85.120 **Displacement of implanted electronic neurostimulator of brain electrode (lead)** A, A

● T85.121 **Displacement of implanted electronic neurostimulator of peripheral nerve electrode (lead)** A, A
Displacement of electrode (lead) for cranial nerve neurostimulators
Displacement of electrode (lead) for gastric neurostimulator
Displacement of electrode (lead) for sacral nerve neurostimulator
Displacement of electrode (lead) for vagal nerve neurostimulators

● T85.122 **Displacement of implanted electronic neurostimulator of spinal cord electrode (lead)** A, A

● T85.123 **Displacement of implanted electronic neurostimulator, generator** A, A
Displacement of implanted electronic neurostimulator generator, brain, peripheral, gastric, spinal
Displacement of implanted electronic sacral neurostimulator, pulse generator or receiver

● T85.128 **Displacement of other implanted electronic stimulator of nervous system** A, A

● T85.19 **Other mechanical complication of implanted electronic stimulator of nervous system**
Leakage of implanted electronic stimulator of nervous system
Obstruction (mechanical) of implanted electronic stimulator of nervous system
Perforation of implanted electronic stimulator of nervous system
Protrusion of implanted electronic stimulator of nervous system

● T85.190 **Other mechanical complication of implanted electronic neurostimulator of brain electrode (lead)** A, A

● T85.191 **Other mechanical complication of implanted electronic neurostimulator of peripheral nerve electrode (lead)** A, A
Other mechanical complication of electrode (lead) for cranial nerve neurostimulators
Other mechanical complication of electrode (lead) for gastric neurostimulator
Other mechanical complication of electrode (lead) for sacral nerve neurostimulator
Other mechanical complication of electrode (lead) for vagal nerve neurostimulators

● T85.192 **Other mechanical complication of implanted electronic neurostimulator of spinal cord electrode (lead)** A, A

● T85.193 **Other mechanical complication of implanted electronic neurostimulator, generator** A, A
Other mechanical complication of implanted electronic neurostimulator generator, brain, peripheral, gastric, spinal
Other mechanical complication of implanted electronic sacral neurostimulator, pulse generator or receiver

● T85.199 **Other mechanical complication of other implanted electronic stimulator of nervous system** A, A

● T85.2 **Mechanical complication of intraocular lens** (Ex) PDX 1995

X● T85.21 **Breakdown (mechanical) of intraocular lens** A

X● T85.22 **Displacement of intraocular lens** A
Malposition of intraocular lens

X● T85.29 **Other mechanical complication of intraocular lens** A
Obstruction (mechanical) of intraocular lens
Perforation of intraocular lens
Protrusion of intraocular lens

● T85.3 **Mechanical complication of other ocular prosthetic devices, implants and grafts** (Ex) PDX 1996
Excludes2 other complications of corneal graft (T86.84-)

● T85.31 **Breakdown (mechanical) of other ocular prosthetic devices, implants and grafts**

● T85.310 **Breakdown (mechanical) of prosthetic orbit of right eye** A

● T85.311 **Breakdown (mechanical) of prosthetic orbit of left eye** A

● T85.318 **Breakdown (mechanical) of other ocular prosthetic devices, implants and grafts**

● T85.32 **Displacement of other ocular prosthetic devices, implants and grafts**
Malposition of other ocular prosthetic devices, implants and grafts

● T85.320 **Displacement of prosthetic orbit of right eye** A

● T85.321 **Displacement of prosthetic orbit of left eye** A

● T85.328 **Displacement of other ocular prosthetic devices, implants and grafts**

● T85.39 **Other mechanical complication of other ocular prosthetic devices, implants and grafts**
Obstruction (mechanical) of other ocular prosthetic devices, implants and grafts
Perforation of other ocular prosthetic devices, implants and grafts
Protrusion of other ocular prosthetic devices, implants and grafts

● T85.390 **Other mechanical complication of prosthetic orbit of right eye** A

● T85.391 **Other mechanical complication of prosthetic orbit of left eye** A

● T85.398 **Other mechanical complication of other ocular prosthetic devices, implants and grafts**

● T85.4 **Mechanical complication of breast prosthesis and implant** (Ex) PDX 1997

X● T85.41 **Breakdown (mechanical) of breast prosthesis and implant** A

X● T85.42 **Displacement of breast prosthesis and implant** A
Malposition of breast prosthesis and implant

X● T85.43 **Leakage of breast prosthesis and implant** A

X● T85.44 **Capsular contracture of breast implant** A

X● T85.49 **Other mechanical complication of breast prosthesis and implant** A
Obstruction (mechanical) of breast prosthesis and implant
Perforation of breast prosthesis and implant
Protrusion of breast prosthesis and implant

● T85.5 **Mechanical complication of gastrointestinal prosthetic devices, implants and grafts** (Ex) PDX 1998

● T85.51 **Breakdown (mechanical) of gastrointestinal prosthetic devices, implants and grafts**

● T85.510 **Breakdown (mechanical) of bile duct prosthesis** A

● T85.511 **Breakdown (mechanical) of esophageal anti-reflux device** A

● T85.518 **Breakdown (mechanical) of other gastrointestinal prosthetic devices, implants and grafts** A

● T85.52 **Displacement of gastrointestinal prosthetic devices, implants and grafts**
Malposition of gastrointestinal prosthetic devices, implants and grafts

● T85.520 **Displacement of bile duct prosthesis** A

● T85.521 **Displacement of esophageal anti-reflux device** A

● T85.528 **Displacement of other gastrointestinal prosthetic devices, implants and grafts** A

● T85.59 **Other mechanical complication of gastrointestinal prosthetic devices, implants and**
Obstruction, mechanical of gastrointestinal prosthetic devices, implants and grafts
Perforation of gastrointestinal prosthetic devices, implants and grafts
Protrusion of gastrointestinal prosthetic devices, implants and grafts

● T85.590 **Other mechanical complication of bile duct prosthesis** A

● T85.591 **Other mechanical complication of esophageal anti-reflux device** A

● T85.598 **Other mechanical complication of other gastrointestinal prosthetic devices, implants and grafts** A

● T85.6 **Mechanical complication of other specified internal and external prosthetic devices, implants and grafts**
Coding Clinic: 2016, Q4, P71

● T85.61 **Breakdown (mechanical) of other specified internal prosthetic devices, implants and grafts**

● T85.610 **Breakdown (mechanical) of cranial or spinal infusion catheter** A (Ex) PDX 1999
Breakdown (mechanical) of epidural infusion catheter
Breakdown (mechanical) of intrathecal infusion catheter
Breakdown (mechanical) of subarachnoid infusion catheter
Breakdown (mechanical) of subdural infusion catheter

● T85.611 **Breakdown (mechanical) of intraperitoneal dialysis catheter** A, A, D, S (Ex) PDX 2000
Excludes1 mechanical complication of vascular dialysis catheter (T82.4-)

● T85.612 **Breakdown (mechanical) of permanent sutures** A (Ex) PDX 2001
Excludes1 mechanical complication of permanent (wire) suture used in bone repair (T84.1-T84.2)

● T85.613 **Breakdown (mechanical) of artificial skin graft and decellularized allodermis** A (Ex) PDX 2002
Failure of artificial skin graft and decellularized allodermis
Non-adherence of artificial skin graft and decellularized allodermis
Poor incorporation of artificial skin graft and decellularized allodermis
Shearing of artificial skin graft and decellularized allodermis

● T85.614 **Breakdown (mechanical) of insulin pump** A (Ex) PDX 2003

● T85.615 **Breakdown (mechanical) of other nervous system device, implant or graft** A, A (Ex) PDX 2001
Breakdown (mechanical) of intrathecal infusion pump

● T85.618 **Breakdown (mechanical) of other specified internal prosthetic devices, implants and grafts** A (Ex) PDX 2001

● **T85.62 Displacement of other specified internal prosthetic devices, implants and grafts**
Malposition of other specified internal prosthetic devices, implants and grafts

● **T85.620 Displacement of cranial or spinal infusion catheter** A (Ex) PDX 1999
Displacement of epidural infusion catheter
Displacement of intrathecal infusion catheter
Displacement of subarachnoid infusion catheter
Displacement of subdural infusion catheter

● **T85.621 Displacement of intraperitoneal dialysis catheter** A, A, D, S (Ex) PDX 2000
Excludes1 mechanical complication of vascular dialysis catheter (T82.4-)

● **T85.622 Displacement of permanent sutures** A (Ex) PDX 2001
Excludes1 mechanical complication of permanent (wire) suture used in bone repair (T84.1-T84.2)

● **T85.623 Displacement of artificial skin graft and decellularized allodermis** A (Ex) PDX 2002
Dislodgement of artificial skin graft and decellularized allodermis

● **T85.624 Displacement of insulin pump** A (Ex) PDX 2003

● **T85.625 Displacement of other nervous system device, implant or graft** A, A (Ex) PDX 2001
Displacement of intrathecal infusion pump

● **T85.628 Displacement of other specified internal prosthetic devices, implants and grafts** A (Ex) PDX 2001
Coding Clinic: 2015, Q1, P15

● **T85.63 Leakage of other specified internal prosthetic devices, implants and grafts**

● **T85.630 Leakage of cranial or spinal infusion catheter** A (Ex) PDX 1999
Leakage of epidural infusion catheter
Leakage of intrathecal infusion catheter
Leakage of subdural infusion catheter
Leakage of subarachnoid infusion catheter
Coding Clinic: 2022, Q3, P24

● **T85.631 Leakage of intraperitoneal dialysis catheter** A, A, D, S (Ex) PDX 2000
Excludes1 mechanical complication of vascular dialysis catheter (T82.4)

● **T85.633 Leakage of insulin pump** A (Ex) PDX 2003

● **T85.635 Leakage of other nervous system device, implant or graft** A, A (Ex) PDX 2001
Leakage of intrathecal infusion pump

● **T85.638 Leakage of other specified internal prosthetic devices, implants and grafts** A (Ex) PDX 2001

● **T85.69 Other mechanical complication of other specified internal prosthetic devices, implants and grafts**
Obstruction, mechanical of other specified internal prosthetic devices, implants and grafts
Perforation of other specified internal prosthetic devices, implants and grafts
Protrusion of other specified internal prosthetic devices, implants and grafts

● **T85.690 Other mechanical complication of cranial or spinal infusion catheter** A (Ex) PDX 1999
Other mechanical complication of epidural infusion catheter
Other mechanical complication of intrathecal infusion catheter
Other mechanical complication of subarachnoid infusion catheter
Other mechanical complication of subdural infusion catheter

● **T85.691 Other mechanical complication of intraperitoneal dialysis catheter** A, A, D, S (Ex) PDX 2000
Excludes1 mechanical complication of vascular dialysis catheter (T82.4)

● **T85.692 Other mechanical complication of permanent sutures** A (Ex) PDX 2001
Excludes1 mechanical complication of permanent (wire) suture used in bone repair (T84.1-T84.2)

● **T85.693 Other mechanical complication of artificial skin graft and decellularized allodermis** A (Ex) PDX 2002

● **T85.694 Other mechanical complication of insulin pump** A (Ex) PDX 2003

● **T85.695 Other mechanical complication of other nervous system device, implant or graft** A, A (Ex) PDX 2001
Other mechanical complication of intrathecal infusion pump

● **T85.698 Other mechanical complication of other specified internal prosthetic devices, implants and grafts** A (Ex) PDX 2001
Mechanical complication of nonabsorbable surgical material NOS

● **T85.7 Infection and inflammatory reaction due to other internal prosthetic devices, implants and grafts**
Use additional code to identify infection
Coding Clinic: 2016, Q4, P72

X● **T85.71 Infection and inflammatory reaction due to peritoneal dialysis catheter** A, A, D, S (Ex) PDX 2001

X● **T85.72 Infection and inflammatory reaction due to insulin pump** A, A (Ex) PDX 2004

● **T85.73 Infection and inflammatory reaction due to nervous system devices, implants and graft** (Ex) PDX 2004

● **T85.730 Infection and inflammatory reaction due to ventricular intracranial (communicating) shunt** A, A

● **T85.731 Infection and inflammatory reaction due to implanted electronic neurostimulator of brain, electrode (lead)** A, A

CHAPTER 19 (S00-T88)

● T85.732 **Infection and inflammatory reaction due to implanted electronic neurostimulator of peripheral nerve, electrode (lead)** A, A
Infection and inflammatory reaction due to electrode (lead) for cranial nerve neurostimulators
Infection and inflammatory reaction due to electrode (lead) for gastric neurostimulator
Infection and inflammatory reaction due to electrode (lead) for sacral nerve neurostimulator
Infection and inflammatory reaction due to electrode (lead) for vagal nerve neurostimulators

● T85.733 **Infection and inflammatory reaction due to implanted electronic neurostimulator of spinal cord, electrode (lead)** A, A

● T85.734 **Infection and inflammatory reaction due to implanted electronic neurostimulator, generator** A, A
Generator pocket infection

● T85.735 **Infection and inflammatory reaction due to cranial or spinal infusion catheter** A, A
Infection and inflammatory reaction due to epidural catheter
Infection and inflammatory reaction due to intrathecal infusion catheter
Infection and inflammatory reaction due to subarachnoid catheter
Infection and inflammatory reaction due to subdural catheter

● T85.738 **Infection and inflammatory reaction due to other nervous system device, implant or graft** A, A
Infection and inflammatory reaction due to intrathecal infusion pump

X● T85.79 **Infection and inflammatory reaction due to other internal prosthetic devices, implants and grafts** A, A (Ex) PDX 2004
Coding Clinic: 2023, Q2, P28; 2022, Q2, P8; 2016, Q4, P72

● T85.8 **Other specified complications of internal prosthetic devices, implants and grafts, not elsewhere classified** (Ex) PDX 2004
Coding Clinic: 2016, Q4, P72

● T85.81 **Embolism due to internal prosthetic devices, implants and grafts, not elsewhere classified**

● T85.810 **Embolism due to nervous system prosthetic devices, implants and grafts** A, D, A

● T85.818 **Embolism due to other internal prosthetic devices, implants and grafts**

● T85.82 **Fibrosis due to internal prosthetic devices, implants and grafts, not elsewhere classified**

● T85.820 **Fibrosis due to nervous system prosthetic devices, implants and grafts** A, D, A

● T85.828 **Fibrosis due to other internal prosthetic devices, implants and grafts**

● T85.83 **Hemorrhage due to internal prosthetic devices, implants and grafts, not elsewhere classified**

● T85.830 **Hemorrhage due to nervous system prosthetic devices, implants and grafts** A, D, A

● T85.838 **Hemorrhage due to other internal prosthetic devices, implants and grafts**

● T85.84 **Pain due to internal prosthetic devices, implants and grafts, not elsewhere classified**

● T85.840 **Pain due to nervous system prosthetic devices, implants and grafts** A, D, A

● T85.848 **Pain due to other internal prosthetic devices, implants and grafts**

● T85.85 **Stenosis due to internal prosthetic devices, implants and grafts, not elsewhere classified**

● T85.850 **Stenosis due to nervous system prosthetic devices, implants and grafts** A, D, A

● T85.858 **Stenosis due to other internal prosthetic devices, implants and grafts**

● T85.86 **Thrombosis due to internal prosthetic devices, implants and grafts, not elsewhere classified**

● T85.860 **Thrombosis due to nervous system prosthetic devices, implants and grafts** A, D, A

● T85.868 **Thrombosis due to other internal prosthetic devices, implants and grafts**
Coding Clinic: 2024, Q2, P7

● T85.89 **Other specified complication of internal prosthetic devices, implants and grafts, not elsewhere classified**
Coding Clinic: 2024, Q2, P8; 2016, Q4, P72

● T85.890 **Other specified complication of nervous system prosthetic devices, implants and grafts** A, D, A

● T85.898 **Other specified complication of other internal prosthetic devices, implants and grafts**
Coding Clinic: 2024, Q2, P8

X● T85.9 **Unspecified complication of internal prosthetic device, implant and graft**
Complication of internal prosthetic device, implant and graft NOS

OGCR Section I.C.19.g.3.

Organ Transplant Complications
Transplant Complications
(a) Transplant complications other than kidney
Codes under category T86, Complications of transplanted organs and tissues, are for use for both complications and rejection of transplanted organs. A transplant complication code is only assigned if the complication affects the function of the transplanted organ. Two codes are required to fully describe a transplant complication: the appropriate code from category T86 and a secondary code that identifies the complication.
Pre-existing conditions or conditions that develop after the transplant are not coded as complications unless they affect the function of the transplanted organs.
See I.C.21 for transplant organ removal status.
See I.C.2 for malignant neoplasm associated with transplanted organ.

● T86 **Complications of transplanted organs and tissue**
Use additional code to identify other transplant complications, such as:
graft-versus-host disease (D89.81-)
malignancy associated with organ transplant (C80.2)
post-transplant lymphoproliferative disorders (PTLD) (D47.Z1)

● T86.0 Complications of bone marrow transplant (Ex) PDX 574
T86.00 Unspecified complication of bone marrow transplant
T86.01 Bone marrow transplant rejection
T86.02 Bone marrow transplant failure
T86.03 Bone marrow transplant infection
T86.09 Other complications of bone marrow transplant
Coding Clinic: 2023, Q3, P20

● T86.1 Complications of kidney transplant (Ex) PDX 2005
T86.10 Unspecified complication of kidney transplant
T86.11 Kidney transplant rejection
T86.12 Kidney transplant failure
Coding Clinic: 2013, Q1, P24
T86.13 Kidney transplant infection
Use additional code to specify infection
T86.19 Other complication of kidney transplant
Coding Clinic: 2019, Q2, P7

● T86.2 Complications of heart transplant (Ex) PDX 2006
Excludes1 complication of:
artificial heart device (T82.5-)
heart-lung transplant (T86.3-)
T86.20 Unspecified complication of heart transplant
T86.21 Heart transplant rejection
T86.22 Heart transplant failure
T86.23 Heart transplant infection
Use additional code to specify infection
● T86.29 Other complications of heart transplant
T86.290 Cardiac allograft vasculopathy
Excludes1 atherosclerosis of coronary arteries (I25.75-, I25.76-, I25.81-)
T86.298 Other complications of heart transplant

● T86.3 Complications of heart-lung transplant (Ex) PDX 2006
T86.30 Unspecified complication of heart-lung transplant
CC when PDx is its own CC
T86.31 Heart-lung transplant rejection
CC when PDx is its own CC
T86.32 Heart-lung transplant failure
CC when PDx is its own CC
T86.33 Heart-lung transplant infection
Use additional code to specify infection
CC when PDx is its own CC
T86.39 Other complications of heart-lung transplant
CC when PDx is its own CC

● T86.4 Complications of liver transplant (Ex) PDX 2007
T86.40 Unspecified complication of liver transplant
T86.41 Liver transplant rejection
T86.42 Liver transplant failure
T86.43 Liver transplant infection
Use additional code to identify infection, such as:
Cytomegalovirus (CMV) infection (B25.-)
T86.49 Other complications of liver transplant

● T86.5 Complications of stem cell transplant (Ex) PDX 2008
Complications from stem cells from peripheral blood
Complications from stem cells from umbilical cord

● T86.8 Complications of other transplanted organs and tissues
● T86.81 Complications of lung transplant (Ex) PDX 2009
Excludes1 complication of heart-lung transplant (T86.3-)
T86.810 Lung transplant rejection
T86.811 Lung transplant failure
T86.812 Lung transplant infection
Use additional code to specify infection
T86.818 Other complications of lung transplant
Coding Clinic: 2019, Q2, P7
T86.819 Unspecified complication of lung transplant
● T86.82 Complications of skin graft (allograft) (autograft) (Ex) PDX 2010
Excludes2 complication of artificial skin graft (T85.693)
T86.820 Skin graft (allograft) rejection
T86.821 Skin graft (allograft) (autograft) failure
T86.822 Skin graft (allograft) (autograft) infection
Use additional code to specify infection
T86.828 Other complications of skin graft (allograft) (autograft)
T86.829 Unspecified complication of skin graft (allograft) (autograft)
● T86.83 Complications of bone graft (Ex) PDX 2011
Excludes2 mechanical complications of bone graft (T84.3-)
T86.830 Bone graft rejection
T86.831 Bone graft failure
T86.832 Bone graft infection
Use additional code to specify infection
T86.838 Other complications of bone graft
Coding Clinic: 2023, Q1, P31
T86.839 Unspecified complication of bone graft
● T86.84 Complications of corneal transplant
Excludes2 mechanical complications of corneal graft (T85.3-)
● T86.840 Corneal transplant rejection (Ex) PDX 2012
T86.8401 Corneal transplant rejection, right eye
T86.8402 Corneal transplant rejection, left eye
T86.8403 Corneal transplant rejection, bilateral
T86.8409 Corneal transplant rejection, unspecified eye
● T86.841 Corneal transplant failure (Ex) PDX 2012
T86.8411 Corneal transplant failure, right eye
T86.8412 Corneal transplant failure, left eye
T86.8413 Corneal transplant failure, bilateral
T86.8419 Corneal transplant failure, unspecified eye

CHAPTER 19 (S00-T88)

T86.842 Corneal transplant infection (Ex) PDX 2013
Use additional code to specify infection
T86.8421 Corneal transplant infection, right eye
T86.8422 Corneal transplant infection, left eye
T86.8423 Corneal transplant infection, bilateral
T86.8429 Corneal transplant infection, unspecified eye

T86.848 Other complications of corneal transplant (Ex) PDX 2013
T86.8481 Other complications of corneal transplant, right eye
T86.8482 Other complications of corneal transplant, left eye
T86.8483 Other complications of corneal transplant, bilateral
T86.8489 Other complications of corneal transplant, unspecified eye

T86.849 Unspecified complication of corneal transplant (Ex) PDX 2013
T86.8491 Unspecified complication of corneal transplant, right eye
T86.8492 Unspecified complication of corneal transplant, left eye
T86.8493 Unspecified complication of corneal transplant, bilateral
T86.8499 Unspecified complication of corneal transplant, unspecified eye

T86.85 Complication of intestine transplant (Ex) PDX 543
T86.850 Intestine transplant rejection
T86.851 Intestine transplant failure
T86.852 Intestine transplant infection
Use additional code to specify infection
T86.858 Other complications of intestine transplant
T86.859 Unspecified complication of intestine transplant

T86.89 Complications of other transplanted tissue (Ex) PDX 2014
Transplant failure or rejection of pancreas
T86.890 Other transplanted tissue rejection
T86.891 Other transplanted tissue failure
T86.892 Other transplanted tissue infection
Use additional code to specify infection
T86.898 Other complications of other transplanted tissue
T86.899 Unspecified complication of other transplanted tissue

T86.9 Complication of unspecified transplanted organ and tissue (Ex) PDX 543
T86.90 Unspecified complication of unspecified transplanted organ and tissue
T86.91 Unspecified transplanted organ and tissue rejection
T86.92 Unspecified transplanted organ and tissue failure
T86.93 Unspecified transplanted organ and tissue infection
Use additional code to specify infection
T86.99 Other complications of unspecified transplanted organ and tissue

T87 Complications peculiar to reattachment and amputation

T87.0 Complications of reattached (part of) upper extremity (Ex) PDX 2015
T87.0X Complications of reattached (part of) upper extremity
T87.0X1 Complications of reattached (part of) right upper extremity
T87.0X2 Complications of reattached (part of) left upper extremity
T87.0X9 Complications of reattached (part of) unspecified upper extremity

T87.1 Complications of reattached (part of) lower extremity (Ex) PDX 2016
T87.1X Complications of reattached (part of) lower extremity
T87.1X1 Complications of reattached (part of) right lower extremity
T87.1X2 Complications of reattached (part of) left lower extremity
T87.1X9 Complications of reattached (part of) unspecified lower extremity

T87.2 Complications of other reattached body part (Ex) PDX 2017

T87.3 Neuroma of amputation stump
T87.30 Neuroma of amputation stump, unspecified extremity
T87.31 Neuroma of amputation stump, right upper extremity
T87.32 Neuroma of amputation stump, left upper extremity
T87.33 Neuroma of amputation stump, right lower extremity
T87.34 Neuroma of amputation stump, left lower extremity

T87.4 Infection of amputation stump (Ex) PDX 2018
T87.40 Infection of amputation stump, unspecified extremity
T87.41 Infection of amputation stump, right upper extremity
T87.42 Infection of amputation stump, left upper extremity
T87.43 Infection of amputation stump, right lower extremity
T87.44 Infection of amputation stump, left lower extremity

T87.5 Necrosis of amputation stump
T87.50 Necrosis of amputation stump, unspecified extremity
T87.51 Necrosis of amputation stump, right upper extremity
T87.52 Necrosis of amputation stump, left upper extremity
T87.53 Necrosis of amputation stump, right lower extremity
T87.54 Necrosis of amputation stump, left lower extremity

● **T87.8 Other complications of amputation stump**

T87.81 Dehiscence of amputation stump

T87.89 Other complications of amputation stump
Amputation stump contracture
Amputation stump contracture of next proximal joint
Amputation stump flexion
Amputation stump edema
Amputation stump hematoma
Excludes2 phantom limb syndrome (G54.6-G54.7)
Coding Clinic: 2022, Q3, P11

T87.9 Unspecified complications of amputation stump

● **T88 Other complications of surgical and medical care, not elsewhere classified**
Excludes2 complication following infusion, transfusion and therapeutic injection (T80.-)
complication following procedure NEC (T81.-)
complications of anesthesia in labor and delivery (O74.-)
complications of anesthesia in pregnancy (O29.-)
complications of anesthesia in puerperium (O89.-)
complications of devices, implants and grafts (T82-T85)
complications of obstetric surgery and procedure (O75.4)
dermatitis due to drugs and medicaments (L23.3, L24.4, L25.1, L27.0-L27.1)
poisoning and toxic effects of drugs and chemicals (T36-T65 with fifth or sixth character 1-4)
specified complications classified elsewhere

The appropriate 7th character is to be added to each code from category T88

A	initial encounter
D	subsequent encounter
S	sequela

X● **T88.0 Infection following immunization** A (Ex) PDX 1400
Sepsis following immunization
Coding Clinic: 2019, Q1, P14;2018, Q4, P90

X● **T88.1 Other complications following immunization, not elsewhere classified** A (Ex) PDX 2019
Generalized vaccinia
Rash following immunization
Excludes1 vaccinia not from vaccine (B08.011)
Excludes2 anaphylactic shock due to serum (T80.5-)
other serum reactions (T80.6-)
postimmunization arthropathy (M02.2)
postimmunization encephalitis (G04.02)
postimmunization fever (R50.83)

X● **T88.2 Shock due to anesthesia** A (Ex) PDX 1971
Use additional code for adverse effect, if applicable, to identify drug (T41.- with fifth or sixth character 5)
Excludes1 complications of anesthesia (in):
labor and delivery (O74.-)
pregnancy (O29.-)
puerperium (O89.-)
postprocedural shock NOS (T81.1-)

X● **T88.3 Malignant hyperthermia due to anesthesia**
A (Ex) PDX 2020
Use additional code for adverse effect, if applicable, to identify drug (T41.- with fifth or sixth character 5)

X● **T88.4 Failed or difficult intubation**

● **T88.5 Other complications of anesthesia**
Use additional code for adverse effect, if applicable, to identify drug (T41.- with fifth or sixth character 5)
Coding Clinic: 2016, Q4, P72

X● **T88.51 Hypothermia following anesthesia**

X● **T88.52 Failed moderate sedation during procedure**
Failed conscious sedation during procedure
Excludes2 personal history of failed moderate sedation (Z92.83)

X● **T88.53 Unintended awareness under general anesthesia during procedure**
Excludes2 personal history of unintended awareness under general anesthesia (Z92.84)
Coding Clinic: 2016, Q4, P72-73

X● **T88.59 Other complications of anesthesia**

X● **T88.6 Anaphylactic reaction due to adverse effect of correct drug or medicament properly administered**
A (Ex) PDX 2021
Anaphylactic shock due to adverse effect of correct drug or medicament properly administered
Anaphylactoid reaction NOS
Use additional code for adverse effect, if applicable, to identify drug (T36-T50 with fifth or sixth character 5)
Excludes1 anaphylactic reaction due to serum (T80.5-)
anaphylactic shock or reaction due to adverse food reaction (T78.0-)
Coding Clinic: 2020, Q1, P18

X● **T88.7 Unspecified adverse effect of drug or medicament**
Drug hypersensitivity NOS
Drug reaction NOS
Use additional code for adverse effect, if applicable, to identify drug (T36-T50 with fifth or sixth character 5)
Excludes1 specified adverse effects of drugs and medicaments (A00-R94 and T80-T88.6, T88.8)

X● **T88.8 Other specified complications of surgical and medical care, not elsewhere classified**
Use additional code to identify the complication
Coding Clinic: 2022, Q2, P8

X● **T88.9 Complication of surgical and medical care, unspecified**

CHAPTER 19 (S00-T88)

CHAPTER 20

EXTERNAL CAUSES OF MORBIDITY (V00-Y99)

OGCR Chapter-Specific Coding Guidelines

20. Chapter 20: External Causes of Morbidity (V00-Y99)
The external causes of morbidity codes should never be sequenced as the first-listed or principal diagnosis.

External cause codes are intended to provide data for injury research and evaluation of injury prevention strategies. These codes capture how the injury or health condition happened (cause), the intent (unintentional or accidental; or intentional, such as suicide or assault), the place where the event occurred the activity of the patient at the time of the event, and the person's status (e.g., civilian, military).

There is no national requirement for mandatory ICD-10-CM external cause code reporting. Unless a provider is subject to a state-based external cause code reporting mandate or these codes are required by a particular payer, reporting of ICD-10-CM codes in Chapter 20, External Causes of Morbidity, is not required. In the absence of a mandatory reporting requirement, providers are encouraged to voluntarily report external cause codes, as they provide valuable data for injury research and evaluation of injury prevention strategies.

a. General External Cause Coding Guidelines

1) Used with any code in the range of A00.0-T88.9, Z00-Z99
An external cause code may be used with any code in the range of A00.0-T88.9, Z00-Z99, classification that represents a health condition due to an external cause. Though they are most applicable to injuries, they are also valid for use with such things as infections or diseases due to an external source, and other health conditions, such as a heart attack that occurs during strenuous physical activity.

2) External cause code used for length of treatment
Assign the external cause code, with the appropriate 7th character (initial encounter, subsequent encounter or sequela) for each encounter for which the injury or condition is being treated.

Most categories in Chapter 20 have a 7th character requirement for each applicable code. Most categories in this chapter have three 7th character values: A, initial encounter, D, subsequent encounter and S, sequela. While the patient may be seen by a new or different provider over the course of treatment for an injury or condition, assignment of the 7th character for external cause should match the 7th character of the code assigned for the associated injury or condition for the encounter.

3) Use the full range of external cause codes
Use the full range of external cause codes to completely describe the cause, the intent, the place of occurrence and if applicable, the activity of the patient at the time of the event, and the patient's status, for all injuries, and other health conditions due to an external cause.

4) Assign as many external cause codes as necessary
Assign as many external cause codes as necessary to fully explain each cause. If only one external code can be recorded, assign the code most related to the principal diagnosis.

5) The selection of the appropriate external cause code
The selection of the appropriate external cause code is guided by the Alphabetic Index of External Causes and by Inclusion and Exclusion notes in the Tabular List.

6) External cause code can never be a principal diagnosis
An external cause code can never be a principal (first-listed) diagnosis.

7) Combination external cause codes
Certain of the external cause codes are combination codes that identify sequential events that result in an injury, such as a fall which results in striking against an object. The injury may be due to either event or both. The combination external cause code used should correspond to the sequence of events regardless of which caused the most serious injury.

8) No external cause code needed in certain circumstances
No external cause code from Chapter 20 is needed if the external cause and intent are included in a code from another chapter (e.g., T36.0X1- Poisoning by penicillins, accidental (unintentional)).

b. Place of Occurrence Guideline
Codes from category Y92, Place of occurrence of the external cause, are secondary codes for use after other external cause codes to identify the location of the patient at the time of injury or other condition.

Generally, a place of occurrence code is assigned only once, at the initial encounter for treatment. However, in the rare instance that a new injury occurs during hospitalization, an additional place of occurrence code may be assigned. No 7th characters are used for Y92. Only one code from Y92 should be recorded on a medical record.

Do not use place of occurrence code Y92.9 if the place is not stated or is not applicable.

c. Activity Code
Assign a code from category Y93, Activity code, to describe the activity of the patient at the time the injury or other health condition occurred.

An activity code is used only once, at the initial encounter for treatment. Only one code from Y93 should be recorded on a medical record.

The activity codes are not applicable to poisonings, adverse effects, misadventures or sequela.

Do not assign Y93.9, Unspecified activity, if the activity is not stated.

A code from category Y93 is appropriate for use with external cause and intent codes if identifying the activity provides additional information about the event.

d. Place of Occurrence, Activity, and Status Codes Used with Other External Cause Code
When applicable, place of occurrence, activity, and external cause status codes are sequenced after the main external cause code(s). Regardless of the number of external cause codes assigned, there should be only one place of occurrence code, one activity code, and one external cause status code assigned to an encounter.

e. If the Reporting Format Limits the Number of External Cause Codes

If the reporting format limits the number of external cause codes that can be used in reporting clinical data, report the code for the cause/intent most related to the principal diagnosis. If the format permits capture of additional external cause codes, the cause/intent, including medical misadventures, of the additional events should be reported rather than the codes for place, activity, or external status.

f. Multiple External Cause Coding Guidelines

More than one external cause code is required to fully describe the external cause of an illness or injury. The assignment of external cause codes should be sequenced in the following priority:

If two or more events cause separate injuries, an external cause code should be assigned for each cause. The first-listed external cause code will be selected in the following order:

External codes for child and adult abuse take priority over all other external cause codes.

See Section I.C.19., Child and Adult abuse guidelines.

External codes for terrorism events take priority over all other external cause codes except child and adult abuse.

External cause codes for cataclysmic events take priority over all other external cause codes except child and adult abuse and terrorism.

External cause codes for transport accidents take priority over all other external cause codes except cataclysmic events, child and adult abuse and terrorism.

Activity and external cause status codes are assigned following all causal (intent) external cause codes.

The first-listed external cause code should correspond to the cause of the most serious diagnosis due to an assault, accident, or self-harm, following the order of hierarchy listed above.

g. Child and Adult Abuse Guideline

Adult and child abuse, neglect and maltreatment are classified as assault. Any of the assault codes may be used to indicate the external cause of any injury resulting from the confirmed abuse.

For confirmed cases of abuse, neglect and maltreatment, when the perpetrator is known, a code from Y07, Perpetrator of maltreatment and neglect, should accompany any other assault codes.

See Section I.C.19. Adult and child abuse, neglect and other maltreatment

h. Unknown or Undetermined Intent Guideline

If the intent (accident, self-harm, assault) of the cause of an injury or other condition is unknown or unspecified, code the intent as accidental intent. All transport accident categories assume accidental intent.

1) Use of undetermined intent

External cause codes for events of undetermined intent are only for use if the documentation in the record specifies that the intent cannot be determined.

i. Sequelae (Late Effects) of External Cause Guidelines

1) Sequelae external cause codes

Sequela are reported using the external cause code with the 7th character "S" for sequela. These codes should be used with any report of a late effect or sequela resulting from a previous injury.

See Section I.B.10. Sequela, (Late Effects).

2) Sequela external cause code with a related current injury

A sequela external cause code should never be used with a related current nature of injury code.

3) Use of sequela external cause codes for subsequent visits

Use a late effect external cause code for subsequent visits when a late effect of the initial injury is being treated. Do not use a late effect external cause code for subsequent visits for follow-up care (e.g., to assess healing, to receive rehabilitative therapy) of the injury when no late effect of the injury has been documented.

j. Terrorism Guidelines

1) Cause of injury identified by the Federal Government (FBI) as terrorism

When the cause of an injury is identified by the Federal Government (FBI) as terrorism, the first-listed external cause code should be a code from category Y38, Terrorism. The definition of terrorism employed by the FBI is found at the inclusion note at the beginning of category Y38. Use additional code for place of occurrence (Y92.-). More than one Y38 code may be assigned if the injury is the result of more than one mechanism of terrorism.

2) Cause of an injury is suspected to be the result of terrorism

When the cause of an injury is suspected to be the result of terrorism a code from category Y38 should not be assigned. Suspected cases should be classified as assault.

3) Code Y38.9, Terrorism, secondary effects

Assign code Y38.9, Terrorism, secondary effects, for conditions occurring subsequent to the terrorist event. This code should not be assigned for conditions that are due to the initial terrorist act.

It is acceptable to assign code Y38.9 with another code from Y38 if there is an injury due to the initial terrorist event and an injury that is a subsequent result of the terrorist event.

k. External cause status

A code from category Y99, External cause status, should be assigned whenever any other external cause code is assigned for an encounter, including an Activity code, except for the events noted below. Assign a code from category Y99, External cause status, to indicate the work status of the person at the time the event occurred. The status code indicates whether the event occurred during military activity, whether a non-military person was at work, whether an individual including a student or volunteer was involved in a non-work activity at the time of the causal event.

A code from Y99, External cause status, should be assigned, when applicable, with other external cause codes, such as transport accidents and falls. The external cause status codes are not applicable to poisonings, adverse effects, misadventures or late effects.

Do not assign a code from category Y99 if no other external cause codes (cause, activity) are applicable for the encounter.

An external cause status code is used only once, at the initial encounter for treatment. Only one code from Y99 should be recorded on a medical record.

Do not assign code Y99.9, Unspecified external cause status, if the status is not stated.

CHAPTER 2Ø

EXTERNAL CAUSES OF MORBIDITY (VØØ-Y99)

Note: This chapter permits the classification of environmental events and circumstances as the cause of injury, and other adverse effects. Where a code from this section is applicable, it is intended that it shall be used secondary to a code from another chapter of the Classification indicating the nature of the condition. Most often, the condition will be classifiable to Chapter 19, Injury, poisoning and certain other consequences of external causes (SØØ-T88). Other conditions that may be stated to be due to external causes are classified in Chapters 1 to 18. For these conditions, codes from Chapter 2Ø should be used to provide additional information as to the cause of the condition.

This chapter contains the following blocks:

VØØ-X58	Accidents
VØØ-V99	Transport accidents
VØØ-VØ9	Pedestrian injured in transport accident
V1Ø-V19	Pedal cycle rider injured in transport accident
V2Ø-V29	Motorcycle rider injured in transport accident
V3Ø-V39	Occupant of three-wheeled motor vehicle injured in transport accident
V4Ø-V49	Car occupant injured in transport accident
V5Ø-V59	Occupant of pick-up truck or van injured in transport accident
V6Ø-V69	Occupant of heavy transport vehicle injured in transport accident
V7Ø-V79	Bus occupant injured in transport accident
V8Ø-V89	Other land transport accidents
V9Ø-V94	Water transport accidents
V95-V97	Air and space transport accidents
V98-V99	Other and unspecified transport accidents
WØØ-X58	Other external causes of accidental injury
WØØ-W19	Slipping, tripping, stumbling and falls
W2Ø-W49	Exposure to inanimate mechanical forces
W5Ø-W64	Exposure to animate mechanical forces
W65-W74	Accidental non-transport drowning and submersion
W85-W99	Exposure to electric current, radiation and extreme ambient air temperature and pressure
XØØ-XØ8	Exposure to smoke, fire and flames
X1Ø-X19	Contact with heat and hot substances
X3Ø-X39	Exposure to forces of nature
X5Ø	Overexertion and strenuous or repetitive movements
X52, X58	Accidental exposure to other specified factors
X71-X83	Intentional self-harm
X92-YØ9	Assault
Y21-Y33	Event of undetermined intent
Y35-Y38	Legal intervention, operations of war, military operations, and terrorism
Y62-Y84	Complications of medical and surgical care
Y62-Y69	Misadventures to patients during surgical and medical care
Y7Ø-Y82	Medical devices associated with adverse incidents in diagnostic and therapeutic use
Y83-Y84	Surgical and other medical procedures as the cause of abnormal reaction of the patient, or of later complication, without mention of misadventure at the time of the procedure
Y9Ø-Y99	Supplementary factors related to causes of morbidity classified elsewhere

ACCIDENTS (VØØ-X58)

TRANSPORT ACCIDENTS (VØØ-V99)

Note: This section is structured in 12 groups. Those relating to land transport accidents (VØØ-V89) reflect the victim's mode of transport and are subdivided to identify the victim's 'counterpart' or the type of event. The vehicle of which the injured person is an occupant is identified in the first two characters since it is seen as the most important factor to identify for prevention purposes. A transport accident is one in which the vehicle involved must be moving or running or in use for transport purposes at the time of the accident.

Use additional code to identify:
- Airbag injury (W22.1)
- Type of street or road (Y92.4-)
- Use of cellular telephone and other electronic equipment at the time of the transport accident (Y93.C-)

Excludes1
- agricultural vehicles in stationary use or maintenance (W31.-)
- assault by crashing of motor vehicle (YØ3.-)
- automobile or motor cycle in stationary use or maintenance - code to type of accident
- crashing of motor vehicle, undetermined intent (Y32)
- intentional self-harm by crashing of motor vehicle (X82)

Excludes2 transport accidents due to cataclysm (X34-X38)

Note: Definitions related to transport accidents:

(a) A transport accident (VØØ-V99) is any accident involving a device designed primarily for, or used at the time primarily for, conveying persons or good from one place to another.

(b) A public highway [trafficway] or street is the entire width between property lines (or other boundary lines) of land open to the public as a matter of right or custom for purposes of moving persons or property from one place to another. A roadway is that part of the public highway designed, improved and customarily used for vehicular traffic.

(c) A traffic accident is any vehicle accident occurring on the public highway [i.e., originating on, terminating on, or involving a vehicle partially on the highway]. A vehicle accident is assumed to have occurred on the public highway unless another place is specified, except in the case of accidents involving only off-road motor vehicles, which are classified as nontraffic accidents unless the contrary is stated.

(d) A nontraffic accident is any vehicle accident that occurs entirely in any place other than a public highway.

(e) A pedestrian is any person involved in an accident who was not at the time of the accident riding in or on a motor vehicle, railway train, streetcar or animal-drawn or other vehicle, or on a pedal cycle or animal. This includes, a person changing a tire, working on a parked car, or a person on foot. It also includes the user of a pedestrian conveyance such as a baby stroller, ice-skates, skis, sled, roller skates, a skateboard, nonmotorized or motorized wheelchair, motorized mobility scooter, or nonmotorized scooter.

(f) A driver is an occupant of a transport vehicle who is operating or intending to operate it.

(g) A passenger is any occupant of a transport vehicle other than the driver, except a person traveling on the outside of the vehicle.

(h) A person on the outside of a vehicle is any person being transported by a vehicle but not occupying the space normally reserved for the driver or passengers, or the space intended for the transport of property. This includes a person travelling on the bodywork, bumper, fender, roof, running board or step of a vehicle, as well as, hanging on the outside of the vehicle.

(i) A pedal cycle is any land transport vehicle operated solely by nonmotorized pedals including a bicycle or tricycle.

(j) A pedal cyclist is any person riding a pedal cycle or in a sidecar or trailer attached to a pedal cycle.

(k) A motorcycle is a two-wheeled motor vehicle with one or two riding saddles and sometimes with a third wheel for the support of a sidecar. The sidecar is considered part of the motorcycle. This includes a moped, motor scooter, or motorized bicycle.

(l) A motorcycle rider is any person riding a motorcycle or in a sidecar or trailer attached to the motorcycle.

(m) A three-wheeled motor vehicle is a motorized tricycle designed primarily for on-road use. This includes a motor-driven tricycle, a motorized rickshaw, or a three-wheeled motor car.

(n) A car [automobile] is a four-wheeled motor vehicle designed primarily for carrying up to 7 persons. A trailer being towed by the car is considered part of the car. It does not include a van or minivan—see definition (o)

(o) A pick-up truck or van is a four or six-wheeled motor vehicle designed for carrying passengers as well as property or cargo weighing less than the local limit for classification as a heavy goods vehicle, and not requiring a special driver's license. This includes a minivan and a sport-utility vehicle (SUV).

(p) A heavy transport vehicle is a motor vehicle designed primarily for carrying property, meeting local criteria for classification as a heavy goods vehicle in terms of weight and requiring a special driver's license.

(q) A bus (coach) is a motor vehicle designed or adapted primarily for carrying more than 10 passengers, and requiring a special driver's license.

(r) A railway train or railway vehicle is any device, with or without freight or passenger cars coupled to it, designed for traffic on a railway track. This includes subterranean (subways) or elevated trains.

(s) A streetcar is a device designed and used primarily for transporting passengers within a municipality, running on rails, usually subject to normal traffic control signals, and operated principally on a right-of-way that forms part of the roadway. This includes a tram or trolley that runs on rails. A trailer being towed by a streetcar is considered part of the streetcar.

(t) A special vehicle mainly used on industrial premises is a motor vehicle designed primarily for use within the buildings and premises of industrial or commercial establishments. This includes battery-powered airport passenger vehicles or baggage/mail trucks, forklifts, coal-cars in a coal mine, logging cars and trucks used in mines or quarries.

(u) A special vehicle mainly used in agriculture is a motor vehicle designed specifically for use in farming and agriculture (horticulture), to work the land, tend and harvest crops and transport materials on the farm. This includes harvesters, farm machinery and tractor and trailers.

(v) A special construction vehicle is a motor vehicle designed specifically for use on construction and demolition sites. This includes bulldozers, diggers, earth levellers, dump trucks, backhoes, front-end loaders, pavers, and mechanical shovels.

(w) A special all-terrain vehicle is a motor vehicle of special design to enable it to negotiate over rough or soft terrain, snow or sand. Examples of special design are high construction, special wheels and tires, tracks, and support on a cushion of air. This includes snow mobiles, all-terrain vehicles (ATV), and dune buggies. It does not include passenger vehicle designated as sport utility vehicles (SUV).

(x) A watercraft is any device designed for transporting passengers or goods on water. This includes motor or sail boats, ships, and hovercraft.

(y) An aircraft is any device for transporting passengers or goods in the air. This includes hot-air balloons, gliders, helicopters and airplanes.

(z) A military vehicle is any motorized vehicle operating on a public roadway owned by the military and being operated by a member of the military.

PEDESTRIAN INJURED IN TRANSPORT ACCIDENT (V00-V09)

Includes person changing tire on transport vehicle
person examining engine of vehicle broken down in (on side of) road

Excludes1 fall due to non-transport collision with other person (W03)
pedestrian on foot falling (slipping) on ice and snow (W00.-)
struck or bumped by another person (W51)

● **V00 Pedestrian conveyance accident**

Use additional place of occurrence and activity external cause codes, if known (Y92.-, Y93.-)

Excludes1 collision with another person without fall (W51)
fall due to person on foot colliding with another person on foot (W03)
fall from non-moving wheelchair, nonmotorized scooter and motorized mobility scooter without collision (W05.-)
pedestrian (conveyance) collision with other land transport vehicle (V01-V09)
pedestrian on foot falling (slipping) on ice and snow (W00.-)

The appropriate 7th character is to be added to each code from category V00

A initial encounter
D subsequent encounter
S sequela

● **V00.0 Pedestrian on foot injured in collision with pedestrian conveyance**

X● **V00.01 Pedestrian on foot injured in collision with roller-skater**

X● **V00.02 Pedestrian on foot injured in collision with skateboarder**

● **V00.03 Pedestrian on foot injured in collision with standing micro-mobility pedestrian conveyance**

V00.031 Pedestrian on foot injured in collision with rider of standing electric scooter

V00.038 Pedestrian on foot injured in collision with rider of other standing micro-mobility pedestrian conveyance
Pedestrian on foot injured in collision with rider of hoverboard
Pedestrian on foot injured in collision with rider of segway

X● **V00.09 Pedestrian on foot injured in collision with other pedestrian conveyance**

● **V00.1 Rolling-type pedestrian conveyance accident**

Excludes1 accident with baby stroller (V00.82-)
accident with wheelchair (powered) (V00.81-)
accident with motorized mobility scooter (V00.83-)

● **V00.11 In-line roller-skate accident**

● **V00.111 Fall from in-line roller-skates**

● **V00.112 In-line roller-skater colliding with stationary object**

● **V00.118 Other in-line roller-skate accident**

Excludes1 roller-skater collision with other land transport vehicle (V01-V09 with 5th character 1)

- V00.12 Non-in-line roller-skate accident
  - V00.121 Fall from non-in-line roller-skates
  - V00.122 Non-in-line roller-skater colliding with stationary object
  - V00.128 Other non-in-line roller-skating accident
    - **Excludes1** roller-skater collision with other land transport vehicle (V01-V09 with 5th character 1)
- V00.13 Skateboard accident
  - V00.131 Fall from skateboard
  - V00.132 Skateboarder colliding with stationary object
  - V00.138 Other skateboard accident
    - **Excludes1** skateboarder collision with other land transport vehicle (V01-V09 with 5th character 2)
- V00.14 Scooter (nonmotorized) accident
  - **Excludes1** motor scooter accident (V20-V29)
  - V00.141 Fall from scooter (nonmotorized)
  - V00.142 Scooter (nonmotorized) colliding with stationary object
  - V00.148 Other scooter (nonmotorized) accident
    - **Excludes1** scooter (non-motorized) collision with other land transport vehicle (V01-V09 with fifth character 9)
- V00.15 Heelies accident
  - Rolling shoe
  - Wheeled shoe
  - Wheelies accident
  - V00.151 Fall from heelies
  - V00.152 Heelies colliding with stationary object
  - V00.158 Other heelies accident
- V00.18 Accident on other rolling-type pedestrian conveyance
  - V00.181 Fall from other rolling-type pedestrian conveyance
  - V00.182 Pedestrian on other rolling-type pedestrian conveyance colliding with stationary object
  - V00.188 Other accident on other rolling-type pedestrian conveyance
- V00.2 Gliding-type pedestrian conveyance accident
  - V00.21 Ice-skates accident
    - V00.211 Fall from ice-skates
    - V00.212 Ice-skater colliding with stationary object
    - V00.218 Other ice-skates accident
      - **Excludes1** ice-skater collision with other land transport vehicle (V01-V09 with 5th character 9)
  - V00.22 Sled accident
    - V00.221 Fall from sled
    - V00.222 Sledder colliding with stationary object
    - V00.228 Other sled accident
      - **Excludes1** sled collision with other land transport vehicle (V01-V09 with 5th character 9)
  - V00.28 Other gliding-type pedestrian conveyance accident
    - V00.281 Fall from other gliding-type pedestrian conveyance
    - V00.282 Pedestrian on other gliding-type pedestrian conveyance colliding with stationary object
    - V00.288 Other accident on other gliding-type pedestrian conveyance
      - **Excludes1** gliding-type pedestrian conveyance collision with other land transport vehicle (V01-V09 with 5th character 9)
- V00.3 Flat-bottomed pedestrian conveyance accident
  - V00.31 Snowboard accident
    - V00.311 Fall from snowboard
    - V00.312 Snowboarder colliding with stationary object
    - V00.318 Other snowboard accident
      - **Excludes1** snowboarder collision with other land transport vehicle (V01-V09 with 5th character 9)
  - V00.32 Snow-ski accident
    - V00.321 Fall from snow-skis
      - Coding Clinic: 2015, Q1, P12
    - V00.322 Snow-skier colliding with stationary object
    - V00.328 Other snow-ski accident
      - **Excludes1** snow-skier collision with other land transport vehicle (V01-V09 with 5th character 9)
  - V00.38 Other flat-bottomed pedestrian conveyance accident
    - V00.381 Fall from other flat-bottomed pedestrian conveyance
    - V00.382 Pedestrian on other flat-bottomed pedestrian conveyance colliding with stationary object
    - V00.388 Other accident on other flat-bottomed pedestrian conveyance
- V00.8 Accident on other pedestrian conveyance
  - V00.81 Accident with wheelchair (powered)
    - V00.811 Fall from moving wheelchair (powered)
      - **Excludes1** fall from non-moving wheelchair (W05.0)
    - V00.812 Wheelchair (powered) colliding with stationary object
    - V00.818 Other accident with wheelchair (powered)
  - V00.82 Accident with baby stroller
    - V00.821 Fall from baby stroller
    - V00.822 Baby stroller colliding with stationary object
    - V00.828 Other accident with baby stroller

● **V00.83 Accident with motorized mobility scooter**

● **V00.831 Fall from motorized mobility scooter**

Excludes1 fall from non-moving motorized mobility scooter (W05.2)

● **V00.832 Motorized mobility scooter colliding with stationary object**

● **V00.838 Other accident with motorized mobility scooter**

● **V00.84 Accident with standing micro-mobility pedestrian conveyance**

V00.841 Fall from standing electric scooter

V00.842 Pedestrian on standing electric scooter colliding with stationary object

V00.848 Other accident with standing micro-mobility pedestrian conveyance

Accident with hoverboard
Accident with segway

● **V00.89 Accident on other pedestrian conveyance**

● **V00.891 Fall from other pedestrian conveyance**

● **V00.892 Pedestrian on other pedestrian conveyance colliding with stationary object**

● **V00.898 Other accident on other pedestrian conveyance**

Excludes1 other pedestrian (conveyance) collision with other land transport vehicle (V01-V09 with 5th character 9)

● **V01 Pedestrian injured in collision with pedal cycle**

The appropriate 7th character is to be added to each code from category V01

A	initial encounter
D	subsequent encounter
S	sequela

● **V01.0 Pedestrian injured in collision with pedal cycle in nontraffic accident**

X● **V01.00 Pedestrian on foot injured in collision with pedal cycle in nontraffic accident**

Pedestrian NOS injured in collision with pedal cycle in nontraffic accident

X● **V01.01 Pedestrian on roller-skates injured in collision with pedal cycle in nontraffic accident**

X● **V01.02 Pedestrian on skateboard injured in collision with pedal cycle in nontraffic accident**

● **V01.03 Pedestrian on standing micro-mobility pedestrian conveyance injured in collision with pedal cycle in nontraffic accident**

V01.031 Pedestrian on standing electric scooter injured in collision with pedal cycle in nontraffic accident

V01.038 Pedestrian on other standing micro-mobility pedestrian conveyance injured in collision with pedal cycle in nontraffic accident

Pedestrian on hoverboard injured in collision with pedal cycle in nontraffic accident
Pedestrian on segway injured in collision with pedal cycle in nontraffic accident

X● **V01.09 Pedestrian with other conveyance injured in collision with pedal cycle in nontraffic accident**

Pedestrian with baby stroller injured in collision with pedal cycle in nontraffic accident
Pedestrian in wheelchair (powered) injured in collision with pedal cycle in nontraffic accident
Pedestrian in motorized mobility scooter injured in collision with pedal cycle in nontraffic accident
Pedestrian on ice-skates injured in collision with pedal cycle in nontraffic accident
Pedestrian on nonmotorized scooter injured in collision with pedal cycle in nontraffic accident
Pedestrian on sled injured in collision with pedal cycle in nontraffic accident
Pedestrian on snowboard injured in collision with pedal cycle in nontraffic accident
Pedestrian on snow-skis injured in collision with pedal cycle in nontraffic accident

● **V01.1 Pedestrian injured in collision with pedal cycle in traffic accident**

X● **V01.10 Pedestrian on foot injured in collision with pedal cycle in traffic accident**

Pedestrian NOS injured in collision with pedal cycle in traffic accident

X● **V01.11 Pedestrian on roller-skates injured in collision with pedal cycle in traffic accident**

X● **V01.12 Pedestrian on skateboard injured in collision with pedal cycle in traffic accident**

● **V01.13 Pedestrian on standing micro-mobility pedestrian conveyance injured in collision with pedal cycle in traffic accident**

V01.131 Pedestrian on standing electric scooter injured in collision with pedal cycle in traffic accident

V01.138 Pedestrian on other standing micro-mobility pedestrian conveyance injured in collision with pedal cycle in traffic accident

Pedestrian on hoverboard injured in collision with pedal cycle in traffic accident
Pedestrian on segway injured in collision with pedal cycle in traffic accident

X● **V01.19 Pedestrian with other conveyance injured in collision with pedal cycle in traffic accident**

Pedestrian with baby stroller injured in collision with pedal cycle in traffic accident
Pedestrian in wheelchair (powered) injured in collision with pedal cycle in traffic accident
Pedestrian in motorized mobility scooter injured in collision with pedal cycle in traffic accident
Pedestrian on ice-skates injured in collision with pedal cycle in traffic accident
Pedestrian on nonmotorized scooter injured in collision with pedal cycle in traffic accident
Pedestrian on sled injured in collision with pedal cycle in traffic accident
Pedestrian on snowboard injured in collision with pedal cycle in traffic accident
Pedestrian on snow-skis injured in collision with pedal cycle in traffic accident

V01.9 Pedestrian injured in collision with pedal cycle, unspecified whether traffic or nontraffic accident

X **V01.90 Pedestrian on foot injured in collision with pedal cycle, unspecified whether traffic or nontraffic accident**
Pedestrian NOS injured in collision with pedal cycle, unspecified whether traffic or nontraffic accident

X **V01.91 Pedestrian on roller-skates injured in collision with pedal cycle, unspecified whether traffic or nontraffic accident**

X **V01.92 Pedestrian on skateboard injured in collision with pedal cycle, unspecified whether traffic or nontraffic accident**

V01.93 Pedestrian on standing micro-mobility pedestrian conveyance injured in collision with pedal cycle, unspecified whether traffic or nontraffic accident

V01.931 Pedestrian on standing electric scooter injured in collision with pedal cycle, unspecified whether traffic or nontraffic accident

V01.938 Pedestrian on other standing micro-mobility pedestrian conveyance injured in collision with pedal cycle, unspecified whether traffic or nontraffic accident
Pedestrian on hoverboard injured in collision with pedal cycle, unspecified whether traffic or nontraffic accident
Pedestrian on segway injured in collision with pedal cycle, unspecified whether traffic or nontraffic accident

X **V01.99 Pedestrian with other conveyance injured in collision with pedal cycle, unspecified whether traffic or nontraffic accident**
Pedestrian with baby stroller injured in collision with pedal cycle, unspecified whether traffic or nontraffic accident
Pedestrian in wheelchair (powered) injured in collision with pedal cycle, unspecified whether traffic or nontraffic accident
Pedestrian in motorized mobility scooter injured in collision with pedal cycle, unspecified whether traffic or nontraffic accident
Pedestrian on ice-skates injured in collision with pedal cycle unspecified, whether traffic or nontraffic accident
Pedestrian on nonmotorized scooter injured in collision with pedal cycle, unspecified whether traffic or nontraffic accident
Pedestrian on sled injured in collision with pedal cycle unspecified, whether traffic or nontraffic accident
Pedestrian on snowboard injured in collision with pedal cycle, unspecified whether traffic or nontraffic accident
Pedestrian on snow-skis injured in collision with pedal cycle, unspecified whether traffic or nontraffic accident

V02 Pedestrian injured in collision with two- or three-wheeled motor vehicle

The appropriate 7th character is to be added to each code from category V02

A initial encounter
D subsequent encounter
S sequela

V02.0 Pedestrian injured in collision with two- or three-wheeled motor vehicle in nontraffic accident

X **V02.00 Pedestrian on foot injured in collision with two- or three-wheeled motor vehicle in nontraffic accident**
Pedestrian NOS injured in collision with two- or three-wheeled motor vehicle in nontraffic accident

X **V02.01 Pedestrian on roller-skates injured in collision with two- or three-wheeled motor vehicle in nontraffic accident**

X **V02.02 Pedestrian on skateboard injured in collision with two- or three-wheeled motor vehicle in nontraffic accident**

V02.03 Pedestrian on standing micro-mobility pedestrian conveyance injured in collision with two- or three-wheeled motor vehicle in nontraffic accident

V02.031 Pedestrian on standing electric scooter injured in collision with two- or three-wheeled motor vehicle in nontraffic accident

V02.038 Pedestrian on other standing micro-mobility pedestrian conveyance injured in collision with two- or three-wheeled motor vehicle in nontraffic accident
Pedestrian on hoverboard injured in collision with two-or three wheeled motor vehicle in nontraffic accident
Pedestrian on segway injured in collision with two- or three-wheeled motor vehicle in nontraffic accident

X **V02.09 Pedestrian with other conveyance injured in collision with two- or three-wheeled motor vehicle in nontraffic accident**
Pedestrian with baby stroller injured in collision with two- or three-wheeled motor vehicle in nontraffic accident
Pedestrian on ice-skates injured in collision with two- or three-wheeled motor vehicle in nontraffic accident
Pedestrian in wheelchair (powered) injured in collision with two- or three-wheeled motor vehicle in nontraffic accident
Pedestrian in motorized mobility scooter injured in collision with two- or three-wheeled motor vehicle in nontraffic accident
Pedestrian on nonmotorized scooter injured in collision with two- or three-wheeled motor vehicle in nontraffic accident
Pedestrian on sled injured in collision with two- or three-wheeled motor vehicle in nontraffic accident
Pedestrian on snowboard injured in collision with two- or three-wheeled motor vehicle in nontraffic accident
Pedestrian on snow-skis injured in collision with two- or three-wheeled motor vehicle in nontraffic accident

● **V02.1 Pedestrian injured in collision with two- or three-wheeled motor vehicle in traffic accident**

X● **V02.10 Pedestrian on foot injured in collision with two- or three-wheeled motor vehicle in traffic accident**

Pedestrian NOS injured in collision with two- or three-wheeled motor vehicle in traffic accident

X● **V02.11 Pedestrian on roller-skates injured in collision with two- or three-wheeled motor vehicle in traffic accident**

X● **V02.12 Pedestrian on skateboard injured in collision with two- or three-wheeled motor vehicle in traffic accident**

● **V02.13 Pedestrian on standing micro-mobility pedestrian conveyance injured in collision with two- or three-wheeled motor vehicle in traffic accident**

V02.131 Pedestrian on standing electric scooter injured in collision with two- or three-wheeled motor vehicle in traffic accident

V02.138 Pedestrian on other standing micro-mobility pedestrian conveyance injured in collision with two- or three-wheeled motor vehicle in traffic accident

Pedestrian on hoverboard injured in collision with two-or three wheeled motor vehicle in traffic accident

Pedestrian on segway injured in collision with two- or three-wheeled motor vehicle in traffic accident

X● **V02.19 Pedestrian with other conveyance injured in collision with two- or three-wheeled motor vehicle in traffic accident**

Pedestrian with baby stroller injured in collision with two- or three-wheeled motor vehicle in traffic accident

Pedestrian in wheelchair (powered) injured in collision with two- or three-wheeled motor vehicle in traffic accident

Pedestrian in motorized mobility scooter injured in collision with two- or three-wheeled motor vehicle in traffic accident

Pedestrian on ice-skates injured in collision with two- or three-wheeled motor vehicle in traffic accident

Pedestrian on nonmotorized scooter injured in collision with two- or three-wheeled motor vehicle in traffic accident

Pedestrian on sled injured in collision with two- or three-wheeled motor vehicle in traffic accident

Pedestrian on snowboard injured in collision with two- or three-wheeled motor vehicle in traffic accident

Pedestrian on snow-skis injured in collision with two- or three-wheeled motor vehicle in traffic accident

● **V02.9 Pedestrian injured in collision with two- or three-wheeled motor vehicle, unspecified whether traffic or nontraffic accident**

X● **V02.90 Pedestrian on foot injured in collision with two- or three-wheeled motor vehicle, unspecified whether traffic or nontraffic accident**

Pedestrian NOS injured in collision with two- or three-wheeled motor vehicle, unspecified whether traffic or nontraffic accident

X● **V02.91 Pedestrian on roller-skates injured in collision with two- or three-wheeled motor vehicle, unspecified whether traffic or nontraffic accident**

X● **V02.92 Pedestrian on skateboard injured in collision with two- or three-wheeled motor vehicle, unspecified whether traffic or nontraffic accident**

● **V02.93 Pedestrian on standing micro-mobility pedestrian conveyance injured in collision with two-or three-wheeled motor vehicle, unspecified whether traffic or nontraffic accident**

V02.931 Pedestrian on standing electric scooter injured in collision with two- or three wheeled motor vehicle, unspecified whether traffic or nontraffic accident

V02.938 Pedestrian on other standing micro-mobility pedestrian conveyance injured in collision with two- or three wheeled motor vehicle, unspecified whether traffic or nontraffic accident

Pedestrian on hoverboard injured in collision with two-three-wheeled motor vehicle, unspecified whether traffic or nontraffic accident

Pedestrian on segway injured in collision with two- or three wheeled motor vehicle, unspecified whether traffic or nontraffic accident

X● **V02.99 Pedestrian with other conveyance injured in collision with two- or three-wheeled motor vehicle, unspecified whether traffic or nontraffic accident**

Pedestrian with baby stroller injured in collision with two- or three-wheeled motor vehicle, unspecified whether traffic or nontraffic accident

Pedestrian in wheelchair (powered) injured in collision with two- or three-wheeled motor vehicle, unspecified whether traffic or nontraffic accident

Pedestrian in motorized mobility scooter injured in collision with two- or three-wheeled motor vehicle, unspecified whether traffic or nontraffic accident

Pedestrian on ice-skates injured in collision with two- or three-wheeled motor vehicle, unspecified whether traffic or nontraffic accident

Pedestrian on nonmotorized scooter injured in collision with two- or three-wheeled motor vehicle, unspecified whether traffic or nontraffic accident

Pedestrian on sled injured in collision with two- or three-wheeled motor vehicle, unspecified whether traffic or nontraffic accident

Pedestrian on snowboard injured in collision with two- or three-wheeled motor vehicle, unspecified whether traffic or nontraffic accident

Pedestrian on snow-skis injured in collision with two- or three-wheeled motor vehicle, unspecified whether traffic or nontraffic accident

V03 Pedestrian injured in collision with car, pick-up truck or van

The appropriate 7th character is to be added to each code from category V03

A	initial encounter
D	subsequent encounter
S	sequela

V03.0 Pedestrian injured in collision with car, pick-up truck or van in nontraffic accident

X **V03.00 Pedestrian on foot injured in collision with car, pick-up truck or van in nontraffic accident**

Pedestrian NOS injured in collision with car, pick-up truck or van in nontraffic accident

X **V03.01 Pedestrian on roller-skates injured in collision with car, pick-up truck or van in nontraffic accident**

X **V03.02 Pedestrian on skateboard injured in collision with car, pick-up truck or van in nontraffic accident**

V03.03 Pedestrian on standing micro-mobility pedestrian conveyance injured in collision with car, pick-up or van in nontraffic accident

V03.031 Pedestrian on standing electric scooter injured in collision with car, pick-up or van in nontraffic accident

V03.038 Pedestrian on other standing micro-mobility pedestrian conveyance injured in collision with car, pick-up or van in nontraffic accident

Pedestrian on hoverboard injured in collision with car, pick-up or van in nontraffic accident

Pedestrian on segway injured in collision with car, pick-up or van in nontraffic accident

X **V03.09 Pedestrian with other conveyance injured in collision with car, pick-up truck or van in nontraffic accident**

Pedestrian with baby stroller injured in collision with car, pick-up truck or van in nontraffic accident

Pedestrian in wheelchair (powered) injured in collision with car, pick-up truck or van in nontraffic accident

Pedestrian in motorized mobility scooter injured in collision with car, pick-up truck or van in nontraffic accident

Pedestrian on ice-skates injured in collision with car, pick-up truck or van in nontraffic accident

Pedestrian on nonmotorized scooter injured in collision with car, pick-up truck or van in nontraffic accident

Pedestrian on sled injured in collision with car, pick-up truck or van in nontraffic accident

Pedestrian on snowboard injured in collision with car, pick-up truck or van in nontraffic accident

Pedestrian on snow-skis injured in collision with car, pick-up truck or van in nontraffic accident

V03.1 Pedestrian injured in collision with car, pick-up truck or van in traffic accident

X **V03.10 Pedestrian on foot injured in collision with car, pick-up truck or van in traffic accident**

Pedestrian NOS injured in collision with car, pick-up truck or van in traffic accident

X **V03.11 Pedestrian on roller-skates injured in collision with car, pick-up truck or van in traffic accident**

X **V03.12 Pedestrian on skateboard injured in collision with car, pick-up truck or van in traffic accident**

V03.13 Pedestrian on standing micro-mobility pedestrian conveyance injured in collision with car, pick-up or van in traffic accident

V03.131 Pedestrian on standing electric scooter injured in collision with car, pick-up or van in traffic accident

V03.138 Pedestrian on other standing micro-mobility pedestrian conveyance injured in collision with car, pick-up or van in traffic accident

Pedestrian on hoverboard injured in collision with car, pick-up or van in traffic accident

Pedestrian on segway injured in collision with car, pick-up or van in traffic accident

X **V03.19 Pedestrian with other conveyance injured in collision with car, pick-up truck or van in traffic accident**

Pedestrian with baby stroller injured in collision with car, pick-up truck or van in traffic accident

Pedestrian in wheelchair (powered) injured in collision with car, pick-up truck or van in traffic accident

Pedestrian in motorized mobility scooter injured in collision with car, pick-up truck or van in traffic accident

Pedestrian on ice-skates injured in collision with car, pick-up truck or van in traffic accident

Pedestrian on nonmotorized scooter injured in collision with car, pick-up truck or van in traffic accident

Pedestrian on sled injured in collision with car, pick-up truck or van in traffic accident

Pedestrian on snowboard injured in collision with car, pick-up truck or van in traffic accident

Pedestrian on snow-skis injured in collision with car, pick-up truck or van in traffic accident

V03.9 Pedestrian injured in collision with car, pick-up truck or van, unspecified whether traffic or nontraffic accident

X **V03.90 Pedestrian on foot injured in collision with car, pick-up truck or van, unspecified whether traffic or nontraffic accident**

Pedestrian NOS injured in collision with car, pick-up truck or van, unspecified whether traffic or nontraffic accident

X **V03.91 Pedestrian on roller-skates injured in collision with car, pick-up truck or van, unspecified whether traffic or nontraffic accident**

X **V03.92 Pedestrian on skateboard injured in collision with car, pick-up truck or van, unspecified whether traffic or nontraffic accident**

● V03.93 **Pedestrian on standing micro-mobility pedestrian conveyance injured in collision with car, pick-up or van, unspecified whether traffic or nontraffic accident**

V03.931 **Pedestrian on standing electric scooter injured in collision with car, pick-up or van, unspecified whether traffic or nontraffic accident**

V03.938 **Pedestrian on other standing micro-mobility pedestrian conveyance injured in collision with car, pick-up or van, unspecified whether traffic or nontraffic accident**

Pedestrian on hoverboard injured in collision with car, pick-up or van, unspecified whether traffic or nontraffic accident

Pedestrian on segway injured in collision with car, pick-up or van, unspecified whether traffic or nontraffic accident

X● V03.99 **Pedestrian with other conveyance injured in collision with car, pick-up truck or van, unspecified whether traffic or nontraffic accident**

Pedestrian with baby stroller injured in collision with car, pick-up truck or van, unspecified whether traffic or nontraffic accident

Pedestrian in wheelchair (powered) injured in collision with car, pick-up truck or van, unspecified whether traffic or nontraffic accident

Pedestrian in motorized mobility scooter injured in collision with car, pick-up truck or van, unspecified whether traffic or nontraffic accident

Pedestrian on ice-skates injured in collision with car, pick-up truck or van, unspecified whether traffic or nontraffic accident

Pedestrian on nonmotorized scooter injured in collision with car, pick-up truck or van, unspecified whether traffic or nontraffic accident

Pedestrian on sled injured in collision with car, pick-up truck or van in nontraffic accident

Pedestrian on snowboard injured in collision with car, pick-up truck or van, unspecified whether traffic or nontraffic accident

Pedestrian on snow-skis injured in collision with car, pick-up truck or van, unspecified whether traffic or nontraffic accident

● V04 **Pedestrian injured in collision with heavy transport vehicle or bus**

Excludes1 pedestrian injured in collision with military vehicle (V09.01, V09.21)

The appropriate 7th character is to be added to each code from category V04

A	initial encounter
D	subsequent encounter
S	sequela

● V04.0 **Pedestrian injured in collision with heavy transport vehicle or bus in nontraffic accident**

X● V04.00 **Pedestrian on foot injured in collision with heavy transport vehicle or bus in nontraffic accident**

Pedestrian NOS injured in collision with heavy transport vehicle or bus in nontraffic accident

X● V04.01 **Pedestrian on roller-skates injured in collision with heavy transport vehicle or bus in nontraffic accident**

X● V04.02 **Pedestrian on skateboard injured in collision with heavy transport vehicle or bus in nontraffic accident**

● V04.03 **Pedestrian on standing micro-mobility pedestrian conveyance injured in collision with heavy transport vehicle or bus in nontraffic accident**

V04.031 **Pedestrian on standing electric scooter injured in collision with heavy transport vehicle or bus in nontraffic accident**

V04.038 **Pedestrian on other standing micro-mobility pedestrian conveyance injured in collision with heavy transport vehicle or bus in nontraffic accident**

Pedestrian on hoverboard injured in collision with heavy transport vehicle or bus in nontraffic accident

Pedestrian on segway injured in collision with heavy transport vehicle or bus in nontraffic accident

X● V04.09 **Pedestrian with other conveyance injured in collision with heavy transport vehicle or bus in nontraffic accident**

Pedestrian with baby stroller injured in collision with heavy transport vehicle or bus in nontraffic accident

Pedestrian in wheelchair (powered) injured in collision with heavy transport vehicle or bus in nontraffic accident

Pedestrian in motorized mobility scooter injured in collision with heavy transport vehicle or bus in nontraffic accident

Pedestrian on ice-skates injured in collision with heavy transport vehicle or bus in nontraffic accident

Pedestrian on nonmotorized scooter injured in collision with heavy transport vehicle or bus in nontraffic accident

Pedestrian on sled injured in collision with heavy transport vehicle or bus in nontraffic accident

Pedestrian on snowboard injured in collision with heavy transport vehicle or bus in nontraffic accident

Pedestrian on snow-skis injured in collision with heavy transport vehicle or bus in nontraffic accident

● V04.1 **Pedestrian injured in collision with heavy transport vehicle or bus in traffic accident**

X● V04.10 **Pedestrian on foot injured in collision with heavy transport vehicle or bus in traffic accident**

Pedestrian NOS injured in collision with heavy transport vehicle or bus in traffic accident

X● V04.11 **Pedestrian on roller-skates injured in collision with heavy transport vehicle or bus in traffic accident**

X● V04.12 **Pedestrian on skateboard injured in collision with heavy transport vehicle or bus in traffic accident**

● V04.13 **Pedestrian on standing micro-mobility pedestrian conveyance injured in collision with heavy transport vehicle or bus in traffic accident**

V04.131 **Pedestrian on standing electric scooter injured in collision with heavy transport vehicle or bus in traffic accident**

V04.138 **Pedestrian on other standing micro-mobility pedestrian conveyance injured in collision with heavy transport vehicle or bus in traffic accident**
Pedestrian on hoverboard injured in collision with heavy transport vehicle or bus in traffic accident
Pedestrian on segway injured in collision with heavy transport vehicle or bus in traffic accident

X● V04.19 **Pedestrian with other conveyance injured in collision with heavy transport vehicle or bus in traffic accident**
Pedestrian with baby stroller injured in collision with heavy transport vehicle or bus in traffic accident
Pedestrian in wheelchair (powered) injured in collision with heavy transport vehicle or bus in traffic accident
Pedestrian in motorized mobility scooter injured in collision with heavy transport vehicle or bus in traffic accident
Pedestrian on ice-skates injured in collision with heavy transport vehicle or bus in traffic accident
Pedestrian on nonmotorized scooter injured in collision with heavy transport vehicle or bus in traffic accident
Pedestrian on sled injured in collision with heavy transport vehicle or bus in traffic accident
Pedestrian on snowboard injured in collision with heavy transport vehicle or bus in traffic accident
Pedestrian on snow-skis injured in collision with heavy transport vehicle or bus in traffic accident

● V04.9 **Pedestrian injured in collision with heavy transport vehicle or bus, unspecified whether traffic or nontraffic accident**

X● V04.90 **Pedestrian on foot injured in collision with heavy transport vehicle or bus, unspecified whether traffic or nontraffic accident**
Pedestrian NOS injured in collision with heavy transport vehicle or bus, unspecified whether traffic or nontraffic accident

X● V04.91 **Pedestrian on roller-skates injured in collision with heavy transport vehicle or bus, unspecified whether traffic or nontraffic accident**

X● V04.92 **Pedestrian on skateboard injured in collision with heavy transport vehicle or bus, unspecified whether traffic or nontraffic accident**

● V04.93 **Pedestrian on standing micro-mobility pedestrian conveyance injured in collision with heavy transport vehicle or bus, unspecified whether traffic or nontraffic accident**

V04.931 **Pedestrian on standing electric scooter injured in collision with heavy transport vehicle or bus, unspecified whether traffic or nontraffic accident**

V04.938 **Pedestrian on other standing micro-mobility pedestrian conveyance injured in collision with heavy transport vehicle or bus, unspecified whether traffic or nontraffic accident**
Pedestrian on hoverboard injured in collision with heavy transport vehicle or bus, unspecified whether traffic or nontraffic accident
Pedestrian on segway injured in collision with heavy transport vehicle or bus, unspecified whether traffic or nontraffic accident

X● V04.99 **Pedestrian with other conveyance injured in collision with heavy transport vehicle or bus, unspecified whether traffic or nontraffic accident**
Pedestrian with baby stroller injured in collision with heavy transport vehicle or bus, unspecified whether traffic or nontraffic accident
Pedestrian in wheelchair (powered) injured in collision with heavy transport vehicle or bus, unspecified whether traffic or nontraffic accident
Pedestrian in motorized mobility scooter injured in collision with heavy transport vehicle or bus, unspecified whether traffic or nontraffic accident
Pedestrian on ice-skates injured in collision with heavy transport vehicle or bus, unspecified whether traffic or nontraffic accident
Pedestrian on nonmotorized scooter injured in collision with heavy transport vehicle or bus, unspecified whether traffic or nontraffic accident
Pedestrian on sled injured in collision with heavy transport vehicle or bus, unspecified whether traffic or nontraffic accident
Pedestrian on snowboard injured in collision with heavy transport vehicle or bus, unspecified whether traffic or nontraffic accident
Pedestrian on snow-skis injured in collision with heavy transport vehicle or bus, unspecified whether traffic or nontraffic accident

● V05 **Pedestrian injured in collision with railway train or railway vehicle**

The appropriate 7th character is to be added to each code from category V05

A	initial encounter
D	subsequent encounter
S	sequela

● V05.0 **Pedestrian injured in collision with railway train or railway vehicle in nontraffic accident**

X● V05.00 **Pedestrian on foot injured in collision with railway train or railway vehicle in nontraffic accident**
Pedestrian NOS injured in collision with railway train or railway vehicle in nontraffic accident

X● V05.01 **Pedestrian on roller-skates injured in collision with railway train or railway vehicle in nontraffic accident**

X● V05.02 **Pedestrian on skateboard injured in collision with railway train or railway vehicle in nontraffic accident**

● V05.03 **Pedestrian on standing micro-mobility pedestrian conveyance injured in collision with railway train or railway vehicle in nontraffic accident**

V05.031 **Pedestrian on standing electric scooter injured in collision with railway train or railway vehicle in nontraffic accident**

V05.038 **Pedestrian on other standing micro-mobility pedestrian conveyance injured in collision with railway train or railway vehicle in nontraffic accident**
Pedestrian on hoverboard injured in collision with railway train or railway vehicle in nontraffic accident
Pedestrian on segway injured in collision with railway train or railway vehicle in nontraffic accident

X● **VØ5.09 Pedestrian with other conveyance injured in collision with railway train or railway vehicle in nontraffic accident**
Pedestrian with baby stroller injured in collision with railway train or railway vehicle in nontraffic accident
Pedestrian in wheelchair (powered) injured in collision with railway train or railway vehicle in nontraffic accident
Pedestrian in motorized mobility scooter injured in collision with railway train or railway vehicle in nontraffic accident
Pedestrian on ice-skates injured in collision with railway train or railway vehicle in nontraffic accident
Pedestrian on nonmotorized scooter injured in collision with railway train or railway vehicle in nontraffic accident
Pedestrian on sled injured in collision with railway train or railway vehicle in nontraffic accident
Pedestrian on snowboard injured in collision with railway train or railway vehicle in nontraffic accident
Pedestrian on snow-skis injured in collision with railway train or railway vehicle in nontraffic accident

● **VØ5.1 Pedestrian injured in collision with railway train or railway vehicle in traffic accident**

X● **VØ5.10 Pedestrian on foot injured in collision with railway train or railway vehicle in traffic accident**
Pedestrian NOS injured in collision with railway train or railway vehicle in traffic accident

X● **VØ5.11 Pedestrian on roller-skates injured in collision with railway train or railway vehicle in traffic accident**

X● **VØ5.12 Pedestrian on skateboard injured in collision with railway train or railway vehicle in traffic accident**

● **VØ5.13 Pedestrian on standing micro-mobility pedestrian conveyance injured in collision with railway train or railway vehicle in traffic accident**

VØ5.131 Pedestrian on standing electric scooter injured in collision with railway train or railway vehicle in traffic accident

VØ5.138 Pedestrian on other standing micro-mobility pedestrian conveyance injured in collision with railway train or railway vehicle in traffic accident
Pedestrian on hoverboard injured in collision with railway train or railway vehicle in traffic accident
Pedestrian on segway injured in collision with railway train or railway vehicle in traffic accident

X● **VØ5.19 Pedestrian with other conveyance injured in collision with railway train or railway vehicle in traffic accident**
Pedestrian with baby stroller injured in collision with railway train or railway vehicle in traffic accident
Pedestrian in wheelchair (powered) injured in collision with railway train or railway vehicle in traffic accident
Pedestrian in motorized mobility scooter injured in collision with railway train or railway vehicle in traffic accident
Pedestrian on ice-skates injured in collision with railway train or railway vehicle in traffic accident
Pedestrian on nonmotorized scooter injured in collision with railway train or railway vehicle in traffic accident
Pedestrian on sled injured in collision with railway train or railway vehicle in traffic accident
Pedestrian on snowboard injured in collision with railway train or railway vehicle in traffic accident
Pedestrian on snow-skis injured in collision with railway train or railway vehicle in traffic accident

● **VØ5.9 Pedestrian injured in collision with railway train or railway vehicle, unspecified whether traffic or nontraffic accident**

X● **VØ5.90 Pedestrian on foot injured in collision with railway train or railway vehicle, unspecified whether traffic or nontraffic accident**
Pedestrian NOS injured in collision with railway train or railway vehicle, unspecified whether traffic or nontraffic accident

X● **VØ5.91 Pedestrian on roller-skates injured in collision with railway train or railway vehicle, unspecified whether traffic or nontraffic accident**

X● **VØ5.92 Pedestrian on skateboard injured in collision with railway train or railway vehicle, unspecified whether traffic or nontraffic accident**

● **VØ5.93 Pedestrian on standing micro-mobility pedestrian conveyance injured in collision with railway train or railway vehicle, unspecified whether traffic or nontraffic accident**

VØ5.931 Pedestrian on standing electric scooter injured in collision with railway train or railway vehicle, unspecified whether traffic or nontraffic accident

VØ5.938 Pedestrian on other standing micro-mobility pedestrian conveyance injured in collision with railway train or railway vehicle, unspecified whether traffic or nontraffic accident
Pedestrian on hoverboard injured in collision with railway train or railway vehicle, unspecified whether traffic or nontraffic accident
Pedestrian on segway injured in collision with railway train or railway vehicle, unspecified whether traffic or nontraffic accident

X● **V05.99 Pedestrian with other conveyance injured in collision with railway train or railway vehicle, unspecified whether traffic or nontraffic accident**
Pedestrian with baby stroller injured in collision with railway train or railway vehicle, unspecified whether traffic or nontraffic
Pedestrian in wheelchair (powered) injured in collision with railway train or railway vehicle, unspecified whether traffic or nontraffic
Pedestrian in motorized mobility scooter injured in collision with railway train or railway vehicle, unspecified whether traffic or nontraffic
Pedestrian on ice-skates injured in collision with railway train or railway vehicle, unspecified whether traffic or nontraffic
Pedestrian on nonmotorized scooter injured in collision with railway train or railway vehicle, unspecified whether traffic or nontraffic
Pedestrian on sled injured in collision with railway train or railway vehicle, unspecified whether traffic or nontraffic
Pedestrian on snowboard injured in collision with railway train or railway vehicle, unspecified whether traffic or nontraffic
Pedestrian on snow-skis injured in collision with railway train or railway vehicle, unspecified whether traffic or nontraffic

● **V06 Pedestrian injured in collision with other nonmotor vehicle**
Includes collision with animal-drawn vehicle, animal being ridden, nonpowered streetcar
Excludes1 pedestrian injured in collision with pedestrian conveyance (V00.0-)
The appropriate 7th character is to be added to each code from category V06

A	initial encounter
D	subsequent encounter
S	sequela

● **V06.0 Pedestrian injured in collision with other nonmotor vehicle in nontraffic accident**

X● **V06.00 Pedestrian on foot injured in collision with other nonmotor vehicle in nontraffic accident**
Pedestrian NOS injured in collision with other nonmotor vehicle in nontraffic accident

X● **V06.01 Pedestrian on roller-skates injured in collision with other nonmotor vehicle in nontraffic accident**

X● **V06.02 Pedestrian on skateboard injured in collision with other nonmotor vehicle in nontraffic accident**

● **V06.03 Pedestrian on standing micro-mobility pedestrian conveyance injured in collision with other nonmotor vehicle in nontraffic accident**

V06.031 Pedestrian on standing electric scooter injured in collision with other nonmotor vehicle in nontraffic accident

V06.038 Pedestrian on other standing micro-mobility pedestrian conveyance injured in collision with other nonmotor vehicle in nontraffic accident
Pedestrian on hoverboard injured in collision with other nonmotor vehicle in nontraffic accident
Pedestrian on segway injured in collision with other nonmotor vehicle in nontraffic accident

X● **V06.09 Pedestrian with other conveyance injured in collision with other nonmotor vehicle in nontraffic accident**
Pedestrian with baby stroller injured in collision with other nonmotor vehicle in nontraffic accident
Pedestrian in wheelchair (powered) injured in collision with other nonmotor vehicle in nontraffic accident
Pedestrian in motorized mobility scooter injured in collision with other nonmotor vehicle in nontraffic accident
Pedestrian on ice-skates injured in collision with other nonmotor vehicle in nontraffic accident
Pedestrian on nonmotorized scooter injured in collision with other nonmotor vehicle in nontraffic accident
Pedestrian on sled injured in collision with other nonmotor vehicle in nontraffic accident
Pedestrian on snowboard injured in collision with other nonmotor vehicle in nontraffic accident
Pedestrian on snow-skis injured in collision with other nonmotor vehicle in nontraffic accident

● **V06.1 Pedestrian injured in collision with other nonmotor vehicle in traffic accident**

X● **V06.10 Pedestrian on foot injured in collision with other nonmotor vehicle in traffic accident**
Pedestrian NOS injured in collision with other nonmotor vehicle in traffic accident

X● **V06.11 Pedestrian on roller-skates injured in collision with other nonmotor vehicle in traffic accident**

X● **V06.12 Pedestrian on skateboard injured in collision with other nonmotor vehicle in traffic accident**

● **V06.13 Pedestrian on standing micro-mobility pedestrian conveyance injured in collision with other nonmotor vehicle in traffic accident**

V06.131 Pedestrian on standing electric scooter injured in collision with other nonmotor vehicle in traffic accident

V06.138 Pedestrian on other standing micro-mobility pedestrian conveyance injured in collision with other nonmotor vehicle in traffic accident
Pedestrian on hoverboard injured in collision with other nonmotor vehicle in traffic accident
Pedestrian on segway injured in collision with other nonmotor vehicle in traffic accident

X● **V06.19 Pedestrian with other conveyance injured in collision with other nonmotor vehicle in traffic accident**
Pedestrian with baby stroller injured in collision with other nonmotor vehicle in nontraffic accident
Pedestrian in wheelchair (powered) injured in collision with other nonmotor vehicle in traffic accident
Pedestrian in motorized mobility scooter injured in collision with other nonmotor vehicle in traffic accident
Pedestrian on ice-skates injured in collision with other nonmotor vehicle in traffic accident
Pedestrian on nonmotorized scooter injured in collision with other nonmotor vehicle in traffic accident
Pedestrian on sled injured in collision with other nonmotor vehicle in traffic accident
Pedestrian on snowboard injured in collision with other nonmotor vehicle in traffic accident
Pedestrian on snow-skis injured in collision with other nonmotor vehicle in traffic accident

● **V06.9 Pedestrian injured in collision with other nonmotor vehicle, unspecified whether traffic or nontraffic accident**

X● **V06.90 Pedestrian on foot injured in collision with other nonmotor vehicle, unspecified whether traffic or nontraffic accident**

Pedestrian NOS injured in collision with other nonmotor vehicle, unspecified whether traffic or nontraffic accident

X● **V06.91 Pedestrian on roller-skates injured in collision with other nonmotor vehicle, unspecified whether traffic or nontraffic accident**

X● **V06.92 Pedestrian on skateboard injured in collision with other nonmotor vehicle, unspecified whether traffic or nontraffic accident**

● **V06.93 Pedestrian on standing micro-mobility pedestrian conveyance injured in collision with other nonmotor vehicle, unspecified whether traffic or nontraffic accident**

V06.931 Pedestrian on standing electric scooter injured in collision with other nonmotor vehicle, unspecified whether traffic or nontraffic accident

V06.938 Pedestrian on other standing micro-mobility pedestrian conveyance injured in collision with other nonmotor vehicle, unspecified whether traffic or nontraffic accident

Pedestrian on hoverboard injured in collision with other nonmotor, unspecified whether traffic or nontraffic accident

Pedestrian on segway injured in collision with other nonmotor vehicle, unspecified whether traffic or nontraffic accident

X● **V06.99 Pedestrian with other conveyance injured in collision with other nonmotor vehicle, unspecified whether traffic or nontraffic accident**

Pedestrian with baby stroller injured in collision with other nonmotor vehicle, unspecified whether traffic or nontraffic accident

Pedestrian in wheelchair (powered) injured in collision with other nonmotor vehicle, unspecified whether traffic or nontraffic accident

Pedestrian in motorized mobility scooter injured in collision with other nonmotor vehicle, unspecified whether traffic or nontraffic accident

Pedestrian on ice-skates injured in collision with other nonmotor vehicle, unspecified whether traffic or nontraffic accident

Pedestrian on nonmotorized scooter injured in collision with other nonmotor vehicle, unspecified whether traffic or nontraffic accident

Pedestrian on sled injured in collision with other nonmotor vehicle, unspecified whether traffic or nontraffic accident

Pedestrian on snowboard injured in collision with other nonmotor vehicle, unspecified whether traffic or nontraffic accident

Pedestrian on snow-skis injured in collision with other nonmotor vehicle, unspecified whether traffic or nontraffic accident

● **V09 Pedestrian injured in other and unspecified transport accidents**

The appropriate 7th character is to be added to each code from category V09

A	initial encounter
D	subsequent encounter
S	sequela

● **V09.0 Pedestrian injured in nontraffic accident involving other and unspecified motor vehicles**

X● **V09.00 Pedestrian injured in nontraffic accident involving unspecified motor vehicles**

X● **V09.01 Pedestrian injured in nontraffic accident involving military vehicle**

X● **V09.09 Pedestrian injured in nontraffic accident involving other motor vehicles**

Pedestrian injured in nontraffic accident by special vehicle

X● **V09.1 Pedestrian injured in unspecified nontraffic accident**

● **V09.2 Pedestrian injured in traffic accident involving other and unspecified motor vehicles**

X● **V09.20 Pedestrian injured in traffic accident involving unspecified motor vehicles**

X● **V09.21 Pedestrian injured in traffic accident involving military vehicle**

X● **V09.29 Pedestrian injured in traffic accident involving other motor vehicles**

X● **V09.3 Pedestrian injured in unspecified traffic accident**

X● **V09.9 Pedestrian injured in unspecified transport accident**

PEDAL CYCLE RIDER INJURED IN TRANSPORT ACCIDENT (V10-V19)

Includes any non-motorized vehicle, excluding an animal-drawn vehicle, or a sidecar or trailer attached to the pedal cycle

Excludes2 rupture of pedal cycle tire (W37.0)

● **V10 Pedal cycle rider injured in collision with pedestrian or animal**

Excludes1 pedal cycle rider collision with animal-drawn vehicle or animal being ridden (V16.-)

The appropriate 7th character is to be added to each code from category V10

A	initial encounter
D	subsequent encounter
S	sequela

X● **V10.0 Pedal cycle driver injured in collision with pedestrian or animal in nontraffic accident**

X● **V10.1 Pedal cycle passenger injured in collision with pedestrian or animal in nontraffic accident**

X● **V10.2 Unspecified pedal cyclist injured in collision with pedestrian or animal in nontraffic accident**

X● **V10.3 Person boarding or alighting a pedal cycle injured in collision with pedestrian or animal**

X● **V10.4 Pedal cycle driver injured in collision with pedestrian or animal in traffic accident**

X● **V10.5 Pedal cycle passenger injured in collision with pedestrian or animal in traffic accident**

X● **V10.9 Unspecified pedal cyclist injured in collision with pedestrian or animal in traffic accident**

● **V11 Pedal cycle rider injured in collision with other pedal cycle**

The appropriate 7th character is to be added to each code from category V11

A	initial encounter
D	subsequent encounter
S	sequela

X● **V11.0** **Pedal cycle driver injured in collision with other pedal cycle in nontraffic accident**

X● **V11.1** **Pedal cycle passenger injured in collision with other pedal cycle in nontraffic accident**

X● **V11.2** **Unspecified pedal cyclist injured in collision with other pedal cycle in nontraffic accident**

X● **V11.3** **Person boarding or alighting a pedal cycle injured in collision with other pedal cycle**

X● **V11.4** **Pedal cycle driver injured in collision with other pedal cycle in traffic accident**

X● **V11.5** **Pedal cycle passenger injured in collision with other pedal cycle in traffic accident**

X● **V11.9** **Unspecified pedal cyclist injured in collision with other pedal cycle in traffic accident**

● **V12 Pedal cycle rider injured in collision with two- or three-wheeled motor vehicle**

The appropriate 7th character is to be added to each code from category V12

A	initial encounter
D	subsequent encounter
S	sequela

X● **V12.0** **Pedal cycle driver injured in collision with two- or three-wheeled motor vehicle in nontraffic accident**

X● **V12.1** **Pedal cycle passenger injured in collision with two- or three-wheeled motor vehicle in nontraffic accident**

X● **V12.2** **Unspecified pedal cyclist injured in collision with two- or three-wheeled motor vehicle in nontraffic accident**

X● **V12.3** **Person boarding or alighting a pedal cycle injured in collision with two- or three-wheeled motor vehicle**

X● **V12.4** **Pedal cycle driver injured in collision with two- or three-wheeled motor vehicle in traffic accident**

X● **V12.5** **Pedal cycle passenger injured in collision with two- or three-wheeled motor vehicle in traffic accident**

X● **V12.9** **Unspecified pedal cyclist injured in collision with two- or three-wheeled motor vehicle in traffic accident**

● **V13 Pedal cycle rider injured in collision with car, pick-up truck or van**

The appropriate 7th character is to be added to each code from category V13

A	initial encounter
D	subsequent encounter
S	sequela

X● **V13.0** **Pedal cycle driver injured in collision with car, pick-up truck or van in nontraffic accident**

X● **V13.1** **Pedal cycle passenger injured in collision with car, pick-up truck or van in nontraffic accident**

X● **V13.2** **Unspecified pedal cyclist injured in collision with car, pick-up truck or van in nontraffic accident**

X● **V13.3** **Person boarding or alighting a pedal cycle injured in collision with car, pick-up truck or van**

X● **V13.4** **Pedal cycle driver injured in collision with car, pick-up truck or van in traffic accident**

X● **V13.5** **Pedal cycle passenger injured in collision with car, pick-up truck or van in traffic accident**

X● **V13.9** **Unspecified pedal cyclist injured in collision with car, pick-up truck or van in traffic accident**

● **V14 Pedal cycle rider injured in collision with heavy transport vehicle or bus**

Excludes1 pedal cycle rider injured in collision with military vehicle (V19.81)

The appropriate 7th character is to be added to each code from category V14

A	initial encounter
D	subsequent encounter
S	sequela

X● **V14.0** **Pedal cycle driver injured in collision with heavy transport vehicle or bus in nontraffic accident**

X● **V14.1** **Pedal cycle passenger injured in collision with heavy transport vehicle or bus in nontraffic accident**

X● **V14.2** **Unspecified pedal cyclist injured in collision with heavy transport vehicle or bus in nontraffic accident**

X● **V14.3** **Person boarding or alighting a pedal cycle injured in collision with heavy transport vehicle or bus**

X● **V14.4** **Pedal cycle driver injured in collision with heavy transport vehicle or bus in traffic accident**

X● **V14.5** **Pedal cycle passenger injured in collision with heavy transport vehicle or bus in traffic accident**

X● **V14.9** **Unspecified pedal cyclist injured in collision with heavy transport vehicle or bus in traffic accident**

● **V15 Pedal cycle rider injured in collision with railway train or railway vehicle**

The appropriate 7th character is to be added to each code from category V15

A	initial encounter
D	subsequent encounter
S	sequela

X● **V15.0** **Pedal cycle driver injured in collision with railway train or railway vehicle in nontraffic accident**

X● **V15.1** **Pedal cycle passenger injured in collision with railway train or railway vehicle in nontraffic accident**

X● **V15.2** **Unspecified pedal cyclist injured in collision with railway train or railway vehicle in nontraffic accident**

X● **V15.3** **Person boarding or alighting a pedal cycle injured in collision with railway train or railway vehicle**

X● **V15.4** **Pedal cycle driver injured in collision with railway train or railway vehicle in traffic accident**

X● **V15.5** **Pedal cycle passenger injured in collision with railway train or railway vehicle in traffic accident**

X● **V15.9** **Unspecified pedal cyclist injured in collision with railway train or railway vehicle in traffic accident**

● **V16 Pedal cycle rider injured in collision with other nonmotor vehicle**

Includes collision with animal-drawn vehicle, animal being ridden, streetcar

The appropriate 7th character is to be added to each code from category V16

A	initial encounter
D	subsequent encounter
S	sequela

X● **V16.0** **Pedal cycle driver injured in collision with other nonmotor vehicle in nontraffic accident**

X● **V16.1** **Pedal cycle passenger injured in collision with other nonmotor vehicle in nontraffic accident**

X● **V16.2** **Unspecified pedal cyclist injured in collision with other nonmotor vehicle in nontraffic accident**

X● **V16.3** **Person boarding or alighting a pedal cycle injured in collision with other nonmotor vehicle in nontraffic accident**

X● **V16.4** **Pedal cycle driver injured in collision with other nonmotor vehicle in traffic accident**

X● **V16.5 Pedal cycle passenger injured in collision with other nonmotor vehicle in traffic accident**

X● **V16.9 Unspecified pedal cyclist injured in collision with other nonmotor vehicle in traffic accident**

● **V17 Pedal cycle rider injured in collision with fixed or stationary object**

The appropriate 7th character is to be added to each code from category V17

A initial encounter
D subsequent encounter
S sequela

X● **V17.0 Pedal cycle driver injured in collision with fixed or stationary object in nontraffic accident**

X● **V17.1 Pedal cycle passenger injured in collision with fixed or stationary object in nontraffic accident**

X● **V17.2 Unspecified pedal cyclist injured in collision with fixed or stationary object in nontraffic accident**

X● **V17.3 Person boarding or alighting a pedal cycle injured in collision with fixed or stationary object**

X● **V17.4 Pedal cycle driver injured in collision with fixed or stationary object in traffic accident**

X● **V17.5 Pedal cycle passenger injured in collision with fixed or stationary object in traffic accident**

X● **V17.9 Unspecified pedal cyclist injured in collision with fixed or stationary object in traffic accident**

● **V18 Pedal cycle rider injured in noncollision transport accident**

Includes fall or thrown from pedal cycle (without antecedent collision)
overturning pedal cycle NOS
overturning pedal cycle without collision

The appropriate 7th character is to be added to each code from category V18

A initial encounter
D subsequent encounter
S sequela

X● **V18.0 Pedal cycle driver injured in noncollision transport accident in nontraffic accident**

X● **V18.1 Pedal cycle passenger injured in noncollision transport accident in nontraffic accident**

X● **V18.2 Unspecified pedal cyclist injured in noncollision transport accident in nontraffic accident**

X● **V18.3 Person boarding or alighting a pedal cycle injured in noncollision transport accident**

X● **V18.4 Pedal cycle driver injured in noncollision transport accident in traffic accident**

X● **V18.5 Pedal cycle passenger injured in noncollision transport accident in traffic accident**

X● **V18.9 Unspecified pedal cyclist injured in noncollision transport accident in traffic accident**

● **V19 Pedal cycle rider injured in other and unspecified transport accidents**

The appropriate 7th character is to be added to each code from category V19

A initial encounter
D subsequent encounter
S sequela

● **V19.0 Pedal cycle driver injured in collision with other and unspecified motor vehicles in nontraffic accident**

X● **V19.00 Pedal cycle driver injured in collision with unspecified motor vehicles in nontraffic accident**

X● **V19.09 Pedal cycle driver injured in collision with other motor vehicles in nontraffic accident**

● **V19.1 Pedal cycle passenger injured in collision with other and unspecified motor vehicles in nontraffic accident**

X● **V19.10 Pedal cycle passenger injured in collision with unspecified motor vehicles in nontraffic accident**

X● **V19.19 Pedal cycle passenger injured in collision with other motor vehicles in nontraffic accident**

● **V19.2 Unspecified pedal cyclist injured in collision with other and unspecified motor vehicles in nontraffic accident**

X● **V19.20 Unspecified pedal cyclist injured in collision with unspecified motor vehicles in nontraffic accident**
Pedal cycle collision NOS, nontraffic

X● **V19.29 Unspecified pedal cyclist injured in collision with other motor vehicles in nontraffic accident**

X● **V19.3 Pedal cyclist (driver) (passenger) injured in unspecified nontraffic accident**
Pedal cycle accident NOS, nontraffic
Pedal cyclist injured in nontraffic accident NOS

● **V19.4 Pedal cycle driver injured in collision with other and unspecified motor vehicles in traffic accident**

X● **V19.40 Pedal cycle driver injured in collision with unspecified motor vehicles in traffic accident**

X● **V19.49 Pedal cycle driver injured in collision with other motor vehicles in traffic accident**

● **V19.5 Pedal cycle passenger injured in collision with other and unspecified motor vehicles in traffic accident**

X● **V19.50 Pedal cycle passenger injured in collision with unspecified motor vehicles in traffic accident**

X● **V19.59 Pedal cycle passenger injured in collision with other motor vehicles in traffic accident**

● **V19.6 Unspecified pedal cyclist injured in collision with other and unspecified motor vehicles in traffic accident**

X● **V19.60 Unspecified pedal cyclist injured in collision with unspecified motor vehicles in traffic accident**
Pedal cycle collision NOS (traffic)

X● **V19.69 Unspecified pedal cyclist injured in collision with other motor vehicles in traffic accident**

● **V19.8 Pedal cyclist (driver) (passenger) injured in other specified transport accidents**

X● **V19.81 Pedal cyclist (driver) (passenger) injured in transport accident with military vehicle**

X● **V19.88 Pedal cyclist (driver) (passenger) injured in other specified transport accidents**

X● **V19.9 Pedal cyclist (driver) (passenger) injured in unspecified traffic accident**
Pedal cycle accident NOS

MOTORCYCLE RIDER INJURED IN TRANSPORT ACCIDENT (V20-V29)

Includes electric bicycle
e-bike
e-bicycle
moped motorcycle with sidecar motorized bicycle
motor scooter

Excludes1 three-wheeled motor vehicle (V30-V39)

● **V20 Motorcycle rider injured in collision with pedestrian or animal**

Excludes1 motorcycle rider collision with animal-drawn vehicle or animal being ridden (V26.-)

The appropriate 7th character is to be added to each code from category V20

A initial encounter
D subsequent encounter
S sequela

X● **V20.0 Motorcycle driver injured in collision with pedestrian or animal in nontraffic accident**

X● **V20.01 Electric (assisted) bicycle driver injured in collision with pedestrian or animal in nontraffic accident**

X● **V20.09 Other motorcycle driver injured in collision with pedestrian or animal in nontraffic accident**

CHAPTER 20 (V00-Y99)

X● V20.1 Motorcycle passenger injured in collision with pedestrian or animal in nontraffic accident

X● V20.11 Electric (assisted) bicycle passenger injured in collision with pedestrian or animal in nontraffic accident

X● V20.19 Other motorcycle passenger injured in collision with pedestrian or animal in nontraffic accident

X● V20.2 Unspecified motorcycle rider injured in collision with pedestrian or animal in nontraffic accident

X● V20.21 Unspecified electric (assisted) bicycle rider injured in collision with pedestrian or animal in nontraffic accident

X● V20.29 Unspecified rider of other motorcycle injured in collision with pedestrian or animal in nontraffic accident

X● V20.3 Person boarding or alighting a motorcycle injured in collision with pedestrian or animal

X● V20.31 Person boarding or alighting an electric (assisted) bicycle injured in collision with pedestrian or animal

X● V20.39 Person boarding or alighting other motorcycle injured in collision with pedestrian or animal

X● V20.4 Motorcycle driver injured in collision with pedestrian or animal in traffic accident

X● V20.41 Electric (assisted) bicycle driver injured in collision with pedestrian or animal in traffic accident

X● V20.49 Other motorcycle driver injured in collision with pedestrian or animal in traffic accident

X● V20.5 Motorcycle passenger injured in collision with pedestrian or animal in traffic accident

X● V20.51 Electric (assisted) bicycle passenger injured in collision with pedestrian or animal in traffic accident

X● V20.59 Other motorcycle passenger injured in collision with pedestrian or animal in traffic accident

X● V20.9 Unspecified motorcycle rider injured in collision with pedestrian or animal in traffic accident

X● V20.91 Unspecified electric (assisted) bicycle rider injured in collision with pedestrian or animal in traffic accident

X● V20.99 Unspecified rider of other motorcycle injured in collision with pedestrian or animal in traffic accident

● V21 Motorcycle rider injured in collision with pedal cycle

The appropriate 7th character is to be added to each code from category V21

A	initial encounter
D	subsequent encounter
S	sequela

X● V21.0 Motorcycle driver injured in collision with pedal cycle in nontraffic accident

X● V21.01 Electric (assisted) bicycle driver injured in collision with pedal cycle in nontraffic accident

X● V21.09 Other motorcycle driver injured in collision with pedal cycle in nontraffic accident

X● V21.1 Motorcycle passenger injured in collision with pedal cycle in nontraffic accident

X● V21.11 Electric (assisted) bicycle passenger injured in collision with pedal cycle in nontraffic accident

X● V21.19 Other motorcycle passenger injured in collision with pedal cycle in nontraffic accident

X● V21.2 Unspecified motorcycle rider injured in collision with pedal cycle in nontraffic accident

X● V21.21 Unspecified electric (assisted) bicycle rider injured in collision with pedal cycle in nontraffic accident

X● V21.29 Unspecified rider of other motorcycle injured in collision with pedal cycle in nontraffic accident

X● V21.3 Person boarding or alighting a motorcycle injured in collision with pedal cycle

X● V21.31 Person boarding or alighting an electric (assisted) bicycle injured in collision with pedal cycle

X● V21.39 Person boarding or alighting other motorcycle injured in collision with pedal cycle

X● V21.4 Motorcycle driver injured in collision with pedal cycle in traffic accident

X● V21.41 Electric (assisted) bicycle driver injured in collision with pedal cycle in traffic accident

X● V21.49 Other motorcycle driver injured in collision with pedal cycle in traffic accident

X● V21.5 Motorcycle passenger injured in collision with pedal cycle in traffic accident

X● V21.51 Electric (assisted) bicycle passenger injured in collision with pedal cycle in traffic accident

X● V21.59 Other motorcycle passenger injured in collision with pedal cycle in traffic accident

X● V21.9 Unspecified motorcycle rider injured in collision with pedal cycle in traffic accident

X● V21.91 Unspecified electric (assisted) bicycle rider injured in collision with pedal cycle in traffic accident

X● V21.99 Unspecified rider of other motorcycle injured in collision with pedal cycle in traffic accident

● V22 Motorcycle rider injured in collision with two- or three-wheeled motor vehicle

The appropriate 7th character is to be added to each code from category V22

A	initial encounter
D	subsequent encounter
S	sequela

X● V22.0 Motorcycle driver injured in collision with two- or three-wheeled motor vehicle in nontraffic accident

X● V22.01 Electric (assisted) bicycle driver injured in collision with two- or three-wheeled motor vehicle in nontraffic accident

X● V22.09 Other motorcycle driver injured in collision with two- or three-wheeled motor vehicle in nontraffic accident

X● V22.1 Motorcycle passenger injured in collision with two- or three-wheeled motor vehicle in nontraffic accident

X● V22.11 Electric (assisted) bicycle passenger injured in collision with two- or three-wheeled motor vehicle in nontraffic accident

X● V22.19 Other motorcycle passenger injured in collision with two- or three-wheeled motor vehicle in nontraffic accident

X● V22.2 Unspecified motorcycle rider injured in collision with two- or three-wheeled motor vehicle in nontraffic accident

X● V22.21 Unspecified electric (assisted) bicycle rider injured in collision with two- or three-wheeled motor vehicle in nontraffic accident

X● V22.29 Unspecified rider of other motorcycle injured in collision with two- or three-wheeled motor vehicle in nontraffic accident

X● V22.3 Person boarding or alighting a motorcycle injured in collision with two- or three-wheeled motor vehicle

X● V22.31 Person boarding or alighting an electric (assisted) bicycle injured in collision with two- or three-wheeled motor vehicle

X● V22.39 Person boarding or alighting other motorcycle injured in collision with two- or three-wheeled motor vehicle

X● **V22.4 Motorcycle driver injured in collision with two- or three-wheeled motor vehicle in traffic accident**

X● **V22.41 Electric (assisted) bicycle driver injured in collision with two- or three-wheeled motor vehicle in traffic accident**

X● **V22.49 Other motorcycle driver injured in collision with two- or three-wheeled motor vehicle in traffic accident**

X● **V22.5 Motorcycle passenger injured in collision with two- or three-wheeled motor vehicle in traffic accident**

X● **V22.51 Electric (assisted) bicycle passenger injured in collision with two- or three-wheeled motor vehicle in traffic accident**

X● **V22.59 Other motorcycle passenger injured in collision with two- or three-wheeled motor vehicle in traffic accident**

X● **V22.9 Unspecified motorcycle rider injured in collision with two- or three-wheeled motor vehicle in traffic accident**

X● **V22.91 Unspecified electric (assisted) bicycle rider injured in collision with two- or three-wheeled motor vehicle in traffic accident**

X● **V22.99 Unspecified rider of other motorcycle injured in collision with two- or three-wheeled motor vehicle in traffic accident**

● **V23 Motorcycle rider injured in collision with car, pick-up truck or van**

The appropriate 7th character is to be added to each code from category V23

A	initial encounter
D	subsequent encounter
S	sequela

X● **V23.0 Motorcycle driver injured in collision with car, pick-up truck or van in nontraffic accident**

X● **V23.01 Electric (assisted) bicycle driver injured in collision with car, pick-up truck or van in nontraffic accident**

X● **V23.09 Other motorcycle driver injured in collision with car, pick-up truck or van in nontraffic accident**

X● **V23.1 Motorcycle passenger injured in collision with car, pick-up truck or van in nontraffic accident**

X● **V23.11 Electric (assisted) bicycle passenger injured in collision with car, pick-up truck or van in nontraffic accident**

X● **V23.19 Other motorcycle passenger injured in collision with car, pick-up truck or van in nontraffic accident**

X● **V23.2 Unspecified motorcycle rider injured in collision with car, pick-up truck or van in nontraffic accident**

X● **V23.21 Unspecified electric (assisted) bicycle rider injured in collision with car, pick-up truck or van in nontraffic accident**

X● **V23.29 Unspecified rider of other motorcycle injured in collision with car, pick-up truck or van in nontraffic accident**

X● **V23.3 Person boarding or alighting a motorcycle injured in collision with car, pick-up truck or van**

X● **V23.31 Person boarding or alighting an electric (assisted) bicycle injured in collision with car, pick-up truck or van**

X● **V23.39 Person boarding or alighting other motorcycle injured in collision with car, pick-up truck or van**

X● **V23.4 Motorcycle driver injured in collision with car, pick-up truck or van in traffic accident**

X● **V23.41 Electric (assisted) bicycle driver injured in collision with car, pick-up truck or van in traffic accident**

X● **V23.49 Other motorcycle driver injured in collision with car, pick-up truck or van in traffic accident**

X● **V23.5 Motorcycle passenger injured in collision with car, pick-up truck or van in traffic accident**

X● **V23.51 Electric (assisted) bicycle passenger injured in collision with car, pick-up truck or van in traffic accident**

X● **V23.59 Other motorcycle passenger injured in collision with car, pick-up truck or van in traffic accident**

X● **V23.9 Unspecified motorcycle rider injured in collision with car, pick-up truck or van in traffic accident**

X● **V23.91 Unspecified electric (assisted) bicycle rider injured in collision with car, pick-up truck or van in traffic accident**

X● **V23.99 Unspecified rider of other motorcycle injured in collision with car, pick-up truck or van in traffic accident**

● **V24 Motorcycle rider injured in collision with heavy transport vehicle or bus**

Excludes1 motorcycle rider injured in collision with military vehicle (V29.818)

The appropriate 7th character is to be added to each code from category V24

A	initial encounter
D	subsequent encounter
S	sequela

X● **V24.0 Motorcycle driver injured in collision with heavy transport vehicle or bus in nontraffic accident**

X● **V24.01 Electric (assisted) bicycle driver injured in collision with heavy transport vehicle or bus in nontraffic accident**

X● **V24.09 Other motorcycle driver injured in collision with heavy transport vehicle or bus in nontraffic accident**

X● **V24.1 Motorcycle passenger injured in collision with heavy transport vehicle or bus in nontraffic accident**

X● **V24.11 Electric (assisted) bicycle passenger injured in collision with heavy transport vehicle or bus in nontraffic accident**

X● **V24.19 Other motorcycle passenger injured in collision with heavy transport vehicle or bus in nontraffic accident**

X● **V24.2 Unspecified motorcycle rider injured in collision with heavy transport vehicle or bus in nontraffic accident**

X● **V24.21 Unspecified electric (assisted) bicycle rider injured in collision with heavy transport vehicle or bus in nontraffic accident**

X● **V24.29 Unspecified rider of other motorcycle injured in collision with heavy transport vehicle or bus in nontraffic accident**

X● **V24.3 Person boarding or alighting a motorcycle injured in collision with heavy transport vehicle or bus**

X● **V24.31 Person boarding or alighting an electric (assisted) bicycle injured in collision with heavy transport vehicle or bus**

X● **V24.39 Person boarding or alighting other motorcycle injured in collision with heavy transport vehicle or bus**

X● **V24.4 Motorcycle driver injured in collision with heavy transport vehicle or bus in traffic accident**

X● **V24.41 Electric (assisted) bicycle driver injured in collision with heavy transport vehicle or bus in traffic accident**

X● **V24.49 Other motorcycle driver injured in collision with heavy transport vehicle or bus in traffic accident**

X● **V24.5 Motorcycle passenger injured in collision with heavy transport vehicle or bus in traffic accident**

X● **V24.51 Electric (assisted) bicycle passenger injured in collision with heavy transport vehicle or bus in traffic accident**

X● **V24.59 Other motorcycle passenger injured in collision with heavy transport vehicle or bus in traffic accident**

X● V24.9 Unspecified motorcycle rider injured in collision with heavy transport vehicle or bus in traffic accident

X● V24.91 Unspecified electric (assisted) bicycle rider injured in collision with heavy transport vehicle or bus in traffic accident

X● V24.99 Unspecified rider of other motorcycle injured in collision with heavy transport vehicle or bus in traffic accident

● V25 Motorcycle rider injured in collision with railway train or railway vehicle

The appropriate 7th character is to be added to each code from category V25

A	initial encounter
D	subsequent encounter
S	sequela

X● V25.0 Motorcycle driver injured in collision with railway train or railway vehicle in nontraffic accident

X● V25.01 Electric (assisted) bicycle driver injured in collision with railway train or railway vehicle in nontraffic accident

X● V25.09 Other motorcycle driver injured in collision with railway train or railway vehicle in nontraffic accident

X● V25.1 Motorcycle passenger injured in collision with railway train or railway vehicle in nontraffic accident

X● V25.11 Electric (assisted) bicycle passenger injured in collision with railway train or railway vehicle in nontraffic accident

X● V25.19 Other motorcycle passenger injured in collision with railway train or railway vehicle in nontraffic accident

X● V25.2 Unspecified motorcycle rider injured in collision with railway train or railway vehicle in nontraffic accident

X● V25.21 Unspecified electric (assisted) bicycle rider injured in collision with railway train or railway vehicle in nontraffic accident

X● V25.29 Unspecified rider of other motorcycle injured in collision with railway train or railway vehicle in nontraffic accident

X● V25.3 Person boarding or alighting a motorcycle injured in collision with railway train or railway vehicle

X● V25.31 Person boarding or alighting an electric (assisted) bicycle injured in collision with railway train or railway vehicle

X● V25.39 Person boarding or alighting other motorcycle injured in collision with railway train or railway vehicle

X● V25.4 Motorcycle driver injured in collision with railway train or railway vehicle in traffic accident

X● V25.41 Electric (assisted) bicycle driver injured in collision with railway train or railway vehicle in traffic accident

X● V25.49 Other motorcycle driver injured in collision with railway train or railway vehicle in traffic accident

X● V25.5 Motorcycle passenger injured in collision with railway train or railway vehicle in traffic accident

X● V25.51 Electric (assisted) bicycle passenger injured in collision with railway train or railway vehicle in traffic accident

X● V25.59 Other motorcycle passenger injured in collision with railway train or railway vehicle in traffic accident

X● V25.9 Unspecified motorcycle rider injured in collision with railway train or railway vehicle in traffic accident

X● V25.91 Unspecified electric (assisted) bicycle rider injured in collision with railway train or railway vehicle in traffic accident

X● V25.99 Unspecified rider of other motorcycle injured in collision with railway train or railway vehicle in traffic accident

● V26 Motorcycle rider injured in collision with other nonmotor vehicle

Includes collision with animal-drawn vehicle, animal being ridden, streetcar

The appropriate 7th character is to be added to each code from category V26

A	initial encounter
D	subsequent encounter
S	sequela

X● V26.0 Motorcycle driver injured in collision with other nonmotor vehicle in nontraffic accident

X● V26.01 Electric (assisted) bicycle driver injured in collision with other nonmotor vehicle in nontraffic accident

X● V26.09 Other motorcycle driver injured in collision with other nonmotor vehicle in nontraffic accident

X● V26.1 Motorcycle passenger injured in collision with other nonmotor vehicle in nontraffic accident

X● V26.11 Electric (assisted) bicycle passenger injured in collision with other nonmotor vehicle in nontraffic accident

X● V26.19 Other motorcycle passenger injured in collision with other nonmotor vehicle in nontraffic accident

X● V26.2 Unspecified motorcycle rider injured in collision with other nonmotor vehicle in nontraffic accident

X● V26.21 Unspecified electric (assisted) bicycle rider injured in collision with other nonmotor vehicle in nontraffic accident

X● V26.29 Unspecified rider of other motorcycle injured in collision with other nonmotor vehicle in nontraffic accident

X● V26.3 Person boarding or alighting a motorcycle injured in collision with other nonmotor vehicle

X● V26.31 Person boarding or alighting an electric (assisted) bicycle injured in collision with other nonmotor vehicle

X● V26.39 Person boarding or alighting other motorcycle injured in collision with other nonmotor vehicle

X● V26.4 Motorcycle driver injured in collision with other nonmotor vehicle in traffic accident

X● V26.41 Electric (assisted) bicycle driver injured in collision with other nonmotor vehicle in traffic accident

X● V26.49 Other motorcycle driver injured in collision with other nonmotor vehicle in traffic accident

X● V26.5 Motorcycle passenger injured in collision with other nonmotor vehicle in traffic accident

X● V26.51 Electric (assisted) bicycle passenger injured in collision with other nonmotor vehicle in traffic accident

X● V26.59 Other motorcycle passenger injured in collision with other nonmotor vehicle in traffic accident

X● V26.9 Unspecified motorcycle rider injured in collision with other nonmotor vehicle in traffic accident

X● V26.91 Unspecified electric (assisted) bicycle rider injured in collision with other nonmotor vehicle in traffic accident

X● V26.99 Unspecified rider of other motorcycle injured in collision with other nonmotor vehicle in traffic accident

● **V27 Motorcycle rider injured in collision with fixed or stationary object**

The appropriate 7th character is to be added to each code from category V27

A	initial encounter
D	subsequent encounter
S	sequela

X● **V27.0 Motorcycle driver injured in collision with fixed or stationary object in nontraffic accident**

X● **V27.01 Electric (assisted) bicycle driver injured in collision with fixed or stationary object in nontraffic accident**

X● **V27.09 Other motorcycle driver injured in collision with fixed or stationary object in nontraffic accident**

X● **V27.1 Motorcycle passenger injured in collision with fixed or stationary object in nontraffic accident**

X● **V27.11 Electric (assisted) bicycle passenger injured in collision with fixed or stationary object in nontraffic accident**

X● **V27.19 Other motorcycle passenger injured in collision with fixed or stationary object in nontraffic accident**

X● **V27.2 Unspecified motorcycle rider injured in collision with fixed or stationary object in nontraffic accident**

X● **V27.21 Unspecified electric (assisted) bicycle rider injured in collision with fixed or stationary object in nontraffic accident**

X● **V27.29 Unspecified rider of other motorcycle injured in collision with fixed or stationary object in nontraffic accident**

X● **V27.3 Person boarding or alighting a motorcycle injured in collision with fixed or stationary object**

X● **V27.31 Person boarding or alighting an electric (assisted) bicycle injured in collision with fixed or stationary object**

X● **V27.39 Person boarding or alighting other motorcycle injured in collision with fixed or stationary object**

X● **V27.4 Motorcycle driver injured in collision with fixed or stationary object in traffic accident**

X● **V27.41 Electric (assisted) bicycle driver injured in collision with fixed or stationary object in traffic accident**

X● **V27.49 Other motorcycle driver injured in collision with fixed or stationary object in traffic accident**

X● **V27.5 Motorcycle passenger injured in collision with fixed or stationary object in traffic accident**

X● **V27.51 Electric (assisted) bicycle passenger injured in collision with fixed or stationary object in traffic accident**

X● **V27.59 Other motorcycle passenger injured in collision with fixed or stationary object in traffic accident**

X● **V27.9 Unspecified motorcycle rider injured in collision with fixed or stationary object in traffic accident**

X● **V27.91 Unspecified electric (assisted) bicycle rider injured in collision with fixed or stationary object in traffic accident**

X● **V27.99 Unspecified rider of other motorcycle injured in collision with fixed or stationary object in traffic accident**

● **V28 Motorcycle rider injured in noncollision transport accident**

Includes fall or thrown from motorcycle (without antecedent collision)
overturning motorcycle NOS
overturning motorcycle without collision

The appropriate 7th character is to be added to each code from category V28

A	initial encounter
D	subsequent encounter
S	sequela

X● **V28.0 Motorcycle driver injured in noncollision transport accident in nontraffic accident**

X● **V28.01 Electric (assisted) bicycle driver injured in noncollision transport accident in nontraffic accident**

X● **V28.09 Other motorcycle driver injured in noncollision transport accident in nontraffic accident**

X● **V28.1 Motorcycle passenger injured in noncollision transport accident in nontraffic accident**

X● **V28.11 Electric (assisted) bicycle passenger injured in noncollision transport accident in nontraffic accident**

X● **V28.19 Other motorcycle passenger injured in noncollision transport accident in nontraffic accident**

X● **V28.2 Unspecified motorcycle rider injured in noncollision transport accident in nontraffic accident**

X● **V28.21 Unspecified electric (assisted) bicycle rider injured in noncollision transport accident in nontraffic accident**

X● **V28.29 Unspecified rider of other motorcycle injured in noncollision transport accident in nontraffic accident**

X● **V28.3 Person boarding or alighting a motorcycle injured in noncollision transport accident**

X● **V28.31 Person boarding or alighting an electric (assisted) bicycle injured in noncollision transport accident**

X● **V28.39 Person boarding or alighting other motorcycle injured in noncollision transport accident**

X● **V28.4 Motorcycle driver injured in noncollision transport accident in traffic accident**

X● **V28.41 Electric (assisted) bicycle driver injured in noncollision transport accident in traffic accident**

X● **V28.49 Other motorcycle driver injured in noncollision transport accident in traffic accident**

X● **V28.5 Motorcycle passenger injured in noncollision transport accident in traffic accident**

X● **V28.51 Electric (assisted) bicycle passenger injured in noncollision transport accident in traffic accident**

X● **V28.59 Other motorcycle passenger injured in noncollision transport accident in traffic accident**

X● **V28.9 Unspecified motorcycle rider injured in noncollision transport accident in traffic accident**

X● **V28.91 Unspecified electric (assisted) bicycle rider injured in noncollision transport accident in traffic accident**

X● **V28.99 Unspecified rider of other motorcycle injured in noncollision transport accident in traffic accident**

● V29 Motorcycle rider injured in other and unspecified transport accidents

The appropriate 7th character is to be added to each code from category V29

A	initial encounter
D	subsequent encounter
S	sequela

Coding Clinic: 2015, Q3, P20

● V29.0 Motorcycle driver injured in collision with other and unspecified motor vehicles in nontraffic accident

● V29.00 Motorcycle driver injured in collision with unspecified motor vehicles in nontraffic accident

● V29.001 Electric (assisted) bicycle driver injured in collision with unspecified motor vehicles in nontraffic accident

● V29.008 Other motorcycle driver injured in collision with unspecified motor vehicles in nontraffic accident

● V29.09 Motorcycle driver injured in collision with other motor vehicles in nontraffic accident

● V29.091 Electric (assisted) bicycle driver injured in collision with other motor vehicles in nontraffic accident

● V29.098 Other motorcycle driver injured in collision with other motor vehicles in nontraffic accident

● V29.1 Motorcycle passenger injured in collision with other and unspecified motor vehicles in nontraffic accident

● V29.10 Motorcycle passenger injured in collision with unspecified motor vehicles in nontraffic accident

● V29.101 Electric (assisted) bicycle passenger injured in collision with unspecified motor vehicles in nontraffic accident

● V29.108 Other motorcycle passenger injured in collision with unspecified motor vehicles in nontraffic accident

● V29.19 Motorcycle passenger injured in collision with other motor vehicles in nontraffic accident

● V29.191 Electric (assisted) bicycle passenger injured in collision with other motor vehicles in nontraffic accident

● V29.198 Other motorcycle passenger injured in collision with other motor vehicles in nontraffic accident

● V29.2 Unspecified motorcycle rider injured in collision with other and unspecified motor vehicles in nontraffic accident

● V29.20 Unspecified motorcycle rider injured in collision with unspecified motor vehicles in nontraffic accident

Motorcycle collision NOS, nontraffic

● V29.201 Unspecified electric (assisted) bicycle rider injured in collision with unspecified motor vehicles in nontraffic accident

● V29.208 Unspecified rider of other motorcycle injured in collision with unspecified motor vehicles in nontraffic accident

Motorcycle collision NOS, nontraffic

● V29.29 Unspecified motorcycle rider injured in collision with other motor vehicles in nontraffic accident

● V29.291 Unspecified electric (assisted) bicycle rider injured in collision with other motor vehicles in nontraffic accident

● V29.298 Unspecified rider of other motorcycle injured in collision with other motor vehicles in nontraffic accident

X● V29.3 Motorcycle rider (driver) (passenger) injured in unspecified nontraffic accident

Motorcycle accident NOS, nontraffic

Motorcycle rider injured in nontraffic accident NOS

X● V29.31 Electric (assisted) bicycle (driver) (passenger) injured in unspecified nontraffic accident

X● V29.39 Other motorcycle (driver) (passenger) injured in unspecified nontraffic accident

Motorcycle accident NOS, nontraffic

Motorcycle rider injured in nontraffic accident NOS

● V29.4 Motorcycle driver injured in collision with other and unspecified motor vehicles in traffic accident

● V29.40 Motorcycle driver injured in collision with unspecified motor vehicles in traffic accident

● V29.401 Electric (assisted) bicycle driver injured in collision with unspecified motor vehicles in traffic accident

● V29.408 Other motorcycle driver injured in collision with unspecified motor vehicles in traffic accident

● V29.49 Motorcycle driver injured in collision with other motor vehicles in traffic accident

● V29.491 Electric (assisted) bicycle driver injured in collision with other motor vehicles in traffic accident

● V29.498 Other motorcycle driver injured in collision with other motor vehicles in traffic accident

● V29.5 Motorcycle passenger injured in collision with other and unspecified motor vehicles in traffic accident

● V29.50 Motorcycle passenger injured in collision with unspecified motor vehicles in traffic accident

● V29.501 Electric (assisted) bicycle passenger injured in collision with unspecified motor vehicles in traffic accident

● V29.508 Other motorcycle passenger injured in collision with unspecified motor vehicles in traffic accident

● V29.59 Motorcycle passenger injured in collision with other motor vehicles in traffic accident

● V29.591 Electric (assisted) bicycle passenger injured in collision with other motor vehicles in traffic accident

● V29.598 Other motorcycle passenger injured in collision with other motor vehicles in traffic accident

● V29.6 Unspecified motorcycle rider injured in collision with other and unspecified motor vehicles in traffic accident

● V29.60 Unspecified motorcycle rider injured in collision with unspecified motor vehicles in traffic accident

Motorcycle collision NOS (traffic)

● V29.601 Unspecified electric (assisted) bicycle rider injured in collision with unspecified motor vehicles in traffic accident

● V29.608 Unspecified rider of other motorcycle injured in collision with unspecified motor vehicles in traffic accident

Motorcycle collision NOS (traffic)

● V29.69 Unspecified motorcycle rider injured in collision with other motor vehicles in traffic accident

● V29.691 Unspecified electric (assisted) bicycle rider injured in collision with other motor vehicles in traffic accident

● V29.698 Unspecified rider of other motorcycle injured in collision with other motor vehicles in traffic accident

● **V29.8 Motorcycle rider (driver) (passenger) injured in other specified transport accidents**

● **V29.81 Motorcycle rider (driver) (passenger) injured in transport accident with military vehicle**

● **V29.811 Electric (assisted) bicycle rider (driver) (passenger) injured in transport accident with military vehicle**

● **V29.818 Rider (driver) (passenger) of other motorcycle injured in transport accident with military vehicle**

● **V29.88 Motorcycle rider (driver) (passenger) injured in other specified transport accidents**

● **V29.881 Electric (assisted) bicycle rider (driver) (passenger) injured in other specified transport accidents**

● **V29.888 Rider (driver) (passenger) of other motorcycle injured in other specified transport accidents**

X● **V29.9 Motorcycle rider (driver) (passenger) injured in unspecified traffic accident**

Motorcycle accident NOS

X● **V29.91 Electric (assisted) bicycle rider (driver) (passenger) injured in unspecified traffic accident**

X● **V29.99 Rider (driver) (passenger) of other motorcycle injured in unspecified traffic accident**

Motorcycle accident NOS

OCCUPANT OF THREE-WHEELED MOTOR VEHICLE INJURED IN TRANSPORT ACCIDENT (V30-V39)

Includes motorized tricycle
motorized rickshaw
three-wheeled motor car

Excludes1 all-terrain vehicles (V86.-)
motorcycle with sidecar (V20-V29)
vehicle designed primarily for off-road use (V86.-)

● **V30 Occupant of three-wheeled motor vehicle injured in collision with pedestrian or animal**

Excludes1 three-wheeled motor vehicle collision with animal-drawn vehicle or animal being ridden (V36.-)

The appropriate 7th character is to be added to each code from category V30

A	initial encounter
D	subsequent encounter
S	sequela

X● **V30.0 Driver of three-wheeled motor vehicle injured in collision with pedestrian or animal in nontraffic accident**

X● **V30.1 Passenger in three-wheeled motor vehicle injured in collision with pedestrian or animal in nontraffic accident**

X● **V30.2 Person on outside of three-wheeled motor vehicle injured in collision with pedestrian or animal in nontraffic accident**

X● **V30.3 Unspecified occupant of three-wheeled motor vehicle injured in collision with pedestrian or animal in nontraffic accident**

X● **V30.4 Person boarding or alighting a three-wheeled motor vehicle injured in collision with pedestrian or animal**

X● **V30.5 Driver of three-wheeled motor vehicle injured in collision with pedestrian or animal in traffic accident**

X● **V30.6 Passenger in three-wheeled motor vehicle injured in collision with pedestrian or animal in traffic accident**

X● **V30.7 Person on outside of three-wheeled motor vehicle injured in collision with pedestrian or animal in traffic accident**

X● **V30.9 Unspecified occupant of three-wheeled motor vehicle injured in collision with pedestrian or animal in traffic accident**

● **V31 Occupant of three-wheeled motor vehicle injured in collision with pedal cycle**

The appropriate 7th character is to be added to each code from category V31

A	initial encounter
D	subsequent encounter
S	sequela

X● **V31.0 Driver of three-wheeled motor vehicle injured in collision with pedal cycle in nontraffic accident**

X● **V31.1 Passenger in three-wheeled motor vehicle injured in collision with pedal cycle in nontraffic accident**

X● **V31.2 Person on outside of three-wheeled motor vehicle injured in collision with pedal cycle in nontraffic accident**

X● **V31.3 Unspecified occupant of three-wheeled motor vehicle injured in collision with pedal cycle in nontraffic accident**

X● **V31.4 Person boarding or alighting a three-wheeled motor vehicle injured in collision with pedal cycle**

X● **V31.5 Driver of three-wheeled motor vehicle injured in collision with pedal cycle in traffic accident**

X● **V31.6 Passenger in three-wheeled motor vehicle injured in collision with pedal cycle in traffic accident**

X● **V31.7 Person on outside of three-wheeled motor vehicle injured in collision with pedal cycle in traffic accident**

X● **V31.9 Unspecified occupant of three-wheeled motor vehicle injured in collision with pedal cycle in traffic accident**

● **V32 Occupant of three-wheeled motor vehicle injured in collision with two- or three-wheeled motor vehicle**

The appropriate 7th character is to be added to each code from category V32

A	initial encounter
D	subsequent encounter
S	sequela

X● **V32.0 Driver of three-wheeled motor vehicle injured in collision with two- or three-wheeled motor vehicle in nontraffic accident**

X● **V32.1 Passenger in three-wheeled motor vehicle injured in collision with two- or three-wheeled motor vehicle in nontraffic accident**

X● **V32.2 Person on outside of three-wheeled motor vehicle injured in collision with two- or three-wheeled motor vehicle in nontraffic accident**

X● **V32.3 Unspecified occupant of three-wheeled motor vehicle injured in collision with two- or three-wheeled motor vehicle in nontraffic accident**

X● **V32.4 Person boarding or alighting a three-wheeled motor vehicle injured in collision with two- or three-wheeled motor vehicle**

X● **V32.5 Driver of three-wheeled motor vehicle injured in collision with two- or three-wheeled motor vehicle in traffic accident**

X● **V32.6 Passenger in three-wheeled motor vehicle injured in collision with two- or three-wheeled motor vehicle in traffic accident**

X● **V32.7 Person on outside of three-wheeled motor vehicle injured in collision with two- or three-wheeled motor vehicle in traffic accident**

X● **V32.9 Unspecified occupant of three-wheeled motor vehicle injured in collision with two- or three-wheeled motor vehicle in traffic accident**

● V33 **Occupant of three-wheeled motor vehicle injured in collision with car, pick-up truck or van**

The appropriate 7th character is to be added to each code from category V33

A	initial encounter
D	subsequent encounter
S	sequela

X● V33.0 **Driver of three-wheeled motor vehicle injured in collision with car, pick-up truck or van in nontraffic accident**

X● V33.1 **Passenger in three-wheeled motor vehicle injured in collision with car, pick-up truck or van in nontraffic accident**

X● V33.2 **Person on outside of three-wheeled motor vehicle injured in collision with car, pick-up truck or van in nontraffic accident**

X● V33.3 **Unspecified occupant of three-wheeled motor vehicle injured in collision with car, pick-up truck or van in nontraffic accident**

X● V33.4 **Person boarding or alighting a three-wheeled motor vehicle injured in collision with car, pick-up truck or van**

X● V33.5 **Driver of three-wheeled motor vehicle injured in collision with car, pick-up truck or van in traffic accident**

X● V33.6 **Passenger in three-wheeled motor vehicle injured in collision with car, pick-up truck or van in traffic accident**

X● V33.7 **Person on outside of three-wheeled motor vehicle injured in collision with car, pick-up truck or van in traffic accident**

X● V33.9 **Unspecified occupant of three-wheeled motor vehicle injured in collision with car, pick-up truck or van in traffic accident**

● V34 **Occupant of three-wheeled motor vehicle injured in collision with heavy transport vehicle or bus**

Excludes1 occupant of three-wheeled motor vehicle injured in collision with military vehicle (V39.81)

The appropriate 7th character is to be added to each code from category V34

A	initial encounter
D	subsequent encounter
S	sequela

X● V34.0 **Driver of three-wheeled motor vehicle injured in collision with heavy transport vehicle or bus in nontraffic accident**

X● V34.1 **Passenger in three-wheeled motor vehicle injured in collision with heavy transport vehicle or bus in nontraffic accident**

X● V34.2 **Person on outside of three-wheeled motor vehicle injured in collision with heavy transport vehicle or bus in nontraffic accident**

X● V34.3 **Unspecified occupant of three-wheeled motor vehicle injured in collision with heavy transport vehicle or bus in nontraffic accident**

X● V34.4 **Person boarding or alighting a three-wheeled motor vehicle injured in collision with heavy transport vehicle or bus**

X● V34.5 **Driver of three-wheeled motor vehicle injured in collision with heavy transport vehicle or bus in traffic accident**

X● V34.6 **Passenger in three-wheeled motor vehicle injured in collision with heavy transport vehicle or bus in traffic accident**

X● V34.7 **Person on outside of three-wheeled motor vehicle injured in collision with heavy transport vehicle or bus in traffic accident**

X● V34.9 **Unspecified occupant of three-wheeled motor vehicle injured in collision with heavy transport vehicle or bus in traffic accident**

● V35 **Occupant of three-wheeled motor vehicle injured in collision with railway train or railway vehicle**

The appropriate 7th character is to be added to each code from category V35

A	initial encounter
D	subsequent encounter
S	sequela

X● V35.0 **Driver of three-wheeled motor vehicle injured in collision with railway train or railway vehicle in nontraffic accident**

X● V35.1 **Passenger in three-wheeled motor vehicle injured in collision with railway train or railway vehicle in nontraffic accident**

X● V35.2 **Person on outside of three-wheeled motor vehicle injured in collision with railway train or railway vehicle in nontraffic accident**

X● V35.3 **Unspecified occupant of three-wheeled motor vehicle injured in collision with railway train or railway vehicle in nontraffic accident**

X● V35.4 **Person boarding or alighting a three-wheeled motor vehicle injured in collision with railway train or railway vehicle**

X● V35.5 **Driver of three-wheeled motor vehicle injured in collision with railway train or railway vehicle in traffic accident**

X● V35.6 **Passenger in three-wheeled motor vehicle injured in collision with railway train or railway vehicle in traffic accident**

X● V35.7 **Person on outside of three-wheeled motor vehicle injured in collision with railway train or railway vehicle in traffic accident**

X● V35.9 **Unspecified occupant of three-wheeled motor vehicle injured in collision with railway train or railway vehicle in traffic accident**

● V36 **Occupant of three-wheeled motor vehicle injured in collision with other nonmotor vehicle**

Includes collision with animal-drawn vehicle, animal being ridden, streetcar

The appropriate 7th character is to be added to each code from category V36

A	initial encounter
D	subsequent encounter
S	sequela

X● V36.0 **Driver of three-wheeled motor vehicle injured in collision with other nonmotor vehicle in nontraffic accident**

X● V36.1 **Passenger in three-wheeled motor vehicle injured in collision with other nonmotor vehicle in nontraffic accident**

X● V36.2 **Person on outside of three-wheeled motor vehicle injured in collision with other nonmotor vehicle in nontraffic accident**

X● V36.3 **Unspecified occupant of three-wheeled motor vehicle injured in collision with other nonmotor vehicle in nontraffic accident**

X● V36.4 **Person boarding or alighting a three-wheeled motor vehicle injured in collision with other nonmotor vehicle**

X● V36.5 **Driver of three-wheeled motor vehicle injured in collision with other nonmotor vehicle in traffic accident**

X● V36.6 **Passenger in three-wheeled motor vehicle injured in collision with other nonmotor vehicle in traffic accident**

X● V36.7 **Person on outside of three-wheeled motor vehicle injured in collision with other nonmotor vehicle in traffic accident**

X● V36.9 **Unspecified occupant of three-wheeled motor vehicle injured in collision with other nonmotor vehicle in traffic accident**

● V37 Occupant of three-wheeled motor vehicle injured in collision with fixed or stationary object

The appropriate 7th character is to be added to each code from category V37

A	initial encounter
D	subsequent encounter
S	sequela

X● **V37.0** **Driver of three-wheeled motor vehicle injured in collision with fixed or stationary object in nontraffic accident**

X● **V37.1** **Passenger in three-wheeled motor vehicle injured in collision with fixed or stationary object in nontraffic accident**

X● **V37.2** **Person on outside of three-wheeled motor vehicle injured in collision with fixed or stationary object in nontraffic accident**

X● **V37.3** **Unspecified occupant of three-wheeled motor vehicle injured in collision with fixed or stationary object in nontraffic accident**

X● **V37.4** **Person boarding or alighting a three-wheeled motor vehicle injured in collision with fixed or stationary object**

X● **V37.5** **Driver of three-wheeled motor vehicle injured in collision with fixed or stationary object in traffic accident**

X● **V37.6** **Passenger in three-wheeled motor vehicle injured in collision with fixed or stationary object in traffic accident**

X● **V37.7** **Person on outside of three-wheeled motor vehicle injured in collision with fixed or stationary object in traffic accident**

X● **V37.9** **Unspecified occupant of three-wheeled motor vehicle injured in collision with fixed or stationary object in traffic accident**

● V38 Occupant of three-wheeled motor vehicle injured in noncollision transport accident

Includes fall or thrown from three-wheeled motor vehicle
overturning of three-wheeled motor vehicle NOS
overturning of three-wheeled motor vehicle without collision

The appropriate 7th character is to be added to each code from category V38

A	initial encounter
D	subsequent encounter
S	sequela

X● **V38.0** **Driver of three-wheeled motor vehicle injured in noncollision transport accident in nontraffic accident**

X● **V38.1** **Passenger in three-wheeled motor vehicle injured in noncollision transport accident in nontraffic accident**

X● **V38.2** **Person on outside of three-wheeled motor vehicle injured in noncollision transport accident in nontraffic accident**

X● **V38.3** **Unspecified occupant of three-wheeled motor vehicle injured in noncollision transport accident in nontraffic accident**

X● **V38.4** **Person boarding or alighting a three-wheeled motor vehicle injured in noncollision transport accident**

X● **V38.5** **Driver of three-wheeled motor vehicle injured in noncollision transport accident in traffic accident**

X● **V38.6** **Passenger in three-wheeled motor vehicle injured in noncollision transport accident in traffic accident**

X● **V38.7** **Person on outside of three-wheeled motor vehicle injured in noncollision transport accident in traffic accident**

X● **V38.9** **Unspecified occupant of three-wheeled motor vehicle injured in noncollision transport accident in traffic accident**

● V39 Occupant of three-wheeled motor vehicle injured in other and unspecified transport accidents

The appropriate 7th character is to be added to each code from category V39

A	initial encounter
D	subsequent encounter
S	sequela

● **V39.0** **Driver of three-wheeled motor vehicle injured in collision with other and unspecified motor vehicles in nontraffic accident**

X● **V39.00** **Driver of three-wheeled motor vehicle injured in collision with unspecified motor vehicles in nontraffic accident**

X● **V39.09** **Driver of three-wheeled motor vehicle injured in collision with other motor vehicles in nontraffic accident**

● **V39.1** **Passenger in three-wheeled motor vehicle injured in collision with other and unspecified motor vehicles in nontraffic accident**

X● **V39.10** **Passenger in three-wheeled motor vehicle injured in collision with unspecified motor vehicles in nontraffic accident**

X● **V39.19** **Passenger in three-wheeled motor vehicle injured in collision with other motor vehicles in nontraffic accident**

● **V39.2** **Unspecified occupant of three-wheeled motor vehicle injured in collision with other and unspecified motor vehicles in nontraffic accident**

X● **V39.20** **Unspecified occupant of three-wheeled motor vehicle injured in collision with unspecified motor vehicles in nontraffic accident**

Collision NOS involving three-wheeled motor vehicle, nontraffic

X● **V39.29** **Unspecified occupant of three-wheeled motor vehicle injured in collision with other motor vehicles in nontraffic accident**

X● **V39.3** **Occupant (driver) (passenger) of three-wheeled motor vehicle injured in unspecified nontraffic accident**

Accident NOS involving three-wheeled motor vehicle, nontraffic

Occupant of three-wheeled motor vehicle injured in nontraffic accident NOS

● **V39.4** **Driver of three-wheeled motor vehicle injured in collision with other and unspecified motor vehicles in traffic accident**

X● **V39.40** **Driver of three-wheeled motor vehicle injured in collision with unspecified motor vehicles in traffic accident**

X● **V39.49** **Driver of three-wheeled motor vehicle injured in collision with other motor vehicles in traffic accident**

● **V39.5** **Passenger in three-wheeled motor vehicle injured in collision with other and unspecified motor vehicles in traffic accident**

X● **V39.50** **Passenger in three-wheeled motor vehicle injured in collision with unspecified motor vehicles in traffic accident**

X● **V39.59** **Passenger in three-wheeled motor vehicle injured in collision with other motor vehicles in traffic accident**

● **V39.6** **Unspecified occupant of three-wheeled motor vehicle injured in collision with other and unspecified motor vehicles in traffic accident**

X● **V39.60** **Unspecified occupant of three-wheeled motor vehicle injured in collision with unspecified motor vehicles in traffic accident**

Collision NOS involving three-wheeled motor vehicle (traffic)

X● **V39.69** **Unspecified occupant of three-wheeled motor vehicle injured in collision with other motor vehicles in traffic accident**

● V39.8 Occupant (driver) (passenger) of three-wheeled motor vehicle injured in other specified transport accidents

X● V39.81 Occupant (driver) (passenger) of three-wheeled motor vehicle injured in transport accident with military vehicle

X● V39.89 Occupant (driver) (passenger) of three-wheeled motor vehicle injured in other specified transport accidents

X● V39.9 Occupant (driver) (passenger) of three-wheeled motor vehicle injured in unspecified traffic accident
Accident NOS involving three-wheeled motor vehicle

CAR OCCUPANT INJURED IN TRANSPORT ACCIDENT (V40-V49)

Includes a four-wheeled motor vehicle designed primarily for carrying passengers
automobile (pulling a trailer or camper)

Excludes1 bus (V50-V59)
minibus (V50-V59)
minivan (V50-V59)
motorcoach (V70-V79)
pick-up truck (V50-V59)
sport utility vehicle (SUV) (V50-V59)

● V40 Car occupant injured in collision with pedestrian or animal

Excludes1 car collision with animal-drawn vehicle or animal being ridden (V46.-)

The appropriate 7th character is to be added to each code from category V40

A initial encounter
D subsequent encounter
S sequela

X● V40.0 Car driver injured in collision with pedestrian or animal in nontraffic accident

X● V40.1 Car passenger injured in collision with pedestrian or animal in nontraffic accident

X● V40.2 Person on outside of car injured in collision with pedestrian or animal in nontraffic accident

X● V40.3 Unspecified car occupant injured in collision with pedestrian or animal in nontraffic accident

X● V40.4 Person boarding or alighting a car injured in collision with pedestrian or animal

X● V40.5 Car driver injured in collision with pedestrian or animal in traffic accident

X● V40.6 Car passenger injured in collision with pedestrian or animal in traffic accident

X● V40.7 Person on outside of car injured in collision with pedestrian or animal in traffic accident

X● V40.9 Unspecified car occupant injured in collision with pedestrian or animal in traffic accident

● V41 Car occupant injured in collision with pedal cycle

The appropriate 7th character is to be added to each code from category V41

A initial encounter
D subsequent encounter
S sequela

X● V41.0 Car driver injured in collision with pedal cycle in nontraffic accident

X● V41.1 Car passenger injured in collision with pedal cycle in nontraffic accident

X● V41.2 Person on outside of car injured in collision with pedal cycle in nontraffic accident

X● V41.3 Unspecified car occupant injured in collision with pedal cycle in nontraffic accident

X● V41.4 Person boarding or alighting a car injured in collision with pedal cycle

X● V41.5 Car driver injured in collision with pedal cycle in traffic accident

X● V41.6 Car passenger injured in collision with pedal cycle in traffic accident

X● V41.7 Person on outside of car injured in collision with pedal cycle in traffic accident

X● V41.9 Unspecified car occupant injured in collision with pedal cycle in traffic accident

● V42 Car occupant injured in collision with two- or three-wheeled motor vehicle

The appropriate 7th character is to be added to each code from category V42

A initial encounter
D subsequent encounter
S sequela

X● V42.0 Car driver injured in collision with two- or three-wheeled motor vehicle in nontraffic accident

X● V42.1 Car passenger injured in collision with two- or three-wheeled motor vehicle in nontraffic accident

X● V42.2 Person on outside of car injured in collision with two- or three-wheeled motor vehicle in nontraffic accident

X● V42.3 Unspecified car occupant injured in collision with two- or three-wheeled motor vehicle in nontraffic accident

X● V42.4 Person boarding or alighting a car injured in collision with two- or three-wheeled motor vehicle

X● V42.5 Car driver injured in collision with two- or three-wheeled motor vehicle in traffic accident

X● V42.6 Car passenger injured in collision with two- or three-wheeled motor vehicle in traffic accident

X● V42.7 Person on outside of car injured in collision with two- or three-wheeled motor vehicle in traffic accident

X● V42.9 Unspecified car occupant injured in collision with two- or three-wheeled motor vehicle in traffic accident

● V43 Car occupant injured in collision with car, pick-up truck or van

The appropriate 7th character is to be added to each code from category V43

A initial encounter
D subsequent encounter
S sequela

● V43.0 Car driver injured in collision with car, pick-up truck or van in nontraffic accident

X● V43.01 Car driver injured in collision with sport utility vehicle in nontraffic accident

X● V43.02 Car driver injured in collision with other type car in nontraffic accident

X● V43.03 Car driver injured in collision with pick-up truck in nontraffic accident

X● V43.04 Car driver injured in collision with van in nontraffic accident

● V43.1 Car passenger injured in collision with car, pick-up truck or van in nontraffic accident

X● V43.11 Car passenger injured in collision with sport utility vehicle in nontraffic accident

X● V43.12 Car passenger injured in collision with other type car in nontraffic accident

X● V43.13 Car passenger injured in collision with pick-up truck in nontraffic accident

X● V43.14 Car passenger injured in collision with van in nontraffic accident

● V43.2 Person on outside of car injured in collision with car, pick-up truck or van in nontraffic accident

X● V43.21 Person on outside of car injured in collision with sport utility vehicle in nontraffic accident

X● V43.22 Person on outside of car injured in collision with other type car in nontraffic accident

X● V43.23 Person on outside of car injured in collision with pick-up truck in nontraffic accident

X● V43.24 Person on outside of car injured in collision with van in nontraffic accident

● V43.3 Unspecified car occupant injured in collision with car, pick-up truck or van in nontraffic accident

X● V43.31 Unspecified car occupant injured in collision with sport utility vehicle in nontraffic accident

X● V43.32 Unspecified car occupant injured in collision with other type car in nontraffic accident

X● V43.33 Unspecified car occupant injured in collision with pick-up truck in nontraffic accident

X● V43.34 Unspecified car occupant injured in collision with van in nontraffic accident

● V43.4 Person boarding or alighting a car injured in collision with car, pick-up truck or van

X● V43.41 Person boarding or alighting a car injured in collision with sport utility vehicle

X● V43.42 Person boarding or alighting a car injured in collision with other type car

X● V43.43 Person boarding or alighting a car injured in collision with pick-up truck

X● V43.44 Person boarding or alighting a car injured in collision with van

● V43.5 Car driver injured in collision with car, pick-up truck or van in traffic accident

X● V43.51 Car driver injured in collision with sport utility vehicle in traffic accident

X● V43.52 Car driver injured in collision with other type car in traffic accident

X● V43.53 Car driver injured in collision with pick-up truck in traffic accident

X● V43.54 Car driver injured in collision with van in traffic accident

● V43.6 Car passenger injured in collision with car, pick-up truck or van in traffic accident

X● V43.61 Car passenger injured in collision with sport utility vehicle in traffic accident

Coding Clinic: 2015, Q1, P5-7

X● V43.62 Car passenger injured in collision with other type car in traffic accident

X● V43.63 Car passenger injured in collision with pick-up truck in traffic accident

X● V43.64 Car passenger injured in collision with van in traffic accident

● V43.7 Person on outside of car injured in collision with car, pick-up truck or van in traffic accident

X● V43.71 Person on outside of car injured in collision with sport utility vehicle in traffic accident

X● V43.72 Person on outside of car injured in collision with other type car in traffic accident

X● V43.73 Person on outside of car injured in collision with pick-up truck in traffic accident

X● V43.74 Person on outside of car injured in collision with van in traffic accident

● V43.9 Unspecified car occupant injured in collision with car, pick-up truck or van in traffic accident

X● V43.91 Unspecified car occupant injured in collision with sport utility vehicle in traffic accident

X● V43.92 Unspecified car occupant injured in collision with other type car in traffic accident

X● V43.93 Unspecified car occupant injured in collision with pick-up truck in traffic accident

X● V43.94 Unspecified car occupant injured in collision with van in traffic accident

● V44 Car occupant injured in collision with heavy transport vehicle or bus

Excludes1 car occupant injured in collision with military vehicle (V49.81)

The appropriate 7th character is to be added to each code from category V44

A initial encounter
D subsequent encounter
S sequela

X● V44.0 Car driver injured in collision with heavy transport vehicle or bus in nontraffic accident

X● V44.1 Car passenger injured in collision with heavy transport vehicle or bus in nontraffic accident

X● V44.2 Person on outside of car injured in collision with heavy transport vehicle or bus in nontraffic accident

X● V44.3 Unspecified car occupant injured in collision with heavy transport vehicle or bus in nontraffic accident

X● V44.4 Person boarding or alighting a car injured in collision with heavy transport vehicle or bus

X● V44.5 Car driver injured in collision with heavy transport vehicle or bus in traffic accident

X● V44.6 Car passenger injured in collision with heavy transport vehicle or bus in traffic accident

X● V44.7 Person on outside of car injured in collision with heavy transport vehicle or bus in traffic accident

X● V44.9 Unspecified car occupant injured in collision with heavy transport vehicle or bus in traffic accident

● V45 Car occupant injured in collision with railway train or railway vehicle

The appropriate 7th character is to be added to each code from category V45

A initial encounter
D subsequent encounter
S sequela

X● V45.0 Car driver injured in collision with railway train or railway vehicle in nontraffic accident

X● V45.1 Car passenger injured in collision with railway train or railway vehicle in nontraffic accident

X● V45.2 Person on outside of car injured in collision with railway train or railway vehicle in nontraffic accident

X● V45.3 Unspecified car occupant injured in collision with railway train or railway vehicle in nontraffic accident

X● V45.4 Person boarding or alighting a car injured in collision with railway train or railway vehicle

X● V45.5 Car driver injured in collision with railway train or railway vehicle in traffic accident

X● V45.6 Car passenger injured in collision with railway train or railway vehicle in traffic accident

X● V45.7 Person on outside of car injured in collision with railway train or railway vehicle in traffic accident

X● V45.9 Unspecified car occupant injured in collision with railway train or railway vehicle in traffic accident

● V46 Car occupant injured in collision with other nonmotor vehicle

Includes collision with animal-drawn vehicle, animal being ridden, streetcar

The appropriate 7th character is to be added to each code from category V46

A initial encounter
D subsequent encounter
S sequela

X● V46.0 Car driver injured in collision with other nonmotor vehicle in nontraffic accident

X● V46.1 Car passenger injured in collision with other nonmotor vehicle in nontraffic accident

X● V46.2 Person on outside of car injured in collision with other nonmotor vehicle in nontraffic accident

X● V46.3 Unspecified car occupant injured in collision with other nonmotor vehicle in nontraffic accident

X● V46.4 Person boarding or alighting a car injured in collision with other nonmotor vehicle

X● V46.5 Car driver injured in collision with other nonmotor vehicle in traffic accident

X● V46.6 Car passenger injured in collision with other nonmotor vehicle in traffic accident

X● V46.7 Person on outside of car injured in collision with other nonmotor vehicle in traffic accident

X● V46.9 Unspecified car occupant injured in collision with other nonmotor vehicle in traffic accident

● V47 Car occupant injured in collision with fixed or stationary object

The appropriate 7th character is to be added to each code from category V47

A	initial encounter
D	subsequent encounter
S	sequela

Coding Clinic: 2016, Q4, P73

X● V47.0 Car driver injured in collision with fixed or stationary object in nontraffic accident

X● V47.1 Car passenger injured in collision with fixed or stationary object in nontraffic accident

X● V47.2 Person on outside of car injured in collision with fixed or stationary object in nontraffic accident

X● V47.3 Unspecified car occupant injured in collision with fixed or stationary object in nontraffic accident

X● V47.4 Person boarding or alighting a car injured in collision with fixed or stationary object

X● V47.5 Car driver injured in collision with fixed or stationary object in traffic accident

X● V47.6 Car passenger injured in collision with fixed or stationary object in traffic accident

X● V47.7 Person on outside of car injured in collision with fixed or stationary object in traffic accident

X● V47.9 Unspecified car occupant injured in collision with fixed or stationary object in traffic accident

● V48 Car occupant injured in noncollision transport accident

Includes overturning car NOS
overturning car without collision

The appropriate 7th character is to be added to each code from category V48

A	initial encounter
D	subsequent encounter
S	sequela

X● V48.0 Car driver injured in noncollision transport accident in nontraffic accident

X● V48.1 Car passenger injured in noncollision transport accident in nontraffic accident

X● V48.2 Person on outside of car injured in noncollision transport accident in nontraffic accident

X● V48.3 Unspecified car occupant injured in noncollision transport accident in nontraffic accident

X● V48.4 Person boarding or alighting a car injured in noncollision transport accident

X● V48.5 Car driver injured in noncollision transport accident in traffic accident

X● V48.6 Car passenger injured in noncollision transport accident in traffic accident

X● V48.7 Person on outside of car injured in noncollision transport accident in traffic accident

X● V48.9 Unspecified car occupant injured in noncollision transport accident in traffic accident

● V49 Car occupant injured in other and unspecified transport accidents

The appropriate 7th character is to be added to each code from category V49

A	initial encounter
D	subsequent encounter
S	sequela

● V49.0 Driver injured in collision with other and unspecified motor vehicles in nontraffic accident

X● V49.00 Driver injured in collision with unspecified motor vehicles in nontraffic accident

X● V49.09 Driver injured in collision with other motor vehicles in nontraffic accident

● V49.1 Passenger injured in collision with other and unspecified motor vehicles in nontraffic accident

X● V49.10 Passenger injured in collision with unspecified motor vehicles in nontraffic accident

X● V49.19 Passenger injured in collision with other motor vehicles in nontraffic accident

● V49.2 Unspecified car occupant injured in collision with other and unspecified motor vehicles in nontraffic accident

X● V49.20 Unspecified car occupant injured in collision with unspecified motor vehicles in nontraffic accident
Car collision NOS, nontraffic

X● V49.29 Unspecified car occupant injured in collision with other motor vehicles in nontraffic accident

X● V49.3 Car occupant (driver) (passenger) injured in unspecified nontraffic accident
Car accident NOS, nontraffic
Car occupant injured in nontraffic accident NOS

● V49.4 Driver injured in collision with other and unspecified motor vehicles in traffic accident

X● V49.40 Driver injured in collision with unspecified motor vehicles in traffic accident

X● V49.49 Driver injured in collision with other motor vehicles in traffic accident

● V49.5 Passenger injured in collision with other and unspecified motor vehicles in traffic accident

X● V49.50 Passenger injured in collision with unspecified motor vehicles in traffic accident

X● V49.59 Passenger injured in collision with other motor vehicles in traffic accident

● V49.6 Unspecified car occupant injured in collision with other and unspecified motor vehicles in traffic accident

X● V49.60 Unspecified car occupant injured in collision with unspecified motor vehicles in traffic accident
Car collision NOS (traffic)

X● V49.69 Unspecified car occupant injured in collision with other motor vehicles in traffic accident

● V49.8 Car occupant (driver) (passenger) injured in other specified transport accidents

X● V49.81 Car occupant (driver) (passenger) injured in transport accident with military vehicle

X● V49.88 Car occupant (driver) (passenger) injured in other specified transport accidents

X● V49.9 Car occupant (driver) (passenger) injured in unspecified traffic accident
Car accident NOS
Coding Clinic: 2015, Q1, P11

OCCUPANT OF PICK-UP TRUCK OR VAN INJURED IN TRANSPORT ACCIDENT (V50-V59)

Includes a four- or six-wheel motor vehicle designed primarily for carrying passengers and property but weighing less than the local limit for classification as a heavy goods vehicle
minibus
minivan
sport utility vehicle (SUV)
truck
van

Excludes1 heavy transport vehicle (V60-V69)

V50 Occupant of pick-up truck or van injured in collision with pedestrian or animal

Excludes1 pick-up truck or van collision with animal-drawn vehicle or animal being ridden (V56.-)

The appropriate 7th character is to be added to each code from category V50

A	initial encounter
D	subsequent encounter
S	sequela

X **V50.0 Driver of pick-up truck or van injured in collision with pedestrian or animal in nontraffic accident**

X **V50.1 Passenger in pick-up truck or van injured in collision with pedestrian or animal in nontraffic accident**

X **V50.2 Person on outside of pick-up truck or van injured in collision with pedestrian or animal in nontraffic accident**

X **V50.3 Unspecified occupant of pick-up truck or van injured in collision with pedestrian or animal in nontraffic accident**

X **V50.4 Person boarding or alighting a pick-up truck or van injured in collision with pedestrian or animal**

X **V50.5 Driver of pick-up truck or van injured in collision with pedestrian or animal in traffic accident**

X **V50.6 Passenger in pick-up truck or van injured in collision with pedestrian or animal in traffic accident**

X **V50.7 Person on outside of pick-up truck or van injured in collision with pedestrian or animal in traffic accident**

X **V50.9 Unspecified occupant of pick-up truck or van injured in collision with pedestrian or animal in traffic accident**

V51 Occupant of pick-up truck or van injured in collision with pedal cycle

The appropriate 7th character is to be added to each code from category V51

A	initial encounter
D	subsequent encounter
S	sequela

X **V51.0 Driver of pick-up truck or van injured in collision with pedal cycle in nontraffic accident**

X **V51.1 Passenger in pick-up truck or van injured in collision with pedal cycle in nontraffic accident**

X **V51.2 Person on outside of pick-up truck or van injured in collision with pedal cycle in nontraffic accident**

X **V51.3 Unspecified occupant of pick-up truck or van injured in collision with pedal cycle in nontraffic accident**

X **V51.4 Person boarding or alighting a pick-up truck or van injured in collision with pedal cycle**

X **V51.5 Driver of pick-up truck or van injured in collision with pedal cycle in traffic accident**

X **V51.6 Passenger in pick-up truck or van injured in collision with pedal cycle in traffic accident**

X **V51.7 Person on outside of pick-up truck or van injured in collision with pedal cycle in traffic accident**

X **V51.9 Unspecified occupant of pick-up truck or van injured in collision with pedal cycle in traffic accident**

V52 Occupant of pick-up truck or van injured in collision with two- or three-wheeled motor vehicle

The appropriate 7th character is to be added to each code from category V52

A	initial encounter
D	subsequent encounter
S	sequela

X **V52.0 Driver of pick-up truck or van injured in collision with two- or three-wheeled motor vehicle in nontraffic accident**

X **V52.1 Passenger in pick-up truck or van injured in collision with two- or three-wheeled motor vehicle in nontraffic accident**

X **V52.2 Person on outside of pick-up truck or van injured in collision with two- or three-wheeled motor vehicle in nontraffic accident**

X **V52.3 Unspecified occupant of pick-up truck or van injured in collision with two- or three-wheeled motor vehicle in nontraffic accident**

X **V52.4 Person boarding or alighting a pick-up truck or van injured in collision with two- or three-wheeled motor vehicle**

X **V52.5 Driver of pick-up truck or van injured in collision with two- or three-wheeled motor vehicle in traffic accident**

X **V52.6 Passenger in pick-up truck or van injured in collision with two- or three-wheeled motor vehicle in traffic accident**

X **V52.7 Person on outside of pick-up truck or van injured in collision with two- or three-wheeled motor vehicle in traffic accident**

X **V52.9 Unspecified occupant of pick-up truck or van injured in collision with two- or three-wheeled motor vehicle in traffic accident**

V53 Occupant of pick-up truck or van injured in collision with car, pick-up truck or van

The appropriate 7th character is to be added to each code from category V53

A	initial encounter
D	subsequent encounter
S	sequela

X **V53.0 Driver of pick-up truck or van injured in collision with car, pick-up truck or van in nontraffic accident**

X **V53.1 Passenger in pick-up truck or van injured in collision with car, pick-up truck or van in nontraffic accident**

X **V53.2 Person on outside of pick-up truck or van injured in collision with car, pick-up truck or van in nontraffic accident**

X **V53.3 Unspecified occupant of pick-up truck or van injured in collision with car, pick-up truck or van in nontraffic accident**

X **V53.4 Person boarding or alighting a pick-up truck or van injured in collision with car, pick-up truck or van**

X **V53.5 Driver of pick-up truck or van injured in collision with car, pick-up truck or van in traffic accident**

X **V53.6 Passenger in pick-up truck or van injured in collision with car, pick-up truck or van in traffic accident**

X **V53.7 Person on outside of pick-up truck or van injured in collision with car, pick-up truck or van in traffic accident**

X **V53.9 Unspecified occupant of pick-up truck or van injured in collision with car, pick-up truck or van in traffic accident**

● V54 **Occupant of pick-up truck or van injured in collision with heavy transport vehicle or bus**

Excludes1 occupant of pick-up truck or van injured in collision with military vehicle (V59.81)

The appropriate 7th character is to be added to each code from category V54

A	initial encounter
D	subsequent encounter
S	sequela

X● V54.0 **Driver of pick-up truck or van injured in collision with heavy transport vehicle or bus in nontraffic accident**

X● V54.1 **Passenger in pick-up truck or van injured in collision with heavy transport vehicle or bus in nontraffic accident**

X● V54.2 **Person on outside of pick-up truck or van injured in collision with heavy transport vehicle or bus in nontraffic accident**

X● V54.3 **Unspecified occupant of pick-up truck or van injured in collision with heavy transport vehicle or bus in nontraffic accident**

X● V54.4 **Person boarding or alighting a pick-up truck or van injured in collision with heavy transport vehicle or bus**

X● V54.5 **Driver of pick-up truck or van injured in collision with heavy transport vehicle or bus in traffic accident**

X● V54.6 **Passenger in pick-up truck or van injured in collision with heavy transport vehicle or bus in traffic accident**

X● V54.7 **Person on outside of pick-up truck or van injured in collision with heavy transport vehicle or bus in traffic accident**

X● V54.9 **Unspecified occupant of pick-up truck or van injured in collision with heavy transport vehicle or bus in traffic accident**

● V55 **Occupant of pick-up truck or van injured in collision with railway train or railway vehicle**

The appropriate 7th character is to be added to each code from category V55

A	initial encounter
D	subsequent encounter
S	sequela

X● V55.0 **Driver of pick-up truck or van injured in collision with railway train or railway vehicle in nontraffic accident**

X● V55.1 **Passenger in pick-up truck or van injured in collision with railway train or railway vehicle in nontraffic accident**

X● V55.2 **Person on outside of pick-up truck or van injured in collision with railway train or railway vehicle in nontraffic accident**

X● V55.3 **Unspecified occupant of pick-up truck or van injured in collision with railway train or railway vehicle in nontraffic accident**

X● V55.4 **Person boarding or alighting a pick-up truck or van injured in collision with railway train or railway vehicle**

X● V55.5 **Driver of pick-up truck or van injured in collision with railway train or railway vehicle in traffic accident**

X● V55.6 **Passenger in pick-up truck or van injured in collision with railway train or railway vehicle in traffic accident**

X● V55.7 **Person on outside of pick-up truck or van injured in collision with railway train or railway vehicle in traffic accident**

X● V55.9 **Unspecified occupant of pick-up truck or van injured in collision with railway train or railway vehicle in traffic accident**

● V56 **Occupant of pick-up truck or van injured in collision with other nonmotor vehicle**

Includes collision with animal-drawn vehicle, animal being ridden, streetcar

The appropriate 7th character is to be added to each code from category V56

A	initial encounter
D	subsequent encounter
S	sequela

X● V56.0 **Driver of pick-up truck or van injured in collision with other nonmotor vehicle in nontraffic accident**

X● V56.1 **Passenger in pick-up truck or van injured in collision with other nonmotor vehicle in nontraffic accident**

X● V56.2 **Person on outside of pick-up truck or van injured in collision with other nonmotor vehicle in nontraffic accident**

X● V56.3 **Unspecified occupant of pick-up truck or van injured in collision with other nonmotor vehicle in nontraffic accident**

X● V56.4 **Person boarding or alighting a pick-up truck or van injured in collision with other nonmotor vehicle**

X● V56.5 **Driver of pick-up truck or van injured in collision with other nonmotor vehicle in traffic accident**

X● V56.6 **Passenger in pick-up truck or van injured in collision with other nonmotor vehicle in traffic accident**

X● V56.7 **Person on outside of pick-up truck or van injured in collision with other nonmotor vehicle in traffic accident**

X● V56.9 **Unspecified occupant of pick-up truck or van injured in collision with other nonmotor vehicle in traffic accident**

● V57 **Occupant of pick-up truck or van injured in collision with fixed or stationary object**

The appropriate 7th character is to be added to each code from category V57

A	initial encounter
D	subsequent encounter
S	sequela

X● V57.0 **Driver of pick-up truck or van injured in collision with fixed or stationary object in nontraffic accident**

X● V57.1 **Passenger in pick-up truck or van injured in collision with fixed or stationary object in nontraffic accident**

X● V57.2 **Person on outside of pick-up truck or van injured in collision with fixed or stationary object in nontraffic accident**

X● V57.3 **Unspecified occupant of pick-up truck or van injured in collision with fixed or stationary object in nontraffic accident**

X● V57.4 **Person boarding or alighting a pick-up truck or van injured in collision with fixed or stationary object**

X● V57.5 **Driver of pick-up truck or van injured in collision with fixed or stationary object in traffic accident**

X● V57.6 **Passenger in pick-up truck or van injured in collision with fixed or stationary object in traffic accident**

X● V57.7 **Person on outside of pick-up truck or van injured in collision with fixed or stationary object in traffic accident**

X● V57.9 **Unspecified occupant of pick-up truck or van injured in collision with fixed or stationary object in traffic accident**

V58 Occupant of pick-up truck or van injured in noncollision transport accident

Includes overturning pick-up truck or van NOS
overturning pick-up truck or van without collision

The appropriate 7th character is to be added to each code from category V58

A initial encounter
D subsequent encounter
S sequela

V58.0 **Driver of pick-up truck or van injured in noncollision transport accident in nontraffic accident**

V58.1 **Passenger in pick-up truck or van injured in noncollision transport accident in nontraffic accident**

V58.2 **Person on outside of pick-up truck or van injured in noncollision transport accident in nontraffic accident**

V58.3 **Unspecified occupant of pick-up truck or van injured in noncollision transport accident in nontraffic accident**

V58.4 **Person boarding or alighting a pick-up truck or van injured in noncollision transport accident**

V58.5 **Driver of pick-up truck or van injured in noncollision transport accident in traffic accident**

V58.6 **Passenger in pick-up truck or van injured in noncollision transport accident in traffic accident**

V58.7 **Person on outside of pick-up truck or van injured in noncollision transport accident in traffic accident**

V58.9 **Unspecified occupant of pick-up truck or van injured in noncollision transport accident in traffic accident**

V59 Occupant of pick-up truck or van injured in other and unspecified transport accidents

The appropriate 7th character is to be added to each code from category V59

A initial encounter
D subsequent encounter
S sequela

V59.0 **Driver of pick-up truck or van injured in collision with other and unspecified motor vehicles in nontraffic accident**

V59.00 **Driver of pick-up truck or van injured in collision with unspecified motor vehicles in nontraffic accident**

V59.09 **Driver of pick-up truck or van injured in collision with other motor vehicles in nontraffic accident**

V59.1 **Passenger in pick-up truck or van injured in collision with other and unspecified motor vehicles in nontraffic accident**

V59.10 **Passenger in pick-up truck or van injured in collision with unspecified motor vehicles in nontraffic accident**

V59.19 **Passenger in pick-up truck or van injured in collision with other motor vehicles in nontraffic accident**

V59.2 **Unspecified occupant of pick-up truck or van injured in collision with other and unspecified motor vehicles in nontraffic accident**

V59.20 **Unspecified occupant of pick-up truck or van injured in collision with unspecified motor vehicles in nontraffic accident**

Collision NOS involving pick-up truck or van, nontraffic

V59.29 **Unspecified occupant of pick-up truck or van injured in collision with other motor vehicles in nontraffic accident**

V59.3 **Occupant (driver) (passenger) of pick-up truck or van injured in unspecified nontraffic accident**

Accident NOS involving pick-up truck or van, nontraffic

Occupant of pick-up truck or van injured in nontraffic accident NOS

V59.4 **Driver of pick-up truck or van injured in collision with other and unspecified motor vehicles in traffic accident**

V59.40 **Driver of pick-up truck or van injured in collision with unspecified motor vehicles in traffic accident**

V59.49 **Driver of pick-up truck or van injured in collision with other motor vehicles in traffic accident**

V59.5 **Passenger in pick-up truck or van injured in collision with other and unspecified motor vehicles in traffic accident**

V59.50 **Passenger in pick-up truck or van injured in collision with unspecified motor vehicles in traffic accident**

V59.59 **Passenger in pick-up truck or van injured in collision with other motor vehicles in traffic accident**

V59.6 **Unspecified occupant of pick-up truck or van injured in collision with other and unspecified motor vehicles in traffic accident**

V59.60 **Unspecified occupant of pick-up truck or van injured in collision with unspecified motor vehicles in traffic accident**

Collision NOS involving pick-up truck or van (traffic)

V59.69 **Unspecified occupant of pick-up truck or van injured in collision with other motor vehicles in traffic accident**

V59.8 **Occupant (driver) (passenger) of pick-up truck or van injured in other specified transport accidents**

V59.81 **Occupant (driver) (passenger) of pick-up truck or van injured in transport accident with military vehicle**

V59.88 **Occupant (driver) (passenger) of pick-up truck or van injured in other specified transport accidents**

V59.9 **Occupant (driver) (passenger) of pick-up truck or van injured in unspecified traffic accident**

Accident NOS involving pick-up truck or van

OCCUPANT OF HEAVY TRANSPORT VEHICLE INJURED IN TRANSPORT ACCIDENT (V60-V69)

Includes 18 wheeler
armored car
panel truck

Excludes1 bus
motorcoach

V60 Occupant of heavy transport vehicle injured in collision with pedestrian or animal

Excludes1 heavy transport vehicle collision with animal-drawn vehicle or animal being ridden (V66.-)

The appropriate 7th character is to be added to each code from category V60

A initial encounter
D subsequent encounter
S sequela

V60.0 **Driver of heavy transport vehicle injured in collision with pedestrian or animal in nontraffic accident**

V60.1 **Passenger in heavy transport vehicle injured in collision with pedestrian or animal in nontraffic accident**

V60.2 **Person on outside of heavy transport vehicle injured in collision with pedestrian or animal in nontraffic accident**

V60.3 **Unspecified occupant of heavy transport vehicle injured in collision with pedestrian or animal in nontraffic accident**

V60.4 **Person boarding or alighting a heavy transport vehicle injured in collision with pedestrian or animal**

V60.5 **Driver of heavy transport vehicle injured in collision with pedestrian or animal in traffic accident**

CHAPTER 20 (V00-Y99)

X● V60.6 Passenger in heavy transport vehicle injured in collision with pedestrian or animal in traffic accident

X● V60.7 Person on outside of heavy transport vehicle injured in collision with pedestrian or animal in traffic accident

X● V60.9 Unspecified occupant of heavy transport vehicle injured in collision with pedestrian or animal in traffic accident

● V61 Occupant of heavy transport vehicle injured in collision with pedal cycle

The appropriate 7th character is to be added to each code from category V61

A initial encounter
D subsequent encounter
S sequela

X● V61.0 Driver of heavy transport vehicle injured in collision with pedal cycle in nontraffic accident

X● V61.1 Passenger in heavy transport vehicle injured in collision with pedal cycle in nontraffic accident

X● V61.2 Person on outside of heavy transport vehicle injured in collision with pedal cycle in nontraffic accident

X● V61.3 Unspecified occupant of heavy transport vehicle injured in collision with pedal cycle in nontraffic accident

X● V61.4 Person boarding or alighting a heavy transport vehicle injured in collision with pedal cycle while boarding or alighting

X● V61.5 Driver of heavy transport vehicle injured in collision with pedal cycle in traffic accident

X● V61.6 Passenger in heavy transport vehicle injured in collision with pedal cycle in traffic accident

X● V61.7 Person on outside of heavy transport vehicle injured in collision with pedal cycle in traffic accident

X● V61.9 Unspecified occupant of heavy transport vehicle injured in collision with pedal cycle in traffic accident

● V62 Occupant of heavy transport vehicle injured in collision with two- or three-wheeled motor vehicle

The appropriate 7th character is to be added to each code from category V62

A initial encounter
D subsequent encounter
S sequela

X● V62.0 Driver of heavy transport vehicle injured in collision with two- or three-wheeled motor vehicle in nontraffic accident

X● V62.1 Passenger in heavy transport vehicle injured in collision with two- or three-wheeled motor vehicle in nontraffic accident

X● V62.2 Person on outside of heavy transport vehicle injured in collision with two- or three-wheeled motor vehicle in nontraffic accident

X● V62.3 Unspecified occupant of heavy transport vehicle injured in collision with two- or three-wheeled motor vehicle in nontraffic accident

X● V62.4 Person boarding or alighting a heavy transport vehicle injured in collision with two- or three-wheeled motor vehicle

X● V62.5 Driver of heavy transport vehicle injured in collision with two- or three-wheeled motor vehicle in traffic accident

X● V62.6 Passenger in heavy transport vehicle injured in collision with two- or three-wheeled motor vehicle in traffic accident

X● V62.7 Person on outside of heavy transport vehicle injured in collision with two- or three-wheeled motor vehicle in traffic accident

X● V62.9 Unspecified occupant of heavy transport vehicle injured in collision with two- or three-wheeled motor vehicle in traffic accident

● V63 Occupant of heavy transport vehicle injured in collision with car, pick-up truck or van

The appropriate 7th character is to be added to each code from category V63

A initial encounter
D subsequent encounter
S sequela

X● V63.0 Driver of heavy transport vehicle injured in collision with car, pick-up truck or van in nontraffic accident

X● V63.1 Passenger in heavy transport vehicle injured in collision with car, pick-up truck or van in nontraffic accident

X● V63.2 Person on outside of heavy transport vehicle injured in collision with car, pick-up truck or van in nontraffic accident

X● V63.3 Unspecified occupant of heavy transport vehicle injured in collision with car, pick-up truck or van in nontraffic accident

X● V63.4 Person boarding or alighting a heavy transport vehicle injured in collision with car, pick-up truck or van

X● V63.5 Driver of heavy transport vehicle injured in collision with car, pick-up truck or van in traffic accident

X● V63.6 Passenger in heavy transport vehicle injured in collision with car, pick-up truck or van in traffic accident

X● V63.7 Person on outside of heavy transport vehicle injured in collision with car, pick-up truck or van in traffic accident

X● V63.9 Unspecified occupant of heavy transport vehicle injured in collision with car, pick-up truck or van in traffic accident

● V64 Occupant of heavy transport vehicle injured in collision with heavy transport vehicle or bus

Excludes1 occupant of heavy transport vehicle injured in collision with military vehicle (V69.81)

The appropriate 7th character is to be added to each code from category V64

A initial encounter
D subsequent encounter
S sequela

X● V64.0 Driver of heavy transport vehicle injured in collision with heavy transport vehicle or bus in nontraffic accident

X● V64.1 Passenger in heavy transport vehicle injured in collision with heavy transport vehicle or bus in nontraffic accident

X● V64.2 Person on outside of heavy transport vehicle injured in collision with heavy transport vehicle or bus in nontraffic accident

X● V64.3 Unspecified occupant of heavy transport vehicle injured in collision with heavy transport vehicle or bus in nontraffic accident

X● V64.4 Person boarding or alighting a heavy transport vehicle injured in collision with heavy transport vehicle or bus while boarding or alighting

X● V64.5 Driver of heavy transport vehicle injured in collision with heavy transport vehicle or bus in traffic accident

X● V64.6 Passenger in heavy transport vehicle injured in collision with heavy transport vehicle or bus in traffic accident

X● V64.7 Person on outside of heavy transport vehicle injured in collision with heavy transport vehicle or bus in traffic accident

X● V64.9 Unspecified occupant of heavy transport vehicle injured in collision with heavy transport vehicle or bus in traffic accident

● **V65 Occupant of heavy transport vehicle injured in collision with railway train or railway vehicle**

The appropriate 7th character is to be added to each code from category V65

A	initial encounter
D	subsequent encounter
S	sequela

X● **V65.0 Driver of heavy transport vehicle injured in collision with railway train or railway vehicle in nontraffic accident**

X● **V65.1 Passenger in heavy transport vehicle injured in collision with railway train or railway vehicle in nontraffic accident**

X● **V65.2 Person on outside of heavy transport vehicle injured in collision with railway train or railway vehicle in nontraffic accident**

X● **V65.3 Unspecified occupant of heavy transport vehicle injured in collision with railway train or railway vehicle in nontraffic accident**

X● **V65.4 Person boarding or alighting a heavy transport vehicle injured in collision with railway train or railway vehicle**

X● **V65.5 Driver of heavy transport vehicle injured in collision with railway train or railway vehicle in traffic accident**

X● **V65.6 Passenger in heavy transport vehicle injured in collision with railway train or railway vehicle in traffic accident**

X● **V65.7 Person on outside of heavy transport vehicle injured in collision with railway train or railway vehicle in traffic accident**

X● **V65.9 Unspecified occupant of heavy transport vehicle injured in collision with railway train or railway vehicle in traffic accident**

● **V66 Occupant of heavy transport vehicle injured in collision with other nonmotor vehicle**

Includes collision with animal-drawn vehicle, animal being ridden, streetcar

The appropriate 7th character is to be added to each code from category V66

A	initial encounter
D	subsequent encounter
S	sequela

X● **V66.0 Driver of heavy transport vehicle injured in collision with other nonmotor vehicle in nontraffic accident**

X● **V66.1 Passenger in heavy transport vehicle injured in collision with other nonmotor vehicle in nontraffic accident**

X● **V66.2 Person on outside of heavy transport vehicle injured in collision with other nonmotor vehicle in nontraffic accident**

X● **V66.3 Unspecified occupant of heavy transport vehicle injured in collision with other nonmotor vehicle in nontraffic accident**

X● **V66.4 Person boarding or alighting a heavy transport vehicle injured in collision with other nonmotor vehicle**

X● **V66.5 Driver of heavy transport vehicle injured in collision with other nonmotor vehicle in traffic accident**

X● **V66.6 Passenger in heavy transport vehicle injured in collision with other nonmotor vehicle in traffic accident**

X● **V66.7 Person on outside of heavy transport vehicle injured in collision with other nonmotor vehicle in traffic accident**

X● **V66.9 Unspecified occupant of heavy transport vehicle injured in collision with other nonmotor vehicle in traffic accident**

● **V67 Occupant of heavy transport vehicle injured in collision with fixed or stationary object**

The appropriate 7th character is to be added to each code from category V67

A	initial encounter
D	subsequent encounter
S	sequela

X● **V67.0 Driver of heavy transport vehicle injured in collision with fixed or stationary object in nontraffic accident**

X● **V67.1 Passenger in heavy transport vehicle injured in collision with fixed or stationary object in nontraffic accident**

X● **V67.2 Person on outside of heavy transport vehicle injured in collision with fixed or stationary object in nontraffic accident**

X● **V67.3 Unspecified occupant of heavy transport vehicle injured in collision with fixed or stationary object in nontraffic accident**

X● **V67.4 Person boarding or alighting a heavy transport vehicle injured in collision with fixed or stationary object**

X● **V67.5 Driver of heavy transport vehicle injured in collision with fixed or stationary object in traffic accident**

X● **V67.6 Passenger in heavy transport vehicle injured in collision with fixed or stationary object in traffic accident**

X● **V67.7 Person on outside of heavy transport vehicle injured in collision with fixed or stationary object in traffic accident**

X● **V67.9 Unspecified occupant of heavy transport vehicle injured in collision with fixed or stationary object in traffic accident**

● **V68 Occupant of heavy transport vehicle injured in noncollision transport accident**

Includes overturning heavy transport vehicle NOS
overturning heavy transport vehicle without collision

The appropriate 7th character is to be added to each code from category V68

A	initial encounter
D	subsequent encounter
S	sequela

X● **V68.0 Driver of heavy transport vehicle injured in noncollision transport accident in nontraffic accident**

X● **V68.1 Passenger in heavy transport vehicle injured in noncollision transport accident in nontraffic accident**

X● **V68.2 Person on outside of heavy transport vehicle injured in noncollision transport accident in nontraffic accident**

X● **V68.3 Unspecified occupant of heavy transport vehicle injured in noncollision transport accident in nontraffic accident**

X● **V68.4 Person boarding or alighting a heavy transport vehicle injured in noncollision transport accident**

X● **V68.5 Driver of heavy transport vehicle injured in noncollision transport accident in traffic accident**

X● **V68.6 Passenger in heavy transport vehicle injured in noncollision transport accident in traffic accident**

X● **V68.7 Person on outside of heavy transport vehicle injured in noncollision transport accident in traffic accident**

X● **V68.9 Unspecified occupant of heavy transport vehicle injured in noncollision transport accident in traffic accident**

● **V69 Occupant of heavy transport vehicle injured in other and unspecified transport accidents**

The appropriate 7th character is to be added to each code from category V69

A	initial encounter
D	subsequent encounter
S	sequela

● **V69.0 Driver of heavy transport vehicle injured in collision with other and unspecified motor vehicles in nontraffic accident**

X● **V69.00 Driver of heavy transport vehicle injured in collision with unspecified motor vehicles in nontraffic accident**

X● **V69.09 Driver of heavy transport vehicle injured in collision with other motor vehicles in nontraffic accident**

● **V69.1 Passenger in heavy transport vehicle injured in collision with other and unspecified motor vehicles in nontraffic accident**

X● **V69.10 Passenger in heavy transport vehicle injured in collision with unspecified motor vehicles in nontraffic accident**

X● **V69.19 Passenger in heavy transport vehicle injured in collision with other motor vehicles in nontraffic accident**

● **V69.2 Unspecified occupant of heavy transport vehicle injured in collision with other and unspecified motor vehicles in nontraffic accident**

X● **V69.20 Unspecified occupant of heavy transport vehicle injured in collision with unspecified motor vehicles in nontraffic accident**

Collision NOS involving heavy transport vehicle, nontraffic

X● **V69.29 Unspecified occupant of heavy transport vehicle injured in collision with other motor vehicles in nontraffic accident**

X● **V69.3 Occupant (driver) (passenger) of heavy transport vehicle injured in unspecified nontraffic accident**

Accident NOS involving heavy transport vehicle, nontraffic

Occupant of heavy transport vehicle injured in nontraffic accident NOS

● **V69.4 Driver of heavy transport vehicle injured in collision with other and unspecified motor vehicles in traffic accident**

X● **V69.40 Driver of heavy transport vehicle injured in collision with unspecified motor vehicles in traffic accident**

X● **V69.49 Driver of heavy transport vehicle injured in collision with other motor vehicles in traffic accident**

● **V69.5 Passenger in heavy transport vehicle injured in collision with other and unspecified motor vehicles in traffic accident**

X● **V69.50 Passenger in heavy transport vehicle injured in collision with unspecified motor vehicles in traffic accident**

X● **V69.59 Passenger in heavy transport vehicle injured in collision with other motor vehicles in traffic accident**

● **V69.6 Unspecified occupant of heavy transport vehicle injured in collision with other and unspecified motor vehicles in traffic accident**

X● **V69.60 Unspecified occupant of heavy transport vehicle injured in collision with unspecified motor vehicles in traffic accident**

Collision NOS involving heavy transport vehicle (traffic)

X● **V69.69 Unspecified occupant of heavy transport vehicle injured in collision with other motor vehicles in traffic accident**

● **V69.8 Occupant (driver) (passenger) of heavy transport vehicle injured in other specified transport accidents**

X● **V69.81 Occupant (driver) (passenger) of heavy transport vehicle injured in transport accidents with military vehicle**

X● **V69.88 Occupant (driver) (passenger) of heavy transport vehicle injured in other specified transport accidents**

X● **V69.9 Occupant (driver) (passenger) of heavy transport vehicle injured in unspecified traffic accident**

Accident NOS involving heavy transport vehicle

BUS OCCUPANT INJURED IN TRANSPORT ACCIDENT (V70-V79)

Includes motorcoach

Excludes1 minibus (V50-V59)

● **V70 Bus occupant injured in collision with pedestrian or animal**

Excludes1 bus collision with animal-drawn vehicle or animal being ridden (V76.-)

The appropriate 7th character is to be added to each code from category V70

A	initial encounter
D	subsequent encounter
S	sequela

X● **V70.0 Driver of bus injured in collision with pedestrian or animal in nontraffic accident**

X● **V70.1 Passenger on bus injured in collision with pedestrian or animal in nontraffic accident**

X● **V70.2 Person on outside of bus injured in collision with pedestrian or animal in nontraffic accident**

X● **V70.3 Unspecified occupant of bus injured in collision with pedestrian or animal in nontraffic accident**

X● **V70.4 Person boarding or alighting from bus injured in collision with pedestrian or animal**

X● **V70.5 Driver of bus injured in collision with pedestrian or animal in traffic accident**

X● **V70.6 Passenger on bus injured in collision with pedestrian or animal in traffic accident**

X● **V70.7 Person on outside of bus injured in collision with pedestrian or animal in traffic accident**

X● **V70.9 Unspecified occupant of bus injured in collision with pedestrian or animal in traffic accident**

● **V71 Bus occupant injured in collision with pedal cycle**

The appropriate 7th character is to be added to each code from category V71

A	initial encounter
D	subsequent encounter
S	sequela

X● **V71.0 Driver of bus injured in collision with pedal cycle in nontraffic accident**

X● **V71.1 Passenger on bus injured in collision with pedal cycle in nontraffic accident**

X● **V71.2 Person on outside of bus injured in collision with pedal cycle in nontraffic accident**

X● **V71.3 Unspecified occupant of bus injured in collision with pedal cycle in nontraffic accident**

X● **V71.4 Person boarding or alighting from bus injured in collision with pedal cycle**

X● **V71.5 Driver of bus injured in collision with pedal cycle in traffic accident**

X● **V71.6 Passenger on bus injured in collision with pedal cycle in traffic accident**

X● **V71.7 Person on outside of bus injured in collision with pedal cycle in traffic accident**

X● **V71.9 Unspecified occupant of bus injured in collision with pedal cycle in traffic accident**

● **V72 Bus occupant injured in collision with two- or three-wheeled motor vehicle**

The appropriate 7th character is to be added to each code from category V72

A	initial encounter
D	subsequent encounter
S	sequela

X● **V72.0** Driver of bus injured in collision with two- or three-wheeled motor vehicle in nontraffic accident

X● **V72.1** Passenger on bus injured in collision with two- or three-wheeled motor vehicle in nontraffic accident

X● **V72.2** Person on outside of bus injured in collision with two- or three-wheeled motor vehicle in nontraffic accident

X● **V72.3** Unspecified occupant of bus injured in collision with two- or three-wheeled motor vehicle in nontraffic accident

X● **V72.4** Person boarding or alighting from bus injured in collision with two- or three-wheeled motor vehicle

X● **V72.5** Driver of bus injured in collision with two- or three-wheeled motor vehicle in traffic accident

X● **V72.6** Passenger on bus injured in collision with two- or three-wheeled motor vehicle in traffic accident

X● **V72.7** Person on outside of bus injured in collision with two- or three-wheeled motor vehicle in traffic accident

X● **V72.9** Unspecified occupant of bus injured in collision with two- or three-wheeled motor vehicle in traffic accident

● **V73 Bus occupant injured in collision with car, pick-up truck or van**

The appropriate 7th character is to be added to each code from category V73

A	initial encounter
D	subsequent encounter
S	sequela

X● **V73.0** Driver of bus injured in collision with car, pick-up truck or van in nontraffic accident

X● **V73.1** Passenger on bus injured in collision with car, pick-up truck or van in nontraffic accident

X● **V73.2** Person on outside of bus injured in collision with car, pick-up truck or van in nontraffic accident

X● **V73.3** Unspecified occupant of bus injured in collision with car, pick-up truck or van in nontraffic accident

X● **V73.4** Person boarding or alighting from bus injured in collision with car, pick-up truck or van

X● **V73.5** Driver of bus injured in collision with car, pick-up truck or van in traffic accident

X● **V73.6** Passenger on bus injured in collision with car, pick-up truck or van in traffic accident

X● **V73.7** Person on outside of bus injured in collision with car, pick-up truck or van in traffic accident

X● **V73.9** Unspecified occupant of bus injured in collision with car, pick-up truck or van in traffic accident

● **V74 Bus occupant injured in collision with heavy transport vehicle or bus**

Excludes1 bus occupant injured in collision with military vehicle (V79.81)

The appropriate 7th character is to be added to each code from category V74

A	initial encounter
D	subsequent encounter
S	sequela

X● **V74.0** Driver of bus injured in collision with heavy transport vehicle or bus in nontraffic accident

X● **V74.1** Passenger on bus injured in collision with heavy transport vehicle or bus in nontraffic accident

X● **V74.2** Person on outside of bus injured in collision with heavy transport vehicle or bus in nontraffic accident

X● **V74.3** Unspecified occupant of bus injured in collision with heavy transport vehicle or bus in nontraffic accident

X● **V74.4** Person boarding or alighting from bus injured in collision with heavy transport vehicle or bus

X● **V74.5** Driver of bus injured in collision with heavy transport vehicle or bus in traffic accident

X● **V74.6** Passenger on bus injured in collision with heavy transport vehicle or bus in traffic accident

X● **V74.7** Person on outside of bus injured in collision with heavy transport vehicle or bus in traffic accident

X● **V74.9** Unspecified occupant of bus injured in collision with heavy transport vehicle or bus in traffic accident

● **V75 Bus occupant injured in collision with railway train or railway vehicle**

The appropriate 7th character is to be added to each code from category V75

A	initial encounter
D	subsequent encounter
S	sequela

X● **V75.0** Driver of bus injured in collision with railway train or railway vehicle in nontraffic accident

X● **V75.1** Passenger on bus injured in collision with railway train or railway vehicle in nontraffic accident

X● **V75.2** Person on outside of bus injured in collision with railway train or railway vehicle in nontraffic accident

X● **V75.3** Unspecified occupant of bus injured in collision with railway train or railway vehicle in nontraffic accident

X● **V75.4** Person boarding or alighting from bus injured in collision with railway train or railway vehicle

X● **V75.5** Driver of bus injured in collision with railway train or railway vehicle in traffic accident

X● **V75.6** Passenger on bus injured in collision with railway train or railway vehicle in traffic accident

X● **V75.7** Person on outside of bus injured in collision with railway train or railway vehicle in traffic accident

X● **V75.9** Unspecified occupant of bus injured in collision with railway train or railway vehicle in traffic accident

● **V76 Bus occupant injured in collision with other nonmotor vehicle**

Includes collision with animal-drawn vehicle, animal being ridden, streetcar

The appropriate 7th character is to be added to each code from category V76

A	initial encounter
D	subsequent encounter
S	sequela

X● **V76.0** Driver of bus injured in collision with other nonmotor vehicle in nontraffic accident

X● **V76.1** Passenger on bus injured in collision with other nonmotor vehicle in nontraffic accident

X● **V76.2** Person on outside of bus injured in collision with other nonmotor vehicle in nontraffic accident

X● **V76.3** Unspecified occupant of bus injured in collision with other nonmotor vehicle in nontraffic accident

X● **V76.4** Person boarding or alighting from bus injured in collision with other nonmotor vehicle

X● **V76.5** Driver of bus injured in collision with other nonmotor vehicle in traffic accident

X● **V76.6** Passenger on bus injured in collision with other nonmotor vehicle in traffic accident

X● **V76.7** Person on outside of bus injured in collision with other nonmotor vehicle in traffic accident

X● **V76.9** Unspecified occupant of bus injured in collision with other nonmotor vehicle in traffic accident

● V77 Bus occupant injured in collision with fixed or stationary object
The appropriate 7th character is to be added to each code from category V77
A initial encounter
D subsequent encounter
S sequela

X● V77.0 Driver of bus injured in collision with fixed or stationary object in nontraffic accident

X● V77.1 Passenger on bus injured in collision with fixed or stationary object in nontraffic accident

X● V77.2 Person on outside of bus injured in collision with fixed or stationary object in nontraffic accident

X● V77.3 Unspecified occupant of bus injured in collision with fixed or stationary object in nontraffic accident

X● V77.4 Person boarding or alighting from bus injured in collision with fixed or stationary object

X● V77.5 Driver of bus injured in collision with fixed or stationary object in traffic accident

X● V77.6 Passenger on bus injured in collision with fixed or stationary object in traffic accident

X● V77.7 Person on outside of bus injured in collision with fixed or stationary object in traffic accident

X● V77.9 Unspecified occupant of bus injured in collision with fixed or stationary object in traffic accident

● V78 Bus occupant injured in noncollision transport accident
Includes overturning bus NOS
overturning bus without collision
The appropriate 7th character is to be added to each code from category V78
A initial encounter
D subsequent encounter
S sequela

X● V78.0 Driver of bus injured in noncollision transport accident in nontraffic accident

X● V78.1 Passenger on bus injured in noncollision transport accident in nontraffic accident

X● V78.2 Person on outside of bus injured in noncollision transport accident in nontraffic accident

X● V78.3 Unspecified occupant of bus injured in noncollision transport accident in nontraffic accident

X● V78.4 Person boarding or alighting from bus injured in noncollision transport accident

X● V78.5 Driver of bus injured in noncollision transport accident in traffic accident

X● V78.6 Passenger on bus injured in noncollision transport accident in traffic accident

X● V78.7 Person on outside of bus injured in noncollision transport accident in traffic accident

X● V78.9 Unspecified occupant of bus injured in noncollision transport accident in traffic accident

● V79 Bus occupant injured in other and unspecified transport accidents
The appropriate 7th character is to be added to each code from category V79
A initial encounter
D subsequent encounter
S sequela

● V79.0 Driver of bus injured in collision with other and unspecified motor vehicles in nontraffic accident

X● V79.00 Driver of bus injured in collision with unspecified motor vehicles in nontraffic accident

X● V79.09 Driver of bus injured in collision with other motor vehicles in nontraffic accident

● V79.1 Passenger on bus injured in collision with other and unspecified motor vehicles in nontraffic accident

X● V79.10 Passenger on bus injured in collision with unspecified motor vehicles in nontraffic accident

X● V79.19 Passenger on bus injured in collision with other motor vehicles in nontraffic accident

● V79.2 Unspecified bus occupant injured in collision with other and unspecified motor vehicles in nontraffic accident

X● V79.20 Unspecified bus occupant injured in collision with unspecified motor vehicles in nontraffic accident
Bus collision NOS, nontraffic

X● V79.29 Unspecified bus occupant injured in collision with other motor vehicles in nontraffic accident

X● V79.3 Bus occupant (driver) (passenger) injured in unspecified nontraffic accident
Bus accident NOS, nontraffic
Bus occupant injured in nontraffic accident NOS

● V79.4 Driver of bus injured in collision with other and unspecified motor vehicles in traffic accident

X● V79.40 Driver of bus injured in collision with unspecified motor vehicles in traffic accident

X● V79.49 Driver of bus injured in collision with other motor vehicles in traffic accident

● V79.5 Passenger on bus injured in collision with other and unspecified motor vehicles in traffic accident

X● V79.50 Passenger on bus injured in collision with unspecified motor vehicles in traffic accident

X● V79.59 Passenger on bus injured in collision with other motor vehicles in traffic accident

● V79.6 Unspecified bus occupant injured in collision with other and unspecified motor vehicles in traffic accident

X● V79.60 Unspecified bus occupant injured in collision with unspecified motor vehicles in traffic accident
Bus collision NOS (traffic)

X● V79.69 Unspecified bus occupant injured in collision with other motor vehicles in traffic accident

● V79.8 Bus occupant (driver) (passenger) injured in other specified transport accidents

X● V79.81 Bus occupant (driver) (passenger) injured in transport accidents with military vehicle

X● V79.88 Bus occupant (driver) (passenger) injured in other specified transport accidents

X● V79.9 Bus occupant (driver) (passenger) injured in unspecified traffic accident
Bus accident NOS

OTHER LAND TRANSPORT ACCIDENTS (V80-V89)

● V80 Animal-rider or occupant of animal-drawn vehicle injured in transport accident
The appropriate 7th character is to be added to each code from category V80
A initial encounter
D subsequent encounter
S sequela

● V80.0 Animal-rider or occupant of animal drawn vehicle injured by fall from or being thrown from animal or animal-drawn vehicle in noncollision accident

● V80.01 Animal-rider injured by fall from or being thrown from animal in noncollision accident

● V80.010 Animal-rider injured by fall from or being thrown from horse in noncollision accident

● V80.018 Animal-rider injured by fall from or being thrown from other animal in noncollision accident

X● **V80.02** **Occupant of animal-drawn vehicle injured by fall from or being thrown from animal-drawn vehicle in noncollision accident**
Overturning animal-drawn vehicle NOS
Overturning animal-drawn vehicle without collision

● **V80.1** **Animal-rider or occupant of animal-drawn vehicle injured in collision with pedestrian or animal**
Excludes1 animal-rider or animal-drawn vehicle collision with animal-drawn vehicle or animal being ridden (V80.7)

X● **V80.11** **Animal-rider injured in collision with pedestrian or animal**

X● **V80.12** **Occupant of animal-drawn vehicle injured in collision with pedestrian or animal**

● **V80.2** **Animal-rider or occupant of animal-drawn vehicle injured in collision with pedal cycle**

X● **V80.21** **Animal-rider injured in collision with pedal cycle**

X● **V80.22** **Occupant of animal-drawn vehicle injured in collision with pedal cycle**

● **V80.3** **Animal-rider or occupant of animal-drawn vehicle injured in collision with two- or three-wheeled motor vehicle**

X● **V80.31** **Animal-rider injured in collision with two- or three-wheeled motor vehicle**

X● **V80.32** **Occupant of animal-drawn vehicle injured in collision with two- or three-wheeled motor vehicle**

● **V80.4** **Animal-rider or occupant of animal-drawn vehicle injured in collision with car, pick-up truck, van, heavy transport vehicle or bus**
Excludes1 animal-rider injured in collision with military vehicle (V80.910)
occupant of animal-drawn vehicle injured in collision with military vehicle (V80.920)

X● **V80.41** **Animal-rider injured in collision with car, pick-up truck, van, heavy transport vehicle or bus**

X● **V80.42** **Occupant of animal-drawn vehicle injured in collision with car, pick-up truck, van, heavy transport vehicle or bus**

● **V80.5** **Animal-rider or occupant of animal-drawn vehicle injured in collision with other specified motor vehicle**

X● **V80.51** **Animal-rider injured in collision with other specified motor vehicle**

X● **V80.52** **Occupant of animal-drawn vehicle injured in collision with other specified motor vehicle**

● **V80.6** **Animal-rider or occupant of animal-drawn vehicle injured in collision with railway train or railway vehicle**

X● **V80.61** **Animal-rider injured in collision with railway train or railway vehicle**

X● **V80.62** **Occupant of animal-drawn vehicle injured in collision with railway train or railway vehicle**

● **V80.7** **Animal-rider or occupant of animal-drawn vehicle injured in collision with other nonmotor vehicles**

● **V80.71** **Animal-rider or occupant of animal-drawn vehicle injured in collision with animal being ridden**

● **V80.710** **Animal-rider injured in collision with other animal being ridden**

● **V80.711** **Occupant of animal-drawn vehicle injured in collision with animal being ridden**

● **V80.72** **Animal-rider or occupant of animal-drawn vehicle injured in collision with other animal-drawn vehicle**

● **V80.720** **Animal-rider injured in collision with animal-drawn vehicle**

● **V80.721** **Occupant of animal-drawn vehicle injured in collision with other animal-drawn vehicle**

● **V80.73** **Animal-rider or occupant of animal-drawn vehicle injured in collision with streetcar**

● **V80.730** **Animal-rider injured in collision with streetcar**

● **V80.731** **Occupant of animal-drawn vehicle injured in collision with streetcar**

● **V80.79** **Animal-rider or occupant of animal-drawn vehicle injured in collision with other nonmotor vehicles**

● **V80.790** **Animal-rider injured in collision with other nonmotor vehicles**

● **V80.791** **Occupant of animal-drawn vehicle injured in collision with other nonmotor vehicles**

● **V80.8** **Animal-rider or occupant of animal-drawn vehicle injured in collision with fixed or stationary object**

X● **V80.81** **Animal-rider injured in collision with fixed or stationary object**

X● **V80.82** **Occupant of animal-drawn vehicle injured in collision with fixed or stationary object**

● **V80.9** **Animal-rider or occupant of animal-drawn vehicle injured in other and unspecified transport accidents**

● **V80.91** **Animal-rider injured in other and unspecified transport accidents**

● **V80.910** **Animal-rider injured in transport accident with military vehicle**

● **V80.918** **Animal-rider injured in other transport accident**

● **V80.919** **Animal-rider injured in unspecified transport accident**
Animal rider accident NOS

● **V80.92** **Occupant of animal-drawn vehicle injured in other and unspecified transport accidents**

● **V80.920** **Occupant of animal-drawn vehicle injured in transport accident with military vehicle**

● **V80.928** **Occupant of animal-drawn vehicle injured in other transport accident**

● **V80.929** **Occupant of animal-drawn vehicle injured in unspecified transport accident**
Animal-drawn vehicle accident NOS

● **V81** **Occupant of railway train or railway vehicle injured in transport accident**
Includes derailment of railway train or railway vehicle
person on outside of train
Excludes1 streetcar (V82.-)
The appropriate 7th character is to be added to each code from category V81

A	initial encounter
D	subsequent encounter
S	sequela

X● **V81.0** **Occupant of railway train or railway vehicle injured in collision with motor vehicle in nontraffic accident**
Excludes1 occupant of railway train or railway vehicle injured due to collision with military vehicle (V81.83)

X● **V81.1** **Occupant of railway train or railway vehicle injured in collision with motor vehicle in traffic accident**
Excludes1 occupant of railway train or railway vehicle injured due to collision with military vehicle (V81.83)

X● **V81.2** **Occupant of railway train or railway vehicle injured in collision with or hit by rolling stock**

X● **V81.3** **Occupant of railway train or railway vehicle injured in collision with other object**
Railway collision NOS

X● **V81.4** **Person injured while boarding or alighting from railway train or railway vehicle**

CHAPTER 20 (V00-Y99)

X● V81.5 **Occupant of railway train or railway vehicle injured by fall in railway train or railway vehicle**

X● V81.6 **Occupant of railway train or railway vehicle injured by fall from railway train or railway vehicle**

X● V81.7 **Occupant of railway train or railway vehicle injured in derailment without antecedent collision**

● V81.8 **Occupant of railway train or railway vehicle injured in other specified railway accidents**

X● V81.81 **Occupant of railway train or railway vehicle injured due to explosion or fire on train**

X● V81.82 **Occupant of railway train or railway vehicle injured due to object falling onto train**

Occupant of railway train or railway vehicle injured due to falling earth onto train
Occupant of railway train or railway vehicle injured due to falling rocks onto train
Occupant of railway train or railway vehicle injured due to falling snow onto train
Occupant of railway train or railway vehicle injured due to falling trees onto train

X● V81.83 **Occupant of railway train or railway vehicle injured due to collision with military vehicle**

X● V81.89 **Occupant of railway train or railway vehicle injured due to other specified railway accident**

X● V81.9 **Occupant of railway train or railway vehicle injured in unspecified railway accident**

Railway accident NOS

● V82 **Occupant of powered streetcar injured in transport accident**

Includes interurban electric car
person on outside of streetcar
tram (car)
trolley (car)

Excludes1 bus (V70-V79)
motorcoach (V70-V79)
nonpowered streetcar (V76.-)
train (V81.-)

The appropriate 7th character is to be added to each code from category V82

A initial encounter
D subsequent encounter
S sequela

X● V82.0 **Occupant of streetcar injured in collision with motor vehicle in nontraffic accident**

X● V82.1 **Occupant of streetcar injured in collision with motor vehicle in traffic accident**

X● V82.2 **Occupant of streetcar injured in collision with or hit by rolling stock**

X● V82.3 **Occupant of streetcar injured in collision with other object**

Excludes1 collision with animal-drawn vehicle or animal being ridden (V82.8)

X● V82.4 **Person injured while boarding or alighting from streetcar**

X● V82.5 **Occupant of streetcar injured by fall in streetcar**

Excludes1 fall in streetcar:
while boarding or alighting (V82.4)
with antecedent collision (V82.0-V82.3)

X● V82.6 **Occupant of streetcar injured by fall from streetcar**

Excludes1 fall from streetcar:
while boarding or alighting (V82.4)
with antecedent collision (V82.0-V82.3)

X● V82.7 **Occupant of streetcar injured in derailment without antecedent collision**

Excludes1 occupant of streetcar injured in derailment with antecedent collision (V82.0-V82.3)

X● V82.8 **Occupant of streetcar injured in other specified transport accidents**

Streetcar collision with military vehicle
Streetcar collision with train or nonmotor vehicles

X● V82.9 **Occupant of streetcar injured in unspecified traffic accident**

Streetcar accident NOS

● V83 **Occupant of special vehicle mainly used on industrial premises injured in transport accident**

Includes battery-powered airport passenger vehicle
battery-powered truck (baggage) (mail)
coal-car in mine
forklift (truck)
logging car
self-propelled industrial truck
station baggage truck (powered)
tram, truck, or tub (powered) in mine or quarry

Excludes1 special construction vehicles (V85.-)
special industrial vehicle in stationary use or maintenance (W31.-)

The appropriate 7th character is to be added to each code from category V83

A initial encounter
D subsequent encounter
S sequela

X● V83.0 **Driver of special industrial vehicle injured in traffic accident**

X● V83.1 **Passenger of special industrial vehicle injured in traffic accident**

X● V83.2 **Person on outside of special industrial vehicle injured in traffic accident**

X● V83.3 **Unspecified occupant of special industrial vehicle injured in traffic accident**

X● V83.4 **Person injured while boarding or alighting from special industrial vehicle**

X● V83.5 **Driver of special industrial vehicle injured in nontraffic accident**

X● V83.6 **Passenger of special industrial vehicle injured in nontraffic accident**

X● V83.7 **Person on outside of special industrial vehicle injured in nontraffic accident**

X● V83.9 **Unspecified occupant of special industrial vehicle injured in nontraffic accident**

Special-industrial-vehicle accident NOS

● V84 **Occupant of special vehicle mainly used in agriculture injured in transport accident**

Includes self-propelled farm machinery
tractor (and trailer)

Excludes1 animal-powered farm machinery accident (W30.8-)
contact with combine harvester (W30.0)
special agricultural vehicle in stationary use or maintenance (W30.-)

The appropriate 7th character is to be added to each code from category V84

A initial encounter
D subsequent encounter
S sequela

X● V84.0 **Driver of special agricultural vehicle injured in traffic accident**

X● V84.1 **Passenger of special agricultural vehicle injured in traffic accident**

X● V84.2 **Person on outside of special agricultural vehicle injured in traffic accident**

X● V84.3 **Unspecified occupant of special agricultural vehicle injured in traffic accident**

X● V84.4 **Person injured while boarding or alighting from special agricultural vehicle**

X● V84.5 **Driver of special agricultural vehicle injured in nontraffic accident**

X● V84.6 **Passenger of special agricultural vehicle injured in nontraffic accident**

X● **V84.7 Person on outside of special agricultural vehicle injured in nontraffic accident**

X● **V84.9 Unspecified occupant of special agricultural vehicle injured in nontraffic accident**
Special-agricultural vehicle accident NOS

● **V85 Occupant of special construction vehicle injured in transport accident**

Includes bulldozer
digger
dump truck
earth-leveller
mechanical shovel
road-roller

Excludes1 special industrial vehicle (V83.-)
special construction vehicle in stationary use or maintenance (W31.-)

The appropriate 7th character is to be added to each code from category V85

A	initial encounter
D	subsequent encounter
S	sequela

X● **V85.0 Driver of special construction vehicle injured in traffic accident**

X● **V85.1 Passenger of special construction vehicle injured in traffic accident**

X● **V85.2 Person on outside of special construction vehicle injured in traffic accident**

X● **V85.3 Unspecified occupant of special construction vehicle injured in traffic accident**

X● **V85.4 Person injured while boarding or alighting from special construction vehicle**

X● **V85.5 Driver of special construction vehicle injured in nontraffic accident**

X● **V85.6 Passenger of special construction vehicle injured in nontraffic accident**

X● **V85.7 Person on outside of special construction vehicle injured in nontraffic accident**

X● **V85.9 Unspecified occupant of special construction vehicle injured in nontraffic accident**
Special-construction-vehicle accident NOS

● **V86 Occupant of special all-terrain or other off-road motor vehicle, injured in transport accident**

Excludes1 special all-terrain vehicle in stationary use or maintenance (W31.-)
sport-utility vehicle (V50-V59)
three-wheeled motor vehicle designed for on-road use (V30-V39)

The appropriate 7th character is to be added to each code from category V86

A	initial encounter
D	subsequent encounter
S	sequela

● **V86.0 Driver of special all-terrain or other off-road motor vehicle injured in traffic accident**

X● **V86.01 Driver of ambulance or fire engine injured in traffic accident**

X● **V86.02 Driver of snowmobile injured in traffic accident**

X● **V86.03 Driver of dune buggy injured in traffic accident**

X● **V86.04 Driver of military vehicle injured in traffic accident**

X● **V86.05 Driver of 3- or 4-wheeled all-terrain vehicle (ATV) injured in traffic accident**

X● **V86.06 Driver of dirt bike or motor/cross bike injured in traffic accident**

X● **V86.09 Driver of other off-road special all-terrain or other off-road vehicle injured in traffic accident**
Driver of go cart injured in traffic accident
Driver of golf cart injured in traffic accident

● **V86.1 Passenger of special all-terrain or other off-road motor vehicle injured in traffic accident**

X● **V86.11 Passenger of ambulance or fire engine injured in traffic accident**

X● **V86.12 Passenger of snowmobile injured in traffic accident**

X● **V86.13 Passenger of dune buggy injured in traffic accident**

X● **V86.14 Passenger of military vehicle injured in traffic accident**

X● **V86.15 Passenger of 3- or 4-wheeled all-terrain vehicle (ATV) injured in traffic accident**

X● **V86.16 Passenger of dirt bike or motor/cross bike injured in traffic accident**

X● **V86.19 Passenger of other off-road special all-terrain or other off-road off-road motor vehicle injured in traffic accident**
Passenger of go cart injured in traffic accident
Passenger of golf cart injured in traffic accident

● **V86.2 Person on outside of special all-terrain or other off-road motor vehicle injured in traffic accident**

X● **V86.21 Person on outside of ambulance or fire engine injured in traffic accident**

X● **V86.22 Person on outside of snowmobile injured in traffic accident**

X● **V86.23 Person on outside of dune buggy injured in traffic accident**

X● **V86.24 Person on outside of military vehicle injured in traffic accident**

X● **V86.25 Person on outside of 3- or 4-wheeled all-terrain vehicle (ATV) injured in traffic accident**

X● **V86.26 Person on outside of dirt bike or motor/cross bike injured in traffic accident**

X● **V86.29 Person on outside of other special all-terrain or other off-road motor vehicle injured in traffic accident**
Person on outside of go cart in traffic accident
Person on outside of golf cart injured in traffic accident

● **V86.3 Unspecified occupant of special all-terrain or other off-road motor vehicle injured in traffic accident**

X● **V86.31 Unspecified occupant of ambulance or fire engine injured in traffic accident**

X● **V86.32 Unspecified occupant of snowmobile injured in traffic accident**

X● **V86.33 Unspecified occupant of dune buggy injured in traffic accident**

X● **V86.34 Unspecified occupant of military vehicle injured in traffic accident**

X● **V86.35 Unspecified occupant of 3- or 4-wheeled all-terrain vehicle (ATV) injured in traffic accident**

X● **V86.36 Unspecified occupant of dirt bike or motor/cross bike injured in traffic accident**

X● **V86.39 Unspecified occupant of other special all-terrain or other off-road motor vehicle injured in traffic accident**
Unspecified occupant of go cart injured in traffic accident
Unspecified occupant of golf cart injured in traffic accident

● **V86.4 Person injured while boarding or alighting from special all-terrain or other off-road motor vehicle**

X● **V86.41 Person injured while boarding or alighting from ambulance or fire engine**

X● **V86.42 Person injured while boarding or alighting from snowmobile**

X● **V86.43 Person injured while boarding or alighting from dune buggy**

X● **V86.44 Person injured while boarding or alighting from military vehicle**

X● **V86.45 Person injured while boarding or alighting from a 3- or 4-wheeled all-terrain vehicle (ATV)**

CHAPTER 20 (V00-Y99)

X● V86.46 **Person injured while boarding or alighting from a dirt bike or motor/cross bike**

X● V86.49 **Person injured while boarding or alighting from other special all-terrain or other off-road motor vehicle**
Person injured while boarding or alighting from go cart
Person injured while boarding or alighting from golf cart

● V86.5 **Driver of special all-terrain or other off-road motor vehicle injured in nontraffic accident**

X● V86.51 **Driver of ambulance or fire engine injured in nontraffic accident**

X● V86.52 **Driver of snowmobile injured in nontraffic accident**

X● V86.53 **Driver of dune buggy injured in nontraffic accident**

X● V86.54 **Driver of military vehicle injured in nontraffic accident**

X● V86.55 **Driver of 3- or 4-wheeled all-terrain vehicle (ATV) injured in nontraffic accident**

X● V86.56 **Driver of dirt bike or motor/cross bike injured in nontraffic accident**

X● V86.59 **Driver of other off-road special all-terrain or other off-road motor vehicle injured in nontraffic accident**
Driver of go cart injured in nontraffic accident
Driver of golf cart injured in nontraffic accident

● V86.6 **Passenger of special all-terrain or other off-road motor vehicle injured in nontraffic accident**

X● V86.61 **Passenger of ambulance or fire engine injured in nontraffic accident**

X● V86.62 **Passenger of snowmobile injured in nontraffic accident**

X● V86.63 **Passenger of dune buggy injured in nontraffic accident**

X● V86.64 **Passenger of military vehicle injured in nontraffic accident**

X● V86.65 **Passenger of 3- or 4-wheeled all-terrain vehicle (ATV) injured in nontraffic accident**

X● V86.66 **Passenger of dirt bike or motor/cross bike injured in nontraffic accident**

X● V86.69 **Passenger of other special all-terrain or other off-road vehicle injured in nontraffic accident**
Passenger of go cart injured in nontraffic accident
Passenger of golf cart injured in nontraffic accident

● V86.7 **Person on outside of special all-terrain or other off-road motor vehicle injured in nontraffic accident**

X● V86.71 **Person on outside of ambulance or fire engine injured in nontraffic accident**

X● V86.72 **Person on outside of snowmobile injured in nontraffic accident**

X● V86.73 **Person on outside of dune buggy injured in nontraffic accident**

X● V86.74 **Person on outside of military vehicle injured in nontraffic accident**

X● V86.75 **Person on outside of 3- or 4-wheeled all-terrain vehicle (ATV) injured in nontraffic accident**

X● V86.76 **Person on outside of dirt bike or motor/cross bike injured in nontraffic accident**

X● V86.79 **Person on outside of other special all-terrain or other off-road motor vehicles injured in nontraffic accident**
Person on outside of go cart injured in nontraffic accident
Person on outside of golf cart injured in nontraffic accident

● V86.9 **Unspecified occupant of special all-terrain or other off-road motor vehicle injured in nontraffic accident**

X● V86.91 **Unspecified occupant of ambulance or fire engine injured in nontraffic accident**

X● V86.92 **Unspecified occupant of snowmobile injured in nontraffic accident**

X● V86.93 **Unspecified occupant of dune buggy injured in nontraffic accident**

X● V86.94 **Unspecified occupant of military vehicle injured in nontraffic accident**

X● V86.95 **Unspecified occupant of 3- or 4-wheeled all-terrain vehicle (ATV) injured in nontraffic accident**

X● V86.96 **Unspecified occupant of dirt bike or motor/cross bike injured in nontraffic accident**

X● V86.99 **Unspecified occupant of other special all-terrain or other off-road motor vehicle injured in nontraffic accident**
Off-road motor-vehicle accident NOS
Other motor-vehicle accident NOS
Unspecified occupant of go cart injured in nontraffic accident
Unspecified occupant of golf cart injured in nontraffic accident
Unspecified occupant of race car injured in nontraffic accident

● V87 **Traffic accident of specified type but victim's mode of transport unknown**

Excludes1 collision involving:
pedal cycle (V10-V19)
pedestrian (V01-V09)

The appropriate 7th character is to be added to each code from category V87

A initial encounter
D subsequent encounter
S sequela

X● V87.0 **Person injured in collision between car and two- or three-wheeled powered vehicle (traffic)**

X● V87.1 **Person injured in collision between other motor vehicle and two- or three-wheeled motor vehicle (traffic)**

X● V87.2 **Person injured in collision between car and pick-up truck or van (traffic)**

X● V87.3 **Person injured in collision between car and bus (traffic)**

X● V87.4 **Person injured in collision between car and heavy transport vehicle (traffic)**

X● V87.5 **Person injured in collision between heavy transport vehicle and bus (traffic)**

X● V87.6 **Person injured in collision between railway train or railway vehicle and car (traffic)**

X● V87.7 **Person injured in collision between other specified motor vehicles (traffic)**

X● V87.8 **Person injured in other specified noncollision transport accidents involving motor vehicle (traffic)**

X● V87.9 **Person injured in other specified (collision) (noncollision) transport accidents involving nonmotor vehicle (traffic)**

● V88 **Nontraffic accident of specified type but victim's mode of transport unknown**

Excludes1 collision involving:
pedal cycle (V10-V19)
pedestrian (V01-V09)

The appropriate 7th character is to be added to each code from category V88

A initial encounter
D subsequent encounter
S sequela

X● V88.0 **Person injured in collision between car and two- or three-wheeled motor vehicle, nontraffic**

X● V88.1 **Person injured in collision between other motor vehicle and two- or three-wheeled motor vehicle, nontraffic**

X● V88.2 **Person injured in collision between car and pick-up truck or van, nontraffic**

X● **V88.3 Person injured in collision between car and bus, nontraffic**

X● **V88.4 Person injured in collision between car and heavy transport vehicle, nontraffic**

X● **V88.5 Person injured in collision between heavy transport vehicle and bus, nontraffic**

X● **V88.6 Person injured in collision between railway train or railway vehicle and car, nontraffic**

X● **V88.7 Person injured in collision between other specified motor vehicle, nontraffic**

X● **V88.8 Person injured in other specified noncollision transport accidents involving motor vehicle, nontraffic**

X● **V88.9 Person injured in other specified (collision) (noncollision) transport accidents involving nonmotor vehicle, nontraffic**

● **V89 Motor- or nonmotor-vehicle accident, type of vehicle unspecified**

The appropriate 7th character is to be added to each code from category V89

A	initial encounter
D	subsequent encounter
S	sequela

X● **V89.0 Person injured in unspecified motor-vehicle accident, nontraffic**
Motor-vehicle accident NOS, nontraffic

X● **V89.1 Person injured in unspecified nonmotor-vehicle accident, nontraffic**
Nonmotor-vehicle accident NOS (nontraffic)

X● **V89.2 Person injured in unspecified motor-vehicle accident, traffic**
Motor-vehicle accident [MVA] NOS
Road (traffic) accident [RTA] NOS

X● **V89.3 Person injured in unspecified nonmotor-vehicle accident, traffic**
Nonmotor-vehicle traffic accident NOS

X● **V89.9 Person injured in unspecified vehicle accident**
Collision NOS

WATER TRANSPORT ACCIDENTS (V90-V94)

● **V90 Drowning and submersion due to accident to watercraft**

Excludes1 civilian water transport accident involving military watercraft (V94.81-)
fall into water not from watercraft (W16.-)
military watercraft accident in military or war operations (Y36.0-, Y37.0-)
water-transport–related drowning or submersion without accident to watercraft (V92.-)

The appropriate 7th character is to be added to each code from category V90

A	initial encounter
D	subsequent encounter
S	sequela

● **V90.0 Drowning and submersion due to watercraft overturning**

X● **V90.00 Drowning and submersion due to merchant ship overturning**

X● **V90.01 Drowning and submersion due to passenger ship overturning**
Drowning and submersion due to ferry-boat overturning
Drowning and submersion due to liner overturning

X● **V90.02 Drowning and submersion due to fishing boat overturning**

X● **V90.03 Drowning and submersion due to other powered watercraft overturning**
Drowning and submersion due to hovercraft (on open water) overturning
Drowning and submersion due to jet ski overturning

X● **V90.04 Drowning and submersion due to sailboat overturning**

X● **V90.05 Drowning and submersion due to canoe or kayak overturning**

X● **V90.06 Drowning and submersion due to (nonpowered) inflatable craft overturning**

X● **V90.08 Drowning and submersion due to other unpowered watercraft overturning**
Drowning and submersion due to windsurfer overturning

X● **V90.09 Drowning and submersion due to unspecified watercraft overturning**
Drowning and submersion due to boat NOS overturning
Drowning and submersion due to ship NOS overturning
Drowning and submersion due to watercraft NOS overturning

● **V90.1 Drowning and submersion due to watercraft sinking**

X● **V90.10 Drowning and submersion due to merchant ship sinking**

X● **V90.11 Drowning and submersion due to passenger ship sinking**
Drowning and submersion due to ferry-boat sinking
Drowning and submersion due to liner sinking

X● **V90.12 Drowning and submersion due to fishing boat sinking**

X● **V90.13 Drowning and submersion due to other powered watercraft sinking**
Drowning and submersion due to hovercraft (on open water) sinking
Drowning and submersion due to jet ski sinking

X● **V90.14 Drowning and submersion due to sailboat sinking**

X● **V90.15 Drowning and submersion due to canoe or kayak sinking**

X● **V90.16 Drowning and submersion due to (nonpowered) inflatable craft sinking**

X● **V90.18 Drowning and submersion due to other unpowered watercraft sinking**

X● **V90.19 Drowning and submersion due to unspecified watercraft sinking**
Drowning and submersion due to boat NOS sinking
Drowning and submersion due to ship NOS sinking
Drowning and submersion due to watercraft NOS sinking

● **V90.2 Drowning and submersion due to falling or jumping from burning watercraft**

X● **V90.20 Drowning and submersion due to falling or jumping from burning merchant ship**

X● **V90.21 Drowning and submersion due to falling or jumping from burning passenger ship**
Drowning and submersion due to falling or jumping from burning ferry-boat
Drowning and submersion due to falling or jumping from burning liner

X● **V90.22 Drowning and submersion due to falling or jumping from burning fishing boat**

X● **V90.23 Drowning and submersion due to falling or jumping from other burning powered watercraft**
Drowning and submersion due to falling and jumping from burning hovercraft (on open water)
Drowning and submersion due to falling and jumping from burning jet ski

X● **V90.24 Drowning and submersion due to falling or jumping from burning sailboat**

X● **V90.25 Drowning and submersion due to falling or jumping from burning canoe or kayak**

CHAPTER 20 (V00-Y99)

X● V90.26 Drowning and submersion due to falling or jumping from burning (nonpowered) inflatable craft

X● V90.27 Drowning and submersion due to falling or jumping from burning water-skis

X● V90.28 Drowning and submersion due to falling or jumping from other burning unpowered watercraft
Drowning and submersion due to falling and jumping from burning surf-board
Drowning and submersion due to falling and jumping from burning windsurfer

X● V90.29 Drowning and submersion due to falling or jumping from unspecified burning watercraft
Drowning and submersion due to falling or jumping from burning boat NOS
Drowning and submersion due to falling or jumping from burning ship NOS
Drowning and submersion due to falling or jumping from burning watercraft NOS

● V90.3 Drowning and submersion due to falling or jumping from crushed watercraft

X● V90.30 Drowning and submersion due to falling or jumping from crushed merchant ship

X● V90.31 Drowning and submersion due to falling or jumping from crushed passenger ship
Drowning and submersion due to falling and jumping from crushed ferry-boat
Drowning and submersion due to falling and jumping from crushed liner

X● V90.32 Drowning and submersion due to falling or jumping from crushed fishing boat

X● V90.33 Drowning and submersion due to falling or jumping from other crushed powered watercraft
Drowning and submersion due to falling and jumping from crushed hovercraft
Drowning and submersion due to falling and jumping from crushed jet ski

X● V90.34 Drowning and submersion due to falling or jumping from crushed sailboat

X● V90.35 Drowning and submersion due to falling or jumping from crushed canoe or kayak

X● V90.36 Drowning and submersion due to falling or jumping from crushed (nonpowered) inflatable craft

X● V90.37 Drowning and submersion due to falling or jumping from crushed water-skis

X● V90.38 Drowning and submersion due to falling or jumping from other crushed unpowered watercraft
Drowning and submersion due to falling and jumping from crushed surf-board
Drowning and submersion due to falling and jumping from crushed windsurfer

X● V90.39 Drowning and submersion due to falling or jumping from crushed unspecified watercraft
Drowning and submersion due to falling and jumping from crushed boat NOS
Drowning and submersion due to falling and jumping from crushed ship NOS
Drowning and submersion due to falling and jumping from crushed watercraft NOS

● V90.8 Drowning and submersion due to other accident to watercraft

X● V90.80 Drowning and submersion due to other accident to merchant ship

X● V90.81 Drowning and submersion due to other accident to passenger ship
Drowning and submersion due to other accident to ferry-boat
Drowning and submersion due to other accident to liner

X● V90.82 Drowning and submersion due to other accident to fishing boat

X● V90.83 Drowning and submersion due to other accident to other powered watercraft
Drowning and submersion due to other accident to hovercraft (on open water)
Drowning and submersion due to other accident to jet ski

X● V90.84 Drowning and submersion due to other accident to sailboat

X● V90.85 Drowning and submersion due to other accident to canoe or kayak

X● V90.86 Drowning and submersion due to other accident to (nonpowered) inflatable craft

X● V90.87 Drowning and submersion due to other accident to water-skis

X● V90.88 Drowning and submersion due to other accident to other unpowered watercraft
Drowning and submersion due to other accident to surf-board
Drowning and submersion due to other accident to windsurfer

X● V90.89 Drowning and submersion due to other accident to unspecified watercraft
Drowning and submersion due to other accident to boat NOS
Drowning and submersion due to other accident to ship NOS
Drowning and submersion due to other accident to watercraft NOS

● V91 Other injury due to accident to watercraft

Includes any injury except drowning and submersion as a result of an accident to watercraft

Excludes1 civilian water transport accident involving military watercraft (V94.81-)
military watercraft accident in military or war operations (Y36, Y37.-)

Excludes2 drowning and submersion due to accident to watercraft (V90.-)

The appropriate 7th character is to be added to each code from category V91

A	initial encounter
D	subsequent encounter
S	sequela

● V91.0 Burn due to watercraft on fire

Excludes1 burn from localized fire or explosion on board ship without accident to watercraft (V93.-)

X● V91.00 Burn due to merchant ship on fire

X● V91.01 Burn due to passenger ship on fire
Burn due to ferry-boat on fire
Burn due to liner on fire

X● V91.02 Burn due to fishing boat on fire

X● V91.03 Burn due to other powered watercraft on fire
Burn due to hovercraft (on open water) on fire
Burn due to jet ski on fire

X● V91.04 Burn due to sailboat on fire

X● V91.05 Burn due to canoe or kayak on fire

X● V91.06 Burn due to (nonpowered) inflatable craft on fire

X● V91.07 Burn due to water-skis on fire

X● V91.08 Burn due to other unpowered watercraft on fire

X● V91.09 Burn due to unspecified watercraft on fire
Burn due to boat NOS on fire
Burn due to ship NOS on fire
Burn due to watercraft NOS on fire

● **V91.1 Crushed between watercraft and other watercraft or other object due to collision**
Crushed by lifeboat after abandoning ship in a collision
Note: Select the specified type of watercraft that the victim was on at the time of the collision.

X● **V91.10 Crushed between merchant ship and other watercraft or other object due to collision**

X● **V91.11 Crushed between passenger ship and other watercraft or other object due to collision**
Crushed between ferry-boat and other watercraft or other object due to collision
Crushed between liner and other watercraft or other object due to collision

X● **V91.12 Crushed between fishing boat and other watercraft or other object due to collision**

X● **V91.13 Crushed between other powered watercraft and other watercraft or other object due to collision**
Crushed between hovercraft (on open water) and other watercraft or other object due to collision
Crushed between jet ski and other watercraft or other object due to collision

X● **V91.14 Crushed between sailboat and other watercraft or other object due to collision**

X● **V91.15 Crushed between canoe or kayak and other watercraft or other object due to collision**

X● **V91.16 Crushed between (nonpowered) inflatable craft and other watercraft or other object due to collision**

X● **V91.18 Crushed between other unpowered watercraft and other watercraft or other object due to collision**
Crushed between surfboard and other watercraft or other object due to collision
Crushed between windsurfer and other watercraft or other object due to collision

X● **V91.19 Crushed between unspecified watercraft and other watercraft or other object due to collision**
Crushed between boat NOS and other watercraft or other object due to collision
Crushed between ship NOS and other watercraft or other object due to collision
Crushed between watercraft NOS and other watercraft or other object due to collision

● **V91.2 Fall due to collision between watercraft and other watercraft or other object**
Fall while remaining on watercraft after collision
Note: Select the specified type of watercraft that the victim was on at the time of the collision.
Excludes1 crushed between watercraft and other watercraft and other object due to collision (V91.1-)
drowning and submersion due to falling from crushed watercraft (V90.3-)

X● **V91.20 Fall due to collision between merchant ship and other watercraft or other object**

X● **V91.21 Fall due to collision between passenger ship and other watercraft or other object**
Fall due to collision between ferry-boat and other watercraft or other object
Fall due to collision between liner and other watercraft or other object

X● **V91.22 Fall due to collision between fishing boat and other watercraft or other object**

X● **V91.23 Fall due to collision between other powered watercraft and other watercraft or other object**
Fall due to collision between hovercraft (on open water) and other watercraft or other object
Fall due to collision between jet ski and other watercraft or other object

X● **V91.24 Fall due to collision between sailboat and other watercraft or other object**

X● **V91.25 Fall due to collision between canoe or kayak and other watercraft or other object**

X● **V91.26 Fall due to collision between (nonpowered) inflatable craft and other watercraft or other object**

X● **V91.29 Fall due to collision between unspecified watercraft and other watercraft or other object**
Fall due to collision between boat NOS and other watercraft or other object
Fall due to collision between ship NOS and other watercraft or other object
Fall due to collision between watercraft NOS and other watercraft or other object

● **V91.3 Hit or struck by falling object due to accident to watercraft**
Hit or struck by falling object (part of damaged watercraft or other object) after falling or jumping from damaged watercraft
Excludes2 drowning or submersion due to fall or jumping from damaged watercraft (V90.2-, V90.3-)

X● **V91.30 Hit or struck by falling object due to accident to merchant ship**

X● **V91.31 Hit or struck by falling object due to accident to passenger ship**
Hit or struck by falling object due to accident to ferry-boat
Hit or struck by falling object due to accident to liner

X● **V91.32 Hit or struck by falling object due to accident to fishing boat**

X● **V91.33 Hit or struck by falling object due to accident to other powered watercraft**
Hit or struck by falling object due to accident to hovercraft (on open water)
Hit or struck by falling object due to accident to jet ski

X● **V91.34 Hit or struck by falling object due to accident to sailboat**

X● **V91.35 Hit or struck by falling object due to accident to canoe or kayak**

X● **V91.36 Hit or struck by falling object due to accident to (nonpowered) inflatable craft**

X● **V91.37 Hit or struck by falling object due to accident to water-skis**
Hit by water-skis after jumping off of waterskis

X● **V91.38 Hit or struck by falling object due to accident to other unpowered watercraft**
Hit or struck by surf-board after falling off damaged surf-board
Hit or struck by object after falling off damaged windsurfer

X● **V91.39 Hit or struck by falling object due to accident to unspecified watercraft**
Hit or struck by falling object due to accident to boat NOS
Hit or struck by falling object due to accident to ship NOS
Hit or struck by falling object due to accident to watercraft NOS

● **V91.8 Other injury due to other accident to watercraft**

X● **V91.80 Other injury due to other accident to merchant ship**

X● **V91.81 Other injury due to other accident to passenger ship**
Other injury due to other accident to ferry-boat
Other injury due to other accident to liner

X● **V91.82 Other injury due to other accident to fishing boat**

X● **V91.83 Other injury due to other accident to other powered watercraft**
Other injury due to other accident to hovercraft (on open water)
Other injury due to other accident to jet ski

CHAPTER 20 (V00-Y99)

X● V91.84 Other injury due to other accident to **sailboat**

X● V91.85 Other injury due to other accident to **canoe or kayak**

X● V91.86 Other injury due to other accident to (nonpowered) **inflatable craft**

X● V91.87 Other injury due to other accident to **water-skis**

X● V91.88 Other injury due to other accident to **other unpowered watercraft**
Other injury due to other accident to surf-board
Other injury due to other accident to windsurfer

X● V91.89 Other injury due to other accident to **unspecified** watercraft
Other injury due to other accident to boat NOS
Other injury due to other accident to ship NOS
Other injury due to other accident to watercraft NOS

● **V92 Drowning and submersion due to accident on board watercraft, without accident to watercraft**

Excludes1 civilian water transport accident involving military watercraft (V94.81-)
drowning or submersion due to accident to watercraft (V90-V91)
drowning or submersion of diver who voluntarily jumps from boat not involved in an accident (W16.711, W16.721)
fall into water without watercraft (W16.-)
military watercraft accident in military or war operations (Y36, Y37)

The appropriate 7th character is to be added to each code from category V92

A	initial encounter
D	subsequent encounter
S	sequela

● **V92.0 Drowning and submersion due to fall off watercraft**
Drowning and submersion due to fall from gangplank of watercraft
Drowning and submersion due to fall overboard watercraft
Excludes2 hitting head on object or bottom of body of water due to fall from watercraft (V94.0-)

X● V92.00 **Drowning and submersion due to fall off merchant ship**

X● V92.01 **Drowning and submersion due to fall off passenger ship**
Drowning and submersion due to fall off ferry-boat
Drowning and submersion due to fall off liner

X● V92.02 **Drowning and submersion due to fall off fishing boat**

X● V92.03 **Drowning and submersion due to fall off other powered watercraft**
Drowning and submersion due to fall off hovercraft (on open water)
Drowning and submersion due to fall off jet ski

X● V92.04 **Drowning and submersion due to fall off sailboat**

X● V92.05 **Drowning and submersion due to fall off canoe or kayak**

X● V92.06 **Drowning and submersion due to fall off (nonpowered) inflatable craft**

X● V92.07 **Drowning and submersion due to fall off water-skis**
Excludes1 drowning and submersion due to falling off burning water-skis (V90.27)
drowning and submersion due to falling off crushed water-skis (V90.37)
hit by boat while water-skiing NOS (V94.-)

X● V92.08 **Drowning and submersion due to fall off other unpowered watercraft**
Drowning and submersion due to fall off surf-board
Drowning and submersion due to fall off windsurfer
Excludes1 drowning and submersion due to fall off burning unpowered watercraft (V90.28)
drowning and submersion due to fall off crushed unpowered watercraft (V90.38)
drowning and submersion due to fall off damaged unpowered watercraft (V90.88)
drowning and submersion due to rider of nonpowered watercraft being hit by other watercraft (V94.-)
other injury due to rider of nonpowered watercraft being hit by other watercraft (V94.-)

X● V92.09 **Drowning and submersion due to fall off unspecified watercraft**
Drowning and submersion due to fall off boat NOS
Drowning and submersion due to fall off ship
Drowning and submersion due to fall off watercraft NOS

● **V92.1 Drowning and submersion due to being thrown overboard by motion of watercraft**
Excludes1 drowning and submersion due to fall off surf-board (V92.08)
drowning and submersion due to fall off water-skis (V92.07)
drowning and submersion due to fall off windsurfer (V92.08)

X● V92.10 **Drowning and submersion due to being thrown overboard by motion of merchant ship**

X● V92.11 **Drowning and submersion due to being thrown overboard by motion of passenger ship**
Drowning and submersion due to being thrown overboard by motion of ferry-boat
Drowning and submersion due to being thrown overboard by motion of liner

X● V92.12 **Drowning and submersion due to being thrown overboard by motion of fishing boat**

X● V92.13 **Drowning and submersion due to being thrown overboard by motion of other powered watercraft**
Drowning and submersion due to being thrown overboard by motion of hovercraft

X● V92.14 **Drowning and submersion due to being thrown overboard by motion of sailboat**

X● V92.15 **Drowning and submersion due to being thrown overboard by motion of canoe or kayak**

X● V92.16 **Drowning and submersion due to being thrown overboard by motion of (nonpowered) inflatable craft**

X● V92.19 **Drowning and submersion due to being thrown overboard by motion of unspecified watercraft**
Drowning and submersion due to being thrown overboard by motion of boat NOS
Drowning and submersion due to being thrown overboard by motion of ship NOS
Drowning and submersion due to being thrown overboard by motion of watercraft NOS

● V92.2 **Drowning and submersion due to being washed overboard from watercraft**
Code first any associated cataclysm (X37.Ø-)

X● V92.2Ø **Drowning and submersion due to being washed overboard from merchant ship**

X● V92.21 **Drowning and submersion due to being washed overboard from passenger ship**
Drowning and submersion due to being washed overboard from ferry-boat
Drowning and submersion due to being washed overboard from liner

X● V92.22 **Drowning and submersion due to being washed overboard from fishing boat**

X● V92.23 **Drowning and submersion due to being washed overboard from other powered watercraft**
Drowning and submersion due to being washed overboard from hovercraft (on open water)
Drowning and submersion due to being washed overboard from jet ski

X● V92.24 **Drowning and submersion due to being washed overboard from sailboat**

X● V92.25 **Drowning and submersion due to being washed overboard from canoe or kayak**

X● V92.26 **Drowning and submersion due to being washed overboard from (nonpowered) inflatable craft**

X● V92.27 **Drowning and submersion due to being washed overboard from water-skis**
Excludes1 drowning and submersion due to fall off water-skis (V92.Ø7)

X● V92.28 **Drowning and submersion due to being washed overboard from other unpowered watercraft**
Drowning and submersion due to being washed overboard from surf-board
Drowning and submersion due to being washed overboard from windsurfer

X● V92.29 **Drowning and submersion due to being washed overboard from unspecified** watercraft
Drowning and submersion due to being washed overboard from boat NOS
Drowning and submersion due to being washed overboard from ship NOS
Drowning and submersion due to being washed overboard from watercraft NOS

● V93 **Other injury due to accident on board watercraft, without accident to watercraft**
Excludes1 civilian water transport accident involving military watercraft (V94.81-)
other injury due to accident to watercraft (V91.-)
military watercraft accident in military or war operations (Y36, Y37.-)
Excludes2 drowning and submersion due to accident on board watercraft, without accident to watercraft (V92.-)

The appropriate 7th character is to be added to each code from category V93

A initial encounter
D subsequent encounter
S sequela

● V93.Ø **Burn due to localized fire on board** watercraft
Excludes1 burn due to watercraft on fire (V91.Ø-)

X● V93.ØØ **Burn due to localized fire on board merchant vessel**

X● V93.Ø1 **Burn due to localized fire on board passenger vessel**
Burn due to localized fire on board ferry-boat
Burn due to localized fire on board liner

X● V93.Ø2 **Burn due to localized fire on board fishing boat**

X● V93.Ø3 **Burn due to localized fire on board other powered watercraft**
Burn due to localized fire on board hovercraft
Burn due to localized fire on board jet ski

X● V93.Ø4 **Burn due to localized fire on board sailboat**

X● V93.Ø9 **Burn due to localized fire on board unspecified watercraft**
Burn due to localized fire on board boat NOS
Burn due to localized fire on board ship NOS
Burn due to localized fire on board watercraft NOS

● V93.1 **Other burn on board watercraft**
Burn due to source other than fire on board watercraft
Excludes1 burn due to watercraft on fire (V91.Ø-)

X● V93.1Ø **Other burn on board merchant vessel**

X● V93.11 **Other burn on board passenger vessel**
Other burn on board ferry-boat
Other burn on board liner

X● V93.12 **Other burn on board fishing boat**

X● V93.13 **Other burn on board other powered watercraft**
Other burn on board hovercraft
Other burn on board jet ski

X● V93.14 **Other burn on board sailboat**

X● V93.19 **Other burn on board unspecified watercraft**
Other burn on board boat NOS
Other burn on board ship NOS
Other burn on board watercraft NOS

● V93.2 **Heat exposure on board watercraft**
Excludes1 exposure to man-made heat not aboard watercraft (W92)
exposure to natural heat while on board watercraft (X3Ø)
exposure to sunlight while on board watercraft (X32)
Excludes2 burn due to fire on board watercraft (V93.Ø-)

X● V93.2Ø **Heat exposure on board merchant ship**

X● V93.21 **Heat exposure on board passenger ship**
Heat exposure on board ferry-boat
Heat exposure on board liner

X● V93.22 **Heat exposure on board fishing boat**

X● V93.23 **Heat exposure on board other powered watercraft**
Heat exposure on board hovercraft

X● V93.24 **Heat exposure on board sailboat**

X● V93.29 **Heat exposure on board unspecified** watercraft
Heat exposure on board boat NOS
Heat exposure on board ship NOS
Heat exposure on board watercraft NOS

● V93.3 **Fall on board watercraft**
Excludes1 fall due to collision of watercraft (V91.2-)

X● V93.3Ø **Fall on board merchant ship**

X● V93.31 **Fall on board passenger ship**
Fall on board ferry-boat
Fall on board liner

X● V93.32 **Fall on board fishing boat**

X● V93.33 **Fall on board other powered watercraft**
Fall on board hovercraft (on open water)
Fall on board jet ski

X● V93.34 **Fall on board sailboat**

X● V93.35 **Fall on board canoe or kayak**

X● V93.36 **Fall on board (nonpowered) inflatable craft**

X● V93.38 **Fall on board other unpowered watercraft**

X● V93.39 **Fall on board unspecified** watercraft
Fall on board boat NOS
Fall on board ship NOS
Fall on board watercraft NOS

● **V93.4 Struck by falling object on board watercraft**
Hit by falling object on board watercraft
Excludes1 struck by falling object due to accident to watercraft (V91.3)

X● **V93.40 Struck by falling object on merchant ship**

X● **V93.41 Struck by falling object on passenger ship**
Struck by falling object on ferry-boat
Struck by falling object on liner

X● **V93.42 Struck by falling object on fishing boat**

X● **V93.43 Struck by falling object on other powered watercraft**
Struck by falling object on hovercraft

X● **V93.44 Struck by falling object on sailboat**

X● **V93.48 Struck by falling object on other unpowered watercraft**

X● **V93.49 Struck by falling object on unspecified watercraft**

● **V93.5 Explosion on board watercraft**
Boiler explosion on steamship
Excludes2 fire on board watercraft (V93.Ø-)

X● **V93.5Ø Explosion on board merchant ship**

X● **V93.51 Explosion on board passenger ship**
Explosion on board ferry-boat
Explosion on board liner

X● **V93.52 Explosion on board fishing boat**

X● **V93.53 Explosion on board other powered watercraft**
Explosion on board hovercraft
Explosion on board jet ski

X● **V93.54 Explosion on board sailboat**

X● **V93.59 Explosion on board unspecified watercraft**
Explosion on board boat NOS
Explosion on board ship NOS
Explosion on board watercraft NOS

● **V93.6 Machinery accident on board watercraft**
Excludes1 machinery explosion on board watercraft (V93.4-)
machinery fire on board watercraft (V93.Ø-)

X● **V93.6Ø Machinery accident on board merchant ship**

X● **V93.61 Machinery accident on board passenger ship**
Machinery accident on board ferry-boat
Machinery accident on board liner

X● **V93.62 Machinery accident on board fishing boat**

X● **V93.63 Machinery accident on board other powered watercraft**
Machinery accident on board hovercraft

X● **V93.64 Machinery accident on board sailboat**

X● **V93.69 Machinery accident on board unspecified watercraft**
Machinery accident on board boat NOS
Machinery accident on board ship NOS
Machinery accident on board watercraft NOS

● **V93.8 Other injury due to other accident on board watercraft**
Accidental poisoning by gases or fumes on watercraft

X● **V93.8Ø Other injury due to other accident on board merchant ship**

X● **V93.81 Other injury due to other accident on board passenger ship**
Other injury due to other accident on board ferry-boat
Other injury due to other accident on board liner

X● **V93.82 Other injury due to other accident on board fishing boat**

X● **V93.83 Other injury due to other accident on board other powered watercraft**
Other injury due to other accident on board hovercraft
Other injury due to other accident on board jet ski

X● **V93.84 Other injury due to other accident on board sailboat**

X● **V93.85 Other injury due to other accident on board canoe or kayak**

X● **V93.86 Other injury due to other accident on board (nonpowered) inflatable craft**

X● **V93.87 Other injury due to other accident on board water-skis**
Hit or struck by object while waterskiing

X● **V93.88 Other injury due to other accident on board other unpowered watercraft**
Hit or struck by object while surfing
Hit or struck by object while on board windsurfer

X● **V93.89 Other injury due to other accident on board unspecified watercraft**
Other injury due to other accident on board boat NOS
Other injury due to other accident on board ship NOS
Other injury due to other accident on board watercraft NOS

● **V94 Other and unspecified water transport accidents**
Excludes1 military watercraft accidents in military or war operations (Y36, Y37)

The appropriate 7th character is to be added to each code from category V94

A	initial encounter
D	subsequent encounter
S	sequela

X● **V94.Ø Hitting object or bottom of body of water due to fall from watercraft**
Excludes2 drowning and submersion due to fall from watercraft (V92.Ø-)

● **V94.1 Bather struck by watercraft**
Swimmer hit by watercraft

X● **V94.11 Bather struck by powered watercraft**

X● **V94.12 Bather struck by nonpowered watercraft**

● **V94.2 Rider of nonpowered watercraft struck by other watercraft**

X● **V94.21 Rider of nonpowered watercraft struck by other nonpowered watercraft**
Canoer hit by other nonpowered watercraft
Surfer hit by other nonpowered watercraft
Windsurfer hit by other nonpowered watercraft

X● **V94.22 Rider of nonpowered watercraft struck by powered watercraft**
Canoer hit by motorboat
Surfer hit by motorboat
Windsurfer hit by motorboat

● **V94.3 Injury to rider of (inflatable) watercraft being pulled behind other watercraft**

X● **V94.31 Injury to rider of (inflatable) recreational watercraft being pulled behind other watercraft**
Injury to rider of inner-tube pulled behind motor boat

X● **V94.32 Injury to rider of non-recreational watercraft being pulled behind other watercraft**
Injury to occupant of dingy being pulled behind boat or ship
Injury to occupant of life-raft being pulled behind boat or ship

X● **V94.4 Injury to barefoot water-skier**
Injury to person being pulled behind boat or ship

● **V94.8 Other water transport accident**

● **V94.81 Water transport accident involving military watercraft**

● **V94.81Ø Civilian watercraft involved in water transport accident with military watercraft**
Passenger on civilian watercraft injured due to accident with military watercraft

V94.811 Civilian in water injured by military watercraft

V94.818 Other water transport accident involving military watercraft

X V94.89 Other water transport accident

X V94.9 Unspecified water transport accident
Water transport accident NOS

AIR AND SPACE TRANSPORT ACCIDENTS (V95-V97)

Excludes1 military aircraft accidents in military or war operations (Y36, Y37)

V95 Accident to powered aircraft causing injury to occupant

The appropriate 7th character is to be added to each code from category V95

A	initial encounter
D	subsequent encounter
S	sequela

V95.0 Helicopter accident injuring occupant

X V95.00 Unspecified helicopter accident injuring occupant

X V95.01 Helicopter crash injuring occupant

X V95.02 Forced landing of helicopter injuring occupant

X V95.03 Helicopter collision injuring occupant
Helicopter collision with any object, fixed, movable or moving

X V95.04 Helicopter fire injuring occupant

X V95.05 Helicopter explosion injuring occupant

X V95.09 Other helicopter accident injuring occupant

V95.1 Ultralight, microlight or powered-glider accident injuring occupant

X V95.10 Unspecified ultralight, microlight or powered-glider accident injuring occupant

X V95.11 Ultralight, microlight or powered-glider crash injuring occupant

X V95.12 Forced landing of ultralight, microlight or powered-glider injuring occupant

X V95.13 Ultralight, microlight or powered-glider collision injuring occupant
Ultralight, microlight or powered-glider collision with any object, fixed, movable or moving

X V95.14 Ultralight, microlight or powered-glider fire injuring occupant

X V95.15 Ultralight, microlight or powered-glider explosion injuring occupant

X V95.19 Other ultralight, microlight or powered-glider accident injuring occupant

V95.2 Other private fixed-wing aircraft accident injuring occupant

X V95.20 Unspecified accident to other private fixed-wing aircraft, injuring occupant

X V95.21 Other private fixed-wing aircraft crash injuring occupant

X V95.22 Forced landing of other private fixed-wing aircraft injuring occupant

X V95.23 Other private fixed-wing aircraft collision injuring occupant
Other private fixed-wing aircraft collision with any object, fixed, movable or moving

X V95.24 Other private fixed-wing aircraft fire injuring occupant

X V95.25 Other private fixed-wing aircraft explosion injuring occupant

X V95.29 Other accident to other private fixed-wing aircraft injuring occupant

V95.3 Commercial fixed-wing aircraft accident injuring occupant

X V95.30 Unspecified accident to commercial fixed-wing aircraft injuring occupant

X V95.31 Commercial fixed-wing aircraft crash injuring occupant

X V95.32 Forced landing of commercial fixed-wing aircraft injuring occupant

X V95.33 Commercial fixed-wing aircraft collision injuring occupant
Commercial fixed-wing aircraft collision with any object, fixed, movable or moving

X V95.34 Commercial fixed-wing aircraft fire injuring occupant

X V95.35 Commercial fixed-wing aircraft explosion injuring occupant

X V95.39 Other accident to commercial fixed-wing aircraft injuring occupant

V95.4 Spacecraft accident injuring occupant

X V95.40 Unspecified spacecraft accident injuring occupant

X V95.41 Spacecraft crash injuring occupant

X V95.42 Forced landing of spacecraft injuring occupant

X V95.43 Spacecraft collision injuring occupant
Spacecraft collision with any object, fixed, moveable or moving

X V95.44 Spacecraft fire injuring occupant

X V95.45 Spacecraft explosion injuring occupant

X V95.49 Other spacecraft accident injuring occupant

X V95.8 Other powered aircraft accidents injuring occupant

X V95.9 Unspecified aircraft accident injuring occupant
Aircraft accident NOS
Air transport accident NOS

V96 Accident to nonpowered aircraft causing injury to occupant

The appropriate 7th character is to be added to each code from category V96

A	initial encounter
D	subsequent encounter
S	sequela

V96.0 Balloon accident injuring occupant

X V96.00 Unspecified balloon accident injuring occupant

X V96.01 Balloon crash injuring occupant

X V96.02 Forced landing of balloon injuring occupant

X V96.03 Balloon collision injuring occupant
Balloon collision with any object, fixed, moveable or moving

X V96.04 Balloon fire injuring occupant

X V96.05 Balloon explosion injuring occupant

X V96.09 Other balloon accident injuring occupant

V96.1 Hang-glider accident injuring occupant

X V96.10 Unspecified hang-glider accident injuring occupant

X V96.11 Hang-glider crash injuring occupant

X V96.12 Forced landing of hang-glider injuring occupant

X V96.13 Hang-glider collision injuring occupant
Hang-glider collision with any object, fixed, moveable or moving

X V96.14 Hang-glider fire injuring occupant

X V96.15 Hang-glider explosion injuring occupant

X V96.19 Other hang-glider accident injuring occupant

V96.2 Glider (nonpowered) accident injuring occupant

X V96.20 Unspecified glider (nonpowered) accident injuring occupant

X V96.21 Glider (nonpowered) crash injuring occupant

X V96.22 Forced landing of glider (nonpowered) injuring occupant

X● V96.23 Glider (nonpowered) collision injuring occupant
Glider (nonpowered) collision with any object, fixed, moveable or moving

X● V96.24 Glider (nonpowered) fire injuring occupant

X● V96.25 Glider (nonpowered) explosion injuring occupant

X● V96.29 Other glider (nonpowered) accident injuring occupant

X● V96.8 Other nonpowered-aircraft accidents injuring occupant
Kite carrying a person accident injuring occupant

X● V96.9 Unspecified nonpowered-aircraft accident injuring occupant
Nonpowered-aircraft accident NOS

● V97 Other specified air transport accidents
The appropriate 7th character is to be added to each code from category V97

A	initial encounter
D	subsequent encounter
S	sequela

X● V97.0 Occupant of aircraft injured in other specified air transport accidents
Fall in, on or from aircraft in air transport accident
Excludes1 accident while boarding or alighting aircraft (V97.1)

X● V97.1 Person injured while boarding or alighting from aircraft

● V97.2 Parachutist accident

X● V97.21 Parachutist entangled in object
Parachutist landing in tree

X● V97.22 Parachutist injured on landing

X● V97.29 Other parachutist accident

● V97.3 Person on ground injured in air transport accident

X● V97.31 Hit by object falling from aircraft
Hit by crashing aircraft
Injured by aircraft hitting house
Injured by aircraft hitting car

X● V97.32 Injured by rotating propeller

X● V97.33 Sucked into jet engine

X● V97.39 Other injury to person on ground due to air transport accident

● V97.8 Other air transport accidents, not elsewhere classified
Excludes1 aircraft accident NOS (V95.9)
exposure to changes in air pressure during ascent or descent (W94.-)

● V97.81 Air transport accident involving military aircraft

● V97.810 Civilian aircraft involved in air transport accident with military aircraft
Passenger in civilian aircraft injured due to accident with military aircraft

● V97.811 Civilian injured by military aircraft

● V97.818 Other air transport accident involving military aircraft

X● V97.89 Other air transport accidents, not elsewhere classified
Injury from machinery on aircraft

OTHER AND UNSPECIFIED TRANSPORT ACCIDENTS (V98-V99)

Excludes1 vehicle accident, type of vehicle unspecified (V89.-)

● V98 Other specified transport accidents
The appropriate 7th character is to be added to each code from category V98

A	initial encounter
D	subsequent encounter
S	sequela

X● V98.0 Accident to, on or involving cable-car, not on rails
Caught or dragged by cable-car, not on rails
Fall or jump from cable-car, not on rails
Object thrown from or in cable-car, not on rails

X● V98.1 Accident to, on or involving land-yacht

X● V98.2 Accident to, on or involving ice yacht

X● V98.3 Accident to, on or involving ski lift
Accident to, on or involving ski chair-lift
Accident to, on or involving ski-lift with gondola

X● V98.8 Other specified transport accidents

X● V99 Unspecified transport accident
The appropriate 7th character is to be added to code V99

A	initial encounter
D	subsequent encounter
S	sequela

OTHER EXTERNAL CAUSES OF ACCIDENTAL INJURY (W00-X58)

SLIPPING, TRIPPING, STUMBLING AND FALLS (W00-W19)

Excludes1 assault involving a fall (Y01-Y02)
fall from animal (V80.-)
fall (in) (from) machinery (in operation) (W28-W31)
fall (in) (from) transport vehicle (V01-V99)
intentional self-harm involving a fall (X80-X81)

Excludes2 at risk for fall (history of fall) Z91.81
fall (in) (from) burning building (X00.-)
fall into fire (X00-X04, X08)

● W00 Fall due to ice and snow
Includes pedestrian on foot falling (slipping) on ice and snow
Excludes1 fall on (from) ice and snow involving pedestrian conveyance (V00.-)
fall from stairs and steps not due to ice and snow (W10.-)
The appropriate 7th character is to be added to each code from category W00

A	initial encounter
D	subsequent encounter
S	sequela

X● W00.0 Fall on same level due to ice and snow
Coding Clinic: 2016, Q2, P5

X● W00.1 Fall from stairs and steps due to ice and snow

X● W00.2 Other fall from one level to another due to ice and snow

X● W00.9 Unspecified fall due to ice and snow

● W01 Fall on same level from slipping, tripping and stumbling
Includes fall on moving sidewalk
Excludes1 fall due to bumping (striking) against object (W18.0-)
fall in shower or bathtub (W18.2-)
fall on same level NOS (W18.30)
fall on same level from slipping, tripping and stumbling due to ice or snow (W00.0)
fall off or from toilet (W18.1-)
slipping, tripping and stumbling NOS (W18.40)
slipping, tripping and stumbling without falling (W18.4-)
The appropriate 7th character is to be added to each code from category W01

A	initial encounter
D	subsequent encounter
S	sequela

X● W01.0 Fall on same level from slipping, tripping and stumbling without subsequent striking against object
Falling over animal

● W01.1 Fall on same level from slipping, tripping and stumbling with subsequent striking against object

X ● **W01.10 Fall on same level from slipping, tripping and stumbling with subsequent striking against unspecified object**

● **W01.11 Fall on same level from slipping, tripping and stumbling with subsequent striking against sharp object**

● **W01.110 Fall on same level from slipping, tripping and stumbling with subsequent striking against sharp glass**

● **W01.111 Fall on same level from slipping, tripping and stumbling with subsequent striking against power tool or machine**

● **W01.118 Fall on same level from slipping, tripping and stumbling with subsequent striking against other sharp object**

● **W01.119 Fall on same level from slipping, tripping and stumbling with subsequent striking against unspecified sharp object**

● **W01.19 Fall on same level from slipping, tripping and stumbling with subsequent striking against other object**

● **W01.190 Fall on same level from slipping, tripping and stumbling with subsequent striking against furniture**

Coding Clinic: 2021, Q1, P5

● **W01.198 Fall on same level from slipping, tripping and stumbling with subsequent striking against other object**

X ● **W03 Other fall on same level due to collision with another person**

Fall due to non-transport collision with other person

Excludes1 collision with another person without fall (W51)
crushed or pushed by a crowd or human stampede (W52)
fall involving pedestrian conveyance (V00-V09)
fall due to ice or snow (W00)
fall on same level NOS (W18.30)

The appropriate 7th character is to be added to code W03

- A initial encounter
- D subsequent encounter
- S sequela

Coding Clinic: 2015, Q1, P9-10; 2012, Q4, P108

X ● **W04 Fall while being carried or supported by other persons**

Accidentally dropped while being carried

The appropriate 7th character is to be added to code W04

- A initial encounter
- D subsequent encounter
- S sequel

● **W05 Fall from non-moving wheelchair, nonmotorized scooter and motorized mobility scooter**

Excludes1 fall from moving wheelchair (powered) (V00.811)
fall from moving motorized mobility scooter (V00.831)
fall from nonmotorized scooter (V00.141)

The appropriate 7th character is to be added to each code from category W05

- A initial encounter
- D subsequent encounter
- S sequela

X ● **W05.0 Fall from non-moving wheelchair**

Coding Clinic: 2019, Q2, P27

X ● **W05.1 Fall from non-moving nonmotorized scooter**

X ● **W05.2 Fall from non-moving motorized mobility scooter**

X ● **W06 Fall from bed**

The appropriate 7th character is to be added to code W06

- A initial encounter
- D subsequent encounter
- S sequela

X ● **W07 Fall from chair**

The appropriate 7th character is to be added to code W07

- A initial encounter
- D subsequent encounter
- S sequela

X ● **W08 Fall from other furniture**

The appropriate 7th character is to be added to code W08

- A initial encounter
- D subsequent encounter
- S sequela

● **W09 Fall on and from playground equipment**

Excludes1 fall involving recreational machinery (W31)

The appropriate 7th character is to be added to each code from category W09

- A initial encounter
- D subsequent encounter
- S sequela

X ● **W09.0 Fall on or from playground slide**

X ● **W09.1 Fall from playground swing**

X ● **W09.2 Fall on or from jungle gym**

X ● **W09.8 Fall on or from other playground equipment**

● **W10 Fall on and from stairs and steps**

Excludes1 fall from stairs and steps due to ice and snow (W00.1)

The appropriate 7th character is to be added to each code from category W10

- A initial encounter
- D subsequent encounter
- S sequela

X ● **W10.0 Fall (on) (from) escalator**

X ● **W10.1 Fall (on) (from) sidewalk curb**

X ● **W10.2 Fall (on) (from) incline**

Fall (on) (from) ramp

X ● **W10.8 Fall (on) (from) other stairs and steps**

X ● **W10.9 Fall (on) (from) unspecified stairs and steps**

X ● **W11 Fall on and from ladder**

The appropriate 7th character is to be added to code W11

- A initial encounter
- D subsequent encounter
- S sequela

X ● **W12 Fall on and from scaffolding**

The appropriate 7th character is to be added to code W12

- A initial encounter
- D subsequent encounter
- S sequela

● **W13 Fall from, out of or through building or structure**

The appropriate 7th character is to be added to each code from category W13

- A initial encounter
- D subsequent encounter
- S sequela

CHAPTER 20 (V00-Y99)

X● **W13.Ø Fall from, out of or through balcony**
Fall from, out of or through railing

X● **W13.1 Fall from, out of or through bridge**

X● **W13.2 Fall from, out of or through roof**

X● **W13.3 Fall through floor**

X● **W13.4 Fall from, out of or through window**
Excludes2 fall with subsequent striking against sharp glass (WØ1.11Ø-)

X● **W13.8 Fall from, out of or through other building or structure**
Fall from, out of or through viaduct
Fall from, out of or through wall
Fall from, out of or through flag-pole

X● **W13.9 Fall from, out of or through building, not otherwise specified**
Excludes1 collapse of a building or structure (W2Ø.-)
fall or jump from burning building or structure (XØØ.-)

X● **W14 Fall from tree**
The appropriate 7th character is to be added to code W14

A	initial encounter
D	subsequent encounter
S	sequela

X● **W15 Fall from cliff**
The appropriate 7th character is to be added to code W15

A	initial encounter
D	subsequent encounter
S	sequela

● **W16 Fall, jump or diving into water**
Excludes1 accidental non-watercraft drowning and submersion not involving fall (W65-W74)
effects of air pressure from diving (W94.-)
fall into water from watercraft (V9Ø-V94)
hitting an object or against bottom when falling from watercraft (V94.Ø)
Excludes2 striking or hitting diving board (W21.4)
The appropriate 7th character is to be added to each code from category W16

A	initial encounter
D	subsequent encounter
S	sequela

● **W16.Ø Fall into swimming pool**
Fall into swimming pool NOS
Excludes1 fall into empty swimming pool (W17.3)

● **W16.Ø1 Fall into swimming pool striking water surface**

● **W16.Ø11 Fall into swimming pool striking water surface causing drowning and submersion**
Excludes1 drowning and submersion while in swimming pool without fall (W67)

● **W16.Ø12 Fall into swimming pool striking water surface causing other injury**

● **W16.Ø2 Fall into swimming pool striking bottom**

● **W16.Ø21 Fall into swimming pool striking bottom causing drowning and submersion**
Excludes1 drowning and submersion while in swimming pool without fall (W67)

● **W16.Ø22 Fall into swimming pool striking bottom causing other injury**

● **W16.Ø3 Fall into swimming pool striking wall**

● **W16.Ø31 Fall into swimming pool striking wall causing drowning and submersion**
Excludes1 drowning and submersion while in swimming pool without fall (W67)

● **W16.Ø32 Fall into swimming pool striking wall causing other injury**

● **W16.1 Fall into natural body of water**
Fall into lake
Fall into open sea
Fall into river
Fall into stream

● **W16.11 Fall into natural body of water striking water surface**

● **W16.111 Fall into natural body of water striking water surface causing drowning and submersion**
Excludes1 drowning and submersion while in natural body of water without fall (W69)

● **W16.112 Fall into natural body of water striking water surface causing other injury**

● **W16.12 Fall into natural body of water striking bottom**

● **W16.121 Fall into natural body of water striking bottom causing drowning and submersion**
Excludes1 drowning and submersion while in natural body of water without fall (W69)

● **W16.122 Fall into natural body of water striking bottom causing other injury**

● **W16.13 Fall into natural body of water striking side**

● **W16.131 Fall into natural body of water striking side causing drowning and submersion**
Excludes1 drowning and submersion while in natural body of water without fall (W69)

● **W16.132 Fall into natural body of water striking side causing other injury**

● **W16.2 Fall in (into) filled bathtub or bucket of water**

● **W16.21 Fall in (into) filled bathtub**
Excludes1 fall into empty bathtub (W18.2)

● **W16.211 Fall in (into) filled bathtub causing drowning and submersion**
Excludes1 drowning and submersion while in filled bathtub without fall (W65)

● **W16.212 Fall in (into) filled bathtub causing other injury**

● **W16.22 Fall in (into) bucket of water**

● **W16.221 Fall in (into) bucket of water causing drowning and submersion**

● **W16.222 Fall in (into) bucket of water causing other injury**

● **W16.3 Fall into other water**
Fall into fountain
Fall into reservoir

● **W16.31 Fall into other water striking water surface**

● **W16.311 Fall into other water striking water surface causing drowning and submersion**
Excludes1 drowning and submersion while in other water without fall (W73)

● **W16.312 Fall into other water striking water surface causing other injury**

● **W16.32 Fall into other water striking bottom**

● **W16.321 Fall into other water striking bottom causing drowning and submersion**
Excludes1 drowning and submersion while in other water without fall (W73)

● **W16.322 Fall into other water striking bottom causing other injury**

● **W16.33 Fall into other water striking wall**

● **W16.331 Fall into other water striking wall causing drowning and submersion**
Excludes1 drowning and submersion while in other water without fall (W73)

● **W16.332 Fall into other water striking wall causing other injury**

● **W16.4 Fall into unspecified water**

X● **W16.41 Fall into unspecified water causing drowning and submersion**

X● **W16.42 Fall into unspecified water causing other injury**

● **W16.5 Jumping or diving into swimming pool**

● **W16.51 Jumping or diving into swimming pool striking water surface**

● **W16.511 Jumping or diving into swimming pool striking water surface causing drowning and submersion**
Excludes1 drowning and submersion while in swimming pool without jumping or diving (W67)

● **W16.512 Jumping or diving into swimming pool striking water surface causing other injury**

● **W16.52 Jumping or diving into swimming pool striking bottom**

● **W16.521 Jumping or diving into swimming pool striking bottom causing drowning and submersion**
Excludes1 drowning and submersion while in swimming pool without jumping or diving (W67)

● **W16.522 Jumping or diving into swimming pool striking bottom causing other injury**

● **W16.53 Jumping or diving into swimming pool striking wall**

● **W16.531 Jumping or diving into swimming pool striking wall causing drowning and submersion**
Excludes1 drowning and submersion while in swimming pool without jumping or diving (W67)

● **W16.532 Jumping or diving into swimming pool striking wall causing other injury**

● **W16.6 Jumping or diving into natural body of water**
Jumping or diving into lake
Jumping or diving into open sea
Jumping or diving into river
Jumping or diving into stream

● **W16.61 Jumping or diving into natural body of water striking water surface**

● **W16.611 Jumping or diving into natural body of water striking water surface causing drowning and submersion**
Excludes1 drowning and submersion while in natural body of water without jumping or diving (W69)

● **W16.612 Jumping or diving into natural body of water striking water surface causing other injury**

● **W16.62 Jumping or diving into natural body of water striking bottom**

● **W16.621 Jumping or diving into natural body of water striking bottom causing drowning and submersion**
Excludes1 drowning and submersion while in natural body of water without jumping or diving (W69)

● **W16.622 Jumping or diving into natural body of water striking bottom causing other injury**

● **W16.7 Jumping or diving from boat**
Excludes1 fall from boat into water - see watercraft accident (V9Ø-V94)

● **W16.71 Jumping or diving from boat striking water surface**

● **W16.711 Jumping or diving from boat striking water surface causing drowning and submersion**

● **W16.712 Jumping or diving from boat striking water surface causing other injury**

● **W16.72 Jumping or diving from boat striking bottom**

● **W16.721 Jumping or diving from boat striking bottom causing drowning and submersion**

● **W16.722 Jumping or diving from boat striking bottom causing other injury**

● W16.8 Jumping or diving into other water
Jumping or diving into fountain
Jumping or diving into reservoir

● W16.81 Jumping or diving into other water striking water surface

● W16.811 Jumping or diving into other water striking water surface causing drowning and submersion
Excludes1 drowning and submersion while in other water without jumping or diving (W73)

● W16.812 Jumping or diving into other water striking water surface causing other injury

● W16.82 Jumping or diving into other water striking bottom

● W16.821 Jumping or diving into other water striking bottom causing drowning and submersion
Excludes1 drowning and submersion while in other water without jumping or diving (W73)

● W16.822 Jumping or diving into other water striking bottom causing other injury

● W16.83 Jumping or diving into other water striking wall

● W16.831 Jumping or diving into other water striking wall causing drowning and submersion
Excludes1 drowning and submersion while in other water without jumping or diving (W73)

● W16.832 Jumping or diving into other water striking wall causing other injury

● W16.9 Jumping or diving into unspecified water

X● W16.91 Jumping or diving into unspecified water causing drowning and submersion

X● W16.92 Jumping or diving into unspecified water causing other injury

● W17 Other fall from one level to another
The appropriate 7th character is to be added to each code from category W17

A	initial encounter
D	subsequent encounter
S	sequela

X● W17.0 Fall into well

X● W17.1 Fall into storm drain or manhole

X● W17.2 Fall into hole
Fall into pit

X● W17.3 Fall into empty swimming pool
Excludes1 fall into filled swimming pool (W16.0-)

X● W17.4 Fall from dock

● W17.8 Other fall from one level to another

X● W17.81 Fall down embankment (hill)

X● W17.82 Fall from (out of) grocery cart
Fall due to grocery cart tipping over

X● W17.89 Other fall from one level to another
Fall from cherry picker
Fall from lifting device
Fall from mobile elevated work platform [MEWP]
Fall from sky lift
Coding Clinic: 2015, Q2, P6

● W18 Other slipping, tripping and stumbling and falls
The appropriate 7th character is to be added to each code from category W18

A	initial encounter
D	subsequent encounter
S	sequela

● W18.0 Fall due to bumping against object
Striking against object with subsequent fall
Excludes1 fall on same level due to slipping, tripping, or stumbling with subsequent striking against object (W01.1-)

X● W18.00 Striking against unspecified object with subsequent fall

X● W18.01 Striking against sports equipment with subsequent fall

X● W18.02 Striking against glass with subsequent fall

X● W18.09 Striking against other object with subsequent fall

● W18.1 Fall from or off toilet

X● W18.11 Fall from or off toilet without subsequent striking against object
Fall from (off) toilet NOS

X● W18.12 Fall from or off toilet with subsequent striking against object

X● W18.2 Fall in (into) shower or empty bathtub
Excludes1 fall in full bathtub causing drowning or submersion (W16.21-)

● W18.3 Other and unspecified fall on same level

X● W18.30 Fall on same level, unspecified

X● W18.31 Fall on same level due to stepping on an object
Fall on same level due to stepping on an animal
Excludes1 slipping, tripping and stumbling without fall due to stepping on animal (W18.41)

X● W18.39 Other fall on same level

● W18.4 Slipping, tripping and stumbling without falling
Excludes1 collision with another person without fall (W51)

X● W18.40 Slipping, tripping and stumbling without falling, unspecified

X● W18.41 Slipping, tripping and stumbling without falling due to stepping on object
Slipping, tripping and stumbling without falling due to stepping on animal
Excludes1 slipping, tripping and stumbling with fall due to stepping on animal (W18.31)

X● W18.42 Slipping, tripping and stumbling without falling due to stepping into hole or opening

X● W18.43 Slipping, tripping and stumbling without falling due to stepping from one level to another

X● W18.49 Other slipping, tripping and stumbling without falling

X● W19 Unspecified fall
Accidental fall NOS
The appropriate 7th character is to be added to code W19

A	initial encounter
D	subsequent encounter
S	sequela

CHAPTER 20 (V00-Y99)

EXPOSURE TO INANIMATE MECHANICAL FORCES (W20-W49)

Excludes1 assault (X92-Y09)
contact or collision with animals or persons (W50-W64)
exposure to inanimate mechanical forces involving military or war operations (Y36.-, Y37.-)
intentional self-harm (X71-X83)

Coding Clinic: 2022, Q4, P45; 2021, Q2, P5; 2016, Q4, P129; 2012, Q4, P95

● **W20 Struck by thrown, projected or falling object**

Code first any associated:
cataclysm (X34-X39)
lightning strike (T75.00)

Excludes1 falling object in machinery accident (W24, W28-W31)
falling object in transport accident (V01-V99)
object set in motion by explosion (W35-W40)
object set in motion by firearm (W32-W34)
struck by thrown sports equipment (W21.-)

The appropriate 7th character is to be added to each code from category W20

A	initial encounter
D	subsequent encounter
S	sequela

X● **W20.0 Struck by falling object in cave-in**
Excludes2 asphyxiation due to cave-in (T71.21)

X● **W20.1 Struck by object due to collapse of building**
Excludes1 struck by object due to collapse of burning building (X00.2, X02.2)

X● **W20.8 Other cause of strike by thrown, projected or falling object**
Excludes1 struck by thrown sports equipment (W21.-)

● **W21 Striking against or struck by sports equipment**

Excludes1 assault with sports equipment (Y08.0-)
striking against or struck by sports equipment with subsequent fall (W18.01)

The appropriate 7th character is to be added to each code from category W21

A	initial encounter
D	subsequent encounter
S	sequela

● **W21.0 Struck by hit or thrown ball**
X● **W21.00 Struck by hit or thrown ball, unspecified type**
X● **W21.01 Struck by football**
X● **W21.02 Struck by soccer ball**
X● **W21.03 Struck by baseball**
X● **W21.04 Struck by golf ball**
X● **W21.05 Struck by basketball**
X● **W21.06 Struck by volleyball**
X● **W21.07 Struck by softball**
X● **W21.09 Struck by other hit or thrown ball**

● **W21.1 Struck by bat, racquet or club**
X● **W21.11 Struck by baseball bat**
X● **W21.12 Struck by tennis racquet**
X● **W21.13 Struck by golf club**
X● **W21.19 Struck by other bat, racquet or club**

● **W21.2 Struck by hockey stick or puck**
● **W21.21 Struck by hockey stick**
● **W21.210 Struck by ice hockey stick**
● **W21.211 Struck by field hockey stick**
● **W21.22 Struck by hockey puck**
● **W21.220 Struck by ice hockey puck**
● **W21.221 Struck by field hockey puck**

● **W21.3 Struck by sports foot wear**
X● **W21.31 Struck by shoe cleats**
Stepped on by shoe cleats
X● **W21.32 Struck by skate blades**
Skated over by skate blades
X● **W21.39 Struck by other sports foot wear**

X● **W21.4 Striking against diving board**
Use additional code for subsequent falling into water, if applicable (W16.-)

● **W21.8 Striking against or struck by other sports equipment**
X● **W21.81 Striking against or struck by football helmet**
X● **W21.89 Striking against or struck by other sports equipment**

X● **W21.9 Striking against or struck by unspecified sports equipment**

● **W22 Striking against or struck by other objects**

Excludes1 striking against or struck by object with subsequent fall (W18.09)

The appropriate 7th character is to be added to each code from category W22

A	initial encounter
D	subsequent encounter
S	sequela

● **W22.0 Striking against stationary object**
Excludes1 striking against stationary sports equipment (W21.8)
X● **W22.01 Walked into wall**
X● **W22.02 Walked into lamppost**
X● **W22.03 Walked into furniture**
● **W22.04 Striking against wall of swimming pool**
● **W22.041 Striking against wall of swimming pool causing drowning and submersion**
Excludes1 drowning and submersion while swimming without striking against wall (W67)
● **W22.042 Striking against wall of swimming pool causing other injury**
X● **W22.09 Striking against other stationary object**

● **W22.1 Striking against or struck by automobile airbag**
X● **W22.10 Striking against or struck by unspecified automobile airbag**
X● **W22.11 Striking against or struck by driver side automobile airbag**
X● **W22.12 Striking against or struck by front passenger side automobile airbag**
X● **W22.19 Striking against or struck by other automobile airbag**

X● **W22.8 Striking against or struck by other objects**
Striking against or struck by object NOS
Excludes1 struck by thrown, projected or falling object (W20.-)

CHAPTER 20 (V00-Y99)

●W23 **Caught, crushed, jammed or pinched in or between objects**
Excludes1 injury caused by cutting or piercing instruments (W25-W27)
injury caused by firearms malfunction (W32.1, W33.1-, W34.1-)
injury caused by lifting and transmission devices (W24.-)
injury caused by machinery (W28-W31)
injury caused by nonpowered hand tools (W27.-)
injury caused by transport vehicle being used as a means of transportation (V01-V99)
injury caused by struck by thrown, projected or falling object (W20.-)
The appropriate 7th character is to be added to each code from category W23
A initial encounter
D subsequent encounter
S sequela

X● W23.0 **Caught, crushed, jammed, or pinched between moving objects**
X● W23.1 **Caught, crushed, jammed, or pinched between stationary objects**
X● W23.2 **Caught, crushed, jammed or pinched between a moving and stationary object**

●W24 **Contact with lifting and transmission devices, not elsewhere classified**
Excludes1 transport accidents (V01-V99)
The appropriate 7th character is to be added to each code from category W24
A initial encounter
D subsequent encounter
S sequela

X● W24.0 **Contact with lifting devices, not elsewhere classified**
Contact with chain hoist
Contact with drive belt
Contact with pulley (block)
X● W24.1 **Contact with transmission devices, not elsewhere classified**
Contact with transmission belt or cable

X●W25 **Contact with sharp glass**
Code first any associated:
injury due to flying glass from explosion or firearm discharge (W32-W40)
transport accident (V00-V99)
Excludes1 fall on same level due to slipping, tripping and stumbling with subsequent striking against sharp glass (W01.110-)
striking against sharp glass with subsequent fall (W18.02-)
Excludes2 glass embedded in skin (W45.-)
The appropriate 7th character is to be added to code W25
A initial encounter
D subsequent encounter
S sequela

●W26 **Contact with other sharp objects**
Excludes2 sharp object(s) embedded in skin (W45.-)
The appropriate 7th character is to be added to each code from category W26
A initial encounter
D subsequent encounter
S sequela

Coding Clinic: 2016, Q4, P73

X● W26.0 **Contact with knife**
Excludes1 contact with electric knife (W29.1)
X● W26.1 **Contact with sword or dagger**
X● W26.2 **Contact with edge of stiff paper**
Paper cut
Coding Clinic: 2016, Q4, P73
X● W26.8 **Contact with other sharp object(s), not elsewhere classified**
Contact with tin can lid
Coding Clinic: 2016, Q4, P73
X● W26.9 **Contact with unspecified sharp object(s)**
Coding Clinic: 2016, Q4, P73

●W27 **Contact with nonpowered hand tool**
The appropriate 7th character is to be added to each code from category W27
A initial encounter
D subsequent encounter
S sequela

X● W27.0 **Contact with workbench tool**
Contact with auger
Contact with axe
Contact with chisel
Contact with handsaw
Contact with screwdriver
X● W27.1 **Contact with garden tool**
Contact with hoe
Contact with nonpowered lawn mower
Contact with pitchfork
Contact with rake
X● W27.2 **Contact with scissors**
X● W27.3 **Contact with needle (sewing)**
Excludes1 contact with hypodermic needle (W46.-)
X● W27.4 **Contact with kitchen utensil**
Contact with fork
Contact with ice-pick
Contact with can-opener NOS
X● W27.5 **Contact with paper-cutter**
X● W27.8 **Contact with other nonpowered hand tool**
Contact with nonpowered sewing machine
Contact with shovel

X●W28 **Contact with powered lawn mower**
Powered lawn mower (commercial) (residential)
Excludes1 contact with nonpowered lawn mower (W27.1)
Excludes2 exposure to electric current (W86.-)
The appropriate 7th character is to be added to code W28
A initial encounter
D subsequent encounter
S sequela

●W29 **Contact with other powered hand tools and household machinery**
Excludes1 contact with commercial machinery (W31.82)
contact with hot household appliance (X15)
contact with nonpowered hand tool (W27.-)
exposure to electric current (W86)
The appropriate 7th character is to be added to each code from category W29
A initial encounter
D subsequent encounter
S sequela

X● W29.0 **Contact with powered kitchen appliance**
Contact with blender
Contact with can-opener
Contact with garbage disposal
Contact with mixer
X● W29.1 **Contact with electric knife**
X● W29.2 **Contact with other powered household machinery**
Contact with electric fan
Contact with powered dryer (clothes) (powered) (spin)
Contact with washing-machine
Contact with sewing machine

X● W29.3 Contact with powered garden and outdoor hand tools and machinery
Contact with chainsaw
Contact with edger
Contact with garden cultivator (tiller)
Contact with hedge trimmer
Contact with other powered garden tool
Excludes1 contact with powered lawn mower (W28)

X● W29.4 Contact with nail gun

X● W29.8 Contact with other powered hand tools and household machinery
Contact with do-it-yourself tool NOS

● W30 Contact with agricultural machinery
Includes animal-powered farm machine
Excludes1 agricultural transport vehicle accident (V01-V99)
explosion of grain store (W40.8)
exposure to electric current (W86.-)

The appropriate 7th character is to be added to each code from category W30

A	initial encounter
D	subsequent encounter
S	sequela

X● W30.0 Contact with combine harvester
Contact with reaper
Contact with thresher

X● W30.1 Contact with power take-off devices (PTO)

X● W30.2 Contact with hay derrick

X● W30.3 Contact with grain storage elevator
Excludes1 explosion of grain store (W40.8)

● W30.8 Contact with other specified agricultural machinery

X● W30.81 Contact with agricultural transport vehicle in stationary use
Contact with agricultural transport vehicle under repair, not on public roadway
Excludes1 agricultural transport vehicle accident (V01-V99)

X● W30.89 Contact with other specified agricultural machinery

X● W30.9 Contact with unspecified agricultural machinery
Contact with farm machinery NOS

● W31 Contact with other and unspecified machinery
Excludes1 contact with agricultural machinery (W30.-)
contact with machinery in transport under own power or being towed by a vehicle (V01-V99)
exposure to electric current (W86)

The appropriate 7th character is to be added to each code from category W31

A	initial encounter
D	subsequent encounter
S	sequela

X● W31.0 Contact with mining and earth-drilling machinery
Contact with bore or drill (land) (seabed)
Contact with shaft hoist
Contact with shaft lift
Contact with undercutter

X● W31.1 Contact with metalworking machines
Contact with abrasive wheel
Contact with forging machine
Contact with lathe
Contact with mechanical shears
Contact with metal drilling machine
Contact with milling machine
Contact with power press
Contact with rolling-mill
Contact with metal sawing machine

X● W31.2 Contact with powered woodworking and forming machines
Contact with band saw
Contact with bench saw
Contact with circular saw
Contact with molding machine
Contact with overhead plane
Contact with powered saw
Contact with radial saw
Contact with sander
Excludes1 nonpowered woodworking tools (W27.0)

X● W31.3 Contact with prime movers
Contact with gas turbine
Contact with internal combustion engine
Contact with steam engine
Contact with water driven turbine

● W31.8 Contact with other specified machinery

X● W31.81 Contact with recreational machinery
Contact with roller-coaster

X● W31.82 Contact with other commercial machinery
Contact with commercial electric fan
Contact with commercial kitchen appliances
Contact with commercial powered dryer (clothes) (powered) (spin)
Contact with commercial washing-machine
Contact with commercial sewing machine
Excludes1 contact with household machinery (W29.-)
contact with powered lawn mower (W28)

X● W31.83 Contact with special construction vehicle in stationary use
Contact with special construction vehicle under repair, not on public roadway
Excludes1 special construction vehicle accident (V01-V99)

X● W31.89 Contact with other specified machinery

X● W31.9 Contact with unspecified machinery
Contact with machinery NOS

● W32 Accidental handgun discharge and malfunction
Includes accidental discharge and malfunction of gun for single hand use
accidental discharge and malfunction of pistol
accidental discharge and malfunction of revolver
handgun discharge and malfunction NOS
Excludes1 accidental airgun discharge and malfunction (W34.010, W34.110)
accidental BB gun discharge and malfunction (W34.010, W34.110)
accidental pellet gun discharge and malfunction (W34.010, W34.110)
accidental shotgun discharge and malfunction (W33.01, W33.11)
assault by handgun discharge (X93)
handgun discharge involving legal intervention (Y35.0-)
handgun discharge involving military or war operations (Y36.4-)
intentional self-harm by handgun discharge (X72)
Very pistol discharge and malfunction (W34.09, W34.19)

The appropriate 7th character is to be added to each code from category W32

A	initial encounter
D	subsequent encounter
S	sequela

X● W32.0 Accidental handgun discharge

X● W32.1 Accidental handgun malfunction
Injury due to explosion of handgun (parts)
Injury due to malfunction of mechanism or component of handgun
Injury due to recoil of handgun
Powder burn from handgun

CHAPTER 20 (V00-Y99)

W33 Accidental rifle, shotgun and larger firearm discharge and malfunction

Includes rifle, shotgun and larger firearm discharge and malfunction NOS

Excludes1 accidental airgun discharge and malfunction (W34.010, W34.110)
accidental BB gun discharge and malfunction (W34.010, W34.110)
accidental handgun discharge and malfunction (W32.-)
accidental pellet gun discharge and malfunction (W34.010, W34.110)
assault by rifle, shotgun and larger firearm discharge (X94)
firearm discharge involving legal intervention (Y35.0-)
firearm discharge involving military or war operations (Y36.4-)
intentional self-harm by rifle, shotgun and larger firearm discharge (X73)

The appropriate 7th character is to be added to each code from category W33

A initial encounter
D subsequent encounter
S sequela

W33.0 Accidental rifle, shotgun and larger firearm discharge

X **W33.00 Accidental discharge of unspecified larger firearm**
Discharge of unspecified larger firearm NOS

X **W33.01 Accidental discharge of shotgun**
Discharge of shotgun NOS

X **W33.02 Accidental discharge of hunting rifle**
Discharge of hunting rifle NOS

X **W33.03 Accidental discharge of machine gun**
Discharge of machine gun NOS

X **W33.09 Accidental discharge of other larger firearm**
Discharge of other larger firearm NOS

W33.1 Accidental rifle, shotgun and larger firearm malfunction
Injury due to explosion of rifle, shotgun and larger firearm (parts)
Injury due to malfunction of mechanism or component of rifle, shotgun and larger firearm
Injury due to piercing, cutting, crushing or pinching due to (by) slide trigger mechanism, scope or other gun part
Injury due to recoil of rifle, shotgun and larger firearm
Powder burn from rifle, shotgun and larger firearm

X **W33.10 Accidental malfunction of unspecified larger firearm**
Malfunction of unspecified larger firearm NOS

X **W33.11 Accidental malfunction of shotgun**
Malfunction of shotgun NOS

X **W33.12 Accidental malfunction of hunting rifle**
Malfunction of hunting rifle NOS

X **W33.13 Accidental malfunction of machine gun**
Malfunction of machine gun NOS

X **W33.19 Accidental malfunction of other larger firearm**
Malfunction of other larger firearm NOS

W34 Accidental discharge and malfunction from other and unspecified firearms and guns

The appropriate 7th character is to be added to each code from category W34

A initial encounter
D subsequent encounter
S sequela

W34.0 Accidental discharge from other and unspecified firearms and guns

X **W34.00 Accidental discharge from unspecified firearms or gun**
Discharge from firearm NOS
Gunshot wound NOS
Shot NOS
Coding Clinic: 2015, Q1, P17

W34.01 Accidental discharge of gas, air or spring-operated guns

W34.010 Accidental discharge of airgun
Accidental discharge of BB gun
Accidental discharge of pellet gun

W34.011 Accidental discharge of paintball gun
Accidental injury due to paintball discharge

W34.018 Accidental discharge of other gas, air or spring-operated gun

X **W34.09 Accidental discharge from other specified firearms**
Accidental discharge from Very pistol [flare]

W34.1 Accidental malfunction from other and unspecified firearms and guns

X **W34.10 Accidental malfunction from unspecified firearms or gun**
Firearm malfunction NOS

W34.11 Accidental malfunction of gas, air or spring-operated guns

W34.110 Accidental malfunction of airgun
Accidental malfunction of BB gun
Accidental malfunction of pellet gun

W34.111 Accidental malfunction of paintball gun
Accidental injury due to paintball gun malfunction

W34.118 Accidental malfunction of other gas, air or spring-operated gun

X **W34.19 Accidental malfunction from other specified firearms**
Accidental malfunction from Very pistol [flare]

X **W35 Explosion and rupture of boiler**

Excludes1 explosion and rupture of boiler on watercraft (V93.4)

The appropriate 7th character is to be added to code W35

A initial encounter
D subsequent encounter
S sequela

W36 Explosion and rupture of gas cylinder

The appropriate 7th character is to be added to each code from category W36

A initial encounter
D subsequent encounter
S sequela

X **W36.1 Explosion and rupture of aerosol can**

X **W36.2 Explosion and rupture of air tank**

X **W36.3 Explosion and rupture of pressurized-gas tank**

X **W36.8 Explosion and rupture of other gas cylinder**

X **W36.9 Explosion and rupture of unspecified gas cylinder**

W37 Explosion and rupture of pressurized tire, pipe or hose

The appropriate 7th character is to be added to each code from category W37

A initial encounter
D subsequent encounter
S sequela

X **W37.0 Explosion of bicycle tire**

X **W37.8 Explosion and rupture of other pressurized tire, pipe or hose**

CHAPTER 20 (V00-Y99)

X● W38 Explosion and rupture of other specified pressurized devices

The appropriate 7th character is to be added to code W38

A	initial encounter
D	subsequent encounter
S	sequela

X● W39 Discharge of firework

The appropriate 7th character is to be added to code W39

A	initial encounter
D	subsequent encounter
S	sequela

● W40 Explosion of other materials

Excludes1 assault by explosive material (X96)
explosion involving legal intervention (Y35.1-)
explosion involving military or war operations (Y36.0-, Y36.2-)
intentional self-harm by explosive material (X75)

The appropriate 7th character is to be added to each code from category W40

A	initial encounter
D	subsequent encounter
S	sequela

X● W40.0 Explosion of blasting material
Explosion of blasting cap
Explosion of detonator
Explosion of dynamite
Explosion of explosive (any) used in blasting operations

X● W40.1 Explosion of explosive gases
Explosion of acetylene
Explosion of butane
Explosion of coal gas
Explosion in mine NOS
Explosion of explosive gas
Explosion of fire damp
Explosion of gasoline fumes
Explosion of methane
Explosion of propane

X● W40.8 Explosion of other specified explosive materials
Explosion in dump NOS
Explosion in factory NOS
Explosion in grain store
Explosion in munitions

Excludes1 explosion involving legal intervention (Y35.1-)
explosion involving military or war operations (Y36.0-, Y36.2-)

X● W40.9 Explosion of unspecified explosive materials
Explosion NOS

● W42 Exposure to noise

The appropriate 7th character is to be added to each code from category W42

A	initial encounter
D	subsequent encounter
S	sequela

X● W42.0 Exposure to supersonic waves

X● W42.9 Exposure to other noise
Exposure to sound waves NOS

● W44 Foreign body entering into or through a natural orifice

Excludes2 contact with other sharp objects (W26)
contact with sharp glass (W25)
foreign body or object entering through skin (W45)

The appropriate 7th character is to be added to each code from category W44

A	initial encounter
D	subsequent encounter
S	sequela

X● W44.A Battery entering into or through a natural orifice

W44.A0 Battery unspecified, entering into or through a natural orifice

W44.A1 Button battery entering into or through a natural orifice

W44.A9 Other batteries entering into or through a natural orifice
Cylindrical battery

X● W44.B Plastic entering into or through a natural orifice

W44.B0 Plastic object unspecified, entering into or through a natural orifice

W44.B1 Plastic bead entering into or through a natural orifice

Excludes2 Plastic jewelry entering into or through a natural orifice (W44.B4)

W44.B2 Plastic coin entering into or through a natural orifice

W44.B3 Plastic toy and toy part entering into or through a natural orifice

W44.B4 Plastic jewelry entering into or through a natural orifice

Excludes2 Plastic bead entering into or through a natural orifice (W44.B1)

W44.B5 Plastic bottle entering into or through a natural orifice

W44.B9 Other plastic object entering into or through a natural orifice

X● W44.C Glass entering into or through a natural orifice

W44.C0 Glass unspecified, entering into or through a natural orifice

W44.C1 Sharp glass entering into or through a natural orifice
Glass shard entering into or through a natural orifice

W44.C2 Intact glass entering into or through a natural orifice
Intact glass bottle entering into or through a natural orifice

X● W44.D Magnetic metal entering into or through a natural orifice

W44.D0 Magnetic metal object unspecified, entering into or through a natural orifice

W44.D1 Magnetic metal bead entering into or through a natural orifice

W44.D2 Magnetic metal coin entering into or through a natural orifice

W44.D3 Magnetic metal toy entering into or through a natural orifice

W44.D4 Magnetic metal jewelry entering into or through a natural orifice

W44.D9 Other magnetic metal objects entering into or through a natural orifice

X● W44.E Non-magnetic metal entering into or through a natural orifice

W44.E0 Non-magnetic metal object unspecified, entering into or through a natural orifice

W44.E1 Non-magnetic metal bead entering into or through a natural orifice

W44.E2 Non-magnetic metal coin entering into or through a natural orifice

W44.E3 **Non-magnetic metal toy entering into or through a natural orifice**

W44.E4 **Non-magnetic metal jewelry entering into or through a natural orifice**

W44.E9 **Other non-magnetic metal objects entering into or through a natural orifice**
Bottle cap entering into or through a natural orifice
Can lid entering into or through a natural orifice
Pull tab entering into or through a natural orifice

X● **W44.F Objects of natural or organic material entering into or through a natural orifice**

W44.F0 **Objects of natural or organic material unspecified, entering into or through anatural orifice**

W44.F1 **Bezoar entering into or through a natural orifice**

W44.F2 **Rubber band entering into or through a natural orifice**

W44.F3 **Food entering into or through a natural orifice**

W44.F4 **Insect entering into or through a natural orifice**

W44.F9 **Other object of natural or organic material, entering into or through a natural orifice**

X● **W44.G Other non-organic objects entering into or through a natural orifice**

W44.G0 **Other non-organic objects unspecified, entering into or through a natural orifice**

W44.G1 **Audio device entering into or through a natural orifice**
Ear buds
Hearing aids

W44.G2 **Combination metal and plastic toy and toy part entering into or through natural orifice**

W44.G3 **Combination metal and plastic jewelry entering into or through a natural orifice**

W44.G9 **Other non-organic objects entering into or through a natural orifice**

X● **W44.H Other sharp object entering into or through a natural orifice**

W44.H0 **Other sharp object unspecified, entering into or through a natural orifice**

W44.H1 **Needle entering into or through a natural orifice**
Dart entering into or through a natural orifice
Hypodermic needle entering into or through a natural orifice
Safety pin entering into or through a natural orifice
Sewing needle entering into or through a natural orifice

W44.H2 **Knife, sword or dagger entering into or through a natural orifice**

W44.8 **Other foreign body entering into or through a natural orifice**

W44.9 **Unspecified foreign body entering into or through a natural orifice**
Foreign body NOS entering into or through a natural orifice

● **W45 Foreign body or object entering through skin**

Includes foreign body or object embedded in skin
nail embedded in skin

Excludes2 contact with hand tools (nonpowered) (powered) (W27-W29)
contact with other sharp object(s) (W26.-)
contact with sharp glass (W25.-)
struck by objects (W20-W22)

The appropriate 7th character is to be added to each code from category W45

A	initial encounter
D	subsequent encounter
S	sequela

X● **W45.0 Nail entering through skin**

X● **W45.8 Other foreign body or object entering through skin**
Splinter in skin NOS

● **W46 Contact with hypodermic needle**

The appropriate 7th character is to be added to each code from category W46

A	initial encounter
D	subsequent encounter
S	sequela

X● **W46.0 Contact with hypodermic needle**
Hypodermic needle stick NOS

X● **W46.1 Contact with contaminated hypodermic needle**

● **W49 Exposure to other inanimate mechanical forces**

Includes exposure to abnormal gravitational [G] forces
exposure to inanimate mechanical forces NEC

Excludes1 exposure to inanimate mechanical forces involving military or war operations (Y36.-, Y37.-)

The appropriate 7th character is to be added to each code from category W49

A	initial encounter
D	subsequent encounter
S	sequela

● **W49.0 Item causing external constriction**

X● **W49.01 Hair causing external constriction**

X● **W49.02 String or thread causing external constriction**

X● **W49.03 Rubber band causing external constriction**

X● **W49.04 Ring or other jewelry causing external constriction**

X● **W49.09 Other item causing external constriction**

X● **W49.9 Exposure to other inanimate mechanical forces**

EXPOSURE TO ANIMATE MECHANICAL FORCES (W50-W64)

Excludes1 toxic effect of contact with venomous animals and plants (T63.-)

● **W50 Accidental hit, strike, kick, twist, bite or scratch by another person**

Includes hit, strike, kick, twist, bite, or scratch by another person NOS

Excludes1 assault by bodily force (Y04)
struck by objects (W20-W22)

The appropriate 7th character is to be added to each code from category W50

A	initial encounter
D	subsequent encounter
S	sequela

X● **W50.0 Accidental hit or strike by another person**
Hit or strike by another person NOS

X● **W50.1 Accidental kick by another person**
Kick by another person NOS

X● **W50.2 Accidental twist by another person**
Twist by another person NOS
Coding Clinic: 2015, Q1, P8

X● **W50.3 Accidental bite by another person**
Human bite
Bite by another person NOS

X● **W50.4 Accidental scratch by another person**
Scratch by another person NOS

CHAPTER 20 (V00-Y99)

X● **W51 Accidental striking against or bumped into by another person**

Excludes1 assault by striking against or bumping into by another person (Y04.2)
fall due to collision with another person (W03)

The appropriate 7th character is to be added to code W51

A initial encounter
D subsequent encounter
S sequela

X● **W52 Crushed, pushed or stepped on by crowd or human stampede**

Crushed, pushed or stepped on by crowd or human stampede with or without fall

The appropriate 7th character is to be added to code W52

A initial encounter
D subsequent encounter
S sequela

● **W53 Contact with rodent**

Includes contact with saliva, feces or urine of rodent

The appropriate 7th character is to be added to each code from category W53

A initial encounter
D subsequent encounter
S sequela

● **W53.0 Contact with mouse**
X● **W53.01 Bitten by mouse**
X● **W53.09 Other contact with mouse**
● **W53.1 Contact with rat**
X● **W53.11 Bitten by rat**
X● **W53.19 Other contact with rat**
● **W53.2 Contact with squirrel**
X● **W53.21 Bitten by squirrel**
X● **W53.29 Other contact with squirrel**
● **W53.8 Contact with other rodent**
X● **W53.81 Bitten by other rodent**
X● **W53.89 Other contact with other rodent**

● **W54 Contact with dog**

Includes contact with saliva, feces or urine of dog

The appropriate 7th character is to be added to each code from category W54

A initial encounter
D subsequent encounter
S sequela

X● **W54.0 Bitten by dog**
X● **W54.1 Struck by dog**
Knocked over by dog
X● **W54.8 Other contact with dog**

● **W55 Contact with other mammals**

Includes contact with saliva, feces or urine of mammal
Excludes1 animal being ridden - see transport accidents
bitten or struck by dog (W54)
bitten or struck by rodent (W53.-)
contact with marine mammals (W56.X-)

The appropriate 7th character is to be added to each code from category W55

A initial encounter
D subsequent encounter
S sequela

● **W55.0 Contact with cat**
X● **W55.01 Bitten by cat**
X● **W55.03 Scratched by cat**
X● **W55.09 Other contact with cat**
● **W55.1 Contact with horse**
X● **W55.11 Bitten by horse**
X● **W55.12 Struck by horse**
X● **W55.19 Other contact with horse**
● **W55.2 Contact with cow**
Contact with bull
X● **W55.21 Bitten by cow**
X● **W55.22 Struck by cow**
Gored by bull
X● **W55.29 Other contact with cow**
● **W55.3 Contact with other hoof stock**
Contact with goats
Contact with sheep
X● **W55.31 Bitten by other hoof stock**
X● **W55.32 Struck by other hoof stock**
Gored by goat
Gored by ram
X● **W55.39 Other contact with other hoof stock**
● **W55.4 Contact with pig**
X● **W55.41 Bitten by pig**
X● **W55.42 Struck by pig**
X● **W55.49 Other contact with pig**
● **W55.5 Contact with raccoon**
X● **W55.51 Bitten by raccoon**
X● **W55.52 Struck by raccoon**
X● **W55.59 Other contact with raccoon**
● **W55.8 Contact with other mammals**
X● **W55.81 Bitten by other mammals**
X● **W55.82 Struck by other mammals**
X● **W55.89 Other contact with other mammals**

● **W56 Contact with nonvenomous marine animal**

Excludes1 contact with venomous marine animal (T63.-)

The appropriate 7th character is to be added to each code from category W56

A initial encounter
D subsequent encounter
S sequela

● **W56.0 Contact with dolphin**
X● **W56.01 Bitten by dolphin**
X● **W56.02 Struck by dolphin**
X● **W56.09 Other contact with dolphin**
● **W56.1 Contact with sea lion**
X● **W56.11 Bitten by sea lion**
X● **W56.12 Struck by sea lion**
X● **W56.19 Other contact with sea lion**
● **W56.2 Contact with orca**
Contact with killer whale
X● **W56.21 Bitten by orca**
X● **W56.22 Struck by orca**
X● **W56.29 Other contact with orca**
● **W56.3 Contact with other marine mammals**
X● **W56.31 Bitten by other marine mammals**
X● **W56.32 Struck by other marine mammals**
X● **W56.39 Other contact with other marine mammals**
● **W56.4 Contact with shark**
X● **W56.41 Bitten by shark**
X● **W56.42 Struck by shark**
X● **W56.49 Other contact with shark**
● **W56.5 Contact with other fish**
X● **W56.51 Bitten by other fish**
X● **W56.52 Struck by other fish**
X● **W56.59 Other contact with other fish**

●W56.8 Contact with other nonvenomous marine animals
X●W56.81 Bitten by other nonvenomous marine animals
X●W56.82 Struck by other nonvenomous marine animals
X●W56.89 Other contact with other nonvenomous marine animals

X●W57 Bitten or stung by nonvenomous insect and other nonvenomous arthropods
Excludes1 contact with venomous insects and arthropods (T63.2-, T63.3-, T63.4-)
The appropriate 7th character is to be added to code W57

A	initial encounter
D	subsequent encounter
S	sequela

●W58 Contact with crocodile or alligator
The appropriate 7th character is to be added to each code from category W58

A	initial encounter
D	subsequent encounter
S	sequela

●W58.0 Contact with alligator
X●W58.01 Bitten by alligator
X●W58.02 Struck by alligator
X●W58.03 Crushed by alligator
X●W58.09 Other contact with alligator
●W58.1 Contact with crocodile
X●W58.11 Bitten by crocodile
X●W58.12 Struck by crocodile
X●W58.13 Crushed by crocodile
X●W58.19 Other contact with crocodile

●W59 Contact with other nonvenomous reptiles
Excludes1 contact with venomous reptile (T63.0-, T63.1-)
The appropriate 7th character is to be added to each code from category W59

A	initial encounter
D	subsequent encounter
S	sequela

●W59.0 Contact with nonvenomous lizards
X●W59.01 Bitten by nonvenomous lizards
X●W59.02 Struck by nonvenomous lizards
X●W59.09 Other contact with nonvenomous lizards
Exposure to nonvenomous lizards
●W59.1 Contact with nonvenomous snakes
X●W59.11 Bitten by nonvenomous snake
X●W59.12 Struck by nonvenomous snake
X●W59.13 Crushed by nonvenomous snake
X●W59.19 Other contact with nonvenomous snake
●W59.2 Contact with turtles
Excludes1 contact with tortoises (W59.8-)
X●W59.21 Bitten by turtle
X●W59.22 Struck by turtle
X●W59.29 Other contact with turtle
Exposure to turtles
●W59.8 Contact with other nonvenomous reptiles
X●W59.81 Bitten by other nonvenomous reptiles
X●W59.82 Struck by other nonvenomous reptiles
X●W59.83 Crushed by other nonvenomous reptiles
X●W59.89 Other contact with other nonvenomous reptiles

X●W60 Contact with nonvenomous plant thorns and spines and sharp leaves
Excludes1 contact with venomous plants (T63.X7-)
The appropriate 7th character is to be added to code W60

A	initial encounter
D	subsequent encounter
S	sequela

●W61 Contact with birds (domestic) (wild)
Includes contact with excreta of birds
The appropriate 7th character is to be added to each code from category W61

A	initial encounter
D	subsequent encounter
S	sequela

●W61.0 Contact with parrot
X●W61.01 Bitten by parrot
X●W61.02 Struck by parrot
X●W61.09 Other contact with parrot
Exposure to parrots
●W61.1 Contact with macaw
X●W61.11 Bitten by macaw
X●W61.12 Struck by macaw
X●W61.19 Other contact with macaw
Exposure to macaws
●W61.2 Contact with other psittacines
X●W61.21 Bitten by other psittacines
X●W61.22 Struck by other psittacines
X●W61.29 Other contact with other psittacines
Exposure to other psittacines
●W61.3 Contact with chicken
X●W61.32 Struck by chicken
X●W61.33 Pecked by chicken
X●W61.39 Other contact with chicken
Exposure to chickens
●W61.4 Contact with turkey
X●W61.42 Struck by turkey
X●W61.43 Pecked by turkey
X●W61.49 Other contact with turkey
●W61.5 Contact with goose
X●W61.51 Bitten by goose
X●W61.52 Struck by goose
X●W61.59 Other contact with goose
●W61.6 Contact with duck
X●W61.61 Bitten by duck
X●W61.62 Struck by duck
X●W61.69 Other contact with duck
●W61.9 Contact with other birds
X●W61.91 Bitten by other birds
X●W61.92 Struck by other birds
X●W61.99 Other contact with other birds
Contact with bird NOS

●W62 Contact with nonvenomous amphibians
Excludes1 contact with venomous amphibians (T63.81-T63.83)
The appropriate 7th character is to be added to each code from category W62

A	initial encounter
D	subsequent encounter
S	sequela

X●W62.0 Contact with nonvenomous frogs
X●W62.1 Contact with nonvenomous toads
X●W62.9 Contact with other nonvenomous amphibians

X● W64 Exposure to other animate mechanical forces

Includes exposure to nonvenomous animal NOS

Excludes1 contact with venomous animal (T63.-)

The appropriate 7th character is to be added to code W64

A initial encounter
D subsequent encounter
S sequela

ACCIDENTAL NON-TRANSPORT DROWNING AND SUBMERSION (W65-W74)

Excludes1 accidental drowning and submersion due to fall into water (W16.-)
accidental drowning and submersion due to water transport accident (V9Ø.-, V92.-)

Excludes2 accidental drowning and submersion due to cataclysm (X34-X39)

X● W65 Accidental drowning and submersion while in bathtub

Excludes1 accidental drowning and submersion due to fall in (into) bathtub (W16.211)

The appropriate 7th character is to be added to code W65

A initial encounter
D subsequent encounter
S sequela

X● W67 Accidental drowning and submersion while in swimming pool

Excludes1 accidental drowning and submersion due to fall into swimming pool (W16.Ø11, W16.Ø21, W16.Ø31)
accidental drowning and submersion due to striking into wall of swimming pool (W22.Ø41)

Coding Clinic: 2Ø23, Q1, P26

The appropriate 7th character is to be added to code W67

A initial encounter
D subsequent encounter
S sequela

X● W69 Accidental drowning and submersion while in natural water

Accidental drowning and submersion while in lake
Accidental drowning and submersion while in open sea
Accidental drowning and submersion while in river
Accidental drowning and submersion while in stream

Excludes1 accidental drowning and submersion due to fall into natural body of water (W16.111, W16.121, W16.131)

The appropriate 7th character is to be added to code W69

A initial encounter
D subsequent encounter
S sequela

X● W73 Other specified cause of accidental non-transport drowning and submersion

Accidental drowning and submersion while in quenching tank
Accidental drowning and submersion while in reservoir

Excludes1 accidental drowning and submersion due to fall into other water (W16.311, W16.321, W16.331)

The appropriate 7th character is to be added to code W73

A initial encounter
D subsequent encounter
S sequela

X● W74 Unspecified cause of accidental drowning and submersion

Drowning NOS

The appropriate 7th character is to be added to code W74

A initial encounter
D subsequent encounter
S sequela

EXPOSURE TO ELECTRIC CURRENT, RADIATION AND EXTREME AMBIENT AIR TEMPERATURE AND PRESSURE (W85-W99)

Excludes1 exposure to:
failure in dosage of radiation or temperature during surgical and medical care (Y63.2-Y63.5)
lightning (T75.Ø-)
natural cold (X31)
natural heat (X3Ø)
natural radiation NOS (X39)
radiological procedure and radiotherapy (Y84.2)
sunlight (X32)

X● W85 Exposure to electric transmission lines

Broken power line

The appropriate 7th character is to be added to code W85

A initial encounter
D subsequent encounter
S sequela

● W86 Exposure to other specified electric current

The appropriate 7th character is to be added to each code from category W86

A initial encounter
D subsequent encounter
S sequela

X● W86.Ø Exposure to domestic wiring and appliances

X● W86.1 Exposure to industrial wiring, appliances and electrical machinery

Exposure to conductors
Exposure to control apparatus
Exposure to electrical equipment and machinery
Exposure to transformers

X● W86.8 Exposure to other electric current

Exposure to wiring and appliances in or on farm (not farmhouse)
Exposure to wiring and appliances outdoors
Exposure to wiring and appliances in or on public building
Exposure to wiring and appliances in or on residential institutions
Exposure to wiring and appliances in or on schools

● W88 Exposure to ionizing radiation

Excludes1 exposure to sunlight (X32)

The appropriate 7th character is to be added to each code from category W88

A initial encounter
D subsequent encounter
S sequela

X● W88.Ø Exposure to X-rays

X● W88.1 Exposure to radioactive isotopes

X● W88.8 Exposure to other ionizing radiation

● W89 Exposure to man-made visible and ultraviolet light

Includes exposure to welding light (arc)

Excludes2 exposure to sunlight (X32)

The appropriate 7th character is to be added to each code from category W89

A initial encounter
D subsequent encounter
S sequela

X● W89.Ø Exposure to welding light (arc)

X● W89.1 Exposure to tanning bed

X● W89.8 Exposure to other man-made visible and ultraviolet light

X● W89.9 Exposure to unspecified man-made visible and ultraviolet light

CHAPTER 2Ø (VØØ-Y99)

● **W90 Exposure to other nonionizing radiation**
Excludes2 exposure to sunlight (X32)
The appropriate 7th character is to be added to each code from category W90
A initial encounter
D subsequent encounter
S sequela

X● **W90.0 Exposure to radiofrequency**
X● **W90.1 Exposure to infrared radiation**
X● **W90.2 Exposure to laser radiation**
X● **W90.8 Exposure to other nonionizing radiation**

X● **W92 Exposure to excessive heat of man-made origin**
The appropriate 7th character is to be added to code W92
A initial encounter
D subsequent encounter
S sequela

● **W93 Exposure to excessive cold of man-made origin**
The appropriate 7th character is to be added to each code from category W93
A initial encounter
D subsequent encounter
S sequela

● **W93.0 Contact with or inhalation of dry ice**
X● **W93.01 Contact with dry ice**
X● **W93.02 Inhalation of dry ice**
● **W93.1 Contact with or inhalation of liquid air**
X● **W93.11 Contact with liquid air**
Contact with liquid hydrogen
Contact with liquid nitrogen
X● **W93.12 Inhalation of liquid air**
Inhalation of liquid hydrogen
Inhalation of liquid nitrogen
X● **W93.2 Prolonged exposure in deep freeze unit or refrigerator**
X● **W93.8 Exposure to other excessive cold of man-made origin**

● **W94 Exposure to high and low air pressure and changes in air pressure**
The appropriate 7th character is to be added to each code from category W94
A initial encounter
D subsequent encounter
S sequela

X● **W94.0 Exposure to prolonged high air pressure**
● **W94.1 Exposure to prolonged low air pressure**
X● **W94.11 Exposure to residence or prolonged visit at high altitude**
X● **W94.12 Exposure to other prolonged low air pressure**
● **W94.2 Exposure to rapid changes in air pressure during ascent**
X● **W94.21 Exposure to reduction in atmospheric pressure while surfacing from deep-water diving**
X● **W94.22 Exposure to reduction in atmospheric pressure while surfacing from underground**
X● **W94.23 Exposure to sudden change in air pressure in aircraft during ascent**
X● **W94.29 Exposure to other rapid changes in air pressure during ascent**
● **W94.3 Exposure to rapid changes in air pressure during descent**
X● **W94.31 Exposure to sudden change in air pressure in aircraft during descent**
X● **W94.32 Exposure to high air pressure from rapid descent in water**
X● **W94.39 Exposure to other rapid changes in air pressure during descent**

X● **W99 Exposure to other man-made environmental factors**
The appropriate 7th character is to be added to code W99
A initial encounter
D subsequent encounter
S sequela

EXPOSURE TO SMOKE, FIRE AND FLAMES (X00-X08)

Excludes1 arson (X97)
Excludes2 explosions (W35-W40)
lightning (T75.0-)
transport accident (V01-V99)

● **X00 Exposure to uncontrolled fire in building or structure**
Includes conflagration in building or structure
Code first any associated cataclysm
Excludes2 exposure to ignition or melting of nightwear (X05)
exposure to ignition or melting of other clothing and apparel (X06.-)
exposure to other specified smoke, fire and flames (X08.-)
The appropriate 7th character is to be added to each code from category X00
A initial encounter
D subsequent encounter
S sequela

X● **X00.0 Exposure to flames in uncontrolled fire in building or structure**
Coding Clinic: 2016, Q2, P5-6; 2015, Q1, P19
X● **X00.1 Exposure to smoke in uncontrolled fire in building or structure**
X● **X00.2 Injury due to collapse of burning building or structure in uncontrolled fire**
Excludes1 injury due to collapse of building not on fire (W20.1)
X● **X00.3 Fall from burning building or structure in uncontrolled fire**
X● **X00.4 Hit by object from burning building or structure in uncontrolled fire**
X● **X00.5 Jump from burning building or structure in uncontrolled fire**
X● **X00.8 Other exposure to uncontrolled fire in building or structure**

● **X01 Exposure to uncontrolled fire, not in building or structure**
Includes exposure to forest fire
The appropriate 7th character is to be added to each code from category X01
A initial encounter
D subsequent encounter
S sequela

X● **X01.0 Exposure to flames in uncontrolled fire, not in building or structure**
X● **X01.1 Exposure to smoke in uncontrolled fire, not in building or structure**
X● **X01.3 Fall due to uncontrolled fire, not in building or structure**
X● **X01.4 Hit by object due to uncontrolled fire, not in building or structure**
X● **X01.8 Other exposure to uncontrolled fire, not in building or structure**

● X02 Exposure to controlled fire in building or structure

Includes exposure to fire in fireplace exposure to fire in stove

The appropriate 7th character is to be added to each code from category X02

A	initial encounter
D	subsequent encounter
S	sequela

X● X02.0 Exposure to flames in controlled fire in building or structure

X● X02.1 Exposure to smoke in controlled fire in building or structure

X● X02.2 Injury due to collapse of burning building or structure in controlled fire

Excludes1 injury due to collapse of building not on fire (W20.1)

X● X02.3 Fall from burning building or structure in controlled fire

X● X02.4 Hit by object from burning building or structure in controlled fire

X● X02.5 Jump from burning building or structure in controlled fire

X● X02.8 Other exposure to controlled fire in building or structure

● X03 Exposure to controlled fire, not in building or structure

Includes exposure to bon fire exposure to camp fire exposure to trash fire

The appropriate 7th character is to be added to each code from category X03

A	initial encounter
D	subsequent encounter
S	sequela

X● X03.0 Exposure to flames in controlled fire, not in building or structure

Coding Clinic: 2015, Q1, P19

X● X03.1 Exposure to smoke in controlled fire, not in building or structure

X● X03.3 Fall due to controlled fire, not in building or structure

X● X03.4 Hit by object due to controlled fire, not in building or structure

X● X03.8 Other exposure to controlled fire, not in building or structure

X● X04 Exposure to ignition of highly flammable material

Exposure to ignition of gasoline
Exposure to ignition of kerosene
Exposure to ignition of petrol

Excludes2 exposure to ignition or melting of nightwear (X05)
exposure to ignition or melting of other clothing and apparel (X06)

The appropriate 7th character is to be added to code X04

A	initial encounter
D	subsequent encounter
S	sequela

Coding Clinic: 2016, Q2, P4

X● X05 Exposure to ignition or melting of nightwear

Excludes2 exposure to uncontrolled fire in building or structure (X00.-)
exposure to uncontrolled fire, not in building or structure (X01.-)
exposure to controlled fire in building or structure (X02.-)
exposure to controlled fire, not in building or structure (X03.-)
exposure to ignition of highly flammable materials (X04.-)

The appropriate 7th character is to be added to code X05

A	initial encounter
D	subsequent encounter
S	sequela

● X06 Exposure to ignition or melting of other clothing and apparel

Excludes2 exposure to uncontrolled fire in building or structure (X00.-)
exposure to uncontrolled fire, not in building or structure (X01.-)
exposure to controlled fire in building or structure (X02.-)
exposure to controlled fire, not in building or structure (X03.-)
exposure to ignition of highly flammable materials (X04.-)

The appropriate 7th character is to be added to each code from category X06

A	initial encounter
D	subsequent encounter
S	sequela

X● X06.0 Exposure to ignition of plastic jewelry

X● X06.1 Exposure to melting of plastic jewelry

X● X06.2 Exposure to ignition of other clothing and apparel

X● X06.3 Exposure to melting of other clothing and apparel

● X08 Exposure to other specified smoke, fire and flames

The appropriate 7th character is to be added to each code from category X08

A	initial encounter
D	subsequent encounter
S	sequela

● X08.0 Exposure to bed fire

Exposure to mattress fire

X● X08.00 Exposure to bed fire due to unspecified burning material

X● X08.01 Exposure to bed fire due to burning cigarette

Coding Clinic: 2015, Q1, P19

X● X08.09 Exposure to bed fire due to other burning material

● X08.1 Exposure to sofa fire

X● X08.10 Exposure to sofa fire due to unspecified burning material

X● X08.11 Exposure to sofa fire due to burning cigarette

X● X08.19 Exposure to sofa fire due to other burning material

● X08.2 Exposure to other furniture fire

X● X08.20 Exposure to other furniture fire due to unspecified burning material

X● X08.21 Exposure to other furniture fire due to burning cigarette

X● X08.29 Exposure to other furniture fire due to other burning material

X● X08.8 Exposure to other specified smoke, fire and flames

CHAPTER 20 (V00-Y99)

CONTACT WITH HEAT AND HOT SUBSTANCES (X1Ø-X19)

Excludes1 exposure to excessive natural heat (X3Ø)
exposure to fire and flames (XØØ-XØ8)

● **X1Ø Contact with hot drinks, food, fats and cooking oils**
The appropriate 7th character is to be added to each code from category X1Ø
A initial encounter
D subsequent encounter
S sequela

X● **X1Ø.Ø Contact with hot drinks**
X● **X1Ø.1 Contact with hot food**
X● **X1Ø.2 Contact with fats and cooking oils**

● **X11 Contact with hot tap-water**
Includes contact with boiling tap-water
contact with boiling water NOS
Excludes1 contact with water heated on stove (X12)
The appropriate 7th character is to be added to each code from category X11
A initial encounter
D subsequent encounter
S sequela

X● **X11.Ø Contact with hot water in bath or tub**
Excludes1 contact with running hot water in bath or tub (X11.1)
X● **X11.1 Contact with running hot water**
Contact with hot water running out of hose
Contact with hot water running out of tap
X● **X11.8 Contact with other hot tap-water**
Contact with hot water in bucket
Contact with hot tap-water NOS

X● **X12 Contact with other hot fluids**
Contact with water heated on stove
Excludes1 hot (liquid) metals (X18)
The appropriate 7th character is to be added to code X12
A initial encounter
D subsequent encounter
S sequela

● **X13 Contact with steam and other hot vapors**
The appropriate 7th character is to be added to each code from category X13
A initial encounter
D subsequent encounter
S sequela

X● **X13.Ø Inhalation of steam and other hot vapors**
X● **X13.1 Other contact with steam and other hot vapors**

● **X14 Contact with hot air and other hot gases**
The appropriate 7th character is to be added to each code from category X14
A initial encounter
D subsequent encounter
S sequela

X● **X14.Ø Inhalation of hot air and gases**
X● **X14.1 Other contact with hot air and other hot gases**

● **X15 Contact with hot household appliances**
Excludes1 contact with heating appliances (X16)
contact with powered household appliances (W29.-)
exposure to controlled fire in building or structure due to household appliance (XØ2.8)
exposure to household appliances electrical current (W86.Ø)
The appropriate 7th character is to be added to each code from category X15
A initial encounter
D subsequent encounter
S sequela

X● **X15.Ø Contact with hot stove (kitchen)**
X● **X15.1 Contact with hot toaster**
X● **X15.2 Contact with hotplate**
X● **X15.3 Contact with hot saucepan or skillet**
Contact with hot cooking pan
Contact with hot cooking pot
X● **X15.8 Contact with other hot household appliances**
Contact with cooker
Contact with kettle
Contact with light bulbs

X● **X16 Contact with hot heating appliances, radiators and pipes**
Excludes1 contact with powered appliances (W29.-)
exposure to controlled fire in building or structure due to appliance (XØ2.8)
exposure to industrial appliances electrical current (W86.1)
The appropriate 7th character is to be added to code X16
A initial encounter
D subsequent encounter
S sequela

X● **X17 Contact with hot engines, machinery and tools**
Excludes1 contact with hot heating appliances, radiators and pipes (X16)
contact with hot household appliances (X15)
The appropriate 7th character is to be added to code X17
A initial encounter
D subsequent encounter
S sequela

X● **X18 Contact with other hot metals**
Contact with liquid metal
The appropriate 7th character is to be added to code X18
A initial encounter
D subsequent encounter
S sequela

X● **X19 Contact with other heat and hot substances**
Excludes1 objects that are not normally hot, e.g., an object made hot by a house fire (XØØ-XØ8)
The appropriate 7th character is to be added to code X19
A initial encounter
D subsequent encounter
S sequela

EXPOSURE TO FORCES OF NATURE (X30-X39)

X● **X30 Exposure to excessive natural heat**
Exposure to excessive heat as the cause of sunstroke
Exposure to heat NOS
Excludes1 excessive heat of man-made origin (W92)
exposure to man-made radiation (W89)
exposure to sunlight (X32)
exposure to tanning bed (W89)
The appropriate 7th character is to be added to code X30

A	initial encounter
D	subsequent encounter
S	sequela

X● **X31 Exposure to excessive natural cold**
Excessive cold as the cause of chilblains NOS
Excessive cold as the cause of immersion foot or hand
Exposure to cold NOS
Exposure to weather conditions
Excludes1 cold of man-made origin (W93.-)
contact with or inhalation of dry ice (W93.-)
contact with or inhalation of liquefied gas (W93.-)
The appropriate 7th character is to be added to code X31

A	initial encounter
D	subsequent encounter
S	sequela

X● **X32 Exposure to sunlight**
Excludes1 man-made radiation (tanning bed) (W89)
Excludes2 radiation-related disorders of the skin and subcutaneous tissue (L55-L59)
The appropriate 7th character is to be added to code X32

A	initial encounter
D	subsequent encounter
S	sequela

X● **X34 Earthquake**
Excludes2 tidal wave (tsunami) due to earthquake (X37.41)
The appropriate 7th character is to be added to code X34

A	initial encounter
D	subsequent encounter
S	sequela

X● **X35 Volcanic eruption**
Excludes2 tidal wave (tsunami) due to volcanic eruption (X37.41)
The appropriate 7th character is to be added to code X35

A	initial encounter
D	subsequent encounter
S	sequela

● **X36 Avalanche, landslide and other earth movements**
Includes victim of mudslide of cataclysmic nature
Excludes1 earthquake (X34)
Excludes2 transport accident involving collision with avalanche or landslide not in motion (V01-V99)
The appropriate 7th character is to be added to each code from category X36

A	initial encounter
D	subsequent encounter
S	sequela

X● **X36.0 Collapse of dam or man-made structure causing earth movement**
X● **X36.1 Avalanche, landslide, or mudslide**

● **X37 Cataclysmic storm**
The appropriate 7th character is to be added to each code from category X37

A	initial encounter
D	subsequent encounter
S	sequela

X● **X37.0 Hurricane**
Storm surge
Typhoon
X● **X37.1 Tornado**
Cyclone
Twister
X● **X37.2 Blizzard (snow) (ice)**
X● **X37.3 Dust storm**
● **X37.4 Tidalwave**
X● **X37.41 Tidal wave due to earthquake or volcanic eruption**
Tidal wave NOS
Tsunami
X● **X37.42 Tidal wave due to storm**
X● **X37.43 Tidal wave due to landslide**
X● **X37.8 Other cataclysmic storms**
Cloudburst
Torrential rain
Excludes2 flood (X38)
X● **X37.9 Unspecified cataclysmic storm**
Storm NOS
Excludes1 collapse of dam or man-made structure causing earth movement (X36.0)

X● **X38 Flood**
Flood arising from remote storm
Flood of cataclysmic nature arising from melting snow
Flood resulting directly from storm
Excludes1 collapse of dam or man-made structure causing earth movement (X36.0)
tidal wave NOS (X37.41)
tidal wave caused by storm (X37.42)
The appropriate 7th character is to be added to code X38

A	initial encounter
D	subsequent encounter
S	sequela

● **X39 Exposure to other forces of nature**
The appropriate 7th character is to be added to each code from category X39

A	initial encounter
D	subsequent encounter
S	sequela

● **X39.0 Exposure to natural radiation**
Excludes1 contact with and (suspected) exposure to radon and other naturally occurring radiation (Z77.123)
exposure to man-made radiation (W88-W90)
exposure to sunlight (X32)
X● **X39.01 Exposure to radon**
X● **X39.08 Exposure to other natural radiation**
X● **X39.8 Other exposure to forces of nature**

CHAPTER 20 (V00-Y99)

OVEREXERTION AND STRENUOUS OR REPETITIVE MOVEMENTS (X50)

●**X50 Overexertion and strenuous or repetitive movements**

The appropriate 7th character is to be added to each code from category X50

A	initial encounter
D	subsequent encounter
S	sequela

Coding Clinic: 2016, Q4, P73-74

X● **X50.0 Overexertion from strenuous movement or load**
Lifting heavy objects
Lifting weights
Coding Clinic: 2016, Q4, P74

X● **X50.1 Overexertion from prolonged static or awkward postures**
Prolonged bending
Prolonged kneeling
Prolonged reaching
Prolonged sitting
Prolonged standing
Prolonged twisting
Static bending
Static kneeling
Static reaching
Static sitting
Static standing
Static twisting

X● **X50.3 Overexertion from repetitive movements**
Use of hand as hammer
Excludes2 Overuse from prolonged static or awkward postures (X50.1)
Coding Clinic: 2016, Q4, P74

X● **X50.9 Other and unspecified overexertion or strenuous movements or postures**
Contact pressure
Contact stress

ACCIDENTAL EXPOSURE TO OTHER SPECIFIED FACTORS (X52, X58)

X●**X52 Prolonged stay in weightless environment**
Weightlessness in spacecraft (simulator)

The appropriate 7th character is to be added to code X52

A	initial encounter
D	subsequent encounter
S	sequela

X●**X58 Exposure to other specified factors**
Accident NOS
Exposure NOS

The appropriate 7th character is to be added to code X58

A	initial encounter
D	subsequent encounter
S	sequela

INTENTIONAL SELF-HARM (X71-X83)

Purposely self-inflicted injury
Suicide (attempted)

●**X71 Intentional self-harm by drowning and submersion**

The appropriate 7th character is to be added to each code from category X71

A	initial encounter
D	subsequent encounter
S	sequela

X● **X71.0 Intentional self-harm by drowning and submersion while in bathtub A, D, S**

X● **X71.1 Intentional self-harm by drowning and submersion while in swimming pool A, D, S**

X● **X71.2 Intentional self-harm by drowning and submersion after jump into swimming pool A, D, S**

X● **X71.3 Intentional self-harm by drowning and submersion in natural water A, D, S**

X● **X71.8 Other intentional self-harm by drowning and submersion A, D, S**

X● **X71.9 Intentional self-harm by drowning and submersion, unspecified A, D, S**

X●**X72 Intentional self-harm by handgun discharge A, D, S**
Intentional self-harm by gun for single hand use
Intentional self-harm by pistol
Intentional self-harm by revolver
Excludes1 Very pistol (X74.8)

The appropriate 7th character is to be added to code X72

A	initial encounter
D	subsequent encounter
S	sequela

●**X73 Intentional self-harm by rifle, shotgun and larger firearm discharge**
Excludes1 airgun (X74.01)

The appropriate 7th character is to be added to each code from category X73

A	initial encounter
D	subsequent encounter
S	sequela

X● **X73.0 Intentional self-harm by shotgun discharge A, D, S**

X● **X73.1 Intentional self-harm by hunting rifle discharge A, D, S**

X● **X73.2 Intentional self-harm by machine gun discharge A, D, S**

X● **X73.8 Intentional self-harm by other larger firearm discharge A, D, S**

X● **X73.9 Intentional self-harm by unspecified larger firearm discharge A, D, S**

●**X74 Intentional self-harm by other and unspecified firearm and gun discharge**

The appropriate 7th character is to be added to each code from category X74

A	initial encounter
D	subsequent encounter
S	sequela

● **X74.0 Intentional self-harm by gas, air or spring-operated guns**

X● **X74.01 Intentional self-harm by airgun A, D, S**
Intentional self-harm by BB gun discharge
Intentional self-harm by pellet gun discharge

X● **X74.02 Intentional self-harm by paintball gun A, D, S**

X● **X74.09 Intentional self-harm by other gas, air or spring-operated gun A, D, S**

X● **X74.8 Intentional self-harm by other firearm discharge A, D, S**
Intentional self-harm by Very pistol [flare] discharge

X● **X74.9 Intentional self-harm by unspecified firearm discharge A, D, S**

X●**X75 Intentional self-harm by explosive material A, D, S**

The appropriate 7th character is to be added to code X75

A	initial encounter
D	subsequent encounter
S	sequela

X●**X76 Intentional self-harm by smoke, fire and flames A, D, S**

The appropriate 7th character is to be added to code X76

A	initial encounter
D	subsequent encounter
S	sequela

CHAPTER 20 (V00-Y99)

X77 Intentional self-harm by steam, hot vapors and hot objects

The appropriate 7th character is to be added to each code from category X77

A	initial encounter
D	subsequent encounter
S	sequela

X **X77.0** Intentional self-harm by steam or hot vapors A, D, S

X **X77.1** Intentional self-harm by hot tap water A, D, S

X **X77.2** Intentional self-harm by other hot fluids A, D, S

X **X77.3** Intentional self-harm by hot household appliances A, D, S

X **X77.8** Intentional self-harm by other hot objects A, D, S

X **X77.9** Intentional self-harm by unspecified hot objects A, D, S

X78 Intentional self-harm by sharp object

The appropriate 7th character is to be added to each code from category X78

A	initial encounter
D	subsequent encounter
S	sequela

X **X78.0** Intentional self-harm by sharp glass A, D, S

X **X78.1** Intentional self-harm by knife A, D, S

X **X78.2** Intentional self-harm by sword or dagger A, D, S

X **X78.8** Intentional self-harm by other sharp object A, D, S

Coding Clinic: 2022, Q1, P27

X **X78.9** Intentional self-harm by unspecified sharp object A, D, S

X **X79 Intentional self-harm by blunt object A, D, S**

The appropriate 7th character is to be added to code X79

A	initial encounter
D	subsequent encounter
S	sequela

X **X80 Intentional self-harm by jumping from a high place A, D, S**

Intentional fall from one level to another

The appropriate 7th character is to be added to code X80

A	initial encounter
D	subsequent encounter
S	sequela

X81 Intentional self-harm by jumping or lying in front of moving object

The appropriate 7th character is to be added to each code from category X81

A	initial encounter
D	subsequent encounter
S	sequela

X **X81.0** Intentional self-harm by jumping or lying in front of motor vehicle A, D, S

X **X81.1** Intentional self-harm by jumping or lying in front of (subway) train A, D, S

X **X81.8** Intentional self-harm by jumping or lying in front of other moving object A, D, S

X82 Intentional self-harm by crashing of motor vehicle

The appropriate 7th character is to be added to each code from category X82

A	initial encounter
D	subsequent encounter
S	sequela

X **X82.0** Intentional collision of motor vehicle with other motor vehicle A, D, S

X **X82.1** Intentional collision of motor vehicle with train A, D, S

X **X82.2** Intentional collision of motor vehicle with tree A, D, S

X **X82.8** Other intentional self-harm by crashing of motor vehicle A, D, S

X83 Intentional self-harm by other specified means

Excludes1 intentional self-harm by poisoning or contact with toxic substance - see Table of Drugs and Chemicals

The appropriate 7th character is to be added to each code from category X83

A	initial encounter
D	subsequent encounter
S	sequela

X **X83.0** Intentional self-harm by crashing of aircraft A, D, S

X **X83.1** Intentional self-harm by electrocution A, D, S

X **X83.2** Intentional self-harm by exposure to extremes of cold A, D, S

X **X83.8** Intentional self-harm by other specified means A, D, S

ASSAULT (X92-Y09)

Includes homicide injuries inflicted by another person with intent to injure or kill, by any means

Excludes1 injuries due to legal intervention (Y35.-)
injuries due to operations of war (Y36.-)
injuries due to terrorism (Y38.-)

X92 Assault by drowning and submersion

The appropriate 7th character is to be added to each code from category X92

A	initial encounter
D	subsequent encounter
S	sequela

X **X92.0** Assault by drowning and submersion while in bathtub

X **X92.1** Assault by drowning and submersion while in swimming pool

X **X92.2** Assault by drowning and submersion after push into swimming pool

X **X92.3** Assault by drowning and submersion in natural water

X **X92.8** Other assault by drowning and submersion

X **X92.9** Assault by drowning and submersion, unspecified

X **X93 Assault by handgun discharge**

Assault by discharge of gun for single hand use
Assault by discharge of pistol
Assault by discharge of revolver

Excludes1 Very pistol (X95.8)

The appropriate 7th character is to be added to code X93

A	initial encounter
D	subsequent encounter
S	sequela

X94 Assault by rifle, shotgun and larger firearm discharge

Excludes1 airgun (X95.01)

The appropriate 7th character is to be added to each code from category X94

A	initial encounter
D	subsequent encounter
S	sequela

X **X94.0** Assault by shotgun

X **X94.1** Assault by hunting rifle

X **X94.2** Assault by machine gun

X **X94.8** Assault by other larger firearm discharge

X **X94.9** Assault by unspecified larger firearm discharge

● **X95 Assault by other and unspecified firearm and gun discharge**
The appropriate 7th character is to be added to each code from category X95

A	initial encounter
D	subsequent encounter
S	sequela

● **X95.0 Assault by gas, air or spring-operated guns**
X● **X95.01 Assault by airgun discharge**
Assault by BB gun discharge
Assault by pellet gun discharge
X● **X95.02 Assault by paintball gun discharge**
X● **X95.09 Assault by other gas, air or spring-operated gun**
X● **X95.8 Assault by other firearm discharge**
Assault by very pistol [flare] discharge
X● **X95.9 Assault by unspecified firearm discharge**
Coding Clinic: 2023, Q3, P8,12; 2016, Q3, P24

● **X96 Assault by explosive material**
Excludes1 incendiary device (X97)
terrorism involving explosive material (Y38.2-)
The appropriate 7th character is to be added to each code from category X96

A	initial encounter
D	subsequent encounter
S	sequela

X● **X96.0 Assault by antipersonnel bomb**
Excludes1 antipersonnel bomb use in military or war (Y36.2-)
X● **X96.1 Assault by gasoline bomb**
X● **X96.2 Assault by letter bomb**
X● **X96.3 Assault by fertilizer bomb**
X● **X96.4 Assault by pipe bomb**
X● **X96.8 Assault by other specified explosive**
X● **X96.9 Assault by unspecified explosive**

X● **X97 Assault by smoke, fire and flames**
Assault by arson
Assault by cigarettes
Assault by incendiary device
The appropriate 7th character is to be added to code X97

A	initial encounter
D	subsequent encounter
S	sequela

● **X98 Assault by steam, hot vapors and hot objects**
The appropriate 7th character is to be added to each code from category X98

A	initial encounter
D	subsequent encounter
S	sequela

X● **X98.0 Assault by steam or hot vapors**
X● **X98.1 Assault by hot tap water**
X● **X98.2 Assault by hot fluids**
X● **X98.3 Assault by hot household appliances**
X● **X98.8 Assault by other hot objects**
X● **X98.9 Assault by unspecified hot objects**

● **X99 Assault by sharp object**
Excludes1 assault by strike by sports equipment (Y08.0-)
The appropriate 7th character is to be added to each code from category X99

A	initial encounter
D	subsequent encounter
S	sequela

X● **X99.0 Assault by sharp glass**
X● **X99.1 Assault by knife**
X● **X99.2 Assault by sword or dagger**
X● **X99.8 Assault by other sharp object**
X● **X99.9 Assault by unspecified sharp object**
Assault by stabbing NOS

X● **Y00 Assault by blunt object**
Excludes1 assault by strike by sports equipment (Y08.0)
The appropriate 7th character is to be added to code Y00

A	initial encounter
D	subsequent encounter
S	sequela

X● **Y01 Assault by pushing from high place**
The appropriate 7th character is to be added to code Y01

A	initial encounter
D	subsequent encounter
S	sequela

● **Y02 Assault by pushing or placing victim in front of moving object**
The appropriate 7th character is to be added to each code from category Y02

A	initial encounter
D	subsequent encounter
S	sequela

X● **Y02.0 Assault by pushing or placing victim in front of motor vehicle**
X● **Y02.1 Assault by pushing or placing victim in front of (subway) train**
X● **Y02.8 Assault by pushing or placing victim in front of other moving object**

● **Y03 Assault by crashing of motor vehicle**
The appropriate 7th character is to be added to each code from category Y03

A	initial encounter
D	subsequent encounter
S	sequela

X● **Y03.0 Assault by being hit or run over by motor vehicle**
X● **Y03.8 Other assault by crashing of motor vehicle**

● **Y04 Assault by bodily force**
Excludes1 assault by:
submersion (X92.-)
use of weapon (X93-X95, X99, Y00)
The appropriate 7th character is to be added to each code from category Y04

A	initial encounter
D	subsequent encounter
S	sequela

X● **Y04.0 Assault by unarmed brawl or fight**
X● **Y04.1 Assault by human bite**
X● **Y04.2 Assault by strike against or bumped into by another person**
X● **Y04.8 Assault by other bodily force**
Assault by bodily force NOS

OGCR Section I.C.19.f.

Adult and child abuse, neglect and other maltreatment

Sequence first the appropriate code from categories T74 or T76 for abuse, neglect and other maltreatment, followed by any accompanying mental health or injury code(s).

If the documentation in the medical record states abuse or neglect it is coded as confirmed (T74.-). It is coded as suspected if it is documented as suspected (T76.-).

For cases of confirmed abuse or neglect an external cause code from the assault section (X92-Y09) should be added to identify the cause of any physical injuries. A perpetrator code (Y07) should be added when the perpetrator of the abuse is known. For suspected cases of abuse or neglect, do not report external cause or perpetrator code.

If a suspected case of abuse, neglect or mistreatment is ruled out during an encounter code Z04.71, Encounter for examination and observation following alleged physical adult abuse, ruled out, or code Z04.72, Encounter for examination and observation following alleged adult rape, should be used, not a code from T76.

If a suspected case of alleged rape or sexual abuse is ruled out during an encounter code Z04.41, Encounter for examination and observation following alleged adult rape or code Z04.42, Encounter for examination and observation following alleged child rape should be used, not a code from T76.

● **Y07 Perpetrator of assault, maltreatment and neglect**

Note: Codes from this category are for use only in cases of confirmed abuse (T74.-)

Selection of the correct perpetrator code is based on the relationship between the perpetrator and the victim

Includes perpetrator of abandonment
perpetrator of emotional neglect
perpetrator of mental cruelty
perpetrator of physical abuse
perpetrator of physical neglect
perpetrator of sexual abuse
perpetrator of torture

Coding Clinic: 2016, Q4, P129

● **Y07.0 Spouse or partner, perpetrator of maltreatment and neglect**
Spouse or partner, perpetrator of maltreatment and neglect against spouse or partner

● **Y07.01 Husband, perpetrator of maltreatment and neglect**

Y07.010 Husband, current, perpetrator of maltreatment and neglect

Y07.011 Husband, former, perpetrator of maltreatment and neglect

● **Y07.02 Wife, perpetrator of maltreatment and neglect**

Y07.020 Wife, current, perpetrator of maltreatment and neglect

Y07.021 Wife, former, perpetrator of maltreatment and neglect

● **Y07.03 Male partner, perpetrator of maltreatment and neglect**
Male intimate or dating partner, perpetrator of maltreatment and neglect

Y07.030 Male partner, current, perpetrator of maltreatment and neglect

Y07.031 Male partner, former, perpetrator of maltreatment and neglect

● **Y07.04 Female partner, perpetrator of maltreatment and neglect**
Female intimate or dating partner, perpetrator of maltreatment and neglect

Y07.040 Female partner, current, perpetrator of maltreatment and neglect

Y07.041 Female partner, former, perpetrator of maltreatment and neglect

● **Y07.05 Non-binary partner, perpetrator of maltreatment and neglect**
Gender non-conforming partner, perpetrator of maltreatment and neglect

Y07.050 Non-binary partner, current, perpetrator of maltreatment and neglect

Y07.051 Non-binary partner, former, perpetrator of maltreatment and neglect

● **Y07.1 Parent (adoptive) (biological), perpetrator of maltreatment and neglect**

Y07.11 Biological father, perpetrator of maltreatment and neglect

Y07.12 Biological mother, perpetrator of maltreatment and neglect

Y07.13 Adoptive father, perpetrator of maltreatment and neglect

Y07.14 Adoptive mother, perpetrator of maltreatment and neglect

● **Y07.4 Other family member, perpetrator of maltreatment and neglect**

● **Y07.41 Sibling, perpetrator of maltreatment and neglect**

Excludes1 stepsibling, perpetrator of maltreatment and neglect (Y07.435, Y07.436)

Y07.410 Brother, perpetrator of maltreatment and neglect

Y07.411 Sister, perpetrator of maltreatment and neglect

● **Y07.42 Foster parent, perpetrator of maltreatment and neglect**

Y07.420 Foster father, perpetrator of maltreatment and neglect

Y07.421 Foster mother, perpetrator of maltreatment and neglect

● **Y07.43 Stepparent or stepsibling, perpetrator of maltreatment and neglect**

Y07.430 Stepfather, perpetrator of maltreatment and neglect

Y07.432 Male friend of parent (co-residing in household), perpetrator of maltreatment and neglect

Y07.433 Stepmother, perpetrator of maltreatment and neglect

Y07.434 Female friend of parent (co-residing in household), perpetrator of maltreatment and neglect

Y07.435 Stepbrother, perpetrator or maltreatment and neglect

Y07.436 Stepsister, perpetrator of maltreatment and neglect

● **Y07.44 Child, perpetrator of maltreatment and neglect**
Adopted child, perpetrator of maltreatment and neglect
Biological child, perpetrator of maltreatment and neglect
Daughter, perpetrator of maltreatment and neglect
Foster child, perpetrator of maltreatment and neglect
In-law child, perpetrator of maltreatment and neglect
Non-binary child, perpetrator of maltreatment and neglect
Son, perpetrator of maltreatment and neglect
Stepchild, perpetrator of maltreatment and neglect

● Y07.45 **Grandchild, perpetrator of maltreatment and neglect**
Adopted grandchild, perpetrator of maltreatment and neglect
Biological grandchild, perpetrator of maltreatment and neglect
Foster grandchild, perpetrator of maltreatment and neglect
Granddaughter, perpetrator of maltreatment and neglect
Grandson, perpetrator of maltreatment and neglect
In-law grandchild, perpetrator of maltreatment and neglect
Non-binary grandchild, perpetrator of maltreatment and neglect
Step grandchild, perpetrator of maltreatment and neglect

● Y07.46 **Grandparent, perpetrator of maltreatment and neglect**
Grandfather, perpetrator of maltreatment and neglect
Grandmother, perpetrator of maltreatment and neglect
Non-binary grandparent, perpetrator of maltreatment and neglect

● Y07.47 **Parental sibling, perpetrator of maltreatment and neglect**
Aunt, perpetrator of maltreatment and neglect
Non-binary parental sibling, perpetrator of maltreatment and neglect
Uncle, perpetrator of maltreatment and neglect

● Y07.49 **Other family member, perpetrator of maltreatment and neglect**
Y07.490 **Male cousin, perpetrator of maltreatment and neglect**
Y07.491 **Female cousin, perpetrator of maltreatment and neglect**
Y07.499 **Other family member, perpetrator of maltreatment and neglect**

● Y07.5 **Non-family member, perpetrator of maltreatment and neglect**
Y07.50 **Unspecified non-family member, perpetrator of maltreatment and neglect**

● Y07.51 **Daycare provider, perpetrator of maltreatment and neglect**
Y07.510 **At-home childcare provider, perpetrator of maltreatment and neglect**
Y07.511 **Daycare center childcare provider, perpetrator of maltreatment and neglect**
Y07.512 **At-home adultcare provider, perpetrator of maltreatment and neglect**
Y07.513 **Adultcare center provider, perpetrator of maltreatment and neglect**
Y07.519 **Unspecified daycare provider, perpetrator of maltreatment and neglect**

● Y07.52 **Healthcare provider, perpetrator of maltreatment and neglect**
Y07.521 **Mental health provider, perpetrator of maltreatment and neglect**
Y07.528 **Other therapist or healthcare provider, perpetrator of maltreatment and neglect**
Nurse perpetrator of maltreatment and neglect
Occupational therapist perpetrator of maltreatment and neglect
Physical therapist perpetrator of maltreatment and neglect
Speech therapist perpetrator of maltreatment and neglect
Y07.529 **Unspecified healthcare provider, perpetrator of maltreatment and neglect**

Y07.53 **Teacher or instructor, perpetrator of maltreatment and neglect**
Coach, perpetrator of maltreatment and neglect

Y07.54 **Acquaintance or friend, perpetrator of maltreatment and neglect**

Y07.59 **Other non-family member, perpetrator of maltreatment and neglect**

Y07.6 **Multiple perpetrators of maltreatment and neglect**

Y07.9 **Unspecified perpetrator of maltreatment and neglect**

● Y08 **Assault by other specified means**
The appropriate 7th character is to be added to each code from category Y08

A	initial encounter
D	subsequent encounter
S	sequela

● Y08.0 **Assault by strike by sport equipment**
X● Y08.01 **Assault by strike by hockey stick**
X● Y08.02 **Assault by strike by baseball bat**
X● Y08.09 **Assault by strike by other specified type of sport equipment**

● Y08.8 **Assault by other specified means**
X● Y08.81 **Assault by crashing of aircraft**
X● Y08.89 **Assault by other specified means**

● Y09 **Assault by unspecified means**
Assassination (attempted) NOS
Homicide (attempted) NOS
Manslaughter (attempted) NOS
Murder (attempted) NOS

EVENT OF UNDETERMINED INTENT (Y21-Y33)

Undetermined intent is only for use when there is specific documentation in the record that the intent of the injury cannot be determined. If no such documentation is present, code to accidental (unintentional)

● Y21 **Drowning and submersion, undetermined intent**
The appropriate 7th character is to be added to each code from category Y21

A	initial encounter
D	subsequent encounter
S	sequela

X● Y21.0 **Drowning and submersion while in bathtub, undetermined intent**
X● Y21.1 **Drowning and submersion after fall into bathtub, undetermined intent**
X● Y21.2 **Drowning and submersion while in swimming pool, undetermined intent**
X● Y21.3 **Drowning and submersion after fall into swimming pool, undetermined intent**
X● Y21.4 **Drowning and submersion in natural water, undetermined intent**
X● Y21.8 **Other drowning and submersion, undetermined intent**
X● Y21.9 **Unspecified drowning and submersion, undetermined intent**

X● Y22 **Handgun discharge, undetermined intent**
Discharge of gun for single hand use, undetermined intent
Discharge of pistol, undetermined intent
Discharge of revolver, undetermined intent
Excludes2 very pistol (Y24.8)
The appropriate 7th character is to be added to code Y22

A	initial encounter
D	subsequent encounter
S	sequela

Y23 Rifle, shotgun and larger firearm discharge, undetermined intent

Excludes2 airgun (Y24.0)

The appropriate 7th character is to be added to each code from category Y23

A initial encounter
D subsequent encounter
S sequela

X Y23.0 Shotgun discharge, undetermined intent
X Y23.1 Hunting rifle discharge, undetermined intent
X Y23.2 Military firearm discharge, undetermined intent
X Y23.3 Machine gun discharge, undetermined intent
X Y23.8 Other larger firearm discharge, undetermined intent
X Y23.9 Unspecified larger firearm discharge, undetermined intent

Y24 Other and unspecified firearm discharge, undetermined intent

The appropriate 7th character is to be added to each code from category Y24

A initial encounter
D subsequent encounter
S sequela

X Y24.0 Airgun discharge, undetermined intent
BB gun discharge, undetermined intent
Pellet gun discharge, undetermined intent
X Y24.8 Other firearm discharge, undetermined intent
Paintball gun discharge, undetermined intent
Very pistol [flare] discharge, undetermined intent
X Y24.9 Unspecified firearm discharge, undetermined intent

X Y25 Contact with explosive material, undetermined intent

The appropriate 7th character is to be added to code Y25

A initial encounter
D subsequent encounter
S sequela

X Y26 Exposure to smoke, fire and flames, undetermined intent

The appropriate 7th character is to be added to code Y26

A initial encounter
D subsequent encounter
S sequela

Y27 Contact with steam, hot vapors and hot objects, undetermined intent

The appropriate 7th character is to be added to each code from category Y27

A initial encounter
D subsequent encounter
S sequela

X Y27.0 Contact with steam and hot vapors, undetermined intent
X Y27.1 Contact with hot tap water, undetermined intent
X Y27.2 Contact with hot fluids, undetermined intent
X Y27.3 Contact with hot household appliance, undetermined intent
X Y27.8 Contact with other hot objects, undetermined intent
X Y27.9 Contact with unspecified hot objects, undetermined intent

Y28 Contact with sharp object, undetermined intent

The appropriate 7th character is to be added to each code from category Y28

A initial encounter
D subsequent encounter
S sequela

X Y28.0 Contact with sharp glass, undetermined intent
X Y28.1 Contact with knife, undetermined intent
X Y28.2 Contact with sword or dagger, undetermined intent
X Y28.8 Contact with other sharp object, undetermined intent
X Y28.9 Contact with unspecified sharp object, undetermined intent

X Y29 Contact with blunt object, undetermined intent

The appropriate 7th character is to be added to code Y29

A initial encounter
D subsequent encounter
S sequela

X Y30 Falling, jumping or pushed from a high place, undetermined intent

Victim falling from one level to another, undetermined intent

The appropriate 7th character is to be added to code Y30

A initial encounter
D subsequent encounter
S sequela

X Y31 Falling, lying or running before or into moving object, undetermined intent

The appropriate 7th character is to be added to code Y31

A initial encounter
D subsequent encounter
S sequela

X Y32 Crashing of motor vehicle, undetermined intent

The appropriate 7th character is to be added to code Y32

A initial encounter
D subsequent encounter
S sequela

X Y33 Other specified events, undetermined intent

The appropriate 7th character is to be added to code Y33

A initial encounter
D subsequent encounter
S sequela

LEGAL INTERVENTION, OPERATIONS OF WAR, MILITARY OPERATIONS, AND TERRORISM (Y35-Y38)

Y35 Legal intervention

Includes any injury sustained as a result of an encounter with any law enforcement official, serving in any capacity at the time of the encounter, whether on-duty or off-duty. Includes: injury to law enforcement official, suspect and bystander

The appropriate 7th character is to be added to each code from category Y35

A initial encounter
D subsequent encounter
S sequela

Y35.0 Legal intervention involving firearm discharge
Y35.00 Legal intervention involving unspecified firearm discharge
Legal intervention involving gunshot wound
Legal intervention involving shot NOS
Y35.001 Legal intervention involving unspecified firearm discharge, law enforcement official injured
Y35.002 Legal intervention involving unspecified firearm discharge, bystander injured
Y35.003 Legal intervention involving unspecified firearm discharge, suspect injured

CHAPTER 20 (V00-Y99)

Y35.009 Legal intervention involving unspecified firearm discharge, unspecified person injured

Y35.01 Legal intervention involving injury by machine gun

Y35.011 Legal intervention involving injury by machine gun, law enforcement official injured

Y35.012 Legal intervention involving injury by machine gun, bystander injured

Y35.013 Legal intervention involving injury by machine gun, suspect injured

Y35.019 Legal intervention involving injury by machine gun, unspecified person injured

Y35.02 Legal intervention involving injury by handgun

Y35.021 Legal intervention involving injury by handgun, law enforcement official injured

Y35.022 Legal intervention involving injury by handgun, bystander injured

Y35.023 Legal intervention involving injury by handgun, suspect injured

Y35.029 Legal intervention involving injury by handgun, unspecified person injured

Y35.03 Legal intervention involving injury by rifle pellet

Y35.031 Legal intervention involving injury by rifle pellet, law enforcement official injured

Y35.032 Legal intervention involving injury by rifle pellet, bystander injured

Y35.033 Legal intervention involving injury by rifle pellet, suspect injured

Y35.039 Legal intervention involving injury by rifle pellet, unspecified person injured

Y35.04 Legal intervention involving injury by rubber bullet

Y35.041 Legal intervention involving injury by rubber bullet, law enforcement official injured

Y35.042 Legal intervention involving injury by rubber bullet, bystander injured

Y35.043 Legal intervention involving injury by rubber bullet, suspect injured

Y35.049 Legal intervention involving injury by rubber bullet, unspecified person injured

Y35.09 Legal intervention involving other firearm discharge

Y35.091 Legal intervention involving other firearm discharge, law enforcement official injured

Y35.092 Legal intervention involving other firearm discharge, bystander injured

Y35.093 Legal intervention involving other firearm discharge, suspect injured

Y35.099 Legal intervention involving other firearm discharge, unspecified person injured

Y35.1 Legal intervention involving explosives

Y35.10 Legal intervention involving unspecified explosives

Y35.101 Legal intervention involving unspecified explosives, law enforcement official injured

Y35.102 Legal intervention involving unspecified explosives, bystander injured

Y35.103 Legal intervention involving unspecified explosives, suspect injured

Y35.109 Legal intervention involving unspecified explosives, unspecified person injured

Y35.11 Legal intervention involving injury by dynamite

Y35.111 Legal intervention involving injury by dynamite, law enforcement official injured

Y35.112 Legal intervention involving injury by dynamite, bystander injured

Y35.113 Legal intervention involving injury by dynamite, suspect injured

Y35.119 Legal intervention involving injury by dynamite, unspecified person injured

Y35.12 Legal intervention involving injury by explosive shell

Y35.121 Legal intervention involving injury by explosive shell, law enforcement official injured

Y35.122 Legal intervention involving injury by explosive shell, bystander injured

Y35.123 Legal intervention involving injury by explosive shell, suspect injured

Y35.129 Legal intervention involving other explosives, unspecified person injured

Y35.19 Legal intervention involving other explosives

Legal intervention involving injury by grenade

Legal intervention involving injury by mortar bomb

Y35.191 Legal intervention involving other explosives, law enforcement official injured

Y35.192 Legal intervention involving other explosives, bystander injured

Y35.193 Legal intervention involving other explosives, suspect injured

Y35.199 Legal intervention involving other explosives, unspecified person injured

Y35.2 Legal intervention involving gas

Legal intervention involving asphyxiation by gas

Legal intervention involving poisoning by gas

Y35.20 Legal intervention involving unspecified gas

Y35.201 Legal intervention involving unspecified gas, law enforcement official injured

Y35.202 Legal intervention involving unspecified gas, bystander injured

Y35.203 Legal intervention involving unspecified gas, suspect injured

Y35.209 Legal intervention involving unspecified gas, unspecified person injured

Y35.21 Legal intervention involving injury by tear gas

Y35.211 Legal intervention involving injury by tear gas, law enforcement official injured

Y35.212 Legal intervention involving injury by tear gas, bystander injured

Y35.213 Legal intervention involving injury by tear gas, suspect injured

Y35.219 Legal intervention involving injury by tear gas, unspecified person injured

Y35.29 Legal intervention involving other gas
Y35.291 Legal intervention involving other gas, law enforcement official injured
Y35.292 Legal intervention involving other gas, bystander injured
Y35.293 Legal intervention involving other gas, suspect injured
Y35.299 Legal intervention involving other gas, unspecified person injured

Y35.3 Legal intervention involving blunt objects
Legal intervention involving being hit or struck by blunt object
Y35.30 Legal intervention involving unspecified blunt objects
Y35.301 Legal intervention involving unspecified blunt objects, law enforcement official injured
Y35.302 Legal intervention involving unspecified blunt objects, bystander injured
Y35.303 Legal intervention involving unspecified blunt objects, suspect injured
Y35.309 Legal intervention involving unspecified blunt objects, unspecified person injured
Y35.31 Legal intervention involving baton
Y35.311 Legal intervention involving baton, law enforcement official injured
Y35.312 Legal intervention involving baton, bystander injured
Y35.313 Legal intervention involving baton, suspect injured
Y35.319 Legal intervention involving baton, unspecified person injured
Y35.39 Legal intervention involving other blunt objects
Y35.391 Legal intervention involving other blunt objects, law enforcement official injured
Y35.392 Legal intervention involving other blunt objects, bystander injured
Y35.393 Legal intervention involving other blunt objects, suspect injured
Y35.399 Legal intervention involving other blunt objects, unspecified person injured

Y35.4 Legal intervention involving sharp objects
Legal intervention involving being cut by sharp objects
Legal intervention involving being stabbed by sharp objects
Y35.40 Legal intervention involving unspecified sharp objects
Y35.401 Legal intervention involving unspecified sharp objects, law enforcement official injured
Y35.402 Legal intervention involving unspecified sharp objects, bystander injured
Y35.403 Legal intervention involving unspecified sharp objects, suspect injured
Y35.409 Legal intervention involving unspecified sharp objects, unspecified person injured
Y35.41 Legal intervention involving bayonet
Y35.411 Legal intervention involving bayonet, law enforcement official injured
Y35.412 Legal intervention involving bayonet, bystander injured
Y35.413 Legal intervention involving bayonet, suspect injured
Y35.419 Legal intervention involving bayonet, unspecified person injured
Y35.49 Legal intervention involving other sharp objects
Y35.491 Legal intervention involving other sharp objects, law enforcement official injured
Y35.492 Legal intervention involving other sharp objects, bystander injured
Y35.493 Legal intervention involving other sharp objects, suspect injured
Y35.499 Legal intervention involving other sharp objects, unspecified person injured

Y35.8 Legal intervention involving other specified means
Y35.81 Legal intervention involving manhandling
Y35.811 Legal intervention involving manhandling, law enforcement official injured
Y35.812 Legal intervention involving manhandling, bystander injured
Y35.813 Legal intervention involving manhandling, suspect injured
Y35.819 Legal intervention involving manhandling, unspecified person injured
Y35.83 Legal intervention involving a conducted energy device
Electroshock device (taser)
Stun gun
Y35.831 Legal intervention involving a conducted energy device, law enforcement official injured
Y35.832 Legal intervention involving a conducted energy device, bystander injured
Y35.833 Legal intervention involving a conducted energy device, suspect injured
Y35.839 Legal intervention involving a conducted energy device, unspecified person injured
Y35.89 Legal intervention involving other specified means
Y35.891 Legal intervention involving other specified means, law enforcement official injured
Y35.892 Legal intervention involving other specified means, bystander injured
Y35.893 Legal intervention involving other specified means, suspect injured
Coding Clinic: 2018, Q1, P5
Y35.899 Legal intervention involving other specified means, unspecified person injured

Y35.9 Legal intervention, means unspecified
X Y35.91 Legal intervention, means unspecified, law enforcement official injured
X Y35.92 Legal intervention, means unspecified, bystander injured
X Y35.93 Legal intervention, means unspecified, suspect injured
X Y35.99 Legal intervention, means unspecified, unspecified person injured

CHAPTER 20 (V00-Y99)

● Y36 Operations of war

Includes injuries to military personnel and civilians caused by war, civil insurrection, and peacekeeping missions

Excludes1 injury to military personnel occurring during peacetime military operations (Y37.-)
military vehicles involved in transport accidents with non-military vehicle during peacetime (V09.01, V09.21, V19.81, V29.818, V39.81, V49.81, V59.81, V69.81, V79.81)

The appropriate 7th character is to be added to each code from category Y36

A	initial encounter
D	subsequent encounter
S	sequela

● **Y36.0 War operations involving explosion of marine weapons**
Weapons and military watercraft

● **Y36.00 War operations involving explosion of unspecified marine weapon**
War operations involving underwater blast NOS

● **Y36.000 War operations involving explosion of unspecified marine weapon, military personnel**

● **Y36.001 War operations involving explosion of unspecified marine weapon, civilian**

● **Y36.01 War operations involving explosion of depth-charge**

● **Y36.010 War operations involving explosion of depth-charge, military personnel**

● **Y36.011 War operations involving explosion of depth-charge, civilian**

● **Y36.02 War operations involving explosion of marine mine**
War operations involving explosion of marine mine, at sea or in harbor

● **Y36.020 War operations involving explosion of marine mine, military personnel**

● **Y36.021 War operations involving explosion of marine mine, civilian**

● **Y36.03 War operations involving explosion of sea-based artillery shell**

● **Y36.030 War operations involving explosion of sea-based artillery shell, military personnel**

● **Y36.031 War operations involving explosion of sea-based artillery shell, civilian**

● **Y36.04 War operations involving explosion of torpedo**

● **Y36.040 War operations involving explosion of torpedo, military personnel**

● **Y36.041 War operations involving explosion of torpedo, civilian**

● **Y36.05 War operations involving accidental detonation of onboard marine weapons**

● **Y36.050 War operations involving accidental detonation of onboard marine weapons, military personnel**

● **Y36.051 War operations involving accidental detonation of onboard marine weapons, civilian**

● **Y36.09 War operations involving explosion of other marine weapons**

● **Y36.090 War operations involving explosion of other marine weapons, military personnel**

● **Y36.091 War operations involving explosion of other marine weapons, civilian**

● **Y36.1 War operations involving destruction of aircraft**

● **Y36.10 War operations involving unspecified destruction of aircraft**

● **Y36.100 War operations involving unspecified destruction of aircraft, military personnel**

● **Y36.101 War operations involving unspecified destruction of aircraft, civilian**

● **Y36.11 War operations involving destruction of aircraft due to enemy fire or explosives**
War operations involving destruction of aircraft due to air to air missile
War operations involving destruction of aircraft due to explosive placed on aircraft
War operations involving destruction of aircraft due to rocket propelled grenade [RPG]
War operations involving destruction of aircraft due to small arms fire
War operations involving destruction of aircraft due to surface to air missile

● **Y36.110 War operations involving destruction of aircraft due to enemy fire or explosives, military personnel**

● **Y36.111 War operations involving destruction of aircraft due to enemy fire or explosives, civilian**

● **Y36.12 War operations involving destruction of aircraft due to collision with other aircraft**

● **Y36.120 War operations involving destruction of aircraft due to collision with other aircraft, military personnel**

● **Y36.121 War operations involving destruction of aircraft due to collision with other aircraft, civilian**

● **Y36.13 War operations involving destruction of aircraft due to onboard fire**

● **Y36.130 War operations involving destruction of aircraft due to onboard fire, military personnel**

● **Y36.131 War operations involving destruction of aircraft due to onboard fire, civilian**

● **Y36.14 War operations involving destruction of aircraft due to accidental detonation of onboard munitions and explosives**

● **Y36.140 War operations involving destruction of aircraft due to accidental detonation of onboard munitions and explosives, military personnel**

● **Y36.141 War operations involving destruction of aircraft due to accidental detonation of onboard munitions and explosives, civilian**

● **Y36.19 War operations involving other destruction of aircraft**

● **Y36.190 War operations involving other destruction of aircraft, military personnel**

● **Y36.191 War operations involving other destruction of aircraft, civilian**

● **Y36.2 War operations involving other explosions and fragments**

Excludes1 war operations involving explosion of aircraft (Y36.1-)
war operations involving explosion of marine weapons (Y36.0-)
war operations involving explosion of nuclear weapons (Y36.5-)
war operations involving explosion occurring after cessation of hostilities (Y36.8-)

● **Y36.20 War operations involving unspecified explosion and fragments**
War operations involving air blast NOS
War operations involving blast NOS
War operations involving blast fragments NOS
War operations involving blast wave NOS
War operations involving blast wind NOS
War operations involving explosion NOS
War operations involving explosion of bomb NOS

● **Y36.200 War operations involving unspecified explosion and fragments, military personnel**

● **Y36.201 War operations involving unspecified explosion and fragments, civilian**

● **Y36.21 War operations involving explosion of aerial bomb**

● **Y36.210 War operations involving explosion of aerial bomb, military personnel**

● **Y36.211 War operations involving explosion of aerial bomb, civilian**

● **Y36.22 War operations involving explosion of guided missile**

● **Y36.220 War operations involving explosion of guided missile, military personnel**

● **Y36.221 War operations involving explosion of guided missile, civilian**

● **Y36.23 War operations involving explosion of improvised explosive device [IED]**
War operations involving explosion of person-borne improvised explosive device [IED]
War operations involving explosion of vehicle-borne improvised explosive device [IED]
War operations involving explosion of roadside improvised explosive device [IED]

● **Y36.230 War operations involving explosion of improvised explosive device [IED], military personnel**

● **Y36.231 War operations involving explosion of improvised explosive device [IED], civilian**

● **Y36.24 War operations involving explosion due to accidental detonation and discharge of own munitions or munitions launch device**

● **Y36.240 War operations involving explosion due to accidental detonation and discharge of own munitions or munitions launch device, military personnel**

● **Y36.241 War operations involving explosion due to accidental detonation and discharge of own munitions or munitions launch device, civilian**

● **Y36.25 War operations involving fragments from munitions**

● **Y36.250 War operations involving fragments from munitions, military personnel**

● **Y36.251 War operations involving fragments from munitions, civilian**

● **Y36.26 War operations involving fragments of improvised explosive device [IED]**
War operations involving fragments of person-borne improvised explosive device [IED]
War operations involving fragments of vehicle-borne improvised explosive device [IED]
War operations involving fragments of roadside improvised explosive device [IED]

● **Y36.260 War operations involving fragments of improvised explosive device [IED], military personnel**

● **Y36.261 War operations involving fragments of improvised explosive device [IED], civilian**

● **Y36.27 War operations involving fragments from weapons**

● **Y36.270 War operations involving fragments from weapons, military personnel**

● **Y36.271 War operations involving fragments from weapons, civilian**

● **Y36.29 War operations involving other explosions and fragments**
War operations involving explosion of grenade
War operations involving explosions of land mine
War operations involving shrapnel NOS

● **Y36.290 War operations involving other explosions and fragments, military personnel**

● **Y36.291 War operations involving other explosions and fragments, civilian**

● **Y36.3 War operations involving fires, conflagrations and hot substances**
War operations involving smoke, fumes, and heat from fires, conflagrations and hot substances
Excludes1 war operations involving fires and conflagrations aboard military aircraft (Y36.1-)
war operations involving fires and conflagrations aboard military watercraft (Y36.Ø-)
war operations involving fires and conflagrations caused indirectly by conventional weapons (Y36.2-)
war operations involving fires and thermal effects of nuclear weapons (Y36.53-)

● **Y36.30 War operations involving unspecified fire, conflagration and hot substance**

● **Y36.300 War operations involving unspecified fire, conflagration and hot substance, military personnel**

● **Y36.301 War operations involving unspecified fire, conflagration and hot substance, civilian**

● **Y36.31 War operations involving gasoline bomb**
War operations involving incendiary bomb
War operations involving petrol bomb

● **Y36.310 War operations involving gasoline bomb, military personnel**

● **Y36.311 War operations involving gasoline bomb, civilian**

● **Y36.32 War operations involving incendiary bullet**

● **Y36.320 War operations involving incendiary bullet, military personnel**

● **Y36.321 War operations involving incendiary bullet, civilian**

● **Y36.33 War operations involving flamethrower**

● **Y36.330 War operations involving flamethrower, military personnel**

● **Y36.331 War operations involving flamethrower, civilian**

● **Y36.39 War operations involving other fires, conflagrations and hot substances**

● **Y36.390 War operations involving other fires, conflagrations and hot substances, military personnel**

● **Y36.391 War operations involving other fires, conflagrations and hot substances, civilian**

● **Y36.4 War operations involving firearm discharge and other forms of conventional warfare**

● **Y36.41 War operations involving rubber bullets**

● **Y36.410 War operations involving rubber bullets, military personnel**

● **Y36.411 War operations involving rubber bullets, civilian**

CHAPTER 2Ø (VØØ-Y99)

● Y36.42 War operations involving firearms pellets
● Y36.42Ø War operations involving firearms pellets, military personnel
● Y36.421 War operations involving firearms pellets, civilian
● Y36.43 War operations involving other firearms discharge
War operations involving bullets NOS
Excludes1 war operations involving munitions fragments (Y36.25-)
war operations involving incendiary bullets (Y36.32-)
● Y36.43Ø War operations involving other firearms discharge, military personnel
● Y36.431 War operations involving other firearms discharge, civilian
● Y36.44 War operations involving unarmed hand to hand combat
Excludes1 war operations involving combat using blunt or piercing object (Y36.45-)
war operations involving intentional restriction of air and airway (Y36.46-)
war operations involving unintentional restriction of air and airway (Y36.47-)
● Y36.44Ø War operations involving unarmed hand to hand combat, military personnel
● Y36.441 War operations involving unarmed hand to hand combat, civilian
● Y36.45 War operations involving combat using blunt or piercing object
● Y36.45Ø War operations involving combat using blunt or piercing object, military personnel
● Y36.451 War operations involving combat using blunt or piercing object, civilian
● Y36.46 War operations involving intentional restriction of air and airway
● Y36.46Ø War operations involving intentional restriction of air and airway, military personnel
● Y36.461 War operations involving intentional restriction of air and airway, civilian
● Y36.47 War operations involving unintentional restriction of air and airway
● Y36.47Ø War operations involving unintentional restriction of air and airway, military personnel
● Y36.471 War operations involving unintentional restriction of air and airway, civilian
● Y36.49 War operations involving other forms of conventional warfare
● Y36.49Ø War operations involving other forms of conventional warfare, military personnel
● Y36.491 War operations involving other forms of conventional warfare, civilian
● Y36.5 War operations involving nuclear weapons
War operations involving dirty bomb NOS
● Y36.5Ø War operations involving unspecified effect of nuclear weapon
● Y36.5ØØ War operations involving unspecified effect of nuclear weapon, military personnel
● Y36.5Ø1 War operations involving unspecified effect of nuclear weapon, civilian
● Y36.51 War operations involving direct blast effect of nuclear weapon
War operations involving blast pressure of nuclear weapon
● Y36.51Ø War operations involving direct blast effect of nuclear weapon, military personnel
● Y36.511 War operations involving direct blast effect of nuclear weapon, civilian
● Y36.52 War operations involving indirect blast effect of nuclear weapon
War operations involving being thrown by blast of nuclear weapon
War operations involving being struck or crushed by blast debris of nuclear weapon
● Y36.52Ø War operations involving indirect blast effect of nuclear weapon, military personnel
● Y36.521 War operations involving indirect blast effect of nuclear weapon, civilian
● Y36.53 War operations involving thermal radiation effect of nuclear weapon
War operations involving direct heat from nuclear weapon
War operation involving fireball effects from nuclear weapon
● Y36.53Ø War operations involving thermal radiation effect of nuclear weapon, military personnel
● Y36.531 War operations involving thermal radiation effect of nuclear weapon, civilian
● Y36.54 War operation involving nuclear radiation effects of nuclear weapon
War operation involving acute radiation exposure from nuclear weapon
War operation involving exposure to immediate ionizing radiation from nuclear weapon
War operation involving fallout exposure from nuclear weapon
War operation involving secondary effects of nuclear weapons
● Y36.54Ø War operation involving nuclear radiation effects of nuclear weapon, military personnel
● Y36.541 War operation involving nuclear radiation effects of nuclear weapon, civilian
● Y36.59 War operation involving other effects of nuclear weapons
● Y36.59Ø War operation involving other effects of nuclear weapons, military personnel
● Y36.591 War operation involving other effects of nuclear weapons, civilian
● Y36.6 War operations involving biological weapons
● Y36.6X War operations involving biological weapons
● Y36.6XØ War operations involving biological weapons, military personnel
● Y36.6X1 War operations involving biological weapons, civilian
● Y36.7 War operations involving chemical weapons and other forms of unconventional warfare
Excludes1 war operations involving incendiary devices (Y36.3-, Y36.5-)
● Y36.7X War operations involving chemical weapons and other forms of unconventional warfare
● Y36.7XØ War operations involving chemical weapons and other forms of unconventional warfare, military personnel

● Y36.7X1 **War operations involving chemical weapons and other forms of unconventional warfare, civilian**

● Y36.8 **War operations occurring after cessation of hostilities**
War operations classifiable to categories Y36.Ø-Y36.8 but occurring after cessation of hostilities

● Y36.81 **Explosion of mine placed during war operations but exploding after cessation of hostilities**

● Y36.81Ø **Explosion of mine placed during war operations but exploding after cessation of hostilities, military personnel**

● Y36.811 **Explosion of mine placed during war operations but exploding after cessation of hostilities, civilian**

● Y36.82 **Explosion of bomb placed during war operations but exploding after cessation of hostilities**

● Y36.82Ø **Explosion of bomb placed during war operations but exploding after cessation of hostilities, military personnel**

● Y36.821 **Explosion of bomb placed during war operations but exploding after cessation of hostilities, civilian**

● Y36.88 **Other war operations occurring after cessation of hostilities**

● Y36.88Ø **Other war operations occurring after cessation of hostilities, military personnel**

● Y36.881 **Other war operations occurring after cessation of hostilities, civilian**

● Y36.89 **Unspecified war operations occurring after cessation of hostilities**

● Y36.89Ø **Unspecified war operations occurring after cessation of hostilities, military personnel**

● Y36.891 **Unspecified war operations occurring after cessation of hostilities, civilian**

● Y36.9 **Other and unspecified war operations**

X● Y36.9Ø **War operations, unspecified**

X● Y36.91 **War operations involving unspecified weapon of mass destruction [WMD]**

X● Y36.92 **War operations involving friendly fire**

● Y37 **Military operations**

Includes Injuries to military personnel and civilians occurring during peacetime on military property and during routine military exercises and operations

Excludes1 military aircraft involved in aircraft accident with civilian aircraft (V97.81-)
military vehicles involved in transport accident with civilian vehicle (VØ9.Ø1, VØ9.21, V19.81, V29.818, V39.81, V49.81, V59.81, V69.81, V79.81)
military watercraft involved in water transport accident with civilian watercraft (V94.81-)
war operations (Y36.-)

The appropriate 7th character is to be added to each code from category Y37

A	initial encounter
D	subsequent encounter
S	sequela

● Y37.Ø **Military operations involving explosion of marine weapons**

● Y37.ØØ **Military operations involving explosion of unspecified marine weapon**
Military operations involving underwater blast NOS

● Y37.ØØØ **Military operations involving explosion of unspecified marine weapon, military personnel**

● Y37.ØØ1 **Military operations involving explosion of unspecified marine weapon, civilian**

● Y37.Ø1 **Military operations involving explosion of depth-charge**

● Y37.Ø1Ø **Military operations involving explosion of depth-charge, military personnel**

● Y37.Ø11 **Military operations involving explosion of depth-charge, civilian**

● Y37.Ø2 **Military operations involving explosion of marine mine**
Military operations involving explosion of marine mine, at sea or in harbor

● Y37.Ø2Ø **Military operations involving explosion of marine mine, military personnel**

● Y37.Ø21 **Military operations involving explosion of marine mine, civilian**

● Y37.Ø3 **Military operations involving explosion of sea-based artillery shell**

● Y37.Ø3Ø **Military operations involving explosion of sea-based artillery shell, military personnel**

● Y37.Ø31 **Military operations involving explosion of sea-based artillery shell, civilian**

● Y37.Ø4 **Military operations involving explosion of torpedo**

● Y37.Ø4Ø **Military operations involving explosion of torpedo, military personnel**

● Y37.Ø41 **Military operations involving explosion of torpedo, civilian**

● Y37.Ø5 **Military operations involving accidental detonation of onboard marine weapons**

● Y37.Ø5Ø **Military operations involving accidental detonation of onboard marine weapons, military personnel**

● Y37.Ø51 **Military operations involving accidental detonation of onboard marine weapons, civilian**

● Y37.Ø9 **Military operations involving explosion of other marine weapons**

● Y37.Ø9Ø **Military operations involving explosion of other marine weapons, military personnel**

● Y37.Ø91 **Military operations involving explosion of other marine weapons, civilian**

● Y37.1 **Military operations involving destruction of aircraft**

● Y37.1Ø **Military operations involving unspecified destruction of aircraft**

● Y37.1ØØ **Military operations involving unspecified destruction of aircraft, military personnel**

● Y37.1Ø1 **Military operations involving unspecified destruction of aircraft, civilian**

● Y37.11 **Military operations involving destruction of aircraft due to enemy fire or explosives**
Military operations involving destruction of aircraft due to air to air missile
Military operations involving destruction of aircraft due to explosive placed on aircraft
Military operations involving destruction of aircraft due to rocket propelled grenade [RPG]
Military operations involving destruction of aircraft due to small arms fire
Military operations involving destruction of aircraft due to surface to air missile

CHAPTER 2Ø (VØØ-Y99)

Y37.110 Military operations involving destruction of aircraft due to enemy fire or explosives, military personnel

Y37.111 Military operations involving destruction of aircraft due to enemy fire or explosives, civilian

Y37.12 Military operations involving destruction of aircraft due to collision with other aircraft

Y37.120 Military operations involving destruction of aircraft due to collision with other aircraft, military personnel

Y37.121 Military operations involving destruction of aircraft due to collision with other aircraft, civilian

Y37.13 Military operations involving destruction of aircraft due to onboard fire

Y37.130 Military operations involving destruction of aircraft due to onboard fire, military personnel

Y37.131 Military operations involving destruction of aircraft due to onboard fire, civilian

Y37.14 Military operations involving destruction of aircraft due to accidental detonation of onboard munitions and explosives

Y37.140 Military operations involving destruction of aircraft due to accidental detonation of onboard munitions and explosives, military personnel

Y37.141 Military operations involving destruction of aircraft due to accidental detonation of onboard munitions and explosives, civilian

Y37.19 Military operations involving other destruction of aircraft

Y37.190 Military operations involving other destruction of aircraft, military personnel

Y37.191 Military operations involving other destruction of aircraft, civilian

Y37.2 Military operations involving other explosions and fragments

Excludes1 military operations involving explosion of aircraft (Y37.1-)
military operations involving explosion of marine weapons (Y37.0-)
military operations involving explosion of nuclear weapons (Y37.5-)

Y37.20 Military operations involving unspecified explosion and fragments
Military operations involving air blast NOS
Military operations involving blast NOS
Military operations involving blast fragments NOS
Military operations involving blast wave NOS
Military operations involving blast wind NOS
Military operations involving explosion NOS
Military operations involving explosion of bomb NOS

Y37.200 Military operations involving unspecified explosion and fragments, military personnel

Y37.201 Military operations involving unspecified explosion and fragments, civilian

Y37.21 Military operations involving explosion of aerial bomb

Y37.210 Military operations involving explosion of aerial bomb, military personnel

Y37.211 Military operations involving explosion of aerial bomb, civilian

Y37.22 Military operations involving explosion of guided missile

Y37.220 Military operations involving explosion of guided missile, military personnel

Y37.221 Military operations involving explosion of guided missile, civilian

Y37.23 Military operations involving explosion of improvised explosive device [IED]
Military operations involving explosion of person-borne improvised explosive device [IED]
Military operations involving explosion of vehicle-borne improvised explosive device [IED]
Military operations involving explosion of roadside improvised explosive device [IED]

Y37.230 Military operations involving explosion of improvised explosive device [IED], military personnel

Y37.231 Military operations involving explosion of improvised explosive device [IED], civilian

Y37.24 Military operations involving explosion due to accidental detonation and discharge of own munitions or munitions launch device

Y37.240 Military operations involving explosion due to accidental detonation and discharge of own munitions or munitions launch device, military personnel

Y37.241 Military operations involving explosion due to accidental detonation and discharge of own munitions or munitions launch device, civilian

Y37.25 Military operations involving fragments from munitions

Y37.250 Military operations involving fragments from munitions, military personnel

Y37.251 Military operations involving fragments from munitions, civilian

Y37.26 Military operations involving fragments of improvised explosive device [IED]
Military operations involving fragments of person-borne improvised explosive device [IED]
Military operations involving fragments of vehicle-borne improvised explosive device [IED]
Military operations involving fragments of roadside improvised explosive device [IED]

Y37.260 Military operations involving fragments of improvised explosive device [IED], military personnel

Y37.261 Military operations involving fragments of improvised explosive device [IED], civilian

Y37.27 Military operations involving fragments from weapons

Y37.270 Military operations involving fragments from weapons, military personnel

Y37.271 Military operations involving fragments from weapons, civilian

Y37.29 Military operations involving other explosions and fragments
Military operations involving explosion of grenade
Military operations involving explosions of land mine
Military operations involving shrapnel NOS

Y37.290 Military operations involving other explosions and fragments, military personnel

● Y37.291 **Military operations involving other explosions and fragments, civilian**

● Y37.3 **Military operations involving fires, conflagrations and hot substances**

Military operations involving smoke, fumes, and heat from fires, conflagrations and hot substances

Excludes1 military operations involving fires and conflagrations aboard military aircraft (Y37.1-)
military operations involving fires and conflagrations aboard military watercraft (Y37.0-)
military operations involving fires and conflagrations caused indirectly by conventional weapons (Y37.2-)
military operations involving fires and thermal effects of nuclear weapons (Y36.53-)

● Y37.30 **Military operations involving unspecified fire, conflagration and hot substance**

● Y37.300 **Military operations involving unspecified fire, conflagration and hot substance, military personnel**

● Y37.301 **Military operations involving unspecified fire, conflagration and hot substance, civilian**

● Y37.31 **Military operations involving gasoline bomb**

Military operations involving incendiary bomb
Military operations involving petrol bomb

● Y37.310 **Military operations involving gasoline bomb, military personnel**

● Y37.311 **Military operations involving gasoline bomb, civilian**

● Y37.32 **Military operations involving incendiary bullet**

● Y37.320 **Military operations involving incendiary bullet, military personnel**

● Y37.321 **Military operations involving incendiary bullet, civilian**

● Y37.33 **Military operations involving flamethrower**

● Y37.330 **Military operations involving flamethrower, military personnel**

● Y37.331 **Military operations involving flamethrower, civilian**

● Y37.39 **Military operations involving other fires, conflagrations and hot substances**

● Y37.390 **Military operations involving other fires, conflagrations and hot substances, military personnel**

● Y37.391 **Military operations involving other fires, conflagrations and hot substances, civilian**

● Y37.4 **Military operations involving firearm discharge and other forms of conventional warfare**

● Y37.41 **Military operations involving rubber bullets**

● Y37.410 **Military operations involving rubber bullets, military personnel**

● Y37.411 **Military operations involving rubber bullets, civilian**

● Y37.42 **Military operations involving firearms pellets**

● Y37.420 **Military operations involving firearms pellets, military personnel**

● Y37.421 **Military operations involving firearms pellets, civilian**

● Y37.43 **Military operations involving other firearms discharge**

Military operations involving bullets NOS

Excludes1 military operations involving munitions fragments (Y37.25-)
military operations involving incendiary bullets (Y37.32-)

● Y37.430 **Military operations involving other firearms discharge, military personnel**

● Y37.431 **Military operations involving other firearms discharge, civilian**

● Y37.44 **Military operations involving unarmed hand to hand combat**

Excludes1 military operations involving combat using blunt or piercing object (Y37.45-)
military operations involving intentional restriction of air and airway (Y37.46-)
military operations involving unintentional restriction of air and airway (Y37.47-)

● Y37.440 **Military operations involving unarmed hand to hand combat, military personnel**

● Y37.441 **Military operations involving unarmed hand to hand combat, civilian**

● Y37.45 **Military operations involving combat using blunt or piercing object**

● Y37.450 **Military operations involving combat using blunt or piercing object, military personnel**

● Y37.451 **Military operations involving combat using blunt or piercing object, civilian**

● Y37.46 **Military operations involving intentional restriction of air and airway**

● Y37.460 **Military operations involving intentional restriction of air and airway, military personnel**

● Y37.461 **Military operations involving intentional restriction of air and airway, civilian**

● Y37.47 **Military operations involving unintentional restriction of air and airway**

● Y37.470 **Military operations involving unintentional restriction of air and airway, military personnel**

● Y37.471 **Military operations involving unintentional restriction of air and airway, civilian**

● Y37.49 **Military operations involving other forms of conventional warfare**

● Y37.490 **Military operations involving other forms of conventional warfare, military personnel**

● Y37.491 **Military operations involving other forms of conventional warfare, civilian**

● Y37.5 **Military operations involving nuclear weapons**

Military operation involving dirty bomb NOS

● Y37.50 **Military operations involving unspecified effect of nuclear weapon**

● Y37.500 **Military operations involving unspecified effect of nuclear weapon, military personnel**

● Y37.501 **Military operations involving unspecified effect of nuclear weapon, civilian**

● Y37.51 **Military operations involving direct blast effect of nuclear weapon**

Military operations involving blast pressure of nuclear weapon

● Y37.510 **Military operations involving direct blast effect of nuclear weapon, military personnel**

● Y37.511 **Military operations involving direct blast effect of nuclear weapon, civilian**

● Y37.52 **Military operations involving indirect blast effect of nuclear weapon**
Military operations involving being thrown by blast of nuclear weapon
Military operations involving being struck or crushed by blast debris of nuclear weapon

● Y37.520 **Military operations involving indirect blast effect of nuclear weapon, military personnel**

● Y37.521 **Military operations involving indirect blast effect of nuclear weapon, civilian**

● Y37.53 **Military operations involving thermal radiation effect of nuclear weapon**
Military operations involving direct heat from nuclear weapon
Military operation involving fireball effects from nuclear weapon

● Y37.530 **Military operations involving thermal radiation effect of nuclear weapon, military personnel**

● Y37.531 **Military operations involving thermal radiation effect of nuclear weapon, civilian**

● Y37.54 **Military operation involving nuclear radiation effects of nuclear weapon**
Military operation involving acute radiation exposure from nuclear weapon
Military operation involving exposure to immediate ionizing radiation from nuclear weapon
Military operation involving fallout exposure from nuclear weapon
Military operation involving secondary effects of nuclear weapons

● Y37.540 **Military operation involving nuclear radiation effects of nuclear weapon, military personnel**

● Y37.541 **Military operation involving nuclear radiation effects of nuclear weapon, civilian**

● Y37.59 **Military operation involving other effects of nuclear weapons**

● Y37.590 **Military operation involving other effects of nuclear weapons, military personnel**

● Y37.591 **Military operation involving other effects of nuclear weapons, civilian**

● Y37.6 **Military operations involving biological weapons**

● Y37.6X **Military operations involving biological weapons**

● Y37.6X0 **Military operations involving biological weapons, military personnel**

● Y37.6X1 **Military operations involving biological weapons, civilian**

● Y37.7 **Military operations involving chemical weapons and other forms of unconventional warfare**
Excludes1 military operations involving incendiary devices (Y36.3-, Y36.5-)

● Y37.7X **Military operations involving chemical weapons and other forms of unconventional warfare**

● Y37.7X0 **Military operations involving chemical weapons and other forms of unconventional warfare, military personnel**

● Y37.7X1 **Military operations involving chemical weapons and other forms of unconventional warfare, civilian**

● Y37.9 **Other and unspecified military operations**

X● Y37.90 **Military operations, unspecified**

X● Y37.91 **Military operations involving unspecified weapon of mass destruction [WMD]**

X● Y37.92 **Military operations involving friendly fire**

● Y38 **Terrorism**
These codes are for use to identify injuries resulting from the unlawful use of force or violence against persons or property to intimidate or coerce a government, the civilian population, or any segment thereof, in furtherance of political or social objective
Use additional code for place of occurrence (Y92.-)
The appropriate 7th character is to be added to each code from category Y38

A	initial encounter
D	subsequent encounter
S	sequela

● Y38.0 **Terrorism involving explosion of marine weapons**
Terrorism involving depth-charge
Terrorism involving marine mine
Terrorism involving mine NOS, at sea or in harbor
Terrorism involving sea-based artillery shell
Terrorism involving torpedo
Terrorism involving underwater blast

● Y38.0X **Terrorism involving explosion of marine weapons**

● Y38.0X1 **Terrorism involving explosion of marine weapons, public safety official injured**

● Y38.0X2 **Terrorism involving explosion of marine weapons, civilian injured**

● Y38.0X3 **Terrorism involving explosion of marine weapons, terrorist injured**

● Y38.1 **Terrorism involving destruction of aircraft**
Terrorism involving aircraft burned
Terrorism involving aircraft exploded
Terrorism involving aircraft being shot down
Terrorism involving aircraft used as a weapon

● Y38.1X **Terrorism involving destruction of aircraft**

● Y38.1X1 **Terrorism involving destruction of aircraft, public safety official injured**

● Y38.1X2 **Terrorism involving destruction of aircraft, civilian injured**

● Y38.1X3 **Terrorism involving destruction of aircraft, terrorist injured**

● Y38.2 **Terrorism involving other explosions and fragments**
Terrorism involving antipersonnel (fragments) bomb
Terrorism involving blast NOS
Terrorism involving explosion NOS
Terrorism involving explosion of breech block
Terrorism involving explosion of cannon block
Terrorism involving explosion (fragments) of artillery shell
Terrorism involving explosion (fragments) of bomb
Terrorism involving explosion (fragments) of grenade
Terrorism involving explosion (fragments) of guided missile
Terrorism involving explosion (fragments) of land mine
Terrorism involving explosion of mortar bomb
Terrorism involving explosion of munitions
Terrorism involving explosion (fragments) of rocket
Terrorism involving explosion (fragments) of shell
Terrorism involving shrapnel
Terrorism involving mine NOS, on land
Excludes1 terrorism involving explosion of nuclear weapon (Y38.5)
terrorism involving suicide bomber (Y38.81)

● Y38.2X **Terrorism involving other explosions and fragments**

● Y38.2X1 **Terrorism involving other explosions and fragments, public safety official injured**

● Y38.2X2 **Terrorism involving other explosions and fragments, civilian injured**

● Y38.2X3 **Terrorism involving other explosions and fragments, terrorist injured**

● Y38.3 **Terrorism involving fires, conflagration and hot substances**
Terrorism involving conflagration NOS
Terrorism involving fire NOS
Terrorism involving petrol bomb
Excludes1 terrorism involving fire or heat of nuclear weapon (Y38.5)

● Y38.3X **Terrorism involving fires, conflagration and hot substances**

● Y38.3X1 **Terrorism involving fires, conflagration and hot substances, public safety official injured**

● Y38.3X2 **Terrorism involving fires, conflagration and hot substances, civilian injured**

● Y38.3X3 **Terrorism involving fires, conflagration and hot substances, terrorist injured**

● Y38.4 **Terrorism involving firearms**
Terrorism involving carbine bullet
Terrorism involving machine gun bullet
Terrorism involving pellets (shotgun)
Terrorism involving pistol bullet
Terrorism involving rifle bullet
Terrorism involving rubber (rifle) bullet

● Y38.4X **Terrorism involving firearms**

● Y38.4X1 **Terrorism involving firearms, public safety official injured**

● Y38.4X2 **Terrorism involving firearms, civilian injured**

● Y38.4X3 **Terrorism involving firearms, terrorist injured**

● Y38.5 **Terrorism involving nuclear weapons**
Terrorism involving blast effects of nuclear weapon
Terrorism involving exposure to ionizing radiation from nuclear weapon
Terrorism involving fireball effect of nuclear weapon
Terrorism involving heat from nuclear weapon

● Y38.5X **Terrorism involving nuclear weapons**

● Y38.5X1 **Terrorism involving nuclear weapons, public safety official injured**

● Y38.5X2 **Terrorism involving nuclear weapons, civilian injured**

● Y38.5X3 **Terrorism involving nuclear weapons, terrorist injured**

● Y38.6 **Terrorism involving biological weapons**
Terrorism involving anthrax
Terrorism involving cholera
A serious, often deadly, infectious disease of the small intestine
Terrorism involving smallpox

● Y38.6X **Terrorism involving biological weapons**

● Y38.6X1 **Terrorism involving biological weapons, public safety official injured**

● Y38.6X2 **Terrorism involving biological weapons, civilian injured**

● Y38.6X3 **Terrorism involving biological weapons, terrorist injured**

● Y38.7 **Terrorism involving chemical weapons**
Terrorism involving gases, fumes, chemicals
Terrorism involving hydrogen cyanide
Terrorism involving phosgene
Terrorism involving sarin

● Y38.7X **Terrorism involving chemical weapons**

● Y38.7X1 **Terrorism involving chemical weapons, public safety official injured**

● Y38.7X2 **Terrorism involving chemical weapons, civilian injured**

● Y38.7X3 **Terrorism involving chemical weapons, terrorist injured**

● Y38.8 **Terrorism involving other and unspecified means**

● Y38.80 **Terrorism involving unspecified means**
Terrorism NOS

● Y38.81 **Terrorism involving suicide bomber**

● Y38.811 **Terrorism involving suicide bomber, public safety official injured**

● Y38.812 **Terrorism involving suicide bomber, civilian injured**

● Y38.89 **Terrorism involving other means**
Terrorism involving drowning and submersion
Terrorism involving lasers
Terrorism involving piercing or stabbing instruments

● Y38.891 **Terrorism involving other means, public safety official injured**

● Y38.892 **Terrorism involving other means, civilian injured**

● Y38.893 **Terrorism involving other means, terrorist injured**

● Y38.9 **Terrorism, secondary effects**
Note: This code is for use to identify conditions occurring subsequent to a terrorist attack not those that are due to the initial terrorist attack.

● Y38.9X **Terrorism, secondary effects**

● Y38.9X1 **Terrorism, secondary effects, public safety official injured**

● Y38.9X2 **Terrorism, secondary effects, civilian injured categories**

COMPLICATIONS OF MEDICAL AND SURGICAL CARE (Y62-Y84)

Includes complications of medical devices surgical and medical procedures as the cause of abnormal reaction of the patient, or of later complication, without mention of misadventure at the time of the procedure

MISADVENTURES TO PATIENTS DURING SURGICAL AND MEDICAL CARE (Y62-Y69)

Excludes1 surgical and medical procedures as the cause of abnormal reaction of the patient, without mention of misadventure at the time of the procedure (Y83-Y84)

● Y62 **Failure of sterile precautions during surgical and medical care**

Y62.0 **Failure of sterile precautions during surgical operation**

Y62.1 **Failure of sterile precautions during infusion or transfusion**

Y62.2 **Failure of sterile precautions during kidney dialysis and other perfusion**

Y62.3 **Failure of sterile precautions during injection or immunization**

Y62.4 **Failure of sterile precautions during endoscopic examination**

Y62.5 **Failure of sterile precautions during heart catheterization**

Y62.6 **Failure of sterile precautions during aspiration, puncture and other catheterization**

Y62.8 **Failure of sterile precautions during other surgical and medical care**

Y62.9 **Failure of sterile precautions during unspecified surgical and medical care**

● Y63 **Failure in dosage during surgical and medical care**
Excludes2 accidental overdose of drug or wrong drug given in error (T36-T50)

Y63.0 **Excessive amount of blood or other fluid given during transfusion or infusion**

Y63.1 **Incorrect dilution of fluid used during infusion**

Y63.2 **Overdose of radiation given during therapy**

Y63.3 **Inadvertent exposure of patient to radiation during medical care**

Y63.4 **Failure in dosage in electroshock or insulin-shock therapy**

CHAPTER 20 (V00-Y99)

Y63.5 Inappropriate temperature in local application and packing

Y63.6 Underdosing and nonadministration of necessary drug, medicament or biological substance

Y63.8 Failure in dosage during other surgical and medical care

Y63.9 Failure in dosage during unspecified surgical and medical care

● Y64 Contaminated medical or biological substances

Y64.0 Contaminated medical or biological substance, transfused or infused

Y64.1 Contaminated medical or biological substance, injected or used for immunization

Y64.8 Contaminated medical or biological substance administered by other means

Y64.9 Contaminated medical or biological substance administered by unspecified means
Administered contaminated medical or biological substance NOS

● Y65 Other misadventures during surgical and medical care

Y65.0 Mismatched blood in transfusion

Y65.1 Wrong fluid used in infusion

Y65.2 Failure in suture or ligature during surgical operation

Y65.3 Endotracheal tube wrongly placed during anesthetic procedure

Y65.4 Failure to introduce or to remove other tube or instrument

● Y65.5 Performance of wrong procedure (operation)

● Y65.51 Performance of wrong procedure (operation) on correct patient
Wrong device implanted into correct surgical site
Excludes1 performance of correct procedure (operation) on wrong side or body part (Y65.53)
MCE: Wrong procedure performed

● Y65.52 Performance of procedure (operation) on patient not scheduled for surgery
Performance of procedure (operation) intended for another patient
Performance of procedure (operation) on wrong patient
MCE: Wrong procedure performed

● Y65.53 Performance of correct procedure (operation) on wrong side or body part
Performance of correct procedure (operation) on wrong side
Performance of correct procedure (operation) on wrong site
MCE: Wrong procedure performed

Y65.8 Other specified misadventures during surgical and medical care
Coding Clinic: 2019, Q2, P24

Y66 Nonadministration of surgical and medical care
Premature cessation of surgical and medical care
Excludes1 DNR status (Z66)
palliative care (Z51.5)

Y69 Unspecified misadventure during surgical and medical care

MEDICAL DEVICES ASSOCIATED WITH ADVERSE INCIDENTS IN DIAGNOSTIC AND THERAPEUTIC USE (Y70-Y82)

Includes breakdown or malfunction of medical devices (during use) (after implantation) (ongoing use)

Excludes2 later complications following use of medical devices without breakdown or malfunctioning of device (Y83-Y84)
misadventure to patients during surgical and medical care, classifiable to (Y62-Y69)
surgical and other medical procedures as the cause of abnormal reaction of the patient, or of later complication, without mention of misadventure at the time of the procedure (Y83-Y84)

● Y70 Anesthesiology devices associated with adverse incidents

Y70.0 Diagnostic and monitoring anesthesiology devices associated with adverse incidents

Y70.1 Therapeutic (nonsurgical) and rehabilitative anesthesiology devices associated with adverse incidents

Y70.2 Prosthetic and other implants, materials and accessory anesthesiology devices associated with adverse incidents

Y70.3 Surgical instruments, materials and anesthesiology devices (including sutures) associated with adverse incidents

Y70.8 Miscellaneous anesthesiology devices associated with adverse incidents, not elsewhere classified

● Y71 Cardiovascular devices associated with adverse incidents

Y71.0 Diagnostic and monitoring cardiovascular devices associated with adverse incidents

Y71.1 Therapeutic (nonsurgical) and rehabilitative cardiovascular devices associated with adverse incidents

Y71.2 Prosthetic and other implants, materials and accessory cardiovascular devices associated with adverse incidents

Y71.3 Surgical instruments, materials and cardiovascular devices (including sutures) associated with adverse incidents

Y71.8 Miscellaneous cardiovascular devices associated with adverse incidents, not elsewhere classified

● Y72 Otorhinolaryngological devices associated with adverse incidents

Y72.0 Diagnostic and monitoring otorhinolaryngological devices associated with adverse incidents

Y72.1 Therapeutic (nonsurgical) and rehabilitative otorhinolaryngological devices associated with adverse incidents

Y72.2 Prosthetic and other implants, materials and accessory otorhinolaryngological devices associated with adverse incidents

Y72.3 Surgical instruments, materials and otorhinolaryngological devices (including sutures) associated with adverse incidents

Y72.8 Miscellaneous otorhinolaryngological devices associated with adverse incidents, not elsewhere classified

● Y73 Gastroenterology and urology devices associated with adverse incidents

Y73.0 Diagnostic and monitoring gastroenterology and urology devices associated with adverse incidents

Y73.1 Therapeutic (nonsurgical) and rehabilitative gastroenterology and urology devices associated with adverse incidents

Y73.2 Prosthetic and other implants, materials and accessory gastroenterology and urology devices associated with adverse incidents

Y73.3 Surgical instruments, materials and gastroenterology and urology devices (including sutures) associated with adverse incidents

Y73.8 Miscellaneous gastroenterology and urology devices associated with adverse incidents, not elsewhere classified

● **Y74** General hospital and personal-use devices associated with adverse incidents
- Y74.0 Diagnostic and monitoring general hospital and personal-use devices associated with adverse incidents
- Y74.1 Therapeutic (nonsurgical) and rehabilitative general hospital and personal-use devices associated with adverse incidents
- Y74.2 Prosthetic and other implants, materials and accessory general hospital and personal-use devices associated with adverse incidents
- Y74.3 Surgical instruments, materials and general hospital and personal-use devices (including sutures) associated with adverse incidents
- Y74.8 Miscellaneous general hospital and personal-use devices associated with adverse incidents, not elsewhere classified

● **Y75** Neurological devices associated with adverse incidents
- Y75.0 Diagnostic and monitoring neurological devices associated with adverse incidents
- Y75.1 Therapeutic (nonsurgical) and rehabilitative neurological devices associated with adverse incidents
- Y75.2 Prosthetic and other implants, materials and neurological devices associated with adverse incidents
- Y75.3 Surgical instruments, materials and neurological devices (including sutures) associated with adverse incidents
- Y75.8 Miscellaneous neurological devices associated with adverse incidents, not elsewhere classified

● **Y76** Obstetric and gynecological devices associated with adverse incidents
- Y76.0 Diagnostic and monitoring obstetric and gynecological devices associated with adverse incidents
- Y76.1 Therapeutic (nonsurgical) and rehabilitative obstetric and gynecological devices associated with adverse incidents
- Y76.2 Prosthetic and other implants, materials and accessory obstetric and gynecological devices associated with adverse incidents
- Y76.3 Surgical instruments, materials and obstetric and gynecological devices (including sutures) associated with adverse incidents
- Y76.8 Miscellaneous obstetric and gynecological devices associated with adverse incidents, not elsewhere classified

● **Y77** Ophthalmic devices associated with adverse incidents
- Y77.0 Diagnostic and monitoring ophthalmic devices associated with adverse incidents
- ● Y77.1 Therapeutic (nonsurgical) and rehabilitative ophthalmic devices associated with adverse incidents
  - Y77.11 Contact lens associated with adverse incidents
    - Rigid gas permeable contact lens associated with adverse incidents
    - Soft (hydrophilic) contact lens associated with adverse incidents
  - Y77.19 Other therapeutic (nonsurgical) and rehabilitative ophthalmic devices associated with adverse incidents
- Y77.2 Prosthetic and other implants, materials and accessory ophthalmic devices associated with adverse incidents
- Y77.3 Surgical instruments, materials and ophthalmic devices (including sutures) associated with adverse incidents
- Y77.8 Miscellaneous ophthalmic devices associated with adverse incidents, not elsewhere classified

● **Y78** Radiological devices associated with adverse incidents
- Y78.0 Diagnostic and monitoring radiological devices associated with adverse incidents
- Y78.1 Therapeutic (nonsurgical) and rehabilitative radiological devices associated with adverse incidents
- Y78.2 Prosthetic and other implants, materials and accessory radiological devices associated with adverse incidents
- Y78.3 Surgical instruments, materials and radiological devices (including sutures) associated with adverse incidents
- Y78.8 Miscellaneous radiological devices associated with adverse incidents, not elsewhere classified

● **Y79** Orthopedic devices associated with adverse incidents
- Y79.0 Diagnostic and monitoring orthopedic devices associated with adverse incidents
- Y79.1 Therapeutic (nonsurgical) and rehabilitative orthopedic devices associated with adverse incidents
- Y79.2 Prosthetic and other implants, materials and accessory orthopedic devices associated with adverse incidents
- Y79.3 Surgical instruments, materials and orthopedic devices (including sutures) associated with adverse incidents
- Y79.8 Miscellaneous orthopedic devices associated with adverse incidents, not elsewhere classified

● **Y80** Physical medicine devices associated with adverse incidents
- Y80.0 Diagnostic and monitoring physical medicine devices associated with adverse incidents
- Y80.1 Therapeutic (nonsurgical) and rehabilitative physical medicine devices associated with adverse incidents
- Y80.2 Prosthetic and other implants, materials and accessory physical medicine devices associated with adverse incidents
- Y80.3 Surgical instruments, materials and physical medicine devices (including sutures) associated with adverse incidents
- Y80.8 Miscellaneous physical medicine devices associated with adverse incidents, not elsewhere classified

● **Y81** General- and plastic-surgery devices associated with adverse incidents
- Y81.0 Diagnostic and monitoring general- and plastic-surgery devices associated with adverse incidents
- Y81.1 Therapeutic (nonsurgical) and rehabilitative general- and plastic-surgery devices associated with adverse incidents
- Y81.2 Prosthetic and other implants, materials and accessory general- and plastic-surgery devices associated with adverse incidents
- Y81.3 Surgical instruments, materials and general- and plastic-surgery devices (including sutures) associated with adverse incidents
- Y81.8 Miscellaneous general- and plastic-surgery devices associated with adverse incidents, not elsewhere classified

● **Y82** Other and unspecified medical devices associated with adverse incidents
- Y82.8 Other medical devices associated with adverse incidents
- Y82.9 Unspecified medical devices associated with adverse incidents

SURGICAL AND OTHER MEDICAL PROCEDURES AS THE CAUSE OF ABNORMAL REACTION OF THE PATIENT, OR OF LATER COMPLICATION, WITHOUT MENTION OF MISADVENTURE AT THE TIME OF THE PROCEDURE (Y83-Y84)

Excludes1 misadventures to patients during surgical and medical care, classifiable to (Y62-Y69)

Excludes2 breakdown or malfunctioning of medical device (after implantation) (during procedure) (ongoing use) (Y70-Y82)

● **Y83** Surgical operation and other surgical procedures as the cause of abnormal reaction of the patient, or of later complication, without mention of misadventure at the time of the procedure
- Y83.0 Surgical operation with transplant of whole organ as the cause of abnormal reaction of the patient, or of later complication, without mention of misadventure at the time of the procedure
- Y83.1 Surgical operation with implant of artificial internal device as the cause of abnormal reaction of the patient, or of later complication, without mention of misadventure at the time of the procedure

CHAPTER 20 (V00-Y99)

Y83.2 Surgical operation with anastomosis, bypass or graft as the cause of abnormal reaction of the patient, or of later complication, without mention of misadventure at the time of the procedure

Y83.3 Surgical operation with formation of external stoma as the cause of abnormal reaction of the patient, or of later complication, without mention of misadventure at the time of the procedure

Y83.4 Other reconstructive surgery as the cause of abnormal reaction of the patient, or of later complication, without mention of misadventure at the time of the procedure

Y83.5 Amputation of limb(s) as the cause of abnormal reaction of the patient, or of later complication, without mention of misadventure at the time of the procedure

Y83.6 Removal of other organ (partial) (total) as the cause of abnormal reaction of the patient, or of later complication, without mention of misadventure at the time of the procedure

Y83.8 Other surgical procedures as the cause of abnormal reaction of the patient, or of later complication, without mention of misadventure at the time of the procedure
Coding Clinic: 2023, Q2, P14

Y83.9 Surgical procedure, unspecified as the cause of abnormal reaction of the patient, or of later complication, without mention of misadventure at the time of the procedure

● Y84 Other medical procedures as the cause of abnormal reaction of the patient, or of later complication, without mention of misadventure at the time of the procedure

Y84.0 Cardiac catheterization as the cause of abnormal reaction of the patient, or of later complication, without mention of misadventure at the time of the procedure

Y84.1 Kidney dialysis as the cause of abnormal reaction of the patient, or of later complication, without mention of misadventure at the time of the procedure

Y84.2 Radiological procedure and radiotherapy as the cause of abnormal reaction of the patient, or of later complication, without mention of misadventure at the time of the procedure
Coding Clinic: 2019, Q1, P21; 2017, Q1, P34

Y84.3 Shock therapy as the cause of abnormal reaction of the patient, or of later complication, without mention of misadventure at the time of the procedure

Y84.4 Aspiration of fluid as the cause of abnormal reaction of the patient, or of later complication, without mention of misadventure at the time of the procedure

Y84.5 Insertion of gastric or duodenal sound as the cause of abnormal reaction of the patient, or of later complication, without mention of misadventure at the time of the procedure

Y84.6 Urinary catheterization as the cause of abnormal reaction of the patient, or of later complication, without mention of misadventure at the time of the procedure

Y84.7 Blood-sampling as the cause of abnormal reaction of the patient, or of later complication, without mention of misadventure at the time of the procedure

Y84.8 Other medical procedures as the cause of abnormal reaction of the patient, or of later complication, without mention of misadventure at the time of the procedure
Coding Clinic: 2024, Q1, P26; 2023, Q2, P28; 2021, Q1, P5

Y84.9 Medical procedure, unspecified as the cause of abnormal reaction of the patient, or of later complication, without mention of misadventure at the time of the procedure

SUPPLEMENTARY FACTORS RELATED TO CAUSES OF MORBIDITY CLASSIFIED ELSEWHERE (Y90-Y99)

Note: These categories may be used to provide supplementary information concerning causes of morbidity. They are not to be used for single-condition coding.

● Y90 Evidence of alcohol involvement determined by blood alcohol level
Code first any associated alcohol related disorders (F10)
Coding Clinic: 2024, Q2, P10

Y90.0 Blood alcohol level of less than 20 mg/100 ml

Y90.1 Blood alcohol level of 20-39 mg/100 ml

Y90.2 Blood alcohol level of 40-59 mg/100 ml

Y90.3 Blood alcohol level of 60-79 mg/100 ml

Y90.4 Blood alcohol level of 80-99 mg/100 ml

Y90.5 Blood alcohol level of 100-119 mg/100 ml

Y90.6 Blood alcohol level of 120-199 mg/100 ml

Y90.7 Blood alcohol level of 200-239 mg/100 ml

Y90.8 Blood alcohol level of 240 mg/100 ml or more

Y90.9 Presence of alcohol in blood, level not specified

OGCR Section I.C.20.b.

Place of Occurrence Guideline

Codes from category Y92, Place of occurrence of the external cause, are secondary codes for use after other external cause codes to identify the location of the patient at the time of injury or other condition.

Generally, a place of occurrence code is assigned only once, at the initial encounter for treatment. However, in the rare instance that a new injury occurs during hospitalization, an additional place of occurrence code may be assigned. No 7th characters are used for Y92.

Only one code from Y92 should be recorded on a medical record.

Do not use place of occurrence code Y92.9 if the place is not stated or is not applicable.

● Y92 Place of occurrence of the external cause
The following category is for use, when relevant, to identify the place of occurrence of the external cause. Use in conjunction with an activity code.
Place of occurrence should be recorded only at the initial encounter for treatment

● Y92.0 Non-institutional (private) residence as the place of occurrence of the external cause
Excludes1 abandoned or derelict house (Y92.89)
home under construction but not yet occupied (Y92.6-)
institutional place of residence (Y92.1-)

● Y92.00 Unspecified non-institutional (private) residence as the place of occurrence of the external cause

Y92.000 Kitchen of unspecified non-institutional (private) residence as the place of occurrence of the external cause

Y92.001 Dining room of unspecified non-institutional (private) residence as the place of occurrence of the external cause

Y92.002 Bathroom of unspecified non-institutional (private) residence as the place of occurrence of the external cause

Y92.003 Bedroom of unspecified non-institutional (private) residence as the place of occurrence of the external cause

Y92.007 Garden or yard of unspecified non-institutional (private) residence as the place of occurrence of the external cause

Y92.008 Other place in unspecified non-institutional (private) residence as the place of occurrence of the external cause

Y92.009 Unspecified place in unspecified non-institutional (private) residence as the place of occurrence of the external cause
Home (NOS) as the place of occurrence of the external cause
Coding Clinic: 2021, Q2, P5

● **Y92.01** **Single-family non-institutional (private) house as the place of occurrence of the external cause**
Farmhouse as the place of occurrence of the external cause
Excludes1 barn (Y92.71)
chicken coop or hen house (Y92.72)
farm field (Y92.73)
orchard (Y92.74)
single family mobile home or trailer (Y92.02-)
slaughter house (Y92.86)

Y92.010 **Kitchen of single-family (private) house as the place of occurrence of the external cause**

Y92.011 **Dining room of single-family (private) house as the place of occurrence of the external cause**

Y92.012 **Bathroom of single-family (private) house as the place of occurrence of the external cause**

Y92.013 **Bedroom of single-family (private) house as the place of occurrence of the external cause**

Y92.014 **Private driveway to single-family (private) house as the place of occurrence of the external cause**

Y92.015 **Private garage of single-family (private) house as the place of occurrence of the external cause**

Y92.016 **Swimming pool in single-family (private) house or garden as the place of occurrence of the external cause**

Y92.017 **Garden or yard in single-family (private) house as the place of occurrence of the external cause**

Y92.018 **Other place in single-family (private) house as the place of occurrence of the external cause**

Y92.019 **Unspecified place in single-family (private) house as the place of occurrence of the external cause**

● **Y92.02** **Mobile home as the place of occurrence of the external cause**

Y92.020 **Kitchen in mobile home as the place of occurrence of the external cause**

Y92.021 **Dining room in mobile home as the place of occurrence of the external cause**

Y92.022 **Bathroom in mobile home as the place of occurrence of the external cause**

Y92.023 **Bedroom in mobile home as the place of occurrence of the external cause**

Y92.024 **Driveway of mobile home as the place of occurrence of the external cause**

Y92.025 **Garage of mobile home as the place of occurrence of the external cause**

Y92.026 **Swimming pool of mobile home as the place of occurrence of the external cause**

Y92.027 **Garden or yard of mobile home as the place of occurrence of the external cause**

Y92.028 **Other place in mobile home as the place of occurrence of the external cause**

Y92.029 **Unspecified place in mobile home as the place of occurrence of the external cause**

● **Y92.03** **Apartment as the place of occurrence of the external cause**
Condominium as the place of occurrence of the external cause
Co-op apartment as the place of occurrence of the external cause

Y92.030 **Kitchen in apartment as the place of occurrence of the external cause**

Y92.031 **Bathroom in apartment as the place of occurrence of the external cause**

Y92.032 **Bedroom in apartment as the place of occurrence of the external cause**

Y92.038 **Other place in apartment as the place of occurrence of the external cause**

Y92.039 **Unspecified place in apartment as the place of occurrence of the external cause**

● **Y92.04** **Boarding-house as the place of occurrence of the external cause**

Y92.040 **Kitchen in boarding-house as the place of occurrence of the external cause**

Y92.041 **Bathroom in boarding-house as the place of occurrence of the external cause**

Y92.042 **Bedroom in boarding-house as the place of occurrence of the external cause**

Y92.043 **Driveway of boarding-house as the place of occurrence of the external cause**

Y92.044 **Garage of boarding-house as the place of occurrence of the external cause**

Y92.045 **Swimming pool of boarding-house as the place of occurrence of the external cause**

Y92.046 **Garden or yard of boarding-house as the place of occurrence of the external cause**

Y92.048 **Other place in boarding-house as the place of occurrence of the external cause**

Y92.049 **Unspecified place in boarding-house as the place of occurrence of the external cause**

● **Y92.09** **Other non-institutional residence as the place of occurrence of the external cause**

Y92.090 **Kitchen in other non-institutional residence as the place of occurrence of the external cause**

Y92.091 **Bathroom in other non-institutional residence as the place of occurrence of the external cause**

Y92.092 **Bedroom in other non-institutional residence as the place of occurrence of the external cause**

Y92.093 **Driveway of other non-institutional residence as the place of occurrence of the external cause**

Y92.094 **Garage of other non-institutional residence as the place of occurrence of the external cause**

Y92.095 **Swimming pool of other non-institutional residence as the place of occurrence of the external cause**

Y92.096 **Garden or yard of other non-institutional residence as the place of occurrence of the external cause**

Y92.098 **Other place in other non-institutional residence as the place of occurrence of the external cause**

Y92.099 **Unspecified place in other non-institutional residence as the place of occurrence of the external cause**
Coding Clinic: 2017, Q2, P10

● Y92.1 Institutional (nonprivate) residence as the place of occurrence of the external cause

Y92.10 Unspecified residential institution as the place of occurrence of the external cause

● Y92.11 Children's home and orphanage as the place of occurrence of the external cause

Y92.110 Kitchen in children's home and orphanage as the place of occurrence of the external cause

Y92.111 Bathroom in children's home and orphanage as the place of occurrence of the external cause

Y92.112 Bedroom in children's home and orphanage as the place of occurrence of the external cause

Y92.113 Driveway of children's home and orphanage as the place of occurrence of the external cause

Y92.114 Garage of children's home and orphanage as the place of occurrence of the external cause

Y92.115 Swimming pool of children's home and orphanage as the place of occurrence of the external cause

Y92.116 Garden or yard of children's home and orphanage as the place of occurrence of the external cause

Y92.118 Other place in children's home and orphanage as the place of occurrence of the external cause

Y92.119 Unspecified place in children's home and orphanage as the place of occurrence of the external cause

● Y92.12 Nursing home as the place of occurrence of the external cause

Home for the sick as the place of occurrence of the external cause

Hospice as the place of occurrence of the external cause

Y92.120 Kitchen in nursing home as the place of occurrence of the external cause

Y92.121 Bathroom in nursing home as the place of occurrence of the external cause

Y92.122 Bedroom in nursing home as the place of occurrence of the external cause

Y92.123 Driveway of nursing home as the place of occurrence of the external cause

Y92.124 Garage of nursing home as the place of occurrence of the external cause

Y92.125 Swimming pool of nursing home as the place of occurrence of the external cause

Y92.126 Garden or yard of nursing home as the place of occurrence of the external cause

Y92.128 Other place in nursing home as the place of occurrence of the external cause

Y92.129 Unspecified place in nursing home as the place of occurrence of the external cause

Coding Clinic: 2017, Q2, P10

● Y92.13 Military base as the place of occurrence of the external cause

Excludes1 military training grounds (Y92.83)

Y92.130 Kitchen on military base as the place of occurrence of the external cause

Y92.131 Mess hall on military base as the place of occurrence of the external cause

Y92.133 Barracks on military base as the place of occurrence of the external cause

Y92.135 Garage on military base as the place of occurrence of the external cause

Y92.136 Swimming pool on military base as the place of occurrence of the external cause

Y92.137 Garden or yard on military base as the place of occurrence of the external cause

Y92.138 Other place on military base as the place of occurrence of the external cause

Y92.139 Unspecified place military base as the place of occurrence of the external cause

● Y92.14 Prison as the place of occurrence of the external cause

Y92.140 Kitchen in prison as the place of occurrence of the external cause

Y92.141 Dining room in prison as the place of occurrence of the external cause

Y92.142 Bathroom in prison as the place of occurrence of the external cause

Y92.143 Cell of prison as the place of occurrence of the external cause

Y92.146 Swimming pool of prison as the place of occurrence of the external cause

Y92.147 Courtyard of prison as the place of occurrence of the external cause

Y92.148 Other place in prison as the place of occurrence of the external cause

Y92.149 Unspecified place in prison as the place of occurrence of the external cause

● Y92.15 Reform school as the place of occurrence of the external cause

Y92.150 Kitchen in reform school as the place of occurrence of the external cause

Y92.151 Dining room in reform school as the place of occurrence of the external cause

Y92.152 Bathroom in reform school as the place of occurrence of the external cause

Y92.153 Bedroom in reform school as the place of occurrence of the external cause

Y92.154 Driveway of reform school as the place of occurrence of the external cause

Y92.155 Garage of reform school as the place of occurrence of the external cause

Y92.156 Swimming pool of reform school as the place of occurrence of the external cause

Y92.157 Garden or yard of reform school as the place of occurrence of the external cause

Y92.158 Other place in reform school as the place of occurrence of the external cause

Y92.159 Unspecified place in reform school as the place of occurrence of the external cause

● Y92.16 School dormitory as the place of occurrence of the external cause

Excludes1 reform school as the place of occurrence of the external cause (Y92.15-)
school buildings and grounds as the place of occurrence of the external cause (Y92.2-)
school sports and athletic areas as the place of occurrence of the external cause (Y92.3-)

Y92.160 Kitchen in school dormitory as the place of occurrence of the external cause

Y92.161 **Dining room** in school dormitory as the place of occurrence of the external cause

Y92.162 **Bathroom** in school dormitory as the place of occurrence of the external cause

Y92.163 **Bedroom** in school dormitory as the place of occurrence of the external cause

Y92.168 **Other place** in school dormitory as the place of occurrence of the external cause

Y92.169 **Unspecified** place in school dormitory as the place of occurrence of the external cause

● Y92.19 **Other specified residential institution** as the place of occurrence of the external cause

Y92.190 **Kitchen** in other specified residential institution as the place of occurrence of the external cause

Y92.191 **Dining room** in other specified residential institution as the place of occurrence of the external cause

Y92.192 **Bathroom** in other specified residential institution as the place of occurrence of the external cause

Y92.193 **Bedroom** in other specified residential institution as the place of occurrence of the external cause

Y92.194 **Driveway** of other specified residential institution as the place of occurrence of the external cause

Y92.195 **Garage** of other specified residential institution as the place of occurrence of the external cause

Y92.196 **Pool** of other specified residential institution as the place of occurrence of the external cause

Y92.197 **Garden or yard** of other specified residential institution as the place of occurrence of the external cause

Y92.198 **Other place** in other specified residential institution as the place of occurrence of the external cause

Coding Clinic: 2017, Q2, P11

Y92.199 **Unspecified** place in other specified residential institution as the place of occurrence of the external cause

Coding Clinic: 2017, Q2, P10

● Y92.2 **School, other institution and public administrative area as the place of occurrence of the external cause**

Building and adjacent grounds used by the general public or by a particular group of the public

Excludes1 building under construction as the place of occurrence of the external cause (Y92.6)

residential institution as the place of occurrence of the external cause (Y92.1)

school dormitory as the place of occurrence of the external cause (Y92.16-)

sports and athletics area of schools as the place of occurrence of the external cause (Y92.3-)

● Y92.21 **School** (private) (public) (state) as the place of occurrence of the external cause

Y92.210 **Daycare center** as the place of occurrence of the external cause

Y92.211 **Elementary school** as the place of occurrence of the external cause

Kindergarten as the place of occurrence of the external cause

Y92.212 **Middle school** as the place of occurrence of the external cause

Y92.213 **High school** as the place of occurrence of the external cause

Coding Clinic: 2012, Q4, P108

Y92.214 **College** as the place of occurrence of the external cause

University as the place of occurrence of the external cause

Y92.215 **Trade school** as the place of occurrence of the external cause

Y92.218 **Other school** as the place of occurrence of the external cause

Y92.219 **Unspecified** school as the place of occurrence of the external cause

Y92.22 **Religious institution** as the place of occurrence of the external cause

Church as the place of occurrence of the external cause

Mosque as the place of occurrence of the external cause

Synagogue as the place of occurrence of the external cause

● Y92.23 **Hospital** as the place of occurrence of the external cause

Excludes1 ambulatory (outpatient) health services establishments (Y92.53-)

home for the sick as the place of occurrence of the external cause (Y92.12-)

hospice as the place of occurrence of the external cause (Y92.12-)

nursing home as the place of occurrence of the external cause (Y92.12-)

Y92.230 **Patient room** in hospital as the place of occurrence of the external cause

Y92.231 **Patient bathroom** in hospital as the place of occurrence of the external cause

Y92.232 **Corridor** of hospital as the place of occurrence of the external cause

Y92.233 **Cafeteria** of hospital as the place of occurrence of the external cause

Y92.234 **Operating room** of hospital as the place of occurrence of the external cause

Y92.238 **Other place** in hospital as the place of occurrence of the external cause

Y92.239 **Unspecified** place in hospital as the place of occurrence of the external cause

● Y92.24 **Public administrative building** as the place of occurrence of the external cause

Y92.240 **Courthouse** as the place of occurrence of the external cause

Y92.241 **Library** as the place of occurrence of the external cause

Y92.242 **Post office** as the place of occurrence of the external cause

Y92.243 **City hall** as the place of occurrence of the external cause

Y92.248 **Other** public administrative building as the place of occurrence of the external cause

● Y92.25 **Cultural building** as the place of occurrence of the external cause

Y92.250 **Art gallery** as the place of occurrence of the external cause

Y92.251 **Museum** as the place of occurrence of the external cause

Y92.252 **Music hall** as the place of occurrence of the external cause

Y92.253 **Opera house** as the place of occurrence of the external cause

Y92.254 **Theater** (live) as the place of occurrence of the external cause

Y92.258 **Other** cultural public building as the place of occurrence of the external cause

Y92.26 **Movie house or cinema** as the place of occurrence of the external cause

Y92.29 **Other specified public building** as the place of occurrence of the external cause

Assembly hall as the place of occurrence of the external cause

Clubhouse as the place of occurrence of the external cause

● Y92.3 **Sports and athletics area** as the place of occurrence of the external cause

● Y92.31 **Athletic court** as the place of occurrence of the external cause

Excludes1 tennis court in private home or garden (Y92.09)

Y92.310 **Basketball** court as the place of occurrence of the external cause

Y92.311 **Squash** court as the place of occurrence of the external cause

Y92.312 **Tennis** court as the place of occurrence of the external cause

Y92.318 **Other** athletic court as the place of occurrence of the external cause

● Y92.32 **Athletic field** as the place of occurrence of the external cause

Y92.320 **Baseball** field as the place of occurrence of the external cause

Y92.321 **Football** field as the place of occurrence of the external cause

Y92.322 **Soccer** field as the place of occurrence of the external cause

Y92.328 **Other** athletic field as the place of occurrence of the external cause

Cricket field as the place of occurrence of the external cause

Hockey field as the place of occurrence of the external cause

● Y92.33 **Skating rink** as the place of occurrence of the external cause

Y92.330 **Ice** skating rink (indoor) (outdoor) as the place of occurrence of the external cause

Y92.331 **Roller** skating rink as the place of occurrence of the external cause

Y92.34 **Swimming pool** (public) as the place of occurrence of the external cause

Excludes1 swimming pool in private home or garden (Y92.016)

Y92.39 **Other specified** sports and athletic area as the place of occurrence of the external cause

Golf-course as the place of occurrence of the external cause

Gymnasium as the place of occurrence of the external cause

Riding-school as the place of occurrence of the external cause

Stadium as the place of occurrence of the external cause

● Y92.4 **Street, highway and other paved roadways as the place of occurrence of the external cause**

Excludes1 private driveway of residence (Y92.014, Y92.024, Y92.043, Y92.093, Y92.113, Y92.123, Y92.154, Y92.194)

● Y92.41 **Street and highway** as the place of occurrence of the external cause

Y92.410 **Unspecified** street and highway as the place of occurrence of the external cause

Road NOS as the place of occurrence of the external cause

Y92.411 **Interstate** highway as the place of occurrence of the external cause

Freeway as the place of occurrence of the external cause

Motorway as the place of occurrence of the external cause

Y92.412 **Parkway** as the place of occurrence of the external cause

Y92.413 **State road** as the place of occurrence of the external cause

Y92.414 **Local residential or business street** as the place of occurrence of the external cause

Y92.415 **Exit ramp or entrance ramp** of street or highway as the place of occurrence of the external cause

● Y92.48 **Other paved roadways** as the place of occurrence of the external cause

Y92.480 **Sidewalk** as the place of occurrence of the external cause

Y92.481 **Parking lot** as the place of occurrence of the external cause

Y92.482 **Bike path** as the place of occurrence of the external cause

Y92.488 **Other** paved roadways as the place of occurrence of the external cause

● Y92.5 **Trade and service area** as the place of occurrence of the external cause

Excludes1 garage in private home (Y92.015)
schools and other public administration buildings (Y92.2-)

● Y92.51 **Private commercial establishments** as the place of occurrence of the external cause

Y92.510 **Bank** as the place of occurrence of the external cause

Y92.511 **Restaurant or café** as the place of occurrence of the external cause

Y92.512 **Supermarket, store or market** as the place of occurrence of the external cause

Y92.513 **Shop** (commercial) as the place of occurrence of the external cause

● Y92.52 **Service areas** as the place of occurrence of the external cause

Y92.520 **Airport** as the place of occurrence of the external cause

Y92.521 **Bus station** as the place of occurrence of the external cause

Y92.522 **Railway station** as the place of occurrence of the external cause

Y92.523 **Highway rest stop** as the place of occurrence of the external cause

Y92.524 **Gas station** as the place of occurrence of the external cause

Petroleum station as the place of occurrence of the external cause

Service station as the place of occurrence of the external cause

● **Y92.53 Ambulatory health services establishments** as the place of occurrence of the external cause

Y92.530 Ambulatory surgery center as the place of occurrence of the external cause

Outpatient surgery center, including that connected with a hospital as the place of occurrence of the external cause

Same day surgery center, including that connected with a hospital as the place of occurrence of the external cause

Y92.531 Health care provider office as the place of occurrence of the external cause

Physician office as the place of occurrence of the external cause

Y92.532 Urgent care center as the place of occurrence of the external cause

Y92.538 Other ambulatory health services establishments as the place of occurrence of the external cause

Coding Clinic: 2019, Q1, P21

Y92.59 Other trade areas as the place of occurrence of the external cause

Office building as the place of occurrence of the external cause

Casino as the place of occurrence of the external cause

Garage (commercial) as the place of occurrence of the external cause

Hotel as the place of occurrence of the external cause

Radio or television station as the place of occurrence of the external cause

Shopping mall as the place of occurrence of the external cause

Warehouse as the place of occurrence of the external cause

● **Y92.6 Industrial and construction area** as the place of occurrence of the external cause

Y92.61 Building [any] under construction as the place of occurrence of the external cause

Y92.62 Dock or shipyard as the place of occurrence of the external cause

Dockyard as the place of occurrence of the external cause

Dry dock as the place of occurrence of the external cause

Shipyard as the place of occurrence of the external cause

Y92.63 Factory as the place of occurrence of the external cause

Factory building as the place of occurrence of the external cause

Factory premises as the place of occurrence of the external cause

Industrial yard as the place of occurrence of the external cause

Y92.64 Mine or pit as the place of occurrence of the external cause

Mine as the place of occurrence of the external cause

Y92.65 Oil rig as the place of occurrence of the external cause

Pit (coal) (gravel) (sand) as the place of occurrence of the external cause

Y92.69 Other specified industrial and construction area as the place of occurrence of the external cause

Gasworks as the place of occurrence of the external cause

Power-station (coal) (nuclear) (oil) as the place of occurrence of the external cause

Tunnel under construction as the place of occurrence of the external cause

Workshop as the place of occurrence of the external cause

● **Y92.7 Farm** as the place of occurrence of the external cause

Ranch as the place of occurrence of the external cause

Excludes1 farmhouse and home premises of farm (Y92.01-)

Y92.71 Barn as the place of occurrence of the external cause

Y92.72 Chicken coop as the place of occurrence of the external cause

Hen house as the place of occurrence of the external cause

Y92.73 Farm field as the place of occurrence of the external cause

Y92.74 Orchard as the place of occurrence of the external cause

Y92.79 Other farm location as the place of occurrence of the external cause

● **Y92.8 Other places** as the place of occurrence of the external cause

● **Y92.81 Transport vehicle** as the place of occurrence of the external cause

Excludes1 transport accidents (V00-V99)

Y92.810 Car as the place of occurrence of the external cause

Y92.811 Bus as the place of occurrence of the external cause

Y92.812 Truck as the place of occurrence of the external cause

Y92.813 Airplane as the place of occurrence of the external cause

Y92.814 Boat as the place of occurrence of the external cause

Y92.815 Train as the place of occurrence of the external cause

Y92.816 Subway car as the place of occurrence of the external cause

Y92.818 Other transport vehicle as the place of occurrence of the external cause

● **Y92.82 Wilderness area**

Y92.820 Desert as the place of occurrence of the external cause

Y92.821 Forest as the place of occurrence of the external cause

Y92.828 Other wilderness area as the place of occurrence of the external cause

Swamp as the place of occurrence of the external cause

Mountain as the place of occurrence of the external cause

Marsh as the place of occurrence of the external cause

Prairie as the place of occurrence of the external cause

● **Y92.83 Recreation area** as the place of occurrence of the external cause

Y92.830 Public park as the place of occurrence of the external cause

Y92.831 Amusement park as the place of occurrence of the external cause

Y92.832 Beach as the place of occurrence of the external cause

Seashore as the place of occurrence of the external cause

Y92.833 Campsite as the place of occurrence of the external cause

Y92.834 Zoological garden (zoo) as the place of occurrence of the external cause

Y92.838 Other recreation area as the place of occurrence of the external cause

Y92.84 Military training ground as the place of occurrence of the external cause

Y92.85 Railroad track as the place of occurrence of the external cause

Y92.86 **Slaughter house as the place of occurrence of the external cause**

Y92.89 **Other specified places as the place of occurrence of the external cause**
Derelict house as the place of occurrence of the external cause

OGCR Section I.C.20.b.

Do not use place of occurrence code Y92.9 if the place is not stated or is not applicable.

Y92.9 **Unspecified place or not applicable**

OGCR See Section I.C.2Ø.c.

Activity Code

Assign a code from category Y93, Activity code, to describe the activity of the patient at the time the injury or other health condition occurred.

An activity code is used only once, at the initial encounter for treatment. Only one code from Y93 should be recorded on a medical record.

The activity codes are not applicable to poisonings, adverse effects, misadventures or sequela.

Do not assign Y93.9, Unspecified activity, if the activity is not stated.

A code from category Y93 is appropriate for use with external cause and intent codes if identifying the activity provides additional information about the event.

● Y93 **Activity codes**

Note: Category Y93 is provided for use to indicate the activity of the person seeking healthcare for an injury or health condition, such as a heart attack while shoveling snow, which resulted from, or was contributed to, by the activity. These codes are appropriate for use for both acute injuries, such as those from Chapter 19, and conditions that are due to the long-term, cumulative effects of an activity, such as those from Chapter 13. They are also appropriate for use with external cause codes for cause and intent if identifying the activity provides additional information on the event. These codes should be used in conjunction with codes for external cause status (Y99) and place of occurrence (Y92).

This section contains the following broad activity categories:

Y93.Ø Activities involving walking and running
Y93.1 Activities involving water and water craft
Y93.2 Activities involving ice and snow
Y93.3 Activities involving climbing, rappelling, and jumping off
Y93.4 Activities involving dancing and other rhythmic movement
Y93.5 Activities involving other sports and athletics played individually
Y93.6 Activities involving other sports and athletics played as a team or group
Y93.7 Activities involving other specified sports and athletics
Y93.A Activities involving other cardiorespiratory exercise
Y93.B Activities involving other muscle strengthening exercises
Y93.C Activities involving computer technology and electronic devices
Y93.D Activities involving arts and handcrafts
Y93.E Activities involving personal hygiene and interior property and clothing maintenance
Y93.F Activities involving caregiving
Y93.G Activities involving food preparation, cooking and grilling
Y93.H Activities involving exterior property and land maintenance, building and construction
Y93.I Activities involving roller coasters and other types of external motion
Y93.J Activities involving playing musical instrument
Y93.K Activities involving animal care
Y93.8 Activities, other specified
Y93.9 Activity, unspecified

● Y93.Ø **Activities involving walking and running**
Excludes1 Activity, walking an animal (Y93.K1)
Activity, walking or running on a treadmill (Y93.A1)

Y93.Ø1 **Activity, walking, marching and hiking**
Activity, walking, marching and hiking on level or elevated terrain
Excludes1 activity, mountain climbing (Y93.31)

Y93.Ø2 **Activity, running**

● Y93.1 **Activities involving water and water craft**
Excludes1 activities involving ice (Y93.2-)

Y93.11 **Activity, swimming**

Y93.12 **Activity, springboard and platform diving**

Y93.13 **Activity, water polo**

Y93.14 **Activity, water aerobics and water exercise**

Y93.15 **Activity, underwater diving and snorkeling**
Activity, SCUBA diving

Y93.16 **Activity, rowing, canoeing, kayaking, rafting and tubing**
Activity, canoeing, kayaking, rafting and tubing in calm and turbulent water

Y93.17 **Activity, water skiing and wake boarding**

Y93.18 **Activity, surfing, windsurfing and boogie boarding**
Activity, water sliding

Y93.19 **Activity, other involving water and watercraft**
Activity involving water NOS
Activity, parasailing
Activity, water survival training and testing

● Y93.2 **Activities involving ice and snow**
Excludes1 activity, shoveling ice and snow (Y93.H1)

Y93.21 **Activity, ice skating**
Activity, figure skating (singles) (pairs)
Activity, ice dancing
Excludes1 activity, ice hockey (Y93.22)

Y93.22 **Activity, ice hockey**

Y93.23 **Activity, snow (alpine) (downhill) skiing, snowboarding, sledding, tobogganing and snow tubing**
Excludes1 activity, cross country skiing (Y93.24)

Y93.24 **Activity, cross country skiing**
Activity, nordic skiing

Y93.29 **Activity, other activity involving ice and snow**
Activity, activity involving ice and snow NOS

● Y93.3 **Activities involving climbing, rappelling and jumping off**
Excludes1 activity, hiking on level or elevated terrain (Y93.Ø1)
activity, jumping rope (Y93.56)
activity, trampoline jumping (Y93.44)

Y93.31 **Activity, mountain climbing, rock climbing and wall climbing**

Y93.32 **Activity, rappelling**

Y93.33 **Activity, BASE jumping**
Activity, building, Antenna, Span, Earth jumping

Y93.34 **Activity, bungee jumping**

Y93.35 **Activity, hang gliding**

Y93.39 **Activity, other activity involving climbing, rappelling and jumping off**

● Y93.4 **Activities involving dancing and other rhythmic movement**
Excludes1 activity, martial arts (Y93.75)

Y93.41 **Activity, dancing**
Coding Clinic: 2Ø12, Q4, P1Ø8

Y93.42 **Activity, yoga**

Y93.43 Activity, gymnastics
Activity, rhythmic gymnastics
Excludes1 activity, trampolining (Y93.44)
Y93.44 Activity, trampolining
Y93.45 Activity, cheerleading
Y93.49 Activity, other involving dancing and other rhythmic movements

● **Y93.5 Activities involving other sports and athletics played individually**
Excludes1 activity, dancing (Y93.41)
activity, gymnastic (Y93.43)
activity, trampolining (Y93.44)
activity, yoga (Y93.42)
Y93.51 Activity, roller skating (inline) and skateboarding
Y93.52 Activity, horseback riding
Y93.53 Activity, golf
Y93.54 Activity, bowling
Y93.55 Activity, bike riding
Y93.56 Activity, jumping rope
Y93.57 Activity, non-running track and field events
Excludes1 activity, running (any form) (Y93.02)
Y93.59 Activity, other involving other sports and athletics played individually
Excludes1 activities involving climbing, rappelling, and jumping (Y93.3-)
activities involving ice and snow (Y93.2-)
activities involving walking and running (Y93.0-)
activities involving water and watercraft (Y93.1-)

● **Y93.6 Activities involving other sports and athletics played as a team or group**
Excludes1 activity, ice hockey (Y93.22)
activity, water polo (Y93.13)
Y93.61 Activity, American tackle football
Activity, football NOS
Y93.62 Activity, American flag or touch football
Y93.63 Activity, rugby
Y93.64 Activity, baseball
Activity, softball
Y93.65 Activity, lacrosse and field hockey
Coding Clinic: 2015, Q1, P9
Y93.66 Activity, soccer
Y93.67 Activity, basketball
Coding Clinic: 2019, Q4, P18
Y93.68 Activity, volleyball (beach) (court)
Y93.6A Activity, physical games generally associated with school recess, summer camp and children
Activity, capture the flag
Activity, dodge ball
Activity, four square
Activity, kickball
Y93.69 Activity, other involving other sports and athletics played as a team or group
Cricket

● **Y93.7 Activities involving other specified sports and athletics**
Y93.71 Activity, boxing
Y93.72 Activity, wrestling
Y93.73 Activity, racquet and hand sports
Activity, handball
Activity, racquetball
Activity, squash
Activity, tennis
Y93.74 Activity, frisbee
Activity, ultimate frisbee
Y93.75 Activity, martial arts
Activity, combatives
Y93.79 Activity, other specified sports and athletics
Excludes1 sports and athletics activities specified in categories Y93.0-Y93.6

● **Y93.A Activities involving other cardiorespiratory exercise**
Activities involving physical training
Y93.A1 Activity, exercise machines primarily for cardiorespiratory conditioning
Activity, elliptical and stepper machines
Activity, stationary bike
Activity, treadmill
Y93.A2 Activity, calisthenics
Activity, jumping jacks
Activity, warm up and cool down
Y93.A3 Activity, aerobic and step exercise
Y93.A4 Activity, circuit training
Y93.A5 Activity, obstacle course
Activity, challenge course
Activity, confidence course
Y93.A6 Activity, grass drills
Activity, guerilla drills
Y93.A9 Activity, other involving other cardiorespiratory exercise
Excludes1 activities involving cardiorespiratory exercise specified in categories Y93.0-Y93.7

● **Y93.B Activity involving other muscle strengthening exercises**
Y93.B1 Activity, exercise machines primarily for muscle strengthening
Y93.B2 Activity, push-ups, pull-ups, sit-ups
Y93.B3 Activity, free weights
Activity, barbells
Activity, dumbbells
Y93.B4 Activity, pilates
Y93.B9 Activity, other involving other muscle strengthening exercises
Excludes1 activities involving muscle strengthening specified in categories Y93.0-Y93.A

● **Y93.C Activities involving computer technology and electronic devices**
Excludes1 activity, electronic musical keyboard or instruments (Y93.J-)
Y93.C1 Activity, computer keyboarding
Activity, electronic game playing using keyboard or other stationary device
Y93.C2 Activity, hand held interactive electronic device
Activity, cellular telephone and communication device
Activity, electronic game playing using interactive device
Excludes1 activity, electronic game playing using keyboard or other stationary device (Y93.C1)
Y93.C9 Activity, other involving computer technology and electronic devices

● **Y93.D Activities involving arts and handcrafts**
Excludes1 activities involving playing musical instrument (Y93.J-)
Y93.D1 Knitting and crocheting
Y93.D2 Sewing
Y93.D3 Furniture building and finishing
Furniture repair
Y93.D9 Activity, other involving arts and handcrafts

CHAPTER 20 (V00-Y99)

● Y93.E Activities involving personal hygiene and interior property and clothing maintenance
  Excludes1 activities involving cooking and grilling (Y93.G-)
  activities involving exterior property and land maintenance, building and construction (Y93.H-)
  activity involving caregiving (Y93.F-)
  activity, dishwashing (Y93.G1)
  activity, food preparation (Y93.G1)
  activity, gardening (Y93.H2)

Y93.E1 Activity, personal bathing and showering

Y93.E2 Activity, laundry

Y93.E3 Activity, vacuuming

Y93.E4 Activity, ironing

Y93.E5 Activity, floor mopping and cleaning

Y93.E6 Activity, residential relocation
  Activity, packing up and unpacking involved in moving to a new residence

Y93.E8 Activity, other personal hygiene activity

Y93.E9 Activity, other household maintenance

● Y93.F Activities involving person providing caregiving
  Activity involving the provider of caregiving

Y93.F1 Activity, caregiving involving bathing

Y93.F2 Activity, caregiving involving lifting
  Coding Clinic: 2016, Q4, P74

Y93.F9 Activity, other caregiving

● Y93.G Activities involving food preparation, cooking and grilling

Y93.G1 Activity, food preparation and clean up
  Activity, dishwashing

Y93.G2 Activity, grilling and smoking food

Y93.G3 Activity, cooking and baking
  Activity, use of stove, oven and microwave oven

Y93.G9 Activity, other activity involving cooking and grilling

● Y93.H Activities involving property and land maintenance, building and construction

Y93.H1 Activity, digging, shoveling and raking
  Activity, dirt digging
  Activity, raking leaves
  Activity, snow shoveling

Y93.H2 Activity, gardening and landscaping
  Activity, pruning, trimming shrubs, weeding

Y93.H3 Activity, building and construction

Y93.H9 Activity, other activity involving property and land maintenance, building and construction

● Y93.I Activities involving roller coasters and other types of external motion

Y93.I1 Activity, rollercoaster riding

Y93.I9 Activity, other involving external motion

● Y93.J Activities involving playing musical instrument
  Activity involving playing electric musical instrument

Y93.J1 Activity, piano playing
  Activity, musical keyboard (electronic) playing

Y93.J2 Activity, drum and other percussion instrument playing

Y93.J3 Activity, string instrument playing

Y93.J4 Activity, winds and brass instrument playing

● Y93.K Activities involving animal care
  Excludes1 activity, horseback riding (Y93.52)

Y93.K1 Activity, walking an animal

Y93.K2 Activity, milking an animal

Y93.K3 Activity, grooming and shearing an animal

Y93.K9 Activity, other activity involving animal care

● Y93.8 Other activity
  Coding Clinic: 2016, Q4, P74

Y93.81 Activity, refereeing a sports activity

Y93.82 Activity, spectator at an event

Y93.83 Activity, rough housing and horseplay
  Coding Clinic: 2015, Q1, P8

Y93.84 Activity, sleeping

Y93.85 Activity, choking game
  Activity, blackout game
  Activity, fainting game
  Activity, pass out game
  Coding Clinic: 2016, Q4, P74-76

Y93.89 Activity, other specified

OGCR See Section I.C.20.c.

Do not assign Y93.9, Unspecified activity, if the activity is not stated.

● Y93.9 Activity, unspecified

Y95 Nosocomial condition

● Y99 External cause status

Note: A single code from category Y99 should be used in conjunction with the external cause code(s) assigned to a record to indicate the status of the person at the time the event occurred.

Coding Clinic: 2016, Q4, P74

Y99.Ø Civilian activity done for income or pay
  Civilian activity done for financial or other compensation
  Excludes1 military activity (Y99.1)
  volunteer activity (Y99.2)

Y99.1 Military activity
  Excludes1 activity of off duty military personnel (Y99.8)

Y99.2 Volunteer activity
  Excludes1 activity of child or other family member assisting in compensated work of other family member (Y99.8)

Y99.8 Other external cause status
  Activity NEC
  Activity of child or other family member assisting in compensated work of other family member
  Hobby not done for income
  Leisure activity
  Off-duty activity of military personnel
  Recreation or sport not for income or while a student
  Student activity
  Excludes1 civilian activity done for income or compensation (Y99.Ø)
  military activity (Y99.1)
  Coding Clinic: 2012, Q4, P1Ø8

Y99.9 Unspecified external cause status

CHAPTER 21

FACTORS INFLUENCING HEALTH STATUS AND CONTACT WITH HEALTH SERVICES (Z00-Z99)

OGCR Chapter-Specific Coding Guidelines

21. **Chapter 21: Factors influencing health status and contact with health services (Z00-Z99)**

Note: The chapter specific guidelines provide additional information about the use of Z codes for specified encounters.

a. **Use of Z codes in any healthcare setting**

Z codes are for use in any healthcare setting. Z codes may be used as either a first-listed (principal diagnosis code in the inpatient setting) or secondary code, depending on the circumstances of the encounter. Certain Z codes may only be used as first-listed or principal diagnosis.

b. **Z Codes indicate a reason for an encounter**

Z codes are not procedure codes. A corresponding procedure code must accompany a Z code to describe any procedure performed.

c. **Categories of Z Codes**

1) **Contact/Exposure**

Category Z20 indicates contact with, and suspected exposure to, communicable diseases. These codes are for patients who do not show any sign or symptom of a disease but are suspected to have been exposed to it by close personal contact with an infected individual or are in an area where a disease is epidemic.

Category Z77, Other contact with and (suspected) exposures hazardous to health, indicates contact with and suspected exposures hazardous to health.

Contact/exposure codes may be used as a first-listed code to explain an encounter for testing, or, more commonly, as a secondary code to identify a potential risk.

2) **Inoculations and vaccinations**

Code Z23 is for encounters for inoculations and vaccinations. It indicates that a patient is being seen to receive a prophylactic inoculation against a disease. Procedure codes are required to identify the actual administration of the injection and the type(s) of immunizations given. Code Z23 may be used as a secondary code if the inoculation is given as a routine part of preventive health care, such as a well-baby visit.

3) **Status**

Status codes indicate that a patient is either a carrier of a disease or has the sequelae or residual of a past disease or condition. This includes such things as the presence of prosthetic or mechanical devices resulting from past treatment. A status code is informative, because the status may affect the course of treatment and its outcome. A status code is distinct from a history code. The history code indicates that the patient no longer has the condition.

A status code should not be used with a diagnosis code from one of the body system chapters, if the diagnosis code includes the information provided by the status code. For example, code Z94.1, Heart transplant status, should not be used with a code from subcategory T86.2, Complications of heart transplant. The status code does not provide additional information. The complication code indicates that the patient is a heart transplant patient.

For encounters for weaning from a mechanical ventilator, assign a code from subcategory J96.1, Chronic respiratory failure, followed by code Z99.11, Dependence on respirator [ventilator] status.

The status Z codes/categories are:

Z14 Genetic carrier
Genetic carrier status indicates that a person carries a gene, associated with a particular disease, which may be passed to offspring who may develop that disease. The person does not have the disease and is not at risk of developing the disease.

Z15 Genetic susceptibility to disease Genetic susceptibility indicates that a person has a gene that increases the risk of that person developing the disease.

Codes from category Z15 should not be used as principal or first-listed codes. If the patient has the condition to which he/she is susceptible, and that condition is the reason for the encounter, the code for the current condition should be sequenced first. If the patient is being seen for follow-up after completed treatment for this condition, and the condition no longer exists, a follow-up code should be sequenced first, followed by the appropriate personal history and genetic susceptibility codes. If the purpose of the encounter is genetic counseling associated with procreative management, code Z31.5, Encounter for genetic counseling, should be assigned as the first-listed code, followed by a code from category Z15. Additional codes should be assigned for any applicable family or personal history.

Z16 Resistance to antimicrobial drugs
This code indicates that a patient has a condition that is resistant to antimicrobial drug treatment. Sequence the infection code first.

Z17 Estrogen receptor status

Z18 Retained foreign body fragments

Z19 Hormone sensitivity malignancy status

Z21 Asymptomatic HIV infection status This code indicates that a patient has tested positive for HIV but has manifested no signs or symptoms of the disease.

Z22 Carrier of infectious disease Carrier status indicates that a person harbors the specific organisms of a disease without manifest symptoms and is capable of transmitting the infection.

Z28.3 Underimmunization status

Z33.1 Pregnant state, incidental This code is a secondary code only for use when the pregnancy is in no way complicating the reason for visit. Otherwise, a code from the obstetric chapter is required.

Z66 Do not resuscitate

This code may be used when it is documented by the provider that a patient is on do not resuscitate status at any time during the stay.

Z67 Blood type

Z68 Body mass index (BMI)
BMI codes should only be assigned when the associated diagnosis (such as overweight or obesity) meets the definition of a reportable diagnosis (see Section III, Reporting Additional Diagnoses). Do not assign BMI codes during pregnancy. See Section I.B.14 for BMI documentation by clinicians other than the patient's provider.

Z74.01 Bed confinement status

Z76.82 Awaiting organ transplant status

Z78 Other specified health status

Code Z78.1, Physical restraint status, may be used when it is documented by the provider that a patient has been put in restraints during the current encounter. Please note that this code should not be reported when it is documented by the provider that a patient is temporarily restrained during a procedure.

Z79 Long-term (current) drug therapy

Codes from this category indicate a patient's continuous use of a prescribed drug (including such things as aspirin therapy) for the long-term treatment of a condition or for prophylactic use. It is not for use for patients who have addictions to drugs. This subcategory is not for use of medications for detoxification or maintenance programs to prevent withdrawal symptoms in patients with drug dependence (e.g., methadone maintenance for opiate dependence). Assign the appropriate code for the drug dependence instead.

Assign a code from Z79 if the patient is receiving a medication for an extended period as a prophylactic measure (such as for the prevention of deep vein thrombosis) or as treatment of a chronic condition (such as arthritis) or a disease requiring a lengthy course of treatment (such as cancer). Do not assign a code from category Z79 for medication being administered for a brief period of time to treat an acute illness or injury (such as a course of antibiotics to treat acute bronchitis).

Z88 Allergy status to drugs, medicaments and biological substances Except: Z88.9, Allergy status to unspecified drugs, medicaments and biological substances status

Z89 Acquired absence of limb

Z90 Acquired absence of organs, not elsewhere classified

Z91.0- Allergy status, other than to drugs and biological substances

Z92.82 Status post administration of tPA (rtPA) in a different facility within the last 24 hours prior to admission to a current facility Assign code Z92.82, Status post administration of tPA (rtPA) in a different facility within the last 24 hours prior to admission to current facility, as a secondary diagnosis when a patient is received by transfer into a facility and documentation indicates they were administered tissue plasminogen activator (tPA) within the last 24 hours prior to admission to the current facility. This guideline applies even if the patient is still receiving the tPA at the time they are received into the current facility. The appropriate code for the condition for which the tPA was administered (such as cerebrovascular disease or myocardial infarction) should be assigned first. Code Z92.82 is only applicable to the receiving facility record and not to the transferring facility record.

Z93 Artificial opening status
Z94 Transplanted organ and tissue status
Z95 Presence of cardiac and vascular implants and grafts
Z96 Presence of other functional implants
Z97 Presence of other devices
Z98 Other postprocedural states

Assign code Z98.85, Transplanted organ removal status, to indicate that a transplanted organ has been previously removed. This code should not be assigned for the encounter in which the transplanted organ is removed. The complication necessitating removal of the transplant organ should be assigned for that encounter.

See Section I.C.19. for information on the coding of organ transplant complications.

Z99 Dependence on enabling machines and devices, not elsewhere classified

Note: Categories Z89-Z90 and Z93-Z99 are for use only if there are no complications or malfunctions of the organ or tissue replaced, the amputation site or the equipment on which the patient is dependent.

4) History (of)

There are two types of history Z codes, personal and family. Personal history codes explain a patient's past medical condition that no longer exists and is not receiving any treatment, but that has the potential for recurrence, and therefore may require continued monitoring.

Family history codes are for use when a patient has a family member(s) who has had a particular disease that causes the patient to be at higher risk of also contracting the disease.

Personal history codes may be used in conjunction with follow-up codes and family history codes may be used in conjunction with screening codes to explain the need for a test or procedure. History codes are also acceptable on any medical record regardless of the reason for visit. A history of an illness, even if no longer present, is important information that may alter the type of treatment ordered.

The history Z code categories are:

Z80 Family history of primary malignant neoplasm
Z81 Family history of mental and behavioral disorders
Z82 Family history of certain disabilities and chronic diseases (leading to disablement)
Z83 Family history of other specific disorders
Z84 Family history of other conditions
Z85 Personal history of malignant neoplasm
Z86 Personal history of certain other diseases
Z87 Personal history of other diseases and conditions
Z91.4- Personal history of psychological trauma, not elsewhere classified
Z91.5 Personal history of self-harm
Z91.81 History of falling
Z91.82 Personal history of military deployment
Z92 Personal history of medical treatment Except: Z92.Ø, Personal history of contraception Except: Z92.82, Status post administration of tPA (rtPA) in a different facility within the last 24 hours prior to admission to a current facility

5) Screening

Screening is the testing for disease or disease precursors in seemingly well individuals so that early detection and treatment can be provided for those who test positive for the disease (e.g., screening mammogram).

The testing of a person to rule out or confirm a suspected diagnosis because the patient has some sign or symptom is a diagnostic examination, not a screening. In these cases, the sign or symptom is used to explain the reason for the test.

A screening code may be a first-listed code if the reason for the visit is specifically the screening exam. It may also be used as an additional code if the screening is done during an office visit for other health problems. A screening code is not necessary if the screening is inherent to a routine examination, such as a pap smear done during a routine pelvic examination.

Should a condition be discovered during the screening then the code for the condition may be assigned as an additional diagnosis.

The Z code indicates that a screening exam is planned. A procedure code is required to confirm that the screening was performed.

The screening Z codes/categories:

Z11 Encounter for screening for infectious and parasitic diseases
Z12 Encounter for screening for malignant neoplasms
Z13 Encounter for screening for other diseases and disorders Except: Z13.9, Encounter for screening, unspecified
Z36 Encounter for antenatal screening for mother

6) Observation

There are three observation Z code categories. They are for use in very limited circumstances when a person is being observed for a suspected condition that is ruled out. The observation codes are not for use if an injury or illness or any signs or symptoms related to the suspected condition are present. In such cases the diagnosis/symptom code is used with the corresponding external cause code.

The observation codes are to be used as principal diagnosis only. The only exception to this is when the principal diagnosis is required to be a code from category Z38, Liveborn infants according to place of birth and type of delivery. Then a code from category ZØ5, Encounter for observation and evaluation of newborn for suspected diseases and conditions ruled out, is sequenced after the Z38 code. Additional codes may be used in addition to the observation code but only if they are unrelated to the suspected condition being observed.

Codes from subcategory ZØ3.7 Encounter for suspected maternal and fetal conditions ruled out, may either be used as a first-listed or as an additional code assignment depending on the case. They are for use in very limited circumstances on a maternal record when an encounter is for a suspected maternal or fetal condition that is ruled out during that encounter (for example, a maternal or fetal condition may be suspected due to an abnormal test result). These codes should not be used when the condition is confirmed. In those cases, the confirmed condition should be coded. In addition, these codes are not for use if an illness or any signs or symptoms related to the suspected condition or problem are present. In such cases the diagnosis/symptom code is used.

Additional codes may be used in addition to the code from subcategory ZØ3.7, but only if they are unrelated to the suspected condition being evaluated.

Codes from subcategory ZØ3.7 may not be used for encounters for antenatal screening of mother. *See Section I.C.21. Screening.*

For encounters for suspected fetal condition that are inconclusive following testing and evaluation, assign the appropriate code from category O35, O36, O4Ø or O41.

The observation Z code categories:

ZØ3 Encounter for medical observation for suspected diseases and conditions ruled out
ZØ4 Encounter for examination and observation for other reasons Except: ZØ4.9, Encounter for examination and observation for unspecified reason
ZØ5 Encounter for observation and evaluation of newborn for suspected diseases and conditions ruled out

7) Aftercare

Aftercare visit codes cover situations when the initial treatment of a disease has been performed and the patient requires continued care during the healing or recovery phase, or for the long-term consequences of the disease. The aftercare Z code should not be used if treatment is directed at a current, acute disease. The diagnosis code is to be used in these cases.

Exceptions to this rule are codes Z51.Ø, Encounter for antineoplastic radiation therapy, and codes from subcategory Z51.1, Encounter for antineoplastic chemotherapy and immunotherapy. These codes are to be first-listed, followed by the diagnosis code when a patient's encounter is solely to receive radiation therapy, chemotherapy, or immunotherapy for the treatment of a neoplasm. If the reason for the encounter is more than one type of antineoplastic therapy, code Z51.Ø and a code from subcategory Z51.1 may be assigned together, in which case one of these codes would be reported as a secondary diagnosis.

The aftercare Z codes should also not be used for aftercare for injuries. For aftercare of an injury, assign the acute injury code with the appropriate 7th character (for subsequent encounter).

The aftercare codes are generally first-listed to explain the specific reason for the encounter. An aftercare code may be used as an additional code when some type of aftercare is provided in addition to the reason for admission and no diagnosis code is applicable. An example of this would be the closure of a colostomy during an encounter for treatment of another condition.

Aftercare codes should be used in conjunction with other aftercare codes or diagnosis codes to provide better detail on the specifics of an aftercare encounter visit, unless otherwise directed by the classification. Should a patient receive multiple types of antineoplastic therapy during the same encounter, code Z51.Ø, Encounter for antineoplastic radiation therapy, and codes from subcategory Z51.1, Encounter for antineoplastic chemotherapy and immunotherapy, may be used together on a record. The sequencing of multiple aftercare codes depends on the circumstances of the encounter.

Certain aftercare Z code categories need a secondary diagnosis code to describe the resolving condition or sequelae. For others, the condition is included in the code title.

Additional Z code aftercare category terms include fitting and adjustment, and attention to artificial openings.

Status Z codes may be used with aftercare Z codes to indicate the nature of the aftercare. For example code Z95.1, Presence of aortocoronary bypass graft, may be used with code Z48.812, Encounter for surgical aftercare following surgery on the circulatory system, to indicate the surgery for which the aftercare is being performed. A status code should not be used when the aftercare code indicates the type of status, such as using Z43.Ø, Encounter for attention to tracheostomy, with Z93.Ø, Tracheostomy status.

The aftercare Z category/codes:

Z42	Encounter for plastic and reconstructive surgery following medical procedure or healed injury
Z43	Encounter for attention to artificial openings
Z44	Encounter for fitting and adjustment of external prosthetic device
Z45	Encounter for adjustment and management of implanted device
Z46	Encounter for fitting and adjustment of other devices
Z47	Orthopedic aftercare
Z48	Encounter for other postprocedural aftercare
Z49	Encounter for care involving renal dialysis
Z51	Encounter for other aftercare and medical care

8) Follow-up

The follow-up codes are used to explain continuing surveillance following completed treatment of a disease, condition, or injury. They imply that the condition has been fully treated and no longer exists. They should not be confused with aftercare codes, or injury codes with a 7th character for subsequent encounter, that explain ongoing care of a healing condition or its sequelae. Follow-up codes may be used in conjunction with history codes to provide the full picture of the healed condition and its treatment. The follow-up code is sequenced first, followed by the history code.

A follow-up code may be used to explain multiple visits. Should a condition be found to have recurred on the follow-up visit, then the diagnosis code for the condition should be assigned in place of the follow-up code.

The follow-up Z code categories:

ZØ8	Encounter for follow-up examination after completed treatment for malignant neoplasm
ZØ9	Encounter for follow-up examination after completed treatment for conditions other than malignant neoplasm
Z39	Encounter for maternal postpartum care and examination

9) Donor

Codes in category Z52, Donors of organs and tissues, are used for living individuals who are donating blood or other body tissue. These codes are only for individuals donating for others, not for self-donations. They are not used to identify cadaveric donations.

1Ø) Counseling

Counseling Z codes are used when a patient or family member receives assistance in the aftermath of an illness or injury, or when support is required in coping with family or social problems.

The counseling Z codes/categories:

Z3Ø.Ø-	Encounter for general counseling and advice on contraception
Z31.5	Encounter for procreative genetic counseling
Z31.6-	Encounter for general counseling and advice on procreation
Z32.2	Encounter for childbirth instruction
Z32.3	Encounter for childcare instruction
Z69	Encounter for mental health services for victim and perpetrator of abuse
Z7Ø	Counseling related to sexual attitude, behavior and orientation
Z71	Persons encountering health services for other counseling and medical advice, not elsewhere classified
Z76.81	Expectant mother prebirth pediatrician visit

11) Encounters for Obstetrical and Reproductive Services

See Section I.C.15. Pregnancy, Childbirth, and the Puerperium, for further instruction on the use of these codes.

Z codes for pregnancy are for use in those circumstances when none of the problems or complications included in the codes from the Obstetrics chapter exist (a routine prenatal visit or postpartum care). Codes in category Z34, Encounter for supervision of normal pregnancy, are always first listed and are not to be used with any other code from the OB chapter.

Codes in category Z3A, Weeks of gestation, may be assigned to provide additional information about the pregnancy. Category Z3A codes should not be assigned for pregnancies with abortive outcomes (categories OØØ-OØ8), elective termination of pregnancy (code Z33.2), nor for postpartum conditions, as category Z3A is not applicable to these conditions. The date of the admission should be used to determine weeks of gestation for inpatient admissions that encompass more than one gestational week.

The outcome of delivery, category Z37, should be included on all maternal delivery records. It is always a secondary code. Codes in category Z37 should not be used on the newborn record.

Z codes for family planning (contraceptive) or procreative management and counseling should be included on an obstetric record either during the pregnancy or the postpartum stage, if applicable.

Z codes/categories for obstetrical and reproductive services:

Z3Ø	Encounter for contraceptive management
Z31	Encounter for procreative management
Z32.2	Encounter for childbirth instruction
Z32.3	Encounter for childcare instruction
Z33	Pregnant state
Z34	Encounter for supervision of normal pregnancy
Z36	Encounter for antenatal screening of mother
Z3A	Weeks of gestation
Z37	Outcome of delivery
Z39	Encounter for maternal postpartum care and examination
Z76.81	Expectant mother prebirth pediatrician visit

12) Newborns and Infants

See Section I.C.16. Newborn (Perinatal) Guidelines, for further instruction on the use of these codes.

Newborn Z codes/categories:

Z76.1	Encounter for health supervision and care of foundling
ZØØ.1-	Encounter for routine child health examination
Z38	Liveborn infants according to place of birth and type of delivery

13) Routine and administrative examinations

The Z codes allow for the description of encounters for routine examinations, such as, a general check-up, or, examinations for administrative purposes, such as, a pre-employment physical. The codes are not to be used if the examination is for diagnosis of a suspected condition or for treatment purposes. In such cases the diagnosis code is used. During a routine exam, should a diagnosis or condition be discovered, it should be coded as an additional code. Pre-existing and chronic conditions and history codes may also be included as additional codes as long as the examination is for administrative purposes and not focused on any particular condition.

Some of the codes for routine health examinations distinguish between "with" and "without" abnormal findings. Code assignment depends on the information that is known at the time the encounter is being coded. For example, if no abnormal findings were found during the examination, but the encounter is being coded before test results are back, it is acceptable to assign the code for "without abnormal findings." When assigning a code for "with abnormal findings," additional code(s) should be assigned to identify the specific abnormal finding(s).

Pre-operative examination and pre-procedural laboratory examination Z codes are for use only in those situations when a patient is being cleared for a procedure or surgery and no treatment is given.

The Z codes/categories for routine and administrative examinations:

Z00	Encounter for general examination without complaint, suspected or reported diagnosis
Z01	Encounter for other special examination without complaint, suspected or reported diagnosis
Z02	Encounter for administrative examination Except: Z02.9, Encounter for administrative examinations, unspecified
Z32.0-	Encounter for pregnancy test

14) Miscellaneous Z codes

The miscellaneous Z codes capture a number of other health care encounters that do not fall into one of the other categories. Certain of these codes identify the reason for the encounter; others are for use as additional codes that provide useful information on circumstances that may affect a patient's care and treatment.

Prophylactic Organ Removal

For encounters specifically for prophylactic removal of an organ (such as prophylactic removal of breasts due to a genetic susceptibility to cancer or a family history of cancer), the principal or first-listed code should be a code from category Z40, Encounter for prophylactic surgery, followed by the appropriate codes to identify the associated risk factor (such as genetic susceptibility or family history).

If the patient has a malignancy of one site and is having prophylactic removal at another site to prevent either a new primary malignancy or metastatic disease, a code for the malignancy should also be assigned in addition to a code from subcategory Z40.0, Encounter for prophylactic surgery for risk factors related to malignant neoplasms. A Z40.0 code should not be assigned if the patient is having organ removal for treatment of a malignancy, such as the removal of the testes for the treatment of prostate cancer.

Miscellaneous Z codes/categories:

Z28	Immunization not carried out Except: Z28.3, Underimmunization status
Z29	Encounter for other prophylactic measures
Z40	Encounter for prophylactic surgery
Z41	Encounter for procedures for purposes other than remedying health state Except: Z41.9, Encounter for procedure for purposes other than remedying health state, unspecified
Z53	Persons encountering health services for specific procedures and treatment, not carried out
Z55	Problems related to education and literacy
Z56	Problems related to employment and unemployment
Z57	Occupational exposure to risk factors
Z58	Problems related to physical environment
Z59	Problems related to housing and economic circumstances
Z60	Problems related to social environment
Z62	Problems related to upbringing
Z63	Other problems related to primary support group, including family circumstances
Z64	Problems related to certain psychosocial circumstances
Z65	Problems related to other psychosocial circumstances
Z72	Problems related to lifestyle Note: These codes should be assigned only when the documentation specifies that the patient has an associated problem
Z73	Problems related to life management difficulty
Z74	Problems related to care provider dependency Except: Z74.01, Bed confinement status
Z75	Problems related to medical facilities and other health care
Z76.0	Encounter for issue of repeat prescription
Z76.3	Healthy person accompanying sick person
Z76.4	Other boarder to healthcare facility
Z76.5	Malingerer [conscious simulation]
Z91.1-	Patient's noncompliance with medical treatment and regimen
Z91.83	Wandering in diseases classified elsewhere
Z91.84-	Oral health risk factors
Z91.89	Other specified personal risk factors, not elsewhere classified

See Section I.B.14 for Z55-Z65 Persons with potential health hazards related to socioeconomic and psychosocial circumstances, documentation by clinicians other than the patient's provider.

15) Nonspecific Z codes

Certain Z codes are so non-specific, or potentially redundant with other codes in the classification, that there can be little justification for their use in the inpatient setting. Their use in the outpatient setting should be limited to those instances when there is no further documentation to permit more precise coding. Otherwise, any sign or symptom or any other reason for visit that is captured in another code should be used.

Nonspecific Z codes/categories:

Z02.9	Encounter for administrative examinations, unspecified
Z04.9	Encounter for examination and observation for unspecified reason
Z13.9	Encounter for screening, unspecified
Z41.9	Encounter for procedure for purposes other than remedying health state, unspecified
Z52.9	Donor of unspecified organ or tissue
Z86.59	Personal history of other mental and behavioral disorders
Z88.9	Allergy status to unspecified drugs, medicaments and biological substances status
Z92.0	Personal history of contraception

16) Z Codes That May Only Be Principal/First-Listed Diagnosis

The following Z codes/categories may only be reported as the principal/first-listed diagnosis, except when there are multiple encounters on the same day and the medical records for the encounters are combined:

Z00	Encounter for general examination without complaint, suspected or reported diagnosis Except: Z00.6
Z01	Encounter for other special examination without complaint, suspected or reported diagnosis
Z02	Encounter for administrative examination
Z03	Encounter for medical observation for suspected diseases and conditions ruled out
Z04	Encounter for examination and observation for other reasons
Z33.2	Encounter for elective termination of pregnancy
Z31.81	Encounter for male factor infertility in female patient
Z31.83	Encounter for assisted reproductive fertility procedure cycle
Z31.84	Encounter for fertility preservation procedure
Z34	Encounter for supervision of normal pregnancy
Z39	Encounter for maternal postpartum care and examination
Z38	Liveborn infants according to place of birth and type of delivery
Z40	Encounter for prophylactic surgery
Z42	Encounter for plastic and reconstructive surgery following medical procedure or healed injury
Z51.0	Encounter for antineoplastic radiation therapy
Z51.1-	Encounter for antineoplastic chemotherapy and immunotherapy
Z52	Donors of organs and tissues Except: Z52.9, Donor of unspecified organ or tissue
Z76.1	Encounter for health supervision and care of foundling
Z76.2	Encounter for health supervision and care of other healthy infant and child
Z99.12	Encounter for respirator [ventilator] dependence during power failure

CHAPTER 21

FACTORS INFLUENCING HEALTH STATUS AND CONTACT WITH HEALTH SERVICES (Z00-Z99)

Note: Z codes represent reasons for encounters. A corresponding procedure code must accompany a Z code if a procedure is performed. Categories Z00-Z99 are provided for occasions when circumstances other than a disease, injury or external cause classifiable to categories A00-Y89 are recorded as "diagnoses" or "problems." This can arise in two main ways:

(a) When a person who may or may not be sick encounters the health services for some specific purpose, such as to receive limited care or service for a current condition, to donate an organ or tissue, to receive prophylactic vaccination (immunization), or to discuss a problem which is in itself not a disease or injury.

(b) When some circumstance or problem is present which influences the person's health status but is not in itself a current illness or injury.

This chapter contains the following blocks:

Z00-Z13	Persons encountering health services for examination
Z14-Z15	Genetic carrier and genetic susceptibility to disease
Z16	Resistance to antimicrobial drugs
Z17	Estrogen, and other hormones and factors receptor status
Z18	Retained foreign body fragments
Z19	Hormone sensitivity malignancy status
Z20-Z29	Persons with potential health hazards related to communicable diseases
Z30-Z39	Persons encountering health services in circumstances related to reproduction
Z40-Z53	Encounters for other specific health care
Z55-Z65	Persons with potential health hazards related to socioeconomic and psychosocial circumstances
Z66	Do not resuscitate status
Z67	Blood type
Z68	Body mass index (BMI)
Z69-Z76	Persons encountering health services in other circumstances
Z77-Z99	Persons with potential health hazards related to family and personal history and certain conditions influencing health status

PERSONS ENCOUNTERING HEALTH SERVICES FOR EXAMINATIONS (Z00-Z13)

Note: Nonspecific abnormal findings disclosed at the time of these examinations are classified to categories R70-R94.

Excludes1 examinations related to pregnancy and reproduction (Z30-Z36, Z39.-)

● **Z00 Encounter for general examination without complaint, suspected or reported diagnosis**

Excludes1 encounter for examination for administrative purposes (Z02.-)

Excludes2 encounter for pre-procedural examinations (Z01.81-)
special screening examinations (Z11-Z13)

● **Z00.0 Encounter for general adult medical examination**
Encounter for adult periodic examination (annual) (physical) and any associated laboratory and radiologic examinations

Excludes1 encounter for examination of sign or symptom - code to sign or symptom
general health check-up of infant or child (Z00.12.-)

Coding Clinic: 2016, Q4, P131

● **Z00.00 Encounter for general adult medical examination without abnormal findings** A
Encounter for adult health check-up NOS
Coding Clinic: 2017, Q4, P95; 2016, Q1, P37

● **Z00.01 Encounter for general adult medical examination with abnormal findings** A
Use additional code to identify abnormal findings
Coding Clinic: 2016, Q1, P36

● **Z00.1 Encounter for newborn, infant and child health examinations**

● **Z00.11 Newborn health examination**
Health check for child under 29 days old
Use additional code to identify any abnormal findings

Excludes1 health check for child over 28 days old (Z00.12-)

● **Z00.110 Health examination for newborn under 8 days old** N
Health check for newborn under 8 days old

● **Z00.111 Health examination for newborn 8 to 28 days old** N
Health check for newborn 8 to 28 days old
Newborn weight check

● **Z00.12 Encounter for routine child health examination**
Immunizations appropriate for age
Health check (routine) for child over 28 days old
Routine developmental screening of infant or child
Routine vision and hearing testing

Excludes1 health check for child under 29 days old (Z00.11-)
health supervision of foundling or other healthy infant or child (Z76.1-Z76.2)
newborn health examination (Z00.11-)

● **Z00.121 Encounter for routine child health examination with abnormal findings** P
Use additional code to identify abnormal findings
Coding Clinic: 2017, Q4, P95; 2016, Q1, P34-35

● **Z00.129 Encounter for routine child health examination without abnormal findings** P
Encounter for routine child health examination NOS
Coding Clinic: 2016, Q1, P34

● **Z00.2 Encounter for examination for period of rapid growth in childhood** P

● **Z00.3 Encounter for examination for adolescent development state** P
Encounter for puberty development state

● **Z00.5 Encounter for examination of potential donor of organ and tissue**

Z00.6 Encounter for examination for normal comparison and control in clinical research program
Examination of participant or control in clinical research program

● **Z00.7 Encounter for examination for period of delayed growth in childhood**

● **Z00.70 Encounter for examination for period of delayed growth in childhood without abnormal findings** P

● **Z00.71 Encounter for examination for period of delayed growth in childhood with abnormal findings** P
Use additional code to identify abnormal findings

● **Z00.8 Encounter for other general examination**
Encounter for health examination in population surveys

Z01 Encounter for other special examination without complaint, suspected or reported diagnosis

Includes routine examination of specific system

Note: Codes from category Z01 represent the reason for the encounter. A separate procedure code is required to identify any examinations or procedures performed.

Excludes1 encounter for examination for administrative purposes (Z02.-)
encounter for examination for suspected conditions, proven not to exist (Z03.-)
encounter for laboratory and radiologic examinations as a component of general medical examinations (Z00.0-)
encounter for laboratory, radiologic and imaging examinations for sign(s) and symptom(s) - code to the sign(s) or symptom(s)

Excludes2 screening examinations (Z11-Z13)

Z01.0 Encounter for examination of eyes and vision

Excludes1 examination for driving license (Z02.4)

Z01.00 Encounter for examination of eyes and vision without abnormal findings
Encounter for examination of eyes and vision NOS

Z01.01 Encounter for examination of eyes and vision with abnormal findings
Use additional code to identify abnormal findings
Coding Clinic: 2016, Q4, P21

Z01.02 Encounter for examination of eyes and vision following failed vision screening

Excludes1 encounter for examination of eyes and vision with abnormal findings (Z01.01)
encounter for examination of eyes and vision without abnormal findings (Z01.00)

Z01.020 Encounter for examination of eyes and vision following failed vision screening without abnormal findings

Z01.021 Encounter for examination of eyes and vision following failed vision screening with abnormal findings
Use additional code to identify abnormal findings

Z01.1 Encounter for examination of ears and hearing

Z01.10 Encounter for examination of ears and hearing without abnormal findings
Encounter for examination of ears and hearing NOS
Coding Clinic: 2016, Q4, P25

Z01.11 Encounter for examination of ears and hearing with abnormal findings
Coding Clinic: 2016, Q3, P18

Z01.110 Encounter for hearing examination following failed hearing screening
Coding Clinic: 2016, Q3, P18-19

Z01.118 Encounter for examination of ears and hearing with other abnormal findings
Use additional code to identify abnormal findings
Coding Clinic: 2016, Q3, P17

Z01.12 Encounter for hearing conservation and treatment

Z01.2 Encounter for dental examination and cleaning

Z01.20 Encounter for dental examination and cleaning without abnormal findings
Encounter for dental examination and cleaning NOS

Z01.21 Encounter for dental examination and cleaning with abnormal findings
Use additional code to identify abnormal findings

Z01.3 Encounter for examination of blood pressure

Z01.30 Encounter for examination of blood pressure without abnormal findings
Encounter for examination of blood pressure NOS

Z01.31 Encounter for examination of blood pressure with abnormal findings
Use additional code to identify abnormal findings

Z01.4 Encounter for gynecological examination

Excludes2 pregnancy examination or test (Z32.0-)
routine examination for contraceptive maintenance (Z30.4-)

Z01.41 Encounter for routine gynecological examination
Encounter for general gynecological examination with or without cervical smear
Encounter for gynecological examination (general) (routine) NOS
Encounter for pelvic examination (annual) (periodic)
Use additional code:
for screening for human papillomavirus, if applicable (Z11.51)
for screening vaginal pap smear, if applicable (Z12.72)
to identify acquired absence of uterus, if applicable (Z90.71-)

Excludes1 gynecologic examination status-post hysterectomy for malignant condition (Z08)
screening cervical pap smear not a part of a routine gynecological examination (Z12.4)

Z01.411 Encounter for gynecological examination (general) (routine) with abnormal findings
Use additional code to identify any abnormal findings

Z01.419 Encounter for gynecological examination (general) (routine) without abnormal findings

Z01.42 Encounter for cervical smear to confirm findings of recent normal smear following initial abnormal smear

Z01.8 Encounter for other specified special examinations

Z01.81 Encounter for preprocedural examinations
Encounter for preoperative examinations
Encounter for radiological and imaging examinations as part of preprocedural examination

Z01.810 Encounter for preprocedural cardiovascular examination

Z01.811 Encounter for preprocedural respiratory examination

Z01.812 Encounter for preprocedural laboratory examination
Blood and urine tests prior to treatment or procedure
Coding Clinic: 2023, Q2, P4; 2021, Q1, P38

Z01.818 Encounter for other preprocedural examination
Encounter for preprocedural examination NOS
Encounter for examinations prior to antineoplastic chemotherapy

Z01.82 Encounter for allergy testing

Excludes1 encounter for antibody response examination (Z01.84)

Z01.83 Encounter for blood typing
Encounter for Rh typing

● **Z01.84** **Encounter for antibody response examination**
Encounter for immunity status testing
Excludes1 encounter for allergy testing (Z01.82)

● **Z01.89** **Encounter for other specified special examinations**

● **Z02** **Encounter for administrative examination**

● **Z02.0** **Encounter for examination for admission to educational institution**
Encounter for examination for admission to preschool (education)
Encounter for examination for re-admission to school following illness or medical treatment

Z02.1 **Encounter for pre-employment examination**

● **Z02.2** **Encounter for examination for admission to residential institution**
Excludes1 examination for admission to prison (Z02.89)

Z02.3 **Encounter for examination for recruitment to armed forces**

● **Z02.4** **Encounter for examination for driving license**

● **Z02.5** **Encounter for examination for participation in sport**
Excludes1 blood-alcohol and blood-drug test (Z02.83)

● **Z02.6** **Encounter for examination for insurance purposes**

● **Z02.7** **Encounter for issue of medical certificate**
Excludes1 encounter for general medical examination (Z00-Z01, Z02.0-Z02.6, Z02.8-Z02.9)

● **Z02.71** **Encounter for disability determination**
Encounter for issue of medical certificate of incapacity
Encounter for issue of medical certificate of invalidity

● **Z02.79** **Encounter for issue of other medical certificate**

● **Z02.8** **Encounter for other administrative examinations**

Z02.81 **Encounter for paternity testing**

● **Z02.82** **Encounter for adoption services**

Z02.83 **Encounter for blood-alcohol and blood-drug test**
Use additional code for findings of alcohol or drugs in blood (R78.-)

Z02.84 **Encounter for child welfare exam**
Encounter for child welfare screening exam
Excludes2 encounter for examination and observation for alleged child physical abuse(Z04.72)
encounter for examination and observation for alleged child rape (Z04.42)

● **Z02.89** **Encounter for other administrative examinations**
Encounter for examination for admission to prison
Encounter for examination for admission to summer camp
Encounter for immigration examination
Encounter for naturalization examination
Encounter for premarital examination
Excludes1 health supervision of foundling or other healthy infant or child (Z76.1-Z76.2)

● **Z02.9** **Encounter for administrative examinations, unspecified**

OGCR Section II.C.21.c.6.

Observation

There are three observation Z code categories. They are for use in very limited circumstances when a person is being observed for a suspected condition that is ruled out. The observation codes are not for use if an injury or illnesses or any signs or symptoms related to the suspected condition are present. In such cases the diagnosis/symptom code is used with the corresponding external cause code.

The observation codes are to be used as principal diagnosis only. The only exception to this is when the principal diagnosis is required to be a code from category Z38, Liveborn infants according to place of birth and type of delivery. Then a code from category Z05, Encounter for observation and evaluation of newborn for suspected diseases and conditions ruled out, is sequenced after the Z38 code. Additional codes may be used in addition to the observation code but only if they are unrelated to the suspected condition being observed.

Codes from subcategory Z03.7 Encounter for suspected maternal and fetal conditions ruled out, may either be used as a first listed or as an additional code assignment depending on the case. They are for use in very limited circumstances on a maternal record when an encounter is for a suspected maternal or fetal condition that is ruled out during that encounter (for example, a maternal or fetal condition may be suspected due to an abnormal test result). These codes should not be used when the condition is confirmed. In those cases, the confirmed condition should be coded. In addition, these codes are not for use if an illness or any signs or symptoms related to the suspected condition or problem are present. In such cases the diagnosis/symptom code is used.

Additional codes may be used in addition to the code from subcategory Z03.7, but only if they are unrelated to the suspected condition being evaluated.

Codes from subcategory Z03.7 may not be used for encounters for antenatal screening of mother. *See Section I.C.21. Screening.*

For encounters for suspected fetal condition that are inconclusive following testing and evaluation, assign the appropriate code from category O35, O36, O40 or O41.

The observation Z code categories:

Z03 Encounter for medical observation for suspected diseases and conditions ruled out

Z04 Encounter for examination and observation for other reasons Except: Z04.9, Encounter for examination and observation for unspecified reason

Z05 Encounter for observation and evaluation of newborn for suspected diseases and conditions ruled out

● **Z03** **Encounter for medical observation for suspected diseases and conditions ruled out**
This category is to be used when a person without a diagnosis is suspected of having an abnormal condition, without signs or symptoms, which requires study, but after examination and observation, is ruled out. This category is also for use for administrative and legal observation status.
Excludes1 contact with and (suspected) exposures hazardous to health (Z77.-)
encounter for observation and evaluation of newborn for suspected diseases and conditions ruled out (Z05.-)
person with feared complaint in whom no diagnosis is made (Z71.1)
signs or symptoms under study - code to signs or symptoms

Z03.6 **Encounter for observation for suspected toxic effect from ingested substance ruled out**
Encounter for observation for suspected adverse effect from drug
Encounter for observation for suspected poisoning

● **Z03.7 Encounter for suspected maternal and fetal conditions ruled out**
Encounter for suspected maternal and fetal conditions not found
Excludes1 known or suspected fetal anomalies affecting management of mother, not ruled out (O26.-, O35.-, O36.-, O40.-, O41.-)

● **Z03.71 Encounter for suspected problem with amniotic cavity and membrane ruled out** M
Encounter for suspected oligohydramnios ruled out
Encounter for suspected polyhydramnios ruled out

● **Z03.72 Encounter for suspected placental problem ruled out** M

● **Z03.73 Encounter for suspected fetal anomaly ruled out** M
Coding Clinic: 2016, Q4, P6

● **Z03.74 Encounter for suspected problem with fetal growth ruled out** M

● **Z03.75 Encounter for suspected cervical shortening ruled out** M

● **Z03.79 Encounter for other suspected maternal and fetal conditions ruled out** M
Coding Clinic: 2016, Q4, P7

● **Z03.8 Encounter for observation for other suspected diseases and conditions ruled out**

● **Z03.81 Encounter for observation for suspected exposure to biological agents ruled out**

Z03.810 Encounter for observation for suspected exposure to anthrax ruled out

Z03.818 Encounter for observation for suspected exposure to other biological agents ruled out

● **Z03.82 Encounter for observation for suspected foreign body ruled out**
Excludes1 retained foreign body (Z18.-)
retained foreign body in eyelid (H02.81)
residual foreign body in soft tissue (M79.5)
Excludes2 confirmed foreign body ingestion or aspiration including:
foreign body in alimentary tract (T18)
foreign body in ear (T16)
foreign body on external eye (T15)
foreign body in respiratory tract (T17)

● **Z03.821 Encounter for observation for suspected ingested foreign body ruled out**

● **Z03.822 Encounter for observation for suspected aspirated (inhaled) foreign body ruled out**

● **Z03.823 Encounter for observation for suspected inserted (injected) foreign body ruled out**
Encounter for observation for suspected inserted (injected) foreign body in eye ruled out
Encounter for observation for suspected inserted (injected) foreign body in orifice ruled out
Encounter for observation for suspected inserted (injected) foreign body in skin ruled out

● **Z03.83 Encounter for observation for suspected conditions related to home physiologic monitoring device ruled out**
Encounter for observation for apnea alarm without findings
Encounter for observation for bradycardia alarm without findings
Encounter for observation for malfunction of home cardiorespiratory monitor
Encounter for observation for non-specific findings home physiologic monitoring device
Encounter for observation for pulse oximeter alarm without findings
Excludes1 apnea NOS (R06.81)
neonatal bradycardia (P29.12)
newborn apnea (P28.4-)
primary sleep apnea of newborn (P28.3-)
sleep apnea (G47.3-)

Z03.89 Encounter for observation for other suspected diseases and conditions ruled out

● **Z04 Encounter for examination and observation for other reasons**
Includes encounter for examination for medicolegal reasons
This category is to be used when a person without a diagnosis is suspected of having an abnormal condition, without signs or symptoms, which requires study, but after examination and observation, is ruled-out. This category is also for use for administrative and legal observation status.

Z04.1 Encounter for examination and observation following transport accident
Excludes1 encounter for examination and observation following work accident (Z04.2)
Coding Clinic: 2019, Q2, P11

Z04.2 Encounter for examination and observation following work accident

Z04.3 Encounter for examination and observation following other accident

● **Z04.4 Encounter for examination and observation following alleged rape**
Encounter for examination and observation of victim following alleged rape
Encounter for examination and observation of victim following alleged sexual abuse
Coding Clinic: 2016, Q4, P129

Z04.41 Encounter for examination and observation following alleged adult rape A
Suspected adult rape, ruled out
Suspected adult sexual abuse, ruled out

Z04.42 Encounter for examination and observation following alleged child rape P
Suspected child rape, ruled out
Suspected child sexual abuse, ruled out

Z04.6 Encounter for general psychiatric examination, requested by authority

● **Z04.7 Encounter for examination and observation following alleged physical abuse**

Z04.71 Encounter for examination and observation following alleged adult physical abuse A
Suspected adult physical abuse, ruled out
Excludes1 confirmed case of adult physical abuse (T74.-)
encounter for examination and observation following alleged adult sexual abuse (Z04.41)
suspected case of adult physical abuse, not ruled out (T76.-)

CHAPTER 21 (Z00-Z99)

Z04.72 **Encounter for examination and observation following alleged child physical abuse** P
Suspected child physical abuse, ruled out
Excludes1 confirmed case of child physical abuse (T74.-)
encounter for examination and observation following alleged child sexual abuse (Z04.42)
suspected case of child physical abuse, not ruled out (T76.-)

● Z04.8 **Encounter for examination and observation for other specified reasons**
Encounter for examination and observation for request for expert evidence

Z04.81 **Encounter for examination and observation of victim following forced sexual exploitation**

Z04.82 **Encounter for examination and observation of victim following forced labor exploitation**

Z04.89 **Encounter for examination and observation for other specified reasons**

● Z04.9 **Encounter for examination and observation for unspecified reason**
Encounter for observation NOS

● Z05 **Encounter for observation and evaluation of newborn for suspected diseases and conditions ruled out**
This category is to be used for newborns, within the neonatal period (the first 28 days of life), who are suspected of having an abnormal condition, but without signs or symptoms, and which, after examination and observation, is ruled out.
Coding Clinic: 2022, Q1, P17-18; 2019, Q2, P11; 2016, Q4, P54, 77, 126-127, 130

Z05.0 **Observation and evaluation of newborn for suspected cardiac condition ruled out** N

Z05.1 **Observation and evaluation of newborn for suspected infectious condition ruled out** N
Coding Clinic: 2019, Q2, P11

Z05.2 **Observation and evaluation of newborn for suspected neurological condition ruled out** N

Z05.3 **Observation and evaluation of newborn for suspected respiratory condition ruled out** N

● Z05.4 **Observation and evaluation of newborn for suspected genetic, metabolic or immunologic condition ruled out**

Z05.41 **Observation and evaluation of newborn for suspected genetic condition ruled out** N
Coding Clinic: 2016, Q4, P55

Z05.42 **Observation and evaluation of newborn for suspected metabolic condition ruled out** N

Z05.43 **Observation and evaluation of newborn for suspected immunologic condition ruled out** N

Z05.5 **Observation and evaluation of newborn for suspected gastrointestinal condition ruled out** N

Z05.6 **Observation and evaluation of newborn for suspected genitourinary condition ruled out** N

● Z05.7 **Observation and evaluation of newborn for suspected skin, subcutaneous, musculoskeletal and connective tissue condition ruled out**

Z05.71 **Observation and evaluation of newborn for suspected skin and subcutaneous tissue condition ruled out** N

Z05.72 **Observation and evaluation of newborn for suspected musculoskeletal condition ruled out** N

Z05.73 **Observation and evaluation of newborn for suspected connective tissue condition ruled out** N

● Z05.8 **Observation and evaluation of newborn for other specified suspected condition ruled out** N
Coding Clinic: 2022, Q1, P17-18

Z05.81 **Observation and evaluation of newborn for suspected condition related to home physiologic monitoring device ruled out**
Encounter for observation of newborn for apnea alarm without findings
Encounter for observation of newborn for bradycardia alarm without findings
Encounter for observation of newborn for malfunction of home cardiorespiratory monitor
Encounter for observation of newborn for non-specific findings home physiologic monitoring device
Encounter for observation of newborn for pulse oximeter alarm without findings
Excludes1 encounter for observation for suspected conditions related to home physiologic monitoring device ruled out (Z03.83)
neonatal bradycardia (P29.12)
other newborn apnea (P28.4-)
primary sleep apnea of newborn (P28.3-)

Z05.89 **Observation and evaluation of newborn for other specified suspected condition ruled out**

Z05.9 **Observation and evaluation of newborn for unspecified suspected condition ruled out** N

OGCR See Section II.C.21.c.8.

The follow-up codes are used to explain continuing surveillance following completed treatment of a disease, condition, or injury. They imply that the condition has been fully treated and no longer exists. They should not be confused with aftercare codes, or injury codes with 7th character "D," that explain ongoing care of a healing condition or its sequelae. Follow-up codes may be used in conjunction with history codes to provide the full picture of the healed condition and its treatment. The follow-up code is sequenced first, followed by the history code.

A follow-up code may be used to explain multiple visits. Should a condition be found to have recurred on the follow-up visit, then the diagnosis code for the condition should be assigned in place of the follow-up code.

The follow-up Z code categories:
Z08 Encounter for follow-up examination after completed treatment for malignant neoplasm
Z09 Encounter for follow-up examination after completed treatment for conditions other than malignant neoplasm
Z39 Encounter for maternal postpartum care and examination

● Z08 **Encounter for follow-up examination after completed treatment for malignant neoplasm**
Medical surveillance following completed treatment
Use additional code to identify any acquired absence of organs (Z90.-)
Use additional code to identify the personal history of malignant neoplasm (Z85.-)
Excludes1 aftercare following medical care (Z43-Z49, Z51)

● Z09 **Encounter for follow-up examination after completed treatment for conditions other than malignant neoplasm**
Medical surveillance following completed treatment
Use additional code to identify any applicable history of disease code (Z86.-, Z87.-)
Excludes1 aftercare following medical care (Z43-Z49, Z51)
surveillance of contraception (Z30.4-)
surveillance of prosthetic and other medical devices (Z44-Z46)
Coding Clinic: 2022, Q3, P4; 2021, Q1, P33; 2017, Q1, P9; 2015, Q1, P8

OGCR Section II.C.21.c.5.

Screening

Screening is the testing for disease or disease precursors in seemingly well individuals so that early detection and treatment can be provided for those who test positive for the disease (e.g., screening mammogram).

The testing of a person to rule out or confirm a suspected diagnosis because the patient has some sign or symptom is a diagnostic examination, not a screening. In these cases, the sign or symptom is used to explain the reason for the test.

A screening code may be a first listed code if the reason for the visit is specifically the screening exam. It may also be used as an additional code if the screening is done during an office visit for other health problems. A screening code is not necessary if the screening is inherent to a routine examination, such as a pap smear done during a routine pelvic examination.

Should a condition be discovered during the screening then the code for the condition may be assigned as an additional diagnosis.

The Z code indicates that a screening exam is planned. A procedure code is required to confirm that the screening was performed.

The screening Z codes/categories:

Z11 Encounter for screening for infectious and parasitic diseases
Z12 Encounter for screening for malignant neoplasms
Z13 Encounter for screening for other diseases and disorders
Except: Z13.9, Encounter for screening, unspecified
Z36 Encounter for antenatal screening for mother

● Z11 Encounter for screening for infectious and parasitic diseases
Screening is the testing for disease or disease precursors in asymptomatic individuals so that early detection and treatment can be provided for those who test positive for the disease.
Excludes1 encounter for diagnostic examination - code to sign or symptom

● **Z11.0 Encounter for screening for intestinal infectious diseases**
Encounter for screening for active tuberculosis disease

● **Z11.1 Encounter for screening for respiratory tuberculosis**

● **Z11.2 Encounter for screening for other bacterial diseases**

● **Z11.3 Encounter for screening for infections with a predominantly sexual mode of transmission**
Excludes2 encounter for screening for human immunodeficiency virus [HIV] (Z11.4)
encounter for screening for human papillomavirus (Z11.51)

● **Z11.4 Encounter for screening for human immunodeficiency virus [HIV]**

● **Z11.5 Encounter for screening for other viral diseases**
Excludes2 encounter for screening for viral intestinal disease (Z11.0)

● **Z11.51 Encounter for screening for human papillomavirus (HPV)**
Coding Clinic: 2023, Q2, P3

● **Z11.52 Encounter for screening for COVID-19**
Coding Clinic: 2023, Q2, P4; 2021, Q1, P37, 42

● **Z11.59 Encounter for screening for other viral diseases**
Coding Clinic: 2021, Q1, P37

● **Z11.6 Encounter for screening for other protozoal diseases and helminthiases**
Diseases or infestations caused by parasitic worms
Excludes2 encounter for screening for protozoal intestinal disease (Z11.0)

Z11.7 Encounter for testing for latent tuberculosis infection

● **Z11.8 Encounter for screening for other infectious and parasitic diseases**
Encounter for screening for chlamydia
Encounter for screening for rickettsial
Encounter for screening for spirochetal
Encounter for screening for mycoses

● **Z11.9 Encounter for screening for infectious and parasitic diseases, unspecified**

● **Z12 Encounter for screening for malignant neoplasms**
Screening is the testing for disease or disease precursors in asymptomatic individuals so that early detection and treatment can be provided for those who test positive for the disease.
Use additional code to identify any family history of malignant neoplasm (Z80.-)
Excludes1 encounter for diagnostic examination - code to sign or symptom

● **Z12.0 Encounter for screening for malignant neoplasm of stomach**

● **Z12.1 Encounter for screening for malignant neoplasm of intestinal tract**

● **Z12.10 Encounter for screening for malignant neoplasm of intestinal tract, unspecified**

● **Z12.11 Encounter for screening for malignant neoplasm of colon**
Encounter for screening colonoscopy NOS
Coding Clinic: 2018, Q1, P7; 2017, Q1, P8-9

● **Z12.12 Encounter for screening for malignant neoplasm of rectum**

● **Z12.13 Encounter for screening for malignant neoplasm of small intestine**

● **Z12.2 Encounter for screening for malignant neoplasm of respiratory organs**

● **Z12.3 Encounter for screening for malignant neoplasm of breast**

● **Z12.31 Encounter for screening mammogram for malignant neoplasm of breast**
Excludes1 inconclusive mammogram (R92.2)
Coding Clinic: 2023, Q4, P44; 2015, Q1, P24

● **Z12.39 Encounter for other screening for malignant neoplasm of breast**

● **Z12.4 Encounter for screening for malignant neoplasm of cervix**
Encounter for screening pap smear for malignant neoplasm of cervix
Excludes1 when screening is part of general gynecological examination (Z01.4-)
Excludes2 encounter for screening for human papillomavirus (Z11.51)

Z12.5 Encounter for screening for malignant neoplasm of prostate

● **Z12.6 Encounter for screening for malignant neoplasm of bladder**

● **Z12.7 Encounter for screening for malignant neoplasm of other genitourinary organs**

● **Z12.71 Encounter for screening for malignant neoplasm of testis**

● **Z12.72 Encounter for screening for malignant neoplasm of vagina**
Vaginal pap smear status - post hysterectomy for non-malignant condition
Use additional code to identify acquired absence of uterus (Z90.71-)
Excludes1 vaginal pap smear status - post hysterectomy for malignant conditions (Z08)

● **Z12.73 Encounter for screening for malignant neoplasm of ovary**

● **Z12.79 Encounter for screening for malignant neoplasm of other genitourinary organs**

● **Z12.8 Encounter for screening for malignant neoplasm of other sites**

● **Z12.81 Encounter for screening for malignant neoplasm of oral cavity**

● **Z12.82 Encounter for screening for malignant neoplasm of nervous system**

● **Z12.83 Encounter for screening for malignant neoplasm of skin**

Z12.89 Encounter for screening for malignant neoplasm of other sites
Coding Clinic: 2021, Q1, P15

Z12.9 Encounter for screening for malignant neoplasm, site unspecified

Z13 Encounter for screening for other diseases and disorders
Screening is the testing for disease or disease precursors in asymptomatic individuals so that early detection and treatment can be provided for those who test positive for the disease.
Excludes1 encounter for diagnostic examination - code to sign or symptom

Z13.0 Encounter for screening for diseases of the blood and blood-forming organs and certain disorders involving the immune mechanism

Z13.1 Encounter for screening for diabetes mellitus

Z13.2 Encounter for screening for nutritional, metabolic and other endocrine disorders

Z13.21 Encounter for screening for nutritional disorder

Z13.22 Encounter for screening for metabolic disorder

Z13.220 Encounter for screening for lipoid disorders
Encounter for screening for cholesterol level
Encounter for screening for hypercholesterolemia
Encounter for screening for hyperlipidemia

Z13.228 Encounter for screening for other metabolic disorders

Z13.29 Encounter for screening for other suspected endocrine disorder
Excludes2 encounter for screening for diabetes mellitus (Z13.1)

Z13.3 Encounter for screening examination for mental health and behavioral disorders

Z13.30 Encounter for screening examination for mental health and behavioral disorders, unspecified

Z13.31 Encounter for screening for depression
Encounter for screening for depression, adult
Encounter for screening for depression for child or adolescent

Z13.32 Encounter for screening for maternal depression
Encounter for screening for perinatal depression

Z13.39 Encounter for screening examination for other mental health and behavioral disorders
Encounter for screening for alcoholism
Encounter for screening for intellectual disabilities

Z13.4 Encounter for screening for certain developmental disorders in childhood P
Encounter for development testing of infant or child
Encounter for screening for developmental handicaps in early childhood
Excludes2 encounter for routine child health examination (Z00.12-)

Z13.40 Encounter for screening for unspecified developmental delays

Z13.41 Encounter for autism screening

Z13.42 Encounter for screening for global developmental delays (milestones)
Encounter for screening for developmental handicaps in early childhood

Z13.49 Encounter for screening for other developmental delays

Z13.5 Encounter for screening for eye and ear disorders
Excludes2 encounter for general hearing examination (Z01.1-)
encounter for general vision examination (Z01.0-)
Coding Clinic: 2016, Q3, P17

Z13.6 Encounter for screening for cardiovascular disorders

Z13.7 Encounter for screening for genetic and chromosomal anomalies
Excludes1 genetic testing for procreative management (Z31.4-)

Z13.71 Encounter for nonprocreative screening for genetic disease carrier status

Z13.79 Encounter for other screening for genetic and chromosomal anomalies

Z13.8 Encounter for screening for other specified diseases and disorders
Excludes2 screening for malignant neoplasms (Z12.-)

Z13.81 Encounter for screening for digestive system disorders

Z13.810 Encounter for screening for upper gastrointestinal disorder

Z13.811 Encounter for screening for lower gastrointestinal disorder
Excludes1 encounter for screening for intestinal infectious disease (Z11.0)

Z13.818 Encounter for screening for other digestive system disorders

Z13.82 Encounter for screening for musculoskeletal disorder

Z13.820 Encounter for screening for osteoporosis

Z13.828 Encounter for screening for other musculoskeletal disorder

Z13.83 Encounter for screening for respiratory disorder NEC
Excludes1 encounter for screening for respiratory tuberculosis (Z11.1)

Z13.84 Encounter for screening for dental disorders

Z13.85 Encounter for screening for nervous system disorders

Z13.850 Encounter for screening for traumatic brain injury

Z13.858 Encounter for screening for other nervous system disorders

Z13.88 Encounter for screening for disorder due to exposure to contaminants
Excludes1 those exposed to contaminants without suspected disorders (Z57-Z77.-)

Z13.89 Encounter for screening for other disorder
Encounter for screening for genitourinary disorders

Z13.9 Encounter for screening, unspecified

GENETIC CARRIER AND GENETIC SUSCEPTIBILITY TO DISEASE (Z14-Z15)

Z14 Genetic carrier

Z14.0 Hemophilia A carrier

Z14.01 Asymptomatic hemophilia A carrier

Z14.02 Symptomatic hemophilia A carrier

Z14.1 Cystic fibrosis carrier

Z14.8 Genetic carrier of other disease

Z15 Genetic susceptibility to disease
Excludes1 chromosomal anomalies (Q90-Q99)
Includes confirmed abnormal gene
Use additional code, if applicable, for any associated family history of the disease (Z80-Z84)

Z15.0 Genetic susceptibility to malignant neoplasm

Code first if applicable, any current malignant neoplasm (C00-C75, C81-C96)

Use additional code, if applicable, for any personal history of malignant neoplasm (Z85.-)

Z15.01 Genetic susceptibility to malignant neoplasm of breast

Z15.02 Genetic susceptibility to malignant neoplasm of ovary

Z15.03 Genetic susceptibility to malignant neoplasm of prostate

Z15.04 Genetic susceptibility to malignant neoplasm of endometrium

Z15.09 Genetic susceptibility to other malignant neoplasm

Coding Clinic: 2021, Q1, P15

Z15.1 Genetic susceptibility to epilepsy and neurodevelopmental disorders

Code also, if applicable, related disorders such as:
- developmental and epileptic encephalopathy (G93.45)
- developmental disorder of speech and language (F80.-)
- developmental disorders of scholastic skills (F81.-)
- epilepsy, by specific type (G40.-)
- intellectual disabilities (F70-F79)
- other neurodevelopmental disorder (F88)
- pervasive developmental disorders (F84.-)

Z15.2 Genetic susceptibility to obesity

Code also, if applicable, any associated manifestations, such as:
- other obesity (E66.8-)
- polyphagia (R63.2)

Use Additional code to identify body mass index (BMI), if known (Z68.-)

Z15.8 Genetic susceptibility to other disease

Z15.81 Genetic susceptibility to multiple endocrine neoplasia [MEN]

Excludes1 multiple endocrine neoplasia [MEN] syndromes (E31.2-)

Z15.89 Genetic susceptibility to other disease

RESISTANCE TO ANTIMICROBIAL DRUGS (Z16)

Z16 Resistance to antimicrobial drugs

Note: The codes in this category are provided for use as additional codes to identify the resistance and non-responsiveness of a condition to antimicrobial drugs.

Code first the infection

Excludes1 Methicillin resistant Staphylococcus aureus infection (A49.02)
Methicillin resistant Staphylococcus aureus pneumonia (J15.212)
Sepsis due to Methicillin resistant Staphylococcus aureus (A41.02)

Z16.1 Resistance to beta lactam antibiotics (Ex) No exclusions

Z16.10 Resistance to unspecified beta lactam antibiotics

Z16.11 Resistance to penicillins
Resistance to amoxicillin
Resistance to ampicillin

Z16.12 Extended spectrum beta lactamase (ESBL) resistance

Excludes2 Methicillin resistant Staphylococcus aureus infection in diseases classified elsewhere (B95.62)

Z16.13 Resistance to carbapenem

Z16.19 Resistance to other specified beta lactam antibiotics
Resistance to cephalosporins

Z16.2 Resistance to other antibiotics (Ex) No exclusions

Z16.20 Resistance to unspecified antibiotic
Resistance to antibiotics NOS

Z16.21 Resistance to vancomycin

Z16.22 Resistance to vancomycin related antibiotics

Z16.23 Resistance to quinolones and fluoroquinolones

Z16.24 Resistance to multiple antibiotics

Z16.29 Resistance to other single specified antibiotic
Resistance to aminoglycosides
Resistance to macrolides
Resistance to sulfonamides
Resistance to tetracyclines

Z16.3 Resistance to other antimicrobial drugs (Ex) No exclusions

Excludes1 resistance to antibiotics (Z16.1-, Z16.2-)

Z16.30 Resistance to unspecified antimicrobial drugs
Drug resistance NOS

Z16.31 Resistance to antiparasitic drug(s)
Resistance to quinine and related compounds

Z16.32 Resistance to antifungal drug(s)

Z16.33 Resistance to antiviral drug(s)

Z16.34 Resistance to antimycobacterial drug(s)
Resistance to tuberculostatics

Z16.341 Resistance to single antimycobacterial drug
Resistance to antimycobacterial drug NOS

Z16.342 Resistance to multiple antimycobacterial drugs

Z16.35 Resistance to multiple antimicrobial drugs

Excludes1 Resistance to multiple antibiotics only (Z16.24)

Z16.39 Resistance to other specified antimicrobial drug

ESTROGEN, AND OTHER HORMONES AND FACTORS RECEPTOR STATUS (Z17)

Z17 Estrogen, and other hormones and factors receptor status

Note: Use one code, as available, for each receptor: Z17.0, Z17.1, Z17.2-. Z17.3-

Code first malignant neoplasm of breast (C50.-)

Code first malignant neoplasm, such as:
- *malignant neoplasm of ovary (C56.-)*

Z17.0 Estrogen receptor positive status [ER+]

Coding Clinic: 2022, Q3, P15

Z17.1 Estrogen receptor negative status [ER-]

Z17.2 Progesterone receptor status

Z17.21 Progesterone receptor positive status
PR+

Z17.22 Progesterone receptor negative status
PR-

Z17.3 Human epidermal growth factor 2 receptor

Z17.31 Human epidermal growth factor receptor 2 positive status
HER2+

Z17.32 Human epidermal growth factor receptor 2 negative status
HER2-

Z17.4 Combined receptor status

Note: Assign a code from subcategory Z17.4- when only a combined receptor status is documented

Z17.41 Hormone receptor positive
HR+

Z17.410 Hormone receptor positive with human epidermal growth factor receptor 2 positive status
HR+ with HER2+

Z17.411 Hormone receptor positive with human epidermal growth factor receptor 2 negative status
HR+ with HER2-

CHAPTER 21 (Z00-Z99)

▶● **Z17.42 Hormone receptor negative**
▶HR-

▶● **Z17.420 Hormone receptor negative with human epidermal growth factor receptor 2 positive status**
▶HR- with HER2+

▶● **Z17.421 Hormone receptor negative with human epidermal growth factor receptor 2 negative status**
▶HR- with HER2-
▶TNBC
▶Triple negative breast cancer

RETAINED FOREIGN BODY FRAGMENTS (Z18)

● **Z18 Retained foreign body fragments**

Includes embedded fragment (status)
embedded splinter (status)
retained foreign body status

Excludes1 artificial joint prosthesis status (Z96.6-)
foreign body accidentally left during a procedure (T81.5-)
foreign body entering through orifice (T15-T19)
in situ cardiac device (Z95.-)
organ or tissue replaced by means other than transplant (Z96.-, Z97.-)
organ or tissue replaced by transplant (Z94.-)
personal history of retained foreign body fully removed Z87.821
superficial foreign body (non-embedded splinter) - code to superficial foreign body, by site

● **Z18.0 Retained radioactive fragments**

● **Z18.01 Retained depleted uranium fragments**

● **Z18.09 Other retained radioactive fragments**
Other retained depleted isotope fragments
Retained nontherapeutic radioactive fragments

● **Z18.1 Retained metal fragments**

Excludes1 retained radioactive metal fragments (Z18.01-Z18.09)

● **Z18.10 Retained metal fragments, unspecified**
Retained metal fragment NOS

● **Z18.11 Retained magnetic metal fragments**

● **Z18.12 Retained nonmagnetic metal fragments**

● **Z18.2 Retained plastic fragments**
Acrylics fragments
Diethylhexylphthalates fragments
Isocyanate fragments

● **Z18.3 Retained organic fragments**

● **Z18.31 Retained animal quills or spines**

● **Z18.32 Retained tooth**

● **Z18.33 Retained wood fragments**

● **Z18.39 Other retained organic fragments**

● **Z18.8 Other specified retained foreign body**

● **Z18.81 Retained glass fragments**

● **Z18.83 Retained stone or crystalline fragments**
Retained concrete or cement fragments

● **Z18.89 Other specified retained foreign body fragments**
Coding Clinic: 2016, Q3, P24

● **Z18.9 Retained foreign body fragments, unspecified material**

HORMONE SENSITIVITY MALIGNANCY STATUS (Z19)

● **Z19 Hormone sensitivity malignancy status**

Code first malignant neoplasm —*see* Table of Neoplasms, by site, malignant
Coding Clinic: 2016, Q4, P129

Z19.1 Hormone sensitive malignancy status
Coding Clinic: 2016, Q4, P76

Z19.2 Hormone resistant malignancy status
Castrate resistant prostate malignancy status
Coding Clinic: 2016, Q4, P76

PERSONS WITH POTENTIAL HEALTH HAZARDS RELATED TO COMMUNICABLE DISEASES (Z20-Z29)

● **Z20 Contact with and (suspected) exposure to communicable diseases**

Excludes1 carrier of infectious disease (Z22.-)
diagnosed current infectious or parasitic disease - see Alphabetic Index

Excludes2 personal history of infectious and parasitic diseases (Z86.1-)

Coding Clinic: 2021, Q1, P37

● **Z20.0 Contact with and (suspected) exposure to intestinal infectious diseases**

Z20.01 Contact with and (suspected) exposure to intestinal infectious diseases due to Escherichia coli (E. coli)

● **Z20.09 Contact with and (suspected) exposure to other intestinal infectious diseases**

● **Z20.1 Contact with and (suspected) exposure to tuberculosis**

● **Z20.2 Contact with and (suspected) exposure to infections with a predominantly sexual mode of transmission**

● **Z20.3 Contact with and (suspected) exposure to rabies**

● **Z20.4 Contact with and (suspected) exposure to rubella**

Z20.5 Contact with and (suspected) exposure to viral hepatitis

Z20.6 Contact with and (suspected) exposure to human immunodeficiency virus [HIV]

Excludes1 asymptomatic human immunodeficiency virus [HIV]
HIV infection status (Z21)

● **Z20.7 Contact with and (suspected) exposure to pediculosis, acariasis and other infestations**

● **Z20.8 Contact with and (suspected) exposure to other communicable diseases**

● **Z20.81 Contact with and (suspected) exposure to other bacterial communicable diseases**

● **Z20.810 Contact with and (suspected) exposure to anthrax**

Z20.811 Contact with and (suspected) exposure to meningococcus

● **Z20.818 Contact with and (suspected) exposure to other bacterial communicable diseases**

● **Z20.82 Contact with and (suspected) exposure to other viral communicable diseases**

Z20.820 Contact with and (suspected) exposure to varicella

● **Z20.821 Contact with and (suspected) exposure to Zika virus**

● **Z20.822 Contact with and (suspected) exposure to COVID-19**
Contact with and (suspected) exposure to SARS-CoV-2
Coding Clinic: 2023, Q2, P3-4; 2022, Q2, P28,29; 2021, Q4, P109; 2021, Q1, P37-39, 42

Z20.828 Contact with and (suspected) exposure to other viral communicable diseases
Coding Clinic: 2022, Q3, P4; 2021, Q1, P37-39; 2016, Q4, P6-7, 121

● **Z20.89 Contact with and (suspected) exposure to other communicable diseases**

● **Z20.9 Contact with and (suspected) exposure to unspecified communicable disease**

CHAPTER 21 (Z00-Z99)

Z21 Asymptomatic human immunodeficiency virus [HIV] infection status
HIV positive NOS
Code first Human immunodeficiency virus [HIV] disease complicating pregnancy, childbirth and the puerperium, if applicable (O98.7-)
Excludes1 acquired immunodeficiency syndrome (B20)
contact with human immunodeficiency virus [HIV] (Z20.6)
exposure to human immunodeficiency virus [HIV] (Z20.6)
human immunodeficiency virus [HIV] disease (B20)
inconclusive laboratory evidence of human immunodeficiency virus [HIV] (R75)
MCE: Questionable admission when principal dx
Coding Clinic: 2022, Q1, P37; 2019, Q1, P10-11

Z22 Carrier of infectious disease
Includes colonization status
suspected carrier
Excludes2 carrier of viral hepatitis (B18.-)
Z22.0 Carrier of typhoid
Z22.1 Carrier of other intestinal infectious diseases
Z22.2 Carrier of diphtheria
Z22.3 Carrier of other specified bacterial diseases
Z22.31 Carrier of bacterial disease due to meningococci
Z22.32 Carrier of bacterial disease due to staphylococci
Z22.321 Carrier or suspected carrier of Methicillin susceptible Staphylococcus aureus
MSSA colonization
Z22.322 Carrier or suspected carrier of Methicillin resistant Staphylococcus aureus
MRSA colonization
Z22.33 Carrier of bacterial disease due to streptococci
Z22.330 Carrier of Group B streptococcus
Excludes1 Carrier of streptococcus group B (GBS) complicating pregnancy, childbirth and the puerperium (O99.82-)
Z22.338 Carrier of other streptococcus
Z22.34 Carrier of Acinetobacter baumannii
Z22.340 Carrier of carbapenem-resistant Acinetobacter baumannii
Z22.341 Carrier of carbapenem-sensitive Acinetobacter baumannii
Z22.349 Carrier of Acinetobacter baumannii, unspecified
Z22.35 Carrier of Enterobacterales
Carrier of E. coli
Carrier of K. pneumoniae
Z22.350 Carrier of carbapenem-resistant Enterobacterales
Z22.358 Carrier of other Enterobacterales
Carrier of carbapenem-sensitive Enterobacterales
Carrier of ESBL-producing Enterobacterales
Carrier of extended-spectrum beta-lactamase producing Enterobacterales
Z22.359 Carrier of Enterobacterales, unspecified
Z22.39 Carrier of other specified bacterial diseases
Z22.4 Carrier of infections with a predominantly sexual mode of transmission
Z22.6 Carrier of human T-lymphotropic virus type-1 [HTLV-1] infection
Z22.7 Latent tuberculosis
Latent tuberculosis infection (LTBI)
Excludes1 nonspecific reaction to cell mediated immunity measurement of gamma interferon antigen response without active tuberculosis (R76.12)
nonspecific reaction to tuberculin skin test without active tuberculosis (R76.11)
Z22.8 Carrier of other infectious diseases
Z22.9 Carrier of infectious disease, unspecified

Z23 Encounter for immunization
Code first any routine childhood examination
Note: Procedure codes are required to identify the types of immunizations given.
Code also, if applicable, encounter for immunization safety counseling (Z71.85)

Z28 Immunization not carried out and underimmunization status
Includes vaccination not carried out
Code also, if applicable, encounter for immunization safety counseling (Z71.85)
Z28.0 Immunization not carried out because of contraindication
Z28.01 Immunization not carried out because of acute illness of patient
Z28.02 Immunization not carried out because of chronic illness or condition of patient
Z28.03 Immunization not carried out because of immune compromised state of patient
Z28.04 Immunization not carried out because of patient allergy to vaccine or component
Z28.09 Immunization not carried out because of other contraindication
Z28.1 Immunization not carried out because of patient decision for reasons of belief or group pressure
Immunization not carried out because of religious belief
Z28.2 Immunization not carried out because of patient decision for other and unspecified reason
Z28.20 Immunization not carried out because of patient decision for unspecified reason
Z28.21 Immunization not carried out because of patient refusal
Z28.29 Immunization not carried out because of patient decision for other reason
Z28.3 Underimmunization status
Coding Clinic: 2021, Q4, P110
Use additional code, if applicable, to identify:
immunization not carried out because of contraindication (Z28.0-)
immunization not carried out because of patient decision for other and unspecified reason (Z28.2-)
immunization not carried out because of patient decision for reasons of belief or group pressure (Z28.1)
immunization not carried out for other reason (Z28.8-)
Z28.31 Underimmunization for COVID-19 status
Note: These codes should not be used for individuals who are not eligible for the COVID-19 vaccines, as determined by the healthcare provider.
Z28.310 Unvaccinated for COVID-19
Z28.311 Partially vaccinated for COVID-19
Z28.39 Other underimmunization status
Delinquent immunization status
Lapsed immunization schedule status
Z28.8 Immunization not carried out for other reason
Z28.81 Immunization not carried out due to patient having had the disease

Z28.82 **Immunization not carried out because of caregiver refusal**
Immunization not carried out because of guardian refusal
Immunization not carried out because of parent refusal
Excludes1 immunization not carried out because of caregiver refusal because of religious belief (Z28.1)

Z28.83 **Immunization not carried out due to unavailability of vaccine**
Delay in delivery of vaccine
Lack of availability of vaccine
Manufacturer delay of vaccine

Z28.89 **Immunization not carried out for other reason**

Z28.9 **Immunization not carried out for unspecified reason**

Z29 **Encounter for other prophylactic measures**
Excludes1 desensitization to allergens (Z51.6)
prophylactic surgery (Z40.-)
Coding Clinic: 2016, Q4, P130

Z29.1 **Encounter for prophylactic immunotherapy**
Encounter for administration of immunoglobulin
Coding Clinic: 2016, Q4, P78-79

Z29.11 **Encounter for prophylactic immunotherapy for respiratory syncytial virus (RSV)**

Z29.12 **Encounter for prophylactic antivenin**

Z29.13 **Encounter for prophylactic Rho(D) immune globulin**
Coding Clinic: 2019, Q3, P5

Z29.14 **Encounter for prophylactic rabies immune globin**

Z29.3 **Encounter for prophylactic fluoride administration**
Coding Clinic: 2016, Q4, P79

Z29.8 **Encounter for other specified prophylactic measures**
Coding Clinic: 2022, Q2, P27; 2016, Q4, P79

Z29.81 **Encounter for HIV pre-exposure prophylaxis**
Code also, if applicable, risk factors for HIV, such as:
contact with and (suspected) exposure to human immunodeficiency virus [HIV](Z20.6)
high risk sexual behavior (Z72.5-)

Z29.89 **Encounter for other specified prophylactic measures**

Z29.9 **Encounter for prophylactic measures, unspecified**
Coding Clinic: 2016, Q4, P79

PERSONS ENCOUNTERING HEALTH SERVICES IN CIRCUMSTANCES RELATED TO REPRODUCTION (Z30-Z39)

Z30 **Encounter for contraceptive management**

Z30.0 **Encounter for general counseling and advice on contraception**

Z30.01 **Encounter for initial prescription of contraceptives**
Excludes1 encounter for surveillance of contraceptives (Z30.4-)

Z30.011 **Encounter for initial prescription of contraceptive pills**

Z30.012 **Encounter for prescription of emergency contraception**
Encounter for postcoital contraception

Z30.013 **Encounter for initial prescription of injectable contraceptive**

Z30.014 **Encounter for initial prescription of intrauterine contraceptive device**
Excludes1 encounter for insertion of intrauterine contraceptive device (Z30.430, Z30.432)

Z30.015 **Encounter for initial prescription of vaginal ring hormonal contraceptive**
Coding Clinic: 2016, Q4, P78

Z30.016 **Encounter for initial prescription of transdermal patch hormonal contraceptive device**
Coding Clinic: 2016, Q4, P78

Z30.017 **Encounter for initial prescription of implantable subdermal contraceptive**
Coding Clinic: 2016, Q4, P78

Z30.018 **Encounter for initial prescription of other contraceptives**
Encounter for initial prescription of barrier contraception
Encounter for initial prescription of diaphragm

Z30.019 **Encounter for initial prescription of contraceptives, unspecified**

Z30.02 **Counseling and instruction in natural family planning to avoid pregnancy**

Z30.09 **Encounter for other general counseling and advice on contraception**
Encounter for family planning advice NOS

Z30.2 **Encounter for sterilization**
Coding Clinic: 2021, Q3, P13

Z30.4 **Encounter for surveillance of contraceptives**

Z30.40 **Encounter for surveillance of contraceptives, unspecified**

Z30.41 **Encounter for surveillance of contraceptive pills**
Encounter for repeat prescription for contraceptive pill

Z30.42 **Encounter for surveillance of injectable contraceptive**

Z30.43 **Encounter for surveillance of intrauterine contraceptive device**

Z30.430 **Encounter for insertion of intrauterine contraceptive device**

Z30.431 **Encounter for routine checking of intrauterine contraceptive device**

Z30.432 **Encounter for removal of intrauterine contraceptive device**

Z30.433 **Encounter for removal and reinsertion of intrauterine contraceptive device**
Encounter for replacement of intrauterine contraceptive device

Z30.44 **Encounter for surveillance of vaginal ring hormonal contraceptive device**
Coding Clinic: 2016, Q4, P78

Z30.45 **Encounter for surveillance of transdermal patch hormonal contraceptive device**
Coding Clinic: 2016, Q4, P78

Z30.46 **Encounter for surveillance of implantable subdermal contraceptive**
Encounter for checking, reinsertion or removal of implantable subdermal contraceptive
Coding Clinic: 2016, Q4, P78

Z30.49 **Encounter for surveillance of other contraceptives**
Encounter for surveillance of barrier contraception
Encounter for surveillance of diaphragm

Z30.8 **Encounter for other contraceptive management**
Encounter for postvasectomy sperm count
Encounter for routine examination for contraceptive maintenance
Excludes1 sperm count following sterilization reversal (Z31.42)
sperm count for fertility testing (Z31.41)

Z30.9 **Encounter for contraceptive management, unspecified**

CHAPTER 21 (Z00-Z99)

● **Z31 Encounter for procreative management**
Excludes2 complications associated with artificial fertilization (N98.-)
female infertility (N97.-)
male infertility (N46.-)

Z31.0 Encounter for reversal of previous sterilization

● **Z31.4 Encounter for procreative investigation and testing**
Excludes1 postvasectomy sperm count (Z30.8)

● **Z31.41 Encounter for fertility testing**
Encounter for fallopian tube patency testing
Encounter for sperm count for fertility testing

● **Z31.42 Aftercare following sterilization reversal**
Sperm count following sterilization reversal

● **Z31.43 Encounter for genetic testing of female for procreative management**
Use additional code for recurrent pregnancy loss, if applicable (N96, O26.2-)
Excludes1 nonprocreative genetic testing (Z13.7-)

● **Z31.430 Encounter of female for testing for genetic disease carrier status for procreative management**

● **Z31.438 Encounter for other genetic testing of female for procreative management**

● **Z31.44 Encounter for genetic testing of male for procreative management**
Excludes1 nonprocreative genetic testing (Z13.7-)

● **Z31.440 Encounter of male for testing for genetic disease carrier status for procreative management**

● **Z31.441 Encounter for testing of male partner of patient with recurrent pregnancy loss** A

● **Z31.448 Encounter for other genetic testing of male for procreative management** A

● **Z31.49 Encounter for other procreative investigation and testing**

● **Z31.5 Encounter for procreative genetic counseling**

● **Z31.6 Encounter for general counseling and advice on procreation**

● **Z31.61 Procreative counseling and advice using natural family planning**

● **Z31.62 Encounter for fertility preservation counseling**
Encounter for fertility preservation counseling prior to cancer therapy
Encounter for fertility preservation counseling prior to surgical removal of gonads

● **Z31.69 Encounter for other general counseling and advice on procreation**

● **Z31.7 Encounter for procreative management and counseling for gestational carrier**
Excludes1 pregnant state, gestational carrier (Z33.3)
Coding Clinic: 2016, Q4, P78

● **Z31.8 Encounter for other procreative management**

● **Z31.81 Encounter for male factor infertility in female patient**

● **Z31.82 Encounter for Rh incompatibility status**
Coding Clinic: 2015, Q3, P40

● **Z31.83 Encounter for assisted reproductive fertility procedure cycle**
Patient undergoing in vitro fertilization cycle
Use additional code to identify the type of infertility
Excludes1 pre-cycle diagnosis and testing - code to reason for encounter
Coding Clinic: 2022, Q2, P15,16

● **Z31.84 Encounter for fertility preservation procedure**
Encounter for fertility preservation procedure prior to cancer therapy
Encounter for fertility preservation procedure prior to surgical removal of gonads

● **Z31.89 Encounter for other procreative management**

● **Z31.9 Encounter for procreative management, unspecified**

● **Z32 Encounter for pregnancy test and childbirth and childcare instruction**

● **Z32.0 Encounter for pregnancy test**

Z32.00 Encounter for pregnancy test, result unknown
Encounter for pregnancy test NOS

Z32.01 Encounter for pregnancy test, result positive M

Z32.02 Encounter for pregnancy test, result negative

● **Z32.2 Encounter for childbirth instruction**

● **Z32.3 Encounter for childcare instruction**
Encounter for prenatal or postpartum childcare instruction

● **Z33 Pregnant state**

● **Z33.1 Pregnant state, incidental** M
Pregnancy NOS
Pregnant state NOS
Excludes1 complications of pregnancy (O00-O9A)
pregnant state, gestational carrier (Z33.3)

Z33.2 Encounter for elective termination of pregnancy M
Excludes1 early fetal death with retention of dead fetus (O02.1)
late fetal death (O36.4)
spontaneous abortion (O03)
Coding Clinic: 2023, Q2, P15; 2016, Q4, P130

● **Z33.3 Pregnant state, gestational carrier**
Excludes1 encounter for procreative management and counseling for gestational carrier (Z31.7)
Coding Clinic: 2016, Q4, P78

● **Z34 Encounter for supervision of normal pregnancy**
Excludes1 any complication of pregnancy (O00-O9A)
encounter for pregnancy test (Z32.0-)
encounter for supervision of high risk pregnancy (O09.-)
Coding Clinic: 2016, Q4, P6

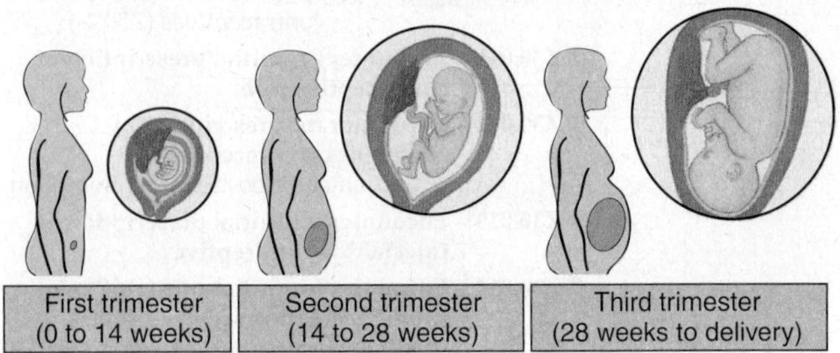

Figure 21-1 Trimesters. (From Shiland, Betsy J. Medical Terminology & Anatomy for ICD-10 Coding, ed 2, Mosby, 2015)

CHAPTER 21 (Z00-Z99)

- **Z34.0** Encounter for supervision of normal first pregnancy
  - **Z34.00** Encounter for supervision of normal first pregnancy, unspecified trimester M
  - **Z34.01** Encounter for supervision of normal first pregnancy, first trimester M
  - **Z34.02** Encounter for supervision of normal first pregnancy, second trimester M
  - **Z34.03** Encounter for supervision of normal first pregnancy, third trimester M
- **Z34.8** Encounter for supervision of other normal pregnancy
  - **Z34.80** Encounter for supervision of other normal pregnancy, unspecified trimester M
  - **Z34.81** Encounter for supervision of other normal pregnancy, first trimester M
  - **Z34.82** Encounter for supervision of other normal pregnancy, second trimester M
  - **Z34.83** Encounter for supervision of other normal pregnancy, third trimester M
- **Z34.9** Encounter for supervision of normal pregnancy, unspecified
  - **Z34.90** Encounter for supervision of normal pregnancy, unspecified, unspecified trimester M
  - **Z34.91** Encounter for supervision of normal pregnancy, unspecified, first trimester M
  - **Z34.92** Encounter for supervision of normal pregnancy, unspecified, second trimester M
  - **Z34.93** Encounter for supervision of normal pregnancy, unspecified, third trimester M

Z36 **Encounter for antenatal screening of mother**

Includes Encounter for placental sample (taken vaginally)
Screening is the testing for disease or disease precursors in asymptomatic individuals so that early detection and treatment can be provided for those who test positive for the disease.

Excludes1 diagnostic examination - code to sign or symptom
encounter for suspected maternal and fetal conditions ruled out (Z03.7-)
suspected fetal condition affecting management of pregnancy - code to condition in Chapter 15

Excludes2 abnormal findings on antenatal screening of mother (O28.-)
genetic counseling and testing (Z31.43-, Z31.5)
routine prenatal care (Z34)

- **Z36.0** Encounter for antenatal screening for chromosomal anomalies M
- **Z36.1** Encounter for antenatal screening for raised alphafetoprotein level M
  Encounter for antenatal screening for elevated maternal serum alphafetoprotein level
- **Z36.2** Encounter for other antenatal screening follow-up M
  Non-visualized anatomy on a previous scan
- **Z36.3** Encounter for antenatal screening for malformations M
  Screening for a suspected anomaly
- **Z36.4** Encounter for antenatal screening for fetal growth retardation M
  Intrauterine growth restriction (IUGR)/small-for-dates
- **Z36.5** Encounter for antenatal screening for isoimmunization M
- **Z36.8** Encounter for other antenatal screening
  - **Z36.81** Encounter for antenatal screening for hydrops fetalis M
  - **Z36.82** Encounter for antenatal screening for nuchal translucency M
  - **Z36.83** Encounter for fetal screening for congenital cardiac abnormalities M
  - **Z36.84** Encounter for antenatal screening for fetal lung maturity M
  - **Z36.85** Encounter for antenatal screening for Streptococcus B M
  - **Z36.86** Encounter for antenatal screening for cervical length M
    Screening for risk of pre-term labor
  - **Z36.87** Encounter for antenatal screening for uncertain dates
  - **Z36.88** Encounter for antenatal screening for fetal macrosomia M
    Screening for large-for-dates
  - **Z36.89** Encounter for other specified antenatal screening M
  - **Z36.8A** Encounter for antenatal screening for other genetic defects M
- **Z36.9** Encounter for antenatal screening, unspecified M

Z3A **Weeks of gestation**

Note: Codes from category Z3A are for use, only on the maternal record, to indicate the weeks of gestation of the pregnancy, if known.

Code first obstetric condition or encounter for delivery (O09-O60, O80-O82)

Coding Clinic: 2022, Q2, P3-4; 2016, Q4, P130; 2013, Q2, P33

- **Z3A.0** Weeks of gestation of pregnancy, unspecified or less than 10 weeks
  - **Z3A.00** Weeks of gestation of pregnancy not specified M
  - **Z3A.01** Less than 8 weeks gestation of pregnancy M
  - **Z3A.08** 8 weeks gestation of pregnancy M
  - **Z3A.09** 9 weeks gestation of pregnancy M
- **Z3A.1** Weeks of gestation of pregnancy, weeks 10-19
  - **Z3A.10** 10 weeks gestation of pregnancy M
  - **Z3A.11** 11 weeks gestation of pregnancy M
  - **Z3A.12** 12 weeks gestation of pregnancy M
  - **Z3A.13** 13 weeks gestation of pregnancy M
  - **Z3A.14** 14 weeks gestation of pregnancy M
  - **Z3A.15** 15 weeks gestation of pregnancy M
  - **Z3A.16** 16 weeks gestation of pregnancy M
    Coding Clinic: 2016, Q4, P5
  - **Z3A.17** 17 weeks gestation of pregnancy M
  - **Z3A.18** 18 weeks gestation of pregnancy M
    Coding Clinic: 2019, Q2, P11
  - **Z3A.19** 19 weeks gestation of pregnancy M
- **Z3A.2** Weeks of gestation of pregnancy, weeks 20-29
  - **Z3A.20** 20 weeks gestation of pregnancy M
    Coding Clinic: 2016, Q4, P6
  - **Z3A.21** 21 weeks gestation of pregnancy M
  - **Z3A.22** 22 weeks gestation of pregnancy M
    Coding Clinic: 2016, Q4, P6
  - **Z3A.23** 23 weeks gestation of pregnancy M
  - **Z3A.24** 24 weeks gestation of pregnancy M
  - **Z3A.25** 25 weeks gestation of pregnancy M
  - **Z3A.26** 26 weeks gestation of pregnancy M
  - **Z3A.27** 27 weeks gestation of pregnancy M
  - **Z3A.28** 28 weeks gestation of pregnancy M
  - **Z3A.29** 29 weeks gestation of pregnancy M
- **Z3A.3** Weeks of gestation of pregnancy, weeks 30-39
  - **Z3A.30** 30 weeks gestation of pregnancy M
  - **Z3A.31** 31 weeks gestation of pregnancy M
  - **Z3A.32** 32 weeks gestation of pregnancy M
    Coding Clinic: 2016, Q4, P6
  - **Z3A.33** 33 weeks gestation of pregnancy M
  - **Z3A.34** 34 weeks gestation of pregnancy M
  - **Z3A.35** 35 weeks gestation of pregnancy M
  - **Z3A.36** 36 weeks gestation of pregnancy M
  - **Z3A.37** 37 weeks gestation of pregnancy M
  - **Z3A.38** 38 weeks gestation of pregnancy M
    Coding Clinic: 2016, Q2, P34
  - **Z3A.39** 39 weeks gestation of pregnancy M

CHAPTER 21 (Z00-Z99)

● Z3A.4 Weeks of gestation of pregnancy, weeks 40 or greater
- ● Z3A.40 40 weeks gestation of pregnancy M
- ● Z3A.41 41 weeks gestation of pregnancy M
- ● Z3A.42 42 weeks gestation of pregnancy M
- ● Z3A.49 Greater than 42 weeks gestation of pregnancy M

● Z37 Outcome of delivery

This category is intended for use as an additional code to identify the outcome of delivery on the mother's record. It is not for use on the newborn record.

Excludes1 stillbirth (P95)

- ● Z37.0 Single live birth M
  - Coding Clinic: 2016, Q2, P34
- ● Z37.1 Single stillbirth M
- ● Z37.2 Twins, both liveborn M
- ● Z37.3 Twins, one liveborn and one stillborn M
- ● Z37.4 Twins, both stillborn M
- ● Z37.5 Other multiple births, all liveborn
  - ● Z37.50 Multiple births, unspecified, all liveborn M
  - ● Z37.51 Triplets, all liveborn M
  - ● Z37.52 Quadruplets, all liveborn M
  - ● Z37.53 Quintuplets, all liveborn M
  - ● Z37.54 Sextuplets, all liveborn M
  - ● Z37.59 Other multiple births, all liveborn M
- ● Z37.6 Other multiple births, some liveborn
  - ● Z37.60 Multiple births, unspecified, some liveborn M
  - ● Z37.61 Triplets, some liveborn M
  - ● Z37.62 Quadruplets, some liveborn M
  - ● Z37.63 Quintuplets, some liveborn M
  - ● Z37.64 Sextuplets, some liveborn M
  - ● Z37.69 Other multiple births, some liveborn M
- ● Z37.7 Other multiple births, all stillborn M
- ● Z37.9 Outcome of delivery, unspecified M
  - Multiple birth NOS
  - Single birth NOS

● Z38 Liveborn infants according to place of birth and type of delivery

This category is for use as the principal code on the initial record of a newborn baby. It is to be used for the initial birth record only. It is not to be used on the mother's record.

Coding Clinic: 2017, Q2, P6-7; 2016, Q4, P126-127, 130; 2015, Q2, P15

- ● Z38.0 Single liveborn infant, born in hospital
  - Single liveborn infant, born in birthing center or other health care facility
  - Coding Clinic: 2017, Q2, P5-7
  - Z38.00 Single liveborn infant, delivered vaginally N
    - Coding Clinic: 2021, Q4, P23; 2018, Q4, P26; 2016, Q4, P7, 55
  - Z38.01 Single liveborn infant, delivered by cesarean N
    - Coding Clinic: 2017, Q2, P7; 2016, Q3, P18
- Z38.1 Single liveborn infant, born outside hospital N
- Z38.2 Single liveborn infant, unspecified as to place of birth N
  - Single liveborn infant NOS
- ● Z38.3 Twin liveborn infant, born in hospital
  - Z38.30 Twin liveborn infant, delivered vaginally N
  - Z38.31 Twin liveborn infant, delivered by cesarean N
- Z38.4 Twin liveborn infant, born outside hospital N
- Z38.5 Twin liveborn infant, unspecified as to place of birth N
- ● Z38.6 Other multiple liveborn infant, born in hospital
  - Z38.61 Triplet liveborn infant, delivered vaginally N
  - Z38.62 Triplet liveborn infant, delivered by cesarean N
  - Z38.63 Quadruplet liveborn infant, delivered vaginally N
  - Z38.64 Quadruplet liveborn infant, delivered by cesarean N
  - Z38.65 Quintuplet liveborn infant, delivered vaginally N
  - Z38.66 Quintuplet liveborn infant, delivered by cesarean N
  - Z38.68 Other multiple liveborn infant, delivered vaginally N
  - Z38.69 Other multiple liveborn infant, delivered by cesarean N
- Z38.7 Other multiple liveborn infant, born outside hospital N
- Z38.8 Other multiple liveborn infant, unspecified as to place of birth N

● Z39 Encounter for maternal postpartum care and examination
- Z39.0 Encounter for care and examination of mother immediately after delivery M
  - Care and observation in uncomplicated cases when the delivery occurs outside a healthcare facility
  - **Excludes1** care for postpartum complication - see Alphabetic index
  - Coding Clinic: 2021, Q3, P13
- ● Z39.1 Encounter for care and examination of lactating mother M
  - Encounter for supervision of lactation
  - **Excludes1** disorders of lactation (O92.-)
- ● Z39.2 Encounter for routine postpartum follow-up M

ENCOUNTERS FOR OTHER SPECIFIC HEALTH CARE (Z40-Z53)

Categories Z40-Z53 are intended for use to indicate a reason for care. They may be used for patients who have already been treated for a disease or injury, but who are receiving aftercare or prophylactic care, or care to consolidate the treatment, or to deal with a residual state

Excludes2 follow-up examination for medical surveillance after treatment (Z08-Z09)

● Z40 Encounter for prophylactic surgery

Excludes1 organ donations (Z52.-)
therapeutic organ removal - code to condition

Coding Clinic: 2016, Q4, P79

- ● Z40.0 Encounter for prophylactic surgery for risk factors related to malignant neoplasms
  - Admission for prophylactic organ removal
  - Use additional code to identify risk factor
  - Z40.00 Encounter for prophylactic removal of unspecified organ
  - Z40.01 Encounter for prophylactic removal of breast
  - Z40.02 Encounter for prophylactic removal of ovary(s)
    - Encounter for prophylactic removal of ovary(s) and fallopian tube(s)
  - Z40.03 Encounter for prophylactic removal of fallopian tube(s)
  - Z40.09 Encounter for prophylactic removal of other organ
- ● Z40.8 Encounter for other prophylactic surgery
- ● Z40.9 Encounter for prophylactic surgery, unspecified

● Z41 Encounter for procedures for purposes other than remedying health state
- Z41.1 Encounter for cosmetic surgery
  - Encounter for cosmetic breast implant
  - Encounter for cosmetic procedure
  - **Excludes1** encounter for plastic and reconstructive surgery following medical procedure or healed injury (Z42.-)
    encounter for post-mastectomy breast implantation (Z42.1)
- Z41.2 Encounter for routine and ritual male circumcision
- ● Z41.3 Encounter for ear piercing
- Z41.8 Encounter for other procedures for purposes other than remedying health state
- ● Z41.9 Encounter for procedure for purposes other than remedying health state, unspecified

Z42 Encounter for plastic and reconstructive surgery following medical procedure or healed injury

Excludes1 encounter for cosmetic plastic surgery (Z41.1)
encounter for plastic surgery for treatment of current injury - code to relevent injury

Z42.1 Encounter for breast reconstruction following mastectomy A

Excludes1 deformity and disproportion of reconstructed breast (N65.1-)

Z42.8 Encounter for other plastic and reconstructive surgery following medical procedure or healed injury

Coding Clinic: 2017, Q1, P42

Z43 Encounter for attention to artificial openings

Includes closure of artificial openings
passage of sounds or bougies through artificial openings
reforming artificial openings
removal of catheter from artificial openings
toilet or cleansing of artificial openings

Excludes1 complications of external stoma (J95.Ø-, K94.-, N99.5-)

Excludes2 fitting and adjustment of prosthetic and other devices (Z44-Z46)

Z43.Ø Encounter for attention to tracheostomy

Z43.1 Encounter for attention to gastrostomy (Ex) PDX 2023

Excludes2 artificial opening status only, without need for care (Z93.-)

Z43.2 Encounter for attention to ileostomy

Coding Clinic: 2016, Q3, P5

Z43.3 Encounter for attention to colostomy

Z43.4 Encounter for attention to other artificial openings of digestive tract

Z43.5 Encounter for attention to cystostomy

Z43.6 Encounter for attention to other artificial openings of urinary tract

Encounter for attention to nephrostomy
Encounter for attention to ureterostomy
Encounter for attention to urethrostomy

Z43.7 Encounter for attention to artificial vagina

Z43.8 Encounter for attention to other artificial openings

Z43.9 Encounter for attention to unspecified artificial opening

Z44 Encounter for fitting and adjustment of external prosthetic device

Includes removal or replacement of external prosthetic device

Excludes1 malfunction or other complications of device - see Alphabetical Index presence of prosthetic device (Z97.-)

Z44.Ø Encounter for fitting and adjustment of artificial arm

Z44.ØØ Encounter for fitting and adjustment of unspecified artificial arm

Z44.ØØ1 Encounter for fitting and adjustment of unspecified right artificial arm

Z44.ØØ2 Encounter for fitting and adjustment of unspecified left artificial arm

Z44.ØØ9 Encounter for fitting and adjustment of unspecified artificial arm, unspecified arm

Z44.Ø1 Encounter for fitting and adjustment of complete artificial arm

Z44.Ø11 Encounter for fitting and adjustment of complete right artificial arm

Z44.Ø12 Encounter for fitting and adjustment of complete left artificial arm

Z44.Ø19 Encounter for fitting and adjustment of complete artificial arm, unspecified arm

Z44.Ø2 Encounter for fitting and adjustment of partial artificial arm

Z44.Ø21 Encounter for fitting and adjustment of partial artificial right arm

Z44.Ø22 Encounter for fitting and adjustment of partial artificial left arm

Z44.Ø29 Encounter for fitting and adjustment of partial artificial arm, unspecified arm

Z44.1 Encounter for fitting and adjustment of artificial leg

Z44.1Ø Encounter for fitting and adjustment of unspecified artificial leg

Z44.1Ø1 Encounter for fitting and adjustment of unspecified right artificial leg

Z44.1Ø2 Encounter for fitting and adjustment of unspecified left artificial leg

Z44.1Ø9 Encounter for fitting and adjustment of unspecified artificial leg, unspecified leg

Z44.11 Encounter for fitting and adjustment of complete artificial leg

Z44.111 Encounter for fitting and adjustment of complete right artificial leg

Z44.112 Encounter for fitting and adjustment of complete left artificial leg

Z44.119 Encounter for fitting and adjustment of complete artificial leg, unspecified leg

Z44.12 Encounter for fitting and adjustment of partial artificial leg

Z44.121 Encounter for fitting and adjustment of partial artificial right leg

Z44.122 Encounter for fitting and adjustment of partial artificial left leg

Z44.129 Encounter for fitting and adjustment of partial artificial leg, unspecified leg

Z44.2 Encounter for fitting and adjustment of artificial eye

Excludes1 mechanical complication of ocular prosthesis (T85.3)

Z44.2Ø Encounter for fitting and adjustment of artificial eye, unspecified

Z44.21 Encounter for fitting and adjustment of artificial right eye

Z44.22 Encounter for fitting and adjustment of artificial left eye

Z44.3 Encounter for fitting and adjustment of external breast prosthesis

Excludes1 complications of breast implant (T85.4-)
encounter for adjustment or removal of breast implant (Z45.81-)
encounter for initial breast implant insertion for cosmetic breast augmentation (Z41.1)
encounter for breast reconstruction following mastectomy (Z42.1)

Z44.3Ø Encounter for fitting and adjustment of external breast prosthesis, unspecified breast

Z44.31 Encounter for fitting and adjustment of external right breast prosthesis

Z44.32 Encounter for fitting and adjustment of external left breast prosthesis

Z44.8 Encounter for fitting and adjustment of other external prosthetic devices

Z44.9 Encounter for fitting and adjustment of unspecified external prosthetic device

Z45 Encounter for adjustment and management of implanted device

Includes removal or replacement of implanted device

Excludes1 malfunction or other complications of device - see Alphabetical Index

Excludes2 encounter for fitting and adjustment of non-implanted device (Z46.-)

Z45.Ø Encounter for adjustment and management of cardiac device

CHAPTER 21 (ZØØ-Z99)

- Z45.01 **Encounter for adjustment and management of cardiac pacemaker**
  - Encounter for adjustment and management of cardiac resynchronization therapy pacemaker (CRT-P)
  - **Excludes1** encounter for adjustment and management of automatic implantable cardiac defibrillator with synchronous cardiac pacemaker (Z45.02)
  - Z45.010 **Encounter for checking and testing of cardiac pacemaker pulse generator [battery]**
    - Encounter for replacing cardiac pacemaker pulse generator [battery]
    - MCE: Questionable admission when principal dx
  - Z45.018 **Encounter for adjustment and management of other part of cardiac pacemaker**
    - **Excludes1** presence of other part of cardiac pacemaker (Z95.0)
    - **Excludes2** presence of prosthetic and other devices (Z95.1-Z95.5, Z95.811-Z97)
    - MCE: Questionable admission when principal dx
- Z45.02 **Encounter for adjustment and management of automatic implantable cardiac defibrillator**
  - Encounter for adjustment and management of automatic implantable cardiac defibrillator with synchronous cardiac pacemaker
  - Encounter for adjustment and management of cardiac resynchronization therapy defibrillator (CRT-D)
  - MCE: Questionable admission when principal dx
  - Coding Clinic: 2024, Q1, P22,23
- Z45.09 **Encounter for adjustment and management of other cardiac device**
  - MCE: Questionable admission when principal dx

Z45.1 **Encounter for adjustment and management of infusion pump**

Z45.2 **Encounter for adjustment and management of vascular access device**
- Encounter for adjustment and management of vascular catheters
- **Excludes1** encounter for adjustment and management of renal dialysis catheter (Z49.01)

Z45.3 **Encounter for adjustment and management of implanted devices of the special senses**
- Z45.31 **Encounter for adjustment and management of implanted visual substitution device**
- Z45.32 **Encounter for adjustment and management of implanted hearing device**
  - **Excludes1** encounter for fitting and adjustment of hearing aid (Z46.1)
  - Z45.320 **Encounter for adjustment and management of bone conduction device**
  - Z45.321 **Encounter for adjustment and management of cochlear device**
  - Z45.328 **Encounter for adjustment and management of other implanted hearing device**

Z45.4 **Encounter for adjustment and management of implanted nervous system device**
- Z45.41 **Encounter for adjustment and management of cerebrospinal fluid drainage device**
  - Encounter for adjustment and management of cerebral ventricular (communicating) shunt
- Z45.42 **Encounter for adjustment and management of neuropacemaker**
  - Encounter for adjustment and management of brain neurostimulator
  - Encounter for adjustment and management of gastric neurostimulator
  - Encounter for adjustment and management of peripheral nerve neurostimulator
  - Encounter for adjustment and management of sacral nerve neurostimulator
  - Encounter for adjustment and management of spinal cord neurostimulator
  - Encounter for adjustment and management of vagus nerve neurostimulator
- Z45.49 **Encounter for adjustment and management of other implanted nervous system device**

Z45.8 **Encounter for adjustment and management of other implanted devices**
- Z45.81 **Encounter for adjustment or removal of breast implant**
  - Encounter for elective implant exchange (different material) (different size)
  - Encounter for removal of tissue expander with or without synchronous insertion of permanent implant
  - **Excludes1** complications of breast implant (T85.4-)
    - encounter for initial breast implant insertion for cosmetic breast augmentation (Z41.1)
    - encounter for breast reconstruction following mastectomy (Z42.1)
  - Z45.811 **Encounter for adjustment or removal of right breast implant**
  - Z45.812 **Encounter for adjustment or removal of left breast implant**
  - Z45.819 **Encounter for adjustment or removal of unspecified breast implant**
- Z45.82 **Encounter for adjustment or removal of myringotomy device (stent) (tube)**
- Z45.89 **Encounter for adjustment and management of other implanted devices**

Z45.9 **Encounter for adjustment and management of unspecified implanted device**

Z46 Encounter for fitting and adjustment of other devices

- **Includes** removal or replacement of other device
- **Excludes1** malfunction or other complications of device - see Alphabetical Index
- **Excludes2** encounter for fitting and management of implanted devices (Z45.-)
  - issue of repeat prescription only (Z76.0)
  - presence of prosthetic and other devices (Z95-Z97)

Z46.0 **Encounter for fitting and adjustment of spectacles and contact lenses**

Z46.1 **Encounter for fitting and adjustment of hearing aid**
- **Excludes1** encounter for adjustment and management of implanted hearing device (Z45.32-)

Z46.2 **Encounter for fitting and adjustment of other devices related to nervous system and special senses**
- **Excludes2** encounter for adjustment and management of implanted nervous system device (Z45.4-)
  - encounter for adjustment and management of implanted visual substitution device (Z45.31)

Z46.3 **Encounter for fitting and adjustment of dental prosthetic device**
- Encounter for fitting and adjustment of dentures

Z46.4 **Encounter for fitting and adjustment of orthodontic device**

Z46.5 Encounter for fitting and adjustment of other gastrointestinal appliance and device
Excludes1 encounter for attention to artificial openings of digestive tract (Z43.1-Z43.4)

Z46.51 Encounter for fitting and adjustment of gastric lap band

Z46.59 Encounter for fitting and adjustment of other gastrointestinal appliance and device

Z46.6 Encounter for fitting and adjustment of urinary device
Excludes2 attention to artificial openings of urinary tract (Z43.5, Z43.6)

Z46.8 Encounter for fitting and adjustment of other specified devices

Z46.81 Encounter for fitting and adjustment of insulin pump
Encounter for insulin pump instruction and training
Encounter for insulin pump titration

Z46.82 Encounter for fitting and adjustment of non-vascular catheter

Z46.89 Encounter for fitting and adjustment of other specified devices
Encounter for fitting and adjustment of wheelchair

Z46.9 Encounter for fitting and adjustment of unspecified device

Z47 Orthopedic aftercare
Excludes1 aftercare for healing fracture - code to fracture with 7th character D

Z47.1 Aftercare following joint replacement surgery
Use additional code to identify the joint (Z96.6-)
Coding Clinic: 2020, Q1, P23-24

Z47.2 Encounter for removal of internal fixation device
Excludes1 encounter for adjustment of internal fixation device for fracture treatment - code to fracture with appropriate 7th character
encounter for removal of external fixation device - code to fracture with 7th character D
infection or inflammatory reaction to internal fixation device (T84.6-)
mechanical complication of internal fixation device (T84.1-)

Z47.3 Aftercare following explantation of joint prosthesis
Aftercare following explantation of joint prosthesis, staged procedure
Encounter for joint prosthesis insertion following prior explantation of joint prosthesis
Coding Clinic: 2020, Q1, P23; 2015, Q1, P17

Z47.31 Aftercare following explantation of shoulder joint prosthesis
Excludes1 acquired absence of shoulder joint following prior explantation of shoulder joint prosthesis (Z89.23-)
shoulder joint prosthesis explantation status (Z89.23-)

Z47.32 Aftercare following explantation of hip joint prosthesis
Excludes1 acquired absence of hip joint following prior explantation of hip joint prosthesis (Z89.62-)
hip joint prosthesis explantation status (Z89.62-)
Coding Clinic: 2015, Q1, P17

Z47.33 Aftercare following explantation of knee joint prosthesis
Excludes1 acquired absence of knee joint following prior explantation of knee prosthesis (Z89.52-)
knee joint prosthesis explantation status (Z89.52-)

Z47.8 Encounter for other orthopedic aftercare

Z47.81 Encounter for orthopedic aftercare following surgical amputation
Use additional code to identify the limb amputated (Z89.-)

Z47.82 Encounter for orthopedic aftercare following scoliosis surgery

Z47.89 Encounter for other orthopedic aftercare
Coding Clinic: 2015, Q1, P8

Z48 Encounter for other postprocedural aftercare
Excludes1 encounter for aftercare following injury - code to Injury, by site, with appropriate 7th character for subsequent encounter
encounter for follow-up examination after completed treatment (Z08-Z09)
Excludes2 encounter for attention to artificial openings (Z43.-)
encounter for fitting and adjustment of prosthetic and other devices (Z44-Z46)

Z48.0 Encounter for attention to dressings, sutures and drains
Excludes1 encounter for planned postprocedural wound closure (Z48.1)

Z48.00 Encounter for change or removal of nonsurgical wound dressing
Encounter for change or removal of wound dressing NOS

Z48.01 Encounter for change or removal of surgical wound dressing
Coding Clinic: 2019, Q2, P33; 2015, Q4, P38

Z48.02 Encounter for removal of sutures
Encounter for removal of staples
Coding Clinic: 2015, Q1, P6

Z48.03 Encounter for change or removal of drains

Z48.1 Encounter for planned postprocedural wound closure
Excludes1 encounter for attention to dressings and sutures (Z48.0-)

Z48.2 Encounter for aftercare following organ transplant

Z48.21 Encounter for aftercare following heart transplant (Ex) PDX 2024
CC when PDx is its own CC

Z48.22 Encounter for aftercare following kidney transplant (Ex) PDX 2025
CC when PDx is its own CC

Z48.23 Encounter for aftercare following liver transplant (Ex) PDX 2026
CC when PDx is its own CC

Z48.24 Encounter for aftercare following lung transplant (Ex) PDX 2027
CC when PDx is its own CC

Z48.28 Encounter for aftercare following multiple organ transplant

Z48.280 Encounter for aftercare following heart-lung transplant (Ex) PDX 2028
CC when PDx is its own CC

Z48.288 Encounter for aftercare following multiple organ transplant

Z48.29 Encounter for aftercare following other organ transplant

Z48.290 Encounter for aftercare following bone marrow transplant (Ex) PDX 2029
CC when PDx is its own CC

Z48.298 Encounter for aftercare following other organ transplant

Z48.3 Aftercare following surgery for neoplasm
Use additional code to identify the neoplasm

Z48.8 Encounter for other specified postprocedural aftercare

● Z48.81 Encounter for surgical aftercare following surgery on specified body systems
These codes identify the body system requiring aftercare. They are for use in conjunction with other aftercare codes to fully explain the aftercare encounter. The condition treated should also be coded if still present.
Excludes1 aftercare for injury - code the injury with 7th character D
aftercare following surgery for neoplasm (Z48.3)
Excludes2 aftercare following organ transplant (Z48.2-)
orthopedic aftercare (Z47.-)

Z48.810 Encounter for surgical aftercare following surgery on the sense organs

Z48.811 Encounter for surgical aftercare following surgery on the nervous system
Excludes2 encounter for surgical aftercare following surgery on the sense organs (Z48.810)

Z48.812 Encounter for surgical aftercare following surgery on the circulatory system
Coding Clinic: 2012, Q4, P96

Z48.813 Encounter for surgical aftercare following surgery on the respiratory system
Coding Clinic: 2019, Q2, P33

Z48.814 Encounter for surgical aftercare following surgery on the teeth or oral cavity

Z48.815 Encounter for surgical aftercare following surgery on the digestive system
Coding Clinic: 2015, Q4, P38

Z48.816 Encounter for surgical aftercare following surgery on the genitourinary system
Excludes1 encounter for aftercare following sterilization reversal (Z31.42)

Z48.817 Encounter for surgical aftercare following surgery on the skin and subcutaneous tissue
Coding Clinic: 2015, Q1, P6

Z48.89 Encounter for other specified surgical aftercare

● Z49 Encounter for care involving renal dialysis
Code also associated end stage renal disease (N18.6)

● Z49.0 Preparatory care for renal dialysis
Encounter for dialysis instruction and training

● Z49.01 Encounter for fitting and adjustment of extracorporeal dialysis catheter
Removal or replacement of renal dialysis catheter
Toilet or cleansing of renal dialysis catheter

● Z49.02 Encounter for fitting and adjustment of peritoneal dialysis catheter

● Z49.3 Encounter for adequacy testing for dialysis

● Z49.31 Encounter for adequacy testing for hemodialysis

● Z49.32 Encounter for adequacy testing for peritoneal dialysis
Encounter for peritoneal equilibration test

● Z51 Encounter for other aftercare and medical care
Code also condition requiring care
Excludes1 follow-up examination after treatment (Z08-Z09)
Coding Clinic: 2017, Q1, P49; 2016, Q4, P130

Z51.0 Encounter for antineoplastic radiation therapy
Coding Clinic: 2017, Q4, P103

● Z51.1 Encounter for antineoplastic chemotherapy and immunotherapy
Excludes2 encounter for chemotherapy and immunotherapy for nonneoplastic condition-code to condition

Z51.11 Encounter for antineoplastic chemotherapy
Coding Clinic: 2022, Q1, P16; 2015, Q3, P19

Z51.12 Encounter for antineoplastic immunotherapy
Coding Clinic: 2024, Q1, P24

Z51.5 Encounter for palliative care
Coding Clinic: 2022, Q1, P19; 2017, Q1, P48-49

● Z51.6 Encounter for desensitization to allergens
Coding Clinic: 2016, Q4, P77-79

● Z51.8 Encounter for other specified aftercare
Excludes1 holiday relief care (Z75.5)

Z51.81 Encounter for therapeutic drug level monitoring
Code also any long-term (current) drug therapy (Z79.-)
Excludes1 encounter for blood-drug test for administrative or medicolegal reasons (Z02.83)

● Z51.89 Encounter for other specified aftercare
MCE: This code may be considered "acceptable" when a secondary diagnosis is also coded on the record.
Coding Clinic: 2012, Q4, P96-97

▶ Z51.A Encounter for sepsis aftercare

● Z52 Donors of organs and tissues
Includes autologous and other living donors
Excludes1 cadaveric donor - omit code
examination of potential donor (Z00.5)
Coding Clinic: 2012, Q4, P100

● Z52.0 Blood donor

● Z52.00 Unspecified blood donor

● Z52.000 Unspecified donor, whole blood

● Z52.001 Unspecified donor, stem cells

● Z52.008 Unspecified donor, other blood

● Z52.01 Autologous blood donor

● Z52.010 Autologous donor, whole blood

● Z52.011 Autologous donor, stem cells

● Z52.018 Autologous donor, other blood

● Z52.09 Other blood donor
Volunteer donor

● Z52.090 Other blood donor, whole blood

● Z52.091 Other blood donor, stem cells

● Z52.098 Other blood donor, other blood

● Z52.1 Skin donor

Z52.10 Skin donor, unspecified

Z52.11 Skin donor, autologous

Z52.19 Skin donor, other

● Z52.2 Bone donor

Z52.20 Bone donor, unspecified

Z52.21 Bone donor, autologous

Z52.29 Bone donor, other

Z52.3 Bone marrow donor

Z52.4 Kidney donor

Z52.5 Cornea donor

Z52.6 Liver donor
Coding Clinic: 2012, Q4, P100

● Z52.8 Donor of other specified organs or tissues

● Z52.81 Egg (Oocyte) donor

● Z52.810 Egg (Oocyte) donor under age 35, anonymous recipient
Egg donor under age 35 NOS

CHAPTER 21 (Z00-Z99)

Z52.811 Egg (Oocyte) donor under age 35, designated recipient

Z52.812 Egg (Oocyte) donor age 35 and over, anonymous recipient
Egg donor age 35 and over NOS

Z52.813 Egg (Oocyte) donor age 35 and over, designated recipient

Z52.819 Egg (Oocyte) donor, unspecified

Z52.89 Donor of other specified organs or tissues

Z52.9 Donor of unspecified organ or tissue
Donor NOS

Z53 Persons encountering health services for specific procedures and treatment, not carried out

Z53.0 Procedure and treatment not carried out because of contraindication

Z53.01 Procedure and treatment not carried out due to patient smoking

Z53.09 Procedure and treatment not carried out because of other contraindication

Z53.1 Procedure and treatment not carried out because of patient's decision for reasons of belief and group pressure

Z53.2 Procedure and treatment not carried out because of patient's decision for other and unspecified reasons

Z53.20 Procedure and treatment not carried out because of patient's decision for unspecified reasons

Z53.21 Procedure and treatment not carried out due to patient leaving prior to being seen by health care provider

Z53.29 Procedure and treatment not carried out because of patient's decision for other reasons

Z53.3 Procedure converted to open procedure
Coding Clinic: 2016, Q4, P79

Z53.31 Laparoscopic surgical procedure converted to open procedure
Coding Clinic: 2016, Q4, P100

Z53.32 Thoracoscopic surgical procedure converted to open procedure

Z53.33 Arthroscopic surgical procedure converted to open procedure

Z53.39 Other specified procedure converted to open procedure

Z53.8 Procedure and treatment not carried out for other reasons

Z53.9 Procedure and treatment not carried out, unspecified reason

PERSONS WITH POTENTIAL HEALTH HAZARDS RELATED TO SOCIOECONOMIC AND PSYCHOSOCIAL CIRCUMSTANCES (Z55-Z65)

Z55 Problems related to education and literacy
Excludes1 disorders of psychological development (F80-F89)

Z55.0 Illiteracy and low-level literacy

Z55.1 Schooling unavailable and unattainable

Z55.2 Failed school examinations

Z55.3 Underachievement in school

Z55.4 Educational maladjustment and discord with teachers and classmates

Z55.5 Less than a high school diploma
No general equivalence degree (GED)

Z55.6 Problems related to health literacy
Difficulty understanding health related information
Difficulty understanding medication instructions
Problem completing medical forms

Z55.8 Other problems related to education and literacy
Problems related to inadequate teaching

Z55.9 Problems related to education and literacy, unspecified
Academic problems NOS

Z56 Problems related to employment and unemployment
Excludes2 occupational exposure to risk factors (Z57.-)
problems related to housing and economic circumstances (Z59.-)

Z56.0 Unemployment, unspecified

Z56.1 Change of job A

Z56.2 Threat of job loss

Z56.3 Stressful work schedule

Z56.4 Discord with boss and workmates

Z56.5 Uncongenial work environment
Difficult conditions at work

Z56.6 Other physical and mental strain related to work

Z56.8 Other problems related to employment

Z56.81 Sexual harassment on the job

Z56.82 Military deployment status
Individual (civilian or military) currently deployed in theater or in support of military war, peacekeeping and humanitarian operations

Z56.89 Other problems related to employment

Z56.9 Unspecified problems related to employment
Occupational problems NOS

Z57 Occupational exposure to risk factors

Z57.0 Occupational exposure to noise

Z57.1 Occupational exposure to radiation

Z57.2 Occupational exposure to dust

Z57.3 Occupational exposure to other air contaminants

Z57.31 Occupational exposure to environmental tobacco smoke
Excludes2 exposure to environmental tobacco smoke (Z77.22)

Z57.39 Occupational exposure to other air contaminants

Z57.4 Occupational exposure to toxic agents in agriculture
Occupational exposure to solids, liquids, gases or vapors in agriculture

Z57.5 Occupational exposure to toxic agents in other industries
Occupational exposure to solids, liquids, gases or vapors in other industries

Z57.6 Occupational exposure to extreme temperature

Z57.7 Occupational exposure to vibration

Z57.8 Occupational exposure to other risk factors

Z57.9 Occupational exposure to unspecified risk factor

Z58 Problems related to physical environment
Excludes2 occupational exposure (Z57.-)

Z58.6 Inadequate drinking-water supply
Lack of safe drinking water
Excludes2 deprivation of water (T73.1)

Z58.8 Other problems related to physical environment

Z58.81 Basic services unavailable in physical environment
Unable to obtain internet service, due to unavailability in geographic area
Unable to obtain telephone service, due to unavailability in geographic area
Unable to obtain utilities, due to inadequate physical environment

Z58.89 Other problems related to physical environment

Z59 Problems related to housing and economic circumstances
Excludes2 problems related to upbringing (Z62.-)

Z59.0 Homelessness (Ex) No exclusions

Z59.00 Homelessness unspecified

Z59.01 Sheltered homelessness
Doubled up
Living in a shelter such as: motel, scattered site housing, temporary or transitional living situation

Z59.02 Unsheltered homelessness
Residing in place not meant for human habitation such as: abandoned buildings, cars, parks, sidewalk
Residing on the street

CHAPTER 21 (Z00-Z99)

● Z59.1 **Inadequate housing**

~~Excludes1 problems related to the natural and physical environment (Z77.1-)~~

▶ **Excludes1** problems related to the natural and physical environment (Z77.1-)

● Z59.10 **Inadequate housing, unspecified**
Inadequate housing NOS

● Z59.11 **Inadequate housing environmental temperature**
Lack of air conditioning
Lack of heating

● Z59.12 **Inadequate housing utilities**
Lack of electricity services
Lack of gas services
Lack of oil services
Lack of water services
Excludes2 basic services unavailable in physical environment (Z58.81)
lack of adequate food (Z59.4-)
other problems related to housing and economic circumstances (Z59.8-)

● Z59.19 **Other inadequate housing**
Pest infestation
Restriction of space
Technical defects in home preventing adequate care
Unsatisfactory surroundings

● Z59.2 **Discord with neighbors, lodgers and landlord**

● Z59.3 **Problems related to living in residential institution**
Boarding-school resident
Excludes1 institutional upbringing (Z62.22)

● Z59.4 **Lack of adequate food**
Excludes2 deprivation of food (T73.0)
effects of hunger (T73.0)
inappropriate diet or eating habits (Z72.4)
malnutrition (E40-E46)

● Z59.41 **Food insecurity**

● Z59.48 **Other specified lack of adequate food**
Inadequate food
Lack of food

● Z59.5 **Extreme poverty**

● Z59.6 **Low income**

● Z59.7 **Insufficient social insurance and welfare support**

● Z59.71 **Insufficient health insurance coverage**
Inadequate social insurance
Insufficient social insurance
No health insurance coverage

● Z59.72 **Insufficient welfare support**
Inadequate welfare support

● Z59.8 **Other problems related to housing and economic circumstances**

● Z59.81 **Housing instability, housed**
Foreclosure on home loan
Past due on rent or mortgage
Unwanted multiple moves in the last 12 months

● Z59.811 **Housing instability, housed, with risk of homelessness**
Imminent risk of homelessness

● Z59.812 **Housing instability, housed, homelessness in past 12 months**

● Z59.819 **Housing instability, housed unspecified**
Excludes2 extreme poverty (Z59.5)
financial insecurity (Z59.86)
low income (Z59.6)
material hardship due to limited financial resources, not elsewhere classified (Z59.87)

● Z59.82 **Transportation insecurity**
Excessive transportation time
Inaccessible transportation
Inadequate transportation
Lack of transportation
Unaffordable transportation
Unreliable transportation
Unsafe transportation
Excludes2 unavailability and inaccessibility of healthcare facilities (Z75.3)

● Z59.86 **Financial insecurity**
Bankruptcy
Burdensome debt
Economic strain
Financial strain
Money problems
Running out of money
Unable to make ends meet
Excludes2 extreme poverty (Z59.5)
low income (Z59.6)
material hardship, not elsewhere classified (Z59.87)

● Z59.87 **Material hardship due to limited financial resources, not elsewhere classified**
Material deprivation due to limited financial resources
Unable to obtain adequate childcare due to limited financial resources
Unable to obtain adequate clothing due to limited financial resources
Unable to obtain adequate utilities due to limited financial resources
Unable to obtain basic needs due to limited financial resources
Excludes2 extreme poverty (Z59.5)
financial insecurity, not elsewhere classified (Z59.86)
low income (Z59.6)

● Z59.89 **Other problems related to housing and economic circumstances**
Foreclosure on loan
Isolated dwelling
Problems with creditors

● Z59.9 **Problem related to housing and economic circumstances, unspecified**

● Z60 **Problems related to social environment**

● Z60.0 **Problems of adjustment to life-cycle transitions**
Empty nest syndrome
Phase of life problem
Problem with adjustment to retirement [pension]

● Z60.2 **Problems related to living alone**

● Z60.3 **Acculturation difficulty**
Problem with migration
Problem with social transplantation

● Z60.4 **Social exclusion and rejection**
Exclusion and rejection on the basis of personal characteristics, such as unusual physical appearance, illness or behavior.
Social isolation
Excludes1 target of adverse discrimination such as for racial or religious reasons (Z60.5)

● Z60.5 **Target of (perceived) adverse discrimination and persecution**
Excludes1 social exclusion and rejection (Z60.4)

● Z60.8 **Other problems related to social environment**
Inadequate social support
Lack of emotional support

● Z60.9 **Problem related to social environment, unspecified**

Z62 Problems related to upbringing

Includes current and past negative life events in childhood
current and past problems of a child related to upbringing

Excludes2 maltreatment syndrome (T74.-)
problems related to housing and economic circumstances (Z59.-)

Z62.0 Inadequate parental supervision and control

Z62.1 Parental overprotection

Z62.2 Upbringing away from parents

Excludes1 problems with boarding school (Z59.3)

Z62.21 Child in welfare custody P
Child in foster care
Child in welfare guardianship

Z62.22 Institutional upbringing
Child living in group home
Child living in orphanage
Code also, if applicable, child in welfare custody (Z62.21)

Z62.23 Child in custody of non-parental relative
Child in care of non-parental family member
Child in custody of grandparent
Child in kinship care
Guardianship by non-parental relative
Code also, if applicable, child in welfare custody (Z62.21)

Z62.24 Child in custody of non-relative guardian
Code also, if applicable, child in welfare custody (Z62.21)

Z62.29 Other upbringing away from parents

Z62.3 Hostility towards and scapegoating of child P

Z62.6 Inappropriate (excessive) parental pressure

Z62.8 Other specified problems related to upbringing

Code also, if applicable:
absence of family member (Z63.3-)
disappearance and death of family member (Z63.4)
disruption of family by separation and divorce (Z63.5)
other specified problems related to primary support group (Z63.8)
other stressful life events affecting family and household (Z63.7-)

Z62.81 Personal history of abuse in childhood
Personal history of abuse in adolescence

Z62.810 Personal history of physical and sexual abuse in childhood

Excludes1 current child physical abuse (T74.12, T76.12)
current child sexual abuse (T74.22, T76.22)

Z62.811 Personal history of psychological abuse in childhood

Excludes1 current child psychological abuse (T74.32, T76.32)

Z62.812 Personal history of neglect in childhood

Excludes1 current child neglect (T74.02, T76.02)

Z62.813 Personal history of forced labor or sexual exploitation in childhood

Z62.814 Personal history of child financial abuse

Excludes1 current child financial abuse (T74.A2)

Z62.815 Personal history of intimate partner abuse in childhood

Excludes2 adult and child abuse, neglect and other maltreatment, confirmed (T74.-)

Z62.819 Personal history of unspecified abuse in childhood

Excludes1 current child abuse NOS (T74.92, T76.92)

Z62.82 Parent-child conflict

Z62.820 Parent-biological child conflict
Parent-child problem NOS

Z62.821 Parent-adopted child conflict

Z62.822 Parent-foster child conflict

Z62.823 Parent-step child conflict

Z62.83 Non-parental relative or guardian-child conflict

Z62.831 Non-parental relative-child conflict
Grandparent-child conflict
Kinship-care child conflict
Non-parental relative legal guardian-child conflict
Other relative-child conflict

Excludes1 group home staff-child conflict (Z62.833)

Z62.832 Non-relative guardian-child conflict

Excludes1 group home staff-child conflict (Z62.833)

Z62.833 Group home staff-child conflict

Z62.89 Other specified problems related to upbringing

Z62.890 Parent-child estrangement NEC

Z62.891 Sibling rivalry

Z62.892 Runaway [from current living environment]
Child leaving living situation without permission

Z62.898 Other specified problems related to upbringing

Z62.9 Problem related to upbringing, unspecified

Z63 Other problems related to primary support group, including family circumstances

Excludes2 maltreatment syndrome (T74.-, T76)
parent-child problems (Z62.-)
problems related to negative life events in childhood (Z62.-)
problems related to upbringing (Z62.-)

Z63.0 Problems in relationship with spouse or partner
Relationship distress with spouse or intimate partner

Excludes1 counseling for spousal or partner abuse problems (Z69.1)
counseling related to sexual attitude, behavior, and orientation (Z70.-)

Z63.1 Problems in relationship with in-laws

Z63.3 Absence of family member

Excludes1 absence of family member due to disappearance and death (Z63.4)
absence of family member due to separation and divorce (Z63.5)

Z63.31 Absence of family member due to military deployment
Individual or family affected by other family member being on military deployment

Excludes1 family disruption due to return of family member from military deployment (Z63.71)

Z63.32 Other absence of family member

Z63.4 Disappearance and death of family member
Assumed death of family member
Bereavement

Z63.5 Disruption of family by separation and divorce
Marital estrangement

Z63.6 Dependent relative needing care at home

Z63.7 **Other stressful life events affecting family and household**

Z63.71 **Stress on family due to return of family member from military deployment**
Individual or family affected by family member having returned from military deployment (current or past conflict)

Z63.72 **Alcoholism and drug addiction in family**

Z63.79 **Other stressful life events affecting family and household**
Anxiety (normal) about sick person in family
Health problems within family
Ill or disturbed family member
Isolated family

Z63.8 **Other specified problems related to primary support group**
Family discord NOS
Family estrangement NOS
High expressed emotional level within family
Inadequate family support NOS
Inadequate or distorted communication within family

Z63.9 **Problem related to primary support group, unspecified**
Relationship disorder NOS

Z64 **Problems related to certain psychosocial circumstances**

Z64.0 **Problems related to unwanted pregnancy**

Z64.1 **Problems related to multiparity**

Z64.4 **Discord with counselors**
Discord with probation officer
Discord with social worker

Z65 **Problems related to other psychosocial circumstances**

Z65.0 **Conviction in civil and criminal proceedings without imprisonment**

Z65.1 **Imprisonment and other incarceration**

Z65.2 **Problems related to release from prison**

Z65.3 **Problems related to other legal circumstances**
Arrest
Child custody or support proceedings
Litigation
Prosecution

Z65.4 **Victim of crime and terrorism**
Victim of torture

Z65.5 **Exposure to disaster, war and other hostilities**
Excludes1 target of perceived discrimination or persecution (Z60.5)

Z65.8 **Other specified problems related to psychosocial circumstances**
At risk for feeling loneliness
Religious or spiritual problem

Z65.9 **Problem related to unspecified psychosocial circumstances**

DO NOT RESUSCITATE STATUS (Z66)

Z66 **Do not resuscitate**
DNR status

BLOOD TYPE (Z67)

Z67 **Blood type**
Coding Clinic: 2015, Q3, P40

Z67.1 **Type A blood**

Z67.10 **Type A blood, Rh positive**

Z67.11 **Type A blood, Rh negative**

Z67.2 **Type B blood**

Z67.20 **Type B blood, Rh positive**

Z67.21 **Type B blood, Rh negative**

Z67.3 **Type AB blood**

Z67.30 **Type AB blood, Rh positive**

Z67.31 **Type AB blood, Rh negative**

Z67.4 **Type O blood**

Z67.40 **Type O blood, Rh positive**

Z67.41 **Type O blood, Rh negative**

Z67.9 **Unspecified blood type**

Z67.90 **Unspecified blood type, Rh positive**

Z67.91 **Unspecified blood type, Rh negative**
Coding Clinic: 2015, Q3, P40

▶Z67.A **Duffy phenotype**

▶Z67.A1 **Duffy null**
▶Duffy phenotype Fy(a-b-)

▶Z67.A2 **Duffy a positive**
▶Duffy phenotype Fy(a+b-)

▶Z67.A3 **Duffy b positive**
▶Duffy phenotype Fy(a-b+)

▶Z67.A4 **Duffy a and b positive**
▶Duffy phenotype Fy(a+b+)

BODY MASS INDEX [BMI] (Z68)

OGCR Section I.B.14.

General Coding Guidelines

14. Documentation for BMI, Depth of Non-pressure ulcers, Pressure Ulcer Stages, Coma Scale, and NIH Stroke Scale

For the Body Mass Index (BMI), depth of non-pressure chronic ulcers, pressure ulcer stage, coma scale, and NIH stroke scale (NIHSS) codes, code assignment may be based on medical record documentation from clinicians who are not the patient's provider (i.e., physician or other qualified healthcare practitioner legally accountable for establishing the patient's diagnosis), since this information is typically documented by other clinicians involved in the care of the patient (e.g., a dietitian often documents the BMI, a nurse often documents the pressure ulcer stages, and an emergency medical technician often documents the coma scale). However, the associated diagnosis (such as overweight, obesity, acute stroke, or pressure ulcer) must be documented by the patient's provider. If there is conflicting medical record documentation, either from the same clinician or different clinicians, the patient's attending provider should be queried for clarification.

The BMI, coma scale, and NIHSS codes should only be reported as secondary diagnoses.

Z68 **Body mass index [BMI]**
Kilograms per meters squared
Note: BMI adult codes are for use for persons 20 years of age or older.
BMI pediatric codes are for use for persons 2-19 years of age.
These percentiles are based on the growth charts published by the Centers for Disease Control and Prevention (CDC)
Coding Clinic: 2018, Q4, P81; 2016, Q4, P129

Z68.1 **Body mass index [BMI] 19.9 or less, adult** (Ex) PDX 2030 A
Coding Clinic: 2017, Q1, P39

Z68.2 **Body mass index [BMI] 20-29, adult**

Z68.20 **Body mass index [BMI] 20.0-20.9, adult** A

Z68.21 **Body mass index [BMI] 21.0-21.9, adult** A

Z68.22 **Body mass index [BMI] 22.0-22.9, adult** A

Z68.23 **Body mass index [BMI] 23.0-23.9, adult** A

Z68.24 **Body mass index [BMI] 24.0-24.9, adult** A

Z68.25 **Body mass index [BMI] 25.0-25.9, adult** A

Z68.26 **Body mass index [BMI] 26.0-26.9, adult** A

Z68.27 **Body mass index [BMI] 27.0-27.9, adult** A

Z68.28 **Body mass index [BMI] 28.0-28.9, adult** A

Z68.29 **Body mass index [BMI] 29.0-29.9, adult** A

Z68.3 **Body mass index [BMI] 30-39, adult**

Z68.30 **Body mass index [BMI] 30.0-30.9, adult** A

Z68.31 **Body mass index [BMI] 31.0-31.9, adult** A

Z68.32 **Body mass index [BMI] 32.0-32.9, adult** A

Z68.33 **Body mass index [BMI] 33.0-33.9, adult** A

Z68.34 **Body mass index [BMI] 34.0-34.9, adult** A

Z68.35 **Body mass index [BMI] 35.0-35.9, adult** A
Coding Clinic: 2022, Q3, P6

Z68.36 **Body mass index [BMI] 36.0-36.9, adult** A

Z68.37 **Body mass index [BMI] 37.0-37.9, adult** A

- **Z68.38 Body mass index [BMI] 38.0-38.9, adult** A
- **Z68.39 Body mass index [BMI] 39.0-39.9, adult** A

Z68.4 Body mass index [BMI] 40 or greater, adult (Ex) PDX 2031

- **Z68.41 Body mass index [BMI] 40.0-44.9, adult** A
- **Z68.42 Body mass index [BMI] 45.0-49.9, adult** A
- **Z68.43 Body mass index [BMI] 50.0-59.9, adult** A
- **Z68.44 Body mass index [BMI] 60.0-69.9, adult** A
- **Z68.45 Body mass index [BMI] 70 or greater, adult** A

Z68.5 Body mass index [BMI] pediatric (Ex) PDX 2031
Coding Clinic: 2018, Q4, P81

- **Z68.51 Body mass index [BMI] pediatric, less than 5th percentile for age**
  Coding Clinic: 2018, Q4, P82
- **Z68.52 Body mass index [BMI] pediatric, 5th percentile to less than 85th percentile for age**
- **Z68.53 Body mass index [BMI] pediatric, 85th percentile to less than 95th percentile for age**
- **Z68.54 Body mass index [BMI] pediatric, 95th percentile for age to less than 120% of the 95th percentile for age**
- **Z68.55 Body mass index [BMI] pediatric, 120% of the 95th percentile for age to less than 140% of the 95th percentile for age**
- **Z68.56 Body mass index [BMI] pediatric, greater than or equal to 140% of the 95th percentile for age**

PERSONS ENCOUNTERING HEALTH SERVICES IN OTHER CIRCUMSTANCES (Z69-Z76)

Z69 Encounter for mental health services for victim and perpetrator of abuse

Includes counseling for victims and perpetrators of abuse

Z69.0 Encounter for mental health services for child abuse problems

Z69.01 Encounter for mental health services for parental child abuse

Z69.010 Encounter for mental health services for victim of parental child abuse P
Encounter for mental health services for victim of child abuse by parent
Encounter for mental health services for victim of child neglect by parent
Encounter for mental health services for victim of child psychological abuse by parent
Encounter for mental health services for victim of child sexual abuse by parent

Z69.011 Encounter for mental health services for perpetrator of parental child abuse
Encounter for mental health services for perpetrator of parental child neglect
Encounter for mental health services for perpetrator of parental child psychological abuse
Encounter for mental health services for perpetrator of parental child sexual abuse

Excludes1 encounter for mental health services for non-parental child abuse (Z69.02-)

Z69.02 Encounter for mental health services for non-parental child abuse

Z69.020 Encounter for mental health services for victim of non-parental child abuse P
Encounter for mental health services for victim of non-parental child neglect
Encounter for mental health services for victim of non-parental child psychological abuse
Encounter for mental health services for victim of non-parental child sexual abuse

Z69.021 Encounter for mental health services for perpetrator of non- parental child abuse
Encounter for mental health services for perpetrator of non-parental child neglect
Encounter for mental health services for perpetrator of non-parental child psychological abuse
Encounter for mental health services for perpetrator of non-parental child sexual abuse

Z69.1 Encounter for mental health services for spousal or partner abuse problems

Z69.11 Encounter for mental health services for victim of spousal or partner abuse
Encounter for mental health services for victim of spouse or partner neglect
Encounter for mental health services for victim of spouse or partner psychological abuse
Encounter for mental health services for victim of spouse or partner violence, physical

Z69.12 Encounter for mental health services for perpetrator of spousal or partner abuse
Encounter for mental health services for perpetrator of spouse or partner neglect
Encounter for mental health services for perpetrator of spouse or partner psychological abuse
Encounter for mental health services for perpetrator of spouse or partner violence, physical
Encounter for mental health services for perpetrator of spouse or partner violence, sexual

Z69.8 Encounter for mental health services for victim or perpetrator of other abuse

Z69.81 Encounter for mental health services for victim of other abuse
Encounter for mental health services for victim of non-spousal adult abuse
Encounter for mental health services for victim of spouse or partner violence, sexual
Encounter for rape victim counseling

Z69.82 Encounter for mental health services for perpetrator of other abuse
Encounter for mental health services for perpetrator of non-spousal adult abuse

Z70 Counseling related to sexual attitude, behavior and orientation

Includes encounter for mental health services for sexual attitude, behavior and orientation

Excludes2 contraceptive or procreative counseling (Z30-Z31)

Z70.0 Counseling related to sexual attitude

Z70.1 Counseling related to patient's sexual behavior and orientation
Patient concerned regarding impotence
Patient concerned regarding non-responsiveness
Patient concerned regarding promiscuity
Patient concerned regarding sexual orientation

Z70.2 Counseling related to sexual behavior and orientation of third party
Advice sought regarding sexual behavior and orientation of child
Advice sought regarding sexual behavior and orientation of partner
Advice sought regarding sexual behavior and orientation of spouse

Z70.3 Counseling related to combined concerns regarding sexual attitude, behavior and orientation

Z70.8 Other sex counseling
Encounter for sex education

Z70.9 Sex counseling, unspecified

● **Z71 Persons encountering health services for other counseling and medical advice, not elsewhere classified**

Excludes2 contraceptive or procreation counseling (Z30-Z31)
sex counseling (Z70.-)

● **Z71.0 Person encountering health services to consult on behalf of another person**
Person encountering health services to seek advice or treatment for non-attending third party
Excludes2 anxiety (normal) about sick person in family (Z63.7)
expectant (adoptive) parent(s) pre-birth pediatrician visit (Z76.81)

● **Z71.1 Person with feared health complaint in whom no diagnosis is made**
Person encountering health services with feared condition which was not demonstrated
Person encountering health services in which problem was normal state
"Worried well"
Excludes1 medical observation for suspected diseases and conditions proven not to exist (Z03.-)
Coding Clinic: 2016, Q4, P7

● **Z71.2 Person consulting for explanation of examination or test findings**

● **Z71.3 Dietary counseling and surveillance**
Use additional code for any associated underlying medical condition
Use additional code to identify body mass index (BMI), if known (Z68.-)

● **Z71.4 Alcohol abuse counseling and surveillance**
Use additional code for alcohol abuse or dependence (F10.-)

● **Z71.41 Alcohol abuse counseling and surveillance of alcoholic**

● **Z71.42 Counseling for family member of alcoholic**
Counseling for significant other, partner, or friend of alcoholic

● **Z71.5 Drug abuse counseling and surveillance**
Use additional code for drug abuse or dependence (F11-F16, F18-F19)

● **Z71.51 Drug abuse counseling and surveillance of drug abuser**

● **Z71.52 Counseling for family member of drug abuser**
Counseling for significant other, partner, or friend of drug abuser

● **Z71.6 Tobacco abuse counseling**
Use additional code for nicotine dependence (F17.-)

● **Z71.7 Human immunodeficiency virus [HIV] counseling**

● **Z71.8 Other specified counseling**
Excludes2 counseling for contraception (Z30.0-)

● **Z71.81 Spiritual or religious counseling**

● **Z71.82 Exercise counseling**

Z71.83 Encounter for nonprocreative genetic counseling
Excludes1 counseling for procreative genetics (Z31.5)
counseling for procreative management (Z31.6)

● **Z71.84 Encounter for health counseling related to travel**
Encounter for health risk and safety counseling for (international) travel
Code also, if applicable, encounter for immunization (Z23)
Excludes2 encounter for administrative examination (Z02.-)
encounter for other special examination without complaint, suspected or reported diagnosis (Z01.-)

● **Z71.85 Encounter for immunization safety counseling**
Encounter for vaccine product safety counseling
Code also, if applicable, encounter for immunization (Z23)
Code also, if applicable, immunization not carried out (Z28.-)
Excludes1 encounter for health counseling related to travel (Z71.84)

● **Z71.87 Encounter for pediatric-to-adult transition counseling**
Code also chronic condition, if applicable, such as:
autism spectrum disorder (F84.0)
congenital malformations of the circulatory system (Q20-Q28)
cystic fibrosis (E84-)
sickle-cell disorder (D57-)

● **Z71.88 Encounter for counseling for socioeconomic factors**

● **Z71.89 Other specified counseling**

● **Z71.9 Counseling, unspecified**
Encounter for medical advice NOS

● **Z72 Problems related to lifestyle**
Excludes2 problems related to life-management difficulty (Z73.-)
problems related to socioeconomic and psychosocial circumstances (Z55-Z65)
Coding Clinic: 2016, Q4, P130

● **Z72.0 Tobacco use**
Tobacco use NOS
Excludes1 history of tobacco dependence (Z87.891)
nicotine dependence (F17.2-)
tobacco dependence (F17.2-)
tobacco use during pregnancy (O99.33-)

● **Z72.3 Lack of physical exercise**

● **Z72.4 Inappropriate diet and eating habits**
Excludes1 behavioral eating disorders of infancy or childhood (F98.2.-F98.3)
eating disorders (F50.-)
lack of adequate food (Z59.48)
malnutrition and other nutritional deficiencies (E40-E64)

● **Z72.5 High risk sexual behavior**
Promiscuity
Excludes1 paraphilias (F65)

● **Z72.51 High risk heterosexual behavior**

● **Z72.52 High risk homosexual behavior**

● **Z72.53 High risk bisexual behavior**

● **Z72.6 Gambling and betting**
Excludes1 compulsive or pathological gambling (F63.0)

● **Z72.8 Other problems related to lifestyle**

● **Z72.81 Antisocial behavior**
Excludes1 conduct disorders (F91.-)

Z72.810 Child and adolescent antisocial behavior P
Antisocial behavior (child) (adolescent) without manifest psychiatric disorder
Delinquency NOS
Group delinquency
Offenses in the context of gang membership
Stealing in company with others
Truancy from school

Z72.811 Adult antisocial behavior A
Adult antisocial behavior without manifest psychiatric disorder

● **Z72.82 Problems related to sleep**

Z72.820 Sleep deprivation
Lack of adequate sleep
Excludes1 insomnia (G47.Ø-)

● **Z72.821 Inadequate sleep hygiene**
Bad sleep habits
Irregular sleep habits
Unhealthy sleep wake schedule
Excludes1 insomnia (F51.Ø-, G47.Ø-)

● **Z72.823 Risk of suffocation (smothering) under another while sleeping**
Child-caregiver co-sleeping
Infant bed-sharing

● **Z72.89 Other problems related to lifestyle**
Self-damaging behavior

● **Z72.9 Problem related to lifestyle, unspecified**

● **Z73 Problems related to life management difficulty**
Excludes2 problems related to socioeconomic and psychosocial circumstances (Z55-Z65)

● **Z73.Ø Burn-out**

● **Z73.1 Type A behavior pattern**

● **Z73.2 Lack of relaxation and leisure**

● **Z73.3 Stress, not elsewhere classified**
Physical and mental strain NOS
Excludes1 stress related to employment or unemployment (Z56.-)

● **Z73.4 Inadequate social skills, not elsewhere classified**

● **Z73.5 Social role conflict, not elsewhere classified**

● **Z73.6 Limitation of activities due to disability**
Excludes1 care-provider dependency (Z74.-)

● **Z73.8 Other problems related to life management difficulty**

● **Z73.81 Behavioral insomnia of childhood**

● **Z73.81Ø Behavioral insomnia of childhood, sleep-onset association type** P

● **Z73.811 Behavioral insomnia of childhood, limit setting type** P

● **Z73.812 Behavioral insomnia of childhood, combined type** P

● **Z73.819 Behavioral insomnia of childhood, unspecified type** P

● **Z73.82 Dual sensory impairment**

● **Z73.89 Other problems related to life management difficulty**

● **Z73.9 Problem related to life management difficulty, unspecified**

● **Z74 Problems related to care provider dependency**
Excludes2 dependence on enabling machines or devices NEC (Z99.-)

● **Z74.Ø Reduced mobility**

● **Z74.Ø1 Bed confinement status**
Bedridden

● **Z74.Ø9 Other reduced mobility**
Chairridden
Reduced mobility NOS
Excludes2 wheelchair dependence (Z99.3)

● **Z74.1 Need for assistance with personal care**

● **Z74.2 Need for assistance at home and no other household member able to render care**

● **Z74.3 Need for continuous supervision**

● **Z74.8 Other problems related to care provider dependency**

● **Z74.9 Problem related to care provider dependency, unspecified**

● **Z75 Problems related to medical facilities and other health care**

● **Z75.Ø Medical services not available in home**
Excludes1 no other household member able to render care (Z74.2)

● **Z75.1 Person awaiting admission to adequate facility elsewhere**

● **Z75.2 Other waiting period for investigation and treatment**

● **Z75.3 Unavailability and inaccessibility of health care facilities**
Excludes1 bed unavailable (Z75.1)

● **Z75.4 Unavailability and inaccessibility of other helping agencies**

● **Z75.5 Holiday relief care**

● **Z75.8 Other problems related to medical facilities and other health care**

● **Z75.9 Unspecified problem related to medical facilities and other health care**

● **Z76 Persons encountering health services in other circumstances**

● **Z76.Ø Encounter for issue of repeat prescription**
Encounter for issue of repeat prescription for appliance
Encounter for issue of repeat prescription for medicaments
Encounter for issue of repeat prescription for spectacles
Excludes2 issue of medical certificate (ZØ2.7)
repeat prescription for contraceptive (Z3Ø.4-)

Z76.1 Encounter for health supervision and care of foundling

● **Z76.2 Encounter for health supervision and care of other healthy infant and child** P
Encounter for medical or nursing care or supervision of healthy infant under circumstances such as adverse socioeconomic conditions at home
Encounter for medical or nursing care or supervision of healthy infant under circumstances such as awaiting foster or adoptive placement
Encounter for medical or nursing care or supervision of healthy infant under circumstances such as maternal illness
Encounter for medical or nursing care or supervision of healthy infant under circumstances such as number of children at home preventing or interfering with normal care

Z76.3 Healthy person accompanying sick person

Z76.4 Other boarder to healthcare facility
Excludes1 homelessness (Z59.Ø-)

Z76.5 Malingerer [conscious simulation]
Person feigning illness (with obvious motivation)
Excludes1 factitious disorder (F68.1-, F68.A)
peregrinating patient (F68.1-)

● **Z76.8 Persons encountering health services in other specified circumstances**

● **Z76.81 Expectant parent(s) prebirth pediatrician visit**
Pre-adoption pediatrician visit for adoptive parent(s)

● **Z76.82 Awaiting organ transplant status**
Patient waiting for organ availability

● **Z76.89 Persons encountering health services in other specified circumstances**
Persons encountering health services NOS
Coding Clinic:2Ø22, Q3, P7

CHAPTER 21 (ZØØ-Z99)

PERSONS WITH POTENTIAL HEALTH HAZARDS RELATED TO FAMILY AND PERSONAL HISTORY AND CERTAIN CONDITIONS INFLUENCING HEALTH STATUS (Z77-Z99)

Code also any follow-up examination (Z08-Z09)

● **Z77 Other contact with and (suspected) exposures hazardous to health**

Includes contact with and (suspected) exposures to potential hazards to health

Excludes2 contact with and (suspected) exposure to communicable diseases (Z20.-)
exposure to (parental) (environmental) tobacco smoke in the perinatal period (P96.81)
newborn affected by noxious substances transmitted via placenta or breast milk (P04.-)
occupational exposure to risk factors (Z57.-)
retained foreign body (Z18.-)
retained foreign body fully removed (Z87.821)
toxic effects of substances chiefly nonmedicinal as to source (T51-T65)

● **Z77.0 Contact with and (suspected) exposure to hazardous, chiefly nonmedicinal, chemicals**

● **Z77.01 Contact with and (suspected) exposure to hazardous metals**

● **Z77.010 Contact with and (suspected) exposure to arsenic**

● **Z77.011 Contact with and (suspected) exposure to lead**

● **Z77.012 Contact with and (suspected) exposure to uranium**

Excludes1 retained depleted uranium fragments (Z18.01)

● **Z77.018 Contact with and (suspected) exposure to other hazardous metals**

Contact with and (suspected) exposure to chromium compounds
Contact with and (suspected) exposure to nickel dust

● **Z77.02 Contact with and (suspected) exposure to hazardous aromatic compounds**

● **Z77.020 Contact with and (suspected) exposure to aromatic amines**

● **Z77.021 Contact with and (suspected) exposure to benzene**

● **Z77.028 Contact with and (suspected) exposure to other hazardous aromatic compounds**

Aromatic dyes NOS
Polycyclic aromatic hydrocarbons

● **Z77.09 Contact with and (suspected) exposure to other hazardous, chiefly nonmedicinal, chemicals**

● **Z77.090 Contact with and (suspected) exposure to asbestos**

● **Z77.098 Contact with and (suspected) exposure to other hazardous, chiefly nonmedicinal, chemicals**

Dyes NOS

● **Z77.1 Contact with and (suspected) exposure to environmental pollution and hazards in the physical environment**

● **Z77.11 Contact with and (suspected) exposure to environmental pollution**

● **Z77.110 Contact with and (suspected) exposure to air pollution**

● **Z77.111 Contact with and (suspected) exposure to water pollution**

● **Z77.112 Contact with and (suspected) exposure to soil pollution**

● **Z77.118 Contact with and (suspected) exposure to other environmental pollution**

● **Z77.12 Contact with and (suspected) exposure to hazards in the physical environment**

● **Z77.120 Contact with and (suspected) exposure to mold (toxic)**

● **Z77.121 Contact with and (suspected) exposure to harmful algae and algae toxins**

Contact with and (suspected) exposure to (harmful) algae bloom NOS
Contact with and (suspected) exposure to blue-green algae bloom
Contact with and (suspected) exposure to brown tide
Contact with and (suspected) exposure to cyanobacteria bloom
Contact with and (suspected) exposure to Florida red tide
Contact with and (suspected) exposure to pfiesteria piscicida
Contact with and (suspected) exposure to red tide

● **Z77.122 Contact with and (suspected) exposure to noise**

● **Z77.123 Contact with and (suspected) exposure to radon and other naturally occurring radiation**

Excludes2 radiation exposure as the cause of a confirmed condition (W88-W90, X39.0-)
radiation sickness NOS (T66)

● **Z77.128 Contact with and (suspected) exposure to other hazards in the physical environment**

● **Z77.2 Contact with and (suspected) exposure to other hazardous substances**

● **Z77.21 Contact with and (suspected) exposure to potentially hazardous body fluids**

● **Z77.22 Contact with and (suspected) exposure to environmental tobacco smoke (acute) (chronic)**

Exposure to second hand tobacco smoke (acute) (chronic)
Passive smoking (acute) (chronic)

Excludes1 nicotine dependence (F17.-)
tobacco use (Z72.0)

Excludes2 occupational exposure to environmental tobacco smoke (Z57.31)

● **Z77.29 Contact with and (suspected) exposure to other hazardous substances**

Coding Clinic: 2016, Q2, P34

● **Z77.9 Other contact with and (suspected) exposures hazardous to health**

● **Z78 Other specified health status**

Excludes2 asymptomatic human immunodeficiency virus [HIV] infection status (Z21)
postprocedural status (Z93-Z99)
sex reassignment status (Z87.890)

● **Z78.0 Asymptomatic menopausal state** A

Menopausal state NOS
Postmenopausal status NOS

Excludes2 symptomatic menopausal state (N95.1)

● **Z78.1 Physical restraint status**

Excludes1 physical restraint due to a procedure - omit code

● **Z78.9 Other specified health status**

Z79 Long term (current) drug therapy

Includes long term (current) drug use for prophylactic purposes

Code also any therapeutic drug level monitoring (Z51.81)

Excludes2 drug abuse and dependence (F11-F19)
drug use complicating pregnancy, childbirth, and the puerperium (O99.32-)

Coding Clinic: 2024, Q2, P26

Z79.0 Long term (current) use of anticoagulants and antithrombotics/antiplatelets

Excludes2 long term (current) use of aspirin (Z79.82)

Coding Clinic: 2021, Q1, P12-13

Z79.01 Long term (current) use of anticoagulants

Coding Clinic: 2023, Q2, P28; 2022, Q2, P17; 2021, Q1, P5

Z79.02 Long term (current) use of antithrombotics/antiplatelets

Z79.1 Long term (current) use of non-steroidal anti-inflammatories (NSAID)

Excludes2 long term (current) use of aspirin (Z79.82)

Z79.2 Long term (current) use of antibiotics

Z79.3 Long term (current) use of hormonal contraceptives

Long term (current) use of birth control pill or patch

Z79.4 Long term (current) use of insulin

Excludes2 long-term (current) use of injectable non-insulin antidiabetic drugs (Z79.85)
long term (current) use of oral hypoglycemic drugs (Z79.84)
long term (current) use of oral antidiabetic drugs (Z79.84)

Z79.5 Long term (current) use of steroids

Z79.51 Long term (current) use of inhaled steroids

Z79.52 Long term (current) use of systemic steroids

Z79.6 Long term (current) use of immunomodulators and immunosuppressants

Excludes2 long term (current) use of steroids (Z79.5-)
long term (current) use of agents affecting estrogen receptors and estrogen levels (Z79.81-)

Z79.60 Long term (current) use of unspecified immunomodulators and immunosuppressants

Z79.61 Long term (current) use of immunomodulator

Long term (current) use of apremilast
Long term (current) use of immunomodulatory imide drug
Long term (current) use of lenalidomide
Long term (current) use of pomalidomide

Z79.62 Long term (current) use of immunosuppressant

Z79.620 Long term (current) use of immunosuppressive biologic

Long term (current) use of adalimumab
Long term (current) use of etanercept
Long term (current) use of infliximab
Long term (current) use of monoclonal antibodies

Z79.621 Long term (current) use of calcineurin inhibitor

Long term (current) use of cyclosporine
Long term (current) use of tacrolimus

Z79.622 Long term (current) use of Janus kinase inhibitor

Long term (current) use of tofacitinib

Z79.623 Long term (current) use of mammalian target of rapamycin (mTOR) inhibitor

Long term (current) use of sirolimus

Z79.624 Long term (current) use of inhibitors of nucleotide synthesis

Long term (current) use of azathioprine
Long term (current) use mycophenolate
Long term (current) use of purine synthesis (IMDH) inhibitors

Z79.63 Long term (current) use of chemotherapeutic agent

Z79.630 Long term (current) use of alkylating agent

Long term (current) use of chlorambucil
Long term (current) use of cisplatin
Long term (current) use of cyclophosphamide

Z79.631 Long term (current) use of antimetabolite agent

Long term (current) use of 5-fluorouracil
Long term (current) use of 6-mercaptopurine
Long term (current) use of cytarabine
Long term (current) use of methotrexate

Z79.632 Long term (current) use of antitumor antibiotic

Long term (current) use of bleomycin
Long term (current) use of doxorubicin
Long term (current) use of mitomycin C

Z79.633 Long term (current) use of mitotic inhibitor

Long term (current) use of paclitaxel
Long term (current) use of plant alkaloids
Long term (current) use of vinblastine
Long term (current) use of vincristine

Z79.634 Long term (current) use of topoisomerase inhibitor

Long term (current) use of etoposide
Long term (current) use of irinotecan
Long term (current) use of topotecan

Z79.64 Long term (current) use of myelosuppressive agent

Long term (current) use of hydroxyurea

Z79.69 Long term (current) use of other immunomodulators and immunosuppressants

CHAPTER 21 (Z00-Z99)

● Z79.8 Other long term (current) drug therapy

● Z79.81 Long term (current) use of agents affecting estrogen receptors and estrogen levels

Code first, if applicable:
malignant neoplasm of breast (C5Ø.-)
malignant neoplasm of prostate (C61)

Use additional code, if applicable, to identify:
estrogen receptor positive status (Z17.Ø)
family history of breast cancer (Z8Ø.3)
genetic susceptibility to malignant neoplasm (cancer) (Z15.Ø-)
personal history of breast cancer (Z85.3)
personal history of prostate cancer (Z85.46)
postmenopausal status (Z78.Ø)

Excludes1 hormone replacement therapy (Z79.89Ø)

● Z79.81Ø **Long term (current) use of selective estrogen receptor modulators (SERMs)**
Long term (current) use of raloxifene (Evista)
Long term (current) use of tamoxifen (Nolvadex)
Long term (current) use of toremifene (Fareston)
Coding Clinic: 2022, Q3, P15

● Z79.811 **Long term (current) use of aromatase inhibitors**
Long term (current) use of anastrozole (Arimidex)
Long term (current) use of exemestane (Aromasin)
Long term (current) use of letrozole (Femara)

● Z79.818 **Long term (current) use of other agents affecting estrogen receptors and estrogen levels**
Long term (current) use of estrogen receptor downregulators
Long term (current) use of fulvestrant (Faslodex)
Long term (current) use of gonadotropin-releasing hormone (GnRH) agonist
Long term (current) use of goserelin acetate (Zoladex)
Long term (current) use of leuprolide acetate (leuprorelin) (Lupron)
Long term (current) use of megestrol acetate (Megace)

Z79.82 **Long term (current) use of aspirin**

● Z79.83 **Long term (current) use of bisphosphonates**
Coding Clinic: 2016, Q4, P42

● Z79.84 **Long term (current) use of oral hypoglycemic drugs**
Long term (current) use of oral antidiabetic drugs

Excludes2 long-term (current) use of injectable non-insulin antidiabetic drugs (Z79.85)
long term (current) use of insulin (Z79.4)

Coding Clinic: 2016, Q4, P76, 121-122, 126

● Z79.85 **Long-term (current) use of injectable non-insulin antidiabetic drugs**

Excludes2 long term (current) use of insulin (Z79.4)
long term (current) use of oral hypoglycemic drugs (Z79.84)

● Z79.89 Other long term (current) drug therapy

● Z79.89Ø **Hormone replacement therapy**

Z79.891 **Long term (current) use of opiate analgesic**
Long term (current) use of methadone for pain management

Excludes1 methodone use NOS (F11.9-)
use of methodone for treatment of heroin addiction (F11.2-)

Z79.899 **Other long term (current) drug therapy**
Coding Clinic: 2023, Q3, P17-18; 2015, Q4, P34, Q3, P21

● Z8Ø **Family history of primary malignant neoplasm**

● Z8Ø.Ø **Family history of malignant neoplasm of digestive organs**
Conditions classifiable to C15-C26
Coding Clinic: 2018, Q1, P7

● Z8Ø.1 **Family history of malignant neoplasm of trachea, bronchus and lung**
Conditions classifiable to C33-C34

● Z8Ø.2 **Family history of malignant neoplasm of other respiratory and intrathoracic organs**
Conditions classifiable to C3Ø-C32, C37-C39

● Z8Ø.3 **Family history of malignant neoplasm of breast**
Conditions classifiable to C5Ø.-

● Z8Ø.4 **Family history of malignant neoplasm of genital organs**
Conditions classifiable to C51-C63

● Z8Ø.41 **Family history of malignant neoplasm of ovary**

● Z8Ø.42 **Family history of malignant neoplasm of prostate**

● Z8Ø.43 **Family history of malignant neoplasm of testis**

● Z8Ø.49 **Family history of malignant neoplasm of other genital organs**

● Z8Ø.5 **Family history of malignant neoplasm of urinary tract**
Conditions classifiable to C64-C68

● Z8Ø.51 **Family history of malignant neoplasm of kidney**

● Z8Ø.52 **Family history of malignant neoplasm of bladder**

● Z8Ø.59 **Family history of malignant neoplasm of other urinary tract organ**

● Z8Ø.6 **Family history of leukemia**
Conditions classifiable to C91-C95

● Z8Ø.7 **Family history of other malignant neoplasms of lymphoid, hematopoietic and related tissues**
Conditions classifiable to C81-C9Ø, C96.-

● Z8Ø.8 **Family history of malignant neoplasm of other organs or systems**
Conditions classifiable to CØØ-C14, C4Ø-C49, C69-C79

● Z8Ø.9 **Family history of malignant neoplasm, unspecified**
Conditions classifiable to C8Ø.1

● Z81 **Family history of mental and behavioral disorders**

● Z81.Ø **Family history of intellectual disabilities**
Conditions classifiable to F7Ø-F79

● Z81.1 **Family history of alcohol abuse and dependence**
Conditions classifiable to F1Ø.-

● Z81.2 **Family history of tobacco abuse and dependence**
Conditions classifiable to F17.-

● Z81.3 **Family history of other psychoactive substance abuse and dependence**
Conditions classifiable to F11-F16, F18-F19

● Z81.4 **Family history of other substance abuse and dependence**
Conditions classifiable to F55

● Z81.8 **Family history of other mental and behavioral disorders**
Conditions classifiable elsewhere in FØ1-F99

CHAPTER 21 (ZØØ-Z99)

Z82 Family history of certain disabilities and chronic diseases (leading to disablement)

Z82.0 Family history of epilepsy and other diseases of the nervous system
Conditions classifiable to GØØ-G99

Z82.1 Family history of blindness and visual loss
Conditions classifiable to H54.-

Z82.2 Family history of deafness and hearing loss
Conditions classifiable to H90-H91

Z82.3 Family history of stroke
Conditions classifiable to I60-I64

Z82.4 Family history of ischemic heart disease and other diseases of the circulatory system
Conditions classifiable to IØØ-I5A, I65-I99

Z82.41 Family history of sudden cardiac death

Z82.49 Family history of ischemic heart disease and other diseases of the circulatory system

Z82.5 Family history of asthma and other chronic lower respiratory diseases
Conditions classifiable to J40-J47
Excludes2 family history of other diseases of the respiratory system (Z83.6)

Z82.6 Family history of arthritis and other diseases of the musculoskeletal system and connective tissue
Conditions classifiable to MØØ-M99

Z82.61 Family history of arthritis

Z82.62 Family history of osteoporosis

Z82.69 Family history of other diseases of the musculoskeletal system and connective tissue

Z82.7 Family history of congenital malformations, deformations and chromosomal abnormalities
Conditions classifiable to QØØ-Q99

Z82.71 Family history of polycystic kidney

Z82.79 Family history of other congenital malformations, deformations and chromosomal abnormalities

Z82.8 Family history of other disabilities and chronic diseases leading to disablement, not elsewhere classified

Z83 Family history of other specific disorders
Excludes2 contact with and (suspected) exposure to communicable disease in the family (Z2Ø.-)

Z83.Ø Family history of human immunodeficiency virus [HIV] disease
Conditions classifiable to B2Ø

Z83.1 Family history of other infectious and parasitic diseases
Conditions classifiable to AØØ-B19, B25-B94, B99

Z83.2 Family history of diseases of the blood and blood-forming organs and certain disorders involving the immune mechanism
Conditions classifiable to D5Ø-D89

Z83.3 Family history of diabetes mellitus
Conditions classifiable to EØ8-E13

Z83.4 Family history of other endocrine, nutritional and metabolic diseases
Conditions classifiable to EØØ-EØ7, E15-E88

Z83.41 Family history of multiple endocrine neoplasia [MEN] syndrome

Z83.42 Family history of familial hypercholesterolemia
Coding Clinic: 2Ø16, Q4, P77

Z83.43 Family history of other disorder of lipoprotein metabolism and other lipidemias

Z83.43Ø Family history of elevated lipoprotein(a)
Family history of elevated Lp(a)

Z83.438 Family history of other disorder of lipoprotein metabolism and other lipidemia
Family history of familial combined hyperlipidemia

Z83.49 Family history of other endocrine, nutritional and metabolic diseases

Z83.5 Family history of eye and ear disorders

Z83.51 Family history of eye disorders
Conditions classifiable to HØØ-H53, H55-H59
Excludes2 family history of blindness and visual loss (Z82.1)

Z83.511 Family history of glaucoma

Z83.518 Family history of other specified eye disorder

Z83.52 Family history of ear disorders
Conditions classifiable to H6Ø-H83, H92-H95
Excludes2 family history of deafness and hearing loss (Z82.2)

Z83.6 Family history of other diseases of the respiratory system
Conditions classifiable to JØØ-J39, J6Ø-J99
Excludes2 family history of asthma and other chronic lower respiratory diseases (Z82.5)

Z83.7 Family history of diseases of the digestive system
Conditions classifiable to D12, KØØ-K93

Z83.71 Family history of colonic polyps
Excludes2 family history of malignant neoplasm of digestive organs (Z8Ø.Ø)
Coding Clinic: 2Ø21, Q1, P15

Z83.71Ø Family history of adenomatous and serrated polyps
Conditions classifiable to D12.-
Family history of tubular adenoma polyps
Family history of tubulovillous adenoma polyps
Family history of villous adenoma polyps

Z83.711 Family history of hyperplastic colon polyps

Z83.718 Other family history of colon polyps
Family history of inflammatory colon polyps

Z83.719 Family history of colon polyps, unspecified
Family history of colon polyps NOS

Z83.72 Family history of familial adenomatous polyposis

Z83.79 Family history of other diseases of the digestive system

Z84 Family history of other conditions

Z84.Ø Family history of diseases of the skin and subcutaneous tissue
Conditions classifiable to LØØ-L99

Z84.1 Family history of disorders of kidney and ureter
Conditions classifiable to NØØ-N29

Z84.2 Family history of other diseases of the genitourinary system
Conditions classifiable to N3Ø-N99
Coding Clinic: 2Ø16, Q4, P77

Z84.3 Family history of consanguinity

Z84.8 Family history of other specified conditions

Z84.81 Family history of carrier of genetic disease
Coding Clinic: 2Ø21, Q1, P15

Z84.82 Family history of sudden infant death syndrome
Family history of SIDS

Z84.89 Family history of other specified conditions

Z85 Personal history of malignant neoplasm

Code first any follow-up examination after treatment of malignant neoplasm (Z08)

Use additional code to identify:
alcohol use and dependence (F10.-)
exposure to environmental tobacco smoke (Z77.22)
history of tobacco dependence (Z87.891)
occupational exposure to environmental tobacco smoke (Z57.31)
tobacco dependence (F17.-)
tobacco use (Z72.0)

Excludes2 personal history of benign neoplasm (Z86.01-)
personal history of carcinoma-in-situ (Z86.00-)

Coding Clinic: 2022, Q3, P28

Z85.0 Personal history of malignant neoplasm of digestive organs

Z85.00 Personal history of malignant neoplasm of unspecified digestive organ

Z85.01 Personal history of malignant neoplasm of esophagus
Conditions classifiable to C15

Z85.02 Personal history of malignant neoplasm of stomach

Z85.020 Personal history of malignant carcinoid tumor of stomach
Conditions classifiable to C7A.092

Z85.028 Personal history of other malignant neoplasm of stomach
Conditions classifiable to C16

Z85.03 Personal history of malignant neoplasm of large intestine

Z85.030 Personal history of malignant carcinoid tumor of large intestine
Conditions classifiable to C7A.022-C7A.025, C7A.029

Z85.038 Personal history of other malignant neoplasm of large intestine
Conditions classifiable to C18

Z85.04 Personal history of malignant neoplasm of rectum, rectosigmoid junction, and anus

Z85.040 Personal history of malignant carcinoid tumor of rectum
Conditions classifiable to C7A.026

Z85.048 Personal history of other malignant neoplasm of rectum, rectosigmoid junction, and anus
Conditions classifiable to C19-C21

Z85.05 Personal history of malignant neoplasm of liver
Conditions classifiable to C22

Z85.06 Personal history of malignant neoplasm of small intestine

Z85.060 Personal history of malignant carcinoid tumor of small intestine
Conditions classifiable to C7A.01-

Z85.068 Personal history of other malignant neoplasm of small intestine
Conditions classifiable to C17

Z85.07 Personal history of malignant neoplasm of pancreas
Conditions classifiable to C25

Z85.09 Personal history of malignant neoplasm of other digestive organs

Z85.1 Personal history of malignant neoplasm of trachea, bronchus and lung

Z85.11 Personal history of malignant neoplasm of bronchus and lung

Z85.110 Personal history of malignant carcinoid tumor of bronchus and lung
Conditions classifiable to C7A.090

Z85.118 Personal history of other malignant neoplasm of bronchus and lung
Conditions classifiable to C34

Z85.12 Personal history of malignant neoplasm of trachea
Conditions classifiable to C33

Z85.2 Personal history of malignant neoplasm of other respiratory and intrathoracic organs

Z85.20 Personal history of malignant neoplasm of unspecified respiratory organ

Z85.21 Personal history of malignant neoplasm of larynx
Conditions classifiable to C32

Z85.22 Personal history of malignant neoplasm of nasal cavities, middle ear, and accessory sinuses
Conditions classifiable to C30-C31

Z85.23 Personal history of malignant neoplasm of thymus

Z85.230 Personal history of malignant carcinoid tumor of thymus
Conditions classifiable to C7A.091

Z85.238 Personal history of other malignant neoplasm of thymus
Conditions classifiable to C37

Z85.29 Personal history of malignant neoplasm of other respiratory and intrathoracic organs

Z85.3 Personal history of malignant neoplasm of breast
Conditions classifiable to C50.-

Z85.4 Personal history of malignant neoplasm of genital organs
Conditions classifiable to C51-C63

Z85.40 Personal history of malignant neoplasm of unspecified female genital organ

Z85.41 Personal history of malignant neoplasm of cervix uteri

Z85.42 Personal history of malignant neoplasm of other parts of uterus

Z85.43 Personal history of malignant neoplasm of ovary

Z85.44 Personal history of malignant neoplasm of other female genital organs
Coding Clinic: 2024, Q2, P11,12

Z85.45 Personal history of malignant neoplasm of unspecified male genital organ

Z85.46 Personal history of malignant neoplasm of prostate
Coding Clinic: 2023, Q2, P5

Z85.47 Personal history of malignant neoplasm of testis

Z85.48 Personal history of malignant neoplasm of epididymis

Z85.49 Personal history of malignant neoplasm of other male genital organs

Z85.5 Personal history of malignant neoplasm of urinary tract
Conditions classifiable to C64-C68

Z85.50 Personal history of malignant neoplasm of unspecified urinary tract organ

Z85.51 Personal history of malignant neoplasm of bladder

Z85.52 Personal history of malignant neoplasm of kidney

Excludes1 personal history of malignant neoplasm of renal pelvis (Z85.53)

Z85.520 Personal history of malignant carcinoid tumor of kidney
Conditions classifiable to C7A.093

Z85.528 Personal history of other malignant neoplasm of kidney
Conditions classifiable to C64

Z85.53 Personal history of malignant neoplasm of renal pelvis

Z85.54 Personal history of malignant neoplasm of ureter

Z85.59 Personal history of malignant neoplasm of other urinary tract organ

Z85.6 Personal history of leukemia
Conditions classifiable to C91-C95
Excludes1 leukemia in remission C91.0-C95.9 with 5th character 1

Z85.7 Personal history of other malignant neoplasms of lymphoid, hematopoietic and related tissues

Z85.71 Personal history of Hodgkin lymphoma
Conditions classifiable to C81

Z85.72 Personal history of non-Hodgkin lymphomas
Conditions classifiable to C82-C85
Coding Clinic: 2022, Q3, P28

Z85.79 Personal history of other malignant neoplasms of lymphoid, hematopoietic and related tissues
Conditions classifiable to C88-C90, C96
Excludes1 multiple myeloma in remission (C90.01)
plasma cell leukemia in remission (C90.11)
plasmacytoma in remission (C90.21)

Z85.8 Personal history of malignant neoplasms of other organs and systems
Conditions classifiable to C00-C14, C40-C49, C69-C75, C7A.098, C76-C79

Z85.81 Personal history of malignant neoplasm of lip, oral cavity, and pharynx
Conditions classifiable to C00-C14

Z85.810 Personal history of malignant neoplasm of tongue

Z85.818 Personal history of malignant neoplasm of other sites of lip, oral cavity, and pharynx

Z85.819 Personal history of malignant neoplasm of unspecified site of lip, oral cavity, and pharynx

Z85.82 Personal history of malignant neoplasm of skin

Z85.820 Personal history of malignant melanoma of skin
Conditions classifiable to C43
Coding Clinic: 2022, Q3, P9

Z85.821 Personal history of Merkel cell carcinoma
Conditions classifiable to C4A

Z85.828 Personal history of other malignant neoplasm of skin
Conditions classifiable to C44

Z85.83 Personal history of malignant neoplasm of bone and soft tissue
Conditions classifiable to C40-C41; C45-C49

Z85.830 Personal history of malignant neoplasm of bone

Z85.831 Personal history of malignant neoplasm of soft tissue
Excludes2 personal history of malignant neoplasm of skin (Z85.82-)

Z85.84 Personal history of malignant neoplasm of eye and nervous tissue
Conditions classifiable to C69-C72

Z85.840 Personal history of malignant neoplasm of eye

Z85.841 Personal history of malignant neoplasm of brain

Z85.848 Personal history of malignant neoplasm of other parts of nervous tissue

Z85.85 Personal history of malignant neoplasm of endocrine glands
Conditions classifiable to C73-C75

Z85.850 Personal history of malignant neoplasm of thyroid

Z85.858 Personal history of malignant neoplasm of other endocrine glands
Coding Clinic: 2024, Q2, P10

Z85.89 Personal history of malignant neoplasm of other organs and systems
Conditions classifiable to C7A.098, C76, C77-C79

Z85.9 Personal history of malignant neoplasm, unspecified
Conditions classifiable to C7A.00, C80.1

Z86 Personal history of certain other diseases
Code first any follow-up examination after treatment (Z09)

Z86.0 Personal history of in-situ and benign neoplasms and neoplasms of uncertain behavior
Excludes2 personal history of malignant neoplasms (Z85.-)

Z86.00 Personal history of in-situ neoplasm
Conditions classifiable to D00-D09

Z86.000 Personal history of in-situ neoplasm of breast
Conditions classifiable to D05

Z86.001 Personal history of in-situ neoplasm of cervix uteri
Conditions classifiable to D06
Personal history of cervical intraepithelial neoplasia III [CIN III]

Z86.002 Personal history of in-situ neoplasm of other and unspecified genital organs
Conditions classifiable to D07
Personal history of high-grade prostatic intraepithelial neoplasia III [HGPIN III]
Personal history of vaginal intraepithelial neoplasia III [VAIN III]
Personal history of vulvar intraepithelial neoplasia III [VIN III]

Z86.003 Personal history of in-situ neoplasm of oral cavity, esophagus and stomach
Conditions classifiable to D00

Z86.004 Personal history of in-situ neoplasm of other and unspecified digestive organs
Conditions classifiable to D01
Personal history of anal intraepithelial neoplasia (AIN III)

Z86.005 Personal history of in-situ neoplasm of middle ear and respiratory system
Conditions classifiable to D02

Z86.006 Personal history of melanoma in-situ
Conditions classifiable to D03
Excludes2 sites other than skin - code to personal history of in-situ neoplasm of the site

Z86.007 Personal history of in-situ neoplasm of skin
Conditions classifiable to D04
Personal history of carcinoma in situ of skin

Z86.008 Personal history of in-situ neoplasm of other site
Conditions classifiable to D09

CHAPTER 21 (Z00-Z99)

Z86.01 Personal history of benign neoplasm
Coding Clinic: 2017, Q1, P14

Z86.010 Personal history of colon polyps
- Personal history of colorectal polyps
- Personal history of rectal polyps

Coding Clinic: 2021, Q1, P15; 2017, Q1, P9, P14

Z86.0100 Personal history of colon polyps, unspecified
- Personal history of colon polyps NOS

Z86.0101 Personal history of adenomatous and serrated colon polyps
- Personal history of tubular adenoma polyps
- Personal history of sessile adenomatous colon polyp
- Personal history of sessile serrated colon polyp
- Personal history of tubulovillous adenoma polyps
- Personal history of villous adenoma polyps
- Personal history of traditional serrated adenoma polyps

Z86.0102 Personal history of hyperplastic colon polyps

Z86.0109 Personal history of other colon polyps

Z86.011 Personal history of benign neoplasm of the brain

Z86.012 Personal history of benign carcinoid tumor

Z86.018 Personal history of other benign neoplasm
Coding Clinic: 2017, Q1, P14

Z86.03 Personal history of neoplasm of uncertain behavior

Z86.1 Personal history of infectious and parasitic diseases
Conditions classifiable to A00-B89, B99
Excludes1 personal history of infectious diseases specific to a body system sequelae of infectious and parasitic diseases (B90-B94)
Coding Clinic: 2016, Q4, P5

Z86.11 Personal history of tuberculosis

Z86.12 Personal history of poliomyelitis

Z86.13 Personal history of malaria

Z86.14 Personal history of Methicillin resistant Staphylococcus aureus infection
Personal history of MRSA infection

Z86.15 Personal history of latent tuberculosis infection

Z86.16 Personal history of COVID-19
Excludes1 post COVID-19 condition (U09.9)
Coding Clinic: 2022, Q3, P4; 2021, Q4, P103-105, 107-108; 2021, Q1, P34-35, 40-42, 44, 46

Z86.19 Personal history of other infectious and parasitic diseases
Coding Clinic: 2021, Q1, P34-35, 40-41

Z86.2 Personal history of diseases of the blood and blood-forming organs and certain disorders involving the immune mechanism
Conditions classifiable to D50-D89

Z86.3 Personal history of endocrine, nutritional and metabolic diseases
Conditions classifiable to E00-E88

Z86.31 Personal history of diabetic foot ulcer
Excludes2 current diabetic foot ulcer (E08.621, E09.621, E10.621, E11.621, E13.621)

Z86.32 Personal history of gestational diabetes
Personal history of conditions classifiable to O24.4-
Excludes1 gestational diabetes mellitus in current pregnancy (O24.4-)

Z86.39 Personal history of other endocrine, nutritional and metabolic disease
Coding Clinic: 2020, Q1, P13

Z86.5 Personal history of mental and behavioral disorders
Conditions classifiable to F40-F59

Z86.51 Personal history of combat and operational stress reaction A

Z86.59 Personal history of other mental and behavioral disorders

Z86.6 Personal history of diseases of the nervous system and sense organs
Conditions classifiable to G00-G99, H00-H95

Z86.61 Personal history of infections of the central nervous system
Personal history of encephalitis
Personal history of meningitis

Z86.69 Personal history of other diseases of the nervous system and sense organs
Coding Clinic: 2016, Q4, P25

Z86.7 Personal history of diseases of the circulatory system
Conditions classifiable to I00-I99
Excludes2 old myocardial infarction (I25.2)
personal history of anaphylactic shock (Z87.892)
postmyocardial infarction syndrome (I24.1)

Z86.71 Personal history of venous thrombosis and embolism

Z86.711 Personal history of pulmonary embolism

Z86.718 Personal history of other venous thrombosis and embolism

Z86.72 Personal history of thrombophlebitis

Z86.73 Personal history of transient ischemic attack (TIA), and cerebral infarction without residual deficits
Personal history of prolonged reversible ischemic neurological deficit (PRIND)
Personal history of stroke NOS without residual deficits
Excludes1 personal history of traumatic brain injury (Z87.820)
sequelae of cerebrovascular disease (I69.-)
Coding Clinic: 2023, Q1, P37; 2012, Q4, P3

Z86.74 Personal history of sudden cardiac arrest
Personal history of sudden cardiac death successfully resuscitated
Coding Clinic: 2024, Q1, P27

Z86.79 Personal history of other diseases of the circulatory system
Coding Clinic: 2022, Q2, P15; 2020, Q1, P13

Z87 Personal history of other diseases and conditions
Code first any follow-up examination after treatment (Z09)

Z87.0 Personal history of diseases of the respiratory system
Conditions classifiable to J00-J99

Z87.01 Personal history of pneumonia (recurrent)

Z87.09 Personal history of other diseases of the respiratory system

Z87.1 Personal history of diseases of the digestive system
Conditions classifiable to K00-K93

Z87.11 Personal history of peptic ulcer disease

Z87.19 Personal history of other diseases of the digestive system
Coding Clinic: 2017, Q1, P14

Z87.2 Personal history of diseases of the skin and subcutaneous tissue
Conditions classifiable to L00-L99
Excludes2 personal history of diabetic foot ulcer (Z86.31)

Z87.3 Personal history of diseases of the musculoskeletal system and connective tissue
Conditions classifiable to M00-M99
Excludes2 personal history of (healed) traumatic fracture (Z87.81)

Z87.31 Personal history of (healed) nontraumatic fracture

Z87.310 Personal history of (healed) osteoporosis fracture
Personal history of (healed) fragility fracture
Personal history of (healed) collapsed vertebra due to osteoporosis

Z87.311 Personal history of (healed) other pathological fracture
Personal history of (healed) collapsed vertebra NOS
Excludes2 personal history of osteoporosis fracture (Z87.310)

Z87.312 Personal history of (healed) stress fracture
Personal history of (healed) fatigue fracture

Z87.39 Personal history of other diseases of the musculoskeletal system and connective tissue

Z87.4 Personal history of diseases of genitourinary system
Conditions classifiable to N00-N99

Z87.41 Personal history of dysplasia of the female genital tract
Excludes1 personal history of intraepithelial neoplasia III of female genital tract (Z86.001, Z86.008)
personal history of malignant neoplasm of female genital tract (Z85.40-Z85.44)

Z87.410 Personal history of cervical dysplasia

Z87.411 Personal history of vaginal dysplasia

Z87.412 Personal history of vulvar dysplasia

Z87.42 Personal history of other diseases of the female genital tract

Z87.43 Personal history of diseases of male genital organs

Z87.430 Personal history of prostatic dysplasia
Excludes1 personal history of malignant neoplasm of prostate (Z85.46)

Z87.438 Personal history of other diseases of male genital organs

Z87.44 Personal history of diseases of urinary system
Excludes1 personal history of malignant neoplasm of cervix uteri (Z85.41)

Z87.440 Personal history of urinary (tract) infections

Z87.441 Personal history of nephrotic syndrome

Z87.442 Personal history of urinary calculi
Personal history of kidney stones

Z87.448 Personal history of other diseases of urinary system

Z87.5 Personal history of complications of pregnancy, childbirth and the puerperium
Conditions classifiable to O00-O9A
Excludes2 recurrent pregnancy loss (N96)

Z87.51 Personal history of pre-term labor
Excludes1 current pregnancy with history of pre-term labor (O09.21-)

Z87.59 Personal history of other complications of pregnancy, childbirth and the puerperium
Personal history of trophoblastic disease

Z87.6 Personal history of certain (corrected) conditions arising in the perinatal period
Conditions classifiable to P00-P96
Excludes1 personal history of (corrected) congenital malformations (Z87.7-)

Z87.61 Personal history of (corrected) necrotizing enterocolitis of newborn

Z87.68 Personal history of other (corrected) conditions arising in the perinatal period

Z87.7 Personal history of (corrected) congenital malformations
Conditions classifiable to Q00-Q89 that have been repaired or corrected
Excludes1 congenital malformations that have been partially corrected or repair but which still require medical treatment - code to condition
Excludes2 other postprocedural states (Z98.-)
personal history of medical treatment (Z92.-)
presence of cardiac and vascular implants and grafts (Z95.-)
presence of other devices (Z97.-)
presence of other functional implants (Z96.-)
transplanted organ and tissue status (Z94.-)

Z87.71 Personal history of (corrected) congenital malformations of genitourinary system

Z87.710 Personal history of (corrected) hypospadias

Z87.718 Personal history of other specified (corrected) congenital malformations of genitourinary system

Z87.72 Personal history of (corrected) congenital malformations of nervous system and sense organs

Z87.720 Personal history of (corrected) congenital malformations of eye

Z87.721 Personal history of (corrected) congenital malformations of ear

Z87.728 Personal history of other specified (corrected) congenital malformations of nervous system and sense organs

Z87.73 Personal history of (corrected) congenital malformations of digestive system

Z87.730 Personal history of (corrected) cleft lip and palate

Z87.731 Personal history of (corrected) tracheoesophageal fistula or atresia

Z87.732 Personal history of (corrected) persistent cloaca or cloacal malformations

Z87.738 Personal history of other specified (corrected) congenital malformations of digestive system

Z87.74 Personal history of (corrected) congenital malformations of heart and circulatory system

Z87.75 Personal history of (corrected) congenital malformations of respiratory system

Z87.76 Personal history of (corrected) congenital malformations of integument, limbs and musculoskeletal system

Z87.760 Personal history of (corrected) congenital diaphragmatic hernia or other congenital diaphragm malformations

Z87.761 Personal history of (corrected) gastroschisis

Z87.762 Personal history of (corrected) prune belly malformation

Z87.763 Personal history of other (corrected) congenital abdominal wall malformations

Z87.768 Personal history of other specified (corrected) congenital malformations of integument, limbs and musculoskeletal system

Z87.79 Personal history of other (corrected) congenital malformations

Z87.790 Personal history of (corrected) congenital malformations of face and neck

Z87.798 Personal history of other (corrected) congenital malformations

Z87.8 Personal history of other specified conditions

Excludes2 personal history of self harm (Z91.5-)

Z87.81 Personal history of (healed) traumatic fracture

Excludes2 personal history of (healed) nontraumatic fracture (Z87.31-)

Z87.82 Personal history of other (healed) physical injury and trauma

Conditions classifiable to S00-T88, except traumatic fractures

Z87.820 Personal history of traumatic brain injury

Excludes1 personal history of transient ischemic attack (TIA), and cerebral infarction without residual deficits (Z86.73)

Z87.821 Personal history of retained foreign body fully removed

Z87.828 Personal history of other (healed) physical injury and trauma

Z87.89 Personal history of other specified conditions

Z87.890 Personal history of sex reassignment

Z87.891 Personal history of nicotine dependence

Excludes1 current nicotine dependence (F17.2-)

Coding Clinic: 2017, Q2, P27

Z87.892 Personal history of anaphylaxis

Code also allergy status such as:
allergy status to drugs, medicaments and biological substances (Z88.-)
allergy status, other than to drugs and biological substances (Z91.0-)

Z87.898 Personal history of other specified conditions

Coding Clinic: 2013, Q1, P21

Z88 Allergy status to drugs, medicaments and biological substances

Excludes2 allergy status, other than to drugs and biological substances (Z91.0-)

Z88.0 Allergy status to penicillin

Z88.1 Allergy status to other antibiotic agents

Z88.2 Allergy status to sulfonamides

Coding Clinic: 2015, Q3, P23

Z88.3 Allergy status to other anti-infective agents

Z88.4 Allergy status to anesthetic agent

Z88.5 Allergy status to narcotic agent

Z88.6 Allergy status to analgesic agent

Z88.7 Allergy status to serum and vaccine

Z88.8 Allergy status to other drugs, medicaments and biological substances

Z88.9 Allergy status to unspecified drugs, medicaments and biological substances

Z89 Acquired absence of limb

Includes amputation status
postprocedural loss of limb
post-traumatic loss of limb

Excludes1 acquired deformities of limbs (M20-M21)
congenital absence of limbs (Q71-Q73)

Z89.0 Acquired absence of thumb and other finger(s)

Z89.01 Acquired absence of thumb

Z89.011 Acquired absence of right thumb

Z89.012 Acquired absence of left thumb

Z89.019 Acquired absence of unspecified thumb

Z89.02 Acquired absence of other finger(s)

Excludes2 acquired absence of thumb (Z89.01-)

Z89.021 Acquired absence of right finger(s)

Z89.022 Acquired absence of left finger(s)

Z89.029 Acquired absence of unspecified finger(s)

Z89.1 Acquired absence of hand and wrist

Z89.11 Acquired absence of hand

Z89.111 Acquired absence of right hand

Z89.112 Acquired absence of left hand

Z89.119 Acquired absence of unspecified hand

Z89.12 Acquired absence of wrist

Disarticulation at wrist

Z89.121 Acquired absence of right wrist

Z89.122 Acquired absence of left wrist

Z89.129 Acquired absence of unspecified wrist

Z89.2 Acquired absence of upper limb above wrist

Z89.20 Acquired absence of upper limb, unspecified level

Z89.201 Acquired absence of right upper limb, unspecified level

Z89.202 Acquired absence of left upper limb, unspecified level

Z89.209 Acquired absence of unspecified upper limb, unspecified level

Acquired absence of arm NOS

Z89.21 Acquired absence of upper limb below elbow

Z89.211 Acquired absence of right upper limb below elbow

Z89.212 Acquired absence of left upper limb below elbow

Z89.219 Acquired absence of unspecified upper limb below elbow

Z89.22 Acquired absence of upper limb above elbow

Disarticulation at elbow

Z89.221 Acquired absence of right upper limb above elbow

Z89.222 Acquired absence of left upper limb above elbow

Z89.229 Acquired absence of unspecified upper limb above elbow

Z89.23 Acquired absence of shoulder
Acquired absence of shoulder joint following explantation of shoulder joint prosthesis, with or without presence of antibiotic-impregnated cement spacer
- **Z89.231 Acquired absence of right shoulder**
- **Z89.232 Acquired absence of left shoulder**
- **Z89.239 Acquired absence of unspecified shoulder**

Z89.4 Acquired absence of toe(s), foot, and ankle

Z89.41 Acquired absence of great toe
- **Z89.411 Acquired absence of right great toe**
- **Z89.412 Acquired absence of left great toe**
- **Z89.419 Acquired absence of unspecified great toe**

Z89.42 Acquired absence of other toe(s)
Excludes2 acquired absence of great toe (Z89.41-)
- **Z89.421 Acquired absence of other right toe(s)**
- **Z89.422 Acquired absence of other left toe(s)**
- **Z89.429 Acquired absence of other toe(s), unspecified side**

Z89.43 Acquired absence of foot
- **Z89.431 Acquired absence of right foot**
- **Z89.432 Acquired absence of left foot**
- **Z89.439 Acquired absence of unspecified foot**

Z89.44 Acquired absence of ankle
Disarticulation of ankle
- **Z89.441 Acquired absence of right ankle**
- **Z89.442 Acquired absence of left ankle**
- **Z89.449 Acquired absence of unspecified ankle**

Z89.5 Acquired absence of leg below knee

Z89.51 Acquired absence of leg below knee
- **Z89.511 Acquired absence of right leg below knee**
- **Z89.512 Acquired absence of left leg below knee**
- **Z89.519 Acquired absence of unspecified leg below knee**

Z89.52 Acquired absence of knee
Acquired absence of knee joint following explantation of knee joint prosthesis, with or without presence of antibiotic-impregnated cement spacer
- **Z89.521 Acquired absence of right knee**
- **Z89.522 Acquired absence of left knee**
- **Z89.529 Acquired absence of unspecified knee**

Z89.6 Acquired absence of leg above knee

Z89.61 Acquired absence of leg above knee
Acquired absence of leg NOS
Disarticulation at knee
- **Z89.611 Acquired absence of right leg above knee**
- **Z89.612 Acquired absence of left leg above knee**
- **Z89.619 Acquired absence of unspecified leg above knee**

Z89.62 Acquired absence of hip
Acquired absence of hip joint following explantation of hip joint prosthesis, with or without presence of antibiotic-impregnated cement spacer
Disarticulation at hip
- **Z89.621 Acquired absence of right hip joint**
- **Z89.622 Acquired absence of left hip joint**
- **Z89.629 Acquired absence of unspecified hip joint**

Z89.9 Acquired absence of limb, unspecified

Z90 Acquired absence of organs, not elsewhere classified
Includes postprocedural or post-traumatic loss of body part NEC
Excludes1 congenital absence - see Alphabetical Index
Excludes2 postprocedural absence of endocrine glands (E89.-)

Z90.0 Acquired absence of part of head and neck
- **Z90.01 Acquired absence of eye**
- **Z90.02 Acquired absence of larynx**
- **Z90.09 Acquired absence of other part of head and neck**
  Acquired absence of nose
  Excludes2 teeth (K08.1)

Z90.1 Acquired absence of breast and nipple
- **Z90.10 Acquired absence of unspecified breast and nipple**
- **Z90.11 Acquired absence of right breast and nipple**
- **Z90.12 Acquired absence of left breast and nipple**
- **Z90.13 Acquired absence of bilateral breasts and nipples**
  Coding Clinic: 2022, Q3, P8

Z90.2 Acquired absence of lung [part of]

Z90.3 Acquired absence of stomach [part of]

Z90.4 Acquired absence of other specified parts of digestive tract

Z90.41 Acquired absence of pancreas
Code also exocrine pancreatic insufficiency (K86.81)
Use additional code to identify any associated:
diabetes mellitus, postpancreatectomy (E13.-)
insulin use (Z79.4)
- **Z90.410 Acquired total absence of pancreas**
  Acquired absence of pancreas NOS
- **Z90.411 Acquired partial absence of pancreas**
  Coding Clinic: 2024, Q2, P10

Z90.49 Acquired absence of other specified parts of digestive tract

Z90.5 Acquired absence of kidney

Z90.6 Acquired absence of other parts of urinary tract
Acquired absence of bladder

Z90.7 Acquired absence of genital organ(s)
Excludes1 personal history of sex reassignment (Z87.890)
Excludes2 female genital mutilation status (N90.81-)

Z90.71 Acquired absence of cervix and uterus
- **Z90.710 Acquired absence of both cervix and uterus**
  Acquired absence of uterus NOS
  Status post total hysterectomy
- **Z90.711 Acquired absence of uterus with remaining cervical stump**
  Status post partial hysterectomy with remaining cervical stump
- **Z90.712 Acquired absence of cervix with remaining uterus**

Z90.72 Acquired absence of ovaries
- **Z90.721 Acquired absence of ovaries, unilateral**
- **Z90.722 Acquired absence of ovaries, bilateral**

Z90.79 Acquired absence of other genital organ(s)
Coding Clinic: 2023, Q2, P5

Z90.8 Acquired absence of other organs
- **Z90.81 Acquired absence of spleen**
- **Z90.89 Acquired absence of other organs**
  Coding Clinic: 2023, Q3, P13

CHAPTER 21 (Z00-Z99)

● Z91 **Personal risk factors, not elsewhere classified**
Excludes2 contact with and (suspected) exposures hazardous to health (Z77.-)
exposure to pollution and other problems related to physical environment (Z77.1-)
female genital mutilation status (N90.81-)
occupational exposure to risk factors (Z57.-)
personal history of physical injury and trauma (Z87.81, Z87.82-)

● Z91.0 **Allergy status, other than to drugs and biological substances**
Excludes2 allergy status to drugs, medicaments, and biological substances (Z88.-)

● Z91.01 **Food allergy status**
Excludes2 food additives allergy status (Z91.02)

● Z91.010 **Allergy to peanuts**

● Z91.011 **Allergy to milk products**
Excludes1 lactose intolerance (E73.-)

● Z91.012 **Allergy to eggs**

● Z91.013 **Allergy to seafood**
Allergy to shellfish
Allergy to octopus or squid ink

● Z91.014 **Allergy to mammalian meats**
Allergy to beef
Allergy to lamb
Allergy to pork
Allergy to red meats

● Z91.018 **Allergy to other foods**
Allergy to nuts other than peanuts

● Z91.02 **Food additives allergy status**

● Z91.03 **Insect allergy status**

● Z91.030 **Bee allergy status**

● Z91.038 **Other insect allergy status**

● Z91.04 **Nonmedicinal substance allergy status**

● Z91.040 **Latex allergy status**
Latex sensitivity status

● Z91.041 **Radiographic dye allergy status**
Allergy status to contrast media used for diagnostic X-ray procedure

● Z91.048 **Other nonmedicinal substance allergy status**

● Z91.09 **Other allergy status, other than to drugs and biological substances**

● Z91.1 **Patient's noncompliance with medical treatment and regimen**
Code also, if applicable, to identify underdosing of specific drug (T36-T50 with final character 6)
Excludes2 caregiver noncompliance with patient's medical treatment and regimen (Z91.A-)

● Z91.11 **Patient's noncompliance with dietary regimen**
Code also, if applicable, food insecurity (Z59.4-)

● Z91.110 **Patient's noncompliance with dietary regimen due to financial hardship**

● Z91.118 **Patient's noncompliance with dietary regimen for other reason**
Inability to comply with dietary regimen

● Z91.119 **Patient's noncompliance with dietary regimen due to unspecified reason**

● Z91.12 **Patient's intentional underdosing of medication regimen**
Code first underdosing of medication (T36-T50) with fifth or sixth character 6
Excludes1 ~~adverse effect of prescribed drug taken as directed - code to adverse effect~~
poisoning (overdose) - code to poisoning

● Z91.120 **Patient's intentional underdosing of medication regimen due to financial hardship**

● Z91.128 **Patient's intentional underdosing of medication regimen for other reason**

● Z91.13 **Patient's unintentional underdosing of medication regimen**
Code first underdosing of medication (T36-T50) with fifth or sixth character 6
Excludes1 ~~adverse effect of prescribed drug taken as directed - code to adverse effect~~
poisoning (overdose) - code to poisoning

● Z91.130 **Patient's unintentional underdosing of medication regimen due to age-related debility**

● Z91.138 **Patient's unintentional underdosing of medication regimen for other reason**

● Z91.14 **Patient's other noncompliance with medication regimen**
▶ *Code first if applicable, adverse effect of underdosing (T36-T50)*
Patient's underdosing of medication NOS
Coding Clinic: 2022, Q1, P36

● Z91.141 **Patient's other noncompliance with medication regimen due to financial hardship**

● Z91.148 **Patient's other noncompliance with medication regimen for other reason**

● Z91.15 **Patient's noncompliance with renal dialysis**

● Z91.151 **Patient's noncompliance with renal dialysis due to financial hardship**

● Z91.158 **Patient's noncompliance with renal dialysis for other reason**

● Z91.19 **Patient's noncompliance with other medical treatment and regimen**
Patient's nonadherence to medical treatment

● Z91.190 **Patient's noncompliance with other medical treatment and regimen due to financial hardship**

● Z91.198 **Patient's noncompliance with other medical treatment and regimen for other reason**
Coding Clinic: 2024, Q1, P24

● Z91.199 **Patient's noncompliance with other medical treatment and regimen due to unspecified reason**

● Z91.4 **Personal history of psychological trauma, not elsewhere classified**

● Z91.41 **Personal history of adult abuse**
Excludes2 personal history of abuse in childhood (Z62.81-)

● Z91.410 **Personal history of adult physical and sexual abuse** A
Excludes1 current adult physical abuse (T74.11, T76.11)
current adult sexual abuse (T74.21, T76.11)

● Z91.411 **Personal history of adult psychological abuse** A

● Z91.412 **Personal history of adult neglect** A
Excludes1 current adult neglect (T74.01, T76.01)

● Z91.413 **Personal history of adult financial abuse**

● Z91.414 **Personal history of adult intimate partner abuse**

● Z91.419 **Personal history of unspecified adult abuse** A

Z91.42 Personal history of forced labor or sexual exploitation

Z91.49 Other personal history of psychological trauma, not elsewhere classified

Z91.5 Personal history of self-harm

Code also mental health disorder, if known

Z91.51 Personal history of suicidal behavior

Personal history of parasuicide
Personal history of self-poisoning
Personal history of suicide attempt

Z91.52 Personal history of nonsuicidal self-harm

Personal history of nonsuicidal self-injury
Personal history of self-inflicted injury without suicidal intent
Personal history of self-mutilation

Z91.8 Other specified personal risk factors, not elsewhere classified

Z91.81 History of falling

At risk for falling

Z91.82 Personal history of military deployment A

Individual (civilian or military) with past history of military war, peacekeeping and humanitarian deployment (current or past conflict)
Returned from military deployment

Excludes2 personal history of military service (Z91.85)

Z91.83 Wandering in diseases classified elsewhere

Code first underlying disorder such as:
Alzheimer's disease (G30.-)
autism or pervasive developmental disorder (F84.-)
intellectual disabilities (F70-F79)
unspecified dementia with behavioral disturbance (F03.9-, F03.A-, F03.B-, F03.C-)

Z91.84 Oral health risk factors

Z91.841 Risk for dental caries, low

Z91.842 Risk for dental caries, moderate

Z91.843 Risk for dental caries, high

Z91.849 Unspecified risk for dental caries

Z91.85 Personal history of military service

Excludes2 personal history of military deployment(Z91.82)
personal history of serving in the armed forces
personal history of veteran

Z91.89 Other specified personal risk factors, not elsewhere classified

Increased risk for social isolation
Coding Clinic: 2017, Q1, P46

Z91.A Caregiver's noncompliance with patient's medical treatment and regimen

Z91.A1 Caregiver's noncompliance with patient's dietary regimen

Caregiver's inability to comply with patient's dietary regimen

Code also, if applicable, food insecurity (Z59.4-)

Z91.A10 Caregiver's noncompliance with patient's dietary regimen due to financial hardship

Z91.A18 Caregiver's noncompliance with patient's dietary regimen for other reason

Z91.A2 Caregiver's intentional underdosing of patient's medication regimen

Code first underdosing of medication (T36-T50) with fifth or sixth character 6

Z91.A20 Caregiver's intentional underdosing of patient's medication regimen due to financial hardship

Z91.A28 Caregiver's intentional underdosing of medication regimen for other reason

Z91.A3 Caregiver's unintentional underdosing of patient's medication regimen

Code first underdosing of medication (T36-T50) with fifth or sixth character 6

Z91.A4 Caregiver's other noncompliance with patient's medication regimen

Caregiver's underdosing of patient's medication NOS

Z91.A41 Caregiver's other noncompliance with patient's medication regimen due to financial hardship

Z91.A48 Caregiver's other noncompliance with patient's medication regimen for other reason

Z91.A5 Caregiver's noncompliance with patient's renal dialysis

Z91.A51 Caregiver's noncompliance with patient's renal dialysis due to financial hardship

Z91.A58 Caregiver's noncompliance with patient's renal dialysis for other reason

Z91.A9 Caregiver's noncompliance with patient's other medical treatment and regimen

Caregiver's nonadherence to patient's medical treatment

Z91.A91 Caregiver's noncompliance with patient's other medical treatment and regimen due to financial hardship

Z91.A98 Caregiver's noncompliance with patient's other medical treatment and regimen for other reason

Z92 Personal history of medical treatment

Excludes2 postprocedural states (Z98.-)

Z92.0 Personal history of contraception

Excludes1 counseling or management of current contraceptive practices (Z30.-)
long term (current) use of contraception (Z79.3)
presence of (intrauterine) contraceptive device (Z97.5)

Z92.2 Personal history of drug therapy

Excludes2 long term (current) drug therapy (Z79.-)

Z92.21 Personal history of antineoplastic chemotherapy

Z92.22 Personal history of monoclonal drug therapy

▶ **Excludes2** personal history of immune checkpoint inhibitor therapy (Z92.26)

Z92.23 Personal history of estrogen therapy

Z92.24 Personal history of steroid therapy

Z92.240 Personal history of inhaled steroid therapy

Z92.241 Personal history of systemic steroid therapy

Personal history of steroid therapy NOS

Z92.25 Personal history of immunosuppression therapy

Excludes2 personal history of steroid therapy (Z92.24)

Z92.26 ▶ **Personal history of immune checkpoint inhibitor therapy**

▶ Personal history of ICI drug therapy

Z92.29 Personal history of other drug therapy

CHAPTER 21 (Z00-Z99)

- Z92.3 Personal history of irradiation
  Personal history of exposure to therapeutic radiation
  Excludes1 exposure to radiation in the physical environment (Z77.12)
  occupational exposure to radiation (Z57.1)
- Z92.8 Personal history of other medical treatment
  Coding Clinic: 2016, Q4, P72
  - Z92.81 Personal history of extracorporeal membrane oxygenation (ECMO)
  - Z92.82 Status post administration of tPA (rtPA) in a different facility within the last 24 hours prior to admission to current facility
    Code first condition requiring tPA administration, such as:
    acute cerebral infarction (I63.-)
    acute myocardial infarction (I21.-, I22.-)
  - Z92.83 Personal history of failed moderate sedation
    Personal history of failed conscious sedation
    Excludes2 failed moderate sedation during procedure (T88.52)
  - Z92.84 Personal history of unintended awareness under general anesthesia
    Excludes2 unintended awareness under general anesthesia during procedure (T88.53)
    Coding Clinic: 2016, Q4, P72, 77
  - Z92.85 Personal history of cellular therapy
    ▶ **Excludes2** personal history of immune checkpoint inhibitor therapy (Z92.26)
    - Z92.850 Personal history of Chimeric Antigen Receptor T-cell therapy
      Personal history of CAR T-cell therapy
    - Z92.858 Personal history of other cellular therapy
    - Z92.859 Personal history of cellular therapy, unspecified
  - Z92.86 Personal history of gene therapy
  - Z92.89 Personal history of other medical treatment
    Coding Clinic: 2020, Q1, P18
- Z93 Artificial opening status
  Excludes1 artificial openings requiring attention or management (Z43.-)
  complications of external stoma (J95.0-, K94.-, N99.5-)
  - Z93.0 Tracheostomy status
  - Z93.1 Gastrostomy status
  - Z93.2 Ileostomy status
  - Z93.3 Colostomy status
    ▶Ileal pouch status
    ▶Kock pouch status
  - Z93.4 Other artificial openings of gastrointestinal tract status
  - Z93.5 Cystostomy status
    - Z93.50 Unspecified cystostomy status
    - Z93.51 Cutaneous-vesicostomy status
    - Z93.52 Appendico-vesicostomy status
    - Z93.59 Other cystostomy status
  - Z93.6 Other artificial openings of urinary tract status
    Nephrostomy status
    Ureterostomy status
    Urethrostomy status
  - Z93.8 Other artificial opening status
  - Z93.9 Artificial opening status, unspecified
- Z94 Transplanted organ and tissue status
  Includes organ or tissue replaced by heterogenous or homogenous transplant
  Excludes1 complications of transplanted organ or tissue - see Alphabetical Index
  Excludes2 presence of vascular grafts (Z95.-)
  - Z94.0 Kidney transplant status Ex: PDX 2032
  - Z94.1 Heart transplant status Ex: PDX 2033
    Excludes1 artificial heart status (Z95.812)
    heart-valve replacement status (Z95.2-Z95.4)
  - Z94.2 Lung transplant status Ex: PDX 2034
  - Z94.3 Heart and lungs transplant status Ex: PDX 2033
    CC when PDx is its own CC
  - Z94.4 Liver transplant status Ex: PDX 2035
  - Z94.5 Skin transplant status
    Autogenous skin transplant status
  - Z94.6 Bone transplant status
  - Z94.7 Corneal transplant status
  - Z94.8 Other transplanted organ and tissue status
    - Z94.81 Bone marrow transplant status Ex: PDX 2036
    - Z94.82 Intestine transplant status Ex: PDX 2037
    - Z94.83 Pancreas transplant status Ex: PDX 2038
    - Z94.84 Stem cells transplant status Ex: PDX 2039
    - Z94.89 Other transplanted organ and tissue status
  - Z94.9 Transplanted organ and tissue status, unspecified
- Z95 Presence of cardiac and vascular implants and grafts
  Excludes2 complications of cardiac and vascular devices, implants and grafts (T82.-)
  - Z95.0 Presence of cardiac pacemaker
    Presence of cardiac resynchronization therapy (CRT-P) pacemaker
    Excludes1 adjustment or management of cardiac device (Z45.0-)
    adjustment or management of cardiac pacemaker (Z45.0)
    presence of automatic (implantable) cardiac defibrillator with synchronous cardiac pacemaker (Z95.810)
    Coding Clinic: 2019, Q1, P33
  - Z95.1 Presence of aortocoronary bypass graft
    Presence of coronary artery bypass graft
  - Z95.2 Presence of prosthetic heart valve
    Presence of heart valve NOS
  - Z95.3 Presence of xenogenic heart valve
  - Z95.4 Presence of other heart-valve replacement
  - Z95.5 Presence of coronary angioplasty implant and graft
    Excludes1 coronary angioplasty status without implant and graft (Z98.61)
  - Z95.8 Presence of other cardiac and vascular implants and grafts
    - Z95.81 Presence of other cardiac implants and grafts Ex: PDX 2033
      - Z95.810 Presence of automatic (implantable) cardiac defibrillator
        Presence of automatic (implantable) cardiac defribrillator with synchronous cardiac pacemaker
        Presence of cardiac resynchronization therapy defibrillator (CRT-D)
        Presence of cardioverter-defribillator (ICD)
        Coding Clinic: 2022, Q2, P15
      - Z95.811 Presence of heart assist device
      - Z95.812 Presence of fully implantable artificial heart
      - Z95.818 Presence of other cardiac implants and grafts

CHAPTER 21 (Z00-Z99)

▶ New ➡ Revised ~~deleted~~ Deleted Excludes 1 Excludes 2 Includes Use additional Code first Code also Key words
OGCR Official Guidelines ● Unacceptable Principal Diagnosis X Assign placeholder X ● Use Additional Character(s) ◗ Manifestation Code Coding Clinic

Z95.82 Presence of other vascular implants and grafts
- Z95.820 Peripheral vascular angioplasty status with implants and grafts
  - **Excludes1** peripheral vascular angioplasty without implant and graft (Z98.62)
- Z95.828 Presence of other vascular implants and grafts
  - Presence of intravascular prosthesis NEC

Z95.9 Presence of cardiac and vascular implant and graft, unspecified

Z96 Presence of other functional implants

Excludes2 complications of internal prosthetic devices, implants and grafts (T82-T85)
fitting and adjustment of prosthetic and other devices (Z44-Z46)

Z96.0 Presence of urogenital implants

Z96.1 Presence of intraocular lens
- Presence of pseudophakia

Z96.2 Presence of otological and audiological implants
- Z96.20 Presence of otological and audiological implant, unspecified
- Z96.21 Cochlear implant status
- Z96.22 Myringotomy tube(s) status
- Z96.29 Presence of other otological and audiological implants
  - Presence of bone-conduction hearing device
  - Presence of eustachian tube stent
  - Stapes replacement

Z96.3 Presence of artificial larynx

Z96.4 Presence of endocrine implants
- Z96.41 Presence of insulin pump (external) (internal)
- Z96.49 Presence of other endocrine implants

Z96.5 Presence of tooth-root and mandibular implants

Z96.6 Presence of orthopedic joint implants
- Z96.60 Presence of unspecified orthopedic joint implant
- Z96.61 Presence of artificial shoulder joint
  - Z96.611 Presence of right artificial shoulder joint
  - Z96.612 Presence of left artificial shoulder joint
  - Z96.619 Presence of unspecified artificial shoulder joint
- Z96.62 Presence of artificial elbow joint
  - Z96.621 Presence of right artificial elbow joint
  - Z96.622 Presence of left artificial elbow joint
  - Z96.629 Presence of unspecified artificial elbow joint
- Z96.63 Presence of artificial wrist joint
  - Z96.631 Presence of right artificial wrist joint
  - Z96.632 Presence of left artificial wrist joint
  - Z96.639 Presence of unspecified artificial wrist joint
- Z96.64 Presence of artificial hip joint
  - Hip-joint replacement (partial) (total)
  - Z96.641 Presence of right artificial hip joint
    - Coding Clinic: 2016, Q3, P17
  - Z96.642 Presence of left artificial hip joint
    - Coding Clinic: 2015, Q1, P16
  - Z96.643 Presence of artificial hip joint, bilateral
  - Z96.649 Presence of unspecified artificial hip joint
- Z96.65 Presence of artificial knee joint
  - Z96.651 Presence of right artificial knee joint
  - Z96.652 Presence of left artificial knee joint
    - Coding Clinic: 2019, Q3, P16
  - Z96.653 Presence of artificial knee joint, bilateral
  - Z96.659 Presence of unspecified artificial knee joint
- Z96.66 Presence of artificial ankle joint
  - Z96.661 Presence of right artificial ankle joint
  - Z96.662 Presence of left artificial ankle joint
  - Z96.669 Presence of unspecified artificial ankle joint
- Z96.69 Presence of other orthopedic joint implants
  - Z96.691 Finger-joint replacement of right hand
  - Z96.692 Finger-joint replacement of left hand
  - Z96.693 Finger-joint replacement, bilateral
  - Z96.698 Presence of other orthopedic joint implants

Z96.7 Presence of other bone and tendon implants
- Presence of skull plate

Z96.8 Presence of other specified functional implants
- Z96.81 Presence of artificial skin
- Z96.82 Presence of neurostimulator
  - Presence of brain neurostimulator
  - Presence of gastric neurostimulator
  - Presence of peripheral nerve neurostimulator
  - Presence of sacral nerve neurostimulator
  - Presence of spinal cord neurostimulator
  - Presence of vagus nerve neurostimulator
- Z96.89 Presence of other specified functional implants

Z96.9 Presence of functional implant, unspecified

Z97 Presence of other devices

Excludes2 fitting and adjustment of prosthetic and other devices (Z44-Z46)
presence of cerebrospinal fluid drainage device (Z98.2)

Z97.0 Presence of artificial eye

Z97.1 Presence of artificial limb (complete) (partial)
- Z97.10 Presence of artificial limb (complete) (partial), unspecified
- Z97.11 Presence of artificial right arm (complete) (partial)
- Z97.12 Presence of artificial left arm (complete) (partial)
- Z97.13 Presence of artificial right leg (complete) (partial)
- Z97.14 Presence of artificial left leg (complete) (partial)
- Z97.15 Presence of artificial arms, bilateral (complete) (partial)
- Z97.16 Presence of artificial legs, bilateral (complete) (partial)

Z97.2 Presence of dental prosthetic device (complete) (partial)
- Presence of dentures (complete) (partial)

Z97.3 Presence of spectacles and contact lenses

Z97.4 Presence of external hearing-aid

Z97.5 Presence of (intrauterine) contraceptive device
- **Excludes1** checking, reinsertion or removal of implantable subdermal contraceptive (Z30.46)
  checking, reinsertion or removal of intrauterine contraceptive device (Z30.43-)

Z97.8 Presence of other specified devices

Z98 Other postprocedural states

Excludes2 aftercare (Z43-Z49, Z51)
follow-up medical care (Z08-Z09)
postprocedural complication - see Alphabetical Index

Z98.0 Intestinal bypass and anastomosis status
- **Excludes2** bariatric surgery status (Z98.84)
  gastric bypass status (Z98.84)
  obesity surgery status (Z98.84)

- Z98.1 **Arthrodesis status**
- Z98.2 **Presence of cerebrospinal fluid drainage device**
  - Presence of CSF shunt
- Z98.3 **Post therapeutic collapse of lung status**
  - *Code first underlying disease*
- Z98.4 **Cataract extraction status**
  - Use additional code to identify intraocular lens implant status (Z96.1)
  - **Excludes1** aphakia (H27.0)
  - Z98.41 **Cataract extraction status, right eye**
  - Z98.42 **Cataract extraction status, left eye**
  - Z98.49 **Cataract extraction status, unspecified eye**
- Z98.5 **Sterilization status**
  - **Excludes1** female infertility (N97.-)
    male infertility (N46.-)
  - Z98.51 **Tubal ligation status**
  - Z98.52 **Vasectomy status** A
- Z98.6 **Angioplasty status**
  - Z98.61 **Coronary angioplasty status**
    - **Excludes1** coronary angioplasty status with implant and graft (Z95.5)
    - Coding Clinic: 2022, Q4, P23
  - Z98.62 **Peripheral vascular angioplasty status**
    - **Excludes1** peripheral vascular angioplasty status with implant and graft (Z95.820)
- Z98.8 **Other specified postprocedural states**
  - Coding Clinic: 2016, Q4, P76
  - Z98.81 **Dental procedure status**
    - Z98.810 **Dental sealant status**
    - Z98.811 **Dental restoration status**
      - Dental crown status
      - Dental fillings status
    - Z98.818 **Other dental procedure status**
  - Z98.82 **Breast implant status**
    - **Excludes1** breast implant removal status (Z98.86)
    - Coding Clinic: 2022, Q3, P8
  - Z98.83 **Filtering (vitreous) bleb after glaucoma surgery status**
    - **Excludes1** inflammation (infection) of postprocedural bleb (H59.4-)
  - Z98.84 **Bariatric surgery status**
    - Gastric banding status
    - Gastric bypass status for obesity
    - Obesity surgery status
    - **Excludes1** bariatric surgery status complicating pregnancy, childbirth, or the puerperium (O99.84)
    - **Excludes2** intestinal bypass and anastomosis status (Z98.0)
    - Coding Clinic: 2020, Q1, P12
  - Z98.85 **Transplanted organ removal status**
    - Transplanted organ previously removed due to complication, failure, rejection or infection
    - **Excludes1** encounter for removal of transplanted organ - code to complication of transplanted organ (T86.-)
  - Z98.86 **Personal history of breast implant removal**
  - Z98.87 **Personal history of in utero procedure**
    - Z98.870 **Personal history of in utero procedure during pregnancy**
      - **Excludes2** complications from in utero procedure for current pregnancy (O35.7)
        supervision of current pregnancy with history of in utero procedure during previous pregnancy (O09.82-)
    - Z98.871 **Personal history of in utero procedure while a fetus**
  - Z98.89 **Other specified postprocedural states**
    - Coding Clinic: 2016, Q4, P76
    - Z98.890 **Other specified postprocedural states**
      - Personal history of surgery, not elsewhere classified
      - Coding Clinic: 2023, Q3, P13
    - Z98.891 **History of uterine scar from previous surgery**
      - **Excludes1** Maternal care due to uterine scar from previous surgery (O34.2-)
      - Coding Clinic: 2016, Q4, P52, P76

Z99 **Dependence on enabling machines and devices, not elsewhere classified**

Coding Clinic: 2020, Q1, P11

- Z99.0 **Dependence on aspirator**
- Z99.1 **Dependence on respirator** Ex PDX 1061
  - Dependence on ventilator
  - Z99.11 **Dependence on respirator [ventilator] status**
    - Coding Clinic: 2018, Q1, P14; 2015, Q1, P21
  - Z99.12 **Encounter for respirator [ventilator] dependence during power failure**
    - **Excludes1** mechanical complication of respirator [ventilator] (J95.850)
- Z99.2 **Dependence on renal dialysis**
  - Hemodialysis status
  - Peritoneal dialysis status
  - Presence of arteriovenous shunt for dialysis
  - Renal dialysis status NOS
  - **Excludes1** encounter for fitting and adjustment of dialysis catheter (Z49.0-)
  - **Excludes2** noncompliance with renal dialysis (Z91.15-)
  - Coding Clinic: 2022, Q3, P16; 2016, Q1, P13
- Z99.3 **Dependence on wheelchair**
  - Wheelchair confinement status
  - *Code first cause of dependence, such as:*
    muscular dystrophy (G71.0-)
    obesity (E66.-)
- Z99.8 **Dependence on other enabling machines and devices**
  - Z99.81 **Dependence on supplemental oxygen**
    - Dependence on long-term oxygen
  - Z99.89 **Dependence on other enabling machines and devices**
    - Dependence on machine or device NOS
    - Coding Clinic: 2020, Q1, P11

CHAPTER 21 (Z00-Z99)

CHAPTER 22

CODES FOR SPECIAL PURPOSES (U00-U85)

Note: Codes from this chapter are for use on newborn records only, never on maternal records.

This chapter contains the following blocks:

U00-U49	Provisional assignment of new diseases of uncertain etiology or emergency use

PROVISIONAL ASSIGNMENT OF NEW DISEASES OF UNCERTAIN ETIOLOGY OR EMERGENCY USE (U00-U49)

U07 Emergency use of U07

U07.0 Vaping-related disorder

Dabbing related lung damage
Dabbing related lung injury
E-cigarette, or vaping, product use associated lung injury [EVALI]
Electronic cigarette related lung damage
Electronic cigarette related lung injury

Use additional code to identify manifestations, such as:
abdominal pain (R10.84)
acute respiratory distress syndrome (J80)
diarrhea (R19.7)
drug-induced interstitial lung disorder (J70.4)
lipoid pneumonia (J69.1)
weight loss (R63.4)

U07.1 COVID-19 (Ex) PDX 2022

Use additional code to identify pneumonia or other manifestations

Use Additional code, if applicable, for associated conditions such as:
COVID-19 associated coagulopathy (D68.8)
disseminated intravascular coagulation (D65)
hypercoagulable states (D68.69)
thrombophilia (D68.69)

Excludes1 coronavirus as the cause of diseases classified elsewhere (B97.2-)
pneumonia due to SARS-associated coronavirus (J12.81)

Coding Clinic: 2022, Q2, P29; 2021, Q4, P109; 2021, Q1, P31-33, 36, 39-40, 47, 49

● **U09 Post COVID-19 condition**

U09.9 Post COVID-19 condition, unspecified

Note: This code enables establishment of a link with COVID-19.

This code is not to be used in cases that are still presenting with active COVID-19. However, an exception is made in cases of re-infection with COVID-19, occurring with a condition related to prior COVID-19.

Post-acute sequela of COVID-19

Code first the specific condition related to COVID-19 if known, such as:
chronic respiratory failure (J96.1-)
loss of smell (R43.8)
loss of taste (R43.8)
multisystem inflammatory syndrome (M35.81)
pulmonary embolism (I26.-)
pulmonary fibrosis (J84.10)

Coding Clinic: 2021, Q4, P102-104,106

CHAPTER 22 (U00-U85)